REPRODUCTIVE AND DEVELOPMENTAL TOXICOLOGY

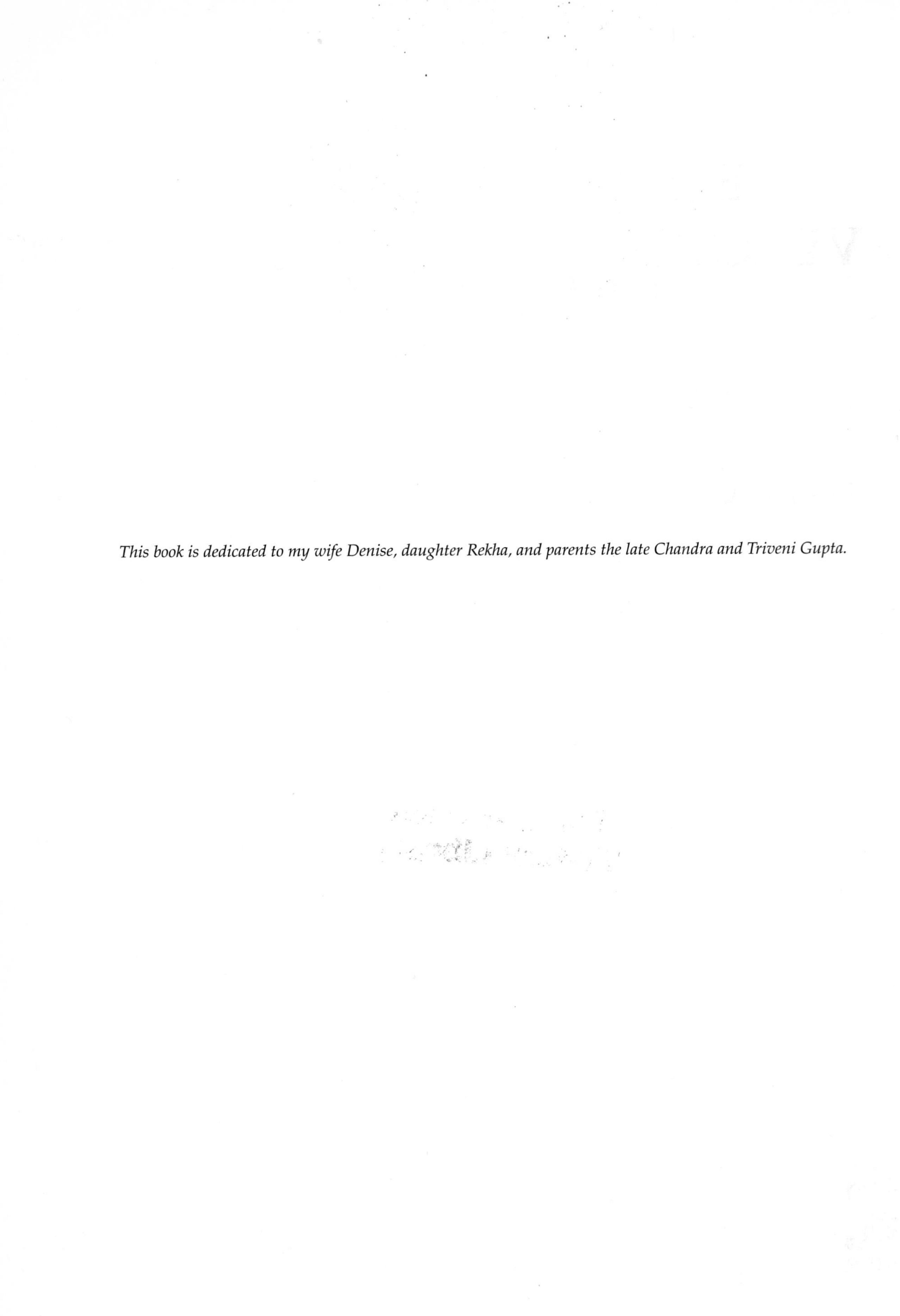

This book is dedicated to my wife Denise, daughter Rekha, and parents the late Chandra and Triveni Gupta.

REPRODUCTIVE AND DEVELOPMENTAL TOXICOLOGY

Edited by

RAMESH C. GUPTA, DVM, MVSc, PhD, DABT, FACT, FATS

Professor and Head, Toxicology Department
Breathitt Veterinary Center
Murray State University
Hopkinsville, Kentucky
USA

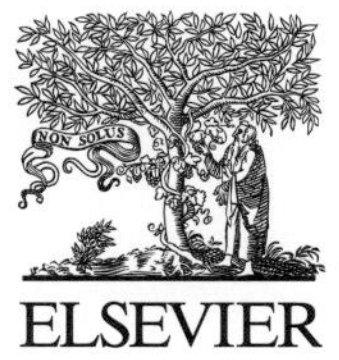

AMSTERDAM • BOSTON • HEIDELBERG • LONDON • NEW YORK • OXFORD
PARIS • SAN DIEGO • SAN FRANCISCO • SINGAPORE • SYDNEY • TOKYO
Academic Press is an imprint of Elsevier

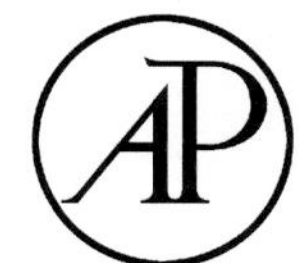

Academic Press is an imprint of Elsevier
32 Jamestown Road, London NW1 7BY, UK
30 Corporate Drive, Suite 400, Burlington, MA 01803, USA
525 B Street, Suite 1800, San Diego, CA 92101-4495, USA

First edition 2011

British Library Cataloguing-in-Publication Data
A catalogue record for this book is available from the British Library

Library of Congress Cataloging-in-Publication Data
A catalog record for this book is available from the Library of Congress

ISBN : 978-0-12-382032-7

Typeset by TNQ Books and Journals

Printed and bound in United States of America

11 12 13 14   10 9 8 7 6 5 4 3 2 1

Contents

Section 9 Phytotoxicants

Section 10 Biotoxins

Section 11 Special Topics

Section 12 Endocrine Disruption, Mutagenicity, Carcinogenicity, Infertility and Teratogenicity

Section 13 Toxicologic Pathology

Section 14 Placental Toxicity

Foreword

This book, *Reproductive and Developmental Toxicology*, presents one of the most comprehensive and thorough treatments of the complex discipline of toxicological phenomena in reproducing and developing organisms available. The focus is obviously often on human species, which is quite understandable, but the book also covers other species, from organisms used for toxicology testing to related aspects of wildlife species. The book surveys a large number of different chemicals, from pharmaceuticals to environmental pollutants, and various experimental systems at all levels of biological organization. We anticipate that this book will be heavily used as a handbook for critically evaluated information that may be not so easily available from other sources.

There are several reasons why such a wide and thorough collection of authoritative reviews and surveys is useful, even imperative. The first reason is the very extraordinary nature of the subject: the developing organism and its creation. Adults of reproducing age "get the ball rolling", so to speak, but by no means is the new organism a small adult. It could even be said that there is no such thing as a developing organism, but an organism that is constantly and often rapidly changing, with various and variable characteristics at each point in time. It is a moving target for research and the dimension of time has always to be taken into consideration.

Development is manifest at all levels of inquiry: expression of genetic programs at specified stages, consequent changes in the patterns of nucleic acid messages, proteins, enzyme activities, signal transduction systems and so on, as well as formation and modification of anatomical structures and physiological functions. And ultimately, this finely tuned marvel of creation of a new individual could be disrupted at any stage of development, in various ways and by various forces, by physical, chemical and biological insults. The grand goal of the research on reproductive and developmental toxicology is to understand the interplay between exogenous, potentially harmful factors and endogenous, intrinsic molecular, physiological and anatomical determinants, which may ultimately result in derangements in reproduction and development. The epitome of such a deranged development was the thalidomide catastrophe about 50 years ago, which had and still has far-reaching consequences in basic research, drug development and regulatory pharmacology and toxicology.

As toxicologists and pharmacologists, we used to think that chemicals most often cause their effects via specific target molecules, receptors, enzymes, regulatory factors and so on. However, the appearance of such targets in the developing organism depends on developmental programs, which dictate appearance and disappearance of specific molecular effectors and modifiers. Consequently, if a specific target is still "sleeping" at a certain stage in development, a chemical affecting that specific target does not cause an effect. Toxicity mechanisms elucidated in adults do not necessarily apply in developing organisms.

A developing organism does not exist on its own; it is dependent on its mother, and there are unique structures such as yolk sac and placenta taking care of certain functions during pregnancy. The placenta both connects and separates mother and fetus, and after birth its function has been fulfilled. From a toxicological point of view, the placenta has a central function: it controls the movement and access of chemicals from mother to fetus. Although we know now that the placenta is not a barrier in the old meaning of the word, we still use this misnomer. It is imperative to understand the role of the placenta in the kinetics and dynamics of chemicals, because only then we can fully assess potential hazards and risks to a developing organism.

Up to this day many, perhaps most, reproductive and developmental toxicants have been detected after human exposures. However, the best way to avoid such tragedies should be prevention: to detect potential developmental toxicity in animals before human exposures. Since the thalidomide tragedy, drugs and many other chemicals with intended or unintended human exposures have had to be screened in animal experiments. Recently also a few *in vitro* testing systems have been validated for the same purposes. Animal experiments have their own drawbacks, including sometimes very large and partially unknown or unexplained interspecies differences, and increasingly influential ethical issues. The main problem of *in vitro* testing systems is that they can never represent the whole complex organism, only some rather limited processes, and thus they need extensive validation to be reliable indicators for developmental hazards and risks. A significant way to avoid difficulties inherent in animal or *in vitro* studies is the thorough characterization of physiological and pathological development and the identification of rate-limiting processes and mechanisms via which toxicants may affect normal development.

The most important humane reason to emphasize the significance of continuous research in reproductive and developmental toxicity is the simple fact that damage in early life, if permanent, will be with the affected individual for the rest of their life. This is also the principal reason why research efforts have to be directed towards preventive, anticipatory tools and actions. The ultimate goal is to prevent the exposure of reproducing adults and developing individuals to potentially harmful toxicants by reliable and predictive toxicity testing, which employs the most modern *in silico, in vitro, ex vivo* (and *in vivo*, if possible and necessary) tools in an integrated framework of hazard identification and risk assessment.

Olavi Pelkonen, MD, PhD
Professor of Pharmacology (emeritus),
University of Oulu, Oulu, Finland

List of Contributors

Margaret R. Adams, BS
Center for Molecular Neuroscience, Department of Pediatrics, Vanderbilt University Medical Center, Nashville, TN, USA

Manoj Aggarwal, BVSc, MVSc, PhD
Bernburg, Germany; Human Health Assessment, Dow AgroSciences, European Development Centre, Abingdon, Oxon, UK

Tausif Ahmed, PhD
Department of DMPK and Toxicology, Sai Advantium Pharma Ltd, Hinjewadi, Pune, India

Patrick Allard, PhD
Department of Genetics, Harvard Medical School, Boston, MA, USA

Arturo Anadón, DVM, PhD, DipECVPT
Department of Toxicology and Pharmacology, Faculty of Veterinary Medicine, Universidad Complutense de Madrid, Madrid, Spain

Gregory J. Anger, MSc
Department of Pharmaceutical Sciences, Faculty of Pharmacy, University of Toronto, Toronto, Ontario, Canada

Anthony E. Archibong, PhD
Department of Physiology, Meharry Medical College, Nashville, TN, USA

Michael Aschner, PhD
Department of Pediatrics, Vanderbilt University Medical Center, Nashville, TN, USA

Daiana S. Avila, PhD
Department of Pediatrics, Vanderbilt University Medical Center, Nashville, TN, USA

Debasis Bagchi, PhD, MACN, CNS, MAIChE
Department of Pharmacology and Pharmaceutical Sciences, University of Houston College of Pharmacy, Houston, TX, USA

Manashi Bagchi, PhD, FACN
NutriToday, Boston, MA, USA

Norman J. Barlow, DVM, PhD, MBA, MLD
Preclinical Safety - Disposition, Safety and Animal Research, sanofi-aventis US, Bridgewater, NJ, USA

Dana Boyd Barr, PhD
Emory University, Rollins School of Public Health, Atlanta, GA, USA

Sudheer Beedanagari, PhD
Lexicon Pharmaceuticals, The Woodlands, TX, USA

Karyn Bischoff, DVM, MS, DABVT
Cornell University, New York State Animal Health Diagnostic Center, Ithaca, NY, USA

William M. Bracken, PhD, DABT
Preclinical Safety, Global Pharmaceutical R&D, Abbott Laboratories, Abbott Park, IL, USA

Rich M. Breyer, PhD
Vanderbilt University School of Medicine, Nashville, TN, USA

Susan Bright, DVM
Food and Drug Administration, Center for Veterinary Medicine, Office of Surveillance and Compliance, Rockville, MD, USA

Kaylon L. Bruner-Tran, PhD
Women's Reproductive Health Research Center, Department of Obstetrics and Gynecology, Vanderbilt University School of Medicine, Nashville, TN, USA

Shilpa Buch, PhD
Department of Pharmacology and Experimental Neuroscience, Nebraska Medical Center, University of Nebraska Medical Center, Omaha, NE, USA

Brian Buckley, PhD
Environmental and Occupational Health Science Institute, Rutgers University, Piscataway, NJ, USA

Steven J. Bursian, PhD
Department of Animal Science, Michigan State University, East Lansing, MI, USA

Edward W. Carney, PhD
The Dow Chemical Company, Midland, MI, USA

Victor Castellano, DVM, PhD
Department of Toxicology and Pharmacology, Faculty of Veterinary Medicine, Universidad Complutense de Madrid, Madrid, Spain

Sudipta Chakraborty, BS
Center for Molecular Neuroscience, Department of Pediatrics, Vanderbilt University Medical Center, Nashville, TN, USA

Jing Chen, PhD
Department of Environmental and Occupational Health Sciences University of Washington, Seattle, WA, USA

Sanika Chirwa, MD, PhD
Department of Neuroscience and Pharmacology, Meharry Medical College; Department of Pharmacology, Vanderbilt University, Nashville, TN, USA

Rajani Choudhuri, PhD
Radiation Biology Branch, NCI, National Institutes of Health, Bethesda, MD, USA

Supratim Choudhuri, PhD
US Food and Drug Administration, Center for Food Safety and Applied Nutrition, Office of Food Additive Safety, Division of Biotechnology and GRAS Notice Review, College Park, MD, USA

Jane K. Cleal, PhD
Developmental Origins of Health and Disease, School of Medicine, University of Southampton, Southampton General Hospital, Southampton, UK

Monica P. Colaiácovo, PhD
Department of Genetics, Harvard Medical School, Boston, MA, USA

Robert W. Coppock, DVM, DABVT, PhD, DABT
Toxicologist & Associates Ltd, Vegreville, AB, USA

Lucio G. Costa, PhD, ATS
Department of Environmental and Occupational Health Sciences, University of Washington, Seattle, WA, USA, and Department of Human Anatomy, Pharmacology and Forensic Science, University of Parma, Italy

Maged M. Costantine, MD
Department of Obstetrics and Gynecology, University of Texas Medical Branch, Galveston, TX, USA

Tirupapuliyur V. Damodaran, PhD
Department of Biology, North Carolina Central University, Durham, NC, USA

Rosane Souza Da Silva, PhD
Laboratory of Neurochemistry and Psychopharmacology, Department of Cellular and Molecular Biology, Pontifícia Universidade Católica do Rio Grande do Sul, Brazil

T. Zane Davis, PhD
US Department of Agriculture-Agricultural Research Service, Poisonous Plant Research Laboratory, Logan, UT, USA

Marta Di Carlo, PhD
Istituto di Biomedicina ed Immunologia Molecolare "Alberto Monroy", Palermo, Italy

John D. Doherty, PhD, DABT
Health Effects Division, Office of Chemical Safety and Pollution Prevention, USEPA, Washington DC, USA

José L. Domingo, PhD
Laboratory of Toxicology and Environmental Health, School of Medicine, Universitat "Rovira i Virgili", Reus, Catalonia, Spain

Margitta M. Dziwenka, DVM
Toxicologist & Associates Ltd, Vegreville, AB, USA

Per Eriksson, PhD
Department of Physiology and Developmental Biology, Environmental Toxicology, Uppsala University, Sweden

Carmen Estevan Martínez, PhD Environmental Sciences
Unidad de Toxicología y Seguridad Química, Instituto de Bioingeniería, Universidad Miguel Hernández de Elche, Spain

Timothy J. Evans, DVM, MS, PhD, DABVT, DACT
Department of Veterinary Pathobiology, Veterinary Medical Diagnostic Laboratory, College of Veterinary Medicine, University of Missouri-Columbia, MO, USA

Bengt Fadeel, MD, PhD
Division of Molecular Toxicology, Institute of Environmental Medicine, Karolinska Institutet, Stockholm, Sweden

Ali S. Faqi, DVM, PhD, DABT
Developmental & Reproductive Toxicology, MPI Research, Inc., Mattawan, MI, USA

Marcelo Farina, PhD
Departamento de Bioquímica, CCB, Universidade Federal de Santa Catarina, Florianópolis, Santa Catarina, Brazil

Suzanne E. Fenton, PhD
National Toxicology Program, National Institute of Environmental Health Sciences, Research Triangle Park, NC, USA.

Maureen H. Feuston, PhD
Disposition, Safety and Animal Research, sanofi-aventis US, Bridgewater, NJ, USA

John Flaskos, Bsc, Msc, PhD
Laboratory of Biochemistry and Toxicology, Faculty of Veterinary Medicine, Aristotle University of Thessaloniki, Thessaloniki, Greece

Swaran J. S. Flora, MSc, PhD, FABT
Division of Pharmacology and Toxicology, Defence Research and Development Establishment, Gwalior, India

Vekataseshu K. Ganjam, BSc, BVSc, MS, PhD, MA(Penn, hc)
Departments of Biomedical Science and Veterinary Medicine and Surgery, University of Missouri-Columbia, MO

Dale R. Gardner, PhD
US Department of Agriculture-Agricultural Research Service, Poisonous Plant Research Laboratory, Logan, UT, USA

Ramesh C. Garg, BVSc, PhD, DABT
Preclinical Safety, Global Pharmaceutical R&D, Abbott Laboratories, Abbott Park, IL, USA

Vincent F. Garry, MD, MS, DABT
University of Minnesota Medical School, Minneapolis, MN, USA

Janee Gelineau-van Waes, PhD, DVM
Department of Pharmacology, Creighton University School of Medicine, Omaha, NE, USA

Gennaro Giordano, PhD
Department of Environmental and Occupational Health Sciences, University of Washington, Seattle, WA, USA

Scott Glaberman, PhD
US Environmental Protection Agency, National Center for Environmental Assessment, Washington DC, USA

Keith M. Godfrey, MD, PhD
MRC Lifecourse Epidemiology Unit, School of Medicine, University of Southampton, and Southampton NIHR Nutrition, Diet & Lifestyle Biomedical Research Unit, Southampton General Hospital, Southampton, UK

Marina Guizzetti, PhD
Department of Psychiatry, University of Illinois at Chicago, and Jesse Brown VA Medical Center, Chicago, IL, USA

Kavita Gulati, MSc, PhD
Department of Pharmacology, Vallabhbhai Patel Chest Institute, University of Delhi, Delhi, India

Mary Gulumian, BSc, MSc, PhD
National Institute for Occupational Health and the University of the Witwatersrand, Johannesburg, South Africa

P. K. Gupta, BVSc, MSc, VM & AH, PhD, PGDCA, FNA VSc, FASc AW, FST, FAEB, FACVT
Former Head of the Division of Pharmacology and Toxicology, and WHO Advisor, Rajender Nagar, Bareilly, UP, India

Ramesh C. Gupta, DVM, MVSc, PhD, DABT, FACT, FATS
Professor and Head, Toxicology Department, Breathitt Veterinary Center, Murray State University, Hopkinsville, KY, USA

Sharon M. Gwaltney-Brant, DVM, PhD, DABVT, DABT
Adjunct Faculty, Department of Veterinary Biosciences, College of Veterinary Medicine, University of Illinois, Urbana, IL, USA

Jeffery O. Hall, DVM, PhD
Utah State Veterinary Diagnostic Laboratory, Utah State University, Logan, UT, USA

Xiaodong Han, PhD
Immunology and Reproduction Biology Laboratory, Medical School, Nanjing University, Nanjing, Jiangsu, China

Deborah K. Hansen, PhD
Division of Personalized Nutrition and Medicine, FDA/ National Center for Toxicological Research, Jefferson, AR, USA

Alan J. Hargreaves, BSc, PhD
School of Science and Technology, Nottingham Trent University, Clifton Lane, Nottingham, UK

Alan M. Hoberman, PhD, DABT, Fellow ATS
Site Operations & Toxicology, Preclinical Services, Charles River Laboratories, Horsham, PA, USA

Darryl B. Hood, PhD
Department of Neuroscience and Pharmacology, Environmental-Health Disparities and Medicine, Center for Molecular and Behavioral Neuroscience, Meharry Medical College, Nashville, TN, USA

Karin Sørig Hougaard, BM, MSc, PhD
National Research Centre for the Working Environment, Copenhagen, Denmark

Amy L. Inselman, PhD
Division of Personalized Nutrition and Medicine, FDA/National Center for Toxicological Research, Jefferson, AR, USA

William A. Irwin, PhD, DABT
Health Effects Division, Office of Chemical Safety and Pollution Prevention, USEPA, Washington DC, USA

Valerian E. Kagan, PhD, DSc
Department of Environmental and Occupational Health, University of Pittsburgh, Pittsburgh, PA, USA

Starling Kalpana, BVSc, MVSc, PhD
Indian Veterinary Research Institute, National Referral Laboratory (Chemical Residues), Izatnagar, Bareilly, UP, India

Anumantha G. Kanthasamy, PhD
Department of Biomedical Sciences, Iowa Center for Advanced Neurotoxicology, Iowa State University, Ames, IA, USA

Arthi Kanthasamy, PhD
Department of Biomedical Sciences, Iowa Center for Advanced Neurotoxicology, Iowa State University, Ames, IA, USA

Vesa Karttunen, MSc
Faculty of Health Sciences, University of Eastern Finland, Kuopio, Finland

Habibeh Khoshbouei, PharmD, PhD
Department of Physiology, Meharry Medical College, Nashville, TN, USA

Hyung Sik Kim, PhD
College of Pharmacy, Pusan National University, Busan, Korea

Prasada Rao S. Kodavanti, PhD
Neurotoxicology Branch, Toxicity Assessment Division, National Health and Environmental Effects Research Laboratory, Office of Research and Development, US Environmental Protection Agency, Research Triangle Park, NC, USA

Katarina Koprivsek, MD, PhD
Diagnostic Imaging Centre, Institute for Oncology, Institutski put, Sremska Kamenica, Serbia

Dusko Kozic, MD, PhD
Diagnostic Imaging Centre, Institute for Oncology, Kamenicki put, Sremska Kamenica, Serbia

Kannan Krishnan, PhD, ATS, DABT
Département de Santé Environnementale et Santé au Travail, Faculté de Médecine & École de Santé Publique, Université de Montréal, Canada

Shaila Kulkarni, MS
Immunotoxicology, Mechanistic and Predictive Toxicology, Merck Research Laboratories, Summit, NJ, USA

Maria Kummu, MSc
Institute of Biomedicine, Department of Pharmacology and Toxicology, University of Oulu, Finland

Byung Mu Lee, DrPH
Division of Toxicology, College of Pharmacy, Sungkyunkwan University, Suwon, Korea

Rohan M. Lewis, PhD
Developmental Origins of Health and Disease, School of Medicine, University of Southampton, Southampton General Hospital, Southampton, UK

Dongmei Li, PhD
Immunology and Reproduction Biology Laboratory, Medical School, Nanjing University, Nanjing, Jiangsu, China

Xin Li, BS
Neuroscience Graduate Program, Vanderbilt University Medical Center, Nashville, TN, USA

Marja-Liisa Lindbohm, PhD
Finnish Institute of Occupational Health, Helsinki, Finland

Jarkko Loikkanen, PhD
Faculty of Health Sciences, University of Eastern Finland, Kuopio, Finland

Jan L. Lyche, DVM, PhD, ERT (European Registered Toxicologist)
Norwegian School of Veterinary Science, Department of Food Safety and Infection Biology, Oslo, Norway

Robert MacPhail, PhD
Toxicology Assessment Division, National Health and Environmental Effects Research Laboratory, US Environmental Protection Agency, Research Triangle Park, NC, USA

Brinda Mahadevan, PhD
Genetic Toxicology, Mechanistic and Predictive Toxicology, Merck Research Laboratories, Summit, NJ, USA

Susan L. Makris, MS
US Environmental Protection Agency, National Center for Environmental Assessment, Washington DC, USA

Jitendra K. Malik, BVSc, MVSc, PhD, FST
Indian Veterinary Research Institute, National Referral Laboratory (Chemical Residues), Izatnagar, Bareilly, UP, India

Maria Rosa Martínez-Larrañaga, DSc, PhD
Department of Toxicology and Pharmacology, Faculty of Veterinary Medicine, Universidad Complutense de Madrid, Madrid, Spain

Jerrold S. Meyer, PhD
Department of Psychology, Neuroscience and Behavior Program, University of Massachusetts, Amherst, MA, USA

Dejan Milatovic, PhD
Vanderbilt University, Department of Pediatrics, Nashville, TN, USA

Thomas J. Montine, MD, PhD
University of Washington School of Medicine, Seattle, WA, USA

Inbal Mor, PhD
Department of Biological Chemistry, The Hebrew University of Jerusalem, Jerusalem, Israel

Michelle Mostrom, DVM, MS, PhD, DABT, DABVT
North Dakota State University – Veterinary Diagnostic Laboratory Department, Fargo, ND, USA

Päivi Myllynen, MD, PhD
Institute of Biomedicine, Department of Pharmacology and Toxicology, University of Oulu, Finland

Jayaprakash Narayana Kolla, PhD
Cellular and Molecular Biology Division, Laila Impex R&D Center, Jawahar Autonagar, Vijayawada, India

Tultul Nayyar, PhD
Meharry Medical College School of Medicine, Nashville, TN, USA

John L. Newsted, PhD
Cardno ENTRIX, Okemos, MI, USA

Mingwei Ni, MD
Department of Pharmacology, Vanderbilt University Medical Center, Nashville, TN, USA

Efstathios Nikolaidis, DVM, PhD
Laboratory of Pharmacology, Veterinary School, Aristotle University of Thessaloniki, Thessaloniki, Greece

Aleksandra Novakov Mikic, MD, PhD
Department of Obstetrics and Gynaecology, Clinical Centre of Vojvodina, Novi Sad, Serbia

Meliton N. Novilla, DVM, MS, PhD, DACVP
Purdue University School of Veterinary Medicine, Shin Nippon Biomedical Laboratories, Everett, WA, USA

Kevin G. Osteen, PhD
Women's Reproductive Health Research Center, Department of Obstetrics and Gynecology, Vanderbilt University School of Medicine, Nashville, TN, USA

Vidhu Pachauri, MPharma
Division of Pharmacology and Toxicology, Defence Research and Development Establishment, Gwalior, India

Stephanie Padilla, PhD
Integrated Systems Toxicology Division, National Health and Environmental Effects Research Laboratory, US Environmental Protection Agency, Research Triangle Park, NC, USA

Carlos M. Palmeira, PhD
Center for Neuroscience and Cell Biology, Department of Life Sciences, University of Coimbra, Coimbra, Portugal

David Pamies, PhD
Unidad de Toxicología y Seguridad Química, Instituto de Bioingeniería, Universidad Miguel Hernández de Elche, Spain

Kip E. Panter, PhD
US Department of Agriculture-Agricultural Research Service, Poisonous Plant Research Laboratory, Logan, UT, USA

Heidi Partanen, MSc
Faculty of Health Sciences, University of Eastern Finland, Kuopio, Finland

Sangeeta Patel, PhD
Product Solutions, Davis, CA, USA

Brian J. Piper, PhD
Methamphetamine Abuse Research Center, Department of Behavioral Neuroscience, Oregon Health Science University, Portland, OR, USA

Micheline Piquette-Miller, PhD
Department of Pharmaceutical Sciences, Faculty of Pharmacy, University of Toronto, Toronto, Ontario, Canada

Vadim Popov, PhD
Research Institute of Hygiene, Occupational Pathology and Human Ecology Federal State Unitary Enterprise, Federal Medical Biological Agency of Russia, St Petersburg, Russia

M. Margaret Pratt, PhD
National Center for Environmental Assessment, Office of Research and Development, US Environmental Protection Agency, Washington, DC, USA

Galina Protasova, PhD (Medicine)
Research Institute of Hygiene, Occupational Pathology and Human Ecology Federal State Unitary Enterprise, Federal Medical Biological Agency of Russia, St Petersburg, Russia

João Ramalho-Santos, PhD
Center for Neuroscience and Cell Biology, Department of Life Sciences, University of Coimbra, Coimbra, Portugal

Aramandla Ramesh, PhD
Department of Biochemistry & Cancer Biology, Meharry Medical College, Nashville, TN USA

Eva Ramos, DPharm, PhD
Department of Toxicology and Pharmacology, Faculty of Veterinary Medicine, Universidad Complutense de Madrid, Madrid, Spain

Arunabha Ray, MD, PhD
Department of Pharmacology, Vallabhbhai Patel Chest Institute, University of Delhi, Delhi, India

Kausik Ray, PhD
Laboratory of Cellular Biology, NIDCD, National Institutes of Health, Bethesda, MD, USA

Stephen J. Renaud, PhD
Institute for Reproductive Health and Regenerative Medicine, Department of Pathology and Laboratory Medicine, University of Kansas Medical Center, Kansas City, KS, USA

Bashir M. Rezk, PhD
Department of Urology, Tulane University, Health Sciences Center, New Orleans, LA, USA

Ronald T. Riley, PhD
Toxicology and Mycotoxin Research Unit, United States Department of Agriculture, Agricultural Research Service, Athens, GA, USA

Drucilla J. Roberts, MD
Massachusetts General Hospital, Department of Pathology, Boston, MA, USA

Noemi Robles, PhD
Institut de Neurociències, Departament de Bioquímica i Biologia Molecular, Facultat de Medicina, Universitat Autònoma de Barcelona, Barcelona, Spain

João Batista Teixeira da Rocha, PhD
Departamento de Química, Centro de Ciências Naturais e Exatas, Universidade Federal de Santa Maria, Santa Maria–RS, Brazil

Lu Rongzhu, PhD
Department of Preventive Medicine, School of Medical Science and Laboratory Medicine, Jiangsu University, Zhenjiang, Jiangsu, China

Josefa Sabriá, PhD
Institut de Neurociències, Departament de Bioquímica i Biologia Molecular, Facultat de Medicina, Universitat Autònoma de Barcelona, Barcelona, Spain

Magdalini Sachana, DVM, MSc, PhD
Laboratory of Biochemistry and Toxicology, Faculty of Veterinary Medicine, Aristotle University of Thessaloniki, Thessaloniki, Greece

Markku Sallmén, PhD
Finnish Institute of Occupational Health, Helsinki, Finland

Ana Paula Marreilha dos Santos, PhD
i-Med-UL, Faculdade de Farmácia da Universidade de Lisboa, Lisbon, Portugal

Kai M. Savolainen, MD, PhD
Nanosafety Research Centre, Finnish Institute of Occupational Health, Helsinki, Finland

Geetu Saxena, MSc, PhD
Division of Pharmacology and Toxicology, Defence Research and Development Establishment, Gwalior, India

Manu Sebastian, DVM, MS, PhD, Dipl ACVP, Dipl ABT
College of Physicians and Surgeons Columbia University, New York, NY, USA

Helmut Segner, PhD
Centre for Fish and Wildlife Health, University of Berne, Berne, Switzerland

Krishanu Sengupta, PhD, FACN
Cellular and Molecular Biology Division, Laila Impex R&D Center, Jawahar Autonagar, Vijayawada, India

Kathleen T. Shiverick, PhD
Department of Pharmacology and Therapeutics, University of Florida, Gainesville, FL, USA

Elina Sieppi, MSc
Institute of Biomedicine, Department of Pharmacology and Toxicology, University of Oulu, Finland

Suresh Sikka, PhD, HCLD
Department of Urology, Tulane University, Health Sciences Center, New Orleans, LA, USA

Michael J. Soares, PhD
Institute for Reproductive Health and Regenerative Medicine, Department of Pathology and Laboratory Medicine, University of Kansas Medical Center, Kansas City, KS, USA

Miguel Angel Sogorb, PhD
Unidad de Toxicología y Seguridad Química, Instituto de Bioingeniería, Universidad Miguel Hernández de Elche, Spain

Offie P. Soldin, PhD
Departments of Oncology, Medicine and Physiology and Biophysics, Lombardi Comprehensive Cancer Center, Georgetown University Medical Center, Washington DC, USA

Chunjuan Song, MS
Department of Biomedical Sciences, Iowa Center for Advanced Neurotoxicology, Iowa State University, Ames, IA, USA

Hermona Soreq, PhD
Department of Biological Chemistry, The Hebrew University of Jerusalem, Jerusalem, Israel

Tammy E. Stoker, PhD
Endocrine Toxicology Branch, Toxicity Assessment Division National Health and Environmental Effects Research Laboratory, Office of Research and Development, US Environmental Protection Agency, Research Triangle Park, NC, USA

Teruo Sugawara, MD, PhD
Health Services Center, Otaru University of Commerce, Otaru, Hokkaido, Japan

David T. Szabo, PhD
Curriculum in Toxicology, University of North Carolina in Chapel Hill, and Integrated Systems Toxicology Division, Phamacokinetics Branch, National Health and Environmental Effects Research Laboratory, Office of Research and Development, US Environmental Protection Agency, Research Triangle Park, NC, USA

Helena Taskinen, MD
Faculty of Medicine, Hjelt Institute, University of Helsinki, Finland and Finnish Institute of Occupational Health, Helsinki, Finland

Peter Truran, PhD
Center for the Philosophy of Science, University of Minnesota, Minneapolis, MN, USA

Kirsi H. Vähäkangas, MD, PhD
Faculty of Health Sciences, University of Eastern Finland, Kuopio, Finland

Subrahmanyam Vangala, PhD
Department of DMPK and Toxicology, Sai Advantium Pharma Ltd, Hinjewadi, Pune, India

Neil Vargesson, BSc (Hons), PhD
School of Medical Sciences, Institute of Medical Sciences, University of Aberdeen, Foresterhill, Aberdeen, Scotland, UK

Jenni Veid, MSc
Faculty of Health Sciences, University of Eastern Finland, Kuopio, Finland

Henrik Viberg, PhD
Department of Physiology and Developmental Biology, Environmental Toxicology, Uppsala University, Sweden

Eugenio Vilanova, PhD
Unidad de Toxicología y Seguridad Química, Instituto de Bioingeniería, Universidad Miguel Hernández de Elche, Spain

Kenneth A. Voss, PhD
Toxicology and Mycotoxin Research Unit, United States Department of Agriculture, Agricultural Research Service, Athens, GA, USA

Suryanarayana V. Vulimiri, BVSc, PhD, DABT
National Center for Environmental Assessment, Office of Research and Development, US Environmental Protection Agency, Washington DC, USA

Etsuko Wada, MD, PhD
Department of Degenerative Neurological Diseases, National Institute of Neuroscience, National Center of Neurology and Psychiatry, Tokyo, Japan and Core Research for Evolutional Science and Technology, Japan Science and Technology Agency, Saitama, Japan

Keiji Wada, MD, PhD
Department of Degenerative Neurological Diseases, National Institute of Neuroscience, National Center of Neurology and Psychiatry, Tokyo, Japan and Core Research for Evolutional Science and Technology, Japan Science and Technology Agency, Saitama, Japan

Pralhad Wangikar, MVSc, PhD, DABT
Department of DMPK and Toxicology, Sai Advantium Pharma Ltd, Hinjewadi, Pune, India

Kevin D. Welch, PhD
US Department of Agriculture-Agricultural Research Service, Poisonous Plant Research Laboratory, Logan, UT, USA

Honghong Yao, PhD
Department of Pharmacology and Experimental Neuroscience, Nebraska Medical Center, University of Nebraska Medical Center, Omaha, NE, USA

Zhaobao Yin, MD, PhD
Vanderbilt University, Department of Pediatrics, Nashville, TN, USA

Xiaoyou Ying, BEng, MSc, PhD
Biomarkers, Bioimaging and Biological Assays - Disposition, Safety and Animal Research, sanofi-aventis US, Bridgewater, NJ, USA

Shirley Zafra-Stone, BS
Product Solutions, Davis, CA, USA

Snjezana Zaja-Milatovic, MSc
Vanderbilt University School of Medicine, Nashville, TN, USA

Matthew J. Zwiernik, PhD
Department of Animal Science, Michigan State University, East Lansing, MI, USA

Section 1

General

CHAPTER

1

Introduction

Ramesh C. Gupta

INTRODUCTION

Unsuccessful conception and adverse pregnancy outcomes have likely occurred since the inception of life. The etiology of such disappointing events can often be attributed to common factors such as malnutrition, hyperthermia, or a stressful environment at home or at the workplace. In addition, exposure to biotoxins, chemical toxicants, radiation or multiple factors seems to be involved in infertility, miscarriage and birth defects. A single factor or a combination of these factors can exert deleterious effects on male and/or female reproductive performance and on the mother, placenta or conceptus after conception. Homeostatic maintenance of human and animal/wildlife species requires proper function of the male and female reproductive systems, and development of offspring.

Reproductive and developmental toxicology is a very complex subject because of continuous changes taking place in the mother, placenta and the unborn. Exposure of the developing organism to chemicals can occur *in utero* or through the mother's milk or contaminated food. In general, it is believed that developing organisms are more sensitive than adults to the toxic effects of chemicals because of limited defense and detoxifying mechanisms. In particular, the nervous and reproductive systems may be more vulnerable to the toxic insult of chemicals due to incomplete blood–brain and blood–testes barriers. Compelling evidence suggests that *in utero* or early postnatal exposure to chemicals not only damages the developing organism, but can predispose an individual for the development of devastating diseases like diabetes, metabolic syndrome, Alzheimer's or Parkinson's in later life.

Toxicological problems related to reproductive and developmental systems have been recognized for centuries, but this area of toxicology has received enormous attention since the thalidomide incident. During the period of 1957–1961, thousands of pregnant women around the world received thalidomide for morning sickness. More than 10,000 children, exposed *in utero* to thalidomide during the first trimester of gestation, were born with a variety of severe birth defects, mainly phocomelia and amelia. Other anomalies related to thalidomide syndrome involved eyes, ears and the central nervous system. From this tragedy, with exhaustive efforts over half a century, scientists learned that: (1) wide species differences exist due to unknown factors, (2) the period of exposure is crucial for expression of teratogenicity, and (3) thalidomide exerts multifaceted effects through multiple mechanisms, although, we are still far from understanding the exact mechanism of teratogenicity. Presently, thalidomide and its analogs are available on the market for indications in leprosy, Crohn's disease, HIV, multiple myeloma and vascular disorder, but of course not prescribed for women who are pregnant or trying to get pregnant.

In another incident, methylmercury was involved in Minamata disease in Japan affecting approximately 3,000 people after consumption of contaminated fish during the late 1950s to the mid-1960s. In the early 1970s, more than 10,000 people died and 100,000 suffered permanent brain damage in Iraq by consuming "wonder wheat" imported from Mexico that was treated with methylmercury as a fungicide. In both incidents, offspring of mothers exposed to methylmercury suffered from severe malformations, cognitive impairment, and behavioral disorders, including "quiet baby syndrome". Because of the catastrophic effects of Minamata disease, the Japanese government has established the "National Institute for Minamata Disease" for biomonitoring and surveillance of mercury exposure to avoid future cases.

Following the thalidomide tragedy, drug safety efforts were intensified throughout the world; however, although presently more than 80,000 chemicals are on the market, used alone or in combinations, only 200 of them have been tested for toxicity and safety. Developmental and reproductive toxicity testing (DART) in animals has been a vital component of the drug development process for humans since the late 1940s. Currently, this set of non-clinical studies in animals is required for drug approval by regulatory agencies, such as the US Food and Drug Administration (FDA), the Organization for Economic and Cooperative Development (OECD), the Japan Pharmaceutical Manufacturers Association (JPMA), and other such agencies in many countries. Currently, many associations (the Pharmaceutical Manufacturers Association, the European Federation of Pharmaceutical Industries Association, and the Japan Pharmaceutical Manufacturers Association), professional organizations (the Society of Toxicology and its specialty section on Reproductive and Developmental Toxicology, the Teratology Society and the International Federation of Teratology Societies) and regulatory agencies (primarily

Reproductive and Developmental Toxicology, Edited by Ramesh C. Gupta
ISBN: 978-0-12-382032-7

from the USA, Europe, and Japan) are actively engaged in drug safety to avoid reproductive and developmental effects. In this context, the International Federation of Pharmaceutical Manufacturers Association (IFPMA) plays a pivotal role in bringing together the regulatory authorities of the USA, Europe, Japan and elsewhere. In the USA, agencies including the Consumer Product Safety Commission, the US Environmental Protection Agency, the US Food and Drug Administration, the US Department of Agriculture, the Agency for Toxic Substance and Disease Registry, the National Toxicology Program, the National Institute of Environmental Health Sciences, the National Institute for Occupational Safety and Health and the Occupational Safety and Health Administration, and in Europe the OECD and REACH (Registration, Evaluation, Authorization and Restriction of Chemicals), play pivotal roles in safety evaluation of non-pharmaceutical chemicals.

It is worth mentioning that developmental and reproductive toxicity risk assessment criteria differ from country to country, and the International Conference on Harmonization (ICH) and related agencies take an active part in dealing with such disparities. The objective of all these regulatory agencies is to identify reproductive and developmental hazards and to ensure the safety of drugs and chemicals.

This book, *Reproductive and Developmental Toxicology*, provides extensive coverage of safety evaluation of new pharmaceutical compounds and risk characterization of chemicals using the guidelines of the agencies listed above.

The complexity of reproductive and developmental toxicity involves many variables, including species, gender, developmental stage, diet, genetic polymorphisms, environmental and many other factors. Pregnant women, the unborn, infants and toddlers constitute unique populations with greater vulnerability in terms of sensitivity to chemicals. Even functional foods including black tea, coffee, etc. can cause developmental effects if consumed in excess during gestation.

It is well established that environmental and genetic factors in relation to chemical toxicity have changed significantly in the last 50 years. This is partly due to the flood of chemicals (therapeutic drugs, industrial chemicals and environmental pollutants), greenhouse gases and global warming. Alcohol, smoke, illicit drugs and anticonvulsants are among the most frequently encountered reproductive and developmental toxicants. These substances, along with many others, cross the placental barrier easily and can lead to a variety of effects, including intrauterine growth restriction (IUGR), preterm birth and spontaneous abortion.

Environmental contaminants, such as PCBs and brominated flame retardants, and recently bisphenol A, phthalates, perfluorooctanoic acid, pesticides, lead in toys (toxic toys), cadmium and zinc in imported jewelry, and high levels of cadmium in drinking glasses and dishes, have raised serious concerns about adverse health effects in general and reproductive and developmental effects in particular. The current concern about "Toxic Childhood" in "Toxic America" is real and the community as a whole has no choice but to face the challenges of the 21st century to minimize chemical exposure.

Each year approximately 3% of babies in the USA are born with birth defects that are life-threatening. One of the most common human birth defects is neural tube defects (NTDs), due to failure of neural tube closure, often resulting in anencephaly, exencephaly and spina bifida. Although, the etiology of NTDs is complex, chemical agents (antiepileptic drugs, thalidomide, folate antagonists, etc.), in addition to genetic and environmental factors, appear to be involved.

Today's advanced technologies allow biomonitoring of chemical (therapeutic and environmental concern) residues at parts per billion or parts per trillion in biological tissues and fluids. In recent investigations, 10,000 babies were examined and more than 200 chemicals were found in the umbilical cord. On the one hand, the presence of a chemical in the cord blood does not prove the chemical is harmful to the unborn; on the other hand, its harmful effects cannot be ruled out unless proven safe based on toxicity testing. In essence, every chemical is safe unless proven toxic. Molecular toxicology offers novel biomarkers and sensitive endpoints of cellular and molecular damage (biochemical, neurochemical or histopathological) to the fetus that are particularly useful in reproductive and developmental toxicity and safety testing. *In vitro*, *in vivo* and *in silico* models, national and international guidelines for toxicity testing, and international harmonization in risk assessment criteria are necessary for the safety evaluation of chemicals and drugs. Pharmacokinetics/toxicokinetics and physiologically based pharmacokinetics of drugs/toxicants seem to differ substantially in male vs. female, and more so in pregnant vs. non-pregnant; and therefore special attention should be paid when dealing with pregnancies, and fetal, neonatal and pediatric populations. Current technologies such as ultrasound, MRI and micro-CT imaging aid in an early diagnosis of any malformations in embryonic-fetal development.

Reproductive and Developmental Toxicology is the single most comprehensive resource on this subject, comprised of more than 80 chapters, which are arranged into 15 sections. The book is prepared with a user-friendly format for academia, pharmaceutical industries and regulatory/governmental agencies. Standalone chapters are provided on major topics, so the reader can easily find the required information. The volume covers many novel topics related to reproductive and developmental toxicants, especially topics of current concern, such as endocrine disruptors, pesticides, industrial solvents, metals, bisphenol A, phthalates, nanoparticles, nutraceuticals, pharmaceuticals, phytoestrogens, mycotoxins and zootoxins. Ten chapters are offered in Section XI on special topics, including stem cells, toxicogenomics, metabolomics, epigenetic regulation, cell signaling mechanisms, neuroinflammation, and mitochondrial dysfunction in reproductive and developmental toxicity. Multiple chapters offer state-of-the-art techniques, including ultrasound, magnetic resonance and micro-CT imaging for prenatal diagnosis of developmental anomalies. Atlas-style coverage of toxicologic pathology is presented for testing and screening of chemicals having the potential for reproductive and developmental toxicity. Since the placenta is the key to the success of pregnancy, extensive coverage of placental toxicity is provided with five chapters, dealing with placentation in humans and rodent species, placental role in fetal programming and biocommunication between mother and fetus, placental structure, function and barrier, significance of transporters and other molecular mechanisms in the feto-placental unit, and toxicologic pathology of a variety of drugs, chemicals and biotoxins. Finally, the last section of the book offers multiple chapters describing reproductive and developmental toxicity and endocrine disruption in domestic, wildlife and aquatic species.

The contributors of this book are highly qualified and considered authorities in toxicology in general and reproductive and developmental toxicology in particular. Their hard work and dedication to this book is greatly appreciated. The editor expresses his gratitude to Robin B. Doss and Kristie M. Rohde for technical assistance, Alexandre Katos for the cover design and Denise M. Gupta for indexing. Last but not least, the editor immensely appreciates the tireless efforts of publishing editors April Graham, Nancy Maragioglio and Kirsten Chrisman at Academic Press/ Elsevier for their various roles in the preparation of this book.

CHAPTER

2

Reproductive anatomy and physiology

Timothy J. Evans and Vekataseshu K. Ganjam

INTRODUCTION

In order for one to fully appreciate how xenobiotics can adversely affect reproductive function, including development, it is necessary to have some understanding of the coordinated sequence of events and physiological processes involved. Normal reproduction will be reviewed in this chapter to provide anatomical and physiological bases for the discussions of specific mechanisms of action and reproductive toxicants in the other chapters of this book. Although the emphasis of this chapter will be on human reproduction, many of the same principles are applicable to reproductive processes in other mammals, as well as other classes of vertebrates.

Unfortunately, space constraints limit the amount of information which can be presented in this chapter, and many of the presented topics cannot be discussed at great length. If additional information is required for better understanding of the subject matter, there are several excellent textbooks which provide an overview, including detailed illustrations, of the basic reproductive anatomy and physiology of humans (Berne et al., 2004; Netter, 1997; Piñón, 2002), as well as animals (Senger, 2007). There are also a number of book chapters in other toxicology texts which cover this information, as it applies directly to exposures to toxicants (Evans, 2007; Foster and Gray, 2008). Other references can be consulted for more in-depth discussion of specific cells or organs involved in the reproductive process (De Jonge and Barratt, 2006; Payne and Hardy, 2007; Skinner and Griswold, 2005). The reader is also directed to references cited in this chapter (many of which are available online) in order to gain additional insight into the specific topics being discussed.

IMPORTANT DEFINITIONS AND CONCEPTS

Reproduction

Reproduction in humans, as well as domestic, wild and laboratory vertebrates, encompasses the wide range of physiological processes and the associated behaviors and anatomical structures necessary for the birth of the next generation of a given species (Evans, 2007; Senger, 2007). Those physiological processes involved specifically in human reproduction are illustrated in Figure 2.1 and generally include the following (Evans, 2007):

1. Gametogenesis (production of sperm or ova) and the pre- and peripubertal changes leading up to its onset.
2. Release of gametes (i.e., sperm transport/maturation, libido/courtship, penile erection, intromission/copulation, emission and ejaculation of semen, and ovulation of an oocyte).
3. Formation of the zygote (i.e., sperm storage, capacitation, and processes leading to fertilization or union of a single sperm with an egg).
4. Embryonic and fetal development during pregnancy or gestation (i.e., activities related to the initiation and progression of zygote cleavage, blastocyst formation, separation of the germ layers, placentation, neurulation and organogenesis.
5. Parturition or "birth" of a single or multiple offspring.
6. Lactogenesis and lactation for the postpartum nutrition of offspring.

All of these processes are potential targets for reproductive toxicants present in the environment, workplace or home.

Hormones and hormone receptors

The term "hormone" classically refers to a substance which is secreted into the circulation by a ductless gland and which alters the function of its target cells (Hodgson *et al.*, 2000). While the traditional "endocrine" aspect of hormone action involves organ-to-organ signaling (and in the case of mammalian pregnancy animal-to-animal signaling), it is recognized that hormones can also be involved in "paracrine" (cell-to-cell) communication and signaling pathways within the same cell in which they were produced ("autocrine" function) (Evans, 2007). In vertebrates there are a wide variety of different hormones involved in reproductive function. The major reproductive hormones are generally grouped according to their basic molecular structure and include amino acid derivatives (e.g., dopamine or prolactin inhibitory factor and melatonin); peptides (e.g., oxytocin, adrenocorticotropin hormone or ACTH, corticotropin releasing factor or hormone or CRF/CRH, gonadotropin releasing hormone or GnRH, and

Reproductive and Developmental Toxicology, Edited by Ramesh C. Gupta
ISBN: 978-0-12-382032-7

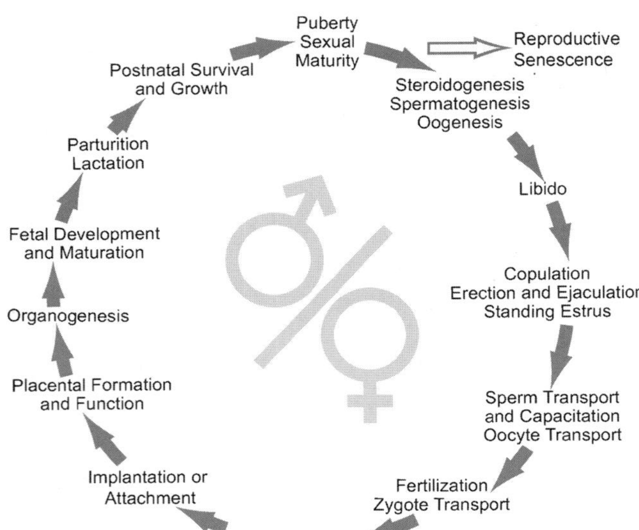

FIGURE 2.1 The continuum of developmental stages and reproductive functions taking place in males and/or females, as well as the embryo and fetus, are shown schematically and illustrate the complexity of reproduction in mammalian species, especially in humans, where additional behavioral, psychological, social and environmental factors, as well as eventual senescence, can come into play. This figure was adapted, with permission, from Evans (2007). Modifications and artwork were courtesy of Don Connor and Howard Wilson.

thyrotropin releasing hormone or TRH); proteins (e.g., activin, inhibin, insulin-like growth factors, prolactin and relaxin); glycoproteins (e.g., follicle-stimulating hormone or FSH, luteinizing hormone or LH, and thyroid-stimulating hormone or TSH or thyrotropin); steroids (e.g., androgens, estrogens and progestagens); and eicosanoids, which include prostaglandins.

The actions of hormones on their targets are generally mediated through receptors which initiate or inhibit some sort of signal transduction pathway or are required for hormone-induced alterations in gene expression. Hormone–receptor interactions can be modulated by a number of factors, including the amount of hormone present, the affinity of the hormone for the receptor, receptor density and occupancy and interactions with other hormones, receptors and hormone-receptor complexes, as well as a variety of endogenous co-activators and inhibitors (Bigsby *et al.*, 2005; Evans, 2007; Genuth, 2004a). It should be evident from the topics covered in this textbook that various xenobiotics are also capable, under certain exposure conditions, of modulating the interactions between endogenous hormones and their receptors.

Gonadal steroid hormones and their "nuclear" receptors

As has been reviewed by the authors previously (Evans *et al.*, 1997), the basic structure of steroid hormones consists of four rings labeled as A, B, C and D. The various members of this hormone class differ from one another with respect to the location of double bonds and types of functional groups attached to the ring structure. The major gonadal steroids are also referred to as the "sex" steroids and include androgens (i.e., androstenedione, testosterone and dihydrotestosterone, which is the 5α-reductase conversion product of testosterone in the testes and selected non-gonadal tissues), estrogens (i.e., estradiol and estrone) and, for the purposes of this chapter, progesterone and other endogenous progestagens. Mineralocorticoids, glucocorticoids and progestagens are all 21-carbon compounds. Androgens are 19-carbon compounds, and estrogens contain 18 carbons. In the classical Δ^4 biosynthetic pathway for endogenous steroids, cholesterol is the steroid precursor, and the rate-limiting step in steroidogenesis is cholesterol transfer within the mitochondria, which is mediated by steroidogenic acute regulatory protein (Stocco, 2007). Cholesterol is cleaved and converted to the progestagen, prenenolone, which is converted to progesterone by 3β-hydroxysteroid dehydrogenase. Androstenedione is synthesized from progesterone by the actions of several enzymes, including 17-hydroxylase, and can be converted to testosterone by 17β-hydroxysteroid dehydrogenase. Androgens are converted to estrogens by aromatase, a member of the cytochrome P450 (CYP) family of enzymes. Androstenedione is converted to estrone, and testosterone is converted by aromatase to estradiol. It is also possible in the Δ^4 steroidogenesis pathway for estradiol to be synthesized from estrone via the actions of 17β-hydroxysteroid dehydrogenase (Evans *et al.*, 1997).

In appropriate cell types, mineralocorticoids and glucocorticoids can be synthesized from progesterone. Interestingly, both of these types of steroid hormones can also interact with the promiscuous mineralocorticoid receptor. Isoforms of 11β-hydroxysteroid dehydrogenase are present in many different cell types to regulate the relative proportions of the active and inactive forms of glucocorticoids (i.e., cortisol and cortisone, respectively, in humans). This regulation is important from the perspective of mineralocorticoid activity, as well as the modulation of the adverse effects of glucocorticoids on reproduction and other physiological processes (Hardy and Ganjam, 1997).

The gonadal steroids facilitate the development and regulation of reproductive function in humans and animal species, in large part by interacting with (i.e., functioning as ligands for) receptors which are members of the steroid/thyroid ("nuclear") receptor superfamily, the largest family of transcription factors in eukaryotic systems (Evans, 2007; Genuth, 2004a; Tsai and O'Malley, 1994). Receptors in this superfamily are large oligomeric proteins (Genuth, 2004a), which generally consist of six domains (A/B, C, D, E and F) (Tsai and O'Malley, 1994). Although specific portions of the gonadal steroid nuclear receptor molecules can interact with a variety of co-activators as well as inhibitors, the most important domains of these receptors are generally considered to be those involved in transactivation (N-terminal A/B domain; also C-terminus in estrogen receptors); DNA-binding and hormone–receptor complex dimerization (middle portion containing two helical zinc fingers; C domain); and hormone (ligand) binding (C-terminus; E domain) (Bigsby *et al.*, 2005; Genuth, 2004a). While androgen, estrogen and progesterone receptors, which are members of the steroid/thyroid superfamily, are often thought of as being exclusively nuclear in their location, these receptors can also be located in the cytoplasm of some cells. Cytoplasmic and nuclear gonadal steroid receptors can be bound to a variety of different heat shock proteins, which interact with the receptor's hormone-binding domain. Heat shock proteins can act as "blocking" molecules and are displaced by hormones binding to the receptors (Bigsby *et al.*, 2005; Genuth, 2004a) or as "chaperones" involved in receptor turnover and "trafficking" of these receptors between the nucleus and cytoplasm (Evans, 2007).

There is reportedly a single type of androgen receptor which is a member of the steroid/thyroid superfamily. In contrast, there are two types of nuclear estrogen receptors

(ERα and ERβ), which are the products of distinct genes on separate chromosomes (O'Donnell *et al.*, 2001). ERα and ERβ differ in their amino acid structure, tissue distribution, affinity for selective ER modulators (SERMs) and their role in female (Britt and Findlay, 2002) as well as, somewhat surprisingly, male fertility (Evans, 2007; Hess, 2003; O'Donnell *et al.*, 2001). The nuclear progesterone receptor also has two isoforms, progesterone receptor A and progesterone receptor B (PRA and PRB, respectively), which differ slightly in their amino acid sequences and their interactions with co-activators, but, unlike ERα and ERβ, PRA and PRB are the product of a single gene (Brayman *et al.*, 2006).

Genomic and non-genomic mechanisms of action of gonadal steroid hormones

Traditionally, the receptor-mediated reproductive effects of gonadal steroids were thought to occur almost exclusively through interactions between homodimers of the hormone–nuclear receptor complexes and specific regions of DNA upstream from the basal promoter of a given gene, referred to as hormone response elements (HREs) or, more specifically, androgen and estrogen response elements (ARE and ERE, respectively) (Genuth, 2004a; Tsai and O'Malley, 1994). It is now understood that these "genomic" effects of gonadal steroids and their nuclear receptors, which involve alterations in gene transcription, can, in some instances, involve heterodimers of different nuclear steroid–receptor complexes, indirect binding of hormone–receptor complexes to DNA via proteins within a preformed transcriptional complexes and even ligand (hormone)-independent "activation" of nuclear gonadal steroid receptor molecules (Bigsby *et al.*, 2005; O'Donnell *et al.*, 2001; Thomas and Khan, 2005). In addition, it is also apparent that gonadal steroids can affect cellular function by non-genomic mechanisms of action involving changes in intracellular concentrations of ions, cAMP and its second messengers, and the mitogen-activated protein (MAP) kinase pathway. These non-genomic mechanisms are independent of the somewhat "time-consuming" alterations in gene expression traditionally associated with gonadal steroids and occur rapidly within seconds or minutes (O'Donnell *et al.*, 2001; Thomas and Khan, 2005). While the rapid, non-genomic effects of gonadal steroids most likely involve receptors bound to the plasma membrane, the specific identity and classification of these receptors remain unclear and might involve a number of different receptor types (Evans, 2007; O'Donnell *et al.*, 2001; Razandi *et al.*, 1999; Thomas and Khan, 2005; Warner and Gustafsson, 2006).

REVIEW OF NORMAL HUMAN REPRODUCTION

Historical perspectives and complexity of reproductive function

It should be evident from a review of Figures 2.2A, 2.2B and 2.2C that for well over 200 years the basic anatomical components required for human reproduction have been fairly well recognized and their primary functions understood. However, it has only been more recently that we have gained a more accurate understanding of the specific cellular, hormonal and molecular aspects involved in this process. Figure 2.1 demonstrates how reproduction is a complex and dynamic process involving precise coordination and integration of the functions of multiple organs within the body. The production of viable and functional gametes and their transport and union to form a zygote which develops into a healthy and fertile individual require that many stringent physiological and metabolic needs be met. A thorough understanding of the mechanisms involved in reproduction is absolutely essential in order to recognize which steps in the reproductive process are most susceptible to the adverse effects of potential toxicants.

Relevance of a basic understanding of human reproductive anatomy and physiology

It is necessary, from a clinical perspective, to identify what constitutes "normal" reproduction in order to recognize abnormal reproductive behaviors, function and morphologic changes in humans, as well as in wild, domestic and laboratory animals. It is also critical that one be able to understand the pathophysiological basis for reproductive abnormalities. Impaired reproductive function in humans associated with exposure to toxic amounts of xenobiotics necessitates the use of diagnostic, therapeutic and prognostic procedures, which require a thorough knowledge of normal reproductive anatomy and physiology (Evans, 2007). In addition, if we are to develop animal models for human reproductive diseases or are to extrapolate results of toxicology experiments performed with laboratory animals to human exposures to the same xenobiotics, we need to understand how human anatomy and/or reproductive physiology differs from that of the animals being used for modeling.

Neuroendocrine control of reproduction

In humans and animals alike, visual, olfactory, auditory and other sensory data are integrated within the brain and are reflected in endocrine events. The neuroendocrine functions of the pineal gland, hypothalamus and pituitary gland play an important role in the integration of the body's physiological processes, including reproduction, and are potential targets for toxicants (i.e., dioxins). The proper function of the hypothalamic–pituitary–gonadal axis facilitates development of the reproductive tract and endocrine regulation of spermatogenesis in the male and the menstrual or estrous cycle in the female. The onset of puberty and sexual behavior in males and females, the ability to achieve erection and ejaculation in males, and the normal progression of gestation, parturition and lactation in females are also facilitated by the secretions of the hypothalamus and pituitary gland (Evans, 2007; Evans *et al.*, 1997; Senger, 2007).

The hormones involved in the neuroendocrine control of reproduction are produced in several regions of the brain. Melatonin is produced in the pineal gland. The major hormones of reproductive interest which are of hypothalamic origin are dopamine, CRF, GnRH and TRH. Oxytocin is released from the posterior pituitary (neurohypophysis), and ACTH, FSH, LH, prolactin and TSH are synthesized and released from the anterior pituitary (adenohypophysis) (Evans, 2007; Evans *et al.*, 1997). The production and release of these hormones are regulated by various positive and negative feedback loops (Figure 2.3), which are potentially susceptible to the effects of hormonally active xenobiotics.

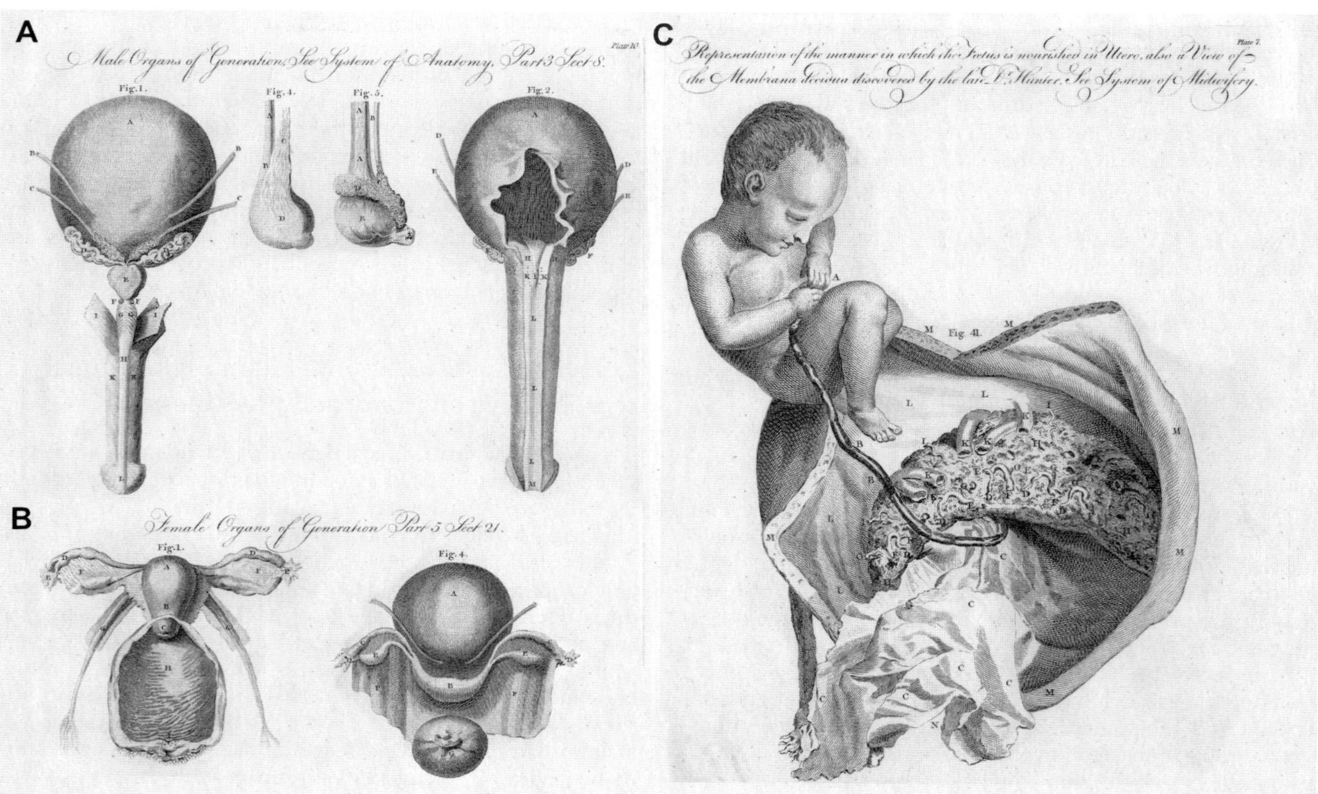

FIGURE 2.2 An artist's renderings, which were obviously not drawn to scale and which were published in the *Modern Universal Dictionary of Arts and Sciences* (also referred to as *Hall's Encyclopedia*) in or around 1798, show the male and female "organs of generation" and a representation of the "manner in which fetus is nourished *in utero*" in **A**, **B** and **C**, respectively. While, unfortunately, the original legends for these drawings were not available for review of the terminology, it should be clear, despite some departures from our current understanding, that there was a basic comprehension and appreciation of reproductive anatomy at the time and that people were keenly interested in learning more about these physiological processes. This figure will be explained in quite some detail, as it provides a historical basis for the extensive, subsequent investigation of the cellular, as well as subcellular and molecular processes involved in mammalian and, more specifically, human reproductive function. In **A**, the key anatomical components being demonstrated in Fig. 1 are posterior views of the urinary bladder (A), showing the entry of the ureters (B) into the bladder; the ductuli or ducti deferens (C) and their expanded distal extremities (i.e., the ampullae), which are considered accessory sex glands in men; and the other male accessory sex glands, including the seminal vesicles (D), the prostate gland (E) and bulbourethral or Cowper's glands (F). The position of the seemingly erect penis (most likely straightened for display purposes), with the foreskin and, possibly, the fascial and portions of the muscular layers removed, is not one which would be observed *in situ* (image of *in situ* anatomical arrangement not shown). If the pelvis were present, the pelvic urethra would form an approximately 90° angle with the penile or cavernous urethra and would be directed away from the reader. The "penile" structures shown from an inferior view include the bulbus urethrae covered by the bulbocavernosus muscles (G); the corpus spongiosum, which surrounds the penile urethra (H); the paired ischiocavernosus muscles (I); what appear to be the penile corpora cavernosa (K); and the distal end of the urethra surrounded by the glans. In Fig. 2 of **A**, the urinary bladder (A) and the ureters, ductuli deferens and seminiferous vesicles (D, E and F, respectively) are observed from an anterior view, and the "penile" structures in this image, which would be directed towards the reader in the presence of a pelvis, can be evaluated from a superior view. Important structures on the floor of the penile urethra (L), which terminates at the external urethral orifice located within the glans (M), include the seminal colliculus and the orifices of the ejaculatory ducts (I), as well as the multiple orifices of the prostate gland (K). The testis (D) in Fig. 4 appears to be covered by an intact parietal tunica vaginalis (i.e., a protective connective tissue structure which has internal or visceral and external or parietal components), with the cremaster muscle (C) and components of the spermatic cord (A and B) shown. The parietal tunica vaginalis appears to have been removed from the testis (E) in Fig. 5, which is viewed from the lateral perspective, showing portions of the epididymis (C and D), as well as the vascular components of the spermatic cord (A) and the ductus deferens (B). In **B**, the key anatomical components of the female reproductive tract and nearby organs are shown from frontal (Fig. 1) and posterior perspectives (Fig. 4). The fundus (A), body (B) and cervix or internal cervical os (C) of the simplex human uterus are illustrated in Fig. 1 and connect with the uterine or Fallopian tube or oviduct (D) and its terminal infundibulum, with the associated fimbriae and ostium (E) above, and with the vagina (H) below. The urethral orifice and the associated openings of various ducts and what is most likely the clitoris are indicated by I and K, respectively. The round ligament is denoted by G. In Fig. 4, it should be noted that the reproductive tract lies below the urinary bladder (A) and above the rectum (G). The tubular genitalia, including the uterus (B), the body of the uterine tube (C), and the oviduct's terminal infundibulum, with its fimbriae (D), are all suspended within the broad ligament (F in both Fig. 1 and Fig. 4), along with the ovaries (E). As was customary for the particular time period in which it was drawn, **C** shows an extremely mature fetus (A) exhibiting some developmental characteristics more typical of older children or, even, young adults than neonates. This meticulously drawn illustration clearly shows the umbilical cord (B), the amnion (C) and the discoid placenta with its decidual (maternal) and chorionic (fetal) components. The detail in this drawing implies a reasonable understanding of the importance of the placenta and its circulation for fetal nourishment and well-being. Modifications of figures were performed by Howard Wilson and Don Connor.

Puberty and sexual maturity

The onset of puberty

The onset and completion of puberty are potential targets for a variety of reproductive toxicants, and, depending on the toxicant, these events can be hastened or delayed. Puberty in male and female offspring, especially in domestic animals, implies reproductive competence and corresponds to the onset of normal spermatogenesis in the male and reproductive cyclicity in the female. In females of domestic animal species, puberty can be defined by the age at first estrus or ovulation or even the age at which pregnancy can be maintained safely (Evans *et al.*, 1997; Senger, 2007). In the male of most animal species,

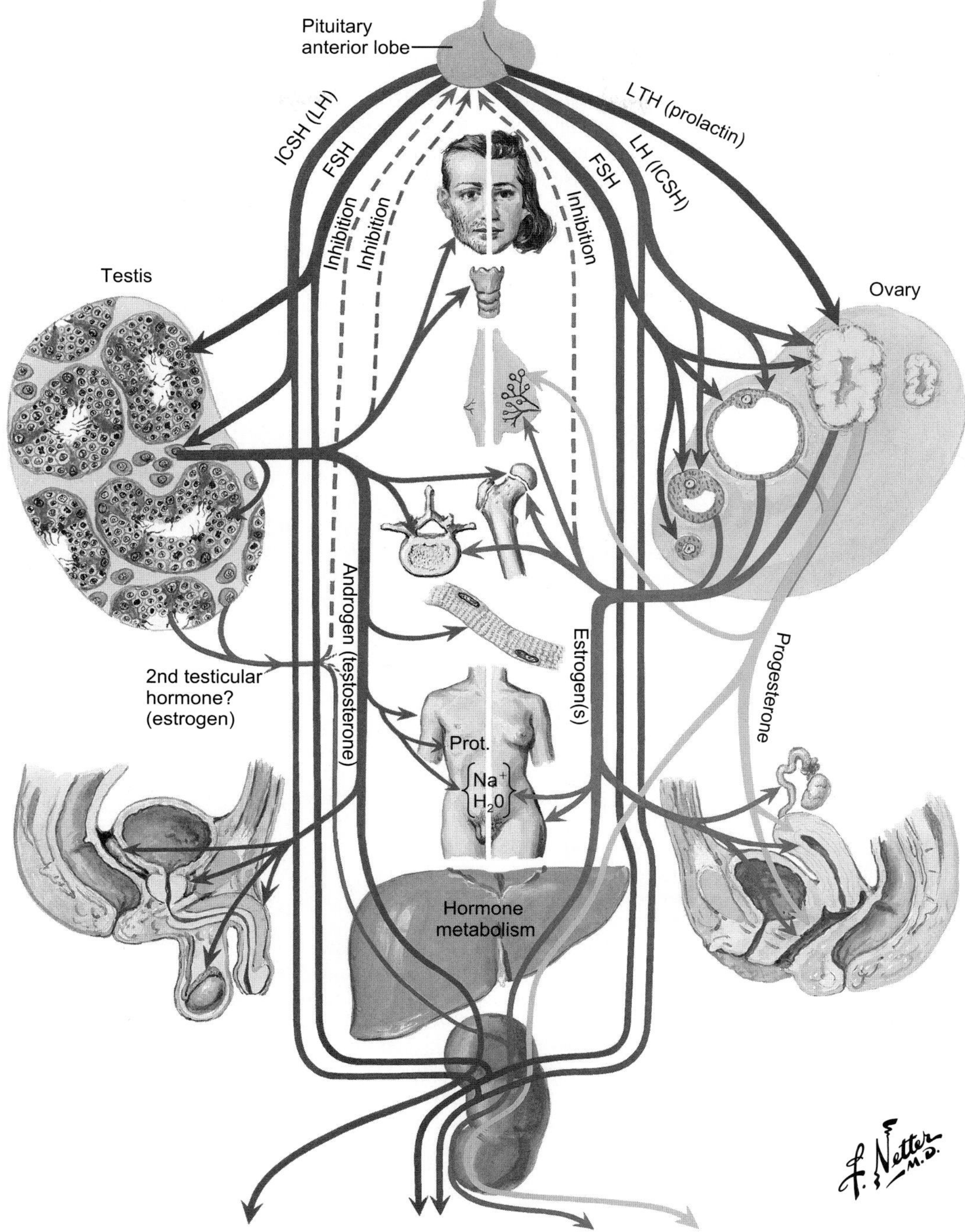

FIGURE 2.3 The basic gonadal steroidogenic pathways, target sites, feedback loops and routes of excretion for the adult male and female human are summarized in this figure. Positive and negative feedback mechanisms involving gonadal steroids help maintain an endocrine environment which is conducive to normal male and female reproductive function. Figure was obtained, with permission, from Netter (1997). Please refer to color plate section.

the age at the time of preputial separation in some species and the acquisition of the ability to ejaculate or the age at the first appearance of spermatozoa in the ejaculate or urine, as well as the production of threshold concentrations of fertile sperm in the ejaculate, have all been used as indicators of puberty (Senger, 2007). Species, nutritional status, environmental and social factors, pheromones and photoperiod in short- or long-day breeders can all influence the age of onset of puberty in animal species (Evans, 2007; Senger, 2007).

In humans, some of the processes by which girls and boys change in appearance and become sexually mature men and women are unique to higher primates. Pubertal development in humans generally takes place in stages and over a longer period of time than in most other animal species (Foster and Gray, 2008; Marshall and Tanner, 1969, 1970). Marshall and Tanner (1969) defined the stages of puberty in girls based on thelarche (i.e., the first stages of breast development), adrenarche, which has been found to be associated with the secretion of androgens (i.e., dehydoepiandrosterone or DHEA and its sulfated conjugate or DHEAS), which induce the growth of pubic hair and alter the composition of sweat gland secretions (Foster and Gray, 2008), and menarche (i.e., the occurrence of the first menses or sloughing of the endometrial lining in response to cyclic endocrine alterations), which is used by some investigators as a single indicator of puberty. On average, girls begin early breast development by nine or ten years of age, although normally developing girls have been reported to start this process as late as 12 or 13 years of age. Many girls experience menarche between 11.5 and 15.5 years of age and are thought to be sexually mature by the time they reach 14 to 16 years of age (Genuth, 2004b). Similar to puberty in girls, the stages of puberty in boys (Marshall and Tanner, 1970) have been described, at least in part, in terms of the growth of pubic hair related to adrenarche, where, as in girls, adrenarche is associated with phenotypic responses to the androgenic secretions of the zona reticularis portion of the adrenal gland, which develops independent of the maturation of the hypothalamic–pituitary–gonadal axis. The progression of puberty in boys is also evaluated by assessing gonadal and penile growth and development, which unlike adrenarche is dependent on the hypothalamic–pituitary–gonadal axis. On average, boys begin pubertal development by the time they are 10 to 11 years of age, with pubic hair developing between 12 and 16 years of age (Genuth, 2004b). While "full" reproductive function in males is usually achieved by 15 to 17 years of age, this is subject to some variation and is not the same as "maximum reproductive function". In addition to the visual assessment of various physical characteristics related to sexual maturity, the progression of puberty in humans can also be assessed by measurement of serum concentrations of estradiol and testosterone, as well as other estrogens and androgens (Foster and Gray, 2008; Genuth, 2004b).

The endocrinology of puberty

From an endocrine perspective, puberty is associated with maturation of the hypothalamic–pituitary–gonadal axis and the ability of the hypothalamus to release enough GnRH to induce gonadotropin production by the anterior pituitary gland (Evans, 2007; Genuth, 2004b; Senger, 2007). This endocrine milestone is brought about by the postnatal developmental changes which allow the hypothalamus to overcome the negative feedback of testicular androgens and estrogens in males and which facilitate the ovary's ability to produce sufficient estrogens to induce the preovulatory surge of GnRH in females (Evans, 2007; Senger, 2007). Many of the endocrine changes which come into play with the onset of puberty are also involved in the transition from anestrus to the ovulatory season in seasonally polyestrous female animals (Evans, 2007).

Normal male reproductive anatomy and physiology

Developmental perspectives

While the mechanisms of sexual differentiation will be covered in greater detail later in this chapter, it is important to note, as male and, subsequently, female reproductive anatomy and physiology are reviewed, that there is an "undifferentiated" stage during development (Figure 2.4A), where the male fetus is internally and externally indistinguishable from the female fetus. A complex set of structural modifications (Figures 2.5A and 2.5B) result in what is seen internally, with respect to the testes and excurrent duct system (Figure 2.4A), as well as externally for penile and scrotal morphology (Figure 2.4B).

Reproductive anatomy of the male

Anatomical structures associated with reproduction in the male usually include, especially in mammals, paired testes (i.e., male gonads) positioned outside the abdominal cavity in most species; an excurrent duct system (i.e., efferent ductules, paired epididymidies, ducti deferens and urethra); accessory sex glands (i.e., ampullae, seminal vesicles, prostate and bulbourethral glands); a scrotum and its associated thermoregulatory functions to protect the testes from mechanical and thermal insult; and some form of copulatory organ or penis with a mechanism for protrusion, erection, emission of glandular secretions and sperm into the urethra and ejaculation of semen from the urethra at the time of orgasm (Figure 2.2A). The primary functions of the testis (testicle) are spermatogenesis or production of male gametes (sperm or spermatozoa) and steroidogenesis (production of androgens and estrogens). Unlike the female in which oogonia are no longer replicating and the full complement of potential oocytes is present at birth, spermatogonia are proliferating and differentiating into spermatozoa continuously, and the testis is organized in such a way as to maximize sperm production (Evans, 2007; Foster and Gray, 2008; Senger, 2007). Figure 2.2A clearly shows the primary anatomical components of the male reproductive tract, and, while the names and understanding of the underlying cellular and molecular processes taking place in these tissues have changed over the last 200 years, the appearance of these structures and how they are presented in anatomical illustrations has essentially remained unchanged.

Testicular structure

Taking a closer look at the human testis, it is evident that the testis is divided into lobules of parenchyma consisting of tubular and interstitial compartments (Evans, 2007; Netter, 1997; Senger, 2007). The structural and functional units within the tubular compartment are the seminiferous tubules (Figures 2.6A and 2.6B), which, depending on the species, comprise approximately 80% of the adult testis (Genuth, 2004b). As shown in Figure 2.6A, seminiferous tubules form highly convoluted loops (tubulus contortus) which begin and end with straight portions (tubulus rectus) that connect to the rete tubules (Genuth, 2004b; Netter, 1997; Senger, 2007). In some species, such as the human, the rete tubules coalesce in a fibrous region of the testis referred to as the mediastinum, which joins with septal projections of the tunica albuginea, part of the testicular capsule. The rete tubules join with the efferent ductules, which attach to the epididymidis, which leads into the ductus deferens or vas deferens.

Within the seminiferous tubules are germ cells at various stages of differentiation and Sertoli cells, which provide germ cells with structural support and nutrients, as well as regulatory and paracrine factors (Foster and Gray, 2008) (Figure 2.6B). Tight junctions (junctional complexes) between adjacent Sertoli cells divide the seminiferous epithelium into basal and adluminal compartments, with Sertoli cells anchored to the basement membrane and surrounding the developing populations of germ cells (Evans, 2007; Foster

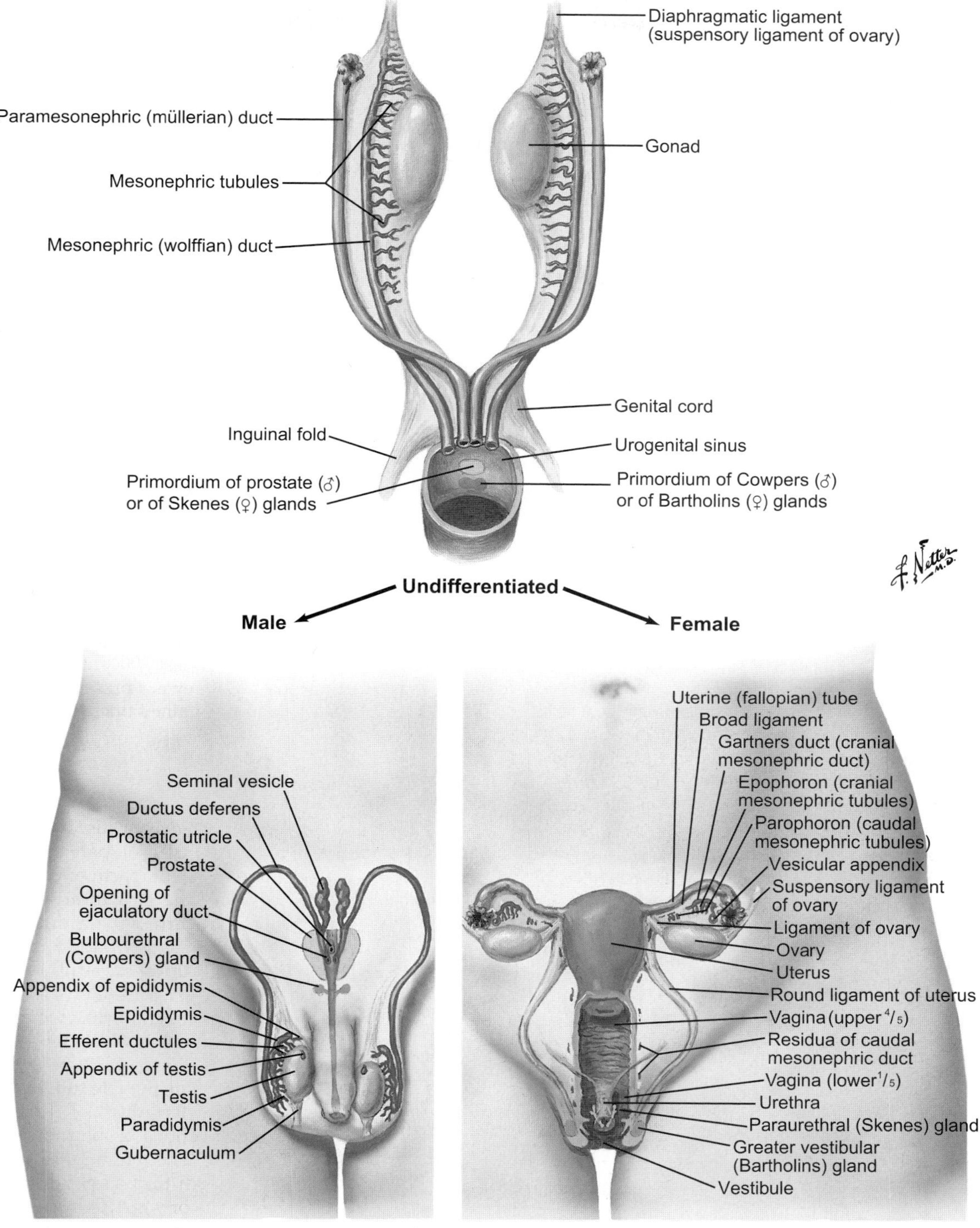

FIGURE 2.4 The "undifferentiated" stage observed in the fetus, regardless of genotypic sex, early in gestation prior to gonadal sexual differentiation, as well as the gonads, internal genitalia and other associated anatomical structures of the sexually mature male and female are shown in **A**. **B** (page 14) illustrates the standard sequence of events in the development of the external genitalia of men and women, as well as other mammalian species. The failure of the urethral groove to close at any point during this sequence results in various degrees of hypospadias, which is a relatively common congenital birth defect in male offspring and one which has been induced in laboratory species by prenatal exposure to a number of xenobiotics. Figures were obtained, with permission, from Netter (1997). Please refer to color plate section.

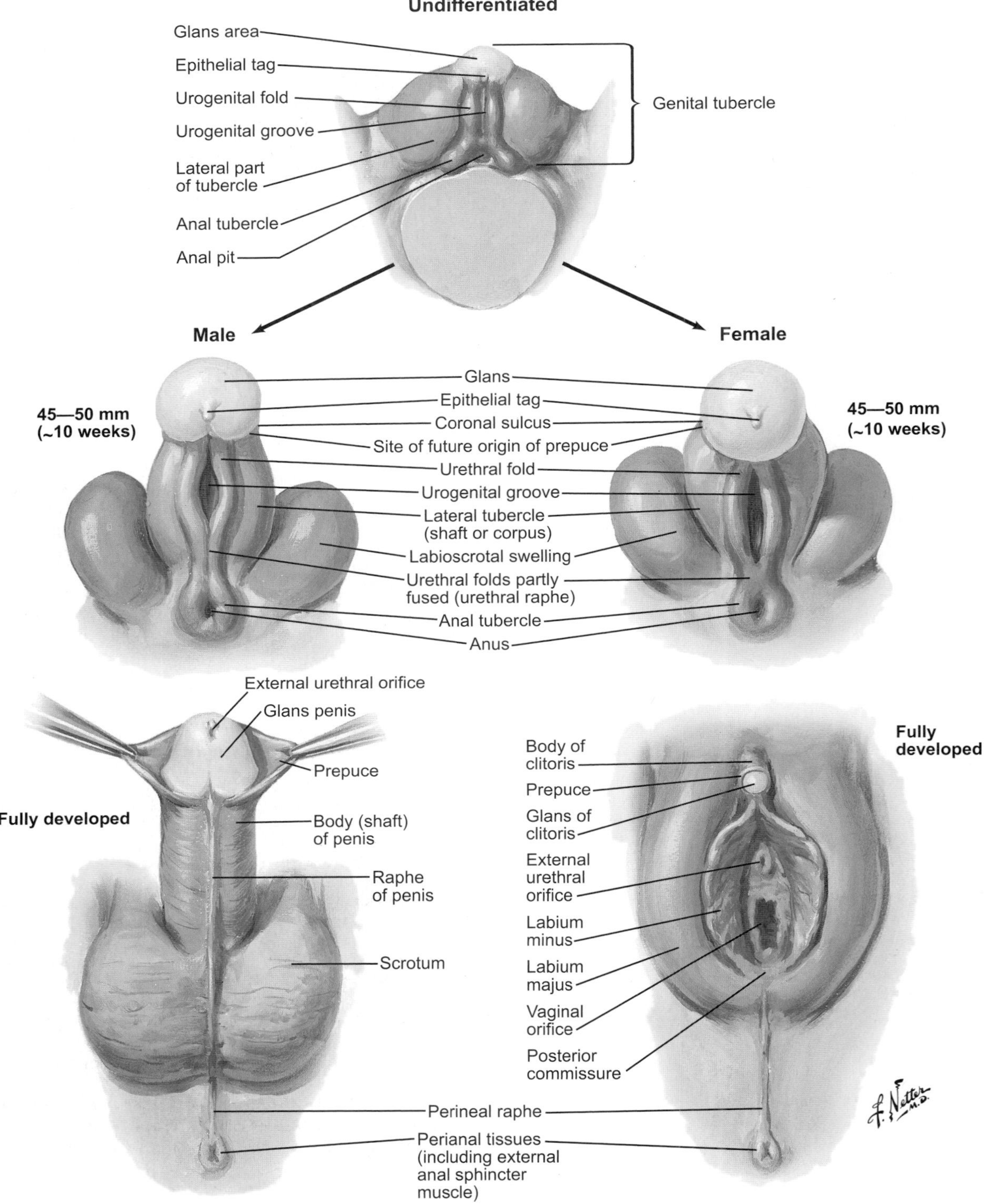

FIGURE 2.4—Cont'd

and Gray, 2008; Genuth, 2004b; Senger, 2007). The seminiferous tubules are surrounded by peritubular myoid cells which participate in important cell–cell interactions with Sertoli cells, the junctional complexes of which form the "blood–testis barrier" or "Sertoli cell barrier" to prevent free exchange of large proteins and some xenobiotics between the blood and the fluid within the seminiferous tubules (Hess and França, 2005; Senger, 2007). It should be noted from Figure 2.6B that, as expected, the appearance of the seminiferous tubules changes as male offspring mature postnatally.

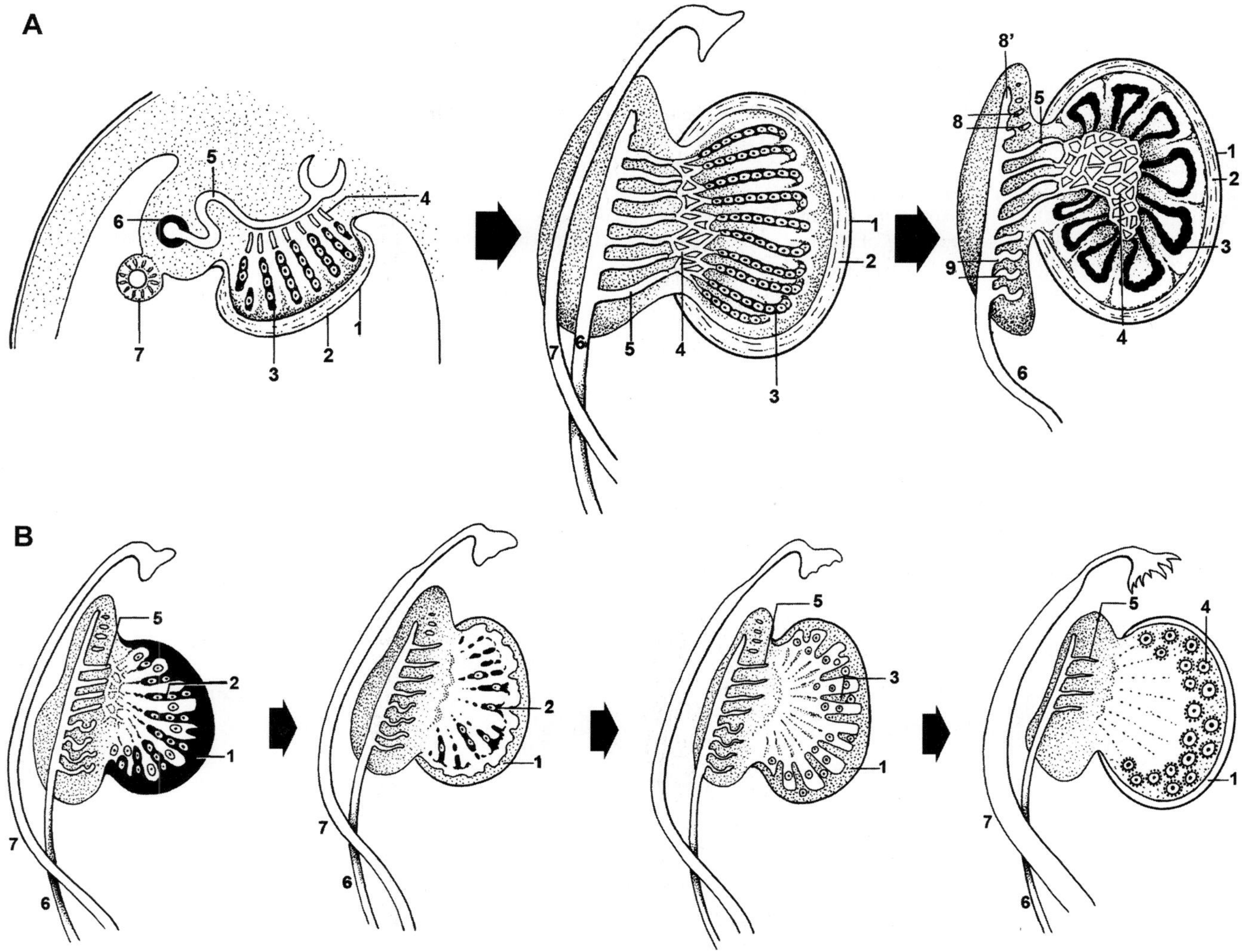

FIGURE 2.5 The initial stages in the development of the testis and the formation of the excurrent duct system are shown in **A**. The initial formation of the tunica albuginea isolates the epithelial cords from the surface epithelium, and the epithelial cords, rete testis and mesonephric tubules (also referred to as the mesonephric ductules or mesonephric duct system) subsequently interconnect. The epithelial cords (sex cords) will eventually become the seminiferous tubules, and the mesonephric ductules will be incorporated into the formation of the excurrent duct system. (1) Celomic epithelium; (2) tunica albuginea; (3) epithelial cords (future seminiferous tubules); (4) rete testis; (5) mesonephric tubules (later efferent ductules); (6) mesonephric duct (future epididymis (proximal portion contiguous with mesonephric tubules and ductus deferens (distal portion)); (7) paramesonephric duct; (8) cranial remnant of mesonephric duct system (aberrant ductules); (8′) remnant of mesonephric duct (appendix of epididymis); and (9) caudal remnant of mesonephric duct (paradidymis). The initial stages in the development of the ovary and the formation of paramesonephric ducts are shown in **B**. The epithelial cords (sex cords) penetrate and then regress within the developing ovary, eventually fragmenting and organizing into cell clusters which consist of a single oocyte surrounded by a layer of granulosa cells (primordial follicles). The paramesonephric ducts undergo further development and differentiation, and the mesonephric duct system begins to regress. (1) Celomic epithelium; (2) epithelial cords which initially penetrate then regress and fragment; (3) early formation of future cortical region; (4) primordial follicles; (5) regressing mesonephric tubules; (6) mesonephric duct which will eventually regress; and (7) paramesonephric duct which will undergo further development and differentiation into the major female tubular genitalia. This figure was adapted, with permission, from Gupta (2007). Modifications were courtesy of Don Connor and Howard Wilson.

Within the interstitial compartment, the primary cellular components are the Leydig or interstitial cells, and capillaries, lymphatic vessels and connective tissue are also present in this portion of the testicular parenchyma (Evans, 2007; Senger, 2007). The Leydig cells are homologous to the theca interna cells in the ovary and produce testosterone (also estrogen in some species). There are species differences with respect to the abundance of Leydig cells in the interstitium, and these differences are important to recognize when reporting Leydig or interstitial cell hyperplasia in response to toxicant exposure. It should also be noted that Leydig and, to a lesser extent, Sertoli cells contain enzymes involved in xenobiotic biotransformation, and the synthesis of toxic metabolites can actually occur within the testis, in close proximity to the target cells for a given reproductive toxicant.

Excurrent duct system

The excurrent duct system for each testis consists of the efferent ductules, the epididymal duct and the ductus deferens. This duct system functions to conduct spermatozoa, rete fluid and some testicular secretory products away from the testis and eventually into the pelvic urethra (Senger, 2007). The reabsorption of fluid by a species-variable number of efferent ductules is essential for normal testicular function (Hess, 2003; O'Donnell *et al.*, 2001), and these tubules terminate by joining a single highly coiled epididymal duct, commonly referred to as the epididymidis or epididymis. Depending on the species, the epididymidis is generally subdivided into the initial segment, head (caput), body (corpus) and tail (cauda), with the various portions sometimes being further subdivided (França *et al.*, 2005; Senger, 2007). The primary functions of the epididymidis are transport and sustenance of sperm; reabsorption and secretion of fluid (initial segment and head, respectively); spermatozoal acquisition of motility and fertile potential (i.e., sperm maturation); recognition and elimination of defective spermatozoa; sperm storage prior to ejaculation; and secretory contributions to the seminal fluid (Evans, 2007; Sutovsky *et al.*, 2001). The epididymal transit time varies somewhat with species, but is generally approximately 7 to 14 days in length, depending on several factors, including ejaculation frequency. The ductus deferens conducts spermatozoa matured in the epididymidis to the pelvic urethra which helps to form the penis.

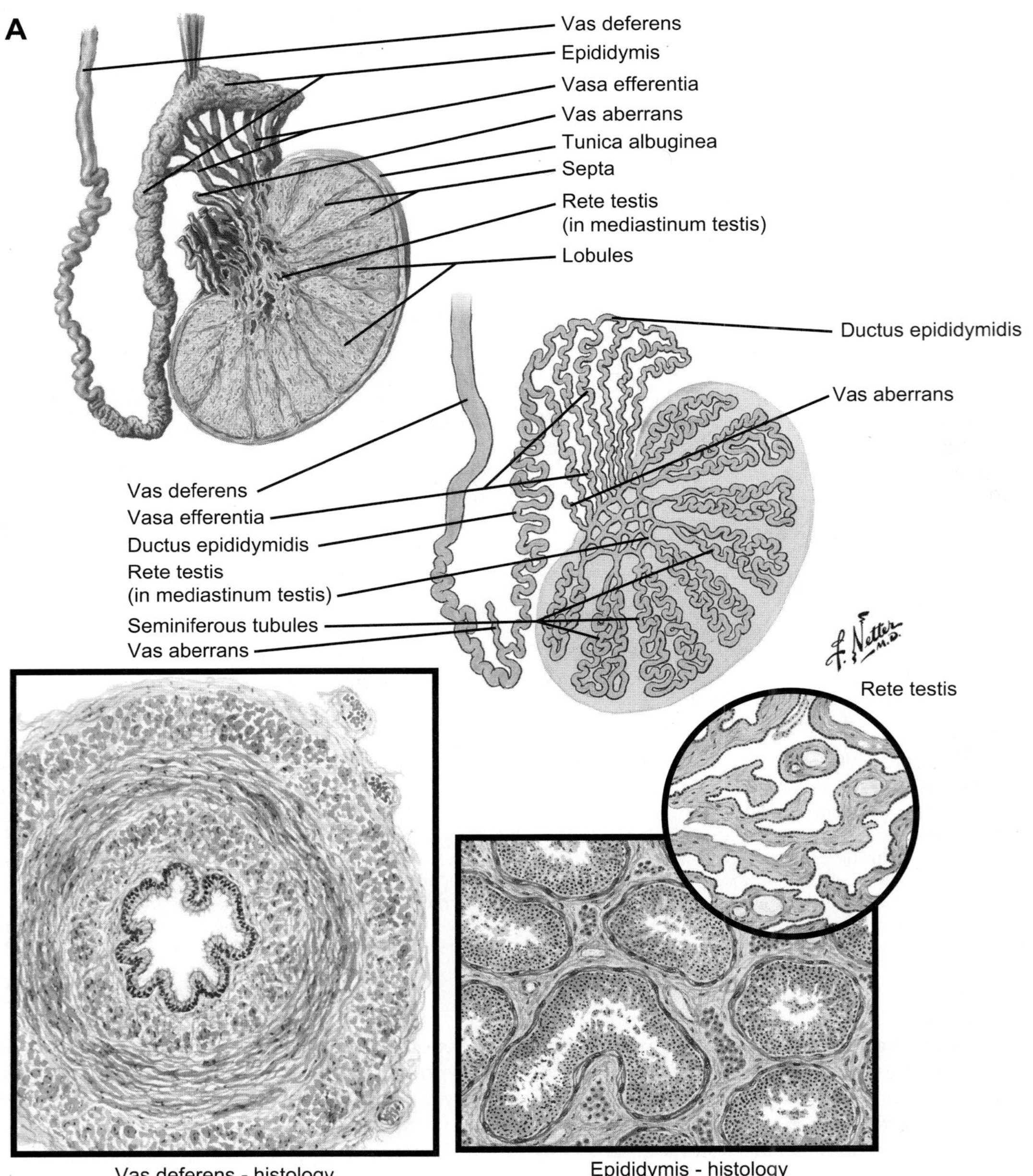

FIGURE 2.6 The structural relationships between the tunica albuginea, septa, lobules of testicular parenchyma, the mediastinum testis and the excurrent duct system within the testes of humans are shown in **A**. **A** also illustrates the sequential transport of sperm through the loops of the seminiferous tubules, rete testis and the excurrent duct system, which includes the efferent ductules (vasa efferentia), epididymidis (epididymis) and ductus deferens (vas deferens) and shows cross-sections of the rete testis, epididymis and ductus deferens within the mature human testis. The structural and functional units within the tubular compartment are the seminiferous tubules, and the complex nature of the association between Sertoli cells and developing germ cells within the seminiferous epithelium of the human testis, including during various stages of sexual maturity, are shown in **B**. Figures were obtained and modified, with permission, from Netter (1997).

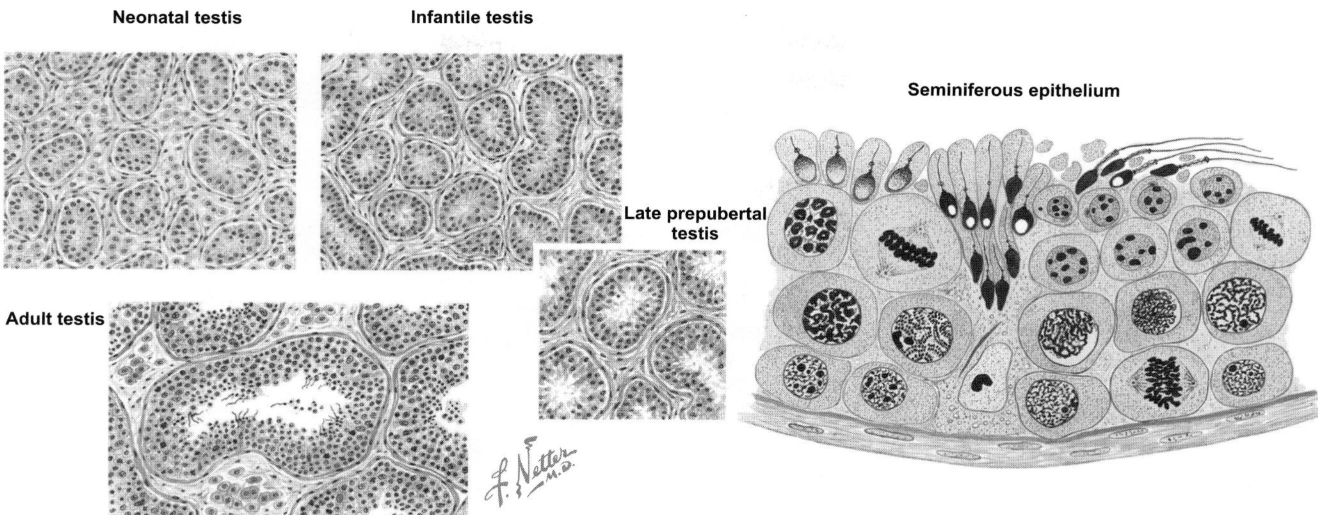

FIGURE 2.6—Cont'd

Accessory sex glands

There are a number of accessory sex glands (the complement of which varies with species) that contribute to the composition of the seminal fluid in mammals. In humans, these glands include the ampullae, seminal vesicles (vesicular glands), prostate and bulbourethral glands (Haschek *et al.*, 2010; Senger, 2007) (Figures 2.2A and 2.7). Laboratory rodents (i.e., mice and rats) have an additional gland referred to as the preputial gland, which appears to have a role in the production of pheromone (Haschek *et al.*, 2010). These accessory sex glands in the male are generally considered to be androgen dependent, with the conversion of testosterone to DHT occurring in the prostate and seminal vesicles of many species (Evans, 2007; Senger, 2007). The weights of the accessory sex glands can be used as an indirect measure of testosterone concentrations or exposure to antiandrogens (Foster and Gray, 2008; Haschek *et al.*, 2010). The human prostate gland is particularly susceptible to the development of benign prostatic hypertrophy (BPH) and various neoplasias, so that familiarity with its internal and external structure can be very useful when evaluating xenobiotic-induced alterations (Figure 2.7).

External genitalia

The external genitalia of the male consist of the copulatory organ or penis, the prepuce or foreskin, which protects the penis from environmental and mechanical injury, and the scrotum for testes positioned outside the abdominal cavity. In humans, the foreskin is frequently removed shortly after birth by circumcision. Penile structure is extremely species variable, with some species even having a special penile bone (i.e., os penis), but the shaft of the penis generally consists of erectile tissue (corpus cavernosum and corpus spongiosum) which surrounds the pelvic urethra. The development of the external genitalia follows a standard sequence of events, and the failure of the urethral groove to close at any point during this sequence results in various degrees of hypospadias (Figure 2.4B). As shown in Figure 2.4B, the glans penis is homologous to the female clitoris, and stimulation of the glans is the primary factor involved in the initiation of ejaculation (Netter, 1997; Senger, 2007). The scrotum protects the testes from mechanical injury and, in conjunction with the tunica dartos, cremaster muscle and pampiniform plexus, plays a major thermoregulatory role with respect to temperature-sensitive, testicular spermatogenesis (Senger, 2007). In some species of wildlife (e.g., elephants and marine mammals), the testes are positioned intra-abdominally.

Spermatogenesis

Spermatozoa are highly specialized haploid cells equipped with a self-powered flagellum to facilitate motility, as well as an acrosome to mediate penetration of the zona pellucida. Spermatogenesis takes place within the seminiferous tubules and consists of all the changes germ cells undergo in the seminiferous epithelium in order to produce adequate numbers of viable spermatozoa each day and to continuously replace spermatogonial stem cells (Evans, 2007; Foster and Gray, 2008). Spermatogenesis provides for genetic diversity and ensures that germ cells are in an immunologically favored site (Senger, 2007). The duration of spermatogenesis varies with species but generally ranges between 4 and 8 weeks (approximately 30 to 60 days) in domestic and laboratory animals and is approximately 75 days (almost 11 weeks) in humans. It is important to keep in mind the durations of spermatogenesis and epididymal sperm transport in a given species, as well as the normal, species-specific number of spermatozoa produced daily by the testes, when determining the period of toxicant exposure relative to the appearance of abnormal spermatozoa in an ejaculate and when assessing the severity and reversibility of toxicant-induced damage to sperm precursors within the testes (Evans, 2007).

Spermatogenesis can be subdivided into three phases or stages referred to as "proliferation", "meiosis" and "differentiation". During each of these phases, sperm precursors or male germ cells (spermatogonia, spermatocytes or spermatids) undergo specific, stepwise changes as they develop

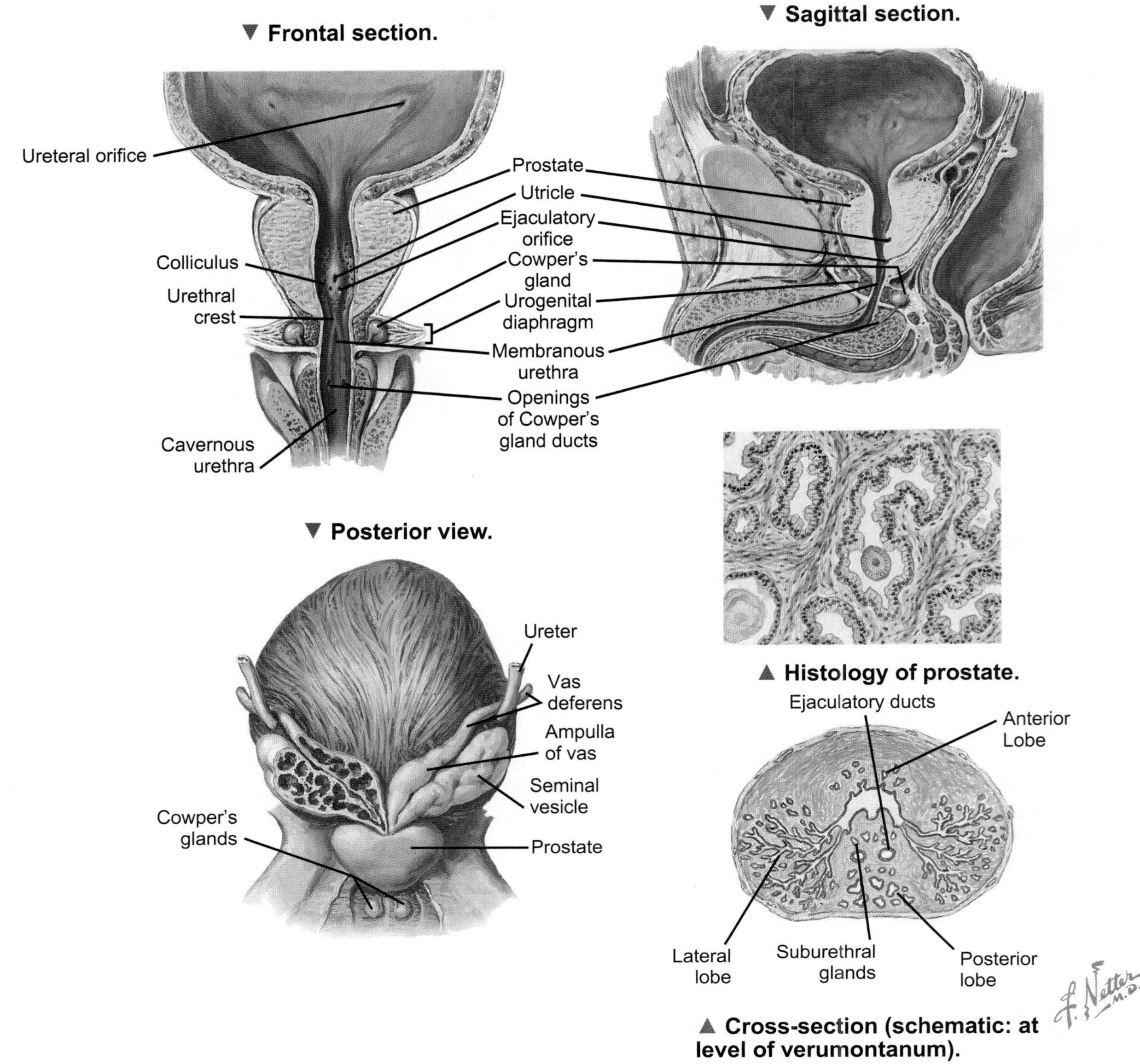

FIGURE 2.7 The anatomical relationships between the accessory sex glands in sexually mature men and the histological appearance of the human prostate gland are shown. Figure was obtained, with permission, from Netter (1997).

into spermatozoa which will eventually be released into the excurrent duct system. Each of these phases involves a different type of germ cell undergoing a different developmental process, and, as such, these phases have the potential to differ in their susceptibility to the mechanisms of action of various reproductive toxicants (Evans, 2007; Foster and Gray, 2008).

Proliferation (mitosis or spermatocytogenesis)

The "proliferation" phase of spermatogenesis has also been referred to as "mitosis" or "spermatocytogenesis" and occurs within the basal compartment of the seminiferous tubule. Proliferation denotes all of the mitotic divisions involving spermatogonia (Foster and Gray, 2008; Senger, 2007). A large number of B-spermatogonia result from the mitoses of several generations of spermatogonia (e.g., A_1, A_2, A_3, A_4 and I; some species variations in nomenclature) (Genuth, 2004b; Senger, 2007). Stem cell renewal is accomplished during proliferation by the reversion of some spermatogonia to more primitive germ cells (Senger, 2007). Germ cell mitosis during spermatogenesis ends with the transformation of B-spermatogonia into primary spermatocytes, and this process is particularly susceptible to toxicants, such as chemotherapeutic agents and radiation, which target rapidly dividing cells (Evans, 2007).

Meiosis

"Meiosis" takes place within the adluminal compartment of the seminiferous tubules and involves the participation of primary and secondary spermatocytes in a total of two meiotic divisions. The chromosomal reduplication, synapsis and cross-over, as well as cellular division and separation, which occur during this phase of spermatogenesis, are extremely complex and guarantee genetic diversity (Genuth, 2004b; Senger, 2007). The meiosis phase of spermatogenesis is considered by some to be most susceptible to toxic insult and ends with the production of haploid round spermatids.

Differentiation (spermiogenesis)

Spermatozoa have been aptly characterized as "sophisticated, self-propelled packages of DNA and enzymes" (Senger, 2007). "Differentiation" or "spermiogenesis" involves all the changes occurring within the adluminal compartment, which transform round spermatids into spermatozoa possessing an acrosome for penetration of the zona pellucida and a tail or flagellum to facilitate motility (Genuth, 2004b). Differentiation can be subdivided into the "Golgi", "cap", "acrosomal" and "maturation" phases, which correspond respectively to acrosomal vesicle formation; spreading of the acrosomal vesicle over the nucleus; elongation of the nucleus and cytoplasm; and final assembly involving the formation of the postnuclear cap organization of the tail components (Senger, 2007). Following the nuclear and cytoplasmic reorganization which characterizes the changes to germ cells during spermiogenesis, differentiated spermatozoa are released from Sertoli cells into the lumen of the seminiferous tubules by a process referred to as "spermiation". The complex signaling pathways and genomic imprinting involved in regulating the differentiation of round spermatids into spermatozoa are potential targets for endocrine disrupting chemicals (EDCs) or endocrine disruptors (Evans, 2007; Foster and Gray, 2008).

The cycle of the seminiferous epithelium

In most sexually mature mammals, spermatozoa are produced continuously, with the entry of germ cells into the proliferation phase of spermatogenesis occurring in a coordinated cyclic manner (Foster and Gray, 2008; Genuth, 2004b). Spermatogonia A in a given region of the seminiferous tubule commit to proliferate in a synchronous manner, with cohorts of their progeny germ cells (cellular generations) connected by intercellular bridges and developing and differentiating in unison. Including spermatogonia A, four or five generations or concentric layers of sperm precursors are present in each cross-section of the seminiferous tubules (Figure 2.6B). The cycle of the seminiferous epithelium in most mammals is characterized by germ cells in each spermatogenic phase associating with contiguous generations in a repeatable pattern of specific cellular associations or "stages" (Foster and Gray, 2008; França *et al.*, 2005). There is generally only one stage per seminiferous tubular cross-section section in subprimates, and each stage transitions into the next at predictable intervals (Senger, 2007). At any given point along a seminiferous tubule, the entire cycle of the seminiferous epithelium occurs over a set time interval closely associated with the spermatogonial turnover rate for that particular mammalian species. The number and durations of the various stages of the cycle of the seminiferous epithelium vary with species, and various classification schemes have been used, based on the morphological characteristics of the spermatid nucleus or the development of the acrosomic system. In subprimates, sequential stages are arranged along the length of the seminiferous tubule in consecutive order, forming a "spermatogenic wave" (Haschek *et al.*, 2010; Senger, 2007). The progeny of one spermatogonium A will progress through approximately 4.5 cycles of the seminiferous epithelium before being released into the lumen of the seminiferous tubule and progressing through the rete testis into the excurrent duct system. An understanding of the cycle of the seminiferous epithelium is very useful for the evaluation of the effects of xenobiotics on spermatogenesis and for the determination of the populations of germ cells most susceptible to a given toxicant.

Male reproductive physiology

Gonadal steroid synthesis in the testes

The endocrine events which regulate spermatogenesis and sexual behavior in males are very distinct from those which take place in females. The primary gonadal steroids produced by the testes are androgens, testosterone and DHT, which are also produced from testosterone in selected nongonadal tissues, and estrogens (primarily estradiol in most species), which are now recognized as playing essential roles in male reproductive development and function (Hess, 2003; O'Donnell *et al.*, 2001). Leydig cells in the interstitium synthesize pregnenolone and then progesterone from cholesterol and convert progesterone to testosterone under the influence of LH (Genuth, 2004b; Senger, 2007). The site of estrogen synthesis (i.e., aromatase activity) varies with the age and species of animal. In the male fetus, postnatal immature male and, in some species, the adult male, Sertoli cells within the seminiferous tubules play a major role in the aromatase-mediated conversion of testosterone to estradiol under the influence of FSH. In many mammals, however, Leydig cells in the fetal testis and, especially, the postnatal immature testis gradually begin to synthesize estrogens, and, at sexual maturity, a major portion of the estrogens in these species are produced by aromatase activity in the Leydig cells, under the influence of LH rather than FSH (Hess, 2003; O'Donnell, 2001; Payne, 2007). More recently, germ cells have been identified as another potential source of estrogen in the testis, and it is possible that germ cell-derived estrogens play major roles in regulating male reproductive function (Hess, 2003).

Endocrine regulation of spermatogenesis

The basic gonadal steroidogenic pathways, target sites, feedback loops and routes of excretion for the adult male human are summarized in Figure 2.3. While the female hypothalamus has both fully developed tonic and surge centers for GnRH release (especially prior to ovulation), the hypothalamic GnRH surge center in the male is diminished, and the anterior pituitary gland of the male does not experience surges in GnRH stimulation. This sex-specific alteration in the hypothalamus facilitates the normal endocrine milieu which maintains continuous spermatogenesis and stimulates normal sexual behavior. The tonic pulsatile release of GnRH induces the anterior pituitary to produce pulses of LH and FSH several times during the day and facilitates adequate LH-dependent testosterone production and, depending on the species, normal FSH-dependent Sertoli function, both of which are essential for spermatogenesis to occur continuously in the seminiferous tubules. In some species, FSH is primarily required for the onset of puberty and the initiation of spermatogenesis, with many of the functions of FSH in the immature male being taken over by testosterone in the sexually mature animal (Evans, 2007). Testosterone stimulates Sertoli cells to produce several androgen-regulated proteins (including androgen-binding protein) which are required for spermatogenesis. Estrogens are required for various aspects of the normal development and function of Sertoli cells and germ cells within the seminiferous tubules. Xenobiotics which mimic or inhibit the actions of estradiol within the testis can disrupt normal spermatogenesis.

Positive and negative feedback loops involved in male reproduction

Positive and negative feedback mechanisms involving gonadal steroids help maintain an endocrine environment which is conducive to normal male reproductive function (Figure 2.3). In addition to these feedback loops, the Sertoli cell can produce activin and inhibin which respectively increase and decrease the secretion of FSH by gonadotropes and, in some species, GnRH release from the hypothalamus (Haschek *et al.*, 2010). Testosterone, DHT and estradiol all provide negative feedback to the hypothalamus with respect to GnRH release, and testosterone can also directly inhibit LH secretion by gonadotropes (Haschek *et al.*, 2010; Senger, 2007). Xenoestrogens and xenoandrogens have the potential to disturb the hypothalamic–pituitary–gonadal axis (O'Donnell *et al.*, 2001). Antiandrogens and a variety of other xenobiotics can interfere with this feedback loop, resulting in excessive secretion of LH and Leydig or interstitial cell hyperplasia (Evans, 2007; Foster and Gray, 2008).

Epididymal and accessory sex gland function

Epididymal development and function are dependent on the proper balance of androgenic and estrogenic stimulation and are required for normal male reproductive function and fertility. The accessory sex glands are considered to be primarily androgen dependent, and the secretions of these glands, as well as those of the epididymidis, are important components of seminal fluid. Conversion of testosterone to DHT can generally occur in the epididymidis, prostate and seminal vesicles. Hormonally active xenobiotics, which alter the normal endocrine events associated with epididymal and accessory gland development and function, can have adverse effects on male fertility (Evans, 2007).

Sexual behavior, erection, emission and ejaculation

Sexual behavior is mediated by estradiol in postnatal males and females. The conversion of the steadily produced testosterone in the male to estradiol in the brain (plus the effects of estrogens of testicular origin) results in the male being sexually receptive most of the time (Evans, 2007; Senger, 2007). Adequate libido and sexual receptivity, as well as adequate concentrations of testosterone, are necessary for erection of the penis, which is required for intromission during copulation (Sikka, *et al.*, 2005). Olfactory (detection of pheromones), auditory and visual stimuli play roles in facilitating cholinergic and NANC (non-adrenergic/non-cholinergic) parasympathetic neuron-mediated penile erection, which, especially in men and stallions, requires a significant amount of nitric oxide-associated vasodilation and vascular engorgement. During copulation, the events which lead to emission of the secretions of the accessory sex glands and sperm (i.e., semen) into the urethra and the ejaculation of semen from the urethra at the time of orgasm generally involve tactile stimuli to the glans penis, stimulation by sympathetic neurons and spinal reflexes.

Normal female reproductive anatomy and physiology

Developmental perspectives

Similar to the male, there is an "undifferentiated" stage during development (Figure 2.4A), where the female fetus is internally and externally indistinguishable from the male fetus. What is eventually observed internally (Figure 2.4A) as well as externally (Figure 2.4B) in the female is due to a complex set of structural modifications (Figure 2.5B), resulting in the formation of the ovary and the internal tubular genitalia.

Reproductive anatomy of the female

Although there are some distinct morphological differences between species (e.g., simplex uterus in primates, duplex cervices in rabbits), the female reproductive tract, as shown for humans in Figure 2.2B, generally consists of paired ovaries, the "tubular genitalia", which include the paired oviducts (uterine tubes), the contiguous uterus, cervix, vagina, vestibule and vulva. In species other than humans and other higher primates, there are also separate uterine horns of varying lengths and degrees of curvature, which connect with the uterus (Evans, 2007; Senger, 2007). As in the male, the organs involved in female reproductive function have been well recognized for over 200 years and are physiologically and morphologically dynamic. They function to produce the oocyte, facilitate its fertilization, provide an environment for embryonic and fetal development, and transport the fetus from the maternal to the external environment. Variations in size, appearance, location and function of the female reproductive organs depend on the endocrine milieu dictated by the effects of sexual maturation, stage of the estrous or menstrual cycle, gestational hormone production of maternal, fetal and/or placental origin, exposure to exogenous hormonally active agents or HAAs (sometimes used interchangeably with EDCs or endocrine disruptors) and seasonal influences (Evans, 2007; Foster and Gray, 2008; Netter, 1997; Senger, 2007).

The primary functions of the ovary are oogenesis or production of female gametes (oocytes or ova) and steroidogenesis (production of estrogens and progesterone). The ovaries of most domestic mammals consist of a peripheral parenchymatous zone (cortex), containing various stages of follicular and luteal gland development and a central vascular zone (medulla), comprised of collagenous connective tissue rich in blood vessels (Evans, 2007; Foster and Gray, 2008; Genuth, 2004b; Senger, 2007). The structural and functional unit of the ovary is the

Regulation of follicle and endometrial development and pregnancy

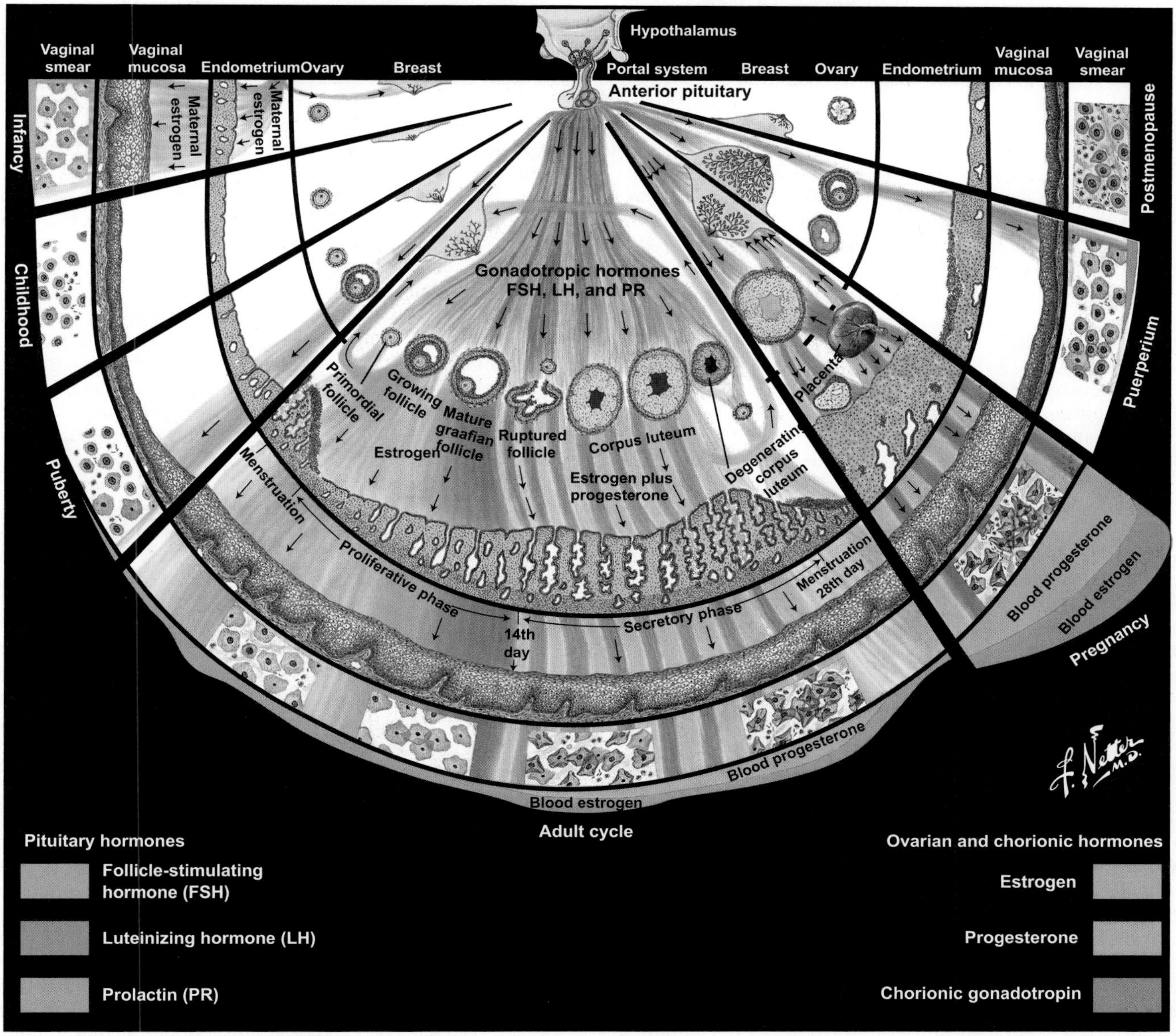

FIGURE 2.8 In humans, chemical exposures can take place over an entire lifetime, and early xenobiotic exposures have the potential to affect reproductive events occurring later in life. This figure clearly and comprehensively summarizes all of the anatomical and physiological reproductive changes which can take place in women's lives between infancy and menopause, including those associated with puberty and the various stages of the menstrual cycle, as well as periods of pregnancy and lactation. The transition between the various aspects of a woman's reproductive activity involves alterations in anterior pituitary hormone secretion and structural and functional modifications in the ovaries, endometrium, vaginal epithelium and the mammary glands. Figure was obtained, with permission, from Netter (1997). Please refer to color plate section.

follicle (Figure 2.8). Follicles are classified as primordial, primary (some become atretic), secondary and tertiary (i.e., antral) follicles based on their stage of development (Evans, 2007).

A primary oocyte surrounded by a single, flattened cell layer is a primordial follicle. A basal lamina separates the single layer of what will become granulosa cells from the adjacent stromal tissue which eventually develops into the theca cells (theca interna and theca externa). The granulosa cells are homologous to the Sertoli cells in the testis, and the theca interna cells are the female equivalent of the Leydig cells (Evans, 2007; Senger, 2007). Following the appropriate endocrine stimulation, primordial follicles are recruited to undergo possible further differentiation into estrogen-producing antral (i.e., tertiary) follicles and ultimately ovulation, which results in the release of a secondary oocyte (primary oocyte in dogs) and formation of a corpus luteum (CL) which produces progesterone.

Female reproductive physiology

Females are born with a finite pool of primordial follicles (up to hundreds of thousands), and reproductive cyclicity (i.e., estrous or menstrual cycles) provides females with repeated opportunities for the establishment of pregnancy.

The majority of mammalian species (subprimates) have estrous cycles, which reflect the physiologic changes occurring between successive ovulations and/or periods of sexual receptivity (estrus) (Senger, 2007). Humans and non-human primates experience menstrual rather than estrous cycles and do not have defined periods of sexual receptivity (i.e., estrus). As illustrated in Figure 2.8, unlike the estrous cycles in subprimates, the reproductive cycle in menstruating animals is divided into phases (i.e., menses, proliferative and secretory phases), which are defined based on the physiological state of the uterine endometrium, rather than on the predominant ovarian structures (i.e., estrous cycles) (Genuth, 2004b; Netter, 1997; Senger, 2007).

The estrous cycle

The follicular and luteal phases of the estrous cycle describe the predominant ovarian structures and the corresponding gonadal steroid concentrations which result from the follicular secretion of estrogens or the luteal secretion of progesterone, respectively (Evans, 2007; Senger, 2007). Both the follicular and luteal phases can generally be further subdivided into two stages each, proestrus and estrus (sexual receptivity) for the follicular phase and metestrus and diestrus (sexual non-receptivity) for the luteal phase. Proestrus represents the period of transition from the diestrous dominance of progesterone to the dominance of estrogens during estrus, while metestrus represents the opposite shift in the endocrine milieu (estrogen dominance to progesterone dominance).

The menstrual cycle

The reader is directed to Figure 2.8 in order to best understand the sequence of the morphological and endocrine events which take place during the menstrual cycle in women, which is generally 28 days in duration. As mentioned earlier, the menstrual cycle is defined in terms of phases corresponding to events occurring within the endometrium, rather than within the ovary; however, an effort will be made here to discuss also ovarian events taking place at the same time as the endometrial changes so one can understand the correlations between the estrous and menstrual cycles. At the beginning of menses, follicles develop under the influence of FSH (i.e., follicular phase begins), with minimal LH secretion, thereby reflecting anterior pituitary sensitivity to GnRH (Genuth, 2004b). As tertiary follicles develop, more estrogens are produced, and the endometrium enters the proliferative stage. Estrogens provide negative feedback for FSH secretion and positive feedback for LH release by the anterior pituitary. The increasing amount of LH and decreasing FSH results in ovulation about midway through the cycle (i.e., day 14), and the follicle begins to undergo luteinization and forms corpus luteum, which produces progesterone, as well as estrogen (i.e., luteal phase begins) (Genuth, 2004b). The secretory phase of the endometrium begins as the corpus luteum forms and secretes progesterone and estrogens. In response to feedback loops involving this secreted progesterone and estrogens, the relative proportions of FSH and LH secreted by the anterior pituitary change, with subtle decreases in the amounts of progesterone and estrogens produced by the corpus luteum observed. During the late secretory phase of the endometrium, the absence of a conceptus in the uterus results in the regression of the corpus luteum (i.e., luteolysis), a precipitous decrease in the secretion of progesterone and estrogens, the local production and subsequent release of leukotrienes and prostaglandins within the endometrium, and the subsequent cascade of vascular events which result in the sloughing of the endometrium accompanied by bleeding, which are characteristic of menses (Figure 2.8) (Genuth, 2004b; Netter, 1997).

Follicular development

The general sequence of endocrine and morphologic changes occurring during the estrous and menstrual cycles involves a variety of positive and negative feedback loops affecting the hypothalamic–pituitary–gonadal axis and leads to the development of antral follicles, the primary source of estrogens, and, eventually, the formation of corpora lutea, which produce progesterone (Figures 2.3 and 2.8). When females are exhibiting reproductive cyclicity, there are cyclic alterations in the pattern of hypothalamic GnRH secretion from the tonic and surge centers, which interact with the anterior pituitary to influence the relative amounts of FSH and LH secreted by anterior pituitary gonadotropes. Over the course of sequential ovulatory cycles, many (up to several hundred or more, depending on the species) primordial follicles leave the reserve pool in a cyclic fashion (under the influence of FSH) and enter the active pool of follicles (primary follicles) undergoing growth and differentiation (folliculogenesis) and eventually atresia or ovulation (Evans *et al.*, 1997; Senger, 2007). The oocyte in the developing follicle grows in size, the zona pellucida is formed and the granulosa cells surrounding the oocyte undergo mitosis and further differentiation. As shown in Figure 2.8, a primary follicle is transformed into a secondary follicle when there are several layers of granulosa cells. Preantral follicles (primary and secondary follicles) become antral (tertiary) follicles, when fluid from the granulosa cells of secondary follicles coalesces to form an antrum (Evans, 2007).

Cyclic increases in FSH concentrations facilitate recruitment of antral follicles. Granulosa cells can produce activin which is thought to provide positive feedback to the anterior pituitary, further increasing gonadotropic FSH secretion (Evans, 2007; Senger, 2007). Recruited antral follicles, which are gonadotropin sensitive, undergo several waves of follicular development beginning in metestrus and ending in proestrus. In subprimates, the final wave of one or more dominant follicles, destined for ovulation, rather than atresia, produces the large amounts of estrogens typical of estrus and required for sexual receptivity and the preovulatory estrous surges in GnRH and LH secretion in subprimates.

Ovarian follicular synthesis of estrogens

The production of estrogens (predominantly estradiol) by antral follicles is accomplished by a mechanism termed the "two-cell or two-gonadotropin model", which can vary somewhat between species (Evans, 2007; Senger, 2007). Cells from the theca interna and/or granulosa cells (depending on the species) produce progesterone from pregnenolone synthesized from cholesterol and, under the influence of relatively low concentrations of LH, theca interna cells convert this progesterone into androgens and, ultimately, testosterone. In granulosa cells (reportedly theca interna cells in some species), the release of FSH from the anterior pituitary induces aromatase mediated conversion of testosterone produced in the theca cells into estradiol. Stimulation of aromatase activity by xenobiotics can have an overall estrogenic effect on exposed animals (increased production of estradiol).

The effects of estrogenic feedback on the hypothalamic–pituitary–gonadal axis

Increasing concentrations of estrogens associated with estrus alter the hypothalamic GnRH secretory pattern or act on the anterior pituitary itself (Figures 2.3 and 2.8) and decrease pituitary secretion of FSH, while greatly increasing the amount of LH produced and released by the anterior pituitary gland (preovulatory LH surge). Although inhibin produced by granulosa cells further decreases FSH secretion, dominant follicles surviving to estrus do not undergo atresia because of an enhanced sensitivity to basal (FSH) levels. Xenoestrogens have the potential to either imitate or inhibit these estradiol feedback mechanisms in sexually mature females, depending on amount of estrogenic xenobiotic, the endocrine milieu at the time of the exposure and the relative binding affinity of the xenobiotic for estrogen receptors.

Ovulation

The granulosa cells in the one or more dominant follicles (Graafian follicles) cease to divide shortly prior to ovulation and undergo further differentiation, with increased numbers (i.e., upregulation) of LH receptors responsive to the estrogen-induced preovulatory LH surge (Evans *et al.*, 1997; Senger, 2007). As LH increases, granulosa cells (theca interna cells in some species) continue to convert pregnenolone to progesterone, but estradiol production decreases, resulting in a slight preovulatory decline in estradiol. The preovulatory LH surge is associated with increased follicular pressure, degeneration of theca cells and weakening of the follicular wall, completion of the first meiotic division within the oocyte (end of meiotic inhibition except in dogs and foxes) and, finally, ovulation of a secondary oocyte arrested in metaphase II. In felids, ferrets, mink, camelids and rabbits, the preovulatory LH surge is induced by copulation (intromission or vaginal stimulation in most induced ovulators; seminal fluid in camelids). Toxicants which interfere with copulation or sexual contact in these species can interfere with the ovulatory process (Evans, 2007).

Formation and function of a corpus luteum (CL)

Following ovulation, a cascade of endocrine changes takes place in the female subprimate which facilitates the transition from sexual receptivity to non-receptivity. Once an ovulation occurs, blood concentrations of follicular estradiol and inhibin return to their basal levels, and granulosa cells continue their growth, differentiation and increased production and release of progesterone (luteinization) under the influence of LH (Evans *et al.*, 1997; Senger, 2007). The functional ovarian structure which eventually develops from each ovulated follicle is a corpus luteum (often abbreviated CL), which is comprised of large and small luteal cells derived from the granulosa and theca interna cells (granulosa cells in horses), respectively. In most species, luteal cells are responsive to LH and produce progesterone until, shortly before the usual end of diestrus in non-pregnant animals (i.e., late secretory phase in higher primates), the corpus luteum undergoes luteolysis. While the induction of luteolysis is an intraovarian event in higher primates, luteal regression in non-pregnant subprimates is mediated by oxytocin-stimulated production of the luteolysin, prostaglandins $F_{2\alpha}$ ($PGF_{2\alpha}$). Xenobiotics, which can cause endometritis or mimic the actions of oxytocin or $PGF_{2\alpha}$, such as endotoxin or lipopolysaccharide (LPS), can be associated with premature luteolysis. Conversely, toxicants with the opposite oxytocin/$PGF_{2\alpha}$-related effects would be expected to disrupt normal reproductive cyclicity by prolonging the lifespan of the CL and causing a prolonged diestrus or pseudopregnancy (e.g., xenoestrogens in swine) (Evans, 2007).

Species of animals can vary in the number of fertile ovulations and, therefore, corpora lutea which are characteristically associated with each estrous cycle. Monotocous mammalian species usually only ovulate a single secondary oocyte each estrous cycle. The ovaries of litter-bearing (polytocous) mammals generally develop multiple follicles which mature, ovulate and form functional corpora lutea.

Summary of the effects of estrogens and progesterone during the female reproductive cycle

The endocrine changes which occur during the estrous cycle are reflected in behavior and the size, morphology, position and function of the tubular genitalia. As noted in Figures 2.3 and 2.8, estrogens have multiple effects on the female reproductive tract, as well as organ systems, which include: (1) interactions with the hypothalamus and anterior pituitary to alter the patterns of GnRH and gonadotropin secretion which govern follicular development and ovulation; (2) facilitation of sexual receptivity, especially in subprimates; (3) increased blood flow to the reproductive tract; (4) genital swelling; (5) leukocytosis; (6) mucosal secretion and myometrial tone; (7) proliferation and/or keritinization of luminal and/or glandular epithelium within the tubular genitalia; (8) altered electrical conductivity of mucosal secretions; (9) the initiation of the growth of endometrial and mammary glands; and (10) regulation of bone metabolism (Evans, 2007; Senger, 2007). Like estrogens, progesterone also has several effects on the reproductive tract of the female, but the effects of progesterone generally oppose those of estrogens, favoring pregnancy maintenance and sexual non-receptivity, especially in subprimates, over ovulation and appropriately timed sexual receptivity associated with estrogenic stimulation. Progesterone is generally associated with negative feedback to the hypothalamus and anterior pituitary gland which limits GnRH and gonadotropin secretion. Sexual receptivity in subprimates and myometrial contractility and tone are diminished in an endocrine environment dominated by progesterone, while mammary and endometrial gland development and secretion are promoted. Toxicants which disrupt the communication and coordination between the ovary and the other parts of the reproductive tract (e.g., xenoestrogens, xenoandrogens and antiestrogens) will alter the appearance and function of the reproductive organs and can interfere with survival of the oocyte, embryo and/or fetus (Evans, 2007).

Oocyte/sperm transport, normal capacitation of sperm and fertilization

Transport of the ovulated oocyte

The primary reproductive organs involved in the transport of ovulated secondary oocytes (primary oocytes in the bitch) are the oviducts or uterine tubes. Each oviduct consists of an infundibulum, isthmus and ampulla, which have some distinct differences in structure, as well as function (Evans *et al.*, 1997). The ovulated ovum enters the funnel-like opening to infundibulum and is transported to the ampulla or ampullary–isthmic junction for fertilization. Unlike spermatozoa which can generally survive for several days in the oviduct, secondary oocytes usually, depending on the species, are viable for 12 to 24 hours (Evans, 2007; Genuth, 2004b). The appropriate endocrine environment is required for adequate oviductal entry and transport of ovulated oocytes to the site of fertilization. Delayed transport of oocytes within the uterine tubes can result in the death of ova before contact can be made with fertile spermatozoa.

Transport and capacitation of spermatozoa

Transport of spermatozoa

During mammalian copulation, mature sperm stored in the caudae epididymidies travel through the ductus deferens and penile urethra to be ejaculated into the anterior vagina, cervix or uterine body of the female reproductive tract, depending on the species. Spermatozoa can be lost from the female reproductive tract by retrograde loss and phagocytosis by leukocytes (Senger, 2007). Contractions of the smooth muscle within the tubular genitalia (muscularis), as well as interactions involving components of the seminal fluid and luminal secretions of the female reproductive tract, facilitate the transport of sperm to the oviducts (uterine tubes) where, depending on the species, fertilization takes place in the ampulla or at the junction of the ampulla and the isthmus (ampullary–isthmic junction) (Genuth, 2004b; Senger, 2007). While sperm can be rapidly transported to the ampullary–isthmic junction or ampullae of the oviducts (uterine tubes) within minutes of natural or artificial insemination, the relatively slow, sustained transport of motile sperm from reservoirs of spermatozoa in the cervix and uterotubal junctions is the primary mechanism by which the viable sperm that can participate in fertilization actually enter the oviducts (Senger, 2007). Xenobiotics which interfere with the endocrine milieu required for appropriate muscularis contractility and the cervical and uterine mucosal secretions which facilitate sperm transport (e.g., phytoestrogens in sheep) can prevent spermatozoa from getting to the site of fertilization in a timely manner (Evans, 2007).

Capacitation of spermatozoa

Spermatozoa can generally survive in the oviducts (uterine tubes) for several days following insemination. Ejaculated sperm are not competent either to bind to the zona pellucida or to undergo the acrosomal (acrosome) reaction, both of which are required for fertilization of ova by mature spermatozoa. Sperm must be capacitated in order to interact with the ovum. The capacitation process involves calcium influx and biochemical changes to the sperm plasma membrane which result in the "removal" or modification of epididymal and seminal plasma proteins and the exposure of the surface molecules required for spermatozoal binding to the zona pellucida of the ovulated secondary oocyte (Genuth, 2004b; Senger, 2007). Depending on the species and, to some extent, the site of their deposition, spermatozoa become capacitated within the cervix, uterus and/or the oviduct or uterine tube (Senger, 2007).

Fertilization

Fertilization of secondary oocytes by capacitated sperm is a complex process involving a cascade of events which prevents fertilization of an ovum by more than one sperm (polyspermy) and ends in the fusion of the male and female pronuclei (syngamy). In the oviductal ampulla or at the ampullary–isthmic junction, the motility of capacitated sperm becomes hyperactive, facilitating the precise sequence of events which includes the following in their respective order: (1) sperm binding to the zona pellucida of the oocyte involving interactions between species-specific sperm and oocyte proteins; (2) the sperm acrosomal reaction, which results in the release of acrosomal enzymes and exposure of the equatorial segment of the sperm plasma membrane; (3) acrosomal enzyme-associated penetration of zona pellucida by a single spermatozoon; (4) fusion of the plasma membrane of the sperm at its equatorial segment with the plasma membrane of the oocyte; (5) membrane fusion-associated sperm engulfment and the oocyte cortical reaction, which prevents additional oocyte zona binding and membrane fusion (i.e., polyspermy prevention); (6) female pronucleus formation and completion of meiosis; (7) decondensation within the sperm nucleus and male pronucleus formation; and (8) the fusion of male and female pronuclei or syngamy which produces a zygote ready to undergo embryogenesis (Evans, 2007; Genuth, 2004b; Senger, 2007). From the complexity of the fertilization process, it should be apparent that toxicants which result in direct, subtle aberrations in sperm and oocyte formation and maturation can have profound, indirect effects on gamete formation and, potentially, even later downstream changes in embryonic development.

Important aspects of normal embryonic and fetal development

Historical perspective

It should be very evident from Figure 2.2C that, although the depicted newborn has some adult-like qualities, there was a basic understanding of the processes involved in fetal development and nutrition, as well as parturition several hundred years ago. What has really changed over the last century is our understanding of early embryonic development and the signaling pathways which result in the establishment of healthy pregnancies and the delivery of normally developed neonates.

Blastocyst formation and differentiation of the germ cell layers

In order for a zygote to develop into a viable offspring, multiple steps involving cellular division, migration, differentiation and organization must take place. Embryonic

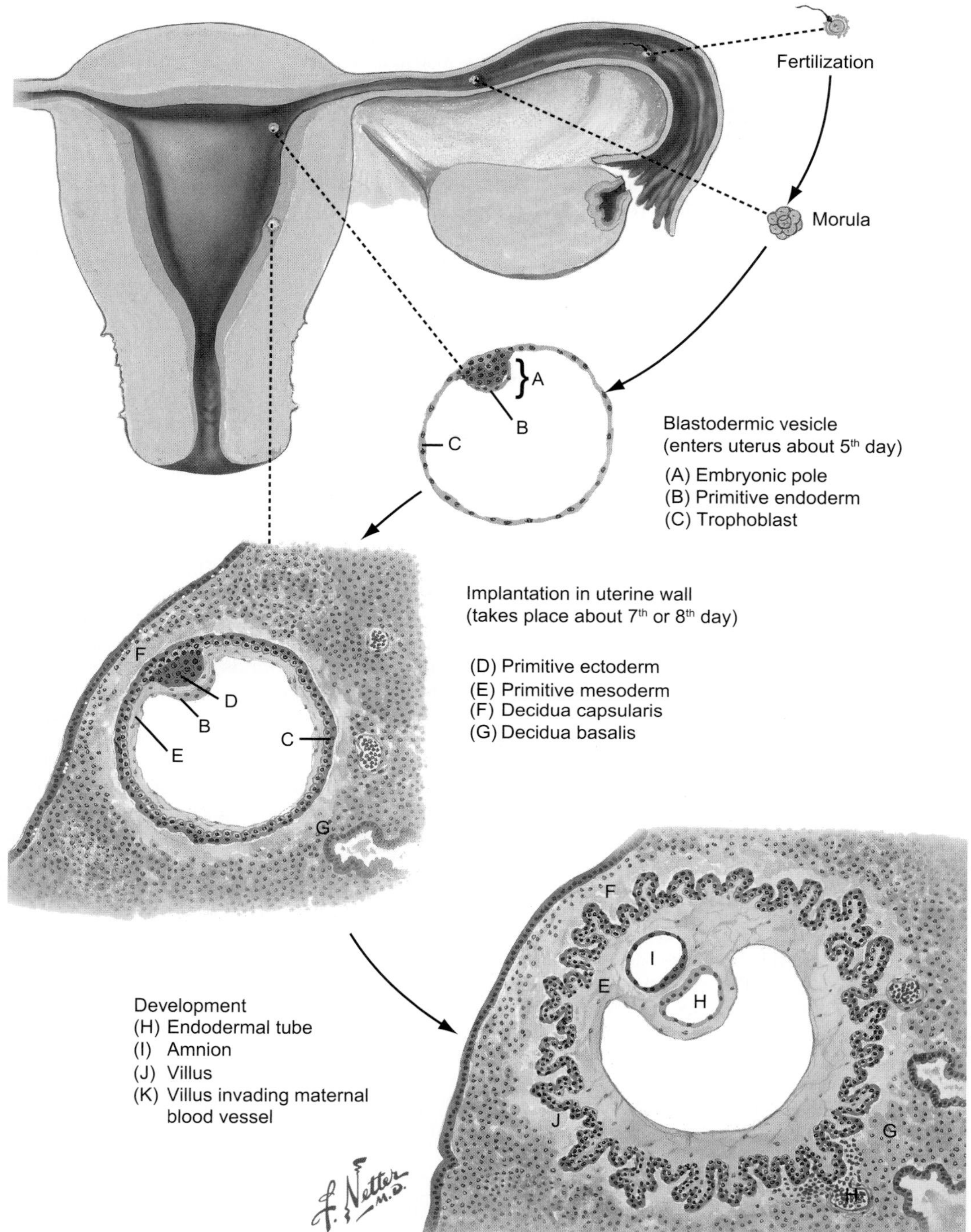

FIGURE 2.9 The series of developmental events associated with embryogenesis in humans, which occur after fertilization, including implantation and initial formation of the amnion and chorionic villi, are shown. Figure was obtained and modified, with permission, from Netter (1997).

and fetal survival requires that these various steps take place in a precise order and at set times during the gestation of each species. Within 24 hours following fertilization, the zygote located in the oviduct begins to divide, within the confines of the zona pellucida, into multiple blastomeres, which ultimately form a ball of cells referred to as the morula (Evans, 2007; Senger, 2007). As shown in Figure 2.9, a fluid-filled cavity (blastocoele) develops within the developing embryo, and the newly formed blastocyst, which is divided into cells forming either the inner cell mass (future embryo proper) or the trophoblast (future chorion), enters the uterus. In humans, the entry of the blastocyst or blastodermic vesicle into the uterus generally occurs on day 5 after ovulation and "hatches" from the zona pellucida on approximately day 6 (Evans, 2007; Genuth, 2004b; Netter, 1997).

"Maternal recognition of pregnancy" and implantation

The conceptus and, in most cases, the trophoblastic cells of most mammalian embryos, other than those for which the timing of luteolysis and duration of pregnancy are very similar to one another (i.e., dogs and cats), must produce some signal to prevent luteolysis (i.e., entry into the next estrus or, in the case of higher primates, menses) and to maintain luteal phase progesterone concentrations until an alternative source of progestagens develops (Evans, 2007; Senger, 2007). In subprimates, this process, which is also referred to as "maternal recognition of pregnancy", involves species-specific embryo–endometrium interactions which prevent the production or redirect the release of endometrial $PGF_{2\alpha}$. Embryonic production of species-specific interferon-τ, o-IFN-τ- and b-IFN-τ, prevents luteolysis in sheep and cattle, respectively, by inhibiting the synthesis of $PGF_{2\alpha}$. In swine, estrogen secretion by porcine embryos appears to prevent luteolysis by redirecting the release of $PGF_{2\alpha}$ away from the ovarian circulation. Embryonic intrauterine migration appears to prevent luteolysis and maintain luteal production of progesterone in equids.

Higher primates, such as humans, present a different set of circumstances, with respect to "maternal recognition of pregnancy" and maintenance of the corpus luteum. In these species, the endometrium does not appear to have an essential role in luteolysis, and the regulation of luteal regression appears to be an intraovarian event. Therefore, the blastocysts of higher primates must produce some "signal", which directly interacts with the maternal ovaries, in order to facilitate "maternal recognition of pregnancy" and prevent luteolysis. It is interesting to note that the embryos of these species of "higher" mammals undergo true implantation within the maternal endometrium, rather than the "attachment" which is observed in large domestic mammals, and that specialized cells involved in implantation play a pivotal role in preventing luteolysis.

Shortly after entry into the uterus during the secretory phase of the menstrual cycle, the human blastocyst attaches to the pregravid endometrium (i.e., the early decidua or the hormonally stimulated lining of the endometrium which will eventually form the maternal component of the placenta) (Netter, 1997). Very soon thereafter, in the mid- to late-secretory phase (i.e., luteal phase), fibroblast-type, stromal cells, located near uterine blood vessels, increase in size and accumulate glycogen and lipid to form decidual cells, which are only maintained if pregnancy occurs. By approximately day 7 or 8 after ovulation, the blastocyst has penetrated the luminal epithelium of the uterus, and the invasive capabilities of the trophoblastic cells of the blastocyst, specifically the syncytiotrophoblasts, have enabled the implantation of the blastocyst within the endometrium, surrounded by decidual cells (Figure 2.9) (Foster and Gray, 2008; Netter, 1997). On day 9 after ovulation, the syncytiotrophoblastic cells begin to secrete human chorionic gonadotropin (hCG) which, because of its LH-like activity, "rescues" the corpus luteum from luteolysis and increases the luteal production of progesterone, as well as estrogens. The increased secretion of these hormones, especially progesterone, stimulates widespread "decidualization" of the uterine stroma and atrophy of endometrial glands (Foster and Gray, 2008; Genuth, 2004b; Netter, 1997). Concurrent with these events, the syncytiotrophoblasts continue their invasion of the endometrium and, in particular, the uterine vasculature, to provide for the future nourishment and growth of the developing embryo and fetus. In other species of animals (e.g., rodents) where there is also actual implantation versus simple "attachment" of the embryo, the same, basic sequence of events (i.e., attachment to the endometrium, epithelial penetration, decidualization, and trophoblastic invasion into the uterine vasculature) also take place, including the production of chorionic gonadotropin and placental lactogen.

Formation of the extraembryonic membranes

Concepts and definitions

Most mammalian species are "eutherian", and during pregnancy form a placenta which is comprised of both maternal and fetal components. The term "decidua" is generally used in reference to humans and higher primates and can be used to refer to the lining of the endometrium which is shed during menses. However, "decidua" is used more frequently in connection with the maternal portion of the placenta which is shed at birth. The portion of the decidua which interdigitates with the trophoblast and, eventually, the chorion, is referred to as the decidua basalis. This portion of the deciduas provides nourishment to the embryo until formal connections to maternal vascular channels are established and a single, central circulation is formed (Genuth, 2004b). The portion of the decidua which surrounds the human embryo and, later, the fetus is the decidua capsularis. The decidua vera or decidua parietalis refers to the rest of the endometrial lining which is shed at birth but which does not interact with the trophoblatic cells or chorion (Figure 2.9) (Netter, 1997).

The yolk sac, amnion, allantois and chorion are the extraembryonic membranes formed by the mammalian embryo (Senger, 2007). While the yolk sac in most mammalian species normally undergoes regression (early in pregnancy in higher primates; later in rodents and rabbits), the allantois and chorion generally fuse to form the allantochorion, and the fluid-filled amnion provides a shock-absorbing, aquatic environment to facilitate fetal development and transport (Evans, 2007; Foster and Gray, 2008; Senger, 2007). The allantochorionic membrane is the fetal contribution to the placenta and the chorionic villi are the structures which interdigitate with various layers of the maternal endometrium which are maintained during pregnancy (Evans, 2007; Foster and Gray, 2008; Senger, 2007). In higher primates, the placental circulation and hemotrophic nutrition are established very early.

Placental types

Mammalian placentation can be classified according to the degree of intimacy between the maternal and fetal circulations (i.e., the number of tissue layers separating maternal and fetal blood) and by the pattern of distribution of the chorionic villi on the surface of the placenta facing the maternal endometrium. Epitheliochorial placentae have a total of six layers separating the maternal and fetal circulations and are observed in a variety of species, including equids and swine. Ruminant placentation is described as syndesmochorial because of the transient erosion and regrowth of the maternal epithelium, which results in the intermittent exposure of maternal endothelium (capillaries) to chorionic epithelium (Foster and Gray, 2008; Senger, 2007). Canine and feline placentas are classified as endotheliochorial, and the hemochorial placentation reported in primates and rodents has essentially only chorionic epithelium separating the maternal blood from that of the fetus. Interestingly, rabbit placentation undergoes a transition during gestation and is generally classified as hemoendothelial by the end of the pregnancy (Rozman and Klaassen, 2001), while the placentation of rodents is also often categorized as hemoendothelial because of attenuation of the chorion (Foster and Gray, 2008). The placenta of each species is associated with a typical distribution of the chorionic villi, classified as being diffuse (e.g., equids and swine), cotyledonary (e.g., ruminants), zonary (e.g., dogs and cats) or discoid (e.g., primates and rodents).

Placental function

The placenta (1) acts as an attachment between the fetal and maternal systems; (2) functions as a transient endocrine organ; (3) plays essential roles in the exchange of gases, nutrients and metabolic wastes between the maternal and fetal circulations; and (4) acts to protect the fetus from physical, mechanical and/or, potentially, chemical harm (Evans, 2007; Senger, 2007). In polytocous species, each fetus has its own placenta. Although the term "implantation" is frequently used to describe the appropriately timed attachment of the extraembryonic membranes to the endometrium, as has been discussed previously, only the conceptuses of primate and rodent species undergo true implantation (Evans, 2007; Senger, 2007).

The "placental barrier"

The placenta has often been referred to as a "barrier" which protects the fetus from toxicants, infectious disease and the attack by the mother's immune system. Multidrug resistance protein, as well as enzymes involved in the biotransformation of xenobiotics, have also been found to be components of this maternal–fetal complex (Rozman and Klaassen, 2001).

However, xenobiotics can cross the placenta by a variety of different mechanisms, including simple (i.e., passive) diffusion, facilitated diffusion and active transport, as well as pinocytosis and phagocytosis of some nutrients or toxicants resembling these nutrients. While the passage of materials across the placenta has been traditionally thought of as primarily being a function of the intimacy (i.e., number of tissue layers) between the maternal and fetal circulations, especially with respect to maternal immunoglobulins which cross hemoendothelial and hemo- and endotheliochorial placentae but not those types of placentae having more layers, the number of layers of tissue separating the maternal from the fetal circulation is only one of many placental- or xenobiotic-related factors influencing the accessibility of toxicants to the fetal circulation. While the placentae of most species very effectively prevent the passage of molecules with weights greater than 1,000 Da, most xenobiotics have molecular weights less than or equal to 500 Da, thereby somewhat limiting the impact of molecular size on the transfer of many xenobiotics across the placenta (Evans, 2007; Foster and Gray, 2007; Senger, 2007). Additional, placenta-related factors, such as surface area, the presence of specific carrier systems and membrane lipid-protein content, and xenobiotic-associated factors, including degree of ionization, lipid solubility and protein binding, also affect how likely it is that a given toxicant will cross the placenta.

Sex determination and sexual differentiation of reproductive function

Germ layer differentiation leads to organogenesis and the transformation of an embryo into the fetus which continues to grow and develop for the remainder of pregnancy. With respect to reproductive toxicity in non-rodent mammals, the organogenic and other developmental processes occurring during the first trimester of pregnancy are especially susceptible to the teratogenic effects of xenobiotics. The abnormalities induced by a teratogen are dependent on the specific developmental processes or signaling pathways targeted by that toxicant and the timing of the exposure. Sexual differentiation is a developmental process which is particularly susceptible to xenobiotic-induced abnormalities and is described in some detail.

Genotypic sex and development of the primitive sex cords

The genotypic sex of a mammalian conceptus is determined at fertilization by the sex chromosome (X or Y) contributed by the sperm, which, in combination with the X chromosome in the ovum, denotes either a genotypically female (XX) or a male (XY) zygote. During early gestation in most species, the primordial germ cells arise from the epithelium of the embryonic yolk sac and migrate through the developing mesentery to the gonadal (genital) ridge (testicular or ovarian anlage) in its position contiguous with the mesonephros (Evans, 2007; Senger, 2007). Germ cells and stimulated somatic cells proliferate and organize into primitive sex cords within undifferentiated (bipotential) gonads, which have the potential to develop into either ovaries or testes (Figure 2.4A) (Basrur, 2006; Senger, 2007).

Gonadal sex determination and phenotypic sexual differentiation

Development of a phenotypically male or female mammalian fetus occurs during the first trimester of pregnancy in most species and consists of the determination of gonadal sex followed by the further development and differentiation of either the mesonephric or the paramesonephric ducts and regression of the other duct system. The selection of the mesonephric or paramesonephric ducts for retention and further differentiation results in the formation of genitalia (phenotypic sex) appropriate for either the male or female gonads, respectively (Genuth, 2004b). Gonadal sex determination and phenotypic sexual differentiation are dependent on complex and carefully timed signaling events and are extremely susceptible to disruption by xenobiotics. Toxicants which alter epigenetic programming or mimic or inhibit endogenous hormones can have potentially deleterious effects on sexual development (Basrur, 2006). Xenobiotic-induced abnormalities in phenotypic sexual differentiation can arise from defects in testicular formation, defects in androgen production and defects in androgenic action (Basrur, 2006; Hughes *et al.*, 2006). While some toxicant-induced abnormalities in sexual differentiation can be very obvious, such as hermaphroditism or the presence of ovotestes, pseudohermaphroditism (i.e., differences in gonadal and phenotypic sex), hypospadias (feminized external genitalia; failure of urethral fold fusion) (Figure 2.4B) and cryptorchidism (failure of testicular descent), other, more subtle effects can be related to functional, rather than structural abnormalities. In order to identify the steps in gonadal sex determination and phenotypic sexual differentiation most likely to be targeted by the effects of endocrine disruptors and other reproductive toxicants, it is important to understand how these processes are initiated within the fetus and how they impact subsequent fetal development.

For the last several decades, the model for gonadal sex determination and phenotypic sexual differentiation has been based on the premise that a "testis determining factor" (TDF), which is encoded for by a gene on the Y chromosome (i.e., sex-determining region of the Y or SRY located on the distal part of the short arm of the human Y chromosome), dictates that a gonad differentiates into a testis and initiates the cascade of endocrine changes which results in a phenotypically male fetus exhibiting a developed mesonephric duct system and regressed paramesonephric ducts (Figures 2.4A and 2.5A) (Basrur, 2006; Genuth, 2004b; Senger, 2007). It is now also known that a gene identical to the SRY gene or linked to it encodes for a histocompatibility antigen commonly referred to as H-Y antigen, which also plays a role in determining that the gonadal sex will be male (i.e., a testis will form) when the Y chromosome is present (barring any gene translocations) in mammals (Genuth, 2004b). Without the determination that the gonads will develop into testes, the "default" or "constitutive" pathway is followed and ovarian gonads are formed in association with a developed paramesonephric duct system and regressed mesonephric ducts (Figures 2.4A and 2.5B) (Basrur, 2006; Genuth, 2004b; Senger, 2007).

While this model has been useful to explain rather complex developmental processes, it should be kept in mind that other toxicant-susceptible mechanisms might also play a role in gonadal sex determination and sexual differentiation. It is apparent that very precise, sex-specific patterns of germline epigenetic programming and interactions with somatic cells take place during the early stages of sexual differentiation (Anway and Skinner, 2006). Recent data have suggested that these signaling pathways are susceptible to epigenetic modifications induced by some antiandrogens (Anway *et al.*, 2005; Anway and Skinner, 2006). It has also been suggested that gonadal sex determination involves other genes on both sex and autosomal chromosomes that might be targeted by reproductive toxicants (Basrur, 2006; Genuth, 2004b).

Development of the male phenotype

Once previously undifferentiated gonads commit to testes development (TDF present), a coordinated series of endocrine-induced morphologic changes takes place, resulting in both a genotypically and phenotypically male fetus (Figures 2.4A, 2.4B and 2.5A). The sequence of signaling and developmental changes, which result in male sexual differentiation, include the following: (1) Sertoli cell development and secretion of anti-Müllerian hormone (AMH) or Müllerian inhibiting substance (MIS); (2) AMH-induced regression of the paramesonephric (Müllerian) ducts and differentiation of Leydig cells capable of producing testosterone; (3) testosterone-facilitated development of the mesonephric or Wolffian ducts; (4) differentiation of the mesonephric ducts into the rete testes, efferent ductules, epididymidies and ducti deferens; (5) development of primordial accessory sex glands and the formation of external genitalia from primordial; and (6) in most species (some exceptions in wildlife species) testicular descent of the intra-abdominal testes into their extra-abdominal position in the scrotum, prior to or very shortly after birth (some species) (Basrur, 2006; Edwards *et al.*, 2006; Genuth, 2004b; Senger, 2007).

Development of the female phenotype

If the previously undifferentiated gonads do not commit to testes development (TDF absent), ovaries are formed and a cascade of morphologic changes occurs in the absence of AMH and testosterone stimulation, resulting in a genotypically and phenotypically female fetus (Figures 2.4A, 2.4B and 2.5B). This sequence of "default" or "constitutive" morphologic and endocrine alterations results in the following sequence of developmental events: (1) regression of mesonephric (Wolffian ducts); (2) differentiation of the paramesonephric (Müllerian) ducts into the oviducts (uterine tubes), uterine horns, uterine body, cervix and anterior vagina; (3) remodeling of the ovary into its typical parenchymal and cortical structure; (4) cortical development of primordial follicles, with primary oocytes arrested in meiosis and surrounded by future granulosa and theca interna cells; and (5) development of the caudal vagina and vulva from the urogenital sinus (external genitalia primordia) (Basrur, 2006; Edwards *et al.*, 2006; Evans 2007; Genuth, 2004b; Senger; 2003).

Sexual differentiation of the brain

Sex-specific endocrine patterns and the resulting gender appropriate sexual behaviors in animals are necessary for fertile copulations to occur and require that the brain also undergo prenatal (postnatal in some species) sexual differentiation. Although large amounts of estradiol defeminize the brain; alpha-fetoprotein prevents most of the endogenous estrogens in the female fetus from crossing the blood–brain barrier. The brain remains inherently female under the influence of minimal amounts of estradiol, and both the GnRH tonic and surge centers are maintained within the hypothalamus of the female fetus in this low estradiol environment (Ford and D'Occhio, 1989; Senger, 2007). Testosterone produced by the fetal testes crosses the blood–brain barrier and is converted to estradiol within the brain, and, as a result of this estradiol synthesis, the hypothalamic GnRH surge center in the male fetus is minimized.

While the differentiation of male sexual behavior in large domestic animals generally involves prenatal defeminization, especially in species having longer gestations, it should be noted that postnatal defeminization of the brain occurs in both male swine and rodents (Ford and D'Occhio, 1989). There is also evidence to suggest that the males of some species with prenatal defeminization of the brain might also require postnatal exposure to androgens for maximum masculinization of the brain (Senger, 2007). Depending on the timing of exposure, xenoestrogens and, possibly, some xenoandrogens, which cross the placenta and the blood–brain barrier, have the potential to have profound effects on sexual differentiation of the brain and future reproductive function.

The endocrinology of pregnancy

Gestational hormones

Pregnancy begins with fertilization of the oocyte within the oviduct (uterine tube), followed by the first cleavage of the zygote, and terminates with parturition. Although the endocrine physiology and duration of mammalian pregnancy are very species specific and are characterized by a great deal of interspecies variation, the overall goals during the entire gestation for all pregnant mammals, their embryo(s) and, eventually, the maternal–fetal–placental unit are the same. A uterine environment conducive to embryonic and fetal development must be facilitated and the pregnancy (pregnancies in polytocous animals) must be maintained for the entire normal gestational length. The primary hormones involved in establishing the proper uterine environment and maintaining pregnancy are progesterone secreted by the maternal ovary and/or the placenta, as well as, in some species, a variety of placental progestagens. In addition, a variety of other endogenous hormones of maternal, fetal and/or placental origin (depending on the species and gender of the offspring), including androgens, estrogens, prolactin, placental lactogen, human, rat and equine chorionic gonadotropins (i.e., hCG, rCG, and eCG, respectively) and relaxin, also have important gestational functions. Normal embryonic and fetal development requires that gestational hormones, especially endogenous androgens and estrogens, be synthesized and secreted in sufficient quantities and at the appropriate times during pregnancy. The proper reproductive development of the female fetus is primarily dependent on exposure to estrogens at specific times during gestation. However, the male fetus must have appropriately timed exposure to normal amounts of both androgens and estrogens for normal development of the reproductive tract and optimal adult reproductive performance (Hess, 2003). Depending on the timing of exposure, endocrine disrupting chemicals (i.e., EDCs or HAAs), especially those which function as gonadal steroid receptor agonists and antagonists, can potentially interfere with normal gestational signaling and sexual differentiation.

Some species of mammals, such as dogs, cats, camelids, goats, swine, rodents and rabbits, depend solely on luteal progesterone secretion for the maintenance of pregnancy (Evans, 2007; Foster and Gray, 2008; Senger, 2007). The placenta takes over progesterone-associated pregnancy maintenance in sheep at approximately 50 days post-conception and between the sixth and eighth month of gestation in cattle. The uterofetoplacental unit of the mare begins to produce a unique assortment of progestagens classified as 5α-pregnanes, beginning at about day 70 of pregnancy.

The approximate length of gestation in women is 38 weeks or approximately 40 weeks after the last normal menses. In humans, circulating hCG concentrations reach a peak by 9 to 12 weeks after ovulation and then slowly stabilize to concentrations maintained throughout the remainder of gestation. By 6 weeks after ovulation, the syncytiotrophoblasts in the placenta begin to synthesize progesterone, and the placenta replaces the corpus luteum as the major source of progestagens in pregnant women after 12 weeks. Likewise, estrogens are also produced by the placenta, but the mother and fetus must both provide steroid hormone precursors for this biosynthetic pathway (Genuth, 2004b).

Parturition

Physiology of parturition

Parturition constitutes transport of the fetus and its associated membranes from the maternal to the external environment, and represents transition of the fetus to a neonate. Maturation of the fetal hypothalamic–pituitary–adrenal axis plays an important role in the cascade of neural and endocrine events which eventually lead to parturition and/or which facilitate fetal maturation in most mammalian species, including humans (Evans, 2007; Senger, 2007). While the specific events which initiate parturition in humans are still not very well defined and might involve locally mediated events within the uterofetoplacental unit, it is very clear from studies in ruminants that maturation of the fetal hypothalamic–pituitary–adrenal axis and the release of cortisol are the key events directly involved in the initiation of labor in those species. Fetal CRF stimulates the release of ACTH from the fetal pituitary, and ACTH, in turn, stimulates fetal secretion of cortisol by the adrenal glands. Elevations in fetal cortisol (fetal LH may be involved as well) activate placental steroidogenic enzyme systems, resulting in decreased progestagen and elevated estrogens prior to parturition (Evans, 2007; Genuth, 2004b; Senger, 2007). The increase in the placental estrogen:progestagen ratio facilitates several important processes (e.g., cervical softening, upregulation of myometrial oxytocin receptors, uterine synthesis of $PGF_2\alpha$ and increased blood flow to the gravid uterus and placenta), which prepare the uterus for parturition. In many mammalian species, the aforementioned shift in placental steroidogenesis results not only in an increased placental estrogen:progestagen ratio but also in a precipitous drop in circulating concentrations of progestagens. While the placental estrogen:progestagen ratio increases in pregnant women and most likely plays a role in the cascade of events leading to parturition, the systemic concentrations of progestagens do not drop in humans, as they do in other species. Based on the proposed mechanism for the onset of parturition, xenobiotic exposure causing maternal and/or fetal stress could be associated with abortion or premature parturition, and, similarly, the parenteral administration of glucocorticoids to some species (i.e., sheep and cattle) could be used in protocols to induce abortion or parturition.

Normal parturition approaches as neural signals caused by fetal movements and myometrial contractions, along with elevated basal levels of oxytocin and increased secretion of $PGF_2\alpha$ bring about the first stage of labor. A rapid increase in oxytocin and $PGF_2\alpha$ secretion leads to rupture of the allantochorionic membrane and the commencement of the second stage of labor. Secretion of oxytocin and catecholamines can also play a role in stimulating uterine contractions via oxytocin and α-adrenergic receptors. Strong myometrial contractions result in the delivery of offspring, as well as the expulsion of the fetal membranes plus, depending on the species, the decidua during the third stage of labor (Evans, 2007; Senger, 2007).

The mammary glands

Anatomy

The mammary glands or breasts are important for the production of colostrum (i.e., first milk produced after birth) and subsequent lactation for the nutrition and growth of

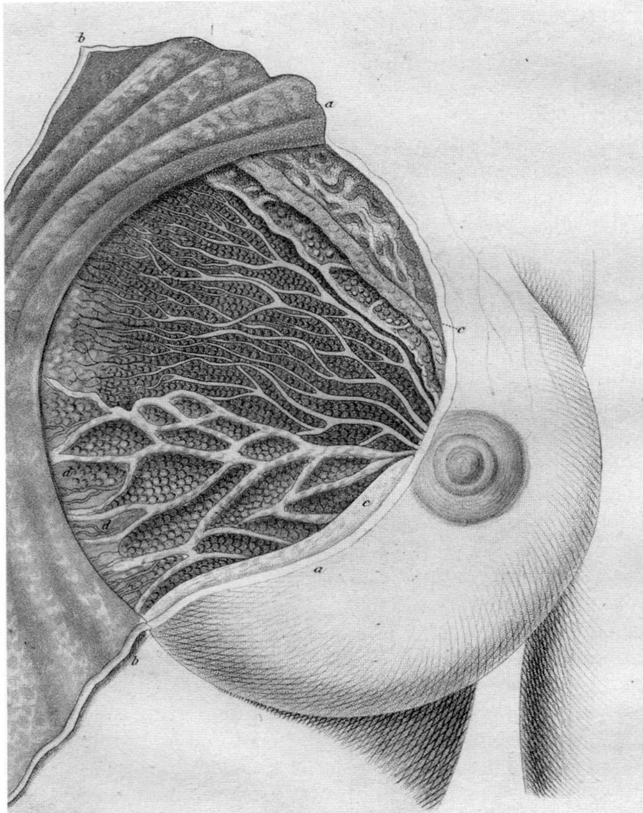

FIGURE 2.10 Although drawn almost 200 years ago, the depiction of the frontal section of the mammary gland of a non-pregnant woman clearly shows the different types of tissue composing the human breast and demonstrates the degree of understanding of the anatomical structures involved in lactation which existed at that time. Figure was adapted from *Dictionnaire Pittoresque d'Histoire Naturelle et des Phenomenes de la Nature* by Felix Edward Guerin-Meneville (c. 1839). Modifications were courtesy of Howard Wilson and Don Connor.

the neonate. The glandular portions of the breasts can also be affected by neoplasia. Figure 2.10 shows the mammary glands of a non-pregnant woman. It is evident from this image drawn almost 200 years ago, that, like other aspects of human reproduction, there was a fairly good understanding of the anatomical structures involved in lactation.

Physiology of lactation

Lactogenesis

Appropriately timed lactogenesis is critical for survival of mammalian offspring. Lactogenesis is a two-stage process involving (1) the enzymatic and cytologic differentiation of the alveolar cells within the mammary gland and (2) the copious secretion of milk, which is distinct from the colostral sequestration of antibodies (Tucker, 1994). Growth hormone, aldosterone, prostaglandins, insulin, estrogens, progestagens, placental lactogens (if present) and prolactin are required for the first stage of lactogenesis, which generally occurs during the last trimester of pregnancy (Evans, 2007; Tucker, 1994). Large increases in pulsatile prolactin secretion by lactotropes in the anterior pituitary are necessary for the initiation of the second stage of lactogenesis, which generally occurs in close temporal association with the endocrine milieu of parturition, which is characterized by a precipitous drop in progestagen and estrogen concentrations. Oxytocin, the secretion of which by the posterior pituitary gland is stimulated by the suckling reflex, is very effective at causing milk ejection, in large part because of its effects on myoepithelial cells.

In the females of many species, circulating concentrations of prolactin are elevated above basal levels for a month or two after parturition. It should be of interest to note that reproductive function is suppressed in several mammalian species, including humans, by prolactin-induced suppression of LH secretion and insensitivity to FSH (Genuth, 2004b). A placental lactogen performs many of the same endocrine functions as prolactin and is secreted during gestation in several species, including women (Evans, 2007).

Control of prolactin secretion

Lactotropic prolactin secretion is tonically inhibited by dopamine secreted by hypothalamic neurons belonging to either the tuberoinfundibular or tuberohypophysial dopaminergic systems (TIDA and THDA, respectively) (Evans, 2007; Neill and Nagy, 1994). Vasoactive intestinal peptide (VIP) and TRH are thought to act as prolactin releasing factors and can interfere with the dopamine-associated tonic inhibition of prolactin release. Oxytocin, in conjunction with the suckling reflex, will increase pituitary lactotropic production and secretion of prolactin, as well as cause milk ejection. In species strictly dependent on prolactin for lactogenesis, toxicants which mimic dopamine and tonically inhibit prolactin secretion pose a risk to fetal survival.

Reproductive senescence

Women and the females of some other mammalian species are known to undergo reproductive senescence. In humans this process generally begins at approximately 50 years of age and is associated with dysregulation of the hypothalamic–pituitary–gonadal axis and lower circulating estrogen concentrations, as well as decreased amounts of steroids in the brain (Foster and Gray, 2008). In women, there is usually a gradual transition from regular to irregular menstrual cycles, followed by the cessation of cyclicity (i.e., menopause) and, ultimately, infertility (Foster and Gray, 2008; Yin and Gore, 2006). Unfortunately, this transition is often associated with changes in behavior, mood swings, malaise and increased risk for the development of osteoporosis. It is currently thought that age-related alterations in the morphology and function of the GnRH neurosecretory system within the hypothalamus play an important role in the onset of menopause in women (Yin and Gore, 2006). There is increasing evidence that males can also experience a similar age-related process, which is referred to as andropause and is associated with decreased circulating concentrations of androgens.

CONCLUDING REMARKS AND FUTURE DIRECTIONS

The purpose of this chapter was to acquaint the reader with the basic anatomical and physiological aspects of reproductive function. Reproduction is a complex process required for species survival. There are stringent physiological and metabolic requirements for: (1) the production of viable and functional male and female gametes; (2) their transport and union to form a zygote; (3) the multiplication and differentiation of the cells within the embryonic vesicle; (4) formation of the placenta to provide nourishment for the developing embryo/fetus; and ultimately, (5) the development of a healthy and fertile member of the species. For well over 200 years, the basic anatomical components required for human reproduction have been fairly well recognized and their primary functions understood. As scientific investigation has progressed, a great deal has been learned about the specific cellular, hormonal and, even, molecular processes which are the bases for the complex and dynamic processes involved in human reproduction (Figure 2.1).

It is important to understand that exposures to potential toxicants will have different reproductive outcomes depending on the timing and developmental stage when an organism is exposed, as well as the dosage and duration of the toxicant exposure. In humans, exposure to reproductive toxicants can be accidental or occupational over a very short period of time, or chemical exposures can take place over an entire lifetime. While pre- and postnatal development, gametogenesis and sexual function in men can all be adversely affected by exposures to potential toxicants, the target organs and functions in women are generally more diverse and dynamic. Figure 2.8 clearly shows all of the anatomical and physiological reproductive changes which can take place in women's lives between infancy and menopause, including during periods of pregnancy and lactation. A basic understanding of these processes is necessary as one investigates specific reproductive toxicants.

There is currently increasing societal concern that sublethal chemical exposures have the potential to impact human and animal reproductive function. To facilitate sound experimental designs and accurate risk assessment, it is important to be able to recognize subtle and not-so-subtle xenobiotic-induced adverse reproductive effects in experimental animals, as well as variations in reproductive endpoints within human and animal populations. We cannot, nor would we want to, live in a chemical-free world. However, we should have a thorough enough comprehension of all of the various developmental, physiological and behavioral aspects of reproductive function to evaluate the safety of xenobiotics and their mixtures at current levels of environmental, occupational and domestic exposures and make sound stewardship, lifestyle and policy decisions.

REFERENCES

Anway MD, Cupp AS, Uzumcu M, Skinner MK (2005) Epigenetic transgenerational actions of endocrine disruptor and male fertility. *Science* **308:** 1466–9.

Anway MD, Skinner MK (2006) Epigenetic transgenerational actions of endocrine disruptors. *Endocrinology* **147 (Supplement):** S43–9.

Basrur PK (2006) Disrupted sex differentiation and feminization of man and domestic animals. *Environ Res* **100:** 18–38.

Berne RM, Levy MN, Koeppen BM, Stanton BA (eds.) (2004) *Physiology*, 5th edition, Mosby, Inc., St. Louis, pp. 719–42.

Bigsby RM, Mercado-Feliciano M, Mubiru J (2005) Molecular mechanisms of estrogen dependent processes. In *Endocrine Disruptors: Effects on Male and Female Reproductive Systems*, 2nd edition (Naz RK, ed.). CRC Press and Taylor & Francis Group, LLC, Boca Raton, pp. 217–47.

Brayman MJ, Julian J, Mulac-Jericevic B, Conneely OM., Edwards DP, Carson DD (2006) Progesterone receptor isoforms A and B differentially regulate MUC1 expression in uterine epithelial cells. *Mol Endocrinol* **20:** 2278–91.

Britt KL, Findlay JK (2002) Estrogen actions in the ovary revisited. *J Endocrinology* **175:** 269–76.

De Jonge C, Barratt C (eds.) (2006) *The Sperm Cell*. Cambridge University Press, New York.

Edwards TM, Moore BC, Guillette LJ Jr (2006) Reproductive dysgenesis in wildlife: a comparative view. *Int J Androl* **29:** 109–19.

Evans TJ (2007) Reproductive toxicity and endocrine disruption. In *Veterinary Toxicology: Basic and Clinical Principles* (Gupta, RC, ed.). Academic Press/Elsevier, Inc., New York, pp. 206–44.

Evans TJ, Constantinescu GM, Ganjam VK (1997) Clinical reproductive anatomy and physiology of the mare. In *Current Therapy in Large Animal Theriogenology* (Younquist RS, ed.). W.B. Saunders, Philadelphia, pp. 43–68.

Ford JJ, D'Occhio MJ (1989) Differentiation of sexual behavior in cattle, sheep and swine. *J Anim Sci* **67:** 1816–23.

Foster PMD, Gray LE Jr (2008) Toxic responses of the reproductive system. In *Casarett &Doull's Toxicology: The Basic Science of Poisons*, 7th edition (Klaassen CD, ed.). McGraw-Hill, New York, pp. 761–806.

França LR, Avelar GF, Almeida FFL. (2005) Spermatogenesis and sperm transit through the epididymis in mammals with emphass on pigs. *Theriogenology* **63:** 300–18.

Genuth SM (2004a) General principles of endocrine physiology. In *Physiology*, 5th edition (Berne RM, Levy MN, Koeppen BM, Stanton BA, eds.). Mosby, Inc., St. Louis, pp. 719–42.

Genuth SM (2004b) The reproductive glands. In *Physiology*, 5th edition (Berne RM, Levy MN, Koeppen BM, Stanton BA, eds.). Mosby, Inc., St. Louis, pp. 920–78.

Gupta RC (ed.) (2007) *Veterinary Toxicology: Basic and Applied Principles*. Academic Press/Elsevier, Inc., New York, pp. 206–44.

Hardy MP, Ganjam VK (1997) Stress, 11beta-HSD, and Leydig cell function. *J Androl* **18:** 475–9.

Haschek WM, Rousseaux CG, Wallig MA (2010) *Fundamentals of Toxicologic Pathology*, 2nd edition. Academic Press-Elsevier, New York, pp. 553–97.

Hess RA (2003) Estrogen in the adult male reproductive tract: a review. *Reprod Biol Endocrinol* **1:** 52–65.

Hess RA, França LR (2005) Structure of the Sertoli cell. In *Sertoli Cell Biology* (Skinner MK, Griswold MD, eds.). Elsevier-Academic Press, New York, pp. 19–40.

Hodgson E, Mailman RB, Chambers JE, Dow RE (eds.) (2000) *Dictionary of Toxicology*, 2nd edition. Grove's Dictionaries Inc., New York.

Hughes IA, Martin H, Jääskeläinen J (2006) Genetic mechanisms of fetal male undermasculinization: a background to the role of endocrine disruptors. *Environ Res* **100:** 44–9.

Marshall WA, Tanner JM (1969) Variations in the pattern of pubertal changes in girls. *Arch Dis Child* **44:** 291–303.

Marshall WA, Tanner JM (1970) Variations in the pattern of pubertal changes in boys. *Arch Dis Child* **45:** 13–23.

Neill JD, Nagy GM (1994) Prolactin secretion and its control. In *The Physiology of Reproduction*, 2nd edition (Knobil E, Neill JD, eds.). Raven Press, New York, pp. 1833–60.

Netter FH (1997) *The Netter Collection of Medical Illustrations, Volume 2, Reproductive System*. Sunders Elsevier, Philadelphia.

O'Donnell L, Robertson KM, Jones ME, Simpson ER (2001) Estrogen and spermatogenesis. *Endocrine Rev* **22:** 229–318.

Payne AH (2007) Steroidogenic enzymes in Leydig cells. In *The Leydig Cell in Health and Disease* (Payne AH, Hardy MP, eds.). Human Press, Tottawa, NJ, pp. 157–71.

Payne AH, Hardy MP (eds.) (2007) *The Leydig Cell in Health and Disease*. Humana Press, Tottawa, NJ.

Piñón R Jr (2002) *The Biology of Human Reproduction*. University Science Books, Sausolito, CA.

Razandi M, Pedram A, Greene GL, Levin ER (1999) Cell membrane and nuclear estrogen receptors (ERs) originate from a single transcript: studies of ERα and ERβ expressed in Chinese hamster ovary cells. *Mol Endocrinol* **13:** 307–19.

Rozman KK, Klaassen CD (2001). Absorption, distribution and excretion of toxicants. In *Casarett &Doull's Toxicology: The Basic Science of Poisons*, 6th edition (Klaassen CD, ed.). McGraw-Hill, New York, pp. 107–32.

Senger PL (2007) *Pathways to Pregnancy and Parturition*, 2nd revised edition. Current Conceptions, Inc., Moscow, ID.

Sikka SC, Kendirci M, Naz R (2005) Endocrine disruptors and male infertility. In *Endocrine Disruptors: Effects on Male and Female Reproductive Systems*, 2nd edition (Naz RK, ed.). CRC Press and Taylor & Francis Group, LLC, Boca Raton, pp. 291–312.

Skinner MK, Griswold MD (eds.) (2005) *Sertoli Cell Biology*. Elsevier-Academic Press, New York.

Stocco DM (2007) The role of StAR in Leydig cell steroidogenesis. In *The Leydig Cell in Health and Disease* (Payne AH, Hardy MP, eds.). Human Press, Tottawa, NJ, pp. 149–55.

Sutovsky P, Moreno R, Ramahlho-Santos J, Dominko T, Thompson W (2001) A putative, ubiquitin-dependent mechanism for the recognition and elimination of defective spermatozoa in the mammalian epididymis. *J Cell Science* **114:** 1665–75.

Thomas P, Khan IA (2005) Disruption of nongenomic steroid actions on gametes and serotonergic pathways controlling reproductive neuroendocrine function by environmental chemicals. In *Endocrine Disruptors: Effects on Male and Female Reproductive Systems*, 2nd edition (Naz RK, ed.). CRC Press and Taylor & Francis Group, LLC, Boca Raton, pp. 3–45.

Tsai MJ, O'Malley BW. (1994) Molecular mechanisms of action of steroid/thyroid receptor superfamily members. *Ann Rev Biochem* **63:** 451–86.

Tucker A (1994) Lactation and its hormonal control. In *The Physiology of Reproduction*, 2nd edition (Knobil E, Neill JD, eds.). Raven Press, New York, pp. 1065–98.

Warner M, Gustafsson J-A (2006) Nongenomic effects of estrogen: why all the uncertainty? *Steroids* **71:** 91–5.

Yin W, Gore AC (2006) Neuroendocrine control of reproductive aging: roles of GnRH neurons. *Reproduction* **131:** 403–14.

CHAPTER

3

Bio-communication between mother and offspring

Etsuko Wada and Keiji Wada

INTRODUCTION

Living organisms, including humans, survive under a wide range of environmental conditions. Recently, it has become evident that such environmental conditions have far greater influence on fetal and neonatal development than one might imagine. At early developmental stages, not only inherited genetic factors but also the maternal environment, such as nutritional status and the living environment, affect the formation of neural network and physiological responses in the offspring. Furthermore, these influences can produce irreversible changes and increase the risk of disease in later life in the offspring; this is called fetal programming (Wu *et al.*, 2004). For instance, Barker (1997) reported an association between maternal nutrition and disease in the offspring in later life, including coronary heart disease, diabetes and hypertension. Individuals prenatally exposed to the Dutch winter famine of 1944–1945 had higher rates of low birth weight, insulin resistance and vascular disease than those not exposed (Lumey, 1998). Such epidemiological analyses have indicated the association between maternal conditions during pregnancy and impairment of the offspring in later life. However, these studies have not investigated the molecular basis of such maternal influences. This has now begun to be addressed using animal models. Recent studies in rodents have indicated that the maternal conditions, including the nutritional, psychiatric and physical states, affect neural development, metabolism and behavior in the offspring.

With changes in maternal status, certain bioactive substances are transferred from mother to offspring via the placenta or milk and affect the offspring's development. Recently, Kodomari *et al.* (2009a) reported that maternal acyl ghrelin, which is increased by repeated restraint stress, is transported across the placenta, resulting in increased acyl ghrelin in the fetus. Even under normal conditions, some bioactive substances have been shown to be transported from mother to fetus via the placenta and influence fetal development. Similarly, physiological responses in the pregnant mother can be affected by bioactive substances from the fetus or placenta. For example, fetal oxytocin transferred into the mother's circulation induces myocardial contraction of the uterus prior to parturition (Schriefer *et al.*, 1982). These bioactive substances, such as peptides, hormones and growth factors, play important roles in the development of the offspring as well as maternal physiological responses. In addition, these substances are important in the understanding of the molecular basis of the mutual influences between the mother and her offspring. We termed such molecular "conversations" between mother and offspring "bio-communication" (Tozuka *et al.*, 2009a). Clarifying the mechanisms that regulate bio-communication will improve our understanding of normal development and brain function as well as developmental disorders.

Over the past two decades, the number of reports using two generations (dam and offspring) of experimental animals has increased remarkably. Because this research spans the fields of pediatrics, nutrition, neuroscience and psychiatry, only a few reviews have comprehensively summarized the bio-communication between mother and offspring. In this chapter, we provide an overview of previous investigations that have demonstrated maternal influences on the development of the offspring and the transportation of bioactive substances between mother and offspring.

MATERNAL INFLUENCES ON THE DEVELOPMENT OF THE OFFSPRING

This section of the chapter describes the influence of maternal nutritional status (overnutrition, undernutrition) and living environment (enrichment, maternal care) on the development of the offspring. Common maternal situations and their possible effects on the offspring are summarized in Table 3.1.

Maternal nutritional status: overnutrition

While more than one million people die of starvation every year, the increased prevalence of obesity and its related metabolic disorders is considered a major health issue worldwide.

Reproductive and Developmental Toxicology, Edited by Ramesh C. Gupta
ISBN: 978-0-12-382032-7

TABLE 3.1 Maternal situations and possible effects on their offspring

Maternal situations	Effects	References
Nutritional status		
Overnutrition (high fat diet)	Metabolic disturbance	Srinivasan *et al.*, 2006; Férézou-Viala *et al.*, 2007; Chang *et al.*, 2008
	Transplacental transfer	Jones *et al.*, 2009
	Leptin sensitivity	Férézou-Viala *et al.*, 2007
	Gene expression of orexigenic peptide	Chang *et al.*, 2008
	Lipid peroxidation	Tozuka *et al.*, 2009b
	Postnatal hippocampal neurogenesis	Tozuka *et al.*, 2009b
	Learning and memory	Tozuka *et al.*, 2010
Undernutrition (diet restriction)	Intrauterine growth retardation	Woodall *et al.*, 1996
	Hypertension	Langley-Evans *et al.*, 1994
	Glucose metabolism, Insulin resistance	Zambrano *et al.*, 2006
	Postnatal leptin surge	Yura *et al.*, 2005
	Emotional behavior, Activity	Simonson *et al.*, 1971
	HPA axis	Vieau *et al.*, 2007
	Growth, Emotional behavior, Activity	Kumon *et al.*, 2010
Living environment		
Environmental enrichment	Learning and memory	Kiyono *et al.*, 1985
	Stress response	Welberg *et al.*, 2006
	Retinal development	Sale *et al.*, 2007
	Hippocampal prolifereation	Maruoka *et al.*, 2009
Exercise (running, swimming)	Neurogenesis	Brown *et al.*, 2003; Lee *et al.*, 2006; Bick-Sander *et al.*, 2006
	Learning/memory	Parnpiansil *et al.*, 2003; Lee *et al.*, 2006; Kim *et al.*, 2007
Maternal care	Glucocorticoid feedback sensitivity	Liu *et al.*, 1997
	DNA methylation, Gene expression	Weaver *et al.*, 2004, 2006
	Cognitive function	Liu *et al.*, 2000
	Anxiety behavior	Weaver *et al.*, 2006
Maternal deprivation	Neurogenesis	Kikusui *et al.*, 2009
	Stress hormone, Growth factor	Daniels *et al.*, 2009
Stress	Stress hormone, Fear memory	Griffin *et al.*, 2003
	Lower birth weight	Van den Hove *et al.*, 2006
	Learning/memory	Cherian *et al.*, 2009
	HPA axis, Anxiety behavior	Brunton and Russell, 2010

Abbreviation: HPA, hypothalamic–pituitary–adrenal

For instance, in the United States, the prevalence of overweight or obesity among adults aged at least 20 years in 1999–2002 was more than 60% (Hedley *et al.*, 2004). The greater numbers of overweight individuals in adulthood are consistent with a remarkable increase in the prevalence of obesity among pregnant women (Yeh and Shelton, 2005). Overweight during pregnancy is known to increase the risk of various impairments, including pregnancy-related hypertension, gestational diabetes and obstetric complications (Hincz *et al.*, 2009). In addition, recent animal studies have indicated that maternal obesity and related metabolic disorders cause long-term physiological and behavioral changes in the offspring.

In many animal studies, female mice fed a high fat diet (HFD) have been used as an animal model of maternal overnutrition. Maternal HFD causes increased body weight, food intake and circulating levels of free fatty acids, triglycerides, insulin, glucose and leptin in adult offspring (Srinivasan *et al.*, 2006; Férézou-Viala *et al.*, 2007; Chang *et al.*, 2008). Although the mechanisms underlying fetal overgrowth were not evident, a recent study indicated that a maternal HFD increased transplacental transport of glucose and neutral amino acids *in vivo*, and increased protein expression of their transporters in microvillous plasma membranes (Jones *et al.*, 2009). In the hypothalamus of offspring from HFD dams, leptin resistance and increased gene expression of orexigenic peptides, including galanin and orexin, were observed (Férézou-Viala *et al.*, 2007; Chang *et al.*, 2008).

Recently, Tozuka *et al.* (2009b, 2010) demonstrated that a maternal HFD before mating and throughout pregnancy and lactation affected hippocampal formation in the young offspring. Offspring from HFD dams (HFD offspring) showed increased peroxidized lipid accumulation and decreased postnatal neurogenesis in the dentate gyrus of the hippocampus (Tozuka *et al.*, 2009b). In addition, expression of brain-derived neurotrophic factor (Bdnf) in the hippocampus of HFD offspring was lower than that in offspring from mothers fed a normal diet. It is known that Bdnf plays important roles in dendritic arborization and spatial learning and memory (Gao *et al.*, 2009; Taliaz *et al.*, 2010). In young HFD offspring, impairment of dendritic arborization of hippocampal new neurons and acquisition of spatial learning and memory were observed (Tozuka *et al.*, 2010).

Maternal nutritional status: undernutrition

It is well established that sufficient nutrition supplied from the mother is critical for the growth and development of the fetus. Previous epidemiological and animal studies have presented that maternal undernutrition during pregnancy causes intrauterine growth retardation (IUGR), with subsequent long-term health consequences. In humans, maternal undernutrition caused IUGR and low birth weight, potentially increasing the risk of emotional and behavioral problems and low social competency (Wu *et al.*, 2004; Dahl *et al.*, 2006). Moreover maternal undernutrition during pregnancy resulted in placental insufficiency and epigenetic changes leading to an increased predisposition to diabetes and cardiovascular disease in adult offspring (Le Clair *et al.*, 2009). These results are supported by numerous studies using animal models. For example, in rats, maternal nutritional restriction during pregnancy produced not only IUGR in the offspring (Woodall *et al.*, 1996), but also hypertension and deregulation of glucose metabolism and insulin resistance in later life (Langley-Evans *et al.* 1994; Zambrano *et al.*, 2006). Plasma leptin levels rise transiently during the neonatal period; this is called a "neonatal leptin surge" and it is involved in the formation of energy-regulation circuits (Ahima *et al.*, 1998). Yura *et al.* (2005) have reported that intrauterine undernutrition advances the leptin surge and alters hypothalamic energy regulation in mice. Furthermore, maternal undernutrition during gestation resulted in heightened emotional behavior and decreased activity in the offspring (Simonson *et al.*, 1971). In addition, fetuses from pregnant rats that received 50% food restriction during the final week of gestation showed reduced hypothalamic–pituitary–adrenal axis function and greater transplacental transfer of glucocorticoids (Vieau *et al.*, 2007).

Because developmental processes such as neurogenesis, neuronal migration and axonal projection take place in the central nervous system during the early postnatal period, the maternal nutritional state during lactation is also critical for the pups. Recently, Kumon *et al.* (2010) investigated the influence of maternal undernutrition during lactation on the development of the pups, using 70% food-restricted mice. Findings revealed that the offspring from dietary-restricted dams had a smaller body size than those from control dams from 1 to 10 weeks of age, though they did not when they were older. In addition, the offspring from dietary-restricted dams showed decreased locomotor activity and increased anxiety behavior compared with those in the offspring from control dams.

Maternal living environment: environmental enrichment

In experiments with rodents, environmental enrichment (EE) consists of a large cage containing motor activities and objects for sensory and cognitive stimulation and novelty recognition (Petrosini *et al.*, 2009). Previous studies using adult rodents have demonstrated that EE increases cell proliferation and neurogenesis in the adult dentate gyrus and affects emotional behaviors such as anxiety- and depression-like behaviors (Benaroya-Milshtein *et al.*, 2004; Hattori *et al.*, 2007; Leal-Galicia *et al.*, 2007). Kiyono *et al.* (1985) demonstrated that maternal EE also affected the development of the offspring. Maternal EE during pregnancy can facilitate the postnatal learning abilities of the offspring. In addition, a recent study demonstrated that EE during pregnancy affects prenatal hippocampal neuronal proliferation and locomotor activity in adult female offspring (Maruoka *et al.*, 2009).

Maternal living environment: maternal care

Recently, it has been reported that maternal behavior alters gene expression as a consequence of DNA methylation, thereby affecting behavior in the offspring. Licking and grooming (LG) and arched-back nursing (ABN) are commonly observed as maternal behaviors in untreated rats. There are two naturally occurring variants in maternal behavior: high frequency LG-ABN and low frequency LG-ABN (L LG-ABN). In adult offspring suckled by L LG-ABN dams, elevation of cytosine methylation across the glucocorticoid receptor gene promoter and decreased glucocorticoid receptor gene expression in the hippocampus were observed (Weaver *et al.*, 2004). Furthermore, these offspring showed alterations in glucocorticoid feedback sensitivity and anxiety-mediated behavior (Liu *et al.*, 1997; Weaver *et al.*, 2006). Recently, alterations in DNA methylation have been reported in patients with Rett syndrome and other forms of mental retardation (Amir *et al.*, 1999; Urdinguio *et al.*, 2009). Moreover, aberrant DNA methylation is becoming increasingly recognized as being important in neurodegenerative disorders (Urdinguio *et al.*, 2009). Further analysis is needed to investigate whether epigenetic modifications produced by environmental changes during early development can predispose to neuropsychiatric disorders in later life.

TRANSPORTATION OF BIOACTIVE SUBSTANCES BETWEEN MOTHER AND OFFSPRING

Transportation via the placenta

With changes in the maternal state, even under normal physiological conditions, bioactive substances, including peptides, hormones and growth factors, are transferred between mother and offspring via the placenta. Such biological substances play an important role in fetal development as well as maternal physiological responses. To find novel transportable bioactive substances is important to understand the early development of the offspring as well as the mechanisms of influence between mother and offspring. Some of the bioactive substances transported from mother to fetus or from fetus to mother are summarized in Table 3.2.

Acyl ghrelin

Acyl ghrelin is an endogenous ligand for the growth hormone secretagogue receptor (Ghsr) and stimulates growth hormone secretion from the pituitary gland (Kojima *et al.*, 1999). Several studies have investigated the transfer of acyl ghrelin across the placenta from mother to fetus, and the effects of maternal ghrelin on fetal development in rodents (Nakahara *et al.*, 2006; Yuzuriha *et al.*, 2007; Kodomari *et al.*, 2009a). Ghrelin has been shown to cross the placenta to the fetus, and chronic ghrelin treatment in pregnant rats resulted in a significant increase in the birthweight of newborn pups compared with that of control pups (Nakahara *et al.*, 2006). Ghrelin administration to pregnant mice was also shown to inhibit malformation of the fetal neural tube induced by overexpression of peptide YY (Yuzuriha *et al.*, 2007). Moreover, when ghrelin was administered to pregnant mice,

TABLE 3.2 Bioactive substances between mother and offspring via placenta, and their possible effects

Bioactive substances	Effects	References
From mother to fetus	**Effects on offspring**	
Corticosterone	ND	Zarrow *et al.*, 1970; Montano *et al.*, 1993
Epidermal growth factor (EGF)	ND	Popliker *et al.*, 1987
Transforming growth factor-β1 (TGF-β1)	Cardiac development	Letterio *et al.*, 1994
Vasoactive intestinal peptide (VIP)	Early post-implantation development	Hill *et al.*, 1996; Spong *et al.*, 1999
Oxytocin	Transient inhibitory switch in GABA signaling	Malek *et al.*, 1996; Tyzio *et al.*, 2006
Serotonin	Cardiac development	Côté *et al.*, 2007; Fligny *et al.*, 2008
Ghrelin	Birth weight of new born pups	Nakahara *et al.*, 2006
	Neural tube formation in peptide YY overexpressed mice	Yuzuriha *et al.*, 2007
	Stress response, Hypothalamic gene expression	Kodomari *et al.*, 2009a
Brain-derived neurotrophic factor (BDNF)	ND	Kodomari *et al.*, 2009b
From fetus to mother	**Effects on mother**	
Oxytocin	Induce myocardial contraction of uterus	Malek *et al.*, 1996; Schriefer *et al.*, 1982

ND: not described in the listed reference

adult offspring exhibited suppression of exploratory behavior similar to that of acute stressed mice in the open field test. Basal corticotropin-releasing hormone plasma levels were greater in offspring from ghrelin-treated dams, and did not change in response to acute restraint stress. Reduced *Ghsr* and neuropeptide Y mRNA expression was observed in the hypothalamus of adult offspring. In addition, under physiological conditions, increased maternal ghrelin plasma levels occurring because of repeated restraint stress to the dam caused an increase in fetal plasma acyl ghrelin levels (Kodomari *et al.*, 2009a).

Brain-derived neurotrophic factor

Brain-derived neurotrophic factor (Bdnf), a neurotrophin, is a critical regulator of neural development (Lewin and Barde, 1996). Kodomari *et al.* (2009b) demonstrated the placental permeability of Bdnf using homozygous Bdnf gene-null ($Bdnf^{-/-}$) fetuses (Conover *et al.*, 1995) crossed between heterozygous ($Bdnf^{+/-}$) mice that produce the Bdnf protein. In the brain of $Bdnf^{-/-}$ fetuses at embryonic day (E) 13.5–14.5, Bdnf protein was detected at levels comparable to those in wild-type fetuses, although Bdnf mRNA was not expressed. After E 17.5, Bdnf protein in $Bdnf^{-/-}$ fetal brain was still detectable but its levels were significantly decreased below those in wild-type brain. In addition, when recombinant Bdnf protein was injected into pregnant dams carrying E 14.5 embryos, Bdnf protein levels in fetal brains were increased in a dose-dependent manner. These results suggest that maternal Bdnf reaches the fetal brain across the utero–placental barrier and might contribute to fetal development (Kodomari *et al.*, 2009b).

Transportation via maternal milk

Maternal milk supplies various bioactive substances to the pups, including growth factors and hormones for normal development and immunoglobulin to protect against infection. The major nutrients also have specific biological activities, even the digested small peptides in milk. Because it is difficult to obtain sufficient volumes for analysis from rodents, most studies have been performed using human or bovine milk. Some of the bioactive substances in maternal milk are summarized in Table 3.3.

TABLE 3.3 Bioactive substances in maternal milk

Bioactive substances	References
Peptides/Hormones	
Corticosterone	Yeh, 1984
Ghrelin	Aydin *et al.*, 2006
Leptin	Woliński and Zabielski, 2005
β-Endorphin	Zanardo *et al.*, 2001
TGF-β1	Letterio *et al.*, 1994
Digested milk proteins	
β-Lactotensin	Yamauchi *et al.*, 2003a,b
Casoxin C	Takahashi *et al.*, 1997
β-Casomorphin	Sakaguchi *et al.*, 2003, 2006

β-Lactotensin

Recently the four-residue bioactive peptide β-lactotensin (β-LT; His-Ile-Arg-Leu) was isolated from a chymotrypsin digest of bovine β-lactoglobulin (Yamauchi *et al.*, 2003a). β-Lactoglobulin is the major whey protein of cow's milk and is present in many other mammalian species. Oral administration of β-LT reduces serum cholesterol in mice fed a high cholesterol diet (Yamauchi *et al.*, 2003b). Interestingly, improvement of hypercholesterolemia was mediated via the neurotensin receptor subtype 2, which is expressed abundantly in astrocytes (Kamichi *et al.*, 2005).

CONCLUDING REMARKS AND FUTURE DIRECTIONS

This chapter described recent investigations that demonstrate the influence of bio-communication between a mother and her offspring. During the early development of the fetus and neonate, peripheral organs as well as the nervous system are sensitive to the environment or bioactive substances. Certain maternal bioactive substances influence peripheral organs (Table 3.2). Moreover, neurons are neither the sole target nor the sole effector cells of bio-communication. To understand the molecular basis of bio-communication, influences on all parts of the body, including the vascular system and the neural network including glial cells, should be considered.

In this research field, many animal studies have used rodent models. Although rodent models are beneficial in many ways, there are anatomical differences between rodents and humans. The laboratory mouse and laboratory rat have three layers of trophoblast between the maternal blood space and fetal vessels, whereas humans have only one layer (Enders, 1965). Therefore, the permeability of bioactive substances through the trophoblast in the placenta might differ between rodents and humans. Furthermore, the social environment, including maternal behavior, is quite different between human society and rodent models. Further studies with non-human primate models are required.

Elucidating the molecular basis of bio-communication will improve our understanding of neural development. Moreover, further studies will reveal whether defects in bio-communication increase the risk of psychiatric and neurodegenerative disorders, and whether prophylactically improving bio-communication can reduce this risk.

REFERENCES

Ahima RS, Prabakaran D, Flier JS (1998) Postnatal leptin surge and regulation of circadian rhythm of leptin by feeding. Implications for energy homeostasis and neuroendocrine function. *J Clin Invest* **101:** 1020–7.

Amir RE, Van den Veyver IB, Wan M, Tran CQ, Francke U, Zoghbi HY (1999) Rett syndrome is caused by mutations in X-linked MECP2, encoding methyl-CpG-binding protein 2. *Nat Genet* **23:** 185–8.

Aydin S, Ozkan Y, Kumru S (2006) Ghrelin is present in human colostrum, transitional and mature milk. *Peptides* **27:** 878–82.

Barker DJ (1997) Maternal nutrition, fetal nutrition, and disease in later life. *Nutrition* **13:** 807–13.

Benaroya-Milshtein N, Hollander N, Apter A, Kukulansky T, Raz N, Wilf A, Yaniv I, Pick CG (2004) Environmental enrichment in mice decreases anxiety, attenuates stress responses and enhances natural killer cell activity. *Eur J Neurosci* **20:** 1341–7.

Bick-Sander A, Steiner B, Wolf SA, Babu H, Kempermann G (2006) Running in pregnancy transiently increases postnatal hippocampal neurogenesis in the offspring. *Proc Natl Acad Sci USA* **103:** 3852–7.

Brown J, Cooper-Kuhn CM, Kempermann G, Van Praag H, Winkler J, Gage FH, Kuhn HG (2003) Enriched environment and physical activity stimulate hippocampal but not olfactory bulb neurogenesis. *Eur J Neurosci* **17:** 2042–6.

Brunton PJ, Russell JA (2010) Prenatal social stress in the rat programmes neuroendocrine and behavioural responses to stress in the adult offspring: sex specific effects. *J Neuroendocrinol* **22:** 258–71.

Chang GQ, Gaysinskaya V, Karatayev O, Leibowitz SF (2008) Maternal high-fat diet and fetal programming: increased proliferation of hypothalamic peptide-producing neurons that increase risk for overeating and obesity. *J Neurosci* **28:** 12107–19.

Cherian SB, Bairy KL, Rao MS (2009) Chronic prenatal restraint stress induced memory impairment in passive avoidance task in post weaned male and female Wistar rats. *Indian J Exp Biol* **47:** 893–9.

Conover JC, Erickson JT, Katz DM, Bianchi LM, Poueymirou WT, McClain J, Pan L, Helgren M, Ip NY, Boland P, et al. (1995) Neuronal deficits, not involving motor neurons, in mice lacking BDNF and/or NT4. *Nature* **375:** 235–8.

Côté F, Fligny C, Bayard E, Launay JM, Gershon MD, Mallet J, Vodjdani G (2007) Maternal serotonin is crucial for murine embryonic development. *Proc Natl Acad Sci USA* **104:** 329–34.

Dahl LB, Kaaresen PI, Tunby J, Handegard BH, Kvernmo S, Ronning JA (2006) Emotional, behavioral, social, and academic outcomes in adolescents born with very low birth weight. *Pediatrics* **118:** e449–59.

Daniels WM, Fairbairn LR, van Tilburg G, McEvoy CR, Zigmond MJ, Russell VA, Stein DJ (2009) Maternal separation alters nerve growth factor and corticosterone levels but not the DNA methylation status of the exon 1(7) glucocorticoid receptor promoter region. *Metab Brain Dis* **24:** 615–27.

Enders AC (1965) A comparative study of the fine structure of the trophoblast in several hemochorial placentas. *Am J Anat* **116:** 29–67.

Férézou-Viala J, Roy AF, Serougne C, Gripois D, Parquet M, Bailleux V, Gertler A, Delplanque B, Djiane J, Riottot M, Taouis M (2007) Long-term consequences of maternal high-fat feeding on hypothalamic leptin sensitivity and diet-induced obesity in the offspring. *Am J Physiol Regul Integr Comp Physiol* **293:** R1056–62.

Fligny C, Fromes Y, Bonnin P, Darmon M, Bayard E, Launay JM, Cote F, Mallet J, Vodjdani G (2008) Maternal serotonin influences cardiac function in adult offspring. *FASEB J* **22:** 2340–9.

Gao X, Smith GM, Chen J (2009) Impaired dendritic development and synaptic formation of postnatal-born dentate gyrus granular neurons in the absence of brain-derived neurotrophic factor signaling. *Exp Neurol* **215:** 178–90.

Griffin WC, 3rd, Skinner HD, Salm AK, Birkle DL (2003) Mild prenatal stress in rats is associated with enhanced conditioned fear. *Physiol Behav* **79:** 209–15.

Hattori S, Hashimoto R, Miyakawa T, Yamanaka H, Maeno H, Wada K, Kunugi H (2007) Enriched environments influence depression-related behavior in adult mice and the survival of newborn cells in their hippocampi. *Behav Brain Res* **180:** 69–76.

Hedley AA, Ogden CL, Johnson CL, Carroll MD, Curtin LR, Flegal KM (2004) Prevalence of overweight and obesity among US children, adolescents, and adults, 1999–2002. *J Am Med Assoc* **291:** 2847–50.

Hill JM, McCune SK, Alvero RJ, Glazner GW, Henins KA, Stanziale SF, Keimowitz JR, Brenneman DE (1996) Maternal vasoactive intestinal peptide and the regulation of embryonic growth in the rodent. *J Clin Invest* **97:** 202–8.

Hincz P, Borowski D, Krekora M, Podciechowski L, Horzelski W, Wilczynski J (2009) Maternal obesity as a perinatal risk factor. *Ginekol Pol* **80:** 334–7.

Jones HN, Woollett LA, Barbour N, Prasad PD, Powell TL, Jansson T (2009) High-fat diet before and during pregnancy causes marked up-regulation of placental nutrient transport and fetal overgrowth in C57/BL6 mice. *FASEB J* **23:** 271–8.

Kamichi S, Wada E, Aoki S, Sekiguchi M, Kimura I, Wada K (2005) Immunohistochemical localization of gastrin-releasing peptide receptor in the mouse brain. *Brain Res* **1032:** 162–70.

Kikusui T, Ichikawa S, Mori Y (2009) Maternal deprivation by early weaning increases corticosterone and decreases hippocampal BDNF and neurogenesis in mice. *Psychoneuroendocrinology* **34:** 762–72.

Kim H, Lee SH, Kim SS, Yoo JH, Kim CJ (2007) The influence of maternal treadmill running during pregnancy on short-term memory and hippocampal cell survival in rat pups. *Int J Dev Neurosci* **25:** 243–9.

Kiyono S, Seo ML, Shibagaki M, Inouye M (1985) Facilitative effects of maternal environmental enrichment on maze learning in rat offspring. *Physiol Behav* **34:** 431–5.

Kodomari I, Maruoka T, Yamauchi R, Wada E, Wada K (2009a) Ghrelin alters postnatal endocrine secretion and behavior in mouse offspring. *Neurochem Int* **54:** 222–8.

Kodomari I, Wada E, Nakamura S, Wada K (2009b) Maternal supply of BDNF to mouse fetal brain through the placenta. *Neurochem Int* **54:** 95–8.

Kojima M, Hosoda H, Date Y, Nakazato M, Matsuo H, Kangawa K (1999) Ghrelin is a growth-hormone-releasing acylated peptide from stomach. *Nature* **402:** 656–60.

Kumon M, Yamamoto K, Takahashi A, Wada K, Wada E (2010) Maternal dietary restriction during lactation influences postnatal growth and behavior in the offspring of mice. *Neurochem Int* **57:** 235–47.

Langley-Evans SC, Phillips GJ, Jackson AA (1994) *In utero* exposure to maternal low protein diets induces hypertension in weanling rats, independently of maternal blood pressure changes. *Clin Nutr* **13:** 319–24.

Le Clair C, Abbi T, Sandhu H, Tappia PS (2009) Impact of maternal undernutrition on diabetes and cardiovascular disease risk in adult offspring. *Can J Physiol Pharmacol* **87:** 161–79.

Leal-Galicia P, Saldivar-Gonzalez A, Morimoto S, Arias C (2007) Exposure to environmental enrichment elicits differential hippocampal cell proliferation: role of individual responsiveness to anxiety. *Dev Neurobiol* **67:** 395–405.

Lee HH, Kim H, Lee JW, Kim YS, Yang HY, Chang HK, Lee TH, Shin MC, Lee MH, Shin MS, Park S, Baek S, Kim CJ (2006) Maternal swimming during pregnancy enhances short-term memory and neurogenesis in the hippocampus of rat pups. *Brain Dev* **28:** 147–54.

Letterio JJ, Geiser AG, Kulkarni AB, Roche NS, Sporn MB, Roberts AB (1994) Maternal rescue of transforming growth factor-beta 1 null mice. *Science* **264:** 1936–8.

Lewin GR, Barde YA (1996) Physiology of the neurotrophins. *Annu Rev Neurosci* **19:** 289–317.

Liu D, Diorio J, Day JC, Francis DD, Meaney MJ (2000) Maternal care, hippocampal synaptogenesis and cognitive development in rats. *Nat Neurosci* **3:** 799–806.

Liu D, Diorio J, Tannenbaum B, Caldji C, Francis D, Freedman A, Sharma S, Pearson D, Plotsky PM, Meaney MJ (1997) Maternal care, hippocampal glucocorticoid receptors, and hypothalamic–pituitary–adrenal responses to stress. *Science* **277:** 1659–62.

Lumey LH (1998) Reproductive outcomes in women prenatally exposed to undernutrition: a review of findings from the Dutch famine birth cohort. *Proc Nutr Soc* **57:** 129–35.

Malek A, Blann E, Mattison DR (1996) Human placental transport of oxytocin. *J Matern Fetal Med* **5:** 245–55.

Maruoka T, Kodomari I, Yamauchi R, Wada E, Wada K (2009) Maternal enrichment affects prenatal hippocampal proliferation and open-field behaviors in female offspring mice. *Neurosci Lett* **454:** 28–32.

Montano MM, Wang MH, vom Saal FS (1993) Sex differences in plasma corticosterone in mouse fetuses are mediated by differential placental transport from the mother and eliminated by maternal adrenalectomy or stress. *J Reprod Fertil* **99:** 283–90.

Nakahara K, Nakagawa M, Baba Y, Sato M, Toshinai K, Date Y, Nakazato M, Kojima M, Miyazato M, Kaiya H, Hosoda H, Kangawa K, Murakami N (2006) Maternal ghrelin plays an important role in rat fetal development during pregnancy. *Endocrinology* **147:** 1333–42.

Parnpiansil P, Jutapakdeegul N, Chentanez T, Kotchabhakdi N (2003) Exercise during pregnancy increases hippocampal brain-derived neurotrophic factor mRNA expression and spatial learning in neonatal rat pup. *Neurosci Lett* **352:** 45–8.

Petrosini L, De Bartolo P, Foti F, Gelfo F, Cutuli D, Leggio MG, Mandolesi L (2009) On whether the environmental enrichment may provide cognitive and brain reserves. *Brain Res Rev* **61:** 221–39.

Popliker M, Shatz A, Avivi A, Ullrich A, Schlessinger J, Webb CG (1987) Onset of endogenous synthesis of epidermal growth factor in neonatal mice. *Dev Biol* **119:** 38–44.

Sakaguchi M, Koseki M, Wakamatsu M, Matsumura E (2006) Effects of systemic administration of beta-casomorphin-5 on learning and memory in mice. *Eur J Pharmacol* **530:** 81–7.

Sakaguchi M, Murayama K, Jinsmaa Y, Yoshikawa M, Matsumura E (2003) Neurite outgrowth-stimulating activities of beta-casomorphins in Neuro-2a mouse neuroblastoma cells. *Biosci Biotechnol Biochem* **67:** 2541–7.

Sale A, Cenni MC, Ciucci F, Putignano E, Chierzi S, Maffei L (2007) Maternal enrichment during pregnancy accelerates retinal development of the fetus. *PLoS One* 2: e1160.

Schriefer JA, Lewis PR, Miller JW (1982) Role of fetal oxytocin in parturition in the rat. *Biol Reprod* **27:** 362–8.

Simonson M, Stephan JK, Hanson HM, Chow BF (1971) Open field studies in offspring of underfed mother rats. *J Nutr* **101:** 331–5.

Spong CY, Lee SJ, McCune SK, Gibney G, Abebe DT, Alvero R, Brenneman DE, Hill JM (1999) Maternal regulation of embryonic growth: the role of vasoactive intestinal peptide. *Endocrinology* **140:** 917–24.

Srinivasan M, Katewa SD, Palaniyappan A, Pandya JD, Patel MS (2006) Maternal high-fat diet consumption results in fetal malprogramming predisposing to the onset of metabolic syndrome-like phenotype in adulthood. *Am J Physiol Endocrinol Metab* E792–9.

Takahashi M, Moriguchi S, Suganuma H, Shiota A, Tani F, Usui H, Kurahashi K, Sasaki R, Yoshikawa M (1997) Identification of casoxin C, an ileum-contracting peptide derived from bovine kappa-casein, as an agonist for C3a receptors. *Peptides* **18:** 329–36.

Taliaz D, Stall N, Dar DE, Zangen A (2010) Knockdown of brain-derived neurotrophic factor in specific brain sites precipitates behaviors associated with depression and reduces neurogenesis. *Mol Psychiatry* **15:** 80–92.

Tozuka Y, Kumon M, Wada E, Onodera M, Mochizuki H, Wada K (2010) Diet-induced maternal obesity decreases hippocampal BDNF production and impairs spatial learning performance in young mouse offspring. *Neurochem Intl*. Submitted.

Tozuka Y, Wada E, Wada K (2009a) "Bio-communication" between mother and offspring: lessons from animals and new perspectives for brain science. *J Pharmacol Sci* **110:** 127–32.

Tozuka Y, Wada E, Wada K (2009b) Diet-induced obesity in female mice leads to peroxidized lipid accumulations and impairment of hippocampal neurogenesis during the early life of their offspring. *FASEB J* **23:** 1920–34.

Tyzio R, Cossart R, Khalilov I, Minlebaev M, Hubner CA, Represa A, Ben-Ari Y, Khazipov R (2006) Maternal oxytocin triggers a transient inhibitory switch in GABA signaling in the fetal brain during delivery. *Science* **314:** 1788–92.

Urdinguio RG, Sanchez-Mut JV, Esteller M (2009) Epigenetic mechanisms in neurological diseases: genes, syndromes, and therapies. *Lancet Neurol* **8:** 1056–72.

Van den Hove DL, Steinbusch HW, Scheepens A, Van de Berg WD, Kooiman LA, Boosten BJ, Prickaerts J, Blanco CE (2006) Prenatal stress and neonatal rat brain development. *Neuroscience* **137:** 145–55.

Vieau D, Sebaai N, Leonhardt M, Dutriez-Casteloot I, Molendi-Coste O, Laborie C, Breton C, Deloof S, Lesage J (2007) HPA axis programming by maternal undernutrition in the male rat offspring. *Psychoneuroendocrinology* 32 **Suppl 1:** S16–20.

Weaver IC, Cervoni N, Champagne FA, D'Alessio AC, Sharma S, Seckl JR, Dymov S, Szyf M, Meaney MJ (2004) Epigenetic programming by maternal behavior. *Nat Neurosci* **7:** 847–54.

Weaver IC, Meaney MJ, Szyf M (2006) Maternal care effects on the hippocampal transcriptome and anxiety-mediated behaviors in the offspring that are reversible in adulthood. *Proc Natl Acad Sci USA* **103:** 3480–5.

Welberg L, Thrivikraman KV, Plotsky PM (2006) Combined pre- and postnatal environmental enrichment programs the HPA axis differentially in male and female rats. *Psychoneuroendocrinology* **31:** 553–64.

Woli ski J, Zabielski R (2005) Presence of leptin in mammalian colostrum and milk and in artificial milk formulas. *Med Wieku Rozwoj* **9:** 629–36.

Woodall SM, Breier BH, Johnston BM, Gluckman PD (1996) A model of intrauterine growth retardation caused by chronic maternal undernutrition in the rat: effects on the somatotrophic axis and postnatal growth. *J Endocrinol* **150:** 231–42.

Wu G, Bazer FW, Cudd TA, Meininger CJ, Spencer TE (2004) Maternal nutrition and fetal development. *J Nutr* **134:** 2169–72.

Yamauchi R, Ohinata K, Yoshikawa M (2003b) Beta-lactotensin and neurotensin rapidly reduce serum cholesterol via NT2 receptor. *Peptides* **24:** 1955–61.

Yamauchi R, Usui H, Yunden J, Takenaka Y, Tani F, Yoshikawa M (2003a) Characterization of beta-lactotensin, a bioactive peptide derived from bovine beta-lactoglobulin, as a neurotensin agonist. *Biosci Biotechnol Biochem* **67:** 940–3.

Yeh J, Shelton JA (2005) Increasing prepregnancy body mass index: analysis of trends and contributing variables. *Am J Obstet Gynecol* **193:** 1994–8.

Yeh KY (1984) Corticosterone concentrations in the serum and milk of lactating rats: parallel changes after induced stress. *Endocrinology* **115:** 1364–70.

Yura S, Itoh H, Sagawa N, Yamamoto H, Masuzaki H, Nakao K, Kawamura M, Takemura M, Kakui K, Ogawa Y, Fujii S (2005) Role of premature leptin surge in obesity resulting from intrauterine undernutrition. *Cell Metab* **1:** 371–8.

Yuzuriha H, Inui A, Asakawa A, Ueno N, Kasuga M, Meguid MM, Miyazaki J, Ninomiya M, Herzog H, Fujimiya M (2007) Gastrointestinal hormones (anorexigenic peptide YY and orexigenic ghrelin) influence neural tube development. *FASEB J* **21:** 2108–12.

Zambrano E, Bautista CJ, Deas M, Martinez-Samayoa PM, Gonzalez-Zamorano M, Ledesma H, Morales J, Larrea F, Nathanielsz PW (2006) A low maternal protein diet during pregnancy and lactation has sex- and window of exposure-specific effects on offspring growth and food intake, glucose metabolism and serum leptin in the rat. *J Physiol* **571:** 221–30.

Zanardo V, Nicolussi S, Carlo G, Marzari F, Faggian D, Favaro F, Plebani M (2001) Beta endorphin concentrations in human milk. *J Pediatr Gastroenterol Nutr* **33:** 160–4.

Zarrow MX, Philpott JE, Denenberg VH (1970) Passage of 14C-4-corticosterone from the rat mother to the fetus and neonate. *Nature* **226:** 1058–9.

C H A P T E R

4

Pharmacokinetics in pregnancy

Gregory J. Anger, Maged M. Costantine and Micheline Piquette-Miller

INTRODUCTION

Prescription and over-the-counter (OTC) drug use during pregnancy is necessary for many women. A study of approximately 20,000 US and Canadian women found that the average participant used 2.3 drugs during the course of their pregnancy and 28% of participants used four or more (Mitchell *et al.*, 2001). For some, this is because women often enter into pregnancy with pre-existing medical conditions that require ongoing or intermittent pharmacotherapy such as asthma, hypertension, epilepsy, HIV infection and various psychiatric disorders. For others, this is because the state of pregnancy itself can give rise to new medical conditions such as nausea and vomiting and gestational diabetes. The principal concern of prescribing physicians is often whether or not pharmacologic agents will cause harm to the fetus (i.e., teratogenic effects). This concern rose to prominence primarily as a result of the thalidomide disaster. Marketed for use in morning sickness, the drug thalidomide was found to be a potent teratogen capable of producing a variety of birth defects relating to development (McBride, 1961). In line with the clinical focus, determining the teratogenicity of new drugs dominates the objectives of pregnancy-relevant experiments conducted throughout drug development. This comes at the expense of valuable pharmacokinetic (PK) studies, which are seldom performed premarketing. Physicians lacking adequate PK information typically prescribe the standard adult dose in pregnancy but this can be, as is the case with other special patient populations, either inadequate or excessive depending on a variety of factors. When inadequate, both mother and fetus may experience increased morbidity while unnecessarily exposing the fetus to drug(s). The purpose of this chapter is to provide a general overview of some of the factors that affect pharmacokinetics in pregnancy. The issues surrounding the way PK information is obtained in pregnancy are also discussed.

FACTORS AFFECTING PHARMACOKINETICS IN PREGNANCY

Pharmacokinetic information describes how a drug is absorbed, distributed, metabolized and eliminated by the body and how these processes impact plasma drug concentrations. Sex differences in various PK parameters have been consistently demonstrated since the 1930s (Curry, 2001; Czerniak, 2001). It is, therefore, not surprising that differences also exist between pregnant and non-pregnant women. A wide array of physiological and hormonal change occurs during pregnancy; most begins early in the first trimester and increases linearly until the end of the third trimester/parturition (Dawes and Chowienczyk, 2001).

Absorption

The rise in progesterone that accompanies pregnancy delays gastric emptying and small intestine motility by approximately 30–50% with corresponding alterations to bioavailability parameters like maximum concentration (C_{max}) and time to maximum concentration (T_{max}) (Parry *et al.*, 1970). These effects would likely be most pronounced in the third trimester when progesterone levels are at their peak (Dawood, 1976). While decreased C_{max} and T_{max} is less of a concern with repeated dosing regimens, alterations in these parameters could impact the efficacy of oral drugs that are taken as a single dose, such as analgesic and anti-emetic drugs, because a rapid onset of action is typically desired (Dawes and Chowienczyk, 2001).

Maternal disease as well as the action(s) of some drugs may further affect absorption. Nausea and vomiting of pregnancy (NVP) decreases absorption and results in lower plasma drug concentrations. For this reason, patients with NVP are routinely advised to take their medications when nausea is minimal (i.e., during the evening hours). Also, opioid use during labor more or less arrests gastrointestinal motility (Clements *et al.*, 1978). This delays small intestine absorption of drugs taken during labor and can lead to greatly elevated plasma drug levels postpartum. Gastrointestinal motility remains delayed during the immediate postpartum period. Finally, iron and other metal supplements as well as antacids may compound changes to absorption in pregnancy by chelating co-administered drugs, which decreases their absorption (Garnett *et al.*, 1980; Carter *et al.*, 1981).

Outside of C_{max} and T_{max} alterations, few studies have documented clinically meaningful changes in drug absorption during pregnancy.

Reproductive and Developmental Toxicology, Edited by Ramesh C. Gupta
ISBN: 978-0-12-382032-7

Distribution

During pregnancy, there is an increase in total body weight (Table 4.1). Much of this body weight increase is due to a 6–8 L increase in the volume of water found in intravascular (i.e., plasma) and extravascular (i.e., tissues such as the breasts, fetus, placenta and amniotic fluid) compartments (Reynolds, 1998; Dawes and Chowienczyk, 2001). Increased water within the body creates a larger volume of distribution (V_d) for drugs that are hydrophilic. In addition, an increase in body fat means that there is also a larger V_d for lipophilic drugs. For some drugs, a larger V_d could necessitate a higher initial and maintenance dose to obtain therapeutic plasma concentrations.

During pregnancy, there is also a decrease in the concentration of several plasma proteins with the capacity to bind drugs because the above-mentioned increase in intravascular water results in hemodilution. The majority of drugs used clinically bind to plasma proteins to some degree so that the total plasma drug concentration can be divided into a fraction that is bound and therefore inactive and a fraction that is free and therefore active. To become clinically relevant, changes in plasma protein binding of highly protein bound drugs need not be extreme. To put things into perspective, if a drug is 99% bound to albumin in non-pregnant patients but 98% bound to albumin in pregnant patients then the active fraction of the drug in pregnancy is effectively double.

The most clinically relevant plasma protein decrease occurs with albumin, which transitions from an average concentration of 42 g/L in non-pregnant women to 36 g/L by the second trimester (Frederiksen, 2001). Digoxin, midazolam, phenytoin and a multitude of other acidic drugs that are utilized during pregnancy are primarily bound to albumin. While most plasma proteins exhibit decreased concentrations during pregnancy, there are exceptions. For example, in response to elevated estrogen, plasma thyroxine-binding globulin increases during pregnancy (Glinoer, 1997). For women on levothyroxine (LT4) for hypothyroidism, upward dosage adjustments are required to compensate for the decrease in free T4 created by increased thyroxine-binding globulin (Mandel *et al.*, 1990).

Metabolism

Drug metabolism is another PK parameter that is altered in pregnancy and these alterations are highly linked, as was the case with absorption, to elevated sex hormones. In general, drug metabolism occurs through phase I metabolism, which involves oxidation, reduction or hydrolysis, and/or phase II metabolism, which involves conjugation of polar bodies (e.g., glucuronidation, acetylation, methylation and sulfation). Both types of metabolic processes play an important role in altering drugs so that they obtain a polarity that is conducive to excretion. Phase I and phase II metabolism have also been found to exhibit a mixture of increased and decreased activity during pregnancy. With regards to phase I, the family of oxidative liver enzymes known as cytochrome P450 (CYP450) enzymes represents a major route of drug metabolism for many drugs. In particular, CYP3A4 has been found to exhibit a broad substrate specificity that includes many drugs used in pregnant women. Nifedipine, carbamazepine, midazolam and the anti-retroviral drugs saquinavir, indinavir, lopinavir and ritonavir are examples of CYP3A4 substrates (Schwartz, 2003; Mattison and Zajicek, 2006). Both the activity and abundance of CYP3A4 is increased in pregnancy and corresponding increases in the clearance of its substrates have been demonstrated (Little, 1999). In the case of anti-retroviral drugs, failure to maintain therapeutic plasma concentrations during pregnancy not only has a negative impact on the mother's health (i.e., increased viral load and resistance formation) but also increases the chances of vertical HIV transmission. Levels of CYP2D6 also increase in the majority of pregnant women and there is a corresponding increase in the metabolism of substrates like dextromethorphan and the antidepressants fluoxetine and nortriptyline (Wadelius *et al.*, 1997; Tracy *et al.*, 2005). In addition to metabolizing drugs to promote clearance, CYP2D6 plays an important role in the metabolism of several opioid analgesics, such as codeine, hydrocodone, oxycodone and tramadol, to their active chemical forms. Frequently used for the management of maternal pain, some pregnant patients may require a lower dose of these drugs to prevent active metabolite toxicities. Dosage adjustments would be particularly likely in pregnant patients who exhibit the "ultrarapid metabolizer" or "extensive metabolizer" CYP2D6 phenotype.

With regards to phase II metabolism, the activities of important conjugating enzymes, such as uridine 5′-diphospho-glucuronosyltransferase (UGT) 1A4, are altered during pregnancy. Oral clearance of the UGT1A4 substrate lamotrigine significantly increases in pregnancy (Pennell, 2003; de Haan *et al.*, 2004). Alterations in phase II enzymes may also work in concert with alterations in phase I enzymes to produce atypical effects. An example of this is the decreased clearance of caffeine observed in pregnancy that is the result, in part, of a decrease in the activity of its metabolizers: CYP1A2 (phase I) and N-acetyltransferase 2 (phase II) (Tsutsumi *et al.*, 2001). Metabolism through either phase I or phase II enzymes in pregnancy may be further enhanced by a rise in hepatic blood flow, occurring in the third trimester, which serves to increase the amount of drug available to the liver for metabolism (Nakai *et al.*, 2002).

TABLE 4.1 Weight gain in pregnancy

Tissue or fluid	10 weeks (g)	20 weeks (g)	30 weeks (g)	40 weeks (g)
Fetus	5	300	1,500	3,400
Placenta	20	170	300	650
Amniotic fluid	30	350	750	800
Uterus	140	320	600	970
Breasts	45	180	360	405
Blood	100	600	1,300	1,450
Extravascular fluid	0	30	80	1,480
Maternal fat stores	310	2,050	3,480	3,345
Total	650	4,000	8,500	12,500

Adapted from Cunningham *et al.*, 2001.

Renal excretion

Drug elimination also changes during pregnancy due to a significant increase in renal excretion. During pregnancy, there is an increase in the flow of blood to various organs including a 50–80% increase in effective renal plasma flow which results in a corresponding 40–65% increase in the glomerular filtration rate (Conrad, 2004). This increase in renal clearance can have notable effects on drugs that are eliminated by the kidneys. Increases in elimination rates that range from 20 to 60% have been reported for ampicillin, cefuroxime, cephradine, cefazolin, piperacillin, atenalol, digoxin, lithium and many others (reviewed in Anderson, 2005).

THE FETAL COMPARTMENT

A discussion of PK in pregnancy would be incomplete without some mention of the fetal compartment. Comprised of the placenta, fetus and amniotic fluid, the fetal compartment represents a space into which drug may distribute that, for obvious reasons, is unique to the pregnant state. Drugs that easily cross the placenta to enter the fetal compartment are generally small (less than 500 daltons), non-ionized and unbound to plasma protein. They also tend not to be substrates for the myriad of drug efflux transporters present in the placenta's apical membrane (reviewed in Syme *et al.*, 2004). While some drugs are much more extensively distributed to the fetus than others, it is generally acknowledged that the fetal compartment will be exposed to all drugs that are consumed by the mother during pregnancy. The fetal compartment is not passive in its handling of drugs as they are often subject to metabolism by placental and fetal tissues and/or concentrated within this compartment.

Drug metabolism within the fetal compartment

It has been established that drugs may be subject to metabolism by placental and fetal tissues. In the placenta, the presence and activity of a variety of CYP450 and UGT enzymes has been documented. CYP1A1, 1B1, 2E1, 2F1, 3A4, 3A5, 3A7 and 4B1 mRNA and/or protein have been detected, in a variety of studies, in both first trimester and term human placenta (summarized in Syme *et al.*, 2004). UGT2B4, 2B7, 2B10, 2B11 and 2B15 have also been detected in both first trimester and term human placenta while UGT1A isoforms have been detected only in the former (Collier *et al.*, 2002a,b). In terms of UGT activity, Collier *et al.* demonstrated that the clearance of 4-methylumbelliferone, a "non-specific" UGT substrate, by placental microsomes, derived from 25 placentas, ranged from 7.5 to 43% of female human liver values (Collier *et al.*, 2002a). Metabolism may also occur within the fetal liver. In the fetus, the presence and activity of CYP450 and UGT enzymes have been documented but levels are considerably lower than those found in pregnant women. One of the dominant CYP450 isoforms within the fetal liver is CYP3A7. In comparison to CYP3A4, which is the dominant CYP3A isoform in adults, CYP3A7 exhibits significantly reduced metabolic capabilities (Williams *et al.*, 2002). The clinical significance of drug metabolism in placental and fetal tissues has not yet been determined. At present, it is believed to have a minimal impact on the pharmacokinetic parameters of the mother. For example, in a study of zidovudine metabolism in pregnant baboons, Garland and colleagues estimated that placental and fetal clearance (mL/min) was approximately 5% and 15% of the maternal clearance rate, respectively (Garland *et al.*, 1998).

Drug accumulation within the fetal compartment

It is possible for drugs to accumulate within the fetal compartment because the ionization and protein binding capacities of the fetal compartment differ from that of the maternal central compartment. As mentioned, non-ionized drugs cross into the fetal compartment much more easily than ionized drugs; however, the fetal circulation is normally 0.1 to 0.15 pH points lower than the maternal circulation and drugs may, therefore, be ionized after crossing. Drugs that become ionized after crossing could accumulate within the fetal compartment as their ionization state would now disfavor passive diffusion across the placenta (Figure 4.1A). This effect, called ion trapping, would be most pronounced in cases of fetal acidosis, a condition that is associated with fetal hypoxia (Brown *et al.*, 1976; Kennedy *et al.*, 1979; Pickering *et al.*, 1981). Similar to ion trapping, accumulation within the fetal compartment can occur when the tissue or plasma protein-binding capacity is higher in the fetus than in the mother (Figure 4.1B).

MATERNAL DISEASE AND OBSTETRICAL COMPLICATIONS

Studies in non-pregnant participants have clearly demonstrated that disease can have clinically significant effects on PK. For example, in the late 1970s and early 1980s, decreased theophylline clearance was observed in children with viral infections of the upper respiratory tract and adults after influenza vaccination (Chang *et al.*, 1978; Renton *et al.*, 1980). Subsequent studies linked these findings to the altered expression of drug transporters and CYP450 metabolic enzymes that we now know accompany inflammation (reviewed in Morgan *et al.*, 2008). As previously mentioned, women often enter into pregnancy with pre-existing medical conditions or develop conditions during the course of their pregnancy. Many of these conditions are associated with inflammation, such as diabetes mellitus and chorioamnionitis, and this means that they could potentially compound the PK changes that are associated with pregnancy itself (Rodriguez-Moran and Guerrero-Romero, 1999, 2003; Døllner *et al.*, 2002). Studies with pregnant rats have demonstrated that lipopolysaccharide-induced systemic inflammation can decrease the expression of drug transporters and metabolic enzymes in both the maternal liver and the placenta, with corresponding changes to maternal PK and fetal exposure, but clinical confirmation is currently lacking (Petrovic *et al.*, 2008).

Dysregulation of drug transporters and metabolic enzymes is not the only route by which maternal disease could alter PK. Maternal obesity, despite being associated with systemic inflammation as well, is more likely to contribute to PK variability by increasing the V_d of lipophilic drugs than by promoting the dysregulation of drug transporters and metabolic enzymes. Maternal diabetes mellitus, also associated with systemic inflammation, can induce hyperlipidemia and data from both clinical studies in non-pregnant patients and preclinical studies in pregnant rats suggest that this alters the plasma protein binding of a variety of drugs (Spector *et al.*, 1973; Chauvelot-Moachon *et al.*, 1988; Anger and Piquette-Miller, 2010). As with inflammation's effects, clinical confirmation of maternal obesity and

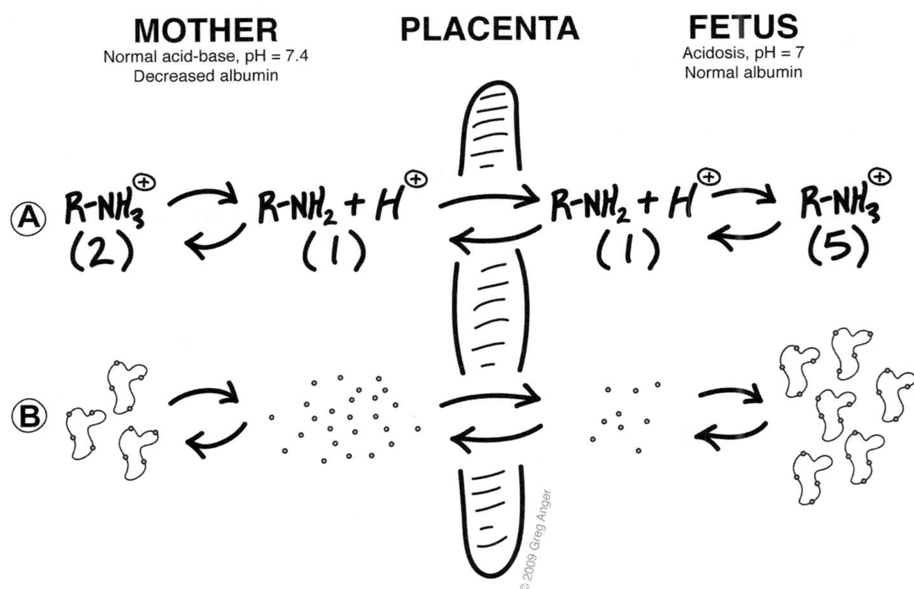

FIGURE 4.1 Mechanisms of drug accumulation within the fetal compartment. Only drug molecules that are non-ionized and unbound to plasma proteins can passively diffuse across the placenta. **A**. The fetal circulation is more acidic than the maternal circulation and, consequently, basic drugs may become ionized after they cross the placenta and circulate in this compartment. In this situation, drugs could accumulate within the fetal compartment because more drug is able to transfer across the placenta from mother to fetus than from fetus to mother. This phenomenon is called ion trapping. **B**. When the concentration of plasma proteins, such as albumin, are higher in the fetus than in the mother, drugs may be retained within the former due to a higher degree of protein binding. In this situation, as with ion trapping, more drug is free to transfer across the placenta from mother to fetus than from fetus to mother. In this figure, $R\text{-}NH_3$ represents a hypothetical basic drug with a pK_A that is approximately 7.7 and the globular "Y" shapes represent plasma proteins.

diabetes-induced hyperlipidemia's effects on PK in pregnancy is currently lacking.

At present, the vast majority of data concerned with the impact of maternal disease on PK in pregnancy is limited to preclinical studies employing animal models of disease. While a complete account of these data is beyond the scope of this chapter, it should be noted that maternal disease probably represents a largely overlooked source of PK variability in pregnancy. As preclinical evidence mounts, for a variety of common maternal diseases, innovative clinical study designs will be required to distinguish PK variability introduced by disease from variability introduced by pregnancy.

The use of tocolytic therapy for the prevention of preterm labor is one area of maternal–fetal medicine where PK information has proven useful in generating hypotheses regarding adverse effects and dosage adjustments. In practice, the use of tocolytics to treat this obstetrical complication should be individualized and based on maternal condition, potential maternal and fetal adverse effects and gestational age (Tan *et al.*, 2006). Indomethacin, a non-selective cyclo-oxygenase enzyme inhibitor that is used to arrest preterm labour, is known to cause fetal vasoconstriction leading to premature closure of the ductus arteriosus, decreased urine production and oligohydramnios. These effects are more pronounced if the drug is used after 32 weeks and are considered reversible if used before 32 weeks of gestation (Gordon and Samuels, 1995; Vermillion and Robinson, 2005). Indomethacin is 90% bound to albumin and crosses the placenta so that the fetal umbilical artery serum concentrations equilibrate with maternal serum levels within 5 hours of dosing. Two hours after dosing, fetal blood levels are 50% of maternal blood levels (Moise *et al.*, 1990). The half-life ($t_{1/2}$) of indomethacin is much longer in the fetal circulation (14.7 hours) than in the maternal circulation (2.2 hours) and this is likely due to the immaturity of fetal hepatic metabolism (Moise *et al.*, 1990; Tsatsaris *et al.*, 2004). These PK properties are believed to play a role in the high rate of fetal adverse effects.

Another class of tocolytics includes the dihydropyridine calcium channel blockers, such as nifedipine. Following oral administration, nifedipine is rapidly and nearly completely (approximately 90%) absorbed from the gastrointestinal tract. Despite this high absorption rate, however, bioavailability is low because first-pass metabolism (the metabolism that occurs in the intestinal walls and liver before a drug reaches systemic circulation) results in 40% of the drug being converted into inactive metabolites by oxidative pathways (Tsatsaris *et al.*, 2004). Additionally, nifedipine clearance increases and C_{max} and $t_{1/2}$ are decreased during pregnancy. Thus, to have the same therapeutic effect in pregnant patients as in non-pregnant patients, the dosage in pregnant patients should be higher and the interval time shorter.

ORIGINS OF THE KNOWLEDGE GAP

The changes to PK parameters during pregnancy that are presented in this chapter should illustrate that PK information is necessary if physicians are to make evidence-based dosage recommendations. A meta-analysis conducted to determine whether pregnancy was associated with alterations to the PK profile of a variety of drugs found that the AUC of 29% of drugs that were examined increased while that of 41% decreased (Little, 1999). This illustrates that alterations in PK parameters do not apply only to a few select drugs but are likely to impact a wide array of drugs that are used in pregnancy.

Drugs are often approved by regulatory agencies on the basis of clinical trials that are devoid of pregnant participants. In the USA, standard reproductive toxicology studies are performed in animals and are used to assign a category in a labeling subsection concerned with birth defects and other effects on reproduction and pregnancy. Instituted by the US FDA in 1979, the information provided by category assignment is generally considered vague and hard to apply (Frederiksen, 2002). On the basis of demonstrated safety and efficacy in the general public and reproductive toxicity studies, physicians typically prescribe drugs to pregnant patients based on their own relative assessment of the risks and benefits. Given that most drugs lack clear, evidence-based dosage adjustment guidelines for pregnancy, physicians tend not to deviate from the standard adult dose even when efficacy is questioned.

The major difficulty in establishing PK information in pregnancy stems from a lack of well-controlled clinical trials as few drugs are specifically targeted for the pregnant population. Often, safety information is first acquired from clinical reports of atypical drug actions in pregnant patients (e.g., poor efficacy, adverse drug reactions, etc.). In most cases, collaborative teams of clinicians and academic scientists will then work to explain the phenomenon in a process that generates invaluable PK data. This process can, however, take too long to generate the kind of information that will aid in creating dosing recommendations. Moreover, the ethics of this are questionable since pregnant women are theoretically required to undergo an atypical drug experience before clinicians are alerted and this process is initiated. Furthermore, this assumes that clinicians will then take the initiative to either inform the scientific community or strike the collaborations required to examine the drug further.

Ethical and legal considerations are among the most commonly cited reasons for excluding pregnant women from clinical trials. Clinical research in Europe and North America has not always been monitored as closely as it is today and examples of unethical conduct are all too abundant. One example is the infamous Tuskegee Syphilis Study conducted by the US Public Health Service from 1932 to 1972. In this study, the effects of tertiary syphilis were monitored in a group of African Americans who were not informed of the purpose of the study and were not encouraged to take penicillin once it was proven to be an effective method of treating the disease in 1945. Examples such as this highlight the fact that it is unethical to conduct clinical research using coercion and deception and without obtaining informed consent. Regulations such as those established by the World Medical Association's *Declaration of Helsinki* in 1964 were born of unethical practices such as these and included specific guidelines for clinical research in vulnerable populations such as children, the mentally disabled, prisoners and pregnant women. In the case of pregnant women, however, the vulnerable entity was the unborn fetus and drug developers and regulatory agencies responded by not only excluding pregnant women but all women of childbearing age. This response was codified in 1977 for women of childbearing age when the FDA formally restricted this group from participation in phase one and two clinical trials (CDER, 1977).

One argument against this standard is that by excluding pregnant mothers from clinical trials, an information gap is created that actually makes prescribing medications much more dangerous for both the mother and the vulnerable fetus. For the mother, an improper dose could be administered, resulting in either poor efficacy when plasma concentrations are too low or possible adverse drug reactions when they are too high. For certain disorders, this can have dire consequences for the mother that directly impacts the fetus. For example, epilepsy is a neurological disorder that requires treatment throughout pregnancy. Failure to properly manage seizures not only results in harm to the mother but also substantially increases the risk of miscarriage. A review of studies published on anticonvulsant use in pregnancy found that 30–50% of epileptic women on anticonvulsants experience an increase in seizure frequency while pregnant (Sawle, 2000). While the sleep disturbances that occur during pregnancy are likely to contribute to this rise, alterations to PK have been linked to the decreased efficacy of anticonvulsant drugs like carbamazepine and phenytoin during pregnancy (Yerby *et al.*, 1990). Evidence-based dosage adjustments for anticonvulsants are now commonly implemented in pregnancy (Pennell, 2003).

The fear of litigation is another factor in the pharmaceutical industry's reluctance to conduct controlled clinical trials in pregnant women for the purposes of obtaining PK data. It is a common legal strategy for those seeking reparations for injuries to target those from which they stand to gain the most. In this case, that means the "deep pockets" of drug developers. Given the preponderance of lawsuits (many of which are class action) that follow most drug-related injuries, it is not surprising that drug developers typically view introducing a drug into pregnant women as risky and avoid doing so whenever possible. It stands to reason, however, that performing studies in the context of a controlled clinical trial and in a relatively small group of pregnant women is less risky than leaving it at the discretion of individual prescribing practices in the general pregnant population. A fear of litigation should not be the sole basis for excluding pregnant women in clinical trials if the appropriate reproductive toxicology studies have been performed and there is no other reason to suspect teratogenicity.

CONCLUDING REMARKS, CURRENT INITIATIVES AND FUTURE DIRECTIONS

A number of steps have been taken in recent years by various regulatory agencies and the scientific community to address this issue. In 1993, the FDA acknowledged the need to begin obtaining more detailed information for drugs that could be taken by pregnant women. This was done first by removing the 1977 restrictions as well as the publication of "Guideline for the Study and Evaluation of Gender Differences in the Clinical Evaluation of Drugs" (FDA, 1993). Shortly thereafter, the FDA established the *Office of Women's Health* and has continued to formalize its new stance by way of inclusions in the *Modernization Act* (FDAMA) of 1997 and several additions to titles 21 and 45 of the US *Code of Federal Regulations* in the late 1990s and early 2000s. Several guidance documents have also been released on topics such as the establishment of pregnancy exposure registries and, of relevance to this discussion, pharmacokinetic studies in pregnancy. In the latter document, guidance is provided for industry on all aspects of clinical trial design in pregnant subjects with topics ranging from appropriate control selection to data analysis. One problem with these initiatives, at least with respect to pregnant women, is that they make inclusion in clinical trials compulsory only for drug candidates that specifically target this demographic or for which there is a high probability that its use in pregnant women will be prevalent. The vast majority of FDA guidance on the issue comes in the form of recommendations. Since delaying the release of a blockbuster drug can translate to lost sales on the order of millions of dollars per day, additional studies to refine dosage recommendations in pregnancy are unlikely to be performed with sufficient frequency premarketing if they are not made compulsory or some form of incentive is provided.

One possible incentive could be the extension of patent privileges in exchange for detailed PK data in pregnancy as is done already for certain drugs in pediatric populations. A variety of medical conditions, ranging from pain to diabetes mellitus, are present in both children and adults yet treated with drugs that are tested in and labeled solely for adult populations. In order to increase the formal study of drugs in pediatric populations, a *Pediatric Exclusivity Provision* was included in the FDAMA. The provision allows for an additional 6 months of exclusive marketing rights to be added to pre-existing patent protection if studies are conducted that determine uses and doses in children (FDA, 2001). This provision provides the necessary incentive required for the pharmaceutical industry to conduct studies of this nature and has resulted in a dramatic increase in the amount of pediatric information included in product labeling. For example, the anti-HIV drug abacavir was tested in children prior to its approval at the request of the FDA. Once approved, dosing information was available that made abacavir an important option for HIV-positive individuals that are 3 months to 12 years of age which is a population with limited therapeutic choices (FDA, 2001). Therefore, a similar provision could be used to increase the availability of PK information for drugs used in pregnancy.

Steps to address this issue would ideally occur premarketing but phase IV clinical trials represent an option that could attract greater participation from drug developers while still increasing the speed at which information becomes available. This option is noted in the FDA guidance document "Guidance for Industry – Pharmacokinetics in Pregnancy – Study Design, Data Analysis, and Impact on Dosing and Labeling". While this document focuses on the inclusion of pregnant women in phase III of development, it states that it anticipates the majority of PK studies in pregnant women will likely occur in the post-marketing period with pregnant women who have already been prescribed the drug as therapy by their own physician (CDER, 2004). Drugs that lack PK data could be flagged for immediate investigation in the first wave of pregnant patients to consume it. As opposed to the current standard of monitoring adverse drug reactions through methods like pregnancy exposure registries, drug developers could initiate PK studies in this population and then compare data to subsequent measurements taken postpartum.

One final step that is being taken to improve our understanding of PK in pregnancy involves the consideration of known alterations to physiology that occur during pregnancy throughout the drug development process. A drug developer's decision to include or exclude pregnant women in trials is then based on models that consider the unique physiology of pregnancy and the properties of the drug in question. For example, it has previously been stated that drugs that are substrates for CYP3A4 and CYP2D6 are metabolized faster during pregnancy. The inclusion of pregnant women in clinical trials for drugs that are substrates of significantly altered CYP450 enzymes should, therefore, be considered when it is reasonable to assume pregnant women would eventually use them. This same approach could be used to predict the likelihood of fetal accumulation and potential teratogenic effects (Gedeon and Koren, 2006). Modeling all of the above-mentioned alterations to absorption, distribution, metabolism and elimination, however, is a highly complex undertaking. Advances in physiologically based pharmacokinetic (PBPK) modeling have been made but the extensive bioinformatics expertise that is required and the fact that the predictive validity of this approach has not yet been demonstrated remain hurdles. The PBPK computer model for human pregnancy by Luecke and colleagues, consisting of 27 maternal compartments and 16 fetal compartments, provides an example of the complexity involved with such modeling (Luecke *et al.*, 1994). Stage of gestation (i.e., early versus late) and maternal disease are difficult to incorporate into these models and both of these variables can have a significant impact on PK in pregnancy for reasons outlined above.

In summary, it is unreasonable to assume that the majority of women will be able to stop the consumption of prescription and OTC drugs for the duration of their pregnancy. Women enter into pregnancy with pre-existing disorders and/or develop disorders that demand pharmacotherapy; however, the efficacy of these drugs is altered in many cases because of changes in physiology that ultimately affect PK. As has been described, many of these changes make the absorption, distribution, metabolism and elimination of drugs sufficiently different to warrant dosage adjustment. Steps currently being taken by various regulatory agencies and the scientific community to address this issue have been discussed and common themes involve a need to use binding guidelines and incentives with drug developers and a need to promote more phase IV trials with pregnant women when data are not available prior to marketing. Known modifications to PK parameters could also be considered when deciding whether PK studies in pregnant women are warranted. Pregnant women and their physicians are routinely making risk versus benefit analyses with respect to established and new drugs. With new drugs, for which PK data are often sparse or non-existent, evidence-based dosing decisions of benefit to both mother and fetus are difficult and options in the pharmacopoeia are effectively limited because of this. Future efforts must continue to encourage the production of PK information for as wide an array of drugs as possible if women are to benefit from the same therapeutic effects when pregnant as they do when not.

REFERENCES

Anderson GD (2005) Pregnancy-induced changes in pharmacokinetics: a mechanistic-based approach. *Clin Pharmacokin* **44:** 989–1008.

Anger GJ, Piquette-Miller M (2010) Impact of hyperlipidemia on plasma protein binding and hepatic drug transporter and metabolic enzyme regulation in a rat model of gestational diabetes. *J Pharmacol Exp Therap.* In press.

Brown WU, Bell GC, Alper MH (1976) Acidosis, local anesthetics, and the newborn. *Obstet Gynecol* **48:** 27–30.

Carter BL, Garnett WR, Pellock JM, Stratton MA, Howell JR (1981) Effect of antacids on phenytoin bioavailability. *Ther Drug Monit.* **3:** 333–40.

CDER (1977) Guidance for industry: general considerations for the clinical evaluation of drugs. *US Department of Health, Education, and Welfare*: 1–15.

CDER (2004) Guidance for industry: pharmacokinetics in pregnancy – study design, data analysis, and impact on dosing and labeling. *US Department of Health and Human Services*: 1–17.

Chang K, Bell T, Lauer B, Chai H (1978) Altered theophylline pharmacokinetics during acute respiratory viral illness. *Lancet* **1:** 1132–3.

Chauvelot-Moachon L, Tallet F, Durlach-Misteli C, Giroud JP (1988) Delipidation of alpha 1-acid glycoprotein. Propranolol binding to this glycoprotein and its modification by extracted material and exogenous lipids. *J Pharmacol Methods* **20:** 15–28.

Clements JA, Heading RC, Nimmo WS, Prescott LF (1978) Kinetics of acetaminophen absorption and gastric emptying in man. *Clin Pharmacol Ther* **24:** 420–31.

Collier AC, Ganley NA, Tingle MD, Blumenstein M, Marvin KW, Paxton JW, Mitchell MD, Keelan JA (2002a) UDP-glucuronosyltransferase activity, expression and cellular localization in human placenta at term. *Biochem Pharmacol* **63:** 409–19.

Collier AC, Tingle MD, Paxton JW, Mitchell MD, Keelan JA (2002b) Metabolizing enzyme localization and activities in the first trimester human placenta: the effect of maternal and gestational age, smoking and alcohol consumption. *Human Repro* **17:** 2564–72.

Conrad KP (2004) Mechanisms of renal vasodilation and hyperfiltration during pregnancy. *J Soc Gynecol Invest* **11:** 438–48.

Cunningham F, Gant N, Leveno K, Gilstrap L, Hauth J, Wentstrom K (2001) Chapter 8: Maternal adaptations to pregnancy, in *Williams Obstetrics*, McGraw-Hill, New York.

Curry B (2001) Animal models used in identifying gender-related differences. *Int J Toxicol* **20:** 153–60.

Czerniak R (2001) Gender-based differences in pharmacokinetics in laboratory animals. *Int J Toxicol* **20:** 161–3.

Dawes M, Chowienczyk PJ (2001) Pharmacokinetics in pregnancy. *Best Practice and Res Clin Obstet Gynaecol* **15:** 819–26.

Dawood MY (1976) Circulating maternal serum progesterone in high-risk pregnancies. *Am J Obstet Gynecol* **125:** 832–40.

de Haan G, Edelbroek P, Segers J, Engelsman M, Lindhout D, Devile-Notschaele M, Augustijn P (2004) Gestation-induced changes in lamotrigine pharmacokinetics: a monotherapy study. *Neurology* **63:** 571–3.

Døllner H, Vatten L, Halgunset J, Rahimipoor S, Austgulen R (2002) Histologic chorioamnionitis and umbilical serum levels of pro-inflammatory cytokines and cytokine inhibitors. *BJOG* **109:** 534–9.

FDA (1993) Guideline for the study and evaluation of gender differences in the clinical evaluation of drugs; notice. *Fed Regist* **58:** 39406–16.

FDA (2001) The pediatric exclusivity provision – January 2001; status report to congress. *US Department of Health and Human Services*: 1–57.

Frederiksen MC (2001) Physiologic changes in pregnancy and their effect on drug disposition. *Seminars in Perinatology* **25:** 120–3.

Frederiksen MC (2002) The drug development process and the pregnant woman. *J Midwifery Women's Health* **47:** 422–5.

Garland M, Szeto HH, Daniel SS, Tropper PJ, Myers MM, Stark RI (1998) Placental transfer and fetal metabolism of zidovudine in the baboon. *Pediatr Res* **44:** 47–53.

Garnett WR, Carter BL, Pellock JM (1980) Effect of calcium and antacids on phenytoin bioavailability. *Arch Neurol* **37:** 467.

Gedeon C, Koren G (2006) Designing pregnancy centered medications: drugs which do not cross the human placenta. *Placenta* **27:** 861–8.

Glinoer D (1997) The regulation of thyroid function in pregnancy: pathways of endocrine adaptation from physiology to pathology. *Endocr Rev* **18:** 404–33.

Gordon MC, Samuels P (1995) Indomethacin. *Clin Obstetr Gynecol* **38:** 697–705.

Kennedy RL, Erenberg A, Robillard JE, Merkow A, Turner T (1979) Effects of changes in maternal–fetal pH on the transplacental equilibrium of bupivacaine. *Anesthesiology* **51:** 50–4.

Little BB (1999) Pharmacokinetics during pregnancy: evidence-based maternal dose formulation. *Obstetr Gynecol* **93:** 858–68.

Luecke RH, Wosilait WD, Pearce BA, Young JF (1994) A physiologically based pharmacokinetic computer model for human pregnancy. *Teratology* **49:** 90–103.

Mandel SJ, Larsen PR, Seely EW, Brent GA (1990) Increased need for thyroxine during pregnancy in women with primary hypothyroidism. *New England J Med* **323:** 91–6.

Mattison D, Zajicek A (2006) Gaps in knowledge in treating pregnant women. *Gen Med* **3:** 169–82.

McBride W (1961) Thalidomide and congenital abnormalities. *Lancet* **278:** 1358.

Mitchell AA, Hernandez-Diaz S, Louik C, Werler MM (2001) Medication use in pregnancy: 1976–2000. *Pharmacoepidemiol Drug Safety* **10:** S146.

Moise KJ, Ou CN, Kirshon B, Cano LE, Rognerud C, Carpenter RJ (1990) Placental transfer of indomethacin in the human pregnancy. *Am J Obstetr Gynecol* **162:** 549–54.

Morgan E, Goralski K, Piquette-Miller M, Renton K, Robertson G, Chaluvadi M, Charles K, Clarke S, Kacevska M, Liddle C, Richardson T, Sharma R, Sinal C (2008) Regulation of drug-metabolizing enzymes and transporters in infection, inflammation, and cancer. *Drug Metabol Dispos* **36:** 205–16.

Nakai A, Sekiya I, Oya A, Koshino T, Araki T (2002) Assessment of the hepatic arterial and portal venous blood flows during pregnancy with Doppler ultrasonography. *Arch Gynecol Obstetr* **266:** 25–9.

Parry E, Shields R, Turnbull AC (1970) Transit time in the small intestine in pregnancy. *J Obstetr Gynaecol Brit Commonwealth* **77:** 900–901.

Pennell PB (2003) Antiepileptic drug pharmacokinetics during pregnancy and lactation. *Neurology* **61:** S35–S42.

Petrovic V, Wang J, Piquette-Miller M (2008) Effect of endotoxin on the expression of placental drug transporters and glyburide disposition in pregnant rats. *Drug Metabol Dispos* **36:** 1944–50.

Pickering B, Biehl D, Meatherall R (1981) The effect of foetal acidosis on bupivacaine levels in utero. *Canadian Anaesthetists' Soc J* **28:** 544–9.

Renton K, Gray J, Hall R (1980) Decreased elimination of theophylline after influenza vaccination. *Canadian Med Assoc J* **123:** 288–90.

Reynolds F (1998) Pharmacokinetics, in *Clinical Physiology in Obstetrics* (Chamberlain G and Pipkin FB, eds.), pp. 239–60, Blackwell Sciences, Ltd, London.

Rodriguez-Moran M, Guerrero-Romero F (1999) Increased levels of C-reactive protein in noncontrolled type II diabetic subjects. *J Diabetes Complications* **13:** 211–15.

Rodriguez-Moran M, Guerrero-Romero F (2003) Elevated concentrations of C-reactive protein in subjects with type 2 diabetes mellitus are moderately influenced by glycemic control. *J Endocrinol Invest* **26:** 216–21.

Sawle G (2000) Epilepsy and anticonvulsant drugs, in *Prescribing in Pregnancy* (Rubin P, ed.), pp. 112–26, BMJ Books, London.

Schwartz JB (2003) The influence of sex on pharmacokinetics. *Clin Pharmacokin* **42:** 107–121.

Spector AA, Santos EC, Ashbrook JD, Fletcher JE (1973) Influence of free fatty acid concentration on drug binding to plasma albumin. *Ann New York Acad Sci* **226:** 247–58.

Syme MR, Paxton JW, Keelan JA (2004) Drug transfer and metabolism by the human placenta. *Clin Pharmacokin* **43:** 487–514.

Tan TC, Devendra K, Tan LK, Tan HK (2006) Tocolytic treatment for the management of preterm labour: a systematic review. *Singapore Med J* **47:** 361–6.

Tracy TS, Venkataramanan R, Glover DD, Caritis SN (2005) Temporal changes in drug metabolism (CYP1A2, CYP2D6 and CYP3A Activity) during pregnancy. *Am J Obstetr Gynecol* **192:** 633–9.

Tsatsaris V, Cabrol D, Carbonne B (2004) Pharmacokinetics of tocolytic agents. *Clin Pharmacokin* **43:** 833–44.

Tsutsumi K, Kotegawa T, Matsuki S, Tanaka Y, Ishii Y, Kodama Y, Kuranari M, Miyakawa I, Nakano S (2001) The effect of pregnancy on cytochrome P4501A2, xanthine oxidase, and N-acetyltransferase activities in humans. *Clin Pharmacol Ther* **70:** 121–5.

Vermillion ST, Robinson CJ (2005) Antiprostaglandin drugs. *Obstetr Gynecol Clin North America* **32:** 501–17.

Wadelius M, Darj E, Frenne G, Rane A (1997) Induction of CYP2D6 in pregnancy. *Clin Pharmacol Ther* **62:** 400–7.

Williams JA, Ring BJ, Cantrell VE, Jones DR, Eckstein J, Ruterbories K, Hamman MA, Hall SD, Wrighton SA (2002) Comparative metabolic capabilities of CYP3A4, CYP3A5, and CYP3A7. *Drug Metabol Dispos* **30:** 883–91.

Yerby MS, Friel PN, McCormick K, Koerner M, Van Allen M, Leavitt AM, Sells CJ, Yerby JA (1990) Pharmacokinetics of anticonvulsants in pregnancy: alterations in plasma protein binding. *Epilepsy Res* **5:** 223–8.

C H A P T E R

5

PBPK models in reproductive and developmental toxicology

Kannan Krishnan

INTRODUCTION

The elucidation of the mode of action of reproductive and developmental toxicants requires a better understanding of their pharmacokinetics and the potential toxic moiety at the site of action. The measurement of the concentration of the putative toxic moiety as a function of time in the target site is not always possible for all species, exposure routes, dose levels and exposure scenarios. Therefore, the development of quantitative models to predict the tissue dose and kinetics of chemicals and their metabolites as a function of species, lifestage, test system (e.g., *in vitro*), exposure route and exposure scenario is of utmost importance. In this regard, the mechanism-based mathematical models have a unique role to play; they not only facilitate the integration of the current knowledge to identify data gaps but also permit the evaluation of the "if...then" type of questions to design new experiments (Krishnan and Andersen, 2007). In planning the new experiments, it is critically useful to be able to forecast the blood and tissue concentrations in the exposed animal (particularly in the target site such as the fetus) as a function of time, such that appropriate sampling times and volumes can be chosen. In other terms, quantitative mechanistic models such as the physiologically based pharmacokinetic (PBPK) models are of potential use in efficiently determining the sacrifice/sampling times at which the chemical concentrations would still be above the limit of detection (LOD) of the analytical method, as well as be adequately representative of critical portions of the time-course curve to facilitate the calculation of dose metrics (e.g., AUC as a measure of internal exposure) during a specific window of susceptibility for risk assessment applications (Welsch *et al.*, 1995; Gargas *et al.*, 2000). Similarly, when limited or no *in vivo* data on the toxic moiety and mode of action are available for reproductive and developmental toxicants (RDTs), the PBPK models can be of particular use in predicting kinetics and dose to target in intact animals on the basis of *in vitro* data (Van Ommen *et al.*, 1995; Quick and Shuler, 2000; MacGregor *et al.*, 2001; Hissink *et al.*, 2002; Kamgang *et al.*, 2008).

The peer-reviewed literature contains examples of the use of PBPK models to estimate dose to the fetus at critical times during gestation, and as well as in developing organisms exposed via lactation. The PBPK model-derived estimates of internal dose have been evaluated for correlation with developmental effects (e.g., area under the concentration vs time curve (AUC), maximal concentration (C_{max})) (Mattison and Sandler, 1994). By uniquely incorporating quantitative changes in maternal and embryo/fetal tissue weights and blood flows associated with gestation, PBPK models allow the simulation of concentration profiles that may correlate with the final outcomes. When combined with biologically based pharmacodynamic models, the PBPK models are useful not only in determining the toxicologically equivalent doses of systemically acting RDTs for different exposure routes but also for simulating the time-course of toxicological responses on the basis of known or hypothesized mode of action (Young *et al.*, 1997). This chapter provides an outline of the process of developing PBPK models, as well as their implementation for evaluating RDTs.

PBPK MODELING: BASIC CONCEPTS AND TOOLS

Physiologically based pharmacokinetic (PBPK) models are quantitative descriptions of the interplay among the key determinants of absorption, distribution, metabolism and excretion (ADME) of chemicals in biota. The conceptual representation of a PBPK model (Figure 5.1) depicts the working hypothesis or the current state of knowledge of the investigator regarding the ADME and mode of action of the chemical being investigated. While choosing the compartments to be represented in the model, consideration should be given to the following aspects:

- Target site (e.g., fetus)
- Portals of entry (e.g., lung, GI tract, placenta)

Reproductive and Developmental Toxicology, Edited by Ramesh C. Gupta
ISBN: 978-0-12-382032-7

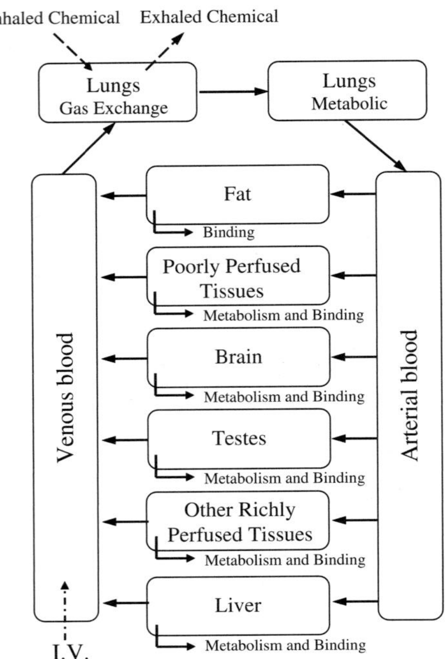

FIGURE 5.1 Conceptual representation of a physiologically based pharmacokinetic model for ethylene oxide. Reproduced with permission from Krishnan *et al.* (1992).

- Metabolism and excretion sites (e.g., metabolic clearance, lactation, urinary excretion)
- Lipophilicity consideration (e.g., adipose tissue), and
- Mass balance

On the basis of these considerations, the number and nature of the compartments constituting the PBPK model are defined (Krishnan and Andersen, 2007). Subsequently, each tissue compartment is described with a mass balance differential equation based on clearance terms in terms of volume per unit time. The PBPK models essentially are physiological clearance models facilitating the simulation of the pharmacokinetics of compounds. The clearance terms are reflective of the influx, efflux, metabolic and other processes occurring in the tissues. Accordingly, a generic mass balance differential equation (MBDE) would be as follows:

$$dAt/dt = \text{Influx} - \text{Efflux} - \text{Metabolism} - \text{Other CL processes} \quad (1)$$

where dAt/dt = rate of change in the amount of chemical in tissue t.

Notationally, the above equation can be written as follows:

$$\frac{dA_t}{dt} = Cl_u C_a - Cl_e C_{vt} - Cl_m C_a - Cl_f C_a \quad (2)$$

where Cl = clearance and C = concentration. The subscripts a, e, f, m and u represent arterial, efflux, metabolic, other and uptake (influx).

Considering the fundamental processes of tissue uptake (i.e., influx and efflux), they are described in PBPK models as per Fick's law of simple diffusion, which states that the rate of change in the amount of a chemical is proportional to its concentration gradient:

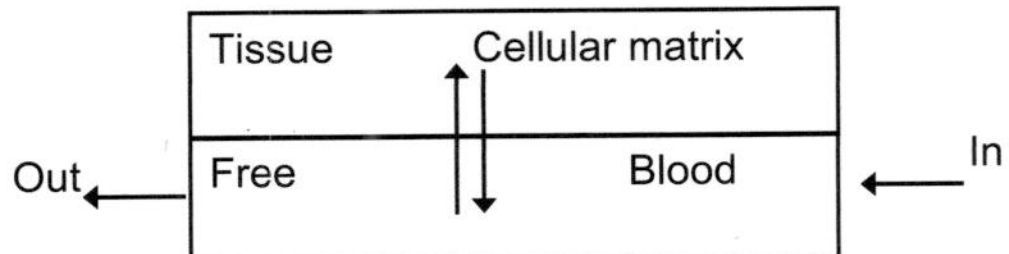

FIGURE 5.2 Schematic representation of chemical movement through a tissue compartment in PBPK models.

$$\frac{dA_t}{dt} \infty \Delta C \quad (3)$$

For high molecular weight compounds diffusion is often the rate-limiting process such that their flux through the subcompartments (i.e., cellular matrix (dA_{cm}/dt) and tissue blood (dA_{tb}/dt)) needs to be considered (Figure 5.2). The computation under this condition is based on the use of separate equations for the cellular matrix and tissue blood subcompartments.

For cellular matrix subcompartment:

$$\frac{dA_{cm}}{dt} = PA_t\left(C_{vt} - \frac{C_t}{P_t}\right) \quad (4)$$

For tissue blood subcompartment:

$$\frac{dA_{tb}}{dt} = Q_t(C_a - C_{vt}) - PA_t\left(C_{vt} - \frac{C_t}{P_t}\right) \quad (5)$$

where PA_t = permeation coefficient–surface area cross-product for the tissue (t), Q_t = tissue blood flow rate, C_t = concentration in tissue t, C_{vt} = chemical concentration in venous blood leaving tissue t, and P_t = tissue:blood partition coefficient for tissue t.

If the diffusion of a chemical from tissue blood to cellular matrix is slow with respect to tissue perfusion rate, both equations are necessary. On the other hand, if tissue blood flow (i.e., perfusion) is slow with respect to diffusion, the tissues are described as homogeneous, well-mixed compartments such that the rate of change in the amount of chemical in the tissue can be described with a single equation for the whole tissue mass as follows (Krishnan and Andersen, 2007):

$$\frac{dA_t}{dt} = Q_t(C_a - C_{vt}) \quad (6)$$

where C_a = chemical concentration in arterial blood entering the tissue compartment.

In order to solve the above equations and determine the temporal values of concentration of chemicals and their metabolites in blood and tissues, knowledge of the following parameters are required: physiological, biochemical and physicochemical. The physiological parameters correspond to the volumes and blood perfusion rates for various tissues and tissue compartments; physicochemical parameters represent the blood:air and tissue:blood partition coefficients; and biochemical parameters refer to the metabolic constants (V_{max}: maximal velocity, K_m: Michaelis affinity parameter, $CL_{int} = V_{max}/K_m$) as well as protein-binding parameters specific to each tissue, lifestage and species. Whereas physiological parametrer databases for PBPK modeling in developing animals have become available (Price *et al.*, 2003b; Gentry *et al.*, 2004), the other parameters are frequently estimated either *in vivo* or *in vitro* (reviewed in Krishnan and Andersen,

TABLE 5.1 Examples of software for PBPK modeling

Software
ACSL-X-treme®
BASICA
Excel®
Madonna®
Matlab®
ModelMaker®
ScoP®
Simusolv®
STELLA®

1998, 2007). To a limited extent, *in silico* approaches may be of use in providing initial estimates of partition coefficients and metabolic parameters (Béliveau *et al.*, 2003, 2005).

The PBPK model, comprising algebraic equations and integration algorithms along with the input parameter values, is written and solved using simulation software or packages (Table 5.1). Several of these are essentially computer programming packages that are commercially available and have features apt for efficient and rapid construction of PBPK models. Spreadsheets such as Microsoft Excel® can also be used for developing and for transparently evaluating the "working" of PBPK models (Haddad *et al.*, 1996).

Once the model compartments are identified, the equations written, and input parameters defined, the model simulations can be obtained and compared with experimental data. The PBPK models, as other mechanistic models, are simplified representations of the system under study, and as such only account for those determinants and processes that are hypothesized to be critical by the investigator(s). When there is a high degree of concordance between model predictions and diverse sets of experimental data, there is greater confidence regarding the predictive capability of the model (Chiu *et al.*, 2007). Meaningful comparisons of PBPK model simulations with experimental data can be performed by visual inspection, statistical tests or discrepancy indices. It is important to ensure that such comparisons and evaluations be done to facilitate confident application of these models in developmental and reproductive toxicology.

PBPK MODELING IN REPRODUCTIVE AND DEVELOPMENTAL TOXICOLOGY

PBPK models used in reproductive and developmental toxicology invoke different levels of complexity (in terms of the number and nature of the compartments) depending upon the intended application. A key question in this regard is whether the kinetics of parent chemical and/or metabolite is to be simulated during a specific day or during a particular window of exposure. If the simulations of chemical concentrations are to be obtained for the reproductive organ in adult animals or humans, then model structures similar to Figure 5.2 have been used. Here the male reproductive organ (testes) is isolated from the richly perfused tissues compartment, and characterized individually with knowledge of its volume, blood flow rate as well as the testes:blood partition coefficient (e.g., Krishnan *et al.*, 1992; Campbell, 2009).

Since the magnitude of metabolism in the reproductive organs is often minor in terms of their impact on the overall kinetics of chemicals, these organs are not routinely represented as a separate compartment. The reproductive organs, as well as other internal organs, are richly perfused and thus are frequently represented as a single lumped compartment. In this regard, Maruyama *et al.* (2003), developing a PBPK model for polychloro dibenzo-pdioxin and dioxin-like polychlorinated biphenyls to simulate concentrations in human fetuses, assumed that the fetal concentrations would be the same as that of the richly perfused tissues. Accordingly, these authors used a PBPK model that contained liver, kidney, fat, blood, muscle and richly perfused tissues and skin as the compartments, for obtaining simulations of use in the conduct of a reproductive risk assessment for the Japanese population. This approach is justified when the lumped tissues exhibit the same time constants (i.e., volume × partition coefficient/blood flow) because they would be anticipated to display similar kinetic curves and therefore there is no gain in representing each one of them separately.

In the case of developing organisms, PBPK models are constructed either for simulating chemical kinetics on a particular day of gestation, or for generating simulations covering the whole perinatal period. PBPK models developed for a particular gestation day have often focused on latter periods of gestation in mice, rats and rabbits, and have relied on a single set of physiological parameter estimates for the mother and the fetus or embryo (Olanoff and Anderson, 1980; Gabrielsson and Paalzow, 1983; Gabrielsson *et al.*, 1984, 1985; Terry *et al.*, 1995; Kim *et al.*, 1996; Ward *et al.*, 1997; Gabrielsson and Groth, 1998; Hays *et al.*, 2000; Kawamoto *et al.*, 2007; Thrall *et al.*, 2009). A PBPK model for simulating the kinetics of TCDD associated with developmental exposures developed by Emond *et al.* (2004) consists of four compartments (liver, fat, placenta and rest of body) for the dam and one compartment for fetuses (Figure 5.3). This simple model does not describe blood flow to fetuses but describes chemical transfer on the basis of simple diffusional clearance between the placental and fetal compartments. Dynamics of the growth of the various compartments, including the placenta and fetus, were described quantitatively on the basis of experimental data obtained from the literature. The weights of these latter compartments in PBPK models are frequently expressed as a fraction of the mother's body weight. Following the inclusion of MBDEs for the placental and fetal compartments, the PBPK model can be used for simulating the profile of chemical kinetics in the fetal compartment for maternal exposures during that particular day of gestation.

In the developmental PBPK models, the rate of change in the amount of chemical in the placental (dA_{pla}/dt) and fetal (dA_{fet}/dt) compartments has been described as follows (Fisher *et al.*, 1989):

$$dA_{pla}/dt = Q_{pla}(C_a - C_{pla}/P_{pla}) - dA_{fet}/dt \tag{7}$$

$$dA_{fet}/dt = Q_{fet}(C_{pla}/P_{pla} \times P_1/P - C_{fet}/P_{fet}) \tag{8}$$

where Q_{pla} = blood flow to placenta, Q_{fet} = blood flow to fetus/embryo, C_{pla} = concentration in placenta, C_{fet} = concentration in the fetus/embryo, P_{pla} = placenta:blood partition coefficient, P_{fet} = fetal blood:air partition coefficient, and P = maternal blood:air partition coefficient (Krishnan and Andersen, 1998).

This PBPK modeling framework can be extended to account for the dynamics of growing a fetus or embryo during the entire length of pregnancy, and to simulate the kinetics of

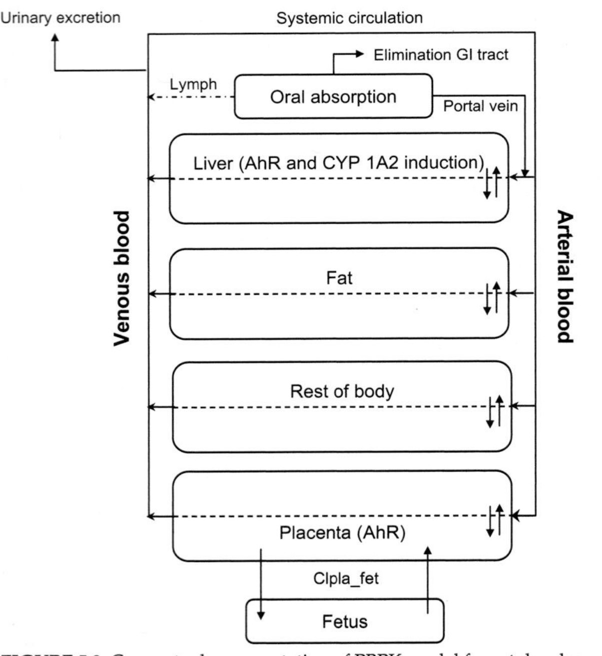

FIGURE 5.3 Conceptual representation of PBPK model for rat developmental exposure to TCDD. Reproduced with permission from Emond *et al.* (2004).

chemicals in the fetus (Figure 5.4). For this purpose then, the model should account for the temporal change in the numeric values of the various parameters (e.g., volumes of tissues and blood flows) related to the various model compartments (i.e., maternal tissues, placenta and fetus). For example, the growth of the human embryo or fetus has been modeled using the Verhulst logistic equation, a polynomial equation, or Gompertz equation (Wosilait *et al.*, 1992). Alternatively, based on the available experimental data on physiological parameters, mathematical relationships can be developed and integrated within the PBPK models (O'Flaherty *et al.*, 1992, 1995). Such relationships may be developed either for the entire growth curve with a single smoothing equation, or with several regression equations each of which describes a segment of the growth curve. In this regard, body weight (*BW*) of the fetus/embryo, has been modeled using the Gompertz equation (Corley *et al.*, 2003):

$$BW(t) = 0.001374 \times \exp\{(0.19741/0.013063)(1 - \exp[-0.013063 \times t])\} \quad (9)$$

Similarly, the fetal organ weights (*W*) can be computed as a function of fetal body weight using the following general equation:

$$W = a \times (BW)^b \quad (10)$$

where a and b are constants specific for each organ, as listed in Table 5.2.

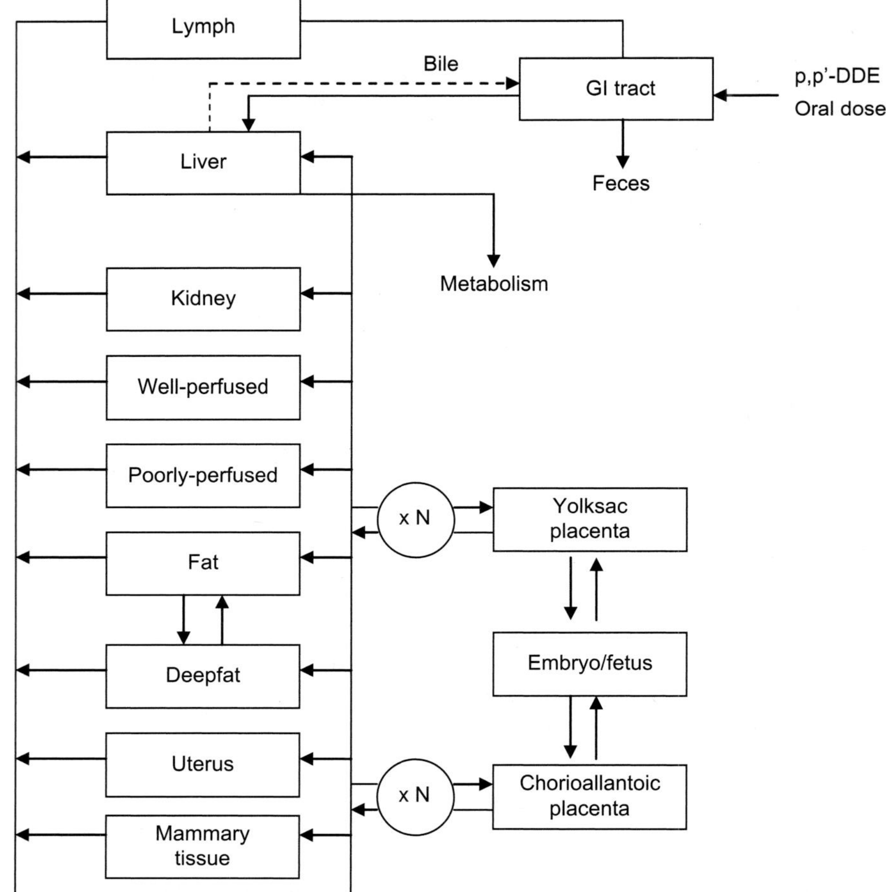

FIGURE 5.4 Diagrammatic representation of the PBPK model for gestation. Reproduced with permission from You *et al.* (1999).

A review of the quantitative approaches for computing physiological parameters as well as the alternative structures for modeling of a number of chemicals and drugs during pregnancy and lactation have been presented by Corley *et al.* (2003).

TABLE 5.2 Allometric parameters for fetal organs and tissues subject to change during pregnancy

Fetal organs/tissues	a	b
Adrenal	0.007467	0.8902
Bone	0.05169	0.9288
Bone marrow	0.01425	0.9943
Brain	0.1871	0.9585
Fat	0.1803	−0.9422
Heart	0.01012	0.9489
Kidney	0.004203	1.255
Liver	0.06050	0.9737
Lung	0.09351	1.552
Pancreas	0.1883	0.3854
Plasma	0.06796	0.9729
Skeletal muscle	0.02668	1.234
Spleen	0.0001302	1.204
Thymus	0.001218	1.093
Thyroid	0.006470	1.023

The constants *a* and *b* are used in the following equation $W_{tissue} = aW_{body}^{b}$. A third constant *c* (=0.2332, −0.02127, −0.059545 or 0.02909, respectively) is used in the case of fat, kidney, lung and spleen to accommodate growth rate differences in these organs and total weight of human embryo/fetus (Luecke *et al.*, 1995)

The dynamic developmental PBPK model has been used to simulate the concentration profiles of a number of chemicals in the maternal tissues as well as embryo or fetus during pregnancy, from conception to parturition (O'Flaherty *et al.*, 1992, 1995; Clarke *et al.*, 1993; Terry *et al.*, 1995; Luecke *et al.*, 1997; Ward *et al.*, 1997; Clewell *et al.*, 2003, 2008). In developing the dynamic PBPK models for the mother and fetus, depending upon the intended application of the model, the fetus has either been described as a single homogeneous compartment or as a network of several appropriate tissue compartments to facilitate the simulation of the tissue dosimetry of chemicals (Figure 5.4 vs. Figure 5.5). The fetus compartment in turn may correspond to a single compartment representing the entire litter (e.g., 13 fetuses in a litter) (Yoon *et al.*, 2009).

Figure 5.6 presents sample simulations obtained with a developmental PBPK model. Here, the PBPK model simulation is compared to experimental data on the kinetics of 2-methoxyethanol in maternal plasma as well as that of its metabolite 2-methoxy acetic acid in maternal plasma, embryo and embryonic fluid, following a single gavage dose of 250 mg/kg to mice on gestational day 11 (Clarke *et al.*, 1993). Using such a dynamic PBPK modeling approach, O'Flaherty *et al.* (1992) successfully simulated the kinetics of weak acids in mouse, rat and monkey, during the entire period of gestation including the organogenesis. These simulations illustrate the usefulness of PBPK models in conducting extrapolation of fetal tissue concentrations from one

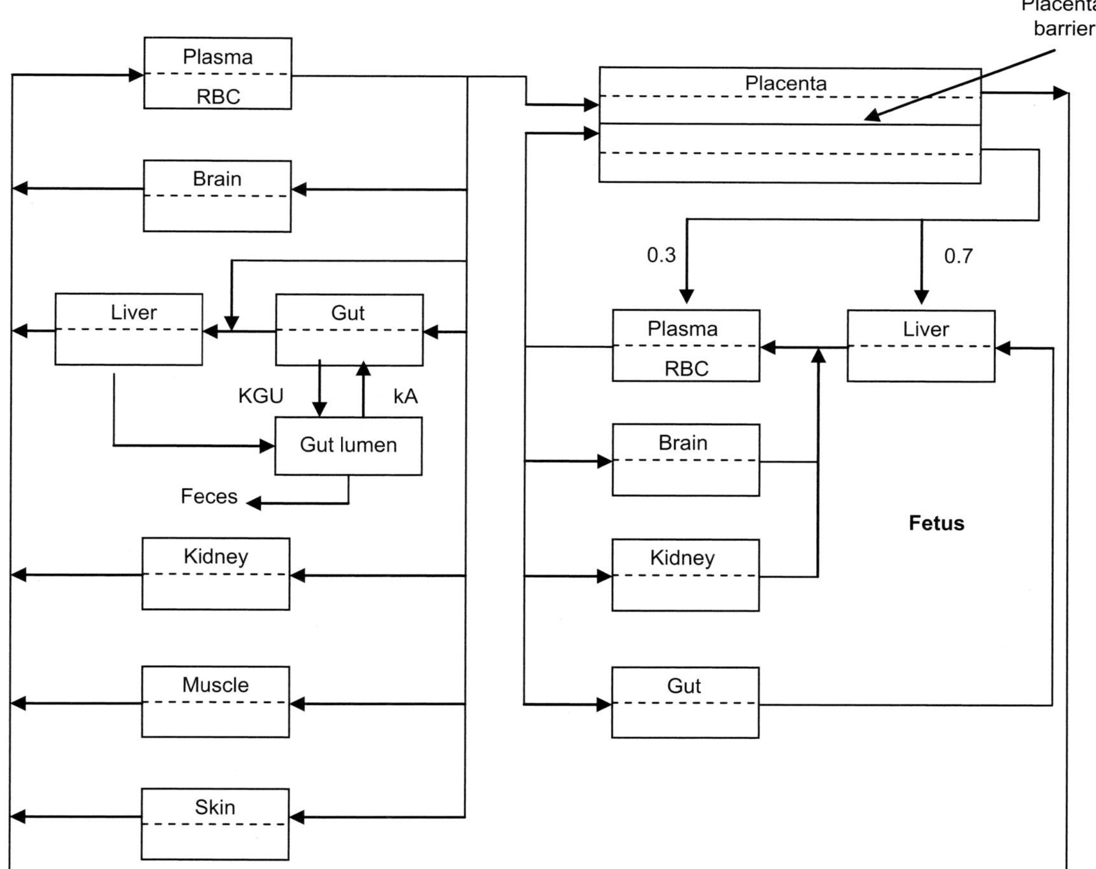

FIGURE 5.5 PBPK model for methyl mercury transport in the pregnant rat and fetus. kB, kA, and KGU are rate constants for biliary secretion, gut absorption, and gut cell shedding, respectively. Reproduced with permission from Gray (1995).

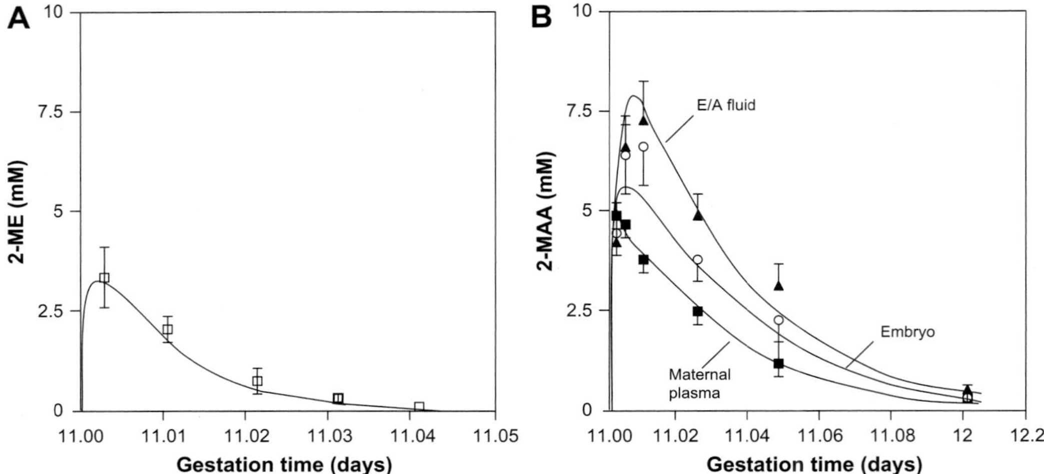

FIGURE 5.6 Kinetic profiles of 2-methoxyethanol (2-ME) and its metabolite 2-methoxy acetic acid (2-MAA) following bolus gavage of 250 mg 2-ME • kg^{-1} to mice on GD 11. Curves represent the model simulations of experimental data points which are the mean ± SD of three to seven animals. Reproduced with permission from Clarke *et al.* (1993).

developmental stage to another. When temporal changes in the model parameters are accounted for, the PBPK model can be used to simulate the concentration profiles of chemicals on any particular day of gestation (Gray, 1995; Terry *et al.*, 1995: Luecke *et al.*, 1997; Gargas *et al.*, 2000). This aspect of PBPK modeling has important implications with regard to the risk assessment of developmental toxicants as well as the elucidation of the pharmacokinetic mechanisms of toxicity.

Similar to the dynamic modeling of physiological and metabolic changes during the prenatal period, the changes during the postnatal period have also been captured within the PBPK framework (Farris *et al.*, 1993; You *et al.*, 1999; Nong *et al.*, 2006; Nong and Krishnan, 2007). Furthermore, the postnatal PBPK models take into account the direct and indirect exposure pathways of relevance to the infants. In this regard, physiologically based descriptions of the nursing mother and the nursed infant can be constructed and interconnected to simulate tissue dose of breast milk-driven chemicals in infants. The combined description of the mother and pup requires that the ADME processes and determinants be characterized for each of them as a function of time (Figure 5.7). The resulting PBPK model can simulate the kinetics of chemicals in the pup following the ingestion of milk from mother exposed to the contaminant in an exposure medium (Fisher *et al.*, 1990: Byczkowski *et al.*, 1994).

For simulating lactational transfer of contaminants, two alternative approaches have been employed in PBPK models. The first approach computes the milk concentration (C_{mlk}) on the basis of the rate of change in the quantity of chemical in the milk (dA_{mk}/dt) and mammary gland (dA_{mg}/dt) compartments as follows (Krishnan and Andersen, 1998):

$$dA_{mg}/dt = Q_{mg}(C_a - C_{mlk}/P_{mlk}) - Q_{mlk}C_{mlk} \tag{11}$$

$$dA_{mk}/d_t = Q_{mlk}C_{mlk} - Q_{skl}C_{mlk} \tag{12}$$

where Q_{skl} = suckling rate of the infant, Q_{mlk} = rate of milk production and P_{mlk} = milk:blood partition coefficient of the chemical.

The second approach calculates the concentration in milk as a function of the mammary gland concentration at the time of milk production; it therefore considers the milk and the mammary tissue as pertaining to the same compartment. The mass balance differential equation describing this phenomenon (dA_{mk}/dt) is as follows:

$$dA_{mk}/dt = Q_{mlk}(C_a - C_{mlk}/P_{mlk}) - Q_{skl}C_{mlk} \tag{13}$$

Integrating these descriptions along with the MBDEs for the various tissue compartments of the mother and infant (or dam and pup), simulations of kinetics of RDTs can be obtained. Such an approach has been used to simulate the tissue dose in pups (or infants) resulting from the lactational transfer of chemicals from dams (or mothers) exposed to volatile organic chemicals in inhaled air (Shelley *et al.*, 1988; Fisher *et al.*, 1990, 1997). For the simulation of the kinetics in toddlers and teenagers, the appropriate direct exposure routes can be considered in the PBPK model. In this case, by accounting for the age-related change in physiological parameters and metabolic rates (Alcorn and McNamara, 2002a,b; Price *et al.*, 2003a,b), the PBPK models facilitate simulation of the kinetics and tissue dose of chemicals in children. Figure 5.8 presents the inhalation pharmacokinetics of furan in children of various age groups in comparison with the adult. Here, the PBPK model structure and equations are the same for children of all ages and adults; however, the numerical values of input parameters are not.

PBPK MODEL APPLICATIONS IN REPRODUCTIVE AND DEVELOPMENTAL TOXICOLOGY

The applications of PBPK models in toxicology, including developmental and reproductive toxicology, have been reviewed by Corley *et al.* (2003), Reddy *et al.* (2005) and Krishnan and Andersen (1998, 2010). Lipscomb and Ohanian (2006) present a number of case studies of chemical risk assessments in which PBPK models have been evaluated and/or used for replacing the default interspecies uncertainty and intraspecies variability factors. This is feasible because they permit

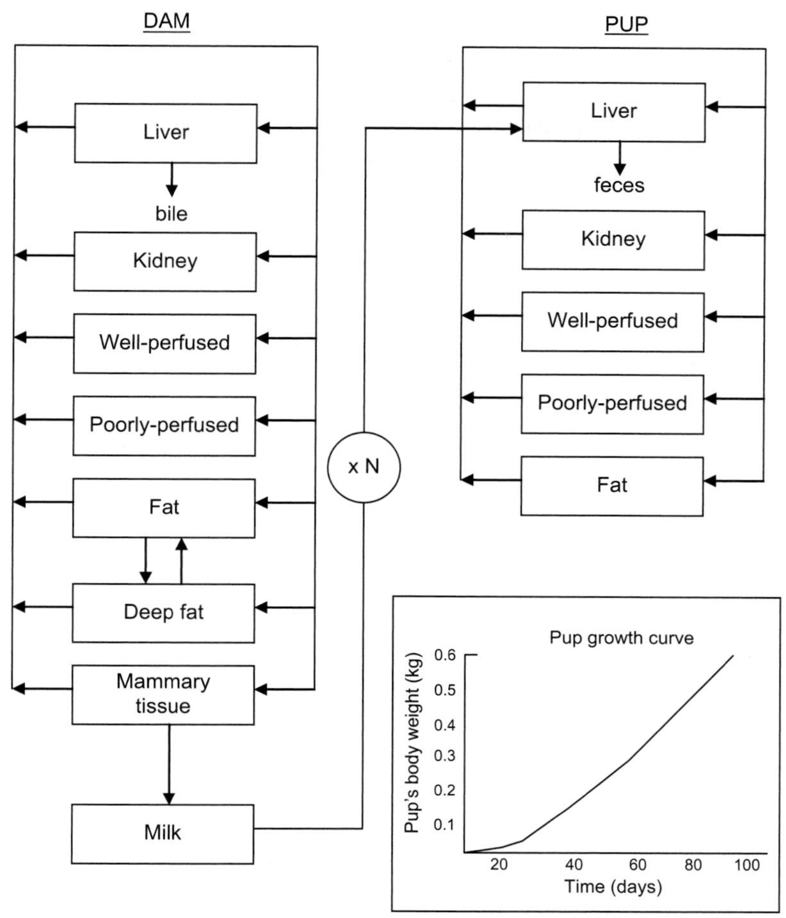

FIGURE 5.7 Diagrammatic representation of the PBPK model for the lactating dam and nursing pup. The insert shows the body growth curve of the pups used in the model. Reproduced with permission from You *et al.* (1999).

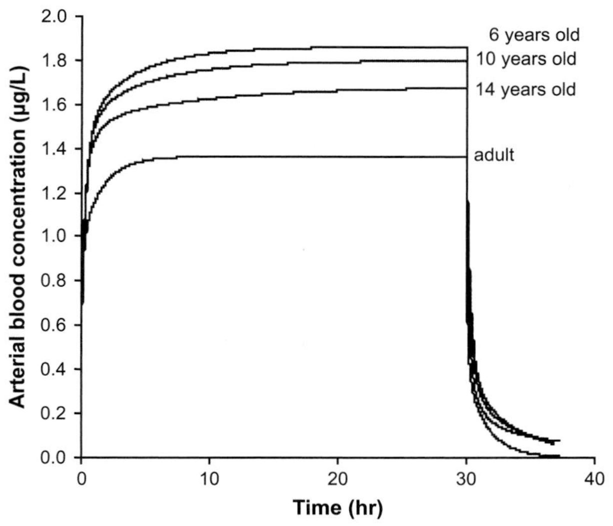

FIGURE 5.8 PBPK model simulations of the arterial blood concentration of furan following inhalation exposure. Reproduced with permission from Price *et al.* (2003a).

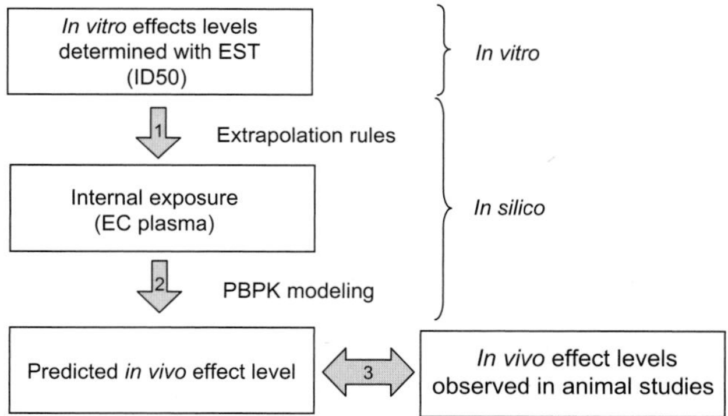

FIGURE 5.9 An integrated approach including *in vitro* toxicity test (EST) and *in silico* methods (extrapolation rules and PBPK models) to predict *in vivo* effect levels. Reproduced with permission from Verwei *et al.* (2006).

the simulation of change in tissue dose during the various life stages. In this context, PBPK models have been applied to compare the maternal and fetal/neonatal blood and tissue dose metrics during pregnancy and lactation using six chemicals representative of a variety of physicochemical properties (isopropanol, vinyl chloride, methylene chloride, perchloroethylene, nicotine and TCDD) (Gentry *et al.*, 2003). A systematic analysis using the PBPK models indicated that the blood concentrations were lower in neonates during lactation than in the fetus during gestation; however, compared to the maternal exposure, fetal/neonatal exposure ranged from approximately twice as great (TCDD) to several orders of magnitude lower (for isopropanol) (Gentry *et al.*,

2003). These models are useful not only in estimating the age-dependent differences in tissue dosimetry, but also for identifying appropriate dose metrics for use in dose–response assessment (Krishnan and Andersen, 2010).

Another application of the PBPK models that will continue to expand in the future relates to *in vitro–in vivo* extrapolation. The newer toxicity testing paradigm of the US National Academy of Sciences (2007) insists upon the importance and role of *in vitro* tests. For interpretation of such tests, the development of modeling tools is inevitable. An example of the application of PBPK models to interpret *in vitro* tests with developmental toxicants is that of Verwei *et al.* (2006). Here, the *in vitro–in vivo* extrapolation capacity of the PBPK models was coupled with the results of embryonic stem cell test, to predict the corresponding *in vivo* doses and classify compounds on the basis of *in vivo* embryotoxic potency. First, the relevant (unbound) plasma concentration corresponding to the *in vitro* concentrations are determined, and then the dose level corresponding to the target plasma level is determined using PBPK models as illustrated in Figure 5.9 (Verwei *et al.*, 2006).

Finally, the PBPK models can be used as a tool in planning and refining reproductive and developmental toxicology studies. An example would be the study of Faber *et al.* (2006), in which the PBPK model was used to conduct a route-to-route extrapolation to overcome a potential difficulty in the conduct of continuous exposures of the dams. Specifically, in case of inhalation reproductive toxicity studies, inhalation exposures cannot normally be continued from gestation day 20 through lactation day 4. Removal of the dam to the exposure chambers during this period of parturition and early lactation could result in severe stress to the offsprings resulting in increased pup mortality. Therefore, as an alternative these authors used the PBPK model to determine the inhalation-equivalent dose to be given orally to the dams, on the basis of equivalent AUC (Faber *et al.*, 2006). This unique application of PBPK modeling in the design of two-generation reproductive toxicity studies ensures that the treatment is continued through the critical period of early lactation.

CONCLUDING REMARKS AND FUTURE DIRECTIONS

PBPK modeling involves mathematical description of the interrelationships among critical parameters that determine the behavior of the system under study. These quantitative biological models are unique tools useful for simulating the appropriate dose metrics of reproductive and developmental toxicants. The motivation for the use of PBPK models in developmental and reproductive toxicology research is to uncover the biological determinants of tissue dose to the developing animal, and occasionally to refine the experimental protocol. These models then become an essential part of any systematic approach to characterizing how DRTs gain entry into, distribute within, and are eliminated from the body. As the interest and use in such models continue to increase, it is important to develop appropriate approaches to evaluate them. In this regard, the process should focus on the following specific aspects: (1) model purpose, (2) model structure, (3) mathematical representation, (4) parameter estimation, (5) computer implementation, (6) predictive capacity, and (7) specialized analyses (i.e., sensitivity, variability and uncertainty analyses) (Clark *et al.*, 2004; Chiu *et al.*, 2007; Clewell *et al.*, 2007).

REFERENCES

Alcorn J, McNamara PJ (2002a) Ontogeny of hepatic and renal systemic clearance pathways in infants: Part I. *Clin Pharmacokinet* **41:** 959–98.

Alcorn J, McNamara PJ (2002b) Ontogeny of hepatic and renal systemic clearance pathways in infants: Part II. *Clin Pharmacokinet* **41:** 1077–94.

Béliveau M, Lipscomb J, Tardif R, Krishnan K (2005) Quantitative structure–property relationships for interspecies extrapolation of the inhalation pharmacokinetics of organic chemicals. *Chem Res Toxicol* **18:** 475–85.

Béliveau M, Tardif R, Krishnan K (2003) Quantitative structure–property relationships for physiologically based pharmacokinetic modeling of volatile organic chemicals in rats. *Toxicol Appl Pharmacol* **189:** 221–32.

Byczkowski JZ, Kinkead ER, Leahy HF, Randall GM, Fisher JW (1994) Computer simulation of the lactational transfer of tetrachloroethylene in rats using a physiologically based model. *Toxicol Appl Pharmacol* **125(2):** 228–36.

Campbell A (2009) Development of PBPK model of molinate and molinate sulfoxide in rats and humans. *Regul Toxicol Pharmacol* **53(3):** 195–204.

Chiu WA, Barton HA, DeWoskin RS, Schlosser P, Thompson CM, Sonawane B, Lipscomb JC, Krishnan K (2007) Evaluation of physiologically based pharmacokinetic models for use in risk assessment. *J Appl Toxicol* **27:** 218–37.

Clarke DO, Elswick BA, Welsch F, Conolly RB (1993) Pharmacokinetics of 2-methoxyethanol and 2-methoxyacetic acid in the pregnant mouse: a physiologically based mathematical model. *Toxicol Appl Pharmacol* **121(2):** 239–52.

Clark LH, Setzer RW, Barton HA (2004) Framework for evaluation of physiologically-based pharmacokinetic models for use in safety or risk assessment. *Risk Anal* **24(6):** 1697–717.

Clewell RA, Merrill EA, Yu KO, Mahle DA, Sterner TR, Mattie DR, Robinson PJ, Fisher JW, Gearhart JM (2003) Predicting fetal perchlorate dose and inhibition of iodide kinetics during gestation: a physiologically-based pharmacokinetic analysis of perchlorate and iodide kinetics in the rat. *Toxicol Sci* **73:** 235–55.

Clewell RA, Merrill EA, Gearhart JM, Robinson PJ, Sterner TR, Mattie DR, Clewell HJ III (2007) Perchlorate and radioiodide kinetics across life stages in the human: using PBPK models to predict dosimetry and thyroid inhibition and sensitive subpopulations based on developmental stage. *J Toxicol Environ Health* A **70:** 408–28.

Clewell RA, Kremer JJ, Williams CC, Campbell JL Jr, Andersen ME, Borghoff SJ (2008) Tissue exposures to free and glucuronidated monobutylyphthalate in the pregnant and fetal rat following exposure to di-n-butylphthalate: evaluation with a PBPK model. *Toxicol Sci* **103(2):** 241–59.

Corley RA, Mast TJ, Carney EW, Rogers JM, Daston GP (2003). Evaluation of physiologically based models of pregnancy and lactation for their application in children's health risk assessments. *Crit Rev Toxicol* **33:** 137–211.

Emond C, Birnbaum LS, DeVito MJ (2004) Physiologically based pharmacokinetic model for developmental exposures to TCDD in the rat. *Toxicol Sci* **80(1):** 115–33.

Faber WD, Roberts LS, Stump DG, Tardif R, Krishnan K, Tort M, Dimond S, Dutton D, Moran E, Lawrence W (2006) Two generation reproduction study of ethylbenzene by inhalation in Crl-CD rats. *Birth Defects Res B Dev Reprod Toxicol* **77(1):** 10–21.

Farris FF, Dedrick RL, Allen PV, Smith JC (1993) Physiological model for the pharmacokinetics of methyl mercury in the growing rat. *Toxicol Appl Pharmacol* **119(1):** 74–90.

Fisher J, Mahle D, Bankston L, Greene R, Gearhart J (1997) Lactational transfer of volatile chemicals in breast milk. *Am Ind Hyg Assoc J* **58(6):** 425–31.

Fisher JW, Whittaker TA, Taylor DH, Clewell HJ 3rd, Andersen ME (1989) Physiologically based pharmacokinetic modeling of the pregnant rat: a multiroute exposure model for trichloroethylene and its metabolite, trichloroacetic acid. *Toxicol Appl Pharmacol* **99(3):** 395–414.

Fisher JW, Whittaker TA, Taylor DH, Clewell HJ 3rd, Andersen ME (1990) Physiologically based pharmacokinetic modeling of the lactating rat and nursing pup: a multiroute exposure model for trichloroethylene and its metabolite, trichloroacetic acid. *Toxicol Appl Pharmacol* **102(3):** 497–513.

Gabrielsson JL, Groth T (1998) An extended physiological pharmacokinetic model of methadone disposition in the rat: validation and sensitivity analysis. *J Pharmacokinet Biopharm* **16(2):** 183–201.

Gabrielsson JL, Johansson P, Bondesson U, Paalzow LK (1985) Analysis of methadone disposition in the pregnant rat by means of a physiological flow model. *J Pharmacokinet Biopharm* **13(4):** 355–72.

Gabrielsson JL, Paalzow LK, Nordström L (1984) A physiologically based pharmacokinetic model for theophylline disposition in the pregnant and nonpregnant rat. *J Pharmacokinet Biopharm* **12(2):** 149–65.

Gabrielsson JL, Paalzow LK (1983) A physiological pharmacokinetic model for morphine disposition in the pregnant rat. *J Pharmacokinet Biopharm* **11(2):** 147–63.

Gargas ML, Tyler TR, Sweeney LM, Corley RA, Weitz KK, Mast TJ, Paustenbach DJ, Hays SM (2000) A toxicokinetic study of inhaled ethylene glycol ethyl ether acetate and validation of a physiologically based pharmacokinetic model for rat and human. *Toxicol Appl Pharmacol* **165:** 63–73.

Gentry PR, Covington TR, Clewell HJ III (2003) Evaluation of the potential impact of pharmacokinetic differences on tissue dosimetry in offspring during pregnancy and lactation. *Regul Toxicol Pharmacol* **38:** 1–16.

Gentry PR, Haber LT, McDonald TB, Zhao Q, Covington T, Nance P, Clewell HJ III, Lipscomb JC (2004) Data for physiologically based pharmacokinetic modeling in neonatal animals: physiological parameters in mice and Sprague–Dawley rats. *J Child Health* **2:** 363–411.

Gray DG (1995) A physiologically based pharmacokinetic model for methyl mercury in the pregnant rat and fetus. *Toxicol Appl Pharmacol* **132(1):** 91–102.

Haddad S, Pelekis M, Krishnan K (1996) A methodology for solving physiologically based pharmacokinetic models without the use of simulation softwares. *Toxicol Lett* **85:** 113–26.

Hays SM, Elswick BA, Blumenthal GM, Welsch F, Conolly RB, Gargas ML (2000) Development of a physiologically based pharmacokinetic model of 2-methoxyethanol and 2-methoxyacetic acid disposition in pregnant rats. *Toxicol Appl Pharmacol* **163(1):** 67–74.

Hissink EM, Bogaards JJP, Freidig AP, Commandeur JNM, Vermeulen NPE, van Bladeren PJ (2002) The use of in vitro metabolic parameters and physiologically based pharmacokinetic (PBPK) modeling to explore the risk assessment of trichloroethylene. *Environ Toxicol Pharmacol* **11:** 259–71.

Kamgang F, Peyret T, Krishnan K (2008) An intergrated QSPR-PBPK modeling approach for the in vitro–in vito extrapolation of pharmacokinetics in rats. *SAR and QSAR in Environ Res* **19(7–8):** 1–12.

Kawamoto Y, Matsuyama W, Wada M, Hishikawa J, Chan MP, Nakayama A, Morisawa S (2007) Development of a physiologically based pharmacokinetic model for bisphenol A in pregnant mice. *Toxicol Appl Pharmacol* **224(2):** 182–91.

Kim CS, Binienda Z, Sandberg JA (1996) Construction of a physiologically based pharmacokinetic model for 2,4-dichlorophenoxyacetic acid dosimetry in the developing rabbit brain. *Toxicol Appl Pharmacol* **136(2):** 250–9.

Krishnan K, Gargas ML, Fennell TR, Andersen ME (1992) A physiologically based description of ethylene oxide dosimetry in the rat. *Toxicol Ind Health* **8:** 121–40.

Krishnan K, Andersen ME (1998) Physiologically based pharmacokinetic models in the risk assessment of developmental neurotoxicants. In *Handbook of Developmental Neurotoxicology* (Slikker W, Chang LW, eds.). San Diego, Academic Press, pp. 709–25.

Krishnan K, Andersen ME (2007) Physiologically based pharmacokinetic and toxicokinetic models. In *Principles and Methods of Toxicology* (Hayes AW, ed.). Boca Raton, CRC Press, pp. 231–92.

Krishnan K, Andersen ME (2010) *Quantitative Modeling in Toxicology*. Wiley, Chichester, UK.

Lipscomb JC, Ohanian GW (2006) *Toxicokinetics and Risk Assessment*. Informa Healthcare, New York.

Luecke RH, Wosilait WD, Pearce BA, Young JF (1995) Mathematical representation of organ growth in the human embryo/fetus. *Int J Bio-Med Comp* **39:** 337–47.

Luecke RH, Wosilait WD, Pearce BA, Young JF (1997) A computer model and program for xenobiotic disposition during pregnancy. *Comput Methods Programs Biomed* **53(3):** 201–24.

MacGregor JT, Collins JM, Sugiyama Y, Tyson CA, Dean J, Smith L, Andersen M, Curren RD, Houston JB, Kadlubar FF, Kedderis GL, Krishnan K, Li AP, Parchment RE, Thummel K, Tomaszewski JE, Ulrich R, Vickers AE, Wrighton SA (2001) In vitro human tissue models in risk assessment: report of a consensus-building workshop. *Toxicol Sci* **59(1):** 17–36.

Maruyama W, Yoshida K, Tanaka T, Nakanishi J (2003) Simulation of dioxin accumulation in human tissues and analysis of reproductive risk. *Chemosphere* **53(4):** 301–13.

Mattison DR, Sandler JD (1994) Summary of the workshop on issues in risk assessment: quantitative methods for developmental toxicology. *Risk Anal* **14:** 595–604.

National Academy of Sciences (2007) *Toxicity Testing in the 21st Century: A Vision and a Strategy*. National Research Council, Washington DC.

Nong A, McCarver DG, Hines RN, Krishnan K (2006) Modeling interchild differences in pharmacokinetics on the basis of subject-specific data on physiology and hepatic CYP2E1 levels: a case study with toluene. *Toxicol Appl Pharmacol* **214(1):** 78–87.

Nong A, Krishnan K (2007) Estimation of interindividual pharmacokinetic variability factor for inhaled volatile organic chemicals using a probability-bounds approach. *Regul Toxicol Pharmacol* **48(1):** 93–101.

O'Flaherty EJ, Nau H, McCandless D, Beliles RP, Schreiner CM, Scott WJ Jr (1995) Physiologically based pharmacokinetics of methoxyacetic acid: dose-effect considerations in C57BL/6 mice. *Teratology* **52(2):** 78–89.

O'Flaherty EJ, Scott W, Schreiner C, Beliles RP (1992) A physiologically based kinetic model of rat and mouse gestation: disposition of a weak acid. *Toxicol Appl Pharmacol* **112(2):** 245–56.

Olanoff LS, Anderson JM (1980) Controlled release of tetracycline – III: A physiological pharmacokinetic model of the pregnant rat. *J Pharmacokinet Biopharm* **8(6):** 599–620.

Price K, Haddad S, Krishnan K (2003a) Physiological modeling of age-specific changes in the pharmacokinetics of organic chemicals in children. *J Toxicol Environ Health* A **66:** 417–33.

Price PS, Conolly RB, Chaisson K, Gross EA, Young JS, Mathis ET, Tedder DR (2003b) Modeling interindividual variation in physiological factors used in PBPK models of humans. *Crit Rev Toxicol* **33:** 469–503.

Quick DJ, Shuler ML (2000) Use of in vitro data for construction of a physiologically based pharmacokinetic model for naphthalene in rats and mice to probe species differences. *Biotechnol Progr* **15:** 540–55.

Reddy MB, Yang RSH, Clewell HJ III, Andersen ME (2005) *Physiologically-based Pharmacokinetic Modelling. Science and Applications.* Wiley Interscience, Hoboken, NJ, 420 pp.

Shelley ML, Andersen ME, Fisher JW (1988) An inhalation distribution model for the lactating mother and nursing child. *Toxicol Lett* **43(1–3):** 23–9.

Terry KK, Elswick BA, Welsch F, Conolly RB (1995) Development of a physiologically based pharmacokinetic model describing 2-methoxyacetic acid disposition in the pregnant mouse. *Toxicol Appl Pharmacol* **132(1):** 103–14.

Thrall KD, Sasser LB, Creim JA, Gargas ML, Kinzell JH, Corley RA (2009) Studies supporting the development of a physiologically based pharmacokinetic (PBPK) model for methyl iodide: pharmacokinetics of sodium iodide (NaI) in pregnant rabbits. *Inhal Toxicol* **21(6):** 519–23.

Van Ommen B, de Jongh J, van de Sandt J, Blaauboer B, Hissink E, Bogaards J, van Bladeren P (1995) Computer-aided biokinetic modelling combined with in vitro data. *Toxicol in Vitro* **9:** 537–42.

Verwei M, van Burgsteden JA, Krul CA, van de Sandt JJ, Freidig AP (2006) Prediction of in vivo embryotoxic effect levels with a combination of in vitro studies and PBPK modelling. *Toxicol Lett* **165:** 79–87.

Ward KW, Blumenthal GM, Welsch F, Pollack GM (1997) Development of a physiologically based pharmacokinetic model to describe the disposition of methanol in pregnant rats and mice. *Toxicol Appl Pharmacol* **145(2):** 311–22.

Welsch F, Blumenthal GM, Conolly RB (1995) Physiologically based pharmacokinetic models applicable to organogenesis: extrapolation between species and potential use in prenatal toxicity risk assessments. *Toxicol Lett* **82–83:** 539–47.

Wosilait WD, Luecke RH, Young JF (1992) A mathematical analysis of human embryonic and fetal growth data. *Growth Dev Aging* **56(4):** 249–57.

Yoon M, Nong A, Clewell HJ 3rd, Taylor MD, Dorman DC, Andersen ME (2009) Evaluating placental transfer and tissue concentrations of manganese in the pregnant rat and fetuses after inhalation exposures with a PBPK model. *Toxicol Sci* **112:** 44–58.

You L, Gazi E, Rchibeque-Engle S, Casanova M, Conolly RB, Heck HA (1999) Transplacental and lactational transfer of p,p′-DDE in Sprague–Dawley rats. *Toxicol Appl Pharmacol* **157:** 134–44.

Young JF, Branham WS, Sheehan DM, Baker ME, Wosilait WD, Luecke RH (1997) Physiological "constants" for PBPK models for pregnancy. *J Toxicol Environ Health* **52:** 385–401.

C H A P T E R

6

Transfer of drugs and xenobiotics through milk

Arturo Anadón, Maria Rosa Martínez-Larrañaga, Eva Ramos and Victor Castellano

INTRODUCTION

Breast milk remains the best source of infant nutrition, but constant surveillance is needed to keep it pure. Breastfeeding offers many advantages to neonates (1 day–1 month) and infants (1 month–2 years), and provides a range of benefits for growth, immunity and development. The composition of human milk varies at different stages of lactation, distinct times of the day, during each feed and even between breasts, contains powerful growth- and immune-enhancing factors, and suckling is considered as the best and only source of nutrition necessary for the infant during the first 6 months of life. Drugs, non-medicinal substances and xenobiotics in milk, if the level is high enough or if the infant is sensitive enough, interact at many possible physiological levels.

Numerous studies have associated breastfeeding with potential medical and social benefits, which include decreased mortality and morbidity in infants from infectious and other diseases (i.e., lower rates of gastrointestinal disease, anemia, respiratory ailments and otitis media), influenced brain development, increased resistance to chronic diseases (e.g., asthma, allergies and diabetes) and decreased incidence of cancer and osteoporosis in the mothers.

The breasts begin to develop at puberty. This development is stimulated by the estrogens of the monthly female sexual cycle. Estrogens stimulate growth of the breasts' mammary glands plus fat is deposited to give the breast mass. In addition, far greater growth occurs during the high estrogenic state of pregnancy, and only then does the glandular tissue become completely developed for the production of milk.

Nursing women also benefit from breastfeeding. Breastfeeding increases maternal levels of oxytocin, resulting in decreased postpartum bleeding uterine involution. The act of breastfeeding is associated with increased maternal infant bonding and maternal sense of fulfillment and self-worth. Increased oxytocin and prolactin in the mother induce feelings of relaxation and well-being.

On the other hand, it is well known that many women require treatments during pregnancy and some of them need to continue treatment postpartum, and wish to breastfeed. Almost all lactating women receive some medications immediately postpartum and during breastfeeding. Women may choose to formulate or interrupt their own drug therapy for fear of exposure of their infant to drugs in their milk. When chronic medications are required by lactating women (e.g., epilepsy and hyperthyroidism), it may be more difficult to discontinue therapy. In these cases, women are more likely (when compared to acute therapy, e.g. therapy with antibiotics) to continue medication and default to formula feeding. The presence of adverse events reported in the literature, or the theoretical risks of adverse events, does not automatically suggest contraindication, although a cautious approach may be required (e.g., monitoring the infant for physical/behavioral changes). Although the majority of medications taken by lactating women have been shown not to cause overt adverse events in the suckling infant, there is diminutive epidemiological data regarding the probability of the adverse effects of maternal drugs on breastfed infants (Anderson *et al.*, 2003).

For drugs, infant dosage is also affected by drug infant clearance, infant suckling pattern, milk composition, maternal dosage, drug half-life, feed timing and the maternal pharmacokinetics. Infant clearance of the drug greatly influences infant plasma concentration. Figure 6.1 shows the drug transfer into milk, the capacity of the infant to eliminate drug and/or resulting consequence of the drug on the infant. Drug clearance is generally decreased in neonates and premature infants, especially in the early neonatal period (Ito and Koren, 1994). It is predicted to be approximately 10% of the maternal clearance in preterm infants, 33% at birth in term infants, increasing to 100% by 6 months (Wojnar-Horton *et al.*, 1997).

This chapter describes the principles of drug transfer mechanisms into milk as well as the potential adverse effects in suckling neonates and infants. Not only are drugs covered, but also non-medicinal substances, drugs of abuse and environmental chemical pollutants which constitute other important groups potentially contaminating human milk. The main principles of drug excretion into breast milk and the different determinants of the age-dependent factors affecting gastrointestinal absorption and the resulting pharmacokinetics outcomes relative to adult levels are discussed. Risk assessment of maternal drug treatment and exposure to the substances or contaminants during breastfeeding are presented but there is lack of data on long-term adverse outcomes in infants.

Reproductive and Developmental Toxicology, Edited by Ramesh C. Gupta
ISBN: 978-0-12-382032-7

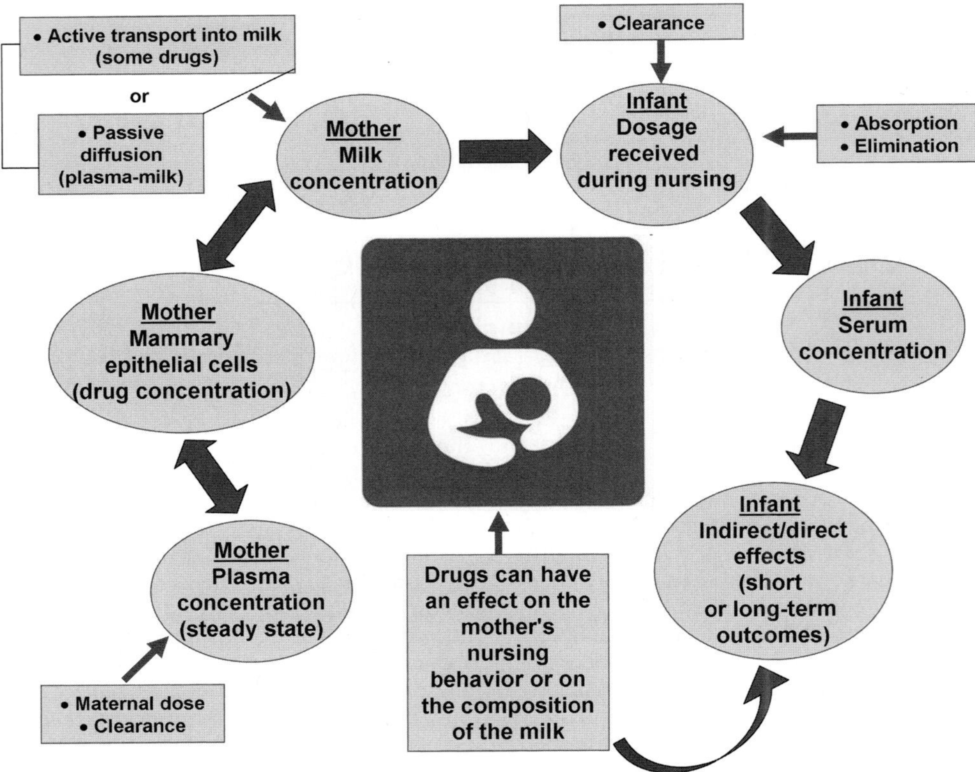

FIGURE 6.1 Infant drug exposure through breastfeeding. Please refer to color plate section.

DRUG EXCRETION INTO BREAST MILK

Maternal pharmacokinetics in the postpartum period

The characteristics of the drug itself, and its absorption, distribution, metabolism and excretion, should be taken into consideration when dealing with drug excretion in milk.

There is a large inter-individual variability in maternal pharmacokinetics during postpartum and various factors influence the capacity of an individual to metabolize drugs. One of the most important factors is the genetically determined oxidative capacity of liver enzymes. For instance, many psychotropic drugs are metabolized by the cytochrome P450 (CYP) enzymes CYP1A2, CYP2C19, CYP2D6 and CYP3A4 (Lacroix *et al.*, 1997). The activities of CYP2C19 and CYP2D6 are bimodally distributed within the population, and an individual can thus be classified as either an "extensive" metabolizer (EM) or a "poor" metabolizer (PM) based on the activity of each of these enzymes. Depending on race, the prevalence of CYP2C19 PMs varies between 4 and 20%, while the prevalence of CYP2D6 PMs varies between 1 and 7% (Lacroix *et al.*, 1997; Kraus *et al.*, 1993). If the mother, the infant or both are PMs and a standard maternal dose of a drug metabolized by the CYP enzyme is given, this will result in a high concentration of drug in the plasma of the breastfed infant, with the associated risk of adverse drug reactions. CYP1A2 and CYP3A4 exhibit considerable inter-individual variation in their activities, although no genetic polymorphisms have been demonstrated. For all isozymes, inhibition may take place during simultaneous treatment with other drugs.

Drug medications interfering with milk production

Drugs including bromocriptine, estradiol, oral contraceptives in large doses, levodopa and the antidepressant trazodone could suppress or inhibit lactation. Contraindicated drugs in this period include anticancer drugs, therapeutic doses of radiopharmaceuticals, ergot and its derivatives (e.g., methysergide), lithium, chloramphenicol, atropine, thiouracil, iodides and mercurials. Those drugs should not be used in nursing mothers or nursing should be stopped if any of these drugs is essential. Other drugs to be avoided in the lack of studies on their excretion in breast milk are: (1) those with long half-lives; (2) those that are potent toxins to the bone marrow; and (3) those given in high doses for the long term. However, drugs that are so poorly absorbed orally that they are given (to the mother) parenterally pose no threat to the infant, who would receive the drug orally but not absorb it.

The American Academy of Pediatrics (2001) addressed some considerations before prescribing drugs to lactating women (Table 6.1).

Drugs that decrease lactation

Although estrogen and progesterone are essential for the physical development of the breast during pregnancy, both

TABLE 6.1 Prescription of drugs to lactating woman

1. Is drug therapy really necessary? If drugs are required, consultation between the pediatrician and the mother's physician can be most useful in determining what options to choose.
2. The safest drug should be chosen, for example acetaminophen rather than aspirin for analgesia.
3. If there is a possibility that a drug may present a risk to the infant, consideration should be given to measurement of blood concentrations in the nursing infant.
4. Drug exposure to the nursing infant may be minimized by having the mother take the medication just after she has breastfed the infant or just before the infant is due to have a lengthy sleep period.

hormones inhibit the secretion of milk. Controversially, the hormone prolactin has exactly the opposite effect on milk, acting on the mother's breasts to keep the mammary glands secreting milk into the alveoli for the subsequent nursing periods (Guyton and Hall, 2006).

The most sensitive time for suppression is early postpartum before the mother's milk supply is established. Waiting as long as possible (weeks to months) prior to use is recommended. All mothers should be informed that in some cases reduced milk supply may result and they should be observed for such changes (Hale, 2003).

Since infant weight gain and development are directly related to milk production, the potential problems associated with reduced milk supply are of much magnitude.

Some medications are well known to decrease lactation. Drugs that may potentially inhibit milk production include estrogens (Sweezy, 1992), progestagens, ergot alkaloids (e.g., bromocriptine, carbergoline and ergotamine), pseudoephedrine (Hale, 2002) and to a slight degree alcohol (Hale, 2002; Neville and Walsh, 1996). The antidepressant bupropion may reduce milk supply and caution is recommended (Briggs *et al.*, 1993).

Drugs that increase lactation

Among the factors that control milk production, the pituitary hormone prolactin is perhaps the most important. The prolactin acts on the mother's breasts to keep the mammary glands secreting milk into the alveoli for subsequent nursing. In addition, the placenta secretes large quantities of human chorionic somatomammotropin, which probably has lactogenic properties, thus supporting the prolactin from the mother's pituitary during pregnancy (Guyton and Hall, 2006). Although prolactin levels must be enhanced in milk, absolute levels of prolactin are not necessarily related to the lactation level (Chatterton *et al.*, 2000). In some mothers with preterm infants, prolactin levels may not be sufficient to support adequate lactation or their ductal tissue has not developed appropriately; in those patients, the most common dopamine antagonists to be used are domperidone, metoclopramide, risperidone and phenothiazine neuroleptics which may stimulate lactation. It is known that dopamine can decrease prolactin secretion by as much as 10-fold. In essence, antenatal prolactin levels are quite high and subsequently over the next 6 months descend significantly almost to normal ranges, even though the quantity of milk production is virtually unchanged (Kauppila *et al.*, 1983; Petraglia *et al.*, 1985).

The breast contains secretory lobules, alveoli and lactiferous ducts (milk ducts) that constitute its mammary gland. The mammary gland secretes milk into the alveoli where there are milk secreting epithelial cells. The milk is secreted continuously into the alveoli of the breast, but milk does not flow easily from the alveoli into the ductal system and, therefore, does not continually leak from the breast nipples. Instead, the milk must be ejected from the alveoli into the ducts before the infant can obtain it. This is caused by a combined neurogenic and hormonal reflex that involves the posterior pituitary hormones oxytocin, as follows (Guyton and Hall, 2006).

Overall, in lactating mothers there are several drugs that should be used with caution and labels should be checked for warnings against use and for special guidelines for nursing mothers: (1) propylthiouracil and phenylbutazone can be given to nursing mothers without any adverse effects on their infants, but methimazole is contraindicated; (2) neuroleptics and antidepressants, sedatives and tranquilizers must be used with caution and the dosing controlled; (3) low dose, single-hormone contraceptives can be used; high dose contraceptives may suppress lactation; (4) metronidazole use depends on the age of the infant and maternal dosing; (5) nursing infants should be closely observed with prolonged use of any drug by their mother to be sure there are no changes in feeding or sleeping patterns; and (6) vaccines are not contraindicated while mothers are lactating.

Passage of medications into the mother's milk and drug transport

Human milk is a biological fluid synthesized in the mammary tissue by cellular mechanisms delicately designed to provide the infant with the precise quantitative and qualitative growth- and immune-enhancing factors, while at the same time enhancing mother–child bonding. Drugs and other chemicals transferring into breast milk are determined by factors such as ionization, plasma protein binding, molecular weight, drug lipophilicity and its pharmacokinetics in the mother (Schanker, 1963). Biochemical characteristics of milk including lower pH and higher lipid contents compared to plasma contribute to this phenomenon (Atkinson *et al.*, 1988; Bailey and Ito, 1997). The factors responsible for the transfer of compounds into the milk are listed in Table 6.2.

Drugs pass into milk by five identified pathways. Passive diffusion (appears to account for most of the drugs), carrier mediated transport system and active transport, pinocytosis and reverse pinocytosis (Ito and Alcorn, 2003). It is presumed that the body is a single compartment and the blood is distributed in the compartment uniformly. An important characteristic of the drug is the volume of distribution (V_d) which can be calculated (V_d is the total amount of drug in the body/concentration of drug in the plasma). Thus, drugs with a large volume of distribution do not get into the breast milk in any amount as compared to drugs with a low volume of distribution which enter into the milk from the plasma in higher quantities.

The usual route is probably transcellular diffusion, in which small molecules (molecular weight 100–200) are dragged along with water flow (hydrostatic or osmotic pressure differences). Compounds of a larger molecular weight might enter into the milk through intercellular diffusion,

TABLE 6.2 Transfer of drugs into breast milk

Drug pharmacokinetics in mother is affected by	
Plasma protein binding	Drugs with high plasma protein binding are less likely to be transferred into breast milk.
Ionization	Most drugs are weak acids or bases that are present in solution as both non-ionized and ionized species. The non-ionized molecules are usually lipid soluble and can diffuse across the milk–plasma membrane.
Acidity	Basic drugs are more likely to be transferred into breast milk due to milk being more acidic (pH 6.8–7.2) than plasma (pH 7.4). *Acid drugs*: barbiturates, diuretics (chlorothiazide, hydrochlorothiazide), non-steroidal anti-inflammatory agents (NSAIDs), penicillins, phenytoin, sulfonamides. *Basic drugs*: alkaloids, antidepressants, antihistamines, antipsychotics, erythromycin, isoniazid, lincomycin, lithium, metronidazole, quinine, thiouracil.
Degree of lipophilicity	Milk contains more lipid than plasma, thus drugs with high lipid solubility tend to be concentrated in breast milk.
Molecular weight	The lower the molecular weight, the more easily the drugs will be transferred.

thus avoiding the alveolar cell entirely. The molecular shape will also determine its passage. Passive diffusion could occur from interstitial water from the base of the cell. Ionophore diffusion might facilitate the transfer of charged ions and other substances that might be bound to carrier proteins. Lipid soluble substances, as well as non-ionized compounds, are readily transported; the lipid soluble substances of a small molecular weight and no electrical charge will appear in milk at concentrations very similar to the simultaneous maternal plasma concentration (e.g., ethyl alcohol) (Kesaniemi, 1974).

The drug characteristics to be considered significant include: route of administration, absorption rate, half-life or peak serum time, dissociation constant and volume of distribution. So, the transfer of a drug is influenced by the molecule size, its ionization and the pH of the substrate (i.e., plasma, milk), the solubility in water and in lipids, and the protein binding. The non-ionized fraction of any molecule is transferred rapidly across the milk–plasma membrane; the concentration of weak bases in milk tends to be higher than that of weak acids. Moreover, the concentrations of weak bases tend to be higher in milk with a low pH than in milk with a high pH.

The solubility of a compound in water and in lipid is a conclusive factor for its transfer throughout lactation. This is an important peculiarity because the alveolar and epithelial layer of the breast is a lipid barrier that is most permeable in the first few days of lactation, when colostrum is being produced.

Not all drugs enter into the breast milk (e.g., insulin and epinephrine). Caffeine and theophylline are not well excreted and may be accumulated by the infant, causing hyperirritability. Other limitations to mothers are alcohol intake, which should be limited to no more than 0.5 g/kg body weight/day, and refraining from smoking during breastfeeding – mothers should not breastfeed infants within 2 h of smoking.

Drug milk-to-plasma (M/P) ratio

The excretory properties of a drug into breast milk are often presented as the comparison between drug concentrations in a mother's milk and that simultaneously in plasma, called the M/P ratio. Equations have been formulated to predict infant dose using the M/P ratio, which if not known can be predicted utilizing pK_A, plasma protein binding and octanol/water partition coefficients, and estimated infant clearance of the drug.

The same assumptions should be applied to excretion of drugs in breast milk. Since milk is more acidic than plasma, basic compounds may be slightly concentrated in this fluid, and the concentration of acidic compounds in the milk is lower than in plasma. Non-electrolytes (e.g., ethanol, urea) readily enter breast milk and reach the same concentration as in plasma, independent of the pH of milk (Atkinson *et al.*, 1988).

The maternal drug plasma concentration is an important determinant of how much drug is available for excretion into milk. Because diffusion occurs along a concentration gradient, high maternal plasma/serum levels will produce high milk levels. The drug serum/plasma concentration is determined not only by the maternal dose but also by ability of the mothers to metabolize the drug. The ability to metabolize a drug is genetically determined, so there are "poor" or "slow" drug metabolizers in a given population. The ratio of "poor/slow" to "normal" metabolizers might be as high as 1–10 for some substances, so drug concentrations in milk in these subjects will be much higher than predicted (Berlin, 2004).

The daily amount of milk consumed by an infant is about 150 ml/kg/day. Many scientists use this value to estimate the weight-adjusted dose consumed by a nursing infant, to make a prediction on the relative safety of a drug during breastfeeding.

Ion trapping might occur during the transfer of a drug from maternal plasma to milk. Breast milk is slightly acidic as compared to plasma, so the acid/base characteristics of a drug as mentioned previously are of importance. All acid–base chemicals exist in equilibrium between their ionized and non-ionized forms. This equilibrium is an important determinant of how much drug can be reached in milk (e.g., the equilibrium for acidic drugs will favour ionization in the relatively alkaline plasma and, thus, less will be available for transport into milk). When transport does occur, the equilibrium obtained in milk will favour the non-ionized form because of the relatively acidic milk, so the drug will be transported back into the plasma. This reverse "ion trapping" in plasma for acidic drugs will, in general, result in drug M/P ratios of <1.0.

The contrary is true for basic drugs. In this case, the relatively acidic milk shifts the equilibrium to the ionized form, thereby trapping the drug and producing drug M/P ratios of >1.0.

Beardmore *et al.* (2002) made a compilation of studies examining the transfer of antihypertensive medications to breast milk. The M/P concentration ratio is used to compare the studies as a method of correlating the data (Bailey and Ito, 1977) using the following criteria: (1) an M/P ratio >1.0 indicates that the concentration of the drug in breast milk is greater than that in the maternal plasma, indicating that the drug is freely excreted into breast milk; (2) an M/P ratio of 0.5–1.0 indicates some excretion; (3) M/P <0.5 indicates limited excretion; and (4) an M/P <0.1 indicates none or negligible. The data compilation found that the M/P ratios varied widely across the beta-blocker family, the beta-blockers with low protein binding having the highest M/P ratios. The angiotensin-converting enzyme (ACE) inhibitors, methyldopa and some calcium blockers had low M/P ratios. The data available indicate that AEC inhibitors, metyldopa and beta-blockers all appear to be safe treatment of hypertension in a nursing mother (Beardmore *et al.*, 2002).

Most drugs for which data are available have a milk to-plasma ratio of ≤1; about 25% have ratios of >1 and about 15% have ratios of >2 (Ito and Koren, 1994). Although an appropriately derived M/P ratio is useful for understanding the amount of the drug in breast milk, its importance is often overemphasized. For instance, a ratio of >1 indicates that the drug is concentrated in breast milk, but this information may be clinically irrelevant (Ito, 2000).

Because the milk concentrations for most drugs are less than or equal to the maternal plasma concentration, the total exposure of the nursing infant is usually <1% of the maternal dose (Berlin, 2004). It is important to stress that these data are mostly from studies using a single maternal dose and do not reflect the quantitative transport in mothers on chronic drug therapy with steady-state plasma concentrations.

Drug dose received by the infant (level of exposure)

The M/P ratio for drugs has been studied for an important number of medications. The M/P ratio compares drug concentration in breast milk simultaneously with the maternal plasma. It assumes that the relationship between the two remains constant, but in most cases it does not. Thus, the M/P ratio is often calculated from the average concentrations in the blood and milk over a longer period of several hours. These average concentrations are the area under the respective concentration curves (area under curve, or AUC), which are constructed from individual concentrations. This calculation is preferred due to the M/P values they establish and are more representative.

Nevertheless, there are considerable variations in the M/P ratios calculated, not only between different studies and subjects, but also in the same mother; the colostrum has different concentrations than the milk some weeks later, and the first milk of a breastfeed is different from a sample taken later in the same feed. Colostrum is the fluid secreted during the last few days before parturition and the first few days after parturition and contains essentially the same concentration of proteins and lactose as milk, but it has almost no fat, and its maximum rate of production is about 1/100 the subsequent rate of milk production (Guyton and Hall, 2006). M/P ratio is a time-dependent parameter, influenced by factors such as maternal pharmacokinetics and compositional changes of milk. It has been proposed that the ratio can be predicted from the physicochemical characteristics of the drug that is mainly transferred into milk by passive diffusion (Atkinson and Begg, 1990; Fleisaker *et al.*, 1987).

The M/P ratio is not suitable for comparison of drug risks. An M/P ratio of 1.0 assumes that the levels are the same in both plasma and milk. The clinical significance of M/P ratios is often misunderstood; for example, an M/P ratio of ≥1 can suggest a misleadingly high potential for adverse effects in the nursing infant, but if plasma levels are trivial, milk levels are as well (Lawrence and Schaefer, 2007). For instance, if isoniazid is given to the mother at therapeutic dosage, plasma concentration is typically 6 μg/ml. If the M/P ratio is 1, an infant consuming 240 ml of milk will ingest only 1.4 mg/feeding, much less than the infant dose for isoniazid (i.e. 10–20 mg/kg). Thus, problems are uncommon unless milk concentrations are high or a drug is highly potent or toxic even in low concentrations or has cumulative effects because of the infant's immature drug metabolizing and excretion capacities.

Low M/P ratios of <1 indicate that there is no accumulation in the breast milk. However, significant concentrations in the milk can be reached even with low M/P ratios when there is a high maternal plasma value. On the other hand, relevant or even toxic amounts of drug cannot necessarily be assumed from a high M/P ratio with those drugs where the concentration in the maternal serum is very limited because of a high volume of distribution typical for the particular drug. In such a case, even an M/P ratio of 8, which indicates a relative accumulation in the milk compared to the maternal plasma, means only a limited concentration of the medication in the milk, and consequently only a limited relative dosage.

Amount of medication in milk and relative dose

If the concentration of a drug in breast milk over time is known, it can estimate the amount of the drug which the infant would consume via the milk per unit of time by assuming intake of a specific amount of milk (e.g., 150 ml/kg body weight/day) (Ito, 2000).

The amount of milk produced daily is between 500 and 900 ml. This amount is achieved about 4 days after birth. As basis for calculation, the average daily amount per kg body weight that the infant takes in, rather than the individual total amount of milk consumed, is used. An average infant receives about 150 ml/kg per day. If, for example, the milk concentration of a drug is 50 μg/l, the breastfed infant receives: 50 μg/l × 0.15 l/kg daily = 7.5 μg/kg daily (Lawrence and Schaefer, 2007).

Exposure index

This estimated dose is then compared with the therapeutic doses of the drug and expressed in terms of the exposure index, which is directly proportional to the M/P ratio and inversely proportional to the rate of infant drug clearance. This parameter is indicative of the amount of the drug in the breast milk that the infant ingests and is expressed as a percentage of the therapeutic (or equivalent) dose for the infant.

"Exposure index" has been proposed as a concept linking M/P ratio, milk intake and the infant drug clearance to a time-averaged drug exposure level of the breastfed infant:

$$\text{Exposure index}\,(\%) = 100 \times \text{M/P ratio} \times A\,/\,\text{infant drug clearance}$$

where A is milk intake (150 ml/kg/day = 0.1 ml/kg/min), and clearance is expressed as ml/kg/min (Ito, 2000; Ito and Koren, 1994).

This parameter is conceptually equivalent to the infant drug dose in milk that is expressed as a percentage of the infant therapeutic dose (i.e., established or theoretical). Alternatively, it can be viewed as a mean steady-state serum drug concentration of the breastfed infant (which is achieved after exposure to the drug in milk) expressed as a percentage of the corresponding therapeutic serum level (i.e., established or theoretical). Because of its hyperbolic relation to infant drug clearance, the "exposure index" becomes very high at a low clearance (e.g., 1 ml/kg/min) (Ito and Koren, 1994). Also, M/P ratio may have substantial impact on the exposure level, if the infant drug clearance is sufficiently low. Hence, both the mechanisms governing drug transfer into milk and infant pharmacokinetics including drug clearance are important determinants of the exposure levels.

Since the M/P ratio and the rate of clearance specify a hyperbolic function that defines an exposure infant level, then drugs with low rates of clearance are likely to result in a higher level of exposure and also large variations in those levels, depending on the M/P ratio. On the other hand, if the clearance rate of the drug is sufficiently high, even a high M/P ratio will not result in a substantial level of exposure, and changes in the rate of drug clearance and the M/P ratio will have less influence on exposure levels. For the infant, the drug clearance rate is more important in determining the degree of exposure than is the drug M/P ratio.

For most drugs, the dose below which there is no clinical effect in infants is unknown. This uncertainty can be overcome by arbitrarily defining as safe a value of no more than 10% of the therapeutic dose for infants (or the adult dose standardized by weight if the therapeutic dose for infants is unknown) (Bennett, 1996). If the dose received in breast milk is <10% of the therapeutic dose, or if the exposure index is <10%, the degree of exposure to the drug in breast milk is considered clinically not relevant. However, there are exceptions to this approach (e.g., in infants with glucose-6-phosphate dehydrogenase deficiency, in whom drug-induced hemolysis may occur at very low plasma concentrations of certain drugs).

Relative dose

Relative dose is the proportion of the maternal dosage per kg body weight that the breastfed infant takes in from the milk per kg of his/her body weight (i.e., the percentage of the maternal weight-related dosage):

$$\text{Relative dosage}\,(\%) = \frac{\text{dosage via mother's milk/kg}}{\text{maternal dosage/kg}} \times 100$$

Assuming that the maternal daily drug dosage is 150 mg (=150,000 μg), the mother weighs 60 kg and the infant takes in 7.5 μg/kg daily, then the relative dosage is:

$$\text{Relative dosage}\,(\%) = \frac{7.5\ \mu\text{g/kg daily}}{150{,}000\ \mu\text{g daily}/60} \times 100 = 0.3\,\%$$

Compared to the M/P ratio, the "relative dose" is more appropriate for estimating the exposure risk for the child via breast milk because it considers the distribution volume of the drug (Lawrence and Schaefer, 2007).

DRUG DISPOSITION IN THE INFANT

Postnatal changes in body composition, extent of the binding to plasma proteins and tissue components, and hemodynamic factors (cardiac output, tissue perfusion and membrane permeability) may alter distribution characteristics in the developing infant. The apparent volume of distribution (V_d) provides a useful marker to assess age-related changes in drug distribution. Developmental changes in V_d may also relate to postnatal enhancements in hemodynamic parameters, changes in membrane permeabilities and maturation of carrier-mediated transport systems and changes in tissue binding affinities or capacities since newborns and young infants have significantly greater liver, kidney and brain masses relative to total body mass (Assael, 1982; Alcorn and McNamara, 2003).

The drug parameters and the dose in serum of the mother, the level in the milk, and the infant characteristics are essential. The exposure of a suckling infant to a drug is not only related to the dose ingested, but is also dependent on the drug kinetics in the infant. The age and maturity of the infant is therefore a critical factor to take into account in the risk–benefit assessment of drug exposure through breast milk.

The volume of distribution of drugs may change rapidly during the neonatal period due to alterations in total body water content and changes in protein binding. Several drugs are less bound to plasma proteins in neonates than in adults, which is most likely due to qualitative and quantitative differences in albumin and to the displacement of the drug from binding sites by endogenous substances such as bilirubin (Morselli *et al.*, 1980). Because the blood–brain barrier is not fully developed in neonates, drug passage into the CNS is generally facilitated.

The infant dose will vary depending on the maturity of hepatic and renal function, the time of breastfeeding post-maternal dosing, and the maternal metabolic rate.

Gastrointestinal biotransformation and transport in the newborn and infant

Bacterial flora, mainly located in the ileum and colon, may influence the extent of drug absorption due to its influence on gastrointestinal motility and ability to metabolize compounds. At birth, infant gastrointestinal flora is very immature and little information is available on the effect of postnatal maturation of bacterial flora on bioavailability (Simon and Gorbach, 1984; Anadón *et al.*, 2010). In general, the bacterial flora of the infant gastrointestinal tract approaches adult populations by 4 years of age.

The proximal small intestine is the main absorptive site and site for significant first-pass effects for many orally administered compounds. In the adult, the small intestinal mucosa functionally expresses a limited number of phase I and phase II enzymes and their expression has led to significant inter- and intra-individual variability in oral drug bioavailability (Obach *et al.*, 2001). Cytochrome P450 (CYP) 3A4 is the predominant CYP enzyme expressed in enterocytes, and CYP2C has the second highest expression levels (Zhang *et al.*, 1999). Very low activity levels for CYP1A1 and CYP2D6 were detected in intestinal microsomes (Madani *et al.*, 1999).

Little is known about the developmental changes in drug absorption from the gastrointestinal tract. The absorption from the gastrointestinal tract of the infant is dependent on the drug bioavailability, the effect of gastric pH and gastric enzymes and the presence of food. In most cases, irregular motility and slow gastric emptying may affect the rate, but not the degree, of drug absorption (Morselli *et al.*, 1980).

Hepatic biotransformation in the fetus and neonate

Each liver enzyme system matures at a different rate in the developing infant. Thus, different substrates are metabolized at different points in maturation. The activities of the hepatic biotransformation enzymes are low in the neonate, particularly in premature neonates.

The various liver enzyme systems in the liver mature at different rates in the developing infant. There are two examples: (1) while glucuronyl transferase activity is mature enough to metabolize bilirubin 3 days after term, it cannot safely degrade chloramphenicol until at least day 10. Hepatic enzyme immaturity is even more pronounced in premature infants. Premature and full-term infants have a diminished capacity to metabolize medications for at least the first 2 weeks of life; (2) a reduced capacity to form hydroxylated derivatives of diazepam, together with a relatively good ability to demethylate the drug, has been observed in both pre- and full-term neonates (Morselli, 1976; Morselli *et al.*, 1980).

In neonates, the ability to perform conjugation reactions is impaired to an even greater extent than the oxidative metabolic capacity. Drugs that form glucuronides without any major alternative metabolic pathway, such as oxazepam, have elimination half-lives that are 3 to 4 times longer in neonates than in adults. Although the glucuronide conjugation system generally is thought to mature very slowly, a full-term neonate seems to be able to handle oxazepam efficiently less than 1 week postnatally (Morselli, 1976; Kanto, 1982).

Reduced conjugating activity contributes to hyperbilirubinemia and the risk of bilirubin-induced encephalopathy. It is also the basis for the increased toxicity in the neonate of drugs such as chloramphenicol and certain opioids. A poorly developed blood–brain barrier, weak biotransformation activity and immature mechanisms for excretion combine to make the fetus and neonate very vulnerable to toxic effects of drugs. The capacity for biotransformation increases during the early months of postnatal life, although the pattern for different enzymes is variable. Cytochrome P450 enzymes are usually near adult activities after a few months, whereas phase II enzymes develop more slowly.

At a given intake and a concentration of drug in milk, lower clearance causes higher drug exposure levels of the breastfed infant. Overall, clearance values are lower in neonates and young infants due to immaturity of drug elimination systems, although variations exist between drugs in their development patterns of clearance because the ontogeny of each elimination system has its own time profile of development.

Renal excretion

The anatomical and functional immaturity of the newborn kidney leads to reduced renal clearances of compounds during the early postnatal period. Differences in the rate of development of glomerular filtration and tubular transport function and the potential for the induction or inhibition of renal glomerular and tubule transport function (van den Anker *et al.*, 1995) may have variable and complex effects on renal elimination (Alcorn and McNamara, 2003).

Between 28 and 34 weeks of gestational age, the glomerular filtration rate (GFR) is approximately 25% that of the rate in adults. Thereafter, GFR gradually increases, until adult values are reached by 2 to 5 months of age. Tubular function is even more impaired in neonates compared with adults, and reduced tubular function may persist up until 6 to 9 months of age (Morselli *et al.*, 1980; Blumer and Reed, 1992). However, renal excretion is of minor importance, for instance in the elimination of psychotropic drugs, with the exception of lithium.

While the ratio of kidney weight to body mass in infants is twice that in adults, the newborn kidney is functionally immature. With a glomerular filtration rate only 30–40% of adult values and tubular secretion 20–30% of adult function, renal excretion is considerably diminished. Consequently, compounds eliminated through the kidney tend to accumulate in the infant, causing toxic exposure over time. For full-term infants, the glomerular filtration rate seen in adults is achieved between the second and fifth months of life (Murray and Segar, 1994).

Immune system in neonates

Breast milk contains several components that provide specific immunity and affect the maturation of the infant's immune system. Between those components protecting the infant against infections there are antibodies, viable lymphocytes, lactoferrin (an iron-chelating protein), lysozyme and oligosaccharides (Goldman, 1993) as well as several cytokines and chemokines (Böttcher, 2000). For newborns, the immune system is not fully developed and is influenced by maternal immunity, both transplacentally and via the breast milk.

Drug passage into the central nervous system

Since the newborn blood–brain barrier (BBB) is also immature, lipid soluble agents can be 10–30 times more concentrated in the CSF than in serum and may be higher in infants for a given plasma concentration compared to adults. Because body fat storage sites are limited in the neonate, central nervous system (CNS) concentrations of lipid soluble substances are greater in newborns than in older infants (Mortola, 1989).

There is a special concern about the vulnerability of the developing CNS. This concern with exogenous substances in the infant's formula is not confined only to breast milk. A recent example of this is the addition of long-chain polyunsaturated fatty acids, such as arachidonic acid (ARA) and docosahexaenoic acid (DHA), to commercial formulas;

the recommendations of these long-chain polyunsaturated fatty acids in pregnancy, lactating period and first year of life have been reviewed recently (e.g., a supplemented amount of 0.5% DHA commercial formulas for infants should not be exceeded due to the long effect of these doses) (Campoy *et al.*, 2010).

DRUGS THAT SHOULD BE USED WITH CAUTION

Analgesics

Analgesics are the most commonly used medications in breastfeeding mothers (e.g., ibuprofen, ketorolac, naproxen, indomethacin, morphine, methadone, meperidine and fentanyl). Of the NSAID family, ibuprofen and ketorolac are perhaps ideal agents, with low relative infant doses (<0.6%). The short-term use of naproxen is suitable, although bleeding, hemorrhage and acute anemia were reported in a 7-day-old infant.

Narcotic analgesics (e.g., codeine, morphine, meperidine and methadone) in therapeutic doses in the treatment of opiate addiction can be excreted in breast milk at very low concentrations that minimally affect infants in single doses because they are used in pregnant patients. However, in mothers taking repeated doses, particularly when they are narcotic addicts using high doses, significant amounts are excreted in milk, affecting the breastfed infants and causing withdrawal symptoms when a feeding is missed. For that reason, chronic narcotic users should not breastfeed. Methadone concentrations in breast milk ranged from 27 to 260 g/L in patients receiving 25 to 180 ml/day (McCarthy and Posey, 2000). Morphine does not appear in high concentrations in breast milk and the published data vary. Codeine and hydrocodone are most commonly used opiate analgesics in breastfeeding mothers and codeine produces sedation and apnea; the relative infant dose is 1.4% (Bennett, 1996). Meperidine is used in the perinatal period and is obstetrical; it is metabolized to normeperidine (half-life, 62–73 hours). Small but significant amounts of parent and metabolite are transferred into breast milk and produce changes in neurocognitive function (Wittels *et al.*, 1990). Low-dose methadone therapy (20 mg/day) does not pose an appreciable risk to breastfed infants. Among breastfeeding women who are receiving more that 20 mg/day, methadone concentrations should be monitored in breast milk and plasma of infants (Ito, 2000). However, because the absolute dose received by the infant is dependent on the maternal dose rate, the risk–benefit ratio should be considered for each individual case. High doses of methadone (> 40 mg daily) received via milk are unlikely to be sufficient to prevent the neonate abstinence syndrome (Begg *et al.*, 2001).

Hale (2003) reported that the residues of newer COX2 inhibitors, such as celecoxib and valdecoxib, are quite low in the breast milk (<200 μg/l). These may prove to be useful and suitable alternatives to the older NSAIDs.

Antibiotics

One of the most common classes of medications used in breastfeeding mothers are antibiotics. The vast majority of antibiotics have been studied and data levels in breast milk are available. Antibiotics generally can be taken by nursing mothers without significant adverse effects on their infants. However, because almost all antibiotics are excreted in milk, infants may rarely develop hypersensibility, diarrhea or candidiasis. In general, for neonates the only reported side effects include occasional changes in gut flora, although these are rare. Practically all of the penicillins and cephalosporins produce only trace levels in breast milk. Some changes in infant intestinal flora could be expected.

Usually the concentration of tetracyclines in breast milk is low. The bioavailability of these products is poor in milk due to their precipitation by calcium in milk (i.e., chelation); absorption by nursing infants is generally too low to cause adverse effects. However, lipophilic drugs such as minocycline and doxycycline are greatly absorbed orally and not affected by food. Short-term administration of these compounds for up to 3 weeks is permissible. By contrast, long-term use, such as for acne, is not recommended in breastfeeding mothers (Hale, 2003).

The fluoroquinolones are somewhat controversial. Although the dose received via breast milk is far too low to induce artropathy, pseudomembranous colitis (which can occur with any antibiotic) has been reported (Anadón and Martínez-Larrañaga, 1992). Studies undertaken with new fluoroquinolones suggest that ofloxacin concentrations in breast milk are probably lowest, although ciprofloxacin has been approved for use in breastfeeding mothers. Nalidixic acid, sulfonamides and other oxidant drugs can cause hemolysis in G6PD-deficient infants whether breastfed or not (Giamarellou *et al.*, 1989). In addition cyprofloxacin may have metabolic interactions with other drugs (Anadón *et al.*, 1990).

Metronidazole is a commonly used antimicrobial in pediatric patients and is significantly excreted in breast milk. Relative infant doses are moderate, approximately 9–13% of the maternal dose. High maternal oral doses may potentially generate high levels in breast milk. In these patients, a brief interruption of breastfeeding is recommended for 12 to 24 h. Following an oral dose of 400 mg three times daily, C_{max} concentrations in breast milk average 15.5 mg/l (Passmore *et al.*, 1988).

Erythromycin and azithromycin levels in breast milk are quite low. Erythromycin doses of 2 g daily produce milk levels varying from 1.6 to 3.2 mg/l of milk (Knowles, 1972).

Acyclovir levels in breast milk are also low, and the oral bioavailability in an infant is likely low as well (Taddio *et al.*, 1994).

The use of antifungals (e.g., nistatin, miconazol, fluconazole) in breastfeeding mothers is increasing. The transfer of fluconazole is reported to be approximately 12% of the maternal dose, still considerably less than the clinical dose commonly used in neonates. While there are some risks of elevated liver enzymes, none have been reported following exposure to fluconazole in breast milk (Livingston and Stringer, 1999).

Cardiovascular drugs

Atenolol, a beta-blocking agent used to control hypertension, is mainly eliminated through glomerular filtration. There is a case report of significant beta-blockade in a neonate breastfed by a woman on atenolol after delivery (Schimmel *et al.*, 1989). Atenolol is also known to accumulate in milk (M/P ratio of ≈2). In addition to its relatively high excretion into milk, immaturity of renal function of infant was probably one of the contributing factors to toxicity in this case.

Propranolol, digitalis, metoprolol, captopril and diuretics that are slightly acidic have low concentrations in milk.

Steroidal hormonal drugs

Hormones, when given to nursing mothers in large doses, can achieve high concentrations in milk, which represents a hazard to those hormones that can be orally absorbed by the infant.

Ethinyl estradiol and mestranol are also excreted into breast milk. They can reduce milk production and also reduce levels of pyridoxine (vitamin B_6) in the milk.

Corticosteroids, when given to the mother in large doses for weeks or months, can achieve high concentrations in milk and risk suppressing growth and interfering with endogenous corticosteroid production in the infant. A few days of treatment, however, are apparently safe, and the infant is automatically weaned off them as the mother decreases her dose.

Antiepileptics

Barbiturates and phenytoin in nursing mothers can induce microsomal oxidizing enzymes in infants, enhancing the degradation of endogenous steroids, but in small maternal doses are usually safe.

Psychoactive drugs

This is a concern, especially for psychoactive medications, even without apparent immediate clinical effects. Without the data, it is impossible to interpret and assess clinical significance of any amounts of drug excreted into milk and ingested by the infant. Although all psychotropic drugs that have been studied are excreted into breast milk, there is limited information on the practical impact of the, often very low, milk level found (Spigset and Hägg, 1998).

Sedatives and hypnotics

Most of the benzodiazepine anxiolytics have been studied in breastfeeding mothers. Levels of diazepam, lorazepam and midazolam are quite low and are not of concern for infants. Diazepam excreted in breast milk, with multiple maternal doses, can cause lethargy, drowsiness and loss of weight in breastfed infants. For infants, metabolism of diazepam is slow. Since diazepam, after initial metabolism, is conjugated with glucuronic acid, competition with bilirubin for glucuronic acid may predispose infants <1 month to hyperbilirubinemia. The use of phenothiazine sedatives (e.g., promethazine, chlorpromazine) may increase sleep apnea (Kahn *et al.*, 1985) and the risk of sudden infant death syndrome (Cantu, 1989); these substances should be avoided in breastfeeding mothers if possible.

The transfer of phenobarbital is moderate. Maternal plasma levels should be closely monitored and kept in the normal range to prevent higher transfer to the infant. It can be suggested that infant plasma levels are approximately 30–40% of the maternal plasma levels in term infants.

Antidepressants

A high prevalence of psychiatric disease either prenatal or postnatal is present in mothers. Serotonin reuptake inhibitors (SSRIs) are used increasingly in a number of mothers delivering and breastfeeding infants. Early postpartum sleep deprivation and stress are normal and antidepressants are required. Sertraline and paroxetine are transferred into breast milk in minimal quantities and no side effects have been reported in breastfed infants.

Numerous case reports of colic, prolonged crying, vomiting, tremulousness and other symptoms have been reported following the use of fluoxetine in breastfeeding mothers (Hale *et al.*, 2001). Neonatal withdrawal symptoms characterized by poor adaptation, jitteriness, irritability and poor gaze control after pregnancy exposure to selective SSRIs have been reported for fluoxetine, sertraline and paroxetine (Nulman *et al.*, 1997)

Anticoagulants

Warfarin and dicoumarol can be given cautiously to nursing mothers, but at very large doses could cause hemorrhage. In very young infants, dicoumarol can cause hyperbilirubinemia, which might lead to kernicterus. Heparin does not pass into milk. Low molecular weight heparin when used for thromboprophylaxis during pregnancy and puerperium may induce clinically relevant effects on the nursing infant (Richter *et al.*, 2001).

Antihypertensives

The use of antihypertensives in breastfeeding mothers, particularly those with preterm infants, requires a higher degree of care.

Beta-blockers

Beta-blockers and their excretion into breast milk have been the most studied of all the antihypertensive drugs during the lactation period. The level of transfer into breast milk differs markedly among beta-blockers, as they are all weak bases but differ in lipid solubility and protein binding.

The wide-ranging excretory properties of the beta-blocker family into breast milk are consistent with a prediction based on their plasma protein binding. Metoprolol, nadolol, acebutolol, sotalol and atenolol exhibit low protein binding resulting in increased availability of the drug for diffusion into breast milk, whereas oxprenolol, dilevalol, mepindolol and propranolol have high protein binding resulting in low diffusion into breast milk.

Metoprolol, nadolol, acebutolol, sotalol and atenolol have the highest M/P ratios of the beta-blockers, each averaging >1, with reports of M/P ratios as high as 9.2 for acebutolol. This indicates that these drugs are freely excreted into breast milk and therefore will be ingested by the breastfed infant. Several beta-blockers (e.g., atenolol and acebutolol) have produced in breastfed infants the following clinical effects: cyanosis, bradycardia and hypotension (Boutroy *et al.*, 1986). This is because the infant dose (calculated for an infant consuming 1,000 mL of milk per day) is significantly less than the therapeutic dose for children despite the excretion into breast milk. Also, in the studies where the infants were breastfed and the infants' plasma was tested, the drug levels in the plasma were immeasurable or very low except for two case studies, on atenolol and labetalol, where significant levels of these drugs were detected. In contrast, oxprenolol, dilevalol, metoprolol, mepindolol, propranolol and labetalol have lower M/P ratios, indicating greater safety profiles in the breastfeeding mother. When considering which antihypertensive is suitable, it is preferable to choose a beta-blocker with a lower M/P ratio to reduce the risk of beta blockade in the infant. This is particularly relevant if either the mother or infant has impaired renal or hepatic function.

Calcium channel blockers

Based on the limited evidence available on the excretion of calcium channel blockers into breast milk, the dihydropyridines nitrendipine and nimodipine have minimal excretion into breast milk, making them safe for use in a breastfeeding mother. Nifedipine and diltiazem concentration in breast milk is quite low. The M/P ratio of verapamil varied from low to high (Hale, 2003).

Methyldopa

Data on methyldopa indicate limited excretion into breast milk, and therefore it can be concluded that therapeutic maternal doses are safe during lactation (White *et al.*, 1985).

Angiotensin-converting enzyme (ACE) inhibitors

ACE inhibitors are highly potent and potentially dangerous in the early postpartum period, particularly in infants who are borderline hypotensive. These substances should not be used in breastfeeding mothers until their infants can maintain adequate control of their blood pressure. Minimal amounts of ACE inhibitors are transferred into breast milk. They display the lowest M/P ratio of any of the groups of antihypertensive medications, being the safest group of antihypertensive drugs for breastfeeding mothers.

ACE inhibitor protein binding in plasma varies (captopril 30%, enalapril 60%). These values are lower than for the beta-blockers with low M/P ratios, suggesting that protein binding is not the only factor limiting the transfer of ACE inhibitors into breast milk. The concentration in breast milk of enalapril and its active metabolite, enalaprilat, has been compared (Hale, 2002). Enalapril was found to be more efficiently excreted into breast milk than enalaprilat, although both displayed low M/P ratios. ACE activity was found to be normal in breast milk, while maternal serum ACE activity was markedly depressed after treatment with enalapril (Rush *et al.*, 1989).

For the breastfed infant of a mother being treated with a short-acting ACE inhibitor there have been no reports of adverse effects and therefore this is a safe choice of antihypertensive medication during breastfeeding. Data for long-acting ACE inhibitors are not available.

Potential improvement of study of antihypertensive drugs in breastfeeding women

The ideal study would be one in which a standard continuous dose of a drug is administered to a group of women at the same stage of lactation, that is ideally testing at <1 week, 2–3 weeks and 8–12 weeks postpartum. Plasma and milk samples should be taken at the same time, at both the beginning and end of each feed. Samples should be collected hourly for up to 12 h. The area under the concentration–time profiles should be measured over the whole dose interval. Since current data suggest that most antihypertensive medication will not affect the infant, the infant should be breastfed as normal while under close clinical surveillance, and biochemical monitoring should be used to detect the concentration of the drug in the milk and the infant serum concentration of the drug. The concentration of most drugs in breast milk and serum can be accurately determined by high performance liquid chromatography or capillary gas chromatography (Beardmore *et al.*, 2002).

NON-MEDICINAL SUBSTANCES

Illicit drugs

Because most drugs of abuse are neuroleptics, they pass readily into the brain and the breast milk compartment. Most of these drugs are recommended during the interruption of breastfeeding after use. The most dangerous compounds are hallucinogens such as LSD and phencyclidine (also known as PCP or angel dust) (recommended interruption 48 hours and 1–2 weeks, respectively) (Hale, 2003). Mothers who are drug-screen positive for these substances must be strongly warned that these agents are the most dangerous of this group and pose significant hazard to their infants.

Amphetamines and methylphenidate pass into breast milk, but the levels may not be high enough to pose a major hazard to most infants, although this is as yet unclear.

Cocaine-induced toxicity in a 2-week-old infant who was breastfed showed extreme irritability, tremulousness, vomiting and diarrhea (Chasnoff *et al.*, 1987). The child's mother was abusing cocaine intranasally; its residue in breast milk has never been reported. Cocaine undoubtedly enters breast milk avidly, but as yet there are no data.

Marijuana has been studied in moderate smokers. Thus far, neurobehavioral effects on infants have not been reported. Marijuana passes rapidly out of the plasma compartment and enters adipose tissue. Because of this rapid redistribution, levels in breast milk are apparently low (Perez-Reyes and Wall, 1982; Tennes *et al.*, 1985). Exposure to marijuana through breast milk may delay the motor development of infants (Astley and Little, 1990).

Heroin has not been well studied. While it is metabolized to its active metabolite, morphine, and morphine is considered a good analgesic for breastfeeding mothers, the major problem with heroine is the dose. The dose of heroine used by some addicts is extraordinarily large. Hence, levels of morphine in breast milk could be potentially quite high and therefore hazardous. Mothers should be warned that these drugs enter breast milk readily, that their infants will drug-screen positive for weeks and that the dose in breast milk could be potentially fatal in some cases.

Tetrahydrocannabinol, the most psychoactive component of marijuana, is highly bound to lipoproteins, and excretion into breast milk is very low in animals. Yet, nursing mothers should avoid marijuana since the plasma half-life in humans may be as long as 2 days. Cocaine persists in the milk for up to 24h, thus, mothers using either should pump or discard milk for 24h.

ENVIRONMENTAL POLLUTANTS

Maternal exposure to insecticides or to other chemical pollutants is rarely a contraindication to nursing unless the exposure is excessive.

Persistent organic pollutants (POPs) in breast milk

The presence of toxic chemicals in human milk raises a series of important concerns for pediatric practice, for the practice of women's and children's health, and for the environmental health research community, and has also gained attention from national and international regulatory agencies. Landrigan *et al.* (2002) have stated that information on the following is lacking: contaminants, consistent protocols and toxicokinetic data, data on health outcomes and evidence-based health standards. With regard to the lack of toxicokinetic data, it is known that women may be exposed to lipophilic chemicals from various sources including air, food, water and occupational and household environments. Lipophilic chemicals can be stored and accumulated over time in body fat, have the capacity to pass through the placental barrier and into the fetal blood stream, can sometimes reach higher umbilical blood levels than in maternal blood and can also be mobilized into milk during lactation. Generally, chemicals enter breast milk by passive transfer from plasma, and their concentration in milk is proportional to their solubility and lipophilicity. Twenty percent or more of maternal body burden of some persistent pollutants, such as PCBs, can be transferred during 6 months of lactation (Niessen *et al.*, 1984).

The WHO Regional Office for Europe initiated a series of international studies on the concentrations of polychlorinated dioxins (PCDDs), furans (PCDFs) and polychlorinated biphenyls (PCBs) in human milk. The first round of studies took place in 1987–1988, and the health risks to infants were reassessed at a consultation in 1988 on the basis of the results. As the measured intakes found were the first to have been reported for many years and for many countries, the consultation recommended that the studies be repeated at 5-year intervals, in order to define the trends in intake. The second round of studies was performed in 1993, involving 19 countries in which samples could be collected and analytical data produced by the agreed deadline (WHO, 1996). Collection of samples for the third round began in 2000, the bulk of the samples being collected in 2001.

In 1998, the Global Environment Monitoring System, Food Contamination Monitoring and Assessment Programme assessed the risk of selected organochlorine contaminants in breast milk. Data on breast milk levels of DDT complex, hexachlorobenzene (HCB), γ-hexachlorocyclohexane (γ-HCH; lindane), isomeric mixtures of HCH (aldrin and dieldrin) and PCBs indicated that the reported levels of residues in human milk of the HCH isomers aldrin and dieldrin were close to reference intake values. DDT was reported in higher concentrations in developing countries, and HCB levels were high in industrialized countries. The levels of PCBs in breast milk raised greatest concern. In industrialized countries, concentrations exceeded the reference intake of 1 μg/kg of body weight; however, levels over time were stable or only slowly decreased (Pronczuk *et al.*, 2002).

On May 22, 2001, the USA and 119 other nations signed an international treaty in Stockholm (known also as "Stockholm Convention") to phase out use and production of 12 POPs worldwide (i.e., aldrin, chlordane, DDT, dieldrin, endrin, hepatchlor, HCB, mirex, toxaphene, PCBs, PCDDs and PCDFs) and established a procedure to add other chemicals to the list of banned pollutants. The treaty also promotes action to minimize the release of biologically persistent industrial by-products such as dioxins and furans. Over the last several decades, individual nations have banned certain chemicals, effectively reducing the threat that these chemicals pose. For example, the USA has banned DDT and PCBs. Countries that have banned certain POPs are likely to have lower levels of pollutants in mother's milk. However, even with the signing of the treaty, newly emerging hazards such as polybrominated diphenyl ethers (PBDEs) and nonyl phenols must be monitored (Hooper and McDonald, 2000). POPs are chemical substances that remain intact in the environment for long periods, become widely distributed geographically, accumulate in the fatty tissue of living organisms and are toxic to humans and wildlife. POPs are lipophilic compounds resistant to both physicochemical and biological degradation: they accumulate in biological organisms and subsequently in humans via food. Levels of chemical contaminants in human milk fat are a good indicator of potential future public health and environmental problems. This is also relevant in measuring the developmental exposure of unborn children.

Contamination of human milk is widespread and is the consequence of inadequately controlled pollution of the environment by toxic chemicals. PCBs, DDT and its metabolites, dioxins, dibenzofurans (PBDEs) and heavy metals, are among the toxic chemicals most often found in human milk (Hooper and McDonald, 2000). These compounds are encountered to varying extents among women in industrialized and non-developed countries. Some of the highest levels of contaminants are seen among women in agricultural areas of the developing countries where pesticides are extensively used and among women living in remote areas who eat a diet rich in seal, whale and other species high on the marine food chain that accumulate heavy burdens of POPs.

A few European countries (e.g., Sweden and Germany) have systematic breast milk monitoring programs that have tested considerable numbers of women over time; however, most countries have done little monitoring for metal, pesticides or industrial chemicals in breast milk. In the USA the objectives and goals of a breast milk monitoring program for women are as follows: (1) Information should be obtained on women from diverse geographic regions of the USA and from different socio-economic and demographic backgrounds. Samples should be collected from both rural and urban locations. (2) Previous studies should be extended by testing for an increased number of environmental chemicals in breast milk (e.g., certain heavy metals as well as other chemicals with significant lipid solubility and long biological half-life).

(3) Longitudinal information should be obtained during the course of lactation so that the decrease in concentration of the chemical over time can be assessed. Lactating women should be enrolled in the study on a longitudinal basis, donating samples on a monthly basis (or more frequently in the first 2 months) and then every 2–3 months if lactation continues. Recruitment of participants may be aided by lactation consultants. (4) Harmonization of sampling and analysis protocols should be promoted to improve the comparability of the results (LaKind *et al.*, 2001).

One study performed in Uppsala County (Sweden) shows that the concentrations of some non-, mono- and di-ortho PCB congeners are strongly associated with mother's milk concentrations of PCB/PCDD/PCDF TEQs in primiparas (Glynn *et al.*, 2001)

The "Stockholm Convention" requires that parties phase out or ban the production, use, import and export of unintentionally produced POPs, with the exception of DDT, which will be permitted for vector control according to WHO guidelines until feasible alternatives have been found. For unintentionally produced POPs, namely dioxins and furans, parties should minimize and eliminate emissions from anthropogenic sources where possible.

The "Stockholm Convention" also requires the Conference of Parties to evaluate its effectiveness, starting 4 years after its entry into force. To facilitate this evaluation, the Conference of Parties should initiate arrangements to provide itself with comparable monitoring data on the presence of POPs and their regional and global environmental transport. The first evaluation took place in 2008 and should be a baseline for future evaluations. It was focus on core data from appropriate matrices, such as air and human tissues (blood and/or human milk), and rely extensively on existing programmes global monitoring of POPs (e.g., the Arctic Monitoring and Assessment Programme, the Global Air Passive Sampling project and the WHO Global Survey of Human Milk for POPs. The aim was to provide core data for the 12 POPs from all five United Nations regions. Strategic arrangements and partnerships should be established, involving the health sector.

European Union (EU) Regulation (EC) No. 850/2004 of the European Parliament and of the Council of April 29, 2004 on persistent organic pollutants and amending Directive 79/117/EEC entered into force on May 20, 2004 (L 158, 30.4.2004). This implements the provisions of the "Stockholm Convention". Dioxins, PCDFs and PCBs are listed as unintentionally released POPs, the release of which should be continuously and cost-effectively reduced as quickly as possible. The links between the exposure of children to POPs and their health effects are specifically addressed by the EU Science, Children, Awareness, EU Legislation and Continuous Evaluation (SCALE) initiative and the Children's Environment and Health Action Plan for Europe indicator RPG IV. Policy action should follow from these European strategies that takes into account children's sensitivity to these pollutants (WHO, 2007).

The indicator shows clear differences in POP levels between European countries. For dioxins the differences were initially as much as 3–10-fold. It also shows a decrease in most countries, especially in those with the highest initial levels. This results from abolishment at source (i.e., bans on their production and use and improved waste incinerators). The levels of pesticide POPs are very low, but some newer compounds have emerged (polybrominated and polyfluorinated compounds); although these are still present at reasonably low levels, they need to be monitored.

Unlike other POPs, PBDEs are not restricted or banned from use in most countries. Most studies had found that higher levels of PCDD/furans, PCBs and organochloride pesticides were strongly correlated with increased maternal age and primiparity, but only weakly correlated with decreased maternal body mass index and education level. The difference in associations between PBDEs and POPs may reflect different exposure pathways, toxicokinetics or the effects of restrictions and bans, and differences in bioavailability, bioaccumulation, biotransformation and half-lives in biota (Chao *et al.*, 2010).

Other xenobiotic contaminants

Several studies have provided evidence on the transfer of heavy metals (e.g., lead, cadmium, mercury) into mothers' breast milk to breastfeed infants. Other contaminants such as aflatoxins and ochratoxin A have also been found in breast milk. With those levels of contaminants the potential intakes were calculated for the newborn (Turconi *et al.*, 2004).

Other xenobiotic contaminants such as diesters of phthalic acid, commonly known as phthalates, a group of industrial chemicals with many commercial uses such as solvents, additives and plasticizers, could be found in breast milk especially DBP and DEHP because of their ubiquitous presence in the environment.

Risk assessment

The risk assessment methods generally do not consider chemical exposures to infants via mother's milk and therefore need to be expanded. Traditional risk assessment is normally based on adult body weights and food consumption data (Sonawane, 1995). The level of risk to infants and children of exposure to chemical contaminants in human milk depends on each mother's food consumption patterns, the nature and levels of chemical residues in her milk and the toxicological potency of those chemicals. A comprehensive analysis of the potential health risks to infants and children exposed to chemicals from breast milk will require consideration of all these factors as well as of the unique vulnerabilities of infants and children. Infants and children may exhibit unique susceptibilities to the toxic effects of chemicals because they are undergoing rapid tissue growth and development (Landrigan, 1999). In addition, infants and children consume much greater quantities of milk fat and certain foods than those adults on a body weight basis, and therefore they may be subjected to proportionately higher levels of exposure to certain chemicals.

Among the POPs, dioxins (polychlorinated dibenzo-p-dioxins) and dioxin-like chemicals (including polychlorinated dibenzofurans and dioxin-like polychlorinated biphenyls) seem to have the lowest safety margin and to be the most likely group to cause adverse effects in humans (Van Leuwen and Malisch, 2002).

Lorber and Phillips (2002) used a one-compartment, first-order pharmacokinetics model to predict the infant body burdens of dioxin-like compounds that result from breastfeeding. They predict that the body burden of the formula-fed infants will remain below 10 ppt TEQ lipid during the first year compared to the current adult average body burden of 25 ppt TEQ lipid. These authors found that an infant who had been breastfed for 1 year had an accumulated dose six times higher than a 1-year-old infant who had not been breastfed. For a 70-year lifetime, individuals who had been breastfed had an accumulated dose 3–18% higher than individuals who had not been breastfed.

CONCLUDING REMARKS AND FUTURE DIRECTIONS

The presence of drugs, non-medicinal substances and xenobiotics in milk, at high levels or when the infant is sensitive enough, interact at many possible physiological levels. Usually, most drugs administered to the lactating mother will appear in milk in concentrations similar to maternal plasma concentrations. Premature infants presenting an anatomical and functional immaturity of the organs and other biochemical and physiological processes involved in drug pharmacokinetics is further exacerbated. So, functional immaturity of pharmacokinetics processes (i.e., absorption, distribution, metabolism and excretion) contribute to the several responses observed between neonates, infants and adults. Postnatal maturation of pharmacokinetics processes has significant implications with respect to systemic exposure levels and the safety and/or efficacy of a drug in the neonate and young infant.

The use of medications in breastfeeding mothers always requires a significant assessment of risk versus benefit. The enormous benefits of breastfeeding are well known, but the risks of most medications used in breastfeeding should be taken in consideration. Unfortunately, there is a lack of epidemiological data on the probability of adverse effects in breastfed neonates and infants, despite the existing information on the toxicokinetics of drugs and xenobiotics in breast milk.

An assessment of the therapeutic efficacy or toxic susceptibility of a newborn to an exposure will require a careful consideration of the developmental aspects of pharmacokinetics processes. In general, the combined effects of age-related changes in each pharmacokinetics process on plasma levels of a specific compound could be difficult to understand. Clinical studies encompassing neonates and infants within narrow postnatal-age groups are needed to enhance the pharmacokinetics and clinical consequences of postnatal maturation of pharmacokinetics processes. Such information will help to establish more effective guidelines to predict an exposure outcome in a newborn or infant and to ensure safe exposures to therapeutic or inadvertent compounds such as the environmental contaminants that require biological monitoring.

Adverse events caused by such exposure are very rare and almost always occur in the infant less than 6 months of age. Long-term studies should be done to measure any possible neurobehavioral or developmental effects.

Analgesics, antibiotics, cardiovascular drugs, steroidal hormones drugs, antiepileptics, psychoactive drugs, anticoagulants, non-medical substances such as drugs of abuse, among others, require careful assessment of risk. Drugs such as beta-blockers, salicylates, lithium, antineoplastic agents and drugs of abuse should be avoided in the newborn and in infants less than 6 months of age.

The finding of toxic chemicals in breast milk raises a series of important issues for pediatric practice, for the practice of public health and for the environmental health research community.

On the whole levels in human milk fat are a good indicator of potential future public health and environmental problems. Exposure varies significantly based on local chemical use and on the dietary habits of the population under study. This measure is also relevant in the developmental exposure of unborn children.

Although research has provided information on the different types of chemicals to be found in breast milk and on the toxicological aspects of many of these chemicals, there are few data on parameters related to infant exposure via breastfeeding, including those with a time-dependent nature.

Major concern has been expressed on the presence of environmental contaminants such as pesticides, heavy metals (e.g., lead, cadmium, mercury) and POPs in breast milk and their potential effects on infant health and development. In some instances, mothers with known or suspected high levels of contaminants in breast milk due to acute or chronic exposure have been advised to reduce or interrupt breastfeeding. It is also known that workers exposed to PCBs, women consuming high animal and vegetable diets in highly polluted areas or cooking with oil contaminated with PCBs and other polychlorinated compounds have been advised to reduce or interrupt breastfeeding. Exposure to PCBs and dioxins has been associated with a greater susceptibility to infectious diseases in infants and a lower prevalence of allergic reactions.

Comprehensive breast milk monitoring with standardized protocols for specimen collection and analysis must be expanded worldwide. Another need is to study lactating women prospectively to determine rates of decrease in concentrations of chemicals over the course of lactation. It has been recommended that women should donate milk samples on a monthly basis (or more frequently in the first 2 months) and then every 2–3 months if lactation continues.

Dioxins and dioxin-like chemicals (including polychlorinated dibenzofurans and dioxin-like polychlorinated biphenyls) seem to have the lowest margin of safety and probably is the main group to cause adverse effects in humans.

ACKNOWLEDGMENT

This work was supported by the *Comunidad de Madrid* and the *Ministerio de Educación y Ciencia*, Projects Ref. S2009/AGR-1469, and Consolider-Ingenio 2010 Ref. CSD/2007/00063 (FUN-C-FOOD), Madrid, Spain.

REFERENCES

Alcorn J, McNamara, PJ (2003) Pharmacokinetics in the newborn. *Adv Drug Delivery Rev* **55:** 667–86.

American Academy of Pediatrics (2001) The transfer of drugs and other chemicals into human milk. *Pediatrics* **108(3):** 776–89.

Anadón A, Martínez-Larrañaga MR, Caballero V, Castellano V (2010). Chapter 2. Assessment of prebiotics and probiotics: an overview. In *Bioactive Foods in Promoting Health: Probiotics and Prebiotics* (Watson R, Preedy VR, eds.). Elsevier Inc., Academic Press, pp. 19–41 (ISBN: 978-0-12-374938-3).

Anadón A, Martínez-Larrañaga MR, Fernández MC, Diaz MJ, Bringas P (1990) The effect of ciprofloxacin on antipyrine pharmacokinetics and metabolism in rat. *Antimicrob Agents Chemother* **34(11):** 2148–51.

Anadón A, Martínez-Larrañaga MR (1992) Pharmacology and toxicology of quinolones. In *Recent Developments in Therapeutic Drug Monitoring and Clinical Toxicology* (Sunshine I, ed.). Marcel Dekker, Inc., New York. Chapter 30, pp. 193–8 (ISBN: 0-8247-8586-X).

Anderson PO, Pochop SL, Manoguerra AS (2003) Adverse drug reaction in breastfed infants: less than imagined. *Clin Pediatrics* **42:** 325–40.

Assael BM (1982) Pharmacokinetics and drug distribution during postnatal development. *Pharmacol Ther* **18:** 159–97.

Astley SJ, Little RE (1990) Maternal marijuana use during lactation and infant development at one year. *Neurotoxicol Teratol* **12:** 161–8.

Atkinson HC, Begg EJ (1990) Prediction of drug distribution into human milk from physicochemical characteristics. *Clin Pharmacokinet* **18:** 151–67.

Atkinson HC, Begg EJ, Darlow BA (1988) Drugs in milk: clinical pharmacokinetic considerations. *Clin Pharmacokinet* **14:** 217–40.

Bailey B, Ito S (1997) Breast-feeding and maternal drug use. *Pediatr Clin North Am* **44:** 41–54.

Beardmore KS, Morris JM, Gallery EDM (2002) Excretion of antihypertensive medication into human breast milk: a systematic review. *Hypertens Pregnancy* **21:** 85–95.

Begg EJ, Malpas TJ, Hackett LP, Ilett KF (2001) Distribution of R- and S-methadone into human milk during multiple, medium to high oral dosing. *Br J Pharmacol* **52:** 681–5.

Bennett PN (1996) *Drugs and Human Lactation*, 2nd edition. Elsevier, Amsterdam.

Berlin CM (2004) The excretion of drugs and chemicals in human milk. In *Neonatal and Pediatric Pharmacology* (Yaffe SJ, Aranda JV, eds.), 3rd edition. Williams & Wilkins, Lippincott, Philadelphia, pp. 187–96.

Blumer JL, Reed MD (1992) Principles of neonatal pharmacology. In *Pediatric Pharmacology* (Yaffe SJ, Aranda, JV, eds.). W.B. Saunders, Philadelphia, pp. 164–77.

Böttcher MF (2000) Cytokines and chemokines in breast milk from allergic and non-allergic mothers. *Allergy Clin Immunol Int* **12:** 153–60.

Boutroy MJ, Bianchetti G, Dubruc C, Vert P, Morselli PL (1986) To nurse when receiving acebutolol: is it dangerous for the neonate? *Eur J Clin Pharmacol* **30:** 737–9.

Briggs GG, Samson JH, Ambrose PJ, Schroeder DH (1993) Excretion of bupropion in beast milk. *Ann Pharmacother* **27:** 431–3.

Campoy C, Cabero L, Sanjurjo P, Serra L, Anadón A, Morán J, Fraga JM (2010) Update of knowledge, recommendations and full consensus about the role of long chain polyunsaturated fatty acids in pregnancy, lactating period and first year of life. *Med Clin (Barcelona)* **135:** 75–82.

Cantu TG (1989) Phenothiazines and sudden infant death syndrome. *DICP* **23:** 795–6.

Chao HA, Chen C-C, Chang C-M, Koh T-W, Chang-Chien G-P, Ouyang E, Lin S-L, Shy C-G, Chen F-A, Cho H-R (2010). Concentrations of polybrominated diphenyl ethers in breast milk correlated to maternal age, education level, and occupational exposure. *J Hazardous Mat* **175:** 492–500.

Chasnoff IJ, Lewis DE, Squires L (1987) Cocaine intoxication in a breast-fed infant. *Pediatrics* **80:** 836–8.

Chatterton RT Jr, Hill PD, Algad JC, Hodges KR, Belknap SM, Zinaman MJ (2000) Relation of plasma oxytocin and prolaction concentrations to milk production in mothers of preterm infants: influence of stress. *J Clin Endocrinol Metab* **85:** 3661–8.

Fleishaker JC, Desai N, McNamara PJ (1987) Factors affecting the milk-to-plasma drug concentration ratio in lactating woman: physical interactions with protein and fat. *J Pharm Sci* **76:** 189–93.

Giamarellou H., Kolokythas E, Petrikkos G, Gazis J, Aravantinos D, Sfikakis P (1989) Pharmacokinetics of three newer quinolones in pregnant and lactating women. *Am J Med* **87:** 49S–51S.

Glynn AW, Atuma S, Aune M, Darnerud PO, Cnattingius S (2001) Polychlorinated biphenyl congeners as markers of toxic equivalents of polychlorinated biphenyls, dibenzo-*p*-dioxins and dibenzofurans in breast milk. *Environ Res Sec* A **86:** 217–28.

Goldman AS (1993) The immune system of human milk: antimicrobial, anti-inflammatory and immunomodulating properties. *Pediatr Infect Dis J* **12:** 664–71.

Guyton AC, Hall, JE (2006) *Textbook of Medical Physiology*, 11th edition. Elsevier Saunders, Philadelphia, Pennsylvania.

Hale TW (2002) *Medications and Mothers' Milk*, 10th edition. Amarillo, Texas, Pharmasoft.

Hale TW (2003) Medications in breastfeeding mothers of preterm infants. *Pediatr Ann* **32:** 337–47.

Hale TW, Shum S, Grossber M (2001) Fluoxetine toxicity in a breastfed infant. *Clin Pediatr (Phila)* **40:** 681–4.

Hooper K, McDonald TA (2000) The PBDEs: an emerging environmental challenge and another reason for breast-milk monitoring programs. *Environ Health Perspect* **108:** 387–92.

Ito S (2000) Drug therapy for breast-feeding women. *New Engl J Med* **343:** 118–26.

Ito S, Alcorn J (2003) Xenobiotic transporter expression and function in the mammary gland. *Adv Drug Deliver Rev* **55:** 653–65.

Ito S, Koren GA (1994) Novel index for expressing exposure of the infant to drugs in breast milk. *Br J Clin Pharmacol* **38:** 99–102.

Kahn A, Hasaerts D, Blum D (1985) Phenothiazine-induced sleep apneas in normal infants. *Pediatrics* **75:** 844–7.

Kanto JH (1982) Use of benzodiazepines during pregnancy, labour and lactation, with particular reference to pharmacokinetic considerations. *Drugs* **23:** 354–80.

Kauppila A, Arvela P, Koivisto M, Kivinen S, Ylikorkala O, Pelkonen O (1983) Metoclopramide and breast feeding: transfer into milk and the newborn. *Eur J Clin Pharmacol* **25:** 819–23.

Kesaniemi YA (1974) Ethanol and acetaldehyde in the milk and peripheral blood of lactating women after ethanol administration. *J Obstet Gynaecol Br Commonw* **81:** 301–10.

Knowles JA (1972) Drugs in milk. *Pediatr Currents* **21:** 28–32.

Kraus DM, Fischer JH, Reitz SJ, Kecskes SA, Yeh TF, McCulloch KM, Tung EC, Cwik MJ (1993) Alterations in teophylline metabolism during the first year of life. *Clin Pharmacol Ther* **54:** 351–9.

Lacroix D, Sonnier M, Moncion A, Cheron G, Cresteil T (1997) Expression of CYP3A in human liver: evidence that the shift between CYP3A7 and CP3A4 occurs immediately after birth. *Eur J Biochem* **257:** 625–34.

LaKind JS, Berlin CM, Naiman DQ (2001) Infant exposure to chemicals in breast milk in the United States: what we need to learn from a breast milk monitoring program. *Environ Health Perspect* **109:** 75–88.

Landrigan PJ (1999) Risk assessment for children and other sensitive populations. *Ann N Y Acad Sci* **895:** 1–9.

Landrigan PJ, Sonawane B, Mattison D, McCally M, Garg A (2002) Chemical contaminants in breast milk and their impacts on children's health: an overview. *Environ Health Perspect* **110:** A313–15.

Lawrence R, Schaefer C (2007) General commentary on drug therapy and drug risk during lactation. In *Drugs During Pregnancy and Lactation. Treatment Option and Risk Assessment* (Schaefer C, Peters P, Miller RK, eds.). Elsevier-Academic Press, Amsterdam, pp. 609–20.

Livingston V, Stringer J (1999) The treatment of *Staphyloccocus aureus* infected sore nipples: a randomized comparative study. *J Human Lact* **15:** 241–6.

Lorber M, Phillips L (2002) Infant exposure to dioxin-like compounds in breast milk. *Environ Health Perspect* **110:** A325–32.

Madani S, Paine MF, Lewis L, Thummel KE, Shen DD (1999) Comparison of CYP2D6 content and metoprolol oxidation between microsomes isolated from human livers and small intestines. *Pharm Res* **16:** 1199–205.

McCarthy JJ, Posey BL (2000) Methadone levels in human milk. *J Human Lact* **16:** 115–20.

Morselli PL (1976) Clinical pharmacokinetics in neonates. *Clin Pharmacokinet* **1:** 81–9.

Morselli PL, Franco-Morselli R, Bossi L (1980) Clinical pharmacokinetics in newborns and infants. *Clin Pharmacokinet* **5:** 485–527.

Mortola J (989) The use of psychotropic agents in pregnancy and lactation. *Psychiatr Clin North Am* **12:** 69–87.

Murray L, Segar D (1994) Drug therapy during pregnancy and lactation. *Emerg Med Clin North Am* **12:** 129–49.

Neville MC, Walsh CT (1996) Effects of drugs on milk secretion and composition. In *Drugs and Human Lactation* (Bennett PN, eds.). Elsevier, Amsterdam, pp. 15–46.

Niessen KH, Ramolla J, Binder M, Brugmann G, Hofmann U (1984) Chlorinated hydrocarbons in adipose tissue of infants and toddlers: inventory and studies on their association with intake of mothers' milk. *Eur J Pediatr* **142:** 238–43.

Nulman I, Rovet J, Stwart DE, Wolpin J, Gardner HA, Theis JGW, Kuln N, Koren G (1997) Neurodevelopment of children exposed in utero to antidepressant drugs. *N Engl J Med* **336:** 258–62.

Obach RS, Zhang QY, Dunbar D, Kaminsky LS (2001) Metabolic characterization of the major human small intestinal cytochrome p450s. *Drug Metab Dispos* **29:** 347–52.

Passmore CM, McElnay JC, Rainey EA, D'Arcy PF (1988) Metronidazole excretion in human milk and its effect on the suckling neonate. *Br J Clin Pharmacol* **26:** 45–51.

Perez-Reyes M, Wall ME (1982) Presence of delta9-tetrahydrocannabinol in human milk. *N Engl J Med* **307:** 819–20.

Petraglia F, De LV, Sardelli S, Pieroni ML, D'Antona N, Genazzani AR (1985) Domperidone in defective and insufficient lactation. *Eur J Obstet Gynecol Reprod Biol* **19:** 281–7.

Pronczuk J, Akre J, Moy G, Vallenas C (2002) Global perspectives in breast milk contamination: infectious and toxic hazards. *Environ Health Perspect* **110:** A349–51.

Richter C, Sitzmann J, Lang P, Weitzel H, Huch A, Huch R (2001). Excretion of low weight heparin in human milk. *Br J Clin Pharmacol* **52:** 708–10.

Rush JE, Snyder DL, Barrish A, Hichens M, Comment on Huttunen K, Gronhagen-Riska C, Fyhrquist F (1989) Enalapril treatment of a nursing mother with slightly impaired renal function. *Clin Nephrol* **35:** 234–9.

Schanker LS (1963) Passage of drugs across body membranes. *Pharmacol Rev* **14:** 501–30.

Schimmel MS, Eidelman AI, Wilschanski MA, Shaw D, Ogilvie RJ, Koren G (1989) Toxic effects of atenolol consumed during breast feeding, *J Pediatr* **114:** 476–8.

Simon SL, Gorbach SL (1984) Intestinal flora in health and disease. *Gastroenterology* **86:** 174–93.

Sonawane BR (1995) Chemical contaminants in human milk: an overview. *Environ Health Perspect* **103 (Suppl 6):**197–205.

Spigset O, Hägg S (1998) Excretion of psychotropic drugs into breast milk. *Drug Ther* **9:** 111–34.

Sweezy SR (1992) Contraception for the post-partum woman. *NAACOGS Clin Issu Perinat Women's Health Nurs* **3:** 209–26.

Taddio A, Klein J, Koren G (1994) Acyclovir excretion in human breast milk. *Ann Pharmacother* **28:** 585–7.

Tennes K, Avitable N, Blackard C, Boyles C, Hassoun B, Holmes L, Kreye M (1985) Marijuana: prenatal and postnatal exposure in the human. *NIDA Res Monogr* **59:** 48–60.

Turconi G, Guarcello M, Livieri C, Comizzoli S, Maccarini L, Castellazzi AM, Pietri A, Piva G, Roggi C (2004) Evaluation of xenobiotics in human milk and ingestion by the newborn. An epidemiological survey in Lombardy (Northern Italy). *Eur J Nutr* **43:** 191–7.

van den Anker JN, Schoemaker RC, Hop WC, van der Heijden BJ, Weber A, Sauer PJ, Neijens HJ, de Groot R (1995) Ceftazidime pharmacokinetics in preterm infants: effects of renal function and gestational age. *Clin Pharmacol Ther* **58:** 650–9.

Van Leuwen FXR, Malisch R (2002) Results of the third round of the WHO-coordinated exposure study on the levels of PCBs, PCDDs and PCDFs in human milk. *Organohalogen Comp* **56:** 311–16.

White WB, Andreoli JW, Cohn RD (1985) Alpha-methyldopa disposition in mothers with hypertension and in their breast-fed infants. *Clin Pharmacol Ther* **37:** 387–90.

WHO (1996) Levels of PCBs, PCDDs and PCDFs in human milk. *Environmental Health in Europe* (No. 3), Bilthoven: WHO European Centre for Environment and Health.

WHO (2007) Persistent organic pollutants (POPs) in human milk. ENHIS, Fact Sheet No. 4.3, May. Code: RPG4 Food Ex2.

Wittels B, Scott DT, Sinatra RS (1990) Exogenous opioids in human breast milk and acute neonatal neurobehaviour: a preliminary study. *Anesthesiology* **73:** 864–9.

Wojnar-Horton RE, Kristensen JH, Yapp P, Ilett KF, Dusci LJ, Hackett LP (1977) Methadone distribution and excretion into breast milk of clients in a methadone maintenance programme. *Br J Clin Pharmacol* **44:** 543–7.

Zhang QY, Dunbar D, Ostrowska A, Zeisloft S, Yang LS, Kaminsky LS (1999) Characterization of human small intestinal cytochromes P-450. *Drug Metab Dispos* **27:** 804–9.

Section 2

Safety Evaluation and Toxicity Testing Models

CHAPTER

7

Postmarket surveillance and regulatory considerations in reproductive and developmental toxicology: an FDA perspective

Susan Bright

Disclaimer. No official support or endorsement of this material by the Food and Drug Administration is intended or should be inferred.

INTRODUCTION

Brief history of the Food and Drug Administration

The US Food and Drug Administration (FDA) is a regulatory, science-based federal agency responsible for protecting and promoting the public health through the monitoring and regulation of a number of items necessary for the health and well-being of consumers. The FDA's jurisdiction includes most food products (other than meat and poultry), human and animal drugs, medical devices, veterinary devices, therapeutic agents of biologic origin, radiation-emitting products for consumer, medical and occupational use, cosmetics and animal feed. Recently, tobacco products have also come under the purview of the FDA. The history of the FDA can be traced back to the latter part of the 19th century, when Harvey Washington Wiley, chief chemist of the US Department of Agriculture (USDA) Division of Chemistry, began conducting research into the misbranding and adulteration of food and drug products in US commerce. Wiley published the Division's findings and lobbied for new federal laws to set uniform standards for food and drugs entering into interstate commerce. This came at a time when the American public had already been awakened to hazards in the marketplace by journalists such as Upton Sinclair, who in 1906 published the novel *The Jungle*, which exposed appalling conditions in the US meat packing industry. The resulting public uproar contributed in part to the passage a few months later of the 1906 Food and Drugs Act and the Meat Inspection Act. The Food and Drugs Act prohibited the interstate transport of adulterated or misbranded food, drink and drugs, and was administered by the USDA's Bureau of Chemistry. The Bureau of Chemistry's regulatory powers were reorganized under a new USDA body, the Food, Drug, and Insecticide organization, which later was shortened to the Food and Drug Administration. The Food and Drugs Act was replaced by broader legislation, in light of the "Elixir Sulfanilamide" tragedy, in which over 100 people died after using a drug formulated with a toxic solvent (diethylene glycol). The new Food, Drug and Cosmetic Act was signed into law by President Franklin D. Roosevelt in 1938. This law significantly increased regulatory authority over drugs by mandating a premarket review of the safety of all new drugs, as well as banning false therapeutic claims in drug labeling. The law also authorized inspections of factories and expanded enforcement powers, in addition to setting new regulatory standards for foods, and brought cosmetics and therapeutic devices under federal regulatory authority. In 1940, the FDA was transferred from the USDA to the Department which would ultimately become today's Department of Health and Human Services (DHHS).

By 1959, concerns were brought to the forefront by Senator Estes Kefauver about pharmaceutical industry practices, such as high cost and uncertain efficacy of many drugs. A tragedy involving thalidomide pushed Congress to lend support to expansion of FDA authority. The use of thalidomide, marketed in Europe for the treatment of nausea during pregnancy, led to thousands of European babies being born deformed. The drug had not been approved in the USA, but trial samples had been sent to American doctors during clinical investigations of the drug, a process which at the time was entirely without regulation. The thalidomide tragedy prompted the passage of the 1962 Kefauver-Harris Amendment to the Food, Drug and Cosmetic Act. Now the law required that all new drug applications demonstrate substantial evidence of the drug's efficacy for a specific indication, in addition to the existing requirement for premarket demonstration of safety. Drugs approved between 1938 and 1962 were also subject to FDA review of efficacy. The 1962 amendments also placed some restrictions on drug advertising and expanded the FDA's authority to inspect drug manufacturing facilities.

Prior to the 1906 passage of the Food and Drugs Act, Congress enacted the Biologics Control Act of 1902, which gave the

Reproductive and Developmental Toxicology, Edited by Ramesh C. Gupta
ISBN: 978-0-12-382032-7

government control over production processes used for biological products, such as vaccines, serum and antitoxins. This Act was also brought about by a tragedy involving the death of 13 children who had been given diphtheria antitoxin derived from a horse infected with tetanus. The horse serum was manufactured locally, with no central or uniform production controls. The Biologics Control Act required that manufacturers of vaccines be licensed annually for the manufacture and sale of vaccines, serum and antitoxins. Manufacturing facilities were also required to undergo inspections. In addition, all product labels were required to include the product name, expiration date, address and license number of the manufacturer. Today, biologics are regulated under the Public Health Service Act (PHS Act) which provides for their licensing, as well as under provisions of the Food, Drug and Cosmetic Act.

Medical devices were subject to policing by the FDA between 1938 and the early 1970s. The Agency could bring charges against products that were found to be adulterated or misbranded, but no requirement for premarket testing, review or approval existed at the time. In 1972 and 1973 pacemaker failures began to be reported, and in 1975, certain intrauterine shield devices caused thousands of reported injuries. These incidents helped reinforce the need for medical device regulation, and the Medical Device Amendments were passed in 1976. Medical devices were now subject to classification requirements, and Class III device manufacturers were required to notify the FDA prior to marketing. In addition, good manufacturing practice (GMP) regulations were authorized.

Under the Food, Drug and Cosmetic Act of 1938, manufacturers of human or animal drugs only had to demonstrate that their products were safe. The 1962 amendments to this Act required their products also be shown effective; however, the 1962 amendments generally did not distinguish between human and animal drugs. In 1968, Congress passed legislation to strengthen provisions of the Act that pertained to regulation of animal drugs. The Animal Drugs Amendments of 1968 required that animal drugs, medicated feeds and food additives be safe for the animal for which they were intended for use; and for food-producing animals, safe for human consumption and safe for the environment. Effectiveness studies were also required (FDA, 2009a).

The FDA is made up of six centers:

- **Center for Drug Evaluation and Research (CDER)** – regulates prescription and over-the-counter drugs intended for human use
- **Center for Biologics Evaluation and Research (CBER)** – regulates biological products intended for human use, such as vaccines, blood and blood components and gene therapy products
- **Center for Devices and Radiological Health (CDRH)** – regulates medical devices and radiation-emitting products
- **Center for Veterinary Medicine (CVM)** – regulates drugs, devices and feed intended for use in animals
- **Center for Food Safety and Nutrition (CFSAN)** – regulates most foods (except meat and poultry), food additives, infant formulas, dietary supplements and cosmetics
- **Center for Tobacco Products (CTP)** – regulates cigarettes, cigarette tobacco and smokeless tobacco

In addition, the FDA includes a research center, the National Center for Toxicological Research (NCTR), and two offices – the Office of Regulatory Affairs (ORA) which conducts inspections and enforces FDA regulations, and the Office of the Commissioner (OC) which provides leadership and direction to all of the FDA.

The National Center for Toxicological Research (NCTR), established by executive order in 1971, is an important research component of the FDA that plays a critical role in the FDA's and the DHHS' mission to promote and protect public health. NCTR – in partnership with researchers from elsewhere in the FDA, other government agencies, academia and industry – provides innovative technology, methods development, vital scientific training and technical expertise. The unique scientific expertise of the NCTR is critical in supporting FDA product centers and their regulatory roles. The NCTR conducts FDA mission-critical, peer-reviewed, critical path research targeted to developing a scientifically sound basis for regulatory decisions and reducing risks associated with FDA-regulated products. Research is aimed at evaluating the biological effects of potentially toxic chemicals or microorganisms, defining the complex mechanisms that govern their toxicity, understanding critical biological events in the expression of toxicity, and developing methods to improve assessment of human exposure, susceptibility and risk. Customized assessment of chemicals of vital interest to the FDA involves the coordination of expertise in the areas of biochemical and molecular markers of safety and toxicity, neurotoxicology, microbiology, chemistry, genetic or reproductive/developmental toxicology and systems-biology assessments for characterizing biomarkers. The NCTR has developed and is standardizing technologies, such as genomics, proteomics, metabolomics and nanotechnology, to identify and characterize early biomarkers of toxicity using quantitative risk assessment methods. The NCTR also represents the FDA on key committees of the National Toxicology Program (NTP), a program that evaluates the effects of chemicals on health. Of particular application to reproductive and developmental toxicity assessments, the NCTR maintains an endocrine disruptor knowledge database (EDKB) program, a major element of which has been the development of computer-based predictive models to predict affinity for binding of compounds to estrogen and androgen nuclear receptor proteins (FDA, 2009b).

Overview of the FDA's postmarket surveillance and pharmacovigilance

The safety of the medical products regulated by the FDA has been a key focus of the Agency since it was established more than a century ago as the nation's first consumer protection agency. Drugs are approved after the FDA determines in the premarket phase that a product's benefits outweigh the risks associated with its labeled use for the intended population. Although the FDA has a rigorous preapproval process for drugs, well-conducted, randomized, controlled clinical trials cannot uncover every safety problem, nor are they expected to do so. In most cases, clinical trials are not large enough, diverse enough or long enough in duration to provide all of the information on a product's performance and safety. In addition, clinical trials are unlikely to reliably detect rare, serious adverse events that occur with long latency or in subpopulations that have not participated in studies. Furthermore, as new medical products enter the market, the potential for interactions with other drugs, biologics, medical devices and foods increases. Additional information about medical product safety can be obtained during post-approval use.

The use of medical products brings both benefits and risks. Although marketed medical products are required by federal law to be safe for their intended use, safety does not mean zero risk. A safe product is one that has acceptable risks, given the magnitude of the benefit expected in a specific population and within the context of alternatives available. The FDA carefully considers all of the available safety information submitted to the agency during the pre-approval process. However, unexpected and sometimes serious safety problems can emerge once a product goes on the market and is used by millions of people.

A cornerstone of the FDA's safety surveillance and monitoring efforts are regulations that require firms who market medical products to report to the FDA adverse medical events associated with the product's use that are reported to the firm. Usually firms learn of these adverse events from health professionals or patients who experience serious problems that they suspect are associated with the drugs and medical devices they prescribe, dispense or use. Healthcare professionals and patients may also inform the FDA directly about these events. Case reports published in the medical literature and results of post-approval and other clinical studies are also important to the FDA's safety surveillance and monitoring efforts. In recent years, rapid scientific advances as well as advances in information technology have created new opportunities for monitoring the performance of medical products, including active surveillance methods.

The monitoring of the safety of marketed medical products is known as pharmacovigilance, defined by the WHO as "the science and activities relating to the detection, assessment, understanding, and prevention of adverse effects or any other drug-related problems" (WHO, 2006). Pharmaceutical companies have obligations to collect all data relevant to the safety of their products and submit such data to regulatory agencies in line with guidance and legislation. Regulators monitor these data for signals but also collect and screen safety data on medical products for signal detection independently of pharmaceutical companies. A signal is defined by the WHO as reported information on a possible causal relationship between an adverse event and a drug, the relationship being unknown or incompletely documented previously. Usually more than a single report is required to generate a signal, depending upon the seriousness of the event and the quality of the information (WHO, 2006). Historically, most safety signals come from spontaneously reported adverse drug experiences, but major safety issues may be detected from any relevant data sources. Underreporting occurs with most adverse event reporting systems. The frequency of reporting for a given medical product varies over time, with time from first marketing, and with periods of media activity surrounding a product. Given the variability in reporting and the many factors that affect reporting, it is well accepted that reporting rates cannot be used to reliably estimate incidence rates, and that comparison of reporting rates between products or between countries may not be reliable. Generally, spontaneous adverse event reports are examined by systematic manual review of every report received. As an aid to signal detection, screening algorithms based on automated signal detection systems have been explored. These methods are referred to as data mining. The aim of these statistical aids is to provide the means of comparing the frequency of a product–event combination with all other such combinations in a database under consideration, with the potential for early detection of signals of potential product–event associations. Signals are then confirmed ideally with epidemiologic investigations.

In the postmarketing phase of a product's lifecycle, once a safety issue has been identified, and evaluation has resulted in a judgment that the product may in fact pose a significant threat to public health, a thorough risk–benefit assessment should be conducted. Risk–benefit assessments consider the disease or condition being treated, the population being treated, the purpose of the intervention (treatment, prevention, etc.), availability of therapeutic alternatives, the frequency of the adverse event and the overall adverse event profile of the product. After a risk–benefit assessment is conducted, some action may be necessary to either increase the benefit of the product or reduce the risk. These actions may include healthcare practitioner and consumer education, or on occasion, restricting the use of a product. If the overall balance of risks and benefits is determined to be negative, then the product may be withdrawn, unless risk minimization strategies can reasonably be put into effect that would change the overall risk–benefit balance.

In addition to passive and active postmarket surveillance activities, postmarketing study commitments may be required of or agreed to by a sponsor, which are conducted after the FDA has approved a product for marketing. The FDA uses postmarketing study commitments to gather additional information about a product's safety, efficacy or optimal use. Agreements with sponsors to conduct postmarketing studies can be reached either before or after FDA has granted approval to a sponsor to market a product. The Food and Drug Administration Modernization Act of 1997 (FDAMA) amended the Food, Drug and Cosmetic Act by adding a new section 506B (21 USC 356b). This section provides additional authority for monitoring the progress of postmarketing studies that drug and biologic applicants have agreed to conduct to address safety concerns. Congress enacted this section in response to concerns expressed by the Food and Drug Administration and the public about the timeliness of completing postmarketing studies and about the need to update drug labeling with information obtained from such studies. This provision requires sponsors of approved drugs and biologics to report to the FDA annually on the progress of their postmarketing study commitments. In addition, the FDA publishes annually in the Federal Register a report that provides information on the status of postmarketing studies that sponsors have agreed to conduct and for which annual reports have been submitted. The FDA also provides basic information about the status of each postmarketing study commitment to the public on the FDA website (FDA, 2009c).

This chapter describes postmarket surveillance and pharmacovigilance activities which the FDA conducts to monitor the safety of drugs and vaccines intended for use in humans and drugs intended for use in animals. Information about the FDA's postmarket surveillance activities regarding food safety and medical devices are beyond the scope of this chapter, but may be found on the FDA's website (www.fda.gov). Throughout this chapter, reference may be made to the Code of Federal Regulations (CFR) and certain guidance documents. The Code of Federal Regulations (CFR) is a codification of the general and permanent rules published in the Federal Register by the Executive departments and agencies of the federal government. Title 21 of the CFR is reserved for rules of the Food and Drug Administration. Each title (or volume) of the CFR is revised once each calendar year. A revised Title 21 is issued on approximately April 1 of each year and is usually available on the FDA's website several months later. Guidance documents represent the FDA's current thinking on a particular subject. These documents are prepared for FDA review staff and regulated industry to provide guidelines for the processing, content and evaluation or approval of applications and also for the design, production, manufacturing and testing of regulated products. They also establish policies intended to achieve consistency in the FDA's regulatory approach and establish inspection and enforcement procedures. Because guidance documents are not regulations or laws, they are not enforceable, either through administrative actions or through the courts. An alternative approach may be used if such approach satisfies the requirements of the applicable statute, regulations or both.

DRUGS INTENDED FOR USE IN HUMANS

Human drugs are approved and monitored by the FDA's Center for Drug Evaluation and Research (CDER). Among the CDER's regulatory activities are reviewing new drug applications for brand name, innovator pharmaceuticals and for generic pharmaceuticals; enforcement of regulations governing the manufacture of pharmaceutical products, the promotion and advertising of prescription drugs, and drug experience reporting by firms marketing drugs; taking action against drugs marketed without approval; and collecting and analyzing safety data about marketed pharmaceuticals.

One of the CDER's primary objectives is to ensure that prescription and over-the-counter (OTC) medications are safe and effective when used as directed. All drugs have risks, and healthcare professionals and patients must balance the risks and benefits of a drug when making decisions about medical therapy. The FDA monitors and reviews available safety information related to marketed drugs throughout each product's lifecycle. When a drug is approved, the product labeling includes, among other things, available information about the benefits and risks of the drug.

After drug approval, the FDA may learn of new, or more frequent, serious adverse drug experiences from post-approval clinical studies or from clinical use. For example, additional adverse drug experiences may be identified as a drug is more widely used and under more diverse conditions. 21 CFR 314.80 defines an "adverse drug experience" as "any adverse event associated with the use of a drug in humans, whether or not considered drug related, including the following: an adverse event occurring in the course of the use of a drug product in professional practice; an adverse event occurring from drug overdose whether accidental or intentional; an adverse event occurring from drug abuse; an adverse event occurring from drug withdrawal; and any failure of expected pharmacological action". Further, this regulation defines a "serious adverse drug experience" as "any adverse drug experience occurring at any dose that results in any of the following outcomes: death, a life-threatening adverse drug experience, inpatient hospitalization or prolongation of existing hospitalization, a persistent or significant disability/incapacity, or a congenital anomaly/birth defect. Important medical events that may not result in death, be life-threatening, or require hospitalization may be considered a serious adverse drug experience when, based upon appropriate medical judgment, they may jeopardize the patient or subject and may require medical or surgical intervention to prevent one of the outcomes listed in this definition...." An "unexpected adverse drug experience" is "any adverse drug experience that is not listed in the current labeling for the drug product. This includes events that may be symptomatically and pathophysiologically related to an event listed in the labeling, but differ from the event because of greater severity or specificity...'unexpected,' as used in this definition, refers to an adverse drug experience that has not been previously observed (i.e., included in the labeling) rather than from the perspective of such experience not being anticipated from the pharmacological properties of the pharmaceutical product."

The FDA depends upon the recognition and voluntary reporting of adverse events by healthcare providers and patients, and on the mandatory reporting of adverse events by firms holding approved drug applications, drugs manufacturers, and drug distributors as required by law and regulation. Unsolicited reports from healthcare professionals or consumers received by the FDA are called spontaneous reports. Spontaneous reports of adverse drug reactions, medication errors and product quality problems are sent directly to the FDA through the MedWatch program or through the application holders to the FDA. Application holders are required to report adverse experiences that they learn about to the FDA under 21 CFR 314.80 as described above. Adverse experiences that are both serious and unexpected, whether foreign or domestic, must be reported as soon as possible but not later than 15 calendar days of initial receipt of the information. Application holders must promptly investigate all adverse experiences that are the subject of these postmarketing 15-day reports and submit follow-up reports within 15 calendar days of receipt of new information, or as requested by the FDA. Fifteen-day Alert reports based on information from the scientific literature are required to be accompanied by a copy of the published article. Firms that are identified on the drug label as its manufacturer or distributor are also required to report serious and unexpected adverse events that they learn about, either by notifying the FDA or the drug's application holder. Adverse events that are not serious and unexpected are reported in periodic adverse drug experience reports, which are submitted by the application holder at quarterly intervals for the first 3 years after approval, then annually. Adverse experiences are also reported from postmarketing studies.

The FDA began to computerize the storage of adverse event reports in 1967, and the data were entered into the Spontaneous Reporting System (SRS). The SRS was replaced in 1997 by a computerized database (AERS – Adverse Event Reporting System) to support its postmarketing safety surveillance programs for all approved human drug and therapeutic biologic products (other than vaccines). Adverse events in AERS are coded to terms in the Medical Dictionary for Regulatory Activities (MedDRA, 2010). In 1993, the FDA launched its MedWatch Adverse Event Reporting Program, to facilitate and support the voluntary adverse event reporting process by healthcare professionals and consumers. MedWatch also helps provide timely information about safety alerts, recalls, market withdrawals and drug labeling changes (FDA, 2010a). Voluntary reporting is conducted on a single, one-page reporting form (Form FDA 3500). Another form (FDA 3500a) is provided for use by mandatory reporters.

The FDA receives nearly 1,000 spontaneous reports of adverse events daily. Adverse drug event reports are evaluated by clinical safety reviewers in the CDER. Features of the AERS database system facilitate the review of AE reports.

For example, in a primary triage process, the AERS program screens incoming reports and alerts safety reviewers to serious and unlabeled events, and serious medical events known to be drug related (toxic epidermal necrolysis, etc.). In a secondary triage process, signals are identified based on overall counts for each risk category associated with all adverse event reports received for a given drug. The AERS can also generate periodic reports and perform active queries to aid in investigating signals found from initial screening. When potential signals are identified, a case series is assembled, and the safety reviewers may look for common trends and potential risk factors.

AERS data do have limitations. First, there is no certainty that the reported event was actually due to the product. The FDA does not require that a causal relationship between a product and event be proven, and reports do not always contain enough detail to properly evaluate an event. Further, the FDA does not receive all adverse event reports that occur with a product. Many factors can influence whether or not an event will be reported, such as the time a product has been marketed and publicity about an event. Therefore, the AERS cannot be used to calculate the incidence of an adverse event in the US population. Since 1998, the FDA has explored various automated Bayesian data mining techniques to augment its ability to monitor the safety of drugs and biologics. Data mining involves the automated computer generation of drug-adverse event signals by comparing the frequency of reports with what would be expected if all drugs and adverse events were expected to follow certain patterns. Data mining has the goal of distinguishing the more important or stronger signals, and to facilitate identification of drug-adverse event combinations that warrant further in-depth investigation.

The Sentinel Initiative is a national strategy for monitoring drug and medical product safety, with a primary goal of increasing active surveillance for safety problems instead of relying only on passive surveillance through spontaneous adverse event reporting. Government and commercial databases (e.g., managed care organizations, prescription benefit management companies) are used in the Sentinel Initiative to conduct population surveillance and identify safety issues in groups of patients rather than relying on isolated individual case reports. In this way, a systematic approach using data from several sources can be used to monitor the effects of drugs in populations, identify safety problems and the need for drug use modifications or restrictions, while facilitating an evidence-based approach to adverse drug event monitoring.

Once investigation and confirmation of a signal occurs, the FDA may initiate various regulatory actions, depending upon the seriousness of the adverse event, and taking into consideration the availability and acceptability of alternative therapies. Regulatory interventions may include changes in labeling approved for practitioners; patient/consumer-directed information (e.g., Medication Guides); issuance of "Dear Doctor" letters; drug name or packaging changes, or rarely, restricted use or distribution of a drug (see discussion of RiskMAPs and REMS below), or even withdrawal of a medical product from the market. Applicants may be asked by the FDA to distribute a "Dear Doctor" (or "Dear Health Care Practitioner") letter in order to disseminate information concerning a significant hazard to health, to announce important changes in drug package labeling or to correct prescription drug advertising or labeling. Applicants may distribute these letters for a variety of other reasons as well.

Historically, the information from adverse drug experience reports, along with data from formal clinical studies and from the medical and scientific literature, have made up the primary data source upon which the FDA's postmarketing safety surveillance depends. A report issued by the Institute of Medicine (IOM) in 2006 to the US Congress made several recommendations about how the FDA could improve its drug safety program (IOM, 2006). The IOM recommended several actions to address certain problems and provided the impetus for the FDA to enhance postmarketing surveillance. The FDA and the Agency for Healthcare Research and Quality (AHRQ) conducted a workshop in 2007 about the implementation of risk minimization action plans (RiskMAPs) to support quality use of pharmaceuticals. The goal of the workshop was to obtain input from stakeholders about useful mechanisms application holders can take to minimize the risks of medications with unusual safety and patient monitoring concerns. The FDA's authority to require holders of applications for human drugs to implement RiskMAPs was established in the Food and Drug Administration Amendments Act (FDAAA) of 2007, which calls them Risk Evaluation and Mitigation Strategies (REMS). The simplest REMS involve enhanced patient and healthcare provider education and risk communication strategies. Other components of REMS may include informed consent forms; limiting prescribing to practitioners with special training or certification; limiting use of the drug to hospitals or other healthcare settings; limiting dispensing of drugs to patients with documentation of particular laboratory results; and enrollment of patients into registries and other special monitoring programs (FDA, 2007). The need for REMS may be determined by the FDA at the time of drug approval, or after approval as safety issues emerge in the postmarketing period. REMS must be assessed at specified intervals. One of the most common reasons for REMS is when the drug is a teratogen. A list of currently approved risk evaluation mitigation strategies is available on the FDA's website (FDA CDER, 2010). The FDA also conducts regular, biweekly screening of the AERS database and posts a quarterly report on the AERS website describing any new safety information or potential signal of a serious risk identified by the AERS within the past quarter.

For many years, the FDA has provided information on drug risks and benefits to healthcare professionals and patients when that information has generated a specific concern or prompted a regulatory action, such as a revision to the drug product's labeling. More recently, the FDA has begun taking a more comprehensive approach to making information on potential drug risks available to the public earlier, in some cases while the Agency is still evaluating whether any regulatory action is warranted. In 2005, the FDA created an independent Drug Safety Oversight Board to enhance oversight of drug safety decision making within the CDER. As new information related to a marketed drug becomes available, the Agency reviews the data and evaluates whether there is a potential drug safety concern. When a potential drug safety concern arises, relevant scientific experts within the Agency engage in a prompt review and analysis of available data. Often, there is a period of uncertainty while the FDA evaluates the new safety information to determine whether there is an important drug safety issue related to a specific drug or drug class and whether regulatory action is appropriate. During this period, the FDA also is actively engaged in scientific efforts to gather additional safety information. The Drug Safety Oversight Board may be consulted and provide recommendations to the Director of the Center for Drug Evaluation and Research regarding the management and communication of an emerging drug safety issue. The FDA also may consult an Advisory Committee regarding an emerging drug safety issue. Sponsors are also evaluating the new safety information and providing the results of their analyses to the FDA during this time. As additional data relevant to an emerging drug safety issue become available (e.g., data from an ongoing study or data from available clinical databases), such data are considered in the analysis and decision-making process. Upon evaluation of additional data, further regulatory action, such as a revision to product labeling or initiation of REMS, may be appropriate.

As the CDER evaluates an emerging drug safety issue to determine whether regulatory action is warranted, information may be communicated to the public at appropriate points in the decision-making process. The FDA considers many factors in the course of evaluating an emerging drug safety concern and deciding when information should be made available to the public (FDA CDER, 2007a). These factors include, but are not limited to, reliability of the data, magnitude of the risk, seriousness of the event relative to the disease being treated, plausibility of a causal relationship between the use of the drug and the adverse events, extent of patient exposure and disproportionate impact on vulnerable populations (children, elderly, etc.). The FDA uses a broad range of methods to communicate drug safety information to the public. Certain forms of communication are targeted to specific audiences (e.g., healthcare professionals or patients). Others are directed at more than one group to ensure widespread dissemination of information about important drug safety issues.

The FDA issues Public Health Advisories (PHAs) to provide information regarding important public health issues to the general public, including patients and healthcare professionals. For example, PHAs may highlight important safety information about a drug, inform the public about the status of the FDA's evaluation of an emerging drug safety issue, announce the implementation of an REMS program for a drug, or advise the public regarding a manufacturer's suspension of marketing of a drug due to safety concerns. For example, a PHA was released by the FDA in 2007 after it had received new information about a rare but serious side effect in nursing infants whose mothers take codeine. Reports of morphine overdoses in nursing infants were published in the scientific literature and it was found that some women are ultra-rapid metabolizers of codeine, which is metabolized to morphine (Koren *et al.*, 2006). Nursing mothers taking codeine may have higher than normal levels of morphine in breast milk which is subsequently ingested by their infant and may result in life-threatening morphine overdose in the infant. The FDA issued a PHA to inform nursing mothers and prescribing healthcare professionals about the dangers of potential morphine overdose in nursing infants, and the FDA requested that manufacturers of prescription codeine-containing products include information in labeling about differences in codeine metabolism and potential concerns with breastfeeding (FDA CDER, 2007b).

PHAs are sometimes issued in conjunction with other drug safety communications, such as Alerts on Patient Information Sheets and Healthcare Professional Sheets. In 2005, the FDA began posting Patient Information Sheets when important new information regarding the safety of a marketed drug came to the attention of the FDA. These sheets include an Alert when appropriate, to communicate an emerging drug safety issue. Alerts may describe newly observed, serious adverse events that may be associated with the drug, information about how such adverse events may be prevented and information regarding serious adverse events that may be associated with use of the drug in populations in which the drug was not previously studied.

FDA-approved drug product labeling is the primary source of information about a drug's safety and effectiveness, and it summarizes the essential scientific information needed for the safe and effective use of the drug. Labeling for prescription drug products is directed to healthcare professionals, but may include sections that are intended for patients and that also must be FDA-approved. For some prescription drugs, such as oral contraceptives and estrogens, the FDA long ago determined that the safe and effective use of the drug required additional labeling in non-technical language to be distributed directly to patients by their healthcare provider or pharmacist (21 CFR 310.501 and 310.515). These patient package inserts also may be provided voluntarily by manufacturers for other drugs and are regulated by the FDA as product labeling.

In some cases, the FDA has required patient labeling in non-technical language in the form of Medication Guides (MedGuides). These have been required for certain prescription drugs that pose a serious and significant public health concern and for which FDA-approved patient information is necessary for a patient's safe and effective use of the product. MedGuides are required if the FDA determines that one or more of the following circumstances exists: patient labeling could help prevent serious adverse effects; a drug product has serious risk(s) of which patients should be made aware because information concerning the risk(s) could affect a patient's decision to use, or to continue to use, the product; or patient adherence to directions for use is crucial to the drug's effectiveness (21 CFR 208.1). Drugs that are prescribed with Medication Guides are listed on the FDA's website. Over-the-counter (OTC) drugs bear a "Drug Facts" label that conveys information in a clear, standardized format to enable patient self-selection of an appropriate drug and enhance the safe and effective use of the drug by consumers.

The premarket approval process for new drugs is a complex process which is described in depth on the FDA's website and in various guidance documents. The FDA has published guidances for reviewers specific to human reproduction including "Reviewer Guidance – Evaluating the Risks of Drug Exposure in Human Pregnancies" (FDA, CDER/CBER, 2005). This guidance is intended to help FDA staff evaluate human fetal outcome data generated after medical product exposures during pregnancy. The goal of such evaluations is to assist in the development of product labeling that is useful to medical care providers when caring for patients who are pregnant or planning pregnancy. Whether a drug causes abnormal development or not depends not only on the physical and chemical nature of the drug, but also on the dose, duration, frequency, route of exposure and gestational timing involved. Pregnant women are rarely included in clinical trials of new drug products. There may be inadvertent pregnancy exposures during clinical trials, but available data are usually not sufficient to permit adequate statistical analysis of outcomes. The only data on fetal effects initially available in drug labeling usually comes from animal reproductive toxicology studies, the results of which may or may not be relevant to safety in humans.

Because little is known before marketing about a drug's teratogenic potential, postmarketing surveillance of drug use in pregnancy is critical to the detection of drug-induced fetal effects. Some drugs may induce teratogenic effects that are not clinically evident until many years after birth, such as the reproductive tract abnormalities associated with diethylstilbestrol (DES) exposure *in utero*. When making a determination about whether and how human pregnancy data should be included in drug labeling, the FDA considers effects such as background prevalence of adverse pregnancy outcomes, timing and intensity of exposure, variability of responses and class effects, among others. Information on human gestational drug exposures will emerge during the postmarketing phase for most drug products. In addition, postmarketing pregnancy registries are being increasingly used proactively to monitor for major fetal effects. Sponsors of new drug applications may develop pregnancy exposure registries, either on their own initiative or when requested by the FDA as a postmarketing commitment. In 2002, the FDA published industry guidance on establishing pregnancy exposure registries to encourage the development of epidemiologically sound, written study protocols (FDA, CDER/CBER, 2002). A list of current pregnancy exposure registries enrolling women is available on the FDA's website (FDA, 2010b). If there is an increased risk associated with the use of the drug during pregnancy, the labeling should describe the specific abnormality, the incidence, seriousness, reversibility of the abnormality and the effect of dose, duration of exposure and timing of gestational exposure on the likelihood of risk. The labeling should also include and be routinely updated with data from ongoing studies, such as from pregnancy exposure registries.

Under the current labeling system, information about a drug's effects on reproduction, pregnancy and teratogenic effects gathered from pre-approval developmental and reproductive toxicity studies is included in product labeling. The current regulations provide that, unless a drug is not absorbed systemically and is not known to have a potential for indirect harm to a fetus, a "Pregnancy" subsection must be included within the "Use in Specific Populations" section of the labeling. The "Pregnancy" subsection must contain information on the drug's teratogenic effects and other effects on reproduction and pregnancy. When available, a description of human studies with the drug and data on its effects on later growth, development and functional maturation of the child must also be included. The regulations require that each product be classified under one of five pregnancy categories (A, B, C, D or X) on the basis of risk of reproductive and developmental adverse effects or, for certain categories, on the basis of such risk weighed against potential benefit. Pregnancy categories are described in Table 7.1.

Additionally, with regard to labor, delivery and lactation, regulations at 21 CFR 201.57(c)(9) and 201.80 (f)(7) and (8) specify statements that must be included in the "Use in Specific Populations" of drug labeling in some circumstances.

The FDA has proposed updating its approach to pregnancy and lactation labeling. Under the Proposed Rule on Pregnancy and Lactation Labeling issued in May 2008, the present "Labor and Delivery" section would be eliminated, and both the "Pregnancy" and "Lactation" subsections would consist of three principal components: the risk summary, clinical considerations and data sections. A summary of this proposed rule can be reviewed on the FDA's website (FDA CDER, 2009). At the time this chapter was written in June 2010, this rule had not yet been finalized and was therefore not in effect.

In December 2009, the FDA announced the formation of a new research program called the Medication Exposure in Pregnancy Risk Evaluation Program (MEPREP) which will fund research to study the effects of prescription medications used during pregnancy. The program is a collaboration among researchers at the FDA and the HMO Research Network Center for Education and Research in Therapeutics (CERT), Kaiser Permanente's multiple research centers and Vanderbilt University (FDA, 2009d). About two-thirds of women who deliver a baby have taken at least one prescription medication during pregnancy according to a journal article published in the *American Journal of Obstetrics and Gynecology* (Andrade *et al.*, 2004). There are very few clinical trials that test the safety of medications in pregnancy due to concerns about the health of the mother and child. To overcome the challenges presented by the lack of clinical trial data about the use of medications during pregnancy, the research program will link healthcare information for mothers and their babies in each of the participating research sites. Collectively, the 11 participating sites have healthcare information for about 1 million births over a 7-year time period (2001–2007). Many of the mothers associated with these births likely used medication during their pregnancies and now the FDA and participating researchers have a systematic and timely way of retrieving information from this network. A Steering Committee composed of representatives from each participating site and the FDA oversees MEPREP activities and provides scientific leadership for the program. The investigators participating in the program have collaborated on studies related to medication use during pregnancy and birth outcomes, as well as studies on the effects of antidepressant medications, antibiotics and cardiovascular medications on birth defects and perinatal outcomes. Results of these studies will provide valuable information for patients and physicians when making important decisions about medication use during pregnancy.

VACCINES INTENDED FOR USE IN HUMANS

The Center for Biologics Evaluation and Research (CBER) has the mission to protect and enhance the public health through the regulation of biological and related products including blood, vaccines, allergenics, tissues, and cellular and gene therapies. Biological products, in contrast to drugs, many of which are chemically synthesized, are derived from living sources (such as humans, animals and microorganisms), may not be easily identified or characterized, and many are manufactured using biotechnology. These products often represent cutting-edge biomedical research and may offer very effective means to treat a variety of medical illnesses and conditions that presently have few or no other treatment options. The CBER regulates an array of diverse and complex biological products, both investigational and licensed, including allergenics (patch tests and extracts used to diagnose and treat allergic conditions); blood and blood components used for transfusion, clotting factors and immunoglobulins; human tissues for transplantation and cellular products such as human stem cells; gene therapy products; vaccines; certain

TABLE 7.1 Pregnancy categories and required label statements (21 CFR 201.57(c)(9)(i))

Pregnancy Category A	If adequate and well-controlled studies in pregnant women have failed to demonstrate a risk to the fetus in the first trimester of pregnancy (and there is no evidence of a risk in later trimesters), the labeling must state: Studies in pregnant women have not shown that (*name of drug*) increases the risk of fetal abnormalities if administered during the first (*second, third, or all*) trimester(s) of pregnancy. If this drug is used during pregnancy, the possibility of fetal harm appears remote. Because studies cannot rule out the possibility of harm, however, (*name of drug*) should be used during pregnancy only if clearly needed. If animal reproduction studies are also available and they fail to demonstrate a risk to the fetus, the labeling must also state: Reproduction studies have been performed in (*kinds of animal(s)*) at doses up to (*x*) times the human dose and have revealed no evidence of impaired fertility or harm to the fetus due to (*name of drug*).
Pregnancy Category B	Reproduction studies have been performed in (*kind(s) of animal(s)*) at doses up to (*x*) times the human dose and have revealed no evidence of impaired fertility or harm to the fetus due to (*name of drug*). There are, however, no adequate and well-controlled studies in pregnant women. Because animal reproduction studies are not always predictive of human response, this drug should be used in pregnancy only if clearly needed. If animal reproduction studies have shown an adverse effect (other than decrease in fertility), but adequate and well-controlled studies in pregnant women have failed to demonstrate a risk to the fetus during the first trimester of pregnancy (and there is no evidence of a risk in later trimesters), the labeling must state: Reproduction studies in (*kind(s) of animal(s)*) have shown (*describe findings*) at (*x*) times the human dose. Studies in pregnant women, however, have not shown that (*name of drug*) increases the risk of abnormalities when administered during the first (*second, third, or all*) trimester(s) of pregnancy. Despite the animal findings, it would appear that the possibility of fetal harm is remote, if the drug is used during pregnancy. Nevertheless, because the studies in humans cannot rule out the possibility of harm, (*name of drug*) should be used during pregnancy only if clearly needed.
Pregnancy Category C	If animal reproduction studies have shown an adverse effect on the fetus, if there are no adequate and well-controlled studies in humans, and if the benefits from the use of the drug in pregnant women may be acceptable despite its potential risks, the labeling must state: Pregnancy Category C. (*Name of drug*) has been shown to be teratogenic (or to have an embryocidal effect or other adverse effect) in (*name(s) of species*) when given in doses (*x*) times the human dose. There are no adequate and well-controlled studies in pregnant women. (*Name of drug*) should be used during pregnancy only if the potential benefit justifies the potential risk to the fetus. If there are no animal reproduction studies and no adequate and well-controlled studies in humans, the labeling must state: Pregnancy Category C. Animal reproduction studies have not been conducted with (*name of drug*). It is also not known whether (*name of drug*) can cause fetal harm when administered to a pregnant woman or can affect reproduction capacity. (*Name of drug*) should be given to a pregnant woman only if clearly needed.
Pregnancy Category D	If there is positive evidence of human fetal risk based on adverse reaction data from investigational or marketing experience or studies in humans, but the potential benefits from the use of the drug in pregnant women may be acceptable despite its potential risks, the labeling must state: Pregnancy Category D. See "Warnings and Precautions" section (for § 201.57(c)(9)(i)(A)(4)) or Pregnancy Category D. See "Warnings" Section (for § 201.80(f)(6)(i)(d)). Under the "Warnings and Precautions" or "Warnings" section, the labeling must state: (*Name of drug*) can cause fetal harm when administered to a pregnant woman. (*Describe the human data and any pertinent animal data.*) If this drug is used during pregnancy, or if the patient becomes pregnant while taking this drug, the patient should be apprised of the potential hazard to a fetus.
Pregnancy Category X	If studies in animals or humans have demonstrated fetal abnormalities or if there is positive evidence of fetal risk based on adverse reaction reports from investigational or marketing experience, or both, and the risk of the use of the drug in a pregnant woman clearly outweighs any possible benefit, the labeling must state: Pregnancy Category X. See "Contraindications" section. Under "Contraindications," the labeling must state: (*Name of drug*) may (*can*) cause fetal harm when administered to a pregnant woman. (*Describe the human data and any pertinent animal data.*) (*Name of drug*) is contraindicated in women who are or may become pregnant. If this drug is used during pregnancy, or if the patient becomes pregnant while taking this drug, the patient should be apprised of the potential hazard to a fetus.

medical devices used to safeguard blood and blood components from infectious agents, blood-typing reagents and equipment used to collect blood and blood components; as well as xenotransplantation products. This section will focus on vaccines intended for use in humans.

Biological products are licensed under Section 351 of the Public Health Service Act. The CBER evaluates scientific and clinical data, as well as a full description of the manufacturing methods and other information submitted by manufacturers to determine if a product meets the conditions of approval specified in the regulations. The Biologics License Application (BLA) is a request for permission to introduce, or deliver for introduction, a biological product into interstate commerce. Biological products are regulated by the FDA under 21 CFR 600–680. Because many biological products also meet the definition of "drugs" under the Federal Food, Drug and Cosmetic Act, they are also subject to regulation under 21 CFR Parts 210–211. The CBER works to ensure that manufacturers follow current Good Manufacturing Practices, monitors promotion and advertising, and collects and analyzes safety data about biological products that are already on the market. Adverse events related to biological products other than vaccines are reported to the AERS as described for drugs. Vaccine-related adverse events are reported to the Vaccine Adverse Event Reporting System (VAERS). Biological products intended for veterinary use are regulated under a separate law, the Virus, Serum and Toxin Act, which is administered by the US Department of Agriculture. Blood and most blood products intended for animal use are regulated as drugs by the FDA.

After assessment of premarket data and consideration of all of the other conditions for licensure, as described in 21 CFR 601.20, the CBER makes a decision about approval of a biological product. The CBER's authority resides in the Public Health Service Act and in specific sections of the Federal Food, Drug and Cosmetic Act. The Public Health Service Act also provides authority to suspend licenses in situations where there exists a danger to public health. In addition, this statute allows for the preparation or procurement of products in the event of shortages and critical public health needs, and authorizes the creation and enforcement of regulations to prevent the introduction or spread of communicable diseases in the USA.

The CBER continues to monitor the safety of biological products after they have been approved. Although medical products are required to be safe, safety does not mean zero risk, since most medical products are associated with some level of risk. A safe biological product is one that has reasonable risks, given the patient's condition, the magnitude of the benefit expected and the alternatives available. Manufacturers holding an approved biologics license application are required to report adverse experiences to the FDA under 21 CFR 600.80. Adverse experiences that are both serious and unexpected, whether foreign or domestic, must be reported as soon as possible but not later than 15 calendar days of initial receipt of the information. The manufacturer must promptly investigate all adverse experiences that are the subject of these postmarketing 15-day reports and must submit follow-up reports within 15 calendar days of receipt of new information, or as requested by the FDA. Periodic adverse experience reports are submitted by the manufacturer at quarterly intervals for the first 3 years of licensure, then annually. Adverse experiences are also reported from postmarketing studies.

Vaccines undergo a rigorous review of laboratory and clinical data to ensure the safety, efficacy, purity and potency of these products. Many of these are childhood vaccines that have contributed to a significant reduction of preventable diseases. The prevention of infectious diseases through effective immunization programs is dependent on ensuring the safety of vaccines, as well as successful communication of their risks and benefits. Clinical trials conducted prior to vaccine licensure usually reveal that most adverse events are minor. Rare, serious adverse events are less likely to be detected during the pre-licensure process, even in large clinical trials. If a serious adverse event is found to be causally related to a vaccine, the balance of benefits and risks of vaccination may shift, possibly leading to changes in recommendations for vaccination (Griffin *et al.*, 2009).

The National Childhood Vaccine Injury Act of 1986 mandated reporting of certain adverse events and led to the establishment of the Vaccine Adverse Event Reporting System, or VAERS. The VAERS is a national vaccine safety surveillance program co-sponsored since 1990 by the FDA and the Centers for Disease Control and Prevention (CDC). The purpose of the VAERS is to detect possible signals of adverse events associated with vaccines. The VAERS collects and analyzes information from reports of adverse events that occur after the administration of US licensed vaccines. Reports are accepted from all concerned individuals, including healthcare providers, manufacturers and the public. The VAERS is continually monitored for any unexpected patterns or changes in rates of adverse events. The FDA also analyzes patterns of reporting associated with vaccine lots. The primary objectives of the VAERS are to detect new, unusual, or rare vaccine adverse events; to monitor increases in known adverse events; to determine patient risk factors for particular types of adverse events; to identify vaccine lots with increased numbers or types of reported adverse events; and to assess the safety of newly licensed vaccines. Although the VAERS can rarely provide definitive evidence of causal associations between vaccines and particular risks, its unique role as a national spontaneous reporting system enables the early detection of signals that can then be more rigorously investigated.

VAERS data are used by the CDC, the FDA and other organizations to monitor and study vaccine safety. The CDC and the FDA use VAERS data to respond to public inquiries regarding vaccine safety, and both organizations have published and presented vaccine safety studies based on VAERS data. VAERS data are also used by the CDC's Advisory Committee on Immunization Practices and the Vaccine and Related Biological Products Advisory Committee to evaluate possible adverse events after vaccinations and to develop recommendations for precautions and contraindications to vaccinations. Through continued reporting of adverse events after vaccination to the VAERS by healthcare providers, public health professionals and the public, the system will continue to be able to detect rare but potentially serious consequences of vaccination. The report of an adverse event to the VAERS is not proof that a vaccine caused the event. More than 10 million vaccinations per year are given to children less than 1 year old, usually between 2 months and 6 months of age (FDA CBER, 2009). At this stage of development, infants are at risk for a variety of medical events and serious childhood illnesses. These naturally occurring events include fevers, seizures, sudden infant death syndrome (SIDS), cancer, congenital heart disease, asthma and other conditions. Some infants coincidentally experience an adverse event shortly after a vaccination. In such situations an infection, congenital abnormality, injury or some other provocation may cause the event. Because of such coincidences, it is usually not possible from VAERS data alone to determine whether a particular adverse event resulted from a concurrent condition or from a vaccination – even when the event occurs soon after vaccination.

If VAERS data suggest a possible link between an adverse event and vaccination, the relationship may be further studied in a controlled fashion. Analyzing VAERS reports is a complex task. Children are often administered more than one vaccine at a time, making it difficult to know which vaccine, if any, may have contributed to any subsequent adverse events. While about 85% of adverse events reported to the VAERS are minor (such as mild fevers or redness and swelling at the injection site), the remaining 15% describe more serious events. The more serious events include hospitalizations, life-threatening events and deaths. As part of the VAERS program, the FDA reviews the deaths and other serious reports weekly, and conducts follow-up. In some cases, certain vaccines and potentially associated symptoms will receive more intense follow-up.

In addition to analyzing individual VAERS reports, the FDA also analyzes patterns of reporting associated with vaccine lots. Many complex factors must be considered in comparing reports between different vaccine lots. More reports may be received for a large lot than for a small one simply because more doses of vaccine from the large lot will be given to more individuals. Some lots contain as many as 700,000 doses, while others as few as 20,000 doses. Similarly, more reports will be received for a lot that has been in use for a long time than for a lot that has been in use for a short time. Even among lots of similar size and time in use, some lots will receive more reports than others, simply due to chance. The FDA looks for lots that have received more death reports than would be expected on the basis of such factors as time in use and chance variation as well as any unusual patterns in other serious reports within a lot. If such a lot is detected, further review is conducted to determine if the lot is safe for continued use or if additional FDA actions are needed. The FDA has the authority to recall a vaccine from use in the USA if it represents a risk to the American public.

The process of identifying a new vaccine safety signal requires a combination of clinical insight and epidemiologic knowledge. Several factors may make identification of true signals difficult, for example many vaccines are administered early in life, at a time when "baseline" risk is continually evolving. The evaluation of safety profiles of vaccines may involve comparing the proportions of particular symptoms out of the total number of events for a given vaccine to that observed among reports for another vaccine. This is an example of a proportional reporting rate ratio method and is a widely used measure in vaccine adverse event reporting systems for prospective and retrospective signal generation (Strom and Kimmel, 2006). Signals generated by adverse event reporting systems may need to be confirmed in epidemiologic studies. These studies can have several limitations, including exposure misclassification if there is poor documentation of vaccinations, difficulty in identifying enough cases for a meaningful study due to rare outcome events, difficulty in identifying a comparable control group of unvaccinated people and potential confounding factors, such as age in children. In 1990, the CDC initiated the Vaccine Safety Datalink (VSD) project. This study prospectively collects vaccination, medical outcome and covariate data under a joint protocol with multiple HMOs. Data from the VSD may be used to explore new vaccine safety hypotheses that may arise from medical literature, the VAERS or introduction of new vaccines (CDC, 2010). The FDA, the CDC and other Federal and private partners conduct active surveillance, in addition to full epidemiologic studies, to monitor and improve vaccine safety. The purpose of active safety surveillance is to rapidly identify signals of potential excess risk of adverse outcomes following introduction of a drug or vaccine into clinical practice. Electronic data, including but not limited to claims data, are often used for active surveillance of large medical databases. Once a signal of a potential excess risk is detected by the surveillance system, appropriate epidemiologic studies should be conducted to confirm or refute the association.

The VAERS is subject to the limitations inherent in any passive surveillance system. These limitations include underreporting; differential reporting (increased reporting in the first few years after vaccine licensure, or increased reporting of events occurring soon after vaccination); stimulated reporting (increased reporting after a known or alleged type of adverse event); reporting of coincidental events; poor data quality; and a lack of denominator data (number of doses of vaccines actually administered), so calculation of adverse event incidence rates is not usually possible. Despite the VAERS's limitations, an example of a successful vaccine safety alert provided by the VAERS is that of rotavirus vaccination and risk of intussusception in children. Intussusception had been reported among infant recipients of a rotavirus vaccine, RotaShield®, licensed in August 1998. Fifteen VAERS intussusception reports received between September 1, 1998 and July 7, 1999 were initially analyzed, leading to further investigation involving case-control and retrospective cohort studies. These studies demonstrated a substantially increased frequency of intussusception in the first one to two weeks after vaccination with RotaShield®, compared to infants who did not receive the vaccine. Multiple studies confirmed the association, and the manufacturer voluntarily recalled the vaccine (Zhou *et al.*, 2003).

Another example of how VAERS data may be used to assess safety of certain vaccines is that of the human papillomavirus (HPV) virus vaccine, Gardasil. The FDA approved Gardasil on June 8, 2006. It is approved for females 9–26 years of age to protect against cervical, vulvar and vaginal cancers caused by human papillomavirus (HPV) types 16 and 18 and genital warts caused by HPV types 6 and 11. The CDC's Advisory Committee on Immunization Practices (ACIP) recommended a routine three-dose vaccination series for girls 11 and 12 years of age. The vaccine is also recommended for girls and women aged 13 through 26 years who have not yet been vaccinated or who have not received all three doses. On August 19, 2009, the Journal of the American Medical Association published an article coauthored by the FDA and the CDC that reviewed the safety data for Gardasil for select adverse events that had been reported to the VAERS, from the time period starting from product licensure in June 2006 through December 31, 2008 (Slade *et al.*, 2009). The article describes 12,424 reports of adverse events following Gardasil vaccination. Of these, 772 were reports of serious events (6.2% of the reports) and the remaining 11,652 (93.8%) were classified as non-serious. The Gardasil safety review assessed the following adverse events: local injection site reactions, syncope, dizziness and nausea, headaches, hypersensitivity reactions, such as rashes, hives, itching, anaphylaxis, Guillain-Barré syndrome (GBS), transverse myelitis, motor neuron disease, venous thromboembolic events (VTEs), pancreatitis, autoimmune disorders and deaths. All of these events are included in Gardasil's approved labeling. Based on the review of available information by the FDA and the CDC, it was determined that Gardasil's benefits continue to outweigh its risks. As with all licensed vaccines, the FDA continues to closely monitor the safety of Gardasil.

Registries of people inadvertently exposed to vaccines can contribute to the knowledge base regarding prognosis in these populations, and registries of those with rare adverse events allow exploration of genetic or other predictors of such effects. An example of such a registry is the National Smallpox Vaccine in Pregnancy Registry, established by the CDC in collaboration with the FDA and the Department of Defense in 2003. When the USA implemented civilian and military smallpox vaccination programs in 2003, the National Smallpox Vaccine in Pregnancy Registry was established to better evaluate outcomes after the inadvertent vaccination of pregnant women. Smallpox vaccine is known to cause fetal vaccinia, a very rare but serious complication of exposure to smallpox vaccine during pregnancy. Fewer than 50 cases have been reported, three of which occurred in the USA in 1924, 1959 and 1968. Affected pregnancies have been reported in women vaccinated in all three trimesters, in primary vaccinees and in those being revaccinated, and in non-vaccinated contacts of vaccinees. Because a risk of infection to the fetus is possible, smallpox vaccination is not recommended for pregnant women or anyone with close physical contact to a pregnant woman. To prevent inadvertent exposure of pregnant women to vaccinia virus, screening for pregnancy is a component of smallpox vaccination programs. Women are referred to the registry by vaccine administrators, healthcare providers or state health departments, through self-referral or through reports from the Department of Defense (DoD), the CDC, the FDA and the VAERS (Ryan and Grabenstein, 2003; CDC, 2003). Registry professionals actively follow up with all enrolled women and collect data on pregnancy, birth and infant health outcomes. As of September 2006, pregnancy outcome data were available from 376 women. Most (77%) were vaccinated near the time of conception, before results of a standard pregnancy test would have been positive. To date, outcome evaluations have not revealed higher-than-expected rates of pregnancy loss (11.9%), preterm birth (10.7%) or birth defects (2.8%), compared with those in healthy referent populations. No cases of fetal vaccinia have been identified. The Smallpox Vaccine in Pregnancy Registry continues to actively enroll women and follow infant and early-childhood health outcomes (Ryan and Seward, 2008).

The CBER reviews a broad spectrum of applications for investigational vaccines intended for the prevention and treatment of infectious diseases and indicated for immunization of adolescents and adults. Thus, the target population for vaccines often includes females of childbearing potential who may become pregnant during the vaccination period. A number of vaccines are in clinical development specifically for maternal immunization indications with the goal of preventing infectious disease in the pregnant mother and/or neonate through passive antibody transfer from mother to fetus (FDA CBER, 2000). Unless the vaccine is specifically indicated for maternal immunization, studies are typically not conducted prior to product licensure to determine the vaccine's safety in pregnant women. During clinical development of most vaccines not specifically intended for use during pregnancy, pregnant women are generally ineligible to participate in clinical trials. If pregnancy occurs during a study, treatment is usually discontinued and the woman does not receive additional immunizations. Consequently, there are few clinical data to address reproductive and developmental toxicity of the vaccine in pregnant women or females of childbearing potential at the time of product licensure.

The CDC provides guidelines for the vaccination of pregnant and lactating women. According to the CDC, risk to a developing fetus from vaccination of the mother during pregnancy is primarily theoretical. No evidence exists of risk from vaccinating pregnant women with inactivated virus or bacterial vaccines or toxoids. Live vaccines pose a theoretical risk to the fetus. Benefits of vaccinating pregnant women usually outweigh potential risks when the likelihood of disease exposure is high, when infection would pose a risk to the mother or fetus and when the vaccine is unlikely to cause harm (CDC, 2006). Generally, live-virus vaccines are contraindicated for pregnant women because of the theoretical risk of transmission of the vaccine virus to the fetus. If a live-virus vaccine is inadvertently given to a pregnant woman, or if a woman becomes pregnant within 4 weeks after vaccination, she should be counseled about the potential effects on the fetus, but vaccination is not ordinarily an indication to terminate the pregnancy. Whether live or inactivated vaccines are used, vaccination of pregnant women should be considered on the basis of risks versus benefits – i.e., the risk of the vaccination versus the benefits of protection in a particular circumstance. The CDC also currently recommends prenatal screening for rubella and hepatitis B and prenatal assessment for varicella. See www.cdc.gov/vaccines/pubs/preg-guide.htm for CDC recommendations regarding specific vaccines and prenatal screening.

DRUGS INTENDED FOR USE IN ANIMALS

The Center for Veterinary Medicine (CVM) is responsible for approving drugs for animals, including drugs used in medicated feeds, and for monitoring drugs and feeds intended for use in animals. There are currently no requirements for FDA premarket approval of medical devices intended for animal use. Among the CVM's regulatory activities are reviewing new animal drug applications for brand-name, innovator pharmaceuticals and generic animal pharmaceuticals; enforcement of regulations governing the manufacture of animal pharmaceutical products, the promotion and advertising of prescription animal drugs, and drug experience reporting by firms marketing drugs; taking action against animal drugs marketed without approval; and collecting and analyzing safety data about marketed animal pharmaceuticals. One of the CVM's primary objectives is to ensure that prescription and over-the-counter (OTC) medications intended for animal use are safe and effective when used as directed. All drugs have risks, and healthcare professionals and animal owners must balance the risks and benefits of a drug when making decisions about medical therapy. The FDA monitors and reviews available safety and effectiveness information related to marketed drugs throughout each product's lifecycle. Similar to human drugs, when an animal drug is approved, the product labeling includes, among other things, available information about the benefits and risks of the drug.

The CVM's additional responsibilities include ensuring that food products from treated food-producing animals are safe for human consumption. Part of the pre-approval process for drugs intended for use in food-producing animals includes the determination of safety of drug residues in animal-derived food products. Tolerances for residues of animal drugs in food are codified in 21 CFR Part 556. In addition, pre-approval safety evaluation of certain animal drugs includes a determination of the effects of the animal drug on the environment and on human health in some cases. In support of the drug review function, the CVM's Office of Research conducts studies in animal drug safety and efficacy, antimicrobial resistance mechanisms, metabolism, standardization of test methods and pharmacokinetics/pharmacodynamics. The Office of Research supports compliance programs of the center through the development of analytical methods and evaluation of screening tests for detection of drug residues in imported and domestic food products. It also conducts research to understand the microbiology of animal feeds and the dissemination of resistant bacteria via livestock feeds, and develops methods to detect material prohibited by the BSE (bovine spongiform encephalopathy) feed regulation that could compromise animal feed safety (FDA CVM, 2010).

After drug approval, the FDA may learn of new, or more frequent, serious adverse drug experiences from post-approval clinical studies or from clinical use in animals. For example, additional adverse drug experiences may be identified as a drug is more widely used and under more diverse conditions. Regulations at 21 CFR 514.80 describe the spontaneous reporting obligations for holders of approved new animal drug applications and other firms marketing these products. Definitions in 21 CFR 514.3 for "adverse drug experience", "serious adverse drug experience" and "unexpected adverse drug experience" are similar to the human definitions found in 21 CFR 314.80, with a few exceptions. "Adverse drug experience" as defined in 21 CFR 514.3 is any adverse event associated with the use of a new animal drug, whether or not considered to be drug related, and whether or not the new animal drug was used in accordance with the approved labeling (i.e., used according to label directions or used in an extralabel manner, including but not limited to different route of administration, different species, different indications or other than labeled dosage). Adverse drug experience includes, but is not limited to: an adverse event occurring in animals in the course of the use of an animal drug product by a veterinarian or by a livestock producer or other animal owner or caretaker; failure of a new animal drug to produce its expected pharmacological or clinical effect (lack of expected effectiveness); or an adverse event occurring in humans from exposure during manufacture, testing, handling or use of a new animal drug. "Serious adverse drug experience" as defined by 21 CFR 514.3 is an adverse event that is fatal, or life-threatening, or requires professional intervention, or causes an abortion, or stillbirth, or infertility, or congenital anomaly, or prolonged or permanent disability, or disfigurement. "Unexpected adverse drug experience" has the same definition as found in 21 CFR 314.80.

Reporting of adverse drug events (ADEs) by veterinarians and animal owners is voluntary and mandatory for animal drug application holders and, in the case of serious and unexpected adverse events, manufacturers or distributors named on the label. Application holders send reports directly to the CVM, manufacturers and distributors to the CVM or the application holder. The CVM also accepts electronic submission of adverse event information for veterinary drugs. Electronic submission of adverse event information will be possible through the Electronic Submissions System (ESS) and the Rational Questionnaire (RQ) in the Safety Reporting Portal (SRP), a joint FDA–National Institutes of Health initiative. The SRP was launched on May 24, 2010, and when fully developed, will provide a mechanism for the reporting of certain pre- and postmarket safety data to the Federal government. Currently the SRP website can be used to report safety problems related to foods, including animal feed and animal drugs, as well as adverse events occurring on human gene transfer trials. Consumers can also use the site to report problems with pet foods and pet treats (FDA, 2010c).

When an ADE report arrives at the CVM, it is logged into the center's Document Control Unit, assigned a submission number and forwarded to the CVM's Division of Surveillance for processing. CVM safety reviewers, who are experienced clinical veterinarians, then review the individual ADE reports. The safety reviewers enter all relevant information such as age, breed, history, pre-existing problems and concomitant drugs into a searchable ADE database. The reviewers evaluate each clinical sign reported using a scoring system that is a modified version of the Kramer algorithm. Under the scoring system, information about age, breed, gender, pre-existing conditions and concomitant drugs is considered. A summary causality assessment score for each clinical sign is determined and entered into the database as part of the evaluation process. The summary score corresponds to the strength of the association between the drug and the clinical sign and ranges between −9 and +7. Clinical signs with summary scores of zero or greater are considered possibly, probably, or definitely drug related. Every reported clinical sign is reviewed and evaluated for each of the following criteria in the Kramer algorithm: previous experience with the drug, alternative etiologic candidates, timing of events, evidence of overdose, dechallenge and rechallenge. The primary purpose for maintaining the CVM's ADE database is to provide an early warning or signaling system to the center for adverse effects not detected during premarket testing of FDA-approved animal drugs and for monitoring the performance of drugs used both on and off label (extralabel) in animals. The Animal Medicinal Drug Use Clarification Act of 1994 (AMDUCA) allows veterinarians to prescribe extralabel uses of certain approved animal drugs and approved human drugs for animals under certain conditions. Extralabel use refers to the use of an approved drug in a manner that is not in accordance with the approved label directions. The key constraints of the AMDUCA are that any extralabel use must be by or on the order of a veterinarian within the context of a veterinarian–client–patient relationship, must not result in violative residues in food-producing animals and the use must be in conformance with the implementing regulations published at 21 CFR Part 530.

CVM scientists use the ADE database to make decisions about product safety which may include changes to the label or other regulatory actions. Interventions utilized for human pharmaceuticals may also be used for animal drugs to help enhance safe use; for example, "Dear Doctor" letters, restricted distribution programs under RiskMAPs, and additional labeling components such as Client Information Sheets (similar to human medication guides) may be required. ADE summary reports are posted on the CVM's website and updated at regular intervals. The appropriate use of this website information is to search the active ingredient of a drug to see if particular signs have been reported with their use. Clinical signs for each drug are listed in order of frequency from most frequently observed to least frequently observed. As with other pharmacovigilance databases, for any given ADE report, there is no certainty that the reported drug caused the adverse event. The adverse event may have been related to an underlying disease, using other drugs at the same time, or other non-drug related causes. In addition, the accuracy of information regarding an adverse drug experience depends on the quality of information received from the reporter. Like the CDER, the CVM is also actively exploring various automated Bayesian data mining techniques to augment its ability to monitor the safety of animal drugs.

Just as for human drugs, FDA-approved animal drug product labeling is the primary source of information about a drug's safety and effectiveness, and it summarizes the essential scientific information needed for the safe and effective use of the drug. Labeling for prescription animal drug products is directed to healthcare professionals, but may include sections that are intended for animal owners and that also must be FDA approved. Similar to medication guides for humans which are commonly distributed with human pharmacy prescriptions, the Client Information Sheets may be required by the FDA as part of the approved labeling for animal drugs. These are written in "consumer-friendly" language and provide information in easily understood terms about the benefits and side effects associated with the use of certain drugs. Examples of drugs which include Client Information Sheets as part of the labeling are the non-steroidal anti-inflammatory drugs intended for use in companion animals.

Certain animal drug labels are required to bear specific warnings or precautions as related to potential animal or human reproductive toxicity issues. For example, as the safety of most corticosteroid drugs for use during all stages of pregnancy has not been adequately established in animals, 21 CFR 510.410 requires corticosteroids for oral, injectable and ophthalmic use in animals to contain the following statement: "Warning: Clinical and experimental data have demonstrated that corticosteroids administered orally or by injection to animals may induce the first stage of parturition if used during the last trimester of pregnancy and may precipitate premature parturition followed by dystocia, fetal death, retained placenta, and metritis. Additionally, corticosteroids administered to dogs, rabbits, and rodents during pregnancy have resulted in cleft palate in offspring. Corticosteroids administered to dogs during pregnancy have also resulted in other congenital anomalies, including deformed forelegs, phocomelia, and anasarca." Certain animal drugs may be required to bear warnings or precautions as related to human exposure to the product. For example, Regu-Mate® (altrenogest) Solution 0.22% is indicated to suppress estrus in mares. Suppression of estrus allows for a predictable occurrence of estrus following drug withdrawal. This facilitates the attainment of regular cyclicity during the transition from winter anestrus to the physiological breeding season. Suppression of estrus will also facilitate management of prolonged estrus conditions. Suppression of estrus may be used to facilitate scheduled breeding during the physiological breeding season. The drug label for this product contains specific human warnings regarding the potential effects of exposure to the drug on human reproduction: "Human Warning: Skin contact must be avoided as Regu-Mate® (altrenogest) Solution 0.22% is readily absorbed through unbroken skin. Protective gloves must be worn by all persons handling this product. Pregnant women or women who suspect they are pregnant should not handle Regu-Mate® (altrenogest) Solution 0.22%. Women of childbearing age should exercise extreme caution when handling this product. Accidental absorption could lead to a disruption of the menstrual cycle or prolongation of pregnancy. Direct contact with the skin should therefore be avoided. Accidental spillage on the skin should be washed off immediately with soap and water." There has been no approved human use of this specific product. The information contained in the labeling of this product is extrapolated from data available on other products of the same pharmacological class that have been used in humans. Effects anticipated are due to the progestational activity of altrenogest. Acute effects after a single exposure are possible; however, continued daily exposure has the potential for more untoward effects such as disruption of the menstrual cycle, uterine or abdominal cramping, increased or decreased uterine bleeding, prolongation of pregnancy and headaches.

Presently, animal drug labeling is not required by regulation to contain specific "Pregnancy" or "Lactation" subsections. Drug manufacturers generally will provide any known information, or a statement indicating that use in pregnant or lactating animals has not been evaluated. Drugs reported to be contraindicated during pregnancy in animals include fluoroquinolones, tetracyclines, griseofulvin, pentobarbital, misoprostol, warfarin, diethylstilbestrol, estracypionate, mitotane, stanozolol and testosterone (Evans, 2007).

CVM does not regulate animal vaccines or any other biological products that achieve their primary intended purposes by enhancing or stimulating the animal's immune system, such as bacterins, antisera and some diagnostic kits. These products are regulated by the United States Department of Agriculture (USDA) under the Virus-Serum-Toxin Act (VSTA) through its Center for Veterinary Biologics (CVB). The CVB is charged with ensuring that the veterinary biologics available for the diagnosis, prevention and treatment of animal diseases are pure, safe, potent and effective. The Veterinary Biologics Pharmacovigilance Program is for the ongoing surveillance of adverse events associated with animal vaccines and other biologics, in cooperation with the veterinary profession and the veterinary biologics industry. Information about reporting adverse events related to animal vaccines may be found on the USDA's website, http://www.aphis.usda.gov/animal_health/vet_biologics/.

REFERENCES

Andrade SE, Gurwitz JH, Davis RL, Chan KA, Finkelstein JA, Fortman K, McPhillips H, Raebel MA, Roblin D, Smith DH, Yood MU, Morse AN, Platt R (2004) Prescription drug use in pregnancy. *Am J Obst and Gyn* **191:** 398–407.

CDC (2003) Notice to Readers: National Smallpox Vaccine in Pregnancy Registry. *CDC MMWR* **52(12):** 256.

CDC (2006) General recommendations on immunization: recommendations of the Advisory Committee on Immunization Practices (ACIP). *CDC MMWR* **55 (No. RR-15):** 32–3.

CDC (2010) Vaccine Safety Datalink (VSD) Project. http://www.cdc.gov/vaccinesafetyActvitities/VSD.html (accessed June 2010).

Evans, TJ (2007) Reproductive toxicity and endocrine disruption. In *Veterinary Toxicology: Basic and Clinical Principles* (Gupta, RC, ed.). Elsevier, New York, NY, pp. 206–44.

FDA (2007) U.S. FDA Section 505-1[21 USC §355-1] Risk evaluation and mitigation strategies.

FDA (2008) The Sentinel Initiative: a national strategy for monitoring medical product safety. Rockville, MD. http://www.fda.gov/Safety/FDASentinelInitiative/ucm089474.htm.

FDA (2009a) About FDA. http://www.fda.gov/About FDA/WhatWeDo/History/default.htm.

FDA (2009b) Endocrine Disruptor Knowledge Database. http://www.fda.gov/ScienceResearch/BioinformaticsTools/EndocrineDisruptorKnowledgebase/default.htm.

FDA (2009c) Postmarket Requirements and Commitments. http://www.fda.gov/Drugs/GuidanceComplianceRegulatoryInformation/Post-marketingPhaseIVCommitments/default.htm.

FDA (2009d) Health Organizations to Study Safety of Medications Taken During Pregnancy. http://www.fda.gov/NewsEvents/Newsroom/PressAnnouncements/ucm195934.htm.

FDA (2010a) MedWatch: The FDA Safety Information Adverse Event Reporting Program. http://www.fda.gov/Safety/Medwatch/default.htm.

FDA (2010b) List of Pregnancy Exposure Registries.http://www.fda.gov/ScienceResearch/SpecialTopics/WomensHealthResearch/ucm 13848.htm.

FDA (2010c) Safety Reporting Portal: a new online tool. http://www.fda.gov/NewsEvents/PublicHealthFocus/ucm212845.htm.

FDA CBER (2000) Draft Guidance for Industry: Considerations for Reproductive Toxicity Studies for Preventive Vaccines for Infectious Disease Indications. http://www.fda.gov/BiologicsBloodVaccines/GuidanceComplianceRegulatoryInformation/Guidances/Vaccines/ucm076611.htm

FDA CBER (2009) Vaccine Adverse Events. http://www.fda.gov/BiologicsBloodVaccines/SafetyAvailability/ReportaProblem/VaccineAdverseEvents/default.htm.

FDA CDER (2007a) Guidance: Drug Safety Information – FDA's Communication to the Public, March 2007. http://ww.fda.gov/downloads/Drugs/GuidanceComplianceRegulatoryInformation/Guidances/ucm72281.pdf.

FDA CDER (2007b) Public Health Advisory: Use of Codeine by Some Breastfeeding Mothers May Lead to Life-Threatening Side Effects in Nursing Babies. http://www.fda.gov/Drugs/DrugSafety/PublicHealthAdvisories/ucm054717.htm.

FDA CDER (2009) Summary of Proposed Rule on Pregnancy and Lactation. http://www.fda.gov/Drugs/DevelopmentApprovalProcess/DevelopmentalResources/Labeling/ucm093310.htm.

FDA CDER, Rockville, MD (2010) Approved Risk Evaluation Mitigation Strategies. http://www.fda.gov/Drugs/DrugSafety/PostmarketDrugSafetyInformationforPatientsandProviders/ucm111350.htm.

FDA CDER/CBER (2002) Guidance for Industry: Establishing Pregnancy Exposure Registries. http://www.fda.gov/downloads/Drugs/GuidanceComplianceRegulatoryInformation/Guidances/ucm071639.pdf.

FDA, CDER/CBER (2005) Reviewer Guidance – Evaluating the Risks of Drug Exposure in Human Pregnancies. http://www.fda.gov/downloads/Drugs/GuidanceComplianceRegulatoryInformation/Guidances/ucm071645.pdf.

FDA CVM (2010) Bovine Spongiform Encephalopathy. http://www.fda.gov/AnimalVeterinary/GuidanceComplianceEnforcement/ComplianceEnforcement/BovineSpongiformEncephalopathy/default.htm.

Griffin MR, Braun MM, Bart KJ (2009) What should an ideal vaccine postlicensure safety system be? *Am J Public Hlth* Suppl 2, **99:** S345–50.

IOM (2006) The future of drug safety: promoting and protecting the health of the public. September 22, 2006. http:// www.iom.edu/CMS/3793/26341/37329.aspx.

Koren G, Cairns J, Chitayat D, Gaedigk A, Leeder SJ (2006) Pharmacogenetics of morphine poisoning in a breastfed neonate of a codeine-prescribed mother. *The Lancet* **368 (9536):** 704.

MedDRA, Medical Dictionary for Regulatory Activities Maintenance and Support Services Organization (2010). http://www.meddramsso.com/.

Ryan MA, Grabenstein JD (2003) Women with smallpox vaccine exposure during pregnancy reported to the National Smallpox Vaccine in Pregnancy Registry – United Sates, 2003. *CDC MMWR* **52(17):** 386–8.

Ryan MA, Seward JF (2008) Smallpox vaccine in pregnancy registry team. *Clin Infect Dis* **46 (Suppl. 3):** S221–6.

Slade BA, Leidel L, Vellozzi C, Woo EJ, Hua W, Sutherland A, Izurieta HS, Ball R, Miller N, Braun MM, Markowitz LE, Iskander J (2009) Postlicensure safety surveillance for quadrivalent human papillomavirus recombinant vaccine. *JAMA* **302(7):** 750–7.

Strom BL, Kimmel SE (2006) Special applications of pharmacoepidemiology. In *Textbook of Pharmacoepidemiology*. John Wiley & Sons, West Sussex, England, pp. 411–14.

World Health Organization (WHO) Safety Monitoring of Medical Products: Guidelines for Setting up and Running a Pharmacovigilance Centre. Uppsala Monitoring Centre, Sweden, 2006.

Zhou W, Pool V, Iskander JK, English-Bullard R, Ball R, Wise RP, Haber P, Pless RP, Mootrey G, Ellenberg SS, Braun MM, Chen RT (2003) Surveillance for safety after immunization: Vaccine Adverse Event Reporting System (VAERS) – United States, 1991–2001. *CDC MMWR* **52 (ss01):** 1–24.

C H A P T E R

8

Reproductive and developmental safety evaluation of new pharmaceutical compounds

Ramesh C. Garg, William M. Bracken and Alan M. Hoberman

INTRODUCTION

The term "Pharmaceuticals" usually implies: (1) innovative small molecules, their therapeutically equivalent or generic medicinal products; (2) innovative biopharmaceuticals, medicinal products of biotechnology origin and their biosimilar, follow-on biologics or biogeneric medicinal products; and (3) veterinary pharmaceuticals. This chapter outlines identification, interpretation and communication of potential reproductive and developmental toxicity hazard/risks for new pharmaceutical compounds that could be prescribed as drugs after regulatory approval for specific indication(s) to men and women of various age groups. When prescribed to men and women of reproductive age or to women during pregnancy, the reproductive safety information included on the product label will be a primary source for safety and efficacy of data of interest to physicians and patients. Reproductive safety data based on actual human experiences are always considered more relevant and preferred over data from animals but for new pharmaceuticals, such information is often not available or rare. The initial label information is mainly based on animal studies performed according to internationally recognized guidelines for Development and Reproductive Toxicity (DART) studies in animals. Performing studies to evaluate the reproductive and developmental effects of a test article in healthy men or women would be unethical as consent of the unborn can never be obtained. This information can only be generated in animals. The healthcare professionals usually know that a drug has undergone an approval process by an appropriate regulatory body such as the Food and Drug Administration (FDA) in the USA but very few really know or are familiar with the extent of non-clinical testing that is undertaken by the drug's manufacturer. The non-clinical set of toxicology studies usually includes DART studies to help assure reproductive safety by identifying reproductive hazards for a New Molecular Entity (NME) or a drug. This is considered very important unless the drug is intended for subjects where effects on reproductive functions are not a consideration (e.g., postmenopausal women). As the predictive value of findings observed in animal toxicity studies for use in humans is not always consistent, and at the time of drug approval information relating to effects of the NME in pregnant women is not or rarely available, most drugs are not labeled for use during pregnancy and carry a statement *"Use in pregnancy is not recommended unless the potential benefits justify the potential risks to the fetus."* The purpose of animal toxicity studies including the DART studies is to identify safety hazards and limit the risk of adverse or harmful effects when a new drug is used in human subjects at recommended therapeutic dosages. This information is intended to help the prescribing physician make the best medical decision for the patient, particularly for use of a drug in women of child-bearing potential or in women that may become or are already pregnant.

Identification, interpretation, communication and management of potential reproductive or developmental toxicity-related hazards/risks during the development process of a pharmaceutical compound are discussed in this chapter. In addition to an introduction to the pharmaceutical development process, this required discussions related to current internationally harmonized study guidelines, timing of studies with respect to drug development process, history and evolution of reproductive safety testing guidelines, outlines of commonly used developmental and reproductive toxicity studies, special consideration for evaluating biotherapeutics, regulatory considerations for interpretation of reproductive risks for humans, risk communication, upcoming drug product label changes, and risk management plans for addressing the reproductive risks associated with a newly approved drug product, if any. These are included below.

OVERVIEW OF HUMAN PHARMACEUTICAL DEVELOPMENT PROCESS

An overview of human pharmaceutical development is discussed with respect to both innovator (small and large molecule) and generic (or biosimilar) pharmaceutical compounds intended for human use.

Reproductive and Developmental Toxicology, Edited by Ramesh C. Gupta
ISBN: 978-0-12-382032-7

Innovator pharmaceuticals – small molecules or biotherapeutics

The drug development process for a new, innovator compound (a small molecule or a biotherapeutic drug product) is a long and expensive undertaking in the USA. It carries a substantial risk of failure inherent in rigorous and complex studies that are undertaken during discovery, preclinical and clinical testing of a new drug to assure and protect patient safety.

As summarized in a recent Pharmaceutical Industry Profile 2008 by the Pharmaceutical Research and Manufacturing Association (PhRMA, 2008), it takes many people, ideas, dollars and years with no guarantee of success to develop a drug. On average, researchers spend between 10 and 15 years developing each new potential medicine, yet the odds that any new medicine will make it all the way to the market are slim. A team of chemists, pharmacologists and biologists screen thousands of compounds or create a new one and test them against the target(s) to identify any that has a potential for successful development. In general, for every 5,000 to 10,000 compounds tested, only 250 make it to preclinical stage, just five ever make it to clinical trials stage and only one is ever approved by the FDA. About half of all experimental drugs in phase 3 clinical trials ever become approved medicines. More than $1 billion is spent on research and development for each new drug or biological approval. Only 2 in 10 approved drugs bring in enough revenue to recoup their cost of development. The overall steps involved in the development of a small molecule pharmaceutical are shown in Figure 8.1.

The timing for various non-clinical toxicity studies needed for development of a small molecule or a biotherapeutic innovator drug product extends from discovery phase to the phase 3 clinical development stage as shown in Figure 8.1.

Non-clinical aspects of biotherapeutic development are discussed later in another section of this chapter. As a general introduction, several case studies relating to biotherapeutic development were discussed in a meeting sponsored by the PhRMA and the FDA (2007). The meeting outcome was published recently by Buckley *et al.* (2008) highlighting special considerations needed for developing innovator biotherapeutic drug products. With respect to DART studies for biotherapeutics, participants of the meeting agreed that: (1) rodents and rabbits are the preferred animal models for DART studies as long as they are pharmacologically relevant species and drug exposure can be demonstrated; (2) cohorts of rodents may be used to test different segments of the reproductive lifecycle including embryo–fetal development per International Conference on Harmonization of Technical Requirements for the Registration of Pharmaceuticals for Human Use (ICH) guidance (S5(R2) listed in Table 8.3) to avoid potentially confounding immunogenicity; (3) surrogate molecule strategies (e.g., homologous protein versus clinical candidate) could be considered following careful characterization of the surrogate with regard to comparative affinity, biologic effect and placental transfer properties as well as consideration of impurities; and (4) DART studies could be performed in non-human primates (NHPs); however, issues of low statistical power (resulting from one offspring per mating) and limited historical control data need to be carefully considered to ensure that the use of NHP species would be appropriate. A scientific justification for species selection, study design and strategies for achieving the stated objectives is usually considered appropriate.

Generic drugs

Small molecule

Unlike the New Drug Application (NDA) process that requires extensive safety testing for an innovator compound or NME for approval for marketing, the generic drug applicants only need to demonstrate that their products are pharmaceutically equivalent and bioequivalent to the reference (innovator) product. Pharmaceutically equivalent products have the same active ingredient(s) in the same strength in the same dosage form. The generic drug approval process as revised in 1984 does not require preclinical or clinical data establishing the active ingredient's safety and efficacy (Henderson, 1992; Welage *et al.*, 2001). This is based on the understanding that when a generic drug is pharmaceutically equivalent and bioequivalent, it is expected to

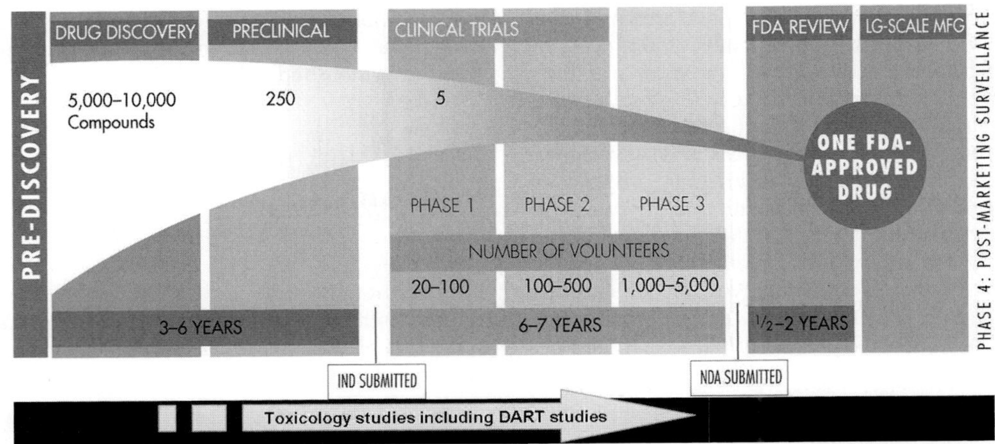

FIGURE 8.1 Drug development, a long, complex and costly process. (Adapted with permission from Profile 2008 – Pharmaceutical Industry, PhRMA, Washington DC, March 2008.)

be therapeutically and toxicologically equivalent. In other words, the assumption is that if the active ingredient has been shown to be safe and effective after it is absorbed into the bloodstream, any product with the same dosage form that gives rise to the same concentrations of active ingredient in the body to the same rate and extent would produce the same biological effect.

Overview of the generic drugs approval process in the USA

The generic drug approval process has been reviewed (Welage *et al.*, 2001) for scientific issues associated with the approval process. In 1984, the Drug Price Competition and Patent Term Restoration Act gave the FDA statutory authority to approve generic versions of innovator drug products approved after 1962 as safe and effective (Henderson, 1992).

Prior to 1984, the generic drug approval process evolved slowly over several decades with varying requirements. In 1970, the FDA established the Abbreviated New Drug Application (ANDA) as a mechanism for review and approval of generic versions of the drug products that had been approved between 1938 and 1962 (Henderson, 1992). For drugs approved after 1962, manufacturers of generic products were required to submit complete safety and efficacy data. Until 1978, manufacturers of generic drugs needed to conduct clinical efficacy and safety trials. After 1978, this requirement was modified but still the manufacturers were required to cite the published reports of such trials for documenting safety and efficacy. Neither of these approaches was considered satisfactory, as the former was quite expensive and the latter required evidence that usually was not available, i.e. data that had not been published.

Biosimilar or biogeneric drugs for biotherapeutics

As summarized by Gottlieb (2008), no formal regulatory process/guidance exists in the USA for bringing these drugs to market. In addition, the current tools available for fully characterizing biotherapeuticss are not well developed in certain cases, especially for proteins that have complex structures or are heavily glycosylated. In addition, using "similar" but not completely "identical" proteins raises concerns about the potential for immunogenicity. The bottom line is that demonstrating therapeutic equivalence and interchangeability for biosimilars is not a straightforward matter. It cannot be based on the same criteria as for conventional small-molecule drugs. The science, while obtainable, is more complex. For example, it is assumed that showing that a biosimilar protein can be safely used interchangeably with an innovator protein would require, at the least, some limited clinical data and interchangeability studies.

Some preclinical studies may be required on a case-by-case basis as noted by Brodniewicz-Proba (2008) with respect to European Medicines Agency's (EMA) recommendations for biosimilar erythropoietin and insulin. For biosimilar erythropoietin, in addition to recommendation for a few *in vivo* and *in vitro* studies, the needed toxicology studies included a 3-month repeated dose and local tolerance studies in at least one species. The reproductive or mutagenicity studies were not included in this recommendation.

DEVELOPMENTAL AND REPRODUCTIVE TOXICITY (DART) STUDIES NEEDED FOR DEVELOPMENT OF INNOVATIVE HUMAN PHARMACEUTICALS

Overview

Recent data from Centers for Disease Control (CDC, 2009) suggests that about 120,000 babies (1 in 33) in the USA are born each year with birth defects, and that birth defects are the leading cause of death during the first year of life (Mathews and MacDorman, 2008). These observations coupled with increased exposure to chronic use of pharmaceuticals for managing health conditions like blood pressure, diabetes, cholesterol, gastro-esophageal reflex, etc., highlight the importance of identifying and characterizing the reproductive risks for all new pharmaceuticals intended for use by the reproductive age population. This risk is broadly divided into two categories, (1) reproductive risks and (2) developmental risks. The reproductive risks are related to interference with or effect on processes like fertility (male and female), parturition and lactation. The developmental risks relate to the fetus and include mortality, dysmorphogenesis (structural alterations), alteration in growth and functional deficits. The historical evolution of reproductive testing guidelines, outlines for DART studies, considerations for testing of biotherapeutics, timing of studies with respect to pharmaceutical development process and related topics are discussed in sections below.

History and evolution of reproductive testing guidelines

Regulatory guidelines were principally the result of three human tragedies. Each of these tragedies resulted from *in utero* exposure to a drug: (1) 1961 – congenital malformations (Lenz, 1961; McBride, 1961); (2) early 1970s – cancer (Herbst *et al.*, 1971); and (3) 1976 – behavioral/functional alterations (Koos and Longo, 1976). The first of these pivotal events completely changed the existent concerns regarding consumption of a medicine and the potential adverse outcomes of a pregnancy. The second raised additional concerns regarding adverse effects of a drug that were the result of *in utero* exposure but were not evident until after puberty. The third resulted in addition of tests for postnatal behavioral changes to the regulations. These events and concerns changed the concepts regarding the ability of agents to affect *in utero* development and refocused the tests from identifying the potential of pharmaceuticals to produce adverse effects on the entire reproductive process to testing for effects on development of the conceptus, in particular, fetal malformations.

In the first half of the 20th century, Warkany (1965) noted that human birth defects were usually considered spontaneous or hereditary events, although diseases and some chemicals, such as alcohol, were considered possibly to affect reproductive performance or the outcome of a given pregnancy. Malnutrition in humans and animals was considered to affect reproduction by potentially reducing fertility or birth weight or by causing abortion or death of the conceptus. Jackson's definitive review (1925) of the effects of malnutrition did not identify congenital malformation as a possible outcome. Measles caused congenital cataracts in humans (Gregg, 1941) and was the first identified malformation that was not due to malnutrition. This causal relationship of maternal measles and congenital malformation was considered unique because of the interrelated maternal disease, and humans were still considered to be unaffected by *in utero* exposure to drugs or chemicals. Not until after World War II, when the effects of malnutrition in Leningrad and Holland were reported (Antonov, 1947; Smith, 1947), was it identified that maternal malnutrition could result in congenital malformations in humans, as well as other unfavorable outcomes including reproductive failure, abnormal or absent menstrual cycles, increased abortion, small birth weight and reduced postnatal survival.

In 1921, an anecdotal report was published that possibly identified a congenital malformation associated with maternal malnutrition (Zilva *et al.*, 1921), rudimentary limbs in four piglets born to a sow fed a deficient diet in a study of "fat-soluble factor". In 1933 and 1935, Hale (Hale, 1933, 1935) published the first definitive demonstration that anophthalmia in piglets was associated with a maternal dietary deficiency (vitamin A). These malformations were caused by vitamin A deficiency, not vitamin A excess, the current human concern (Teratology Society Position Paper, 1987). The first publications of congenital malformations in a conventional laboratory species, the rat, were issued in 1940 and 1941 by Warkany and Nelson (Warkany and Nelson, 1940, 1941) who were also studying agents that might affect nutrition and subsequently affect reproduction.

Government regulatory recommendations regarding testing for effects on reproduction were first issued in 1949 when the staff of the Division of Pharmacology, FDA, recommended a three-generation continuous feeding reproduction study (Lehman *et al.*, 1949). The described multigeneration study was designed to determine the possible cumulative effects of a chemical on three generations from conception to weaning. It was based on the opposite concept to that used as the basis for designing studies of nutritional deprivation, i.e. that it is necessary to deprive an animal of specific nutrients through multiple generations in order to deplete stored nutrients to toxic levels.

In 1959, the FDA issued the first regulatory mandate for reproductive studies (Fitzhugh, 1959), a three-generation evaluation included in the chronic oral toxicity testing profile for a chemical because this reproduction assay was considered to have "special value" in identifying long-term effects of chemicals that: (1) were important food items; (2) might affect the nutrition of the general public; and (3) might be selectively toxic to the sex organs. Remarkably, hazards to development of offspring were still not specifically addressed. These guidelines (Fitzhugh, 1959) continued to be recommended by the FDA until 1966, although they were slightly modified by increasing the group sizes from 8 male and 16 female rodents to 20 rodents of each sex, and increasing the number of litters per group from 10 to 20 (Palmer, 1973) after thalidomide was identified as a human teratogen in 1961 (Lenz, 1961; McBride, 1961).

Thalidomide was the first drug identified to cause congenital malformations in humans (Lenz, 1961; McBride, 1961). Because thalidomide had multiple indications, one of which was treating morning sickness in pregnant women, some 7,000 children that were exposed during the first trimester were born with phocomelia (an interesting review of how thalidomide was identified as a human teratogen is available; Fraser *et al.*, 1988). As would be expected on the basis of the FDA requirements in force at the time the manufacturers provided a submission for marketing to the FDA; Dr. Francis Kelsey (1988), the regulator who reviewed the submission and prevented thalidomide from being marketed in the USA, did not have concerns regarding potential effects on reproduction, rather her concerns were about a side effect of thalidomide, such as peripheral neuritis. Before information about the side effect was provided by the manufacturer, thalidomide was identified as the cause of the phocomelia by Lenz (1961) in Germany and McBride (1961) in Australia, and the course of regulatory concerns was irrevocably altered. From this point on, congenital malformations were the focus of reproductive safety evaluations, and the existing procedures for study designs, data interpretation and labeling of products were modified to address this new concern, with essential obliteration of concerns regarding potential effects of drugs on other reproductive processes or on other aspects of development or survival of the conceptus.

In August 1962, following a grant from the Pharmaceutical Manufacturers Association (PMA), now called the Pharmaceutical Research and Manufacturers of America (PhRMA, the Commission on Drug Safety was formed. The Subcommittee on Teratology was chaired by Josef Warkany, who first identified congenital malformations in a common laboratory species; he invited Dr. James G. Wilson to direct a workshop, held at the University of Florida in February 1964 and attended by 41 participants, 18 observers and 11 faculty members. The results of this workshop (Wilson and Warkany, 1965) and a subsequent PMA-sponsored workshop held in 1965 (Pharmaceutical Manufacturers Association, 1965) provided the basis for "teratology" testing (Christian, 1993) and the guidelines published by the FDA in 1966 (US FDA, 1966), Japan (stated by Tanimura, 1990) and the World Health Organization in 1967.

The FDA replaced the multigeneration study with three nested studies, commonly identified as Segments I, II and III, on the premise that, particularly in evaluations of embryo–fetal toxicity–teratogenicity, interruption of pregnancy prior to term provides more reliable data, and shorter-term evaluations more precisely evaluate effects on fertility, embryo death, malformation incidence and maternal parturition and lactation (Schwetz *et al.*, 1980). The Japanese Ministry of Health and Welfare (MHW) guidelines differed slightly in approach. Postnatal evaluations were part of the embryotoxicity testing design in the temporary guidelines issued by Japan in 1963 (as reported by Tanimura, 1990); in contrast, the FDA did not require postnatal evaluations after weaning, although for drugs intended for long-term, continuous or intermittent use, it was recommended that offspring be reared (untreated) to maturity and examined for possible adverse effects on later development, behavior and reproductive capacity (Palmer, 1981).

In the early 1970s, Herbst *et al.* (1971) identified diethylstilbestrol as a human transplacental carcinogen. Although consideration was given to including a carcinogenicity evaluation as part of the reproduction evaluations (Goldberg, 1974), standard incorporation of this test was generally thought to be neither appropriate nor required (Clegg, 1979; US EPA, Christian and Voytek,1982), with the exception of the specific concerns for direct and indirect food additives (US FDA, 1982, 1993). For food additives, a carcinogenicity study is required that uses animals that are exposed to the agent *in utero*.

In 1976, Koos and Longo (1976) identified that "Minamata" disease, a cerebral palsy-like condition in children, was the result of *in utero* exposure to methyl mercury, and the regulatory requirements for testing pharmaceuticals for marking in Japan (MHW, 1975) Great Britain (the UK) Committee on the Safety of Medicines (CSM, 1974) and Canada (1977) were changed to include "behavioral teratology" testing. Two of the initial efforts at harmonization of these multiple guidelines for various types of agents were those of the Interagency Regulatory Liaison Group (IRLG), comprised of five US regulatory agencies (Consumer Product Safety Commission, US Environmental Protection Agency, Food and Drug Administration (US Department of Human Health and Safety), Food Safety and Quality Service (US Department of Agriculture) and Occupational Safety and Health Administration (US Department of Labor)), and of the Organization of Economic and Cooperative Development (OECD), an international organization then consisting of 26 nations and principally concerned with regulations regarding chemicals. In 1979 to 1980, these efforts (OECD, 1979; IRLG, 1980) assisted in the updating and standardization of testing procedures, but the issued guidelines are usually considered not to provide sufficient information for adequate use internationally.

Attempts to update the European Economic Community (EEC) guidelines (1988) provided the basis for the ICH harmonization process. Beginning in the 1990s (Christian, 1993; D'Arcy *et al.*, 1992), the International Federation of Pharmaceutical Manufacturers Associations (IFPMA) initiated an effort to bring together the regulatory authorities of Europe, Japan and the USA, as well as experts from the pharmaceutical industry in these three major geographical regions. The IFPMA mission was to identify new ways to eliminate redundant technical requirements and expedite global development and availability of new medicines, without sacrificing safeguards on quality, safety or efficacy. The six co-sponsors or "SIX-PAC" of the effort are: the Commission of the European Communities (CEC), the European Federation of Pharmaceutical Industries Associations (EFPIA), the Ministry of Health and Welfare (MHW, Japan), the Japan Pharmaceutical Manufacturers Association (JPMA), the US Food and Drug Administration (FDA) and the Pharmaceutical Manufacturers Association (PMA, USA), now called the Pharmaceutical Research and Manufacturers of America (PhRMA). The results of these efforts have ultimately produced many internationally accepted regulatory requirements.

The ICH guideline on "Detection of Toxicity to Reproduction for Medicinal Products" was the first draft document to be approved (1993). The effort that produced this document was spearheaded by Professor Rolf Bass of the *Bundesgsundheit Institut für Arzeimittel*, Germany (BGA). As noted by Dr. Bass (1993) in his presentation of the document at the Second International Conference on Harmonization (ICH-2) in October 1993, although the ultimate acceptance of this guideline was due to the efforts of the "SIX PAC", many individual scientists in academia, regulatory agencies and industry and other professional organizations, such as the International Federation of Teratology Societies (IFTS), the American, European and Japanese Teratology Societies, and the pharmaceutical industry, contributed to this effort with their personal time and the financial support of their individual affiliations. Additional information regarding the ICH process and this particular effort is available in several publications elsewhere (Christian, 1993; D'Arcy *et al.*, 1992).

Currently, the reproduction and development toxicity studies for pharmaceuticals are performed mainly based on ICH S5 (R2), ICH M3 (R2) and ICH S6 guidance documents as listed in Table 8.3.

Outlines of developmental and reproductive toxicity studies (per ICH guidelines)

Description of existing guidelines

Before the ICH harmonization process that resulted in the ICH reproductive toxicology testing guideline first released in 1993 and last revised November 2005, differences in the multiple guidelines appeared to preclude use of one set of tests for international drug registration. The ICH harmonization effort allows standardization of protocols and deletion of unnecessary procedures.

The guideline divides the reproductive lifecycle into Stages A to F.

ICH Stages

ICH Stage A – Premating to Conception: This ICH Stage evaluates reproductive functions in adult male and female animals, including development and maturation of gametes, mating behavior and fertilization. By convention, it was agreed that pregnancy would be timed on the basis of when spermatozoa are identified in a vaginal smear or a copulatory plug is observed, and that these events would identify day 0 of gestation, even if mating occurred overnight.

ICH Stage B – Conception to Implantation: This ICH Stage examines reproductive functions in the adult female and preimplantation and implantation of the conceptus. Unless other data are provided that prove otherwise, it is assumed that implantation occurs in rats, mice and rabbits approximately on days 6 to 7 of pregnancy (Table 8.1).

ICH Stage C – Implantation to Closure of the Hard Palate: This ICH Stage evaluates adult female reproductive functions, embryonic development and major organ formation. The period of embryogenesis is completed at closure of the hard palate, which, by convention, is considered to occur on days 15 through 18 of pregnancy in rats, mice and hamsters.

ICH Stage D – Closure of the Hard Palate to the End of Pregnancy: Adult female reproductive function continues to be examined in this ICH Stage, as well as fetal development and growth and organ development and growth.

ICH Stage E – Birth to Weaning: Again adult female reproduction function is examined; this ICH Stage also evaluates adaptation of the neonate to extrauterine life, including preweaning development and growth of the neonate. By convention, the day of birth is considered postnatal day 0, unless specified otherwise. It is also noted that when there are delays or accelerations of pregnancy, postnatal age may be optimally based on postcoital age.

ICH Stage F – Weaning to Sexual Maturity: This ICH Stage is generally treated only when the intended use of the pharmaceutical product is in children. The ICH guideline identifies that it may sometimes be appropriate also to treat the neonate during this ICH Stage, in addition to the required evaluations of the offspring. This ICH Stage provides observations of postweaning development and growth,

TABLE 8.1 Reproductive stages/function evaluated in segmented approach of reproductive toxicity testing

Segment/study type	Main reproductive stage evaluated	Gestation day* with respect to mating day as gestation day 0: Rat	Rabbit	Mouse	G. pig	Monkey	Usual observations
Segment 1: Effect on fertility and early embryonic development	Premating to conception	Period					**ICH Stage A:** Adult (male and female) reproductive functions, development and maturation of gametes, mating behavior, fertilization
	Conception to implantation	Gestation day for implantation* 5–6	7.5	7	6	9	**ICH Stage B:** Adult (female) reproductive function, pre-implantation development of embryo and implantation
Segment II: Effect on embryo–fetal development	Implantation to closure of hard palate	Gestation day for closure of hard palate 15	18	15	29	44–45	**ICH Stage C:** Included in both Segment II and Segment III stages. Adult female reproductive functions, embryonic development, major organ formation
Segment III: Effect on pre- and postnatal development *(This segment includes ICH Stage C to F)*	Closure of hard palate to end of pregnancy	Gestation day for parturition* 21–22	30–32	19–20	67–68	166	**ICH Stage D:** Adult female reproductive functions, fetal development and growth, organ development and growth
	Birth to weaning	After the gestational period					**ICH Stage E:** Adult female reproductive functions, neonate adaption to extra-uterine life, pre-weaning development and growth
	Weaning to sexual maturity						**ICH Stage F:** Post-weaning development and growth, adaption to independent life, growth of behavioral and sexual functions

*Data based on DeSesso (1996)

adaptation to independent life and attainment of full sexual development.

The stages of the reproductive cycle indentified in the ICH guideline are combined in various protocols. The most common combinations of these stages relate to the FDA guidelines (1966) for testing drugs and consist of a three-segment design, commonly identified as Segment I (Fertility), Segment II ("Teratology", Embryotoxicity) and Segment III (Perinatal and Postnatal) evaluations. These segments with reproductive phases covered by each segment are shown in Figure 8.2 and Table 8.1. Alternative designs that can combine fertility and embryotoxicity studies and can reduce animal usage and cost are discussed in Barrow (2009).

Fertility Study: (Segment I, ICH Stages A and B): The fertility study is generally performed in the rodent, but can be evaluated in rabbits or NHPs (without actual mating of the monkeys). The appropriate species for all reproductive testing is the one in which the test article is active. The study is designed to detect adverse effects on male and female gametes, mating performance and development of the fertilized ova through implantation. As with all ICH guideline studies, group sizes of 20 pregnancies (minimum 16) are recommended. An equivalent number of male rats should be used, with mating being one male to one female.

A test article should be administered starting two weeks prior to mating to cycling females and sexually mature males. Administration should continue in the female until implantation is complete (days 6–7 in the rat or mouse, with day 0 as the day of mating). Females are then necropsied mid-gestation to determine if viable embryos are present *in utero*. Comparison of corpora lutea counts to implantations allows for calculation of preimplantation loss, an indicator of changes in fertility if reduced in a dose-dependent manner.

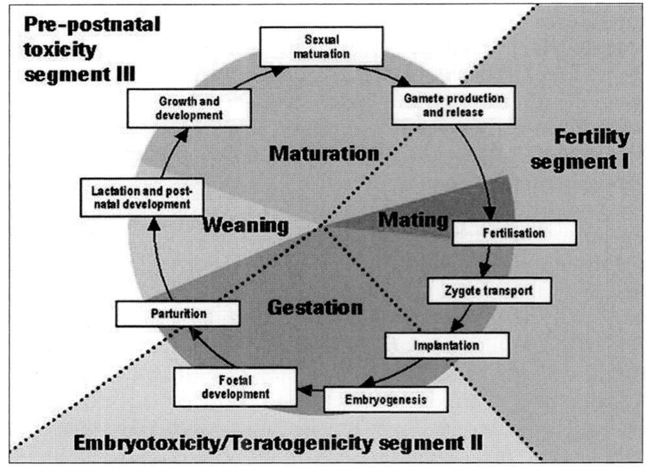

FIGURE 8.2 Segment 1, 2 and 3 studies of drug testing according to ICH. (Adapted with author's permission from Spielmann, 2009.) Please refer to color plate section.

The males are necropsied after mating but are usually continued on study until it has been assured that a sufficient number of pregnancies have occurred. If fertility is low, having the males continued on study allows for a remating with untreated females to establish if the males were the reason for any infertility. Continued dosing of the males also allows for dosing through a spermatogenic cycle (about 8 weeks in the rodent). Male reproductive organs including the testes, epididiymides, seminal vesicles, coagulating gland and prostate are weighed. In both sexes, reproductive organs can be retained for histopathology. Evaluation of sperm parameters including count, motility and morphology can be conducted but in the rodent the value of these evaluations has been questioned due to the large reserve capacity of sperm and the impression that only large reductions in count result in infertility. Sperm evaluations in rabbits and NHP models may be more appropriate.

The dosing period of 2 weeks prior to mating has evolved over the years from a standard 10 weeks period prior to mating in the males based on surveys of past studies that demonstrated 2 weeks to be a sufficient period of dosing in males. This dosing period is only considered appropriate when it has already been established in a general toxicity study of at least 4 weeks in duration that no histopathological changes to the testes (including an observation of the spermatozoa) have occurred. The rationale behind this 2-week dosing period is reviewed in Barrow (2009); however, if histopathological changes in the testes are found or expected based on the mechanism of action of the test article, then a premating dosing period of 10 weeks (spermatogenic cycle, plus capacitation of sperm) prior to mating is deemed necessary. Additionally it is prudent to mate the males to untreated females and females to untreated males to allow for identification of sex-related differences and assure sufficient pregnancies for evaluation of fecundity. Finally, if a 10-week dosing period is used for the males, then incorporation of the fertility evaluation into the 90-day (13-week) study is possible and acceptable.

Embryo–Fetal Development ("Teratology") (ICH Stage C, Segment II): This study is conducted in two species, one rodent and one non-rodent. Two species are tested because: (1) identifying fetal malformations has become the major focus of evaluation, based on an incorrect assumption of mimicry in response across species; and (2) thalidomide did not cause phocomelia in the rat, although it can produce phocomelia in the rabbit (Somers, 1962). Despite Wilson (1973) noting that one cannot assume mimicry of responses across species, and Palmer (1973) identifying that appropriate interpretation of rat data from a two-litter test would have identified that thalidomide was selectively toxic to the development of the conceptuses (i.e., it increased resorption and reduced live litter sizes at dosages that were not toxic to the dams), the rabbit continues generally to be the non-rodent species tested in this assay.

The embryo/fetal toxicity study is commonly perceived as an evaluation of the potential of an agent to malform the conceptus; in contrast to this perception is the fact that this study is actually an evaluation of embryo–fetal (developmental) toxicity and differs from a "teratology" study, in which "pulse" exposure occurs (Johnson and Christian, 1983). In the embryo–fetal toxicity study, pregnant female animals are treated for the period of major organogenesis (embryogenesis), generally defined as the interval between implantation and palate closure, and necropsied shortly before expected parturition. The ovaries are examined for the number of corpora lutea. The uterus is examined for implantation sites, live and dead fetuses and early and late resorptions. The fetuses are weighed, and the fetal sex is identified. In rodent studies, one-third to one-half of the fetuses in each litter are examined for soft tissue alterations by using either Wilson's sectioning technique (Wilson, 1965) or Staples' visceral examination technique (1974) (possibly as adapted by Stuckhardt and Poppe, 1984). The remaining fetuses are stained with alizarin red-S (Staples and Schnell, 1963) and examined for skeletal alterations. In non-rodent studies, all fetuses are examined for soft tissue and skeletal alterations.

Day 0 of presumed gestation is generally recognized as the day spermatozoa, a vaginal or copulatory plug (rodents) or insemination (rabbit) occurs. The period of organogenesis or embryogenesis is identified as days 6 to 15 in the mouse, 6 or 7 through 17 of gestation in the rat and days 6 or 7 to 18 or 19 of gestation in the rabbit. The fetuses are caesarean-delivered one or two days before parturition is expected to occur, i.e. usually on days 20 or 21, 18 and 29 of gestation in the rat, mouse and rabbit, respectively.

The guideline requires 16–20 litters to be evaluated per group. In practice, the minimum requirement is interpreted as 20 litters for rodent studies or 16 litters for rabbit studies. In order to achieve these numbers of litters, about 24 rats or 20 rabbits are mated and dosed per group. A footnote to the guideline states that it may be sufficient to examine the fetuses from just the control and high dose groups, provided that the fetuses from the intermediate dose groups are retained for possible future examination. This option is almost never followed because the data from the intermediate dose groups, while not always essential, invariably add support to the interpretation of the experimental results. In cases where multiple dose groups are not of interest, such as drugs that appear to be completely non-toxic at the highest practicable dose level (e.g., vaccines), then intermediate dose groups are usually omitted from the study design (Barrow, 2009).

Perinatal/Postnatal Evaluation: (ICH Stages C through F, Segment III): The perinatal/postnatal (prenatal/postnatal terminology used in ICH guidelines) evaluation was designed to evaluate the effects of a test article when exposure occurs during embryogenesis through late stages of gestation and through parturition and lactation. Treatment of presumed pregnant rodents begins on day 6 or 7 of gestation and continues through gestation, parturition and a 21-day lactation period. However, the ICH document (ICH, 1993) also notes that lifetime exposure to a drug sometimes occurs, and that there may be drugs that can be more appropriately tested by exposure throughout the entire reproductive life, i.e. through use of a multigeneration study design.

Pup birth and development are monitored, including observations for prolonged gestation, dystocia, postnatal mortality and impaired maternal behavior. At weaning, one male and one female pup are selected from each litter to form the F_1 generation. The dams and non-selected pups are necropsied. The selected F_1-generation pups are not dosed, but their physical development is monitored up to the age of sexual maturity. Behavioral testing (learning, memory and activity) is recommended. The specific testing paradigms are left to the test facility and their previous experience. After attaining sexual maturity, the F_1 pups are paired within each group to evaluate their fertility. The F_1 females are euthanized mid-gestation, a day or two prior to delivery or the pregnant F_1 females may be allowed to give birth and are then necropsied with their pups anytime between day 4 postpartum and weaning. Each of these options is acceptable. When females are necropsied just prior to term (delivery), the F_2 generation can be saved for possible future evaluation.

General considerations defined by ICH S5 (R2)

Rather than a standard "checklist" approach, the ICH guideline (ICH S5 (R2)) emphasizes flexibility in developing the testing strategy. Although the most probable options are identified, the development of the testing strategy is to be based on the following points:

- anticipated drug use especially in relation to reproduction
- the form of the substance and route(s) of administration intended for humans
- making use of any existing data on toxicity, pharmacodynamics, kinetics and similarity to other compounds in structure/activity.

Although the notes in the ICH guideline (ICH S5 (R2)) describe some methods appropriate for use in specific portions of the tests, the document emphasizes that the individual investigator is at liberty to identify the tests used, and that the ICH guideline (ICH S5 (R2)) is a guideline and not a set of rules. The overall aim of the described reproductive toxicity studies is to identify any effect of an active substance on mammalian reproduction, with subsequent comparison of this effect with all other pharmacologic and toxicologic data. The objective is to determine whether human risk of effects on the reproductive process is the same as, increased or reduced, in comparison with the risks of other toxic effects of the agent. The document clearly states that for extrapolation of results of the animal studies, other pertinent information should be used, including human exposure considerations, comparative kinetics and the mechanism of the toxic effect.

Because the objective of these tests is to assess all stages of reproduction, the total exposure period includes mature adults and all stages of development of the offspring, from conception to weaning. Observations should be made over one complete lifecycle (from conception in the first generation through conception and pregnancy in the second generation).

Consideration for performing DART studies for biotherapeutics

The principles for evaluating the effects of biotherapeutics on reproduction and development are similar to those for small molecules. Key differentiating features include higher target (receptor or epitope) specificity in humans for biotherapeutics and limited cross reactivity for traditional toxicology species (rat and rabbit) used for evaluating effects on reproduction and development. Development of immunogenic responses to biotherapeutics introduces concerns for neutralization of therapeutic proteins and potential invalidation of a study due to lack of exposure at the target that are not factors for small molecules. Because of these and other differences, testing strategies for biotherapeutics are less proscriptive and more often case by case where a science-based understanding of the target and animal models dictates the specific strategy.

Biotherapeutics encompass a large variety of platforms that include but are not limited to monoclonal antibodies, recombinant proteins, hybrid protein molecules, fusion proteins, peptides, oligonucleotides, vaccines, gene products and cell-based therapies. Comments within this section focus on monoclonal antibodies but the concepts are applicable to many of these platforms.

For a detailed discussion of considerations in assessing the reproductive and developmental toxicity potential of biotherapeutics the reader is referred to more detailed and recent reviews (Chellman *et al.*, 2009; Martin *et al.*, 2009).

An excellent place to learn the requirements for safety evaluation of biotherapeutics is the ICH guidances S6, M3 (R2) and M5 (R2) as they have specific recommendations related to reproductive and developmental toxicity studies. In conjunction with recent reviews (Chellman *et al.*, 2009; Martin *et al.*, 2009), the ICH guidance provides a nearly complete picture of the study requirements, timing for study conduct relative to stage of clinical development and specific science-based issues that factor into the overall determination of preparedness to initiate reproductive and development toxicity studies for a biotherapeutic. As highlighted in ICH S6, the need for reproductive and developmental studies for biotherapeutics is dependent upon the product, clinical indication and intended patient population. Should public information be available regarding potential reproductive and developmental effects of a particular class of compounds where the only relevant species is a non-human primate, it may be possible to avoid conduct of such studies by mechanistically demonstrating similarity of the test molecule to the pharmacological class. It is also worth noting that ICH S6 is undergoing review based on learnings since its adoption in 1997 and an amended version is expected to be issued.

In keeping with available regulatory guidance, should reproductive and developmental studies be needed, key features to help prepare for and frame the perspective for these studies are highlighted in the following paragraphs.

As with small molecules, evaluation of the full spectrum of reproduction and development toxicity is expected for biotherapeutics. Because of the high degree of target specificity, identifying a relevant species is a critical aspect for the conduct of the studies. A relevant species is defined by ICH S6 as one in which the biotherapeutic is pharmacologically active due to the expression of the receptor or target epitope. Parameters useful in defining species relevance often include receptor (or epitope) binding, density and distribution as well as functional measures related to the pharmacologic action. A combination of *in vitro* and *in vivo* assays is often utilized.

Determination of relevant species for testing of monoclonal antibodies has often relied on expression of the target epitope and demonstration by immunohistochemical techniques that tissue cross reactivity is similar to human tissues. The intent is to be able to account for potential on-target and off-target effects that may occur. The value and relevance of tissue cross reactivity data in selecting relevant species has been questioned and it is recommended that careful consideration be given to whether this information will add significant value to the justification of species relevance before conducting the assays.

If a molecule is enabled to be tested in rats or rabbits, a conventional approach to the conduct of the battery of reproductive and developmental studies addressing fertility, embryo–fetal development and peri-/postnatal development is expected. One species could be considered for embryo–fetal development studies since biotherapeutics are highly specific for their pharmacologic target, reducing the likelihood of off-target effects. Molecule degradation is expected via proteolytic mechanisms and not via phase I/II metabolic pathways as occurs with small molecules further supports the suitability of a single relevant species for these studies.

While testing in two species is preferable, the use of one species for evaluation of embryo–fetal development may be justified, when the biologic activity of the biotherapeutic is well understood or the clinical candidate is only active in one species. Evaluation in a non-relevant species does not provide useful information and is often misleading. It is generally not recommended to use a homologous product as the relevance to the human candidate is usually not well understood. Exceptions to this can be considered on a case-by-case basis, when there is a scientific rationale to support this approach.

When non-human primates are the single relevant species or the species of choice, further considerations should be given to modifying the conventional approach to the characterization of effects on reproduction and development. While conventional fertility studies are possible with non-human primates the modest fertility rate and the high background abortion rate results in a need for large numbers of animals. Alternatively, the potential effects on fertility for both males and females can be evaluated in sexually mature animals by assessing the histopathology of reproductive organs and tissues and monitoring the menstrual cycle during repeat dose studies of 3 months' or longer duration. More specialized measures for male or female reproductive hormones and conventional measures of sperm quality and quantity are often included for higher risk targets.

The approach to the embryo–fetal development study design is influenced by concerns regarding passage of large therapeutic proteins across the placental barrier. Small molecules less than 600 Da freely cross the placenta but higher molecular weight protein therapeutics and immunoglobulins pass the placenta less freely (see references in Kane and Acquah, 2009). Transport of monoclonal antibodies across the placenta may not occur until the second or third trimester raising concern about the *in utero* exposure to the fetus during embryogenesis (GD 20–50 for non-human primates) (Martin *et al.*, 2009). For the conduct of a conventional embryo–fetal development study in non-human primates the dosing duration should be extended from GD 20 through at least GD 90–100 to better optimize exposure. Because of the high background abortion rate and the fetal losses that can occur during late pregnancy of non-human primates, larger numbers of animals are needed to assure an adequate number of fetuses needed for evaluation. Chellman *et al.* (2009) provide specific recommendations for the design and conduct of these studies and the reader is encouraged to seek guidance from this information.

For biotherapeutics where non-human primates are the single relevant species, consideration should be given to conducting a single study where dosing is planned from embryogenesis through natural delivery, with subsequent monitoring during the postnatal phase to assess infant viability, growth and morphology postnatally (Stewart, 2009). This design is identified as the enhanced pre-/postnatal development (ePPND) study. There is a progressive development of offspring data that includes viability and survival, external malformations, skeletal effects and visceral morphology. Monitoring of pharmacological endpoints such as immune function, learning, behavior and memory can be included during the postnatal period and help to define the duration of this observation stage. As described by Stewart (2009), the advantage of the ePPND design is that it allows visualization of the postnatal morphologic consequences of gestational exposure in conjunction with the functional consequences in the same individual animal. Live born infants enter the postnatal and observational phase of the study at the end of which termination of the infants allows full assessment of skeletal morphology using radiography, visceral morphology and histopathology of all or specific organs of interest.

Ongoing dialogue among researchers and regulators regarding the acceptance of the ePPND study design continues. Some concerns remain about the lack of visceral evaluations in newborn fetuses but ultrasound evaluation during gestation or after birth allows for data acquisition to address this concern. The authors are aware of examples in the USA where this design has received acceptance from the FDA as a replacement for separate Seg II and Seg III studies in non-human primates. The reader is encouraged to seek advice from regulatory authorities to further understand the acceptability or specific design considerations for the ePPND. The reader should look for an expected revision to ICH S6 to address this issue and define the acceptability and timing of this study to support development of biotherapeutics.

Timing of DART studies during the drug development process

A summary for timing of various DART studies with respect to the drug development process is included in Table 8.2. This is based on recent ICH guidance (ICH M3 (R2) Step 4, June 2009) proposed for different ICH regions and as adapted by the FDA, January 2010 (Table 8.3).

DART studies are performed at various time-points during clinical development according to regulatory guidelines in different ICH regions. As summarized by Martin *et al.* (2009), regional differences existed in the expected timing of developmental toxicity studies for including Women of Child Bearing Potential (WOCBP) in clinical trials. In Japan, assessment of potential effects on female fertility and embryo–fetal development were required prior to the inclusion of WOCBP in any clinical trial. In the European Union (EU), an assessment of potential effects on embryo–fetal development was expected prior to phase 1 trials and female fertility studies were expected prior to initiation of phase 3. In the USA, WOCBP can be included in early phase 1 clinical trials, without data from animal reproduction studies, provided appropriate precautions are taken to prevent pregnancy. The recommended precautions include pregnancy testing, use of effective birth control measures, and enrollment after confirmation of menstrual cyclicity, with continued monitoring throughout the duration of the clinical trial. To further support this approach, the informed consent statement would include any known pertinent information related to reproductive effects or toxicity.

Per latest ICH M3 (R2) guidance (ICH M3 (R2) Step 4, June 2009) as adapted by the FDA, January 2010, reproduction studies per ICH S5 (R2) are needed to be completed as appropriate for the intended human population. Key points from this guidance are as follows.

Men

Men can be included in phase 1 and 2 clinical trials before the conduct of a male fertility study since an evaluation of the male reproductive organs is performed in the repeated-dose toxicity studies. A male fertility study should be completed before the initiation of large-scale or long duration clinical trials (e.g., phase 3 trials).

TABLE 8.2 Timing of developmental and reproductive toxicity studies with respect to phase of drug development per ICH M3 (R2)

		Data/Information needed for subjects enrollment prior to initiation of clinical trial/event			
Clinical trialsubjects	**ICH region**	**Clinical trial up to 2 weeks**	**Clinical trial over 2 weeks to 3 months**	**Phase 2 over 3 months or phase 3**	**NDA submission**
Male volunteers	USA Europe Japan	Repeat dose toxicity studies with histopathology of testes completed		A male fertility study (Segment I) needed before the initiation of large-scale or long-duration clinical trials	No additional data
Women NOT of child-bearing potential	USA Europe Japan	Repeat dose toxicity studies with evaluation of the female reproductive organs completed			
Pregnant women	USA Europe Japan	All female reproductive toxicity studies ICH S5 (R2) listed in Table 8.3 and standard battery of genotoxicity tests should be completed			
Women of child-bearing potential (WOCBP)	USA	(a) Intensive control of pregnancy risk or (b) when predominance of the disease in women and objective of clinical trial cannot be met without including WOCBP and there are sufficient precautions to prevent pregnancy and (c) there is knowledge of the mechanism of action and type of pharmaceutical agent, and the extent of fetal exposure or there is difficulty of conducting study in appropriate animal model	Preliminary developmental reproductive toxicity data (Segment II) from two animal species if precautions to prevent pregnancy are implemented and less that 150 WOCBP would be exposed to the drug or Definitive developmental reproductive toxicity studies (two species) completed (Segment II)	(1) Definitive reproduction developmental toxicity testing (Segment II) and (2) Female fertility and early embryonic toxicity study (Segment I) completed in addition to data generated in repeat-dose studies	Pre- and postnatal development toxicity study completed (Segment III)
	Europe	As above or definitive non-clinical developmental reproductive toxicity studies (Segment II)	Definitive developmental reproductive toxicity studies (two species) completed (Segment II)	As above	
	Japan	As above or definitive non-clinical developmental reproductive toxicity studies (Segment II)	Definitive developmental reproductive toxicity studies (two species) completed (Segment II)	As above	

Women that are not of child-bearing potential

Women that are not of child-bearing potential (i.e., permanently sterilized, postmenopausal), can be included in clinical trials without reproduction toxicity studies if the relevant repeated-dose toxicity studies (which include an evaluation of the female reproductive organs) have been conducted. The term "postmenopausal" for this purpose has been defined as 12 months with no menses without an alternative medical cause.

Women of child-bearing potential (WOCBP)

WOCBP is the population where a high level of concern exists for the unintentional exposure of an embryo or fetus. The recommendations on timing of reproduction toxicity studies for including WOCBP in clinical trials are now similar in all ICH regions. These are (1) either conduct the needed reproduction toxicity studies to characterize the inherent risk of a drug and take appropriate precautions during exposure of WOCBP in clinical trials or (2) limit the risk by taking precautions to prevent pregnancy during clinical trials. These precautions are explained in the ICH M3 (R2) guidance of June 2009.

In all ICH regions, WOCBP can be included in early clinical trials without non-clinical developmental toxicity studies (e.g., embryo–fetal studies) only under certain circumstances. Examples of circumstances include (1) intensive control of pregnancy risk over a short duration (e.g., 2 weeks), (2) clinical trials where there is a predominance of a disease in women and the objectives of the clinical trial cannot be effectively met without including WOCBP and sufficient precautions to prevent pregnancy as discussed in the

TABLE 8.3 ICH guidelines related to developmental and reproductive toxicity testing of pharmaceuticals

Agency/ Region/Country	Guidance document	Implementation in ICH regions
International Conference on Harmonization (ICH)	**S5(R2)** Detection of Toxicity to Reproduction for Medicinal Products and Toxicity to Male Fertility (core guideline, *Step 5*)	**EU:** September 93, CPMP, issued as CPMP/ICH/386/95 **MHLW:** July 94, PAB/PCD Notification No. 470 **FDA:** September 22, 1994, Published in the Federal Register, Vol. 59, No. 183, pages 48746–48752
	S5(R2) Detection of Toxicity to Reproduction for Medicinal Products and Toxicity to Male Fertility (Addendum, *Step 5*) Addendum dated November 9, 2000 incorporated in November 2005	**EU:** December 95 by CPMP, issued as CPMP/ICH/136/95 – Amended guideline: CPMP/ICH136/95 modification **MHLW:** April 97, PAB/PCD Notification No. 316 – Amended guideline: Adopted December 27, 2000, PMSB/ELD Notification No. 1834 **FDA:** April 5, 1996, Published in the Federal Register, Vol. 61, No. 67, page 15360 – Amended guideline: To be notified per ICH guideline listing of 2005
	S6: Preclinical Safety Evaluation of Biotechnology-Derived Pharmaceuticals (*Step 5*, July 1997)	**EU:** September 97, CPMP, issued as CPMP/ICH/302/95 **MHLW:** February 2000, PAB/PCD, Notification No. 326, 22 **FDA:** November 18, 1997, Published in the Federal Register, Vol. 62, No. 222, page 61515
	S6(R1): Preclinical Safety Evaluation of Biotechnology-Derived Pharmaceuticals (*Step 3*, October 2009) Included for considerations for DART studies for biotechnology-based pharmaceuticals	**EU:** December 2009, Transmission to CHMP and Interested Parties. Deadline for comments: February 2010. Issued as CPMP/ICH/302/95 **MHLW:** March 8, 2010, Released for consultation January 8, 2010 **FDA:** December 17, 2009, Published in the Federal Register, Docket No. FDA-2009-D-0573, Deadline for comments by February 1, 2010
	M3(R2): Guidance on Non-Clinical Safety Studies for the Conduct of Human Clinical Trials and Marketing Authorization for Pharmaceuticals (*Step 5*, June 2009)	**EU:** June 2009, CHMP issued as CPMP/ICH/286/95. Date for coming into operation: December 2009 **MHLW:** To be notified per ICH guideline listing of 2005 **FDA:** January 2010, Revised M3 (R2) guidance issued
	S2(R1): Guidance on Genotoxicity Testing and Data Interpretation for Pharmaceuticals Intended for Human Use; *Step 3*, March 2008 (combines ICH S2A and S2B earlier codes)	**EU:** Transmitted to CHMP and Interested Parties in March 2008, issued as EMEA/CHMP/ICH/126642/2008 **MHLW:** Released for consultation April 1, 2008, PFSB/ELD, deadline for comments April 30, 2008 **FDA:** Published in the Federal Register, March 26, 2008, Vol. 73, No. 59, pages 16024–16025

guidance would be taken. Other circumstances that could be considered may include knowledge of a drug's mechanism of action, the type of pharmaceutical agent and the extent of fetal exposure or the difficulty of conducting developmental toxicity studies in an appropriate animal model. For example, for monoclonal antibodies for which embryo–fetal exposure during organogenesis is understood to be low in humans based on current scientific knowledge, the developmental toxicity studies can be conducted during phase 3. The completed reports should be submitted with the marketing application.

Further, inclusion of WOCBP (up to 150 subjects) receiving investigational treatment for a relatively short duration (up to 3 months) can occur before conduct of definitive reproduction toxicity testing, where appropriate preliminary (dose range-finding) reproduction toxicity data are available from two species, and where precautions to prevent pregnancy in clinical trials as discussed in ICH M3 (R2) guidance (Table 8.3) are used. In the USA, assessment of definitive embryo–fetal development studies can be deferred until before phase 3 for WOCBP using precautions to prevent pregnancy as discussed above. In the EU and Japan, other than the situations described in the preceding paragraphs, definitive non-clinical developmental toxicity studies should be completed before exposure of WOCBP.

In all ICH regions, WOCBP can be included in repeated-dose phase 1 and 2 trials before conduct of the female fertility study since an evaluation of the female reproductive organs is performed in the repeated-dose toxicity studies. Non-clinical studies that specifically address female fertility should be completed to support inclusion of WOCBP in large-scale or long-duration clinical trials (e.g., phase 3 trials).

In all ICH regions, the pre- and postnatal development toxicity study (called peri- and postnatal per original FDA guideline) should be completed prior to submitting for marketing approval. All female reproduction toxicity studies per ICH S5 (R2) and the standard battery of genotoxicity tests per ICH S2 (R1) guideline listed in Table 8.3 should be completed before inclusion of WOCBP in any clinical trial, not using highly effective birth control (as discussed above) or whose pregnancy status is unknown.

If pregnant women need to be included in clinical trials, data from all female reproduction toxicity studies per ICH S5 (R2) and the standard battery of genotoxicity tests per ICH S2 (R1) guideline listed in Table 8.3 should be available for toxicity hazard evaluation. In addition, safety data from previous human exposure (if available) should be evaluated.

Options to improve detection and interpretation of reproductive hazards

Assessment of developmental immune function for F1 generation in peri-postnatal (1CH-2) study if any evidence for immune system related effect occurred in adults

Because the developing human (embryo, fetus, newborn and infant) has been shown to be more sensitive to immunotoxicants, Barrow (2009) has suggested that an assessment of developmental immunotoxicity should be included in any future revision of the reproductive testing guidelines. The current ICH M3 (R2) guidelines of June 2009 (Table 8.3) suggest that all new human pharmaceuticals should be evaluated for a potential to produce immunotoxicity, as part of a standard repeat dose toxicity study that includes immune-related endpoints or in a separate immunotoxicity study that is conducted as appropriate based on a weight-of-evidence basis. To evaluate effects on the developing immune system, one approach is to include developmental immunotoxicity endpoints in a pre- and postnatal reproduction toxicity study, if the new drug candidate has or is suspected to have affected the maternal/adult animal immune functions. Where maternal/adult animal immune functions are affected, it is likely that F1 subjects may also be affected if there was an evidence of *in utero* or neonatal drug exposure to the fetus or newborn. Holsapple (2003) and Barrow (2003) have reviewed the scope of including immunotoxicity evaluation in the pre- and postnatal study. The ILSI/HESI workshop conclusions (Holsapple, 2003) indicate that a variety of techniques are available for assessing immunosuppression in adult animal models but emphasized uncertainty about the application of these techniques to a developing animal, particularly if the data are to be used for regulatory risk assessment purposes. Despite the options of including histopathology examination of the lymphoid organs/tissues, immunophenotyping of lymphocyte subsets, immunoglobin and cytokine measurements and T-cell-dependent antigen response (TDAR) to sheep red blood cells or keyhole limpet hemocyanin (KLH) antigens as the endpoints for immunosuppression (Barrow and Ravel, 2005), it is still the prevailing opinion that more research is required to devise and validate methods to detect adverse effects on the immune system (Barrow, 2009).

Measurement of fetal/neonatal drug exposure

The current ICH guidelines, S5 (R2) or S3A do not recommend an assessment of fetal exposure data as (1) effects induced by a drug in the fetus are an indirect evidence of fetal exposure and (2) it does not help in direct extrapolation to human risk since blood is not easily obtainable from human fetuses. Still, fetal exposure data can be helpful in certain pharmaceutical development situations. Toxicologists working on early discovery stage compounds may find such information as value added. For example, if a lead compound has been determined to be associated with adverse fetal effects and the backup discovery compound is not, availability of fetal drug exposure would allow one to interpret if the negative results for the backup compound are due to a lack of placental drug transfer or due to the backup compound being not associated with a direct effect on the fetus despite the evidence of fetal drug exposure. On the other hand, the observation of fetal effects without an evidence of fetal drug exposure would suggest potential involvement of maternally associated pharmacological or related effects for the induction of fetal effects. This topic has been recently discussed by Wise *et al.* (2009). Sampling strategies for accomplishing toxicokinetics in pregnant animals and fetuses have been discussed by Weir (2006). For neonates also, the toxicokinetic data are not required per latest ICH guidelines mentioned above. If it is considered value-added information, the blood samples can be collected in rat from culled neonates on postnatal day (PND) 4 of the pre- and postnatal toxicity study. This information can be helpful to assess the magnitude of plasma exposure in neonates that would be associated with adverse effects such as mortality or poor growth.

Ovarian follicle counting

Ovarian follicle counting is not usually required or done for pharmaceuticals but is discussed here for general information. Ovarian follicle quantitation has been reviewed in detail by Heindel (1999). This endpoint has been included in EPA's TSCA/FIFRA guidelines (USEPA, 1998) for chemical or pesticide compounds but ICH has not included this for routine testing in its core and amended S5 (R2) guideline listed in Table 8.3. The EPA guidance recommends collection of ovaries for possible histopathology examination. The follicle count in ovaries can be performed on a case-by-case basis particularly when the NME is expected to affect the male or female sex hormones, or where the pituitary–hypothalamic axis is anticipated to be affected.

The conventional qualitative measures of reproductive toxicity in females, including reduced fertility, abnormal maternal behavior, clinical signs (e.g., weight loss), or problems in lactation in dams or altered reproductive outcome, embryo toxicity, etc. do provide good estimates for effect on fertility but lack a quantitative estimate as is done for evaluation of male fertility by including sperm count, morphology and motility. Inclusion of ovarian follicle counting can provide the quantitative estimate for females as well. One advantage of such a quantitative estimate is to get an idea of the long-term effect of the drug. By counting the type (size) of follicles affected or destroyed one can estimate if the drug's effect is temporary or long term. If the compound destroys the mature (antral) follicles, the effect can be interpreted as temporary infertility (as replacement of the damaged mature follicles is expected through recruitment from the pool of immature (small and growing) follicles). If the compound depletes or destroys the small and growing follicles, this may lead to permanent infertility and earlier reproductive senescence, e.g. accelerated menopause because the finite number of the progenitor oocytes cannot be replaced. With respect to size of the follicles, Heindel (1999) has recommended assessment of three types of follicles: (1) small follicle: consisting of an isolated oocyte or an oocyte surrounded by a partial or unbroken single layer of granulosa cells, mean diameter 20 μm; (b) growing follicle: an oocyte surrounded by a multilayered, solid mantle of granulosa cells, mean diameter 20–70 μm; (c) antral/large/mature/primordial follicle: a central oocyte and a fluid-filled space bordered by hundreds of layered granulosa cells, mean diameter of more than 70 μm.

For a detailed review of methodology, including tissue processing, selection of ovarian sections, follicle counting and relationship between follicle counting and functional outcome, the reader is referred to the article by Heindel

(1999). Serial ovary sections from 10 to 20 animals per group are considered the standard procedure for counting follicles (Collins, 2006). This has traditionally been performed manually using hematoxylin and eosin (H&E) stained sections but recently Picut *et al.* (2008) have described immunohistochemical semi-automated methods, such as cytochrome P450 1B1 (CYP1B1) and proliferating cell nuclear antigen (PCNA), that yield accurate and consistent counts.

Ovarian follicle counts are considered a sensitive and quantitative measure for female reproductive toxicity (Bolon *et al.*, 1997) but species differences can be observed in case of specific compounds. Information from ovarian follicle counts is used in conjunction with information from other endpoints measuring effects on female fertility. With cyclophosphamide, the number of mature (primordial) follicles is decreased in mature C57BL/6N and DBA/2N mice but not in immature or adult Sprague-Dawley rats (Jarrell *et al.*, 1987; Shiromizu *et al.*, 1984). Recently, Muhammad *et al.* (2009) reported that in the case of 4-vinylcyclohexene diepoxide (VCD), usually the primordial follicles are destroyed selectively in young rats, but at higher dose (80 mg/kg), VCD destroyed both primordial and primary follicles (small and growing) to a similar extent in both adult and peripubertal Sprague-Dawley rats. This indicates that differences in dose and age of rat or mice may affect the findings related to ovarian follicle count in certain cases. Overall, this parameter is considered a value-added tool for estimating reproductive toxicity related to ovarian function, particularly for compounds that may have a potential to disrupt the pituitary–hypothalamic axis or have a direct adverse effect on the ovaries.

Reversibility of effects on female fertility, where observed

In cases where drugs, such as hormonal compounds, are expected to adversely impact the estrous cyclicity or other fertility related endpoints, it is value-added to assess recovery from such effects by allowing two breeding cycles. In such cases, a larger number of females need to be included in each group during the first breeding cycle so that an adequate number of F_0 females exposed to the test drug (until gestation day 6) can be allowed to deliver and be maintained until postnatal days 2 to 4 and the rest necropsied or subjected to C-section per protocol. These F_0 females are allowed to deliver, and after a reasonable recovery period (could vary depending on dose and type of compound), when estrous cyclicity has been resumed and two estrous cycles (10 days) have successfully been completed, can be bred again with healthy males for the second breeding cycle. As the second breeding cycle is for a recovery phase, there is no drug treatment during premating, mating or postmating periods of the second breeding cycle. The animals are then examined at C-section for terminal evaluations as done for part of the females during the first breeding cycle. The dose with full recovery in the second breeding cycle can allow one to estimate the extent of recovery for disrupted reproductive functions after the drug exposure.

Modern imaging procedures for morphological examination of fetuses

Already practical for non-human primate fetuses, ultrasound can be conducted as often as necessary (typically every two weeks) throughout pregnancy to evaluate fetal viability, fetal length, long bone length, circumference (head, abdomen), biparietal diameter, and/or occipitofrontal diameter (Chellman *et al.*, 2009). The use of the most sophisticated ultrasound (3D) can also provide excellent images of the near term fetus and allow evaluation for major and minor malformations. The mother can then be allowed to deliver providing a postnatal period for evaluation of maternal interaction, behavioral assessment of the offspring and a general evaluation of growth.

Micro-computed tomography (micro-CT) has recently been adapted for routine evaluation of skeletal specimens from rodents and rabbits (Wise *et al.*, 2009). Over the next few years it is expected that micro-CT will continue to develop to allow routine evaluations of gross, soft tissue and skeletal tissue. The current methods of fresh visceral dissection (Staples' technique) or free-hand razor-blade sectioning of fetuses (Wilson's technique) will be eliminated. The advantage of micro-CT or other imaging techniques would be the availability of the data for future review online as well as the ability to analyze bone density, lengths of bones and volumes of organs. For further details of micro-CT readers are referred to Chapter 82.

Eventually Positron Emission Tomography (PET) imaging should allow real-time evaluation of fetal development *in utero*. Such techniques will become practical only after the cost of the PET equipment comes down and the appropriate computational programs are developed for routine use in the laboratory.

INTERPRETATION OF HUMAN RISK FROM THE REPRODUCTIVE AND DEVELOPMENTAL TOXICITY STUDIES IN ANIMALS

Overview

The question of consistent interpretation of animal data for human risk assessment has been the subject of several scientific workshops. In 1981, the Interagency Regulatory Liaison Group (IRLG) sponsored a workshop and identified a task group for developing criteria to support consistent interpretation of DART studies for human risk assessment (IRLG, 1986). At the time the relevance and predictability of animal teratology data to humans was not clear, even when testing guidelines were established for animal reproduction and teratology studies for substances regulated by the FDA (Frankos, 1985). The extrapolation of data from animals to humans is further complicated by background or spontaneous incidence of birth defects or malformations in humans as discussed earlier in this chapter. In view of this, the proposed rule for pregnancy labeling (US FDA, 2008) now requires a general statement about background risk to make the healthcare provider and the patient aware of the background incidence. Because of limitations in predictability of human risk from animal data, the proposed rule for pregnancy labeling suggests the use of standardized risk statements to convey risk based on animal data with inclusion of narrative statements based on risk from human data where available. While predictability of teratogenesis findings from animals to humans varies, integrated knowledge of animal species used for reproductive toxicology studies and certain principles of reproductive toxicology do provide some basis for expected human risk.

Overall, it can be emphasized that animal data can only predict that a hazard/risk exists. In considering this assumption, however, the FDA does not assume that responses in animal models reflect exactly what will occur in humans (Collins, 2006). There are several differences between animal models of reproductive and developmental toxicity and human reproduction that support the FDA's cautious position for extrapolation of animal data to humans (Frankos, 1985). These include: (1) physiological and biochemical differences that relate to absorption, metabolism and excretion of the compound; (2) variability in placental barriers; (3) differences in susceptibility to chemical interactions at the cellular, tissue and organ system levels; (4) variability in background incidence of disease; and (5) variability in gestational development sequence.

Current FDA approach for human reproductive risk assessment when only animal data are available

In April 2000, a conference was held in Washington DC to review a regulator's approach to evaluating animal reproductive toxicology data. The objective of this meeting was to develop a consistent approach to interpretation of animal data for human risk assessment. Based on recommendations from this meeting and other related input, a draft guidance document was published by the FDA in October 2001 (US FDA, 2001) for integration of animal study results for a comprehensive assessment of human reproductive and developmental risks. This draft is not final but highlights current thinking of the agency on this topic.

As summarized by Collins (2006), the overall approach is to integrate non-clinical toxicology data from general, reproductive, developmental, toxicokinetic and metabolism studies and from all available clinical studies and then evaluate a drug's potential to increased risk related to adverse developmental or reproductive outcomes in humans. For this purpose, two broad categories of animal toxicity data, (1) reproductive and (2) developmental, have been considered. In the reproductive category, classes of toxicity evaluated include toxic effect on fertility, parturition and lactation. In the development toxicity category, classes of toxicity evaluated include mortality, dysmorphogenesis, alterations to growth and functional toxicities. Each class of toxicity should be assessed for a positive signal to influence human risk. A decision algorithm was proposed in the draft guidance and was considered an important "tool" for this assessment. Based on diagrammatic presentation, this tool has been referred to as "the wedge" for human risk assessment.

Predictive value of animal DART studies for effects in humans

As discussed above, positive findings from animal DART studies would indicate that a hazard/risk exists but may not indicate that an exact response would be produced in humans. The teratogenic findings in humans associated with thalidomide left an impression that human teratogenicity could not be predicted based on animal studies. This assertion is only partly true because a good amount of animal data has provided reasonably relevant information for human risk assessment, where reproductive effects or malformations noted in animals have been observed in humans. Such information has been compiled by Koren (1998) and does suggest that every drug since the thalidomide incident that has been found to be teratogenic in humans has caused similar or related teratogenic effects in animals also (Table 8.4). This does not mean that all drugs that are teratogenic in animals will produce similar effects in humans but it is encouraging that, to date, a second thalidomide incident has not occurred. Based on animal data, regulatory authorities could require risk management plans from the drug sponsor to further reduce the likelihood of another thalidomide-like incident.

At the same time there are drugs that have shown teratogenic effects in initial animal studies but were not found to be teratogenic in later animal studies or in humans at clinically recommended doses. Examples include glucocorticoids, benzodiazepines, salicylates, oral contraceptives and bendectin (Table 8.5). These examples suggest that not all drugs teratogenic in some animal studies result in malformations in humans at clinical doses.

REPRODUCTIVE RISKS COMMUNICATION AND MANAGEMENT

Product label as an effective communication tool

Overview

The product label is a tool to communicate prescribing information to the healthcare provider to assure safe and effective use of the drug in patients. The general goals of a product label are to communicate and educate the clinician, pharmacist, nurse, patient or any other healthcare professional with information that would permit best usage of the drug and avoid any potential adverse effects associated with the drug, including reproductive and pregnancy risks. Information about the drug's effect on reproduction, pregnancy and teratogenic/developmental effects is initially based on results from animal DART studies and is later updated with human-based information. For a US drug product label, reproduction related information is presently included as "Impairment of Fertility" under the label section, "Nonclinical Toxicology". The pregnancy or developmental effects-related information is included under the heading "Pregnancy" under the label section "Use in Specific Populations".

Pregnancy categories

In 1979, the FDA began grouping prescription drugs into five pregnancy categories – A, B, C, D and X – to describe and communicate risks when drugs are used during pregnancy. This was based on a similar system that was introduced in Sweden one year earlier that was based on risks related to reproduction and fetal development, or on the basis of risks weighed against potential benefits. There have been questions related to pregnancy categories as not depicting the true risk and may vary in different countries. One characteristic of the FDA definitions of the pregnancy categories is that the FDA requires a relatively large amount of high quality data on a drug for it to be

TABLE 8.4 Teratogenic effects of drugs in humans that were signaled by animal studies

Drugs	Effects in animals	Effects in humans
Angiotensin-converting enzyme inhibitors	Stillbirths and increased fetal loss in sheep and rabbits (Pipkin *et al.*, 1980)	Prolonged renal failure and hypotension in the newborn, decreased skull ossification, hypocalvaria and renal tubular dysgenesis (Rosa *et al.*, 1989)
Carbamazepine	Cleft palate, dilated cerebral ventricles, and growth retardation in mice (Sullivan and McEllhatton, 1977)	Neural-tube defects (Rosa, 1991)
Cocaine	Dose-dependent decrease in uterine blood flow, fetal hypoxia, hypertension, and tachycardia in sheep (Wood *et al.*, 1987); reduced fetal weight, fetal edema and increased resorption in rats and mice (Fantel and Macphail, 1982)	Growth retardation involving weight, length and head circumference (Weathers *et al.*, 1993); placental abruption (Lutiger *et al.*, 1991; Chasnoff, 1992) and uterine rupture
Ethanol	Microencephaly, growth deficiency and limb anomalies in dogs, chickens and mice (Ellis and Pick, 1980; Shoemaker *et al.*, 1980; Sulik *et al.*, 1981)	Fetal alcohol syndrome: prenatal and postnatal growth deficiency, CNS[a] anomalies (microcephaly, behavioral abnormalities and mental retardation), characteristic pattern of facial features (shorter palpebral fissure, hypoplastic philtrum and flattened maxilla), and major organ-system malformations (Clarren, 1981); with age facial features may become less distinctive, but short stature, microcephaly and behavioral abnormalities persist (Streissguth, 1991)
Isotretinoin	CNS, head, limb and cardiovascular defects in rats and rabbit (Fantel *et al.*, 1977)	Retinoid embryopathy resulting in some or all of the following abnormalities (Lammer *et al.*, 1985): CNS defects (hydrocephalus, optic nerve blindness, retinal defects, microphthalmia, posterior fossa defects, cortical and cerebellar defects); craniofacial defects (microtia or anotia, low set ears, hypertelorism, depressed nasal bridge, microcephaly, micrognathia and agenesis or stenosis of external ear canals); cardiovascular defects (transposition of greater vessels, tetralogy of Fallot and ventricular or atrial septal defects); thymic defects (ectopia and hypoplasia or aplasia); and miscellaneous defects (limb reduction, decreased muscle tone, spontaneous abortion and behavioral abnormalities)
Lithium	Heart defects in rats (Wilby *et al.*, 1987)	Ebstein's anomaly and other heart defects (Nora *et al.*, 1974; Jacobson *et al.*, 1992)
Methyl mercury	CNS abnormalities in rats (Tatetsu, 1968); growth retardation, major disturbances, microencephaly and brain lesions in rhesus monkeys (Dougherty *et al.*, 1974)	Fetal Minimata disease: diffuse neuronal disintegration with gliosis, cerebral palsy, microcephaly strabismus, blindness, speech disorders, motor impairment, abnormal reflexes and mental retardation (Matsumoto *et al.*, 1965)
Phenytoin	Cleft palate, micromelia, renal defects, and hydrocephalus in rabbits, mice and rat (McLain and Langhoff, 1979; Finnell, 1981; Harbison, 1969)	Fetal hydantoin syndrome (Hanson and Smith, 1975): prenatal and postnatal growth deficiency, motor or mental deficiency, short nose with broad nasal bridge, microcephaly, hypertelorism, strabismus, epicanthus, wide fontanelles, low set or abnormally formed ears, positional deformities of limbs, hypoplasia of nails and distal phalanges, hypospadias, hernia, webbed neck, low hairline, impaired neurodevelopment and low performance scores on tests of intelligence (Scolnik *et al.*, 1994)
Thalidomide[b]	Limb-shortening defects in rabbits, the most sensitive species (Fratta *et al.*, 1965)	Limb-shortening defects (McBride, 1961), loss of hearing, abducens paralysis, facial paralysis, anotia, renal malformations, congenital heart disease
Valproic acid	Exencephaly in hamsters and mice (Nau, 1986; Finnel *et al.*, 1988)	Neural-tube defects (Jager-Roman *et al.*, 1986; Lammer *et al.*, 1987)
Warfarin[b]	Maxillonasal hypoplasia and skeletal anomalies in rats (Howe and Webster, 1992)	Fetal warfarin syndrome: skeletal defects (nasal hypoplasia and stippled epiphyses), limb hypoplasia (particularly in distal digits), low birth weights (<10th percentile), hearing loss and ophthalmic anomalies (Hall *et al.*, 1980), CNS defects with exposure after first trimester; dorsal midline dysplasia (agenesis of corpus callosum and Dandy–Walker malformations) or ventral midline dysplasia (optic atrophy) (Schardein, 1993)

[a] CNS denotes central nervous system
[b] Initial studies in animals failed to show teratogenicity; hence, documentation in humans preceded that in animals
Adapted with permission from *The New Eng J Med* for using data from Koren *et al.* (1998)

TABLE 8.5 Common drugs initially thought to be teratogenic but subsequently proved safe

Drugs	Initial evidence of risk	Subsequent evidence of safety (no teratogenic finding)
Diazepam[a]	Oral cleft (Saxen, 1975)	No increase in risk in large cohort or case-control studies (Rosenberg *et al.*, 1983; Shiono and Mills, 1984; Czeizel, 1987)
Oral contraceptives	Birth defects involving the vertebrae, anus, heart, trachea, esophagus, kidney and limbs (Nora *et al.*, 1978); masculinizing effects on female fetuses resulting in pseudohermaphrodism (Schardein, 1980)	No association between first-trimester exposure to oral contraceptives and malformations in general or external genital malformations in two meta-analyses (Bracken, 1990; Raman-Wilms *et al.*, 1995)
Spermicides	Limb defects, tumors, Down's syndrome and hypospadias (Jick *et al.*, 1981)	No increase in risk in meta-analysis (Einarson, 1990)
Salicylates	Cleft palate (Walker, 1971) and congenital heart disease	No increase in large cohort studies (Werler *et al.*, 1971; Slone *et al.*, 1976)
Bendectin (doxylamine plus pyridoxine)	Cardiac and limb defects (Dickson, 1977; Donnai and Harris, 1978)	No increase in risk in two meta-analyses (Einarson *et al.*, 1988; McKeigue *et al.*, 1994)

[a] Diazepam taken near term may cause the neonatal withdrawal syndrome or cardiorespiratory instability
Adapted with permission from the *New England Journal of Medicine* for using data from Koren *et al.* (1998)

defined as Pregnancy Category A as compared to some other countries. Table 8.6 lists criteria for assignment of pregnancy categories in the USA and Australia. Many of the drugs that would be considered Pregnancy Category A in other countries are allocated to be Category C by the FDA.

For newly approved drugs in the USA, to communicate lack of data in humans, the majority of new drugs approved for marketing carry a statement that reads: "*There are, however, no adequate and well-controlled studies in pregnant women. Because animal reproductive studies are not always predictive of human response, this drug should be used during pregnancy only if clearly needed.*"

Overview of FDA's proposed rule for changes in communicating pregnancy risks

The system of using pregnancy categories has not changed in the USA since being established in 1979. This system has served well for general risk evaluation but has not been without issues related to interpretation. Over the years the FDA has received comments that the system has led to inaccurate and an overly simplified view of prescribing risks during pregnancy. In view of this, the FDA, after careful and extended evaluation, proposed a new rule in 2008 to address changes in labeling related to pregnancy and lactation. This new rule is entitled: "*Content and Format of Labeling for Human Prescription Drugs and Biological Products; Requirements for Pregnancy and Lactation Labeling*" (US FDA, 2008).

The FDA proposed two major subsections, "Pregnancy" and "Lactation," which would be subsections 8.1 and 8.2 under the section "Use in Specific Populations" in the new label. These major subsections would replace the existing "Pregnancy", "Labor and Delivery" and "Nursing Mothers" sections of the current FDA drug label. The proposed rule also would eliminate the current alphabetical (A, B, C, D and X) categorization of pregnancy risk. Instead, the pregnancy subsection would have five principal components: (1) *Pregnancy exposure registry*, (2) *General statement about background risk*, (3) *Fetal risk summary*, (4) *Clinical considerations* and (5) *a data section*. Details on preparing the contents of the Pregnancy section can be found in the FDA proposed rule (US FDA, 2008).

The "*Fetal Risk Summary*" information related to use of more understandable terminology has been summarized here since some of the terminology is highly technical and unfamiliar to most healthcare providers. The FDA is proposing to use simpler terminology so that pregnancy labeling based on the proposed rule would be more easily understood. With this objective in mind, birth defects usually referred to as developmental toxicities by reproductive toxicologists are divided into four types of effect: (1) dysmorphogenesis, (2) developmental mortality, (3) functional toxicity and (4) alterations to growth. Accordingly, the proposed rule uses "*developmental abnormalities*" for developmental toxicities; "*structural anomalies*" for dysmorphogenesis, which includes malformations, deformations and disruptions; "*fetal and infant mortality*" for developmental mortality, which includes miscarriage, stillbirth and neonatal death; and "*impaired physiologic function*" for functional toxicity, which includes outcomes such as deafness, endocrinopathy, neurodevelopmental effects and impairment of reproductive function. The proposed rule retains the term "*alterations to growth*", which includes outcomes such as growth retardation, excessive growth and early maturation because this term is not as technical as the others.

The FDA believes that a label must contain the section for "pregnancy" and both human and animal data should be discussed. It is important for pregnancy labeling to describe, to the extent possible, all recognized potential adverse outcomes to the fetus associated with drug use during pregnancy. Whenever possible, labeling must be based on data derived from human experience. In "*Fetal Risk Summary*" the summary must state whether it is based on human or animal data, and must present human data before the animal data.

Management of reproductive risks after drug approval

A Risk Management Program/Plan (RMP) is important particularly for drugs that have a potential for adverse reproductive risks including but not limited to fetal malformations, fetal or neonatal growth or pregnancy maintenance. For such drugs, the hazard is usually indicated by animal testing and actual human data are sparse or lacking at the time of drug

TABLE 8.6 Differences in pregnancy categories for pharmaceuticals in selected countries

Pregnancy categories and description	
USA	**Australia**
A: Adequate and well-controlled studies have failed to demonstrate a risk to the fetus in the first trimester of pregnancy (and there is no evidence of risk in later trimesters).	**A:** Drugs which have been taken by a large number of pregnant women and women of child-bearing age without an increase in the frequency of malformations or other direct or indirect harmful effects on the fetus having been observed.
B: Animal reproduction studies have failed to demonstrate a risk to the fetus and there are no adequate and well-controlled studies in pregnant women OR Animal studies have shown an adverse effect, but adequate and well-controlled studies in pregnant women have failed to demonstrate a risk to the fetus in any trimester.	**B1:** Drugs which have been taken by only a limited number of pregnant women and women of child-bearing age, without an increase in the frequency of malformation or other direct or indirect harmful effects on the human fetus having been observed. Studies in animals have not shown evidence of an increased occurrence of fetal damage. **B2:** Drugs which have been taken by only a limited number of pregnant women and women of child-bearing age, without an increase in the frequency of malformation or other direct or indirect harmful effects on the human fetus having been observed. Studies in animals are inadequate or may be lacking, but available data show no evidence of an increased occurrence of fetal damage. **B3:** Drugs which have been taken by only a limited number of pregnant women and women of child-bearing age, without an increase in the frequency of malformation or other direct or indirect harmful effects on the human fetus having been observed. Studies in animals have shown evidence of an increased occurrence of fetal damage, the significance of which is considered uncertain in humans.
C: Animal reproduction studies have shown an adverse effect on the fetus and there are no adequate and well-controlled studies in humans, but potential benefits may warrant use of the drug in pregnant women despite potential risks.	**C:** Drugs which, owing to their pharmaceutical effects, have caused or may be suspected of causing, harmful effects on the human fetus or neonate without causing malformations. These effects may be reversible.
D: There is positive evidence of human fetal risk based on adverse reaction data from investigational or marketing experience or studies in humans, but potential benefits may warrant use of the drug in pregnant women despite potential risks.	**D:** Drugs which have caused or are suspected to have caused or may be expected to cause an increased incidence of human fetal malformations or irreversible damage. These drugs may also have adverse pharmacological effects.
X: Studies in animals or humans have demonstrated fetal abnormalities and/or there is positive evidence of human fetal risk based on adverse reaction data from investigational or marketing experience, and the risks involved in use of the drug in pregnant women clearly outweigh potential benefits.	**X:** Drugs that have such a high risk of causing permanent damage to the fetus that they should NOT be used in pregnancy or when there is a possibility of pregnancy.

approval. Regulatory agencies are emphasizing risk monitoring to better evaluate the safety of drug use in humans. The RMP is usually designed and implemented by the drug sponsor in consultation and advice from the regulatory agency. The features of an RMP can vary with respect to drug class, potential for adverse effects, intended patient population and extent of drug usage. The RMP developed for Accutane is used here as an example where pregnancy prevention was vital for avoiding potential teratogenic effects in targeted users of the drug (Brinker *et al.*, 2005). The Accutane RMP included:

- **Prescriber registration and education:** Prior to writing any prescriptions, the prescribers were required to read the SMART "Guide to Best Practices" provided by the manufacturer and then signed and returned along with a letter of understanding attesting their knowledge of the measures to minimize fetal exposure to Accutane. Prescribers were encouraged to attend Accutane educational programs related to pregnancy prevention. The prescribers were then eligible to receive Accutane qualification stickers that would be attached to the prescription forms.
- **Patient registration and education and informed consent:** For female patients this involved (1) being educated about the teratogenic effects of Accutane, signing of the consent statement indicating that they understood the risks associated with use of Accutane during pregnancy and taking an initial (screening) pregnancy test; (2) receiving counsel from the prescriber for sexually active women to select and use two forms of effective contraception measures simultaneously for at least 1 month prior to initiation, during and for 1 month following discontinuation of Accutane therapy; (3) arranging a follow-up (confirmatory) pregnancy test within 7 days of actually initiating the treatment.
- **Restricted and documented dispensing:** Pharmacists were to dispense Accutane only on presentation of a prescription with a "qualification sticker" and dispense only for 30 days along with a copy of the FDA-approved "Accutane Medication Guide". Requests for refills without a new prescription, electronic, telephonic or mail prescriptions were not to be honored.

In addition to the above pregnancy prevention measures used for Accutane, related general steps that could be part of an RMP on a wider scale may include:

- **Pregnancy registry and follow-up:** This is to track and monitor women who have or may have been exposed to a drug with potential for adverse reproductive or developmental effects during pregnancy. Such women are followed during pregnancy, delivery and after delivery for any effects related to structural or functional deficits in the baby at birth or at a later stage during growing years.
- **Monitoring effectiveness of the program:** The Risk Management Program is evaluated for compliance, effectiveness and could be modified as needed to achieve optimal outcome with respect to safety of the unborn.

CONCLUDING REMARKS AND FUTURE DIRECTIONS

DART testing of pharmaceuticals in the 21st century is likely to focus on two major areas: (1) development and validation of new tests using emerging technologies and (2) refinement of the currently used *in vivo* test for better identification and prediction of reproductive hazard/risks.

Early identification of potential toxicological risks during drug discovery and the screening stage of drug development is an important objective for advancing only the most promising compounds to preclinical and clinical phase of drug development. Due to relatively larger numbers of compounds evaluated during the early stages of drug discovery the rapid turnaround of toxicity test results, good predictivity of the test results for humans, cost effectiveness and ability to use small amounts of test compound have been the key requirements for such testing.

Development and validation of new DART tests using emerging technologies

Current status

The need for *in vitro* tests for reproductive and developmental toxicity was indentified as early as the 1970s. Work relating to use of rat whole-embryo culture for this purpose dates back to this period (New, 1978). Many potential models, such as hydra regeneration, chick embryo neural retina cells, embryonic palatal mesenchyme cells, mouse ovarian tumor cell attachment, chick embryo, whole rat embryos *in vitro*, whole mouse embryos, mouse palatal cultures, mouse limb bud reaggregates, embryonic stem cells and rabbit whole embryo culture have been investigated and were recently reviewed (Chapin *et al.*, 2008).

In an earlier review of *in vitro* assays for developmental toxicity (Daston, 1996) a case was made that these models are capable of distinguishing between toxicants and non-toxicants nearly 80% of the time. The European Center for the Validation of Alternative Methods (ECVAM) also evaluated three *in vitro* embryotoxicity tests (the Embryonic Stem Cell Test using two permanent mouse cell lines, 3T3 fibroblasts and embryonic stem cell line D3 – mEST; the MicroMass test using undifferentiated mesenchyme cells of early rat embryo limb – MM test; and the postimplantation rat Whole-Embryo Culture assay – WEC test) and indicated there was acceptable scientific validation for the predictivity of these assays relative to *in vivo* tests (Balls and Hellsten, 2002).

In vitro *test gaining wider scientific attention*

A steering committee sponsored by the Developmental and Reproductive Toxicology Technical Committee of the Health and Environmental Science Institute (HESI), a part of the International Life Science Institute (ILSI), summarized information for three types of *in vitro* developmental toxicity assays (Chapin *et al.*, 2008). These assays included Whole-Embryo Culture (WEC), mouse Embryonic Stem Cell Test (mEST) and Zebrafish assay. These assays were considered promising for further refinement; however, several tasks were identified that were needed to address the challenges encountered.

Current usage of in vitro *tests*

As indicated above, significant progress has been made during the last 30 years to develop and validate *in vitro* tests for identification of developmental toxicity risks, with newly developed assays employing more recent innovation (zebrafish and mEST) but still these tests are in their infancy and need further improvement (Chapin *et al.*, 2008).

Following recognition by ECVAM, the mEST *in vitro* test has been used by some pharmaceutical and chemical companies for priority setting for early stage compounds (Horie *et al.*, 2007; Whitlow *et al.*, 2007). In a recent commentary on the path forward for developmental and reproductive toxicity testing, Spielmann (2009) has indicated that even though mEST has not yet been accepted for regulatory purposes, it is the most advanced and promising *in vitro* test. Recently, Pfizer used mEST for testing 63 compounds (Paquette *et al.*, 2008), and reported that overall performance of the test was considered good (accuracy of 75%) but there was lower predictive value for low risk compounds and that the false positive rate was nearly 40%. Future work in this area is expected to result in more predictable tests but complicating factors such as (1) complexity of the mammalian reproductive cycle, (2) the role of pharmacokinetics and drug metabolism during *in vivo* testing and (3) instances where developmental effects occur later in life or during the next generation as well as some fetal effects being related to the maternal health effects (indirect influence on the fetus) remain to be addressed.

Modern imaging procedures for morphological examination of fetuses

As discussed in an earlier section of this chapter, techniques like ultrasound (already practical for non-human primate fetuses), micro-computed tomography (micro-CT) and Positron Emission Tomography (PET) imaging should allow real-time evaluation of fetal development *in utero*. Such techniques will become more common with moderation in cost of equipments needed and availability of staff trained in performing the procedures.

In conclusion, a significant progress has been made during the last 50 years with respect to reproductive and developmental toxicity testing for pharmaceuticals. With international guidelines harmonized, several new technologies for *in vitro* models made available, regulatory requirements made clear and overall reproductive hazard identification improved for human pharmaceuticals, a "thalidomide"-like tragedy has not been repeated so far and is not expected to occur in the future. Animal studies are still expected to provide the key data for regulatory risk assessment for humans for several years to come particularly with respect to use of drugs in women of child-bearing potential.

REFERENCES

Antonov AN (1947) Children born during the siege of Leningrad in 1942. *J Pediatr* **30:** 250–9.

Balls M, Hellsten E (2002) The use of scientifically validated *in vitro* tests for embryotoxicity. *ATLA* **30:** 265–73.

Barrow PC (2003) Reproductive toxicology studies and immunotherapeutics. *Toxicology* **185:** 205–12.

Barrow PC (2009) Reproductive toxicity testing for pharmaceuticals under ICH. *Reprod Toxicol* **28:** 172–9.

Barrow PC, Ravel G (2005) Immune assessment in developmental and juvenile toxicology: practical considerations for the regulatory safety testing of pharmaceuticals. *Reg Toxicol Pharmacol* **43:** 35–44.

Bass R (1993) Report on Progress Since ICH-1, The Second International Conference on

Bolon B, Bucci TJ, Warbritton AR, Chen JJ, Mattison DR, Heindel JJ (1997) Differential follicle counts as a screen chemically-induced ovarian toxicity in mice: results from continuous breeding bioassays. *Fund Appl Toxicol* **39:** 1–10.

Bracken MB (1990) Oral contraceptives and congenital malformations in offspring: a review and meta-analysis of the prospective studies. *Obstet Gynecol* **76:** 552–7.

Brinker A, Kornegay C, Nourjah P (2005) Trends on adherence to a revised risk management program designed to decrease or eliminate isotretinoin-exposed pregnancies. *Arch Dermatol* **141:** 563–9.

Brodniewicz-Proba T (2008) The scope and requirements related to preclinical and clinical studies of a new medicinal product, including biotechnological and biosimilar products. *Acta Polaniae Pharmaceutica – Drug Research* **65:** 641–5.

Buckley LA, Benson K, Davis-Bruno K, Dempster M, Finch GL, Harlow P, Haggerty HG, Hart T, Kinter L, Leighton JK, McNulty J, Roskos L, Saber H, Stauber A, Tabrizi M (2008) Nonclinical aspects of biopharmaceutical development: discussion of case studies at a PhRMA-FDA workshop. *Int J Toxicol* **27:** 303–12.

Canada (1977) Health Protection Branch, *The Testing of Chemicals for Carcinogenicity, Mutagenicity and Teratogenicity*, Ministry of Health and Welfare, Canada.

Centers for Disease Control and Prevention (CDC) (2009) Birth Defects, March 11, 2009, cited in *March of Dimes: Pregnancy & Newborn Health Education Center, Quick Reference: Fact Sheet*, June 2009.

Chapin R, Augustine-Rauch K, Beyer B, Daston G, Finnell R, Flynn T, Hunter S, Mirkes P, O'Shea KS, Piersma A, Sandler D, Vanparys P, Maele-Fabrey GV (2008) State of the art in developmental toxicity screening methods and a way forward: a meeting report addressing embryonic stem cells, whole embryo culture and zebrafish. *Birth Defect Res (Part B)* **83:** 446–56.

Chasnoff IJ (1992) Cocaine, pregnancy and the growing child. *Curr Probl Pediatr* **22:** 302–21.

Chellman GJ, Bussiere JL, Makori N, Martin PL, Ooshima Y, Weinbauer GF (2009) Developmental and reproductive toxicology studies in nonhuman primates. *Birth Defect Res (Part B)* **86:** 446–62.

Christian MS (1993) Harmonization of reproductive guidelines: a perspective from the International Federation of Teratology Societies. *J Am Coll Toxicol* **11(3):** 299–302.

Clarren SK (1981) Recognition of fetal alcohol syndrome. *JAMA* **245:** 2436–9.

Clegg DJ (1979) Animal reproduction and carcinogenicity studies in relation to human safety evaluations. *Devel Toxicol Environ Sci* **4:** 45–59.

Collins TFX (2006) History and evolution of reproductive and developmental toxicology guidelines. *Current Pharma Design* **12:** 1449–65.

Committee on the Safety of Medicines (CSM) (1974) *Notes for Guidance on Reproduction Studies*. Department of Health and Social Security, Great Britain.

Czeizel A (1987) Lack of evidence of teratogenicity of benzodiazepine drugs in Hungary. *Reprod Toxicol* **1:** 183–8.

D'Arcy PF, Harron DWG (eds.) (1992) Topic 2: Reproductive toxicology. In *Proceedings of the First International Conference on Harmonisation*. The Queen's University of Belfast, p. 255.

Daston GP (1996) The theoretical and empirical case for in vitro developmental toxicity screens, and potential applications. *Teratology* **53:** 339–44.

DeSesso JM (1996) Comparative embryology. In *Handbook of Developmental Toxicology* (Hood RD, ed.). CRC Press, New York, pp. 111–74.

Dickson JH (1977) Congenital deformities associated with Bendectin. *Can Med Assoc J* **117:** 691–2.

Donnai D, Harris R (1978) Unusual fetal malformations after antiemetics in pregnancy. *BMJ* **1:** 691–2.

Dougherty WJ, Coulston F, Golberg L (1974) Toxicity of methylmercury in pregnant rhesus monkeys. *Toxicol Appl Pharmacol* **29:** 138 abstract.

Einarson TR, Koren G, Mattice D, Schechter-Tsafriri O (1990) Maternal spermicide use and adverse reproductive outcome: a meta analysis. *Am J Obstet Gynecol* **162:** 655–60.

Einarson TR, Leeder JS, Koren G (1988) A method for meta-analysis of epidemiological studies. *Drug Intell Clin Pharm* **22:** 813–24.

Ellis FW, Pick JR (1980) An animal model of the fetal alcohol syndrome in beagles. *Alcohol Clin Exp Res* **4:** 123–34.

European Economic Community (1988) The Rules Governing Medicinal Products in the European Community, Vol. III, Guidelines on the Quality, Safety and Efficacy of Medicinal Products for Human Use. Office of Official Publications of the European Communities, Brussels.

Fantel AG, Macphail BJ (1982) The teratogenicity of cocaine. *Teratology* **26:** 17–19.

Fantel AG, Shepard TH, Newell-Morris LL, Moffett BC (1977) Teratogenic effects of retinoic acid in pigtail monkeys (Macaca nemestrina). I. General Features. *Teratology* **15:** 65–71.

Finnell RH (1981) Phenytoin-induced teratogenesis: a mouse model. *Science* **211:** 483–4.

Finnell RH, Bennett GD, Karras SB, Mohl VK (1988) Common hierarchies of susceptibilities to the induction of neural tube defect in mouse embryo by valproic acid and its 4-propyl-4- pentenoic acid metabolite. *Teratology* **38:** 313–20.

Fitzhugh OG (1959) Chronic oral toxicity. In *Appraisal of the Safety of Chemicals in Foods, Drugs and Cosmetics*. Association of Food and Drug Officials of the United States, Austin, Texas, 36.

Frankos VH (1985) FDA perspectives on the use of teratology data for human risk assessment. *Fund Appl Toxicol* **5:** 615–25.

Fraser FC, Lenz W, Warkany J, Kelsey FO, Heshka T, Stevens TD, Brent RL, Holmes LB (1988) Thalidomide symposium; thalidomide retrospective: what did we learn? Paper presented at the 26th Annual Meeting of the Teratology Society, July 6–10, 1986, Boston, MA. *Teratology* **38:** 201–2.

Fratta ID, Sigg EB, Maiorana K (1965) Teratogenic effects of thalidomide in rabbits, rats, hamsters, and mice. *Toxicol Appl Pharmacol* **7:** 268–86.

Goldberg L (ed.) (1974) Recommendations of a conference as stated by the conference chairman. In *Carcinogenesis Testing of Chemicals*. CRC Press, Cleveland, pp. 123.

Gottlieb S (2008) Biosimilars: policy, clinical and regulatory considerations. *Am J Health Syst Pharm* **65:** S2–8.

Gregg NM (1941) Congenital cataract following German measles in mothers. *Trans Ophthalmol Soc Austral* **3:** 35–46.

Hale F (1933) Pigs born without eyeballs. *J Heredity* **24:** 105–6.

Hale F (1935) The relation of vitamin A to anophthalmos in pigs. *Am J Ophthamol* **18:** 1087–93.

Hall JG, Pauli RM, Wilson KM (1980) Maternal and fetal sequelae of anticoagulation during pregnancy. *Am J Med* **68:** 122–40.

Hanson JW, Smith DW (1975) The fetal hydantoin syndrome. *J Pediatr* **87:** 285–90.

Harbison RD (1969) Studies on the mechanism of teratogenic action and neonatal pharmacology of diphenylhydantoin (PhD thesis. Iowa State University, Iowa, USA).

Harmonisation, Orlando, Florida, October 27–9, 1993.

Heindel JJ (1999) VII Oocyst quantitation and ovarian histology. In *An Evaluation and Interpretation of Reproductive Endpoints for Human Health Risk Assessment*. Washington DC, Int Life Sci Institute 57–74.

Henderson JD (1992) Current issues in bioequivalence determination. *Appl Clin Trials* **1:** 44–9.

Herbst AL, Ulfelder H, Poskanzer DC (1971) Adenocarcinoma of the vagina: association of maternal stilbestrol therapy with tumor appearance in young women. *New Eng J Med* **284:** 878–81.

Holsapple MP (2003) Developmental immunotoxicity testing: a review. *Toxicology* **185:** 193–203.

Horie N, Higuchi H, Kawamura S, Saito K, Suzuki N (2007) Safety evaluation study using embryonic stem (ES) cells. *Sumitomo Kagaku* **2007-I:** 1–7 (abstract).

Howe AM, Webster WS (1992) The warfarin embryopathy: a rat model showing maxillonasal hypoplasia and other skeletal disturbances. *Teratology* **46:** 379–90.

Interagency Regulatory Liaison Group (1986) Interagency regulatory liaison group workshop on reproductive toxicity risk assessment. *Environ Hlth Pers* **66**: 193–221.

Interagency Regulatory Liaison Group (IRLG) (1980) Recommended guideline for teratogenicity studies in the rat, mouse, hamster or rabbit, April.

International Conference on Harmonisation of Technical Requirements for the Registration of Pharmaceuticals for Human Use. *ICH Harmonised Tripartite Guideline; Detection of Toxicity to Reproduction for Medicinal Products*, June 24, 1993. Presented at The Second International Conference on Harmonisation, Orlando, Florida, October 27–9, 1993.

Jackson CM (1925) *Effects of Inanition and Malnutrition upon Growth and Structure*. P. Blakiston's Son & Co., Philadelphia.

Jacobson SJ, Jones K, Johnson K, Ceolin L, Kaur P, Sahn D, Donnenfeld AE, Rieder M, Santelli R, Smythe J, Pastuszak, Einarson T, Koren G (1992) Prospective multicenter study of pregnancy outcome after lithium exposure during first trimester. *Lancet* **339**: 530–3.

Jager-Roman E, Deichi A, Jakob S, Hartmann A, Koch S, Rating D, Steldinger R, Nau H, Helge H (1986) Fetal growth, major malformations, and minor anomalies in infants born to women receiving valproic acid. *J Pediatr* **108**: 997–1004.

Jarrell J, Young Lai EV, Barr R, McMahon A, Belbeck L, O'Connell G (1987) Ovarian toxicity of cyclophosphamide alone and in combination with ovarian irradiation in the rats. *Cancer Res* **47**: 2340–3.

Jick H, Walker AM, Rothman KL, Hunter JR, Holmes LB, Watkins RN, D'Ewart DC, Danford A, Madsen S (1981) Vaginal spermicides and congenital disorders. *JAMA* **245**: 1329–32.

Johnson EM, Christian MS (1983) When is a teratology study not an evaluation of teratogenicity? *J Am Coll Toxicol* **3**: 431–4.

Kane SV, Acquah LA (2009) Placental transport of immunoglobulins: a clinical review for gastroenterologists who prescribe therapeutic monoclonal antibodies to women during conception and pregnancy. *The Am J Gastroenterol* **104**: 228–33.

Kelsey FO (1988) Thalidomide update: regulatory aspects. *Teratology* **38**: 221–6.

Koos BJ, Longo L (1976) Mercury toxicity in pregnant women, fetus and newborn infant. *Am J Obstet Gynecol* **126**: 390–409.

Koren G, Pastuszak A, Ito S (1998) Drugs in pregnancy. *N Eng J Med* **338**: 1128–37.

Lammer EJ, Chen DJ, Hoar RM, Agnish ND, Benke PJ, Braun JT, Curry CJ, Fernhoff PM, Grix AW, Lott IT, Richard JM, Sun SC (1985) Retinoic acid embryopathy. *N Eng J Med* **313**: 837–41.

Lammer EJ, Sever LE, Oakley GP Jr (1987) Teratogen update: valproic acid. *Teratology* **35**: 465–73.

Lehman AJ, Laug EP, Woodard G, Draize JH, Fitzhugh OG, Nelson AA (1949) Procedures for the appraisal of the toxicity of chemicals in foods. *Food Drug Cosmet Law J* **4**: 412–34.

Lenz W (1961) Kindliche missbildungen nach medikament wahrend der draviditat? *Deutsch Med Wochenschr* **86**: 2555.

Lutiger B, Graham K, Einarson TR, Koren G (1991) Relationship between gestational cocaine use and pregnancy outcome: meta-analysis. *Teratology* **44**: 405–14.

Martin PL, Breslin W, Rocca M, Wright D, Cavagnaro J (2009) Considerations in assessing the developmental and reproductive toxicity potential of biopharmaceuticals *Birth Defect Res (Part B)* **86**: 176–203.

Mathews TJ, MacDorman MF (2008) Infant mortality statistics from the 2005 period linked birth/infant death data set. *National Vital Statistics Reports*, volume **57**: July 30, 2008. Cited in *March of Dimes: Pregnancy & Newborn Health Education Center, Quick Reference: Fact Sheet*, June 2009.

Matsumoto H, Koya G, Takeuchi T (1965) Fetal Minamata disease: a neuropathological study of two cases of intrauterine intoxication by a methylmercury compound. *J Neuropathol Exp Neurol* **24**: 563–74.

McBride WG (1961) Thalidomide and congenital abnormalities. *Lancet* **278**: 1358.

McKeigue PM, Lamm SH, Linn S, Kutcher JS (1994) Bendectin and birth defects. I. A meta-analysis of the epidemiological studies. *Teratology* **50**: 27–37.

McLain RM, Langhoff L (1979) Teratogenicity of diphenylhydantoin in New Zealand white rabbits. *Toxicol Appl Pharmacol* **48**: A32 (abstract).

Ministry of Health and Welfare, Japan (MHW), *On Animal Experimental Methods for Testing the Effects of Drugs on Reproduction*, Notification No. 529 of the Pharmaceutical Affairs Bureau, Ministry of Health and Welfare, March 31, 1975.

Muhammad FS, Goode AK, Kock ND, Arifin EA, Cline JM, Adams MR, Hoyer PB, Christian PJ, Isom S, Japlan JR, Appt SE (2009) Effect of 4-vinylcyclohexene diepoxide on peripubertal and adult Sprague-Dawley rats: ovarian, clinical, and pathologic outcomes. *Comp Med* **59**: 46–59.

Nau H (1986) Species differences in pharmacokinetics and drug teratogenesis. *Environ Health Perspect* **70**: 113–29.

New DA (1978) Whole-embryo culture and the study of mammalian embryo during organogenesis. *Biol Rev Camb Philos Soc* **53**: 81–122.

Nora JJ, Nora AH, Blu J, Ingram J, Fountain A, Peterson M, Lortscher RH, Kimberling WJ (1978) Exogenous progestogen and estrogen implicated in birth defects. *JAMA* **240**: 837–43.

Nora JJ, Nora AH, Toews JM (1974) Lithium Ebstein's anomaly, and other congenital heart defects. *Lancet* **304**: 594–5.

Organization for Economic Cooperation and Development (OECD): Final Report-OECD short-term and long-term toxicology groups. *Teratogenicity* December 31, 1979, 110.

Palmer AK (1973) Some thoughts on reproductive studies for safety evaluations. *Proc Euro Soc Study Drug Tox* **14**: 79–90.

Palmer AK (1981) Regulatory requirements for reproductive toxicology: theory and practice. In *Developmental Toxicology* (Kimmel CA, Buelke-Sam J, eds). Raven Press, New York, pp. 259.

Paquette JA, Kumpf SW, Streck RD, Thompson JJ, Chapin RE, Stedman DB (2008) Assessment of the embryonic stem cell test and application and use in the pharmaceutical industry. *Birth Defect Res (Part B)* **83**: 104–11.

Pharmaceutical Manufacturers Association (PMA) (1965) *Second Workshop in Teratology. Supplement to the Teratology Workshop Manual* (A collection of lectures and demonstrations from the Second Workshop in Teratology held January 25–30, 1965, Berkeley, California), Pharmaceutical Manufacturers Association, Washington DC.

Pharmaceutical Research and Manufacturers of America (2008) *Pharmaceutical Industry Profile 2008*, Washington, DC: PhRMA, March 2008.

Picut CA, Swanson CL, Scully KL, Roseman VC, Parker RF, Remick AK (2008) Ovarian follicle count using proliferating cell nuclear antigen (PCNA) and semi-automated image analysis in rats. *Toxicol Pathol* **36**: 674–9.

Pipkin FB, Turner SR, Symonds EM (1980) Possible risk with captopril in pregnancy: some animal data. *Lancet* **1**: 1256.

Ramen-Wilms L, Tseng AL, Wighardt S, Einarson TR, Koren G (1995) Fetal genital effects of first trimester sex hormones exposure: a meta analysis. *Obstet Gynec* **85**: 141–9.

Rosa FW (1991) Spina bifida in infants of women treated with carbamazepine during pregnancy. *N Engl J Med* **324**: 674–7.

Rosa FW, Bosco LA, Graham CF, Milstien JB, Michael D, Creamer J (1989) Neonatal anuria with maternal angiotensin-converting enzyme inhibition. *Obstet Gynecol* **74**: 371–4.

Rosenberg L, Mitchell AA, Parsells JL, Pashayan H, Luvik C, Shapiro S (1983) Lack of relation of oral clefts to diazepam use during pregnancy. *N Engl J Med* **309**: 1282–5.

Saxen I (1975) Association between oral cleft and drugs taken during pregnancy. *Int J Epidemiol* **4**: 37–44.

Schardein JL (1980) Congenital abnormalities and hormones during pregnancy: a clinical review. *Teratology* **22**: 251–70.

Schardein JL (1993) *Chemically Induced Birth Defects*, 2nd ed. rev. New York, Marcel Dekker.

Schwetz BA, Rao KS, Park CN (1980) Insensitivity of test for reproductive problems. *J Environ Pathol Toxicol* **3**: 81–98.

Scolnik D, Nulman I, Rovet J, Gladstone D, Czuchta D, Gardner HA, Gladstone R, Ashby P, Weksberg R, Einarson T, Koren G (1994) Neurodevelopment of children exposed in utero to phenytoin and carbamazepine monotherapy. *JAMA* **271**: 767–70.

Shiono PH, Mills JL (1984) Oral clefts and diazepam use during pregnancy. *N Engl J Med* **311**: 919–20.

Shiromizu K, Thorgeirsson S, Mattison D (1984) Effect of cyclophosphamide on oocyte and follicle number in Sprague-Dawley rats, C57BL/6N and DBA/2N mice. *Pediatr Pharmacol* **4**: 213–321.

Shoemaker WJ, Koda LY, Shoemaker CA, Bloom FE (1980) Ethanol effects in chick embryo: cerebellar Purkinje neurons. *Neurobehav Toxicol* **2**: 239–42.

Slone D, Siskind V, Heinonen OP, Monson RR, Kaufman DW, Shapiro S (1976) Aspirin and congenital malformations. *Lancet* **307**: 1373–5.

Smith CA (1947) Effects of maternal undernutrition upon the newborn infant in Holland (1944–1945). *J Pediatr* **30**: 229–43.

Somers GF (1962) Letter to the editor. *Lancet* **1**: 912.

Spielmann H (2009) The way forward in reproductive/developmental toxicity testing. *ATLA* **37**: 641–56.

Staples RE (1974) Detection of visceral alterations in mammalian fetuses. Presented at the Teratology Soc 14th Annual Meeting, Vancouver, Canada. *Teratology* **9**: A37–8 (abstract).

Staples RE, Schnell JL (1964) Refinement in rapid clearing technique in the KOH-alizarin red S method for fetal bone. *Stain Technol* **39**: 61–3.

Stewart J (2009) Developmental toxicity testing of monoclonal antibodies: an enhanced pre- and postnatal study design option. *Reprod Toxicol* **28(2):** 220–5.

Streissguth AP, Aase JM, Clarren SK, Randels SP, LaDue RA, Smith DF (1991) Fetal alcohol syndrome in adolescents and adults. *JAMA* **265:** 1961–7.

Stuckhardt JL, Poppe PM (1984) Fresh visceral examination of rat and rabbit fetuses used in teratogenicity testing. *Teratogenesis, Carcinogenesis and Mutagenesis* **4:** 181–8.

Sulik KK, Johnston MC, Webb MA (1981) Fetal alcohol syndrome: embryogenesis in a mouse model. *Science* **214:** 936–8.

Sullivan FM, McElhatton PR (1977) A comparison of the teratogenic activity of the antiepileptic drugs carbamazepine, clonazepam, ethosuximide, phenobarbital, phenytoin and pyrimidone in mice. *Toxicol Appl Pharmacol* **40:** 365–78.

Tanimura T (1990) Japanese perspectives on the reproductive and developmental toxicity evaluation of pharmaceuticals. *J Amer Coll Toxicol* **9:** 27–37.

Tatetsu M (1968) Experimental manifestation of "congenital minamata disease". *Psychiatr Neurol Jpn* **70:** 162.

Teratology Society, Teratology Society position paper (1987) Recommendations for vitamin A use during pregnancy. *Teratology* **35:** 269–75.

US Environmental Protection Agency (1998) Health effects test guidelines (OPPTS 870.3800). Reproductive infertility effects. Available at: http://www.epa.gov/docs/OPPTS_Harmonized/870_Health_Effects_Test_Guidelines/Drafts/870.3800.txt.html.

US Environmental Protection Agency (EPA), Christian MS, Voytek PE (1982) *In Vivo Reproductive and Mutagenicity Tests*, US Environmental Protection Agency, Washington DC. National Technical Information Service, US Department of Commerce, Springfield, VA 22161.

US Food and Drug Administration (1966) Guidelines for reproduction studies for safety evaluation of drugs for human use. Washington DC, FDA, 5 pp.

US Food and Drug Administration (2001) Reviewer Guidance: integration of study results to assess concerns about human reproductive and developmental toxicities. Draft Guidance Rockville, MD, Center for Drug Evaluation and Research.

US Food and Drug Administration (2008) Proposed Rule: contents and format of labeling for human prescription drug and biological products; requirements for pregnancy and lactation labeling. *Federal Register* **73:** Number 104, Thursday May 29, 2009.

US Food and Drug Administration (FDA) (1982) *Toxicological Principles and Procedures for Priority Based Assessment of Food Additives (Red Book)*. Guidelines for Reproduction Testing with a Teratology Phase, Bureau of Foods, US Food and Drug Administration, Washington, DC, p. 80.

US Food and Drug Administration (FDA) (1993) *Draft – Toxicological Principles for the Safety Assessment of Direct Food Additives and Color Additives Used in Food (Red Book II)*. Guidelines for Reproduction and Developmental Toxicity Studies, Center for Food Safety and Applied Nutrition, US Food and Drug Administration, Washington DC, p. 123.

Walker BE (1971) Induction of cleft palate in rats with antiinflammatory drugs. *Teratology* **4:** 39–42.

Warkany J (1965) Development of experimental mammalian teratology. In *Teratology Principles and Techniques* (Wilson JG, Warkany J, eds.). University of Chicago Press, p. 1.

Warkany J, Nelson RC (1940) Appearance of skeletal abnormalities in the offspring of rats reared on a deficient diet. *Science* **92:** 383–4.

Warkany J, Nelson RC (1941) Skeletal abnormalities in offspring of rats reared on deficient diets. *Anat Rec* **79:** 83–100.

Weathers WT, Crane MM, Sauvain KJ, Blackhurst DW (1993) Cocaine use in women from defined population: prevalence at delivery and effect on growth in infants. *Pediatrics* **91:** 350–4.

Welage LS, Kirking DM, Ascione FJ, Gaither CA (2001) Understanding the scientific issues embedded in the generic drug approval process. *J Am Pharm Assn* **41:** 856–67.

Werler MM, Mitchell AA, Shapiro S (1989) The relation of aspirin use during the first trimester of pregnancy to congenital cardiac defects. *N Engl J Med* **321:** 1639–42.

Whitlow S, Burgin H, Clemann N (2007) The embryonic stem cell test for the early selection of pharmaceutical compounds. *ALTEX* **24:** 3–6.

Wier P (2006) Use of toxicokinetics in developmental and reproductive toxicology. In *Developmental and Reproductive Toxicology* (Hood RD, ed.). CRC, Taylor & Francis Group, Boca Raton, London, New York, 2nd edition, pp. 571–97.

Wilby OK, Tesh SA, Ross FW, Tesh JM (1987) Effects of lithium on development in vitro and in vivo in the rat. *Teratology* **35:** 69 (abstract).

Wilson JG (1965) Methods for administering agents and detecting malformations in experimental animals. In *Teratology, Principles and Techniques.* University of Chicago Press, Chicago, p. 262.

Wilson JG (1973) Principles of teratology. In *Environment and Birth Defects.* Academic Press, New York, p. 11.

Wilson JG, Warkany J (1965) *Teratology: Principles and Techniques* (Lectures and demonstrations given at the First Workshop in Teratology, University of Florida, February 2–8, 1964). University of Chicago Press, Chicago.

Wise DL, Buschmann J, Feuston MH, Fisher JE, Hew KW, Hoberman AM, Lerman SA, Ooshima Y, Stump DG (2009) Embryo–fetal developmental toxicity study design for pharmaceuticals. *Birth Defect Res (Part B)* **86:** 418–28.

Wood JR Jr, Plessinger MA, Clark KE (1987) Effect of cocaine on uterine blood flow and fetal oxygenation. *JAMA* **257:** 957–61.

World Health Organization (WHO) (1967) Principles for the testing of drugs for teratogenicity. *WHO Tech. Rept. Series*, No. 364, Geneva.

Zilva SS, Goulding J, Brummond JC, Coward KH (1921) The relation of the fat-soluble factor to rickets and growth in pigs. *Biochem J* **15:** 427–37.

CHAPTER

9

Relevance of animal testing and sensitivity of endpoints in reproductive and developmental toxicity

Efstathios Nikolaidis

INTRODUCTION

Reproductive toxicity has been defined as "any effect of chemicals that would interfere with reproductive ability or capacity", with subsequent effects on lactation and the development of the offspring (UNECE, 2004). The reproductive cycle is perhaps one of the most complex processes of biological functions, making it extremely difficult, if not impossible, to model the whole cycle in one *in vitro* system that would detect the effects of an exogenous substance on all aspects of mammalian reproduction. The answer to this complexity is the breaking down of this cycle into its biological components, which can then be studied separately or together. This can lead to a better understanding of the biological activity and the underlying mechanism of the specific substance. In this context, reproductive toxicity is defined as the adverse effects of a substance on any part of this reproductive cycle, including the impairment of the reproductive function in males and females, as well as the effects on the fetus or offspring.

Developmental toxicity has been defined by the Globally Harmonized System (GHS) as the "adverse effects induced during pregnancy, or as a result of parental exposure", which "can be manifested at any point in the life span of the organism" (UNECE, 2004).

Therefore, developmental toxicity may result from exposure to specific exogenous substances before conception in either parent, exposure during gestation or exposure during postnatal development from birth to sexual maturation. Endpoints for developmental toxicity include a wide range of effects, such as spontaneous abortions, stillbirths, malformations, early postnatal mortality, reduced birth weight leading to structural abnormality, altered growth, functional deficiency and death of the developing organism (EPA, 1991).

The use of animal models to assess hazard and risk to humans from exogenous substances continues to be the standard for protecting human health. On this basis, we currently rely on animal tests to predict the potential of chemicals to cause reproductive harm in humans. Animal tests assessing reproductive toxicity are designed to examine the entire reproductive cycle, either as a series of single tests that evaluate specific stages of the reproductive cycle (reproduction/fertility, prenatal development, postnatal development), or as a protocol (two-generation test). These tests evaluate structure and function from gametogenesis through embryonic and postnatal development to adulthood.

Standardized protocols for testing potentially hazardous chemicals to ensure the application of sound scientific methods and generation of high quality data that are critical for assessing human hazards and risks have been developed and implemented through many guidelines from various international organizations.

The aim of toxicity testing in animals is to identify possible adverse effects resulting from exposure to an exogenous substance and to develop dose–response relationships that will allow evaluation of responses at other exposures and extrapolation to human toxicity. Animal reproductive and developmental toxicity tests should minimize variance and bias and resolve the problem of false-positive and false-negative results. In order to assess reproductive toxicity animal tests must be designed to cover the entire reproductive cycle. A series of tests can be performed to evaluate specific stages of the reproductive cycle (reproduction, fertility, prenatal development, postnatal development), or a single protocol test can be conducted (two-generation test). As mentioned previously, in the area of reproductive and developmental toxicity, animal tests are the current tool to predict the potential for chemicals to cause reproductive deficits in humans. This goal, however, must be weighed in light of constraints on costs, ethics and resources. Animal studies are expensive and in most cases may not provide information on the proper mechanism of action. Testing for reproductive toxicity is animal intensive. Moreover, the experimental assessment of reproductive toxicity is regarded as one of the most costly evaluations to conduct. The total number of animals used in Europe for reproductive toxicology testing in 1999 was about 113,000 animals (EU COM, 2003). The European Union has enacted a new chemical regulation called

Reproductive and Developmental Toxicology, Edited by Ramesh C. Gupta
ISBN: 978-0-12-382032-7

REACH (Registration, Evaluation and Authorization of Chemicals) (Höfer *et al.*, 2006; Lilienblum *et al.*, 2008; Scialli, 2008), according to which registration of existing chemicals, i.e. those marketed before 1981, will take place. As toxicological information is lacking for most of these chemicals, it is expected that this information will be required for about 30,000 substances. In Europe, reproductive toxicity studies and cancer bioassays have so far been applied only to a few new chemicals, and thus the prediction is that animal use in these tests is going to be high. In order to counterbalance this need, REACH strongly promotes alternative methods to traditional *in vivo* testing.

Animal studies ideally should provide clear data pointing to evidence of specific reproductive toxicity in the absence of other, systemic, toxic effects. If developmental toxicity occurs together with other toxic effects in the female, the potential influence of the generalized adverse effects should also be assessed to the greatest extent possible. Ideally, the species of choice should have the same pharmacokinetic profile as in humans. It is thus apparent that the selection of the most sensitive species for evaluating the safety of the substance is important.

CHOICE OF ANIMAL TEST MODELS

The ICH Harmonized Tripartite Guideline (ICH, 1993) states: "In choosing an animal species and strain for reproductive toxicity testing, care should be given to select a relevant model" and continues: "If it can be shown – by means of kinetic, pharmacological and toxicological data – that the species selected is a relevant model for the human, a single species can be sufficient. There is little value in using a second species if it does not show the same similarities to humans. Advantages and disadvantages of species (strains) should be considered in relation to the substance to be tested, the selected study design and to the subsequent interpretation of the results."

The laboratory rat has been, and continues to be, a mainstay in reproductive and developmental toxicity studies. The rat is the most commonly used species for testing, while mice and rabbits are also used. If another mammalian species other than the rat is used, it is urged, in most test guidelines, that there should be a justification for its selection and a description of the modifications that will be necessary (EPA, 1982; OECD, 1983, 1984a). In all studies, healthy parental animals, which have not been subjected to previous experimental procedures, must be used. For certain studies, it is also stated that strains with low fecundity or well-known high incidence of developmental defects should not be used (OECD, 2001b, 2008a, 2009a). The main advantages of the rat as a test species for reproductive and developmental toxicity tests, of course, are that it is inexpensive when compared to bigger mammals and, also, that it produces a satisfactory number of offspring. The rat is very useful in teratology studies because of its short reproductive cycle, large litter size and relatively few spontaneous congenital anomalies. A disadvantage is that the rat and small rodents do not provide enough quantities of test material during sampling and must frequently be euthanized. The rabbit has certain advantages as a non-rodent and second model in reproductive and developmental toxicity studies (Foote and Carney, 2000). It has been well characterized, can provide enough quantities of test material during sampling, semen can be obtained easily and repeatedly and its visceral yolk sac and extra-embryonic membranes resemble the equivalent histological elements in humans more closely than do other rodents. On the other hand, rabbits are more expensive and space consuming and require larger amounts of chemical test compounds. The rabbit is not considered to be suitable for testing of antibiotics and other residues because these substances can often cause diarrhea and general weakening, which in turn can lead to abortion or fetal resorption (Barlow *et al.*, 2002).

The dog has been commonly used as the non-rodent species for reproductive toxicity testing. The dogs used should be of any defined breed but it is common practice to use the beagle. The latter has many advantages, e.g. medium size and length of hair coat, shows adaptability to living in group housing and it is most easily handled. It also has some disadvantages, e.g. the number of litters is not as high as in rodents, it is costly, it needs exercise and has special housing requirements, it varies in body weight and size, it has a natural tendency to vomit and requires larger amounts of test material than rodents and, in addition, its use is ethically questionable. A strong case for favoring the dog as a non-rodent test species is the extensive knowledge on the physiology of its reproductive system (FDA, 1982; OECD, 1998a). Other species, e.g. the swine (Rocca and Wehner, 2009) and mini-pigs (Jorgensen, 1998; Svendsen, 2006), may also be used, especially in cases where traditional animal models are not relevant. The cynomolgus monkey is the non-human primate species used most commonly for reproductive studies (Meyer *et al.*, 2006). Although menstrual cycles and gestation periods are long and affect the length of the studies, the cynomolgus monkeys breed all year round, in contrast to rhesus macaques. However, their pregnancy rate is lower than in rodents and they have only one offspring. Ethical issues demand the use of a minimum number of animals. All reproductive toxicity testing in animals must be performed adhering to the principles of Good Laboratory Practice (FDA, 1987; OECD, 1998d).

NON-MAMMALIAN ANIMAL MODELS

The avian reproduction test (OECD, 1984c) determines mortality in adults, egg production, egg-shell thickness, viability, hatchability of eggs and the effects on young birds. In this test, the birds are fed a diet containing the test substance for 20 weeks at least. Eggs are collected over a 10-week period, incubated and hatched, and the young maintained for observation for 14 days.

The fish short-term reproduction assay (OECD, 2009c) is an *in vivo* screening assay where sexually mature male and spawning female fish are held together and exposed to a chemical during a limited part of their lifecycle (21 days). The recommended species is the fathead minnow *Pimephales promelas*. Two endpoints are measured in males and females as indicators of endocrine activity of a test chemical: vitellogenin and secondary sexual characteristics. Gonads of both sexes are also preserved and histopathology may be evaluated to assess the reproductive fitness of the test animals and to add to the weight of evidence of other endpoints.

The 21-day fish assay (OECD, 2009d) is a short-term screening test for certain endocrine active substances on estrogenic and androgenic activity, and aromatase inhibition.

During this test sexually mature male and spawning female fish are kept together and exposed to a chemical during a 21-day part of their lifecycle. After a 21-day exposure period, vitellogenin is measured in fathead minnow, Japanese medaka and zebrafish. Secondary sex characteristics are measured in the fathead minnow and Japanese medaka only. In particular, the zebrafish (*Danio rerio*) test model is being used more often due to the increasing amount of molecular and genetic information available for this species (Briggs, 2002).

The amphibian metamorphosis assay (OECD, 2009e) recommends the use of the species *Xenopus laevis*. After a 21-day exposure period, the endpoints assessed are the developmental stage, snout-to-vent length and hind limb. The collembolan reproduction test in soil (OECD, 2009f) tests chemicals on effects on the reproduction of collembolans in soil. The parthenogenetic *Folsomia candida* and *Folsomia fimetaria* are the recommended species for use. The duration of a reproduction test is 4 weeks for *F. candida* and 3 weeks for *F. fimetaria*.

The *Daphnia magna* reproduction test (OECD, 1998c) is designed to examine the effects of chemicals on the reproductive output of *Daphnia magna* Straus. The test duration is 21 days. Endpoints include the total number of living offspring produced per parent alive, sex ratio, parent mortality, oxygen concentration, temperature, hardness and pH values and the determination of the concentrations of the test substance.

On a different scale the reproductive status of invertebrates in both freshwater and coastal ecosystems may be assessed for the effects of potential endocrine disruptors in order to develop robust invertebrate chronic test methodologies (Hutchinson, 2007). It is argued that freshwater and saltwater invertebrate species can be used for assessing developmental or reproductive endpoints in current or potential future standard protocols (Mottet and Landolt, 1987; Ballatori and Villalobos, 2002).

ENDPOINTS OF REPRODUCTIVE TOXICITY

The United Nations (UN) Globally Harmonized System of Classification and Labelling of Chemicals (GHS) (UNECE, 2003) has formed a classification system for reproductive toxicity where chemical substances can be included into one of two categories. Evidence from animal tests only place a substance into category 1B.

The two categories (and subcategories) are:

Category 1: Known or presumed human reproductive toxicant.

Category 1A: Known to have produced an adverse effect on reproductive ability or capacity or on development in human. (Evidence mostly from humans.)

Category 1B: Presumed to produce an adverse effect on reproductive ability or capacity or on development in humans. (Evidence mostly from experimental animals.)

Category 2: Suspected human reproductive or developmental toxicant. (Evidence from humans and/or experimental animals, with other information/weight-of-evidence of reproductive or developmental toxicity not sufficient to place the substance in category 1.) Some effects, e.g. reproductive capacity and effects on lactation, are considered a separate hazard category.

The endpoints of reproductive toxicity in test animals tend currently to be categorized according to sex:

Male endpoints for reproductive studies

Male-specific endpoints of reproductive toxicity include: determination of body weight and organ weights (testes, epididymides, seminal vesicles, prostate and pituitary); alterations found by visual examination and histopathology in the male reproductive organs or in related endocrine systems; mating behavior including libido, mounting, erection, intromission and ejaculation; histopathology of the testes, epididymides, seminal vesicles, prostate and pituitary; sperm quality including sperm count, viability, morphology and motility (Morrissey *et al.*, 1988a; Linder *et al.*, 1992); and production of seminal fluid and sperm transport, maturation and storage in the epididymis as well as production and secretion of hormones (levels of LH, FSH, testosterone, estrogen, prolactin, etc.) in the pituitary–hypothalamus–gonadal axis. The effects on normal development of the male can also be investigated, such as testis descent, ano-genital distance and structure of external genitalia.

Testing on males only has been shown in humans (Davis *et al.*, 1992; Colie, 1993; Savitz *et al.*, 1994) to cause adverse effects in offspring, including pre- and postimplantation loss, structural malformations, growth and behavioral deficits. Interestingly, the human male is of low fertility and thus may be at greater risk from reproductive toxicants than are males of the laboratory animal model species used (Working, 1988). Some chemicals reported to cause paternally mediated effects exhibit genotoxic activity and may cause transmissible genetic alterations. Also, other mechanisms of induction of male-mediated effects are also possible, including non-genetic (e.g., presence of drug in seminal fluid) or epigenetic (e.g., effect on imprinted gene expression from the paternal alleles, resulting in loss of gene function). There is a need for clarification of the mechanisms on paternal exposure which are associated with adverse effects on offspring. In general, it is considered that if a test substance is shown to cause a paternally mediated adverse effect on offspring in the test species, that effect should be considered an adverse reproductive effect.

Female endpoints for reproductive studies

Female-specific endpoints of reproductive toxicity include: determination of organ weights (ovary, uterus, vagina, pituitary); alterations found by visual examination and histopathology in the female reproductive organs (ovary, uterus, vagina, pituitary, oviduct, mammary gland); and endpoints reflecting effects on the estrous cycle normality, such as vaginal smear cytology, estrous cycle onset, length and other characteristics, ovarian follicular development and ovulation (Morrissey *et al.*, 1988b). Ovarian follicle biology and toxicology have been reviewed by Crisp (1992). Other possible endpoints include: signs of alterations in sexual behavior, such as vaginal plugs, and in mating behavior, such as lordosis, proceptivity and receptivity (Uphouse and Williams, 1989), and production and secretion of hormones in the pituitary–hypothalamus–gonadal axis (Hong *et al.*, 1985; Hughes, 1988), fertility, gestation length, number of corpora lutea, pre- and postimplantation losses, parturition, lactation, nursing behavior, uterine implantation and decidualization, placentation and senescence (again, vaginal smear cytology and ovarian histology). The effects on normal development of the female can also be investigated, such as vaginal opening, onset of estrous behavior and the normality in the structure of external genitalia.

Suspect reproductive toxins can be tested on laboratory rodents using the qualitative and quantitative parameters for estrous cyclicity (May and Finch, 1988). The reproductive lifecycle of the female is complex and comprises several phases (embryo–fetal, pre-pubertal, cycling adult, pregnant, lactating and reproductively senescent). Quantitative changes in estrous cycles, such as cycle length distribution, indicate more subtle effects in reproductive function and require refined data analysis. The outcome of a pregnancy depends on the function of tolerance mechanisms being uninterrupted, and inhibition of such mechanisms can lead to rejection. The balance of influence that can distinguish between tolerance and rejection is, most importantly, dependent on environmental factors, and is also under the control of maternal and fetal factors (Thellin and Heinen, 2003).

Prenatal or postnatal treatment of females with estrogens or estrogenic pesticides has been implicated in impaired ovulation and sterility (Gorski, 1979). Reproduction is a continuous cycle, but, for the purposes of toxicity testing, it is broadly divided into the above-mentioned phases. Studies should be conducted to show adverse effects occurring during any of these phases. The adult female reproductive system fluctuates with time. In non-pregnant rats, the ovarian and uterine structures (and other reproductive organs) change throughout the estrous cycle. Other changes, not cyclic, normally occur during pregnancy and lactation, and return to cyclic form after the end of lactation. These physiological fluctuations can influence the evaluation of female reproductive endpoints. Knowing the point in the estrous cycle may help in the unbiased evaluation of some endpoints, such as uterine weight and histopathology of the ovary, uterus and vagina (Risk Assessment Forum – EPA, 1996).

Comprehensive multi-generation studies are performed in order to provide information about the effects of exogenous substances on this highly complex reproductive cycle (OECD 415, 1983; OECD 416, 2001b). These studies tend to primarily detect adverse effects on the female fertility, and on offspring survival and development. Adverse alterations in the non-pregnant female reproductive system have been shown at treatment levels below those that resulted in reduced fertility or resulted in adverse effects on the litter (Levier and Jankowiak, 1972; Sonawane and Yaffe, 1983; Cummings and Gray, 1987).

"Couple-mediated" endpoints for reproductive studies

Couple-mediated endpoints are defined reproductive endpoints where both sexes may contribute. Couple-mediated endpoints from reproductive toxicity multi-generation tests include: mating rate, time to mating, time to pregnancy, pregnancy and delivery rate, gestation length, litter size, fetal death rate, offspring gender, birth and postnatal weight, external malformations, offspring survival and reproduction.

Other reproductive points include: ovulation and fertilization rate, pre- and postimplantation loss as well as implantation number, internal malformations and postnatal functional and structural development.

TESTS AND TEST GUIDELINES

There is a plethora of test guidelines that are currently used for the identification of reproductive toxicants. They have been used and evaluated with varying results (Piersma *et al.*, 1995). These guidelines have been designed for the three major key phases of the reproductive cycle and they are:

1. For maturation, including postnatal development, lactation and gamete production and release: OECD TG 415, OECD TG 416, OECD TG 421, OECD TG 422, OECD TG 426, OECD TG 478 and OECD TG 483.
2. For mating, including fertilization and implantation of the embryo: OECD TG 415, OECD TG 416, OECD TG 421 and OECD TG 422.
3. For gestation, including late and early prenatal development: OECD TG 414, OECD TG 415, OECD TG 416, OECD TG 421, OECD TG 422 and OECD TG 426.

Other guidelines

For endpoints concerning effects on the endocrine system the repeated dose 28-day oral toxicity study in rodents (OECD, 2008b).

For endpoints concerning effects on fertility the repeated dose 28-day toxicity study (OECD, 2008b, 1981a,b) and the repeated dose 90-day toxicity study (OECD, 1998b,a, 1981c).

For endpoints concerning genotoxicity and mutagenicity, the mammalian erythrocyte micronucleus test (OECD, 1997a), the mammalian bone marrow chromosomal aberration test (OECD, 1997b), the sex-linked recessive lethal test in *Drosophila melanogaster* (OECD, 1984b), the rodent dominant lethal test (OECD, 1984a), the mammalian spermatogonial chromosome aberration test (OECD, 1997c), the mouse spot test (OECD, 1986a), the mouse heritable translocation assay (OECD, 1986b) and the unscheduled DNA synthesis (UDS) test with mammalian liver cells (OECD, 1997d).

TYPES OF STUDIES

Reproductive toxicity may result from single or repeated doses of a chemical. Since both single and repeated exposures are possible for human exposure, the reproductive toxicity studies must examine both situations possible.

Single-generation reproduction study

The one-generation reproduction toxicity testing was primarily designed to provide general information concerning the effects of a test substance on male and female reproductive performance. In this study the male is exposed to the substance under evaluation for a full cycle of spermatogenesis and epididymal transit time. The female is exposed to the substance for at least two estrous cycles. It is, therefore, evident that the one-generation reproduction toxicity testing does not test for potential effects on all phases of the reproductive cycle. Endpoints include gonadal function, estrous cycle, mating behavior, conception, parturition, lactation and weaning. In addition, it may also provide preliminary information about developmental toxic effects of the test substance, and the endpoints include neonatal morbidity, mortality, behavior and teratogenesis. It may also provide information on the subchronic effects of peri-pubertal and adult animals (OECD, 1983). However, it does not provide information on the F_1 generation, such as structural anomalies or breeding capacity.

All in all, the single-generation reproduction toxicity study has been designed to provide information on basic male and female reproductive functions.

In a single-generation reproduction study, males and females can be exposed during the same or separate trials to determine whether one or both sexes are affected. A well-conducted, single-generation reproductive toxicity study should provide an estimate of a no-observed-adverse-effect level (NOAEL) and an evaluation of adverse effects on reproduction, parturition, lactation and postnatal growth. What has been spotted as a limitation of a single-generation toxicity study is that it provides no information on the breeding capacity of offspring. At an EPA workshop Francis and Kimmel (1988) assessed the value of the single-generation reproductive toxicity study and came to the conclusion that it was "insufficient to identify all potential reproductive toxicants, because it would exclude detection of effects caused by prenatal and postnatal exposures (including the pre-pubertal period) as well as effects on germ cells that could be transmitted to and expressed in the next generation" (EPA, 1996).

Other short-term reproductive toxicity studies have been designed using the National Toxicology Program's (NTP) short-term reproductive and developmental toxicity screen protocol (Harris *et al.*, 1992). They are designed to distinguish between potent and less effective compounds, thus, providing preliminary data on the reproductive and developmental toxicity of chemicals on which there are little or no data available. The results can be used to screen chemicals for subsequent studies, for finding of doses that will be applied to other test strategies and to assess the relative toxicities of structurally related chemicals.

The uterotrophic bioassay in rodents (OECD, 2007b) and the Hershberger bioassay in rats (OECD, 2009b) are short-term *in vivo* screening tests that originated in the 1930s. The uterotrophic bioassay is based on the increase in uterine weight or uterotrophic response of the rodent for the *in vivo* screening of estrogen agonists and antagonists. The Hershberger bioassay uses the accessory tissues of the male reproductive tract. The castrated peripubertal male is the subject of the Hershberger bioassay using as endpoint the changes in the weight of five androgen-dependent tissues.

Extended one-generation reproductive toxicity study

The ILSI Agricultural Chemical Safety Assessment Project has proposed an extended one-generation study (Cooper *et al.*, 2006) in an effort to highlight toxicological endpoints and exposure durations that are relevant for risk assessment. The approach includes a rat reproduction and developmental study with an increased number of endpoints and a rabbit developmental study. This flexible study addresses the main limitation of OECD TG 415 by incorporating additional postnatal evaluations, e.g. functional observations, and by using an extended (to PND day 70) F_1 generation dosing period to address developmental neurotoxicity. The proposed extended one-generation reproductive toxicity study is designed to provide an evaluation of the pre- and postnatal effects of chemicals on development as well as a thorough evaluation of systemic toxicity in pregnant and lactating females and young and adult offspring. The key aim is the examination in detail of certain developmental endpoints, such as offspring viability, developmental status at birth, neonatal health and physical and functional development until adulthood. The assessment of these endpoints will help to identify specific target organs in the offspring. It will also provide information on the effects of a test substance on the integrity and performance of the adult male and female reproductive systems. The endpoints considered in the draft proposal for the extended one-generation reproductive toxicity study (OECD, 2008a, 2009a) can be the gonadal function, estrous cycle, epididymal sperm maturation, mating behavior, conception, pregnancy, parturition and lactation. Furthermore, the information obtained from the developmental neurotoxicity and developmental immunotoxicity assessments will characterize potential effects in those systems. The data derived from these tests are expected to allow the determination of no-observed adverse-effect levels (NOAELs) and of lowest-observed-adverse-effect levels (LOAELs), in order to identify effects detected in previous repeat-dose studies and to serve as a guide for further testing (OECD, 2009a). Spielmann and Vogel proposed to reduce reproductive toxicity testing under REACH, by limiting fertility testing to an extended one-generation study (Spielmann and Vogel, 2006). Finally, endpoints such as reproductive organ histopathology and sperm parameters (andrology) are considered more sensitive than fertility, suggesting that second breeding can be avoided (OECD, 2008a).

Multi-generation reproduction study

A 1987 US EPA workshop emphasized the value of the multi-generation reproduction study in the detection of potential adverse effects on the offspring and on reproductive functions, e.g. transmissible germ cell (Francis and Kimmel, 1988).

Multi-generation reproduction studies assess the potential of an agent to induce adverse effects on the male and female reproductive system as well as in the embryo and in the neonate (Lamb, 1988, 1989). There are some published guidelines on multi-generation reproductive assays by different organizations (EPA, 1998a,b; FDA, 2000; OECD, 2001b). The multi-generation reproduction study treats male and female test animals for a period of 10 weeks, while exposure continues for all generations in the study through lactation or treatment.

The OECD two-generation reproduction toxicity study and the proposal for an updated two-generation reproduction toxicity study (OECD, 2001b) aim to provide general information about the effects of a test substance on the male and female reproductive systems, including gonadal function, the estrous cycle, mating behavior, conception, gestation, parturition, lactation and weaning, and the growth and development of the offspring. The two-generation reproduction toxicity study may also provide information on the effects of the test substances on neonatal morbidity and mortality, can supply preliminary data on prenatal and postnatal developmental toxicity and can be used as a guide for further tests. Beyond examining the F_1 generation, the two-generation reproduction toxicity study aims to assess the integrity and performance of the male and female reproductive systems as well as the growth and development of the F_2 generation.

Multi-generation reproduction studies include reproduction endpoints such as libido, deviation from normal estrous cyclicity, effects on germ cells, gametogenesis, fertilization, implantation, embryonic, fetal and neonatal growth, development, parturition, lactation, post-weaning growth and maturity. Other endpoints may include development of the reproductive system as well as organ weights of the reproductive organs, brain, spleen and thymus. No sperm endpoints have given consistently highly predictive results (Clark *et al.*, 1992).

The multi-generation studies are quite elaborate and provide information on toxicity manifestation throughout the entire reproductive cycle, although they do not evaluate reproductive senescence and gross anomalies of the offspring. Because of its study design, a multi-generation reproduction study can provide data that cannot be derived from many other standard testing strategies.

Reproductive Assessment by Continuous Breeding Study (RACB)

The US National Toxicology Program (NTP) has developed a reproductive toxicity study protocol for evaluating toxicity through a reproductive assessment by a continuous breeding (RACB) study design (Lamb, 1989; Morrissey *et al.*, 1989; Gulati *et al.*, 1991; Chapin and Sloane, 1997; Chapin *et al.*, 1997, 1998). The protocol was originally developed for mice as a faster and more cost-effective alternative to the conventional regulatory reproductive toxicity studies, but it also has been used successfully with rats (Gulati *et al.*, 1991). In the above protocol, prenatally treated mice are housed as breeding pairs in individual cages and allowed to mate continuously with untreated male mice. The total number of offspring is measured by removing the female when noticeably pregnant and then returning the female to the cage with the male immediately after delivery in order to establish a pattern of repetitive breeding. Exposure to the test substance (usually in feed or drinking water) is continued throughout the study. This type of protocol allows the examination of pups from each generation and emphasizes the delayed effects on fertility and reproductive performance, which can be more severe the longer the exposure of parental animals, or develop small but biologically important decrements in successive litters in the treated animals. As in the standard multi-generation protocol, the endpoints are fertility, pups per litter, pup weight, survival, etc. The RACB does not give information on specific male and female reproductive effects unless cross-breeding of control and treated males and females is done following the 14-week mating trial. It also does not provide information on effects in the second generation unless F_1 pups are raised to breeding age and mated to produce a second generation as in the multi-generation study design. The difference between an RACB study and the multi-generation reproduction study is that time is a factor between litters. The RACB allows more than one litter to be examined per generation and can give an indication of subfertility and infertility. The RACB study shows the effects on fertility and reproduction throughout breeding generations which otherwise would not be apparent.

Dominant lethal study

The dominant lethal study protocol is designed to mate treated and control males with untreated females. Subsequently, females are examined in order to determine the numbers of corpora lutea as well as the number of implantations in the uterus. All implants are then characterized as normal fetuses, dead fetuses or early or late resorptions and fetal weights are recorded. Dominant lethality is then determined by measuring both pre- and postimplantation embryonic losses (OECD, 1984a,b,c; EPA, 1996, 1998b). Serial mating makes it possible to assess the sensitive stages of spermatogenesis and susceptible cell types. The dominant lethal study assesses primarily the effects of chemicals suspected to be reproductive toxicants on fertility by continuous breeding and repeated dose toxicity testing by subjecting the gonads to pathological examination. The male dominant lethal test identifies mutagenic effects in the male spermatogenic process that are lethal to the offspring; it is considered a means to identify chromosome breakage and possibly other mutagenic effects (Green *et al.*, 1985; Jha and Bharti, 2002). The dominant lethal test can detect changes in non-genetic reproductive functions, such as libido and germ cell cytotoxicity and can also be used in the female to detect analogous effects on oogenesis (Generoso and Piegorsch, 1993; Christian, 1996). After all, dominant lethal mutations were shown in female guinea pigs and hamsters quite early in reproductive toxicity studies (Caine and Lyon, 1979). Dominant lethal mutations, congenital malformations and heritable translocations in mice are associated to heritable damage (Pacchierotti *et al.*, 1998; Anderson, 2001) as well as to male-mediated developmental toxicity (Anderson, 2005). The various stages of spermatogenesis differ in sensitivity to toxic effects and, in addition, each toxic substance can affect different sperm cell populations (Parvinen, 1982; Toppari and Parvinen, 1985).

The dominant lethal study *in vivo* test is not considered relevant for the purposes of the cosmetic industry mainly because there is a barrier that is formed by the tight junctions between the Sertoli cells; mature germ cells can be protected from chemical effects, thus making redundant the need for additional tests that are designed to detect germ cell mutagenicity, such as the dominant lethal test or the mammalian spermatogonial aberration test (Bremer *et al.*, 2005). Other *in vivo* tests that should be removed from the recommended test list of the cosmetic industry, because they are not relevant (Maurici *et al.*, 2005), are the rodent dominant lethal test (OECD, 1984a), the mouse heritable translocation assay (OECD, 1986b), the specific locus test (OECD, 1986a), the mouse spot test, the mammalian spermatogonial chromosome aberration test (OECD, 1997c) and the sex-linked recessive lethal test in *Drosophila melanogaster* (OECD, 1984b).

The mammalian spermatogonial chromosome aberration test (OECD, 1997c) aims to identify substances that cause structural aberrations in mammalian spermatogonial cells. Animals are exposed to the test substance by the appropriate route of exposure. Prior to sacrifice, at certain times after treatment, animals are treated with a metaphase-arresting agent. Chromosome preparations are then made from germ cells and stained, while metaphase cells are analyzed for chromosome aberrations.

The mammalian chromosome aberration test (OECD, 1997e) has been suggested as an alternative *in vitro* test (Lilienblum *et al.*, 2008). Other examples of *in vivo* heritable germ cell mutagenicity tests are the mouse heritable translocation assay (OECD, 1986b) and the mouse-specific locus test.

Total reproductive capacity

A procedure that was first used to measure the long-term reproductive performance of female mice exposed to ionizing radiations, because of the high sensitivity of immature oocytes of irradiated female mice (Russell *et al.*, 1959), was also adopted in order to study the effects of chemicals (Generoso *et al.*, 1971; Generoso and Cosgrove, 1973). In female mice and other female mammalian species, a finite number of germ cells are formed before birth. Female fetuses, therefore, are particularly susceptible to chemicals that can affect these germ cells, since no new germ cells develop after birth. In the total reproductive capacity study female animals are exposed to a test substance for a short period *in utero* (McLachlan *et al.*, 1981) or postnatally (Generoso *et al.*, 1971) and subsequently mate with a single male in a continuous breeding study design. The endpoints include the numbers of litters and offspring. The total reproductive capacity assessment procedure for female mice is simple and requires few animals when compared to other studies. The aim of the total reproductive capacity test is to evaluate female reproductive capacity specifically and the test does not assess the general reproductive functions, although it can be readily included in other test strategies, which include other tests, such as those for carcinogenicity and teratogenicity (Witt and Bishop, 1996). In addition, it is possible to screen chemicals for a wide range of toxicity effects (Bishop *et al.*, 1997).

Finally, both the dominant lethal and total reproductive capacity studies have not shown any effects in the case of some chemicals, such as the case of dihydroergotoxine mesylate (Matter *et al.*, 1978) and vinyl chloride, although this compound has been shown to be a mutagen and carcinogen in many other test systems (Thornton *et al.*, 2002).

THE PATH TO ALTERNATIVE TESTS AND CONCLUSIONS

In vitro models for the detection of reproductive and developmental toxicants have been developing over the last few decades. However, the establishment of the European Centre for Validation of Alternative Methods (ECVAM) in the early 1990s, in order to ensure that all the aspects of the 3 "R"s (replacement, reduction and refinement) (Russell and Burch, 1959) are put more vigorously to use has changed the picture. There are now three tests validated by the ECVAM Scientific Advisory Committee (ESAC) (Balls and Hellsten, 2002; Worth and Balls, 2002; Spielmann *et al.*, 2006): the micromass embryotoxicity assay (MM), the whole (rat postimplantation) embryo culture (WEC) embryotoxicity assay, and the embryonic stem cell test (EST). Moreover, a workshop by the Interagency Coordinating Committee on the Validation of Alternative Methods (ICCVAM) and the NTP Interagency Center for the Evaluation of Alternative Toxicological Methods (NICEATM) reviewed the Frog Embryo Teratogenesis Assay: Xenopus (FETAX) as an alternative test for assessing developmental toxicants and although this test did not receive a validation, it is still considered worthy of further attention (Brown *et al.*, 1995; Fort *et al.*, 1998, 2004).

The micromass assay (MM) has been developed after the technique was devised to study the development and differentiation of cultured chick embryo limb cells (Umansky, 1966). It was later designed to use central nervous system (CNS) cell culture (Flint, 1983) and limb bud cells (Flint and Orton, 1984). The limb micromass test system has also been recently adapted to using rabbits (Hansen *et al.*, 2001).

In the micromass assay, the undifferentiated mesenchyme cells of limb buds will form foci of differentiating chondrocytes in micromass culture. The limb bud micromass culture system uses rat limb buds that are then harvested on gestation day 14. Under culture conditions, mesenchymal cells in the limb bud will differentiate into chondrocytes. The chondrocytes are then identified by light microscopy. The criterion is that if a substance decreases chondrocytes without an effect on overall cell number and viability, it may be considered to have selective effects on embryonic development. The micromass test is an experimentally validated test which is more useful for identifying strongly embryotoxic chemicals and needs some further improvement in the future (Spielmann *et al.*, 2004).

The whole embryo culture assay (WEC) assesses developmental toxicity by using embryo cultures derived from mice, rats or rabbits. Embryos are dissected free from maternal tissue and cultured in medium for 24–48 hours. The endpoints assessed after the incubation period are embryonic growth, dysmorphogenic effects, differentiation, yolk sac circulation and vascularization, and effects on hematopoiesis. Although rat and mouse whole embryo culture is the most common (New, 1978; Brown and Fabro, 1981; Sadler *et al.*, 1982), rabbit whole embryo culture has been developed and can also be used (Naya *et al.*, 1991; Ninomiya *et al.*, 1993).

The embryonic stem cell test (EST) is an *in vitro* assay designed to provide mechanistic data. It focuses on target-aimed tests and involves the differentiation of murine embryonic stem cells into neurons. The embryonic stem cell test which is performed according to an updated version of INVITTOX Protocol 113 (Bremer *et al.*, 2005) is comprised of a cytotoxicity test using the mouse embryonic stem (ES) cell line, D3, cells of the differentiated mouse fibroblast cell line, 3T3, and a differentiation assay using D3 cells. The EST represents specific cellular differentiation pathways. Endpoints which characterize the embryotoxic potential of chemicals are: (1) inhibition of the differentiation of ES cells into cardiomyocytes (ID50); (2) decrease in the viability of 3T3 cells (IC503T3 MTT cytotoxicity test); and (3) decrease in the viability of ES cells (IC50D3 MTT test). As embryonic stem cells possess the capacity to differentiate *in vitro* into a variety of cell lineages, additional tissue-specific endpoints can be used (zur Nieden *et al.*, 2004; Seiler *et al.*, 2006, Lilienblum *et al.*, 2008). Information obtained suggests that *in vitro* embryonic stem cell differentiation may resemble closely the processes that take place during *in vivo* embryogenesis, and, therefore, may be an appropriate model for the embryo with respect to developmental toxicity testing. A clear advantage, from an ethical perspective, is that unlike other *in vitro* protocols, which require the use of donor animals for test tissue, embryonic stem cell lines are immortal, thus requiring no further animal use. All the validation projects of the prediction models showed that the EST provides a high accuracy (Bremer *et al.*, 2005). Human embryonic stem cells seem to have a place in the embryonic stem cell test strategies (Thomson *et al.*, 1998). Furthermore, there is a continuous effort to design xeno-free human embryonic stem cell cultures which will stop the necessity for animal use (Goodman, 2002).

All these three tests are strategies that aim to replace the OECD TG 414 (OECD, 2001a). The MM test examines the differentiation of limb bud cells into cartilage-producing chondrocytes, the WEC assay is a developmental system with a very narrow period of embryo–fetal development and the EST represents cardiomyocyte and other specific cellular differentiation pathways (Spielmann *et al.*, 2006). In order to assess embryotoxic potential, the EST, the WEC and the MM tests are immediate tests. The EST is the only one of the three which could have a relatively high throughput, without using large numbers of pregnant animals (Worth and Balls, 2002) and although the micromass and whole embryo cultures require donor animals, the numbers used are dramatically reduced when compared to comparable *in vivo* studies. The predictive performance of these validated assays for the compound classes tested has been characterized as satisfactory and they are considered better suited for distinguishing between strong and non-/weak embryotoxicants (Genschow *et al.*, 2004).

The *in vitro* chromosome aberration test (CAT) (OECD, 1997e) and the *in vitro* micronucleus test (MNT) were compared in many previous studies and showed a high correlation (Shelby and Witt, 1995; Ogura *et al.*, 1996; Miller *et al.*, 1997, 1998). After recommendations by an expert working group on genotoxicity and mutagenicity (Maurici *et al.*, 2005), a retrospective validation of the above two tests, initiated under the coordination of ECVAM, concluded that the *in vitro* MNT is reliable and relevant and can therefore be used as an alternative method to the *in vitro* CAT (Corvi *et al.*, 2008).

ECVAM, in an effort to reduce the high impact of reproductive toxicity studies on the number of animals used and to stimulate further development and optimization of *in vitro* models for toxicological safety testing, went a step further than the three validated tests, and started an integrated project "ReProTect" (Bremer *et al.*, 2005; Hareng *et al.*, 2005) in 2004 that was originally designed to have a time span of five years; it encompasses several research areas, namely male and female fertility, implantation and prenatal development. In this strategy new technologies such as sensor technologies, *in silico* approaches – (Q)SARs (Netzeva *et al.*, 2005), grouping or read-across methods (toxicological properties of substances are based on similarities to other well-studied structurally related substances) (Fabjan *et al.*, 2006; Scialli, 2008), and pattern-based methods (e.g., toxicogenomics, proteomics and metabonomics) – will be integrated with multiple *in vitro* models. This integration will help assess the entire mammalian reproductive cycle including further developmental endpoints. In addition, knowledge generated throughout this process will be used to validate further new tests in the future.

Traditional animal reproductive and developmental toxicity tests will evaluate the endpoints of an exposure to a substance but will not illustrate how this result occurred. These endpoints when evaluated, of course, correspond to relevant biological processes in humans. Animal testing cannot predict human reproductive hazard unless the physiological differences in reproductive processes between man and the common test species are demonstrated at the mechanistic level. Here is where the *in vitro* models are very important, because they are most suitable for elucidating potential mechanisms. Indeed, compared to the *in vitro* tests assays, the reproductive and developmental toxicity animal tests are ill-suited for identifying relevant mechanisms of action. On the other hand, the *in vitro* assays are more appropriate for characterizing the mechanism of action of a tested substance as well as for investigating the basic biology of the reproductive cycle. Modeling the reproductive cycle to the extent that non-animal assays can predict human reproductive risk is the most challenging future task of alternative reproductive and developmental toxicity testing. It is also becoming clearer that no single reproductive endpoint in any laboratory animal model can serve as a totally accurate indicator of reproductive risk in humans. In contrast, the integrated projects seem to carry more hope for the future. This shift to a new paradigm needs to be implemented carefully and supported by robust validation data, while trying to minimize variance, bias and the potential for false-positive and false-negative results (Gibb, 2008; Hoffman *et al.*, 2008; Holsapple *et al.*, 2009). After all, tests should aim at establishing reproductive and/or developmental endpoints and exposure durations that are relevant for risk assessment.

REFERENCES

Anderson D (2001) Genetic and reproductive toxicity of butadiene and isoprene. *Chem-Biol Interact* **135–6:** 65–80.

Anderson D (2005) Male-mediated developmental toxicity. *Toxicol Appl Pharm* **207:** 506–13.

Ballatori N, Villalobos AR (2002) Defining the molecular and cellular basis of toxicity using comparative models. *Toxicol Appl Pharm* **183:** 207–20.

Balls M, Hellsten E (2002) Statement of the scientific validity of the embryonic stem cell test (EST) – an in vitro test for embryotoxicity. Statement of the scientific validity of the micromass test – an in vitro test for embryotoxicity. Statement of the scientific validity of the postimplantation rat whole embryo culture assay – an in vitro test for embryotoxicity. In ECVAM News and Views. *ATLA* **30:** 265–73.

Barlow SM, Greig JB, Bridges JW, Carere A, Carpy AJM, Galli CL, Kleiner J, Knudsen I, Koeter HBWM, Levey LS, Madsen C, Mayer S, Narbonne J-F, Pfannkuch F, Prodanchuk MG, Smith MR, Steinberg P (2002) Hazard identification by methods of animal based toxicology. *Food Chem Toxicol* **40:** 145–91.

Bishop JB, Morris RW, Seely JC, Hughes LA, Cain KT, Generoso WM (1997) Alteration in the reproductive patterns of female mice exposed to xenobiotics. *Fundam Appl Toxicol* **40:** 191–204.

Bremer S, Balduzzi D, Cortvrindt R, Daston G, Eletti B, Galli A, Huhtaniemi I, Laws S, Lazzari G, Liminga U, Smitz J, Spano M, Themmen A, Tilloy A, Waalkens-Behrends I (2005) The Effects of Chemicals on Mammalian Fertility: The Report and Recommendations of ECVAM Workshop 53 – The First Strategic Workshop of the EU ReProTect Project. *ATLA* **33:** 391–416.

Briggs JP (2002) The zebrafish: a new model organism for integrative physiology. *Am J Physiol Regul Integr Comp Physiol* **282:** R3–R9.

Brown NA, Fabro S (1981) Quantitation of rat embryonic development in vitro: a morphological scoring system. *Teratology* **24:** 65–78.

Brown NA, Spielmann H, Bechter R, Flint OP, Freeman RJ, Jelinek RJ, Koch E, Nau H, Newall DR, Palmer AK, Renault JY, Repetto MF, Vogel R, Wiger R (1995) Screening chemicals for reproductive toxicity: the current alternatives. The Report and Recommendations of an ECVAM/ETS Workshop (ECVAM Workshop 12). *ATLA* **23:** 868–82.

Caine A, Lyon MF (1979) Reproductive capacity and dominant lethal mutations in female guinea-pigs and djungarian hamsters following x-rays or chemical mutagens. *Mutat Res* **59:** 231–44.

Chapin RE, Sloane RA (1997) Reproductive assessment by continuous breeding: evolving study design and summaries of ninety studies. *Environ Health Perspect* **105 (Suppl. 1):** 199–205.

Chapin RE, Sloane RA, Haseman JK (1997) The relationships among reproductive endpoints in Swiss mice, using the reproductive assessment by Continuous Breeding database. *Fundam Appl Toxicol* **38(2):** 129–42.

Chapin RE, Sloane RA, Haseman JK (1998) Reproductive endpoints in general toxicity studies: are they predictive? *Reprod Toxicol* **12(4):** 489–94.

Christian M (1996) Review of reproductive and developmental toxicity of 1,3-butadiene. *Toxicology* **113:** 137–43.

Clark CR, Ferguson PW, Katchen MA, Craig DK (1992) Two-generation reproduction study of hydrated shale oil vapors. *Fundam Appl Toxicol* **18:** 227–32.

Colie CF (1993) Male mediated teratogenesis. *Reprod Toxicol* **7(1):** 3–9.

Cooper RL, Lamb IV JC, Barlow SM, Bentley K, Brady AM, Doerrer NG, Eisenbrandt DL, Fenner-Crisp PA, Hines RN, Irvine LF, Kimmel CA, Koeter H, Li AA, Makris SL, Sheets LP, Speijers G, Whitby KE (2006) A tiered approach to life stages testing for agricultural chemical safety assessment. *Crit Rev Toxicol* **36:** 69–98.

Corvi R, Albertini S, Hartung T, Hoffmann S, Maurici D, Pfuhler S, van Benthem J, Vanparys P (2008) ECVAM retrospective validation of in vitro micronucleus test (MNT). *Mutagenesis* **23(4):** 271–83.

Crisp TM (1992) Organization of the ovarian follicle and events in its biology: oogenesis, ovulation or atresia. *Mutat Res* **296:** 89–106.

Cummings AM, Gray LE (1987) Methoxychlor affects the decidual cell response of the uterus but not other progestational parameters in female rats. *Toxicol Appl Pharmacol* **90:** 330–6.

Davis DL, Friedler G, Mattison D, Morris R (1992) Male-mediated teratogenesis and other reproductive effects: biologic and epidemiologic findings and a plea for clinical research. *Reprod Toxicol* **6(4):** 289–92.

EPA (US Environmental Protection Agency) (1982) Reproductive and Fertility Effects. Pesticide Assessment Guidelines, Subdivision F. Hazard Evaluation: Human and Domestic Animals. Office of Pesticides and Toxic Substances, Washington DC. EPA-540/9-82-025.

EPA (US Environmental Protection Agency) (1991) Guidelines for Developmental Toxicity Risk Assessment. Risk Assessment Forum, US Environmental Protection Agency, Washington DC. EPA/600/FR-91/001.

EPA (US Environmental Protection Agency) (1996) Guidelines for Reproductive Toxicity Risk Assessment. Risk Assessment Forum, US Environmental Protection Agency, Washington DC. EPA/630/R-96/009.

EPA (US Environmental Protection Agency) (1998a) Health Effects Test Guidelines OPPTS 870.5450 Rodent Dominant Lethal Assay. EPA 712-C-98-227. Office of Prevention, Pesticides and Toxic Substances, US Environmental Protection Agency. [Online] Available: http://www.epa.gov/ocspp/pubs/frs/publications/Test_Guidelines/series870.htm

EPA (US Environmental Protection Agency) (1998b) Health Effects Test Guidelines OPPTS 870.3800 Reproduction and Fertility Effects. EPA 712-C-98-208. Office of Prevention, Pesticides and Toxic Substances, US Environmental Protection Agency. Washington DC. EPA 712-C-98-208.

EU COM, Commission of the European Communities (2003) Report from the Commission to the Council and the European Parliament – Third Report from the Commission to the Council and the European Parliament on the Statistics on the Number of Animals Used for Experimental and other Scientific Purposes in the Member States of the European Union. COM/2003/0019 final, Brussels.

Fabjan E, Hulzebos E, Mennes W, Piersma AH (2006) A category approach for reproductive effects of phthalates. *Crit Rev Toxicol* **36(9):** 695–726.

FDA (US Food and Drug Administration) (1982) Toxicological Principles for the Safety Assessment of Direct Food Additives and Color Additives Used in Food: Guidelines for Long-Term Toxicity Studies in the Dog. Appendix II, 42–52.

FDA (US Food and Drug Administration) (1987) Good Laboratory Practice Regulations for Nonclinical Laboratory Studies, Regulatory Program 21CFR 58. US Food and Drug Administration, Washington DC.

FDA (US Food and Drug Administration) (2000) Toxicological Principles for the Safety Assessment of Food Ingredients, Redbook 2000: IV.C.9.a. Guidelines for reproduction studies. College Park, MD.

Flint OP (1983) A micromass culture method for rat embryonic neural cells. *J Cell Sci* **61:** 247–62.

Flint OP, Orton TC (1984) An in vitro assay for teratogens with cultures of rat embryo midbrain and limb bud cells. *Toxicol Appl Pharmacol* **76:** 383–95.

Foote RH, Carney EW (2002) The rabbit as a model for reproductive and developmental toxicity studies. *Reprod Toxicol* **14:** 477–93.

Fort DJ, Stover EL, Bantle JA, Rayburn JR, Hull MA, Finch RA, Burton DT, Turley SD, Dawson DA, Linder G, Buchwalter D, Kumsher-King M, Gaudet-Hull AM (1998) Phase III interlaboratory study of FETAX, Part 2: Interlaboratory validation of an exogenous metabolic activation system for frog embryo teratogenesis assay – Xenopus (FETAX). *Drug Chem Toxicol* **21(1):** 1–14.

Fort DJ, Rogers RL, Thomas JH, Buzzard BO, Noll AM, Spaulding CD (2004) Comparative sensitivity of Xenopus tropicalis and Xenopus laevis as test species for the FETAX model. *J Appl Toxicol* **24:** 443–57.

Francis EZ, Kimmel GL (1988) Proceedings of the Workshop on One- versus Two-Generation Reproductive Effects Studies. *Int J Toxicol* **7(7):** 911–25.

Generoso WM, Cosgrove GE (1973) Total reproductive capacity in female mice: chemical effects and their analysis. In *Chemical Mutagens: Principles and Methods for their Detection*, Vol. 3 (Hollaender A, ed.). Plenum, New York, pp. 241–58.

Generoso WM, Piegorsch WW (1993) Dominant lethal tests in male and female mice. In *Methods in Toxicology: Male Reproductive Toxicology* (Chapin RE, Heindel J, ed.). Academic Press, San Diego, pp. 124–39.

Generoso WM, Stout SK, Huff SW (1971) Effects of alkylating chemicals on reproductive capacity of adult female mice. *Mutat Res* **13:** 171–84.

Genschow E, Spielmann H, Scholz G, Pohl I, Seiler A, Clemann N, Bremer S, Becker K (2004) Validation of the embryonic stem cell test in the international ECVAM validation study on three in vitro embryotoxicity tests. *ATLA* **32:** 209–44.

Gibb S (2008) Toxicity testing in the 21st century: a vision and a strategy. *Reprod Toxicol* **25:** 136–8.

Goodman S (2002) Race is on to find alternative tests. *Nature* **418(6894):** 116.

Gorski RA (1979) The neuroendocrinology of reproduction: an overview. *Biol Reprod* **20:** 111–27.

Green S, Auletta A, Fabricant R, Kapp M, Sheu C, Springer J, Whitfield B (1985) Current status of bioassays in genetic toxicology: the dominant lethal test. *Mutat Res* **154:** 49–67.

Gulati DK, Hope E, Teague J, Chapin RE (1991) Reproductive toxicity assessment by continuous breeding in Sprague-Dawley rats: a comparison of two study designs. *Fundam Appl Toxicol* **17(2):** 270–9.

Hansen JM, Carney EW, Harris C (2001) Altered differentiation in rat and rabbit limb bud micromass cultures by glutathione modulating agents. *Free Radic Biol Med* **31(12):** 1582–92.

Hareng L, Pellizzer C, Bremer S, Schwarz M, Hartung T (2005) The Integrated Project ReProTect: a novel approach in reproductive toxicity hazard assessment. *Reprod Toxicol* **20:** 441–52.

Harris MW, Chapin RE, Lockhart AC, Jokinen MP (1992) Assessment of a short-term reproductive and developmental toxicity screen. *Fundam Appl Toxicol* **19(2):** 186–96.

Hoffmann S, Edler L, Gardner I, Gribaldo L, Hartung H, Klein C, Liebsch M, Sauerland S, Schechtman L, Stammati A, Nikolaidis E (2008) Points of reference in the validation process: the report and recommendations of ECVAM workshop 66. *ATLA* **36:** 343–52.

Holsapple MP, Afshari CA, Lehman-McKeeman LD (2009) The "vision" for toxicity testing in the 21st century: promises and conundrums. *Toxicol Sci* **107(2):** 307–8.

Höfer T, Gerner I, Gundert-Remy U, Liebsch M, Schulte A, Spielmann H, Vogel R, Wettig K (2004) Animal testing and alternative approaches for the human health risk assessment under the proposed new European chemicals regulation. *Arch Toxicol* **78:** 549–64.

Hong JS, Hudson PM, Yoshikawa K, Ali SF, Manson GA (1985) Effects of chlordecone administration on brain and pituitary peptide systems. *Neurotoxicology* **6(1):** 167–82.

Hughes CL (1988) Effects of phytoestrogens on GnRH-induced luteinizing hormone secretion of ovariectomized rats. *Reprod Toxicol* **1(3):** 179–81.

Hutchinson TH (2007) Small is useful in endocrine disrupter assessment – four key recommendations for aquatic invertebrate research. *Ecotoxicology* **16:** 231–8.

ICH (1993) International Conference on Harmonisation of Technical Requirements for Registration of Pharmaceuticals for Human Use, ICH Harmonised Tripartite Guideline. Detection of toxicity to reproduction for medicinal products, S5A. Endorsed at Step 4 of the ICH process on June 24, 1993 by the ICH Steering Committee.

Jha AM, Bharti MK (2002) Mutagenic profiles of carbazole in the male germ cells of Swiss albino mice. *Mutat Res* **500:** 97–101.

Jørgensen KD (1998) Minipig in reproduction toxicology. *Scand J Lab Anim Sci Suppl 1*: 63–75.

Lamb JC (1988) Fundamentals of male reproductive toxicity testing. In *Physiology and Toxicology of Male Reproduction* (Lamb IV, JC, Foster PMD, eds.). Academic Press, New York, pp. 137–53.

Lamb JC (1989) Design and use of multigeneration breeding studies for identification of reproductive toxicants. In *Toxicology of the Male and Female Reproductive Systems* (Working PK, ed.). Hemisphere Publishing, New York, pp. 131–55.

Levier RR, Jankowiak ME (1972) The hormonal and antifertility activity of 2,6-cis-diphenylhexamethylcyclotetrasiloxane in the female rat. *Biol Reprod* **7:** 260–6.

Lilienblum W, Dekant W, Foth H, Gebel T, Hengstler JG, Kahl R, Kramer PJ, Schweinfurth H, Wollin KM (2008) Alternative methods to safety studies in experimental animals: role in the risk assessment of chemicals under the new European Chemicals Legislation (REACH). *Arch Toxicol* **82:** 211–36.

Linder RE, Strader LF, Slott VL, Suarez JD (1992) Endpoints of spermatoxicity in the rat after duration exposures to fourteen reproductive toxicants. *Reprod Toxicol* **6:** 491–505.

Matter BE, Tsuchimoto T, Deyssenroth H (1978) Failure to detect dominant-lethal mutations and effects on reproductive capacity in mice exposed to dihydroergotoxine mesylate. *Arzneimittel-Forsc* **28(12):** 2286–90.

Maurici D, Aardema M, Corvi R, Kleber M, Krul C, Laurent C, Loprieno N, Pasanen M, Pfuhler S, Phillips B, Sabbioni E, Sanner T, Vanparys P (2005) Genotoxicity and mutagenicity in alternative (non-animal) methods for cosmetics testing: current status and future prospects (Eskes C and Zuang V, eds.). *ATLA* **33 (Suppl. 1):** 117–30.

May PC, Finch CE (1988) Aging and responses to toxins in female reproductive functions. *Reprod Toxicol* **1(3):** 223–8.

McLachlan JA, Newbold RR, Korach KS, Lamb JC, Suzuki Y (1981). Transplacental toxicology: prenatal factors influencing postnatal fertility. In *Developmental Toxicology* (Kimmel CA, Buelke-Sam J, eds.). Raven Press, New York, pp. 213–32.

Meyer JK, Fitzsimmons D, Hastings TF, Chellman GJ (2006) Methods for the prediction of breeding success in male cynomolgus monkeys (Macaca fascicularis) used for reproductive toxicology studies. *J Am Assoc Lab Anim Sci* **45(2):** 31–6.

Miller B, Albertini S, Locher F, Thybaud V, Lorge E (1997) Comparative evaluation of the in vitro micronucleus test and the in vitro chromosome aberrations test: industrial experience. *Mutat Res* **392:** 45–59.

Miller B, Pötter-Locher F, Seelbach A, Stopper H, Utesch D, Madle S (1998) Evaluation of the in vitro micronucleus test as an alternative to the in vitro chromosome aberrations assay: position of the GUM working group on the in vitro micronucleus test. *Mutat Res* **410(1):** 81–116.

Morrissey RE, Lamb JC, Morris RW, Chapin RE, Gulati DK, Heindel JJ (1989) Results and evaluations of 48 continuous breeding reproduction studies conducted in mice. *Fundam Appl Toxicol* **13:** 747–77.

Morrissey RE, Lamb JC, Schwetz BA, Teague JL, Morris RW (1988a) Association of sperm, vaginal cytology, and reproductive organ weight data with results of continuous breeding reproduction studies in Swiss (CD-1) mice. *Fundam Appl Toxicol* **11(2):** 359–71.

Morrissey RE, Schwetz BA, Lamb JC, Ross MD, Teague JL, Morris RW (1988b) Evaluation of rodent sperm, vaginal cytology, and reproductive organ weight data from National Toxicology Program 13-week studies. *Fundam Appl Toxicol* **11(2):** 343–58.

Mottet NK, Landolt ML (1987) Advantages of using aquatic animals for biomedical research on reproductive toxicology. *Environ Health Perspect* **71:** 69–75.

Naya M, Kito Y, Eto K, Deguchi T (1991) Development of rabbit whole embryo culture during organogenesis. *Cong Anom* **31:** 153–6.

Netzeva TI, Worth A, Aldenberg T, Benigni R, Cronin MT, Gramatica P, Jaworska JS, Kahn S, Klopman G, Marchant CA, Myatt G, Nikolova-Jeliazkova N, Patlewicz GY, Perkins R, Roberts D, Schultz T, Stanton DW, van de Sandt JJ, Tong W, Veith G, Yang C (2005) Current status of methods for defining the applicability domain of (quantitative) structure-activity relationships. The report and recommendations of ECVAM Workshop 52. *ATLA* **33(2):** 155–73.

New DAT (1978) Whole-embryo culture and the study of mammalian embryos during organogenesis. *Biol Rev* **53:** 81–122.

Ninomiya H, Kishida K, Ohno Y, Tsurumi K, Ero K (1993) Effects of trypan blue on rat and rabbit embryos cultured in vitro. *Toxic in Vitro* **7:** 707–17.

OECD (Organisation for Economic Cooperation and Development) (1981a) Repeated dose dermal toxicity: 21/28-day study. OECD guidance 410 adopted 12-05-1981.

OECD (Organisation for Economic Cooperation and Development) (1981b) Subchronic inhalation toxicity: 28/14-day study. OECD guidance 411 adopted 12-05-1981.

OECD (Organisation for Economic Cooperation and Development) (1981c) Repeated dose inhalation toxicity: 90-day study. OECD guidance 412 adopted 12-05-1981.

OECD (Organisation for Economic Cooperation and Development) (1983) One-generation reproduction toxicity study. OECD guidance 415 adopted 26-05-1983.

OECD (Organisation for Economic Cooperation and Development) (1984a) Genetic toxicology: rodent dominant lethal test. OECD guidance 478 adopted 4-04-1984.

OECD (Organisation for Economic Cooperation and Development) (1984b) Sex-linked recessive lethal test in Drosophila melanogaster. OECD guidance 477 adopted 4-04-1984.

OECD (Organisation for Economic Cooperation and Development) (1984c) Avian reproduction test. OECD guidance 206 adopted 4-04-1984.

OECD (Organisation for Economic Cooperation and Development) (1986a) Mouse spot test. OECD guidance 484 adopted 23-10-1986.

OECD (Organisation for Economic Cooperation and Development) (1986b) Mouse heritable translocation assay. OECD guidance 485 adopted 23-10-1986.

OECD (Organisation for Economic Cooperation and Development) (1995) Reproduction/Developmental toxicity screening test. OECD guidance 421 adopted 27-07-1995.

OECD (Organisation for Economic Cooperation and Development) (1996) Combined repeated dose toxicity study with the reproduction/developmental toxicity screening test. OECD guidance 422 adopted 22-03-1996.

OECD (Organisation for Economic Cooperation and Development) (1997a) Mammalian erythrocyte micronucleus test. OECD guidance 474 adopted 21-07-1997.

OECD (Organisation for Economic Cooperation and Development) (1997b) Mammalian bone marrow chromosomal aberration test. OECD guidance 475 adopted 21-07-1997.

OECD (Organisation for Economic Cooperation and Development) (1997c) Mammalian spermatogonial chromosome aberration test. OECD guidance 483 adopted 21-07-1997.

OECD (Organisation for Economic Cooperation and Development) (1997d) Unscheduled DNA synthesis (UDS) test with mammalian liver cells. OECD guidance 486 adopted 21-07-1997.

OECD (Organisation for Economic Cooperation and Development) (1997e) In vitro mammalian chromosome aberration test. OECD guidance 473 adopted 21-07-1997.

OECD (Organisation for Economic Cooperation and Development) (1998a) Repeated dose 90-day toxicity study in non-rodents. OECD guidance 409 adopted 21-09-1998.

OECD (Organisation for Economic Cooperation and Development) (1998b) Repeated dose 90-day toxicity study in rodents. OECD guidance 408 adopted 21-09-1998.

OECD (Organisation for Economic Cooperation and Development) (1998c) Daphnia magna reproduction test. OECD guidance 211 adopted 21-09-1998.

OECD (Organisation for Economic Cooperation and Development) (1998d) OECD Principles on good laboratory practice (as revised in 1997). ENV/MC/CHEM(98)17.

OECD (Organisation for Economic Cooperation and Development) (2001a) Prenatal developmental toxicity study. OECD guidance 414 adopted 22-01-2001.

OECD (Organisation for Economic Cooperation and Development) (2001b) Two-generation reproduction toxicity study. OECD guidance 416 adopted 22-01-2001.

OECD (Organisation for Economic Cooperation and Development) (2007a) Developmental neurotoxicity study. OECD guidance 426 adopted 16-10-2007.

OECD (Organisation for Economic Cooperation and Development) (2007b) Uterotrophic bioassay in rodents: a short-term screening test for oestrogenic properties. OECD guidance 440 adopted 16-10-2007.

OECD (Organisation for Economic Cooperation and Development) (2008a) Draft extended one-generation reproductive toxicity test guideline. OECD merged draft new guideline version 4, 18-06-2008.

OECD (Organisation for Economic Cooperation and Development) (2008b) Repeated dose 28-day oral toxicity study in rodents. OECD guidance 407 adopted 3-10-2008.

OECD (Organisation for Economic Cooperation and Development) (2009a) Draft proposal for an extended one-generation reproductive toxicity study. OECD draft new guideline, 28-10-2009.

OECD (Organisation for Economic Cooperation and Development) (2009b) Hershberger bioassay in rats: a short-term in vivo screening test for (anti) androgenic properties. OECD guidance 441 adopted 7-9-2009.

OECD (Organisation for Economic Cooperation and Development) (2009c) Fish short term reproduction assay. OECD guidance 229 adopted 7-9-2009.

OECD (Organisation for Economic Cooperation and Development) (2009d) 21-day fish assay: a short-term screening for oestrogenic and androgenic activity, and aromatase inhibition. OECD guidance 230 adopted 7-9-2009.

OECD (Organisation for Economic Cooperation and Development) (2009e) The amphibian metamorphosis assay. OECD guidance 231 adopted 7-9-2009.

OECD (Organisation for Economic Cooperation and Development) (2009f) Collembolan reproduction test in soil. OECD guidance 232 adopted 7-9-2009.

Ogura H, Takeuchi T, Morimoto K (1996) A comparison of the 8-hydroxydeoxyguanosine, chromosome aberrations and micronucleus techniques for the assessment of the genotoxicity of mercury compounds in human blood lymphocytes. *Mutat Res* **340:** 175–82.

Pacchierotti F, Adler ID, Anderson D, Brinkworth M, Demopoulos NA, Lahdetie J, Osterman-Golkar S, Peltonen K, Russo A, Tates A, Waters R (1998) Genetic effects of 1,3-butadiene and associated risk for heritable damage. *Mutat Res* **397:** 93–115.

Parvinen M (1982) Regulation of the seminiferous epithelium. *Endocr Rev* **3(4):** 404–17.

Piersma AH, Verhoef A, Dortant PM (1995) Evaluation of the OECD 421 reproductive toxicity screening test protocol using 1-(butylcarbamoyl)-2-benzimidazolecarbamate (benomyl). *Teratogen Carcinogen Mutagen* **15:** 93–100.

Risk Assessment Forum, US Environmental Protection Agency (1996) Guidelines for reproductive toxicity risk assessment, October 31, 1996. Fed Regist, 61(212): 56274–322.

Rocca MS, Wehner NG (2009) The guinea pig as an animal model for developmental and reproductive toxicology studies. *Birth Defects Res (Part B)* **86:** 92–7.

Russell WM, Burch RL (1959) *The Principles of Humane Experimental Technique.* Methuen, London.

Russell LB, Stelzner KF, Russell WL (1959) Influence of dose rate on radiation effect on fertility of female mice. *Proc Soc Exp Biol Med* **102:** 471–9.

Sadler TW, Horton WE, Warner CW (1982) Whole embryo culture: a screening technique for teratogens. *Teratog Carcinog Mutagen* **2:** 243–53.

Savitz DA, Sonnenfeld NL, Olshan AF (1994) Review of epidemiologic studies of paternal occupational exposure and spontaneous abortion. *Am J Ind Med* **25(3):** 361–83.

Scialli AR (2008) The challenge of reproductive and developmental toxicology under REACH. *Regul Toxicol Pha* **51:** 244–50.

Seiler A, Buesen R, Hayess K, Schlechter K, Visan A, Genschow E, Slawik B, Spielmann H (2006) Current status of the embryonic stem cell test: the use of recent advances in the weld of stem cell technology and gene expression analysis. *ALTEX* **23 (Suppl.):** 393–9.

Shelby MD, Witt KL (1995) Comparison of results from mouse bone marrow chromosome aberration and micronucleus tests. *Environ Mol Mutagen* **25:** 302–13.

Sonawane BR, Yaffe SJ (1983) Delayed effects of drug exposure during pregnancy: reproductive function. *Biol Res Pregnancy* **4:** 48–55.

Spielmann H, Genschow E, Brown NA, Piersma AH, Verhoef A, Spanjersberg MQ, Huuskonen H, Paillard F, Seiler A (2004) Validation of the rat limb bud micromass test in the international ECVAM validation study on three in vitro embryotoxicity tests. *ATLA* **32(3):** 245–74.

Spielmann H, Vogel R (2006) REACH testing requirements must not be driven by reproductive toxicity testing in animals. *ATLA* **34:** 365–6.

Spielmann H, Seiler A, Bremer S, Hareng L, Hartung T, Ahr H, Faustman E, Haas U, Moffat GJ, Nau H, Vanparys P, Piersma A, Sintes JR, Stuart J (2006) The practical application of three validated in vitro embryotoxicity tests. The report and recommendations of an ECVAM/ZEBET workshop (ECVAM Workshop 57). *ATLA* **34:** 527–38.

Svendsen O (2006) The minipig in toxicology. *Exp Toxicol Pathol* **57:** 335–9.

Thellin O, Heinen E (2003) Pregnancy and the immune system: between tolerance and rejection. *Toxicology* **185:** 179–84.

Thomson JA, Itskovitz-Eldor J, Shapiro SS, Waknitz MA, Swiergiel JJ, Marshall VS, *et al.* (1998) Embryonic stem cell lines derived from human blastocysts. *Science* **282(5391):** 1145–7.

Thornton SR, Schroeder RE, Robison RL, Rodwell DE, Penney DA, Nitschke KD, Sherman WK (2002) Embryo–fetal developmental and reproductive toxicology of vinyl chloride in rats. *Toxicol Sci* **68:** 207–19.

Toppari J, Parvinen M (1985) In vitro differentiation of rat seminiferous tubular segments from defined stages of the epithelial cycle. Morphologic and immunolocalization analysis. *J Androl* **6:** 334–43.

Umansky R (1966) The effect of cell population density on the developmental fate of reaggregating mouse limb bud mesenchyme. *Dev Biol* **13:** 31–56.

United Nations Economic Commission for Europe (UNECE) (2003) Globally Harmonized System of Classification and Labelling of Chemicals (GHS). UN ST/SG/AC.10/30, United Nations Publications sales no. E.03.II.E.25. United Nations, New York/Geneva.

United Nations Economic Commission for Europe (UNECE) (2004) Globally Harmonized System of Classification and Labelling of Chemicals (GHS). Part 3. Health and environmental hazards. Chapter 3.7. Reproductive Toxicity. United Nations, New York/Geneva.

Uphouse L, Williams J (1989) Sexual behavior of intact female rats after treatment with o,p′-DDT or p,p′-DDT. *Reprod Toxicol* **3(1):** 33–41.

Witt KL, Bishop JB (1996) Mutagenicity of anticancer drugs in mammalian germ cells. *Mutat Res* **355(1-2):** 209–34.

Working PK (1988) Male Reproductive toxicology: comparison of the human to animal models. *Environ Health Perspect* **77:** 37–44.

Worth AP, Balls M (eds.) (2002) Alternative (non-animal) methods for chemicals testing current status and future prospects. *ATLA* **30 (Suppl. 1):** 1–125.

Zur Nieden NI, Kempka G, Ahr HJ (2004) Molecular multiple endpoint embryonic stem cell test – a possible approach to test for the teratogenic potential of compounds. *Toxicol Appl Pharmacol* **194:** 257–69.

C H A P T E R

10

OECD guidelines and validated methods for *in vivo* testing of reproductive toxicity

Carmen Estevan Martínez, David Pamies, Miguel Angel Sogorb and Eugenio Vilanova

INTRODUCTION

The OECD Guidelines for Testing of Chemicals are a package of protocols and methods aimed at producing a toxicity test sufficiently well designed to enable it to be carried out in a similar manner in different countries and to produce results that will be fully acceptable to different regulatory bodies. Guidelines in this chapter are described for educational purposes only. Therefore, the official original and updated guidelines must be followed if intended for performing assays for regulatory purposes. The reproductive toxicity guidelines characterize the adverse effects against the reproductive system attributable to the exposure to chemicals for two purposes: (1) hazard characterization and (2) risk characterization. The reproduction/developmental studies, included in the OECD Guidelines, are relevant in the risk characterization of chemicals. The endpoints evaluated in these protocols and the no-observed-adverse-effect levels (NOAELs) obtained are taken into consideration not only for the reproductive toxicity testing but also for the risk assessment of general systemic effects. For example, the NOAEL of systemic maternal toxicity in the teratogenicity study is frequently considered for risk characterization in short-term scenarios.

The results from these methods are recorded for the evaluation of multiple endpoints. Some of them describe the effects on the developmental process. The reproductive toxicity tests are relevant in the classification of substances. In the European Union, the substances classified as CMR (carcinogenic, mutagenic, reprotoxic) have strong restrictions in their use independently of the potential risk. The NOAEL obtained from the teratogenicity study is used in the classification and labeling of the substances. Also, the data of effects in the reproductive organs or systems obtained from studies of subchronic repeated dose are considered in the decisions for classification and labeling.

In general, the severity of effects on endpoints relevant to development or fertility should be evaluated relative to the systemic general toxicity effects. The teratogenicity studies relevant to humans are not interpretable for secondary effects of maternal toxicity just because they are observed at the same dose. However, in the fertility studies, the data are more relevant if there is no effect to parental toxicity (either the male or females in the F_0). If the development or fertility impairment is observed at the same dose causing significant systemic parental effects, it should be clarified that the effects are not secondary to the parental damage. Further mechanistic studies or additional ad hoc studies may be needed for better interpretation.

The criteria for interpreting the relationship between parental toxicity and effects on development or fertility are frequently a matter of discussion among experts in agencies making decisions for regulatory process. Table 10.1 summarizes the methods adopted by the OECD regarding reproductive toxicity. Method OECD 414 studies the effects of the exposure to substances during the gestation process for the evaluation of the effects in development. This test describes the prenatal effects in the implantation and organogenesis in test animals (rats/rabbits) and also the maternal effects produced during pregnancy.

In order to evaluate fertility in parental generation and prenatal and postnatal systemic effects in the first generation, method OECD 415 studies the toxicity to one generation in the rat or mouse. The exposure starts in the parental generation before mating to observe effects in spermatogenesis or the estrous cycle. After mating, only the pregnant female is exposed to the substance during gestation until the end of the nursing period.

A more complete method, OECD 416, not only describes the systemic effects on the first generation but also the fertility and functionality of their reproductive system to produce a second generation. The exposure to parental generation starts before mating so as to detect effects on the fertility and it lasts during mating, gestation and weaning of the F_1 generation. The F_1 offspring is administered the test substance during its growth, adulthood, mating and gestation of the F_2 generation until it is weaned.

Method OECD 421 is a screening test to detect postnatal effects due to prenatal exposure, usually in rats. It is also aimed to be used as a range-finding study for more detailed

Reproductive and Developmental Toxicology, Edited by Ramesh C. Gupta
ISBN: 978-0-12-382032-7

TABLE 10.1 This table shows a summary of the reproductive toxicity protocols validated by the OECD and compares the different endpoints evaluated on each

OECD	Date (adopted)	EPA no.	EU	Species	Number and sex of animals	Dosage	Administration	Endpoints
414	2001	870.3700	B.31	rat/rabbit	20 females per concentration	3 concentration + control	Oral	– litters with implants – litters with live fetuses
415	1983		B.34	rat/mouse	20 females per concentration	3 concentration + control	Oral	– fertility – gestation – viability index – body weight – necropsy
416	2001	870.3800	B.35	rat	20 pregnant females per concentration	3 concentration + control – males during spermatogenesis – females during several estrus cycles	Oral	F_1 – growth – development – reproductive system F_2 – growth – development
421	1995	870.3550		rat	8 pregnant females per concentration	3 concentration + control 2 weeks prior to mating Males total of 28 days Females until day 3 postpartum	Oral	– gross lesions – identified target organs – infertility – clinical abnormalities – affected reproductive and litter performance – body weight changes – effects on mortality
422	1996	870.3650		rat	8 pregnant females per concentration	3 concentration + control 54 days approximately	Oral	– live births and postimplantation loss; – pups with abnormalities, runts; – time of death during the study or whether animals survived to termination; – implantations, corpora lutea, litter size and weights
426	2007	870.6300		rat	20 litters per concentration	3 concentration + control administered daily to mated females from the time of implantation (gestation day 6) throughout lactation (PND 21)	Oral	– body weight and clinical observations – brain weight – neuropathology – sexual maturation – other developmental landmarks (eye opening, incisor eruptions) – behavioral ontogeny – motor activity (including habituation) – motor and sensory function – learning and memory

tests. In this protocol, males are exposed during approximately 4 weeks (2 weeks before mating and 2 weeks postmating). Females are exposed 2 weeks before mating and then during pregnancy until weaning of the pups. The effects observed include fertility of the parental generation and systemic effects on the parental and first generation.

A combined method, using method OECD 421 and repeated dose toxicity studies, described in the protocol OECD 422 for simultaneous evaluation, entails the effects of a repeated exposure with a screening test of reproductive/developmental toxicity. As a screening test its results are of limited use; it is mainly used as a preliminary study to establish doses for further studies.

Method OECD 426 describes the neurotoxic effects of the test substance produced during the development of an organism. The females of the parental generation are dosed, from implantation (approximately day 6 after mating) to weaning of the first generation (day 21 after birth). This procedure allows the pups to be exposed during the neurological developmental process (pre- and postnatally) and evaluate the effects produced by the test substance to the fetus and newborns.

Apart from these validated methods, there are some other methods (developmental immunotoxicity and one-generation extended reproduction toxicity study) that have not been validated yet by the regulatory agencies.

A method that has not been adopted yet by the OECD consists of the extension of the one-generation reproduction toxicity study (OECD 415) up to the sexual maturity of the first generation. This method does not imply the gestation of a second generation but a detailed study by histological and functional analysis of the first generation in order to detect any reasons for infertility and gestation of a new generation. The method for evaluating the developmental immunotoxicity has not been adapted by any international agency but it has been proposed by some committees and expert groups. It is based on the different immune response capacity by adult or developing organisms against chemicals. However, in the OECD there are no technical guidelines dedicated to immunotoxicity, either in developmental or in adult animals. Moreover, there are no legal requirements for the evaluation of developmental immunotoxicity, so it is improbable that this method will be adopted in the next few years.

Below, the methods adapted by the OECD and some other protocols are described in detail, including the general principles of the study, the main aspects of the procedure, the endpoints and the observations, data reporting and criteria for interpreting results, and summarizing the guidelines. This summary must not be used as an actual protocol to be performed for regulatory purposes. The original full OECD Guidelines must be used.

METHOD OECD 414 (PRENATAL DEVELOPMENTAL TOXICITY)

Among the methods for testing developmental toxicity, OECD guideline 414 (OECD, 2001a) provides general information concerning the effects of prenatal exposure on the pregnant test animal and on the developing organism. This protocol has its equivalents in the Environmental Protection Agency (EPA, number 870.3700) and in the European Union Test Method B.31. This includes the assessment of maternal effects as well as death, structural abnormalities or altered growth in the fetus. Although functional deficits are important parts of development, they are not included in these guidelines. Testing for these deficiencies and other postnatal effects are evaluated in the two-generation reproductive toxicity study (OECD, 2001b) and the developmental neurotoxicity study (OECD, 2007).

The preferred rodent species is the rat and the preferred non-rodent species is the rabbit. The test substance is administered to pregnant animals at least from implantation (day 5 after mating) to one day prior to the day of scheduled labor. The test examines the period of organogenesis (from day 5 to 15 in rats and 6 to 18 in rabbits) and also effects from preimplantation, through the entire period of gestation to the day before caesarean section. A tested substance or vehicle is usually administered orally by intubation. At least three dose levels and a concurrent control are used. Each test and control group contains a sufficient number of females to result in approximately 20 female animals (Table 10.1) with implantation sites at necropsy. Groups with fewer than 16 animals with implantation sites may be inappropriate. Dose levels should be selected taking into account any existing toxicity data. The highest dose should produce developmental and/or maternal toxicity (mild clinical signs or a decrease in body weight) but not death or severe suffering.

Clinical observations are made and recorded once a day, preferably at the same time(s) each day taking into consideration the peak period of anticipated effects after dosing. Animals are weighed on day 0, on the first day of dosing, every 3 days during the dosing period and on the day of scheduled labor. Food consumption is also recorded at 3-day intervals and should coincide with days of body weight determination. Females should be killed 1 day prior to the expected day of delivery. Females showing signs of abortion or premature delivery prior to scheduled kill should be sacrificed and subjected to a macroscopic examination. At the time of termination or death, the dam is examined macroscopically for structural abnormalities or pathological changes (caesarean section and subsequent fetal analyses).

Uterine contents

Immediately after termination or as soon as possible after death, the uterus is removed and the pregnancy status of the animals is ascertained. Uteri that appear non-gravid are further examined. Gravid uteri including the cervix are weighed, except from animals found dead during the study. The number of corpora lutea (indication of implants) for pregnant animals is determined. The uterine contents are examined for numbers of embryonic or fetal deaths and viable fetuses.

Examination of fetuses

The sex and body weight of each fetus are determined. Each fetus is examined for external skeletal and soft tissue alterations (e.g., variations and malformations or anomalies). For rats, half of each litter is prepared and examined for skeletal alterations. For rabbits, all fetuses are examined for soft tissue and skeletal alterations. The bodies of these fetuses are evaluated by dissection for soft tissue alterations, which include procedures for further evaluation of internal cardiac structure. The heads of one-half of the fetuses examined are removed and processed for evaluation of soft tissue alterations (including eyes, brain, nasal passages and tongue), using standard serial sectioning methods. The bodies of these fetuses and the remaining intact fetuses are processed and examined for skeletal alterations.

Data reporting

Data are reported in tabular form, showing for each test group the number of animals at the start of the test, the number of animals found dead during the test or killed for humane reasons, the time of any death or humane sacrifice, the number of pregnant females, the number of animals showing signs of toxicity, a description of the signs of toxicity observed, including time of onset, duration, and severity of any toxic effects, the types of fetal observations, and all relevant litter data.

Endpoints

Litters with implants are evaluated for developmental endpoints: number of corpora lutea as an indication of implantations, number and percent of live and dead fetuses and resorptions and number and percent of pre- and postimplantation losses. Litters with live fetuses are examined for the following developmental endpoints: number and percent of live offspring, sex ratio, fetal body weight, preferably by sex and combined; external, soft tissue and skeletal malformations and other relevant alterations, total number and percent of fetuses and litters with any external, soft tissue or skeletal alteration, and types and incidences of individual anomalies and other relevant alterations.

Interpretation of results

A prenatal developmental toxicity study provides information on the effects of repeated oral exposure to a substance during pregnancy. The results of the study should be interpreted in conjunction with the findings of subchronic, reproduction, toxicokinetic and other studies. Since emphasis is placed on general toxicity and developmental toxicity endpoints, the results of the study allow for the discrimination between developmental effects occurring in the absence of general toxicity and those which are only expressed at levels that are also toxic to the maternal animal.

METHOD OECD 415 (ONE-GENERATION REPRODUCTION TOXICITY STUDY)

This protocol (OECD, 1983) has equivalence in the European Test Method B.34.

Principles of the test

This test guideline is designed to provide general information concerning the effects of the tested substance on male and female reproductive performance, such as gonadal function, estrous cycle, mating behavior, conception, parturition, lactation and weaning. The study also provides information about developmental effects, such as neonatal morbidity, mortality, behavior and teratogenesis.

This test is designed for use with rat or mouse. Males of parental generation (F_0) are dosed during growth and for at least one spermatogenic cycle (approximately 56 days in the mouse and 70 days in the rat) in order to elicit any adverse effect on spermatogenesis by the tested substance. Females of the parental generation are dosed for at least two complete estrous cycles (4 to 5 days) in order to elicit any adverse effects on estrus by the test substance. The animals are then mated. The test substance is administered to both sexes during the mating period and thereafter only to females during pregnancy and for the duration of the nursing period.

At least three treatment groups and a control group are used (Table 10.1). Each test and control group should contain a sufficient number of animals to yield about 20 pregnant females at or near term. Ideally, the highest dose level should induce toxicity but not mortality in the parental animals, the intermediate dose should induce minimal toxic effects attributable to the tested substance and the lowest dose should not induce any observable adverse effects on the parents or offspring.

The objective is to produce enough pregnancies and offspring to assure a meaningful evaluation of the potential of the substance to affect fertility, pregnancy and maternal behavior in parental generation animals and suckling, growth and development of the F_1 offspring from conception to weaning. Daily dosing of the parental males begins when they are about 5 to 9 weeks old. In rats dosing is continued for 10 weeks prior to the mating period (for mice, 8 weeks). Males are killed and examined either at the end of the mating period or may be retained on test diet for the possible production of a second litter. For parental females, dosing begins after at least 5 days of acclimatization and continues for at least 2 weeks prior to mating. Daily dosing of the parental females continues throughout the 3-week mating period, pregnancy and up to the weaning of the F_1 offspring.

Animals dosed during the fertility study are allowed to litter normally and rear their progeny to the stage of weaning without standardization. If standardization is carried out, the following procedure is suggested: on day 4 after birth, the size of each litter may be adjusted by eliminating extra pups by selection to yield, as nearly as possible, four males and four females per litter.

Endpoints

Behavioral changes, such as signs of difficulty or prolonged parturition and all signs of toxicity, including mortality, are recorded. During pre-mating and mating periods and optionally during pregnancy, food consumption is measured weekly. After parturition, and during lactation, food consumption measurements are made on the same day as the litters are weighed. Parental generation is weighed on the first day of dosing and weekly thereafter. Each litter is examined as soon as possible after delivery to establish the number and sex of pups, stillbirths, live births and the presence of gross anomalies. Dead pups and pups killed at day 4 are preserved and studied for possible defects. Live pups are counted and litters weighed on the morning after birth and on days 4 and 7 and then weekly until termination of the study, when animals are weighed individually. Physical or behavioral abnormalities observed in the dams or offspring are recorded.

At the time of sacrifice or death the animals of the parental generation are examined macroscopically for structural abnormalities or pathological chances, with special attention to the organs of the reproductive system. The ovaries, uterus, cervix, vagina, testes, epididymides, seminal vesicles, prostate, coagulating gland, pituitary gland and target organs of all parental animals are preserved for examination. These organs are microscopically examined in all high dose and control animals and in animals which die during the study. Organs showing abnormalities in these animals are then examined in all other parental animals. In these instances microscopic examination is made of all tissues showing gross pathological changes. Reproductive organs of animals suspected of infertility may be subjected to microscopic examination.

Data reporting

Data are summarized in tabular form, showing for each test group the number of animals at the start of the test, the number of fertile males, the number of pregnant females, the types of changes and the percentage of animals displaying each type of change (fertility, clinical abnormalities, body weight changes, effects on mortality and any other toxic effects).

Interpretation of the results

This reproductive toxicity study provides information on the effects of repeated oral exposure to a substance. The results of the study should be interpreted in conjunction with the findings of subchronic, teratogenic (see comments for OECD 414 guideline above) and other studies. Extrapolation of the results of the study to humans is valid to a limited degree, although it provides useful information on no-effect levels and permissible human exposure.

METHOD OECD 416 (TWO-GENERATION REPRODUCTION TOXICITY STUDY)

The protocol for studying the effects of a chemical substance in a two-generation study has been adopted by different agencies. The OECD adopted it in 2001 as method 416 (OECD, 2001b), while the EPA named it 870.3800 and the European Union as B.35. This test is designed to provide general information concerning the effects of a tested substance on the integrity and performance of the male and female reproductive systems, including gonadal function, the estrus cycle, mating behavior, conception, gestation, parturition, lactation and weaning, and the growth and development of the offspring. The study also provides information about the effects on the first generation (F_1) including neonatal morbidity, mortality and preliminary data on prenatal and postnatal developmental toxicity. In addition to studying growth and development of the F_1 generation (Table 10.1), the test is also intended to assess the integrity and performance of the male and female reproductive systems as well as growth and development of the second generation (F_2).

The tested substance is administered in graduated doses (at least three doses and a control) to groups of males and females. The rat is the preferred species for testing. Males of the parental generation are dosed during growth and for at least one complete spermatogenic cycle (approximately 56 days in the mouse and 70 days in the rat) in order to elicit any adverse effects on spermatogenesis. Effects on sperm are determined by some sperm parameters (e.g., sperm morphology and motility) and in tissue preparation and detailed histopathology. Females of the parental generation are dosed during growth and for several complete estrus cycles in order to detect adverse effects on estrus cycle normality produced by the substance. The tested substance is administered to parental animals during their mating, during the resulting pregnancies and through the weaning of their F_1 offspring. At weaning the administration of the substance is continued to F_1 offspring during their growth into adulthood, mating, gestation, until the F_2 generation is weaned.

Each test and control group should contain a sufficient number of animals to yield preferably not less than 20 pregnant females at or near parturition. The objective is to produce enough pregnancies to assure a meaningful evaluation of the potential of the substance to affect fertility, pregnancy and maternal behavior and suckling, growth and development of the F_1 offspring from conception to maturity, and the development of their offspring (F_2) to weaning.

Dosing

Daily dosing of the parental males and females begins when they are 5 to 9 weeks old. Daily dosing of the F_1 males and females begins at weaning. During the lactation period, direct exposure of the F_1 pups to the test substance may already occur. For both sexes (F_0 and F_1), dosing continues for at least 10 weeks before the mating period. Dosing is continued in both sexes during the 2-week mating period. Males are humanely killed and examined when they are no longer needed for assessment of reproductive effects. For parental females, dosing continues throughout pregnancy and up to weaning of the F_1 offspring. Treatment of F_0 and F_1 males and females continues until termination.

Observations

This method studies different endpoints related to sperm parameters, observations of the offspring, physical development, functional investigations and pathological changes with special attention to the organs of the reproductive system. For the sperm parameters, the effects on spermatogenesis are evaluated by histopathological examination of testis and epididymis. Sperm evaluation for abnormalities is conducted in control and high dose F_0 and F_1 males; or in all males in each dose group when there are evidences from other studies of possible effects on spermatogenesis. If the sperm evaluation parameters have already been examined as part of a systemic toxicity study of at least 90 days (in subchronic or chronic repeated dose testing), they need not necessarily be repeated in the two-generation study.

For observations of the offspring, physical development of the offspring is recorded mainly by body weight gain. Other physical parameters give supplementary information, but these data are evaluated in the context of data on sexual maturation (age and body weight at vaginal opening or balano-preputial separation), and functional investigations (motor activity, sensory function, reflex ontogeny) of the F_1 offspring. The age of vaginal opening and preputial separation should be determined for F_1 weanlings selected for mating. Ano-genital distance should be measured at postnatal day 0 in F_2 pups if triggered by alterations in F_1 sex ratio or timing of sexual maturation.

All parental animals (F_0 and F_1), all pups with external abnormalities or clinical signs, and at least one randomly selected pup/sex/litter from both the F_1 and F_2 generation, are examined macroscopically for any structural abnormalities or pathological changes with special attention to the organs of the reproductive system. The uteri of all primiparous females are examined, in a manner which does not compromise histopathological evaluation, for the presence and number of implantation sites.

At the time of termination, body weight and the weight of organs of all F_0 and F_1 parental animals are determined (uterus, ovaries; testes, epididymis (total and caudal); prostate; seminal vesicles with coagulating glands and their fluids; brain, liver, kidneys, spleen, pituitary, thyroid and adrenal glands and known target organs). Terminal body weights for F_1 and F_2 pups that are selected for necropsy are determined and the organs (brain, spleen and thymus) from one selected pup/sex/litter are weighed.

Parameters observed in a prenatal developmental toxicity study (OECD, 2001a) about implantation and development of the fetus are also evaluated and described in the OECD TG 416 for two-generation reproduction toxicity.

Reporting of data

The evaluation of the data provided in this test includes the relationship, or lack, between the dose of the tested substance and the presence or absence, incidence and severity of abnormalities, including gross lesions, identified target organs, including necropsy and microscopic findings, affected fertility, clinical abnormalities, affected reproductive and litter performance, body weight changes, effects on mortality and any other toxic effects. A two-generation reproduction toxicity study provides information on the effects of repeated exposure to a substance during all phases of the reproductive cycle. In particular, the study provides information on the reproductive parameters, and on development, growth and survival of offspring. The results of the study should be interpreted in conjunction with the findings of subchronic, prenatal developmental and toxicokinetic and other available studies.

METHOD OECD 421 (REPRODUCTION/ DEVELOPMENTAL TOXICITY SCREENING TEST)

The test is used as part of a set of initial screening tests for existing chemicals for which little or no toxicological information is available, as a dose range finding study for more extensive reproduction/developmental studies. The OECD Guideline 421 (OECD, 1995) was adopted by the EPA as Method 870.3550. This test does not provide complete information on all aspects of reproduction and development. It offers only limited means of detecting postnatal manifestations of prenatal exposure, or effects that may be induced during postnatal exposure. Due to the relatively small numbers of animals, the selectivity of the endpoints and the short duration of the study, this method does not provide evidence for definite claims of no effects. As a consequence, negative data do not indicate absolute safety with respect to reproduction and development. This information may provide some reassurance if actual exposures were clearly less than the dose related to the NOAEL of repeated dose subchronic or chronic dose studies.

Principle of the test

Males should be dosed for a minimum of 4 weeks, including the day before scheduled labor. This includes a minimum of 2 weeks prior to mating, during the mating period and, approximately, 2 weeks post-mating. In view of the limited pre-mating dosing period in males, fertility may not be a particular sensitive indicator of testicular toxicity. Therefore, a detailed histological examination of the testes is essential. The combination of a pre-mating dosing period of 2 weeks and subsequent mating/fertility observations with an overall dosing period of at least 4 weeks, followed by detailed histopathology of the male gonads, is considered sufficient to enable detection of the majority of effects on male fertility and spermatogenesis.

This guideline is designed for performing the test with rats. Females should be dosed throughout the study. This includes 2 weeks prior to mating (with the objective of covering at least two complete estrous cycles), the variable time to conception, the duration of pregnancy and at least 4 days after delivery, up to and including the day before scheduled labor. Duration of study, following acclimatization, is approximately 54 days (at least 14 days pre-mating, (up to) 14 days mating, 22 days gestation, 4 days of lactation), as indicated in Figure 10.1, but it depends on female performance.

The guideline recommends the test substance to be administered orally, daily for 7 days a week, and each group should start with at least 10 animals of each sex. Except in the case of marked toxic effects, it is expected that this will provide at least eight pregnant females per group, which is the minimum acceptable number per group. At least three test groups and a control group are used. Two- to four-fold intervals are frequently optimal for setting the descending dose levels.

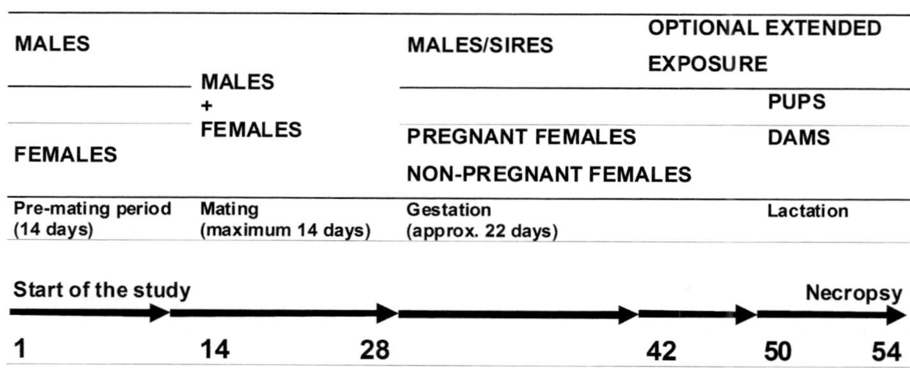

FIGURE 10.1 Temporal schedule for the Method OECD 421, indicating the period (days) of exposure.

Dosing of both sexes begins at least 2 weeks prior to mating and mating begins soon after the animals have attained full sexual maturity (10–12 weeks of age). Dosing is continued in both sexes during the mating period. Males should further be dosed after the mating period at least until the minimum total dosing period of 28 days (Table 10.1) has been completed. Parental female dosing should continue throughout pregnancy and at least up to, and including, day 3 postpartum. For studies where the test substance is administered by inhalation or by the dermal route, dosing is continued at least up to, and including, day 19 of gestation.

Observations

Food consumption and body weight are evaluated in males and females the first day of dosing, at least weekly during the test and at termination. Adult animals are examined macroscopically for abnormalities or pathological changes. Special attention is paid to the organs of the reproductive system. The number of implantation sites is recorded. The counting of corpora lutea is strongly recommended for estimating successful implantations over total implantations in order to deduce the number of implantation losses. The testes and epididymides of all male adult animals are weighed. Dead pups and pups killed at day 4 postpartum are carefully examined externally for gross abnormalities. The ovaries, testes, epididymides, accessory sex organs and all organs showing macroscopic lesions of all adult animals are preserved.

Detailed histological examination is performed on the ovaries, testes and epididymides (with detailed study on stages of spermatogenesis and histopathology of interstitial testicular cell structure) of the animals of the highest dose group and the control group. Examinations are extended to the animals of other dosage groups when changes are seen in the highest dose group.

Data reporting

The evaluation includes the relationship between the dose of the test substance and the presence or absence, incidence and severity of abnormalities, including gross lesions, identified target organs, infertility, clinical abnormalities, affected reproductive and litter performance, body weight changes, effects on mortality and any other toxic effects. Because of the short period of treatment of the male, the histopathology of the testis and epididymis should be considered along with the fertility data, when assessing male reproductive effects.

The results that are reported from this test include body weight and food consumption changes; toxic response data by sex and dose, including fertility, gestation and other signs of toxicity; gestation length, toxic or other effects on reproduction, offspring, postnatal growth, etc.; nature, severity and duration of clinical observations; number of live births and postimplantation loss; number of pups with grossly visible abnormalities, number of runts; time of death; number of implantations, corpora lutea, litter size and litter weights; organ weight data for the parental animals; necropsy findings; microscopic findings of the male genital tract and in other tissues and absorption data.

METHOD OECD 422 (COMBINED REPEATED DOSE TOXICITY STUDY WITH THE REPRODUCTION/ DEVELOPMENTAL TOXICITY SCREENING TEST)

This protocol (OECD, 1996) has also been adopted by the Environmental Protection Agency as 870.3650. This test is intended for identification of possible health hazards likely to arise from repeated exposure over a relatively limited period of time. The method comprises a reproduction/developmental toxicity screening test and, therefore, is also used to provide initial information on possible effects on male and female reproductive performance such as gonadal function, mating behavior, conception, development of the conceptus and parturition. This test does not provide complete information on all aspects of reproduction and development. It only offers limited means of detecting postnatal manifestations of prenatal exposure, or effects that may have been induced during postnatal exposure. It can also be used as a dose range finding study for more extensive reproduction/developmental studies. In this test, the dosing period is longer than in a conventional 28-day repeated dose study. However, it uses fewer animals of each sex per group.

Principle of the test

This study is designed for use with rats. The tested substance is administered orally to at least three test groups of males and females and a control. Males are dosed for a minimum of 4 weeks (2 weeks before mating, during the mating period and approximately 2 weeks post-mating). In view of the limited pre-mating dosing period in males, fertility may not be a particularly sensitive indicator of testicular toxicity. Therefore, a detailed histological examination of the testes is essential. The combination of a pre-mating dosing period of 2 weeks and subsequent mating/fertility observations with an overall dosing period of at least 4 weeks, followed by detailed histopathology of the male gonads, is considered sufficient to enable detection of the majority of effects on male fertility and spermatogenesis.

Females are dosed throughout the study. This includes 2 weeks prior to mating (to cover at least two complete estrous cycles), the time to conception, the duration of pregnancy and at least 4 days after delivery, up to and including the day before scheduled labor.

Procedure

The guideline recommends each group to start with at least 10 animals of each sex. Except in the case of marked toxic effects, it is expected that this will provide at least eight pregnant females per group which normally is the minimum acceptable number of pregnant females per group. The objective is to produce enough pregnancies and offspring to assure a meaningful evaluation of the potential of the substance to affect fertility, pregnancy, maternal and suckling behavior, and growth and development of the F_1 offspring from conception to day 4 postpartum. Two- to four-fold intervals are frequently optimum for the dosing.

The animals are dosed with the test substance daily for 7 days a week.

After animals of both sexes have been acclimatized for at least 5 days, 2 weeks prior to mating, dosing begins. Mating begins soon after the animals have attained full sexual maturity (10–12 weeks of age). Males are dosed after the mating period at least until a minimum total dosing period of 28 days (Table 10.1). Daily dosing of the parental females continues throughout pregnancy and at least up to, and including, day 3 postpartum or the day before sacrifice.

Observations

General clinical observations are made daily. Once before the first exposure and at least once a week thereafter, detailed clinical observations are made in all animals. Changes in skin, fur, eyes, mucous membranes, occurrence of secretions and excretions, sensory reactivity to stimuli and autonomic activity (e.g., lacrimation, piloerection, pupil size, unusual respiratory pattern) is evaluated. The duration of gestation should be recorded and is calculated from day 0 of pregnancy. Each litter is examined as soon as possible and live pups are counted and sexed, and litters are weighed within 24 hours of parturition. Males and females are weighed on the first day of dosing, weekly thereafter and at termination. Food consumption is measured weekly.

Hematological examinations are made in five males and five females randomly selected from each group and the following parameters are measured: hematocrit, hemoglobin concentration, erythrocyte count, total and differential leukocyte count, platelet count and a measure of blood clotting time/potential. Clinical biochemistry determinations to investigate major toxic effects in tissues and, specifically, effects on kidney and liver, are performed on blood samples obtained from the selected five males and five females of each group. Other determinations should be carried out if the known properties of the test substance may, or are suspected to, affect the metabolic profiles.

All adult animals in the study are subjected to a full, detailed, gross necropsy which includes careful examination of the external surface of the body, all orifices and the cranial, thoracic and abdominal cavities and their contents. Special attention is paid to the organs of the reproductive system. The testes and epididymides of all adult males are weighed and the ovaries, testes, epididymides, accessory sex organs and all organs showing macroscopic lesions of all adult animals are preserved. For five adult males and females, randomly selected from each group, the liver, kidneys, adrenals, thymus, spleen, brain and heart are trimmed of any adherent tissue, as appropriate, and their wet weight taken as soon as possible after dissection. Of the selected males and females, the following tissues are also preserved: all gross lesions, brain (representative regions including cerebrum, cerebellum and pons), spinal cord, stomach, small and large intestines, liver, kidneys, adrenals, spleen, heart, thymus, thyroid, trachea and lungs, uterus, urinary bladder, lymph nodes (preferably one lymph node covering the route of administration and another one distant from the route of administration to cover systemic effects), peripheral nerve (sciatic or tibial) preferably in close proximity to the muscle, and a section of bone marrow (or, alternatively, a fresh mounted marrow aspirate). These examinations should be extended to animals of other dosage groups, if treatment-related changes are observed in the highest dose group.

Data reporting

Due to the limited dimensions of the study, statistical analysis in the form of tests for "significance" is of limited value for many endpoints, especially reproductive endpoints. The findings of this toxicity study are evaluated in terms of the observed effects, necropsy and microscopic findings. The evaluation includes the relationship between the dose of the tested substance and the presence or absence, incidence and severity of abnormalities, including gross lesions, identified target organs, infertility, clinical abnormalities, affected reproductive and litter performance, body weight changes, effects on mortality and any other toxic effects. Because of the short period of treatment of the male, the histopathology of the testis and epididymis must be considered along with the fertility data, when assessing male reproduction effects.

The test report must include body weight changes, food consumption, toxic response data by sex and dose, including fertility, gestation and any other signs of toxicity, gestation length, toxic or other effects on reproduction, offspring, postnatal growth, nature, severity and duration of clinical observations, sensory activity, grip strength and motor activity assessments, hematological and clinical biochemistry tests, number of live births and postimplantation loss, number of pups with grossly visible abnormalities, number of runts, time of death during the study or whether animals survived to termination, number of implantations, corpora lutea (recommended), litter size and litter weights at the time of recording, body and organ weight data for the parental animals; necropsy findings, histopathological findings, absorption data and statistical treatment of results.

The study provides an evaluation of reproduction/developmental toxicity associated with administration of repeated doses. In particular, since emphasis is placed on general toxicity and reproduction/developmental toxicity endpoints, the results of the study allow for the discrimination between reproductive/developmental effects occurring in the absence of general toxicity and those which are only expressed at levels that are also toxic to parent animals. It could provide an indication of the need to conduct further investigations and could provide guidance in the design of subsequent studies and for justification of waiving full studies.

The experimental schedule for the study duration of this test is similar to that shown in method 421 (see Figure 10.1), with a maximum duration of the study of 54 days.

METHOD OECD 426 (DEVELOPMENTAL NEUROTOXICITY STUDY)

Developmental neurotoxicity studies are designed to provide data, including dose–response characterization, on the potential functional and morphological effects on the developing nervous system of the offspring that may arise from exposure in uterus and during early life. A developmental neurotoxicity study can be conducted as a separate study, incorporated into a reproductive toxicity and/or adult neurotoxicity study, or added onto a prenatal developmental toxicity study.

This method was adopted by the OECD as Guideline 426 (OECD, 2007) and by the EPA as Method 870.6300.

Procedure

The preferred test species is the rat while other species can be used when appropriate. Each test and control group should contain a sufficient number of pregnant females to be exposed to the test substance to ensure that an adequate number of offspring (20 litters are recommended per dose level) is produced for neurotoxicity evaluation. On or before postnatal day (PND) 4, the size of each litter should be adjusted by eliminating extra pups by random selection to yield a uniform litter size for all litters. The litter size should not exceed the average litter size for the strain of rodents used (8–12).

At least three dose levels and a concurrent control should be used. The highest dose level should be chosen with the aim of inducing some maternal toxicity and may be limited to 1,000 mg/kg body weight. The tested substance (or vehicle) should be administered by the most relevant route to potential human exposure, and based on available metabolism and distribution information in the test animals. The tested substance (or vehicle) should, at least, be administered daily to mated females from the time of implantation (gestation day 6) throughout lactation (PND 21), so that the pups are exposed to the test substance during pre- and postnatal neurological development (Table 10.2).

TABLE 10.2 Timing of the assessment of physical and developmental landmarks, and functional/behavioral endpoints (number of times when measurements are performed) for OECD Guideline 426

	Age periods		
	Pre-weaning	**Adolescence**	**Young adults**
Endpoints			
Physical and developmental landmarks			
Body weight and clinical observations	weekly	at least every two weeks	at least every two weeks
Brain weight	PND 22		at termination
Neuropathology	PND 22		at termination
Sexual maturation	–	as appropriate	–
Other developmental landmarks	as appropriate	–	–
Functional/behavioral endpoints			
Behavioral ontogeny		at least two measures	
Motor activity (including habituation)	1–3 times	–	once
Motor and sensory function	–	once	once
Learning and memory	–	once	once

Observations

During the treatment and observation periods, detailed clinical observations are conducted periodically (a minimum of twice during the gestational and the lactational dosing period) using at least 10 dams per dose level. Clinical observations include changes in skin, fur, eyes, mucous membranes, occurrence of secretions and autonomic activity (lacrimation, piloerection, pupil size, unusual respiratory pattern and/or mouth breathing and any unusual signs of urination or defecation). Unusual responses with respect to body position, activity level (decreased or increased exploration of the standard area), coordination, posture, reactivity to environmental stimuli, presence of clonic or tonic movements, convulsions, tremors, stereotypies, bizarre behavior (biting or excessive licking, self-mutilation, walking backwards, vocalization) or aggression should be recorded.

Signs of toxicity should be recorded, including the day of onset, time of day, degree and duration. Animals are weighed at the time of dosing at least once a week throughout the study, on or near the day of delivery, and on PND 21. For gavage studies dams should be weighed at least twice weekly. Food consumption is measured weekly at a minimum during gestation and lactation.

For the offspring (at least one pup/sex/litter), during the treatment and observation periods, detailed clinical observations are conducted. The observations should be the same as for the dams. Changes in pre-weaning landmarks of development (pinna unfolding, eye opening, incisor eruption) are highly correlated with body weight, so this may be the best indicator of physical development.

Neuropathological evaluation of the offspring is conducted using tissues from animals. For offspring killed through PND 22, brain tissues should be evaluated; for animals killed at termination (PND 70), both central nervous system (CNS) tissues and peripheral nervous system (PNS) tissues are evaluated. All gross abnormalities appearing at the time of necropsy should be noted. Tissue samples taken should represent all major regions of the nervous system. The purposes of the qualitative examination are to identify regions within the nervous system exhibiting evidence of neuropathological alterations, types of neuropathological alterations resulting from exposure to the test substance and to determine the range of severity of the neuropathological alterations. Morphometric (quantitative) evaluation should be performed as these data may assist in the detection of a treatment-related effect and are valuable in the interpretation of treatment-related differences in brain weight or morphology.

Neuropathological evaluation should include an examination for indications of developmental damage to the nervous system, in addition to the cellular alterations. Some significant changes are alterations in the gross size or shape of the olfactory bulbs, cerebrum or cerebellum; alterations in the relative size of various brain regions, including changes in the size of regions resulting from the loss or persistence of normally transient populations of cells or axonal projections; alterations in proliferation, migration and differentiation, as indicated by areas of excessive apoptosis or necrosis, clusters or dispersed populations of ectopic, disoriented or malformed neurons or alterations in the relative size of various layers of cortical structures; alterations in patterns of myelination, including an overall size reduction or altered staining of myelinated structures; evidence of hydrocephalus, in particular enlargement of the ventricles, stenosis of the cerebral aqueduct and thinning of the cerebral hemispheres. For each type of lesion, the characteristics used to define each severity grade should be described, indicating the features used to differentiate each grade. The frequency of each type of lesion and its severity grade should be recorded and a statistical analysis should be performed to evaluate the nature of a dose–response relationship.

Data and reporting

A developmental neurotoxicity study provides information on the effects of repeated exposure to a substance during prenatal and early postnatal development. Since emphasis is placed on both general toxicity and developmental neurotoxicity endpoints, the results of the study allow for the discrimination between neurodevelopmental effects occurring in the absence of general maternal toxicity, and those which are only expressed at levels that are also toxic to the maternal animal.

The test report for this test should include the following results (Table 10.2): number of animals at the start and at the end of the study; number of animals and litters used for each test method; identification number of each animal; litter size and mean weight at birth by sex; body weight and body weight change data, including terminal body weight for dams and offspring; food consumption data, and water consumption data if appropriate; toxic response data by sex and dose level, including signs of toxicity or mortality, including time and cause of death; detailed description of clinical observations; score on each developmental landmark (weight, sexual maturation and behavioral ontogeny); detailed description of all behavioral, functional, neuropathological, neurochemical, electrophysiological findings by sex; necropsy findings; brain weights; diagnoses derived from neurological signs and lesions, including naturally occurring diseases or conditions; images of exemplar findings; low power images to assess homology of sections used for morphometry; absorption and metabolism data; statistical treatment of results and list of study personnel.

The discussion of results in the report must contain dose–response information, by sex and group; relationship of any other toxic effects to a conclusion about the neurotoxic potential of the test chemical, by sex and group, impact of toxicokinetic information on the conclusions, similarities of effects to any known neurotoxicants, data supporting the reliability and sensitivity of the test method, relationships between neuropathological and functional effects and NOAEL or benchmark dose for dams and offspring, by sex and group.

OTHER METHODS NOT INCLUDED IN THE OECD

Developmental immunotoxicity

The Agricultural Chemical Safety Assessment (ACSA) Technical Committee developed in 1999 a database for developmental immunotoxicity. The developing immune system can be significantly more sensitive than the adult immune system to xenobiotic-induced insult (Dietert and Holsapple, 2007). There are distinct differences between the immune system surrounding birth and that in the mature adult as well as differences in the nature of immunotoxic changes based on age. Immunosuppression is not the only concern. Immunotoxic changes that increase the risk for allergic or autoimmune responses should also be considered. Therefore, researchers should not assume that immunotoxicity assays validated for adult exposure assessment are inherently the most predictive for developmental immunotoxicology (DIT) evaluation. Many of those adult-based protocols were developed solely to detect immunosuppression, whereas DIT concerns include shifts in immune balance. However, majority of participants at the April 2008 ECETOC-ECVAM expert workshop (ECETOC-ECVAM, 2008) believe it is premature to include a DIT module in the enhanced one-generation technical guideline for the following reasons: no regulatory data requirement for DIT exists anywhere in the world, and only a handful of ad hoc "special studies" have been requested to date. Only recently one pesticide regulator has codified a requirement for an adult immunotoxicity study, so no contribution can be claimed to further international harmonization of hazard and risk assessment approaches. No standardized or validated methodology or OECD technical guidelines currently exist for the evaluation of immunotoxicity in either adult or developing animals, although discussions among experts have taken place (Holsapple *et al.*, 2005). Although an enhanced one-generation study would be suited for general use, DIT data are of dubious relevance outside the pesticides sector (Vogel *et al.*, 2010).

One-generation extended reproduction toxicity study

This method has been proposed by different groups (Reuter *et al.*, 2003; Vogel *et al.*, 2010) in order to produce a more efficient protocol for testing the reproductive/developmental effects of chemical substances using one generation. This proposal uses a smaller number of animals, with benefits in economic effort and also ethically.

Previous evaluations of multi-generational tests (Reuter *et al.*, 2003; Cooper *et al.*, 2006; Myers *et al.*, 2008) show that in nearly all cases, the effects produced by the chemical had already been shown in the first generation and only in a minimal number of cases had the effect been visible in the second generation.

This method consists of the extension of the one-generation study (OECD 415) with detailed evaluation of different endpoints in F_1 generation. The F_1 generation is examined for functional, histological and pathological changes in its system and most exhaustively in the reproductive organs. Although this proposed method has not been approved by official organisms, it has already been used by industry. The benefits from using this method have been stated before and are related to the reduction in the number of animals and ethical reasons. Some of the arguments stated by industry for avoiding the use of this method are the expensive costs of detailed and exhaustive examinations of histopathology and functional changes in the animals.

CONCLUDING REMARKS AND FUTURE DIRECTIONS

Different organizations at international levels (OECD, EPA, EU) have developed *in vivo* protocols for testing the reproductive toxicity of chemicals. These protocols are used all over the world and have been previously validated, so they are considered reliable. The endpoints evaluated in those methods cover toxicity in the fertility in the parental generation to effects in the developmental process and include the birth of new generations of animals. The evaluation of the adverse effects produced on these tests provides useful information for the characterization of the toxic potential of a chemical. New protocols are being developed in order to reduce the number of animals used in the assessment and to improve the predictability for identification of human health hazards.

REFERENCES

Cooper RL, Lamb JC, Barlow SM, Bentley K, Brady AM, Doerrer NG, Eisenbrandt DL, Fenner-Crisp PA, Hines RN, Irvine LF, Kimmel CA, Koeter H, Li AA, Makris SL, Sheets LP, Speijers G, Whitby KE (2006) A tiered approach to life stages testing for agricultural chemical safety assessment. *Crit Rev Toxicol* **36:** 69–98.

Dietert RR, Holsapple MP (2007) Methodologies for developmental immunotoxicity (DIT) testing. *Methods* **47:** 123–31.

ECETOC-ECVAM (European Centre for Ecotoxicology and Toxicology of Chemicals and European Centre for the Validation of Alternative Methods). Report of the Workshop on Triggering and Waiving Criteria for the Extended One-Generation Reproduction Toxicity Study (2008) Barza d'Ispra, Workshop Report No. 12, 2008.

Holsapple MP, Burns-Naas LA, Hastings KL, Ladics GS, Lavin AL, Makris SL, Yang Y, Luster MI (2005) Proposed testing framework for developmental immunotoxicology (DIT). *Toxicol Sci* **83:** 18–24.

Myers DP, Willoughby CR, Bottomley AM, Buschmann J (2008) An analysis of the results from two-generation reproduction toxicity studies to assess the value of the second (F1) generation of the detection of adverse treatment-related effects on reproductive performance. *Reprod Toxicol* **26:** 47–50.

OECD (Organisation for Economic Cooperation and Development) (2001a) Prenatal developmental toxicity study. OECD guidance 414 adopted 22-01-2001.

OECD (Organisation for Economic Cooperation and Development) (1983) One-generation reproduction toxicity study. OECD guidance 415 adopted 23-05-1983.

OECD (Organisation for Economic Cooperation and Development) (2001b) Two-generation reproduction toxicity study. OECD guidance 416 adopted 22-01-2001.

OECD (Organisation for Economic Cooperation and Development) (1995) Reproduction/Developmental toxicity screening test. OECD guidance 421 adopted 27-07-1995.

OECD (Organisation for Economic Cooperation and Development) (1996) One-generation reproduction toxicity study. OECD guidance 422 adopted 22-03-1996.

OECD (Organisation for Economic Cooperation and Development) (2007) One-generation reproduction toxicity study. OECD guidance 426 adopted 16-10-2007.

Reuter U, Heinrich-Hirsch B, Hellwig J, Holzum B, Welsch F. (2003) Evaluation of OECD screening tests 421 (reproduction/developmental toxicity screening test) and 422 (combined repeated dose toxicity study with the reproduction/developmental toxicity screening test). *Regul Toxicol Pharmacol* **38:** 17–26.

Vogel R, Seidle T, Spielmann H (2010) A modular one-generation reproduction study as a flexible testing system for regulatory safety assessment. *Reprod Toxicol* **29:** 242–5.

C H A P T E R

11

Mechanism-based models in reproductive and developmental toxicology

David Pamies, Carmen Estevan Martínez, Miguel A. Sogorb and Eugenio Vilanova

INTRODUCTION

The term reproductive toxicology is defined as the adverse effect either on fertility of parental generation or on the development of the progeny. The term developmental toxicology is defined as the adverse effects on the developing organism from the moment of conception to the time of sexual maturation and therefore developmental toxicology can be considered as part of reproductive toxicology. The term embryotoxicity is defined as the toxic effects in progeny in the first period of pregnancy between conception and the fetal stage and therefore is included within developmental toxicology and by extension also within reproductive toxicology. Finally, the term teratogenicity is defined as the structural malformations or defects in offspring after the period of embryogenesis and is considered as a developmental toxicology effect.

It seems obvious that the complexity of the reproductive process cannot be studied with a single *in vitro* model and therefore it is necessary to split the whole process into certain steps (maturation of gamete, fertilization, implantation, embryogenesis, fetogenesis, etc.). This chapter will be mainly focused on the study of the currently available models for testing developmental toxicity (embryotoxicity and teratogenicity). Other parts of the processes such as infertility, endocrine disruption, mutagenicity of germinal cells, etc. are already covered in other chapters of this book.

THE NECESSITY OF ALTERNATIVE MODELS FOR TESTING REPRODUCTIVE AND DEVELOPMENTAL TOXICOLOGY

The OECD has several validated guidelines for *in vivo* studies of reproductive toxicology (covering in the same assay therefore fertility and developmental issues) and for *in vivo* studies of developmental toxicology (covering teratogenicity, since the exposure starts after embryogenesis). These guidelines are discussed in detail in the previous chapter of this book. However, it needs to be mentioned that there are no guidelines for testing only *in vivo* embryotoxicity. This is a relevant gap because a guideline for this purpose would allow the detection of developmental toxins in early stages of development without waiting for teratogenicity.

Regulations in all developed countries require *in vivo* studies regarding the toxicity to reproduction in order to perform the necessary risk assessment before registration and authorization of the use of chemicals with medium and high volume of production. Regulations also concern the use of a large number of animals with the corresponding ethical, logistical and economic implications. Höfer and coworkers (2004) have estimated the number of animals needed to perform a basic set of assays for testing toxicity to reproduction. This number would include a total of 3,910 vertebrates according to the following scheme: 150 animals (either rats or rabbits) for developmental studies (OECD Guideline 414); 560 animals (rats) for reproduction/developmental toxicity screening test (OECD Guideline 421); and 3,200 animals (rats) for the two-generation reproduction toxicity study (OECD Guideline 416). According to data published by Fleischer (2004), obtained from a survey performed among laboratories in the European Union and Switzerland, the cost of this set of assays would reach €446,000.00. Rovida and Hartung (2009) have estimated that the area of reproductive toxicology would demand 90% of animals and 70% of the economical cost of assays for registration.

Taking into consideration the figures outlined in the above paragraph it is easy to understand that the use of fast, safe and reliable alternative models for testing reproductive toxicology would be highly appreciated by the industry. These models might be especially relevant for the process of massive high throughput screening performed in the early stages of developing molecules as biocides, cosmetics, food additives, etc. Also, other potential applications of these alternative models would be (Spielman, 2005): (1) to compare the developmental toxicity potential of a new chemical that is only a slight modification of an existing chemical that has

Reproductive and Developmental Toxicology, Edited by Ramesh C. Gupta
ISBN: 978-0-12-382032-7

already been tested *in vivo*; and (2) evaluating compounds for which testing is not routinely performed, usually since the anticipated exposure is very low.

The next section describes the main alternative models for testing developmental toxicity. These models are divided between validated models (whole-embryo culture test (WEC), micromass test (MM) and embryonic stem cell test (EST)) and those that are not currently validated (although have proven scientific validity) as is the case of zebrafish, frog embryo teratogenesis assay (FETAX), *in silico* models for predicting embryotoxicity, *in vitro* cellular models different from the EST method, and methods using fragments of embryos.

VALIDATED ALTERNATIVE MODELS FOR TESTING DEVELOPMENTAL TOXICOLOGY

Between 1996 and 2000 the European Centre for Validation of Alternative Methods (ECVAM) sponsored prevalidation and validation studies of the WEC, MM and EST methods. These three methods reduce, refine and/or replace the use of animals and therefore fit within the philosophy of alternative methods. WEC uses whole rat embryos with 10 days of gestation that are further exposed *in vitro* to the tested chemical during 48 hours, while MM and EST are methods based on the determination of the effects of the chemical on differentiation of cells from two different sources: embryos (in the case of MM) or embryonic stem cells (in the case of EST). These three methods also share a common approach based on obtaining records for their respective endpoints and further analysis of these records with validated statistical functions that allow assignment of the tested chemicals to the following three categories: non-, weakly or strongly embryotoxic. The ECVAM Scientific Advisory Committee has endorsed the scientific validity of the three methods: EST and WEC were considered to be scientifically validated for distinguishing among non-, weak and strong embryotoxins, whereas MM was considered scientifically validated for identifying only strongly embryotoxic chemicals (ESAC, 2002).

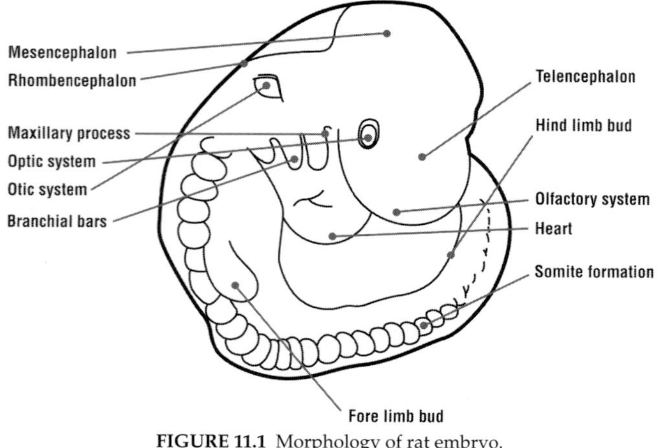

FIGURE 11.1 Morphology of rat embryo.

Whole-embryo culture test (WEC)

The embryotoxicity testing in postimplantation rat or mouse whole-embryo culture (WEC) is intended to identify substances with the capability of inducing malformations resulting in embryotoxicity and it is proposed to be used within the context of OECD Guideline 414 for testing teratogenicity (ECVAM, 2006a).

The rationale of this study is based on the *in vitro* exposure of embryos during the time where major aspects of organogenesis occur, as in the case of heart development, closure of the neural tube, and the development of ear and eye, branchial bars and limb buds. Therefore, it is assumed that interferences during this period may lead to general retardation of growth and development or to specific malformations.

Basic procedure

Rat or mouse embryos are *in vitro* cultured for 48 hours starting on day 9.5 of gestation in the presence of the tested substance. After 48 hours each embryo (Figure 11.1) is transferred to a Petri dish and scored according to the parameters described in Table 11.1. These parameters include records about growth (yolk sac diameter, crown–rump length and head length), function (heartbeat, yolk sac circulation and allantoic circulation), morphology (final minus initial somite number) and malformations (as indicated in Table 11.1 from A through R). The assay is performed in two steps. The first one is a range finding test carried out using three embryos per concentration and using ten-fold concentration intervals. In the second step the highest ineffective concentration and a concentration which results in at least a 50% reduction of control total morphological scores (estimated as is indicated in Table 11.1), as well as two intermediate concentrations, are tested to a total of seven embryos per concentration. The assay is considered valid when it meets the following criteria: (1) a maximum rate of malformed embryos in the control group of 15% (1 out of 7); (2) a positive control of 5-fluoracil (0.03, 0.1, and 0.3 mg/ml) and a negative control of penicillin G (1 mg/ml) are run together with the main assay.

The WEC can be considered an alternative model because the number of animals needed is lower than its *in vivo* equivalent OECD Guideline 414 (therefore causing a reduction in the number of needed animals) and refines the animal suffering since the exposure is performed *in vitro*.

Endpoints of the assay and prediction model

The results of a prevalidation study performed with six chemicals of well-known *in vivo* embryotoxic potential and four independent laboratories were analyzed in order to create a biostatistically based prediction model (PM) to identify the embryotoxic potential (non-, weakly and strongly embryotoxic) of the tested chemicals.

Two PMs (PM1 and PM2) were created using linear discriminant analysis (Genschow *et al.*, 2000). PM1 was developed during the prevalidation study and showed poorer results than the EST test (see detailed explanation about EST test in another section of this chapter). Because PM1 took into consideration parameters exclusively focused on differentiation and development but no measures of cytotoxicity, the PM2 was further developed with the aim of improving the performance of PM1 by including cytotoxicity data with 3T3 fibroblast coming from the EST test (Genschow *et al.*, 2002).

The PMs of the WEC test are displayed in Table 11.2 and include the following endpoints: (1) $IC_{NOEC\ TMS}$, which describes the lowest assayed concentration that has no effect on the total morphological score (TMS) estimated as shown in Table 11.1; (2) $IC_{50\ MAL}$, which is the concentration at which 50% of all tested embryos are malformed; (3) IC_{MAX}, obtained as the lowest assayed concentration at which a maximum malformation rate is obtained; and (4) $IC_{50\ 3T3}$, which corresponds with the concentration which causes 50% of reduction in viability of 3T3 mouse fibroblasts after 10 days of exposure in conditions described for EST assay.

The analysis of these endpoints allowed the creation of three lineal discrimination functions for each of the PMs. The relationships among these three functions allow for the classification of the tested chemical as non-, weakly or strongly embryotoxic according to criteria showed in Table 11.3.

Performance of the WEC test

After the prevalidation study a blind validation study was boarded by the participating laboratories adding 14 new compounds (thus for a total of 20 compounds) to the list of tested chemicals. Because the test chemicals were assigned to only three categories of embryotoxicity, 33% of correct classifications might be expected by chance. In consideration of this the criteria for evaluating the results of the validation study were established as stated in Table 11.4.

All strongly embryotoxic chemicals could be identified (precision) and correctly predicted (predictivity) with PM2 (Table 11.4). The predictivity for non-embryotoxic and weakly embryotoxic chemicals ranged between 56 and 76% for both PM1 and PM2, while these same records for precision ranged between 45 and 80% (Table 11.4). Applying the

TABLE 11.1 Parameters to score after exposure of rat or mouse embryos in the WEC assay

Growth parameters		Malformations (0 for normal/1 for malformed)
Yolk sac diameter (mm)		Yolk sac vessel defect
Crown–rump length (mm)		Allantois not fused with ectoplacental cone
Head length (mm)		Allantois large size
Functional parameters (1 for normal/0 for abnormal)		Flexion deficient
		Pericardiac sac wide, filled with fluid
Yolk sac circulation		Heart ventrally turned
Allantois circulation		Posterior neuropore open
Heartbeat		Dorsal midline irregular
Somite development		Prosencephalon open
Final somite number		Rhomboencephalon narrow
Final–initial somite number		Cranial neural folds suture line irregular
Morphological scores		Head small and bent backwards
A	Yolk sac blood vessels	Craniofacial appearance abnormal
B	Allantois	Neural tube haemorrhagic
C	Flexion	Rhombencephalon large and transparent
D	Heart	Rhombencephalon narrow
E	Caudal neural tube	Otic vesicles deformed
F	Hind brain	Optic vesicles deformed
G	Mid brain	Branchial bars deformed
H	Fore brain	Maxillary process swollen
J	Otic system	Mandibular processes unapproached
K	Optic system	Mandibular process deformed
L	Olfactory system	Somites small
M	Branchial bars	Somites irregular
N	Maxillary process	Tail kinked
P	Mandibular process	Rail short and thickened
Q	Fore limb	Subcutaneous blisters
R	Hind limb	Haemorrhages
Total Morphological Score (A + B + C + ... + R)		Other

Taken from official validated protocol available in the European Centre for Validation of Alternative Methods (ECVAM)

TABLE 11.2 Linear discriminant functions for the prediction of embryotoxicity in the three validated methods

(a) Prediction model of the embryonic stem cell test (EST)

$$\text{Function I} = 5.92 \log(IC_{50\ 3T3}) + 3.50 \log(IC_{50\ D3}) - 5.31\frac{IC_{50\ 3T3} - ID_{50}}{IC_{50\ 3T3}} - 15.7$$

$$\text{Function II} = 3.65 \log(IC_{50\ 3T3}) + 2.39 \log(IC_{50\ D3}) - 2.03\frac{IC_{50\ 3T3} - ID_{50}}{IC_{50\ 3T3}} - 6.85$$

$$\text{Function III} = -0.125 \log(IC_{50\ 3T3}) - 1.92 \log(IC_{50\ D3}) + 1.50\frac{IC_{50\ 3T3} - ID_{50}}{IC_{50\ 3T3}} - 2.67$$

(b) Prediction model number 1 of the whole embryonic test (WEC)

$$\text{Function I} = 18.08 \log(IC_{50\ Mal}) - 11.56 \log(IC_{NOEC\ TMS}) - 10.19$$

$$\text{Function II} = 21.55 \log(IC_{50\ Mal}) - 15.31 \log(IC_{NOEC\ TMS}) - 10.65$$

$$\text{Function III} = 8.70 \log(IC_{50\ Mal}) - 8.53 \log(IC_{NOEC\ TMS}) - 2.53$$

(c) Prediction model number 2 of the whole embryonic test (WEC)

$$\text{Function I} = 21\frac{IC_{50\ 3T3} - IC_{NOEC\ TMS}}{IC_{50\ 3T3}} + 15.37 \log(IC_{max}) - 23.58$$

$$\text{Function II} = 27\frac{IC_{50\ 3T3} - IC_{NOEC\ TMS}}{IC_{50\ 3T3}} + 17.71 \log(IC_{max}) - 32.37$$

$$\text{Function III} = 9.3\frac{IC_{50\ 3T3} - IC_{NOEC\ TMS}}{IC_{50\ 3T3}} + 4.21 \log(IC_{max}) - 4.23$$

(d) Prediction model of the micromass test (MM)

$$\text{Function I} = 6.65 \times \log(ID_{50}) - 9.49$$

$$\text{Function II} = 6.16 \times \log(ID_{50}) - 8.29$$

$$\text{Function III} = -1.31 \times \log(ID_{50}) - 1.42$$

Abbreviations: $IC_{50\ 3T3}$ = Concentration that reduces viability of 3T3 cells to 50% after exposure according to the protocol; $IC_{50\ D3}$ = Concentration that reduces viability of D3 cells to 50% after exposure according to the protocol; ID_{50} = Concentration that reduces to 50% the differentiation of either D3 cells to cardiomyocytes (EST) or primary culture of limb bud cells to cartilage (MM) after exposure according to the respective EST and MM protocols; $IC_{50\ Mal}$ = Concentration at which 50% of exposed embryos display malformations; $IC_{NOEC\ TMS}$ = The lowest concentration without observed effect on the total morphological score (see Table 11.1); IC_{max} = The lowest concentration that causes the maximum malformation rate.

two PMs to the results obtained in the WEC test provided a maximal overall accuracy (the proportion of correct outcomes of the method independently of the category of the tested chemical) of 80% correct prediction of embryotoxic potential *in vivo* (Table 11.4).

Based on the successful outcome of the validation study the ECVAM Scientific Advisory Committee has endorsed the WEC as a scientifically validated test since it yields reproducible results, the correlation between *in vivo* and *in vitro* data was good and the test proved applicable to testing a diverse group of chemicals of different embryotoxic potentials (ESAC, 2002). Therefore, the WEC test is ready to be considered for regulatory purposes.

The micromass test (MM)

This method uses rat micromass cultures of limb bud and detects the inhibition of cell differentiation and growth, which are parameters suitable for testing teratogenicity. This is because this method is also intended to be used within the context of OECD Guideline 414 (ECAVM, 2006b).

This method is based on the capability of the primary culture of limb bud cells of mammalian origin to reproduce cartilage histogenesis, a fundamental step in the morphogenesis of the skeleton, cell proliferation and differentiation, cell to cell communication and cell to extracellular matrix interactions. Therefore, interference in these basic cell developmental functions may result in teratogenic consequences.

TABLE 11.3 The embryotoxic potential classification criteria according to prediction models displayed in Table 11.2 for EST, WEC and MM methods

Classification	Requirements
Strong embryotoxicity	Function III > Function II and Function III > Function I
Weak embryotoxicity	Function II > Function III and Function II > Function I
No embryotoxicity	Function I > Function III and Function I > Function II

Basic procedure

Embryos are obtained from Wistar rats on day 14 of gestation and the limb buds (Figure 11.1) are isolated. A primary culture of these cells is generated with tripsin and the cells are next seeded in 96-well plates. The cells are further exposed to the tested compound during 5 days and finally the number of differentiated cells is determined with alcian blue (a cartilage-specific proteoglycan stain). The test is performed in two steps. Initially, a range-finding study is performed using as highest concentration the limit of solubility of the tested chemical (or alternatively a maximum concentration of 1 mg/ml) plus seven additional concentrations separated by a dilution factor of 10. This range-finding experiment allows selection of the relevant concentration range and a final experiment must be further performed using eight different dilutions (with a maximum dilution factor of 1.5). The quality criteria of the experiments require that there must be at least three concentrations within the range of 90 to 10% of control differentiation values and a positive (5-fluoracil) and a negative (penicillin-G) control must be included. For each chemical two independent experiments meeting these quality controls are required, although these two experiments do not necessarily have to use exactly the same concentrations.

As in the case of WEC, the MM also can be considered an alternative model because the number of animals needed is lower than its *in vivo* equivalent OECD Guideline 414 and reduces animal suffering since the exposure is performed in primary cultures and not in the whole animal.

Endpoints of the assay and prediction model

During the prevalidation study performed with six chemicals a discriminate PM was developed using two endpoints, the cytotoxicity and the inhibition of the differentiation of the MM cultures. A further refinement of the PM determined that the concentration that inhibited 50% of cell differentiation to cartilage (ID_{50}) was enough to discriminate among the three categories of embryotoxic potential on the basis of the three lineal functions displayed in Table 11.2 according to the criteria shown in Table 11.3 (Genschow *et al.*, 2000).

TABLE 11.4 Results of the validation study of EST, MM and WEC protocols

	WEC PM1	WEC PM2	MM	EST
Predictivity for non-embryotoxic (%)	56 (insufficient)	70 (sufficient)	57 (insufficient)	72 (sufficient)
Predictivity for weakly embryotoxic (%)	75 (good)	76 (good)	71 (sufficient)	70 (sufficient)
Predictivity for strongly embryotoxic (%)	79 (good)	100 (excellent)	100 (excellent)	100 (excellent)
Precision for non-embryotoxic (%)	70 (sufficient)	80 (good)	80 (good)	70 (sufficient)
Precision for weakly embryotoxic (%)	45 (insufficient)	65 (sufficient)	60 (insufficient)	83 (good)
Precision for strongly embryotoxic (%)	94 (excellent)	100 (excellent)	69 (sufficient)	81 (good)
Total accuracy (%)	**68 (good)**	**80 (good)**	**70 (sufficient)**	**78 (good)**
Assessment	**Rate of correct classifications**			
By chance	=33%			
Insufficient	<65%			
Sufficient	≥65%			
Good	≥75%			
Excellent	≥85%			

Taken from Glenschow *et al.* (2002)

Performance of the MM test

The predictivity of MM for strongly embryotoxic chemicals was 100%; however, predictivity was insufficient (only 57%) and good (71%) for non- and weakly embryotoxic, respectively (Table 11.4). The precision of the MM ranged between 60 and 80% for weakly and non-embryotoxic chemicals, being the accuracy of the method (for all chemicals) of 70% (Table 11.4).

Based on these results the ECVAM Scientific Advisory Committee agreed with the conclusion that the MM test is scientifically validated for identifying strongly embryotoxic chemicals and that it is ready to be considered for regulatory purposes (ESAC, 2002). Therefore, the main difference with the WEC test is that the MM test is suitable for testing only strongly embryotoxic chemicals, while WEC can be used for testing all three categories.

The embryonic stem cell test (EST)

In this method the embryotoxic potential of chemicals is determined by the evaluation of the inhibition of the differentiation of mouse embryonic stem cells belonging to the D3 line and the inhibition of growth of these D3 cells and also of mouse fibroblast belonging to the 3T3 line. As in the case of WEC and MM the EST test is also proposed to be used within the context of the OECD Guideline 414 for testing developmental toxicity (ECVAM, 2006c).

Two permanent cell lines are used in the EST test; D3 cells represent embryonic tissues while adult tissues are represented by 3T3 cells. EST is the only validated embryotoxicity test that totally eliminates the use of animals. D3 cells can be maintained in the undifferentiated stage in the presence of the cytokine leukemia inhibition factor. When released from this leukemia inhibition factor the embryonic stem cells form embryonic bodies and differentiate into the major embryonic cell lineages. This test is based on the determination of the inhibition of the differentiation of the embryonic stem cells and on the differences in the sensitivity between embryonic and adult cells against a cytotoxic insult.

Basic procedure for the differentiation assay

Seven to eight concentrations with a 1.2–3-fold dilution factor covering the relevant range of cytotoxicity must be tested in each experiment. On day 0 a suspension of 37,500 D3 cells/ml is prepared in culture medium (in absence of leukemia inhibition factor and containing the appropriate concentration of the chemical) and 20 μl of this suspension (thus containing 750 D3 cells) is dispensed on the inner side of a 100 mm Petri dish. At least 24 drops per tested concentration must be prepared. The lid is carefully turned into its regular position and put on the top of the Petri dish filled with 5 ml of phosphate buffer saline. These hanging drops are incubated until day 3 when they are gently transferred to a 60 mm Petri dish with 5 ml of culture medium containing freshly prepared tested chemical. On day 5, the embryonic bodies are transferred to a 24-well plate (one embryonic body per well containing 1 ml of fresh medium with the tested chemical in each well). Finally, on day 10 the embryonic bodies should be differentiated into contractile cardiomyocytes and the number of beating embryonic bodies is determined under light microscopy. The assay is acceptable when at least 21 of the 24 control embryonic bodies are beating after the differentiation period; the negative control (1 mg penicillin/ml) has been differentiated in the same proportion as the controls; and a concentration of 5-fluoracil (the positive control) between 48 and 60 ng/ml is able to inhibit 50% of the differentiation. At least two independent experiments meeting these quality criteria must be run to validate the results.

Basic procedure for the cytotoxicity assay

The cytotoxicity of D3 and 3T3 cells must be initially assayed in a range-finding study covering from the highest soluble concentration plus a series of eight dilutions each with a factor of 10. The main experiment is performed with seven concentrations covering the relevant range of doses determined in the range-finding experiment. The experiment starts seeding 500 D3 or 3T3 cells on 96-well plates with medium without leukemia inhibition factor and with the appropriate concentration of the tested chemical. The seeded cells are incubated during 10 days with changing of medium at the same points that the differentiation test (days 3 and 5). The viability of the exposed cells is tested on day 10 with the MTT (thiazolyl blue formazan) assay. MTT is based on the colorimetric determination of formazan formed in the mitochondria using MTT as substrate. The amount of formed formazan directly relates with the amount of viable cells there is in the medium, which is a reflection of both mitochondrial integrity and the level of functionality of the mitochondrial dehydrogenases (Borenfreud *et al.*, 1988). At least two independent assays might be performed meeting the following quality criteria: (1) concentration of 5-fluoracil (positive control) exhibits a capability to cause 50% of cytotoxicity ranging between 48–86 ng/ml and 120–500 ng/ml for D3 and 3T3 cells, respectively; (2) the negative control (1 mg penicillin-G/ml) does not affect the viability of the cells (neither D3 nor 3T3).

Endpoints of the assay and prediction model

Three different endpoints were needed to build the three different discriminating functions shown in Table 11.2. These endpoints are (Genschow *et al.*, 2000): ID_{50} as the concentration with the capability to inhibit 50% of the differentiation of D3 cells into beating cardiomyocytes; and $IC_{50\,D3}$ and $IC_{50\,3T3}$ as the concentrations with the capability to reduce to 50% the viability of D3 and 3T3 cells in MTT assay, respectively. These endpoints allow the discrimination of the embryotoxic potential of the tested chemical according to criteria shown in Table 11.3.

Performance of the EST test

The testing of the 20 test chemicals employed in the EST validation study provided 78% accuracy (correct classifications) (Table 11.4) (Genschow *et al.*, 2004). The highest precisions were detected for weak and strong embryotoxic chemicals, which were correctly detected in 83% and 81% of the cases, respectively (Table 11.4). The poorest precision was recorded for detection of non-embryotoxic compounds (70%) (Table 11.4). Finally, the predictivity for strongly embryotoxic chemicals was, as for MM and WEC, 100%, while predictivity for non- and weakly embryotoxic compounds was similar (70 and 72%, respectively) (Table 11.4).

TABLE 11.5 Characteristics of the main embryotoxicity–teratogenicity assays

Assay	Biological tissue	Type of assay	Time of exposure (days)	Technical difficulty	Biotransformation	Animal (mammals) sacrifice	Morphological alterations determination	Throughput capability
EST	Mouse	Cellular assay	10	Medium	NO	NO	NO	High
WEC	Mouse or rat	Whole embryo	2	High	NO	YES	YES	Poor
MM	Rats	Fragment of embryo (cellular assay)	5	Low	NO	YES	NO	Very high
FETAX	Frog	Whole embryo	4	Medium	YES	NO	YES	Medium
Zebrafish	Fish	Whole embryo	2–5	Medium	YES	NO	YES	Medium

The ECVAM Scientific Advisory Committee agreed that EST is a scientifically validated test applicable to testing a diverse group of chemicals of different embryotoxic potentials (ESAC, 2002). EST is also ready to be considered for regulatory purposes since the results obtained in the validation study were highly reproducible and the correlations between *in vivo* and *in vitro* data were good (ESAC, 2002).

Improvements for the EST test

Various studies have proposed improvements for the performance of the EST method. Some of these proposals are: (1) the use of *in vitro* data combined with pharmacokinetic studies (Verwei *et al.*, 2006); (2) the optimization of the culture protocols for D3 cells (De Smedt *et al.*, 2008; Marx-Stoelting *et al.*, 2009); (3) the use of automated image processing systems (Paparella *et al.*, 2002; Peters *et al.*, 2008); (4) the quantification of the differentiation by the expression of the actin and heavy myosin chain genes (Seiler *et al.*, 2004); (5) to split cellular differentiation from cellular proliferation (van Dartel *et al.*, 2009); (6) the quantification of endothelial cell-induced differentiation by means of specific marker genes of this particular lineage (Festag *et al.*, 2007); (7) the quantification of cell differentiation using flux cytometry (Buesen *et al.*, 2009); (8) the substitution of D3 cells for other mouse embryonic stem cells (Marx-Stoelting *et al.*, 2009); (9) substitution of MTT test for other viability tests (Marx-Stoelting *et al.*, 2009); (10) generation of embryonic bodies either by horizontal shaker or in suspension instead of hanging drops (Marx-Stoelting *et al.*, 2009); (11) to reduce to 2 (yes/no) the embryotoxicity categories (Marx-Stoelting *et al.*, 2009); (12) to employ a protocol of sequential differentiation of embryonic stem cells starting in the heart and passing through neurons, bone and finishing in cartilage (Marx-Stoelting *et al.*, 2009); (13) use of transcriptomics (van Dartel *et al.*, 2010a); (14) a reduction of the exposure time combined with the use of transcriptomics (van Dartel *et al.*, 2010b). Finally, the adaptation of the protocol to human embryonic stem cell lines has been also proposed (Adler *et al.*, 2008; Stummann *et al.*, 2009).

Main advantages and disadvantages of the three validated methods

Table 11.5 displays a comparison among the main characteristics of EST, MM and WEC. The two main limitations common to all three methods are the absence of metabolic competence and their incapability to detect teratogenic chemicals with mechanisms acting beyond the initial embryo differentiation steps. The three methods require different levels of technical difficulties, being WEC, the most demanding method, since it manages the highest number of endpoints and requires staff trained in the identification and quantification of the specific embryo malformations displayed in Table 11.1. These technical requirements make the WEC test the less appropriate for massive high throughput screening processes. EST is the method with an intermediate level of technical difficulty because it requires two endpoints and cultures of two different cell lines, while MM requires a single endpoint with only one cell primary culture. It is also remarkable that EST is the only method that does not need the sacrifice of pregnant animals, and WEC is the only method which yields information about the morphological alterations caused by the teratogen.

Optimization of the predictivity of the validated tests

ECVAM has issued certain recommendations in order to overcome some of the above listed limitations. These recommendations include (Spielman *et al.*, 2006):

1. To develop a metabolically competent *in vitro* system to be integrated into the three methods;
2. To integrate protocols for the differentiation of ESC into specific lineages because the current approach (differentiation to beating cardiomyocytes coming from the mesoderm) might not detect embryotoxicity exerted in other cellular lineages as endoderm or ectoderm;
3. To develop additional PM for specific purposes or compound classes;
4. To use more quantitative endpoints for the EST as the use of tissue-specific gene expression markers, immunohistochemical methods or flow cytometry (these approaches would improve the quantification of the alterations in the differentiation regarding the current method based on the simple examination of the beating cardiomyocytes);
5. To create mathematic and pharmacokinetics models to correlate the effective concentrations of test chemicals in the *in vitro* test with the effective concentrations in maternal serum; and
6. To develop and integrate an *in vitro* model for considering the role of the placenta.

Possible future uses for validated embryotoxicity test

On the one hand, the successful improvement of the methods could allow them to be used for regulatory purposes and then a positive result would allow a chemical to be classified as toxic to reproduction without the necessity of animal assays. On the other hand, a negative result with the same method would not rule out the necessity of assays with animals, but would allow these assays to be more directed and therefore would reduce the number of animals employed in the assay.

NON-VALIDATED ALTERNATIVE MODELS FOR TESTING DEVELOPMENTAL TOXICOLOGY

Frog Embryo Teratogenesis Assay (FETAX)

Organogenesis is a process highly conserved in the phylogenetic scale and therefore amphibians can be used as models for testing this process in mammalians. In addition to that, amphibian embryos are very sensitive to chemicals, easily handled in the laboratory and the availability of embryos is not seasonal because ovulation can be induced with chorionic gonadotropin. All these reasons make frog embryos ideal models for testing alterations in the development of vertebrates. Specifically, the first 96 hours of embryonic development in *Xenopus laevis* parallel many of the major processes of human organogenesis (NICEATM, 2000). Nevertheless, other authors suggest that other species of *Xenopus* as *Xenopus tropicalis* can also be effectively used (Fort *et al.*, 2004).

The endpoints for the FETAX assay are (NICEATM, 2000): (1) mortality, expressed as the concentration that causes 50% mortality (LC_{50}); (2) malformations, evaluated and recorded according to the *Atlas of Abnormalities* (Bantle *et al.*, 1998) and expressed as the concentration that causes malformations in 50% of embryos (EC_{50}); (3) grown, estimated as the distance between head and tail; (4) teratogenic index, estimated as the ratio between LC_{50} and EC_{50}; and (5) minimum concentration to inhibit growth. A chemical ranked with a teratogenic index greater than 1.5 is an ideal candidate to be teratogenic in the absence of significant mortality. In the same way, teratogenic hazard is considered to be present when either growth is significantly inhibited at concentrations below 30% of LC_{50} or when the ratio between minimum concentration to inhibit growth and LC_{50} is lower than 0.30.

Seven different concentrations must be assessed in each assay. For each dose group, two dishes containing 25 embryos in 10 ml of test solution are used. Control condition is assayed with four dishes of 25 embryos. The exposure takes place at 24±2°C during 96 h (or until 90% of control embryos reach stage 46 of development). Frog embryos lack metabolic competence and in order to cover this gap the assays are run in two conditions, in absence and in presence of a metabolic activation system (rat liver microsomes and NADPH-generating system). The positive control without metabolic activation is run with 6-aminonicotinamide, which should yield a teratogenic index of around 446; while the positive control with metabolic activation is run with cyclophosphamide, which should cause 100% mortality of embryos after 96 h of exposure to 4 mg/ml. One of the main quality requirements to consider in a valid assay is that mortality and mean of malformations in control embryos should be both lower than 10%.

Several studies of validation for FETAX assays have been run with promising results (Bantle *et al.*, 1996, 1999; Fort *et al.*, 1998, 2000). Nevertheless, the US Environmental Protection Agency (US EPA) asked the Interagency Coordinating Committee on the Validation of Alternative Methods (ICCVAM) to evaluate the FETAX test. In 2000, an expert scientific panel concluded that FETAX is not sufficiently validated or optimized for regulatory use (Minutes..., 2000). Nevertheless and despite this consideration, FETAX is an assay of proven scientific validity and is widely used for identification of hazards to human and environmental health (for recent examples see Bacchetta *et al.*, 2008; Bosisio *et al.*, 2009; Longo *et al.*, 2008).

Developmental toxicity assays with zebrafish

The teleost zebrafish (*Danio rerio*) is a well-known organism frequently used in general and developmental toxicology (Froehlicher *et al.*, 2009), neurotoxicology (Anichtchik *et al.*, 2004; Bretaud *et al.*, 2004; Linney *et al.*, 2004) and also in other basic sciences such as embryology (Ticho *et al.*, 1996). The small size, cheap maintenance, easy conditions for breeding, high nativity rate (a single female can lay up to 400 eggs per week (Laale, 1977)), they spawn throughout the year under laboratory conditions, the transparency of its embryos and the fact they develop outside the mother make zebrafish an excellent model for research (Yang *et al.*, 2009).

The zebrafish was widely introduced into laboratories as a model to study development (Maves and Kimmel, 2005) and neurobiology (Froehlicher *et al.*, 2009) between the end of the 1980s and the start of the 1990s. In a short period of time, the increase of the genetic techniques along with the advantages of this model placed the zebrafish in an ideal position as a model organism for drug target discovery, target validation, drug-finding strategies and toxicological studies (Langheinrich, 2003).

The stages of embryonic development of zebrafish were described in detail more than 30 years ago. These stages highlight the changes of the major developmental processes that occur faster (during the first 3 days after fertilization) in zebrafish than in mammalians. The knowledge regarding zebrafish embryonic development stages together with the availability of its genetic sequence and of a large number of mutants and transgenic lines provides this model with a number of experimental possibilities (Yang *et al.*, 2009).

Zebrafish embryonic development

The development of the embryo in zebrafish is particularly fast. The stages of embryonic development of *Danio rerio* are divided in seven periods (Figure 11.2): the zygote, cleavage, blastula, gastrula, segmentation, pharyngula and hatching periods. The zygote is formed immediately after union of female with male gametes. Cleavage is produced between 45 minutes and 2 hours and consists of a series of mitotic cell differentiation that produces the blastula. The formation of the blastula is produced between 2 and 4 hours and is a hollow structure consisting of a single layer of cells. Gastrula is produced around 10 hours after fertilization and consists of the migration of the cells forming different structures that result in the formation of the three primary germ layers, ectoderm, endoderm and mesoderm. Segmentation is a morphogenetic process where the somites develop and start to be patent the rudiments of the primary organs, the tail bud becomes more prominent and the embryo of zebrafish elongates. The formation of pharyngula starts at 24 hours after fertilization and takes another 24 hours. In this stage all vertebrate embryos show important similitude. However, at this moment the notochord and post-anal tail are developed, along with rapid cerebellar morphogenesis of the metencephalon. Hatching is a period between 48 and 72 hours after fertilization and consists of the formation of the primary organ system, rudiments of the pectoral fins, the jaws and the gills (Kimmel *et al.*, 1995).

The effect produced for the exposition of different chemicals or drugs can be divided into six different phenomena (angiogenesis, hemostasis, apoptosis and proliferation, lipid metabolism, inflammation and neural tolerance) (Langheinrich, 2003).

Advantages of zebrafish endpoints

Zebrafish eggs have the property to remain transparent until 72 hours after fertilization; this allows a better study of embryonic development until the moment when the tissues become denser and pigmentation starts. There are techniques that eliminate some of this pigment, for example use of phenylthiourea or beaching after fixation (Hill *et al.*, 2005). Another major advantage of zebrafish embryos is that they have very high survivability, and are able to survive long periods despite their lack of certain organs, severe dysfunction or some other kind of abnormality, which allows embryologic changes to be observed at very high concentrations without death of the embryo. Another advantage of this model is that it has been demonstrated that zebrafish possess more than 80% of orthologs of human drug targets (Gunnarsson *et al.*, 2008).

Dario rerio embryotoxicity test (DarT)

DarT is based on the study of the effects on embryos as a consequence of their exposure to the tested chemical for 48 h. DarT is considered an *in vitro* test and is accepted as an alternative method to animal experimentation. Twenty embryos per concentration are incubated during 48 hours after fertilization in a 24-well plate with a 12 hour light–dark cycle. After 48 hours of exposure different parameters are analyzed: size of the eggs, position of the eye and the sacculi/otoliths, pigmentation, the tail not detached and the frequency of spontaneous movements (Busquet *et al.*, 2008). A positive control of 3,4-dichloroaniline is run in parallel with the test compound since the effect of this compound on embryo zebrafish development is well known (Nagel *et al.*, 1991).

Variants about the DarT

Certain studies show that teratogenic effects are due to the biotransformation of the chemical in the mother instead of the parental chemical itself (Fantel, 1982; Webster *et al.*, 1997).

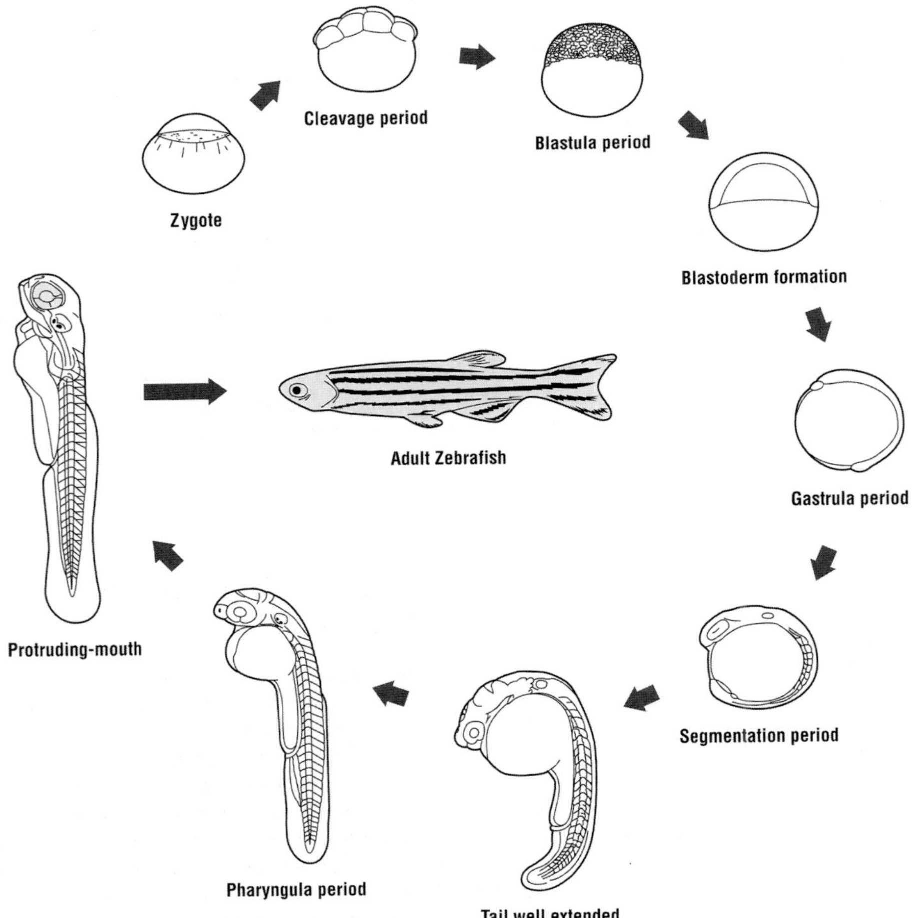

FIGURE 11.2 Embryological stages of zebrafish.

Therefore, the use of a metabolic activation system, such as S9-mix, microsomes, hepatocytes, etc., has been proposed coupled with whole embryo systems (Fantel, 1982). Certain studies try to employ this exogenous metabolic activation with DarT (Busquet *et al.*, 2008; Weigt *et al.*, 2008).

One different approach to DarT is called Gene-*Dar*T (gene expression *Danio rerio* embryo test). This method allows the identification of the teratogenic mechanisms through the analysis of changes in expression of different genes using a 14k zebrafish oligonucleotide microarray.

The model MolDart uses the detection of changes in the expression of specific target genes after 120 hours of exposure (Liedtke *et al.*, 2008). This test system uses developing zebrafish and detects changes in mRNA abundance of selected target genes after exposure for 5 days. The aim of this test system is to allow the detection of multiple effects using biomarker analysis. Feasibility of this assay for detection of estrogenic effects by vitellogenin 1 mRNA induction has been demonstrated (Muncke and Eggen, 2006; Muncke *et al.*, 2007).

The mechanosensory lateral line zebrafish test is normally used in neurotoxicity and yields a very clear idea about the effects of the exposure to chemicals in embryonic development. This method consists of the study of mechanoreceptors found in an interconnected network between head and body. In recent years a large number of genes related to these sensory cells have been reported (Li *et al.*, 2010), which allows the early detection of dysfunctions and problems using molecular approaches. This method may serve as a test for detecting chemicals with effects in the development of neurosensory function, and detection of variations in gene expression can further be used to discern different mechanisms of action of toxic compounds.

Validated versus non-validated models: a comparison

Table 11.5 displays a comparison among the main characteristics of the three validated models (EST, MM and WEC) and non-validated models (FETAX and zebrafish). FETAX and zebrafish are methods that use, as is the case with WEC, a whole embryo and therefore also both allow the identification of the specific malformation caused by exposure to the tested chemical. However, animal models used in FETAX and zebrafish are not mammals and, as in the case of EST, these methods can be considered to suppress the use of superior animals. In close and inverse relationship with the complexity of the animal model is the fact that the number of endpoints to analyze and score (and consequently also the technical difficulty) is lower in FETAX and zebrafish assays than in WEC. FETAX and zebrafish include the possibility of being coupled with an exogenous metabolization source, which is not considered in EST, MM and WEC.

Developmental toxicity assays with cell lines

The cell lines are easy to manipulate in the laboratory, can be stored for long periods of time, and the economical costs of assays performed with cells are lower than those performed with animals. This favors the possibility of developing a battery of tests with different cell lines to mimic the different stages of vertebrate development and testing the effect of chemicals in each of these stages.

Developmental toxicity assays with stem cells

Developmental toxicity assays with stem cells display a prominent position within the available battery of cellular assays since some studies have demonstrated that stem cells can be used to illuminate the processes underlying organogenesis, as has been shown in the case of the heart (Miller *et al.*, 2008). Therefore, the study of the interferences in stem cell differentiation caused by chemicals can be used to detect potential developmental toxicants. An additional advantage of these models is that the genetic molecular approaches allow for an exhaustive analysis of which genes are affected by each substance and subsequently research into the mechanisms of action underlying the teratogenic or embryotoxic effects caused by the assessed chemical.

The Adherent Cell Differentiation and Cytotoxicity (ACDC) assay is a test that establishes a model system that would evaluate the chemical effect using a single cell culture (instead of two as the EST) in order to improve the feasibilities for throughput assays (Barrier *et al.*, 2010). ACDC assay uses quantitative markers for differentiation degree and for cell proliferation. In this assay, pluripotent J1 mouse embryonic stem cells are plated in a 96 multiwell plate and further cultured in differentiation medium for 9 days. After that, each well is assessed for cell number and differentiation to cardiomyocytes (using quantitative in-cell Western analysis for myosin heavy chain protein normalized with cell number). This method has already proved its suitability testing the effects of haloacetic acids and their major metabolites (Jeffay *et al.*, 2010).

The most developed method for testing embryotoxicity using stem cells is the EST method, which was presented and discussed in detail together with a number of proposals for improving its performance elsewhere in this chapter and therefore is not further discussed here.

Developmental toxicity assays with other (non-stem) cell lines

Other cell lines have been used to assess the effect of chemicals on development. Cell lines such as the embryonic carcinoma cells have been used for detecting chemicals that affect embryonic development of specific processes such as neural tube development (Jergil *et al.*, 2009). Other lines such as mouse fibroblastoid L929 have also been used for detecting changes in morphology and proliferation (Walmod *et al.*, 2004).

Developmental toxicity assays with embryo fragments

The use of whole embryos has been already commented on (see sections devoted to the use of rat (WEC), frog (FETAX) and zebrafish (DarT) embryos for testing developmental toxicity) in former sections of this chapter. Another approach to the use of embryos is the use of only certain parts of these embryos. The main inconvenience of these methods is that they do not totally avoid the use of animals and that the technical skills needed for staff involved in the assays should be higher than for methods employing cell cultures. Various *in vitro* systems have been developed using parts of embryos, as is the case of cells derived from embryo rodent midbrain and limb buds (see MM method in another section) (Cicurel and Schmid, 1988; Flint and Orton, 1984). Other methods related to the development of fetal maxillary have shown good capacity to detect changes in normal development of the rodent maxillary fetus region cultured *in vitro* (Kosazuma *et al.*, 2004; Mino *et al.*, 1994; Shiota *et al.*, 1990). Although most studies on this topic are performed on rats, there are other approaches in other animals, such as rabbits (Carney *et al.*, 2008) and mice (Hunter *et al.*, 2006).

In silico methods for testing developmental toxicity

The complexity of the reproductive process makes delicate the development of reliable *in silico* methods for predicting toxicity to embryonic development. Despite these considerations, several methods based on mathematical approaches have been proposed as alternatives to animal experimentation for testing developmental toxicity (Hewitt *et al.*, 2009).

With exception of quantitative structure activity relationships (QSAR) for the variables related to endocrine disruption, and in particular with the estrogen and androgen receptor (Cronin and Worth, 2008), the number of available *in silico* methods for testing toxicity to development is lower than for testing other areas of toxicology. There are a number of reasons for the lack of progress in the development of QSAR for reproductive and developmental toxicology. These include: (1) a perceived lack of high quality toxicity data needed for modeling; (2) the lack of knowledge of modes and mechanisms of action that is required for modeling; (3) the appreciation that reproductive toxicity is a composite effect comprising a number of endpoints, some of them with very specific mechanisms; (4) a perceived difficulty in modeling reproductive toxicology due to a combination of the previous three points; and (5) the QSAR and modeling community has possibly not viewed reproductive toxicity as an area of concern or interest because there are no readily available databases for modeling such as there are in other areas of human and environmental toxicology (Cronin and Worth, 2008). In the next paragraphs we summarize some of the available *in silico* methods for predicting toxicity to reproduction.

The CAESAR developmental toxicity model

The CAESAR (Computer Assisted Evaluation of industrial chemical Substances According to Regulations) developmental toxicity model is based on the next four points: skin sensitization, mutagenicity, carcinogenicity and toxicity to development. The developmental toxicity CAESAR model uses a QSAR model which includes 292 substances classified according to risk factors for the FDA with 13 different descriptors (Benfenati *et al.*, 2009; Kirchmair *et al.*, 2007; Novic and Vracko, 2010). This model is available in a Java-based web application found at http://www.caesar-project.eu

Super-endpoint reproductive toxicity

This is the set of knowledge generated for over 15 years by numerous scientists working on this project (Marchant *et al.*, 2008; White *et al.*, 2003). This system is designed to predict carcinogenicity, mutagenicity, genotoxicity, skin sensitization, teratogenicity, irritation, respiratory sensitization, hepatotoxicity, chromosome damage and ocular toxicity. This predictive system is based on the analysis of the molecular structures of substances and uses a series of algorithms to correlate the structure and the hypothetical mechanism of action of each substance to study. More information about this system is available at https://www.lhasalimited.org/derek/general_information

Toxmatch

Toxmatch is a model designed to find similarities between substances according to chemical structure, and is based on the codification of the substances according to a series of indices of similarity. Some of the parameters used by Toxmatch are the octanol–water partition coefficient, molecular weight, ionization potential, maximum diameter, minimum diameter, molecular surface area, etc. Toxmatch has been developed by the European Commission and is available free at http://ecb.jrc.ec.europa.eu/qsar/qsar-tools/index.php?c=TOXMATCH

COREPA

COREPA software has been developed and commercially distributed by the Laboratory of Mathematical Chemistry of the Bourgas University (Bulgaria). The discrimination parameters used by this method are placed in groups that are considered to have endpoints or similar activities. A detailed Bayesian tree is further used to classify the substances according to their toxic potential (Mekenyan *et al.*, 2003; Serafimova *et al.*, 2007).

CONCLUDING REMARKS AND FUTURE DIRECTIONS

Embryonic development is a very complex process which includes a number of coordinated complex processes in several stages. The alteration of whatever of these processes due to the action of chemicals might potentially suppose an embryotoxic–teratogenic effect. Due to the complexity of the embryonic development the whole process cannot be covered with a single alternative *in vitro* model and therefore the toxicity to development must be studied with a battery of assays covering each of the stages of embryonic development.

To date only three *in vitro* methods (MM, EST and WEC) have been validated by an international agency (ECVAM) in order to be used for testing the embryotoxicity potential of chemicals, although other models such as FETAX and zebrafish have also proved their validity for this purpose. Methods based on the employment of embryos allow the specific malformation expected after exposure to the chemical to be determined, while methods based on cellular systems are more relevant in order to determine the mechanism underlying the adverse observed effect and still display a wide field for improving their prediction capability. *In silico* methods for testing developmental toxicity need further development and improvement although the information obtained through these methods might be used to support other information obtained using embryos or cellular systems.

In conclusion, the analysis and integration of all information collected with this battery of embryotoxicity–teratogenicity assays might be very relevant for risk assessment of chemicals and for their classification and labeling with a strong reduction and refinement in the number of vertebrate animals employed for these purposes in the corresponding *in vivo* assays, although strong efforts are still needed to improve the prediction capability of these testing models.

REFERENCES

Adler S, Lindqvist J, Uddenberg K, Hyllner J, Strehl R (2008) Testing potential developmental toxicants with a cytotoxicity assay based on human embryonic stem cells. *Altern Lab Anim* **36:** 129–40.

Anichtchik OV, Kaslin J, Peitsaro N, Scheinin M, Panula P (2004) Neurochemical and behavioural changes in zebrafish Danio rerio after systemic administration of 6-hydroxydopamine and 1-methyl-4-phenyl-1,2,3,6-tetrahydropyridine. *J Neurochem* **88:** 443–53.

Bacchetta R, Mantecca P, Andrioletti M, Vismara C, Vailati G (2008) Axial-skeletal defects caused by Carbaryl in Xenopus laevis embryos. *Sci Total Environ* **392:** 110–18.

Bantle JA, Dumont JN, Finch RA, Linder G, Fort DJ (1998) *Atlas of Abnormalities: A Guide for the Performance of FETAX*. Oklahoma State University Press (2nd ed.).

Bantle JA, Finch RA, Burton DT, Fort DJ, Dawson DA, Linder G, Rayburn JR, Hull M, Kumsher-King M, Gaudet-Hull AM, Turley SD (1996) FETAX interlaboratory validation study: phase III – Part 1 testing. *J Appl Toxicol* **16:** 517–28.

Barrier M, Jeffay S, Nichols H, Hunter S (2010) Evaluation of a mouse embryonic stem cell adherent cell differentiation and cytotoxicity (ACDC) assay. *The Toxicologist* **114:** 358–9.

Benfenati E, Benigni R, Demarini DM, Helma C, Kirkland D, Martin TM, Mazzatorta P, Ouédraogo-Arras G, Richard AM, Schilter B, Schoonen WG, Snyder RD, Yang C (2009) Predictive models for carcinogenicity and mutagenicity: frameworks, state-of-the-art, and perspectives. *J Environ Sci Health C Environ Carcinog Ecotoxicol Rev* **27:** 57–90.

Borenfreund E, Babich H, Martin-Aguacil N (1988) Comparisons of two in vitro cytotoxicity assays – the neutral red (NR) and tetrazolium MTT tests. *Toxicol in Vitro* **2:** 1–6.

Bosisio S, Fortaner S, Bellinetto S, Farina M, Del Torchio R, Prati M, Gornati R, Bernardini G, Sabbioni E (2009) Developmental toxicity, uptake and distribution of sodium chromate assayed by frog embryo teratogenesis assay-Xenopus (FETAX). *Sci Total Environ* **407:** 5039–45.

Bretaud S, Lee S, Guo S (2004) Sensitivity of zebrafish to environmental toxins implicated in Parkinson's disease. *Neurotoxicol Teratol* **26:** 857–64.

Buesen R, Genschow E, Slawik B, Visan A, Spielmann H, Luch A, Seiler A (2009) Embryonic stem cell test remastered: comparison between the validated EST and the new molecular FACS-EST for assessing developmental toxicity in vitro. *Toxicol Sci* **108:** 389–400.

Busquet F, Nagel R, von Landenberg F, Mueller SO, Huebler N, Broschard TH (2008) Development of a new screening assay to identify proteratogenic substances using zebrafish Danio rerio embryo combined with an exogenous mammalian metabolic activation system (mDarT). *Toxicol Sci* **104:** 177–188. Epub 2008 Mar 28.

Carney EW, Tornesi B, Markham DA, Rasoulpour RJ, Moore N (2008) Species-specificity of ethylene glycol-induced developmental toxicity: toxicokinetic and whole embryo culture studies in the rabbit. *Birth Defects Res B Dev Reprod Toxicol* **83:** 573–81.

Cicurel L, Schmid BP (1988) Postimplantation embryo culture for the assessment of the teratogenic potential and potency of compounds. *Experientia* **44:** 833–40.

Cronin MTD, Worth AP (2008) (Q)SARs for predicting effects relating to reproductive toxicity. *Qsar & Combinatorial Science* **27:** 91–100.

De Smedt A, Steemans M, De Boeck M, Peters AK, van der Leede BJ, Van Goethem F, Lampo A, Vanparys P (2008) Optimisation of the cell cultivation methods in the embryonic stem cell test results in an increased differentiation potential of the cells into strong beating myocard cells. *Toxicol in Vitro* **22:** 1789–96.

ECVAM (European Centre for Validation of Alternative Methods) (2006a) Embryotoxicity Testing in Post-Implantation Embryo Culture – Method of Piersma. Available at: http://ecvam.jrc.ec.europa.eu/

ECVAM (European Centre for Validation of Alternative Methods) (2006b) The Micromass Test – Method of Brown. Available at: http://ecvam.jrc.ec.europa.eu/

ECVAM (European Centre for Validation of Alternative Methods) (2006c) EmbryonicStemCellTest(EST).Availableat:http://ecvam.jrc.ec.europa.eu/

ESAC (European Centre for Validation of Alternative Methods (ECVAM) Scientific Advisory Committee) (2002) The Use of Scientifically-Validated *in Vitro* Tests for Embryotoxicity. Available at: http://ecvam.jrc.ec.europa.eu/

Fantel AG (1982) Culture of whole rodent embryos in teratogen screening. *Teratog Carcinog Mutagen* **2:** 231–42.

Festag M, Viertel B, Steinberg P, Sehner C (2007) An *in vitro* embryotoxicity assay based on the disturbance of the differentiation of murine embryonic stem cells into endothelial cells. II. Testing of compounds. *Toxicol in Vitro* **21:** 1631–40.

Fleischer M (2004) Testing costs and testing capacity according to the REACH requirements – results of a survey of independent and corporate GLP laboratories in the EU and Switzerland. *J Bus Chem* **4:** 96–114.

Flint OP, Orton TC (1984) An in vitro assay for teratogens with cultures of rat embryo midbrain and limb bud cells. *Toxicol Appl Pharmacol* **76:** 383–95.

Fort DJ, Stover EL, Bantle JA, Rayburn JR, Hull MA, Finch RA, Burton DT, Turley SD, Dawson DA, Linder G, Buchwalter D, Dumont JN, Kumsher-King M, Gaudet-Hull AM (1998) Phase III interlaboratory study of FETAX, Part 2: interlaboratory validation of an exogenous metabolic activation system for frog embryo teratogenesis assay-Xenopus (FETAX). *Drug Chem Toxicol* **21:** 1–14.

Fort DJ, Stover EL, Farmer DR, Lemen JK (2000) Assessing the predictive validity of frog embryo teratogenesis assay-Xenopus (FETAX). *Teratog Carcinog Mutagen* **20:** 87–98.

Fort DJ, Rogers RL, Thomas JH, Buzzard BO, Noll AM, Spaulding CD (2004) Comparative sensitivity of Xenopus tropicalis and Xenopus laevis as test species for the FETAX model. *J Appl Toxicol* **24:** 443–57.

Froehlicher M, Liedtke A, Groh KJ, Neuhauss SC, Segner H, Eggen RI (2009) Zebrafish (Danio rerio) neuromast: promising biological endpoint linking developmental and toxicological studies. *Aquat Toxicol* **95:** 307–19.

Genschow E, Scholz G, Brown N, Piersma A, Brady M, Clemann N, Huuskonen H, Paillard F, Bremer S, Becker K, Spielmann H (2000) Development of prediction models for three in vitro embryotoxicity tests in an ECVAM validation study. *In Vitro Mol Toxicol* **13:** 51–66.

Genschow E, Spielmann H, Scholz G, Pohl I, Seiler A, Clemann N, Bremer S, Becker K (2004) Validation of the embryonic stem cell test in the international ECVAM validation study on three in vitro embryotoxicity tests. *Altern Lab Anim* **32:** 209–44.

Genschow E, Spielmann H, Scholz G, Seiler A, Brown N, Piersma A, Brady M, Clemann N, Huuskonen H, Paillard F, Bremer S, Becker K (2002) The ECVAM international validation study on in vitro embryotoxicity tests: results of the definitive phase and evaluation of prediction models. European Centre for the Validation of Alternative Methods. *Altern Lab Anim* **30:** 151–76.

Gunnarsson L, Jauhiainen A, Kristiansson E, Nerman O, Larsson DG (2008) Evolutionary conservation of human drug targets in organisms used for environmental risk assessments. *Environ Sci Technol* **42:** 5807–13.

Hewitt M, Ellison CM, Enoch SJ, Madden JC, Cronin MT (2009) Integrating (Q)SAR models, expert systems and read-across approaches for the prediction of developmental toxicity. *Reprod Toxicol* **30:** 147–60.

Hill AJ, Teraoka H, Heideman W, Peterson RE (2005) Zebrafish as a model vertebrate for investigating chemical toxicity. *Toxicol Sci* **86:** 6–19.

Höfer T, Gerner I, Gundert-Remy U, Liebsch M, Schulte A, Spielmann H, Vogel R, Wettig K (2004) Animal testing and alternative approaches for the human health risk assessment under the proposed new European chemicals regulation. *Arch Toxicol* **78:** 549–64.

Hunter ES 3rd, Blanton MR, Rogers EH, Leonard Mole M, Andrews J, Chernoff N (2006) Short-term exposures to dihaloacetic acids produce dysmorphogenesis in mouse conceptuses in vitro. *Reprod Toxicol* **22:** 443–8.

Jeffay S, Nichols H, Barrier M, Hunter S (2010) Effects of haloacetic acids and their major metabolites in a mouse embryonic stem cell adherent cell differentiation and cytotoxicity (ACDC) assay. *The Toxicologist* **114:** 359.

Jergil M, Kultima K, Gustafson AL, Dencker L, Stigson M (2009) Valproic acid-induced deregulation in vitro of genes associated in vivo with neural tube defects. *Toxicol Sci* **108:** 132–48.

Kimmel CB, Ballard WW, Kimmel SR, Ullmann B, Schilling TF (1995) Stages of embryonic development of the zebrafish.*Dev Dyn* **203:** 253–310.

Kirchmair J, Ristic S, Eder K, Markt P, Wolber G, Laggner C, Langer T (2007) Fast and efficient in silico 3D screening: toward maximum computational efficiency of pharmacophore-based and shape-based approaches. *J Chem Inf Model* **47:** 2182–96.

Kosazuma T, Hashimoto S, Ohno H, Chou MJ, Shiota K (2004) Organ culture of the fetal mouse palate for screening the developmental toxicity of chemicals: a validation study. *Congenit Anom (Kyoto)* **44:** 60–71.

Laale HW (1977) Biology and use of zebrafish, brachydanio-rerio in fisheries research. *J Fish Biol* **10:** 121–73.

Langheinrich U (2003) Zebrafish: a new model on the pharmaceutical catwalk. *Bioessays* **25:** 904–12.

Li H, Kloosterman W, Fekete DM (2010) MicroRNA-183 family members regulate sensorineural fates in the inner ear. *J Neurosci* **30:** 3254–63.

Liedtke A, Muncke J, Rüfenacht K, Eggen RI (2008) Molecular multi-effect screening of environmental pollutants using the MolDarT. *Environ Toxicol* **23:** 59–67.

Linney E, Upchurch L, Donerly S (2004) Zebrafish as a neurotoxicological model. *Neurotoxicol Teratol* **26:** 709–18. Erratum in: *Neurotoxicol Teratol* 2005 **27:** 175.

Longo M, Zanoncelli S, Della Torre P, Rosa F, Giusti A, Colombo P, Brughera M, Mazué G, Olliaro P (2008) Investigations of the effects of the antimalarial drug dihydroartemisinin (DHA) using the Frog Embryo Teratogenesis Assay-Xenopus (FETAX). *Reprod Toxicol* **25:** 433–41.

Marchant CA, Briggs KA, Long A (2008) In silico tools for sharing data and knowledge on toxicity and metabolism: derek for windows, meteor, and vitic. *Toxicol Mech Methods* **18:** 177–87.

Marx-Stoelting P, Adriaens E, Ahr HJ, Bremer S, Garthoff B, Gelbke HP, Piersma A, Pellizzer C, Reuter U, Rogiers V, Schenk B, Schwengberg S, Seiler A, Spielmann H, Steemans M, Stedman DB, Vanparys P, Vericat JA, Verwei M, van der Water F, Weimer M, Schwarz M. (2009) A review of the implementation of the embryonic stem cell test (EST). The report and recommendations of an ECVAM/ReProTect Workshop. *Altern Lab Anim* **37:** 313–28.

Maves L, Kimmel CB (2005) Dynamic and sequential patterning of the zebrafish posterior hindbrain by retinoic acid. *Dev Biol* **285:** 593–605.

Mekenyan O, Dimitrov S, Schmieder P, Veith G (2003) In silico modelling of hazard endpoints: current problems and perspectives. *SAR QSAR Environ Res* **14:** 361–71.

Miller RA, Christoforou N, Pevsner J, McCallion AS, Gearhart JD (2008) Efficient array-based identification of novel cardiac genes through differentiation of mouse ESCs. *PLoS One* **3:** e2176.

Mino Y, Mizusawa H, Shiota K (1994) Effects of anticonvulsant drugs on fetal mouse palates cultured in vitro. *Reprod Toxicol* **8:** 225–30.

Minutes of the Expert Panel Meeting on the Frog Embryo Teratogenesis Assay-Xenopus (FETAX): A Proposed Screening Method for Identifying the Developmental Toxicity Potential of Chemicals and Environmental Samples, May 16–18, 2000. Available at: http://iccvam.niehs.nih.gov/meetings/minutes/fetaxMin.pdf

Muncke J, Eggen RI (2006) Vitellogenin 1 mRNA as an early molecular biomarker for endocrine disruption in developing zebrafish (Danio rerio). *Environ Toxicol Chem* **25:** 2734–41.

Muncke J, Junghans M, Eggen RI (2007) Testing estrogenicity of known and novel (xeno)estrogens in the MolDarT using developing zebrafish (Danio rerio). *Environ Toxicol* **22:** 185–93.

Nagel R, Bresch H, Caspers N, Hansen PD, Markert M, Munk R, Scholz N, ter Höfte BB (1991) Effect of 3,4-dichloroaniline on the early life stages of the zebrafish (Brachydanio rerio): results of a comparative laboratory study. *Ecotoxicol Environ Saf* **21:** 157–64.

NICEATM (National Toxicology Program (NTP) Interagency Center for the Evaluation of Alternative Toxicological Methods) (2000). Background Review Document Frog Embryo Teratogenesis Assay-Xenopus (FETAX) (2000) Available at: http//ecvam.niehs/nih/gov/methods/fetaxdoc/

Novic M, Vracko M (2010) QSAR models for reproductive toxicity and endocrine disruption activity. *Molecules* **15:** 1987–99.

Paparella M, Kolossov E, Fleischmann BK, Hescheler J, Bremer S (2002) The use of quantitative image analysis in the assessment of in vitro embryotoxicity endpoints based on a novel embryonic stem cell clone with endoderm-related GFP expression. *Toxicol in Vitro* **16:** 589–97.

Peters AK, Wouwer GV, Weyn B, Verheyen GR, Vanparys P, Gompel JV (2008) Automated analysis of contractility in the embryonic stem cell test, a novel approach to assess embryotoxicity. *Toxicol in Vitro* **22:** 1948–56.

Rovida C, Hartung T (2009) Re-evaluation of animal numbers and costs for in vivo tests to accomplish REACH legislation requirements for chemicals – a report by the transatlantic think tank for toxicology (t(4)). *ALTEX* **26:** 187–208.

Seiler A, Visan A, Buesen R, Genschow E, Spielmann H (2004) Improvement of an in vitro stem cell assay for developmental toxicity: the use of molecular endpoints in the embryonic stem cell test. *Reprod Toxicol* **18:** 231–40.

Serafimova R, Todorov M, Nedelcheva D, Pavlov T, Akahori Y, Nakai M, Mekenyan O (2007) QSAR and mechanistic interpretation of estrogen receptor binding. *SAR QSAR Environ Res* **18:** 389–421.

Shiota K, Kosazuma T, Klug S, Neubert D (1990) Development of the fetal mouse palate in suspension organ culture. *Acta Anat (Basel)* **137:** 59–64.

Spielmann H (2005) Predicting the risk of developmental toxicity from in vitro assays. *Toxicol Appl Pharmacol* **207(2 Suppl):** 375–80.

Spielmann H, Seiler A, Bremer S, Hareng L, Hartung T, Ahr H, Faustman E, Haas U, Moffat GJ, Nau H, Vanparys P, Piersma A, Sintes JR, Stuart J (2006) The practical application of three validated in vitro embryotoxicity tests. The report and recommendations of an ECVAM/ZEBET workshop (ECVAM workshop 57). *Altern Lab Anim* **34:** 527–38.

Stummann TC, Hareng L, Bremer S (2009) Hazard assessment of methylmercury toxicity to neuronal induction in embryogenesis using human embryonic stem cells. *Toxicology* **257:** 117–26.

Ticho BS, Stainier DY, Fishman MC, Breitbart RE (1996) Three zebrafish MEF2 genes delineate somitic and cardiac muscle development in wild-type and mutant embryos. *Mech Dev* **59:** 205–18.

van Dartel DA, Pennings JL, van Schooten FJ, Piersma AH (2010a) Transcriptomics-based identification of developmental toxicants through their interference with cardiomyocyte differentiation of embryonic stem cells. *Toxicol Appl Pharmacol* **243:** 420–8.

van Dartel DAM, Pennings JLA, de la Fonteyne LJJ, van Herwijnen MH, van Delft JH, van Schooten FJ, Piersma AH (2010b) Monitoring developmental toxicity in the embryonic stem cell test using differential gene expression of differentiation-related genes. *Tox Sci* **16:** 130–9.

van Dartel DA, Zeijen NJ, de la Fonteyne LJ, van Schooten FJ, Piersma AH (2009) Disentangling cellular proliferation and differentiation in the embryonic stem cell test, and its impact on the experimental protocol. *Reprod Toxicol* **28:** 254–61.

Verwei M, van Burgsteden JA, Krul CA, van de Sandt JJ, Freidig AP (2006) Prediction of in vivo embryotoxic effect levels with a combination of in vitro studies and PBPK modelling. *Toxicol Lett* **165:** 79–87.

Walmod PS, Gravemann U, Nau H, Berezin V, Bock E (2004) Discriminative power of an assay for automated in vitro screening of teratogens. *Toxicol in Vitro* **18:** 511–25.

Webster WS, Brown-Woodman PD, Ritchie HE (1997) A review of the contribution of whole embryo culture to the determination of hazard and risk in teratogenicity testing. *Int J Dev Biol* **41:** 329–35.

Weigt S, Busquet F, Landenberg F, Braunbeck T, Huebler N, Broschard TH (2008) Application of human and rat liver microsomes in teratogenicity testing using zebrafish Danio rerio embryos (mDarT). *Toxicol Lett* **180:** S96–7.

White AC, Mueller RA, Gallavan RH, Aaron S, Wilson AG (2003) A multiple in silico program approach for the prediction of mutagenicity from chemical structure. *Mutat Res* **539:** 77–89.

Yang L, Ho NY, Alshut R, Legradi J, Weiss C, Reischl M, Mikut R, Liebel U, Müller F, Strähle U (2009) Zebrafish embryos as models for embryotoxic and teratological effects of chemicals. *Reprod Toxicol* **28:** 245–53.

CHAPTER

12

In vitro embryotoxicity testing

Vadim Popov and Galina Protasova

INTRODUCTION

The presently growing rate of pathologic pregnancy outcomes (pre- and postnatal mortality, spontaneous abortions, congenital developmental abnormalities, functional disorders, mental retardation of children, etc.) is an impact of combined exposure to both exogenous environmental factors of chemical (industrial toxicants, agricultural chemicals, medicines, etc.), physical (radioactive and microwave radiation, light and sound effects, hyper- and hypothermia, etc.) and biological (viral, bacterial or parasitic) origin and endogenous factors of genetic (dominant, recessive, X-chromosome-linked and other mutations) and non-genetic (metabolic disorders, somatic mother's diseases, fetal hypoxia, hyperbilirubinemia, encephalopathy, hydroamnion, placental circulation disorder, etc.) origin. In general, the evidence obtained over the past few decades shows that 2–5% of children have birth defects (BD). In subsequent years, an additional 5–7% of children with BD have been detected, and taking into account children with mental retardation and abnormal behavior, the total number of children with the BD is approximately 10–12% (Swaab and Mirmiran, 1986; Brent, 1987; Fara *et al.*, 1988). However, these figures do not correspond to the entire volume of the actual outcome of pathological pregnancies: this should be added to the high level of prenatal loss (5–7%) and stillbirths (Wilson, 1973; Arima, 1988; Wilcox *et al.*, 1988). Including prenatal losses, the risk of being born with a physically and functionally expressed BD is estimated at 5% (NBDPN, 2008; TERIS, 2010).

Most researchers note a number of reasons for high levels of BD and pre- and postnatal losses, placing particular emphasis on genetic and environmental factors and their combined effects (Wilson, 1973; Bochkov, 1982; Kalter and Warkany, 1983; Brent, 1987; Brown *et al.*, 1995). Brent (1995) and Nelson and Holmes (1986) have analyzed the causes of BD in newborns and found that the share of genetic diseases comprises 10–25%, environmental factors contribute 10% and multifactor unknown effects 65–75%. Clinical observations show that about 9% of diagnosed pregnancies are accompanied by chromosomal disorders, and as a result genetic diseases are revealed in about 1% of newborns.

All kinds of exposures are a serious threat to human reproduction and necessitate comprehensive research and development of methods for revealing, assessing and preventing. Therefore, it should be borne in mind that pathologic pregnancy outcomes are much dependent on occupational and ecological factors. Intensive industrial and agricultural activities have extended the range of contacts of humans and, what is extremely dangerous, women of reproductive age with chemical toxicants. Water, air, soil and foodstuffs containing mixtures of pollutants of unknown composition have transformed, in essence, in multicomponent systems with a definite (indefinite?) toxic (embryotoxic, genotoxic, gonadotoxic) potential. Probably, if exposure to a complex mixture of chemicals in developed industrial and agricultural regions results in a growing rate of unfavorable outcomes of pregnancy, male and female infertility and spermato- and oogenesis pathologies will occur.

Under unfavorable environmental conditions, the task of revealing, assessing and, if possible, predicting the hazard of concrete chemical substances, multicomponent systems and complex exposures on human embryogenesis and genetic apparatus has assumed extreme importance. Successful solution of this task requires maximally full and, at the same time, prompt information. The search for potential inductors of specific diseases, as well as general pathogenic factors responsible for the unfavorable medical ecological situation in one or another region, be they concrete toxicants or multicomponent systems contaminated with xenobiotics, should be performed by an extensive program in terms of various toxicologic–hygienic approaches. At the same time, to assess the reproductive health of a population and its different professional groups requires the application of rapid test systems, which allow potential pathogens to be searched for by multidirectional testing of environmental objects and biosubstrates (blood and its components, tissue fluids, amniotic fluids, etc.) and predicting the potential hazards they pose to the reproductive function of humans, in particular their embryonic development. The aforementioned fact points to the necessity of developing test systems designed to assess the effect of exposure not only to specific chemical substances, but also to a combination of unfavorable factors on human embryogenesis.

IN VITRO MODELS OF EMBRYOTOXICITY TESTING

At present the testing of chemical substances, including drugs, for embryotoxicity (embryolethality, teratogenicity and embryonic growth inhibition) is regulated by international and national guidelines (EPA, 1998, 2000; OECD, 2001; Guidelines

Reproductive and Developmental Toxicology, Edited by Ramesh C. Gupta
ISBN: 978-0-12-382032-7

for the Study of Reproductive of Drugs, 2005) which basically regulate the use of animal testing. This kind of testing is not free of drawbacks, one of which, in particular, is that animal data are hardly extrapolated to human embryogenesis. Analysis of a broad range of animal teratogens (>1,500) and proven human teratogens (about 40) (Shepard and Lemire, 2004) data obtained in animal experiments is hardly appropriate to meet the declared goal of testing, specifically hazard (safety) assessment of toxicants for human embryogenesis. At the same time, there is no doubt that animal data contribute much to the understanding of mechanisms underlying the embryopathogenic effect of test substances.

There has been a tendency over the past decades to replace or complement the standard procedure of embryotoxicity testing of chemicals on pregnant animals by rapid *in vitro* test systems on the basis of cell cultures. This trend was inspired by the advent of short-term test systems for mutagenicity and blastomogenicity assessment of chemical substances with no account for essential differences in the responses of cells and embryos. As a result, specific test systems for cytotoxicity assessment were developed, and cytotoxicity was declared as a universal criterion for embryotoxicity of chemical substances. However, it is quite clear that the developing embryo is not a simple cell community where proliferation and its suppression are the most informative criteria of the effect of the test sample but a developing and self-differentiating system in which cell death far from always disturbs or stops development, at least due to compensatory–reparative processes and because this death is physiologically programmed. In cell test systems, effects on such intrinsic features of embryogenesis as progressive development with tissue and organ cell differentiation over the course of form-building processes, direct and inductive interactions of embryonic tissues, organogenesis and establishment of systems, for example blood circulation system, are not at the forefront of researchers' attention. The effect of exposure in such test systems is impossible to assess in terms of simple embryotoxicity parameters, specifically embryolethality, teratogenicity, stage-, tissue- and organ specificity, irreversibility of pathologic processes or the possibility of their compensation or reparation, etc. Nothing more than certain pathological changes in isolated cells (cell cultures) or specialized (differentiating) tissues (organ cultures) are registered, which, indeed, allows one to judge the possible nature of damage in these structures; however, under the conditions when the compensatory and reparative processes are not expressed, the outcome of the exposure is impossible to interpret unambiguously. It should be specially emphasized that none of the above-mentioned test systems involves full-scale formation of the blood circulation system, which prevents the forming buds (for example in organ culturing) from satisfying trophic and respiratory demands of tissues, especially in-depth ones. Under such conditions, high levels of spontaneous pathology and unpredictable development of marginal and in-depth segments of the explants are generally observed. In our opinion, the most adequate cell model for embryotoxicity screening is embryonic stem cells (ESC) differentiating in different cell lines (Rohwedel *et al.*, 2001; Scholz *et al.*, 1999; Spielmann *et al.*, 1997; Festag *et al.*, 2007a,b; Gordeeva *et al.*, 2005). The cell line differentiation process is accompanied by the recapitulation of consecutive morphogenetic processes at the regulatory level with timely expression of genes corresponding to embryonic development *in vivo*. This is an excellent model for research on the mechanisms of embryogenesis and induced functional teratogenesis. At the same time, it lacks criteria for embryo death and a morphologically expressed teratogenesis. We consider that teratogenicity assessment should be based on a flexible system (array) of various tests on one or two basic models. Such test array should allow its methodical potential and research level to the goal of research and specific properties of the test substance to be adapted (physicochemical properties, metabolic features, kinetics in a body, etc.).

Ideally, such a test system should be designed not only to assess the *embryotoxic activity* of test substances, as is characteristic of most specific test models *in vitro* and even of the standard system of testing on pregnant animals, but also to reveal and assess the *embryotoxic properties* of these substances. This implies that such a test system should allow different ways of assessing the hazard of a chemical substance (CS) including, in particular, teratogenicity testing not only the parent compounds but also their possible biotransformation products, and the possibility for testing the mother's bodily fluids, for example blood, to reveal induced embryotoxic factors and assess their kinetics. The possibility for determining the rate of embryolethal and teratogenic effects and evaluating the period of relative safety of a CS for embryonic development, when the initiated changes in embryonic structures are still possible to compensate, and timely interference by medicine, could minimize or eliminate completely the pathogenic effect of exposure. Naturally, such *in vitro* test system is quite desirable to operate with a whole organism, i.e. a whole embryo, rather than one of its structures. Such models are available and used for embryotoxicity testing of CSs, for example the FETAX (Frog Embryo Teratogenesis Assay: Xenopus) (Fort *et al.*, 1989, 1998, 2001a,b) or CHEST (Chick Embryotoxicity Screening Test) (Jelinek and Marhan, 1994). The above-mentioned assays offer undeniable advantages, but extrapolation of their results, for diverse reasons (species, habitat features, development and metabolism features, etc.), does not assess the real hazard the test substance poses for mammal, and, especially, human embryogenesis, even though these results are quite valuable for assessing the possible pollution of ecosystems, damage of the reproductive function of agricultural animals and poultry, etc.

More attractive test objects are mammal embryos at the stages of cleavage and early organogenesis. Cleavage stage embryos are relatively tolerant to exposures, having fewer degrees of response on exposure: the response is formed by the "all-or-nothing" principle, i.e. either further development or death. Dysmorphogenesis, as the reaction of cleaving embryos to exposure, is disputed by many researches, but even the mentioned set of pathological reactions would suffice to assess the reaction of embryos and, in certain cases, specifics of exposure. At the same time, we consider that the use of these stage embryos, along with early organogenesis ones, will allow more comprehensive embryotoxicity testing.

EARLY MOUSE AND RAT EMBRYOS AS A MODEL FOR EMBRYOTOXICITY TESTING *IN VITRO*

The rapid method complex to estimate the embryotoxic properties of chemicals consists of the usage of two models: mice preimplantation embryos C57Bl/CBA (from cleavage stage up to blastocyst formation, 1–4 days of development) and rat postimplantation embryos (head fold stage – 27–30 pairs of somites, 9.5–11.5 days of development). Mice preimplantation embryos are simultaneously cytological and embryological test models being both few-cells structures or self-determined system and integrated (whole) organisms. Based on the model, it is possible to estimate both cytotoxic and embryotoxic effects after pathogenic influence has occurred. Even though the preimplantation period is considered to be fairly refractory (Wilson, 1973), there is some evidence (Fara *et al.*, 1988; Berry, 1981; Arima, 1988) for high vulnerability of embryos in this period: up to 10% of embryos perish before implantation and up to 70% during implantation and in the early postimplantation period. The threat of embryo damage in the preimplantation period (in humans, 1–7 days of pregnancy) is probably associated with the fact that women are most commonly not aware of the initiated pregnancy and do not protect the embryo from extreme exposures. Consequently, a human fetus requires protection from exposure to pathogenic factors in the preimplantation period, and to include this period in the practice of experimental research on the hazards of environmental factors is a prerequisite for objective assessment of their impact on the course and outcome of pregnancy. Thus, experimental identification of hazards from one or other factors for the earliest stages of embryogenesis can serve prognostic and preventive purposes.

Most information on the pathogenic effects of various factors can be gained by studying embryos developing *in vitro* at the initial organogenesis stages, which are the most sensitive to damaging agents. It is important to mention that the majority of presently known teratogenic fetal syndromes, such as thalidomide, alcohol, phenytoin, diabetes, etc., were induced by exposures during the initial organogenesis stages of the human fetus (Hanson, 1986; Clarren and Smith, 1978; Mille and Stromland, 1999). The high vulnerability of the developing fetus at this embryogenesis stage is due to the high significance for further development of such morphogenetic processes as placentation, providing establishment of chorioallantoic connection; neurulation, providing establishment of the fetal nervous system; and in turn controlling the definitive position of the fetus with respect to embryonic shells; establishment of the vascular system, blood-making processes, respiration, etc. Over this period, one can observe organ anlage and differentiation directly in the culture (fusion of the paired heart rudiments and initiation of heart beating, anlage of fore and hind limbs, head brain segments, auditory and ophthalmic placodes, somitogenesis, etc.).

The use of postimplantation rat embryos allows express assessment of not only embryotoxic, but also potential genotoxic effects of pathogenic factors, by means, in particular, of the most sensitive genotoxicity tests, such as sister chromatide exchange (SCE) frequency assay (Galloway *et al.*, 1980; Popov and Patkin, 1985; Popov *et al.*, 1981a,b, 1998). Simultaneous assessment of these effects in the framework of a single model makes it possible to interrelate the embryotoxic and mutagenic impacts. Naturally, the SCE frequency assay does not exhaust genotoxicity testing approaches; in particular, the micronuclear test can also be used.

DEFINITIONS, REVEALED EFFECTS AND THEIR ASSESSMENT CRITERIA

For an unambiguous understanding of induced embryopathologic processes, it is necessary to give an interpretation of the criteria we use for assessing the revealed effects.

The basic criteria for assessment of the development of cultured embryos under pathogenic exposures include the embryotoxic effect, embryolethal effect, teratogenic effect (dysmorphogenesis), cytotoxic effect, dynamic morphofunctional disorders, and, if required, genotoxic effect.

The *embryotoxic effect* is considered a combination of the embryolethal and teratogenic (dysmorphogenic) effects and dynamic morphofunctional disorders: inhibition of embryonic growth processes, edematous changes, hemorrhages and other changes in embryonic and extra embryonic tissues.

The *embryolethal effect* is identified by the lack of regular heart beating and embryonic and extra embryonic (omphaloid) circulation in cultured early embryos, and also by the observation of a complex of specific pathologies in cleaving embryos, which are incompatible with further development. Quantitatively, this effect is related to the total number of cultured embryos.

The *teratogenic effect* is a stable (irreversible) pathology of embryonal morphogenesis and is identified as a morphologically well-defined irreversible deviation, primarily, deformation of embryonic structures, including their size (hyper-, hypo- or aplasia). Developmental defects can be either compatible (for example, lack of limbs) or incompatible (for example, eventration of the neutral tube, lack of chorioallantoic connection) with further fetal life. As a rule, developmental defects are revealed in live embryos, and, consequently, the teratogenic effect is measured by the number of anomalous embryos among live ones. Developmental defects in dead embryos are described, specifying the stage of embryogenesis termination. For describing pathologies in cleaving embryos, the term dysmorphogenesis is preferred.

Morphofunctional disorders are dynamic pathologic changes in embryonic and extra embryonic structures, which do not necessarily lead to irreversible changes (teratogenic effect) due to the possibility of subsequent compensatory processes. The morphofunctional disorders include local edematous changes, hemorrhages, inhibition of embryonic growth, etc.

Minimal effective embryotoxic concentration (EC_{min}) is the concentration of a test substance, which induces a minimum death of embryos or signs of dysmorphogenesis, unobservable at lower concentrations.

The *cytotoxic effect* is various forms of cellular pathology in cleaving embryos (pycnosis, lysis, proliferation retardation, etc.); the form of manifestation of the toxic effect at the cellular level in cleaving embryos. The extreme manifestation of this effect is the cytostatic action, i.e. cell death.

THE METHODICAL APPROACHES OF TESTING

Based on the technique of *in vitro* cultivation of early embryos, several research groups (Popov, 1981, 1985; Popov *et al.*, 1981 a,b; Popov and Protasova, 2009; ECVAM DB-ALM: INVITTOX protocol, 2002; Klug *et al.*, 1985; Piersma *et al.*, 1995; Schmid *et al.*, 1983) have developed scientific and methodical principles of a system of *in vitro* testing of chemical substances for embryotoxicity. The methodical approaches are combined to form a uniform test system targeted at revealing the *embryotoxic properties* of a test substance, such as:

direct exposure

- morphofunctional assessment of embryo development;
- determination of the minimum effective embryotoxic concentration EC_{min};

- determination of the time–concentration–effect dependence;
- comparison of experimental data with human pharmacokinetics data;
- prognosis for human embryogenesis.

biotransformation
- assessment of the embryotoxicity and genotoxicity of metabolites formed;
- assessment of the metabolic pathway: bioactivation, bioinactivation, non-metabolic inactivation.

detemination of the terms of realization of the embryotoxic effect
- assessment of the rate of formation of irreversible embryopathologic changes.

revelation and assessment of the embryotoxic factors in the blood of treated animals
- study of the dynamics of embryopathogenic factors in the blood of treated animals;
- assessment of the persistence time of a test substance in the blood of treated animals.

The test system can also be targeted at **revealing the embryopathogenic factors in human blood** with the aim, for example, of revealing and assessing the embryotoxic factors in the blood of women of reproductive age exposed to chemical substances

- when subject to therapeutic treatment;
- when occupied in industry or agriculture;
- when living in ecologically unfavorable regions.

These methodical approaches form an experimental basis of a new scientific field – experimental embryotoxicology *in vitro*, combining methods of experimental embryology, specifically *in vitro* development of animal embryos, and toxicological research.

CONCEPTIONS AND PRINCIPLES OF *IN VITRO* EMBRYOTOXICITY TESTING

We consider the system for *in vitro* embryotoxicity testing of chemical substances as a set of task-oriented methodical approaches to assess the hazard of CS for the embryonic development of a chosen model (in our case, pre- and post-implantation embryos) with the aim of revealing the principal embryotoxic properties of a test substance.

The *in vitro* test system represents a flexible system (battery) of different tests in the framework of a single or a few compatible test models. The test system should allow its methodical potential and research level to be varied, depending on the goal of testing and specific properties of the test substance (physicochemical, metabolism, etc.).

The *in vitro* test system makes it possible to gain additional information and should not be considered as an alternative to the standard CS toxicity test on pregnant animals. The basic aim of testing is to give a prognosis of the hazard of a test substance for human embryogenesis. Dealing with one or another test system we should realize its potential and tend, on the one hand, to include it in the most informative tests, but, on the other, not to expect more than it is able to provide. We should bear in mind that

- there are no universal animal testing systems;
- single tests, including specialized, are unable to reflect the entire diversity of embryo responses to exposure;
- the system of testing should include approaches for testing as much as possible developmental processes and allow general conclusions as to the embryo development;
- the test system should allow one not only to assess the embryotoxic activity of a test substance, but also to reveal its *embryotoxic properties*, where activity is only one of these properties;
- the system should allow testing well and poorly water-soluble, as well as gaseous, substances;
- the possibility of using the metabolic activation/inactivation system should be available; the possibility of using the intrinsic metabolic resource of the test model is desirable;
- genetic modifications of the test model are desirable;
- the system should be able to accept human pharmacokinetics/toxicokinetics data and allow the use of human fluids and tissues (blood, amniotic fluids, abortive material, etc.).
- *in vitro* methods allow the embryotoxic activity of a substance to be tested directly on an embryo, irrespective of how the structure and activity of the substance have been modified in the mother's organism. This is quite an important point, since the pharmacokinetics of a substance in a body is not infrequently individual (genetically determined) and reflects the specific features of a species, animal strain and concrete specimen.

THE EVALUATION OF DIRECT EFFECTS ON CULTURED EMBRYOS

This is an ordinary approach, and it is used by everybody who works with cell and tissue cultures. This technique involves direct introduction of a test agent into the culture medium. After incubation, induced effects and toxic and ineffective levels of the test sample are estimated. The work with embryo cultures has certain features which seem to be decisive. Embryo *in vitro* culturing, i.e. in the absence of the mother's organism, makes it possible to assess a direct hazard the test agent poses on the developing fetus, irrespective of possible (genetic or functional) fluctuations of the mother's organism. Direct exposure of *in vitro* cultured embryos allows one:

- to perform morphofunctional assessment of embryo development;
- to determine the threshold and effective concentrations;
- to determine the time–concentration–effect function;
- to compare obtained data with human pharmacokinetics data;
- to give a prognosis for human embryogenesis.

The morphofunctional assessment of embryo development in culture is performed by measuring the principal development parameters related to growth processes (craniocaudal size, total protein content), embryo body differentiation (somitogenesis, development of brain and heart compartments, limb rudiments, vision and hearing organs, hyoid arches, mandibular and maxillary processes, etc.), morphofunctional processes (neurulation, embryo turning, allantoic growth and establishment of chorioallantoic connection, formation of blood islets, vasculogenesis, hematopoiesis, initiation of yolk circulation, etc.). In practice, a semi-quantitative (grade) system is not infrequently used to characterize the degree of development of one or another rudiment or completeness of morphogenetic processes (Brown and Fabro, 1981).

The evaluation of preimplantation embryos is analyzed in terms of the numbers of live, dead and abnormal (dysmorphogenic) ones that have reached certain stages of development. Among the dead include deformed, fragmented nuclei and nuclei with dull cytoplasm. Anomalies have been detected in the continuing development of embryos in culture. After culturing, matured embryos evaluate cell mass, proliferative activity and cell death, expressed by the number of pycnotic nuclei (Mammalian development, 1990).

The result of cultivation allows determination of the effective embryotoxic concentration, threshold concentration (the minimum effective and non-effective) on various (if there is a need) effects (embryolethality, teratogenic effect, growth retardation, the impact on the proliferative activity of cells, the effect on a particular morphogenetic process). We suggest that the effective concentrations derived from experiments on cultured embryos acquire a new meaning *when correlated with the concentrations developed in human (mother's) blood*. In this case, a prognostic parameter appears which allows experimental results to be correlated with a real concentration of a test substance in human blood. The criterion of toxic hazard for human embryo thus becomes the minimum effective embryotoxic concentration EC_{min} determined by *in vitro* experiments, which we consider as a key parameter for extrapolation of experimental results on human embryogenesis.

We compared the EC_{min} values for a series of (1) well-known teratogens, (2) substances that clearly do not possess teratogenic properties, and (3) substances just suspected of teratogenicity – with their concentrations observed in human blood, for example with the therapeutical (C_{ther}) or maximum observed (C_{max}) concentrations. The following regularities were revealed.

The therapeutically and maximum observed concentrations of well-known teratogens (ethanol, phenytoin, valproic acid, diethylstilbestrol, fluorouracil) were higher than the minimum effective embryotoxic concentrations ($EC_{min} \leq C_{ther}$, C_{max}).

1. The minimum effective embryotoxic concentrations of substances with an unproven (but possible) teratogenicity for humans (acetaldehyde, cadmium chloride, salicilates, coffein) are close to the maximum observed concentrations: $EC_{min} \sim C_{max}$.
2. For unlikely teratogens (diazepam, dexamethasone, phenobarbital), $EC_{min} > C_{max}$.

These results show that the EC_{min} values obtained by testing embryo cultures are readily extrapolated to human embryogenesis, thereby predicting the potential hazard in the teratogen–potential teratogen–non-teratogen series. In our opinion, this is a key advantage offered by direct assessment of CS in mammalian embryo cultures: *the effective concentrations determined in vitro acquire a new meaning when correlated with the concentrations developed in human (mother's) blood.* Therefore, the concentrations equal or above EC_{min}, if present in mother's blood, are considered to pose potential hazards to the human fetus. Therefore, substances with $EC_{min} > C_{max}$ are generally not potential teratogens for humans (Popov and Protasova, 2009). It should be noted that both pre- and postimplantation embryos can be cultured both in synthetic media (Biggers *et al.*, 1971, 2005; Mammalian development, 1990; Zusman *et al.*, 1987, 1989; Popov *et al.*, 1981c; Popov, 1981, 1985; Sekirina, 1985; Popov and Protasova, 2009) with added rat or human blood serum and in blood (say, rat) serum, which will allow, to a certain extent, the effect of binding of a test substance with blood proteins to be assessed.

However, one should not overestimate the significance of EC_{min}, if for no other reason than it is not the only parameter related to the effect. One more important parameter is the time during which the embryo is exposed to this concentration. The exposure time sufficient to induce the embryopathogenic effect at a given concentration (T_{min}) can serve as the second most informative and prognostic parameter.

To determine the minimum time required for the development of the embryotoxic effect in cultured embryos, a test agent is introduced in the medium in admittedly effective concentrations (not lower than EC_{min}) determined in direct exposure experiments (see above). After 1–24h embryos should be transferred into a medium free of the test agent and cultured for a preset time. The experimental results allow assessment of the hazard of the concrete concentration of the substance by relating it to the time required for the realization of the embryopathogenic effect (T_{min}). Furthermore, we relate the T_{min} with the half-life of the test substance in humans ($T_{1/2}$) at C_{max}, which allows an optimized prognosis of the teratogenic hazard of the test substance for human embryogenesis (Popov, 2007; Popov and Protasova, 2009).

For example, we present our experiments with ethanol and its immediate metabolite – acetaldehyde (Table 12.1). Ethanol is a well-known human teratogen which induces fetal alcohol syndrome (FAS). At the same time, certain studies indicate FAS due to acetaldehyde. The table contains the ineffective, effective and EC_{min} for ethanol and acetaldehyde (EC_{min} 3mg/ml and 2µg/ml, respectively). The effects of these agents at various concentrations in human blood are shown in the second column of the table. Thus, the EC_{min} of ethanol, derived from *in vitro* experiments, is observed in the blood of humans with a moderate or heavy alcohol intoxication, and the EC_{min} of acetaldehyde is found in the blood of people suffering chronic alcoholism. Thus, the results provide evidence for the compatibility of experimental and real concentrations, and comparison of the rates of realization of the embryotoxic effect of various concentrations of ethanol and acetaldehyde in experiments *in vitro* suggests that to exert an effect the highest concentrations should persist in blood for no shorter than 24h, which is unreal: most ethanol is eliminated from human blood within 6–8h, whereas acetaldehyde rapidly degrades even upon taking a single portion of alcohol. Moreover, alcohol in high concentrations is a threat to human life, whereas acetaldehyde in higher concentrations (110µM, 5µg/ml) may occur in people suffering chronic alcoholism, and as little as 3h will be enough for the agent to damage the fetus. In reality, during the course of treatment of chronic alcoholism with aldehyde dehydrogenase (ALDH) inhibitors, acetaldehyde may persist much longer in blood. It should be mentioned here that FAS is generally induced in women suffering from chronic alcoholism (Jones *et al.*, 1973; Veghelyi *et al.*, 1978; Cumberland and Pratten, 1995).

TABLE 12.1 Minimum times for the realization *in vitro* of the embryolethal and teratogenic effects of various concentrations of ethanol and acetaldehyde in postimplantation rat embryo cultures

Concentration	Effects in humans	Exposure time (h) and embryotoxic effect in vitro (+ yes, – no)				
		1	3	15	24	48
Ethanol						
17 mM (0.8 mg/ml)	Moderate or heavy intoxication	–	–	–	–	–
33 mM (1.5 mg/ml)		–	–	–	–	–
65 mM (3.0 mg/ml) $\mathbf{EC_{min}}$						+
87 mM (4.0 mg/ml)	Coma				+	+
108 mM (5.0 mg/ml)	Death				+	+
Acetaldehyde						
4.5 μM (0.2 μg/ml)	Intoxication	–	–	–	–	–
45 mM (2.0mg/ml) $\mathbf{EC_{min}}$	At chronic alcoholism	–	–	–	–	+
110 μM (5.0 μg/ml)	In women who gave birth to children with FAS	–	+	+	+	+
225 μM (10 μg/ml)	At treatment with ALDH inhibitors	+	+	+	+	+
450 μM (20 μg/ml)		+	+	+	+	+

Thus, knowing the pharmacokinetics of a test agent in humans allows one to use its persistence time in blood, along with concentration, as one of the principal criteria of the hazard of the agent for human embryogenesis. At this time rat embryos should be cultured with agents, after which the embryos should be transferred into a control (agent-free) medium. If this exposure time is sufficient for the test agent to realize its embryotoxic potential (i.e., to induce embryo death or dysmorphogenesis), the agent is unconditionally considered a danger to the human fetus. In an opposite case (i.e., if toxic concentrations of a test agent failed to exert effect within terms characteristic of its kinetics in humans), the agent can be considered potentially (arbitrarily) dangerous, in view of the possible individual metabolism fluctuations, when the persistence time of the agent may prove long enough for it to exhibit embryopathogenic activity. This means that the experiments must have a certain "safety margin" as the highest concentration and duration of exposure.

The experimental results allow us to estimate the risk of a particular concentration of the drug by linking it with the time needed to implement embryopathogenic effect (T_{min}). In the next step we correlate T_{min}, during which EC_{min} produces pathogenic effects in the experiment – with time ($T_{1/2}$) persistence of C_{max} in human blood, which optimizes the prediction of teratogenic activity of a substance for human embryogenesis. Thus, the comparison of experimental data, evaluating the parameter of the concentration–time effect with real parameters for finding the drug in the blood (pharmacokinetics data), allows us to approach the optimum assessment of its risk to human embryogenesis.

Experiments with salicylates and some other substances proved that the experimentally determined EC_{min} and T_{min} do not always provide sufficient information for predicting the hazard of the test substance for human embryogenesis, since the induced effect is strongly dependent on the degree of binding of the test substance with blood proteins. Salicylates are marker teratogens for laboratory animals (Greenaway *et al.*, 1982, 1984; McGarrity *et al.*, 1981), but their teratogenicity for humans is not proven. It is known that sodium salicylates act on an embryo as a whole molecule (McGarrity *et al.*, 1981; Xu *et al.*, 1999), faster conjugates with blood proteins of primates than with those of rodents. The degree of human blood protein binding (BPBhum) of aspirin and salicylates is 73–98%. To find out whether the degree BPB of sodium salicylates is a key parameter (BPBrat controlling the realization of teratogenic effect in rodents, we cultured rat embryos in rat and human blood serum in the presence of sodium salicylates. Our experiments demonstrated (Popov and Protasova, 2009) that the embryotoxic effect in human blood serum was weaker by a factor of 1.8 (46% of embryos affected) than in rat blood serum (82% of embryos affected). These data are direct evidence for a stronger binding of sodium salicylates with human serum proteins (BPBhum > BPBrat), which most probably creates a deficit of the free form of salicylic acid.

Thus, the threshold concentration (EC_{min}) of a toxicant, minimum time required for the realization of its embryopathogenic effect (T_{min}), as well as the degree of its binding with blood proteins are the key parameters for extrapolation of experimental data to humans and prognostic estimates for the teratogenic hazard of this toxicant for human embryogenesis. The experimental values should be correlated with the respective parameters for human blood (C_{ther}, C_{max}, $T_{1/2}$, BPB_{human}). If $EC_{min} \leq C_{max}$, the substance is considered as a potential human teratogen, provided the experimental T_{min} compares with $T_{1/2}$ for humans. Therefore, if $BPB_{human} > BPB_{exp}$, further research is required to determine the ratios of the free and protein-bound forms of the toxicant in animal and human blood.

Biotransformation of toxicants in rat embryo culture

The next test in the system is to evaluate the biotransformation products of the test substance. Biotransformation of the test substance is held directly in the culture medium, adding exogenous metabolic mixture (NADPH- or NAD-dependent oxidation systems), consisting of a microsomal (or cytosol, or postmitochondrial S9) fraction of rat liver homogenates and the necessary cofactors (Fantel *et al.*, 1979; Popov *et al.*, 1981a,b).

Sometimes the biotransformation of drugs is carried out on co-cultivation embryos or embryonic organs with animal hepatocytes (Manson and Simons, 1979; Piersma *et al.*, 1990).

The developed approaches allow research on the following biotransformation pathways *in vitro*:

- metabolic activation of embryotoxic properties of toxicants;
- metabolic inactivation of embryotoxic properties of toxicants;
- non-metabolic inactivation of embryotoxic properties of toxicants.

In a bioactivation study, a test substance is introduced to a concentration maximally non-toxic for cultured embryos, and in bioinactivation study, in an admittedly effective concentration. These two concentrations are determined in experiments on a direct effect of the substance (see above).

Techniques for bioactivation of cyclophosphamide, ethanol, polyaromatic hydrocarbons and other substances are well documented (Fantel *et al.*, 1979; Galloway, 1980; Popov *et al.*, 1981a,b; Juchau, 1989; Miller *et al.*, 1996; Nebert, 2004). Biotransformation results in bioactivation of a substance to teratogenic and, not infrequently, mutagenic products, which provides evidence for the occurrence of biotransformation in culture and for pro-teratogenic properties of the substance.

A more difficult task is to reveal substances whose embryopathogenic properties are inactivated in the course of metabolic detoxication. Metabolic inactivation is the only way to detoxicate chemical substances. The metabolic inactivation of a substance is an ordinary process, but if it is accompanied by the inactivation of teratogenic properties, then, being covert in nature, this process is much more dangerous than the metabolic activation of pro-teratogens. By introducing such substances in pregnant female animals, we face a high risk of observing no symptoms of damage to embryogenesis or observing a minimum embryopathologic effect and thus drawing incorrect conclusions. Experimental *in vitro* and *in vivo* studies on such substances (for instance, cytochalasin D) showed that their embryopathogenicity depends on the activity of the metabolic system of the animal (Fantel, 1981; Harris *et al.*, 1988; Popov and Protasova, 2009).

Biotransformation is sometimes the only way to reveal the teratogenic potential of a preparation. More widely known are the experimental difficulties associated with revealing the teratogenicity of thalidomide, and, probably, the ability to assess the teratogenic properties of this drug can be considered a criterion of the performance of any embryotoxicity testing system. This relates in full measure to a system employing mammalian embryo cultures. The biotransformation of thalidomide with the microsomal or S-9 fraction hepatocytes of rat, mouse or monkey does not provide or provides only a weak specific drug effect – the impact on the development of the limb rudiments (Shepard and Shiota, 1983; Spezia *et al.*, 1999; Yokoyama *et al.*, 1994). Culturing embryos of transgenic mice bearing the CYP1A1 human gene, in the cultural medium containing thalidomide at a concentration of 500 μg/ml, caused a weak limb hypoplasia only (Akita *et al.*, 2005a). With embryos of transgenic mice (11.5–12.5 days of development) bearing a different human gene CYP3A7, in the presence of 250 μg/ml of the drug, limb hypoplasia was already observed in 57% of embryos and the introduction additionally of CYP3A7 human microsomes increased the rate of limb hypoplasias to 80%. These data suggest that the fetal limb pathology might have resulted from thalidomide metabolism directly in fetus tissues, as well as in mother tissues (Akita *et al.*, 2005b). The above experimental results provide evidence for the ability of the used tests to assess the teratogenic potential of studied substances.

A different approach, *non-metabolic inactivation*, was tried on an example of benzotrichloride which is a known carcinogen and mutagen. In these experiments, embryos were introduced in the cultural medium at definite intervals following the introduction of the test substance; the embryotoxic and genotoxic effects (SCE test) were then assessed. Benzotrichloride underwent hydrolysis in aqueous solution and lost its embryotoxic and genotoxic potential (Popov and Protasova, 2009).

REVEALING AND ASSESSING EMBRYOTOXIC FACTORS IN ANIMAL BLOOD

Revealing embryotoxic factors in animal blood after acute exposures: determination of threshold doses

One of the methodical approaches involves embryo culturing in animal blood serum. This approach is based on the ability of early embryos of laboratory rodents for normal development in the blood serum of mammals, such as rats, monkeys, humans, etc. (Klein *et al.*, 1980; Popov *al.*, 1981c; Steel, 1985; Popov and Arkhangel'skaia, 1993), as well as the ability of embryos cultured in serum to react to the presence and level of toxic (embryotoxic) factors in the cultural medium (Dyban *et al.*, 1979; Popov, 1981; Clapper *et al.*, 1986). The toxic factors primarily include a toxicant and its biotransformation products in toxic concentrations, as well as a complex of pathogenic factors developing in the animal blood as a response to exposure of the animal to the toxicant (cell destruction products, free radicals, abnormal levels of enzymes and hormones, etc.). The effects produced by the blood serum of experimental (exposed to a toxicant) animals (rats) and by the same toxicant introduced directly into the cultural medium (direct effect) are generally coincident, provided the test substances do not change their embryotoxic properties as a result of biotransformation. The same relates to the effects observed upon the biotransformation of, for example, pro-teratogens, and also after culturing embryos in animal blood serum (Popov, 1981; Popov *et al.*, 1981a,b; Popov and Protasova, 2009). Revealing embryotoxic factors in animal blood is also a test for embryotoxicity (embryolethality, teratogenicity, growth retardation). This test is quite suitable when the studied substance is insoluble or poorly soluble in water. By single introduction of decreasing doses of a test substance, one can determine in such *in vitro* experiments the threshold doses and compare them with the doses obtained with pregnant animals.

We have also explored the possibility of using other bodily fluids contacting, in one or another way, the developing embryos (amniotic, exocelomic and tissue fluids). It was shown that these fluids are also suitable for revealing embryotoxic factors and assessing their dysmorphogenic potential (Protasova *et al.*, 2007).

Revealing and assessing the embryotoxic factors in animal blood can also be used for (1) study of the dynamics of embryopathogenic factors in animal blood after acute exposure; (2) assessment of the persistence time of toxic concentrations of CS in blood; and (3) assessment of a chronic effect of CS on the embryonic development.

STUDY OF THE DYNAMICS OF EMBRYOTOXIC FACTORS IN ANIMAL BLOOD

A change in the level and composition of pathogenic factors in animal blood (for example, with time after exposure) affects the character and degree of damage of cultured embryos, which allows one to assess, by the biological effect (if revealed), the dynamics of embryopathogenic factors in animal blood.

Figure 12.1 shows a plot of the toxicity of rat blood serums versus time after exposure to a powder and an encapsulated form of endosulfan insecticide. The figure illustrates the sensitivity of the approach: differences in blood saturation with powdered and microencapsulated agent and the dynamics of agent toxicity for cultured embryos, corresponding to the saturation trends. The plot allows one to trace not only the dynamics in the toxicity of factors developed in blood in response to exposure, but also the time of their persistence in blood. Powdered endosulfan very rapidly enters blood, the maximum embryotoxic effect is observed after 6h, high toxicity persists for up to 24h and then rapidly decays. Microencapsulated endosulfan is slowly accumulated in blood, the maximum effect is observed after 24–48h and tends to decay by the 72nd h after exposure. Figure 12.2 shows the dynamics of both the embryolethal and teratogenic effects of blood serums obtained in different times after exposure to the antimalarial agent pyrimethamine. The curve reflecting a combined effect of these two effects (embryotoxic effect) is also given.

We made an attempt to find out the potential of this test for assessing the effect of chronic exposure to CS, using the blood serum of animals administered one or another preparation for a long time, for modeling chronic exposure of embryos. Clearly, embryos of laboratory animals are impossible to subject to chronic exposure. Therefore, the use of blood serum of test animals exposed for a long time to test agents is no more than evidence showing that chronic exposure results in the accumulation in animal blood of embryopathogenic factors. In particular, we performed an assessment of the effect of chronic exposure (2 months) of rats to aqueous extracts of bitumen salt masses (BSM) containing destruction products of sarin, soman and VX. The rat blood serum was used as a cultural medium for cleaving mouse and rat embryos at early stages of organogenesis. The results of this research have been reported in detail in a series of publications (Radilov *et al.*, 2002; Popov *et al.*, 2004).

Human blood serum – an object for embryotoxicity testing

As mentioned above, potential test systems should allow one to assess not only specific chemical effects, but also a combined effect of unfavorable factors of human embryogenesis. The use of *in vitro* testing of the blood serum of laboratory animals, as well as women of reproductive age, occupied in the chemical industry or living in ecologically unfavorable regions, can help in predicting a real hazard of toxicants appearing in human blood and affecting the developing fetus.

The ability of pre- and postimplantation mouse and rat embryos to develop in human blood serum, demonstrated by many investigators (Popov *et al.*, 1981c; Steel, 1985; Klein *et al.*, 1980), has made it possible to initiate research into revealing embryotoxic factors in the blood of women of reproductive age and suffering diseases that pose a risk of unfavorable outcomes of pregnancy (future or present), such as diabetes (Zusman *et al.*, 1987, 1989), epilepsy (Chatot *et al.*, 1984), Chagas disease (Robbins *et al.*, 1991), certain forms of infertility (Hewitt *et al.*, 2000), as well as of women who previously delivered children with neural tube defects (Anwar *et al.*, 1989) or suffering recurrent or late miscarriages (Chavez and McIntyre, 1984). These researches allowed the introduction in environmental hygienic practices of approaches targeted at revealing potential pathogenic factors in the blood of women living in the vicinity of large chemical facilities, working at such facilities, or living in ecologically unfavorable regions (Popov and Arkhangel'skaia, 1991, 1993; Popov and Protasova, 2009; Popov *et al.*, 2010).

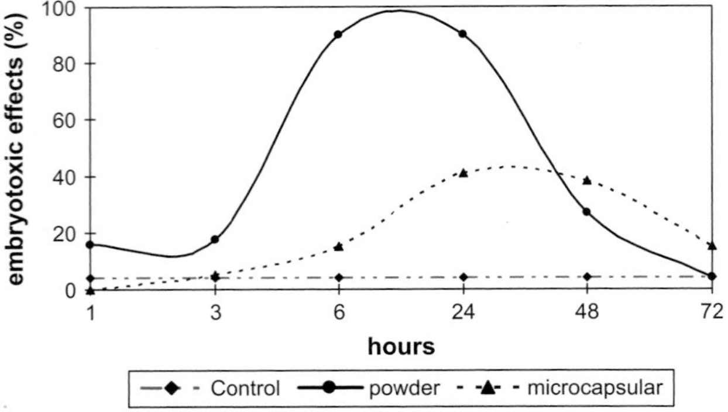

FIGURE 12.1 Dynamics of embryotoxic factors in the blood of rats exposed to powdered and microencapsulated endosulfan (by the results of culturing preimplantation mouse embryos and postimplantation rat embryos in animal blood serum).

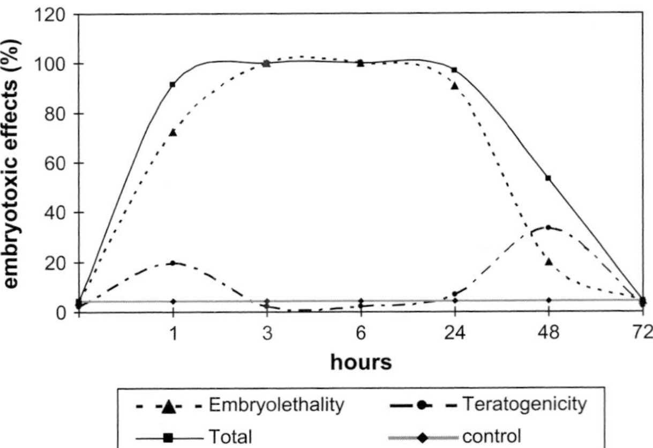

FIGURE 12.2 Dynamics of the embryolethal, teratogenic and combined effects of the blood serum of rats exposed to pyrimethamine (by the results of culturing postimplantation rat embryos).

CONCLUDING REMARKS AND FUTURE DIRECTIONS

Studies are performed using fast methods for revealing and assessing embryotoxic properties of CS, based on two principal models: *in vitro* cultured pre- and postimplantation embryos of laboratory animals (mice or rats). The attractiveness of preimplantation embryos as a model for chemical hazard assessment is associated with a number of reasons. They include (1) the absence of principal differences in the morphogenetic processes that occur in humans and laboratory animals at this stage of embryogenesis, (2) the possibility of full-scale development outside the mother's body throughout the entire preimplantation period, (3) the development rate *in vitro* is virtually the same as *in utero*, and (4) minimal volumes of blood serum (0.01 ml) necessary for embryotoxicity testing. One of the main arguments against serum (animal or human) as a cultural medium is that it, unlike synthetic media, has an unstable composition which may affect embryonic development. However, in our opinion, this is the ability of embryos to react on a varied composition of the cultural medium, which offers an advantage and allows teratogenicity assessment of new components. Our research gave evidence for this possibility. Thus, *in vitro* culturing pre- and postimplantation embryos of laboratory animals at the most pathogen-sensitive stages of embryogenesis (egg cleavage and early organogenesis) was used to reveal embryopathogenic factors in the blood of pregnant women working at chemical enterprises and living in regions endemic for hemolytic disease of newborns. This research demonstrated the possibility of revealing and assessing in early animal embryos cultures of embryopathogenic factors in the blood of women having reproductive complications in the obstetric history, as well as the possibility of predicting unfavorable pregnancy outcomes in women living in regions with a high environmental load (Protasova and Popov, 2002; Popov *et al.*, 2010).

The above-described approaches for the assessment of the teratogenic hazards of chemical substances and of combined exposures are already presently used by many researchers (Fantel *et al.*, 1979; Popov, 1981, 1985, 2007; Popov *et al.*, 1981a,b; Schmid *et al.*, 1983; ECVAM, 2002; Klug *et al.*, 1985; Piersma *et al.*, 1990; Zusman *et al.*, 1987, 1989; Akita *et al.*, 2005a,b). In our work we made an attempt to combine them into a unified system of research, which has formed a field of contemporary embryotoxicology, specifically embryotoxicology *in vitro*.

REFERENCES

Akita M, Kato M, Iwano S, Ishida M, Suzuki S, Katsuki M, Yokoyama A, Kamataki T (2005a) Effects of thalidomide in transgenic mice carrying various human CYP genes, investigated using the whole embryo culture method. *Congenit Anom (Kyoto)*. **45(4):** P. A42–A43.

Akita M, Kato M, Iwano S, Ishida M, Suzuki S, Katsuki M, Yokoyama A, Kamataki T (2005b) Effects of thalidomide in transgenic mice carrying various human CYP genes, investigated using the whole embryo culture method. *Congenit Anom (Kyoto)* **45(4):** P. A43.

Anwar M, MacVicar J, Beck F (1989) Serum from pregnant women carrying a fetus with neural tube defect is teratogenic for rat embryos in culture. *Br J Obstet Gynaecol* **96:** 33–7.

Arima M (1988) Congenital anomalies. Past, present, and future. *Asian Med J* **31:** 308–14.

Berry CL (1981) Congenital malformations. In *Paediatric Pathology* (Berry CL, ed.). Berlin, Heidelberg, New York, Springer Verlag, pp. 67–86.

Biggers JD, McGinnis LK, Lawitts JA (2005) One-step versus two-step culture of mouse preimplantation embryos: is there a difference. *Hum Reprod* **20:** 3376–84.

Biggers JD, Whitten WK, Whittingham DG (1971) The culture of mouse embryos in vitro. In *Methods in Mammalian Embryology* (Daniel JC, ed.). San Francisco, CA, Freeman, pp. 86–116.

Bochkov NP (1982) The role of cytogenetics in evolution of human genetic risk. In *Environmental Mutagens and Cancirogens*. Tokyo-New York, A.R. Liss, pp. 423–9.

Brent RL (1987) Etiology of human birth defects: what are the causes of the large group of birth defects of unknown etiology? In *Developmental Toxicology: Mechanisms and Risk*. Cold Spring, NY, pp. 362–3.

Brent RL (1995) The application of the principles of toxicology and teratology in evaluating the risks of new drugs for treatment of drug addiction in women of reproductive age. *NIDA Res Monogr* **149:** 130–84.

Brown NA, Fabro S (1981) Quantitation of rat embryonic development in vitro: a morphological scoring system. *Teratolology* **24:** 65–78.

Brown NA, Spielmann H, Bechter R, Flint OP, Stuart JF, Jelinek RJ, Koch E, Nau H, Newall DR, Palmer AK, Renault J, Repetto MF, Vogel R, Wiger R (1995) Screening chemicals for reproductive toxicity: the current alternatives. The report and recommendations of an ECVAM//ETS workshop. *ATLA* **23:** 868–82.

Chatot CL, Klein NW, Clapper ML, Resor SR, Singer WD, Russman BS, Holmes GL, Mattson RH, Cramer JA (1984) Human serum teratogenicity studied by rat embryo culture: epilepsy, anticonvulsant drugs, and nutrition. *Epilepsia* **25:** 205–16.

Chavez DJ, McIntyre JA (1984) Sera from women with histories of repeated pregnancy losses cause abnormalities in mouse preimplantation blastocysts. *J Reprod Immunol* **6:** 273–81.

Clapper ML, Clark ME, Klein NW, Kurtz PJ, Carlton BD, Chhabra RS (1986) Cardiovascular defects in rat embryos cultured in serum from rats chronically exposed to phenitoin. *Teratogenesis Carcinog Mutagen* **6:** 151–61.

Clarren SK, Smith DW (1978) The fetal alcohol syndrome. *N Engl J Med* **298:** 1063–7.

Cumberland PF, Pratten MK (1995) Teratogenicity of thalidomide-related compounds in vitro. *Teratology* **51:** 22A.

Dyban AP, Puchkov VF, Popov VB, Golinskiĭ GF (1979) Testing of some chemical environmental pollutants to teratogenicity using mammalian embryos cultivated *in vitro*. *Proceedings of the US-USSR third Joint Symposium on Problems on Environmental Health*, Suzdal, USSR, pp. 300–22.

ECVAM (European Centre for the Validation of Alternative Methods) DB-ALM: INVITTOX protocol (2002) Embryotoxicity Testing in Post-Implantation Embryo Culture – Method of Piersma, INVITTOX No. 123, pp. 1–12.

EPA (Environmental Protection Agency) (1998) Health effects test guidelines OPPTS 870.3700 Prenatal developmental toxicity study. EPA 712-C-98-207.

EPA (Environmental Protection Agency) (2000) Health effects test guidelines OPPTS 870.3550 Reproduction/developmental toxicity screening test. EPA 712-C-00-367.

Fantel AG, Greenaway JC, Juchau MR, Shepard TH (1979) Teratogenic bioactivation of cyclophosphamide in vitro. *Life Sci* **25:** 67–72.

Fantel AG, Greenaway JC, Shepard TH, Juchau MR, Selleck SB (1981) The teratogenicity of cytochalasin D and its inhibition by drug metabolism. *Teratology* **23:** 223–31.

Fara M, Jelinek R, Peterka M, Dostal M, Hrivnakova J (1988) Orofacial clefts. A theoretical basis for their prevention and treatment. *Acta Univ Carol Med Monogr* **124:** 1–143.

Festag M, Sehner C, Steinberg P, Viertel B (2007a) An in vitro embryotoxicity assay based on the disturbance of the differentiation of murine embryonic stem cells into endothelial cells. I: Establishment of the differentiation protocol. *Toxicol in Vitro* **21:** 1619–30.

Festag M, Viertel B, Steinberg P, Sehner C (2007b) An in vitro embryotoxicity assay based on the disturbance of the differentiation of murine embryonic stem cells into endothelial cells. II. Testing of compounds. *Toxicol in Vitro* **21:** 1631–40.

Fort DJ, James BL, Bantle JA (1989) Evaluation of the developmental toxicity of five compounds with the frog embryo teratogenesis assay: Xenopus (FETAX) and a metabolic activation system. *J Appl Toxicol* **9:** 377–88.

Fort DJ, Propst TL, Stover EL, Schrock B, Bantle JA (1998) Evaluation of the developmental toxicity of benzo(a)pyrene and 2-acetylaminofluorene using Xenopus: modes of biotransformation. *Toxicology* **42:** 284–5.

Fort DJ, Rogers RL, Paul RR, Stover EL, Finch RA (2001b) Optimization of an exogenous metabolic activation system for FETAX. II. Preliminary evaluation. *Drug Chem Toxicol* **24:** 117–27.

Fort DJ, Rogers RL, Stover EL, Finch RA (2001a) Optimization of an exogenous metabolic activation system for FETAX. I. Post-isolation rat liver microsome mixtures. *Drug Chem Toxicol* **24:** 103–15.

Galloway SM, Perry PE, Meneses J, Nebert DW, Pedersen RA (1980) Cultured mouse embryos metabolize benzo(a)pyrene during early gestation; genetic differences detectable by sister chromatid exchange. *Proc Natl Acad Sci USA* **77(6):** 3524–8.

Gordeeva OF, Krasnikova NYu, Larionova AV (2005) Comparative studies of transcript profiles of the embryonic stem cells for the development of cellular test-systems of new generation. Bulletin of biotechnology and physical chemical biology named by Yu. *A Ovchinnikov* **1(1):** 79–84.

Greenaway JC, Bark DH, Juchau MR (1984) Embryotoxic effects of salicylates: role of biotransformation. *Toxicol Appl Pharmacol* **74:** 141–9.

Greenaway JC, Shepard TH, Fantel AG, Juchau MR (1982) Sodium salicylate teratogenicity in vitro. *Teratology* **26:** 167–73.

Guidelines for the study of reproductive of drugs (2005) Guidelines for the experimental (preclinical) study of new pharmacological agents (Habriev RU, ed.). M. Medicina, pp. 87–100. Russian.

Hanson JW (1986) Teratogen update: fetal hydantoin effects. *Teratology* **33:** 349–53.

Harris C, Stark KL, Juchau MR (1988) Glutathione status and the incidence of neural tube defects elicited by direct acting teratogens in vitro. *Teratology* **37:** 577–90.

Hewitt MJ, Pratten MK, Regan L, Quenby SM, Baker RN (2000) The use of whole rat embryo culture as a technique for investigating potential serum toxicity in recurrent miscarriage patients. *Hum Reprod* **15:** 2200–4.

Jelinek R, Marhan O (1994) Validation of the chick embryotoxicity screening test (CHEST). A comparative study. *Function Develop Morphol* **4:** 317–25.

Jones RL, Smith DW, Ulleland N, Streissguth AP (1973) Pattern of malformation in offspring of chronic alcoholic mothers. *Lancet* **1:** 1267–71.

Juchau MR (1989) Bioactivation in chemical teratogenesis. *Annu Rev Pharmacol Toxicol* **29:** 165–87.

Kalter H, Warkany J (1983) Congenital malformations: etiologic factors and their role in prevention. *N Engl J Med* **308:** 424–31.

Klein NW, Parker RM, Plenefish JD (1980) In vitro culture of rat embryos on monkey serum: effects of menstrual cycle and thalidomide consumption. *Teratology* **21(2):** 50–51A.

Klug S, Lewandowski C, Nau H, Neubert D (1985) Modification and standardization of the culture of early postimplantation embryos for toxicological studies. *Arch Toxicol* **58:** 84–8.

Mammalian development (1990) A practical approach (M. Monk, ed.). *M. Mir* 406 p.

Manson JM, Simons R (1979) In vitro metabolism of cyclophosphamide in limb bud culture. *Teratology* **19:** 149–58.

McGarrity C, Samani N, Beck F, Gulamhusein A (1981) The effect of sodium salicylate on the rat embryo in culture: an in vitro model for the morphological assessment of teratogenicity. *J Anat* **133:** 257–69.

Mille MT, Stromland K (1999) Teratogen update: thalidomide: a review, with a focus on ocular findings and new potential uses. *Teratology* **60:** 306–21.

Miller MS, Juchau MR, Guengerich FP, Nebert DW, Raucy JL (1996) Drug metabolic enzymes in developmental toxicology. *Fundam Appl Toxicol* **34(2):** 165–75.

NBDPN (2008) Centers for Disease Control and National Birth Defects Prevention Network Preventing Birth Defects. Available at: http://www.nbdpn.org/current/2008pdf/PrevBDBroch.pdf

Nebert DW, Dalton TP, Okey AB, Gonzalez FJ (2004) Role of aryl hydrocarbon receptor-mediated induction of the CYP1 enzymes in environmental toxicity and cancer. *J Biol Chem* **279:** Issue 23, 23847–50.

Nelson K, Holmes LB (1986) Malformations due to spontaneous mutations in newborn infants. *Teratology* **33:** P. 30C.

OECD (Organisation for Economic Cooperation and Development) (2001) Prenatal developmental toxicity study. OECD guidance 414 adopted 22-01-2001.

Piersma AH, Attenon P, Bechter R, Govers MJAP, Krafft N, Schmid BP, Stadler J, Verhoef A, Verseil C (1995) Interlaboratory evaluation of embryotoxicity in the postimplantation rat embryo culture. *Reprod Toxicol* **9:** 275–80.

Piersma AH, Van Aerts L, Verhoef A, Robinson JE, Peters PW (1990) Biotransformation in post-implantation rat embryo culture using maternal hepatocytes in suspension coculture. *Teratology* **41(5):** 585.

Popov VB (1981) Action of cyclophosphamide in a culture of rat postimplantation embryos. *Ontogenez* **12(3):** 251–6. Russian.

Popov VB (1985) Testing chemicals for teratogenicity in the culture of postimplantation rat embryos. In *The General Regulatory and Supervisory Mechanisms of Early Embryogenesis in Mammals Normal and Pathology*. L, pp. 58–69. Russian.

Popov VB (2007) Minimum effective concentration of chemical toxicants in embryotoxical experiments in vitro and its role in predicting the induced human embryo pathogenesis. In *Actual Problems of Chemical Safety in the Russian Federation*. Proceedings. St Petersburg, pp. 180–5. Russian.

Popov VB, Arkhangel'skaia IB (1991) Endogenous factors of blood serum and development in vitro. In *Endocrine Systems and Harmful Environmental Factors*. L, p. 188. Russian.

Popov VB, Arkhangel'skaia IB (1993) Identification and assessment of toxic factors in the blood of people living in ecologically unfavorable regions of the Altai region. In *Nuclear Testing, Environment and Health of the Population of the Altai Region. Barnaul* **3(2):** 49–53. Russian.

Popov VB, Patkin EL (1985) The study of relationships of teratogenic effect and the number of sister chromatid exchanges in the biotransformation of ethanol in the culture of rat embryos. In *The General Regulatory and Supervisory Mechanisms of Early Embryogenesis in Mammals Normal and Pathology*. L, pp. 85–90. Russian.

Popov VB, Protasova GA (2009) Experimental embryotoxicology of chemicals in vitro. Monograph. In *Toxicology, Hygiene, Occupational Pathology when Working with Extremely Hazardous Chemicals*. Information issue **3:** 371 p. Russian.

Popov VB, Protasova GA, Protasova OV, Maximova IA (2010) The elicitation and evaluation of embryopathogenic factors in the blood of pregnant women with the use of the cultures of early embryos of laboratory animals. *Mol Med* **3:** 47–52. Russian.

Popov VB, Protasova GA, Radilov AS (1998) Embryo- and genotoxic effects of two endosulfan forms in the culture of rat and mouse pre- and postimplantation embryos. *Ontogenez* **29(2):**104–12. Russian.

Popov VB, Protasova GA, Shabasheva LV (2004) Developmental and reproductive effects of the chemical weapons destruction end-products (sarin, soman, Vx). Proceedings of 8th International Symposium on Protection against Chemical and Biological Warfare Agents, Gothenburg, Sweden, CD, www.cbwsymp.foi.se

Popov VB, Puchkov VF, Ignat'eva TV (1981c) In vitro development of the postimplantation embryos of laboratory rodents in human blood serum. *Arkh Anat Gistol Embriol* **81(11):** 92–6. Russian.

Popov VB, Vaĭsman BL, Puchkov VF (1981a) Embryotoxic effect of cyclophosphamide after being biotransformed in a culture of postimplantation rat embryos. *Biull Eksp Biol Med* May **91(5):** 613–15. Russian.

Popov VB, Vaisman BL, Puchkov VF, Ignat'eva TV (1981b) Embryotoxic effect of ethanol and its biotransformation products in cultures of postimplantation rat embryos. *Biull Eksp Biol Med* **92(12):** 725–8. Russian.

Protasova GA, Popov VB (2002) Detection and prognostic evaluation of embryotoxic factors in the blood of women from ecologically unfavorable regions. In *Medical and Hygienic Aspects of Working with Highly Hazardous Chemicals*, pp. 349–59. Russian.

Protasova GA, Popov VB, Shabasheva LV (2007) Use of biological fluids of experimental animals to predict the embryotoxic hazard of chemicals. In *Actual Problems of Chemical Safety in the Russian Federation*. Proceedings, pp. 185–91. Russian.

Radilov AS, Popov VB, Protasova GA, Shabasheva LV, Ermolaeva EE (2002) Studies of embryotoxic effects of bitumen-salt masses (BSM) and their aqueous extracts containing GB, GD, or VX two-stage destruction products. *The Toxicologist* **66(1):** Suppl, 235.

Robbins B, Klein NW, Cavalkanti H (1991) Toxicity of sera from individuals with Chagas disease to cultured rat embryos: role of antibodies to laminin. *Teratology* **44(5):** 561–70.

Rohwedel J, Guan K, Hegert C, Wobus AM (2001) Embryonic stem cells as an in vitro model for mutagenicity, cytotoxicity and embryotoxicity studies: present state and future prospects. *Toxicol in Vitro* **5(6):** 741–53.

Schmid BP, Trippmacher A, Bianchi A (1983) Validation of the whole-embryo culture method for in vitro teratogenicity testing. In *Developments and Practice in the Science of Toxicology* (Hayes AW, Schnell RC, Miya TS, eds.). Elsevier, Amsterdam, pp. 563–6.

Scholz G, Pohl I, Genschow E, Klemm M, Spielmann H (1999) Embryotoxicity screening using embryonic stem cells *in vitro*: correlation to *in vivo* teratogenicity. *Cells, Tissues, Organs* **3–4:** 203–11.

Sekirina GG (1985) The development of preimplantation embryos of mice in a medium with heterologous (rat) serum. In *The General Regulatory and Supervisory Mechanisms of Early Embryogenesis in Mammals Normal and Pathology*. L, pp. 31–5. Russian.

Shepard TH, Lemire RJ (2004) *Catalog of Teratogenic Agents*, 11th ed. Baltimore, Johns Hopkins University Press, 552 p.

Shepard TH, Shiota K (1983) Bioactivation of thalidomide by a monkey liver fraction in a rat limb culture system. In *Limb. Development and Regeneration*, Part A 377–85.

Spezia F, Lorenzon G, Fournex R, Vannier B (1999) Action of thalidomide on whole rat embryo cultures with and without S9-mix from various species. *Reprod Toxicol* **5(3):** 269–70.

Spielmann H, Pohl I, Doering B, Liebsch M, Moldenhauer F (1997) The embryonic stem cell test, an in vitro embryotoxicity test using two permanent mouse cell lines: 3T3 fibroblasts and embryonic stem cells. *In Vitro Toxicol* **10:** 119–27.

Steel CE (1985) Human serum as a culture medium for rat embryos. *Experientia* **41(12):** 1601–3.

Swaab DF, Mirmiran H (1986) Functional teratogenic effects of chemicals on the developing brain. Monogram. *Neural Sci* **12:** 45–7.

TERIS (The Teratogen Information System) (2010) http://depts.washington.edu/terisweb/teris/Preamble.htm

Veghelyi P, Osztovics M, Kardos G (1978) The fetal alcohol syndromes: symptoms and pathogenesis. *Acta Paed Acad Acient Hung* **19:** 171–89.

Wilcox AJ, Weinberg CR, O'Connor JF, Baird DD, Schlatterer JP, Canfield RE, Armstrong EG, Nisula BC (1988) Incidence of early loss of pregnancy. *New England J Med* **319:** 189–94.

Wilson JG (1973) *Environmental and Birth Defects*. Academic Press, NY, London, 305 p.

Xu X-M, Sansores-Garcia L, Chen X-M, Matijevic-Aleksic N, Du M, Wu KK (1999) Suppression of inducible cyclooxygenase 2 gene transcription by aspirin and sodium salicylate. *Proc Natl Acad Sci USA* **96(9):** 5292–7.

Yokoyama A, Akita M, Kuroda Y (1994) Effects of thalidomide on cultured rat embryos. *Teratology* **50(6):** 28B.

Zusman I, Yaffe P, Ornoy A (1987) Effects of metabolic factors in the diabetic state on the in vitro development of preimplantation mouse embryos. *Teratology* **35(1):** 77–85.

Zusman I, Yaffe P, Raz I, Baron H, Ornoy A (1989) Effects of human diabetic serum on the in vitro development of early somite rat embryos. *Teratology* **39(1):** 85–92.

C H A P T E R

13

In vitro approaches to developmental neurotoxicity

Lucio G. Costa, Gennaro Giordano and Marina Guizzetti

INTRODUCTION

Neurotoxicity can be defined as any adverse effect on the chemistry, structure or function of the nervous system, during development or at maturity, induced by chemical or physical influences (Costa, 1998). An adverse effect is "any treatment related change which interferes with normal function and compromises adaptation to the environment" (ECETOC, 1992). Thus, most morphological changes such as neuronopathy (a loss of neurons), axonopathy (a degeneration of the neuronal axon), or myelinopathy (a loss of the glial cells surrounding the axon), or other gliopathies, would be considered adverse, even if structural and/or functional changes were mild or transitory. In addition, neurochemical changes, also in the absence of structural damage, should be considered adverse, even if they are reversible. For example, exposure to organophosphorus (OP) insecticides or to certain solvents may cause only transient nervous system effects, but these should be considered neurotoxic, as they lead to impaired function.

The definition of neurotoxicity also indicates a potential difference between the developing and the mature nervous system, to underscore the fact that developmental neurotoxicity is an important aspect of neurotoxicology. Most known human neurotoxicants are indeed developmental neurotoxicants (Grandjean and Landrigan, 2006). In most, but not all cases, the developing nervous system is more sensitive to adverse effects than the adult nervous system, as indicated, for example, by the most deleterious effects of ethanol, methylmercury or lead when exposure occurs *in utero* or during childhood. Furthermore, the blood–brain barrier (BBB), which protects the mature nervous system from the entry of a number of substances, appears to be poorly developed at birth and during the first few years of life (Jensen and Catalano, 1998).

Neurotoxicity can also occur as a result of indirect effects. For example, damage to hepatic, renal, circulatory or pancreatic structures may result in secondary effects on the function and structure of the nervous system, such as encephalopathy or polyneuropathy. Secondary effects would not cause a substance to be considered neurotoxic, though at high enough doses, neurotoxicity could be evident. Thus, for the purpose of this review, a substance is defined as neurotoxic when it or its metabolites produce adverse effects as a result of direct interactions with the nervous system. It should be noted, nevertheless, that some chemicals may have multiple modes of action and affect the nervous system directly and indirectly. For example, several halogenated compounds (e.g., polychlorinated biphenyls (PCB), or polybrominated diphenyl ethers) may interact directly with brain cells, and also affect the development of the nervous system by altering thyroid hormone homeostasis (Costa and Giordano, 2007; Crofton, 2008).

IN VIVO TESTING FOR NEUROTOXICITY AND DEVELOPMENTAL NEUROTOXICITY

Neurotoxic effects can be detected in the course of standard toxicity testing (acute, subacute, subchronic, chronic, developmental/reproductive toxicity) required by regulatory agencies worldwide. However, specific guidelines exist to further probe the potential neurotoxicity of chemicals (OECD, 1997; USEPA, 1998a). Such tests are performed in rodents and are meant to assess specific effects of the tested chemical on the nervous system. The USEPA (United States Environmental Protection Agency) guidelines focus on a functional observational battery, on measurements of motor activity and on neuropathological examinations (USEPA, 1998a). The OECD (Organization for Economic Co-operation and Development) guidelines similarly focus on clinical observations, functional tests (e.g., motor activity, sensory reactivity to stimuli) and on neuropathology (OECD, 1997). These batteries are not meant to provide a complete evaluation of neurotoxicity, but to act as a Tier 1 screening for potential neurotoxicity. If no effects are seen at the appropriate dose level, and if the chemical structure of the substance and/or its metabolites does not suggest concern for potential neurotoxicity, the substance may be considered as not neurotoxic. On the other hand, positive findings can be followed up by further testing (Tier 2) in case of commonly existing substances with commercial

Reproductive and Developmental Toxicology, Edited by Ramesh C. Gupta
ISBN: 978-0-12-382032-7

value or wide exposure; for new chemical entities, development of the molecule may instead be abandoned. The decision to carry out additional studies should be thus made on a case-by-case approach and may depend upon factors such as the intended use of the chemical, the potential of human exposure and its potential to accumulate in biological systems. Such Tier 2 studies may include specialized behavioral tests, electrophysiological and neurochemical measurements and additional morphologic studies. Examples are tests for measuring learning and memory, measurements of nerve conduction velocity and biochemical parameters related to neurotransmission or to indices of cell integrity and functions (Costa, 1998).

The nervous system undergoes gradual development that continues well after birth in both animals and humans. While on one hand, the developing nervous system may more readily adapt to, or compensate for, functional losses as a result of a toxic insult, on the other hand, damage to the nervous system during key periods of brain development may result in long-term, irreversible damage (Costa, 1998). Evidence that developmental exposure to chemicals and drugs may alter behavioral functions in young animals began to emerge in the early 1970s. The field of developmental neurotoxicology thus evolved from the disciplines of neurotoxicology, developmental toxicology and experimental psychology (Makris *et al.*, 2009). In response to this issue, developmental neurotoxicity (DNT) testing guidelines were developed both in the USA and in Europe (USEPA, 1998b; OECD, 2007). Exposure to the test chemicals is from gestational day 6 to postnatal day 10 or 21 to the mother, thus ensuring exposure *in utero* and through maternal milk. Tests involve measurements of developmental landmarks and reflexes, motor activity, auditory startle test, learning and memory tests and neuropathology. As for neurotoxicity testing, DNT testing has been proven to be useful and effective in identifying compounds with developmental neurotoxicity potential (Makris *et al.*, 2009). This is not to say that current DNT testing guidelines cannot be improved; indeed it has been pointed out that they may be overly sensitive and produce a high rate of false positives (Claudio *et al.*, 2000), or, in contrast, that they may be too insensitive and not enough comprehensive (Cory-Slechta *et al.*, 2001). Furthermore, issues have been raised regarding historical control data, toxicokinetic parameters, maternally mediated toxicity vs. direct effects, selection of tests and their analysis and interpretation, and others (Kaufmann, 2003; Li, 2005).

IN VITRO APPROACHES TO DEVELOPMENTAL NEUROTOXICITY

In the past several years, the need to develop acceptable alternatives to conventional animal testing has been increasingly recognized by toxicologists, to address problems related to the escalating costs and time required for toxicity assessments, the increasing number of chemicals being developed and commercialized, the need to respond to recent legislations (e.g., REACH (Registration Evaluation and Authorization of Chemicals) and the Cosmetics Directive (76/768/EEC) in the EU) and efforts aimed at reducing the number of animals used for toxicity testing (Costa, 1998; Harry *et al.*, 1998; Lein *et al.*, 2005; Gartlon *et al.*, 2006; Sunol *et al.*, 2008; Bal-Price *et al.*, 2010). Hence, efforts have been directed toward the development of alternative models, utilizing either mammalian cells in culture or non-mammalian model systems, which could serve as tools for neurotoxicity and developmental neurotoxicity testing. Such *in vitro* testing procedures have two main purposes: (1) investigate mode and/or mechanism of action of chemicals, particularly related to early, upstream events in the neurotoxic process; and (2) screening of chemicals of unknown toxicity to flag compounds for further *in vitro* and *in vivo* studies.

Mammalian cells in culture

Several issues need to be considered when exploring potential *in vitro* cell culture models for neurotoxicity and developmental neurotoxicity. First, the nervous system comprises several types of cells (neurons, astrocytes, oligodendrocytes, Schwann cells, microglia and neural stem (progenitor) cells). Second, there are several different cell models which can be used; in increasing level of complexity they are immortalized cell lines, primary cells, cells in co-culture, aggregating cell cultures and brain slices (Coecke *et al.*, 2006). Each model has its own advantages and disadvantages. For example, a cell line provides a defined and homogeneous population of cells (usually clonal) derived from tumors or using oncogene-containing retroviruses. Cell lines are easy to grow, divide rapidly, are available from various animal species including humans and can be induced to differentiate. On the other hand, transformed cell lines may not exhibit the same phenotype of primary cells or may represent a specific cell subpopulation. There is also increased genetic instability with increased number of passages (Hughes *et al.*, 2007). Additionally, neurites may not represent true axons or dendrites, and cell–cell interactions are missing.

Cells in primary culture, most often isolated from rodent central or peripheral nervous system, have usually the same characteristics and maintain most neurodevelopmental features of brain cells *in situ*. They are relatively easy to prepare and can be obtained from specific brain regions. Limitations include a limited lifespan, variability among different cultures, problems of purity and the need of particular attention during preparation and culturing.

A more complex system, such as aggregating brain cell cultures, has the advantage of providing a three-dimensional cell system containing all cell types and allowing cell–cell interactions, and permits testing of multiple endpoints in different cell types, including, for example, inflammatory responses (Honegger and Monnet-Tschudi, 2001). However, such cultures are difficult to prepare and maintain, there is a notable degree of variability between aggregates and the anatomical organization of the tissue is missing.

Brain slices can be obtained from different brain areas, but are most often isolated from the hippocampus. They conserve the brain area cytoarchitecture and its synaptic organization, as well as cell–cell interactions, and are amenable for complex electrophysiological testing. On the other hand, they can be kept for a limited time in culture, need special care to ensure appropriate oxygen and nutrient supply, and are not amenable to high throughput screening.

Additional issues in the choice of a specific model should also be considered. For example, is it better to use human or animal cell lines? Though the use of human cell lines may be preferred, there is no compelling evidence that they would be more sensitive or predictive of neurotoxicity (McLean *et al.*,

1998; Costa *et al.*, 2007). In most cases, human and animal cell lines appear to respond similarly to neurotoxicants; however, in a few cases, opposite effects have been found (e.g., lead and neurite initiation (Radio and Mundy, 2008)). Are primary cells a better model than cell lines, and do they provide a higher sensitivity? There is a general belief that cells in primary culture may be more sensitive to the effects of neurotoxicants. Though this is true at times, it is not always the case (Gartlon *et al.*, 2006; Costa *et al.*, 2007), and differences are often due to different culturing conditions. Which cell type/brain area should I choose? Cell type and brain area may represent an important determinant in the response to neurotoxicants. For example, cocaine was shown to inhibit neurite outgrowth in neurons from the locus coeruleus, but not of the substantia nigra (Dey *et al.*, 2006). Rodent neural stem cells were found to be two orders of magnitude more sensitive than hippocampal neurons to the toxicity of methylmercury (Tamm *et al.*, 2006). Cerebellar Purkinje neurons were eight-fold more susceptible to the toxicity of PCB126 (a dioxin-like PCB) than cerebellar granule neurons (Costa *et al.*, 2007). Astrocytes, which have higher glutathione content than neurons, are normally more resistant to the toxicity of chemicals that cause oxidative stress (Giordano *et al.*, 2008). Thus, while selection of the appropriate cell model can be driven by specific knowledge or hypotheses in case of mechanistic studies, it remains a primary concern for applications to screening.

Mechanistic studies

In vitro systems are amenable and very useful for mechanistic studies at the cellular and molecular level. As such, they have been used extensively in neurobiology and in neurotoxicology. Because of the complexity of the nervous system, no single *in vitro* preparation can be relied on to detect all possible endpoints. However, depending on the knowledge on the neurotoxicity of a certain compound, and of the specific questions that are being asked, different cellular systems or preparations can be used, and a tiered approach can be applied in this context as well. There are indeed hundreds, if not thousands, of examples in which different cell culture models have been successfully utilized to investigate specific mechanisms of action of neurotoxicants. *In vitro* test systems are amenable to biochemical, molecular, electrophysiologic and morphologic examinations. In the context of mechanistic *in vitro* neurotoxicology and developmental neurotoxicology, one can point to studies investigating mechanisms of neurotoxicant-induced neuronal cell death (Giordano *et al.*, 2007), inhibition of cell proliferation (Guizzetti *et al.*, 2004), inhibition of neurite outgrowth (Das *et al.*, 2004), alteration of signal transduction pathways (Kodavanti and Ward, 2005), modulation of neurotoxicity by cell–cell interactions (Zurich *et al.*, 2004; Giordano *et al.*, 2009) or alterations of inhibitory or excitatory circuitries (Janigro and Costa, 1987). Extrapolation of *in vitro* findings to *in vivo* effects requires important considerations, related for instance to dose selection, role of metabolism and pharmacokinetics, BBB permeability, etc. (Goldoni *et al.*, 2003; Coecke *et al.*, 2006; Bal-Price *et al.*, 2010); however, there is no doubt that *in vitro* systems play the most relevant role in mechanistic neurotoxicology.

Even limited knowledge on mechanism and/or mode of action may lead to the use of *in vitro* methods to screen for a specific neurotoxicity. For example, the acute neurotoxicity of OP compounds is the result of inhibition of the enzyme acetylcholinesterase (AChE), while their delayed neurotoxicity (a polyneuropathy) is attributed instead to irreversible inhibition of another esterase, NTE (neuropathy target esterase) (Lotti and Moretto, 2005). Knowledge of the two neurotoxicity targets has allowed utilization of human neuroblastoma cells *in vitro* to screen OPs for their potential of inducing delayed polyneuropathy (Ehrich *et al.*, 1997). Another example is the use of cerebellar granule neurons (CGNs) from transgenic mice to investigate neurotoxicant-induced oxidative stress. Mice lacking GCLM (the modifier subunit of glutamate cysteine ligase, the first and rate-limiting enzyme in the synthesis of glutathione) have very low glutathione content, and as such should be more susceptible to the toxic effects of chemicals that cause oxidative stress. CGNs from *Gclm*(−/−) mice are indeed more susceptible than their wild-type counterparts to the neurotoxicity of chemicals known to induce oxidative stress, but not to that of other neurotoxicants known to act through other mechanisms (Costa *et al.*, 2010).

Screening

As said, a second primary objective of *in vitro* systems is that of providing a rapid, relatively inexpensive, and reliable way for screening chemicals for potential neurotoxicity and/or developmental neurotoxicity. Screening is by definition a Tier 1 evaluation of chemicals that will be followed by more specific and complex tests, both *in vitro* and *in vivo*. The same general criteria for *in vitro* screening approaches for other endpoints of toxicity also apply to the neurotoxicity screening: (1) low incidence of false positives and false negatives; (2) high correlation with *in vivo* data, i.e. good predictive value; and (3) sensitive, relatively simple, rapid (amenable for medium–high throughput screening), economical and versatile (Costa, 1998).

The choice of one or more *in vitro* models for neurotoxicity screening poses a number of problems, as one has to decide which cell type to use, the degree of model complexity and particularly which endpoints are to be measured. A common belief is that for screening purposes one should examine general cellular processes such as cell viability or proliferation, differentiation of precursors or elaboration of axon or dendrites. However, each possibility requires careful consideration. For example, basic tests of cytotoxicity and viability are common to most cell types and include measurements of cell death, membrane permeability, mitochondrial function, cell growth and reproduction, energy regulation and synthesis of macromolecules. If these endpoints are affected by a chemical in neuronal/glial cells, one cannot conclude that a chemical is neurotoxic, but only that it displays cytotoxicity in these cells (Costa, 1998). For example, Gartlon *et al.* (2006) examined 13 neurotoxic compounds and two non-neurotoxic compounds in undifferentiated or differentiated PC12 cells and in rat cerebellar granule neurons. Though various endpoints were utilized in this study, such as cell viability, ATP depletion, production of reactive oxygen species and cytoskeletal modifications, the system did not provide distinction between cytotoxicity and neurotoxicity.

The use of non-neuronal cell types may provide initial information on whether a chemical may have differential effects, or display different potencies, in neuronal versus non-neuronal cells. For example, a battery of 17 different cell types, including cell lines and primary cells (both neuronal and glial), human and rat cells, nervous system and non-nervous system cells, was utilized to assess the toxicity of known developmental neurotoxicants, such as methylmercury and polychlorinated biphenyls (PCBs) (Costa *et al.*, 2007). Using cell viability and cell proliferation as endpoints, this simple approach flagged out methylmercury as a potential neurotoxicant, as toxicity was greater in neuronal cells than in other cell types; PCB-153 was also flagged out as a potential neurotoxicant, though not specific for neurons, as glial cells were similarly affected (Costa *et al.*, 2007).

Using the more complex model of aggregating cell cultures, van Vliet *et al.* (2008) investigated an *in vitro* metabolomics approach for neurotoxicity testing. A neurotoxic compound, methylmercury, at subcytotoxic concentrations, caused significant changes in the levels of GABA, choline, glutamine, spermine and creatine, while the brain stimulant caffeine altered levels of spermine and creatine only. This profile was mimicked by three other known neurotoxicants (trimethyltin, methylmercury and paraquat), while a series of five non-neurotoxic compounds elicited a metabolomic profile similar to that observed in control cultures. This interesting and novel approach should be further pursued using a larger battery of known neurotoxic and non-neurotoxic compounds, as well as known neuropharmacological agents. These investigators, using the same *in vitro* system, also explored the possibility of electrophysiological measurements by means of a multi-electrode array system (van Vliet *et al.*, 2007). Initial experiments indicated that electrophysiological recordings of evoked field potentials in reaggregating brain cell cultures involve glutamatergic and GABAergic synaptic transmission. Electrophysiological changes in neural activity can be detected before any morphological change occurs, and may thus represent a promising and sensitive approach to detect early effects of chemicals. As expected, however, the test method cannot distinguish between pharmacological actions (e.g., interactions with neurotransmitters or their receptors) and neurotoxicity. Nevertheless, it was found that trimethyltin and methylmercury caused a decrease in field potential amplitude and an irreversible loss of neuronal electric activity at high concentrations. In contrast, the effects of ethanol were fully reversible upon washout. Thus, the simple observation of loss/recovery of electrical function may allow differentiation between neurotoxic or acute pharmacological effects (van Vliet *et al.*, 2007).

Special considerations for developmental neurotoxicity

When the objective is to screen potential developmental neurotoxicants, *in vitro* cell culture models need to represent specific cellular and/or molecular events known to be critical to the development of the nervous system. These include cell proliferation, differentiation of stem cells into neuronal or glial cell types, cell migration, axonal and dendritic outgrowth, formation and pruning of synapses, programmed cell death, ontogeny of neurotransmission and receptors, myelination and development of the blood–brain barrier (Lein *et al.*, 2005). All these endpoints can be measured *in vitro* in different cell models. However, validation of such models for screening purposes for developmental neurotoxicity has only been carried out to a very limited extent. Indeed, the main issue relates to the very limited progress that has been made in the validation process. Over a decade ago we wrote that "the validation process should require the testing, under standardized conditions, of a large number of chemicals, some of which are neurotoxic...and others that are known not to affect the nervous system" (Costa, 1998). A decade later, one can find an almost identical statement "in order to make meaningful comparisons between model systems, a standard set of chemicals should be tested in all models. This reference set should include compounds known to inhibit neurite outgrowth, as well as compounds that are non-toxic..." (Radio *et al.*, 2008). Thus, despite the development of several models and tests of potential usefulness, the lack of validation to determine the rate of false positives/false negatives, and the degree of inter-laboratory variability, has hampered so far the further use of such alternative approaches.

Two models that have been tested to a limited extent, and that appear to be promising, are briefly discussed. Neurite outgrowth is considered an important endpoint for screening of developmental neurotoxicants (Radio and Mundy, 2008). It can be measured in cell lines induced to differentiate by various factors, or in primary cultures or neural stem cells. In a recent study, a subclone of PC12 cells (Neuroscreen-1 (NS-1) cells), induced to differentiate with nerve growth factor, was used to examine the ability of 21 compounds to inhibit neurite outgrowth, as a model to screen for potential developmental neurotoxicants (Radio *et al.*, 2008), with the results shown in Table 13.1. Five chemicals, already known to inhibit neurite outgrowth, tested positive at concentrations devoid of any cytotoxicity. Among non-neurotoxic compounds, 6/8 had no effect on neurite outgrowth, while two increased neurite outgrowth at subcytotoxic concentrations. Among neurotoxic compounds, only two (*trans*-retinoic acid and methylmercury) inhibited neurite outgrowth at subcytotoxic concentrations; two compounds (dexamethasone and cadmium) equally affected cell viability, while one increased neurite outgrowth (amphetamine), and three (lead, valproic acid and diphenylhydantoin) were devoid of effects. If one considers alteration of neurite outgrowth (either inhibition or augmentation) as an index of potential neurotoxicity, this study would provide 2/8 false positives and 3/8 false negatives.

Despite these caveats, the study of Radio *et al.* (2008) is of much interest because it utilized an automated microscopy and image analysis system (high content analysis, HCA), which would allow the screening of a large number of compounds in a reasonable time. The same investigators expanded their work by comparing the effects of 14 chemicals on neurite outgrowth in NS-1 cells and in rat CGNs (Radio *et al.*, 2010). The compounds were a subset of those used in the previous study (Table 13.1), and included seven non-neurotoxic compounds (omeprazole was excluded), five developmentally neurotoxic compounds (cadmium, diphenylhydantoin and dexamethasone were excluded) and two positive controls (UO126 and Bis-I). In general, results in NS-1 confirmed those previously obtained. One exception was dimethylphthalate which did not have any effect on neurite outgrowth in this study. Among neurotoxic compounds and positive controls, results in NS-1 cells were identical to those of the first study (Radio *et al.*, 2008), with the exception of amphetamine which did not affect neurite outgrowth. Overall, these results reveal a notable reproducibility, at least within the same laboratory.

The comparison with CGNs indicated that these cells could detect one more compound (lead acetate) than NS-1 cells, but were less sensitive to the effect of another (*trans*-retinoic

TABLE 13.1 *In vitro* screening of chemicals for effects on neurite outgrowth in a PC-12 cell line (NS-1)

Compound	Use	Effect on neurite outgrowth	Effect on cell viability
Positive controls			
Bis-I	PKC inhibitor	**Inhibition**	No effect
UO1261	MAPK inhibitor	**Inhibition**	No effect
Okaidic acid	Phosphatase inhibitor	**Inhibition**	No effect
Vincristine	Microtubule depolarizing agent	**Inhibition**	No effect
K252a	Tyrosine kinase inhibitor	**Inhibition**	No effect
Non-neurotoxic compounds			
Amoxicillin	Drug (antibiotic)	No effect	No effect
Sorbitol	Sweetener	No effect	No effect
Saccharin	Artificial sweetener	No effect	No effect
Acetominophen	Drug (antipyretic)	No effect	No effect
Dimethyl phthalate	Plasticizer	**Increase**	No effect
Diphenylhydramine	Drug (antihistamine)	No effect	No effect
Omeprazole	Drug (anti-ulcer)	**Increase**	No effect
Glyphosate	Herbicide	No effect	No effect
Developmentally neurotoxic compounds			
Diphenylhydantoin	Drug (anticonvulsant)	No effect	No effect
Trans-retinoic acid	Vitamin (anti-acne)	**Inhibition**	No effect
Valproic acid	Drug (anticonvulsant)	No effect	No effect
Dexamethasone	Synthetic glucocorticoid	**Inhibition**	**Decrease**
Amphetamine	Drug (stimulant)	**Increase**	No effect
Cadmium	Metal	**Inhibition**	**Decrease**
Lead	Metal	No effect	No effect
Methylmercury	Organometal	**Inhibition**	No effect

Adapted from: Radio *et al.* (2008)

acid). In general, based on concentrations, CGNs were more sensitive than NS-1 cells for detecting changes in neurite outgrowth, but neither cell type detected all neurotoxic chemicals, though in both models neurite outgrowth was more sensitive than cell viability. Table 13.2 summarizes the results of these two studies (Radio *et al.*, 2008, 2010). While neurite outgrowth appears to be a useful endpoint for screening of developmental neurotoxicants, these findings also indicate that the effects may be cell specific. Furthermore, given the still high percentage of false negatives (Table 13.2), additional validation studies are certainly needed.

Embryonic stem cells (ESC) and neuroprogenitor cells (NPC) have been proposed as relevant models for screening of developmental neurotoxicants. ESC and NPC can be derived from rodents, and human cells are available commercially (Breier *et al.*, 2010). Breier *et al.* (2008) utilized ReNcell CX (an immortalized neuroprogenitor cell line from 14-week human fetal cortex) to study the neurotoxicity of 16 chemicals (half of which are known neurotoxicants), utilizing cell viability and cell proliferation as endpoints. The assay, which was adapted to high throughput, revealed 2/8 false negatives and 2/8 false positives. It should be noted that both false negatives (valproic acid and 5,5-diphenylhydantoin) and both false positives (diphenhydramine and omeprazole) are pharmaceutical compounds. The reason(s) for such false positive/negative results are not apparent, so far.

NPCs can also be grown as neurospheres; these three-dimensional heterogeneous, self-regulated cellular systems mimic basic processes of brain development. Indeed, proliferation, migration, differentiation and viability can be measured in the same system (Moors *et al.*, 2009). So far, no set of compounds has been tested in this model, but findings with individual compounds are quite promising. For example, both

TABLE 13.2 Effects of chemicals on neurite outgrowth: reproducibility and cell-specific differences

Chemicals	NS-1 (1)	NS-1 (2)	CGNs
Positive controls	5/5 (100%)	2/2 (100%)	2/2 (100%)
DNT	5/8 (62.5%)	2/5 (40%)	3/5 (60%)
Not-DNT	6/8 (75%)	7/7 (100%)	6/7 (85.7%)

NS-1 = Neuroscreen-1 cells (a PC12 cell clone); CGNs (rat cerebellar granule neurons); DNT = developmental neurotoxic. Indicated is the number of tested chemicals that exerted the expected effect. The percentage of false negatives appears to be the highest, as only 40–62.5% of known DNT compounds were detected by the screening.
Adapted from Radio *et al.* (2008, 2010)

lead and ethanol have been found to inhibit cell proliferation, while ethanol and methylmercury inhibit migration. These same compounds, together with PCBs, also affect, in different ways, differentiation (see references in Breier *et al.* 2010).

Non-mammalian models

In the not so distant past, animals other than mammals, with few exceptions such as certain birds or fishes, were not considered ideal for the study of biomedical sciences, because of their phylogenic distance from humans. Yet, several organisms have proven to be of great similitude to humans, and have provided great insights into fundamental biological processes, two excellent examples being the marine snail *Aplysia* and the fly *Drosophila melanogaster*. A number of alternative non-mammalian models are starting to be investigated also in the context of screening for neurotoxic chemicals (Peterson *et al.*, 2008). Zebrafish and the nematode *Caenorhabditis elegans* will be briefly considered here, but others (e.g., sea urchin and *Drosophila*) have also been proposed and utilized to a limited extent (Buznikov *et al.*, 2001; Falugi *et al.*, 2008; Rand, 2010).

Zebrafish

Zebrafish (*Danio rerio*) has been used historically to assess environmental toxicity, and is an approved model for aquatic toxicity testing. The small size, chemical permeability and optical transparency of the zebrafish embryo are also inducive to small molecule screening, and have found application in the area of cardiac toxicity (Zon and Peterson, 2005). The zebrafish is providing an excellent model to study the development of the nervous system (Blader and Strahle, 2000), as it presents many similarities to the mammalian counterpart, including the presence of a BBB (Jeong *et al.*, 2008). More recently, zebrafish have also been proposed as a model for neurotoxicity and developmental neurotoxicity studies that combine cellular, molecular, behavioral and genetic approaches (Lein *et al.*, 2005; Ton *et al.*, 2006; Parng *et al.*, 2007). A few known neurotoxic compounds have been investigated in zebrafish, leading to a proof of concept; for example, 6-hydroxydopamine and MPTP have been shown to c ause a loss of dopaminergic neurons, as seen in mammals (McKinley *et al.*, 2005; Parng *et al.*, 2007). Ethanol, a known human developmental neurotoxicant, has been shown to alter a subset of genes important for brain development (Fan *et al.*, 2010). However, these studies examined only a limited number of chemicals, and did not include any negative controls; thus, validation studies are still required to exploit the full potential of this model.

C. elegans

An even simpler model is represented by the nematode *C. elegans*. It has a very small size (~1 mm), is transparent, has a short lifespan, has simply measurable behaviors and is easily amenable to genetic manipulations. Homologues for 60–80% of human genes have been found in *C. elegans* (Kaletta and Hengartner, 2006). The acute toxicities of several chemicals in worms correlate with those found in rats and mice (Helmke *et al.*, 2010). The structure, metabolism and bioenergetics of *C. elegans* mitochondria are very similar to those of humans, contributing to its potential usefulness in investigating various mechanisms of oxidative stress-mediated toxicity. Its nervous system contains only a few hundred neurons and fewer than 7,000 synapses (White *et al.*, 1986), as well as most neurotransmitters and signaling systems found in humans. The conservation of neuroanatomic, neurochemical and neurophysiological components from nematodes to humans has allowed the study of basic mechanisms of neuronal fate, differentiation and migration, axon guidance and synaptogenesis and axon degeneration (Leung *et al.*, 2008). Mechanistic elucidation of the apoptotic pathways have also been carried out extensively in *C. elegans* (Hengartner and Horvitz, 1994). *C. elegans* has been used over the years to study effects and mechanisms of a number of neurotoxic metals and pesticides, and as a model for studying neurodegenerative diseases (Leung *et al.*, 2008). *C. elegans* has also been recently proposed as a model for high throughput neurotoxicity screening (Leung *et al.*, 2008; Boyd *et al.*, 2010; Helmke *et al.*, 2010). A series of eight compounds were tested utilizing four endpoints (growth, feeding, reproduction and locomotion), but the data are too preliminary to allow any conclusion (Boyd *et al.*, 2010). Nevertheless, evidence accumulated so far suggests that changes in *C. elegans* following chemical exposure appear to be predictive of developmental shifts and/or neurological damage in rodents, highlighting the promise of this worm as an alternative screening model for neurotoxicity and developmental neurotoxicity.

CONCLUDING REMARKS AND FUTURE DIRECTIONS

Neurotoxicity and developmental neurotoxicity are important adverse health effects of hundreds of environmental contaminants and occupational chemicals, natural toxins and pharmaceutical drugs. *In vivo* testing guidelines for neurotoxicity and developmental neurotoxicity have been developed, implemented and validated. Though there is still room for improvements and refinements, these *in vivo* tests have been shown, so far, to provide reliable indications on the potential neurotoxicity of chemical substances. However, such *in vivo* tests are time-consuming, expensive and require the use of a substantial number of animals. Hence, there is a great need to develop alternative models, utilizing mammalian cell preparations of different complexity and/or non-mammalian animal system, as indicated earlier. These alternative tests should serve as Tier 1 tests to allow the screening of compounds whose potential neurotoxicity is unknown. Given the complexity of the nervous system and the multiple facets of possible neurotoxic effects, it is highly unlikely that a single test (as the Ames test for mutagenicity) will cover the spectrum of neurotoxicity or developmental neurotoxicity. Rather, a battery of tests should be considered, which may include some *in vitro* tests with mammalian cells and one or two tests with non-mammalian models. This may be complemented by quantitative structure–activity relationship (QSAR)-based computational approaches. Novel approaches, part of the "omics" technologies, may also find a role in such endeavor. Genomics, proteomics and metabolomics each offer the potential of fingerprinting potential neurotoxic compounds and thus find application to neurotoxicity screening. However, such approaches in this context still need to be developed.

Independent of the chosen approach, the key issue is that it needs to undergo a rigorous validation process. This should include the testing of several known neurotoxicants and developmental neurotoxicants, and of several non-neurotoxicants, to determine the sensitivity and specificity of the test or battery; information on reproducibility and interlaboratory variability are also needed. Key elements of the validation process are the choice of neurotoxic compounds (which ones and how many) and their concentrations to be used in *in vitro* tests. This is particularly challenging for neurotoxicity, as multiple cell types and cellular mechanisms can be targeted by neurotoxicants. As indicated earlier, neurons and various types of glial cells can be affected by neurotoxicants. A chemical may cause a neuronopathy, an axonopathy or affect synaptic transmission; it may alter astrocyte or oligodendrocyte/Schwann cell functions, or act by other mechanisms that may lead to neuro-inflammation. Alternative models for neurotoxicity should thus attempt to mimic several processes that may occur *in vivo*. Similarly, chemicals to be used as positive controls in validation studies should cover most, if not all, of these processes, and would thus need to be several dozens. So far, only 10–20 chemicals have been used in limited validation experiments. The concentration of chemical to be used in these studies is also most relevant. The scenario for neurotoxicity is thus much more complex than that for other target organs of toxicity. For example, it has been shown that hepatotoxicity can be predicted by a few specific features (e.g., mitochondrial damage, oxidative stress, intracellular glutathione), which has allowed the development of potentially highly predictive screening approaches (Xu *et al.*, 2008).

Finally, a battery of alternative testing models for neurotoxicity is not expected to fully replace current *in vivo* animal testing, but would limit such testing only to those compounds for which, for different reasons, additional information on neurotoxicity is deemed important. Without concerted efforts by regulatory agencies, institutions, foundations and private entities worldwide, it is doubtful that such validation process will take place. If so, ten years from now, we will still be discussing perhaps new, sophisticated models that have the potential to serve as screening tools for neurotoxicity, but that would leave this potential still unfulfilled.

REFERENCES

Bal-Price AK, Hogberg HT, Buzanska L, Coecke S (2010) Relevance of *in vitro* neurotoxicity testing for regulatory requirements: challenges to be considered. *Neurotoxicol Teratol* **32:** 36–41.

Blader P, Strahle U (2000) Zebrafish developmental genetics and central nervous system development. *Hum Mol Genet* **9:** 945–51.

Boyd WA, Smith MV, Kissling G, Freedman JH (2010) Medium- and high-throughput screening of neurotoxicants using *C. elegans*. *Neurotoxicol Teratol* **32:** 68–73.

Breier JM, Radio NM, Mundy WR, Shafer TJ (2008) Development of a high-throughput screening assay for chemical effects on proliferation and viability of immortalized human neural progenitor cells. *Toxicol Sci* **105:** 119–33.

Breier JM, Gassmann K, Kayser R, *et al.* (2010) Neural progenitor cells as models for high throughput screens of developmental neurotoxicity: state of the science. *Neurotoxicol Teratol* **32:** 4–15.

Buznikov GA, Nikitina LA, Bezuglov VV, Lauder JM, Padilla S, Slotkin TA (2001) An invertebrate model of the developmental neurotoxicity of insecticides: effects of chlorpyrifos and dieldrin in sea urchin embryos and larvae. *Environ Health Perspect* **109:** 651–61.

Claudio L, Kwa WC, Russell AL, Wallinga D (2000) Testing methods for developmental neurotoxicity of environmental chemicals. *Toxicol Appl Pharmacol* **164:** 1–14.

Coecke S, Eskes C, Gartlon J, *et al.* (2006) The value of alternative testing for neurotoxicity in the context of regulatory needs. *Environ Toxicol Pharmacol* **21:** 153–67.

Cory-Slechta DA, Crofton KM, Foran JA, *et al.* (2001) Methods to identify and characterize developmental neurotoxicity for human health risk assessment. I: Behavioral effects. *Environ Health Perspect* **109 (Suppl 1):** 79–91.

Costa LG, Fattori V, Giordano G, Vitalone A (2007) An *in vitro* approach to assess the toxicity of certain food contaminants: methylmercury and polychlorinated biphenyls. *Toxicology* **237:** 65–76.

Costa LG, Giordano G (2007) Developmental neurotoxicity of polybrominated diphenyl ether (PBDE) flame retardants. *Neurotoxicology* **28:** 1047–67.

Costa LG, Giordano G, Guizzetti M (2010) Predictive models for neurotoxicity assessment. In *Predictive Toxicology in Drug Safety* (Xu JJ, Urban L, eds.). Cambridge University Press. In press.

Costa LG (1998) Neurotoxicity testing: a discussion of *in vitro* alternatives. *Environ Health Perspect* **106 (Suppl. 2):** 505–10.

Crofton KM (2008) Thyroid disrupting chemicals: mechanisms and mixtures. *Int J Androl* **31:** 209–23.

Das KP, Freudenrich TM, Mundy WR (2004) Assessment of PC12 cell differentiation and neurite growth: a comparison of morphological and neurochemical measures. *Neurotoxicol Teratol* **26:** 397–406.

Dey S, Mactutus CF, Booze RM, Snow DM (2006) Specificity of prenatal cocaine on inhibition of locus coeruleus neurite outgrowth. *Neuroscience* **139:** 899–907.

ECETOC (1992) *Evaluation of the Neurotoxic Potential of Chemicals*. Brussels, European Center for Ecotoxicology and Toxicology of Chemicals.

Ehrich M, Correll L, Veronesi B (1997) Acetylcholinesterase and neuropathy target esterase inhibitions in neuroblastoma cells to distinguish organophosphorus compounds causing acute and delayed neurotoxicity. *Fund Appl Toxicol* **38:** 55–63.

Falugi C, Lammerding-Koppel M, Aluigi MG (2008) Sea urchin development: an alternative model for mechanistic understanding of neurodevelopment and neurotoxicity. *Birth Defects Res (Pt C)* **84:** 188–203.

Fan CY, Cowden J, Simmons SO, Padilla S, Ramabhadran R (2010) Gene expression changes in developing zebrafish as potential markers for rapid developmental neurotoxicity screening. *Neurotoxicol Teratol* **32:** 91–8.

Gartlon J, Kinsner A, Bal-Price A, Coecke S, Clothier RH (2006) Evaluation of a proposed *in vitro* test strategy using neuronal and non-neuronal cell systems for detecting neurotoxicity. *Toxicol in Vitro* **20:** 1569–81.

Giordano G, Kavanagh TJ, Costa LG (2009) Mouse cerebellar astrocytes protect cerebellar granule neurons against toxicity of the polybrominated diphenyl ether (PBDE) mixture DE-71. *Neurotoxicology* **30:** 326–9.

Giordano G, Kavanagh TJ, Costa LG (2008) Neurotoxicity of a polybrominated diphenyl ether mixture (DE-71) in mouse neurons and astrocytes is modulated by intracellular glutathione levels. *Toxicol Appl Pharmacol* **232:** 161–8.

Giordano G, White CC, Mohar I, Kavanagh TJ, Costa LG (2007) Glutathione levels modulate domoic acid-induced apoptosis in mouse cerebellar granule cells. *Toxicol Sci* **100:** 433–44.

Goldoni M, Vettori MV, Alinovi R, Caglieri A, Ceccatelli S, Mutti A (2003) Models of neurotoxicity: extrapolation of threshold doses in vitro. *Risk Anal* **23:** 505–14.

Grandjean P, Landrigan PJ (2006) Developmental neurotoxicity of industrial chemicals. *Lancet* **368:** 2167–78.

Guizzetti M, Thompson BD, Kim Y, VanDeMark K, Costa LG (2004) Role of phospholipase D signaling in ethanol induced inhibition of carbachol-stimulated DNA synthesis of 1321N1 astrocytoma cells. *J Neurochem* **90:** 646–53.

Harry GJ, Billingsley M, Bruinink A, *et al.* (1998) *In vitro* techniques for the assessment of neurotoxicity. *Environ Health Perspect* **106 (Suppl. 1):** 131–58.

Helmke KJ, Avila DS, Aschner M (2010) Utility of *Caenorhabditis elegans* in high throughput neurotoxicological research. *Neurotoxicol Teratol* **32:** 62–7.

Hengartner MO, Horvitz HR (1994) Programmed cell death in *Caenorhabditis elegans*. *Curr Op Genet Dev* **4:** 581–6.

Honegger P, Monnet-Tschudi F (2001) Aggregating neural cell cultures. In *Protocols for Neural Cell Cultures* (Fedoroff S, Richardson A, eds.). Humana Press, Ottawa, pp. 199–218.

Hughes P, Marshall D, Reid Y, Parkes H, Gelber C (2007) The costs of using unauthenticated, over-passaged cell lines: how much more data do we need? *BioTechniques* **43:** 575–86.

Janigro D, Costa LG (1987) Effects of trimethyltin on granule cells excitability in the in vitro rat dentate gyrus. *Neurotoxicol Teratol* **9:** 33–8.

Jensen KF, Catalano SM (1998) Brain morphogenesis and developmental neurotoxicology. In *Handbook of Developmental Neurotoxicology* (Slikker W, Chang LW, eds.). Academic Press, San Diego, pp. 3–41.

Jeong JY, Kwon HB, Ahn JC, *et al.* (2008) Functional and developmental analysis of the blood–brain barrier in zebrafish. *Brain Res Bull* **75:** 619–28.

Kaletta T, Hengartner MO (2006) Finding function in novel targets: *C. elegans* as a model organism. *Nat Rev Drug Discovery* **5:** 387–98.

Kaufmann W (2003) Current status of developmental neurotoxicity testing: and industry perspective. *Toxicol Lett* **140–141:** 161–9.

Kodavanti PR, Ward TR (2005) Differential effects of commercial polybrominated diphenyl ether and polychlorinated biphenyl mixtures on intracellular signaling in rat brain *in vitro*. *Toxicol Sci* **85:** 952–62.

Lein P, Silbergeld E, Locke P, Goldberg AM (2005) In vitro and other alternative approaches to developmental neurotoxicity testing (DNT). *Environ Toxicol Pharmacol* **19:** 735–44.

Leung MCK, Williams PL, Benedetto A, *et al.* (2008) *Caenorhabditis elegans*: and emerging model in biomedical and environmental toxicology. *Toxicol Sci* **106:** 5–28.

Li AA (2005) Regulatory developmental neurotoxicology testing: data evaluation for risk assessment purposes. *Environ Toxicol Pharmacol* **19:** 727–33.

Lotti M, Moretto A (2005) Organophosphate-induced delayed polyneuropathy. *Toxicol Rev* **24:** 37–49.

Makris SL, Raffaele K, Allen S, *et al.* (2009) A retrospective performance assessment of the developmental neurotoxicity study in support of OECD test guideline 426. *Environ Health Perspect* **117:** 17–25.

McKinley ET, Baranowski TC, Blavo DO, Cato C, Doan TN, Rubinstein AL (2005) Neuroprotection of MPTP-induced toxicity in zebrafish dopaminergic neurons. *Brain Res Mol Brain Res* **141:** 128–37.

McLean WG, Holme AD, Janneh O, Southgate A, Howard CV, Reed MG (1998) The effect of benomyl on neurite outgrowth in mouse NB2A and human SH-SY5Y neuroblastoma cells *in vitro*. *Neurotoxicology* **19:** 629–32.

Moors M, Rockel TD, Abel J, *et al.* (2009) Human neurospheres as three-dimensional cellular systems for developmental neurotoxicity testing. *Environ Health Perspect* **117:** 1131–8.

OECD (Organization for Economic Co-operation and Development) (1997) Test Guideline 424. OECD Guideline for Testing of Chemicals. Neurotoxicity study in rodents. Paris, OECD.

OECD (Organization for Economic Co-operation and Development) (2007) Test Guideline 426. OECD Guideline for Testing of Chemicals. Developmental neurotoxicity study. Paris, OECD.

Parng C, Roy NM, Ton C, Lin Y, McGrath P (2007) Neurotoxicity assessment using zebrafish. *J Pharmacol Toxicol Meth* **55:** 103–12.

Peterson RT, Nass R, Boyd WA, Freedman JH, Dong K, Narahashi T (2008) Use of non-mammalian alternative models for neurotoxicological study. *Neurotoxicology* **29:** 546–55.

Radio NM, Breier JM, Shafer TJ, Mundy WR (2008) Assessment of chemical effects on neurite outgrowth in PC12 cells using high content screening. *Toxicol Sci* **105:** 106–18.

Radio NM, Mundy WR (2008) Developmental neurotoxicity testing *in vitro*: models for assessing chemical effects on neurite outgrowth. *Neurotoxicology* **29:** 361–76.

Radio NM, Freudenrich TM, Robinette BL, Crofton KM, Mundy WM (2010) Comparison of PC12 and cerebellar granule cell cultures for evaluating neurite outgrowth using high content analysis. *Neurotoxicol Teratol* **32:** 25–35.

Rand MD (2010) Drosophotoxicology: the growing potential for *Drosophila* in neurotoxicology. *Neurotoxicol Teratol* **32:** 74–83.

Sunol C, Babot Z, Fonfria E, *et al.* (2008) Studies with neuronal cells: from basic studies of mechanisms of neurotoxicity to the prediction of chemical toxicity. *Toxicol in Vitro* **22:** 1350–55.

Tamm C, Duckworth J, Hemanson O, Ceccatelli S (2006) High susceptibility of neural stem cells to methylmercury toxic effects on cell survival and neuronal differentiation. *J Neurochem* **97:** 69–78.

Ton C, Lin Y, Willett C (2006) Zebrafish as a model for developmental neurotoxicity testing. *Birth Defects Res (Pt A)* **76:** 553–67.

USEPA (United States Environmental Protection Agency) (1998a) Health Effects Test Guidelines. OPPTS 870.6200. Neurotoxicity screening battery. Washington DC, USEPA.

USEPA (United States Environmental Protection Agency) (1998b) Health Effects Test Guidelines. OPPTS 870.6300. Developmental neurotoxicity study. Washington DC, USEPA.

Van Vliet E, Morath S, Eskes C, *et al.* (2008) A novel metabolomics approach for neurotoxicity testing, proof of principle for methylmercury chloride and caffeine. *Neurotoxicology* **29:** 1–12.

Van Vliet E, Stoppini L, Balestrino M, *et al.* (2007) Electrophysiological recording of re-aggregating brain cell cultures on multi-electrode arrays to detect acute neurotoxic effects. *Neurotoxicology* **28:** 1136–46.

White JG, Southgate J, Thomson JN, Brenner FRS (1986) The structure of the nervous system of the nematode *Caenorhabditis elegans*. *Philos Trans R Soc Lond, B Biol Sci* **314:** 1–340.

Xu JJ, Henstock PV, Dunn MC, Smith AR, Chabot JR, de Graaft D (2008) Cellular imaging predictions of clinical drug-induced liver injury. *Toxicol Sci* **105:** 97–105.

Zon LJ, Peterson RT (2005) In vivo drug discovery in the zebrafish. *Nature Rev Drug Discov* **4:** 35–44.

Zurich MG, Honegger P, Schilter B, Costa LG, Monnet-Tschudi F (2004) Involvement of glial cells in the neurotoxicity of parathion and chlorpyrifos. *Toxicol Sci* **201:** 97–104.

CHAPTER

14

Reproductive and developmental toxicity models in relation to neurodegenerative diseases

Marta Di Carlo

INTRODUCTION

The population of the industrial countries is aging, and an ever-increasing number of people are afflicted with neurodegenerative diseases. Neurodegenerative diseases result from the gradual and progressive loss of neural cells. According to the National Institute of Neurological Disorders and Stroke, there are more than 600 neurologic disorders, with millions of people affected each year. In the USA, it has been calculated that neurodegenerative diseases cost the economy billions of dollars in healthcare each year.

Neurodegeneration and cancer represent opposite ends of an aspect: whereas cancer is an uncontrolled proliferation of cells, neurodegeneration is the result of the death of cells due to direct cell death by necrosis or the delayed process of apoptosis. Known risk factors for neurodegenerative diseases include certain genetic polymorphisms or mutations and increasing age. Other possible causes may include gender, poor education, endocrine conditions, oxidative stress, inflammation, stroke, hypertension, diabetes, smoking, head trauma, depression, infection, tumors, vitamin deficiencies, immune and metabolic conditions, and chemical exposure. Attention is also now being focused on environmental agents' potential for damaging the developing and mature nervous system.

Dysfunction and/or progressive degeneration of subsets of neurons in the brain leads to several human neurodegenerative diseases that can be divided into two groups according to phenotypic effects, although these are not mutually exclusive: (1) conditions causing problems with tremor and movements, such as ataxia; and (2) conditions affecting memory and related to dementia.

These diseases include Parkinson's disease (PD), Alzheimer's disease (AD), frontotemporal dementia with Parkinsonism (FTDP), Huntington's disease (HD), several spinocerebellar ataxias (SCAs) and spinobulbar muscular atrophy (SBMA) diseases, triple nucleotide expansion diseases, and many others. Although most of these diseases are sporadic, familiar forms have also been found, which provide a handle on altered gene function. Some of these diseases are dominant, others recessive, and some are influenced by environmental circumstances. A major pathological characteristic found in most neurodegenerative diseases is the formation of insoluble protein accumulations, suggesting potential common defects in protein folding and degradation (Table 14.1). Although, classically, researchers have modeled human disease in cell lines or mouse, the nematode *Caenorhabditis elegans*, the zebrafish, the fruit fly *Drosophila melanogaster* and the sea urchin, transgenic or not, can offer many advantages to obtain information about the toxic mechanisms underlying human neurodegenerative disease. Moreover, these simple model systems can be easily utilized to test efficacy of putative neuroprotective compounds and can be even utilized in compound screens for therapeutic discovery.

Neurotoxicity is based on protein misfolding

A key molecular pathway implicated in diverse neurodegenerative diseases is the misfolding, aggregation and accumulation of proteins in the brain. Compelling evidence strongly supports the hypothesis that accumulation of misfolded proteins leads to synaptic dysfunction, neuronal apoptosis, brain damage and disease. However, the mechanism by which protein misfolding and aggregation trigger neurodegeneration and the identity of the neurotoxic structure is still unclear. Thus, how and why a physiological protein or peptide becomes a pathological protein is not well understood.

Neurodegenerative diseases such as AD, PD, HD, ALS and prion diseases are increasingly being realized to have common cellular and molecular mechanisms including protein aggregation and inclusion body formations. The aggregates usually consist of fibers containing misfolded proteins with a β-sheet conformation termed amyloid. There is a relationship, even if not perfect, between the cells in which abnormal proteins are deposited and the cells in which degeneration occurs. An explanation is that amyloid plaques and protein aggregates represent an end stage of a molecular cascade of

Reproductive and Developmental Toxicology, Edited by Ramesh C. Gupta
ISBN: 978-0-12-382032-7

TABLE 14.1 A relationship between some aggregated proteins or peptides and diseases

Neurodegenerative diseases	Aggregating protein or peptide
Alzheimer's disease	Amyloid-β peptide
Spongiform encephalopathies	Prion protein
Parkinson's disease	α-Synuclein
Amyotrophic lateral sclerosis	Superoxide dismutase SOOD, TDP-43
Huntington's disease	Huntington with polyQ expansion
Spinocerebellar ataxia	Ataxin with polyQ expansion and josephin
Frontotemporal lobar degeneration	Tau

several steps, and that earlier steps in the cascade may be more directly connected to the pathogenesis than the plaques themselves. Many neurodegenerative diseases can be termed *amyloidosis* because they are caused by the transition of endogenous proteins and peptides from the physiological globular configuration to a pathological fibrillar state and are characterized by the extracellular deposition of fibrillar proteic material (Pepys, 2002). Independently of the nature of the amyloid protein by which they are formed, these fibrils have a common ultrastructure. They grow, unbranched, to a variable length that may reach several microns, with a diameter of 7–10 nm. They are organized in a characteristic helicoidal β-structure and are able to bind to Congo Red dye generating a typical birefringence, a phenomenon which is commonly used as a test to detect their presence.

Of course, the big question not yet answered is: why do peptides, which normally circulate in soluble form in the cerebrospinal fluid (CSF) and in the plasma, become prone to aggregate, forming highly toxic oligomers and protofibrils and in the end mature fibrils accumulating in devasting plaques? The complex process is still not properly understood. It is widely accepted that, in most of the cases, the first step leading to protein aggregation is a partial unfolding of the proteins induced by temperature (de la Fuente *et al.*, 2002; Carrotta *et al.*, 2003; Dobson, 2004; Vetri and Militello, 2005). The partial unfolding of the proteins causes the exposition of sites like hydrophobic surface or thiol groups (SH) that have a dominant role in the aggregation process. Conformational changes lead to an increase in the amount of secondary β-sheet structures, and a decrease in α-helice structures (Dobson, 2004), and this process evolves into an ever larger fibrillar aggregate formation until amyloid plaques are formed (Figure 14.1).

The aggregation of physiologically secreted soluble oligomers and large fibrils has been studied in particular using the amyloid-β, the peptide involved in AD. Amyloid-β-peptide can interact *in vivo* with many different molecules, which could play a significant role in the onset and progress of AD. However, as a starting point, great effort has been spent understanding the mechanism of fibrillogenesis *in vitro* in simple conditions. The effect of sequence on the ability to form fibrils has been studied and has identified a hydrophobic core in the group of residues 17–21 and a major role in the aggregation played by the C-terminus (Tycko, 2003). This explains the seminal role shown by amyloid-β and other shorter peptides with full-length C-terminus, as outlined by examination of deposits in senile plaques. The structural analysis of the end products extracted *in vivo* from the deposited plaques helps to elucidate the amyloid-β aggregation mechanism. In fact, both electron microscopy and X-ray diffraction experiments on *ex vivo* amyloid-β fibrils, together with solid state NMR measured on *in vitro* samples, led to a model for the core structure of an amyloid-β fibril (Tycko, 2003). The search for a feasible model is simplified by the fact that amyloid fibrils are primarily β-sheet structures and by the condition that the β-sheets form a cross-β motif, as clearly indicated by X-ray diffraction data on several amyloid systems (Sunde *et al.*, 1997; Tycko, 2003). amyloid-β molecules self-associate to form a protofilament made from a sequence of peptides stacked and helically wrapped around a principal axis. The amyloid-β molecules are in a hairpin conformation with two β-strands forming separate parallel β-sheets. The cross-β unit is therefore a double-layered β-sheet structure characterized by the typical intra- and intermolecular distances detected by X-ray diffraction (4.7 Å and 10 Å). Data are consistent with a model for amyloid-β peptide fibrils, where two protofilaments pack face-to-face the C-terminus strands of the cross-β units. Dimensions of this filament can be about 5 nm, in agreement with the thinnest fibrils seen by EM microscopy. Mature fibrils can be composed of more filaments and be 1 μm long. Actually this model can be valid for all the fibrils, from a variety of amyloidoses, which yield a diffraction pattern remarkably similar to amyloid-β fibrils (Kirshner *et al.*, 1986). However, it still remains controversial whether the aggregates are more neurotoxic or protective than soluble monomer or intermediate oligomers (Walsh and Selkoe, 2007) but due to misfolding and aggregation the most upstream change that occurs during the neurodegenerative diseases process, inhibition of misfolding/aggregation, is expected to widely suppress multiple downstream pathogenic changes.

Why to use simple model systems

A model organism is a non-human species that is extensively studied to understand particular biological phenomena, with the expectation that discoveries made in the organism model will provide insight into the workings of other organisms. In particular, model organisms are widely used to explore potential causes and treatments for human disease when human experimentation would be unfeasible or unethical. This strategy is made possible by the common descent of all living organisms and the conservation of metabolic and developmental pathways and genetic material over the course of evolution. Studying model organisms can be informative, but care must be taken when generalizing from one organism to another.

The human brain is arguably the most complicated biological entity known. Understanding the processes that maintain the neurons and how we can intervene when these processes are disrupted is not easy. Thus, an efficacious treatment still does not exist. Model systems have been also utilized for studying mechanisms underlying neurodegenerative diseases. The discovery of specific genes and proteins associated with these specific diseases, and the development of new technologies for production of transgenic animals, has helped researchers to overcome the lack of natural models. For this aim cellular, pharmacological and genetic *in vivo* model systems of neurodegenerative diseases have been utilized to obtain key information about the cellular

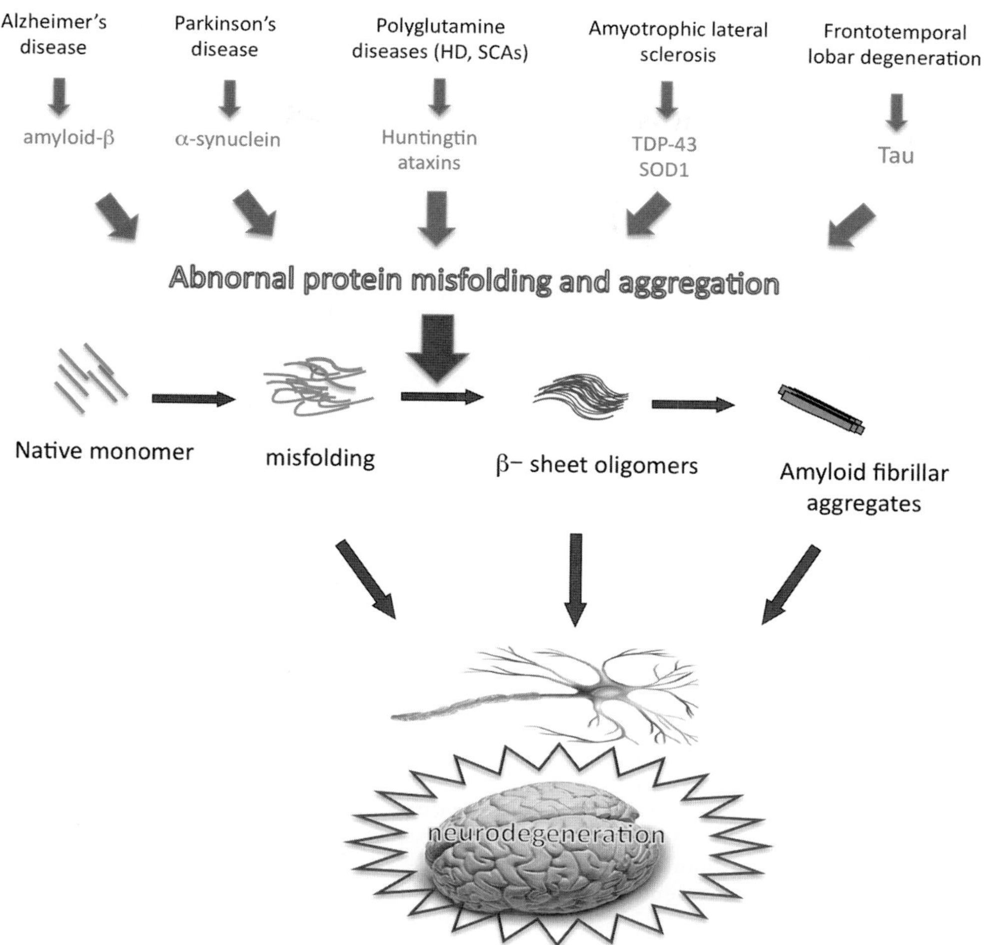

FIGURE 14.1 Protein misfolding and aggregation as the common molecular pathogenesis of neurodegenerative diseases. Some genetic mutations responsible for neurodegenerative diseases render the causative proteins prone to misfold and to form β-sheet-rich oligomers and amyloid fibrillar aggregates, resulting in their accumulation in the affected neurons and eventually leading to degeneration in the brain. This mechanism is retained common to a broad variety of neurodegenerative diseases.

and molecular mechanisms with the possibility of providing the basis for evaluating potential therapeutic interventions. However, the capability to produce transgenic models raises the question: which is the "right" model and can a given model be instructive or possibly misleading? Here, it will be evidenced that evolutionally distant animal models such as *C. elegans*, zebrafish, *Drosophila*, sea urchin can help to understand some aspects of human diseases.

The worm Caenorhabditis elegans *as a model system*

Defining specific mutations in familiar human neurodegenerative diseases has allowed researchers to make transgenic animal models of the diseases through directed genetic approaches. These studies help to address the molecular mechanisms of disease, and provide the foundation toward therapeutics. Modeling human neurodegenerative diseases in invertebrates has revolutionized the field in such a way that both reverse and forward genetic approaches are leading to the discovery of new players in neurodegeneration.

The nematode (roundworm) *Caenorhabditis elegans* (*C. elegans*) is a transgenically useful model with which to study common and fundamental toxic mechanisms underlying human neurodegenerative diseases. *C. elegans* is a free-living nematode about 1 mm in length, which lives in temperate soil environments. Research into the molecular and developmental biology of *C. elegans* was begun in 1974 by Sydney Brenner and it has since been used extensively as a model organism for a variety of reasons. It is a multicellular eukaryotic organism that is simple enough to be studied in great detail. Strains are cheap to breed and can be frozen. When subsequently thawed they remain viable, allowing long-term storage. *C. elegans* is transparent, facilitating the study of cellular differentiation and other developmental processes in the intact organism. The developmental fate of every single somatic cell (959 in the adult hermaphrodite; 1,031 in the adult male) has been mapped out (Sulston and Horvitz, 1977; Kimble and Hirsh, 1979). These patterns of cell lineage are largely invariant between individuals, in contrast to mammals where cell development from the embryo is more largely dependent on cellular cues. In both sexes, a large number of additional cells are naturally eliminated and by observing this phenomenon programmed cell death or apoptosis, one of the most important mechanisms of cell death, was discovered. In 2002, the Nobel Prize for Medicine was awarded to Sydney Brenner, H. Robert Horvitz and John E. Sulston for their work on how *C. elegans* genes cause programmed cell death.

Moreover, *C. elegans* is one of the simplest organisms with a nervous system. In the hermaphrodite, the nervous system comprises 302 neurons (Kosinski and Zaremba, 2007) whose pattern of connectivity has been completely mapped out, and shown to be a small-world network (Watts and Strogatz, 1988). Neuronal classes include chemosensory, mechanosensory and thermosensory types: 75 motor neurons innervate the body wall muscles (excluding the head); 56 of these are cholinergic and 19 are GABAnergic. *C. elegans* larvae contain four serotonergic and eight dopaminergic neurons. Formation, trafficking and release of synaptic vesicles in *C. elegans* is highly conserved, employing many of the same proteins used in mammalian neurons.

In addition, *C. elegans* was the first multicellular organism to have its genome completely sequenced. Clear results concerning this organism have permitted the development of transgenic disease-associated human proteins models (Link, 2006). Concerning neurodegenerative diseases another relevant advantage of *C. elegans* models is their short lifespan, which allows both rapid construction of different transgenic models and quick assessment of experimental interventions or the role of aging in pathological phenotypes. However, some limitations for studying neurodegeneration in *C. elegans* exist. Worms do not have myelination or an active immune system, so they are presumably not appropriate for some neurodegenerative conditions such as multiple sclerosis. Practically, worm neurons are small and difficult to patch clamp, although recordings can be made from single identified neurons (Ramot *et al.*, 2008). RNA interference (RNAi), a particularly useful tool in *C. elegans*, is often ineffective in neurons, necessitating the introduction of additional mutations to enhance neuronal RNAi efficacy.

Transgenic *C. elegans* models have been successively developed for Alzheimer's disease (AD), one of the most studied neurodegenerative diseases, with the aim of understanding the mechanisms underlying amyloid-β peptide (Aβ) toxicity and as a potential use for drug intervention. This peptide is obtained by the processing of its precursor the amyloid precursor protein (APP), a transmembrane protein (Walsh and Selkoe, 2007). The Aβ is the primary component of senile plaques found in the brains of AD patients, and the existence of mutations in the gene encoding APP in a subset of familial AD cases argues for a role for this peptide in this disease. Although the *C. elegans* model obviously lacks the neuronal cognitive complexity of mammals, it turns out to be a valid model to replicate cellular processes that may underlie AD.

Several attempts have been made to obtain a transgenic worm expressing detectable level of human Aβ. Initially to develop a mutant strain by targeting the endogenous APP gene, researchers found that the *C. elegans* genome does include genes that encode proteins related to human APP-*apl-1* (Daigle and Li, 1993). Analogous to human APP, the invertebrate APP-family members are composed of single transmembrane proteins with a large extracellular domain and a short intracellular domain, which can be cleaved to release intracellular and extracellular proteolytic fragments. However, APP-like genes in this nematode do not possess the region encoding the neurotoxic Aβ. So, the first model of AD generated by mutation of endogenous APP cleavage seemed irrelevant. Successively, alternative approaches were utilized to construct transgenic *C. elegans* models, accumulating transgenically expressed Aβ fragments intracellularly in muscle cells, and resulting in an age-dependent paralysis phenotype (Link, 1995; Fay *et al.*, 1998; Link *et al.*, 2001).

In developing the transgenic *C. elegans* model of AD, the minigene construct pCL12 containing the chimeric gene *unc*-54/Aβ1-42 was introduced into the nematode by gonad microinjection to produce Aβ constitutively expressed in the CL2006 strain of *C. elegans* (Link, 1995). Furthermore, CL2006 had the pPD30.38 vector containing the *unc*-54 promoter/enhancer sequence that produces high level muscle-specific gene expression, causing Aβ deposits in the muscle cells of the animals (Link, 1995). To discriminate transgenic nematodes, these transgenes were co-injected with plasmids expressing the dominant morphological marker *rol*-6 (pRF4), which causes the animal to rotate around its longitudinal axis. The resulting movement, due to this roller marker, is a distinctive non-sinusoidal one used to identify those animals maintaining the injected transgenes (Fay *et al.*, 1998). To detect the location of intracellular deposit and the ultrastructure of amyloid fibrils, immuno-electron microscopy and the amyloid-specific dye X-34, an intensely fluorescent Congo red derivative, were employed (Link *et al.*, 2001). This dye has been also utilized to detect amyloid in senile and soluble Aβ in postmortem AD brain tissue (Styren *et al.*, 2000). From the results of immuno-electron microscopy and fluorescence staining, it was found that the amyloid deposits are located intracellularly and that the increased amyloid fibrils in individual worms from mid-larva to adult stages were caused by an increase in the deposit size rather than the emergence of new deposits (Link *et al.*, 2001). Taken together these evidences demonstrated that the construct satisfied the expectations. In particular this transgenic worm was utilized to test whether amyloid fibrils were the toxic species in the *C. elegans* model and for Aβ structure/function. Successively a series of transgenic lines were generated expressing potentially non-amyloidic variant forms of Aβ in which single amino acid substitutions (e.g., Leu, Pro) dramatically reduced amyloid and blocked amyloid formation but it did not reduce toxicity, suggesting that amyloid aggregates are not the real toxic species (Fay *et al.*, 1998).

Transgenic *C. elegans* was also utilized to study the age dependence of AD investigating whether in bacterial deprivation, a form of dietary restriction that extends lifespan, Aβ toxicity can be reduced (Steinkraus *et al.*, 2008). The authors demonstrated that dietary restriction confers a general protective effect against toxicity and promotes longevity by a mechanism involving heat shock factor-1 (hsf-1).

The validity of the *C. elegans* model to study AD comes also from studies that associate learning and behavior of the worm with Aβ toxicity (Nuttley *et al.*, 2002; Zhang *et al.*, 2005). Many nematodes are influenced by food and modify their behaviors in response to the presence or absence of food. Enhanced slowing response, an experience-dependent learning (ESR) behavior, relies on a conserved response to starvation. *C. elegans* behaviors were investigated in relation to phenotype learning-related behavioral changes owing to the introduction of the human Aβ gene in *C. elegans*. It has been demonstrated that the transgenic worms have a significantly decreased lifespan at 23°C, reduced serotonin-stimulated egg laying, impaired associative learning and ESR (Dosanjh *et al.*, 2010).

C. elegans models of α-synuclein toxicity were also constructed to study Parkinson's disease (PD). α-synuclein is a major component of Lewy bodies found in dystrophic dopaminergic neurons in PD, and α-synuclein mutations have been found to be present in a relatively small number of familial PD cases. *C. elegans* models of synucleinopathy have been constructed in different labs with human α-synuclein expression in either dopaminergic neurons or pan-neurons (Lakso *et al.*, 2003; Cao *et al.*, 2005; Kuwahara *et al.*, 2006). The different researcher groups constructed the transgenic models using different promoters, obtaining different phenotypes, but all reported loss of either dopaminergic neuron cell bodies or dendrites when α-synuclein expression is driven by the dopaminergic-specific *dat-1* promoter. Recently the pan-neuronal α-synuclein model has been used in a large-scale feeding RNAi screen to identify enhancers of α-synuclein toxicity, leading to the identification of a number of genes (e.g., *apa-2*, *aps-2*, *eps-8* and *rab-7*) involved in the endocytic pathway and a link between α-synuclein toxicity and intracellular vesicle trafficking has been demonstrated (Kuwahara *et al.*, 2008). Moreover, using a genome-wide RNAi approach, 186 genes were identified that, when suppressed, specifically prevented α-synuclein aggregation (Nollen *et al.*, 2004) suggesting that *C. elegans* is also a suitable model to study protein aggregation, an important component of many neurodegenerative diseases. The identified genes codified for proteins involved in RNA metabolism, protein synthesis, protein folding, protein degradation and protein trafficking.

Polyglutamine (polyQ)-expansion diseases include Huntington's disease (HD) and at least eight other neurodegenerative disorders (Morfini *et al.*, 2005). Disease alleles contain expanded exonic CAG regions that produce expanded polyQ tracts in the expressed protein. In normal proteins, the polyQ tract contains 10–30 residues, whereas longer polyglutamine tracts result in neurodegeneration. Although the mechanisms underlying expanded polyQ toxicity are not fully understood, a hallmark of polyQ-expansion diseases is intracellular aggregation of expanded polyQ proteins (Ross and Poirier, 2004). Taking advantage both of the rapid engineering of transgenic *C. elegans* and its transparency throughout its lifecycle, a series of transgenic lines expressing GFP fused with polyglutamine repeat were generated. These transgenic lines were utilized to examine the toxic effects of short (Q19) and long (Q82) polyglutamine repeat lengths in *C. elegans* body wall muscle cells (Satyal *et al.*, 2000). Expression of GFP-Q82 resulted in aggregate formation and induction of heat shock proteins. Subsequent studies with a series of GFP-polyQ fusions demonstrated a narrow threshold of polyQ repeat size (35–40) for induction of aggregation and toxicity and an age dependence for aggregation was demonstrated.

Different cellular pathways may contribute to the degradation of polyQ proteins and the prevention of intracellular accumulation of polyQ protein aggregates. Proteasomes are responsible for the normal degradation of wild-type polyQ proteins and expanded-polyQ disease proteins (Goldberg, 2003). However, eukaryotic proteasomes may inefficiently digest long-glutamine repeats, suggesting the involvement of other protein degradation systems (Venkartraman *et al.*, 2009). There is increasing evidence that the lysosomal degradation pathway of autophagy may also be important in the degradation of polyQ aggregates (Iwata *et al.*, 2005). Autophagy is the major cellular pathway for the degradation of long-lived proteins and cytoplasmic organelles. During autophagy, cellular components are sequestered into autophagosomes and delivered to lysosomes where they are degraded and recycled (Levine and Klionsky, 2004). Autophagy is induced under starvation conditions and other forms of cellular stress, including the accumulation of intracellular protein aggregates. To have information whether autophagy genes play a role *in vivo* in protecting against disease caused by mutant aggregate-prone, expanded polyQ proteins two models of polyQ-induced toxicity in *C. elegans* were utilized (Jia *et al.*, 2007). It was found that genetic inactivation of autophagy genes accelerates the accumulation of polyQ40 aggregates in *C. elegans* muscle cells and exacerbates polyQ40-induced muscle dysfunction. Autophagy gene inactivation also increases the accumulation of Htn-Q150 aggregates in *C. elegans'* ASH sensory neurons and results in enhanced neurodegeneration.

*The zebrafish (*Danio rerio*) as model system*

The zebrafish is a tropical freshwater fish, a popular aquarium fish and has emerged as an excellent model organism for studies of vertebrate biology. The fish is named because of the five uniform, pigmented, horizontal blue stripes on the side of the body, all of which extend to the end of the caudal fin. External development and optical clarity during embryogenesis allow for visual analyses of early developmental processes, and high fecundity and short generation times facilitate genetic analyses. Large-scale genetic screens have exploited these characteristics with great success, resulting in the identification of more than 500 mutant phenotypes in various aspects of early development. In this way, it is possible to address issues of organogenesis, complex disease and other vertebrate processes on the basis of function, without a previous knowledge of the genes involved. Furthermore, such analysis can serve as a functional complement to the Human Genome Project, which is producing enormous amounts of sequencing information but lacks functional information for many of the identified genes. Orthologs of some human genes are duplicated in the zebrafish genome (Chen *et al.*, 2009), raising the possibility that resulting subfunctionalization may help to dissect the functions of the human genes. Orthologs of genes involved in Parkinsonism, Alzheimer's disease and Huntington's disease are among those identified in zebrafish. Through careful and creative design of screens, any developmental or clinically relevant process can be studied, and zebrafish provides a forward genetic approach for assigning function to genes, and positioning them in developmental and/or disease-related pathways.

As a vertebrate, the basic organization and divisions of the nervous system are similar to those of other vertebrates, including humans. The zebrafish CNS contains specialized neuronal populations of direct relevance to human neurodegenerative diseases, for example dopaminergic neurons (Ma, 2003), cerebellar Purkinje cells (Koulen *et al.*, 2000) and motor neurons (Bai *et al.*, 2006). In addition to neurons, the zebrafish CNS contains oligodendrocytes (Brosamle and Halpern, 2002) and astrocytes (Kawai *et al.*, 2001), the human homologs of which may play central roles in neurodegeneration through critical neural–glial interactions. This anatomic structure permits the use of zebrafish as a model for studying neurodegenerative diseases. Different techniques were utilized to generate transgenic zebrafish starting from microinjection of linearized plasmids or transposons, or producing constructs with appropriate *cis*-acting regulatory elements (Sager *et al.*, 2010).

As a first step towards developing zebrafish models of neurodegenerative disease, the possibility was tested that zebrafish, engineered to express genes associated with neurodegeneration in humans, will develop histological and biochemical abnormalities related to those found in the relevant diseases. This hypothesis was tested by generating transgenic zebrafish expressing appropriate genes in CNS neurons, and then carrying out analysis for evidence of neuronal cell death or dysfunction and histopathological features or biochemical abnormalities resembling the human diseases. The generation of transgenic models relies on the availability of *cis*-acting regulatory elements that drive transgene expression in an appropriate spatial and temporal pattern. For a neurodegenerative disease model, the regulatory elements should have specific properties such as expression in a wide variety of differentiated neurons persisting into adulthood, in order to examine the effects of aging on pathogenesis and disease progression.

Different transgenic zebrafish models have been developed and some of them were used to study the so-called tauopathies. In neurodegenerative diseases tau proteins are displaced from their normal association with microtubules and are found in a hyperphosphorylated state deposited into paired helical filaments (PHFs). PHFs are the hallmark cytoskeletal pathology of these diseases and the degree of PHF is closely correlated with their clinical severity (Kidd, 1963). Since its pathological alteration is strongly correlated with disease progression in AD, frontotemporal dementia (FTD) and other neurodegenerative diseases, tau suppression has been found to improve memory function (Braak and Braak, 1991), thus tau protein is an important target for research and drug development.

Tau phosphorylation has been studied extensively, but several important issues remain unresolved. It is not yet clear which phosphorylation systems actually phosphorylate PHF tau, and it is not completely understood how phosphorylation affects its functional properties and how Tau in neurodegenerative diseases becomes redistributed from its normal concentration in neuronal axons to pathological inclusions in neuronal soma known as neurofibrillary tangles (NFT). In addition, and importantly, mutations in the gene-encoding human tau have been implicated in a variety of hereditary dementias, collectively termed frontotemporal dementia with Parkinsonism linked to chromosome 17 (FTDP-17) (Hutton *et al.*, 1998).

Given the proposed central role of tau in a number of important neurodegenerative conditions, there has been interest in the construction of zebrafish tauopathy models. Initially a transient model, in which a tau-GFP fusion protein was overexpressed in zebrafish larvae using the GATA-2 promoter of tauopathy changes in human disease, was reported. The construct contained an FTDP-17 mutated form of human tau and was developed to study the functional consequences and trafficking patterns in zebrafish neurons (Tomasiewicz *et al.*, 2002). This model had the aim of detecting a hierarchy of events relevant to potential mechanisms of neurodegenerative diseases related to critical early stages in the development of disease. The fusion protein was phosphorylated similar to native tau *in vitro* and showed an expression pattern in tissue culture suggesting interaction with the cytoskeleton. Moreover, cytoskeletal disruption that closely resembled the NFT in human disease was observed.

Stable transgenic zebrafish expressing human 4-repeat tau were subsequently constructed to obtain a tauopathy model (Bai *et al.*, 2007). The zebrafish *eno*2 gene encoding the neuron-specific γ-enolase isoenzyme was identified as a marker of differentiated neurons. Expression of *eno*2 was detected at low levels by 24 h post-fertilization, but the abundance of the mRNA increased substantially in the brain and spinal cord between 60 and 72 h post-fertilization, and expression persisted at high levels into adulthood, in a pan-neuronal pattern. The regulatory region of *eno*2 is complex, there is an untranslated first exon and the first intron contains a CpG island that appears important for promoter activity. A 12 kb fragment of the promoter, including the first intron, was active in driving reporter gene expression in neurons throughout the brain and spinal cord from 48 h post-fertilization through adulthood, including neuronal types relevant to neurodegenerative diseases, such as cerebellar Purkinje cells and cholinergic neurons. The *eno*2 promoter was used to drive overexpression of tau and evidence of tau accumulation within neuronal cell bodies and proximal axons, resembling neurofibrillary tangles, was reported. The construct containing *eno*2 promoter has permitted the study of biochemical and histological changes representative of human diseases which may be provoked in susceptible neuronal populations by expression of mutant transgenes.

More recently, the Gal4–UAS system has been exploited in order to generate a tauopathy model that shows a larval phenotype, with potential application to high throughput screening. Expression of the FTDP-17 tau mutant P301L was driven from a novel bidirectional UAS promoter, allowing simultaneous expression of a separate red fluorescent protein in tau-expressing cells (Paquet *et al.*, 2009). The high levels of mutant tau expression provoked by the *huc:gal4-vp16* driver were sufficient to induce a transient motor phenotype during embryogenesis, caused by a motor axonal outgrowth delay. At later time points, the tau mutant caused enhanced cell death and protein aggregation in the spinal cord. Moreover, rapid progression from early to late pathological tau phosphorylation was seen over the first few days of life; the phosphorylation of tau was reduced by application of GSK3β inhibitors, suggesting that the model may be used to identify other similar pharmacological inhibitors from chemical libraries. Unfortunately, loss of promoter activity prevented the examination of later pathological changes, and so it is unclear whether the phenotype was progressive and age-dependent, or transient. In addition, the *huc* promoter fragment used in this model only induced robust transgene expression in the spinal cord, which is not a prominent site of tauopathy changes in human disease. However, this valuable study showed the utility of the Gal4–UAS system for modeling neurodegeneration in transgenic zebrafish and demonstrated evidence that biochemical changes characteristic of tauopathy, including an orderly acquisition of abnormal phospho-epitopes and conformers, can be obtained in larval zebrafish.

As discussed before, a number of autosomal dominant neurodegenerative diseases, including Huntington's disease and several of the spinocerebellar ataxias, are caused by pathological expansion of a tandem trinucleotide CAG repeat in the relevant gene, resulting in an elongated stretch of glutamine residues in the resulting protein. It is thought that the mechanism of pathogenesis involves a toxic gain of function mediated by the expanded polyglutamine tract, rather than loss of function of the affected gene (Zoghbi and Orr, 2009). Since this general pathogenic mechanism may be shared by these diseases, a polyQ toxicity model in zebrafish would present a possible means to elucidate pathogenesis and perhaps isolate a common treatment for the whole group of conditions.

In the first report of a zebrafish polyQ model, transient expression of GFP-polyQ fusion proteins was achieved by microinjection of plasmids, encoding the fluorescent fusion with polyQ tracts of differing lengths, under transcriptional control of a strong viral promoter (Miller *et al.*, 2005). In human polyQ diseases, there is correlation between the length of the polyQ expansion and the severity of the phenotype, as measured by age of onset or rate of clinical progression. Expression of GFP-polyQ fusion proteins in zebrafish caused a decrease in embryo length and loss of tissue differentiation, resulting in morphological deficits and reduced viability. Although this acute response does not reflect the chronic neurological diseases seen in patients with polyQ expansion mutations, significant overexpression of these artificial proteins would be expected to provoke acute and severe phenotypes. Importantly, however, the model showed two key features of polyQ diseases: (1) there was correlation between the polyQ repeat length and the severity of the morphological phenotype; and (2) GFP-positive inclusion bodies were formed, suggesting the formation of aggregates dependent on the polyQ tract (Miller *et al.*, 2005).

A recent study tested the possibility in cell culture that enhanced autophagy might be efficacious in clearing aggregated Huntington and other substrates from cells (Williams *et al.*, 2008). The identified compounds were then subjected to verification in a novel stable transgenic zebrafish line, expressing a GFP-Huntington 71Q fusion protein under the control of the rhodopsin promoter, leading to aggregation of the fusion protein and loss of rod outer segments and rhodopsin expression from the retina. Several of the compounds identified as reducing aggregation in the cell culture model also prevented formation of aggregates in the zebrafish model, providing validation of the cell culture system, and suggesting that zebrafish models might be useful in the future for primary screens of therapeutic compounds.

The fruit fly Drosophila melanogaster *as a model system*

Drosophila melanogaster is a small, common fly found near unripe and rotted fruit. Wild-type fruit flies have brick red eyes, are yellow-brown in color, and have transverse black rings across their abdomen. They exhibit sexual dimorphism: females are about 2.5 millimeters long; males are slightly smaller and the back of their bodies is darker. Males are easily distinguished from females based on color differences, with a distinct black patch at the abdomen, less noticeable in recently emerged flies and the sexcombs.

Drosophila melanogaster is one of the most studied organisms in biological research, particularly in genetics and developmental biology, for several reasons: (1) it is small and easy to grow in the laboratory and their morphology is easy to identify once they are anesthetized; (2) care and culture requires the minimum of equipment and space even when using large cultures and the overall cost is low; (3) it has a short generation time (about 10 days at room temperature) so several generations can be studied within a few weeks; (4) it has a high fecundity (females lay up to 100 eggs per day, and perhaps 2,000 in a lifetime) and the developmental period varies with temperature; and (5) males and females are readily distinguished and virgin females are easily isolated, facilitating genetic crossing.

Drosophila has been in use for over a century to study genetics and lends itself well to behavioral studies. Thomas Hunt Morgan was the preeminent biologist studying *Drosophila* early in the 1900s. Morgan was the first to discover sex-linkage and genetic recombination, which placed this small fly in the forefront of genetic research. Due to its small size, ease of culture and short generation time, geneticists have been using *Drosophila* ever since. It is one of the few organisms whose entire genome is known and many genes have been identified.

The biological similarities between humans and *Drosophila* have been exploited with great success in the field of neurodegenerative disease (Jeibmann and Paulus, 2009). The principal reason behind this is that the fly has a brain, containing approximately 200,000 neurones, and like the vertebrate central nervous system, it is composed of a series of functionally specialized substructures. The primary sources of sensory input are visual and olfactory, and these are processed in the optic and antennal lobes, respectively. The mushroom bodies deal with memory, and the central complex provides the motor output, once sensory integration is complete. The neurons are very similar to their human equivalents in terms of their shape, synaptic intercommunications and biochemical signatures. These functional and structural similarities allow the construction of fly models of human diseases. These models typically involve transgenic flies expressing a human gene bearing a known dominant mutation or expressing a targeted loss-of-function mutation generated in the fly orthologs of these genes (for reviews see Cellotto and Palladino, 2005; Lessing and Bonini, 2009; Moloney *et al.*, 2010). There are now fly models for Alzheimer's disease (Iijima *et al.*, 2004), Huntington's disease (Jackson *et al.*, 1998; Kazemi-Esfarjani and Benzer, 2000), a range of related polyQ expansion disorders (Warrick *et al.*, 1999), transthyretin-linked amyloid polyneuropathy (Pokrzywa *et al.*, 2007), Parkinson's disease (Feany and Bender, 2000), motor neurone disease (Watson *et al.*, 2008) and spinal muscular atrophy (Chan *et al.*, 2003).

Parkinson's disease, as already mentioned, is a common neurodegenerative condition that can result from several distinct genetic mutations and specific environmental conditions. The effects of α-synuclein and parkin mutations have been studied in the *Drosophila* model. Important hallmarks of PD are the appearance of filamentous Lewy body and Lewy neurite inclusions and the selective loss of dopaminergic cells in the substantia nigra. α-synuclein is a known component of these inclusions, and mutations in α-synuclein are known to cause familial PD. Flies overexpressing wild-type or mutant (i.e., A30P or A53T) α-synuclein reveal progressive loss of dopaminergic cells in the brain (Feany and Bender, 2000). Transgenic α-synuclein flies, wild type or mutant, also exhibit progressive locomotor impairment, summarizing several key features of PD.

Autosomal recessive juvenile-onset Parkinson's disease (AR-JP) begins at youth and is a severe form of the disease, resulting from the loss-of-function mutation of parkin. The parkin protein functions as an E3-ubiquitin protein ligase, suggesting that the inability to target proteins for ubiquitin proteolytic degradation may be a direct cause of PD. Consistent with this hypothesis, several components of Lewy body inclusions are known targets of parkin. Flies lacking parkin function have reduced longevity, locomotor impairment, male sterility, muscle degeneration, mitochondrial impairment and selective dopaminergic cell loss (Greene *et al.*, 2003).

Drosophila polyQ disease models have been also constructed. In flies, we know that expression of polyQ alone (Kazemi-Esfarjani and Benzer, 2000) or in the context of known human disease proteins such as Huntington's (Jackson *et al.*, 1998), ataxin-1 (Fernandez-Funez *et al.*, 2000) and ataxin-3 (Warrick *et al.*, 1998) all result in neurodegeneration. The dominant nature of these conditions allows one to express a polyQ-bearing transgene and to observe a phenotype without removing the function of the fly orthologs. The eye is an ideal place to express these genes for several reasons: (1) the eye is not an essential tissue; (2) degeneration of the eye cells cause a rough appearance that can be readily observed; and (3) the eye is composed of photoreceptor cells organized into ommatidia, and quantitative measure of cell loss can be obtained by counting the number of photoreceptors remaining per ommatidium. Studies utilizing *Drosophila* transgenic models of this human disease have confirmed that important pathogenic features are conserved between flies and humans. The threshold for pathogenicity of polyQ length is similar for flies and humans: more than 40 (Andrew *et al.*, 1997). Additionally, in flies, as in humans, the phenotypes are progressive and increased severity is associated with increased polyQ length. Another hallmark of polyQ disease is the presence of inclusions, formed from aggregated polyQ proteins with other cellular proteins. Fly models of these diseases form inclusion bodies, the cellular components including polyQ proteins, chaperones, [cAMP response element binding protein (CREB)-binding protein] (CBP), and ubiquitin, similar to the constituent proteins found in human inclusion bodies. Despite the different etiologies of these genetic disorders, the affected genes produce an aberration in the nervous system of the fly that is similar to the aberration in the human CNS. The common modes of pathogenesis suggest a high degree of conservation in the processes that maintain neural function with age and argue that mechanistic advances made in *Drosophila* will be directly relevant to the human condition.

Other neurodegenerative mutants involved in some biochemical processes have been identified. Two examples are superoxide dismutase 1 (*SOD1*) and *Drosophila* adenosine deaminase that acts on RNA mutants (*dADAR*). *SOD1*, also termed Cu/Zn SOD, is a broadly expressed cytosolic enzyme that catalyzes the destruction of toxic superoxides. Reactive oxygen species (ROS) cause cellular stress (i.e., damage to lipids, proteins and DNA) and have been implicated in disease pathogenesis and aging. *SOD1* mutant flies exhibit reduced longevity and neurodegeneration (Phillips *et al.*, 1995). Mutations in human *SOD1* are known to cause ALS (Deng *et al.*, 1993) suggesting these flies could be used to model this disease condition. Adenosine-to-inosine (A-to-I) RNA editing is a post-transcriptional process that modifies pre-mRNA transcripts, often altering the coding potential of the processed transcripts. Although not exclusive to the nervous system, RNA editing of many ion channel or receptor transcripts has been described, and it has been hypothesized that the process contributes significantly to the protein diversity required for complex neural function in animals (Hoopengardner *et al.*, 2003). Consistent with this hypothesis dADAR is enriched in the *Drosophila* nervous system, and dADAR null mutations result in flies with severe behavioral impairment (Palladino *et al.*, 2000). Studies of dADAR-null flies also led to the discovery that RNA editing is required for the maintenance of neural integrity during the aging process in flies. The mechanism of neuropathogenesis in dADAR mutants is complicated because of numerous affected targets; however, loss of ion homeostasis, altered neural signaling and ROS-dependent mechanisms have been suggested (Chen *et al.*, 2004).

Fly models of Alzheimer's disease are also available to the community and are providing new insights into disease mechanisms, and assisting in the identification of novel targets for therapy (Moloney *et al.*, 2009). A particularly model of Aβ toxicity has been achieved by creating transgenic flies that carry gal4-driven constructs encoding human APP and human beta-site APP-cleaving enzyme 1 (BACE1). When expressed in the brain, human APP is cleaved by the transgenic human BACE1 and then by endogenous *Drosophila* γ-secretase, resulting in the generation of the Aβ peptide (Greeve *et al.*, 2004). This relatively complex model is ideal for the assessment of modulators of BACE1 or APP metabolism, but, in some respects, is less easy to handle than models in which the Aβ sequence is fused downstream of a secretion signal peptide (Finelli *et al.*, 2004; Crowther *et al.*, 2005; Stokin *et al.*, 2008). In these latter models, the expressed peptide has its signal peptide cleaved off as Aβ enters the secretory pathway and a proportion of the peptide is subsequently released from the cell. However, the degree of intracellular Aβ accumulation correlates with early phenotypes such as locomotor dysfunction and severity, and immunogold electron microscopy reveals that the peptides localize to the endoplasmic reticulum (ER), Golgi and lysosomes, but not the nucleus or mitochondria (Iijima *et al.*, 2008). This finding suggests that the potentially reversible early phenotypes in AD could be mediated by the intracellular accumulation and aggregation of Aβ.

Although studies on Aβ can help to understand one crucial aspect of AD pathogenesis, to investigate the role of tau is also of great importance. The tauopathies are a set of human neurodegenerative diseases related to AD, often presenting as fronto-temporal dementia, which are characterized by prominent intracellular accumulations of the microtubule binding protein tau (Lee *et al.*, 2001). Familial tauopathies are caused either by deregulated mRNA splicing and the consequent accumulation of a particular tau isoform, or alternatively by an underlying genetic mutation (Goedert and Jakes, 2005). Fly models allow one to investigate both the mechanism of neurodegeneration in these tauopathies and the role of tau in AD. The fly tauopathy models that have been generated thus far are tau-overexpression models. Although wild-type human tau is neurotoxic when overexpressed in neuronal tissues, the rough eye and longevity phenotypes in *Drosophila* model systems are more severe when disease-related variants of tau are expressed (Shulman and Feany, 2003), even when tau does not form neurofibrillary tangles (Wittmann *et al.*, 2001). Moreover, flies overexpressing wild-type human tau can be induced to form intracellular inclusions that resemble neurofibrillary tangles, when glycogen synthase kinase 3β (GSK3β) activity is increased (Jackson *et al.*, 2002). This finding is concordant with the known pathways of tau toxicity that seem to require hyperphosphorylation of tau to speed aggregation.

The sea urchin Paracentrotus lividus *and* Spherechinus granularis *as model systems*

Sea urchin is a useful model system for studying many problems in early animal development, and recently it has been used for the identification of specific pathways involved in human pathology or as an indicative tool for pharmacological evaluation.

Historically, sea urchin was a key system in elucidating a variety of classic developmental problems, including the mechanisms of fertilization, egg activation, animal/vegetal axis formation, cleavage, gastrulation and the regulation of differentiation in the early embryo. Gametes can be obtained easily, sterility is not required and the eggs and early embryos of many species are beautifully transparent. The early development of sea urchin embryos is also highly synchronous, thus when a batch of eggs is fertilized all of the resulting embryos typically develop on the same schedule, making possible biochemical and molecular studies of early embryos. Moreover, the sea urchin occupies a key phylogenetic position as the only non-chordate deuterostome and the results obtained on this embryo can be extrapolated and compared to those of higher eukaryotes such as mammals.

By microscopy inspection it is easy to follow fertilization and all the developmental stages from cleavage until the larval form called pluteus (Giudice, 1973). As soon as a sperm meets the egg, it releases the content of "cortical granules" which include enzymes that release a membrane tied to the surface. This membrane initially looks like bubbles on the surface, which is necessary for preventing "polyspermy". Soon after fertilization, one can observe the "sperm aster", and the female pronucleus in the center of the zygote and cleavage starts. Sea urchin is perhaps the best organism exhibiting one of the most important steps of embryogenesis: gastrulation. During this moment the vegetal-most region of the blastula, the last undifferentiated embryonal stage, invaginates as a single epithelial layer to form a pit, which then elongates until it crosses the blastocoel cavity, extending into a thin tube, called archenteron, that will be the intestine. In the site at which gastrulation begins, the anus will be formed, hence the term "deuterostomes" used to describe the echinoderms and related phyla. During archenteron elongation, cells, called primary mesenchyme cells, rearrange and begin to form the skeletal rods that will define the pluteus. The first skeletal rudiments appear on the vegetal side of the embryo, one each on left and right sides. These have a distinctive refractility, and are always tri-radiate in normal embryos. They consist of calcite crystals secreted intracellularly within a syncytium made by fusion of the primary mesenchyme cells. Moreover, nervous systems begin to be present with some neurons and neurites at late gastrula, and at pluteus ganglia, neurons and neuritis are present in the structure called ciliary band, in the esophagus, and in the intestine (Nakajima *et al.*, 2004). Further, several clusters of neurons with associated neuropil are organized as ganglia, the largest of which is the apical organ. In the early larva, the apical organ is composed of 4–6 bilaterally positioned sensory cells containing serotonin, a central cluster of 10–12 neurons and several non-neural supporting cells (Figure 14.2).

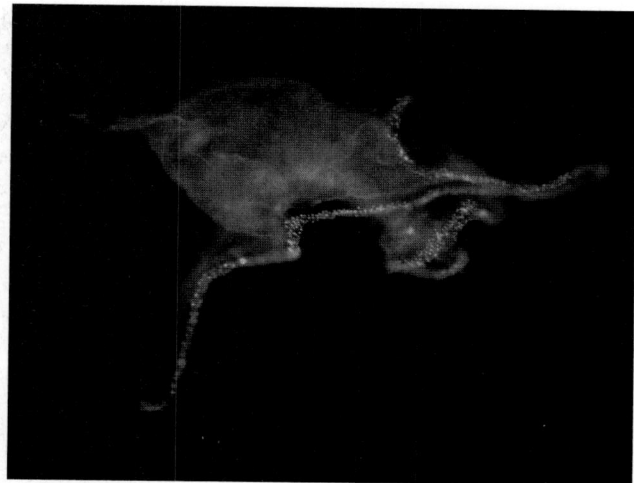

FIGURE 14.2 Sea urchin larval nervous system. Immunohistochemistry of *Paracentrotus lividus* pluteus incubated with anti-serotonin.

All these morphological events that appear perfectly synchronous in sea urchin embryo cultures are perturbed when they are exposed to toxic agents such as metals or teratogens and neurotoxicants and their adverse effects produce uniform phenotypes for a given toxicant and critical exposure period (Buznikov, 1983). Moreover, the *Strongylocentrotus purpuratus* sea urchin genome has been sequenced and about 7,000 genes in common with humans, including genes associated with pathologies such as Parkinson's, Alzheimer's and Huntington's diseases, as well as muscular dystrophy, were found (Sodergren *et al.*, 2006). Despite having no eyes, nose or ears, the sea urchin has genes similar to those used for vision, hearing and smell in humans. Further, mechanisms that are involved in normal or altered cell homeostasis common to humans have been identified. For example, the neurodegeneration process leads to apoptosis, a cell death mechanism well conserved and studied in sea urchin (Voronina and Wessel, 2001; Agnello and Roccheri, 2010). Even though the simple sea urchin model has been the least employed for studying neurodegeneration, a few papers regarding principally Aβ toxicity reveal that this model can be utilized for identification of specific pathways involved in death mechanisms or as an indicative tool for pharmacological evaluation of novel therapeutic agents.

Using a recombinant Aβ42 (rAβ42) and *Paracentrotus lividus* sea urchin embryo the structure–activity relation between different aggregation forms and toxicity was investigated (Carrotta *et al.*, 2006). A preliminary biophysical work was done to stabilize different rAβ42 aggregation forms under two conditions: small oligomers at physiological pH and larger aggregates at low pH; these different aggregation forms were verified by dynamic light scattering measures. It was observed that, in comparison with acid solution (aggregate form), neutral solution (oligomer form) significantly increased the level of toxicity on sea urchin embryos, indicating that the state of Aβ assembly appears to influence their biological activities. The presence of small oligomers stabilized at pH 7 brings malformation and complete interruption of the embryo's development at the pathologically occluded blastula state after 48 h. At the same stage, larger aggregates of rAβ42, stabilized at pH 3, allow some embryos to reach normal development or the more advanced (though pathologically) occluded prism state. The results supported the belief that early symptoms of AD can be the effect of cellular malfunctioning due to pathologically small oligomers of Aβ peptides. Regarding the possible mechanism the authors suggest that small oligomers might be more diffusible with respect to larger aggregates or fibrils and can easily be inserted into the extracellular space or in the lipid bilayer, or can be internalized within the cells of the developing embryos, altering their vital functions. In contrast, preformed larger aggregates or fibrils in sea urchin could mimic the extracellular plaques of AD in neurons and compromise cell–cell interaction and all the processes related to cellular membrane.

Moreover, an antigen related to the human APP, the protein produced *in vivo* by proteolitic cleavage of the Aβ peptide, called PlAPP, was identified in sea urchin embryo

(Pellicanò *et al.*, 2009). This antigen, after the gastrula stage, as occurs in the human brain, is processed producing a polypeptide of about 10 kDa, suggesting that some molecules and pathways involved in the degenerative process could be conserved during evolution. Thus, sea urchin could be a valid model to understand the different steps or molecules underlining the cytotoxicity of Aβ. In particular sea urchin has permitted one to find a relation between Aβ aggregation forms and different apoptotic pathway activations (Pellicanò *et al.*, 2009). Aβ aggregates, indeed, induce apoptosis by extrinsic pathway activation, whereas oligomers induce apoptosis both by extrinsic and intrinsic pathway activation. Moreover, involvement in apoptosis via the intrinsic pathway of an organelle such as mitochondria, pivotal in controlling cell life and death, can explain the major toxicity of oligomers with respect to aggregates (Carrotta *et al.*, 2006; Picone *et al.*, 2009).

Using a different sea urchin species, *Sphaerechinus granularis*, the critical periods in which different types of anomalies are evoked by Aβ were examined, and, importantly, the role played by acetylcholine (ACh) and other neurotransmitters such as serotonin (5HT) and cannabinoids as potential protectants was established (Buznikov *et al.*, 2008a). The outcomes identified in morphological studies of this type can be used for guiding mechanistic evaluations of the biochemical and molecular mechanisms that underlie both damage by amyloid and protection provided by neurotransmitter analogs.

Sphaerechinus granularis embryo was employed to evaluate the developmental abnormalities caused by administration of exogenous APP96–110 in sea urchin embryos and larvae, which, like the developing mammalian brain, utilize acetylcholine and other neurotransmitters as morphogens and the effects were compared to those of Aβ, the neurotoxic APP fragment contained within neurodegenerative plaques in Alzheimer's disease (Buznikov *et al.*, 2008b). Although both peptides elicited dysmorphogenesis, Aβ was far more potent; in addition, whereas Aβ produced abnormalities at developmental stages ranging from early cleavage divisions to the late pluteus, APP96–110 effects were restricted to the intermediate, mid-blastula stage. For both agents, anomalies were prevented or reduced by addition of lipid-permeable analogs of acetylcholine, serotonin or cannabinoids; physostigmine, a carbamate-derived cholinesterase inhibitor, was also effective. In contrast, agents that act on NMDA receptors (memantine) or α-adrenergic receptors (nicergoline), and are therapeutic in Alzheimer's disease, were themselves embryotoxic, as was tacrine, a cholinesterase inhibitor from a different chemical class than physostigmine. Protection was also provided by agents acting downstream from receptor-mediated events: increasing cyclic AMP with caffeine or isobutylmethylxanthine, or administering the antioxidant α-tocopherol, were all partially effective.

CONCLUDING REMARKS AND FUTURE PERSPECTIVES

C. elegans, zebrafish, *Drosophila*, sea urchin, together with other non-human model systems not discussed here, summarize some features of human neurological diseases and will continue to be used to elucidate mechanistic details and provide the basis for evaluating drug therapies.

Many of the common neurodegenerative diseases show a high degree of heritability and some of the risk factors are genetic. Heritability depends on a large number of genes, each of which provides a small contribution to disease risk. The current generation of genome-wide association studies is designed to detect these small contributions by exhaustively linking single nucleotide polymorphisms (SNPs) with risk for disease across a large number of loci per individual. These data, helped by statistical analysis, could permit one to identify large numbers of genes that are involved in pathogenesis. The number of possible human modifier genes could be high and it will be necessary to focus detailed studies on those genes that play fundamental roles in the disease process. The simple model systems could allow the assessment of the pathological importance of large numbers of possible modifier genes particularly where orthologs exist. Genes that are found to have a functional importance in simple model systems, as well as showing linkage to disease in humans, will be of particular interest for future detailed studies. Moreover, fundamentally important gene products will be the targets for a new generation of therapeutic compounds for the treatment, or even prevention, of neurodegenerative diseases. Genetic screens, indeed, can help to define new neuroprotective pathways.

REFERENCES

Agnello M, Roccheri MC (2010) Apoptosis: focus on sea urchin development. *Apotosis* **15:** 322–30.

Andrew SE, Goldberg YP, Hayden MR (1997) Rethinking genotype and phenotype correlations in polyglutamine expansion disorders. *Hum Mol Genet* **6:** 2005–10.

Bai Q, Garver JA , Hukriede NA, Burton EA (2007) Generation of a transgenic zebrafish model of tauopathy using a novel promoter element derived from the zebrafish eno2 gene. *Nucleic Acids Research* **35:** 6501–16.

Bai Q, Mullett SJ, Garver JA, Hinkle DA, Burton EA (2006) Zebrafish DJ-1 is evolutionarily conserved and expressed in dopaminergic neurons. *Brain Res* **1113:** 33–44.

Braak H, Braak E (1991) Neuropathological staging of Alzheimer-related changes. *Acta Neuropathol* **82:** 239–59.

Brenner S (1974) The genetics of *Caenorhabditis elegans*. *Genetics* **77:** 71–94.

Brosamle C, Halpern ME (2002) Characterization of myelination in the developing zebrafish. *Glia* **39:** 47–57.

Buznikov GA (1983) Sea urchin embryos as a test system to detect embryotoxicity of chemical compounds. *Biol Int* **8:** 5–8.

Buznikov GA, Nikitina LA, Bezuglov VV, Milosević I, Lazarević L, Rogac L, Ruzdijić S, Slotkin TA, Rakić LM (2008a) Sea urchin embryonic development provides a model for evaluating therapies against beta-amyloid toxicity. *Brain Res Bull* **75:** 94–100.

Buznikov GA, Nikitina LA, Seidler FJ, Slotkin TA, Bezuglov VV, Milosević I, Lazarević L, Rogac L, Ruzdijić S, Rakić LM (2008b) Amyloid precursor protein 96-110 and beta-amyloid 1-42 elicit developmental anomalies in sea urchin embryos and larvae that are alleviated by neurotransmitter analogs for acetylcholine, serotonin and cannabinoids. *Neurotoxicol Teratol* **30:** 503–9.

Cao S, Gelwix CC, Caldwell KA, Caldwell GA (2005) Torsin-mediated protection from cellular stress in the dopaminergic neurons of *Caenorhabditis elegans*. *J Neurosci* **25:** 3801–12.

Carrotta R, Arleth L, Pedersen JS, Bauer R (2003) Small-angle x-ray scattering studies of metastable intermediates of beta-lactoglobulin isolated after heat-induced aggregation. *Biopolymers* **70:** 377–90.

Carrotta R, Di Carlo M, Manno M, Montana G, Picone P, Romancino D, San Biagio PL (2006) Toxicity of recombinant beta-amyloid prefibrillar oligomers on the morphogenesis of the sea urchin *Paracentrotus lividus*. *FASEB J* **20:** 1916–24.

Celotto AM, Palladino MJ (2005) Drosophila: a "model" model system to study neurodegeneration. *Mol Interv* **5:** 292–303.

Chan YB, Miguel-Aliaga I, Franks C, Thomas N, Trülzsch B, Sattelle DB, Davies KE, van den Heuvel M (2003) Neuromuscular defects in a Drosophila survival motor neuron gene mutant. *Hum Mol Genet* **12:** 1367–76.

Chen L, Rio DC, Haddad GG, Ma E (2004) Regulatory role of dADAR in ROS metabolism in *Drosophila* CNS. *Brain Res Mol Brain Res* **131:** 93–100.

Chen M, Martins RN, Lardelli M (2009) Complex splicing and neural expression of duplicated tau genes in zebrafish embryos. *J Alzheimers Dis* **18:** 305–17.

Crowther DC, Kinghorn KJ, Miranda E, Page R, Curry JA, Duthie FA, Gubb DC, Lomas DA (2005) Intraneuronal Abeta, non-amyloid aggregates and neurodegeneration in a Drosophila model of Alzheimer's disease. *Neuroscience* **132:** 123–35.

Daigle I, Li C (1993) apl-1, a Caenorhabditis elegans gene encoding a protein related to the human beta-amyloid protein precursor. *Proc Natl Acad Sci USA* **90:** 12045–9.

de la Fuente MA, Singh H, Hemar Y (2002) Recent advances in the characterization of heat induced aggregates and intermediates of whey proteins. *Trends Food Sci Tech* **13:** 262–74.

Deng HX, Hentati A, Tainer JA, Iqbal Z, Cayabyab A, Hung WY, Getzoff ED, Hu P, Herzfeldt B, Roos RP (1993) Amyotrophic lateral sclerosis and structural defects in Cu, Zn superoxide dismutase. *Science* **261:** 1047–51.

Dobson CM (2004) Principles of protein folding, misfolding and aggregation. *Semin Cell Dev Biol* **15:** 3–16.

Dosanjh LE, Brown MK, Rao G, Link CD, Luo Y (2010) Behavioral phenotyping of a transgenic Caenorhabditis elegans expressing neuronal amyloid-beta. *J Alzheimers Dis* **19:** 681–90.

Fay DS, Fluet A, Johnson CJ, Link CD (1998) *In vivo* aggregation of beta-amyloid peptide variants. *J Neurochem* **71:** 1616–25.

Feany MB, Bender WW (2000) A *Drosophila* model of Parkinson's disease. *Nature* **404:** 394–8.

Fernandez-Funez P, Nino-Rosales ML, de Gouyon B, She WC, Luchak JM, Martinez P, Turiegano E, Benito J, Capovilla M, Skinner PJ, McCall A, Canal I, Orr HT, Zoghbi HY, Botas J (2000) Identification of genes that modify ataxin-1-induced neurodegeneration. *Nature* **408:** 101–6.

Finelli A, Kelkar A, Song HJ, Yang H, Konsolaki M (2004) A model for studying Alzheimer's Abeta42-induced toxicity in Drosophila melanogaster. *Mol Cell Neurosci* **26:** 365–75.

Giudice G (1973) *Developmental Biology of the Sea Urchin Embryo*. Academic Press, New York and London.

Goedert M and Jakes R (2005) Mutations causing neurodegenerative tauopathies. *Biochim Biophys Acta* **1739:** 240–50.

Goldberg AL (2003) Protein degradation and protection against misfolded or damaged proteins. *Nature* **426:** 895–9.

Greene JC, Whitworth AJ, Kuo I, Andrews LA, Feany MB, Pallanck LJ (2003) Mitochondrial pathology and apoptotic muscle degeneration in *Drosophila* parkin mutants. *Proc Natl Acad Sci USA* **100:** 4078–83.

Greeve I, Kretzschmar D, Tschäpe JA, Beyn A, Brellinger C, Schweizer M, Nitsch RM, Reifegerste R (2004) Age-dependent neurodegeneration and Alzheimer-amyloid plaque formation in transgenic *Drosophila*. *J Neurosci* **24:** 3899–906.

Hoopengardner B, Bhalla T, Staber C, Reenan R (2003) Nervous system targets of RNA editing identified by comparative genomics. *Science* **301:** 832–6.

Hutton M, Lendon CL, Rizzu P, Baker M, Froelich S, Houlden H, Pickering-Brown S, *et al.* (1998) Association of missense and 5′-splice-site mutations in tau with the inherited dementia FTDP-17. *Nature* **393:** 702–5.

Iijima K, Chiang HC, Hearn SA, Hakker I, Gatt A, Shenton C, Granger L, Leung A, Iijima-Ando K, Zhong Y (2008) Abeta42 mutants with different aggregation profiles induce distinct pathologies in *Drosophila*. *PLoS ONE* **3:** e1703.

Iijima K, Liu HP, Chiang AS, Hearn SA, Konsolaki M, Zhong Y (2004) Dissecting the pathological effects of human Ab40 and Ab42 in Drosophila: a potential model for Alzheimer's disease. *Proc Natl Acad Sci USA* **101:** 6623–8.

Iwata A, Christianson JC, Bucci M, Ellerby LM, Nukina N, Forno LS, Kopito RR (2005) Increased susceptibility of cytoplasmic over nuclear polyglutamine aggregates to autophagic degradation. *Proc Natl Acad Sci USA* **102:** 13135–40.

Jackson GR, Salecker I, Dong X, Yao X, Arnheim N, Faber PW, MacDonald ME, Zipursky SL (1998) Polyglutamine-expanded human Huntington transgenes induce degeneration of *Drosophila* photoreceptor neurons. *Neuron* **21:** 633–42.

Jackson GR, Wiedau-Pazos M, Sang TK, Wagle N, Brown CA, Massachi S, Geschwind DH (2002) Human wild-type tau interacts with wingless pathway components and produces neurofibrillary pathology in *Drosophila*. *Neuron* **34:** 509–19.

Jeibmann A, Paulus W (2009) *Drosophila melanogaster* as a model organism of brain diseases. *Int J Mol Sci* **10:** 407–40.

Jia K, Hart AC, Levine B (2007) Autophagy Genes Protect Against Disease Caused by Polyglutamine Expansion Proteins in *Caenorhabditis elegans*. *Autophagy* **3:** 21–5.

Kawai H, Arata N, Nakayasu H (2001) Three-dimensional distribution of astrocytes in zebrafish spinal cord. *Glia* **36:** 406–13.

Kazemi-Esfarjani P, Benzer S (2000) Genetic suppression of polyglutamine toxicity in Drosophila. *Science* **287:** 1837–40.

Kidd M (1963) Paired helical filaments in electron microscopy of Alzheimer's disease. *Nature* **197:** 192–3.

Kimble J, Hirsh D (1979) The postembryonic cell lineages of the hermaphrodite and male gonads in Caenorhabditis elegans. *Dev Biol* **70:** 396–417.

Kirschner DA, Abraham C, Selkoe DJ (1986) X-ray diffraction from intraneuronal paired helical filaments and extraneuronal amyloid fibers in Alzheimer disease indicates cross-beta conformation. *Proc Natl Acad Sci USA* **83:** 503–7.

Kosinski RA, Zaremba M (2007) Dynamics of the model of the Caenorhabditis elegans neural network. *Acta Physica Polonica* **38:** 202.

Koulen P, Janowitz T, Johnston LD, Ehrlich BE (2000) Conservation of localization patterns of IP(3) receptor type 1 in cerebellar Purkinje cells across vertebrate species. *J Neurosci Res* **61:** 493–9.

Kuwahara T, Koyama A, Gengyo-Ando K, Masuda M, Kowa H, Tsunoda M, Mitani S, Iwatsubo T (2006) Familial Parkinson mutant alphasynuclein causes dopamine neuron dysfunction in transgenic *C. elegans*. *J Biol Chem* **281:** 334–40.

Kuwahara T, Koyama A, Koyama S, Yoshina S, Ren CH, Kato T, Mitani S, Iwatsubo T (2008) A systematic RNAi screen reveals involvement of endocytic pathway in neuronal dysfunction in alpha-synuclein transgenic *C. elegans*. *Hum Mol Genet* **17:** 2997–3009.

Lakso M, Vartiainen S, Moilanen AM, Sirvio J, Thomas JH, Nass R, Blakely RD, Wong G (2003) Dopaminergic neuronal loss and motor deficits in *Caenorhabditis elegans* overexpressing human alpha-synuclein. *J Neurochem* **86:** 165–72.

Lee VM, Goedertand YM, Trojanowski JQ (2001) Neurodegenerative tauopathies. *Annu Rev Neurosci* **24:** 1121–59.

Lessing D, Bonini NM (2009) Maintaining the brain: insight into human neurodegeneration from Drosophila melanogaster mutants. *Nat Rev Genet* **10:** 359–70.

Levine B, Klionsky DJ (2004) Development by self-digestion: molecular mechanisms and biological functions of autophagy. *Dev Cell* **6:** 463–77.

Link CD (1995) Expression of human beta-amyloid peptide in transgenic *Caenorhabditis elegans*. *Proc Natl Acad Sci USA* **92:** 9368–72.

Link CD, Johnson CJ, Fonte V, Paupard M, Hall DH, Styren S, Mathis CA, Klunk WE (2001) Visualization of fibrillar amyloid deposits in living, transgenic *Caenorhabditis elegans* animals using the sensitive amyloid dye, X-34. *Neurobiol Aging* **22:** 217–26.

Link CD (2006) *C. elegans* models of age-associated neurodegenerative diseases: lessons from transgenic worm models of Alzheimer's disease. *Exp Geront* **41:** 1007–13.

Ma PM (2003) Catecholaminergic systems in the zebrafish. IV. Organization and projection pattern of dopaminergic neurons in the diencephalon. *J Comp Neurol* **460:** 13–37.

Miller VM, Nelson RF, Gouvion CM, Williams A, Rodriguez-Lebron E, Harper SQ, Davidson BL, Rebagliati MR, Paulson HL (2005) CHIP suppresses polyglutamine aggregation and toxicity in vitro and in vivo. *J Neurosci* **25:** 9152–61.

Moloney A, Sattelle DB, Lomas DA, Crowther DC (2010) Alzheimer's disease: insights from Drosophila melanogaster models. *Trends Biochem Sci* **35:** 228–35.

Morfini G, Pigino G, Brady ST (2005) Polyglutamine expansion diseases: failing to deliver. *Trends Mol Med* **11:** 64–70.

Nakajima Y, Kaneko H, Murray G, Burke RD (2004) Divergent patterns of neural development in larval echinoids and asteroids. *Evol Dev* **6:** 95–104.

Nollen EA, Garcia SM, van Haaften G, Kim S, Chavez A, Morimoto RI, Plasterk RH (2004) Genome-wide RNA interference screen identifies previously undescribed regulators of polyglutamine aggregation. *Proc Natl Acad Sci USA* **101:** 6403–8.

Nuttley WM, Atkinson-Leadbeater KP, Van Der Kooy D (2002) Serotonin mediates food-odor associative learning in the nematode *Caenorhabditis elegans*. *Proc Natl Acad Sci USA* **99:** 12449–54.

Palladino MJ, Keegan LP, O'Connell MA, Reenan RA (2000) A-to-I pre-mRNA editing in Drosophila is primarily involved in adult nervous system function and integrity. *Cell* **102:** 437–49.

Paquet D, Bhat R, Sydow A, Mandelkow EM, Berg S, Hellberg S, Falting J, Distel M, Koster RW, Schmid B, Haass C (2009) A zebrafish model of tauopathy allows in vivo imaging of neuronal cell death and drug evaluation. *J Clin Invest* **119:** 1382–95.

Pellicanò M, Picone P, Cavalieri V, Carrotta R, Spinelli G, Di Carlo M (2009) The sea urchin embryo: a model to study Alzheimer's beta amyloid induced toxicity. *Arch Biochem Biophys* **483:** 120–6.

Pepys MB (2002) Pathogenesis, diagnosis and treatment of systematic amyloidosis. *Philos Trans R Soc Lond B Biol Sci* **356:** 203–10.

Phillips JP, Tainer JA, Getzoff ED, Boulianne GL, Kirby K, Hilliker AJ (1995) Subunit-destabilizing mutations in Drosophila copper/zinc superoxide dismutase: neuropathology and a model of dimer dysequilibrium. *Proc Natl Acad Sci USA* **92:** 8574–8.

Picone P, Carrotta R, Montana G, Nobile MR, San Biagio PL, Di Carlo M (2009) Abeta oligomers and fibrillar aggregates induce different apoptotic pathways in LAN5 neuroblastoma cell cultures. *Biophys J* **96:** 4200–11.

Pokrzywa M, Dacklin I, Hultmark D, Lundgren E (2007) Misfolded transthyretin causes behavioral changes in a Drosophila model for transthyretin-associated amyloidosis. *Eur J Neurosci* **26:** 913–24.

Ramot D, MacInnis BL, Goodman MB (2008) Bidirectional temperature sensing by a single thermosensory neuron in *C. elegans*. *Nat Neurosci* **11:** 908–15.

Ross CA, Poirier MA (2004) Protein aggregation and neurodegenerative disease. *Nat Med* **10 (Suppl.):** S10–S17.

Sager JJ, Bai Q, Burton EA (2010) Transgenic zebrafish models of neurodegenerative diseases. *Brain Struct Funct* **214:** 285–302.

Satyal SH, Schmidt E, Kitagawa K, Sondheimer N, Lindquist S, Kramer JM, Morimoto RI (2000) Polyglutamine aggregates alter protein folding homeostasis in *Caenorhabditis elegans*. *Proc Natl Acad Sci USA* **97:** 5750–5.

Shulman JM, Feany MB (2003) Genetic modifiers of tauopathy in *Drosophila*. *Genetics* **165:** 1233–42.

Sodergren E, Weinstock GM, Davidson EH, Cameron RA, Gibbs RA, Angerer RC, *et al.* (2006) The genome of the sea urchin *Strongylocentrotus purpuratus*. *Science* **314:** 941–52.

Steinkraus KA, Smith ED, Davis C, Carr D, Pendergrass WR, Sutphin GL, Kennedy BK, Kaeberlein M (2008) Dietary restriction suppresses proteotoxicity and enhances longevity by an *hsf-1*-dependent mechanism in *Caenorhabditis elegans*. *Aging Cell* **7:** 394–404.

Stokin GB, Almenar-Queralt A, Gunawardena S, Rodrigues EM, Falzone T, Kim J, Lillo C, Mount SL, Roberts EA, McGowan E, Williams DS, Goldstein LS (2008) Amyloid precursor protein-induced axonopathies are independent of amyloid-beta peptides. *Hum Mol Genet* **17:** 3474–86.

Styren SD, Hamilton RL, Styren GC, Klunk WE (2000) X-34, a fluorescent derivative of Congo red: a novel histochemical stain for Alzheimer's disease pathology. *J Histochem Cytochem* **48:** 1223–32.

Sulston JE, Horvitz HR (1977) Post-embryonic cell lineages of the nematode, *Caenorhabditis elegans*. *Dev Biol* **56:** 110–56.

Sunde M, Serpell LC, Bartlam M, Fraser PE, Pepys MB, Blake CCF (1997) Common core structure of amyloid fibrils by synchrotron X-ray diffraction. *J Mol Biol* **273:** 729–39.

Tomasiewicz HG, Flaherty DB, Soria JP, Wood JG (2002) Transgenic Zebrafish model of neurodegeneration. *J Neurosci Res* **70:** 734–45.

Tycko R (2003) Insights into the amyloid folding problem from solid-state NMR. *Biochemistry* **42:** 3151–9.

Venkatraman P, Wetzel R, Tanaka M, Nukina N, Goldberg AL, Anichtchik O, Toleikyte G, Kaslin J, Panula P (2009) Eukaryotic proteasomes cannot digest polyglutamine sequences and release them during degradation of polyglutamine-containing proteins. *Mol Cell* **14:** 95–104.

Vetri V, Militello V (2005) Thermal induced conformational changes involved in the aggregation pathways of beta-lactoglobulin. *Biophys Chem* **113:** 83–91.

Voronina E, Wessel GM (2001) Apoptosis in sea urchin oocytes, eggs, and early embryos. *Mol Reprod Dev* **60:** 553–61.

Walsh DM, Selkoe DJ (2007) A-beta oligomers a decade of discovery. *J Neurochem* **101:** 1172–84.

Warrick JM, Chan HY, Gray-Board GL, Chai Y, Paulson HL, Bonini NM (1999) Suppression of polyglutamine-mediated neurodegeneration in Drosophila by the molecular chaperone HSP70. *Nat Genet* **23:** 425–8.

Warrick JM, Paulson HL, Gray-Board GL, Bui QT, Fischbeck KH, Pittman RN, Bonini NM (1998) Expanded polyglutamine protein forms nuclear inclusions and causes neural degeneration in *Drosophila*. *Cell* **93:** 939–49.

Watson MR, Lagow RD, Xu K, Zhang B, Bonini NM (2008) A *Drosophila* model for amyotrophic lateral sclerosis reveals motor neuron damage by human SOD1. *J Biol Chem* **283:** 24972–81.

Watts DJ, Strogatz SH (1998) Collective dynamics of "small-world network". *Nature* **393:** 440–42.

Williams A, Sarkar S, Cuddon P, Ttofi EK, Saiki S, Siddiqi FH, Jahreiss L, Fleming A, Pask D, Goldsmith P, O'Kane CJ, Floto RA, Rubinsztein DC (2008) Novel targets for Huntington's disease in an mTOR-independent autophagy pathway. *Nat Chem Biol* **4:** 295–305.

Wittmann CW, Wszolek MF, Shulman JM, Salvaterra PM, Lewis J, Hutton M, Feany MB (2001) Tauopathy in Drosophila: neurodegeneration without neurofibrillary tangles. *Science* **293:** 711–14.

Zhang Y, Lu H, Bargmann CI (2005) Pathogenic bacteria induce aversive olfactory learning in Caenorhabditis elegans. *Nature* **438:** 179–84.

Zoghbi HY, Orr HT (2009) Pathogenic mechanisms of a polyglutamine-mediated neurodegenerative disease, spinocerebellar ataxia type 1. *J Biol Chem* **284:** 7425–9.

C H A P T E R

15

Using zebrafish to assess developmental neurotoxicity

Stephanie Padilla and Robert MacPhail

INTRODUCTION

It is widely accepted that the developing nervous system is especially vulnerable to a variety of chemicals, including drugs and environmental contaminants. It is also clear that our understanding of the risks from chemical exposures during development is rudimentary, and that the resources required for remedying the situation are legion. As a result, increasing attention is being directed toward alternative test methods including *in vitro* preparations, computational (*in silico*) models and *in vivo* model (or alternative) organisms. In particular, zebrafish have become a popular test species in toxicology, pharmacology and biomedical research. This chapter addresses several issues, results and research needs regarding the use of zebrafish to assess developmental neurotoxicity. Particular attention is given to using zebrafish to screen groups of chemicals for developmental neurotoxicity. Considerable advances have been made in understanding the basic biology of nervous system development in zebrafish, in techniques for rapidly evaluating the effect of chemical exposures on nervous system development, and notably to a lesser extent in understanding the significance of results for predicting human effects. This chapter was written as an introduction to the use of zebrafish in developmental neurotoxicology, and to encourage the use of this model either for screening or mechanistic purposes. We have endeavored to make the reader aware of significant research findings, and to offer a balanced view of the advantages and limitations in using zebrafish as a model for investigating developmental neurotoxicity. Although zebrafish are being used increasingly to discover the mechanistic underpinnings of many human diseases, it will become clear that an extensive program of research is required before zebrafish can become a realistic substitute for mammalian tests of developmental neurotoxicity.

EARLY DEVELOPMENT

Early development requires the coordinated, time-dependent participation of numerous genetic, biochemical and morphological processes that mold the physiology and behavior of an organism. These processes initially prepare the organism for adaptation to its environment. The environment, of course, plays an important role and must be conducive to the developing organism. Disruption of developmental processes, or degradation of the environment, can lead to adverse consequences for the organism's adaptation and survival.

Development also involves rapid changes in all organ systems, and it is these transitions that may make the organism uniquely vulnerable to adverse events. This is particularly true for the nervous system: no other organ system can match its cellular and molecular complexity, its distribution throughout the body and the functions it serves in regulating the body and promoting adaptation. The myriad events required to build a functioning nervous system offer almost unlimited opportunities for disruption by numerous variables including nutrition, stress, hormones, drugs and environmental contaminants.

VULNERABILITY OF THE DEVELOPING NERVOUS SYSTEM

The adverse effects of alcohol on the developing organism have been known for centuries (reviewed in Calhoun and Warren, 2007). In more recent times the effects were rediscovered and labeled Fetal Alcohol Syndrome (Jones and Smith, 1973). Offspring of mothers that had consumed alcohol had notable facial malformations and, importantly, faulty cognitive function. Malformations and faulty cognitive development were also found in the offspring of mothers that had consumed fish contaminated with methylmercury (Amin-Zaki *et al.*, 1981; Kurland *et al.*, 1960). Perinatal lead exposure was also linked conclusively to faulty cognitive function and behavioral disorders in the 1970s (Needleman *et al.*, 1979). More recently, concerns have grown over the possible adverse developmental effects of the environmentally persistent polychlorinated biphenyls (PCBs) and the brominated flame retardants (polybrominated diphenyl ethers or PBDEs) (Costa *et al.*, 2008; Kodavanti, 2005). Both PCBs and PBDEs are notable in that a major target appears to be the thyroid gland, which is critical for normal development (Kodavanti, 2005; Schreiber *et al.*, 2010).

Reproductive and Developmental Toxicology, Edited by Ramesh C. Gupta
ISBN: 978-0-12-382032-7

Environmental contaminants are not alone is selectively attacking the developing nervous system. A number of drugs, in addition to ethanol, also cause adverse effects on development including nicotine, cocaine and anticonvulsants such as valproate (Ornoy, 2009; Slotkin, 1998; Costa *et al.*, 2004).

ADVERSE EFFECTS PRODUCED BY DEVELOPMENTAL NEUROTOXICANTS

Early exposure to several drugs and environmental contaminants can cause adverse effects on a number of basic neurobiological functions, including sensory, motor and cognitive. These adverse effects have frequently been identified first in humans, then later "confirmed" in laboratory studies using mammalian (typically rodent) models. As a result, laboratory testing for developmental neurotoxicity often involves a series of tests with rodents that evaluate sensory and motor function, and some aspect(s) of cognitive function. There are numerous tests that can be applied in these studies (reviewed in Weiss and Cory-Slechta, 2001). For example, sensory function can be evaluated simply (but crudely) by gauging the reaction of a rat to a sudden snap of the finger or a tail pinch. More sophisticated tests are available to measure sensory integrity, including thresholds that capitalize on the sensory startle reflex response or a previously learned operant response. Many tests are also available for evaluating motor function including measurements of general motor activity, or balance, endurance and grip strength. A substantial number of tests have been used to study learning, motivation, memory and attention in the laboratory. In all cases the tests vary in the degree of instrumentation, the amount of training required of the test subject, the measurement scale(s) and amount of data that are generated (MacPhail and Tilson, 1995).

The tests mentioned above concentrate on evaluating developmental neurotoxicity based on an organism's behavior. To a large extent behavior represents the final common pathway of all nervous system activity, making it a good apical endpoint for screening. It should therefore be clear that neurotoxicity may also be manifest at morphological, biochemical or physiological levels of nervous-system organization (NRC, 1992). Morphological alterations were once considered the "gold standard" of toxicity, and changes in morphology are still taken as incontrovertible evidence of an adverse effect. The advent of immunohistological stains has sharpened our understanding of the architecture of the nervous system and has revealed structural changes, for example in neuronal patterning, that could not be detected using traditional histopathological methods (Jensen, 1995). Biochemical assays of nervous system development have been used extensively. For example, enzymes involved in neurotransmitter synthesis and metabolism frequently have been used in evaluating damage to the nervous system following toxicant (and drug) exposure (e.g., tyrosine hydroxylase or cholinesterase activity). Changes in neurotransmitter levels have also been used as indicators of nervous system damage (e.g., dopamine, serotonin). Isolation and identification of specific nervous system proteins and gene products have advanced our understanding of the sites of action of toxicants in the nervous system (Manzo *et al.*, 1996; O'Callaghan and Sriram, 2005). Electrophysiological measurements have also been used to evaluate neurotoxicity, with notable advances in our understanding of ion channels as targets for neurotoxicants (Narahashi *et al.*, 2007).

ALTERNATIVE ANIMAL MODELS

Almost without exception, the above methods for assessing neurotoxicity have been applied in studies on the developing, as well as the adult, mammalian nervous system. But must we use the mammalian nervous system to predict toxicity to humans? Perhaps one of the most exciting new developments is the discovery of conserved biological processes extending to what were until recently considered "lower" organisms or alternative species.

Three events have led to the popularity of alternative species. First, molecular biology has revealed the basic concordance of cellular events in a wide range of "lower" species including yeast, worms, flies and fishes. Second, the concordance has been verified with advances in genetics and pathway analyses. As a result, these alternative species are now being used increasingly in probing the basic processes of life and disease. Third, the size and speed of development of these organisms has made them even more attractive for use. It should be noted, however, that although yeast, worms, flies and fishes are often labeled alternative species, it is better to consider them complementary species (Cerutti and Levin, 2006), whose role in biomedical science is steadily growing, and whose application in fathoming basic biology, health and disease is yet to be fully appreciated.

PRACTICAL CONSIDERATIONS IN ZEBRAFISH NEUROTOXICOLOGICAL RESEARCH

Zebrafish represent an attractive complementary species for developmental neurotoxicity assessments. The fish are small, allowing large laboratory colonies of subjects. It is not difficult to set up a breeding colony; detailed guidance is available in the literature (Westerfield, 2000) and on the internet (www.zfin.org). Breeding can be accomplished with ease, producing literally hundreds of embryos each day. Development takes place rapidly without any parental influence. The liver matures early allowing the embryo to metabolize many protoxicants into the active metabolite(s). Up until approximately 6 days post-fertilization (dpf) the embryo feeds on its yolk, thereby eliminating the need for nutritional supplementation. The embryos are transparent, allowing detailed non-invasive observation of the development of organ systems and processes. In order to highlight specific areas of the nervous system, many stains or vital dyes may be used. Mutant or reporter strains may be easily obtained through the central repository at the Zebrafish International Resource Center in Eugene, Oregon (http://zebrafish.org). In addition, genetic selection and modification via morpholino knockdown has become an increasingly important strategy in studies of basic biology and disease processes (see examples below). In the context of chemical screening, the small size of the larvae allows housing, exposure and testing in the small wells of a microtiter plate, and the use of small quantities of chemicals for investigation. This latter point is especially germane for

A

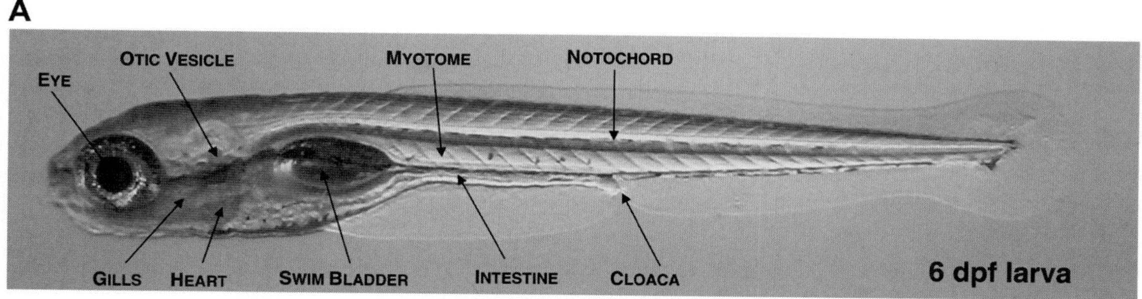

B

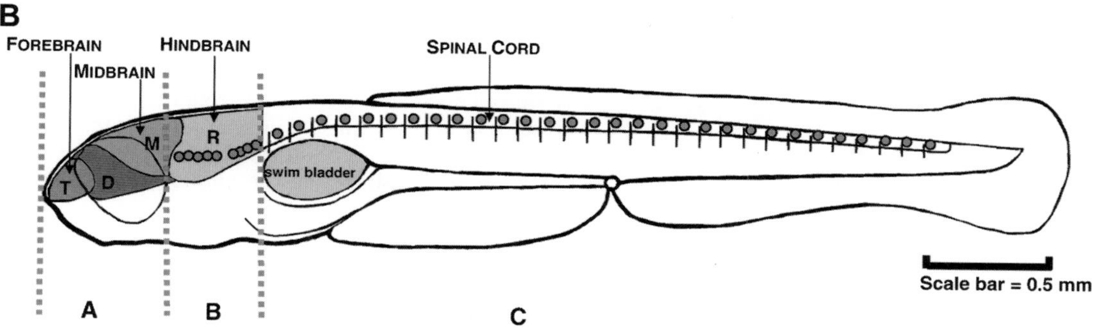

FIGURE 15.1 Photograph and schematic depicting the major anatomical features of the 6-day-old zebrafish larva. T: telencephalon; D: diencephalon; M: mesencephalon; and R: rhombencephalon. Vertical red dotted lines represent convenient dissection locations for obtaining fore- and mid-brain vs hindbrain samples using the eye and swim bladder as landmarks. Filled red circles represent the superior and inferior serotonergic raphe neurons in the hindbrain and the ventromedial serotonergic neurons in the spinal cord. Reprinted from Airhart *et al.* (2007), with permission from Elsevier. Please refer to color plate section.

certain types of chemicals whose cost can be prohibitive for large-scale mammalian testing. Lastly, the embryo soon transitions to a larva that in a few days displays sensory, motor and cognitive functions that allow detailed investigation of the behavioral dimensions of susceptibility to chemical exposures. For a clear, concise review of the early development of the zebrafish nervous system, see Guo (2009). A zebrafish larva and its landmark structures are depicted in Figure 15.1.

While zebrafish offer many advantages as a model species, they have limitations. The most important limitation for toxicity studies is the dosing scenario. The most convenient way to expose an embryo is to simply place it in a solution of the chemical; however, the actual dose that reaches the embryo is unknown. A number of investigators have measured the internal dose using radiolabeled compounds or analytical methods, and the one conclusion from these studies is that the "dose" to the embryo/larva is rarely identical to the nominal concentration in the surrounding water (Huang *et al.*, 2010; Schreiber *et al.*, 2009; Thomas *et al.*, 2009). It would be highly desirable to use a physical characteristic(s) of the chemical to at least estimate "dose" to the embryo/larva. The Log P (octanol:water partition coefficient) would seem to be an ideal candidate. Although there are formulae using the Log P to calculate bioaccumulation of a chemical in an organism (Connell and Hawker, 1988; Arnot *et al.*, 2009), there is, as yet, no way to calculate reliably the bioavailability of the chemical in the zebrafish embryo/larvae using different exposure scenarios, so one has to rely on analytical means if the actual dose that is delivered must be determined. Moreover, for the first 2 to 3 days the embryo is encased in a chorion, which may serve as an additional barrier to some chemicals. Embryos can be dechorionated either mechanically or with a pronase solution, but this dechorionation may affect the integrity and behavior of the embryos. In fact, changes in reflex behavior have been noted in dechorionated embryos (Saint-Amant and Drapeau, 1998; Thomas *et al.*, 2009). Dechorionation also eliminates the possibility of determining the effect of a chemical on hatching. Additionally, it should be obvious that chemicals need to be water soluble, although some investigators have overcome this obstacle by injecting the toxicant directly into the yolk. The main route of exposure early in development (the first 5 days) is likely dermal, as the gills are not functioning and the animal is not feeding.

The small size of zebrafish and the rapid pace at which they develop pose some challenges. Biochemical or genetic analyses often require pooling of embryos or larvae because they are so small. Embedding and sectioning of the embryos and larvae are also challenging, and the size of the larvae greatly constrains the types of recording equipment that can be used for testing and evaluation. In addition, development proceeds rapidly. By 6dfp larval swimming and vision are well developed, as are the major organ systems, as well as the neuronal pathways and neurotransmitters in the peripheral and central nervous system including the spinal cord. The rapid pace of development places a premium on the timing of observations post-fertilization in order to record developmental landmarks, such that a few hours can make a significant difference in the developmental stage or, perhaps, in sensitivity to toxicants.

ZEBRAFISH AS A MODEL OF DEVELOPMENTAL NEUROTOXICITY

Zebrafish have been used for the last 30 years to study the basics of neurodevelopment. Elegant work has been published on the development of the nervous system (Strähle and Blader, 1994; Blader and Strähle, 2000; Kimmel, 1993; Kimmel

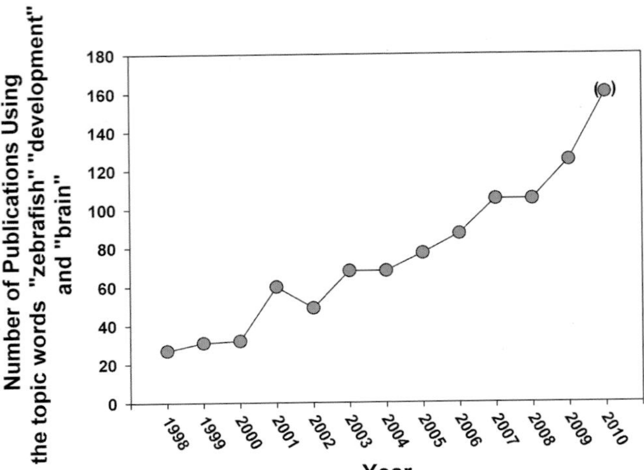

FIGURE 15.2 The annual number of publications in PubMed (http://www.ncbi.nlm.nih.gov/sites/entrez?db=pubmed) that were identified using the keywords "zebrafish", "brain" and "development". The total for 2010 is an estimate based on publications in the first quarter.

et al., 1991; Wullimann *et al.*, 1999; Mueller and Wullimann, 2003), neuronal pathfinding (e.g., Struermer, 1988; Baier, 2000; Baier *et al.*, 1996, 1994), myelination (Buckley *et al.*, 2010; Jung *et al.*, 2010; Kirby *et al.*, 2006; Monk and Talbot, 2009) and the genetic or structural basis of nervous system function (Fadool and Dowling, 2008; Fetcho *et al.*, 2008; Fetcho and Liu, 1998; Fetcho and O'Malley, 1997). As testimony to their rapid rise in popularity, the number of papers published annually has quadrupled in the last 10 years (Figure 15.2), and the rate is not yet slowing. The study of zebrafish nervous system development is a fast growing area. It would benefit the developmental neurotoxicity research community to be a participant in this upwelling of knowledge rather than a bystander.

Even though there has been rapid progress in understanding zebrafish neurodevelopment, our understanding of the effects of toxic compounds on development has not progressed as swiftly. Many have expressed an opinion that zebrafish would be appropriate for modeling diseases (Tropepe and Sive, 2003; Shin and Fishman, 2002; Pogoda *et al.*, 2006; Penberthy *et al.*, 2002; Patton and Zon, 2001; Panula *et al.*, 2006), for general toxicity testing (Zhang *et al.*, 2009; Yang *et al.*, 2009; Teraoka *et al.*, 2003; Rubinstein, 2006; Pichler *et al.*, 2003; Parng *et al.*, 2002; Markou *et al.*, 2009; Hill *et al.*, 2005), and specifically for developmental neurotoxicity testing (Brannen *et al.*, 2010; Guo 2004, 2009; Lammer *et al.*, 2009; Linney *et al.*, 2004; Peterson *et al.*, 2008; Ton *et al.*, 2006). Table 15.1 summarizes a number of relevant publications that used zebrafish to study developmental neurotoxicity. These papers were chosen because the researchers investigated a compound or compounds that were known to be neurotoxic, or they used endpoints that indicated the compound affected the developing nervous system. Also, the papers in Table 15.1 used chemical exposure durations of more than 10 hours during development, and the endpoint(s) were more specific indicators for neurotoxicity than, for example, spinal curvature, which is a common malformation in developing zebrafish. We cannot claim that this table is comprehensive in either its content or details, but it is included so readers may have a reference resource for finding information on endpoints or chemicals of interest. Note that the majority of the studies in Table 15.1 have been published in the last 10, if not the last 5, years, reinforcing the notion that developmental neurotoxicity assessment in zebrafish is still in its infancy. Also, when reviewing the studies one is struck that there is no consistent protocol for study design. For example, there are wide variations in the duration of exposure, whether the animals are dosed individually or in groups, whether the chemical is renewed daily or not, the "window" of exposure, how soon after exposure the animal is assessed, and the method of statistical analysis. In many studies it is also difficult to assess how the degree of overt toxicity (lethality or malformations) compares with the degree of neurotoxicity, which is extremely important for classifying the toxicity profile of the compound. It is difficult to know if a compound is truly neurotoxic or if that neurotoxicity is "contaminated" by many other effects. For example, if zebrafish show both decreased activity and pericardial edema after exposure to a toxicant during development, is the decreased activity a neurotoxic effect or due simply to the animals' inability to move efficiently because of the edema?

THE IMPORTANCE OF SCREENS

More recently, studies in zebrafish have emerged that are designed for rapid assessment of the potential of large numbers of chemicals to perturb the developing nervous system. These studies employ what are properly referred to as neurotoxicity screens.

In virtually all areas of biomedical science there are many times when a relatively rapid response to a question is desired. For example, one may want to know whether a new drug offers promise in treating a disease, or whether a mutant organism has a defect needed to investigate the etiology of a disease. In toxicology, quick answers may be needed regarding the potential adverse effect of a chemical. The need for "quick" or preliminary answers regarding chemical toxicity is especially important when it comes to environmental chemicals. Although estimates vary, it is generally accepted that there are tens of thousands of commercial chemicals, yet toxicity data are available on an exceedingly small fraction (Grandjean and Landrigan, 2006; Judson *et al.*, 2009). Grandjean and Landrigan (Figure 15.3) estimated that the "chemical universe" consists of about 80,000 chemicals, of which 1/8 or 10,000 chemicals have been demonstrated in the laboratory to be neurotoxic, and yet there appear to be only five confirmed developmental neurotoxicants in humans. This is not a comment on the scarcity of developmentally neurotoxic chemicals in the chemical universe, but rather on the lack of testing for developmental neurotoxicity. The authors concluded that with so many of the 80,000 compounds already demonstrated to have neurotoxic potential, it was highly likely that many must also be developmentally neurotoxic. Screening methods may therefore be useful in providing preliminary data on toxicity, and in identifying and prioritizing chemicals for in-depth follow-up investigations.

Screening methods may be distinguished on the basis of whether they focus on an endpoint of concern or a mechanism of toxicity. For example, the observation that numerous compounds impair vision may justify a screening test for deficits in visual function. On the other hand, visual impairment can be due to any number of reasons, and if the underlying

TABLE 15.1 Developmental neurotoxicological investigations in zebrafish

Toxin, toxicant, drug	Nervous system toxicity finding	Reference(s)
Arsenite	Decreased reflexive movement, disordered axonal outgrowth	Li *et al.* (2009)
Bifenthrin	Changes in locomotor activity	Jin *et al.* (2009)
Caffeine	Disorganized muscle fibers, reduced tactile sensitivity, secondary motor axon defects, neuromuscular junction defects	Chen *et al.* (2008)
Cadmium	Notochord defects, motor axon defects	Hen Chow and Cheng (2003)
Cadmium	Less distinct mid-hindbrain boundary, decreased neuronal differentiation, decreased axonogenesis	Chow *et al.* (2009)
Cadmium	Small eyes, visual impairment, decreased neuronal differentiation in retina, impaired retinal ganglion cell formation and lack of cone photoreceptors	Chow *et al.* (2009)
Cartap	Abnormal notochord	Zhou *et al.* (2009)
p-Chlorophenylalanine (serotonin synthesis inhibitor)	No effect on neurotransmitter levels, no effect on motor activity	Sallinen *et al.* (2009a)
Chlorpyrifos	Spatial discrimination impairment; altered response latency; altered startle response	Levin *et al.* (2003), Eddins *et al.* (2010), Levin *et al.* (2004)
Chlorpyrifos	Increased tail coilings, altered locomotor activity	Selderslaghs *et al.* (2010)
Cimetidine (histamine H_2 receptor antagonist)	Decreased locomotor activity	Peitsaro *et al.* (2007)
Clorgyline (MAO inhibitor)	Decreased locomotor activity	Sallinen *et al.* (2009a)
Copper	Decreased number of neuromasts	Johnson *et al.* (2007)
Cyclopamine	Malformed notochord	Loucks and Ahlgren (2009)
Deprenyl	Decreased MAO activity, altered levels of neurotransmitters, decreased locomotor activity, altered vertical place preference	Sallinen *et al.* (2009a)
Domoic acid	Elevated sensitivity to pentylenetetrazole-induced seizures	Tiedeken and Ramsdell (2007)
Endosulfan I and Endosulfan sulfate	Decreased sensitivity to touch	Stanley *et al.* (2009)
Ethanol	Cyclopia, duplicated notochord	Laale (1971)
Ethanol	CNS cell death, skeletal defects, changes in learning and memory, changes in startle response	Loucks and Carvan (2004), Carvan *et al.* (2004)
Ethanol	Cyclopia, impaired lamination of optic tectum, delay of retinal lamination	Arenzana *et al.* (2006)
Ethanol	Underdevelopment of the optic nerve; decreased growth of the photoreceptor outer segment; increased visual threshold; impaired photoreceptor function	Matsui *et al.* (2006)
Ethanol	Decreased eye area; decreased volume of retinal layers: photoreceptor, inner nuclear and ganglionic	Dlugos and Rabin (2007)
Ethanol	Reduced eye size; reduced lens size; disrupted retinal cell differentiation	Kashyap *et al.* (2007)
Ethanol	Malformed notochord	Loucks and Ahlgren (2009)
Ethanol	Altered locomotor activity	Peng *et al.* (2009)
Ethanol	Decreased touch response, motor neuron axon defects	Sylvain *et al.* (2010)
Fipronil	Decreased touch response, abnormal notochord, abnormal muscle morphology	Stehr *et al.* (2006)
Fluoxetine (serotonin reuptake inhibitor)	Persistent decreased locomotor activity	Airhart *et al.* (2007)
Fluvoxamine (serotonin reuptake inhibitor)	Decreased motor activity	Sallinen *et al.* (2009a)
Forskolin	Malformed notochord	Loucks and Ahlgren (2009)
4-Hydroxy androstenedione (aromatase inhibitor)	Neurodevelopmental landmarks (eye movement, righting response, touch response, fin movement) were absent or delayed. Effects were mitigated by addition of estrogen	Nelson *et al.* (2008)
6-Hydroxydopamine	Decreased tyrosine hydroxylase positive neurons, increased oxidative stress biomarker (nitrotyrosine) in brain	Parng *et al.* (2007)
Immepip (histamine H_3 receptor agonist)	Decreased locomotor activity	Peitsaro *et al.* (2007)
Lithium	Loss of anterior CNS	Macdonald *et al.* (1994), van de Water *et al.* (2001)
Metam sodium	Malformed notochord	Tilton *et al.* (2008), Tilton and Tanguay (2008)
β-*N*-Methylamino-L-alanine (BMAA)	Increased incidence of clonus-like convulsions	Purdie *et al.* (2009a, b)

(Continued)

TABLE 15.1 Developmental neurotoxicological investigations in zebrafish—*Cont'd*

Toxin, toxicant, drug	Nervous system toxicity finding	Reference(s)
Methyl mercury	Decreased locomotor activity, impaired prey capture	Samson *et al.* (2001)
Methyl mercury	Negative: no effect on brain expression of some genes	Gonzalez *et al.* (2005)
Methyl mercury	Depressed escape response, decreased learning and memory	Weber (2006), Weber *et al.* (2008), Smith *et al.* (2010)
MPTP	Changes in locomotor activity, fewer dopaminergic neurons	Bretaud *et al.* (2004)
MPTP	Neuronal loss in ventral diencephalon	McKinley *et al.* (2005)
MPTP	Decreased tyrosine hydroxylase, increased swimming bouts	Thirumalai and Cline (2008)
MPTP	Decreased tyrosine hydroxylase or dopamine transporter positive neurons in ventral diencephalon	Chen *et al.* (2009)
MPTP	Decreased locomotor activity, selective decrease in tyrosine hydroxylase positive neurons	Sallinen *et al.* (2009b)
MPP^+	Decreased locomotor activity, selective decrease in tyrosine hydroxylase positive neurons	Sallinen *et al.* (2009b)
Nicotine	Delayed development and pathfinding error of the secondary spinal motorneurons	Svoboda *et al.* (2002), Welsh *et al.* (2009)
Nicotine	Increased startle response	Eddins *et al.* (2010)
Paraquat	No changes in locomotor activity, no changes in dopaminergic neurons	Bretaud *et al.* (2004)
Perfluorooctanesulfonic acid (PFOS)	Increased locomotor activity	Huang *et al.* (2010)
Pilocarpine (cholinergic agonist)	Increased startle response	Eddins *et al.* (2010)
Polychlorinated biphenyls (Aroclor 1254)	Decreased serotonin levels; decreased neuronal outgrowth	Kreiling *et al.* (2007)
Pyrethroid pesticides (permethrin, resmethrin, bifenthrin, deltamethrin, cypermethrin, λ-cyhalothrin)	Craniofacial abnormalities, spasms	DeMicco *et al.* (2010)
Pyrilamine (histamine H_1 receptor antagonist)	Decreased locomotor activity	Peitsaro *et al.* (2007)
Retinoic acid	Perturbed development of caudal midbrain, caudal hindbrain and some cranial ganglia	Hill *et al.* (1995), Holder and Hill (1991)
Rotenone	No changes in locomotor activity, no changes in dopaminergic neurons	Bretaud *et al.* (2004)
Saxitoxin	Reversible paralysis; persistently impaired growth and survival	Lefebvre *et al.* (2004)
Silver nitrate	Decreased locomotor activity	Powers *et al.* (2010)
Sodium benzoate	Decreased tyrosine hydroxylase or dopamine transporter positive neurons in ventral diencephalon; decreased locomotor activity, decreased touch response	Chen *et al.* (2009), Tsay *et al.* (2007)
Tamoxifen (estrogen receptor blocker)	Decreased eye size and decreased thickness of the inner plexiform layer in the retina; mitigated by the addition of estrogen	Hamad *et al.* (2007)
Taxol (mitotic inhibitor)	Increased brain apoptosis	Parng *et al.* (2007)
TCDD	Increased brain necrosis	Henry *et al.* (1997)
TCDD	Increased apoptosis in optic tectum, secondary to decreased blood flow	Dong *et al.* (2001, 2002, 2004)
TCDD	Brain volume decrease, decreased neuronal number	Hill *et al.* (2003)
2,2′,4,4′-Tetrabromodiphenyl ether (PBDE 47)	Impaired cerebrospinal fluid flow	Lema *et al.* (2007)
Thalidomide	Reduced otic vesicle size	Ito *et al.* (2010)
Thioperamide (histamine H_3 receptor antagonist)	Decreased locomotor activity	Peitsaro *et al.* (2007)

reason (mechanism) is known, then a more targeted screening test could conceivably be developed. It is generally the case, however, and certainly in developmental neurotoxicology, that the mechanism of action of most toxic compounds is unknown. As a result, most screening tests evaluate endpoints of concern, and this will likely be the preferred course until sufficient knowledge is gained regarding the mechanisms of developmental neurotoxicity.

SCREENING APPROACHES USING LARVAL ZEBRAFISH: SOME BASIC PRINCIPLES

There have been numerous publications on the virtues of using zebrafish in at least three screening contexts: (1) environmental chemicals; (2) pharmaceuticals; and (3) mutations

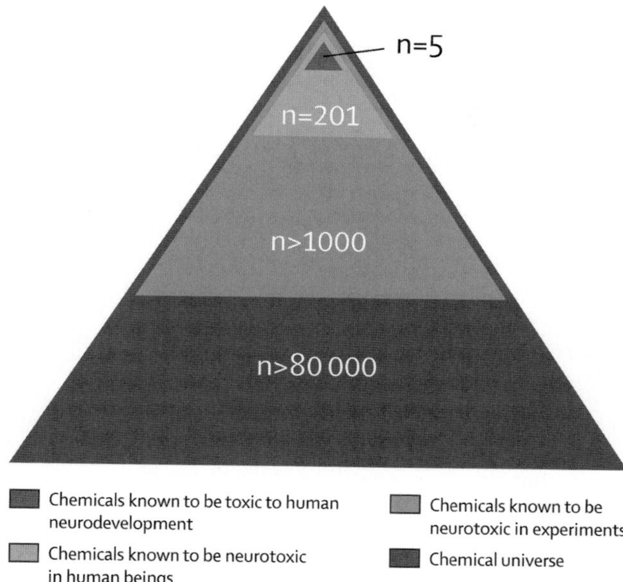

FIGURE 15.3 A large chemical universe has not been systematically tested for human neurodevelopmental toxicity. Reprinted from Grandjean and Landrigan (2006), with permission from Elsevier.

(Lieschke and Currie, 2007; Rubinstein, 2006; Parng *et al.*, 2002; Patton and Zon, 2001; Yang *et al.*, 2009; Brittijn *et al.*, 2009; Embry *et al.*, 2010; Love *et al.*, 2004; Kari *et al.*, 2007; Redfern *et al.*, 2008; Chow *et al.*, 2009; David and Pancharatna, 2008; Brannen *et al.*, 2010), and some specifically in the realm of screening for neurotoxicity (Best and Alderton, 2008; Guo, 2009; Linney *et al.*, 2004; Peterson *et al.*, 2008; Ton *et al.*, 2006; Bang *et al.*, 2002; Froehlicher *et al.*, 2009). Screening for both environmental chemicals and pharmaceuticals has been undertaken for better understanding their potential adverse effects; screening pharmaceuticals has also been undertaken to identify new candidates for medication. Screening for mutations has been primarily conducted to identify genes that may be involved in development and in disease. There is a growing body of literature on screening results, involving a number of chemical compounds and endpoints. An exhaustive review of this literature is beyond the scope of this chapter, making it necessary to highlight only a few studies that have focused on some aspect of developmental neurotoxicity in the context of chemical screening. These studies also highlight some of the considerations that are critical in developing and evaluating a screening assay.

Regardless of the endpoint, a common strategy in evaluating the utility of a screening assay is to test a number of compounds (a training set) that are considered known "positives" and those that are considered known "negatives", in other words, compounds that do and do not affect the endpoint of interest. This strategy has been employed by a few investigators in assessing the developmental neurotoxicity of chemicals (Ton *et al.*, 2006), including focused investigations of chemicals that may affect the development of the lateral line (Chiu *et al.*, 2008; Ton and Parng, 2005). Selecting the positives and negatives involves a number of considerations, but generally they are selected on the basis of a review of the scientific literature involving humans and/or laboratory mammalian test species. To date, the majority of studies include more positives than negatives.

Once selected, the compounds may or may not be tested in a blinded fashion. This may involve a single dose/concentration or a range of concentrations. Criteria are developed for determining whether a compound has an effect or not, and then the results are tallied in a two-by-two matrix that compares outcomes against expectations. The screen should be able to identify correctly both the positives and the negatives. Correct identification of positives is considered "hits" and the percentage of hits vs. "misses" (in other words the positives that were not identified) formally defines the sensitivity of the screening assay. Correspondingly, the correct identification of negatives are considered "correct rejections" and the percentage of these correct rejections versus "false alarms" (or the negatives that were not identified as such) formally defines the specificity of the assay. The accuracy of the assay is then defined as the joint probability of hits and correct rejections. Swets provides an authoritative review of the sensitivity, specificity and accuracy of test methods and their use in decision making (Swets, 1988; Swets *et al.*, 2000). It should be obvious that for a useful assay, hits should exceed misses and correct rejections should exceed false alarms. But by how much should hits or correct rejections exceed misses or false alarms? Answering this question involves an entirely new realm of considerations, but suffice it to note that the European Center for the Validation of Alternative Methods (ECVAM) and the Organization of Economic Development and Cooperation (OECD) consider the accuracy of an assay of >65% as "sufficient", >75% as "good" and >85% as "excellent" (Anonymous, 2005; Genschow *et al.*, 2002).

ZEBRAFISH DEVELOPMENTAL NEUROTOXICITY TESTING: SCREENING LARGE NUMBERS OF CHEMICALS

There are a few examples in the literature of screens for various aspects of developmental neurotoxicity (Chiu *et al.*, 2008; Kokel *et al.*, 2010; Ou *et al.*, 2009; Richards *et al.*, 2008; Scheil and Köhler, 2009; Ton *et al.*, 2006; Ton and Parng, 2005; Winter *et al.* 2008; Berghmans *et al.* 2008; Yang *et al.*, 2009, 2007; Rihel *et al.*, 2010). Some used a training set of chemicals, whereas others assessed large numbers of chemicals with unknown effects. We highlight a few examples below.

One of the first microarray analyses of developmental toxicant exposure in zebrafish included many neurotoxic chemicals (Yang *et al.*, 2007), but no negative chemicals. Although developmental exposure to these chemicals tended to produce similar morphological changes in the zebrafish larvae, the gene expression changes were specific to each chemical, and predictable dose-related changes were apparent at low doses relative to morphological changes.

Richards and coworkers (2008) developed a screen for visual defects in larval zebrafish. The assay used the optomotor response, or the movement of a larva in a lane in the same direction as a striped pattern. Exposure to 27 chemicals (19 positives and 8 negatives) occurred between 3 and 8 dpf with assessment on the last day of exposure. Assay sensitivity (proportion of positives that were detected as positives) was 68%, specificity (proportion of negatives detected as negatives) was 75% and accuracy (% total correct) was 70%. Discussion focused on possible reasons for less than 100% accuracy including poor penetrability of the chemicals into the larvae and confounding effects due to chemical-induced locomotor decreases. In a related investigation using a similar experimental design (Berghmans *et al.*, 2008), using 1 negative, and 7 positives, the optomotor response in larval zebrafish at 8 dpf correctly identified the one negative compound (aspirin), and 5 of the 7 positive compounds (i.e., sensitivity = 71%).

One area where many investigators have used zebrafish in neurotoxicity screening is ototoxicity (Chiu *et al.*, 2008; Coffin *et al.*, 2010; Ou *et al.*, 2009; Ton and Parng, 2005). In most of these studies, the embryos/larvae were exposed to the chemical in question only during a short period during neuromast development in the lateral line. The neuromasts are structurally similar to mammalian hair cells, and visualization of the neuromasts is relatively easy because of the availability of specific vital dyes and stains. Not only have these investigators found that there is concordance between chemicals that cause hair cell damage in humans and those that cause neuromast damage in zebrafish, but through screening of libraries of thousands of compounds, they have also been able to identify FDA pharmaceuticals which protect hair cells from chemically induced damage (Coffin *et al.*, 2010; Ou *et al.*, 2009). Moreover, a unique aspect of these studies is that a small number of the ototoxic and otoprotective chemicals identified in the zebrafish screens were then applied to explant cultures of mammalian (mature mouse) utricle hair cells. It was found that the chemicals had the expected effect: either toxic to the mammalian hair cells if they were toxic to the zebrafish neuromasts (Chiu *et al.*, 2008) or protective of neomycin-induced hair cell damage in the mammalian utricle if they had been protective of neomycin-induced neuromast damage in the zebrafish (Coffin *et al.*, 2010; Ou *et al.*, 2009). These results are significant as a proof-of-principle, but it should be clear that an *in vitro* preparation of mouse tissue is still far removed from a demonstration of concordant effects in humans.

Assessing the rest/wake locomotor states in 4-day larval zebrafish for 72 hours, Rihel and coworkers (2010) tested 3,968 compounds and found that 13.7% (547) altered the behavioral phenotype (degree of locomotor activity and diurnal variation in activity). Using hierarchical clustering, they found that the larval zebrafish behavior phenotype could accurately group the neuroactive compounds according to their mechanism of action. Therefore, a relatively simple behavioral assessment in zebrafish larvae was able to classify accurately human bioactive drugs. It is difficult, however, to know if these investigators were testing the effects of the drugs on development of the nervous system because exposure and testing took place after much of the zebrafish nervous system had developed. It is likely, therefore, that the drugs produced differences in behavioral patterns due to their acute effects.

In a related study, the effects measured were obviously acute because testing took place in a short period (30 seconds) and mainly neuroactive drugs were used (Kokel *et al.*, 2010). A total of 13,976 chemicals from various libraries were tested using the pattern of locomotor activity in response to a bright light in 30-hour-old embryos. They also found that hierarchical clustering of the patterns of effects in zebrafish tended to group chemicals with similar functions or mechanisms of action that occur in mammals. Novel molecules were identified that clustered with known molecules. For example, a novel molecule clustered with the MAO inhibitors, and when tested *in vitro*, was found to be a potent MAO inhibitor, thereby reinforcing the notion that a behavioral test in zebrafish may be able to screen chemicals for desired neuroactive properties. Kokel and coworkers concluded that "functionally related molecules cause similar phenotypes, and behavioral barcodes may be used to sort molecules with different cellular targets into common pathways".

Winter and coworkers (2008) developed a screen for seizure liability in larval zebrafish. This is another screening study that is not technically a developmental toxicity study because the larvae were only exposed and tested on day 6. Larvae were exposed acutely to a range of doses of 25 chemicals (17 positives, 8 negatives) and seizures were measured as rapid locomotion over a 1-hour period. Sensitivity of the assay was 77%, specificity was 63% and accuracy was 72%. Possible reasons for less than 100% accuracy offered were (1) bioavailability of the chemical (this includes both water solubility as well as penetration into the embryo); (2) the possibility that dopaminergically active drugs may confound the locomotor-based assay; and (3) species difference in sensitivities.

Screening for developmental neurotoxicity is gaining traction. Although it is becoming clear that zebrafish larvae respond to neuroactive drug classes in ways resembling mammalian responses, very few studies have screened large numbers of chemicals for specific effects on the development of the nervous system.

THE ZEBRAFISH/HUMAN CONNECTION

Despite some notable successes in screening drugs with acute effects, why would developmental neurotoxicity studies in zebrafish embryos/larvae be predictive of human toxicity? For one, there are already numerous examples of zebrafish being used to model human diseases (reviewed by Dodd *et al.*, 2000; Xu and Zon, 2010), the functional organization of the vertebrate nervous system (Fetcho, 2007; Fetcho and Liu, 1998) or left–right asymmetry phenotypes in mammals (Bisgrove *et al.*, 2003). Second, in a survey of the 1,318 human drug targets, Gunnarsson *et al.* (2008) found that zebrafish possessed orthologs for 86% of the targets. Third, in the last 5 years, substantial proof has arisen that zebrafish and mammalian neurodevelopment are quite similar. To cite only a few examples, the same gene (*Foxg1*) is required for both mouse and zebrafish olfactory development (Duggan *et al.*, 2008); zebrafish show changes in developmental sensitivity to hair-cell death caused by neomycin treatment – a pattern of sensitivity similar to that seen in mammals (Murakami *et al.*, 2003); the morpholino knockdown of the gene implicated in human familial Parkinson's disease (*pink1*) causes disorganized dopaminergic neuronal development and altered locomotor activity in zebrafish (Anichtchik *et al.*, 2008; Xi *et al.*, 2010); and a microarray analysis of the "addiction" pathways of adult zebrafish to either ethanol or nicotine shows considerable similarity with those in mammals (Kily *et al.*, 2008). Moreover, it is especially interesting to note that some aspects of the zebrafish and human genomes are similar (Postlethwait *et al.*, 2009), and interchangeable, as highly conserved non-coding elements in human genes will regulate gene expression in zebrafish when transfected during development (Navratilova *et al.*, 2009; Ragvin *et al.*, 2010).

The above examples show the similarities between the zebrafish and mammalian function and development, but recently, another pattern of discovery is emerging. Zebrafish are now being used to discover novel pathways or mechanisms of toxicity, and possible treatments for various human diseases. Because of the ease of manipulating the zebrafish genome, the zebrafish model has unlocked hitherto unknown roles of various genes in the etiology of human disease and toxicant action. The pattern of discovery is commonly as follows: (1) a gene is first identified as associated with the development of a human condition, usually through epidemiological studies; (2) the ortholog for that gene is identified in zebrafish; (3) using that ortholog, a knockdown is constructed in zebrafish embryos; and (4) the phenotype and rescue characteristics in zebrafish are noted. For example, it has been shown that a transcription factor (*IRX3*) that had been associated with diabetes and obesity in mammals is intimately involved in the development of the insulin producing cells in the zebrafish pancreas, thereby opening up new avenues of research and treatment for both obesity and type 2 diabetes (Ragvin *et al.*, 2010). Further, in a recent study on thalidomide toxicity, Ito and coworkers (2010) showed that knocking down various components of the hypothesized thalidomide toxicity pathway elicited a phenotype in zebrafish similar to that produced by thalidomide treatment, thereby providing strong evidence to support their proposed mechanism of toxicity. Using the same type of approach to study the molecular underpinnings of schizophrenia, Wood and coworkers (2009) studied the function of the schizophrenia candidate genes *DISC1* (disrupted-in-schizophrenia 1) and *NRG1* (neuregulin 1) in the nervous system development of zebrafish using knockdown technology. Interestingly, they found that both genes were involved in oligodendrocyte development, as well as the development of a subclass of cerebellar neurons, and produced similar phenotypes in the nervous system. This role had been previously implicated for *NRG1*, but was unknown for *DISC1*, enabling the authors to note pathway connections between these two key schizophrenia-associated genes. It appears that zebrafish are emerging as the new, improved version of the laboratory rat or mouse.

CONCLUDING REMARKS AND FUTURE DIRECTIONS

The use of zebrafish in developmental neurotoxicology, and more broadly in developmental biology, is based on a firm theoretical and empirical foundation. The theoretical justification lies, of course, with the tenets of evolution and the essential conservation of physiological processes and functions throughout the animal kingdom. We can only speculate about Darwin's pleasure over the use of zebrafish embryos and larvae in understanding human health and disease. The empirical foundation derives from two pillars. The first is the highly conserved nature of human drug targets in zebrafish. The second pillar comes from recent studies using zebrafish to screen chemicals with known effects in humans. Although the literature is still sparse, there are enough data to demonstrate the utility of zebrafish in identifying chemicals that have known effects in the human population and, to a lesser extent, in identifying chemicals that are known *not* to have effects in humans.

The demonstration that chemicals known to cause toxicity in humans can also cause toxicity in developing zebrafish indicates the potential utility of the model for screening and mechanistic studies. Showing, however, that what happens in humans can also occur in zebrafish does not mean the reverse is proven. In this regard, and despite good reason for optimism, there has yet to be an unequivocal demonstration of the utility of zebrafish tests for either predicting human disease or identifying therapeutic interventions.

The growth in popularity of zebrafish as an experimental subject has been nothing short of phenomenal. In addition to their use in biology, their popularity has quickly spread to genetics, medicine, pharmacology and toxicology. From our perspective, their application in studies on environmental chemicals and nervous system development has been particularly beneficial (Table 15.1). The field, however, is still in its early stages, but this review has indicated the wealth of information is expanding rapidly. We anticipate major advances in the use of zebrafish in developmental neurotoxicology, in both screening chemicals for adverse health effects and in unraveling the mechanisms of toxicant effects on the nervous system.

ACKNOWLEDGMENT

Our thanks to Deborah L. Hunter for helping organize the references.

This manuscript has been reviewed by the National Health and Environmental Effects Research Laboratory and approved for publication. Approval does not signify that the contents reflect the views of the Agency, nor does mention of trade names or commercial products constitute endorsement or recommendation for use.

REFERENCES

Airhart MJ, Lee DH, Wilson TD, Miller BE, Miller MN, Skalko RG (2007) Movement disorders and neurochemical changes in zebrafish larvae after bath exposure to fluoxetine (PROZAC). *Neurotoxicol Teratol* **29:** 652–64.

Amin-Zaki L, Majeed MA, Greenwood MR, Elhassani SB, Clarkson TW, Doherty RA (1981) Methylmercury poisoning in the Iraqi suckling infant: a longitudinal study over five years. *J Appl Toxicol* **1:** 210–14.

Anichtchik O, Diekmann H, Fleming A, Roach A, Goldsmith P, Rubinsztein DC (2008) Loss of PINK1 function affects development and results in neurodegeneration in zebrafish. *J Neurosci* **28:** 8199–207.

Anonymous (2005) Guidance document on the validation and international acceptance of new or updated test methods for hazard identification. In *Environmental Health and Safety Monograph Series on Test and Assessment*, pp. 1–96. Organisation for Economic Cooperation and Development, No. 34.

Arenzana FJ, Carvan MJ 3rd, Aijon J, Sanchez-Gonzalez R, Arevalo R, Porteros A (2006) Teratogenic effects of ethanol exposure on zebrafish visual system development. *Neurotoxicol Teratol* **28:** 342–8.

Arnot JA, Arnot M, Mackay D, Couillard Y, Macdonald D, Bonnell M, Doyle P (2010) Molecular size cut-off criteria for screening bioaccumulation potential: fact or fiction? *Integr Environ Assess Manag* **6**: 210–14.

Baier H (2000) Zebrafish on the move: towards a behavior-genetic analysis of vertebrate vision. *Curr Opin Neurobiol* **10:** 451–5.

Baier H, Klostermann S, Trowe T, Karlstrom RO, Nusslein-Volhard C, Bonhoeffer F (1996) Genetic dissection of the retinotectal projection. *Development* **123:** 415–25.

Baier H, Rotter S, Korsching S (1994) Connectional topography in the zebrafish olfactory system: random positions but regular spacing of sensory neurons projecting to an individual glomerulus. *Proc Natl Acad Sci USA* **91:** 11646–50.

Bang PI, Yelick PC, Malicki JJ, Sewell WF (2002) High-throughput behavioral screening method for detecting auditory response defects in zebrafish. *J Neurosci Methods* **118:** 177–87.

Berghmans S, Butler P, Goldsmith P, Waldron G, Gardner I, Golder Z, Richards FM, Kimber G, Roach A, Alderton W, Fleming A (2008) Zebrafish based assays for the assessment of cardiac, visual and gut function – potential safety screens for early drug discovery. *J Pharmacol Toxicol Methods* **58:** 59–68.

Best JD, Alderton WK (2008) Zebrafish: an *in vivo* model for the study of neurological diseases. *Neuropsychiatr Dis Treat* **4:** 567–76.

Bisgrove BW, Morelli SH, Yost HJ (2003) Genetics of human laterality disorders: insights from vertebrate model systems. *Annu Rev Genomics Hum Genet* **4:** 1–32.

Blader P, Strähle U (2000) Zebrafish developmental genetics and central nervous system development. *Hum Mol Genet* **9:** 945–51.

Brannen KC, Panzica-Kelly JM, Danberry TL, Augustine-Rauch KA (2010) Development of a zebrafish embryo teratogenicity assay and quantitative prediction model. *Birth Def Res Part B* **89:** 66–77.

Bretaud S, Lee S, Guo S (2004) Sensitivity of zebrafish to environmental toxins implicated in Parkinson's disease. *Neurotoxicol Teratol* **26:** 857–64.

Brittijn SA, Duivesteijn SJ, Belmamoune M, Bertens LF, Bitter W, de Bruijn JD, Champagne DL, Cuppen E, Flik G, Vandenbroucke-Grauls CM, Janssen RA, de Jong IM, de Kloet ER, Kros A, Meijer AH, Metz JR, van der Sar AM, Schaaf MJ, Schulte-Merker S, Spaink HP, Tak PP, Verbeek FJ, Vervoordeldonk MJ, Vonk FJ, Witte F, Yuan H, Richardson MK (2009) Zebrafish development and regeneration: new tools for biomedical research. *Int J Dev Biol* **53:** 835–50.

Buckley CE, Marguerie A, Alderton WK, Franklin RJ (2010) Temporal dynamics of myelination in the zebrafish spinal cord. *Glia* **58:** 802–12.

Calhoun F, Warren K (2007) Fetal alcohol syndrome: historical perspectives. *Neurosci Biobehav Rev* **31:** 168–71.

Carvan MJ 3rd, Loucks E, Weber DN, Williams FE (2004) Ethanol effects on the developing zebrafish: neurobehavior and skeletal morphogenesis. *Neurotoxicol Teratol* **26:** 757–68.

Cerutti D, Levin ED (2006) Cognitive impairment models using complementary species. In *Animal Models of Cognitive Impairment* (Levin ED, Buccafusco JJ, eds.), pp. 315–42. Taylor and Francis, New York.

Chen Q, Huang NN, Huang JT, Chen S, Fan J, Li C, Xie FK (2009) Sodium benzoate exposure downregulates the expression of tyrosine hydroxylase and dopamine transporter in dopaminergic neurons in developing zebrafish. *Birth Defects Res B Dev Reprod Toxicol* **86:** 85–91.

Chen YH, Huang YH, Wen CC, Wang YH, Chen WL, Chen LC, Tsay HJ (2008) Movement disorder and neuromuscular change in zebrafish embryos after exposure to caffeine. *Neurotoxicol Teratol* **30:** 440–7.

Chiu LL, Cunningham LL, Raible DW, Rubel EW, Ou HC (2008) Using the zebrafish lateral line to screen for ototoxicity. *J Assoc Res Otolaryngol* **9:** 178–90.

Chow ES, Hui MN, Cheng CW, Cheng SH (2009) Cadmium affects retinogenesis during zebrafish embryonic development. *Toxicol Appl Pharmacol* **235:** 68–76.

Coffin AB, Ou H, Owens KN, Santos F, Simon JA, Rubel EW, Raible DW (2010) Chemical screening for hair cell loss and protection in the zebrafish lateral line. *Zebrafish* **7:** 3–11.

Connell DW, Hawker DW (1988) Use of polynomial expressions to describe the bioconcentration of hydrophobic chemicals by fish. *Ecotoxicol Environ Saf* **16:** 242–57.

Costa LG, Giordano G, Tagliaferri S, Caglieri A, Mutti A (2008) Polybrominated diphenyl ether (PBDE) flame retardants: environmental contamination, human body burden and potential adverse health effects. *Acta Biomed* **79:** 172–83.

Costa LG, Steardo L, Cuomo V (2004) Structural effects and neurofunctional sequelae of developmental exposure to psychotherapeutic drugs: experimental and clinical aspects. *Pharmacol Rev* **56:** 103–47.

David A, Pancharatna K (2010) Effects of acetaminophen (paracetamol) in the embryonic development of zebrafish, *Danio rerio*. *J Appl Toxicol* **29:** 597–602.

DeMicco A, Cooper KR, Richardson JR, White LA (2010) Developmental neurotoxicity of pyrethroid insecticides in zebrafish embryos. *Toxicol Sci* **113:** 177–86.

Dlugos CA, Rabin RA (2007) Ocular deficits associated with alcohol exposure during zebrafish development. *J Comp Neurol* **502:** 497–506.

Dodd A, Curtis PM, Williams LC, Love DR (2000) Zebrafish: bridging the gap between development and disease. *Hum Mol Genet* **9:** 2443–9.

Dong W, Teraoka H, Kondo S, Hiraga T (2001) 2,3,7,8-tetrachlorodibenzo-p-dioxin induces apoptosis in the dorsal midbrain of zebrafish embryos by activation of aryl hydrocarbon receptor. *Neurosci Lett* **303:** 169–72.

Dong W, Teraoka H, Tsujimoto Y, Stegeman JJ, Hiraga T (2004) Role of aryl hydrocarbon receptor in mesencephalic circulation failure and apoptosis in zebrafish embryos exposed to 2,3,7,8-tetrachlorodibenzo-p-dioxin. *Toxicol Sci* **77:** 109–16.

Dong W, Teraoka H, Yamazaki K, Tsukiyama S, Imani S, Imagawa T, Stegeman JJ, Peterson RE, Hiraga T (2002) 2,3,7,8-tetrachlorodibenzo-p-dioxin toxicity in the zebrafish embryo: local circulation failure in the dorsal midbrain is associated with increased apoptosis. *Toxicol Sci* **69:** 191–201.

Duggan CD, DeMaria S, Baudhuin A, Stafford D, Ngai J (2008) Foxg1 is required for development of the vertebrate olfactory system. *J Neurosci* **28:** 5229–39.

Eddins D, Cerutti D, Williams P, Linney E, Levin ED (2010) Zebrafish provide a sensitive model of persisting neurobehavioral effects of developmental chlorpyrifos exposure: comparison with nicotine and pilocarpine effects and relationship to dopamine deficits. *Neurotoxicol Teratol* **32:** 99–108.

Embry MR, Belanger SE, Braunbeck TA, Galay-Burgos M, Halder M, Hinton DE, Leonard MA, Lillicrap A, Norberg-King T, Whale G (2010) The fish embryo toxicity test as an animal alternative method in hazard and risk assessment and scientific research. *Aquat Toxicol* **97:** 79–87.

Fadool JM, Dowling JE (2008) Zebrafish: a model system for the study of eye genetics. *Prog Retin Eye Res* **27:** 89–110.

Fetcho JR (2007) The utility of zebrafish for studies of the comparative biology of motor systems. *J Exper Zool (Mol Dev Evol)* **308B:** 550–62.

Fetcho JR, Higashijima S, McLean DL (2008) Zebrafish and motor control over the last decade. *Brain Res Rev* **57:** 86–93.

Fetcho JR, Liu KS (1998) Zebrafish as a model system for studying neuronal circuits and behavior. *Ann NY Acad Sci* **860:** 333–45.

Fetcho JR, O'Malley DM (1997) Imaging neuronal networks in behaving animals. *Curr Opin Neurobiol* **7:** 832–8.

Froehlicher M, Liedtke A, Groh KJ, Neuhauss SC, Segner H, Eggen RI (2009) Zebrafish (*Danio rerio*) neuromast: promising biological endpoint linking developmental and toxicological studies. *Aquat Toxicol* **95:** 307–19.

Genschow E, Spielmann H, Scholz G, Seiler A, Brown N, Piersma A, Brady N, Clemann N, Huuskonen H, Paillard F, Bremer S, Becker K (2002) The ECVAM international validation study on *in vitro* embryotoxicity tests: results of the definitive phase and evaluation of prediction models, Vol. 30, pp. 151–76. European Centre for the Validation of Alternative Methods. ALTLA-Alternatives to Laboratory Animals.

Gonzalez P, Dominique Y, Massabuau JC, Boudou A, Bourdineaud JP (2005) Comparative effects of dietary methylmercury on gene expression in liver, skeletal muscle, and brain of the zebrafish (*Danio rerio*). *Environ Sci Technol* **39:** 3972–80.

Grandjean P, Landrigan PJ (2006) Developmental neurotoxicity of industrial chemicals. *Lancet* **368:** 2167–78.

Gunnarsson L, Jauhiainen A, Kristiansson E, Nerman O, Larsson DG (2008) Evolutionary conservation of human drug targets in organisms used for environmental risk assessments. *Environ Sci Technol* **42:** 5807–13.

Guo S (2004) Linking genes to brain, behavior and neurological diseases: what can we learn from zebrafish? *Genes Brain Behav* **3:** 63–74.

Guo S (2009) Using zebrafish to assess the impact of drugs on neural development and function. *Expert Opin Drug Discov* **4:** 715–26.

Hamad A, Kluk M, Fox J, Park M, Turner JE (2007) The effects of aromatase inhibitors and selective estrogen receptor modulators on eye development in the zebrafish (*Danio rerio*). *Curr Eye Res* **32:** 819–27.

Hen Chow ES, Cheng SH (2003) Cadmium affects muscle type development and axon growth in zebrafish embryonic somitogenesis. *Toxicol Sci* **73:** 149–59.

Henry TR, Spitsbergen JM, Hornung MW, Abnet CC, Peterson RE (1997) Early life stage toxicity of 2,3,7,8–tetrachlorodibenzo-*p*-dioxin in zebrafish (*Danio rerio*). *Toxicol Appl Pharmacol* **142:** 56–68.

Hill A, Howard CV, Strahle U, Cossins A (2003) Neurodevelopmental defects in zebrafish (*Danio rerio*) at environmentally relevant dioxin (TCDD) concentrations. *Toxicol Sci* **76:** 392–9.

Hill AJ, Teraoka H, Heideman W, Peterson RE (2005) Zebrafish as a model vertebrate for investigating chemical toxicity. *Toxicol Sci* **86:** 6–19.

Hill J, Clarke JD, Vargesson N, Jowett T, Holder N (1995) Exogenous retinoic acid causes specific alterations in the development of the midbrain and hindbrain of the zebrafish embryo including positional respecification of the Mauthner neuron. *Mech Dev* **50:** 3–16.

Holder N, Hill J (1991) Retinoic acid modifies development of the midbrain-hindbrain border and affects cranial ganglion formation in zebrafish embryos. *Development* **113:** 1159–70.

Huang H, Huang C, Wang L, Ye X, Bai C, Simonich MT, Tanguay RL, Dong Q (2010) Toxicity, uptake kinetics and behavior assessment in zebrafish embryos following exposure to perfluorooctanesulphonicacid (PFOS). *Aquat Toxicol*, doi:10.1016/j.aquatox.2010.1002.1003.

Ito T, Ando H, Suzuki T, Ogura T, Hotta K, Imamura Y, Yamaguchi Y, Handa H (2010) Identification of a primary target of thalidomide teratogenicity. *Science* **327:** 1345–50.

Jensen K (1995) Neuroanatomical techniques for labeling neurons and their utility in neurotoxicology. In *Neurotoxicology: Approaches and Methods* (Slikker Jr W, Chang LW, eds.), pp. 27–66. Academic Press, New York.

Jin M, Zhang X, Wang L, Huang C, Zhang Y, Zhao M (2009) Developmental toxicity of bifenthrin in embryo-larval stages of zebrafish. *Aquat Toxicol* **95:** 347–54.

Johnson A, Carew E, Sloman KA (2007) The effects of copper on the morphological and functional development of zebrafish embryos. *Aquat Toxicol* **84:** 431–38.

Jones KL, Smith DW (1973) Recognition of the fetal alcohol syndrome in early infancy. *Lancet* **302:** 999–1001.

Judson R, Richard A, Dix DJ, Houck K, Martin M, Kavlock R, Dellarco V, Henry T, Holderman T, Sayre P, Tan S, Carpenter T, Smith E (2009) The toxicity data landscape for environmental chemicals. *Environ Health Perspect* **117:** 685–95.

Jung SH, Kim S, Chung AY, Kim HT, So JH, Ryu J, Park HC, Kim CH (2010) Visualization of myelination in GFP-transgenic zebrafish. *Dev Dyn* **239:** 592–7.

Kari G, Rodeck U, Dicker AP (2007) Zebrafish: an emerging model system for human disease and drug discovery. *Clin Pharmacol Ther* **82:** 70–80.

Kashyap B, Frederickson LC, Stenkamp DL (2007) Mechanisms for persistent microphthalmia following ethanol exposure during retinal neurogenesis in zebrafish embryos. *Vis Neurosci* **24:** 409–21.

Kily LJ, Cowe YC, Hussain O, Patel S, McElwaine S, Cotter FE, Brennan CH (2008) Gene expression changes in a zebrafish model of drug dependency suggest conservation of neuro-adaptation pathways. *J Exp Biol* **211:** 1623–34.

Kimmel CB (1993) Patterning the brain of the zebrafish embryo. *Annu Rev Neurosci* **16:** 707–32.

Kimmel CB, Hatta K, Eisen JS (1991) Genetic control of primary neuronal development in zebrafish. *Development* **Suppl. 2:** 47–57.

Kirby BB, Takada N, Latimer AJ, Shin J, Carney TJ, Kelsh RN, Appel B (2006) *In vivo* time-lapse imaging shows dynamic oligodendrocyte progenitor behavior during zebrafish development. *Nat Neurosci* **9:** 1506–11.

Kodavanti PR (2005) Neurotoxicity of persistent organic pollutants: Possible mode(s) of action and further considerations. *Dose Response* **3:** 273–305.

Kokel D, Bryan J, Laggner C, White R, Cheung CY, Mateus R, Healey D, Kim S, Werdich AA, Haggarty SJ, Macrae CA, Shoichet B, Peterson RT (2010) Rapid behavior-based identification of neuroactive small molecules in the zebrafish. *Nat Chem Biol* **6:** 231–7.

Kreiling JA, Creton R, Reinisch C (2007) Early embryonic exposure to polychlorinated biphenyls disrupts heat-shock protein 70 cognate expression in zebrafish. *J Toxicol Environ Health A* **70:** 1005–13.

Kurland LT, Faro SN, Siedler H (1960) Minamata disease. The outbreak of a neurologic disorder in Minamata, Japan, and its relationship to the ingestion of seafood contaminated by mercuric compounds. *World Neurol* **1:** 370–95.

Laale HW (1971) Ethanol induced notochord and spinal cord duplications in the embryo of the zebrafish, *Brachydanio rerio*. *J Exp Zool* **177:** 51–64.

Lammer E, Kamp HG, Hisgen B, Koch M, Reinhard D, Salinas ER, Wendler K, Zok S, Braunbeck T (2009) Development of a flow-through system for the fish embryo toxicity test (FET) with the zebrafish (*Danio rerio*). *Toxicol in Vitro* **23:** 1436–42.

Lefebvre KA, Trainer VL, Scholz NL (2004) Morphological abnormalities and sensorimotor deficits in fish exposed to dissolved saxitoxin. *Aquat Toxicol* **66:** 159–70.

Lema SC, Schultz IR, Scholz NL, Incardona JP, Swanson P (2007) Neural defects and cardiac arrhythmia in fish larvae following embryonic exposure to 2,2′,4,4′-tetrabromodiphenyl ether (PBDE 47). *Aquat Toxicol* **82:** 296–307.

Levin ED, Chrysanthis E, Yacisin K, Linney E (2003) Chlorpyrifos exposure of developing zebrafish: effects on survival and long-term effects on response latency and spatial discrimination. *Neurotoxicol Teratol* **25:** 51–7.

Levin ED, Swain HA, Donerly S, Linney E (2004) Developmental chlorpyrifos effects on hatchling zebrafish swimming behavior. *Neurotoxicol Teratol* **26:** 719–23.

Li D, Lu C, Wang J, Hu W, Cao Z, Sun D, Xia H, Ma X (2009) Developmental mechanisms of arsenite toxicity in zebrafish (*Danio rerio*) embryos. *Aquat Toxicol* **91:** 229–37.

Lieschke GJ, Currie PD (2007) Animal models of human disease: zebrafish swim into view. *Nat Rev Genet* **8:** 353–67.

Linney E, Upchurch L, Donerly S (2004) Zebrafish as a neurotoxicological model. *Neurotoxicol Teratol* **26:** 709–18.

Loucks E, Carvan MJ 3rd (2004) Strain-dependent effects of developmental ethanol exposure in zebrafish. *Neurotoxicol Teratol* **26:** 745–55.

Loucks EJ, Ahlgren SC (2009) Deciphering the role of Shh signaling in axial defects produced by ethanol exposure. *Birth Defects Res A Clin Mol Teratol* **85:** 556–67.

Love DR, Pichler FB, Dodd A, Copp BR, Greenwood DR (2004) Technology for high-throughput screens: the present and future using zebrafish. *Curr Opin Biotechnol* **15:** 564–71.

Macdonald R, Xu Q, Barth KA, Mikkola I, Holder N, Fjose A, Krauss S, Wilson SW (1994) Regulatory gene expression boundaries demarcate sites of neuronal differentiation in the embryonic zebrafish forebrain. *Neuron* **13:** 1039–53.

MacPhail RC, Tilson HA (1995) Behavioral screening tests: past, present and future. In *Neurotoxicology: Approaches and Methods* (Chang LW, Slikker W Jr, eds.), pp. 231–8. Academic Press, New York.

Manzo L, Artigas F, Martinez E, Mutti A, Bergamaschi E, Nicotera P, Tonini M, Candura SM, Ray DE, Costa LG (1996) Biochemical markers of neurotoxicity. A review of mechanistic studies and applications. *Hum Exp Toxicol* **15 (Suppl. 1):** S20–S35.

Markou A, Chiamulera C, Geyer MA, Tricklebank M, Steckler T (2009) Removing obstacles in neuroscience drug discovery: the future path for animal models. *Neuropsychopharmacology* **34:** 74–89.

Matsui JI, Egana AL, Sponholtz TR, Adolph AR, Dowling JE (2006) Effects of ethanol on photoreceptors and visual function in developing zebrafish. *Invest Ophthalmol Vis Sci* **47:** 4589–97.

McKinley ET, Baranowski TC, Blavo DO, Cato C, Doan TN, Rubinstein AL (2005) Neuroprotection of MPTP-induced toxicity in zebrafish dopaminergic neurons. *Brain Res Mol Brain Res* **141:** 128–37.

Monk KR, Talbot WS (2009) Genetic dissection of myelinated axons in zebrafish. *Curr Opin Neurobiol* **19:** 486–90.

Mueller T, Wullimann MF (2003) Anatomy of neurogenesis in the early zebrafish brain. *Brain Res Dev Brain Res* **140:** 137–55.

Murakami SL, Cunningham LL, Werner LA, Bauer E, Pujol R, Raible DW, Rubel EW (2003) Developmental differences in susceptibility to neomycin-induced hair cell death in the lateral line neuromasts of zebrafish (*Danio rerio*). *Hear Res* **186:** 47–56.

Narahashi T, Zhao X, Ikeda T, Nagata K, Yeh JZ (2007) Differential actions of insecticides on target sites: basis for selective toxicity. *Hum Exp Toxicol* **26:** 361–6.

Navratilova P, Fredman D, Hawkins TA, Turner K, Lenhard B, Becker TS (2009) Systematic human/zebrafish comparative identification of cis-regulatory activity around vertebrate developmental transcription factor genes. *Dev Biol* **327:** 526–40.

Needleman HL, Gunnoe C, Leviton A, Reed R, Peresie H, Maher C, Barrett P (1979) Deficits in psychologic and classroom performance of children with elevated dentine lead levels. *N Engl J Med* **300:** 689–95.

Nelson BP, Henriet RP, Holt AW, Bopp KC, Houser AP, Allgood OE Jr, Turner JE (2008) The role of estrogen in the developmental appearance of sensory-motor behaviors in the zebrafish (*Danio rerio*): the characterization of the "listless" model. *Brain Res* **1222:** 118–28.

NRC (1992) National Research Council. Environmental Neurotoxicology. National Academy Press, Washington DC.

O'Callaghan JP, Sriram K (2005) Glial fibrillary acidic protein and related glial proteins as biomarkers of neurotoxicity. *Expert Opin Drug Saf* **4:** 433–42.

Ornoy A (2009) Valproic acid in pregnancy: how much are we endangering the embryo and fetus? *Reprod Toxicol* **28:** 1–10.

Ou HC, Cunningham LL, Francis SP, Brandon CS, Simon JA, Raible DW, Rubel EW (2009) Identification of FDA-approved drugs and bioactives that protect hair cells in the zebrafish (*Danio rerio*) lateral line and mouse (*Mus musculus*) utricle. *Assoc Res Otolaryngol* **10:** 191–203.

Panula P, Sallinen V, Sundvik M, Kolehmainen J, Torkko V, Tiittula A, Moshnyakov M, Podlasz P (2006) Modulatory neurotransmitter systems and behavior: towards zebrafish models of neurodegenerative diseases. *Zebrafish* **3:** 235–47.

Parng C, Roy NM, Ton C, Lin Y, McGrath P (2007) Neurotoxicity assessment using zebrafish. *J Pharmacol Toxicol Methods* **55:** 103–12.

Parng C, Seng WL, Semino C, McGrath P (2002) Zebrafish: a preclinical model for drug screening. *Assay Drug Dev Technol* **1:** 41–8.

Patton EE, Zon LI (2001) The art and design of genetic screens: zebrafish. *Nat Rev Genet* **2:** 956–66.

Peitsaro N, Sundvik M, Anichtchik OV, Kaslin J, Panula P (2007) Identification of zebrafish histamine H1, H2 and H3 receptors and effects of histaminergic ligands on behavior. *Biochem Pharmacol* **73:** 1205–14.

Penberthy WT, Shafizadeh E, Lin S (2002) The zebrafish as a model for human disease. *Front Biosci* **7:** d1439–d1453.

Peng J, Wagle M, Mueller T, Mathur P, Lockwood BL, Bretaud S, Guo S (2009) Ethanol-modulated camouflage response screen in zebrafish uncovers a novel role for cAMP and extracellular signal-regulated kinase signaling in behavioral sensitivity to ethanol. *J of Neuroscience* **29:** 8408–18.

Peterson RT, Nass R, Boyd WA, Freedman JH, Dong K, Narahashi T (2008) Use of non-mammalian alternative models for neurotoxicological study. *Neurotoxicology* **29:** 546–55.

Pichler FB, Laurenson S, Williams LC, Dodd A, Copp BR, Love DR (2003) Chemical discovery and global gene expression analysis in zebrafish. *Nat Biotechnol* **21:** 879–83.

Pogoda HM, Sternheim N, Lyons DA, Diamond B, Hawkins TA, Woods IG, Bhatt DH, Franzini-Armstrong C, Dominguez C, Arana N, Jacobs J, Nix R, Fetcho JR, Talbot WS (2006) A genetic screen identifies genes essential for development of myelinated axons in zebrafish. *Dev Biol* **298:** 118–31.

Postlethwait JH, Woods IG, Ngo-Hazelett P, Yan Y-L, Kelly PD, Chu F, Huang H, Hill-Force A, Talbot WS (2009) Zebrafish comparative genomics and the origins of vertebrate chromosomes. *Genome Research* **10:** 1890–902.

Powers CM, Yen J, Linney EA, Seidler FJ, Slotkin TA (2010) Silver exposure in developing zebrafish (*Danio rerio*): Persistent effects on larval behavior and survival. *Neurotoxicol Teratol* **32:** 391–7.

Purdie EL, Metcalf JS, Kashmiri S, Codd GA (2009a) Toxicity of the cyanobacterial neurotoxin β-*N*-methylamino-L-alanine to three aquatic animal species. *Amyotrophic Lateral Sclerosis* **2:** 67–70.

Purdie EL, Samsudin S, Eddy FB, Codd GA (2009b) Effects of the cyanobacterial neurotoxin β-*N*-methylamino-L-alanine on the early-life stage development of zebrafish (*Danio rerio*). *Aquat Toxicol* **95:** 279–84.

Ragvin A, Moro E, Fredman D, Navratilova P, Drivenes O, Engstrom PG, Alonso ME, Mustienes Ede L, Skarmeta JL, Tavares MJ, Casares F, Manzanares M, van Heyningen V, Molven A, Njolstad PR, Argenton F, Lenhard B, Becker TS (2010) Long-range gene regulation links genomic type 2 diabetes and obesity risk regions to HHEX, SOX4, and IRX3. *Proc Natl Acad Sci USA* **107:** 775–80.

Redfern WS, Waldron G, Winter MJ, Butler P, Holbrook M, Wallis R, Valentin JP (2008) Zebrafish assays as early safety pharmacology screens: paradigm shift or red herring? *J Pharmacol Toxicol Methods* **58:** 110–17.

Richards FM, Alderton WK, Kimber GM, Liu Z, Strang I, Redfern WS, Valentin JP, Winter MJ, Hutchinson TH (2008) Validation of the use of zebrafish larvae in visual safety assessment. *J Pharmacol Toxicol Methods* **58:** 50–8.

Rihel J, Prober DA, Arvanites A, Lam K, Zimmerman S, Jang S, Haggarty SJ, Kokel D, Rubin LL, Peterson RT, Schier AF (2010) Zebrafish behavioral profiling links drugs to biological targets and rest/wake regulation. *Science* **327:** 348–51.

Rubinstein AL (2006) Zebrafish assays for drug toxicity screening. *Expert Opin Drug Metab Toxicol* **2:** 231–40.

Saint-Amant L, Drapeau P (1998) Time course of the development of motor behaviors in the zebrafish embryo. *J Neurobiol* **37:** 622–32.

Sallinen V, Sundvik M, Reenila I, Peitsaro N, Khrustalyov D, Anichtchik O, Toleikyte G, Kaslin J, Panula P (2009a) Hyperserotonergic phenotype after monoamine oxidase inhibition in larval zebrafish. *J Neurochem* **109:** 403–15.

Sallinen V, Torkko V, Sundvik M, Reenila I, Khrustalyov D, Kaslin J, Panula P (2009b) MPTP and MPP+ target specific aminergic cell populations in larval zebrafish. *J Neurochem* **108:** 719–31.

Samson JC, Goodridge R, Olobatuyi F, Weis JS (2001) Delayed effects of embryonic exposure of zebrafish (*Danio rerio*) to methylmercury (MeHg). *Aquat Toxicol* **51:** 369–76.

Scheil V, Köhler H-R (2009) Influence of nickel chloride, chlorpyrifos, and imidacloprid in combination with different temperatures on the embyogenesis of the zebrafish *Danio rerio*. *Arch Environ Contam Toxicol* **56:** 238–43.

Schreiber R, Altenburger R, Paschke A, Schuurmann G, Küster E (2009) A novel *in vitro* system for the determination of bioconcentration factors and the internal dose in zebrafish (*Danio rerio*) eggs. *Chemosphere* **77:** 928–33.

Schreiber T, Gassmann K, Gotz C, Hubenthal U, Moors M, Krause G, Merk HF, Nguyen NH, Scanlan TS, Abel J, Rose CR, Fritsche E (2010) Polybrominated diphenyl ethers induce developmental neurotoxicity in a human in vitro model: evidence for endocrine disruption. *Environ Health Perspect* **118:** 572–8.

Selderslaghs IW, Hooyberghs J, De Coen W, Witters HE (2010) Locomotor activity in zebrafish embryos: a new method to assess developmental neurotoxicity. *Neurotoxicol Teratol*, doi: 10.1016/j.ntt.2010.03.002.

Shin JT and Fishman MC (2002) From zebrafish to human: modular medical models. *Annu Rev Genomics Hum Genet* **3:** 311–40.

Slotkin TA (1998) Fetal nicotine or cocaine exposure: which one is worse? *J Pharmacol Exp Ther* **285:** 931–45.

Smith LE, Carvan MJ 3rd, Dellinger JA, Ghorai JK, White DB, Williams FE, Weber DN (2010) Developmental selenomethionine and methylmercury exposures affect zebrafish learning. *Neurotoxicol Teratol* **32:** 246–55.

Stanley KA, Curtis LR, Simonich SL, Tanguay RL (2009) Endosulfan I and endosulfan sulfate disrupts zebrafish embryonic development. *Aquat Toxicol* **95:** 355–61.

Stehr CM, Linbo TL, Incardona JP, Scholz NL (2006) The developmental neurotoxicity of fipronil: notochord degeneration and locomotor defects in zebrafish embryos and larvae. *Toxicol Sci* **92:** 270–8.

Strähle U, Blader P (1994) Early neurogenesis in the zebrafish embryo. *FASEB J* **8:** 692–8.

Struermer CAO (1988) Retinotopic organization of the developing retinotectal projection in the zebrafish embryo. *Journal of Neuroscience* **8:** 4513–30.

Svoboda KR, Vijayaraghavan S, Tanguay RL (2002) Nicotinic receptors mediate changes in spinal motoneuron development and axonal pathfinding in embryonic zebrafish exposed to nicotine. *J Neurosci* **22:** 10731–41.

Swets JA (1988) Measuring the accuracy of diagnostic systems. *Science* **240:** 1285–93.

Swets JA, Dawes RM, Monahan J (2000) Better decisions through science. *Sci Am* **283:** 82–7.

Sylvain NJ, Brewster DL, Ali DW (2010) Zebrafish embryos exposed to alcohol undergo abnormal development of motor neurons and muscle fibers. *Neurotoxicol Teratol* **32:** 472–80.

Teraoka H, Dong W, Hiraga T (2003) Zebrafish as a novel experimental model for developmental toxicology. *Congenit Anom (Kyoto)* **43:** 123–32.

Thirumalai V, Cline HT (2008) Endogenous dopamine suppresses initiation of swimming in prefeeding zebrafish larvae. *J Neurophysiol* **100:** 1635–48.

Thomas LT, Welsh L, Galvez F, Svoboda KR (2009) Acute nicotine exposure and modulation of a spinal motor circuit in embryonic zebrafish. *Toxicol Appl Pharmacol* **239:** 1–12.

Tiedeken JA, Ramsdell JS (2007) Embryonic exposure to domoic acid increases the susceptibility of zebrafish larvae to the chemical convulsant pentylenetetrazole. *Environ Health Perspect* **115:** 1547–52.

Tilton F, La Du JK, Tanguay RL (2008) Sulfhydryl systems are a critical factor in the zebrafish developmental toxicity of the dithiocarbamate sodium metam (NaM). *Aquat Toxicol* **90:** 121–7.

Tilton F, Tanguay RL (2008) Exposure to sodium metam during zebrafish somitogenesis results in early transcriptional indicators of the ensuing neuronal and muscular dysfunction. *Toxicol Sci* **106:** 103–12.

Ton C, Lin Y, Willett C (2006) Zebrafish as a model for developmental neurotoxicity testing. *Birth Defects Research (Part A)* **76:** 553–67.

Ton C, Parng C (2005) The use of zebrafish for assessing ototoxic and otoprotective agents. *Hear Res* **208:** 79–88.

Tropepe V, Sive HL (2003) Can zebrafish be used as a model to study the neurodevelopmental causes of autism? *Genes Brain Behav* **2:** 268–81.

Tsay HJ, Wang YH, Chen WL, Huang MY, Chen YH (2007) Treatment with sodium benzoate leads to malformation of zebrafish larvae. *Neurotoxicol Teratol* **29:** 562–9.

van de Water S, van de Wetering M, Joore J, Esseling J, Bink R, Clevers H, Zivkovic D (2001) Ectopic Wnt signal determines the eyeless phenotype of zebrafish masterblind mutant. *Development* **128:** 3877–88.

Weber DN (2006) Dose-dependent effects of developmental mercury exposure on C-start escape responses of larval zebrafish *Danio rerio*. *J Fish Biology* **69:** 75–94.

Weber DN, Connaughton VP, Dellinger JA, Klemer D, Udvadia A, Carvan MJ 3rd (2008) Selenomethionine reduces visual deficits due to developmental methylmercury exposures. *Physiol Behav* **93:** 250–60.

Weiss B, Cory-Slechta DA (2001) Assessment of behavioral toxicity. In *Principles and Methods of Toxicology* (Hayes WW, ed.), pp. 1451–528. Taylor and Francis, Philadelphia.

Welsh L, Tanguay RL, Svoboda KR (2009) Uncoupling nicotine mediated motoneuron axonal pathfinding errors and muscle degeneration in zebrafish. *Toxicol Appl Pharmacol* **237:** 29–40.

Westerfield M (2000) *The Zebrafish Book: A Guide for the Laboratory Use of Zebrafish (Danio rerio)*. University of Oregon Press, Eugene.

Winter MJ, Redfern WS, Hayfield AJ, Owen SF, Valentin JP, Hutchinson TH (2008) Validation of a larval zebrafish locomotor assay for assessing the seizure liability of early-stage development drugs. *J Pharmacol Toxicol Methods* **57:** 176–87.

Wood JD, Bonath F, Kumar S, Ross CA, Cunliffe VT (2009) Disrupted-in-schizophrenia 1 and neuregulin 1 are required for the specification of oligodendrocytes and neurones in the zebrafish brain. *Hum Mol Genet* **18:** 391–404.

Wullimann MF, Puelles L, Wicht H (1999) Early postembryonic neural development in the zebrafish: a 3-D reconstruction of forebrain proliferation zones shows their relation to prosomeres. *Eur J Morphol* **37:** 117–21.

Xi Y, Ryan J, Noble S, Yu M, Yilbas AE, Ekker M (2010) Impaired dopaminergic neuron development and locomotor function in zebrafish with loss of pink1 function. *Eur J Neurosci* **31:** 623–33.

Xu C, Zon LI (2010) The zebrafish as a model for human disease. In *Fish Physiology* (Perry SF, Ekker M, Farrell AP, Brauner CJ, eds.), Vol. 29, pp. 345–65. Academic Press.

Yang L, Ho NY, Alshut R, Legradi J, Weiss C, Reischl M, Mikut R, Liebel U, Muller F, Strähle U (2009) Zebrafish embryos as models for embryotoxic and teratological effects of chemicals. *Reproductive Toxicology* **28:** 245–53.

Yang L, Kemadjou JR, Zinsmeister C, Bauer M, Legradi J, Muller F, Pankratz M, Jakel J, Strähle U (2007) Transcriptional profiling reveals barcode-like toxicogenomic responses in the zebrafish embryo. *Genome Biol* **8:** R227.

Zhang CX, Panzica-Kelly J, Augustine-Rauch K (2009) Way forward essay on current and future state of developmental toxicology assays. In *Toxicity Endpoints & Tests*, AltTox.org.

Zhou S, Dong Q, Li S, Guo J, Wang X, Zhu G (2009) Developmental toxicity of cartap on zebrafish embryos. *Aquat Toxicol* **95:** 339–46.

C H A P T E R

16

Caenorhabditis elegans as a model to assess reproductive and developmental toxicity

Daiana S. Avila, Margaret R. Adams, Sudipta Chakraborty and Michael Aschner

INTRODUCTION

The challenge of assessing the environmental and public health impacts of human activities requires a comprehensive approach that integrates both chemical analysis and biomonitoring. Monitoring and understanding the impacts of various toxic agents have required increasingly sensitive sublethal assays using multiple organisms belonging to different levels of biological organization, structure and functionality. In this context, the usefulness of the nematode, *Caenorhabditis elegans* (*C. elegans*), has been extensively demonstrated in several fields of scientific research, including toxicology. Due to evolutionary conservation, the mechanisms underlying toxicity in nematodes are likely to have parallels in other organisms, including humans.

The developmental and reproductive processes in the nematode, *C. elegans*, are widely known to be invariant at standard conditions. For this reason, alterations in these parameters can be safely used as biomarkers. Several researchers have shown, over the past three decades, that toxic agents may cause decreased lifespan, cellular alterations, neurodegeneration, genotoxic effects, reproductive delay and even decreased progeny in *C. elegans*, events very similar to those observed in mammals. These parallel results occur due to the approximately 80% homology of the genome between this species of nematode and mammals. For this reason, *C. elegans* has been validated and used as a model to predict the effects of toxicants in superior vertebrates. This chapter describes the detailed methodologies that have been employed to evaluate toxicological endpoints, and the accomplishments of investigative researchers in toxicology regarding the use of the nematode to assess reproductive and developmental toxicity.

BACKGROUND ON C. *ELEGANS*

The free-living soil nematode *C. elegans* has been a workhorse for biological exploration since its initial use in the 1970s as a model to study the genetic control of development (Brenner, 2009). Since then, its use has prospered due to a multitude of advantages that *C. elegans* provides. Some of these advantages include its size (adults are approximately 1 mm in length), rapid lifecycle (approximately 3 days at 20°C to reach adulthood, see Figure 16.1), short lifespan (~18 days), ability to self-fertilize, large brood size (>300 offspring per hermaphrodite) and the ease with which it can be genetically manipulated (Leung *et al.*, 2008). Because the only requirements for growth and reproduction are ambient temperature, humid environment, atmospheric oxygen and bacteria as food, *C. elegans* is particularly inexpensive and easy to maintain in a laboratory.

There are two sexes, male and hermaphrodite. The hermaphrodite can reproduce by self-fertilization, generating only hermaphrodites with the same genetic code as the progenitor, whereas cross-fertilization produces males and hermaphrodites in equal proportions. This sexual organization is particularly valuable for genetic analysis. Further, the worm's transparency facilitates the visualization and monitoring of cellular processes and has permitted the recording and determination of the complete pattern of cell divisions that generate the 959 somatic cells in the adult hermaphrodite and the 1,031 in the adult male (Sulston *et al.*, 1983). Despite this simplicity, there is a high degree of differentiation once the worms have developed muscle cells, a hypodermis, intestine, gonads, glands, excretory system and a nervous system, which contains 302 neurons and their connecting synapses (White *et al.*, 1976; Sulston, 1983).

Furthermore, the *C. elegans* genome has been intensively studied. The complete cell lineage map, knockout (KO) mutant libraries and established genetic methodologies such as mutagenesis, transgenesis and RNA interference (RNAi) provide a variety of options to manipulate and study molecular processes in the worm. In addition, the generation of transgenic worms expressing the green florescent protein (GFP) in tagged proteins has proven to be a very useful means to observe, *in vivo*, both cells and pathways (Chalfie *et al.*, 1994).

Reproductive and Developmental Toxicology, Edited by Ramesh C. Gupta
ISBN: 978-0-12-382032-7

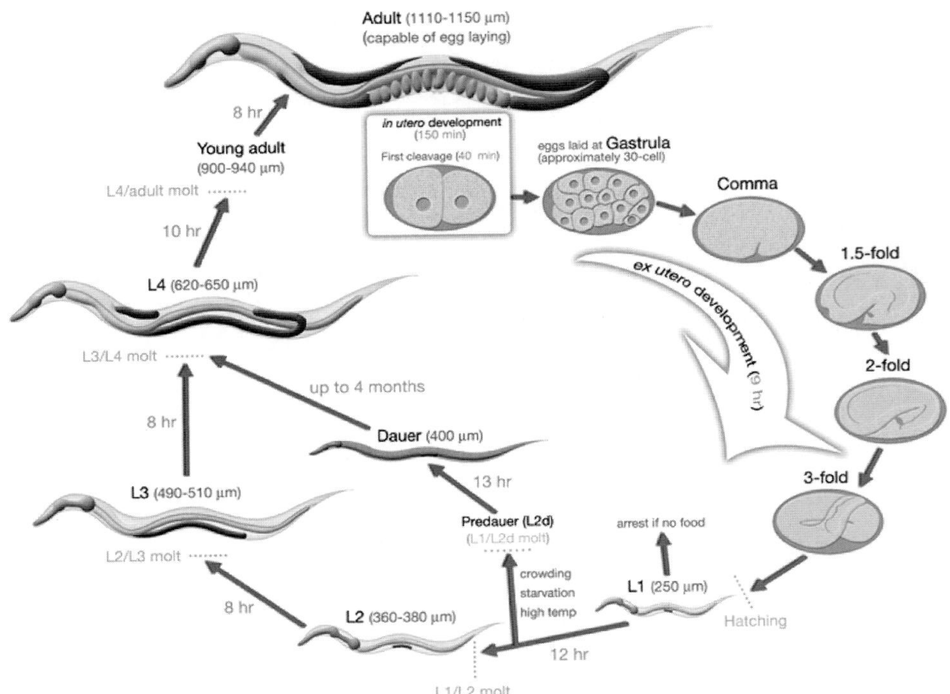

FIGURE 16.1 The development in *C. elegans* (From Altun and Hall, 2008).

The development

The *C. elegans* development is represented in Figure 16.1. Mature oocytes pass through the spermatheca and become fertilized, either by the hermaphodite's own or male sperm. The zygote develops a tough, chitinous shell and a viteline membrane, which render the egg particularly impermeable to most solutes and able to survive outside the uterus. Normally, eggs are held in the uterus for the first few cleavages and then deposited through the vulva at about the time of gastrulation, which is approximately 3 hours after fertilization. During embryogenesis, cell proliferation, organogenesis and morphogenesis occur, ultimately culminating in the first-stage larva. Growth during postembryonic development is continuous; meanwhile the germ line proliferates to fill the gonad (Schedl, 1997), and the number of somatic cell nuclei increases from 558 to 959 in adult hermaphrodites.

During the next 50 hours, larval development proceeds through three additional larval stages, L2, L3 and L4. About 10% of the cells in the L1 stage are somatic blast cells that undergo further cell division during larval development, contributing to the hypodermis, nervous system, musculature and somatic gonadal structures. Several proteins are differentially expressed among the larval stages and also between the larval and adult stages. For example, the amount of the Cu^{2+}/Zn^{2+} superoxide dismutase (SOD) and an aspartyl proteinase are highest in the first larval stage (L1) and decrease during the ontogenesis from the first larval stage to the adult (Madi *et al.*, 2003).

Gonadogenesis, a process which confers reproductive capability, is completed during the L4 stage, and at this point, the worm is considered to be a young adult. The entire lifecycle, from an egg to an adult producing more eggs, takes just 3.5 days at 20°C. With adequate food throughout the cycle, under standardized conditions, the average lifespan of a wild-type animal is approximately 18 days after worms reach adulthood. In the absence of food and at high population density, an alternative stage, the dauer, is formed at the L2/L3 molt. It is a specialized L3 stage that does not feed, is resistant to desiccation and can survive for up to 3 months without further development (Hope, 1999).

The reproduction

The hermaphrodite reproductive system (Figure 16.2A) consists of a symmetrically arranged bilobed gonad, with one lobe extending anteriorly and the other posteriorly from the center of the animal. Each lobe is U-shaped, comprising a distal (to the uterus) ovary and a proximal oviduct and spermatheca. The ovaries are syncytial, with germ-line nuclei, partially segregated by membranes, surrounding a central cytoplasmic core. Moving proximally from the distal tip, the nuclei are first mitotic, and then progress to meiotic prophase, reaching diakinesis in the oviduct prior to fertilization. At the end of each lobe, individual nuclei become almost completely enclosed by membranes to form oocytes, which enlarge and then mature as they pass down the oviduct. However, the oocytes maintain contact with the syncytium until close to the time of fertilization. The oviduct in each lobe terminates at the spermatheca carrying, in a young adult, about 150 ameboid sperm. The spermathecae connect to a common uterus, which contains fertilized eggs in the early stages of embryogenesis. The uterus opens to the exterior through a vulva, which protrudes visibly from the ventral surface of the adult (Kimble and Ward, 1988).

The male gonad is a single lobed (Figure 16.2B), U-shaped structure, extending anteriorly from its distal end and then looping posteriorly and connecting with the cloaca near the tail. At its distal end, the germ-line nuclei are mitotic. Meiotic

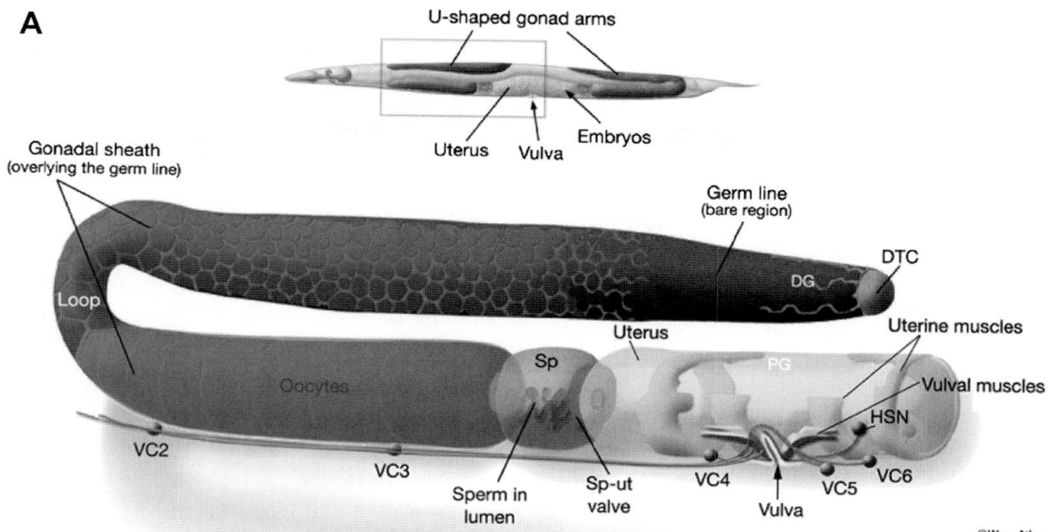

FIGURE 16.2A The hermaphrodite reproductive system in *C. elegans* (From Altun and Hall, 2008).

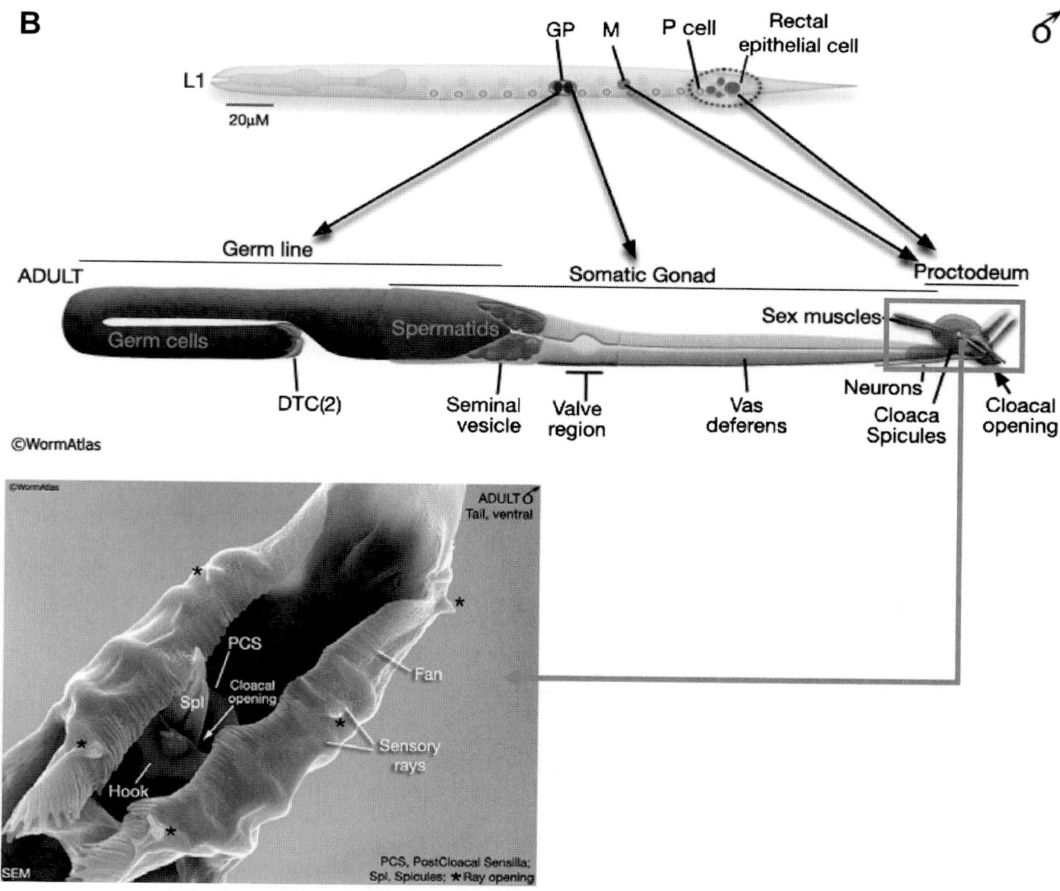

FIGURE 16.2B The male reproductive system in *C. elegans* (From Lints and Hall, 2005).

cells in progressively later stages of spermatogenesis are distributed sequentially along the gonad from the distal end to the seminal vesicle. Two meiotic divisions occur to produce the mature spermatids, which are stored in the seminal vesicle and released during copulation through a vas deferens to the cloaca (Kimble and Ward, 1988).

The male tail has specialized neurons, muscles and hypodermal structures for mating that give it a distinctly different appearance from that of the hermaphrodite. The male tail is fan shaped with 18 sensory rays. At the base of the tail are two spicules, which are inserted into the hermaphrodite vulva during copulation to aid in the transfer of sperm (Hope, 1999).

C. *ELEGANS* AND TOXICITY

During the late 1990s, *C. elegans* began to emerge as the nematode species of choice for toxicity studies based on the tremendous body of knowledge developed by basic scientists using this model organism for biological studies. Over time, a variety of toxicants have been tested and endpoints have been assessed, including the use of transgenic strains of *C. elegans* with specific biomarkers (Candido and Jones, 1996; Chu *et al.*, 2005; Roh *et al.*, 2006), growth and reproduction (Anderson *et al.*, 2001; Hoss and Weltje, 2007), feeding (Boyd *et al.*, 2003), and movement (Anderson *et al.*, 2004), just to name a few.

The toxicological studies regarding development and reproduction in *C. elegans* have been more focused on environmental toxicants such as metals and pesticides in the later part of this chapter. To date, only limited research exploring the effects of pharmacological drugs and other toxicants has been carried out in *C. elegans*. Of particular importance, several authors have demonstrated that growth and reproduction in *C. elegans* are much more sensitive parameters of adverse response than lethality for some toxicants, such as in the exposure to polycyclic aromatic hydrocarbons (PAHs) (Sese *et al.*, 2009).

C. *elegans* and developmental toxicity

As described earlier, the developmental stages in *C. elegans* are very short, and its molecular and morphological pathways are well reported. Hence, in this model, it is very easy to assess alterations in development caused by toxicants. Several assays and techniques have been developed and improved, such as the high throughput screenings described in the later part of this chapter.

Developmental parameters are based on alterations in worm size and in the various transformations that take place as eggs progress through all four larval stages to become mature adults over a certain period of time. Classical endpoints are assessed to determine toxicity throughout development, including body size, lifespan and developmental progress, all of which are often reduced or delayed by toxicants (Kumar *et al.*, 2010; Au *et al.*, 2009; Helmcke *et al.*, 2009; Lagido *et al.*, 2009) (Table 16.1). Associating these parameters with both genetic and molecular analyses is a proven and valuable approach for discovering and elucidating mechanisms that underlie developmental toxicity. For example, using whole genome microarray, Cui *et al.* (2007) demonstrated that several genes, particularly the metallothioneins, were differentially regulated after exposure to cadmium, alterations that may shed new light on why this metal causes developmental delay in *C. elegans* (Cui *et al.*, 2007).

The *C. elegans* vulva is an elegant model for dissecting a gene regulatory network (GRN) that directs postembryonic organogenesis. The mature vulva consists of seven cell types (vulA, vulB1, vulB2, vulC, vulD, vulE and vulF), each with its own unique pattern of spatial and temporal gene expression (Sternberg, 2005). When a toxicant causes vulval defects, one phenotype that has been observed is a hermaphrodite incapable of laying eggs or one that displays morphological defects such as a protruding vulva and eversion of the vulva (Sternberg, 2005). The mechanisms that underlie toxicant-induced vulval alterations are hypothesized to be related to apoptosis of the germ lines or modifications in the genes that regulate vulva formation during development (Kumar *et al.*, 2010; Ririe *et al.*, 2008).

The nervous system as a parameter of developmental toxicity

The adult *C. elegans* has 302 neurons in two independent nervous systems: 282 in the somatic nervous system and 20 in the pharyngeal nervous system (Boyd *et al.*, 2010a,b). There are approximately 6,500 chemical synapses, 900 gap junctions and 1,500 neuromuscular junctions. These nervous systems control locomotion, feeding, defecation, reproduction and environmental sensing (temperature, chemicals, odorants and food) (Hope, 1999). Hence, alterations in any of these functions may be indicators of neurotoxicity.

In order to evaluate neurotoxicity in *C. elegans*, researchers have employed several approaches, including the assessment of behavioral tasks and neuronal imaging, using the GFP reporter in specific neurons. Foraging for food, for example, is essential for growth and development, and it is

TABLE 16.1 Endpoints used to determine developmental toxicity in *C. elegans*

Endpoint	Principle	Reference
Lifespan	Synchronized worms are transferred to FUdR-NGM seeded plates, and the viability of adult worms is scored every day.	Harada *et al.* (2007)
Vulva development	The development of the vulva is observed under the microscope, based on gross morphology; it is used to evaluate organogenesis in *C. elegans*.	Kumar *et al.* (2010)
Body size or growth rate	Synchronized worms are mounted in agarose slides containing anesthetic and photographed. Software such as Open Lab ver.2.2.5 can determine body length.	Fujiwara *et al.* (2002)
Developmental progress/ larval arrest	By considering body length of the worms and the characteristics of each stage, the development stage ratio of a toxicant-exposed population can be determined.	Helmcke *et al.* (2009)
Body bends	It is used to measure locomotor activity. Animals are placed individually in a plate, and the body bend movement is scored after exposure to toxicants.	Tsalik and Hobert (2003)
Chemotaxis assay	It is used to evaluate the memory of the worms after exposure to a toxicant; worms are conditioned to some chemoattractant for a period of time; after removal and washes, the worm migration to the attractant is measured while a different chemical is also present in the plate.	Lin *et al.* (2006)

primarily controlled by serotoninergic and dopaminergic signaling pathways (Sze *et al.*, 2000; Hills *et al.*, 2004). Therefore, the reduced feeding behavior indicated by reduced pharyngeal pumping in chlorpyrifos-exposed worms (Boyd *et al.*, 2009) elucidates the observed reduced size and developmental delay, supporting the relationship between the nervous system and development in *C. elegans* (Ruan *et al.*, 2009). Similarly, locomotion, which is mostly regulated by the cholinergic system, is decreased by several toxicants (Boyd *et al.*, 2010a,b; Wang and Wang, 2008b; Wang *et al.*, 2009a; Xing *et al.*, 2009a), as is associative learning behavior (Wang and Xing, 2008), outcomes which may have indirect effects on development and reproduction.

Neuronal morphology has been observed using GFP constructs in toxicant-exposed worms. Du and Wang (2008) demonstrated γ-aminobutyric acid (GABA)-ergic motor neuron degeneration in L4 worms treated with different metals. Neurodegeneration in dopaminergic neurons was observed using P_{DAT-1} (dopamine transporter)::GFP transgenic worms exposed to 6-hydroxydopamine (OHDA), 1-methyl-4-phenyl-1,2,3,6-tetrahydropyridine (MPTP) and manganese (Mn) (Nass *et al.*, 2002; Nass and Blakely, 2003; Settivari *et al.*, 2009).

C. *elegans* and reproductive toxicity

Because of its simple reproductive system, large brood size and the fact that several genes involved in the process have been extensively described, the reproductive process in *C. elegans* can be easily evaluated using low or high throughput techniques. The most common endpoints evaluated are brood size, generation time, fertility rate and egg-laying (Table 16.2). High-throughput analysis facilitates the screening of toxicants (Boyd *et al.*, 2010a), and molecular analysis helps to clarify the mechanisms responsible for such effects. For instance, microarray has been applied to profile gene expression in worms with reproductive impairment caused by toxicants (Kim and Choung, 2009; Menzel *et al.*, 2009).

Nervous system and reproductive toxicity

Several studies have shown that some reproductive endpoints are controlled by the nervous system. *C. elegans* egg-laying, for instance, is mediated by hermaphrodite-specific neurons that release serotonin, acethylcoline or neuropeptides, which innervate the vulval muscles and drive egg-laying (Trent *et al.*, 1983; Bany *et al.*, 2003). Several neurotoxicants, such as metals (Roh *et al.*, 2009; Xing *et al.*, 2009c), pesticides (Ruan *et al.*, 2009) and 5-fluorouracil (Kumar *et al.*, 2010) have been reported to cause egg-laying defects.

In the male, the entire machinery and its own mating behavior are controlled by the nervous system. *C. elegans* male mating behavior comprises a series of steps: response to contact with the hermaphrodite, backing along her body, turning around her head or tail, location of the vulva, insertion of the two copulatory spicules into the vulva and sperm transfer (Barr and Garcia, 2006). Every step is controlled by different sensory neurons and hence toxicants that cause neurotoxicological effects may affect male reproduction. For example, Lopes *et al.* (2008) demonstrated that levamisole, a nematicide that targets the nicotinergic acethylcoline receptor, impairs reproduction and mating by reducing the encounters between hermaphrodites and males (Lopes *et al.*, 2008).

MOLECULAR AND CELLULAR BASIS OF DEVELOPMENTAL AND REPRODUCTIVE TOXICITY IN C. *ELEGANS*

The *C. elegans* genome was the first completely sequenced genome of a multicellular organism (Consortium TCeS, 1998). Since the genome was first published, a plethora of molecular techniques have been developed for genetic manipulation and cellular and molecular observation that are particularly valuable for toxicological studies. A high density map of polymorphism for the wild-type *C. elegans* facilitates the mapping of genetic mutations, giving researchers the ability to link molecular mechanisms to genetic susceptibility to toxicants. Techniques for site direct mutagenesis, RNAi gene knockdown and transgene introduction enable the manipulation of gene expression at the level of the single gene or single cell in *C. elegans*, thereby allowing researchers to investigate the implications of a single gene in a toxicant response. *C. elegans*-specific microarrays allow for the examination of the genome-wide effects of a particular toxicant as well as high throughput techniques such as the automated behavioral and genetic screening of toxicant effects. Even before the *C. elegans* genome was sequenced, researchers investigated the normal and abnormal development of the nematode, creating both an extensive cell lineage map for the worm (Sulston, 1983) and a complete serial electron microscopy

TABLE 16.2 Endpoints used to assess reproductive toxicity in C. *elegans*

Endpoint	Principle	Reference
Generation time	The time from P_0 egg to the first F_1 egg is monitored.	Wang *et al.* (2007)
Brood size	Nematodes are monitored and transferred to a new plate every 1.5 days, and the total number of eggs released is counted.	Guo *et al.* (2009)
Egg laying	The number of laid eggs from one exposed worm is scored during a certain period of time.	Collins *et al.* (2008)
Male mating behavior	A male is placed in a drop with a hermaphrodite, and the encounter rate is scored after exposure to the toxicant.	Lopes *et al.* (2008)
Fertility rate	The number of offspring from hatched fertilized eggs from toxicant-exposed worms is scored. This parameter can be scored not only for the 1st generation, but also for the 2nd and 3rd ones.	Harada *et al.* (2007)

(EM) reconstruction of the worm (Hall, 1995), establishing a foundation for cell fate analysis to investigate toxicant effects on a variety of developmental endpoints. Newer molecular techniques, paired with extensive knowledge of the normal worm, position *C. elegans* as a strong candidate for modeling reproductive toxicity.

Transgenic worms as bioindicators for environmental toxicant exposure

Transgenic *C. elegans* have been employed as biomarkers of a variety of environmental exposures and provide valuable insight regarding the molecular bases of cellular stress and toxicity. As a complement to more traditional toxicological parameters such as motion, feeding, growth rate and fecundity, the examination of transgenic *C. elegans* as bioindicators often enables researchers to gain information regarding the molecular response pathways involved in a particular toxicant exposure. Transgenic strains of *C. elegans* suitable for use as bioindicators are generated by creating a reporter gene with a stress inducible promoter and then integrating the gene into the worm either as an extra chromosomal array or as a stable insertion into the existing genome. Commonly used reporter genes include the *lacZ* gene from *Escherichia coli*, the *luc* gene from firefly luciferase and the green florescent protein (GFP) gene from the jellyfish. The LacZ reporter line was the first version of transgenic *C. elegans* to be created, but has become less common in toxicological research recently because of the permeabilization and sacrifice of animals necessary for substrate exposure and subsequent colometric analysis (Candido and Jones, 1996). However, worms of this strain are still useful because they give a more precise readout of gene expression (as units of LacZ activity) then GFP expression.

GFP has become a very useful reporter gene in *C. elegans* because the nematodes' translucent body plan allows for GFP transgene expression to be recorded in live animals without the addition of a substrate. Common stress-inducible promoters include promoters for genes in the heat shock protein (HSP) family, metalothioneins, glutathione-s-transferase (GST) and superoxide dismutase (SOD). Ideal stress-inducible promoters are associated with normal gene products that are basically undetectable (Candido and Jones, 1996) and are strictly and rapidly induced upon exposure to a stressor. These model limitations for promoter selection allow the transgenic expression of the reporter gene to be read as a selective response to the stressor.

Transgenic *C. elegans* have been used to investigate the molecular mechanisms involved in a number of toxicant responses with a variety of paradigms. For example, strains carrying a transgene with a promoter for *hsp-16* driving a variety of reporter genes have been used to investigate the effects of fungicides (Jones *et al.*, 1996), bacterial toxins (Bischof *et al.*, 2008), microwaves (Daniells *et al.*, 1998), immunological stress (Nowell *et al.*, 2004), redox quinones (Link *et al.*, 1999) and microwave radiation (David *et al.*, 2003), as well as a variety of pesticides and heavy metals. Strains carrying a transgene with an *hsp-16* promoter have been used to examine toxicant environmental contamination in both soil and water (Boyd *et al.*, 2003) considering that the nematode is a soil-dwelling organism. Transgenic *C. elegans* reporter strains expressing full length HSP-16 fused with GFP have also been generated. HSP-16 fused with GFP can be used to measure molecular level responses and compensations following toxicant exposure (Roh *et al.*, 2007). Transgenic *C. elegans* represent a valuable tool for preliminary investigation and screening of the molecular mechanisms involved in toxicant response.

Analyzing cellular specificity of toxicants using *C. elegans*

Light microscopy is another valuable tool for the examination of toxicant effects in *C. elegans* because the worm maintains a transparent body throughout development and displays a variety of cell or cell-type specific markers. Subcellular effects of toxicants can also be observed using light microscopy in *C. elegans*. Subcellular markers, such as Mitotracker, permit the examination of mitochondrial morphology in live animals (Wang *et al.*, 2002). Nuclear markers are also available for evaluating the effects of genomic morphology, such as synaptonemal complexes (Goldstein, 2001) and terminal deoxynucleotidyl transferase-mediated dUTP nick-end labeling (TUNEL) assay (Wang *et al.*, 2002).

Electron microscopy (EM) is another useful tool for identifying the cellular and subcellular targets of a toxicant. EM is especially helpful when cellular structure is suspected to be affected by a toxicant, but it can also be used to examine subcellular effects at the level of the organelles or membranes. EM has been used to assess the effects of endogenous proteins such as tau (Miyasaka *et al.*, 2005) and alpha-synuclein (Berkowitz *et al.*, 2008), as well as metal toxicity (Au *et al.*, 2009; Settivari *et al.*, 2009; Wang *et al.*, 2009a).

Toxicity testing using *C. elegans* high throughput techniques

High-throughput screening is feasible with *C. elegans* because the nematode is suited to both the aquatic and terrestrial lifestyles, produces a large number of offspring, and has a short reproductive cycle. Once a large population of worms is obtained, there are a variety of high throughput methods that can be utilized to examine toxicant effects (Helmcke *et al.*, 2010).

A variety of computer-based assays have been developed to assess outcomes of toxicant exposure in *C. elegans*. Computer-based assays can give automated readouts of the effects of toxicants on movement and transgenic-fluorescence, as well as relevant developmental and reproductive endpoints such as egg-laying, dauer formation and lifespan. *C. elegans* swimming behavior (thrashing) can be measured using a variety of automated programs (Buckingham and Sattelle, 2009) and has been used to investigate the effects of methylmercury (MeHg) toxicity (Helmcke *et al.*, 2009). Reproductive endpoints such as egg-laying can also be measured using chitinase enzyme and plate-reader computer-based assays for high throughput of reproductive specific endpoints (Kaletta and Hengartner, 2006). Innovations for measuring fluorescence have also been developed to aid in the larger volume examination of toxicant effects. Fluorescence dyes such as SYTOX green fluorescent dye allow for multi-well plate examination of toxicity using *C. elegans* (Gill *et al.*, 2003).

The COPAS biosorter represents a recent advance in computerized worm manipulation enabling high throughput sorting and plating of large numbers of worms. The COPAS biosorter is a modified cell sorter akin to devices associated with flow cytometry. In addition to assisting with the simple manipulation of worms, the biosorter provides a mechanism for examining more traditional toxicological endpoints such as size and stage, as well as more complex endpoints, such as subcellular localization and gene expression assays using transgenic reporter and transgenic expression strains (Rohde *et al.*, 2007).

Genome-wide screens for molecular contributors to toxicity

Genome-wide screening using *C. elegans* is a classical approach for studying the functional repercussions of a gene in a given molecular response, and such screening is particularly valuable for investigating the molecular basis of toxicity. Forward and reverse genetic screens using *C. elegans* permit the examination of single gene contributions to toxicant responses. Forward genetics starts with a phenotype of interest and seeks to find mutants of that phenotype for analysis. In contrast, reverse genetics starts with a gene sequence and seeks to find animals that display mutations in the gene of interest. The aim of both techniques is to relate genotype to phenotype. However, forward genetics starts with the phenotype, whereas reverse genetics starts with the genotype. In the latter, the functional study of a gene starts with the gene sequence rather than a mutant phenotype, and a gene's function is altered and the effect on the development or behavior of the organism is assessed. In addition, gene expression analysis using microarray or proteomics approaches allows for the examination of more global effects of a toxicant and can implicate multiple pathways for investigation in a toxicant response.

DNA microarrays provide a rapid, economical and precise assessment of the level of expression of essentially every *C. elegans* gene. These microarrays have been used in toxicology to identify up- and downregulated genes after they have been exposed to a particular toxicant. Investigating these alterations may lead to greater understanding regarding their effects on development and reproduction in worms. For example, using this approach, Roh *et al.* demonstrated that the decreased reproduction potential caused by silver nanoparticles is associated with an increase in *sod-3* and *daf-12* genes, which may be related to the oxidative stress caused by the toxicant (Roh *et al.*, 2009). Microarrays offer basic predictions and interpretations of potential mechanisms of toxicity, but they need to be complemented by PCR and by the use of mutants to strengthen the resulting data.

In *C. elegans*, the major reverse genetic approaches include RNAi and the use of deletion mutants for the disruption of specific genes or molecules of interest. RNAi uses double-stranded RNA to knock down the expression of a particular gene. The RNAi protocols are incredibly simple, requiring expression of the double-stranded constructs in the *E. coli* food source and then simply feeding the RNAi to the nematode. RNAi libraries are readily available, containing RNAi targeted to almost every gene in *C. elegans*, and they can be helpful in determining the likely result(s) of loss of function for the targeted gene. RNAi libraries can also be used to conduct genome-wide RNAi screens for genes involved in protection against or perpetuation of the toxicant response by examining the toxicant endpoint in the presence or absence of the RNAi for a specific gene. Genome-wide RNAi screens have been employed to study the regulation of endogenous toxins such as protein aggregations (Nollen *et al.*, 2004; van Ham *et al.*, 2008). Pairing high throughput toxicant-related phenotypic endpoints with RNAi could be a potential strategy for examining the effects of reproductive toxicants, although this method has not been employed to date.

Forward genetic mutagenesis screens are conducted by mutagenizing a population of animals, choosing animals with phenotypes of interest, i.e. those displaying fertility defects, and then determining the particular genetic identity by cloning the mutated gene. A forward genetic screen (see above) for *C. elegans* mutants with impaired fertilization revealed a variety of proteins necessary for sperm and egg combinations in the nematode and offered insights regarding mammalian infertility (Singson, 2001). Forward genetic screens can be paired with toxicant response by examining phenotypes in the mutagenized populations that are specific to the toxicant exposure. However, this approach is limited by the specific toxicant phenotype responses, and may result in many false positives when multiple pathways are targeted by a toxicant. *C. elegans* is particularly useful in forward genetic screening because the genome is sequenced and mapping of a mutation is relatively simple.

DEVELOPMENTAL AND REPRODUCTIVE TOXICITY CAUSED BY METALS

Cadmium

Cadmium (Cd) is a non-essential, toxic heavy metal that occurs naturally in the environment. Given its properties, this transition metal has been highly commercialized, particularly in the metal coating, plastics, battery and pigment industries (Swain *et al.*, 2004). Such commercial utilization and its bio-availability have made Cd a significant environmental pollutant. Cd has several adverse effects on the development and reproduction of *C. elegans*. Studies have shown that upon exposure to 100 μM Cd, nematodes failed to progress past the L1–L2 larval stage. Exposure to lower doses of Cd (20 μM) led to a decrease in the proportion of adults present, and this effect was accompanied by an increase in the proportion of nematodes in the L4 larval stage (Lagido *et al.*, 2009). Similar effects have been observed in lifespan assays, with worms exposed to 30 μM Cd exhibiting premature death and reduction in median survival time of approximately 1.5 days (Swain *et al.*, 2004). Reproduction in *C. elegans* is also affected by exposure to Cd. It has been shown that brood size is decreased in a dose-dependent fashion, with 50 μM and 100 μM Cd exposure producing 83% and 92% reduction in brood size, respectively. Further, the increase in generation time in *C. elegans* was found to be dose-dependent, with lengthening by 15–40% with 30 μM and 75 μM Cd exposures, respectively (Swain *et al.*, 2004).

Moreover, normal apoptosis during early development is not a requisite for oogenesis in *C. elegans*; however, if inhibited, the number of progeny produced is decreased (Gumienny *et al.*, 1999). The nematodes possess in their germ lines two U-shaped gonad arms that unite at a common uterus. Upon exposure to Cd, a dose-dependent increase in apoptotic cells was observed in the gonad arms, affirming Cd-induced germ-line apoptosis. However, upon exposure to higher doses (50–100 μM Cd), the number of germ cell corpses produced was significantly decreased, demonstrating an inhibition in normal germ-line apoptosis and a decrease in the total number of germ cells produced (Wang *et al.*, 2008). In addition, metal-related proteins are also affected by Cd exposure in the nematode. *C. elegans* that possess a defect in phytochelatin (metal-binding peptide) synthesis (*pcs1* mutants) and transport (*hmt-1* mutants) exhibit enhanced Cd toxicity (Vatamaniuk *et al.*, 2001, 2005), which is also magnified in wild-type worms that are subjected to both knockout and knockdown of the metallothionein genes by RNAi (Swain *et al.*, 2004). Similarly, the cadmium resistant 1 (*cdr-1*) gene confers resistance to Cd toxicity (Liao *et al.*, 2002). The inhibition of two homologs of *cdr-1*, namely *cdr-4* and *cdr-6*, resulted in the absence of Cd and a significant decrease in the worm's lifespan; this effect could not be rescued by the addition of Cd (Dong *et al.*, 2008).

Zinc

Unlike Cd, zinc (Zn) is an essential metal for survival and is one of the most highly abundant metals in animals, playing critical physiological roles in various enzymatic activities and signaling processes (Bruinsma *et al.*, 2008). However, excess Zn can be toxic. *C. elegans* has been beneficial in characterizing excess Zn toxicity, revealing novel information about its mechanistic effects on development and reproduction in the nematode. For example, it has been shown that in the absence of supplemental dietary Zn, 100% of wild-type worms developed at a normal rate, falling to 0%, upon exposure to 0.2 mM supplemental Zn (Bruinsma *et al.*, 2008). The nematodes that exhibited this developmental delay (animals not progressing to the adult stage within 4 days) also displayed a prolonged L1 larval stage. Moreover, with higher doses of supplemental Zn, a significant proportion of the exposed animals arrested at the L1 larval stage, displaying an LC_{50} of 0.2 mM Zn (Bruinsma *et al.*, 2008). In 2004, Yoder and his colleagues characterized the function of *sur-7*, a member of the CDF-1 cation diffusion facilitator protein family. *cdf-1* is a positive regulator of Ras signaling, and its loss-of-function resulted in increased cytosolic Zn concentrations (Bruinsma *et al.*, 2002). Subsequently, it was found that *sur-7* mutant worms displayed heightened sensitivity to increased Zn^{2+} doses when compared to wild-type worms, and their progeny revealed enhanced sensitivity to increased Zn^{2+} doses as assayed by the rate of developmental maturation or the percentage of worms reaching egg-laying maturity (Yoder *et al.*, 2004).

Although Zn is not necessarily a significant environmental pollutant, with the advent of nanoparticle (NP) usage, several groups have recently investigated the effects of Zn oxide particles in *C. elegans*. The potential toxicity in *C. elegans* of zinc oxide (ZnO) nanoparticles (NPs) compared to aqueous zinc chloride ($ZnCl_2$) was investigated in transgenic strains. An *mtl-2::GFP* (metallothionein-2) transgenic strain was used in order to enable transgene expression as an endpoint of toxicity, given that exposure to metal ions has been previously shown to induce transgene expression in a dose-dependent manner (Ma *et al.*, 2009). Worms displayed a significant decrease in the average number of offspring with increased doses of exposure to either ZnO-NPs (zinc oxide nanoparticles) or $ZnCl_2$ (10–200 mg Zn/L), although no significant difference was seen between ZnO-NPs and $ZnCl_2$. Similarly, ZnO-NPs increased transgene expression in a dose-dependent fashion in a manner analogous to $ZnCl_2$, demonstrating that reproduction was more severely affected than survival or behavior, having the lowest EC_{50} values compared to the other endpoints of toxicity (Ma *et al.*, 2009).

Lead and mercury

Lead (Pb) is another heavy metal of neurotoxic concern. Pb toxicity arises mostly from its ability to impair the normal functioning of enzymes and structural proteins. The toxicant's effects are largely attributable to lead's ability to compete with or mimic calcium (Needleman, 2004). Environmental exposure to Pb is widespread, as it is abundant in manufacturing, building construction and industrial materials. Although environmental exposure is more prevalent in adults, Pb toxicity in children is also of significant concern because children exhibit higher sensitivity to Pb (Needleman, 2004). Similarly, mercury (Hg) exposure affects the developing nervous system in a more severe fashion than it does in adults (Myers *et al.*, 2009).

Using a 4-hour exposure assay, younger *C. elegans* larvae (in the L1–L3 larval stages) exhibited more severe lethality to metals as compared to L4 and young adult worms (Xing *et al.*, 2009c). The effects were particularly severe with Pb and Hg exposure over chromium (Cr) and Cd; lethality in L1 worms after a 4-hour exposure was comparable to 24-hour exposure in young adult animals. Lethality in the 4-hour assay ranked as follows: Hg > Pb > Cr > Cd (Xing *et al.*, 2009c). Upon further inspection of the effects of Pb and Hg, it was found that both cholinergic transmission and GABAergic neuronal survival during development were largely spared. However, both Pb and Hg caused a significant increase in neuronal loss, and dorsal and ventral cord gaps were seen in L1–L3 worms when compared to untreated worms. Such changes, however, were not significant in L4 and young adult worms unless they were treated with doses of 50 and 100 μM Pb and Hg. Additionally, L1–L3 worms showed partial resistance to aldicarb and levamisole when compared to controls, indicating impaired cholinergic transmission (Xing *et al.*, 2009b).

Furthermore, L1 worms exposed to methylmercury (MeHg) were more sensitive to toxicity as compared to L4 worms. This sensitivity, along with Hg accumulation in the worms, was dose-dependent. Although it did not alter the brood size of *C. elegans*, treatment with MeHg led to the retardation of larval development. Both L1 and L4 worms treated with MeHg arrested at their larval stage, while untreated control worms developed normally (Helmcke *et al.*, 2009). Similarly, treatment of nematodes with Pb did not significantly affect the brood size when compared to untreated worms, although Pb exposure slightly increased the body length (Roh *et al.*, 2006). In addition, Guo *et al.* (2009) noted that Hg more severely decreased brood size and increased generation time as compared to Pb, Cd and Cr. Hg exposure not only induced the most severe reproductive toxicity among the metals examined, but L1 worms were the most sensitive to Hg toxicity when compared to worms in later larval stages as well as adult nematodes (Guo *et al.*, 2009), findings which are consistent with observations in mammalian systems and the heightened sensitivity of the developing organism to this metal.

Manganese

Manganese (Mn) is an essential trace element that is a vital co-factor for many enzymes. Despite its essentiality, excess Mn is toxic. Exposures to high levels of Mn occur largely in occupational cohorts, such as in miners, welders and other industrial workers. Following an acute, 30-minute Mn exposure, wild-type *C. elegans* exhibited lethality at doses above 10 mM, and the LD_{50} was 47 mM Mn (Au *et al.*, 2009). Moreover, developmental delay was observed upon Mn exposure. Twenty-four hours post-treatment with 35 mM Mn, 83% of surviving worms were arrested at the L1 larval stage, while only 13% of control worms were arrested at the same stage, with most moving on to the L2 larval stage (Au *et al.*, 2009). Mn-treated worms were also 30% shorter in body length than were controls. These dose-dependent effects corresponded to an increase in vacuolization in the epidermis, excretory cell and gut, all tissues vital for *C. elegans* survival (Au *et al.*, 2009). Moreover, prolonged (48 h) vs. shorter (6 h) exposure to high Mn doses (75 or 200 μM/L) induced more severe, highly significant deficits in reproduction, development and lifespan (Xiao *et al.*, 2009). Due to Mn's high prevalence in the environment, as well as its ability to produce a Parkinsonian-like syndrome, referred to as manganism, further studies investigating developmental and reproductive toxicity in *C. elegans* are well warranted and should reveal important information regarding the mechanisms of Mn-induced neurotoxicity.

Other metals

The effects of exposure to other metals, such as copper (Cu), cobalt (Co), barium (Ba), nickel (Ni), aluminum (Al) and iron (Fe) have also been examined in *C. elegans*. Exposures to high doses of the essential metal Cu led to a significant decrease in brood size and a significant increase in generation time in both wild type and worms exposed to *cutc-1* (a putative copper transporter) RNAi (Calafato *et al.*, 2008). Also, both the protruding vulva (pvl) and bag of worms (egl) phenotypes were noted in worms subjected to *cutc-1* RNAi in the presence of $CuSO_4$ (Calafato *et al.*, 2008). On the other hand, transgenic worms expressing the human beta amyloid (Aβ) peptide implicated in Alzheimer's disease exhibited increased resistance to Cu toxicity as compared to wild-type worms, along with a small but significant increase in median and total lifespan upon $CuCl_2$ exposure (Minniti *et al.*, 2009).

Co is another essential trace element that is toxic at excess levels of exposure, whether dietary or environmental. Generation time and brood size were lengthened or reduced compared to controls, respectively, in *C. elegans* exposed to $CoCl_2$; these effects were only partially recovered in the F_1 progeny (Wang *et al.*, 2007). Additionally, body size in co-exposed worms was significantly decreased as compared to controls, with F_1 progeny displaying more severe decreases; vulva morphological abnormalities were also present and passed on to progeny of Co-exposed worms (Wang *et al.*, 2007). Similar reproductive effects were seen in worms exposed to Ba, characterized by significant reduction in maximum lifespan (by almost 4 days) when compared to untreated worms (Wang and Wang, 2008b). Further, both developmental and reproductive toxicity in worms was also affected by Ni exposure. Brood size was markedly reduced, and body size was significantly increased in a dose-dependent manner in Ni-exposed worms with rescue in F_1 progeny occurring only at the lowest exposures (Wang and Wang, 2008a).

Al exposure also produced damaging effects on reproductive behavior and development in the nematode. Brood size, body size and generation time were impaired upon exposure to low Al doses, with higher doses more prominently increasing the generation time in the worms. Additionally, the effects upon higher Al exposures were transferable to the progeny, with generation time defects being much stronger in the progeny than in their exposed parents (Wang *et al.*, 2009b). Moreover, exposure to $AlCl_3$ led to a dose-dependent decrease in the number of eggs per worm and subsequent number of offspring per worm. The toxicity to $AlCl_3$ was significantly higher than the toxicity produced by Al_2O_3 NPs or bulk Al_2O_3. These findings are consistent with a lower LC_{50} value for survival that most likely corresponds to higher toxicity arising from the Al ions (Wang *et al.*, 2009a). Analogous to Al, Fe exposure also affected body size, brood size and generation time in *C. elegans* in a dose-dependent manner, and these effects were passed on to the progeny of Fe-exposed worms (Hu *et al.*, 2008).

Depleted uranium (DU) is a by-product of the enrichment process of naturally occurring uranium, is highly dense and is used in armor, ammunition and radiation shielding (Aschner and Jiang, 2009). However, experiments employing worms expressing either pan-neural GFP (NW1229 strain) or GFP in their dopaminergic neurons (BY250 strain) showed that a dose-dependent increase in DU accumulation did not result in neurodegeneration in the worm (Jiang *et al.*, 2007). Furthermore, DU exposure seemed to induce expression of metallothionein genes in *C. elegans*, with *mtl-1* and *mtl-2* KO strains showing increased susceptibility to DU toxicity when compared to wild-type worms (Jiang *et al.*, 2009). *mtl-1* also appeared to be the most important isoform in mediating uranium accumulation in the worms (Jiang *et al.*, 2009).

DEVELOPMENTAL AND REPRODUCTIVE TOXICITY CAUSED BY PESTICIDES

Over the past several decades, pesticide use has been tightly examined and carefully regulated due to a multitude of toxic effects on both humans and animals. Depending on the structure and mechanism of action, pesticides can be categorized into various chemical families, such as organochlorines, pyrethroids, organophosphates, carbamates and rotenoids, just to name a few. Organochlorine (OC) pesticides, like DDT, are extremely noxious and are no longer widely used due to persistence in the environment and heavy bioaccumulation (Kutz *et al.*, 1991). Following a ban on DDT use, the synthetic pyrethroid pesticides became more popular, due to effective pest control with lower mammalian toxicity. These pesticides work by causing the repetitive discharging of nerve fibers followed by paralysis of the fibers from a constant open state of sodium channels, compared to the disturbance of the nerve fibers' sodium/potassium balance, which is the operative mechanism in OCPs (Yamamoto, 1970). However, OCPs have been mostly replaced by organophosphate (OP) pesticides and carbamates, both of which function by inactivating acetylcholinesterase, an enzyme that is necessary for proper nerve function. The inhibition of acetylcholinesterase causes an accumulation of acetylcholine, leading not only to arrested movement, but an overall impaired nervous system and potentially subsequent cell death (Costa, 2006). Aldicarb is a known carbamate that functions as an acetylcholinesterase inhibitor. Its mechanism of action has been examined using various *C. elegans* strains with mutated genes that would lead to a decrease in the build-up of acetycholine. *cha-1* (choline acetyltransferase gene), *ric-1* (newly identified resistance to acetylcholinesterase inhibitor gene involved in synaptic function) and *snt-1* (synaptotagmin gene) mutant strains were extremely resistant to aldicarb exposure, with growth rates almost unaffected even at the highest concentrations (Nguyen *et al.*, 1995).

Moreover, dichlorvos, fensulfothion, methidathion, methyl parathion and parathion are all known OP pesticides that produce toxicity phenotypes in *C. elegans*. These pesticides have subsequently also been shown to significantly inhibit cholinesterase activity, while demeton-S-methyl sulfone has failed to inhibit acetylcholinesterase activity (Cole *et al.*, 2004). Out of several OP pesticides tested in *C. elegans*, dichlorvos has been found to be the most toxic, with an LC_{50} of 0.039 mM, while acephate and methamidophos have an LC_{50} in the range of 400–500 mM (Rajini *et al.*, 2008). Dichlorvos also leads to a dose-dependent inhibition in feeding, with a complete halt after just 4 hours of exposure. Dichlorvos and fenamiphos were found to induce expression in several genes related both to cell death and detoxification in nematodes that failed to develop from L4 larvae into early gravid adults upon exposure to OP (Lewis *et al.*, 2009). Many of the detoxification genes which were induced encode cytochrome P450 monooxygenases or UDP-glucuronosyl/glucosyltransferases; the cell death-associated effects included downregulation of the anti-apoptotic map-2 metalloprotease gene and increased levels of NEX-1 apoptotic engulfment protein (Lewis *et al.*, 2009).

Chlorpyrifos is another OP pesticide that is known to cause developmental delays. Control-untreated nematodes have been found to exhibit normal maturation from the L1 larval stage to adult by 60 hours. Exposure to sublethal doses, however, induced a dose-dependent decrease in growth, with higher doses (75 μM) completely inhibiting worms from developing past the L2 larval stage. Nematodes exposed to lower doses at or below 30 μM developed abnormally, but appeared starved and thinner as compared to untreated worms (Boyd *et al.*, 2009). Chlorpyrifos also increased the amount of time needed to reach the next developmental stage, with an increased duration spent in L2 and L3 stages, and a delay at the L3/L4 molt stage. Overall, these younger L2 and L3 stage worms were more susceptible to toxicity than were later larval and young adult stage worms (Boyd *et al.*, 2009). Moreover, exposure to this pesticide significantly decreased the total number of eggs and worms in the L1–L3 and L4 stages as compared to control, untreated worms (Roh and Choi, 2008). With regard to reproduction, chlorpyrifos caused an increase in generation time and a decrease in brood size, and its effects on reproduction were more significant than the effects induced by the other four tested pesticides, imidacloprid, buprofezin, cyhalothrin and glyphosate (Ruan *et al.*, 2009).

Phosphine is a commonly used insecticide in noxious gas form that protects stored products from pest infestation, utilizing oxygen for its toxic effects. Exposure to phosphine prevents egg development, and phosphine-resistant mutant worms (*pre-33*) have been shown to display a higher LC_{50} (2.31 mg/l) as compared to wild-type worms (LC_{50} = 0.26 mg/l) exposed to phosphine (Cheng *et al.*, 2003). These mutant worms also had an extended average life expectancy which was 12.5–25.3% greater than that of the wild-type worms (Cheng *et al.*, 2003). The mechanism behind phosphine toxicity is still not clearly understood, although recent evidence points to a possible connection to impaired iron homeostasis. Phosphine seemed to stimulate the release of iron from ferritin, with RNAi-induced inhibition of ferritin-2 gene expression in *C. elegans* increasing susceptibility to phosphine toxicity. This sensitivity to toxicity was also significantly affected upon iron overload in the worms (Cha'on *et al.*, 2007).

Additionally, many other pesticides also produce detrimental effects on development and reproduction in *C. elegans*. For example, buprofezin exposure for 24 hours induced a more significant increase in generation time in nematodes in a dose-dependent manner than did a longer 72-hour exposure (Ruan *et al.*, 2009). Moreover, nematodes exposed during 20 generations to the pesticide levamisole exhibited decreased survival, fecundity and male frequency (dropping 30% to 0%) as compared to untreated controls. This drop in male frequency within 10 generations could be attributed to a decrease in the number of encounters between males and hermaphrodites due to the influence of levamisole on mobility (Lopes *et al.*, 2008). Remarkably, the worms displayed experimental evolution to this pesticide, with the male frequency increasing by generation 20 (Lopes *et al.*, 2008). Paraquat, a reactive oxygen species (ROS)-generating pesticide, also poses a major health concern to humans, as it is heavily used in the farming industry in bulk supply. Upon paraquat treatment, wild-type worms have been shown to retain their ability to lay eggs, but their F_1 progeny arrested in the L1 larval stage (Kim and Sun, 2007). However, a mutation in *C. elegans* daf-2 (encoding an insulin/insulin-like growth factor 1 receptor-like molecule) conferred sensitivity to paraquat toxicity when compared to wild-type treated worms, with an almost 300% increase in mean survival time (Kim and Sun, 2007). In contrast, inactivation of the *daf-18* gene (*C. elegans* homolog of the PTEN tumor suppressor) actually conferred paraquat sensitivity to the worms. These data implicate the insulin/IGF-1-like signaling pathway in the regulation of oxidative stress, as illuminated by paraquat exposure in *C. elegans* (Kim and Sun, 2007).

CONCLUDING REMARKS AND FUTURE DIRECTIONS

This chapter has described the achievements realized in the field of toxicology through the use of the nematode *C. elegans* as an animal model. Of particular importance, the chapter has described the effects of some toxicants in the development and reproduction of *C. elegans* by assessing specific endpoints which provide a means for evaluating and predicting the toxicity in vertebrates.

Toxicological studies using *C. elegans* date back to the 1990s. The field is relatively new, accounting for the fact that little research with this particular species has been carried out with emphasis on the relationship between environmental exposures and genetics. Nevertheless, considering that *C. elegans* mimics toxicological outcomes in mammals (Helmcke *et al.*, 2009, 2010; Leung *et al.*, 2008; Steinberg *et al.*, 2008) and given the need for alternative models, this model will likely become more prevalent in years to come. Furthermore, as *C. elegans* readily and easily allows for the use of high throughput techniques, screening for several toxicants will become faster and more consistent. Endpoints to assess development and reproduction have been proven to be reliable tools in toxicology. Emerging techniques have been currently applied to previously established toxicant endpoints in *C. elegans*, providing new insights into the molecular mechanisms involved in the toxicant response. Efforts to attain basic knowledge about the toxicant response mechanism(s) in *C. elegans* will greatly enhance the transition to high throughput experimental design through the development of defined phenotypic models of toxicant response in conjunction with genetic manipulation strategies. In the coming years, combining basic toxicological experimentation and investigation with newer genetic and high throughput methods will make *C. elegans* an invaluable tool for examining the molecular and cellular mechanisms of toxicity.

ACKNOWLEDGMENTS

This chapter was supported in part by NIEHS R01 10563 and R01 07331 and the Stahlman Chair in Neuroscience (Michael Aschner) and NIEHS T32 ES007028, Training Program in Environmental Toxicology (Margaret Adams).

REFERENCES

Altun ZF, Hall DH (2008) Handbook of *C. elegans* Anatomy http://www.wormatlas.org/hermaphrodite/hermaphroditehomepage.htm. In *WormAtlas* (Altun ZF, Herndon LA, Crocker C, Lints R, Hall, DH, eds.).

Anderson GL, Boyd WA, Williams PL (2001) Assessment of sublethal endpoints for toxicity testing with the nematode *Caenorhabditis elegans*. *Environ Toxicol Chem* **20:** 833–8.

Anderson GL, Cole RD, Williams PL (2004) Assessing behavioral toxicity with *Caenorhabditis elegans*. *Environ Toxicol Chem* **23:** 1235–40.

Aschner M, Jiang GC (2009) Toxicity studies on depleted uranium in primary rat cortical neurons and in *Caenorhabditis elegans*: what have we learned? *J Toxicol Environ Health B Crit Rev* **12:** 525–39.

Au C, Benedetto A, Anderson J, Labrousse A, Erikson K, Ewbank JJ, Aschner M (2009) SMF-1, SMF-2 and SMF-3 DMT1 orthologues regulate and are regulated differentially by manganese levels in C. elegans. *PLoS One* **4:** e7792.

Bany IA, Dong MQ, Koelle MR (2003) Genetic and cellular basis for acetylcholine inhibition of *Caenorhabditis elegans* egg-laying behavior. *J Neurosci* **23:** 8060–9.

Barr MM, Garcia LR (2006) Male mating behavior. *WormBook*: 1–11.

Berkowitz LA, Hamamichi S, Knight AL, Harrington AJ, Caldwell GA, Caldwell KA (2008) Application of a *C. elegans* dopamine neuron degeneration assay for the validation of potential Parkinson's disease genes. *J Vis Exp* pii: 835. doi 10.3791/835.

Bischof LJ, Kao CY, Los FC, Gonzalez MR, Shen Z, Briggs SP, van der Goot FG, Aroian RV (2008) Activation of the unfolded protein response is required for defenses against bacterial pore-forming toxin in vivo. *PLoS Pathog* **4:** e1000176.

Boyd WA, Cole RD, Anderson GL, Williams PL (2003) The effects of metals and food availability on the behavior of *Caenorhabditis elegans*. *Environ Toxicol Chem* **22:** 3049–55.

Boyd WA, McBride SJ, Rice JR, Snyder DW, Freedman JH (2010a) A high-throughput method for assessing chemical toxicity using a *Caenorhabditis elegans* reproduction assay. *Toxicol Appl Pharmacol* **245:** 153–9.

Boyd WA, Smith MV, Kissling GE, Freedman JH (2010b) Medium- and high-throughput screening of neurotoxicants using *C. elegans*. *Neurotoxicol Teratol* **32:** 68–73.

Boyd WA, Smith MV, Kissling GE, Rice JR, Snyder DW, Portier CJ, Freedman JH (2009) Application of a mathematical model to describe the effects of chlorpyrifos on *Caenorhabditis elegans* development. *PLoS One* **4:** e7024.

Brenner S. (2009) In the beginning was the worm. *Genetics* **182:** 413–15.

Bruinsma JJ, Jirakulaporn T, Muslin AJ, Kornfeld K (2002) Zinc ions and cation diffusion facilitator proteins regulate Ras-mediated signaling. *Dev Cell* **2:** 567–78.

Bruinsma JJ, Schneider DL, Davis DE, Kornfeld K (2008) Identification of mutations in *Caenorhabditis elegans* that cause resistance to high levels of dietary zinc and analysis using a genomewide map of single nucleotide polymorphisms scored by pyrosequencing. *Genetics* **179:** 811–28.

Buckingham SD, Sattelle DB (2009) Fast, automated measurement of nematode swimming (thrashing) without morphometry. *BMC Neurosci* **10:** 84.

Calafato S, Swain S, Hughes S, Kille P, Sturzenbaum SR (2008) Knock down of *Caenorhabditis elegans* cutc-1 exacerbates the sensitivity toward high levels of copper. *Toxicol Sci* **106:** 384–91.

Candido EP, Jones D (1996) Transgenic *Caenorhabditis elegans* strains as biosensors. *Trends Biotechnol* **14:** 125–29.

Cha'on U, Valmas N, Collins PJ, Reilly PE, Hammock BD, Ebert PR (2007) Disruption of iron homeostasis increases phosphine toxicity in *Caenorhabditis elegans*. *Toxicol Sci* **96:** 194–201.

Chalfie M, Tu Y, Euskirchen G, Ward WW, Prasher DC (1994) Green fluorescent protein as a marker for gene expression. *Science* **263:** 802–5.

Cheng Q, Valmas N, Reilly PE, Collins PJ, Kopittke R, Ebert PR (2003) *Caenorhabditis elegans* mutants resistant to phosphine toxicity show increased longevity and cross-resistance to the synergistic action of oxygen. *Toxicol Sci* **73:** 60–5.

Chu KW, Chan SK, Chow KL (2005) Improvement of heavy metal stress and toxicity assays by coupling a transgenic reporter in a mutant nematode strain. *Aquat Toxicol* **74:** 320–32.

Cole RD, Anderson GL, Williams PL (2004) The nematode *Caenorhabditis elegans* as a model of organophosphate-induced mammalian neurotoxicity. *Toxicol Appl Pharmacol* **194:** 248–56.

Collins JJ, Evason K, Pickett CL, Schneider DL, Kornfeld K (2008) The anticonvulsant ethosuximide disrupts sensory function to extend C. elegans lifespan. *PLoS Genet* **4:** e1000230.

Consortium TCeS (1998) Genome sequence of the nematode *C. elegans*: a platform for investigating biology. *Science* **282:** 2012–18.

Costa LG (2006) Current issues in organophosphate toxicology. *Clin Chim Acta* **366:** 1–13.

Cui Y, McBride SJ, Boyd WA, Alper S, Freedman JH (2007) Toxicogenomic analysis of *Caenorhabditis elegans* reveals novel genes and pathways involved in the resistance to cadmium toxicity. *Genome Biol* **8:** R122.

Daniells C, Duce I, Thomas D, Sewell P, Tattersall J, de Pomerai D (1998) Transgenic nematodes as biomonitors of microwave-induced stress. *Mutat Res* **399:** 55–64.

David HE, Dawe AS, de Pomerai DI, Jones D, Candido EP, Daniells C (2003) Construction and evaluation of a transgenic hsp16-GFP-lacZ *Caenorhabditis elegans* strain for environmental monitoring. *Environ Toxicol Chem* **22:** 111–18.

Dong J, Boyd WA, Freedman JH (2008) Molecular characterization of two homologs of the *Caenorhabditis elegans* cadmium-responsive gene cdr-1: cdr-4 and cdr-6. *J Mol Biol* **376:** 621–33.

Fujiwara M, Sengupta P, McIntire SL (2002) Regulation of body size and behavioral state of *C. elegans* by sensory perception and the EGL-4 cGMP-dependent protein kinase. *Neuron* **36:** 1091–102.

Gill MS, Olsen A, Sampayo JN, Lithgow GJ (2003) An automated high-throughput assay for survival of the nematode *Caenorhabditis elegans*. *Free Radic Biol Med* **35:** 558–65.

Goldstein B (2001) On the evolution of early development in the Nematoda. *Philos Trans R Soc Lond B Biol Sci* **356:** 1521–31.

Gumienny TL, Lambie E, Hartwieg E, Horvitz HR, Hengartner MO (1999) Genetic control of programmed cell death in the *Caenorhabditis elegans* hermaphrodite germline. *Development* **126:** 1011–22.

Guo Y, Yang Y, Wang D (2009) Induction of reproductive deficits in nematode *Caenorhabditis elegans* exposed to metals at different developmental stages. *Reprod Toxicol* **28:** 90–5.

Hall DH (1995) Electron microscopy and three-dimensional image reconstruction. *Methods Cell Biol* **48:** 395–436.

Harada H, Kurauchi M, Hayashi R, Eki T (2007) Shortened lifespan of nematode *Caenorhabditis elegans* after prolonged exposure to heavy metals and detergents. *Ecotoxicol Environ Saf* **66:** 378–83.

Helmcke KJ, Avila DS, Aschner M (2010) Utility of *Caenorhabditis elegans* in high throughput neurotoxicological research. *Neurotoxicol Teratol* **32:** 62–7.

Helmcke KJ, Syversen T, Miller DM, 3rd, Aschner M (2009) Characterization of the effects of methylmercury on *Caenorhabditis elegans*. *Toxicol Appl Pharmacol* **240:** 265–72.

Hills T, Brockie PJ, Maricq AV (2004) Dopamine and glutamate control area-restricted search behavior in *Caenorhabditis elegans*. *J Neurosci* **24:** 1217–25.

Hope IA (1999) *C. elegans – A practical Approach*. New York, Oxford University Press.

Hoss S, Weltje L (2007) Endocrine disruption in nematodes: effects and mechanisms. *Ecotoxicology* **16:** 15–28.

Hu YO, Wang Y, Ye BP, Wang DY (2008) Phenotypic and behavioral defects induced by iron exposure can be transferred to progeny in *Caenorhabditis elegans*. *Biomed Environ Sci* **21:** 467–73.

Jadhav KB, Rajini PS (2009) Evaluation of sublethal effects of dichlorvos upon *Caenorhabditis elegans* based on a set of end points of toxicity. *J Biochem Mol Toxicol* **23:** 9–17.

Jiang GC, Hughes S, Sturzenbaum SR, Evje L, Syversen T, Aschner M (2009) *Caenorhabditis elegans* metallothioneins protect against toxicity induced by depleted uranium. *Toxicol Sci* **111:** 345–54.

Jiang GC, Tidwell K, McLaughlin BA, Cai J, Gupta RC, Milatovic D, Nass R, Aschner M (2007) Neurotoxic potential of depleted uranium effects in primary cortical neuron cultures and in *Caenorhabditis elegans*. *Toxicol Sci* **99:** 553–65.

Jones D, Stringham EG, Babich SL, Candido EP (1996) Transgenic strains of the nematode C. elegans in biomonitoring and toxicology: effects of captan and related compounds on the stress response. *Toxicology* **109:** 119–27.

Kaletta T, Hengartner MO (2006) Finding function in novel targets: *C. elegans* as a model organism. *Nat Rev Drug Discov* **5:** 387–98.

Kim SJ, Choung SY (2009) Whole genomic expression analysis of octachlorostyrene-induced chronic toxicity in *Caenorhabditis elegans*. *Arch Pharm Res* **32:** 1585–92.

Kim Y, Sun H (2007) Functional genomic approach to identify novel genes involved in the regulation of oxidative stress resistance and animal lifespan. *Aging Cell* **6:** 489–503.

Kimble J, Ward S (1988) Germ-line development and fertilization. In *The Nematode C. elegans* (Wood WB, ed.). New York, Cold Spring Harbor Laboratory Press.

Kumar S, Aninat C, Michaux G, Morel F (2010) Anticancer drug 5-fluorouracil induces reproductive and developmental defects in *Caenorhabditis elegans*. *Reprod Toxicol* **219:** 415–20.

Kutz FW, Wood PH, Bottimore DP (1991) Organochlorine pesticides and polychlorinated biphenyls in human adipose tissue. *Rev Environ Contam Toxicol* **120:** 1–82.

Lagido C, McLaggan D, Flett A, Pettitt J, Glover LA (2009) Rapid sublethal toxicity assessment using bioluminescent Caenorhabditis elegans, a novel whole-animal metabolic biosensor. *Toxicol Sci* **109:** 88–95.

Leung MC, Williams PL, Benedetto A, Au C, Helmcke KJ, Aschner M, Meyer JN (2008) *Caenorhabditis elegans*: an emerging model in biomedical and environmental toxicology. *Toxicol Sci* **106:** 5–28.

Lewis JA, Szilagyi M, Gehman E, Dennis WE, Jackson DA (2009) Distinct patterns of gene and protein expression elicited by organophosphorus pesticides in *Caenorhabditis elegans*. *BMC Genomics* **10:** 202.

Liao VH, Dong J, Freedman JH (2002) Molecular characterization of a novel, cadmium-inducible gene from the nematode *Caenorhabditis elegans*: a new gene that contributes to the resistance to cadmium toxicity. *J Biol Chem* **277:** 42049–59.

Lin L, Wakabayashi T, Oikawa T, Sato T, Ogurusu T, Shingai R (2006) *Caenorhabditis elegans* mutants having altered preference of chemotaxis behavior during simultaneous presentation of two chemoattractants. *Biosci Biotechnol Biochem* **70:** 2754–8.

Link CD, Cypser JR, Johnson CJ, Johnson TE (1999) Direct observation of stress response in *Caenorhabditis elegans* using a reporter transgene. *Cell Stress Chaperones* **4:** 235–42.

Lints R, Hall DH (2005) Handbook of C. elegans Male Anatomy http://www.wormatlas.org/male/malehomepage.htm. In *WormAtlas* (Altun ZF, Herndon LA, Crocker C, Lints R, Hall, DH, eds.).

Lopes PC, Sucena E, Santos ME, Magalhaes S (2008) Rapid experimental evolution of pesticide resistance in *C. elegans* entails no costs and affects the mating system. *PLoS One* **3:** e3741.

Ma H, Bertsch PM, Glenn TC, Kabengi NJ, Williams PL (2009) Toxicity of manufactured zinc oxide nanoparticles in the nematode *Caenorhabditis elegans*. *Environ Toxicol Chem* **28:** 1324–30.

Madi A, Mikkat S, Ringel B, Thiesen HJ, Glocker MO (2003) Profiling stage-dependent changes of protein expression in *Caenorhabditis elegans* by mass spectrometric proteome analysis leads to the identification of stage-specific marker proteins. *Electrophoresis* **24:** 1809–17.

Menzel R, Swain SC, Hoess S, Claus E, Menzel S, Steinberg CE, Reifferscheid G, Sturzenbaum SR (2009) Gene expression profiling to characterize sediment toxicity – a pilot study using *Caenorhabditis elegans* whole genome microarrays. *BMC Genomics* **10:** 160.

Minniti AN, Rebolledo DL, Grez PM, Fadic R, Aldunate R, Volitakis I, Cherny RA, Opazo C, Masters C, Bush AI, Inestrosa NC (2009) Intracellular amyloid formation in muscle cells of Abeta-transgenic *Caenorhabditis elegans*: determinants and physiological role in copper detoxification. *Mol Neurodegener* **4:** 2.

Miyasaka T, Ding Z, Gengyo-Ando K, Oue M, Yamaguchi H, Mitani S, Ihara Y (2005) Progressive neurodegeneration in C. elegans model of tauopathy. *Neurobiol Dis* **20:** 372–83.

Myers GJ, Thurston SW, Pearson AT, Davidson PW, Cox C, Shamlaye CF, Cernichiari E, Clarkson TW (2009) Postnatal exposure to methyl mercury from fish consumption: a review and new data from the Seychelles Child Development Study. *Neurotoxicology* **30:** 338–49.

Nass R, Blakely RD (2003) The *Caenorhabditis elegans* dopaminergic system: opportunities for insights into dopamine transport and neurodegeneration. *Annu Rev Pharmacol Toxicol* **43:** 521–44.

Nass R, Hall DH, Miller DM 3rd, Blakely RD (2002) Neurotoxin-induced degeneration of dopamine neurons in *Caenorhabditis elegans*. *Proc Natl Acad Sci USA* **99:** 3264–9.

Needleman H (2004) Lead poisoning. *Annu Rev Med* **55:** 209–22.

Nguyen M, Alfonso A, Johnson CD, Rand JB (1995) *Caenorhabditis elegans* mutants resistant to inhibitors of acetylcholinesterase. *Genetics* **140:** 527–35.

Nollen EA, Garcia SM, van Haaften G, Kim S, Chavez A, Morimoto RI, Plasterk RH (2004) Genome-wide RNA interference screen identifies previously undescribed regulators of polyglutamine aggregation. *Proc Natl Acad Sci USA* **101:** 6403–8.

Rajini PS, Melstrom P, Williams PL (2008) A comparative study on the relationship between various toxicological endpoints in *Caenorhabditis elegans* exposed to organophosphorus insecticides. *J Toxicol Environ Health A* **71:** 1043–50.

Ririe TO, Fernandes JS, Sternberg PW (2008) The *Caenorhabditis elegans* vulva: a post-embryonic gene regulatory network controlling organogenesis. *Proc Natl Acad Sci USA* **105:** 20095–9.

Roh JY, Choi J (2008) Ecotoxicological evaluation of chlorpyrifos exposure on the nematode *Caenorhabditis elegans*. *Ecotoxicol Environ Saf* **71:** 483–9.

Roh JY, Jung IH, Lee JY, Choi J (2007) Toxic effects of di(2-ethylhexyl)phthalate on mortality, growth, reproduction and stress-related gene expression in the soil nematode *Caenorhabditis elegans*. *Toxicology* **237:** 126–33.

Roh JY, Lee J, Choi J (2006) Assessment of stress-related gene expression in the heavy metal-exposed nematode *Caenorhabditis elegans*: a potential biomarker for metal-induced toxicity monitoring and environmental risk assessment. *Environ Toxicol Chem* **25:** 2946–56.

Roh JY, Sim SJ, Yi J, Park K, Chung KH, Ryu DY, Choi J (2009) Ecotoxicity of silver nanoparticles on the soil nematode *Caenorhabditis elegans* using functional ecotoxicogenomics. *Environ Sci Technol* **43:** 3933–40.

Rohde CB, Zeng F, Gonzalez-Rubio R, Angel M, Yanik MF (2007) Microfluidic system for on-chip high-throughput whole-animal sorting and screening at subcellular resolution. *Proc Natl Acad Sci USA* **104:** 13891–5.

Ruan QL, Ju JJ, Li YH, Liu R, Pu YP, Yin LH, Wang DY (2009) Evaluation of pesticide toxicities with differing mechanisms using *Caenorhabditis elegans*. *J Toxicol Environ Health A* **72:** 746–51.

Schedl T (1997) Developmental genetics of the germ line. In *C. elegans II* (Riddle DL, Blumenthal T, Meyer BJ, Priess JR, eds.). New York, Cold Spring Harbor Laboratory Press, pp. 191–213.

Sese BT, Grant A, Reid BJ (2009) Toxicity of polycyclic aromatic hydrocarbons to the nematode *Caenorhabditis elegans*. *J Toxicol Environ Health A* **72:** 1168–80.

Settivari R, Levora J, Nass R (2009) The divalent metal transporter homologues SMF-1/2 mediate dopamine neuron sensitivity in *Caenorhabditis elegans* models of manganism and parkinson disease. *J Biol Chem* **284:** 35758–68.

Singson A (2001) Every sperm is sacred: fertilization in *Caenorhabditis elegans*. *Dev Biol* **230:** 101–9.

Steinberg CE, Sturzenbaum SR, Menzel R (2008) Genes and environment – striking the fine balance between sophisticated biomonitoring and true functional environmental genomics. *Sci Total Environ* **400:** 142–61.

Sternberg PW (2005) Vulval development. *WormBook*: 1–28.

Sulston JE (1983) Neuronal cell lineages in the nematode *Caenorhabditis elegans*. *Cold Spring Harb Symp Quant Biol* **48 (Pt 2):** 443–52.

Sulston JE, Schierenberg E, White JG, Thomson JN (1983) The embryonic cell lineage of the nematode *Caenorhabditis elegans*. *Dev Biol* **100:** 64–119.

Swain SC, Keusekotten K, Baumeister R, Sturzenbaum SR (2004) *C. elegans* metallothioneins: new insights into the phenotypic effects of cadmium toxicosis. *J Mol Biol* **341:** 951–9.

Sze JY, Victor M, Loer C, Shi Y, Ruvkun G (2000) Food and metabolic signalling defects in a *Caenorhabditis elegans* serotonin-synthesis mutant. *Nature* **403:** 560–4.

Trent C, Tsuing N, Horvitz HR (1983) Egg-laying defective mutants of the nematode *Caenorhabditis elegans*. *Genetics* **104:** 619–47.

Tsalik EL, Hobert O (2003) Functional mapping of neurons that control locomotory behavior in *Caenorhabditis elegans*. *J Neurobiol* **56:** 178–97.

van Ham TJ, Thijssen KL, Breitling R, Hofstra RM, Plasterk RH, Nollen EA (2008) *C. elegans* model identifies genetic modifiers of alpha-synuclein inclusion formation during aging. *PLoS Genet* **4:** e1000027.

Vatamaniuk OK, Bucher EA, Sundaram MV, Rea PA (2005) CeHMT-1, a putative phytochelatin transporter, is required for cadmium tolerance in *Caenorhabditis elegans*. *J Biol Chem* **280:** 23684–90.

Vatamaniuk OK, Bucher EA, Ward JT, Rea PA (2001) A new pathway for heavy metal detoxification in animals. Phytochelatin synthase is required for cadmium tolerance in *Caenorhabditis elegans*. *J Biol Chem* **276:** 20817–20.

Wang D, Wang Y (2008a) Nickel sulfate induces numerous defects in *Caenorhabditis elegans* that can also be transferred to progeny. *Environ Pollut* **151:** 585–92.

Wang D, Xing X (2008) Assessment of locomotion behavioral defects induced by acute toxicity from heavy metal exposure in nematode *Caenorhabditis elegans*. *J Environ Sci (China)* **20:** 1132–7.

Wang DY, Wang Y (2008b) Phenotypic and behavioral defects caused by barium exposure in nematode *Caenorhabditis elegans*. *Arch Environ Contam Toxicol* **54:** 447–53.

Wang DY, Yang YC, Wang Y (2009a) Aluminium toxicosis causing transferable defects from exposed animals to their progeny in *Caenorhabditis elegans*. *Zhonghua Yu Fang Yi Xue Za Zhi* **43:** 45–51.

Wang H, Wick RL, Xing B (2009b) Toxicity of nanoparticulate and bulk ZnO, Al2O3 and TiO2 to the nematode *Caenorhabditis elegans*. *Environ Pollut* **157:** 1171–7.

Wang S, Tang M, Pei B, Xiao X, Wang J, Hang H, Wu L (2008) Cadmium-induced germline apoptosis in *Caenorhabditis elegans*: the roles of HUS1, p53, and MAPK signaling pathways. *Toxicol Sci* **102:** 345–51.

Wang X, Yang C, Chai J, Shi Y, Xue D (2002) Mechanisms of AIF-mediated apoptotic DNA degradation in *Caenorhabditis elegans*. *Science* **298:** 1587–92.

Wang Y, Xie W, Wang D (2007) Transferable properties of multi-biological toxicity caused by cobalt exposure in *Caenorhabditis elegans*. *Environ Toxicol Chem* **26:** 2405–12.

White JG, Southgate E, Thomson JN, Brenner S (1976) The structure of the ventral nerve cord of *Caenorhabditis elegans*. *Philos Trans R Soc Lond B Biol Sci* **275:** 327–48.

Xiao J, Rui Q, Guo Y, Chang X, Wang D (2009) Prolonged manganese exposure induces severe deficits in lifespan, development and reproduction possibly by altering oxidative stress response in *Caenorhabditis elegans*. *J Environ Sci (China)* **21:** 842–8.

Xing X, Guo Y, Wang D (2009a) Using the larvae nematode *Caenorhabditis elegans* to evaluate neurobehavioral toxicity to metallic salts. *Ecotoxicol Environ Saf* **72:** 1819–23.

Xing X, Rui Q, Wang D (2009b) Lethality toxicities induced by metal exposure during development in nematode *Caenorhabditis elegans*. *Bull Environ Contam Toxicol* **83:** 530–6.

Xing XJ, Rui Q, Du M, Wang DY (2009c) Exposure to lead and mercury in young larvae induces more severe deficits in neuronal survival and synaptic function than in adult nematodes. *Arch Environ Contam Toxicol* **56:** 732–41.

Yamamoto Y (1970) Mode of action of pyrethroids, nicotinoids, and rotenoids. *Annual Review of Entomology* **15:** 275–82.

Yoder JH, Chong H, Guan KL, Han M (2004) Modulation of KSR activity in *Caenorhabditis elegans* by Zn ions, PAR-1 kinase and PP2A phosphatase. *EMBO J* **23:** 111–19.

CHAPTER

17

A primate as an animal model for reproductive and developmental toxicity testing

Ali S. Faqi

INTRODUCTION

Macaque monkeys are native to Asia and Africa belonging to the genus *Macaca*, family Cercopithecidae. The non-human primates are used in many areas of biomedical research where their similarities to humans make them exclusively valuable animal models. Rhesus macaques are the most studied non-human primate, both in the field and in laboratory setting. The rhesus monkey exhibits breeding seasonality of reproductive activity for both sexes with females becoming reproductively active in response to an environmental cue and males becoming sexually active in response to ovulating females (Herndon, 2005). The female rhesus tends to conceive on the first ovulatory cycle of the season, and the best predictor of the timing of ovulation in a particular female is its reproductive outcome in the previous year (Gordon, 1981). The occurrence of ovulation and conception in the female rhesus monkey (*Macaca mulatta*) under natural conditions is seasonal and peaks during the months of October to March. Such seasonality in reproduction suggests dependence on environmental factors like photoperiod, temperature and rainfall (Ghosh and Sengupta, 1992).

The macaque monkeys exhibit marked similarities to humans in almost all aspects of their anatomy, endocrinology and physiology (Shimizu, 2008). Striking similarities between the Rhesus monkey and human species in changing follicular population distributions related to reproductive senescence was observed and this led to the conclusion that the macaque species are considered to be the most appropriate model for reproductive ageing studies as their menstrual cycling, hormonal secretion patterns and morphological characteristics of the reproductive organs are similar to those of the human female (Nichols *et al.*, 2005; Walker and Herndon, 2008). Old macaque monkeys (20–25 years old) frequently exhibit marked cyclic irregularity and display endocrine and ovarian changes at menopause similar to those in menopausal women (Dierschke, 1985; Brodie *et al.*, 1989). In addition, genetic similarity, relatively long lives and similar reproductive endocrinology suggest that non-human primates (NHPs) are likely candidates as models of skeletal and reproductive aging in humans. The physiology of the menstrual cycle of old world monkeys (Cercopithecidea) closely resembles that of the human and the endometrium of the cynomolgus monkey represents the general pattern of the development, structure and function of the endometrium of old world non-human primates and human beings (Van Esch *et al.*, 2008).

The ovarian cycle in various macaque species shows close similarities to that in women. However, primates display considerable differences from other mammalian species, in particular rodents or ruminants in terms of ovarian cycle characteristics and regulation. Regardless of whether conception occurs or not primates have a comparatively long lifespan of the corpus luteum (about 2 weeks or longer) and if a pregnancy is established, the corpus luteum has an extended duration of function and delayed luteal regression to permit implantation and the luteal–placental shift. Unlike in rodents, prolactin is not considered to play a decisive role during the luteal phase, and luteolysis does not involve a uterine signal (Weinbauer *et al.*, 2008b). The endometrium undergoes dramatic morphologic and functional changes in both the human and the macaque monkey during the menstrual cycle. The sequential events that take place in the endometrium are mainly due to the ovarian steroids, namely, estradiol and progesterone and their respective receptors (Van Esch *et al.*, 2008).

Normal predictive values for a variety of growth parameters including gestational sac, greatest length, biparietal diameter and femur length have been calculated by multiple regression analysis. No significant differences in size during the embryonic and early fetal periods were observed, but a greater acceleration of growth in the rhesus beginning at approximately gestation day (GD) 100–110 was reported when observations during the embryonic and fetal periods in both rhesus monkeys and humans have been compared with diagnostic ultrasound. In addition, analysis of embryonic and fetal heart rates indicates no differences between the two species (Tarantal and Hendrickx, 2005).

Black and Lane (2002) reported that several species of NHP exhibit changes in bone and reproduction that are comparable to those known to occur in humans. Also Hendrickx *et al.* (2000) reported that embryonic exposure to triamcinolone acetonide, a potent corticosteroid, during critical periods of thymus

Reproductive and Developmental Toxicology, Edited by Ramesh C. Gupta
ISBN: 978-0-12-382032-7

development caused marked hypoplasia, depletion of thymic lymphocytes and reduction of epithelial elements suggesting that several macaque species are appropriate animal models for preclinical safety assessment of immunomodulatory drugs.

Moreover, the general process of spermatogenesis in the cynomolgus monkey is considered to be highly comparable to that in humans which makes non-human primates very suitable as models to study the effects on the male reproductive system. The male cynomolgus is considered to be a good model of male fertility in specific cases (Ehmcke *et al.*, 2006).

The non-human primate as an animal model for the study of developmental toxicity was recognized following the thalidomide tragedy. Since that time they have played important roles in both testing of drugs for human safety and as models for studying specific malformations commonly observed in children. Macaque monkeys were reported to act almost identically to thalidomide in humans (Wilson and Gavan, 1967).

The preclinical safety testing of biotherapeutics poses a particular challenge in selecting a relevant animal species for use in toxicology studies. A number of factors should be considered when determining the relevant species for the safety testing of biotechnology-derived pharmaceuticals. This should include comparisons of target sequence homology between species followed by cell-based assays to make qualitative and quantitative cross-species comparisons of relative target binding affinities and receptor/legend occupancy and kinetics (ICH S6 [R1], 2009). The determination of a relevant species selection defined in the regulatory framework for the mAb is the one in which the test compound is pharmacologically active due to the expression of the epitope and demonstrates a similar tissue cross-reactivity profile as for humans (ICH S6 [R1], 2009). Accurate prediction on the target effects of mAbs requires testing in a species which shows cross-reactivity as these compounds are highly specific to their targets. Because of the restricted reactivity of human-specific mAb, non-human primates are the only available species for efficacy and safety studies (Jonker, 1990; Chapman *et al.*, 2007).

Indeed NHPs are most frequently used for developmental and reproductive toxicity testing when commonly used rodents and/or rabbits are not pharmacologically relevant species. Several other reasons why the cynomolgus monkey (*Macaca fascicularis*) may be used as an alternative species in developmental and reproductive testing include (1) when the compound is not tolerated in rats and rabbits, (2) when teratogenicity is not only observed in rats or rabbits, (3) when the metabolism in rats and rabbits is completely different from that in humans, and (4) when hormonal compounds are tested (De Ruk and Van Esch, 2008). Although safety testing in preclinical studies represents one of the major uses of non-human primates, in reality only few compounds are tested in NHPs. The NHP are not used as a second species for safety testing; they are only used in circumstances where no alternative methods are available and when testing is considered essential for safety assessment. The *Macaca fascicularis*, the crab eating macaque and cynomolgus monkey are the most commonly used macaques in biomedical research. The cynomolgus monkeys offer several advantages as an animal model for developmental and reproductive toxicity testing. They are not seasonal breeders and therefore readily available for use anytime throughout the year. In addition historical control data for teratogenicity and developmental and reproductive toxicity are available for this species.

There are several published scientific papers and a book chapter that could be used as an aid to design the NHP DART studies (Weinbauer *et al.*, 2008a; Chellman *et al.*, 2009); nevertheless the need for an additional tool was felt necessary. Consequently this chapter was composed with the goal of providing the scientific community involved in conducting, monitoring or reviewing these types of studies with a better tool that depicts the regulatory and the scientific aspects as well as the technical challenges implicated in designing and executing the NHP DART studies.

IMMUNOGENICITY

Immunogenicity has the potential to be a significant obstacle in the development of successful biological drugs. Many of the protein therapeutics elicit immune response when administered to patients (Schellekens, 2002). Similarly as human proteins are foreign to animals, it is common for animals to develop anti-drug antibodies (ADA), which can lead to increased clearance of the biopharmaceuticals, yielding exposure reduction and overestimating safety. In some cases, the formation of neutralizing and non-neutralizing antibodies reduces drug efficacy and potency. In general, immune responses to biological products tend to induce less severe adverse effects, resulting mostly in affecting efficacy of the product; but it has been shown that immune responses to certain biotechnology products can have serious clinical consequences in humans (Casadevall *et al.*, 2002). Because of this serious clinical consequence regulatory agencies will expect, prior to marketing, detailed clinical evaluation of the potential for immunogenicity. Depending on the product, a substantial postmarketing commitment to monitor immunogenicity in the relevant clinical setting may be demanded as well (Chamberlain and Mire-Sluis, 2003). The immunogenicity assessment of protein therapeutics has received significant attention, from both the industry and regulatory authorities. Preclinical immunogenicity testing has been limited to monitoring antibody formation in rodents and NHPs. There are currently no animal models available to predict reliably the potential for a protein therapeutic to induce an immunogenic response in man (ICH S6 [R1], 2009). However, specialized animal models including genetically engineered mice and MHC-defined primates clinically mimic critical aspects of the human immune response, such as tolerance and T-reportoire, and may therefore justify their high costs of development (Chirino *et al.*, 2004).

DEVELOPMENTAL AND REPRODUCTIVE TOXICITY STUDIES

Evaluation of developmental and reproductive toxicology (DART) endpoints is an integral part of the safety assessment for compounds with potential use in women of child-bearing age, or females that might be exposed during pregnancy. Developmental toxicity is defined as the study of adverse effects on the developing organism that may result from exposure prior to conception (either parent), during prenatal development or postnatally to the time of sexual maturation (US EPA, 1991). It is reported that 50.7% of congenital malformations were estimated to have genetic or multifactorial causes, while 43.2% remain unknown; 3.2% were associated with exposure to exogenous agents and 2.9% to uterine factors (Nelson and Holmes, 1989). The most common manifestations of developmental toxicants in animals and humans include (1) intrauterine growth retardation or death, (2) structural abnormality, (3) altered growth, and (4) functional deficiency (US EPA, 1991). This emphasizes that structural malformations are not the only possible outcome after the fetus is exposed to a developmental toxicant; indeed, it is known that in many cases the outcomes are interrelated. For example, at a relatively high dose of a developmental toxicant, the conceptus might suffer a high level of cell death that cannot be fixed by available repair and compensatory mechanisms. This, in turn could result in growth retardation and death of the conceptus, if the induced cell death is widespread, and if the cell death compromises organ systems essential for viability of the conceptus, respectively. Also particular malformations and functional disorders might occur at lower doses; however, the outcome, or combination of outcomes, will depend on the dose, the chemical characteristics of the developmental toxicant and the developmental stage of the conceptus at the time of exposure (National Research Council, 2000).

We currently rely on animal testing to predict the potential for small molecules/biologics or chemicals to cause developmental toxicity in humans. Rats, mice and rabbits are the most relevant species used in developmental toxicity testing.

The ICH S5(R2) document entitled "Detection of Toxicity to Reproduction for Medicinal Products" describes that developmental and reproductive toxicity studies be performed to evaluate the potential adverse effects of a drug product on different segments of the reproductive cycle, defined as stages A–F. The studies are designed to identify the effects of drugs on mammalian reproduction and include exposure of mature adults, as well as all stages of development from conception to sexual maturity. The required developmental and reproductive toxicity studies are dictated by the clinical indication and intended patient population and because many biopharmaceuticals are species specific, they may induce immunogenicity and have a longer half-life; consequently alternate approaches may be needed to evaluate DART potential. For successful preclinical development, the most relevant species should be used in safety testing. A relevant species is defined as one in which the antibody is pharmacologically active and the target antigen is present or expressed and the tissue cross-reactivity profile is similar to humans (Chapman *et al.*, 2007).

The regulatory agencies around the world including the Food and Drug Administration (FDA) generally require developmental and reproductive toxicity testing of all new drugs to be used by women of child-bearing age or men of reproductive potential.

According to the International Conference for Harmonization (ICH S5 R2) guideline for the "Detection of toxicity to reproduction for medicinal products" the developmental and reproductive toxicity testing should entail the following assessments:

1. Study of fertility and early embryonic developmental to implantation (ICH 4.1.1).
2. Study for effects on pre- and postnatal development, including maternal function (ICH 4.1.2).
3. Study for effects on embryo–fetal development (ICH 4.1.3).

In small molecules rodents and/or rabbits are the most commonly used species for these studies. There are differences in the opinions of the regulatory authorities in the USA, Europe and Japan regarding the nature and amount of data from reproductive toxicity tests that should be available at the various stages of clinical development.

When ICH M3 was developed in 1997, there were several issues that were not harmonized. These include, but are not limited to, the timing of non-clinical safety studies for the conduct of clinical trials and the timing of each of the developmental and reproductive toxicity studies to conduct each phase of the clinical trials. However, the revised ICH M3 (R2) (2009) provides guidance with regard to timing of non-clinical studies for biotechnology-derived products relative to clinical development. The guidance document stresses that when the NHP is the only relevant species, the assessments of male and female fertility can be integrated in repeated toxicity studies of at least 3 months' duration in sexually mature animals. It also indicates that for monoclonal antibodies, for which embryo–fetal exposure during organogenesis is understood to be low in humans based on current scientific knowledge, the developmental toxicity studies can be conducted during Phase III and the final reports should be submitted with the marketing application. ICH M3 (R2) also states that for other biological compounds where embryo–fetal exposure is shown to be low during the period of organogenesis, the same timing for testing applies. This implies that despite the expected low maternal transfer of mAb or other biological compounds with lower exposure during the period of organogenesis in primate embryo–fetal development studies, it is still important to use study design that could detect hazards during the early embryonic development. Based on the pattern of placental transfer of IgG in humans, Pentšuk *et al.* (2009) recommended a study design that allows detection of both the indirect effects in early gestation plus the effects of direct fetal exposure in mid and late exposure. Such a study design characterized as an enhanced pre- and postnatal development was described by Stewart (2009). This design is particularly relevant to the risk assessment of mAbs where fetal exposure to maternal IgG increases as pregnancy progresses and where morphologic examination of a preterm fetus may not be adequate to reveal the presence of adverse effects on functional development of key target organs.

FERTILITY STUDY IN NHP

Fertility testing comprises evaluation of adverse effects on libido, sexual behavior, spermatogenesis, oogenesis, fertilization and implantation. According to the ICH M3 (R2) guidance, fertility assessment can be done in a rodent species for products where rodents are relevant species; however, depending on the nature of the compound the study is required to address the potential for immunogenicity. But when NHP is the only relevant species, the fertility assessment will be integrated in repeated dose toxicity studies of at least 3 months' duration using sexually mature NHPs. In contrast to rodent fertility study, it is recognized that mating is not practical for NHPs mainly due to low spontaneous conception rate (approx. 45%), litter size of usually one and the impossibility of assessing implantation sites. Because of these limitations, the fertility assessment in NHPs is focused on effects on reproductive potential rather than fertility *per se*.

Female fertility assessment

In female fertility assessment only sexually mature females and those who are regularly cycling should be used. A standalone female fertility study design or incorporation of female fertility parameters into a >3 month repeated toxicity study is illustrated in Figure 17.1. To assure sexual maturity a minimum age of ≥3 years with a body weight of 2.5 kg is recommended (Chellman *et al.*, 2009). The cynomolgus monkey has a menstrual cycle of 28–32 days' duration and a pre-study cycle monitoring of 2–3 months is necessary to select females with regular menstrual cycle prior to inclusion in the study. The number of animals per group should be at least eight for 3–4 groups with five females per group sacrificed at terminal necropsy and the remaining three animals per group used as a recovery. The duration of dosing should be at least 2–3 menstrual cycles. Parameters investigated include monitoring of menstrual cycle, weekly body weight, qualitative food consumption, clinical observations, TK and anti-drug antibody (ADA) determination, histopathology and hormone analysis such as ovarian hormones (progesterone and estrogen). Moreover, if needed, FSH, LH and inhibin A and B can also be analyzed and evaluated. Measurement of inhibin A and B to evaluate follicular and luteal phase can also be determined. Inhibins are important biomarkers of ovarian functions in monkeys and humans (Fraser and Lunn, 1999) and the macaques seem to be suitable models, because the expression of inhibin and activin subunits in their ovaries is similar to that in the human (Schwall *et al.*, 1990).

The ovarian cycle can also be traced by examining daily vaginal smears. Each female monkey is monitored daily using vaginal swabs to determine the onset, duration of menstrual bleeding, alteration and to allow the correlation with hormonal data. Chellman *et al.* (2009) in an excellent review elucidated the need for two study designs for blood schedule intended for hormonal analysis in female fertility testing. For designs incorporated into a chronic toxicity study, blood schedule for hormonal analysis would be three times per week for approximately 6 weeks conducted once during each phase of the study (pretreatment, dosing and recovery). For standalone designs blood collection is recommended to be every 2 days during follicular phase to ensure capture of the estrogen and LH peak and every 3 days during the luteal phase. It is therefore important that the study is scheduled with respect to the stage of menstrual cycle of the females to avoid collecting hormone samples from females with different menstrual cycle stages leading to the generation of data that is difficult to interpret. To circumvent such a problem at

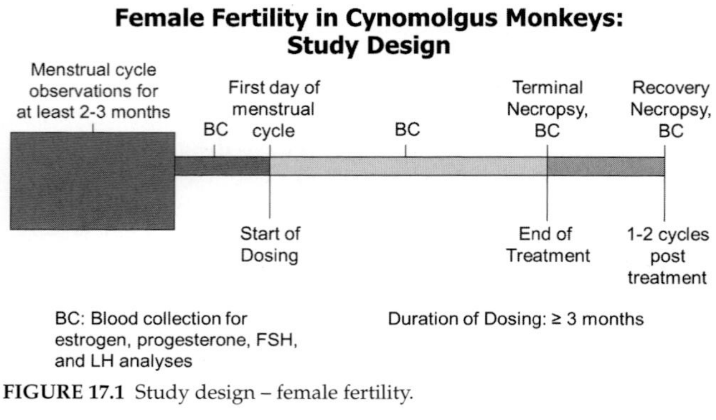

FIGURE 17.1 Study design – female fertility.

the end of the study it becomes essential to understand the hormonal regulation of the ovarian cycle to better interpret the hormone data. The menstrual cycle of mammals represents the integration of three very different cycles: (1) the ovarian cycle, the function of which is to produce a mature egg and release an oocyte, (2) the uterine cycle, the function of which is to provide the appropriate environment for implantation in the event of fertilization, and (3) the cervical cycle, the function of which is to allow sperm to enter the female reproductive tract only at the appropriate time as the cervix produces "fertile" cervical fluids that promote sperm movement and longevity. These three functions are integrated through the hormones of the pituitary, hypothalamus and ovary. In the adult ovary, folliculogenesis starts when follicles leave the pool of resting follicles to enter the growth phase. From there, the early growing follicle undergoes a developmental process including a dramatic course of cellular proliferation and differentiation. In primates, only one follicle commonly reaches the pre-ovulatory stage every cycle; most follicles fail to complete this maturation scheme, dying in a process termed atresia. Follicular growth and development are brought about by the combined action of FSH and LH on the follicular cells. The gonadotropin releasing hormone (GnRH), also called luteinizing hormone releasing hormone (LHRH), plays a key role in the regulation of mammalian reproduction. GnRH is secreted from the hypothalamus and stimulates the synthesis and release of the gonadotropic hormones LH and FSH from the pituitary gland. LH acts on ovarian theca cells which are the endocrine cells associated with ovarian follicles that play an essential role in fertility by producing the androgen substrate required for ovarian estrogen biosynthesis. Within the follicle, androgens act on the somatic granulosa cells and are converted by them into estradiol. FSH acts directly on the granulosa cells to stimulate follicular growth. Estrogens exert a positive feedback effect on gonadotropin release prior to ovulation and provoke the ovulatory LH peak, whereas during the postovulatory luteal phase and in the early follicular phase, estrogens inhibit gonadotropin levels. During the luteal phase, LH stimulates progesterone production leading to further negative feedback effects on gonadotropin secretion and, along with estrogen, is believed to result in the luteal inhibition of early follicular development (Figure 17.2; Weinbauer *et al.*, 2008b).

At necropsy anatomic pathology assessments, including macroscopic and microscopic pathology evaluation with special emphasis on female reproductive organs and additional tissues as needed, shall be conducted. TK studies are conducted in order to understand exposure, to allow cross-species comparisons and to predict margins of safety for clinical trials based on exposure. Toxicokinetic (TK) and ADA scheduled bleeding would be the first day and last day of dosing. The ADA screening is based on assessment to what extent antibody results are needed for the correct interpretation of the exposure and toxicity data.

Male fertility assessment

Males are particularly used in studies involving compounds that are developed in the field of male contraception and hormone therapy. The male fertility study can be conducted as a standalone study or the fertility endpoints can be incorporated into a >3 month repeated toxicity study (Figure 17.3).

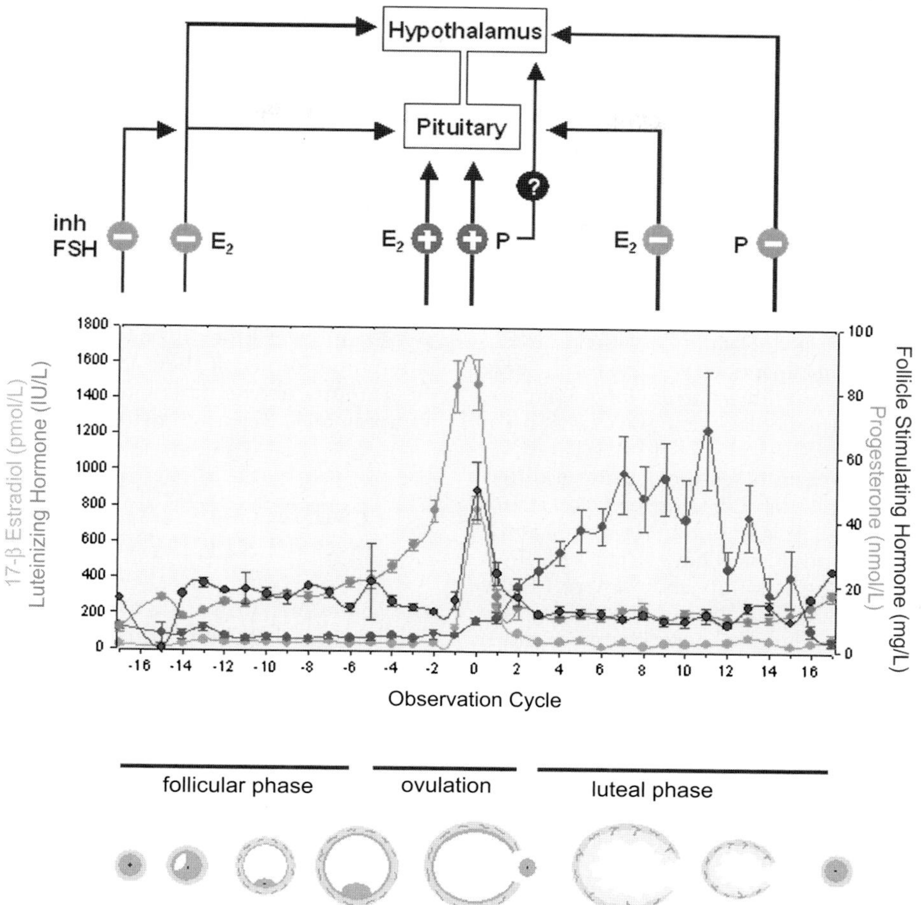

FIGURE 17.2 Endocrine profiles of estradiol (E2), LH, FSH and progesterone (P) during the ovarian cycle in the cynomolgus monkey and presumed feedback actions of ovarian hormones. The day of ovulation is denoted as zero, and days for follicular and luteal phases are counted relative to ovulation time point. Endocrine data represent $M \pm SD$ of 44 animals except for FSH with data from 14 animals. During ovulation, ovarian steroids are assumed to exert primarily a direct and positive feedback effect on pituitary gonadotropin secretion, whereas negative feedback actions occur during the follicular and luteal phases. Adapted from Weinbauer *et al.* (2008b) with permission.

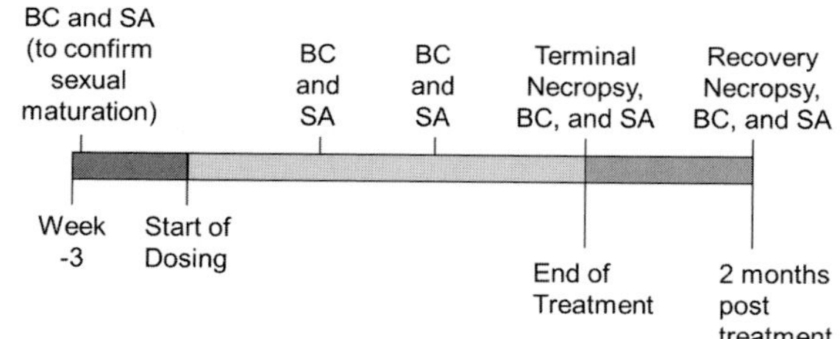

FIGURE 17.3 Study design – male fertility.

As in female fertility only sexually mature males should be used due to the small group sizes used and the difficulties of assessing pubertal status at the start of the study. Routinely it is common that animals of different maturity are assigned to dose groups in a non-random manner which makes differentiation of possible treatment-induced testicular toxicity from immaturity-related effects at the end of the study very difficult (Dreef *et al.*, 2007).

In male fertility studies, five animals per group at the end of dosing with 3–4 groups are considered to be appropriate. However, for biologics the use of two dose levels and a control may be sufficient. At least 60 days of dosing is required to address possible effects on all germ cells (Chellman *et al.*, 2009). The intention is to dose the animals for a complete spermatogenesis, the duration of which is estimated to be of 40–46 days in cynomolgus monkeys (Aslam *et al.*, 1999). A variety of parameters are routinely evaluated for male fertility, most of which correspond to clinical endpoints examined in human. These include testicular volume, ejaculate weight, sperm assessments including motility, morphology, sperm count, serum testosterone and histopathology of male reproductive organs such as testis and epididymis. In addition parameters such as daily sperm production, spermatogenesis staging and reproductive hormones (FSH, LH and inhibin) may be evaluated as needed.

Testicular volume is determined by measuring the length and the width of the testis in anesthetized animals and the following formula of an ellipsoid body is used to calculate the testicular volume (Kamischke *et al.*, 2002):

$$V(\mathrm{mL}) = w^2 \times 1 \times \pi / 6$$

Testicular volume can also be assessed by using an orchidometer. The orchidometer is a non-invasive measurement of testicular volume and was found to be a reasonable predictor of testicular weight and to rapidly measure of total testicular volume (Ku *et al.*, 2009). In a field investigation study performed in a Chinese breeding facility Korte *et al.* (1995) concluded that body weight, age, testicular volume and serum testosterone can be used as a good indicator of sexual maturation in males. Mature males are defined to be 4–5 years old with a body weight of >4.5 kg, a combined testicular volume of >10 mL and testosterone level of >15–20 mmol/L. However, prior to the inclusion of the male in the study the presence of sperm in the ejaculate should be confirmed. Data on variation in ejaculate quality showed that primate species with relatively large testes also produced ejaculates with relatively large volumes, high sperm counts, high sperm motility and more motile sperm (Moller, 2006).

Sperm is collected for sperm assessment using a different technique. In the authors' lab the direct penile electroejaculation technique is used. It is important to note that the technique used to collect sperm may have a marked effect on sperm viability, morphology, motility and number. Ideally the method used for semen collection should be repeatable and reliable and should not influence sperm characteristics.

Routinely the sperm number is determined in the hemocytometer chamber and the motility is quantified by computer assisted analysis (CASA) which produces reproducible and reliable results. The CASA analysis of sperm morphology is an integral part of a routine semen examination. Morphological changes in sperm tail are the most obvious abnormality observed in cynomolgus monkeys. Figure 17.4 depicts normal and some sperm tail abnormalities in cynomolgus monkeys.

However, the usefulness of sperm morphology assessment as a predictor of infertility has often been challenged due to different classification systems, slide preparation techniques and inconsistency of analyses within and between laboratories (Ombelet *et al.*, 1995). Histopathology is considered as the most sensitive endpoint for detecting testicular toxicity. However, identification and interpretation of chemically induced morphological changes in the testis require fundamental knowledge of spermatogenesis and its dynamics and regulation. Moreover, the ability to identify tubular stages of the spermatogenic cycle is essential to perform histopathological examination and to interpret the morphological changes observed.

Spermatogenesis in cynomolgus monkey is controlled by a complex hormonal interrelationship with testosterone and FSH acting directly on spermatogenesis in the Sertoli cells, while LH acts directly via testosterone produced by Leydig cells (Weinbauer and Nielschlag, 1998).

Determination of hormone levels is important to determine the effect of the protein therapeutics on fertility. Serum testosterone should be measured routinely, whereas the investigation of other hormones like LH and FSH should only be performed if there is an effect on testosterone and other reproductive parameters. Mating is conducted for approximately 8 h each day for 3 days.

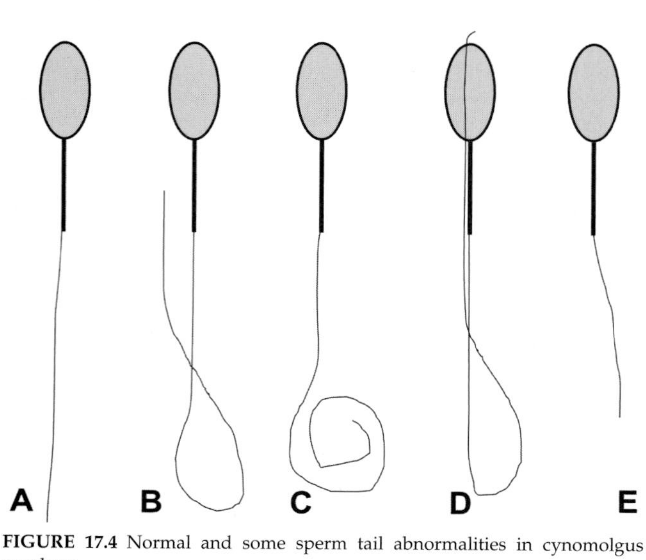

FIGURE 17.4 Normal and some sperm tail abnormalities in cynomolgus monkeys.

EMBRYO–FETAL DEVELOPMENT STUDY (ICH 4.1.3)

The non-human primate as an animal model for the study of developmental toxicity was recognized following the thalidomide tragedy. Table 17.1 illustrates key female reproductive parameters in NHPs and humans.

The objective of the embryo–fetal development study is to detect the adverse effects on the pregnant female and the developing embryo and fetus exposed during the period of organogenesis. In rodents and rabbits, this requires the investigation between implantation and closure of the hard palate; however, in cynomolgus monkeys the examination begins from the period of postimplantation to the closure of the hard palate. Sexually mature, female *Macaca nemestrina* macaques are used. The animals are handled humanely, and experiments performed within the National Institutes of Health's animal use guidelines. Ultrasounds are performed once as a part of pre-screening prior to breeding, after breeding and during gestation. The purpose of this pre-screening ultrasound is to evaluate reproductive organs, to ensure normal anatomy for the establishment and/or maintenance of pregnancy. The use of ultrasound postbreeding provides an efficient method of pregnancy detection, and

TABLE 17.1 Comparison of key female reproductive parameters in NHPs and humans

Parameters	Cynomolgus	*Human*
Puberty/sexual maturation (years)	2.5–4	*10–18*
Seasonality	All year – no seasonality	*All year – no seasonality*
Menstrual cycle length (days)	28–32	*28–30*
Ovulation period	Day 11–14	*Day 13–15*
Implantation window	Day 9–15	*Day 6–13*
Gestation length	160 (134–184 range observed extremes)	*280 (range of 259–294)*
Organogenesis	Weeks 3–7 (GD 20–50)	*Weeks 3–8*
Mean weight of offspring at term	Mean: 350 (range 325–375 g)	*Mean: 3400 g*
Number of offspring	*1 (twins frequency, 0.1%)*	*1 (twins frequency, 0.1%)*

Modified from Van Esch *et al.* (2008)

monitoring of the fetus during gestation. Vaginal bleeding is a common finding in macaques in early pregnancy, and can occur at the same time menses is expected, thus preventing the use of this finding to determine the pregnancy.

The study design for embryo–fetal development study in NHP includes monitoring of menstrual cycle, weekly body weight, qualitative food consumption, clinical observations, toxicokinetics (TK), hematology and clinical chemistry, anti-drug antibody determination and maternal immunological evaluation (Figure 17.5). Monitoring of the menstrual period for at least 3 months prior to mating is desirable. This is essential to estimate the ovulation period and critical to determine the optimal time of mating. Daily vaginal examinations are performed in order to detect the first day of menstrual bleeding which is considered day 1 of the cycle. Selection of dose levels poses a challenge in designing a proper developmental reproductive toxicity study. Usually a range-finding study is conducted in rodents prior to planning the definitive embryo–fetal developmental toxicity study. The main purpose of a range-finding study is to determine the dose levels for a subsequent developmental toxicity study. At least three dose levels and a concurrent control are used. Unless limited by physical or chemical properties, the high dose is selected to produce minimal maternal toxicity, including marginal but significant reduction of body weight, decreased weight gain or specific organ toxicity, and at the most produces no more than 10% mortality. The mid dose should produce minimal observable toxic effects. The low dose is expected to generally produce a no-observed-adverse-effect level (NOAEL) for maternal and developmental effects. Information on developmental effects may be of limited value or difficult to interpret if doses that cause excessive maternal toxicity are employed. The adequate dose limit under most circumstances should be 1,000 mg/kg/day (ICH S5, 1994).

For biologics two treatment groups and a control are considered acceptable. Dose selection is usually driven from general toxicity studies, but a range-finding study in pregnant females using ($n=5$/group) may be conducted (Chellman *et al.*, 2009). It might be possible to conduct the embryo–fetal development study using a control group and one dose group, provided there is a scientific justification for the dose level selected. An example of an appropriate scientific justification would be a monoclonal antibody which binds a soluble target and the clinical dosing regimen is intended to saturate target binding. If such a saturation of target binding can be demonstrated in the animal species selected and there is an up to 10-fold exposure multiple over therapeutic drug levels, a single dose level and control group would provide adequate evidence of a hazard to embryo–fetal development (ICH S6 [R1], 2009).

Due to large number of spontaneous abortions in cynomolgus monkeys, 12–14 pregnancies per group are considered to be sufficient. It is crucial to take into account the pregnancy loss (spontaneous abortion) when planning for group size in developmental toxicity testing. Females are bred mid cycle to proven male breeders 1–8 h/day for 3 consecutive days with the second day of mating considered to be gestation day (GD) 0. The pregnancy is confirmed on GD 18–20 using ultrasound. Pregnant animals are dosed from GD 20 to 50 and c-section is performed on GD 100. An ultrasound showing the presence of gestational sac confirms the pregnancy. The gestational sac is the earliest sonographic finding in pregnancy for cynomolgus monkeys. It does not correspond to specific anatomic structures, but is an ultrasonic finding characteristic of early pregnancy. Pregnancy status is monitored by ultrasound every 2 weeks beginning GD 18–50 and monthly from GD 51 to GD 100 under slight sedation. Due to a potential increase of fetal exposure to maternal IgG on late gestation (Buse, 2005), study designs that allow detection of both the indirect effects in early gestation plus the effects of direct fetal exposure in mid and late gestation are recommended for developmental toxicity of mAbs (Pentšuk and Van der Laan, 2009). As a result dosing should be extended to GD 90 or 100 for mABs (Chellmann *et al.*, 2009). Therapeutic mAbs are most commonly of the IgG1 subclass, which is transported most efficiently to the fetus. In all animal species used for testing developmental toxicity with the exceptions of rodents, fetal exposure to IgG is very low during the period of organogenesis (GD 20–50), but this increases during the second half of gestation to a point where the neonate is born with an IgG1 concentration similar to the mother (Pentšuk and Van der Laan, 2009). A placental transfer study can be conducted if there is a concern that the protein therapeutic may cross the placental barrier. Animals receive a single dose of the test article on GD 100 followed by the c-section at the half-life of the compound. Maternal blood can be collected at c-section; blood from umbilical cord or amniotic fluid can be analyzed to determine the concentration levels of the test article. Generally, the requirements for therapeutic proteins with respect to evaluating the toxicokinetics of the compound are the same as for small molecules, but specific considerations are needed related to the inherent characteristics of proteins. It is very important to determine exposure to the test agent; possible days of sampling are GD 20, GD 50, GD 100 or GD 140, with minimal sampling time points on each day as follows: prior to dosing, 6, and 24 hours post-dosing. For some agents that may elicit an immunogenic response, it may also be important to obtain blood samples for analysis of neutralizing antibodies to the test agent. This is intended to help determine if the compound is immunogenic and to consider potential impacts on the toxicokinetic parameters (Chellman *et al.*, 2009). Hematology and clinical chemistry are important tools for monitoring the onset, course and severity of the toxicity of the test article. It should be designed to meet specific study objectives. Potential hematological effects of the test compounds are identified primarily by evaluations of red blood cells (RBC), white blood cells (WBC), platelets in peripheral blood and evaluation of the bone marrow. The clinical pathology parameters should be fully considered at the time of protocol preparation to ensure these can be addressed.

Embryo-Fetal Development in Cynomolgus Monkey: Study Design

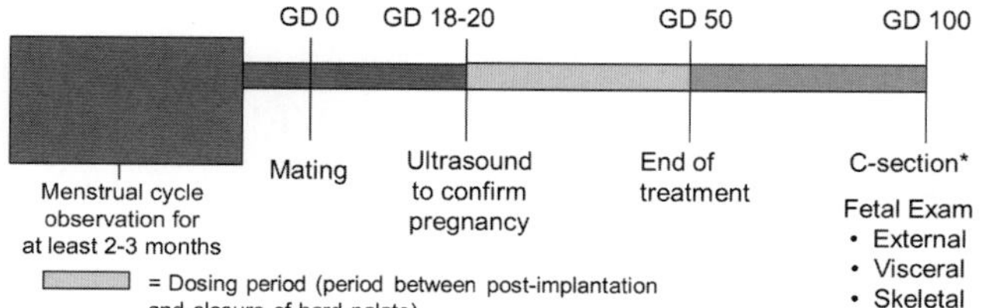

*C-section includes evaluations of amniotic fluid (volume, clarity), placenta (weight, number of disks, diameter of disk(s), appearance of maternal and fetal surfaces, location of cord insertion), and umbilical cord (length).

Note: Biopharmaceuticals (e.g. monoclonal antibodies) may require extended dosing up through GD 100 or later, C-section would then occur between GD 120 and 140.

FIGURE 17.5 Study design – embryo–fetal developmental toxicity.

On GD 100 cesarean section is performed and should the pregnant female show evidence of premature parturition, the fetus may be harvested prior to GD 100. Prior to gestation day 100, spontaneous loss may occur. Spontaneous loss can result in resorptions, early embryonic death (Figure 17.6) and or/abortions. Signs of looming abortion include the presence of heavy intrauterine bleeding and echogenic hematomas with or without the presence of viable fetus. Spontaneous abortion is defined as loss of an embryo or fetus on or prior to GD 100. The term is inclusive for both the embryonic loss and fetal death, which are defined as:

1. **Embryonic loss:** death and/or resorption of an embryo with no evidence of expulsion prior to completion of organogenesis period at GD 50
2. **Fetal death:** death of the fetus *in utero*, as indicated by either the absence of fetal heart beat or expulsion of the fetus after GD 50

At c-section (GD 100) anesthesia is induced and maintained and the animal is positioned in dorsal recumbency when performing c-section. A ventral midline laparotomy is then performed to expose the uterus. The body of the uterus is incised and the fetus and placenta identified and extricated. After evaluation of viability, each fetus will be euthanized by an intraperitoneal injection of sodium pentobarbital. When practical, the uterine incision will be closed in two layers, the second an inverting layer with absorbable suture. The abdomen may be lavaged with warm sterile 0.9% NaCl solution if gross contamination with uterine fluids occurred. The abdominal wall will be closed using an interrupted pattern with absorbable suture. The subcutaneous tissues and skin will be apposed in a routine manner, and the skin closed with skin glue or skin staples. Fetuses are evaluated for external, skeletal and soft-tissue anomalies.

Each fetus is weighed and the sex is determined by measuring ano-genital distance. The fetus is individually examined externally and the evaluation proceeds in an orderly manner as in rodents and rabbit fetuses. External examination may include measurements of crown–rump length, head circumference and long bone length. Fresh fetal dissection is performed for internal organ examination and this may include collection of fetal organs and histopathology and/or immunohistopathology evaluation of selected organs. Fetuses are stained with alizarin red for skeletal evaluation. To ensure all bones are seen clearly after staining, any remaining adipose tissue from the fetuses will be removed prior to the evaluation. For c-section performed late in pregnancy X-ray may be used for skeletal evaluation. For alizarin red staining the fetus is skinned, eviscerated and tagged prior to staining with alizarin red (Dawson, 1926). The procedure is similar to the one used to stain rats and rabbits with slight modification and involves placing the fetus in plastic containers filled with 95% of isopropyl alcohol for a minimum of 2 weeks. The alcohol is then drained off; the fetuses rinsed with tap water, drained and then placed in a 2% potassium hydroxide (KOH) solution for 24 hours in rats and up to 8 days in rabbits. The KOH is then drained off and fetuses are placed in 0.5% KOH and alizarin red solution (25 mg/L) for the same period of time as the 2% KOH. The staining solution is then poured off and replaced with 25% glycerin for 1 week, and is then placed in 1:1 solution of 70% ethanol/99.5 glycerin; the fetal skeleton can remain in this solution ad infinitum for evaluation and storage. The

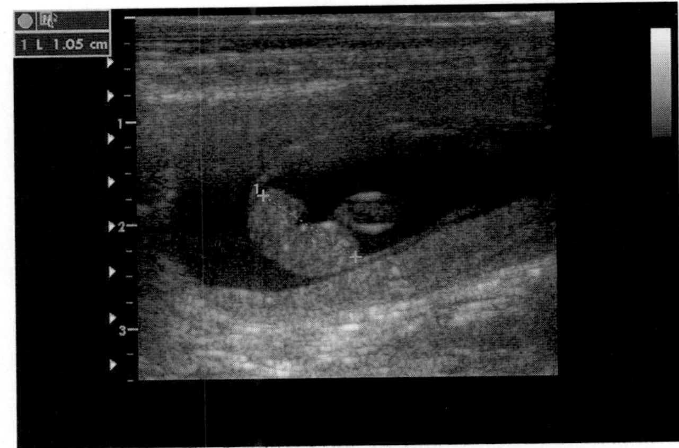

FIGURE 17.6 Ultrasound showing an embryonic death.

skeletal evaluation of fetal NHP poses some new difficulties. The amount of cleared tissue remaining after maceration is significant and needs to be carefully removed prior to the examination. This requires removal with patience and care to avoid damaging some of the skeletal structure. Also the position of the foramen magnum makes the attachment of the vertebral column to the base of the skull rather cumbersome compared to rat/rabbit fetuses. This requires also some careful manipulation to observe the cranial structure. Each fetus is individually examined for skeletal evaluation and the evaluation proceeds in an orderly manner from head to tail (Figure 17.7). The bones for each vertebra and the digits on the forepaws and hindpaws are counted and examined for abnormalities (Figures 17.8 and 17.9): Any deviations from the normal development of the bone and cartilage are recorded and classified into developmental malformations and variations. Table 17.2 shows skeletal enumerations by species.

The external, visceral and skeletal findings are classified as malformations or variations. A malformation is defined as a permanent (or irreversible) change in the species under investigation that is likely to affect survival or health, and variation is defined as a change that occurs within the normal population under investigation and is unlikely to adversely affect survival or health. This change may include a delay in growth or morphogenesis that has otherwise followed a normal pattern of development (Chahoud *et al.*, 1999). Background data collected between 1983 and 1996 showed that the malformation rate for the cynomolgus monkey was low (0.3%) and most of the observed malformations affected the musculoskeletal and cardiovascular systems, while a smaller number of defects were observed in the gastrointestinal, urogenital, endocrine and central nervous systems (Peterson, 1997).

PRE- AND POSTNATAL DEVELOPMENT, INCLUDING MATERNAL FUNCTION (ICH 4.1.2)

The primary focus for pre- and postnatal development, including maternal function study is to detect adverse effects on the pregnant/lactating female and development of the embryo/fetus and the offspring following exposure of the female to the test compound from implantation through weaning, with follow-up of the offspring through

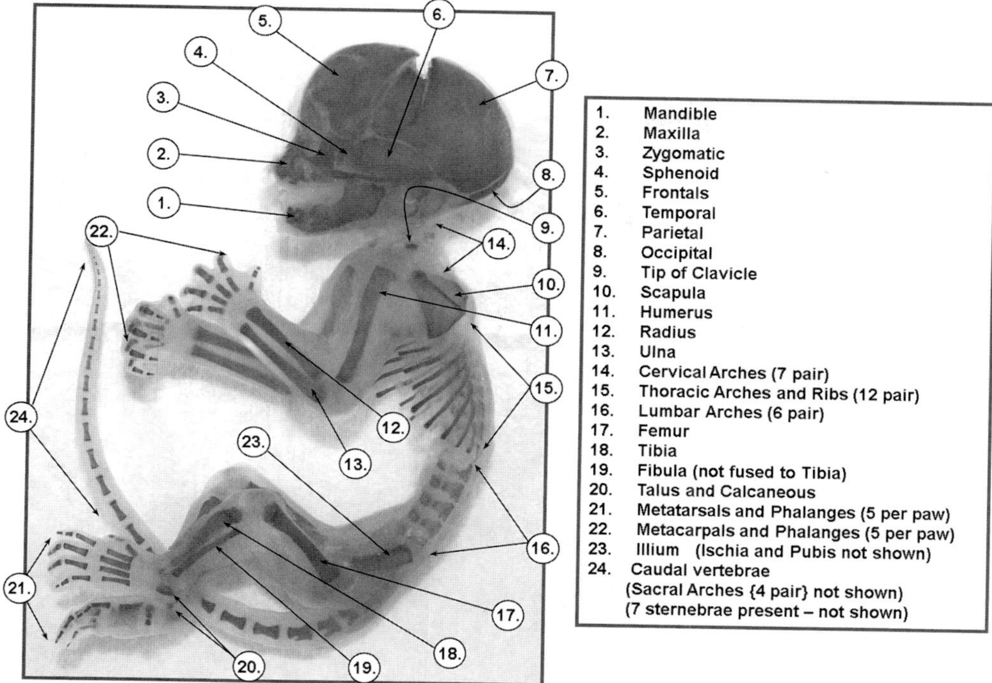

FIGURE 17.7 Alizarin stained fetal skeletal of cynomolgus monkey (GD 100). Please refer to color plate section.

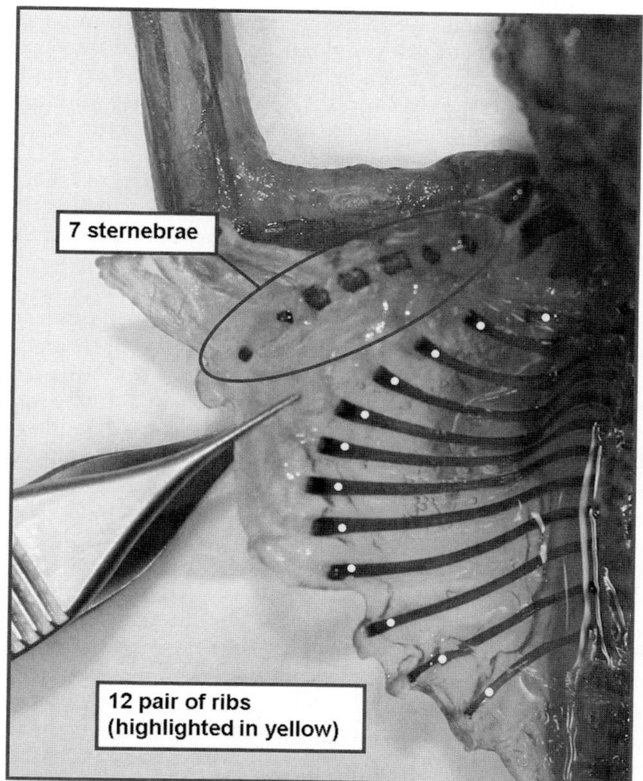

FIGURE 17.8 Fetus with normal sternebrae and ribs. Please refer to color plate section.

one generation. The rat is the species normally used for this type of study. In rats the F_1 evaluations include sexual maturation, neurobehavioral and fertility assessments. In cynomolgus monkeys sexual maturation does not occur until 3–6 years, therefore, it is unrealistic to follow up the offspring through sexual maturation and subsequently mating to assess fertility as this will take over 6 years of study duration. Because of these difficulties, Stewart (2009) proposed a study design that combines the embryo–fetal development study with the pre- and postnatal development (PPND) study into a single study called "enhanced" pre- and postnatal development (ePPND) study design in the cynomolgus monkey where a single cohort of animals is exposed throughout gestation and allowed to give birth naturally. This study design is particularly relevant for monoclonal antibodies where fetal exposure to maternal IgG is known to increase as pregnancy progresses and morphologic examination of a preterm fetus may not be adequate to reveal the presence of adverse effects on functional development of key target organs. This combined study design offers several advantages including the reduced use of animal number, economy and saving in time. However, the disadvantage is that if there is an increase in spontaneous abortions during the early or late of stage of gestation, then large animals may be needed to ensure a sufficient number of neonates for evaluation (Chellman *et al.*, 2009). The study design for the ePPD is illustrated in Figure 17.10. Selection of the animals in the study is similar to the procedure adapted in the embryo–fetal development study. Usually sexually mature animals are used in the study. Due to the large number of spontaneous abortions in cynomolgus monkeys, 16–20 pregnancies per group are considered to be sufficient. Dosing begins usually on GD 20 and continues through delivery, and infants are subsequently evaluated for growth and development.

Sex is determined on day 1 of birth. Although c-section is not performed to assess fetal morphology, early delivery and stillborn infants should be assessed for abnormalities. An ultrasound on late pregnancy should generate information

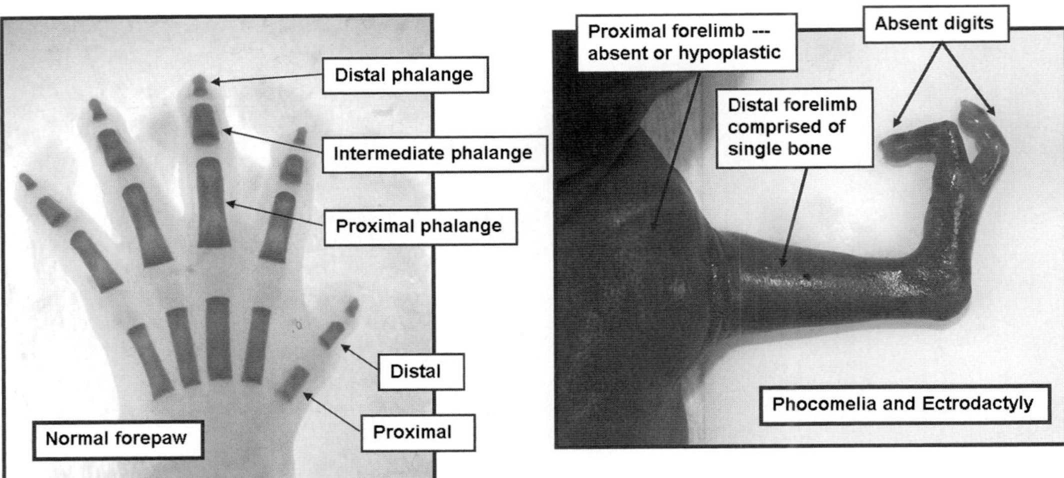

FIGURE 17.9 Normal forepaw, phocomelia and ectrodactyly.

TABLE 17.2 Skeletal enumeration: comparison between species

	Species			
	Primate	Rat	Rabbit	Canine
Cervical vertebrae	7	7	7	7
Sternebrae	7	6	6	8
Thoracic vertebrae and rib pairs	12	13	12	13
Lumbar vertebrae	6	6	7	7
Sacral vertebrae	4	4	4	3
Forepaws[a] (digits)	5	5	5	5
Hindpaws[a] (digits)	5	5	4	4

[a]Presence or absence of a dewclaw is considered normal and is not scored

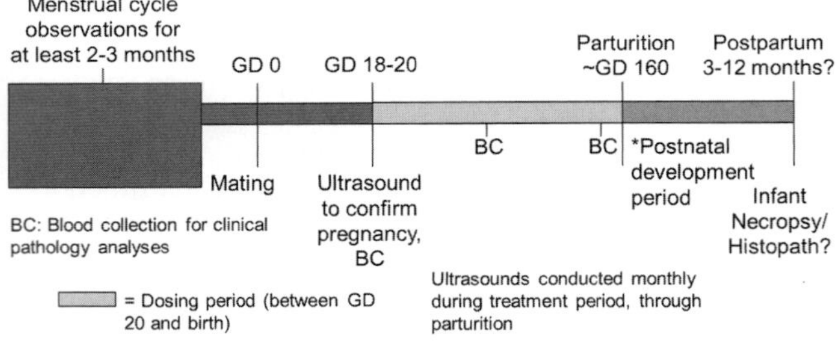

FIGURE 17.10 Study design: enhanced pre- and postnatal development (ePPD).

such as placental location, cervical softening and cervical length and fetal position status. Delivery can be expected within 24–48 hours if the cervix is found to be completely dilated. The day of parturition is considered to be Lactation Day (LD) 0 or Postnatal Day (PND) 0. After birth and during postnatal development the infant undergoes a series of postnatal assessments. The duration of postnatal assessment is variable, but may continue up to 6–9 months to assess specific functionality tailored to address particular concerns of the test article. Body weight is collected weekly or monthly and clinical signs of toxicity are observed twice daily in infants. Blood collection for clinical pathology can be performed monthly. There are several behavioral and functional development assays for neonatal NHP. The behavioral assessment panel available for the NHP is based primarily on the best known tool for assessing human neonates, known as the Brazelton Newborn Assessment Scale (BNAS) (Brazelton, 1984). Some of the available test battery for assessment of behavioral and functional development in cynomolgus monkey infant that is assessed on LD 1 and 7 includes clasp support, dorsireflex, grasp support, glabellar tap, rooting and the suckling reflex, moro reflex and visual following. Papillary reflex is assessed on PND 1 and 7 and if negative the test is repeated on PND 14. Grip strength is performed on PND 28. For learning ability the test is performed at the age of 6 and 9 months (Weinbauer *et al.*, 2008a).

In addition mother–infant interaction could be performed (beginning approximately at 3 months postpartum); immunophenotyping and functional assessment of the immune system could be performed in infants 3–4 months old. Mother–infant interactions can be assessed via video recording; separation and reunion of mother–infant are scored and which party initiates the interaction and how the other party reacts are scored as well. Differences in parenting style and hormonal variables in abusive and non-abusive rhesus macaque mothers were studied by Maestripieri and Magna (2000) during the first 2 months of lactation. They found that abusive mothers were more protective and more rejecting of their infants than non-abusive mothers, particularly in the first month. It was concluded that though pregnancy or lactation hormones are unlikely to be one of the main determinants of abusive behavior, endocrine variables may interact with personality characteristics or environmental factors in causing this phenomenon.

The functional assessment of the immune system involves several tests such as T-cell dependent antibody response (TDAR), NK-cell activity test and lymphocyte proliferation test. At the end of the study, F_1 animals undergo full necropsy; however, there is no consensus in the industry whether full histopathological evaluation should be performed at the terminal necropsy of the infants or not.

CONCLUDING REMARKS AND FUTURE DIRECTIONS

The preclinical safety testing of biotherapeutics poses a particular challenge in selecting a relevant animal species for use in toxicology studies. The most important consideration in species selection for biologics is to determine whether the drug is pharmacologically active in the preclinical species. This is very important because biotherapeutics are highly targeted and rarely, if ever, demonstrate off-target toxicity. The non-human primates are often the only relevant species that can be used to assess the safety of a biotherapeutics. Evaluation of developmental and reproductive toxicology (DART) endpoints is an integral part of the safety assessment for compounds with potential use in women of child-bearing age, or females that might be exposed during pregnancy. The non-human primate as animal models for the study of developmental toxicity was recognized following the thalidomide tragedy. Since then they have played important roles in both testing of drugs for human safety and as models for studying specific malformations commonly observed in children. Although safety testing in preclinical studies represents one of the major uses of non-human primates, in reality only few compounds are tested in NHPs. The NHP primates are not used as a second species for safety testing; they are only used in circumstances where no alternative methods are available and when testing is considered essential for safety assessment. Due to the technical, logistical challenges and the need of using fewer animals and based on the pattern of placental transfer of IgG in humans study, the trend in the future for mAbs will be the use of ePPD study design or a similar design that allows detection of both the indirect effects in early gestation plus the effects of direct fetal exposure in mid and late exposure which is particularly relevant to the risk assessments of mAbs.

ACKNOWLEDGMENT

I would like to thank Ms. Laura Ott and Mr. Steve Magness for their technical contribution to this project.

REFERENCES

Aslam H, Rosiepen G, Krishnamurthy H, Arslan M, Clemen G, Nieschlag E, Weinbauer GF (1999) The cycle duration of the seminiferous epithelium remains unaltered during GnRH antagonist-induced testicular involution in rats and monkeys. *J Endocrinol* **161(2):** 281-8.

Black A, Lane MA (2002) Nonhuman primate models of skeletal and reproductive aging. *Gerontology* **48(2):** 72–80.

Brazelton TB (1984) *Neonatal Behavioral Assessment Scale,* 2nd edition. Lippincott, Philadelphia.

Brodie AM, Hammond JO, Ghosh M, Meyer K, Albrecht ED (1989) Effect of treatment with aromatase inhibitor 4-hydroxandrostenedione on the non-human primate menstrual cycle. *Cancer Res* **49:** 4780–4.

Buse E (2005) Development of the immune system in the cynomolgus monkey: the appropriate model in human targeted toxicology? *J Immunotoxicol* **2(4):** 211-16.

Casadevall N, Nataf J, Viron B, Kolta A, Kiladjian JJ, Martin-Dupont P, Michaud P, Papo T, Ugo V, Teyssandier I, Varet B, Mayeux P (2002) Pure red-cell aplasia and antierythropoietin antibodies in patients treated with recombinant erythropoietin. *New Eng J* **346:** 469–75.

Chahoud I, Buschmann J, Clark R, Druga A, Falka H, Faqi A, Hansen E, Heinrich-Hisrch B, Hellwig J, Link W, Paumgarten F, Pfeil R, Platzek T, Scialli A, Seed J, Stahlmann R, Ulbrich B, Wu X, Yasuda M, Younes M, Solecki R (1999) Classificatory terms in developmental toxicology: need for harmonization. *Reprod Toxicol* **13:** 77–82.

Chamberlain P, Mire-Sluis AR (2003) An Overview of scientific and regulatory issues for the immunogenicity of biological products. In *Immunogenicity of Therapeutic Biological Products* (Brown F, Mire-Sluis AR, eds.). *Dev Biol.* Basel, Karger **112:** 3–11.

Chapman K, Pullen N, Graham M, Ragan I (2007) Preclinical safety testing of monoclonal antibodies: the significance of species relevance. *Nat Rev Drug Discov* **6:** 120–6.

Chellman GJ, Bussiere JL, Makori N, Martin PL, Ooshima Y, Weinbauer GF (2009) Developmental and reproductive toxicology studies in nonhuman primates. *Birth Defects Res B Dev Reprod Toxicol* **86(6)**: 446-62.

Chirino AJ, Ary ML, Marshall SA (2004) Minimizing the immunogenicity of protein therapeutics. Minimizing the immunogenicity of protein therapeutics. *Drug Discov Today* **9(2):** 82–90.

Dawson AB (1926) Note on the staining of skeleton of cleared specimens with Alizarin Red S. *Stain Technol* **1:** 123–4.

De Ruk E, Van Esch E (2008) The macaque placenta – a mini-review. *Toxicol Pathol* **36:** 108S–118S.

Dierschke DJ (1985) Temperature changes suggestive of hot flashes in rhesus monkeys: preliminary observations. *J Med Primatol* **14:** 271–80.

Dreef HC, Van Esch E, De Rijk EP (2007) Spermatogenesis in the cynomolgus monkey (*Macaca fascicularis*): a practical guide for routine morphological staging. *Toxicol Pathol* **35:** 395–404.

Ehmcke J, Wistuba J, Schlatt S (2006) Spermatogonial stem cells: questions, models and perspectives. *Hum Reprod Update* **12(3):** 275–82.

Fraser HM, Lunn SF (1999) Nonhuman primates and female reproductive medicine. In *Reproduction in Nonhuman Primates* (Weinabuaer GF, Korte R, eds.). Waxmann, Munster, pp. 27–59.

Ghosh D, Sengupta J (1992) Patterns of ovulation, conception and pre-implantation embryo development during the breeding season in rhesus monkeys kept under semi-natural conditions. *Acta Endocrinologica* **127(2):** 168–73.

Gordon TP (1981) Reproductive behavior in the Rhesus monkey: social and endocrine variables. *Am Zool* **21(1):** 185-95.

Hendrickx AG, Makori N, Peterson N (2000) Nonhuman primates: their role in assessing developmental effects of immunomodulatory agents. Hum Exp Toxicol **19:** 219–25.

Herndon, JG (2005). Seasonal breeding in rhesus monkeys: influence of the behavioral environment. *Am J Primatol* **5(3):** 197–204.

ICH S6 [R1] (2009) Preclinical Safety Evaluation of Biotechnology-Derived Pharmaceuticals, ICH S6 (R1), Current Step 2 version Parent Guideline dated July 16, 1997; Addendum dated October 29, 2009.

International Conference on Harmonization (ICH): Harmonized Tripartite Guideline "Detection of Toxicity to Reproduction for Medicinal Products" (59 FR 48746, September 22, 1994), http://www.fda.gov/cder/guidance/s5a.pdf

Jonker M (1990) The importance of non-human primates for preclinical testing of immunosuppressive monoclonal antibodies. *Semin Immunol* **2(6):** 427–36.

Kamischke A, Weinbauer G, Neischlag E (2002) Scrotal and transrectal ultrasonography in nonhuman primates. In: *Primate Models in Pharmaceutical Drug Development* (Korte R, Vogel F and Weinbauer G, eds). Waxmann Publishing Company, Munster, pp. 23–34.

Korte F, Vogel U, Zühlke W, Hofmann A (1995) Risk of invalid toxicity studies in the non-human primate due to improper selection of mature male animals. *Toxicologist* **15:** 248.

Ku W, Pagliusi F, Foley G, Roesler A, Zimmerman T (2009) A simple orchidometric method for the preliminary assessment of maturity status in male cynomolgus monkeys (*Macaca fascicularis*) used for nonclinical safety studies. *J Pharmacol Toxicol Methods* **61(1):** 32–7.

Maestripieri D, Megna NL (2000) Hormones and behavior in rhesus macaque abusive and nonabusive mothers. 2. Mother–infant interactions. *Physiol Behav* **71(1-2):** 43–9.

Moller AP (2006) Ejaculate quality, testes size and sperm competition in primates. *J Human Evolution* **17(5):** 479–88.

National Research Council (2000) Scientific Frontiers in Developmental Toxicity Risk Assessment. National Academy Press (Committee on Developmental Toxicology, Based on Environmental Studies and Toxicology, National Research Council), Washington DC, p. 361.

Nelson K, Holmes LB (1989) Malformations due to presumed spontaneous mutations in newborn infants. *N Engl J Med* **320**: 19–23.

Nichols SM, Bavister BD, Brenner CA, Didier PJ, Harrison RM, Kubisch HM (2005) Ovarian senescence in the rhesus monkey (Macaca mulatta). *Human Repro* **20(1):** 79–83.

Ombelet W, Menkveld R, Kruger TF, Steeno O (1995) Sperm morphology assessment: historical review in relation to fertility. *Human Repro Update* **1(6):** 543–57.

Pentšuk N, Van der Laan JW (2009) An interspecies comparison of placental antibody transfer: new insights into developmental toxicity testing of monoclonal antibodies. *Birth Defects Res (Part B)* **86:** 328–44.

Peterson PE, Short JJ, Tarara R, Valverde C, Rothgarn E, Hendrickx AG (1997) Frequency of spontaneous congenital defects in rhesus and cynomolgus macaques. *J Med Primatol* **26(5):** 267–75.

Schellekens H (ed.) (2002) Immunogenicity of therapeutic proteins: clinical implications and future prospects. *Clin Ther* **24:** 1720–40.

Schwall RH, Mason AJ, Wilcox JS, Bassett SG, Zeleznik AJ (1990) Localization of inhibin/activin subunit mRNAs within the primate ovary. *Mol Endocrinol* **4:** 75–9.

Shimizu K (2008) Reproductive hormones and the ovarian cycle in macaques. *J Mammal Ova Res* **25(3):** 122–6.

Stewart J (2009) Developmental toxicity testing of monoclonal antibodies: an enhanced pre- and postnatal study design option. *Repro Toxicol* **28(2):** 220–5.

Tarantal AF, Hendrickx AG (2005) Prenatal growth in the cynomolgus and rhesus macaque (Macaca fascicularis and Macaca mulatta): a comparison by ultrasonography. *Am J Primatol* **15(4):** 309–23.

US EPA (1991) Guidelines for developmental toxicity risk assessment. *Fed Reg* **56(234):** 63798–826.

Van Esch E, Buse E, Weinbauer GF, Cline JM (2008) The macaque endometrium, with special reference to the cynomolgus monkey (*Macaca fascicularis*). *Toxicol Pathol* **36:** 67S–100S.

Walker ML, Herndon JG (2008) Menopause in nonhuman primates? *Biol Repro* **79:** 398–406.

Weinbauer G, Nielschlag E (1998) The role of testosterone in spermatogenesis. In *Testosterone: Action, Deficiency, Substitution*, 2nd edition (Nielschlag, E., Behre HM, eds.). Springer, Berlin, Heidelberg, New York, pp. 143–68.

Weinbauer GF, Frings W, Fuchs A, Niehaus M, Osterburg I (2008a) Reproductive/developmental toxicity assessment of biopharmaceuticals in nonhuman primates. In *Preclinical Safety Evaluation of Biopharmaceuticals: A Science-based Approach to Facilitating Clinical Trials* (Cavagnaro J, ed.). John Wiley & Sons, Inc.

Weinbauer GF, Niehoff M, Niehaus M, Srivastav SH, Fuchs A, Van Esch E, Cline JM (2008b) Physiology and endocrinology of the ovarian cycle in macaques. *Toxicol Pathol* **36:** 7S–23S.

Wilson JG, Gavan JA (1967) Congenital malformations in nonhuman primates: spontaneous and experimentally induced. *Anat Rec* **158(1):** 99–109.

CHAPTER

18

Developmental immunotoxicity testing

Susan L. Makris and Scott Glaberman

Disclaimer. The views expressed in this chapter are those of the authors and do not necessarily reflect the views or policies of the US Environmental Protection Agency.

INTRODUCTION

A great deal of concern has been expressed regarding the need for the identification and characterization of the potential for developmental immunotoxicity following exposures to environmental contaminants, including pesticides, industrial chemicals and pollutants (NRC, 1993). Within the past several decades, an ever-growing body of research has identified developmental immunotoxicity outcomes for a broad list of substances. These include metals (arsenic, cadmium, lead, manganese and mercury), polycyclic aromatic hydrocarbons, polycyclic chlorinated biphenyls, dioxin, tributyltins, environmental tobacco smoke, atrazine and bisphenol-A (Dietert and Dietert, 2007).

Developmental immunotoxicity is defined as adverse effects on immune system structure or function following exposures occurring during pre- and/or postnatal ontogeny. Some outcomes may be expressed immediately; others may be observed at a later time point or life stage. The developing immune system is generally considered to be of equal or greater sensitivity to perturbation than that of the mature individual. Age-related differences in susceptibility to developmental immunotoxicants may be expressed qualitatively or quantitatively. Some effects may be transient, while others may be permanent, and there can be a range of severity of effects.

DEVELOPMENT OF THE IMMUNE SYSTEM

Development of the vertebrate immune system involves a complex series of events spanning many organs, tissues and cell types. There is growing consensus that disruption of this process at any number of stages can result in severe or persistent effects on postnatal immune system function. Concern for developmental immunotoxicants has stimulated numerous articles and several consensus workshops aimed at reforming testing protocols so that they can adequately evaluate these effects (Holsapple, 2002; Luster *et al.*, 2003; Holsapple *et al.*, 2005). This chapter is aimed at providing a foundation for understanding why developmental toxicity is a concern and how existing and prospective frameworks are aimed at addressing this issue.

In order to evaluate existing and potential developmental immunotoxicity testing (DIT) schemes, we must first consider the cascade of developmental events that may lead to immune dysfunction if disturbed. While we are ultimately concerned with toxicity to humans, the majority of immunology data comes from rodents, especially mice, as well as from several other model vertebrate species. In this chapter, the initial goal is to provide a background of immune ontogeny in rodents and humans. In most cases, the sequence of developmental events is similar between the two groups. However, since rodent gestation is vastly shorter than in humans – approximately 21 days and 40 weeks, respectively – special attention is paid to relative rather than absolute differences in timing. Developmental landmarks are given in gestational days (GD) or weeks (GW), as well as postnatal days (PND) or weeks (PNW). More detailed comparisons of immune development between model vertebrate species can be found elsewhere (Barnett, 1996; Holladay and Smialowicz, 2000; Felsburg, 2002; Landreth, 2002; West, 2002; Holsapple *et al.*, 2003b; Landreth and Dodson, 2005; Dietert and Piepenbrink, 2006; Burns-Naas *et al.*, 2008).

Immune organs and cells

Immune cells and organs function in an integrated manner, and therefore at least some knowledge of the various immune system components is helpful for assessing potential targets of immunotoxicity. Leukocytes are the major class of immune cells, and together with erythrocytes they derive from the same set of totipotent hematopoietic stem cells (HSC) (Micklem *et al.*, 1966; Prchal *et al.*, 1978). HSC have the capacity for self-renewal and give rise to a series of increasingly lineage-restricted cell lines. Lymphoid stem cells are one of the two main HSC subsets, and ultimately differentiate into B and T lymphocytes and natural killer (NK) cells. Myeloid stem cells, on the other hand, give rise to monocytes,

Reproductive and Developmental Toxicology, Edited by Ramesh C. Gupta
ISBN: 978-0-12-382032-7

dendritic cells, granulocytes (basophils, eosinophils, and neutrophils), mast cells, as well as erythrocytes and platelets. The bone marrow and thymus are considered the two primary immune organs in mammals, providing the essential microenvironment for the differentiation and maturation of immune cells. The bone marrow is the main site of hematopoiesis in adults, including all the major blood cell types, while the thymus is responsible for T-cell development. There are also several peripheral immune organs and tissues including the spleen, lymph nodes and gut-associated lymphoid tissue (GALT). They are often populated by mature immune cells and serve as centers of pathogen defense and reactivity.

Hematopoietic stem cell development and migration

During ontogeny, uncommitted hematopoietic precursors first appear in the yolk sac (R: GD 7, H: GW 2–3) (Moore and Metcalf, 1970; Tavian *et al.*, 1999; Cumano and Godin, 2007) and are found soon after in the intraembryonic tissue surrounding the heart (R: GD 8; H: GW 4–6) (Muller *et al.*, 1994; Tavian *et al.*, 1999; Cumano and Godin, 2001). The latter site is now viewed to be the definitive source of HSC for the developing fetus (Cumano and Godin, 2001). HSC then migrate to the fetal liver (R: GD 10; H: GW 5–6) and spleen (R: GD 13; H: GW 10–12), where they accumulate and begin differentiating into lineage-restricted stem cells, which have the capacity to self-renew, as well as progenitor cells, which can proliferate but not self-renew (Hann *et al.*, 1983; Tavassoli, 1991; Godin *et al.*, 1999; Holt and Jones, 2000; Cumano and Godin, 2001). At this point, the liver serves as the primary hematopoietic organ and the source of HSC and progenitor cells to the primary and secondary immune organs and tissues, where they eventually mature into the full range of lymphoid and myeloid cell lines (Tavassoli, 1991). A key difference between rodent and human immune development is that, in the former, the central hematopoietic role of the liver continues until around the end of gestation (GD 18), when it rapidly shifts toward metabolic function (Owen *et al.*, 1974, 1977). Conversely, in humans, hematopoiesis begins transitioning from the liver to the bone marrow at around GW 11–12, and the bone marrow is nearly completely responsible for hematopoiesis by GW 20, well before parturition (Tavassoli and Yoffey, 1983; Cooper and Nisbet-Brown, 1993; Rolink *et al.*, 1993). The spleen plays a minor role in gestational hematopoiesis compared to the liver, but it functions well into postnatal life and can serve as a reservoir of HSC following damage to the bone marrow (Landreth and Dodson, 2004).

Bone marrow and leukocyte development

The bone marrow is the focal site of hematopoiesis in adult life and is the primary source of uncommitted stem cells as well as myeloid and lymphoid precursors (Cumano and Godin, 2001). It is also inhabited by several other cell types that are essential for hematopoiesis, particularly fibroblastic stromal cells and endothelial cells. They provide the necessary microenvironment, including expression of cytokines (e.g., GM-SF, IL7) and adhesion molecules (CD44, VCAM-1), which allow immune cells to differentiate and mature (Mudry *et al.*, 2000; Banfi *et al.*, 2001). When the bone marrow is sufficiently developed, it is colonized by HSC and precursors primarily from the fetal liver and rapidly assumes hematopoietic function thereafter. Once leukocytes reach maturity in the bone marrow, they migrate to the secondary immune organs via the blood.

Since the bone marrow develops much earlier in humans than in rodents relative to parturition, the developmental timing of various leukocyte progenitors differs between these groups. In rodents, pro-/pre-B lymphocytes (surface IgM^{-}) are detected in the fetal liver at approximately GD 11–14 where they expand until the end of gestation. B cells first appear in the bone marrow at GD 19, which is around the time of birth, and continue to increase in numbers during the first several months of postnatal life (Velardi and Cooper, 1984). In humans, on the other hand, pro-/pre-B cells are already found in the fetal liver of humans by GW 8 and become abundant in the bone marrow between GW 16 and 20, which is approximately halfway through gestation (Andersson *et al.*, 1981; Holladay and Smialowicz, 2000; Holt and Jones, 2000). Nevertheless, most B cells produced in the human bone marrow before birth are relatively immature and do not express the various immunoglobulin types that are required for host defense. Also, surface marker data from the CD5 antigen show that human B-cell populations or subtypes change dramatically between neonate and adult stages (Hannet *et al.*, 1992). Thus, while B-cell development at parturition is further along in humans than in rodents, additional events during the first months or years of life are still necessary to reach full immunocompetence.

Likewise, expression patterns of immunoglobulins (Ig) are also immature at birth in humans. Although Ig molecules have been detected quite early in development (e.g., IgM/IgE at GW 10–12), their levels fluctuate throughout gestation and are very low at parturition (Miller *et al.*, 1973; Holladay and Smialowicz, 2000; Holt and Jones, 2000). Adult levels of IgM, IgG and IgA are not reached until 1–2, 5–6 and 10–12 years, respectively (de Muralt, 1978; Miyawaki *et al.*, 1981; Vetro and Bellanti, 1989).

Other important activities in the bone marrow exhibit similar timing differences between rodents and humans. In the former, production of granulocytes begins to accelerate in the bone marrow around the time of birth, while in humans, granulocytes begin developing long before parturition, but remain functionally immature and in low numbers (Holladay and Smialowicz, 2000). Erythropoietic activity also begins postnatally in the mouse bone marrow, but well before birth in humans. In humans, there is a steep decline in NK cell abundance after birth (de Vries *et al.*, 2000). This suggests that these cells play an important role during pregnancy. This is not the case in rodents.

Thymus and T-cell development

The thymus is the major site of T-lymphocyte development in mammals. Notable events in T-cell maturation include positive and negative selection of thymocytes, formation and expression of a diverse T-cell receptor (TcR) repertoire, and expression of surface markers that represent various stages of lineage commitment (e.g., Thy1, CD2, CD3, CD4, CD8). The thymus contains two regions, the cortex and the medulla. The cortex is the major site of cell proliferation as well as positive selection. During positive selection, thymocytes interact closely with cortical epithelial cells and undergo apoptosis if they fail to recognize self-derived peptides paired with major histocompatibility complex (MHC) receptor molecules. Negative selection, on the other hand, occurs primarily at the cortico-medullary boundary, and involves removal of thymocytes that react with self-peptide fragments (Janeway *et al.*, 2005).

The thymus begins forming early in development and is immediately colonized by uncommitted stem cells and T-lymphocyte progenitors from the fetal liver or bone marrow (R: GD 9–11; H: GW 9) (Kay *et al.*, 1962; Owen and Raff, 1970; Velardi and Cooper, 1984; Adkins *et al.*, 1987; Haynes *et al.*, 1988; von Gaudecker, 1991). Shortly after, thymocytes begin expressing CD4 and CD8 membrane molecules (R: GD 13–14; H: GW 10) as well as functional TcR (R: GD 16–17; H: GW 9–10) (Lobach and Haynes, 1987; Tentori *et al.*, 1988; Teh, 1993; Ridge *et al.*, 1996; Holladay and Smialowicz, 2000). Around this time, cortical and medullary compartments form in the thymus (R: GD 13–14; H: GW 11–14) (Holsapple *et al.*, 2004). In humans, positive and negative selection have both largely completed before birth, while it continues in rodents throughout the first few weeks of neonatal life. Finally, mature $CD4^+$ or $CD8^+$ thymocytes begin leaving the thymus for the periphery (R: around birth; H: GW 13) (Bogue *et al.*, 1992).

The delay in thymus and T-cell development in rodents as compared to humans parallels the situation in the bone marrow. Most key lymphocyte developmental processes take place in the first trimester in humans, but in the second half of gestation in rodents. Moreover, the human thymus is fully formed at birth, while in rodents it continues to develop postnatally for several weeks (Janeway *et al.*, 2005).

Thymus size and cellularity are at their maximum just after parturition and the organ significantly involutes when sexual maturity is reached (R: PNW 8–10; H: 10–12 years). Consequently, removal of the thymus in adults does not significantly affect cell-mediated immune function (Janeway *et al.*, 2005). Cell-mediated immunity persists in adults because T cells are often long-lived cells and most immune functions consist of further division of available T cells or activation of circulating T memory cells. More in-depth information about the process and timing of rodent and human T-cell development can be found elsewhere (West, 2002).

Peripheral immune organs and maturation of immune system

Lymphocytes mostly develop in the bone marrow and thymus, but complete their functional maturation in the periphery, where they come in contact with antigens. This generally occurs after birth when the host is exposed to antigenic environment. The peripheral immune organs include the spleen, lymph nodes and gut associated lymphoid tissues, which include Peyer's patches, lamina propria and appendix. All of these begin forming around the same time (R: GD 10–15; H: GW 8–14) (Landreth and Dodson, 2004; Leibnitz, 2004).

During the first month of life in rodents, there is significant maturation of the immune system. At this point, there is clear response to antigens and an array of different antibodies are produced (Raff, 1970). Humans are already fairly mature at birth, but T-cell activity and inflammatory responses, and antibody production are still at lower levels than in adults (Peakman *et al.*, 1992; Leibnitz, 2004).

Th1/Th2 balance

Three main types of T helper cells develop in the fetus that have different functions and are associated with different cytokines. Th1 cells are generally involved in cell-mediated immunity, including "removal of malignant or afflicted cells", and secrete IL-2, IFN-γ and TNF-β (Mosmann and Coffman, 1989). Th2 cells are more involved in the proliferation of B cells in response to extracellular antigens and are associated with IL-4, IL-5, IL-6 and IL-10. Th17 cells secrete IL-17, which promotes proinflammatory pathways and the migration of neutrophils into tissues (Bettelli *et al.*, 2008). Special focus has been placed on balance in number and function of Th1 and Th2 subsets before and after parturition. It is hypothesized that Th1 activity is generally suppressed in mother and fetus during gestation in order to minimize allogeneic rejection (von Freeden *et al.*, 1991; Adkins *et al.*, 2001). At birth, this typically becomes more balanced, since both pathways are necessary to deal with the diverse antigens in the external environment. However, there is growing evidence that disruption of certain events during pregnancy can delay or exaggerate this transition leading to short-term or long-term immune dysfunction (Holt and Sly, 2002). Continued overemphasis of Th2 activity has been linked to atopy, eczema and asthma, and is associated with activity of IgE, which is a product of Th2-mediated B-cell function (Humbert *et al.*, 1999). On the other hand, a skew toward Th1 function after birth is related to organ-specific autoimmune diseases such as multiple sclerosis and type 1 diabetes (Kidd, 2003). It should be noted that the significance of the Th1/Th2 paradigm is still being unraveled, and its role in immune dysfunction is under active debate (Kidd, 2003).

DEVELOPMENTAL IMMUNOTOXICITY TESTING PARADIGM

Developmental immunotoxicity is an issue of importance for the hazard screening and risk assessment of environmental chemicals. The need for DIT screening was raised by the National Research Council in the landmark report on "Pesticides in the Diets of Infants and Children" (NRC, 1993). Consideration of DIT in risk assessment was further influenced by the passage of the Food Quality Protection Act (FQPA), an amendment to the Federal Insecticide, Fungicide and Rodenticide Act (1996). The FQPA mandated the characterization of risk to infants and children for pesticides with tolerances and required the application of a 10-fold safety factor when toxicity and exposure data were insufficient to fully assess safety. Further emphasis was given to the adequacy of children's health risk assessment for environmental chemicals in an Executive order signed into law by President Clinton in 1998. This law mandated that all federal agencies address risks to children. To date, no standard guideline protocol has been implemented by EPA or OECD for developmental immunotoxicity testing, either for pharmaceuticals or environmental chemicals. However, numerous discussions on this topic have been held by interagency participants in a public forum, and three collaborative scientific workshops have been conducted with the goal and intent of addressing the best approaches and methods for the assessment of DIT (Table 18.1). They incorporated information from a previous US EPA effort addressing critical windows of susceptibility,

TABLE 18.1 Select historical landmarks in the development of a framework for DIT assessment of environmental toxicants (Burns-Naas *et al.*, 2008)

Year	Event	Impact/Conclusions	Reference
1993	NRC publication: *Pesticides in the Diet of Infants and Children*	Recommended testing; acknowledged age-related susceptibility and recommended DIT assessment	NRC, 1993
1996	EPA legislation: Food Quality Protection Act; Safe Drinking Water Act Amendment	Required characterization of susceptibility and assessment of risk for infants and children	USEPA, 1996
1997	Executive Order 13045	Required federal agencies to address risks to children	Federal Register Vol. 62, No. 78 April 23, 1997
2001	ILSI/HESI DIT workshop	Proposed approaches to DIT testing; identified issues for further resolution	Holsapple, 2003a
2001	NIEHS/NIOSH DIT workshop	Defined appropriate experimental design for DIT testing, including limitations and data gaps	Luster *et al.*, 2003
2003	ILSI/HESI DIT workshop	Proposed framework for DIT testing	Holsapple *et al.*, 2005

NRC = National Research Council of the National Academies of Science
ILSI/HESI = International Life Science Institute, Health and Environmental Science Institute
NIEHS = National Institute of Environmental Health Science
NIOSH = National Institute of Occupational Safety and Health

which focused on the timing of perturbation for the development of various organ systems, including the immune system (Dietert and Dietert, 2007; Holladay and Smialowicz, 2000). The subsequent DIT workshops addressed a framework for testing, developing scientific consensus on general approaches and on specific issues, characterizing normal immune system development in humans and test animal models, and identifying critical windows of developmental exposure for the perturbation of immune system structure or function (Holsapple, 2002; Luster *et al.*, 2003; Holsapple *et al.*, 2005).

The workshop efforts, which addressed testing needs for both pharmaceutical and environmental chemicals, focused on the development of a protocol that could be used to screen offspring for immunosuppressive effects following chemical exposure during immune system development (Burns-Naas *et al.*, 2008). A DIT study can be conducted independently, or to reduce the use of test animals and refine the testing paradigm it may be possible to incorporate DIT assessments into another protocol, e.g. a reproduction study.

In a typical standalone DIT screening study (Figure 18.1), maternal rats would be administered a test substance from at least the time of implantation (approximately gestation

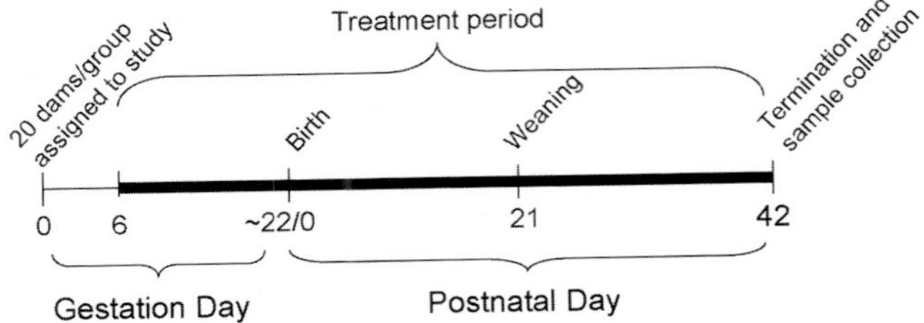

FIGURE 18.1 Developmental immunotoxicity study (From Holsapple *et al.*, 2005).

TABLE 18.2 Recommended DIT study endpoints

General observations	Immune system assessments (at approx. PND 42)
Body weight	Complete total and differential blood cell count
Survival	Organ weights (thymus, spleen and lymph nodes)
Clinical observations	Primary antibody response to a T-dependent antigen
Macroscopic pathology	Functional test of Th1 immunity (e.g., cytotoxic T lymphocyte or delayed hypersensitivity response)

day 6) to parturition and into the lactation period. It is critical to the sensitivity and veracity of the study that the offspring be continuously treated during all critical phases of immune system development. Therefore, test substance administration would be scheduled to continue in the offspring, whether via maternal milk (as confirmed by pharmacokinetic data) and/or directly to the offspring by the most appropriate method, through the time of weaning (i.e., PND 21) and until approximately PND 42. By that age, the offspring would be sexually mature young adults with a fully functional immune system; at that time, the offspring would be terminated for evaluation of immune system organs, tissues and function. Endpoints recommended by workshop participants for evaluation in a DIT study are summarized in Table 18.2. These endpoints, considered together, assess the primary aspects of immune system development in the rodent.

Since the workshops on DIT testing were conducted, another protocol has been proposed that also addressed DIT assessment. The concept of an extended one-generation reproduction study was raised in an International Life Sciences Institute (ILSI) Agricultural Chemical Safety Association (ACSA) effort (Cooper *et al.*, 2006) that focused on creating an alternative reproductive/developmental toxicity screening study that maximized the amount of relevant information generated across specific critical and potentially susceptible life stages. Additional goals of the effort were to reduce the number of animals and other resources required and limit the redundancy that inevitably arose when utilizing multiple study protocols for toxicological screening. As a result of extensive discussion and international efforts to further develop this study design for regulatory purposes, a collaborative OECD/EPA draft extended one-generation study design has been released for review and comment (OECD, 2009). This study, which is illustrated in Figure 18.2, is conducted using three cohorts of F_1 animals. In Cohort 1, reproductive and developmental endpoints are assessed. Cohort 1 animals are exposed to the test substance for

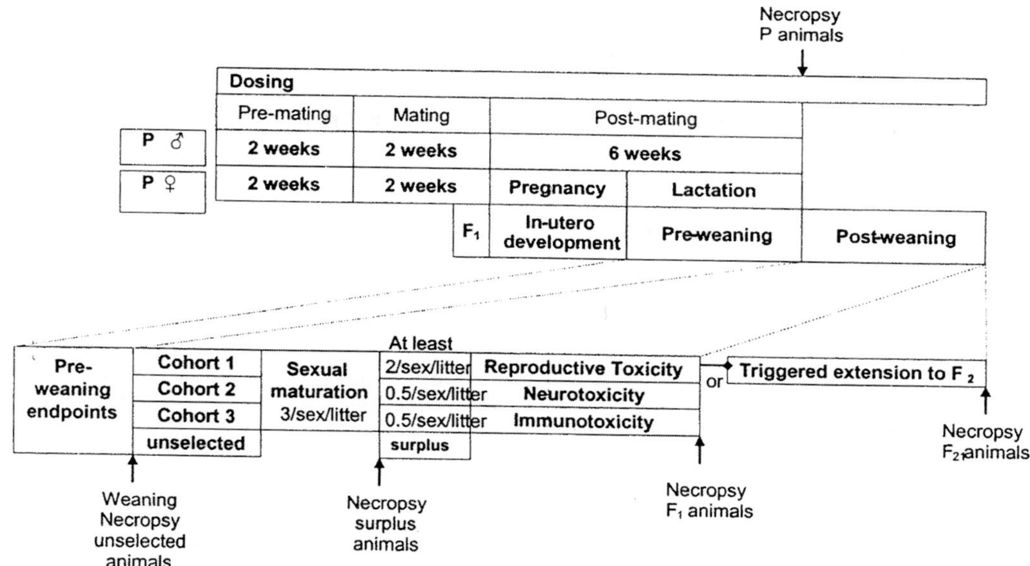

FIGURE 18.2 Extended one-generation reproduction study (From OECD, 2009).

approximately 13 weeks, and this cohort may be extended to include an F_2 generation, dependent upon available background data and/or observations recorded during the in-life phase of the study. Cohort 2 assesses the potential impact of the test substance on the developing nervous system, while Cohort 3 assesses the potential impact on the developing immune system. In concept, this extended one-generation study might, in some situations, replace the two-generation reproduction and fertility effects study and the standalone guideline developmental neurotoxicity study in a future regulatory context. The inclusion of a developmental immunotoxicity cohort is unique and important because (1) as mentioned above, there is currently no standalone EPA or OECD DIT study guideline, although a framework for this type of study has been developed (Holsapple, 2002; Luster *et al.*, 2003; Holsapple *et al.*, 2005; Burns-Nass *et al.*, 2008), and (2) the assessment of developmental immunotoxicity is recognized as important to the adequate evaluation of children's health risk (Dietert and Piepenbrink, 2006; Dietert and Dietert, 2007; Makris *et al.*, 2008). Another important aspect of the extended one-generation reproduction study is the explicit directive to consider toxicokinetic (TK) data in designing the study, selecting dose levels and interpreting results. While the collection and use of TK data in studies that include early life stage exposures have been encouraged for many years (Barton *et al.*, 2006), inclusion in the extended one-generation study protocol provides additional prominence to the concept. The extended one-generation reproduction study protocol also includes enhanced assessment of endocrine endpoints, including thyroid hormone levels (which are not evaluated in the typical two-generation reproduction study).

ISSUES FOR RISK ASSESSMENT

Based upon evidence that the developing immune system is more sensitive to toxic insult than the mature immune system, the use of a developmental screening paradigm to characterize potential immunosuppression may be preferable to the use of a protocol that includes only adult animals (Dietert and Piepenbrink, 2006; Luebke *et al.*, 2006). It is also noted that this study design does not evaluate other perturbations of immune function that are important to human health risk assessment (e.g., asthma, autoimmunity and hypersensitivity), nor does it assess latent responses to developmental insult (e.g., in elderly animals). Nevertheless, the DIT study assesses both structural and functional alterations to the developing immune system, utilizing a juvenile animal model, and thus is unique and valuable to children's health risk assessment.

In conducting risk assessments for environmental toxicants, developmental endpoints, whether structural or functional, can be considered in hazard characterization and dose–response analysis, and integrated with exposure information in risk characterization. By definition, this includes developmental immunotoxicity endpoints (Kimmel *et al.*, 2005). Developmental toxicity data can be used in setting reference doses (RfDs) for oral exposures or reference concentrations (RfCs) for inhalation exposures in human health risk assessment for environmental toxicants. Reference values are derived from studying no-observed-adverse-effect-levels (NOAELs) or benchmark dose lower confidence limits (BMDLs) that define a point of departure for health effects that are not assumed to have a linear low dose response relationship (i.e., most non-cancer health effects and carcinogens that act via indirect mechanisms). In calculating the reference values, uncertainty factors are applied as deemed appropriate to address animal to human extrapolation (which may be divided into toxicokinetic and toxicodynamic components), within human variability, the lack of an NOAEL and use of the lowest-observed-adverse-effect level (LOAEL), the use of a subchronic study to set a chronic reference value when no chronic study is available, and a database factor to account for missing data that are considered essential in characterizing risk. The application of an additional 10-fold FQPA factor is required for pesticides, but this may be revised (reduced, removed or sometimes even increased) on the basis of the quality and extent of toxicity and exposure data relevant to children's health risk assessment.

Thus, DIT data can impact the risk calculations in either of two ways. First, endpoints and doses from a DIT study could be used as the critical effect in calculating reference values. Alternatively, for a chemical with identified immunotoxic potential, the presence or absence of an adequate assessment of developmental immunotoxic hazard and/or dose–response might affect the determination of the uncertainty factors used in reference value calculations. For example, a database uncertainty factor might be applied (or an FQPA factor retained) to address the lack of a developmental immunotoxicity study; careful consideration of the overall toxicology database is critical to determining the need for and the magnitude of such an uncertainty factor.

CONCLUDING REMARKS AND FUTURE DIRECTIONS

In conclusion, the need for an adequate assessment of developmental immunotoxicity has long been recognized. The complexity and timing of development of the mammalian immune system, reviewed above, presents challenges in the construction of a predictive testing paradigm for developmental immunotoxicity. A protocol for the evaluation of immune suppression following exposures during immune system ontogeny in the rodent has been developed through the efforts of several workshops. This testing paradigm could be implemented, either through a standalone study or as a segment of a generational study. Data resulting from such testing are applicable to risk assessment.

REFERENCES

Adkins B, Bu Y, Guevara P (2001) The generation of Th memory in neonates versus adults: prolonged primary Th2 effector function and impaired development of Th1 memory effector function in murine neonates. *J Immunol* **166:** 918–25.

Adkins B, Mueller C, Okada CY, Reichert RA, Weissman IL, Spangrude GJ (1987) Early events in T-cell maturation. *Annu Rev Immunol* **5:** 325–65.

Andersson U, Bird AG, Britton BS, Palacios R (1981) Humoral and cellular immunity in humans studied at the cell level from birth to two years of age. *Immunol Rev* **57:** 1–38.

Banfi A, Bianchi G, Galotto M, Cancedda R, Quarto R (2001) Bone marrow stromal damage after chemo/radiotherapy: occurrence, consequences and possibilities of treatment. *Leuk Lymphoma* **42:** 863–70.

Barnett JB (1996) Developmental immunotoxicology. In *Experimental Immunotoxicology* (Holsapple MP, Smialowicz RJ, eds.). CRC Press, Boca Raton, FL, pp. 47–62.

Barton HA, Pastoor TP, Baetcke K, Chambers JE, Diliberto J, Doerrer NG, Driver JH, Hastings CE, Iyengar S, Krieger R, Stahl B, Timchalk C (2006) The acquisition and application of absorption, distribution, metabolism, and excretion (ADME) data in agricultural chemical safety assessments. *Crit Rev Toxicol* **36:** 9–35.

Bettelli E, Korn T, Oukka M, Kuchroo, VK (2008) Induction and effector functions of T(H)17 cells. *Nature* **453:** 1051–7.

Bogue M, Gilfillan S, Benoist C, Mathis D (1992) Regulation of N-region diversity in antigen receptors through thymocyte differentiation and thymus ontogeny. *Proc Natl Acad Sci USA* **89:** 11011–15.

Burns-Naas LA, Hastings KL, Ladics GS, Makris SL, Parker GA, Holsapple MP (2008) What's so special about the developing immune system? *Int J Toxicol* **27:** 223–54.

Cooper EL, Nisbet-Brown E (1993) *Developmental Immunology*. Oxford University Press, New York.

Cooper RL, Lamb JC, Barlow SM, Bentley K, Brady AM, Doerrer NG, Eisenbrandt DL, Fenner-Crisp PA, Hines RN, Irvine L, Kimmel CA, Koeter H, Li AA, Makris SL, Sheets L, Speijers GJA, Whitby K (2006) A tiered approach to life stages testing for agricultural chemical safety assessment. *Crit Rev Toxicol* **36:** 69–98.

Cumano A, Godin I (2001) Pluripotent hematopoietic stem cell development during embryogenesis. *Curr Opin Immunol* **13:** 166–71.

Cumano A, Godin I (2007) Ontogeny of the hematopoietic system. *Annu Rev Immunol* **25:** 745–85.

de Muralt G (1978) Maturation of cellular and humoral immunity. In *Perinatal Physiology* (Stave U, ed.). Plenum, New York, p. 267.

de Vries E, de Bruin-Versteeg S, Comans-Bitter WM, de Groot R, Hop WC, Boerma GJ, Lotgering FK, van Dongen JJ (2000) Longitudinal survey of lymphocyte subpopulations in the first year of life. *Pediatr Res* **47:** 528–37.

Dietert RR, Dietert JM (2007) Early-life immune insult and developmental immunotoxicity (DIT)-associated diseases: potential of herbal- and fungal-derived medicinals. *Curr Med Chem* **14:** 1075–85.

Dietert RR, Piepenbrink MS (2006) Perinatal immunotoxicity: why adult exposure assessment fails to predict risk. *Environ Health Perspect* **14(4):** 477–83.

Felsburg PJ (2002) Overview of immune system development in the dog: comparison with humans. *Human Exp Toxicol* **21:** 487–92.

Godin I, Garcia-Porrero JA, Dieterlen-Lievre F, Cumano A (1999) Stem cell emergence and hemopoietic activity are incompatible in mouse intraembryonic sites. *J Exp Med* **190:** 43–52.

Hann IM, Bodger MP, Hoffbrand AV (1983) Development of pluripotent hematopoietic progenitor cells in the human fetus. *Blood* **62:** 118–23.

Hannet I, Erkeller-Yuksel F, Lydyard P, Deneys V, DeBruyere M (1992) Developmental and maturational changes in human blood lymphocyte subpopulations. *Immunol Today* **13:** 215, 218.

Haynes BF, Martin ME, Kay HH, Kurtzberg J (1988) Early events in human T cell ontogeny. Phenotypic characterization and immunohistologic localization of T cell precursors in early human fetal tissues. *J Exp Med* **168:** 1061–80.

Holladay SD, Smialowicz RJ (2000) Development of the murine and human immune system: differential effects of immunotoxicants depend on time of exposure. *Environ Health Perspect* **108 (Suppl. 3):** 463–73.

Holsapple MP (2002) Developmental immunotoxicology and risk assessment: a workshop summary. *Human Exp Toxicol* **21:** 473–8.

Holsapple MP, Burns-Naas LA, Hastings KL, Ladics GS, Lavin AL, Makris SL, Yang Y, Luster MI (2003a) A proposed testing framework for developmental immunotoxicology (DIT). *Toxicol Sci* **83(1):** 83–4.

Holsapple, MP, Paustenbach DJ, Charnley G, West LJ, Luster MI, Dietert RR, Burns-Naas LA (2004) Symposium summary: children's health risk – what's so special about the developing immune system? *Toxicol Appl Pharmacol* **199:** 61–70.

Holsapple MP, West LJ, Landreth KS (2003b) Species comparison of anatomical and functional immune system development. *Birth Defects Res B Dev Reprod Toxicol* **68:** 321–34.

Holt PG, Jones CA (2000) The development of the immune system during pregnancy and early life. *Allergy* **55:** 688–97.

Holt PG, Sly PD (2002) Interactions between RSV infection, asthma, and atopy: unraveling the complexities. *J Exp Med* **196:** 1271–5.

Humbert M, Menz G, Ying S, Corrigan CJ, Robinson DS, Durham SR, Kay AB (1999) The immunopathology of extrinsic (atopic) and intrinsic (non-atopic) asthma: more similarities than differences. *Immunol Today* **20:** 528–33.

Janeway C, Travers P, Walport M, Shlomchik M (2005) *Immunobiology: The Immune System in Health and Disease*. Garland Science Publishing, New York.

Kay HE, Playfair JH, Wolfendale M, Hopper PK (1962) Development of the thymus in the human foetus and its relation to immunological potential. *Nature* **196:** 238–40.

Kidd P (2003) Th1/Th2 balance: the hypothesis, its limitations, and implications for health and disease. *Altern Med Rev* **8:** 223–46.

Kimmel CA, King MD, Makris SL (2005) Risk assessment perspectives for developmental immunotoxicity. In *Developmental Immunotoxicology* (Holladay SD, ed.). CRC Press, Washington DC.

Landreth K, Dodson S (2004) Development of the rodent immune system. In *Developmental Immunotoxicology* (Holladay SD, ed.). CRC Press, Boca Raton, FL, pp. 3–19.

Landreth K, Dodson S (2005) Development of the rodent immune system. In *Developmental Immunotoxicology* (Holladay SD, ed.). CRC Press, Boca Raton, FL, pp. 3–19.

Landreth KS (2002) Critical windows in development of the rodent immune system. *Human Exp Toxicol* **21:** 493–8.

Leibnitz R (2004) Development of the human immune system. In *Developmental Immunotoxicology* (Holladay SD, ed.). CRC Press, Boca Raton, FL, pp. 21–42.

Lobach DF, Haynes BF (1987) Ontogeny of the human thymus during fetal development. *J Clin Immunol* **7:** 81–97.

Luebke RW, Chen DH, Dietert R, Yang Y, King M, Luster MJ (2006) The comparative immunotoxicity of five selected compounds following developmental or adult exposure. *J Toxicol Environ Health Crit Rev* **9(1):** 1–26.

Luster MI, Dean JH, Germolec DR (2003) Consensus workshop on methods to evaluate developmental immunotoxicity. *Environ Health Perspect* **111:** 579–83.

Makris S, Thompson CM, Euling SY, Selevan SG, Sonawane B (2008) A lifestage-specific approach to hazard and dose-response characterization for children's health risk assessment. *Birth Defects Res Part B* **83:** 530–46.

Micklem HS, Ford CE, Evans EP, Gray J (1966) Interrelationships of myeloid and lymphoid cells: studies with chromosome-marked cells transfused into lethally irradiated mice. *Proc R Soc Lond B Biol Sci* **165:** 78–102.

Miller DL, Hiravonen T, Gitlin D (1973) Synthesis of IgE by the human conceptus. *J Allergy Clin Immunol* **52:** 182–8.

Miyawaki T, Moriya N, Nagaoki T, Taniguchi N (1981) Maturation of B-cell differentiation ability and T-cell regulatory function in infancy and childhood. *Immunol Rev* **57:** 61–87.

Moore MA, Metcalf D (1970) Ontogeny of the haemopoietic system: yolk sac origin of in vivo and in vitro colony forming cells in the developing mouse embryo. *Br J Haematol* **18:** 279–96.

Mosmann TR, Coffman RL (1989) TH1 and TH2 cells: different patterns of lymphokine secretion lead to different functional properties. *Annu Rev Immunol* **7:** 145–73.

Mudry RE, Fortney JE, York T, Hall BM, Gibson LF (2000) Stromal cells regulate survival of B-lineage leukemic cells during chemotherapy. *Blood* **96:** 1926–32.

Muller AM, Medvinsky A, Strouboulis J, F. Grosveld F, Dzierzak E (1994) Development of hematopoietic stem cell activity in the mouse embryo. *Immunity* **1:** 291–301.

NRC (National Research Council) (1993) *Pesticides in the Diets of Infants and Children*. Washington, DC: National Academy Press.

OECD (2009) Draft extended one-generation reproductive toxicity test guideline. OECD guideline for the testing of chemicals. Draft version 28, October 2009. Paris, France. Available: http://www.oecd.org/document/55/0,3343,en_2649_34377_2349687_1_1_1_1,00.html

Owen JJ, Cooper MD, Raff MC (1974) In vitro generation of B lymphocytes in mouse foetal liver, a mammalian "bursa equivalent". *Nature* **249:** 361–3.

Owen JJ, Jordan RK, Robinson JH, Singh U, Willcox HN (1977) In vitro studies on the generation of lymphocyte diversity. *Cold Spring Harb Symp Quant Biol* **41 (Pt 1):** 129–37.

Owen JJ, Raff MC (1970) Studies on the differentiation of thymus-derived lymphocytes. *J Exp Med* **132:** 1216–32.

Peakman M, Buggins AG, Nicolaides KH, Layton DM, Vergani D (1992) Analysis of lymphocyte phenotypes in cord blood from early gestation fetuses. *Clin Exp Immunol* **90:** 345–50.

Prchal JT, Throckmorton DW, Carroll AJ 3rd, Fuson EW, Gams RA, Prchal JF (1978) A common progenitor for human myeloid and lymphoid cells. *Nature* **274:** 590–1.

Raff MC (1970) Two distinct populations of peripheral lymphocytes in mice distinguishable by immunofluorescence. *Immunology* **19:** 637–50.

Ridge JP, Fuchs EJ, Matzinger P (1996) Neonatal tolerance revisited: turning on newborn T cells with dendritic cells. *Science* **271:** 1723–6.

Rolink A, Haasner D, Nishikawa S, Melchers F (1993) Changes in frequencies of clonable pre B cells during life in different lymphoid organs of mice. *Blood* **81:** 2290–300.

Tavassoli M (1991) Embryonic and fetal hemopoiesis: an overview. *Blood Cells* **17:** 269–86.

Tavassoli M, Yoffey JM (1983) *Bone Marrow: Structure and Function*. Alan R. Liss, New York.

Tavian M, Hallais MF, Peault B (1999) Emergence of intraembryonic hematopoietic precursors in the pre-liver human embryo. *Development* **126:** 793–803.

Teh H-S (1993) T cell development and repertoire selection. In *Developmental Immunology* (Cooper E, Nisbet-Brown E, eds.). Oxford University Press, New York, p. 217.

Tentori L, Pardoll DM, Zuniga JC, Hu-Li J, Paul WE, Bluestone JA, Kruisbeek AM (1988) Proliferation and production of IL-2 and B cell stimulatory factor 1/IL-4 in early fetal thymocytes by activation through Thy-1 and CD3. *J Immunol* **140:** 1089–94.

Velardi A, Cooper MD (1984) An immunofluorescence analysis of the ontogeny of myeloid, T, and B lineage cells in mouse hemopoietic tissues. *J Immunol* **133:** 672–7.

Vetro SW, Bellanti JA (1989) Fetal and neonatal immunoincompetence. *Fetal Ther* **4 (Suppl. 1):** 82–91.

von Freeden U, Zessack N, van Valen F, Burdach S (1991) Defective interferon gamma production in neonatal T cells is independent of interleukin-2 receptor binding. *Pediatr Res* **30:** 270–5.

von Gaudecker B (1991) Functional histology of the human thymus. *Anat Embryol (Berl)* **183:** 1–15.

West LJ (2002) Defining critical windows in the development of the human immune system. *Human Exp Toxicol* **21:** 499–505.

C H A P T E R

19

In vitro biomarkers of developmental neurotoxicity

Magdalini Sachana, John Flaskos and Alan J. Hargreaves

INTRODUCTION

This chapter provides an overview of the endpoint measurements used in studying developmental neurotoxicity by alternative to animal approaches and, more specifically, by applying *in vitro* models. Among the cellular models currently available to investigate the chemical effects on nervous system development are: transformed cell lines of human or animal origin, fetal or neonatal primary cultures mainly of rodents, embryonic stem cells or neuroprogenitor cells and brain cells from aborted fetuses. In these *in vitro* systems, a significant number of complex processes of nervous system development can be modeled and effectively assessed. Here, we review some of the most important markers of developmental neurotoxicity associated with cell proliferation, apoptosis, differentiation and synaptogenesis. Furthermore, transcription factors and signaling pathways as well as cytoskeletal proteins are included and analyzed for their potential use as endpoints of developmental neurotoxicity.

The above markers are discussed in relation to methylmercury (MeHg), lead, arsenic, ethanol, toluene and polychlorinated biphenyls (PCBs), six well-documented developmental neurotoxicants (DNTs) (Grandjean and Landrigan, 2006). Additionally, chlorpyrifos (CPF), diazinon (DZN) and polybrominated diphenyl ethers (PBDEs), which are identified as potential developmentally neurotoxic for humans (Grandjean and Landrigan, 2006), are also included.

This chapter summarizes existing *in vitro* studies on the field of developmental neurotoxicity, especially focusing on endpoints that may be potentially used for screening purposes, tailored to the particularities of the developing nervous system. Each endpoint is described separately in relation to developing brain and its validity is discussed in light of available information gleaned from *in vivo* studies investigating developmental neurotoxicants (DNTs).

CELL PROLIFERATION AND APOPTOSIS

Cell proliferation and apoptotic cell death are essential events that take place during neurodevelopment. For this reason cell death has long been a primary endpoint for many *in vitro* studies of developmental neurotoxicity of industrial chemicals or environmental pollutants. Indeed, many DNTs cause reduction in cell number in specific brain areas, which is manifested as microencephaly in humans and animal models (something that will be discussed separately for each DNT), justifying further the choice of this endpoint in cultured cells.

Apoptosis and necrosis are the best defined types (Type I and II, respectively) of cell death characterized by different morphological and biochemical aspects (Golstein and Kroemer, 2006; Blomgren *et al.*, 2007). Necrosis is thought to be mainly an uncontrolled form of cell death with obvious plasma membrane rupture, enlargement of mitochondria, disintegration and subsequent local inflammation. On the other hand, apoptosis is a regulated type of cell death defined by chromatin condensation and fragmentation, cell shrinkage and blebbing of the plasma membrane. Apoptotic cells are recognized and eliminated by phagocytes with no effect on neighboring cells. Here, we review *in vitro* studies investigating the induction of apoptosis or necrosis by DNTs based on the morphological criteria stated above, as well as on the determination of DNA fragmentation by agarose gel electrophoresis in the case of apoptosis.

It is thought that neuronal and glial cells are overproduced during development and that the excess cells are removed by apoptosis (Sastry and Rao, 2000; Madden and Cotter, 2008), which is considered vital to the pre- and postnatal development of the brain. The problem rises when these brain cells, already susceptible to apoptosis due to overexpression of large numbers of effectors of this developmental cell death program, are accidentally exposed to DNTs causing further exaggeration of this death machinery by triggering different cell death pathways and resulting in complex biochemical alterations and morphological manifestations (Blomgren *et al.*, 2007). It should also be mentioned that disruption of either the grade or the timing of apoptosis in brain can modify not only cell number but also patterns of neuronal connectivity, leading to functional alterations often in the absence of apparent pathological findings (Sastry and Rao, 2000).

It has been suggested that an insult by a toxin during the postnatal period, when synaptogenesis is at its peak, could generate the suicide signal. For the execution of this signal,

Reproductive and Developmental Toxicology, Edited by Ramesh C. Gupta
ISBN: 978-0-12-382032-7

several cell death pathways could be activated separately or simultaneously. These are based on: (1) the release of cytochrome *c* from mitochondria and its corresponding effectors (caspases); (2) excessive intracellular calcium levels; (3) disruption of potassium and chloride homeostasis (not covered in the present review); and (4) oxidative stress mediated mainly by reactive oxygen species (ROS) (Blomgren *et al.*, 2007).

Caspase-3 is the most abundant effector caspase in the developing brain as well as a potent effector of apoptosis triggered via several different pathways and is one of the most important caspases activated downstream of cytochrome *c* in the intrinsic apoptosis pathways. Assays of caspase-3 activation as an early marker of the development of apoptosis induced by DNTs *in vitro* are of particular interest in this chapter.

Calcium ions play important roles in the regulation of neurotransmission and the developmental cell death program. Excessive calcium levels can damage neurons, even causing cell death by apoptosis and is briefly discussed here in relation to DNTs (see Orrenius *et al.*, 2003, for review). Calcium overload can activate Ca^{2+}-dependent proteases that regulate apoptosis or elevate the generation of ROS that can trigger cytochrome *c* release and subsequent caspase activation (Green and Reed, 1998). Furthermore, cross-talk between caspase-3 and calpains, which are calcium activated cysteine proteases, has been shown recently (Blomgren *et al.*, 2007).

The immature brain is particularly sensitive to oxidative stress, possibly due to its high availability in free iron for the catalytic formation of hydroxyl radicals and the limited antioxidant capacity (Gupta, 2004). Oxidative stress refers to the cytotoxic consequences of ROS and the tripeptide glutathione (GSH; γ-glutamyl-cysteinylglycine) is a major defense mechanism against ROS. When ROS production overrides cellular scavenging systems, it induces cellular damage by affecting DNA, proteins and membrane lipids but most importantly it can modulate the release of proapoptotic factors leading to cellular demise (Blomgren *et al.*, 2007).

Apart from cell death, cell proliferation is used as an endpoint in many studies of developmental neurotoxicology. In the immature nervous system, alterations in cell cycle length can influence development and function of the brain (Salomoni and Calegari, 2010). Although not the only cell proliferation endpoint, the effects of DNTs on cell cycle will be a major focus in this section.

Over the last two decades, there has been a great surge of interest in the effects of DNTs on apoptosis and cell proliferation *in vitro*. In this section, we focus mainly on the general cytotoxicity, apoptosis, necrosis and oxidative stress induced by DNTs mainly in cellular systems, with special emphasis on experimental approaches that use these endpoints to further establish biologically plausible links between the molecular actions of DNTs and their effects in exposed humans and animal models.

Heavy metals

Mercury

The main pathological finding after developmental exposure to MeHg in both humans and animal models is brain atrophy due to cell loss (Burbacher *et al.*, 1990). It is therefore not surprising that a significant number of *in vitro* studies deal with this injurious effect of methylmercury (MeHg). This has been part of the basis for a growing interest in the elucidation of the molecular mechanisms underlying the developmental neurotoxicity of MeHg.

Basal cytotoxicity studies conducted in a variety of cellular models aided enormously in this effort. The LC_{50} ranges for a variety of mammalian primary neuronal cultures, and neuronotypic cell lines are between approximately 1 and 10 μM (Kromidas *et al.*, 1990; Sarafian and Verity, 1991; Kunimoto *et al.*, 1992; Park *et al.*, 1996; Sakamoto *et al.*, 1996; Ou *et al.*, 1997; Miura *et al.*, 1999; Gasso *et al.*, 2001; Sanfeliu *et al.*, 2001; de Melo Reis *et al.*, 2007).

MeHg has been reported to trigger either dose-dependent necrosis after acute treatment of cerebellar granule cells (CGCs) from 8-day-old rats (0.5–10 μM for 1 h) or time-dependent apoptosis (6–18 h) with 1 μM (Castoldi *et al.*, 2000). In mouse HT22 hippocampal cells, MeHg (2–4 μM) caused a significant increase in apoptosis and necrosis after 24 h exposure (Tofighi *et al.*, 2010). Previously, Kunimoto (1994) showed MeHg-induced apoptosis CGCs at lower concentrations (0.1 and 0.3 μM) and longer incubation time (72 h). Furthermore, the concentration of 2 μM MeHg produced apoptosis in mouse CGCs over 2 days' exposure (Buleit and Cui, 1998). Chromatin condensation and DNA fragmentation in CGCs treated with increasing doses of MeHg (0.1–1.5 μM) for 24 h revealed apoptosis not related to activation of caspase-3 but of calpain (Dare *et al.*, 2000; Sakaue *et al.*, 2005). Similarly, caspase-independent apoptosis and associated activation of calpains was found in HT 22 cells exposed to MeHg (Tofighi *et al.*, 2010). Conversely, primary culture of rat cerebrocortical neurons from 17-day-old rat embryos treated with 100 nM MeHg exhibited apoptosis after 3 days' incubation accompanied by activation of caspase-3 (Fujimura *et al.*, 2009). However, MeHg-induced apoptosis has been reported to be caspase-independent in rat and mice CGCs, after acute or long-term MeHg exposure to 1 μM and 300 nM, respectively (Dare *et al.*, 2001a; Vendrell *et al.*, 2007). This supports the notion that differently regulated mechanisms are utilized during MeHg-induced apoptosis depending on the *in vitro* system used.

Elevated expression of genes related to apoptosis was recorded by transcriptional profiling of rat pheochromocytoma PC12 cells exposed to 1 μM for 24 h (Wilke *et al.*, 2003). In the same cell line, MeHg exposure revealed chromatin condensation, DNA fragmentation and decreased cell body area (Miura *et al.*, 1999; Parran *et al.*, 2001). Apart from PC12 cells, neuroblastoma cell lines such as SH-SY5Y and C-1300 cells were found to undergo apoptosis after MeHg treatment (Miura *et al.*, 1999; Toimela and Tahti, 2004).

Recently, the vulnerability of neural stem cells (NSCs) to MeHg has been investigated by using primary cultures of cortical NSCs (cNCSs) and murine C17.2 NSC line (Tamm *et al.*, 2006). Interestingly, MeHg doses previously used to induce apoptosis in other *in vitro* models (Dare *et al.*, 2000, 2001a) proved to be highly cytotoxic in NSCs. Furthermore, cNSCs appeared to need 10-fold lower concentration of MeHg (0.05 μM) to reveal 15–20% apoptotic cells compared to the cell line (0.5 μM) (Tamm *et al.*, 2006). Similar MeHg concentration also caused inhibition of proliferation and induction of apoptosis in human HUCB-NSC line by immunocytochemical expression of specific markers (Buzanska *et al.*, 2009). These pioneering works laid the ground for further investigation of the neurodevelopmental effects of biologically relevant concentrations of MeHg in these dynamic and highly sensitive *in vitro* systems.

Notably, research conducted on GT1-7 hypothalamic neuronal cell line revealed that exposure to 10 μM MeHg for 3 h results in 20% cell death strongly associated with increased generation of ROS rather than with the reduction of glutathione (GSH), pointing out the key role of oxidative stress in MeHg-induced developmental neurotoxicity (Sarafian *et al.*, 1994). In PC12 cells, levels of lipid peroxidation increased significantly after exposure to 0.5 μM MeHg (Vettori *et al.*, 2006). In the same cell line, as well as in rat dissociated sensory neurons from embryonic rat pup dorsal root ganglia, treatment with 1 μM MeHg for 6 h caused increased expression of oxidative stress associated genes (Wilke *et al.*, 2003). Under the same experimental conditions, MeHg-induced membrane lipoperoxidation or ROS generation have also been detected in CGCs after acute or chronic exposure to MeHg (Sarafian and Verity, 1991; Ali *et al.*, 1992; Oyama *et al.*, 1994; Verity *et al.*, 1994; Yee and Choi, 1996; Mundy and Freudenrich, 2000; Vendrell *et al.*, 2007). Indeed, antioxidants/oxygen radical scavengers appeared to provide partial protection against MeHg neurotoxicity in cultured neurons, mainly by reversing the oxidative stress indicators rather than inhibiting cell loss (Sarafian and Verity, 1991; Park *et al.*, 1996; Dare *et al.*, 2000). Oyama *et al.* (1994) demonstrated that ROS formation by MeHg was significantly inhibited in the absence of extracellular Ca^{2+}. However, a more recent study showed that none of the tested compounds that interfere with Ca^{2+} homeostasis decreased ROS generation mediated by MeHg (Gasso *et al.*, 2001). Recently, CGCs derived from mice with genetically altered low glutathione levels showed increased sensitivity to MeHg compared to wild-type cells, revealing the oxidative stress involvement in MeHg-induced cytotoxicity (Costa *et al.*, 2007).

MeHg (2 and 4 μM) exposure over a period of 0–48 h caused a dose- and time-dependent inhibition of cell cycling in primary embryonic CNS cells in culture related to upregualtion of the Gadd genes, which play important role in cell cycle arrest (Ponce *et al.*, 1994; Ou *et al.*, 1997). Time-dependent changes in the cell cycle occurred in PC12 cells treated with 3 μM MeHg, resulting in G2/M phase arrest (Miura *et al.*, 1999). Increased expression of genes associated with cell cycling was revealed when the same cell line was exposed to 1 μM MeHg for 24 h (Wilke *et al.*, 2003). MeHg was also a strong inhibitor of [methyl-^{3}H]-thymidine incorporation into DNA, suggesting the importance of cell cycle regulation as a sensitive *in vitro* endpoint of MeHg neurotoxicity (Costa *et al.*, 2007).

It has been suggested that astrocytes are more resistant than neurons to MeHg-induced cell death (Toimela and Tahti, 2004; Costa *et al.*, 2007; Crespo-Lopez *et al.*, 2007). For example, primary astrocyte cultures from human fetal brain were more resistant to MeHg cytoxicity (LC_{50} 8.1 μM for 24 h) than neurons (LC_{50} 6.5 μM) (Sanfeliu *et al.*, 2001). However, using an immature three-dimensional cell culture system of fetal rat telencephalon, apoptosis occurred in astrocytes rather than in neurons at low concentrations of MeHg (1 μM) after chronic exposure (10 d) (Monnet-Tschudi, 1998). Similarly, Dare *et al.* (2001b) identified MeHg-induced apoptosis in D384 human astrocytoma cells but failed to detect caspase activation at (1 μM) (for 24 h). Apoptosis was, also, the only detectable type of cell death in rat C6 glioma cells, a model expressing both oligodendrocytic and astrocytic markers, treated with MeHg (Belletti *et al.*, 2002). High levels of ROS formation in C6 cells and cerebral cortical astrocytes obtained from newborn rats were one of the earliest measurable effects in conjunction with oxidative DNA damage (Belletti *et al.*, 2002; Shanker *et al.*, 2004). MeHg-induced ROS generation has been found to be attenuated by antioxidants (Shanker and Aschner, 2003; Shanker *et al.*, 2005), whereas another study showed astrocytes to be not as responsive to antioxidant treatment (Sanfeliu *et al.*, 2001). Taken together, these studies indicate that glial cells may play a significant role in MeHg-induced developmental neurotoxicity.

Microglial cells have also been found to be targeted by MeHg, which subsequently alters homeostasis of the brain microenvironment (Monnet-Tschudi *et al.*, 1996; Nishioku *et al.*, 2000). Early experimentation on aggregating brain cell cultures showed microglial activation by low concentrations of MeHg, as an early sign of toxicity (Monnet-Tschudi *et al.*, 1996), whereas recent work on primary cultured cerebral microglia obtained from new born rats showed MeHg-induced apoptosis associated with DNA fragmentation and caspase-3 activation (Nishioku *et al.*, 2000).

Lead

Lead, another ubiquitous environmental pollutant, has detrimental effects on developing brain by decreasing neuronal cell number (Verina *et al.*, 2007) and causing intellectual impairment (Bellinger and Needleman, 2003).

In one of the first *in vitro* studies addressing the neurotoxicity of lead, rat primary hippocampal neurons, rat B50 and mouse N1E-115 neuroblastoma cell lines were challenged with a range of concentrations up to 1 mM and neuron viability was found to be affected differently, with B50 cells to demonstrate increased resistance (Audesirk *et al.*, 1991). This altered neuronal survival status by lead was further investigated in newborn rat CGCs in culture by applying low concentrations (down to 1 μM) and revealing DNA fragmentation and involvement of apoptotic death (Oberto *et al.*, 1996). Increased LDH release was noted in rat NSCs at concentrations above 10 μM; however, at lower and environmentally relevant concentrations (0.1–1 μM) lead reduced cell proliferation without causing cell death (Huang and Schneider, 2004). In human SH-SY5Y neurobalstoma cells, lead caused a dose-dependent inhibition of cell proliferation as determined by MTT reduction assay, after exposure to 0.01–10 μM for 48 h (Suresh *et al.*, 2006; Chetty, 2007). This neurotoxicity was partly attributed to apoptosis due to activation of caspase-3 (Suresh *et al.*, 2006; Chetty, 2007). Apoptosis has also been suggested as the cause of lead-induced cell death in neuron-like PC12 cells treated with 3, 30 or 90 μM for 24 h, as demonstrated by DNA fragmentation (Sharifi and Mousavi, 2008). Shorter incubation time (4 h) of the same cell line after exposure to lead (1–100 μM) also revealed a concentration-dependent reduction in viability (MTS assay) and elevated caspase-3 activity for the higher dose (Penugonda *et al.*, 2006). Using as little as 0.1 μM lead, Xu *et al.* (2006) showed significant activation of caspase-3, DNA fragmentation and apoptosis-related cell death in PC12 cells.

Recent findings laid the ground for the concept that lead not only induces cell death but also poses trophic effects by promoting the survival of cells in rat primary cortical precursors (Davidovics and DiCicco-Bloom, 2005). Interestingly, pharmacologically relevant lead concentrations (3 and 30 μM) for up to 4 days elevated cell numbers without increasing DNA synthesis, suggesting a novel mechanism by which the metal elicits neurotoxicity in developing brain. However, the same study also showed enhanced cell death at higher concentrations (90 μM), in agreement with the previous reports.

Lead-induced oxidative stress has been studied in PC12 cells (Jadhav *et al.*, 2000; Chen *et al.*, 2003; Sharifi *et al.*, 2005; Penugonda *et al.*, 2006), E 14 mesencephalic cells (Scortegagna *et al.*, 1998), mouse hypothalamic GT-17 cells and neuroblastoma cells (Naarala *et al.*, 1995; Aimo and Oteiza, 2006). The concentrations associated with elevated NO production and generation of ROS were as little as 1 μM up to 100 μM lead (Jadhav *et al.*, 2000; Chen *et al.*, 2003; Sharifi *et al.*, 2005; Penugonda *et al.*, 2006). The global concentration of intracellular oxidants increased in human neuroblastoma IMR-32 cells after exposure to lead (Aimo and Oteiza, 2006). However, exposure of human SH-SY5Y neurobalstoma cells and mouse hypothalamic GT-17 cells to lead had no effect on the production of ROS (Naarala *et al.*, 1995). Interestingly, when Naarala *et al.* (1995) measured the total soluble lead in the incubation medium by atomic absorption spectrometry, it revealed that the actual concentration was between 10 and 20 μM instead of 1 mM. This and other studies raised concerns about the binding properties of this metal and the real dose that actually causes developmental neurotoxicity at the cellular level. Some of the experimental approaches used lead concentrations equivalent to those measured in blood of children with cognitive deficits (10–60 μg/dl) corresponding to 0.5–3 μM free ionic lead in cell culture, without addressing the binding issue (Bellinger and Needleman, 2003; Canfield *et al.*, 2003; Davidovics and DiCicco-Bloom, 2005).

Unlike neuronal cells, the different glial cell types do not all appear to be affected in the same way by lead. For example, astroglia were found to be resistant to lead toxicity, whereas oligodendroglia demonstrated significantly reduced viability and proliferation over a wide range of concentrations (Tiffany-Castiglioni *et al.*, 1989; Opanashuk and Finkelstein, 1995). Indeed, oligodendrocyte progenitor cells (OPCs) from 2-day-old rats exposed to lead for 24 h showed dose-dependent cell death and caspase-3 activation for doses of 10–20 μM (Deng and Poretz, 2002). Whereas a treatment of as low as 1 μM of lead in the same *in vitro* system can interfere with cell proliferation after acute exposure (Deng and Poretz, 2002) and the viability of cell numbers after chronic exposure (above 3 days) (Deng *et al.*, 2002). Moreover, 10 μM lead had no effect on cell growth or apoptosis of human U-373MG glioblastoma cells despite the increased expression of tumor necrosis factor-α (TNF-α) (Cheng *et al.*, 2002), revealing the necessity for further studies to this direction.

Arsenic

Arsenic, an environmental contaminant, has been recently described as a potential DNT based on epidemiological and *in vivo* studies (Rodriguez *et al.*, 2002; Dakeishi *et al.*, 2006; von Ehrenstein *et al.*, 2007). The focus of this section is on the cytotoxicity induced by the different forms of arsenic detected in the environment and no attempt has been made to cover the apoptotic and anti-cancer properties of arsenic trioxide.

Human fetal brain explants exposed to 0.3 ppm sodium arsenite for up to 18 d demonstrated reduced cell viability by Trypan-blue exclusion (Chattopadhyay *et al.*, 2002). Similar effects were observed when arsenic was administered to pregnant rats and explants prepared from newborn and post-gestational rat brain. However, only the human fetal brain and rat neonatal brain explants showed signs of apoptosis by microscopy. In primary astroglia cultures from 3-day-old rat pups, exposure to the inorganic but not the organic arsenicals resulted in elevated cell death and DNA damage (Jin *et al.*, 2004). In contrast, treatment of rodent primary neonatal cerebellar, cortical neurons and PC12 and SH-SY5Y neuroblastoma cells with arsenic, both in its inorganic or organic form, at environmentally relevant concentrations reduced cell viability and caused apoptosis (Namgung and Xia, 2000, 2001; Namgung *et al.*, 2001; Wong *et al.*, 2005; Cai *et al.*, 2006; vanVliet *et al.*, 2007; Cai and Xia, 2008; Watcharasit *et al.*, 2008). On the other hand, studies on neuroblastoma cell lines, embryonic primary cortical neurons and embryonic primary rat midbrain neuroepithelial cells failed to demonstrate apoptosis following exposure to trivalent arsenite (Mangesdorf *et al.*, 2002; Sidhu *et al.*, 2006; Shavali and Sens, 2008).

The involvement of cell cycle perturbation in arsenite-induced neurodevelopmental toxicity has been also studied, revealing a dose-dependent inhibition of cell cycle progression and cytostasis (Sidhu *et al.*, 2006). Furthermore, arsenite at low concentrations appeared to induce oxidative stress in human fetal brain and rat neonatal brain explants (Chattopadhyay *et al.*, 2002), as well as in mesencephalic cell line 1RB3AN27 (Felix *et al.*, 2005). Arsenite-induced oxidative stress has also been found in cultured rat astrocytes followed by increased GSH content and hydrogen peroxide production (Sagara *et al.*, 1996), whereas the involvement of ROS in arsenic-induced oxidative stress has been studied in the glutamate-resistant HT22 hippocampal nerve cell line (Dargusch and Schubert, 2002).

The above studies project a complex picture of arsenic-induced cell death depending on the cell type, concentration and method of evaluation, emphasizing the importance of continuing research in this area.

Organic solvents

Ethanol

Ethanol is a well-known developmental neurotoxicant associated with severe morphological, mental and behavioral deficits in children due to maternal alcohol abuse mainly during pregnancy (Guerri *et al.*, 2009). In humans and animal models, developmental exposure to ethanol caused microencephaly (Guerri *et al.*, 2009) due to decreased cell number in various brain regions and specific neuronal cell populations. Similarly, ethanol exposure reduced cell numbers in neuronal primary and organotypic brain slice cultures (Pantazis *et al.*, 1993; Chen and Sulik, 1996; Collins *et al.*, 1998; Mitchell *et al.*, 1999b; de la Monte *et al.*, 2001; Jacobs and Miller, 2001; Vaudry *et al.*, 2002; Moulder *et al.*, 2002; Siler-Marsiglio *et al.*, 2004b; Nowoslawski *et al.*, 2005; Watts *et al.*, 2005; Vaudry *et al.*, 2005; Ke *et al.*, 2009) and cell lines (Pantazis *et al.*, 1992; Oberdoerster *et al.*, 1998; Luo *et al.*, 1999; Li *et al.*, 2000; Kang *et al.*, 2005; Meng *et al.*, 2006).

Luo and Miller (1997b) reported no change in cell viability after exposure of three neuroblastoma cell lines to 87 mM ethanol, possibly due to interactions of this developmental neurotoxin and serum factors. Similar antagonistic interactions among ethanol and trophic factors have been observed by others (Luo *et al.*, 1997; Oberdoerster *et al.*, 1998; Vaudry *et al.*, 2002; Chen *et al.*, 2006).

Acute treatment of cells with physiologically relevant concentrations of ethanol had no significant effect on cell number of neuronal or astrocytic populations (Crews *et al.*, 1999; Hao *et al.*, 2003; Lamarche *et al.*, 2003; Kane *et al.*, 2008). However, a concentration-dependent cell loss at relatively high ethanol doses has been reported (Pantazis *et al.*, 1993; Saito *et al.*, 1999; McAlhany *et al.*, 2000; Vaudry *et al.*, 2002; Lamarche *et al.*, 2003), especially after long acute exposure (Mitchell *et al.*, 1999b).

The above-mentioned decrease in cell number could be due to either augmentation of cell death or decreased proliferation. Cell proliferation has been found to be altered by ethanol in both *in vivo* and *in vitro* studies (Guerri *et al.*, 1990; Pantazis *et al.*, 1992; Luo and Miller, 1997b,a; Jacobs and Miller, 2001; Lamarche *et al.*, 2003). Notably, short exposure to ethanol caused cell cycle delays in PC12 cells (Luo *et al.*, 1999) and accumulation of human SK-N-MC cells in the sub-G1 phase (Jang *et al.*, 2001), whereas, cell proliferation was demonstrated to be dose dependent in PC12 cells (Pantazis *et al.*, 1992; Oberdoerster *et al.*, 1998).

Jacobs and Miller (2001) found an increase in the length of the cell cycle and of the S phase in chronic ethanol treated neocortical neurons in culture, similar to Li *et al.* (2001a) who used neonatal cerebellar granule progenitors (CGPs). This is supported by another study demonstrating that alteration in protein expression of early cell cycle regulators is associated with reduced proliferation in ethanol treated E14 dorsal root ganglia neuronal stem cells and whole embryo cultures (Antony *et al.*, 2008). The cell cycle of astrocytes in culture was also found to be disturbed by ethanol at high concentrations of ethanol (100–200 mM) (Guerri *et al.*, 1990; Holownia *et al.*, 1997), but not at low concentrations (10 mM) (Guizzetti and Costa, 1996).

Cell death could be the other reason for cell number reduction, which is associated with apoptosis or necrosis. Although the ethanol-induced cell death in whole fetal brain has been suggested to be mediated by apoptotic mechanisms (Ramachandran *et al.*, 2003; Druse *et al.*, 2005, 2006, 2007) most reports were unable to distinguish between effects on neuronal and glial cell populations. In addition, because of the complexity of the animal models, researchers were unable to establish the mechanism underlying the cell loss. Therefore, a significant number of *in vitro* studies have been conducted to address this problem in primary neurons and neuronotypic cell lines, revealing ethanol-induced apoptotic cell death (De *et al.*, 1994; Bhave and Hoffman, 1997; Leisi, 1997; Castoldi *et al.*, 1998; Oberdoerster *et al.*, 1998; Oberdoerster and Rabin, 1999a,b; Saito *et al.*, 1999; McAlhany *et al.*, 2000; Thibault *et al.*, 2000; Jacobs and Miller, 2001; Jang *et al.*, 2001; Vaudry *et al.*, 2002; Lamarche *et al.*, 2003; Ramachandran *et al.*, 2003; Heaton *et al.*, 2004; Siler-Marsiglio *et al.*, 2004b; Takadera and Ohyashiki, 2004; Druse *et al.*, 2005, 2006, 2007; Kang *et al.*, 2005; Nowoslawski *et al.*, 2005; Watts *et al.*, 2005; Chen *et al.*, 2006; Meng *et al.*, 2006; Zhong *et al.*, 2006; Antonio and Druse, 2008; Antony *et al.*, 2008; Cherian *et al.*, 2008; Maffi *et al.*, 2008; Liu *et al.*, 2010).

Furthermore, delayed apoptosis was found in proliferating CGPs (Li *et al.*, 2001a) compared to post-mitotic CGCs, where apoptosis occurs rapidly (Castoldi *et al.*, 1998; Zhang *et al.*, 1998). Conversely, no apoptotic cells were detected in primary culture of neonatal rat astroglial cells exposed to similar doses of ethanol that induce apoptosis in neurons (Halownia *et al.*, 1997), whereas, recently, Pascual *et al.* (2003) demonstrated that ethanol exposed fetal astrocytes undergo apoptotic cell death.

Proapototic proteins can be released due to oxidative stress induced by increased levels of ROS. Indeed, ethanol was demonstrated to cause elevation of ROS formation, after a short (2 h) (Ramachandran *et al.*, 2003) or long incubation (4 d) (Liu *et al.*, 2010) in cultured fetal cortical neurons and PC12 cells, leading to a cascade of mitochondria associated effects and finally in apoptotic death. The increased levels of free radicals and the protective effect of antioxidants against ethanol-induced apoptosis in cultured primary neuronal cells and neurotypic cell lines were also shown in several studies (Chen and Sulik, 1996; Chandler *et al.*, 1997; Mitchell *et al.*, 1999a,b; Li *et al.*, 2000, 2001b; de la Monte *et al.*, 2001; Siler-Marsiglio *et al.*, 2004a,b; Ku *et al.*, 2006; Meng *et al.*, 2006; Chen *et al.*, 2008; Sheth *et al.*, 2009).

Evidence for involvement of GSH in protection from ethanol-mediated apoptosis was obtained using the same embryonic cortical neurons, revealing the important role of oxidative stress in developmental neurotoxicity of ethanol (Ramachandran *et al.*, 2003; Watts *et al.*, 2005; Maffi *et al.*, 2008; Liu *et al.*, 2010). However, *in vivo* exposure to ethanol failed to induce ROS generation, in cultured cerebellar granule neurons (CGNs) obtained from treated 14-day-old rat pups (Kane *et al.*, 2008). On the other hand, ethanol caused a concentration-dependent increase in ROS formation and exhaustion of GSH content in astrocytes in culture (Montoliu *et al.*, 1995). Finally, there have been reports on the protective role of astrocytes against ethanol-induced oxidative injury to neurons (Gonthier *et al.*, 2004; Watts *et al.*, 2005; Rathinam *et al.*, 2006).

A closer look at Table 19.1, which describes most of the cell culture studies investigating the ethanol-induced developmental cytotoxicity, cell cycle retardation, apoptosis and oxidative stress available in the literature, reveals that most studies have been conducted in primary cell cultures rather than immortal cell lines. And it seems that there is a good agreement in the findings derived from both parts, revealing the importance of this kind of approach for the elucidation of the mechanisms underlying the developmental neurotoxicity of ethanol.

Toluene

Like ethanol, toluene has also been reported to cause growth retardation and microcephaly in newborns. In an animal study, exposure of pregnant rats to toluene led to the birth of pups with reduced number of cortical neurons; however, it is not known whether such alteration is due to increased apoptosis or reduced neurogenesis (Gospe and Zhou, 2000). Consecutive toluene treatment (1–5 mM for 3 days) of hippocampal neurons prepared from embryonic day 18 rats failed to reveal any cytotoxic effect (Lin *et al.*, 2002). However, some studies suggest the involvement of glia in the developmental neurotoxicity of toluene (Hansson *et al.*, 1988; Gospe and Zhou, 2000; Costa *et al.*, 2002). Toluene was found to inhibit proliferation without causing cytotoxicity in human astrocytoma cells and cortical astrocytes (Burry *et al.*, 2003). Furthermore, exposure of cultured rat neonatal cortical astrocytes to relevant high concentration of toluene (40 mM) for over 7 h was associated with caspase-3-dependent apoptosis (Lin *et al.*, 2002).

TABLE 19.1 Effects of ethanol on cell proliferation and apoptosis *in vitro*

In vitro model	Effects	References
Primary cell cultures		
Neuronal		
Cerebral cortical neurons from fetal rats at 17 to 19 days of gestation 16 to 17 days of gestation	Cell death Inhibition of cell proliferation Apoptosis Oxidative stress	Takadera *et al.*, 1990 Ahern *et al.*, 1994 Seabold *et al.*, 1998 Jacobs and Miller, 2001 Ramachandran *et al.*, 2003 Takadera and Ohyashiki, 2004 Watts *et al.*, 2005 Cherian *et al.*, 2008 Maffi *et al.*, 2008 Liu *et al.*, 2010
Cerebral cortical neurons from: 1-day-old rat pups	Cell death	Chandler *et al.*, 1993 Chandler *et al.*, 1997
Cerebellar granule cells (CGCs) from: 7- to 8-day-old rat pups 9- to 10-day-old rat pups	Cell death Apoptosis Oxidative stress	Iorio *et al.*, 1993 Pantazis *et al.*, 1993 Pantazis *et al.*, 1995 Luo *et al.*, 1997 Castoldi *et al.*, 1998 Pantazis *et al.*, 1998 Zhang *et al.*, 1998 Oberdoerster and Rabin, 1999a Heaton *et al.*, 2004 Siler-Marsiglio *et al.*, 2004a Siler-Marsiglio *et al.*, 2004b
CGCs from: 6- to 7-day-old mice pups	Cell death Apoptosis	Vaudry *et al.*, 2005 Nowoslawski *et al.*, 2005
Cerebellar granule neurons (CGNs) from: 6- to 8-day-old rat pups 4- and 14-day-old rat pups (*in vivo* exposure)	Cell death Apoptosis Oxidative stress	Bhave and Hoffman, 1997 Leisi, 1997 Saito *et al.*, 1999 Bhave *et al.*, 2000 de la Monte *et al.*, 2001 Vaudry *et al.*, 2002 Zhong *et al.*, 2006 Kane *et al.*, 2008 Ke *et al.*, 2009
Hypothalamic neurons from fetal rats at: 18 to 21 days of gestation	Apoptosis	De *et al.*, 1994 Chen *et al.*, 2006
Neural crest cell (NCC) from fetal mice at: 8 days of gestation	Cell death Oxidative stress	Chen and Sulik, 1996
Biogenic amine neurons (serotonin and dopamine) from fetal rats at: 14 days of gestation	Cell death	Crews *et al.*, 1999
Organotypic entorhinal/hippocampal slice cultures from: 8- to 10-day-old rat pups	Cell death	Collins *et al.*, 1998
Hippocampal neurons from fetal rats at: 18 days of gestation	Cell death Oxidative stress	Mitchell *et al.*, 1999a Mitchell *et al.*, 1999b
Hippocampal neurons from: 1- to 3-day-old rat pups	Cell death	Moulder *et al.*, 2002
Hemispheres neuron cultures from fetal rats at: 18 days of gestation	Cell death Apoptosis	Lamarche *et al.*, 2003
Rhombencephalic neurons from fetal rats at: 14 days of gestation	Apoptosis	Druse *et al.*, 2005, 2006, 2007 Antonio and Druse, 2008
Glial		
Cerebral cortical astrocytes from fetal rats at: 21 days of gestation	Cell death Inhibition of cell proliferation Apoptosis Oxidative stress	Guerri *et al.*, 1990 Montoliu *et al.*, 1995 Guizzetti and Costa, 1996 Pascual *et al.*, 2003
Cerebral cortical astrocytes and oligodendrocytes from: newborn rat pups	Inhibition of cell proliferation Necrosis	Holownia *et al.*, 1997
Cerebral cortical astrocytes from: 1- to 2-day-old rat pups 4- to 5-day-old rat pups	Inhibition of cell proliferation Oxidative stress	Luo and Miller, 1999a Gonthier *et al.*, 2004 Watts *et al.*, 2005

TABLE 19.1 Effects of ethanol on cell proliferation and apoptosis in vitro—Cont'd

In vitro model	Effects	References
Cerebral cortical astrocytes from: 2-day-old rat pups Co-culture with cortical neurons from fetal rats at: 16 to 17 days of gestation	Apoptosis Oxidative stress	Watts *et al.*, 2005 Rathinam *et al.*, 2006
Cell lines		
Neuronotypic		
Rat pheochromocytoma PC12 cells	Cell death Inhibition of cell proliferation Apoptosis Oxidative stress	Pantazis *et al.*, 1992 Oberdoerster *et al.*, 1998 Li *et al.*, 1999 Luo *et al.*, 1999 Oberdoerster and Rabin, 1999b Li *et al.*, 2000, 2001b Meng *et al.*, 2006 Krzyzanski *et al.*, 2007 Liu *et al.*, 2010
Rat B104 neuroblastoma cells	Cell death Inhibition of cell proliferation	Luo and Miller 1997a, 1999b
Human SH-SY5Y neuroblastoma cells	Inhibition of cell proliferation Apoptosis Oxidative stress	Luo and Miller, 1997b Thibault *et al.*, 2000 Chen *et al.*, 2008
Human SK-N-SH neuroblastoma cells	Inhibition of cell proliferation Apoptosis Necrosis	Luo and Miller, 1997b McAlhany *et al.*, 2000
Human IMR32 neuroblastoma cells	Inhibition of cell proliferation	Luo and Miller, 1997b
Human SK-N-MC neuroblastoma cells	Apoptosis	Jang *et al.*, 2001
Murine N2a neuroblastoma cells	Apoptosis	Kang *et al.*, 2005
Murine hippocampal neuroblastoma cell line HT22	Oxidative stress	Ku *et al.*, 2006
Murine HN2-5 hippocampal-derived cell line	Oxidative stress	Sheth *et al.*, 2009
Gliotypic		
Rat C6 glioma cells	Proliferation	Luo and Miller, 1996

Pesticides

There is growing body of epidemiological evidence that organophosphates (OPs) and in particular chlorpyrifos (CPF) induce developmental neurotoxicity, as demonstrated in a recent review by Eaton *et al.* (2008). Furthermore, both prenatal and postnatal administration of CPF were found to cause significant brain loss by reducing cell density, as indicated by diminished DNA concentration, something that can even continue into adolescence and adulthood (Campbell *et al.*, 1997; Qiao *et al.*, 2002, 2003). Another OP, diazinon (DZN), increased or decreased cell number, depending on the brain area and elevated cell density, when administered in rat pups; however, it is unclear to what extent it can cause developmental neurotoxicity (Slotkin *et al.*, 2008a).

The developmental neurotoxicity of CPF has been recently reviewed and summarized in a comprehensive table, where all *in vitro* models as well as the endpoints used to study CPF-induced cytotoxicity, apoptosis and oxidative stress are available (Eaton *et al.*, 2008). Briefly, the IC_{50} values were found to be 12 μM and 2.5 μM for CPF and CPF-oxon (CPO), respectively, in mouse CGNs (Giordano *et al.*, 2007). Interestingly, the IC_{50} value (290 μM) of CPO in PC12 cells was considerably higher than the one established in primary cells (Li and Casida, 1998). In rat C6 glioma cells the IC_{50} value for CPO was 267 μM, whereas rat CG-4 oligodendrocyte progenitor cells showed that the IC_{50} value for CPO was 125 μM (Li and Casida, 1998; Saulsbury *et al.*, 2009).

Apoptosis was studied in newborn and embryonic rat cortical neurons after exposure to CPF (30 μM), revealing higher sensitivity of embryonic neurons to CPF-induced nuclear fragmentation and condensation (Caughlan *et al.*, 2004). In the same study, the oxon-metabolite of CPF (20 μM) was found to be slightly more potent than the parent compound (50 μM) in inducing neonatal cortical neuron apoptosis (Caughlan *et al.*, 2004). However, recent findings suggest that CPF (100 μM) and CPO (1–10 μM for 3–7 days) induce necrosis rather than apoptosis in mixed cortical cell cultures from fetal mice and rat hippocampal slices, respectively (Prendergast *et al.*, 2007; Rush *et al.*, 2010).

High concentrations of CPF (100 μM) were also needed for the detection of apoptotic signals in astrocytes isolated from second semester human fetal brains treated for 2 weeks, although as little as 0.2 μM could cause increased LDH release in the same *in vitro* system (Mense *et al.*, 2006). CPF (60 and 120 μM) caused nuclear condensation and fragmentation and caspase activation in cultured oligodendrocyte progenitor cells, though this was not blocked by a pan-caspase inhibitor (Saulsbury *et al.*, 2009). Studies on mouse embryo blastomeres also demonstrated that CPF is capable of inducing apoptosis (Grennlee *et al.*, 2004). Earlier work on whole rat embryo culture showed apoptosis within the neuroepithelium in embryos exposed to CPF (Roy *et al.*, 1998). DZN

(30 μM) exposure of fetal mixed cortical cells showed nuclear condensation and fragmentation, whereas a non-selective caspase inhibitor attenuated DZN-induced apoptosis (Rush *et al.*, 2010). Caspase activation and induction of apoptosis have also been noted in human NTera2-clone D1 neuronal precursor cells exposed to DZN (Aluigi *et al.*, 2010). Moreover, DZN-induced apoptosis was found in differentiated PC12 cells by TUNEL staining (Sadri *et al.*, 2010).

Studies with PC12 cells suggested that CPF can elicit cell injury through production of oxidative stress measured by DNA-single strand breaks and ROS generation (Bagchi *et al.*, 1995; Crumpton *et al.*, 2000a; Geter *et al.*, 2008). In the same *in vitro* model, there have been a number of studies investigating the CPF-induced oxidative stress through evaluation of lipid peroxidation (Qiao *et al.*, 2005; Slotkin *et al.*, 2007; Slotkin and Seidler, 2010). The same research group reported that CPF and DZN had a significant effect on the expression of oxidative stress-related genes in PC12 cells (Slotkin and Seidler, 2009a). Previously, both OPs and their oxygen analogs (1 μM) were found to increase ROS formation and lipid peroxidation in CGNs (Giordano *et al.*, 2007). In glia-like models, acute CPF treatment of C6 cells elicited increase of ROS generation, especially in differentiated cells (Garcia *et al.*, 2001). Using CG-4 cells, it was demonstrated that CPF-induced injury is associated with induction of oxidative stress that can be attenuated by antioxidant treatment (Saulsbury *et al.*, 2009).

PCBs

Recently, epidemiological studies suggested that perinatal PCB exposure impairs learning and memory, decreases IQ scores and causes attention deficits in children (Seegal, 1996; Weisglas-Kuperus, 1998; Ribas-Fito *et al.*, 2001), in agreement with neurobehavioral studies conducted in non-human primates and rodents (Tilson *et al.*, 1990; Tilson and Kodavanti, 1998). However, all these neurobehavioral alterations occur in the absence of pathological findings in the brain (Brouwer *et al.*, 1999), supporting the notion that PCB-induced cognitive deficits mirror delicate organizational deficiencies in the brain, which attracted the most attention and laid the ground for cellular studies (Seegal, 1996; Gilbert *et al.*, 2000). PCB mixture Aroclor 1254 (10 μM) and PCB congeners 47 (1 μM), but not 77 (1 μM), induced apoptosis in primary embryonic hippocampal but not in cortical neurons from rats pups (Howard *et al.*, 2003). Similarly, Inglefield *et al.* (2001) showed that the loss of cell viability induced by Aroclor 1254 in developing neocortical cells in culture occurred through a non-poptotic mechanism. By contrast, two other PCB commercial mixtures, Aroclor 1248 and Aroclor 1260, managed to increase the apoptotic nuclear staining and to show DNA fragmentation in primary cortical neurons of rat embryonic origin (Sánchez-Alonso *et al.*, 2004).

Upon treatment of human neuroblastoma SK-N-MC cells with PCB 52, time- and dose-dependent cell cytotoxicity was observed (Hwang *et al.*, 2001). In addition, as little as 15 μg/ml of PCB 52 resulted in condensation of chromatin and an apoptotic DNA ladder (Hwang *et al.*, 2001). In mouse HT22 hippocampal cells, 24 h exposure to PCB 153 and 126 caused a significant elevation of both apoptosis and necrosis (Tofighi *et al.*, 2010). PCB 153 was also studied on human SH-SY5Y neuroblastoma cell line and showed induction of apoptosis associated with increased expression of mRNA and protein levels of cytochrome *c* (He *et al.*, 2009). In the same study, PCB 153 treatment failed to alter intracellular calcium homeostasis. On the other hand, one study using PC12 cells showed that the PCB congener 2, 2′, 4, 6′-TeCB increases calcium levels and induces calcium influx (Shin *et al.*, 2002). The same congener at 50 μM diminished cell viability and caused DNA fragmentation in a time-dependent manner in PC12 cells, whereas, 3,3′,4,4′-TeCB failed to do so. Moreover, PCB congener 2,4,4′ was found to be extremely neurotoxic in CGCs derived from 7- to 14-day-old pups and to cause late elevation of intracellular free calcium (Carpenter *et al.*, 1997). Remarkably, inhibition of PCB-induced increase of intracellular calcium resulted in the reduction of human SH-SY5Y neuroblastoma cell death evoked by exposure to PCBs (Magi *et al.*, 2005; Canzoniero *et al.*, 2006).

Exposure of neonatal rat CGCs to Aroclor 1254, 1242 and PCB 153 but not PCB 126 induced a concentration-dependent increase in cell loss and ROS generation, after acute exposure (24 h) to a wide range of doses (6.5–50 μM) (Mariussen *et al.*, 2002). Voie and Fonnum (2000) have also reported that the PCB congener 2,2′-DCB activates ROS formation in rat brain synaptosomes. Furthermore, Howard *et al.* (2003) suggested that the proapoptotic activity of Aroclor 1254 and PCB 47 require elevation of ROS generation. The involvement of oxidative stress in PCB neurotoxicity was even more strengthened by demonstrating the sensitivity of CGCs of mice origin with genetically determined low glutathione levels exposed to PCB 153 and 126, compared to wild-type cells (Costa *et al.*, 2007). However, a recent study using the HT22 cell line suggested that oxidative stress has no involvement in PCB 153 and 126 neurotoxic effects (Tofighi *et al.*, 2010).

PBDEs

PBDEs represent another category of environmental pollutant that alters learning and memory processes (Eriksson *et al.*, 2001; Viberg *et al.*, 2003; Dufault *et al.*, 2005), without causing pathological damage in the brain. Hence, the elucidation of the mechanism of action of PBDEs relies on well-designed *in vitro* studies, aiming to reveal what really happens at a molecular level.

The effects of a number of PBDEs in mouse CGCs were studied, revealing that all of them are cytotoxic and induce apoptotic cell death to different degrees with PBDE-100 being the most potent congener followed by PBDE-47, -99, -153 and finally -209 (Huang *et al.*, 2010). PBDE-47-induced apoptosis as determined by flow cytometry in human SH-SY5Y neuroblastoma cells and primary cultured neonatal rat hippocampal neurons (He *et al.*, 2008a,b). In the same primary cell culture, PBDE-209 caused a concentration-dependent increase in cell death and apoptotic cells (Chen *et al.*, 2010). Another study also indicated that there was a dose–effect relationship between DE-71 (a penta-BDE mixture) concentration and apoptotic cell death in mouse CGCs, especially in those derived from hippocampus (Giordano *et al.*, 2008). Interestingly, Reistad *et al.* (2006) reported on DE-71-induced apoptosis in rat CGCs independent of increased caspase-3 activity. No apparent increase of the same intracellular effector was also found in cultures of prenatal (GD17) rat cortical cells treated with high concentration of PBDE-99 that displayed high mortality rates (Alm *et al.*, 2008). By contrast, Yu *et al.* (2008) reported on DE-71-induced apoptosis in human neuroblastoma cell line, SK-N-SH, through a caspase activation pathway.

Fetal human neural progenitor cells exposed to low concentrations (0.1–10 μM) of PBDE-47 and -99 for long incubation time revealed no effect on cell proliferation and calcium levels (Schreiber *et al.*, 2010). On the other hand, as little as 1 μM PBDE-47 increased calcium levels and induced apoptosis in a human neuroblastoma cell line, showing a positive correlation between these two endpoints (He *et al.*, 2009). Dingemans *et al.* (2008) also demonstrated altered calcium homeostasis by PBDE-47 in PC12 cells. Consistently, PBDE-209 and DE-71 did increase calcium ion content in cultured hippocampal neurons and SK-N-SH neuroblastoma cells, respectively (Yu *et al.*, 2008; Chen *et al.*, 2010).

PBDE-100, -47, -99, -153 and -209 were found to cause oxidative stress through elevation of ROS levels in mouse CGCs (Huang *et al.*, 2010). ROS levels were enhanced by PBDE-47 treatment in primary rat hippocampal neurons and SH-SY5Y neuroblastoma cells (He *et al.*, 2008a,b; Gao *et al.*, 2009). Neonatal rat hippocampal cells exposed to PBDE-209 (10, 30 or 50 μg/ml) also showed elevation of ROS formation (Chen *et al.*, 2010). An elegant recent study has even shown that DE-71 causes increase not only in ROS but also in lipid peroxidation, which was more pronounced in CGCs obtained from glutathione-depleted mice than from wild-type mice. No induction of ROS generation was found after exposure of human neuroblastoma cells to the mixture DE-71 (Yu *et al.*, 2008). Reistad *et al.* (2006) similarly failed to detect any elevation of ROS in primary rat CGCs. Recently, high (15 and 20 μM) but not low concentrations (1 and 5 μM) of PBDE-47 and -99 induced significant enhancement of ROS levels by using human neuroblastoma SK-N-MC cell line (Tagliaferri *et al.*, 2010). Interestingly, the same study showed that combined exposure to low but not high concentrations caused increased ROS formation. Again, astrocytes appeared to be more resistant than neurons to developmental neurotoxicity of PBDEs (Giraldo *et al.*, 2008; Giordano *et al.*, 2009). However, human 132-1N1 astrocytoma cells like neuronal-type cell lines were found to undergo apoptosis after treatment with PBDE-99 (Madia *et al.*, 2004).

NEURITE OUTGROWTH

Neurite outgrowth is a marker of neuronal differentiation that has been widely employed in toxicological studies. It is a morphological marker that is determined with the aid of a microscope, although in a few cases it has been determined biochemically by measuring the ratio of membrane protein to total protein or DNA (Qiao *et al.*, 2003; Slotkin *et al.*, 2006, 2008a). In the majority of studies, neurite outgrowth has been measured following the *in vitro* addition of the toxic agent to a culture system. In a few instances, outgrowth has been assessed after administration of the agent to developing animals. In almost all cases, culture systems employed in neurite outgrowth toxicological studies are cell cultures. Both primary neuronal cell cultures and neuronotypic cell lines have been used. In a few notable cases, outgrowth has been assessed in gliotypic cell lines as an index of glial cell differentiation. A comprehensive review of available data concerning six of the most well-established DNTs *in vivo* (mercury, lead, arsenic, ethanol, PCBs/dioxins and organophosphate esters) indicates that these substances do also disrupt *in vitro* the process of neurite outgrowth. Remarkably, in almost all cases involving primary cell cultures, an inhibitory effect has been obtained. On the other hand, in cell lines, data are not as consistent. Thus, whereas an inhibitory effect has been demonstrated in many cases, in certain instances, a stimulatory action on neurite outgrowth has been recorded. This has been mainly noted for the PC12 cell line. This excessive neurite outgrowth has been interpreted as being indicative of premature *in vivo* neuronal differentiation that could, similarly to neurite outgrowth inhibition, harm the developing nervous system by disturbing the normal, balanced neural developmental pattern. This peculiar response of PC12 cells should be borne in mind in toxicological studies using neurite outgrowth as differentiation marker.

When using neurite outgrowth disruption as an index of *in vivo* developmental neurotoxicity, it should be pointed out that the effects obtained depend not only on the type of culture system employed, as highlighted in several studies, such as that of Audesirk *et al.* (1991), but also depend on a number of additional factors. Thus, within the same cell culture type, both the magnitude (Crumpton *et al.*, 2001) and the direction (Parran *et al.*, 2001) of changes in neurite outgrowth are dependent on the stage of differentiation at which the cultured cells are present at the time of their exposure to the developmental neurotoxicant. Indeed, there is a difference in the response of cells that are already differentiated and cells that have not been previously exposed to the differentiating agent. In addition, neurite outgrowth effects appear to depend on the concentration of the developmental neurotoxicant employed. This is illustrated in studies with lead, where different concentrations of this chemical have been found to exert different effects on neurite outgrowth assessed in both primary cultures (Kern *et al.*, 1993) and cell lines (Crumpton *et al.*, 2001).

The outcome of a toxicological study using neurite outgrowth as a marker seems also to depend to some extent on what exactly has been counted. A review of the literature shows that there is a wide variety of relevant parameters that have been assessed. Such parameters, among others, include total neurite length per cell, number of neurites per cell, total number of neurites longer than two cell body diameters, number of neurites longer than 10 μm, branch points per cell, fragments per cell, fragment length per cell, etc. The use of fully automated technology adopted recently (Radio *et al.*, 2008) allows rapid and precise counting of these constituent measures of neurite outgrowth.

All of the factors outlined above can lead to considerable variability in neurite outgrowth data and should be taken into account in studies using this endpoint as an *in vitro* developmental neurotoxicity marker. A central issue that remains unresolved is the extent to which neurite outgrowth constitutes a valid marker for *in vivo* developmental neurotoxicity. Thus, in a number of cell culture studies a range of exogenous substances of widely differing structures have been shown to interfere with neurite outgrowth but still their *in vivo* developmental neurotoxicity is not known (Abdulla and Campbell, 1993; Axelrad *et al.*, 2003). It is, therefore, important to establish in future studies whether compounds that have been shown to affect neurite outgrowth *in vitro* are indeed capable of inducing neurodevelopmental toxicity *in vivo* following prenatal or postnatal administration. On the other hand, compounds may be DNTs *in vivo* without having an effect on neurite outgrowth, as they may disrupt other important developmental processes, such as neuronal migration, myelination, etc.

Heavy metals

Mercury

The particular toxicity of mercury to the developing nervous system was established several decades ago as a result of the tragic poisoning incidents in Japan (Takeuchi *et al.*, 1959) and Iraq (Bakir *et al.*, 1973) and, also, thanks to several *in vivo* experimental studies in a number of different animal species including humans (Choi *et al.*, 1978). In response to this, a number of *in vitro* studies have been undertaken to assess the effect of mercury on the processes of neurite outgrowth. For this purpose, both primary cultures and cell lines have been employed. Most studies have used MeHg, as this compound is known to be *in vivo* more toxic than inorganic mercury. However, a recent study has also assessed the neurite outgrowth effect of ethyl mercury thiosalicylate (thimerosal) (Lawton *et al.*, 2007). Knowledge of the developmental neurotoxic potential of this compound is important, as it is present in several vaccines that may be administered to infants. All studies on MeHg, conducted in several cell culture systems, indicate that this compound, at submicromolar or low micromolar concentrations, inhibits neurite outgrowth under a variety of conditions. Thus, inhibition of neurite outgrowth has been demonstrated in both embryonic sensory (Nakada *et al.*, 1981; Soderstrom and Ebendal, 1995) and sympathetic (Soderstrom and Ebendal, 1995) dorsal root ganglia. Similarly, in cultures of embryonic forebrain neurons, subcytotoxic concentrations of MeHg (0.25 and 0.5 μM) inhibited neurite outgrowth by 50% (Heidemann *et al.*, 2001). The potent inhibitory properties of MeHg have also been demonstrated in cell lines. In mouse N2a neuroblastoma cells MeHg, at a subcytotoxic concentration of 1 μM, inhibited within 4 hours neurite outgrowth by more than 50% (Lawton *et al.*, 2007). Interestingly, this concentration inhibited with the same potency also the outgrowth of processes from cultured rat C6 glioma cells, indicating that MeHg effects on the differentiation of the nervous system may be more extensive than previously thought. Neurite inhibition by MeHg has been systematically studied in PC12 cells. MeHg, at concentrations of 0.3–3 μM, decreased total neurite outgrowth, although it had no effect on the extent of neurite branching (Parran *et al.*, 2001). However, some of these effects were noted at concentrations affecting cell viability. More potent and differentiation-specific effects were, however, noted in PC12 cells that were already in a fully differentiated state. In this case, MeHg inhibited neurite outgrowth, with an IC_{50} value as low as 0.03 μM, as well as neurite branching. These effects were confirmed in a subsequent study by the same research group (Parran *et al.*, 2003). A more recent study from this group, employing a more technologically advanced system to quantify neurite outgrowth, established that MeHg also inhibited neurite outgrowth in a subclone of PC12 cells, the NS-1 cell line, with a significant effect being noted at a concentration as low as 1 nM, a level 1,000-fold higher than that affecting cell viability (Radio *et al.*, 2008).

In contrast to the MeHg studies showing consistently inhibitory effects on neurite outgrowth, available data on the effects of inorganic mercury, in the form of $HgCl_2$, are contradictory, with both decreases and increases in neurite outgrowth being recorded. Thus, $HgCl_2$ inhibited neurite outgrowth in cultures of embryonic sensory dorsal root ganglia, albeit with a potency 25 times lower than that of MeHg in the same culture system (Nakada *et al.*, 1981). An inhibitory effect was also noted in human SKNSH neuroblastoma cells, where a concentration of $HgCl_2$ as low as 0.1 nM caused a significant 19% neurite outgrowth inhibition (Abdulla and Campbell, 1995). In PC12 cells, on the other hand, data are not as consistent and this could be, at least partly, related to the different differentiation states in which the PC12 cells were at the time of $HgCl_2$ exposure. Thus, addition of $HgCl_2$, at concentrations of 0.3 and 0.5 μM to undifferentiated cells in the presence of NGF produced a marked increase in neurite outgrowth (Rossi *et al.*, 1993). Similarly, $HgCl_2$ concentrations of 0.1–3 μM that did not affect cell viability increased neurite outgrowth as well as the extent of neurite branching (Parran *et al.*, 2001). In contrast, addition of $HgCl_2$, in the same study, to fully differentiated PC12 cells at subcytotoxic concentrations as low as 0.03 μM, exerted an inhibitory effect on neurite outgrowth and, also, did not affect neurite branching.

Particularly interesting are the results of a recent study of the effects of ethyl mercury thiosalicylate (thimerosal) on neurite outgrowth, in view of the use of this compound as an additive in a number of vaccines and topical medications that can be given to infants. According to the obtained data, this compound, at a subcytotoxic concentration of 1 μM, was able to interfere with neurite/extension outgrowth in both neuronotypic (N2a) and gliotypic (C6) cell lines, causing more than 50% inhibition after as early as 4 hours' exposure (Lawton *et al.*, 2007). Comparison of the potency of thimerosal to that of MeHg under identical conditions in fact indicates that thimerosal may be more potent in its neurite-inhibitory effect in N2a cells, raising concern about its *in vivo* developmental neurotoxic potential.

Lead

The ability of lead to induce developmental neurotoxicity *in vivo* is well documented both epidemiologically and experimentally. *In vitro* studies assessing the effect of lead on neurite outgrowth have been mostly conducted before the last decade and nearly half of them have come from the same research group. Both primary cell cultures and cell lines have been employed. All studies using primary cultures have demonstrated a neurite outgrowth inhibitory effect, whereas results with cell lines are not as consistent with more recent studies in PC12 cells showing an increase or no effect. In several cases, effects have been noted at submicromolar concentrations similar to those found in the CSF of humans with no known history of occupational lead exposure. In fact, some researchers have observed a stronger effect at the lower lead concentrations used.

In an earlier study lead was found to inhibit neurite outgrowth in cultures of dorsal root ganglion neurons, although it was less potent than mercury and arsenic (Windebank, 1986). Evidence that lead exerts a potent inhibitory effect on neurite outgrowth in primary cultures has also come from subsequent studies with embryonic hippocampal and cortical neurons. Thus, in hippocampal neurons lead effects were noted at concentrations as low as 25 nM (Audesirk *et al.*, 1991), with a concentration of 0.1 μM causing up to 30% neurite inhibition (Kern and Audesirk, 1995). A similar effect was also noted by the same research group in embryonic motor cortical neurons (Kern *et al.*, 1993). In contrast, studies with cell lines have yielded contradictory data. Thus, in the human IMR32 neuroblastoma cell line, lead was found to inhibit neurite outgrowth (Gotti *et al.*, 1987), whereas in another neuroblastoma cell line, the mouse N1E-115 cell line, a neurite outgrowth stimulatory effect was demonstrated (Audesirk *et al.*, 1991). Two more recent studies have shown independently that lead exerts a stimulatory effect on neurite outgrowth in the PC12 cell line (Williams *et al.*, 2000; Crumpton *et al.*, 2001). Importantly, this effect is noted at lead concentrations of 0.1 μM or less and includes increases in the extent of neurite branching. The neurite outgrowth promoting property of lead was also noted in already differentiated PC12 cells, although this effect was 4–20 times less robust than in PC12 cells not previously exposed to NGF. On the other hand, in a more recent study using fully automated technology for the quantification of neurite outgrowth, lead, at non-cytotoxic concentrations of 1 nM to 100 μM, failed to have an effect in a PC12 cell clone, the NS-1 cell line (Radio *et al.*, 2008).

Arsenic

Although there is growing evidence that arsenic exposure can induce neurotoxic effects in children and adolescents (Wang *et al.*, 2004; Wasserman *et al.*, 2004), the effect of this metal on the process of neurite outgrowth has not been adequately investigated. In fact, in one study the assessment of the effect of arsenic on the differentiation of the human neuroblastoma cell line IMR-32 has been conducted not in the context of developmental neurotoxicity but for the pharmacological purpose of assessing the ability of this chemical to interfere with the development of neuroblastoma tumors (Cheung *et al.*, 2007). In this study, arsenic treatment induced the extension of short processes, but, as there were no significant increases in the expression of neurofilament proteins, it was inferred that only minimal differentiation occurred. A recent study that has assessed the *in vitro* effects of arsenic in the context of developmental neurotoxicity, however, demonstrated that this chemical (in the form of sodium arsenite) interfered, in PC12 cells, with the initial stages of neurite outgrowth, affecting, among others, the length of the longest neurite, the proportion of cells with long neurites, the neurite width and the extent of neurite branching (Frankel *et al.*, 2009). Neurite outgrowth and branching was also reduced in PC12 cells already bearing some neurites, indicating that arsenic can also affect the later stages of differentiation and neurite elongation.

Organic solvents

Ethanol

The predominant involvement of the CNS in the characteristic pattern of abnormalities noted in the fetus as a result of maternal alcohol consumption during pregnancy has long been a witness to the developmental neurotoxic potential of ethanol. Accordingly, several studies have assessed the effect of this compound on the process of neurite outgrowth *in vitro*. The majority of studies indicate that ethanol can interfere with neurite outgrowth. However, the nature of the effect varies and seems to depend on the culture system employed. In most culture systems an inhibitory ethanol effect on neurite outgrowth has been demonstrated, although in some cases an enhancement of neurite outgrowth has been shown and there are, also, reports of no ethanol effects. Moreover, it is worth noting that a number of investigations have employed ethanol concentrations that may not be physiologically relevant (>50 mM). Both primary cultures and cell lines have been used.

The sensitivity of the process of neurite outgrowth to ethanol was noted in chick embryonic neuroblast-enriched cultures, where there was a profound decrease in both neurite number and length (Kentroti and Vernadakis, 1991). Ethanol also inhibited neurite outgrowth in cultures of dorsal root ganglion neurons, where its effect is prevented by high NGF levels (Heaton *et al.*, 1993). In this culture system, neurite inhibition was also caused by acetaldehyde, the primary metabolite of ethanol *in vivo* (Bradley *et al.*, 1995). In cultures of postnatal cerebellar neurons ethanol also displayed an inhibitory effect on neurite outgrowth. This effect was specific as it concerned only neurite outgrowth mediated by the neural cell adhesion molecule L1 and not outgrowth mediated by laminin or N-cadherin (Bearer *et al.*, 1999). The neurite inhibitory effect of ethanol also extends to cultures of embryonic neurons from the cerebral cortex. Significantly, this effect was noted at ethanol concentrations as low as 4.5 μM (Bingham *et al.*, 2004). A concentration of 45 μM was even capable of affecting dendritic branching. The latter effect was decreased by a number of growth factors and estrogen (Barclay *et al.*, 2005). In more complex culture systems, e.g. embryonic spinal cord-muscle or fetal septal-hippocampal co-cultured explants, ethanol caused loss of target-oriented neurite outgrowth (Heaton *et al.*, 1995).

The ability of ethanol to influence neurite outgrowth has been also assessed in neuroblastoma cell lines. Although in earlier studies neurite outgrowth from mouse N2a neuroblastoma cells was unaffected by ethanol treatment (Leskawa *et al.*, 1995), recently a neurite outgrowth inhibitory effect in this culture system was noted (Chen *et al.*, 2009). Neurite inhibition was reversed by cyanine-3-glucoside. An inhibitory effect of ethanol was also shown recently in human neuroblastoma cells (Hellman *et al.*, 2009), where the morphological effect was accompanied by decreased expression of neuronal marker proteins.

In contrast to these studies showing inhibitory effects of ethanol on the process of neurite outgrowth, in some investigations a neurite-promoting action has been demonstrated, in line with some data indicating that in some brain regions ethanol enhances the development of dendrites (Messing *et al.*, 1991). Thus, in cultures of embryonic cerebellar macroneurons ethanol enhanced neurite outgrowth by inducing significant increases in the percentage of neurite-bearing cells, the total neuritic length per cell, the length of the longest neurite in each cell and the mean number of neurite branches (Zou *et al.*, 1993). Similarly, a neurite-promoting effect was noted in the PC12 cell line. In these cells, ethanol enhanced NGF- and basic FGF-induced neurite outgrowth (Roivainen *et al.*, 1993; Furuya *et al.*, 2002), and this effect was further increased by docosahexaenoic acid (Furuya *et al.*, 2002).

The effect of ethanol on the development of extensions from glial cells has not been studied. However, neurite outgrowth was perturbed in rhombencephalic neuronal cultures grown in conditioned media produced by ethanol-treated cultured cortical astrocytes, as the latter lack essential neurotrophic factors (Kim and Druse, 1996).

Pesticides

A rapidly growing body of data over the last decade, both experimental and epidemiological, indicate that organophosphate (OP) esters are capable of inducing developmental neurotoxicity *in vivo* (Flaskos and Sachana, in press). The biggest volume of this evidence involves two widely used phosphorothionate pesticides (CPF and DZN). Accordingly, there have been a number of studies that have assessed *in vitro* the ability of these compounds to affect the process of neurite outgrowth. Both primary cell cultures and cell lines have been employed for this purpose. Remarkably, in almost all cases, both OPs have been found to exert an inhibitory effect on neurite outgrowth. It is worth noting that even when neurite outgrowth has been assessed after the *in vivo* OP administration to developing animals by biochemical means, an inhibitory effect of CPF and DZN has been demonstrated (Qiao *et al.*, 2003; Slotkin *et al.*, 2006).

The effect of CPF has been studied in primary cultures of embryonic sympathetic neurons derived from superior cervical ganglia (Howard *et al.*, 2005) as well as in cultures of sensory neurons derived from embryonic dorsal root ganglia (Yang *et al.*, 2008). In both systems, CPF, at a concentration as low as 1 nM, inhibited the outgrowth of axonal length, although it had no effect on the number of these processes. CPF also impaired neurite outgrowth in cell lines. Thus, exposure of PC12 cells to CPF inhibited NGF-induced differentiation (Song *et al.*, 1998; Das and Barone, 1999). CPF, at low micromolar concentrations, also caused rapid inhibition of neurite outgrowth in cultures of mouse N2a neuroblastoma cells (Sachana *et al.*, 2001, 2005; Axelrad *et al.*, 2003). An inhibitory effect under somewhat different exposure conditions was also noted in another neuroblastoma cell line, the mouse N-18 neuroblastoma cells (Henschler *et al.*, 1992), although this effect in a subsequent study was only noted at cytotoxic CPF levels (Schmuck and Ahr, 1997).

The effect of DZN on neurite outgrowth has only been assessed in cultures of N2a cells. In these cells, this OP, at low micromolar concentrations, inhibited neurite outgrowth (Axelrad *et al.*, 2003; Flaskos *et al.*, 2007).

Particularly important for the assessment of the *in vivo* developmental neurotoxic potential of OPs has been the demonstration that certain major *in vivo* metabolites of both CPF and DZN can also directly inhibit neurite outgrowth in a number of different culture systems. Thus, the oxon metabolite of CPF, CPO, at concentrations as low as 0.001 and 0.01 nM, inhibited axonal outgrowth in cultures of embryonic superior cervical (Howard *et al.*, 2005) and dorsal root (Yang *et al.*, 2008) ganglia, respectively. Similarly, the oxon metabolite of DZN, DZO, also impaired, at submicromolar concentrations, neurite outgrowth in the N2a cell line (Sidiropoulou *et al.*, 2009a). In all these cell culture systems, the neurite-inhibiting potency of the oxon metabolites was in fact 10–1,000 times greater than that of the parent pesticides. Even trichloropyridinol, a CPF metabolite generally considered as toxicologically innocuous, interfered, at biologically relevant levels, with neurite outgrowth in primary cultures of embryonic sympathetic neurons (Howard *et al.*, 2005).

OPs have also been found to be capable of interfering with the development of extensions from cultured differentiating rat C6 glioma cells, in line with growing evidence showing the ability of these compounds to disrupt normal development of glial cells *in vivo* (Flaskos and Sachana, in press). In an earlier study, a number of OPs, including CPF, were noted to inhibit extension outgrowth from C6 cells exposed to the OP for 20 days (Henschler *et al.*, 1992). A more recent study, using much shorter exposure times and subcytotoxic concentrations of OPs that lay within the range of expected fetal exposures in agricultural settings, indicated that both CPF and CPO were capable of impairing extension outgrowth in differentiating C6 cells (Sachana *et al.*, 2008). Interestingly, an inhibitory effect on extension outgrowth from C6 cells was also induced by DZO (Sidiropoulou *et al.*, 2009b), but not by the parent compound (Flaskos *et al.*, 2007).

PCBs/Dioxins

In a recent study, 2,3,7,8-tetrachlorodibenzo-p-dioxin (TCDD), at a subcytotoxic concentration as low as 5 nM, was able to inhibit neurite outgrowth in cultures of differentiating human SH-SY5Y neuroblastoma cells (Jung *et al.*, 2009), in line with the ability of this compound to induce developmental neurotoxicity *in vivo*.

NEUROTRANSMISSION/ SYNAPTOGENESIS

The life of a neurotransmitter consists of a number of separate events including its synthesis, storage, release, receptor binding, uptake and degradation. Most of these processes occur at or near the synapse and, thus, the development of neurotransmitter systems is closely related to synaptogenesis. Synaptogenesis is a long developmental process involving synapse formation, synapse maintenance (stabilization) and activity-dependent synapse refinement and elimination, and is important for the establishment of the neuronal network and the precision of brain circuitry (Cohen-Cory, 2002). Thus, any toxic insult on the development of neurotransmitter systems may have severe repercussions on the progression of neuronal development.

Each of the processes in the life of a neurotransmitter can be the specific target of developmental neurotoxic action and can be studied using a range of different approaches and methods of assessment. In addition, each of these processes involves the coordinated participation of a wide variety of distinct molecules. Due to the existence of several neurotransmitter systems, the diversity of approaches adopted (biochemical, molecular, electrophysiological, morphological, etc.) and the large number of distinct molecules required, there is an abundance of neurotransmitter-related parameters that have been studied as indices of developmental neurotoxicity. For reasons of space, as an indication, only the biochemical/molecular parameters that have been used as markers of the developmental neurotoxicity of mercury and lead will be reviewed. Studies of the effects of mercury and lead following *in vivo* animal exposure will also be included in several cases in order to indicate the extent to which the *in vitro* biochemical markers reflect analogous *in vivo* phenomena.

Heavy metals

Mercury

All studies on the effects of mercury on neurotransmission have involved MeHg. Due to its highly reactive nature,

MeHg exerts its neurotoxicity via a large number of distinct mechanisms involving a multitude of separate targets (Aschner *et al.*, 2000; Limke *et al.*, 2004), some of which are related to neurotransmission. Biochemical studies employing both homogenates and synaptosomal preparations from whole brain or specific brain regions have shown that MeHg increases neurotransmitter release (Bondy *et al.*, 1979; Minnema *et al.*, 1989), decreases neurotransmitter uptake (Rajanna and Hobson, 1985; O'Kusky, 1989) and alters neurotransmitter turnover (Kobayashi *et al.*, 1980; Bartolome *et al.*, 1982). In addition, it influences the availability of transmitter precursors (Bondy *et al.*, 1979; O'Kusky, 1989) as well as the activities of enzymes involved in the synthesis and degradation of transmitters (Tsuzuki, 1981; Omata *et al.*, 1982). Moreover, biochemical investigations indicate that binding to neurotransmitter receptors is also interfered with (Komulainen *et al.*, 1995; Castoldi *et al.*, 1996). However, all the above studies have employed brain preparations from animals exposed to mercury postdevelopmentally and, thus, the extent to which the various biochemical measures of transmitter synthesis, release, receptor binding, uptake, metabolism and turnover used above can constitute useful *in vitro* markers of MeHg developmental neurotoxicity is not clear. Some of the limited developmentally relevant data available indicate that MeHg affects biochemical measures of catecholaminergic neurotransmission. Thus, neonatal administration of this chemical to animals induces changes in the synaptosomal uptake and the turnover of both norepinephrine and dopamine (Bartolome *et al.*, 1982). Similarly, MeHg affects the expression of the catecholamine biosynthetic enzyme tyrosine hydroxylase (as determined by immunocytochemistry) in cultures of mouse embryonic ventral mesencephalic cells (Gotz *et al.*, 2002). MeHg also affects the development of biochemical parameters of the glutamatergic system. Thus, at submicromolar concentrations, it inhibits N-methyl-D-aspartate (NMDA)-specific [^{3}H]-glutamate receptor binding to neonatal brain synaptosomes (Rajanna *et al.*, 1997). Interestingly, the potency of this inhibition is more than 70 times greater than that noted in the adult brain under identical conditions. Interference with the developing glutamatergic system is also shown in *in vitro* experiments with astrocytes. Thus, MeHg inhibits uptake of L-glutamate in neonatal cortical astrocyte cultures and increases efflux of glutamate from preloaded astrocytes (Aschner *et al.*, 1993). These effects lead to an excessive elevation of glutamate levels in the synaptic fluid resulting in MeHg excitotoxicity (Aschner *et al.*, 2000).

Lead

The long-established adverse effects of lead on cognition, learning and behavior noted in epidemiological and experimental behavioral studies indicate that this chemical interferes with neurotransmission. In addition, there is now a considerable body of evidence from biochemical/histochemical, morphometric and electrophysiological studies which demonstrates that lead exerts toxic effects on the cholinergic, catecholaminergic, serotonergic and, particularly, the glutamatergic neurotransmitter systems. Biochemical studies have determined a wide range of neurotransmission-related parameters, but several of these studies have involved lead exposure of adult animals. Accordingly, only biochemical studies of direct developmental relevance will be reviewed here.

Perinatal exposure of chemicals to lead induces a reduction in the neonatal activity of choline acetylcholinesterase (ChAT) in the medial septum and the hippocampus, with the effects in the two brain regions persisting for 2 and 3 months, respectively (Bourjeily and Suszkiw, 1997). A considerable decrease in ChAT activity has also been noted in lead-exposed PC12 cells, and this is accompanied by a reduction in ChAT mRNA levels (Tian *et al.*, 2000). In contrast, ChAT activity is unaltered by lead treatment in cholinergic SN56 neuroblastoma cells (Jankowska-Kulawy *et al.*, 2008). Among other cholinergic neurotransmission parameters assessed, hippocampal hemicholinium-3 binding exhibits a large and lasting (6-month) decrease after perinatal lead exposure (Bourjeily and Suszkiw, 1997) and there is also a reduction in acetylcholine content in lead-treated SN56 cells (Jankowska-Kulawy *et al.*, 2008). On the other hand, neither AChE activity nor muscarinic receptor density (as measured by [^{3}H]-quinuclidinyl benzylate binding to membrane fractions) are affected in lead-exposed cultures of embryonic neural retina (Luo and Berman, 1997).

A number of biochemical studies indicate that exposure to lead during development leads to disruption of monoaminergic (catecholaminergic and, possibly, serotonergic) neurotransmission. Levels of the serotonin (5-HT) metabolite, 5-hydroxyindoloacetic acid (5-HIAA), determined by liquid chromatography, are reduced in several brain regions after developmental lead exposure of animals, whereas dopamine turnover is decreased in the frontal cortex and the nucleus accumbens (Lasley *et al.*, 1984). Interference with the developing dopaminergic system in nucleus accumbens by lead is also evidenced by alterations in dopamine receptor number (as measured by standard receptor binding assays) in tissue homogenates (Cory-Slechta *et al.*, 1993). Furthermore, developmental exposure of animals to lead induces significant decreases in the levels of dopamine in nucleus accumbens and hypothalamus and, also, affects the levels of the dopamine metabolites, homovanillic acid and 3,4-dihydroxy phenylacetic acid (Kala and Jadhav, 1995). Under these conditions, lead also affects the serotonergic system, as evidenced by decreases in both 5-HT and 5-HIAA in seven brain regions. The reduction in dopamine content can be, at least partly, attributed to an effect on tyrosine hydroxylase, the key regulatory enzyme in dopamine synthesis. Thus, exposure of developing animals to lead produces in whole brain homogenates a significant reduction in the activity of tyrosine hydroxylase, assayed by a radioisotopic method using [^{3}H]-tyrosine, and also causes a decrease in enzyme protein levels, as determined by Western blot analysis (Jadhav and Ramesh, 1997). A significant inhibition of tyrosine hydroxylase activity is also noted following *in vitro* exposure to lead of whole brain homogenates from developing animals.

Of all the effects of lead on neurotransmitter systems, it is its action on the glutamatergic system that has received the greatest attention. Indeed, a wide range of studies indicate that a principal target for lead-induced neurotoxicity is the NMDA subtype of glutamate receptor and it is lead's effects on this receptor during development that are related to the ability of this chemical to interfere with synaptic plasticity and induce cognitive and behavioral deficits (Marchetti, 2003). Depending on the approach followed, a number of different parameters have been employed as indices of NMDA receptor function. In the case of biochemical studies, many earlier investigations have used the binding of [^{3}H]-MK-801, a potent and selective non-competitive NMDA receptor antagonist, as a marker of NMDA receptor activity. A review of available data indicates that developmental exposure to lead both *in vitro* and *in vivo* usually reduces [^{3}H]-MK-801 binding. Thus, *in vitro* exposure of cortical membranes to lead inhibits [^{3}H]-MK-801 binding. Importantly, this inhibition is significantly higher in membranes prepared from neonatal animals than from adults (Guilarte and Miceli, 1992). A similar result has been obtained using [^{3}H]-glutamate instead of [^{3}H]-MK-801 as a ligand (Rajanna *et al.*, 1997). Inhibition of [^{3}H]-MK-801 binding to membranes from neonatal animals following *in vitro* lead exposure is also noted in the hippocampus, where, in fact, the inhibitory effect is four-fold stronger than in the cortex (Guilarte and Miceli, 1992). In addition, inhibition of [^{3}H]-MK-801 binding after *in vitro* developmental exposure occurs in the forebrain (Schulte *et al.*, 1995). A reduction in NMDA receptor activity is also found after *in vivo* exposure of developing animals to lead. Thus, lead-exposed neonatal animals exhibit a significant decrease in the number of [^{3}H]-MK-801 binding sites in the cortex, whereas exposure of adult animals has no effect (Guilarte and Miceli, 1992). In contrast, [^{3}H]-MK-801 binding after *in vivo* lead administration in the forebrain is slightly increased (Schulte *et al.*, 1995). A difference in response to neonatal lead exposure is also noted between the hippocampus and the cerebellum, with the number of [^{3}H]-MK-801 binding sites increasing during development in the former and decreasing in the latter (Guilarte, 1997).

The NMDA receptors are tetrameric complexes consisting of different subunits, which have different functions and follow different patterns of expression during development (Wenzel *et al.*, 1997). Later biochemical studies have, thus, assessed the developmental neurotoxicity of lead in terms of its effects on the expression of specific NMDA receptor (NR) subunits. Use of this parameter as a biochemical marker for the developmental neurotoxicity of lead has been quite popular with relevant assessments performed both at the mRNA level (using RT-PCR or *in situ* hybridization histochemistry) and the protein level (using Western blot analysis). Developmental exposure of animals to lead causes a reduction in the protein levels of the NR2A subunit in the hippocampus (Nihei and Guilarte, 1999), which concurs with previous findings of reduced hippocampal NR2A mRNA levels (Guilarte and McGlothan, 1998). In contrast, there are no changes in the mRNA and protein levels of this subunit in the cerebral cortex. The reduction in hippocampal NR2A protein levels is not always apparent, although the finding of a lead-induced reduction in the hippocampal NR2A mRNA levels has been confirmed (Nihei *et al.*, 2000). Developmental exposure of animals to lead also reduces in the hippocampus the mRNA and the protein levels of the NR1 receptor subunit, a constituent of all NMDA receptors (Nihei *et al.*, 2000). The reduction in the mRNA levels of NR1 subunit is mainly due to a decrease in the levels of the NR1-4 and NR1-2 splice variants (Guilarte and McGlothan, 2003). This affects the targeting of NMDA receptor complexes to the synapse and their cell surface expression and ultimately results in reduced synaptic plasticity.

The above changes in the mRNA and/or protein levels of the NMDA receptor subunits induced by lead during development lead to alterations in the subunit composition of NMDA receptor complexes. Using [^{3}H]-ifenprodil, a non-competitive NMDA receptor antagonist, with a 400-fold selectivity for NR1/NR2B relative to NR1/NR2A receptor complexes, developmental lead exposure has been shown to increase the proportion of NR2B-containing complexes in the hippocampus and the cerebral cortex (Toscano *et al.*, 2002). Lead may, thus, prevent or delay the switching of NR2B- to NR2A-containing NMDA receptor complexes that normally occurs during development, and this has been suggested to lead to reduced synaptic plasticity.

The effects of lead on NMDA receptor subunit gene expression have been studied also in cultured neurons. Exposure of cultures of primary neuronal cells isolated from the hippocampus of neonatal animals to lead causes a reduction in the levels of mRNA and protein of both the NR1 and NR2B subunits, as determined by RT-PCR and Western blotting, respectively (Lau *et al.*, 2002). In contrast, in cultures of neonatal cortical neurons, lead increases the mRNA and protein levels of the NR2B subunit and has no effect on the expression of the NR1 subunit, indicating differential responses of the hippocampus and the cerebral cortex. On the other hand, in embryonic cultures of primary neuronal cells isolated from the whole brain, lead causes a marked decrease in the protein levels of all NMDA receptor subunits assessed (NR1, NR2A and NR2B) (Xu *et al.*, 2006).

Apart from these parameters, which are related to specific neurotransmitter systems, lead also targets a number of molecules that are generally essential for neurotransmission. Particular attention has been paid to a number of proteins important in vesicular neurotransmitter release. Thus, lead alters the normal calcium-binding characteristics of the synaptic vesicle protein synaptotagmin I (Bouton *et al.*, 2001). Lead also affects vesicle mobilization by influencing the activity of synapsin I (Suszkiw, 2004). In addition, lead exposure of cultured hippocampal neurons during synaptogenesis has been recently found to cause the loss of synaptophysin and synaptobrevin, two proteins also involved in vesicular release (Neal *et al.*, in press). Lead targets also the neural cell adhesion molecule (NCAM), a substance involved in synapse formation, selection and stabilization. Thus, lead exposure of developing animals inhibits the removal of sialic acid from NCAM, a process which normally occurs during development and which is responsible for increased cell adhesion and the stabilization of the synaptic network (Regan, 1989).

CYTOSKELETON

The cytoskeleton is a complex interconnected protein filamentous meshwork, comprising three distinct interconnected arrays of microtubules (MTs), microfilaments (MFs) and intermediate filaments (IFs). It plays a key role role in a variety of developmentally important phenomena in the nervous system, including the regulation of mitosis, cell differentiation, cell migration and neurite outgrowth (Hargreaves, 1997). These roles, in turn, are dependent on the regulation of the integrity of the cytoskeleton. MTs and microfilaments are formed by the polymerization of tubulin dimers or actin monomers in a nucleotide-dependent fashion (Hargreaves, 1997). In mammalian cells, MTs exhibit a property known as dynamic instability, whereby some MT subpopulations may rapidly shrink while others undergo rapid growth, maintaining a constant polymer mass (Mitchison and Kirschner, 1988). GTP binding is required for MT assembly, its hydrolysis to GDP occurs shortly after incorporation of tubulin dimers and the growing ends of MTs are stabilized by a 'cap' of tubulin subunits with non-hydrolyzed GTP (Carlier *et al.*, 1984). MF assembly and dynamics, on the other hand, are dependent on the binding and hydrolysis of ATP, respectively (Gungabissoon and Bamburg, 2003).

In neural development, MTs and MFs or their functions modulated by interactions with a number of accessory proteins can stabilize, destabilize, act as motor proteins or link MTs and MFs to other cytoskeletal elements and membranes. Developmentally important MT-associated proteins (MAPs) include MAP 1b, MAP 2, tau and stathmin which stabilize growth cones, dendritic and axonal MTs in developing neurons or increase MT dynamics by upregulating GTP hydrolysis at the GTP cap, respectively (Kosik and Finch, 1987; Mack *et al.*, 2000; Ohkawa *et al.*, 2007). The binding of MAPs to MTs is regulated by various protein kinases including MT affinity regulating kinases (MARKs), calmodulin kinase, etc., (Biernat *et al.*, 2002; Ohkawa *et al.*, 2007). The motor proteins kinesin and dynein also play key roles in the regulation of MT-dependent phenomena, including formation of the mitotic spindle, chromosome alignment/segregation, intracellular transport (e.g., axonal transport) and neurite outgrowth (Schliwa and Woehlke, 2003). As the roles of MTs are dependent on the correct regulation of MT dynamics and MAP interaction, neurotoxins that interfere with this process might be potential developmental toxins.

Of the actin binding proteins, cofilin is of particular neurodevelopmental importance as it regulates actin dynamics in the growth cone of developing neurites, the binding of which is blocked when phosphorylated by the neurodevelopmentally important LIM kinase and Slingshot phosphatase (Endo *et al.*, 2003). The dynamic properties of MFs are closely regulated throughout neural development, enabling them to perform key developmental functions such as the formation of the contractile ring at the end of mitosis, the regulation of cell migration and growth cone advance.

IFs are biochemically much more stable than MTs and MFs. Thus they play a more structural or supportive role. However, like MTs and MFs they are modulated to some degree by their phosphorylation state (Omary *et al.*, 2006). IFs specific to the nervous system include:

- Glial fibrillary acidic protein (GFAP) and peripherin, which are found mainly in astrocytes and peripheral neurons, respectively.
- Neurofilaments (NFs) which comprise a triplet of polypeptides known as the neurofilament heavy (NFH; 200 kDa), medium (NFM; 120–150 kDa) and light (NFL; 70 kDa) chains, which are found in most neurons and enriched in axons.

In summary, the complexity and developmental importance of the cytoskeleton makes it a likely target for DNTs. Indeed, *in vitro* toxicity studies have shown that a variety of cytoskeletal proteins may be targeted by DNTs. This can occur in a number of ways, which are summarized in Table 19.2. The rest of this section will focus on cytoskeletal targets identified in cellular studies of neural cell differentiation.

Heavy metals

Reduced phosphorylation state of ADF/cofilin, but no change in the levels of total cofilin or actin, was demonstrated in proteomic studies of differentiating primary cultures of mouse CGCs exposed to subcytotoxic levels of MeHg chloride (Vendrell *et al.*, 2010). This would potentially result in enhanced binding of cofilin to actin and increased microfilament dynamics.

TABLE 19.2 Ways in which developmental neurotoxins can target the cytoskeleton

Target	Characteristics of toxic agent
Core protein	1. Agents that may bind directly to the polymer-forming subunit and interfere with dynamics, integrity or assembly the network. 2. Agents that affect the expression of nerve-specific cytoskeletal core proteins, such as β-type III tubulin, GFAP and NFs.
Cytoskeleton associated proteins	Agents that affect the protein levels and/or gene expression of regulatory proteins such as MAPs and ABPs.
Phosphorylation status of cytoskeletal proteins	Agents that affect the activities of kinases that modulate the binding of regulatory proteins and/or core proteins.
Free SH groups	Agents that block -SH groups directly or induce their oxidation indirectly.

Various studies on mitotic tumor cell lines and purified MT suggested that MeHg was capable of disrupting the MT network and preventing MT assembly, respectively (Vogel *et al.*, 1985; Miura *et al.*, 1999). Using *in vitro* development assays, MT disruption was found in cultured cells induced to differentiate into a neuronal phenotype (Graff *et al.*, 1997) and the immunological detection of neuron-specific β-tubulin was applied to demonstrate the disruption of MTs and reduced numbers of neurons in MeHg-treated neural stem cells (Tamm *et al.*, 2006).

Studies with organic lead compounds have also shown disruption of the MT network using polymerization assays with purified MTs and *in vitro* cellular models, suggesting a direct interaction that disrupts the assembly and/or distribution of MTs (Zimmermann *et al.*, 1985a). Zimmermann *et al.* (1985b) also found that triethyl lead had a direct effect on purified NFs and disrupted NFs in cultured cells, although no such effect has yet been reported for MeHg. Furthermore, these authors detected no obvious effect on the MF network (Zimmermann *et al.*, 1985a), suggesting that the two heavy metals may have some differences in their cytoskeletal toxicity.

It is known that many heavy metals are capable of disrupting the cytoskeleton in non-neural cultured cells (Chou, 1989) although not all of them have been tested in developing neural cell models. However, the recent demonstration that sublethal levels of arsenic inhibits the outgrowth of neurites by differentiating PC12 cells (Frankel *et al.*, 2009) suggests that cytoskeletal organization is a likely target for this toxin in developing neurons.

In a further report it was also suggested that measurement of the levels of mRNA corresponding to specific cytoskeletal proteins could be a very sensitive method for detecting exposure to neurodevelopmentally toxic metals using *in vitro* models (Hogberg *et al.*, 2010). However, it should be borne in mind that a detectable (or lack of) effect using this approach may not necessarily reflect the same change at the protein level and is unable to demonstrate changes due to post-translational modifications such as proteolytic degradation, phosphorylation, etc.

Organic solvents

Solvents such as ethanol and toluene have also been shown to disrupt cytoskeletal proteins in cultured neural cells. For example, microfilament disassembly was shown to be involved in the ability of ethanol to inhibit NMDA receptor activity in primary neural cultures (Popp and Dertien, 2008). Toluene is also known to disrupt NMDA receptor activity but a similar effect on microfilaments has not yet been demonstrated (Bale *et al.*, 2007). On the other hand, the enhancement of neurite outgrowth in differentiating PC12 cells by chronic ethanol exposure was associated with increased MT polymerization though the precise mechanism remains unknown (Reiter-Funk and Dohrman, 2005). In a study with cultured mouse embryo cells, the ability of toluene to inhibit astrocyte differentiation was demonstrated by reduced GFAP expression following chromic exposure to environmentally relevant levels of solvent (Yamaguchi *et al.*, 2002). By contrast, ethanol exposure was found to increase GFAP expression in cultured differentiating neural stem cells, consistent with enhanced differentiation/proliferation of astrocytes under the conditions tested (Tateno *et al.*, 2005).

Pesticides

Exposure of differentiating neuronal and/or glial cells to sublethal neurite inhibitory concentrations of the DZN and CPF has been shown to affect the levels of cytoskeletal proteins. At a molecular level, exposure to both agents had no effect on MT organization or the levels of tubulin, but did cause reduced reactivity of antibodies with MAP1B and NFH, in addition to NFH aggregation in the cell body (Sachana *et al.*, 1999, 2001, 2005; Flaskos *et al.*, 2007). Furthermore, although DZN had no effect on the levels of actin detected on Western blots, it induced upregulation of the ABP cofilin, which regulates MF dynamics in the advancing growth cone (Harris *et al.*, 2009). The levels of phosphorylated cofilin (p-cofilin) detected immunologically were also upregulated but to a significantly lower extent than total cofilin, suggesting a reduction in the overall level of cofilin phosphorylation and increased MF dynamics under these experimental conditions. It is not yet known whether CPF induces the same effects. The neurite inhibitory effects of CPF on differentiating C6 glioma cells were associated with reduced levels of MAP1B but not MAP 2c (transiently expressed during early development) or tubulin (Sachana *et al.*, 2008).

However, studies of the effects of the acutely toxic (in terms of acetylcholinesterase activity inhibition) oxon metabolites of DZN and CPF on C6 cell differentiation suggest that *both* agents inhibit astrocyte differentiation, as determined by reduced levels of the astrocyte marker GFAP (Sidiropoulou *et al.*, 2009b). In both cases, impaired neurite outgrowth was associated with reduced levels of antibody reactivity with α-tubulin and MAP1B, suggesting reduced synthesis and/or increased degradation of these MT proteins (Sachana *et al.*, 2008; Sidiropoulou *et al.*, 2009b). In contrast, the levels of MAP 2c in CPO- (Sachana *et al.*, 2008) and DZO- (Sidiropoulou *et al.*, 2009b) treated cells were not significantly affected. The validity of the neural cytoskeleton as a target for CPF and CPO was further strengthened by the demonstration of a direct binding interaction of both compounds with tubulin and by their ability to inhibit MT assembly and to interfere with kinesin-dependent MT motility assays *in vitro* (Gearhart *et al.*, 2007; Prendergast *et al.*, 2007). In differentiating N2a cells, neurite inhibitory concentrations of DZO had no effect on tubulin or NFH levels but did induce increased phosphorylation of NFH; data for CPO are not yet available (Sidiropoulou *et al.*, 2009a). These data suggest that, while cytoskeletal changes may represent good biomarkers of effect in cellular models of development, chemically related compounds may affect these proteins differently in a manner concomitant with their potency as a developmental toxin.

PCBs

Few studies have been published showing direct effects of PCBs on the neural cytoskeleton using *in vitro* models. However, the ability of sublethal concentrations of several PCBs to (1) inhibit differentiation, induce cellular hypertrophy and to impair the formation of contractile filaments in a differentiating skeletal muscle myocyte cell line (Coletti *et al.*, 2001), (2) perturb calcium homeostasis in cultured rat CGCs (Kodavanti *et al.*, 1993), and (3) promote neurite outgrowth in differentiating PC12 cells (Angus and Contreras, 1994) imply underlying molecular effects on cytoskeletal targets.

TRANSCRIPTION FACTORS AND SIGNALING PATHWAYS

Neural development and the complexity of the nervous system are dependent on a complex series of events involving numerous transcription factors (TFs) and the co-ordinated activation/inactivation of various cell signaling pathways at different stages (Jessel, 2000; Bertrand *et al.*, 2002). TFs are proteins that bind to specific regions of genes in a manner that regulates their transcription. Neural TFs may be inducible (e.g., Fos, Jun, etc.), which require some form of stimulation (e.g., extracellular receptor mediated signaling) or constitutive, in that they are expressed in quiescent or unstimulated cells (e.g., CREB, ATF, etc.); these TFs are thought to regulate the expression of the former (Herdegen and Leah, 1998). Jun, Fos and Sox families of transcription factors are known to play a variety of roles in stem cell maintenance, the generation of neuronal and glial cells, and terminal differentiation (Herdegen and Leah, 1998; Wegner and Stolt, 2005). The induced expression of these TFs leads to the upregulation of genes involved in the subsequent stages of neural development.

Signaling pathways are involved in the induction of neurite outgrowth *in vitro* (e.g., by NGF), which is dependent on the sustained activation of extracellular receptor mitogen-activated protein kinase (MAP kinase) ERK 1/2 (Das *et al.*, 2004), a major convergence point for other signaling pathways of importance to neural cell proliferation, differentiation and survival (Perron and Bixby, 1999). ERK 1/2 phosphorylates a wide range of substrates including cytoskeletal proteins (e.g., NF-H), and can initiate a chain of events leading to the activation of TFs such as c-FOS, though its overall effect depends on the length of time it remains activated, the effects of regulatory phosphatases and its interaction with other proteins (Shaul and Seger, 2007).

Neural cell morphogenesis and cell migration are dependent on extracellular factors (e.g., cell contact, chemotaxis, neurotrophins, etc.) that regulate the above-mentioned signal transduction cascades involved in the control of neurite outgrowth and neuronal growth cone advance. These pathways control the activities of numerous other downstream signaling molecules such as calmodulin kinase, protein kinase C, MARK kinase and small GTPases such as Rho, Rac and cdc42 (Strittmatter, 1996; Brouns *et al.*, 2000; Biernat *et al.*, 2002), which initiate rapid changes in the organization and dynamics of cytoskeletal networks either by direct binding, phosphorylation of cytoskeletal substrates and/or the production of 2nd messengers (e.g., Ca^{2+}) that bind to and modulate cytoskeletal proteins at critical stages of neural development (Li *et al.*, 2003; Dave *et al.*, 2009).

The signaling pathways and transcription factors mentioned here is not an exhaustive list but give a clear idea of how signaling events and transcription factors collectively regulate the process of neural development. Thus, DNT-induced changes in TFs and signaling pathways are of great interest to *in vitro* developmental toxicologists, and will be the main focus of the rest of this section.

Heavy metals

Lead has been shown to disrupt the binding of TF Sp1 to DNA *in vivo* and in both mitotic and differentiating PC12 cells; it also affects the expression of other TFs including the immediate early genes c-fos and c-jun and erg, via disruption of ERK 1/2 and PKC activities (Zawia *et al.*, 1998; Bressler *et al.*, 1999; Crumpton *et al.*, 2001; Atkins *et al.*, 2003). This suggests that exposure to lead can be effectively monitored by the disruption of these transcription factors and cell signaling events, although it has been suggested that many of the effects of lead may be due to the interaction of lead with Ca^{2+} and zinc binding proteins, including PKC and zinc finger TFs (Godwin, 2001).

Mercury chloride was found to inhibit neurotrophin-induced janus tyrosine kinase/signal transducer activators of transcription (Jak-STAT) signaling in BE(2)-C human neuroblastoma cells at sublethal concentrations, an effect linked to oxidative stress (Monroe and Halvorsen, 2006). Bland and Rand (2006), on the other hand, showed that MeHg chloride was capable of activating the Notch receptor signaling pathway in cultured Drosophila cells resulting in the upregulation of TFs, by activation of a specific protease. As Notch receptor signaling is influential in the regulation of cell fate decisions, cell migration, proliferation and neurite outgrowth in developing neurons (Artavanis-Tsakonas *et al.*, 2001), it may be that this and related cell fate determining receptor pathways can be affected by mercury in mammalian systems. A broader effect of mercury on TF expression is further suggested by the ability of nM levels of MeHg chloride to inhibit the expression of Sox 10 in cultured CGCs (Bal-Price *et al.*, 2009), which is important for stem cell maintenance. Furthermore, the possibility that mercury might be able to bind directly to both zinc finger and non-zinc finger TFs such as Sp1 and AP-2, respectively, was demonstrated in a study by Rodgers *et al.* (2000), in which TF binding to DNA was inhibited in binding assays performed in the presence of mercuric ions *in vitro*. Other metal compounds such as arsenic have also been shown to disrupt the cytoskeleton or induce apoptosis by the activation of p38 and JNK MAP kinases and/or glycogen synthase kinase 3β in different cellular systems (Namgung and Xia, 2001; DeFuria and Shea, 2007).

Organic solvents

Disruption of signaling pathways has also been demonstrated in ethanol-treated cultured rat CGCs, in which solvent induced cell death was ablated by the activation of either the nitric oxide-cGMP or the PI3-K pathway by NMDA receptor agonists and neurotrophins, respectively (Heaton *et al.*, 2000; Pantazis *et al.*, 2001). The ability of ethanol to induce neurite outgrowth in PC12 cells was found to involve the activation of ERK 1/2 and PKC (Roivainen *et al.*, 1994). However, it is interesting to note that, while toluene demonstrated the ability to reduce human neuroblastoma cell viability by disrupting Ca^{2+} homeostasis, it had no effect on the activation status of either ERK 1/2 or p38 MAP kinase or JNK pathways, though PI3-K and PKC were not measured (McDermott *et al.*, 2007). A study of solvent effects on developmentally regulated and/or stress-induced TFs may help to establish comprehensive toxicity profiles for these agents.

Pesticides

Subcholinergic levels of CPF were found to impair the expression of transcription factor Sp1 and adenylyl cyclase activity in differentiating PC12 and C6 cells (Crumpton *et al.*, 2000b; Garcia *et al.*, 2001). Exposure of differentiating PC12 cells to CPF and to a lesser extent DZ resulted in the altered regulation of genes associated with the PKC pathway, suggesting some differences between the mechanisms of toxicity of these two OP pesticides (Slotkin and Seidler, 2009b), although more work is needed to confirm these effects at the protein level. Caughlan *et al.* (2004) demonstrated that the induction of apoptosis in rat cortical neurons by subcholinergic levels of CPF was associated with increased activation of ERK 1/2, p38 MAP kinase and JNK and that embryonic cells were more sensitive than postnatal cells, indicating that this OP is capable of disrupting the activities of a range of signaling pathways important in the regulation of neuronal cell development and survival. Developmental signaling disruption by DZ and CPF is further supported by microarray studies showing altered regulation of genes for a variety of neurotrophins, their receptors and components of their signaling pathways Slotkin *et al.* (2008b). However, as altered gene expression does not always reflect protein levels and enzyme activities, further work to identify changes at the protein level would be worthwhile. In this respect, the altered phosphorylation status of cofilin and NF-H in N2a cells exposed to DZ and DZO, respectively (Harris *et al.*, 2009; Sidiropoulou *et al.*, 2009a), indicates potential downstream consequences of such signaling events. The application of Western blotting analysis using phospho-specific antibodies that recognize activated or inactivated signaling molecules and/or antibody arrays directed at signaling pathways would go some way to achieving this end.

PCBs and PBDEs

This group of compounds has been shown to interact with the ligand-activated aryl hydrocarbon receptor in mouse CGCs; the ligand bound receptor migrates to the nucleus and binds to the nuclear translocator protein Arnt which then interacts with dioxin responsive elements to regulate transcription (Williamson *et al.*, 2005). It has also been shown that, while *in vivo* effects may involve reduced levels of circulating thyroid hormone (T3), some PCBs directly disrupt thyroid hormone T3 receptor mediated differentiation pathways in cultured normal human progenitor cells (Fritsche *et al.*, 2005). This suggests that *in vitro* studies of PCB effects on T3-responsive TFs might reveal potentially useful DNT markers. However, the induction of increased c-Jun expression in mitotic PC12 cells by nM levels of hydroxylated-PCB but not T3 suggests that T3 responsive TFs and signaling pathways are not necessarily the only ones affected by PCB exposure (Shimokawa *et al.*, 2006). Disruption of Ca^{2+} homeostasis and intracellular signaling pathways were also identified as potential biomarkers of toxicity in this cellular system and in primary cultures of neonatal rat hippocampal neurons and rat brain extracts treated with PBDEs and PCBs (Kodavanti and Ward, 2005; Chen *et al.*, 2010), suggesting that major disruption of signaling pathways and second messenger levels are useful markers for these groups of compounds in developmental neurotoxicity models *in vitro*, though the efficacy of individual compounds may vary with specific endpoints. Differential effects of PCBs and PBDEs on protein kinase C and the phosphatidylinositol 3 kinase (PI3-K) signaling pathway were further suggested in a study of PBDE-99 and Aroclor 1254 toxicity in cultured human astroglial cells (Madia *et al.*, 2004).

CONCLUDING REMARKS AND FUTURE DIRECTIONS

Although there is only a handful of chemicals that have been firmly identified as DNTs, the studies reviewed in this chapter indicate that there are a large number of molecules and processes that are affected. Each one of these chemicals, indeed, interferes separately with several distinct developmental processes and induces changes in many different parameters. In several cases, these changes that have been recorded *in vitro* appear to mirror analogous phenomena occurring *in vivo*, so that the parameters involved can be used as valid *in vitro* markers of developmental neurotoxicity. This multitude of valid *in vitro* markers provides valuable insights into possible mechanisms of actions. Equally important, these *in vitro* markers, if judiciously selected, can be efficiently exploited for screening purposes. Use of these *in vitro* markers is, indeed, particularly important, since the application of *in vivo* screening tests is not appropriate for the large number of chemicals that need to be evaluated for developmental neurotoxicity, as *in vivo* tests are laborious, time-consuming, costly and involve the use and sacrifice of live (pregnant and young) animals. Thus, the use of an appropriate battery of *in vitro* markers can greatly assist the process of the initial screening to identify chemicals with developmental neurotoxicity potential before subsequent *in vivo* testing is applied.

A battery of markers recently proposed as potentially suitable for initial screening for developmental neurotoxicity includes the expression (mRNA levels) of a total of eight genes specific for three cell types (neuronal, glial and neuronal precursor cells) and related to different critical stages of development (Bal-Price *et al.*, 2010). These markers are determined in an *in vitro* system of primary neuronal cultures of CGCs prepared from 7-day-old rat pups. Critical to development of efficient *in vitro* screening systems is the rapid generation of new *in vitro* markers of developmental neurotoxicity. The latter process can now be greatly accelerated through the application of the -omics technologies in the context of developmental neurotoxicity, as recently performed in cultures of both primary neuronal cells (Vendrell *et al.*, 2010) and neuronal cell lines (Harris *et al.*, 2009). It is hoped that the conduction of further studies using such technologies in the near future will contribute towards the incorporation of more suitable, mechanistically based *in vitro* markers in the initial screening of DNTs, thus accelerating the whole process of regulatory developmental neurotoxicity evaluation.

REFERENCES

Abdulla EM, Campbell IC (1993) Use of neurite outgrowth as an in vitro method of assessing neurotoxicity. *Ann NY Acad Sci* **697:** 276–9.

Ahern KB, Lustig HS, Greenberg DA (1994) Enhancement of NMDA toxicity and calcium responses by chronic exposure of cultured cortical neurons to ethanol. *Neurosci Lett* **165:** 211–14.

Aimo L, Oteiza PI (2006) Zinc deficiency increases the susceptibility of human neuroblastoma cells to lead-induced activator protein-1 activation. *Toxicol Sci* **91:** 184–91.

Ali SF, LeBel CP, Bondy SC (1992) Reactive oxygen species formation as a biomarker of methylmercury and trimethyltin neurotoxicity. *Neurotoxicology* **13:** 637–48.

Alm H, Kultima K, Scholz B, Nilsson A, Andren PE, Fex-Svenningsen A, Dencker L, Stigson M (2008) Exposure to brominated flame retardant PBDE-99 affects cytoskeletal protein expression in the neonatal mouse cerebral cortex. *Neurotoxicology* **29:** 628–37.

Aluigi MG, Guida C, Falugi C (2010) Apoptosis as a specific biomarker of diazinon toxicity in NTera2-D1 cells. *Chem Biol Interact*. In press.

Angus WG, Contreras ML (1994) The effects of Arochlor 1254 on undifferentiated and NGF-stimulated differentiating PC12 cells. *Neurotoxicology* **15:** 809–17.

Antonio AM, Druse MJ (2008) Antioxidants prevent ethanol-associated apoptosis in fetal rhombencephalic neurons. *Brain Res* **1204:** 16–23.

Antony B, Zhou, FC, Ogawa T, Goodlett CR, Ruiz J (2008) Alcohol exposure alters cell cycle and apoptotic events during early neurulation. *Alcohol Alcohol* **43:** 261–73.

Artavanis-Tsakonas S, Delidakis C, Fehon RG (1991) The Notch locus and the cell biology of neuroblast segregation. *Ann Rev Cell Biol* **7:** 427–52.

Aschner M, Du Y-L, Gannon M, Kimelberg HK (1993) Furosemide treatment reverses methylmercury-induced increases in excitatory amino acid efflux from rat primary astrocyte cultures. *Brain Res* **602:** 181–6.

Aschner M, Yao CP, Allen JW, Tan KH (2000) Methylmercury alters glutamate transport in astrocytes. *Neurochem Int* **37:** 199–206.

Atkins DS, Basha MR, Zawia NH (2003) Intracellular signaling pathways involved in mediating the effects of lead on the transcription factor Sp1. *Int J Dev Neurosci* **21:** 235–44.

Audesirk T, Audesirk G, Ferguson C, Shugarts D (1991) Effects of inorganic lead on the differentiation and growth of cultured hippocampal and neuroblastoma cells. *Neurotoxicology* **12:** 529–38.

Axelrad JC, Howard CV, McLean WG (2003) The effects of acute pesticide exposure on neuroblastoma cells chronically exposed to diazinon. *Toxicology* **185:** 67–78.

Bagchi D, Bagchi M, Hassoun EA, Stohs SJ (1995) In vitro and in vivo generation of reactive oxygen species, DNA damage and lactate dehydrogenase leakage by selected pesticides. *Toxicology* 104: 129–40.

Bakir F, Damluji SF, Amin-Zaki L, Murtadha M, Khalidi A, al-Rawi NY, Tikriti S, Dahahir HI, Clarkson TW, Smith JC, Doherty RA (1973) Methylmercury poisoning in Iraq. *Science* **181:** 230–41.

Bal-Price AK, Hogberg HT, Buzanska L, Lenas P, van Vliet E, Hortung T (2010) In vitro developmental neurotoxicity (DNT) testing: relevant models and endpoints. *Neurotoxicology* **31:** 545–54.

Bale AS, Jackson MD, Krantz QT, Benignus VA, Bushnell PJ, Shafer TJ, Boyes WK (2007) Evaluating the NMDA-glutamate receptor as a site of action for toluene, in vivo. *Toxicol Sci* **98:** 159–66.

Barclay DC, Hallbergson AF, Montague JR, Mudd LM (2005) Reversal of ethanol toxicity in embryonic neurons with growth factors and estrogen. *Brain Res Bull* **67:** 459–65.

Bartolome J, Trepanier P, Chait EA, Seidler FJ, Deskin R, Slotkin TA (1982) Neonatal methylmercury poisoning in the rat: effects on development of central catecholamine neurotransmitter systems. *Toxicol Appl Pharmacol* **65:** 92–9.

Bearer CF, Swick AR, O'Riordan MA, Cheng G (1999) Ethanol inhibits L1-mediated neurite outgrowth in postnatal rat cerebellar granule cells. *J Biol Chem* **247:** 13264–70.

Belletti S, Orlandini G, Vettori MV, Mutti A, Uggeri J, Scandroglio R, Alinovi R, Gatti R (2002) Time course assessment of methylmercury effects on C6 glioma cells: submicromolar concentrations induce oxidative DNA damage and apoptosis. *J Neurosci Res* **70:** 703–11.

Bellinger DC, Needleman HL (2003) Intellectual impairment and blood lead levels. *N Engl J Med* **349:** 500–2.

Bertrand N, Castro DS, Guillemot F (2002) Proneural genes and the specification of neural cell types. *Nat Rev Neurosci* **3:** 517–30.

Bhave SV, Hoffman PL (1997) Ethanol promotes apoptosis in cerebellar granule cells by inhibiting the trophic effect of NMDA. *J Neurochem* **68:** 578–86.

Bhave SV, Snell LD, Tabakoff B, Hoffman PL (2000) Chronic ethanol exposure attenuates the anti-apoptotic effect of NMDA in cerebellar granule neurons. *J Neurochem* **75:** 1035-44.

Biernat J, Wu YZ, Timm T, Zheng-Fischöfer Q, Mandelkow E, Meijer L, Mandelkow EM (2002) Protein kinase MARK/PAR-1 is required for neurite outgrowth and establishment of neurite polarity. *Mol Biol Cell* **13:** 4013–28.

Bingham SM, Mudd LM, Lopez TF, Montague JR (2004) Effects of ethanol on cultured embryonic neurons from the cerebral cortex of the rat. *Alcohol* **32:** 129–35.

Bland C, Rand MD (2006) Methyl mercury induces activation of Notch signaling. *Neurotoxicology* **27:** 982–91.

Blomgren K, Leist M, Groc L (2007) Pathological apoptosis in the developing brain. *Apoptosis* **12:** 993–1010.

Bondy SC, Anderson CL, Harrington ME, Prasad KN (1979) The effects of organic and inorganic lead and mercury on neurotransmitter high-affinity transport and release mechanisms. *Environ Res* **19:** 102–11.

Bourjeily N, Suszkiw JB (1997) Developmental cholinotoxicity of lead: loss of septal cholinergic neurons and long-term changes in cholinergic innervation of the hippocampus in perinatally lead-exposed rats. *Brain Res* **771:** 319–28.

Bouton CM, Frelin LP, Forde CE, Arnold Godwin H, Pevsner J (2001) Synaptotagmin I is molecular target for lead. *J Neurochem* **76:** 1724–35.

Bradley DM, Paiva M, Tonjes LA, Heaton MB (1995) In vitro comparison of the effects of ethanol and acetaldehyde on dorsal root ganglion neurons. *Alcohol Clin Exp Res* **19:** 1345–50.

Bressler J, Kim KA, Chakraborti T, Goldstein G (1999) Molecular mechanisms of lead neurotoxicity. *Neurochem Res* **24:** 595–600.

Brouns MR, Matheson SF, Ho KQ, Delalle I, Caviness Jr VS, Silver J, Bronson RT, Settleman J (2000) The adhesion signalling molecule p190 RhoGAP is required for morphogenetic processes in neural development. *Development* **127:** 4891–903.

Brouwer A, Longnecker MP, Bimbaum LS, Cogliano J, Kostyniak P, Moore J, Schantz S, Winnek G (1999) Characterization of potential endocrine-related health effects at low-dose levels of exposure to PCBs. *Environ Health Perspect* **107:** 639–49.

Bulleit RF, Cui H (1998) Methylmercury antagonizes the survival promoting activity of insulin-like growth factor on developing cerebella granule neurons. *Toxicol Appl Pharmacol* **153:** 161–8.

Burbacher TM, Rodier PM, Weiss B (1990) Methylmercury developmental neurotoxicity: a comparison of effects in humans and animals. *Neurotoxicol Teratol* **12:** 191–202.

Burry M, Guizzetti M, Oberdoerster J, Costa LG (2003) Developmental neurotoxicity of toluene: in vivo and in vitro effects on astroglial cells. *Dev Neurosci* **25:** 14–19.

Buzanska L, Sypecka J, Nerini-Molteni S, Compagnoni A, Hogberg HT, del Torchio R, Domanska-Janik K, Zimmer J, Coecke S (2009) A human stem cell-based model for identifying adverse effects of organic and inorganic chemicals on the developing nervous system. *Stem Cells* **27:** 2591–601.

Cai B, Chang SH, Becker BB, Bonni A, Xia Z (2006) p38 MAP kinase mediates apoptosis through phosphorylation of BimEL at Ser-65. *J Biol Chem* **281:** 25215–22.

Cai B, Xia Z (2008) p38 MAP kinase mediates arsenite-induced apoptosis through FOXO3a activation and induction of Bim transcription. *Apoptosis* **13:** 803–10.

Campbell CG, Seidler FJ, Slotkin TA (1997) Chlorpyrifos interferes with cell development in rat brain regions. *Brain Res Bull* **43:** 179–89.

Canfield RL, Henderson CR, Cory-Slechta DA, Cox C, Jusko TA, Lanphear BP (2003) Intellectual impairment in children with blood concentrations below 10μg per deciliter. *N Engl J Med* **348:** 1517–26.

Canzoniero LM, Adornetto A, Secondo A, Magi S, Dell'aversano C, Scorziello A, Amoroso S, Di Renzo G (2006) Involvement of the nitric oxide/protein kinase G pathway in polychlorinated biphenyl-induced cell death in SH-SY5Y neuroblastoma cells. *J Neurosci Res* **84:** 692–7.

Carlier MF, Hill TL, Chen YD (1984) Interference of GTP hydrolysis in the mechanism of microtubule assembly: an experimental study. *Proc Natl Acad Sci* **81:** 771–5.

Carpenter DO, Stoner CR, Lawrence DA (1997) Flow cytometric measurements of neuronal death triggered by PCBs. *Neurotoxicology* **18:** 507–13.

Castoldi AF, Candura SM, Costa P, Manzo L, Costa LG (1996) Interaction of mercury compounds with muscarinic receptor subtypes in the rat brain. *Neurotoxicology* **17:** 735–42.

Castoldi AF, Barni S, Randine G, Costa LG, Manzo L (1998) Ethanol selectively interferes with the trophic action of NMDA and carbachol on cultured cerebellar granule neurons undergoing apoptosis. *Develop Brain Res* **111:** 279–89.

Castoldi AF, Barni S, Turin I, Gandini C, Manzo L (2000) Early acute necrosis, delayed apoptosis and cytoskeletal breakdown in cultured cerebellar granule neurons exposed to methylmercury. *J Neurosci Res* **59:** 775–87.

Caughlan A, Newhouse K, Namgung U, Xia Z (2004) Chlorpyrifos induces apoptosis in rat cortical neurons that is regulated by a balance between p38 and ERK/JNK MAP kinases. *Toxicol Sci* **78:** 125–34.

Chandler LJ, Newsom H, Sumners C, Crews F (1993) Chronic ethanol exposure potentiates NMDA excitotoxicity in cerebral cortical neurons. *J Neurochem* **60:** 1578–81.

Chandler JL, Sutton G, Norwiid D, Sumners C, Crews FT (1997) Chronic alcohol increases N-methyl-D-aspartate-stimulated nitric oxide formation but not receptor density in cultured cortical neurons. *Mol Pharmacol* **51:** 733–40.

Chattopadhyay S, Bhaumik S, Chaudhury AN, Gupta SD (2002) Arsenic induced changes in growth development and apoptosis in neonatal and adult brain cells in vivo and in tissue culture. *Toxicol Lett* **128:** 73–84.

Chen CP, Kuhn P, Chaturvedi K, Boyadjieva N, Sarkar DK (2006) Ethanol induces apoptotic death of developing β-endorphin neurons via suppression of cyclic adenosine monophosphate production and activation of transforming growth factor-β1-linked apoptotic signaling. *Mol Pharmacol* **69:** 706–17.

Chen G, Ma C, Bower KA, Shi X, Ke Z, Luo J (2008) Ethanol promotes endoplasmic reticulum stress-induced neuronal death: involvement of oxidative stress. *J Neurosci Res* **86:** 937–46.

Chen G, Bower KA, Xu M, Ding M, Shi X, Ke ZJ, Luo J (2009) Cyanidin-3-glucoside reverses ethanol-induced inhibition of neurite outgrowth: role of glycogen synthase kinase 3 beta. *Neurotox Res* **15:** 321–31.

Chen J, Liufu C, Sun W, Sun X, Chen D (2010) Assessment of the neurotoxic mechanisms of decabrominated diphenyl ether (PBDE-209) in primary cultured neonatal rat hippocampal neurons includes alterations in second messenger signaling and oxidative stress. *Toxicol Lett* **192:** 431–9.

Chen L, Yang X, Jiao H, Zhao B (2003) Tea catechins protect against lead-induced ROS formation, mitochondrial dysfunction and calcium dysregulation in PC12 cells. *Chem Res Toxicol* **16:** 1155–61.

Chen L, Chetty CS, Vemuri MC, Camleadell K, Suresh C (2005) Lead-induced cell death of human neuroblastoma cells involves GSH deprivation. *Cell Mol Biol Lett* **10:** 413–23.

Chen S, Sulik K (1996) Free radicals and ethanol-induced cytotoxicity in neural crest cells. *Alcohol Clin Exp Res* **20:** 1071–6.

Cheng Y-J, Yang B-C, Hsieh W-C, Huang B-M, Liu M-Y (2002) Enhancement of TNF-α expression does not trigger apoptosis upon exposure of glial cells to lead and lipopolysaccharide. *Toxicology* **178:** 183–91.

Cherian PP, Schenker S, Henderson GI (2008) Ethanol mediated DNA damage and PARP-1 apoptotic responses in cultured fetal cortical neurons. *Alcohol Clin Exp Res* **32:** 1884–92.

Chetty CS, Vemuri MC, Reddy GR, Suresh C (2007) Protective effect of 17-beta-estrodiol in human neuroblastoma models of lead exposure. *Neurotoxicology* **28:** 396–401.

Cheung WMW, Chu PWK, Kwong YL (2007) Effects of arsenic trioxide on the cellular proliferation of human neuroblastoma cells. *Cancer Lett* **246:** 122–8.

Choi BH, Lapham LW, Amin-Zaki L, Saleem T (1978) Abnormal neuronal migration, deranged cerebral cortical organization, and diffuse white matter astrocytosis of human fetal brain: a major effect of methylmercury poisoning in utero. *J Neuropathol Exp Neurol* **37:** 719–33.

Chou IN (1989) Distinct cytoskeletal injuries induced by As, Cd, Co, Cr and Ni compounds. *Biomed Environ Sci* **2:** 358–65.

Cohen-Cory S (2002) The developing synapse: construction and modulation of synaptic structures and circuits. *Science* **298:** 770–6.

Coletti D, Palleschi S, Silvestroni L, Cannavò A, Vivarelli E, Molinaro M, Adamo S (2001) Polychlorobiphenyls inhibit skeletal muscle differentiation in culture. *Toxicol Appl Pharmacol* **175:** 226–33.

Collins MA, Zou JY, Neafsey EJ (1998) Brain damage due to episodic alcohol exposure *in vivo* and *in vitro*: furosemide neuroprotection implicates edema based mechanism. *FASEB J* **12:** 221–30.

Cory-Slechta DA, Widzowski DV, Pokora MJ (1993) Functional alterations in dopamine systems assessed using drug discrimination procedures. *Neurotoxicology* **14:** 105–14.

Costa LG, Guizzetti M, Burry M, Oberdoerster J (2002) Developmental neurotoxicity: do similar phenotypes indicate a common mode of action? A comparison of fetal alcohol syndrome, toluene embryopathy and maternal phenylketonuria. *Toxicol Lett* **127:** 197–205.

Costa LG, Fattori V, Giordano G, Vitalone A (2007) An in vitro approach to assess the toxicity of certain food contaminants: methylmercury and polychlorinated biphenyls. *Toxicology* **237:** 65–76.

Crespo-Lopez ME, Lima de Sa A, Herculano AM, Rodriguez Burbano R, Do Nascimento JL (2007) Methylmercury genotoxicity: a novel effect in human cell lines of the central nervous system. *Environ Int* **33:** 141–6.

Crews FT, Waage HG, Wilkie MB, Lauder JM (1999) Ethanol pretreatment enhances NMDA excitotoxicity in biogenic amine neurons: protection by brain derived neurotrophic factors. *Alcohol Clin Exp Res* **23:** 1834–42.

Crumpton TL, Seidler FJ, Slotkin TA (2000a) Is oxidative stress involved in the developmental neurotoxicity of chlorpyrifos? *Dev Brain Res* **121:** 189–95.

Crumpton TL, Seidler FJ, Slotkin TA (2000b) Developmental toxicity of chlorpyrifos in vivo and in vitro: effects on nuclear transcription factors involved in cell replication and differentiation. *Brain Res* **857:** 87–98.

Crumpton T, Atkins DS, Zawia NH, Barone S Jr (2001) Lead exposure in pheochromocytoma (PC12) cells alters neural differentiation and Sp1 DNA-binding. *Neurotoxicology* **22:** 49–62.

Dakeishi M, Murata K, Grandjean P (2006) Long-term consequences of arsenic poisoning during infancy due to contaminated milk powder. *Environ Health* **5:** 31.

Dare E, Gotz ME, Zhivotovsky B, Manzo L, Ceccatelli S (2000) Antioxidants J811 and 17beta-estradiol protect cerebellar granule cells from methylmercury-induced apoptotic cell death. *J Neurosci Res* **62:** 557–65.

Dare E, Gorman AM, Ahlbom E, Gotz ME, Momoi T, Ceccatelli S (2001a) Apoptotic morphology does not always require caspase activity in rat cerebellar granule neurons. *Neurotox Res* **3:** 501–14.

Dare E, Li W, Zhivotovsky B, Yuan X, Ceccatelli S (2001b) Methylmercury and H_2O_2 provoke lysosomal damage in human astrocytoma D384 cells followed by apoptosis. *Free Radic Biol Med* **30:** 1347–56.

Dargusch R, Schubert D (2002) Specificity of resistance to oxidative stress. *J Neurochem* **81:** 1394–400.

Das KP, Barone S Jr (1999) Neuronal differentiation in PC12 cells is inhibited by chlorpyrifos and its metabolites: is acetylcholinesterase inhibition the site of action? *Toxicol Appl Pharmacol* **160:** 217–30.

Das KP, Freudenrich TM, Mundy WR (2004) Assessment of PC12 cell differentiation and neurite outgrowth: a comparison of morphological and neurochemical measures. *Neurotoxicol Teratol* **26:** 397–406.

Dave RH, Saengsawang W, Yu JZ, Donati R, Rasenick MM (2009) Heterotrimeric G-proteins interact directly with cytoskeletal proteins to modify microtubule-dependent cellular processes. *Neurosignals* **17:** 100–8.

Davidovics Z, DiCicco-Bloom E (2005) Moderate lead exposure elicits neurotrophic effects in cerebral cortical precursor cell in culture. *J Neurosci Res* **80:** 817–25.

De A, Boyadjieva NI, Pastorcic M, Reddy BV, Sarkar DK (1994) Cyclic AMP and ethanol interact to control apoptosis and differentiation in hypothalamic b-endorphin neurons. *J Biol Chem* **269:** 26697–705.

DeFuria J, Shea TB (2007) Arsenic inhibits neurofilament transport and induces perikaryal accumulation of phosphorylated: Roles of JNK and GSK-3β. *Brain Res* **1181:** 74–82.

de la Monte SM, Neely TR, Cannon J, Wands JR (2001) Ethanol impairs insulin stimulated mitochondrial function in cerebellar granular neurons. *Cell Mol Life Sci* **58:** 648–59.

deMelo Reis RA, Herculano AM, da Silva MC, dos Santos RM, do Nascimento JL (2007) In vitro toxicity induced by methylmercury on sympathetic neurons is reverted by L-cysteine or glutathione. *Neurosci Res* **58:** 278–84.

Deng W, McKinnon RD, Poretz RD (2002) Lead exposure delays the differentiation of oligodendroglial progenitors in vitro. *Brain Res* **929:** 87–95.

Deng W, Poretz RD (2002) Protein kinase C activation is required for the lead-induced inhibition of proliferation and differentiation of cultured oligodendroglial progenitor cells. *Brain Res* **929:** 87–95.

Dingemans MML, de Groot A, van Kleef RGDM, Bergman A, van den Berg M, Vijverberg HPM, Westerink RHS (2008) Hydroxylation increases the neurotoxic potential of BDE-47 to affect exocytosis and calcium homeostasis in PC12 cells. *Environ Health Perspect* **116:** 637–43.

Druse MJ, Tajuddin NF, Gillespie RA, Dickson E, Atieh M, Pietrzak CA, Le PT (2005) Signaling pathways involved with serotonin1A agonist-mediated neuroprotection against ethanol-induced apoptosis of fetal rhombencephalic neurons. *Brain Res Dev Brain Res* **159:** 18–28.

Druse MJ, Tajuddin NF, Gillespie RA, Le P (2006) The effects of ethanol and the serotonin1A agonist ipsapirone on the expression of the serotonin1 A receptor and several antiapoptotic proteins in fetal rhombencephalic neurons. *Brain Res* **1092:** 79–86.

Druse M, Gillespie RA, Tajuddin NF, Rich M (2007) S100B-mediated protection against the pro-apoptotic effects of ethanol on fetal rhombencephalic neurons. *Brain Res* **1150:** 46–54.

Dufault C, Poles G, Driscoll LL (2005) Brief postnatal PBDE exposure alters learning and the cholinergic modulation of attention in rats. *Toxicol Sci* **88:** 172–80.

Eaton DL, Daroff RB, Autrup H, Bridges J, Buffler P, Costa LG, Coyle J, McKhann G, Mobley WC, Nadel L, Neubert D, Schulte-Hermann R, Spencer PS (2008) Review of the toxicology of chlorpyrifos with an emphasis on human exposure and neurodevelopment. *Crit Rev Toxicol* **38:** 1–125.

Endo M, Ohashi K, Sasaki Y, Goshima Y, Niwa R, Uemura T, Mizuno K (2003) Control of growth cone motility and morphology by LIM kinase and Slingshot via phosphorylation and dephosphorylation of cofilin. *J Neurosci* **23:** 2527–37.

Eriksson P, Jakobsson E, Fredriksson A (2001) Brominated flame retardants: a novel class of developmental neurotoxicants in our environment? *Environ Health Perspect* **109:** 903–8.

Felix K, Manna SK, Wise K, Barr J, Ramesh GT (2005) Low levels of arsenite activates nuclear factor-kappaB and activator protein-1 in immortalized mesencephalic cells. *J Biochem Mol Toxicol* **19:** 67–77.

Flaskos J, Harris W, Sachana M, Munoz D, Tack J, Hargreaves AJ (2007) The effects of diazinon and cypermethrin on the differentiation of neuronal and glial cell lines. *Toxicol Appl Pharmacol* **219:** 172–80.

Flaskos J, Sachana M (2010) Developmental neurotoxicity of anticholinesterase pesticides. In *Anticholinesterase Pesticides: Metabolism, Neurotoxicity and Epidemiology* (Gupta RC, Satoh T, eds.). John Wiley and Sons, New Jersey. In press.

Frankel S, Concannon J, Brusky K, Pietrowicz E, Giorgianni S, Thompson WD, Currie DA (2009) Arsenic exposure disrupts neurite growth and complexity in vitro. *Neurotoxicology* **30:** 529–37.

Fritsche E, Cline JE, Nguyen NH, Scanlan TS, Abel J (2005) Polychlorinated biphenyls disturb differentiation of normal human neural progenitor cells: Clue for involvement of thyroid hormone receptors. *Env Health Perspect* **113:** 871–6.

Fujimura M, Usuki F, Sawada M, Rostene W, Godefroy D, Takashima A (2009) Methylmercury exposure downregulates the expression of Racl and leads to neuritic degeneration and ultimately apoptosis in cerebrocortical neurons. *Neurotoxicology* **30:** 16–22.

Furuya H, Watanabe T, Sugioka Y, Inagaki Y, Okazaki I (2002) Effect of ethanol and docosahexaenoic acid on nerve growth factor-induced neurite formation and neuron specific growth-associated protein gene expression in PC12 cells. *Nihon Arukoru Yakubutsu Igakkai Zasshi* **37:** 513–22.

Gao P, He P, Wang A, Xia T, Xu B, Xu Z, Niu Q, Guo LG, Chen X (2009) Influence of PCB153 on oxidative DNA damage and DNA repair-related gene expression induced by PBDE-47 in human neuroblastoma cells in vitro. *Toxicol Sci* **107:** 165–70.

Garcia SJ, Seidler FJ, Crumpton TL, Slotkin TA (2001) Does the developmental neurotoxicity of chlorpyrifos involve glial targets? Macromolecule synthesis, adenylyl cyclase signaling, nuclear transcription factors, and formation of reactive oxygen in C6 glioma cells. *Brain Res* **891:** 54–68.

Gasso S, Cristofol RM, Selema G, Rosa R, Rodriguez-Farre E, Sanfeliu C (2001) Antioxidant compounds and Ca^{2+} pathway blockers differentially protect against methylmercury and mercuric chloride neurotoxicity. *J Neurosci Res* **66:** 135–45.

Gearhart D, Sickles DW, Buccafusco JJ, Prendergast M, Terry AV (2007) Chlorpyrifos, chlorpyrifos-oxon and diisopropylfluorophosphate inhibit kinesin-dependent microtubule motility. *Toxicol Appl Pharmacol* **218:** 20–9.

Geter DR, Kan HL, Lowe ER, Rick DL, Charles GD, Gollapudi BB, Mattsson JL (2008) Investigations of oxidative stress, antioxidant response, and protein binding in chlorpyrifos exposed rat neuronal PC12 cells. *Toxicol Mech Methods* **18:** 17–23.

Gilbert ME, Mundy WR, Crofton KM (2000) Spatial learning and long-term potentiation in the dentate gyrus of the hippocampus in animals developmentally exposed to Aroclor 1254. *Toxicol Sci* **57:** 102–11.

Giordano G, Afsharinejad Z, Guizzetti M, Vitalone A, Kavanagh TJ, Costa LG (2007) Organophosphorus insecticides chlorpyrifos and diazinon and oxidative stress in neuronal cells in a genetic model of glutathione deficiency. *Toxicol Appl Pharmacol* **219:** 181–9.

Giordano G, Kavanagh TJ, Costa LG (2008) Neurotoxicity of a polybrominated diphenyl ether mixture (DE-71) in mouse neurons and astrocytes is modulated by intracellular glutathione levels. *Toxicol Appl Pharmacol* **232:** 161–8.

Giordano G, Kavanagh TJ, Costa LG (2009) Mouse cerebellar astrocytes protect cerebellar granule neurons against toxicity of the polybrominated diphenyl ether (PBDE) mixture DE-71. *Neurotoxicology* **30:** 326–9.

Godwin HA (2001) The biological chemistry of lead. *Curr Opin Chem Biol* **5:** 223–7.

Golstein P, Kroemer G (2006) Cell death by necrosis: towards molecular definition. *Trends in Biochem Sci* **32:** 37–43.

Gonthier B, Signorini-Allibe N, Soubeyran A, Eysseric H, Lamarche F, Barret L (2004) Ethanol can modify the effects of certain free radical-generating systems on astrocytes. *Alcohol Clin Exp Res* **28:** 526–34.

Gospe SM, Zhou SS (2000) Prenatal exposure to toluene results in abnormal neurogenesis and migration in rat somatosensory cortex. *Pediatr Res* **47:** 362–8.

Gotti C, Cabrini D, Sher E, Clementi F (1987) Effects of long-term in vitro exposure to aluminum, cadmium or lead on differentiation and cholinergic receptor expression in a human neuroblastoma cell line. *Cell Biol Toxicol* **3:** 431–40.

Gotz ME, Koutsilieri E, Riederer P, Ceccatelli S, Dare E (2002) Methylmercury induces neurite degeneration in primary culture of mouse dopaminergic mesencephalic cells. *J Neural Transm* **109:** 597–605.

Graff RD, Falconer MM, Brown DL, Reuhl KR (1997) Altered sensitivity of posttranslationally modified microtubules to methylmercury in differentiating embryonal carcinoma-derived neurons. *Toxicol Appl Pharmacol* **144:** 215–24.

Grandjean P, Landrigan PJ (2006) Developmental neurotoxicity of industrial chemicals. *Lancet* **368:** 2167–78.

Green DR, Reed JC (1998) Mitochondria and apoptosis. *Science* **281:** 1309–12.

Grennlee AR, Ellis TM, Berg RL (2004) Low-dose agrochemicals and lawn-care pesticides induce developmental toxicity in murine preimplantation embryos. *Environ Health Perspect* **112:** 703–9.

Guerri C, Saez R, Sancho-Tello M, Martin De Aquilera E, Renau-Piqueras J (1990) Ethanol alters astrocyte development: a study of critical periods using primary cultures. *Neurochem Res* **15:** 559–65.

Guerri C, Bazinet A, Riley EP (2009) Foetal alcohol spectrum disorders and alterations in brain and behaviour. *Alcohol Alcohol* **44:** 108–14.

Guilarte TR, Miceli RC (1992) Age-dependent effects of lead on [3H]MK–801 binding to the NMDA receptor-gated ionophore: in vitro and in vivo studies. *Neurosci Lett* **148:** 27–30.

Guilarte TR (1997) Pb^{2+} inhibits NMDA receptor function at high and low affinity sites: developmental and regional brain expression. *Neurotoxicology* **18:** 43–51.

Guilarte TR, McGlothan JL (1998) Hippocampal NMDA receptor mRNA undergoes subunit specific changes during developmental lead exposure. *Brain Res* **790:** 98–107.

Guilarte TR, McGlothan JL (2003) Selective decrease in NR1 subunit splice variant mRNA in the hippocampus of Pb^{2+}-exposed rats: implications for synaptic targeting and cell surface expression of NMDAR complexes. *Brain Res Mol Brain Res* **113:** 37–43.

Guizzetti M, Costa LG (1996) Inhibition of muscarinic receptor-stimulated glial cell proliferation by ethanol. *J Neurochem* **67:** 2236–45.

Gungabissoon RA, Bamburg JR (2003) Regulation of growth cone actin dynamics by ADF/cofilin. *J Histochem Cytochem* **51:** 411–20.

Gupta RC (2004) Brain regional heterogeneity and toxicological mechanisms of organophosphates and carbamates. *Toxicol Mechan Methods* **14:** 103–43.

Hansson E, Von Euler G, Fuxe K, Hansson T (1988) Toluene induces changes in the morphology of astroglia and neurons in striatal primary cell cultures. *Toxicology* **49:** 155–63.

Hao HN, Parker GC, Zhao J, Barami K, Lyman WD (2003) Human neural stem cells are more sensitive than astrocytes to ethanol exposure. *Alcohol Clin Exp Res* **27:** 1310–17.

Hargreaves AJ (1997) The cytoskeleton as a target in cell toxicity. *Adv Mol Cell Biol* **20:** 119–44.

Harris W, Sachana M, Flaskos W, Hargreaves AJ (2009) Proteomic analysis of differentiating neuroblastoma cells treated with sub-lethal neurite inhibitory concentrations of diazinon: identification of novel biomarkers of effect. *Toxicol Appl Pharmacol* **240:** 159–65.

He P, He W, Wang A, Xia T, Xu B, Zhang M, Chen X (2008a) PBDE-47-induced oxidative stress, DNA damage and apoptosis in primary cultured hippocampal neurons. *Neurotoxicology* **29:** 124–9.

He P, Wang AG, Xia T, Gao P, Niu Q, Guo LG, Xu B-Y, Chen X-M (2009) Mechanism of the neurotoxic effect of PBDE-47 and interaction of PBDE-47 and PCB153 in enhancing toxicity in SH-SY5Y cells. *Neurotoxicology* **30:** 10–15.

He W, He P, Wang A, Xia T, Xu B, Chen X (2008b) Effects of PBDE-47 on cytotoxicity and genotoxicity in human neuroblastoma cells in vitro. *Mutat Res* **649:** 62–70.

Heaton MB, Paiva M, Swanson DJ, Walker DW (1993) Modulation of ethanol neurotoxicity by nerve growth factor. *Brain Res* **620:** 78–85.

Heaton MB, Carlin M, Paiva M, Walker DW (1995) Perturbation of target-directed neurite outgrowth in embryonic CNS co-cultures grown in the presence of ethanol. *Brain Res Dev Brain Res* **89:** 270–80.

Heaton MB, Kim DS, Paiva M (2000) Neurotrophic factor protection against ethanol toxicity in cerebellar granule cells requires phosphatidylinositol 3-kinase activation. *Neurosci Lett* **291:** 121–5.

Heaton MB, Madorsky I, Paiva M, Siler-Marsiglio KI (2004) Vitamin E amelioration of ethanol neurotoxicity involves modulation of apoptosis-related protein levels in neonatal rat cerebellar granule cells. *Dev Brain Res* **150:** 117–24.

Heidemann SR, Lamoureux P, Atchison WD (2001) Inhibition of axonal morphogenesis by nonlethal, submicromolar concentrations of methylmercury. *Toxicol Appl Pharmacol* **174:** 49–59.

Hellmann J, Rommelspacher H, Wernicke C (2009) Long-term ethanol exposure impairs neuronal differentiation of human neuroblastoma cells involving neurotrophin-mediated intracellular signaling and in particular protein kinase C. *Alcohol Clin Exp Res* **33:** 538–50.

Henschler D, Schmuck G, Van Aerssen M, Schiffmann D (1992) The inhibitory effect of neuropathic organophosphate esters on neurite outgrowth in cell cultures: a basis for screening for delayed neurotoxicity *Toxicol In Vitro* **6:** 327–35.

Herdegen T, Leah JD (1998) Inducible and constitutive transcription factors in the mammalian nervous system: control of gene expression by Jun, Fos and Krox, and CREB/ATF proteins. *Brain Res Rev* **28:** 370–490.

Hogberg HT, Kinsner-Ovaskainen A, Coecke S, Hartung T, Bal-Price AK (2010) mRNA expression is a relevant tool to identify developmental neurotoxicants using an in vitro approach. *Toxicol Sci* **113:** 95–115.

Holownia A, Ledig M, Menez JF (1997) Ethanol-induced cell death in cultured rat astroglia. *Neurotox Teratol* **19:** 141–6.

Howard AS, Fitzpatrick R, Pessah I, Kostyniak P, Lein PJ (2003) Polychlorinated biphenyls induce caspase-dependent cell death in cultured embryonic rat hippocampal but not cortical neurons via activation of the ryanodine receptor. *Toxicol Appl Pharmacol* **190:** 72–86.

Howard AS, Bucelli R, Jett DA, Bruun D, Yang D, Lein PJ (2005). Chlorpyrifos exerts opposing effects on axonal and dendritic growth in primary neuronal cultures. *Toxicol Appl Pharmacol* **207:** 112–24.

Huang F, Schneider JS (2004) Effects of lead exposure on proliferation and differentiation of neural stem cells derived from different regions of embryonic rat brain. *Neurotoxicology* **25:** 1001–12.

Huang SC, Giordano G, Costa LG (2010) Comparative cytotoxicity and intracellular accumulation of five polybrominated diphenyl ether congeners in mouse cerebellar granule neurons. *Toxicol Sci* **114:** 124–32.

Hwang S-G, Lee H-C, Lee D-W, Kim Y-S, Joo W-H, Cho Y-K, Moon J-Y (2001) Induction of apoptotic cell death by a p53-independent pathway in neuronal SK-N-MC cells after treatment with 2,2′, 5,5′-tetrachlorobiphenyl. *Toxicology* **165:** 179–88.

Inglefield JR, Mundy WR, Shafer TJ (2001) Inositol 1,4,5-triphosphate receptor-sensitive Ca^{2+} release, store-operated Ca^{2+} entry, and cAMP responsive element binding protein phosphorylation in developing cortical cells following exposure to polychlorinated biphenyls. *J Pharmacol Exp Ther* **297:** 762–73.

Iorio KR, Tabakoff B, Hoffman PL (1993) Glutamate-induced neurotoxicity is increased in cerebellar granule cells exposed chronically to ethanol. *Eur J Pharmacol* **248:** 209–12.

Jacobs JS, Miller MW (2001) Proliferation and death of cultured fetal neocortical neurons: effects of ethanol on the dynamics of cell growth. *J Neurocytol* **30:** 391–401.

Jadhav AL, Ramesh GT (1997) Pb-induced alterations in tyrosine hydroxylase activity in rat brain. *Mol Cell Biochem* **175:** 137–41.

Jadhav AL, Ramesh GT, Gunasekar PG (2000) Contribution of protein kinase C and glutamate in Pb^{+2}-induced cytotoxicity. *Toxicol Lett* **115:** 89–98.

Jang MH, Shin MC, Kim YJ, Chung JH, Yim SV, Kim EH, Kim Y, Kim CJ (2001) Protective effects of puerariae flos against ethanol-induced apoptosis on human neuroblastoma cell line SK-N-MC. *Jpn J Pharmacol* **87:** 338–42.

Jankowska-Kulawy A, Gul-Hinc S, Blelarczyk H, Suszkiw JB, Pawelczyk T, Dys A, Szutowicz A (2008) Effects of lead on cholinergic SN56 neuroblastoma cells. *Acta Neurobiol Exp* **68:** 453–62.

Jessell TM (2000) Neuronal specification in the spinal cord: inductive signals and transcriptional codes. *Nat Rev Gen* **1:** 20–9.

Jin Y, Sun G, Li X, Li G, Lu C, Qu L (2004) Study on the toxic effects induced by different arsenicals in primary cultured rat astroglia. *Toxicol Appl Pharmacol* **196:** 396–403.

Jung JE, Moon JY, Ghil SH, Yoo BS (2009) 2,3,7,8-Tetrachlorodibenzo-p-dioxin (TCDD) inhibits neurite outgrowth in differentiating human SH-SY5Y neuroblastoma cells. *Toxicol Lett* **188:** 153–6.

Kala SV, Jadhav AL (1995) Region-specific alterations in dopamine and serotonin metabolism in brains of rats exposed to low levels of lead. *Neurotoxicology* **16:** 297–308.

Kane CJM, Chang JY, Roberson PK, Garg TK, Han L (2008) Ethanol exposure of neonatal rats does not increase biomarkers of oxidative stress in isolated cerebellar granule neurons. *Alcohol* **42:** 29–36.

Kang K, Oh YK, Choue R, Kang SJ (2005) Scutellariae radix extracts suppress ethanol-induced caspase-11 expression and cell death in N2a cells. *Mol Brain Res* **142:** 139–45.

Ke ZJ, Wang X, Fan Z, Luo J (2009) Ethanol promotes thiamine deficiency-induced neuronal death: involvement of double-stranded RNA-activated protein kinase. *Alcohol Clin Exp Res* **33:** 1097–103.

Kentroti S, Vernadakis A (1991) Correlation between morphological and biochemical effects of ethanol on neuroblast-enriched cultures derived from three-day-old chick embryos. *J Neurosci Res* **30:** 484–92.

Kern M, Audesirk G (1995) Inorganic lead may inhibit neurite development in cultured rat hippocampal neurons through hyperphosphorylation. *Toxicol Appl Pharmacol* **134:** 111–23.

Kern M, Audesirk T, Audesirk G (1993) Effects of inorganic lead on the differentiation and growth of cortical neurons in culture. *Neurotoxicology* **14:** 319–27.

Kim JA, Druse MJ (1996) Deficiency of essential neurotrophic factors in conditioned media produced by ethanol-exposed cortical astrocytes. *Brain Res Dev Brain Res* **96:** 1–10.

Kobayashi H, Yuyama A, Matsusaka N, Takeno K, Yanagiya I (1980) Effect of methylmercury on brain acetylcholine concentrations and turnover in mice. *Toxicol Appl Pharmacol* **54:** 1–8.

Kodavanti PR, Shin DS, Tilson HA, Harry GJ (1993) Comparative effects of two polychlorinated biphenyl congeners on calcium homeostasis in rat cerebellar granule cells. *Toxicol Appl Pharmacol* **123:** 97–106.

Kodavanti PRS, Ward TR (2005) Differential effects of commercial polybrominated diphenyl ether and polychlorinated biphenyl mixtures on intracellular signaling in rat brain in vitro. *Toxicol Sci* **85:** 952–62.

Komulainen H, Keranen A, Saano V (1995) Methylmercury modulates GABAA receptor complex differentially in rat cortical and cerebellar membranes in vitro. *Neurochem Res* **20:** 659–62.

Kosik KS, Finch EA (1987) MAP2 and tau segregate into dendritic and axonal domains after the elaboration of morphologically distinct neurites: an immunocytochemical study of cultured rat cerebrum. *J Neurosci* **7:** 3142–53.

Kromidas L, Trombetta LD, Jamall IS (1990) The protective effects of glutathione against methylmercury cytotoxicity. *Toxicol Lett* **51:** 67–80.

Krzyzanski W, Oberdoerster J, Rabin RA (2007) Mechanism of ethanol enhancement of apoptosis and caspase activation in serum-deprived PC12 cells *Life Sci* **81:** 756–64.

Ku BM, Joo Y, Mun J, Roh GS, Kang SS, Cho GJ, Choi WS, Kim HJ (2006) Heme oxygenase protects hippocampal neurons from ethanol-induced neurotoxicity. *Neurosci Lett* **405:** 168–71.

Kunimoto M (1994) Methylmercury induces apoptosis of rat cerebellar neurons in primary culture. *Biochem Biophys Res Commun* **204:** 310–17.

Kunimoto M, Aoki Y, Shibata K, Miura T (1992) Differential cytotoxic effects of methylmercury and organotin compounds on mature and immature neuronal cells and non-neuronal cells in vitro. *Toxicol in Vitro* **6:** 349–55.

Lamarche F, Gonthier B, Signorini N, Eysseric H, Barret L (2003) Acute exposure of cultured neurones to ethanol results in reversible DNA single-strand breaks; whereas chronic exposure causes loss of cell viability. *Alcohol Alcohol* **38:** 550–8.

Lasley SM, Greenland RD, Minnema DJ, Michaelson IA (1984) Influence of chronic inorganic lead exposure on regional dopamine and 5-hydroxytryptamine turnover in rat brain. *Neurochem Res* **9:** 1675–88.

Lau WK, Yeung CW, Lui PW, Cheung LH, Poon NT, Yung KKL (2002) Different trends in modulation of NMDAR1 and NMDAR2B gene expression in cultured cortical and hippocampal neurons after lead exposure. *Brain Res* **932:** 10–24.

Lawton M, Iqbal M, Kontovraki M, Lloyd Mills C, Hargreaves AJ (2007) Reduced tubulin tyrosination as an early marker of mercury toxicity in differentiating N2a cells. *Toxicol in Vitro* **212:** 1258–61.

Leisi P (1997) Ethanol-exposed central neurons fail to migrate and undergo apoptosis. *J Neurosci Res* **48:** 439–48.

Leskawa KC, Maddox T, Webster KA (1995) Effects of ethanol on neuroblastoma cells in culture: role of gangliosides in neuritogenesis and substrate adhesion. *J Neurosci Res* **42:** 377–84.

Li C, Xiang T, Tang M, Yong W, Yan D, Deng H, Wang H, Wang M, Chen J, Ruan D (2008) Involvement of cyclin D1/CDk4 and pRb mediated by PI3K/AKT pathway activation in Pb^{+2}-induced neuronal death in cultured hippocampal neurons. *Toxicol Appl Pharmacol* **229:** 351–61.

Li Q, Ho CS, Marinescu V, Bhatti H, Bokoch GM, Ernst SA, Holz RW, Stuenkel EL (2003) Facilitation of Ca^{2+}-dependent exocytosis by Rac-1 GTPase in bovine chromaffin cells. *J Physiol* **550:** 431–45.

Li Y, King MA, Grimes J, Smith N, De Fiebre CM, Meyer EM (1999) α7 nicotinic receptor-mediated protection against ethanol-induced cytotoxicity in PC12 cells. *Brain Res* **816:** 225–8.

Li Y, King MA, Meyer EM (2000) α7 nicotinic receptor-mediated protection against ethanol-induced oxidative stress and cytotoxicity in PC12 cells. *Brain Res* **861:** 165–7.

Li Z, Lin H, Zhu Y, Wang M, Luo J (2001a) Disruption of cell cycle kinetics and cyclin-dependent kinase system by ethanol in cultured cerebellar granule progenitors. *Brain Res Dev Brain Res* **132:** 47–58.

Li Y, Walker DW, King MA (2001b) Peroxide mediates ethanol-induced cytotoxicity in PC12 cells. *Free Radic Biol Med* **30:** 389–92.

Li W, Casida JE (1998) Organophosphorus neuropathy target esterase inhibitors selectively block outgrowth of neurite-like and cell processes in cultured cells. *Toxicol Lett* **98:** 139–46.

Limke TL, Heidemann SR, Atchison WD (2004) Disruption of intraneuronal divalent cation regulation by methylmercury: are specific targets involved in altered neuronal development and cytotoxicity in methylmercury poisoning? *Neurotoxicology* **25:** 741–60.

Lin HJ, Shaffer KM, Chang YH, Barker JL, Pancrazio JJ, Stenger DA, Ma W (2002) Acute exposure of toluene transiently potentiates p42/44 mitogen activated protein kinase (MAPK) activity in cultured rat cortical astrocytes. *Neurosci Lett* **332:** 103–6.

Liu L, Cao JX, Sun B, Li HL, Xia Y, Wu Z, Tang CL, Hu J (2010) Mesenchymal stem cells inhibition of chronic ethanol-induced oxidative damage via upregulation of phosphatidylinositol-3-kinase/Akt and modulation of extracellular signal-regulated kinase 1/2 activation in PC12 cells and neurons. *Neuroscience* **167:** 1115–24.

Luo J, West JR, Pantazis NJ (1997) Nerve growth factor and basic fibroblast growth factor protect rat cerebellar granule cells in culture against ethanol-induced cell death. *Alcohol Clin Exp Res* **21:** 1108–20.

Luo J, Miller MW (1996) Ethanol inhibits bFGF-mediated proliferation of C6 glioma cells. *J Neurochem* **67:** 1448–56.

Luo J, Miller MW (1997a) Basic fibroblast growth factor- and platelet-derived growth factor-mediated cell proliferation in B104 neuroblastoma cells: Effect of ethanol on cell cycle kinetics. *Brain Res* **770:** 139–50.

Luo J, Miller MW (1997b) Differential sensitivity of human neuroblastoma cell lines to ethanol: Correlations with their proliferative responses to mitogenic growth factors and expression of growth factor receptors. *Alcohol Clin Exp Res* **21:** 1186–94.

Luo J, Miller MW (1999a) Platelet-derived growth factor-mediated signal transduction underlying astrocyte proliferation: Site of ethanol action. *J Neurosci* **19:** 10014–25.

Luo J, Miller MW (1999b) Transforming growth factor beta1-regulated cell proliferation and expression of neural cell adhesion molecule in B104 neuroblastoma cells: differential effects of ethanol. *J Neurochem* **72:** 2286–93.

Luo J, West JR, Cook RT, Pantazis NJ, (1999) Ethanol induced cell death and cell cycle delay in cultures of pheochromocytoma (PC12) cells. *Alcohol Clin Exp Res* **23:** 644–56.

Luo ZD, Berman HA (1997) The influence of Pb^{2+} on expression of acetylcholinesterase and acetylcholine receptor. *Toxicol Appl Pharmacol* **145:** 237–45.

Mack TGA, Koester MP, Pollerberg GE (2000) The microtubule-associated protein MAP1B is involved in local stabilization of turning growth cones. *Mol Cell Neurosci* **15:** 51–65.

Madden SD, Cotter TG (2008) Cell death in brain development and degeneration: control of caspase expression may be key! *Mol Neurobiol* **37:** 1–6.

Madia F, Giordano G, Fattori V, Vitalone A, Branchi I, Capone F, Costa LG (2004) Differential in vitro neurotoxicity of the flame retardant PBDE-99 and of the PCB Aroclor 1254 in human astrocytoma cells. *Toxicol Lett* **154:** 11–21.

Maffi SK, Rathinam ML, Cherian PP, Pate W, Hamby-Mason R, Schenker S, Henderson GI (2008) Glutathion content as a potential mediator of the vulnerability of cultured fetal cortical neurons to ethanol-induced apoptosis. *J Neurosci Res* **86:** 1064–76.

Magi S, Castaldo P, Carrieri G, Scorziello A, Di Renzo GF, Amoroso S (2005) Involvement of Na^+–Ca^{2+} exchanger in intracellular Ca^{2+} increase and neuronal injury induced by polychlorinated biphenyls in human neuroblastoma SH-SY5Y cells. *J Pharmacol Exp Ther* **315:** 291–6.

Mangesdorf T, Althausen S, Paschen W (2002) Genes associated with pro-apoptotic and protective mechanisms are affected differently on exposure of neuronal cell cultures to arsenite. No indication for endoplasmic reticulum stress despite activation of grp78 and gadd153 expression. *Brain Res Mol Brain Res* **104:** 227–39.

Marchetti C (2003) Molecular targets of lead in brain neurotoxicity. *Neurotox Res* **5:** 221–36.

Mariussen E, Myhre O, Reistad T, Fonnum F (2002) The polychlorinated biphenyl mixture aroclor 1254 induces death of rat cerebellar granule cells: the involvement of the *N*-methyl-D-aspartate receptor and reactive oxygen species. *Toxicol Appl Pharmacol* **179:** 137–44.

McAlhany RE Jr, West JR, Miranda RC (2000) Glial-derived neurotrophic factor (GDNF) prevents ethanol-induced apoptosis and JUN kinase phosphorylation. *Dev Brain Res* **119:** 209–16.

McDermott C, Allshire A, van Pelt FNAM, Heffron JJA (2007) Sub-chronic toxicity of low concentrations of industrial volatile organic pollutants in vitro. *Toxicol Appl Pharmacol* **219:** 85–94.

McFarlane Abdulla E, Calaminici M, Campbell IC (1995) Comparison of neurite outgrowth with neurofilament protein subunit levels in neuroblastoma cells following mercuric oxide exposure. *Clin Exp Pharmacol Physiol* **22:** 362–3.

Meng XF, Zou XJ, Peng B, Shi J, Guan XM, Zhang C (2006) Inhibition of ethanol-induced toxicity by tanshinone IIA in PC12 cells. *Acta Pharmacol Sin* **27:** 659–64.

Mense SM, Sengupta A, Lan C, Zhou M, Bentsman G, Volsky DJ, Whyatt RM, Perera FP, Zhang L (2006) The common insecticides cyfluthrin and chlorpyrifos alter the expression of a subset of genes with diverse functions in primary human astrocytes. *Toxicol Sci* **93:** 125–35.

Messing RO, Henteleff M, Park JJ (1991) Ethanol enhances growth factor-induced neurite formation in PC12 cells. *Brain Res* **565:** 301–11.

Minnema DJ, Cooper GP, Greenland RD (1989) Effects of methylmercury on neurotransmitter release from rat brain synaptosomes.*Toxicol Appl Pharmacol* **99:** 510–21.

Mitchell JJ, Paiva M, Heaton MB (1999a) Vitamin E and β-carotene protect against ethanol combined with ischemia in an embryonic rat hippocampal culture model of fetal alcohol syndrome. *Neurosci Lett* **263:** 189–92.

Mitchell JJ, Paiva M, Heaton MB (1999b) The antioxidants vitamine E and β-carotene protect against ethanol-induced neurotoxicity in embryonic rat hippocampal cultures. *Alcohol* **17:** 163–8.

Mitchison T, Kirschner M (1988) Cytoskeletal dynamics and nerve growth. *Neuron* **1:** 761–72.

Miura K, Koide N, Himeno S, Nakagawa I, Imura N (1999) The involvement of microtubular disruption in methylmercury-induced apoptosis in neuronal and nonneuronal cell lines. *Toxicol Appl Pharmacol* **160:** 279–88.

Monnet-Tschudi F (1998) Induction of apoptosis by mercury compounds depends on maturation and is not associated with microglial activation. *J Neurosci Res* **53:** 361–7.

Monnet-Tschudi F, Zurich MG, Honegger P (1996) Comparison of the developmental effects of two mercury compounds on glial cells and neurons in aggregate cultures of rat telencephalon. *Brain Res* **741:** 52–9.

Monroe RK, Halvorsen SW (2006) Mercury abolishes neurotrophic factor-stimulated Jak-STAT signalling in nerve cells by oxidative stress. *Toxicol Sci* **94:** 129–38.

Montoliu C, Sancho-Tello M, Azorin I, Burgal M, Valles S, Renau-Piqueras J, Guerri C (1995) Ethanol increases cytochrome P4502E1 and induces oxidative stress in astrocytes. *J Neurochem* 65: 2561–70.

Moulder KL, Fu T, Melbostad H, Cormier RJ, Isenberg KE, Zorumski CF, Mennerick S (2002) Ethanol-induced death of postnatal hippocampal neurons. *Neurobiol Dis* **10:** 396–409.

Mundy WR, Freudenrich TM (2000) Sensitivity of immature neurons in culture to metal-induced changes in reactive oxygen species and intracellular free calcium. *Neurotoxicology* **21:** 1135–44.

Naarala JT, Loikkanen JJ, Ruotsalainen MH, Savolainen KM (1995) Lead amplifies glutamate-induced oxidative stress. *Free Rad Biol Med* **5:** 689–93.

Nakada S, Saito H, Imura N (1981) Effect of methylmercury and inorganic mercury on the nerve growth factor-induced neurite outgrowth in chick embryonic sensory ganglia. *Toxicol Lett* **8:** 23–8.

Namgung U, Xia Z (2000) Arsenite-induced apoptosis in cortical neurons is mediated by c-Jun N-terminal protein kinase 3 and p38 mitogen activated protein kinases. *J Neurosci* **20:** 6442–51.

Namgung U, Xia Z (2001) Arsenic induces apoptosis in rat cerebellar neurons via activation of JNK3 and p38 MAP kinases. *Toxicol Appl Pharmacol* **174:** 130–8.

Namgung U, Kim DH, Lim SR, Xia Z (2001) Blockade of calcium entry accelerates arsenite-mediated apoptosis in rat cerebellar granule cells. *Mol Cells* **15:** 256–61.

Neal AP, Stansfield KH, Worley PF, Thompson RE, Guilarte TR (2010) Lead exposure during synaptogenesis alters vesicular proteins and impairs vesicular release: potential role of NMDA receptor-dependent BDNF signalling. *Toxicol Sci* doi:10.1093/toxsci/kfq111.

Nihei MK, Guilarte TR (1999) NMDAR-2A subunit protein expression is reduced in the hippocampus of rats exposed to Pb^{2+} during development. *Mol Brain Res* **66:** 42–9.

Nihei MK, Desmond NL, McGlothan JL, Kuhlmann AC, Guilarte TR (2000) N-methyl-D-aspartate receptor subunit changes are associated with lead-induced deficits of long-term potentiation and spatial learning. *Neuroscience* **99:** 233–42.

Nishioku T, Takai N, Miyamoto K, Murao K, Hara C, Yamamoto K, Nakanishi H (2000) Involvement of caspase 3-like protease in methylmercury-induced apoptosis of primary cultured rat cerebral microglia. *Brain Res* **871:** 160–4.

Nowoslawski L, Klocke BJ, Roth KA (2005) Molecular regulation of acute ethanol-induced neuron apoptosis. *J Neuropathol Exp Neurol* **64:** 490–7.

Oberdoerster J, Kamer AR, Rabin RA (1998) Differential effect of ethanol on PC12 cell death. *J Pharmacol Exp Ther* **287:** 359–65.

Oberdoerster J, Rabin RA (1999a) Enhanced caspase activity during ethanol induced apoptosis in rat cerebellar granule cells. *Eur J Pharmacol* **385:** 273–82.

Oberdoerster J, Rabin RA (1999b) NGF-differentiated and undifferentiated PC12 cells vary in induction of apoptosis by ethanol. *Life Sci* **64:** 267–72.

Oberto A, Marks N, Evans HL, Guidotti A (1996) Lead (Lead+2) promotes apoptosis in newborn rat cerebellar neurons: pathological implications. *J Pharmacol Exp Ther* **279:** 435–42.

Ohkawa N, Fujitani K, Tokunaga E, Furuya S, Inokuchi K (2007) The microtubule destabilizer stathmin mediates the development of dendritic arbors in neuronal cells. *J Cell Sci* **120:** 1447–56.

O'Kusky JR (1989) Methylmercury-induced movement and postural disorders in developing rat: high-affinity uptake of choline, glutamate, and γ-aminobutyric acid in the cerebral cortex and caudate-putamen. *J Neurochem* **53:** 999–1006.

Olivieri G, Brack Ch, Müller-Spahn F, Stähelin HB, Herrmann M, Renard P, Brockhaus M, Hock C (2000) Mercury induces cell cytotoxicity and oxidative stress and increases β-amyloid and tau phosphorylation in SHSY5Y neuroblastoma cells. *J Neurochem* **74:** 231–6.

Omary MB, Ku NO, Tao GZ, Toivola DM, Liao J (2006) 'Heads and tails' of intermediate filament phosphorylation: multiple sites and functional insights. *TIBS* **31:** 383–94.

Omata S, Hirakawa E, Daimaon Y, Uchiyama M, Nakashita H, Horigome T, Sugano I, Sugano H (1982) Methylmercury induced changes in the activities of neurotransmitter enzymes in nervous tissues of the rat. *Arch Toxicol* **51:** 285–94.

Opanashuk LA, Finkelstein JN (1995) Relationship of lead-induced proteins to stress response proteins in astroglial cells. *J Neurosci Res* **42:** 623–32.

Orrenius S, Zhivotovsky B, Nicotera P (2003) Regulation of cell death: the calcium-apoptosis link. *Nat Rev Mol Cell Biol* **4:** 552–65.

Ou YC, Thompson SA, Kirchner SC, Kavanagh TJ, Faustman EM (1997) Induction of growth arrest and DNA damage-inducible genes Gadd45 and Gadd153 in primary rodent embryonic cells following exposure to methylmercury. *Toxicol Appl Pharmacol* **147:** 31–8.

Oyama Y, Tomiyoshi F, Ueno S, Furukawa K, Chikahisa L (1994) Methylmercury-induced augmentation of oxidative metabolism in cerebellar neurons dissociated from the rats: its dependence on intracellular Ca^{+2}. *Brain Res* **660:** 154–7.

Pantazis NJ, Dohrman DP, Luo J, Goodlett CR (1992) Alcohol reduces the number of pheochromocytoma (PC12) cells in culture. *Alcohol* **9:** 171–80.

Pantazis NJ, Dohrman DP, Goodlett CR, Cook RT, West JR (1993) Vulnerability of cerebellar granule cells to alcohol-induced cell death diminishes with time in culture. *Alcohol Clin Exp Res* **17:** 1014–21.

Pantazis NJ, Dohrman DP, Luo J, Thomas JD, Goodlett CR West JR (1995) NMDA prevents alcohol-induced neuronal cell death of cerebellar granule cells in culture. *Alcoholism Clin Exp Res* **19:** 846–53.

Pantazis NJ, West JR Dai D (1998) The nitric oxide-cyclic GMP pathway plays an essential role in both promoting cell survival of cerebellar granule cells in culture and protecting cells against ethanol neurotoxicity. *J Neurochem* **70:** 1826–38.

Pantazis NJ, West JR, Dai D (2001) The nitric oxide-cyclic GMP pathway plays an essential role in both promoting cell survival of cerebellar granule cells in culture and protecting the cells against ethanol neurotoxicity. *J Neurochem* **70:** 1826–38.

Park ST, Lim KT, Chung YT, Kim SU (1996) Methylmercury-induced neurotoxicity in cerebral neuron culture is blocked by antioxidants and NMDA receptor antagonists. *Neurotoxicology* **17:** 37–45.

Parran DK, Mundy WR, Barone S Jr (2001) Effects of methylmercury and mercuric chloride on differentiation and cell viability in PC12 cells. *Toxicol Sci* **59:** 278–90.

Parran DK, Barone S Jr, Mundy WR (2003) Methylmercury decreases NGF-induced TrkA autophosphorylation and neurite outgrowth in PC12 cells. *Dev Brain Res* **141:** 71–81.

Pascual M, Valles SL, Renau-Piqueras J, Guerri C (2003) Ceramide pathways modulate ethanol-induced cell death in astrocytes. *J Neurochem* **87:** 1535–45.

Penugonda S, Mare S, Lutz P, Banks WA, Ercal N (2006) Potentiation of lead-induced cell death in PC12 cells by glutamate: protection by N-acetylcysteine amide (NACA), a novel thiol antioxidant. *Toxicol Appl Pharmacol* **216:** 197–205.

Perron JC, Bixby JL (1999) Distinct neurite outgrowth signalling pathways converge on ERK activation. *Mol Cell Neurosci* **13:** 362–78.

Ponce RA, Kavanagh TJ, Mottet NK, Whittaker SG, Faustman EM (1994) Effects of methyl mercury on the cell cycle of primary rat CNS cells in vitro. *Toxicol Appl Pharmacol* **127:** 83–90.

Popp RL, Dertien JS (2008) Actin depolymerisation contributes to ethanol inhibition of NMDA receptors in primary cultured cerebellar granule neurons. *Alcohol* **42:** 525–39.

Prendergast MA, Self RL, Smith KJ, Chayoumi L, Mullins MM, Butler TR, Buccafusco JJ, Gearhart DA, Terry AV Jr (2007) Microtubule-associated targets in chlorpyrifos oxon hippocampal neurotoxicity. *Neuroscience* **146:** 330–9.

Qiao D, Seidler FJ, Padilla S, Slotkin TA (2002) Developmental neurotoxicity of chlorpyrifos: what is the vulnerable period? *Environ Health Perspect* **110:** 1097–103.

Qiao D, Seidler FJ, Tate CA, Cousins MM, Slotkin TA (2003). Fetal chlorpyrifos exposure: adverse effects on brain cell development and cholinergic biomarkers emerge postnatally and continue into adolescence and adulthood. *Environ Health Perspect* **111:** 536–44.

Qiao D, Seidler FJ, Slotkin TA (2005) Oxidative mechanisms contributing to the developmental neurotoxicity of nicotine and chlorpyrifos. *Toxicol Appl Pharmacol* **206:** 17–26.

Radio NM, Breier JM, Shafer TJ, Mundy WR (2008) Assessment of chemical effects on neurite outgrowth in PC12 cells using high content screening. *Toxicol Sci* **105:** 106–18.

Rajanna B, Hobson M (1985) Influence of mercury on uptake of [^{3}H]dopamine and [^{3}H]norepinephrine by rat brain synaptosomes. *Toxicol Lett* **27:** 7–14.

Rajanna B, Rajanna S, Hall E, Yallapragada PR (1997) In vitro metal inhibition of N-methyl-D-aspartate specific glutamate receptor binding in neonatal and adult rat brain. *Drug Chem Toxicol* **20:** 21–9.

Ramachandran V, Watts LT, Maf SK, Chen JJ, Schenker S, Henderson G (2003) Ethanol-induced oxidative stress precedes mitochondrially mediated apoptotic death of cultured fetal cortical neurons. *J Neurosci Res* **74:** 577–88.

Rathinam ML, Watts LT, Stark AA, Mahimainathan L, Stewart J, Schenker S, Henderson GI (2006) Astrocyte control of fetal cortical neuron glutathione homeostasis: up-regulation by ethanol. *J Neurochem* **96:** 1289–300.

Regan CM (1989) Lead-impaired neurodevelopment. Mechanisms and threshold values in the rodent. *Neurotoxicol Teratol* **11:** 533–7.

Reistad T, Fonnum F, Mariussen E (2006) Neurotoxicity of the pentabrominated diphenyl ether mixture, DE-71, and hexabromocyclododecane (HBCD) in rat cerebellar granule cells in vitro. *Arch Toxicol* **80:** 785–96.

Reiter-Funk MC, Dohrman DP (2005) Chronic ethanol exposure increases microtubule content in PC12 cells. *BMC Neurosci* **6:** 16.

Ribas-Fito N, Sala M, Kogevinas M, Sunyer J (2001) Polychlorinated biphenyls (PCBs) and neurological development in children: a systematic review. *J Epidemiol Community Health* **55:** 537–46.

Rodgers JS, Hocker JR, Hanas RJ, Nwosu EC, Hanas JS (2000) Mercuric on inhibition of eukaryotic transcription factor binding to DNA. *Biochem Pharmacol* **61:** 1543–50.

Rodriguez VM, Carrizales L, Mendoza MS, Fajardo OR, Giordano M (2002) Effects of sodium arsenite exposure on development and behaviour in rat. *Neurotoxicol Teratol* **24:** 743–50.

Roivainen R, McMahon T, Messing RO (1993) Protein kinase C isozymes that mediate enhancement of neurite outgrowth by ethanol and phorbol esters in PC12 cells. *Brain Res* **624:** 85–93.

Roivainen R, Hundel B, Messing RO (1994) Ethanol enhances growth factor activation of mitogen-activated protein kinase by a protein kinase C-dependent mechanism. *Proc Natl Acad Sci* **92:** 1891–5.

Rossi AD, Larsson O, Manzo L, Orrenius S, Vahter M, Berggren P-O, Nicotera P (1993) Modifications of Ca^{2+} signalling by inorganic mercury in PC12 cells. *FASEB* **7:** 1507–14.

Roy TS, Andrews JE, Seidler FJ, Slotkin TA (1998) Chlorpyrifos elicits mitotic abnormalities and apoptosis in neuroepithelium of cultured rat embryos. *Teratology* **58:** 62–8.

Rush T, Liu XQ, Hjelmhaug J, Lobner D (2010) Mechanisms of chlorpyrifos and diazinon induced neurotoxicity in cortical culture. *Neuroscience* **166:** 899–906.

Sachana M, Flaskos J, Alexaki E, Glynn P, Hargreaves AJ (2001) The toxicity of chlorpyrifos towards differentiating mouse N2a neuroblastoma cells. *Toxicology in Vitro* **15:** 369–72.

Sachana M, Flaskos J, Hargreaves AJ (2005) Effects of chlorpyrifos and chlorpyrifos-methyl on the outgrowth of axon-like processes, tubulin and GAP-43 in N2a cells. *Toxicol Mech Methods* **15:** 405–10.

Sachana M, Flaskos J, Sidiropoulou E, Yavari CA, Hargreaves AJ (2008) Inhibition of extension outgrowth in differentiating rat C6 glioma cells by chlorpyrifos and chlorpyrifos oxon: effects on microtubule proteins. *Toxicol in Vitro* **22:** 1387–91.

Sadri S, Bahrami F, Khazaei M, Hashemi M, Asgari A (2010) Cannabinoid receptor agonist WIN-55,212-2 protects differentiated PC12 cells from organophosphorus-induced apoptosis. *Int J Toxicol* **29:** 201–8.

Sagara J, Makino N, Bannai S (1996) Glutathione efflux from cultured astrocytes. *J Neurochem* **66:** 1876–81.

Saito M, Saito M, Berg MJ, Guidotti A, Marks N (1999) Gangliosides attenuate ethanol-induced apoptosis in rat cerebellar granule neurons. *Neurochem Res* **24:** 1107–15.

Sakamoto M, Ikegami N, Nakano A (1996) Protective effects of Ca^{+2} channel blockers against methyl mercury toxicity. *Pharmacol Toxicol* **78:** 193–9.

Sakaue M, Okazaki M, Hara S (2005) Very low levels of methylmercury induce cell death of cultured rat cerebellar neurons via calpain activation. *Toxicology* **213:** 97–106.

Salomoni P, Calegari F (2010) Cell cycle control of mammalian neural stem cells: putting a speed limit on G1. *TICB* doi: 10.1016/j.tcb.2010.01.006.

Sánchez-Alonso JA, López-Aparicio P, Recio MN, Pérez-Albarsanz MA (2004) Polychlorinated biphenyl mixture (Aroclors) induce apoptosis via Bcl-2, Bax and caspase-3 proteins in neuronal cell cultures. *Toxicol Lett* **153:** 311–26.

Sanfeliu C, Sebastia J, Ki SU (2001) Methylmercury neurotoxicity in cultures of human neurons, astrocytes, neuroblastoma cells. *Neurotoxicology* **22:** 317–27.

Sarafian TA, Verity MA (1991) Oxidative stress underlying methyl mercury neurotoxicity. *Int J Dev Neurosci* **9:** 147–53.

Sarafian T, Vartavarian L, Kane DJ, Bredesen DE, Verity MA (1994). Bcl-2 expression decreases methyl mercury-induced free-radical generation and cell killing in a neural cell line. *Toxicol Lett* **74:** 149–55.

Sastry PS, Rao KS (2000) Apoptosis and the nervous system. *J Neurochem* **74:** 1–20.

Saulsbury MD, Heylinger SO, Wang K, Johnson DJ (2009) Chlorpyrifos induces oxidative stress in oligodendrocyte progenitor cells. *Toxicology* **259:** 1–9.

Schliwa M, Woehlke G (2003) Molecular motors. *Nature* **422:** 759–65.

Schmuck G, Ahr HJ (1997) In vitro method for screening organophosphate-induced delayed polyneuropathy. *Toxicol in Vitro* **11:** 263–70.

Schreiber T, Gassmann K, Gotz C, Hubenthal U, Moors M, Krause G, Merk HF, Nguyen NH, Scanlan TS, Abel J, Rose CR, Fritsche E (2010) Polybrominated diphenyl ethers induce developmental neurotoxicity in a human in vitro model: evidence for endocrine disruption. *Environ Health Perspect* **118:** 572–8.

Schulte S, Muller WE, Friedberg KD(1995) In vitro and in vivo effects of lead on specific 3H-MK-801 binding to NMDA-receptors in the brain of mice. *Neurotoxicology* **16:** 309–17.

Scortegagna M, Hanbauer I (1997) The effect of lead exposure and serum deprivation on mesencephalic primary cultures. *Neurotoxicology* **18:** 331–9.

Scortegagna M, Chikhale E, Hanbauer I (1998) Lead exposure increases oxidative stress in serum deprived E14 mesencephalic cultures. *Restor Neurol Neurosci* **18:** 331–9.

Seabold G, Luo J, Miller MW (1998) Effect of ethanol on neurotrophin-mediated cell survival and receptor expression in cortical neuronal cultures. *Dev Brain Res* **128:** 139–45.

Seegal RF (1996) Epidemiological and laboratory evidence of PCB-induced neurotoxicity. *Crit Rev Toxicol* **26:** 709–37.

Shang-Zhi X, Rajanna B (2006) Glutamic acid reverses Pb^{2+}-induced reductions of NMDA receptor subunits in vitro. *Neurotoxicology* **27:** 169–75.

Shanker G, Aschner M (2003) Methylmercury-induced reactive oxygen species formation in neonatal cerebral astrocytic cultures is attenuated by antioxidants. *Mol Brain Res* **110:** 85–91.

Shanker G, Aschner JL, Syversen T, Aschner M (2004) Free radical formation in cerebral cortical astrocytes in culture induced by methylmercury. *Mol Brain Res* **128:** 48–57.

Shanker G, Syversen T, Aschner JL, Aschner M (2005) Modulatory effect of glutathione status and antioxidants on methylmercury induced free radical formation in primary cultures of cerebral astrocytes. *Mol Brain Res* **137:** 11–22.

Sharifi AM, Mousavi SH, Bakhshayesh M, Tehrani FK, Mahmoudian M, Oryan S (2005) Studying of correlation between lead-induced cytotoxicity and nitric oxide production in PC12 cells. *Toxicol Lett* **160:** 43–8.

Sharifi AM, Mousavi SH (2008) Studying the effects of lead on DNA fragmentation and proapoptotic bax and antiapoptotic bcl-2 protein expression in PC12 cells. *Toxicol Mech Methods* **18:** 75–9.

Shaul YD, Seger R (2007) The MEK/ERK cascade: from signalling specificity to diverse functions. *Biochim Biophys Acta* **1773:** 1213–26.

Shavali S, Sens DA (2008) Synergistic neurotoxic effects of arsenic and dopamine in human dopaminergic neuroblastoma SH-SY5Y cells. *Toxicol Sci* **102:** 254–61.

Sheth DS, Tajuddin NF, Druse MJ (2009) Antioxidant neuroprotection against ethanol-induced apoptosis in HN2-5 cells. Brain Res **1285:** 14–21.

Shimokawa N, Miyazaki W, Iwasaki T, Koibuchi N (2006) Low dose hydroxylated PCB induces c-Jun expression in PC12 cells. *Neurotoxicology* **27:** 176–83.

Shin KJ, Chung C, Hwang YA, Kim SH, Han MS, Ryu SH, Suh PG (2002) Phospholipase A2-mediated Ca^{2+} influx by 2,2′,4,6-tetrachlorobiphenyl in PC12 cells. *Toxicol Appl Pharmacol* **178:** 37–43.

Sidhu JS, Ponce RA, Vredevoogd MA, Yu X, Gribble E, Hong S-W, Schneider E, Faustman EM (2006) Cell cycle inhibition by sodium arsenite in primary embryonic rat midbrain neuroepithelial cells. *Toxicol Sci* **89:** 475–84.

Sidiropoulou E, Sachana M, Flaskos J, Harris W, Hargreaves AJ, Woldehiwet Z (2009a) Diazinon oxon affects the differentiation of mouse N2a neuroblastoma cells. *Arch Toxicol* **83:** 373–80.

Sidiropoulou E, Sachana M, Flaskos J, Harris W, Hargreaves AJ, Woldehiwet Z (2009b) Diazinon oxon interferes with the differentiation of rat C6 glial cells. *Toxicol in Vitro* **23:** 1548–52.

Siler-Marsiglio KI, Paiva M, Madorsky I, Serrano Y, Neeley A, Heaton MB (2004a) Protective mechanisms of pycnogenol in ethanol-insulted cerebellar granule cells. *Int J Neurobiol* **61:** 267–76.

Siler-Marsiglio KI, Shaw G, Heaton MB (2004b) Pycnogenol and vitamin E inhibit ethanol-induced apoptosis in cerebellar granule cells. *J Neurobiol* **59:** 261–71.

Slotkin TA, Bodwell BE, Levin ED, Seidler FJ (2008a) Neonatal exposure to low doses of diazinon: long-term effects on neuronal cell development and acetylcholine system. *Environ Health Perspect* **116:** 340–8.

Slotkin TA, Levin ED, Seidler FJ (2006) Comparative developmental neurotoxicity of organophosphate insecticides: effects on brain development are separable from systemic toxicity. *Environ Health Perspect* **114:** 746–51.

Slotkin TA, MacKillop EA, Ryde IT, Tate CA, Seidler FJ (2007) Screening for developmental neurotoxicity using PC12 cells: comparisons of organophosphates with a carbamate, an organochlorine and divalent nickel. *Environ Health Perspect* **115:** 93–101.

Slotkin TA, Seidler FJ, Fumagalli F (2008b) Targeting of neurotrophic factors, their receptors and signalling pathways in the developmental neurotoxicity of organophosphates in vivo and in vitro. *Brain Res Bull* **76:** 424–38.

Slotkin TA, Seidler FJ (2009a) Oxidative and excitatory mechanisms of developmental neurotoxicity: transcriptional profiles for chlorpyrifos, diazinon, dieldrin, and divalent nickel in PC12 cells. *Environ Health Perspect* **117:** 587–96.

Slotkin TA, Seidler FJ (2009b) Protein kinase C is a target for diverse developmental neurotoxicants: transcriptional responses to chlorpyrifos, diazinon, dieldrin and divalent nickel in PC12 cells. *Brain Res* **1263:** 23–32.

Slotkin TA, Seidler FJ (2010) Oxidative stress from diverse developmental neurotoxicants: antioxidants protect against lipid peroxidation without preventing cell loss. *Neurotoxicol Teratol* **32:** 124–31.

Soderstrom S, Ebendal T (1995) In vitro toxicity of methyl mercury: effects on nerve growth factor (NGF)-responsive neurons and on NGF synthesis in fibroblasts. *Toxicol Lett* **75:** 133–44.

Song X, Violin JD, Seidler FJ, Slotkin TA (1998) Modeling the developmental neurotoxicity of chlorpyrifos in vitro: macromolecule synthesis in PC12 cells. *Toxicol Appl Pharmacol* **151:** 182–91.

Strittmatter SM (1996) Signal transduction at the neuronal growth cone. *The Neuroscientist* **2:** 83–6.

Suresh C, Dennis AO, Heinz J, Vemuri MC, Chetty CS (2006) Melatonin protection against lead-induced changes in human neuroblastoma cell cultures. *Int J Toxicol* **25:** 459–64.

Suszkiw JB (2004) Presynaptic disruption of transmitter release by lead. *Neurotoxicology* **25:** 599–604.

Tagliaferri S, Caglieri A, Goldoni M, Pinelli S, Alinovi R, Poli D, Pellacani C, Giordano G, Mutti A, Costa LG (2010) Low concentrations of the brominated flame retardants BDE-47 and BDE-99 induce synergistic oxidative stress-mediated neurotoxicity in human neuroblastoma cells. *Toxicol in Vitro* **24:** 116–22.

Takadera T, Ohyashiki T (2004) Glycogen synthase kinase-3 inhibitors prevent caspase-dependent apoptosis induced by ethanol in cultured rat cortical neurons. *Eur J Pharmacol* **499:** 239–45.

Takadera T, Suzuki R, Mohri T (1990) Protection by ethanol of cortical neurons from N-methyl-d-aspartate-induced neurotoxicity is associated with blocking calcium influx. *Brain Res* **537:** 109–14.

Takeuchi T, Kambara T, Marikawa N, Matsumoto H, Shiraishi Y, Ito H (1959) Pathological observation of the Minamata disease. *Acta Pathol Jpn* **9:** 768–83.

Tamm C, Duckworth J, Hermanson O, Ceccatelli S (2006) High susceptibility of neural stem cells to methylmercury toxicity: effects on cell survival and neuronal differentiation. *J Neurochem* **97:** 69–78.

Tateno M, Ukai W, Yamamoto M, Hashimoto E, Ikeda H, Saito T (2005) The effect of ethanol on cell fate determination of neural stem cells. *Alcohol Clin Exp Res* **29:** 225S–229S.

Thibault C, Lai C, Wilke N, Duong B, Olive MF, Rahman S, Dong H, Hodge CW, Lockhart DJ, Miles MF (2000) Expression profiling of neural cells reveals specific patterns of ethanol-responsive gene expression. *Mol Pharmacol* **52:** 1593–600.

Tian X, Sun X, Suszkiw JB (2000) Upregulation of tyrosine hydroxylase and downregulation of choline acetyltranferase in lead-exposed PC12 cells: the role of PKC activation. *Toxicol Appl Pharmacol* **167:** 246–52.

Tiffany-Castiglioni E, Zmudiazinonki J, Bratton GR (1989) Cellular targets of lead neurotoxicity: in vitro models. *Toxicology* **15:** 303–15.

Tilson HA, Jacobson JL, Rogan WJ (1990) Polychlorinated biphenyls and the developing nervous system: cross-species comparisons. *Neurotoxicol Teratol* **12:** 239–48.

Tilson HA, Kodavanti PR (1998) The neurotoxicity of polychlorinated biphenyls. *Neurotoxicology* **19:** 517–25.

Tofighi R, Johansson C, Goldoni M, Ibrahim WN, Gogvadze V, Mutti A, Ceccatelli S (2010) Hippocampal neurons exposed to the environmental contaminants methylmercury and polychlorinated biphenyls undergo cell death via parallel activation of calpains and lysosomal proteases. *Neurotox Res* doi 10.1007/s12640-010-9159-1.

Toimela T, Tahti H (2004) Mitochondrial viability and apoptosis induced by aluminium, mercuric mercury and methylmercury in cell lines of neural origin. *Arch Toxicol* **78:** 565–74.

Toscano CD, Hashemzadeh-Gargari H, McGlothan JL, Guilarte TR (2002) Developmental Pb^{2+} exposure alters NMDAR subtypes and reduces CREB phosphorylation in the rat brain. *Brain Res Dev Brain Res* **139:** 217–26.

Tsuzuki Y (1981) Effects of chronic methylmercury exposure on activities of neurotransmitter enzymes in rat cerebellum. *Toxicol Appl Pharmacol* **60:** 379–81.

vanVliet E, Eskes C, Stingele S, Garlton J, Price A, Farina M, Ponti J, Hartung T, Sabbioni E, Coecke S (2007) Development of a mechanistically-based genetically engineered PC12 cell system to detect p53-mediated cytotoxicity. *Toxicol in Vitro* **21:** 698–705.

Vaudry D, Rousselle C, Basille M, Falluel-Morel A, Pamantung TF, Fontaine M, Fournier A, Vaudry H, Gonzalez B (2002) Pituitary adenylate cyclase-activating polypeptide protects rat cerebellar granule neurons against ethanol-induced apoptotic cell death. *Proc Natl Acad Sci* **99:** 6398–403.

Vaudry D, Hamelink C, Damadzic R, Eskay RL, Gonzalez B, Eiden LE (2005) Endogenous PACAP acts as a stress response peptide to protect cerebellar neurons from ethanol or oxidative insult. *Peptides* **26:** 2518–24.

Vendrell I, Carrascal M, Vilaro MT, Abián J, Rodrıgues-Farre E, Suñol C (2007) Cell viability and proteomic analysis in cultured neurons exposed to methylmercury. *Hum Exp Toxicol* **26:** 263–72.

Vendrell I, Carrascal M, Campos F, Abián J, Suñol C (2010) Methylmercury disrupts the balance between phosphorylated and non-phosphorylated cofilin in primary cultures of mice cerebellar granule cells. A proteomic study. *Toxicol Appl Pharmacol* **242:** 109–18.

Verina T, Rohde CA, Guilarte TR (2007) Environmental lead exposure during early life alters granule cell neurogenesis and morphology in the hippocampus of young adult rats. *Neuroscience* **145:** 1037–47.

Verity MA, Sarafian T, Pacifici EH, Sevanian A (1994) Phospholipase A2 stimulation by methyl mercury in neuron culture. *J Neurochem* **62:** 705–14.

Vettori MV, Goldoni M, Caglieri A, Poli D, Folesani G, Ceccatelli S, Mutti A (2006). Antagonistic effects of methyl-mercury and PCB153 on PC12 cells after combined and simultaneous exposure. *Food Chem Toxicol* **44:** 1505–12.

Viberg H, Fredriksson A, Eriksson P (2003) Neonatal exposure to polybrominated diphenyl ether (PBDE 153) disrupts spontaneous behaviour, impairs learning and memory, and decreases hippocampal cholinergic receptors in adult mice. *Toxicol Appl Pharmacol* **192:** 95–106.

Vogel DG, Margolis RL, Mottet NK (1985) The effects of methyl mercury binding to microtubules. *Toxicol Appl Pharmacol* **80:** 473–86.

Voie OA, Fonnum F (2000) Effect of polychlorinated biphenyls on production of reactive oxygen species (ROS) in rat synaptosomes. *Arch Toxicol* **73:** 588–93.

von Ehrenstein O, Poddar S, Yuan Y, Mazumder DG, Eskenazi B, Basu A, Hira-Smith M, Ghosh N, Lahiri S, Haque R, Ghosh A, Kalman D, Das S, Smith AH (2007) Children's intellectual function in relation to arsenic exposure. *Epidemiology* **18:** 44–51.

Wang CH, Hsiao CK, Chen CL, Hsu LI, Chiou HY, Chen SY, Hsueh YM, Wu MM, Chen CJ (2004) A review of the epidemiologic literature on the role of environmental arsenic exposure and cardiovascular diseases. *Toxicol Appl Pharmacol* **222:** 315–26.

Wasserman GA, Liu X, Parvez F, Ahsan H, Factor-Litvak P, van Geen A, Slavkovich V, Lolacono NJ, Cheng Z, Hussain I, Momotaj H, Graziano JH (2004) Warer arsenic exposure and children's intellectual function in Araihazar, Bagladesh. *Environ Health Perspect* **112:** 1329–33.

Watcharasit P, Thiantanawat A, Satayavivad J (2008) GSK3 promotes arsenite-induced apoptosis via facilitation of mitochondria disruption. *J Appl Toxicol* **28:** 466–74.

Watts LT, Rathinam ML, Schenker S, Henderson GI (2005) Astrocytes protect neurons from ethanol-induced oxidative stress and apoptotic death. *J Neurosci Res* **80:** 655–66.

Wegner M, Stolt CC (2005) From stem cells to neurons and glia: a soxist's view of neural development. *TINS* **28:** 583–8.

Weisglas-Kuperus N (1998) Neurodevelopmental, immunological and endocrinological indices of perinatal human exposure to PCBs and dioxins. *Chemosphere* **37:** 1845–53.

Wenzel A, Fritschy JM, Mohler H, Benke D (1997) NMDA receptor heterogeneity during postnatal development of the rat brain: differential expression of the NR2A, NR2B, and NR2C subunit proteins. *J Neurochem* **68:** 469–78.

Wilke RA, Kolbert CP, Rahimi RA, Windebank AJ (2003) Methylmercury induces apoptosis in cultured rat dorsal root ganglion neurons. *Neurotoxicology* **24:** 369–78.

Williams TM, Ndifor AM, Near JT, Reams-Brown RR (2000) Lead enhances NGF-induced neurite outgrowth in PC12 cells by potentiating ERK/MAPK activation. *Neurotoxicology* **21:** 1081–9.

Williamson MA, Gasiewicz TA, Opanashuk LA (2005) Aryl hydrocarbon receptor expression and activity in cerebellar granule neuroblasts: Implications for development and dioxin toxicity. *Toxicol Sci* **83:** 340–8.

Windebank AJ (1986) Specific inhibition of myelination by lead in vitro: comparison with arsenic, thallium, and mercury. *Exp Neurol* **94:** 203–12.

Wong HK, Fricker M, Wyttenbach A, Villunger A, Michalak EM, Strasser A, Tolkovsky AM (2005) Mutually exclusive subsets of BH3-only proteins are activated by the p53 and c-Jun N-terminal kinase/c-Jun signaling pathways during cortical neuron apoptosis induced by arsenite. *Mol Cell Biol* **25:** 8732–47.

Xu J, Ji L-D, Xu L-H (2006) Lead-induced apoptosis in PC12 cells: involvement of p53, Bcl-2 family and caspase-3. *Toxicol Lett* **166:** 160–7.

Yamaguchi H, Kidachi Y, Ryoyama K (2002) Toluene at environmentally relevant low levels disrupts differentiation of astrocytes precursor cells. *Arch Env Health* **57:** 232–8.

Yang D, Howard A, Bruun D, Ajua-Alemanj M, Pickart C, Lein PJ (2008) Chlorpyrifos and chlorpyrifos-oxon inhibit axonal growth by interfering with the morphogenic activity of acetylcholinesterase. *Toxicol Appl Pharmacol* **228:** 32–41.

Yee S, Choi BH (1996) Oxidative stress in neurotoxic effects of methylmercury poisoning. *Neurotoxicology* **17:** 17–26.

Yu K, He Y, Yeung LW, Lam PK, Wu RS, Zhou B (2008) DE-71-induced apoptosis involving intracellular calcium and the Bax-mitochondria-caspase protease pathway in human neuroblastoma cells in vitro. *Toxicol Sci* **104:** 341–51.

Zawia NH, Sharan R, Brydie M, Oyama T, Crumpton T (1998) Sp1 as a target for metal-induced perturbations of transcriptional regulation of developmental brain gene expression. *Dev Brain Res* **107:** 291–8.

Zhang FX, Rubin R, Rooney TA (1998) Ethanol induces apoptosis in cerebellar granule neurons by inhibiting insulin-like growth factor 1 signaling. *J Neurochem* **71:** 196–204.

Zhong J, Yang X, Yao W, Lee W (2006) Lithium protects ethanol-induced neuronal apoptosis. *Biochem Biophys Res Commun* **350:** 905–10.

Zimmermann HP, Doenges KH, Roderer G (1985a) Interaction of triethyl lead chloride with microtubules in vitro and in mammalian cells. *Exp Cell Res* **156:** 140–52.

Zimmermann HP, Plagens U, Traub P (1985b) Influence of triethyl lead on neurofilaments in vivo and in vitro. *Neurotoxicology* **8:** 569–77.

Zou J, Rabin RA, Pentney RJ (1993) Ethanol enhances neurite outgrowth in primary cultures of rat cerebellar macroneurons. *Brain Res Dev Brain Res* **72:** 75–84.

CHAPTER

20

In vivo biomarkers and biomonitoring in reproductive and developmental toxicity

Dana Boyd Barr and Brian Buckley

INTRODUCTION

Pesticides are broadly defined by the United States Federal Insecticide, Fungicide and Rodenticide Act (FIFRA) as a substance or mixture intended to prevent, destroy, repel or mitigate any pest including insects, rodents and weeds (Laws, 1991). They include not only insecticides but also herbicides, fungicides, disinfectants and growth regulators. Pesticides have been used in some crude form since early times, but the modern use of synthetic pesticides began in the early to mid-20th century. Currently, there is a catalogue of over 800 pesticides formulated in 21,000 different products that are registered with the US Environmental Protection Agency (EPA) for use in the USA (Barr *et al.*, 1999).

Accurately assessing exposure to pesticides is critical in determining health outcomes that are associated with exposures and for evaluating the success of risk mitigation strategies. Biomonitoring is an important tool that can be used to evaluate human exposure to pesticides by measuring the levels of pesticides, pesticide metabolites or altered biological structures or functions in biological specimens or tissue (Barr *et al.*, 1999; Barr and Needham, 2002). These measurements in biological media reflect human exposure to pesticides through all relevant routes, and can therefore be used to monitor aggregate and cumulative exposures. Aggregate pesticide exposure is defined as exposure to a single pesticide from all sources, across all routes and pathways. Cumulative pesticide exposure is defined as exposure to multiple pesticides that can cause the same toxic effect via a common biochemical mechanism. The complexity of aggregate and cumulative pesticide exposures often obscures the linkages between exposure measurements and potential human health effects. Therefore, biomonitoring offers a means to clarify these critical relationships. However, careful interpretation of biomonitoring data is necessary to accurately assess human exposure to pesticides and the associated human health risks (Barr and Angerer, 2006).

Many public health benefits have been realized by the use of synthetic pesticides. For instance, the supply of food has become safer and more plentiful and the occurrence of vector-borne disease has been dramatically reduced. Despite the obvious benefits of pesticides, their potential impact on the environment and public health is substantial. In 1997, the US EPA public sales and usage report estimates that over 5.5 billion pounds of pesticide-active ingredients were applied worldwide. In the USA, about 75% of the pesticides are used for agricultural purposes with the remaining amount used in residential applications. The EPA estimates that about 85% of US households store and use pesticides for their home. With the widespread use of pesticides, it is virtually impossible to avoid exposure at some level.

Although epidemiologic studies have been conducted to determine if any relationship exists between pesticide exposure and disease, many lack integral components of the risk assessment equation. In 1995, noted epidemiologist Roy Shore wrote "the single greatest weakness of epidemiologic risk assessment is that individual [or population *sic*] quantitative exposure information is very often limited or missing in occupational and environmental studies" (Shore, 1995). In the past several decades, researchers have proposed to fill these missing data gaps using biological monitoring of specific markers related to exposures.

Biomarkers for monitoring toxicant exposures, including pesticides, are typically divided into three broad categories (Barr *et al.*, 1999):

1. *Biomarkers of exposure* include measurements of pesticides, pesticide metabolites and modified molecules or cells (e.g., DNA and protein adducts) in biological tissues/fluids (e.g., blood) or excreta (e.g., urine). These biological measurements are directly related to the dose of a pesticide and are a function of pesticide exposure.
2. *Biomarkers of effect* include measurements of biochemical, physiological or behavioral alterations that are a consequence of pesticide exposure. Some examples of biomarkers of effect include biological measurements of endogenous and inflammatory responses, measurements of DNA, protein, cell, tissue and organ damage/modification, and observations of tumors or cancer cell clusters.

Reproductive and Developmental Toxicology, Edited by Ramesh C. Gupta
ISBN: 978-0-12-382032-7

These biological measurements reflect exposure and biological effect, but are often difficult to ascribe to a specific pesticide exposure event.

3. *Biomarkers of susceptibility* include measurements of an individual's inherent ability to respond to pesticide exposures. These measurements include observations of molecular properties and functions, such as genetic polymorphisms and enzyme activities, which can affect the rates of pesticide absorption, distribution, metabolism and elimination, along with an individual's biochemical disposition towards disease progression or repair. Biomarkers of susceptibility are affected by a suite of exogenous and endogenous sources, and therefore may be difficult to link to a specific pesticide exposure event.

Biomarkers of exposure provide information on the dose of a toxicant which, in turn, can be related to the exposure. Biomarkers of susceptibility indicate the variables that affect an individual's response to a particular toxicant. Biomarkers of effect provide information on an event, usually in the preclinical stage, occurring at a target site after exposure that directly correlates to manifestation of disease. In general, as the biomarker approaches the actual manifestation of disease, data indicating a relationship or lack thereof between exposure to a toxicant and development of disease are considered more solid. For this chapter, we concentrate on biomarkers of exposure.

Biomarkers of exposure can be further divided into two groups: (1) internal or absorbed dose, and (2) biologically effective dose. Because human exposure to these pesticides is multi-media and multi-route and varies with the use of pesticides, environmental monitoring of exposure, which determines the potential dose, must account for all media and routes in order to accurately calculate individual exposures. Conversely, biomarkers of internal dose integrate all pathways of exposure by estimating the amount of a pesticide that is absorbed into the body via measurements of the pesticide, its metabolite or its reaction product in biological media (e.g., urine, blood, saliva, meconium, breast milk, etc.). The biologically effective dose is the amount of a toxicant that has interacted with a target site and altered a physiological function. An example is a site-specific DNA adduct of a toxicant or inhibited cholinesterase enzymes. These biomarkers may be spontaneously repaired or may lead to the development of disease, but very often are difficult to measure.

The purpose of this chapter is to provide an overview of the state-of-the-science for pesticide biomonitoring research. We first present the fundamental concepts and primary uses of biomonitoring, and then highlight the major criteria required for the selection and use of biomarkers in population-based exposure studies. Next we focus on factors that affect the use and interpretation of biomarkers of exposure for current-use pesticides. We conclude by identifying critical data gaps and research needs in the field of biomonitoring; the consideration of these factors in future studies will better inform assessments of exposure, dose and risk.

Biomarkers of exposure from samples of human tissue, fluids and excreta offer qualitative or quantitative evidence of pesticide exposure. These measurements are particularly useful in exposure research because they can highlight population-based exposure trends and improve estimates of pesticide exposure and dose.

BIOMONITORING OF EXPOSURE TO PESTICIDES

Pesticides can be divided into two large categories depending upon their environmental and biological persistence (Table 20.1) (Barr and Needham, 2002). *Persistent pesticides*, which include organochlorine (OC) pesticides, are environmentally persistent and tend to persist and bioaccumulate in wildlife and in humans. Because of their environmental persistence, they are often called "legacy pesticides". *Non-persistent pesticides* tend to biodegrade in the environment with exposure to light and water and metabolize quickly in humans, and then are excreted in the urine. Non-persistent pesticides include most of the currently used pesticides in the USA. However, even though they are considered non-persistent, in indoor environments they can persist for months or even years and a portion of these pesticides, especially the chlorinated pesticides, bioaccumulate in adipose tissue.

Persistent pesticides

Organochlorine (OC) pesticides were used extensively in the USA as insecticides in the mid-20th century. OC pesticides include the cyclodienes, hexachlorocyclohexane isomers and DDT and its analogues. Nine of the organochlorine pesticides as well as polychlorinated dibenzo-p-dioxins, furans and biphenyls were the subject of the Stockholm Convention on Persistent Organic Pollutants (POPs), which called for an immediate ban on the production, import, export and use of most of these POPs as well as disposal guidelines. DDT was given a health-related exemption for the control of malaria-carrying mosquitoes. These nine pesticides are aldrin, chlordane, DDT, dieldrin, endrin, heptachlor, hexachlorobenzene, mirex and toxaphene. These pesticides are measured either directly or as a more persistent metabolite, typically in blood serum. Aldrin is measured as its primary metabolite, dieldrin. Chlordane and heptachlor are generally used together and are monitored as their metabolites, oxychlordane and heptachlor epoxide, as well as their commercial by-product, trans-nonachlor. DDT is sometimes measured as DDT but more generally as its biodegraded product and metabolite, DDE. The measurement of toxaphene in biological samples is the most complex because it is a mixture of chlorinated camphenes, some of which have long biologic half-lives. In the USA only three OC pesticides are still in use (i.e., dicofol, lindane and endosulfan); however, these four tend to be much less persistent than those falling under the Stockholm treaty. Even though these compounds are, for the most part, no longer used, the OC pesticides will continue to be monitored in the ecosystems, including humans. The reasons for this are their toxicity (known animal toxicity, known and suspected human toxicity) and the possibilities of human exposure, primarily via the food chain.

Non-persistent pesticides

Non-persistent pesticides are also called contemporary pesticides or current-use pesticides. The development and production of these pesticides escalated after the more persistent pesticides were banned in the mid-1970s. By nature, these pesticides do not persist appreciably in the environment; most decompose within several weeks with exposure to sunlight

TABLE 20.1 Common pesticides, their classes and metabolites (if applicable). The selectivity of the measurement for the target pesticide is indicated

Pesticide family	Biomarker	Matrix	Specificity*
Organochlorine insecticides	Hexachlorobenzene	Serum	1
	beta-Hexachlorocyclohexane	Serum	2
	gamma-Hexachlorocyclohexane	Serum	1
	Pentachlorophenol	Urine	1
	p,p′-Dichlorodiphenyltrichloroethane (DDE)	Serum	2
	1,1′-(2,2-dichloroethenylidene)-bis[4-chlorobenzene] (DDT)	Serum	1
	Oxychlordane	Serum	2
	Heptachlor epoxide	Serum	2
	trans-Nonachlor	Serum	2
	Mirex	Serum	1
	Dieldrin	Serum	1
	Endrin	Serum	3
Organophosphate insecticides	Dimethylphosphate	Urine	3, 4
	Dimethylthiophosphate	Urine	3, 4
	Dimethyldithiophosphate	Urine	3, 4
	Diethylphosphate	Urine	3, 4
	Diethylthiophosphate	Urine	3, 4
	Diethyldithiophosphate	Urine	3, 4
	Malathion dicarboxylic acid	Urine	3, 4
	para-Nitrophenol	Urine	3, 4
	3,5,6-Trichloro-2-pyridinol	Urine	3, 4
	2-Isopropyl-4-methyl-6-hydroxypyrimidine	Urine	3, 4
Pyrethroid insecticides	4-Fluoro-3-phenoxybenzoic acid	Urine	2
	cis-3-(2,2-Dichlorovinyl)-2,2-dimethylcyclopropane carboxylic acid	Urine	3
	trans-3-(2,2-Dichlorovinyl)-2,2-dimethylcyclopropane carboxylic acid	Urine	3
	cis-3-(2,2-Dibromovinyl)-2,2-dimethylcyclopropane carboxylic acid	Urine	2
	3-Phenoxybenzoic acid	Urine	3
Carbamate insecticides	2-Isopropoxyphenol	Urine	2
	Carbofuranphenol	Urine	3
Herbicides	2,4,5-Trichlorophenoxyacetic acid	Urine	1
	2,4-Dichlorophenoxyacetic acid	Urine	1
	2,4-Dichlorophenol	Urine	4
	Alachlor mercapturate	Urine	2
	Atrazine mercapturate	Urine	2
	Acetochlor mercapturate	Urine	2
	Metolachlor mercapturate	Urine	2
Other pesticides	N,N-Diethyl-3-methylbenzamide	Urine	1
	ortho-Phenylphenol	Urine	1
	2,5-Dichlorophenol	Urine	2

*1 Parent pesticide measured
2 Metabolite or contaminant measured but is reflective of the parent pesticide
3 Reflective of class exposure to pesticides; not indicative of a single pesticide
4 Reflective of exposure to pesticide and non-pesticide chemicals (e.g., other chemicals or degradates)

and water. In addition, these pesticides tend not to bioaccumulate; therefore, they are typically metabolized and excreted from the body in a few days. The contemporary pesticides are structurally diverse and have varied mechanisms of action. Organophosphates, carbamates, synthetic pyrethroids, phenoxyacid herbicides, triazine herbicides, chloroacetanilide herbicides are among the classes included in this pesticide grouping.

Insecticides

Organophosphates

Organophosphate pesticides (OP) are comprised of a phosphate (or thio- or dithio-phosphate) moiety and an organic moiety. In most cases, the phosphate moiety is O,O-dialkyl substituted. These pesticides are potent cholinesterase inhibitors. They can reversibly or irreversibly bind covalently with the serine residue in the active site of acetyl cholinesterase and prevent its natural function in catabolism of neurotransmitters. This action is not unique to insects, but can produce the same effects in wildlife and humans.

Once human exposure occurs, OP insecticides are usually metabolized to the more reactive oxon form which may bind to cholinesterase or be hydrolyzed to a dialkyl phosphate and a hydroxylated organic moiety specific to the pesticide. As a result of binding to cholinesterase, the organic portion of the molecule is released. The cholinesterase-bound phosphate group may be "aged" by the loss of the O,O-dialkyl groups, or may be hydrolyzed to regenerate the active enzyme. These metabolites and hydrolysis products are then excreted in the urine, either in free form or bound to sugars or sulfates. Alternatively, the intact pesticide may undergo hydrolysis prior to any conversion to the oxon form and the polar metabolites are excreted. In any instance, a series of polar metabolites are excreted in the urine.

Six dialkyl phosphate (DAP) metabolites of OP pesticides are the most commonly measured using biomonitoring. The data generated from these analyses do not provide unequivocal identification of a single pesticide, but rather a cumulative index of exposure to most of the members of the class of OP insecticides. It is important to note that DAPs are possible metabolites of some industrial chemicals and pharmaceuticals, but it is generally believed that most urinary DAP results from OP exposure or exposure to OP hydrolysis products in the environment.

Pesticide-specific metabolites of OPs are also frequently measured. The most common metabolite measured is 3,5,6-trichloropyridinol (3,5,6-TCPy), a metabolite of chlorpyrifos. Specific malathion metabolites, malathion dicarboxylic acid and α and β isomers of malathion monocarboxylic acid, have also been measured. Other less frequently measured specific OP metabolites include 2-isopropyl-4-methyl-6-hydroxypyrimidine (IMPY), a metabolite of diazinon, and 4-nitrophenol, which is a metabolite of methyl and ethyl parathion, EPN and other non-OP pesticide chemicals.

Several methods have been reported that measure the intact OP pesticides in blood, serum or plasma. The vast majority of these methods were developed for forensic applications or for diagnosis of acute pesticide intoxication. Most of these methods lack the sensitivity and/or the selectivity to measure pesticides in blood or blood products resulting from incidental exposures.

Carbamates

Carbamate insecticides have the same mechanism of toxicity action as the OP insecticides, except their effects are more reversible and less severe. The most popular of these pesticides for residential uses are carbaryl (Sevin®) and propoxur (Baygon®). Many carbamates such as aldicarb and methomyl are also used in agricultural applications. Carbaryl exposure has been estimated based upon urinary measurements of 1-naphthol, its most abundant metabolite. However, 1-naphthol, as well as 2-naphthol, is a metabolite also of naphthalene, a ubiquitous polyaromatic hydrocarbon. Thus, the measurement of 1-naphthol does not distinguish these two sources. Measurement of other less abundant metabolites of carbaryl, such as 4-hydroxycarbarylglucuronide, may help to circumvent this problem. Indirectly, researchers have examined the correlation of the prevalence of 2-naphthol and 1-naphthol in order to discern the contributions of carbaryl and naphthalene exposure (Meeker *et al.*, 2007).

Other carbamate metabolites that have been measured in urine include benomyl, carbofuran, carbosulfan, propoxur, aldicarb and pirimicarb. In addition, several carbamates have been measured in serum and plasma. The carbamates, in general, are particularly unstable in blood so sometimes their metabolites must be measured as well. For instance, carbaryl is hydrolyzed rapidly in blood to its major metabolite, 1-naphthol; therefore, 1-naphthol is usually measured in serum or plasma. In addition, a propoxur metabolite, 2-isopropoxyphenol, can be successful quantified in serum or plasma. Methomyl was measured in the whole blood of a pilot who died during aerial application of the pesticide.

Pyrethrins and pyrethroids

Pyrethrins are naturally occurring chemicals that are produced by chrysanthemums which exhibit a pesticidal effect on insects. Natural pyrethrins are comprised of many isomeric forms and are usually classified as the pyrethrin I and II isomer sets. Synthetic pyrethroids are synthetic chemicals that are produced to mimic the effective action of natural pyrethrins. Their chemical structures are typically comprised of a chrysanthemic acid analogue that is esterified most often with a ringed structure. Pyrethroids are non-systemic pesticides that have contact and stomach action. Some pyrethroids also have a slight repellent effect. In most formulations, piperonyl butoxide is added as a synergist. In the past several years, the use of synthetic pyrethroids has escalated as the use of the more toxic OP and carbamate insecticides has been curtailed. Many products such as Raid® brand pesticides that are commonly found in retail stores for home use contain pyrethroids such as permethrin and deltamethrin for eliminating household pests such as ants and spiders.

During metabolism of the pyrethroids, the chrysanthemic acid ester is usually cleaved via esterase or mixed function oxidase activity and any resulting alcohol moieties are converted to their corresponding acids. These metabolites are partly conjugated to glucuronide and both the conjugates and free acids are excreted in the urine.

Several methods exist for the measurement of synthetic pyrethroid metabolites in human urine. The metabolites of permethrin, cypermethrin, deltamethrin and cyfluthrin are most commonly measured. 3-Phenoxybenzoic acid (3PBA) is a metabolite that is common to as many as 20 synthetic pyrethroids. It has been measured alone or as a part of a suite of pyrethroid metabolites. Other more specific metabolites of synthetic pyrethroids have also been measured in urine. *Cis*- and *trans*-isomers of 2,2-dichlorovinyl-2,2-dimethylcyclopropane-1-carboxylic acid (*cis*- and *trans*-DCCA) are metabolites of permethrin, cypermethrin and cyfluthrin; *cis*-2,2-dibromovinyl-2,2-dimethylcyclopropane-1-carboxylic acid (DBCA) is a metabolite of deltamethrin; and 4-fluoro-3-phenoxybenzoic acid (4F3PBA) is a metabolite of cyfluthrin.

Synthetic pyrethroids have also been measured in serum and plasma. Leng *et al.* (1997) observed a dramatic decrease in the concentrations of permethrin and several other pyrethroids in spiked serum (60 μg/L) when stored at 4°C over 8 days. By adding 1% formic acid before storing the spiked serum, the deterioration, presumably due to esterase activity, was diminished for permethrin and markedly reduced for the other pyrethroids. Barr *et al.* (2002) did not observe this decrease in permethrin concentrations in spiked serum (50 and 15 pg/g) stored at −70°C over 4 months. However, more variability was observed in the analysis of permethrin isomers in these stored serum samples after about 1 month and other pesticides that are metabolized via esterase activity (i.e., carbamates and some reactive OPs) did show marked decreases. This area warrants further investigation if serum measurements continue to be made.

Herbicides

Triazines

Triazines are pre- and post-emergence herbicides used to control broad-leafed weeds and some annual grasses. These herbicides inhibit the photosynthetic electron transport in certain plants. Human exposure to triazines has been linked with the development of ovarian cancer. The chemical structures of triazine herbicides are permutations of alkyl substituted 2,4-diamines of chlorotriazine. Upon entering the body, they are metabolized via the glutathione detoxification pathway or by simple dealkylation. For glutathione detoxification, the chlorine atom on the triazine herbicide is subject to an enzymatic-catalyzed substitution by the free -SH on the internal cysteine residue of the glutathione tripeptide. The terminal peptides are enzymatically cleaved and the cysteine is N-acetylated. The mercapturate and dealkylation metabolites are then excreted into the urine.

Atrazine is the most studied triazine herbicide. It was also the single most heavily applied pesticide in the USA in 1997 and is currently the second most abundantly applied pesticide. Although dealkylated metabolites can also be formed in the environment and dominate in environmental exposures, atrazine mercapturate was identified as the major human metabolite of occupational exposure to atrazine (Barr *et al.*, 2007). Dealkylated metabolites of triazine herbicides can be formed and excreted in the urine. These metabolites are not specific for a single triazine, but provide class exposure information. Triazines can also be measured as the intact pesticide in blood products.

Phenoxyacids

Phenoxyacid herbicides are post-emergence growth inhibitors used to eliminate unwanted foliage or weeds. The most common phenoxyacid herbicides are 2,4-dichlorophenoxyacetic acid (24D) and 2,4,5-trichlorophenoxyacetic acid (245T). These two herbicides were combined in equal proportions to make Agent Orange, the herbicide applied in the jungles of Vietnam, Laos and Cambodia along with agricultural regions of Vietnam in the late 1960s and early 1970s during the Vietnam War. Because it was contaminated with the highly toxic and persistent 2,3,7,8-tetrachlorodibenzo-p-dioxin along with other chlorinated dioxins and furans, 245T has been banned for most applications. Although 24D also contains small amounts of persistent chlorinated dioxins and furans, it is still the most abundantly applied residential pesticide. In its ester or salt forms, it is commonly found in home and garden stores in combination with other herbicides such as dicamba or mecoprop for application on lawns.

24D is excreted in the urine as the unmetabolized intact pesticide and its esters are hydrolyzed to 24D prior to excretion. In addition to 24D, mecoprop, MCPA (2-methyl-4-chlorophenoxyacetic acid) and 245T have been measured in urine.

Chloroacetanilides

Chloroacetanilides are pre-emergence systemic herbicides that work by preventing protein synthesis and root elongation in plants. The herbicides are N,N-disubstituted anilines. The individual chloroacetanilides usually differ by their alkyl substituents on the aniline ring. Metolachlor and alachlor are two of the most abundantly applied herbicides in the USA. Although detailed metabolism has not been studied on many herbicides in this class, Coleman *et al.* (2000) observed that many of them, with the unusual exception of metolachlor, form diethylaniline or methylethylaniline intermediates human liver microsomes that are capable of reacting with biomolecules. The author suggests two possible mechanisms for the formation of these reactive intermediates: (1) cytochrome P450-mediated formation of the N-monosubstituted acetamide followed by arylamidase reaction, or (2) glutathione conjugation and subsequent amide hydrolysis. In humans, the major urinary metabolites of alachlor, metolachlor and acetachlor have been identified as their mercapturates (Driskell *et al.*, 1996; Driskell and Hill, 1997; Barr *et al.*, 2007). These metabolites are not inconsistent with the suggested metabolic pathways. In addition, some of the intact chloroacetanilide pesticides have been measured in serum and plasma.

Other herbicides

Other herbicides that do not conveniently fit into any other category have also been measured in humans. Dicamba, which is often used in conjunction with 24D in garden applications, has been measured in urine. Additionally, paraquat and diquat have been measured in urine, blood and serum. Chlorthal-dimethyl and trifluralin have been measured in plasma and serum.

Fungicides

Fungicides, although widely used, are not the most common class of pesticides typically measured in humans. Hexachlorobenzene is an industrial chemical and also a fungicide; it was discussed with the organochlorine pesticides. Pentachlorophenol (PCP) has also been widely used as a preventive fungicide, insecticide and herbicide. Previously, it was commonly applied on wood products to prevent termite infestation and mildew development. Many methods have been reported that measure PCP in serum, plasma and urine.

Metabolites of alkylene bisdithiocarbamates have also been measured in humans. Ethylene bisdithiocarbamates, such as maneb, mancozeb and ziram, are metabolized to ethylenethiourea (ETU). ETU itself has been shown to be carcinogenic and a thyroid hormone inhibitor in animals. It is also used as an accelerator in rubber production (Nebbia and Fink-Gremmels, 1996; Brucker-Davis, 1998).

Other fungicides that have been measured in biological matrices include captan, folpet, dichloran, chlorothalonil, metalaxyl and vinclozolin. Captan and folpet have been measured as their major metabolites, tetrahydrophthalimide (THPI) and phthalimide (PI), respectively, in urine and serum samples. In addition, dichloran, chlorothalonil and metalaxyl have been measured in serum and plasma. Vinclozolin metabolites have been measured by base hydrolysis to 3,5-dichloroaniline and the measurement of 3,5-dichloroaniline.

Other pesticides

Chlordimeform and chlorobenzilate are acaricides. The major urinary metabolite of chlordimeform, chlorotoluidine and the major metabolite of chlorobenzilate, p,p′-dichlorobenzophenone have been quantified in urine.

para-Dichlorobenzene and naphthalene are fumigants that are used as insecticides or disinfectants. The major urinary metabolites of both pesticides, 2,5-dichlorophenol and 1- and 2-naphthol, respectively, have been measured in urine. In addition, *para*-dichlorobenzene has been measured in whole blood using purge and trap with gas chromatography-high resolution mass spectrometry.

DEET (diethyl-m-toluamide) is commonly used as a mosquito repellent in commercially available formulations such as OFF®. DEET can be measured directly in blood or as a series of metabolites in urine.

CONTINUAL EVOLUTION OF BIOMONITORING METHODS

Although much research has provided methods for measuring a variety of pesticides in biological matrices, there is still much work left to be done. As pesticides are banned or their use is limited, manufacturers are compelled to create and mass produce effective yet less toxic pesticides. As this occurs, there will be a gradual yet steady shift in the pesticides used worldwide, most assuredly accompanied by a transitional lag in developing countries. In essence, this leaves researchers performing biological monitoring of exposure in a perpetual state of method development in an effort to keep up with the growing and changing face of pesticides. In our modern generation, most pesticide methods use some combination of chromatography for separation of the pesticides or metabolites with mass spectrometry for detection. High performance liquid chromatography, ultra-performance liquid chromatography and gas chromatography are typically interfaced with single-stage quadrupole mass spectrometers (MS), triple quadrupole mass spectrometer for tandem MS applications (MS/MS), ion trap MS for multiple stages of mass spectrometry (MS^n), time-of-flight mass spectrometers and high resolution mass spectrometers (Barr and Needham, 2002). These are all very sensitive and selective analytical platforms that also allow the use of isotope dilution calibration which improves the accuracy, precision and sensitivity of the measurements. Other detectors such as nitrogen phosphorus and electron capture detectors are also still in use.

Matrix considerations

The choice of matrix for biomonitoring of the persistent pesticides is usually fairly straightforward. Most of the persistent pesticides are best measured in serum, plasma or other lipophilic matrices such as breast milk as their biological half lives are quite long. Since these pesticides are inherently lipophilic, they tend to sequester into the fat stores of the body; therefore, their concentration in serum, plasma or breast milk is dependent upon the lipid content of the matrix. For this reason, persistent pesticide levels, like other persistent organic pollutants, are often normalized on the lipid content of the individual sample. This is especially useful for inter-person sample comparisons.

A small portion of persistent pesticides may be metabolized and excreted, at a fairly steady state, in urine over a long time span, depending largely on the pesticide half-life. These metabolites can be measured in urine; however, the data must generally be corrected for urine dilution if a 24-hour sample is not obtained (see discussion below for more details).

Unfortunately, because of the long half-lives of persistent pesticides, it is usually difficult or impossible to distinguish recent exposures from exposures that occurred decades ago. One possible indicator of a recent exposure may be a level elevated above the range that is normally seen.

The choice of matrix for biomonitoring for the contemporary or non-persistent pesticides is dependent upon a number of variables including the toxicokinetics of the pesticide, the availability of the matrix, the ease of matrix manipulation and the LOD of the analytical method. Contemporary pesticides are usually monitored in urine and less frequently in blood.

Measuring the internal dose of toxicants in blood has several advantages over measuring it in urine. Generally, the parent compound, instead of a metabolite, can be directly monitored in blood products such as whole blood, plasma or serum; therefore, the development of a blood measurement technique may not require detailed information on the metabolism.

Because blood is a regulated fluid (i.e., the volume does not vary with water intake or other factors), no corrections for dilution are necessary. As with the persistent pesticides, dependent upon the lipophilicity of the pesticide, lipid corrections may be necessary for inter-sample comparisons; however, this is usually not necessary with contemporary pesticides. Blood concentrations of the toxicant are often at a maximum directly following exposure, so the preferred time range for sampling may be clearer than with urine. However, blood concentrations of toxicants may vary with the exposure route; ingested toxicants usually require more time to reach the blood stream than inhaled or dermally absorbed doses. Furthermore, blood measurements are more likely than urine measurements to reflect the dose available for the target site since the measured dose has not yet been eliminated from the body.

The major disadvantages of blood measurements are the venipuncture required to obtain the sample and the low toxicant concentrations. Unfortunately, the invasive nature of venipuncture sampling limits researchers' ability to obtain samples from children or, in some instances, to get high participation rates in large-scale studies. In addition, when samples can be obtained, the amount of blood available to perform the analysis is often limited; therefore, ultrasensitive analytical techniques may be required. For non-persistent pesticides, analysis of blood is further complicated by the inherently low toxicant concentrations that are generally present in blood (ng/L or parts per trillion) when compared with urinary metabolite concentrations (μg/L or parts per billion).

An obvious advantage of biological monitoring in urine is its ease of availability. This is especially advantageous when multiple samples are required or when biological monitoring of children is necessary. Generally, the participation rate in large-scale studies is higher when urine samples are requested instead of blood.

Another advantage of urine is the amount of sample available for analysis. The analysis is not usually limited by the volume of sample available, except perhaps with very small children; therefore, less sensitive instruments could be used by compensating for the decreased instrument sensitivity with increased sample. The analysis of urine is further enhanced because the concentrations of toxicants or metabolites are higher in urine than in blood due to their relatively rapid metabolism and excretion. However, an increase in the sample size is generally accompanied by an increase in background noise of the sample.

Because urine analyses usually require the measurement of a metabolite instead of the parent pesticide, detailed information regarding the toxicant's metabolism is necessary to determine the appropriate biomarker of exposure. Unfortunately, detailed metabolic information is sometimes not available for pesticides, and in many cases where it is available, the reported metabolism applies only to a particular species of animals. In these cases, studies to determine the major human metabolites of the pesticides must be conducted or the best available information on animal metabolism must be used. Unfortunately, when animal metabolic information is used in developing an analytical method, the metabolite may not be detected in human samples. In these cases, these data do not necessarily indicate low or no internal dose of the toxicant; they may also indicate the wrong metabolite was monitored.

Because urine is a non-regulated body fluid, the concentration of toxicants or metabolites may vary, even if the internal dose remains constant (Barr *et al.*, 2004, 2005). For this reason, either 24-hour urine samples must be obtained for analysis or "spot" or "grab" samples must be corrected for dilution. Because 24-hour urine samples are usually not practical, "spot" or "grab" samples or, for more concentrated samples, first morning voids are generally obtained, and their concentrations are normalized on the creatinine concentration, specific gravity or osmolality of the urine. However, these correction methods do not necessarily correct for urine dilution because the metabolites may not be treated similarly to creatinine in the body and because creatinine excretion can vary based upon several factors including seasonal variations and those related to muscle mass such as age, weight, sex and pregnancy. This problem with creatinine correction is highlighted when comparing adult metabolite levels to children metabolite levels. The inherently lower creatinine concentrations in children may cause the dilution to be "overcorrected" which, in turn, may give the false appearance of elevated levels (when compared to adults) in children. However, to date, creatinine correction is the most widely accepted method for normalizing urine metabolite concentrations.

In some cases, particular metabolites may originate from more than one pesticide, which inhibits specific identification of the source of the original exposure. One example of a non-specific metabolite is a dialkylphosphate, which may be derived from a variety of organophosphate pesticides. Dialkylphosphate concentrations provide non-specific information about exposure to a class of pesticides instead of a single compound. Such information is certainly useful when determining exposure prevalence to most members of a class of compounds; however, it may not accurately reflect the toxicity associated with the exposure. An exception to this may be when the non-specific metabolite is the toxic compound, such as with ethylene thiourea (ETU) metabolites of dithiocarbamates.

Although saliva has been used as a matrix for biomonitoring other xenobiotics, very little work has focused on saliva as a matrix for pesticide measurements. Measurements of pesticides in saliva or oral fluids have been performed using immunoassay. Where saliva measurements are shown to correlate with plasma or serum measurements, saliva may be a good matrix for biomonitoring of pesticides (Wessels *et al.*, 2003).

Saliva measurements offer several distinct advantages. Saliva is likely to be a much cleaner matrix than urine or serum, since those compounds that cannot easily diffuse across cell membranes will be excluded from this matrix. In addition, saliva is plentiful with the average adult secreting from 500 to 1500 mL/day and collection is easy, non-invasive and does not require privacy. To avoid the unpleasantness of spitting, some commercially available collection tubes include a cotton or polyfiber plug which may be chewed for several minutes to collect saliva. Using these special saliva tubes, collection may be done independently and shipped to the researcher. Biomonitoring of pesticides in saliva is an area worth more development.

A limitation in measuring non-persistent chemicals as a whole is the transient nature of the pesticides in the body. In most instances, measurements in urine, blood or saliva will only be indicative of recent exposure. If sampling is not timed correctly, an exposure event might even be totally missed. As more interest has been directed toward children, both pre- and postnatal, and the potential relationship between pesticide exposures and developmental effects (e.g., decreased physiological and psychological development, congenital defects, etc.), the transient exposure information severely limits these studies. In fact, measurement of a short-lived biomarker over time usually demonstrates a great deal of intraindividual variability in exposure, and consequently in excretion (Figure 20.1).

Measurements in meconium offer a potential solution to this problem in studies observing *in utero* exposure effects (Whyatt and Barr, 2001; Whyatt *et al.*, 2009). Meconium is a greenish-black tar-like substance that begins to accumulate in the intestines of a fetus during the second trimester of pregnancy and is expelled shortly after birth as the newborn's first few bowel movements. Theoretically for xenobiotics that cross the placental barrier and enter the fetus, a portion may be partitioned either as the parent compound or a metabolite

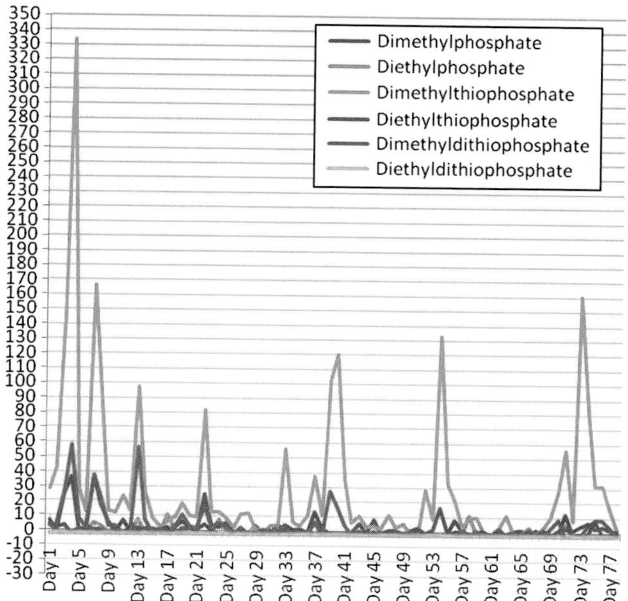

FIGURE 20.1 The intraperson temporal (over 71 days) variability of excretion of six dialkylphosphate metabolites of OP pesticides is shown. Please refer to color plate section.

into the meconium while the remainder is mostly metabolized and excreted into the amniotic fluid. Those metabolites that end up in the amniotic fluid can be swallowed or inhaled by the fetus and again a portion partitioned into the meconium. This cycle may continue until birth; thereby allowing a cumulative dosimeter of *in utero* exposure. Meconium has primarily been used to measure fetal exposure to illicit drugs, nicotine and alcohol. However, more recently, it has been explored as a potential matrix for biomonitoring fetal pesticide exposure. These initial studies show promising potential for using meconium measurements in epidemiologic studies. However, more work needs to be done in calibrating levels in meconium with known levels of exposure.

BIOMARKER SELECTION AND USE

Biomarkers of exposure should be, at a minimum, sensitive, specific, valid, biologically relevant and easy to collect (i.e., practical) in order to be useful as a surveillance tool and for improving quantitative estimates of exposure and dose. Here we examine against these criteria the most commonly used biomarkers of pesticide exposure. Table 20.1 lists pesticide biomarkers, grouped by pesticide class, that have been commonly measured in the literature. We indicate which provide qualitative information on the criteria listed above for each pesticide and matrix. Some pesticide or metabolite measurements may be more meaningful in one matrix as opposed to another. These data all come into consideration when determining the appropriate uses for biomonitoring data.

Sensitivity

Low frequencies of detection of pesticide biomarkers can be an indication of infrequent and/or low level pesticide exposures, or an indication of insufficiently sensitive analytical methods. To be a useful biomarker, the marker should be able to be measured at low dose exposures and should vary consistently and quantitatively with respect to exposure (Wessels *et al.*, 2003). Despite advances in analytical techniques that have allowed the measurement of pesticides at ultra-trace levels, sensitivity issues still can hinder the widespread detection of pesticides. In CDC's most recent NER, only six of 45 pesticides or metabolites measured had frequencies of detection greater than 60%. These data either indicate that the methods are not adequately sensitive enough to detect the biomarkers or that the exposures are so low that they cannot be detected. For some chemicals, the latter seems true as the method sensitivities have not changed over time although the frequencies of detection have. For other analytes though, the former may be true. Several computational methods can be used to impute values for measurements that fall below the analytical limit of detection (LOD) (e.g., LOD divided by 2 or LOD divided by the square root of 2). Discussions of the most appropriate ways to treat values below the analytical LOD have been published; however, this is still a topic of much debate.

Specificity

A useful pesticide biomarker should be specific for a parent compound of interest. Specific pesticide biomarkers can be used to assess aggregate exposure, since the biomarker measurement reflects exposure to one parent compound from all exposure sources and through all exposure routes. Table 20.1 shows the number of pesticide biomarkers that are selective for exposure to a single chemical, a single class or multiple chemicals/classes. In many cases, measured pesticide *metabolites* are not specific biomarkers because they are common to multiple parent compounds. This situation is clearly demonstrated with the six dialkyl phosphate metabolites of OP insecticides, which include dimethylphosphate (DMP), dimethylthiophosphate (DMTP), dimethyldithiophosphate (DMDTP), diethylphosphate (DEP), diethylthiophosphate (DETP) and diethyldithiophosphate (DEDTP). These six metabolites can be produced from the metabolism of several different OP insecticides (e.g., chlorpyrifos, diazinon, malathion and parathion). Therefore, when using these biomarkers to assess exposure, the relative contribution from each OP insecticide must be known to accurately quantify the contribution from a single parent compound.

While non-specific pesticide biomarkers are not ideal for assessing aggregate exposure, they can be useful for assessing cumulative exposure, which involves exposure to multiple parent compounds involving a common mechanism of toxicity. In a case study of the CHAMACOS cohort (Castorina *et al.*, 2003), the six non-specific dialkyl metabolites of OP insecticides (i.e., DMP, DMTP, DMDTP, DEP, DETP and DEDTP) were measured in the urine of 446 pregnant women to assess cumulative OP insecticide exposures. Here, OP insecticide cumulative dose equivalents (calculated using the relative potency factor (RPF = the ratio of the toxic potency of a given chemical to that of an index chemical) of each relevant OP insecticide in the cumulative assessment group) were calculated using non-specific biomarker measurements to assess exposure risks for the pregnant women (Castorina *et al.*, 2003). This application demonstrates the utility of non-specific biomarkers for the assessment of cumulative exposure and dose.

Validity

A selected biomarker of pesticide exposure should be a valid indicator of an underlying exposure event. That is, a biomarker measurement should accurately reflect the magnitude of exposure to a specific pesticide. Unfortunately, many pesticides break down in the environment to produce degradates that are chemically equivalent to biological metabolites. Therefore, biomarker levels can reflect exposure to the parent pesticides and to their environmental degradates. For example, the OP insecticide chlorpyrifos can degrade in the environment to 3,5,6-trichloro-2-pyridinol (TCPy), which is commonly measured as a urinary biomarker of chlorpyrifos exposure. In residential settings, exposures to chlorpyrifos and TCPy can occur from several sources such as soil, dust, air and food, and through several routes including inhalation, ingestion and dermal contact (Morgan *et al.*, 2005). This information, combined with the fact that toxicological research has shown that rats orally exposed to TCPy excreted all of it unchanged in their urine (Busby-Hjerpe *et al.* 2010; Timchalk *et al.*, 2007), indicates that humans likely excrete in their urine substantial amounts of unchanged TCPy as a function of environmental TCPy exposure. This scenario, particularly in residential settings, can lead to an overestimation of exposure to the parent compound when relying on biological *metabolites* as urinary biomarkers of exposure. This issue is widely applicable in pesticide biomonitoring research, because any pesticide that is hydrolytically metabolized in the body is likely to degrade into the metabolite in the environment.

Biological relevance

A biomarker of exposure ideally should be relevant to the exposure–effect continuum. In other words, the most useful biomarkers not only reflect pesticide exposures, but increase our knowledge of the underlying biological events that lead to potential health effects (Schulte and Talaska, 1995). We discussed in the previous section that TCP is a commonly measured urinary metabolite of chlorpyrifos. Although not specific to chlorpyrifos, DEP and DETP can also be measured in the urine to assess environmental chlorpyrifos exposure. However, each of these urinary metabolites is the result of detoxifying biochemical reactions (Timchalk *et al.*, 2007). Since the *in vivo* toxicity of chlorpyrifos is a result of bioactivation into chlorpyrifos-oxon (CPO), the measurement of CPO in a biological matrix is presumably more biologically relevant than that of a detoxified compound (Timchalk *et al.*, 2007). Thus, provided that adequate analytical techniques exist, and the stability of the chemical in the matrix is sufficient, the measurement of a biologically relevant compound is preferable compared to the measurement of detoxification products. Currently CPO is difficult to measure in samples of human blood (Timchalk *et al.*, 2002). However, by measuring products of both activation and detoxification, the underlying biological processes of the exposure–effect continuum may be better explained. Additionally, the measurement of multiple compounds can be useful in identifying factors that may confound biomarker measurements (e.g., environmental metabolite residues and metabolic variations) (Timchalk *et al.*, 2007).

Feasibility

To be useful in large-scale studies, biomarkers should be easy to obtain, store and analyze (Metcalf and Orloff, 2004; NRC, 2006). As previously mentioned, biomarkers of exposure can be measured in samples of human tissues or fluids, and in samples of human excreta. In large pesticide biomonitoring studies, blood and urine are the most commonly used human tissues/fluids and excreta, respectively, because they are relative to other matrices (e.g., breast milk, adipose tissue, cord blood, feces), abundant in supply, collected using relatively non-invasive techniques (particularly urine) and can be analyzed using well-established methods. Biomarkers, whether parent compounds, metabolites or adducts, may not be stable in a biological matrix (or in a sample preparation matrix (e.g., solvent)) if archived prior to analysis. Additionally, samples that are inappropriately collected or stored can be subject to chemical contamination. Any changes for which biomarker levels are not adjusted (i.e., loss due to instability or increase due to contamination) will influence chemical measurements and ultimately lead to inaccurate estimates of exposure and dose.

Another major issue of feasibility in biomonitoring studies is the collection of biological samples from sensitive subpopulations, such as children. Children may be more highly exposed to pesticides than adults, due to obvious differences in diet, environment and daily activities. Increased exposure can have a particularly large impact on children considering their smaller body masses, immature physiological systems and rapid physical development (Needham and Sexton, 2000; O'Rourke *et al.*, 2000). Therefore, it is important to better understand children's exposure to pesticides using biomonitoring. One of the main difficulties in using biomonitoring to assess pesticide exposures in children is the logistics of sample collection. For children that are able to provide blood or urine samples, it may be difficult to acquire the volume necessary for chemical analysis. In addition, urine collection for very young children may require alternative approaches such as using urine bonnets (collection devices placed under toilet seats), disposable diapers or diapers with removable inserts (Hu *et al.*, 2004).

Uses of biomonitoring data

Biomonitoring data can be used for a variety of applications ranging from risk assessment to assessing the effectiveness of exposure mitigation strategies. A list of potential applications of biomonitoring data is given in Table 20.2.

Biomonitoring is commonly used as a surveillance tool to identify baseline exposure levels in a population, trends in exposure levels over time and unique subpopulations with higher exposure levels. Multiple biomonitoring studies have been conducted in the USA and other countries to evaluate human exposure to pesticides. Several of these studies have focused on exposure to specific pesticides within particular subpopulations, including pregnant women (e.g., the Center for the Health Assessment of Mothers and Children of Salinas (CHAMACOS) study (Castorina *et al.*, 2003) and the German Environmental Survey for Children (GerES IV) (Becker *et al.*, 2008)). However, the Centers for Disease Control and Prevention's (CDC) ongoing National Health and Nutrition Examination Survey (NHANES) is the most comprehensive source of pesticide biomonitoring data, providing thousands of yearly measurements of individual pesticide or metabolite measurements along with a multitude of demographic and health data. The NER, a publication of the demographically stratified NHANES data, allows scientists and health officials to evaluate the specific pesticides to which the US population is commonly exposed, to track trends in exposure levels over time and to set priorities on human exposure and human health research efforts (CDC, 2002, 2003, 2005).

Numerous biomarkers are measured in the ongoing NHANES study to assess human exposure to OC insecticides, OP insecticides, carbamate insecticides, pyrethroid insecticides and a variety of herbicides. Many OC insecticides for which biomarkers are measured (e.g., hexachlorobenzene and dichlorodiphenyltrichloroethane (DDT)) are no longer in use, or have restricted use in the USA. However, because of their relatively high persistence in the environment and in the body, these biomarkers can still be measured in human specimens such as blood. Unlike the persistent OC insecticides, many current-use OP insecticides (e.g., chlorpyrifos and malathion), carbamate insecticides (e.g., carbofuran and propoxur), pyrethroid insecticides (e.g., permethrin and deltamethrin) and herbicides (e.g., 2,4-dichlorophenoxyacetic acid (2,4-D) and atrazine) are environmentally and biologically non-persistent (although some of their degradates may remain in the environment for a longer period of

TABLE 20.2 Information required to interpret biomonitoring data for a given application. With increasing information, the uncertainty of the use of the biomonitoring data decreases

Question	Biomarkers of exposure	Biomarkers of susceptibility	Biomarkers of effect
Identify chemicals in the body?	Measurements	No	No
Assess exposure? (individual or population)	Measurements; PK (human) or animal (with knowledge of applicability to humans); timing of exposure; information on contribution from other sources of chemical/metabolite (specific measurements preferred); rate of intake; rate of uptake; to determine average exposure over a given time period, multiple measurements may be required	No	Depending upon the sensitivity and selectivity of the marker: measurements; proportion of chemicals exposed that are related to marker; rate of intake of each chemical; PK of each chemical; rate of uptake of each chemical
Assess internal dose? (individual or population)	Measurements, PK (human) or animal (with knowledge of applicability to humans), information on contribution from other sources of chemical/metabolite (specific measurements preferred); timing of exposure; to determine average exposure over a given time period, multiple measurements may be required	No	Depending upon the sensitivity and specificity of the marker: measurements; proportion of chemicals exposed that are related to marker; rate of intake of each chemical; PK of each chemical
Trends in exposure?	Measurements; comparable populations; information on contribution from other sources of chemical/metabolite (specific measurements preferred)	No	Depending upon the sensitivity and specificity of the marker: measurements; comparable populations
Determine baseline levels?	Measurements; representative population	No	Measurements; representative population; preferably also pre-exposure individual baseline
Determine highly exposed populations?	Measurements; reference levels; appropriate statistical power; information on contribution from other sources of chemical/metabolite (specific measurements preferred)	No	Depending upon the sensitivity and specificity of the marker: measurements; reference levels; appropriate statistical power (exposure may be defined as class exposure or individual chemical exposure)
Translate to adverse effect?	Measurement; measurement in the system the effect was observed; defined effect; if effect determined from dosed animal, also need PK and dose; pharmacodynamics	Measurement; dose assessment; defined effect; measurements of confounders	Measurement; defined effect; measurement in the system effect was observed; pharmacodynamics
Assess population variability?	Measurement; measurement in the system the effect was observed; defined effect; if effect determined from dosed animal, also need PK and dose; pharmacodynamics	Measurement; defined relationship to exposure and/or outcome	n/a

Risk assessment?	Exposure assessment; hazard identification; dose–response relationship between chemical and disease or outcome	Other contributing genetic factors; biomarker of exposure assessment; hazard id; dose–response relationship	Assess exposure; identify hazard; dose–response relationship between biomarker and disease or outcome
Risk management?	Risk assessment; cross-sectional measurements of exposure in population; trends in exposure; information to mitigate exposure (e.g., primary route of exposure); evaluation of risk vs. cost (e.g., financial cost, burden to population) to reduce risk	Other contributing genetic factors; biomarker of exposure assessment; hazard id; dose–response relationship	Risk assessment; cross-sectional measurements of exposure in population; trends in exposure; information to mitigate exposure (e.g., primary route of exposure); evaluation of risk vs. cost (e.g., financial cost, burden to population) to reduce risk
Effectiveness of intervention to reduce exposure?	Measurements (pre-intervention and post-intervention); information on contribution from other sources of chemical/metabolite (specific measurements preferred)	No	If appropriate sensitivity and specificity of the marker: measurements (pre-intervention and post-intervention); information on contribution from other sources of chemical/metabolite (specific measurements preferred)
Association with disease or outcome?	Measurement; disease or outcome measurements; appropriate statistical power; information on contribution from other sources of chemical/metabolite (specific measurements preferred); information on confounders; pharmacodynamics; temporal relevance of exposure	Measurement; disease or outcome measurements; appropriate statistical power; information on contribution from other sources of chemical/metabolite (specific measurements preferred); information on confounders	Measurement; disease or outcome measurements; appropriate statistical power; pharmacodynamics; temporal relevance of marker
Prediction of disease or outcome?	Measurement; known association with disease; pharmacodynamics; information on contribution from other sources of chemical/metabolite (specific measurements preferred); information on confounders; temporal relevance of exposure	Biomarker measurement; known association with disease; information on confounders	Measurement; known association with disease; pharmacodynamics; temporal relevance of marker

time). Therefore, biomarkers of these pesticides reflect more recent environmental exposures (i.e., hours or a few days). Since many of these non-persistent pesticides are still in use, biomonitoring can be used to identify the current exposure trends, to aid in the design of mitigation strategies to reduce broad-scale exposures and to assess the effectiveness of exposure-mitigation efforts (CDC, 2005).

Improving estimates of exposure and dose

Biomonitoring data can improve estimates of dose derived from exposure and kinetic models, since biomarker measurements consider all routes of pesticide exposure, and all physical, behavioral and physiological sources of variability. Additionally, biomonitoring data can improve and validate existing exposure and kinetic models that are needed in population exposure studies where biomonitoring data are not available.

Considering the many sources of variability and uncertainty associated with dose estimates from exposure and kinetic models, biomonitoring is now recognized as a valuable quantitative tool that can be used in concert with exposure and kinetic models to improve dose estimates. Moreover, biomonitoring can help explain the relationships between exposure and biomarker measurements using a forward dosimetry approach, and can be used to work backwards from biomarker measurements to exposure estimates using a reverse dosimetry approach. This information can be used to improve the human health risk assessment of pesticides.

Forward dosimetry is an approach that can be used to understand the quantitative relationships between pesticide exposures and observed biomarker concentrations. In forward dosimetry, estimated or measured pesticide concentrations from environmental and personal (non-biological) samples are used as inputs into probabilistic or deterministic exposure models to estimate pesticide dose. The dose estimate (based on aggregate intake) is then compared to a measured biomarker concentration; the results from this comparison provide necessary information regarding the important sources and routes of human exposure to pesticides and can be used to identify missing sources and routes of exposure. This information is valuable for the interpretation of existing biomarker data, and for the design and execution of future population-based exposure studies. Forward dosimetry can also be used to estimate biomarker levels resulting from pesticide exposures at regulatory/guidance levels (e.g., reference doses or concentrations (RfDs and RfCs)) that are considered to be acceptable or safe (Hays *et al.*, 2007). Comparing these estimated values to observed levels from population-based biomonitoring studies is particularly useful for human health risk assessment. To date, few exposure and biomonitoring studies have been designed to use this forward dosimetry approach (Morgan *et al.*, 2005, 2007; Wilson *et al.*, 2007).

Reverse dosimetry (exposure reconstruction) is an approach that can be used to work backwards from biomarker measurements to estimates of human exposure to environmental pesticides. Reverse dosimetry, like forward dosimetry, requires the use of exposure models and kinetic models to address heterogeneity in environmental exposure measurements, and in the rates of toxicokinetics. This method, utilizing modeling results and measurements of biomarkers from observational studies, has the potential to yield exposure estimates that can be compared to regulatory/guidance levels (Hays *et al.*, 2007).

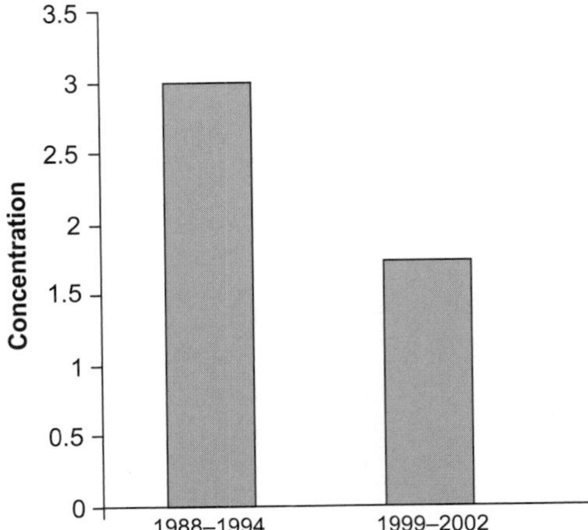

FIGURE 20.2 A temporal trend in a urinary chlorpyrifos metabolite shows a decline in population levels which is consistent with the regulatory limitations put on chlorpyrifos in 2000.

Unfortunately, reverse dosimetry requires the use of numerical model inversion techniques and does not yield a unique solution, but rather a range of potential exposure scenarios (Clewell *et al.*, 2008). Thus, there is uncertainty associated with exposure reconstruction estimates. Reducing uncertainty in exposure estimates will rely on an improved understanding of likely exposure scenarios and the factors affecting variability in toxicokinetic properties. To our knowledge, there are currently no observational studies of environmental pesticide exposure that have been designed to use this approach.

The utility of biomonitoring data depend largely upon the quality of the data being used and the ancillary information available that might assist in the interpretation of those data. For example, in assessing temporal trends in exposures (Figure 20.2), the biomonitoring data alone might be sufficient to appropriately use the data. However, in other applications, such as estimating internal dose, complementary data may be needed. We have summarized potential uses and additional data needed for using the data in Table 20.2.

CONCLUDING REMARKS AND FUTURE DIRECTIONS

Biomonitoring data are useful for a variety of applications from risk assessment to exposure assessment. Biomonitoring methods for pesticides are plenty but they still only touch the tip of the iceberg of available active ingredients that can be measured. Developing methods for measurement of pesticide biomarkers and understanding the resultant data are complex processes that require a great deal of time and intellectual input. Although biomonitoring data are not without their limitations, they still remain a viable tool in environmental public health. With existing data gaps, we may have more uncertain estimates of risk or health outcomes, but the biomonitoring data at least give us a starting point for our endeavors. When more of the data gaps are filled, less uncertainty exists with interpreting the data. In addition to staying abreast of the pesticides that will influx into the market place and developing appropriate methodology for measurement, we must also strive to fill in these data gaps so we can better interpret the data we generate.

REFERENCES

Barr DB, Allen R, Olsson AO, Bravo R, Caltabiano LM, Montesano A, Nguyen J, Udunka S, Walden D, Walker RD, Weerasekera G, Whitehead RD Jr, Schober SE, Needham LL (2005) Concentrations of selective metabolites of organophosphorus pesticides in the United States population. *Environ Res* **99(3):** 314–26.

Barr DB, Angerer J (2006) Potential uses of biomonitoring data: a case study using the organophosphorus pesticides chlorpyrifos and malathion. *Environ Health Perspect* **114(11):** 1763–9.

Barr DB, Barr JR, Driskell WJ, Hill RH Jr, Ashley DL, Needham LL, Head SL, Sampson EJ (1999) Strategies for biological monitoring of exposure for contemporary-use pesticides. *Toxicol Ind Health* **15(1–2):** 168–79.

Barr DB, Barr JR, Maggio VL, Whitehead RD Jr, Sadowski MA, Whyatt RM, Needham LL (2002) A multi-analyte method for the quantification of contemporary pesticides in human serum and plasma using high-resolution mass spectrometry. *J Chromatogr B Analyt Technol Biomed Life Sci* **778(1–2):** 99–111.

Barr DB, Bravo R, Weerasekera G, Caltabiano LM, Whitehead RD Jr, Olsson AO, Caudill SP, Schober SE, Pirkle JL, Sampson EJ, Jackson RJ, Needham LL (2004) Concentrations of dialkyl phosphate metabolites of organophosphorus pesticides in the U.S. population. *Environ Health Perspect* **112(2):** 186–200.

Barr DB, Hines CJ, Olsson AO, Deddens JA, Bravo R, Striley CA, Norrgran J, Needham LL (2007) Identification of human urinary metabolites of acetochlor in exposed herbicide applicators by high-performance liquid chromatography-tandem mass spectrometry. *J Expo Sci Environ Epidemiol* **17(6):** 559–66.

Barr DB, Needham LL (2002) Analytical methods for biological monitoring of exposure to pesticides: a review. *J Chromatogr B Analyt Technol Biomed Life Sci* **778(1–2):** 5–29.

Barr DB, Panuwet P, Nguyen JV, Udunka S, Needham LL (2007) Assessing exposure to atrazine and its metabolites using biomonitoring. *Environ Health Perspect* **115(10):** 1474–8.

Becker K, Mussig-Zufika M, Conrad A, Ludecke A, Schulz C, Seiwert M, Kolossa-Gehring M (2008) German Environmental Survey for Children 2003/06 (GerES IV): Levels of selected substances in blood and urine of children in Germany (Research Report 202 62 219). Berlin, Germany. Federal Ministry of the Environment.

Brucker-Davis F (1998) Effects of environmental synthetic chemicals on thyroid function. *Thyroid* **8(9):** 827–56.

Busby-Hjerpe AL, Campbell JA, Smith JN, Lee S, Poet TS, Barr DB, Timchalk C (2010) Comparative pharmacokinetics of chlorpyrifos versus its major metabolites following oral administration in the rat. *Toxicology* **268(1–2):** 55–63.

Castorina R, Bradman A, McKone TE, Barr DB, Harnly ME, Eskenazi B (2003) Cumulative organophosphate pesticide exposure and risk assessment among pregnant women living in an agricultural community: a case study from the CHAMACOS cohort. *Environ Health Perspect* **111(13):** 1640–8.

CDC (2002) National Report on Human Exposure to Environmental Chemicals, Centers for Disease Control and Prevention. Available at: www.cdc.gov/exposurereport.

CDC (2003) Second National Report on Human Exposure to Environmental Chemicals, Centers for Disease Control and Prevention. Available at: www.cdc.gov/exposurereport.

CDC (2005) Third National Report on Human Exposure to Environmental Chemicals, Centers for Disease Control and Prevention. Available at: www.cdc.gov/exposurereport.

Clewell HJ, Tan YM, Campbell JL, Andersen ME (2008) Quantitative interpretation of human biomonitoring data. *Toxicol Appl Pharmacol* **231(1):** 122–33.

Coleman S, Linderman R, Hodgson E, Rose RL (2000) Comparative metabolism of chloroacetamide herbicides and selected metabolites in human and rat liver microsomes. *Environ Health Perspect* **108(12):** 1151–7.

Driskell WJ, Hill RH Jr (1997) Identification of a major human urinary metabolite of metolachlor by LC-MS/MS. *Bull Environ Contam Toxicol* **58(6):** 929–33.

Driskell WJ, Hill RH Jr, Shealy DB, Hull RD, Hines CJ (1996) Identification of a major human urinary metabolite of alachlor by LC-MS/MS. *Bull Environ Contam Toxicol* **56(6):** 853–9.

Hays SM, Becker RA, Leung HW, Aylward LL, Pyatt DW (2007) Biomonitoring equivalents: a screening approach for interpreting biomonitoring results from a public health risk perspective. *Regul Toxicol Pharmacol* **47(1):** 96–109.

Hu Y, Beach J, Raymer J, Gardner M (2004) Disposable diaper to collect urine samples from young children for pyrethroid pesticide studies. *J Expo Anal Environ Epidemiol* **14(5):** 378–84.

Laws ER, Hayes WJ (1991) *Handbook of Pesticide Toxicology*. San Diego, CA, Academic Press.

Leng G, Kuhn KH, Idel H (1997) Biological monitoring of pyrethroids in blood and pyrethroid metabolites in urine: applications and limitations. *Sci Total Environ* **199(1–2):** 173–81.

Meeker JD, Barr DB, Serdar B, Rappaport SM, Hauser R (2007) Utility of urinary 1-naphthol and 2-naphthol levels to assess environmental carbaryl and naphthalene exposure in an epidemiology study. *J Expo Sci Environ Epidemiol* **17(4):** 314–20.

Metcalf SW, Orloff KG (2004) Biomarkers of exposure in community settings. *J Toxicol Environ Health A* **67(8–10):** 715–26.

Morgan MK, Sheldon LS, Croghan CW, Jones PA, Chuang JC, Wilson NK (2007) An observational study of 127 preschool children at their homes and daycare centers in Ohio: environmental pathways to cis- and trans-permethrin exposure. *Environ Res* **104(2):** 266–74.

Morgan MK, Sheldon LS, Croghan CW, Jones PA, Robertson GL, Chuang JC, Wilson NK, Lyu CW (2005) Exposures of preschool children to chlorpyrifos and its degradation product 3,5,6-trichloro-2-pyridinol in their everyday environments. *J Expo Anal Environ Epidemiol* **15(4):** 297–309.

Nebbia C, Fink-Gremmels J (1996) Acute effects of low doses of zineb and ethylenethiourea on thyroid function in the male rat. *Bull Environ Contam Toxicol* **56(5):** 847–52.

Needham LL, Sexton K (2000) Assessing children's exposure to hazardous environmental chemicals: an overview of selected research challenges and complexities. *J Expo Anal Environ Epidemiol* **10(6 Pt 2):** 611–29.

NRC (2006) *Human Biomonitoring for Environmental Chemicals*. Washington DC, The National Academies Press.

O'Rourke MK, Lizardi PS, Rogan SP, Freeman NC, Aguirre A, Saint CG (2000) Pesticide exposure and creatinine variation among young children. *J Expo Anal Environ Epidemiol* **10(6 Pt 2):** 672–81.

Schulte PA, Talaska G (1995) Validity criteria for the use of biological markers of exposure to chemical agents in environmental epidemiology. *Toxicology* **101(1–2):** 73–88.

Shore RE (1995) Epidemiologic data in risk assessment – imperfect but valuable. *Am J Public Health* **85(4):** 474–6.

Timchalk C, Busby A, Campbell JA, Needham LL, Barr DB (2007) Comparative pharmacokinetics of the organophosphorus insecticide chlorpyrifos and its major metabolites diethylphosphate, diethylthiophosphate and 3,5,6-trichloro-2-pyridinol in the rat. *Toxicology* **237(1–3):** 145–57.

Timchalk C, Nolan RJ, Mendrala AL, Dittenber DA, Brzak KA, Mattsson JL (2002) A Physiologically based pharmacokinetic and pharmacodynamic (PBPK/PD) model for the organophosphate insecticide chlorpyrifos in rats and humans. *Toxicol Sci* **66(1):** 34–53.

Wessels D, Barr DB, Mendola P (2003) Use of biomarkers to indicate exposure of children to organophosphate pesticides: implications for a longitudinal study of children's environmental health. *Environ Health Perspect* **111(16):** 1939–46.

Whyatt RM, Barr DB (2001) Measurement of organophosphate metabolites in postpartum meconium as a potential biomarker of prenatal exposure: a validation study. *Environ Health Perspect* **109(4):** 417–20.

Whyatt RM., Garfinkel R, Hoepner LA, Andrews H, Holmes D, Williams MK, Reyes A, Diaz D, Perera FP, Camann DE, Barr DB (2009) A biomarker validation study of prenatal chlorpyrifos exposure within an inner-city cohort during pregnancy. *Environ Health Perspect* **117(4):** 559–67.

Wilson NK, Chuang JC, Morgan MK, Lordo RA, Sheldon LS (2007) An observational study of the potential exposures of preschool children to pentachlorophenol, bisphenol-A, and nonylphenol at home and daycare. *Environ Res* **103(1):** 9–20.

Section 3

Nanoparticles and Radiation

CHAPTER

21

Developmental toxicity of engineered nanoparticles

Karin Sørig Hougaard, Bengt Fadeel, Mary Gulumian, Valerian E. Kagan and Kai M. Savolainen

INTRODUCTION

Revolutionary developments of physics, chemistry and material sciences have led to the emergence of nanotechnology – a frontier field of knowledge that deals with nanometer-sized objects. Nanotechnology includes several types of objects – materials, devices and systems – which, due to their "smallness" and unique physico-chemical characteristics, have already started demonstrating a huge impact on engineering, chemistry, medicine and computer technology. Nano-objects have found different applications as diagnostic and therapeutic tools in biomedicine and in numerous consumer products. The applications in biomedicine range from novel approaches to the design of artificial organs and tissues for replacement therapies to nano-robotic biosensors, diagnostic devices and miniscule vehicles for targeted drug delivery (Salata, 2004).

A huge diversity of nanoparticles have been synthesized and manufactured during the last decade. Most commonly, nanoparticles represent the core of nanobiomaterial utilized as a surface for molecular modifications and assembly of additional scaffolds and structures. They may be composed of inorganic materials as well as from differently polymerized and/or condensed carbonaceous structures that can vary from lipid spherical vesicles to cylindrical nanotubes.

Living organisms consist of cells that are typically 5–20 μm in width. However, the subcellular organelles and structures are much smaller and have submicron size dimensions. Even smaller are the proteins with a typical size of just few nanometers, which is comparable with the size of the smallest synthetic nanoparticles. This simple comparison of the metric scale of nanoparticles with molecular devices of cells lends itself to the use of nanoparticles as very small probes that allow us to "spy on" cellular machinery without too much interference. However, it also means that improper interactions of nanoparticles with intracellular components may lead to intricate disturbances of highly coordinated and compartmentalized organization of cells as thermodynamically "opened" systems functioning against the laws of growing entropy dominating in "dead" nature. With this in mind, nanotoxicology can be defined as a new discipline studying the interactions of engineered nanomaterials with cellular and extracellular nanomachineries that lead to interference with and disruption of their normal organization and functions. This definition places a significant emphasis on the specific responses that are directly related to the scaling and dimensions of nanomaterials (Shvedova *et al.*, 2010). In addition to size, other physical and chemical properties of nanomaterials may also induce toxicological outcomes in unanticipated ways. Among these are the unusual electronic propensities of nanoparticles – such as their electron-donating and electron-accepting capacities – important possibly for their toxicological effects. For example, the presence of electron-accepting nanoparticles with metal-like conductivity in mitochondria can lead to their undesirable interactions with electron-transporting components of respiratory chains that are incompatible with the generation of membrane potential and energy-producing functions of mitochondria. This essential coincidence in dimensions as well as potentially very unusual physical and chemical propensities of nanoparticles, particularly their redox properties, suggest that unique interactions of nano-sized materials with biosystems may take place leading to an important conclusion that nanotoxicology cannot be deduced from previous vast experience with studies of toxicological profiles of larger particles, including microparticles.

Nanoparticles naturally exist in the environment from sources such as photochemical and volcanic activities. They are also generated as non-intentional by-products of anthropogenic processes such as combustion, welding fumes and vaporization, and from diesel- and petrol-fuelled vehicles (Broos *et al.*, 2010). Another term used in the literature to describe these types of incidental nanoparticles is "ultrafine" (NIOSH, 2009). Developmental toxicity has been studied for some groups of "incidental" nanoparticles, e.g. diesel exhaust particles. However, most studies investigate whole diesel exhaust, i.e. the combined effects of exhaust gases and particles rather than effects of diesel exhaust particles (Hougaard *et al.*, 2008). This chapter describes the toxicity of engineered nanoparticles and in particular their impact on development.

Reproductive and Developmental Toxicology, Edited by Ramesh C. Gupta
ISBN: 978-0-12-382032-7

CHARACTERISTICS, PRODUCTION AND APPLICATIONS OF SOME ENGINEERED INDUSTRIAL NANOMATERIALS

Engineered nanoparticles are defined by differences in their shape, size, surface charge and chemical composition, mostly due to the mode of their production (Brant *et al.*, 2006). Below we summarize characteristics of some of the most dominant types of engineered nanoparticles currently being fabricated or researched internationally. Altogether, the number of different types of engineered nanoparticles exceeds 100,000 and hence here only a few examples are given.

Carbon nanoparticles

Fullerenes are carbon-based allotropes which are hollow sphere, ellipsoid, tube, or plane shaped. When fullerenes are in the form of spherical cages they are generally regarded as buckyballs, as schematically shown in Figure 21.1. They contain between 28 and more than 100 carbon atoms. The most widely studied form is C_{60}, as it contains 60 carbon atoms and was first synthesized by Kroto *et al.* (1985).

Carbon nanotubes

Fullerenes in cylindrical form are called carbon nanotubes (CNTs) or buckytubes. They were discovered in 1991 by Sumio Iijima (Iijima, 1991). CNTs can also be found in a hexagonal network of carbon atoms as hollow cylinders loaded with a wide variety of molecules as shown in Figure 21.2.

Multiple concentric tubes are referred as multi-wall carbon nanotubes (MWCNTs) with significant diameters up to 20 nm, and length greater than 1 mm (Aitken *et al.*, 2004). MWCNTs are manufactured in the presence of a metal catalyst where the final product content of the metal catalyst depends on the synthesis conditions and effectiveness of the subsequent purification processes. Fe, Ni and Cr are frequently used as catalysts in this process (Bladh *et al.*, 2000).

Carbon fullerenes display unique physical properties such as high tensile strength, flexibility, high conductivity, large surface area, unique electronic properties and potentially high molecular adsorption capacity (Maynard *et al.*, 2004). These properties make them suitable for novel applications in consumer products including cosmetics, lubricants, food supplements, building materials, clothing treatment, electronics and fuel cells (Loutfy *et al.*, 2002). MWCNTs exhibit electrical and thermal stability and remarkable flexibility (Cheng and Zhou, 2003). They are therefore used in novel applications including field-emission displays (FEDs), super tough fibers (Somani *et al.*, 2007) and field-effect transistors (Shimada *et al.*, 2004).

Quantum dots

Quantum dots (QDs) are nanocrystalline semiconductors that emit or absorb light of specific wavelengths depending on their size (Aitken *et al.*, 2004). Generally, QDs are fabricated from group II–VI or group III–V elements of the periodic table. Examples include: indium phosphate (InP), indium arsenate (InAs), gallium arsenate (GaAs), gallium nitride (GaN), zinc sulfide (ZnS), zinc–selenium (ZnSe), cadmium–selenium (CdSe), and cadmium–tellurium (CdTe) metalloid cores (Hines and Guyot-Sionnest, 1996; Dabbousi *et al.*, 1997).

Structurally, QDs for biological applications consists of a metalloid crystalline core, and a "cap" or "shell". For example, CdSe/ZnS will denote QDs with CdSe core and ZnS shell. The purpose of the cap or shell is to shield the core and render the QDs less toxic. The further addition of biocompatible coatings or functional groups can make the QD bioavailable (Delehanty *et al.*, 2009; Medintz and Mattoussi, 2009).

Quantum dots were first developed in the form of semiconductors, insulators, metals, magnetic materials and

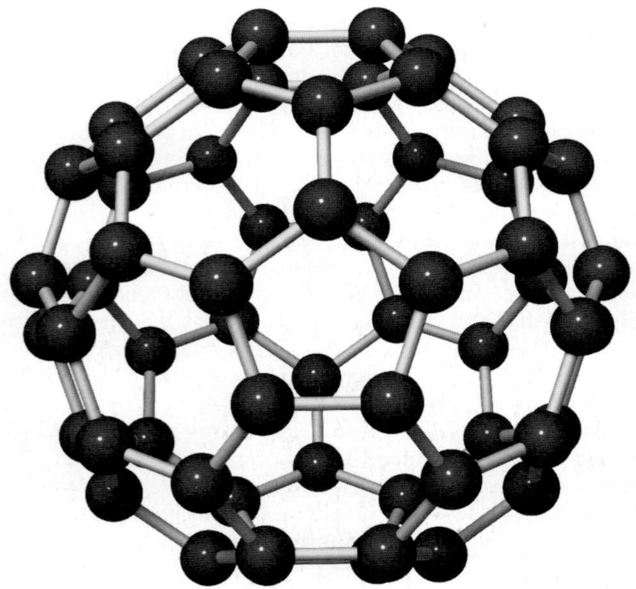

FIGURE 21.1 Schematic presentation of a buckyball (C_{60} fullerene). (Courtesy of Yahachi Saito Laboratory, Nagoya University, Japan; http://www.surf.nuqe.nagoya-u.ac.jp/)

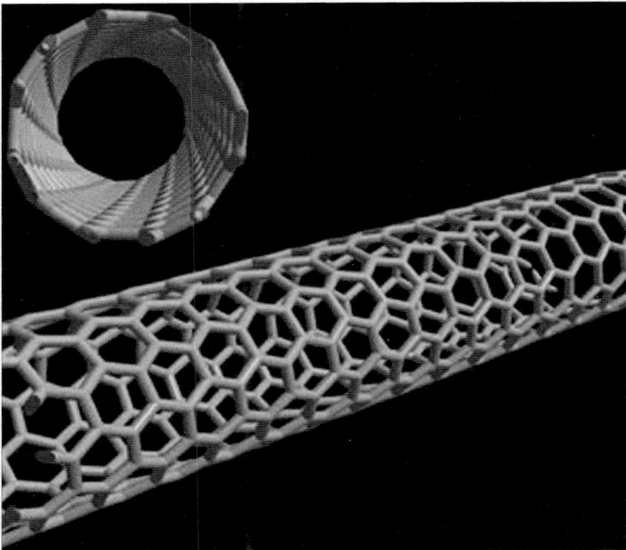

FIGURE 21.2 Schematic presentation of a single-walled carbon nanotube (SWCNT). (Courtesy of R. Bruce Weisman, Rice University; http://www.nsti.org/news/item.html?id=50)

metallic oxides. Their first biological application capability as fluorescent probes in biological staining and diagnostics was demonstrated in 1998 (Bruchez *et al.*, 1998; Chan and Nie, 1998), and thereafter other novel applications such as fluorescent labeling have been found. Within developmental biology, QDs have been investigated for applicability as a fluorescence tracer for oocyte and embryonic maturation analysis (Chan and Shiao, 2008; Hsieh *et al.*, 2009) (as have polystyrene beads; Fynewever *et al.*, 2007).

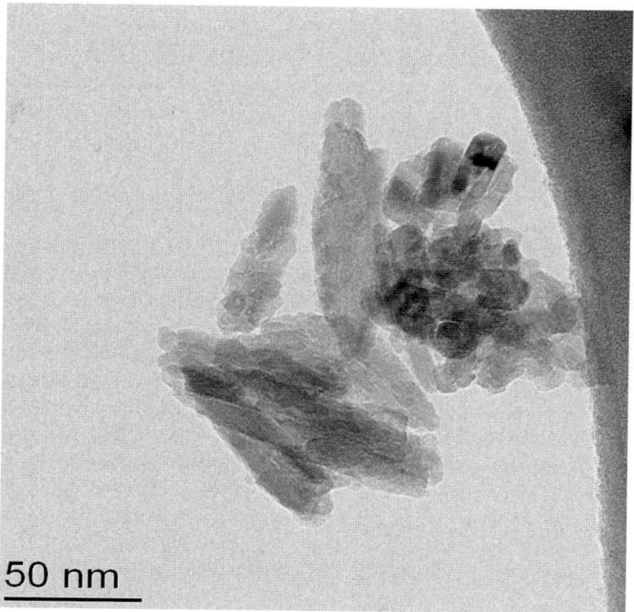

FIGURE 21.3 Transmission electron microscopy image showing typical equidimensional to elongated morphology of TiO_2 crystallites in UV-Titan L181. Bar = 50 nm. Mainly aggregates and agglomerates of TiO_2 crystallites were observed by TEM, with diameters ranging from less than 10 nm to more than 100 nm along the shortest and longest axis. (Courtesy of K.A. Jensen, The National Research Centre for the Working Environment, Denmark, originally published in *Particle and Fibre Toxicology* in Hougaard *et al.*, 2010.)

Inorganic nanoparticles

Inorganic nanoparticles are particles possessing at least one length scale in the nanometer range primarily comprising pure metals, metal oxides or metallic composition. Examples include, among others, gold, silver, aluminum, titanium, silica, tungsten, manganese, copper, molybdenum and palladium nanoparticles (Chen and Mao, 2006; Wang *et al.*, 2006; Murphy *et al.*, 2008).

Gold nanocages for example, are synthesized through the deposition of gold on the surface of silver nanocubes, with the subsequent oxidation and removal of the interior silver (Skrabalak *et al.*, 2008). Silver nanoparticles are synthesized either using traditional – reduction of $AgNO_3$ with $NaBH_4$ – or non-traditional – including high temperature reduction in porous solid matrices, vapor-phase condensation of a metal onto a solid support, laser ablation of a metal target into a suspending liquid, photoreduction of Ag ions and electrolysis of an Ag salt solution – methods (Evanoff and Chumanov, 2005).

Titanium dioxide (TiO_2) nanoparticles are well described and are among the most widely used metal oxide-based nanoparticles (Figure 21.3). The synthesis of titanium dioxide nanoparticles and other nanomaterials has recently been reviewed (Chen and Mao, 2006). Notably, nano-TiO_2 is either available in pure crystalline rutile form (Figure 21.4A), or in pure crystalline form, anatase (Figure 21.4B), or as mixtures of the two crystalline forms, anatase and rutile. In general, anatase nano-TiO_2 is more photocatalytic than the rutile form; on the other hand, nanoscale rutile is less photoreactive than either anatase, rutile mixtures or anatase alone (Sayes *et al.*, 2006).

Mesoporous titanium dioxide (pore diameters between 2 and 50 nm), characterized by high specific surface area, has been reported (Peng *et al.*, 2005). Another example of

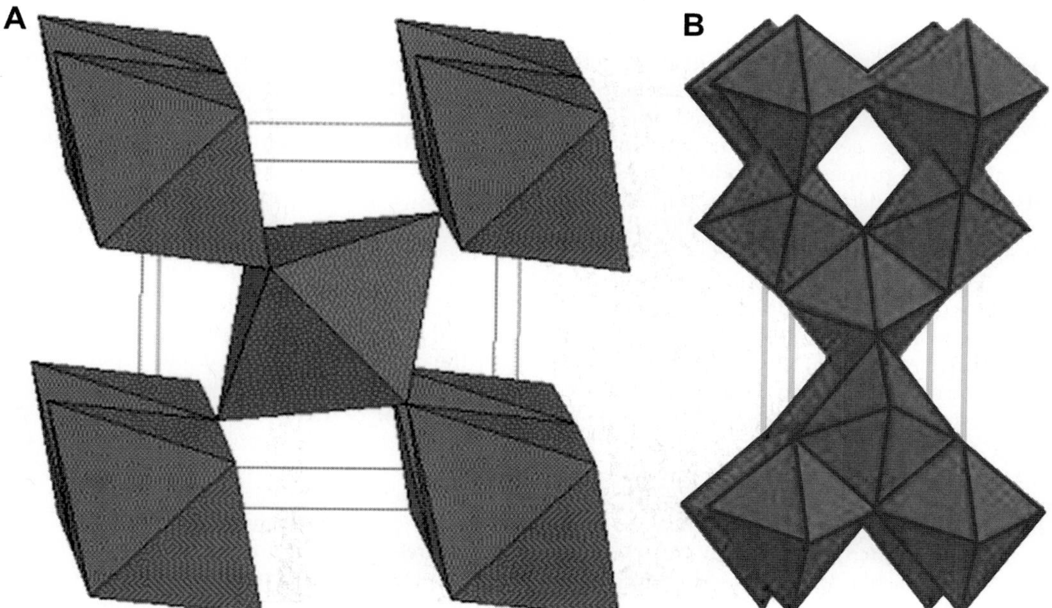

FIGURE 21.4 Polymorphs of TiO_2: (A) rutile; (B) anatase nanoparticles. (Courtesy of Dr. Joseph R. Smith, University of Colorado; http://ruby.colorado.edu/~smyth/min/tic2.html)

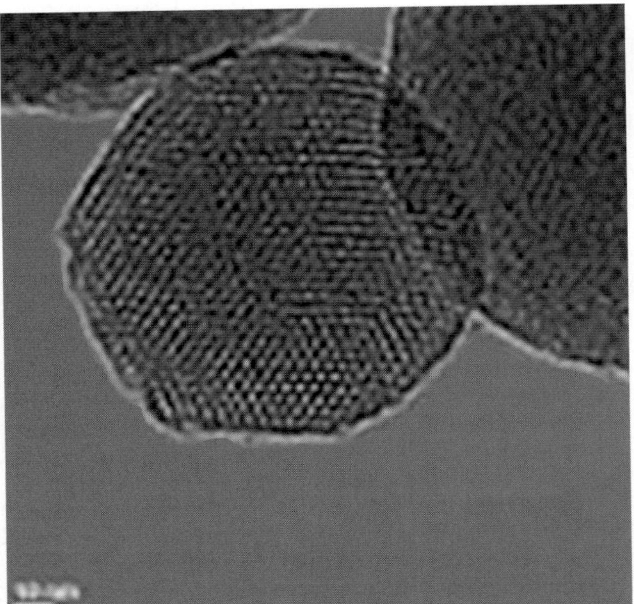

FIGURE 21.5 TEM of a mesoporous silica nanoparticle. (Courtesy of Dr. Victor Lin research group at Iowa State University, USA.)

mesoporous form of nanoparticles is mesoporous silica (Figure 21.5) synthesized using a variety of methodologies including the wet-chemical sol-gel technique involving a chemical solution which acts as the precursor evolving towards the formation of a gel-like diphasic system containing both a liquid and solid phase. The process therefore comprises gelation, precipitation and hydrothermal treatment (Nandiyanto *et al.*, 2009) or a spray drying method (Nandiyanto *et al.*, 2008).

At nanoscale, inorganic nanoparticles display novel mechanical, electrical and other properties owing to dominant quantum effects that do not exist in larger dimensions. Some of these and other properties make them ideal candidates for enhancing cancer detection, cancer treatment, cellular imaging and medical biosensing (Akerman *et al.*, 2002; Hirsch *et al.*, 2003; Ghosh *et al.*, 2008; Lal *et al.*, 2008). Other inorganic nanoparticles are also similarly used for different applications. For example, nanosilver coatings are used on various textiles as well as coatings on certain implants due to their strong antibacterial activity properties. In addition, nanosilver is used for treating wounds and burns, or marketed as a water disinfectant and room spray (Yang *et al.*, 2009).

Nanocrystalline titanium dioxide, when designed appropriately, generates reactive species (RS) efficiently – particularly under ultraviolet (UV) illumination. This capability is exploited in applications ranging from self-cleaning glass to low cost solar cells (Allen *et al.*, 2005), environmental remediation and wastewater purification (Carp *et al.*, 2004; Liu *et al.*, 2006) as well as in cosmetic applications (Diebold, 2003).

Inorganic nanotubes

Following the discovery of carbon nanotubes in 1991, it was recognized that layered metal dichalcogenides such as MoS_2 could also form fullerene and nanotube type structures – and their first successful synthesis was reported in 1992 (Mahalu *et al.*, 1992). The inorganic nanotubes are particularly strong under compression leading to impact-resistant applications such as bulletproof vests. Moreover, they have excellent tribological (lubricating) properties, are resistant to shockwave impact; have a good catalytic reactivity, and high capacity for hydrogen and lithium storage – which suggest a range of promising applications (Kaplan-Ashiri *et al.*, 2006; Tenne *et al.*, 2008).

SPECIAL FEATURES OF NANOMATERIALS IN RELATION TO THEIR TOXICITY: OXIDATIVE STRESS AND BIOPERSISTENCE

Involvement of oxidative stress in toxicity of nanoparticles

Given the unusual redox characteristics of nanoparticles, significant attention has been paid to oxidative stress-based mechanisms of their cytotoxicity. This association of toxic effects of nanoparticles with their ability to initiate the production of reactive oxygen species (ROS) is particularly important in the context of developmental toxicity in different organs, especially in the brain. High oxygen demand along with the abundance of readily oxidizable substrates is required for the normal function of the brain. This necessitates the existence of the complex and multicomponent antioxidant system in the brain for protection against oxidative damage. However, during development, individual components of the antioxidant system are not equally expressed and not always sufficient to fulfill their tasks in a coordinated way. As a result, the developing brain may be more vulnerable to oxidative insults than the adult (Bayir *et al.*, 2006). This results in a developmental "mismatch" in the sequential antioxidant enzyme cascade that is likely to contribute to the vulnerability to free radical toxicity of the immature cerebral white matter, which is "unprepared" for the transition from a hypoxic intrauterine to an oxygen-rich postnatal environment (Folkerth *et al.*, 2004). Brain is not included in the list of five organs – lung, skin, gastro-intestinal tract, nasal olfactory structures and eyes – that represent the major portals through which nanoparticles can enter the body as a result of inadvertent occupational or environmental exposures. However, nanoparticles entering the body through these common routes could translocate into the circulation and travel to distant organs including the cardiovascular system and brain (Oberdörster *et al.*, 2005).

While the association of the toxic effects of nanoparticles with the initiation of oxidative stress is quite justifiable, the causality of the enhanced ROS production in cell damage should be experimentally tested in each case. Excessive oxidative stress has been proposed as a common paradigm for the toxicities of engineered nanoparticles (Xia *et al.*, 2006, 2008; Yang *et al.*, 2009). However, not all studies comply with this general notion (Diaz *et al.*, 2008) thus pointing to the need for additional careful experimental testing of this concept. The two major factors essential for the potential role of nanoparticles in the initiation of oxidative stress are (1) the presence of catalysts, most commonly transition metals, and (2) sources of oxidizing equivalents. Frequently, nanoparticles either directly contain large amounts of metals or the presence of metals is due to the manufacturing process, e.g. as already described for carbon nanotubes (Bladh *et al.*, 2000). These metals could act as potent oxidation catalysts via their propensity to participate in one-electron reduction of oxygen and production of so-called ROS such as superoxide radicals, hydrogen peroxide and hydroxyl radicals (Kagan *et al.*, 2006). The latter can act as an immediate and direct oxidizing entity causing oxidation of biomolecules in cells and tissues. For example, carbon nanotube-induced production of oxygen radicals relevant to the presence of adventitious metals has been well documented in simple model systems. Not surprisingly, accumulation of oxidation products in proteins, DNA and lipids in cells and tissues of animals exposed to carbon nanotubes has been reported by several independent laboratories (Shvedova *et al.*, 2009). Notably, dietary manipulations of anti-/pro-oxidant status of animals achieved by maintaining them on vitamin E-deficient diet have been reported to exacerbate the inflammatory pulmonary response to aspired SWCNT (Shvedova *et al.*, 2007). Oxidative stress is also a potential factor in developmental toxicity of nanoparticles, as investigated *in vitro* for C_{60} (Zhu *et al.*, 2009).

Biopersistence and biodegradation of nanoparticles

High biopersistence of nanomaterials in tissues may be a stumbling block in their biomedical applications. Non-degradable nanomaterials can accumulate in organs and inside cells where they can exert detrimental effects. For example, long-term accumulation of medicinal gold salts in the body has been linked to adverse effects in patients. Carbon nanotubes (CNT) are known to be biopersistent and may remain inside macrophages in the spleen and liver for prolonged periods of time following parenteral administration (Yang *et al.*, 2008). Moreover, SWCNT have been observed in the lungs of exposed mice up to 1 year after pharyngeal administration (Shvedova *et al.*, unpublished observation). Also TiO_2 stays in lung tissue long after exposure. Five days after termination of inhalation exposure, lung tissue from female rats contained 38 mg Ti/kg tissue, only decreasing to 33 mg Ti/kg tissue after 26 days (Hougaard *et al.*, 2010). Furthermore, maternal exposure during gestation to particulate TiO_2 resulted in the presence of particles aggregates in testicle and brain tissue from mouse offspring, up to 6 weeks from birth (Takeda *et al.*, 2009). Biopersistence might therefore be highly relevant for manifestation of developmental toxicity. On the other hand, biodegradation of nanomaterials could also yield adverse responses due to toxic degradation products. For instance, leaching of toxic core components such as cadmium from quantum dots with induction of oxidative stress has been suggested as a mechanism of *in vivo* toxicity of these nanomaterials (Rzigalinski and Strobl, 2009; Hsieh *et al.*, 2009). Biodegradation of nanomaterials thus represents one of the important challenges not only in the field of nanotoxicology but also in nanomedicine, as the safe implementation of nanomaterials for biomedical purposes is contingent upon the controlled degradation and/or clearance of the exogenous nanomaterials from the body. Notably, Park *et al.* (2009b) reported that porous silicon nanoparticles self-destructed in a mouse model into renally cleared components – likely orthosilicic acid – within weeks, with no evidence of toxicity to animal tissues. Moreover, CNT can also undergo biodegradation by a human neutrophil enzyme, myeloperoxidase, thus pointing to possible strategies for the mitigation of unwanted inflammatory responses elicited by CNT in exposed individuals (Kagan *et al.*, 2010).

EXPOSURE AND ASSESSMENT OF EXPOSURE TO ENGINEERED NANOMATERIAL

Factors modifying exposure to engineered nanomaterials

One major uncertainty in interpretation of experimental toxicity studies as well as in risk assessment of engineered nanomaterial arises from lack of systematic knowledge about the physico-chemical characteristics of the material arriving at the major portals through which nanoparticles can enter the body, i.e. lung, skin, gastro-intestinal tract, nasal olfactory structures and eyes. This is true for all forms of particles, whether they exist in the form of macroscopic solid objects, as powders, emulsions or suspensions, or as aerosols (i.e., in the form of airborne particles). All these engineered nanomaterials essentially consist of nanoparticles, or at least nanostructured building blocks such as agglomerates, which have the potential of being released into a transport chain from the "source" to the receiving tissue.

An issue requiring a special and thorough assessment is the possibility of exposure to engineered nanomaterials through products containing engineered nanomaterials. This exposure might take place during any stage of the whole lifecycle of the products. Most products are not likely to cause exposure as long as the engineered nanomaterials are embedded in the polymers or other matrices in a given product (Adlakha-Hutcheon *et al.*, 2009; Kuhlbusch *et al.*, 2009; Nadagouda and Varma, 2009). The situation may change though, when a given material needs further processing, becomes waste or is recycled. The groups at most risk in this kind of context are the workers handling products containing engineered nanomaterials, e.g. in recycling companies (Owen *et al.*, 2009). As more and more consumer products, and even foodstuffs, are enriched with nanoparticulate materials, exposure of the general population also increases. In developmental toxicology this concept is even more complex due to an "extra" barrier between mother and fetus, i.e. the placenta (Saunders, 2009) (Figure 21.6A).

The general release and transport mechanisms are best known for aerosols which are highly dynamic systems, and this information is also relevant to exposure. Nano-aerosols often consist of strongly agglomerated primary particles, already close to the source. This is illustrated by the exposure characteristics from a study in rats of prenatal exposure to a nanoparticulate TiO_2. The exposure atmosphere contained 42 mg/m^3 TiO_2. Average crystallite size of single particles was approximately 21 nm. It is evident, however, from Figure 21.6B that less than 10% of the particles in the chamber air are of this diameter. In fact, 80% of the particles were between 40 and 200 nm, with a major mode of particles of approximately 100 nm. These observations were confirmed by transmission electron micrograph (Figure 21.3) (Hougaard *et al.*, 2010). Depending on their origins and transport history, these nano-structured agglomerates have a potential for subsequent break-up (Rothenbacher *et al.*, 2008).

The tendency of airborne engineered nanomaterials to agglomerate or become attached to the ubiquitous background particles is of special importance because this probably very rapidly changes their typical size-related characteristics. This can be modeled for different scenarios provided that sufficient information can be provided about

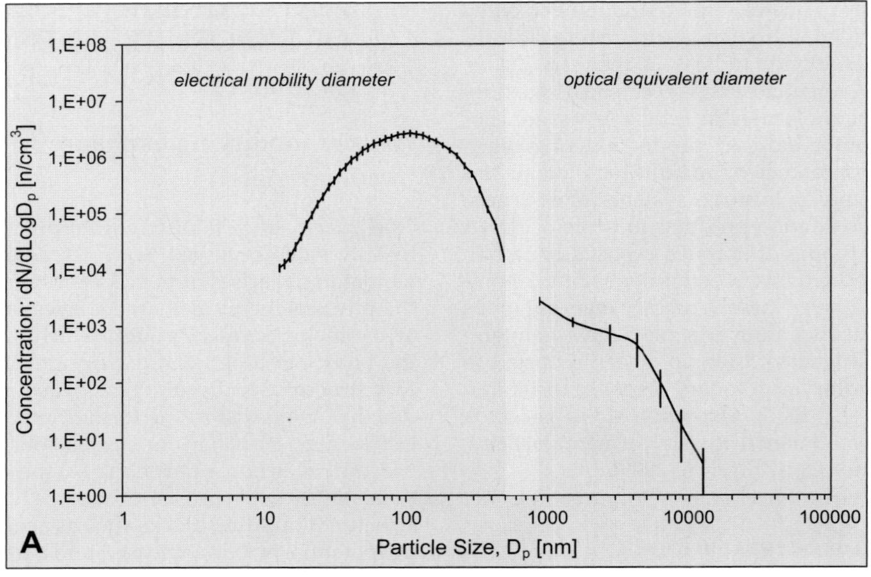

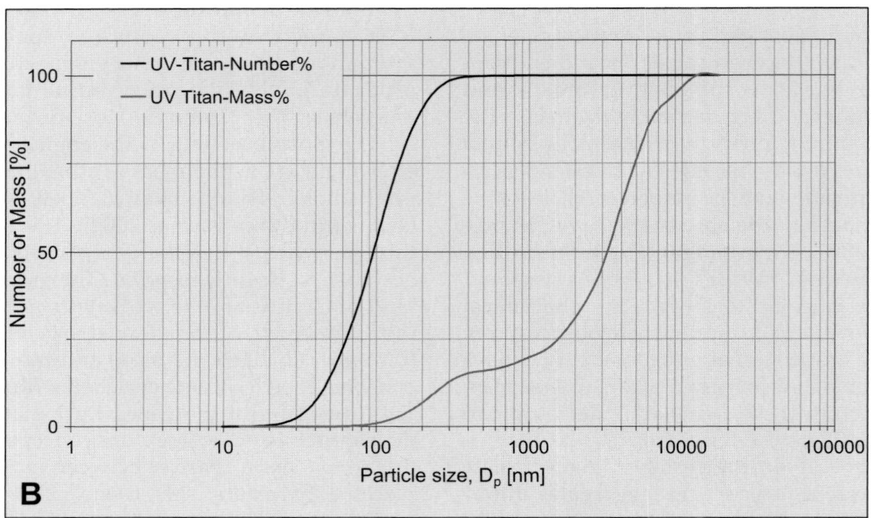

FIGURE 21.6 Characteristics of an exposure atmosphere containing 42 mg/m^3 UV-Titan L181, a TiO_2 particle with an average crystallite size of 21 nm, cf. Figure 21.3. (A) Particle number size distribution of the UV-Titan L181 in the exposure chamber. The major mode of particles was approximately 100 nm (geometric mean number diameter 97 nm), with a coarser size mode of approximately 4 μm. Smaller size modes were observed at ~20 nm and 1 μm. (B) Accumulated number and mass concentration of particle concentrations in the exposure chamber. By number, 80% of the particles were between 40 and 200 nm. (Courtesy of K.A. Jensen, National Research Centre for the Working Environment, Denmark. Originally published in *Particle and Fibre Toxicology* in Hougaard *et al.*, 2010.)

the system (Seipenbusch *et al.*, 2008). The changes in airborne engineered nanomaterials characteristics during transport have several consequences. A change in airborne size will alter the deposition mechanisms for engineered nanomaterials, e.g. in the lungs, and hence the effective dose. It is not known if and how the agglomeration affects toxicological mechanisms. Also, growth and/or attachment of airborne engineered nanomaterials to other particles challenge the established methods for their adequate characterization as does separation and identification of engineered nanomaterials against the background level of particles originating from different sources (Peters *et al.*, 2009). At present, no rapid techniques allow online distinction between background nanoparticles and engineered nanomaterials. The aerosol has to be collected and offline image or compositional analysis must be performed, e.g. by transmission electron microscope (TEM), the gold standard for this type of analysis (Kuhlbusch *et al.*, 2009; Peters *et al.*, 2009).

Assessment of exposure to engineered nanomaterials

Measurement and monitoring of engineered nanomaterials in the air of workers' breathing zones and during inhalation exposure in animal toxicity studies involve capturing the relevant information concerning the amount, i.e. number, surface area or mass concentration, size distribution, as well as shape, composition and chemical reactivity of airborne engineered nanomaterials in a given size class or a broad size range. Selection of the most relevant metric(s) for health-related sampling of engineered nanomaterials is an important component in the development of the concepts, methods and technology for engineered nanomaterials monitoring at workplaces (Maynard, 2002; Maynard *et al.*, 2006; Maynard and Aitken, 2007; Schulte *et al.*, 2008; Seipenbusch *et al.*, 2008). For this purpose, understanding the relationship between engineered nanomaterials metrics and toxicological effects of engineered nanomaterials is necessary but as yet not known. This is because a consensus on the correct metrics to be measured to assess exposure to engineered nanomaterials has not yet been reached internationally (SCENIHR, 2007; OECD, 2008).

The multitude of relevant engineered nanomaterials metrics, in combination with the different possible release mechanisms for engineered nanomaterials into air as well as the poorly defined transport pathways between source and receiving tissue, makes it highly important to establish and define engineered nanomaterials exposure scenarios. For example, it is important to distinguish between fresh engineered nanomaterials and "aged" and "attached" engineered nanomaterials (Hougaard *et al.*, 2008; Seipenbusch *et al.*, 2008).

The current inability to separate engineered nanomaterials from the background nanoparticles by straightforward concentration and size distribution measurements makes it impossible or at least highly problematic to set exposure limits for engineered nanomaterials, e.g. occupational exposure limits (OEL). Harmful health effects, such as increased cardiac and pulmonary mortality, of background nanoparticles or ultrafine particles emphasize the importance of these technologies (Nurkiewicz *et al.*, 2008). This distinction is important to dissect the possible effects of background nanoparticles from those induced by engineered nanomaterials.

Each of the above avenues addresses an important demand: (1) making current engineered nanomaterials monitoring technology more compact, more affordable and more versatile will provide imminent short-term solutions required by toxicologists and the inhalation exposure community; (2) new sensing technology will have a mid-term effect by providing sophisticated measurement options for very small particles which can be adapted to the needs of aerosol monitoring technology; (3) finally, the need for devices capable of capturing entirely new properties will provide new tools to characterize airborne engineered nanomaterials. It will be important for these new devices to provide real-time and online data. However, the foregoing discussion also makes it clear that an ideal, all-purpose monitoring method will only become available (if it ever becomes available) once a clear link between health effects and engineered nanomaterials characteristics is well established for a majority of exposure scenarios; this will only happen after sufficient data have been collected and analyzed.

So far, the available data on exposure to engineered nanomaterials in, e.g., the working environments in which engineered nanomaterials are being synthesized or used, especially TiO_2, suggest that the exposure levels are low, and hence not likely to pose an immediate human hazard. The situation may, however, change when the production volumes increase, and when the portfolio of engineered nanomaterials produced becomes larger (Peters *et al.*, 2009). Under certain circumstances, e.g. when using spray products in confined spaces, exposure levels become very high (Nørgaard *et al.*, 2009).

CROSSING BIOLOGICAL BARRIERS

There is a common assumption that the small size of nanoparticles allows them to easily enter and traverse tissues, cells and organelles since the actual size of engineered nanoparticles is similar to that of many biological molecules and structures (e.g., proteins and viruses). However, nanoparticles may not freely or indiscriminately cross all biological barriers (Fischer and Chan, 2007). These processes may instead be governed by the specific physico-chemical properties of the nanoparticles themselves as well as the identity of the functional molecules added to their surfaces. A case in point, the coating of nanoparticles with the polymer polyethylene glycol prevents their non-selective accumulation in cells of the reticuloendothelial system, which is critical for the targeted delivery of nanoparticles to specific target tissues (Akerman *et al.*, 2002). An increased understanding of the mechanisms that dictate the behavior and fate of nanoparticles upon introduction into the body is important not only for the development of nanoparticles for targeted drug delivery, but also for the prediction of the potential toxicological responses to such nanomaterials. The present chapter describes translocation of nanoparticles across biological barriers, namely the blood–brain barrier, from the lung to blood, and, especially relevant within developmental toxicology, the placenta.

Translocation from lung to blood and across the blood–brain barrier

A major difference compared to larger size particles is the fact that nanoparticles may translocate from the portal of entry (e.g., the respiratory tract) to secondary organs. This makes nanoparticles uniquely suitable for biomedical applications, but it also renders target organs such as the central nervous system (CNS) vulnerable to potential adverse effects. Indeed, Oberdörster *et al.* (2002) demonstrated in a rat model that ultrafine particles, i.e. nano-sized particles that are inhaled, can translocate to extra pulmonary organs such as liver within 4 to 24 h after exposure. A subsequent study showed that both composition of the material and particle size are important determinants of the translocation of nanoparticles from the lungs of rats to the blood and other secondary organs. Hence, significantly less translocation and accumulation in secondary organs was noted for 80 nm than for 20 nm nanoparticles of iridium while such translocation was less pronounced for carbon nanoparticles/aggregates (Kreyling *et al.*, 2009). Moreover, ultrafine particles were also detected in the brain following inhalation. It was concluded that the most likely mechanism is that the particles deposited on the olfactory mucosa of the nasopharyngeal region of the respiratory tract subsequently translocated via the olfactory nerve into the brain (Oberdörster *et al.*, 2004). These studies suggest a novel portal of entry into the CNS for nano-sized particles, circumventing the blood–brain barrier. These findings have potential implications for drug delivery via the nasal route into the CNS, but also suggest that neurotoxic and/or neurodegenerative effects may arise following inhalation of certain nanoparticles (Oberdörster *et al.*, 2009). More recent studies have shown that titanium dioxide nanoparticles administered into the abdominal cavity of mice may translocate to the brain and cause oxidative stress with lipid peroxidation and decreases in anti-oxidant capacities (Ma *et al.*, 2010).

Translocation of particles across the placenta

In order for particles to directly interfere with fetal development, the particles need to gain access to the fetus. This involves passage of the placenta. The placenta is generally considered a barrier between the maternal and fetal compartments, while its major function is to serve as a nutritional interface between mother and fetus, granting passage of nutrients of importance for fetal development and survival. Passage may occur by passive diffusion, active and facilitated transport, endocytosis and filtration. These pathways unfortunately allow several "unwanted" chemicals to pass, for example due to structural similarity with the natural substrates of placental modes of transportation. The resulting effects on the fetus are apparent and described in several chapters throughout this book. Ethanol, thalidomide, organic solvents and pesticides present as sad reminders of xenobiotics that adversely interfere with development once access to the fetal compartment has taken place.

Studies of the passage of engineered nanoparticles across the placenta have just started to emerge, and investigations have been performed in animals as well as human placenta model systems, as summarized in Table 21.1. In a study of prenatal exposure to TiO_2, pregnant mice were exposed by subcutaneous injections on day 3, 7, 10 and 14 of gestation. Particles ranged from 25 to 70 nm in size, and the daily dose was 0.1 mg (total dose amounting to approximately 16 mg/kg). The dams were allowed to litter, and male offspring were euthanized at postnatal day 4 or 6 weeks of age. Thin sections of testis and brain tissue were visualized by field emission-type scanning electron microscopy. Aggregates of TiO_2 nanoparticles (100–200 nm) were observed in testicles and brain as long as 6 weeks after birth (Figure 21.7). The question is therefore not if particles reach the fetus, but rather to which degree transfer takes place, and it depends on physico-chemical properties of the engineered nanoparticles.

In vivo animal studies suggest that a limited fraction of particles in maternal blood transfers to the fetal compartment (Challier *et al.*, 1973). One study in mice reports neither transfer nor placental uptake 24 hours after a single i.v. injection of 2 or 40 nm gold particles, on gestation day 17 (12.1 or 58 μg, respectively) (Sadauskas *et al.*, 2007). Also, titanium was not detected in the liver from offspring of dams exposed by inhalation on gestation days 8–18, to 42 mg/m^3 titanium dioxide particles for 1 hour/day to (21 nm UV-titan L-181, with peak-size of 97 nm). In dams, 33 mg titanium/kg lung tissue were still detectable a month after exposure. The method of detection probably lacked sensitivity to measure very small amounts of titanium in offspring liver tissue (Hougaard *et al.*, 2010). Two other mouse studies observe some presence of gold nanoparticles in uterine contents 24 hour after i.v. administration, i.e. 0.06% for 1.2 nm, 0.018% for 5 nm, 0.005% for 18 and 30 nm gold particles (Takahashi and Matsuoka, 1981; Semmler-Behnke *et al.*, 2007). Translocation thus seems higher for smaller compared to larger nanoparticles, but this is probably a simplified assumption. In-depth analysis of the data (Takahashi and Matsuoka, 1981) indicates that the average concentration of particles in maternal blood rather than particle size determined the amount of transfer. After injection, particles were rapidly withdrawn from the maternal peripheral blood, but at a higher rate of clearance for 30 nm than for 5 nm particles. Furthermore, the number of particles injected was higher for 5 nm than for 30 nm particles. The average remaining concentration in maternal blood was therefore greater for 5 nm than for 30 nm particles. Calculations based on numbers of particles in maternal blood as well as utero-placental blood flow allowed for estimation of the extraction ratio, i.e. the ratio between the amount of particles brought to the utero-placental unit and that deposited in the feto-placental unit. In this study, particle size did not seem a significant determinant of extraction, indicating that smaller particles were not extracted from maternal blood to a higher degree than were larger particles (Takahashi and Matsuoka, 1981).

Differences in placental structure may hamper direct extrapolation of transfer data from animal data to humans. Here, the *ex vivo* perfused human placenta model represents an alternative model, in that some of the complexity of the intact human placenta is maintained. In this model, intact placentas are obtained from uncomplicated term pregnancies and a cotyledon is excised and cannulated for perfusion from both the maternal and the fetal side. A study of nanoparticulate gold, coated with polyethylene glycol, did not demonstrate transport of particles from the maternal to the fetal circulation during the 6 hours of monitoring. Particles were 10 or 30 nm in diameter, but coating with polyethylene glycol added another 10 nm to the particulate diameter. The authors themselves infer that due to the limit of detection by mass spectrometry (ICP-MS), 0.13–0.2% of the particles in the maternal circulation should pass to the fetal unit in order for transfer to be detected (Myllynen *et al.*, 2008a). In the light of transfer rates reported for animal studies, this may not have been the case. An altogether different finding is evident for nano-sized polystyrene beads, also studied in the placental perfusion model (Wick *et al.*, 2010). Here, close to 30% of the polystyrene beads in the maternal circuit transferred to the fetal compartment for particles with diameters of 50 nm and 80 nm within the first hours of exposure. Some transfer (9%) was also evident for 240 nm particles, whereas only 1% of particles with a diameter around 500 nm crossed the placenta (Wick *et al.*, 2010).

That polystyrene beads and gold nanoparticles interact differently with the placental system suggests that the capability for transplacental transfer depends highly on the physico-chemical properties of the nanoparticles. How surface modification of particles influences the movement of particles was studied in mouse blastocysts. Blastocysts were flushed out of the uterine horn 7.5 days after fertilization. Polystyrene particles were injected into the extra embryonic tissue followed by 12 hour incubation. Twenty nanometer particles modified with carboxyl groups on the surface distributed in embryonic and extra embryonic germ layers. Particles with diameters of 100 or 500 nm accumulated in the extra embryonic tissue with no sign of translocation to the embryos. However, when 200 nm polystyrene particles were modified with amine groups, they were able to pass into embryos (Tian *et al.*, 2009). These findings implicate that placental transfer has to be assessed separately for each type of nanoparticle.

At the maternal–fetal interface, placental cells seem to internalize nanoparticles. This has been observed *in vivo* in mice as well as *ex vivo* in the human placental model (Semmler-Behnke *et al.*, 2007; Myllynen *et al.*, 2008; Wick *et al.*, 2010). In the human placenta model, gold particles were primarily located in the syncytiotrophoblast cell layer, when particles had been added to the maternal compartment in the human placenta model. Transmission electron microscopy identified gold particle aggregates in cyncytiotrophoblasts

TABLE 21.1 Passage of engineered nanoparticles across the placenta. Animal and human placenta model studies

Particle type	Size (nm)	Species	Dose (route)	Gestation time and length of exposure	Particle passage	In placenta	Ref.
Animal studies							
Gold (negative surface charge)	1.4 18	Rat	N.s. (i.v.)	N.s. After 24 h	1.4 nm: 0.06% 18 nm: 0.005%	1.4 nm: 3% 18 nm: 0.02%	(Semmler-Behnke *et al.*, 2007)
Gold^{198}	5 30	Rat	0.020 mg (i.v.)	GD 19 After 24 h	5 nm: 0.018% 30 nm: 0.005%	Much more than was actually translocated	(Takahashi and Matsuoka, 1981)
Gold (negative surface charge)	2 40	Mouse	12.1 µg (2 nm) 58.2 µg (40 nm) (i.v.)	GD 16–18 After 24 h	None	None	(Sadauskas *et al.*, 2007)
Latex	6–14 µm	Mouse	N.s. (transcardiac inj.)	Various stages After ½ h Littered offspring (4–9 days)	None Particles were noted in offspring after birth, in dams pretreated with hualuronidase	N.a.	(Kennison *et al.*, 1971)
Perfused human placenta model							
Gold (coated with polyethylene glycol)	10 (20 with PEG) 15 (25 with PEG)	Human	9.1*10^9 particles/ml 2.0*10^9 particles/ml	6 h	None (due to detection limit, 0.13–0.2% of particles should have passed for detection)	Visualized in trophoblastic cell layer	(Myllynen *et al.*, 2008)
Polystyrene	50 80 240 500	Human	Media concentration: 25 µg/mL	6 h	50: 35% 80: 30% 240: 9% 500: 1%	N.a.	(Wick *et al.*, 2010)
In vitro (BeWo cells)							
Gold (coated with polyethylene glycol)	10 (20 with PEG)	Human	Media concentration: 3.6*10.10 particles/mL	48 h	–	Particles were visualized inside cells	(Myllynen *et al.*, 2008)

GD: Gestation day; N.s.: Not stated; N.a.: Not assessed

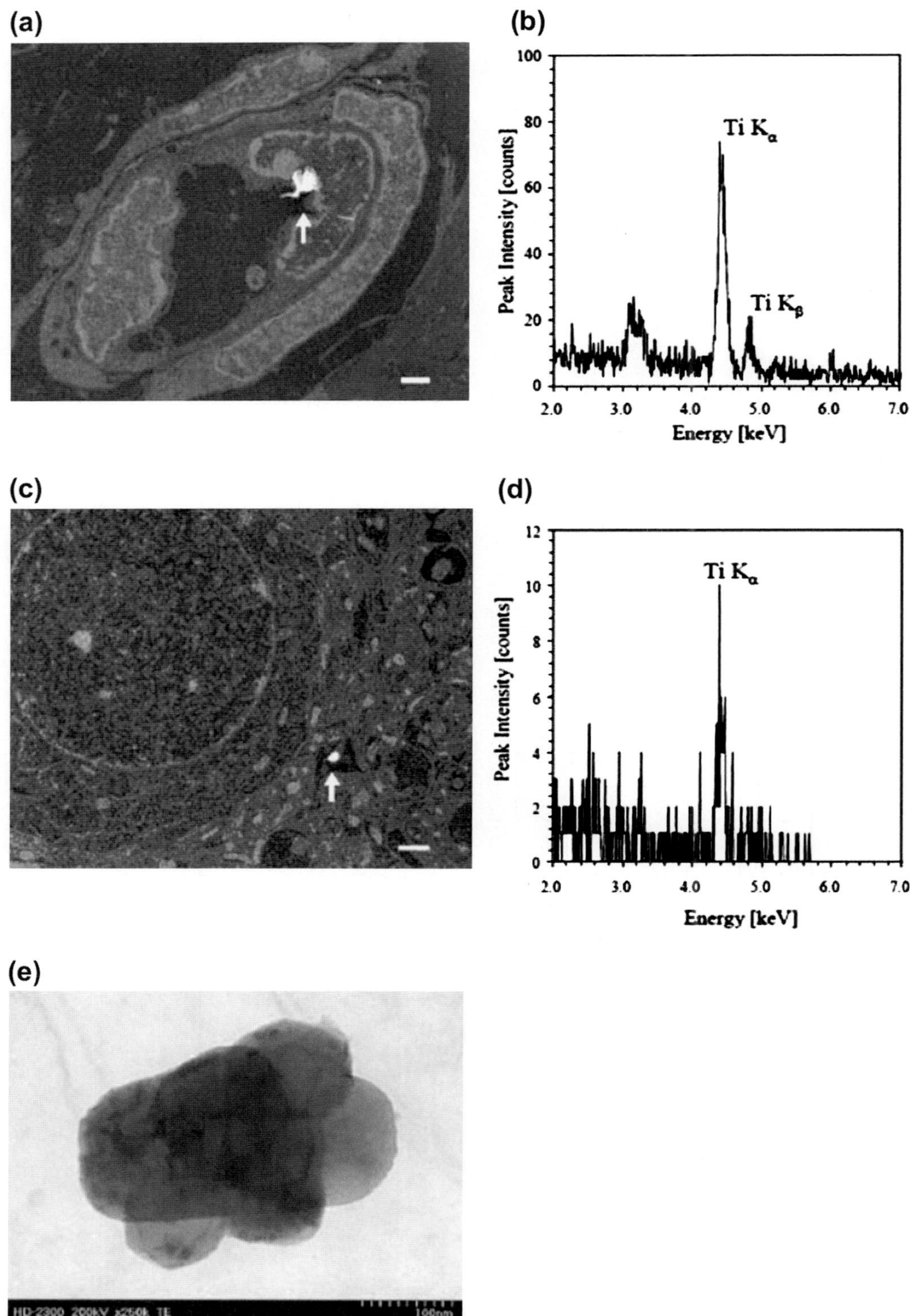

FIGURE 21.7 Detection of TiO_2 nanoparticles in the olfactory bulb and cerebral cortex from 6-week-old offspring of TiO_2-exposed pregnant mice. Photograph demonstrates aggregated TiO_2 nanoparticles (100–200 nm) in endothelial cells of the olfactory bulb (a) and nerve cell fibers in the cerebral cortex (c). Scale bars 1μ. TiO_2 particles are indicated by arrows. Particles were identified as TiO_2 by energy-dispersive X-ray spectroscopy at 15 kV (b) and 7 kV (d) accelerating voltage, 1×10^{-10} A beam and 100 sec measurements. Electron micrograph demonstrates magnified aggregated TiO_2 particles in nerve cells in cerebral cortex (e). (Courtesy of *Journal of Health Science*, Takeda *et al.*, 2009.)

and trophoblasts. BeWo choriocarcinoma cells, a placental cell line that has been widely used as an *in vitro* model for the placenta, also internalized gold nanoparticles coated with polyethyleneglycol (Myllynen *et al.*, 2008).

For studies of placental transfer of particles, it is imperative to evaluate whether the duration of the experiment is sufficient for transport to actually take place, since translocation of particles likely takes longer than does transport of soluble liquids (Saunders, 2009). When the transfer of 5 nm gold particles was assessed in fetuses after maternal administration, radioactivity was detectable in fetuses sacrificed both 1 and 24 hours after injection. In the dams injected with 30 nm particles, radioactivity was only detected in fetuses 24 hours after injection (Takahashi and Matsuoka, 1981).

Transfer of particles across the placenta may increase under some conditions. Inflammation is a condition that has been associated with leakage across endothelial tight junctions, potentially allowing greater passage of nanoparticles (Saunders, 2009). It is therefore interesting that several inflammatory cytokines displayed increased mRNA levels in placentas from pregnant mice exposed to whole diesel exhaust (with a large part of the particles in the nanorange). Unfortunately, correlation of inflammation and particle passage was not attempted (Fujimoto *et al.*, 2005). Some support from the importance of placental integrity in placental transfer comes from an older study, in which pregnant mice were administered hyaluronidase (an enzyme that alters placental permeability), followed by injection of a suspension of 6–14 μm latex particles into the blood. When fetuses were sacrificed soon after injection of particles, particles were not observed in fetal tissue. However, several latex particles were observed in organs of neonates that were delivered 4 to 9 days after maternal treatments (Kennison *et al.*, 1971). Timing of exposure during pregnancy probably plays a role as well, since it is well known that transfer of antibodies, another group of large molecules, primarily takes place during the last trimester in humans (Sidiropoulos *et al.*, 1986). This has yet to be investigated for engineered nanoparticles.

Finally, transfer from mother to offspring of particles or particle-related compounds could potentially take place during lactation, through milk (Tozuka *et al.*, 2004). This has only recently been investigated, by analysis of titanium in milk-filled stomachs from offspring of dams exposed by inhalation to nanoparticulate TiO_2. No titanium was detected in stomach contents a few days after delivery. The limit of detection for titanium in tissues was estimated to be 0.2–5 mg/kg, so transfer of small amounts of titanium would probably not have been detected (Hougaard *et al.*, 2010).

It may be concluded that engineered nanoparticles may indeed pass through the placenta, as has been shown both *in vivo* in animals and *ex vivo* in the human placental perfusion model. The question is to which degree transfer takes place, and how placental transfer depends on physico-chemical properties of the nanoparticles. Transplacental transfer seems to depend highly on the physico-chemical properties of the nanoparticles, including surface coating. Transfer of particles across the placenta has been proposed to increase under some conditions, e.g. inflammatory conditions and timing during pregnancy. This has yet to be investigated. Possibly, placental transfer has to be assessed separately for each type of nanoparticle.

POTENTIAL MECHANISMS OF ACTION IN DEVELOPMENTAL TOXICOLOGY

Maternal exposure to engineered nanoparticles may potentially affect fetal development directly as well as through indirect pathways. It is up for investigation whether particles pass the placenta to any appreciable extent, as discussed above. In the event that engineered nanoparticles actually traverse from the maternal blood to the fetal compartment, particles may reach fetal tissues. Aggregates of TiO_2 particles have been observed in testicle and brain tissue from mice, as long as 6 weeks after their mothers were exposed during gestation to 25–70 nm particles s.c. (Figure 21.7) (Takeda *et al.*, 2009). A direct developmental effect of maternal particle exposure is therefore a definite possibility, although intracellular presence of particles does not necessarily affect the development. The embryonic stem cell test investigates the potential of test compounds to inhibit the differentiation of embryonic stem cells into spontaneously contracting cardiomyocytes. Silica nanoparticles of 10 and 30 nm inhibited differentiation in this test, but particles of 80 and 400 nm did not, even if the largest particles were clearly visible inside vacuoles of the embryoid bodies (Park *et al.*, 2009). It has yet to be investigated whether physical presence of engineered nanoparticles specifically interferes with fetal development.

Toxicity might also occur due to toxic compounds associated with the particles themselves. Biodegradation may cause molecules to dissociate from the core of the engineered particles, enter the maternal blood stream and subsequently traverse the placenta. If titanium dissociates from TiO_2 particles, molecular titanium would probably be able to cross the placenta (Kopf-Maier *et al.*, 1988; Park *et al.*, 2009c; Zhu *et al.*, 2009). For diesel exhaust particles, associated compounds (e.g., polycyclic aromatics) have been postulated to leach from particles to maternal blood, transfer via the placenta or breast milk, and thus gain access to the developing organism (Srivastava *et al.*, 1986; Tozuka *et al.*, 2004). Engineered nanoparticles are often coated or associated with functional chemical groups to add specific properties. Quantum dots often contain cadmium, and toxic effects have been ascribed to leaching of cadmium (Rzigalinski and Strobl, 2009). Since cadmium is a known developmental toxicant (Thompson and Bannigan, 2008), leaching of cadmium presents an additional mechanism by which nanoparticles may influence reproduction and development (Hsieh *et al.*, 2009). However, leaching of carbon from pure carbon particles, such as carbon black, is not expected, indicating that at least for this type of particle, other mechanisms must be present.

It is a question whether nanoparticles need to cross the placenta or even enter the maternal blood stream in order to affect fetal development, or if mediators induced by maternal lung inflammation, such as pro-inflammatory substances (Park *et al.* 2009a), might act as causative factors. Maternal exposure to a single, small dose of nano-sized particles by nasal insufflation produced offspring with increased allergic susceptibility. In this case, transplacental transfer is predicted to be extremely low, considering the dose level and the route of exposure (Fedulov *et al.*, 2008). The mechanism underlying these observations remains undefined (Fedulov and Kobzik, 2008). When exposure takes place through the airways, particles induce an inflammatory response in the lung, as described below. Inflammatory cytokines are able to cross the placenta (Jonakait, 2007) and maternal inflammation may adversely interfere with fetal development (Jonakait 2007; Meyer *et al.*, 2009). Particle-induced inflammation may therefore represent yet another pathway for interference with fetal development (Fedulov *et al.*, 2008). It is therefore intriguing that pregnancy seems to enhance inflammatory response in the lungs following airway exposure to nanoparticles (Fedulov *et al.*, 2008; Lamoureux *et al.*, 2010). Gestational inhalation exposure to diesel exhaust (with a large share of the particles in the nano-range) has furthermore been associated with increased mRNA levels of several inflammatory cytokines in the placentas of mice (Fujimoto *et al.*, 2005).

At the maternal–fetal interface placental cells seem to internalize nanoparticles, as described above. Whether nanoparticles compromise placental function and present a risk for the placenta *per se* warrants further scrutiny. Nano-sized polystyrene beads did not affect viability of placental cotyledons in the human placental perfusion model as judged by several biomarkers. Furthermore, the presence of nanoparticles did not affect the diffusion kinetics of the marker antipyrene. These data indicate that particles did not alter the transfer properties of the placenta (Wick *et al.*, 2010).

An ongoing point of discussion is the most appropriate dose metric for expressing the concentration of nanoparticles in toxicity testing, i.e. weight, volume surface area, number of particles, etc. In the embryonic stem cell test described above, the manufacturer stated that silica particles were 10, 30, 80 and 400 nm in diameter, when in fact they were 11, 34, 34 and 248 nm. The particles were of identical chemical compositions, had been produced by similar processes and dose levels were comparable. Still, the 30 nm particle inhibited differentiation of stem cells whereas the "80" nm did not. Furthermore the 30 nm particle was more cytotoxic than the "80" nm particle. Obviously, primary size is not the only factor determining the toxic properties of nanomaterials (Park *et al.*, 2009c). The involvement of oxidative stress in the toxicity of nanoparticles was discussed earlier in this chapter. Oxidative stress might also be of major importance in developmental toxicity. Data from the zebrafish embryonic toxicity test indicate that oxidative stress associated with exposure to nanoparticles is an important determinant in developmental toxicity. C_{60} and C_{70} fullerenes elicited notable adverse effects on zebrafish embryo survival, hatching and heartbeat. In contrast, fullerol particles, a derivative of C_{60} with several hydroxy groups connected by covalent bonds, left embryos unaffected. Apparently, toxicity of C_{60} derivatives decrease as the number of chemical groups attached to the buckyball increases. Developmental toxicity was also effectively attenuated by co-exposing zebrafish embryos to the antioxidant glutathione (GSH) and C_{60}. The beneficial presence of GSH supports the notion that there might be a free radical-induced toxicity mechanism involved in the developmental toxicity of C_{60} (Usenko *et al.*, 2007; Zhu *et al.*, 2007). Immaturity of the brain antioxidant system early in life (Bayir *et al.*, 2006) might render the developing brain more vulnerable than the adult brain to insults from free radicals generated by engineered nanoparticles.

HEALTH EFFECTS OF ENGINEERED NANOMATERIALS

In toxicology, dose is everything. As stated above, it is still a matter of debate as to what constitutes the most relevant dose metric for nanoscale materials: mass, particle number, surface area or a combination of the above. It is evident that size directly affects the surface to mass ratio (specific surface area) which can have a dramatic impact on surface reactivity/surface chemistry. Moreover, size can govern where and how cells of the immune system react to particles (Fadeel and Garcia-Bennett, 2010). A prevailing view in the field of nanotoxicology is that surface area is an important determinant of toxicity. For instance, Oberdörster *et al.* (1994) reported that following inhalation exposure to 20 nm or 250 nm titanium dioxide particles, the half-times for alveolar clearance of the particles were proportional to the titanium dioxide particle surface area per million macrophages. In a more recent study, Monteiller *et al.* (2007) noted that surface area is a more appropriate dose metric than mass for the pro-inflammatory effects (cytokine secretion) and induction of oxidative stress (glutathione depletion) of TiO_2 and carbon-based particles.

Inflammation

Engineered nanomaterials can exert desirable as well as undesirable effects on the immune system (Dobrovolskaia and McNeil, 2007; Hubbell *et al.*, 2009). Understanding which particle parameters are responsible for which biological effects will greatly advance our ability to harness nanoparticles for therapeutic benefit while at the same time designing materials that are not hazardous to human health.

Our current understanding of nanomaterial-induced toxicity suggests that the induction of oxidative stress may constitute a common pathway of cellular damage (as discussed above). Oxidative stress may somewhat trigger inflammation at the organ and tissue level, and markers of the inflammatory response (for instance, the induction of cytokine genes and secretion of the corresponding cytokines) may also serve as useful indicators of nanotoxicity in cellular models. Inflammation is often thought of as something inherently bad that needs to be dampened. Although this is certainly often the case inflammation is also natural, beneficial and, indeed, essential (Henson, 2005). Inflammation is thus a protective tissue response to injury or irritation, which serves to destroy or wall off both the injurious agent (such as invading microorganisms) and the damaged tissue. The key players in inflammation are the cells of the innate immune system, including neutrophil granulocytes and macrophages, as well as many soluble signaling molecules that orchestrate the inflammatory response. Sometimes the recruitment and accumulation of immune-competent cells leads to the formation of granulomas which serve to encapsulate offending organisms or particles. Neutrophils and macrophages are so-called professional phagocytes that are highly specialized in the disposal of foreign intruders including microorganisms, as well as dying cells and cellular debris. The question as to whether the immune system is also capable of recognizing and responding to nanoparticles is a subject of investigation. The degree of recognition and internalization of nanomaterials by professional phagocytes is likely to influence their biodistribution. Hence, Sadauskas *et al.* (2007) reported that gold nanoparticles (40 nm) injected into mice were taken up primarily by resident macrophages in the liver and secondarily by macrophages in other organs. Also in the fetus, colloidal gold was retained in liver when administered directly into the vitelline vein (Challier *et al.*, 1973). In contrast, inhaled titanium dioxide nanoparticles (20 nm) were shown to escape from clearance by alveolar macrophages in peripheral lung of exposed mice and this phenomenon could potentially explain the translocation of such particles into circulation (Geiser *et al.*, 2008). In addition, the degree of internalization of nanoparticles may determine not only their distribution in the body but also their toxic potential. In support of this notion, Chang *et al.* (2006) reported that the number of internalized quantum dots, i.e. the "intracellular dose" of the nanomaterial, correlates with *in vitro* toxicity. This being said, very recent studies suggest that certain nanoparticles may also damage cells from a distance. Hence, cobalt–chromium nanoparticles with a diameter of approximately 30 nm were shown to damage human fibroblast cells across an intact cellular barrier without having to cross the barrier (Bhabra *et al.*, 2009). The damage was mediated by a novel mechanism involving transmission of purine nucleotides (such as ATP) and the outcome, which included DNA damage without significant cell death, was different from that observed in cells subjected to direct exposure to nanoparticles. In sum, the current literature suggests that nano-sized particles may exert novel toxicities that one may not be able to deduce from studies of larger particles.

Pristine (non-functionalized) carbon nanotubes are not readily taken up by macrophages. However, functionalization of SWCNT with an anionic phospholipid, phosphatidylserine (PS), a known recognition signal for macrophages, targeted the nanotubes to several classes of professional phagocytes, including monocyte-derived macrophages and dendritic cells as well as microglia, the resident macrophages of the brain (Konduru *et al.*, 2009). Moreover, the uptake of PS-coated SWCNT resulted in a reduction of pro-inflammatory cytokine secretion in *in vitro* activated macrophages, with a concomitant increase in the secretion of anti-inflammatory cytokines. This serves to emphasize that the way in which the immune system "sees" a nanoparticle will determine the biological/toxicological outcome.

Allergy

Allergic reactions occur to normally harmless environmental substances known as allergens. Allergy is characterized by excessive activation of mast cells and basophils by IgE antibodies, resulting in an exaggerated inflammatory response. Engineered nanoparticles offer attractive approaches for the modulation of immune responses and are being considered for use in vaccines and in diagnostic tests for allergic reactions (Montanez *et al.*, 2010). In a very recent study, dendritic cells from allergic subjects stimulated *in vitro* with a mixture of biodegradable poly(gamma-glutamic acid) (gamma-PGA) nanoparticles and extract of grass pollen allergen augmented allergen-specific cytokine production and proliferation of autologous memory T cells (Broos *et al.*, 2010). Also TiO_2-particles display adjuvant properties (Larsen *et al.*, 2010).

A number of studies have indicated that engineered nanomaterials may exacerbate allergic responses. For instance, Ryman-Rasmussen *et al.* (2009) demonstrated pulmonary inflammatory responses in ovalbumin (OVA)-sensitized mice with allergic asthma after inhalation of multi-walled carbon nanotubes (MWCNT). The latter studies suggested that pre-existing allergic inflammation may increase the susceptibility for airway fibrosis. In a more recent study, exposure of mice to MWCNT delivered by intra-tracheal instillation was shown to cause pulmonary and systemic immune responses. Total numbers of immune cells in BAL fluid were significantly increased following exposure with increased numbers of neutrophils recovered by lavage. Pro-inflammatory cytokines were also increased in a dose-dependent manner, and B-cell distributions in spleen and blood were increased. The authors concluded that MWCNT may induce allergic responses in mice through B-cell activation and production of IgE (Park *et al.*, 2009a). Moreover, single-walled CNTs (SWCNT) also worsened murine allergic airway inflammation (Nygaard *et al.*, 2009; Inoue *et al.*, 2010). This exacerbation was suggested to occur partly through the inappropriate activation of antigen-presenting cells, including dendritic cells.

To summarize, these examples drawn from studies of immuno-stimulatory effects of nanomaterials illustrate quite well the paradox of engineered nanomaterials: the same unique physical and chemical properties that make these materials so attractive may be associated with their potentially hazardous effects on cells and tissues (Kagan *et al.* 2005). Understanding which parameter(s) trigger the toxic responses and the signaling pathways that are engaged at the cellular level, and modifying the materials in order to mitigate toxicity while at the same time retaining the desirable properties of the materials, remains one of the major challenges in bio-nanotechnology.

Genotoxicity

The number of studies exploring the genotoxic effect of engineered nanomaterials is small in view of the large variety of different engineered nanomaterials already on the market. Recent reviews concluded that information on the genotoxicity of engineered nanomaterials is still inadequate for general conclusions, e.g., on the engineered nanomaterials characteristics critical for genotoxicity (Cunningham, 2007; SCCP, 2007; Gonzalez *et al.*, 2008; Landsiedel *et al.*, 2009). Although models for genotoxicity testing of particles and engineered nanomaterials in particular exist (Speit, 2002; Gonzalez *et al.*, 2008; Landsiedel *et al.*, 2009), it is presently unclear how well standard genotoxicity tests, designed for soluble chemicals, can be used to assess the genotoxicity of engineered nanomaterials. Nor is it known if the existing genotoxicity assays are adequately predictive of the long-term effects of engineered nanomaterials such as carcinogenicity of engineered nanomaterials. A fundamental question is whether *in vivo* tests are preferred instead of *in vitro* tests, considering the possible mechanisms of engineered nanomaterials genotoxicity which may be linked with inflammatory processes (SCCP, 2007). In agreement with previous experience with asbestos fibers, *Salmonella* mutagenicity test does not appear to be responsive to insoluble engineered nanomaterials, probably because of the bacterial cell wall (Kisin *et al.*, 2007; Warheit *et al.*, 2007; Di Sotto *et al.*, 2009; Landsiedel *et al.*, 2009; Wirnitzer *et al.*, 2009; Yoshida *et al.*, 2009). On the other hand, many engineered nanomaterials appear to be positive in tests of DNA damage and micronuclei (Gonzalez *et al.*, 2008; Landsiedel *et al.*, 2009).

Genotoxicity data on CNT, although limited, appear to be primarily positive, which is interesting, considering the recent findings of the carcinogenic potential of MWCNT (Takagi *et al.*, 2008; Sakamoto *et al.*, 2009). More variable results have been obtained on the genotoxicity of other types of engineered nanomaterials. The genotoxicity of nano-sized TiO_2 has been examined in several studies, but the use of different types of TiO_2, various cell systems, and variable assay conditions complicates the comparison of the existing studies (Falck *et al.*, 2009). There is some indication that anatase phase TiO_2, especially, has genotoxic potential *in vitro* (Bhattacharya *et al.*, 2009; Falck *et al.*, 2009; Karlsson *et al.*, 2009).

Carcinogenicity

The carcinogenic effects of persistent particles such as asbestos have been suggested to be due to the local generation of reactive oxygen and nitrogen species in association with emerging inflammation (Takagi *et al.*, 2008). Studies with rats and mice have shown that MWCNT induce oxidative stress, inflammation, granulomas and fibrosis in the lungs (Shvedova *et al.*, 2005; Lam et al., 2006; Li *et al.*, 2007; Muller *et al.*, 2008). Due to these properties of CNT, it has been envisaged for a number of years that engineered nanomaterials with fibrogenic properties could induce cancers. Rodent studies using intraperitoneal exposure to MWCNT indicate that the ability of MWCNT to induce mesotheliomas exceeds that of crocidolite asbestos (Takagi *et al.*, 2008; Sakamoto *et al.*, 2009). In all studies in which MWCNT have been given intraperitoneally (Poland *et al.*, 2008; Takagi *et al.*, 2008; Sakamoto *et al.*, 2009), MWCNT formed agglomerates or bundles, and single MWCNT were not present. This type of agglomeration is typical of MWCNT and SWCNT also in occupational environments when the material exists in aerosol (Maynard *et al.*, 2004). Furthermore, MWCNT induced asbestosis-like pathogenic changes in the mesothelial lining of the abdominal cavity when introduced into the abdominal cavity of mice (Poland *et al.*, 2008). Due to the intraperitoneal route of exposure, these data cannot be used to assess risks of human inhalation exposure to CNT but they may provide useful information for the identification of hazards, i.e. carcinogenic potential of CNT. Whether MWCNT have the ability to induce mesotheliomas also in the thoracic cavity through the relevant exposure route, inhalation, remains to be seen, and is mandatory for reliable assessment of carcinogenic risk. One has to keep in mind that there are about 50,000 different CNT commercially available, and each publication usually only deals with one type of CNT. The carcinogenic potential of engineered nanomaterials in addition to CNT has not been markedly explored.

DEVELOPMENTAL AND REPRODUCTIVE TOXICITY

That the developing fetus may be vulnerable to maternal chemical exposures during pregnancy is apparent from several contributions in this book. Fetal development may also be susceptible to insult from engineered nanoparticles. Nano-sized particles may potentially affect the developing fetus through several pathways, as outlined above. Leaching of coating, core or associated chemicals followed by placental transfer represents one pathway. Although potentially of great importance, this mechanism belongs more within traditional developmental toxicology than within developmental nanotoxicology. Effects of engineered particles *per se* represent another pathway, reflecting the emerging topic of nanotoxicology. For the best elucidation of the latter, the following description of developmental toxicity of engineered nanoparticles focuses on particulate effects, rather than effects of specific chemicals.

Pregnancy and fetal development

The database of developmental effects of nanoparticles is still in the early phase, as only few studies are published. Although easy to record, basic gestational and developmental measures (e.g., maternal weight gain, litter size and birth weights) have only been described for a couple of studies. In one study, mice were exposed by inhalation to titanium dioxide particles (rutile; UV-titan L181) on gestation days 8–18, 1 hour/day to $42\,mg/m^3$ aerosolized powder (Figures 21.3 and 21.6). The rutile particles were produced for use in paints, and particles were therefore modified with Al, Si and Zr, and coated with polyalcohols. Maternal weight gain, length of gestation and number and loss of implantations were similar to control values, as were litter size, offspring body weight and sex ratio. Pup viability during lactation tended to be reduced in TiO_2 litters, but not significantly so. When mature offspring were cross-mated to naïve CBA/J mice, litter size was similar in TiO_2 and control litters in the second generation (Hougaard *et al.*, 2010). Prenatal exposure to carbonaceous nanoparticles by intratracheal instillation ($200\,\mu g$/mouse on gestational days 7 and 14) also left gestational parameters unaffected in mice (Yoshida *et al.*, 2009). Findings in these two studies do not indicate that engineered nanoparticles are fetotoxic as such, at least not when maternal exposure is through the airways. This is supported by a couple of yet unpublished studies from our laboratory, where gestational parameters appear virtually unaffected by exposure to carbonaceous nanoparticles by either inhalation or intratracheal instillation, even at relatively high dose levels (Hougaard, personal communication). One published study does, however, report severe fetal effects. This study exposed pregnant mice ($n = 2$/group) to 25, 50 or 157 mg/kg fullerenes (C60) on gestation day 10 by intraperioneal injection. Embryos were examined 18 hours later. Particles distributed throughout fetuses and yolk sac, and all the fetuses in the exposed groups died. At the higher dose levels, several fetuses also displayed severe abnormalities (Tsuchiya *et al.*, 1996). It is unclear whether bypassing the blood–placenta barrier and the high dose levels contributed to the very severe effects.

Central nervous system

As described under transplacental transport of particles, prenatal exposure on gestation day 3, 7, 10 and 14 by maternal subcutaneous injections to 0.1 mg pure 20–70 nm TiO_2 particles resulted in particle aggregates being detected in cerebral cortex and olfactory bulb in mouse offspring, 6 weeks after birth (Figure 21.7). This indicates that particles are able to pass from the maternal organism to the fetal brain. Brain tissue from exposed offspring furthermore showed significant signs of apoptosis, envisioned by caspase-3 staining of cells and electron microscopy, 6 weeks after birth (Takeda *et al.*, 2009). An almost similar prenatal exposure regimen was associated with alterations in gene expression related to brain development, apoptosis and central neural system function. Unfortunately very limited information was provided on specific gene changes and effective group size was in essence $n = 1$, hampering interpretation of these findings (Shimizu *et al.*, 2009). When the functional implications of prenatal exposure to the UV-titan L181 (details described above) were investigated by use of a neurobehavioral test battery, exposed offspring displayed some neurobehavioral alterations. Exposed male and female offspring tended to avoid the central zone of the open field, and prepulse inhibition of the startle reaction was somewhat changed in exposed female offspring, compared to sham exposed control offspring. Cognitive function was unaffected when assessed in the Morris water maze test (Hougaard *et al.*, 2010). At least hypothetically, immaturity of the antioxidant system renders the developing brain vulnerable to oxidative stress generated by engineered nanoparticles. The observations described above emphasize developmental neurotoxicity as an area of importance in relation to toxicity of nanoparticles.

Reproductive system

As described above, TiO_2 particulate aggregates were also observed in testicular tissue 6 weeks after birth in males exposed during fetal life. Particles were located intracellularly in Leydig and Sertoli cells as well as in spermatids (Figure 21.8). Sperm morphology was similar in control and exposed male offspring at this time point. However, testicular morphology was abnormal in exposed males and daily sperm production was significantly lower in exposed offspring compared to controls (Takeda *et al.*, 2009).

Seminiferous tissue and daily sperm production was also adversely affected after prenatal exposure to nano-sized carbon particles (intratracheal administration of 200 μg at gestation day 7 and 14) (Yoshida *et al.*, 2009). Functional implications of prenatal exposure to TiO_2 particles (UV-titan L181 as described above) were assessed by cross-mating mature offspring to naïve mice. Time-to-delivery of the first F_2 litter was similar for control and exposed female offspring, but was somewhat (but non-significantly) delayed for exposed compared to control male offspring (Hougaard *et al.*, 2010).

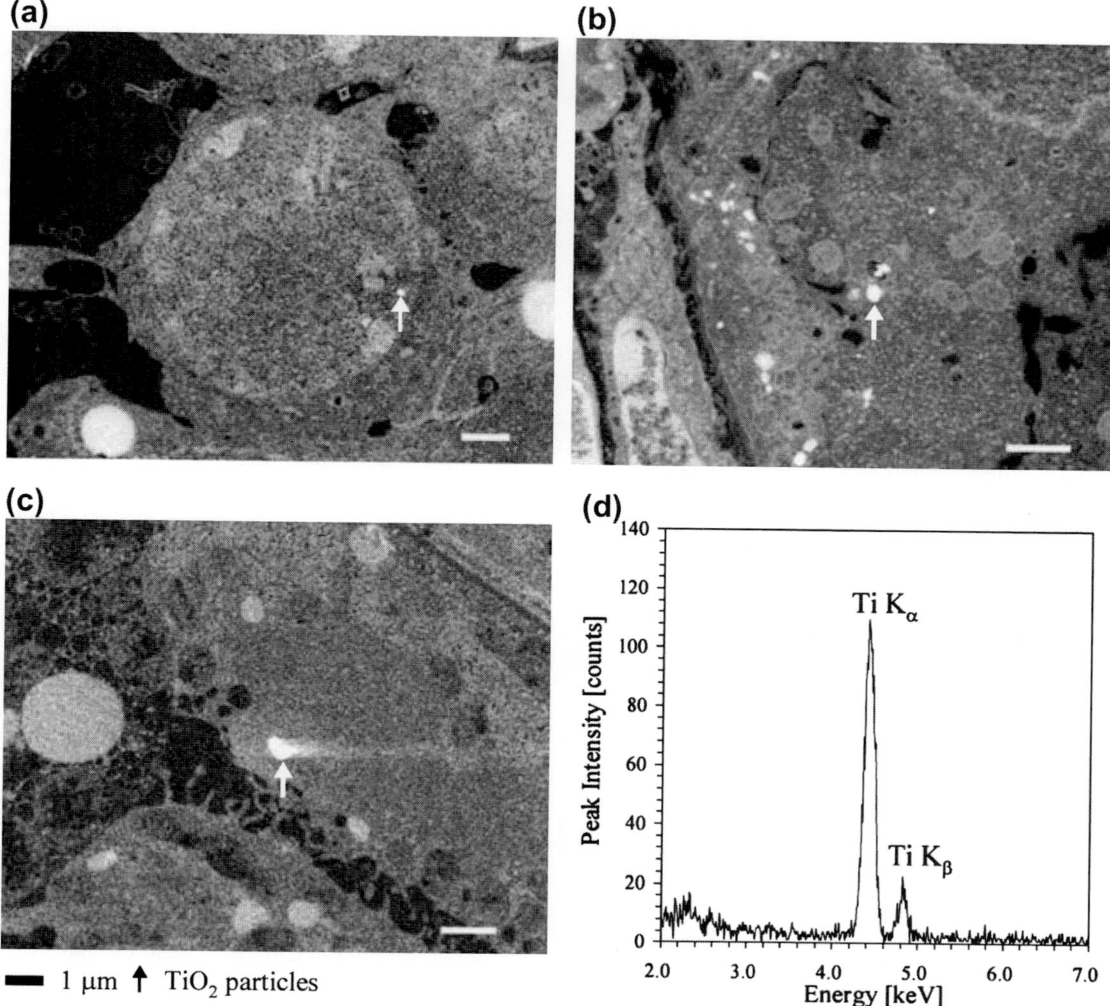

FIGURE 21.8 Detection of TiO_2 nanoparticles in the testis from 6-week-old offspring of TiO_2-exposed pregnant mice. Aggregated TiO_2 particles (100–200 nm) were detected in spermatids (a), Sertoli cells (b) and Leydig cells (c). Scale bars 1μ. TiO_2 particles are indicated by arrows. Particles were identified as TiO_2 by energy-dispersive X-ray spectroscopy at 7 kV accelerating voltage, 1×10^{-10} A beam and 100 sec measurements (d). (Courtesy of *Journal of Health Science*, Takeda *et al.*, 2009.)

Interestingly, carbonaceous nanoparticles were also associated with decreased daily sperm production and damaged sperm producing tissue in male mice when exposure was initiated in adolescence (intratracheal administration of 0.1 mg of 14, 56 or 95 nm carbon black/mouse, once weekly for 10 weeks) (Yoshida *et al.*, 2009). *In vitro*, Leydig cells have been shown to internalize TiO_2 particles (Komatsu *et al.*, 2008).

Female reproductive function has primarily been assessed *in vitro*. Fertilized one-cell mouse embryos developed similarly to controls 2 days after addition of 40–120 nm polystyrene nanoparticles to culture media, but some effect was noted after 6 days. Development was severely hampered when the same procedure was performed with 40 nm carboxylated polyacrylonitrile nanoparticles. Both particle types impaired development when injected directly into the zygote, compared to sham injected control zygotes (Fynewever *et al.*, 2007). *In vitro* exposure of two-cell mouse embryos to 40–120 nm polystyrene-based particles did not interfere statistically significantly with development to the blastocyst stage or with implantation, although a trend towards reduced success for exposed embryos was demonstrated. Smaller particles were actually internalized by embryonic cells (Bosman *et al.*, 2005). Otherwise drastic effects were observed after a 24 hour exposure of oocytes and blastocysts to cadmium containing quantum dots on development, from fertilization to implantation and fetal development. Coating quantum dots with zinc-sulfide circumvented adverse effects to control levels and has been shown to reduce both cytotoxicity and release of Cd by blocking surface oxidation and release of Cd^{2-} ions. Circumvention of reproductive effects by coating quantum dots indicates that cadmium was probably responsible for the developmental effects (Chan and Shiao, 2008; Hsieh *et al.*, 2009).

Immune system

Maternal gestational exposure to very small doses of nanosized particles has been associated with increased allergic susceptibility in the offspring. A single dose of 50 μg nanosized titanium dioxide, carbon black or diesel exhaust particles were administered by nasal insufflation to pregnant mice at gestation day 14. After birth, offspring were sensitized and exposed to aerosolized ovalbumin. Neonates of mothers exposed intranasally to nanoparticles developed a more pronounced asthmatic phenotype than did sham exposed control offspring. Thus, maternal exposure to particles at a dose level and route of exposure of very limited transplacental transfer seemed to promote offspring immune responses to allergen sensitization and challenge (Fedulov *et al.*, 2008). Increased reactivity of the immune systems has also been reported for other prenatal particulate exposures (Watanabe and Ohsawa, 2002; Singh *et al.*, 2003, 2009; Hamada *et al.*, 2007; Penn *et al.*, 2007; Latzin *et al.*, 2009).

In conclusion, data published so far indicate that exposure to engineered particles has the potential to affect reproduction and development. As for other kinds of toxicity, magnitude and type of effect depend on the physico-chemical characteristics of the particles. However, some manifestations of developmental toxicity might be related primarily to a particle effect. Furthermore, the major manifestations of toxicity of engineered nanoparticles might not be malformations or fetotoxicity, but rather functional impairment of the offspring, perhaps even with delayed onset.

RISK ASSESSMENT OF ENGINEERED NANOMATERIALS INCLUDING NOVEL STRATEGIES AND CONTROL BANDING

The number of novel engineered nanomaterials increases rapidly (SCENIHR, 2007; Peters *et al.*, 2009; Schulte *et al.*, 2009; Woodrow Wilson, 2010), and risks and safety of these novel engineered nanomaterials displaying unique properties need to be assessed. For example, the number of different CNT exceeds 50,000 (Schulte *et al.*, 2009). Today, there is no general agreement as to how to assess the risk associated with exposure to engineered nanomaterials, i.e. regarding metrics and toxicity assessment.

A rapid tiered approach based on best available evidence for risk assessment of engineered nanomaterials would thus be important. A validated approach would allow separation of engineered nanomaterials of concern from those of less or of no concern. This would help prioritization of necessary actions to protect workers and consumers from harmful exposure to and effects of engineered nanomaterials. Likewise, a validated approach would also help avoiding misleading generalizations regarding harmfulness of engineered nanomaterials as a single group of materials. Engineered nanomaterials are as different from each other as any other chemicals, even if they share similar characteristics. There have been some attempts to develop tiered safety assessment systems for engineered nanomaterials with a proposed set of *in vitro* methods for the assessment of engineered nanomaterials toxicity (Warheit *et al.*, 2007; Melkonyan and Kozyrev, 2009). Many of these proposals have, however, suffered from shortcomings in delineating the key endpoints to be assessed, or in defining the most suitable specific tests to be used.

Toxicity testing of engineered nanomaterials should preferentially start with careful physico-chemical characterization (Elder *et al.*, 2009). Engineered nanomaterials should be explored for structural alerts or other characteristics associated with harmful effects. Such characteristics may include large surface area, high reactivity or chemical composition. To date, the stage of understanding of the association between such alerts and effects of engineered nanomaterials is still inadequate. Regarding developmental toxicity, mutagenicity and association of particles with already known developmental toxicants would be an obvious trigger, e.g. cadmium in quantum dots (Thompson and Bannigan, 2008). However, such triggers rely rather on a traditional toxicological way of thinking. They do not address the potential specific toxicity of engineered nanoparticles as such for development.

After thorough characterization, engineered nanomaterials can then be investigated in a tiered fashion by first using acellular systems to explore the reactivity of the materials, assisted by high throughput methods to explore effects of engineered nanomaterials at a subcellular level. Testing could then proceed to carefully validated *in vitro* cellular models that would support an evidence-based testing process (Guzelian *et al.*, 2009). Chosen *in vitro* testing methods should address carefully the relevant endpoints such as cytotoxicity, apoptosis, skin and ocular toxicity, genotoxicity, potential carcinogenicity, effects on the immunological system, neuronal cells and the vascular system (a major and already identified challenge for the development of this kind of tiered testing procedure continues to be the validation of *in vitro* testing with appropriate predictive power for *in vivo* effects in whole organisms).

Some endpoints cannot be tested *in vitro* and would therefore require *a priori in vivo* testing. This is certainly true for developmental toxicity and carcinogenicity. In other instances positive and consistent results from validated *in vitro* tests with demonstrated predictive power would lead to higher tier testing procedures with experimental animals. These would consist of lower tiers of short-term studies, and long-term studies with experimental animals would be required less frequently than at present. A pictorial presentation of the proposed tiered testing approach is shown in Figure 21.9.

Reproductive and developmental toxicity are integrated into the nanomaterials research strategy of the US Environmental Protection Agency (US EPA, 2009) and recommended by the Reproductive Health Research Team under the National Occupational Research Agenda (NORA) of the US National Institute for Occupational Safety and Health (NIOSH) (Lawson *et al.*, 2006). However, as this chapter clearly demonstrates, as yet very little is known about developmental toxicity of nanomaterials.

Developmental toxicity cannot be tested *in vitro* and would require *a priori in vivo* testing. It is important to realize that traditional guidelines for developmental toxicity may not suffice for uncovering developmental toxicity of nanoparticles. Although the foundation is as yet very fragile, the true culprits of engineered nanoparticles might not be malformations or fetotoxicity, but rather functional impairment of the offspring, possibly even with delayed onset, e.g. developmental neurotoxicity, increased susceptibility of the offspring to develop allergic disease or decreased fertility (cf. descriptions of developmental and reproductive toxicity earlier in this chapter).

Use of safety and toxicity data of engineered nanomaterials for risk assessment and management

The need for risk assessment of engineered nanomaterials has also generated a need for a novel risk assessment concept.

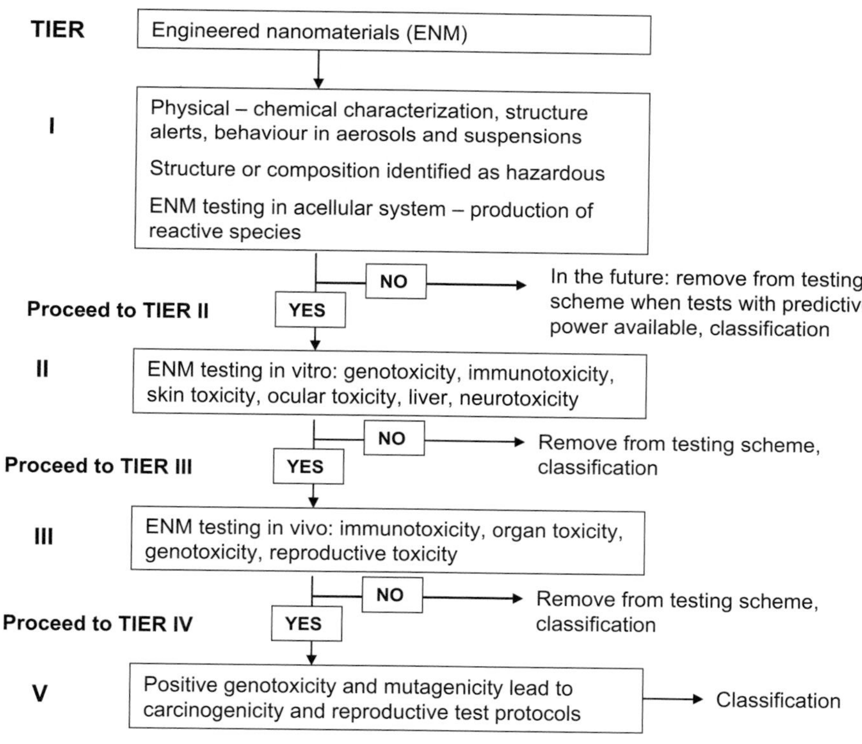

TIERS II, III and IV: Combine with results from exposure assessment data from the field, results from the dustiness test, and modelling in the future.

RISK ASSESSMENT

1. Evaluation of magnitude of risk at different exposure levels, setting of occupational exposure levels (OEL) and other regulatory limits.
2. Based on hazard assessment of ENM; combining the knowledge on experimental levels of exposure to ENM and toxic effects induced by them, and comparing these levels with levels in occupational environments.

FIGURE 21.9 A schematic representation of the proposed tiered testing approach for engineered nanomaterials. (Reprinted with permission from Savolainen *et al.*, 2010.)

Even though the key steps of risk assessment, notably risk identification, risk characterization and exposure assessment followed by overall risk assessment, remains the cornerstone of assessment of safety of engineered nanomaterials, special features of engineered nanomaterials require modifications to the current procedures. However, there are several additional datasets that require special attention the availability of which is essential for the reliable risk assessment of engineered nanomaterials.

Careful material characterization has become a vital part of the risk assessment of engineered nanomaterials beyond the requirements set up for regular chemical compounds. These data should be actively used in the selection of engineered nanomaterials to be tested in higher tiers.

A vital part of the data required and used in any risk assessment is exposure assessment data. The tendency of engineered nanomaterials to coagulate or agglomerate and make aggregates complicates the exposure assessment efforts but these data are an absolute prerequisite for any reliable risk assessment of exposure to engineered nanomaterials. From the risk assessment perspective, information on the cellular level within cells and organisms is also essential; this emphasizes the use of these types of data (Bihari *et al.*, 2008; Seipenbusch *et al.*, 2008).

CONTROL BANDING

In the current situation, where the challenge of engineered nanomaterials flowing into the market dramatically exceeds the results available for reliably engineered nanomaterials risk assessment, other more economical approaches will be sought. Control banding is one highly promising approach which has not been developed for engineered nanomaterials risk assessment but for engineered nanomaterials risk characterization. The goal of control banding is to prevent excessive exposure to compounds such as engineered nanomaterials in a situation in which the amount of knowledge is not sufficient for appropriate risk assessment-based regulatory actions. Control banding enables decisions to be made regarding appropriate levels of control that are product and process based, without complete information on hazard and exposure. The concept allows a pragmatic controlling exposure where limited information is available. In control banding, it is possible to assign an "impact index" to engineered nanomaterials, based on their composition-based hazard and perturbations associated with their nanostructure, i.e. surface area, surface chemistry, shape and particle size. A corresponding "exposure index" can in turn represent the amount of material used and its propensity to become airborne. As with conventional control banding for conventional chemicals, the combination of these two indices could then be linked to specific control bands for engineered nanomaterials (Maynard and Aitken, 2007). Two types of indices are a "severity index", containing, subject to availability, (1) surface chemistry; (2) particle shape; (3) particle diameter; (4) solubility; (5) carcinogenicity; (6) reproductive toxicity; (7) dermal toxicity; and (8) toxicity, including carcinogenicity, reproductive toxicity, genotoxicity and dermal toxicity of parent material, and a "probability index" consisting of factors contributing to likelihood of exposure, notably (1) dustiness; (2) number of employees with similar exposure; (3) frequency of operation; and (4) duration of operation. The overall probability index was calculated based on this information. Linking of these two indices produced a matrix in which the severity and probability of harm could be assessed, and consequently the required control bands (required actions) could be determined, and was (1) adjusting general ventilation; (2) making changes to fume hoods or local exhaust ventilation; (3) considering containment; and (4) seeking specialist advice. It turned out that this approach was useful for assessing risks of engineered nanomaterials operations, and provided recommendations for appropriate engineering controls and facilitated the allocation of resources to the activities that most need them. Hence, control banding may be useful in prioritizing necessary activities required for exposure mitigation.

CONCLUDING REMARKS AND FUTURE DIRECTIONS

Risk assessment of engineered nanomaterials challenges some of the current risk assessment procedures due to the unique nature of material at nanoscale. The fundamental elements of risk assessment are likely to remain and will continue to include the elements carefully designed for other chemicals and particles, notably (1) risk identification; (2) risk characterization; (3) exposure assessment; and (4) overall risk assessment. However, the features of these materials set new challenges, for example characterization of test materials. In addition, it is likely that many of the toxicity tests used today for hazard assessment need to be modified to meet the specific characteristics of these materials. Perhaps the most demanding challenge for risk assessment is the need to develop an intelligent, tiered testing strategy to be able to reduce the amount of resources for engineered nanomaterials risk assessment without jeopardizing the safe use of these unique materials.

Specific challenges of safe use of engineered nanomaterials are capturing more information on the association between engineered nanomaterials metrics and toxicity, measuring technologies and specific toxicity endpoints such as carcinogenicity, genotoxicity and reproductive toxicity.

Specifically for developmental toxicity, data published so far indicate that engineered nanoparticles may indeed pass the placenta. The question is to which degree transfer takes place, and how placental transfer depends on physicochemical properties of the nanoparticles. It has yet to be investigated whether transfer of particles across the placenta increases due to inflammatory conditions. Possibly, placental transfer has to be assessed separately for each type of nanoparticle.

Maternal exposure to engineered nanoparticles may potentially affect fetal development directly as well as through indirect pathways. Toxicity might also occur due to toxic compounds associated with the particles themselves. A true challenge is that nanoparticles might not need to cross the placenta or even enter the maternal blood stream in order to affect fetal development.

Developmental toxicity of nanoparticles might also challenge traditional toxicology in that the true culprits could be functional impairment of the offspring, possibly with delayed onset, rather than malformations or fetotoxicity. Research within developmental toxicity so far bears the impressions of hypothesis generating studies. Most studies did not include maternal and traditional gestational measures (e.g., maternal weight gain, litter size, birth weights) even if these are easy to record. It was often difficult to extract the number of pregnant dams included in each exposure group and if more than one pup per litter was used for investigation of effects, potentially increasing the potential for litter effects. For advice on how to design good studies, researchers may refer to established guidelines, e.g. "Guidance for developmental toxicity risk assessment" from the US EPA (United States Environmental Protection Agency, 1991).

REFERENCES

Adlakha-Hutcheon G, Khaydarov R, Korenstein R, Varma R, Vaseashta A, Stamm H, Abdel-Mottaleb M (2009) Nanomaterials, nanotechnology: applications, consumer products, and benefits. In *Nanomaterials: Risks and Benefits* (Linkov I, Steevens J, eds.). Dordrecht: Springer, pp. 195–207.

Aitken RJ, Creely KS, Tran CL (2004) Nanoparticles: an occupational hygiene review. *Health Safety Executive (HSE)* 1–113.

Akerman ME, Chan WC, Laakkonen P, Bhatia SN, Ruoslahti E (2002) Nanocrystal targeting in vivo. *Proc Natl Acad Sci USA* **99:** 12617–21.

Allen NS, Edge M, Sandoval G, Verran J, Stratton J, Maltby J (2005) Photocatalytic coatings for environmental applications. *Photochem Photobiol* **81:** 279–90.

Bayir H, Kochanek PM, Kagan VE (2006) Oxidative stress in immature brain after traumatic brain injury. *Dev Neurosci* **28:** 420–31.

Bhabra G, Sood A, Fisher B, Cartwright L, Saunders M, Evans WH, Surprenant A, Lopez-Castejon G, Mann S, Davis SA, Hails LA, Ingham E, Verkade P, Lane J, Heesom K, Newson R, Case CP (2009) Nanoparticles can cause DNA damage across a cellular barrier. *Nat Nanotechnol* **4:** 876–83.

Bhattacharya K, Davoren M, Boertz J, Schins RP, Hoffmann E, Dopp E (2009) Titanium dioxide nanoparticles induce oxidative stress and DNA-adduct formation but not DNA-breakage in human lung cells. *Part Fibre Toxicol* **6:** 17.

Bihari P, Vippola M, Schultes S, Praetner M, Khandoga AG, Reichel CA, Coester C, Tuomi T, Rehberg M, Krombach F (2008) Optimized dispersion of nanoparticles for biological in vitro and in vivo studies. *Part Fibre Toxicol* **5:** 14.

Bladh K, Falk LKL, Rohmund F (2000) On the iron-catalyzed growth of single-walled carbon nanotubes and encapsulated metal particles in the gas phase. *Appl Phys A* **70:** 317–22.

Bosman SJ, Nieto SP, Patton WC, Jacobson JD, Corselli JU, Chan PJ (2005) Development of mammalian embryos exposed to mixed-size nanoparticles. *Clin Exp Obstet Gynecol* **32:** 222–4.

Brant JA, Labille J, Bottero JY, Wiesner MR (2006) Characterizing the impact of preparation method on fullerene cluster structure and chemistry. *Langmuir* **22:** 3878–85.

Broos S, Lundberg K, Akagi T, Kadowaki K, Akashi M, Greiff L, Borrebaeck CA, Lindstedt M (2010) Immunomodulatory nanoparticles as adjuvants and allergen-delivery system to human dendritic cells: Implications for specific immunotherapy. *Vaccine*. In press.

Bruchez M Jr, Moronne M, Gin P, Weiss S, Alivisatos AP (1998) Semiconductor nanocrystals as fluorescent biological labels. *Science* **281:** 2013–16.

Carp O, Huisman CL, Reller A (2004) Photoinduced reactivity of titanium dioxide. *Progr Solid State Chem* **32:** 33–177.

Challier JC, Panigel M, Meyer E (1973) Uptake of colloidal 198Au by fetal liver in rat, after direct intrafetal administration. *Int J Nucl Med Biol* **1:** 103–6.

Chan WC, Nie S (1998) Quantum dot bioconjugates for ultrasensitive nonisotopic detection. *Science* **281:** 2016–18.

Chan WH, Shiao NH (2008) Cytotoxic effect of CdSe quantum dots on mouse embryonic development. *Acta Pharmacol Sin* **29:** 259–66.

Chang E, Thekkek N, Yu WW, Colvin VL, Drezek R (2006) Evaluation of quantum dot cytotoxicity based on intracellular uptake. *Small* **2:** 1412–17.

Chen X, Mao SS (2006) Synthesis of titanium dioxide (TiO_2) nanomaterials. *J Nanosci Nanotechnol* **6:** 906–25.

Cheng Y, Zhou O (2003) Electron field emission from carbon nanotubes. *C R Physique* **4:** 1021–33.

Cunningham MJ (2007) Gene–cellular interactions of nanomaterials: genotoxicity to genomics. In *Nanotoxicology – Characterization, Dosing and Health Effects* (Monteiro-Riviere NA, Tran CL, eds.). New York, Informa Healthcare, pp. 173–96.

Dabbousi BO, Rodriguez-Viejo J, Mikulec FV, Heine JR, Mattoussi H, Ober R, Jensen KF, Bawendi MG (1997) (CdSe)ZnS Core–shell quantum dots: synthesis and characterization of a size series of highly luminescent nanocrystallites. *J Phys Chem B* **101:** 9463–75.

Delehanty JB, Mattoussi H, Medintz IL 2009 Delivering quantum dots into cells: strategies, progress and remaining issues. *Anal Bioanal Chem* **393:** 1091–105.

Di Sotto A., Chiaretti M, Carru GA, Bellucci S, Mazzanti G (2009) Multi-walled carbon nanotubes: lack of mutagenic activity in the bacterial reverse mutation assay. *Toxicol Lett* **184:** 192–7.

Diaz B, Sanchez-Espinel C, Arruebo M, Faro J, de ME, Magadan S, Yague C, Fernandez-Pacheco R, Ibarra MR, Santamaria J, Gonzalez-Fernandez A (2008) Assessing methods for blood cell cytotoxic responses to inorganic nanoparticles and nanoparticle aggregates. *Small* **4:** 2025–34.

Diebold U (2003) The surface science of titanium dioxide. *Surface Science Reports* **48:** 53–229.

Dobrovolskaia MA, McNeil SE (2007) Immunological properties of engineered nanomaterials. *Nat Nanotechnol* **2:** 469–78.

Elder A, Lynch I, Grieger K, Chan-Remillard S, Gatti A, Gnewuch H, Kenaway E, Korenstein R, Kuhlbusch T, Linker F, Matias S, Monteiro-Riviere NA, Pinto VRS, Rudnitsky R, Savolainen K, Shvedova AA (2009) Human health risks of engineered nanomaterials: critical knowledge gaps in nanomaterials risk assessment. In *Nanomaterials: Risks and Benefits* (Linkov I, Steevens J, eds.). Dordrecht, Springer, pp. 3–29.

Evanoff JDD, Chumanov G (2005) Synthesis and optical properties of silver nanoparticles and arrays. *Chemphyschem* **6:** 1221–31.

Fadeel B, Garcia-Bennett AE (2010) Better safe than sorry: understanding the toxicological properties of inorganic nanoparticles manufactured for biomedical applications. *Adv Drug Deliv Rev* **62:** 362–74.

Falck GC, Lindberg HK, Suhonen S, Vippola M, Vanhala E, Catalan J, Savolainen K, Norppa H (2009) Genotoxic effects of nanomaterials: induction of DNA damage and micronuclei by TiO_2 in human bronchial epithelial cells. *Hum Exp Toxicol* **28:** 339–52.

Fedulov AV, Kobzik L (2008) Immunotoxicologic analysis of maternal transmission of asthma risk. *J Immunotoxicol* **5:** 445–52.

Fedulov AV, Leme A, Yang Z, Dahl M, Lim R, Mariani TJ, Kobzik L (2008) Pulmonary exposure to particles during pregnancy causes increased neonatal asthma susceptibility. *Am J Respir Cell Mol Biol* **38:** 57–67.

Fischer HC, Chan WC (2007) Nanotoxicity: the growing need for in vivo study. *Curr Opin Biotechnol* **18:** 565–71.

Folkerth RD, Haynes RL, Borenstein NS, Belliveau RA, Trachtenberg F, Rosenberg PA, Volpe JJ, Kinney HC (2004) Developmental lag in superoxide dismutases relative to other antioxidant enzymes in premyelinated human telencephalic white matter. *J Neuropathol Exp Neurol* **63:** 990–9.

Fujimoto A, Tsukue N, Watanabe M, Sugawara I, Yanagisawa R, Takano H, Yoshida S, Takeda K (2005) Diesel exhaust affects immunological action in the placentas of mice. *Environ Toxicol* **20:** 431–40.

Fynewever TL, Agcaoili ES, Jacobson JD, Patton WC, Chan PJ (2007) In vitro tagging of embryos with nanoparticles. *J Assist Reprod Genet* **24:** 61–5.

Geiser M, Casaulta M, Kupferschmid B, Schulz H, Semmler-Behnke M, Kreyling W (2008) The role of macrophages in the clearance of inhaled ultrafine titanium dioxide particles. *Am J Respir Cell Mol Biol* **38:** 371–6.

Ghosh P, Han G, De M, Kim CK, Rotello VM (2008) Gold nanoparticles in delivery applications. *Adv Drug Deliv Rev* **60:** 1307–15.

Gonzalez L, Lison D, Kirsch-Volders M (2008) Genotoxicity of engineered nanomaterials: a critical review. *Nanotechnology* **2:** 252–73.

Guzelian PS, Victoroff MS, Halmes C, James RC (2009) Clear path: towards an evidence-based toxicology (EBT). *Hum Exp Toxicol* **28:** 71–9.

Hamada K, Suzaki Y, Leme A, Ito T, Miyamoto K, Kobzik L, Kimura H (2007) Exposure of pregnant mice to an air pollutant aerosol increases asthma susceptibility in offspring. *J Toxicol Environ Health A* **70:** 688–95.

Henson PM (2005) Dampening inflammation. *Nat Immunol* **6:** 1179–81.

Hines MA, Guyot-Sionnest P (1996) Synthesis and characterization of strongly luminescing ZnS-capped CdSe nanocrystals. *J Phys Chem B* **100:** 468–71.

Hirsch LR, Stafford RJ, Bankson JA, Sershen SR, Rivera B, Price RE, Hazle JD, Halas NJ, West JL (2003) Nanoshell-mediated near-infrared thermal therapy of tumors under magnetic resonance guidance. *Proc Natl Acad Sci USA* **100:** 13549–54.

Hougaard KS, Jackson P, Jensen KA, Sloth JJ, Löschner K, Larsen EH, Birkedal RK, Vibenholt A, Boisen AM, Wallin H, Vogel U (2010) Effects of prenatal exposure to surface-coated nanosized titanium dioxide (UV-Titan). A study in mice. *Part Fibre Toxicol.* **14(7):** 16.

Hougaard KS, Jensen KA, Nordly P, Taxvig C, Vogel U, Saber AT, Wallin H (2008) Effects of prenatal exposure to diesel exhaust particles on postnatal development, behavior, genotoxicity and inflammation in mice. *Part Fibre Toxicol* **5:** 3.

Hsieh MS, Shiao NH, Chan WH (2009) Cytotoxic effects of CdSe quantum dots on maturation of mouse oocytes, fertilization, and fetal development. *Int J Mol Sci* **10:** 2122–35.

Hubbell JA, Thomas SN, Swartz MA (2009) Materials engineering for immunomodulation. *Nature* **462:** 449–60.

Iijima S (1991) Helical microtubules of graphitic carbon. *Nature* **354:** 56–8.

Inoue K, Yanagisawa R, Koike E, Nishikawa M, Takano H (2010) Repeated pulmonary exposure to single-walled carbon nanotubes exacerbates allergic inflammation of the airway: possible role of oxidative stress. *Free Radic Biol Med* **48:** 924–34.

Jonakait GM (2007) The effects of maternal inflammation on neuronal development: possible mechanisms. *Int J Dev Neurosci* **25:** 415–25.

Kagan VE, Bayir H, Shvedova AA (2005) Nanomedicine and nanotoxicology: two sides of the same coin. *Nanomedicine* **1:** 313–16.

Kagan VE, Konduru NV, Feng W, Allen BL, Conroy J, Volkov Y, Vlasova II, Belikova NA, Yanamala N, Kapralov A, Tyurina YY, Shi J, Kisin ER, Murray AR, Franks J, Stolz D, Gou P, Klein-Seetharaman J, Fadeel B, Star A, Shvedova AA (2010) Carbon nanotubes degraded by neutrophil myeloperoxidase induce less pulmonary inflammation. *Nat Nanotechnol* **5:** 354–9.

Kagan VE, Tyurina YY, Tyurin VA, Konduru NV, Potapovich AI, Osipov AN, Kisin ER, Schwegler-Berry D, Mercer R, Castranova V, Shvedova AA (2006) Direct and indirect effects of single walled carbon nanotubes on RAW 264.7 macrophages: role of iron. *Toxicol Lett* **165:** 88–100.

Kaplan-Ashiri I, Cohen SR, Gartsman K, Ivanoskaya V, Heine T, Seifert G, Wiesel I, Wagner HD, Tenne R (2006) On the mechanical behavior of WS_2 nanotubes under axial tension and compression. *Proc Natl Acad Sci USA* **103:** 523–8.

Karlsson HL, Gustafsson J, Cronholm P, Moller L (2009) Size-dependent toxicity of metal oxide particles – a comparison between nano- and micrometer size. *Toxicol Lett* **188:** 112–18.

Kennison RD, Bardawil WA, Mitchell GW Jr (1971) Passage of particles across the mouse placenta. *Surg Forum* **22:** 392–4.

Kisin ER, Murray AR, Keane MJ, Shi XC, Schwegler-Berry D, Gorelik O, Arepalli S, Castranova V, Wallace WE, Kagan VE, Shvedova AA (2007) Single-walled carbon nanotubes: geno- and cytotoxic effects in lung fibroblast V79 cells. *J Toxicol Environ Health A* **70:** 2071–9.

Komatsu T, Tabata M, Kubo-Irie M, Shimizu T, Suzuki K, Nihei Y, Takeda K (2008) The effects of nanoparticles on mouse testis Leydig cells in vitro. *Toxicol in Vitro* **22:** 1825–31.

Konduru NV, Tyurina YY, Feng W, Basova LV, Belikova NA, Bayir H, Clark K, Rubin M, Stolz D, Vallhov H, Scheynius A, Witasp E, Fadeel B, Kichambare PD, Star A, Kisin ER, Murray AR, Shvedova AA, Kagan VE (2009) Phosphatidylserine targets single-walled carbon nanotubes to professional phagocytes in vitro and in vivo. *PLoS One* **4:** e4398.

Kopf-Maier P, Brauchle U, Heussler A (1988) Transplacental passage of titanium after treatment with titanocene dichloride. *Toxicology* **48:** 253–60.

Kreyling WG, Semmler-Behnke M, Seitz J, Scymczak W, Wenk A, Mayer P, Takenaka S, Oberdörster G (2009) Size dependence of the translocation of inhaled iridium and carbon nanoparticle aggregates from the lung of rats to the blood and secondary target organs. *Inhal Toxicol* **21 (Suppl. 1):** 55–60.

Kroto HW, Heath JR, O'Brien SC, Curl RF, Smalley RE (1985) C_{60}: Buckminsterfullerene. *Nature* **318:** 162–3.

Kuhlbusch T, Fissan H, Asbach C (2009) Nanotechnologies and environmental risks: measurement technologies and strategies. In *Nanomaterials: Risks and Benefits* (Linkov I, Steevens J, eds.). Dordrecht, Springer, pp. 233–43.

Lal S, Clare SE, Halas NJ (2008) Nanoshell-enabled photothermal cancer therapy: impending clinical impact. *Acc Chem Res* **41:** 1842–51.

Lam CW, James JT, McCluskey R, Arepalli S, Hunter RL (2006) A review of carbon nanotube toxicity and assessment of potential occupational and environmental health risks. *Crit Rev Toxicol* **36:** 189–217.

Lamoureux DP, Kobzik L, Fedulov AV (2010) Customized PCR-array analysis informed by gene-chip microarray and biological hypothesis reveals pathways involved in lung inflammatory response to titanium dioxide in pregnancy. *J Toxicol Environ Health A* **73:** 596–606.

Landsiedel R, Kapp MD, Schulz M, Wiench K, Oesch F (2009) Genotoxicity investigations on nanomaterials: methods, preparation and characterization of test material, potential artifacts and limitations – many questions, some answers. *Mutat Res* **681:** 241–58.

Larsen ST, Roursgaard M, Jensen KA, Nielsen GD (2010) Nano titanium dioxide particles promote allergic sensitization and lung inflammation in mice. *Basic Clin Pharmacol Toxicol* **106:** 114–17.

Latzin P, Roosli M, Huss A, Kuehni CE, Frey U (2009) Air pollution during pregnancy and lung function in newborns: a birth cohort study. *Eur Respir J* **33:** 594–603.

Lawson CC, Grajewski B, Daston GP, Frazier LM, Lynch D, McDiarmid M, Murono E, Perreault SD, Robbins WA, Ryan MA, Shelby M, Whelan EA (2006) Workgroup report: implementing a national occupational reproductive research agenda – decade one and beyond. *Environ Health Perspect* **114:** 435–41.

Li JG, Li WX, Xu JY, Cai XQ, Liu RL, Li YJ, Zhao QF, Li QN (2007) Comparative study of pathological lesions induced by multiwalled carbon nanotubes in lungs of mice by intratracheal instillation and inhalation. *Environ Toxicol* **22:** 415–21.

Liu Z, He Y, Li F, Liu Y (2006) Photocatalytic treatment of RDX wastewater with nano-sized titanium dioxide. *Environ Sci Pollut Res Int* **13:** 328–32.

Loutfy RO, Lowe TP, Moravesky AP, Katagiri S (2002) Commercial production of fullerenes and carbon nanotubes. In *Perspectives of Fullerene Nanotechnology*. Netherlands, Springer.

Ma L, Liu J, Li N, Wang J, Duan Y, Yan J, Liu H, Wang H, Hong F (2010) Oxidative stress in the brain of mice caused by translocated nanoparticulate TiO_2 delivered to the abdominal cavity. *Biomaterials* **31:** 99–105.

Mahalu D, Margulis L, Wold A, Tenne R (1992) Preparation of WSe2 surfaces with high photoactivity. *Phys Rev B Condens Matter* **45:** 1943–6.

Maynard AD (2002) Experimental determination of ultrafine TiO_2 de-agglomeration in surrogate pulmonary surfactant – preliminary results. *Ann Occup Hyg* **46:** 197–202.

Maynard AD, Aitken R (2007) Assessing exposure to airborne nanomaterials: current abilities and future requirements. *Nanotoxicology* **1:** 26–41.

Maynard AD, Aitken RJ, Butz T, Colvin V, Donaldson K, Oberdörster G, Philbert MA, Ryan J, Seaton A, Stone V, Tinkle SS, Tran L, Walker NJ, Warheit DB (2006) Safe handling of nanotechnology. *Nature* **444:** 267–9.

Maynard AD, Baron PA, Foley M, Shvedova AA, Kisin ER, Castranova V (2004) Exposure to carbon nanotube material: aerosol release during the handling of unrefined single-walled carbon nanotube material. *J Toxicol Environ Health A* **67:** 87–107.

Medintz IL, Mattoussi H (2009) Quantum dot-based resonance energy transfer and its growing application in biology. *Phys Chem Chem Phys* **11:** 17–45.

Melkonyan M, Kozyrev S (2009) The current state-of-the-art in the area of nanotechnology risk assessment in Russia. In *Nanomaterials: Risks and Benefits* (Linkov I, Steevens J, eds.). Dordrecht, Springer, pp. 309–15.

Meyer U, Feldon J, Fatemi SH (2009) In vivo rodent models for the experimental investigation of prenatal immune activation effects in neurodevelopmental brain disorders. *Neurosci Biobehav Rev* **33:** 1061–79.

Montanez MI, Ruiz-Sanchez AJ, Perez-Inestrosa E (2010) A perspective of nanotechnology in hypersensitivity reactions including drug allergy. *Curr Opin Allergy Clin Immunol.* In press.

Monteiller C, Tran L, MacNee W, Faux S, Jones A, Miller B, Donaldson K (2007) The pro-inflammatiory effects of low-toxicity low-solubility particles, nanoparticles and fine particles, on epithelial cells in vitro: the role of surface area. *Occup Environ Med* **64:** 609–15.

Muller J, Decordier I, Hoet PH, Lombaert N, Thomassen L, Huaux F, Lison D, Kirsch-Volders M (2008) Clastogenic and aneugenic effects of multi-wall carbon nanotubes in epithelial cells. *Carcinogenesis* **29:** 427–33.

Murphy CJ, Gole AM, Stone JW, Sisco PN, Alkilany AM, Goldsmith EC, Baxter SC (2008) Gold nanoparticles in biology: beyond toxicity to cellular imaging. *Acc Chem Res* **41:** 1721–30.

Myllynen PK, Loughran MJ, Howard CV, Sormunen R, Walsh AA, Vahakangas KH (2008) Kinetics of gold nanoparticles in the human placenta. *Reprod Toxicol* **26:** 130–7.

Nadagouda MN, Varma R (2009) Risk reduction via greener synthesis of noble metal nanostructures. In *Nanomaterials: Risks and Benefits* (Linkov I, Steevens J, eds.). Dordrecht, Springer, pp. 209–17.

Nandiyanto ABD, Iskandar F, Okuyama K (2008) Nano-sized polymer particle-facilitated preparation of mesoporous silica particles using a spray method. *Chemistry Letters* **37:** 1040.

Nandiyanto ABD, Kim S-GFI, Okuyama K (2009) Synthesis of silica nanoparticles with nanometer-size controllable mesopores and outer diameters. *Microporous and Mesoporous Materials* **120:** 447–53.

NIOSH (2009) Current Intelligence Bulletin 60: Interim Guidance for Medical Screening and Hazard Surveillance for Workers Potentially Exposed to Engineered Nanoparticles. Ref Type: Report.

Nørgaard AW, Jensen KA, Janfelt C, Lauritzen FR, Clausen PA, Wolkoff P (2009) Release of VOCs and particles during use of nanofilm spray products. *Environ Sci Technol* **43:** 7824–30.

Nurkiewicz TR, Porter DW, Hubbs AF, Cumpston JL, Chen BT, Frazer DG, Castranova V (2008) Nanoparticle inhalation augments particle-dependent systemic microvascular dysfunction. *Part Fibre Toxicol* **5:** 1.

Nygaard UC, Hansen JS, Samuelsen M, Alberg T, Marioara CD, Lovik M (2009) Single-walled and multi-walled carbon nanotubes promote allergic immune responses in mice. *Toxicol Sci* **109:** 113–23.

Oberdörster G, Elder A, Rinderknecht A (2009) Nanoparticles and the brain: cause for concern? *J Nanosci Nanotechnol* **9:** 4996–5007.

Oberdörster G, Ferin J, Lehnert BE (1994) Correlation between particle size, in vivo particle persistence, and lung injury. *Environ Health Perspect* **102 (Suppl. 5):** 173–9.

Oberdörster G, Oberdörster E, Oberdörster J (2005) Nanotoxicology: an emerging discipline evolving from studies of ultrafine particles. *Environ Health Perspect* **113:** 823–39.

Oberdörster G, Sharp Z, Atudorei V, Elder A, Gelein R, Kreyling W, Cox C (2004) Translocation of inhaled ultrafine particles to the brain. *Inhal Toxicol* **16:** 437–45.

Oberdörster G, Sharp Z, Atudorei V, Elder A, Gelein R, Lunts A, Kreyling W, Cox C (2002) Extrapulmonary translocation of ultrafine carbon particles following whole-body inhalation exposure of rats. *J Toxicol Environ Health* **45:** 1531–43.

OECD. OECD Quantitative Structure Activity Relationships [(Q)SARs] Project (2008) OECD Environment Directorate. Report.

Owen R, Crane M, Grieger K, Handy R, Linkov I, Depkedge M (2009) Strategic approaches for the management of environmental risk uncertainties posed by nanomaterials. In *Nanomaterials: Risks and Benefits* (Linkov I, Steevens J, eds.). Dordrecht, Springer, pp. 369–84.

Park EJ, Cho WS, Jeong J, Yi J, Choi K, Park K (2009a) Pro-inflammatory and potential allergic responses resulting from B cell activation in mice treated with multi-walled carbon nanotubes by intratracheal instillation. *Toxicology* **259:** 113–21.

Park JH, Gu L, von MG, Ruoslahti E, Bhatia SN, Sailor MJ (2009b) Biodegradable luminescent porous silicon nanoparticles for in vivo applications. *Nat Mater* **8:** 331–6.

Park MV, Annema W, Salvati A, Lesniak A, Elsaesser A, Barnes C, McKerr G, Howard CV, Lynch I, Dawson KA, Piersma AH, de Jong WH (2009c) In vitro developmental toxicity test detects inhibition of stem cell differentiation by silica nanoparticles. *Toxicol Appl Pharmacol* **240:** 108–16.

Peng T, Zhao D, Dai K, Shi W, Hirao K (2005) Synthesis of titanium dioxide nanoparticles with mesoporous anatase wall and high photocatalytic activity. *J Phys Chem B* **109:** 4947–52.

Penn AL, Rouse RL, Horohov DW, Kearney MT, Paulsen DB, Lomax L (2007) In utero exposure to environmental tobacco smoke potentiates adult responses to allergen in BALB/c mice. *Environ Health Perspect* **115:** 548–55.

Peters TM, Elzey S, Johnson R, Park H, Grassian VH, Maher T, O'Shaughnessy P (2009) Airborne monitoring to distinguish engineered nanomaterials from incidental particles for environmental health and safety. *J Occup Environ Hyg* **6:** 73–81.

Poland CA, Duffin R, Kinloch I, Maynard A, Wallace WA, Seaton A, Stone V, Brown S, MacNee W, Donaldson K (2008) Carbon nanotubes introduced into the abdominal cavity of mice show asbestos-like pathogenicity in a pilot study. *Nat Nanotechnol* **3:** 423–8.

Rothenbacher S, Messerer A, Kasper G (2008) Fragmentation and bond strength of airborne diesel soot agglomerates. *Part Fibre Toxicol* **5:** 9.

Ryman-Rasmussen JP, Tewksbury EW, Moss OR, Cesta MF, Wong BA, Bonner JC. (2009) Inhaled multiwalled carbon nanotubes potentiate airway fibrosis in murine allergic asthma. *Am J Resp Cell Mol Biol* **40:** 349–58.

Rzigalinski BA, Strobl JS (2009) Cadmium-containing nanoparticles: perspectives on pharmacology and toxicology of quantum dots. *Toxicol Appl Pharmacol* **238:** 280–8.

Sadauskas E, Wallin H, Stoltenberg M, Vogel U, Doering P, Larsen A, Danscher G (2007) Kupffer cells are central in the removal of nanoparticles from the organism. *Part Fibre Toxicol* **4:** 10.

Sakamoto Y, Nakae D, Fukumori N, Tayama K, Maekawa A, Imai K, Hirose A, Nishimura T, Ohashi N, Ogata A (2009) Induction of mesothelioma by a single intrascrotal administration of multi-wall carbon nanotube in intact male Fischer 344 rats. *J Toxicol Sci* **34:** 65–76.

Salata O (2004) Applications of nanoparticles in biology and medicine. *J Nanobiotechnol* **2:** 3.

Saunders M (2009) Transplacental transport of nanomaterials. *Wiley Interdiscip Rev Nanomed Nanobiotechnol* **1:** 671–84.

Savolainen K, Alenius H, Norppa H, Pylkkänen L, Tuomi T, Kasper G (2010) Risk assessment of engineered nanomaterials and nanotechnologies – a review. *Toxicology* **269:** 92–104.

Sayes CM, Wahi R, Kurian PA, Liu Y, West JL, Ausman KD, Warheit DB, Colvin VL (2006) Correlating nanoscale titania structure with toxicity: a cytotoxicity and inflammatory response study with human dermal fibroblasts and human lung epithelial cells. *Toxicol Sci* **92:** 174–85.

SCCP (2007) Opinion on safety of nanomaterials in cosmetic products. European Commission, Health and Consumer Protection DG, Brussels. Scientific Committee on Consumer Products. Ref Type: Electronic Citation.

SCENIHR (2007) Opinion on the appropiateness of the risk assessment methodology in accordance with the technical guidance documents for new and existing substances for assessing the risks of nanomaterials. European Commission, Health and Consumer Protection DG, Brussels. Scientific Committee on Emerging and Newly-Identified Health Risks. Ref Type: Electronic Citation.

Schulte PA, Schubauer-Berigan MK, Mayweather C, Geraci CL, Zumwalde R, McKernan JL (2009) Issues in the development of epidemiologic studies of workers exposed to engineered nanoparticles. *J Occup Environ Med* **51:** 323–35.

Schulte PA, Trout D, Zumwalde RD, Kuempel E, Geraci CL, Castranova V, Mundt DJ, Mundt KA, Halperin WE (2008) Options for occupational health surveillance of workers potentially exposed to engineered nanoparticles: state of the science. *J Occup Environ Med* **50:** 517–26.

Seipenbusch M, Binder A, Kasper G (2008) Temporal evolution of nanoparticle aerosols in workplace exposure. *Ann Occup Hyg* **52:** 707–16.

Semmler-Behnke M, Fertsch S, Schmid G, Wenk A, Keryling WG (2007) Uptake of 1.4 nm versus 18 nm gold particles by secondary target organs is size dependent in control and pregnant rats after intratracheal or intravenous application. *Nanotoxicology Abstract Book*, 14. Ref Type: Abstract.

Shimada T, Sugai T, Ohno Y, Kishimoto S, Mizutani T, Yoshida H, Okazaki T, Shinohara H (2004) Double-wall carbon nanotube field-effect transistors: ambipolar transport characteristics. *Appl Phys Lett* **84:** 2412–14.

Shimizu M, Tainaka H, Oba T, Mizuo K, Umezawa M, Takeda K (2009) Maternal exposure to nanoparticulate titanium dioxide during the prenatal period alters gene expression related to brain development in the mouse. *Part Fibre Toxicol* **6:** 20.

Shvedova AA, Kagan VE, Fadeel B (2010) Close encounters of the small kind: adverse effects of man-made materials interfacing with the nano-cosmos of biological systems. *Annu Rev Pharmacol Toxicol* **50:** 63–88.

Shvedova AA, Kisin ER, Mercer R, Murray AR, Johnson VJ, Potapovich AI, Tyurina YY, Gorelik O, Arepalli S, Schwegler-Berry D, Hubbs AF, Antonini J, Evans DE, Ku BK, Ramsey D, Maynard A, Kagan VE, Castranova V, Baron P (2005) Unusual inflammatory and fibrogenic pulmonary responses to single-walled carbon nanotubes in mice. *Am J Physiol Lung Cell Mol Physiol* **289:** L698–L708.

Shvedova AA, Kisin ER, Murray AR, Gorelik O, Arepalli S, Castranova V, Young SH, Gao F, Tyurina YY, Oury TD, Kagan VE (2007) Vitamin E deficiency enhances pulmonary inflammatory response and oxidative stress induced by single-walled carbon nanotubes in C57BL/6 mice. *Toxicol Appl Pharmacol* **221:** 339–48.

Shvedova AA, Kisin ER, Porter D, Schulte P, Kagan VE, Fadeel B, Castranova V (2009) Mechanisms of pulmonary toxicity and medical applications of carbon nanotubes: two faces of Janus? *Pharmacol Ther* **121:** 192–204.

Sidiropoulos D, Herrmann U Jr, Morell A, von MG, Barandun S (1986) Transplacental passage of intravenous immunoglobulin in the last trimester of pregnancy. *J Pediatr* **109:** 505–8.

Singh SP, Barrett EG, Kalra R, Razani-Boroujerdi S, Langley RJ, Kurup V, Tesfaigzi Y, Sopori ML (2003) Prenatal cigarette smoke decreases lung cAMP and increases airway hyperresponsiveness. *Am J Respir Crit Care Med* **168:** 342–7.

Singh SP, Mishra NC, Rir-Sima-Ah J, Campen M, Kurup V, Razani-Boroujerdi S, Sopori ML (2009) Maternal exposure to secondhand cigarette smoke primes the lung for induction of phosphodiesterase-4D5 isozyme and exacerbated Th2 responses: rolipram attenuates the airway hyperreactivity and muscarinic receptor expression but not lung inflammation and atopy. *J Immunol* **183:** 2115–21.

Skrabalak SE, Chen J, Sun Y, Lu X, Au L, Cobley CM, Xia Y (2008) Gold nanocages: synthesis, properties, and applications. *Acc Chem Res* **41:** 1587–95.

Somani PR, Somani SP, Lau SP, Flahaut E, Tanemura M, Umeno M (2007) Field electron emission of double walled carbon nanotube film prepared by drop casting method. *Solid-State Electronics* **51:** 788–92.

Speit G (2002) Appropriate in vitro test conditions for genotoxicity testing of fibers. *Inhal Toxicol* **14:** 79–90.

Srivastava VK, Chauhan SS, Srivastava PK, Kumar V, Misra UK (1986) Fetal translocation and metabolism of PAH obtained from coal fly ash given intratracheally to pregnant rats. *J Toxicol Environ Health* **18:** 459–69.

Takagi A, Hirose A, Nishimura T, Fukumori N, Ogata A, Ohashi N, Kitajima S, Kanno J (2008) Induction of mesothelioma in p53+/− mouse by intraperitoneal application of multi-wall carbon nanotube. *J Toxicol Sci* **33:** 105–16.

Takahashi S, Matsuoka O (1981) Cross placental transfer of (1981) Au-colloid in near term rats. *J Radiat Res (Tokyo)* **22:** 242–9.

Takeda K, Suzuki K, Ishihara A, Kubo-Irie M, Fujimoto R, Tabata M, Oshio S, Nihei Y, Ihara T, Sugamata M (2009) Nanoparticles transferred from pregnant mice to their offspring can damage the genital and cranial nerve systems. *J Health Sci* **55:** 95–102.

Tenne R, Remskar M, Enyashin A, Seifert G (2008) Inorganic nanotubes and fullerene-like structures. In *Carbon Nanotubes* (Jorio A, Dresselhaus G, Dresselhaus MS, eds.). Berlin Heidelberg, Springer-Verlag, pp. 631–71.

Thompson J, Bannigan J (2008) Cadmium: toxic effects on the reproductive system and the embryo. *Reprod Toxicol* **25:** 304–15.

Tian F, Razansky D, Estrada GG, Semmler-Behnke M, Beyerle A, Kreyling W, Ntziachristos V, Stoeger T (2009) Surface modification and size dependence in particle translocation during early embryonic development. *Inhal Toxicol* **21:** 92–6.

Tozuka Y, Watanabe N, Osawa M, Toriba A, Kizu R, Hayakawa K (2004) Transfer of polycyclic aromatic hydrocarbons to fetuses and breast milk of rats exposed to diesel exhaust. *J Health Sci* **50:** 497–502.

Tsuchiya T, Oguri I, Yamakoshi YN, Miyata N (1996) Novel harmful effects of [60]fullerene on mouse embryos in vitro and in vivo. *FEBS Lett* **393:** 139–45.

United States Environmental Protection Agency (1991) Guidelines for developmental toxicity risk assessment. *Fed Regist* **56:** 63798–826.

US Environmental Protection Agency. Nanomaterials Research Strategy. EPA 620/K-09/011 (2009) Washington DC. Office of Research and Development, US Environmental Protection Agency. Ref Type: Report.

Usenko CY, Harper SL, Tanguay RL (2007) In vivo evaluation of carbon fullerene toxicity using embryonic zebrafish. *Carbon NY* **45:** 1891–8.

Wang H, Brandl DW, Le F, Nordlander P, Halas NJ (2006) Nanorice: a hybrid plasmonic nanostructure. *Nano Lett* **6:** 827–32.

Warheit DB, Hoke RA, Finlay C, Donner EM, Reed KL, Sayes CM (2007) Development of a base set of toxicity tests using ultrafine TiO_2 particles as a component of nanoparticle risk management. *Toxicol Lett* **171:** 99–110.

Watanabe N, Ohsawa M (2002) Elevated serum immunoglobulin E to Cryptomeria japonica pollen in rats exposed to diesel exhaust during fetal and neonatal periods. *BMC Pregnancy Childbirth* **2:** 2–11.

Wick P, Malek A, Manser P, Meili D, Maeder-Althaus X, Diener L, Diener PA, Zisch A, Krug HF, von MU (2010) Barrier capacity of human placenta for nanosized materials. *Environ Health Perspect* **118:** 432–6.

Wirnitzer U, Herbold B, Voetz M, Ragot J (2009) Studies on the in vitro genotoxicity of baytubes, agglomerates of engineered multi-walled carbon-nanotubes (MWCNT). *Toxicol Lett* **186:** 160–5.

Woodrow Wilson. Woodrow Wilson International Centre for Scholars (2010) Ref Type: Electronic Citation.

Xia T, Kovochich M, Brant J, Hotze M, Sempf J, Oberley T, Sioutas C, Yeh JI, Wiesner MR, Nel AE (2006) Comparison of the abilities of ambient and manufactured nanoparticles to induce cellular toxicity according to an oxidative stress paradigm. *Nano Lett* **6:** 1794–807.

Xia T, Kovochich M, Liong M, Madler L, Gilbert B, Shi H, Yeh JI, Zink JI, Nel AE (2008) Comparison of the mechanism of toxicity of zinc oxide and cerium oxide nanoparticles based on dissolution and oxidative stress properties. *ACS Nano* **2:** 2121–34.

Yang H, Liu C, Yang D, Zhang H, Xi Z (2009) Comparative study of cytotoxicity, oxidative stress and genotoxicity induced by four typical nanomaterials: the role of particle size, shape and composition. *J Appl Toxicol* **29:** 69–78.

Yang HL, Lin JC, Huang C (2009) Application of nanosilver surface modification to RO membrane and spacer for mitigating biofouling in seawater desalination. *Water Res.* **43:** 3777–86.

Yang ST, Wang X, Jia G, Gu Y, Wang T, Nie H, Ge C, Wang H, Liu Y (2008) Long-term accumulation and low toxicity of single-walled carbon nanotubes in intravenously exposed mice. *Toxicol Lett* **181:** 182–9.

Yoshida S, Hiyoshi K, Oshio S, Takano H, Takeda K, Ichinose T (2009) Effects of fetal exposure to carbon nanoparticles on reproductive function in male offspring. *Fertil Steril* **93:** 1695–9.

Zhu X, Wang J, Zhang X, Chang Y, Chen Y (2009) The impact of ZnO nanoparticle aggregates on the embryonic development of zebrafish (Danio rerio). *Nanotechnology* **20:** 195103.

Zhu X, Zhu L, Li Y, Duan Z, Chen W, Alvarez PJ (2007) Developmental toxicity in zebrafish (Danio rerio) embryos after exposure to manufactured nanomaterials: buckminsterfullerene aggregates (nC60) and fullerol. *Environ Toxicol Chem* **26:** 976–9.

CHAPTER

22

Effects of radiation on the reproductive system

Kausik Ray and Rajani Choudhuri

INTRODUCTION

The effects of radiation on the reproductive system in humans have been extensively explored through events in which a large number of the population were exposed (Harley, 2001, 2008). Many of these studies are now well known, such as the case of radium dial painters, survivors of the atomic bomb, workers and residents around Chernobyl and uranium miners exposed to radon soil gas, and to the short-lived radon daughter isotopes. Occupational hazards are also well documented in reproductive epidemiological research when workers are exposed to high doses of ionizing radiation accidentally during their occupation as compared to environmental radiation exposure. Also, radiotherapy treatment of cancer patients leads to radiation-induced hazards that can have a profound effect on reproductive function. The effects of radiation have been known since the 1920s and the reproductive systems of both males and females are highly sensitive to radiation. A large number of experimental data are available on the adverse effects of radiation on the male and female reproductive systems of various animal species and from reproductive data on human beings. The biological response to radiation varies among different tissues and organs and the total dose and number of fractions are important determinants of the radiobiological effect. However, the concept of dose–response and time–response applies to radiation-induced toxicity just like any other branch of toxicology (Harley, 2008). This chapter will provide an overview of radiation dose and risk, the reproductive consequences of exposure to radiation, some historical perspectives and new details on involvements of novel regulatory inputs in reproductive functions as potential targets to preserve fertility after radiation exposure.

RADIATION DOSE AND RISK

A radiation dose to tissue is expressed as *absorbed energy per unit tissue mass*. The unit of radiation dose is the *gray* (Gy), which is quantified as 1 joule/kg. The older unit *rad* is also used (1 rad = 0.01 Gy). The harmful effects of radiation depend upon the absorbed dose (energy). Radiation hits an absorbing medium and transfers or deposits the energy to the medium. The rate at which energy (E) is transferred to the absorbing medium per unit distance (l) traversed by the radiation is called *linear energy transfer* or LET (L). It is quantified as $L = dE/dl$; if the distance traversed is measured in mm, then $L = keV/mm$. Therefore, high LET radiations, such as α-particles, neutrons, heavy ions, pions (also known as pi mesons) will lose, i.e. deposit in the absorbing medium, greater amounts of energy than low LET radiations, such as γ-rays, X-rays, electrons. When living tissue is exposed to radiation, the energy deposited to the tissue causes ionizations and generates free radicals which, in turn, cause macromolecular damage. Thus, high LET radiations can be more destructive to biological materials than low LET radiations if they penetrate the tissue equally because at the same dose, low LET radiations induce the same number of radicals more sparsely within a cell, whereas high LET radiations transfer most of their energy to a small region of the cell. Ironically, because the high LET radiations deposit a greater amount of energy to the absorbing medium, they are not able to penetrate the medium far enough. If humans are exposed to high LET radiations, the radiation will deposit more energy at the skin surface and thus may not be able to penetrate deep into the tissue. Thus, in order for the alpha emitters to be very damaging, they have to be inhaled or ingested. The localized DNA damage caused by dense ionizations from high LET radiations is more difficult to repair than the diffuse DNA damage caused by the sparse ionizations from low LET radiations.

An absorbed dose of 1 Gy generates about 2×10^5 ionizations within the mammalian cell. Approximately 1% of these ionizations occur in the DNA itself (Adams and Cox, 1997), which can cause DNA damage. Each tract from X-irradiation of gamma rays results in about 70 events across the width of the nucleus for ~0.5 rads (5 mGy). Alternatively, a 400 MeV alpha track may produce as many as 30,000 events across the same nucleus for ~300 rads (3 Gy). Within the nucleus even low LET gamma radiation may produce some microregions of relatively dense ionizations in the DNA region. The threshold is very low for some single strand breaks (Panajotovic *et al.*, 2006 cited in Harley, 2008). DNA damage involves both single-strand and double-strand breaks, and most of these lesions are repaired within a few hours. Single-strand breaks, which are more frequently caused by low LET radiations, are more readily repaired than double-strand breaks.

Reproductive and Developmental Toxicology, Edited by Ramesh C. Gupta
ISBN: 978-0-12-382032-7

Double-strand breaks are also more detrimental to maintaining genome integrity.

Ionizing radiation results in the generation of free radicals, which causes oxidative stress in the cell/tissue. These free radicals cause severe damage to cellular macromolecules including nuclear DNA (Wu *et al.*, 1999; Spitz *et al.*, 2004). A cell's oxidative status plays an important role not only at the time of radiation exposure, but also long after exposure. Radiation exposure may produce free radicals for several minutes or even hours after exposure (Spitz *et al.*, 2004). At the cytological level an extension of radiation-induced DNA damage is chromosome breakage. Radiation can induce aberrant intrachromosomal crossing-over that involves one or both chromatids. Radiation can also induce non-disjunction of homologous chromosomes resulting in trisomy in the F_1 offsprings, as well as other chromosomal aberrations, such as translocations and deletions (Adams and Cox, 1997). Chromosomal breaks have been shown to occur at a higher frequency in certain fragile sites. In other words, depending on the energy, radiation can cause increased genomic instability. Thus, radiation exposure can cause severe damage to the reproductive tissues resulting in infertility, mutation that can be passed on to the next generation or miscarriage in the case of pregnant women.

RADIATION EXPOSURE AND GENETICS HAZARDS

Possible genetic effects of radiation exposure on future generations are real concerns for men and women who have had radiation exposures. Radiation exposures may impact the development of sperm and eggs (ova) or may potentially expose the fetus or embryo to radiation that lead to birth defects and genetic diseases. Many diagnostic procedures expose women who are pregnant to X-rays, computerized tomography (CT or CAT) scans, fluoroscopy or radiation therapy, or an administered radioactive material. Most diagnostic procedures expose the fetus to less than 5 rad or 50 mSv and this level of radiation exposure is believed not to increase reproductive risks such as birth defects or miscarriage. Various published reports suggest an increased incidence of birth defects or miscarriage is above 20 rad or 200 mSv and correlate with higher radiation doses (Wo and Viswanathan, 2009). Diagnostic X-ray studies may involve direct radiation exposure of the developing fetus. In this scenario, the X-ray beam may or may not be directed toward the embryo or ovary. Since radiation therapy treatment for cancer involves very high doses of radiation, in the thousands of rad, it is very likely that the fetus will be affected if radiation therapy is initiated to the woman during pregnancy. Irrespective of these radiation exposure risk factors, it is important to realize that a woman who begins pregnancy has a reproductive risk of 3% for major birth defects in the embryo and 15% for miscarriage, depending on the family history and her own reproductive health. Similarly, men exposed to radiation therapy and receiving large doses of radiation may have exposed the testes to radiation. The concern is whether testicular radiation exposure and, therefore, exposure to the sperm will result in birth defects. The risk from radiation exposure of sperm prior to conception has been studied in two large populations. In one study, thousands of patients who were exposed to radiation in Hiroshima and Nagasaki in Japan and had families were studied for incidence of genetic diseases and other reproductive effects. After 50 years of studying this population, there has been little demonstrable increase in genetic diseases and thus the risk of radiation-induced genetic damage is too small to be detected (Neel *et al.*, 1990; Otake *et al.*, 1990). In another large study, families of several thousand individuals who have survived cancer and received large doses of radiation in childhood, adolescence or early adulthood have been studied by the National Cancer Institute in collaboration with three hospital-based registries and two population-based registries (Byrne *et al.*, 1998). These family members demonstrated no increase in birth defects and miscarriages. These studies provide reassurance that radiation treatment did not have an increased incidence in genetic disease or birth defects in the next generation. A massive international study is now under way on the possible genetic effects of radiation exposure on future generations (University of Oklahoma, October 8, 2009; Genetic effects of radiation: study will help understand radiation exposure in cancer survivors and their children; retrieved May 20, 2010, from http://www.sciencedaily.com/releases/2009/10/091007171739.htm). This study combines cancer survivors in the USA and Scandinavia, and examines potential genetic consequences of reproductive organs exposed to curative therapy by drugs or radiation. In these studies, the scientists will determine whether radiation or chemotherapy before conception increases the occurrence of birth defects, cancer, DNA damage, stillbirths and genetic defects such as Down's syndrome.

The accident at the Chernobyl nuclear power station on April 26, 1986 was the most serious accidental release of radiation in the 20th century. Release of radiation and radioactive materials into the atmosphere produced the most serious atmospheric contamination over more than 100,000 square km of territories in Ukraine, Belorussia and Russia. Twenty-four years after the accident, the areas contaminated by radionuclides show complex medical and demographical conditions compared to unaffected neighboring areas. These complex medical issues include lower birth rates, relatively higher number of stillborns and high infant mortality. The UN, WHO, International Atomic Energy Agency and government organizations from Russia, Belarus and Ukraine undertook a major study and in 2005 released their findings. They found no evidence of an increased risk of birth defects or other reproductive effects in areas contaminated by radiation. This study was highly criticized and controversy surrounding the true toll of fallout from the Chernobyl disaster has been questioned in several studies. A comprehensive survey of 688 pregnant women and their babies was carried out over an 8-year period (Kulakov *et al.*, 1993). The results showed that the health of mothers, fetuses and children were significantly influenced by the radiation. Although the female reproductive system remained relatively intact, adaptational and pathological abnormalities of various organs and body systems of pregnant women and children caused complex patterns of bodily dysfunction. Similar patterns of general deterioration of the health of mothers and children in all polluted areas of Ukraine, Belorussia and Russia were observed. Fetoplacental disorders also caused long-term and chronic diseases in the newborns. Hyperproduction of red blood cells and hemoglobin in response to stress was seen in babies in their first year of life following the accident. Even after 4 years since the accident, erythropenia, monoblastosis, anisocytosis and poikilocytosis were found in the newborns and these changes were progressive. Some recent studies have also found continuing health effects and a rise in birth defects in regions most affected by this catastrophe (Kozenko and Chudley, 2010; Wertelecki, 2010). Therefore, it is important to re-evaluate the health effects of the Chernobyl nuclear disaster and continue more comprehensive studies to understand whether the Chernobyl disaster and birth defects are linked.

RADIATION EXPOSURE AND HYPOTHALAMUS–PITUITARY–GONADAL (HPG) AXIS DYSFUNCTION

Morphological features of the hypothalamus and pituitary gland are similar for males and females across species. Reproduction in both the male and female is controlled by a complex series of hormonal interactions that begin in the hypothalamus–pituitary–gonadal (HPG) axis located at the base of the brain. Normal function of the hormonal circuit of the HPG axis is crucial for the maturation of the reproductive organs and functions in both sexes, as well as the maintenance of gonadal hormone production and gametogenesis in adult life. The medial basal hypothalamus in humans contains an interconnected group of secretory neurons that produce gonadotropin-releasing hormone (GnRH) with periodic pulsatile release of GnRH. The anterior pituitary lobe is composed of a heterogeneous population of cells arranged in irregular cords and masses. A subpopulation of glandular cells (10% or so) constitutes gonadotroph cells and are of special interest for this chapter as these cells secrete hormones called gonadotropins including luteinizing hormone (LH) and follicle-stimulating hormone (FSH). In response to GnRH, the pituitary gland secretes the gonadotropins, LH and FSH, in a pulsatile manner. These gonadotropins act together and in turn induce testicular and ovarian production of sex steroid hormones and gametogenesis. The timely secretion of gonadal sex steroids is also essential for the initiation of puberty and the post-pubertal maintenance of secondary sexual characteristics, among other features. Figure 22.1 illustrates the normal HPG axis and negative feedback controls by gonadal steroid hormones. It has been known for many years that the HPG axis is susceptible to negative feedback regulation from the gonads by sex steroids. With gonadal dysfunction, that is, testicular or ovarian failure, the loss of negative feedback by testosterone or estradiol causes high concentrations of gonadotropins (LH and FSH). In contrast, abnormalities of the hypothalamus or pituitary result in low concentrations of both gonadotropins and sex hormones. However, the mediator (s) of steroid hormone feedback has remained elusive for many years, as GnRH neurons do not possess estrogen receptor alpha (ERα), progesterone receptor

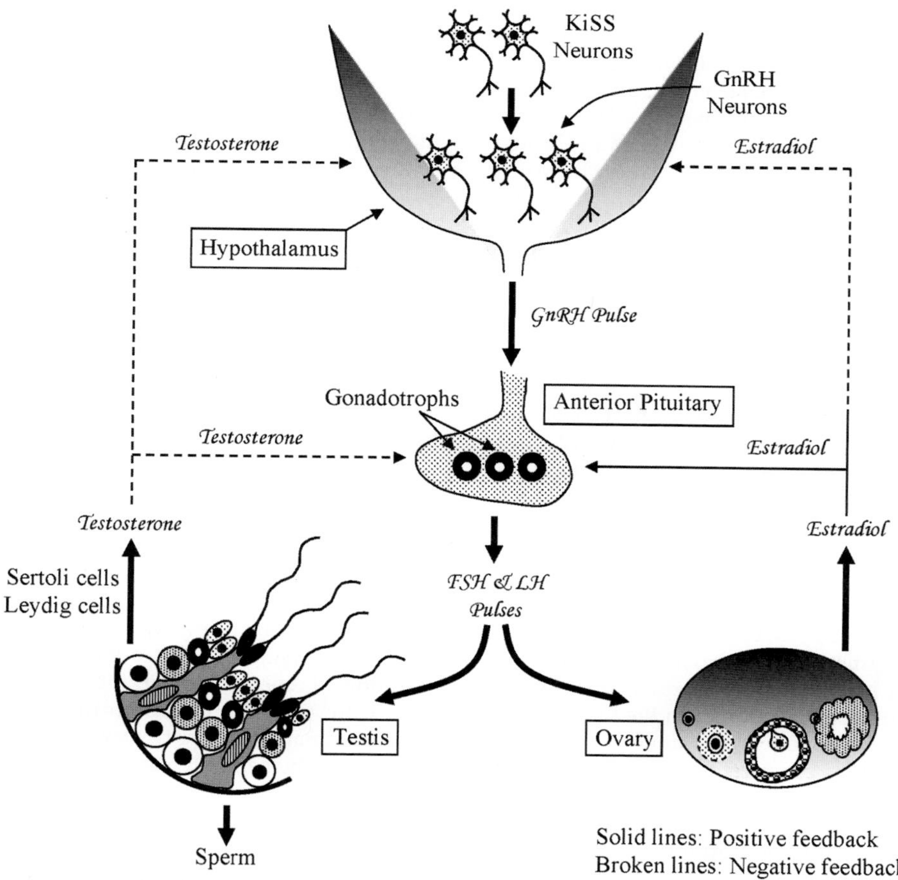

FIGURE 22.1 Schematic representation of the hypothalamus–pituitary–gonadal (HPG) axis. Negative feedback of testosterone and estradiol on the HPG axis decreases FSH and LH release. In males, LH stimulates testosterone production from the Leydig cells in the testes, and FSH along with testosterone promotes spermatogenesis. In males, Leydig cells release androgens of which testosterone plays a critical role in sperm production. Androgen synthesis in Leydig cells is controlled by LH with negative feedback of testosterone on the HPG axis. In females, FSH promotes ovarian follicle development and LH promotes ovulation and formation of corpus luteum. An estradiol peak stimulates pulsatile LH release which results in ovulation.

(PR) and androgen receptor (AR) that are known to play roles in feedback regulation. Therefore, neurons upstream of the GnRH neurons which may contain these receptors have been sought as possible mediators of steroid effects on the GnRH neuron. A breakthrough in understanding the regulation of GnRH synthesis and secretion has been made by the discovery of the G-protein-coupled receptor GPR54 or KiSS1R and its ligand, kisspeptin, a product of the KiSS-1 gene, implicated as masterpieces in the neuroendocrine control of the HPG axis (de Roux *et al.*, 2003; Seminara *et al.*, 2003). Since then the KiSS-1/GPR54 system has been found to play an important role in triggering puberty in humans and experimental animals (Gottsh *et al.*, 2004; Kauffman *et al.*, 2007; Gianetti and Seminara, 2008). Kisspeptin neurons express ERα, PR and AR and therefore relay feedback effects on the GnRH neuron. Regulation of KiSS-1 expression is a likely mediator of negative feedback in mammals and evidence now suggests that sex steroids can negatively regulate KiSS-1 expression (Smith *et al.*, 2006; Adachi *et al.*, 2007; Rance, 2008).

In humans, the gonadal endocrine system is active *in utero* before entering a state of quiescence. The reactivation of the GnRH pulsatory release system is the earliest detectable event at puberty but the suppression and then rekindling of this system at puberty are critical enigma of reproductive biology. Although these basic principles of this complex regulatory circuit have been known for a long time, new details about involvements of novel regulatory inputs and the genes responsible are emerging rapidly. Regulatory molecules such as KAL1, NELF, FGFR1, PROK1 and PROK2 have been identified which are essential for the embryonic migration of GnRH neurons to the hypothalamus from the olfactory placode. Humans with genetic defects in these molecules fail to enter puberty (Cadman *et al.*, 2007). Recent studies through a combination of human and mouse genetics also identified a large number of genes that are potentially involved in sex determination, fertility and in the HPG axis (Crowley *et al.*, 2008). Moreover, several single gene disorders affect HPG function and fertility in humans (Achermann and Jameson, 1999; Huhtaniemi and Alevizaki, 2007; Plant, 2008). Although a detailed discussion of these genetic disorders is beyond the scope of this chapter, it is important to know that these disorders have provided insight into many genes that might regulate reproductive function. It should be emphasized that radiation exposure does not create new mutations in humans but increases the frequency of mutations occurring naturally in the general population. Thus radiation-induced mutations affecting the endocrine regulation of the HPG axis are rare; however, they should be known and kept in mind.

Radiation damage is a potent cause of dysfunction in the HPG and subtle to severe abnormalities in HPG axis function are frequently seen in cancer survivors who have received prophylactic or therapeutic cranial irradiation. In therapeutic cranial irradiation, such damage may occur in cases where the hypothalamus and pituitary fall within the radiotherapy field. Deficiency of one or more hypothalamic releasing hormones and anterior pituitary hormones has been reported following therapeutic cranial irradiation for nasopharyngeal tumors, primary brain tumors, tumors involving HPA and solid tumors of the face and neck. Anterior pituitary hormone deficiencies represent the most common complications of successful cancer therapy in both children and adults. Such deficiencies exert negative effects on body image, growth, skeletal health, sexual function and other aspects of quality of life. For the sake of simplicity, we will focus only on radiation-induced hormone deficiencies related to HPG dysfunction and effects on the reproductive system. Clinical studies provide sufficient evidence that radiation inflicts damage to both hypothalamus and pituitary and results in multiple hormone deficiencies (Samaan *et al.*, 1982; Constine *et al.*, 1993; Agha *et al.*, 2005). Some studies have suggested that the hypothalamus is affected by radiation damage with doses less than 40 Gy, whereas other studies support the opposite scenario, suggesting radiation-induced damage to the pituitary occurs even at lower doses and that the pituitary might be the predominant site of radiation damage (Ogilvy-Stuart and Shalet, 1993). Gonadotropin deficiency is unusual after a low dose of radiation therapy (i.e., below 40 Gy) but an increased incidence of gonadotropin deficiency is seen after intensive radiation schedules. Gonadotropin deficiency can be detected by GnRH testing which can help to distinguish between hypothalamic and pituitary causes for such a condition. Severe gonadotropin impairment is associated with reduced circulating sex hormone levels, by normal or low normal basal LH and/or FSH levels, with reduced circulating sex hormone concentrations and impaired fertility. Gonadotropin deficiency can delay puberty onset and progression but it occurs more frequently in adults than children. Repeated intermittent infusions of GnRH might restore pituitary responsiveness and prolonged treatment can potentially restore gonadal function and fertility.

Early and precocious puberty occurs in some children receiving cranial irradiation for brain tumors and acute lymphoblastic leukemia. By definition, precocious puberty means development of any secondary sexual characteristic before the age of 8 years in girls and 9 years in boys. Radiation doses below 50 Gy can cause premature activation of the HPG, and result in precocious puberty. Radiation doses of 25–50 Gy results in precocious puberty in both boys and girls equally. Lower doses (18–24 Gy), however, give rise to precocious puberty almost exclusively in girls (Leiper *et al.*, 1983, 1987). Radiation-induced precocious puberty might be caused by damage to the inhibitory feedback system in the HPG thereby prematurely reactivating GnRH release from hypothalamic neurons with increased frequency and amplitude of GnRH pulsatile secretion. Patients who develop precocious puberty remain at risk of delayed gonadotropin deficiency, especially those who received radiation doses in excess of 30 Gy (Brauner *et al.*, 1983).

RADIATION EFFECTS ON MALE REPRODUCTIVE SYSTEM

The testicle is one of the most radiosensitive organs and the damage depends on the radiation dose. Thus, an understanding of the process of spermatogenesis is essential to appreciate radiation effects on the testis. Figure 22.2 shows a diagrammatic view of the testis and spermatogenesis process inside the seminiferous tubule of the testis. The Sertoli cells and the germinal cells (precursors of spermatocytes) are the major components of seminiferous tubules, also known as the sperm-producing tubules. These seminiferous tubules are surrounded by a basement membrane from the bulk of the testis and drain into the vas deferens. The basement membranes of the seminiferous tubules consist of germinal stem cells (spermatogonia). Diploid spermatogonia divide by mitosis to produce more spermatogonia or differentiate into

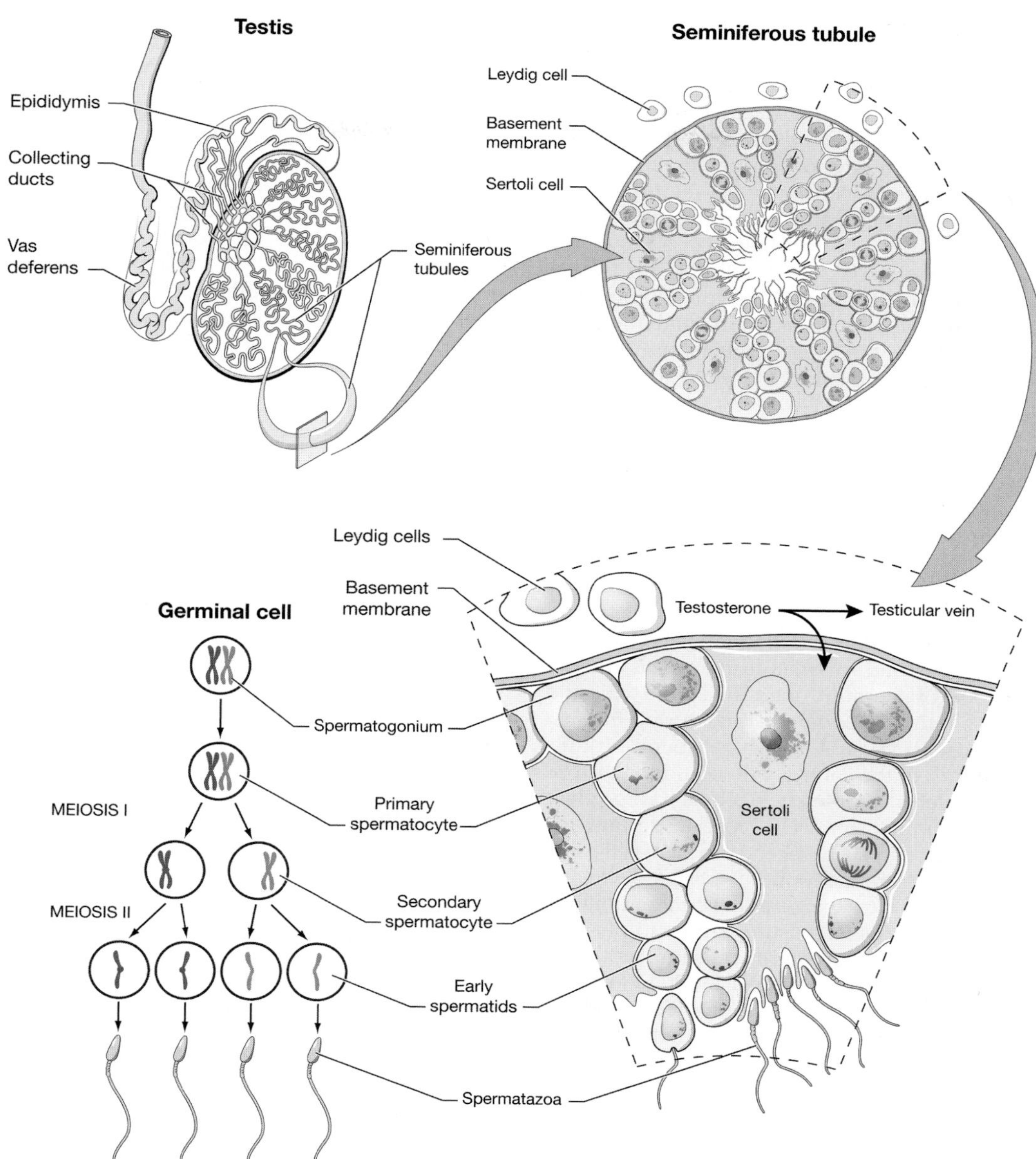

FIGURE 22.2 Schematic representation of male testis and spermatogenesis. Spermatogenesis is initiated in the male testis with the beginning of puberty. This comprises the development of the spermatogonia (former primordial germ cells) up to sperm cells. The gonadal cords that are solid in the juvenile testis develop a lumen with the start of puberty. They then gradually transform themselves into spermatic canals that eventually reach a length of roughly 50–60 cm. They are termed convoluted seminiferous tubules. As shown, germinal epithelium within seminiferous tubules exhibits two differing cell populations: some are Sertoli cells and the great majority are the germ cells in various stages of division and differentiation shown here in greatly simplified manner.

spermatocyte. Meiosis of each spermatocyte produces four haploid spermatids that take 3 weeks to complete in man. Then the spermatids differentiate into sperm losing most of their cytoplasmic content in the process. Sertoli cells span the thickness of the tubule wall and at their base they are connected to adjacent Sertoli cells through tight junctions. These tight junctions form a blood–testis barrier and help to protect maturing sperm from potential toxins and leakage out of the tubule. Sertoli cells organize and nurture waves of spermatogenesis. Leydig cells lie between the tubules and hence are termed interstitial cells and comprise less than 5% of testicular volume. The primary function of the Leydig cells is to synthesize and release androgens of which testosterone is the most important sex steroid for the potency and quantity of sperm production. Testosterone diffuses into the seminiferous tubules to maintain spermatogenesis. Through the testicular vein testosterone also enters the blood stream. The importance of FSH in the development and maturation of the seminiferous tubules and of LH or maternal hCG on the proliferation, differentiation and testosterone production of the Leydig cells has been well documented. Leydig cell steroidogenesis is controlled primarily by LH with negative feedback of testosterone on the HPG axis (Figure 22.1). FSH acts on Sertoli cells to stimulate protein synthesis and production of testicular fluid. Thus, the action of testosterone and FSH on Sertoli cells is synergistic allowing spermatogenesis to be completed.

Although, the number of human cases is not significantly large and individuals show a degree of variation in their responses to irradiation, a number of general principles emerge on radiation effects on human fertility from reports on therapeutic exposure and deliberate experimental exposure in animals. In males, fractioned irradiation of the testes may be more harmful than acute, at least up to a total dose of about 600 Gy. Fractioned doses greater than 35 Gy cause a complete lack of semen or aspermia, the time taken for recovery increases with dose, and after more than 200 Gy aspermia may be permanent. No proliferation occurs after irradiation of either Leydig or Sertoli cells because these lethally irradiated cells die during cell division. Differentiating spermatogonia are also very sensitive to irradiation and after doses as low as 1 Gy both their numbers and those of their daughter cells (spermatocytes) are severely reduced (Ash, 1980; Clifton and Brenner, 1983). The doses of irradiation that are needed to destroy spermatocytes are higher than for spermatogonia. Usually 2–3 Gy results in the blockage of cell division and maturation process and resultant decrease in spermatid number. Though the mature spermatids show no significant damage at this dose after 4–6 Gy the resultant sperms are significantly decreased in number signifying covert spermatid damage. Due to this radiosensitivity of spermatogonia, spermatocytes and spermatids, the sperm disappears from the testis after irradiation. The combined lifespan of spermatocytes and spermatids in humans is about 46 days and transport of sperm through the epididymis and vas deferens takes another 4–12 days. Thus, during the first 4 weeks after low dose irradiation (1.5–2 Gy), sperm production remains about 50% of the control values and then drops dramatically and depletes completely. Recovery takes place from the surviving germinal stem cells (type A spermatogonia) and cell division by mitosis to regenerate stem cell numbers. Differentiation of spermatogonia to spermatocyte and later to spermatids repopulates the germinal epithelium with germ cells. With a single dose exposure, return to pre-irradiation sperm concentrations and germ cell numbers takes place within 9–18 months after less than 1 Gy, 30 months for 2–3 Gy and 5 or more years after 4–6 Gy. Studies in rodents similarly indicate a depletion of primary spermatocytes and significant decrease in spermatids by day 28 post-irradiation to 1 Gy of γ-irradiation. In adult mice exposed to 300 R X-irradiation, the spermatogonial population was selectively killed except for the radio-resistant type A spermatogonial stem cells. It was proposed that these stem cells preferentially survived irradiation doses that killed other spermatogonia because they were long cycling (prolonged G1 or "A-phase" portion of cell cycle) and irradiation injury prematurely triggered from A-phase into DNA synthesis (S phase), thereby initiating restoration of germ cell population (Huckins and Oakberg, 1978).

In childhood, neither the threshold dose of irradiation to damage the germinal cells, nor the dose required to cause irreversible damage are quite well known. With doses of direct testicular irradiation of 24–25 Gy, the germinal epithelium is completed ablated, and Leydig cell function is seriously affected in most patients. Ten of 12 boys showed evidence of Leydig cell dysfunction 10 months to 8.5 years after testicular irradiation (Brauner *et al.*, 1983; Leiper *et al.*, 1983). Similar findings were reported that showed Leydig cell failure occurs soon after irradiation, with no evidence of recovery up to 5 years after irradiation (Shalet *et al.*, 1985). In general, the degree of testicular damage to the germinal epithelium and Leydig cell is dependent on the radiation dose and the age and puberty stage of boys.

FEMALE REPRODUCTIVE FUNCTIONS AND RADIATION EFFECTS

For women exposed to radiation during diagnostic procedures or when undergoing chemotherapy and radioactive therapy in the treatment of cancer and other illnesses, the major side effects of these treatments are ovarian failure and infertility. Particularly for women of child-bearing age, the potential negative effects of radiation exposure on the reproductive system can be life changing. Ovarian toxicity is an important and common long-term side effect of curative chemotherapy and radiotherapy. Information on the effects of irradiation on the ovary has been acquired from women receiving the treatment for malignancies and accidental exposure such as the nuclear explosions of Hiroshima and Nagasaki. In many of these patients, who were young with expectations of a normal reproductive life, premature menopause and sterilization may have impacted their quality of life dramatically. The ovaries are exposed to significant doses of radiation when radiotherapy is used to treat pelvic and abdominal diseases, such as cervical and rectal cancer. When pelvic lymph nodes are irradiated for hematological malignancies such as Hodgkin's disease, in many patients before or at child-bearing age, direct irradiation to the ovaries is sometimes unavoidable.

The function of the ovaries is to house the egg-containing (oocyte) ovarian follicles. The maturation stages of an ovarian follicle are shown in Figure 22.3. In prenatal life the oogonia undergo mitosis and are highly susceptible to radiation. As the cells pass through meiotic cell division resistance to radiation-induced cell death decreases. Human oocytes enter a prolonged resting stage after birth till puberty which terminates shortly after ovulation. The central dogma is that the ovaries of a newborn girl contain a finite number of oocytes usually in the millions and during menstrual cycle many years later each follicle will mature through a biological process called folliculogenesis. The validity of this dogma has been challenged in recent studies arguing support for the possibility that adult females replenish their oocyte reserve (Tilly *et al.*, 2009). The concept that females, like males, have the capacity to renew their primordial germ cell pool during adult life has many implications and replicative germ cells responsible for maintaining oocyte output during postnatal life could become a new therapeutic target (Tilly and Rueda, 2008). This treatment perhaps can rescue ovarian function and fertility in female cancer patients after cytotoxic and radiation treatments.

Assessing the extent of radiation-induced damage of the primordial oocytes and predicting the impact on fertility have been challenging. The degree of impairment is related to the total radiation dose, fractionation schedule and age at the time of radiation treatment. Generally, the higher number of follicles in the pre-puberty ovary makes it less vulnerable to apoptosis than the ovary of women in late reproductive life (Wallace *et al.*, 2005), but the risk of ovarian insufficiency after abdominal radiotherapy is still high in younger women. It has been estimated that a total ovarian radiation dose of 60 cGy has no deleterious effect. A dose of 150 cGy has no deleterious effect in young women but there was some risk for women older than 40. At a dose of 250–500 cGy, in women aged 15–40, 60% experienced permanent sterility, and the remainder may suffer temporary amenorrhea, whereas women older than 40 may become

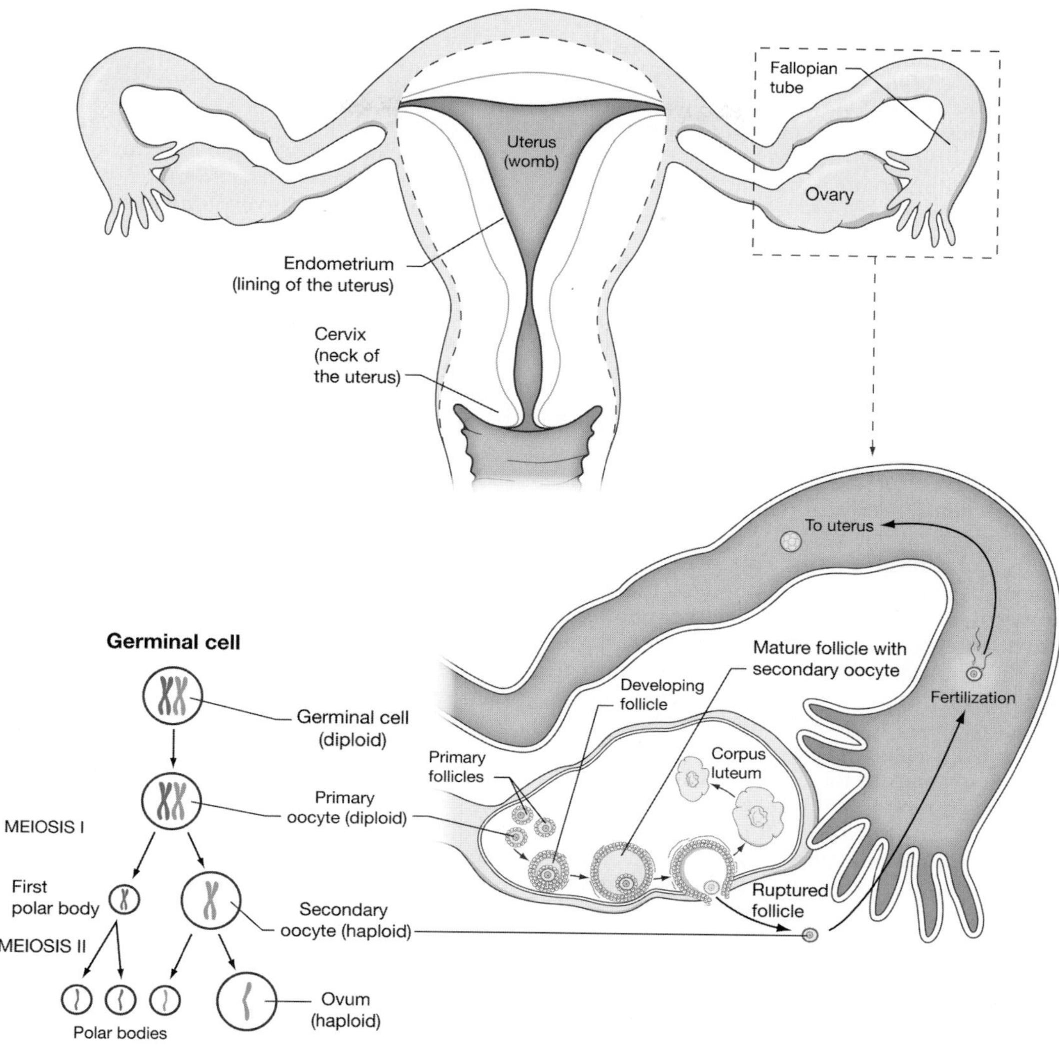

FIGURE 22.3 Schematic representation of female reproductive organ and oogenesis. In contrast to males, the initial steps in egg production occur prior to birth. Diploid stem cells called oogonia divide by mitosis to produce more oogonia and primary oocytes. By the time the fetus is 20 weeks old, the process reaches its peak and by the time of birth, 1–2 million of these cells remain in the ovaries. Each has initiated the first meiotic division (meiosis I), but has not completed it. No further development occurs until sexual maturity. At the time of sexual maturity, the primary oocytes recommence their development, usually one at a time and once a month. The primary oocyte grows much larger and completes the meiosis I, forming a large secondary oocyte and a small polar body that receives little more than one set of chromosomes. Which chromosomes end up in the egg and which in the polar body is entirely a matter of chance. In humans (and most vertebrates), the first polar body does not go on to meiosis II, but the secondary oocyte does proceed as far as metaphase of meiosis II and then stops. Only if fertilization occurs will meiosis II ever be completed. Completion of meiosis II converts the secondary oocyte into a fertilized egg or zygote (and also a second polar body). As in the diagram for spermatogenesis, the behavior of the chromosomes shown in this diagram is greatly simplified.

100% permanently sterilized (Damewood and Grochow, 1986). Because ovarian follicles are remarkably vulnerable to DNA damage, irradiation results in ovarian atrophy and reduced follicle stores. After irradiation, damaged oocytes either undergo repair or are eliminated from the ovary by cell death and phagocytosis. On the cellular level, oocytes show rapid onset of pyknosis, chromosome condensation and disruption of nuclear envelope. Also, the susceptibility to radiation-induced cell death depends on the developmental stage of the germ cell at the time of exposure. The radiosensitivity of the oocytes varies during the growth phase and is age dependent. In women, primordial oocytes are more resistant than oocytes in growing follicles but still highly susceptible to the damage caused by radiotherapy. This is probably because of the risk of undergoing induced apoptosis. A number of studies have examined the ovarian histology following chemotherapy and radiotherapy treatments. The general observation is ovarian atrophy, a reduced follicle store, and apoptosis associated cell destruction (Perez *et al.*, 1997). Recent studies have initiated mapping of the cell death (apoptosis) signaling pathways underlying germ cell destruction by chemotherapy/radiotherapy, and identifying key genes and proteins as potential inhibitors to block the path of primordial follicular destruction. Ovarian follicles are remarkably vulnerable to ionizing radiation since it can cause DNA damage. A number of studies have examined the ovarian histology after chemotherapy and radiotherapy treatments and investigated the mechanisms of such damage. Histological studies have shown that chemotherapy/radiotherapy induces pre-granulosa cell nuclear swelling, primordial follicle disruption, disappearance of the lumen and oocytes. Follicular cells exhibited marked swelling and cell death or apoptosis following radiation. Studies are under way to determine the apoptosis signaling pathways underlying germ cell destruction by chemotherapy and genes or proteins as potential inhibitors to block the path of primordial follicle destruction.

In the hope of finding treatments to preserve fertility of women undergoing cancer therapy, chemical and genetic manipulations are being investigated to reduce gonadotoxic effects of the drugs and radiation. Several options exist for preservation of ovarian steroid secretion and fertility in female cancer patients, although some are not applicable to children (Meirow, 1999; Meirow and Nugent, 2001). Co-treatment with GnRH during the course of treatment with chemotherapy has been proposed as a way of diminishing the loss of follicles in the ovaries. Clinical studies in patients during chemotherapy for malignant and non-malignant conditions receiving GnRH agonist have shown a protective effect of GnRH agonist (Blumenfeld, 2001). Unlike the protective effect shown by the chemotherapy drug, following radiation the follicle counts were not preserved in GnRH agonist-treated monkeys (Ataya *et al.*, 1995). More studies are needed to understand the mechanism of primordial follicle destruction, the mechanism by which GnRH agonist renders its protective effect and how inhibition of the HPG axis may prevent ovaries from damage. The technique of moving the ovaries out of the field of radiation, known as oophoropexy, may be considered in cases of women receiving pelvic and abdominal irradiation but the long-term effect remains uncertain. Another option is cryopreservation of the oocytes and embryos. Although the initial results were disappointing, using the vitrification technique, survival rates after freezing and thawing show clinical outcomes similar to those obtained with fresh oocytes (Cobo *et al.*, 2008). Similarly cryopreservation of fertilized embryos is a well-established technique and babies are born each year as a result of frozen embryo replacements (Andersson *et al.*, 2008).

A successful term pregnancy will depend not only on ovarian function but also on a normally functioning HPG axis and a uterine environment that is not only receptive to implantation but also able to accommodate normal growth of the fetus. Again, the degree of damage to the uterus depends on the total radiation dose and the site of irradiation. In young women who have been exposed to radiotherapy below the diaphragm for childhood cancer, the reproductive problems often include significantly impaired development of the uterus and blood flow, and highly reduced uterus size that can lead to uterine dysfunction (Critchley *et al.*, 1992; Bath *et al.*, 1999; Larsen *et al.*, 2004). It is also likely that radiation damage to the uterine musculature and vasculature adversely affects prospects of pregnancy in adult women. Long-term surviving women with total body irradiation in childhood are at risk of premature labor, low birth weight infants and early pregnancy loss if pregnancy is achieved (Holm *et al.*, 1999). Sex steroid hormone replacement in physiological doses can significantly increase uterine volume and endometrial thickness and re-establish uterine blood flow; however, a successful pregnancy outcome is by no means ensured. The uterine factor remains a concern for women who survived childhood cancer with total body irradiation in childhood.

CONCLUDING REMARKS AND FUTURE DIRECTIONS

The gonads are highly sensitive to the effects of radiation exposure with resultant temporary or permanent defects on fertility depending on the dose of exposures. Genetic studies in a large population exposed to a nuclear explosion such as Hiroshima and Nagaski point to the fact that lethal doses of emitted irradiation may render the surviving population sterile but may not increase genetic or birth defects. In addition to the radiation effect on germ cells, sex steroid hormone production may also be impaired. In the adults this will result in symptoms of sex steroid deficiency and in young children pubertal development would either not occur or be arrested. Radiation exposure of cranial parts may have effects on the timing of the onset of puberty or on the HPG axis and control of gonadotropin secretion, with subsequent infertility and sex steroid deficiency. For the near future, research in reproductive sciences is likely to identify novel modes or mechanisms of action and biochemical pathways that are altered following radiation exposure. Several studies are asking the question whether oocytes can be generated from stem or progenitor cell sources. Since the initial publication in 2003 that mouse embryonic stem (ES) cells could spontaneously form oocytes contained within follicles or follicle-like structures (Hübner *et al.*, 2003), several laboratories have reported similar observations (Novak *et al.*, 2006; Kerkis *et al.*, 2007). Furthermore, male germ cells have been generated from mouse ES cells (Geijsen *et al.*, 2004; Kerkis *et al.*, 2007) and from bone marrow of men (Lee *et al.*, 2007). While additional studies are needed, the ultimate goal of producing fertilization competent oocytes and viable offspring using female germ line or somatic stem cell-based technologies may not be so far away. There is also no doubt that further investigations of the complex reproductive regulatory circuitry, chemical and genetic manipulations have the potential to better preserve fertility of men and women undergoing cancer therapy and reduce the gonadotoxic effects of radiation.

ACKNOWLEDGMENT

This work was supported by the intramural program of NIDCD.

REFERENCES

Achermann JC, Jameson JL (1999) Fertility and infertility: genetic contributions from the hypothalamic–pituitary gonadal axis. *Mol Endocrinol* **13:** 812–18.

Adachi S, Yamada S, Takatsu Y, *et al.* (2007) Involvement of anteroventral periventricular metastin/kispeptin neurons in estrogen positive feedback action on luteinizing hormone release in female rats. *J Repro Dev* **53:** 367–78.

Adams GE, Cox R (1997) Radiation carcinogenesis. In *Cellular and Molecular Biology of Cancer*, 3rd ed. (Franks LM, Teich NM, eds.). Oxford University Press, Oxford, pp. 130–50.

Agha A, Sherlock M, Brennan S, *et al.* (2005) Hypothalamic–pituitary dysfunction after irradiation of non-pituitary brain tumors in adults. *J Clin Endocrinol Metab* **90:** 6355–60.

Andersson RA, Wallace WHB, Baird DT (2008) Ovarian cryopreservation for fertility preservation: indications and outcomes. *Reproduction* **136:** 681–9.

Ash P (1980) The influence of radiation on fertility in man. *Br J Radiol* **53:** 271–8.

Ataya K, Pydyn E, Ramahi-Ataya A, Orton CG (1995b) Is radiation-induced ovarian failure in rhesus monkeys preventable by luteinizing hormone-releasing hormone agonists?: preliminary observations. *J Clin Endocrinol Metab* **80:** 790–5.

Bath LE, Critchley HO, Chambers SE, Anderson RA, Kelnar CJ, Wallace WH (1999) Ovarian and uterine characteristics after total body irradiation in childhood and adolescence: response to sex steroid replacement. *Br J Obstet Gynaecol* **106:** 1265–72.

Blumenfeld Z (2001) Ovarian rescue/protection from chemotherapeutic agents (1). *J Soc Gynecol Investig* **8:** S60–S64.

Brauner R, Czernichow P, Cramer P, Schaison G, Rappaport R (1983) Leydig cell function in children after direct testicular irradiation for acute lymphoblastic leukaemia. *N Engl J Med* **309:** 25–8.

Byrne J, Rasmussen SA, Steinhorn SC, Connelly RR, Myers MH, Lynch CF, Flannery J, Austin DF, Holmes FF, Holmes GE, Strong LC, Mulvihill JJ (1998) Genetic disease in offspring of long-term survivors of childhood and adolescent cancer. *Am J Hum Genet* **62:** 45–52.

Cadman SM, Kim SH, Hu Y, González-Martínez D, Bouloux PM (2007) Molecular pathogenesis of Kallmann's syndrome. *Hormone Res* **67:** 231–42.

Clifton DK, Brenner WJ (1983) The effect of testicular x-irradiation on spermatogenesis in man. A comparison with the mouse. *J Androl* **4:** 387–92.

Cobo A, Domingo J, Perez S, Crespo J, Remohí J, Pellicer A (2008) Vitrification: an effective new approach to oocyte banking and preserving fertility in cancer patients. *Clin Transl Oncol* **10:** 268–73.

Constine LS, Woolf PD, Cann D, Mick G, McCormick K, Raubertas RF, Rubin P (1993) Hypothalamic–pituitary dysfunction after radiation for brain tumors. *N Engl J Med* **328:** 87–94.

Critchley HO, Wallace WH, Shalet SM, Mamtora H, Higginson J, Anderson DC (1992) Abdominal irradiation in childhood: the potential for pregnancy. *Br J Obstet Gynaecol* **99:** 392–4.

Crowley WF Jr, Pitteloud N, Seminara S (2008) New genes controlling human reproduction and how you find them. *Trans Am Clin Climatol Assoc* **119:** 29–37.

Damewood MD, Grochow LB (1986) Prospects for fertility after chemotherapy or radiation for neoplastic disease. *Fertil Steril* **45:** 443–59.

de Roux N, Genin E, Carel JC, Matsuda F, Chaussain JL, Milgrom E (2003) Hypogonadotropic hypogonadism due to loss of function of the KiSS1-derived peptide receptor GPR54. *Proc Natl Acad Sci USA* **100:** 10972–6.

Geijsen N, Horoschak M, Kim K, Gribnau J, Eggan K, Daley GQ (2004) Derivation of embryonic germ cells and male gametes from embryonic stem cells. *Nature* **427:** 148–54.

Gianetti E, Seminara S (2008) Kisspeptin and KISS1R: a critical pathway in the reproductive system. *Reproduction* **136:** 295–301.

Gottsch ML, Cunningham MJ, Smith JT, Popa SM, Acohido BV, Crowley WF, Seminara S, Clifton DK, Steiner RA (2004) A role of Kisspeptins in the regulation of gonadotropin secretion in the mouse. *Endocrinology* **145:** 4073–7.

Harley NH (2001) Toxic effects of radiation and radioactive materials. In *Casarett and Doull's Toxicology: The Basic Science of Poisons, 6th ed.* (Klaassen CD, ed.). New York, NY, McGraw Hill Inc., pp. 917–42.

Harley NH (2008) Health effects of radiation and radioactive materials. In *Casarett and Doull's Toxicology: The Basic Science of Poisons*, 7th ed. (Klaassen CD ed.). New York, NY, McGraw Hill Medical, pp. 1053–82.

Holm K, Nysom K, Brocks V, Hertz H, Jacobsen N, Müller, J (1999) Ultrasound B-mode changes in the uterus and ovaries and Doppler changes in the uterus after total body irradiation and allogenic bone marrow transplantation in childhood. *Bone Marrow Transp* **23:** 259–63.

Hübner K, Fuhrmann G, Christenson LK, Kehler J, Reinbold R, De La Fuente R, Wood J, Strauss JF 3rd, Boiani M, Schöler HR (2003) Derivation of oocytes from mouse embryonic stem cells. *Science* **300:** 1251–6.

Huckins C, Oakberg EF (1978) Morphological and quantitative analysis of spermatogonia in mouse testis using whole mounted seminiferous tubules. II. The irradiated testes. *Anat Rec* **192:** 529–42.

Huhtaniemi I, Alevizaki M (2007) Mutations along the hypothalamus–pituitary gonadal axis affecting male reproduction. *Repro Bio Med* **15:** 622–32.

Kauffman AS, Clifton DK, Steiner RA (2007) Emerging ideas about Kisspeptin-GPR54 signaling in the neuroendocrine regulation of reproduction. *Trends Neurosc* **30:** 504–11.

Kerkis A, Fonseca SA, Serafirm RC, Lavagnolli TM, Abdelmassih S, Abdelmassih R, Kerkis I (2007) In vitro differentiation of male mouse embryonic stem cells into both presumptive sperm cells and oocytes. *Cloning Stem Cells* **9:** 535–48.

Kozenko M, Chudley AE (2010) Genetic implications and health consequences following Chernobyl nuclear accident. *Clin Genet* **77:** 221–6.

Kulakov VI, Sokur TN, Volobuev AI, Tzibulskaya IS, Malisheva VA, Zikin BI, Ezova LC, Belyaeva LA, Bonartzev PD, Speranskaya NV, *et al.* (1993). Female reproductive function in areas affected by radiation after the Chernobyl power station accident. *Environ Health Perspect* **101 (Suppl. 2):** 117–23.

Larsen EC, Schmiegelow K, Rechnitzer C, Loft A, Müller J, Andersen AN (2004) Radiotherapy at a young age reduces uterine volume of childhood cancer survivors. *Acta Obstet Gynecol Scand* **83:** 96–102.

Lee HJ, Selesniemi K, Niikura Y, Niikura T, Klein R, Dombkowski DM, Tilly JL (2007) Bone marrow transplantation generates immature oocytes and rescues long-term fertility in a preclinical mouse model of chemotherapy-induced premature ovarian failure. *J Clin Oncol* **25:** 3198–204.

Leiper AD, Grant DB, Chessells JM (1983) The effect of testicular irradiation on Leydig cell function in prepubertal boys with acute lymphoblastic leukaemia. *Arch Dis Child* **58:** 906–10.

Leiper AD, Stanhope R, Kitching P, Chessells JM (1987) Precocious and premature puberty associated with treatment of acute lymphoblastic leukaemia. *Arch Dis Child* **62:** 1107–12.

Meirow D (1999) Ovarian injury and modern options to preserve fertility in female cancer patients treated with high dose radio-chemotherapy for hemato-oncological neoplasias and other cancers. *Leuk Lymphoma* **33:** 65–76.

Meirow D, Nugent D (2001) The effects of radiotherapy and chemotherapy on female reproduction. *Human Reprod Update* **7:** 535–43.

Neel JV, Schull WJ, Awa AA, Satoh C, Kato H, Otake M, Yoshimoto Y (1990) The children of parents exposed to atomic bombs: estimates of the genetic doubling dose of radiation for humans. *Am J Hum Genet* **46:** 1053–72.

Novak I, Lightfoot DA, Wang H, Eriksson A, Mahdy E, Höög C (2006) Mouse embryonic stem cells form follicle-like ovarian structures but do not progress through meiosis. *Stem Cells* **8:** 1931–6.

Ogilvy-Stuart AL, Shalet SM (1993) Effect of radiation on the human reproductive system. *Environ Health Perspect* **101 (Suppl. 2):** 109–16.

Otake M, Schull WJ, Neel JV (1990) Congenital malformations, stillbirths, and early mortality among the children of atomic bomb survivors: a reanalysis. *Radiat Res* **122:** 1–11.

Perez GI, Knudson CM, Leykin L, Korsmeyer SJ, Tilly JL (1997) Apoptosis-associated signaling pathways are required for chemotherapy-mediated female germ cell destruction. *Nature Med* **3:** 1228–32.

Plant TM (2008) Hypothalamic control of the pituitary–gonadol axis in higher primates: key advances over the last two decades. *J Neuroendocrinol* **20:** pp. 719–26.

Rance NE (2009) Menopause and the human hypothalamus: evidence for the role of kisspeptin/neurokinin B neuron in the regulation of estrogen negative feedback. *Peptides* **30:** 111–22.

Samaan NA, Vieto R, Schultz PN, *et al.* (1982) Hypothalamic, pituitary and thyroid dysfunction after radiotherapy to the head and neck. *Int J Radiat Oncol Biol Phys* **8:** 1857–67.

Seminara SB, Messager S, Chatzidaki EE, *et al.* (2003) The GPR54 gene as a regulator of puberty. *New Eng J Med* **349:** 1614–27.

Shalet SM, Horner A, Ahmed SR, Morris-Jones PH (1985) Leydig cell damage after testicular irradiation for lymphoblastic leukaemia. *Med Pediatr Oncol* **13:** 65–8.

Smith JT, Clifton DK, Steiner RA (2006) Regulation of the neuroendocrine reproductive axis by kisspeptin-GPR54 signaling. *Reproduction* **131:** 623–30.

Spitz DR, Azzam EI, Li JJ, Gius D (2004) Metabolic oxidation/reduction reactions and cellular responses to ionizing radiation: a unifying concept in stress response biology. *Cancer Metas Rev* **23:** 311–22.

Tilly JL, Niikura Y, Rueda BR (2009) The current status of evidence for and against postnatal oogenesis in mammals: a case of ovarian optimism versus pessimism? *Biol Reprod* **80:** 2–12.

Tilly JL, Rueda BR (2008) Stem cell contribution to ovarian development, function, and disease. *Endocrinology* **149:** 4307–11.

Wallace TH, Thomson AB, Saran F, Kelsey TW (2005) Predicting age of ovarian failure after radiation to a field that includes the ovaries. *Int J Radiat Oncol Biol Phys* **62:** 738–44.

Wertelecki W (2010) Malformations in a Chernobyl-impacted region. *Pediatrics* **125:** e836–e843.

Wo JY, Viswanathan AN (2009) Impact of radiotherapy on fertility, pregnancy, and neonatal outcomes in female cancer patients. *Int J Radiation Oncology Biol Phys* **73:** 1304–12.

Wu LJ, Randers-Pehrson G, Xu A, Waldren CA, Geard CR, Yu Z, Hei TK (1999) Targeted cytoplasmic irradiation with alpha particles induces mutations in mammalian cells. *Proc Natl Acad Sci USA* **96:** 4959–64.

Section 4

Gases and Solvents

CHAPTER

23

Reproductive and developmental toxicology: toxic solvents and gases

Suryanarayana V. Vulimiri, M. Margaret Pratt, Shaila Kulkarni, Sudheer Beedanagari and Brinda Mahadevan

Disclaimer. The views expressed in this chapter are those of the authors and do not necessarily reflect the views or policies of the US Environmental Protection Agency.

INTRODUCTION

Reproductive dysfunctions and developmental effects, including birth defects, are a great public health concern. The occurrence of developmental defects has been known since ancient times; however, only in the 19th and 20th centuries have efforts been undertaken to methodically investigate their etiological factors. Xenobiotics can induce adverse effects by targeting several stages of the reproductive and developmental processes which are controlled by several factors, including those of genetic origin. Any deviation from this well-conserved process is likely to generate abnormalities and affect normal functioning, including reproductive capacity. In the early 1960s, the phase of modern developmental toxicology was initiated when there was a report of developmental abnormalities, such as phocomelia, associated with the use of thalidomide, a sedative which was prescribed to pregnant women in Europe and Australia. As a result of this tragedy the regulatory community has expanded its traditional approaches to include the currently practiced endpoint toxicity testing for drugs and pharmaceutical agents. This was followed by the US Food and Drug Administration (FDA) developing a set of three assays to evaluate the effects of xenobiotics on the reproductive cycle of experimental animals. Also, the US Environmental Protection agency (USEPA) developed risk assessment guidelines for developmental (EPA, 1991) and reproductive toxicity (EPA, 1996).

In both sexes, infertility can occur as a result of toxic exposures. Toxicity of the male reproductive system, indicating infertility, is evaluated by clinical measurement of several sperm parameters such as total counts or concentration, motility and morphology. In males, toxicity can also be indicated by reduced libido. Also, since reproductive toxicants frequently target a particular stage of spermatogenesis, histopathological evaluation of testis in experimental animals might provide additional predictors of infertility (Russell *et al.*, 1990). For female reproductive toxicology, hormonal regulation of the estrous cycle is important since many chemicals are known to affect the estrous cycle by depleting the primordial follicles and prematurely inducing menopause. In women, reproductive toxicities can be evidenced by aberrations in menstrual and ovarian cycles, altered fecundity (defined as reproductive potential and measured by time to pregnancy) and incidence of adverse pregnancy outcomes (e.g., spontaneous abortion, stillbirth, congenital malformation or low birth weight). Toxicity to the fetus can result in developmental or teratogenic defects such as prenatal and postnatal death, structural abnormalities (e.g., neural tube and heart defects), altered growth (e.g., low birth weight) or functional deficiencies (e.g., mental retardation or delayed neurodevelopmental ontogeny). For the neonate, toxicants may also cause postnatal development perturbations (e.g., occurrence of childhood cancer). In addition, gene mutations, maternal metabolic imbalances, infections and exposure to harmful physical (e.g., radiation) or chemical (occupational, therapeutic or environmental) agents are known etiological contributors to reproductive and developmental toxicities (Mitchell *et al.*, 2004). Several of the adverse pregnancy outcomes described above were observed following exposures during the critical period of organogenesis such as the first trimester of pregnancy. For the organ systems that are not fully developed at birth (e.g., the reproductive system and the neurological system), adverse effects on development can occur with postnatal exposures.

Various classes of toxic solvents and gases are known to cause both reproductive and developmental effects in animals and humans (Table 23.1). About one-third of the tested industrial solvents are developmental toxicants in laboratory animals via inhalation and dermal routes, suggesting that they may have strong developmental toxicity potential in humans via the same routes of exposure (Schardein, 2000). In this chapter we focus on those chemicals that have high potential for human exposure, e.g. widely distributed or easily absorbed, and those that are components of environmental mixtures and/or reactive agents. We therefore confine our

Reproductive and Developmental Toxicology, Edited by Ramesh C. Gupta
ISBN: 978-0-12-382032-7

TABLE 23.1 Selected toxic solvents and gases causing reproductive/developmental toxicity in humans/experimental animals

Chemical agent(s)	Type	Class	Products/Uses
Carbon tetrachloride (CCl_4)	Solvents	Chlorinated hydrocarbon	Synthesis of fluorocarbons; refrigerant, dry-cleaning agent, grain fumigant, antihelminthic
Tetrachloroethylene or perchloroethylene (PCE or PERC)	Solvents	Chloroethane family	Dry cleaning, industrial metal cleaning; chemical intermediate
Trichloroethylene (TCE)	Solvents	Chloroethane family	Vapor degreasing of fabricated metal parts; solvent; low-temperature heat transfer fluid
Chloroform ($CHCl_3$)	Solvents	Chlorinated hydrocarbon	Synthesis of fluorocarbons for use in refrigerants, propellants, plastics; in floor polishes, adhesives; as fumigant
Methylene chloride (dichloromethane)	Solvents	Chloromethane family	Solvent degreaser; co-solvent or vapor pressure depressant in hair sprays, insecticides, spray paints, pharmaceuticals; in food extraction, urethane foam blowing and surface treatment including paint stripping
Isoamyl nitrite, isobutyl nitrite	Solvents	Aliphatic nitrites	Room deodorizers (inhalant recreational drugs)
Toluene, benzene, xylene	Solvents	Aromatic hydrocarbons	Glues and cleaners
Butane, propane, gasoline	Solvents	Aliphatic hydrocarbons	Fuels, cigarette lighters
Acetone	Solvents	Ketones	Glues and nail-polish removers
Kerosene and jet fuels	Solvents	Aliphatic and aromatic hydrocarbons	Domestic energy sources and aviation fuels
Formaldehyde	Gas	Aldehydes	Manufacture of plastics and resins; used in wood products, construction materials; preservation of human and animal body/tissues, embalming
Nitrous oxide	Gas	Oxide of nitrogen	Propellant in food dispenser (e.g., whipped cream); anesthetic and analgesic
Ethylene oxide	Gas	Epoxide	Sterilant for medical, dental and scientific supplies; used in the production of ethylene glycol, glycol ethers and ethanolamines
Enflurane, halothane, isoflurane	Gas	Halogenated ethers and hydrocarbons	Inhalation anesthetics

Adapted from Hooper *et al.* (1992)

report to selected solvents/gases from the list of potential priority reproductive/developmental toxicants (Hooper *et al.*, 1992), including carbon tetrachloride, tetrachloroethylene, toluene, styrene, benzene, gasoline, kerosene and jet fuels and formaldehyde. In addition, with practical limits to the number and scope of areas that could be addressed for each individual reproductive or developmental toxicant, we address the agents mentioned above, realizing that such agents can arise from varying sources – which can be anthropogenic and/or natural – having extensive chemical structural diversity. Hence, if the information is available in published literature, we have garnered and incorporated the historical background, toxicokinetics, mechanism of action, general toxicity, and reproductive and developmental toxicity of selected individual solvents and gases. Wherever possible/applicable we have highlighted the magnitude and severity of exposure to these selected compounds within the priority list of agents. This overview is not a comprehensive literature review of original publications, but deliberately intended to be informative based on secondary sources of information.

CARBON TETRACHLORIDE (CASRN 56-23-5)

Carbon tetrachloride (CCl_4) is a colorless, highly volatile liquid with a sweetish (ethereal) odor similar to chloroform. It decomposes to highly toxic fumes of phosgene upon heating. Carbon tetrachloride is primarily used in the production of chlorofluorocarbons that are used as refrigerants. It has also been used as an antihelminthic, insecticide dispersant, dry-cleaning agent, fabric-spotting fluid, grain-fumigant and fire extinguisher (NTP, 2005a). It is still used as a fire extinguisher; however, it is not permitted in products for household use. As a solvent it is used in the production of plastics and resins, as a foam blowing agent and as an aerosol propellant. In the USA large-scale production of CCl_4 began in 1907. The fumigation process was the major occupational risk of human exposure to CCl_4. The USEPA banned its use as a grain fumigant in 1985 (NTP, 2005a).

Carbon tetrachloride is rapidly absorbed via oral (gastrointestinal tract) and inhalation (lungs) routes and to a lesser extent via the dermal (skin) route both in humans and animals. Following absorption, carbon tetrachloride rapidly diffuses from the blood to different internal organs (e.g., liver, kidney, brain) with peak concentrations reached within 1–6 hours depending on the duration of exposure and concentration. A fraction of the chemical accumulates in adipose tissue (Sanzgiri *et al.*, 1997).

CCl_4 is metabolized primarily by cytochrome (CYP) P450 enzyme isoform 2E1 (CYP2E1) forming trichloromethyl ($\bullet CCl_3$) radical and with further oxidation to trichloromethyl peroxy ($\bullet O{-}O{-}CCl_3$) free radicals. The trichloromethylperoxyl radical can react further to form phosgene, which may be detoxified by reaction with water to produce carbon dioxide or conjugated with reduced glutathione (GSH) or cysteine (Manibusan *et al.*, 2007). Under anaerobic conditions, CCl_4 is converted to chloroform and dichlorocarbene. In humans and experimental animals, CCl_4 is rapidly eliminated by passive diffusion primarily through exhaled breath, with a smaller fraction eliminated in urine and feces (IARC, 1979).

The free radicals generated by CCl_4 metabolism attack polyunsaturated fatty acids in cell membranes forming fatty acid-free radicals and induce lipid peroxidation with the production of reactive aldehydes (e.g., formaldehyde, acetaldehyde, crotonaldehyde, etc.). Reactive aldehydes quench thiols (e.g., GSH) affecting the glutathione pathway and causing oxidative stress (Manibusan *et al.*, 2007). Several reactive aldehydes (e.g., 4-hydroxynonenal and malondialdehyde) and free radicals generated during CCl_4 metabolism induce DNA strand breaks and promutagenic DNA lesions, which contribute to the genotoxicity of CCl_4. Lipid peroxidation also causes cell membrane disruption leading to increased cell membrane permeability, enzyme leakage and disruption of calcium homeostasis. This in turn activates cellular proteases and phospholipases causing phospholipid and protein degradation leading to cytotoxicity and an inflammatory response. Genotoxicity can also contribute to cytotoxicity leading to apoptosis or necrosis. Cytotoxicity is followed by cellular regeneration and proliferation which, when coupled with increased oxidative and lipid peroxidative DNA damage, could overcome the DNA repair mechanisms leading to increased mutagenicity and hepatocarcinogenesis (Manibusan *et al.*, 2007).

Human exposure to high levels of carbon tetrachloride is likely to occur during the production and fumigation process, from accidental spills and leaks during transportation, etc. (NTP, 2005a). Exposure via inhalation and ingestion is harmful and sometimes fatal with amounts as low as 2–3 mL (45–68 mg/kg based on reference adult body weight of 70 kg) and skin contact causes dermatitis (Ruprah *et al.*, 1985). In humans, acute symptoms after CCl_4 exposure are independent of the route of intake and are characterized by gastrointestinal and neurological symptoms, such as nausea, vomiting, headache, dizziness, dyspnea and death. Long-term exposure to CCl_4 causes renal and hepatotoxicity, central nervous system (CNS) disturbance, and damage to eyes, skin and lungs; causing several molecular changes such as cytotoxicity, regenerative proliferation and overwhelmed DNA repair in liver eventually may lead to hepatocarcinogenesis (Anonymous, 1992).

To date, there are no human data reporting reproductive effects after inhalation exposure to CCl_4. However, animal studies provide evidence for CCl_4-induced reproductive and/or developmental toxicity following either oral or inhalation exposure. For example, pregnant rats exposed to CCl_4 by gavage during gestation days (GD) 6–19 have shown clear maternal toxicity, decrease in maternal hormone (e.g., progesterone and luteinizing hormone) levels, full-litter resorption or pregnancy loss, retarded fetal growth and occasional dose-related piloerection and kyphosis (Schwetz *et al.*, 1974; Narotsky and Kavlock, 1995; Narotsky *et al.*, 1997a,b; Nagano *et al.*, 2007). In male mice subchronic inhalation exposure to CCl_4 has been shown to cause testicular atrophy, while intraperitoneal exposure in rats causes degeneration of testicular germinal epithelium (Adams *et al.*, 1952; Chatterjee, 1966; Kalla and Bansal, 1975). In a three-generation inhalation study, exposure to CCl_4 caused decreased fertility in rats, and male mice have shown elevated absolute and relative testicular weights; in female mice deposition of ceroid in the ovaries has been reported (Chatterjee, 1966).

With regard to developmental toxicity there are no studies reporting developmental effects in humans after inhalation exposure to carbon tetrachloride, except one study where an increased risk of small-for-gestational-age live born babies has been observed in women exposed to CCl_4 during their second or third trimester of pregnancy (Seidler *et al.*, 1999). However, two rodent studies reported developmental toxicity of CCl_4 given either by inhalation (Wilson, 1954) or by gavage (Schwetz *et al.*, 1974). Although these studies did not show any gross anomalies and CCl_4 has not been shown to be teratogenic, significant dose-dependent reductions in fetal body weight and crown–rump length and a significant delay in the ossification of sternebrae have been observed in fetuses at high doses.

TETRACHLOROETHYLENE (CASRN 127-18-4)

Tetrachloroethylene or perchloroethylene (PCE or PERC) is a non-flammable, colorless volatile liquid with ether-like odor. It is mostly miscible with organic compounds such as alcohol, ether, benzene, etc., and is less soluble in water. PCE is used primarily as a solvent in dry cleaning, textile processing and metal-cleaning operations. It is also used as an industrial solvent for fats, oils, tars, rubber, gums and as a metal cleaning and degreasing agent. PCE is also used as an antihelminthic for hookworms, and as a grain protectant and fumigant (NTP, 2005b; Gold *et al.*, 2008). Tetrachloroethylene has been detected in both ground and surface water, in the air, soil, food and breast milk. Human exposure to PCE occurs primarily through inhalation, ingestion of contaminated water and to a smaller extent through dermal absorption from water during bathing, showering or swimming (NTP, 2005b).

A large portion of PCE produced in several industrial operations is released into air, and has been detected in rural (in parts per trillion (ppt) range), urban and industrial areas (in ppt to parts per billion (ppb) range). A small portion of PCE is also formed during chlorination of water. Inhalation and ingestion of contaminated water and food are the primary routes of human exposure to PCE (Gold *et al.*, 2008). Tetrachloroethylene has also been detected in several other sources such as surface and ground water, commercial deionized charcoal-filtered water and some foods (e.g., fresh bread, fats, oils, fruits and vegetables). Personnel working in dry-cleaning, metal degreasing and fluorocarbon production facilities are exposed to PCE and often the highest exposures are possible during the loading and unloading of dry-cleaning equipment. Also, personnel working with dry-cleaners are a source of exposure to family members. PCE exposure is also possible from coin-operated laundromats which house dry-cleaners and from freshly dry-cleaned clothing that is stored in closets (NTP, 2005b).

Humans are exposed to tetrachloroethylene by inhalation, ingestion and dermal contact, with the pulmonary route being the primary one in humans. Although pulmonary absorption is rapid, it takes several hours to attain tissue equilibrium. Further, absorption into systemic circulation is proportional to the ventilation rate, duration of exposure and the concentration in the ambient air to which humans are exposed. Gastrointestinal absorption following ingestion of PCE is rapid and complete. Dermal contact with the pure solvent, vapor or solvent mixture results in PCE rapidly reaching the blood stream. Since tetrachloroethylene is lipophilic, it can be found accumulated in adipose tissue and also in brain and liver. Continuous occupational exposure (5 days/week) leads to accumulation in body fat until it reaches a steady state within 3–4 weeks and is released slowly over a period of time. Human exposure to PCE has reportedly resulted in ~120-fold higher concentration in the brain when compared to that of the lungs and one study found brain concentrations ~3–8 times higher than those reported in other organs. PCE has been shown to cross both the blood–brain and the placenta barriers. PCE is eliminated through breast milk, thus newborn babies can be exposed to PCE while nursing (Gold *et al.*, 2008).

In both humans and experimental animals, tetrachloroethylene is metabolized by two pathways. The major pathway is oxidative metabolism through CYP2E1, which primarily occurs in liver and extra hepatic tissues, such as brain and, to a lesser degree, in lung. Trichloroacetic acid is the major urinary metabolite of PCE in all species, while dichloroacetic acid and few other metabolites have been measured in some species. Oxalic acid has been identified as a major metabolite in rats. In the second metabolic pathway, which takes place primarily in the liver, PCE is conjugated by GSH which is mediated by glutathione-S-transferase (GST), forming tetrachlorovinyl glutathione (TCVG), an important pathway for bioactivation rather than detoxification. Further, TCVG is transported to kidneys where it undergoes enzymatic removal of glycine and glutamine from the TCVG conjugate resulting in the formation of trichlorovinyl cysteine. The metabolites of PCE generated through oxidative and conjugative pathways, respectively, have been shown to be involved in hepatic and renal toxicity (Lash and Parker, 2001).

Inhalation exposure of mice to PCE has been shown to cause hepatic leukocytic infiltration, centrilobular necrosis, bile stasis, mitotic alteration and renal tubular cell karyomegaly at low concentrations (<200 ppm). Exposure at high doses (400 ppm) causes reduced survival of male rats partially due to increased incidence of mononuclear cell leukemia. Early deaths in mice may have been related to the development of hepatocellular carcinomas.

In general, the epidemiologic studies on tetrachloroethylene do not present quantitative information on level of exposure and maternal toxicity or affecting fetal development (Gold *et al.*, 2008). In most cases exposure data has been derived from self-reported information provided by study subjects in questionnaires or interviews. In humans exposed to PCE as a pure solvent or in a mixture there have been reports of adverse effects on reproductive and developmental toxicity such as increased risk of spontaneous abortion, still birth and congenital anomalies. High levels of PCE detected in dry-cleaning facilities has been associated with decreased potential for pregnancy among the wives of the workers (Eskenazi *et al.*, 1991a) and affected semen quality in men (Eskenazi *et al.*, 1991b).

When compared to women working in the laundry or non-operator dry-cleaning industry, the wives of dry-cleaners or current or former female employees in the dry-cleaning industry had an increased risk of spontaneous abortions while working any time during pregnancy or during the three months before conception (Bosco *et al.*, 1987; Olsen *et al.*, 1990; Windham *et al.*, 1991; Doyle *et al.*, 1997). These studies minimized the potential for bias by using pregnancy as the unit of analysis, adjusting for previous pregnancy loss (Doyle *et al.*, 1997), and also examined the relationship between spontaneous abortion and occupational exposure to PCE (Bosco *et al.*, 1987; Olsen *et al.*, 1990). A study of Finnish workers that reported spontaneous abortion as the most significant observation following high exposures during the first trimester of pregnancy also reported low birth weight and congenital anomalies (Olsen *et al.*, 1990). Other studies reported delayed conception and hormonal imbalance (Rachootin and Olsen, 1983), low birth weights and oral cleft palate defects in the offspring born to parents who were exposed to PCE through drinking water (Bove *et al.*, 1995). Maternal organic solvent exposure, in particular to PCE, has been shown to cause deficits in neurobehavioral parameters and visual system functioning of their children at young age, suggesting vulnerability of the developing fetus to solvent exposure (Till *et al.*, 2001a,b, 2003; Laslo-Baker *et al.*, 2004).

In animal studies, inhalation exposure to PCE has been shown to cause sperm head abnormalities in male mice (Beliles, 2002), decreased fetal weight, delayed ossification, skeletal retardations and malformations in fetuses as well as maternal toxicity in pregnant rats, mice and rabbits (Schwetz *et al.*, 1975; Nelson *et al.*, 1979; Szakmáry *et al.*, 1997). Exposure by gavage to PCE between 10 and 16 days postnatally has been associated with altered behavior at 60 days of age affecting the spontaneous motor activity, as measured by locomotion, rearing and total activity in mice (Fredriksson *et al.*, 1993).

STYRENE (CASRN 100-42-5)

Styrene is a colorless to yellowish viscous liquid with a sweet, sharp odor. Styrene is insoluble in water, soluble in acetone, diethyl ether and ethanol and very soluble in benzene and petroleum ether. Styrene, produced naturally by plants, bacteria and fungi, was first isolated in 1831 by distillation of storax, a natural balsam from trees of the genus *Liquidambar*. Commercial production of styrene via dehydrogenation of ethylbenzene began in Germany in 1925. Production of styrene in the USA alone has recently been measured in the tens of billions of pounds. It is used in the manufacture of polystyrene and copolymers which are used as packaging materials, insulation for electrical uses in homes and other buildings, in making fiberglass, plastic pipes, automobile parts, drinking cups and other "food-use" items as well as carpet backing. Styrene is also present in combustion products such as cigarette smoke and automobile exhaust. The general population is primarily exposed to low levels of styrene in ambient air, drinking water and by consuming food contained in styrene-based packaging material. The greatest styrene exposure occurs among occupationally exposed workers in the reinforced plastics industry (IARC, 2002; ATSDR, 2007b).

Inhalation is considered the major route of styrene exposure for humans with 60 to 70% of inhaled styrene being rapidly absorbed. The primary metabolic pathway involves the oxidation of styrene to styrene 7,8-oxide by several CYP isoforms followed by subsequent hydrolysis to styrene glycol. More than 95% of the absorbed styrene is eliminated in the urine as mandelic and phenylglyoxylic acids (Cruzan *et al.*, 2002). In experimental animals, styrene is also rapidly metabolized to styrene 7,8-oxide following absorption by oral, dermal or inhalation exposure. Interspecies differences exist in the rates of metabolism of styrene by liver and lung tissue. Metabolism of styrene 7,8-oxide can proceed via epoxide hydrolase (EH)-mediated hydrolysis or through glutathione *S*-transferase (GST)-mediated conjugation with GSH. Conversion of styrene to phenylacetaldehyde and other ring-opened metabolites provides additional pathways for styrene and styrene 7,8-oxide metabolism (Sumner and Fennell, 1994). Stable products representing each of these pathways are eliminated in the urine.

One potential mode of action for styrene toxicity involves induction of cytotoxicity by its metabolite styrene 7,8-oxide which in turn stimulates cell replication and proliferation. Repeated exposure to styrene progressively results in focal crowding of bronchiolar cells, bronchiolar and bronchio-alveolar hyperplasia in the lungs of mice but not rats (Cruzan *et al.*, 1997, 1998, 2001; Cohen *et al.*, 2002).

A second mode of action for styrene-induced carcinogenicity involves DNA reactivity by forming stable N^2 and O^6 adducts of deoxyguanosine in human lymphocytes and cultured mammalian cells resulting in genotoxicity. Styrene 7,8-oxide enantiomers, but not styrene itself, are DNA reactive. The O^6 adduct of styrene 7,8-oxide is relatively persistent and often detectable in the peripheral blood lymphocytes of workers exposed to styrene (IARC, 2002).

Styrene has been shown to induce neurotoxicity among workers from the reinforced plastics industry, primarily affecting the CNS with toxic symptoms such as decreased color discrimination, vestibular effects, hearing impairment, delays in reaction time, impaired performance on tests measuring attention and memory as well as symptoms of neurotoxicity similar to drunkenness (ATSDR, 2007b).

In humans, there was no evidence for an association between workplace exposure to styrene and reproductive toxicities such as spontaneous abortions, malformations or decreased male fecundity (NTP-CERHR, 2006). One reproductive toxicity study in female workers from the plastic manufacturing industry exposed to 13 or 52 ppm styrene has been negative for menstrual disorders (Lemasters *et al.*, 1985), while another study has shown increased frequency of spontaneous abortions and a decreased frequency of births in humans (Lemasters *et al.*, 1989). However, these studies do not have the exposure data and have confounding factors which make the studies inconclusive. Thus, occupational exposure studies have examined the reproductive and developmental toxicity of styrene; these studies did not find statistically significant alterations in the occurrence of stillbirths, infant deaths, malformations or birth weight (Harkonen *et al.*, 1984; Ahlborg *et al.*, 1987; Lemasters *et al.*, 1989). The National Toxicology Program's Center for the Evaluation of Risks to Human Reproduction (NTP-CERHR) expert panel evaluating these data concluded that the human studies were not sufficient to evaluate developmental toxicity due to the low statistical power of the studies and the lack of adequate information on exposure (NTP-CERHR, 2006).

In general, animal studies have not found styrene-related developmental effects following inhalation exposure (rats, mice, rabbits or hamsters) or oral exposure (rats); additionally, no reproductive toxic effects were observed in a rat two-generation study. The NTP-CERHR expert panel determined that there was sufficient animal data to conclude that styrene does not cause reproductive toxicity in rats following inhalation or oral exposure or in rabbits following inhalation exposure (NTP-CERHR, 2006). No studies were found that examined styrene toxicity subsequent to the exposure of young laboratory animals.

TOLUENE (CASRN 108-88-3)

Toluene is an aromatic hydrocarbon (a methyl substituted benzene derivative), which occurs as a clear colorless volatile liquid and possesses a pungent, benzene-like odor. Toluene is water insoluble, but is miscible with other organic solvents. It is routinely added to gasoline as an additive along with benzene and xylene to increase the octane rating. Toluene occurs naturally in crude oil. It is produced in the process of making gasoline and other fuels from crude oil, in making coke from coal and as a by-product in the manufacture of styrene and benzene. Toluene is also used in paints, coatings, inks, adhesives, fingernail polish and cleaners as well as in leather tanning processes and in the production of rubber, nylon, plastics and polyurethanes. Toluene was once used as a medicinal anthelmintic agent against round worms and hookworms (ATSDR, 2000; EPA, 2005).

A ubiquitous solvent, incidental exposure to low concentrations of toluene in both the home and workplace is common. The major source of environmental exposure to toluene occurs through its release during the production, transport and use of gasoline. Toluene has been detected in soil and as a contaminant in drinking water supplies in the close proximity of the underground storage tanks for fuel products or near some of the hazardous waste sites. It has also been detected in smoke from cigarettes and wood. Because of its neurotoxic effects, the Occupational Safety and Health Administration (OSHA) promulgated an 8-hour permissible exposure limit (PEL) of 200 ppm in 1993 and later in 2000 the American Conference of Governmental Industrial Hygienists (ACGIH) recommending a time-weighted average (TWA) of 50 ppm (ATSDR, 2000). Very high concentrations of toluene in binge patterns of exposure rapidly yield high peak blood toluene concentrations presenting relatively greater risk (Hannigan and Bowen, 2010).

Toluene is readily absorbed through the respiratory and gastrointestinal tracts and, to a lesser extent, through the skin. Respiratory tract being the primary route of exposure, inhaled toluene vapors are rapidly absorbed through the lungs and are widely distributed to highly perfused and fatty tissues (Hannigan and Bowen, 2010).

The majority of inhaled toluene is detoxified and excreted following initial hydroxylation to benzyl alcohol primarily by CYP2E1, followed by oxidation to benzoic acid (ATSDR, 2000). Most of the benzoic acid is conjugated to glycine to form hippuric acid, the main metabolite of toluene found in urine and blood and a primary biomarker of exposure. A minor CYP-related pathway mediated by CYP1A2, 2B2 or 2E1 involves a transient epoxidation of the aromatic ring to form either *o*- or *p*-cresol. The cresols may undergo a variety of conjugation reactions, forming mainly sulfates and glucuronides. Glutathione conjugation may also occur resulting in S-benzylglutathione and S-benzylmercapturic acid (conjugation to benzyl alcohol), or S-*p*-toluylglutathione and S-*p*-toluylmercaptic acid (conjugation to the epoxidated ring) (Nakajima *et al.*, 1992).

In females of reproductive age, toluene-based solvents are the most commonly abused solvents (Kuczkowski, 2007). Women occupationally exposed to toluene did not differ from unexposed controls on menstrual cycle irregularities (Ng *et al.*, 1992a), but reported significantly higher incidence of spontaneous abortions (Taskinen *et al.*, 1989; Ng *et al.*, 1992b). However, the data were inconsistent due to a small sample size and paucity of data on exposure levels. Reduced fecundity was noted in occupationally exposed women, as compared to controls, and among females as compared to male personnel working with toluene or other solvents. The relationship between prenatal toluene exposure in humans and reproductive factors, including fetal growth and birth weight, is unclear. The clinical manifestations of toluene abuse-related embryopathy have not been clearly discriminated from the effects of other exposures (Hannigan and Bowen, 2010). For example, outcomes common to both toluene and alcohol abuse include prematurity, pre- and/or postnatal growth restriction, craniofacial and/or other organ system malformations, developmental delays and perinatal death (Hannigan and Bowen, 2010).

Most of the evidence for reproductive disruption following toluene exposure comes from studies in animal models. In female rats inhalation exposure to toluene has been shown to cause a dose-dependent increase in litters with runts having morphological anomalies (Bowen *et al.*, 2005), fewer pups (Bowen *et al.*, 2007), structural variations in ovarian follicles (Tap *et al.*, 1996) and induction of spontaneous abortion in rabbits (Ungvary and Tatrai, 1985); and in males, sperm abnormalities (Ono *et al.*, 1996) have been observed. Toluene exposure also has been shown to induce several developmental effects such as brain development (Slomianka *et al.*, 1990), increased morphological anomalies and skeletal growth retardation in rats and mice (Hudak and Ungvary, 1978; Ungvary and Tatrai, 1985). Also, prenatal exposure of pregnant rats to toluene by gavage has been shown to cause abnormal neuronal proliferation and migration in the brain of pups without affecting the brain weight (Gospe and Zhou, 2000).

BENZENE (CASRN 608-93-5)

Benzene, also known as benzol, is an aromatic hydrocarbon which occurs as a clear, colorless liquid with a sweet odor. It is a highly volatile and flammable liquid with poor water solubility. Benzene is found as a pollutant in air, soil and water. It occurs naturally as a product of pyrolysis, mostly through anthropogenic sources. Cigarette smoke is one of the major sources of benzene exposure and smokers, in general, are exposed to 10 times more benzene than non-smokers. Benzene is commercially produced from coal and petroleum. It ranks in the top 20 chemicals for production volume in the USA (ATSDR, 2007a). It is used as a starting material or intermediate in the production of plastics, resins, synthetic fiber dyes, detergents, drugs and pesticides (ATSDR, 2007a). Though naturally present in gasoline, benzene has been used as a fuel additive in amounts that vary depending on the formulation requirements of the producer (NTP, 2005c). The use of benzene as a solvent has declined in recent years following its classification as a hazardous compound and carcinogen (ATSDR, 2007a). Almost half the human exposure to benzene occurs from cigarette smoke; other sources include fuel evaporation from auto service stations, exhaust from automobiles, industrial emissions and natural processes. Hence, there continues to be a greater potential for human exposure to benzene, particularly in industrialized countries (NTP, 2005c).

Human exposure to benzene predominantly occurs through inhalation, although oral and dermal routes of exposure are also important (NTP, 2005c). Owing to its high volatility, a significant amount of benzene evaporates before being absorbed through the skin (ATSDR, 2007a). In humans, women were found to absorb higher levels than men. After absorption benzene is rapidly distributed throughout the body, and due to its high lipophilicity, it accumulates in fatty tissues of different organs (ATSDR, 2007a).

Metabolism of benzene is essential to induce toxicity. Liver is the major organ for benzene metabolism wherein CYP2E1 oxidizes benzene to benzene oxide and several reactive metabolites which are capable of disrupting different cellular biochemical pathways inducing a wide range of toxic effects (Snyder, 2004; Rappaport *et al.*, 2010). Benzene oxide exists in equilibrium with its tautomer oxepin and is spontaneously converted to phenol, a major product of metabolism, which is either excreted as glucuronide or sulfate conjugates or further metabolized to catechol and hydroquinone that will be ultimately metabolized to highly reactive metabolites 1-2 benzoquinone and 1,4-benzoquinone, respectively, by myeloperoxidase. Benzene oxide may also react with GSH forming phenylmercapturic acid, which is converted to benzene dihydrodiol by epoxide hydrolase with subsequent conversion to catechol. Alternatively, benzoic acid may undergo an iron-catalyzed, ring-opening reaction to form trans,trans-muconaldehyde with subsequent metabolism to trans,trans-muconic acid. Metabolism of benzene in humans and several animal species is similar; at low levels of exposure, benzene is metabolized rapidly and excreted, while at higher doses, owing to the saturation of the metabolic pathways, the unmetabolized parent compound accumulates in fatty tissues and/or is excreted through exhaled air (Snyder, 2004; Rappaport *et al.*, 2010; Smith, 2010).

Workers from a wide range of industries, such as petroleum, rubber, paint, shoe making, printing solvent and other industries, have a potential to be occupationally exposed to benzene as well as from a mixture of aromatic hydrocarbons containing benzene. Hence, it is difficult to separate the toxic effects of benzene from those of the other chemicals (Snyder, 2004). In both humans and animal models, benzene most commonly affects peripheral blood and bone marrow resulting in several hematotoxicities, including leucopenia, lymphocytopenia, anemia, granulocytosis and reticulocytosis (ATSDR, 2007a). Benzene exposure is highly correlated with the development of several cancers, including acute myelogenous leukemia, non-Hodgkin's lymphoma and multiple myeloma in both humans and animal models (Schnatter *et al.*, 2005). Although the results on DNA adduct formation by benzene or its metabolites are conflicting (Whysner *et al.*, 2004), other genotoxic endpoints (e.g., chromosomal abnormalities) have been reported. Benzene has also been shown to produce neurotoxicity, but only at very high doses (ATSDR, 2007a).

Epidemiological studies showing reproductive and developmental effects of benzene exposure in humans are limited. The most common reproductive symptoms of benzene exposure in women include menstrual disorders, both temporal and functional, and, in men, a decrease in sperm count, motility and concentration as well as decreased semen volume (Yin *et al.*, 1987; Huang, 1991; De Celis *et al.*, 2000; Xing *et al.*, 2010). Similar to reproductive toxicity studies, the available literature on developmental toxicity of benzene in humans is also limited and inconclusive. However, the limited number of studies available suggests that benzene does interfere with human reproduction and fertility.

In contrast, extensive literature is available in multiple animal species on benzene-induced reproductive and developmental toxic effects, although multiple-generation reproductive toxicity studies are not currently available, making it difficult to assess the long-term effects of benzene exposure on the reproductive system. In male rodents, benzene exposure has been shown to cause decreased organ weight for rat testis (Wolf *et al.*, 1956) and reduced normal sperm count, increase in abnormal sperm counts and testicular atrophy in mice (Ward *et al.*, 1985). The common developmental effects of benzene reported in several rodent studies include reduced fetal body and liver weights and skeletal abnormalities (Green *et al.*, 1978; Coate *et al.*, 1984; Kuna *et al.*, 1992).

GASOLINE (CASRN 8006-61-9)

Gasoline, also known as gas (USA), petrol (Commonwealth countries) and benzin (Germany), is primarily used as motor fuel in combustion engines. It is a liquid mixture of aliphatic hydrocarbons derived from fractional distillation of petroleum which is then combined with additives such as isooctane and aromatic hydrocarbons (e.g., toluene and benzene) to boost the octane rating of gasoline and to prevent engines from "knocking". Gasoline contains several other additives including ethanol, methanol, formaldehyde, xylene, 1,3-butadiene, methyl tertiary butyl ether (MTBE) and hexane. Gasoline is also used as a diluent for paints, as a finishing agent and as an industrial solvent (Sittig, 1984). The anti-knock additives (e.g., aromatic hydrocarbons) present in gasoline are euphorigenic in nature, and are considered to be hazardous substances. Unleaded gasoline contains at least 15 hazardous chemicals including, by volume, benzene (~5%), toluene (35%), naphthalene (~1%), trimethylbenzene (~7%), methyl tertiary butyl ether (MTBE) (~18%, in some states) and about 10 others. Although lead was added to gasoline starting in the 1920s as an anti-knock agent, its use has been phased out due in part to its incompatibility with catalytic converters, which were mandatory on all automobiles manufactured after 1975, and also owing to its hazardous nature. Gasoline combustion is a source of pollutant gases such as carbon dioxide, nitrogen oxides and carbon monoxides, some of which can react with sunlight to produce photochemical smog (Sittig, 1984). Historically, gasoline has been used as an effective treatment for lice. It is also used for removing grease stains from clothing.

Human exposure to gasoline occurs primarily by inhalation. Due to its widespread availability, it is abused by "gasoline sniffers" worldwide. Inhalation exposure data on gasoline is available for personnel working in gas filling and/or service stations. The highest internal levels of gasoline have been measured in sniffers who use it for euphoric effects (Grandjean and Grandjean, 1984; NESCAUM, 1989). Gasoline additives with higher blood/gas coefficients have higher rates of absorption than compounds with lower coefficients. In humans and animals, absorption of ingested gasoline is complete due to high lipophilicity of hydrocarbons and the large surface area of the gastrointestinal tract which provides a long residence time. Dermal absorption of gasoline is lesser compared to oral exposure, and it is known that aromatic hydrocarbons more readily penetrate the skin than do aliphatic hydrocarbons (NESCAUM, 1989). There are limited data on gasoline distribution in humans following ingestion or inhalation. In one case of human fatality due to accidental ingestion of gasoline, the highest concentrations of the solvent were detected in the liver, gastric walls and lungs (324–663 ppm), while brain, bile and kidney had 48–52 ppm and blood from brain, lungs and heart showed 29–52 ppm (Camevale *et al.*, 1983).

Metabolism of gasoline is not well understood, but it is assumed that gasoline components induce mixed function oxidase activities in humans and rats (Harman *et al.*, 1981). There is no conclusive data on the elimination of gasoline following oral, dermal or inhalation exposures.

Inhalation of gasoline vapors targets the CNS and, depending on the duration and dose, the symptoms range from eye irritation, dizziness, headaches, giddiness, euphoria, vertigo, blurred vision, nausea, numbness, drowsiness, anesthesia and coma. In gasoline sniffers, neurological symptoms indicative of inhalation exposure have been observed. High concentrations of gasoline exposure cause asphyxia followed by CNS depression, respiratory failure, cardiac sensitization to circulating catecholamines leading to a fatal arrhythmia and death (Polkis, 1976). Studies in rats and monkeys showed inconsistent adverse respiratory effects with intermediate exposure to gasoline (Kuna and Ulrich, 1984). In rats, a 12-week inhalation study with gasoline caused the development of pulmonary lesions consistent with fibrosing alveolitis (Lykke *et al.*, 1979). Chronic inhalation exposure of unleaded gasoline to rats and mice did not affect brain weight and histopathology of the spinal cord and peripheral nerves; however, multifocal pulmonary inflammatory response has been observed. Rats, but not mice, appear to be susceptible to the pulmonary irritating effects of gasoline (MacFarland *et al.*, 1984). Exposure of gasoline specifically results in nephropathy in male rats. It has been hypothesized that a metabolite of gasoline binds to α2u-globulin in male rat kidney forming a complex, and the inability of lysosomes to catabolize these complexes results in their accumulation which upon lysis causes the release of lysosomal enzymes leading to cytotoxicity and cell death (Swenberg *et al.*, 1989).

There is limited evidence on the reproductive/developmental toxicity of gasoline in humans (ATSDR, 1995b). One study has shown an increased risk of spontaneous abortion in pregnant women with exposure to gasoline and other petrochemicals (Xu *et al.*, 1998). Traffic constables exposed to unleaded gasoline exhaust showed high blood lead (PbB) levels (48.5 μg/100 dL of blood) which were associated with sperm abnormalities such as reduced sperm count and motility (Eibensteiner *et al.*, 2005). In a small Native American community, chronic inhalation exposure of pregnant mothers to gasoline was shown to induce congenital CNS defects in two of the children exposed *in utero*, who displayed severe growth retardation and minor developmental anomalies (Hunter *et al.*, 1979). However, these results could not be confirmed owing to small sample size, absence of data on exposure levels and confounding factors such as concomitant exposure to alcohol and lead which may have also contributed to the developmental defects in these children.

However, a developmental toxicity study in rats exposed up to 1,600 ppm gasoline by inhalation did not induce developmental defects in the offspring (Litton Bionetics, 1978). In albino rats, inhalation exposure to gasoline has been associated with a significant decrease in serum reproductive hormones in both sexes (Ugwoke *et al.*, 2005). In contrast, in a two-generation toxicity study in rats exposed by inhalation to gasoline up to 20,000 mg/m^3, no significant reproductive or developmental toxic effects were observed. However, systemic kidney toxicity in male rats consistent with an α2u-globulin-mediated process was observed (McKee *et al.*, 2000).

Neither developmental toxicity nor any adverse reproductive effects were observed in pregnant rats exposed to unleaded gasoline vapor from day 6 through 19 of gestation (Roberts *et al.*, 2001). Also, mice which received inhalation exposure to unleaded gasoline reported no evidence of dominant lethal effects on sperm morphology and no significant increase in pre- or postimplantation loss of embryos in mated female mice (Litton Bionetics, 1980). Even a higher dose of inhalation exposure to unleaded gasoline vapor (~2,056 ppm) did not produce developmental toxicity in mice (Roberts *et al.*, 2001). Overall, animal studies on reproductive and developmental toxicity of gasoline were negative, while there were limited studies in humans.

KEROSENE AND JET FUELS

Kerosene, also known as paraffin or paraffin oil, is a clear, flammable liquid distilled from petroleum. It is a blend of different hydrocarbons and is less volatile than gasoline. Kerosene is predominantly used as a fuel in jet engines and rockets, but it is also used as a solvent for greases and insecticides (CONCAWE, 1995). The blend of kerosene used for jet fuel consists of 20% aromatic hydrocarbons ranging from C9 to C16. Various jet fuels are formulated to have high flash points for safe refueling, low freezing point for high altitude flying and a high degree of hydrophobicity (Ritchie *et al.*, 2003).

Abraham Gesner, a Canadian geologist, first distilled kerosene from coal in 1846 and kerosene lamps were thereafter widely used before being superseded by light bulbs. Kerosene is widely used as a home heating fuel for both portable and installed heaters and in developing countries it is used in cooking stoves. The first jet propulsion (JP) fuels were based on kerosene or a gasoline–kerosene mixture, and newer jet fuels are still kerosene based. Several jet fuel formulations, including JP-5, JP-8, JP-4 and JP-7, are routinely used in the military and are blended with other chemicals. More than a million military and civilian personnel in the USA are occupationally exposed to JP-8 every year (Ritchie *et al.*, 2003).

Except for a single case report that JP-4 can be absorbed following inhalation exposure in humans, no other studies were located that evaluated the absorption of JP-4 and JP-7 in humans or animals (Stoica *et al.*, 2001). Studies on distribution or metabolism of these fuels are lacking. The limited data describing kerosene metabolism suggest that kerosene is removed from circulation via the liver and lungs. Although much more information is available regarding the individual components of these mixtures (Ritchie *et al.*, 2003), there is very limited literature describing the mechanism of action of either jet fuels or kerosene.

Lungs and skin are the most common target organs for kerosene toxicity (Nessel, 1999). High inhalation exposure to kerosene can induce CNS depression, characterized by ataxia, hypoactivity and prostration. Severe to mild skin irritation has been seen with straight run kerosene, hydrodesulferized kerosene, cracked kerosene, jet fuel A and jet A-1 (ATSDR, 1995a, 1998; CONCAWE, 1995).

There is limited literature available on the reproductive and developmental toxicity of kerosene-based jet fuels in humans. One study did not find significant differences in sperm parameters in USAF personnel exposed to JP-4/JP-8 and other hydrocarbons compared to unexposed controls (Lemasters *et al.*, 1999). However, a study in children who had intrauterine exposure to jet fuels when their mothers were pregnant showed an increased risk for the development of brain tumors (Bunin *et al.*, 1994). Studies on reproductive effects following inhalation exposure to JP-4 or JP-7 in humans are lacking (ATSDR, 1995a). Current literature studies on JP-8 and other jet fuels are limited for the assessment of reproductive and developmental toxicity risk to humans.

Although animal studies on the reproductive effects of JP-7 were not reported, in one chronic study in mice exposed to 1,000 or 5,000 mg/m^3 of JP-4 which caused testicular atrophy 12 months after the end of exposure period, while this exposure did not adversely affect the testis in rats (Bruner *et al.*, 1993). Inhalation studies in monkeys, dogs and rats to intermediate levels of JP-4 did not find adverse respiratory clinical signs or lung histopathological changes and no reproductive or developmental effects have been observed (Davies, 1964; Air Force, 1974, 1980). However, one study with JP-8 given undiluted by gavage to rats for 90 days at several doses (0, 750, 1,500 or 3,000 mg/kg) reported an increase in relative testicular weights without any observable histopathological changes (Mattie *et al.*, 1991). Dermal exposure of rats to hydrodesulferized kerosene at 494 mg/kg/day for 8 weeks did not result in pathological changes in the reproductive organs of the first generation of pups and no excessive anomalies were found (Schreiner *et al.*, 1997). In summary, no well-conducted reproductive and developmental toxicity studies exist to evaluate human health risk of acute or chronic exposure to kerosene and jet fuels.

FORMALDEHYDE (CASRN 50-00-0)

Formaldehyde is an aliphatic aldehyde, and is a highly reactive and flammable chemical. It can readily undergo polymerization and can form explosive mixtures with air. Pure formaldehyde is a colorless gas at room temperature with a strong, pungent, suffocating and highly irritating aroma. It is readily soluble in water, alcohols, ether and other polar solvents. Formalin is a 37% aqueous solution of formaldehyde and 12–15% methanol (NTP, 2005d).

Although Aleksandr Butlerov first synthesized formaldehyde in 1859, it was identified in 1867 by August Wilhelm von Hofmann as the product formed when methanol and air were passed over a heated platinum spiral, a method still used as the basis for the industrial production of formaldehyde today. Since the early 1900s formaldehyde has been produced commercially, and ranks in the top 25 highest volume chemicals produced in the USA. In recent years more than 11 billion pounds were produced annually in the USA compared to 43 billion pounds worldwide (NTP, 2005d). Formaldehyde is used primarily in the production of phenol- or urea-formaldehyde resins, plastics and chemical intermediates that go into building construction, in textile treatments, decorative laminates, molding compounds, etc. People working in the resin, construction, textile industries are exposed to formaldehyde gas by inhalation or by dermal absorption. In addition, formaldehyde is used as a preservative for specimens or cadavers in pathology and anatomy labs and morgues (Tang *et al.*, 2009). Health care professionals (pathologists, technicians and students), embalmers and morticians are exposed to formaldehyde at the workplace while handling specimens or cadavers preserved in formalin. Sources of environmental exposure include off-gassing from mobile homes as seen among the displaced victims of Hurricane Katrina in 2005, automobile exhaust and environmental tobacco smoke (Tang *et al.*, 2009).

Formaldehyde exposure can occur via inhalation, ingestion, as well as dermal routes. Of these, inhalation is predominant with most of the inhaled formaldehyde being absorbed from the upper respiratory tract. It is quickly absorbed into circulation, where it binds reversibly to glutathione (GSH) forming the non-enzymatic hemiacetal adduct, S-(hydroxymethyl) glutathione (HMGSH). This adduct is oxidized by formaldehyde dehydrogenase (FDH) to S-formylglutathione, which is further metabolized by S-formylglutathione hydrolase to formate releasing free GSH (Thompson *et al.*, 2010). Formate can enter the one-carbon pool and metabolically incorporate into proteins and nucleic acids or can be metabolized to CO_2 and water. A very small amount of formaldehyde is produced endogenously during normal physiological processes and is similarly cleared. Formate is excreted in urine while CO_2 is removed in the exhaled air (Thompson *et al.*, 2010).

Formaldehyde exposure increases airway inflammation, induces sensitization and reduces pulmonary function (McGwin *et al.*, 2010). Inhaled formaldehyde causes a direct exposure at the portal of entry with nasal passages where it binds covalently to cellular macromolecules, forming DNA–protein crosslinks and DNA adducts (Liu *et al.*, 2006). With chronic exposure this results in increased squamous cell metaplasia, decreased mucociliary clearance, induction of cytotoxicity and cell proliferation, eventually inducing nasopharyngeal cancers in both exposed human populations and experimental rodents (Bachand *et al.*, 2010). Direct inhalation exposure to formaldehyde causes sensory irritation of the eyes, nose and throat of individuals working in industries or in personnel working in anatomy/pathology labs. Long-term exposure causes increased respiratory symptoms such as asthma, especially in children (McGwin *et al.*, 2010).

Formaldehyde inhalation exposure has been associated with adverse developmental and reproductive outcomes in both epidemiologic studies and experimental animal studies. Epidemiological studies reported spontaneous abortion in women occupationally exposed to formaldehyde; increased time to pregnancy, congenital malformations and low birth weights have been reported (Taskinen *et al.*, 1999). Among women working in a wood-processing industry, more than a three-fold increased risk of spontaneous abortion, ~50% incidence of reduced fertility (delayed conception or an increased time to pregnancy) and an increased risk for endometriosis have been reported, although early studies did not show differences in formaldehyde-induced reproductive toxicity between exposed and unexposed populations (reviewed in (Tang *et al.*, 2009)).

Several rodent studies have demonstrated reproductive and developmental toxicity effects with inhalation or gavage exposure to formaldehyde. Consistent with endometriosis observed in women in one epidemiological report (Taskinen *et al.*, 1999), studies in female mice have shown that exposure to formaldehyde causes weight loss, increased mortality, resorption and endometrial and ovarian hyperplasia (Maronpot *et al.*, 1986). In several studies involving rats, maternal exposure to formaldehyde has been associated with early fetal death. In female rats, increases in ovary weight, number of ovulating cells and changes in blood levels of gonadotropins have been observed, suggesting a possible role of formaldehyde in stimulating the hypothalamus–pituitary–gonadal axis (Kitaev *et al.*, 1984). Repeat inhalation exposure to formaldehyde in male rats reportedly caused reproductive system toxicity as reflected by degeneration of seminiferous tubules, decrease in testes weight, alterations in sperm measures, decreased testosterone levels, alterations in trace metals in the testes and/or dominant lethal effects (Özen *et al.*, 2002, 2005; Golalipour *et al.*, 2007) as well as an increase in abnormal sperm count (Xing *et al.*, 2007).

There is limited information from occupational studies regarding the affect of formaldehyde exposure on developmental endpoints such as congenital malformations and low birth weight. Observed developmental outcomes include fetal loss, structural alterations, growth retardation, and delays in functional development. One study found an association between formaldehyde exposure and congenital anomalies in three of the 34 cases from a Finnish Registry (Hemminki *et al.*, 1985). However, in a case-control study involving laboratory technicians, no association was observed between formaldehyde exposure and congenital anomalies. In experimental animals, inhalation exposure of formaldehyde has been shown to cause lowered fetal weight gain, a decrease in the number of fetuses per dam, decreased organ weight, increased kidney and liver toxicity and undescended testis in males (Gofmekler, 1968; Gofmekler and Bonashevskaia, 1969; Saillenfait *et al.*, 1989; Martin, 1990; Thrasher and Kilburn, 2001). In neonatal rats, exposure to formaldehyde (6,000 or 12,000 ppb, 5 days for 9 weeks from postnatal day 0 to 30) by inhalation has been associated with alterations in brain structure (Aslan *et al.*, 2006; Sarsilmaz *et al.*, 2007), and brain chemistry (Songur *et al.*, 2008).

CONCLUDING REMARKS AND FUTURE DIRECTIONS

This chapter has focused on the reproductive and developmental toxicity of several commonly used solvents that are easily volatilized so that inhalation is a primary route of exposure as summarized in Table 23.2. In general, chlorinated solvents appear to vary in their reproductive and developmental toxic effects in humans. The limited available evidence suggests an increased risk of small-for-gestational-age live born babies in women exposed to CCl_4. In contrast, the dry cleaning solvent PCE has been associated with increased risks of spontaneous abortions, time to pregnancy and decrease in fertility in women who were directly employed or whose spouses were working in the dry-cleaning industry. Men working in these facilities have shown abnormal sperm morphology and other reproductive dysfunctions. Styrene is a component of many household and commercial products worldwide. It is, therefore, crucial to have an understanding of the consequences of exposure to these products. Most case studies to date have focused on the toxic effects on the individual who received the styrene exposure; however, based on available published data, certainly there is a need for information from long-term, low levels of exposure of styrene and other industrial solvents used in many consumer products. Toluene, due to its widespread use in industrial processes and, particularly, in products of commercial or household use, has been associated with spontaneous abortions in women with no developmental effects observed. More studies are needed to better understand the effects of toluene exposure before and during pregnancy. Menstrual

TABLE 23.2 Summary of the effects of selected toxic solvents and gases on reproductive and developmental toxicity in humans and experimental animals

Chemical agent	Species	Reproductive toxicity	Developmental toxicity
Carbon tetrachloride	Human	None	↑ risk of small-for-gestational-age live born babies
	Experimental animals	Rats F: ↓ in fecundity and fertility; ↓ LH, progesterone levels; full litter resorption; M: testicular degeneration; Mice M: testicular atrophy	Retarded fetal development and litter growth
Tetrachloroethylene	Human	F: ↓ fertility; spontaneous abortions, delayed conception, hormonal imbalance; M: sperm abnormalities, ↑ ALH	Low birth weight, congenital anomalies; oral cleft defects
	Experimental animals	Rats F: maternal toxicity; ↑ resorption; M: sperm head abnormalities; Mice and rabbits F: maternal toxicity	Rats: skeletal retardations and total malformations; ↓ postnatal survival; Mice: ↓ fetal weight; delayed ossification; postnatal neurodevelopmental toxicity
Styrene	Human	Spontaneous abortions and decreased male fecundity	Malformations
	Experimental animals	Rats F: maternal toxicity; M: degeneration of seminiferous tubules; ↓ sperm counts;	Rats: ↑neonatal deaths and developmental toxicity
Toluene	Human	↑incidence of spontaneous abortions	None
	Experimental animals	Rats F: ↑litters with ruts; structural variations in ovaries; M: ↓ sperm counts and epididymal weights; Mice: maternal mortality; Rabbits: abortion	Rats: morphological anomalies; ↑neonatal mortality and fetal skeletal retardation or anomalies; Mice: retardation of fetal skeletal development; abnormal neuronal proliferation and migration in the brain of pups
Benzene	Human	F: hypermenorrhea, ovarian hypofunction, menstrual cycle disturbances, spontaneous abortions and premature births	↑intrauterine fetal asphyxia with ↑duration of exposure
	Experimental animals	Rats F: ↓ BW and BWG; Mice M: ↓sperm count; ↑ in abnormal sperm forms; testicular atrophy	Rats: ↓ BW and length; ↑in skeletal retardations and malformations; Rabbits: skeletal variations
Gasoline	Human	F: ↑risk of spontaneous abortions; M: sperm abnormalities	Childhood abnormalities (one study)
	Experimental animals	Rats M: hyaline droplet nephropathy	None
Kerosene and jet fuels	Human	None	None
	Experimental animals	Rats F: ↑cystic mammary hyperplasia; M: ↑cystic degeneration of prostrate and testicular atrophy; Mice M: ↑testicular atrophy	Rats F and M: ↓FW
Formaldehyde	Human	Spontaneous abortions, ↑time to pregnancy	Fetal loss, structural alterations, growth retardation and functional development delays
	Experimental animals	Rats F: ↑pregnancy duration, ovary weight, LH and FSH levels; M: ↓ serum testosterone levels and seminiferous tubule diameter and germ cells; arrested spermatogenesis; Mice F:↑ resorption; M: abnormal sperm	Rats: ↑number of degenerating embryos; delayed ossification; unossified sternebrae; alteration in brain structure and chemistry of postnatally exposed pups; Mice: ↓ live fetuses

F, female; M, male; LH, luteinizing hormone; ALH, amplitude of lateral head displacement; FSH, follicle stimulating hormone; BW, body weight; BWG, body weight gain; FW, fetal weight

cycle disturbances, spontaneous abortions and premature births have been reported in women exposed to volatile solvent mixtures that include benzene and limited developmental effects have been documented. More studies are needed to understand the contribution of benzene, as well as its interaction with other components, to the toxic responses following exposure to benzene-containing complex mixtures. Gasoline exposure has been shown to induce spontaneous abortions in women and sperm abnormalities in men. However, most of the available data describes acute gasoline toxicity following ingestion. Inhalation is an important exposure route, particularly during the fueling of automobiles. Because metabolism and biotransformation of the blended agents likely varies between species, identification of relevant animal models to study these issues is critical. Based on currently available, very limited data, kerosene and jet fuels do not appear to cause significant reproductive and developmental effects in humans.

Formaldehyde, a toxic gas, has been associated with spontaneous abortions and increased time to pregnancy in occupationally exposed women; it was also shown to induce developmental defects in some epidemiological studies. Toluene, benzene and formaldehyde reportedly induce neurodevelopmental toxicity in neonate animal models. A major limitation of most human studies is that, with the exception of PCE, most of the exposures are chemical exposures to complex mixtures. Therefore, in order to better understand the potential for reproductive and developmental toxicity risks, it is important both to gather more information on individual chemicals and to have more detailed information regarding the composition of and response to complex solvent/volatile mixtures to which people are exposed.

ACKNOWLEDGMENTS

The authors would like to thank Dr. Bob Sonawane of the US Environmental Protection Agency, Washington DC, for the critical review of the manuscript and helpful discussions.

REFERENCES

Adams EM, Spencer HC, Rowe VK, Mc CD, Irish DD (1952) Vapor toxicity of carbon tetrachloride determined by experiments on laboratory animals. *AMA Arch Ind Hyg Occup Med* **6:** 50–66.

Ahlborg G Jr, Bjerkedal T, Egenaes J (1987) Delivery outcome among women employed in the plastics industry in Sweden and Norway. *Am J Ind Med* **12:** 507–17.

Air Force (1974) Chronic inhalation toxicity of "JP-4 jet fuel", *Toxic hazards research unit annual technical report* AMRL-TR-74-78, pp. 5–26, Aerospace Medical Research Laboratory, AD, Air Force Systems Command, Wright-Patterson Air Force Base, OH.

Air Force (1980) Evaluation of the toxic effect of a 90-day continuous inhalation exposure to petroleum JP-4 vapor, *Toxic hazards research unit annual technical report* AMRL-TR-80-79, pp. 32–45, Aerospace Medical Research Laboratory, AD, Air Force Systems Command, Wright-Patterson Air Force Base, OH.

Anonymous (1992) Carbon tetrachloride toxicity. Agency for Toxic Substances and Disease Registry. *Am Fam Physician* **46:** 1199–207.

Aslan H, Songur A, Tunc AT, Ozen OA, Bas O, Yagmurca M, Turgut M, Sarsilmaz M, Kaplan S (2006) Effects of formaldehyde exposure on granule cell number and volume of dentate gyrus: a histopathological and stereological study. *Brain Res* **1122:** 191–200.

ATSDR (Agency for Toxic Substances and Disease Registry) (1995a) Toxicological Profile for Jet fuels JP-4 and JP-7. 150, US Department of Health and Human Services, Public Health Service: Atlanta, GA.

ATSDR (Agency for Toxic Substances and Disease Registry) (1995b) Toxicological profile for automotive gasoline. US Department of Health and Human Services, Public Health Service: Atlanta, GA.

ATSDR (Agency for Toxic Substances and Disease Registry) (1998) Toxicological Profile for Jet fuels JP-5 and JP-8. 200, US Department of Health and Human Services, Public Health Service: Atlanta, GA.

ATSDR (Agency for Toxic Substances and Disease Registry) (2000) Toxicological Profile for Toluene. Public Health Service, US Department of Health and Human Services: Atlanta, GA.

ATSDR (Agency for Toxic Substances and Disease Registry) (2007a) Toxicological Profile for Benzene. US Department of Health and Human Services, Public Health Service: Atlanta, GA.

ATSDR (Agency for Toxic Substances and Disease Registry) (2007b) Draft Toxicological Profile for Styrene. US Department of Health and Human Services, Public Health Service: Atlanta, GA.

Bachand AM, Mundt KA, Mundt DJ, Montgomery RR (2010) Epidemiological studies of formaldehyde exposure and risk of leukemia and nasopharyngeal cancer: a meta-analysis. *Crit Rev Toxicol* **40:** 85–100.

Beliles RP (2002) Concordance across species in the reproductive and developmental toxicity of tetrachloroethylene. *Toxicol Ind Health* **18:** 91–106.

Bosco MG, Figa-Talamanca I, Salerno S (1987) Health and reproductive status of female workers in dry cleaning shops. *Int Arch Occup Environ Health* **59:** 295–301.

Bove FJ, Fulcomer MC, Klotz JB, Esmart J, Dufficy EM, Savrin JE (1995) Public drinking water contamination and birth outcomes. *Am J Epidemiol* **141:** 850–62.

Bowen SE, Hannigan JH, Irtenkauf S (2007) Maternal and fetal blood and organ toluene levels in rats following acute and repeated binge inhalation exposure. *Reprod Toxicol* **24:** 343–52.

Bowen SE, Batis JC, Mohammadi MH, Hannigan JH (2005) Abuse pattern of gestational toluene exposure and early postnatal development in rats. *Neurotoxicol Teratol* **27:** 105–16.

Bruner RH, Kinkead ER, O'Neill TP, Flemming CD, Mattie DR, Russell CA, Wall HG (1993) The toxicologic and oncogenic potential of JP-4 jet fuel vapors in rats and mice: 12-month intermittent inhalation exposures. *Fundam Appl Toxicol* **20:** 97–110.

Bunin GR, Buckley JD, Boesel CP, Rorke LB, Meadows AT (1994) Risk factors for astrocytic glioma and primitive neuroectodermal tumor of the brain in young children: a report from the Children's Cancer Group. *Cancer Epidemiol Biomarkers Prev* **3:** 197–204.

Camevale A, Chiarotti M, De Giovanni N (1983) Accidental death by gasoline ingestion: case report and toxicological study. *Am J Forensic Med Pathol* **4:** 153–7.

Chatterjee A (1966) Testicular degeneration in rats by carbon tetrachloride intoxication. *Experientia* **22:** 395–6.

Coate WB, Hoberman AM, Durloo RS (1984) Inhalation teratology study of benzene in rats. *Adv Mod Environ Toxicol* **6:** 187–98.

Cohen JT, Carlson G, Charnley G, Coggon D, Delzell E, Graham JD, Greim H, Krewski D, Medinsky M, Monson R, Paustenbach D, Petersen B, Rappaport S, Rhomberg L, Ryan PB, Thompson K (2002) A comprehensive evaluation of the potential health risks associated with occupational and environmental exposure to styrene. *J Toxicol Environ Health B Crit Rev* **5:** 1–265.

CONCAWE (1995) Kerosines/Jet Fuels, Product Dossier No. 94/106, Brussels, Belgium.

Cruzan G, Carlson GP, Johnson KA, Andrews LS, Banton MI, Bevan C, Cushman JR (2002) Styrene respiratory tract toxicity and mouse lung tumors are mediated by CYP2F-generated metabolites. *Regul Toxicol Pharmacol* **35:** 308–19.

Cruzan G, Cushman JR, Andrews LS, Granville GC, Miller RR, Hardy CJ, Coombs DW, Mullins PA (1997) Subchronic inhalation studies of styrene in CD rats and CD-1 mice. *Fundam Appl Toxicol* **35:** 152–65.

Cruzan G, Cushman JR, Andrews LS, Granville GC, Johnson KA, Hardy CJ, Coombs DW, Mullins PA, Brown WR (1998) Chronic toxicity/oncogenicity study of styrene in CD rats by inhalation exposure for 104 weeks. *Toxicol Sci* **46:** 266–81.

Cruzan G, Cushman JR, Andrews LS, Granville GC, Johnson KA, Bevan C, Hardy CJ, Coombs DW, Mullins PA, Brown WR (2001) Chronic toxicity/oncogenicity study of styrene in CD-1 mice by inhalation exposure for 104 weeks. *J Appl Toxicol* **21:** 185–98.

Davies NE (1964) Jet fuel intoxication. *Aerosp Med* **35:** 481–2.

De Celis R, Feria-Velasco A, Gonzalez-Unzaga M, Torres-Calleja J, Pedron-Nuevo N (2000) Semen quality of workers occupationally exposed to hydrocarbons. *Fertil Steril* **73:** 221–8.

Doyle P, Roman E, Beral V, Brookes M (1997) Spontaneous abortion in dry cleaning workers potentially exposed to perchloroethylene. *Occup Environ Med* **54:** 848–53.

Eibensteiner L, Del Carpio Sanz A, Frumkin H, Gonzales C, Gonzales GF (2005) Lead exposure and semen quality among traffic police in Arequipa, Peru. *Int J Occup Environ Health* **11:** 161–6.

EPA (Environmental Protection Agency) (1991) Guidelines for developmental toxicity risk assessment. *Fed Reg* **56:** 63798–826, Washington DC.

EPA (Environmental Protection Agency) (1996) Reproductive toxicity risk assessment guidelines. *Fed Reg* **61:** 56273–322, Washington DC.

EPA (Environmental Protection Agency) (2005) Toxicological review of toluene. 179, EPA/635/R-05/004, Washington DC.

Eskenazi B, Fenster L, Hudes M, Wyrobek AJ, Katz DF, Gerson J, Rempel DM (1991a) A study of the effect of perchloroethylene exposure on the reproductive outcomes of wives of dry-cleaning workers. *Am J Ind Med* **20:** 593–600.

Eskenazi B, Wyrobek AJ, Fenster L, Katz DF, Sadler M, Lee J, Hudes M, Rempel DM (1991b) A study of the effect of perchloroethylene exposure on semen quality in dry cleaning workers. *Am J Ind Med* **20:** 575–91.

Fredriksson A, Danielsson BR, Eriksson P (1993) Altered behaviour in adult mice orally exposed to tri- and tetrachloroethylene as neonates. *Toxicol Lett* **66:** 13–19.

Gofmekler VA (1968) [The embryotropic action of benzene and formaldehyde in experimental administration by inhalation]. *Gig Sanit* **33:** 12–16.

Gofmekler VA, Bonashevskaia TI (1969) [A study of the experimental teratogenic effect of formaldehyde, based on data of morphological studies]. *Gig Sanit* **34:** 92–4.

Golalipour MJ, Azarhoush R, Ghafari S, Gharravi AM, Fazeli SA, Davarian A (2007) Formaldehyde exposure induces histopathological and morphometric changes in the rat testis. *Folia Morphol (Warsz)* **66:** 167–71.

Gold LS, De Roos AJ, Waters M, Stewart P (2008) Systematic literature review of uses and levels of occupational exposure to tetrachloroethylene. *J Occup Environ Hyg* **5:** 807–39.

Gospe SM Jr, Zhou SS (2000) Prenatal exposure to toluene results in abnormal neurogenesis and migration in rat somatosensory cortex. *Pediatr Res* **47:** 362–8.

Grandjean P, Grandjean EC (1984). *Biological Effects of Organo-Lead Compounds*. Boca Raton, FL, CRC Press, pp. 220–37.

Green JD, Leong BK, Laskin S (1978) Inhaled benzene fetotoxicity in rats. *Toxicol Appl Pharmacol* **46:** 9–18.

Hannigan JH, Bowen SE (2010) Reproductive toxicology and teratology of abused toluene. *Syst Biol Reprod Med* **56:** 184–200.

Harkonen H, Lehtniemi A, Aitio A (1984) Styrene exposure and the liver. *Scand J Work Environ Health* **10:** 59–61.

Harman AW, Frewin DB, Priestly BG (1981) Induction of microsomal drug metabolism in man and in the rat by exposure to petroleum. *Br J Ind Med* **38:** 91–7.

Hemminki K, Kyyronen P, Lindbohm ML (1985) Spontaneous abortions and malformations in the offspring of nurses exposed to anaesthetic gases, cytostatic drugs, and other potential hazards in hospitals, based on registered information of outcome. *J Epidemiol Community Health* **39:** 141–7.

Hooper K, LaDou J, Rosenbaum JS, Book SA (1992) Regulation of priority carcinogens and reproductive or developmental toxicants. *Am J Ind Med* **22:** 793–808.

Huang XY (1991) [Influence on benzene and toluene to reproductive function of female workers in leather shoe-making industry]. *Zhonghua Yu Fang Yi Xue Za Zhi* **25:** 89–91.

Hudak A, Ungvary G (1978) Embryotoxic effects of benzene and its methyl derivatives: toluene, xylene. *Toxicology* **11:** 55–63.

Hunter AG, Thompson D, Evans JA (1979) Is there a fetal gasoline syndrome? *Teratology* **20:** 75–9.

IARC (International Agency for Research on Cancer) (1979) Carbon tetrachloride. *IARC Monogr Eval Carcinog Risk Chem Hum* **20:** 371–99, Lyon, France.

IARC (International Agency for Research on Cancer) (2002) Some traditional herbal medicines, some mycotoxins, naphthalene and styrene, *IARC Monogr Eval Carcinog Risks Hum* **82:** 437–522, Lyons, France.

Kalla NR, Bansal MP (1975) Effect of carbon tetrachloride on gonadal physiology in male rats. *Acta Anat (Basel)* **91:** 380–5.

Kitaev EM, Savchenko ON, Lovchikov VA, Altukhov VV, Vishniakov Iu S (1984) Embryonic development and various indicators of reproductive function in rats after inhalation of formaldehyde in the preimplantation phase. *Akush Ginekol (Mosk)*: 49–52.

Kuczkowski KM (2007) The effects of drug abuse on pregnancy. *Curr Opin Obstet Gynecol* **19:** 578–85.

Kuna RA, Ulrich CE (1984) Subchronic inhalation toxicity of two motor fuels. *J Am Coll Toxicol* **3:** 217–29.

Kuna RA, Nicolich MJ, Schroeder RE (1992) A female rat fertility study with inhaled benzene. *Am Coll Toxicol* **11:** 275–82.

Lash LH, Parker JC (2001) Hepatic and renal toxicities associated with perchloroethylene. *Pharmacol Rev* **53:** 177–208.

Laslo-Baker D, Barrera M, Knittel-Keren D, Kozer E, Wolpin J, Khattak S, Hackman R, Rovet J, Koren G (2004) Child neurodevelopmental outcome and maternal occupational exposure to solvents. *Arch Pediatr Adolesc Med* **158:** 956–61.

Lemasters GK, Hagen A, Samuels SJ (1985) Reproductive outcomes in women exposed to solvents in 36 reinforced plastics companies. I. Menstrual dysfunction. *J Occup Med* **27:** 490–4.

Lemasters GK, Samuels SJ, Morrison JA, Brooks SM (1989) Reproductive outcomes of pregnant workers employed at 36 reinforced plastics companies. II. Lowered birth weight. *J Occup Med* **31:** 115–20.

Lemasters GK, Olsen DM, Yiin JH, Lockey JE, Shukla R, Selevan SG, Schrader SM, Toth GP, Evenson DP, Huszar GB (1999) Male reproductive effects of solvent and fuel exposure during aircraft maintenance. *Reprod Toxicol* **13:** 155–66.

Litton Bionetics (1978) Teratology study in rats: unleaded gasoline. *Final report submitted to American Petroleum Institute*, Litton Bionetics, Inc., Kensington, MD, Washington DC.

Litton Bionetics (1980) Mutagenicity evaluation of gasoline, API PS-6 fuel in the mouse dominant lethal assay. *Final report submitted to American Petroleum Institute*, Litton Bionetics, Inc., Kensington, MD, Washington DC.

Liu Y, Li CM, Lu Z, Ding S, Yang X, Mo J (2006) Studies on formation and repair of formaldehyde-damaged DNA by detection of DNA–protein crosslinks and DNA breaks. *Front Biosci* **11:** 991–7.

Lykke AW, Stewart BW, O'Connell PJ, Le Mesurier SM (1979) Pulmonary responses to atmospheric pollutants. I: An ultrastructural study of fibrosing alveolitis evoked by petrol vapour. *Pathology* **11:** 71–80.

MacFarland HN, Ulrich CE, Holdsworth CE, Kitchen DN, Halliwell WH, Blum SC (1984) A chronic inhalation study with unleaded gasoline vapor. *J Am Coll Toxicol* **3:** 231–48.

Manibusan MK, Odin M, Eastmond DA (2007) Postulated carbon tetrachloride mode of action: a review. *J Environ Sci Health C Environ Carcinog Ecotoxicol Rev* **25:** 185–209.

Maronpot RR, Miller RA, Clarke WJ, Westerberg RB, Decker JR, Moss OR (1986) Toxicity of formaldehyde vapor in B6C3F1 mice exposed for 13 weeks. *Toxicology* **41:** 253–66.

Martin WJ (1990) A teratology study of inhaled formaldehyde in the rat. *Reprod Toxicol* **4:** 237–9.

Mattie DR, Alden CL, Newell TK, Gaworski CL, Flemming CD (1991) A 90-day continuous vapor inhalation toxicity study of JP-8 jet fuel followed by 20 or 21 months of recovery in Fischer 344 rats and C57BL/6 mice. *Toxicol Pathol* **19:** 77–87.

McGwin G, Lienert J, Kennedy JI (2010) Formaldehyde exposure and asthma in children: a systematic review. *Environ Health Perspect* **118:** 313–17.

McKee RH, Trimmer GW, Whitman FT, Nessel CS, Mackerer CR, Hagemann R, Priston RA, Riley AJ, Cruzan G, Simpson BJ, Urbanus JH (2000) Assessment in rats of the reproductive toxicity of gasoline from a gasoline vapor recovery unit. *Reprod Toxicol* **14:** 337–53.

Mitchell A, Bakshi K, Kimmel C, Buck G, Feuston M, Foster PM, Friedman J, Holson J, Hughes C, Moore J, Schwetz B, Scialli A, Scott W, Vorhees C, Zirkin B (2004) Evaluating chemical and other agent exposures for reproductive and developmental toxicity. *J Toxicol Environ Health A* **67:** 1159–314.

Nagano K, Sasaki T, Umeda Y, Nishizawa T, Ikawa N, Ohbayashi H, Arito H, Yamamoto S, Fukushima S (2007) Inhalation carcinogenicity and chronic toxicity of carbon tetrachloride in rats and mice. *Inhal Toxicol* **19:** 1089–103.

Nakajima T, Wang RS, Elovaara E, Park SS, Gelboin HV, Vainio H (1992) A comparative study on the contribution of cytochrome P450 isozymes to metabolism of benzene, toluene and trichloroethylene in rat liver. *Biochem Pharmacol* **43:** 251–7.

Narotsky MG, Kavlock RJ (1995) A multidisciplinary approach to toxicological screening: II. Developmental toxicity. *J Toxicol Environ Health* **45:** 145–71.

Narotsky MG, Brownie CF, Kavlock RJ (1997a) Critical period of carbon tetrachloride-induced pregnancy loss in Fischer-344 rats, with insights into the detection of resorption sites by ammonium sulfide staining. *Teratology* **56:** 252–61.

Narotsky MG, Pegram RA, Kavlock RJ (1997b) Effect of dosing vehicle on the developmental toxicity of bromodichloromethane and carbon tetrachloride in rats. *Fundam Appl Toxicol* **40:** 30–6.

Nelson BK, Taylor BJ, Setzer JV, Hornung RW (1979) Behavioral teratology of perchloroethylene in rats. *J Environ Pathol Toxicol* **3:** 233–50.

NESCAUM (1989) Air toxic committee. Evaluation of the Health Effects from Exposure of Gasoline and Gasoline Vapors. Northeast States for Coordinated Air Use Management, Final Report.

Nessel CS (1999) A comprehensive evaluation of the carcinogenic potential of middle distillate fuels. *Drug Chem Toxicol* **22:** 165–80.

Ng TP, Foo SC, Yoong T (1992a) Menstrual function in workers exposed to toluene. *Br J Ind Med* **49:** 799–803.

Ng TP, Foo SC, Yoong T (1992b) Risk of spontaneous abortion in workers exposed to toluene. *Br J Ind Med* **49:** 804–8.

NTP-CERHR (National Toxicology Program-Center for the Evaluation of Risks to Human Reproduction) (2006) NTP-CERHR Monograph on the Potential Human Reproductive and Developmental Effects of Styrene. NIH Publication No. 06-4475, CERHR, NTP, US Department of Health and Human Services: Research Triangle Park, NC.

NTP (National Toxicology Program) (2005a) Carbon tetrachloride CAS No. 56-23-5. *Report on Carcinogens, Eleventh Edition*, 1–2, US Department of Health and Human Services, Public Health Service, National Toxicology Program: Research Triangle Park, NC.

NTP (National Toxicology Program) (2005b) Tetrachloroethylene (Perchloroethylene) CAS No. 127-18-4. *Report on Carcinogens, Eleventh Edition*, 1–2, US Department of Health and Human Services, Public Health Service, National Toxicology Program: Research Triangle Park, NC.

NTP (National Toxicology Program) (2005c) Benzene CAS No. 71-43-2. *Report on Carcinogens, Eleventh Edition*, 1–2, US Department of Health and Human

Services, Public Health Service, National Toxicology Program: Research Triangle Park, NC.

NTP (National Toxicology Program) (2005d) Formaldehyde (gas) CAS No. 50-00-0. *Report on Carcinogens, Eleventh Edition*, 1–2, US Department of Health and Human Services, Public Health Service, National Toxicology Program: Research Triangle Park, NC.

Olsen J, Hemminki K, Ahlborg G, Bjerkedal T, Kyyronen P, Taskinen H, Lindbohm ML, Heinonen OP, Brandt L, Kolstad H, Halvorsen BA, Egenaes J (1990) Low birthweight, congenital malformations, and spontaneous abortions among dry-cleaning workers in Scandinavia. *Scand J Work Environ Health* **16:** 163–8.

Ono A, Sekita K, Ogawa Y, Hirose A, Suzuki S, Saito M, Naito K, Kaneko T, Furuya T, Kawashima K, Yasuhara K, Matsumoto K, Tanaka S, Inoue T, Kurokawa Y (1996) Reproductive and developmental toxicity studies of toluene. II. Effects of inhalation exposure on fertility in rats. *J Environ Pathol Toxicol Oncol* **15:** 9–20.

Özen OA, Yaman M, Sarsilmaz M, Songur A, Kus I (2002) Testicular zinc, copper and iron concentrations in male rats exposed to subacute and subchronic formaldehyde gas inhalation. *J Trace Elem Med Biol* **16:** 119–22.

Özen OA, Akpolat N, Songur A, Kus I, Zararsiz I, Ozacmak VH, Sarsilmaz M (2005) Effect of formaldehyde inhalation on Hsp70 in seminiferous tubules of rat testes: an immunohistochemical study. *Toxicol Ind Health* **21:** 249–54.

Polkis A (1976) Death resulting from gasoline "sniffing": a case report. *J Forensic Sci* **16:** 43–6.

Rachootin P, Olsen J (1983) The risk of infertility and delayed conception associated with exposures in the Danish workplace. *J Occup Med* **25:** 394–402.

Rappaport SM, Kim S, Lan Q, Li G, Vermeulen R, Waidyanatha S, Zhang L, Yin S, Smith MT, Rothman N (2010) Human benzene metabolism following occupational and environmental exposures. *Chem Biol Interact* **184:** 189–95.

Ritchie G, Still K, Rossi J 3rd, Bekkedal M, Bobb A, Arfsten D (2003) Biological and health effects of exposure to kerosene-based jet fuels and performance additives. *J Toxicol Environ Health B Crit Rev* **6:** 357–451.

Roberts L, White R, Bui Q, Daughtrey W, Koschier F, Rodney S, Schreiner C, Steup D, Breglia R, Rhoden R, Schroeder R, Newton P (2001) Developmental toxicity evaluation of unleaded gasoline vapor in the rat. *Reprod Toxicol* **15:** 487–94.

Ruprah M, Mant TG, Flanagan RJ (1985) Acute carbon tetrachloride poisoning in 19 patients: implications for diagnosis and treatment. *Lancet* **1:** 1027–9.

Russell LD, Ettlin RA, Sinha Hikim AP, Clegg ED (1990) *Histological and Histopathological Evaluation of the Testis*. Clearwater, FL, Cache River Press.

Saillenfait AM, Bonnet P, de Ceaurriz J (1989) The effects of maternally inhaled formaldehyde on embryonal and foetal development in rats. *Food Chem Toxicol* **27:** 545–8.

Sanzgiri UY, Srivatsan V, Muralidhara S, Dallas CE, Bruckner JV (1997) Uptake, distribution, and elimination of carbon tetrachloride in rat tissues following inhalation and ingestion exposures. *Toxicol Appl Pharmacol* **143:** 120–9.

Sarsilmaz M, Kaplan S, Songur A, Colakoglu S, Aslan H, Tunc AT, Ozen OA, Turgut M, Bas O (2007) Effects of postnatal formaldehyde exposure on pyramidal cell number, volume of cell layer in hippocampus and hemisphere in the rat: a stereological study. *Brain Res* **1145:** 157–67.

Schardein JL (2000) *28. Industrial Solvents*, 3rd ed., revised and expanded. *Chemically Induced Birth Defects*. New York, Marcel Dekker, Inc., pp. 909–40.

Schnatter AR, Rosamilia K, Wojcik NC (2005) Review of the literature on benzene exposure and leukemia subtypes. *Chem Biol Interact* **153–154:** 9–21.

Schreiner C, Bui Q, Breglia R, Burnett D, Koschier F, Podhasky P, Lapadula L, White R, Feuston M, Krueger A, Rodriquez S (1997) Toxicity evaluation of petroleum blending streams: reproductive and developmental effects of hydrodesulfurized kerosine. *J Toxicol Environ Health* **52:** 211–29.

Schwetz BA, Leong BK, Gehring PJ (1974) Embryo- and fetotoxicity of inhaled carbon tetrachloride, 1,1-dichloroethane and methyl ethyl ketone in rats. *Toxicol Appl Pharmacol* **28:** 452–64.

Schwetz BA, Leong KJ, Gehring PJ (1975) The effect of maternally inhaled trichloroethylene, perchloroethylene, methyl chloroform, and methylene chloride on embryonal and fetal development in mice and rats. *Toxicol Appl Pharmacol* **32:** 84–96.

Seidler A, Raum E, Arabin B, Hellenbrand W, Walter U, Schwartz FW (1999) Maternal occupational exposure to chemical substances and the risk of infants small-for-gestational-age. *Am J Ind Med* **36:** 213–22.

Sittig M (1984) *Handbook of Toxic and Hazardous Chemicals and Carcinogens*, 2nd ed. Park Ridge, NJ, Noyes Publicatons, pp. 470–1.

Slomianka L, Edelfors S, Ravn-Jonsen A, Rungby J, Danscher G, West MJ (1990) The effect of low-level toluene exposure on the developing hippocampal region of the rat: histological evidence and volumetric findings. *Toxicology* **62:** 189–202.

Smith MT (2010) Advances in understanding benzene health effects and susceptibility. *Annu Rev Public Health* **31:** 133–48 2 pp following 48.

Snyder R (2004) Xenobiotic metabolism and the mechanism(s) of benzene toxicity. *Drug Metab Rev* **36:** 531–47.

Songur A, Sarsilmaz M, Ozen O, Sahin S, Koken R, Zararsiz I, Ilhan N (2008) The effects of inhaled formaldehyde on oxidant and antioxidant systems of rat cerebellum during the postnatal development process. *Toxicol Mech Methods* **18:** 569–74.

Stoica BA, Boulares AH, Rosenthal DS, Iyer S, Hamilton ID, Smulson ME (2001) Mechanisms of JP-8 jet fuel toxicity. I. Induction of apoptosis in rat lung epithelial cells. *Toxicol Appl Pharmacol* **171:** 94–106.

Sumner SJ, Fennell TR (1994) Review of the metabolic fate of styrene. *Crit Rev Toxicol* **24 (Suppl.):** S11–S33.

Swenberg JA, Short B, Borghoff S, Strasser J, Charbonneau M (1989) The comparative pathobiology of alpha 2u-globulin nephropathy. *Toxicol Appl Pharmacol* **97:** 35–46.

Szakmáry É, Ungváry G, Tátrai E (1997) The offspring-damaging effect of tetrachloroethylene in rats, mice, and rabbits. *Central Eur J Occup Environ Med* **3:** 31–9.

Tang X, Bai Y, Duong A, Smith MT, Li L, Zhang L (2009) Formaldehyde in China: production, consumption, exposure levels, and health effects. *Environ Int* **35:** 1210–24.

Tap O, Solmaz S, Polat S, Mete UO, Ozbilgin MK, Kaya M (1996) The effect of toluene on the rat ovary: an ultrastructural study. *J Submicrosc Cytol Pathol* **28:** 553–8.

Taskinen H, Anttila A, Lindbohm ML, Sallmen M, Hemminki K (1989) Spontaneous abortions and congenital malformations among the wives of men occupationally exposed to organic solvents. *Scand J Work Environ Health* **15:** 345–52.

Taskinen HK, Kyyronen P, Sallmen M, Virtanen SV, Liukkonen TA, Huida O, Lindbohm ML, Anttila A (1999) Reduced fertility among female wood workers exposed to formaldehyde. *Am J Ind Med* **36:** 206–12.

Thompson CM, Ceder R, Grafstrom RC (2010) Formaldehyde dehydrogenase: beyond phase I metabolism. *Toxicol Lett* **193:** 1–3.

Thrasher JD, Kilburn KH (2001) Embryo toxicity and teratogenicity of formaldehyde. *Arch Environ Health* **56:** 300–11.

Till C, Koren G, Rovet JF (2001a) Prenatal exposure to organic solvents and child neurobehavioral performance. *Neurotoxicol Teratol* **23:** 235–45.

Till C, Westall CA, Rovet JF, Koren G (2001b) Effects of maternal occupational exposure to organic solvents on offspring visual functioning: a prospective controlled study. *Teratology* **64:** 134–41.

Till C, Rovet JF, Koren G, Westall CA (2003) Assessment of visual functions following prenatal exposure to organic solvents. *Neurotoxicology* **24:** 725–31.

Ugwoke CC, Nwobodo ED, Unekwe P, Odike M, Chukwumai ST, Amilo G (2005) The reproductive dysfunction effects of gasoline inhalation in albino rats. *Niger J Physiol Sci* **20:** 54–7.

Ungvary G, Tatrai E (1985) On the embryotoxic effects of benzene and its alkyl derivatives in mice, rats and rabbits. *Arch Toxicol Suppl* **8:** 425–30.

Ward CO, Kuna RA, Snyder NK, Alsaker RD, Coate WB, Craig PH (1985) Subchronic inhalation toxicity of benzene in rats and mice. *Am J Ind Med* **7:** 457–73.

Whysner J, Reddy MV, Ross PM, Mohan M, Lax EA (2004) Genotoxicity of benzene and its metabolites. *Mutat Res* **566:** 99–130.

Wilson JG (1954) Influence on the offspring of altered physiologic states during pregnancy in the rat. *Ann NY Acad Sci* **57:** 517–25.

Windham GC, Shusterman D, Swan SH, Fenster L, Eskenazi B (1991) Exposure to organic solvents and adverse pregnancy outcome. *Am J Ind Med* **20:** 241–59.

Wolf MA, Rowe VK, McCollister DD, Hollingsworth RL, Oyen F (1956) Toxicological studies of certain alkylated benzenes and benzene; experiments on laboratory animals. *AMA Arch Ind Health* **14:** 387–98.

Xing C, Marchetti F, Li G, Weldon RH, Kurtovich E, Young S, Schmid TE, Zhang L, Rappaport S, Waidyanatha S, Wyrobek AJ, Eskenazi B (2010) Benzene exposure near the U.S. permissible limit is associated with sperm aneuploidy. *Environ Health Perspect* **118:** 833–9.

Xing S-Y, Ye L, Wang N-N (2007) Toxic effect of formaldehyde on reproduction and heredity in male mice. *J Jilin Univ* **33:** 716–18.

Xu X, Cho SI, Sammel M, You L, Cui S, Huang Y, Ma G, Padungtod C, Pothier L, Niu T, Christiani D, Smith T, Ryan L, Wang L (1998) Association of petrochemical exposure with spontaneous abortion. *Occup Environ Med* **55:** 31–6.

Yin SN, Li GL, Hu YT, Zhang XM, Jin C, Inoue O, Seiji K, Kasahara M, Nakatsuka H, Ikeda M (1987) Symptoms and signs of workers exposed to benzene, toluene or the combination. *Ind Health* **25:** 113–30.

Section 5

Smoking, Alcohol, and Drugs of Abuse and Addiction

CHAPTER

24

Cigarette smoking and reproductive and developmental toxicity

Kathleen T. Shiverick

INTRODUCTION

This chapter describes the major observations and principal controversies relating to the effects of cigarette smoking and the constituents of tobacco on female and male reproduction and the development of offspring. Maternal exposure is assessed relative to specific tobacco-related chemicals and the impact of mutagenic products on potential reproductive targets. Important new information is being learned from clinical *in vitro* fertilization and assisted reproduction technologies which has allowed a more thorough analysis of successful pregnancy cycles and the negative consequences of smoking. Lastly, increased emphasis is being placed on smoking cessation during pregnancy using pharmacological intervention with nicotine replacement.

HISTORICAL BACKGROUND

The landmark publication of the first United States (US) Surgeon General's Report on Smoking and Health in 1964 identified the causal relationship of smoking to lung cancer in men (USDHHS, 2004). Studies have demonstrated a strong relationship between tobacco smoke, carcinogen–DNA adduct formation, smoke exposure and cancer risk. Presently there is sufficient scientific evidence to causally link tobacco use to cancers at 18 different organ sites (American Cancer Society, 2009; IARC, 2004; USDHHS, 2004). In the USA, tobacco causes nearly 30% of all cancer deaths. In addition, tobacco causes many other diseases and adverse health conditions, including cardiovascular and respiratory disease. According to a Centers for Disease Control and Prevention (CDC) report, 44 million adults, more than 20% of the population, were current smokers, including almost as many women as men (CDC, 2009).

Cigarette smoke is known to be a complex mixture of more than 4,000 chemicals containing at least 60 toxicants, including nicotine, cadmium, polycyclic aromatic hydrocarbons (PAHs), nitroso compounds and aromatic amines (Table 24.1) (Rodgman and Perfetti, 2009; Hecht, 2008). Nicotine is the major constituent of tobacco smoke that is known to cause addiction (Alouf *et al.*, 2006). Secondhand smoke, also referred to as environmental tobacco smoke, is now recognized to cause disease and premature death in non-smoking adults and children. Secondhand smoke is composed of sidestream smoke given off by the burning end of a tobacco product as well as exhaled mainstream smoke from the smoker. Sidestream smoke contains more than 50 cancer-causing chemicals, some of which occur in proportionately higher levels than mainstream smoke (CDC, 2008). The Environmental Protection Agency (EPA) has now classified secondhand smoke as a carcinogen because of concerns regarding adverse health effects on both adults and the children of smokers (EPA, 1993). In 2006 the US Surgeon General concluded that there is no safe level of exposure to secondhand tobacco smoke and that the only way to fully protect nonsmokers from secondhand smoke exposure is to eliminate smoking in indoor spaces (USDHHS, 2006).

Approximately 30% of reproductive age women and 35% of reproductive age men in the USA smoke cigarettes. Maternal smoking during pregnancy is known to be associated with adverse pregnancy outcomes, including low birth weight, premature delivery, spontaneous abortion, placental abruption, perinatal mortality and ectopic pregnancy (for review: Shiverick and Salafia, 1999; Cnattingius, 2004; Practice Committee of the American Society for Reproductive Medicine, 2008; Rogers, 2008; Cooper and Moley, 2008; Viswanath *et al.*, 2010). According to the American Lung Association, maternal smoking accounts for up to 15% of all preterm deliveries, 20–30% of all low birth weight babies and approximately 10% of all stillborn births (http://www.lungusa.org/site/, May 2007). The adverse effect of cigarette smoking on female fertility has been clearly documented in several systematic reviews of multiple observational studies of natural conception (Hughes and Brennan, 1996; Augood *et al.*, 1998; Hull *et al.*, 2000). The negative association between smoking and live birth rates was dose dependent with number of cigarettes smoked, which supports a causal relationship. Active smoking by either partner has been found to delay conception.

A number of mechanisms have been implicated in the smoking-related loss of fertility. First, smoking accelerates

Reproductive and Developmental Toxicology, Edited by Ramesh C. Gupta
ISBN: 978-0-12-382032-7

TABLE 24.1 Constituents of cigarette smoke

Tobacco smoke contains >4,000 chemicals, including:
Acetaldehyde
Acrolein
4-Aminobiphenyl
Benzene
Benz(a)anthracene
Benzo(a)pyrene
1,3-Butadiene
Cadmium
Carbon monoxide
Chromium VI
Formaldehyde
Hydrazine
Methyl chloride
2-Naphthylamine2-naphthylamine
Nicotine
NNK (4-[methyl-nitrosamino]-1-[3-pyridyl]-1-butanone)
Phenol
Potassium cyanide
Styrene
Toluene

the loss of ovarian follicles and may advance the time of menopause by 1 to 4 years (Mattison *et al.*, 1989; Baron *et al.*, 1990; Cooper *et al.*, 1995; Shiverick and Salafia, 1999). Many studies show a direct interference with intrafollicular processes such as steroid hormone production and oocyte maturation, or altered pituitary output of gonadotropins (FSH and luteinizing hormone) (Kondoh *et al.*, 2002; Paszkowski *et al.*, 2002; Smida *et al.*, 2004). Advancements in the field of *in vitro* fertilization (IVF) have provided more detailed information on the effects of cigarette smoking on the process of conception (for review: Soares and Melo, 2008; Practice Committee of the American Society for Reproductive Medicine, 2008). Recent studies have been able to analyze conception through ovarian follicular development and steroidogenesis, oocyte quality and quantity, fertilization, embryo quality and implantation because of the continued monitoring and analysis of gametes and embryos during the IVF process. The outcome of assisted reproduction technology (ART) cycles show that smokers require nearly twice the number of IVF attempts to conceive as non-smokers (El-Nemr *et al.*, 1998; Cooper *et al.*, 1995; Sharara *et al.*, 1994). Objective data have been collected on the presence of heavy metals, PAHs, and nicotine in follicular fluid as well as serum and urine. Neal *et al.* (2005) more recently found that exposure to passive smoke was as harmful as active smoking to pregnancy rates in patients undergoing IVF, even with similar fertilization rates and embryo quality.

Second, smoking is associated with increased risks of ectopic pregnancy and spontaneous abortion through mechanisms related to altered tubal function and uterine receptiveness. Recent studies have implicated oocyte pick-up and transport in the fallopian tube as factors involved in the adverse effects of cigarette smoke constituents (Knoll and Talbot, 1998; Talbot, 2008), which may underlie the increased risk of ectopic pregnancy (Saraiya *et al.*, 1998). Smoking is further associated with increased spontaneous miscarriage in both natural and ART cycles (Hughes and Brennan, 1996; Ness *et al.*, 1999; Winter *et al.*, 2002). Interestingly, the effects of smoking on the uterus have been less well documented. Smokers have as much as a 50% lower risk of endometrial cancer compared with non-smokers, as well as a decreased incidence of endometriosis and uterine fibroids (Baron *et al.*, 1990; Shiverick and Slafia, 1999). Although factors such as weight, diet, parity, alcohol use and early menopause in smokers may exert an anti-estrogenic effect, post-menopausal women who smoke still exhibit a substantially lowered risk of endometrial cancer (Franks *et al.*, 1987). Thus, cigarette smoke is seemingly 'protective' against benign and malignant uterine disorders, while at the same time being associated with impaired implantation and pregnancy rate.

Third, gamete mutagenesis is another mechanism whereby smoking may adversely affect fertility and reproductive outcomes. Gene damage to human gametes and embryos is linked to exposure to cigarette smoke (Zenzes, 2000), including altered meiotic maturation of oocytes (Zenzes *et al.*, 1997) and DNA adducts in sperm (Zenzes *et al.*, 1999). In men, the effects of smoking on semen have been reported as reductions in sperm density and motility, as well as function (Sofikitis *et al.*, 2000).

Infants born to mothers who smoke are frequently premature and smaller than infants of non-smokers, even after adjustment for gestational age. In addition, there are increased postnatal morbidity and mortality relating to deficits in pulmonary function and neurocognitive development (Naeye, 1992; MacDorman *et al.*, 1997). More recent studies now recognize additional adverse outcomes of maternal cigarette smoking to include childhood cancer, as well as obesity, high blood pressure and diabetes later in life (Rogers, 2008; Salihu and Wilson, 2007). Lastly, it is reported that more than 70% of women who smoke continue to do so throughout their pregnancy (http://www.lungusa.org/site/, May 2007; Doherty *et al.*, 2009). Given the combined number of women who actively smoke cigarettes during pregnancy as well as those exposed passively to environmental tobacco smoke (ETS), it is estimated that about 2 million babies are born each year that have been exposed to cigarette smoke *in utero* (Byrd and Howard, 1995). For this reason, a major effort has been initiated to facilitate smoking cessation by providing education and monitoring to eliminate exposure to tobacco smoke in both women and men (Shiverick and Salafia, 1999; Practice Committee of the American Society for Reproductive Medicine, 2008). When behavioral approaches fail to be successful, then pharmacologic agents are recommended to achieve tobacco smoking cessation, with nicotine replacement therapy (NRT) being the most common approach.

PHARMACOKINETICS/ TOXICOKINETICS

Cigarette smoke is known to be a complex colloid containing more than 4,000 chemicals (Hecht, 2008; Rogers, 2008; Rodgman and Perfetti, 2009). Some of these chemicals originate in the cigarette itself, while others are produced during burning or are added to the cigarette during manufacture to improve flavor. Table 24.1 lists some of the 60 toxic compounds that have been identified in tobacco smoke, including nicotine, cadmium, polycyclic aromatic hydrocarbons (PAHs), nitroso compounds and aromatic amines. Nicotine is the major constituent known to cause addiction (Alouf *et al.*, 2006). Mean concentrations of benzo(a)pyrene, a major PAH, and declared tar, nicotine and carbon monoxide levels per cigarette have been documented in 35 major brands (Kaiserman and Rickert, 1992). Carbon monoxide in cigarette smoke is rapidly absorbed and binds to hemoglobin, forming carboxyhemoglobin in both maternal and fetal blood. Nicotine and carbon monoxide rapidly cross the placental barrier, and levels in the fetus can become higher than those in the maternal compartment with chronic exposure. Cadmium, a heavy metal, is also important because it accumulates in the placenta and may play a role in intrauterine growth restriction (Eisenmann and Miller, 1996). However, most of the chemicals in smoke have not yet been analyzed for their toxicological properties, and smoke probably contains many toxicants that are as yet unidentified.

Burning a cigarette produces two major classes of smoke. Mainstream smoke is the bolus of smoke inhaled by an active smoker, while sidestream smoke burns off the end of a cigarette. The 2006 US Surgeon General's Report reviewed the health consequences of involuntary exposure to tobacco smoke (USDHHS, 2006). Environmental tobacco smoke is composed of sidestream smoke plus the smoke that an active smoker exhales. Thus, sidestream smoke is inhaled by both active and passive smokers. While the chemical composition of both types of smoke is similar, the concentration of individual components varies in each type (EPA, 1993). Sidestream smoke contains more than 50 cancer-causing chemicals, some of which occur in higher levels than mainstream smoke (Neal *et al.*, 2005). This difference in concentrations is partially due to the fact that mainstream smoke is sometimes filtered whereas sidestream smoke is not filtered. While concentrations of toxicants in sidestream smoke tend to be higher than in mainstream smoke, the concentration of sidestream smoke inhaled by a smoker varies with the degree of its dilution in air before inhalation occurs.

Nicotine

Nicotine and its primary metabolite, cotinine, have been measured in multiple body fluids and specimens from smokers, those exposed to secondhand tobacco smoke, users of smokeless tobacco and people undergoing nicotine replacement therapy (NRT) (for review: Rogers, 2008). As the serum half-life of nicotine is only 2 hours compared with 16 hours for cotinine, levels of cotinine are used as a more sensitive and reliable indicator for daily smoke exposure. Cotinine concentrations in serum, urine, hair and saliva are commonly used as biomarkers of recent tobacco exposure in epidemiological studies. In pregnant women, cotinine levels in maternal and neonatal hair show significant differences between active smokers, passive smokers and non-smokers (Eliopoulos *et al.*, 1996), and cotinine concentrations in maternal urine are inversely related to infant birth size (Wang *et al.*, 1997). In a meta-analysis, Florescu *et al.* (2007) proposed reference values for cotinine in hair of women of reproductive age, pregnant women, their children and neonates. Reference values are defined for hair cotinine (ng/mg) that distinguish between active smokers, those passively exposed to secondhand smoke and unexposed non-smokers. In this regard, epidemiological research into the effects of cigarette smoking has been limited in that assessment of exposure in many studies is based on self-reported smoking patterns. It is recognized that questionnaire-based assessments can introduce ascertainment bias into the data in the direction of underreporting of tobacco use.

PAHs and nitrosamines

In cigarette smoke, the two major classes of mutagenic agents are PAHs and nitrosamines (Hecht, 2008). Levels of PAHs, especially benzo(a)pyrene (BaP), are present in concentrations 10-fold higher in sidestream than mainstream smoke (Lodovici *et al.*, 2004). Cigarette use during pregnancy has been related to the presence of smoking and benzo(a)pyrene-related DNA adducts in human term placentas (Everson *et al.*, 1986; Manchester *et al.*, 1988), indicating environmental exposure that damages human DNA. Potent tobacco-related carcinogens also cross the placenta based upon evidence that 4-aminobiphenyl binds covalently to fetal hemoglobin in significantly higher concentrations in smokers (Myers *et al.*, 1996), and a derivative of the carcinogen NNK was found in the urine of infants born to smokers (Hecht *et al.*, 1998). The presence of NNK, the tobacco-specific carcinogenic nitrosamine 4-(methyl-nitrosamino)-1-(3-pyridyl)-1-butanone, in cervical mucous of smokers (Prokopczyk *et al.*, 1997) was linked with findings of DNA damage in cervical epithelium and cervical dysplasia, as well as increased risk for cervical cancer in smokers (Winkelstein, 1990; Simons *et al.*, 1993). Moreover, tobacco smoke induces placental and fetal enzyme systems capable of bioactivation of pro-carcinogens to carcinogenic and mutagenic products (Pasanen *et al.*, 1988; Sanyal *et al.*, 1993).

Testing tobacco products *in vitro*

This was recently reviewed by Andreoli *et al.* (2003) and Talbot (2008). Smoke solutions and condensates are usually prepared from cigarettes smoked in a smoking machine using a protocol established by the Federal Trade Commission/International Organization for Standardization (FTC/ISO). A standard protocol involves a 35ml puff of 2sec duration every minute (Group, 2007); however, other smoking machine protocols have been developed to reflect variations in inhalation patterns with different tobacco products. For *in vitro* exposures, a commonly used method involves collection of smoke on a glass surface or filter, then extraction and testing of the condensate. Solutions of tobacco smoke can be prepared by drawing smoke through culture medium which is then tested at various doses (Knoll and Talbot, 1998). Solutions from whole smoke can be tested, or the particulate phase and gas phase can be collected and assayed separately. Alternatively, smoke can be drawn directly over cultured cells or culture medium can be exposed to smoke for variable lengths of time to produce smoke conditioned medium (Vidal *et al.*, 2006). The advantage of using a smoking machine to create solutions and condensates for *in vitro* testing is that the test solutions can be more accurately controlled, and concentrations of nicotine or PAHs in smoke solutions and condensates can be measured, which enables *in vitro* experiments to be done using quantified exposures. However, any effect observed *in vitro* needs to be confirmed *in vivo* since toxicants in smoke may be metabolized to a non-toxic form or, alternatively, activated to a harmful form *in vivo*.

MECHANISMS OF ACTION

Of the 60 toxic compounds identified in tobacco smoke, clear mechanisms of action are known for nicotine, carbon monoxide and polycyclic aromatic hydrocarbons (PAHs). Other constituents of tobacco and tobacco smoke may exert teratogenicity or fetotoxicity in laboratory animals, but whether they contribute to the developmental toxicity of tobacco or tobacco smoke in humans is unknown. A greater understanding of the molecular pathways underlying tobacco carcinogens will be based on new technologies and systems biology approaches such as genomics, epigenomics, transcriptomics, proteomics and metabolomics.

Nicotine

Nicotine is a major constituent of tobacco smoke and the developmental toxicity of nicotine has been reviewed recently (Pauly and Slotkin, 2008; Bruin *et al.*, 2010). The effects of nicotine on the development of the central nervous system are the subject of another chapter in this book. Nicotine binds to nicotinic cholinergic receptors which activate important signal transduction pathways in many developing organs and tissues in addition to the central nervous system (Bruin *et al.*, 2010). Nicotine is clearly a neuroteratogen and is the most likely cause of cognitive, emotional and behavioral problems seen in children of smokers. The development of other organs, including the lung, is also adversely affected by nicotine.

Carbon monoxide

Carbon monoxide in cigarette smoke is rapidly absorbed and binds to hemoglobin, forming carboxyhemoglobin in both maternal and fetal blood. Carboxyhemoglobin formation will result in fetal hypoxia, which, if severe enough, is teratogenic and fetotoxic.

PAHs

There are many known carcinogens in tobacco, but direct links to specific carcinogens have not been established for most. The two major classes of mutagenic agents are PAHs and nitrosamines (Hecht, 2008). Smoking also induces epigenetic effects that contribute to carcinogenesis (Schwartz *et al.*, 2007). The reproductive and developmental toxicity of specific PAHs is the subject of other chapters in this book. Research has elucidated many biological mechanisms by which tobacco use and smoke exposure lead to cancer. For example, tobacco carcinogens are metabolically activated in humans to forms that bind to DNA and create DNA adducts, which then cause mutations in genes such as the important growth-regulatory genes *ras* and *p53* (Hecht, 2008). The PAH family is a class of compounds formed by the incomplete combustion of fossil fuels and organic matter (Sagredo *et al.*, 2006). Benzo(a)pyrene (BaP) is a PAH that is a ubiquitous environmental pollutant that possesses potent mutagenic properties. BaP is known to cause the formation of DNA adducts and is primarily activated by P450 enzymes, most notably CYP1A1 and CYP1B1, which are regulated by the Aryl hydrocarbon receptor (AhR) pathway. Upon exposure to BaP, the AhR is bound by BaP and translocates to the nucleus, where it binds the AhR nuclear translocator and transcriptionally activates genes containing the xenobiotic response element in their promoter regions (Sagredo *et al.*, 2006). Ovarian follicles of women exposed to cigarette smoke have detectable levels of BaP in follicular fluid (Neal *et al.*, 2007). The follicles are also known to express the AhR (Thompson *et al.*, 2005) and are susceptible to BaP exposure.

Genetic factors

Wang *et al.* (2002) reported that the effects of maternal smoking on infant birth weight were influenced by specific metabolic gene polymorphisms of the mother. Specifically, a subgroup of pregnant women with the cytochrome P450 1A1 (*CYPIA1*) Mspl variant genotype and/or the glutathione *S*-transferase theta 1 (*GSTT1*) deletion genotype were particularly susceptible to the adverse effects of smoking during pregnancy. The greatest reduction in birth weight and gestational length was observed in infants whose smoking mother had one of these polymorphisms. Thus, evidence indicates that the maternal genotype can play a role in cigarette smoke-induced effects on birth weight and gestational duration.

TOXICITY

The adverse effects of cigarette smoking on female and male reproduction and prenatal and postnatal development are summarized in Table 24.2.

Fertility

Hughes and Brennan (1996) conducted a meta-analysis to assess the effects of female and male smoking on natural and assisted fertilization. In 13 studies of natural conception, all but one demonstrated a negative association between smoking and time to conception and live birth rate. Smoking one pack of cigarettes per day and starting to smoke before

TABLE 24.2 Effects of cigarette smoking on reproduction and development

Effects on the female
Decreased fertility
Ectopic pregnancy
Placental abruption
Placenta previa
Spontaneous abortion
Effects on the child
Malformations
Stillbirth
Preterm delivery
Low birth weight (<2,500 g)
Decreased birth weight
Respiratory deficits
SIDS (sudden infant death syndrome)
Asthma
Cognitive deficits
Behavior problems
Attention deficit disorders
Cancer
Effects on the male
Decreased fertility
Decreased sperm density
Decreased sperm motility

18 years of age were further associated with an increased risk of infertility, providing evidence of dose- and age-related effects on natural fertility (Laurent *et al.*, 1992). Furthermore, fertility is lower in women with sidestream smoke exposure (Neal *et al.*, 2005) which suggests that chemicals present in environmental tobacco smoke are also reproductive toxicants. In assisted reproduction cycles, ovarian function can be assessed by measuring blood steroid hormone levels, oocyte numbers and oocyte quality following the administration of a known stimulatory dose of gonadotropins. A meta-analysis of seven studies of subfertile women undergoing assisted reproductive technologies showed small but consistent reductions in pregnancy rates among smokers (Hughes and Brennan, 1996). Recent assisted reproduction studies have begun to identify differential effects of smoking on ovarian function compared to implantation and the maintenance of pregnancy (for review: Shiverick and Salafia, 1999; Soares and Melo, 2008; Practice Committee of the American Society for Reproductive Medicine, 2008). Despite substantial variability in clinical parameters for assisted reproductive cycles, some interesting themes have developed from studies on the influence of tobacco use on fertility. First, smoking is related to a prolonged and dose-dependent adverse effect on ovarian function in past and current smokers. Second, smoking has a more transient effect on implantation and ongoing pregnancy in that current smokers had a markedly decreased pregnancy rate after treatment cycle when compared to non-smokers, as well as to women who quit smoking before initiating treatment.

TABLE 24.3 Targets of cigarette smoke in females and males: *in vitro* assays

Ovary
Fetal ovary organ culture
Ovarian follicle explant
Cumulus expansion
In vitro steroidogenesis
Human oocytes and cumulus from IVF
Oviduct
Infundibular explant assay
Cilliary beat frequency
Oocyte pick-up rate
Adhesion assay
Muscle contraction rate
Uterus
In vitro contraction
Uterine microvascular assays
Placenta
Placental explants
In vitro perfusion
Placental microsomes
In vitro steroidogenesis

Ovarian function

Tobacco smoke has been causally linked to impairments in many functions of the ovary: steroidogenesis, folliculogenesis, gametogenesis and ovulation and corpus luteum function. The effects of smoke and its constituents on oocytes have been studied extensively both *in vivo* and *in vitro*. IVF laboratories have provided human oocytes for *in vitro* assessment of smoke's effects on oocyte quality and ability to be fertilized. In these studies, the material used comes from documented smokers or non-smokers and evaluations are done *in vitro* following removal from the patient. As summarized in Table 24.3, *in vitro* assays include fetal ovary organ culture, ovarian follicular explants, cumulus expansion, steroidogenesis and assessment of oocytes and cumulus cells from *in vitro* fertilization patients.

Ovarian follicle depletion

It is well accepted that menopause occurs 1 to 4 years earlier in smoking women than in non-smokers. The dose-dependent nature of the effect is evidence that smoking accelerates ovarian follicular depletion and may lead to diminished ovarian reserve at earlier reproductive ages (Practice Committee of the American Society for Reproductive Medicine, 2008). Mean basal FSH levels are significantly higher in young smokers than in non-smokers (Cooper *et al.*, 1995; El-Nemr *et al.*, 1998). Basal FSH levels were 66% higher in active smokers than in non-smokers and 39% higher in passive smokers than in non-smokers (Cooper *et al.*, 1995; Cooper and Moley, 2008). Urinary estrogen excretion during the luteal phase in smokers is only about one-third that observed in non-smokers. Mean gonadotropin dose requirements for smokers receiving stimulation for IVF are higher when compared to those of non-smoking women. In the clomiphene citrate challenge test (CCCT), a higher prevalence of abnormal results was found in smokers than in age-matched non-smokers, providing further evidence that smoking has adverse effects on ovarian reserve (Sharara *et al.*, 1994). The detrimental effect of smoking becomes more detectable in older women undergoing treatment, suggesting that the effects of smoking and advancing age may synergize to accelerate the rate of oocyte depletion (Sharara *et al.*, 1994; Hughes and Brennan, 1996; Zenzes *et al.*, 1997).

Evidence now clearly shows that specific chemicals in cigarette smoke can accelerate follicular depletion and the loss of reproductive function. In animal models, cigarette smoke extracts cause ovarian atresia in rodents (Mattison *et al.*, 1989). A recent study further showed that cigarette smoke exposure in mice, at exposure concentrations representative of human exposure, induced a significant reduction in the number of primordial follicles, but not growing or antral follicles compared with controls (Tuttle *et al.*, 2009). A potential toxin to the ovary is the heavy metal cadmium which is present in high concentrations in tobacco and accumulates in ovarian tissue of smokers (Varga *et al.*, 1993). In rats, cadmium is a potent ovarian toxin associated with alterations in the meiotic maturation of oocytes (Watanabe and Endo, 1982). Both cadmium and cotinine levels in ovarian follicular fluid aspirated from women at time of egg retrieval in IVF cycles were correlated with the level of cigarette smoking (Zenzes *et al.*, 1995, 1997). All women known to be exposed to passive smoke also had detectable follicular fluid cotinine levels, though at lower concentrations.

PAHs present in cigarette smoke represent another potential source of chemicals toxic to the ovary. The prototype PAHs 7,12-dimethylbenz(a)anthracene (DMBA) and benzo(a)pyrene (BaP) cause oocyte destruction in mice and alter the formation of corpora lutea (Mattison *et al.*, 1989). In this regard, BaP was detected as a DNA adduct in granulosa-lutein cells of women undergoing IVF who were exposed to cigarette smoke (Zenzes *et al.*, 1998). A more recent study of women undergoing IVF found that BaP is detectable in the serum and follicular fluid of smokers (Neal *et al.*, 2007), and it was present in significantly higher levels in follicular fluid with active smoking compared to sidestream-exposed or non-smoking controls (Neal *et al.*, 2008). In addition, levels of BaP were significantly higher in the follicular fluid of women who did not conceive compared to those that became pregnant. Other PAHs known to be present in cigarette smoke were also detectable in both serum and follicular fluid of IVF patients, but with less frequency compared to BaP, and no differences were found associated with active smoking (Neal *et al.*, 2008). Moreover, in the rat ovarian follicle assay, BaP, inhibited FSH-stimulated follicular growth at concentrations present in follicular fluid of women who smoke (Neal *et al.*, 2007).

Evidence further indicates that PAHs can activate the same cell death regulatory pathways utilized by ovarian cells under normal physiological conditions. *In vitro* studies demonstrated that DMBA caused oocyte destruction involving a dose-dependent induction of programmed cell death (apoptosis) in germ cells, as well as in mouse granulosa cells (Perez *et al.*, 1997). The observation that mouse oocytes deficient in expression of Bax, a key regulatory gene in the apoptotic pathway, were resistant to DMBA toxicity is further evidence that PAH-mediated oocyte destruction involves activation of genes involved in programmed cell death. Using gene expression profiling with both large-scale and targeted microarray analysis, Pru *et al.* (2009) recently showed in mice that DMBA upregulates ovarian expression of a large cassette of proapoptotic genes that function at multiple steps of the cell death signaling pathway. Ovarian expression of p53 was increased by DMBA treatment, as well as several proapoptotic genes that are known transcriptional targets of p53; in addition, mice lacking functional p53 are resistant to the ovotoxic effects of *in vivo* PAH exposure.

Smoking appears to impair angiogenesis during maturation of human oocytes through increased levels in follicular fluid of a soluble truncated form of vascular endothelial growth factor fms-like tyrosine receptor 1 (sVEGFR-1, or sFlt-1) (Motejlek *et al.*, 2006). This soluble receptor binds to VEGF-A and inhibits its binding with the normal form of the transmembrane receptor. Self-reported smoking was confirmed in this study by the finding of nearly 30 times the cotinine levels in the follicular fluid from the smokers compared with non-smokers.

Ovarian steroidogenesis

There is evidence for acute and chronic inhibition of steroidogenic function and estrogen synthesis by cigarette smoke and its constituents. Several mechanisms have been proposed for tobacco effects on steroid hormone synthesis in the ovary. *In vitro* exposure to extracts of cigarette smoke and nicotine produced a direct inhibition of granulosa cell aromatase activity (Barbieri *et al.*, 1986; Vidal *et al.*, 2006). In addition, nicotine and cotinine directly inhibited aromatase in human trophoblasts in culture in a dose-dependent fashion, and both aromatase activity and cytochrome P-450 aromatase concentration in term placentae from smokers were significantly decreased (Kitawaki *et al.*, 1993). In a bovine model, both theca interna and granulosa cells were cultured *in vitro* and treated with nicotine or cotinine (Sanders *et al.*, 2002). Androstenedione secretion (a precursor of estradiol) by theca interna cells was inhibited by treatment with nicotine but not with cotinine. In a hamster model, transplanted ovarian grafts exposed to nicotine had a significant amount of granulosa cell apoptosis in a dose-dependent fashion (Bordel *et al.*, 2006). Further information on steroidogenesis has recently been reviewed (Mlynarcikova *et al.*, 2005). It has been proposed that inhibition of granulosa–luteal cell function may lead to corpus luteal deficiency which could underlie the increase in early pregnancy loss observed in smokers. In this context, nicotine has been shown to reduce progesterone production from human luteal cells *in vitro* (Miceli *et al.*, 2005). In addition, smoking appears to affect steroid hormone metabolism. Placental microsomes of smokers have increased 2- and 4-hydroxylation of estradiol (Juchau *et al.*, 1982). The observation that the 2-hydroxylation of estradiol is increased in smokers led to the proposal that increased catechol estrogen formation is a mechanism for the anti-estrogenic effect of smoking (Tankó and Christiansen, 2004).

Oocyte maturation

IVF laboratories have provided human oocytes for assessment of smoke's effects on oocyte quality and ability to be fertilized. Both chromosomal and DNA damage to human germ cells may result from tobacco smoke exposure. In oocytes from IVF patients, the proportion of diploid oocytes was found to increase with the number of cigarettes smoked per day, suggesting that smoking may disrupt function of the meiotic spindle in humans (Zenzes *et al.*, 1995). In an animal model, nicotine has also been shown to block hamster oocytes in metaphase I of meiosis by alteration of spindle formation (Racowsky *et al.*, 1989). Cadmium, when injected into hamsters, caused a significant increase in oocytes without a polar body and many oocytes were found to be diploid (Watanabe and Endo, 1982).

Cumulus expansion normally occurs in ovarian follicles before ovulation of the oocyte, and the cumulus complex (OCC) is necessary for successful ovulation and pick-up of oocytes by the oviduct (Talbot, 2008). The effect of cigarette smoke on cumulus expansion has been studied *in vitro* using FSH-induced expansion in a porcine model exposed to varying doses of cadmium, anabasine or nicotine, all components of cigarette smoke (Vrsanská *et al.*, 2003; Mlynarcikova *et al.*, 2005). Treated OCC failed to expand as much as untreated controls, and hyaluronic acid synthesis was impaired. Interestingly, treatment with BaP impairs cumulus expansion in isolated rat follicle culture experiments (Neal *et al.*, 2007). In women undergoing IVF procedures, cumulus cells showed more DNA damage in smokers than in non-smokers (Sinkó *et al.*, 2005). In addition, zona pellucida thickness has also been found to be thicker around oocytes from active and passive smokers (Shiloh *et al.*, 2004).

Oviduct/fallopian tube

There is increasing evidence that smoking may alter fertility by effects on uterine–fallopian tube functions which mediate gamate and conceptus transport (for review: Talbot, 2008). Women who smoked more than 20 cigarettes daily had a significantly increased risk for ectopic pregnancy compared to non-smokers (Saraiya *et al.*, 1998). Nicotine administered to rhesus monkeys significantly altered oviductal tone and contraction amplitude (Neri and Marcus, 1972). While entire oviducts are difficult to culture for long periods of time *in vitro*, Talbot and co-workers have used cultured explants of the hamster infundibulum to monitor the effects of tobacco smoke and its constituents on ciliary beat frequency, adhesion of the OCC to the cilia of the oviduct, oocyte pick-up rate and smooth muscle contraction rate. An inhibitory effect of smoke solutions was demonstrated on ciliary beat frequency and oocyte pick-up rate that was correlated to the presence of potassium cyanide at relevant concentrations (Knoll and Talbot, 1998; Talbot *et al.*, 1998). Whole mainstream smoke and its fractions significantly inhibited ciliary beating, while whole sidestream smoke solutions slightly stimulated beat frequency (Knoll and Talbot, 1998). OCC pick-up rate was inhibited in a dose-dependent manner by both mainstream and sidestream smoke solutions, and at equivalent doses, sidestream smoke was more potent than mainstream smoke. Whole mainstream smoke solutions and their particulate and gas phase fractions inhibited OCC pick-up rate and increased adhesion when either the infundibulum or OCC was pretreated with smoke solution (Gieseke and Talbot, 2005). When infundibula were treated with mainstream or sidestream smoke solutions from traditional commercial cigarettes, both types of smoke from all but one brand significantly inhibited oviductal muscle contraction (Riveles *et al.*, 2007). Thus, innovative new models are providing evidence that smoking may impair fertility through alterations in utero-tubal motility or the rate of oocyte, sperm or conceptus transport, factors which may underlie the reported increase in risk for ectopic pregnancy and tubal infertility in smoking women (Saraiya *et al.*, 1998).

Uterus and implantation

There is some evidence for direct effects of constituents of cigarette smoke on uterine tissue. Smoking increased the resting tone of the uterus and the amplitude of uterine contraction in monkeys (Neri and Marcus, 1972). A more recent study on rat and human myometrium found that *in vitro* exposure to a cigarette smoke solution increased contractile force in response to oxytocin (Nakamoto *et al.*, 2006). Real-time PCR further showed that expression levels of the oxytocin receptor were significantly higher in smoke-treated uteri of both species. Thus, chemicals in smoke may make the uterus more responsive to oxytocin, which could contribute to preterm deliveries often seen in women who smoke. Several groups have used uterine strips to assess the effects of nicotine on uterine muscle contraction. Treatment of uteri from non-pregnant rabbits with nicotine leads to an increase in amplitude of electrical field stimulation evoked contraction (Nas *et al.*, 2007).

Interestingly, less is known regarding the effects of smoking on the response of the human uterine endometrium to steroid hormones or on the ability of the conceptus to implant. It is well accepted that smokers have as much as a 50% lower risk of uterine endometrial cancer compared with non-smokers, as well as a decreased incidence of uterine endometriosis and fibroids (Baron *et al.*, 1990; Baron, 1996), which may reflect an anti-estrogenic effect of smoking. At the same time, nicotine administration to rats produced an adverse effect on the decidualization process (Card and Mitchel, 1978), as well as delayed implantation and altered spacing of implantation sites (Yoshinaga *et al.*, 1979). These nicotine effects, however, may also reflect delayed utero-tubal transport or altered steroid hormone levels in pregnant rats. Other studies have found an effect of the PAH benzo(a)pyrene on uterine endometrial cells (Shiverick and Salafia, 1999). Exposure of human endometrial adenocarcinoma cells to benzo(a) pyrene markedly decreased proliferation, cell attachment and invasion of basement membrane (McGarry *et al.*, 2002). The benzo(a)pyrene-mediated alterations in attachment were linked to a loss of cell surface expression of receptors for epidermal growth factor (EGF) and decreased levels of E-cadherin, a cell adhesion molecule essential for cell to cell communication. In this model, the benzo(a)pyrene-mediated loss of cell adhesion molecules serves as a biomarker for alterations in uterine epithelial cell polarization, which may have an impact on trophoblast implantation. Lastly, human studies of IVF and GIFT in women have reported lower implantation rates and more cycles with failed fertilization in smokers compared to non-smokers (Cooper *et al.*, 1995; Hughes and Brennan, 1996). Importantly, Soares *et al.* (2007) was the first clinical study to demonstrate that cigarette smoking affects uterine receptiveness in which oocytes from smokers had lower pregnancy rates and an increased twin gestation rate.

Male reproduction

Both chromosomal and DNA damage to male germ cells may result from tobacco smoke exposure (Zenzes, 2000; Yauk *et al.*, 2007). The prevalence of Y chromosome disomy in sperm was found to correlate with urinary cotinine concentrations (Rubes *et al.*, 1998). Evidence further suggests that gene damage in sperm may relate to direct binding of benzo(a)pyrene or its intermediates to DNA (Zenzes *et al.*, 1999). Cigarette smoke contains reactive oxygen species (ROS) that help produce adducts and are mutagenic in their own right. Nuclear DNA damage and mitochondrial and cytoskeletal aberrations have been shown to result directly from oxidative stress in gametes. These mechanisms are further supported by the detection of increased benzo(a)pyrene adducts in embryos from smokers compared to non-smokers, indicating transmission of modified DNA originating from parental smoking (Zenzes *et al.*, 1999).

The effects of smoking and passive smoke on various semen parameters have been also evaluated (Vine, 1996; Zenzes *et al.*, 1999; Hull *et al.*, 2000). Reductions in sperm density and motility have been demonstrated, some of which was dose dependent. In a Danish study of healthy men, increased smoking was correlated with reductions in sperm concentration, semen volume, total sperm count and percentage of motile spermatozoa (Ramlau-Hansen *et al.*, 2007). Concentrations of cadmium, lead, malondialdehyde, protein carbonyls and ROS levels in the semen of infertile smokers were significantly higher than in samples from fertile men and non-smoking infertile patients (Kiziler *et al.*, 2007). In addition, the concentration of ascorbic acid, glutathione-S-transferase and reduced glutathione in semen were significantly reduced in smokers (Mostafa *et al.*, 2006). High concentrations of cotinine in semen were associated with an impairment in the process of human spermatozoa membrane maturation, which leads to reduced sperm head permeability and activation (Sofikitis *et al.*, 2000). In addition, studies of sperm in smoking and non-smoking men from infertile couples found increased rates of DNA fragmentation in sperm swim-up samples from smokers (Sepaniak *et al.*, 2006; Viloria *et al.*, 2007).

Studies of natural conception in couples with a smoking male partner have demonstrated a significant reduction in fertility when the number of cigarettes smoked per day was 15 or more, which was associated with an increased time to pregnancy (Hull *et al.*, 2000). Other studies sought to determine if male tobacco consumption leads to a worse prognosis of IVF cycles due to compromised sperm quality. Couples with a male smoker were reported to have a diminished probability of achieving a 12-week pregnancy (Joesbury *et al.*, 1998). In addition, male smokers have a decreased success rate for IVF and intracytoplasmic sperm injection (ICSI) (Zitzmann *et al.*, 2003). In this regard, animal models allow for control over confounding variables that are difficult to eliminate in clinical studies, such as passive female smoke exposure. In rats, male exposure to cigarette smoke resulted in a secretory deficiency of Sertoli and Leydig cells and impaired epididymal maturation (Kapawa *et al.*, 2004). Marked reductions of fertility (*in vivo*) and *in vitro* fertilizing capacity with conventional IVF were observed. In addition, a reduced implantation potential of embryos obtained from "smoking" male rats was observed with two different fertilization techniques used (either conventional IVF or ICSI).

In summary, genetic abnormalities such as aneuploidy and DNA damage are more often seen in spermatozoa from smokers. Tobacco smoking has been associated with reduced sperm production, increased oxidative stress and reduced sperm membrane maturation and capacitation. In IVF cycles, couples with a male smoker have a diminished probability of having an ongoing pregnancy beyond the first trimester. Although it is very difficult in humans to control the concomitant effect of passive smoking on the female partner, studies in animals show that cigarette smoke reduces sperm maturation and fertilizing capacity, and that embryos obtained have lower implantation potential.

Early pregnancy

Smoking is associated with an increase in spontaneous miscarriage in both natural and assisted conception cycles (Hughes and Brennan, 1996; Ness *et al.*, 1999; Winter *et al.*, 2002; Jauniaux and Burton, 2007; Doherty *et al.*, 2009). The increased miscarriage rate among mothers who smoke may be as high as 33%. Evidence supports several hypotheses to explain associations between maternal smoking and fetoplacental alterations. First, the vasoconstrictive properties of some components of cigarette smoke such as nicotine, carbon monoxide and cyanide may lead to placental insufficiency and embryonic and fetal growth restriction and demise. Doppler studies suggest that cigarette smoke increases resistance in fetoplacental circulation, but reduces resistance in uteroplacental vessels. In this respect, placentae of smokers have morphological features consistent with underperfusion (Naeye, 1992; Jauniaux and Burton, 2007). Second, chemicals within tobacco smoke exert direct toxic effects on fetal and placental cells as evidenced by the presence of altered enzyme expression and the presence of protein and DNA adducts (Everson *et al.*, 1986; Manchester *et al.*, 1988; Pasanen *et al.*, 1988; Sanyal *et al.*, 1993; Myers *et al.*, 1996). Third, smoking induces fetal hypoxia through diffusion of carbon monoxide, nicotine and thiocyanate across the placenta. The enhanced ability of fetal hemoglobin to form carboxy-hemoglobin decreases the fetal transport of oxygen.

Placental trophoblast invasion and proliferation

Numerous studies have shown that placentas in pregnant women are targets of cigarette smoke (Salafia and Shiverick, 1999; Shiverick and Salafia, 1999; Zdravkovic *et al.*, 2005; Jauniaux and Burton, 2007). Because placentas are readily available from hospitals, many *in vitro* studies have been done using human placental tissue. The most important smoking-induced placental pathologies are placental abruption and placenta previa. Jauniaux and Burton (2007) have described increased syncytial necrosis and increased thickness of the syncytio/cytotrophoblast membrane in early pregnancy in mothers who smoke. During early pregnancy, stem cells either fuse to form the syncytium or aggregate to form cell columns that first adhere to and then invade the uterus. Experimental data indicate that smoking appears to induce a generalized dysfunction of both villous and invasive trophoblasts in early pregnancy. Chorionic villi from women who smoked more than 20 cigarettes per day have morphologically defective floating and anchoring villi which were characterized by a decreased number of Ki67 positive cells, indicative of decreased mitotic activity in the cytotrophoblasts of the villi (Genbacev *et al.*, 1997, 2000). Biochemical markers of placental function show that maternal levels of estriol, estradiol, human chorionic gonadotropin (hCG) and human placental lactogen (hPL) were lower in smokers compared to non-smokers (Bernstein *et al.*, 1989). As described above, placental aromatase activity has been found to be decreased *in vivo* in smokers, as well as *in vitro* by exposure to nicotine and cotinine (Barbieri *et al.*, 1986; Kitawaki *et al.*, 1993). When chorionic villi from non-smokers were exposed to nicotine *in vitro*, there was a dose-related inhibition of cell column formation and reduced invasion of basement membrane, which was related to decreased synthesis and activation of the 92 kDa Type IV collagenase (Genbacev *et al.*, 1997). The heavy metal cadmium is a known placental toxin in both animals and humans, and placental levels of cadmium are increased in smokers (Eisenmann and Miller, 1996). In the perfused human placenta model, cadmium produced ultrastructural changes and decreased the secretion of hCG.

A consistent finding has been the presence of smoking-related alterations in placental receptors for EGF, a potent mitogen and differentiation factor for trophoblasts. Placentae from smokers show a marked decrease in EGF receptor tyrosine kinase activity, whereas insulin receptor phosphorylation was normal or increased (Lucier *et al.*, 1987; Wang *et al.*, 1988). Exposure of human placental cells in primary culture to PAHs directly resulted in concentration-dependent loss of EGF-receptor binding and kinase activity, which was greatest in cells from first trimester placentae (Guyda *et al.*, 1990). Further studies with human trophoblastic choriocarcinoma cell lines have shown that the benzo(a)pyrene-mediated loss of EGF receptors is linked not only with decreased trophoblast proliferation and hCG secretion (Zhang *et al.*, 1995), but also with decreased expression of the proto-oncogene c-myc, whereas TGF-B1 expression is increased (Zhang and Shiverick, 1997). Thus, evidence is mounting to indicate that constituents of tobacco smoke have the potential to alter trophoblast gene expression in the direction of downmodulation of positive regulators (EGF-R, c-myc) and upmodulation of negative regulators (TGF-B1) of trophoblast function.

Nicotine was subsequently identified as a major chemical in smoke contributing to inhibition of mitosis in cultured anchoring villi *in vitro* through decreased expression of cell cycle markers and decreased incorporation of BrdU (Genbacev *et al.*, 2000). The expression of two markers characteristic of normal cytotrophoblast differentiation (fibronectin and its α5β1 integrin receptor) were also reduced during *in vitro* exposure to nicotine. In a subsequent study by this group, L-selectin, which functions initially in attachment of the embryo to the uterus and later in attaching anchoring villi to the endometrium, was examined in smokers and non-smokers (Zdravkovic *et al.*, 2005). Immunohistochemical results showed less L-selectin in villi of smokers. In video microscopy of *in vitro* cultures, nicotine was further shown to inhibit outgrowth of cytotrophoblasts from cell columns in anchoring villi. The above studies together demonstrate that nicotine impairs growth, differentiation and attachment of cytotrophoblasts and thereby produces important harmful effects on human placentas.

Given the evidence that oxygen tension determines whether cells proliferate or invade, it is likely that smoking-induced hypoxia may be a factor in altered trophoblast differentiation. In this respect, alterations in trophoblast differentiation along invasive or proliferative pathways may explain the changes in endocrine function as well as vascular morphology that are observed in smokers.

Effects of maternal smoking on progeny

There is strong evidence to support a causal relationship between maternal cigarette smoking and fetal growth retardation (Salihu and Wilson, 2007; Rogers, 2008). The relationship includes significant reduction in growth of head circumference, abdominal circumference and femur length, with the largest reduction in size observed for femur length (Jaddoe *et al.*, 2007). It has been estimated there is a 27 g reduction in birth weight for each cigarette smoked per day during the third trimester of pregnancy (Bernstein *et al.*, 2005). In addition, prenatal smoking is reported to be associated with a 20–30% greater risk for stillbirth, a 40% increase in the risk for infant death and a two-fold increase in the incidence of SIDS (Salihu and Wilson, 2007), as well as impaired cognitive and behavioral development (DiFranza *et al.*, 2004). In addition, new evidence is accumulating that links cigarette smoke exposure *in utero* with the development of a variety of disease pathologies in the older offspring including certain childhood cancers (i.e., leukemias, lymphomas and central nervous system tumors) (Ng *et al.*, 2005), respiratory disorders (Penn *et al.*, 2007), type 2 diabetes and obesity (Oken *et al.*, 2005). Relative to human exposures, benzo(a)pyrene (BaP) DNA adducts were detected in the serum of smoking mothers and their prenatally exposed newborns, and adducts were observed at a higher percentage in the neonate compared with the directly exposed mothers (Perera *et al.*, 2004).

Ovarian oocyte depletion

It has been known for many years that cigarette smoke contains ovotoxicants, including PAHs that when injected into mice cause loss of young oocytes (Mattison *et al.*, 1989). Moreover, treatment of pregnant mice with PAHs or cigarette smoke reduces the number of oocytes in their female offspring. Fetal ovarian organ culture was used to study the mechanism of action of PAHs on oocyte survival (Matikainen *et al.*, 2002). DMBA treated ovaries showed a marked increase in immunoreactivity of Bax, a proapoptotic factor. An *in vivo* follow-up study found that Bax mutant fetuses exposed to PAHs were born with a normal number of oocytes in contrast to wild-type controls which had Bax and lost oocytes in response to PAH treatment (Matikainen *et al.*, 2002).

Sudden infant death syndrome

Sudden infant death syndrome (SIDS) is characterized by the unexpected and unexplained death of a seemingly healthy infant (Shah *et al.*, 2006). The etiology of SIDS has not been clearly defined, but known risk factors include maternal smoking. Evidence indicates a two-fold increase in risk among mothers who smoked during pregnancy. Although the mechanism by which maternal smoking increases the risk of SIDS is unknown, numerous hypotheses have been proposed, including brainstem alterations of the fetus and altered lung growth leading to impaired function postnatally (Matturri *et al.*, 2006).

Childhood asthma

Epidemiological studies have revealed a strong link between CS exposure *in utero* and the development of asthma in offspring (Cook and Strachan, 1999). A cross-sectional study that investigated the respiratory health of school-aged children found that maternal smoking while pregnant was associated with asthma and a number of asthma-related symptoms (e.g., wheezing) (Gilliland *et al.*, 2001). As mothers who smoke during pregnancy are not likely to stop after the baby is born, however, it is very difficult to distinguish asthma-related effects due to pre- vs. postnatal exposure to cigarette smoke. Thus, animal models in which smoke exposures can be limited to defined periods of time are useful. In this regard, a number of studies have investigated the effects of *in utero* exposure to environmental tobacco smoke (ETS) in conjunction with allergen sensitization on asthma-related effects in a murine model. Obviously, more studies are needed to understand the mechanisms by which interactive effects between airway modifying factors might occur.

Childhood cancer

Epidemiological evidence indicates an association between prenatal cigarette smoke exposure and subsequent development of certain childhood cancers (i.e., central nervous system tumors, leukemia and lymphomas) (Schuz *et al.*, 2001). In a mouse model of lymphoma, prenatal exposure to cigarette smoke increased tumor incidence and tumor growth rate in the juvenile male offspring (Ng *et al.*, 2005). Thus, findings from this study provide biological plausibility for the epidemiological findings. In addition, evidence suggests a suppressive effect of prenatal cigarette smoke exposure on tumor surveillance mechanisms in the offspring.

Reproduction in male progeny

An epidemiologic study to identify the cause of decreasing sperm counts in Danish vs. Finnish men first suggested an effect of maternal smoking (Storgaard *et al.*, 2003). The follow-up study based on prospectively collected data that evaluated this association was published in 2007 (Ramlau-Hansen *et al.*, 2007). After adjusting for confounding factors, men whose mothers had smoked more than 10 cigarettes per day had lower sperm densities in adult life than men with non-smoking mothers. Paternal smoking was unrelated to semen parameters of the offspring. One possible pathophysiological process through which *in utero* exposure to tobacco might impair gonadal development and spermatogenesis has been recently proposed. Human fetal germ cells have been shown to have receptors for polycyclic aromatic hydrocarbons (PAHs) and the exposure of embryonic germ cell cultures to PAH results in cell apoptosis (Coutts *et al.*, 2007).

Effects of paternal smoking on progeny

Some evidence exists to support the effect of paternal smoking on offspring. The increase in germ-line heritable DNA sequence mutations in individuals exposed to tobacco smoke was studied in mice (Yauk *et al.*, 2007). Exposed animals had a significantly higher mutation frequency in spermatogonial stem cells, and data suggested that mutations accumulate with extended exposure. This type of mutation may be associated with an increased incidence of genetic diseases among the non-smoking offspring of male smokers. In humans, paternal smoking habit was associated with the risk of childhood cancer, a condition known to be linked to genetic mutations (Sorahan *et al.*, 2001). Thus, paternal smoking may reduce fertility in male descendants, as well as increase the risk of genetic diseases in offspring as a whole.

TREATMENT

The adverse effects of cigarette smoke exposure on human reproductive outcomes are a major scientific and public health concern. An important consideration is that much of the reduced fertility associated with smoking may be reversed within a year of cessation (Hughes and Brennan, 1996; Hughes *et al.*, 2000). When successful, smoking cessation represents an important part of effective treatment for infertility (Practice Committee of the American Society for Reproductive Medicine, 2008). Despite the known risks, women throughout the world continue to smoke during pregnancy. Although the majority of users express a desire to reduce their use or stop entirely, less than 30% quit after learning of their pregnancy in the USA. Adolescents are more likely to smoke during pregnancy than women 20 years and older.

Women interested in smoking cessation during pregnancy have a number of options, including behavioral and pharmacological aids, but nicotine replacement therapy (NRT) is the most common approach (Salihu and Wilson, 2007; Practice Committee of the American Society for Reproductive Medicine, 2008). While NRT avoids exposure to the multitude of toxicants present in tobacco smoke, nicotine itself causes damage to the developing nervous system (Pauly and Slotkin, 2008). Available pharmacologic therapies include NRT in the form of gum and patches as well as nasal sprays and inhalers. The nicotine levels that result from daily inhalation of 10 or more cigarettes are higher than those associated with recommended doses of nicotine gum and patches (Windsor *et al.*, 2000). The finding that salivary cotinine concentrations during transdermal replacement were lower in pregnant women than reported in smoking or non-smoking non-pregnant adults suggests that nicotine may be less rapidly metabolized in pregnant women. Nasal sprays and inhalers have not been studied in pregnancy and are classified as category D agents (indicating adverse effects in animal models). Nicotine gum carries a category C classification and the nicotine patch is a category D agent, despite its reported safety in the limited clinical studies involving pregnant women that have been conducted to date. The only non-nicotine FDA-approved smoking cessation agent is bupropion (Zyban). Bupropion is also available for use as an antidepressant (Wellbutrin), but is marketed differently for smoking cessation.

CONCLUDING REMARKS AND FUTURE DIRECTIONS

Conclusive evidence from animal and human studies demonstrates the adverse effects of cigarette smoke exposure on reproductive and developmental outcomes. In humans, cigarette smoking is a major scientific and public health concern. An important effort is in progress to improve risk assessment through genetic profiles and biomarkers of tobacco exposure, effect, harms and susceptibility in order to identify those individuals who are particularly susceptible to tobacco-induced toxicity. Smoking cessation interventions are an essential approach to reducing and/or preventing exposure to the numerous toxicants in cigarette smoke. Given the known adverse effects of nicotine on brain development observed in human and animal studies, however, safer alternatives for smoking cessation in pregnancy are clearly needed.

Lastly, major initiatives for tobacco control are under way in the USA and internationally (Viswanath *et al.*, 2010). The US Food and Drug Administration (FDA) recently received regulatory authority over tobacco products under the Family Smoking Prevention and Tobacco Control Act of 2009 (FSPTCA). Globally, the World Health Organization (WHO)-led Framework Convention on Tobacco Control (FCTC) is the first health treaty of its kind that addresses the devastating consequences of tobacco use around the world. The FCTC, ratified by 168 countries as of the end of 2009, aims to tackle both the supply and demand sides of tobacco use through evidence-based strategies. The FDA now has the authority to require changes to tobacco products that the agency finds to be appropriate for the protection of the public health.

REFERENCES

Alouf B, Feinson JA, Chidekel AS (2006) Preventing and treating nicotine addiction: a review with emphasis on adolescent health. *Del Med J* **78:** 249–56.

American Cancer Society (2009) Cancer Facts and Figures 2009. *American Cancer Society*, Atlanta, GA.

Andreoli C, Gigante D, Nunziata A (2003) A review of *in vitro* methods to assess the biological activity of tobacco smoke with the aim of reducing the toxicity of smoke. *Toxicol in Vitro* **17:** 587–94.

Andres RL (1996) The association of cigarette smoking with placenta previa and abruptio placenta. *Semin Perinatol* **20:** 154–9.

Augood C, Duckitt K, Templeton AA (1998) Smoking and female infertility: a systematic review and meta-analysis. *Hum Reprod* **13:** 1532–9.

Barbieri RL, McShane PM, Ryan KJ (1986) Constituents of cigarette smoke inhibit human granulosa cell aromatase. *Fertil Steril* **46:** 232–6.

Baron JA (1996) Beneficial effects of nicotine and cigarette smoking: the real, the possible and the spurious. *Br Med Bull* **52:** 58–73.

Baron JA, La Vecchia C, Levi F (1990) The antiestrogenic effect of cigarette smoking in women. *Am J Obstet Gynecol* **162:** 502–14.

Bernstein IM, Mongeon JA, Badger GJ, Solomon L, Heil SH, Higgins ST (2005) Maternal smoking and its association with birth weight. *Obstet Gynecol* **106:** 986–91.

Bernstein L, Pike MC, Lobo RA, Depue RH, Ross RK, Henderson BE (1989) Cigarette smoking in pregnancy results in marked decrease in maternal hCG and estradiol levels. *Br J Obstet Gynaecol* **96:** 92–6.

Bordel R, Laschke MW, Menger MD, Vollmar B (2006) Nicotine does not affect vascularization but inhibits growth of freely transplanted ovarian follicles by inducing granulosa cell apoptosis. *Hum Reprod* **21:** 610–17.

Bruin JE, Gerstein HC, Holloway AC (2010) Long-term consequences of fetal and neonatal nicotine exposure: a critical review. *Toxicol Sci* **116:** 364–74.

Byrd RS, Howard CR (1995) Children's passive and prenatal exposure to cigarette smoke. *Pediatr Ann* **24:** 640–5.

Card JP, Mitchel JA (1978) The effects of nicotine administration on desiduoma induction in the rat. *Biol Reprod* **19:** 326–31.

CDC (Centers for Disease Control and Prevention) (2008) Smoking-attributable mortality, years of potential life lost, and productivity losses – United States, 2000–2004. *MMWR Morb Mortal Wkly Rep* **57:** 1226–8.

CDC (Centers for Disease Control and Prevention) (2009) Cigarette smoking among adults and trends in smoking cessation – United States, 2008. *MMWR Morb Mortal Wkly Rep* **58:** 1227–32.

Cnattingius S (2004) The epidemiology of smoking during pregnancy: smoking prevalence, maternal characteristics, and pregnancy outcomes. *Nicotine Tob Res* **6:** S125–S140.

Cook DG, Strachan DP (1999) Summary of effects of parental smoking and the respiratory health of children and implications for research. *Thorax* **54:** 357–66.

Cooper AR, Moley KH (2008) Maternal tobacco use and its preimplantation effects on fertility: more reasons to stop smoking. *Semin Reprod Med* **26:** 204–12.

Cooper GS, Baird DD, Hulka BS, Weinberg CR, Savitz DA, Hughes Jr CL (1995) Follicle-stimulating hormone concentrations in relation to active and passive smoking. *Obstet Gynecol* **85:** 407–11.

Coutts SM, Fulton N, Anderson RA (2007) Environmental toxicant-induced germ cell apoptosis in the human fetal testis. *Hum Reprod* **22:** 2912–18.

DiFranza JR, Aligne CA, Weitzman M (2004) Prenatal and postnatal environmental tobacco smoke exposure and children's health. *Pediatrics* **113 (4 Suppl.):** 1007–15.

Doherty SP, Grabowski J, Hoffman C, Ng SP, Zelikoff JT (2009) Early life insult from cigarette smoke may be predictive of chronic diseases later in life. *Biomarkers* **14 (Suppl. 1):** 97–101.

Eisenmann CJ, Miller RK (1996) Placental transport metabolism and toxicity of metals. In *Toxicology of Metals* (Chang LW, ed.). CRC Press, Boca Raton, FL, pp. 999–1022.

Eliopoulos C, Klein J, Chitayat D, Greenwald M, Koren **G** (1996) Nicotine and cotinine in maternal and neonatal hair as markers of gestational smoking. *Clin Invest Med* **19:** 231–42.

El-Nemr A, Al-Shawaf T, Sabatini L, Wilson C, Lower AM, Grudzinskas JG (1998) Effect of smoking on ovarian reserve and ovarian stimulation in *in-vitro* fertilization and embryo transfer. *Hum Reprod* **13:** 2192–8.

EPA (Environmental Protection Agency) (1993) EPA Report/600/6-90/006F: respiratory health effects of passive smoking: lung cancer and other disorders. Washington DC.

Everson RB, Randerath E, Santella RM, Cefalo RC, Avitts TA, Randerath K (1986) Detection of smoking-related covalent DNA adducts in human placenta. *Science* **231:** 54–7.

Florescu A, Ferrence R, Einarson TR, Selby P, Kramer M, Woodruff S, Grossman L, Rankin A, Jacqz-Aigrain E, Koren G (2007) Reference values for hair cotinine as a biomarker of active and passive smoking in women of reproductive age, pregnant women, children, and neonates: systematic review and meta-analysis. *Ther Drug Monit* **29:** 437–46.

Franks AL, Kendrick JS, Tyler CW (1987) Postmenopausal smoking, estrogen replacement therapy, and the risk of endometrial cancer. *Am J Obstet Gynecol* **156:** 20–3.

Genbacev O, Bass KE, Joslin RJ, Fisher SJ (1995) Maternal smoking inhibits early human cytotrophoblast differentiation. *Reprod Toxicol* **9:** 245–55.

Genbacev O, McMaster MT, Lazic J, Nedeljkovic S, Cvetkovic M, Joslin R, Fisher SJ (2000) Concordant *in situ* and *in vitro* data show that maternal cigarette smoking negatively regulates placental cytotrophoblast passage through the cell cycle. *Reprod Toxicol* **14:** 495–506.

Genbacev O, Zhou Y, Ludlow JW, Fisher SJ (1997) Regulation of human placental development by oxygen tension. *Science* **277:** 1669–72.

Gieseke C, Talbot P (2005) Cigarette smoke inhibits hamster oocyte pickup by increasing adhesion between the oocyte cumulus complex and oviductal cilia. *Biol Reprod* **73:** 443–51.

Gilliland FD, Li YF, Peters JM (2001) Effects of maternal smoking during pregnancy and environmental tobacco smoke on asthma and wheezing children. *Am J Respir Crit Care Med* **163:** 429–36.

Group WS (2007) *The Scientific Basis of Tobacco Product Regulation*. World Health Organization, Geneva.

Guyda HJ, Mathieu L, Lai W, Manchester D, Wang S-L, Ogilvie S, Shiverick KT (1990) Benzo(a)pyrene inhibits epidermal growth factor binding and receptor autophosphorylation in human placental cell cultures. *Mol Pharmacol* **37:** 137–43.

Hecht SS (2008) Progress and challenges in selected areas of tobacco carcinogenesis. *Chem Res Toxicol* **21:** 160–71.

Hecht SS, Carmella SG, Chen M, Salzberger U, Tollner U, Lackman GM (1998) Metabolites of the tobacco-specific lung carcinogen 4-(methylnitrosamino)-1-(3-pyridyl)-1-butanone (NNK) in the urine of newborns. Abstracts of the *American Chemical Society (ACS) National Meeting*, Boston, 1998, #032.

Hughes EG, Brennan BG (1996) Does cigarette smoking impair natural or assisted fecundity? *Fertil Steril* **66:** 679–89.

Hughes EG, Lamont DA, Beecroft ML, Wilson DM, Brennan BG, Rice SC (2000) Randomized trial of a "stage-of-change" oriented smoking cessation intervention in infertile and pregnant women. *Fertil Steril* **74:** 498–503.

Hull MG, North K, Taylor H, Farrow A, Ford WC (2000) The Avon Longitudinal Study of Pregnancy and Childhood Study Team. Delayed conception and active and passive smoking. *Fertil Steril* **74:** 725–33.

IARC (International Agency for Research on Cancer) Working Group on the Evaluation of Carcinogenic Risks to Humans (2004) IARC Monographs on the Evaluation of Carcinogenic Risks to Humans, Volume 83: Tobacco smoke and involuntary smoking. *IARC* Lyon (France).

Jaddoe VW, Verburg BO, de Ridder MA, Hofman A, Mackenbach JP, Moll HA, Steegers EA, Witteman JC (2007) Maternal smoking and fetal growth characteristics in different periods of pregnancy: the generation R study. *Am J Epidemiol* **165:** 1207–15.

Jauniaux E, Burton GJ (2007) Morphological and biological effects of maternal exposure to tobacco smoke on the feto-placental unit. *Early Hum Dev* **83:** 699–706.

Joesbury K, Edirisinghe W, Phillips MR, Yovich JL (1998) Evidence that male smoking affects the likelihood of a pregnancy following IVF treatment: application of the modified cumulative embryo score. *Hum Reprod* **13:** 1506–13.

Juchau MR, Namkung MJ, Chao ST (1982) Mono-oxygenase induction in the human placenta: interrelationships among position-specific hydroxylations of 17β-estradiol and benzo(a)pyrene. *Drug Metabol Dispos* **10:** 220–4.

Kaiserman MJ, Rickert WS (1992) Carcinogens in tobacco smoke: benzo(a) pyrene from Canadian cigarettes and cigarette tobacco. *Am J Publ Health* **82:** 1023–6.

Kapawa A, Giannakis D, Tsoukanelis K, Kanakas N, Baltogiannis D, Agapitos E, Loutradis D, Miyagawa I, Sofikitis N (2004) Effects of paternal cigarette smoking on testicular function, sperm fertilization capacity, embryonic development, and blastocyst capacity for implantation in rats. *Andrologia* **36:** 57–68.

Kitawaki J, Inoue S, Tamura T, Yamamoto T, Honjo H, Higashiyama T, Osawa Y, Okada H (1993) Cigarette smoking during pregnancy lowers aromatase cytochrome P-450 in the human placenta. *J Steroid Biochem Mol Biol* **45:** 485–91.

Kiziler AR, Aydemir B, Onaran I, Alici B, Ozkara H, Gulyasar T, Akyolcu MC (2007) High levels of cadmium and lead in seminal fluid and blood of smoking men are associated with high oxidative stress and damage in infertile subjects. *Biol Trace Elem Res* **120:** 82–91.

Knoll M, Talbot P (1998) Cigarette smoke inhibits oocyte cumulus complex pick-up by the oviduct *in vitro* independent of ciliary beat frequency. *Reprod Toxicol* **12:** 57–68.

Kondoh M, Araragi S, Sato K (2002) Cadmium induces apoptosis partly via caspase-9 activation in HL-60 cells. *Toxicology* **170:** 111–17.

Lodovici M, Akpan V, Evangelisti C, Dolara P (2004) Sidestream tobacco smoke as the main predictor of exposure to polycyclic aromatic hydrocarbons. *J Appl Toxicol* **24:** 277–81.

Lucier GW, Nelson KG, Everson RB, Wong TK, Philpot RM, Tiernan T, Taylor M, Sunahara GI (1987) Placental markers for human exposure to polychlorinated biphenyls and polychlorinated dibenzoflurans. *Environ Health Perspect* **76:** 79–87.

MacDorman MF, Cnattingius S, Hoffman HJ, Kramer MS, Haglund B (1997) Sudden infant death syndrome and smoking in the United States and Sweden. *Am J Epidemiol* **146:** 249–55.

Manchester DK, Weston A, Choi JS, Trivers GE, Fennessey PB, Quintana E, Farmer PB, Mann DL, Harris CC (1988) Detection of benzo(a)pyrene diol epoxide-DNA adducts in human placenta. *Proc Natl Acad Sci USA* **85:** 9243–7.

Matikainen TM, Moriyama T, Morita Y, Perez GI, Korsmeyer SJ, Sherr DH, Tilly JL (2002) Ligand activation of the aromatic hydrocarbon receptor transcription factor drives Bax-dependent apoptosis in developing fetal ovarian germ cells. *Endocrinology* **143:** 615–20.

Mattison DR, Plowchalk DR, Meadows MJ, Miller MM, Malek A, London S (1989) The effect of smoking on oogenesis, fertilization, and implantation. *Semin Reprod Endocrinol* **7:** 291–304.

Matturri L, Ottaviani G, Lavezzi AM (2006) Maternal smoking and sudden infant death syndrome: epidemiological study related to pathology. *Virchows Arch* 449: 697–706.

McGarry MA, Charles GD, Medrano T, Bubb MR, Grant MB, Campbell-Thompson M, Shiverick KT (2002) Benzo(a)pyrene, but not 2,3,7,8-tetrachlorodibenzo-p-dioxin, alters cell adhesion proteins in human uterine RL95-2 cells. *Biochem Biophys Res Commun* **294:** 101–7.

Miceli F, Minici F, Tropea A, Catino S, Orlando M, Lamanna G, Sagnella F, Tiberi F, Bompiani A, Mancuso S, Lanzone A, Apa R (2005) Effects of nicotine on human luteal cells in vitro: a possible role on reproductive outcome for smoking women. *Biol Reprod* **72:** 628–32.

Mlynarcikova A, Fickova M, Scsukova S (2005) Ovarian intrafollicular processes as a target for cigarette smoke components and selected environmental reproductive disruptors. *Endocr Regul* **39:** 21–32.

Mostafa T, Tawadrous G, Roaia MM, Amer MK, Kader RA, Aziz A (2006) Effect of smoking on seminal plasma ascorbic acid in infertile and fertile males. *Andrologia* **8:** 221–4.

Motejlek K, Palluch F, Neulen J, Grummer R (2006) Smoking impairs angiogenesis during maturation of human oocytes. *Fertil Steril* **86:** 186–91.

Myers SR, Spinnato JA, Pinorini-Godly MT, Cook C, Boles B, Rodgers GC (1996) Characterization of 4-aminobiphenyl-hemoglobin adducts in maternal and fetal blood samples. *J Toxicol Env Health* **47:** 553–6.

Naeye RL (1992) Effects of cigarette smoking on the fetus and neonate. In *Disorders of the Placenta, Fetus and Neonate*. Mosby Year Book, St Louis, p. 88.

Nakamoto T, Yasuda K, Yasuhara M, Nakajima T, Mizokami T, Okada H, Kanzaki H (2006) Cigarette smoke extract enhances oxytocin-induced rhythmic contractions of rat and human preterm myometrium. *Reproduction* **132:** 343–53.

Nas T, Barun S, Oztürk GS, Vural IM, Ercan ZS, Sarioglu Y (2007) Nicotine potentiates the electrical field stimulation-evoked contraction of non-pregnant rabbit myometrium. *Tohoku J Exp Med* **211:** 187–93.

Neal MS, Zhu J, Foster WG (2008) Quantification of benzo(a)pyrene and other PAHs in the serum and follicular fluid of smokers versus non-smokers. *Reprod Toxicol* **25:** 100–6.

Neal MS, Zhu J, Holloway AC, Foster WG (2007) Follicle growth is inhibited by benzo(a)pyrene, at concentrations representative of human exposure, in an isolated rat follicle culture assay. *Hum Reprod* **22:** 961–7.

Neal MS, Hughes EG, Holloway AC, Foster WG (2005) Sidestream smoking is equally as damaging as mainstream smoking on IVF outcomes. *Hum Reprod* **20:** 2531–5.

Neri A, Marcus SL (1972) Effect of nicotine on the motility of the oviducts in the rhesus monkey: a preliminary report. *J Reprod Fertil* **31:** 91–7.

Ness RB, Grisso JA, Hirschinger N, Markovic N, Shaw LM, Day NL, Kline J (1999) Cocaine and tobacco use and the risk of spontaneous abortion. *New Engl J Med* 340: 333–9.

Ng SP, Silverstone AE, Lai ZW, Zelikoff JT (2005) Effects of prenatal exposure to cigarette smoke on offspring tumor susceptibility and associated immune mechanisms. *Toxicol Sci* **89:** 135–44.

Oken E, Huh SY, Taveras EM, Rich-Edwards JW, Gillman MW (2005) Associations of maternal smoking with child adiposity and blood pressure. *Obesity Res* **13:** 2021–8.

Pasanen M, Stenback F, Park SS, Gelboin HV, Pelkonen O (1988) Immunohistochemical detection of human placental cytochrome P-450 associated mono-oxygenase system inducible by maternal cigarette smoking. *Placenta* **9:** 267–75.

Paszkowski T, Clarke RN, Hornstein MD (2002) Smoking induces oxidative stress inside the Graafian follicle. *Hum Reprod* **17:** 921–5.

Pauly JR, Slotkin TA (2008) Maternal tobacco smoking, nicotine replacement and neurobehavioural development. *Acta Paediatr* **97:** 1331–7.

Penn AL, Rouse RL, Horohov DW, Kearney MT, Paulsen DB, Lomax L (2007) *In utero* exposure to environmental tobacco smoke potentiates adult responses to allergen in BALB/c mice. *Environ Health Perspect* **115:** 548–55.

Perera FP, Tang D, Tu YH, Cruz LA, Borjas M, Bernert T (2004) Biomarkers in maternal and newborn blood indicate heightened fetal susceptibility to procarcinogenic DNA damage. *Environ Health Perspect* **112:** 1133–6.

Perez GI, Knudson CM, Brown GAJ, Korsmeyer SJ, Tilly JL (1997) Resistance of bax-deficient mouse oocytes to apoptosis induced by 7,12-dimethylbenz(a) anthracene (DMBA) *in vitro*. *Fund Appl Toxicol: Toxicol* **36:** 250.

Practice Committee of the American Society for Reproductive Medicine (2008) Smoking and infertility. *Fertil Steril* **90 (Suppl. 3):** S254–S259.

Prokopczyk B, Cox JE, Hoffmann D, Waggoner SE (1997) Identification of tobacco-specific carcinogen in the cervical mucous of smokers and nonsmokers. *J Natl Cancer Inst* **89:** 868–73.

Pru JK, Kaneko-Tarui T, Jurisicova A, Kashiwagi A, Selesniemi K, Tilly JL (2009) Induction of proapoptotic gene expression and recruitment of p53 herald ovarian follicle loss caused by polycyclic aromatic hydrocarbons. *Reprod Sci* **16:** 347–56.

Racowsky C, Hendricks RC, Baldwin KV (1989) Direct effects of nicotine on the meiotic maturation of hamster oocytes. *Reprod Toxicol* **3:** 13–21.

Ramlau-Hansen CH, Thulstrup AM, Storgaard L, Toft G, Olsen J, Bonde JP (2007) Is prenatal exposure to tobacco smoking a cause of poor semen quality? A follow-up study. *Am J Epidemiol* **165:** 1372–9.

Riveles K, Tran V, Roza R, Kwan D, Talbot P (2007) Smoke from traditional commercial, harm reduction and research brand cigarettes impairs oviductal functioning in hamsters (*Mesocricetus auratus*) *in vitro*. *Hum Reprod* **22:** 346–55.

Rodgman A, Perfetti TA (2009) *The Chemical Components of Tobacco and Tobacco Smoke*. CRC Press, Taylor and Francis Group, Boca Raton, FL.

Rogers JM (2008) Tobacco and pregnancy: overview of exposures and effects. *Birth Defects Res (Part C)* **84:** 1–14.

Rubes J, Lowe X, Moore D 2nd, Perreault S, Slott V, Evenson D, Selevan SG, Wyrobek AJ (1998) Smoking cigarettes is associated with increased sperm disomy in teenage men. *Fertil Steril* **70:** 715–23.

Sagredo C, Ovrebo S, Haugen A, Fujii-Kuriyama Y, Baera R, Botnen I, Mollerup S (2006) Quantitative analysis of benzo(a)pyrene biotransformation and adduct formation in Ahr knockout mice. *Toxicol Let* **167:** 173–82.

Salafia C, Shiverick K (1999) Cigarette smoking and pregnancy. II. Vascular effects. *Placenta* **20:** 273–9.

Salihu HM, Wilson R (2007) Epidemiology of prenatal smoking and perinatal outcomes. *Early Hum Develop* **83:** 713–20.

Sanders SR, Cuneo SP, Turzillo AM (2002) Effects of nicotine and cotinine on bovine theca interna and granulosa cells. *Reprod Toxicol* **16:** 795–800.

Sanyal MK, Li Y-L, Biggers WJ, Satish J, Barnea EY (1993) Augmentation of polynuclear aromatic hydrocarbon metabolism of human placental tissues of first-trimester pregnancy by cigarette smoke exposure. *Am J Obstet Gynecol* **168:** 1587–97.

Saraiya M, Berg CJ, Kendrick JS, Strauss LT, Atrash HK, Ahn YW (1998) Cigarette smoking as a risk factor for ectopic pregnancy. *Am J Obstet Gynecol* **178:** 493–8.

Schuz J, Kaletsch U, Kaatsch P, Meinert R, Michaelis J (2001) Risk factors for pediatric tumors of the central nervous system: results from a German population-based case–control study. *Med Pediatr Oncol* **36:** 274–82.

Schwartz AG, Prysak GM, Bock CH, Cote ML (2007) The molecular epidemiology of lung cancer. *Carcinogenesis* **28:** 507–18.

Sepaniak S, Forges T, Gerard H, Foliguet B, Bene MC, Monnier-Barbarino P (2006) The influence of cigarette smoking on human sperm quality and DNA fragmentation. *Toxicology* **223:** 54–60.

Shah T, Sullivan K, Carter J (2006) Sudden infant death syndrome and reported maternal smoking during pregnancy. *Am J Public Health* **96:** 1757–9.

Sharara FI, Beatse SN, Leonardi MR, Navot D, Scott Jr RT (1994) Cigarette smoking accelerates the development of diminished ovarian reserve as evidenced by the clomiphene citrate challenge test. *Fertil Steril* **62:** 257–62.

Shiloh H, Lahav-Baratz S, Koifman M, Ishai D, Bidder D, Weiner-Meganzi Z, Dirnfeld M (2004) The impact of cigarette smoking on zona pellucida thickness of oocytes and embryos prior to transfer into the uterine cavity. *Hum Reprod* **19:** 157–9.

Shiverick KT, Salafia C (1999) Cigarette smoking and pregnancy. I. Ovarian, uterine and placental effects. *Placenta* **20:** 265–72.

Simons AM, Phillips DH, Coleman DV (1993) Damage to DNA in cervical epithelium related to smoking tobacco. *Br Med J* **306:** 1444–8.

Sinkó I, Mórocz M, Zádori J, Kokavszky K, Raskó I (2005) Effect of cigarette smoking on DNA damage of human cumulus cells analyzed by comet assay. *Reprod Toxicol* **20:** 65–71.

Smida AD, Valderrama XP, Agostini MC, Furlan MA, Chedrese J (2004) Cadmium stimulates transcription of the cytochrome p450 side chain cleavage gene in genetically modified stable porcine granulosa cells. *Biol Reprod* **70:** 25–31.

Soares SR, Melo MA (2008) Cigarette smoking and reproductive function. *Curr Opin Obstet Gynecol* **20:** 281–91.

Soares SR, Simon C, Remohí J, Pellicer A (2007) Cigarette smoking affects uterine receptiveness. *Hum Reprod* **22:** 543–7.

Sofikitis N, Takenaka M, Kanakas N, Papadopoulos H, Yamamoto Y, Drakakis P, Miyagawa I (2000) Effects of cotinine on sperm motility, membrane function, and fertilizing capacity in vitro. *Urol Res* **28:** 370–5.

Sorahan T, McKinney PA, Mann JR, Lancashire RJ, Stiller CA, Birch JM, Dodd HE, Cartwright RA (2001) Childhood cancer and parental use of tobacco: findings from the inter-regional epidemiological study of childhood cancer (IRESCC). *Br J Cancer* **84:** 141–6.

Storgaard L, Bonde JP, Ernst E, Spano M, Andersen CY, Frydenberg, Olsen J (2003) Does smoking during pregnancy affect sons' sperm counts? *Epidemiology* **14:** 278–86.

Talbot P (2008) *In vitro* assessment of reproductive toxicity of tobacco smoke and its constituents. *Birth Defects Res C* **84:** 61–72.

Talbot P, DiCarlantonio G, Knoll M (1998) Identification of cigarette smoke components that alter functioning of hamster (mesocricetus auratus) oviducts in vitro. *Biol Reprod* **58**, 1047–53.

Tankó LB, Christiansen C (2004) An update on the antiestrogenic effect of smoking: a literature review with implications for researchers and practitioners. *Menopause* **11:** 104–9.

Thompson KE, Bourguet SM, Christian PJ, Benedict JC, Sipes IG, Flaws JA, Hoyer PB (2005) Differences between rats and mice in the involvement of the aryl hydrocarbon receptor in 4-vinylcyclohexene diepoxide-induced ovarian follicle loss. *Toxicol Appl Pharmacol* **203:** 114–23.

Tuttle AM, Stämpfli M, Foster WG (2009) Cigarette smoke causes follicle loss in mice ovaries at concentrations representative of human exposure. *Hum Reprod* **24:** 1452–9.

USDHHS (US Department of Health and Human Services) (2004) The Health Consequences of Smoking: A Report of the Surgeon General. *Office of Public Health and Science*, Atlanta, GA.

USDHHS (US Department of Health and Human Services) (2006) The Health Consequences of Involuntary Exposure to Tobacco Smoke: A Report of the Surgeon General. *Office of Public Health and Science*, Atlanta, GA.

Varga B, Zsolnai B, Paksy K, Maray M, Ungary G (1993) Age dependent accumulation of cadmium in the human ovary. *Reprod Toxicol* **7:** 225–8.

Vidal JD, VandeVoort CA, Marcus CB, Lazarewicz NR, Conley AJ (2006) *In vitro* exposure to environmental tobacco smoke induces CYP1B1 expression in human luteinized granulosa cells. *Reprod Toxicol* **22:** 731–7.

Viloria T, Garrido N, Fernández JL, Remohí J, Pellicer A, Meseguer M (2007) Sperm selection by swim-up in terms of deoxyribonucleic acid fragmentation as measured by the sperm chromatin dispersion test is altered in heavy smokers. *Fertil Steril* **88:** 523–5.

Vine MF (1996) Smoking and male reproduction: a review. *Int J Androl* **19:** 323–37.

Viswanath K, Herbst RS, Land SR, Leischow SJ, Shields PG (2010) Writing Committee for the AACR Task Force on Tobacco and Cancer. Tobacco and cancer: an American Association for Cancer Research policy statement. *Cancer Res* **70:** 3419–30.

Vrsanská S, Nagyová E, Mlynarcíková A, Ficková M, Kolena J (2003) Components of cigarette smoke inhibit expansion of oocyte-cumulus complexes from porcine follicles. *Physiol Res* **52:** 383–7.

Wang S-L, Lucier GW, Everson RB, Sunahara GI, Shiverick KT (1988) Smoking-related alterations in epidermal growth factor and insulin receptors in human placenta. *Mol Pharmacol* **34:** 265–71.

Wang X, Tager IB, van Vunakis H, Speizer FE, Hanrahan JP (1997) Maternal smoking during pregnancy, urine cotinine concentrations, and birth outcomes. A prospective cohort study. *Int J Epidemiol* **26:** 978–88.

Wang X, Zuckerman B, Pearson C, Kaufman G, Chen C, Wang G, Niu T, Wise PH, Bauchner H, Xu X (2002) Maternal cigarette smoking, metabolic gene polymorphism, and infant birth weight. *J Amer Med Assoc* **287:** 195–202.

Watanabe T, Endo A (1982) Chromosome analysis of preimplantation embryos after cadmium treatment of oocytes at meiosis. *J Environ Mutagen* **4:** 563–7.

Windsor R, Oncken C, Henningfield J, Hartmann K, Edwards N (2000) Behavioral and pharmacological treatment methods for pregnant smokers: issues for clinical practice. *J Am Med Womens Assoc* **55:** 304–10.

Winkelstein Jr W (1990) Smoking and cervical cancer – current status: a review. *Am J Epidemiol* **131:** 945–57.

Winter E, Wang J, Davies MJ, Norman R (2002) Early pregnancy loss following assisted reproductive technology treatment. *Hum Reprod* **17:** 3220–3.

Yauk CL, Berndt ML, Williams A, Rowan-Carroll A, Douglas GR, Stämpfli MR (2007) Mainstream tobacco smoke causes paternal germ-line DNA mutation. *Cancer Res* **67:** 5103–6.

Yoshinaga K, Rick C, Krenn J, Pilot RL (1979) Effects of nicotine on early pregnancy in the rat. *Biol Reprod* **20:** 294–303.

Zdravkovic T, Genbacev O, McMaster MT, Fisher SJ (2005) The adverse effects of maternal smoking on the human placenta: a review. *Placenta* **26(Suppl A):** S81–S86.

Zenzes MT (2000) Smoking and reproduction: gene damage to human gametes and embryos. *Hum Reprod Update* **6:** 122–31.

Zenzes MT, Bielecki R, Reed TE (1999) Detection of benzo(a)pyrene diol epoxide-DNA adducts in sperm of men exposed to cigarette smoke. *Fertil Steril* **72:** 330–5.

Zenzes MT, Puy L, Bielecki R, Reed TE (1999) Detection of benzo(a)pyrene diol epoxide-DNA adducts in embryos from smoking couples: evidence for transmission by spermatozoa. *Mol Hum Reprod* **5:** 125–31.

Zenzes MT, Puy LA, Bielecki R (1998) Immunodetection of benzo(a)pyrene adducts in ovarian cells of women exposed to cigarette smoke. *Mol Hum Reprod* **4:** 159–65.

Zenzes MT, Reed TE, Casper RF (1997) Effects of cigarette smoking and age on the maturation of human oocytes. *Hum Reprod* **12:** 1736–41.

Zenzes MT, Wang P, Casper RF (1995) Cigarette smoking may affect meiotic maturation of human oocytes. *Hum Reprod* **10:** 3213–17.

Zhang L, Connor EE, Chegini N, Shiverick KT (1995) Modulation by benzo(a) pyrene of epidermal growth factor receptors, cell proliferation, and secretion of human chorionic gonadotropin in human placental cell lines. *Biochem Pharmacol* **50:** 1171–80.

Zhang L, Shiverick KT (1997) Benzo(a)pyrene, but not 2,3,7,8-tetrachlorodibenzo-p-dioxin, alters cell proliferation and c-myc and growth factor expression in human placental choriocarcinoma JEG-3 cells. *Biochem Biophys Res Comm* **231:** 117–20.

Zitzmann M, Rolf C, Nordhoff V, Schräder G, Rickert-Föhring M, Gassner P, Behre HM, Greb RR, Kiesel L, Nieschlag E (2003) Male smokers have a decreased success rate for *in vitro* fertilization and intracytoplasmic sperm injection. *Fertil Steril* **79:** 1550–4.

CHAPTER

25

Effects of ethanol and nicotine on human CNS development

Noemi Robles and Josefa Sabriá

INTRODUCTION

In humans, central nervous system (CNS) development begins on the 19th day after conception due to the interaction of two of the three primitive cell layers – ectoderm and mesoderm – resulting on the neural plate, which closes over itself forming the neural tube. Once closed, precursor cells undergo a series of genetically programmed phases, briefly: (1) neurogenesis of primitive neurons and glia; (2) migration of neurons to their localization in the neural tube; (3) differentiation process of neurons; (4) axonal pathfinding and synaptogenesis; (5) synaptic refinement and programmed cell death; and (6) axonal myelinization.

Neurodevelopment is not a uniform process; some areas develop at early stages of embryonic state while others mature some years after birth, as a result of the interaction between CNS and experience. The whole process ends at the age of 18–20 years with the maturation and myelinization of the prefrontal cortex (Purves *et al.*, 2008).

During this period, the CNS is extremely vulnerable to adverse events that might occur during pregnancy and childhood or adolescence, such as poor nutritional status of the mother during pregnancy, exposure to viruses or toxic agents, substance abuse either by the pregnant mother or by children/adolescents.

Tobacco and alcoholic beverages are the most commonly consumed substances of abuse, as they are both legal and easily available (see Table 25.1 for main characteristics). When consumed during pregnancy, these substances may cross the placenta and reach the fetus CNS, interfering with its normal development. On the other hand, adolescents tend to consume alcohol and tobacco products at an early age, when the CNS is not yet completely formed and is still vulnerable.

Although this chapter is focused on the effects of nicotine and ethanol during CNS development, it is worth mentioning that both substances might interfere with fertility. Some studies reveal that tobacco consumption reduces the fertilizing capacity of spermatozoids, damaging their DNA and morphology (Arabi, 2004; Taszarek *et al.*, 2005; Gaur *et al.*, 2010). Women smokers find it more difficult to conceive and show the highest rates of spontaneous abortion, ectopic pregnancy or placenta previa.

Similar results have been found for alcohol in relation to morphological alterations in spermatozoids (Gaur *et al.*, 2010). Alcohol could also interfere with the sex-hormonal axes, reducing testosterone production and release in males, and inhibiting ovulation and reducing plasma estradiol and progesterone levels in females (Hadi *et al*, 1987; Emanuele and Emanuele, 1998).

HISTORICAL BACKGROUND

Ethanol

Alcoholic beverages have a history of abuse. There is ample evidence of alcohol consumption in Sumerian, Babylonic and Egyptian cultures (around 4000 BC). Alcohol played a symbolic role in religious ceremonies such as Bacchus/Dionysius worship and in Christianity. In addition to recreational use, alcohol has been used for different purposes, including therapeutic applications as an anesthetic, a disinfectant or mixed with opium as a sedative (Koob and Le Moal, 2005).

Ethanol is the principal psychoactive constituent in alcoholic beverages, so from now on the term *ethanol* will be used instead of *alcohol*. Ethanol is obtained by fermenting grain or fruit, or by distillation; its content in the most common fermented beverages is 4–6% for beer and 12–20% for wine, whereas distilled drinks reach contents of around 40–80% of ethanol.

Effects of ethanol consumption on fetal development are well known. In fact, disorders related to maternal ethanol drinking are categorized as fetal alcohol spectrum disorders (FASD) with an estimated prevalence of 1% of all live births. The most common FASD is the fetal alcohol syndrome (FAS), diagnosed when the following criteria have been confirmed: (1) maternal ethanol exposure; (2) evidence of a characteristic pattern of minor facial abnormalities (two or more: short parpebral fissures, thin vermilion border of the upper lip, smooth philtrum); (3) evidence of prenatal and/or postnatal growth

Reproductive and Developmental Toxicology, Edited by Ramesh C. Gupta
ISBN: 978-0-12-382032-7

TABLE 25.1 Summary of main characteristics of ethanol and nicotine

	Alcohol	Nicotine
Main route of administration	Oral (exclusive)	Smoked (main)
Maximum concentration in blood	30–90 minutes	8 seconds
Half-life in organism	6 hours	2 hours
Metabolization	Liver: – ADH system – MEOS (P450 – CYP2E1) – Catalase Brain: – MEOS (P450 – CYP2E1) – Catalase	Liver: cytochrome P450 (CYP2A6)
Profile	CNS depressor	CNS stimulant
Tolerance	Pharmacological Pharmacodynamical	Pharmacological Pharmacodynamical
Dependence	Yes	Yes
Withdrawal syndrome	Yes	Yes
Sites of action on CNS	– Main: own binding site in $GABA_A$ receptors (allosteric modulator) – No binding site: NMDA receptors, voltage calcium channels – Other systems: serotoninergic, dopaminergic, noradrenergic, histaminergic, cholinergic	– Direct with binding site: nicotinic acetylcholine receptors (agonist) – Indirect as release modulator: dopaminergic system, GABAergic system, glutamatergic system
Behavioral/ cognitive effects	– euphoria – disinhibition – decreased attention – increased reaction time – anxiolysis – sedation – analgesia	– increased concentration – increased attention focusing – anxiolysis – analgesia – activation autonomous nervous system

retardation; (4) evidence of deficient brain growth and/or abnormal morphogenesis (one or more: structural brain abnormalities, head circumference ≤10%). The most common neurophysiological alterations related to FAS/FASD include difficulties with arithmetic and number processing, verbal and non-verbal learning, speech and language delay, attention deficits and altered executive functions (judgment, organization and reasoning). The FAS/FASD distribution scores in IQ, WRAT Arithmetic and Vineland Adaptive Behavior Score scales are left-deviates from normative distributions (Sampson *et al.*, 2000; Manning and Eugene, 2007).

Other FASD are partial FAS (no maternal exposure confirmed and/or not all the criteria for FAS fulfilled), alcohol-related birth defects (normal growth and development but characteristic structural abnormalities) and alcohol-related neurodevelopmental disorder (normal growth and development but characteristic behavioral and cognitive abnormalities).

Nicotine

Nicotine is an alkaloid obtained from the tobacco plant *Nicotiana tabacum*, originating in North and South America, and introduced in Europe in the 16th century. Its use is not only recreational; it has even been used for therapeutic purposes, such as to prevent fatigue, purge nasal passages or treat syphilis (Koob and Le Moal, 2005).

The most common route of administration is inhalation: smoked as cigarettes, cigars or in a pipe. It can also be chewed, sniffed or in patches (e.g., chewing gum, chewing tobacco, dipping tobacco, snuff). This chapter will focus only on nicotine administered via inhalation (smoking).

In the case of tobacco, there is no medical categorization for *in utero* nicotine exposure, although the teratogenic effects of nicotine on fetal development are well known. Maternal smoking is related with a wide range of alterations, such as low weight at birth, high rates of sudden infant death syndrome and neuropsychological disturbances, mainly somatosensory deficits, difficulties in learning, high rates of attention deficit hyperactivity disorder, aggressive and antisocial behavior and anxiety (Ernst *et al.*, 2001).

PHARMACOKINETICS

Ethanol

Ethanol is consumed orally. Its absorption begins in the mouth, although it is mainly absorbed in the small intestine and stomach. Ethanol can be detected in blood 5 minutes after being swallowed, but peak concentration is reached after 30–90 minutes. The extent of absorption may be altered by several factors, such as being ingested on a full stomach, the amount and characteristics of nutritional accompanying components, and in females the phase of menstrual cycle. Once absorbed, it is distributed in all tissues in proportion to their water content; the highest concentrations of ethanol are found in the blood and brain, followed by muscles and fat tissue.

Ethanol is not accumulated in any tissue but eliminated almost entirely by oxidative metabolism in the liver. The main enzymatic pathways involved are alcohol dehydrogenase (ADH), cytochrome P450 (CYP2E1) and catalase (Riveros-Rosas *et al.*, 1997). There are several isoforms of ADH. Under normal physiological conditions, the main isoforms involved in human ethanol metabolism are ADH_{1-3} ($K_m < 5$ mM). ADH converts ethanol to acetaldehyde, a highly toxic metabolite, which is easily distributed throughout the body, both intra- and extracellularly. Acetaldehyde is further converted to acetate by aldehyde dehydrogenase. A small amount of ethanol (10% approximately) is excreted in the urine, the sweat and breath. The whole process of ethanol metabolization may take about 6 hours, depending on age, sex, nutritional state or tolerance to ethanol.

When a huge amount of ethanol is ingested, the ADH system collapses and a second mechanism of oxidation is activated: the system of microsomal ethanol oxidation (MEOS), depending on the cytochrome P450 (specifically the isoenzyme 2E1), which is located in the smooth endoplasmic reticulum. MEOS oxidizes ethanol to acetaldehyde. The K_m of cytochrome P450 for ethanol is 8–10 mM, and its activation increases the ability of the organism to metabolize ethanol which is related to the phenomenon of metabolic tolerance

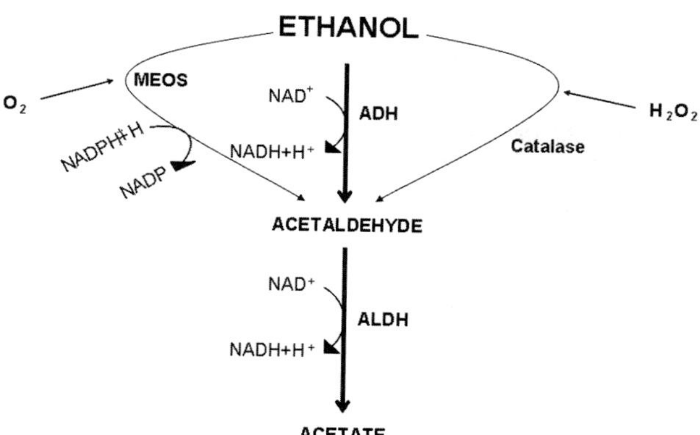

FIGURE 25.1 Primary routes of ethanol metabolism.

developed by chronic drinkers. MEOS is also related to the activation of toxic substrates and an increase in free radicals (see below with more detail).

A third metabolic system involved in the oxidation of ethanol is the catalase of the peroxisomes. This enzyme has a low K_m for ethanol (0.6 mM) and requires the presence of hydrogen peroxide to produce the reaction. Under normal physiological conditions, catalase plays only a minor role in ethanol metabolism.

In the brain, the main metabolic systems involved in ethanol oxidation are the cytochrome P450 and catalase, although some authors have reported the presence of ADH in some regions of rat brain, such as cerebellum and hippocampus (Martínez *et al.*, 2001) (Figure 25.1).

Nicotine

Smoked nicotine is absorbed mainly in the lungs, but also in the mouth; it is then quickly distributed throughout the organism, mainly in the liver, brain, kidneys and spleen. Its absorption depends on pH, chemical compounds of cigarettes or nutritional state. Nicotine reaches the CNS in 8 seconds and its half-life in the organism is roughly 2 hours. It is extensively metabolized to a number of metabolites in the liver, mainly by the cytochrome P450 (isoenzyme CYP2A6 and also CYP2B6). The most important metabolite of nicotine in most mammalian species is the lactam derivative cotinine. In humans, about 70–80% of nicotine is converted to cotinine.

Nicotine can also be metabolized by two non-oxidative pathways, methylation of the pyridine nitrogen giving nicotine isomethonium ion and glucuronidation. Studies using

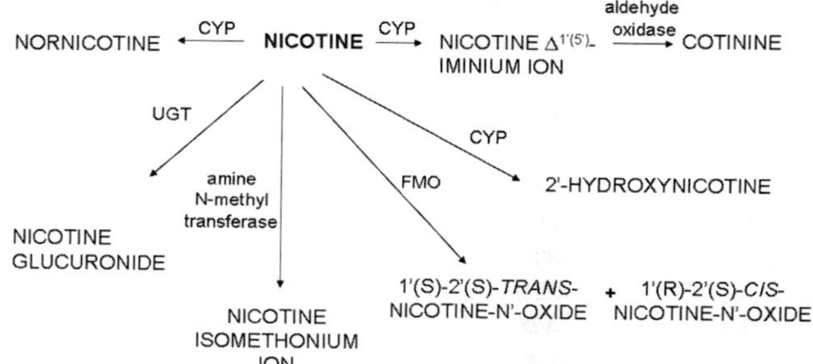

FIGURE 25.2 Primary routes of nicotine metabolism (adaptated from Hukkanen *et al.*, 2005).

animal models and human liver homogenates show that S-adenosyl-L-methionine is the source of the methyl group in a reaction catalyzed by the amine N-methyltransferase. Small amounts of nicotine isomethonium ion have been detected in the urine of smokers.

Nicotine glucuronidation results in an N-quaternary glucuronide in humans. This reaction is catalyzed by uridine diphosphate-glucuronosyltransferase (UGT) enzyme. About 3–5% of nicotine is converted to nicotine glucuronide and excreted in urine in humans (Hukkanen *et al.*, 2005) (Figure 25.2).

MECHANISMS OF ACTION ON BRAIN DEVELOPMENT: *IN UTERO* EXPOSURE

Ethanol

There is a great amount of evidence of the toxicity of ethanol during brain development; in fact, maternal ethanol consumption during pregnancy is considered one of the main causes of impaired cognitive functions and mental retardation.

Some studies reveal that certain brain regions are extremely vulnerable to ethanol exposure, such as neocortex, hippocampus and cerebellum. The extent of brain damage depends on two factors: the dose of ethanol consumed (higher doses, higher damages) and the period of brain development. Most of the alterations observed are mainly produced by the following factors (Nevo and Harmon, 1995; Harper and Matsumoto, 2005):

1. *Effects of acetaldehyde*: this metabolite produces mutagenic and teratogenic effects even at low concentrations. First, the high reactivity of its aldehyde group reacts with the amino and sulfhydryl groups of proteins affecting their synthesis and function, as observed with tubulin. Second, acetaldehyde alters the structure and function of mitochondria, slowing oxidative metabolism. Finally, acetaldehyde may condense with biogenic amines to form tetrahydroisoquinolines, as salsolinol, and β-carbolines and harman, which are highly neurotoxic compounds with potential reinforcement properties at low concentrations.
2. *The participation of the MEOS in the metabolism of ethanol*: this system activates potentially carcinogenic substrates, such as dimethylnitrosamine, or toxic substrates, such as carbon tetrachloride or aminopterin. MEOS also increases the production of free radicals.
3. *Inhibition of excitatory NMDA receptors*: when administered acutely, ethanol selectively and potently inhibits the function of N-methyl-D-aspartate (NMDA) receptors. Additionally, chronic consumption produces a compensatory upregulation of NMDA receptors. This upregulation not only increases vulnerability to cytotoxicity induced by calcium, but also increases glutamatergic activity. Moreover, the enhancement of calcium influx via this receptor interferes with the mitochondrial oxidative metabolism and increases neuronal excitability.
4. *Altered catabolism of homocysteine to methionine*: this process requires the action of folate as cofactor, which is decreased in alcoholism, resulting in an increase of homocysteine. Homocysteine acts as a full or partial agonist of NMDA and glycine receptors, enhancing their functionality.
5. *Reduced availability of trophic factors and impaired function of its receptors (TrkB, TrkA)*: reduction of neurotrophins alters mechanisms of cell survival and apoptosis. This alteration

would hinder the survival of neurons damaged by ethanol as well as facilitate the death of these affected cells.

6. *Induction of oxidative stress and loss of ability to repair DNA damage*: both phenomena precipitate neuronal death processes. Recently, it has been demonstrated that DNA damage in alcoholics is selectively localized in glial cells in the frontal cortex and hippocampus.

All these factors result in brain development disruptions, which have different effects depending on the period of gestation. Fetal ethanol exposure during the first trimester is related with neural tube defects and craniofacial anomalies. In the second gestation trimester, most of the brain areas are under proliferation, migration and differentiation phases, and ethanol could interfere in all these processes, resulting in brain structural abnormalities related to behavioral alterations, such as decreased attention, increase of activity or deficits in reflex development. Finally, given that during the third trimester of gestation synaptogenesis and myelination prevails, ethanol exposure in this period is related to microcephaly and behavioral dysfunctions (Guerri, 1998).

Some studies focused on the effects of ethanol on glial cells (Vallés *et al.*, 1996; Guerri *et al.*, 2001), mainly radial glia and astrocytes. Radial glia cells play a crucial role in migratory phase, guiding with their fibers immature neurons from ventricular zone to their definite localization. Ethanol exposure decreases the number of radial glia cells and alters their morphology. At a biochemical level, ethanol alters most of the molecules involved in cell adhesion and migration and/or their receptors, such as cell adhesion molecules (CAMs), transforming growth factor-β (TGF-β), bone morphogenetic proteins (BMPs) or the glial-derived neurotrophic factor (GDNF). All these alterations result in aberrant patterns of neural migration.

Moreover, as radial glia is the main precursor of astrocytes, ethanol exposure produces a decrease in the astroglial-specific marker glial fibrillary acidic protein (GFAP) and its mRNA levels, which leads to a reduced number of astrocytes found both in *in vivo* and *in vitro* studies.

Specifically, there is a 35% decrease in the number of astrocytes in brains subjected to prenatal ethanol exposure. This subtype of glia is related to several functions such as structural and nutritive support to neurons, regulation of ions and neurotransmitters, involvement in blood–brain barrier or production of growth factors. After prenatal ethanol exposure, in addition to the reduced number of astrocytes, there is evidence of alterations of cytoskeletal protein fibers as GFAP or vimentin, changes in cell membrane glycoproteins and surface membrane proteins.

Moreover, ethanol exposure increases astrocytes' vulnerability to toxicity. First, as astrocytes express the CYP2E1 isoenzyme of P450, they participate in ethanol metabolism through the activation of MEOS, which leads to the generation of free radicals. Second, the exposure of astrocytes to ethanol increases their vulnerability to factors related to cell death, as TNFα.

There are a few secondary factors related to maternal ethanol consumption that could also disrupt normal brain development. These factors are related to nutritional state, as ethanol intake impairs intestinal absorption and therefore is associated with malnutrition. Another factor to be considered is that a great amount of ethanol may induce episodes of ischemia/hypoxia that initiate severe morphological and functional changes, even mechanisms of cell death (Guerri, 1998) (Figure 25.3).

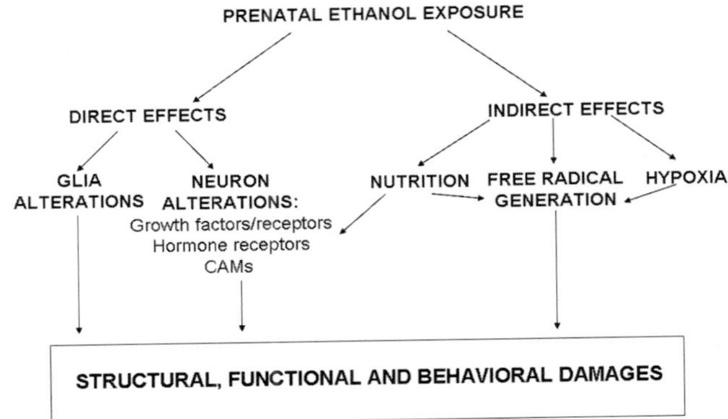

FIGURE 25.3 Direct and indirect effects of ethanol on CNS development during prenatal period (adaptated from Guerri, 1998).

Nicotine

It is accepted that nicotine might play a neuroprotective role in adults, while its presence in developmental periods is linked to neurotoxicity, interfering in brain development in a dose-dependent manner (Ferrea and Winterer, 2009).

Tobacco interferes with offspring through direct and also indirect mechanisms (Ernst *et al.*, 2001; Pauly and Slotkin, 2008). Direct effects are attributed to the action of nicotine on neuronal nicotinic acetylcholine receptors (nnAChRs). These receptors are pentameric ligand-gated cation channels configured by combinations of five α_{2-9} and/or β_{2-4} subunits, each combination with its own pharmacological characteristics. Depending on their subunit composition, nnAChRs can gate both Na^+ and Ca^{2+}. The most common neuronal subtypes in the CNS are the heteropentamer $\alpha_4\beta_2$ and the homopentamer α_7. When nicotine binds to nnAChRs it produces a change in the receptor conformation that leads to the opening of the channel resulting in increased Na^+ or Ca^{2+} ion fluxes, depending on the subunit combination. Heteromeric $\alpha_4\beta_2$ binds nicotine with high affinity and primarily gates Na^+. The homomer α_7 has a low affinity to nicotine, and it has distinct ion selectivity, gating both Na^+ and a large amount of Ca^{2+} (Sharples and Wonnacott, 2001; Barik and Wonnacott, 2009). Immediately after the opening, receptors turn into a desensitized state in which stimulation cannot open the channel. Then the receptors return to their close-resting state. Chronic nicotine exposure produces a permanent desensitization of nnAChRs, which results in an upregulation of neuronal nicotinic receptors in order to compensate the inactivation of the receptors (Wonnacott, 1990; Gaimarri *at al.*, 2007).

In adult brain, nAChRs usually play a role as pre-synaptic and pre-terminal receptors modulating neurotransmitter release and enhancing overall cell excitability, and they are related with learning and memory, regulation of anxiety and modulation of reinforcement pathways. However, during CNS development nnAChRs play a pivotal role in (Dwyer *et al.*, 2009): (1) cell survival and targeting, mainly by means of α_7 subtype and its modulation of Ca^{2+} entry; (2) formation of neural and sensory circuits, due to their ability to generate spontaneous activity; and (3) the regulation of the development of catecholaminergic pathways, controlling their release patterns.

nnAChRs are expressed early during the first trimester of pregnancy, following complex and transient patterns of expression which depend on the brain region and receptor subtype. There is ample evidence of expression of mRNA and binding sites for $\alpha_4\beta_2$ at 6 weeks in spinal cord, pons and medulla; at 8 weeks in cortex, cerebellum and subcortical forebrain; and at 25 weeks in thalamus, hippocampus and basal ganglia. On the other hand, α_7 appears at 5 weeks in midbrain and pons, and later in spinal cord, subcortical forebrain and cortex, approximately at 9 weeks.

Prenatal nicotine exposure results in a permanent desensitization of nnAChRs and their compensatory upregulation, similar to that observed in adults. This effect disrupts normal neurodevelopmental programming processes.

On the other hand, the decrease in the total number of cells after *in utero* nicotine exposure suggests the activation of mechanisms of apoptosis, most of them related with increased intracellular concentrations of calcium, mainly through α_7 receptors. This subtype of receptor has the fastest rate of desensitization, which functionally means that it is the first subtype to recover from the inactivation, so its upregulation could be related with an increased calcium flux and the activation of the apoptotic response.

Another relevant effect to consider is the role of nnAChRs in the formation of catecholaminergic systems, especially dopaminergic pathways. Prenatal nicotine exposure produces alterations in catecholamine levels and their metabolites. These alterations in dopamine projections underlie most of dopamine-dependent diseases commonly present in children exposed to nicotine *in utero*, such as attention deficit hyperactivity disorder or an increased risk of substance abuse during adolescence.

The other main direct effect of tobacco is related to the additive cigarette compounds, most of them toxics such as acetone, ammonia, arsenic, benzene, lead or tar; and with some of the combustion products of tobacco, such as formaldehyde or acetaldehyde, that are able to cross cell membranes and initiate cytotoxic mechanisms. As with ethanol consumption, acetaldehyde resulting from tobacco condenses with amines producing β-carbolines and tetrahydroisoquinolines.

The indirect effects of tobacco that could affect brain development include the poor nutritional status of the mother due to anorexigenic effect of nicotine, carbon monoxide exposure and decreased blood flow to the placenta related with the vasoconstrictive property of nicotine (Figure 25.4).

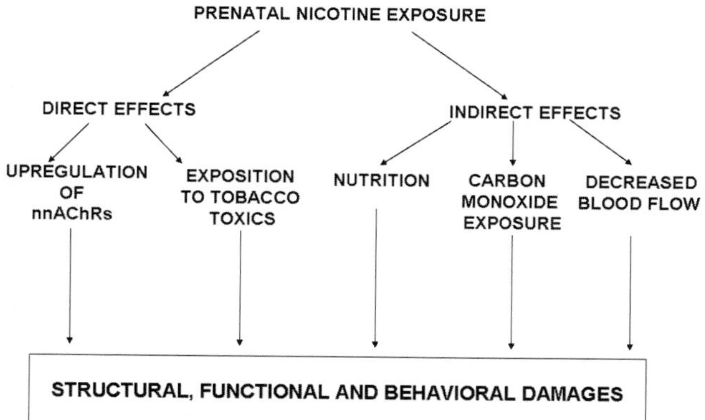

FIGURE 25.4 Direct and indirect effects of nicotine on CNS development during prenatal period.

ETHANOL AND NICOTINE MECHANISMS OF ACTION ON BRAIN DEVELOPMENT: ADOLESCENCE EXPOSURE

During adolescence, brain development completes with synaptic refinement in the prefrontal and temporal cortex, subcortical structures (striatum, thalamus and nucleus accumbens) and in the myelination process. In fact, during this period there is an inverted U-shape pattern of the volume of gray matter and a linear increase in white matter. The other important process occurring during adolescence is the maturation of the reinforcement–dopaminergic pathway (mesolimbic system), related with the motivated behavior.

Mechanism of action of ethanol

Some studies revealed differences in sensitivity to ethanol between adolescents and adults. On the one hand, adolescents are less sensitive to adverse effects of ethanol than adults (e.g., hangover, dysphoria, motor impairment). On the other hand, they are relatively more sensitive to reinforcement properties, such as social facilitation. This lack of sensitivity to negative effects decreases the cues that restrain intake, which results in high amounts of ethanol consumption (Windle *et al.*, 2008).

During adolescence, ethanol disrupts the processes of maturation and myelinization, mainly due to two factors (Guerri and Pascual, 2010; Witt, 2010): (1) NMDA receptor upregulation, which is related with enhanced glutamatergic transmission and increased amount of intracellular Ca^{2+}; and (2) the activation of glial mechanisms of neuroinflammation, such as the release of proinflammatory cytokines (IL-1β or TNFα), activation of cyclooxygenase-2 (COX-2), and an increase in inducible nitric oxide synthase (iNOS) and neural cell death.

Functionally, adolescents who consume ethanol present alterations in learning and memory, which are related with reduced blood oxygen levels in brain areas involved in these processes, as well as structural abnormalities and reduction in the total brain area volume, mainly in the hippocampus (Guerri and Pascual, 2010; Witt, 2010). In this brain region, there is evidence that long-term ethanol consumption inhibits adult neurogenesis, which could also be related with cognitive impairment (Morris *et al.*, 2010).

Finally, some studies have reported gender differences in patterns of neural activity which make women more vulnerable to effects and damages caused by ethanol (Guerri and Pascual, 2010).

Mechanism of action of nicotine

Similar to ethanol, adolescents seem less sensitive to the adverse effects of tobacco than adults. Unfortunately, the role of nnAChRs in neural development has been investigated less during adolescence in comparison with the prenatal phase. However, some studies suggest that the main function of these receptors is the regulation of the formation of the limbic pathways. What it is known for certain is that nicotine intake in adolescents upregulates nnAChRs and induces changes in cholinergic, serotoninergic and catecholaminergic neurotransmission, as it does in adults (Trauth *et al.*, 2001; Slotkin, 2002).

CONCLUDING REMARKS AND FUTURE DIRECTIONS

Exposure to ethanol and nicotine during development of CNS produces a series of disruptions that last for a lifetime. Both drugs act through multiple mechanisms, which imply that these substances have different and complex targets of action. Ethanol and nicotine produce changes at the molecular level and interfere with the structure, connectivity and functionality of genetically programmed neural networks, resulting in cognitive and behavioral impairments. The two most critical periods of CNS development are the gestation time, when the system is beginning to develop and establish the first cell structures and connections, and adolescence, when the CNS is coming to maturity.

Tables 25.2 and 25.3 summarize the main features of this chapter.

This chapter described the effects of tobacco and ethanol on the developing CNS separately, although these two substances of abuse are usually used together. Therefore, in cases of co-abuse the addition of the disruptive mechanisms of both drugs should be considered. Moreover, the two drugs share some cytotoxic mechanisms. One of the most relevant of these mechanisms is the involvement of acetaldehyde, generated during the first step of ethanol metabolism, and during the combustion of tobacco compounds. Another relevant mechanism involves the cholinergic system and nnAChRs; there is evidence that alcohol consumption is able to interact with nnAChRs and regulate their gene expression, in some cases upregulating them the same way as nicotine (Yoshida *et al.*, 1982; Booker and Collins, 1997; Larsson and Engel, 2004; Robles and Sabrià, 2006, 2008; Ribeiro-Carvalho *et al.*, 2008).

TABLE 25.2 Summary of cellular, molecular, physical and behavioral effects of prenatal ethanol exposition

Cellular and molecular neurotoxic mechanisms involved in ethanol effects on CNS development

- Acetaldehyde toxicity
- MEOS toxicity
- Inhibited NMDA receptors
- Altered homocysteine–methionine system
- Reduced trophic factors
- Oxidative stress
- Loose ability to repair DNA damages
- Alterations in molecules involved in cell adhesion and migration: CAMs, TGF-β, BMPs, GDNF
- Alterations in astrocytes: GFAP, vimentin, cell glycoproteins, vulnerability to cell death, activation of neuroinflammatory mechanisms (IL-1β, TNFα, COX-2, iNOS)

Physical and behavioral resulting alterations

Physical alterations	– Short parpebral fissures – Thin vermilion border of the upper lip – Smooth philtrum
Childhood	– Difficulties with arithmetic, verbal and non-verbal learning – Delayed speech and language
Adolescence/young adulthood	– Attention deficits – Disrupted executive functions – Substance abuse predisposition

TABLE 25.3 Cellular molecular, physical and behavioral effects of prenatal nicotine exposition

Cellular and molecular neurotoxic mechanisms involved in nicotine effects on CNS development

- Upregulated nnAChRs
- Acetaldehyde toxicity
- Activation of cytotoxic mechanisms by additive compound of cigarettes and combustion products

Physical and behavioral resulting alterations:

Perinatal effects	– Low weight – Low head circumference
Infancy/toddlerhood (<2 years)	– Motor deficits – Sensory deficits – Verbal comprehension difficulty
Childhood	– Externalizing behavioral problems (oppositional, aggressive, overactive) – Sustained attention difficulty – Memory deficits – Impulsivity
Adolescence/young adulthood	– ADHD – Aggressive and antisocial behavior/criminal behavior – Substance abuse predisposition

Most studies focus on *in utero* exposure, while only a little research is being conducted in perinatal periods. Maternal consumption could interfere in the baby's CNS development even when the placenta union has finished after childbirth. The baby might be further exposed to nicotine/ethanol through breastfeeding, and to the toxic compounds of tobacco by secondhand smoking.

There are no treatments for neuroevolutive diseases produced by ethanol or tobacco exposure. The only course of action is prevention at the early stages of the development. Pregnant women should avoid using these substances at least during pregnancy and preferably also during breastfeeding. The downside of cessation is the appearance of withdrawal symptoms and craving. In the case of nicotine, nicotine replacement therapies (NRT) have been proposed as a preventive treatment option. Some clinical studies have shown that NRT are not completely effective in tobacco cessation and involve certain risks to neurodevelopment (Pauly and Slotkin, 2008). In other cases, partial nicotine agonists can be used, such as cytisine and vereclidine, which have the advantage of agonizing nAChRs without desensitizing receptors. Another advantage of these partial agonists is that they are more selective for the $\alpha_4\beta_2$ subtype, which does not prevent the α_7 subtype from playing its role in cell survival and targeting (Pauly and Slotkin, 2008; Rollema *et al.*, 2009).

The intent of this chapter was to summarize the main effects of ethanol and nicotine consumption over human CNS development, although some results obtained from cell cultures or animal research have been considered. Using animal models is an excellent tool for elucidating the mechanisms underlying the disruptive effects of ethanol and tobacco intake, but they should as much as possible mimic the human patterns of consumption in order to generalize the results. Leaving aside the extreme difficulty of modeling the social factors that affect the onset of ethanol and tobacco consumption, animal models should at least respect the routes of administration and the factors related to consumption. Therefore ethanol consumption models should avoid forced administration, such as intravenous injections, oragastrical tubes or liquid diets. It should also be noted that alcoholic beverages are consumed by their organoleptic characteristics, and that pure ethanol has an aversive taste. Keeping in mind all these aspects, the best option is a voluntary oral administration model (such as the two-bottle choice paradigm), using sweetened drinking solutions (e.g., 10% v/v ethanol + 30% w/v glucose/saccharine).

Designing animal models of tobacco consumption is even more difficult than ethanol. The main problem is that the usual route of administration of nicotine in humans is cigarette smoking, which is almost impossible to model in animals. Animal models of nicotine consumption usually inject nicotine both intravenously and intracerebrally; another option is to implant nicotine minipumps that gradually release the substance into the organism. The pure nicotine administration simplifies the effects of tobacco, as it does not take into account the effects of the additives in cigarettes or the compounds generated by the combustion of cigarettes, which are also highly toxic.

REFERENCES

Arabi M (2004) Nicotinic infertility: assessing DNA and plasma membrane integrity of human spermatozoa. *Andrologia* **36(5):** 305–10.

Barik J, Wonnacott S (2009) Molecular and cellular mechanisms of action of nicotine in the CNS. *Handb Exp Pharmacol* **(192):** 173–207.

Booker TK, Collins AC (1997) Long-term ethanol treatment elicits changes in nicotinic receptor binding in only a few brain regions. *Alcohol* **14:** 131–40.

Dwyer JB, McQuown SC, Leslie FM (2009) The dynamic effects of nicotine on the developing brain. *Pharmacol Ther* **122(2):** 125–39.

Emanuele MA, Emanuele NV (1998) Alcohol's effects on male reproduction. *Alcohol Health Res World* **22(3):** 195–201.

Ernst M, Moolchan ET, Robinson ML (2001) Behavioral and neural consequences of prenatal exposure to nicotine. *J Am Acad Child Adolesc Psychiatry* **40(6):** 630–41.

Ferrea S, Winterer G (2009) Neuroprotective and neurotoxic effects of nicotine. *Pharmacopsychiatry* **42(6):** 255–65.

Gaimarri A, Moretti M, Riganti L, Zanardi A, Clementi F, Gotti C (2007) Regulation of neuronal nicotinic receptor traffic and expression. *Brain Res Rev* **55(1):** 134–43.

Gaur DS, Talekar MS, Pathak VP (2010) Alcohol intake and cigarette smoking: impact of two major lifestyle factors on male fertility. *Indian J Pathol Microbiol* **53(1):** 35–40.

Guerri C (1998) Neuroanatomical and neurophysiological mechanisms involved in central nervous system dysfunctions induced by prenatal alcohol exposure. *Alcohol Clin Exp Res* **22(2):** 304–12.

Guerri C, Pascual M, Renau-Piqueras J (2001) Glia and fetal alcohol syndrome. *Neurotoxicology* **22(5):** 593–9.

Guerri C, Pascual M (2010) Mechanisms involved in the neurotoxic, cognitive, and neurobehavioral effects of alcohol consumption during adolescence. *Alcohol* **44(1):** 15–26.

Hadi HA, Hill JA, Castillo RA (1987) Alcohol and reproductive function: a review. *Obstet Gynecol Surv* **42(2):** 69–74.

Harper C, Matsumoto I (2005) Ethanol and brain damage. *Curr Opin Pharmacol* **5:** 73–8.

Hukkanen J, Jacob P 3rd, Benowitz NL (2005) Metabolism and disposition kinetics of nicotine. *Pharmacol Rev* **57(1):** 79–115.

Koob GF, Le Moal M (2005) *Neurobiology of Addiction*. Amsterdam, Elsevier.

Larsson A, Engel JA (2004) Neurochemical and behavioral studies on ethanol and nicotine interactions. *Neurosci Biobehav Rev* **27(8):** 713–20.

Manning MA, Eugene H (2007) Fetal alcohol spectrum disorders: a practical clinical approach to diagnosis. *Neurosci Biobehav Rev* **31(2):** 230–8.

Martínez SE, Vaglenova J, Sabrià J, Martínez MC, Farrés J, Parés X (2001) Distribution of alcohol dehydrogenase mRNA in the rat central nervous system. Consequences for brain ethanol and retinoid metabolism. *Eur J Biochem* **268(19):** 5045–56.

Morris SA, Eaves DW, Smith AR, Nixon K (2010) Alcohol inhibition of neurogenesis: a mechanism of hippocampal neurodegeneration in an adolescent alcohol abuse model. *Hippocampus* **20(5):** 596–607.

Nevo I, Hamon M (1995). Neurotransmitter and neuromodulatory mechanisms involved in alcohol abuse and alcoholism. *Neurochem Int* **26:** 305–36.

Pauly JR, Slotkin TA (2008) Maternal tobacco smoking, nicotine replacement and neurobehavioural development. *Acta Paediatr* **97(10):** 1331–7.

Purves D, Augustine GJ, Fitzpatrick D, Hall WC, LaMantia AS, McNamara JO, White LE (2008) *Neuroscience*. Sunderland, Sinauer Associates.

Ribeiro-Carvalho A, Lima CS, Filgueiras CC, Manhães AC, Abreu-Villaça Y (2008) Nicotine and ethanol interact during adolescence: effects on the central cholinergic systems. *Brain Res* **26(1232):** 48–60.

Riveros-Rosas H, Julian-Sanchez A, Pinã E (1997) Enzymology of ethanol and acetaldehyde metabolism in mammals. *Arch Med Res* **28(4):** 453–71.

Robles N, Sabriá J (2006) Ethanol consumption produces changes in behavior and on hippocampal alpha7 and alpha4beta2 nicotinic receptors. *J Mol Neurosci* **30(1–2):** 119–20.

Robles N, Sabriá J (2008) Effects of moderate chronic ethanol consumption on hippocampal nicotinic receptors and associative learning. *Neurobiol Learn Mem* **89(4):** 497–503.

Rollema H, Hajós M, Seymour PA, Kozak R, Majchrzak MJ, Guanowsky V, Horner WE, Chapin DS, Hoffmann WE, Johnson DE, McLean S, Freeman J, Williams KE (2009) Preclinical pharmacology of the alpha4beta2 nAChR partial agonist varenicline related to effects on reward, mood and cognition. *Biochem Pharmacol* **78(7):** 813–24.

Sampson PD, Streissguth AP, Bookstein FL, Barr HM (2000) On categorizations in analyses of alcohol teratogenesis. *Environ Health Perspect* **108 (Suppl. 3):** 421–8.

Sharples C, Wonnacott S (2001) Neuronal nicotinic receptors. *Tocris Reviews* **19**.

Slotkin TA (2002) Nicotine and the adolescent brain: insights from an animal model. *Neurotoxicol Teratol* **24(3):** 369–84.

Taszarek H-G, Depa-Martynów M, Derwich K, Pawelczyk L, Jedrzejczak P (2005) [The influence of cigarette smoking on sperm quality of male smokers and nonsmokers in infertile couples]. *Przegl Lek* **62(10):** 978–81.

Trauth JA, Seidler FJ, Ali SF, Slotkin TA (2001). Adolescent nicotine exposure produces immediate and long-term changes in CNS noradrenergic and dopaminergic function. *Brain Res* **892(2):** 269–80.

Vallés S, Sancho-Tello M, Miñana R, Climent E, Renau-Piqueras J, Guerri C (1996) Glial fibrillary acidic protein expression in rat brain and in radial glia culture is delayed by prenatal ethanol exposure. *J Neurochem* **67(6):** 2425–33.

Windle M, Spear LP, Fuligni AJ, Angold A, Brown JD, Pine D, Smith GT, Giedd J, Dahl RE (2008) Transitions into underage and problem drinking: developmental processes and mechanisms between 10 and 15 years of age. *Pediatrics* **121 (Suppl. 4):** S273–S289.

Witt ED (2010) Research on alcohol and adolescent brain development: opportunities and future directions. *Alcohol* **44(1):** 119–24.

Wonnacott S (1990) The paradox of nicotinic acetylcholine receptor upregulation by nicotine. *Trends Pharmaco Sci* **11:** 216–19.

Yoshida K, Engel J, Liljequist S (1982) The effect of chronic ethanol administration of high affinity 3H-nicotinic binding in rat brain. *Naunyn Schmiedebergs Arch Pharmacol* **321:** 74–6.

CHAPTER

26

Developmental neurotoxicity of abused drugs

Jerrold S. Meyer and Brian J. Piper

INTRODUCTION

Substance use during pregnancy is an important issue because of the sensitivity of the developing embryo to various recreational drugs that are less toxic to adults except at extremely high doses. Epidemiological research has identified several important patterns of recreational drug use. Initial experimentation often starts with readily available substances (e.g., inhalants) around the time of puberty and may escalate to more intensive use patterns and/or include illicit drugs (e.g., heroin) during young adulthood. Importantly, a large majority of women who use drugs during pregnancy report either discontinuation or significant reduction in their use after the first trimester when they discover that they are pregnant (e.g., Smith *et al.*, 2008). However, a smaller but significant group continues to abuse substances at very high levels throughout pregnancy. According to the National Survey on Drug Use and Health, in 2007–2008 an estimated 97,000 pregnant women aged 15 to 44 were current users of cannabis and an additional 51,000 were current users of other illicit drugs (e.g., cocaine, heroin, hallucinogens and inhalants) and/or prescription-type psychotherapeutic agents (e.g., pain medications, tranquilizers, sedatives and stimulants) used in a non-medical context (Substance Abuse and Mental Health Services Administration, 2009). From these figures, we can assume that well over 100,000 infants are born each year in the USA that have been exposed *in utero* to substances of abuse other than alcohol and tobacco. While drug abusers often have a preferred drug of choice, the use of multiple substances is the norm rather than the exception, and this caveat frames the interpretation of most investigations with human subjects. Moreover, there is no clear-cut relationship between the legality of specific substance, prevalence of use and the consequences of fetal exposure.

This chapter will focus on the developmental neurotoxicity of illicit drugs. Although alcohol and tobacco are consumed even more widely than the substances discussed below, their effects are described elsewhere in this book. We will use a neurobehavioral teratology framework that has two core tenets. First, the nervous system has a protracted period of developmental susceptibility to disruption of fundamental neurobiological processes. Such processes include the neurogenesis, neuronal differentiation and migration, and synaptogenesis and circuit formation. Second, the most common injuries to the immature nervous system do not produce structural CNS malformations but instead result in functional abnormalities. Deficits in neurobehavior can occur at doses below those known to produce birth defects or other obvious external abnormalities (Vorhees, 1989). Because of the important contributions of laboratory animal research to the field of neurobehavioral teratology, we will first discuss the rationale for and the construction of animal models of developmental neurotoxicity. We will then summarize the human and animal literature on the developmental neurotoxic effects of psychostimulants (cocaine and amphetamine), opiates, cannabinoids, sedative-hypnotic and anxiolytic drugs, hallucinogens and inhalants.

ANIMAL MODELS OF DEVELOPMENTAL NEUROTOXICITY

Rationale for animal models

Human clinical researchers have been studying the neurotoxic effects of prenatal exposure to drugs of abuse for decades. Yet, as we shall see below, the literature that has emerged from this work contains many inconsistencies. It is not difficult to discern why different studies on, for example, the effects of prenatal cocaine exposure on later cognitive development could yield disparate results. Several types of factors can either complicate the interpretation of human fetal exposure studies or act as outright experimental confounds that must be controlled, if possible. The first set of factors is related to the mother's drug-taking habits. Like any group of drug users, pregnant women differ from one another in the amounts of drug they consume and their patterns of consumption, and they may also change their drug-using behavior over the course of pregnancy. In addition, different batches of drug vary in their potency (i.e., percentage of active compound) and purity (i.e., the drug formulation may contain more than one active substance or may

Reproductive and Developmental Toxicology, Edited by Ramesh C. Gupta
ISBN: 978-0-12-382032-7

even be represented by the purveyor as something different than its actual composition). Two other major problems within this category concern polysubstance use and accuracy of estimating drug use during pregnancy.

Pregnant drug-using women frequently consume multiple drugs (Kuczkowski, 2007), some of which are illicit (e.g., cocaine or heroin) and others of which are legal (e.g., alcohol and tobacco). This is a significant potential confounding factor in trying to attribute adverse developmental outcomes to a particular substance that the researchers may be investigating (see later discussion of early studies on so-called "crack babies"). Finally, retrospective studies that recruit women late in their pregnancy or during the postpartum period suffer the problem of inaccuracy of the subjects' recollection of the amounts and patterns of drug use during the 9-month gestational period (known as recall bias). This problem can be significantly reduced by conducting retrospective studies in which women are periodically interviewed over the course of their pregnancy (Richardson and Day, 1991).

The second set of confounding factors is related to other characteristics of the subject population. Even if the drug-using and control groups are as closely matched as possible in age, parity and education (which may be difficult to begin with), there may still be significant differences in amount and quality of prenatal care as well as nutrition. Lack of adequate prenatal care, poor nutrition, as well as use of legal substances such as alcohol and tobacco, can all contribute to being born prematurely and/or being small for one's gestational age. Preterm birth and low birth weight are significant risk factors for poor neurodevelopmental outcomes (Allen, 2008; Yanney and Marlow, 2004), which can complicate the investigator's ability to ascribe such outcomes to the specific molecular actions of an abused drug such as cocaine or heroin on the fetal brain.

Finally, long-term studies of prenatal drug exposure are critical for ascertaining whether offspring are subject to continuing adverse effects as they proceed through infancy, childhood, adolescence and into adulthood. For example, there is growing evidence that use of illicit drugs such as cocaine by pregnant women can affect their offspring not only directly via intrauterine exposure but also by the deleterious effects of the substance on maternal care postpartum (Strathearn and Mayes, 2010). The direct influence of prenatal drug exposure on offspring development can also be confounded by the negative impact of growing up in an impoverished or unstable home environment. Adoption studies or related approaches (e.g., studying subjects raised in a more stable home environment by other family members such as grandparents) may help ameliorate this particular problem to some extent, but such approaches raise new problems that must be dealt with. Even in the types of animal model studies discussed in the next section, procedures such as fostering of prenatal drug-exposed offspring to unexposed mothers play a critical role in experimentally separating the direct influence of the drug on offspring development from potential secondary effects mediated by drug-induced alterations in maternal behavior (i.e., the postnatal environment) (Alleva and Sorace, 2000).

Sophisticated techniques such as stepwise regression analysis have been used in many clinical studies to identify, measure and account for many of the confounding variables mentioned above. However, not all confounds can be handled this way. Moreover, the ability to study the cellular and molecular effects of prenatal drug exposure in humans is limited to what can be obtained through brain imaging methods in living subjects or postmortem analysis of brain tissues from drug-using compared to "control" subjects. Such considerations form the rationale for developing and studying animal models of prenatal drug neurotoxicity. The classic models for such work have relied primarily on rodents (laboratory rats and mice) and on non-human primates (primarily macaque monkeys), the latter being valuable for their more complex brain structure and greater cognitive abilities than rodents. The present chapter will focus on human clinical studies as well as results from these common model organisms. There is also a developmental neurotoxicity literature using birds (drug exposure *in ovo*) and, more recently, zebrafish. However, space limitations preclude a discussion of avian models and the use of zebrafish in developmental neurotoxicity testing is discussed in Chapter 15 of this volume.

Considerations in formulating and evaluating an animal model

Investigators are faced with a number of decisions when formulating or evaluating an animal model of developmental neurotoxicity of an abused drug. These decisions fall into three main categories, each of which will be taken up in turn: (1) species considerations, (2) parameters of drug dosing, and (3) outcome measures to study.

Species considerations

Laboratory rats (*Rattus norvegicus*) and mice (*Mus musculus*) are the most commonly used animals in developmental neurotoxicity studies involving drugs of abuse. Both species are relatively inexpensive, breed readily in the laboratory and have a short gestation period and rapid postnatal development. Investigators using rats or mice can avail themselves of an enormous existing literature on fetal development, neuroanatomy, neurochemistry, molecular genetics and behavioral characteristics of both. Genetic engineering of mice affords an additional powerful tool to examine mechanisms of developmental neurotoxicity, although this approach has not yet been fully exploited by the field. Despite all of the important advantages of using a rodent as opposed to a primate animal model, there are also a few disadvantages that should be kept in mind. First, as mentioned earlier rodents are not as suitable as primates for testing higher cognitive functions. As Merle Paule and his colleagues have elegantly demonstrated, it is possible to design cognitive test batteries that directly probe the same functions in monkeys as in children (Paule *et al.*, 1990), and such test batteries have been used to investigate the effects of prenatal exposure to drugs of abuse as well as other potential toxicants on cognitive function (Morris *et al.*, 1996). Second, because development is so much more rapid in rodents than in humans, it is necessary to adopt an appropriate translational approach in selecting the period of drug administration for modeling human gestational exposure. Early methods for equating brain maturation in rodents (mainly rats) to that of humans relied primarily on neuroanatomical comparisons at specific points in fetal or postnatal development (Clancy *et al.*, 2001, 2007a). However, Clancy and colleagues (2007b) have now developed a web-based neuroinformatics approach to the extrapolation of brain development across 10 different species: hamsters, mice, rats, rabbits, spiny mice, guinea pigs, ferrets, cats, rhesus monkeys and humans (Clancy *et al.*, 2007b). The computational algorithms use days post-conception as the time measure, and separate extrapolations are provided for cortical development, limbic system development and development of non-cortical/non-limbic brain areas. For example, 20 days post-conception in mice (equivalent to roughly 1 day postnatal in this species) translates to approximately 124 days, 90 days and 97 days post-conception for the development of cortical, limbic and non-cortical/non-limbic brain areas respectively in humans. Consequently, administering a drug of abuse to newborn mice can be expected to influence neurodevelopmental events that are occurring during the second trimester of human pregnancy.

Dosing considerations

The use of animal models to study the developmental neurotoxicology of an abused drug requires a consideration of the route of administration of the drug, dose level, pattern of dosing and the period of brain development being targeted. Humans consume drugs of abuse by a wide variety of routes, including oral (p.o.), intravenous (i.v.), intranasal and smoking. In contrast, rodent studies often make use of subcutaneous (s.c.) or intraperitoneal (i.p.) injections for drug delivery because of the relative ease of these methods and, in the case of i.p. administration, relatively rapid absorption. Nevertheless, as seen, for example, in the rat prenatal cocaine literature, models have been developed that make use of other routes of administration such as i.v. (Mactutus *et al.*, 1994) and p.o. (Hutchings *et al.*, 1989). Whatever route of administration is chosen, it is important to consider likely pharmacokinetic differences between the model species (e.g., rats or mice) and humans that encompass differences in metabolic pathways and rates of metabolism. Rodents are often administered higher doses than are consumed by human users because of their greater rates of drug clearance. Investigators may translate doses from humans to animals by a method called interspecies dose scaling (Mahmood, 2005); however, this approach affords only an approximation, and it may not even be appropriate for substances that undergo very different pathways of metabolism in the animal species compared to humans. With respect to dosing pattern, one must decide whether to administer the drug once (or multiple times) daily or intermittently. Regardless of the dosing pattern selected for one's model, at best it will only simulate the consumption pattern of some drug users, not all. Finally, the period of dosing in the model species should be selected so as to coincide with the targeted period of human exposure (as discussed above with respect to cross-species translation). At the same time, it is worth noting that women rarely begin to abuse drugs after they have become pregnant. Yet almost all studies in this field that involve dosing of pregnant animals do not begin such dosing until some time after the animals have mated and pregnancy is under way. This is a frequently unappreciated problem in relating the results of such exposure models to the human clinical situation.

Outcome measures

The final set of considerations in formulating or evaluating an animal model of developmental drug exposure concerns the period(s) of postnatal development to be assessed and the selection of appropriate functional outcome measures. Effects on early postnatal development may be of interest, in which case investigators can look for potential drug-related changes in developmental milestones such as righting reflex, negative geotaxis, rooting reflex, cliff avoidance or startle responses (Alleva and Sorace, 2000; Heyser, 2003; Hill *et al.*, 2007). Several test batteries have been established for rats that screen not only for changes in these developmental milestones but also for later behavioral performance during adolescence and adulthood (Meyer, 1998).

Functional outcome measures suitable for adult animals include tests of anxiety-like behavior, depressive-like behavior and performance on cognitive tasks that assess learning, memory or attention. Anxiety-like behaviors in rodents are commonly assessed using simple tests such as the elevated plus maze, elevated zero maze, emergence test (or a variation called the light–dark test used for mice) and social interaction test (appropriate for rats only) (Bourin *et al.*, 2007; Cryan and Holmes, 2005; Hart *et al.*, 2010; Rodgers, 1997). Tests of depressive-like behaviors include the forced swim test, tail suspension test (mice only) and tests of anhedonia (reduced voluntary consumption of sweet solutions) (Cryan and Holmes, 2005; Cryan, Mombereau *et al.*, 2005; Cryan, Valentino *et al.*, 2005). Despite the widespread use of such tests of anxiety-like and depressive-like behaviors, investigators should be aware of pitfalls that may be associated with interpretation of the results (Bouwknecht and Paylor, 2008; Cryan and Slattery, 2007; Ramos, 2008). Finally, many tests of cognitive function are sensitive to the developmental effects of abused drugs. Such tests include the radial arm maze and Morris water maze to assess spatial navigation learning (Paul *et al.*, 2009) and the 5-choice serial reaction time task to investigate drug-induced alterations in attention and impulsivity (Schwarting, 2009).

Model evaluation

A few basic conclusions can be drawn from the preceding discussion regarding both the rationale for animal models of developmental neurotoxicity and the challenges associated with formulating such models. (1) No animal model of developmental neurotoxicity is perfect. There will always be variation between the parameters of human drug use/abuse and at least some of the parameters of one's animal model. This is especially clear when we are reminded of the variability of drug consumption patterns among the users themselves. (2) Multiple models are needed, encompassing more than one species (e.g., rats, mice and rhesus monkeys), more than one route of administration (particularly if humans take the substance in question by multiple routes), and a range of dosing amounts (modeling low to moderate to heavy drug use) and patterns (e.g., daily or intermittent treatment depending on the substance and the use pattern being modeled). (3) Finally, investigators should be clear about what kind of clinical situation (with respect to drug dosing and use patterns) they are modeling, as well as the strengths and limitations of their chosen model with respect to that situation.

PSYCHOSTIMULANTS

Psychostimulants are compounds that strongly increase psychomotor activity and, in humans, are mood-elevating. Drugs within this category include cocaine, amphetamine and its analogs methamphetamine and 3,4-methylenedioxymethamphetamine (MDMA, or ecstasy), and methylphenidate. Psychostimulants generally have a high potential for abuse and dependence, thereby leading to substantial use by pregnant women. Here we will discuss the neurobehavioral toxicity produced by developmental exposure to cocaine and members of the amphetamine family.

Cocaine

Introduction, pharmacodynamics and pharmacokinetics

Cocaine is an alkaloid found in the leaves of the coca shrub *Erythroxylon coca*, a plant native to South America. Cocaine can be obtained as a free base or as the hydrochloride salt. Cocaine base is smokable, either by a method called freebasing or in the form of crack cocaine, whereas cocaine hydrochloride is water-soluble and is typically ingested by snorting (nasal insufflation) or by intravenous (i.v.) injection. As with drugs of abuse generally, rates of cocaine absorption vary according to the route of administration, with i.v. and smoking yielding rapid absorption and the attaining of peak blood levels, whereas snorting produces somewhat slower absorption. Cocaine elimination is slower in humans than in rodents (half-life values on the order of 90 minutes compared to 15–60 minutes respectively depending on the route of administration; Shuster, 1992). The major molecular targets for cocaine are the plasma membrane transporters for the monoamine neurotransmitters dopamine (DA), serotonin (5-HT) and norepinephrine (NE). Cocaine binds to these transport proteins, thereby inhibiting reuptake and increasing extracellular levels of each transmitter (Ritz *et al.*, 1990).

Developmental neurotoxicology

Scientific studies regarding the developmental neurotoxicity of cocaine date back to 1980, when Shah and colleagues reported that significant amounts of cocaine reach the placenta and fetus following administration to pregnant mice. Around the same time, other studies were beginning to emerge demonstrating that very high doses of cocaine (50–175 mg/kg) given to rodents during the second trimester of pregnancy could result in reduced maternal weight gain, reduced fetal weight, increased rates of fetal resorption and at the highest doses, teratogenic effects (Lee and Chiang, 1985). This work coincided roughly with the widespread introduction of crack cocaine into urban areas around the USA, a consequent upsurge in cocaine addiction, and the first reports in the mid-1980s of pregnancy outcome and offspring development in cocaine-using women. These initial studies found numerous adverse consequences of maternal cocaine use including increased rates of spontaneous abortions, placental abruptions and stillbirths, intrauterine growth retardation and abnormal responses on parts of the Brazelton Neonatal Behavioral Assessment Scale, a standard test of neurobehavioral functioning in neonates (references not cited due to space limitations). Such findings led to dire predictions of a generation of "crack babies" who would flood urban school systems and require millions of dollars of special educational services. However, the initial studies failed to control adequately for various confounding factors such as polysubstance use (particularly alcohol and tobacco) and poor prenatal care within the cocaine-using group. A later review by Frank and colleagues (2001) that controlled for confounding variables found no consistent adverse effects of prenatal cocaine on offspring growth or cognitive development (including language skills) over the first several years of life. On the other hand, Frank *et al.* did find evidence for early (but not later) motor deficits as well as deficits in attention and affect in prenatal cocaine-exposed children.

Other studies have examined the influence of prenatal cocaine in preschool and school-aged children. The most consistent findings from this work are that school-aged offspring of women who had used cocaine during pregnancy exhibit significant deficits on sustained attention tasks and on measures of behavioral self-regulation compared to control offspring (Ackerman *et al.*, 2010; Lester and Lagasse, 2010). Less consistent effects were found with respect to intelligence (IQ and other indices of intellectual ability), language development and school performance. Interestingly, impairments in attentional processing have also been reported for animals exposed to cocaine *in utero* compared to control animals (Gendle *et al.*, 2003; Harvey, 2004). Indeed, based in part on these animal studies, Mayes (2002) has postulated that cocaine exposure during fetal development leads to an abnormal balance between the central dopaminergic and noradrenergic systems, thereby disrupting the normal regulation of arousal and attentional processes by these neurotransmitters.

Structural and functional magnetic resonance imaging (MRI) studies have found various abnormalities in the brains of some infants and children born to cocaine using women, although possible relationships between these abnormalities and behavioral deficits have only been explored in a few cases (Derauf *et al.*, 2009). In addition, animal studies have provided information on neurochemical and cellular changes associated with prenatal cocaine exposure. In a well-characterized rabbit model, prenatal cocaine led to a long-lasting uncoupling of the DA D1 receptor from its signaling pathway in the striatum, frontal cortex and cingulate cortex, dendritic abnormalities in cortical layers III and V pyramidal neurons, and as mentioned above deficits in attentional processing (Harvey, 2004). Similarly, cocaine administration to pregnant rats, mice or non-human primates has been reported to produce a variety of abnormalities in DA neurochemistry, neocortical development and behavior in the offspring (Bhide, 2009; Lidow, 2003). Together, these findings from animal models of *in utero* cocaine exposure complement the human clinical studies and provide insights into neurochemical and cellular changes that may mediate the behavioral abnormalities observed in the offspring of cocaine-using women.

Mechanisms of toxicity

There is clear evidence that the feto-placental unit is sensitive to cocaine (Benveniste *et al.*, 2010), thereby suggesting a potential vulnerability of the fetus to neurodevelopmental perturbations that could adversely affect later behavioral functioning. Such perturbations might occur through a number of possible mechanisms, four of which are mentioned here. First, the monoamine transporters that are blocked by cocaine are expressed in the fetal brain and are capable of binding cocaine and related compounds (Meyer *et al.*, 1993; Shearman *et al.*, 1996). Consequently, cocaine exposure *in utero* could produce long-lasting abnormalities in neural and behavioral functioning by altering neurotransmitter activity during a sensitive developmental period. Second, cocaine is a sympathomimetic compound with the expected vasoconstrictor effects. Thus, some investigators have postulated that maternal cocaine use could produce fetal toxicity due to uteroplacental vasoconstriction leading to fetal hypoxia (Woods, 1998). Third, Lester and Padbury (2009) have proposed that prenatal cocaine exposure could exert long-term effects on neurobehavioral development through fetal programming (i.e., epigenetic modification) of critical genes in stress response systems. Finally, Lee and coworkers (2008) reported evidence that cell proliferation in the fetal brain can be inhibited through a process of oxidative metabolism of cocaine and consequent endoplasmic reticulum (ER) stress in the cells. Few, if any, data are currently available enabling researchers to link any of these mechanisms to specific functional deficits in prenatal cocaine-exposed offspring. However, all four mechanisms are plausible, and it is possible that taken as a whole, the deficits described above stem from complex interactions between altered fetal brain chemistry, uteroplacental vasoconstriction, fetal programming and ER stress.

Amphetamines

Introduction, pharmacodynamics and pharmacokinetics

Amphetamine was first discovered by the Romanian chemist Lazar Edeleanu at the end of the 19th century. This compound was originally used clinically for a variety of purposes including improving breathing, preventing day time sleepiness and weight regulation. More recently, amphetamine is prescribed largely for the treatment of attention deficit hyperactivity disorder (ADHD) with some amount of off-label use in depression and to improve cognition following a stroke. Amphetamine, like cocaine, is a psychomotor stimulant that increases alertness and arousal.

Methamphetamine was first synthesized by Nagayoshi Nagai in 1893. Although therapeutic use of methamphetamine is uncommon due to its abuse potential, this compound is approved for use in ADHD and for the short-term treatment of obesity. Efforts to reduce methamphetamine production by restricting availability of the precursor chemicals ephedrine and pseudoephedrine have led to an unforeseen change in manufacturing facilities from smaller "mom and pop" operations to much larger "super-labs". Methamphetamine is more potent than amphetamine and produces euphoria, increased activity, sexual arousal and occasional paranoia. High or repeated doses can result in stereotyped behavior that may advance to self-injurious behavior.

Methylenedioxymethamphetamine (MDMA, also known as "ecstasy" or "X"), like other members of the amphetamine family, has a relatively brief history. A patent for MDMA was issued to the German pharmaceutical company Merck in 1914, but MDMA did not emerge as a recreational drug until the 1970s. Currently, MDMA is not approved for clinical use although trials are ongoing to determine if MDMA can be used with psychotherapy to reduce anxiety. The subjective effects of MDMA partially overlap with amphetamine to include increased energy but also include a sensation of closeness to others and heightened sensitivity to tactile and auditory stimuli. There is some justification that MDMA does not belong in the stimulant or hallucinogen drug classes. Instead, MDMA may be more appropriately categorized as an entactogen which means "touching within" due to these distinct acute emotional and social effects.

Repeated use of amphetamines rapidly leads to tolerance. Methamphetamine is often used recreationally in "binges" that may last from a few days to a couple of weeks with total daily doses of several grams. In comparison, the recommended starting dose of amphetamine for adults with ADHD is 5 mg with a maximum of 60 mg/day. Methamphetamine is used recreationally in several forms including a powder by nasal insufflation ("snorting") or by mixing with water and i.v. injection. The pure crystalline form of methamphetamine, known as "ice" or "crystal", first emerged in Hawaii in the 1980s and is smoked. "Yaba" is produced in Thailand and has a methamphetamine content of 30–40 mg per pill. Amphetamine is the primary metabolite of methamphetamine and is metabolized in a species-specific fashion with hydroxylation to form 4-hydroxyamphetamine in rats or deamination to form benzoic acid in humans. Ecstasy is predominantly taken orally in capsules that contain 50–200 mg of MDMA. Chemical analysis of pills purported to contain substituted amphetamines reveals quite variable results, particularly for methamphetamine. However, amphetamine is diverted from clinical use and is therefore more commonly available in a pure form. For example, Adderall® contains amphetamine salts *d*- and *l*-amphetamine in a 3:1 ratio and the pills may be crushed and snorted. Although many amphetamine formulations are currently available which attempt to minimize abuse potential, committed substance abusers are quite creative in developing strategies to bypass these.

The distribution and elimination of methamphetamine during pregnancy has been best studied using a sheep model. Intravenous methamphetamine administration to the near-term ewe results in substantial methamphetamine concentrations in the fetus within minutes. Methamphetamine readily accumulates in several tissues including the placenta and fetal lungs, liver, brain and heart. While the maximum methamphetamine plasma concentration is much higher in the ewe than the fetus, the fetus has a longer half-life. MDMA is an extensively metabolized drug with over a dozen metabolites. These breakdown products of MDMA vary considerably between mice, rats and humans.

Amphetamines have a chemical structure similar to DA. After readily crossing the blood–brain barrier, amphetamines act on the monoamine neurotransmitter systems. Like cocaine, amphetamines bind to the plasma membrane transporters for DA, NE and 5-HT, thereby blocking reuptake. Unlike cocaine, however, amphetamines also act as substrates for the transporters, causing transporter reversal and transmitter release from the nerve terminals (Kuczenski and Segal, 1994). Amphetamine and methamphetamine have more potent effects on the DA and NE systems than on 5-HT, whereas the opposite is true for MDMA. The ability of MDMA to induce a subjective state of empathy, a subjective state that is very unlike the profile seen with amphetamine or methamphetamine, may be due to elevations in the peptide oxytocin or the hormone prolactin.

Developmental neurotoxicology

Amphetamines exert direct and indirect effects on the developing offspring. These substances decrease maternal food intake and restrict blood flow to the fetus. Therefore, it may not be surprising that the most consistently identified consequence of prenatal amphetamine or methamphetamine exposure in human or non-human animals is a reduction in body weight and head circumference as well as prematurity (Plessinger, 1998). Further, methamphetamine or MDMA administration to rats causes impairments in spatial memory that are transient when the exposure occurs in adulthood but are extremely long-lasting or even permanent following perinatal exposure (Vorhees *et al.*, 2007). Embryonic exposure to amphetamine or methamphetamine may also disrupt development of the eyes and heart (National Toxicology Program, 2005).

The Infant Development Education and Lifestyle (IDEAL) study is a longitudinal effort that has been following a large cohort of methamphetamine-exposed children from birth. Because the unexposed comparison group is so profoundly different on so many variables (higher socioeconomic status and much lower prenatal alcohol, tobacco and marijuana use), the most conservative interpretation of these findings is that polysubstance/methamphetamine use during pregnancy may be associated with modest indications of neurobehavioral abnormalities during infancy (Smith *et al.*, 2008). However, future reports from this research group may reveal more clear-cut group differences when the exposed children need to respond to the demands of the school environment.

One key finding from the IDEAL study concerns the temporal pattern of *in utero* methamphetamine exposure. Interviews with the women revealed that the majority of users reported stopping smoking methamphetamine by the third trimester of pregnancy. Chemical analysis of the baby's first stool (meconium) determined that most did not contain detectable quantities of methamphetamine or amphetamine (Smith *et al.*, 2008). This result could either be interpreted as evidence that meconium is an insensitive biological matrix to detect maternal methamphetamine drug use or the analytical chemistry corroborated the maternal self-report of substantial reductions in use as the pregnancy progresses. As many recreational drugs including amphetamines are incorporated into the hair (Lee *et al.*, 2009), hair samples, unlike meconium, can be used to quantify maternal substance use patterns over the entire pregnancy. Hair analyses will likely continue to become a more standard feature of human teratology investigations, especially for investigations of controlled substances.

Mechanisms of toxicity

High doses of methamphetamine produce long-term reductions in brain DA and 5-HT levels in adult animals, whereas the embryo is largely resistant to these effects. Similarly, MDMA administration during pregnancy causes reductions in 5-HT and other serotonergic markers in pregnant rats but the offspring are much less likely to exhibit this response (Piper, 2007). The loss of neurotransmitter and other axonal markers (e.g., transporter binding) following treatment with methamphetamine or MDMA is usually interpreted as drug-induced axonal degeneration, although this interpretation has recently been challenged (Biezonski *et al.*, 2010).

The cytochrome P450 family of liver enzymes (especially CYP2D6) is important in the metabolism of amphetamine, methamphetamine and MDMA. These enzymes are expressed at low levels during the first trimester in humans and only gradually become functional postnatally. This immaturity of liver enzymes may be responsible for the paradoxical protection against monoamine neurotoxicity seen during early development because these enzymes are thought by some investigators to be necessary for the production of toxic metabolites (Pizarro *et al.*, 2008). The mechanisms responsible for the aforementioned deficits in spatial memory following exposure to methamphetamine or MDMA during the rodent equivalent of the human third trimester are not known; however, the factors described above for cocaine (alterations in fetal neurochemistry, vasoconstriction of the uteroplacental unit, fetal programming and oxidative stress) are plausible candidates.

Opiates

Introduction, pharmacodynamics and pharmacokinetics

Opiate drugs include naturally occurring alkaloids obtained from the opium poppy (e.g., morphine and codeine) as well as synthetic derivatives such as heroin (diacetylmorphine), hydrocodone and oxycodone. Depending on their physical form, opiate drugs are usually taken by i.v. injection, smoking, snorting or oral administration. These compounds are agonists at opioid receptors, of which the mu receptor plays a particularly important role in opiate reward and addiction (Waldhoer *et al.*, 2004). Opiate pharmacokinetics varies across different compounds and routes of administration, but as an example, morphine reaches peak plasma levels within 30–90 minutes after oral administration and exhibits an elimination half-life of 2–3 hours (Glare and Walsh, 1991). In contrast, the elimination half-life of heroin is approximately 5 minutes when taken by i.v. injection or smoking, which accounts for heroin addicts' need to obtain repeated daily "fixes" of this drug in order to avoid withdrawal. One of the major approaches to the treatment of opiate addicts involves replacement therapy either with the full mu receptor agonist methadone or with the partial agonist buprenorphine. Methadone is currently approved for use in pregnant women, although the safety and efficacy of buprenorphine has also been tested in several clinical studies (Jones *et al.*, 2008). This section of the chapter will describe developmental neurotoxicology studies on morphine, heroin and the opiate replacement drug methadone, as these are the opioids most extensively investigated for their neurodevelopmental effects.

Developmental neurotoxicology

Some of the developmental effects of prenatal opiate exposure are evident at birth. For example, studies of neonates born to women in methadone maintenance programs generally indicate significant intrauterine growth retardation (IUGR) in the drug-exposed group compared to control infants (Hunt *et al.*, 2008; Vance *et al.*, 1997). Babies who are born small for their gestational age are at increased risk for delays in neurological and behavioral development. However, the interpretation of previous findings comparing methadone-exposed with unexposed infants was recently challenged by Liu and coworkers (2010), who reported evidence suggesting that low maternal body mass index is a greater risk factor for IUGR than methadone use by the mother. Moreover, results from the Maternal Lifestyle Study (a large multi-site study of prenatal cocaine- and opiate-exposed offspring) indicate that infants born of opiate-using/-abusing women who were not in a methadone treatment group did not show signs of IUGR (Messinger *et al.*, 2004). It is possible that the intermittent use characteristic of street opiate users has less impact on fetal growth than daily exposure to methadone. Nevertheless, pregnant opiate addicts are still urged to enter a methadone maintenance program due to the other risks to themselves and their unborn child by continuing an uncontrolled opiate-using lifestyle.

Another adverse outcome of repeated opiate exposure *in utero* is the development of physical dependence by the fetus. Thus, offspring of regular opiate users are often born in a state of dependence, regardless of whether the mother is taking a street drug such as heroin, abusing prescription drugs such as morphine or undergoing opioid replacement therapy with methadone or buprenorphine. Consequently, such infants undergo withdrawal after they are born and are no longer receiving transplacental drug exposure. Dependent newborns exhibit a variety of behavioral and autonomic symptoms that together constitute the Neonatal Abstinence Syndrome. Symptoms may include excessive crying, irritability, disrupted sleep patterns, hypertonicity (increased muscle tone), poor feeding, gastrointestinal distress (vomiting or loose stools), tremors and even seizures (Jansson *et al.*, 2009). Severity of this syndrome can be assessed using several scoring systems such as the Finnegan Neonatal Abstinence Scoring System, the Lipsitz Neonatal Drug-Withdrawal Scoring System, the Neonatal Withdrawal Inventory and the Neonatal Narcotic Withdrawal Index. Infants that exhibit high withdrawal scores should be treated in the hospital with appropriate doses of morphine or another opiate drug until they stabilize and their symptoms remit. Anticonvulsant drugs such as barbiturates or benzodiazepines may also be administered if needed. Once the infant has stabilized, medication is gradually tapered until s/he can safely be released from the hospital without the need for further treatment.

Research on the longer-term effects of prenatal opiate exposure on neurobehavioral development has yielded mixed results. Some but not all studies found deficits in psychomotor development in infants exposed to opiates (either methadone or heroin) prenatally compared to unexposed controls (Hunt *et al.*, 2007; Kaltenbach, 1996). Furthermore, even when deficits were observed, they could sometimes be accounted for by statistically controlling for confounding variables (Messinger *et al.*, 2004). Preschool or school-age children who had *in utero* opiate exposure have sometimes been found to suffer deficits in various measures of cognitive functioning (Lester and Lagasse, 2010). However, in most cases there were inadequate controls for confounding variables that likely contributed significantly to the apparent drug effects.

Effects of prenatal opiates on brain structure and function have been assessed by means of neuroimaging in humans and neurochemical measurements in laboratory animals. A structural MRI study by Walhovd and coworkers (2007) on 9- to 14-year-old children reported significant reductions in total brain volume, cortical volume and the volume of several subcortical structures in the opiate-exposed compared to the control group. A second study by the same research group on the same cohort of children found additional group differences in cerebral white matter using diffusion tensor imaging (Walhovd *et al.*, 2010). A number of rodent studies have examined neurochemical and behavioral changes following prenatal exposure to either morphine or heroin. Vathy (2001, 2002) has reviewed evidence that prenatal morphine exerts complex effects on subsequent functioning of the opioidergic, noradrenergic, GABAergic and glutamatergic systems, with functional consequences for the regulation of brain excitability (i.e., seizure susceptibility), sexual behavior and drug reward in rats. Other investigators have shown that prenatal exposure to heroin or morphine in rats or mice gives rise to later deficits in hippocampal-dependent spatial learning and memory. Such effects have been attributed in various studies to abnormal activity of the septo-hippocampal cholinergic system (Yanai *et al.*, 2003), impaired synaptic plasticity in the hippocampal formation (e.g., Niu *et al.*, 2009) or increased apoptotic cell death within the hippocampus (Wang and Han, 2009). Taken together, these preclinical findings indicate that opiates can exert significant neurobehavioral teratogenicity and call for more research on the offspring of opiate-dependent women (Walhovd *et al.*, 2009).

Mechanisms of toxicity

The mechanisms underlying opiate developmental neurotoxicity are poorly understood. Endogenous opioid peptides (endorphins and enkephalins) as well as opioid receptors are known to be expressed during fetal development, thereby providing a substrate for direct actions of maternally ingested opiates on the fetal brain (Sargeant *et al.*, 2008b). One area of research has focused on the developmental effects of exogenous as well as endogenous opioids on cell proliferation and morphogenesis of the brain. Thus, early studies found reduced cell number, packing density and thickness of the primary somatosensory cortex of rats exposed to morphine prenatally (Hammer and Hauser, 1992). These results may be related to the more recent finding of mu opioid receptor expression by neuronal and glial progenitor cells in the developing mouse cortex, and the observation that morphine exposure on embryonic day 15.5 slowed the progression from G_2 to the M phase of the cell cycle in the dorsal telecephalon (Sargeant *et al.*, 2008a). Based on other studies, Yanai and colleagues (2003) have proposed that the influence of prenatal opiate exposure on the septo-hippocampal cholinergic system and on hippocampal-dependent behaviors is mediated by altered opioidergic innervation of the cholinergic system. The relevance of these preclinical findings to humans exposed to opiate drugs *in utero* remains to be determined. Nevertheless, it seems clear that opiates can have an adverse impact on early brain development, and therefore opiate use during pregnancy poses a risk to the later neurobehavioral functioning of the offspring.

Cannabinoids

Introduction, pharmacodynamics and pharmacokinetics

Cannabis sativa (marijuana, weed, ganja) is the illicit substance most frequently used by pregnant women (Muhuri and Gfroerer, 2009). As with other herbal drugs, there are numerous biologically active compounds contained in marijuana but delta^9-tetrahydrocannabinl (THC) is the major psychoactive compound and the one most studied. Smoking of the dried plant produces detectable THC within seconds and peak levels within 10 minutes. In contrast, peak levels are not achieved until 1 hour after oral administration (Grotenherman, 2003). In a rhesus monkey study, THC concentrations were reported to be higher by an order of magnitude in maternal relative to fetal plasma (Bailey *et al.*, 1987). Further, a major metabolite (11-nor-9-carboxy-THC) in adults was undetectable in the fetus, which indicates that either this metabolite does not cross the placenta or that the fetus lacks the liver enzymes necessary for production. Importantly, following maternal administration during lactation, the vast majority of THC is eliminated in the feces and urine but detectable quantities are also present in breast milk (Jakubovic *et al.*, 1974).

Administration of THC to experimental animals results in binding to two cannabinoid receptors denoted CB_1 and CB_2. The CB_1 receptor is responsible for mediating the acute subjective effects induced by marijuana. CB_2 receptors are found in immune cells, spleen and tonsils, and they are also expressed in the nervous system in glial cells (Fernandez-Ruiz *et al.*, 2007). CB_1 receptor distribution differs substantially by age in both humans and experimental animals. In adulthood these receptors are abundant in neurons of the hippocampus, amygdala, cerebellum and striatum, while virtually absent in while matter. In contrast, the late fetal rat brain showed low levels of CB_1 receptor binding in standard locations but substantial amounts in white matter tracts such as the corpus callosum and anterior commissure (Romero *et al.*, 1997). These findings suggest that the central endogenous cannabinoid system may have a different function during development than in adulthood.

Developmental neurotoxicology

There is currently substantial discord between human and animal (primarily rodent) studies regarding the consequences of *in utero* cannabinoid exposure. The general pattern that emerges from a well-designed longitudinal investigation of prenatal marijuana exposure, the Ottawa Prenatal Prospective Study (OPPS), is of exceedingly subtle group differences. For example, during pre-adolescence, the high marijuana exposure group (≥16 joints per week throughout pregnancy) had a mean score on the perceptual organization index of the Weschsler Intelligence Scale for Children that was five points below their unexposed counterparts (Fried and Watkinson, 2000). This subscale measures the child's ability to interpret and organize information presented visually. Importantly, both the marijuana-exposed and unexposed groups from this middle class sample had mean scores that were above the norms for this standardized instrument. The available evidence from the OPPS is that prenatal nicotine, which was used concurrently with marijuana, presents an equivalent or greater risk to the fetus than marijuana (Fried *et al.*, 2001, 2003).

In contrast to the human reports, rodent studies have identified a wide variety of neurochemical effects of *in utero* exposure to cannabinoids. These studies, which have more typically examined the consequences of maternal administration of THC or other cannabinoid agonists rather than the entire *Cannabis sativa* plant, have identified abnormalities in the DA, 5-HT, γ-aminobutyric acid (GABA) and opioid systems (Ramos *et al.*, 2005). Suárez and colleagues (2004) also reported a long-lasting downregulation of glutamate AMPA receptor subunits in the cerebellum of rats exposed to THC both pre- and perinatally. In behavioral studies, differences between exposed and unexposed offspring have been identified with respect to motor activity, learning and memory, and, most consistently, in the response to morphine challenge (Schneider, 2009). The latter finding suggests that maternal cannabinoid use could increase the likelihood of later drug abuse by the offspring.

Mechanisms of toxicity

CB_1 receptors are expressed early in the second trimester in the human brain and have also been found in the placenta at term (Park *et al.*, 2003; Ramos *et al.*, 2005). Two endogenous ligands for this receptor, anandamide and 2-arachdonoylglycerol (2-AG), modulate a variety of key neurodevelopmental processes including cell proliferation and migration, axon guidance, synaptogenesis and myelinogenesis (Ramos *et al.*, 2005; Trezza *et al.*, 2008). Binding of THC to CB_1 receptors could interfere with these processes, thereby altering the maturation of the neurotransmitter systems mentioned earlier.

Nevertheless, a fundamental issue that remains is the substantial discrepancy between investigations showing modest effects following regular marijuana use in humans and pronounced effects in rodents with THC. One possible reason for this discrepancy is the use of relatively high doses in the animal studies that led to reduced maternal weight gain during pregnancy. Consequently, at least in those studies that did not use pair-feeding to control this confound, group differences in offspring neurochemistry may be a by-product of maternal undernutrition. Alternatively, it is possible that one or more of the 70+ cannabinoids naturally occurring in the cannabis plant (for example, cannabidiol) counteract the adverse effects of marijuana-derived THC in humans due to their neuroprotective actions (Schneider, 2009).

Sedative-hypnotic and anxiolytic drugs

Introduction, pharmacodynamics and pharmacokinetics

Sedative-hypnotic and anxiolytic drugs exert a widespread depressant effect on CNS activity. These compounds are used clinically for their sedating, sleep-inducing, anxiolytic, anticonvulsant and muscle relaxant actions. They also have significant abuse potential, which accounts for their inclusion in the present chapter. The two major classes of sedative-hypnotic and anxiolytic drugs that are discussed below are the barbiturates and benzodiazepines (BDZs). Both classes of compounds act primarily on nerve cell membrane ion channels, particularly by enhancing the activity of the inhibitory neurotransmitter GABA at the $GABA_A$ receptor (Coupey, 1997; Smith, 2001). Barbiturates also inhibit the excitatory glutamate AMPA receptor subtype. Most BDZs are long-acting due to a combination of slow clearance and the formation of bioactive metabolites. In contrast, barbiturates vary substantially in their duration of action due largely to differences in lipid solubility. Consequently, it is worth noting that relatively short-acting compounds such as pentobarbital and secobarbital are preferred by barbiturate abusers, whereas virtually all of the human literature on prenatal barbiturate effects has focused on the longer-acting phenobarbital due to its clinical use in the treatment of epilepsy.

Developmental neurotoxicology

A few studies have reported small increases in the risk for birth defects in infants prenatally exposed to phenobarbital or BDZs; however, the evidence is not conclusive at this time (Dean *et al.*, 2002; Einarson, 2009; Iqbal *et al.*, 2002; Perucca, 2005). Of greater concern is the potential for physical dependence in offspring exposed repeatedly to barbiturates or

BDZs *in utero*. The symptoms of withdrawal from these compounds are somewhat similar to those seen in the opiate neonatal abstinence syndrome, although the appearance of symptoms may be delayed due to the longer time required for drug clearance.

Remarkably little attention has been directed to examining the effects of prenatal barbiturate or BDZ exposure on later neurobehavioral functioning. This lack of research is particularly noticeable in recent years, although in the case of barbiturates we can attribute it to the replacement of phenobarbital with later generation antiepileptic medications. The few studies that have been reported suggest the possibility that phenobarbital exposure *in utero* could lead to cognitive deficits later in life (Bromley *et al.*, 2009). However, one major problem with this literature is that many of the offspring studied were exposed to additional anticonvulsant agents such as phenytoin, which makes it difficult to attribute the results specifically to phenobarbital. A few early studies on prenatal BDZ exposure also found evidence for adverse neurobehavioral effects, though again the overall findings are far from conclusive (Cohen and Rosenbaum, 1998).

As we have now seen for several other drugs of abuse, experimental animal studies have found many more significant consequences of prenatal or early postnatal exposure to sedative-hypnotic and anxiolytic drugs. One of the most troubling findings is associated with drug administration during the brain growth spurt, which is a period of intense synaptogenesis marked by rapidly increasing brain weight. The brain growth spurt occurs during the third trimester in humans and in the early postnatal period in rodents. Administration of either barbiturates or BDZs to infant rats during a sensitive period of postnatal development provokes widespread apoptotic cell death (Ikonomidou *et al.*, 2001; Olney *et al.*, 2000). Loss of neurons during the brain growth spurt could obviously have an adverse effect on later neurobehavioral functioning. Whether a similar cell loss occurs in the offspring of women taking barbiturates or BDZs during pregnancy is not known at this time, although it is worth noting that no evidence currently exists for overt brain degeneration in exposed offspring.

Other animal studies have focused on neurochemical and behavioral abnormalities following prenatal barbiturate or BDZ exposure. For example, maternal phenobarbital administration in mice produced aberrant functioning of the cholinergic system and deficits in behaviors dependent on the septo-hippocampal system, effects similar to those previously mentioned for heroin (Rogel-Fuchs *et al.*, 1992). Prenatal exposure to diazepam, a widely prescribed BDZ, led to developmental delays in rats and later alterations in sensitivity to the convulsant drug pentylenetetrazol and in behavioral responses in a social interaction test (Kellogg, 1995; Nicosia *et al.*, 2003). Interestingly, some of these effects were found to be sex specific.

Mechanisms of toxicity

The most likely mechanism underlying the developmental neurotoxicity of barbiturates and BDZs is a direct action on their principal molecular target, the $GABA_A$ receptor. Not only is this receptor expressed in the brain during development, but because of ontogenetic differences in intracellular chloride concentrations, the receptor exerts an excitatory instead of the usual inhibitory effect on neuronal firing (Ben-Ari, 2002). Moreover, GABA itself exerts regulatory effects during development. Consequently, repeated exposure of $GABA_A$ receptors to sedative-hypnotic/anxiolytic drugs could readily perturb the development of many different neural systems. The GABA system itself is likely to be particularly vulnerable to such exposure, as evidenced by the above-mentioned alterations in brain excitability and social interaction behavior, both of which involve GABAergic activity. Kellogg (1999) has discussed potential mechanisms that might underlie sex differences in the long-term effects of prenatal BDZ exposure. The mechanism of barbiturate- and BDZ-induced apoptosis is not yet fully understood, although recently documented changes in drug-induced protein expression are consistent with the involvement of several cell death pathways previously linked to other apoptotic agents (Kaindl *et al.*, 2008).

Hallucinogens

Introduction, pharmacodynamics and pharmacokinetics

The hallucinogens are a large and varied collection of many herbal and synthetic substances that can be loosely categorized based on their neurochemical targets into the following groups: a 5-HT group that includes lysergic acid diethylamide (LSD), psilocybin mushrooms and the peyote cactus; an acetylcholine group that includes plants from the nightshade family; and a glutamate group that includes the dissociative anesthetics ketamine and phencyclidine (PCP). As a result of their pronounced neurodevelopmental effects, the remainder of this section will only focus on the gluatamate receptor antagonists.

Ketamine was synthesized at the Parke-Davis pharmaceutical company by Calvin Stevens and patented by that company in 1966. This compound produces general anesthesia following i.v. doses of 2 mg/kg and is demethylated to form norketamine by CYP3A4 (Sinner and Graf, 2008). Ketamine (known on the street as "special K") is diverted from medical or veterinary use for recreational purposes where it is reported to induce subjective effects such as a dream-like state, out of body experiences, sensations of invulnerability, changes in time and sound perception, and reduced pain sensitivity. Many routes of administration are used, including oral, subcutaneous injection, snorting and smoking. Ketamine is best known as a non-competitive antagonist at glutamate N-methyl-D-aspartic acid (NMDA) receptors, although the compound is not selective and has at least moderate affinity for nicotinic and muscarinic acetylcholine receptors, as well as sigma receptors.

The trade name Serenyl (after serenity) was given to PCP after it was patented by Parke-Davis in 1953. Ironically, PCP was subsequently withdrawn as a human and animal anesthetic because of adverse effects including mania, hallucinations and, later, several highly publicized instances of aggressive behavior. Street names for PCP include "Angel Dust" or, when a nicotine or cannabis cigarette is dipped into a PCP-containing liquid, "embalming fluid" (Kuhn *et al.*, 2003). PCP, like ketamine, is an NMDA antagonist that also has affinity for sigma receptors. The endogenous chemical(s) that binds to the $sigma_1$ or $sigma_2$ receptors are currently unknown, but sigma ligands modulate the activity of the glutamate, NE and DA systems (Skuza and Wedzony, 2004). Peak rates of PCP use in the USA were documented in the late 1970s, with 7% of high-school seniors using this substance in the past year. Even if PCP and ketamine receive very little attention relative other drugs of abuse, the prevalence of their use among young adults continues to be sizeable (Johnson *et al.*, 2009).

Developmental neurotoxicology

Although there have been no long-term controlled investigations on the consequences of prenatal ketamine or PCP exposure in humans, the available evidence from rodents and non-human primates is cause for considerable concern. Administration of ketamine or PCP during the peak of the brain growth spurt causes massive apoptotic neuronal degeneration, even greater than that found with barbiturates and BDZs. This cell loss is especially pronounced in forebrain areas like the frontal cortex, hippocampus and striatum, but is also observed in the cerebellum. Olney and colleagues (2000) have estimated that even brief exposure to an NMDA antagonist causes millions of neurons to die. Moreover, a similar effect has been seen with several other recreational substances, notably alcohol and the inhalant nitrous oxide.

Functional deficits are extremely long-lasting and result from perinatal NMDA antagonist exposure. Persistent deficits in spatial working memory as well as altered NMDA receptor binding have been reported (Sircar, 2003). Abnormalities in the ability to habituate to a novel environment were identified in young adult mice months after exposure to a single relatively low (5 mg/kg) ketamine dose (Viberg *et al.*, 2008). The combination of widespread neuron loss and presumably permanent changes in brain function has prompted some investigators to propose that NMDA receptor inhibition during development is a useful model for understanding the etiology of schizophrenia (Bubeniková-Valesová *et al.*, 2008).

Mechanisms of toxicity

As ketamine is currently in clinical use for obstetrical and surgical purposes, studies of the cellular and molecular mechanisms underlying the drug's apoptotic effects have focused on modeling anesthetic, rather than recreational, exposure. However, this may not be a major concern as the doses used for both purposes are similar. Following NMDA antagonist treatment, there is a compensatory increase in NMDA receptor expression that results in overstimulation of the glutamatergic system by endogenous glutamate. Opening of NMDA receptor channels causes an excessive influx of calcium ions into the neuron, which leads to the production of damaging free radicals, especially superoxide. Finally, recent microarray analyses have determined that ketamine simultaneously downregulates several genes that inhibit apoptosis and upregulates several other pro-apoptotic genes (Shi *et al.*, 2010).

Inhalants

Introduction, pharmacodynamics and pharmacokinetics

Inhalants are an extremely diverse class of compounds that are inexpensive, readily available and legal. These factors contribute to their high prevalence of use, especially among adolescents and young adults. For example, a national survey conducted annually in the USA revealed that approximately one in six eighth-graders had used an inhalant (Johnston *et al.*, 2009). This class includes many common household products including spray paint, varnish, glues, rubber cement, hair spray, nail polish remover, room deodorizers, gasoline, propane and nitrous oxide propellant in food (e.g., whipped cream) dispensers. The remainder of this section will focus on one of the best studied inhalants, the organic solvent toluene.

There are a variety of inhalation strategies that are utilized such as "huffing" (breathing the vapors from a solvent soaked rag), "bagging" (breathing the fumes from a plastic bag), "cuffing" (soaking the cuffs or other clothing with a solvent) or "spraying" (dispensing from a spray can directly into the nose or mouth). The potential reduction in the intake of oxygen is an obvious concern during recreational inhalant use. Abuse involves repeated inhalation of high solvent concentrations (several thousand parts per million) during a short session typically lasting no more than 10 minutes. In contrast, occupational exposure to solvents involves much lower concentrations (100 parts per million) but for periods of hours (Bowen *et al.*, 2006). Hippuric acid is the predominant metabolite of toluene and can be used as an index of maternal use.

Toluene is quickly absorbed by the lungs and readily distributed across the blood–brain barrier or placenta. The distribution and elimination of toluene during gestation has been characterized in mice. Toluene is a low molecular weight substance with high fat solubility. Inhaled toluene and metabolites readily accumulate in the lipid-rich cells of the dam's nervous system, especially the olfactory bulb and cerebellum. These compounds also reach biologically relevant concentrations in the placenta and amniotic fluid. Interestingly, as the embryo has minimal fatty tissue, it has been estimated that the uptake of toluene in the fetus is less than one-twentieth that of the maternal brain (Ghantous and Dannielsson, 1986).

Animal studies have shown that toluene acts on a variety of different ionotropic neurotransmitter receptors. Specifically, this compound enhances the activity of $GABA_A$, glycine and serotonin 5-HT_3 receptors, while inhibiting the activity of NMDA and nicotinic acetylcholine receptors (Bowen *et al.*, 2006). Inhibition of voltage-activated sodium channels in the heart may be responsible for toluene-induced cardiac arrhythmias that can be a fatal consequence of recreational toluene inhalation in adults.

Developmental neurotoxicology

The sequelae of toluene exposure are clearly among the most severe and diffuse of any substance described in this chapter. Infants of mothers who use toluene are at increased risk of premature birth, low birth weight, reduced head circumference, a withdrawal syndrome characterized by excessive high pitched crying, poor feeding and sleep difficulties, and later developmental delays including language impairments and mental retardation (Hannigan and Bowen, 2010). The offspring of mothers who were regular inhalant, but not alcohol, abusers exhibit craniofacial abnormalities that are similar to those found in children with fetal alcohol syndrome. Fetal solvent syndrome includes a small separation between the upper and lower eyelids, a wide nasal bridge, an underdeveloped chin, ear anomalies and blunt fingertips (Arnold *et al.*, 1994; Pearson *et al.*, 1994). These pronounced structural abnormalities have been reproduced by prenatal toluene exposure in rats (Bowen *et al.*, 2009). Animal studies have also noted a blunted response to NMDA agonists and regionally selective alterations in NMDA receptor expression. Overall, investigations with rats and mice have determined that the dosing paradigm is a key variable, with models of recreational exposure producing more severe consequences than models of occupational exposure (Bowen *et al.*, 2006).

Mechanisms of toxicity

The precise mechanisms by which toluene produces neurodevelopmental abnormalities are not well understood. A population of progenitor cells located in the anterior neural ridge is particularly susceptible to alcohol-induced cell death, which in turn mediates subsequent developmental malformations (Sulik, 2005). Due to the substantial overlap in craniofacial teratogenesis between fetal alcohol and fetal solvent syndromes, it is tempting to hypothesize, as Pearson and colleagues (1994) have, that toluene acts similarly to alcohol. Disruption of the *sonic hedgehog* signaling pathway has been linked to the teratogenic effects of alcohol as well as several other substances (Lipinski *et al.*, 2010), thereby warranting future studies to determine whether toluene exerts embryopathic effects by a similar mechanism.

TABLE 26.1 Comparison of drugs of abuse including their typical route(s) of administration and principal mechanisms of action on the nervous system

Drug	Administration route	Mechanisms of action
Cocaine	i.v., smoking, snorting	DA, NE, and 5-HT reuptake blocker
Methamphetamine	smoking, snorting, oral	DA, NE, and 5-HT releaser
MDMA	oral	5-HT, DA, and NE releaser
Opiates	i.v., smoking	Opioid receptor agonists
Cannabinoids	smoking	Cannabinoid receptor agonists
Benzodiazepines and barbiturates	oral	$GABA_A$ receptor positive modulators
Ketamine and PCP	oral, smoking, snorting	NMDA receptor antagonists
Toluene	inhalation	$GABA_A$ receptor positive modulator, NMDA receptor antagonist

CONCLUDING REMARKS AND FUTURE DIRECTIONS

Women who have developed a substance dependence problem often find it difficult to abstain from use of these substances if they become pregnant. As described in this chapter and in Table 26.1, each class of abused drug has its own molecular target(s) and may therefore alter brain development through multiple actions on the fetal–placental unit. However, unlike fetal alcohol syndrome and perhaps also fetal solvent syndrome (described in detail elsewhere in this book), the prevalence and severity of neurobehavioral deficits (particularly long-lasting deficits) in offspring exposed to illicit drug use that can be attributed directly to such exposure remains controversial. Although clinicians may point to specific individuals who have been strongly impacted by their mother's drug use during pregnancy, it is generally much more difficult to demonstrate reliable and persistent drug effects that remain when the typical confounding variables such as quality of prenatal care, use of legal substances like alcohol and tobacco, and so forth, have been statistically eliminated. Indeed, several prominent researchers who have investigated the offspring of cocaine- and/or opiate-using women have argued that prenatal exposure to these drugs should be considered more of a marker for general environmental risk than a risk factor itself (Messinger *et al.*, 2004). Strikingly, animal studies have generally demonstrated much stronger neurochemical and behavioral effects of maternal drug administration than the corresponding human clinical studies. This discrepancy may indicate a significant limitation of the kind of cross-species comparisons inherent in animal models of prenatal drug exposure. However, another important possibility is that the dosing regimens used in typical animal studies produce fetal exposures that are significantly greater than those incurred by most infants of drug-abusing women. Consequently, such studies might yield information on "worst-case" scenarios associated with extreme maternal drug consumption but would fail to model the "typical" outcomes seen in well-controlled clinical studies. As discussed earlier in the chapter, women vary enormously in their patterns of illicit drug use, and interspecies dose scaling is an imprecise tool at best. Nevertheless, we suggest that existing discrepancies between the human and animal literature regarding the developmental neurotoxicity of abused drugs will not be resolved until animal researchers pay more attention to the clinical relevance of their dosing paradigms.

REFERENCES

Ackerman JP, Riggins T, Black MM (2010) A review of the effects of prenatal cocaine exposure among school-aged children. *Pediatrics* **125:** 554–65.

Allen MC (2008) Neurodevelopmental outcomes of preterm infants. *Curr Opin Neurol* **21:** 123–8.

Alleva E, Sorace A (2000) Important hints in behavioural teratology of rodents. *Curr Pharmaceut Des* **6:** 99–126.

Arnold GL, Kirby RS, Langendoerfer S, Wilkins-Haug L (1994) Toluene embryopathy: clinical delineation and developmental follow-up. *Pediatrics* **93:** 216–20.

Bailey JR, Cunny HC, Paule MG, Slikker W (1987) Fetal disposition of delta9-tetrahydrocannabinol (THC) during late pregnancy in the rhesus monkey. *Toxicol Appl Pharmacol* **90:** 315–21.

Ben-Ari Y (2002) Excitatory actions of GABA during development: the nature of the nurture. *Nat Rev Neurosci* **3:** 728–39.

Benveniste H, Fowler JS, Rooney WD, Scharf BA, Backus WW, Izrailtyan I, Knudsen GM, Hasselbalch SG, Volkow ND (2010) Cocaine is pharmacologically active in the nonhuman primate fetal brain. *Proc Natl Acad Sci USA* **107:** 1582–7.

Bhide PG (2009) Dopamine, cocaine and the development of cerebral cortical cytoarchitecture: a review of current concepts. *Semin Cell Dev Biol* **20:** 395–402.

Biezonski DK, Meyer JS (2010) Effects of 3.4-methylenedioxymethamphetamine (MDMA) on serotonin transporter and vesicular monoamine transporter 2 protein and gene expression in rats: implications for MDMA neurotoxicity. *J Neurochem* **112:** 951–62.

Bowen SE, Batis JC, Paez-Martinez N, Cruz SL (2006) The last decade of solvent research in animal models of abuse: mechanistic and behavioral studies. *Neurotoxicol Teratol* **28:** 636–47.

Bourin M, Petit-Demoulière B, Dhonnchadha BN, Hascöet M (2007) Animal models of anxiety in mice. *Fundam Clin Pharmacol* **21:** 567–74.

Bouwknecht JA, Paylor R (2008) Pitfalls in the interpretation of genetic and pharmacological effects on anxiety-like behaviour in rodents. *Behav Pharmacol* **19:** 385–402.

Bowen SE, Irtenkauf S, Hannigan JH, Stefanski AL (2009) Alterations in rat fetal morphology following abuse patterns of toluene exposure. *Reprod Toxicol* **27:** 161–9.

Bromley RL, Baker GA, Meador KJ (2009) Cognitive abilities and behavior of children exposed to antiepileptic drugs *in utero*. *Curr Opin Neurol* **22:** 162–6.

Bubeniková-Valesová V, Horácek J, Vrajová M, Höschi C (2008) Models of schizophrenia in humans and animals based on inhibition of NMDA receptors. *Neurosci Biobehav Rev* **32:** 1014–23.

Clancy B, Darlington RB, Finlay BL (2001) Translating developmental time across mammalian species. *Neuroscience* **105:** 7–17.

Clancy B, Finlay BL, Darlington RB, Anand KJS (2007a) Extrapolating brain development from experimental species to humans. *NeuroToxicology* **28:** 931–7.

Clancy B, Kersh B, Hyde J, Darlington RB, Anand KJ, Finlay BL (2007b) Web-based method for translating neurodevelopment from laboratory species to humans. *Neuroinformatics* **5:** 79–94.

Cohen LS, Rosenbaum JF (1998) Psychotropic drug use during pregnancy: weighing the risks. *J Clin Psychiatry* **59 (Suppl. 2):** 18–28.

Coupey SM (1997) Barbiturates. *Pediatr Rev* **18:** 260–5.

Cryan JF, Holmes A (2005) The ascent of mouse: Advances in modeling human depression and anxiety. *Nat Rev Drug Discov* **4:** 775–90.

Cryan JF, Mombereau C, Vassout A (2005) The tail suspension test as a model for assessing antidepressant activity; Review of pharmacological and genetic studies in mice. *Neurosci Biobehav Rev* **29:** 571–625.

Cryan JF, Slattery DA (2007) Animal models of mood disorders: Recent developments. *Curr Opin Psyciatry* **20: 1–7**

Cryan JF, Valentino RJ, Lucki I (2005) Assessing substrates underlying the behavioral effects of antidepressants using the modified rat forced swimming test. *Neurosci Biobehav Rev* **29:** 547–69.

Dean JCS, Hailey H, Moore SJ, Lloyd DJ, Turnpenny PD, Little J (2002) Long term health and neurodevelopment in children exposed to antiepileptic drugs before birth. *J Med Genet* **39:** 251–9.

Derauf C, Kekatpure M, Neyzi N, Lester B, Kosofsky B (2009) Neuroimaging of children following prenatal drug exposure. *Semin Cell Dev Biol* **20:** 441–54.

Einarson A (2009) Risks/safety of psychotropic medication use during pregnancy. *Can J Clin Pharmacol* **16:** e58–e65.

Fernández-Ruiz J, Romero J, Velasco G, Tolón RM, Ramos JA, Guzmán M (2007) Cannabinoid CB2 receptor: a new target for controlling neural cell survival? *Trends Pharmacol Sci* **28:** 39–45.

Frank DA, Augustyn M, Knight WG, Pell T, Zuckerman B (2001) Growth, development, and behavior in early childhood following prenatal cocaine exposure. A systematic review. *JAMA* **285:** 1613–25.

Fried PA, James DS, Watkinson B (2001) Growth and pubertal milestones during adolescence in offspring prenatally exposed to cigarettes and marihuana. *Neurotoxicol Teratol* **23:** 431–6.

Fried PA, Watkinson B (2000) Visuoperceptual functioning differs in 9- to 12-year-olds prenatally exposed to cigarettes and marihuana. *Neurotoxicol Teratol* **22:** 11–20.

Fried PA, Watkinson B, Gray R (2003) Differential effects on cognitive functioning in 13- to 16-year-olds prenatally exposed to cigarettes and marihuana. *Neurotoxicol Teratol* **25:** 427–36.

Gendle MH, Strawderman MS, Mactutus CF, Booze RM, Levitsky DA, Strupp BJ (2003) Impaired sustained attention and altered reactivity to errors in an animal model of prenatal cocaine exposure. *Dev Brain Res* **147:** 85–96.

Ghantous H, Danielsson BRG (1986) Placental transfer and distribution of toluene, xylene and benzene, and their metabolites during gestation in mice. *Biol Res Pregnancy Perinatol* **7:** 98–105.

Glare PA, Walsh TD (1991) Clinical pharmacokinetics of morphine. *Ther Drug Monit* **13:** 1–23.

Grotenhermen F (2003) Pharmacokinetics and pharmacodyanmics of cannabinoids. *Clin Pharmacokinet* **42:** 327–60.

Hammer RP Jr, Hauser KF (1992) Consequences of early exposure to opioids on cell proliferation and neuronal morphogenesis. In *Development of the Central Nervous System: Effects of Alcohol and Opiates* (Miller MW, ed.). Wiley-Liss, New York, pp. 319–39.

Hannigan JH, Bowen SE (2010) Reproductive toxicology and teratology of abused toluene. *Syst Biol Reprod Med* **56:** 184–200.

Hart PC, Bergner CL, Smolinsky AN, Dufour BD, Egan RJ, Laport JL, Kalueff AV (2010) Experimental models of anxiety for drug discovery and brain research. *Methods Mol Biol* **602:** 299–321.

Harvey JH (2004) Cocaine effects on the developing brain: current status. *Neurosci Biobehav Rev* **27:** 751–64.

Heyser CJ (2003) Assessment of developmental milestones in rodents. *Curr Protocols Neurosci*, Unit 8.18. DOI: 10.1002/0471142301.ns0818s25.

Hill JM, Lim MA, Stone MM (2007) Developmental milestones in the newborn mouse. In *Neuromethods, Vol. 39: Neuropeptide Techniques* (Gozes I, ed.). Humana Press, Totowa, pp. 131–49.

Hunt RW, Tzioumi D, Collins E, Jeffery HE (2008) Adverse neurodevelopmental outcome of infants exposed to opiate in-utero. *Early Hum Dev* **84:** 29–35.

Hutchings DE, Fico TA, Dow-Edwards DL (1989) Prenatal cocaine: maternal toxicity, fetal effects and locomotor activity in rat offspring. *Neurotoxicol Teratol* **11:** 65–9.

Ikonomidou C, Bittigau P, Koch C, Genz K, Hoerster F, Felderhoff-Mueser U, Tenkova T, Dikranian K, Olney JW (2001) Neurotransmitters and apoptosis in the developing brain. *Biochem Pharmacol* **62:** 401–5.

Iqbal MM, Sobhan T, Ryals T (2002) Effects of commonly used benzodiazepines on the fetus, the neonate, and the nursing infant. *Psychiat Serv* **53:** 39–49.

Jakubovic A, Tait RM, McGeer PL (1974) Excretion of THC and its metabolites in ewes' milk. *Toxicol Appl Pharmacol* **28:** 38–43.

Jansson LM, Velez M, Harrow C (2009) The opioid exposed newborn: assessment and pharmacologic management. *J Opioid Manag* **5:** 47–55.

Johnston LD, O'Malley PM, Bachman JG, Schulenberg JE (2009) *Monitoring the Future National survey results on drug use, 1975–2008: Volume I, Secondary school students* (NIH Publication No. 09–7402). National Institute on Drug Abuse, Bethesda.

Jones HE, Martin PR, Heil SH, Kaltenbach K, Selby P, Coyle MG, Stine SM, O'Grady KE, Arria AM, Fischer G (2008) Treatment of opioid-dependent pregnant women: clinical and research issues. *J Subst Abuse Treat* **35:** 245–59.

Kaindl AM, Koppelstaetter A, Nebrich G, Stuwe J, Sifringer M, Zabel C, Klose J, Ikonomidou C (2008) Brief alteration of NMDA or $GABA_A$ receptor-mediated neurotransmission has long term effects on the developing cerebral cortex. *Mol Cell Proteomics* **7:** 2293–310.

Kaltenbach KA (1996) Exposure to opiates: behavioral outcomes in preschool and school-age children. *NIDA Res Monogr* **164:** 230–41.

Kellogg CK (1995) Perinatal benzodiazepine modulation of $GABA_A$ receptor function: influence on adaptive responses. *NIDA Res Monogr* **158:** 202–24.

Kellogg CK (1999) Sex differences in long-term consequences of prenatal diazepam exposure: possible underlying mechanisms. *Pharmacol Biochem Behav* **64:** 673–80.

Kuczenski R, Segal DS (1994) Neurochemistry of amphetamine. In *Amphetamine and its Analogs* (Cho AK, ed.). Academic Press, San Diego, pp. 81–113.

Kuczkowski KM (2007) The effects of drug abuse on pregnancy. *Curr Opin Obstet Gynecol* **19:** 578–85.

Kuhn C, Swartzwelder S, Wilson W (2003) *Buzzed: The Straight Facts about the Most Used and Abused Drugs from Alcohol to Ecstasy*. Norton, New York.

Lee CC, Chiang CN (1985) Maternal–fetal transfer of abused substances: pharmacokinetic and pharmacodynamic data. *NIDA Res Monogr* **60:** 110–47.

Lee C-T, Chen J, Hayashi T, Tsai S-Y, Sanchez JF, Errico SL, Amable R, Su T-P, Lowe RH, Huestis MA, Shen J, Becker KG, Geller HM, Freed WJ (2008) A mechanism for the inhibition of neural progenitor cell proliferation by cocaine. *PLoS Med* **5**: e117. doi:10.1371/journal.pmed.0050117.

Lee S, Han E, Park Y, Choi H, Chung H (2009) Distribution of methamphetamine and amphetamine in drug abusers' head hair. *Forensic Sci Int* **190:** 16–18.

Lester BM, Lagasse LL (2010) Children of addicted women. *J Addict Dis* **29:** 259–76.

Lester BM, Padbury JF (2009) Third pathophysiology of prenatal cocaine exposure. *Dev Neurosci* **31:** 23–35.

Lidow MS (2003) Consequences of prenatal cocaine exposure in nonhuman primates. *Dev Brain Res* **147:** 23–36.

Lipinski RJ, Godin EA, O'Leary-Moore SK, Parnell SE, Sulik KK (2010) Genesis of teratogen-induced holoprosencephaly in mice. *Am J Med Genet* **154C:** 29–42.

Liu AJW, Sithamparanathan S, Jones MP, Cook C-M, Nanan R (2010) Growth restriction in pregnancies of opioid-dependent mothers. *Arch Dis Child Fetal Neonatal Ed* doi:10.1136/adc.2009.163105.

Mactutus CF, Herman AS, Booze RM (1994) Chronic intravenous model for studies of drug (Ab)use in the pregnant and/or group-housed rat: an initial study with cocaine. *Neurotoxicol Teratol* **16:** 183–91.

Mahmood I (2005) *Interspecies Pharmacokinetic Scaling: Principles and Application of Allometric Scaling*. Pine House, Rockville.

Mayes LC (2002) A behavioral teratogenic model of the impact of prenatal cocaine exposure on arousal regulatory systems. *Neurotoxicol Teratol* **24:** 385–95.

Messinger DS, Bauer CR, Das A, Seifer R, Lester BM, Lagasse LL, Wright LL, Shankaran S, Bada HS, Smeriglio VL, Langer JC, Beeghly M, Poole WK (2004) The maternal lifestyle study: cognitive, motor, and behavioral outcomes of cocaine-exposed and opiate-exposed infants through three years of age. *Pediatrics* **113:** 1677–85.

Meyer JS (1998) Behavioral assessment in developmental neurotoxicology. In *Handbook of Developmental Neurotoxicology* (Slikker Jr W, Chang LW, eds.). Academic Press, San Diego, pp. 403–26.

Meyer JS, Shearman LP, Collins LM, Maguire RL (1993) Cocaine binding sites in fetal rat brain: implications for prenatal cocaine action. *Psychopharmacology* **112:** 445–51.

Morris P, Gillam MP, Allen RR, Paule MG (1996) The effect of chronic cocaine exposure during pregnancy on the acquisition of operant behaviors by rhesus monkey offspring. *Neurotoxicol Teratol* **18:** 155–66.

Muhuri PK, Gfroerer JC (2009) Substance use among women: Associations with pregnancy, parenting, and race/ethnicity. *Maternal Child Health J* **13:** 376–85.

National Toxicology Program (2005) NTP-CERHR monograph on the potential human reproductive and developmental effects of amphetamines. *NTP CERHR MON 2005*: vii–III1. http://cerhr.niehs.nih.gov/evals/stimulants/amphetamines/AmphetamineMonograph.pdf.

Nicosia A, Giardina L, Di Leo F, Medico M, Mazzola C, Genazzani AA, Drago F (2003) Long-lasting behavioral changes induced by pre- or neonatal exposure to diazepam in rats. *Eur J Pharmacol* **469:** 103–9.

Niu L, Cao B, Zhu H, Mei B, Wang M, Yang Y, Zhou Y (2009) Impaired in vivo synaptic plasticity in dentate gyrus and spatial memory in juvenile rats induced by prenatal morphine exposure. *Hippocampus* **19:** 649–57.

Olney JW, Farber NB, Wozniak DF, Jevtovic-Todorovic V, Ikonomidou C (2000) Environmental agents that have the potential to trigger massive apoptotic neurodegeneration in the developing brain. *Environ Health Perspect* **108:** 383–8.

Park B, Gibbons HM, Mitchell MD, Glass M (2003) Identification of the CB1 cannabinoid receptor and fatty acid amide hydrolase (FAAH) in the human placenta. *Placenta* **24:** 990–5.

Paul CM, Magda G, Abel S (2009) Spatial memory: Theoretical basis and comparative review on experimental methods in rodents. *Behav Brain Res* **203:** 151-64.

Paule MG, Forrester TM, Maher MA, Cranmer JM, Allen RR (1990) Monkey versus human performance in the NCTR Operant Test Battery. *Neurotoxicol Teratol* **12:** 503–7.

Pearson MA, Hoyme HE, Seaver LH, Rimsza ME (1994) Toluene embryopathy: delineation of the phenotype and comparison with fetal alcohol syndrome. *Pediatrics* **93:** 211–15.

Perucca E (2005) Birth defects after prenatal exposure to antiepileptic drugs. *Lancet Neurol* **4:** 781–6.

Piper BJ (2007) A developmental comparison of the neurobehavioral effects of ecstasy (MDMA). *Neurotoxicol Teratol* **29:** 288–300.

Pizarro N, de la Torre R, Joglar J, Okumura N, Perfetti X, Lau SS, Monks TJ (2008) Serotonergic neurotoxic thioether metabolites of 3,4-methylenedioxymethamphetamine (MDMA, "ecstasy"): synthesis, isolation, and characterization of diasterisomers. *Chem Res* **21:** 2272–9.

Plessinger MA (1998) Prenatal exposure to amphetamines. Risks and adverse outcomes in pregnancy. *Obstet Gynecol Clin North Am* **25:** 19–38.

Ramos A (2008) Animal models of anxiety: do I need multiple tests? *Trends Pharmacol Sci* **29:** 493–8.

Ramos JA, Gómez M, de Miguel R (2005) Effects on development. *Handb Exp Pharmacol* **168:** 643–56.

Richardson GA, Day NL (1991) Maternal and neonatal effects of moderate cocaine use during pregnancy. *Neurotoxicol Teratol* **13:** 455–60.

Ritz MC, Cone EJ, Kuhar MJ (1990) Cocaine inhibition of ligand binding at dopamine, norepinephrine and serotonin transporters: a structure-activity study. *Life Sci* **46:** 635–45.

Rodgers RJ (1997) Animal models of 'anxiety': where next? *Behav Pharmacol* **8:** 477–96.

Rogel-Fuchs Y, Newman ME, Trombka D, Zahalka EA, Yanai J (1992) Hippocampal cholinergic alterations and related behavioral deficits after early exposure to phenobarbital. *Brain Res Bull* **29:** 1–6.

Romero J, Garcia-Palomero E, Berrendero F, Garcia-Gil L, Hernandez ML, Ramos JA, Fernández-Ruiz JJ (1997) Atypical location of cannabinoid receptors in white matter areas during rat brain development. *Synapse* **26:** 317–23.

Sargeant TJ, Day DJ, Miller JH, Steel RWJ (2008a) Acute *in utero* morphine exposure slows G_2/M phase transition in radial glial and basal progenitor cells in the dorsal telencephalon of the E15.5 embryonic mouse. *Eur J Neurosci* **28:** 1060–7.

Sargeant TJ, Miller JH, Day DJ (2008b) Opioidergic regulation of astroglial/neuronal proliferation: where are we now? *J Neurochem* **107:** 883–97.

Schneider M (2009) Cannabis use in pregnancy and early life and its consequences in animal models. *Eur Arch Psychiatry Clin Neurosci* **259:** 383–93.

Schwarting RK (2009) Rodent models of serial reaction time tasks and their implementation in neurobiological research. *Behav Brain Res* **199:** 76–88.

Shah NS, May DA, Yates JD (1980) Disposition of levo-^{3}H-cocaine in pregnant and nonpregnant mice. *Toxicol Appl Pharmacol* **53:** 279–84.

Shearman LP, Collins LM, Meyer JS (1996) Characterization and localization of [^{125}I]RTI-55-labeled cocaine binding sites in fetal and adult rat brain. *J Pharmacol Exp Ther* **277:** 1770–83.

Shi Q, Guo L, Patterson TA, Dial S, Li Q, Sadovova N, Zhang X, Hanig JP, Paule MG, Slikker W Jr, Wang C (2010) Gene expression profiling in the developing rat brain exposed to ketamine. *Neuroscience* **166:** 852–63.

Shuster, L (1992) Pharmacokinetics, metabolism, and disposition of cocaine. In *Cocaine: Pharmacology, Physiology, and Clinical Strategies* (Lakoski JM, Galloway MP, White FJ, eds.). CRC Press, Boca Raton, pp. 1–14.

Sinner B, Graf BM (2008) Ketamine. *Handb Exp Pharmacol* **182:** 313–33.

Sircar R (2003) Postnatal phencyclidine-induced deficit in adult water maze performance is associated with N-methyl-D-aspartate receptor upregulation. *Int J Dev Neurosci* **21:** 159–67.

Skuza G, Wedzony K (2004) Behavioral pharmacology of the sigma receptors. *Pharmacopsychiatry* **37:** S183–S188.

Smith LM, Lagasse LL, Derauf C, Grant P, Shah R, Arria A, Huestis M, Haning W, Strauss A, Grotta SD, Fallone M, Liu J, Lester BM (2008) Prenatal methamphetamine use and neonatal neurobehavioral outcome. *Neurotoxicol Teratol* **30:** 20–28.

Smith TA (2001) Type A γ-aminobutyric acid ($GABA_A$) receptor subunits and benzodiazepine binding: significance to clinical syndromes and their treatment. *Br J Biomed Sci* **58:** 111–21.

Strathearn L, Mayes LC (2010) Cocaine addiction in mothers. Potential effects on maternal care and infant development. *Ann NY Acad Sci* **1187:** 172–83.

Suárez I, Godega G, Fernández-Ruiz J, Ramos JA, Rubio M, Fernández B (2004) Down-regulation of the AMPA glutamate receptor subunits GluR1 and GluR2/3 in the rat cerebellum following pre- and perinatal delta^9-tetrahydocannabinol exposure. *Cerebellum* **3:** 66–74.

Substance Abuse and Mental Health Services Administration (2009) *Results from the 2008 National Survey on Drug Use and Health: National Findings* (Office of Applied Studies, NSDUH Series H-36, HHS Publication No. SMA 09-4434). Rockville.

Sulik KK (2005) Genesis of alcohol-induced craniofacial dysmorphism. *Exp Biol Med* **230:** 366–75.

Trezza V, Cuomo V, Vanderschuren LJ (2008) Cannabis and the developing brain: insights from behavior. *Eur J Pharmacol* **585:** 441–52.

Vance JC, Chant DC, Tudehope DI, Gray PH, Hayes AJ (1997) Infants born to narcotic dependent mothers: physical growth patterns in the first 12 months of life. *J Paediatr Child Health* **33:** 504–8.

Vathy I (2001) Prenatal morphine exposure induces age- and sex-dependent changes in seizure susceptibility. *Prog Neuro-Psychopharmacol Biol Psychiat* **25:** 1203–26.

Vathy I (2002) Prenatal opiate exposure: long-term CNS consequences in the stress system of the offspring. *Psychoneuroendocrinology* **27:** 273–83.

Viberg H, Pontén E, Eriksson P, Gordh T, Fredriksson A (2008) Neonatal ketamine exposure results in changes in biochemical substrates of neuronal growth and synaptogenesis, and alters behavior irreversibly. *Toxicology* **249:** 153–9.

Vorhees CV (1989) Concepts in teratology and developmental toxicology derived from animal research. *Ann NY Acad Sci* **562:** 31–41.

Vorhees CV, Skelton MR, Williams MT (2007) Age-dependent effects of neonatal methamphetamine exposure on spatial learning. *Behav Pharmacol* **18:** 549–62.

Waldhoer M, Bartlett SE, Whistler JL (2004) Opioid receptors. *Annu Rev Biochem* **73:** 953–90.

Walhovd KB, Moe V, Slinning K, Siqveland T, Fjell AM, Bjørnebekk A, Smith L (2009) Effects of prenatal opiate exposure on brain development – a call for attention. *Nat Rev Neurosci* **10:** 390.

Walhovd KB, Moe V, Slinning K, Due-Tønnessen P, Bjørnerud A, Dale AM, van der Kouwe A, Quinn BT, Kosofsky B, Greve D, Fischl B (2007) Volumetric cerebral characteristics of children exposed to opiates and other substances in utero. *NeuroImage* **36:** 1331–44.

Walhovd KB, Westlye LT, Moe V, Slinning K, Due-Tønnessen P, Bjørnerud A, van der Kouwe A, Dale AM, Fjell AM (2010) White matter characteristics and cognition in prenatally opiate- and polysubstance-exposed children: a diffusion tensor imaging study. *Am J Neuroradiol* doi:10.3174/ajnr.A1957.

Wang Y, Han T-Z (2009) Prenatal exposure to heroin in mice elicits memory deficits that can be attributed to neuronal apoptosis. *Neuroscience* **160:** 330–8.

Woods JR (1998) Maternal and transplacental effects of cocaine. *Ann NY Acad Sci* **846:** 1–11.

Yanai J, Huleihel R, Izrael M, Metsuyanim S, Shahak H, Vatury O, Yaniv SP (2003) Functional changes after prenatal opiate exposure related to opiate receptors' regulated alterations in cholinergic innervation. *Int J Neuropsychopharmacol* **6:** 253–65.

Yanney M, Marlow N (2004) Paediatric consequences of fetal growth restriction. *Semin Fetal Neonatal Med* **9:** 411–18.

C H A P T E R

27

Caffeine

Rosane Souza Da Silva

INTRODUCTION

Caffeine-based beverages and foods are widely consumed and considered a harmless habit, although caffeine has powerful effects on a variety of organs, systems and behavior (Fredholm *et al.*, 1999). Caffeine is not a nutrient but a natural chemical present in coffee, soft and cola drinks, chocolate, tea and maté. Xanthines, as caffeine, are also used in the therapeutic field as an adjuvant in analgesics, weight loss products and to treat apnea in infants. The effects of therapeutic doses or normal consumption of caffeine in foods or drinks depend on caffeine exposure; caffeine has quite different effects if given acutely or chronically to an individual.

Caffeine, in concentration ranges for human consumption, acts as a non-specific blocker of the adenosine receptor. Although caffeine intoxication occurs rarely, it can reach toxic doses since heavy caffeine consumption can promote release of calcium from intracellular stores, activate enzymes of the phosphodiesterase family and interfere with activation of neurotransmitter receptors.

Fecundability appears to be affected in individuals who drink coffee and tea, but compounds other than caffeine appear as agents to induce such effects. Caffeine molecules cross biological barriers freely, reaching the fetus during the entire gestation, and can be found in breast milk, reaching breastfeeding neonates. Coffee or caffeine effects have been found to be related to various adverse pregnancy outcomes, including fetal loss, birth defects and fetal growth retardation. The exposure of the fetus to caffeine and its metabolites depends on maternal caffeine metabolism, which shows marked genetic and environmental variation. Concerning environmental variation, there is a strong association between tobacco and caffeine intake, and the interaction of these two xenobiotics is implicated in several effects on reproduction and fetal development.

Findings of caffeine effects on reproduction and fetal development are quite controversial, but in some countries coffee consumption during pregnancy has been subject to preventive action. However, these putative effects of caffeine on reproduction and fetal development have been questioned, and many countries have no regulatory policies against coffee drinking during pregnancy. This chapter describes reproductive and developmental toxicity of caffeine in humans and experimental animals. The chapter has also discussed new insights involved in the later effects of caffeine following its early exposure.

HISTORICAL BACKGROUND

Caffeine is a component of coffee beans (*Coffea arabica* and *Coffea robusta*), tea leaves (*Cammelia thea*) and other plants of the families rubiacea, sterculiacea and theacea. In addition to traditional caffeine-containing products, such as coffee, tea and chocolate, caffeine can be consumed from a variety of non-traditional sources. For example, caffeine is the active compound of energy drinks and has been added to products that individuals already consume such as water, gum, mints and candy. Approximately 90% of adults report regular caffeine use, with an average daily intake of 227 mg (Frary *et al.*, 2005). The main sources of caffeine for adults are coffee (70%), cola drinks (16%) and tea (12%) (Frary *et al.*, 2005).

The USFDA (United States Food and Drug Administration) established that caffeine is generally recognized as safe (GRAS) when used in cola-type beverages up to a level of 0.02% or 200 ppm. The average human caffeine consumption from all sources is about 70 mg/person/day. The daily caffeine consumption of 300 mg from all sources by an adult has been assumed to be safe. However, in some countries the daily caffeine intake can reach up to 400 mg/person.

The results of epidemiological studies suggest that coffee consumption may help prevent several chronic diseases, including type 2 diabetes mellitus, Alzheimer's disease, Parkinson's disease and liver disease (Ross *et al.*, 2000; Van Dam and Feskens, 2002; Homan and Mobarhan, 2006; Arendash and Cao, 2010). Despite coffee consumption being sometimes associated with increases in cardiovascular disease risk factors, including high blood pressure and plasma homocysteine, most evidence suggests that a regular intake of caffeinated coffee does not increase the risk of hypertension and other cardiovascular diseases (Geleijnse, 2008). Caffeine has also been indicated as a cause of spontaneous abortion, intrauterine growth restriction, low birth weight and preterm delivery. However, little or no reproductive adversity has been consistently associated with caffeine consumption (Leviton and Cowan, 2002; CARE Study Group, 2008).

Reproductive and Developmental Toxicology, Edited by Ramesh C. Gupta
ISBN: 978-0-12-382032-7

The most recognized effect of caffeine in humans is its psychostimulant action (Fredholm *et al.*, 1999). Caffeine is a stimulant of central and peripheral nervous systems. The biochemical and physiological mechanisms that underlie caffeine effects in doses of normal human consumption are the unspecific blockage of adenosine receptors (Nehlig *et al.*, 1992). Adenosine receptors are widely expressed in the human body, especially in brain areas, which explains the wide action of caffeine in the whole body. Adenosine, a nucleoside, influences many functions of cardiovascular, cerebral, motor and other systems. Adenosine receptors are prematurely and widely expressed in the fetus (Weaver, 1996). The association of premature expression of biological targets of caffeine and its ability to cross biological barriers pointed out possible effects of caffeine in the development of the fetus from mothers who ingest caffeinated sources. In fact, pharmacological and genetic manipulation of adenosine receptors on early development of rodents showed marked effects on cardiovascular and nervous system and body development. During prenatal life, the adenosinergic system is the dominant humoral regulator of cardiac function, and activation of adenosine A_1 receptors may result in cardiac hypoplasia (Rivkees *et al.*, 2001; Zhao and Rivkees, 2001). In the neonatal period, adenosine A_1 receptors are expressed on axons and growth cones, and their activation can profoundly influence axon and white matter formation (Rivkees *et al.*, 2001; Turner *et al.*, 2001). Ventriculomegaly, reduction in white matter volume and neuronal loss were detected after activation of adenosine receptors subtypes during the first 2 weeks of neonatal life, which suggests that adenosine is involved in neurodevelopment and neuronal death during early development (Rivkees *et al.*, 2001; Turner *et al.*, 2002).

Behavioral effects of early caffeine exposure are also under investigation. Moderate to high doses of caffeine (approximately 100–400 mg) led to increased reports of nervousness, jitteriness, fidgetiness and decreased reports of sluggishness in children and adolescents (Elkins *et al.*, 1981; Rapoport *et al.*, 1981; Bernstein *et al.*, 1994). However, in humans, the investigation of fetal exposure to caffeine and the effects on behavior are quite scarce; however, some reports show no correlation between maternal caffeine exposure and effects on children's behavior (Linnet *et al.*, 2003; Temple, 2009).

TOXICOKINETICS

Caffeine (1,3,7-trimethylxanthine) (Figure 27.1) is a methylxanthine that is rapidly and completely absorbed by the gastrointestinal tract. The moderate lipophilic property of caffeine allows its passage through all biological barriers, which include blood–brain and placental barriers. As a consequence of its poor affinity to serum albumin, caffeine reaches all body compartments through body fluids. Thus, it freely crosses the placenta, which implies that caffeine concentrations in the fetus are near to those in the plasma of the mother. Caffeine reaches a human plasma concentration of 8–10 mg/L between 15 and 120 min after ingestion of 5 to 8 mg/kg (Arnaud and Welsch, 1982). Taking this into account, a cup of coffee containing 0.4 to 2.5 mg/kg will reach a plasma concentration of 0.25 to 2 mg/L (Fredholm *et al.*, 1999). The half-life of caffeine is 4 to 5 h in non-pregnant women but caffeine clearance slows down during pregnancy, and in the second and third trimesters of pregnancy, the half-life of caffeine is tripled in comparison with non-pregnant women (Fredholm *et al.*, 1999; Kot and Daniel, 2008). In neonates, the half-life of caffeine increases because the hepatic system, in order to metabolize caffeine, is still immature until 8 months of age (Björklund *et al.*, 2008). The half-life of caffeine is about 80 ± 23 h for the full-term newborn infant and decreases exponentially as the neonate grows. Caffeine clearance is low in 1-month-old infants (31 ml/kg/h), rising to 331 ml/kg/h in 5- to 6-month-old infants and reaching adult levels of 155 ml/kg/h (Aranda *et al.*, 1979).

Caffeine is mainly metabolized in the liver by hepatic microsomal enzymes. Caffeine products of metabolism are dimethyl and monomethylxanthines, dimethyl and monomethyl uric acids, trimethyl and dimethylallantoin, and uracil derivatives (Arnaud, 1987, 1993). Demethylation and hydroxylation is played by a myriad of enzymes (Figure 27.1). The initial major step of biotransformation is catalyzed by the enzyme family named Cytocrome P450 (CYP450), mainly by the subfamily CYPIA2. This enzyme family promotes demethylation producing paraxanthine (1,7-dimethylxanthine), theophylline (1,3-dimethylxanthine) and theobromine (3,7-dimethylxanthine). The 3-*N*-demethylation played by the CYP1A2 subfamily to produce paraxanthine corresponds to 72–80% of caffeine metabolism (Arnaud and Welsch, 1982; Arnaud, 1993). The CYP1A2 subfamily has a minor participation on 7-*N*-demethylation to produce theophylline; this step being played mostly by CYP2C8, CYP2C9 and CYP3A4 enzyme subfamilies (Kot and Daniel, 2008). C8-hydroxylation to produce 1,3,7-trimethyluric acid is played mainly by CYP3A4 enzymes subfamily and to a lesser extent by CYP2C8, CYP2C9 and CYP2E1 enzyme subfamilies (Kot and Daniel, 2008). Other enzymes play a minor role in the metabolism of caffeine, such as *N*-acetyltransferase 2 (NAT2) and xanthine oxidase, to produce 5-acetylamino-6-formylamino-3-methyluracil (AFMU) and 1-methylurate from caffeine metabolites, respectively (Hakooz, 2009).

Paraxanthine, theobromine and theophylline also have biological activity. In fact, theophylline is approximately three to five times more powerful than caffeine, and paraxanthine has the same potency of caffeine when considering the ability to block adenosine receptors (Fredholm *et al.*, 1999). Theobromine has minor biological effects, but is a precursor of pentoxyphylline, an inhibitor of cytokines with therapeutic action on alcoholic liver disease (Whitfield *et al.*, 2009).

MECHANISM OF ACTION

At normal levels of human consumption, caffeine has adenosine receptors as a target. Caffeine acts as a non-specific blocker of adenosine receptors. The time–spatial distribution of adenosine receptors predicts the tissues affected by caffeine and its metabolites. To understand the widespread effects of caffeine it is essential to be aware of the action of adenosine.

Distribution and signaling of adenosine receptors

Adenosine receptors are A_1, A_{2A}, A_{2B} and A_3 bunched on the P1 purinergic receptors family (Ralevic and Burnstock, 1998). P1 receptors are expressed on the whole body. The high affinity adenosine A_1 receptor is mainly present in brain, spinal cord, testis, heart and autonomic nerve terminals. The adenosine A_{2A}

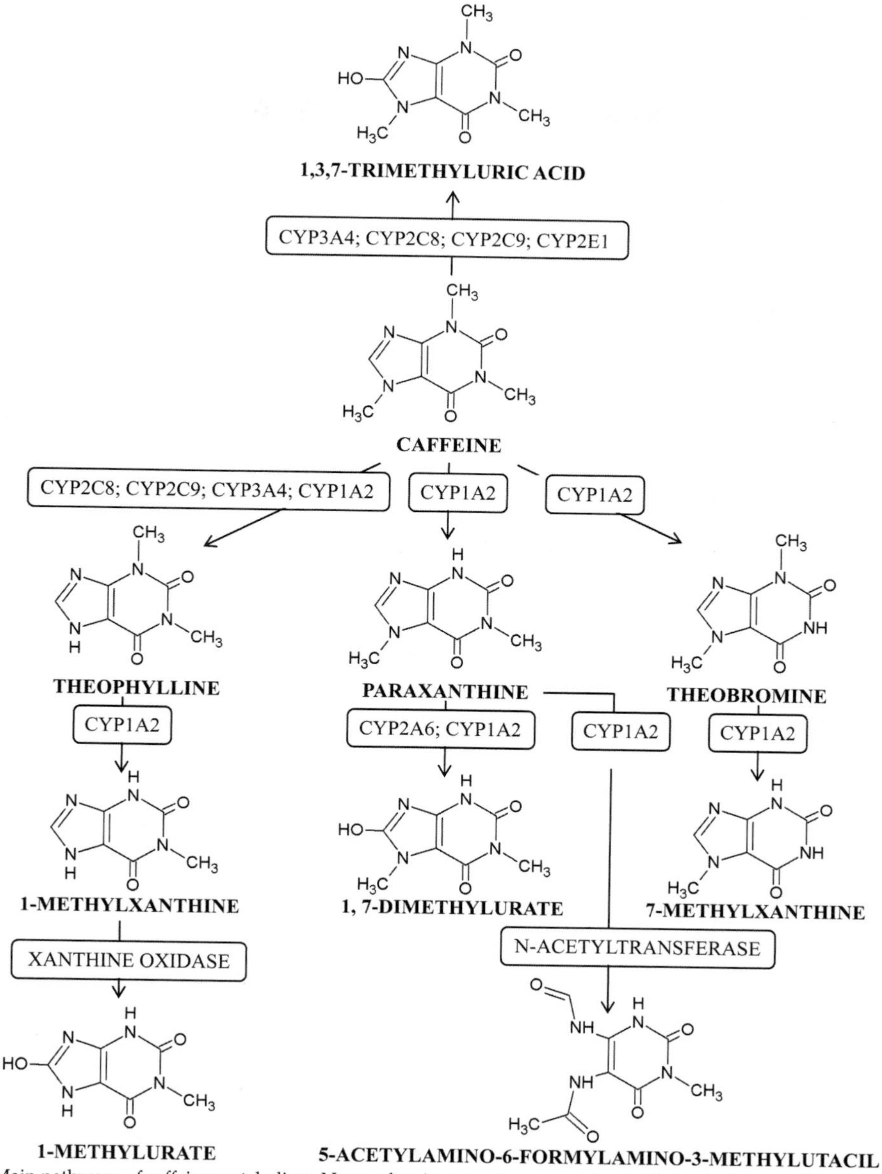

FIGURE 27.1 Main pathways of caffeine metabolism. Name of main enzymes appears inside the boxes. Please refer to color plate section.

receptor is mainly present in the brain, heart, lungs and spleen. The adenosine A_{2B} receptor has its major distribution in the large intestine and bladder, and the adenosine A_3 receptor is present in the lung, liver, brain, testis and heart. Adenosine A_1 and A_{2A} receptors are high affinity receptors being activated by the physiological concentration of adenosine.

Caffeine has different affinities for different adenosine receptors (Table 27.1), and as a result, caffeine produces distinct impacts on tissues depending on the level of expression and the type of adenosine receptors. Despite the highest affinity of caffeine to the adenosine A_{2A} receptor, the most prominent acute effects of caffeine are attributed to adenosine A_1 receptor antagonism. However, chronic caffeine consumption results in the tolerance of adenosine A_1 receptors to caffeine, so that in this condition the effects of caffeine on adenosine A_1 receptors are negligible, and its action on adenosine A_{2A} receptors becomes predominant (Ballari'n *et al.*, 1991; Fredholm *et al.*, 1999).

TABLE 27.1 Caffeine affinity for adenosine receptor

Adenosine receptor subtype	Human (K_D)
A_1	12 μM
A_{2A}	2.4 μM
A_{2B}	13 μM
A_3	80 μM

Data adapted from Fredholm *et al.* (1999)
K_D = Affinity constant

The expression of adenosine receptors during early development is an important support to the correct control of metabolic activity and cellular growth. In rats, the adenosine A_1 receptor is highly present in the primitive myocardial cylinder on GD 8, in the placental mesometrium on GD 10, and in the fetal brain it is initially detected on GD 14 (Weaver, 1996;

Rivkees *et al.*, 2001). Adenosine receptor activation influences cardiac development. Treatment with adenosine receptor agonist during the gestational period reduces ventricular size, thins ventricular walls and promotes intrauterine growth failure (Zhao and Rivkees, 2001).

All adenosine receptors are coupled to the G-protein. Adenosine A_1 and A_3 receptors are coupled to the inhibitory G-protein (G_i and G_o), whereas adenosine A_{2A} and A_{2B} receptors are coupled to the stimulatory G-protein (G_s; for further details, see Sebastião and Ribeiro, 2009). The coupling of adenosine A_{2A} receptor to stimulatory G-protein is mainly observed in peripheral tissues, while in brain regions the coupling is mostly to the G_{olf}-protein (Kull *et al.*, 2000). The adenosine A_3 receptor is also related to the G_q-protein (Abbracchio *et al.*, 1995).

Subsequent to the activation and consequent effects of adenosine receptors on specific G-protein, a number of enzymes and ion channels are affected. Thus, the control exerted by extracellular adenosine through activity of adenylate cyclase manages the cyclic adenosine monophosphate (cAMP) production on intracellular medium, triggering the control of cAMP-dependent enzymes. Different types of ion channels, such as K^+, Na^+ and Ca^{2+} channels, are under direct or indirect adenosine control. Adenosine A_1 receptor activation leads to activation of several types of K^+ channels, inactivation of N-, P- and Q-types of Ca^{2+} channels, activation of phospholipase Cβ, and activation of ERK1/2 (Dunwiddie and Masino, 2001; Fredholm *et al.*, 2005). The endpoint of effects elicited by adenosine on the adenosine A_1 receptor can be hyperpolarization of postsynaptic neurons, reduction of neurotransmitter release, vasoconstriction, bradycardia, inhibition of lipolysis, reduced glomerular filtration, tuberoglomerular feedback, antinociception, reduction of sympathetic and parasympathetic activity, presynaptic inhibition, neuronal hyperpolarization and ischemic preconditioning and behavioral effects (Fredholm *et al.*, 2005; Burnstock, 2008). Adenosine A_{2A} receptor promotes increase of cAMP and control of protein kinase C activity. Major physiological effects of the activating adenosine A_{2A} receptors include facilitation of neurotransmitter release, regulation of sensorimotor integration in basal ganglia, smooth muscle relaxation, anti-inflammatory activity, inhibition of platelet aggregation and polymorphonuclear leukocytes, vasodilatation, protection in ischemic condition and stimulation of sensory nerve activity (Fredholm *et al.*, 2005; Burnstock, 2008). The adenosine A_{2B} receptor has low affinity for adenosine and plays minor functions on normal physiological conditions, such as relaxation of smooth muscle in vasculature and intestine and inhibition of monocyte and macrophage function (Fredholm *et al.*, 2005). The adenosine A_3 receptor has high affinity for adenosine, but has minor impact because a weak expression is observed on the whole body. However, an antitumorigenic action of adenosine A_3 receptor agonists against melanoma, colon and prostate cancers has been shown (Madi *et al.*, 2003; Ohana *et al.*, 2003; Jajoo *et al.*, 2009).

At physiological conditions, adenosine exerts its effects mostly by a balance between adenosine A_1/A_{2A} receptors activation, since they have high affinity by adenosine. The adenosine A_{2B} receptor plays a possible role in allergenic diseases and acts as an anti-inflammatory, while the adenosine A_3 receptor facilitates the release of allergenic mediators (Burnstock, 2008).

Adenosine receptors also can form homo-oligomers and hetero-oligomers as an elegant form to exert modulation upon other systems of neurotransmission (Fredholm *et al.*, 2005). This interaction between neurotransmitter systems has been demonstrated for the adenosine A_1 receptor and $P2Y_1$ receptor (metabotropic ATP receptor), mGlu1 receptor (metabotropic glutamate receptor), μ receptor (opioid receptor), α_1 receptor (adrenergic receptor) and D_1 receptor (dopamine receptor) (Aley and Levine, 1997; Fuxe *et al.*, 1998; Rimondini *et al.*, 1998; Ciruela *et al.*, 2001). The adenosine A_{2A} receptor also forms hetero-oligomers with the D_2 receptor (dopamine receptor) (Fuxe *et al.*, 1998; Rimondini *et al.*, 1998).

Caffeine as a blocker of adenosine function

Caffeine by acting on adenosine receptors alters normal adenosine modulatory action on the above-mentioned physiological functions. Most of the physiological effects of caffeine are played by increased levels of cellular cAMP, which influence cell development, energetic balance, cell survival and other cellular actions. These effects are related to the inhibition of the adenosine A_1 receptor in accordance with its high expression through all tissues. Chronic adenosine receptor antagonism with caffeine promotes upregulation of the adenosine A_1 receptor, while the adenosine A_{2A} receptor seems to be unaltered (Sebastião and Ribeiro, 2009). Consequently, this effect promotes an alteration of the balance between the adenosine A_1/A_{2A} receptors' activation (Ferré *et al.*, 2008).

Caffeine is known to be involved in the control of the phosphorylation state of several phosphoproteins that are targets of protein kinase A, such as DARPP-32 (dopamine- and cyclic AMP-regulated phosphoprotein of 32,000 kDa), phospho-Ser897 NR1, phospho-Ser845 GluR1, phosho-Ser94 spinophilin and phospho-Thr34 (Lindskog *et al.*, 2002; Svenningsson *et al.*, 2005; Sahin *et al.*, 2007).

Caffeine is also known to interact with the dopaminergic system to exert some of its behavioral effects (Cauli and Morelli, 2005; Fredholm and Svenningsson, 2003). This action is likely mediated through inhibition of the adenosine A_{2A} receptor, which is primarily localized in dopamine-rich areas of the brain (Fredholm *et al.*, 1999). The caffeine-induced motor activity is greatly reduced in DARPP-32 knockout mice or mice treated with selective adenosine A_{2A} receptor antagonist. DARPP-32 appears to be an important part of signaling integration between adenosine and dopamine, which is a target of caffeine motor effects (Lindskog *et al.*, 2002). Caffeine is able to directly potentiate dopamine neurotransmission, thereby modulating the rewarding and addicting properties of the nervous system.

As a reflex of blockage of adenosine control of neurotransmitter release, the administration of caffeine promotes release of acetylcholine in the hippocampus and prefrontal cortex and glutamate and dopamine in the nucleus accumbens of rodents (Carter *et al.*, 1995; Acquas *et al.*, 2002; Solinas *et al.*, 2002).

Systemically administered caffeine preferentially activates orexin neurons over non-orexin neurons, which are involved in arousal and could be part of the mechanism of behavioral activation played by caffeine (Murphy *et al.*, 2003). The likely mechanisms to mediate c-Fos expression of orexin neurons after low doses of caffeine can be related to a direct result of caffeine's antagonism of postsynaptic adenosine A_1 receptors present on orexin neurons. As orexin neurons receive glutamatergic input caffeine could also activate orexin neurons by presynaptically disinhibiting the glutamatergic system by adenosine A_1 receptor activation (Murphy *et al.*, 2003).

Long-term consumption of caffeine by rats can induce ventriculomegaly associated to increased production of cerebrospinal fluid, increased expression of Na^+-/K^+-ATPase and increased cerebral blood flow. In contrast to the chronic effects, acute treatment with caffeine decreased the production of cerebrospinal fluid, which is mediated by increased expression of the adenosine A_1 receptor in the choroid plexus of rats chronically treated with caffeine (Han *et al.*, 2007).

Caffeine can elevate plasma levels of stress hormones such as epinephrine, norepinephrine and cortisol, all of which can lead to an increase in blood pressure (Robertson *et al.*, 1979; Lane *et al.*, 1990). However, no association of caffeine with risk of hypertension has been confirmed in studies with large populations (Bonita *et al.*, 2007). The increasing levels of circulating catecholamines induced by caffeine were investigated to interfere with uteroplacental circulation through vasoconstriction (Weathersbee *et al.*, 1977; Kirknen *et al.*, 1983; CARE Study Group, 2008).

Other biological targets of caffeine

Some potential *in vivo* anti-inflammatory function and possible benefits to the heart of caffeine have been suggested in humans. This is because caffeine metabolites are inhibitors of the enzyme poly(ADP-ribose)polymerase-1 in hydrogen peroxide-treated epithelial cells at physiological concentrations (Geraets *et al.*, 2006). Regarding the effects of coffee consumption it is worth attempting to separate the effects of caffeine from the rest of the compounds present in coffee. The diterpene compounds (cafestol and kahweol) are suspected to be two coffee substances which cause the elevation of serum cholesterol. Caffeine itself has no LDL antioxidant activity. However, some of the metabolites of caffeine, namely 1-methylxanthine and 1-methyluric acid, are as effective at preventing LDL oxidation as ascorbic acid at 40 μM (Lee, 2000).

At high levels of caffeine consumption, other biological actions besides adenosine receptor antagonism are present. Caffeine inhibits cyclic nucleotide phosphodiesterases (PDE1, PDE4 and PDE5), promotes calcium release from intracellular stores, inhibits inhibitory $GABA_A$ and glycine receptors, and enhances *N*-methyl-D-aspartate (NMDA) receptor neurotransmission (Daly, 2007; Black *et al.*, 2008).

TOXICITY

Despite its wide availability, caffeine intoxication occurs rarely. Ingestion of caffeine at 20 mg/kg body weight is considered toxic, but patients intoxicated by caffeine appear to survive levels up to 1 mM (Ritchie, 1975). The lethal dose of caffeine consumption has been estimated to be in the range of 150–200 mg/kg (Ritchie, 1975; Rivenes *et al.*, 1997; Rudolph and Knudsen, 2010). In rats, the LD_{50} of caffeine is determined to be 150–265 mg/kg and is assumed to be fairly consistent among several species (Warszawski *et al.*, 1978; Dews, 1982).

The term *caffeinism* was introduced to characterize the symptoms of acute or chronic caffeine intoxication after consumption of high doses (300–800 mg/person/day) (Nehlig and Debry, 1994; Carrillo and Benitez, 1996). These negative symptoms include restlessness, agitation, anxiety, irritability, muscle tremor, palpitations, arrhythmia, tachycardia, diuresis and gastrointestinal disorders. Symptoms of caffeine overdose include headache, nausea, vomiting, hyperventilation, dizziness, anxiety, tinnitus, tremors, excitation and tachycardia. Caffeine overdose may cause hypokalemia, hyponatremia, ventricular arrhythmias, hypertension, followed by hypotension, respiratory failure, seizures, rhabdomyolysis, ventricular fibrillation and finally circulatory collapse.

Toxic concentrations of caffeine are several times higher than the concentration able to block adenosine receptors. To inhibit cyclic nucleotide breakdown through phosphodiesterase inhibition, 20 times higher concentrations of caffeine are required; to block $GABA_A$, 40 times higher concentrations; and to mobilize intracellular calcium depots, 100 times higher concentrations are needed (Fredholm *et al.*, 1999).

Fecundability, pregnancy and caffeine exposure

The consequences of normal caffeine consumption are of minor impact on human health. However, caffeine influences a large number of different physiological functions which can raise concerns about its intake during pregnancy and early development. Adverse reproductive and developmental outcomes, such as delayed conception, stillbirth, anomalies, prematurity and low birth weight have been extensively investigated and attributed to caffeine consumption. However, few studies show a consistent association of caffeine with these outcomes. Since strong evidence exists for caffeine and negative pregnancy outcomes, many health professional organizations advise pregnant women to reduce caffeine intake. Caffeine intake can be frequently associated with tobacco and alcohol, which influence several aspects of pregnancy and serve as confounding factors to the effects of caffeine on reproduction and development in humans.

There are controversial studies regarding the correlation of caffeine intake and infertility. High levels of caffeine intake (>500 mg/day; approximately >5 cups per day) may increase the time to pregnancy, as reported by a 45% increased risk of subfecundity (≥9.5 months to conception) in first pregnancies in the European Study of Infertility and Subfecundity (Bolumar *et al.*, 1997). In contrast, it has been shown that caffeine has no effects on indicators of ovarian age, such as antral follicle count and levels of follicle stimulating hormone (FSH), inhibin B and estradiol (Kinney *et al.*, 2007). Additionally, semen quality also appears not to be affected by caffeine, but high caffeine intake has been associated with higher testosterone levels in men (Ramlau-Hamsen *et al.*, 2008).

The concern about low birth weight has also been extensively investigated but with poorly conclusive studies. Negative effects of caffeine on birth weight often are associated with other drugs or high caffeine intake. Maternal third trimester serum paraxanthine concentration, which reflects caffeine consumption, was associated with a higher risk of reduced fetal growth, but particularly among women who smoked (Klebanoff *et al.*, 2002). No association of fetal growth restriction and maternal caffeine intake has been shown when consumption is less than 100 mg/day (CARE Study Group, 2008). However, caffeine intake of approximately 300 mg/day was associated with fetal growth restriction (Martin and Bracken, 1987; Godel *et al.*, 1992). In some studies, the increased risk of fetal growth restriction is still significant even after taking into account corrections for smoking and alcohol intake (CARE Study Group, 2008).

Taking into consideration the caffeine metabolism as a model to evaluate the risk of spontaneous abortion, lower enzyme activities (CYP1A2, N-acetyltransferase 2 and xanthine oxidase) did not appear to be related to this outcome (Fenster *et al.*, 1998). When genotypes from active enzymes in caffeine metabolism were investigated, no association was found to support the hypothesis that caffeine itself causes stillbirth (Bech *et al.*, 2006).

It is important to mention that a healthy placenta produces a surge of one or more hormones, which in some women produce nausea and a reduced desire for coffee and other strongly flavored beverages. Thus, a woman who has nausea has a healthy placenta and good implantation. If this is true, the unchanged caffeine consumption during the first trimester can indicate diminished placental hormone synthesis and a vulnerable implantation (Stein and Susser, 1991). Preeclampsia, a disorder with prominent cardiovascular manifestations, is a cause of maternal, fetal and infant morbidity and mortality. No conclusive studies have found that chocolate consumption during pregnancy, and in particular the increase in cord serum concentration of theobromine, is associated with reduced occurrence of preeclampsia (Klebanoff *et al.*, 2009).

Currently, there is no evidence that caffeine is teratogenic in humans. Epidemiologic evidence is inadequate to assess the possibility of a small risk of congenital anomalies, such as neural tube defects, resulting from maternal caffeine consumption (Leviton and Cowan, 2002; Browne, 2006; Schmidt *et al.*, 2009).

Animal studies

Negative effects on fertility and birth weight, risk of prematurity and congenital anomalies have been demonstrated in offspring of animals, mainly when given high doses of caffeine (Purves and Sutherland, 1993). Low concentration of caffeine had clearly an inhibitory effect on spermatozoa from mice with reduced number of adenosine A_1 receptors, which could be related to inhibitory effects of caffeine on male fertility (Minelli *et al.*, 2004). Mice lacking the adenosine A_1 receptor are less fertile, implying that the adenosine A_1 receptor, although not indispensable in its capacity to fertilize, is involved in the efficiency of the process (Minelli *et al.*, 2004).

Administration of caffeine to rats in moderate (30 mg/kg/day) or high (60 mg/kg/day) doses throughout gestation resulted in offspring with significant growth retardation in uterus and also with subsequent reduced growth rates. The caffeine-exposed pups grew more slowly resulting in smaller adults (Tye *et al.*, 1993). In rats, it has been shown that a single very high dose of caffeine (120 mg/kg) reduces blood flow to the uterus and deciduas (Kimmel, 1984). In mice, adenosine A_{2A} receptor gene expression in uterus has been shown to be downregulated by maternal caffeine exposure (Momoi *et al.*, 2008). In addition, modest daily maternal caffeine exposure altered regional developing embryonic arterial blood flow and induced intrauterine growth retardation without impacting the maternal cardiovascular function or weight gain in mice. The observed hemodynamic alterations in fetus and uterus of mice after caffeine exposure are mediated by downregulation of adenosine A_{2A} receptors (Momoi *et al.*, 2008). The cardiac system appears as an early target of caffeine action. Mice dams treated with a single dose of caffeine (equivalent to 2 cups of coffee in humans) showed a 38% decrease in cardiac function of their pups in adulthood (Wendler *et al.*, 2009).

The ability of caffeine to cross the blood–brain barrier and its psychoactive action raise concerns about brain development effects of maternal caffeine intake. Long-term consumption of low doses of caffeine, representative of normal human intake, can inhibit hippocampal neurogenesis, astrocytogenesis and hippocampus-dependent learning and memory in rats (Desfrere *et al.*, 2007; Han *et al.*, 2007). In neonate rodents, caffeine in doses that are equal to those consumed by humans do not significantly influence the expression of adenosine receptors in the brain, while adult rodents exposed to high doses of caffeine show increase in adenosine A_1 receptor without changes in mRNA (Johansson *et al.*, 1993; Adén *et al.*, 2000). In addition, rodents with reduced number of adenosine A_1 receptors present a behavioral profile of hyperactivity, quite similar to normal mice exposed perinatally to caffeine (Björklund *et al.*, 2008).

The glutamatergic system can be also affected by chronic caffeine exposure in early life. Rats treated during the gestational and lactational period with caffeine presented markedly reduced response to the classical hyper locomotor effect of MK-801 (dizocilpine maleate), an inhibitor of NMDA glutamate receptor (Da Silva *et al.*, 2005).

RISK ASSESSMENT

Although caffeine has GRAS status from USFDA and falls into the category of functional foods, its risk assessment appears to be complex. This is because it affects multiple physiological functions in several vital organs. Risk assessment of caffeine becomes further complicated when dealing with (1) reproductive and developmental effects, and (2) multiple confounding factors, such as concurrent exposure to smoke, alcohol and other abused drugs.

Caffeine is present in a wide range of dietary products, i.e. coffee, tea, cocoa beverages, energy drinks, chocolate bars, soft drinks, maté, caffeinated water, gums and others. The content of caffeine in coffee ranges from 40 to 180 mg/150 ml, in tea from 24 to 50 mg/150 ml, in soft drinks from 15 to 29 mg/180 ml, in cocoa beverages from 2 to 7 mg/150 ml, in chocolate bars 1 to 36 mg/28 g, in maté approximately 160 mg/L (Fredholm *et al.*, 1999).

Coffee is the most common source of caffeine. There are three main types of coffee according to the preparation method conducted, which are: boiled unfiltered coffee, filtered coffee and decaffeinated coffee, the latter primarily consumed as instant coffee. Three ingredients of coffee have physiological importance, which are caffeine, the diterpene alcohols (cafestol and kahweol), chlorogenic acid and other polyphenols (Gilbert *et al.*, 1976). A cup (150 ml) of home prepared coffee contains between 30 and 175 mg. In specialty coffees consumed usually outside home the range is 18–80 mg/cup and for decaffeinated coffees the average is 5 mg/cup (McCusker *et al.*, 2003). The diterpenoid alcohols are the oils in coffee and their concentration depends on how the coffee is prepared. Filtered coffee has less than 0.1 mg/100 ml (i.e., essentially none) and unfiltered coffee can have between 0.2 and 18 mg/100 ml depending on the method of preparation. Boiled coffee has a higher concentration of coffee oils because of the higher temperature used during its preparation and a longer contact time between the coffee grounds and water.

During pregnancy, caffeine is considered the most consumed xenobiotic. The United Kingdom government's Food

Standards Agency (Committee on Toxicity, 2001) and the USFDA considered that caffeine intake during pregnancy is safe up to 300 mg/person/day. In a study performed in the United Kingdom, the assessment of caffeine exposure by pregnant women showed the profile of caffeine sources during pregnancy: 62% from tea, 14% from coffee, 12% from cola drinks, 8% from chocolate bars, 2% from soft drinks and 2% from other sources such as hot chocolates and energy drinks (CARE Study Group, 2008). In the same study, total caffeine consumption by women was shown to be 238 mg/day before pregnancy, 139 mg/day from week 5 until the third trimester, when it gradually increased to 153 mg/day.

Pregnant women who consume four or more cups of coffee/day do not appear to increase the risk of preterm delivery (Berkowitz *et al.*, 1982; Leviton and Cowan, 2002; Grosso *et al.*, 2006). However, women who consume eight or more cups of coffee/day had nearly double the risk of spontaneous abortion compared to non-consumers of coffee (Tolstrup *et al.*, 2003; Wisborg *et al.*, 2003). Also, it is important to note that reduction of blood flow in placenta was found to be around 25% in pregnant women drinking caffeine (CARE Study Group, 2008).

Early caffeine exposure as a therapeutic measure and risk concern

Caffeine is a powerful respiratory stimulant acting mainly within the CNS. It is administered for several weeks or months as the main therapeutic agent to alleviate the apnea in prematures (Comer *et al.*, 2001). Even at moderate doses, maternal caffeine consumption, in spite of the absence of effects on basal respiratory parameters, may induce a series of subtle developmental alterations that may affect modulation of breathing control in neonates in pathological situations such as hypoxia (Picard *et al.*, 2008). It has been suggested that caffeine exposure may decrease the activity of the O_2-sensing peripheral chemoreceptor pathway and that functional alterations could be associated to increases in adenosine A_{2A} receptor and α_2 $GABA_A$ receptor subunit mRNAs in the medulla (Picard *et al.*, 2008).

Caffeine therapy also promotes successful extubation from invasive positive-pressure ventilation, and decreases the incidence of bronchopulmonary dysplasia (Davis *et al.*, 2010). The recommended dosing for caffeine is a loading dose of 20 mg/kg followed by a 5 mg/kg/day maintenance dose. Routine measurement of steady-state serum caffeine concentrations in infants (24 to 35 weeks gestational age) appears to be not required in the absence of ongoing apnea/hypopnea or signs compatible with toxicity (Millar and Schmidt, 2004; Leon *et al.*, 2007). The methylxanthine therapy for apnea of prematures increases oxygen consumption, but effects on growth, brain development and behavior of infants has been investigated without conclusive results (Millar and Schmidt, 2004).

Cross-sensitization with abused drugs

Cross-sensitization is the process by which taking out one drug enhances the response to other drugs acting at the same neurobiological site. Cross-sensitization is a concern because habitual use of licit drugs, such as caffeine or nicotine, may lead to cross-sensitization to illicit drugs and potentiate substance abuse (Horger *et al.*, 1991, 1992).

Caffeine pretreatment or co-administration increases the rate of cocaine self-administration in rats (Horger *et al.*, 1991; Schenk *et al.*, 1994). In non-human primates, a high dose of caffeine (1 mg/kg) pre-exposure led to an increased number of smoke deliveries (Schenk *et al.*, 1994). Rats pre-exposed to caffeine acquired nicotine self-administration significantly faster than controls (Shoaib *et al.*, 1999). In humans, caffeine and nicotine use have a high rate of co-occurrence (Puccio *et al.*, 1990; Kozlowski *et al.*, 1993; Strain *et al.*, 1994; Swanson *et al.*, 1994). A relationship between caffeine consumption and opiate addiction is suggested on the basis that methylxanthines induce a quasi-morphine withdrawal behavior in rats (Ribeiro *et al.*, 2003). However, this effect was related to PDE inhibition, which occurs in higher concentration than those reached by normal consumption of caffeine by humans (Ribeiro *et al.*, 2003).

The association between caffeine and other substances, such as nicotine and drugs of abuse, may be due to the effects of caffeine on the neural dopamine system, i.e. the neurobiological substrate of reward and reinforcement (Salim *et al.*, 2000; Fuxe *et al.*, 2003; Kudlacek *et al.*, 2003). One potential mechanism is that caffeine primes the dopamine system to respond to cocaine and other drugs of abuse such that drug dependence is established more quickly and perhaps at lower doses (Temple, 2009). Chronic caffeine exposure during adolescence in rats induces long-term cross-sensitization to methylphenidate, a psychostimulant drug used in pediatric and adult human populations to manage the symptoms associated with attention-deficit hyperactivity disorder (ADHD) (Boeck *et al.*, 2009). These authors also demonstrated that the cross-sensitization appears to exist in a DARPP-32-dependent pathway, since the levels of DARPP-32 increased in the striatum and prefrontal cortex.

There is growing body of evidence that caffeine intake and drug addiction are interesting features of possible subtle and prolonged effects of early caffeine exposition. Early exposure to psychostimulant drugs, such as caffeine, can promote neuronal "imprinting", meaning that the early exposure to a psychostimulant drug can result in later additive actions to other psychoactive drugs, as a result of mesolimbic dopamine system activation (Björklund *et al.*, 2008). Perinatal caffeine administration has been linked to enhanced response to cocaine, which displays several features mimicked by deletion of the adenosine A_1 receptor (Björklund *et al.*, 2007). Conversely, the deletion of one copy of the adenosine A_{2A} receptor gene reduces the response to cocaine, which has an interesting feature to treatment of drug addiction (Chen *et al.*, 2000; Björklund *et al.*, 2007).

TREATMENT

As caffeine intoxication occurs rarely and drug dependence or abstinence symptoms are weak or absent, the treatment for caffeine toxicity is poorly developed. Excessive intake of caffeine may produce a life-threatening condition with arrhythmias, pronounced hypokalemia and a risk of ventricular fibrillation. In case of counter-shock resistant ventricular fibrillation, it may be necessary to give a loading dose of an antiarrhythmic drug, such as amiodarone (Rudolph and Knudsen, 2010). Stimulation of enzymes, such as integral membrane protein Na^+-/K^+-ATPase, lowers plasma potassium levels (Holstege and Dobmeier, 2005). This stimulation results in a potassium shift from the blood to intracellular compartments making the membrane potential more negative, which increases the risk for ventricular arrhythmias. Thus, the replacement of serum potassium is important to recover the osmotic and ionic status (Rudolph and Knudsen, 2010). Also, epinephrine and buffer solutions used during resuscitation may further decrease blood potassium levels and should be administered cautiously. Epinephrine can be replaced by other vasopressor drugs, such as vasopressin, without effects on β-receptors. Finally, it is necessary to monitor plasma potassium levels frequently and plasma caffeine values to avoid a risky progress in the post-resuscitation period.

CONCLUDING REMARKS AND FUTURE DIRECTIONS

Caffeine is the most consumed psychostimulant drug with free access to all groups of people through a wide range of dietary and medicinal sources. Caffeine consumption and its effects on fecundability, fetal development and neonatal life have been thoroughly investigated for a long time. In studies with animals, several negative outcomes related to reproduction and development with caffeine exposure are reported. For example, decrease in birth weight, cardiovascular defects and behavioral sensitizations to illicit drugs have been observed. However, no animal study can predict accurately the caffeine effects in humans. Reproductive adversity in human population has no or few consistent association with normal levels of caffeine consumption, despite a vast literature regarding the issue. Even though reproductive-aged women and children are indicated to be at risk, subgroups that may require specific advice on moderating their caffeine intake is yet to be established (CARE Group, 2008; Kuczkowski, 2009).

REFERENCES

Abbracchio MP, Brambilla R, Ceruti S, Kim HO, Von Lubitz DKJE, Jacobson KA, Cattabeni F (1995) G protein-dependent activation of phospholipase C by adenosine A3 receptor in rat brain. *Mol Pharmacol* **48:** 1038–45.

Acquas E, Tanda G, Di Chiara G (2002) Differential effects of caffeine on dopamine and acetylcholine transmission in brain areas of drug-naive and caffeine-pretreated rats. *Neuropsychopharmacology* **27:** 182–93.

Adén U, Leverin AL, Hagberg H, Fredholm BB (2001) Adenosine A(1) receptor agonism in the immature rat brain and heart. *Eur J Pharmacol* **426:** 185–92.

Aley KO, Levine JD (1997) Multiple receptors involved in peripheral alpha 2, mu, and A_1 antinociception, tolerance and withdrawal. *J Neurosci* **17:** 735–44.

Aranda JV, Collinge JM, Zinman R, Watters G (1979) Maturation of caffeine elimination in infancy. *Arch Dis Child* **54:** 946–9.

Arendash GW, Cao C (2010) Caffeine and Coffee as therapeutics against Alzheimer's disease. *J Alzheimers Dis* **20** Suppl 1: S117–26.

Arnaud MJ, Welsch C (1982) Theophylline and caffeine metabolism in man. In *Theophylline and Other Methylxanthines*. Friedr Vieweg and Sons, pp. 135–48.

Arnaud MJ (1987) The pharmacology of caffeine. *Prog Drug Res* **31:** 273–313.

Arnaud MJ (1993) Metabolism of caffeine and other components of coffee. In *Caffeine, Coffee and Health*. Raven Press, pp. 43–95.

Balları'n M, Fredholm BB, Ambrosio S, Mahy N (1991) Extracellular levels of adenosine and its metabolites in the striatum of awake rats: inhibition of uptake and metabolism. *Acta Physiol Scand* **142:** 97–103.

Bech BH, Autrup H, Nohr EA, Henriksen TB, Olsen J (2006) Stillbirth and slow metabolizers of caffeine: comparison by genotypes. *Int J Epidemiol* **35:** 948–53.

Berkowitz GS, Holford TR, Berkowitz RL (1982) Effects of cigarette smoking, alcohol, coffee and tea consumption on preterm delivery. *Early Hum Dev* **7:** 239–50.

Bernstein GA, Carroll ME, Crosby RD, Perwien AR, Go FS, Benowitz NL (1994) Caffeine effects on learning, performance, and anxiety in normal school-age children. *J Am Acad Child Adolesc Psychiatry* **33:** 407–15.

Björklund O, Kahlström J, Salmi P, Ogren SO, Vahter M, Chen JF, Fredholm BB, Daré E (2007) The effects of methylmercury on motor activity are sex of adenosine receptors and caffeine administration. *Toxicology* **241:** 119–33.

Björklund O, Kahlström J, Salmi P, Fredholm BB (2008) Perinatal caffeine, acting on maternal adenosine A (1) receptors, causes long-lasting behavioral changes in mouse offspring. *PLoS One* **3:** e3977.

Black AM, Pandya S, Clark D, Armstrong EA, Yager JY (2008) Effect of caffeine and morphine on the developing pre-mature brain. *Brain Res* **1219:** 136–42.

Boeck CR, Marques VB, Valvassori SS, Constantino LC, Rosa DV, Lima FF, Romano-Silva MA, Quevedo J (2009) Early long-term exposure with caffeine induces cross-sensitization to methylphenidate with involvement of DARPP-32 in adulthood of rats. *Neurochem Int* **55:** 318–22.

Bolumar F, Olsen J, Rebagliato M, Bisanti L (1997) Caffeine intake and delayed conception: a European multicenter study on infertility and subfecundity. European Study Group on Infertility Subfecundity. *Am J Epidemiol* **145:** 324–34.

Bonita JS, Mandarano M, Shuta D, Vinson J (2007) Coffee and cardiovascular disease: in vitro, cellular, animal, and human studies. *Pharmacol Res* **55:** 187–98.

Browne ML (2006) Maternal exposure to caffeine and risk of congenital anomalies: a systematic review. *Epidemiology* **17:** 324–31.

Burnstock G (2008) Purinergic signalling and disorders of the central nervous system. *Nat Rev Drug Discov* **7:** 575–90.

CARE Study Group (2008) Maternal caffeine intake during pregnancy and risk of fetal growth restriction: a large prospective observational study. *BMJ* **337:** a2332.

Carrillo JA, Benitez J (1996) CYP1A2 activity, gender and smoking, as variables influencing the toxicity of caffeine. *Br J Clin Pharmacol* **41:** 605–8.

Carter AJ, O'Connor WT, Carter MJ, Ungerstedt U (1995) Caffeine enhances acetylcholine release in the hippocampus in vivo by a selective interaction with adenosine A1 receptors. *J Pharmacol Exp Ther* **273:** 637–42.

Cauli O, Morelli M (2005) Caffeine and the dopaminergic system. *Behav Pharmacol* **16:** 63–77.

Chen JF, Beilstein M, Xu YH, Turner TJ, Moratalla R, Standaert DG, Aloyo VJ, Fink JS, Schwarzschild MA (2000) Selective attenuation of psychostimulant-induced behavioral responses in mice lacking A (2A) adenosine receptors. *Neuroscience* **97:** 195–204.

Ciruela F, Escriche M, Burgueno J, Angulo E, Casado V, Soloviev MM, Canela EL, Mallol J, Chan WY, Lluis C, Mellhinney RA, Franco R (2001) Metabotropic glutamate 1 alpha and adenosine A1 receptors assemble into functionally interacting complexes. *J Biol Chem* **276:** 18345–51.

Comer AM, Perry CM, Figgitt DP (2001) Caffeine citrate: a review of its use in apnoea of prematurity. *Paediatr Drugs* **3:** 61–79.

Committee on Toxicity (2001) COT statement on the reproductive effects of caffeine. London: Committee on Toxicity of Chemicals in Food, Consumer Products and the Environment. http://cot.food.gov.uk/cotstatements/cot statemenstsyrs/cotstatements2001/caffeine.

Da Silva RS, Hoffman A, de Souza DO, Lara DR, Bonan CD (2005) Maternal caffeine intake impairs MK-801-induced hyperlocomotion in young rats. *Eur J Pharmacol* **509:** 155–9.

Daly JW (2007). Caffeine analogs: biomedical impact. *Cell Mol Life Sci* **64:** 2153–69.

Davis PG, Schmidt B, Roberts RS, Doyle LW, Asztalos E, Haslam R, Sinha S, Tin W; Caffeine for Apnea of Prematurity Trial Group (2010) Caffeine for Apnea of Prematurity trial: benefits may vary in subgroups. *J Pediatr* **156:** 382–7.

Desfrere L, Olivier P, Schwendimann L, Verney C, Gressens P (2007) Transient inhibition of astrocytogenesis in developing mouse brain following postnatal caffeine exposure. *Pediatr Res* **62:** 604–9.

Dews PB (1982) Caffeine. *Annu Rev Nutr* **2:** 323–41.

Dunwiddie TV, Masino SA (2001) The role and regulation of adenosine in the central nervous system. *Annu Rev Neurosci* **24:** 31–55.

Elkins RN, Rapoport JL, Zahn TP, Buchsbaum MS, Weingartner H, Kopin IJ, Langer D, Johnson C (1981) Acute effects of caffeine in normal prepubertal boys. *Am J Psychiatry* **138:** 178–83.

Fenster L, Quale C, Hiatt RA, Wilson M, Windham GC, Benowitz NL (1998) Rate of caffeine metabolism and risk of spontaneous abortion. *Am J Epidemiol* **147:** 503–10.

Ferré S, Ciruela F, Borycz J, Solinas M, Quarta D, Antoniou K, Quiroz C, Justinova Z, Lluis C, Franco R, Goldberg SR (2008) Adenosine A1-A2A receptor heteromers: new targets for caffeine in the brain. *Front Biosci* **13:** 2391–9.

Frary CD, Johnson RK, Wang MQ (2005) Food sources and intakes of caffeine in the diets of persons in the United States. *J Am Diet Assoc* **105:** 110–13.

Fredholm BB, Svenningsson P (2003) Adenosine–dopamine interactions: development of a concept and some comments on therapeutic possibilities. *Neurology* **61:** S5–S9.

Fredholm BB, Bättig K, Holmén J, Nehlig A, Zvartau EE (1999) Actions of caffeine in the brain with special reference to factors that contribute to its widespread use. *Pharmacol Rev* **51:** 83–133.

Fredholm BB, Chen JF, Cunha RA, Svenningsson P, Vaugeois JM (2005) Adenosine and brain function. *Int Rev Neurobiol* **63:** 191–270.

Fuxe K, Ferré S, Zoli M, Agnati LF (1998) Integrated events in central dopamine transmission as analyzed at multiple levels. Evidence for intramembrane adenosine A2A/dopamine D2 and adenosine A1/dopamine D1 receptor interactions in the basal ganglia. *Brain Res Brain Res Rev* **26:** 258–73.

Fuxe, K, Agnati, LF, Jacobsen K, Hillion J, Canals M, Torvinen M, Tinner-Staines B, Staines W, Rosin D, Terasmaa A, Popoli P, Leo G, Vergoni V, Lluis C, Ciruela, F., Franco R, Ferre S (2003) Receptor heteromerization in adenosine A2A receptor signaling: relevance for striatal function and Parkinson's disease. *Neurology* **61:** S19–S23.

Geleijnse JM (2008) Habitual coffee consumption and blood pressure: an epidemiological perspective. *Vasc Health Risk Manag* **4:** 963–70.

Geraets L, Moonen HJ, Wouters EF, Bast A, Hageman GJ (2006) Caffeine metabolites are inhibitors of the nuclear enzyme poly (ADP-ribose) polymerase-1 at physiological concentrations. *Biochem Pharmacol* **72:** 902–10.

Gilbert RM, Marshman JA, Schwieder M, Berg R (1976) Caffeine content of beverages as consumed. *Can Med Assoc J* **114:** 205–8.

Godel JC, Pabst HF, Hodges PE, Johnson KE, Froese GJ, Joffres MR (1992) Smoking and caffeine and alcohol intake during pregnancy in a northern population: effect on fetal growth. *CMAJ* **147:** 181–8.

Grosso LM, Triche EW, Belanger K, Benowitz NL, Holford TR, Bracken MB (2006) Caffeine metabolites in umbilical cord blood, cytochrome P-450 1A2 activity, and intrauterine growth restriction. *Am J Epidemiol* **163:** 1035–41.

Hakooz NM (2009) Caffeine metabolic ratios for the in vivo evaluation of CYP1A2, N-acetyltransferase 2, xanthine oxidase and CYP2A6 enzymatic activities. *Curr Drug Metab* **10:** 329–38.

Han ME, Park KH, Baek SY, Kim BS, Kim JB, Kim HJ, Oh SO (2007) Inhibitory effects of caffeine on hippocampal neurogenesis and function. *Biochem Biophys Res Commun* **356:** 976–80.

Holstege CP, Dobmeier S (2005) Cardiovascular challenges in toxicology emergency. *Med Clin North Am* **23:** 1195–217.

Homan DJ, Mobarhan S (2006) Coffee: good, bad, or just fun? A critical review of coffee's effects on liver enzymes. *Nutr Rev* **64:** 43–6.

Horger BA, Wellman PJ, Morien A, Davies BT, Schenk S (1991) Caffeine exposure sensitizes rats to the reinforcing effects of cocaine. *Neuroreport* **2:** 53–6.

Horger BA, Giles MK, Schenk S (1992) Preexposure to amphetamine and nicotine predisposes rats to self-administer a low dose of cocaine. *Psychopharmacology* **107:** 271–6.

Jajoo S, Mukherjea D, Watabe K, Ramkumar V (2009) Adenosine A (3) receptor suppresses prostate cancer metastasis by inhibiting NADPH oxidase activity. *Neoplasia* **11:** 1132–45.

Johansson B, Ahlberg S, Van der Ploeg I, Brené S, Lindefors N, Persson H, Fredholm BB (1993) Effect of long term caffeine treatment on A1 and A2 adenosine receptor binding and on mRNA levels in rat brain. *Naunyn-Schmiedebergs Arch Pharmacol* **347:** 407–14.

Kimmel CA, Kimmel GL, White CG, Grafton TF, Young JF, Nelson CJ (1984) Blood flow changes and conceptual development in pregnant rats in response to caffeine. *Fundam Appl Toxicol* **4:** 240–7.

Kinney A, Kline J, Kelly A, Reuss ML, Levin B (2007) Smoking, alcohol and caffeine in relation to ovarian age during the reproductive years. *Hum Reprod* **22:** 1175–85.

Kirkinen P, Jouppila P, Koivula A, Vuori J, Puukka M (1983) The effect of caffeine on placental and fetal blood flow in human pregnancy. *Am J Obstet Gynecol* **147:** 939–42.

Klebanoff MA, Levine RJ, Clemens JD, Wilkins DG (2002) Maternal serum caffeine metabolites and small-for-gestational age birth. *Am J Epidemiol* **155:** 32–7.

Klebanoff MA, Zhang J, Zhang C, Levine RJ (2009) Maternal serum theobromine and the development of preeclampsia. *Epidemiology* **20:** 727–32.

Kot M, Daniel WA (2008) Caffeine as a marker substrate for testing cytochrome P450 activity in human and rat. *Pharmacol Rep* **60:** 789–97.

Kozlowski LT, Henningfield JE, Keenan RM, Lei H, Leigh G, Jelinek LC, Pope MA, Haertzen CA (1993) Patterns of alcohol, cigarette, and caffeine and other drug use in two drug abusing populations. *J Subst Abuse Treat* **10:** 171–9.

Kuczkowski KM (2009) Peripartum implications of caffeine intake in pregnancy: is there cause for concern? *Rev Esp Anestesiol Reanim* **56:** 612–15.

Kudlacek O, Just H, Korkhov VM, Vartian N, Klinger M, Pankevych H, Yang Q, Nanoff C, Freissmuth M, Boehm S (2003) The human D2 dopamine receptor synergizes with the A2A adenosine receptor to stimulate adenylyl cyclase inPC12 cells. *Neuropsychopharmacology* **28:** 1317–27.

Kull B, Svenningsson P, Fredholm BB (2000) Adenosine A_{2A} receptors are co-localized with and activate G_{olf} in rat striatum. *Mol Pharmacol* **58:** 63–75.

Lane JD, Adcock RA, Williams RB, Kuhn CM (1990) Caffeine effects on cardiovascular and neuroendocrine responses to acute psychosocial stress and their relationship to level of habitual caffeine consumption. *Psychosom Med* **52:** 320–36.

Lee C (2000) Antioxidant ability of caffeine and its metabolites based on the study of oxygen radical absorbing capacity and inhibition of LDL peroxidation. *Clin Chim Acta* **295:** 141–54.

Leon AE, Michienzi K, Ma CX, Hutchison AA (2007) Serum caffeine concentrations in preterm neonates. *Am J Perinatol* **24:** 39–47.

Leviton A, Cowan L (2002) A review of the literature relating caffeine consumption by women to their risk of reproductive hazards. *Food Chem Toxicol* **40:** 1271–310.

Lindskog M, Svenningsson P, Pozzi L, Kim Y, Fienberg AA, Bibb JA, Fredholm BB, Nairn AC, Greengard P, Fisone G (2002). Involvement of DARPP-32 phosphorylation in the stimulant action of caffeine. *Nature* **418:** 774–8.

Linnet KM, Dalsgaard S, Obel C, Wisborg K, Henriksen TB, Rodriguez A, Kotimaa A, Moilanen I, Thomsen PH, Olsen J, Jarvelin MR (2003) Maternal lifestyle factors in pregnancy risk of attention deficit hyperactivity disorder and associated behaviors: review of the current evidence. *Am J Psychiatry* **160:** 1028–40.

Madi L, Bar-Yehuda S, Barer F, Ardon E, Ochaion A, Fishman P (2003) A3 adenosine receptor activation in melanoma cells: association between receptor fate and tumor growth inhibition. *J Biol Chem* **278:** 42121–30.

Martin TR, Bracken MB (1987) The association between low birth weight and caffeine consumption during pregnancy. *Am J Epidemiol* **126:** 813–21.

McCusker RR, Goldberger BA, Cone EJ (2003) Caffeine content of specialty coffees. *J Anal Toxicol* **27:** 520–2.

Millar D, Schmidt B (2004) Controversies surrounding xanthine therapy. *Semin Neonatol* **9:** 239–44.

Minelli A, Liguori L, Bellazza I, Mannucci R, Johansson B, Fredholm BB (2004) Involvement of A1 adenosine receptors in the acquisition of fertilizing capacity. *J Androl* **25:** 286–92.

Momoi N, Tinney JP, Liu LJ, Elshershari H, Hoffmann PJ, Ralphe JC, Keller BB, Tobita K (2008) Modest maternal caffeine exposure affects developing embryonic cardiovascular function and growth. *Am J Physiol Heart Circ Physiol* **294:** H2248–H2256.

Murphy JA, Deurveilher S, Semba K (2003) Stimulant doses of caffeine induce c-FOS activation in orexin/hypocretin-containing neurons in rat. *Neuroscience* **121:** 269–75.

Nehlig A, Debry G (1994) Potential teratogenic and neurodevelopmental consequences of coffee and caffeine exposure: a review on human and animal data. *Neurotoxicol Teratol* **16:** 531–43.

Nehlig A, Daval JL, Debry G (1992) Caffeine and the central nervous system: mechanisms of action, biochemical, metabolic and psychostimulant effects. *Brain Res Brain Res Rev* **17:** 139–70.

Ohana G, Bar-Yehuda S, Arich A, Madi L, Dreznick Z, Rath-Wolfson L, Silberman D, Slosman G, Fishman P (2003) Inhibition of primary colon carcinoma growth and liver metastasis by the A3 adenosine receptor agonist CF101. *Br J Cancer* **89:** 1552–8.

Picard N, Guénin S, Larnicol N, Perrin Y (2008) Maternal caffeine ingestion during gestation and lactation influences respiratory adaptation to acute alveolar hypoxia in newborn rats and adenosine A2A and GABA A receptor mRNA transcription. *Neuroscience* **156:** 630–9.

Puccio EM, McPhillips JB, Barrett-Connor E, Ganiats TG (1990) Clustering of atherogenic behaviors in coffee drinkers. *Am J Public Health* **80:** 1310–13.

Purves D, Sutherland FM (1993) *Caffeine, Coffee and Health.* Reven Press, pp. 318–42.

Ralevic V, Burnstock G (1998) Receptors for purines and pyrimidines. *Pharmacol Rev* **50:** 413–92.

Ramlau-Hansen CH, Thulstrup AM, Bonde JP, Olsen J, Bech BH (2008) Semen quality according to prenatal coffee and present caffeine exposure: two decades of follow-up of a pregnancy cohort. *Hum Reprod* **23:** 2799–805.

Rapoport JL, Elkins R, Neims A, Zahn T, Berg CJ (1981) Behavioral and autonomic effects of caffeine in normal boys. *Dev Pharmacol Ther* **3:** 74–82.

Ribeiro JA, Sebastião AM, Mendonça A (2003) Participation of adenosine receptors in neuroprotection. *Drugs News Perspect* **16:** 80–6.

Rimondini R, Ferré S, Gimenez-Llort L, Ogren SO, Fuxe K (1998) Differential effects of selective adenosine A1 and A2A receptor agonists on dopamine receptor agonist-induced behavioural responses in rats. *Eur J Pharmacol* **347:** 153–8.

Ritchie JM (1975) The xanthenes. In *The Pharmacological Basis of Therapeutics*. Macmillan, pp. 367–76.

Rivenes SM, Bakerman PR, Miller MB (1997) Intentional caffeine poisoning in an infant. *Pediatrics* **99:** 736–8.

Rivkees SA, Zhao Z, Porter G, Turner C (2001) Influences of adenosine on the fetus and newborn. *Mol Genet Metab* **74:** 160–71.

Robertson D, Johnson GA, Robertson RM, Nies AS, Shand DG, Oates JA (1979) Comparative assessment of stimuli that release neuronal and adrenomedullary catecholamines in man. *Circulation* **59:** 637–43.

Ross GW, Abbott RD, Petrovitch H, Morens DM, Grandinetti A, Tung KH, Tanner CM, Masaki KH, Blanchette PL, Curb JD, Popper JS, White LR (2000) Association of coffee and caffeine intake with the risk of Parkinson disease. *JAMA* **283:** 2674–9.

Rudolph T, Knudsen K (2010) A case of fatal caffeine poisoning. *Acta Anaesthesiol Scand* **54:** 904–5.

Sahin B, Galdi S, Hendrick J, Greene RW, Snyder GL, Bibb JA (2007) Evaluation of neuronal phosphoproteins as effectors of caffeine and mediators of striatal adenosine A2A receptor signaling. *Brain Res* **1129:** 1–14.

Salim H, Ferre S, Dalal A, Peterfreund RA, Fuxe K, Vincent JD, Lledo PM (2000) Activation of adenosine A1 and A2A receptors modulates dopamine D2 receptor-induced responses in stably transfected human neuroblastoma cells. *J Neurochem* **74:** 432–9.

Schenk S, Valadez A, Horger BA, Snow S, Wellman PJ (1994) Interactions between caffeine and cocaine in tests of self-administration. *Behav Pharmacol* **5:** 153–8.

Schmidt RJ, Romitti PA, Burns TL, Browne ML, Druschel CM, Olney RS (2009) National Birth Defects Prevention Study; maternal caffeine consumption and risk of neural tube defects. *Birth Defects Res A Clin Mol Teratol* **85:** 879–989.

Sebastião AM, Ribeiro JA (2009) Adenosine receptors and central nervous system. *Eur J Pharmacol* **623:** 41–6.

Shoaib M, Swanner LS, Yasar S, Goldberg SR (1999) Chronic caffeine exposure potentiates nicotine self-administration in rats. *Psychopharmacology (Berl)* **142:** 327–33.

Solinas M, Ferré S, You ZB, Karcz-Kubicha M, Popoli P, Goldberg S (2002) Caffeine induces dopamine and glutamate release in the shell of the nucleus accumbens. *J Neurosci* **22:** 6321–4.

Stein Z, Susser M (1991) Miscarriage, caffeine, and the epiphenomena of pregnancy: the causal model. *Epidemiology* **2:** 163–7.

Strain EC, Mumford GK, Silverman K, Griffiths RR (1994) Caffeine dependence syndrome. Evidence from case histories and experimental evaluations. *JAMA* **272:** 1043–8.

Svenningsson P, Nairn AC, Greengard P (2005) DARPP-32 mediates the actions of multiple drugs of abuse. *AAPS J* **7:** E353–E360.

Swanson JA, Lee JW, Hopp JW (1994) Caffeine and nicotine: a review of their joint use and possible interactive effects in tobacco withdrawal. *Addict Behav* **19:** 229–56.

Temple JL (2009) Caffeine use in children: what we know, what we have left to learn, and why we should worry. *Neurosci Biobehav Rev* **33:** 793–806.

Tolstrup JS, Kjaer SK, Munk C, Madsen LB, Ottesen B, Bergholt T, Grønbaek M (2003) Does caffeine and alcohol intake before pregnancy predict the occurrence of spontaneous abortion? *Hum Reprod* **18:** 2704–10.

Turner DJ, Segura BJ, Cowles RA, Zhang W, Mulholland MW (2001) Functional overlap of IP (3)- and cADP-ribose-sensitive calcium stores in guinea pig myenteric neurons. *Am J Physiol Gastrointest Liver Physiol* **281:** G208–G215.

Turner CP, Yan H, Schwartz M, Othman T, Rivkees SA (2002) A1 adenosine receptor activation induces ventriculomegaly and white matter loss. *Neuroreport* **13:** 1199–204.

Tye K, Pollard I, Karlsson L, Scheibner V, Tye G (1993) Caffeine exposure in utero increases the incidence of apnea in adult rats. *Reprod Toxicol* **7:** 449–52.

Van Dam RM, Feskens EJ (2002) Coffee consumption and risk of type 2 diabetes mellitus. *Lancet* **360:** 1477–8.

Warszawski D, Gorodischer R, Kaplanski J (1978) Comparative toxicity of caffeine and aminophylline (theophylline ethylenediamine) in young and adult rats. *Biol Neonate* **34:** 68–71.

Weathersbee PS, Olsen LK, Lodge JR (1977) Caffeine and pregnancy. A retrospective survey. *Postgrad Med* **62:** 64–9.

Weaver DR (1996) A1-adenosine receptor gene expression in fetal rat brain. *Brain Res Dev Brain Res* **94:** 205–23.

Wendler CC, Busovsky-McNeal M, Ghatpande S, Kalinowski A, Russell KS, Rivkees SA (2009) Embryonic caffeine exposure induces adverse effects in adulthood. *FASEB J* **23:** 1272–8.

Whitfield K, Rambaldi A, Wetterslev J, Gluud C (2009) Pentoxifylline for alcoholic hepatitis. *Cochrane Database Syst Rev* **4:** CD007339.

Wisborg K, Kesmodel U, Bech BH, Hedegaard M, Henriksen TB (2003) Coffee and stillbirth. *Tidsskr Nor Laegeforen* **123:** 1911.

Zhao Z, Rivkees SA (2001) Inhibition of cell proliferation in the embryonic myocardium by A1 adenosine receptor activation. *Dev Dyn* **221:** 194–200.

Section 6

Food Additives, Nutraceuticals and Pharmaceuticals

CHAPTER

28

Melamine and cyanuric acid

Karyn Bischoff

INTRODUCTION

Melamine (1,3,5-triazine-2,4,6-triamine) is a small nitrogen-rich molecule used in the manufacture of plastics, adhesives, cleaners and yellow dye. Though once considered practically non-toxic based on early laboratory animal studies, significant morbidity and mortality related to crystalluria, nephrolithiasis and nephrotoxicity have resulted from illicit use of melamine as a feed and food ingredient. Melamine and co-contaminant cyanuric acid were responsible for the largest pet food recall in US history in 2007, and similar recalls occurred in Asia and South Africa. One year later, several infants and young children died and many more were sickened in China due to the addition of melamine to baby formula. Although transitional cell carcinoma has been seen in laboratory rats on chronic melamine dosing studies, there is currently no evidence of mutagenic effects or teratogenicity associated with melamine. Developmental effects on the kidneys of exposed children remain to be determined.

HISTORICAL BACKGROUND

Melamine (1,3,5-triazine-2,4,6-triamine), which contains three carbon atoms, six nitrogen atoms and six hydrogen atoms, was first synthesized in the 1830s and has found numerous uses in manufacturing. Melamine is polymerized with formaldehyde to produce a variety of durable resins, adhesives, cleansers and flame retardants. Melamine is also a major ingredient in the pigment Yellow 150, used in textile dyes and inks. Melamine is listed by the Organization for Economic Cooperation and Development (OECD, 2009) as a high production volume chemical. Cyanuric acid, an intermediate produced during melamine manufacture and degradation, is commonly used to stabilize chlorine in swimming pools. Structural formulas of melamine and cyanuric acid are shown in Figure 28.1.

The protein content of foods and feeds is estimated based on the nitrogen content, which is usually measured using the Kjeldahl method. Though considered an illegal adulterant when added to food or feed in the USA, scrap melamine is an inexpensive source of nitrogen. Because melamine is 67% nitrogen based on the molecular weight, its addition to foodstuff increases the nitrogen content and thus the estimated protein content.

Early in 2007, there were several reports of renal failure in cats and dogs consuming commercial pet foods in the USA. Clinical signs included inappetence, vomiting, polyuria, polydipsia and lethargy. Affected animals included cats that were on feeding trials (Cianciolo *et al.*, 2008). The pet food was recalled on March 15 of that year. Melamine was detected in the food 2 weeks later, but the significance was questioned because of melamine's low oral toxicity based on early studies in rodents and dogs. Later, additional contaminants were also detected (Dobson *et al.*, 2008). These contaminants, cyanuric acid, ammelide and ammeline, are intermediates in the production of melamine from urea and in its degradation. The US Food and Drug Administration (FDA) investigation determined that two common pet food ingredients, sold to manufacturers as wheat gluten and rice protein concentrate, were mislabeled by Chinese exporters to avoid inspection. These products actually contained wheat flour and poor quality rice protein mixed with melamine (Osborne *et al.*, 2008). Eventually, >150 pet food products were identified as containing contaminated ingredients and were recalled. Analysis revealed that these products contained up to approximately 3,200 ppm melamine and 600 ppm cyanuric acid (Cianciolo *et al.*, 2008; Skinner *et al.*, 2010). Samples of the imported wheat gluten contained 8.4% melamine, 5.3% cyanuric acid and 2.3 and 1.7% ammelide and ammeline, respectively (Rumbeiha *et al.*, 2010).

Cats and dogs ingesting the contaminated food had evidence of renal failure. Clinical signs included inappetence, vomiting, polyuria, polydipsia and lethargy. Cats had urine specific gravities <1.035 g/ml and elevated serum urea nitrogen and creatinine concentrations. Urinalysis revealed the presence of circular green-brown crystals in urine sediment. Postmortem examination of animals that died typically noted bilateral renomegaly and evidence of uremia. Microscopic lesions were found primarily in the kidneys. Renal tubular necrosis with evidence of rupture and regeneration were present. Distal convoluted tubules contained large golden-brown birefringent crystals (15 to 80 micrometers in diameter) with centrally radiating striations, sometimes in concentric rings, and smaller amorphous crystals (Figure 28.2) (Cianciolo *et al.*, 2008; Thompson *et al.*, 2008). Crystals were spherical with a hedgehog-like appearance on images from scanning electron microscopy (Figure 28.3). Crystals were still present

Reproductive and Developmental Toxicology, Edited by Ramesh C. Gupta
ISBN: 978-0-12-382032-7

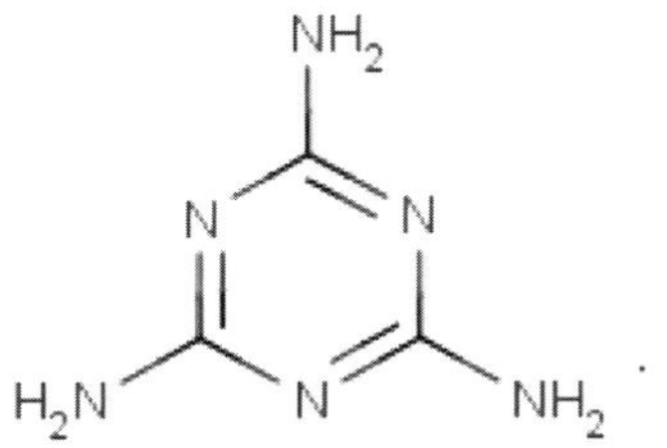

MELAMINE

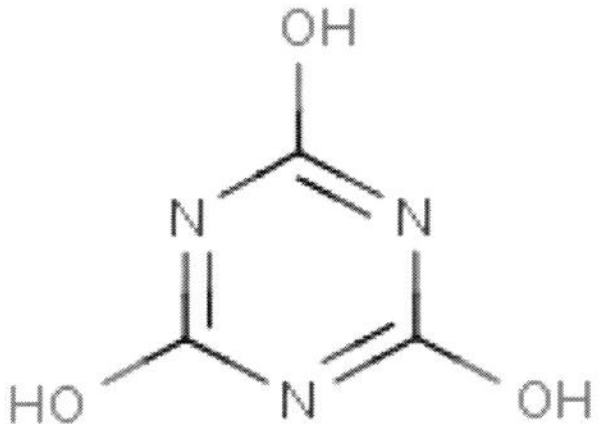

CYANURIC ACID

FIGURE 28.1 Structural formulas of melamine and cyanuric acid.

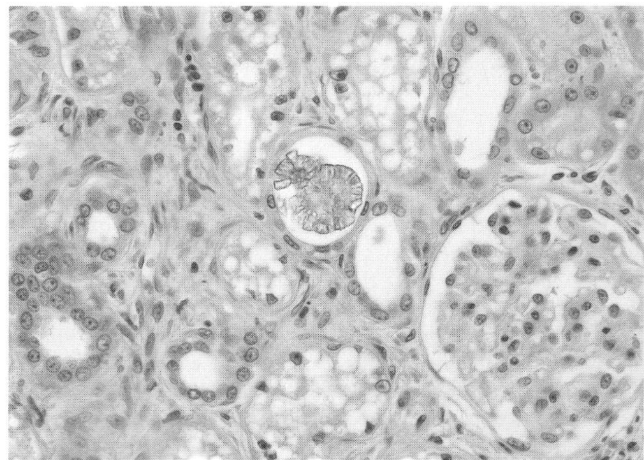

FIGURE 28.2 Crystal in the distal convoluted tubules of a feline kidney. Please note that vacuolation of renal tubular epithelial cells is an expected finding in cats and not related to the pathology of melamine and cyanuric acid. (Photo courtesy of Dr. R. Cianciolo, Comparative Biomedical Sciences North Carolina State University.)

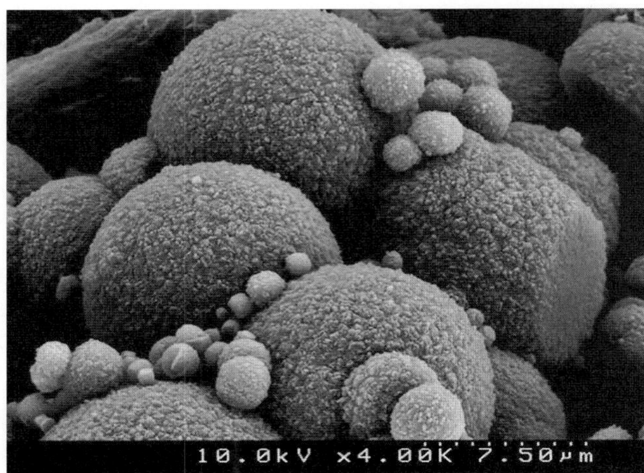

FIGURE 28.3 Scanning electron micrograph of melamine and cyanuric acid crystals from feline urine. (Courtesy of Dr. B. Hoff, University of Guelph.)

in distal convoluted tubules 8 weeks after cessation of exposure to contaminated feed (Cianciolo *et al.*, 2008). Crystals from kidneys and urine contained 70% cyanuric acid and 30% melamine based on infrared spectra (Osborne *et al.*, 2009; Thompson *et al.*, 2008).

There is no way to determine the number of cats and dogs affected by the pet food recalls because the USA lacks central reporting of morbidity and mortality for companion animals. Furthermore, many cats and dogs go without veterinary care or, after death, postmortem examination. Estimates of the numbers of pets affected in the 2007 US outbreak vary depending on the source. A large animal hospital chain estimated 39,000 cats and dogs were affected (Osborne *et al.*, 2009). Analysis of 586 cases reported by veterinarians and accredited veterinary diagnostic laboratories found 451 cases matching the case definition of melamine toxicosis: 65.5% were cats and 34.4% were dogs. Older animals and animals with preexisting conditions were less likely to survive, and 73.3% of affected dogs and 61.5% of affected cats died (Rumbeiha *et al.*, 2010). However, >80% of exposed cats during the original feeding trials survived, suggesting that not all exposed cats become clinically affected (Cianciolo *et al.*, 2008).

Previous outbreaks of renal failure associated with pet food were investigated and determined to be associated with melamine. An incident in 2004 was estimated to have affected more than 6,000 dogs and cats in the Republic of Korea, Japan, Thailand, Malaysia, Singapore, Taiwan and the Philippines. Earlier in 2007, there was a melamine-associated pet food recall in South Africa (Osborne *et al.*, 2009; Yhee *et al.*, 2009). Aside from pet food, feeds for chickens, hogs and fish were also found to be contaminated (Reimschuessel *et al.*, 2009, 2008). Melamine contaminated pet food scraps were fed on hog farms in seven US states and contaminated feeds were traced to 38 poultry farms and at 197 fish hatcheries (Acheson, 2007; Anonymous, 2010). Investigation of renal failure in piglets in Spain between 2003 and 2006 found that the kidneys contained melamine, cyanuric acid and relatively high concentrations of the related contaminants ammelide and ammeline (Gonzalez *et al.*, 2009). Hundreds of fur-bearing raccoon dogs in China died after being fed melamine-contaminated feeds in 2008 (Bhalla *et al.*, 2009).

The 2007 pet food recall was considered a sentinel event by some (Lewin-Smith *et al.*, 2009; Osborne *et al.*, 2009). Indeed one year later melamine contamination of milk-based products, particularly baby formula, was detected in China. Chinese authorities detected melamine concentrations between 2.5 and 2,563 ppm in 13 commercial brands of milk powder and trace contamination in nine others (Bhalla *et al.*, 2009). Approximately 300,000 children may have been affected, more than 52,000 were hospitalized and six died (Gossner *et al.*, 2009). After acknowledging this food-contamination incident, direct communication between the Chinese Ministry of Health and the World Health Organization (WHO) led to information sharing through the WHO/Food and Agricultural Organization International Food Safety authorities Network (INFOSAN). Children in Taiwan, Hong Kong and Macau may also have been affected (Skinner *et al.*, 2010; Reimschuessel *et al.*, 2009; Hau *et al.*, 2009). Due to global marketing of products and ingredients, melamine-contaminated products were found in almost 70 countries, including the USA.

Clinical signs of renal failure in children who consumed contaminated milk products included increased or reduced frequency of urination or anuria, stranguria, hematuria and the presence of stones in the urine, or unexplained crying, but many children were asymptomatic (Wen *et al.*, 2010; Hau *et al.*, 2009; Hu *et al.*, 2010). Studies estimated that renal damage occurred in 0.61 to 8.5% of exposed children (Liu *et al.*, 2010).

The outbreak of melamine-induced nephropathy in children was different from the outbreak in companion animals and livestock in that cyanuric acid and other compounds related to melamine were not important contaminants and were not required for crystal formation. Crystals associated with nephrotoxicosis in these infants contained melamine and uric acid at a molar ratio of 1:1–2, respectively (Skinner *et al.*, 2010; Wen *et al.*, 2010).

PHARMACOKINETICS/ TOXICOKINETICS

Melamine, and its structural analog cyanuric acid, are rapidly absorbed and rapidly excreted almost completely unmetabolized in the urine. Melamine does not accumulate over time in the animal body. Melamine is about 90% eliminated within 1 day by the kidneys (Qin *et al.*, 2010). The half-life for urinary elimination of melamine is 6 hours in dogs (Lipschetz and Stokey, 1945). Therefore, melamine should be almost completely excreted within 2 days of the last exposure; however, crystals were seen microscopically in feline kidneys 8 weeks after dietary exposure to melamine and cyanuric acid (Cianciolo *et al.*, 2008).

Detectable melamine concentrations have been reported in edible tissues from animals. Melamine concentrations in the kidney were higher than concentrations in the skeletal muscle or liver of lambs, and concentrations decreased below 20 ppb 4 days after cessation of exposure. Addition of cyanuric acid to the diet did not affect melamine deposition (Lv *et al.*, 2010). Similarly, highest melamine concentrations were found in the kidneys of chickens fed melamine-containing diets, with lower concentrations in the liver and muscle. Tissue residues were depleted 10 to 20 days after exposure ceased (Bai *et al.*, 2010). Melamine concentrations were detected in catfish and trout within 1 day of dosing, with half-lives in skeletal muscle ranging from 1.5 to 4 days (Reimschuessel, 2009).

Melamine is excreted by dairy cattle into milk, particularly in high producing cattle, though milk yield and composition are otherwise unaffected. Melamine can be detected in milk within 8 hours of exposure and remains detectable until 4 days after cessation of exposure. Transfer efficiency from feed to milk was calculated to be between 0.66 and 0.95% and was not dependent on melamine dose (Shen *et al.*, 2010). Melamine fed to chickens is deposited within eggs within a day or two post-exposure (Chen *et al.*, 2010; Bai *et al.*, 2010). The melamine concentration in eggs is proportional to the dietary concentration; a dietary concentration of 164 ppm could produce an actionable melamine concentration in eggs (2.5 ppm) (Chen *et al.*, 2010).

MECHANISM OF ACTION

Cats and dogs ingesting contaminated food with melamine and cyanuric acid had evidence of renal failure (Dobson *et al.*, 2008). Clinical signs included inappetence, vomiting, polyuria, polydipsia and lethargy. Cats had urine specific gravities <1.035 and elevated serum urea nitrogen and creatinine concentrations. Urinalysis revealed the presence of circular green-brown crystals in urine sediment. Postmortem findings from animals that died typically included bilateral renomegaly and evidence of uremia (Cianciolo *et al.*, 2008; Thompson *et al.*, 2008).

Microscopic lesions were found primarily in the kidneys. Renal tubular necrosis with evidence of rupture and regeneration were present. Distal convoluted tubules contained large golden-brown birefringent crystals (15 to 80 micrometers in diameter, Figure 28.2) with centrally radiating striations, sometimes in concentric rings, and smaller amorphous crystals (Cianciolo *et al.*, 2008; Thompson *et al.*, 2008). Perivascular inflammation of subcapsular veins was reported. Crystals were still present in distal convoluted tubules up to 8 weeks after cessation of exposure (Cianciolo *et al.*, 2008).

Crystals from kidneys and urine contained 70% cyanuric acid and 30% melamine based on infrared spectra results (Osborne *et al.*, 2009; Thompson *et al.*, 2008). Melamine/cyanuric acid crystals could be differentiated from more common types of urinary crystals based on morphology and histochemistry or special staining. Von Kossa stains calcium oxalate and calcium phosphate crystals and Alizarin red S at $4.1 \leq pH \leq 4.3$ stains calcium phosphate crystals only, but neither stains melamine/cyanuric acid crystals. Oil red O, usually used to identify lipids, stains melamine/cyanuric acid crystals but not calcium oxalate or calcium phosphate crystals.

Though previous animal studies found that both melamine and cyanuric acid were relatively non-toxic when given individually, they caused crystal formation in renal tubules when given together. Melamine and cyanuric acid crystallize, forming a lattice structure at the molecular level, at a pH of 5.8 (Osborne *et al.*, 2009; Bhalla *et al.*, 2009). Crystals form in the distal convoluted tubules of the kidneys. Renal pathology is believed to result from intratubular obstruction causing increased intrarenal pressure. This may be the explanation of the hemorrhage and inflammation reported in cats and dogs. Since melamine has diuretic properties, prerenal azotemia could have contributed to the renal pathology (Bhalla *et al.*, 2009).

Clinical signs of renal failure in children that consumed contaminated milk products were relatively subtle and nondescript. The most common symptoms described in these children were increased or reduced frequency of urination or anuria, stranguria and unexplained crying (Hau *et al.*, 2009; Wen *et al.*, 2010). Hematuria and the presence of stones in urine were also reported (Hau *et al.*, 2009). Many children were asymptomatic (Hu *et al.*, 2010). Confirmation of the diagnosis was based on the history of exposure, detection of melamine in the urine by analytical methods, observation of fan-shaped crystals in urine sediment or the presence of uroliths on ultrasound examination (Hau *et al.*, 2009; Wen *et al.*, 2010). Melamine uroliths are radiolucent, therefore radiographs were not helpful. However, uroliths could be seen on computed tomography (Hau *et al.*, 2009; Wen *et al.*, 2010).

Children developed urolithiasis after consuming contaminated formula for 3 to 6 months and almost all were not yet 3 years old. Most affected children were between 6 and 18 months of age (Skinner *et al.*, 2010; Wen *et al.*, 2010). Stones ranged in size from 2 to 18 mm in diameter, and approximately half were <5 mm in diameter. Diameter of the stone was dependent on the concentration of melamine in the diet, but not on the duration of exposure (Hu *et al.*, 2010). Renal calculi were usually bilateral, and calculi were also found in the ureter, unilaterally or bilaterally, and in the urinary bladder (Gao and Shen, 2010; Hau *et al.*, 2009; Wen *et al.*, 2010). A renal biopsy from an affected child had glomerular sclerosis, swelling and necrosis of renal tubular epithelium, tubular dilation with the presence of material consistent with a crystal, and an interstitial lymphoplasmacytic infiltrate. These changes were hypothesized to be due to urinary tract obstruction. Tubular changes resolved after treatment (Sun *et al.*, 2010).

Clinical pathology findings in affected infants included elevated serum potassium, urea nitrogen and creatinine concentrations (Sun *et al.*, 2010). Hematuria and the presence of fan-shaped crystals were reported in urine samples and urine pH ranged from 5.0 to 7.5 (Hau *et al.*, 2009).

Cyanuric acid did not contribute to the formation of urinary calculi in children as it did in companion animals (Gao and Shen, 2010). However, calculi in children were produced by a similar interaction between melamine and uric acid. This interaction has also been reported in poultry (Bai *et al.*, 2010). Humans and most other primates lack the enzyme uricase, which converts uric acid to allantoin (Reimschuessel *et al.*, 2008). Compared to adults, human infants excrete between five and eight times as much uric acid, which may increase their susceptibility to melamine toxicosis (Skinner *et al.*, 2010). Urinary pH <5.5 is associated with the formation of urate crystals and low pH is believed to be involved in melamine/urate crystal formation (Gao and Shen, 2010).

TOXICITY

General toxicity

As mentioned previously, melamine was believed to have a relatively low toxicity based on animal studies. The oral LD_{50} of melamine is 3,200 mg/kg in male rats, 3,800 mg/kg in female rats, 3,300 mg/kg in male mice and 7,000 mg/kg in female mice. Long-term administration of melamine to laboratory rodents at concentrations ranging from 0.225 to 0.9% of the diet produces urolithiasis. Lesions in the urinary bladder, including transitional cell carcinoma, were observed in rats fed diets containing 0.45% melamine (Melnick *et al.*, 1984). Urolithiasis was consistently identified in rats fed diets containing 0.3 to 3.0% melamine (Okumura *et al.*, 1992). Urolithiasis/nephrolithiasis was also a consistent finding in Chinese infants receiving melamine-contaminated powdered milk (Ji *et al.*, 2009; Langman, 2009). Renal cortical fibrosis and lymphoplasmacytic nephritis were reported in female rats fed diets containing 0.45% melamine (Melnick *et al.*, 1984).

Sheep were given single (217 mg/kg) or multiple (200 to 1,351 mg/kg/d for up to 39 days) doses of melamine. Clinical signs, including anorexia, anuria and uremia developed after 5 to 31 days post first exposure in a dose-dependent manner (Clark, 1966). In a study involving dogs fed 125 mg/kg melamine, crystalluria was reported but no other adverse effects were identified (Lipschetz and Stokey, 1945).

Cyanuric acid has similarly low toxicity when given alone. It is known to produce degenerative changes in the kidneys of guinea pigs when given at doses of 30 mg/kg body weight for 6 months, in rats fed a diet containing 8% monosodium cyanurate for 20 weeks, and in dogs fed a diet containing 8% monosodium cyanurate. Lesions included ectasia of the distal collecting tubules and multifocal epithelial cell proliferation (Canelli, 1974). In a 2-year study of rats that were given sodium cyanurate in the drinking water at doses estimated up to 371 mg/kg body weight/day (5,375 mg/L), no substance-related increase in tumor incidence was observed (WHO, 2004). Cyanuric acid is not considered to be carcinogenic or teratogenic (Gossner *et al.*, 2009).

The combination of melamine and cyanuric acid is markedly more toxic to most animals than either compound when given alone. Cats fed diets containing up to 1% melamine or cyanuric acid had no evidence of clinical abnormalities. However, when cats were fed diets containing 0.2% each of melamine and cyanuric acid, they had evidence of acute renal failure within 48 hours. Lesions typical of those associated with the pet food recall were observed (Puschner *et al.*, 2007). In a recent publication, Dobson *et al.* (2008) explained the mode of action by which a combination of melamine and cyanuric acid produced greater toxicity than either compound alone. A pig fed 400 mg/kg melamine and 400 mg/kg cyanuric acid daily had bloody diarrhea within 24 hours, which resolved. Necropsy revealed perirenal edema and round golden-brown crystals with radiating striations in the kidneys. Similar lesions were present in tilapia, rainbow trout and catfish dosed with 400 mg/kg each of melamine and cyanuric acid per day for 3 days, though most of the fish survived the renal damage (Reimschuessel *et al.*, 2008).

Reproductive and developmental toxicity

Neoplasia was associated with the presence of uroliths in the urinary bladders of male rats (Melnick *et al.*, 1984). However, melamine has not been observed to cause mutagenesis. Since the lesions in male rats were associated with the presence of uroliths, the mechanism of carcinogenesis was most likely secondary to epithelial hyperplasia caused by mechanical irritation (Hau *et al.*, 2009; Melnick *et al.*, 1984). Melamine has been classified in carcinogenic risk group 3 (unclassifiable in humans) by the World Health Organization (WHO) (Hau *et al.*, 2009).

Teratogenic effects associated with melamine have not been reported (Wiwanitkit, 2009). However, infants are likely more susceptible to melamine toxicosis than human adults because they excrete between five and eight times as much uric acid, which interacts with melamine to form crystals (Skinner *et al.*, 2010). Preterm infants were more susceptible than full-term infants (Guan *et al.*, 2009; Hard *et al.*, 2009). The long-term effects of melamine exposure in infants remain to be seen. There has been speculation that the developing kidneys may be predisposed to severe intrarenal reflux and secondary fibrosis (Hard *et al.*, 2009). Hypertension, albuminuria and chronic kidney disease are commonly reported in children that have experienced acute renal failure from other causes (Ingelfinger, 2008; Bhalla *et al.*, 2009). To date, there is no evidence that melamine or cyanuric acid is a reproductive and developmental toxicant.

RISK ASSESSMENT

According to the National Institute for Occupational Safety and Health (NIOSH) survey, occupational exposure to melamine may occur through inhalation and dermal contact with this compound at workplaces where melamine is produced and used. The formation of bladder calculi has been identified as the most relevant endpoint, and because the calculi formation is dose dependent or local-concentration dependent, with no signs of significant accumulation, the subchronic studies in rats serve as the basis for the risk assessment (Gossner *et al.*, 2009). Monitoring data indicate that the general population may be exposed to melamine via ingestion of contaminated food. The US FDA estimated a tolerable daily intake (TDI) of 0.36 mg melamine/kg per day. The limit for melamine in food was set as 2.5 ppm, based on a person weighing 60 kg. The allowable limit for infant formula is 1 ppm. The WHO recommended a TDI for 0.2 mg/kg for melamine and 1.5 mg/kg for cyanuric acid. Several national and regional authorities around the world and the WHO have issued preliminary risk assessment and guidance on levels in food, mainly based on information from the 2007 pet food incident, as a first pragmatic approach for public health protection.

TREATMENT

The basic treatment regimens for crystalluria and urolithiasis related to melamine ingestion include fluid therapy and supportive care in both veterinary and pediatric patients (Anonymous, 2007; Wen *et al.*, 2010). Increased water intake and fluid therapy were used to increase urine output. Because low urinary pH is associated with crystal formation in infants, alkalization of the urine was used to maintain urine pH between 6.0 and 7.8 in affected children. Sodium bicarbonate or potassium citrate was added to intravenous fluids for this purpose (Gao and Shen, 2010; Wen *et al.*, 2010). Antispasmodic drugs such as anisodamine or atropine were given to facilitate excretion of uroliths in children and pain management was instituted (Wen *et al.*, 2010; Bhalla *et al.*, 2009). Most children recovered with this conservative management (Gao and Shen, 2010; Wen *et al.*, 2010). However, hemodialysis was required in some patients, as was surgical intervention (Wen *et al.*, 2010). Most children recovered fully, but 12% were found to have renal abnormalities 6 months after treatment (Liu *et al.*, 2010).

CONCLUDING REMARKS AND FUTURE DIRECTIONS

Melamine is produced in large volumes and used around the world for a variety of purposes. Contamination of human food and animal feed with melamine and its analog cyanuric acid in recent years resulted in incidents that led to some of the largest product recalls in recent history. In general, following exposure, these compounds are rapidly absorbed and eliminated with no accumulation and minimal adverse effects in the body, and as a result they are considered chemicals of low toxicity. The combination of melamine and cyanuric acid is markedly more toxic to most animals than either compound when given alone. Kidney is the target organ for melamine, cyanuric acid and related analogs, and toxicosis often occurs due to interaction of these compounds or of melamine with endogenous uric acid. There is no specific antidote for melamine or cyanuric acid toxicity. The formation of bladder calculi has been identified as the most relevant endpoint, and because the calculi formation is dose dependent or local-concentration dependent, with no signs of significant accumulation, the subchronic studies in rats serve as the basis for risk assessment. To date, there is no evidence that melamine and cyanuric acid are reproductive and developmental toxicants or teratogens. Of course, developing infants and neonatal animals appear to be more sensitive than adult humans and adult animals. According to WHO, managing food safety events should be done internationally to prevent multinational consequences expected due to globalized trade. Collaboration between food safety authorities worldwide is needed to efficiently exchange information and to enable tacking and recalling of affected products to ensure food safety and to protect public health.

REFERENCES

Acheson D (2007) Importation of contaminated animal feed ingredients, statement before the House Committee on Agriculture. Washington DC, United States, May 9, 2007.

Anonymous (2007) Specialists confer about the pet food recall. *J Am Vet Med Assoc* **233:** 1603.

Anonymous (2010) Melamine Pet Food Recall – Frequently Asked Questions February 2, 2010. Retrieved July 3, 2010, from United States Food and Drug Administration Department of Health and Human Services: http://www.fda.gov/animalveterinary/safetyhealth/RecallsWithdrawals/ucm129932.htm#AnimalFeed

Bai X, Bai F, Zhang K, Lv X, Qin Y, Li Y, Bai S, Lin S (2010) Tissue deposition and residue depletion in laying hens exposed to melamine-contaminated diets. *J Agric Food Chem* **58:** 5414–20.

Bhalla V, Grimm P, Chertow GM, Pao AC (2009) Melamine nephrotoxicity: an emerging epidemic in an era of globalization. *Kidney Internat* **7:** 774–9.

Canelli E (1974) Chemical, bacteriological, and toxicological properties of cyauric acid and chlorinated isocyanurates as applied to swimming pool disinfection, a review. *Am J Pub Health* **64:** 155–62.

Chen Y, Wenjun Y, Wang Z, Peng Y, Li B, Ahang L, Gong L (2010) Deposition of melamine in eggs from laying hens exposed to melamine contaminated feed. *J Ag Food Chem* **58:** 3512–16.

Cianciolo RE, Bischoff K, Ebel J, Van Winkle TJ, Goldstein RE, Serfilippi LM (2008) Clinicopathologic, histologic, and toxicologic findings in 70 cats inadvertently exposed to pet food contaminated with melamine and cyanuric acid. *J Am Vet Med Assoc* **333:** 729–37.

Clark R (1966) Melamine crystalluria in sheep. *J S Afr Vet Med Assoc* **37:** 349–51.

Dobson RLM, Motlagh S, Quijano M, Cambron RT, Baker TR, *et al.* (2008) Identification and characterization of toxicity of contaminants in pet food leading to an outbreak of renal toxicity in cats and dogs. *Toxicol Sci* **106:** 251–62.

Gao J, Shen Y (2010) Therapeutic effects of potassium sodium, hydrogen citrate on melamine-induced urinary calculi in China. *Chin Med J* **123:** 1112–16.

Gonzalez J, Puschner B, Pérez V, Ferreras MC, Delgado L, Mu oz M, Pérez C, Reyes LE, Velasco J, Fernández V, Garcia-Marin JF (2009) Nephrotoxicosis in Iberian piglets subsequent to exposure to melamine and derivatives in Spain between 2003 and 2006. *J Vet Diag Invest* **21:** 558–36.

Gossner CME, Schlundt J, Embarek PB, Hird S, *et al.* (2009) The melamine incident: implications for international food and feed safety. *Env Health Perspect* **117:** 1803–8.

Guan N, Fab Q, Ding J, Zhao Y, Lu J, Ai Y, Xu G, Zhu S, Yao C, Jiang L, Miao J, Zhang H, Zhao D (2009) Melamine-contaminated powdered formula and urolithiasis in young children. *New England J Med* **360:** 1067–74.

Hard GC, Flake GP, Sills RC (2009) Re-evaluation of kidney histopathology from 13-week toxicity and two-year carcinogenicity studies of melamine in the F344 rat: morphologic evidence of retrograde nephropathy. *Vet Pathol* **46:** 1248–57.

Hau AK, Kwan TH, Kam-tao P (2009) Melamine toxicity in the kidney. *J Am Soc Nephrol* **20:** 245–50.

Hu P, Ling L, Hu B, Zhang CR (2010) The size of melamine-induced stones is dependent on the melamine content of the formula fed, but not the duration of exposure. *Ped Nephrol* **25:** 565–6.

Ingelfinger J (2008) Melamine and global implications of food contamination. *New England J Med* **359:** 2745–8.

Ji K, Zhu S, Liu Z (2009) Melamine-contaminated powdered formula and urolithiasis. *New England J Med* **360:** 2675.

Langman CB (2009) Melamine, powdered milk, and nephrolithiasis in Chinese infants. *New England J Med* **360:** 1139–41.

Lewin-Smith MR, Kalasinsky V, Mullick FG, Thompson ME (2009) Melamine-containing crystals in the urinary tracts of domestic animals: sentinel event? *Arch Pathol Lab Med* **133:** 341–2.

Lipschitz WL, Stokey E (1945) The mode of action of three new diuretics: melamine, adenine, and formoguanamine. *J Pharm Exp Therap* **82:** 235–348.

Liu JM, Ren A, Yang L, Gao J, Pei L, Ye R, Qu Q, Zheng X (2010) Urinary tract abnormalities in Chinese rural children who consumed melamine-contaminated dairy products: a population-based screening and follow-up study. *Can Med Assoc J* **182:** 439–43.

Lv X, Wang J, Wu L, Qiu J, Li J, Wu Z, Qin Y (2010) Tissue deposition and residue depletion in lambs exposed to melamine and cyanuric acid-contaminated diets. *J Agric Food Chem* **58:** 943–8.

Melnick RL, Boorman GA, Haseman JK, Montali RJ, Huff J (1984) Urolithiasis and bladder carcinogenicity of melamine in rodents. *Toxicol Appl Pharmacol* **72:** 292–303.

Okumura M, Hasegawa R, Shirai T, Ito M, Yamada S, Fukushima S (1992) Relationship between calculus formation and carcinogenesis in the urinary bladder of rats administered the non-genotoxic agents, thymine or melamine. *Carcinogenesis* **13:** 1043–5.

Organization for Economic Cooperation and Development (2009) The 2007 OECD list of high production volume chemicals. Series on Testing and Assessment No. 112. http://www.oecd.org/dataoecd/32/9/43947965.pdf (accessed November 3, 2009).

Osborne CA, Lulich JP, Ulrich LK (2008) Melamine and cyanuric acid-induced crystaluria, uroliths, and nephrotoxicity in dogs and cats. *Vet Clin North Am Small Animal* **39:** 1–14.

Puschner B, Poppenga R, Lowenstine L, Filigenzi MS, Pesavento PA (2007) Assessment of melamine and cyanuric acid toxicity in cats. *J Vet Diagn Invest* **19:** 616–24.

Qin Y, Lv X, Li J, Qi G, Diao Q, Liu G, Xue M, Wang J, Tong J, Zhang L, Zhang K (2010) Assessment of melamine contamination in crop, soil, and water in China and risks of melamine accumulation in animal tissues and products. *Environment Internat* **36:** 446–52.

Reimschuessel R, Evans E, Andersen WC, Turnipseed SB, Karbiwnyk CM, Mayer TD, Nochetto C, Rummel NG, Gleseker CM (2009) Residue depletion of melamine and cyanuric acid in catfish and rainbow trout following oral administration. *Vet Pharmacol Ther* **33:** 172–82.

Reimschuessel R, Gieseker CM, Miller RA, Ward J, Boehmer J, Rummel N, Heller DN, Nochetto C, Turnipseed SB, Karbiwnyk CM, Satzger D, Crowe JB, Wilber NR, Reinhard MK, Roberts JF, Witkowski MR (2008) Evaluation of the renal effects of experimental feeding of melamine and cyanuric acid to fish and pigs. *Am J Vet Res* **69:** 1217–28.

Rumbeiha WK, Agnew D, Maxie G, Hoff B, Page C, Curran P, Powers B (2010) Analysis of a survey database of pet food-induced poisoning in North America. *J Med Toxicol* **6:** 172–84.

Shen JS, Wang JQ, Wei HY, Bu DP, Sun P, Zhou LY (2010) Transfer efficiency of melamine from feed to milk in lactating dairy cows fed with different doses of melamine. *J Dairy Sci* **93:** 2060–6.

Skinner CG, Thomas JD, Osterloh JD (2010) Melamine toxicity. *J Med Toxicol* **6:** 50–5.

Sun N, Shen Y, He LJ (2010) Histopathological features of the kidney after acute renal failure from melamine. *New England J Med* **362:** 662.

Thompson ME, Lewin-Smith MR, Kalasinsky K, Pizzolato KM, Fleetwood ML, McElhaney MR, Johnson TO (2008) Characterization of melamine-containing and calcium oxalate crystals in three dogs with suspected pet food-induced nephrotoxicosis. *Vet Pathol* **55:** 417–26.

Wen JG, Li ZZ, Zhang H, Wang Y, Rui FZ, Yang L, Chen Y, Wang JX, Zhang SJ (2010) Melamine related bilateral renal calculi in 50 children: single center experience in clinical diagnosis and treatment. *J Urology* **183:** 1533–8.

WHO (2004) Sodium dichloroisocyanurate. In *Safety Evaluation of Certain Food Additives and Contaminants*. WHO Food Additives Series No. 52. Geneva: World Health Organization.

Wiwanitkit V (2009) Melamine: problems in obstetrics. *Arch Gynecol Obstet* **280:** 345–6.

Yhee JY, Brown CA, Yu CH, Kim JH, Poppenga R, Sur JH (2009) Retrospective study of melamine/cyanuric acid-induced renal failure in dogs in Korea between 2003 and 2004. *Vet Pathol* **46:** 348–54.

CHAPTER

29

Ionophores

Meliton N. Novilla

INTRODUCTION

Ionophores play a significant role in improving the health and feed efficiency in livestock and poultry production. Of the two major subclasses, carboxylic ionophores which form zwitterionic complexes with cations and promote electrically neutral cation exchange diffusion are used since they are better tolerated than the highly toxic neutral ionophores which form charged complexes capable of perturbing biologic membranes and action potentials. Presently, seven carboxylic ionophores are marketed in the USA and around the world for use as anticoccidial drugs for poultry and/or growth promotants in ruminants.

These include monensin (Coban, Rumensin, Rumensin CRC), lasalocid (Avatec, Bovatec), salinomycin (Bio-cox, Sacox), narasin (Monteban, Maxiban), maduramicin (Cygro), laidlomycin (Cattlyst) and semduramycin (Aviax). Structural formulas of these ionophores are shown in Figure 29.1. Before these ionophores were legally marketed for use in food producing animals, sponsors had to demonstrate to the regulatory agencies that each drug was safe and effective in the target animal species, safe for humans consuming edible products from treated animals and safe for the environment (USFDA, 2000, 1986, 1982).

For the purposes of this chapter, monensin is emphasized since more investigational laboratory and field studies as well as information and reports of adverse reactions are available on monensin relative to the other ionophores. This is because of monensin's long-standing and widespread use in food animals, being the first marketed carboxylic ionophore of veterinary importance. Large numbers of preclinical safety and toxicity studies have been submitted in support of registration and marketing approvals in the USA and other countries (Novilla, 2007). The conduct of these studies which started in the early 1960s and led to a stepwise understanding and characterization of the toxicity/safety profile of monensin, roughly conformed to the typical toxicology flowchart (Figure 29.2).

PHARMACOKINETICS, PHARMACOLOGY AND MECHANISM OF ACTION

Carboxylic ionophores, such as monensin, are used as anticoccidial drugs and for growth efficiency enhancement in several target animal species (Shumard and Callender, 1968; Anderson *et al.*, 1976; Pressman, 1976; Stockdale, 1981; Watkins *et al.*, 1986; Jeffers *et al.*, 1988). In cattle, monensin improves the efficiency of rumen fermentation by reducing energy and waste gas losses associated with formation of volatile fatty acids (VFA) (Corah, 1991; Goodrich *et al.*, 1984; Bergen and Bates, 1984; Baile *et al.*, 1979; Richardson *et al.*, 1976). In converting carbohydrates to VFAs, monensin increases the amount of propionic acid produced and reduces the quantities of acetic and butyric acids, resulting in substantial energy savings. Further, the use of monensin in cattle rations, which has been shown to reduce emissions of methane and ammonia, contributes to air and water quality and benefits the environment (Tedeschi *et al.*, 2003). In dairy cattle, monensin use has been associated with improved efficiency, increased milk yield with a reduced fat content, as well as improved health (reduced bloat and reduced ketosis) (Duffield *et al.*, 2003, 2002, 1999; Heuer *et al.*, 2001; Mackintosh *et al.*, 2002; McGuffey *et al.*, 2001; Hayes *et al.*, 1996). When administered before parturition, monensin has shown positive effects on energy metabolism in early lactation, including reduced blood ketones, increases in serum glucose, reduced incidence and duration of subclinical ketosis, clinical ketosis and abomasal displacement.

At the cellular level, monensin and other ionophores facilitate transport of ions across biologic membranes (Pressman, 1976; Pressman and Fahim, 1982; Mollenhauer *et al.*, 1990). The ionophoric activity may alter normal concentration gradients and forms the basis for the functional, metabolic and organic changes associated with this class of compounds. Ionophores have different complexation affinities. For instance, monensin complexes more readily with Na^+ than K^+ or Ca^{2+}, while lasalocid, a divalent ionophore, forms complexes with Ca^{2+} and Mg^{2+} and primary amines, including catecholamines (Figure 29.3).

Ionophores directly affect the asexual and sexual developmental stages of eimerian coccidia by causing the normal transport of Na^+ and K^+ ions to fail (Smith and Galloway, 1983; Smith *et al.*, 1981). Similar events occur in bacteria because monensin causes egress of potassium out of the cell and ingress of hydrogen ions into the cell.

The organisms utilize energy to maintain cellular homeostasis but when energy is exhausted, they swell, rupture and die (Figure 29.4). Excessive ionophore concentrations similarly affect host cells, which may result in the ionophore toxic

Reproductive and Developmental Toxicology, Edited by Ramesh C. Gupta
ISBN: 978-0-12-382032-7

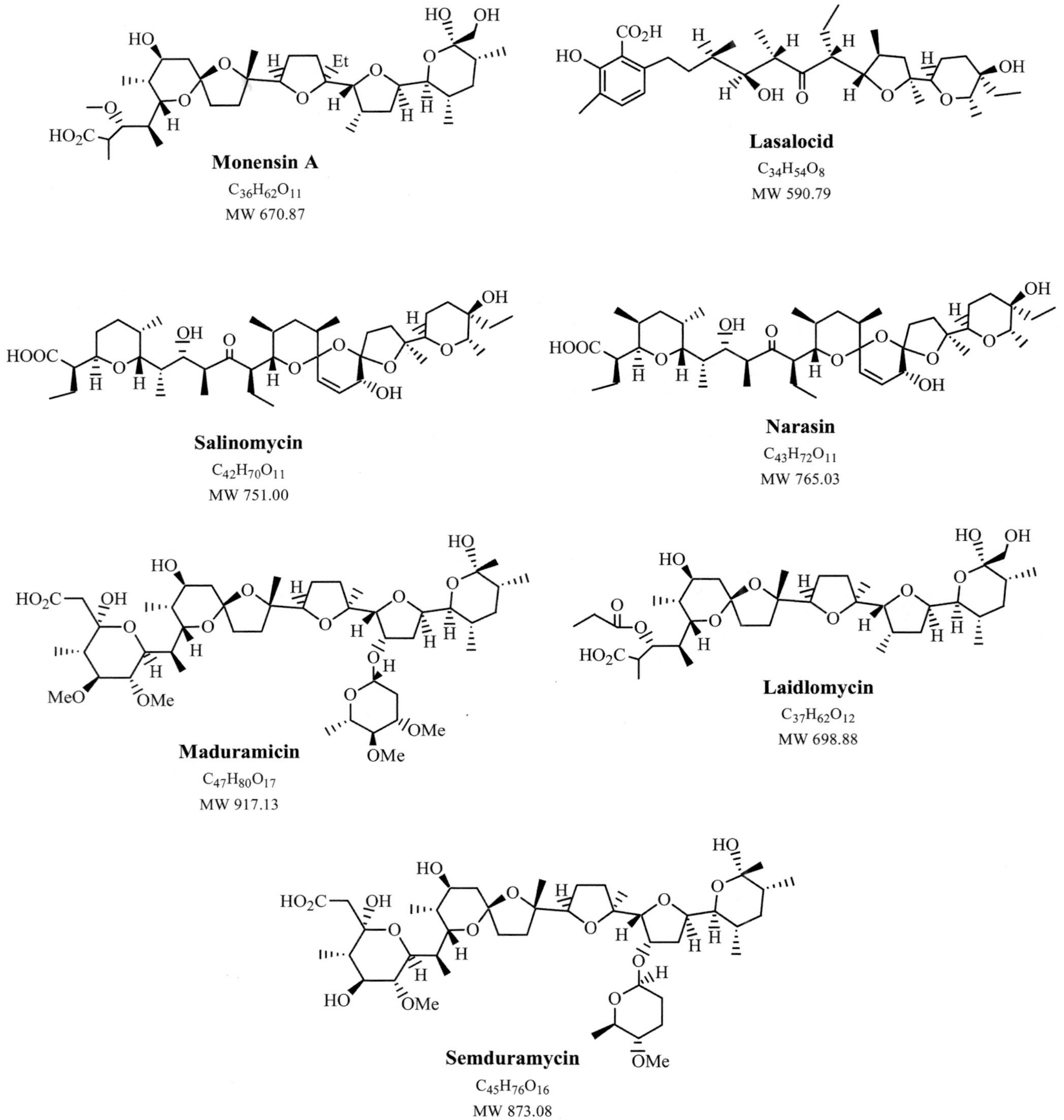

Monensin A
$C_{36}H_{62}O_{11}$
MW 670.87

Lasalocid
$C_{34}H_{54}O_8$
MW 590.79

Salinomycin
$C_{42}H_{70}O_{11}$
MW 751.00

Narasin
$C_{43}H_{72}O_{11}$
MW 765.03

Maduramicin
$C_{47}H_{80}O_{17}$
MW 917.13

Laidlomycin
$C_{37}H_{62}O_{12}$
MW 698.88

Semduramycin
$C_{45}H_{76}O_{16}$
MW 873.08

FIGURE 29.1 Structures of carboxylic ionophores.

syndrome (Novilla and Folkerts, 1986; Novilla, 1992). Monensin was reported to shorten the duration of the action potential and suppressed the pacemaker potential in cardiac tissue (Sutko *et al.*, 1977; Tsuchida and Otomo, 1990). These membrane current effects were related to transmembrane alterations in the gradients of Na^+ and K^+ ions and to increased intracellular Ca^{2+} following the increase in cytoplasmic Na^+ concentration, probably via Na^+/Ca^{2+} exchange mechanism. Alterations in the concentrations of Ca^{2+} and other cations extracellularly as well as changes in their intracellular distribution have been associated with changes in subcellular organelles and cell damage (Shier and Dubardieu, 1992; Calo *et al.*, 2002; Sandercock and Mitchell, 2003).

By immunohistochemistry staining, monensin treatment was shown to increase Na^+/K^+-ATPase and Ca^{2+}-ATPase activities in the heart and skeletal muscle of chickens given 4-, 15- and 40 mg/kg by oral gavage while reduced staining patterns for both enzymes occurred at doses of 100 and 150 mg/kg, associated with physical signs of toxicity and death (Calo *et al.*, 2002).

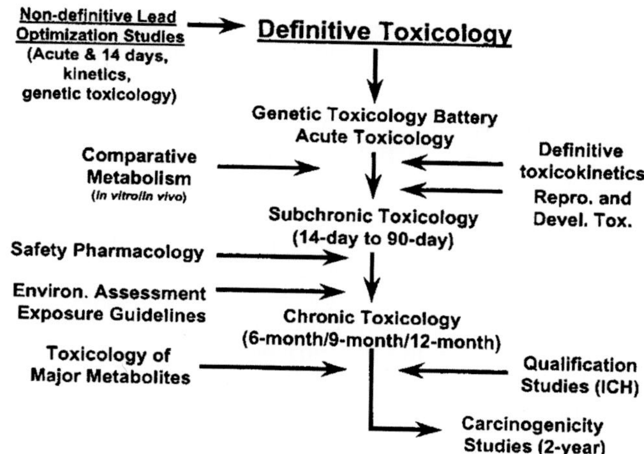

FIGURE 29.2 Typical toxicology profile. From Dorato and Engelhardt (2005).

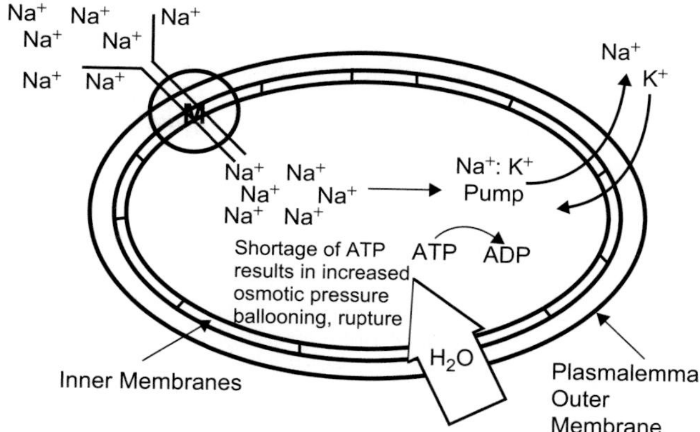

FIGURE 29.4 Effect of ionophores on ion and water dynamics in the coccidia. M = monensin. From Thomas *et al.* (1985) Elanco Animal Health.

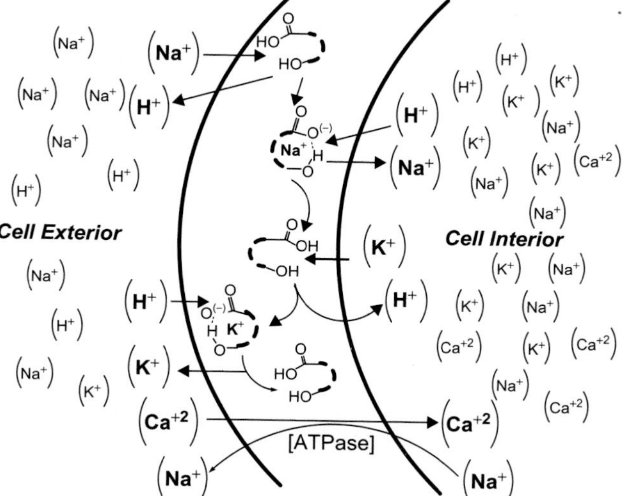

FIGURE 29.3 Diagram of cation ion exchange diffusion across plasma membranes facilitated by monensin. Large arrows indicate major transport activity.

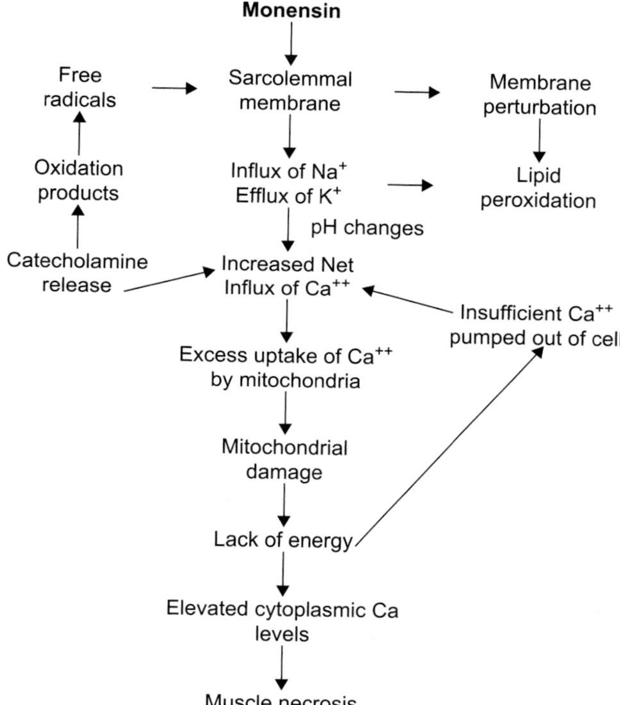

FIGURE 29.5 Probable sequence of events induced by monensin in muscle cells. Adapted from Novilla and Folkerts (1986).

Heart and skeletal muscles have been identified as the primary target organs of toxicity in laboratory animals and domestic livestock given large doses of monensin and other ionophores by oral or parenteral routes (Todd *et al.*, 1984; Novilla and Folkerts, 1986; Novilla and Todd, 1991; Van Vleet *et al.*, 1991; Dowling, 1992; Matsuoka *et al.*, 1996). The development of muscle lesions varies among species. For monensin-induced toxicosis, the heart is primarily affected in horses, skeletal muscle in pigs and dogs, and there is about equal tissue predilection in rats, chickens and cattle (Van Vleet *et al.*, 1991; Novilla, 1992; Novilla and Folkerts, 1986). Morphologic effects induced by toxic doses of monensin include degeneration, necrosis and repair of cardiac and skeletal muscle fibers, and secondary lesions of congestive heart failure. The steps involved in monensin-induced muscle necrosis are shown in Figure 29.5.

The pharmacodynamics of monensin, related to potential effects on the other organ systems, has been evaluated both *in vitro* and *in vivo* (Novilla, 2007). Studies targeting other specific organ systems of laboratory animals indicated that monensin at a dose of 10 mg/kg orally produced no effect on the central, peripheral and autonomic nervous systems or the respiratory and digestive systems (Novilla, 2004). Although acute systemic exposure of humans to significant doses of monensin is unlikely during its manufacture and use in livestock and poultry husbandry, these studies are considered relevant to the overall safety of monensin. They provide insight into the secondary pharmacological actions of the compound and support the margin of safety for exposure in humans handling monensin and premixes (i.e., in accordance with label instructions or ingestion of residues in livestock and poultry products).

The pharmacokinetics of monensin following oral administration has been evaluated in cattle and rats. Several studies with both 14C-monensin and unlabeled compound have shown that following oral administration in cattle and other species, monensin is rapidly absorbed and extensively metabolized by the liver. Most of the administered monensin and its metabolites are excreted via bile into the gastrointestinal tract and this accounts for the extremely low plasma levels of monensin (Donoho, 1984). The metabolite pattern for monensin is similar in cattle, chickens, rats, turkeys, sheep and pigs (Davison, 1984; Donoho, 1984; Atef *et al.*, 1993). Monensin and five metabolites were identified in liver, bile and/or feces from monensin-treated steers and dairy cows. Metabolite characterization studies indicated that hydroxylation (*o*-demethylation and oxidation) was the primary degradative metabolic pathway of monensin resulting in low concentrations of a large number of polar metabolites in the feces of ^{14}C-monensin-dosed animals. Studies have also shown that metabolite M-1 (*o*-desmethyl monensin) was 20 times less potent in biological activity than parent monensin, the marker residue. Hence, the suspected first step in monensin metabolism appears to eliminate most of its biological activity.

Based on radiolabeled studies in steers and dairy cows, the liver had the highest total monensin residue following zero withdrawal (Donoho *et al.*, 1978; Herberg *et al.*, 1978; Donoho, 1984; Kennington *et al.*, 1995). Monensin does not accumulate in tissues of animals even when given toxic doses (Donoho, 1984; Atef *et al.*, 1993). However, simultaneous use of drugs shown to depress metabolism of monensin and other ionophores has resulted in toxic interactions (Anadon and Reeve-Johnson, 1999; Basaraba *et al.*, 1999; Broz and Frigg, 1987; Umemura *et al.*, 1984; Wanner, 1984; Weisman *et al.*, 1984, 1983; Frigg *et al.*, 1983; Stanfield and Lamont, 1981; Meingassner *et al.*, 1979). Feeding of muscle, liver and other viscera from cattle provided dietary levels of 165 ppm monensin (five times the approved use level) to rats and dogs for 3 months, produced no adverse effects (Gossett *et al.*, 1975). In cattle administered ^{14}C-monensin, residues of radioactivity depleted rapidly from the tissues. There were no residues in edible tissues of growing cattle following treatment at 0.9 mg monensin/kg body weight for 28 days (Coyle and Walker, 2005).

Thus, exposure of humans to residues of monensin from animals treated according to the label instructions will be very limited and will be due primarily to the parent compound. Furthermore, the extremely low concentrations of residues present in meat, milk and eggs intended for human consumption are of no safety concern because of the sufficient margin of safety demonstrated in the toxicology studies.

IONOPHORE TOXIC SYNDROME

In general, the marketed carboxylic ionophore products have been found to be safe and effective in the target animal species within the approved dosage ranges (Novilla, 2007). However, overdosage, misuse and drug interactions have resulted in the ionophore toxic syndrome. The toxicology of monensin has been extensively studied in several laboratory, domestic and wildlife animals and its toxicity profile is well established (Condon and McKenzie, 2002; Baird *et al.*, 1997; Matsuoka *et al.*, 1996; Dowling, 1992; Ficken *et al.*, 1989; Potter *et al.*, 1984; Schweitzer *et al.*, 1984; Todd *et al.*, 1984; Confer *et al.*, 1983;Van Vleet *et al.*, 1983a,b,c; Amend *et al.*, 1981; Hanrahan *et al.*, 1981; Wilson, 1980; Whitlock *et al.*, 1978). Monensin toxicity is characterized clinically by anorexia, diarrhea, dyspnea, depression, ataxia, recumbency and death and pathologically by degeneration, necrosis and repair of heart and skeletal muscles.

Dose levels have been identified at which monensin can be administered daily for long periods without producing harmful effects. The monensin oral NOELs were approximately 2 to 3.8 mg/kg in rats and 5 mg/kg/day in dogs after subchronic oral dosing of 3 months, 1.25 mg/kg/day in dogs after chronic oral dosing for 1 year, and 1.4 mg/kg/day in rats and 1.3 mg/kg/day in mice after chronic oral dosing for 2 years (Novilla, 2004).

At the approved use and dose ranges, monensin has been found to be safe and effective in the target animal species, including broiler chickens, feedlot cattle, pasture and range cattle, reproducing beef cows, replacement dairy heifers and lactating dairy cows. In addition, laboratory and field reports have claimed control of toxoplasmosis in sheep (Buxton *et al.*, 1988), disseminated visceral coccidiosis in cranes (Carpenter and Novilla, 1992), and swine dysentery (Kyriakis, 1989).

Collectively, toxicity and safety studies indicate that the greatest risk of monensin toxicity occurs when animals are provided monensin-containing feed for the first time. Under both laboratory and field conditions, a typical ionophore toxic syndrome is observed following feed mixing errors and misuse, usually greater than 3× the maximum recommended levels. The organs damaged by toxic doses of monensin are striated (cardiac and skeletal) muscles (Todd *et al.*, 1984; Van Vleet *et al.*, 1991; Dowling, 1992). The other six ionophores produced similar cardiac and skeletal muscle lesions (Novilla, 2007; Novilla and Folkerts, 1986). Additionally, peripheral nerve lesions have been described following toxic doses of lasalocid (Safran *et al.*, 1993; Shlosberg *et al.*, 1985), narasin (Novilla *et al.*, 1994) and salinomycin (Van der Linde-Sipman *et al.*, 1999). There were no direct treatment-related lesions induced by any of the ionophores in reproductive organs and tissues.

Data on target organ toxicity are presented as background to considerations of the reproductive and developmental toxicity of ionophores and health risks in humans from exposure to residues in meat, milk and eggs produced by target animal species. Some human exposure to monensin is expected to occur even with rigorous use of safety equipment during manufacturing and with standard precautions during handling of the monensin active ingredient and formulated products. The occurrence of eye and skin irritation following monensin exposure suggests that monensin and other ionophores should be handled carefully. However, the results of safety and toxicity studies indicate that multiple low-level exposures are not likely to produce adverse effects in humans (Dorato, 2000a,b; Novilla, 2004).

The information presented below was gleaned from published laboratory and field experiences with monensin in target and non-target animal species and available reviews and expert reports submitted in support of product registrations (Potter *et al.*, 1984; Dorato, 2000a,b; Novilla, 2004).

TOXICITY AND SAFETY STUDIES IN CATTLE

Acute toxicity study in beef cattle

Fifteen Hereford cross steers and heifers with a body weight range of 272 to 338 kg were allotted 5/treatment group and administered mycelial monensin in 5% aqueous acacia suspension at doses of 12.5, 22.4, or 39.8 mg/kg body weight by gavage. Another group of four similar animals were gavaged with solvent extracted mycelia, free of monensin, equal in total mycelial weight to the high monensin dose. Fourteen-day death losses were 0/5, 3/5 and 2/5, respectively, for the 12.5, 22.4 and 39.8 mg/kg groups. No cattle treated with the monensin-free mycelia died. In this study, the median lethal dose (LD50) of monensin was calculated to be 35.8 mg/kg ± 13.5 mg/kg. Clinical signs of intoxication consisting of anorexia, diarrhea and slight depression occurred as early as day 1 post-treatment (PT). By day 5 PT, labored breathing and moderate to severe depression were observed but by day 10 animals were consuming feed normally. All surviving cattle were apparently normal by day 12 PT. There were no pathologic findings in control animals administered monensin-free mycelia. Striated muscle lesions of necrosis and fibroplasia in the heart and necrosis and regeneration in skeletal muscles were found in several monensin-treated animals.

Multiple dose gavage toxicity study in steers

Thirty steers were dosed with aqueous suspensions of mycelial monensin for 7 consecutive days at doses of 0, 400, 600, 1,000, 2,000 and 4,000 mg monensin activity/head/day which was equivalent to approximately 0, 1.6, 2.4, 3.9, 7.6 and 15.5 mg/kg body weight. The occurrence of clinical signs and death was dose and time related. During the 7-day treatment period, three steers from the 2,000 mg group died, two on day 5 and one on day 7 while four steers from the 4,000 mg group died, two on day 4, one each on day 5 and 6. The LD_0 (dose in which no deaths occurred) was estimated to be 1,000 mg/head or 3.9 mg/kg body weight/day. Pathologic evaluation of animals from this study confirmed the presence of cardiac and skeletal muscle lesions similar to those observed in experimentally induced and confirmed field cases of monensin toxicosis (Van Vleet *et al.*, 1983c; Schweitzer *et al.*, 1984; Potter *et al.*, 1984).

Acute tolerance study in lactating dairy cattle

Groups of 2-year-old primiparous and 3-year-old multiparous (second lactation) Holstein cows were given bolus doses of 0, 1 or 10 mg monensin/kg body weight daily. The low dose is approximately equivalent to the maximum approved inclusion rate of monensin in beef cattle feeds of 33 ppm (30 grams/US ton). Bolus dosing, chosen to deliver defined daily doses of monensin and avoid potential confounding effects of altered dietary intake, was scheduled for 21 days. Dosing was shortened to 14 days because all cows from the 10 mg/kg group were removed due to the anorexia criteria. As per protocol, a cow was removed from the study, euthanized and necropsied when it consumed <10% of its pretreatment average consumption of the total mixed ration (TMR) for three consecutive days.

Similar to the control cows, the animals administered 1 mg/kg/day for 14 days did not display any signs of toxicity and appeared normal. Clinical signs of toxicity were apparent in all 10 mg/kg treated cows and included anorexia, lethargy, diarrhea, sunken eyes and a gaunt appearance. In addition there was a severe drop in milk production. By study day 4, seven of the eight cows produced 7.5 kg of milk or less and half of the cows did not produce enough milk for meters to register. A previous field report of toxicosis in dairy cattle (Wentink and Vente, 1981) presented with similar clinical signs and a three-fold decrease in milk production after 2 days of exposure to 366 ppm monensin in the feed (equivalent to 6.5 mg/kg body weight).

In the acute tolerance study, treatment-related lesions were found only in the 10 mg/kg group and consisted of inflammation of the rumen, reticulum and omasum, cardiotoxicosis and toxic myopathy with no involvement of reproductive tissues. The clinical signs and pathologic findings were consistent with those observed in previous experimental studies and confirmed field cases of toxicosis in beef and dairy cattle (Potter *et al.*, 1984; Schweitzer *et al.*, 1984; VanVleet *et al.*, 1983c; Wentink and Vente, 1981). Bolus dosing of 1 mg/kg body weight daily for 14 days was well tolerated by lactating dairy cattle.

This series of studies documented the acute toxic syndrome induced by monensin in beef and dairy cattle. Although the median lethal dose of 26.6 mg monensin/kg body weight was published, a higher estimate of the LD_{50} for cattle of 50 to 80 mg/kg may be more appropriate (Van Vleet *et al.*, 1983c). This would provide a wider margin of safety between maximum daily efficacious dose (approximately 1 mg/kg) and the single dose necessary to produce death. In common with other species tested, cattle develop anorexia when given toxic levels of monensin, hence the greatest risk of intoxication is from the first exposure. Compared to beef cattle, dairy cattle appear to be more tolerant to toxic levels of monensin, probably due to a higher metabolic rate during lactation.

TOXICITY AND SAFETY STUDIES IN CHICKENS

Single- and repeated-dose toxicity studies were conducted with crystalline or mycelial monensin to determine the safety of monensin in chickens. The median lethal dose of monensin in broiler chickens, reported to be 200 mg monensin/kg body weight, was an average derived from pharmacology experiments conducted during the late 1970s. The estimated median lethal dose in the series of trials ranged between 142 and 479 mg monensin/kg body weight. In a more recent study, median lethal dose values calculated for males, females and combined sexes were 203, 226 and 214 mg monensin/kg body weight. There was no evidence of monensin toxicity in broiler chickens administered 63 mg/kg by oral gavage. These acute toxicity trials showed no substantial differences in estimated median lethal dose values between mycelial and crystalline monensin. The latest LD_{50} value of 214 mg monensin/kg is consistent with the published average value of 200 mg monensin/kg. The latest LD_{50} value is equivalent to 2,500 ppm monensin in the final feed or 20-fold higher than the maximum approved level of 125 ppm monensin in complete feed when fed to broiler chickens consuming about 8% of their body weight as feed. Seven-week-old broiler chickens administered single oral doses of crystalline monensin of 150, 200 or 250 mg/kg body weight manifested extreme weakness, anorexia, paralysis and death, gross lesions of emaciation, generalized congestion, heart enlargement and hydropericardium and histologic changes of cardiac and skeletal muscle degeneration and necrosis (Hanrahan *et al.*,1981).

A series of full grow-out trials in broiler chickens with various lots of monensin, including production lots of premixes made with either crystalline or mycelial monensin, demonstrated safety of 121 ppm monensin in complete feeds. Further, feeding of 121 ppm monensin to replacement chickens was found to be safe.

TOXICITY AND SAFETY STUDIES IN PIGS

Acute toxicity in growing pigs

Sixty pigs of mixed sex ranging in weight from 8 to 25 kg were administered mycelial monensin doses of 4, 6, 10 and 16 mg monensin/kg to determine the median lethal dose. Signs of intoxication were diarrhea and ataxia, which occurred the first day following dosage. Three pigs developed bluish discoloration of the skin. Of the 17 pigs that died, 15 died the first day following treatment; the other two died on day 7. Recovery from toxic effects began as early as day 3. From the 7-day death losses, the LD_{50} and LD_0 values were 16.8 and <4 mg monensin/kg, respectively. Ten weanling pigs given mycelial monensin as a single oral dose of 40 mg/kg body weight developed striated muscle lesions concentrated in skeletal muscles and the atrial myocardium (Van Vleet *et al.*, 1983b).

Subchronic feeding study in growing/finishing pigs

Finishing swine weighing between 21.4 and 32.8 kg were allotted to four treatment groups of five barrows and five gilts each. The pigs were fed mycelial monensin in a complete feed at concentrations of 0, 50, 150 and 500 ppm monensin for 111 days. Four of 10 pigs receiving 500 ppm died within the first 10 days of the experiment. The cause of death was undetermined for two of the pigs that died. The other two pigs were diagnosed as having a degenerative myopathy. All remaining monensin-treated pigs survived the test period with no untoward reactions. A comparison of average daily weight gain values for control and treated swine showed that average daily gain was depressed for only the 500 pm group and weight gain was slightly increased for the 50 and 150 ppm doses. In this experiment, the 500 ppm monensin concentration in feed was toxic to finishing swine, but the 50 and 150 ppm concentrations produced no adverse effects.

TOXICITY STUDIES IN LABORATORY ANIMALS

A full series of acute toxicity studies was performed with crystalline or mycelial monensin in five species of laboratory animals. Additional studies were also conducted to evaluate the safety of monensin to workers involved in the manufacturing process. All the relevant routes of potential human exposure were represented in these studies (Dorato, 2002a,b; Novilla, 2004). Results of the single-dose toxicity studies indicate a high potential for producing acute toxicity in humans or non-target animals from accidental ingestion of monensin and premix formulations. There was no significant difference in the acute toxic response to either crystalline or mycelial form of monensin or in median lethal dose values between the unformulated mycelia and monensin premix formulations, based on monensin activity. Oral monensin doses of 10 mg/kg given by capsule produced repeated vomition in the dog, and higher doses (≥110 mg monensin/kg) induced vomition in monkeys.

From the subchronic and chronic toxicity studies, monensin levels to which animals could be exposed for long periods of time were identified. Target organs damaged by toxic doses of monensin were the cardiac and skeletal muscles (Todd *et al.*, 1984). There were no direct treatment-related lesions in reproductive organs and tissues in any of the above studies.

REPRODUCTIVE AND DEVELOPMENTAL TOXICITY

Multigeneration reproduction studies in rats

Crystalline or mycelial monensin was administered continuously as a component of the diet to four successive generations of rats. Monensin levels of 0, 2.5, 12.5 and 25 ppm as crystalline monensin and 0, 33, 50 and 80 ppm as mycelial monensin were used. The reproductive performance of the adults and the health status and condition of delivered offspring of all generations were evaluated. The F_{1a} offspring were assigned to the 2-year chronic and oncogenic studies. The progeny of the F_2 generation were evaluated for teratogenic defects by macroscopic and microscopic examinations for visceral and skeletal abnormalities (Figure 29.6).

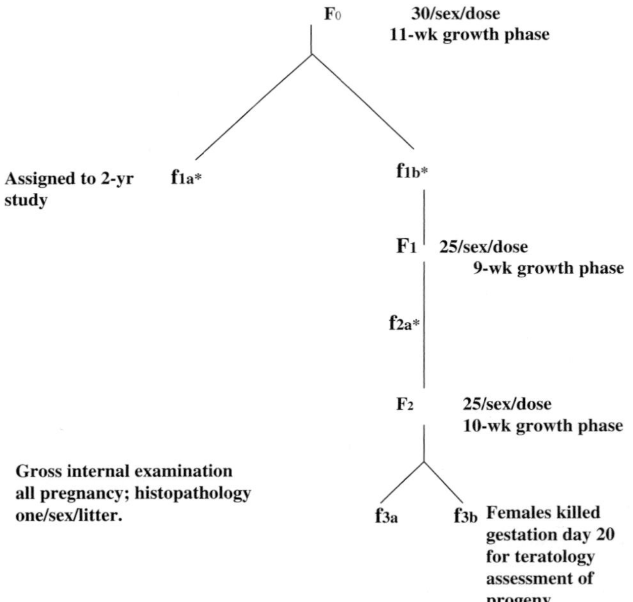

FIGURE 29.6 Treatment and testing protocol for multigeneration reproduction study of monensin in Wistar rats. *Gross internal examination of one·sex^{-1}·litter^{-1}. From Todd *et al.* (1984).

The reproductive capacity through four generations including fertility, litter size, gestation length, parent and progeny survival, and sex distribution was unaffected by any form of monensin treatment. The only treatment-related effect was a slight decrease in body weight gain and lowered body weight noted in each generation administered mycelial monensin. There was no evidence of teratogenicity in the progeny from F_2 parents treated with either crystalline or mycelial monensin.

Marked reductions in growth of the maternal and filial generation of rats fed monensin at 300 ppm but not at 100 ppm were reported by De Sousa Spinosa *et al.* (1999). Findings at the 300 ppm monensin level were attributed to maternal toxicity. However, the most consistent clinical sign of intolerance to feeding of ionophore-medicated complete feed is a dose-dependent anorexia. This may be severe enough in animals that survive acute toxic effects during subacute to chronic feeding studies to result in poor growth due to undernutrition or malnutrition. Kohrs *et al.* (1976) reported that inadequate protein consumption during pregnancy in rats, rabbits, cats and dogs can result in poor reproductive efficiency and decreased birth weight of offspring. In addition, restricting protein intake to 3% of the total energy intake in pregnant rhesus monkeys resulted in major fetal and perinatal problems. For these reasons, it would be more appropriate to consider observations at 300 ppm monensin and above to be due to nutritional deprivation rather than direct reproductive toxicity induced by the ionophore. It is noteworthy that findings at the 100 ppm level are relatively consistent with no adverse developmental effects at the high dose of 80 ppm monensin tested in the studies conducted by Eli Lilly and Company (Todd *et al.*, 1984). It can be concluded that monensin at dietary levels in rats up to 80 ppm did not adversely affect reproductive processes and was not teratogenic to offspring. This dose provided approximately 4 to 8 mg monensin/kg/day which would be very much in excess of monensin residue levels in poultry and cattle products intended for human consumption.

Teratological study in rabbits

For the rabbit teratology study, groups of 25 (control) and 15 (monensin-treated) pregnant Dutch Belted rabbits were given daily oral doses of 0, 0.076, 0.38 or 0.76 mg/kg of monensin on gestation days 6 through 18. On gestation day 28, the females were killed and evaluated for reproductive performance, and the fetuses were examined for abnormalities.

Treatment-related maternal toxicity was indicated by a reduction in mean daily food consumption in all groups after dosing was initiated. However, anorexia was more marked at the high dose. Deaths or abortions of six control and four monensin-treated females occurred independently of treatment. Monensin treatment had no effect on the reproductive parameters and indices. Fetal viability, sex distribution and weight were normal. Developmental deviations were observed in a relatively small number of progeny with no evidence of treatment relationship. Based on this study, monensin administered orally to pregnant rabbits at doses up to 0.76 mg/kg on gestation days 6 through 18 affected neither the reproductive performance of the doe nor the development of the fetus.

REPRODUCTION SAFETY IN CATTLE

Breeding bulls

Groups of growing Hereford and Holstein bulls were fed 0, 200 or 600 mg monensin/head/day supplement or pair fed a complete ration containing 0 or 90 g of monensin/ton up to breeding weight and age. Feed intake of bulls fed 0, 200 or 600 mg monensin/head/day was similar. Feed consumption of pair fed bulls fed a complete ration containing 90 g of monensin/ton was similar to controls fed no monensin. Animals receiving 200 of 600 mg/day had equal or greater rates of body weight gain compared to controls. Monensin had no apparent effect on scrotal circumference, testicular consistency, libido, semen quality or sperm morphology.

In the breeding phase of this study, semen from 15 Hereford and 15 Holstein bulls fed 0, 200 or 600 mg monensin/head/day or pair fed a complete ration containing either 0 or 90 g/ton throughout the growing and semen collection periods was used to artificially inseminate 226 mixed breed cows which had not received monensin. The percentage of cows conceiving (88%) was excellent and similar for all monensin treatment groups. The data indicate that the feeding of monensin to bulls up to 600 mg/head/day or 90 g/ton of feed (3 times the maximum approved inclusion rate) had no effect on semen quality.

Dairy replacement heifers

Sixty dairy replacement heifers were given 0, 200 or 600 mg monensin/head/day in the same TMR and provided at equal amounts up to breeding weight and age. Average daily gains for the 0, 200 and 600 mg/day groups were 0.60, 0.69 and 0.69 kg/day, respectively. The average day of trial to first estrus was similar for all heifers. When compared to controls, average conception date for heifers fed 200 and 600 mg of monensin/head/day, respectively, was 28 and 34 days sooner. Conception rate was excellent for all treatment groups of heifers. Data from this study indicated that feeding monensin up to 600 mg/head/day was safe for growing, dairy replacement heifers.

Breeding and pregnant beef heifers

Ninety-six Hereford heifers, allotted by weight to four groups of 24 animals each, were fed TMR containing 0, 200, 600 or 1,000 mg monensin/head/day. Dietary treatments continued as heifers progressed through estrus, breeding, gestation, calving and re-breeding. Monensin fed to beef heifers at the rate of 200 mg/head/day was safe and beneficial in maintaining growth rate with less feed used. The higher levels of 600 and 1,000 mg/head/day, three- and five-fold higher than the approved use level, produced dose-related decreases in feed intake and body weight gain but did not impair reproduction.

Breeding and pregnant beef cows

One hundred, 3- to 8-year-old, pregnant crossbred beef cows were equally allotted to five treatment groups as follows: 0 mg monensin in 0.45 kg feed supplement/day; 200 mg monensin in 0.45 kg supplement/day; 600 mg monensin in 0.45 kg supplement/day; 1,000 mg monensin in 0.45 kg supplement/day; and 1,000 mg monensin in 2.27 kg supplement/day. Monensin supplements were fed at half the designated dose levels for the first 5 days of the trial. Supplements were fed from the last trimester of pregnancy, through gestation, until the end of breeding. Cows were initially kept in a dry lot and fed hay; later they were turned out to pasture. The trial ended with the collection of conception data by palpation and collection of final body weight data (day 187).

Where the supplement was fed at 0.45 kg/day, intake decreased with increasing monensin concentration. The group receiving the highest concentration of monensin (1,000 mg in 0.45 kg supplement) consumed the least amount of supplement (0.06 kg/head/day) and the greatest amount of hay (10.5 kg/head/day). The treatment group allocated 2.27 kg supplement/day consumed 1.4 kg supplement/head/day and the least amount of hay (5.5 kg/head/day). Initial and final body weights of cows, birth weights of calves, number of live calves, and pregnancy rates were all similar among the treatment groups. There were no mortalities or abortions that could be clinically correlated with the feeding of monensin containing supplements. The data indicated that monensin was safe for reproducing beef cows.

Lactating dairy cattle

A study was conducted to determine effects of a simulated 10 times overdose (OD) of the highest dose of monensin used in the field trials (24 ppm) to support the registration of monensin for lactating dairy cattle in the USA and Canada. Prior to the OD, a total of 22 cows were fed either 0 ($n=11$) or 24 ($n=11$) ppm dry matter (DM) of a total mixed ration (TMR) for 4 weeks. On the day following completion of the pre-OD period, all the cows were fed a TMR containing 240 ppm monensin for 3 days (OD period). At the day 4 feeding, cows were switched to TMRs containing monensin concentrations of either 0 or 24 ppm for 25 days (recovery period). During the OD period, dry matter intake (DMI) over all cows declined significantly from the pre-OD period. Cows fed the 0 ppm monensin TMR pre-OD had lower mean DMI than cows fed 24 ppm. The initial exposure to monensin in the OD period was calculated in excess of 4,400 mg on day 1 and further exposure declined with reduced feed intake. During the recovery period, DMI increased with higher values in cows receiving 24 ppm pre-OD compared to the 0 ppm pre-OD cows.

Most cows showed no clinical effects of the overdose at 22 to 32 hours post-initiation of OD. In a few animals, early clinical signs were diarrhea (3/22), sunken eyes (4/22), slight depression (5/22) and gaunt appearance (lack of fill) in the left flank (2/22). By 46 to 56 hours, 20 of 22 cows had diarrhea, 11 of 22 had depression, 8 of 22 had sunken eyes, and 7 of 22 had lack of fill in the left flank. Diarrhea became severe at 70 to 80 hours and was the only sign observed 24 hours after the third day of OD feeding in 19 of 22 cows. Production parameters were also affected during the OD period; in particular mean daily milk yield was significantly reduced, continuing to day 7 of the recovery period. No other significant treatment-related effects were observed.

This series of safety and toxicity studies documented the toxic syndrome induced by monensin in beef and dairy cattle. Although the median lethal dose of 26.4 mg monensin/kg body weight was published (Potter *et al.*, 1984), a higher estimate of the LD_{50} for cattle (range 50–80 mg/kg body weight) may be more appropriate (Van Vleet *et al.*, 1983c). This would provide a wider margin of safety between maximum daily efficacious dose (approximately 1 mg/kg) and the single dose necessary to produce death. In common with other species tested, cattle developed anorexia when given toxic levels of monensin, hence the greatest risk of intoxication is from the first exposure (Potter *et al.*, 1984). Compared to beef cattle, dairy cattle appear to be more tolerant to toxic levels of monensin, probably due to the higher metabolic rate during lactation.

Field experience trials in lactating dairy cattle provided 300 mg/day monensin via an intraruminal controlled-release capsule (Abe *et al.*, 1994; Hayes *et al.*, 1996; Lean *et al.*, 1994) indicated that conception rates and calving-to-conception or calving-to-heat intervals were not different from control cows. In a study over two lactations, the reproductive performance of dairy cows given 300 ppm monensin in TMR did not differ from the control group during the first lactation but was clearly superior during the second lactation (Phipps *et al.*, 2000). From a series of nine registration trials with monensin fed at the inclusion rates of 0, 7, 15 and 22 g/ton in a TMR to primiparous and multiparous dairy cows, McClary *et al.* (2008) reported the following: (1) services per conception, days open and calving interval were increased and first service conception rate was reduced in the 22 g/ton group compared to controls in lactation 1; (2) pregnancy rates and successful calving rates were similar for all treatment groups; (3) incidence of metritis, cystic ovaries and retained fetal membranes were increased in some treated groups compared to controls; (4) no difference in survival rate between treated and control cows; and (5) all measures of reproductive efficiency for all doses were well within accepted industry standards. There are no published reports on reproductive performance of heifers derived from monensin-medicated cows. However, livestock producers have not reported reproductive problems following the use of monensin in beef and dairy replacement heifers in Canada since 1994 and in reproducing beef cows and replacement beef and dairy heifers in the USA since 1987 and 1983, respectively.

REPRODUCTIVE SAFETY IN NON-TARGET ANIMAL SPECIES

Growing and breeding pigs

One hundred and forty-four crossbred pigs, averaging 35 kg in weight, were randomly assigned to 24 pens of six pigs each and provided either 0 or 100 ppm monensin-medicated feed until finishing time. At the end of the growing/finishing trial, 18 control and 18 treated gilts were retained and maintained on their respective treatments through breeding, gestation, farrowing and lactation. Gilts were transferred to earthen lots and estrus cycles were observed. After approximately 12 weeks, each gilt was moved to a farrowing crate facility on day 16 of estrus. Each gilt was inseminated on the first day of standing heat and re-inseminated daily while she remained in standing heat. Breeding was continued through two heat cycles (approximately 42 days). Percent conception was slightly higher in the monensin-treated gilts than in controls. At 60 days of gestation, one monensin-treated pig was killed *in extremis* because of severe lameness unrelated to monensin treatment. Twelve apparently normal fetuses were found at necropsy. Other reproductive parameters were similar between the monensin-treated and the control groups. Results indicate that monensin at 100 ppm in complete feed (>3 times the approved cattle use level) can be fed safely to growing and reproducing pigs.

Sows and gilts

Sixteen crossbred gilts and 12 crossbred sows were divided into two groups and provided either 0 or 100 ppm monensin in the feed. All sows and gilts were artificially inseminated on the first day of standing heat and each successive day of standing heat during one estrous cycle. Treatment continued through 114 days of gestation and 28 days of lactation. Reproductive parameters were similar for both treatment groups. Monensin had no effects on conception rate, litter size at birth, survival of pigs or growth rate of offspring to weaning.

Broiler breeder and layer chickens

In a preliminary study to evaluate the effects of prolonged monensin feeding in broiler-type chickens, 280 females and 28 males of Vantress X Arbor breeding were fed 0 or 118 ppm monensin throughout developmental and production phases. Production parameters evaluated included egg production, fertility or hatchability and feed per 24-ounce-dozen eggs. No adverse treatment effects on these parameters were observed. Compared to controls, monensin-fed birds showed definite improvement in feed required per 24-ounce-dozen eggs produced. For the subsequent studies, decreasing levels of monensin were fed to 610 males and 164 females (Cobb strain) during brooding, rearing and developmental periods in a 391 day trial. At 1 day of age, the males were randomly placed in four pens (41 birds/pen) while the females were placed in four (102/pen) and two (101/pen) pens. Two male and three female pens received the basal (non-medicated) ration. The other pens were fed monensin according to the following schedule: (1) days 1 through 40, 132 ppm monensin; (2) days 41 through 82, 110 ppm monensin; (3) days 83 through 139, 88 ppm monensin; and (4) days 140 through 391, 0 ppm monensin (non-medicated laying ration). During the prelaying period (days 0 through 139), monensin-fed females gained more weight and had higher mortality than controls but the opposite was true for males. Feed conversion values were better for treated males relative to controls but were similar for females. During the production phase, there were no significant differences between birds previously fed monensin and those that had not been fed monensin with regard to mortality, percent live hen days, average egg weight, percent production and feed conversion. No significant treatment-related differences in percent fertility or percent of eggs incubated that hatched were observed. However, monensin had a highly significant positive effect on the percent hatch of fertile eggs. In a replicated study, White Leghorn males and females were fed only 121 ppm monensin from 1 to 140 days of age. Results indicated no treatment-related effect on growth, feed efficiency, livability, subsequent egg production and reproductive performance.

In contrast to growing birds, older sexually mature birds have been reported to be more susceptible to monensin toxicity than younger birds. Feeding 200 ppm monensin to 25-week-old commercial laying hens decreased food consumption, egg production and egg weight (Ruff and Jensen, 1997). Jones *et al.* (1990) reported that feeding broiler breeders at 40% egg production with 100 ppm monensin for 10 consecutive days was associated with reduced fertility for days 3 to 14 of withdrawal period. Egg production and hatchability of fertile eggs were not affected.

The apparent greater susceptibility of older chickens has been ascribed to be due, in part, to the large amount of feed consumed at any one feeding. Other factors are also known to modulate the response to monensin and other ionophores, including age, sex, selenium–vitamin E status, nitrates, dietary potassium and concomitant use of incompatible feed additives or drugs given via the drinking water (Stuart, 1978; Meingassner *et al.*, 1979; Stanfield and Lamont, 1981; Van Vleet *et al.*, 1983a; Frigg *et al.*, 1983; Weisman *et al.*, 1983, 1984; Umemura *et al.*, 1984; Wanner, 1984; Van Vleet, 1986; Broz and Frigg, 1987; Basaraba *et al.*, 1999; Lin, 1995; Anadon and Reeve-Johnson, 1999).

RISK ASSESSMENT

Among the domestic species of animals, horses appear to be the most sensitive, cattle intermediate and poultry the least sensitive to monensin toxicosis. Clinical effects were usually delayed one to several days, depending on the dose, and some were reversible even with continued monensin administration. In repeated-dose toxicity studies, monensin levels to which animals could be exposed daily for long periods of time without producing harmful effects have been identified. Target animal safety and toxicity studies indicated that it is safe to provide broiler and replacement chickens up to 121 ppm in complete feed, feedlot cattle up to 40 ppm monensin in total mixed ration (TMR), growing pasture cattle up to 200 mg/head/day and to dairy cattle 22 ppm in TMR or up to 400 mg/day via the controlled release capsule (CRC).

In breeding animals, monensin did not affect reproductive performance through four generations of rats and was not teratogenic in either rats or rabbits. Although maternal toxicity was produced at high oral doses in rats and rabbits, the doses used were very much in excess of monensin residue levels that have been found in meat, milk and eggs from beef and dairy cattle and chickens, respectively. In these target animal species, monensin produced no adverse effects on fertility and reproduction and did not harm the offspring.

The primary target organs of monensin toxicity were the cardiac and skeletal muscles. The monensin oral no observed effect levels (NOELs) were approximately 2 to 3.8 mg/kg in rats and 5 mg/kg/day in dogs after subchronic oral dosing of 3 months, 1.25 mg/kg/day in dogs after chronic oral dosing for 1 year and 1.4 mg/kg/day in rats and 1.3 mg/kg/day in mice after chronic oral dosing for 2 years. Earlier, the lowest NOEL of 1.25 mg monensin/kg in the dog was proposed to calculate the acceptable daily intake (ADI) of possible monensin residues in livestock and poultry products intended for human consumption (Novilla, 2004). More recently, CVMP and the EFSA FEEDAP Panel (EMEA, 2007) considered the acute pharmacological effects on the cardiovascular system in dogs to be more relevant, and chose the lower NOEL of 0.345 mg/kg given as a single oral dose. Using an uncertainty factor of 100 from the NOEL of 0.345 mg/kg resulted in the pharmacological ADI of 3.45 μg/kg body weight, i.e. 207 μg/person. For the benefit of harmonization the NOEL was rounded to 0.3 mg/kg and the overall ADI for monensin was calculated to 3 μg/kg body weight, i.e. 180 μg/person.

Based on maximum residue limits (MRLs) established by the FEEDAP Panel of the EFSA for chicken tissues and the CVMP MRLs for milk and the consideration of 50% activity of monensin metabolites, the theoretical maximum daily intake from chicken tissue and milk represents 82% of the ADI. Since the total monensin-derived residue was lower than the ADI, food products from monensin-treated animals are safe for human consumption.

CONCLUDING REMARKS AND FUTURE DIRECTIONS

The toxicology studies conducted with ionophores impact most directly on the safety to target animal species; to humans involved in the manufacture, shipping, feed preparation and administration to the target species; and to the general population who could be exposed to residues in food.

Ionophore toxicity in animal species results from overdosage, misuse and drug–drug interaction. In common with all the vertebrate species tested, the toxic syndrome is characterized clinically by anorexia, diarrhea, dyspnea, depression, ataxia, recumbency and death, and pathologically by degeneration, necrosis and repair of heart and skeletal muscles with secondary lesions of congestive heart failure. Peripheral neuropathy has been reported with lasalocid, salinomycin and narasin but not with monensin, laidlomycin, maduramicin and semduramycin.

The toxicity profile of monensin has been investigated extensively in several species of animals. Horses appear to be the most sensitive, cattle intermediate and poultry the least sensitive of the domestic species. In target animal species, it is safe to provide broiler and replacement chickens up to 121 ppm monensin in complete feed, feedlot cattle up to 40 ppm in total mixed ration (TMR), growing pasture cattle up to 200 mg/head/day and 22 ppm in TMR to dairy cattle or up to 400 mg/day via the controlled release capsule (CRC).

Animals given acutely toxic doses of monensin orally manifested similar clinical signs of toxicity including anorexia, diarrhea, hypoactivity, leg weakness, ataxia, depression and recumbency. Clinical effects were usually delayed one to several days, depending on the dose, and some were reversible even with continued monensin administration. In repeated-dose toxicity studies, monensin levels to which animals could be exposed daily for long periods of time without producing harmful effects have been identified.

There were no monensin-induced lesions in reproductive tissues and organs of rats from several studies, varying from 3 months to 2 years in duration. In these studies, rats were given monensin dietary doses up to 500 ppm for 3 months and 80 ppm for 2 years. These doses (approximately 30 and 5 mg/kg body weight, respectively) are higher than the anticipated 1 mg/kg intake for dairy cattle provided TMR containing 24 ppm monensin.

Safety studies conducted in growing and reproducing beef and dairy bulls, dairy replacement heifers and breeding and pregnant beef and dairy cows indicated that monensin caused no adverse effects on fertility and reproduction and did not harm the offspring. The number of calves born alive and their live weights were not affected by monensin treatment.

Monensin's lack of reproductive toxicity and teratogenic potential was suggested by the results of multigeneration reproduction and teratology studies in rats. Reproductive performance of parents and health status of offspring were not adversely affected through four generations of rats maintained continuously on diets containing either crystalline or mycelial monensin. There was also no evidence of teratogenicity in rats or rabbits. Although maternal toxicity was produced at high oral doses in rats and rabbits, the doses used were very much in excess of monensin residue levels in meat, milk and eggs from monensin treated animals. Since the total monensin-derived residue in cattle tissues and milk and chicken eggs was lower than the ADI, food products from monensin-treated animals are safe for human consumption. Based on the foregoing, it can be concluded that potential low residues of marketed ionophores do not pose a reproductive hazard to women of child-bearing potential or teratogenic risk to human fetuses whose mothers consume meat, milk and egg products from treated animals.

Some unintentional exposure to ionophores is expected to occur in the work place during the manufacture of premixes and the mixing and handling of medicated complete feeds. However, with the use of personal safety equipment and close adherence to GMPs and label instructions, exposure of humans to systemic levels high enough to produce any of the toxic effects is very unlikely during manufacturing or handling of bulk drug, premixes or formulated feeds. Small amounts of residues will also be ingested by people consuming meat and other foods derived from animals fed ionophore-medicated feeds. The results of the subchronic and chronic toxicity studies with the marketed ionophores, typified by monensin, indicate that multiple low-level exposures are not likely to produce adverse effects in humans.

No studies have been reported in which humans were intentionally exposed to ionophores. Nonetheless, monensin and other ionophores have been tested in *in vitro* and *in vivo* animal models for the treatment of human malaria (Adovelande and Schrevel, 1996; Gumila *et al.*, 1997), mycobacteriosis (Brumbaugh *et al.*, 2000), lead poisoning (Hamidinia *et al.*, 2002) and as potentiators for immunotoxin and anticancer drugs for man (Shaik *et al.*, 2001; Griffin *et al.*, 1993). Assuming that the above uses of monensin would pass clinical trials and given regulatory approval, the potential benefits to humankind should far outweigh the risks of the low-level human exposures. It cannot be overemphasized that therapeutic doses for humans would be many fold lower than the single and repeated doses that produced toxicosis in the target animals.

REFERENCES

Abe N, Lean IJ, Rabiee A, Porter J, Graham C (1994) Effects of sodium monensin on reproductive performance of dairy cattle. II. Effects on metabolites in plasma, resumption of ovarian cyclicity and oestrus in lactating cows. *Aust Vet J* **71:** 277–81.

Adovelande JB, Schrevel J (1996) Carboxylic ionophores in malaria chemotherapy: the effects of monensin and Nigericin *Plasmodium falciparum in vitro* and *Plasmodium vinckelpetteri in vivo*. *Pharmacol Lett* **59:** 309–15.

Amend JF, Mallon FM, Wren WB, Ramos AS (1981) Equine monensin toxicosis: some experimental clinicopathologic observations. *Comp Cont Ed* **11:** S173–83.

Anadon A, Reeve-Johnson L (1999) Macrolide antibiotics, drug interactions and microsomal enzymes: implications for veterinary medicine. *Res Vet Sci* **66:** 197–203.

Anderson WI, Reid WM, McDougald LR (1976) Efficacy of monensin against turkey coccidiosis in laboratory and floor pen experiments. *Avian Dis* **20:** 387–94.

Atef M, Ramadan A, Abo El-Sooud K (1993) Pharmacokinetic profile and tissue distribution of monensin in broiler chickens. *Brit Poultry Sci* **34:** 195–203.

Baile CA, McLaughlin CL, Potter EL, Chalupa W (1979) Feeding behavior changes of cattle during introduction of monensin with roughage or concentrate diets. *J Anim Sci* **48:** 1501–8.

Baird DJ, Caldow GL, Peek IS, Grant DA (1997) Monensin toxicity in a flock of ostriches. *Brit Poultry Sci* **34:** 624–6.

Basaraba RJ, Oehme FW, Vorhies MW, Stokka GL (1999) Toxicosis in cattle from concurrent feeding of monensin and dried distillers grains contaminated with macrolide antibiotics. *J Vet Diagn Invest* **11:** 79–86.

Bergen WG, Bates DB (1984) Ionophores: their effect on production efficiency and mode of action. *J Anim Sci* **58:** 1465–83.

Broz J, Frigg M (1987) Incompatibility between lasalocid and chloramphenicol in broiler chicks after long term administration. *Vet Res Comm* **11:** 159–72.

Brumbaugh GW, Edwards JF, Roussel Jr AJ, Thomson TD (2000) Effect of monensin sodium on histological lesions of naturally occurring bovine paratuberculosis. *J Comp Path* **123:** 22–8.

Buxton D, Blewett DA, Trees AJ, McGolgan C, Finlayson J (1988) Further studies in the use of monensin in the control of experimental ovine toxoplasmosis. *J Comp Path* **98:** 225–35.

Calo M, Lo Cascio P, Licata P, Richetti A, Zaccone G, Naccari F (2002) Effects of monensin on Na^{+}-ATPAse and Ca^{++}-ATPase activities in chick skeletal muscle and myocardium after subacute treatment. *Eur J Histochem* **46:** 309–15.

Carpenter JW, Novilla MN (1992) Safety and physiologic effects of the anticoccidial drugs monensin and clasuril in sandhill cranes (*Grus canadensis*). *J Zoo Wild Med* **23:** 214–21.

Condon FP, McKenzie RA (2002) Fatal monensin toxicity in a dog after chewing a bovine ruminal slow-release device. *Aust Vet Pract* **32:** 179–80.

Confer AW, Reavis DI, Panciera RJ (1983) Light and electron microscopic changes in cardiac and skeletal muscle of sheep with experimental monensin toxicosis. *Vet Pathol* **20:** 590–602.

Corah LR (1991) Polyether ionophores – effect on rumen function in feedlot cattle. *Vet Clinics North America* **7:** 127–32.

Coyle D, Walker A (2005) A study to determine the residues of monensin in edible tissues of growing cattle following treatment at 0.9 mg monensin/kg body weight for 28 days. Submitted to the European Medicines Agency CVMP by Elanco Animal Health, Division of Eli Lilly and Company, Indianapolis, IN, USA.

Davison KL (1984) Monensin absorption and metabolism in calves and chickens. *J Agric Food Chem* **32:** 1273–7.

De Sousa Spinosa H, Nicolau AA, Maruo VM, Bernardi MM (1999) Effects of monensin feeding during development on female rats and their offspring. *Neurotoxicol Teratol* **21:** 467–70.

Donoho A, Manthey J, Occolowitz J, Zornes L (1978) Metabolism of monensin in the steer and rat. *J Agric Food Chem* **26:** 1090–5.

Donoho AL (1984) Biochemical studies on the fate of monensin in animals and in the environment. *J Anim Sci* **58:** 1528–39.

Dorato MA (2000a) Expert report on Safety Documentation of Elancoban for Poultry (Monensin sodium). Submitted to the European Medicines Agency CVMP by Elanco Animal Health, Division of Eli Lilly and Company, Indianapolis, IN, USA.

Dorato MA (2000b) Expert report on Safety Documentation of Romensin for Cattle (Monensin sodium). Submitted to the European Medicines Agency CVMP by Elanco Animal Health, Division of Eli Lilly and Company, Indianapolis, IN, USA.

Dorato MA, Engelhardt JA (2005) The no-observed-adverse-effect level in drug safety evaluations: use, issues, and definitions(s). *Regulatory Toxicol Pharmacol* **42:** 265–74.

Dowling L (1992) Ionophore toxicity in chickens: a review of pathology and diagnosis. *Avian Pathol* **21:** 355–68.

Duffield T, Bagg R, DesCoteaux L, Bouchard E, Brodeur M, DuTremblay D, Keefe G, LeBlanc S, Dick P (2002) Prepartum monensin for the reduction of energy associated disease in postpartum cows. *J Dairy Sci* **85:** 397–5.

Duffield T, LeBlanc S, Bagg R, Leslie K, Ten Hag J, Dick P (2003) Effect of monensin controlled release capsule on metabolic parameters in transition dairy cows. *J Dairy Sci* **86:** 1171–6.

Duffield TF, Sandals DK, Leslie E, Lissemore K, McBride BW, Lumsden JH, Dick P, Bagg R (1999) Effect of monensin for the prevention of subclinical ketosis in lactating dairy cows. *J Dairy Sci* **81:** 2866–73.

EMEA (2007) Summary Report Monensin. (Cattle, including dairy cows) Committee for Medicinal Products for Veterinary Use. EMEA/CVMP/185123/2007-Final, pp. 1–9. Accessed online at http://www.emea.europa.eu/pdfs/vet/mrls/monensin.pdf

Ficken MD, Wages DP, Gonder E (1989) Monensin toxicity in turkey breeder hens. *Avian Dis* **33:** 186–90.

Frigg M, Broz J, Weber G (1983) Compatibility studies of ionophore anticoccidials with various antibiotics and chemoterapeutics in broiler chicks. *Archiv fur Geflugelkunde* **47:** 213–20.

Goodrich EA (1984) Influence of monensin on the performance of cattle. *J Anim Sci* **58:** 1484–98.

Gossett FO, Gibson WR, Koenig GR, Marroquin F, Young SS, Worth HM, Morton DM (1975) Dietary relay studies in dogs and rats to evaluate the safety of tissues from cattle fed Rumensin® (mycelial monensin sodium). Lilly Research Laboratories. Submitted to the European Medicines Agency CVMP by Elanco Animal Health, Division of Eli Lilly and Company, Indianapolis, IN, USA.

Griffin T, Ryback ME, Recht, L, Singh M, Raso V (1993) Potentiation of antitumor immunotoxins by liposomal monensin. *J Natl Cancer Inst* **85:** 292–8.

Gumila C, Ancelin ML, Jeminet G, Vial HJ (1997) Characterization of the potent antimalarial activities of ionophore compounds. *Antimicrob Agents Chemother* **41:** 523–9.

Hamidinia SA, Shimelis OI, Tan B, Erdahl WL, Chapman CJ, Renkes GD, Taylor RW, Pfeiffer DR (2002). Monensin mediates a rapid and selective transport of Pb^{2+} possible application of monensin for the treatment of Pb^{2+} intoxication. *J Biol Chem* **277:** 3811–20.

Hanrahan LA, Corner DE, Naqi SA (1981) Monensin toxicosis in broiler chickens. *Vet Pathol* **18:** 665–71.

Hayes DP, Pfeiffer DU, Williamson NB (1996) Effect of intraruminal monensin capsules on reproductive performance and milk production of dairy cows. *J Dairy Sci* **79:** 1000–8.

Herberg R, Manthey J, Richardson L, Cooley C, Donoho A (1978) Excretion and tissue distribution of ^{14}C monensin in cattle. *J Agric Food Chem* **26:** 1087–90.

Heuer C, Schuken YH, Jonker LJ, Wilkinson JID, Noorhuizen JPTM (2001) Effect of monensin on blood ketone bodies, incidence and recurrence of disease and fertility in dairy cows. *J Dairy Sci* **84:** 1085–97.

Jeffers TK, Tonkinson LV, Camp LJ, Murphy CN, Schlegel BF, Snyder DL, Young DC (1988) Field experience trials comparing narasin and monensin. *Poultry Sci* **67:** 1058–61.

Jones JE, Solis J, Hughes BL, Castaldo DJ, Toler JE (1990) Reproduction responses of broiler breeders to anticoccidial agents. *Poultry Sci* **69:** 27–36.

Kennington AS, Darby JM, Ehrenfried KM, Kiehl DE, Moran JW, Sweeney DJ (1995) [^{14}C]Monensin milk and tissue residues/metabolism in dairy cows. Lilly Research Laboratories. Submitted to the European Medicines Agency CVMP by Elanco Animal Health, Division of Eli Lilly and Company, Indianapolis, IN, USA.

Kohrs MB, Harper AE, Kerr GR (1976) Effects of low protein diet during pregnancy of the rhesus monkey. 1. Reproductive efficiency. *Am J Clin Nutrition* **29:** 136–45.

Kyriakis SC (1989) The effect of monensin against swine dysentery. *Brit Vet J* **143:** 373–7.

Lean IJ, Curtis M, Dyson R, Lowe B (1994) Effects of sodium monensin on reproductive performance of dairy cattle. 1. Effects on conception rates, calving-to-conception intervals, calving-to-heat and milk production in dairy cows. *Aust Vet J* **71:** 273–7.

Lin JA (1995) Mass salinomycin toxicity death due to concomitant use of tiamulin in a broiler breeder flock. *Taiwan J Vet Med Anim Husb* **65:** 339–46.

Mackintosh ED, Phipps RH, Sutton JD, Humphries DJ, Wilkinson JID (2002) Effect of monensin on rumen fermentation and digestion and milk production in lactating dairy cows. *J Anim Feed Sci* **11:** 399–410.

Matsuoka T, Novilla MN, Thomson TD, Donoho AL (1996) Review of monensin toxicosis in horses. *J Equine Vet Sci* **16:** 8–15.

McClary DG, Green HB, Mechor GD, Wilkinson JID (2008) Effect of rumensin on health and reproduction of lactating dairy cows. NADA 095-735. Tech Talk Scientific Update from Elanco Animal Health, Division of Eli Lilly and Company, Indianapolis, IN USA.

McGuffey RK, Richardson LF, Wilkinson JID (2001) Ionophores for dairy cattle: current status and future outlook. *J Dairy Sci* **84:** E194–E203.

Meingassner JG, Schmook FP, Czok R, Mieth H (1979) Enhancement of the anticoccidial activity of polyether antibiotics by tiamulin. *Poultry Sci* **58:** 303–13.

Mollenhauer HH, Morre DJ, Rowe LD (1990) Alteration of intracellular traffic by monensin; mechanism, specificity and relationship to toxicity. *Biochim Biophys Acta* **1031:** 225–46.

Novilla MN (1992) The veterinary importance of the toxic syndrome induced by ionophores. *Vet Hum Toxicol* **34:** 66–70.

Novilla MN (2004) Expert report on the safety file of monensin sodium. Submitted to the European Medicines Agency CVMP by Elanco Animal Health, Division of Eli Lilly and Company, Indianapolis, IN, USA.

Novilla MN (2007) Ionophores. In *Veterinary Toxicology. Basic and Clinical Principles* (Gupta RC, ed.). Academic Press/Elsevier, Amsterdam, pp. 1021–41.

Novilla MN, Folkerts TM (1986) Ionophores: monensin, lasalocid, salinomycin, narasin. In *Current Veterinary Therapy. Food Animal Practice* (Howard JL, ed.). Academic Press, New York, pp. 359–63.

Novilla MN, Owen NV, Todd GC (1994) The comparative toxicology of narasin in laboratory animals. *Vet Hum Toxicol* **36:** 318–23.

Novilla MN, Todd GC (1991) Cardiotoxicity of the ionophores, rat. In *Monographs on Pathology of Laboratory Animals Cardiovascular and Musculoskeletal Systems* (Jones TC, Mohr U, Hunt RD, eds.). Springer Verlag, Berlin, pp. 23–9.

Phipps RH, Wilkinson JID, Jonker LJ, Tarrant M, Jones AK, Hodge A (2000) Effect of monensin on milk production of Holstein-Friesian dairy cows. *J Dairy Sci* **83:** 2789–94.

Potter EL, Van Duyn RL, Cooley CO (1984) Monensin toxicity in cattle. *J Anim Sci* **58:** 1499–511.

Pressman BC (1976) Biological applications of ionophores. *Annu Rev Biochem* **45:** 501–30.

Pressman BC, Fahim NI (1982) Pharmacology and toxicology of the monovalent carboxylic ionophores. *Annu Rev Pharmacol Toxicol* **22:** 465–90.

Richardson LF, Raun AP, Potter EL, Cooley CO, Rathmacher RP (1976) Effect of monensin on rumen fermentation in vitro and in vivo. *J Anim Sci* **43:** 657–64.

Ruff MD, Jensen LS (1977) Production, quality and hatchability of eggs from hens fed monensin. *Poultry Sci* **56:** 1956–9.

Safran N, Aisenber I, Bark H (1993) Paralytic syndrome attributed to lasalocid residues in a commercial ration fed to dogs. *J Am Vet Med Assoc* **202:** 1273–5.

Sandercock DA, Mitchell MA (2003) Myopathy in broiler chickens: a role for Ca^{2+}-activated phospholipase A_2? *Poultry Sci* **82:** 1307–12.

Schweitzer D, Kimberling C, Spraker T, Sterner FE, McChesney AE (1984) Accidental monensin sodium intoxication in feedlot cattle. *J Am Vet Med Assoc* **184:** 1273–6.

Shaik MS, Ikidiobe O, Turnage VD, McSween J, Kannikkanan N, Singh M (2001) Long-circulating monensin nanaoparticles for the potentiation of immunotoxin and anticancer drugs. *J Pharm Pharmacol* **53:** 617–27.

Shier WT, Dubordieu WJ (1992) Sodium- and calcium-dependent steps in the mechanism of neonatal rat cardiac myocyte killing by ionophores. *Toxicol Appl Pharmacol* **116:** 38–46.

Shlosberg A, Weisman Y, Klopper U, Perl S (1985) Neurotoxic action of lasalocid at high doses. *Vet Rec* **117:** 394.

Shumard RF, Callender ME (1968) Monensin, a new biologically active compound. VI. Anticoccidial activity. *Antimicrobial Ag Chemother*: 369–77.

Smith CK, Galloway RB, White SL (1981) Effect of ionophores on survival, penetration, and development of *Eimeria tenella* sporozoites *in vitro*. *J Parasitol* **67:** 511–16.

Smith CK, Galloway RG (1983) Influence of monensin on cation influx and glycolysis of *Eimeria tenella* sporozoites *in vitro*. *J Parasitol* **69:** 666–70.

Stanfield DG, Lamont MN (1981) Monensin-tiamulin interactions ain pigs. *Vet Rec* **109:** 545.

Stockdale PHG (1981) Effects of monensin on coccidiosis in ruminants. *Vet Med Small Anim Clinician*. November 1981, pp. 1575–8.

Stuart JC (1978) An outbreak of monensin poisoning in adult turkeys. *Vet Rec* **102:** 303–4.

Sutko JL, Besch HR Jr, Bailey JC, Zimmerman G, Watanabe AM (1977) Direct effects of the monovalent cation ionophores monensin and nigericin on myocardium. *J Pharmacol Exp Therap* **203:** 685–700.

Tedeschi LO, Fox DG, Tylutki TP (2003). Potential environmental benefits of ionophores in ruminant diets. *J Environmental Quality* **32:** 1591–2.

Thomas EE, Smith CK, McGuffey RK, Quinn ME (1985) Monensin provides coccidiosis control: site and mode of action. Tech Talk Scientific Update from Elanco Animal Health, Division of Eli Lilly and Company, Indianapolis, IN USA.

Todd GC, Novilla MN, Howard LC (1984) Comparative toxicology of monensin sodium in laboratory animals. *J Anim Sci* **58:** 1512–17.

Tsuchida K, Otomo S (1990) Electrophysiological effects of monensin, a sodium ionophore, on cardiac Purkinje fibers. *Eur J Pharmacol* **190:** 313–20.

Umemura T, Nakamura H, Goryo M, Itakura C (1984) Ultrastructural changes of monensin–oleandomycin myopathy in broiler chicks. *Avian Pathol* **13:** 743–51.

US Food and Drug Administration (1982) Toxicologic principles for the safety assessment of direct food additives and color additives used in food. US Food and Drug Administration, Bureau of Foods, Washington DC.

US Food and Drug Administration (1986) General principles for evaluating the safety of compounds used in food-producing animals. *Fed Regist* **52** FR, 49583.

US Food and Drug Administration (2000) Toxicological principles for the safety assessment of food ingredients. *Redbook 2000* FDA Center for Food Safety and Nutrition, Washington DC.

Van der Linde-Sipman JS, Van den Ingh TSGAM, Van ES JJ, Verhagen H, Kerster JGTM, Beynen AC, Plekkringa R (1999) Salinomycin-induced polyneuropathy in cats: morphologic and epidemiologic data. *Vet Pathol* **36:** 152–6.

Van Vleet JF (1986) Interaction of nutritional status and ionophore feed additives in animals. *Proceedings of 6th International Conference on Production Diseases in Farm Animals*, Belfast, Northern Ireland, pp. 268–76.

Van Vleet JF, Amstutz HE, Weirich WE, Rebar AH, Ferrans VJ (1983a) Acute monensin toxicosis in swine: effect of graded doses of monensin and protection of swine by pretreatment with selenium–vitamin E. *Am J Vet Res* **44:** 1460–8.

Van Vleet JF, Amstutz HE, Weirich WE, Rebar AH, Ferrans VJ (1983b) Clinical, and clinicopathologic and pathologic alterations of acute monensin toxicosis in swine. *Am J Vet Res* **44:** 1469–75.

Van Vleet JF, Amstutz HE, Weirich WE, Rebar AH, Ferrans VJ (1983c) Clinical, and clinicopathologic and pathologic alterations in acute monensin toxicosis in cattle. *Am J Vet Res* **44:** 2133–44.

Van Vleet JF, Ferrans VJ, Herman E (1991) Cardiovascular and skeletal muscle system. In *Handbook of Toxicologic Pathology* (Haschek WM, Rousseaux CG, eds.). Academic Press, San Diego, CA, pp. 539–624.

Wanner M (1984) Unvertraglichkeit von Tiamulin und Salinomycinbeim Schwein. *Schweiz Arch Tierheilk* **126:** 521–6.

Watkins LE, Wray MI, Basson RP, Feller DL, Olson RD, Fitzgerald PR, Stromberg BE, Davis GW (1986) The prophylactic effects of monensin fed to cattle inoculated with coccidian oocysts. *Agri-Practice* **7:** 1820.

Weisman J, Herz A, Jegana J, Egyed M, Shlosberg A (1983) The effect of tiamulin administered by different routes and at different ages in turkeys receiving monensin in their feed. *Vet Res Comm* **6:** 189–98.

Weisman J, Shkap I, Egyed M, Shlosberg A (1984) Chloramphenicol-induced monensin toxicity. *Refuah Vet* **41:** 3–6.

Wentink GH, Vente JP (1981) A case of monensin poisoning in dairy cattle [Een geval van monensin-vergiftiging bij mlkvee]. *Tijdschr Diergeneesk* **106:** 623–5.

Whitlock RH, White NA, Rowland GN, Plue R (1978) Monensin toxicosis in horses: clinical manifestations. *Proc Am Soc Equine Practnrs* **24:** 473–86.

Wilson JS (1980) Toxic myopathy in a dog associated with the presence of monensin in dry food. *Can Vet J* **21:** 30–1.

CHAPTER

30

Selected herbal supplements and nutraceuticals

Manashi Bagchi, Sangeeta Patel, Shirley Zafra-Stone and Debasis Bagchi

INTRODUCTION

Recently nutraceutical supplements have gained popularity in both men and women around the world. Women are the main consumers of complementary and alternative medicine, in particular botanical medicine. The desire to have personal control over their health has been cited as the strongest motive for women to use herbal medicine. Another motive is dissatisfaction with conventional treatment and its disregard for a holistic approach, as well as concerns about the side effects of pharmaceutical drugs. These concerns explain, in part, the fact that many women use herbal remedies during pregnancy. A survey of 578 pregnant women in the eastern USA reported that 45% of respondents had used herbal medicines, and a survey of 588 women in Australia revealed that 36% had used at least one herbal product during pregnancy (Dog, 2009). Women probably feel comfortable using herbal remedies because of their perceived safety, easy access and the widespread availability of information about them (i.e., Internet, magazines, books).

While it is true that many botanicals are mild in both treatment effects and side effects, the data regarding the safety of those botanicals used during pregnancy are very limited. There are some herbs that are known teratogens, which should not under any circumstances be taken during pregnancy. Some herbs known to cause problems during pregnancy include, but are not limited to: *Semen crotonis* (Ba Dou), *Semen pharbitidis* (Qian Niu Zi), *Radix euphorbiae* (Da Ji), Mulabris (Ban Mao), *Radix phytolaccae* (Shang Lu), Moschus (She Xiang), *Rhizoma sparganii* (San Leng), *Rhizoma zedoariae* (EZhu), *Hirudo seu Whitmania* (Shui Zhi) and Tabanus (Meng Chong) (Rousseaux and Schachter, 2003). Other herbs are recognized as potentially dangerous to the fetus and should be used with caution. Some of these include, but are not limited to: *Semen persicae* (Taò Ren), *Flos carthami* (Hong Hua), *Radix* and *Rhizomia rhei* (Da Huang), *Fructus aurantii* (Zi Shi), *Radix aconiti* (Fu Zhi), *Rhizoma zingiberis* (Gan Jiang) and *Cortex cinnamomi* (Rou Gui) (Buehler, 2003; Rousseaux and Schachter, 2003). While some dietary supplements are found to be safe, others are reported to cause serious toxicity (Haller *et al.*, 2005). Furthermore, it is important to mention that sometimes these herbal medicines are contaminated with chemicals, drugs and adulterants that have the potential to cause reproductive and developmental effects. In addition, plant misidentification and interaction with other herbal products or pharmaceutical products further raise serious concerns about their safety (Ernst and Thompson, 2001; Singla *et al.*, 2009; Jordan *et al.*, 2010).

It has been pointed out that currently a formal surveillance system for tracking adverse events related to dietary supplements does not currently exist, and as a result reliance on voluntary reporting is the only mechanism for detecting toxic effects of dietary supplements (Haller *et al.*, 2005). Adverse effects of dietary supplements can remain undetected for some time, resulting in sporadic reports of potentially serious toxicity. Evaluation of adverse event reports made through the Food and Drug Administration (FDA) MedWatch system remains one of the few mechanisms for detection of trends in toxic reactions and identification of harmful supplement products. This chapter describes the reproductive and developmental effects of commonly used herbal medicines and nutraceuticals.

CHROMIUM(III) SUPPLEMENTS

Chromium(III) is an essential nutrient necessary for normal carbohydrate and lipid metabolism. There is a growing body of evidence to suggest that chromium may have beneficial effects in the regulation of insulin action, metabolic syndrome and cardiovascular disease. The chromium level in the body decreases with age and studies have indicated that the total dietary intake of chromium may be inadequate in the adult population. Furthermore, subjects with diabetes and cardiovascular disease have been shown to have lower circulating levels of chromium (Anderson, 1998) whereas supplementation with chromium improved blood sugar levels and insulin sensitivity. Although the molecular mechanisms of chromium are not fully understood, several studies suggest that Cr(III) increases insulin binding through increasing the number of insulin receptors and phosphorylation when the chromium is bound to chromodulin, a low molecular weight chromium binding substance (Anderson, 1998).

Chromium picolinate (CrPic) and chromium polynicotinate (CrNic) are two of the most popular dietary supplements and are sold individually or as a component of herbal blends or mixed formula with vitamins, minerals or other

Reproductive and Developmental Toxicology, Edited by Ramesh C. Gupta
ISBN: 978-0-12-382032-7

active ingredients. They are also provided in many food and beverage products, such as nutrition bars and sports drinks. To demonstrate their safety, numerous acute and subchronic toxicity studies have been performed on both Cr(III) complexes. However, it is important to note that reproductive and developmental toxicity studies on Cr(III) supplements are of particular importance since Cr(III) has been recommended for pregnant women who are diagnosed with gestational diabetes.

Pregnancy may increase urinary chromium loss, making pregnant women susceptible to chromium deficiency. Moreover, the results of a study by Jovanovic *et al.* (1999) indicate that chromium supplementation may be useful in the treatment of gestational diabetes, a common pregnancy complication. However, the availability of Cr(III) to the embryo and fetus has not yet been fully determined, so their relative Cr exposure is as yet only speculative.

Chromium(III) picolinate (CrPic)

The dietary supplement CrPic has gained much attention as a safe supplement that reportedly promotes fat loss and muscle enhancement in humans. However, several studies demonstrate that CrPic has been associated with oxidative damage to DNA in rats and mutations and DNA fragmentation in cell cultures. In isolated case reports, CrPic supplementation has been said to cause adverse effects, such as anemia, renal failure, liver dysfunction and neuronal impairment.

In a literature search for reproductive and developmental toxicity studies on CrPic, a few comparative developmental studies against CrPic were found. In an early study using *Drosophila melanogaster*, CrPic at levels of 260 μg Cr/kg food or less were found to lower the success rate of pupation and eclosion and to arrest development of pupae in a concentration-dependent fashion. X-linked lethal analysis indicated that the CrPic greatly enhances the rate of appearance of lethal mutations and dominant female sterility (Hepburn *et al.*, 2003).

In recent studies conducted by Bailey *et al.*, researchers compared the effects of CrPic, chromium(III) chloride ($CrCl_3$) and picolinic acid in mice (Bailey *et al.*, 2006) in which the observed developmental effects were more apparent with CrPic than with picolinic acid. In this study, pregnant CD-1 mice were fed diets containing either 200 mg/kg CrPic, 200 mg/kg $CrCl_3$, 174 mg/kg picolinic acid or diet only (control), for 6–17 gestation days. Dams were sacrificed on gestation day 17, and their litters were examined for adverse effects. Results showed that the incidence of bifurcated cervical arches was significantly increased in fetuses from the CrPic group as compared to the diet-only group. Fetuses in the picolinic acid-treated group had an incidence double that of the control group; however, this increase was not statistically significant. Fetuses in the $CrCl_3$ group did not differ from the controls in any variable examined. No maternal toxicity was observed in any of the treatment groups. Overall, this study showed that high maternal oral exposures to CrPic can cause morphological defects in developing offspring of mice. However, in another comparative study by Bailey *et al.*, results differed and shown that maternal exposure to either $CrCl_3$ or CrPic at the dosages employed did not appear to cause deleterious effects to the developing offspring in mice (Bailey *et al.*, 2008a,b). There was no decrease in fetal weight or significantly increased incidence of skeletal defects observed in the $CrCl_3$ or CrPic exposed fetuses compared to the controls. This was reported to be mainly due to an increased incidence of arch defects in the control offspring. However, further toxicity and safety studies demonstrated it to be GRAS (generally recognized as safe) and can be added to food and beverages.

Chromium(III) polynicotinate

A broad spectrum of research investigations including *in vitro*, *in vivo* and clinical studies demonstrated the beneficial effects of niacin-bound chromium (III) complex (NBC) in attenuating insulin resistance and lowering plasma cholesterol levels, increasing cardioprotective potential and lean body mass. Preuss *et al.* (1997) confirmed that NBC supplementation can overcome sucrose-induced blood pressure elevation in spontaneously hypertensive rats. Furthermore, it decreases oxidative stress and extends average lifespan.

The effect of NBC was recently evaluated in a two-generation reproduction toxicity study. Sprague-Dawley rats (30/sex/group) were maintained on feed containing NBC at dose levels of 0, 4, 15 or 60 ppm for 10 weeks prior to mating, during mating and, for females through gestation and lactation, across two generations. During the period of study, animals were examined daily for signs of clinical toxicity and their body weight and feed consumption were recorded twice a week. For the parents (F_0 and F_1) and the offspring (F_1 and F_{2a}), reproductive parameters such as fertility and mating, gestation, parturition, litters, lactation, sexual maturity and development of offspring were assessed. At termination, necropsy and histopathological examinations were performed on all animals. Dietary exposure of NBC to parental male and female rats of both (F_0 and F_1) the generations during the pre-mating and mating periods, for both sexes, and during gestation and lactation in case of female rats, did not reveal any remarkable incidence of mortality or abnormal clinical signs. Compared to respective controls, NBC exposure did not affect feed consumption or body weight at any of the exposure levels. NBC exposure did not affect reproductive performance as evaluated by sexual maturity, fertility and mating, gestation, parturition, litter properties, lactation and development of the offspring. Based on the results of this study, the parental as well as the offspring no-observed-adverse-effect level (NOAEL) for NBC was determined to be greater than 60 ppm in diet or equivalent to 7.80 and 8.31 mg/kg body weight/day in male and female rats, respectively.

The teratogenic potential of NBC was also evaluated in Sprague-Dawley rats. Due to its potential to affect fat synthesis and reduce food intake, processes which are often crucial in normal fetal development, a teratology study was undertaken as part of a multi-generation reproductive investigation. The animals in this study were selected randomly after weaning from each F_{2b} litter of the F_1 generation from the two-generation reproductive toxicity study. To start the teratology study, Sprague-Dawley rat pups (~30/sex/group) from the F_{2b} generation were allowed to grow up to 10–12 weeks of age before mating. The rats in the treatment group were exposed directly to NBC through feed. The dietary exposure levels were the same as those employed for the two-generation reproductive toxicity study, viz. 4, 15 or 60 ppm. Following mating at maturity, the pregnant rats were observed daily for clinical signs of adverse effects, and body weight and feed consumption were recorded. On day 20 of gestation, animals were subjected to a necropsy and cesarean section to examine the uterus, ovaries and fetuses for assessment of different parameters of pregnancy and embryo–fetal defects. In this study, no indications of maternal toxicity, adverse effects on the parameters evaluated for the gravid uteri, external abnormalities in the fetuses, soft tissue abnormalities in the fetuses or skeletal abnormalities in the fetuses were noted. Based on the results of this developmental toxicity study, NBC was found to be non-teratogenic in Sprague-Dawley rat, at the dietary exposure levels of 4, 15 and 60 ppm, equivalent to the dose levels of 0.50, 2.0 or 8.0 mg/kg/day, respectively.

GINGER (*ZINGIBER OFFICINALE*)

Ginger has been used as a herbal medicine in Asian, Indian and Arabic traditions to treat a wide range of ailments including stomach upset, diarrhea, nausea, arthritis, colic and heart conditions. In addition to these medicinal uses, ginger continues to be valued around the world as an important cooking spice and is believed to help treat the common cold, flu-like symptoms, headaches and even painful menstrual periods. Today, health care professionals commonly recommend it to help prevent or treat nausea and vomiting associated with motion sickness, pregnancy and cancer chemotherapy. Side effects associated with ginger are rare, but if taken in excessive doses the herb may cause mild heartburn, diarrhea and irritation of the mouth.

The important active components of the ginger root are zingerone, shogaols and gingerols, volatile oils that compose 1–3% of the weight of fresh ginger. The chemical structure of zingerone is shown in Figure 30.1. In laboratory animals, the gingerols increase the motility of the gastrointestinal tract and have analgesic, sedative, antipyretic and antibacterial properties (O'Hara *et al.*, 1998).

While ginger appears to be a safe, effective alternative to drug treatment, especially in the treatment of morning sickness, little reproductive and developmental research has been done. Furthermore, some sources indicate that ginger should not be used in pregnancy due to the risk of spontaneous abortion or unspecified adverse fetal outcome (Wilkinson, 2000a). In a developmental study using ginger tea, pregnant Sprague-Dawley rats were administered, from gestation day 6 to 15, 20 g/liter or 50 g/liter ginger tea via their drinking water and then sacrificed at day 20. No maternal toxicity was observed; however, embryonic loss in the treatment groups was double that of the controls ($p<0.05$). No gross morphologic malformations were seen in the treated fetuses. Fetuses exposed to ginger tea were found to be significantly heavier than controls, an effect that was greater in female fetuses and was not correlated with increased placental size. Treated fetuses also had more advanced skeletal development as determined by measurement of sternal and metacarpal ossification centers. The results of this study suggest that *in utero* exposure to ginger tea results in increased early embryo loss with increased growth in surviving fetuses (Wilkinson, 2000b).

Conversely, in a separate teratogenic study, ginger extract was shown to be safe when administered to maternal rats. Ginger extract was administered by oral gavage in concentrations of 100, 333 and 1,000 mg/kg, to three groups of 22 pregnant female rats from days 6 to 15 of gestation. Results show that ginger extract caused neither maternal nor developmental toxicity at daily doses of up to 1,000 mg/kg body weight, when administered to pregnant rats during the period of organogenesis (Weidnera and Sigwart, 2001). The differing results of the above studies may possibly be due to the potential variation of active ingredients between different ginger preparations.

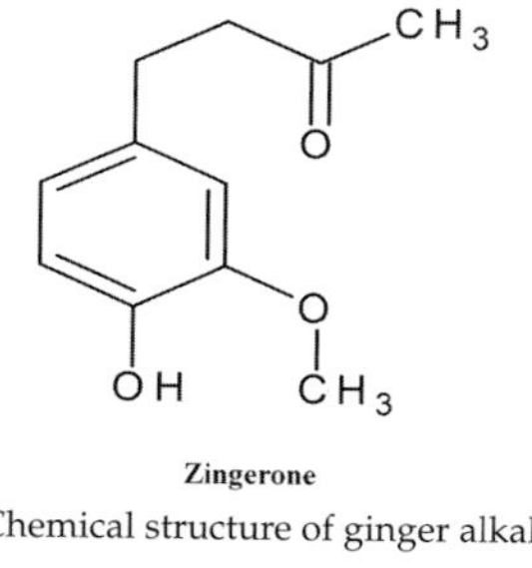

Zingerone

FIGURE 30.1 Chemical structure of ginger alkaloid zingerone.

GENISTEIN

Genistein (5,7-dihydroxy-3-(4-hydroxyphenyl)chromen-4-one) is a phytoestrogen that is found in a wide variety of plant-derived foods especially in soybeans and soy-based foods. Figure 30.2 shows chemical structure of genistein. Genistein and related phytoestrogens are best known as chemopreventive agents for a variety of human diseases and cancers. Soybeans and soy-based foods have been consumed at high levels in several Asian populations for many centuries without any apparent adverse effects. However, there is concern over potential adverse effects due to the estrogenic and other activities of the isoflavones. Isoflavones (genistein, daidzein, glycitein and their conjugated forms) structurally resemble estradiol and have estrogenic activity, but with a binding affinity to the estrogen receptor 100–1,000 times less than estradiol. The reproductive effects of the isoflavones were first noted as a result of infertility in grazing animals, captive cheetahs and California quail (Kaldas and Hughes, 1989; Kurzer and Xu, 1997; Setchell *et al.*, 1987).

Several *in vitro* and *in vivo* studies were conducted by researchers McClain *et al.* (2007) to assess the teratogenic and fetal toxic potential of genistein. Genistein was tested in an *in vitro* rat whole embryo culture assay (WEC), a preliminary screen for fetotoxic and teratogenic potential, over a concentration range from 1 to 100 µg/mL. Treatment-related anomalies were observed at concentrations of 10 µg and at 100 µg/mL all embryos were malformed. Two *in vivo* embryo–fetal developmental safety studies were conducted with genistein by oral administration (gavage and dietary admix) in which there was no evidence for a teratogenic effect.

In an oral (gavage) embryonic and fetal development pilot study, genistein was administered to rats at dose levels of 0, 20, 150 and 1,000 mg/kg/day from days 6 to 20 of

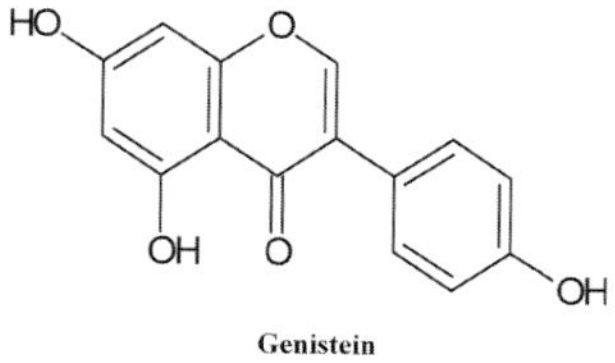

Genistein

FIGURE 30.2 Chemical structure of genistein.

gestation to females that were allowed to litter and rear their offspring up to day 7 of lactation. A slight maternal toxicity at 1,000 mg/kg/day was observed as indicated by decreased body weight and food consumption and at this dose, adverse effects in the pups were observed including increased pup mortality, poor general condition, reduced pup body weights and reduced pup milk uptake. At the high dose of 1,000 mg/kg, no external malformations were noted; however, some minor visceral and skeletal variations were observed. At the low dose of 20 mg/kg/day, an increased mortality, reduced milk uptake, a decreased percent male sex ratio and decreased body weights during lactation were observed. Due to lack of effects at the mid dose and the small number of animals, a relationship to treatment and toxicity was considered unlikely.

In an oral (dietary admix) prenatal developmental safety study, genistein was administered to rats at dose levels of 0, 5, 50, 100 and 500 mg/kg/day from day 5 to 21 of gestation. At 500 mg/kg, maternal body weight and food consumption were markedly reduced. The incidence of resorptions was markedly increased with a corresponding decrease in the number of live fetuses per dam. Fetal body weights were also reduced. No treatment-related teratogenic effects were noted during external, visceral and skeletal examination of fetuses or in body weight normalized anogenital distance.

Based on the studies conducted by McClain *et al.* (2007), it was concluded that genistein has no teratogenic potential *in vivo* at very high doses of up to 1,000 mg/kg/day by oral gavage in the embryo–fetal toxicity pilot study or up to 500 mg/kg/day by dietary admix in the prenatal developmental study even though these doses were maternally toxic and fetal toxic. *In vitro*, studies with genistein had teratogenic potential at high concentrations in the WEC screening assay; however, this was not predictive of the *in vivo* findings. Based on their prenatal development study, the NOAEL for maternal toxicity and adverse effects on embryonic development was considered to be 100 mg/kg/day when administered orally by dietary admixture. Furthermore, genistein is in the list of FDA approved GRAS status.

RESVERATROL

Resveratrol (3,5,4′-trihydroxystilbene) is a natural polyphenol found in grapes and other plants (Baur and Sinclair, 2006). Its chemical structure is shown in Figure 30.3. It is a stilbenoid, a derivate of stilbene, and is produced in plants with the help of the enzyme stilbene synthase. Scientists became interested in exploring potential health benefits of resveratrol in 1992 when its presence was first reported in red wine, leading to speculation that resveratrol might help explain the "French Paradox". More recently, reports on the potential for resveratrol to inhibit the development of cancer and extend lifespan in cell culture and animal models have continued to generate scientific interest. Most resveratrol supplements available in the USA contain extracts of the root of *Polygonum cuspidatum*, also known as Hu Zhang or kojo-kon. Red wine extracts and red grape extracts containing resveratrol and other polyphenols are also available in the USA as dietary supplements. Resveratrol supplements may contain anywhere from 10 to 50 mg of resveratrol, but the effective doses for chronic disease prevention in humans are not known.

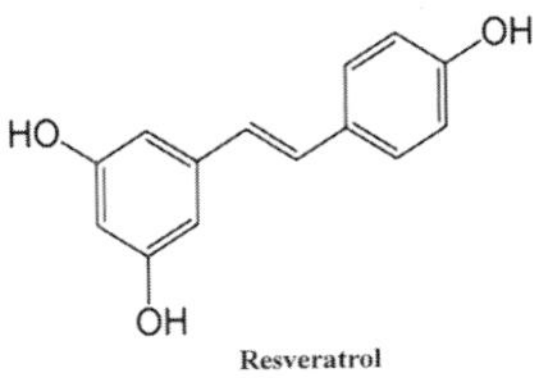

HO OH OH
Resveratrol

FIGURE 30.3 Chemical structure of resveratrol.

The chemical structure of resveratrol is very similar to that of the synthetic estrogen agonist diethylstilbestrol, suggesting that resveratrol might also function as an estrogen agonist. However, in cell culture experiments resveratrol acts as an estrogen agonist under some conditions and an estrogen antagonist under other conditions. In estrogen receptor-positive breast cancer cells, resveratrol acted as an estrogen agonist in the absence of the endogenous estrogen 17beta-estradiol, but acted as an estrogen antagonist in the presence of 17beta-estradiol. At present, it appears that resveratrol has the potential to act as an estrogen agonist or antagonist depending on such factors as cell type, estrogen receptor isoform (ER alpha or ER beta), and the presence of endogenous estrogens.

Published data demonstrates that *in vitro* resveratrol may exhibit weak phytoestrogenic activity (Gehm *et al.*, 1997; Henry and Witt, 2002). In three *in vitro* studies, *trans*-resveratrol was shown to have a low affinity for estrogen receptor binding (approximately 7,000-fold weaker than estrogen) (Li *et al.*, 2004) and to be only weakly active compared to the reference estrogens diethylstilbestrol or estradiol (i.e., the affinity of *trans*-resveratrol is lower than diethylstilbestrol or estradiol, in a yeast hER-a transcription assay and a cos-1 cell transfection assay) (Ashby *et al.*, 1999). As previously indicated, the relevance of *in vitro* assays to *in vivo* conditions is questionable. When administered *in vivo* to female weanling rats for 6 days via gavage, *trans*-resveratrol (0.001, 0.004, 0.01, 0.04 and 0.1 mg/day) did not exhibit estrogenic effects and it was also non-estrogenic in two uterotrophic assays in rats (Ashby *et al.*, 1999). Also, in a recent study using an ovariectomized rat model, the effects of several chemicals suggested to possess phytoestrogenic properties (including *trans*-resveratrol) on bone density was investigated. It was reported that there were no significant changes in bone density between control and *trans*-resveratrol-treated animals. In contrast, in rats exposed to the chemicals genistein and 8-prenylnarigenin there was a statistically significant increase in bone density compared to the control group (Sehmisch *et al.*, 2008). This study provides further evidence that *trans*-resveratrol has low estrogenic potency *in vivo*.

In a reproductive toxicity study, rats were administered trans-resveratrol via gavage at 20 mg/kg for 90 days. *trans*-Resveratrol was shown to significantly reduce the diameter of seminiferous tubules, increase the density of seminiferous tubules and significantly increases sperm count and plasma LH, FSH and testosterone levels (Juan *et al.*, 2005). In another study, *trans*-resveratrol administered at 3 mg/l in drinking water to male and female mice for 4 weeks resulted in a significant decrease in seminal vesicle and spleen weights in male F_0 mice, a significant decrease in seminal vesicle and kidney weights in male F_1 mice and a significant decrease in ovary weight in the female F_0 mice (Kyselova *et al.*, 2003). *trans*-Resveratrol did not affect sperm count and quality or ovarian morphology and was considered to be safe at lower doses. In a very recent study, Svechnikov *et al.* (2009) demonstrated that resveratrol and its analogs structure-dependently attenuated steroidogenesis in Leydig cells through suppression of the expression of StAR and cytochrome P450c17. Moreover, 3,5-diacetyl resveratrol was observed to modulate mitochondrial function in Leydig cells, suppressing polarization of inner mitochondrial membrane and 3,4,4′-trimethoxystilbene stimulated the overall activity of intracellular reductases involved in the reduction of WST-1 to formazan. Thus, the inhibitory actions of resveratrol analogs on steroidogenesis in Leydig cells indicate novel mechanisms of action of these compounds, which may be of potential therapeutic interest, where suppression of androgen action is needed.

GREEN TEA (EGCG)

Green tea and its catechins, (–)-epigallocatechin gallate (EGCG), (–)-epigallocatechin (EGC), (–)-epicatechin gallate (ECG) and (–)-epicatechin (EC), have been demonstrated to have anticancer properties through interactions with multiple biochemical processes. EGCG has been the most extensively studied because of its relatively high abundance and strong epidemiologic evidence for cancer prevention. EGCG have been shown *in vitro* to stimulate apoptosis and cell cycle arrest of various cancer cell lines, including prostate, lymphoma, colon and lung (Mukhtar and Ahmad, 2000).

Little research is available on the effects of green tea and EGCG during pregnancy. Drinking green tea is not encouraged during pregnancy because of the caffeine content, ranging from 14 to 61 mg caffeine per 6–8 ounce serving. This is important because caffeine crosses the placenta and the effects of caffeine on unborn babies are not well known. Although an epidemiology study showed that tea, not caffeine, consumption has been associated with developmental neural tube defects when maternal exposure was high during the preconceptual period (Correa *et al.*, 2000), but the type of tea – green or black – was not specified in this study.

In a study conducted by Isbrucker *et al.* (2006), researchers evaluated the potential effects of EGCG on the fetus. EGCG preparations of >91% purity were administered to pregnant rats during organogenesis and development. In their initial preliminary study using subcutaneous and gavage routes, there was no evidence of any direct embryo–fetal toxicity, although some maternal toxicity was seen. In another recent teratogenicity study, feeding pregnant rats diets supplemented at 1,400, 4,200 or 14,000 ppm during organogenesis was non-toxic to dams or fetuses. A two-generation study in rats fed 1,200, 3,600 or 12,000 ppm EGCG preparation showed no adverse effects on reproduction or fertility. The highest dose reduced the growth rate of offspring, and there was a slight increase in pup loss. A growth effect among pups was also seen at 3,600 ppm, but in the second generation only. The lowest dose was considered the overall NOAEL. As dams consumed twice the amount of feed during the crucial lactation period, the NOAEL was equivalent to 200 mg/kg/day EGCG preparation.

In a recent study by Park *et al.* (2009), the effects of green tea extract on the fetal development and external, visceral and skeletal abnormalities induced by cyclophosphamide were investigated in rats. Pregnant rats were daily administered green tea extract (100 mg/kg) by gavage for 7 days, from the 6th to 12th day of gestation, and intraperitoneally administered with cyclophosphamide (11 mg/kg) 1 h after the final treatment. On the 20th day of gestation, maternal and fetal abnormalities were determined by cesarean section. Cyclophosphamide was found to reduce fetal and placental weights without increasing resorption or death. In addition, it induced malformations in live fetuses; 94.6%, 41.5% and 100% of the external (skull and limb defects), visceral (cleft palate and ureteric dilatation) and skeletal (acrania, vertebral/costal malformations and delayed ossification) abnormalities. When pretreated with green tea extract, cyclophosphamide-induced body weight loss and abnormalities of fetuses were remarkably aggravated. Moreover, repeated treatment with GTE greatly increased mRNA expression and activity of hepatic cytochrome P-450 (CYP) 2B, which metabolizes cyclophosphamide into teratogenic acrolein and cytotoxic phosphoramide mustard, while reducing CYP3A expression (a detoxifying enzyme). The results suggest that repeated intake of green tea extract may aggravate cyclophosphamide-induced body weight loss and malformations of fetuses by modulating CYP2B and CYP3A. Tio International (Japan) has received USFDA GRAS status for its green tea ingredient Suntheanine and is popularly used in food and beverages around the world.

BERBERINE

Berberine, a plant alkaloid, is found in some herbal teas and health-related products. It is a component of goldenseal, a herbal supplement. The chemical structure of berberine alkaloid is shown in Figure 30.4. Berberine chloride dihydrate (BCD) was evaluated for developmental toxicity in rats and mice. BCD was administered in the feed to timed-mated Sprague-Dawley rats (0, 3,625, 7,250 or 14,500 ppm on gestational days 6–20), and Swiss Albino mice (0, 3,500, 5,250 or 7,000 ppm on gestation days 6–17). Ingested doses were 0, 282, 531 and 1,313 mg/kg/day (rats) and 0, 569, 841 and 1,155 mg/kg/day (mice). There were no maternal deaths. The rat maternal LOAEL (low-observed-adverse-effect level), based on reduced maternal weight gain, was 7,250 ppm. The rat developmental toxicity LOAEL, based on reduced fetal body weight per litter, was 14,500 ppm. In the mouse study, equivocal maternal and developmental toxicity LOAELs were 5,250 ppm.

Due to scattering of feed in the high dose groups, a gavage study at 1,000 mg/kg/day was conducted in both species. In rats, maternal, but not fetal, adverse effects were noted. The maternal toxicity LOAEL remained at 7,250 ppm (531 mg/kg/day) based on the feed study and the developmental toxicity NOAEL was raised to 1,000 mg/kg/day BCD based on the gavage study. In the mouse, 33% of the treated females died. Surviving animals had increased relative water intake, and average fetal body weight per litter decreased 5–6% with no change in live litter size. The maternal toxicity LOAEL remained at 5,250 ppm (841 mg/kg/day) BCD, based on increased water consumption. The developmental toxicity LOAEL was raised to 1,000 mg/kg/day BCD based on decreased fetal body weight (Jahnke *et al.*, 2006).

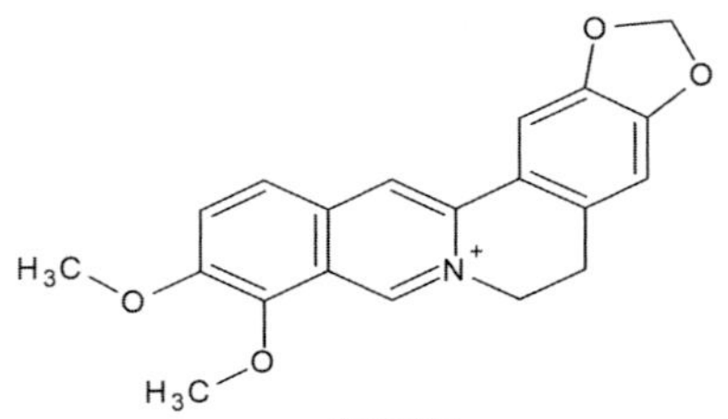

Berberine

FIGURE 30.4 Chemical structure of berberine.

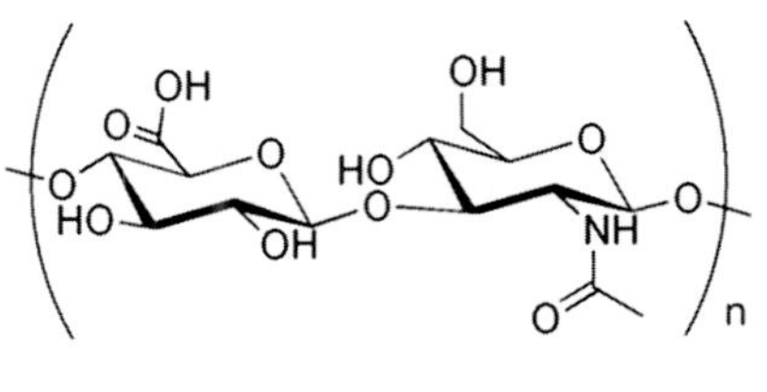

Hyaluronic Acid

FIGURE 30.5 Chemical structure of hyaluronic acid.

GINSENG

The commercially available product "ginseng" usually refers to the dried root of *Panax ginseng*, commonly known as Korean or Asian ginseng. It has been used in traditional Chinese medicine as a way to increase the body's overall resistance to stress and infection. It has been used to treat a variety of disorders including: anemia, insomnia, dyspnea, memory impairment, confusion, decreased libido, chronic fatigue, angina, diabetes mellitus and herpes simplex type-II infections.

Based on strong scientific evidence from a cohort study, *Panax ginseng* was not associated with adverse effects when used during pregnancy. *Panax ginseng* was misreported in the literature as causing androgenization, when, in fact, the case reported was due to an adulterant. There is *in vitro* evidence of teratogenicity with exposure to ginsenosides; however, this evidence is derived from animal embryos and is based on exposure to isolated ginsenosides at much higher levels than achievable through normal consumption in humans. There is also conflicting evidence as to whether or not *Panax ginseng* has estrogenic properties. In lactation, there are no human studies on the safety of *Panax ginseng*, only *in vitro* evidence based on three animal studies reporting minimal risk (Seely *et al.*, 2008).

In a separate study, the effect of ginseng extract on reproductive performance was studied in two generations of Sprague-Dawley rats. Animals of both sexes were fed either control diet or diet supplemented with ginseng extract at dose levels of 1.5, 5 or 15 mg/kg body weight/day. Parameters of reproduction and lactation in the treated groups were comparable to those of the controls for two generations of dams and pups. For F_1 males and females, no treatment-related effects were seen in weekly body weights and food consumption, hematological and clinical chemical data, and ophthalmic, gross and histopathological examinations. The gross autopsies of F_0 and F_2 animals also revealed no significant treatment-related toxicity (Hess *et al.*, 1982).

HYALURONIC ACID

Hyaluronic acid (Figure 30.5), sodium hyaluronate and potassium hyaluronate function in cosmetics as skin conditioning agents at concentrations up to 2%. Hyaluronic acid, primarily obtained from bacterial fermentation and rooster combs, does penetrate to the dermis; is not toxic in a wide range of acute animal toxicity studies, over several species and with different exposure routes; is not immunogenic, nor is it a sensitizer in animal studies; is not a reproductive or developmental toxicant; is not genotoxic; and likely does not play a causal role in cancer metastasis. Rather, increased expression of hyaluronic acid genes may be a consequence of metastatic growth. Widespread clinical use of hyaluronic acid, primarily by injection, has been free of significant adverse reactions and toxicity (Becker *et al.*, 2009). A study in February 2007 in *Food and Chemical Toxicology* has confirmed the safety of oral hyaluronic acid, where no toxicity has been observed, even at a higher dose of 33 times (Schauss *et al.*, 2007).

BOSWELLIA SERRATA

The novel anti-inflammatory properties of the gum resin derived from *Boswellia serrata*, also known as Salai guggal in Ayurvedic medicine, are well recognized and highly recommended for human consumption. The active constituents of the gum resin are boswellic acids. Among the boswellic acids, 3-acetyl-11-keto-beta-boswellic acid (AKBA) potently inhibits 5-lipoxygenase product formation with an IC_{50} of 1.5 μM. The genetic basis of the anti-inflammatory effects of Boswellia was explored in a system of TNFα-induced gene expression in human microvascular endothelial cells. Boswellia significantly prevented the TNFα-induced expression of matrix metalloproteinases and adhesion molecules (ICAM-1 and VCAM-1), and inducible expression of the mediators of apoptosis. With such interesting findings, we plan to determine the broad spectrum safety of Boswellia.

Acute oral, acute dermal, primary skin and eye irritation, and dose-dependent 90-day subchronic toxicity studies were conducted. In safety studies, acute oral LD_{50} of Boswellia was found to be greater than 5,000 mg/kg in both male and female Sprague-Dawley rats. No changes in body weight or adverse effects were observed following necropsy. Acute dermal LD_{50} of Boswellia was found to be >2,000 mg/kg. Primary skin irritation test was conducted with Boswellia on New Zealand albino rabbits and Boswellia was classified as non-irritating. A primary eye irritation test was conducted on rabbits and Boswellia was classified as mildly irritating to the eye. A dose-dependent 90-day subchronic toxicity study demonstrated no significant changes in selected organ weights individually and as percentages of body and brain weights. Boswellia supplementation did not cause changes in hepatic DNA fragmentation on 30, 60 or 90 days of treatment. Hematology, clinical chemistry and histopathological evaluations did not show any adverse effects in all organs tested. Taken together, these results demonstrate the broad spectrum safety of Boswellia (Lalithakumari *et al.*, 2006).

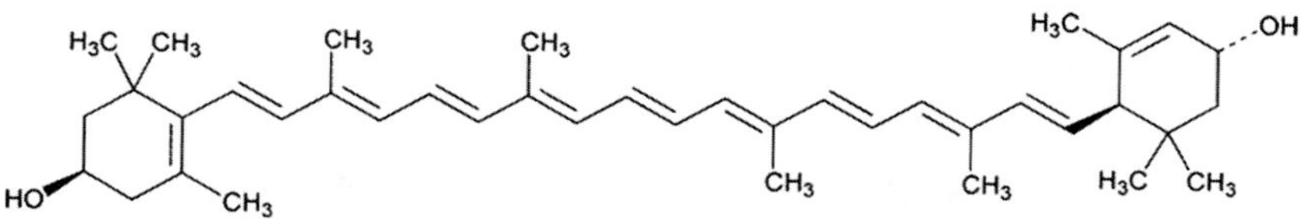

Lutein

FIGURE 30.6 Chemical structure of lutein.

ST. JOHN'S WORT

St. John's wort (*Hypericum perforatum*) is one of the best selling herbal remedies in the USA and Germany for major depression and sleep disorders. More than 25 major clinical trials on St. John's wort involving 5,489 people have been completed in Germany. It has been implicated as an inducer of the P450 enzyme system, and as such may cause increased metabolism of certain drugs, including oral contraceptives. Women using oral contraceptives have been warned against using St. John's wort. Researchers found that in nine of the larger trial, people who took St. John's wort for 4–12 weeks felt significantly better than the placebo group and had fewer side effects. There is enough evidence to suggest from those trials that St. John's wort has a significant anti-depression effect (Aikins, 2002).

POMEGRANATE FRUIT EXTRACT

Pomegranate (*Punica granatum* L.) fruit is widely consumed as fresh fruit and juice. Because of its potential for health benefits, pomegranate fruit extracts have been commonly marketed as dietary supplements in recent years. In traditional medicine pomegranate fruits have been used to treat acidosis, dysentery, microbial infections, diarrhea, helminthiasis, hemorrhage and respiratory pathologies. However, recent investigations have focused mainly on the antioxidant, anti-inflammatory and antibacterial potentials of pomegranate.

Although no reproductive or developmental studies have been done, pomegranate fruit extract has been proven to be safe following subchronic administration in rats. The extract was standardized to 30% punicalagins, the active anomeric ellagitannins responsible for over 50% of the antioxidant potential of the juice. The oral LD_{50} of the extract in rats and mice was found to be greater than 5 g/kg body weight. The intraperitoneal LD_{50} in rats and mice was determined as 217 and 187 mg/kg body weight, respectively. In the subchronic study, Wistar strain rats (10/sex/group) were administered via gavage 0 (control), 60, 240 and 600 mg/kg body weight/day of the extract for 90 days. Two additional groups received 0 and 600 mg/kg/day of the extract for 90 days, followed by a 28-day recovery phase. Compared to the control group, administration of the extract did not result in any toxicologically significant treatment-related changes in clinical observations, ophthalmic examinations, body weights, body weight gains, feed consumption, clinical pathology evaluations and organ weights. The hematology and serum chemistry parameters that showed statistical significant changes compared to control group were within the normal laboratory limits and were considered as biological variations and not the toxic effect of the extract. Terminal necropsy did not reveal any treatment-related gross or histopathology toxicity. Based on the results of this study, the NOAEL for this standardized pomegranate fruit extract was determined as 600 mg/kg body weight/day, the highest dose tested (Patel *et al.*, 2008) and is considered to have broad spectrum of safety.

LUTEIN

In humans, as in plants, the xanthophyll lutein (Figure 30.6) is believed to function in two important ways: first, as a filter of high energy blue light, and second, as an antioxidant that quenches and scavenges photo-induced reactive oxygen species (ROS). Evidence suggests that lutein consumption is inversely related to eye diseases such as age-related macular degeneration and cataracts. This is supported by the finding that lutein (and a stereo isomer, zeaxanthin) are deposited in the lens and the macula lutea, an area of the retina responsible for central and high acuity vision. Human intervention studies show that lutein supplementation results in increased macular pigment and improved vision in patients with age-related macular degeneration and other ocular diseases. Lutein may also serve to protect skin from UV-induced damage and may help reduce the risk of cardiovascular disease.

Crystalline lutein is readily absorbed from foods and from dietary supplements whereas, to enter the bloodstream, lutein esters require prior de-esterification by intestinal enzymes. Unlike the hydrocarbon carotenoids which are mainly found in the LDL fraction, xanthophylls like lutein and zeaxanthin are incorporated into both HDL and LDL. Today, lutein can be obtained from the diet in several different ways, including via supplements, and most recently in functional foods. Animal toxicology studies have been performed to establish lutein's safety as a nutrient. These studies have contributed to the classification of purified crystalline lutein as generally recognized as safe (GRAS). The achievement of GRAS status for purified crystalline lutein allows for the addition of this form into several food and beverage applications. This achievement demonstrates directly to the quality and safety of purified lutein (Alves-Rodrigues and Shao, 2004).

D-RIBOSE

A significant amount of *in vitro*, animal and human research suggests benefits of ribose on cardiac function. Studies have shown that ribose supplementation can enhance cardiac energy levels and support cardiovascular metabolism. Ribose has been shown in clinical trials to enhance the recovery of heart muscle ATP levels and improve myocardial function following exercise. Although no research has been done on the potential reproductive and developmental effects of D-ribose, numerous safe studies have been performed.

A subchronic study of D-ribose evaluated the toxicity in male and female albino Wistar rats. Groups of 20 male and 20 female rats were exposed via the diet to 0%, 5%, 10% or 20% D-ribose, 7 days per week (mean daily intake of 0.0, 3.6, 7.6 and 15.0 g/kg body weight/day in males and 0.0, 4.4, 8.5 and 15.7 g/kg body weight/day in females), for 13 consecutive weeks. Mean feed consumption and feed conversion efficiency values were comparable across all study groups; however, mean body weights of all treated animals were decreased relative to those of controls. Absolute cecal weights were increased in the mid- and high dose animals, and the relative weights were increased in all treated animals. Analysis of microscopic histopathology revealed no evidence of changes that could be attributed to D-ribose treatment. It is scientifically reasonable to conclude that the study supports a concentration of 5% D-ribose in the diet, corresponding to an average daily intake of D-ribose of 3.6 and 4.4 g/kg body weight/day in male and female rats, respectively, as being the absolute NOAEL for this substance (Griffiths *et al.*, 2007). It is widely used in energy beverages and supplements and has an FDA approved GRAS status.

ECHINACEA

In the early 20th century *Echinacea* (*Echinacea angustifolia, E. purpurea* and *E. pallid*) was established as the remedy of choice for cold and flu and was commonly used as an anti-infective until the advent of modern antibiotics. It is now most commonly used as a remedy for viral infections including influenza and the common cold.

There is good scientific evidence from a prospective cohort study that oral consumption of *Echinacea* during the first trimester does not increase the risk for major malformations. Low-level evidence based on expert opinion shows that oral consumption of *Echinacea* in recommended doses is safe for use during pregnancy and lactation. *Echinacea* is non-teratogenic when used during pregnancy. Caution is advised when using *Echinacea* during lactation until further high quality human studies can determine its safety (Perri *et al.*, 2006).

OMEGA-3 AND OMEGA-6 FATTY ACIDS

Omega-3 and omega-6 fatty acids are widely used to improve hormonal systems for men and women, and it also helps in reproduction. They also increase blood flow to the genital region and reproductive organs. For women, these omega supplements help in ovulation and better blood flow to the uterus (Olsen *et al.*, 1992). For men, these omega supplements prevent erectile dysfunction and improve the ability to deliver healthy sperm cells. Studies have shown that men with fertility problems have low levels of omega-3 and -6 fatty acids in their sperm cell membrane (Safarinejad, 2009).

CURCUMIN

Turmeric is a spice derived from the rhizomes of *Circuma longa* and is a polyphenolic compound that gives turmeric its yellow color. The chemical structure of curcumin is shown in Figure 30.7. The reproductive toxicity of curcumin in Wistar rats was studied (Ganiger *et al.*, 2007) to demonstrate safety information for the use of curcumin in humans. The two-generation reproduction study was designed and conducted. Curcumin was mixed in the diet at concentrations of 1,500, 3,000 and 10,000 ppm, fed to three groups of rats, i.e. low, mid- and high dose groups, and studied for two successive generations. A control group received experimental diet without curcumin. No treatment-related toxicity was observed in parental animals. No gross or microscopic changes were observed in any of the organs. None of the reproductive parameters were affected and there were no effects on the offspring other than a small reduction in pre-weaning body weight gain of the F_2 pups at the highest dose level. It was concluded that the NOAEL for reproductive toxicity of curcumin, fed in the diet for two successive generations to rats in this study, was 10,000 ppm, which is equivalent to 847 and 959 mg/kg body weight (bw) per day for male rats and 1,043 and 1,076 for females for F_0 and F_1 generations, respectively (Ganiger *et al.*, 2007).

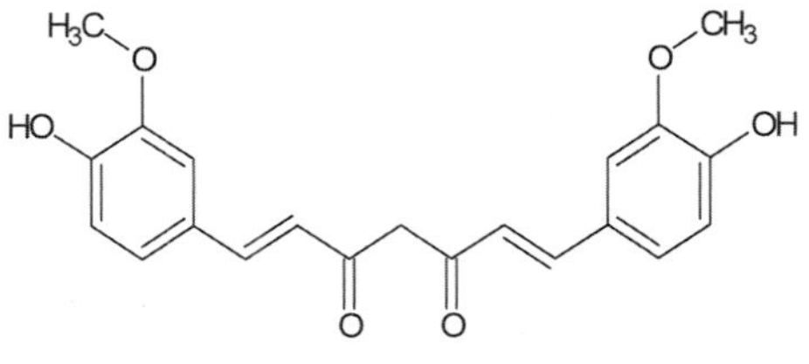

Curcumin

FIGURE 30.7 Chemical structure of curcumin.

CONCLUDING REMARKS AND FUTURE DIRECTIONS

This chapter has described a large number of popular and widely used nutraceutical ingredients, which have been researched and reviewed by the worldwide scientific community. However, proper manufacturing procedures under strict GMP and other regulatory guidelines should be strictly followed to maintain safety, efficacy and functionality. Also, labeling guidelines for all the ingredients should be strictly followed. In future, more human studies, broad spectrum safety and toxicological studies and long-term evaluations are required for human consumption without causing any adverse events.

REFERENCES

Aikins P (2002) St. John's wort and oral contraceptives: reasons for concern? *J Midwifery Womens Health* **47:** 447–50.

Alves-Rodrigues A, Shao A (2004) The science behind lutein. *Toxicol Letters* **150:** 57–83.

Anderson RA, Bryden NA, Polansky MM, Gautschi K (1998) Dietary chromium effects on tissue chromium concentrations and chromium absorption in rats. *J Trace Elements Exp Med* **9:** 11–25.

Ashby J, Tinwell H, Pennie W, Brooks AN, Lefevre PA, Beresford N, Sumpter JP (1999) Partial and weak oestrogenicity of the red wine constituent resveratrol: consideration of its superagonist activity in MCF-7 cells and its suggested cardiovascular protective effects. *J Appl Toxicol* **19:** 39–45.

Bailey MM, Boohaker JG, Jernigan PL, Townsend MB, Sturdivant J, Rasco JF, Vincent JB, Hood RD (2008b) Effects of pre- and postnatal exposure to chromium picolinate or picolinic acid on neurological development in CD-1 Mice. *Bio Trace Element Res* **124:** 70–82.

Bailey MM, Boohaker JG, Sawyer RD, Behling JE, Rasco JF, Jernigan JJ, Hood RD, Vincent JB (2006) Exposure of pregnant mice to chromium picolinate results in skeletal defects in their offspring. *Birth Defects Res Part B. Develop Repro Toxicol* **77:** 244–9.

Bailey MM, Sturdivant J, Jernigant PL, Townsend MB, Bushman J, Ankareddi I, Rasco JF, Hood RD, Vincent JB (2008a) Comparison of the potential for developmental toxicity of prenatal exposure to two dietary chromium supplements, chromium picolinate and [Cr3O(O2CCH2CH3)6(H2O)3] in mice. *Birth Defects Res Part B. Develop Repro Toxicol* **83:** 27–31.

Baur JA, Sinclair DA (2006) Therapeutic potential of resveratrol: the *in vivo* evidence. *Nat Rev Drug Discov* **5:** 493–506.

Becker LC, Bergfeld WF, Belsito DV, Klaassen CD, Marks JG Jr, Shank RC, Slaga TJ, Snyder PW (2009) Cosmetic Ingredient Review Expert Panel, Andersen FA. Final report of the safety assessment of hyaluronic acid, potassium hyaluronate, and sodium hyaluronate. *Int J Toxicol* **28:** 5–67.

Buehler BA (2003) Interactions of herbal products with conventional medicines and potential impact on pregnancy. *Birth Defects Res Part B. Develop Repro Toxicol* **68:** 494–5.

Correa A, Stolley A, Liu Y (2000) Prenatal tea consumption and risks of anencephaly and spina bifida. *Ann Epidemiol* **10:** 476–7.

Dog TL (2009) The use of botanicals during pregnancy and lactation. *Altern Ther Health Med* **15:** 51–8.

Ernst E, Thompson CJ (2001) Heavy metals in traditional Chinese medicines: a systematic review. *Clin Pharmacol Ther* **70:** 497–504.

Ganiger S, Malleshappa HN, Krishnappa H, Rajashekhar G, Ramakrishna Rao V, Sullivan F (2007) A two generation reproductive toxicity study with curcumin, turmeric yellow, in Wistar rats. *Food Chem Toxicol* **45:** 64–9.

Gehm BD, McAndrews JM, Chien PY, Jameson JL (1997) Resveratrol, a polyphenolic compound found in grapes and wine, is an agonist for the estrogen receptor. *Proc Natl Acad Sci USA* **94:** 14138–43.

Griffiths JC, Borzelleca JF, St Cyr J (2007) Sub-chronic (13-week) oral toxicity study with D-ribose in Wistar rats. *Food Chem Toxicol* **45:** 144–52.

Haller CA, Meier KH, Olson KR (2005) Seizures reported in association with use of dietary supplements. *Clin Toxicol* **1:** 23–30.

Henry LA, Witt DM (2002) Resveratrol: phytoestrogen effects on reproductive physiology and behavior in female rats. *Horm Behav* **41:** 220–8.

Hepburn DD, Xiao J, Bindom S, Vincent JB, O'Donnell J (2003) Nutritional supplement chromium picolinate causes sterility and lethal mutations in Drosophila melanogaster. *Proc Natl Acad Sci USA* **100:** 3766–71.

Hess FG Jr, Parent RA, Cox GE, Stevens KR, Becci PJ (1982) Reproduction study in rats of ginseng extract G115 *Food Chem Toxicol* **20:** 189–92.

Isbrucker RA, Edwards JA, Wolz E, Davidovich A, Bausch J (2006) Safety studies on epigallocatechin gallate (EGCG) preparations. Part 3: Teratogenicity and reproductive toxicity studies in rats. *J Food Chem Toxicol* **44:** 651–61.

Jahnke GD, Price CJ, Marr MC, Myers CB, George JD (2006) Developmental toxicity evaluation of berberine in rats and mice. *Birth Defects Res Part B. Develop Repro Toxicol* **77:** 195–206.

Jordan SA, Cunningham DG, Marles RJ (2010) Assessment of herbal medicinal products: Challenges, and opportunities to increase the knowledge base for safety assessment. *Toxicol Appl Pharmacol* **243:** 198–216.

Jovanovic L, Ilic S, Pettitt DJ, Hugo K, Gutierrez M, Bowsher RR, Bastyr EJ (1999) Metabolic and immunologic effects of insulin lispro in gestational diabetes. 3rd. *Diabetes Care* **22:** 1422–7.

Juan ME, Gonzalez-Pons E, Munuera T, Ballester J, Rodriguez-Gil JE, Planas JM (2005) Trans-resveratrol, a natural antioxidant from grapes, increases sperm output in healthy rats. *J Nutr* **135:** 757–60.

Kaldas RS, Hughes CL (1989) Reproductive and general metabolic effects of phytoestrogens in mammals. *Repro Toxicol* **3:** 81–9.

Kurzer MS, Xu X (1997) Dietary phytoestrogens. *Annual Rev Nutr* **17:** 353–81.

Kyselova V, Peknicova J, Buckiova D, Boubelik M (2003) Effects of p-nonylphenol and resveratrol on body and organ weight and in vivo fertility of outbred CD-1 mice. *Reprod Biol Endocrinol* **1:** 1–10.

Lalithakumari K, Krishnaraju AV, Sengupta K, Subbaraju GV, Chatterjee A (2006) Safety and toxicological evaluation of a novel, standardized 3-O-acetyl-11-keto-β-Boswellic acid (AKBA)-enriched Boswellia serrata extract (5-Loxin R). *Toxicol Mech Meth* **16:** 199–226.

Li W, Seifert M, Xu Y, Hock B (2004) Comparative study of estrogenic potencies of estradiol, tamoxifen, bisphenol-A and resveratrol with two in vitro bioassays. *Environ Int* **30:** 329–35.

McClain RM, Wolz E, Davidovich A, Edwards JE, Bausch J (2007) Reproductive safety studies with genistein in rats. *Food Chem Toxicol* **45:** 1319–32.

Mukhtar H, Ahmad N (2000) Tea polyphenols: prevention of cancer and optimizing health. *Am J Clin Nutr* **71:** 1698S–1702S.

O'Hara M, Kiefer D, Farrell K, Kemper K (1998) A review of 12 commonly used medicinal herbs. *Arch Family Med* **7:** 523–36.

Olsen SF, Sorensen JD, Secher NZ, Hedegaard M, Heniriksen TB, Hansen HS, Grant A (1992) Randomized control trial of effect of fish-oil supplementation on pregnancy duration. *Lancet* **339:** 1003–7.

Park D, Jeon JH, Shin S, Joo SS, Kang DH, Moon SH, Jang MJ, Cho YM, Kim JW, Ji HJ, Ahn B, Oh KW, Kim YB (2009) Green tea extract increases cyclophosphamide-induced teratogenesis by modulating the expression of cytochrome P-450 mRNA. *Reprod Toxicol* **27:** 79–84.

Patel C, Dadhaniya P, Hingorani L, Soni MG (2008) Safety assessment of pomegranate fruit extract: acute and subchronic toxicity studies. *Food Chem Toxicol* **46:** 2728–35.

Perri1 D, Dugoua J-J, Mills E, Koren G (2006) Safety and efficacy of echinacea (Echinacea angustifolia, E. purpurea and E. pallida) during pregnancy and lactation. *Can J Clin Pharmacol* **13:** e262–267.

Preuss HG, Grojec PL, Lieberman S, Anderson RA (1997) Effects of different chromium compounds on blood pressure and lipid peroxidation in spontaneously hypertensive rats. *Clin Nephrol* **47:** 325–30.

Rousseaux CG, Schachter H (2003) Regulatory issues concerning the safety, efficacy and quality of herbal remedies Colin G. *Birth Defects Res Part B. Develop Reprod Toxicol* **68:** 505–10.

Safarinejad MR (2009) Efficacy and safety of omega-3 for treatment of early stage Peyronies disease: a prospective, randomized, double-blind placebo-controlled study. *J Sex Med* **6:** 1743–54.

Schauss AG, Markel DJ, Glaza SM, Sorensonet SR (2007) Acute and subchronic oral toxicity studies in rats of a hydrolyzed chicken sterna cartilage preparation. *Food Chem Toxicol* **45:** 315–21.

Seely D, Jean-Jacques Dugoua J-J, Daniel Perri D, Edward Mills M, Gideon Koren G (2008) Safety and efficacy of *Panax ginseng* during pregnancy and lactation. *Can J Clin Pharmcol* **15:** e87–e94.

Sehmisch S, Hammer F, Christoffe J, Seidlova-Wuttke D, Tezval M, Wuttke W, Stuermer KM, Stuermer EK (2008) Comparison of the phytohormones genistein, resveratrol and 8-prenylnaringenin as agents for preventing osteoporosis. *Planta Med* **74:** 794–801.

Setchell KD, Gosselin SJ, Welsh MB, Johnston JO, Balistreri WF, Kramer LW, Dresser BL, Tarr MJ (1987) Dietary estrogens – a probable cause of infertility and liver disease in captive cheetahs. *Gastroenterology* **93:** 225–33.

Singla M, Sahai V, Grewal DS (2009) Neural tube defects and herbal medicines containing lead: a possible relationship. *Medical Hypothesis* **73:** 285–7.

Svechnikov K, Spatafora C, Svechnikova I, Tringali C, Söder O (2009) Effects of resveratrol analogs on steroidogenesis and mitochondrial function in rat Leydig cells *in vitro*. *J Appl Toxicol* **29:** 673–80.

Weidnera MS, Sigwart K (2001) Investigation of the teratogenic potential of a Zingiber officinale extract in the rat. *Repro Toxicol* **15:** 75–80.

Wilkinson JM (2000a) What do we know about herbal morning sickness treatments? A review of the literature. *Midwifery* **16:** 224–8.

Wilkinson JM (2000b) Effect of ginger tea on the fetal development of Sprague-Dawley rats. *Repro Toxicol* **14:** 507–12.

CHAPTER

31

Thalidomide

Neil Vargesson

INTRODUCTION

Thalidomide remains one of the most notorious, and feared, drugs in the world. Its use to treat morning sickness in pregnant women, between 1957 and 1961, resulted in more than 10,000 children being born globally with severe birth defects (Vargesson, 2009). The drug caused limb deformities, but also affected ear, eye, heart, kidney, nerves, genitals and other internal organs; however, limbs were affected in almost every case (Vargesson, 2009). The damage to these tissues occurs in a short time window early in embryonic development. The thalidomide tragedy highlighted species differences in drug action and resulted in legislation that changed the way all drugs were tested for safety and side effects around the world (Lenz, 1988; Kelsey, 1967).

Understanding how thalidomide causes birth defects has been a challenge for many years. This is due in part to thalidomide being a complex drug, requiring breakdown into many active by-products, which have been shown to have a range of actions on the inflammatory pathways, immune system and the vascular system (Franks *et al.*, 2004). Indeed, given this range of actions, thalidomide, and some of its analogs, are now used successfully to treat a wide range of conditions, including leprosy, Crohn's disease, multiple myeloma and HIV, but also some cancers (Gordon and Goggin, 2003). Sadly, however, with its renewed use around the world, children are again being born with thalidomide-induced deformities, which have tragically occurred in South America and Africa as recently as 2005 (Vargesson, 2009). Just how thalidomide causes damage to the embryo has remained a topic of much discussion since the original thalidomide tragedy (Vargesson, 2009). However, in the last few years great strides in the understanding of the teratogenic action of thalidomide have been made. Such work raises the possibility of producing analogs or synthesizing new forms of thalidomide that maintain the clinical benefits but eradicate the teratogenic side effects.

HISTORICAL BACKGROUND

Thalidomide (α-*N*-[phthalimido] glutarimide) was first marketed by the Chemie Grünenthal company in Germany in 1957 (Lenz, 1988; Rajkumar, 2004; Smithells and Newman, 1992). It was advertised as having sedative, hypnotic and anti-emetic actions and thought to have no toxic side effects. Thalidomide was also widely used to treat morning sickness in pregnant women. It was marketed as having no harmful side effects in humans as it was not lethal in overdose experiments in rodents and had no morphological effect on the offspring of rodents (Kelsey, 1967; Lenz, 1988; Vargesson, 2009). It was not until much later that it was realized that thalidomide exhibits species differences in its action and function, for reasons which still remain unclear (Lenz, 1988; Vargesson, 2009). Thalidomide was, by 1961, distributed in 46 countries around the world, including the UK, Ireland, Germany, Sweden, Australia, Japan, Brazil and Canada. The drug was known by a variety of names including Distaval (in the UK and Australia), Contergan (in Germany), Sedalis (in Brazil), Kedavon (in Canada), Isomin (in Japan and Taiwan) and Softenon (in the majority of Europe) (Rajkumar, 2004; Lenz, 1988).

Between 1957 and 1960 an unusually high increase in children being born with severe, rarely seen limb deformities and internal organ problems was observed in Germany, Australia and Britain, which initially confused and concerned physicians (McBride, 1976; Leck and Millar, 1962; Lenz, 1988; Smithells, 1962). It was not until 1961 that a German doctor named Lenz expressed his suspicions that the terrible malformations that were being witnessed were linked to the ingestion of thalidomide by the mothers during their pregnancies (Lenz, 1962; Leck and Millar, 1962; Rajkumar, 2004; Smithells, 1962; Smithells and Newman, 1992). Support for Lenz's argument came soon after, independently, from William McBride, a physician in Australia (McBride, 1961). Due to the important link discovered by Lenz and McBride between thalidomide and malformed babies the withdrawal of the drug from the market began in late 1961, although this was too late to prevent the damage that had already been done to an estimated 10,000 children worldwide (Ances, 2002).

Thalidomide was not formally distributed in the USA between 1957 and 1961 as Dr. Frances Kelsey of the Food and Drug Administration (FDA) denied its approval because of the side effect of peripheral neuropathy that had been experienced in some patients taking thalidomide over a long time period in Germany and Britain and her concerns over its safety during pregnancy (Lenz, 1988; Kelsey, 1967; Miller and Strömland, 1999; Taussig, 1962). Dr. Kelsey was consequently

Reproductive and Developmental Toxicology, Edited by Ramesh C. Gupta
ISBN: 978-0-12-382032-7

given an award for Distinguished Federal Civilian Service by President John F. Kennedy (Rajkumar, 2004).

Following withdrawal of thalidomide from sale in late 1961 the incidence of severe birth defects decreased rapidly, although this happened at different times in different countries (Miller and Strömland, 1999; Smithells and Leck, 1963). For example, in Japan thalidomide was not withdrawn until more than 9 months after it had been withdrawn in some European countries (Miller and Strömland, 1999). This was due to confusion caused due to the different names, and descriptions of the drug's actions, under which thalidomide was prescribed in different countries. This confusion meant, for example, many physicians did not realize that Contergan and Distaval were the same drug and tragically there were some children born more than two years after the withdrawal had began (Taussig, 1962; Smithells and Newman, 1992).

Important lessons were learnt from the thalidomide tragedy. Up to the thalidomide tragedy it was simply assumed the placenta would prevent drugs from reaching the embryo/fetus. The tragedy changed forever the way drug testing is undertaken and established the strict toxicology testing for all drugs used today for adults and children, and really pioneered the toxicology field as we know it today (Kelsey, 1967, 1988). In addition the thalidomide tragedy highlighted species differences that existed in the action, effect and side effects caused by drugs. Thalidomide has little or no effect upon the forming rodent embryo, yet it is highly teratogenic in non-human primates and rabbits (Lenz, 1988). Why thalidomide has little or no effect on early rodent embryos remains unknown. Such findings highlighted additional testing methods required to be used to ensure drug safety. Following the withdrawal of thalidomide new legislation was introduced in many countries with regards to the testing of new drugs and their approval for use in humans, especially those that could come into contact with pregnant women (Kelsey, 1967, 1988).

THALIDOMIDE TODAY

Since being discovered to be effective as a treatment for leprosy in 1965 (Sheskin, 1965; Tseng *et al.*, 1996), the drug is now used around the world again, including the USA (Teo *et al.*, 2002). Thalidomide is used primarily to treat erythema nodosum leprosum (ENL) (a complication of leprosy, a chronic skin and nerve infection caused by *Mycobacterium leprae*) (Teo *et al.*, 2002), and is also used as part of the treatment regime for multiple myeloma – where the bone marrow overproduces white blood cells (Raab *et al.*, 2009). The drug is also used to treat many other conditions including Crohn's disease, HIV, arthritis and some cancers (Ericksson *et al.*, 2001; Franks *et al.*, 2004). Clearly thalidomide is a very useful drug in the clinic.

However, tragically, with the increased use of thalidomide for treatment of ENL/leprosy in South America and Africa, there has been a re-emergence of thalidomide embryopathy in children (Castilla *et al.*, 1996; Schuler-Faccini *et al.*, 2007). This underlines how dangerous thalidomide remains and how strictly its use needs to remain. One of the solutions to reduce and hopefully eradicate such awful side effects is to find a clinically relevant but non-teratogenic analog of thalidomide. Therefore the knowledge of the mechanisms underlying thalidomide embryopathy is crucial to developing a safe, non-teratogenic analog.

THALIDOMIDE EMBRYOPATHY (THALIDOMIDE SYNDROME)

Over 10,000 children were born between 1957 and 1962 with severe birth defects as a direct result of thalidomide exposure *in utero* (Lenz, 1998; Vargesson, 2009). Thalidomide exposure during early embryonic development can affect the limbs, ears, eyes, genitals and many internal organs such as the heart, kidney and intestines, as well as the CNS and nervous system of the embryo, including causing facial palsies (Kajii *et al.*, 1973; Leck and Millar, 1962; McBride, 1976; Miller and Strömland, 1999; Miller *et al.*, 2005; Newman, 1985; Smithells and Newman, 1992). Due to the wide range of conditions this drug caused they are usually referred to as thalidomide embryopathy or thalidomide syndrome (Newman, 1985). The mortality rate for babies, up to their first year, born with thalidomide embryopathy is estimated to be around 40%, likely due to the serious internal malformations such as heart and kidney defects (Lenz, 1988; Smithells and Newman, 1992). Many babies with these serious internal malformations would have miscarried or died *in utero* or soon after birth, and explains why survivors suffer mainly from limb, ear and eye defects and less from internal defects (Vargesson, 2009).

Time-sensitive period of greatest sensitivity upon embryonic morphogenesis

There is a developmental time period during which the human embryo is most sensitive to the teratogenic effects of thalidomide which result in birth defects. This time period is between 20 and 36 days post-fertilization, or 34 to 50 days after the last menstrual period (Lenz and Knapp, 1962; Miller and Strömland, 1999; Smithells and Newman, 1992). Exposure to thalidomide after 36 days post-fertilization has no apparent morphological effect upon the fetus (Newman, 1985). In contrast, thalidomide exposure before the time-sensitive window of development induces miscarriage in humans and rats (James, 1965; Kajii *et al.*, 1973). Estimates suggest there is a significant risk (up to 50%) of subsequent birth defects following thalidomide exposure within the time-sensitive period from just one 50 mg tablet, highlighting the high potency of thalidomide (Newman, 1986; Smithells and Newman, 1992; Miller and Strömland, 1999). The time period of thalidomide sensitivity was determined following interviews with mothers of thalidomide-effected children. Many women knew the exact dates of intake and amount of drug taken and so an accurate correlation could be made to the period of exposure and relationship to anomalies to determine the timing of the induction of deformities (Lenz and Knapp, 1962; Lenz, 1988; Miller and Strömland, 1999). It appears that all the morphological birth defects seen in thalidomide embryopathy can be caused by exposure within this time period. Thalidomide use as a treatment for morning sickness, it was concluded, was the cause of the thalidomide tragedy and the birth defects the drug caused during a short developmental time window (Lenz, 1988). The ears and eyes are affected by the consumption of thalidomide in the first few days of the sensitive period (days 20–24), followed by the upper limb (days 24–31) and the lower limb (day 27–33), respectively (Lenz and Knapp, 1962; Miller and Strömland, 1999). Effects upon the nerves, resulting in facial palsies, hearing loss and autism and epilepsy, can be induced from the start of the time-sensitive window, although the consequence of such nerve damage may not be diagnosed until much later after birth, but can be linked to thalidomide use during the time-sensitive period (Miller and Strömland, 1999; Miller *et al.*, 2005).

Thalidomide was prescribed to relieve the symptoms of morning sickness during pregnancy, typically from week 4 onwards, which correlates with the time-sensitive window when the limbs are first forming. This helps explain why the limbs are the most commonly affected tissue in thalidomide survivors, as the drug was prescribed at a time when limbs are the major tissue forming (Vargesson, 2009). However, recent work has suggested that late fetal exposure to thalidomide can cause some nerve damage in the brain, in areas linked to autism and epilepsy (Hallene *et al.*, 2006). Such findings indicate that there really is no safe time period during pregnancy for thalidomide exposure.

Limb defects

The majority of thalidomide survivors exhibit limb deformities (over 90%; Vargesson, 2009) and are usually reduction defects and most often symmetrical (Kajii *et al.*, 1973; Newman, 1985; Smithells and Leck, 1963; Smithells and Newman, 1992). Defects can be mild affecting only the digits of the hands, or they can be severe, ranging from amelia (complete absence of the limbs) to phocomelia, the most striking deformity, a severe shortening of the limbs (Speirs, 1962; Newman, 1985). Phocomelia itself ranges from the most severe form where the long bones are missing with just a flipper-like structure existing primarily of a handplate articulating directly with the body, to milder forms, where the long bones are shortened but are not absent (Newman, 1985; Henkel and Willert, 1969). The range and type of limb deformities seen following thalidomide exposure exhibit a characteristic pattern. The thumb is the first structure to be affected followed by the radius, humerus and lastly the ulna (Smithells, 1973).

In the lower limb there may also be phocomelia or Amelia; however, abnormalities of the lower limbs are seen less commonly than those of the upper limbs, and lower limb deformities are rarely seen alone (Newman, 1985; Smithells and Leck, 1963; Smithells, 1962). The femur is the bone most often affected in the lower limb and similarly to the ulna the fibula is usually the final bone to remain normal (Smithells and Newman, 1992).

In both the upper and lower limbs the limb girdles are also affected in thalidomide embryopathy. The normal smooth and curved outline of the shoulder becomes sharpened in children with severe upper limb reduction defects as the acromioclavicular joint is more prominent when the shoulder is deformed (Newman, 1985). At the hip the joint may be hypoplastic or completely absent, as is true for the pubic bone (Newman, 1985). The involvement of the limb girdles in thalidomide-induced limb reduction defects is a characteristic of thalidomide embryopathy and in some cases helped physicians to differentiate thalidomide deformities from sporadic or genetic limb defects.

Eye and ear defects

The second commonest group of defects in thalidomide damaged children/adults is seen in the eyes and ears (Miller and Strömland, 1999; Newman, 1985; Smithells, 1973; Smithells and Newman, 1992; Vargesson, 2009). Eye defects include cataracts, microphthalmos (congenital small eye), anophthalmos (absence of eyeball), poor vision, aberrant lacrimation problems and, most commonly, colobomas (deformity of the iris and retina) (Cullen, 1964; Newman, 1985). Ocular defects usually occur unilaterally although there may still be poor vision in the unaffected eye (Smithells, 1973). Thalidomide may also cause abnormalities in eye movement and usually occur in conjunction with ear defects and weakness of the facial muscles (Smithells and Newman, 1992).

Ear defects caused by thalidomide embryopathy are usually symmetrical, ranging from complete absence of the outer ear or pinna (anotia), to part of the outer ear still remaining (microtia) (Cuthbert and Speirs, 1963; Livingstone, 1965; Smithells and Newman, 1992). Anotia is linked to abnormalities of the external auditory meatus and consequently children affected are deaf (Livingstone, 1965). Thalidomide-induced ear defects are also associated with cranial nerve palsies, resulting in facial palsies (Miller and Strömland, 1999; Newman, 1985).

Internal organ defects

Internal organ defects include malformations of the heart, kidneys, genitals and bowel (Smithells and Newman, 1992). The precise incidence of such deformities is unknown as such defects did not always present until later in life. Defects of the heart were thought to be responsible for many of the intrauterine and postnatal deaths. However, many thalidomide survivors do have heart problems which are mainly ventricular and atrial septum defects, as well as pulmonary stenosis and patent ductus arteriosus (Smithells and Newman, 1992; Cuthbert and Speirs, 1963).

The urinary tract and kidneys can also be affected, and horseshoe, hypoplastic, rotated and ectopic malformations of the kidney are seen (Smithells and Newman, 1992; Smithells, 1973). Many of the children affected by thalidomide also suffered from genital defects, both internal and external. Absence of the testes and testicular abnormalities and hypospadias were seen in males, while in females malformations of the uterus and reproductive tract defects were observed (Smithells and Newman, 1992; Chamberlain, 1989). In the bowel thalidomide-induced defects include anorectal stenosis, intestinal atresia, pyloric stenosis and inguinal hernia (Smithells and Newman, 1992; Smithells, 1973; Newman, 1985).

Nerve and CNS defects

Children with thalidomide embryopathy did not appear to suffer from neurological problems and developed into bright and intelligent children (Soules, 1966). However, there is evidence that some thalidomide-damaged children have facial palsies, cranial nerve conduction problems and an increased incidence of autism and epilepsy in later life (Miller and Strömland, 1999; Miller *et al.*, 2005; Smithells and Newman, 1992). Such problems are not diagnosable until later in life. It has been proposed that thalidomide could affect forming nerve pathways during the time window of embryonic sensitivity to thalidomide (Miller *et al.*, 2005) possibly by preventing angiogenesis (Hallene *et al.*, 2006).

Surprisingly, despite the drug's renewed use around the world, it has taken until only very recently to finally understand the teratogenic action of thalidomide.

PHARMACOLOGY

Thalidomide (α-phthalimidoglutarimide) is a derivative of glutamic acid, is odorless, tasteless and white in color and has a melting point of 271°C (Figure 31.1A; McBride, 1976; Strömland and Miller, 1999). Thalidomide possesses a chiral center with an asymmetric carbon atom surrounded by a left-sided phthalimide ring and a right-sided glutarimide ring (Tseng *et al.*, 1996).

Thalidomide can exist in two different isomeric forms, S(−) and R(+), which can interchange spontaneously in body fluids (Franks *et al.*, 2004; Tseng *et al.*, 1996). A racemate mixture of the two thalidomide isomers is used clinically (Eriksson *et al.*, 2001). Each isomer is believed to have different properties: S(−) could be teratogenic and R(+) is a sedative (Franks *et al.*, 2004). As the two isomers can rapidly interchange in physiological pH it is not possible to isolate and treat with just the sedative form of the drug. Thalidomide has a low solubility in water yet is highly unstable and has a half-life of between 5 and 12 hours (Gordon and Goggin, 2003; Lepper *et al.*, 2006; Ericksson *et al.*, 2001). Thalidomide can rapidly hydrolyze in physiological pH in aqueous mediums, which is temperature dependent, into active by-products and this is also how the drug is believed to be primarily eliminated from the body (Ericksson *et al.*, 2001; Franks *et al.*, 2004; Kelsey, 1967; Lepper *et al.*, 2006). Thalidomide can also be actively metabolized by the cytochrome P450 enzyme pathway producing a range of by-products including anti-angiogenic by-products, and is species dependent (Ando *et al.*, 2002; Bauer *et al.*, 1998; Ericksson *et al.*, 2001; Franks *et al.*, 2004; Lepper *et al.*, 2006; Vargesson, 2009). The breakdown of thalidomide results in at least 20 products, one or more of which are thought to be the active metabolite responsible for the detrimental effects of thalidomide (Franks *et al.*, 2004).

In addition synthetic analogs of the drug have been made which are more potent than the original, parent molecule, e.g. lenalidomide which is used to treat multiple myeloma (Galustian and Dalgleish, 2009). Indeed by making substitutions of amino groups or replacing with fluorination groups, greater biological activity can be conferred upon the analogs (Figure 31.1B; Franks *et al.*, 2004; Ng *et al.*, 2003). Over 100 analogs of thalidomide can be made in this way, highlighting the complexity of thalidomide yet also underscoring the many potential therapeutic actions of this drug (Franks *et al.*, 2004).

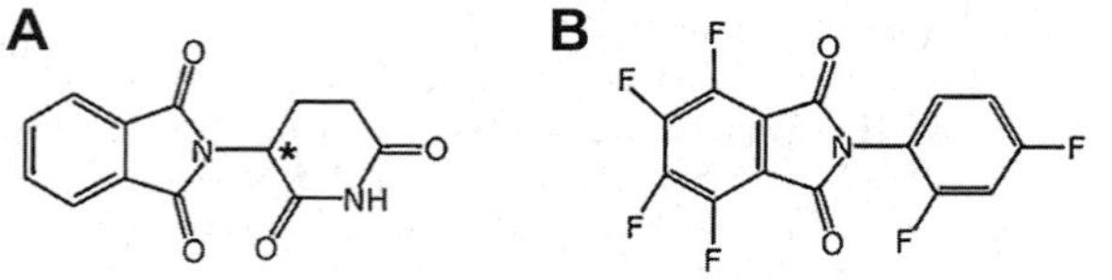

A THALIDOMIDE B CPS49

FIGURE 31.1 Structures of thalidomide and CPS49. Thalidomide (A) is an enantiomer, it can exist in two different chiral states (chiral center indicated by asterisk). (B) CPS49 is an analog based on thalidomide that has been fluorinated to enhance bioactivity.

Anti-inflammatory and immunomodulatory actions

Thalidomide inhibits the production of tumor necrosis factor (TNF)-α by degrading TNF-α mRNA in monocytes and macrophages. TNF-α regulates and controls the inflammatory response by inducing the production of a large range of cytokines, including interleukins and interferon-δ, in response to injury or stimuli. Thalidomide is currently used to target these effectors in inflammatory diseases, including leprosy and Crohn's disease, where the inflammatory response is overactive (Franks *et al.*, 2004; Gordon and Goggin, 2003; Sampaio *et al.*, 1991).

Anti-angiogenic actions

Thalidomide was demonstrated to block angiogenesis (formation of new blood vessels) in a rat cornea assay which led to the hypothesis that the drug's anti-angiogenic effect might be how thalidomide caused limb defects (D'Amato *et al.*, 1994). Since this discovery the drug has been researched as a potential anti-tumor agent (Franks *et al.*, 2004). For these reasons thalidomide is enjoying a renaissance and is used around the world for many clinical applications, indeed it can be a lifesaver.

MECHANISM OF ACTION

How does thalidomide cause the widespread, and sometimes catastrophic, damage to the forming embryo?

Over 30 models/hypotheses of thalidomide's mechanism of action have been proposed since the thalidomide tragedy was first described in 1961. As the limbs are the structures most often affected in survivors of thalidomide embryopathy the possible mechanism(s) by which this arises has been the main focus of research for many years (Figure 31.2; Vargesson, 2009). However, any model or theory of thalidomide action needs also to take into account the other tissues/organs the drug affects (Vargesson, 2009). Models/hypotheses proposed to explain thalidomide-induced defects include DNA mutagenesis, targeting chrondrogenesis, inhibiting growth factor signaling, nerve toxicity, induction of cell death through generation of reactive oxygen species and inhibition of angiogenesis. These have been reviewed previously (Stephens, 1988; Stephens *et al.*, 2000; Stephens and Fillmore, 2000; Vargesson, 2009). To some extent each of these can explain an aspect of thalidomide embryopathy, yet the primary triggering event induced by thalidomide was still missing. Recent advances in pharmacology, molecular biology and imaging now allow this problem to be addressed. Indeed, recent work has uncovered that thalidomide primarily targets rapidly forming, immature, angiogenic blood vessels in the developing limb and embryo (Therapontos *et al.*, 2009; Figure 31.3). These new findings help unite previous data/models of actions into a framework explaining thalidomide teratogenesis (Vargesson, 2009).

Thalidomide prevents limb outgrowth by inhibiting angiogenesis

Thalidomide breaks down into a wide range of metabolites, with anti-inflammatory, immunomodulatory and

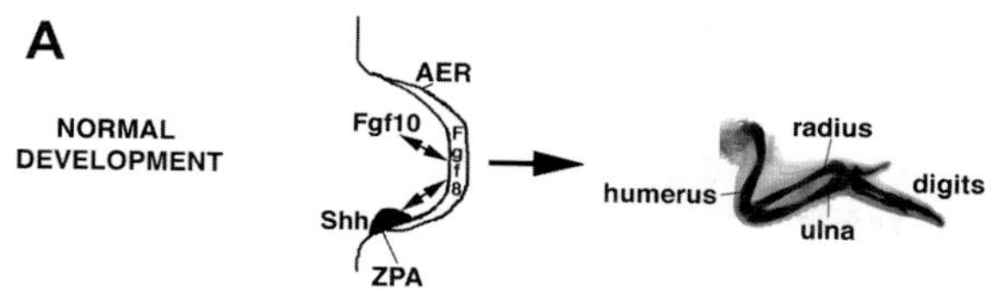

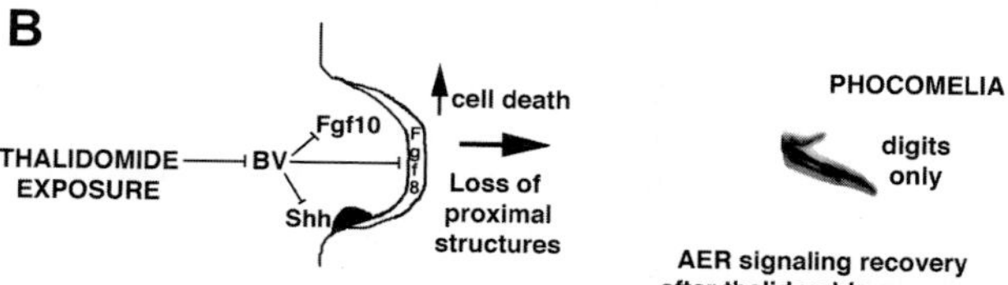

FIGURE 31.2 Limb development and thalidomide-induced phocomelia. (A) Normal limb development. The limb bud grows out from the embryonic flank at day 2.5 in chick embryos and day 23 in humans. The limb elements are specified proximal (humerus/femur) to distal (digits/toes), thus the digits are the last tissues formed. Development and outgrowth is controlled through an interplay of molecules between specialized signaling regions, the apical ectodermal ridge (AER) and the zone of polarizing activity (ZPA). Feedback loops are established between *fgf8* (in the AER) and *fgf10* and *shh* in the mesenchyme. These signaling loops coordinate outgrowth and patterning. Other genes are subsequently activated, including *Hox* genes, which pattern the fine detail of the limb cartilage elements (Tabin and Wolpert, 2007; Towers and Tickle, 2009; Zeller, 2010). (B) Model for thalidomide-induced phocomelia. Blood vessels are inhibited as the limb is growing out from the flank. This results in massive cell death in the mesenchyme of the limb and shuts down the limb signaling and patterning pathways. Loss of the proximal elements of the limb occurs. As the effect of thalidomide wears off, the AER and ZPA can recover and re-establish signaling to the resulting limb bud stump, producing distal structures only.

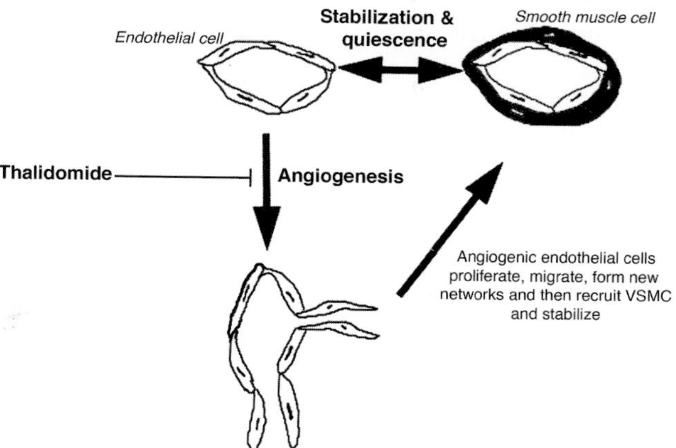

FIGURE 31.3 Angiogenesis and effect of thalidomide. Vessels initially form by a process known as vasculogenesis where endothelial cells coalesce to form a tube through which blood cells will pass. A second process, angiogenesis is where the initial vessels are then elaborated upon to form vascular networks throughout the forming body, organs and tissues. Angiogenesis continues into and throughout adulthood. As vessels are formed they can recruit vascular smooth muscle, this stabilizes the vessel into a mature, quiescent state, others will continue to undergo angiogenesis where the endothelial cells proliferate and migrate into previously avascular regions – such angiogenic vessels do not possess or require to shed existing smooth muscle coats. Many molecules have been shown to regulate and control vessel formation, development, guidance and smooth muscle recruitment, and these molecules include vascular endothelial growth factor and FGFs (Vargesson, 2003). Thalidomide targets the angiogenic, unstable, endothelial cells, preventing proliferation and migration into tissue. In rapidly forming tissues such as the forming limb, such an effect is devastating (Therapontos *et al.*, 2009).

anti-angiogenic actions; which of these actions is responsible for the teratogenic side effects or do they each have a teratogenic consequence? Advances in pharmacology allow the isolation and purification of by-products, and synthesis of analogs to address this question (Franks *et al.*, 2004). Such by-products and analogs can be functionally screened using the developing chick embryo (Therapontos *et al.*, 2009). The chick embryo forms rapidly, is large, development can be imaged, live and *in vivo*, and the effects of the drug upon gene and protein expression can be characterized. In addition the chick embryo has been used for many years to study limb development and has been used as a model to study the effects of thalidomide upon limb development (Boylen *et al.*, 1963; Jurand, 1966; Knobloch *et al.*, 2007; Therapontos *et al.*, 2009; Vargesson, 2009).

Application of thalidomide breakdown products and analogs, with either anti-inflammatory or anti-angiogenic actions, identified that only an anti-angiogenic analog, CPS49, caused limb defects in embryos (Figure 31.4; Therapontos *et al.*, 2009). None of the other by-products tested had any effect upon development, even at very high concentrations (Therapontos *et al.*, 2009). CPS49 is an analog structurally based upon the anti-angiogenic breakdown product of thalidomide, 5′-OH thalidomide (Figure 31.1B; Ng *et al.*, 2003; Vargesson, 2009). Further analysis of CPS49 action and function, in chick and zebrafish embryos, demonstrated that CPS49 rapidly affects, within 2 hours, immature, unstable, highly angiogenic vessels (which do not possess a protective smooth muscle coating) – which are those that are migrating into previously avascular tissues (Figure 31.3; Therapontos *et al.*, 2009). CPS49 causes loss of immature, newly formed vessels within 2 hours, resulting in cell death of surrounding mesenchymal tissue by 6 hours and loss of the major signaling pathways controlling limb outgrowth from 6 hours. Indeed *fgf8* expression in the AER and *fgf10* and *Shh* expression in the underlying mesenchyme were completely absent within 24 hours of exposure – these genes are essential for limb outgrowth and patterning (Therapontos *et al.*, 2009). Loss of *fgf8* expression is also seen in developing limbs of rabbit fetuses exposed to thalidomide (Hansen *et al.*, 2002). In contrast in mature and stable vessels which possess a smooth muscle coat, such as in the head and body, vessels are unaffected – however,

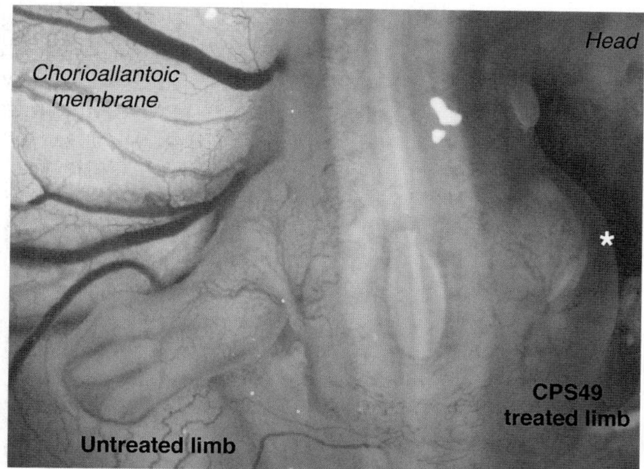

FIGURE 31.4 CPS49 induces limb defects. Chick embryo, 3 days after CPS49 exposure at day 2.5, as the limb is starting to develop. Note the right limb is truncated and just a stump remains (asterisk denotes missing limb). The rest of the embryo appears normal – this is due to vessel immaturity in the limb at the time of drug exposure. Please refer to color plate section.

such vessels can be transiently prevented from undergoing new angiogenesis, but as such vessels are stable and quiescent, the effect is transient until drug activity is eliminated (6–12 hours) (Therapontos *et al.*, 2009; Vargesson, 2009).

CPS49 causes defects in the chick embryo in a time-sensitive manner. When applied as the limbs form, only limb defects were seen, as these vessels are undergoing rapid angiogenesis. Whereas vessels in other regions of the embryo at that time are stable and mature and possess smooth muscle coats (Figure 31.3; Therapontos *et al.*, 2009). However, when CPS49 is applied earlier in embryogenesis, when all vessels are undergoing angiogenesis, and do not possess a smooth muscle coat, the result is lethality. Conversely when applied later in development, when less angiogenesis is occurring, only "mild" limb defects are seen (Therapontos *et al.*, 2009). These results correlate with the damage seen in humans. This confirms that the anti-angiogenic action of thalidomide caused limb defects in forming embryos and, given the essential role angiogenesis plays in normal development, possibly also the other associated thalidomide-induced defects (Vargesson, 2009). Thus, the anti-angiogenic action of thalidomide is responsible for the tissue-specific defects seen in thalidomide embryopathy and the range of defects seen is down to the maturity and stability of the forming vasculature at the time of exposure (Therapontos *et al.*, 2009; Vargesson, 2009).

Vascular smooth muscle cell presence/recruitment is therefore key to protecting vessels from destruction by thalidomide in the embryo (Therapontos *et al.*, 2009). Indeed this appears also to be the case in juvenile and adult mice suffering from hereditary hemorrhagic telangiectasia (HHT) (Lebrin *et al.*, 2010). HHT is a genetic disorder where children and adults suffer from excessive bleeding from the nose and gastrointestinal tract. HHT results in excessive angiogenesis and can lead to arterio-venous malformations, which are potentially life threatening (Lebrin *et al.*, 2010). HHT results from a mutation in the Endoglin gene, an endothelial cell-specific TGFβ-1 receptor, which cannot promote TGFβ signaling. A mouse model of HHT also exhibits excessive angiogenesis. Thalidomide application normalized and stabilized vascular patterns, through induction of PDGF-β from endothelial cells. PDGF-β signals to and recruits pericytes and smooth muscle to the endothelial cell tube (Lebrin *et al.*, 2010; Figure 31.3). This study also confirms that thalidomide in higher doses prevents new vessel formation in mice (Lebrin *et al.*, 2010) confirming the findings of CPS49 in the developing chick embryo (Therapontos *et al.*, 2009). In a separate study, late fetal stage rats exposed to thalidomide exhibit neurological deficits in the brain due to a failure of correct angiogenesis (Hallene *et al.*, 2006).

These findings confirm that thalidomide's anti-angiogenic actions have different consequences depending on developmental stage and timing of exposure. In the embryo, where lots of angiogenesis is required, early drug exposure is devastating, but in the adult, where vascular patterns are established and stable and high amounts of angiogenesis are not normally required, the drug can be therapeutic by inhibiting angiogenesis which could be therapeutic for conditions such as HHT and cancer.

Molecular target of thalidomide

Thalidomide and CPS49 rapidly induce actin stress fibers in the angiogenic endothelial cell, preventing migration and proliferation (Tamilarasan *et al.*, 2006; Therapontos *et al.*, 2009), suggesting targeting of a cytoskeletal component. CPS49 also induces the stress response kinase p38α, leading to endothelial cell death (Warfel *et al.*, 2006). CPS49 and thalidomide also induce mesenchymal cell death (Knobloch *et al.*, 2007; Therapontos *et al.*, 2009) as a result of failed angiogenesis (Therapontos *et al.*, 2009) and loss of cell survival pathways (Knobloch *et al.*, 2007, 2008). However, many molecules have changed expression patterns following thalidomide application, including integrins, vascular endothelial growth factor, PDGFβ, nitric oxide, ceramide, angiopoietins and reactive oxygen species (D'Amato *et al.*, 1994; Hansen and Harris, 2004; Knobloch *et al.*, 2007; Lebrin *et al.*, 2010; Majumder *et al.*, 2009; Neubert *et al.*, 1996; Tamilarasan *et al.*, 2006; Vacca *et al.*, 2005; Yabu *et al.*, 2005). In addition a microarray screen on thalidomide-exposed cynomolgus monkey fetuses demonstrates a very large range of changed gene expression profiles including vasculature markers and actin cytoskeleton markers (1,281 genes upregulated and 1,081 genes downregulated; Ema *et al.*, 2010). The question as to what are the primary molecular targets of thalidomide and what are the secondary effects remains a challenge.

Recently a molecular binding target of thalidomide was identified (Ito *et al.*, 2010). The protein *cereblon* was identified as binding to thalidomide, which is a candidate gene for mental retardation (Ito *et al.*, 2010). *Cereblon* forms part of an E3 ubiquitin ligase complex, which is involved in regulating protein degradation. Thalidomide binds to cereblon inhibiting its function leading to abnormal signaling events (Ito *et al.*, 2010). However, although the identification of a binding target is very exciting, presently, the functional significance of *cereblon* in the cell is not understood and remains to be determined. Whether *cereblon* interacts with blood vessels and/or can act in a time-sensitive manner is also presently unknown. It is likely that other factors are involved, possibly additional or different binding proteins and changes in downstream signaling events contributing to the tissue specificity.

Phocomelia

Perhaps, the most striking and defining characteristic of thalidomide embryopathy are the phocomelic limbs of survivors. Phocomelia is defined as the loss of or severe shortening of the long bones of the limb (upper and/or lower). The majority of thalidomide embryopathy survivors have some form of limb deformity. Current thinking suggests that phocomelia arises due to a loss of cells that should produce the long bones of the limb, early in development (Galloway *et al.*, 2009; Therapontos *et al.*, 2009). Indeed, X-irradiation of early chick limbs results in limbs missing proximal elements (humerus) (Galloway *et al.*, 2009). Furthermore, CPS49 causes vessel loss in the forming chick limb followed by massive mesenchymal cell death and a disruption of limb signaling pathways, resulting in a range of severely truncated limbs with some that look remarkably like phocomelia (Figure 31.2B; Therapontos *et al.*, 2009). The hypothesis is that signaling between the AER and limb mesenchyme recovers, after thalidomide exposure and loss of cell populations destined to form the proximal limb elements, leaving the remaining cells to pattern distal elements under the control of the AER (Figure 31.2B; Therapontos *et al.*, 2009; Vargesson, 2009).

With the recent major advances in understanding thalidomide action, in particular that blood vessels appear to be the primary target tissue, the key now is to identify the precise molecular targets of thalidomide and the sequence of events and effects. There will likely be tissue-specific differences in the downstream signaling changes following thalidomide exposure (Vargesson, 2009). Such an understanding should shed light on improving therapeutic uses for the drug and insight into producing potentially safer forms of the drug.

FRAMEWORK OF THALIDOMIDE TERATOGENICITY

The past few years have seen a leap forward in understanding the mechanisms underlying thalidomide teratogenicity. Recent findings, together with previous research and models, allow the development of a framework of thalidomide action which can be applied to all thalidomide-sensitive tissues (Figure 31.5). Thalidomide breaks down into a range of by-products but it is the anti-angiogenic by-product that causes teratogenesis (Therapontos *et al.*, 2009; Vargesson, 2009). Blood vessels are essential for the development of tissues and organs (Vargesson, 2003). Exposure to thalidomide during periods of rapid angiogenesis and tissue formation results in vascular formation failure, induction of cell death in cells requiring oxygen and nutrients and gene misexpression and ultimately tissue failure and loss of cell types (Therapontos *et al.*, 2009). Such exposure during early limb formation is devastating. If the anti-angiogenic insult occurs earlier in development, when all vessels are angiogenic and all the major tissues and organs are forming, this results in cell death in the tissue concerned and misexpression of signaling pathways. The resulting loss or misdevelopment of tissue may well be lethal, or result in the failure of the correct recruitment and differentiation of other cell types including nerves, neural crest, chrondrocytes, muscle, etc. This would then impact on internal organ function as well as nervous system function, exacerbating the defect in the already damaged tissue (Figure 31.5).

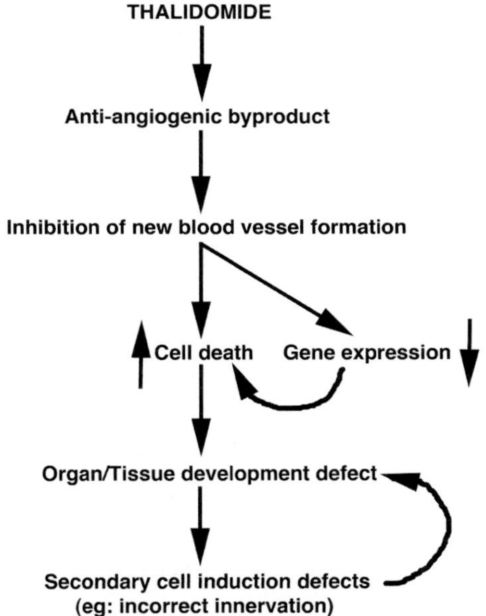

FIGURE 31.5 Framework of thalidomide teratogenicity. Thalidomide is broken down into active by-products. The anti-angiogenic by-product inhibits angiogenesis from existing vessels and also prevents formation of new vessels in tissues and organs. Such an effect causes the death of cells and gene expression and signaling pathway failure, which is also required to maintain cell viability, so gene expression loss will also cause further cell death. Such an event occurring in a rapidly forming tissue, such as a limb, is devastating causing severe deformity and, for example, loss of chrondrogenic cell populations. The malformed tissue/organ would then fail to induce or recruit secondary cell populations, such as nerves, muscle cells, chrondrocytes, etc., resulting in a worsening of the defect.

TOXICITY AND RISK ASSESSMENT

Thalidomide, and its analog lenalidomide, continues to pose a significant risk to the unborn, developing child. For this reason use of thalidomide, and its derivatives, is strictly regulated and requires contraceptives to be taken when being used as a treatment. Patients prescribed thalidomide are usually those with severe debilitating conditions where other normal treatments are unsuccessful. A patient using thalidomide as an anti-tumor agent would be unlikely to be in a position to become pregnant; however, in the case of leprosy and other inflammatory disorders, misuse or misinformed use during pregnancy remains a high risk. Indeed, in South America and Africa, where thalidomide is used widely as a treatment for ENL, there have been multiple recent cases of babies being born with thalidomide embryopathy, some to women who were prescribed the drug for ENL and had either not been warned or not fully understood the warnings of taking the drug during pregnancy, and others to women who had not taken sufficient contraceptive precautions and had fallen pregnant while taking thalidomide (Castilla *et al.*, 1996; Schuler-Faccini *et al.*, 2007; Paumgartten, 2006).

As thalidomide, and its analogs, remains a risk to the unborn child, Celgene, who hold the license to market and distribute thalidomide, and some of its analogs today, has developed the STEPS (System for Thalidomide Education and Prescribing Safety) program as a regulatory guide for the controlled use of thalidomide and is based around the following points (Castaneda *et al.*, 2008):

1. Education of physicians, pharmacists and patients
2. Contraceptive counseling from a physician or other medical professional
3. Pregnancy testing (suggested every 2 weeks) for women of child-bearing age taking thalidomide
4. Informed consent of patients (copies to patient, physician and pharmacist)
5. Managed distribution
6. Mandatory outcomes registry survey

However, long-term thalidomide use has side effects in patients which include constipation and rashes. Perhaps the most infamous side effect from thalidomide use is peripheral neuropathy, where nerve damage occurs causing pain, typically in the extremities (Peltier and Russell, 2006). This side effect has been described since thalidomide was originally marketed (Kelsey, 1967) and remains a problem today (Cundari and Cavaletti, 2009; Peltier and Russell, 2006). How the drug causes peripheral neuropathy remains a mystery. However, patients are advised to stop taking thalidomide if they develop neuropathic symptoms. Clearly a form of the drug that does not have side effects, whether it be peripheral neuropathy or teratogenic, but retains clinical benefits remains the best solution, and given the advances in understanding of the mechanisms underlying teratogenesis and the molecular targets, hopefully in the near future this goal can be achieved.

TREATMENT

Thalidomide was demonstrated to be effective against ENL in the 1960s (Sheskin, 1965), and was shown to be anti-angiogenic in 1994 (D'Amato *et al.*, 1994). Since then thalidomide has been used as a treatment in many inflammatory disorders, as well as an anti-tumor agent, and is currently used to treat a wide range of diseases including: gastrointestinal (Behcet's syndrome, Crohn's disease); rheumatological (discoid lupus erythematosus; rheumatoid arthritis; sarcoidosis); dermatological (leprosy); blood (multiple myeloma; leukemia) and tumors (renal cell carcinoma; malignant gliomas; prostate carcinoma; Kaposi's sarcoma; colorectal carcinoma).

Thalidomide has also been demonstrated to be effective in relieving the symptoms of hereditary hemorrhagic telangiectasia (HHT), a bleeding disorder of the nose and gastrointestinal tract in mice and humans (Lebrin *et al.*, 2010). HHT is another potential use for thalidomide in the clinic.

Given the many breakdown products of thalidomide, the potential to synthesize over a 100 analogs, and the different actions that the drug has been demonstrated to exert, thalidomide is clinically very powerful (Franks *et al.*, 2004). Understanding each of the metabolite's functions should shed light on additional treatment regimens, as well as identify candidate molecules with a single pharmacological action (e.g., solely anti-inflammatory) for the treatment of specific medical conditions thus avoiding contraindications and adverse effects.

CONCLUDING REMARKS AND FUTURE DIRECTIONS

The rising use of thalidomide around the world for the successful treatment of a large range of clinical conditions remains a risk as the drug causes adverse side effects to long-term adult users, and the drug's inadvertent misuse has resulted in new cases of thalidomide embryopathy in Africa and South America. An obvious future direction is the formulation of a form of the drug that maintains the clinical benefits without the side effects. A large range of breakdown products result from non-enzymatic and enzymatic breakdown of thalidomide. Screening of breakdown products and analogs of the drug in the chick embryo has uncovered which part of the drug induces defect, namely the anti-angiogenic action (Therapontos *et al.*, 2009). With the ability to produce a large range of analogs of the drug (Franks *et al.*, 2004) this opens up the possibility of understanding what each of the by-product's functions are. This could uncover new by-products as well as current forms of the drug that could treat existing (and perhaps new) clinical conditions without side effects. Furthermore such an approach should allow a better understanding of the etiology of the actual conditions they are treating, which would help better treat the condition. Together this will shed light on the precise molecular action and consequences of the drug allowing additional drug targets to be identified. Also of interest is to understand the basis of the species differences in thalidomide action. Thalidomide exposure does not cause apparent birth defects in rodents exposed early in development, but can in late fetal stages and in juvenile/adult rodent tissue. An understanding of this will shed additional light on the mechanisms of this drug and further the generation of a safer form of the drug. Together with the very recent advances in understanding of the teratogenic action of the drug, the challenge of producing safe forms of the drug seems achievable.

ACKNOWLEDGMENTS

The author acknowledges The Royal Society, BDF newlife and the University of Aberdeen for financial support for thalidomide research. Thanks also to Eilidh Beaton, Scott McMenemy and Christina Therapontos for discussions on thalidomide.

REFERENCES

Ances BM (2002) New concerns about thalidomide. *Obstetr Gynaecol* **99:** 125–8.

Ando Y, Fuse E, Figg WD (2002) Thalidomide metabolism by the CYP2C subfamily. *Clin Cancer Res* **8:** 1964–73.

Bauer KS, Dixon SC, Figg WD (1998) Inhibition of angiogenesis by thalidomide requires metabolic activation, which is species-dependent. *Biochem Pharmacol* **55:** 1827–34.

Boylen JB, Horne HH, Johnson WJ (1963) Teratogenic effects of thalidomide and related substances. *Lancet* **1:** 552.

Castaneda CP, Zeldis JB, Freeman J, Quigley C, Brandenburg NA, Bwire R (2008) RevAssist: a comprehensive risk minimization programme for preventing fetal exposure to lenalidomide. *Drug Saf* **31:** 743–52.

Castilla EE, Ashton-Prolla P, Barreda-Mejia E, Brunoni D, Cavalcanti DP, Correa-Neto J, Delgadillo JL, Dutra MG, Felix T, Giraldo A, Juarez N, Lopez-Camelo JS, Nazer J, Orioli IM, Paz JE, Pessoto MA, Pina-Neto JM, Quadrelli R, Rittler M, Rueda S, Saltos M, Sánchez O, Schüler L (1996) Thalidomide, a current teratogen in South America. *Teratology* **54:** 273–7.

Chamberlain G (1989) The obstetric problems of the thalidomide children. *Brit Med J* **298:** 6.

Cullen JF (1964) Ocular defects in thalidomide babies. *Bri J Ophthalmol* **48:** 151–3.

Cundari S, Cavaletti G (2009) Thalidomide chemotherapy-induced peripheral neuropathy: actual status and new perspectives with thalidomide analogues derivatives. *Mini Rev Med Chem* **9:** 760–8.

Cuthbert R, Speirs AL (1963) Thalidomide induced malformations – a radiological survey. *Clin Radiology* **XX:** 163–9.

D'Amato RJ, Loughnan MS, Flynn E, Folkman J (1994) Thalidomide is an inhibitor of angiogenesis. *Proc Nat Acad Sci USA* **91:** 4082–5.

Ema M, Ise R, Kato H, Oneda S, Hirose A, Hirata-Koizumi M, Singh AV, Knudsen TB, Ihara T (2010) Fetal malformations and early embryonic gene expression response in cynomolgus monkeys maternally exposed to thalidomide. *Reprod Toxicol* **29:** 49–56.

Eriksson T, Björkman S, Höglund P (2001) Clinical pharmacology of thalidomide. *Eur J Clin Pharmacol* **57:** 365–76.

Franks ME, Macpherson GR, Figg WG (2004) Thalidomide review. *Lancet* **363:** 1802–11.

Galloway JL, Delgado I, Ros MA, Tabin CJ (2009) A reevaluation of x-irradiation-induced phocomelia and proximodistal limb patterning. *Nature* **460:** 400–4.

Galustian C, Dalgleish A (2009) Lenalidomide: a novel anticancer drug with multiple modalities. *Expert Opin Pharmacother* **10:** 125–33.

Gordon JN, Goggin PM (2003) Thalidomide and its derivatives: emerging from the wilderness. *Postgrad Med J* **79:** 127–32.

Hallene KL, Oby E, Lee BJ, Santaguida S, Bassanini S, Cipolla M, Marchi N, Hossain M, Battaglia G, Janigro D (2006) Prenatal exposure to thalidomide, altered vasculogenesis, and CNS malformations. *Neuroscience* **142:** 267–83.

Hansen JM, Gong S-G, Philbert MA, Harris C (2002). Misregulation of gene expression in the redox-sensitive NF-kB-dependent limb outgrowth pathway by thalidomide. *Dev Dyn* **255:** 186–94.

Hansen JM, Harris C (2004) A Novel Hypothesis for thalidomide-induced limb teratogenesis: redox misregulation of the NF-κB pathway. *Antioxid Redox Signal* **6:** 1–14.

Henkel L, Willert H (1969) Dysmelia – a classification and a pattern of malformation in a group of congenital defects of the limbs. *J Bone Joint Surgery* **51:** 399–414.

Ito T, Ando H, Suzuki T, Ogura T, Hotta K, Imamura Y, Yamaguchi Y, Handa H (2010) Identification of a primary target of thalidomide teratogenicity. *Science* **327:** 1345–50.

James WH (1965) Teratogenic properties of thalidomide. *Br Med J* **2:** 1064.

Jurand A (1966) Early changes in limb buds of chick embryos after thalidomide treatment. *J Embryol Exp Morphol* **16:** 289–300.

Kajii T, Kida M, Takahashi K (1973) The effect of thalidomide intake during 113 human pregnancies. *Teratology* **8:** 163–6.

Kelsey FO (1967) Events after thalidomide. *J Dental Res* **46:** 1201–5.

Kelsey FO (1988) Thalidomide update: regulatory aspects. *Teratology* **38:** 221–6.

Knobloch J, Schmitz I, Götz K, Schulze-Osthoff K, Rüther U (2008) Thalidomide induces limb anomalies by PTEN stabilization, Akt suppression, and stimulation of caspase-dependent cell death. *Molec Cell Biol* **28:** 529–38.

Knobloch J, Shaughnessy JD, Rüther U (2007) Thalidomide induces limb deformities by perturbing the Bmp/Dkk1/Wnt signalling pathway. *FASEB J* **21:** 1410–21.

Lebrin F, Srun S, Raymond K, Martin S, van den Brink S, Freitas C, Breant C, Mathivet T, Larriveel B, Thomas J-L, Arthur HM, Westermann CJJ, Disch F, Mager JJ, Snijder RJ, Eichmann A, Mummery C (2010) Thalidomide stimulates vessel maturation and reduces epistaxis in individuals with hereditary hemorrhagic telangiectasia. *Nature Med* **16:** 420–9.

Leck IM, Millar ELM (1962) Incidence of malformations since the introduction of thalidomide. *Br Med J* **2:** 16–20.

Lenz W (1962) Thalidomide and congenital abnormalities. *Lancet* **1:** 271–2.

Lenz W (1988) A short history of thalidomide embryopathy. *Teratology* **38:** 203–15.

Lenz W, Knapp K (1962) Foetal malformations due to thalidomide. *Ger Med Mon* **7:** 253–8.

Lepper ER, Smith NF, Cox MC, Scripture CD, Figg WD (2006) Thalidomide metabolism and hydrolysis: mechanisms and implications. *Curr Drug Metab* **7:** 677–85.

Livingstone G (1965) Congenital ear abnormalities due to thalidomide. *Proc Royal Soc Med Otology Section* **58:** 493–7.

McBride WG (1976) Studies of the etiology of thalidomide dysmorphogenesis. *Teratology* **14:** 71–88.

McBride WG (1961) Thalidomide and congenital malformations. *Lancet* 1358.

Majumder S, Rajaram M, Muley A, Reddy HS, Tamilarasan KP, Kolluru GK, Sinha S, Siamwala JH, Gupta R, Ilavarasan R, Venkataraman S, Sivakumar KC, Anishetty S, Kumar PG, Chatterjee S (2009) Thalidomide attenuates nitric-oxide driven angiogenesis by interacting with soluble guanylyl cyclase. *Br J Pharmacol* **158:** 1720–34.

Miller MT, Strömland K (1999) Teratogen update: thalidomide: a review, with a focus on ocular findings and new potential uses. *Teratology* **60:** 306–21.

Miller MT, Strömland K, Ventura L, Johansson M, Bandim JM, Gillberg C (2005) Autism associated with conditions characterized by developmental errors in early embryogenesis: a mini review. *Int J Dev Neurosci* **23:** 201–19.

Neubert R, Hinz N, Thiel R, Neubert D (1996) Down-regulation of adhesion receptors on cells of primate embryos as a probable mechanism of the teratogenic action of thalidomide. *Life Sci* **58:** 295–316.

Newman CGH (1985) Teratogen update: clinical aspects of thalidomide embryopathy – a continuing preoccupation. *Teratology* **32:** 133–44.

Newman CG (1986) The thalidomide syndrome: risks of exposure and spectrum of malformations. *Clin Perinatol* **13:** 555–73.

Ng SSW, Gutschow M, Weiss M, Hauschildt S, Teubert U, Hecker TK, Luzzio FA, Kruger EA, Eger K, Figg WD (2003) Antiangiogenic activity of N-substituted and tetra-fluorinated thalidomide analogues. *Cancer Res* **63:** 3189–94.

Paumgartten FJR (2006) Thalidomide embryopathy cases in Brazil after 1965. *Rep Tox* **22:** 1–2.

Peltier AC, Russell JW (2006) Advances in understanding drug induced neuropathies. *Drug Saf* **29:** 23–30.

Raab MS, Podar K, Breitkreutz I, Richardson PG, Anderson KC (2009) Multiple myeloma. *Lancet* **374:** 324–39.

Rajkumar SV (2004) Thalidomide: tragic past and promising future. *Mayo Clinic Proc* **79:** 899–903.

Sampaio EP, Sarno EN, Galilly R, Cohn ZA, Kaplan G (1991) Thalidomide selectively inhibits tumor necrosis factor α production by stimulated human monocytes. *J Exp Med* **173:** 699–703.

Schuler-Faccini L, Soares RCF, Sousa AC, Maximino C, Luna E, Schwartz IVD, Waldman C, Castilla EE (2007) New cases of thalidomide embryopathy in Brazil. *Birth Def Res* (Part A) **79:** 671–2.

Sheskin J (1965) Thalidomide in the treatment of lepra reactions. *Clin Pharmacol Ther* **6:** 303–6.

Smithells RW (1962) Thalidomide and malformations in Liverpool. *Lancet* 1270–3.

Smithells RW (1973) Defects and disabilities of thalidomide children. *Brit Med J* **1:** 269–72.

Smithells RW, Leck I (1963) The incidence of limb and ear defects since the withdrawal of thalidomide. *Lancet* 1095–7.

Smithells RW, Newman CG (1992) Recognition of thalidomide defects. *J Med Genet* **29:** 716–23.

Soules BJ (1966) Thalidomide victims in a rehabilitation centre. *Am J Nursing* **66:** 2023–6.

Speirs AL (1962) Thalidomide and congenital abnormalities. *Lancet* 303–5.

Stephens TD, Bunde CJW, Fillmore BJ (2000) Mechanism of action in thalidomide teratogenesis. *Biochem Pharmacol* **59:** 1489–99.

Stephens TD, Fillmore BJ (2000) Hypothesis: thalidomide embryopathy – proposed mechanism of action. *Teratology* **61:** 189–95.

Stephens TD (1988) Proposed mechanisms of action in thalidomide embryopathy. *Teratology* **38:** 229–39.

Tabin C, Wolpert L (2007) Rethinking the proximodistal axis of the vertebrate limb in the molecular era. *Genes Dev* **21:** 1433–42.

Tamilarasan KP, Kolluru GK, Rajaram M, Indhumathy M, Saranya R, Chatterjee S (2006) Thalidomide attenuates nitric oxide mediated angiogenesis by blocking migration of endothelial cells. *BMC Cell Biology* **7:** 1–13.

Taussig HB (1962) Thalidomide and phocomelia. *J Am Acad Paed* **30:** 654–9.

Teo SK, Resztak KE, Scheffler MA, Kook KA, Zeldis JB, Stirling DI, Thomas SD (2002) Thalidomide in the treatment of leprosy. *Microb Infect* **4:** 1193–202.

Therapontos C, Erskine L, Gardner E, Figg WD, Vargesson N (2009) Thalidomide induces limb defects by preventing angiogenic outgrowth during early limb formation. *Proc Natl Acad Sci USA* **106**: 8573–8.

Towers M, Tickle C (2009) Generation of pattern and form in the developing limb. *Int J Dev Biol* **53:** 805–12.

Tseng S, Pak G, Washenik K, Pomeranz MK, Shupack J (1996) Rediscovering thalidomide: a review of its mechanism of action, side effects and potential uses. *J Am Acad Derm* **35:** 969–79.

Vacca A, Scavelli C, Montefusco V, Pietro G, Neri A, Mattioli M, Bicciato S, Nico B, Ribatti D, Dammacco F, Corradini P (2005) Thalidomide downregulates angiogenic genes in bone marrow endothelial cells of patients with active multiple myeloma. *J Clin Oncol* **23:** 5334–46.

Vargesson N (2009) Thalidomide-induced limb defects: resolving a 50 year old puzzle. *BioEssays* **31:** 1327–36.

Vargesson N (2003) Vascularization of the developing chick limb bud: role of the TGFbeta signalling pathway. *J Anat* **202:** 93–103.

Warfel NA, Lepper ER, Zhang C, Figg WD, Dennis PA (2006) Importance of the stress kinase p38alpha in mediating the direct cytotoxic effects of the thalidomide analogue, CPS49, in cancer cells and endothelial cells. *Clin Cancer Res* **12:** 3502–9.

Yabu T, Tomimoto H, Taguchi Y, Yamaoka S, Igarashi Y, Okazaki T (2005) Thalidomide-induced antiangiogenic action is mediated through depletion of VEGF receptors, and is antagonized by spingosine-1-phosphate. *Blood* **106:** 125–34.

Zeller R (2010) The temporal dynamics of vertebrate limb development, teratogenesis and evolution. *Curr Opin Genet Dev*. In press.

Section 7

Metals

C H A P T E R

32

Aluminum

José L. Domingo

INTRODUCTION

Although it is well established that regardless of the host, the route of administration or the speciation, aluminum (Al) is a potent neurotoxicant (Strong and Garruto, 1991; Zatta *et al.*, 1994; Strong *et al.*, 1996), the basis for its toxicity is not quite known yet. In the 1970s, Al was found to be a major causative factor in the development of dialysis encephalopathy (Alfrey *et al.*, 1976). High concentrations of Al were found in plasma and tissue samples of dialyzed and non-dialyzed patients with chronic renal failure (Alfrey *et al.*, 1976; Kaehny *et al.*, 1977; Alfrey, 1985). The toxicity of Al also includes osteomalacia and anemia (Ganrot, 1986). In recent years, numerous investigations have also demonstrated that Al disrupts a wide variety of neurological processes (Savory *et al.*, 2006; Drago *et al.*, 2008; Kumar and Gill, 2009; Lemire *et al.*, 2009). Moreover, Al has been also proposed as a potential contributor to the pathogenesis of serious neurological disorders such as Alzheimer's disease (AD), amyotrophic lateral sclerosis and Parkinsonism-dementia of Guam (McLachlan *et al.*, 1991; Wakayama *et al.*, 1996; Kawahara, 2005; Domingo, 2006; Zatta *et al.*, 2009). In susceptible species, Al induces cytoskeletal changes, in which neurofilaments accumulate in neuronal cell bodies and proximal axonal enlargement (Muma and Singer, 1996; Savory *et al.*, 2006). Although Al has been reported to impact on gene expression, this does not appear to be critical to the induction of cytoskeletal pathology (Strong *et al.*, 1996).

Anyhow, there is unequivocal evidence that Al is a potent neurotoxic agent that induces neurofibrillary degeneration in animal brains after intracerebral Al injections and systemic Al exposure (Strong and Garruto, 1991; Strong *et al.*, 1991, 1996; Struys-Ponsar *et al.*, 1997). However, the association between Al exposure and the pathogenesis of AD and related disorders remains still unproven and questionable (Forbes *et al.*, 1995; Savory *et al.*, 1996; Gupta *et al.*, 2005; Drago *et al.*, 2008; Zatta *et al.*, 2009; Frisardi *et al.*, 2010). In spite of it, a number of reports in the literature strongly suggest that, by limiting human exposure to unnecessarily high Al concentrations, the incidence of AD might be reduced (McLachlan *et al.*, 1991; McLachlan, 1995; Gillette-Guyonnet *et al.*, 2007; Rondeau *et al.*, 2009).

With respect to potential Al toxicity, until recently there was relatively little concern about toxic consequences of Al ingestion because it was assumed that Al was not orally bioavailable. However, in recent decades, it was shown that although the gastrointestinal tract normally represents a major barrier to Al absorption, under some circumstances this barrier might be breached (Alfrey *et al.*, 1976; Alfrey, 1985). Consequently, individuals ingesting large amounts of Al compounds could absorb a definite amount of Al. Aluminum absorption, excretion, tissue retention and deposition all depend on the properties of the Al^{3+} complexes formed with biological ligands. The complexity in the aqueous chemistry of Al also affected Al toxicity studies (Harris *et al.*, 1996).

Normally, mammals maintain very low Al concentrations in their tissues because of a combination of low intestinal uptake and rapid clearance. Notwithstanding, it is well recognized that Al toxicity can occur either if absorption is markedly increased, or renal clearance is impaired. Although most foods contain small but variable amounts of Al, exposure to this metal through the diet is small compared to the quantities of Al in many antacid products, some buffered analgesics, as well as other therapeutic preparations (Domingo, 2001; Reinke *et al.*, 2003). Aluminum-containing antacids are widely used non-prescription medications, which have been administered for many years for the treatment of various gastrointestinal disorders (Reinke *et al.*, 2003). During pregnancy, dyspepsia is a common complaint and antacids are widely used to reduce the dyspeptic symptoms. In most of these drugs, Al is present as Al hydroxide, which has a very low aqueous solubility. However, the consumption of high amounts of Al compounds during pregnancy can mean a potential risk of Al accumulation because of the relatively great number of dietary constituents (ascorbate, citrate, lactate, succinate, etc.), which can enhance the gastrointestinal Al absorption (Domingo *et al.*, 1991a,b, 1994). Until relatively recently, information on human studies to determine whether Al ingestion could have adverse effects on the outcome of pregnancies was very scarce. Weberg *et al.* (1986) reported that since it was not clear whether maternal Al could increase the Al levels in the fetus, high dose antacids should not be consumed during pregnancy. In another study, Golding *et al.* (1991) investigated whether Al sulfate accidentally added to a local water supply (Cornwall, United Kingdom) had adverse embryo–fetal effects in pregnant women. It was concluded that although a lack of major problems associated with fetal exposure to high Al doses was noted, the relatively small number of pregnancies made it

Reproductive and Developmental Toxicology, Edited by Ramesh C. Gupta
ISBN: 978-0-12-382032-7

impossible to say if high doses of Al sulfate could be safe during gestation.

On the other hand, the scientific literature contains rather little information regarding either the experimental embryotoxic and teratogenic potential of Al, or the effects of gestational exposure to Al on the fetus and newborn. In order to obtain an overall understanding of the reproductive and developmental toxicity of Al, an extensive research program on these topics was initiated in our laboratory in the mid-1980s. In this chapter, data about Al-induced embryo–fetal toxicity, the potential reproductive toxicity and the postnatal effects of Al have been discussed.

EMBRYO–FETAL TOXICITY OF ALUMINUM

Nowadays, it is well established that Al may act as an embryo–fetal toxicant depending on the route of exposure and/or the solubility of each specific Al compound. While Al chloride was found to be embryotoxic and teratogenic when given parenterally to rats and mice (Benett *et al.*, 1975; Wide, 1984; Cranmer *et al.*, 1986; Colomina *et al.*, 1998), no evidence of maternal and embryo–fetal toxicity was observed when high doses of Al hydroxide were given to pregnant rats and mice (Domingo *et al.*, 1989; Gómez *et al.*, 1990). Thus, no developmental effects of Al hydroxide were observed when this compound was orally given to rats at 66.5, 133 and 266 mg Al/kg/day (Gómez *et al.*, 1990) or mice at 23, 46 and 92 mg Al/kg/day (Domingo *et al.*, 1989) during organogenesis. In addition, the maternal–placental Al concentrations were not significantly different between control and Al-treated rats, while Al could not be detected in the whole fetuses in any of the groups (Gómez *et al.*, 1990). Those results showed that Al, from Al hydroxide, was very poorly absorbed and did not reach the fetus at levels that might mean a developmental hazard. In mice, the doses of Al hydroxide were equivalent to those consumed by people of 60 kg body weight who ingest 1.4, 2.8 or 5.5 g of Al per day, respectively, which are much higher than the amounts usually ingested for peptic disorders.

In contrast to this, in a previous study, oral administration of Al nitrate nonahydrate (13, 26 and 52 mg Al/kg/day) to pregnant rats on gestation days 6–14 resulted in decreased fetal body weight and increased the incidence and types of external, visceral and skeletal malformations and variations in all the Al-treated groups (Paternain *et al.*, 1988). It was concluded that although embryolethality was not induced in rats by oral Al administration, whereas teratogenic effects might result at Al nitrate doses as high as those administered in that study, which corresponded approximately to 1/20, 1/10 and 1/5 of the acute oral LD_{50} of Al nitrate nonahydrate for adult female rats (Llobet *et al.*, 1995). These data, together with those obtained from studies in which Al hydroxide was given orally to rats and mice (Domingo *et al.*, 1989; Gómez *et al.*, 1990), showed that the Al compound solubility played an essential role in the potential embryo–fetal toxicity of Al.

It has been demonstrated that ingestion of Al hydroxide concurrently with fruit juices or with some common organic constituents of the diet (citrate, ascorbate, lactate, succinate, etc.) caused a marked increase in the gastrointestinal absorption of Al in healthy individuals (Domingo *et al.*, 1991a,b, 1993, 1994; Ogasawara *et al.*, 2002). The presence of Al complexing compounds in the gastrointestinal tract with gastric acid solubilizes Al cations and may thus result in the equilibrium formation of a soluble complex of Al, which by preventing reprecipitation, might result in Al absorption (Domingo *et al.*, 1991a,b, 1993, 1994; Glynn *et al.*, 2001). Taking this into account, we investigated whether the concurrent ingestion of citric, lactic or ascorbic acid and high doses of Al hydroxide could result in developmental toxicity in mammals.

The concurrent oral administration of citric acid (62 mg/kg/day) and Al hydroxide (133 mg Al/kg/day) to rats on gestation days 6–15 did not modify the lack of embryotoxicity and teratogenicity previously reported. However, the incidence of skeletal variations (delayed ossification of occipital and sternebrae) was significantly increased (Gómez *et al.*, 1991). Although not significantly different, the incidence of skeletal variations also increased in fetuses of pregnant mice given oral doses of Al hydroxide (57 mg Al/kg/day) and lactic acid (570 mg/kg/day) on days 6–15 of gestation, in comparison with a group of animals receiving Al hydroxide (57 mg Al/kg/day) only (Colomina *et al.*, 1992). By contrast, no signs of developmental toxicity were observed in mice when Al hydroxide (104 mg Al/kg/day) was given by gavage concurrently with high doses of ascorbic acid (85 mg Al/kg/day) on gestation days 6–15 (Colomina *et al.*, 1994).

EFFECTS OF ALUMINUM ON POSTNATAL DEVELOPMENT AND BEHAVIOR OF THE OFFSPRING

The effects on reproduction, gestation, parturition and lactation of oral Al exposure (0, 13, 26 and 52 mg Al/kg/day given as Al nitrate nonahydrate) were assessed in rats (Domingo *et al.*, 1987a,b). Male rats were orally treated for 60 days prior to mating with mature virgin female rats treated for 14 days prior to mating. Aluminum administration was continued throughout mating, gestation, parturition and weaning of the pups. One-half of the dams in each group were killed on gestation day 13, while the remaining dams were allowed to deliver and wean their offspring. Although no adverse effects on fertility or general reproductive parameters were noted, the survival ratios were higher in the control group. A dose-dependent delay in the growth of the living pups was also observed in all Al-treated groups (Domingo *et al.*, 1987a). The growth of the offspring was also significantly delayed when, in a subsequent experiment, Al nitrate nonahydrate (52 mg Al/kg/day) was given orally to rats from birth throughout lactation (Domingo *et al.*, 1987b).

Yokel (1984, 1985, 1987) reported few effects in the suckling offspring of rabbits whose does received subcutaneous injections of Al lactate at doses of 0.68, 2.7 or 10.8 mg Al/kg/injection, which was attributed to a probable limited distribution of Al into milk, together with a poor gastrointestinal Al absorption (Yokel, 1984; Yokel and McNamara, 1985). These studies, as well as other investigations conducted on rats and mice, indicated that Al was present in the milk of Al-exposed dams, but that it would not readily accumulate in pups during lactation (Golub and Domingo, 1996). By contrast, although in the placenta of pregnant rabbits and mice, Al concentrations were found to be four- to five-fold higher than those found in most fetal or maternal soft tissues of rabbits and mice, accumulation in the placenta did not apparently lessen or prevent Al accumulation in the fetus

(Golub and Domingo, 1996, 1998). This could indicate that the delay on postnatal development following Al exposure was due to an Al accumulation in the fetuses rather than Al absorption from the milk of the dam. However, a lack of remarkable Al transfer with lactation would not necessarily indicate that elevated Al in milk does not cause adverse effects on the offspring. Golub and co-workers (1996) showed that nursing pups of mouse dams fed excess Al in their diet exhibited poor retention of iron and manganese from a milk meal, whereas subcutaneous administration of Al lactate (2.5–10 mg/kg/day) to rats on gestational days 7–15 had no effect on birth weight, mean litter size and the day of eye and ear opening (Gonda *et al.*, 1996). Similar findings were also reported by Yokel (1985) and Muller *et al.* (1990).

On the other hand, a number of studies conducted in rats and mice showed that maternal oral Al exposure could alter performance on a neurobehavioral test battery, specifically impaired negative geotaxis and reduced forelimb and hindlimb grip strength (Bernuzzi *et al.*, 1989a,b; Donald *et al.*, 1989; Golub *et al.*, 1987, 1989, 1992, 1994). A markedly reduced activity level during behavioral testing was reported in adult rats after developmental Al exposure (Muller *et al.*, 1990; Cherroret *et al.*, 1992). However, no deficits in the test of delayed alterations (Golub *et al.*, 1996), in the radial maze (Cherroret *et al.*, 1992) or in the operant light avoidance task (Muller *et al.*, 1990) were found in adult mice and rats exposed to Al during development. Notwithstanding, Gonda *et al.* (1996) reported that although the learning ability of the pups of rats given 9.8 mg/kg/day of Al lactate on gestation days 7–15 was impaired in a passive avoidance task, no effect on the acquisition of a conditioned taste aversion was noted. In turn, Poulos *et al.* (1996) showed that oral Al administration to rats during pregnancy and lactation produced delay in the development of the central nervous system of their pups. The relevance of these findings for children exposed to Al needs to be determined by extending the evaluations to more complex CNS functions, including learning, regulation of arousal and sensory abilities (Golub and Domingo, 1996).

DEVELOPMENTAL EFFECTS OF ALUMINUM AND STRESS

A number of studies in mammals have shown that during pregnancy, maternal stress from restraint, noise, light and heat among others might be associated with adverse effects on embryo–fetal development (Scialli, 1988). Of special concern is the finding that interaction between maternal stress and some chemical teratogens could enhance the developmental toxicity of those chemicals.

Since Al is ubiquitous, exposure to this element is in fact unavoidable. This means that pregnant women may potentially be exposed to Al through food, drinking water, soil ingestion and some medications. Pregnant women may also be concurrently exposed to various types of stress, either at home or in the workplace. Because both Al and maternal stress during pregnancy have been shown to produce adverse developmental effects in mammals, Colomina *et al.* (1998, 1999) investigated the developmental toxicity in mice of a combined exposure to Al and maternal stress. The model stressor used was maternal immobilization. One of the animal models most widely used to examine the effects of maternal stress on the embryo–fetal toxicity of a chemical is restraint. In a first study (Colomina *et al.*, 1998), the potential interaction between Al and maternal restraint stress was assessed in mice. Four groups of plug-positive female mice were given intraperitoneal injections of $AlCl_3$ at 37.5 and 75 mg/kg/day on days 6–15 of gestation. Two of these groups were also subjected to restraint for 2 h/day during the same gestational days. Maternal toxicity was significantly enhanced by restraint stress at 75 mg $AlCl_3$/kg/day. No signs of embryo–fetal toxicity were observed following exposure to Al, maternal restraint or combined Al and restraint. However, a significant decrease in fetal body weight, as well as a significant increase in the number of litters with morphologic defects was observed in the group exposed to 75 mg $AlCl_3$/kg/day plus maternal restraint. These results suggested that maternal stress exacerbated Al-induced maternal and developmental toxicity only at high Al doses, which were also toxic to the dam.

In a subsequent investigation, the potential influence of maternal restraint stress and Al on the postnatal development and behavior of the offspring was assessed (Colomina *et al.*, 1999). On days 6–15 of gestation, two groups of pregnant mice received intraperitoneal injections of $AlCl_3$ at 75 mg/kg/day. One of these groups was also subjected to restraint for 2 h/day during the same days of gestation. The pups were evaluated for physical development, neuromotor maturation and behavior on postnatal days 22, 30 and 60. The results showed that although no significant effects of maternal Al plus restraint on the behavior of the offspring were noted, a significant influence of maternal stress on Al-induced postnatal developmental alterations was observed. These findings were in accordance with the previous results showing that maternal stress could enhance the Al-induced embryo–fetal toxicity in mice (Colomina *et al.*, 1998).

REPRODUCTIVE TOXICITY OF ALUMINUM

Although the knowledge of Al toxicity has markedly improved in recent years, information concerning the reproductive toxicity of this element is still rather limited. Kamboj and Kar (1964) investigated in rats and mice the effects on the testis of 32 water-soluble salts of metals and rare earths, including Al sulfate. A single intratesticular injection of 4.3 mg Al/kg (as Al sulfate) to rats caused focal necrosis of the testes within two days after injection, whereas this dose also destroyed all the spermatozoa within 7 days. A single subcutaneous injection of Al sulfate (4.3 mg Al/kg) had no effect on the weight of the testis in rats, but daily administration of this compound significantly reduced the weight of the testis in mice, although no necrotic changes were seen in the testes of these animals. A single subcutaneous injection of 4.3 mg Al/kg did not alter the histology of the rat testis. However, daily subcutaneous administration of the same dose caused shrinkage of the tubules and spermatogenic arrest at the primary spermatocyte or spermatogonial stages without affecting the interstitium (Kamboj and Kar, 1964). In another study, Krasovskii *et al.* (1979) gave orally Al chloride at 6, 17 and 50 mg Al/kg to rats and guinea pigs, and at 3, 9 and 27 mg Al/kg to rabbits, for 20–30 days (short-term exposure). Aluminum chloride was also given orally at 0.0025, 0.25 and 2.5 mg Al/kg to rats for 6 months (chronic exposure). Short-term Al administration caused slight toxicity to the gonads, whereas the gonadotoxic effect of Al was also weak following chronic exposure. Spermatozoa were only affected at the highest Al dose as shown by changes in their number and in their motility. At that dose, there also was a substantial proliferation of interstitial cells (Leydig cells). In a study performed in our laboratory (1995), adult male mice were intraperitoneally exposed to Al nitrate nonahydrate at doses of 50, 100 and 200 mg/kg/day (3.6, 7.2 and 14.4 mg Al/kg/day) for 4 weeks before mating with untreated females. Reduced body weight was seen in all Al-treated groups of male mice, whereas decreased pregnancy rate was observed in the females mated with males previously exposed to Al nitrate (100 or 200 mg/kg). Necrosis of spermatocytes/spermatids were observed in the testes of mice exposed to 100 and 200 mg/kg of Al nitrate, while decreased testicular and epididymal weights, significant decreases in testicular and spermatid counts, and significant decreases in epididymal sperm counts were also noted at 200 mg/kg. The "no-observable-adverse-effect-level" (NOAEL) was 50 mg/kg/day (3.6 mg Al/kg/day). Taking into account that most of the Al ingested is excreted into urine in individuals with normal renal function, it was concluded that there would be a remarkable safety margin for any adverse reproductive effect in humans due to Al ingestion under the intended conditions of use (Llobet *et al.*, 1995).

In an *in vitro* study using rabbit sperm, Yousef *et al.* (2007) evaluated the cytotoxic effects of different Al concentrations ($AlCl_3$) at 0, 2 and 4 h of incubation on sperm motility and viability, oxidative status and the activities of some antioxidant enzymes. The role of vitamin C (1 mM) or vitamin E (2 mM) was also investigated in counteracting deterioration caused by $AlCl_3$ on the tested parameters. Results revealed that the percentage of motile and viable sperm decreased significantly after $AlCl_3$ treatment at 10, 15 and 20 mM, and the response was both concentration and time dependent. No significant effect from vitamin C or vitamin E on motility and viability was noted. $AlCl_3$ caused deterioration in sperm motility and viability, enhancement of free radicals and alterations in enzymes' activities. The antioxidants revealed protective effects against the cytotoxicity of $AlCl_3$. These results agree well with those of a previous investigation of the same research group, where ascorbic acid significantly increased semen characteristics and seminal plasma enzymes, and decreased the levels of free radicals in male rabbits exposed to $AlCl_3$ (Yousef *et al.*, 2005). Recently, Yousef and Salama (2009) assessed the protective effects of propolis, an important antioxidant, against reproductive toxicity of $AlCl_3$ in male rats. $AlCl_3$ caused a decrease in testes, seminal vesicle and epididymis weights, sperm concentration, motility, testosterone level and the activities of 17-ketosteroid reductase, CAT and GST, and GSH content. In turn, dead and abnormal sperm and testes TBARS concentrations were increased. In the $AlCl_3$-treated group, histopathological examinations revealed apparent alterations in the testes, where Al induced marked lesions in seminiferous tubules. Propolis alone decreased dead and abnormal sperm and TBARS, and increased testosterone, GSH, 17-ketosteroid reductase, CAT and GST. Results showed that propolis antagonized the harmful effects of $AlCl_3$, and therefore it could be effective in protecting against the reproductive toxicity of $AlCl_3$.

PROTECTIVE EFFECTS OF CHELATING AGENTS ON ALUMINUM-INDUCED MATERNAL AND DEVELOPMENTAL TOXICITY

Chelating agents such as desferrioxamine (deferoxamine, DFO) and some 3-hydroxypyridin-4-ones can be effective in reducing Al body burdens (Yokel *et al.*, 1996; Gómez *et al.*, 1998a,b). Taking into account the lack of data on the effects of potential chelation therapies to protect pregnant women, infants and children against Al-induced maternal and/or developmental toxicity, the protective activity of DFO and deferiprone (1,2-dimethyl-3-hydroxypyrid-4-one, L 1) on Al-induced maternal and developmental toxic effects was evaluated in mice.

In a first study, Al chloride was intraperitoneally injected into pregnant mice at 0, 60, 120 and 240 mg/kg/day on gestation days 6–15, while DFO was administered subcutaneously at 40 mg/kg/day on days 6–18 of gestation. In a previous investigation (Bosque *et al.*, 1995), it was reported that the NOAEL for developmental toxicity of parenteral DFO in mice was 176 mg/kg/day. Significant amelioration by DFO of Al-induced maternal toxicity was only noted at 120 mg/kg/day, while no beneficial effects of DFO were observed on fetal body weight, the only embryo–fetal parameter significantly affected by maternal Al exposure (Albina *et al.*, 1999). The unexpected lack of Al-induced embryotoxicity reported in that study could be due to the chelating activity of DFO on $A1^{3+}$ in dam tissues, which would prevent this ion from reaching the embryo. In a second study, a single oral dose of Al nitrate nonahydrate (1,327 mg/kg) was given to mice on gestation day 12, the most sensitive time for Al-induced maternal and developmental toxic effects in this species. At 2, 24, 48 and 72 h thereafter, deferiprone was given by gavage at 0 and 24 mg/kg. Aluminum-induced maternal toxicity was evidenced by significant reductions in body weight gain and food consumption. Developmental toxicity was also evidenced by a significant decrease in fetal weight per litter and an increase in the total number of fetuses and litters showing bone retardation. No beneficial effects of deferiprone on these adverse effects were observed. In contrast, a more pronounced decrease in maternal weight gain, as well as an increase in the number of litters with fetuses showing skeletal variations was noted in the group given Al and deferiprone (Albina *et al.*, 2000).

As both DFO and deferiprone failed to protect against Al-induced maternal and developmental toxicity, subsequent studies investigated whether dietary silicon (Si) could prevent the toxic effects caused by Al in the pregnant animals. The rationale of that study was based on clear evidence showing that oral Si could reduce the gastrointestinal absorption of Al also increasing its elimination (Yokel *et al.*, 1996; Bellés *et al.*, 1998; Exley *et al.*, 2006). The preventive mechanism appears to involve the formation of hydroxyaluminosilicates by the adsorption of silicic acid onto an Al hydroxide template (Harris *et al.*, 1996). On gestation days 6–15, Al nitrate nonahydrate (398 mg/kg/day) was given by gavage to three groups of pregnant mice, which also received Si in drinking water at concentrations of 0, 118 and 236 mg/L on days 7–18 of gestation. Although Si administration at 236 mg/L significantly reduced the percentage of Al-induced maternal deaths, abortions and early deliveries, neither 118 nor 236 mg/L of Si produced significant ameliorations on Al-induced fetotoxicity (Bellés *et al.*, 1999).

Sharma and Mishra (2006) assessed the potential of 4,5-dihydroxy 1,3-benzene disulfonic acid disodium salt (Tiron) and glutathione (GSH) either individually or in combination against Al-induced developmental toxicity in fetuses and sucklings of Wistar rats orally exposed to $AlCl_3$ at 345 mg/kg/day from days 0 to 16 of gestation and 0 to 16 of postpartum. Tiron and GSH were administered at 471 mg/kg/day intraperitoneally and at 100 mg/kg/day orally, respectively, on days 5, 7, 9, 11, 13, 15 and 17 of gestation and postpartum. Aluminum caused reductions in the number of corpora lutea, number of implantation sites, placental and fetal weight and stunted growth. Skeletal malformations were also observed in fetuses. Maternal toxicity was demonstrated by reduction in body weight gain. Induction of oxidative stress was also recorded in the brain of mothers as well as in fetuses and suckling animals after Al exposure. Most parameters responded positively with individual therapy with Tiron. However, more pronounced beneficial effects on the above-described parameters were observed when Tiron was administered in combination with GSH. Treatment with Tiron individually or in combination with glutathione, reduced the accumulation of the Al in almost all the organs studied. It was concluded that chelating agents reduced Al-induced toxicity, Tiron being more effective in reducing blood Al concentration than glutathione when given individually.

CONCLUDING REMARKS AND FUTURE DIRECTIONS

It is well established that Al is a developmental toxicant following parenteral exposure (Domingo, 1987b; Golub and Domingo, 1996). No evidence of embryo–fetal toxicity was observed when high doses of Al hydroxide were given orally to pregnant rats and mice. However, some signs of maternal toxicity and fetotoxicity were found when Al hydroxide was given to mice concurrently with citric or lactic acids, or when Al was administered orally as Al nitrate, lactate or chloride to rats and mice. Therefore, it seems sufficiently demonstrated that oral Al exposure during pregnancy can cause a syndrome including growth retardation, delayed ossification, and malformation at Al doses that also lead to reduced maternal weight gain. The severity of these effects is highly dependent on the chemical form of Al administered. In turn, in the postnatal period, reduced pup weight gain and effects on neuromotor development and behavior can occur as a consequence of maternal and developmental Al exposure.

In a review article written by Borak and Wise (1998), the potential toxicity of Al during pregnancy was minimized by stating that environmental and dietary Al exposures were unlikely to pose risks of Al accumulation to pregnant animals or their fetuses. However, the weight of evidence does not support that statement (Golub and Domingo, 1998). In this context, this chapter provides strong evidence on Al-induced maternal and developmental toxicity in rats and mice.

On the other hand, some attention has also been paid to Al toxicity in infants. Moreno *et al.* (1994) reported that both preterm and full-term neonates were found to be susceptible to Al accumulation in tissues while receiving parenteral nutrition. In turn, Bishop *et al.* (1997) showed that, in preterm implants, prolonged intravenous feeding with solutions containing Al was associated with impaired neurologic development. Bishop *et al.* (1989) had previously shown increased concentrations of Al in the brain of a parenterally led premature infant.

According to the results of most of the above studies, including those on the enhancement of Al absorption from the gastrointestinal tract by certain dietary constituents (ascorbate, citrate, lactate, etc.), the potential effects of maternal stress on Al-induced maternal and developmental toxic effects and the lack of an adequate, safe and effective treatment to protect against these potential adverse effects, suggest the importance of avoiding high dose consumption of Al-containing compounds during gestation and lactation. Data on human studies also agree with this recommendation. Thus, the results of Weberg *et al.* (1986), who performed a small trial to assess whether antacids containing Al were safe during pregnancy, and the findings of Gilbert-Barness *et al.* (1998), based on data related to the death of a 9-year-old girl, who failed to progress developmentally at age 2 months, and whose mother ingested very high amounts of Al hydroxide daily during the entire pregnancy, also support the hypothesis that Al exposure during pregnancy can be a developmental hazard.

REFERENCES

Albina ML, Bellés M, Sánchez DJ, Domingo JL (1999) Prevention by desferrioxamine of aluminum-induced maternal and developmental toxic effects in mice. *Trace Elem Electr* **16:** 192–8.

Albina ML, Bellés M, Sánchez DJ, Domingo JL (2000) Evaluation of the protective activity of deferiprone, an aluminum chelator, on aluminum-induced developmental toxicity in mice. *Teratology* **62:** 86–92.

Alfrey AC, LeGendre GR, Kaehny WD (1976) The dialysis encephalopathy syndrome: possible aluminum intoxication. *N Engl J Med* **294:** 184–8.

Alfrey AC (1985) Gastrointestinal absorption of aluminum. *Clin Nephrol* **24:** S84–7.

Bellés M, Sánchez DJ, Gómez M, Corbella J, Domingo JL (1998) Silicon reduces aluminum accumulation in rats: relevance to the aluminum hypothesis of Alzheimer's disease? *Alzheimer Dis Assoc Disord* **12:** 83–7.

Bellés M, Albina ML, Sánchez DJ, Domingo JL (1999) Lack of protective effects of dietary silicon on aluminum-induced maternal and developmental toxicity in mice. *Pharmacol Toxicol* **85:** 1–6.

Benett RW, Persaud TVN, Moore KL (1975) Experimental studies on the effects of aluminum on pregnancy and fetal development. *Anat Anz Bd* **138:** 365–78.

Bernuzzi V, Desor D, Lehr PR (1989a) Developmental alterations in offspring of female rats orally intoxicated by aluminum chloride or lactate during gestation. *Teratology* **40:** 21–7.

Bernuzzi V, Desor D, Lehr PR (1989b) Effects of postnatal aluminum lactate exposure on neuromotor maturation in the rat. *Bull Environ Contam Toxicol* **42:** 451–5.

Bishop NJ, Robinson MJ, Lendon M, Hewitt CD, Day JP, O'Hara M (1989) Increased concentration of aluminum in the brain of a parenterally fed preterm infant. *Arch Dis Child* **64:** 1316–17.

Bishop NJ, Morley R, Day JP, Lucas A (1997) Aluminum neurotoxicity in preterm infants receiving intravenous feeding solutions. *N Engl J Med* **336:** 1557–61.

Borak J, Wise JP (1998) Does aluminum exposure of pregnant animals lead to accumulation in mothers or their offspring? *Teratology* **57:** 127–39.

Bosque MA, Domingo JL, Corbella J (1995) Assessment of the developmental toxicity of deferoxamine in mice. *Arch Toxicol* **69:** 467–71.

Cherroret G, Bernuzzi V, Desor D, Hutin MF, Burnel D, Lehr PR (1992) Effects of postnatal aluminum exposure on choline acetyltransferase activity and learning abilities in the rat. *Neurotoxicol Teratol* **14:** 259–64.

Colomina MT, Gómez M, Domingo JL, Llobet JM, Corbella J (1992) Concurrent ingestion of lactate and aluminum can result in developmental toxicity in mice. *Res Commun Chem Pathol Pharmacol* **77:** 95–106.

Colomina MT, Gómez M, Domingo JL, Corbella J (1994) Lack of maternal and developmental toxicity in mice given high doses of aluminum hydroxide and ascorbic acid during gestation. *Pharmacol Toxicol* **74:** 236–9.

Colomina MT, Esparza JL, Corbella J, Domingo JL (1998) The effect of maternal restraint on developmental toxicity of aluminum in mice. *Neurotoxicol Teratol* **20:** 651–6.

Colomina MT, Sánchez DJ, Sánchez-Turet M, Domingo JL (1999) Exposure of pregnant mice to aluminum and restraint stress: effects on postnatal development and behaviour of the offspring. *Psychobiology* **27:** 521–9.

Cranmer JM, Wilkins JD, Cannon DJ, Smith L (1986) Fetal–placental–maternal uptake of aluminum in mice following gestational exposure: effect of dose and route of administration. *Neurotoxicology* **7:** 601–8.

Domingo JL (2001) Aluminum: toxicology. In *Encyclopaedia of Food Science, Food Technology and Nutrition*, 2nd edition (Macrae R, Robinson R, Sadler M, eds.). Academic Press, London.

Domingo JL (2006) Aluminum and other metals in Alzheimer's disease: a review of potential therapy with chelating agents. *J Alzheimers Dis* **10:** 331–41.

Domingo JL, Paternain JL, Llobet JM, Corbella J (1987a) The effects of aluminum ingestion on reproduction and postnatal survival in rats. *Life Sci* **41:** 1127–31.

Domingo JL, Paternain JL, Llobet JM, Corbella J (1987b) Effects of oral aluminum administration on prenatal and postnatal progeny development in rats. *Res Commun Chem Pathol Pharmacol* **57:** 129–32.

Domingo JL, Gómez M, Bosque MA, Corbella J (1989) Lack of teratogenicity of aluminum hydroxide in mice. *Life Sci* **45:** 243–7.

Domingo JL, Gómez M, Llobet JM, Corbella J (1991a) Influence of some dietary constituents on aluminum absorption and retention in rats. *Kidney Int* **39:** 598–601.

Domingo JL, Gómez M, Llobet JM, Richart C (1991b) Effect of ascorbic acid on gastrointestinal aluminum absorption. *Lancet* **338:** 1467.

Domingo JL, Gómez M, Sánchez DJ, Llobet JM, Corbella J (1993) Effect of various dietary constituents on gastrointestinal absorption of aluminum from drinking water and diet. *Res Commun Chem Pathol Pharmacol* **79:** 377–80.

Domingo JL, Gómez M, Llobet JM, del Castillo D, Corbella J (1994) Influence of citric, ascorbic and lactic acids on the gastrointestinal absorption of aluminum in uremic rats. *Nephron* **66:** 108–9.

Donald JM, Golub MS, Gershwin ME, Keen CL (1989) Neurobehavioral effects in offspring of mice given excess aluminum in diet during gestation and lactation. *Neurotoxicol Teratol* **11:** 345–51.

Drago D, Bolognin S, Zatta P (2008) Role of metal ions in the abeta oligomerization in Alzheimer's disease and in other neurological disorders. *Curr Alzheimer Res* **5:** 500–7.

Exley C, Korchazhkina O, Job D, Strekopytov S, Polwart A, Crome P (2006) Non-invasive therapy to reduce the body burden of aluminium in Alzheimer's disease. *J Alzheimers Dis* **10:** 17–24.

Forbes WF, Gentleman JF, Maxwell CJ (1995) Concerning the role of aluminum in causing dementia. *Exp Gerontol* **30:** 23–32.

Frisardi V, Solfrizzi V, Capurso C, Kehoe PG, Imbimbo BP, Santamato A, Dellegrazie F, Seripa D, Pilotto A, Capurso A, Panza F (2010) Aluminum in the diet and Alzheimer's disease: from current epidemiology to possible disease-modifying treatment. *J Alzheimers Dis* **20:** 17–30.

Ganrot PO (1986) Metabolism and possible health effects of aluminum. *Environ Health Perspect* **65:** 363–441.

Gilbert-Barness E, Barness L, Wolff J, Harding C (1998) Aluminum toxicity. *Arch Pediatr Adolesc Med* **152:** 511–12.

Gillette Guyonnet S, Andrieu S, Vellas B (2007) The potential influence of silica present in drinking water on Alzheimer's disease and associated disorders. *J Nutr Health Aging* **11:** 119–24.

Glynn AW, Sparén A, Danielsson LG, Sundström B, Jorhem L (2001) The influence of complexing agents on the solubility and absorption of aluminum in rats exposed to aluminum in water. *Food Addit Contam* **18:** 515–23.

Golding J, Rowland A, Greenwood R, Lunt P (1991) Aluminum sulphate in water in north Cornwall and outcome of pregnancy. *Brit J Med* **302:** 1175–7.

Golub MA, Domingo JL (1996) What we know and what we need to know about developmental aluminum toxicity. *J Toxicol Environ Health* **48:** 585–97.

Golub MS, Domingo JL (1998) Fetal aluminum accumulation. *Teratology* **58:** 225–6.

Golub MS, Gershwin ME, Donald JM, Negri S, Keen CL (1987) Maternal and developmental toxicity of chronic aluminum exposure in mice. *Fundam Appl Toxicol* **8:** 346–57.

Golub MS, Donald JM, Gershwin ME, Keen CL (1989) Effects of aluminum ingestion on spontaneous motor activity of mice. *Neurotoxicol Teratol* **11:** 231–5.

Golub MS, Keen CL, Gershwin ME (1992) Neurodevelopmental effects of aluminum in mice: fostering studies. *Neurotoxicol Teratol* **14:** 177–82.

Golub MS, Han B, Keen CL, Gershwin ME (1994) Auditory startle in Swiss Webster mice fed excess aluminum in diet. *Neurotoxicol Teratol* **16:** 423–5.

Golub MS, Han B, Keen CL (1996) Iron and manganese uptake by offspring of lactating mice fed a high aluminum diet. *Toxicology* **109:** 111–18.

Gómez M, Bosque MA, Domingo JL, Llobet JM, Corbella J (1990) Evaluation of the maternal and developmental toxicity of aluminum from high doses of aluminum hydroxide in rats. *Vet Hum Toxicol* **32:** 545–8.

Gómez M, Domingo JL, Llobet JM (1991) Developmental toxicity evaluation of oral aluminum in rats: influence of citrate. *Neurotoxicol Teratol* **13:** 323–8.

Gómez M, Esparza JL, Domingo JL, Corbella J, Singh PK, Jones MM (1998a) Aluminum mobilization: a comparative study of a number of chelating agents in rats. *Pharmacol Toxicol* **82:** 295–300.

Gómez M, Esparza JL, Domingo JL, Singh PK, Jones MM (1998b) Comparative aluminum mobilizing actions of deferoxamine and four 3-hydroxypyridin-4-ones in aluminum-loaded rats. *Toxicology* **130:** 175–81.

Gonda Z, Lehotzky K, Miklósi A (1996) Neurotoxicity induced by prenatal aluminum exposure in rats. *Neurotoxicology* **17:** 459–70.

Gupta VB, Anitha S, Hegde ML, Zecca L, Garruto RM, Ravid R, Shankar SK, Stein R, Shanmugavelu P, Jagannatha Rao KS (2005) Aluminum in Alzheimer's disease: are we still at a crossroad? *Cell Mol Life Sci* **62:** 143–58.

Harris WR, Berthon G, Day JP, Exley C, Flaten TP, Forbes WF, Kiss T, Orvig C, Zatta PF (1996) Speciation of aluminum in biological systems. *J Toxicol Environ Health* **48:** 543–68.

Kaehny WO, Hegg AP, Alfrey AC (1977) Gastrointestinal absorption of aluminum from aluminum-containing antacids. *N Engl J Med* **296:** 1389–90.

Kamboj VP, Kar AB (1964) Antitesticular effect of metallic and rare earth salts. *J Reprod Fertil* **7:** 21–8.

Kawahara M (2005) Effects of aluminum on the nervous system and its possible link with neurodegenerative diseases. *J Alzheimers Dis* **8:** 171–82.

Krasovskii GN, Vasukovich LY, Chariev OG (1979) Experimental study of biological effects of lead and aluminum following oral administration. *Environ Health Perspect* **30:** 47–51.

Kumar V, Gill KD (2009) Aluminum neurotoxicity: neurobehavioral and oxidative aspects. *Arch Toxicol* **83:** 965–78.

Lemire J, Mailloux R, Puiseux-Dao S, Appanna VD (2009) Aluminum-induced defective mitochondrial metabolism perturbs cytoskeletal dynamics in human astrocytoma cells. *J Neurosci Res* **87:** 1474–83.

Llobet JM, Colomina MT, Sirvent JJ, Domingo JL, Corbella J (1995) Reproductive toxicology of aluminum in male mice. *Fundam Appl Toxicol* **25:** 45–51.

McLachlan DRC, Kruck TP, Lukiw WJ, Krishnan SS (1991) Would decreased aluminum ingestion reduce the incidence of Alzheimer's disease? *Can Med Assoc J* **145:** 793–804.

McLachlan DRC (1995) Aluminum and the risk for Alzheimer's disease. *Environmetrics* **6:** 233–75.

Moreno A, Dominguez C, Ballabriga A (1994) Aluminum in the neonate related to parenteral nutrition. *Acta Paediatr* **83:** 25–9.

Muller G, Bernuzzi V, Desor D, Hutin MF, Burnel D, Lehr PR (1990) Developmental alterations in offspring of female rats orally intoxicated by aluminum lactate at different gestation periods. *Teratology* **42:** 253–61.

Muma NA, Singer SM (1996) Aluminum-induced neuropathology: transient changes in microtubule-associated proteins. *Neurotoxicol Teratol* **18:** 679–90.

Ogasawara Y, Sakamoto T, Ishii K, Takahashi H, Tanabe S (2002) Effects of the administration routes and chemical forms of aluminum on aluminum accumulation in rat brain. *Biol Trace Elem Res* **86:** 269–78.

Paternain JL, Domingo JL, Llobet JM, Corbella J (1988) Embryotoxic and teratogenic effects of aluminum nitrate on rats upon oral administration. *Teratology* **38:** 253–7.

Poulos BK, Perazzolo M, Lee VM, Rudelli R, Wisniewski HM, Soifer D (1996) Oral aluminum administration during pregnancy and lactation produces gastric and renal lesions in rat mothers and delay in CNS development of their pups. *Mol Chem Neuropathol* **29:** 15–26.

Reinke CM, Breitkreutz J, Leuenberger H (2003) Aluminum in over-the-counter drugs: risks outweigh benefits? *Drug Saf* **26:** 1011–25.

Rondeau V, Jacqmin-Gadda H, Commenges D, Helmer C, Dartigues JF (2009) Aluminum and silica in drinking water and the risk of Alzheimer's disease or cognitive decline: findings from 15-year follow-up of the PAQUID cohort. *Am J Epidemiol* **169:** 489–96.

Savory J, Herman MM, Ghribi O (2006) Mechanisms of aluminum-induced neurodegeneration in animals: implications for Alzheimer's disease. *J Alzheimers Dis* **10:** 135–44.

Scialli AR (1988) Is stress a developmental toxin? *Reprod Toxicol* **1:** 163–71.

Sharma P, Mishra KP (2006) Aluminum-induced maternal and developmental toxicity and oxidative stress in rat brain: response to combined administration of Tiron and glutathione. *Reprod Toxicol* **21:** 313–21.

Strong MJ, Garruto RM (1991) Potentiation of the neurotoxic induction of experimental chronic neurodegenerative disorders: n-butyl benzene sulfonamide and aluminum chloride. *Neurotoxicology* **12:** 415–26.

Strong MJ, Wolff AV, Wakayama I, Garruto RM (1991) Aluminum-induced myelopathy in rabbits. *Neurotoxicology* **12:** 9–22.

Strong MJ, Garruto RM, Joshi JG, Mundy WR, Shafer T (1996) Can the mechanisms of aluminum neurotoxicity be integrated into a unified scheme? *J Toxicol Environ Health* **48:** 599–613.

Struys-Ponsar C, Kerkhofs A, Gauthier A, Soffié M, van den Bosch de Aguilar Ph (1997) Effects of aluminum exposure on behavioral parameters in the rat. *Pharmacol Biochem Behav* **56:** 643–8.

Wakayama I, Nerurkar VR, Strong MJ, Garruto RM (1996) Comparative study of chronic aluminum-induced neurofilamentous aggregates with intracytoplasmic inclusion of amyotrophic lateral sclerosis. *Acta Neuropathol* **92:** 545–54.

Weberg R, Berstad A, Ladehaug B, Thomassen Y (1986) Are aluminum containing antacids during pregnancy safe? *Acta Pharmacol Toxicol* **59:** S63–S65.

Wide M (1984) Effect of short-term exposure to five industrial metals on the embryonic and fetal development of the mouse. *Environ Res* **33:** 47–53.

Yokel RA (1984) Toxicity of aluminum exposure during lactation to the maternal and suckling rabbit. *Toxicol Appl Pharmacol* **75:** 35–43.

Yokel RA (1985) Toxicity of gestational aluminum exposure to the maternal rabbit and offspring. *Toxicol Appl Pharmacol* **79:** 121–33.

Yokel RA (1987) Toxicity of aluminum exposure to the neonatal and immature rabbit. *Fundam Appl Toxicol* **9:** 795–806.

Yokel RA, McNamara PJ (1985) Aluminum bioavailability and disposition in adult and immature rabbits. *Toxicol Appl Pharmacol* **77:** 344–52.

Yokel RA, Ackrill P, Burgess E, Day JP, Domingo JL, Flaten TP, Savory A (1996) The prevention and treatment of aluminum toxicity including chelation therapy. Status and research needs. *J Toxicol Environ Health* **48:** 667–83.

Yousef MI, El-Morsy AM, Hassan MS (2005) Aluminum-induced deterioration in reproductive performance and seminal plasma biochemistry of male rabbits: protective role of ascorbic acid. *Toxicology* **215:** 97–107.

Yousef MI, Kamel KI, El-Guendi MI, El-Demerdash FM (2007) An in vitro study on reproductive toxicity of aluminum chloride on rabbit sperm: the protective role of some antioxidants. *Toxicology* **239:** 213–23.

Yousef MI, Salama AF (2009) Propolis protection from reproductive toxicity caused by aluminum chloride in male rats. *Food Chem Toxicol* **47:** 1168–75.

Zatta PF, Zambenedetti P, Masiero S (1994) Effects of aluminum lactate on murine neuroblastoma cells. *Neurotoxicology* **15:** 789–98.

Zatta P, Drago D, Bolognin S, Sensi SL (2009) Alzheimer's disease, metal ions and metal homeostatic therapy. *Trends Pharmacol Sci* **30:** 346–55.

C H A P T E R

33

Arsenic, cadmium and lead

Swaran J. S. Flora, Vidhu Pachauri and Geetu Saxena

INTRODUCTION

Metal toxicity has been documented recently as one of the prime mass toxicants especially in the case of occupational and environmental hazards. With the inception of specialized branches like metallotoxicology, a new era of metal toxicity research has begun. However, understanding the mechanisms and establishing the dose–response relationships for metal-induced reproductive and developmental toxicity still remains a challenge for researchers. Metals may cause a wide spectrum of reproductive and developmental adverse effects such as reduced fertility, abortions, retarded growth at the intrauterine cavity, skeletal deformities, malformations and retarded development especially of the nervous system. The type of manifestations, however, mainly depends upon the stage and duration of exposure, and toxicokinetics of the metal which in turn is governed by the metal species and its ability to interfere in the developmental processes. Bioassays in preclinical studies showed teratogenic effects of metal including Al, As, Cd, Co, Cr, Cu, Ga, Hg, Li, Mn, Pb, Zn, etc. in many species. The effects generally observed include fetal death and malformations such as eye defects, cleft palate, anencephaly and skeletal anomalies.

Any teratogen is known to produce toxic manifestations in small doses either directly or injury mediated via systemic toxicity mostly by virtue of high dose effect. Animal experimental results provide information on usually high dose effect on reproductive systems but human evidence is limited. Correlating the two may be difficult since low dose prolonged exposures are more common in the case of humans and possible interspecies variations. Thus, in metal toxicology, unpredictable dose–response relationship and the "no-observable-adverse-effect level" (NOAEL) for most metals remain an important limitation in assessing toxic risks. Moreover in the case of metal toxicity it may not only be the adverse effects of toxic metal *per se* but toxicant-dependent essential metal imbalance that can direct the phenomena. Further physiological and genetic variations including polymorphisms effecting maternal ability to detoxify and eliminate toxic metal from the body cause variations in type and extent of toxicity. For example, arsenic metabolism and, in turn, its toxicity not only varies with species but also greatly differs within the species as evident from human reports. Thus, metal-induced reproductive and developmental toxicity appears to be having multifactorial causations making its mechanistic understanding rather complex. Male or female reproductive health may be retarded depending upon the stage of metal exposure, namely the prenatal, prematurity or maturity stage as well as the route, dose and duration of exposure, the evidence of which is generally animal data driven. Interpreting female fertility defects is very difficult since many factors may influence outcome such as age, ovarian reserves, male reproductive health, hormonal imbalance, genetic malfunctioning or sexually transmitted diseases.

As per the Wilson's principle, toxic manifestations by metal exposure on the fetus greatly depend upon developmental stage at the time of exposure. Toxin exposure at the pre-differentiation stage generally accounts for the "all or none phenomenon" causing embryonic death. At the early differentiation or early organogenesis stage the embryo is most susceptible to malformations; however, organs that show multiphasic development may have more than one susceptible period. Metal exposure during the stage of functional maturity and histogenesis, called late or advanced organogenesis, leads to growth retardations and developmental delays especially neurobehavioral problems.

In the present chapter we will discuss the toxic effects of conventionally known metals such as lead, arsenic and mercury on the reproductive system and developmental processes. The chapter comprises a mechanistic understanding of these toxicities with respect to the toxicokinetics of the metal and related risk assessment.

ARSENIC

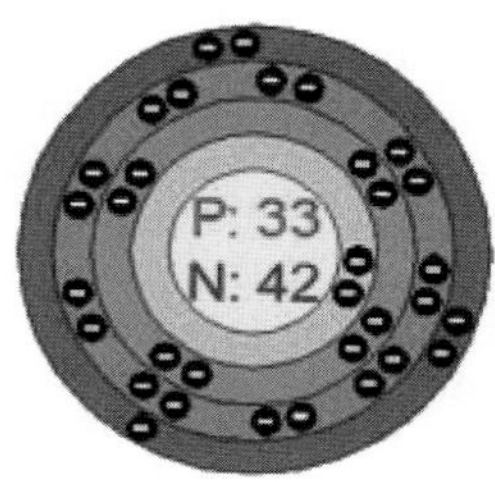

Reproductive and Developmental Toxicology, Edited by Ramesh C. Gupta
ISBN: 978-0-12-382032-7

Name:	Arsenic
Symbol:	As
Atomic number:	33
Atomic mass:	74.9216 amu
Melting point:	817.0°C (1090.15 K, 1502.6°F)
Boiling point:	613.0°C (886.15 K, 1135.4°F)
Number of protons/ electrons:	33
Number of neutrons:	42
Crystal structure:	Rhombohedral
Density @ 293 K:	5.72 g/cm^3
Color:	Gray
Electronic configuration:	[Ar] 4s2 3d10 4p3
Shell structure:	2.8.18.5
Oxidation states:	5, 3, 1,-3

Introduction

Exposure to arsenic is of prime concern due to its vast industrial uses as well as high availability in groundwater. Moreover, awareness regarding its toxic effects is scant. The US Agency for Toxic Substances and Disease Registry (ATSDR) lists more than 20 heavy metals with pronounced toxicity but four are of particular concern to human health; arsenic (As), lead (Pb), cadmium (Cd) and mercury (Hg); out of these four, arsenic is the most common cause of acute heavy metal poisoning and hence ranked number 1 on ATSDR's "top 20 list".

The increasing groundwater levels and high industrial use of arsenic and its related compounds increase the risk of exposure to human beings. The general population is exposed to arsenic via contaminants found in drinking water and food (ATSDR, 2007), while occupational exposure to arsenic usually takes place during mining and smelting operations or manufacturing of arsenic containing compounds in gallium arsenide (GaAs) in the semiconductor, paper, glass industries. According to the guidelines of the World Health Organization, the permissible limit for arsenic in drinking water has reduced from 50 μg/L to 10 μg/L (WHO, 2001, 2004). Although pentavalent arsenic (As^{5+}) is more abundant in the environment, the trivalent form (As^{3+}) is more toxic. Exposure to arsenic may be acute, subchronic or chronic. Acute or high dose exposure of arsenic results in significant and potentially lethal toxicity. In contrast, chronic exposure of arsenic may have more serious effects and leads to mutagenesis, carcinogenesis and/ or apoptotic cell death in various organ systems (Fabiánová *et al.*, 2000).

Arsenic exposure is known to cause toxic effects on various organ systems, for example hepatic, hematopoietic, renal, reproductive, nervous system, etc. (ATSDR, 2000). Reproductive toxicity of arsenic is one of the important areas of research as arsenic tends to cross the placental barrier and induces irreversible defects in the developing progeny (Ferrario *et al.*, 2008). These effects are further enhanced due to the lack of a developed metabolic system as well as naïve immune system. After fertilization, zygote is formed, which passes through different developmental stages, i.e. (1) cleavage, in which the zygote divides to form a ball of cells, the blastula, (2) gastrulation, in which the cell become arranged in three primary germ layers, and (3) organogenesis, in which further cell division and differentiation results in the formation of organs. Thus the exposure of arsenic to the reproductive system of parents, or any of the above-mentioned stages, might have more serious implications on the growing fetus as well as the mother.

Historical background

Over the centuries, arsenic has been used as a pesticide and fungicide. From the 19th century onward, an inorganic compound known as Fowler's solution (1% potassium arsenite solution) was used for the treatment of leukemia, psoriasis, chronic bronchial asthma and as a tonic (Zhao and Chen, 2005). Organic arsenic compounds were used for the treatment of syphilis and trypanosomal infection prior to the introduction of antibiotics. Medical folklore also indicated that various inorganic arsenic-containing tonics were consumed in the therapy of acne, psoriasis, sexual disorders, anemia and rheumatism. Arsenic as copper acetoarsenite was used as a pigment in paints, the best known being "Paris green". Before electricity, coal fires were used for heat and light; these produced hydrogen gas, which when combined with arsenic which was present in "Paris green" of wallpaper formed toxic gas, arsine. A fungus *Scopulariopsis breviculis* present in damp wallpaper also metabolized the arsenic in Paris green to arsine.

Current uses of arsenic are in pesticides (lead arsenate, calcium arsenate and sodium arsenite), herbicides (mono sodium arsenate and cacodylic acid; dimethyl arsenic acid), cotton desiccants (arsenic acid) and wood preservatives (zinc and chromium arsenate). Arsenic is also used as a bronzing and decolorizing agent in the manufacture of glass, and in the production of semiconductors (gallium arsenide, indium arsenide, aluminum gallium arsenide), as a desiccant and defoliant in agriculture, and as a by-product in the smelting of non-ferrous metals, particularly gold and copper, from coal residues (Hall, 2002). In India, herbal medicines are suspected to contain arsenic. Arsenic in homeopathic preparations and for the treatment of hematological malignancies is also being practiced. In Korea, arsenic is prescribed in herbal medicine for hemorrhoids.

Toxicokinetics

Absorption

The majority of arsenic exposures occur via contaminated drinking water. Other routes of exposure are through inhalation, dermal exposure and exposure from food. Systemic absorption via the skin appears to be low. The major site of absorption of arsenic is the small intestine where it is absorbed through an electrogenic process involving a proton gradient. The optimal pH for arsenic absorption is 5.0. Absorption of arsenic in the lungs is dependent on particle size as well as water solubility; respirable particles (0.1–1 μ) are carried further into the lungs and are therefore more likely to be absorbed.

Distribution

A number of factors affect the distribution and retention of arsenic in the system. These include species of arsenic, dose level, methylation capacity, valency form, route of exposure and genetic factors. Both arsenite (As^{3+}) and arsenate (As^{5+}) have a tendency to bind with free sulfhydryl groups; however, As^{3+} has approximately a 10-fold greater affinity than

As^{5+} for sulfhydryl groups. Therefore cellular uptake and retention of As^{5+} is substantially lower than As^{3+}. In terms of cellular efflux of methylated species, dimethyl arsenic (DMA) appears to be more readily excreted than monomethyl arsenic (MMA) (NRC, 2001).

Once absorbed, arsenic rapidly combines with the globin portion of hemoglobin (Hb) and therefore localizes in the blood. The presence of numerous -SH groups containing proteins and low molecular weight compounds such as glutathione (GSH) and cysteine adds to the accumulation of arsenic in blood. The retention of arsenic in the blood varies among species. Arsenic elimination in humans is triphasic with half-life varying from 27 to 86 hours. Among the various species, the retention of arsenic in the blood is comparatively longer in rats because DMA^{III} accumulates in red blood cells, apparently bound to hemoglobin. Recently cysteine-13 residue of the α-chain of Hb has been identified as a binding site of trivalent dimethyl arsenic (DMA^{III}) to rat Hb. The uptake of DMA in blood is dependent on both species and chemical forms. The rate of uptake of DMA^{III} and efflux of pentavalent dimethyl arsenic (DMA^{V}) is greater in hamster RBC than in human. Generally mothers consuming arsenic-contaminated food or water may be more likely to have dimetylated metabolites in the fetus blood (Hall *et al.*, 2007).

The presence of keratin (rich in thiol containing cysteine amino acids) protein in skin, hairs, oral mucosa, etc. provides the binding sites of inorganic arsenic (mainly As^{3+}). The enzyme S-adenosylmethionine (SAM) plays a key role in arsenic methylation. It is known that a decrease in methylation pattern is due to decreased methyltransferase activity (Drobna *et al.*, 2010).

The presence of free -SH groups in tissues is a key factor affecting the retention time and metabolism of arsenic. The retention time for inorganic arsenic varies in different organs; the longest retention of inorganic arsenic in mammalian tissues during experimental studies has been observed in the skin, hair, squamous epithelium of the upper gastrointestinal tract (oral cavity, tongue, esophagus and stomach wall), epididymis, etc. After nine repeated daily doses of radiolabeled arsenic in female B6C3F1, Hughes *et al.* (2003) concluded that accumulation of radioactivity was highest in the bladder, kidney and skin. The loss of radioactivity was greatest in the lungs, but was slowest in the skin. Atomic absorption spectrometry revealed an organ-specific distribution of arsenicals. MMA was detected in all tissues except the bladder, while DMA was found in the highest percentage in the bladder and lung. Inorganic arsenic was predominantly observed in the kidney. Compared to blood and other tissues, the level of arsenic was comparatively lower in blood. Monomethylarsonate preferentially accumulated in the kidney, whereas iAs and dimethylarsonate accumulated in the bladder.

Many studies evidenced the ability of arsenic to cross the placental barrier. In one report, a similar concentration of arsenic was detected in cord blood of fetus and mother (Concha *et al.*, 1998). All forms of arsenic can cross the human placental barrier at all stages of the gestational period and like other organs, As^{3+} has the highest toxic effects followed by MMA^{III}, while MMA^{V} and DMA^{V} do not exert significant effects on human hematopoietic progenitor cells. The marmoset monkey, known for its inability to methylate arsenic, had somewhat less placental transfer after administration of arsenite than mice (Rodriguez *et al.*, 2003). These findings suggest that methylation plays a pivotal role in developmental and/or reproductive toxic effects of arsenic.

Metabolism

Exposures to xenobiotics including arsenic have serious health hazards to humans. The human body has defensive mechanisms to fight against such toxic substances. The metabolism of arsenic is the process of detoxification in which inorganic arsenic is converted into its methylated form and finally excreted from the body. Arsenic metabolism is characterized by two main steps, i.e. (1) reduction reaction of pentavalent to trivalent arsenic and (2) oxidative methylation reaction. To date, two possible metabolic pathways of inorganic arsenic methylation have been proposed: reduction and oxidative methylation. Biomethylation is the main mechanism for the metabolism of inorganic arsenic in which trivalent forms of arsenic are sequentially methylated to form mono-, di- and trimethylated products using SAM as the methyl donor and glutathione (GSH) as an essential cofactor. This involves alternate steps of two-electron reduction followed by oxidative addition of a methyl group (Thomas *et al.*, 2007).

There are various environmental factors that affect arsenic metabolism/methylation, for example dose concentration, age, gender, health status, etc. Methylation capacity might reduce with increasing dosage of arsenic exposure. The level of estrogen in women also plays a key role in arsenic methylation. Estrogen can enhance the *de novo* synthesis of choline via phosphatidylethanolamine methyltransferase upregulation (Fischer *et al.*, 2007). The elevated choline oxidized to betaine which can donate its methyl group to homocysteine to form methionine, which is catalyzed by betaine–homocysteine methyltransferase. This provides an alternative pathway for re-methylation of homocysteine to methionine (Li *et al.*, 2008).

Rats are known to retain arsenic as the red blood cells have high affinity for arsenic, particularly DMA. The whole body retention of inorganic arsenic in rats is known to be 20 times higher than in mice. In spite of the arsenic accumulation in rat erythrocyte, arsenic distributes to other tissue including the fetus.

Mechanism of action

Mechanism for placental transfer

Although many studies report the ability of arsenic and its organic metabolites to cross the placental barrier, the literature about the detailed mechanism of its transportation is scant (Vahter, 2009). Aquaglyceroporins is the group of transport proteins that transports water and other small molecules like urea, glycerol, nitrate, etc. Aquaglyceroporin (AQP7 and AQP9) have been identified as a transporter of inorganic and methylated arsenic and have been mainly found in various tissues like testes, kidneys, adipose tissues, heart, etc. The absence of these aquaglyceroporins in the placental as well as blood–brain barrier raised the question concerning their role in arsenic transportation from mother to fetus. However, some studies suggest the presence of AQP9 in the placenta (Damiano *et al.*, 2006) and hence may have a possible role in arsenic transportation. Another transporter, i.e. glucose transporter 1 (GLUT-1), has also been reported to transport arsenic in various tissues like liver, brain, etc. Since this transporter is also present in the blood–brain barrier as well as placental barrier, it may also provide the transportation facility to arsenic to cross the placental barrier (Liu *et al.*, 2006). In addition, GLUT4 catalyzes the transport of As^{3+} as well as MMA (Vahter, 2009). In contrast to As^{3+}, As^{5+} transfers through the phosphate transporter by virtue of its similarity to the phosphate ion (Rosen and Liu, 2009). Although the role of the above transporters in catalyzing arsenic transportation is well known, sufficient data for placental transport are missing and detailed studies are needed.

Oxidative stress

Another important mechanism for arsenic-induced toxicity is the generation of free radicals which results in oxidative stress in the target organs including reproductive organs and developmental system (Massrieh *et al.*, 2006; He *et al.*, 2007, 2009; Prasenjit *et al.*, 2008). The generation of oxidative stress in arsenic toxicity may be due to (1) the excess free radical formation, (2) inhibition of antioxidant enzymes, (3) autooxidation of accumulated δ-aminolevulinic acid, and (4) enhanced inflammatory response (Fry *et al.*, 2007; Flora *et al.*, 2008, 2009). However, detailed studies are still required to reveal the exact mechanism. Oxidation of As^{3+} to As^{5+} causes the formation of H_2O_2, while disturbance in oxidative phosphorylation by arsenic leads to the formation of superoxide radicals. Other free radicals like singlet oxygen ($^1O_2$), the peroxyl radical (ROO•), nitric oxide (NO•), dimethylarsinic peroxyl radicals ($[(CH_3)_2AsOO\bullet]$) and dimethylarsinic radical $[(CH_3)_2As\bullet]$ have been reported to play an important role in arsenic toxicity (Valko *et al.*, 2006) (Figure 33.1). As stated earlier, DMA is mainly found in fetus, but also plays a crucial role in free radical generation. DMA can react with molecular oxygen and form dimethyl arsenic radicals ($(CH_3)_2As\bullet$) and superoxide anion ($O_2\bullet^-$). This dimethyl

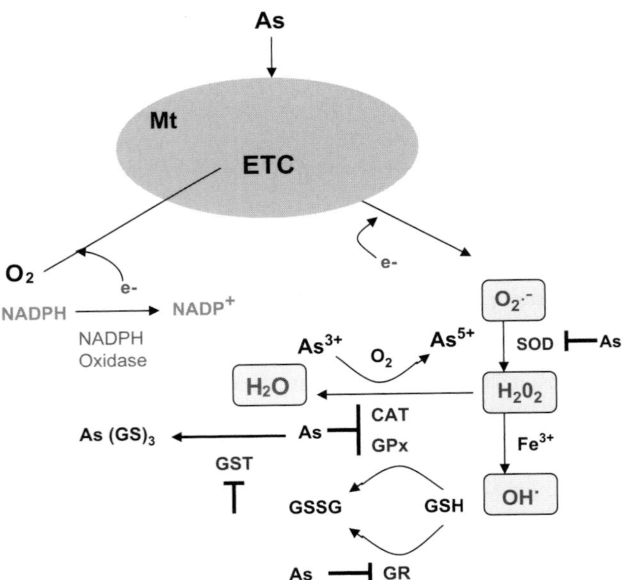

FIGURE 33.1 Arsenic-induced free radical generation and effects on cellular antioxidant defense system. Abbreviations: As^{3+} and As^{5+}: trivalent and pentavalent arsenic; Mt: mitochondria; ETC: electron transport chain; NAPDH and NADP: nicotinamide adenine dinucleotide phosphate reduced and oxidized; SOD: superoxide dismutase; CAT: catalase; GPx: glutathione peroxidase; GST: glutathione-S-transferase; GR: glutathione reductase; GSH and GSSG: reduced and oxidized glutathione; $O_2\bullet^-$: superoxide free radical; H_2O_2: hydrogen peroxide, HO•: hydroxyl radical.

arsenic radical can again react with another oxygen molecule and form dimethyl arsenic peroxyl radicals ($(CH_3)_2AsOO\bullet$) (Kitchin and Ahmed, 2003).

To combat these free radicals, the human body has an antioxidant defense mechanism. Superoxide dismutase (SOD), catalse (CAT), glutathione peroxidase (GPx), glutathione reductase (GR), glutathione-S-transferase (GST) and thioredoxine reductase (TRx) are the important members of this system. Arsenic exposure can alter the activities of these antioxidant enzymes and enhance deleterious effects on free radicals.

Arsenic-induced free radicals result in the oxidation of lipid, protein, DNA and other important biomolecules. Unlike normal somatic cells, sperm cells are abundant in phospholipids, polyunsaturated fatty acids and sterol which makes them susceptible to oxidative damage (Sanocka and Kurpisz, 2004). Apart from this increased oxidative stress-mediated apoptosis, DNA damage could also be a reason behind low sperm count in men (Saleh *et al.*, 2003; Wang *et al.*, 2003; Agarwal and Said, 2005). Reactive oxygen species (ROS) not only have effects on the male reproductive system, they also have effects on the female reproductive system in terms of disturbance in implantation and fertilization of eggs, female infertility and unregulated synthesis of female sex hormones (Agarwal *et al.*, 2005). Although arsenic-induced oxidative stress and the detrimental effects of oxidative stress on male and female reproductive and developmental system are being reported, very few of these suggest the role of arsenic-induced oxidative stress on reproductive and developmental toxicity. Thus it can be hypothesized that generation of oxidative stress in arsenic toxicity is one of the main culprits behind the abnormalities in the above-mentioned organs.

Direct binding with thiol group

Apart from the generation of reactive oxygen species, the direct binding ability of arsenic due to its electrophillic nature helps it to bind with electron-rich -SH groups of proteins, providing another mode of action for its toxic effects. These proteins may be functional or structural in nature. Functional proteins like -SH rich enzymes are inhibited by arsenic, causing malfunctioning in the normal metabolism. Similarly, structural proteins like sperm flagellum and chromatin which are rich in -SH are also highly susceptible to arsenic (Working *et al.*, 1985). Many antioxidants as well as metabolic enzymes with a free sulfhydryl group at their active site are ubiquitous in almost all tissues, which could explain the systemic toxic effects of arsenic as well as its ability to generate oxidative stress (Flora *et al.*, 2008). In contrast to As^{3+}, pentavalent arsenic mimics the phosphate group and hence exerts toxicity during the ATP synthesis process.

Other mechanisms

Arsenic also exerts its toxic effects to the developing fetus by inhibiting enzymes like thioredoxine reductase, methyltransferases and enzymes of the DNA repair mechanism, disturbing the homeostasis of neurotransmitters and hormone secretion, etc. For example, biogenic amines regulate the release of hormones that control spermatogenesis in the male and oogenesis in the female. Arsenic-induced altered

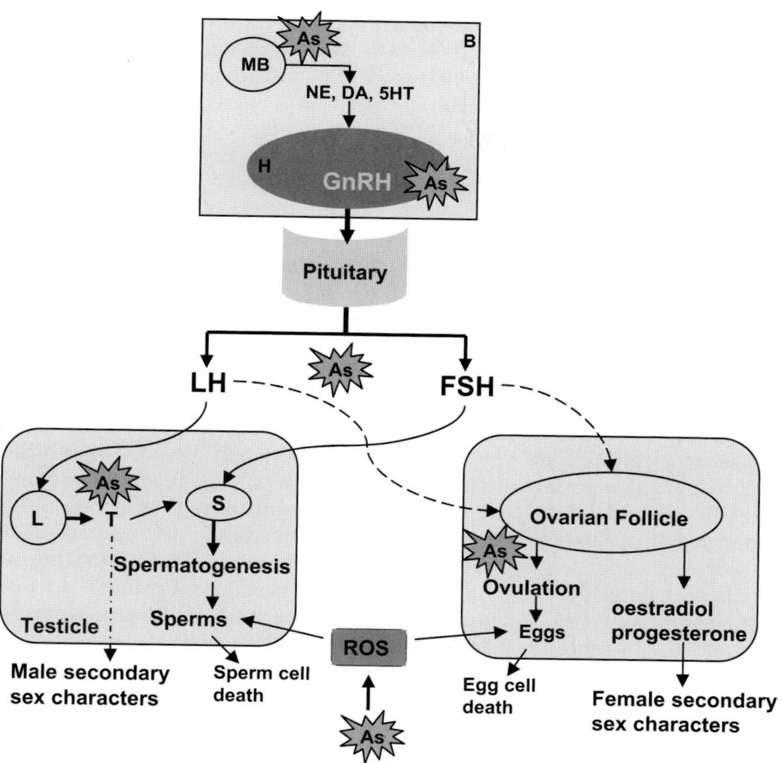

FIGURE 33.2 Possible target site of arsenic on male and female reproductive systems. Abbreviations: As: arsenic; B: brain; MB: midbrain; H: hypothalamus; NE: norepinephrin; DA: dopamine; 5HT: 5-hydroxytryptamine; GnRH: gonadotropic releasing hormone; LH: Luteinizing hormone; FSH: follicular stimulating hormone; L: Leydig cell; T: testesterone; S: Sertoli cell.

synthesis of these biogenic amines may impair the male and female reproductive functions (Jana *et al.*, 2006). Moreover, numerous studies have reported alteration in gene expression patterns of genes involved in reproductive cell formation, reproductive function and synthesis of male and female reproductive hormones. A recent study (Flora and Mehta, 2009) also reported altered gene expression of gene markers of development and differentiation of all germ layers during embryogenesis.

Toxicity

There have been some controversial reports of arsenic-induced reproductive toxicity. While few initial studies concluded the absence of any reproductive malfunctioning, others including a few recent studies have clearly suggested arsenic as a potent reproductive toxicant. In contrast to other organs, animal as well as human data for arsenic-induced reproductive toxicity are still scant. Since arsenic is one of the toxic compounds that can readily cross any barrier like the placental barrier and blood–brain barrier and exerts its toxic effects via various deleterious mechanisms, the toxic effects of arsenic on the reproductive system can be expected. In addition, the growing literature concerning arsenic-induced reproductive and developmental toxicity strongly suggests the multiple organ toxicity of arsenic.

Male reproductive toxicity

Arsenic-induced male reproductive toxicity, including low sperm count, high ROS in testes, abnormal hormonal secretion, male infertility, etc. in various experimental models, has been reported (Chang *et al.*, 2007; Klomberg *et al.*, 2002; Sarkar *et al.*, 2003; Uckun *et al.*, 2002). Male reproductive toxicity following chronic arsenic exposure may be evident by a decrease in absolute testicular weight, decreased sperm count and mortality and abnormal activities of enzymes markers for testicular function, postmeiotic spermatogenesis like sorbitol dehydrogenase (SDH), lactate dehydrogenase (LDH), acid phosphatase (ACP), γ-glutamyltranspeptidase (γ-GT), etc. (Pant *et al.*, 2004). Gonadotropin-releasing hormone secreted by the anterior lobe of the pituitary gland regulates the synthesis of two important gonadotropin hormones, i.e. luteinizing hormone (LH) and follicular stimulating hormone (FSH). Arsenic is reported to cause low plasma levels of these hormones. Although the exact mechanism is still not clear, a few mechanisms such as (1) high corticosterone secretion, (2) altered biogenic amine synthesis, and (3) oxidative stress have been hypothesized (Jana *et al.*, 2006). Since both these hormones play an important role in male hormone testosterone synthesis and spermatogenesis, the decreased levels of these hormones result in low sperm count and male infertility. Arsenic-induced altered variables indicative of oxidative stress like GSH depletion, increased MDA levels and protein carbonyl contents in testes could be another mechanism behind low sperm count (Chang *et al.*, 2007). Apart from targeting polyunsaturated lipid content and -SH groups in sperm, arsenic also targets the testicular enzymes 3β-hydroxysteroid dehydrogenase (3β-HSD) and 17β-HSD that plays an important role in testosterone biosynthesis (Jana *et al.*, 2006). The unaltered activities of these enzymes at transcriptional levels with significant increase in protein carbonyl content again strongly suggest the role of arsenic-induced oxidative stress in male infertility (Chang *et al.*, 2007). Recently ultrastructural analyses of rabbit spermatozoa revealed three types of damage to sperm head membranes in relation to the metal used: acrosome breakage with formation of various sized micro vesicles (arsenic, cadmium, mercury and platinum); a large round hole (arsenic, cadmium and chromium) and numerous folds in the acrosome membrane (vanadium). The data led to the conclusion that arsenic may reduce the sperm motility and probably fertilizing capacity by triggering specific morphological damage to the sperm head (Castellini *et al.*, 2009) (Figure 33.2).

Female reproductive toxicity

Arsenic-induced toxicity to the female reproductive system includes suppression in ovarian steridogenesis, prolonged diestrus, degeneration in cells associated with the female reproductive system (ovarian, follicular and uterine cells), increase in meiotic aberrations in oocytes, and decrease in cleavage and implantation development (Navarro *et al.*, 2004; Wang *et al.*, 2006). Altered neurotransmitter levels like norepinephrin, dopamine and serotonin are also related to arsenic exposure (Tripathi *et al.*, 1997). The abnormal secretion in these neurotransmitters in brain regions could lower gonadotropin secretion that leads to altered levels of gonadotropin hormone secretion. Hypersecretion of serotonin and hyposecretion of norepinephrin levels following arsenic exposure is reported to cause altered gonadotropin signaling while increased secretion of dopamine is associated with arsenic-induced ovarian follicular and uterine cell degeneration (Chattopadhyay *et al.*, 2003). Like the male reproduction system, arsenic exposure to female rats causes decreased plasma levels in LH, FSH and estradiol (Chattopadhyay *et al.*, 2001). In females, gonadotropin hormones play a key role in oogenesis, maturation, ovulation of ovarian follicles and development of the corpus luteum. Low gonadotropin levels could in turn decrease activities of ovarian Δ^5-3β-HSD and 17β-HSD, two important regulatory enzymes for steroidogenesis. Arsenic-induced consistent diestrus can be explained by decreased plasma estradiol level. Apart from this, estradiol has a key role in the regulation of estrous cycles and development of the female reproductive system, and therefore is also called the "hormone of feminine". Thus, following exposure, arsenic disturbs the normal homeostasis of neurotransmitter and hormonal secretion associated with female reproductive function. Although neurotransmitter-dependent altered gonadotropin synthesis is one of the reasons for female reproductive toxicity, the role of oxidative stress could not be ruled out. As discussed above, arsenic is known to cause free radicals elevation which results in uterian cell degeneration (Wang *et al.*, 2006). Arsenic also causes structural damage to the female reproductive organ, evident from the cuboidal-shaped uterine epithelium, dense and irregular-shaped endometrial stroma, loosening of myometrium cell and decreased endometrium thickness. Further, dose-dependent decreases in the level of estradiol and gonadotropin hormone levels were also noted (Akram *et al.*, 2009).

Based upon various reports on arsenic-induced male and female reproductive toxicity, it can be concluded that arsenic has an almost common action on both organs accompanied by altered neurotransmitter secretion, altered gonadotropin levels, increased ROS levels, etc. (Figure 33.2). Based on altered gonadotropin synthesis and the glycoprotein nature of these hormones, it can be hypothesized that (1) arsenic-induced free radicals may participate in oxidative protein damage in the protein part of the gonadotropin hormone and (2) there is arsenic-induced alteration in glycosylation of these hormones. Both of these hypotheses have not yet been proved, thus detailed research could clear the picture about arsenic's mechanism of toxicity.

Developmental toxicity

In contrast to toxic effects on the reproductive system, the effect of arsenic during development of the fetus is widely studied. The placenta is the important structure that transports nutrition from mother to fetus. The presence of arsenic in the placenta showed that it interferes with the nutritional transport that may lead to malnutrition in the developing fetus. In addition, due to arsenic's ability to generate free radicals, it could destroy the placental membrane thus interfering with the communication between the mother and the developing embryo (Massrieh *et al.*, 2006). Thioredoxine reductase is one of the important antioxidant enzymes in the placenta that is inhibited by arsenic, reducing the antioxidant defense system in the placenta (Lu *et al.*, 2007). Blocking of arsenic methylation through peroxidate oxidized adenosine (PAD) significantly increases the toxic effects in terms of mortality of mated male/female mice, litter mortality, litter weight, gross and skeletal effects as compared to arsenic alone (Lammon *et al.*, 2003). Further dietary constituents, especially a protein-rich diet, have the ability to detoxify arsenic exposure directly by interfering in its methylation property or indirectly by enhancing the antioxidant defense system. Based upon this hypothesis, rats exposed to arsenic either alone or with a diet containing different concentrations of protein showed decreased toxic effect with increasing protein concentrations (Lammon and Hood, 2004). In another report, DMA^{III} administration caused significant reduction in litter size and placental weight, while the results were non-significant in DMA^{V} and MMA administration (Irvine *et al.*, 2006). The methylation is also known to play a critical role in arsenic-induced developmental toxicity.

Anemia is one of the common problems which occur in pregnant women and also one of the common causes of fetal and/or mother mortality. Arsenic binds with free thiol groups of the active site of enzyme δ-aminolevulinic acid dehydrogenase (ALAD) which takes part in hemoglobin biosynthesis. The inhibition of this enzyme in arsenic exposure may also increase the vulnerability of pregnant women to anemic conditions (Vahter, 2009). Fetal death and/or other structural malformations are common parameters to assess arsenic-induced developmental toxicity and hence the data regarding this are comparatively easily available. Most of the epidemiological studies in the arsenic-contaminated zone have suggested increased fetal death, fetal structure deformation and increased cases of anemia due to arsenic exposure. Abortions after exposure to arsenic have been reported from the USA (Aschengrau *et al.*, 1989), Hungary (Borzsonyi *et al.*, 1992), north Chile (Hopenhayn-Rich *et al.*, 2000) and Indo-Bangladesh regions (Cherry *et al.*, 2008). These studies clearly indicate and suggest that women from these arsenic-contaminated areas are at risk and need to take necessary precautions during pregnancy.

Unlike earlier data, the exploitation of molecular techniques has made the data about arsenic-induced developmental toxicity more sensitive and reliable. For example, recent studies report the altered gene expression related to (1) oxidant antioxidant homeostasis in the embryo, (2) early and late development stages, apoptosis, inflammation, etc., and (3) estrogen-mediated gene expression. Trophoblast migration is the important event that occurs during placenta formation. Arsenic is reported to block the migration of these cells either by decreasing the expression of the gene of the intracellular protein tyrosine kinase and related genes (Yancy *et al.*, 2005) or by some unknown mechanism (Li and Loch-Caruso, 2007). Fetal exposure to arsenic can enhance the chances of diethylstilbestrol (DES)-induced tumor formation. Gene expression analysis related to estrogen signaling (*ER-α*, *Tff3* and *Agr2* expression), steroid metabolism (*Cyp2a4* and *HSD17β5*) and methionine metabolism (*Bhmt* and *Temt*) in the neonatal adrenal gland could reveal the possible mechanism of action (Liu *et al.*, 2009). The study conducted in Bangkok and arsenic-affected regions in Thailand concludes the impact of prenatal exposure to arsenic on gene expression in newborns. A total of 11 transcripts were mostly affected by arsenic exposure and thus identified as probable biomarkers for prenatal arsenic exposure in newborns. However, these transcripts were markers of inflammation, carcinogenesis, apoptosis, metal exposure, etc. rather than specific arsenic exposure (Fry *et al.*, 2007). Recently Flora and Mehta (2009) studied the expression of about 47 genes, markers for embryonic cell development, its differentiation, apoptosis and cell cycle in human embryonic stem cell-derived embryoid bodies. Arsenic treatment significantly downregulated most of the genes studied: pluripotency (*POU5F1, NANOG, TDGF1*), ectoderm (*NES, NEFH, TUBB3, KRT*), mesoderm (*T, MSX1, ACTC1, CADMIUM34*) and endoderm (*AFP, FOXA2, GATA4* and *ALB*). Apart from affecting the germ layers, a significant decrease in expression was observed for genes of cell cycle (*CCND1, CCRK*) and increased expression of *BAX* and *CASP3* (apoptotic markers). These developmental effects were also validated through *in vivo* study where significant reduction in litter size with increased incidence of visceral and skeletal defects were observed following arsenic exposure.

CADMIUM

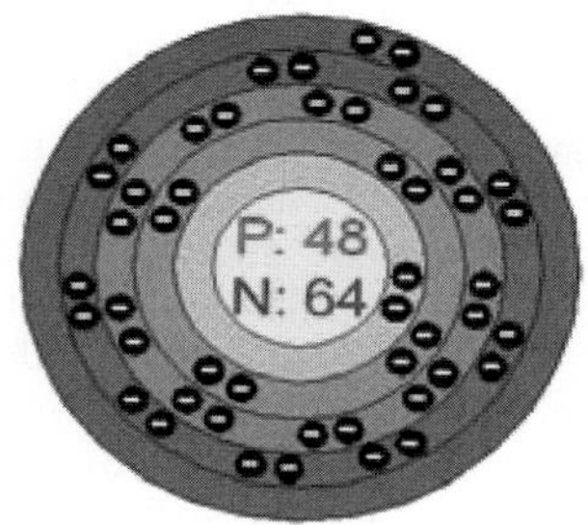

Name:	Cadmium
Symbol:	Cd
Atomic number:	48
Atomic mass:	112.411 amu
Melting point:	320.9°C (594.05 K, 609.62°F)
Boiling point:	765.0°C (1,038.15 K, 1,409.0°F)
Number of protons/ electrons:	48
Number of neutrons:	64
Crystal structure:	Hexagonal
Density @ 293 K:	8.65 g/cm^3
Color:	Silvery
Electronic configuration:	[KR] 5s2 4d10
Shell structure:	2.8.18.18.2
Oxidation states:	2, 1

Introduction

Cadmium occurs naturally in the environment at low levels, usually with zinc, lead and copper ore deposits. It is one of the most toxic industrial and environmental heavy metals because of its long half-life and multifaceted deleterious effects (Domingo, 1994). High cadmium concentrations are often associated with industrial emission sources like mining and smelting operations. Major industrial uses of cadmium are in electroplating, pigments and, particularly, plastics, plastic stabilizers and Ni–Cd rechargeable batteries (Figure 33.3). Manifestations of chronic exposure to cadmium include teratogenic, carcinogenic, hepatotoxic and nephrotoxic effects. Cadmium has a biological half-life of 15–30 years, mainly due to its low rate of excretion from the body, and accumulates over time in the blood, kidneys and liver as well as in the reproductive organs, including the placenta, testes and ovaries.

Historical background

Macroscopic and microscopic changes as an effect of cadmium intoxication in reproductive tissue were first reported nearly a century ago along with testicular necrosis in rats on cadmium injection. Fetal mortality and necrosis of placenta within 24 hours was also demonstrated on maternal administration of cadmium during late gestation. Testicular damage due to cadmium consisted of degeneration of the seminal tubules, interstitial hyperemia and edema with congestion of blood vessels as well as formation of a tumor of the Leydig cell whereas cadmium injection in female rats led to ovarian changes. Cadmium is also embryotoxic and teratogenic in different animal species. Although not much was reported regarding human exposure to cadmium its toxicity is known to occur in humans and since cadmium crosses the human placenta it is retained by the fetus.

Toxicokinetics

Once absorbed, cadmium is rapidly cleared from the blood and concentrates in various tissues especially in the liver and kidneys, causing many metabolic and histological changes, membrane damage and apoptosis. After exposure and uptake into the systemic circulation, cadmium is initially bound to albumin in blood plasma followed by its uptake in blood cells. Cadmium in blood cells is bound partly to a high molecular weight protein and partly to a protein with the same molecular weight as metallothionein. Albumin bound cadmium in plasma is then transported to the liver where the complex undergoes degradation with the release of cadmium, which in turn induces the synthesis of metallothionein (MT). Cadmium-induced MT (Cd-MT) then binds with it and transports the metal to the kidneys for excretion. Cd-MT complex is absorbed by the renal tubules by endocytosis that

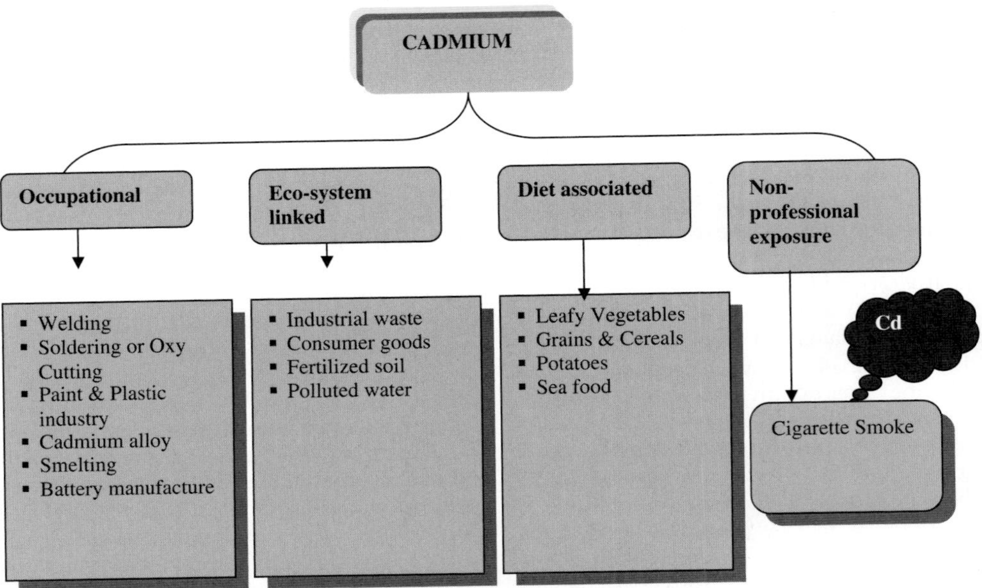

FIGURE 33.3 Various sources of cadmium exposure.

is mediated by ZIP8 transporter, followed by the release of cadmium from MT in the lysosomes of the tubular cells. In humans the half-life of cadmium in kidney is estimated to be 10–40 years. The excretion rate of cadmium in daily urine being very low aids the higher accumulation of cadmium in kidneys following chronic exposure.

It is well known that placentas from smoking mothers have increased pathology and MT induction compared with placentas from non-smoking mothers. It has further been proved that cadmium produced specific toxic responses in 5–8 hours in human placenta under perfusion conditions *in vitro* (Miller *et al.*, 1992). These results were similar in rodents. Moreover, the placenta is reported to accumulate more cadmium than kidneys, although the mechanism was not clear. Furthermore, pregnant and lactating female animals absorb and retain substantially more dietary cadmium than their non-pregnant counterparts (Floris *et al.*, 2000).

Mechanism of action

Interaction of cadmium is particularly strong and has biological implications with polythiol groups. It can form covalent bonding with -SH groups of protein and depletion of cells from major sulfhydryl reserves seems to be an important mechanism of its toxicity. Apart from the -SH groups, cadmium has high affinity for phosphates, cysteinyl and histidyl side chains of proteins, purines, pteridines and porphyrins and thus can non-specifically bind to numerous biological molecules.

The mechanism of cadmium toxicity is believed to involve competition with zinc for divalent cationic sites in metalloenzymes. The occurrence of interactions between cadmium and zinc during pregnancy is very well established. It has been observed that Zn^{2+} antagonizes the action of Cd^{2+} and a high Cd^{2+}/Zn^{2+} ratio is needed for toxicity. Some studies have suggested that the toxic effects of cadmium may be mediated by altered metabolism of zinc (Zn) and copper (Cu). Adequate availability of Zn is essential for normal growth and development. Insufficient Zn or Cu availability in fetal or early postnatal life is teratogenic, retards growth and alters cognitive function. Fetal or neonatal Cu deficiency is also teratogenic, reduces brain catecholamine levels and decreases myelination in the central nervous system. Gestational exposure to oral cadmium levels of >50 ppm in the drinking water results in decreased Zn and Cu levels in the fetal liver, brain, kidney and intestine, as well as in the entire body, and in these tissues of neonates and adult offspring. Cadmium also uses the transport pathways utilized by biologically essential metals like calcium, copper and zinc (Fotakis and Timbrell, 2006) and hence can cause the death of cells via the disruption of important pathways such as the electron transport chain.

Cadmium is an important activator of macrophages, which leads to the secretion of various intracellular mediators and cytokines such as nitric oxide, tumor necrosis factor alpha (TNF-α), interleukin 1 (IL-1), interleukin 6 (IL-6), catalase and other vasoactive amines which are chemotactic (Rikans and Yamano, 2000). Moreover, cadmium can reportedly induce lysosomal, DNA and other cellular damage leading to cell death in hepatoma cell lines (Fotakis *et al.*, 2005). DNA damage induced by cadmium might be due to the formation of reactive oxygen species. Oocyte death was reported to occur preferentially during meiosis-I (Zenzes, 2000). Cellular functions are also affected by cadmium via perturbing signal transductions, such as protein kinase C, mitogen-activated protein kinase and cyclic AMP pathways (Satoh *et al.*, 2003). Exposure to cadmium at relatively high and low levels caused necrosis and apoptosis, respectively, which suggested that the mode of cell death by cadmium was dependent on the exposure level (Satoh *et al.*, 2003).

Metallothioneins (MTs) are members of a family of low molecular weight proteins rich in cysteine that bind with high affinity to cadmium. In rodents, MT-I/II has been localized to spermatogenic and Sertoli cells as well as in interstitial cells. MT-III has also been detected in the testes of humans and rodents. In rats, maternal cadmium exposure produces a decrease in fetal hepatic MT levels with a concomitant

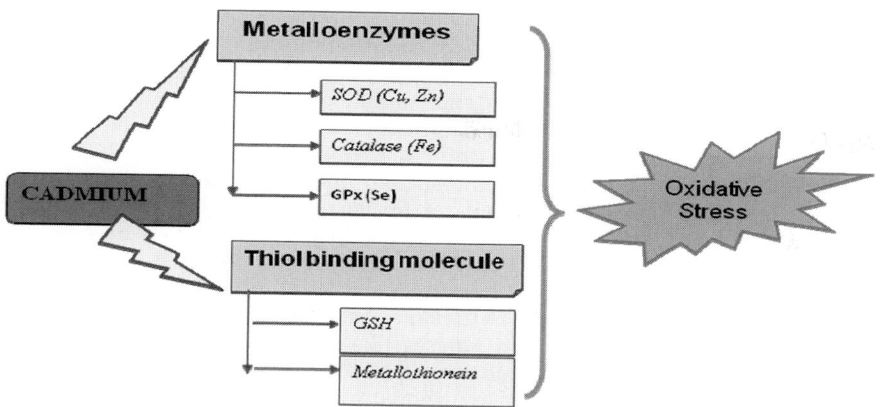

FIGURE 33.4 Mechanism of cadmium-induced oxidative stress.

decrease in Zn concentration. On the other hand, the level of hepatic Zn increases in the rabbit fetus following maternal cadmium exposure, with a concomitant increase in MT. Thus, additional MT not only retains cadmium in the placenta to protect the fetus, but also may affect fetus placental Zn dynamics, which in turn may lead to reduced Zn bioavailability to the fetus and thus contribute to weight impairment.

Oxidative stress

Cadmium may cause prolonged generation of reactive oxygen species which has been proposed to promote necrosis. Oxidative stress is a common factor in about half of the infertile men examined to date, illustrating the importance of cadmium as an inducer of oxidative stress (Tremellen, 2008).

Cadmium is a non-redox metal that adopts a single oxidation state and hence was thought not to be a strong inducer of reactive oxygen species. However, cadmium is known to induce the production of nitric oxide (NO) and hydroxyl radicals (OH•), superoxide anions radicals (O_2•$^-$) and hydrogen peroxide (H_2O_2). It also has the ability to impair the antioxidant defense system when in appreciable levels in the organism. Qanungo and Murherjea (2000) suggested that the placenta is one of the main sources of ROS as it is highly rich in mitochondria. Placental oxidant–antioxidant imbalance may cause the release of lipo-peroxidation products into the circulation with subsequent damage of endothelial cell membranes in several pathological conditions in pregnancy like pre-eclampsia, pregnancy-induced diabetes and hypertension.

Essential metal homeostasis should be also crucial for the development of the fetus–placental unit due to its pleiotropic key role as a cofactor in several enzyme systems. Se and Cu/Zn-dependent enzymes, glutathione peroxidase (GPx) and superoxide dismutase (SOD) constitute one of the main defense mechanisms against effects of ROS. These enzymes may be inhibited by several heavy metals including cadmium (Flora *et al.*, 2008). Therefore, the presence of heavy metals in the placenta may be detrimental for placental GPx and SOD activities and as a result the fetus is subjected to some degree of oxidative stress, which may result in potential damage.

Cadmium is reported to effect acetylcholine release at the neuromuscular junction of frogs and inhibited the activity of some enzymes in the brain. It has been generally accepted that metals deactivate ChEs by binding to their anionic site, thus preventing acetylcholine from binding to ChE and degradation. Perinatal exposure to low doses of lead and cadmium can produce alterations in lipid peroxidation and ultrastructure of rat brain. Important observations included mitochondrial swelling, disruption and partial or total loss of cristae, Nissl body dissolution, degenerated organelles and vacuoles, cytomembrane disappearance and nuclear chromoplasm concentration on cadmium exposure. A general decrease in the activity of SOD, CAT, GPx and AChE and an increase in MDA levels following heavy metal treatment were also observed, demonstrating that cadmium can impair the function and ultrastructure of the central nervous system by producing oxidative stress (Zhang *et al.*, 2009). Increased lipid peroxide (LPO) levels after cadmium administration in liver, kidney, testes and blood of rats has been implicated in cadmium-induced organ damage and dysfunction (Casalino *et al.*, 2002) (Figure 33.4).

The basis of cadmium toxicity is its negative influence on enzymatic systems of cells, resulting from its substitution for divalent mineral elements (Zn^{2+}, Cu^{2+} and Mn^{2+}) in metalloenzymes and its very strong affinity to biological structures containing -SH groups, such as proteins, enzymes and nucleic acids. Thus, decreased SOD activity may imply reduced H_2O_2 production followed by consequent catalase activity decrease, which catalyzes the conversion of H_2O_2 to H_2O and molecular oxygen. It is well known that activity of catalase is directly proportional to the substrate level assumed to be produced by SOD. Cadmium-induced reduction in testicular catalase activity may reflect reduced capacity of testicular mitochondria and microsomes to eliminate H_2O_2 in response to cadmium.

Cadmium binds to cysteine in reduced glutathione (GSH) resulting in the inactivation of GPx, which, therefore, fails to metabolize H_2O_2 to water. There is increasing evidence that cadmium interacts with Se and disrupts GPx activity. In addition, the GSH redox cycle, which includes GSH, GPx and GR, plays an important role in the detoxification of ROS that are generated by cadmium, to protect cells from potential toxicity and carcinogenesis. GSH functions as a direct free radical scavenger, a co-substrate for GPx activity and a co-factor for many enzymes and forms conjugated in endo and xenobiotics reactions (Flora *et al.*, 2009). It is known that the level of free GSH decreases in tissues exposed to cadmium, due to complex formation between cadmium and GSH (cadmium-GS) via a reaction catalyzed by GST (Casalino *et al.*, 2004).

Alternatively, cadmium may alter the protein conformation by interacting with the enzyme, thereby altering its functional activity.

Toxicity

Cadmium is an extremely toxic element. In men, chronic or acute intoxication may lead to critical effects on lung, kidney or bones. This metal is also carcinogenic and is deleterious to the reproductive process, causing retardation of growth, sterility and embryotoxic effects. In cases of humans, exposure to cadmium is often mixed with other entities like cigarette smoke and pollutions from refineries and fossil fuel generators. During pregnancy, exposure to cadmium has been associated with increased incidence of preterm delivery, low birth weight and inhibited IQ development in the postnatal period (Llanos and Ronco, 2009; Tian *et al.*, 2009). A high concentration of placental cadmium has been reported with tobacco usage in pregnant females (Kippler *et al.*, 2010) that has led to detrimental effects on fetal growth and a reduced level of umbilical cord leptin (Röllin *et al.*, 2009). Although no subsequent reports have directly linked declines in leptin with smoking during pregnancy, others have reported definite decreases in peripheral leptin concentrations among mice, men (Stasenko *et al.*, 2009) and non-pregnant women (Jauniaux and Burton, 2007) exposed to tobacco smoke. It has been demonstrated that newborns delivered from mothers who smoked during pregnancy had reduced birth weight, compared to nonsmokers, which was highly correlated with placental levels of cadmium. Tobacco smoke, which is a chief source of cadmium, has been shown to affect neuro-endocrine functions, hypothalamic–pituitary axis, thyroid gland function, adrenal cortical hormone concentrations, glucose regulating hormonal function of pancreas, gastric emptying and bone mass, as well as gonadal and reproductive functions in females, with less dramatic effects in males (Piasek *et al.*, 2001). Although, there are scant reports relating to the testicular function in men exposed to cadmium, Kim and Soh (2009) reported high tissue cadmium levels and some histological changes in testicular autopsy samples from men who had suffered severe cadmium fume poisoning, while Mason (1990) observed reduced sperm production and male infertility in subjects exposed to cadmium.

Male reproductive toxicity

Testicular changes due to cadmium toxicity have been seen in a variety of animal models at different stages of growth and maturity. Cadmium-induced testicular pathogenicity includes severe hemorrhage, edema, necrosis and atrophy, as well as reduction in counts and motility of sperm and decreases in the testosterone concentrations in plasma and testes.

Mammalian testis, due to its unique vascular system, has been postulated to be more susceptible to cadmium (Prozialeck *et al.*, 2008). Apart from high vasculature, genetic factors also make it a major target to cadmium. Recent studies suggest that mice lacking a single locus named "cadmium", displayed cadmium-resistant testis (De Souza *et al.*, 2010). The cadmium gene was identified as the solute-carrier (Slc)39a8gene, encoding the Zrt-, Irt-like protein (ZIP)8, which is most likely responsible for cadmium testicular sensitivity in mice (He *et al.*, 2009). Another potential gene has recently been identified as Ppp3ca, a catalytic subunit of calcineurin (CN), which is calcium/calmodulin-dependent Ser/Thr phosphatase, also known as the isoform of CN (Martin *et al.*, 2002). Ppp3ca was detected in testicular endothelial cells and suggested to be important for spermatogenesis. Cadmium toxicity affecting the blood–testis barrier is regulated by a stress-activated p38MAPK, and inhibition of p38MAPK by SB02190 (inhibitor) could partially block the toxic effects of cadmium (Kusakabe *et al.*, 2008). Apart from p38MAPK, other protein kinases like JNK too are linked with cadmium-induced toxicity (Wong and Cheng, 2005). Numerous reports have shown that cadmium causes disruption of the blood–testis barrier, germ cell loss, testicular edema, hemorrhage and necrosis (Prozialeck *et al.*, 2007; Siu *et al.*, 2009). Cadmium also affects sperm motility activation and movements (Benoff *et al.*, 2009). It is assumed that teleost sperm plasmalemmal structure is highly permeable to metals and thus provides access to metals to bind to flagellum proteins affecting sperm movement symmetry or beat-cross frequency, or bind to enzymes affecting metabolism of the sperm cell. As discussed earlier zinc plays a crucial role in spermatogenesis, sperm motility, antioxidant protection, chromatin condensation and zinc-dependent enzymes and enzymatic activity related to protein phosphorylation. Cadmium, like lead, may compete with zinc and also render its toxic effects on any of the above-mentioned functions.

Female reproductive toxicity

Cadmium is known to adversely affect the maternal–fetal system and the placenta is the primary target where this metal accumulates. Direct cadmium-induced changes include alteration in placental structure, reduction in utero-placental blood flow and congenital developmental abnormalities and ultimately fetal death, whereas indirect effects of accumulated cadmium may alter placental functions such as changes in placental hormone production and transplacental nutrient passage of essential trace elements. These changes, direct or indirect, have unsympathetic impact on human pregnancy and immune processes (Thompson and Bannigan, 2008). Cadmium easily passes the placenta and accumulates in the fetus when administered by intravenous injections.

Exposure to cadmium negatively affected oocyte maturation and caused chromosomal aberrations *in vitro* (Nandi *et al.*, 2010) as well as in hamsters, sheep, cattle and mice *in vivo* (Leoni *et al.*, 2002). Increased embryo lethality and lowered pregnancy rates were not only observed in rats but also *in vitro* exposure of mouse oocytes showed reduced fertilization rates and development to 2-cell stage (Shen *et al.*, 2000). Higher concentrations of cadmium inhibited activity of the P450scc gene, inhibited progesterone synthesis and facilitated changes in cell morphology and cell death. Moreover apart from altering morphology and basic functions of human ovarian granulose cells, cadmium also influences cell–cell contact and the adherence of cells, and consequently can disturb intercellular communication, which in the avascular granulosa layer is a prerequisite for nutrient mediation and signal transmission for the culture period.

Emerging evidence suggests the role of cadmium as an endocrine disruptor in the pituitary (Tsutsumi *et al.*, 2009), ovary (Paksy *et al.*, 1997) and placenta (Lee *et al.*, 2009a). Cadmium accumulates in human placenta with advancing gestation and may disrupt the synthesis and/or release of hormones produced by the trophoblast (Henson and Chedrese, 2004). These hormones include steroids such as progesterone and are necessary for the implantation and maintenance of pregnancy by preserving uterine myometrial quiescence, testosterone and estrogen. Cadmium was shown to inhibit progesterone synthesis in placental tissues presumably through a dose-dependent decline in P450scc and 3β-HSD mRNAs (Kawai *et al.*, 2002). These changes can be induced with very low doses of cadmium that do not cause any morphological changes.

Cadmium has potent estrogen- and androgen-like activities too. It mimics the effects of estrogens by decreasing the level of estrogen receptor (ER) mRNA. Further, it binds with high affinity to hormone-binding domain of estrogen receptor. Cadmium also regulates androgen receptor (AR) gene expression and activity in LNCap cells, a hormone-dependent human prostate cancer cell line, and also mimics androgenic effects in rats and mice. The circadian pattern release of noradrenaline, a regulator of hypothalamus hormone secretion, which resulted in changes in the daily pattern of plasma testosterone and LH levels was also found to be affected by cadmium. In addition, plasma levels of pituitary hormones, e.g. LH, FSH, prolactin and ACTH, were also modified after cadmium exposure.

Lactational transfer of cadmium is an important route of exposure from dams to pups during the lactational period. Although cadmium transfer via the milk has been reported to be low in mice and rats, some studies confirm the importance of lactational transfer of cadmium at low levels (Ishitobi and Watanabe, 2005).

Developmental toxicity

Cadmium has been shown as a developmental toxicant for hamsters, rats, mice and chicks. In rats, hydrocephaly was the most frequent malformation when cadmium was injected i.v. between gestational days 8 and 12, whereas eye defects, gastroschiasis and umbilical hernia were other frequent abnormalities. In hamsters, the type of malformations consisted primarily of craniofacial and limb bud defects. Exposure of pregnant rats with a subcutaneous injection of cadmium at 40 μmol/kg on gestation day 12 resulted in a transient decrease in placental blood flow, while treatment on gestation day 18, with a similar dose of cadmium resulted in 53% fetolethality. Cadmium administration at doses of 40 mg/kg impairs implantation, decreases litter size, produces resorptions and causes fetal or embryonic death. Female offspring that have been exposed *in utero* to cadmium experience an earlier onset of puberty (indicated by earlier vaginal opening) as well as increases in the epithelial area and number of terminal end buds in the mammary glands. It has been shown that just two injections of cadmium at 0.5 μg/kg or 5 μg/kg body weight into dams produce changes in the reproductive organs of the offspring.

The central nervous system of newborn animals is highly susceptible to heavy metals. Cadmium exposure during gestation and early postnatal period may be more toxic to the developing CNS due to lack of functional blood–brain barrier, intense cellular proliferation, differentiation and synaptogenesis. Further, cadmium can disrupt the structural components of the blood–brain barrier by causing injury to endothelial, glial and epithelial cells as well as disrupt the gap junction formations (Virgintino *et al.*, 2004). Apart from this, cadmium also elevates intracellular calcium in neurons and may cause neuronal death (López *et al.*, 2003).

Transplacental transport of cadmium to the fetus appears to be restricted because trophoblasts synthesize metallothionein (MT), which is an important complex protein rich in sulfhydryl groups that binds to cadmium. Cadmium is known to transfer from dams to pups in the first 3 weeks after birth. Cadmium intoxication during pregnancy and lactation has critical effects on the body and brain weights of pups. It may be hypothesized that increased toxic load of cadmium after early developmental exposure (i.e., *in utero* and lactational period) may crush the hepatic bio-transformation enzymes of the F_1 generation in a sex-dependent manner. Further, early developmental exposure to cadmium may alter the sexually dimorphic patterns of hepatic xenobiotic and steroid metabolizing enzyme activities of the F_1 generation in a sex-dependent manner (Pillai *et al.*, 2009).

Studies of occupationally exposed subjects have shown several neurobehavioral effects induced by cadmium, such as lower attention, hypernociception, olfactory dysfunction and memory deficits. Cadmium exposure is also associated with Parkinsonism and amyotrophic lateral sclerosis. At early developmental stage cadmium accumulates primarily at the hypothalamus, and induces alterations on aminergic and aminoacidergic transmitter systems. Cadmium induces several alterations in aspartate, glutamate, glutamine, GABA and taurine levels, and in the daily pattern of hypothalamic amine content (Caride *et al.*, 2009).

In mammals, trophoblast cell differentiation continues throughout embryogenesis along a multilineage pathway and yields several different cell types. During pregnancy several members of the prolactin (PRL)-family of hormones are secreted in rat placental trophoblast, including placental lactogen (PL)-I, -II and -IV, PRL-like protein (PLP)-A, -B, -C, -C-related and -D; and decidual/trophoblast PRL-related protein (d/t PRP). Two morphologically distinct populations of trophoblast cells are seen in the placenta, i.e. trophoblast giant cells and spongiotrophoblast cells, expressing placental PRL-family genes. Placental PRL-family hormones can act as growth promoting agents as they bind growth hormone (GH) or PRL receptors and influence metabolic activities during pregnancy or help in adaptations to physiological stressors, and placental and fetal growth. PL-II has a lactogenic effect on mammary gland growth and directly regulates insulin secretion and β-cell proliferation of maternal islets during the last half of pregnancy in rats. Therefore, it is suggested that cadmium-induced inhibition of PL gene expression leads to the disruption of physiological adaptation and the restriction of placental and fetal growth. Further, E2 and progesterone (P4) are known to stimulate the proliferation of placental trophoblast cells, and exposure to estrogenic chemicals during gestation could impact placental trophoblast cells. A low dose of cadmium (0.2 mg) may significantly reduce the trophoblast cell frequency, placental and fetal weights without the apoptosis or necrosis of placental trophoblast cells induced by a high dose of cadmium (2.0 mg) (Lee *et al.*, 2009b).

Although cadmium has not been studied as extensively as other heavy metals like lead and mercury, it is also an important neurotoxin at developmental stages. Cadmium in general does not cross the placental barrier causing a restricted entry into the fetus when exposure occurs during gestation. Although cadmium was undetected in the brain of offspring exposed during gestation some behavioral alterations have been reported. Entry of cadmium is greatest during neonatal exposure making it the most susceptible to neurotoxic effects of cadmium. Cadmium is known to cause lesions in the sensory ganglia in experimental adult animals. In neonates sensory ganglia are spared and hemorrhagic lesions are found in cerebrum and cerebellum along with caudate-putamen and corpus callosum. During the neonatal stage the blood–brain barrier is still developing and structurally immature capillaries are unable to exclude cadmium from the brain, or entry of cadmium may be facilitated by virtue of physiological and biochemical peculiarities of capillaries related to the metabolic need of rapidly growing brain.

Most of the neuronal damage by cadmium is secondary to vascular insult, i.e. cadmium damages the endothelial cells and choroid plexus. It has also been suggested that cadmium exposure may alter the blood–brain barrier to allow metal gain possibly by depletion of microvessel antioxidants along with lipid peroxidation. Heavy metals are known to cause toxicities by altering essential metal homeostasis. Cadmium can potentially block Ca^{2+}. Cadmium blocks the influx of calcium thereby inhibiting the neurotransmitter release from the synaptic vesicle. This causes a decrease in the end plate potential at the neuromuscular junction. However, at high concentrations (100–500 μM) cadmium solution could increase spontaneous neurotransmitter release. It may be hypothesized that cadmium acts as either a partial blocker and/or an agonist at intracellular sites that normally bind Ca^{2+}. The effect of cadmium on the peripheral nervous system has also been studied. It is reported to suppress adrenergic neurotransmission possibly by inhibiting neurotransmitter release from the presynaptic terminal. However, cadmium shows varied effect with respect to concentration. At concentrations greater than 0.25 μM a similar effect was observed but at low concentrations (0.075–0.25 μM) neurotransmission was enhanced by cadmium. Possibly at low doses of cadmium it inhibits monoamine oxidase and catechol-*o*-methyl transferase enzymes that metabolize catecholamines, thus rendering them available to participate in neurotransmission. Another calcium mimicking mechanism proposed for cadmium toxicity includes dose-dependent inhibition of Ca^{2+}-ATPase activity, interacting with calmodulin, a Ca^{2+} binding protein that regulates several cellular processes. The role of metalloproteins (MT) has also been highlighted in cadmium-induced neurotoxicity. MTs are cysteine-rich proteins that are believed to be involved in homeostasis of essential metals. Cadmium is known to possess high affinity for these proteins that also formulate an important mechanism of detoxifying cadmium by the body. Cadmium levels in the CNS of neonates show negative correlation with expression of MT-III, an MT-isoform that is expressed only in the brain. Moreover, cadmium has been reported to inhibit basal adenylate cyclase activity in homogenates of cerebellum, cerebrum and brain stem, inhibiting methylation of phospholipids in synaptosomal membranes, altering the membrane of phospholipid vesicles, and blocking axonal transport. Finally oxidative stress has also been suggested as an important mechanism responsible for the neurotoxic potential of cadmium.

Human epidemiological studies focusing on the neurotoxic effect of cadmium are rather limited and most have been conducted to identify neurotoxicities of groups of metals and not cadmium alone (Hastings and Miller, 1998).

LEAD

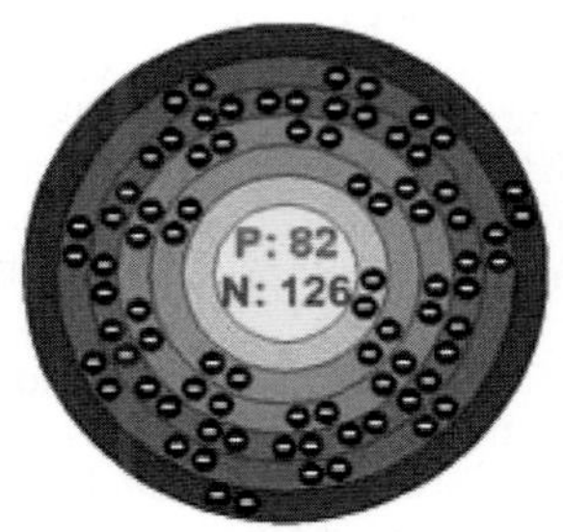

Symbol:	Pb
Atomic number:	82
Atomic mass:	207.2 amu
Melting point:	327.5°C (600.65 K, 621.5°F)
Boiling point:	1740.0°C (2013.15 K, 3164.0°F)
Number of protons/ electrons:	82
Number of neutrons:	125
Crystal structure:	Cubic
Density at 293 K:	11.34 g/cm^3
Color:	Bluish
Electronic configuration:	[Xe].$4f^{14}$.$5d^{10}$.$6s^2$.$6p^2$
Shell structure:	2.8.18.32.18.4
Oxidation states:	2, 4

Introduction

The reproductive toxicity of lead was documented by the Greeks and Romans centuries ago and is known to cause reproductive and developmental toxicity at different levels in an organism. In spite of extensive studies evaluating the pathophysiology of lead toxicity on the reproductive axis, controversy still persists. Whereas the majority of studies suggest that the primary site of lead's toxicity is the central nervous system (CNS), some studies report direct testicular toxicity, and a small number of others question if lead is truly toxic to the reproductive system. This section aims to answer these critical questions.

Lead (Pb), a bluish-gray metal, is distributed in the earth's crust in a large number of minerals. Because of its widespread use over the course of human history, particularly since the advent of the industrial revolution, lead and some of its chemical compounds are nearly ubiquitous in the human environment and can be found in plants, oceans, rivers, drinking water, soil and in various food items. Lead is number 2 on the ATSDR's "top 20 list". Lead accounts for most of the cases of pediatric heavy metal poisoning. It is a very soft metal and was used in pipes, drains and soldering materials for many years. Millions of homes built before 1940 still contain lead (e.g., in painted surfaces), leading to chronic exposure from weathering, flaking, chalking and dust. Every year, industry produces about 2.5 million tons of lead throughout the world. Most of this lead is used for batteries. The remainder is used for cable coverings, plumbing, ammunition and fuel additives. Other uses are as paint pigments and in PVC plastics, X-ray shielding, crystal glass production and pesticides. Target organs are the bones, brain, blood, kidneys and thyroid gland. Lead is now the most widely scattered toxic metal on earth, its toxicity unreduced by the passage of time. Some other equally unsettling facts are as follows:

1. Owing to the short half-life of lead in the blood the period during which lead can be detected in the blood can be far shorter than the duration of its toxic actions in the brain.
2. Once deposited in the brain, lead is eliminated extremely slowly – a brain-half-life of approximately 2 years.
3. Once in the brain, lead cannot be removed by chelation even though BLL have been decreased. It means lead deposited in the brain continues its neurotoxic action. There is still a controversy if the effects of lead on the developing brain eventually are reversed. The disconnection between blood levels of lead (BLL) and brain levels of lead complicates the outcome of treatment.
4. The consequence is that once an elevated blood lead concentration has been detected, it is too late to prevent lead causing brain damage.
5. If we combine all of the above with the recent strong evidence that even very low BLLs can seriously affect brain development and subsequent cognitive function, we are left with a succinct policy conclusion: the only way to prevent fetal and childhood lead poisoning is to prevent lead from ever getting into the bodies of pregnant mothers and their children in the first place.

On the basis of current evidence, Centre for Disease Control (CDC) suggested that blood lead concentrations at or around 10 μg/dL present a public health risk to sensitive populations (such as infants, children and pregnant women [as surrogates for fetuses]). There is growing evidence that even very small exposure to lead can produce subtle effects in humans. Therefore there is the possibility that future guidelines may drop below 10 μg/dL as the mechanisms of lead toxicity become better understood. The adverse effects noted at approximately 10 μg/dL include:

- Impairments of CNS and other organ development in fetuses.
- Impairments in cognitive function and initiation of various behavioral disorders in young children.
- Increases in systolic and diastolic blood pressure in adults including pregnant women.

Lead exerts its toxic effect directly on the developing fetus after gestation begins, and indirectly on paternal or maternal physiology before and during the reproduction process (Ronis *et al.*, 1998). An association between lead exposure and sterility, abortion, stillbirths and neonatal deaths has been established but little evidence is available as to whether subtoxic levels of lead affect fertility or cause fetal injuries in humans. Increase in blood lead reduces semen volume, semen density and counts of total, motile and viable sperm, percentage of progressively motile sperm, levels of zinc, acid phosphatase and citric acid and increase the percentage of pathological sperm (Alexander *et al.*, 1996; Lin *et al.*, 1996). Male reproductive effects may also occur at blood lead levels of 30–40 μg/dL resulting in subclinical suppression of circulating cutinizing and follicle-stimulating hormone and estradiol without overt effects on general health and menstruation.

Abortions, miscarriages and stillbirths have also been reported among women working in lead industries. Prenatal exposure to lead has been associated with toxic effects on the fetus. These include reduced gestational age and birth weight and adversely delayed cognitive development. Significantly, sources of maternal exposure to lead may be current or the result of mobilization from bone stores remaining from previous exposures. Moreover, a significant amount of bone lead is reported to be mobilized, enter the circulation during pregnancy and lactation, and cross the placenta.

Historical background

Lead toxicity has been known for over 2000 years. The early Greeks used lead as a glazing for ceramic pottery and became aware of its harmful effects. Researchers suggest that some Roman emperors became ill, and even died, as a result of lead poisoning from drinking wines contaminated with high levels of lead.

The use of lead has accelerated since the industrial revolution, and particularly since World War II. However, its wide use has resulted in elevated lead concentrations in the ecosystem. In more modern times, the durability of lead made it an excellent paint additive, but its sweetness made it a tempting edible item for young children. Several European countries banned the use of interior lead-based paints in 1909. In 1922, the League of Nations banned lead-based paint, but the USA declined to adopt this rule. In 1943, a report concluded that children eating lead paint chips could suffer from neurological disorders including behavioral, learning and intelligence problems. Finally, in 1971, lead-based paint was phased out in the USA with the passage of the Lead-Based Paint Poisoning Prevention Act. Houses built prior to 1978 may have lead-based paint and this is a particularly serious problem for children living in older housing in large cities. In contrast to popularized reports, there is no persuasive evidence that low-level lead exposure is responsible for any neurobehavioral or intelligence defects. In fact, the bulk of the evidence suggests that there is no adverse impact of low-level lead exposure.

Adverse health effects from exposure to lead are now recognized to be among industrialized society's most important environmental health problems. In the USA, more than 6 million preschool metropolitan children and 400,000 fetuses were believed to have lead concentrations above 10 μg/dL of whole blood. That concentration has been designated by the US Public Health Service as the maximum permissible concentration from the standpoint of protecting the health of children and other sensitive populations, and 20 μg/dL is the concentration at which medical intervention should be considered.

Toxicokinetics

The US Environmental Protection Agency has designed an "Integrated Exposure Uptake Biokinetic Model for Lead in Children" (IEUBK), a detailed, classical compartment model (US EPA, 2002). Foremost is the sensitivity of children to the adverse effects of even low levels of lead exposure and second is dose. There are many reasons why children are more sensitive to lead. Differences in absorption of lead also increase the sensitivity of children. Adults absorb only 5–10% of orally ingested lead, while children absorb approximately 50% and can absorb much more depending on their nutrition. Children and pregnant women will absorb more lead because their bodies have a greater demand for calcium and iron, and the intestine responds by favoring their absorption. Lead mimics calcium and is thus readily absorbed, particularly if a diet is low in calcium and iron. Pregnant women and children in low income families are often in older housing that contains lead and with a poor diet (particularly low calcium) are most vulnerable to the developmental effects of lead.

Lead distributes in several compartments within the body, each with a different half-life. When lead enters the blood stream it attaches to red blood cells and in the blood has a half-life of about 25 days. Lead readily crosses the placenta, thus exposing the developing fetus and fetal nervous system. Lead is also stored in the muscle, where it has a longer half-life of about 40 days. Calcium requirements for children are high mainly because of rapid bone growth. Lead readily substitutes for calcium and is stored in bone. The half-life of lead in the bone is about 20 years. However, if bone turnover is increased, the lead in the bone is mobilized into the blood. This can occur during pregnancy or in older women subject to osteoporosis, which can be caused by decreasing estrogen levels. Considering the short half-life of lead in the blood, tooth lead levels may be an important indicator of childhood lead exposure and a vital marker to use in correlating developmental effects.

Mechanics of action

Mimicking essential metal Ca^{2+}

Toxicity of lead is largely due to its capacity to mimic calcium and substitute it in many of the fundamental cellular processes that are calcium dependent. Lead can cross the cell membrane by various mechanisms that are not clearly understood. Lead transport through the erythrocyte membrane is mediated by the anion exchanger in one direction and by the Ca-ATPase pump in the other. In other tissues, lead permeates the cell membrane through voltage-dependent or other types of calcium channels.

Once inside the cell, lead occupies the calcium binding sites on numerous calcium-dependent proteins, altering their function. Lead binds to calmodulin, a protein that acts as a sensor for free calcium concentration at the synaptic terminal and as a mediator of neurotransmitter release. Furthermore, it alters the functioning of the enzyme protein kinase C, a virtually ubiquitous protein which is of crucial importance in numerous physiological functions. Kinase C is normally activated by modulators exogenous to cells (hormones, neurotransmitters, etc.) through an enzyme chain, in a calcium-dependent manner. Besides many other functions, the activated kinase directly affects the expression of the "Immediate Early Response Genes". Lead has high affinity for the typical calcium-binding sites in this protein; picomolar concentration of lead can replace micromolar calcium concentrations. In model cell systems, it was demonstrated that lead can stimulate gene expression through a protein kinase C-mediated mechanism and it is postulated that this effect may be correlated with alterations in synaptic functioning.

Oxidative stress

Oxidative stress is an important contributor to lead pathogenesis. Lead-induced ROS generation in the biological system is well documented. A number of *in vitro* and *in vivo* studies point to increased production of ROS on lead exposure which induce oxidative damage in several tissues by enhancing lipid per-oxidation through Fenton reaction or by direct participation in free radical-mediated reactions such as inhibition of δ-aminolevulinic acid dehydratase (ALAD) activity or accumulation of ALA, a metabolite that can release Fe^{2+} from ferritin, and induce oxidative damage particularly in the early development. Lead easily crosses the biomembranes to reach the soft tissue cells, and thus accumulates in the ovary, testes and placental tissue as evident from animal experimental data. Lead via ROS generation induces toxicity to the testicular cells causing a decrease in GSH and other antioxidant enzymes like catalase and superoxide dismutase, and increase in lipid peroxidation. However, the effects are dose dependent since acute exposure rather increases the activity of antioxidant defense enzymes unlike in chronic exposures. Further there is enough evidence to suggest that the increase in free radicals along with membrane damage is a major mechanism behind the decreased gonadotropin binding, which leads to reproductive dysfunction. Lead-induced disruption of the prooxidant:antioxidant balance in the brain could also induce injury via oxidative damage to critical biomolecules. The possible involvement of free radical-mediated damage to cell components is supported by several reports.

Risk assessment

Reproductive toxicity resulting from a high dose of lead exposure is well established. Much of the early literature has been focused on increased incidence of spontaneous abortion and stillbirth associated with lead exposure in the workplace. In addition, during 1905 lead was used as an abortifacient in England. These outcomes, which are far less common today, presumably involve some combination of gametotoxic, embryotoxic, fetotoxic and teratogenic effects and define the upper end of the spectrum of reproductive toxicity in humans. Since these earlier reports, industrial exposure of women of child-bearing age was restricted by improved industrial hygiene practices, but a recent US Supreme Court decision ruled exclusion illegal. The decision was based on the premise of equal access to the workplace, not on insufficiency of evidence of toxic harm.

The most common biomarker of lead exposure is the blood lead level, usually measured in micrograms (μg) per one hundredth of a liter of blood (dl) or μg/dl. For example, many regulatory agencies set 40 μg/dl as a level of concern for adult male workers. The decline in acceptable childhood blood levels was a function of research and improved control of lead contamination, such as the removal of lead from gasoline. A blood lead level of 10 μg/dl does not represent a "safe" level, only one where it is prudent to take action to reduce exposure. But it must be noted that a level of 10 μg/dl is considered an action level and does not provide any margin of safety for a child's developing nervous system. Currently, there appears to be no safe level of lead exposure for the developing child.

The nervous system is the most sensitive target of lead poisoning. Fetuses and young children are especially vulnerable to the neurological effects of lead since their blood–brain barrier is immature and brains and nervous systems are still developing. At high levels of lead exposure, brain encephalopathy may occur, possibly resulting in death. It is now generally accepted that for every 10 μg/dl increase in blood lead levels there is a two- to four-point IQ deficit within the range of 5 to 35 μg/dl. Long-term studies of infants and young children exposed to lead showed that as they became older there was an increased likelihood that they would suffer from decreased attention span and reading and learning disabilities.

Toxicity

Male reproductive toxicity

The human male may be more susceptible than the rat to metal toxicity, possibly because of the poorer efficacy of the antioxidant defense system due to lower systemic levels of glutathione, vitamin C and glutathione peroxidase, compared to those in the rat, and greater vulnerability to oxidative damage to sperm DNA and sulfhydryl (-SH) groups required for the maintenance of sperm maturation and motility (Telisman *et al.*, 2007).

Lead toxicity in the male reproductive system is long known despite the controversies on the effect of low to moderate doses or route and duration of exposure involved. High BLL were also associated with delayed puberty onset in a recent prospective study of peripubertal Russian boys (Williams *et al.*, 2010). A positive correlation has been drawn between the blood and seminal plasma lead concentrations, yet seminal plasma lead concentration and male fertility status have not been correlated (Benoff *et al.*, 2000). Human evidence suggests that lead may cause reduced semen quality without any effect on endocrine function (Allouche *et al.*, 2009) as determined by studies of men occupationally exposed to lead (BLL 400 μg/L). Although lead-induced endocrine dysfunctioning is controversial, animal studies support that primary toxicity of lead on the male reproductive system is mediated by disruption of the hypothalamus–pituitary–testicular axis. Various clinical studies on occupationally exposed male human subjects reveal that lead retards semen quality including decreased semen volume, sperm count, sperm motility, abnormal sperm morphology and decreased seminal plasma zinc levels indicative of impaired prostrate secretory function. Controversies still exist due to the shortcomings of these studies, for example inadequate control groups, inclusion of subjects with urinogenital tract infections, etc. However, these toxic effects cannot be denied because animal experimental data correlated well with the human reports. Several animal experimental studies indicate that chronic lead exposure (BLL 400 μg/L) can be associated with decreased intratesticular or epididymal sperm counts, sperm production rate, sperm motility and serum testosterone levels, although mainly without significant effect on male fertility; whereas other studies have shown no significant reproductive effect at comparable blood lead levels (Apostoli *et al.*, 1998; 2007; Flora and Tandon, 1987; Mehta *et al.*, 2006). Lead is also reported to cause reduced sperm count at a low BLL of 240 μg/L and even lower BLLs cause several other effects on semen characteristics in rabbits (Moorman *et al.*, 1998). At low exposures of lead in the human study population (median BLL 49 μg/L; range 11–149 μg/L), a significant lead-related increase in immature sperm concentrations, in percentages of pathologic sperm, wide sperm, round sperm and short sperm, in serum levels of testosterone and estradiol, and decrease in seminal plasma zinc and in serum prolactin has been reported (Telisman *et al.*, 2007). Several other animal and clinical studies demonstrate that toxic effects of lead on the male reproductive system may occur at a concentration range below permissible limits and to which humans may be easily exposed worldwide.

Moreover, BLL is also questioned as an appropriate biomarker for risk assessment in lead toxicity. Since in chronic cases of exposure most lead accumulates in hard tissues and BLL is generally low, other biomarkers need to be validated against risk assessment analysis. The heme biosynthetic pathway is a specific target for lead toxicity. Lead by virtue of thiol-binding affinity inhibits δ-amino-levulanic acid, a crucial enzyme in the heme biosynthetic pathway and has been reported as a highly sensitive biomarker for the presence of lead in the body. In the study described by Telisman *et al.* (2007) immature sperm concentration and sperm morphological abnormalities were found to be better correlated with increase in erythrocyte protoporphyrin and decreased ALAD as compared to BLL, suggesting that these effects may be related to long-term accumulation of lead and biological markers like EP and ALAD and may reflect chronic lead toxicity better. Decrease in ALAD activity was also significantly associated with decreasing size of testes and seminal plasma levels of the lactate dehydrogenase isoenzyme LDH-C4 in another independent study. Besides, seminal plasma lead levels of subjects not occupationally exposed to lead were found to inversely correlate with the fertilizing capacity of sperm (sperm acrosome reaction) and the fertilization rate when using the IVF technique, but also with decreased seminal plasma zinc levels indicative of lead-impaired prostate function (Benoff *et al.*, 2003). Serum levels of sex hormones have also been correlated well with the ALAD inhibition by lead. A significant association was found between decreased serum prolactin, increased serum testosterone and estradiol with respect to increasing BLL (at varying concentrations) and decrease in ALAD activity. Thus, considerable investigations support the potential of ALAD to be employed as a primary biomarker for assessing lead poisoning; however, much validation and dose–response relation needs to be established. Furthermore, serum inhibin B levels could conceivably be used to directly study testicular function, and when combined with FSH measurement, it might be used as an indirect index of the regulation of reproductive hormones. Inhibin A (α–βA) and inhibin B (α–βB) are two kinds of inhibins found in the human body. In men, inhibin B is the major circulating inhibin, and inhibin A is non-detectable. Inhibin B is produced in the testis, principally by the Sertoli cells. Serum inhibin B provides a negative feedback regulating the secretion of pituitary follicle stimulating hormone (FSH) (Meachem *et al.*, 2001). There are, however, not many studies being carried out in this direction and thus requires some detailed investigation.

In some clinical studies seminal plasma lead concentrations were found to be low despite the reported infertility. Since toxic metals are known to cause toxicities mainly via

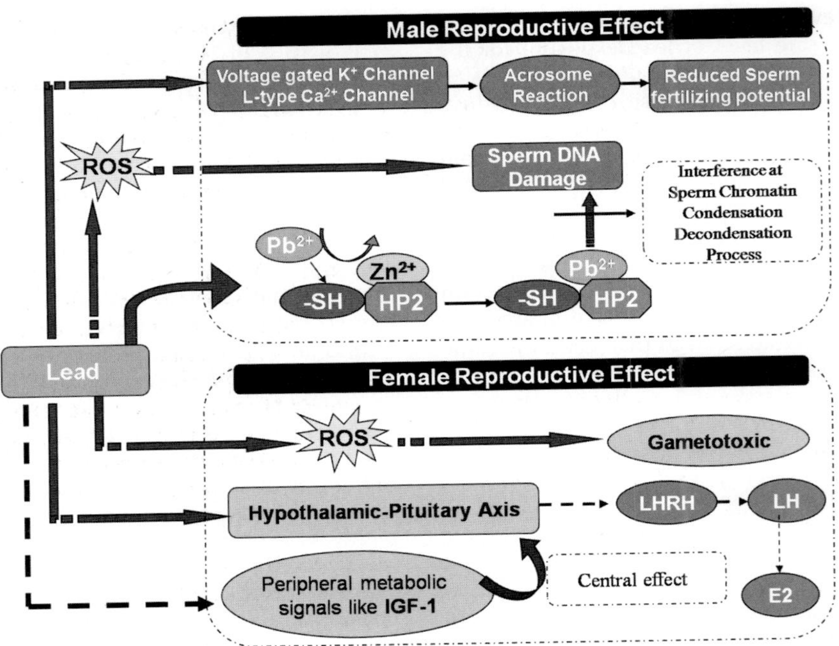

FIGURE 33.5 Proposed mechanisms for lead-induced reproductive toxicity. Abbreviations: -SH: thiol group; HP2: human protamine P2; ROS: reactive oxygen species; LHRH: leutinizing harmone-releasing factor; LH: leutinizing hormone; E2: estradiol; IGF-1: insuline-like growth factor-1.

essential metal imbalance it is important to measure the latter in the same seminal plasma or semen samples. It is previously known that due to similarities of ionic size and normal ionic charge between Pb^{2+}, Ca^{2+} and Zn^{2+}, they mimic the other at various transport sites, physiological reserves and metabolic pathways. Thus, the latter is reported to be an important mechanism in lead-induced toxicities. Lead has high affinity towards zinc binding proteins particularly those rich in sulfhydryl groups. The protective effect of zinc against lead-induced testicular injury in rats and decreased zinc concentrations in seminal plasma and semen that occurs in some forms of infertility provides reasons for the above hypothesis. It may be further explained as, during spermatogenesis, a zinc-containing enzyme, human protamine P2 (HP2), protecting the sperm DNA by binding with the same, thus playing an important role in the sperm chromatin condensation–decondensation process. Lead may compete with or replace zinc in HP2 by binding with its cysteine residue and cause a dose-dependent decrease in extent of HP2-DNA binding in the presence of lead. However, the effect has also been attributed to lead-induced sperm DNA damage affecting sperm chromatin integrity and ultimately infertility (Apostoli *et al.*, 2007; Benoff *et al.*, 2000; Hernandez-Ochoa *et al.*, 2006; Hsu *et al.*, 2009). Lead-induced DNA damage is rather believed to be mediated through oxidative stress. Moreover, spermatozoa are particularly susceptible to oxidative damage because their cell membrane contains large quantities of polyunsaturated fatty acids and their cytoplasm possesses low concentrations of ROS scavenging enzymes. Animal experimentation suggests that testis may be an important target for lead toxicity and even neonatal exposure may be sufficient to reduce fertility in the adult male. It has been suggested that the main mechanism is oxidative stress-induced lipid peroxidation and DNA damage in testicular cells (Pace *et al.*, 2005; Kasperczyk *et al.*, 2008). A summary of proposed mechanisms for lead-induced reproductive toxicity is shown in Figure 33.5.

Besides other mechanisms explaining the male reproductive effect of lead, interference to the ion channel may also be an important explanation. Sperm penetration through the zona pellucid requires acrosome exocytosis induced by sperm–zona binding. The process involves sequential activation of the sperm head-delayed rectifier voltage-gated potassium (K^+) channel and the L-type voltage-dependent Ca^{2+} ion channel. These channels have been reported to interact with metal ions like Pb^{2+} and $cadmium^{2+}$ through distinct binding sites to alter the ion permeation. It is suggested that lead action to reduce human sperm fertilizing potential is mediated by a sperm head voltage-gated K^+ channel that is supported by the fact that lead exposure causes premature acrosome reactions in animal experiments. Since these K^+ channels exist in multiple isoforms helps to explain the varied susceptibility to lead-induced infertility in men.

Lead toxic manifestations in the male reproductive system are reported to be partially reversible either following chelation therapy or after removal of the subject from the exposure site.

Female reproductive toxicity

A positive correlation between lead exposure and abortions by high dose exposure has been known for many years. Epidemiologic studies with lead-exposed women have reported reproductive toxicity in both non-occupational groups and occupational groups. Deficiencies in the design of the studies prevent definitive conclusions, but the studies have helped to direct attention to a potential problem. Very early preimplantation loss can easily go undetected and might occur after moderate dose and perhaps even low dose exposure. With the advent of human chorionic gonadotropin assays, it is now possible to detect the onset of pregnancy and early fetal loss during the first 12 weeks of pregnancy. As mentioned before, interpretation of female reproductive defects is rather complicated due to the various factors involved. Most studies exhibit delay of time-to-pregnancy and abortions as the study endpoint. Analyzing data from the National Natality and Fetal Mortality Survey, which reveals the probability sample of live births and fetal deaths to married women in 1980, suggested that maternal employment in the lead industry could be a risk factor for negative pregnancy outcomes, including stillbirth and preterm birth. Several other prospective studies have examined the issue of the involvement of lead in spontaneous abortion, stillbirth, preterm delivery and low birth weight. Women subjects in Boston, Cleveland, Cincinnati and Port Pirie had average blood lead concentrations of 510 µg/dL during pregnancy; almost all had blood lead concentrations less than 25 µg/dL. The Glasgow and Titova Mitrovica (Wang *et al.*, 2009) cohorts had average blood lead concentrations of about 20 µg/dL. None of these studies reported an association between maternal blood lead concentrations and spontaneous abortion or stillbirth. However, the Cincinnati and Port Pirie studies found a lead-related decrease in duration of pregnancy, and the Glasgow, Cincinnati and Boston studies reported a lead-related decrease in birth weight. The Boston study also found an increased risk of intrauterine growth retardation, low birth weight and small-for-gestational-age deliveries at cord blood lead concentrations of 15 µg/dL or more. The Port Pirie study found that the relative risk of preterm delivery increased 2.8-fold for every 10 µg/dL increase in maternal blood lead. In the Cincinnati study, gestational age was reduced by about 0.6 weeks for each natural log unit increase in blood lead, or by about 1.8 weeks over the entire range of observed blood concentrations. Even after adjustment for the reduced length of pregnancy, the Cincinnati study found reduced infant birth weight (by about 300 g) and birth length (by about 2.5 cm), and the Port Pirie group reported reduced head circumference (by about 0.3 cm). Findings from some of the prospective studies have been extensively reviewed. However, some striking inconsistencies, yet to be explained, characterize the data on the relationship between prenatal lead exposure and fetal growth and maturation. For instance, in the large cohort ($N=907$) of women residing in Kosovo (Factor-Litvak *et al.*, 1991), no associations were seen between mid-pregnancy blood lead concentrations (ranging up to approximately 55 µg/dL) and either infant birth weight or length of gestation.

Animal experimentation reveals that lead exposure in drinking water from the time of weaning may delay the onset of puberty in females. The effect is markedly different and reported to be more profound in cases of low blood lead concentrations as compared to high concentrations indicating difference in mechanism (Iavicoli *et al.*, 2006). Lead-induced delay in the timing of puberty was associated with suppressed serum levels of insulin-like growth factor-1 (IGF-1), luteinizing hormone (LH) and estradiol (E2). Although lead inhibits the basal synthesis of ovarian steroidogenic acute regulatory protein (StAR), it does not alter gonadotropin-stimulated StAR synthesis suggesting that lead-induced estradiol suppression is rather a result of LH suppression (Srivastava *et al.*, 2004). Establishing the mechanism for the effect of lead on puberty, the possibility of systemic effects of lead instead of directly on hypothalamic pituitary axis may not be ruled out. The onset and progression of puberty has been hypothesized to be influenced by metabolic signals of peripheral origin that ultimately act centrally to modify neuronal function causing enhanced secretion of LH-releasing hormone (LHRH). Insulin-like growth factor (IGF-1), a polypeptide mitogen produced mainly by the liver, is regarded as a candidate involved in linking somatic development and activation of reproductive hypothalamus. Interestingly, lead exposure is being associated with decreased circulating levels of IGF-1 in addition to LH and estradiol. *In vitro* studies reveal that IGF-1 of peripheral origin is capable of acting centrally via specific receptors and may stimulate secretion of LHRH from nerve terminals in median eminence of prepubertal female rats via prostraglandin-E2 to accelerate initiation of puberty in two independent studies. Since IGF-1 replacement shows reversal in lead-induced delay in female puberty it has been suggested that lead does not centrally impair the LHRH-releasing system; rather the effect may be due to deficiency in circulating IGF-1 available to the hypothalamus at the time of puberty (Pine *et al.*, 2006). Thus, the mechanism involved may be sequenced as lead-induced deficiency in circulating IGF-1 rendering it unavailable for reproductive hypothalamus activation that causes reduced LHRH release resulting in suppressed LH in the circulation, which in turn decreases serum estradiol.

Lead may also cause delays in vaginal opening as observed in the case of offspring exposed continuously from conception to doses of lead from 25 to 250 ppm. No other effects on fertility or reproductive performance were noted (Wang *et al.*, 2009). When rats were exposed to lead acetate in drinking water *in utero*, prepubertally or postpubertally, the most severe effects were observed in the "*in utero*" exposed group, with delayed vaginal opening and disrupted estrous cycling. In another study female offspring from lead-treated dams had significantly delayed vaginal opening, and 50% of them exhibited prolonged and irregular periods of diestrous, accompanied by absence of observable corpora lutea. The release of gonadotropins revealed irregular patterns of both FSH and LH. Lead may act upon the hypothalamic pituitary axis and on gonadal steroid biosynthesis directly as indicated by animal experimentation. Lead-induced alterations in pubertal progression and hypothalamic–pituitary–ovarian–uterus functions have been confirmed in female monkeys prenatally or postnatally exposed to lead. Blood levels of approximately 350 µg/L resulted in subclinical suppression of circulating LH and FSH and estradiol without producing overt effects on general health and menstruation. The overall results of these investigations suggest that different levels of the hypothalamic–pituitary–gonad axis can be affected by exposure to lead, mainly when structures are undergoing rapid proliferation.

Lead exposure also resulted in slow brain weight development, lowered brain weight and decreased DNA per brain, but no effect on proteins per brain in mice when exposed at premating, prenatally and postnatally when compared to control. Interestingly, it was observed that premating lead exposure animals exhibited significantly increased brain weight and protein but significantly lowered DNA per brain indicating its interference with the developing maternal reproductive systems or on ovulation–fertilization.

Developmental toxicity

Several studies have also searched for evidence of teratogenicity. A retrospective study to understand the association between cord blood lead and major or minor malformations in a cohort of 4,354 infants found a significant increase in

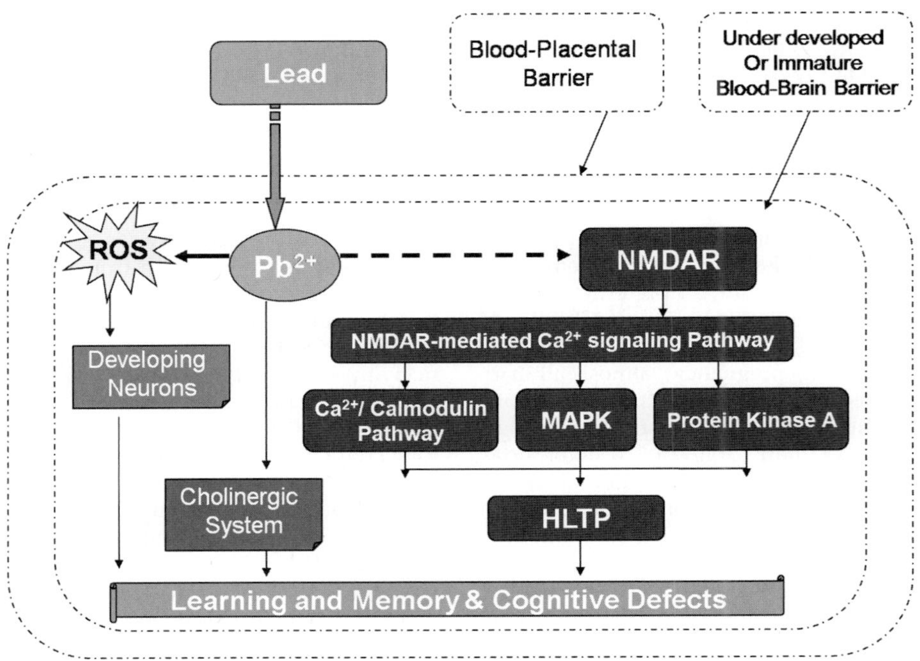

FIGURE 33.6 Possible mechanisms for lead-induced developmental neurotoxicity. Abbreviations: ROS: reactive oxygen species; NMDAR: N-methyl-D-aspartic acid receptor; MAPK: mitogen-activated protein kinase; HLTP: hippocampal long-term potential.

the number of minor anomalies observed per child, but no malformation was found to be associated with lead. Unexpectedly, several other factors, such as premature labor and neonatal respiratory distress, were found to be reduced with increased blood lead. The field study by Needleman *et al.* (2009) is important because the minor anomalies in question might reflect general fetal stress and predict developmental disorders. Evidence is accumulating that relatively small increases in maternal blood lead during pregnancy can be associated with delayed or retarded growth. A study with 260 infants from the Cincinnati prospective lead study experienced retardation in covariate-adjusted growth (Shukla *et al.*, 1989, 1991). More specifically, it found that infants born to women with lead concentrations greater than 8 μg/dL during pregnancy grew at a lower than expected rate if increased lead exposure continued during the first 15 months of life. Conversely, if postnatal lead exposure was small, the infants grew at a higher than expected rate, which suggests a catch-up in growth after fetal growth suppression. No lead-related growth effects were observed in infants born to women with blood lead concentrations less than 8 μg/dL. In a later analysis of stature at 33 months of age a sustained increase in lead exposure above 20 μg/dL throughout the first 33 months of life was associated with reduced stature. However, prenatal exposure was no longer related to stature at 33 months of age. The reported indication of fetal toxicity is consistent with other previously discussed markers of lead-related fetal toxicity. It is also consistent with cross-sectional studies of lead's relation with physical size. Several points emerge from a review of these studies, apart from a lead-related retardation of growth itself. First, the specific manifestations of the fetal insult vary among cohorts and might reflect lead's interaction with such cofactors as adequacy of prenatal care, maternal age, ethnicity and nutritional status. Second, the blood lead concentrations associated with adverse fetal development are low (10–15 μg/dL or even lower) and comparable with those found in a substantial fraction of women of child-bearing age. The validity of the reported association between fetal lead exposure and markers of adverse fetal development is strengthened by the observed negative association between maternal or fetal blood lead concentrations and early physical growth and cognitive development. Thus, the birth-outcome measures, early physical-growth measures and early measures of infant development can be viewed as potentially reflecting the fetal toxicity of lead (Figure 33.6).

In a longitudinal follow-up study (Markowitz and Rosen, 1990), lead-poisoned children showed reduced growth velocity compared with age-matched control subjects. Furthermore, impaired growth velocities in the lead-poisoned children did not change substantially from baseline after chelation therapy. The data on children suggest that endocrinologic disturbances can occur at sensitive points in anthropometric development. Endocrine dysfunction in lead workers with relatively high lead exposure is known. Height in two lead-poisoned children dropped to below the tenth percentile during intoxication; both subjects demonstrated depressed thyroid-stimulating hormone (TSH) responses to thyrotropin-releasing hormone (TRH), and one showed depression in resting TSH concentrations.

Considerable evidence suggests that both prenatal and postnatal lead exposures can induce developmental toxicities in infants. Lead is deposited in the placenta and reported to be higher in occupationally exposed women than unexposed. During pregnancy most lead reaching the fetus is mobilized from the maternal skeleton, absorbed through gastrointestinal tract and transferred through the placenta (Figure 33.6). Low levels of lead in amniotic fluid are reported but cord lead levels are estimated to be around 85% that of maternal blood lead levels. Although early abortions due to low-level lead exposures have been reported its mechanism is not clear. However, reports seem acceptable since independent studies demonstrating gametotoxic effects via DNA damage, hormonal imbalance in both male and female and direct teratogenic effects have been documented. Moreover, lead exposure is reported to cause elevated blood pressure in pregnant women. The latter has direct correlation with vascular effects on the placenta that may be a risk factor for mother and fetus.

In lactating mothers, the source of lead exposure to the infant may be the mother's milk. Lead levels in mother's milk have been reported from various countries and have direct correlation with maternal bone and blood lead levels. A positive correlation has also been drawn between mother's milk lead levels and BLL of breast-fed infants which absorbs most of the milk lead content.

Developmental effects on brain

Lead-induced CNS toxicity has been a major concern in the case of the developing brain. The effects caused in children are difficult to differentiate due to prenatal or postnatal lead exposures. A series of publications exists on the human CNS effects due to lead in children. Referring to the recent independent studies carried out clearly draws an inverse relation of BLL in children between the age of 6 months to 6 years and IQ. Lead-induced injury to the CNS is rather lengthy and does not recover reduced BLL in children with age. The latter was evident from a study done at Port Pirie, Australia, in children that did not show any improvement in IQ when BLL were reduced from 212 μg/L at the age of 2 years to 79 μg/L at age of 11–13 years. Some study reviews deliberate about the relationship between intellectual impairment and BLL in children. It is a possibility that lower BLL has a more profound effect on the brain functions as compared to high lead levels (Koller *et al.*, 2004). Some reviews suggest a supralinear exposure–response relationship stating the possibility of larger IQ loss with BLL changes from 0 to 100 μg/L than from 100 to 200 μg/L (Lanphear *et al.*, 2005).

Non-human primates and rodent models have been used to study the effect of developmental lead exposure on behavioral endpoints. Behavioral studies in animals confirm the developmental neurotoxicity of lead and are easier to correlate with humans due to direct observations and fewer variables involved. However, it does not help to identify the molecular targets of lead in CNS. Behavioral studies in rodents have established the capacity of lead to alter learning and memory. Prenatal and postnatal exposure of lead in the rhesus monkey resulted in impairment of higher-order learning at BLLs of 50 and 70 μg/dl, respectively. Learning a behavioral task greatly depends on normal hippocampus function, thus during its developmental period the brain is highly vulnerable to the presence of lead. Hippocampal long-term potentiation (LTP), a form of synaptic plasticity, is believed to form the cellular basis for learning and memory in the mammalian brain. LTP may be described as a long-lasting increase in synaptic efficacy following brief periods of stimulation of specific synapses. Although LTP is also described in other brain regions, hippocampal LTP has been especially associated with special learning and is dependent upon NMDAR activation. N-methyl-D-aspartate (NMDAR) receptor, an ionotropic receptor that mediates the action of glutamate, is known to play a central role in brain development, learning and memory as well as neurodegenerative diseases. Evidence suggests that lead targets NMDAR and alters those physiological processes that are NMDAR dependent including hippocampus LTP. Lead exposure alters the gene expression of the NMDAR in both the developing and mature brain. Lead exposure induces alterations in the NR1 and NR2A subunit mRNA expressions essentially at the hippocampus region indicating the regional selectivity of the effect of lead. Studying the effect of lead on NR1 splice variants that are most abundantly expressed in the hippocampus also show regional variations. Additionally developmental lead exposure also alters the splicing of the carboxyl terminus cassette (C1 cassette) present at the NR1 splice variant. The C1 cassette is localized in the NR1 splice variant to separate the receptor-rich region in plasma membrane and also provides sequence for phosphorylation by protein kinase C (PKC). These splice variants impart the highest degree of calcium influx and PKC potentiation to NMDAR complexes. Lead exposure during developmental stages causes significant decrease in NR1 splice variants lacking the C1 cassette. Thus, in the hippocampus of adult rats exposed to lead during developmental stages, NMDAR complexes may express as having lower levels of calcium signaling and thus reduced synaptic plasticity. Further, since NMDAR calcium signaling is the most potent activator of neuronal nitric oxide synthase (nNOS), nNOS activity may be reduced in the hippocampus of lead-exposed rats. Nitric oxide, a product of nNOS, is shown to be a neuronal retrograde messenger essential for hippocampal LTP. Thus, lead-induced effects on NR1 splice variants expressed in nNOS positive neurons may decrease NO production and interfere with hippocampal LTP.

Further, as discussed above, it is clear that lead exposure, especially during developmental stages, inhibits NMDAR and alters the ontogeny of its subunit expression. The latter causes interference in the NMDA-mediated calcium signaling pathway that conveys information from synapse to nucleus to activate the expression of genes necessary for learning and memory (Figure 33.6). To understand the details, the transcription of genes essential for learning and memory requires a transcription factor called cyclic-AMP response element binding protein which is stimulated by protein kinase pathways including protein kinase A, mitogen-activated protein kinase (MAPK) and calcium/calmodulin-dependent protein kinase. These kinase pathways are activated by NMDAR–calcium signaling that is targeted by lead toxicity in the developing hippocampus (Toscano and Guilarte, 2005).

In addition, lead disrupts the normal development of the brain causing reduction in cellular development which can be seen at the dendritic, axonal and synaptic level in different brain regions. This reduced neuronal development might reasonably be expected to severely reduce the intellectual potential of the organism. Lead is also capable of reducing neural plasticity and can severely reduce the capacity of cholinergic afferents to sprout new processes. Lead exposure also perturbs the aminergic system in the cortex, cerebellum and hippocampus, thus possibly contributing to the cognitive and behavioral impairments especially in lead-exposed rats at the developmental period (Devi *et al.*, 2005). Lead is therefore capable of reducing neural growth both during development and in adulthood. Diminution in cholinergic functioning may contribute to the reduction in cognitive processing following lead exposure and thus one may consider using cholinergic agonists as therapeutic agents in the treatment of childhood lead poisoning.

THERAPEUTIC STRATEGIES

Antioxidant supplementation

The metal-induced depletion of water-soluble and lipid-soluble antioxidants has led to the increased susceptibility of the tissues to free radical damage. Antioxidants are substances that can prevent or diminish oxidation of bio-molecules by their direct or indirect action. Both enzymatic and non-enzymatic defense mechanisms are present in the cell. The components of these defense systems can be divided into two main groups: antioxidant enzymes including superoxide dismutase (SOD), catalase (CAT) and glutathione peroxidase (GPx) and small endogenous antioxidant molecules such as glutathione (GSH), coenzyme Q (CoQ) and urate. Exogenous antioxidants include tocopherols (vitamin E), ascorbate (vitamin C), vitamin A and carotenoids and some metals, essential for the function of antioxidant enzymes. Glutathione is the most important source of sulfhydryl groups, and glutathione, binding to lead, arsenic and cadmium, is considered to be the first line of defense. *In vivo*, intracellular but not extracellular glutathione is thought to provide the protection against toxicity of these metals. Although no detailed study in humans has been reported for the beneficial effects of vitamin E or C; however, there are enough reports suggesting their role in lead- and arsenic-induced developmental toxicity (Yu *et al.*, 2008; Chang *et al.*, 2007; Chattopadhyay *et al.*, 2001). Vitamin C is essential for testicular differentiation, integrity and steroidogenic functions (Acharya *et al.*, 2008; Luck *et al.*, 1995). Vitamins C and E show protection in rat and mice testes against cadmium-induced oxidative damage (Acharya *et al.*, 2008). Ognjanovi *et al.* (2010) showed increased lipid per oxidation and decreased activities of SOD and catalase in the testis of rats, which was prevented by CoQ and vitamin E.

Zinc and selenium are micronutrients known for their beneficial role in reducing lead-, cadmium- and arsenic-induced reproductive toxicity. Zinc, copper and calcium at 1.0 μg/mL improved maturation rates in oocytes exposed to cadmium (1.0 μg/mL) (Nandi *et al.*, 2010). Zinc also can inhibit the toxicity of cadmium in the human placenta (Miller *et al.*, 1992).

Chelation therapy

Chelation therapy has been the basis for the medical treatment of metal poisoning. Chelating agents have been used clinically as antidotes for acute and chronic metal intoxication. These compounds bind to and enhance the excretion of toxic elements and in some cases they also decrease the metal toxicity by preventing it from binding to cellular target molecules. A number of chelating agents have been suggested for the treatment of metal intoxication. Calcium disodium ethylenediamine tetra-acetic acid ($CaNa_2EDTA$) and meso 2,3-dimercaptosuccinic acid (DMSA) have been the mainstay of chelation therapy for lead poisoning (Flora *et al.*, 1995, 2007). While $CaNa_2EDTA$ needs to be injected intravenously, DMSA could be an oral alternative. DMSA has also been tried successfully in animals and in a few cases of human arsenic poisoning. Although at present there is no specific recommended treatment, it has been shown that systemic cadmium intoxication can be alleviated by administration of dithiocarbamate chelating agents (Jones, 1991).

$CaNa_2EDTA$ is widely used in the clinical cases of lead intoxication. It has been well established that the administration of $CaNa_2EDTA$ during pregnancy can result in teratogenic effects especially when administered between days 11 and 14 at doses comparable to those for humans. Teratogenicity also varies with the route of administration of $CaNa_2EDTA$. Subcutaneous administration of disodium salt at the dose of 375 mg/kg was only maternally toxic, but did not cause any malformation, whereas gavage administration resulted in more signs of toxicity in animal model. Absorption into the circulation, potential interaction with essential trace elements, and the stress associated with the administration of the compound were suggested to be the possible factors involved in the differences in EDTA-induced maternal and developmental toxicity. Teratogenic effects of $CaNa_2EDTA$ too have been reported (Domingo, 1998).

DMSA is a water soluble thiol chelator and was approved by US FDA for the treatment of childhood lead poisoning but is also effective in arsenic poisoning. Maternal and developmental toxicity of DMSA was studied in animal models by Domingo *et al.* (1988) who suggested no observed teratogenic effect level at 410 mg/kg/day. These authors further studied oral administration of DMSA during pregnancy and reported that the drug is embryofetotoxic at levels that did not produce significant maternal toxicity. There is, however, not much data available on the effects of DMSA in pregnant women. Sodium 2,3-dimercaptopropane sulfonate (DMPS) is another thiol chelator and analog of British Anti Lewite (BAL). This is also an effective chelator for lead and arsenic. Information is scarce as far as developmental toxicity of DMPS is concerned. No abnormalities have been reported in pregnant animals treated with this chelator. The NOEL for health hazards to the developing fetuses is 630 mg/kg/day which is much higher than the doses of DMPS given in the treatment of human metal poisoning (Domingo, 1998).

Monoisoamyl dimercaptosuccinic acid (MiADMSA), a monoester of DMSA, has recently been found to be a more effective and promising future chelator against arsenic poisoning. Although studies have been done to generate data for embryo–fetal toxicity there is still no study being performed for its effect during human pregnancy. There has been a recent evaluation of the efficacy of MiADMSA against arsenic and it has been suggested that the results obtained *in vitro* using human embryonic stem (ES) cells were in concordance with the animal model for studying developmental toxicity (Flora and Mehta, 2009).

CONCLUDING REMARKS AND FUTURE DIRECTIONS

The effects of metal-induced reproductive and developmental toxicity have been known for some time but have only been explored recently. The advent of awareness towards environmental, occupational and lifestyle exposure to metals and reports revealing their toxic potential and mechanism is mainly responsible for increasing investigations into their reproductive and developmental effects. Several historic epidemiological studies have investigated the possible correlation between metal exposures, reproductive health and developmental disorders (Figure 33.7). However, it has been only recently that exhaustive research has been conducted by experts to uncover the possible mechanistic aspects that may

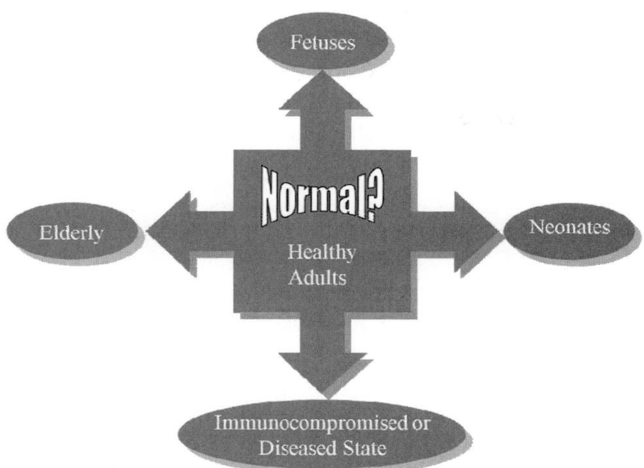

FIGURE 33.7 Populations at risk for metal-induced reproductive and developmental toxicity.

contribute to finding appropriate prophylactic and therapeutic measures. Lead, arsenic and cadmium are rather conventionally known toxic metals extensively used and widely distributed in the environment, geographically or by virtue of its human utility. Reproductive and developmental toxicities of these metals have also been addressed previously by other authors. This chapter compiles the previously known literature with recent updates, including mechanisms of toxicity for each metal, to better understand their effect on male and female reproductive health, and developmental disorders.

The sources of exposure for these three toxic metals are different from each another but toxic manifestation may be similar. Lead and cadmium exposure generally occurs due to occupational reasons or industrial pollution whereas arsenic shows geographical existence in nature. These metals show limited points of similarity that may be of use in finding general prophylactic and therapeutic guidelines as well as specific individual treatment. Lead and cadmium share similar ionic size and charge that allow them to have similar molecular targets to induced toxicity. They both mimic essential ions in the body like Ca^{2+} and Zn^{2+}, which helps them to follow physiological pathways like transport systems and cellular reserves, and allows to interfere with Ca^{2+}- or Zn^{2+}-dependent enzyme functioning and ion channels, etc. The said hypothesis has also been experimentally proven, for example the gametotoxic effect of lead and cadmium. Arsenic and lead, both being thiol-binding metals, also show similar target-binding sites, i.e. protein containing -SH-rich amino acids like the cystein residue. These binding sites and essential metal mimicking not only decide the toxic pathways but also direct the toxicokinetics of these metals to a great extent. For example, lead accumulates in physiologic calcium reservoirs like bones and redistributes during pregnancy thus also affecting its toxicity. Further, lead binds with the cystein residue of HP2 and ALAD enzyme thus exhibiting gametogenesis in the male and affecting the heme biosynthetic pathway development in the fetus, respectively. Besides the specific toxicodynamics of these metals they all are known to induce oxidative stress via ROS generation and interfere with the cellular defense mechanism. Thus, oxidative stress-mediated macromolecule damage (lipid biomembrane, DNA) results in cellular necrosis at high metal concentrations and apoptosis at lower metal concentrations. It is possible, due to the latter, that metals show varied toxicities at different concentration exposures resulting in discrepancies in the literature.

Metal-induced reproductive toxicities are only partially reversible depending upon the extent, duration and time of exposure after removing the subject from the exposure site along with chelation therapy if necessary. However, developmental toxicities are a more serious cause of concern since chelation therapy is contraindicated during pregnancy and developmental abnormalities once established are mostly irreversible. However, other supportive treatments discussed in this chapter, such as antioxidant or essential metal supplementations, etc., may be recommended with experts' suggestions to reduce the chances of metal-induced developmental toxicities.

In conclusion, there is a growing concern within the scientific and governmental regulatory communities regarding the effects of exposures to reproductive toxicants on human fertility. Arsenic, cadmium and lead, ubiquitous heavy metals, are associated with testicular toxicity and impaired fertility leading to adverse reproductive and developmental effects. However, a number of studies available in the literature suggest that there are areas which still need to be explored and critically investigated, including:

1. Several factors restrict the ability of extrapolating animal data to the human situation and these can be attributed to factors like differences in reproductive endpoints between species and also difficulties with comparing exposure assessment.
2. Differences between the toxicokinetics and toxicodynamics of these metals between species are still not well understood.
3. Research on developmental neurotoxicology is needed for metalloids like arsenic and on interaction with essential metals. Much still remains to be learned about the delayed consequences of developmental toxicity in adults as possible causes of neurodegeneration. This research is critical to guide both future research in metals as paradigms of neurotoxic metals and targeted programs of prevention.
4. Further studies are also needed to understand the safety and mechanisms of preventive agents (including chelating drugs) during pregnancy both in animal models and human cases. Studies are also required to improve our understanding of the protective activity of the drugs against the developmental toxicity induced by these compounds and toxic metals.

ACKNOWLEDGMENT

The authors thank Dr. R. Vijayaraghavan, Director of the establishment, for his support and encouragement.

REFERENCES

Acharya UR, Mishra M, Patro J, Panda MK (2008) Effect of vitamins C and E on spermatogenesis in mice exposed to cadmium. *Reprod Toxicol* **25:** 84–8.

Agarwal A, Said TM (2005) Oxidative stress, DNA damage and apoptosis in male infertility: a clinical approach. *BJU Int* **95:** 503–7.

Agarwal A, Gupta S, Sharma RK (2005) Role of oxidative stress in female reproduction. *Reproduct Biol Endocrinol* **3:** 28–49.

Akram Z, Jalali S, Shami SA, Ahmad L, Batool S, Kalsoom O (2009). Adverse effects of arsenic exposure on uterine function and structure in female rat. *Experiment Toxicol Pathol*. In press.

Alexander BH, Checkoway H, van Netten C, Muller CH, Ewers TG, Kaufman JD, Mueller BA, Vaughan TL, Faustman EM (1996) Semen quality of men employed at a lead smelter. *Occup Environ Med* **53:** 411–16.

Allouche L, Hamadouche M, Touabti A (2009) Chronic effects of low lead levels on sperm quality, gonadotropins and testosterone in albino rats. *Exp Toxicol Pathol* **61:** 503–10.

Apostoli P, Telisman S, Sager PR (2007) *Handbook on the Toxicology of Metals*. Academic Press.

Apostoli P, Kiss P, Porru S, Bondle JP, Vanhoome M (1998) Male reproductive toxicity of lead in animals and humans. *Occup Environ Med* **55:** 364–74.

Aschengrau A, Zierler S, Cohen A (1989) Quality of community drinking water and the occurrence of spontaneous abortion. *Arch Environ Health* **44:** 283–90.

ATSDR (Agency for Toxic Substances and Disease Registry) (2000) Toxicological Profile for Arsenic. Atlanta, GA: Agency for Toxic Substances and Disease Registry. Available: http://www.atsdr.cdc.gov/toxprofiles/tp2.html #bookmark06

ATSDR (Agency for Toxic Substances and Disease Registry) (2007) Toxicological Profile for arsenic. Draft for Public Comment. Atlanta GA. Available from: http://www.atsdr.cdc.gov/toxprofiles/tp2.html

Benoff S, Jacob A, Hurley IR (2000) Male infertility and environmental exposure to lead and cadmium. *Human Reproduction Update* **6:** 107–21.

Benoff S, Centola GM, Millan C, Napolitano B, Marmar JL, Hurley IR (2003) Increased seminal plasma lead levels adversely affect the fertility potential of sperm in IVF. *Hum Reprod* **18:** 374–83.

Benoff S, Hauser R, Marmar JL, Hurley IR, Napolitano B, Centola GM (2009) Cadmium concentrations in blood and seminal plasma: correlations with sperm number and motility in three male populations (infertility patients, artificial insemination donors, and unselected volunteers). *Mol Med* **15:** 248–62.

Borzsonyi M, Bereczky A, Rudnai P, Csanady M, Horvath A (1992) Epidemiological studies on human subjects exposed to arsenic in drinking water in southeast Hungary. *Arch Toxicol* **66:** 77–8.

Caride A, Fernández-Pérez B, Cabaleiroa T, Esquifino AI, Lafuente A (2009) Cadmium exposure disrupts GABA and taurine regulation of prolactin secretion in adult male rats. *Toxicol Lett* **185:** 175–9.

Casalino E, Calzaretti G, Sblano C, Landriscina V, Felice Tecce M, Landriscina C (2002) Antioxidant effect of hydroxytyrosol (DPE) and Mn^{2+} in liver of cadmium-intoxicated rats. *Comp Biochem Physiol C Toxicol Pharmacol* **133:** 625–32.

Casalino E, Sblano C, Landriscina V, Calzaretti G, Landriscina C (2004) Rat liver glutathione S-transferase activity stimulation following acute cadmium or manganese intoxication. *Toxicology* **200:** 29–38.

Castellini C, Mourvakia E, Sartini B, Cardinali R, Moretti E, Collode G, Fortanerc S, Sabbionic E, Renieri T (2009) *In vitro* toxic effects of metal compounds on kinetic traits and ultrastructure of rabbit spermatozoa. *Reprod Toxicol* **27:** 46–54.

Chang SI, Jin B, Youn P, Park C, Park JD, Ryu DY (2007) Arsenic-induced toxicity and the protective role of ascorbic acid in mouse testis. *Toxicol Appl Pharmacol* **218:** 196–203.

Chattopadhyay SS, Debnath GJ, Ghosh D (2001) Protection of sodium arsenite-induced ovarian toxicity by coadministration of *L*-ascorbate (vitamin C) in mature Wistar strain rat. *Arch Environ Contam Toxicol* **41:** 83–9.

Chattopadhyay SS, Ghosh P, Ghosh D, Debnath J (2003) Effect of dietary coadministration of sodium selenite on sodium arsenite-induced ovarian and uterine disorders in mature albino rats. *Toxicol Sci* **75:** 412–22.

Cherry N, Shaikh K, McDonald C, Chowdhury Z (2008) Stillbirth in rural Bangladesh: arsenic exposure and other etiological factors: a report from Gonoshasthaya Kendra. *Bull World Health Org* **86:** 172–7.

Concha G, Vogler G, Nermell B, Vahter M (1998) Low-level arsenic excretion in breast milk of native Andean women exposed to high levels of arsenic in the drinking water. *Int Arch Occup Environ Health* **71:** 42–6.

Damiano AE, Zotta E, Ibarra C (2006) Functional and molecular expression of AQP9 channel and UT-A transporter in normal and preeclamptic human placentas. *Placenta* **27:** 1073–81.

De Souza PF, Diamante MA, Dolder H (2010) Testis response to low doses of cadmium in Wistar rats. *Int J Exp Pathol* **91:** 125–31.

Devi CB, Reddy GH, Prasanthi RPJ, Chetty CS, Reddy GR (2005) Developmental lead exposure alters mitochondrial monoamine oxidase and synaptosomal catecholamine levels in rat brain. *Int J Devl Neuroscience* **23:** 375–81.

Domingo JL, Peternain JL, Llobet JM, Corbella J (1988) Developmental toxicity of subcutaneously meso 2,3-dimercaptosuccinic acid in mice. *Fund Appl Toxicol* **11:** 715–22.

Domingo JL (1994) Metal-induced developmental toxicity in mammals: a review. *J Toxicol Environ Health* **42:** 123–41.

Domingo JL (1998) Developmental toxicity of metal chelating agents. *Reprod Toxicol* **12:** 499–510.

Drobna Z, Walton FS, Harmon AW, Thomas DJ, Styblo M (2010) Interspecies differences in metabolism of arsenic by cultured primary hepatocytes. *Toxicol Appl Pharmacol* **245:** 47–56.

Fabiánová E, Hettychová L, Koppová K, Hrubá F, Marko M, Maroni M, Grech G, Bencko V (2000). Health risk assessment for inhalation exposure to arsenic. *Cent Eur J Public Health* **8:** 28–32.

Factor-Litvak P, Graziano JH, Kline JK, Popovac D, Mehmeti A, Ahmedi G, Shrout P, Murphy MJ, Gashi E, Haxhiu R (1991) Prospective study of birthweight and length of gestation in a population surrounding a lead smelter in Kosovo, Yugoslavia. *Int J Epidemiol* **20:** 722–8.

Ferrario D, Croera C, Brustio R, Collotta A, Bowe G, Vahter M, Gribaldo L (2008) Toxicity of inorganic arsenic and its metabolites on haematopoietic progenitors "in vitro": comparison between species and sexes. *Toxicology* **249:** 102–8.

Fischer LM, daCosta KA, Kwock L, Stewart PW, Lu TS (2007) Sex and menopausal status influence human dietary requirements for the nutrient choline. *Am J Clin Nutr* **85:** 1275–85.

Flora SJS, Tandon SK (1987) Influence of calcium disodium edetate on the toxic effect of lead administration in pregnant rats. *Ind J Physiol Pharmacol* **31:** 267–72.

Flora SJS, Mehta A (2009) Monoisoamyl dimercaptosuccinic acid abrogates arsenic-induced developmental toxicity in human embryonic stem cell-derived embryoid bodies: comparison with in vivo studies. *Biochem Pharmacol* **78:** 1340–9.

Flora SJS, Bhattacharya R, Vijayaraghavan R (1995) Combined therapeutic potential of meso 2,3-dimercaptosuccinic acid and calcium disodium edetate on the mobilization and distribution of lead in experimental lead intoxication in rats. *Fund Appl Toxicol* **25:** 233–40.

Flora SJS, Saxena G, Mehta A (2007) Reversal of lead-induced neuronal apoptosis by chelation treatment in rats: role of reactive oxygen species and intracellular Ca^{2+}. *J Pharmacol Exp Ther* **322:** 108–16.

Flora SJS, Mehta A, Mittal M (2008) Heavy metal induced oxidative stress and its possible reversal by chelation therapy. *Ind J Med Res* **128:** 221–43.

Flora SJS, Mittal M, Mishra D (2009) Co-exposure to arsenic and fluoride on oxidative stress, glutathione linked enzymes, biogenic amines and DNA damage in mouse brain. *J Neurol Sci* **285:** 198–205.

Floris B, Bomboi G, Sechi P, Pirino S, Marongiu ML (2000) Cadmium chronic administration to lactating ewes: reproductive performance, cadmium tissue accumulation and placental transfer. *Ann Chem* **90:** 703–8.

Fotakis G, Cemeli E, Anderson D, Timbrell JA (2005) Cadmium chloride-induced DNA and lysosomal damage in a hepatoma cell line. *Toxicol in Vitro* **19:** 481–9.

Fotakis G, Timbrell JA (2006) Role of trace elements in cadmium chloride uptake in hepatoma cell lines. *Toxicol Lett* **164:** 97–103.

Fry RC, Navasumrit P, Valiathan C, Svensson, JP, Hogan1 BJ, Luo M, Bhattacharya S, Kandjanapa K, Soontararuks S, Nookabkaew S, Mahidol C, Ruchirawat M, Samson LD (2007) Activation of iInflammation/NF-jB signaling in infants born to arsenic-exposed mothers. *PLoS Genet* **3:** 2180–9.

Hall AH (2002) Chronic arsenic poisoning. *Toxicol Lett* **128:** 69–72.

Hall M, Gamble M, Slavkovich V, Liu X, Levy D (2007) Determinants of arsenic metabolism: blood arsenic metabolites, plasma folate, cobalamin, and homocysteine concentrations in maternal-newborn pairs. *Environ Health Perspect* **115:** 1503–9.

Hastings L, Miller ML (1998) *Handbook of Developmental Neurotoxicology*. Academic Press, NY.

He W, Greenwell RJ, Brooks DM, Calderon-Garciduenas L, Beall HD, Coffin JD (2007) Arsenic exposure in pregnant mice disrupts placental vasculogenesis and causes spontaneous abortion. *Toxicol Sci* **99:** 244–53.

He L, Wang B, Hay EB, Nebert DW (2009) Discovery of ZIP transporters that participate in cadmium damage to testis and kidney. *Toxicol Appl Pharmacol* **238:** 250–7.

Henson MC, Chedrese PJ (2004). Endocrine disruption by cadmium, a common environmental toxicant with paradoxical effects on reproduction. *Exp Biol Med* **229:** 383–92.

Hernandez-Ochoa I, Sanchez-Gutierrez M, Solis-Heredia MJ, Quintanilla-Vega B (2006) Spermatozoa nucleus takes up lead during the epididymal maturation altering chromatin condensation. *Reprod Toxicol* **21:** 171–8.

Hopenhayn-Rich C, Browning SR, Hertz-Picciotto I, Ferreccio C, Peralta C, Gibb H (2000) Chronic arsenic exposure and risk of infant mortality in two areas of Chile. *Environ Health Perspect* **108:** 667–73.

Hsu P, Chang H, Guo YL, Liu Y, Shih T (2009) Effect of smoking on blood lead levels in workers and role of reactive oxygen species in lead-induced sperm chromatin DNA damage. *Fertility and Sterility* **91:** 1096–103.

Hughes MF, Kenyon EM, Edwards BC, Mitchell CT, Razo LM, Thomas DJ (2003) Accumulation and metabolism of arsenic in mice after repeated oral administration of arsenate. *Toxicol Appl Pharmacol* **191:** 202–10.

Iavicoli I, Garelli G, Stanek EJ, Castellino N, Li Z, Calaabrese EJ (2006) Low doses of dietary lead are associated with a profound reduction in the time to the onset of puberty in female mice. *Reprod Toxicol* **22:** 586–90.

Irvine L, Boyer IJ, DeSesso JM (2006) Monomethylarsonic acid and dimethylarsinic acid: developmental toxicity studies with risk assessment. *Birth Defects Res (Part B)* **77:** 53–68.

Ishitobi H, Watanabe C (2005) Effects of low-dose perinatal cadmium exposure on tissue zinc and copper concentrations in neonatal mice and on the reproductive development of female offspring. *Toxicol Lett* **159:** 38–46.

Jana K, Jana S, Samanta PK (2006) Effects of chronic exposure to sodium arsenite on hypothalamo–pituitary–testicular activities in adult rats: possible an estrogenic mode of action. *Reprod Biol Endocrinol* **4:** 1–13.

Jauniaux E, Burton GJ (2007) Morphological and biological effects of maternal exposure to tobacco smoke on the feto-placental unit. *Early Hum Dev* **83:** 699–706.

Jones MM (1991) New developments in therapeutic chelating agents as antidotes for metal poisoning. *Crit Rev Toxicol* **21:** 209–33.

Kasperczyk A, Kasperczyk S, Horak S, Ostalowska A, Grucka-Mamczar E, Romuk E, Olejek A, Birkner E (2008) Assessment of semen function and lipid peroxidation among lead exposed men. *Toxicology and Applied Pharmacology* **228:** 378–84.

Kawai M, Swan KF, Green AE, Edwards DE, Anderson MB, Henson MC (2002) Placental endocrine disruption induced by cadmium: effects on P450 cholesterol side-chain cleavage and 3beta-hydroxysteroid dehydrogenase enzymes in cultured human trophoblasts. *Biol Reprod* **67:** 178–83.

Kim J, Soh J (2009) Cadmium-induced apoptosis is mediated by the translocation of AIF to the nucleus in rat testes. *Toxicol Lett* **188:** 45–51.

Kippler M, Hoque AM, Raqib R, Ohrvik H, Ekström EC, Vahter M (2010) Accumulation of cadmium in human placenta interacts with the transport of micronutrients to the fetus. *Toxicol Lett* **192:** 162–8.

Kitchin KT, Ahmed S (2003) Oxidative stress as a possible mode of action for arsenic carcinogenesis. *Toxicol Lett* **137:** 3–13.

Klomberg KF, Garland Jr T, Swallow JG, Carter PA (2002) Dominance, plasma testosterone levels, and testis size in house mice artificially selected for high activity levels. *Physiol Behav* **77:** 27–38.

Koller K, Brown T, Spurgeon A, Levy L (2004) Recent developments in low-level lead exposure and intellectual impairment in children. *Environ Health Perspect* **112:** 987–94.

Kusakabe T, Nakajima K, Nakazato K, Suzuki K, Takada H, Satoh T, Oikawa M, Arakawa K, Nagamine T (2008) Changes of heavy metal, metallothionein and heat shock proteins in Sertoli cells induced by cadmium exposure. *Toxicol in Vitro* **22:** 1469–75.

Lammon CA, Hood RD (2004) Effects of protein deficient diets on the developmental toxicity of inorganic arsenic in mice. *Birth Defects Research (Part B)* **71:** 124–34.

Lammon CA, Le XC, Hood RD (2003) Pretreatment with periodate-oxidized adenosine enhances developmental toxicity of inorganic arsenic in mice. *Birth Defects Res (Part B)* **68:** 335–43.

Lanphear BP, Hornung R, Khoury J, Yolton K, Baghurst P, Bellinger DC, Canfield RL, Dietrich KN, Bornschein R, Greene T, Rothenberg SJ, Needleman HL, Schnaas L, Wasserman G, Graziano J, Roberts R (2005) Low-level environmental lead exposure and children's intellectual function: an international pooled analysis. *Environ Health Perspect* **113:** 894–9.

Lee NY, Choi HM, Kang YS (2009a) Choline transport via choline transporter-like protein 1 in conditionally immortalized rat syncytiotrophoblast cell lines TR-TBT. *Placenta* **30:** 368–74.

Lee CK, Lee JT, Yu SJ, Kang SG, Moon CS, Choi YH, Kim JH, Kim DH, Son BC, Lee CH, Kim HD, Ahn JH (2009b) Effects of cadmium on the expression of placental lactogens and Pit-1 genes in the rat placental trophoblast cells. *Mol Cell Endocrinol* **298:** 11–18.

Leoni G, Bogliolo L, Deiana G, Berlinguer F, Rosati I, Pintus PP, Ledda S, Naitana S (2002) Influence of cadmium exposure on in vitro ovine gamete dysfunction. *Reprod Toxicol* **16:** 371–7.

Li CS, Loch-Caruso R (2007) Sodium arsenite inhibits migration of extravillous trophoblast cells *in vitro*. *Reprod Toxicol* **24:** 296–302.

Li L, Ekström EC, Goessler W, Lönnerdal B, Nermell B, Yunus M, Rahman A, El Arifeen S, Persson LA, Vahter M (2008) Nutritional status has marginal influence on the metabolism of inorganic arsenic in pregnant Bangladeshi women. *Environ Health Perspect* **116:** 315–21.

Lin S, Hwang S, Marshall EG, Stone RR, Chen J (1996) Fertility rates among lead workers and professional bus drivers: a comparative study. *Ann Epidemiol* **6:** 201–8.

Liu J, Yua L, Coppina JF, Tokara EJ, Diwanc BA, Waalkesa MP (2009) Fetal arsenic exposure appears to facilitate endocrine disruption by postnatal diethylstilbestrol in neonatal mouse adrenal. *Chem Biol Interact* **182:** 253–8.

Liu Z, Sanchez MA, Jiang X, Boles E, Landfear SM, Rosen BP (2006) Mammalian glucose permease GLUT1 facilitates transport of arsenic trioxide and methylarsonous acid. *Biochem Biophys Res Commun* **351:** 424–30.

Llanos MN, Ronco AM (2009) Fetal growth restriction is related to placental levels of cadmium, lead and arsenic but not with antioxidant activities. *Reprod Toxicol* **27:** 88–92.

López E, Figueroa S, Oset-Gasque MJ, González MP (2003) Apoptosis and necrosis: two distinct events induced by cadmium in cortical neurons in culture. *Br J Pharmacol* **138:** 901–11.

Lu J, Chew EH, Holmgren A (2007) Targeting thioredoxin reductase is a basis for cancer therapy by arsenic trioxide. *Proc Natl Acad Sci* **104:** 12288–93.

Luck MR, Jeyaseelan I, Scholes RA (1995) Ascorbic acid and fertility. *Biol Reprod* **52:** 262–6.

Markowitz ME, Rosen JF (1990) Need for the lead mobilization test in children with lead poisoning. *J Pediatr* **119:** 305–10.

Martin MB, Voeller HJ, Gelmann EP, Lu J, Stoica EG, Hebert EJ, Reiter R, Singh B, Danielsen M, Pentecost E, Stoica A (2002) Role of cadmium in the regulation of AR gene expression and activity. *Endocrinology* **143:** 263–75.

Mason HJ (1990) Occupational cadmium exposure and testicular endocrine function. *Hum Exp Toxicol* **9:** 91–4.

Massrieh W, Derjuga A, Blank V (2006) Induction of endogenous Nrf2/small maf heterodimers by arsenic-mediated stress in placental choriocarcinoma cells. *Antioxid Redox Signal* **8:** 53–9.

Meachem SJ, Nieschlag E, Simoni M (2001) Inhibin B in male reproduction: pathophysiology and clinical relevance. *Eur J Endocrinol* **145:** 561–71.

Mehta A, Pant SC, Flora SJS (2006) Monoisoamyl dimercaptosuccinic acid induced changes in pregnant female rats during late gestation and lactation. *Reprod Toxicol* **21:** 94–103.

Miller R, Faber W, Asai M, Wier P, Di Sant P, Agnese A, Shah Y, Neth N (1992) Placental toxicity of cadmium and retinoids. *Placenta* **13:** 351–67.

Moorman WJ, Skaggs SR, Clark JC, Turner TW, Sharpnack DD, Murrell JA, Simon SD, Chapin RE, Schrader SM (1998) Male reproductive effects of lead, including species extrapolation for the rabbit model. *Reprod Toxicol* **12:** 333–46.

Nandi S, Gupta PS, Selvaraju S, Roy SC, Ravindra JP (2010) Effects of exposure to heavy metals on viability, maturation, fertilization, and embryonic development of buffalo (Bubalus bubalis) oocytes in vitro. *Arch Environ Contam Toxicol* **58:** 194–204.

Navarro PA, Liu L, Keefe DL (2004) *In vivo* effects of arsenite on meiosis, preimplantation development, and apoptosis in the mouse. *Biol Reprod* **70:** 980–5.

Needleman HL (2009) Low level lead exposure: history and discovery. *Ann Epidemiol* **19:** 235–8.

NRC (National Research Council) (2001) *Arsenic in Drinking Water: 2001 Update*. Washington DC: Natl. Acad. Press.

Ognjanović BI, Marković SD, Ethordević NZ, Trbojević IS, Stajn AS, Saičić ZS (2010) Cadmium-induced lipid peroxidation and changes in antioxidant defense system in the rat testes: protective role of coenzyme Q(10) and vitamin E. *Reprod Toxicol* **29:** 191–7.

Pace BM, Lawrence DA, Behr MJ, Parsons PJ, Dias JA (2005) Neonatal lead exposure changes quality of sperm and number of macrophages in testes of BALB/c mice. *Toxicology* **210:** 247–56.

Paksy K, Rajczy K, Forgács Z, Lázár P, Bernard A, Gáti I, Kaáli GS (1997) Effect of cadmium on morphology and steroidogenesis of cultured human ovarian granulosa cells. *J Appl Toxicol* **17:** 321–7.

Pant N, Murty RC, Srivastava SP (2004) Male reproductive toxicity of sodium arsenite in mice. *Human Exp Toxicol* **23:** 399–403.

Piasek M, Blanusa M, Kostial K, Laskey JW (2001) Placental cadmium and progesterone concentrations in cigarette smokers. *Reprod Toxicol* **15:** 673–81.

Pillai P, Patel R, Pandya C, Gupta S (2009) Sex-specific effects of gestational and lactational coexposure to lead and cadmium on hepatic phase I and phase II xenobiotic/steroid-metabolizing enzymes and antioxidant status. *J Biochem Mol Toxicol* **23:** 419–31.

Pine MD, Hiney JK, Dearth RK, Bratton GR, Dees WL (2006) IGF-1 administration to prepubertal female rats can overcome delayed puberty caused by maternal Pb exposure. *Reprod Toxicol* **21:** 104–9.

Prasenjit M, Mahua S, Parames S (2008) Protection of arsenic-induced testicular oxidative stress by arjunolic acid. *Redox Report* **13:** 67–77.

Prozialeck WC, Vaidya VS, Liu J, Waalkes MP, Edwards JR, Lamar PC, Bernard AM, Dumont X, Bonventre JV (2007) Kidney injury molecule-1 is an early biomarker of cadmium nephrotoxicity. *Kidney Int* **72:** 985–93.

Prozialeck WC, Edwards JR, Nebert DW, Woods JM, Barchowsky A, Atchison WD (2008) The vascular system as a target of metal toxicity. *Toxicol Sci* **102:** 207–18.

Qanungo S, Mukherjea M (2000) Ontogenic profile of some antioxidants and lipid peroxidation in human placental and fetal tissues. *Mol Cell Biochem* **215:** 111–19.

Rikans LE, Yamano T (2000) Mechanisms of cadmium-mediated acute hepatotoxicity. *J Biochem Mol Toxicol* **14:** 110–17.

Rodríguez VM, Jiménez-Capdeville ME, Giordano M (2003) The effects of arsenic exposure on the nervous system. *Toxicol Lett* **92:** 1–18.

Röllin HB, Rudge CV, Thomassen Y, Mathee A, Odland JO (2009) Levels of toxic and essential metals in maternal and umbilical cord blood from selected areas of South Africa – results of a pilot study. *J Environ Monit* **11:** 618–27.

Ronis MJ, Badger TM, Shema SJ, Roberson PK, Templer L, Ringer D, Thomas PE (1998) Endocrine mechanisms underlying the growth effects of developmental lead exposure in the rat. *J Toxicol Environ Health A* **54:** 101–20.

Rosen BP, Liu Z (2009) Transport pathways for arsenic and selenium: a minireview. *Environ Int* **35:** 512–15.

Saleh RA, Agarwal A, Nada EA, El-Tonsy MH, Sharma RK, Meyer A, Nelson DR, Thomas AJ (2003) Negative effects of increased sperm DNA damage in relation to seminal oxidative stress in men with idiopathic and male factor infertility. *Fertil Sterl* **79:** 1431–6.

Sanocka D, Kurpisz M (2004) Reactive oxygen species and sperm cells. *Reprod Bio Endocriol* **2:** 1–7.

Sarkar M, Chaudhuri GR, Chattopadhyay A, Biswas NM (2003) Effect of sodium arsenite on spermatogenesis, plasma gonadotrophins and testosterone in rats. *Asian J Androl* **5:** 27–31.

Satoh M, Kaji T, Tohyama C (2003) Low dose exposure to cadmium and its health effects. (3) Toxicity in laboratory animals and cultured cells. *Nippon Eiseigaku Zasshi* **57:** 615–23.

Shen JB, Jiang B, Pappano AJ (2000) Comparison of L-type calcium channel blockade by nifedipine and/or cadmium in guinea pig ventricular myocytes. *J Pharmacol Exp Ther* **294:** 562–70.

Shukla R, Bornschein RL, Dietrich KN, Buncher CR, Berger OG, Hammond PB, Succop PA (1989) Fetal and infant lead exposure: effects on growth in stature. *Pediatrics* **84:** 604–12.

Shukla R, Dietrich KN, Bornschein RL, Berger O, Hammond PB (1991) Lead exposure and growth in the early preschool child: a follow-up report from the Cincinnati Lead Study. *Pediatrics* **88:** 886–92.

Siu ER, Mruk DD, Porto CS, Cheng CY (2009) Cadmium-induced testicular injury. *Toxicol Appl Pharmacol* **238:** 240–9.

Srivastava V, Dearth RK, Hiney JK, Ramirez LM, Bratton GR, Dees WL (2004) The effects of low-level Pb on steroidogenic acute regulatory protein (StAR) in the prepubertal rat ovary. *Toxicol Sci* **77:** 35–40.

Stasenko S, Bradford EM, Piasek M, Henson MC, Varnai VM, Jurasovi J, Kusec V (2009) Metals in human placenta: focus on the effects of cadmium on steroid hormones and leptin. *J Appl Toxicol* **30:** 242–53.

Telisman S, Colak B, Pizent A, Jurasovic J, Cvitkovic P (2007) Reproductive toxicity of low-level lead exposure in men. *Environ Res* **105:** 256–66.

Thomas DJ, Li J, Waters SB, Xing W, Adair BM, Drobna Z, Devesa V, Styblo M (2007) Arsenic (+3 oxidation state) methyltransferase and methylation of arsenicals. *Exp Biol Med* **232:** 3–13.

Thompson J, Bannigan J (2008) Cadmium: toxic effects on the reproductive system and the embryo. *Reprod Toxicol* **25:** 304–15.

Tian LL, Zhao YC, Wang XC, Gu JL, Sun ZJ, Zhang YL, Wang JX (2009) Effects of gestational cadmium exposure on pregnancy outcome and development in the offspring at age 4.5 years. *Biol Trace Elem Res* **24:** 25–9.

Toscano CD, Guilarte TR (2005) Lead neurotoxicity: from exposure to molecular effects. *Brain Research Rev* **49:** 529–54.

Tremellen K (2008) Oxidative stress and male infertility – a clinical perspective. *Hum Reprod Update* **14:** 243–58.

Tripathi, N, Kannan, GM, Pant BP, Jaiswal DK, Malhotra PR, Flora SJS (1997) Arsenic-induced changes in certain neurotransmitter levels and their recoveries following chelation in rat whole brain. *Toxicol Lett* **145:** 1–18.

Tsutsumi R, Hiroi H, Momoeda M, Hosokawa Y, Nakazawa F, Yano T, Tsutsumi O, Taketani Y (2009) Induction of early decidualization by cadmium, a major contaminant of cigarette smoke. *Fertil Steril* **91:** 1614–17.

Uckun FM, Liub XP, D'Cruzc OJ (2002) Human sperm immobilizing activity of aminophenyl arsenic acid and its N-substituted quinazoline, pyrimidine, and purine derivatives: protective effect of glutathione. *Reprod Toxicol* **16:** 57–64.

US EPA (2002) User's Guide for the Integrated Exposure Uptake Biokinetic Model for Lead in Children (IEUBK). Environmental Protection Agency.

Vahter M (2009) Effects of arsenic on maternal and fetal health. *Annu Rev Nutr* **29:** 81–99.

Valko M, Rhodes CJ, Moncol J, Izakovic M, Mazur M (2006) Free radicals, metals and antioxidants in oxidative stress-induced cancer. *Chem Biol Interac* **160:** 1–40.

Virgintino D, Errede M, Robertson D, Capobianco C, Girolamo F, Vimercati A, Bertossi M, Roncali L (2004) Immunolocalization of tight junction proteins in the adult and developing human brain. *Histochem Cell Biol* **122:** 51–9.

Wang X, Sharma RK, Sikka SC, Thomas AJ Jr, Falcone T, Agarwal A (2003) Oxidative stress is associated with increased apoptosis leading to spermatozoa DNA damage in patients with male factor infertility. *Fertil Steril* **80:** 531–5.

Wang A, Holladay SD, Wolf DC, Ahmed SA, Robertson JL (2006) Reproductive and developmental toxicity of arsenic in rodents: a review. *Int J Toxicol* **25:** 319–31.

Wang Y-y, Sui K-x, Li H, Ma, H-y (2009) The effects of lead exposure on placental NF-κB expression and the consequences for gestation. *Repro Toxicol* **27:** 190–5.

WHO (World Health Organization) (2001) *IPCS Environmental Health Criteria 224, Arsenic and Arsenic Compounds*, second edition. International Program on Chemical Safety, WHO, Geneva.

WHO (World Health Organization) (2004) *Guidelines for Drinking-Water Quality*, third edition, Geneva.

Williams PL, Sergeyev O, Lee MM, Korrick SA, Burns JS, Humblet O, Delprato J, Revich B, Hauser R (2010) Blood lead levels and delayed onset of puberty in a longitudinal study of Russian boys. *Pediatrics.* In press.

Wong CH, Cheng CY (2005) The blood–testis barrier: its biology, regulation, and physiological role in spermatogenesis. *Curr Top Dev Biol* **71:** 263–96.

Working PK, Bus JS, Hamm Jr TE (1985) Reproductive effects of inhaled methyl chloride in the male Fischer 344 rat: II. Spermatogonial toxicity and sperm quality. *Toxicol Appl Pharmacol* **77:** 144–57.

Yancy SL, Shelden EA, Gilmont RR, Welsh MJ (2005) Sodium arsenite exposure alters cell migration, focal adhesion localization and decreases tyrosine phosphorylation of focal adhesion kinase in H9C2 myoblasts. *Toxicol Sci* **84:** 278–86.

Yu F, Liao Y, Jin Y, Zhao Y, Ren Y, Lu C, Li G, Li Y, Yang J (2008) Effects of in utero meso-2,3-dimercaptosuccinic acid with calcium and ascorbic acid on lead-induced fetal development. *Arch Toxicol* **82:** 453–9.

Zenzes MT (2000) Smoking and reproduction: gene damage to human gametes and embryos. *Hum Reprod Update* **6:** 122–31.

Zhang YM, Liu XZ, Lu H, Mei L, Liu ZP (2009) Lipid peroxidation and ultrastructural modifications in brain after perinatal exposure to lead and/or cadmium in rat pups. *Biomed Environ Sci* **22:** 423–9.

Zhao WW, Chen SJ (2005) Arsenic treatment for leukemia: new model of human cancer target treatment. *Zhongua Yi Xue Za Zhi* **85:** 439–40.

CHAPTER

34

Manganese

Dejan Milatovic, Ramesh C. Gupta, Zhaobao Yin, Snjezana Zaja-Milatovic and Michael Aschner

INTRODUCTION

Manganese (Mn) is a naturally occurring trace metal commonly found in the environment. It is the twelfth most abundant element in the earth's crust, present in rocks, soil, water and food. It does not occur naturally in a pure state and the most important Mn-containing minerals are oxides, carbonates and silicates (Post, 1999). Mn is utilized in numerous industrial processes including: (1) iron and steel production; (2) manufacture of dry cell batteries; (3) fuel oil additives and antiknock agents; (4) manufacture of glass; (5) production of potassium permanganate and other Mn chemicals; and (6) production of fungicides and tanning of leather (Saric, 1986). Mn is found in drinking water and is naturally present in food with the highest concentrations typically found in nuts, cereals, fruits, vegetables, grains and tea.

Mn is essential for maintaining the proper function and regulation of many biochemical and cellular reactions (Takeda, 2003) critical for humans, animals and plants. It is required for growth and development and plays a role in immune response, blood sugar homeostasis, adenosine triphosphate (ATP) regulation, reproduction, digestion and bone growth (Aschner and Aschner, 2005). Mn is a necessary component of numerous metalloenzymes, such as Mn superoxide dismutase, arginase, phosphoenol-pyruvate decarboxylase and glutamine synthase (Aschner and Aschner, 2005).

Despite its essentiality, Mn is a common environmental contaminant, which can cause toxic effects in humans. The brain, in particular, is highly susceptible to Mn toxicity. Increased concentrations in the brain can occur in a variety of conditions, with contributions to human morbidity stemming from occupational, iatrogenic, medical and environmental exposures (Burton and Guilarte, 2009). Excessive accumulation of Mn in specific brain areas, such as the substantia nigra (SN), the globus pallidus (GP) and the striatum, produce neurotoxicity leading to a degenerative brain disorder, referred to as manganism. It is characterized by clinical signs and morphological lesions similar to those seen in Parkinson's disease (PD) (Racette *et al.*, 2001). Patients suffering from manganism exhibit a signature biphasic model of physical decline comprising an initial phase of psychiatric disturbance and neurological deficits, which are followed by motor deficits, such as akinetic rigidity, dystonia and bradyskinesia (Calne *et al.*, 1994; Olanow, 2004; Dobson *et al.*, 2004).

In addition to neurological effects, Mn accumulation is also associated with reproductive and developmental effects. Some studies reported impaired fertility, impotence and libido in male workers afflicted with clinically identifiable signs of manganism attributed to occupational exposure to Mn for 1–21 days (Emara *et al.*, 1971; Rodier, 1955) and suggested that impaired sexual function in man may be one of the earliest clinical manifestations of Mn toxicity.

Adverse effects of Mn on the developing nervous system are also of special concern. While Mn deficiency may result in birth defects, poor bone formation and increased susceptibility to seizures (Aschner, 2000; Aschner *et al.*, 2002), excessive exposure to Mn in children is associated with a variety of adverse developmental effects, particularly relevant to their behavior and ability to learn and remember (Wasserman *et al.*, 2006). High dose exposure to Mn has been associated with increased fetal brain Mn concentrations (Kontur and Fechter, 1985) although several studies have reported the ability of the placenta to reduce systemic delivery of Mn to the fetal brain. Moreover, Mn plays a role in the modulation of the immune system, and in protein, lipid and carbohydrate metabolism (Addess *et al.*, 1997; Aschner *et al.*, 2002; Fitsanakis and Aschner, 2005; Malecki *et al.*, 1999). This chapter characterizes Mn toxicity effects and addresses future research needs for Mn.

HISTORICAL BACKGROUND

Mn intoxication cases have been described worldwide for almost two centuries. The discovery of the classic features of manganism is credited to James Couper (1837) with his first clear description of the adverse neurological effects of Mn in five Scottish men employed grinding Mn dioxide ore. The most prominent and earliest symptom was described as paraplegia, with lower extremities being markedly more affected than the upper extremities. Facial expression was vacant, with drooling and difficulty speaking. Couper's

Reproductive and Developmental Toxicology, Edited by Ramesh C. Gupta
ISBN: 978-0-12-382032-7

finding appeared about 20 years after James Parkinson's seminal description of "shaking palsy" (Parkinson, 2002) and about the same time as the description of other movement disorders, such as Huntington's chorea in 1842 and Wilson's disease in 1883 (Harper, 2002; Wexler, 2008). As Mn began to be used more widely in the steel alloy industry, more cases with similar symptoms were described (Von Jaksch, 1909) leading to clinical, toxicological and epidemiological evidence that implicated Mn as the cause of this neurological disease (Edsall *et al.*, 1919). Later, psychiatric symptoms, termed *lacura manganica* or "manganese madness", and three clinical phases were described in an extensive study with underground miners (Cotzias, 1958; Rodier, 1955). Prodromal phase was associated with general asthenia, anorexia and apathy. The intermediate phase was characterized by speech disorder, loss of facial expression and clumsy movement. In the established phase, symptoms progressed with obvious gait abnormalities, weakness, tremor and dystonia of the feet and hands (Lucchini *et al.*, 2009).

Since the earlier descriptions, cases of manganism have been reported in many smelters and miners (Schuler *et al.*, 1957; Wang *et al.*, 1989; Lucchini *et al.*, 2009). Manganism has been now described or suspected in a great variety of occupational and non-occupational settings. Subclinical and subfunctional declines in neurophysiological tests, mainly related to motor coordination of fine movements, have been documented not only following acute, high-level exposures, but also in the context of lower-level exposure. Such chronic exposures may progressively extend the site of Mn deposition and toxicity to different brain areas. Therefore, Mn exposure scenarios responsible for the occurrence of manganism in the last century generally have changed from the acute, high-level exposure to chronic exposure to much lower levels. In occupational settings, airborne concentrations of Mn in inhalable particles were often above a full-shift time-weighted average of $1\,mg/m^3$, considered as the minimum level able to cause manganism in susceptible individuals (WHO, 1981). Today, the exposure levels are generally around a time-weighted average value of $200\,\mu g/m^3$ in most ferro-alloy and mining operations (IEH/IOM, 2004). Exposure to Mn has extended to the general environment outside the workplace, with outdoor Mn concentrations approximately $40\,ng/m^3$ in urban areas (EPA, 2003) but can reach $300\,ng/m^3$ in the vicinity of sources such as ferro-alloy facilities and power plants (WHO, 2004). Concern has been also raised regarding the content of Mn in drinking water and the associated neurobehavioral impairment in children (Wasserman *et al.*, 2006; Bouchard *et al.*, 2007). In urban areas of the USA, the median groundwater concentration of Mn was found to be $150\,\mu g/l$, with approximately 3% of the sampled sources from the public water system supplied by groundwater, exceeding the US health reference level of $300\,\mu g/l$ (EPA, 2003).

Mn exposure may start before birth from the maternal exposure throughout inhalation and ingestion of food items from the environmental pollution. Excessive concentration of Mn may cause an overload that is potentially harmful to the fetus (Zota *et al.*, 2009). Postnatal exposure can also be relevant due to a relative high concentration of Mn in formulas (Aschner and Aschner, 2005) and continued exposures during childhood and adulthood from both environmental and occupational exposures.

PHARMACOKINETICS/ PHARMACODYNAMICS

The major routes of intake for Mn in humans are via inhalation and ingestion. Most reports deal with the uptake by inhalation due to the large numbers of occupationally exposed workers. In industrial processes, aerosols are generated containing inorganic Mn species, mainly oxides, which are classified according to the particle size in an inhalable fraction ($\leq 100\,\mu m$ diameter) and a respirable fraction ($\leq 4\,\mu m$) (Gunst *et al.*, 2000). Deposition within the pulmonary airway of the particulates containing Mn is dependent on the size, mass and density of the particle. In general, ultrafine particles that are inhaled are rapidly exhaled without being deposited in the lung, whereas particles ranging from 0.02 to $1\,\mu m$ are preferentially deposited in the lower airway (Pityn *et al.*, 1989; Yu *et al.*, 2000). Larger particles ($>5\,\mu m$), in general, fail to penetrate the smaller branches of the respiratory tract and are mainly deposited in the upper airway. In addition to the site of deposition, several other factors govern the biological availability of inhaled Mn and include the composition of Mn within the particulate matter, the time of exposure within the lung and how efficiently the metal is solubilized by macrophage within the lung. The solubilized metal that is released is presumably transported across the epithelial lining of the lung by transferrin-independent or -dependent processes that are dependent upon the valence state of solubilized Mn. Mn exists in 11 oxidation states (−3 to +7) but only Mn^{2+}, Mn^{3+} and Mn^{4+} are found in both animals and humans. If Mn^{3+} is released, it will bind avidly to transferrin present within the pulmonary fluid, whereas Mn^{2+} will bind to other proteins such as albumin (Wang *et al.*, 2002; Yang *et al.*, 2002).

The rate of clearance of Mn from the lung may influence Mn delivery to the brain and other organs. Mn can enter the CNS through the cerebral spinal fluid and by crossing the capillary endothelial membranes. Mainstream Mn entry into the brain from blood occurs through the capillary endothelial cells of the blood–brain barrier and through the cerebral spinal fluid via the choroid plexuses (Crossgrove and Yokel, 2005). Numerous studies confirmed that Mn is readily taken up within the nasal cavity in presynaptic nerve endings of axonal projections leading from the olfactory (Tjalve and Henriksson, 1999; Fechter *et al.*, 2002; Dobson *et al.*, 2003; Dorman *et al.*, 2002) and trigeminal nerves (Lewis *et al.*, 2005). Mn can cross synapses within the olfactory pathway and will travel along secondary and tertiary neurons to more distal sites within the brain (Tjälve *et al.*, 1996). How Mn crosses the blood–brain barrier (BBB) has been the subject of much investigation and it appears that several pathways are operative, including facilitated diffusion and active transport by DMT-1, ZIP8 and the transferrin receptor system (Aschner *et al.*, 2007). Mn accumulates in multiple brain regions including the basal ganglia, frontal cortex, pre-optic area and hypothalamus, as determined by analytical determination in autopsy samples (Yamada *et al.*, 1986) and by T1-weighted magnetic resonance imaging (MRI) (Aschner and Dorman, 2007). The greatest Mn concentrations accumulate in the globus pallidus. Using inhalation mimicking occupational exposures in humans, Dorman *et al.* (2006a) demonstrated that the globus pallidus in male rhesus monkeys accumulated Mn concentrations in a dose-dependent fashion ranging from 1.6- to 6.0-fold increase relative to control. An intravenous injection paradigm of Mn exposure produced an approximately 5-fold increase in pallidal Mn concentrations in monkeys (Guilarte *et al.*, 2006).

In the brain, Mn is taken up into astrocytes and neurons. Astrocytes serve as the major homeostatic regulator and storage site for Mn in the brain (Aschner *et al.*, 1999). Increased accumulation of Mn in astrocytes may alter release of glutamate and elicit excitatory neurotoxicity (Erikson and Aschner, 2003). Neuronal uptake of Mn involves transferrin (Suarez and Eriksson, 1993) and utilization of specific transporter systems, such as the dopamine transporter (DAT) (Anderson *et al.*, 2007; Chen *et al.*, 2006a). At the cellular level, Mn preferentially accumulates in mitochondria, where it disrupts oxidative phosphorylation and increases the generation of reactive oxygen species (ROS) (Gunter *et al.*, 2006).

Although food and drinking water may contain significant amounts of inorganic Mn, adverse health effects due to ingestion of excess Mn are seldom reported (ATSDR, 2000). However, for patients with total parenteral nutrition, often in combination with liver damage, Mn absorption is high and neurotoxic effects have been reported (Fell *et al.*, 1996). Manganese absorption from the gastrointestinal (GI) tract is complex and influenced not only by the amount of Mn in the diet but also by iron (Fe) and certain other nutrients. In particular, Fe deficiency is a frequent risk factor that can result in increased Mn absorption from the GI tract and enhanced brain delivery of Mn. Divalent Mn absorbed from the GI tract is generally bound to β-globulin and albumin, while trivalent Mn is bound to transferrin. Mn absorption from the GI tract is also dependent upon the age of the individual with neonates having appreciably higher absorption than adults (Dorman *et al.*, 2006b). For example, 20% of ingested Mn has been reported to be retained in term infants who are formula fed (Dorner *et al.*, 1989) versus 3–5% reported in adults. An additional factor that makes the neonate vulnerable to Mn excess is that the brain Mn uptake during the developmental period is relatively high (Aschner *et al.*, 2005).

Rodent studies of enhanced CNS uptake during development have been contradictory. While one study indicates that the amount of Mn that crosses the placenta was not increased by enhanced maternal exposure via diet (Jarvinen and Ahlstrom, 1975), another study indicated increased neonatal brain Mn following chronic high-level exposure of the dam to Mn in drinking water throughout gestation (Kontur and Fechter, 1985). Other studies also showed that, when compared with adults, neonatal rodents attain higher brain Mn levels following similar oral exposures (Dorman *et al.*, 2000; Kontur and Fechter, 1985). This tendency of neonates to attain higher brain Mn concentrations may reflect less than optimal blood–brain barrier, markedly reduced biliary Mn excretion rates and/or increased placental Mn concentration (Aschner *et al.*, 2005). However, an increase in the placental concentrations does not necessary mean higher placental transfer of Mn to the fetus or higher fetal exposure (Dorman *et al.*, 2005; Yoon *et al.*, 2009a). Additionally, brain Mn concentrations are higher in developing animals, suggesting that high amounts of Mn are required for normal brain development in infants (Keen *et al.*, 1986; Takeda *et al.*, 1999). Therefore, whether the relatively higher net increase in brain Mn observed in neonates compared to adults would pose an increased risk for neurotoxicity requires further understanding of the Mn requirements for normal brain development (Yoon *et al.*, 2009b).

MECHANISM OF ACTION

Mn is generally described as neurotoxicant selectively affecting basal ganglia structures. Although it is known that Mn is a cellular toxicant that can impair transport system, enzyme activity and receptor function, the principal manner in which Mn neurotoxicity occurs has not been clearly established (Aschner and Aschner, 1991; Aschner *et al.*, 2007). Early studies on the cellular actions of Mn reported that mitochondria are the principal intracellular repository for the metal (Cotzias and Greenough, 1958). More recent data indicate that mitochondria actively sequester Mn, resulting in rapid inhibition of oxidative phosphorylation (Gavin *et al.*, 1992). Manganese is bound to inner mitochondrial membrane or matrix proteins (Gavin *et al.*, 1990) and thus directly interacts with proteins involved in oxidative phosphorylation. Mn directly inhibits complex II (Singh *et al.*, 1974) and complexes I–IV (Zhang *et al.*, 2003) in brain mitochondria, and suppresses ATP-dependent calcium waves in astrocytes, suggesting that Mn promotes potentially disruptive mitochondrial sequestration of calcium (Tjalkens *et al.*, 2006). Elevated matrix calcium increases the formation of reactive oxygen species (ROS) by the electron transport chain (Kowaltowski *et al.*, 1995) and results in inhibition of aerobic respiration (Kruman and Mattson, 1999). Our recent studies with primary astrocytes and neurons have shown that Mn exposure induces increase in biomarkers of oxidative stress (Milatovic *et al.*, 2007, 2009). We have measured F_2-isoprostanes (F_2-IsoPs) (Morrow and Roberts, 1999; Milatovic and Aschner, 2009), a group of arachidonic acid-derived prostanoid isomers generated by free radical damage due to arachidonic acid and showed that astrocytes exposed to Mn concentrations known to elicit neurotoxic effects (100 μM, 500 μM or 1 mM), induced significant elevations in F_2-IsoPs levels at all investigated exposure times (Figure 34.1). Thus, increases in ROS, which are generated by electron leak from the electron transport chain (ETC) (Turrens and Boveris, 1980), potentially damaging mitochondria directly or through the effects of secondary oxidants like superoxide, H_2O_2 or peroxynitrite ($ONOO^-$), mediate Mn-induced oxidative damage. Moreover, superoxide produced in the mitochondrial electron transport chain may catalyze the transition shift of Mn^{2+} to Mn^{3+} through a set of reactions similar to those mediated by superoxide dismutase and thus lead to the increased oxidant capacity of this metal (Gunter *et al.*, 2006). Consequent oxidative damage produces an array of deleterious effects: it may cause structural and functional derangement of the phospholipids bilayer of membranes, disrupt energy metabolism, metabolite biosynthesis, calcium and iron homeostasis and initiate apoptosis (Uchida, 2003; Attardi and Schatz, 1988; Yang *et al.*, 1997).

Consistent with and preceding the Mn-induced increase in biomarkers of oxidative damage (F_2-IsoPs) (Figure 34.1), our study showed an early decrease in astrocytic ATP levels (Milatovic *et al.*, 2007). As a consequence, ATP depletion or a perturbation in energy metabolism might diminish the ATP-requiring neuroprotective action of astrocytes, such as glutamate and glutamine uptake and free radical scavenging (Rao *et al.*, 2001). In addition, depletion of high energy phosphates may affect intracellular Ca^{2+} in astrocytes through mechanisms involving the disruption of mitochondrial Ca^{2+} signaling. This assertion is supported by data showing that Mn inhibits Na^+-dependent Ca^{2+} efflux (Gavin *et al.*, 1990) and respiration in brain mitochondria (Zhang *et al.*, 2004),

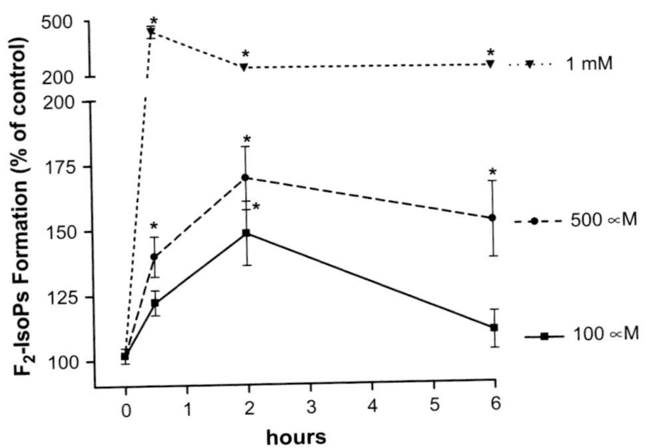

FIGURE 34.1 Effects of $MnCl_2$ on F_2-IsoPs formation in cultured astrocytes. Rat primary astrocyte cultures were incubated at 37°C in the absence or presence of $MnCl_2$ (100 μM, 500 μM or 1 mM), and F_2-IsoPs levels were quantified at 30 min, 2 h and 6 h. Data represent the mean ± SEM from three independent experiments. * Significant difference between values from control and Mn-treated astrocytes (* $p < 0.05$).

both critical for maintaining normal ATP levels and ensuring adequate intermitochondrial signaling. Decrease in ATP following Mn exposure is also associated with excitotoxicity, suggesting a direct effect on astrocytes with subsequent impairment of neuronal function. Mn downregulates the glutamate transporter GLAST in astrocytes (Erikson and Aschner, 2002) and decreases levels of glutamine synthase in exposed primates (Erikson *et al.*, 2008). Studies with a neonatal rat model indicated that both pinacidil, a potassium channel agonist, and nimodipine, a Ca^{2+}channel antagonist, reversed Mn neurotoxicity and loss of glutamine synthase activity, further indicating excitotoxicity in the mechanism of Mn-induced neurotoxicity. Excessive Mn may lead to excitotoxic neuronal injury both by decreased astrocytic glutamate uptake and by loss of ATP-mediated inhibition of glutamatergic synapses.

Another consequence of Mn-associated increased oxidative stress and mitochondrial energy failure is the induction of the mitochondrial permeability transition (MPT), a Ca^{2+}-dependent process characterized by the opening of the permeability transition pore (PTP) in the inner mitochondrial membrane. This process results in increased permeability to protons, ions and other solutes (Zoratti and Szabo, 1995), which subsequently leads to a collapse of the mitochondrial inner membrane potential ($\Delta\Psi_m$). Loss of the $\Delta\Psi_m$ results in colloid osmotic swelling of the mitochondria matrix, movement of metabolites across the inner membrane, defective oxidative phosphorylation, cessation of ATP synthesis and further generation of ROS. We and others have shown a concentration-dependent effect of Mn on the mitochondrial inner membrane potential in cultured astrocytes (Figure 34.2) (Milatovic *et al.*, 2007; Rao and Norenberg, 2004). Studies by Zhang *et al.* (2004) have shown that high levels of Mn chloride (1 mM) cause a significant dissipation of the $\Delta\Psi_m$ in isolated rat brain mitochondria, consistent with induction of the MTP.

Oxidative stress as an important mechanism in Mn-induced neurotoxicity is also confirmed in our *in vivo* model. Analyses of cerebral biomarkers of oxidative damage revealed that one-time challenge of mice with Mn (100 mg/kg) was sufficient to produce significant increases in F_2-IsoPs (Table 34.1) 24 hours following the last injection, respectively. Increased striatal concentrations of ascorbic acid and glutathione (GSH), antioxidants that when increased signal the presence of an elevated burden from ROS, as well as other markers of oxidative stress, have been previously reported (Desole *et al.*, 1994; Dobson *et al.*, 2004; Erikson *et al.*, 2007). Mn-induced decrease in GSH and increased methallothionine was reported in rats (Dobson *et al.*, 2003) and non-human primate studies (Erikson *et al.*, 2007). ROS may act in concert with reactive nitrogen species (RNS) derived from astroglia and microglia to facilitate the Mn-induced degeneration of DAergic neurons. DAergic neurons possess reduced antioxidant capacity, as evidenced by low intracellular GSH, which renders these neurons more vulnerable to oxidative stress and glial activation relative to other cell types (Sloot *et al.*, 1994; Greenamyre *et al.*, 1999). Therefore, the overactivation of glia and release of additional neurotoxic factors may represent a crucial component associated with the degenerative process of DAergic neurons.

In addition to decrease in mitochondrial membrane potential and the depletion of high energy phosphates, Mn-induced ROS generation is also associated with inflammatory responses and release of inflammatory mediators, including prostaglandins. Our studies have confirmed that in parallel with increase in biomarkers of oxidative damage, Mn exposure induced increase in biomarkers of inflammation, prostaglandin E_2 (PGE_2), *in vitro* and *in vivo* (Milatovic *et al.*, 2007, 2009). Results from our *in vivo* study showed that Mn exposure induced time-dependent increase in PGE_2 (Table 34.1). Recent studies have also shown inflammatory response of glial cells following Mn exposure (Chen *et al.*, 2006b; Zhang *et al.*, 2009; Zhao *et al.*, 2009). Mn potentiates lipopolysaccharide-induced increases in proinflammatory cytokines in glial cultures (Filipov *et al.*, 2005) and increase in nitric oxide production (Chang and Liu, 1999). An increase in proinflammatory genes, such as tumor necrosis factor-α, iNOS and activated inflammatory proteins such as P-p38, P-ERK and P-JNK, have been measured in primary rat glial cells after Mn exposure (Chen *et al.*, 2006b). However, data from our study indicate that release of proinflammatory mediators following Mn exposure is not only associated with glial response, but neurons as well, and suggest that these two events are mechanistically related, with neuroinflammation either alone or in combination with activated glial response contributing to oxidative damage and consequent cell injury.

In addition to dysregulation of excitatory glutamatergic neurotransmission, Mn exposure also induces dopaminergic and GABAergic neuronal dysfunction. It is known that *in vitro* Mn can promote autoxidation of dopamine, which leads to the creation of reactive quinones (Miller *et al.*, 1990; Shen and Dryhurst, 1998). However, rodent and non-human primate data offer conflicting evidence on the influence of Mn exposure on catecholamine concentrations (Eriksson *et al.*, 1987a; Olanov *et al.*, 1996; Struve *et al.*, 2007). Additional evidence from non-human primate data suggests an Mn-induced postsynaptic decrease of D2-like dopamine receptor levels (Eriksson *et al.*, 1992). Several rodent studies support an association between Mn exposure and increased brain GABA concentration (Gwiazda *et al.*, 2002; Reaney *et al.*, 2006). However, other rodent studies suggested that Mn decreases striatal and frontal cortex GABA levels (Brouillet *et al.*, 1993; Seth *et al.*, 1981) or no effect of Mn on GABA levels (Bonilla *et al.*, 1994). Additional findings

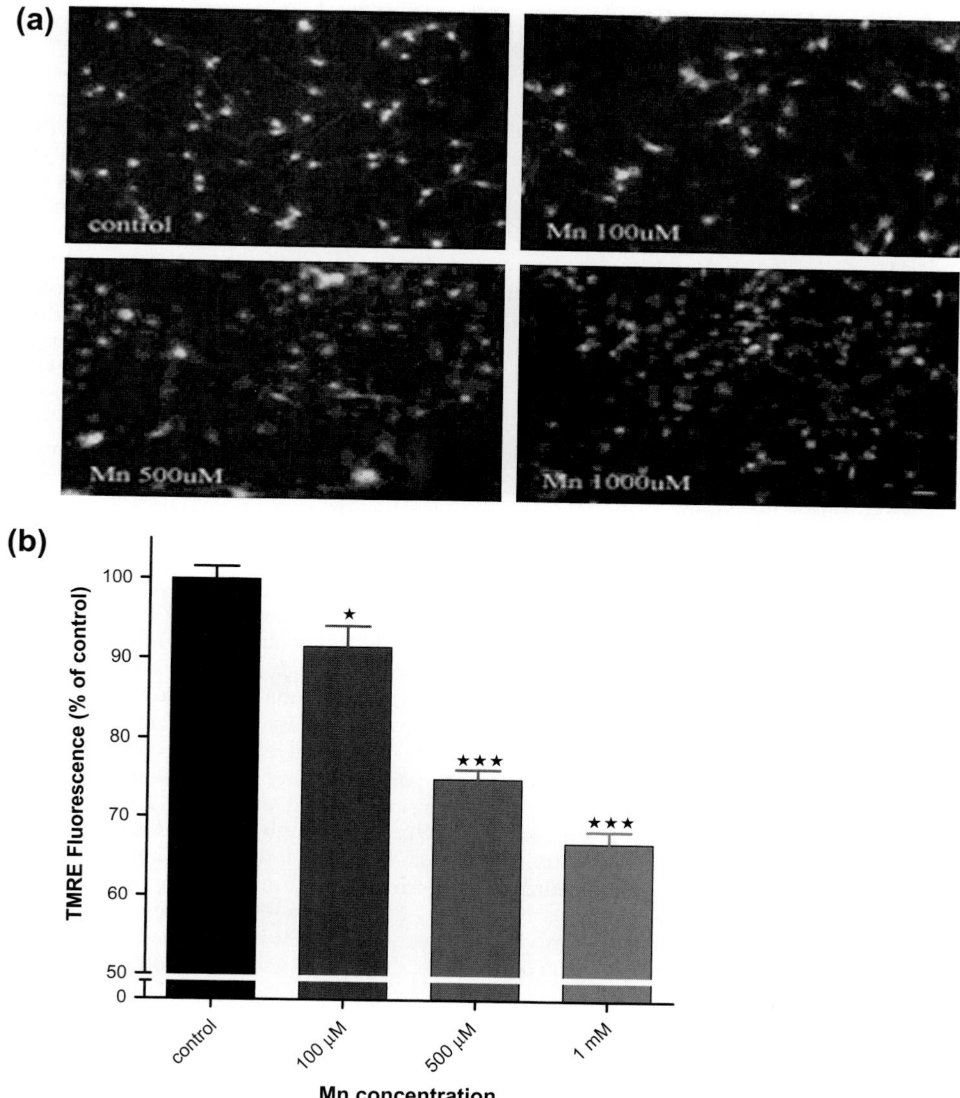

FIGURE 34.2 Quantitation of TMRE fluorescent intensities. Cultured astrocytes were exposed to $MnCl_2$ at various concentrations (0, 100 μM, 500 μM or 1 mM) for 1 h, and the fluorescent images ((A), quantified by using the NIH software, Scion Incorporation) expressed as percent fluorescence change from control (B). Values are expressed as mean ± SEM of 24 random fields in each group. * Significant difference between values from control and Mn-treated astrocytes (* $p<0.05$, *** $p<0.001$).

TABLE 34.1 Cerebral F_2-IsoPs and PGE_2 levels in saline (control) or $MnCl_2$ (100 mg/kg, s.c.) exposed mice. Brains from mice exposed once or three times (day 1, 4 and 7) to $MnCl_2$ were collected 24 h post last injection

Exposure	F_2-IsoPs (ng/g tissue)	PGE_2 (ng/g tissue)
Control (saline)	3.013 + 0.03939	9.488 0.3091
Single Mn	4.302 + 0.3900*	12.03 0.4987*
Multiple Mn	4.211 + 0.4013*	14.22 1.019*

Values of F_2-IsoPs represent mean ± SEM ($n=4$–6)
Significant difference between values from control and Mn-treated mice ($p<0.05$)

also suggest that in the absence of extracellular Ca^{2+}, Mn induces a long-lasting potentiation of acetylcholine (ACh) release from cardiac parasympathetic nerve terminals following titanic nerve stimulation (Kita *et al.*, 1981). In combination with gluatamate-gated cation channel activation, e.g. N-methyl-D-aspartate (NMDA) receptor, secondary excitotoxicity mechanisms play an important role in the development on Mn-induced neurodegeneration.

Several studies have also addressed gene expression changes in Mn-treated cells and animals and complex interaction of Mn with other minerals (Baek *et al.*, 2004; HaMai *et al.*, 2006). Mn-induced expression changes were noted in genes involved in inflammation, DNA replication and repair. Recent work in non-human primates (Guilarte *et al.*, 2008) detected Mn-induced brain gene expression changes associated mainly with genes affecting apoptosis, protein folding and degradation, inflammation and axonal/vesicular transport. In a developmental rat model of chronic Mn toxicity, administration of Mn in drinking water was associated with increased levels of iron, copper, selenium and calcium in various brain regions. The biochemical mechanisms underlying the interaction between Mn and other minerals are unclear.

TOXICITY

Mn toxicity is mostly associated with a neurological disorder referred to as manganism. Symptoms of manganism include irritability, aggressiveness, hallucinations, tremors, difficulty in walking and facial muscle spasm. Some studies also suggest that Mn inhalation can induce cognitive effects, including difficulty with concentration and memory problems (Flynn and Susi, 2009). However, manganism is not only an occupational disease, it is also associated with patients with chronic liver failure (due to impaired biliary excretion of Mn, Hauser *et al.*, 1994), chronic iron deficiency (mostly due to Fe/Mn competition for transporters, Boojar *et al.*, 2002; Roth and Garrick, 2003), subjects on parenteral nutrition (Fell *et al.*, 1996), patients in chronic renal failure undergoing hemodialysis (da Silva *et al.*, 2007; Ohtake *et al.*, 2005) and subjects with genetic deficits affecting Mn homeostasis (Tuschl *et al.*, 2008).

Features of manganism reflect alterations in the integrity of DAergic striatal neurons and DA neurochemistry, including decreased DA transport function and/or striatal DA levels. The striatum is a major recipient structure of neuronal efferents in the basal ganglia. It receives excitatory input from the cortex and dopaminergic input from substantia nigra and projects to the internal segment of the globus pallidus (Dimova *et al.*, 1993; Saka *et al.*, 2002). Nigrostriatal dopamine neurons appear to be particularly sensitive to Mn-induced toxicity (Defazio *et al.*, 1996; Sloot and Gramsbergen, 1994; Sloot *et al.*, 1994). Intense or prolonged Mn exposure in adulthood causes long-term reductions in striatal DA levels and induces a loss of autoreceptor control over DA release (Autissier *et al.*, 1982; Komura and Sakamoto, 1992). Nigrostriatal DA axons synapse onto striatal medium spiny neurons (MSNs), and these neurons have radially projecting dendrites that are densely studded with spines (Wilson and Groves, 1980). Postmortem studies of PD patients have revealed a marked decrease in MSN spine density and dendritic length (Stephens *et al.*, 2005; Zaja-Milatovic *et al.*, 2005). Similar morphological changes in MSNs were seen in animal models of Parkinsonism (Arbuthnott *et al.*, 2000; Day *et al.*, 2006). Our recent study investigated the effects of Mn on degeneration of striatal neurons. Representative images of Golgi impregnated striatal sections with their traced MSNs from control and Mn-exposed animals are presented in Figure 34.3. Images of neurons with Neurolucida-assisted morphometry show that Mn-induced oxidative damage and neuroinflammation targeted the dendritic system with profound dendrite regression of striatal MSNs. While single Mn exposure altered the integrity of the dendritic system and induced significant decrease in spine number (Figure 34.4a) and total dendritic lengths (Figure 34.4b) of MSNs, prolonged Mn exposure led to further reduction in spine number and dendritic length. Our results indicate that MSN neurodegeneration could result from loss of spines, removing the pharmacological target for DA-replacement therapy, without overt MSN death (Stephens *et al.*, 2005; Zaja-Milatovic *et al.*, 2005).

Despite similarities, manganism and PD differ pathologically. In humans and animals with chronic Mn poisoning, lesions are more diffuse, found mainly in the pallidum, caudate nucleus, the putamen and even in the cortex with no effects on the substantia nigra and no Lewy bodies (Pal *et al.*, 1999; Perl and Olanov, 2007). In people with PD, lesions are found in the substantia nigra and other pigmented areas of the brain (Barbeau, 1984) with almost always the presence of Lewy bodies (Calne *et al.*, 1994; Perl and Olanov, 2007). Mn neurotoxicity can continue in the absence of continuing Mn exposure and that a spectrum of response to excess Mn exposure can be seen depending upon dose, duration of exposure and timing of the observation. While some subclinical manifestation of Mn neurotoxicity will resolve, once neuropathology has occurred (in the form of loss of DAergic neurons), then reversal becomes more limited and is restricted to functional compensation.

There is conflicting evidence from human studies for whether occupational exposure to Mn causes adverse reproductive effects. Studies in men occupationally exposed to Mn reported increased sexual dysfunction and reduced sperm quality (Jiang *et al.*, 1996; Wu *et al.*, 1996). Impaired fertility (measured as a decreased number of children/married couples) has been observed in male workers exposed for 1–19 years to Mn dust ($0.97\,mg/m^3$) at levels that did not produce obvious manganism (Lauwerys *et al.*, 1985). This suggests that impaired sexual function in men may be one of the earliest clinical manifestations of manganism, but no dose–response information was presented so it is not possible to define a threshold for this effect. No studies reported reproductive effects in women.

Evidence obtained from laboratory animals indicates that exposure to high levels of Mn may adversely affect sperm quality (Elbetieha *et al.*, 2001; Ponnapakkam *et al.*, 2003a,b) produce decreased testicular weights (Laskey *et al.*, 1982) and impair development of the male reproductive tract. Impaired fertility was observed in male mice exposed to Mn in drinking water for 12 weeks at a daily dose level of 309 mg/kg/day, but not at doses ≤154 mg/kg/day (Elbetieha *et al.*, 2001). At lower dose levels in another study, decreased sperm motility and sperm counts were observed in male CD-1 mice after 43 days of exposure to manganese acetate at doses of 4.6 to 9.6 mg/kg/day, but these doses did not impair the ability of these males to impregnate unexposed females (Ponnapakkam *et al.*, 2003a,b). Szakmary *et al.* (1995) reported that Mn did not result in any reproductive effect in the rabbit when exposed to 11, 22 and 33 mg/kg/day on GDs 6–20. In 13-week dietary studies, no gross or histopathological lesions or organ weight changes were observed in reproductive organs of rats fed up to 618 mg Mn/kg/day or mice fed up with 1,950 mg Mn/kg/day.

There is evidence to suggest that children exposed to high levels of Mn in drinking water may develop a variety of adverse developmental effects, particularly relevant to their behaviors and ability to learn and remember. However, it is not clear whether other genetic or environmental factors are responsible for these changes in the presence of Mn, or whether Mn alone can produce diminished memory, attention deficit and/or hyperactivity. He *et al.* (1994) reported that children exposed to high Mn levels ($0.241 \pm 0.051\,mg/l$ for 3 years in drinking water) performed more poorly on the WHO neurobehavioral score tests than control children. In addition, blood and hair Mn concentrations of exposed children were significantly higher than those of control populations. Zhang *et al.* (1995) reported that the children with increased Mn exposure also performed more poorly in school and their serum levels of serotonin, norepinephrine, dopamine and acetylcholinesterase activity were significantly decreased compared to control. Recent cross-sectional investigation of intellectual functions of 10-year-old children in Bangladesh, who had consumed tube-well water with an average concentration of 793 mg Mn/l, also reported significant decrements

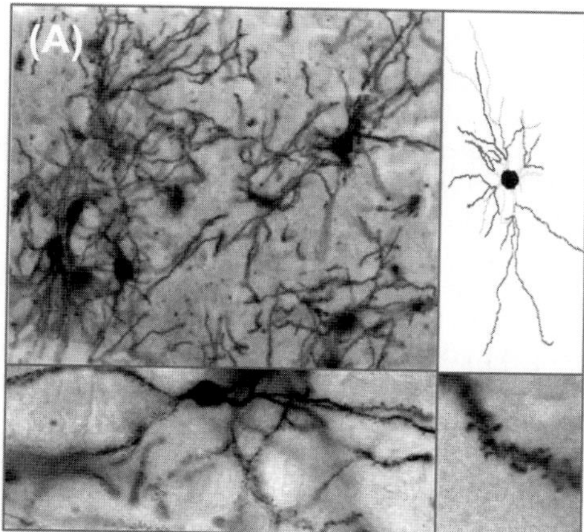

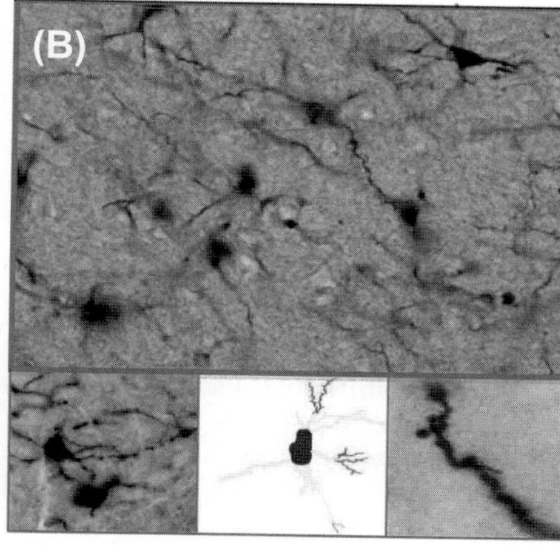

FIGURE 34.3 Photomicrographs of mouse striatal sections with representative tracings of medium spiny neurons (MSNs) from mice treated with saline (control) (A) or $MnCl_2$ (100 mg/kg, s.c.) (B). Brain from mouse exposed three times (day 1, 4 and 7) to $MnCl_2$ was collected 24 h post last injection. Treatment with Mn-induced degeneration of striatal dendritic system, decrease in total number of spines and length of dendrites of MSNs. Tracing and counting are done using a Neurolucida system at 100× under oil immersion (MicroBrightField, VT). Colors indicate the degree of dendritic branching (yellow = 1°, red = 2°, purple = 3°, green = 4°, turquoise = 5°). Please refer to color plate section.

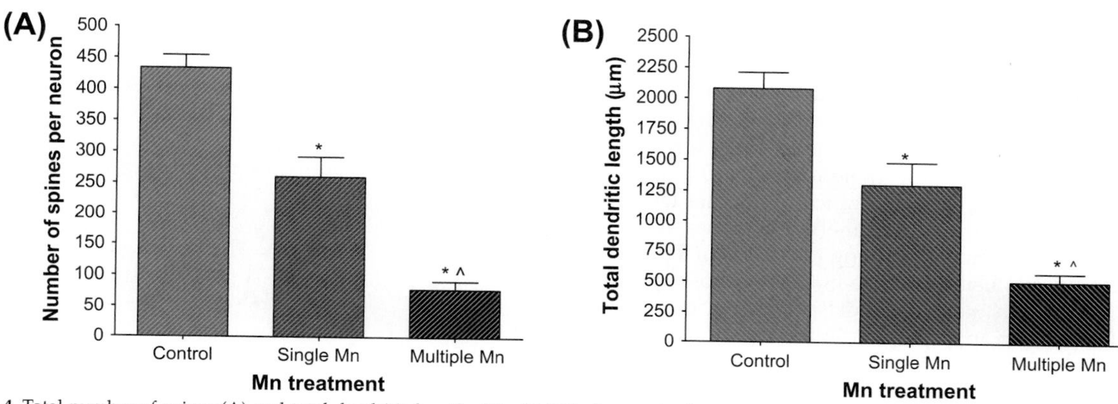

FIGURE 34.4 Total number of spines (A) and total dendritic lengths (B) of MSNs from striatal sections of mice exposed to saline (control), single Mn injection (100 mg/kg, s.c.) or multiple Mn injections (100 mg/kg, s.c.) on day 1, 4 and 7. Mice were sacrificed 24 hours after the last injection. * Significant difference between values from control and Mn-treated mice (* $p < 0.01$). ^ Significant difference between values from single Mn injection vs. multiple (8 days) Mn treatment (^ $p < 0.001$).

in several forms of intellectual performances (Wasserman *et al.*, 2006). A study by Vigeh *et al.* (2008) reported that maternal blood Mn is associated with the risk of intrauterine growth retardation.

Many developmental toxicity studies in animals exposed to Mn have focused on possible effects on reproductive and neurological functions. Several animal studies have shown that Mn exposure decreased the growth of reproductive organs (preputial gland, seminal vesicle and testes) (Gray and Laskey, 1980) with testes weights in males being significantly decreased from controls only when Mn was administered in conjunction with an iron-poor diet (Laskey *et al.*, 1982). Studies in neonatal animals have detected neostructural and neurochemical changes at doses of Mn similar to or slightly above dietary levels (1–10 mg Mn/kg/day) (Chandra and Shukla, 1978; Deskin *et al.*, 1980), suggesting that young animals might be more susceptible to Mn than adults. Another study by Dorman *et al.* (2000) also suggested that neonatal rats are at greater risk than adults for Mn-induced neurotoxicity when compared under similar exposure conditions. Their study showed that oral Mn exposure (11 or 22 mg/kg/day for 21 days) induced a significant increase in amplitude of the acoustic startle reflex and increase in striatal DA and DOPAC concentrations in the high dose-treated neonates. In a similar study, neonatal rats exposed to Mn (0.31 mg Mn/kg/day for 60 days in water) suffered neuronal degeneration and increased brain monoamine oxidase on day 15 and 30 of the study, but did not show any clinical or behavioral signs of neurotoxicity (Chandra and Shukla, 1978). Developmental studies involving the use of laboratory animals have also detected subtle changes in growth (decreased body weight in animals provided with relatively high doses on Mn). These changes were observed both when the animals were exposed while *in utero* and postpartum when animals have already been born.

RISK ASSESSMENT

To assess health risks, qualitative and quantitative health effects information must be related to available exposure information. Exposure guidelines for ambient inhalation exposure to Mn include the US Environmental Protection

Agency reference concentration (RfC) of 0.05 μg/m^3, the World Health Organization (WHO) air quality guideline of 0.15 μg/m^3 and the Agency for Toxic Substances and Disease Registry (ATSDR) minimum risk level of 0.4 μg/m^3. The oral exposure recommendations and guidelines include EPA's oral reference concentration of 0.14 mg/kg/day, EPA's maximum contaminant level (MCL) of 0.05 mg/l in water (based on esthetic properties) and the WHO drinking water guideline of 0.4 mg/l (health-based) (EPA US, 2006).

The most significant exposure for the general population is from food, with an average ingestion rate of 3,800 mg/day (EPA, 1984). Even though gastrointestinal absorption of Mn is low (3–5%), oral exposure is the primary source of absorbed Mn. People ingesting large amounts of food high in Mn have potential for higher-than-usual exposure. This group would include vegetarians who ingest a larger proportion of grains, legumes and nuts in their diets than the average US population, and heavy tea drinkers. In addition to the population with these dietary habits, individuals with iron deficiency show increased rates of Mn absorption. Iron deficiency leads to increased brain Mn concentrations in experimental animals (Aschner and Aschner, 1990). However, in the workplace, exposure to Mn is most likely to occur by inhalation of Mn fumes or Mn-containing dust. This is of concern mainly in the ferromanganese, iron and steel, dry-cell battery, welding, mining and ore processes industries. While airborne Mn levels in a metal-producing plant in the USA were reported as 0.066 mg/m^3 (mean) as respirable dust and 0.18 mg/m^3 in total dust (Gibbs *et al.*, 1999), significantly higher levels of Mn were reported in factories and smelting facilities in China ranging from 0.3 to 2.9 mg/m^3 (Jiang *et al.*, 2007). Thus, for workers in industries using Mn, the major route of exposure is via inhalation from workplace air rather than from food ingestion. In addition, populations living in the vicinity of ferromanganese or iron and steel manufacturing facilities or hazardous waste sites may also be exposed to elevated Mn particulate matter in air or water, although this exposure is likely to be much lower than in the workplace. In comparison to other groups within the general population, persons living close to high density traffic areas, automotive workers and taxi drivers may be exposed to higher concentrations of Mn arising from the combustion of methylcyclopentadienyl manganese tricarbonyl (MMT) because the levels of respirable Mn both indoor and outdoor air near an expressway with high traffic density were shown to be greater than corresponding air samples obtained from a rural location (Bolte *et al.*, 2004).

Mn exposure of children is of particular concern. Mn exposure during a restricted period during early development might induce permanent or irreversible damage to the developing CNS. Previous work comparing the neurotoxic effects of Mn in rats at different ages (Soliman *et al.*, 1995; Vitarella *et al.*, 1996) support concern about greater sensitivity to Mn neurotoxicity during early development. Young children could be at higher risk because of metabolic differences, as suggested by the fact that homeostatic mechanisms for regulating Mn absorption and elimination are not well developed in infants (Lonnerdal, 1989; Bell *et al.*, 1989; Mena, 1981).

The elderly are another population of concern. Over time, Mn body burdens and/or small impairments in neurobehavioral function may accumulate. If neurobehavioral function is already compromised by the normal aging processes or disease states (e.g., preclinical Parkinsonism), the ability to compensate for declines in neurobehavioral function could be eventually overwhelmed by additional insults attributable to Mn (Dawson *et al.*, 1995; Desole *et al.*, 1995).

Another condition able to increase risk of manganism in Mn-exposed individuals may be represented by subclinical impairment of liver function. Mn is almost totally excreted via the biliary system, and therefore any impairment of this pathway is potentially able to cause Mn overload due to insufficient elimination from the body. This is well known in the case of cirrhotic patients showing Mn-related abnormalities, where the liver encephalopathy may be partially explained by excessive Mn in the brain (Rovira *et al.*, 2008).

For assessment of Mn exposure it is important to evaluate biomarkers of exposure, effect and susceptibility. However, reliable exposure biomarkers or specific early biomarkers of effects, such as preclinical neurobehavioral or neurological changes, have not been established for Mn. At present, there is no reliable biomarker of whole body Mn status. Plasma and serum analyses are very variable and generally not good indicators of body stores. Erythrocytes or whole blood Mn concentrations are more accurate and reproducible. A range of 70–280 nmol/l (3.9–15.4 μg/l) in whole blood provides a practical reference for "normal" values. Whole blood Mn also correlates with MRI signal intensity. Brain MRI scans and a battery of specific neurobehavioral tests (Greger, 1998) have been useful in assessing Mn exposure even among industrial workers exposed to airborne Mn (Nelson *et al.*, 1993). These scans also have been successfully used to identify accumulation of Mn in the brains of children exposed to excess Mn (Sahni *et al.*, 2007).

TREATMENT

Treatment of manganism produces various outcomes among patients. Symptom severity increases, and chances of recovery decreases with prolonged Mn exposure; therefore it is important to immediately remove the patient from the source of Mn. Some studies with severe cases of Mn poisoning suggest that chelation therapy may be considered to reduce the body burden of Mn and to alleviate the symptoms. Chelators bind metal ions in a stable form and the compound chelator + metal are then excreted by the urinary and/or biliary routes. Ethylenediaminetatraacetic acid (EDTA) is a polyaminocarboxylic acid that chelates many divalent metals, a property that finds commercial application as a metal sequestrant in food additives. Several studies suggested that EDTA successfully increased Mn excretion in urine and decreased Mn concentration in blood. However, patients did not show significant improvement in their symptoms (Crossgrove and Zheng, 2004; Jiang *et al.*, 2006). Since EDTA cannot effectively chelate and remove Mn ions from brain and damaged neurons, it appears to be of limited therapeutic value for more advanced cases of manganism.

Anti-Parkinsonian drugs, such as levodopa, have been shown to reverse some of the neuromuscular signs of manganism (Ejima *et al.*, 1992). However, this drug can produce a variety of side effects and reports have indicated that levodopa is not effective in improving the symptoms of neurotoxicity in manganism patients (Herrero Hernández *et al.*, 2006), presumably because the nigrostriatal pathway remains intact in manganism. Moreover, levodopa is contraindicated in manganism, as Mn catalyzes autoxidation to toxic quinones and semoquinones (Loyd, 1995; Parenti *et al.*, 1988).

Since Mn has been shown to catalyze the oxidation of dopamine *in vitro* and production of dopamine quinine and hydrogen peroxide, it was also suggested that antioxidants may be effective in suppressing Mn toxicity. In addition, interference with oxidation of Mn may affect cellular uptake, elimination of Mn(III) and neurotoxicity. Further investigation of the inhibition of Mn oxidation as a possible mitigation method should be preceded by additional studies to elucidate the role of Mn in its various oxidation states in normal cell metabolism and to determine whether oxidative stress is a primary mechanism for neurotoxicity by Mn exposure.

CONCLUDING REMARKS AND FUTURE DIRECTIONS

Mn exposure may start before birth from the maternal exposure through inhalation and ingestion of food items from environmental pollution. Postnatal exposure can also be relevant due to a relatively high concentration of Mn in formulas and continued exposure during the childhood and adulthood from both environmental and occupational exposures. Although its accumulation is also associated with reproductive effects, Mn is generally described as neurotoxicant selectively affecting the basal ganglia. Manganism is a medical condition that differs from PD. The dynamic changes of exposures to Mn have led to different situations from the acute high exposure condition that was responsible for the occurrence of manganism to the chronic exposure to much lower levels of Mn, likely not to cause manganism. Cumulative mechanisms of Mn action are not sufficiently known and may vary with environmental factors and individual susceptibilities, including single nucleotide polymorphisms that may alter Mn homeostasis, Mn transport and metabolism. Therefore, further research is required to investigate the direct link between Mn uptake, distribution, accumulation and its downstream target(s), as well as associated clinical manifestations. In addition, there are no conclusive studies on mechanisms associated with the extracellular transport on Mn, mechanistic effects of Mn at the molecular level and its effects on signal transduction pathways, as well as studies on effective diagnosis and treatment of Mn poisoning. Future epidemiological research should assess more clearly the impact of Mn exposure on occupational and community settings.

ACKNOWLEDGMENTS

The authors gratefully acknowledge support by grant from the Department of Defense W81XWH-05-1-0239 (DM, MA) and the National Institute of Environmental Health Science (NIEHS) grant R01 10563 (MA).

REFERENCES

Addess KJ, Basilion JP, Klausner RD, Rouault TA, Pardi A (1997) Structure and dynamics of the iron responsive element RNA: implications for binding of the RNA by iron regulatory binding proteins. *J Mol Biol* **274:** 72–83.

Anderson JG, Cooney PT, Erikson KM (2007) Inhibition of DAT function attenuates manganese accumulation in the globus pallidus. *Environ Toxicol Pharmacol* **23:** 179–84.

Arbuthnott GW, Ingham CA, Wickens JR (2000) Dopamine and synaptic plasticity in the neostriatum. *J. Anat* **196:** 587–96.

Aschner M (2000) Manganese: brain transport and emerging research needs. *Environ Health Perspect* **108:** 429–32.

Aschner M, Aschner JL (1990) Manganese transport across the blood–brain barrier. *Neurotoxicology* **27:** 311–14.

Aschner M, Aschner JL (1991) Manganese neurotoxicity: cellular affects and blood–brain barrier transport. *Neurosci Biobehav Rev* **15:** 333–40.

Aschner JL, Aschner M (2005) Nutritional aspects of manganese homeostasis. *Mol Aspects Med* **26:** 353–62.

Aschner M, Dorman DC (2007) Manganese: pharmacokinetics and molecular mechanisms of brain uptake. *Toxicol Rev* **25:** 147–54.

Aschner M, Erikson KM, Dorman DC (2005) Manganese dosimetry: species differences and implications for neurotoxicity. *Crit Rev Toxicol* **35:** 1–32.

Aschner M, Guilkarte TR, Schneider JS, *et al.* (2007) Manganese: recent advances in understanding its transport and neurotoxicity. *Toxicol Appl Pharmacol* **35:** 1–32.

Aschner M, Shanker G, Erikson K, Yang J, Mutkus LA (2002) The uptake of manganese in brain endothelial cultures. *Neurotoxicology* **23:** 165–8.

Aschner M, Vrana KE, Zheng W (1999) Manganese uptake and distribution in the central nervous system (CNS). *Neurotoxicology* **20:** 173–89.

ATSDR (2000) Toxicological Profile for Manganese, Agency for Toxic Substances and Disease Registry (ATSDR), Atlanta, GA.

Attardi G, Schatz G (1988) Biogenesis of mitochondria. *Annu Rev Cell Biol* **4:** 289–333.

Autissier N, Rochette L, Dumas P, Beley A, Loireau A, Bralet J (1982) Dopamine and norepinephrine turnover in various regions of the rat brain after chronic manganese chloride administration. *Toxicology* **24:** 175–82.

Baek SY, Cho JH, Kim ES, Kim HJ, Yoon S, Kim BS (2004) cDNA array analysis of gene expression profiles in brain of mice exposed to manganese. *Industrial Health* **42:** 315–20.

Barbeau A (1984) Manganese extrapyramidal disorders. *Neurotoxicology* **5:** 13–35.

Bell JG, Keen CL, Lonnerdal B (1989) Higher retention of manganese in suckling than in adult rats is not due to maturational differences in manganese uptake by rat small intestine. *J Toxicol Environ Health* **26:** 387–98.

Bolte S, Normandin L, Kennedy G, *et al.* (2004) Human exposure to respirable manganese in outdoor and indoor air in urban and rural areas. *J Toxicol Environ Health A* **67:** 459–67.

Bonilla E, Arrieta A, Castro F, Davila JO, Quiroz I (1994) Manganese toxicity: free amino acids in the striatum and olfactory bulb of the mouse. *Invest Clin* **35:** 175–81.

Boojar MM, Goodarzi F Basedaghat MA (2002) Long-term follow-up of workplace and well water manganese effects on iron status indexes in manganese miners. *Arch Environ Health* **57:** 519–28.

Bouchard M, Laforest F, Vandelac L, Bellinger D, Mergler D (2007) Hair manganese and hyperactive behaviors: pilot study of school-age children exposed through tap water. *Environ Health Persp* **115:** 122–7.

Brouillet EP, Shinobu L, McGarvey U, Hochberg F, Beal MF (1993) Manganese injection into the rat striatum produces excitotoxic lesions by impairing energy metabolism. *Exp Neurol* **120:** 89–94.

Burton NC, Guilarte TR (2009) Manganese neurotoxicity: lessons learned from longitudinal studies in nonhuman primates. *Environ Health Perspect* **117:** 325–32.

Calne DB, Chu NS, Huang CC, Lu CS, Olanow W (1994) Manganism and idiopathic parkinsonism: similarities and differences. *Neurology* **44:** 1583–6.

Chandra SV, Shukla GS (1978) Manganese encephalopathy in growing rats. *Environ Res* **15:** 28–37.

Chang JY, Liu LZ (1999) Manganese potentiates nitric oxide production by microglia. *Brain Res Mol Brain Res.* **68:** 22–8.

Chen CJ, Ou YC, Lin SY, Liao SL, Chen SY, Chen JH (2006a) Manganese modulates pro-inflammatory gene expression in activated glia. *Neurochem Int* **49:** 62–71.

Chen MK, Lee JS, McGlothan JL, Furukawa E, Adams RJ, Alexander M, *et al.* (2006b) Acute manganese administration alters dopamine transporter levels in the non-human primate striatum. *Neurotoxicology* **27:** 229–36.

Cotzias GC (1958) Manganese in health and disease. *Physiol Rev* **38:** 503–32.

Cotzias GC, Greenough JJ (1958) The high specificity of the manganese pathway through the body. *J Clin Invest* **37:** 1298–305.

Couper J (1837) On the effects of black oxide of manganese when inhaled into the lungs. *British Annals Med Pharmacol* **1:** 41–2.

Crossgrove JS, Yokel RA (2005) Manganese distribution across the blood–brain barrier IV. Evidence of brain influx through store-operated channels. *Neurotoxicology* **26:** 297–307.

Crossgrove J, Zheng W (2004) Manganese toxicity upon overexposure. *NMR Biomed* **17:** 544–53.

da Silva CJ, da Rocha AJ, Jeronymo S, Mendes MF, Milani FT, Maia AC Jr, *et al.* (2007) A preliminary study revealing a new association in patients undergoing maintenance hemodialysis: manganism symptoms and T1 hyperintense changes in the basal ganglia. *Am J Neuroradiol* **28:** 1474–9.

Dawson R, Beal MF, Bondy SC, Di Monte DA, Isom GE (1995) Excitotoxins, aging and environmetal neurotoxins: implications for understanding human neurodegenerative diseases. *Toxicol Appl Pharmacol* **134:** 1–17.

Day M, Wang Z, Ding J, An X, Ingham CA, Shering AF, *et al.* (2006) Selective elimination of glutamatergic synapses on striatopallidal neurons in Parkinson disease models. *Nat Neurosci* **9:** 251–9.

Defazio G, Soleo L, Zefferino R, Livrea P (1996) Manganese toxicity in serumless dissociated mesencephalic and striatal primary culture. *Brain Res Bull* **40:** 257–62.

Deskin R, Bursian SJ, Edens FW (1980) Neurochemical alterations induced by manganese chloride in neonatal rats. *Neurotoxicology* **2:** 65–73.

Desole MS, Esposito E (1995) Cellular defense mechanisms in the striatum of young and aged rats subchronically exposed to manganese. *Neuropharmacology* **34:** 289–95.

Desole MS, Miele M, Esposito G, Migheli R, Fresu L, de Natale G, *et al.* (1994) Dopaminergic system activity and cellular defense mechanisms in the striatum and striatal synaptosomes of the rat subchronically exposed to manganese. *Arch Toxicol* **68:** 566–70.

Dimova R, Vuillet J, Nieoullon A, Kerkeria-Le Goff L (1993) Ultrastructural features of the choline acetyltransferase-containing neurons and relationships with nigral dopaminergic and cortical afferent pathways in the rat striatum. *Neuroscience* **53:** 1059–71.

Dobson AW, Erikson KM, Aschner M (2004) Manganese neurotoxicity. *Ann NY Acad Sci* **1012:** 115–28.

Dobson AW, Weber S, Dorman DC, Lash LK, Erikson KM, Aschner M (2003) Oxidative stress is induced in the rat brain following repeated inhalation exposure to manganese sulfate. *Biol Trace Elem Res* **93:** 113–26.

Dorman DC, Brenneman KA, McElveen AM, Lynch SE, Robers KC, Wong BA (2002) Olfactory transport: a direct route of delivery of inhaled manganese phosphate to the rat brain. *J Toxicol Environ Health A* **65:** 1493–511.

Dorman DC, McElveen AM, Marshall MW, Parkinson CU, James RA, Struve MF, Wong BA (2005) Maternal–fetal distribution of manganese in the rat following inhalation exposure to manganese sulfate. *Neurotoxicology* **26:** 625–32.

Dorman DC, Struve MF, Marshall MW, Parkinson CU, James RA, Wong BA (2006a) Tissue manganese concentrations in young male rhesus monkeys following subchronic manganese sulfate inhalation. *Toxicol Sci* **92:** 201–10.

Dorman DC, Struve MF, Clewell HJ 3rd, Andersen ME (2006b) Application of pharmacokinetic data to the risk assessment of inhaled manganese. *Neurotoxicology* **27:** 752–64.

Dorman DC, Struve MF, Vitarella D, Byerly FL, Goetz J, Miller R (2000) Neurotoxicity of manganese chloride in neonatal and adult CD rats following subchronic (21-day) high-dose oral exposure. *J Appl Toxicol* 20: 179–87.

Dorner K, Dziadzka S, Hohn A, *et al.* (1989) Longitudinal manganese and copper balances in young infants and preterm infants fed on breast-milk and adapted cow's milk formulas. *Br J Nutr* **61:** 559–72.

Edsall DL, Wilbur FP, Drinker CK (1919) The occurrence, course and prevention of chronic manganese poisoning. *J Ind Hyg* **1:** 183–93.

Ejima A, Imamura T, Nakamura S, *et al.* (1992) Manganese intoxication during total parenteral nutrition. *Lancet* **339:** 426.

Elbetieha A, Bataineh H, Darmani H, *et al.* (2001) Effects of long-term exposure to manganese chloride on fertility of male and female mice. *Toxicol Lett* **119:** 193–201.

Emara AM, El-Ghawabi SH, Madkour OI, *et al.* (1971) Chronic manganese poisoning in the dry battery industry. *Br J Ind Med* **28:** 78–82.

EPA (1984) Health assessment document for manganese. Final draft. Cincinnati, OH: US Environmental Protection Agency, Office of Toxic Substances.

EPA (2003) Health effects support document for manganese. EPA822R03003, US Environmental Protection Agency, Washington DC. http://www.epa.gov/safewater/ccl/pdfs/reg_ determine1/support_cc1_magnese_healtheffects.pdf. Accessed July 10, 2009.

EPA (2006) Edition of the drinking water standards and health advisories. Washington DC; US Environmental Protection Agency. EPA 822R06013.

Erikson K, Aschner M (2002) Manganese causes differential regulation of glutamate transporter (GLAST) taurine transporter and metallothionein in cultured rat astrocytes. *Neurotoxicology* **23:** 595–602.

Erikson KM, Aschner M (2003) Manganese neurotoxicity and glutamate-GABA interaction. *Neurochem Int* **43:** 475–80.

Erikson KM, Dorman DC, Lash LH, Aschner M (2007) Manganese inhalation by rhesus monkeys is associated with brain regional changes in biomarkers of neurotoxicity. *Toxicol Sci* **97:** 459–66.

Erikson KM, Dorman DC, Lash LH, Aschner M (2008) Duration of airborne-manganese exposure in rhesus monkeys is associated with brain regional changes in biomarkers of neurotoxicity. *Neurotoxicology* **29:** 377–85.

Eriksson H, Gillberg PG, Aquilonius SM, Hedstrom KG, Heilbronn E (1992) Receptor alterations in manganese intoxicated monkeys. *Arch Toxicol* **66:** 359–64.

Eriksson H, Lenngren S, Heilbronn E (1987) Effect of long-term administration of manganese on biogenic amine levels in discrete striatal regions of rat brain. *Arch Toxicol* **59:** 426–31.

Fechter LD, Johnson DL, Lynch RA (2002) The relationship of particle size to olfactory nerve uptake of a non-soluble form of manganese into brain. *Neurotoxicology* **23:** 177–83.

Fell JM, Reynolds AP, Meadows N, Khan K, Long SG, Quaghebeur G, Taylor WJ, Milla PJ (1996) Manganese toxicity in children receiving long-term parenteral nutrition. *Lancet* **347:** 1218–21.

Filipov NM, Seegal RF, Lawrence DA (2005) Manganese potentiates in vitro production of proinflammatory cytokines and nitric oxide by microglia through a nuclear factor kappa B-dependent mechanism. *Toxicol Sci* **84:** 139–48.

Fitsanakis VA, Aschner M (2005) The importance of glutamate, glycine, and gamma-aminobutyric acid transport and regulation in manganese, mercury and lead neurotoxicity. *Toxicol Appl Pharmacol* 204: 343–54.

Flynn MR, Susi P (2009) Neurological risk associated with manganese exposure from welding operations – a literature review. *Int J Environ Health* **212:** 459–69.

Gavin CE, Gunter KK, Gunter TE (1990) Manganese and calcium efflux kinetics in brain mitochondria. Relevance to manganese toxicity. *The Biochem J* **266:** 329–34.

Gavin CE, Gunter KK, Gunter TE (1992) Mn^{2+} sequestration by mitochondria and inhibition of oxidative phosphorylation. *Toxicol Appl Pharmacol* **115:** 1–5.

Gibbs JP, Crump KS, Houck DP, *et al.* (1999) Focused medical surveillance: a search for subclinical movement disorders in a cohort of U.S. workers exposed to low levels manganese in dust. *Neurotoxicology* **20:** 299–313.

Gray LE, Laskey JW (1980) Multivariate analysis of the toxic effects of manganese on the reproductive physiology and behavior of the male house mouse. *J Toxicol Environ Health* **6:** 861–7.

Greger JL (1998) Dietary standards for manganese: overlap between nutritional and toxicological studies. *J Nutr* **128:** 368S–371S.

Greenamyre JT, MacKenzie G, Peng TI, Stephans SE (1999) Mitochondrial dysfunction in Parkinson's disease. *Biochem Soc Symp* **66:** 85–97.

Guilarte TR, Burton NC, McGlothan JL, *et al.* (2008) Impairment of nigrostriatal dopamine neurotransmission by manganese is mediated by pre-synaptic mechanism(s): implications to manganese-induced parkinsonism. *J Neurochem* **107:** 1236–47.

Guilarte TR, McGlothan JL, Degaonkar M, Chen MK, Barker PB, Syversen T, *et al.* (2006) Evidence for cortical dysfunction and widespread manganese accumulation in the nonhuman primate brain following chronic manganese exposure: a 1H-MRS and MRI study. *Toxicol Sci* **94:** 351–8.

Gunst S, Weinbruch S, Wentzel M, Ortner HM, Skogstad A, Hetland S, Thomassen Y (2000) Chemical composition of individual aerosol particles in workplace air during production of manganese alloys. *J Environ Monit* **1:** 65–71.

Gunter TE, Gavin CE, Aschner M, Gunter KK (2006) Speciation of manganese in cells and mitochondria: a search for the proximal cause of manganese neurotoxicity. *Neurotoxicology* **27:** 765–76.

Gwiazda RH, Lee D, Sheridan J, Smith DR (2002) Low cumulative manganese exposure affects striatal GABA but not dopamine. *Neurotoxicology* **23:** 69–76.

HaMai D, Rinderknecht AL, Guo-Sharman K, Kleinman MT, Bondy SC (2006) Decreased expression of inflammation-related genes following inhalation exposure to manganese. *Neurotoxicology* **27:** 395–401.

Harper PS (2002) Huntington's disease: a historical background. In *Huntington's Disease*, 3rd edition (Bates G, Harper PS, Jones L, eds.). Oxford, Oxford University Press, pp. 3–24.

Hauser RA, Zesiewicz TA, Rosemurgy AS, Martinez C, Olanow CW (1994) Manganese intoxication and chronic liver failure. *Ann Neurol* **36:** 871–5.

He P, Liu D, Zhang G, *et al.* (1994) Effects of high-level manganese sewage irrigation on children's neurobehavior. *Chung Hua Yu Fang I Hsueh Tsa Chih* **28:** 216–18.

Herrero Hernández E, Discalzi G, Valentini C, Venturi F, Chiò A, Carmellino C, *et al.* (2006) Follow-up of patients affected by manganese-induced Parkinsonism after treatment with $CaNa_2EDTA$. *Neurotoxicology* **27:** 333–9.

IEH/IOM (2004) Institute for Environment and Health/Institute of Occupational Medicine Occupational Exposure Limits: criteria document for manganese and inorganic manganese compounds (Web Report W17), Leicester, UK, MRC Institute for Environment and Health. http://www.le.ac.uk/ieh

Jarvinen R, Ahlstrom A (1975) Effect of the dietary manganese level on tissue manganese, iron, copper and zinc concentrations in female rats and their fetuses. *Med Biol* **53:** 93–9.

Jiang Y, Lu J, Xie P, *et al.* (1996) Effects of manganese on the sexual function and reproductive outcome of male exposed workers. *Chi J Ind Hyg Occup Dis* **14:** 271–3.

Jiang YM, Mo XA, Du FQ, Hochberg F, Lilienfeld D, Olanow W, *et al.* (2006) Effective treatment of manganese-induced occupational Parkinsonism with p-aminosalicylic acid: a case of 17-year follow-up study. *J Occup Environ Med* **48:** 644–9.

Jiang Y, Mo X, Du F, *et al.* (2007) Effective treatment of manganese-induced occupational Parkinsonism with p-aminosalicylic acid: a case study of 17-year follow-up study. *J Occup Environ Med* **48:** 644–9.

Keen CL, Bell JG, Lonnerdal B (1986) The effect of age on manganese uptake and retention from milk and infant formulas in rats. *J Nutr* **116:** 395–402.

Kita H, Narira K, Van der Kloot W (1981) Tetanic stimulation increases frequency of miniature end-plate potentials at the frog neuromuscular junction in Mn-, Ni-saline solution. *Brain Res* **205:** 121–2.

Komura J, Sakamoto M (1992) Effects of manganese forms on biogenic amines in the brain and behavioral alterations in the mouse: long-term oral administration of several manganese compounds. *Environ Res* **57:** 34–44.

Kontur PJ, Fechter LD (1985) Brain manganese, catecholamine turnover, and the development of startle in rats prenatally exposed to manganese. *Teratology* **32:** 1–11.

Kowaltowski AJ, Castilho RF, Vercesi AE (1995) Ca^{2+}-induced mitochondrial membrane permeabilization: role of coenzyme Q redox state. *Am J Physiol* **269:** 141–7.

Kruman II, Mattson MP (1999) Pivotal role of mitochondrial calcium uptake in neural cell apoptosis and necrosis. *J Neurochem* **72:** 529–40.

Laskey JW, Rehnberg GL, Hein JF (1982) Effects of chronic manganese (Mn_3O_4) exposure selected reproductive parameters in rats. *J Toxicol Environ Health* **9:** 677–87.

Lauwerys R, Roels H, Genet P, Toussaint G, Bouckaert A, De Cooman S (1985) Fertility of male workers exposed to mercury vapor or to manganese dust: a questionnaire study. *Am J Ind Med* **7:** 171–6.

Lewis J, Bench G, Myers O, Tinner B, Staines W, Barr E, *et al.* (2005) Trigeminal uptake and clearance of inhaled manganese chloride in rats and mice. *Neurotoxicology* **26:** 113–23.

Lloyd RV (1995) Mechanism of the manganese-catalyzed autoxidation of dopamine. *Chem Res Toxicol* **8:** 111–16.

Lonnerdal B (1989) Dietary factors affecting trace element absorption in infants. *Acta Paediatr Scand Suppl* **351:** 109–13.

Lucchini RG, Martin CJ, Doney BC (2009) From manganism to manganese-induced Parkinsonism: a conceptual model based on the evaluation of exposure. *Neuromolec Med* **11:** 311–21.

Malecki EA, Devenyi AG, Beard JL, Connor JR (1999) Existing and emerging mechanisms for transport of iron and manganese to the brain. *J Neurosci Res* **56:** 113–22.

Mena I (1981) Manganese. In *Disorders of Mineral Metabolism* (Bronner F, Coburn JW, eds.). Academic Press, New York, pp. 233–70.

Milatovic D, Aschner M (2009) Measurement of isoprostanes as markers of oxidative stress in neuronal tissue. *Curr Protoc Toxicol* unit **12:** 14: 1–12.

Milatovic D, Yin Z, Gupta RC, Sydoryk M, Albrecht J, Aschner JL, Aschner M (2007) Manganese induces oxidative impairment in cultured rat astrocytes. *Toxicol Sci* **98:** 198–205.

Milatovic D, Zaja-Milatovic S, Gupta RC, Yu Y, Aschner M (2009) Oxidative damage and neurodegeneration in manganese-induced neurotoxicity. *Toxicol Appl Pharmacol* **240:** 219–25.

Miller DM, Buettner GR, Aust SD (1990) Transition metals as catalysts of "autoxidation" reactions. *Free Radic Biol Med* **8:** 95–108.

Morrow JD, Roberts LJ 2nd (1999) Mass spectrometric quantification of F_2-isoprostanes in biological fluids and tissues as measure of oxidant stress. *Methods Enzymol* **300:** 3–12.

Nelson K, Golnick J, Korn T, Angle C (1993) Manganese encephalopathy: utility of early magnetic resonance imaging. *Br J Ind Med* **50:** 510–13.

Ohtake T, Negishi K, Okamoto K, Oka M, Maesato K, Moriya H, *et al.* (2005) Manganese-induced Parkinsonism in a patient undergoing maintenance hemodialysis. *Am J Kidney Dis* **46:** 749–53.

Olanow CW (2004) Manganese-induced parkinsonism and Parkinson's disease. *Ann NY Acad Sci* **1012:** 209–23.

Olanow CW, Good PF, Shinotoh H, Hewitt KA, Vingerhoets F, Snow BJ, Beal MF, Calne DB, Perl DP (1996) Manganese intoxication in the rhesus monkey: a clinical, imaging, pathologic, and biochemical study. *Neurology* **46:** 492–8.

Pal PK, Samii A, Calne DB (1999) Manganese neurotoxicity: a review of clinical features, imaging and pathology. *Neurotoxicology* **20:** 227–38.

Parenti M, Rusconi L, Cappabianca V, Parati EA, Groppetti A (1988) Role of dopamine in manganese neurotoxicity. *Brain Res* **473:** 236–40.

Parkinson J (2002) Neuropsychiatric classics: James Parkinson: an essay on the shaking palsy. *J Neuropsychiatr Clin Neurosci* **14:** 223–36.

Perl DP, Olanow CW (2007) The neuropathology of manganese-induced Parkinsonism. *J Neuropathol Exp Neurol* **66:** 675–82.

Pityn P, Chamberlain MJ, Fraser TM, King M, Morgan WK (1989) The topography of particle deposition in the human lung. *Respir Physiol* **78:** 19–29.

Ponnapakkam TP, Bailey KS, Graves KA, Iszard MB (2003a) Assessment of male reproductive system in CD-1 mice following oral manganese exposure. *Reprod Toxicol* **17:** 547–51.

Ponnapakkam TP, Sam GH, Iszard MB (2003b) Histopathological changes in the testes of the Sprague Dawley rat following orally administered manganese. *Bull Environ Contam Toxicol* **71:** 1151–7.

Post JE (1999) Manganese oxide minerals: crystal structures and economic and environmental significance. *Proc Natl Acad Sci USA* 96: 3447–54.

Racette BA, McGee-Minnich L, Moerlein SM, Mink JW, Videen TO, Perlmutter JS (2001) Welding-related parkinsonism: clinical features, treatment, and pathophysiology. *Neurology* **56:** 8–13.

Rao KV, Norenberg MD (2004) Manganese induces the mitochondrial permeability transition in cultured astrocytes. *J Biol Chem* **279:** 32333–8.

Rao VL, Dogan A, Todd KG, Bowen KK, Kim BT, Rothstein JD, Dempsey RJ (2001) Antisense knockdown of the glial glutamate transporter GLT-1, but not the neuronal glutamate transporter EAAC1, excerbates transient focal cerebral ischemia-induced neuronal damage in rat brain. *J Neurosci* **21:** 1876–83.

Reaney SH, Bench G, Smith DR (2006) Brain accumulation and toxicity of Mn(II) and Mn(III) exposures. *Toxicol Sci* **93:** 114–24.

Rodier J (1955) Manganese poisoning in Moroccan miners. *Br J Ind Med* **12:** 21–35.

Roth JA, Garrick MD (2003) Iron interactions and other biological reactions mediating the physiological and toxic actions of manganese. *Biochem Pharmacol* **66:** 1–13.

Rovira A, Alonso J, Cordoba J (2008) MR imaging findings in hepatic encephalopathy. *AJNR Am J Neuroradiol* **29:** 1612–21.

Sahni V, Léger Y, Panaro L, Allen M, Giffin S, Fury D, Hamm N (2007) Case report: a metabolic disorder presenting as pediatric manganism. *Environ Health Perspect* **115:** 1776–9.

Saka E, Iadarola M, Fitzgerald DJ, Graybiel AM (2002) Local circuit neurons in the striatum regulate neural and behavioral responses to dopaminergic stimulation. *Proc Natl Acad Sci USA* **99:** 9004–9.

Saric M (1986) Manganese. In *Handbook on the Toxicology of Metals,* vol. II: *Specific metals.* Elsevier Science Publishing Co., New York, pp. 354–86.

Schuler P, Oyanguren H, Maturana V, Valenzuela A, Cruz E, Plaza V, Schmidt E, Haddad R (1957) Manganese poisoning: environmental and medical study at a Chilean mine. *Ind Med Surg* **26:** 167–73.

Seth PK, Hong JS, Kilts CD, Bondy SC (1981) Alteration of cerebral neurotransmitter receptor function by exposure of rats to manganese. *Toxicol Lett* **9:** 247–54.

Shen XM, Dryhurst G (1998) Iron- and manganese-catalyzed autoxidation of dopamine in the presence of l-cysteine: possible insights into iron- and manganese-mediated dopaminergic neurotoxicity. *Chem Res Toxicol* **11:** 824–37.

Singh J, Husain R, Tandon SK, Seth PK, Chandra SV (1974) Biochemical and histopathological alterations in early manganese toxicity in rats. *Environ Physiol Biochem* **4:** 16–23.

Sloot WN, Gramsbergen JBP (1994) Axonal transport of manganese and its relevance to selective neurotoxicity in the rat basal ganglia. *Brain Res* **657:** 124–32.

Sloot WN, van der Sluijs-Gelling AJ, Gramsbergen JBP (1994) Selective lesions by manganese and extensive damage by iron after injection into rat striatum or hippocampus. *J Neurochem* **62:** 205–16.

Soliman EF, Slikker W Jr, Ali SF (1995) Manganese-induced oxidative stress as measured by a fluorescent probe: in vitro study. *Neurosci Res Comm* **17:** 185–93.

Stephens B, Mueller AJ, Shering AF, Hood SH, Taggart P, Arbuthnott GW, Bell JE, Kilford L, Kingsbury AE, Daniel SE, Ingham CA (2005) Evidence of a breakdown of corticostriatal connections in Parkinson's disease. *Neuroscience* **132:** 741–54.

Struve MF, McManus BE, Wong BA, Dorman DC (2007) Basal ganglia neurotransmitter concentrations in rhesus monkeys following subchronic manganese sulfate inhalation. *Am J Ind Med* **50:** 772–8.

Suarez N, Eriksson, H (1993) Receptor-mediated endocytosis of a manganese complex of transferrin into neuroblastoma (SHSY5Y) cells in culture. *J Neurochem* **61:** 127–31.

Szakmary E, Ungvary G, Hudak A, *et al.* (1995) Developmental effect of manganese in rat and rabbit. *Cent Eur J Occup Environ Med* **1:** 149–59.

Takeda A (2003) Manganese action in brain function. *Brain Res Rev* **41:** 79–87.

Takeda A, Ishiwatari S, Okada S (1999) Manganese uptake into rat brain during development and aging. *J Neurosci Res* **56:** 93–8.

Tjalkens RB, Zoran MJ, Mohl B, Barhoumi R (2006) Manganese suppresses ATP-dependent intercellular calcium waves in astrocyte networks through alteration of mitochondrial and endoplasmic reticulum calcium dynamics. *Brain Res* **1113:** 210–19.

Tjälve H, Henriksson J (1999) Uptake of metals in the brain via olfactory pathways. *Neurotoxicology* **120:** 181–95.

Tjälve H, Henriksson J, Tallkvist J, Larsson BS, Lindquist NG (1996) Uptake of manganese and cadmium from the nasal mucosa into the central nervous system via olfactory pathways in rats. *Pharmacol Toxicol* **79:** 347–56.

Turrens JF, Boveris A (1980) Generation of superoxide anion by the NADH dehydrogenase of bovine heart mitochondria. *Biochem J* **191:** 421–7.

Tuschl K, Mills PB, Parsons H, Malone M, Fowler D, Bitner-Glindzicz M, Clayton PT (2008) Hepatic cirrhosis, dystonia, polycythaemia and hypermanganesaemia – a new metabolic disorder. *J Inherit Metab Dis* **31:** 151–63.

Uchida K (2003) 4-hyroxy-2-nonenal: a product and mediator of oxidative stress. *Prog Lipid Res* **42:** 318–43.

Vigeh M, Yokoyama K, Ramezanzadeh F, Dahaghin M, Fakhriazad E, Seyedaghamiri Z, Araki S (2008) Blood manganese concentrations and intrauterine growth restriction. *Reprod Toxicol* **25:** 219–23.

Vitarella D, Struve MF, Goetz J, Ledford FI, Miller R, Dorman DC (1996) Comparative neurotoxicity of oral manganese (II) chloride in neonatal and adult CD rats. In *20th Annual Chemical Industry Institute of Toxicology Scientific Open House, 8 October, Research Triangle Park, NC*. Chemical Industry Institute of Toxicology, Research Triangle Park, NC, pp. 46–7.

Von Jaksch R (1909) Ueber gehaufte diffuse Erkrankun-gen des Gehirns und Ruckenmarks, an den Typus der multiplen Sklerose mahnend, welche durch eine besondere Aetiologie gekennzeichnet sind. *Klein Rundsch.* **15:** 729–33 (in German).

Wang X, Ghio AJ, Yang F, Dolan KG, Garrick MD, Piantadosi CA (2002) Iron uptake and Nramp2/DMT1/DCT1 in human bronchial epithelial cells. *Am J Physiol Lung Cell Mol Physiol* **282:** L987–L995.

Wang JD, Huang CC, Hwang YH, Chiang JR, Lin JM, Chen JS (1989) Manganese induced Parkinsonism: an outbreak due to an unrepaired ventilation control system in a ferromanganese smelter. *Br J Ind Med* **46:** 856–9.

Wasserman GA, Liu X, Parvez F, Ahsan H, Levy D, Factor-Litvak P, Kline J, van Geen A, Slavkovich V, LoIacono NJ, Cheng Z, Zheng Y, Graziano JH (2006) Water manganese exposure and children's intellectual function in Araihazar, Bangladesh. *Environ Health Persp* **114:** 124–9.

Wexler A (2008) *The Woman Who Walked into the Sea: Huntington's and the Making of a Genetic Disease* (Wexler A, ed.). Yale University Press, New Haven, pp. 288.

WHO (1981) Manganese. Environmental health criteria 17. World Health Organization, Geneva, Switzerland.

WHO (2004) Manganese in drinking-water. Background document for development of WHO guidelines for drinking-water quality. World Health Organization. WHO/SDE/WSH/03.04/ 104. http://www.who.int/water_sanitation_health/dwq/chemicals/ manganese.pdf. Accessed July 10, 2009.

Wilson P, Groves PM (1980) Fine structure and synaptic connections of the common spiny neuron of the rat neostriatum: a study employing intracellular inject of horseradish peroxidase. *J Comp Neurol* **194:** 599–615.

Wu W, Zhang Y, Zhang F (1996) Studies on semen quality in workers exposed to manganese and electric welding. *Chin J Prev Med* **30:** 266–8.

Yamada M, Ohno S, Okayasu I, Okeda R, Hatakeyama S, Watanabe H, Ushio K, Tsukagoshi H (1986) Chronic manganese poisoning: a neuropathological study with determination of manganese distribution in the brain. *Acta Neuropathologica* **70:** 273–8.

Yang J, Liu X, Bhalla K, Kim CN, Ibrado AM, Cai J, Peng TI, Jones DP, Wang X (1997) Prevention of apoptosis by Bcl-2 release of cytochrome c from mitochondria blocked. *Science* **275:** 1129–32.

Yang F, Wang X, Haile DJ, Piantadosi CA, Ghio AJ (2002) Iron increases expression of iron-export protein MTP1 in lung cells. *Am J Physiol Lung Cell Mol Physiol* **283:** L932–L939.

Yoon M, Nong A, Clewell HJ 3rd, Taylor MD, Dorman DC, Andersen ME (2009a) Evaluating placental transfer and tissue concentrations of manganese in the pregnant rat and fetuses after inhalation exposures with a PBPK model. *Toxicol Sci* **112:** 44–58.

Yoon M, Nong A, Clewell HJ 3rd, Taylor MD, Dorman DC, Andersen ME (2009b) Lactational transfer of manganese in rats: predicting manganese tissue concentration in the dam and pups from inhalation exposure with a pharmacokinetic model. *Toxicol Sci* **112:** 23–43.

Yu IJ, Kim KJ, Chang HK, Song KS, Han KT, Han JH, Maeng SH, Chung YH, Park SH, Chung KH, Han JS, Chung HK (2000) Pattern of deposition of stainless steel welding fume particles inhaled into the respiratory systems of Sprague-Dawley rats exposed to a novel welding fume generating system. *Toxicol Lett* **116:** 103–11.

Zaja-Milatovic S, Milatovic D, Schantz A, Zhang J, Montine K, Montine TJ (2005) Dendritic degeneration in neostriatal medium spiny neurons in late-stage Parkinson disease. *Neurology* **64:** 545–7.

Zhang G, Liu D, He P (1995) Effects of manganese on learning abilities in school children. *Chung Hua Yu Fang I Hsueh Tsa Chih* **29:** 156–8.

Zhang S, Fu J, Zhou Z (2004) In vitro effect of manganese chloride exposure on reactive oxygen species generation and respiratory chain complexes activities of mitochondria isolated from rat brain. *Toxicol in Vitro* **18:** 71–7.

Zhang S, Zhou Z, Fu J (2003) Effect of manganese chloride exposure on liver and brain mitochondria function in rats. *Environ Res* **93:** 149–57.

Zhang P, Wong TA, Lokuta KM, Turner DE, Vujisic K, Liu B (2009) Microglia enhance manganese chloride-induced dopaminergic neurodegeneration: role of free radical generation. *Exp Neurol* **217:** 219–30.

Zhao F, Cai T, Liu M, Zheng G, Luo W, Chen J (2009) Manganese induces dopaminergic neurodegeneration via microglial activation in a rat model of manganism. *Toxicol Sci* **107:** 156–64.

Zoratti M, Szabo I (1995) The mitochondrial permeability transition. *Biochim Biophys Acta* **1241:** 139–76.

Zota AR, Ettinger AS, Bouchard M, Amarasiriwardena CJ, Schwartz J, Hu H, Wright RO (2009) Maternal blood manganese levels and infant birth weight. *Epidemiology* **20:** 367–73.

CHAPTER

35

Mercury

Mingwei Ni, Xin Li, Ana Paula Marreilha dos Santos, Marcelo Farina, João Batista Teixeira da Rocha, Daiana S. Avila, Offie P. Soldin, Lu Rongzhu and Michael Aschner

INTRODUCTION

Human exposure to mercury (Hg) is mainly in the form of methylmercury (MeHg) predominantly from the consumption of fish (Clarkson, 1997; Kamps *et al.*, 1972; Spry and Wiener, 1991). Nearly all fish contain detectable amounts of MeHg (Clarkson *et al.*, 1988). MeHg enrichment in the aquatic food chain is not uniform and is dependent upon water Hg content, bottom sediments, water pH and redox potential, the species, age and size of the particular fish. Furthermore, environmental conditions, such as anoxia, favor the growth of microorganisms and increase the methylation rate of Hg (Boudou *et al.*, 2005) and, by inference, its accumulation in fish. The mechanisms of Hg methylation in oceans and waterways are not fully understood.

The aims of this chapter are to outline the kinetics of organic mercury (MeHg) in humans and the toxic effects of MeHg on the developing fetal central nervous system (CNS) as well as on other organ systems. This chapter describes the differences in MeHg-induced brain damage between the fetus and the adult and highlights several of the proposed mechanisms of MeHg toxicity in the developing organism. The chapter also discusses directions for future studies to address current gaps in the literature, and enhances and expands our knowledge of the underlying mechanisms of MeHg toxicity and its effects upon the environment, animals and humans.

HISTORICAL BACKGROUND

Catastrophic epidemics due to environmental MeHg contamination in Japan (Igata, 1993; Tsubaki *et al.*, 1967) and Sweden (Westoo, 1966) have been previously reported. Exposure was also documented in Iraq, where locals consumed bread prepared from seeds treated with a fungicide containing MeHg (Bakir *et al.*, 1973), causing a large outbreak of human poisoning. Similar incidents have occurred in Pakistan, Guatemala and Ghana (Clarkson *et al.*, 2003). School children living in polluted areas have been found to exhibit diskinesia and intellectual disturbances (Harada, 1964). The initial symptoms of classic congenital Minamata disease due to MeHg exposure were mental retardation, primitive reflexes, coordination disturbance, dysarthria, limb deformation, growth disorder, choreoathetosis and hypersalivation (Harada, 1995). These symptoms occurred at Hg exposure levels exceeding the US EPA reference dose (RfD) of 0.1 μg/kg body weight/day (an exposure without recognized adverse effects). An estimated 8% of US women of child-bearing age have blood Hg concentrations exceeding 5.8 μg/L (level equivalent to the current RfD), the total impact of exposure to Hg upon human populations is of considerable significance and may have tremendous societal consequences, affecting more than 300,000 newborns annually in the USA alone (National Health and Nutrition Examination Survey, 1999–2000). It is reasonable to suggest, considering the magnitude of potential susceptible populations as well as the long latency period for the development of Hg-induced symptoms, that the true number of those affected is even greater than this conservative estimate.

TOXICOKINETICS

The kinetics of MeHg in the human body is summarized in Figure 35.1. MeHg derived from food or occupational exposure is efficiently absorbed (90%) and has a long retention time (half-life of ~70 days). After ingestion, the distribution to the blood compartment is complete within 30 hours, and the blood level accounts for about 7% of the ingested dose (Kershaw *et al.*, 1980). Circulating MeHg accumulates predominantly in red cells where it binds to cysteinyl residues (-SH) on the hemoglobin beta-chain (Doi, 1991), and is then slowly distributed reaching an equilibrium with other tissues at ~4 days (Kershaw *et al.*, 1980).

In the brain, MeHg undergoes slow demethylation and is converted to inorganic mercury (IHg) (Charleston *et al.*, 1995). About 10% mercury is retained in the brain following long-term exposure to MeHg. Accumulated inorganic mercury is deposited in the cortex of the calcarine sulcus of the female *Macaca fascicularis* (Charleston *et al.*, 1995), similar to prolonged subclinical exposure in humans. Mercury is not universally distributed and is deposited in certain

Reproductive and Developmental Toxicology, Edited by Ramesh C. Gupta
ISBN: 978-0-12-382032-7

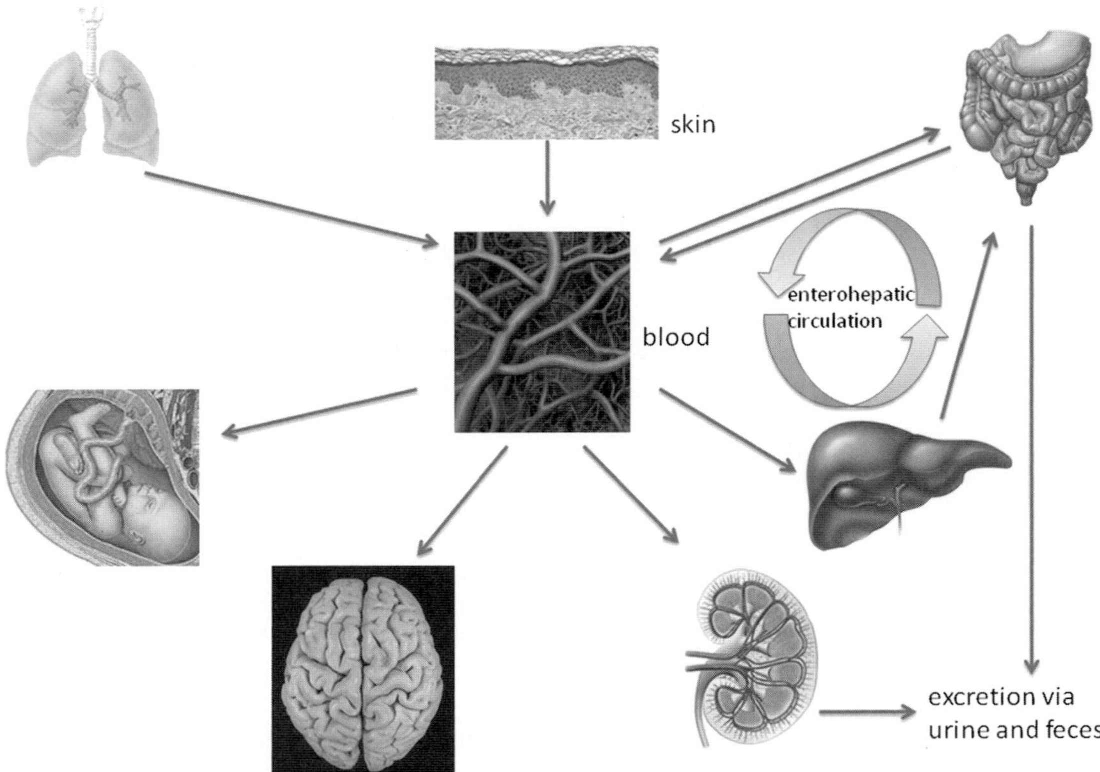

FIGURE 35.1 The distribution of MeHg in the human body. MeHg is readily absorbed by the lung, skin and gastrointestinal tract. Once in the circulation, MeHg predominantly accumulates in red blood cells and is slowly redistributed to other organ systems, including the CNS (major), kidneys and liver. MeHg can cross the placental–blood barrier and it accumulates in the fetus at higher concentrations compared to the mother. Please refer to color plate section.

CNS cell types. Tissue staining following 6 months of exposure to MeHg reveals the largest IHg deposits in astrocytes and microglia. The total mercury accumulation in neurons are significantly lower than those present in the glial cells and increase with length of exposure; virtually all neurons are labeled following 18 months of exposure. In contrast, endothelial cells and pericytes do not contain notable mercury deposits, and deposits in oligodendrocytes are rarely observed. These data are consistent with the hypothesis that the neurotoxicity of MeHg is mediated, at least in part, by glial cells and that glial–neuron interactions play important roles in the process. Notably, staining of mercury deposits in IHg-exposed animals is lower compared to MeHg-exposed animals, supporting the observation that it is the organic form of mercury that more readily crosses the blood–brain barrier (BBB) (Charleston *et al.*, 1995).

MeHg is incorporated into the hair during its formation. The MeHg concentration in blood and hair reflects the body burden, with a blood/hair concentration in humans approximating 1/250 under steady-state conditions (Skerfving, 1974). The net mercury excretion rate in humans is approximately 1% of the body content at non-symptomatic body burden level (Swedish Expert Group, 1971). Most of the MeHg is eliminated through the liver into the bile and through the kidney into the urine. But most MeHg undergoes enterohepatic circulation by reabsorption from the bile in the gut. Slower urine excretion of MeHg in female versus male rats has been reported to result in higher toxicity (Hirayama and Yasutake, 1986). Diet can affect MeHg excretion rate, since certain dietary components can interfere with MeHg reabsorption in the lower part of the intestines, thus breaking up the enterohepatic circulation (Landry *et al.*, 1979).

Approximately 5% of the total MeHg in the maternal blood is found in breast milk (Bakir *et al.*, 1973), but the risk of MeHg exposure to infants through breast-feeding declines rapidly during lactation, which is due to the rapid decrease in mercury transferred through breast milk postpartum and the fast growth of infants after birth (Sakamoto *et al.*, 2002). MeHg crosses the placenta and accumulates in the fetus at concentrations higher than in the mother. For example, neonatal cord blood MeHg is more than twice as high as the level in maternal blood at delivery, but infant blood MeHg levels decrease significantly during the first 13 weeks of the infant's life, and, at 3 months, maternal MeHg concentrations are higher than those of the infant, opposite to the situation at parturition (Sakamoto *et al.*, 2002, 2010). The rapid decline in infant MeHg concentrations postpartum can be explained by lower mercury transfer through breast milk and rapid infant growth after birth.

Hg is covalently bound to the carbon moiety in MeHg (CH_3–Hg^+). The carbon–Hg bond is chemically stable because of the low affinity of Hg for oxygen. MeHg does not exist as a free, unbound cation in biological systems (except an infinitesimal amount as governed by the law of mass action) (Hughes, 1957), and the organic form is highly soluble in organic solvents and lipids. MeHg has a remarkably high affinity for the anionic form of -SH groups (log K, where k is the affinity constant and is on the order of 15–23) (Hughes, 1957). Despite the high thermodynamic stability of the MeHg–SH bond, very rapid exchange of MeHg between -SH groups is known to occur (Rabenstein and Fairhurst, 1975). In cells, MeHg can form a complex with the -SH-containing amino acid cysteine (Bridges and Zalups, 2004). The MeHg–S–Cys complex closely mimics the structure of the neutral amino acid, methionine, and is therefore a substrate of the L-type large neutral amino acid transporter system (LAT1) (Yin *et al.*, 2008). This mimicry is responsible for MeHg uptake into cells. MeHg crosses the placenta via a similar neutral amino acid carrier, accumulating in fetal blood in a time- and dose-dependent manner (Kajiwara *et al.*, 1996).

Overexpression of LAT1 in CHO-k1 cells has been shown to be associated with enhanced uptake of [^{14}C]-MeHg when the cells are treated with L-cysteine, but not with the D-cysteine conjugate. In the presence of excess L-methionine, a substrate for LAT1, L-cysteine-conjugated [^{14}C]-MeHg uptake was significantly attenuated. Knockdown of LAT1 decreases the uptake of L-cysteine-conjugated MeHg and attenuates the effects of MeHg on lactate dehydrogenase (LDH) leakage and CHO-k1 cell viability (Yin *et al.*, 2008). Notably, different neutral amino acids have different suppression effects. For example, the suppression by methionine is not as remarkable as that produced by phenylalanine. This phenomenon could be due to the transient rapid cysteine surge after methionine administration, but not after phenylalanine administration. This newly synthesized cysteine in maternal blood accelerates the mercury uptake across the placenta.

Mechanisms of neurotoxicity

As mentioned previously, MeHg has been found to bind to protein -SH groups of amino acids, such as cysteine, which is also present in glutathione (GSH) (Clarkson, 1993). This affinity for the sulfur and sulfhydryl groups (-SH) is a major factor underlying the biochemical and toxic properties of MeHg and its interference with optimal cell function. A large body of research aimed at deciphering the cellular and molecular mechanisms of MeHg-induced neurotoxicity points to several critical features, namely: (1) inhibition of macromolecule synthesis (DNA, RNA and protein); (2) microtubule disruption; (3) increase in intracellular Ca^{2+} with disturbance of neurotransmitter function; and (4) oxidative stress. Nonetheless, MeHg's primary site of action and the genetic bases of its neurotoxicity have yet to be identified. A brief review outlining the most critical features of the mechanisms involved in MeHg-induced neurotoxicity follows.

MeHg reacts with DNA and RNA, resulting in changes in the secondary structure of these molecules (Gruenwedel and Cruikshank, 1979). Since the 1990s, epidemiological studies have suggested increased genotoxicity in human populations through dietary and occupational exposure (Crespo-Lopez *et al.*, 2009). MeHg inhibits DNA repair mechanisms, thereby leading to genotoxicity. For example, MeHg directly binds to the "zinc finger" core of DNA repair enzymes, affecting their activity. The "zinc finger" proteins contain an atom of zinc and four cysteines and/or histidines. Thus, the high affinity of mercury to sulfhydryl groups on cysteines may deform the structural integrity and activity of these enzymes (Asmuss *et al.*, 2000). MeHg could also give rise to disturbances in protein synthesis (Chang *et al.*, 1972; Choi *et al.*, 1980; Farris and Smith, 1975; Verity *et al.*, 1975). On the other hand, increased protein synthesis due to reactive astrogliosis, has been reported after *in vivo* exposure to MeHg (Brubaker *et al.*, 1973).

The inhibition of the polymerization of tubulin by MeHg is among the major mechanisms of developmental MeHg toxicity (Sager *et al.*, 1982). Microtubular fragmentation has been reported in cultured primary rat cerebellar granular neurons at an MeHg concentration of 0.5–1 μM (Castoldi *et al.*, 2000). Additionally, it has been reported that 4 μM mercury salt, independently of the anion, is capable of inhibiting the polymerization of isolated tubulin in a dose-dependent manner. Further, 0.1 μM mercury salt is sufficient to decrease kinesin-driven motility and to produce a significant increase of micronuclei in V9 hamster lung fibroblasts (Thier *et al.*, 2003). Since microtubules participate in cell division, their fragmentation by MeHg results in antimitotic effects, as well as the inhibition of neuronal migration and the degeneration of neuritis (Choi *et al.*, 1980), all of which are inherent to developmental MeHg exposure outcomes.

MeHg depolarizes the presynaptic membrane, increasing Na^{2+} and decreasing K^{+} ion concentration. This, in turn, causes disruption of Ca^{2+} homeostasis leading to increased intracellular Ca^{2+} concentration (Komulainen and Bondy, 1987; Oyama *et al.*, 1994). Blockers of voltage-dependent Ca^{2+} channels prevent the appearance of neurological signs (Sakamoto *et al.*, 1996). Increased Ca^{2+} concentrations disrupt neurotransmitter signaling. Increased release of dopamine, glutamate, γ-amino butyric acid (GABA), glycine, choline (Bondy *et al.*, 1979) and acetylcholine (Juang, 1976) have been associated with MeHg exposure. Inhibition of the uptake of excitatory amino acids, such as glutamate and aspartate, has also been implicated as a major mechanism of MeHg-induced neurotoxicity (Aschner *et al.*, 1993, 2000). Antagonists of the *N*-methyl-D-aspartic acid receptor have been reported to inhibit the toxic effects of MeHg (Park *et al.*, 1996).

MeHg also alters the cellular energy metabolism. Chen *et al.* (2006) reported that highly enriched Hg concentrations were found in mitochondrial fractions from Hg-exposed porcine cells. Yin *et al.* (2007) demonstrated that MeHg causes a concentration-dependent reduction in the inner mitochondrial membrane potential ($\Delta\Psi m$) of primary cultured astrocytes. MeHg stimulates the ubiquinol:cytochrome C reductase complex (complex III) on the mitochondrial membrane (Yee and Choi, 1996), while inhibiting glutathione peroxidase (GPx) (Farina *et al.*, 2009; Franco *et al.*, 2009), which leads to lipid peroxidation. Fox *et al.* (1975) and Verity *et al.* (1975) further reported that MeHg inhibited state 3 but increases state 4 respiration, inhibiting tricarboxylic acid (TCA) cycle activity and decreasing ATP utilization. In brain tissues, MeHg affects respiratory control in synaptosomes both *in vitro* and *in vivo*. Effects on mitochondrial respiration in the brain have also been reported (Verity *et al.*, 1975; Von Burg and Smith, 1979), causing the inhibition of glycolysis and TCA cycle activity and a decrease in adenosine triphosphate (ATP) utilization. Since the CNS is strictly dependent upon glucose for its energy production, high oxygen utilization and excitability renders it especially susceptible to toxins.

Disruption of redox cellular homeostasis by excess reactive oxygen species (ROS) formation leading to cumulative oxidative stress represents an important feature of MeHg neurotoxicity. MeHg is known to induce oxidative stress (Sarafian, 1999) both *in vitro* and *in vivo* (Ali *et al.*, 1992; Fujimoto *et al.*, 1985; LeBel *et al.*, 1992; Shanker and Aschner, 2003; Yee and Choi, 1994). The production of ROS by MeHg exacerbates toxicity by facilitating cell death via apoptotic pathways. Inhibition of glutathione peroxidase (GPx) by MeHg further potentiates lipid peroxidation. Conversely, several studies have demonstrated partial amelioration of MeHg toxicity in the presence of antioxidants (Gasso *et al.*, 2001; Roos *et al.*, 2009; Sanfeliu *et al.*, 2001; Shanker and Aschner, 2003). A major source of MeHg-increased ROS generation is the mitochondrial electron transport chain. The damaged mitochondrion increases oxidative stress, leading to a decrease in defense mechanisms. It has also been reported that blockage of the mitochondrial transition pore by cyclosporin A in brain synaptosomes decreases MeHg-induced ROS production (Myhre and Fonnum, 2001). MeHg binds to GSH, which is one of the principal endogenous antioxidants, and this binding is responsible for the excretion of MeHg. Thus, decreased GSH levels parallel the increased oxidative stress caused by MeHg (Li *et al.*, 1996; Sternlicht *et al.*, 1994; Vijayalakshmi and Sood, 1994). Upregulation of GSH is neuroprotective against MeHg-induced neurotoxicity (Choi *et al.*, 1996; Farina *et al.*, 2009).

Toxicity

Toxicity in developing brains

The brain is the primary target site for MeHg (ATSDR, 1999), and MeHg effects on the developing CNS are more severe than those in the mature CNS (Atchison, 2005; Hursh *et al.*, 1988). There is usually a latent period of weeks to months between exposure and the onset of symptoms (Clarkson *et al.*, 2003). In less severe cases, psychomotor retardation and increased incidence of seizures have been reported (Marsh *et al.*, 1980). In general, MeHg poisoning results in focal damage in adults and widespread and diffuse damage in the fetal and neonatal brain (Lapham *et al.*, 1995), likely reflecting the dynamic nature of the developing CNS (cell division, migration, differentiation, synaptogenesis). For example, the brain areas most vulnerable to MeHg after adult exposure include the primary sensory and motor cortices, pre- and post-central gyri, the temporal transverse gyrus and the cerebellum (but not Purkinje cells) (Taber and Hurley, 2008). In contrast, upon congenital exposure to MeHg, damage is more widespread, resulting in cortical atrophy, thinning of the corpus collosum and white matter shrinkage. Hematoxylin and eosin stain has established diffuse spongiosus in the deeper layers as well as gliosis with loss of neurons in the upper layers (Davis *et al.*, 1994; Taber and Hurley, 2008).

Because the vulnerability to MeHg poisoning is age-related, with susceptibility decreasing with increasing age, the symptoms of mercury poisoning and mercury deposits are quite different depending on the age at the time of exposure (Taber and Hurley, 2008). Davis *et al.* (1994) followed an entire family chronically exposed to MeHg. An infant exposed to MeHg *in utero* was born mute, blind and with severe mental retardation, quadriparesis, choreoathetosis and seizures. An 8-year-old child in the same family had very similar symptoms. Both died 21 years post-MeHg exposure. In contrast, a 20-year-old child in the same family had a loss of peripheral vision, poor hand coordination and mild cognitive deficits. The parents were reported to be completely asymptomatic (Davis *et al.*, 1994). These results are consistent with previous observations reported by Berlin and Ullberg (1963).

It is likely that unique features of the fetal blood–brain barrier (BBB) contribute to the vulnerability of the fetal brain to MeHg toxicity. The fetal BBB is not fully developed until the middle of the first year of life, resulting in constant exposure to MeHg throughout gestation (Rodier, 1995) and during early postnatal life. It is also likely that, given the immaturity of the CNS, MeHg is not as efficiently excreted from the CNS, as transporters associated with this process are less likely to be fully developed. Furthermore, the increased burden of MeHg in general likely reflects the absence of an efficient mechanism(s) for excretion of MeHg via the bile.

MeHg causes mitotic arrest in developing neurons after prenatal exposure, and the effects of MeHg on neuron proliferation depend on which type of neurons were forming at the time of exposure (Rodier, 1995). It is well known that the generation of neurons continues throughout gestation and well into the first year of life. Typically, a set of neurons destined to be similar in function and morphology is generated in a short period, sometimes within a few days of gestation. In general, large motor neurons are produced first, followed by sensory neurons. Nuclear groups in the brain stem and diencephalon are formed early, but the complex layered structures like the cerebral cortex, cerebellum and hippocampus add more neurons over a long period of time (Rodier, 1995). Therefore, in infants, diffuse neuronal degeneration is detected consistently in these early-formed brain structures.

Further, MeHg causes incomplete or abnormal migration of neurons to the cerebellar and cerebral cortices as well as deranged cortical organization of the cerebrum with regard to heterotopic neurons. Moreover, the laminar cortical pattern of the cerebrum is disturbed, consisting of irregular groupings and deranged alignment of cortical layers. Although the molecular targets of MeHg giving rise to these outcomes are not fully understood, studies on MeHg's effects in the Drosophila model suggest an altered Notch receptor pathway (Bland and Rand, 2006). The Notch receptor pathway is a highly conserved cell–cell signaling mechanism that controls cell fate decision, proliferation, migration and neurite outgrowth during neural development (Bland and Rand, 2006).

Notch receptor activation requires proteolysis by a cell surface disintegrin and metalloproteinase (ADAM), which is required for normal neural development. MeHg exposure promotes activation of ADAM resulting in a concentration- and time-dependent increase in Notch receptor activity (Bland and Rand, 2006). Notably, inorganic mercury is significantly less potent for inducing Notch activity as compared to MeHg, suggesting a mechanism specific to the organic form of mercury.

MeHg also inhibits several fetal brain enzymes. Watanabe and colleagues reported that prenatal MeHg exposure significantly inhibits selenoenzymes, such as glutathione peroxidase (GPx), in fetal mouse brains injected with 3 mgHg/kg of MeHg on gestational day 12–14 (Watanabe *et al.*, 1999b). As a result, glutathione (GSH) is decreased and thiobarbituric acid-reactive substances (TBARS) are increased. Furthermore, lipid peroxidation is increased in fetal brains (Watanabe *et al.*, 1999a).

In addition to its effects on brain structure and brain enzymes, MeHg exposure also affects synaptic transmission. The acute effects of mercury on the amphibian neuromuscular junction have been studied using the isolated sciatic nerve/sartorius muscle preparation. Results have indicated that mercury primarily affects presynaptic neurotransmitter release, but not postsynaptic processes, which include the activation of receptor-associated ionic channels and degradation of chemical transmitters (Atchison, 1988; Cooper and Manalis, 1983). Mercury also disrupts the intracellular buffering of calcium, which further inhibits the calcium-dependent neurotransmitter release (Atchison, 1988; Cooper and Manalis, 1983). Mercury first causes an increase in evoked acetylcholine release followed by a sudden and complete blockade (Atchison, 1988; Cooper and Manalis, 1983).

In all age groups, myelination is greatly inhibited by MeHg. Biopsy of the sural nerve was performed on three patients who died of severe Minamata disease, and the results revealed numerous unmyelinated and poorly myelinated nerve fibers (Takeuchi *et al.*, 1978). The myelinated fibers were scattered irregularly in small numbers or in groups of peculiar features in the intraneural bundle. In addition, abnormally thin or poorly formed myelin sheaths were observed. Regenerated axons were extremely small in size, and sometimes the small axons were lost entirely, leaving only the thin myelin sheaths. MeHg was also reported to inhibit UDP galactose:ceramide galactosyltransferase (CGalT) and 2′,3′-cyclic-nucleotide 3′-phosphodiesterase (CNP), enzymes involved in myelin formation (Grundt and Neskovic, 1985). Notably, MeHg has greater inhibitory effects on myelin formation than diethylmercury, which suggests that different forms of organic mercury produce different effects (Grundt *et al.*, 1980).

Toxicity in other organs/systems

The developing immune system is especially sensitive to the elemental forms of mercury. Occupational studies and animal studies have demonstrated that MeHg affects immune-cell ratios and cellular responses (Committee on the Toxicological Effects of Methylmercury, 2000). MeHg reduces natural killer (NK) cell activity (Ilback *et al.*, 1991) and alters the mitogen response as well as the function of B-cell and T-cell subtypes (Wild *et al.*, 1997). As a result, MeHg-treated animals are more susceptible to viruses and bacterial infections (Ilback *et al.*, 1996). MeHg also induces the autoimmune response by producing antinucleolar antibodies (Hultman and Hansson-Georgiadis, 1999) and anti-DNA antibodies (Cardenas *et al.*, 1993).

Paternal exposure to mercury in humans does not appear to cause infertility or malformations (Alcser *et al.*, 1989), but a study of pregnancy outcomes among the wives of 152 men occupationally exposed to Hg showed an increased incidence of spontaneous abortion (Cordier *et al.*, 1991). At urinary Hg concentration levels exceeding 50 μg/L in male workers, the spontaneous abortion risk in their wives was doubled. In animal tests, MeHg treatment caused abnormal sperm and a low conception rate in monkeys (Mohamed *et al.*, 1987). In a mouse model, MeHg was shown to cause tubular atrophy of the testes (Hirano *et al.*, 1986).

The developing kidney has been found to be more sensitive to organic mercury (Samuels *et al.*, 1982). High mercury exposure results in mild transient proteinuria, gross proteinuria, hematuria, oliguria and acute renal failure. Kidney biopsy specimens from patients with nephrotic syndrome following exposure to metallic mercury demonstrated proximal tubular and glomerular changes, such as necrosis of the tubule epithelium, swollen granular protoplasm and nonstainable nuclei in the kidneys, partially due to mercury accumulation (Hook *et al.*, 1954; Kazantzis *et al.*, 1962). In rodents, MeHg has been shown to cause renal fibrosis (Magos and Butler, 1972), increase renal weight, decrease renal enzymes (Verschuuren *et al.*, 1976a,b) and result in renal hypertrophy (Slotkin *et al.*, 1985). Microscopic examinations reveal cytoplasmic masses in proximal tubules (Fowler, 1972), degeneration of proximal tubules and interstitial fibrosis (Mitsumori *et al.*, 1990).

MeHg also affects other organ systems. It increases the risk for anemia and clotting disorders (Munro and Gummer, 1980). Furthermore, the cardiovascular system appears to be a target for MeHg toxicity in both human beings and animals, with adverse health effects including the following: (1) both elemental and organic forms of Hg alter blood pressure regulation; (2) men with hair Hg concentration exceeding 2 ppm have increased risk of acute myocardial infarction; and (3) prenatal exposure to MeHg is linked to heart rate variability in children (Committee on the Toxicological Effects of Methylmercury, 2000).

RISK ASSESSMENT

The risk and toxicity of MeHg have been analyzed by three epidemiological studies since the EPA's derivation of an RfD in 1995 (NAS, 2000). These longitudinal, developmental studies were conducted in the Seychelles Islands, the Faroe Islands and in New Zealand (http://www.epa.gov/iris/subst/0073.htm). The subjects of the Seychelles longitudinal prospective study were 779 mother–infant pairs from a fish-eating population (Davidson *et al.*, 1998, 1995; Myers *et al.*, 1995, 1997). Infants were followed from birth to 5.5 years of age and assessed at various ages on a number of standardized neuropsychological endpoints. The independent variable was maternal-hair mercury levels. The Faroe Islands study was a longitudinal study of about 900 mother–infant pairs (Grandjean *et al.*, 1997). The main independent variable was cord-blood mercury; maternal-hair mercury was also measured. Children were evaluated at 7 years of age, based on a variety of tasks designed to assess function in specific behavioral domains. The New Zealand study was a prospective case control study of 38 children born to women with hair mercury levels greater than 6 ppm during pregnancy matched with children whose mothers had lower hair mercury levels (Kjellstrom *et al.*, 1989, 1986). At 6 years of age, 237 children were assessed on a number of neuropsychological endpoints similar to those used in the Seychelles study (Kjellstrom *et al.*, 1989). The Seychelles study yielded scant evidence of impairment related to *in utero* MeHg exposure, whereas the other two studies found dose-related effects on a number of neuropsychological endpoints. However, in a 9-year follow-up study of 643 children, the authors of the Seychelles study did not find an association between prenatal MeHg exposure and developmental outcomes (van Wijngaarden *et al.*, 2009). An analysis by Davidson of the same population in a 10.7-year follow-up found a significant association between prenatal exposure to MeHg and impaired visuospatial ability (Davidson *et al.*, 2008). Furthermore, a National Academy of Sciences (NAS) expert panel reviewed the studies and concluded that the weight of the evidence supported adverse health effects due to MeHg exposure (NAS, 2000) and recommended that levels of mercury not to exceed 5.0 μg/L in whole blood or 1.0 μg/g in hair, corresponding to an RfD of 0.1 μg/kg body weight/day.

Various agencies have developed guidelines for "safe" exposure to MeHg, including the EPA (Mahaffey, 1999), the US Agency for Toxic Substances and Disease Registry (ATSDR, 1999), the US Food and Drug Administration (FDA) and the World Health Organization (WHO). These exposure levels range from 0.1 μg/kg body weight/day (EPA) to 0.47 μg/kg body weight/day (WHO, 2000). The range of recommendations is due to varying safety margins, differing emphasis placed on various sources of data, the particular missions of the respective agencies and the unique population that each guideline is intended to protect. All guidelines, however, fall within the same order of magnitude. Although these guidelines may be used as screening tools in risk assessments to evaluate the "safety" of Hg exposures, they are not meant to be distinctive lines above which toxicity will definitely occur. However, as exposure levels increase in multiples of these guidelines, members of the public health community have become increasingly concerned that adverse health consequences may occur (Mahaffey, 1999).

It needs to be emphasized that these levels of exposure to MeHg can be readily attained with only a few meals of fish per week, depending on the source and type of fish. In populations dependent on fish as their source of protein (e.g., in the Faroe Islands), increased hair Hg levels (up to 4.27 ppm) during pregnancy have been shown to be associated with impaired psychomotor test performance of children at 7 years of age (Grandjean *et al.*, 1997). Further, this type of diet led to an average cord-blood MeHg level of 22.9 μg/L and was correlated with neurophysiological and neuropsychological deficits. In a follow-up study in the Faroe Islands, it was reported that similar correlations persisted in 14-year-old children (Debes *et al.*, 2006). In Japan, a strong association between the prevalence of mental retardation and Hg concentration in the umbilical cord was reported both in Minamata (Harada, 1978) and Niigata (Tsubaki and Irukayma, 1977). In another study from New Zealand (Kjellstrom and Kennedy, 1985) maternal hair Hg levels exceeding 6 ppm (range 5–20 ppm) correlated with a deficit in the Denver developmental screening test as well as a neurological screening test in children at 4 years of age. However, an epidemiological study in the province of Quebec, Canada (Keown-Eyssen *et al.*, 1983) indicated no consistent relationship between maternal hair MeHg levels of 24 ppm during pregnancy and developmental outcomes in the female offspring. Also, in the Seychelles study (Davidson *et al.*, 1998; Kjellstrom and Kennedy, 1985; Myers *et al.*, 2003) no adverse effects were detected at a maternal MeHg hair level of 6.8 ppm. The apparent differences in outcomes between the Faroe Islands and Seychelles studies are likely due to numerous factors, extensively reviewed by the NAS (2000), who emphasized that the weight of the evidence supported adverse health effects from MeHg and recommended that levels of Hg not to exceed 5.0 μg/L in whole blood or 1.0 μg/g in hair, corresponding to a reference dose (RfD) of 0.1 μg/kg body weight/day.

TREATMENT

The first step of treatment is to remove patients from the source of exposure. Decontamination requires removal of clothes, flushing eyes and exposed mucosa with saline solution, and washing skin with soap and water. If mercury is swallowed, activated charcoal is used to limit further mercury absorption from the GI system. Patients are given adequate fluids and electrolytes to expedite the excretion of mercury through urine. In severe cases, dialysis could be used. Immediate chelation therapy is the standard of care for patients showing any symptoms of severe mercury poisoning or the patient history suggesting a large total mercury load (Clifton, 2007).

Drug choice in chelation therapy depends on the form of mercury and patient age. In adult patients, acute inorganic mercury poisoning can be treated with dimercaptosuccinic acid (DMSA), 2,3-dimercapto-1-propanesulfonic acid (DMPS), D-penicillamine (DPCN) or dimercaprol (BAL). Of these, only DMSA is currently approved by the FDA for the treatment of children exposed to mercury. However, previous studies found no clear clinical benefit from DMSA treatment in mercury vapor poisoning (Risher and Amler, 2005). DMSA given orally may have fewer side effects and has been reported to be superior to BAL, DPCN and DMPS (Blanuša *et al.*, 2005). Glutathione and alpha-lipoic acid may also be used in mercury poisoning treatment, but they may increase mercury concentrations in the kidney and the brain, although the underlying mechanism is still unknown (Rooney, 2007). Notably, chelation therapy can be hazardous. Baxter and Krenzelok (2008) reported that an incorrect form of EDTA used for chelation therapy caused cardiac arrest in a 5-year-old autistic boy due to irreversible hypocalcemia.

CONCLUDING REMARKS AND FUTURE DIRECTIONS

MeHg is a well-documented neurotoxicant. Studies in children suffering from tragic MeHg poisoning outbreaks in Japan and Iraq have revealed the pronounced susceptibility of the developing brain to MeHg. As a consequence, a plethora of studies have drawn attention to the consequences of prenatal exposure. Previous animal experiments also have shown similar neuromorphological and neurobehavioral alterations induced by MeHg after either acute or chronic exposure. Particular attention was directed to comparative toxicity assessments across species and to the degree of concordance between human and animal data. In general, these studies have established that prenatal MeHg exposure in both humans and laboratory animals leads to diffuse brain damage including reduced brain size, damage to the cortex and basal ganglia, loss of cells, ventricular dilation, ectopic cells, disorganized brain layers and gliosis. The main difference between the human and the monkey in neuropathology is the relative insensitivity of the monkey's cerebellum to MeHg, which represents a major target in humans. Clinical symptoms of prenatal MeHg exposure include blindness, auditory defects, somatosensory impairment, difficulty in learning and delays in social development and in the attainment of cognitive milestones.

Guidelines for exposure to MeHg range from 0.1 μg/kg body weight/day (EPA) to 0.47 ug/kg body weight/day (WHO, 2000). The differences in the guidelines between various regulatory agencies are largely due to the uncertainties intrinsic to human epidemiological studies, including unmeasured confounders and effect modifiers, which could compromise the exposure outcomes. Thus, additional research addressing interspecies comparisons is necessary to determine a more specific standard for critical dose levels of MeHg. An accurate interspecies comparison should take several key factors into account, including the species-related differences in the kinetics of MeHg distribution and its concentration in target organs. Basu *et al.* (2005) studied the inhibitory effects of MeHg on the mACh receptor in the cerebral cortex and further cross-compared the species sensitivity between the human, rat, mouse, mink and river otter. Species sensitivities, irrespective of Hg type and brain region, can be ranked from most to least sensitive as follows: river otter>rat>mink>mouse>humans. Thus, a well-designed comparative study could provide data on interspecies differences and a framework for interpreting results generated from human, murine and wildlife studies.

As a potent environmental pollutant, MeHg reacts with DNA, RNA and proteins. Studies on the potential for toxicogenomic effects of MeHg are sparse, and future studies should focus on the identification of single nucleotide polymorphisms (SNPs) in various genes that will elicit novel information regarding the role of gene and environment interactions and a particular individual's susceptibility to MeHg. Due to the considerable disadvantages inherent in both human epidemiological studies and animal experiments, toxicologists face the major challenge of developing and validating other, more targeted and controlled model systems. For example, using *Caenorhabditis elegans* (*C. elegans*) as the model system in toxicological research is very promising due to this species' simple and well-defined nervous system, its ready visualization through the use of green fluorescent protein (GFP) and its rapid lifecycle (Helmcke *et al.*, 2009). Further improving the *C. elegans* model and developing *in vitro* models will prove of particular import because future toxicological studies will be greatly expanded to cover a much wider range of environments and numbers of species. Additionally, the development of high throughput methods in proteomics, genomics and bioinformatics will lead to better understanding the developmental toxicity of MeHg by the accumulation of vast amounts of valuable toxicological information.

ACKNOWLEDGMENTS

This chapter was supported in part by a grant from NIEHS ES 07331 to MA. OPS is funded in part by a grant from NICHD and by the Office of Research on Women's Health.

REFERENCES

Agency for Toxic Substances and Disease Registry (1999) Toxicological profile for mercury. Agency for Toxic Substances and Disease Registry, Atlanta, GA.

Alcser KH, Brix KA, Fine LJ, Kallenbach LR, Wolfe RA (1989) Occupational mercury exposure and male reproductive health. *Am J Ind Med* **15:** 517–29.

Ali SF, LeBel CP, Bondy SC (1992) Reactive oxygen species formation as a biomarker of methylmercury and trimethyltin neurotoxicity. *Neurotoxicology* **13:** 637–48.

Aschner M, Du YL, Gannon M, Kimelberg HK (1993) Methylmercury-induced alterations in excitatory amino acid transport in rat primary astrocyte cultures. *Brain Res* **602:** 181–6.

Aschner M, Yao CP, Allen JW, Tan KH (2000) Methylmercury alters glutamate transport in astrocytes. *Neurochem Intl* **37:** 199–206.

Asmuss M, Mullenders LH, Hartwig A (2000) Interference by toxic metal compounds with isolated zinc finger DNA repair proteins. *Toxicol Lett* **112–113:** 227–31.

Atchison WD (1988) Effects of neurotoxicants on synaptic transmission: lessons learned from electrophysiological studies. *Neurotoxicol Teratol* **10:** 393–416.

Atchison WD (2005) Is chemical neurotransmission altered specifically during methylmercury-induced cerebellar dysfunction? *Trends Pharmacol Sci* **26:** 549–57.

Bakir F, Damluji SF, Amin-Zaki L, Murtadha M, Khalidi A, al-Rawi NY, Tikriti S, Dahahir HI, Clarkson TW, Smith JC, Doherty RA (1973) Methylmercury poisoning in Iraq. *Science* **181:** 230–41.

Basu N, Stamler CJ, Loua KM, Chan HM (2005) An interspecies comparison of mercury inhibition on muscarinic acetylcholine receptor binding in the cerebral cortex and cerebellum. *Toxicol Appl Pharmacol* **205:** 71–6.

Baxter AJ, Krenzelok EP (2008) Pediatric fatality secondary to EDTA chelation. *Clin Toxicol* **46:** 1083–4.

Berlin M, Ullberg S (1963) Accumulation and retention of mercury in the mouse. I. An autoradiographic study after a single intravenous injection of mercuric chloride. *Arch Environ Health* **6:** 589–601.

Bland C, Rand MD (2006) Methylmercury induces activation of Notch signaling. *Neurotoxicology* **27:** 982–91.

Blanusa M, Varnai VM, Piasek M, Kostial K (2005) Chelators as antidotes of metal toxicity: therapeutic and experimental aspects. *Curr Med Chem* **12:** 2771–94.

Bondy SC, Anderson CL, Harrington ME, Prasad KN (1979) The effects of organic and inorganic lead and mercury on neurotransmitter high-affinity transport and release mechanisms. *Environ Res* **19:** 102–11.

Boudou A, Maury-Brachet R, Coquery M, Durrieu G, Cossa D (2005) Synergic effect of gold mining and damming on mercury contamination in fish. *Environ Sci Technol* **39:** 2448–54.

Bridges CC, Zalups RK (2004) Homocysteine, system b0,+ and the renal epithelial transport and toxicity of inorganic mercury. *Am J Pathol* **165:** 1385–94.

Brubaker PE, Klein R, Herman SP, Lucier GW, Alexander LT, Long MD (1973) DNA, RNA, and protein synthesis in brain, liver, and kidneys of asymptomatic methylmercury treated rats. *Exp Mol Pathol* **18:** 263–80.

Cardenas A, Roels H, Bernard AM, Barbon R, Buchet JP, Lauwerys RR, Rosello J, Hotter G, Mutti A, Franchini I, *et al.* (1993) Markers of early renal changes induced by industrial pollutants. I. Application to workers exposed to mercury vapour. *Br J Ind Med* **50:** 17–27.

Castoldi AF, Barni S, Turin I, Gandini C, Manzo L (2000) Early acute necrosis, delayed apoptosis and cytoskeletal breakdown in cultured cerebellar granule neurons exposed to methylmercury. *J Neurosci Res* **59:** 775–87.

Chang LW, Desnoyers PA, Hartmann HA (1972) Quantitative cytochemical studies of RNA in experimental mercury poisoning. Changes in RNA content. *J Neuropathol Exp Neurol* **31:** 489–501.

Charleston JS, Body RL, Mottet NK, Vahter ME, Burbacher TM (1995) Autometallographic determination of inorganic mercury distribution in the cortex of the calcarine sulcus of the monkey Macaca fascicularis following long-term subclinical exposure to methylmercury and mercuric chloride. *Toxicol Appl Pharmacol* **132:** 325–33.

Chen C, Qu L, Zhao J, Liu S, Deng G, Li B, Zhang P, Chai Z (2006) Accumulation of mercury, selenium and their binding proteins in porcine kidney and liver from mercury-exposed areas with the investigation of their redox responses. *Sci Total Environ* **366:** 627–37.

Choi BH, Cho KH, Lapham LW (1980) Effects of methylmercury on DNA synthesis of human fetal astrocytes: a radioautographic study. *Brain Res* **202:** 238–42.

Choi BH, Yee S, Robles M (1996) The effects of glutathione glycoside in methyl mercury poisoning. *Toxicol Appl Pharmacol* **141:** 357–64.

Clarkson TW, Hursh JB, Sager PR, *et al.* (1988) Mercury. In *Biological Monitoring of Toxic Metals* (Clarkson TW, Hursh JB, Sager PR, eds.). Plenum Press, New York, pp. 199–246.

Clarkson TW (1993) Molecular and ionic mimicry of toxic metals. *Annu Rev Pharmacol Toxicol* **33:** 545–71.

Clarkson TW (1997) The toxicology of mercury. *Crit Rev Clin Lab Sci* **34:** 369–403.

Clarkson TW, Magos L, Myers GJ (2003) The toxicology of mercury – current exposures and clinical manifestations. *N Engl J Med* **349:** 1731–7.

Clifton JC 2nd (2007) Mercury exposure and public health. *Pediatr Clin North Am* **54:** 237–69, viii.

Committee on the Toxicological Effects of Methylmercury, BOESAT, National Research Council (2000) Toxicological Effects of Methylmercury.

Cooper GP, Manalis RS (1983) Influence of heavy metals on synaptic transmission: a review. *Neurotoxicology* **4:** 69–83.

Cordier S, Deplan F, Mandereau L, Hemon D (1991) Paternal exposure to mercury and spontaneous abortions. *Br J Ind Med* **48:** 375–81.

Crespo-Lopez ME, Macedo GL, Pereira SI, Arrifano GP, Picanco-Diniz DL, do Nascimento JL, Herculano AM (2009) Mercury and human genotoxicity: critical considerations and possible molecular mechanisms. *Pharmacol Res* **60:** 212–20.

Davidson PW, Jean Sloane R, Myers GJ, Hansen ON, Huang LS, Georger LA, Cox C, Thurston SW, Shamlaye CF, Clarkson TW (2008) Association between prenatal exposure to methylmercury and visuospatial ability at 10.7 years in the Seychelles child development study. *Neurotoxicology* **29:** 453–9.

Davidson PW, Myers GJ, Cox C, Axtell C, Shamlaye C, Sloane-Reeves J, Cernichiari E, Needham L, Choi A, Wang Y, Berlin M, Clarkson TW (1998) Effects of prenatal and postnatal methylmercury exposure from fish consumption on neurodevelopment: outcomes at 66 months of age in the Seychelles Child Development Study. *J Am Med Assoc* **280:** 701–7.

Davidson PW, Myers GJ, Cox C, Shamlaye CF, Marsh DO, Tanner MA, Berlin M, Sloane-Reeves J, Cernichiari E, Choisy O, *et al.* (1995) Longitudinal neurodevelopmental study of Seychellois children following in utero exposure to methylmercury from maternal fish ingestion: outcomes at 19 and 29 months. *Neurotoxicology* **16:** 677–88.

Davis LE, Kornfeld M, Mooney HS, Fiedler KJ, Haaland KY, Orrison WW, Cernichiari E, Clarkson TW (1994) Methylmercury poisoning: long-term clinical, radiological, toxicological, and pathological studies of an affected family. *Ann Neurol* **35:** 680–8.

Debes F, Budtz-Jorgensen E, Weihe P, White RF, Grandjean P (2006) Impact of prenatal methylmercury exposure on neurobehavioral function at age 14 years. *Neurotoxicol Teratol* **28:** 536–47.

Doi R (1991) Individual difference of methylmercury metabolism in animals and its significance in methylmercury toxicity. In *Advances in Mercury Toxicology* (Suzuki T, Imura N, Clarkson TW, eds.). Plenum Press, New York, London, pp. 77–98.

Farina M, Campos F, Vendrell I, Berenguer J, Barzi M, Pons S, Sunol C (2009) Probucol increases glutathione peroxidase-1 activity and displays long-lasting protection against methylmercury toxicity in cerebellar granule cells. *Toxicol Sci* **112:** 416–26.

Farris FF, Smith JC (1975) In vivo incorporation of 14-C-leucine into brain protein of methylmercury treated rats. *Bull Environ Contam Toxicol* **13:** 451–5.

Fowler BA (1972) The morphologic effects of dieldrin and methyl mercuric chloride on pars recta segments of rat kidney proximal tubules. *Am J Pathol* **69:** 163–78.

Fox JH, Patel-Mandlik K, Cohen MM (1975) Comparative effects of organic and inorganic mercury on brain slice respiration and metabolism. *J Neurochem* **24:** 757–62.

Franco JL, Posser T, Dunkley PR, Dickson PW, Mattos JJ, Martins R, Bainy AC, Marques MR, Dafre AL, Farina M (2009) Methylmercury neurotoxicity is associated with inhibition of the antioxidant enzyme glutathione peroxidase. *Free Radic Biol Med* **47:** 449–57.

Fujimoto Y, Yoshida A, Morisawa K, Ueno T, Fujita T (1985) Enhancement of methyl mercury-induced lipid peroxidation by the addition of ascorbic acid. *Res Commun Chem Pathol Pharmacol* **49:** 267–75.

Gasso S, Cristofol RM, Selema G, Rosa R, Rodriguez-Farre E, Sanfeliu C (2001) Antioxidant compounds and Ca^{2+} pathway blockers differentially protect against methylmercury and mercuric chloride neurotoxicity. *J Neurosci Res* **66:** 135–45.

Grandjean P, Weihe P, White RF, Debes F, Araki S, Yokoyama K, Murata K, Sorensen N, Dahl R, Jorgensen PJ (1997) Cognitive deficit in 7-year-old children with prenatal exposure to methylmercury. *Neurotoxicol Teratol* **19:** 417–28.

Gruenwedel DW, Cruikshank MK (1979) Effect of methylmercury (II) on the synthesis of deoxyribonucleic acid, ribonucleic acid and protein in HeLa S3 cells. *Biochem Pharmacol* **28:** 651–5.

Grundt IK, Neskovic NM (1985) UDPgalactose:ceramide galactosyltransferase and 2′,3′-cyclic-nucleotide 3′-phosphodiesterase activities in rat brain after long-term exposure to methylmercury or triethyllead. *Exp Neurol* **88:** 580–9.

Grundt IK, Stensland E, Syverson TL (1980) Changes in fatty acid composition of myelin cerebrosides after treatment of the developing rat with methylmercury chloride and diethylmercury. *J Lipid Res* **21:** 162–8.

Harada M (1964) Neuropsychiatric disturbances due to organic mercury poisoning during the prenatal period. *Seishin Shinkeigaku Zasshi* **66:** 429–68.

Harada M (1978) Congenital Minamata disease: intrauterine methylmercury poisoning. *Teratology* **18:** 285–8.

Harada M (1995) Minamata disease: methylmercury poisoning in Japan caused by environmental pollution. *Crit Rev Toxicol* **25:** 1–24.

Helmcke KJ, Syversen T, Miller DM 3rd, Aschner M (2009) Characterization of the effects of methylmercury on Caenorhabditis elegans. *Toxicol Appl Pharmacol* **210:** 265–72.

Hirano M, Mitsumori K, Maita K, Shirasu Y (1986) Further carcinogenicity study on methylmercury chloride in ICR mice. *Nippon Juigaku Zasshi* **48:** 127–35.

Hirayama K, Yasutake A (1986) Sex and age differences in mercury distribution and excretion in methylmercury-administered mice. *J Toxicol Environ Health* **18:** 49–60.

Hook O, Lundgren KD, Swensson A (1954) On alkyl mercury poisoning; with a description of two cases. *Acta Med Scand* **150:** 131–7.

Hughes WL (1957) A physicochemical rationale for the biological activity of mercury and its compounds. *Ann NY Acad Sci* **65:** 454–60.

Hultman P, Hansson-Georgiadis H (1999) Methyl mercury-induced autoimmunity in mice. *Toxicol Appl Pharmacol* **154:** 203–11.

Hursh JB, Sichak SP, Clarkson TW (1988) In vitro oxidation of mercury by the blood. *Pharmacol Toxicol* **63:** 266–73.

Igata A (1993) Epidemiological and clinical features of Minamata disease. *Environ Res* **63:** 157–69.

Ilback NG, Sundberg J, Oskarsson A (1991) Methyl mercury exposure via placenta and milk impairs natural killer (NK) cell function in newborn rats. *Toxicol Lett* **58:** 149–58.

Ilback NG, Wesslen L, Fohlman J, Friman G (1996) Effects of methyl mercury on cytokines, inflammation and virus clearance in a common infection (coxsackie B3 myocarditis). *Toxicol Lett* **89:** 19–28.

Juang MS (1976) An electrophysiological study of the action of methylmercuric chloride and mercuric chloride on the sciatic nerve-sartorius muscle preparation of the frog. *Toxicol Appl Pharmacol* **37:** 339–48.

Kajiwara Y, Yasutake A, Adachi T, Hirayama K (1996) Methylmercury transport across the placenta via neutral amino acid carrier. *Arch Toxicol* **70:** 310–14.

Kamps LR, Carr R, Miller H (1972) Total mercury-monomethylmercury content of several species of fish. *Bull Environ Contam Toxicol* **8:** 273–9.

Kazantzis G, Schiller KF, Asscher AW, Drew RG (1962) Albuminuria and the nephrotic syndrome following exposure to mercury and its compounds. *Q J Med* **31:** 403–18.

Keown-Eyssen G, Ruedy J, Neims A (1983) Methylmercury exposure in northern Quebec II. Neurologic findings in children. *Am J Epidemiol* **118:** 470–9.

Kershaw TG, Clarkson TW, Dhahir PH (1980) The relationship between blood levels and dose of methylmercury in man. *Arch Environ Health* **35:** 28–36.

Kjellstrom T, Kennedy P (1985) The association between developmental retardation in children and their prenatal exposure to methylmercury due to maternal fish consumption, SNV-PM. *National Environmental Protection Board Report*, Solna, Sweden.

Kjellstrom T, Kennedy P, Wallis S (1989) Physical and mental development of children with prenatal exposure to mercury from fish. Stage 2. Interviews and psychological tests at age 6, *National Swedish Environmental Board Report*, Solna, Sweden, 3642.

Kjellstrom T, Kennedy P, Wallis S, Mantell C (1986) Physical and mental development of children with prenatal exposure to mercury from fish. Stage 1 Preliminary tests at age 4, Solna, Sweden, 3080.

Komulainen H, Bondy SC (1987) Increased free intrasynaptosomal Ca^{2+} by neurotoxic organometals: distinctive mechanisms. *Toxicol Appl Pharmacol* **88:** 77–86.

Landry TD, Doherty RA, Gates AH (1979) Effects of three diets on mercury excretion after methylmercury administration. *Bull Environ Contam Toxicol* **22:** 151–8.

Lapham LW, Cernichiari E, Cox C, Myers GJ, Baggs RB, Brewer R, Shamlaye CF, Davidson PW, Clarkson TW (1995) An analysis of autopsy brain tissue from infants prenatally exposed to methylmercury. *Neurotoxicology* **16:** 689–704.

LeBel CP, Ali SF, Bondy SC (1992) Deferoxamine inhibits methyl mercury-induced increases in reactive oxygen species formation in rat brain. *Toxicol Appl Pharmacol* **112:** 161–5.

Li S, Thompson SA, Woods JS (1996) Localization of gamma-glutamylcysteine synthetase mRNA expression in mouse brain following methylmercury treatment using reverse transcription in situ PCR amplification. *Toxicol Appl Pharmacol* **140:** 180–7.

Magos L, Butler WH (1972) Cumulative effects of methylmercury dicyandiamide given orally to rats. *Food Cosmet Toxicol* **10:** 513–17.

Mahaffey KR (1999) Methylmercury: a new look at the risks. *Public Health Rep* **114:** 396–9.

Marsh DO, Myers GJ, Clarkson TW, Amin-Zaki L, Tikriti S, Majeed MA (1980) Fetal methylmercury poisoning: clinical and toxicological data on 29 cases. *Ann Neurol* **7:** 348–53.

Mitsumori K, Hirano M, Ueda H, Maita K, Shirasu Y (1990) Chronic toxicity and carcinogenicity of methylmercury chloride in B6C3F1 mice. *Fundam Appl Toxicol* **14:** 179–90.

Mohamed MK, Burbacher TM, Mottet NK (1987) Effects of methyl mercury on testicular functions in Macaca fascicularis monkeys. *Pharmacol Toxicol* **60:** 29–36.

Munro DJ, Gummer WD (1980) Mercury accumulation in biota of Thunder Creek, Saskatchewan. *Bull Environ Contam Toxicol* **25:** 884–90.

Myers GJ, Davidson PW, Cox C, Shamlaye CF, Palumbo D, Cernichiari E, Sloane-Reeves J, Wilding GE, Kost J, Huang LS, Clarkson TW (2003) Prenatal methylmercury exposure from ocean fish consumption in the Seychelles child development study. *Lancet* **361:** 1686–92.

Myers GJ, Davidson PW, Cox C, Shamlaye CF, Tanner MA, Marsh DO, Cernichiari E, Lapham LW, Berlin M, Clarkson TW (1995) Summary of the Seychelles child development study on the relationship of fetal methylmercury exposure to neurodevelopment. *Neurotoxicology* **16:** 711–16.

Myers GJ, Davidson PW, Shamlaye CF, Axtell CD, Cernichiari E, Choisy O, Choi A, Cox C, Clarkson TW (1997) Effects of prenatal methylmercury exposure from a high fish diet on developmental milestones in the Seychelles Child Development Study. *Neurotoxicology* **18:** 819–29.

Myhre O, Fonnum F (2001) The effect of aliphatic, naphthenic, and aromatic hydrocarbons on production of reactive oxygen species and reactive nitrogen species in rat brain synaptosome fraction: the involvement of calcium, nitric oxide synthase, mitochondria, and phospholipase A. *Biochem Pharmacol* **62:** 119–28.

National Academy of Science (2000) Committee on the Toxicological Effects of Methylmercury, Board on Environmental Studies and Toxicology, National Research Council. *Toxicological Effect of Methylmercury*, National Academies Press, Washington DC.

Oyama Y, Tomiyoshi F, Ueno S, Furukawa K, Chikahisa L (1994) Methylmercury-induced augmentation of oxidative metabolism in cerebellar neurons dissociated from the rats: its dependence on intracellular Ca^{2+}. *Brain Res* **660:** 154–7.

Park ST, Lim KT, Chung YT, Kim SU (1996) Methylmercury-induced neurotoxicity in cerebral neuron culture is blocked by antioxidants and NMDA receptor antagonists. *Neurotoxicology* **17:** 37–45.

Rabenstein DL, Fairhurst MT (1975) Nuclear magnetic resonance studies of the solution chemistry of metal complexes. XI. The binding of methylmercury by sulfhydryl-containing amino acids and by glutathione. *J Am Chem Soc* **97:** 2086–92.

Risher JF, Amler SN (2005) Mercury exposure: evaluation and intervention the inappropriate use of chelating agents in the diagnosis and treatment of putative mercury poisoning. *Neurotoxicology* **26:** 691–9.

Rodier PM (1995) Developing brain as a target of toxicity. *Environ Health Perspect* **103 (Suppl. 6):** 73–6.

Rooney JP (2007) The role of thiols, dithiols, nutritional factors and interacting ligands in the toxicology of mercury. *Toxicology* **234:** 145–56.

Roos DH, Puntel RL, Santos MM, Souza DO, Farina M, Nogueira CW, Aschner M, Burger ME, Barbosa NB, Rocha JB (2009) Guanosine and synthetic organoselenium compounds modulate methylmercury-induced oxidative stress in rat brain cortical slices: involvement of oxidative stress and glutamatergic system. *Toxicol in Vitro* **23:** 302–7.

Sager PR, Doherty RA, Rodier PM (1982) Effects of methylmercury on developing mouse cerebellar cortex. *Exp Neurol* **77:** 179–93.

Sakamoto M, Ikegami N, Nakano A (1996) Protective effects of Ca2+ channel blockers against methyl mercury toxicity. *Pharmacol Toxicol* **78:** 193–9.

Sakamoto M, Kubota M, Matsumoto S, Nakano A, Akagi H (2002) Declining risk of methylmercury exposure to infants during lactation. *Environ Res* **90:** 185–9.

Sakamoto M, Murata K, Kubota M, Nakai K, Satoh H (2010) Mercury and heavy metal profiles of maternal and umbilical cord RBCs in Japanese population. *Ecotoxicol Environ Safety* **73:** 1–6.

Samuels ER, Heick HM, McLaine PN, Farant JP (1982) A case of accidental inorganic mercury poisoning. *J Anal Toxicol* **6:** 120–2.

Sanfeliu C, Sebastia J, Ki SU (2001) Methylmercury neurotoxicity in cultures of human neurons, astrocytes, neuroblastoma cells. *Neurotoxicology* **22:** 317–27.

Sarafian TA (1999) Methylmercury-induced generation of free radicals: biological implications. *Met Ions Biol Syst* **36:** 415–44.

Shanker G, Aschner M (2003) Methylmercury-induced reactive oxygen species formation in neonatal cerebral astrocytic cultures is attenuated by antioxidants. *Brain Res Mol Brain Res* **110:** 85–91.

Skerfving S (1974) Methylmercury exposure, mercury levels in blood and hair, and health status in Swedes consuming contaminated fish. *Toxicology* **2:** 3–23.

Slotkin TA, Pachman S, Bartolome J, Kavlock RJ (1985) Biochemical and functional alterations in renal and cardiac development resulting from neonatal methylmercury treatment. *Toxicology* **36:** 231–41.

Spry DJ, Wiener JG (1991) Metal bioavailability and toxicity to fish in low-alkalinity lakes: a critical review. *Environ Pollut* **71:** 243–304.

Sternlicht M, Mirell C, Safarians S, Barsky SH (1994) A novel strategy for the investigation of clonality in precancerous disease states and early stages of tumor progression. *Biochem Biophys Res Commun* **199:** 511–18.

Swedish Expert Group (1971) Methylmercury in fish. A toxicological-epidemiological evaluation of risks. *Nord Hyg Tidskr* **4 (Suppl.):** 9–333.

Taber KH, Hurley RA (2008) Mercury exposure: effects across the lifespan. *J Neuropsychiatry Clin Neurosci* **20:** 389.

Takeuchi T, Eto K, Oyanag S, Miyajima H (1978) Ultrastructural changes of human sural nerves in the neuropathy induced by intrauterine methylmercury poisoning (so-called fetal Minamata disease). *Virchows Arch B Cell Pathol* **27:** 137–54.

Thier R, Bonacker D, Stoiber T, Bohm KJ, Wang M, Unger E, Bolt HM, Degen G (2003) Interaction of metal salts with cytoskeletal motor protein systems. *Toxicol Lett* **140–141:** 75–81.

Tsubaki T, Irukayma K (1977) Methylmercury poisoning in Minamata and Niigata, Japan. In *Minamata Disease* (Tsubaki T, Irukayma K, eds.). Kodansha Ltd Tokyo, Elsevier, Amsterdam.

Tsubaki T, Sato T, Kondo K, Shirakawa K, Kanbayashi K, Hirota K, Yamada K, Murone I (1967) Outbreak of intoxication by organic compounds in Niigata Prefecture. An epidemiological and clinical study. *Jpn J Med Sci Biol* **6:** 132–3.

van Wijngaarden E, Myers GJ, Thurston SW, Shamlaye CF, Davidson PW (2009) Interpreting epidemiological evidence in the presence of multiple endpoints: an alternative analytic approach using the 9-year follow-up of the Seychelles child development study. *Intl Arch Occup Environ Health* **82:** 1031–41.

Verity MA, Brown WJ, Cheung M (1975) Organic mercurial encephalopathy: in vivo and in vitro effects of methyl mercury on synaptosomal respiration. *J Neurochem* **25:** 759–66.

Verschuuren HG, Kroes R, Den Tonkelaar EM, Berkvens JM, Helleman PW, Rauws AG, Schuller PL, Van Esch GJ (1976a) Toxicity of methylmercury chloride in rats I. Short-term study. *Toxicology* **6:** 85–96.

Verschuuren HG, Kroes R, Den Tonkelaar EM, Berkvens JM, Helleman PW, Rauws AG, Schuller PL, Van Esch GJ (1976b) Toxicity of methylmercury chloride in rats. III. Long-term toxicity study. *Toxicology* **6:** 107–23.

Vijayalakshmi K, Sood PP (1994) Ameliorative capacities of vitamins and monothiols post therapy in the restoration of methylmercury altered glutathione metabolism. *Cell Mol Biol (Noisy-le-Grand)* **40:** 211–24.

Von Burg R, Lijoi A, Smith C (1979) Oxygen consumption of rat tissue slices exposed to methylmercury *in vitro*. *Neurosci Lett* **14:** 309–14.

Watanabe C, Kasanuma Y, Dejima Y, Satoh H (1999a) The effect of prenatal methylmercury exposure on the GSH level and lipid peroxidation in the fetal brain and placenta of mice. *Tohoku J Exp Med* **187:** 121–6.

Watanabe C, Yoshida K, Kasanuma Y, Kun Y, Satoh H (1999b) In utero methylmercury exposure differentially affects the activities of selenoenzymes in the fetal mouse brain. *Environ Res* **80:** 208–14.

Westoo G (1966) Determination of methylmercury compounds in foodstuffs. I. Methylmercury compounds in fish, identification and determination. *Acta Chem Scand* **20:** 2131–7.

Wild LG, Ortega HG, Lopez M, Salvaggio JE (1997) Immune system alteration in the rat after indirect exposure to methyl mercury chloride or methyl mercury sulfide. *Environ Res* **74:** 34–42.

WHO (World Health Organization) (2000) Mercury. In *Air Quality Guidelines*. Geneva: WHO.

Yee S, Choi BH (1994) Methylmercury poisoning induces oxidative stress in the mouse brain. *Exp Mol Pathol* **60:** 188–96.

Yee S, Choi BH (1996) Oxidative stress in neurotoxic effects of methylmercury poisoning. *Neurotoxicology* **17:** 17–26.

Yin Z, Jiang H, Syversen T, Rocha JB, Farina M, Aschner M (2008) The methylmercury-L-cysteine conjugate is a substrate for the L-type large neutral amino acid transporter. *J Neurochem* **107:** 1083–90.

Yin Z, Milatovic D, Aschner JL, Syversen T, Rocha JB, Souza DO, Sidoryk M, Albrecht J, Aschner M (2007) Methylmercury induces oxidative injury, alterations in permeability and glutamine transport in cultured astrocytes. *Brain Res* **1131:** 1–10.

C H A P T E R

36

Selenium

T. Zane Davis and Jeffery O. Hall

INTRODUCTION

Selenium (Se) is an essential nutrient that has a relatively narrow window between ingested amounts that result in deficiencies and those that cause toxicoses. Historically, occurrences of livestock disease that is suggestive of chronic selenium poisoning were recorded in the 13th century (Martin, 1973). Marco Polo wrote of such cases in western China in 1295. In 1560, Father Simon Pedro described human cases of presumably chronic selenosis in Colombia (Benavides and Mojica, 1965). A documented record of selenium poisoning in livestock was reported in 1860 by a US Army surgeon (Martin, 1973), when he described a fatal disease of horses that grazed near Fort Randall, South Dakota. It also has been speculated that the horse illness that slowed General Custer's cavalry relief may have been due to selenium, but chronic selenosis generally takes weeks to develop.

The selenium status of an animal depends on the forages or feed that has been ingested, with a very narrow range between selenium deficiency and selenium toxicosis in most species. Selenium deficiencies are very common in areas with low selenium concentrations in the soil and have been historically linked to a variety of clinical effects (McDowell, 2003). However, many of these signs are produced by or in combination with vitamin E deficiency (Oldfield, 2003). Since 1949, vitamin E, cysteine and a "factor 3" were known to protect rats from fatal liver necrosis (Schwarz and Foltz, 1957). After much research, the active, preventive element present in "factor 3" was identified as selenium. Several metabolic diseases were later found to relate to selenium deficiency, including "white muscle disease" (WMD) in calves and lambs (Muth *et al.*, 1958; Godwin and Fraser, 1966), hepatosis dietetica in pigs (Eggert *et al.*, 1957), exudative diathesis in poultry (Patterson *et al.*, 1957), and pancreatic degeneration in poultry (Thompson and Scott, 1969).

Since first identified as an essential nutrient, selenium has been found to act in numerous body systems. In 1973, selenium was identified as an essential component of glutathione peroxidase enzyme (GSH) (Flohe *et al.*, 1973; Rotruck *et al.*, 1973) where selenocysteine is a required component of the active enzyme (Brown and Arthur, 2001). Reduced GSH is a principal physiologic first defense against free radical tissue damage, helping to maintain membrane integrity. Several subclasses of GSH are now recognized (Sunde, 1994; Cohen and Avissar, 1994). Over 30 seleno-proteins have been identified, many of which have vital enzymatic functions (Tiwary, 2004). In addition, selenium plays several roles in normal immune function, reproductive function, hepatic biotransformation reactions, neurotransmitter turnover and anti-carcinogenic functions. Selenium is an essential mineral in humans with added dietary selenium preventing a cardiomyopathy known as "Keshan disease" (Chen, 1986). Selenium supplementation may also play roles in protection against certain types of cancer (Combs, 1997), cardiovascular disease (Duthie *et al.*, 1989) and viral infections (Schrauzer, 1994; Levander, 2000). Because of the essential nature of selenium and environmental occurrences, poisoning cases from both natural plant selenium exposure and nutritional overdoses are common.

HISTORICAL BACKGROUND

Selenium is a metalloid that has an atomic number of 34, an atomic weight of 78.96, four natural oxidation states (–2, 0, +4 and +6) and many different chemical forms in nature. Selenium occurs in the earth's crust most commonly as selenite, selenate and selenides associated with sulfide minerals (NRC, 1983). Many factors dictate the concentration of selenium in plants including but not limited to the type of vegetation, chemical form of selenium in the soil, pH of soil, moisture content of soil and the concentration of selenium in the soil. Selenium is commonly found as water-soluble selenate in well-aerated, alkaline soils and is readily absorbed via the sulfate transporter system by plants, as compared to very poor uptake of selenides and selenite. Some soils also contain selenomethionine from decay of selenium containing vegetation which also is taken up by some plants (Marschner, 1995).

Soils containing high concentrations of selenium are commonly found in many parts of the world. Seleniferous soils are often characterized by alkaline soils that were developed from shales and are located in arid or semi-arid climates. In North America seleniferous soils and forages with high concentrations of selenium have been found in western Canada, Arizona, Colorado, Idaho, Kansas, Nevada, North Dakota, South Dakota, New Mexico and Oklahoma. High soil selenium also occurs in alkaline soils of Algeria,

Reproductive and Developmental Toxicology, Edited by Ramesh C. Gupta
ISBN: 978-0-12-382032-7

Argentina, Australia, Bulgaria, China, Colombia, Ireland, Israel, Mexico, Morocco, New Zealand, South Africa, the former Soviet Union, Spain and Venezuela (NRC, 1983). It must be noted that soil concentrations are not a strict indicator of plant selenium accumulation potential (Lakin, 1961). In fact, Puerto Rico and Hawaii have areas of high selenium soil, but the acid soil type renders it poorly absorbed by plants. Areas that contain soils high in available selenium are often identified by the presence of obligate indicator plants that require high selenium for survival, including *Astragalus* spp., *Oonopsis* spp., *Stanleya pinnata* and *Xylorrhiza* spp. Facultative selenium accumulator plants do not require high selenium for survival but can accumulate high selenium. Obligate selenium accumulator plants can store selenium at concentrations of 3,000 to 10,000 ppm selenium on a dry weight basis (Freeman *et al.*, 2006), while facultative-accumulator plants can contain several hundred to several thousand ppm, and non-accumulator plants growing on the same soil may contain from ten to occasionally a few hundred ppm. The majority of selenium in accumulator plants is found as organic methyl-selenocysteine and selenocystathionine or as inorganic selenate (Shrift and Virupaksha, 1965; Underwood and Suttle, 1999; Pickering *et al.*, 2003; Freeman *et al.*, 2006). The selenium in most plants that grow on normal soils contains <3 mg Se/kg with the predominant forms of selenium being selenate and selenomethionine (Whanger, 2002). Several chemical forms have been reported in non-indicator plants growing on high selenium soils.

Cases of selenium poisoning are usually a result of one of three types of exposure history. First, grazing animals ingest forages that have accumulated selenium in higher concentrations than normal from seleniferous soils. Second, selenium toxicity is from environmental contamination from agricultural drain water, reclaimed soils from phosphate or ore mining, sewage sludge or fly ash. Third, selenosis is caused by accidental overdoses by injection of selenium supplements or by misformulation of feed mixes. With each history of poisoning one may observe subacute, acute or chronic selenosis depending upon the daily dose and duration of exposure.

PHARMACOKINETICS/ TOXICOKINETICS

Absorption

The majority of ingested selenium compounds are absorbed from the duodenum, with lesser amounts in the jejunum and ilium (Whanger *et al.*, 1976; Wright and Bell, 1966). Little to no absorption reportedly occurs from the stomach and rumen. However, one report suggests that minimal absorption of selenomethionine occurs through the rumen wall and into the blood (Hidiroglou and Jenkins, 1973).

The chemical form of selenium greatly impacts overall absorption. Selenite absorption is via passive diffusion through the brush border membranes (Vendeland *et al.*, 1992, 1994). In contrast, selenate has little affinity for the brush border membranes. Selenate is absorbed via a sodium co-transport system that is also utilized by sulfate (Wolffram *et al.*, 1988). Selenium, in the form of seleno-amino acids, selenomethionine and selenocysteine, is absorbed through active amino acid transport mechanisms and is more bioavailable than selenite or selenate (McConnell and Cho, 1967; Ammerman and Miller, 1974; Vendeland *et al.*, 1994). Selenium status is not thought to affect overall absorption, indicating that absorption is not under homeostatic regulation.

In monogastrics, the relative selenium absorption is greater than in ruminants, ranging from 45 to 95% of the dose (Thomson and Stewart, 1974; Furchner *et al.*, 1975; Bopp *et al.*, 1982). Organic forms of selenium are better absorbed than inorganic forms (Robinson *et al.*, 1978). In ruminants, the relative absorption ranges from 29 to 50% (Wright and Bell, 1966; Suttle and Jones, 1989). The decreased absorption in ruminants is due to microbial reduction of selenium forms in the rumen to selenides and elemental selenium which are not bioavailable (Cousins and Cairney, 1961; Whanger *et al.*, 1968; Peter *et al.*, 1982). This reduction in bioavailability is generally exacerbated by high carbohydrate diets, but can be altered by differing rumen microbial populations (Hudman and Glenn, 1984; Koenig *et al.*, 1997). Some rumen microbes more efficiently reduce selenium, while others effectively incorporate it into selenium-containing amino acids. The incorporation of selenium into microbial proteins, as well as systemic absorption, can be competitively inhibited by natural methionine and cysteine (Serra *et al.*, 1996).

Distribution

Tissue distribution is dependent on the chemical form of selenium absorbed. Selenium is generally utilized for synthesis of selenoproteins, incorporated into tissue proteins, or eliminated. Selenomethionine can be non-specifically incorporated into tissue proteins in place of methionine (Awadeh *et al.*, 1998), but selenocysteine is not (Burk *et al.*, 2001), with highest incorporation occurring in tissues with high rates of protein synthesis (Hansson and Jacobsson, 1966). The non-specific incorporation of selenomethionine effectively serves as a pool of selenium reserve with a long biological half-life (Schroeder and Mitchener, 1972). Highest total selenium content is typically found in the kidney and liver, with lesser amounts in all other tissues (Muth *et al.*, 1967; Levander, 1987; Echevarria *et al.*, 1988; Davidson and Kennedy, 1993). Both specific and non-specific selenium incorporation into proteins was greater in supplemented selenium-deficient animals.

Time to peak tissue concentrations are tissue dependent. The peak selenium content of blood, liver, muscle, kidney, spleen and lung was reached within 24 hours after an injection of ^{75}Se as selenite (Muth *et al.*, 1967). In contrast, brain, thymus and reproductive organs do not reach maximal content until much later (Brown and Burk, 1973; McConnell *et al.*, 1979; Smith *et al.*, 1979; Behne *et al.*, 1988).

Selenium is efficiently transferred across the placenta into the fetus during gestation. The overall maternal selenium content is positively correlated with fetal and newborn selenium status (McConnell and Roth, 1964). Newborns get some selenium from milk, with much higher content in colostrums than in milk later in lactation.

Metabolism

Selenite is metabolized in red blood cells to hydrogen selenide (Gasiewicz and Smith, 1978). Sequential methylation reactions result in the formation of monomethyl selenide, dimethyl selenide and trimethyl selenide (Kajander *et al.*, 1991; Itoh and Suzuki, 1997). These reactions utilize

S-adenosylmethionine for methyl groups which are transferred by methyltransferases (Kajander *et al.*, 1991). These sequential reactions can deplete available S-adenosylmethionine, which would limit the degree of methylation. In rats given selenomethionine, trimethyl selenide occurred in the urine more rapidly than in rats given sodium selenite or selenocysteine (Nakamuro *et al.*, 1997), indicating that selenomethionine may be converted to methylselenol, which is easily further methylated.

Selenomethionine is metabolized by demethylation to selenocysteine. This set of pathways is similar to the metabolism of methionine. The selenocysteine is then metabolized by selenocysteine-β-lyase in the liver and kidney to alanine and selenide (Soda *et al.*, 1987).

Elimination

Selenium is primarily excreted in the urine and feces, but the form and extent of elimination by different routes are dose and species dependent. In monogastric animals, urinary elimination predominates, irrespective of the route of exposure (Leng *et al.*, 2000), with less than 10% recovered in feces (Burk *et al.*, 1972). Some literature suggests that urinary eliminated selenium is predominantly metabolites of selenium, with trimethyl selenide predominating at higher doses (McConnell and Roth, 1966; Palmer *et al.*, 1969; Zeisel *et al.*, 1987; Hasegawa *et al.*, 1996; Itoh and Suzuki, 1997), but monomethyl selenide is more abundant at lower doses. Human elimination is tri-exponential for selenite and selenomethionine (Alexander *et al.*, 1987). The terminal elimination phase was 8–20 days and 230 days for selenite and selenomethionine, respectively. Overall selenium retention and maintenance of adequate seleno-enzymes are much longer in animals supplemented with selenomethionine than selenite (Swanson *et al.*, 1991). Elimination rate is dose dependent, with half-lives of 19.5 days and 1.2 days with selenite of 0.1 and 1.0 ppm in the diet, respectively (Burk *et al.*, 1972). Due to non-specific protein incorporation of selenomethionine, urinary and fecal recovery after dosing was less than 30% of that for selenite or selenate (Thomson, 1998).

The literature suggests that the predominant selenium elimination in ruminants is fecal when ingested, but urinary with perenteral administration or in non-ruminating young animals (NRC, 1983). This is actually an error in terminology, as the fecal loss of selenium is primarily in the forms of elemental selenium and precipitated selenides from ruminal reduction (Langlands *et al.*, 1986). Thus, this selenium is just non-absorbed material and not truly being eliminated from the central compartment. However, a small amount of metabolized selenium excesses is excreted in the bile (Cousins and Cairney, 1961). The metabolites eliminated in the urine of ruminants follow a similar pattern to that seen with monogastrics.

Renal selenium elimination is dependent on glomerular filtration and degree of reabsorption. Increasing renal fluid absorption did not increase the selenium content in urine, indicating a tubular reabsorptive process (Oster and Prellwitz, 1990). Thus, dehydration or renal insufficiency would decrease rates of elimination. Excretion and renal clearance rates correlate with creatinine, indicating glomerular filtration is the mechanism of elimination.

Some selenium is eliminated via respired air, but the relative importance of this route is dose dependent. At normal intake, only about 10% or less is eliminated from the respiratory tract (Burk *et al.*, 1972), but as dose increases the percent eliminated in respired air increases (Jacobsson, 1966; McConnell and Roth, 1966). Dimethylselenide and dimethyldiselenide are the predominant forms eliminated in respired air at toxic doses (Jiang *et al.*, 1983). Dimethylselenide predominates when mice were dosed with selenite or selenocysteine, while dimethyldiselenide is most abundant when rats were dosed with selenomethionine. Respiratory elimination is primarily when renal elimination thresholds are maximized, which results in most respiratory elimination occurring in a short time period soon after exposure to toxic doses (McConnell and Roth, 1966; Tiwary *et al.*, 2005).

MECHANISM OF ACTION

Although much research has been conducted with regard to selenium poisoning and a lesser amount on the reproductive effects, the exact mechanism of these toxic effects in the body are still not clearly defined. One theory, especially for acute poisonings, is the depletion of intermediate substrates, such as glutathione and S-adenosylmethionine, which disturbs their respective enzyme activities (Vernie *et al.*, 1978). Another theory is the production of free radicals by reaction of selenium with thiols, causing oxidative tissue damage (Hoffman, 2002; Kaur *et al.*, 2003; Balogh *et al.*, 2004). A third theory is the incorporation of selenium in place of sulfur or seleno-amino acids in place of normal amino acids in proteins, which could disrupt normal cellular functions (Raisbeck, 2000). This is especially likely with the loss of disulfide bridges which provides structural integrity to proteins. Loss of function would also apply to inhibition of DNA methylation by seleno-adenosylmethionine or indirect inhibition by increased S-adenosyl homocysteine content (Hoffman, 1977). It is possible that each of these proposed mechanisms is valid with respect to individual chemical forms or doses of selenium.

It is interesting that predominant sites in which selenium is necessary for adequate health (immune function, reproductive function and antioxidant functions) are also sites in which toxic manifestations of excessive selenium are observed. One could theorize that these sites actively accumulate selenium for function and correspondingly accumulate more of the excess selenium with toxicosis.

GENERAL TOXICITY

Acute oral selenium poisoning occurs with sudden exposure of selenium ranging from 2.2 (Rosenfeld and Beath, 1964) to greater than 20 mg/kg of body weight (Miller and Williams, 1940; Mahan and Moxon, 1984), with age and species being important factors for relative sensitivity. The relative acute toxicity of selenium containing compounds is dependent on their solubility, with poorly soluble selenides and elemental selenium being much less toxic than soluble selenates, selenites and organic selenium (NRC, 2006). Minimum lethal doses for rabbits, rats, dogs and cats is 1.5 to 3 mg/kg body weight (NRC, 1983). The LD_{50} for oral selenite has been estimated to be 1.9 to 8.3 mg/kg body weight in ruminants (Grace, 1994), but other references suggest it to be 9 to 20 mg/kg body weight (Puls, 1994). In poultry, the acute oral LD_{50} of selenium is 33 mg/kg body weight. Injectable selenium is more acutely toxic than oral, with intramuscular LD_{50} of 0.5 mg/kg in lambs (Caravaggi *et al.*, 1970). Subcutaneous LD_{50} of selenium is 1 mg/kg in lambs and 1.9 mg/kg in adult cattle (Grace, 1994).

Clinical manifestation of acute selenium poisoning begins as early as 8–10 hours post-exposure, but can be delayed for up to 36 hours (Franke and Moxon, 1936; NRC, 1983; Raisbeck, 2000; Tiwary, 2004). Early in the clinical syndrome, one can detect the garlicky smell of methylated selenides on the breath. Clinical signs that follow include respiratory distress, restlessness or lethargy, head down, droopy ears, anorexia, gaunt appearance, salivation, watery diarrhea, fever, sweating, tachycardia, teeth grinding, stilted gait, titanic spasms and/or death. Clinical signs tend to progress quickly after first observed. Gross and histologic lesions include systemic congestion, pulmonary edema and petechial hemorrhages in and on the myocardium.

"Blind staggers" has historically been associated with subacute to chronic selenium. However, this association was due to its occurrence in known seleniferous areas. Areas with seleniferous soils also tend to have highly alkaline soils with high potential for excessive sulfur exposure. It has been stated that blind staggers cannot be reproduced with pure selenium compounds alone and likely involves other factors, such as alkaloid poisoning, starvation or polioencephalomalacia (O'Toole and Raisbeck, 1995). However, one can still find references that tie it to selenium (Underwood and Suttle, 1999; NRC, 2006).

Chronic selenosis, often referred to as "alkali disease", is the result of long-term ingestion of seleniferous forages (NRC, 1983, 2006; Raisbeck, 2000). High selenium intake is generally for greater than 30 days and, due to plant selenium content, is usually associated with facultative accumulator plants, not indicator plants, although chronic selenosis can also be reproduced by long-term feeding of high inorganic selenium (Kaur *et al.*, 2003). Calves were chronically poisoned with selenite at 0.25 mg/kg body weight daily for 16 weeks. In a similar study in yearlings, selenite at 0.8 and selenomethionine at 0.28 mg/kg/day resulted in alkali disease (O'Toole and Raisbeck, 1995). However, other studies did not produce alkali disease with selenium doses as high as 11.9 mg/kg of diet in feeders or 118 mg/kg body weight daily for 128 days in dairy cows (Ellis *et al.*, 1997; Lawler *et al.*, 2004). Differences in susceptibility to chronic selenium poisoning may be a product of historical exposure, the form of selenium ingested, nutritional status of the individual and variability in rumen microbial population. Certain microbes can reduce selenium to non-bioavailable forms, resulting in decreased systemic absorption. Pigs develop chronic selenosis with exposure to selenium as low as 8 mg/kg of diet (Goehring *et al*, 1984; Mahan and Magee, 1991; Stowe and Herdt, 1992), while horses exposed to 20 mg Se/kg DM (dry matter) for 3 weeks developed lesions (Stowe and Herdt, 1992).

Clinical signs of chronic selenosis include depression, weakness, emaciation, anemia, hair loss, anorexia, diarrhea, weight loss, lameness and death (Rosenfeld and Beath, 1964; Raisbeck, 2000; O'Toole and Raisbeck, 1995; Underwood and Suttle, 1999). Hoof wall abnormalities are frequently identified in cattle, horses and pigs and include swelling of the coronary band, hoof deformities and/or separation and sloughing of the hoof wall. Hair loss from the base of the tail and switch in cattle, horses and mules is sometimes referred to as "Bobtail disease". Interestingly, sheep do not develop the alopecia or hoof lesions that are seen in cattle, but they have decreased wool growth rates. In pigs, goats and horses, there may be a general alopecia (Franke, 1934). Pigs also develop neurologic signs of paralysis (Goehring *et al.*, 1984; Panter *et al.*, 1996). Pathologic lesions of chronic selenium poisoning are generally related to hoof lesions and to the effects of starvation due to the inability of the poisoned animal to travel to water and forages (Raisbeck, 2000). Lesions of nephritis, hepatic cirrhosis and myocardial necrosis can be expected.

TOXIC EFFECTS OF SELENIUM ON REPRODUCTION

Reduced conception rate/embryo viability

Many species of animals have reduced conception rates when exposed to high concentrations of selenium. Both rats exposed to 3 ppm selenium as seleniferous wheat (Munsell *et al.*, 1936) and mice exposed to 3 ppm selenate in their drinking water (Schroeder and Mitchener, 1972) had abnormally low rates of conception. Decreased conception rates and increased fetal resorption rates in cattle, sheep and horses were observed when they were fed natural diets containing 20–50 mg Se/kg diet (Harr and Muth, 1972). In contrast is a study in pigs, where sows fed a basal diet (0.13 mg Se/kg) supplemented with sodium selenite at 0, 2, 4, 8 or 16 mg/kg from the first estrous cycle though 9 weeks postpartum demonstrated that conception rate, number of offspring and mortality rates of piglets were unaffected by increase of selenium concentration in the feeds (Poulsen *et al.*, 1989). These differences in clinical outcome could simply be due to the differences in chemical form of the selenium.

Embryos of avian species are very sensitive to selenium toxicosis. In one study there was 100% mortality of embryos within 48 hours post-administration of sodium selenite at 0.02 mg per embryo (Szeleszczuk *et al.*, 2004). But, on the opposite end of the scale, eggs also have a very low rate of hatching when hens are fed a diet of very low selenium concentrations (Ort and Latshaw, 1978). One field study demonstrated that egg production and hatchability were decreased when hens were fed a diet with selenium at 1.55 mg Se/kg dry matter (Kinder *et al.*, 1995). Studies with mallard eggs have shown that selenomethionine is more embryotoxic than selenite and its increased toxicity is likely due to its increased accumulation in the eggs (Heinz *et al.*, 1987). Accumulation of the selenium was approximately 10 times greater for groups fed selenomethione in their diet than those fed sodium selenite. When adult ducks were given selenium at 10 mg Se/kg as seleno-DL-methionine, seleno-L-methionine, or selenized yeast, hatching of fertile eggs was significantly lower for ducks fed seleno-DL-methionine or seleno-L-methionine than for controls (Heinz and Hoffman, 1996). Both seleno-L-methionine and seleno-DL-methionine significantly decreased the number of 6-day-old ducklings per hen, and the former also decreased the survival percentage to 6 days old. Recent studies on adverse effects of high dietary selenium on reproduction of birds have been reviewed by Hamilton (2004) and Hoffman (2002).

Abortions/Teratogenesis

Historically, selenium toxicosis has been reported to cause abortion or teratogenesis in many species (Raisbeck, 2000). The reports in mammals have been difficult to prove and there are likely other factors that have in some cases led to misdiagnosis. However, teratogenesis due to selenosis is well documented in avian species. Selenosis in poultry results in birth defects that include deformed or lack of legs, toes, wings, beaks and eyes in the young (Latshaw *et al.*, 2004).

Field and research studies can differ in interpretation of the effects of selenium. Smith *et al.* (1936) reported congenital alkali disease in a 14-day-old colt that was born to a mare that developed clinical signs of selenosis during gestation. The clinical signs observed in the young foal were very similar to those normally observed in adult horses. Malformations of lambs born to ewes that grazed on seleniferous soils were reported by Beath *et al.* (1939). The eyes of the lambs had cystic elevations that protruded through the lids in addition to microphthalmia, rudimentary development and microcorneas. Many of the lambs could not stand because of deformed legs with thickening of the joints. However, different results were observed when yearling ewes were fed high concentrations of sodium selenite (24 mg Se/kg of diet) or *Astragalus bisulcatus* (29 mg Se/kg) as part of an alfalfa pellet for 88 days, as there was no difference in the number of lambs born nor were there any defects (Panter *et al.*, 1995).

Selenium reportedly accumulates to higher concentrations in the fetus at the expense of the dam (Puls, 1994). This is thought to be a protective mechanism to allow neonates to have adequate body reserves to sustain them until they begin eating foods that would contain selenium, as milk has very little selenium. Thus, the higher accumulation of selenium in the fetus may result in abortions, stillbirths or weak/lethargic calves. In a field investigation, Yaeger *et al.* (1998) reported that a 200-cow beef herd in a high selenium region of South Dakota fed alfalfa with elevated selenium concentrations experienced an abortion/stillborn calf rate of 7%. Six of the seven fetuses tested had markedly elevated hepatic selenium concentrations (11.36, 10.8, 6.15, 5.01, 3.59 and 3.33 ppm wet weight; normal range = 0.3–1.2 ppm) while hepatic copper concentrations were within the normal range. Hair sampled from the cows contained 6.01 ± 1.26 ppm dry weight (normal range = 0.50–1.32 ppm). The data reported suggested that subclinical selenium toxicosis in pregnant cows resulted in clinical selenium toxicosis in the developing fetus. However, they reported that in an experiment in which pregnant cows were fed a diet with high concentrations of selenite, they were unable to successfully cause abortions and only one cow in the high dose group had a weak calf that died shortly after birth and had increased hepatic selenium concentration.

Decreased growth rate

The growth rate of neonates is often decreased by high concentrations of selenium in the diet. Schroeder and Mitchener (1972) found that mice that drank selenium-contaminated drinking water had litters with excessive runts (~70%). In a study by Poley *et al.* (1941), chicks that were fed 2, 5 or 8 ppm selenium in their diet were unaffected; however, chicks fed 10 ppm selenium in their ration suffered from reduced growth and in some cases mortality. A similar trend can be seen in pigs, as piglets born from sows fed 8 and 16 mg Se/kg tended to have lower birth weights than the controls, but the differences were not significant (Kim and Mahan, 2001a). Weaning weights of piglets (21 days) tended to be negatively influenced by selenium treatment ($P = 0.08$); however, at 9 weeks of age, piglet body weights and daily feed intakes (from 3 to 9 weeks) were lower in the two highest dose groups compared to the controls. When gilts were fed 0.3, 3, 7 and 10 mg Se/kg of diet as sodium selenite of selenium-enriched yeast from 25 kg body weight through the first parity, both sources of selenium were toxic at the two highest concentrations (Kim and Mahan, 2001b). An interesting observation was that organic selenium had more negative effects on reproductive performance of the gilts during gestation, whereas inorganic selenium was more detrimental to the nursing pigs during lactation. The negative effects of selenium on reproduction may be dependent upon the form of selenium fed to the animals. In field cases where many observations have been linked to excess selenium, the form of selenium is often an organic form. In contrast, when researches have attempted to conduct the studies in a controlled setting they have usually used selenite as the selenium source.

Spermatogenesis

The testis is a specific target of selenium and it appears to be essential for maintaining a normal spermatogenesis and for male fertility. The importance of selenium in male reproduction has been known for decades as selenium imbalances have been known to cause reduced fertility, impaired sperm motility and abnormal tail morphology (Wu *et al.*, 1979; Ursini *et al.*, 1999). Morphological studies of spermatids and spermatozoa have shown that the sperm flagellum (Olson *et al.*, 2004) and altered shape of spermatozoa head (Watanabe and Endo, 1991) were the major targets of selenium deficiency. Rats fed a selenium-deficient diet for several generations suffered from severe testicular atrophy that was reversed by administration of a selenium-adequate diet (Behne *et al.*, 1996).

Nearly all of the selenium in mammalian testis is associated with the enzyme phospholipid hydroperoxide gluthathione peroxidase (PHGPx/GPx4). PHGPx/GPx4 is a large subfamily of the glutathione peroxidases which are antioxidants and act to reduce hydroperoxides while oxidizing glutathione. PHGPx/GPx4 was recently proposed to act with thioredoxin/glutathione reductase by forming a novel disulfide bond formation system at the level of structural components of the sperm (Su, 2005). The plasma protein Selenoprotein I has been shown to be produced in Leydig cells (Koga *et al.*, 1998) and is required for sperm development by the sterility phenotype of the male Sepp 1 knockout mice (Olson *et al.*, 2005). Selenoprotein V has been shown by Northern blot and *in situ* hybridization analysis to be testis specific and its expression is restricted to seminiferous tubules (Kryukov *et al.*, 2003). However, the physiological function of Selenoprotein V remains to be elucidated. Additionally, there are also several other selenoproteins in the testis whose roles remain to be elucidated, including Selenoprotein W, Selenoprotein K, Selenoprotein S and Selenoprotein 15.

As in most tissues, there is a narrow range between selenium deficiency and selenium toxicity in the testis. The effect of selenium-deficient, selenium-adequate and selenium-excess diets on spermatogenesis has been extensively studied in a mouse model and have shown that both a selenium deficiency or excess has resulted in an increase in oxidative stress that negatively affected male germ cell number, differentiation and fertility by affecting redox-sensitive and cell proliferation controlling transcription factors (Boitani and

Puglisi, 2008; Shalini and Bansal 2007, 2005; Kaur and Bansal, 2005). When selenium is administered to selenium-deficient animals, the selenium is supplied to the testis with priority over other tissues (Behne *et al.*, 1982), which could also make them more sensitive to excess.

Secondary effects on reproduction of selenium toxicosis

At least some of the adverse effects on reproduction caused by excess selenium in ruminants are caused by interference with absorption and retention of copper that results in copper deficiency (Amer *et al.*, 1973; Raisbeck, 2000). This effect can be compounded by high sulfur that is often associated with alkaline seleniferous soil and can also cause decreased systemic copper bioavailability. The direct effect of copper deficiency on reproductive performance, plus the negative effects of copper deficiency on immune function can both play a role in the overall syndrome of selenium toxicosis.

The immune system requires selenium for adequate function. In addition, as in the testes, both deficiency and toxicosis result in impaired function of the immune system (Yaeger *et al.*, 1998; Raisbeck, 2000). Impaired immune function can directly affect the fetus or neonate in preventing them from mounting an appropriate response to true pathogens or opportunistic pathogens. In addition, secondary immune compromise in the form of poor maternal immunity can also affect survivability of feti and neonates. As the dam required good immune function to develop good antibody titers, compromised function could result in a lack of adequate maternally provided passive immunity. This lack of or poor passive immunity can render offspring very vulnerable to disease and potential mortality.

TREATMENT

The most effective treatment of selenium toxicosis is to prevent excessive exposure. The maximal tolerable dietary selenium was once set at 2 mg/kg of diet per day for all species, but has now been changed to 5 mg/kg of diet per day for ruminants (NRC, 2006). It has been stated that this new tolerance for ruminants is appropriate for horses as well. Maximum tolerance of 4 mg/kg of diet is used for swine, 3 mg/kg of diet for poultry and 2 mg/kg of diet for fish.

There is no specific mechanism of chelation and removal of selenium in animals. Thus, the primary treatment protocol for both acute and chronic selenium poisoning is supportive care. With chronic poisoning, it is important to understand the long-term therapies necessary to allow an animal with hoof lesions time to re-grow the hoof wall. Especially with organic selenium's incorporation into body proteins, the time necessary to just decrease the body load of selenium, once excessive exposure has stopped, is quite long.

Mild beneficial effects have been reported for some therapies that aim at increasing the rate of elimination and decreasing the tissue injury (Raisbeck, 2000; Casteel and Blodgett, 2004). Use of high dose vitamin E therapy, soon after exposure to toxic doses of selenium, may decrease the potential free radical damage in tissues. Arsanilic acid at 50 to 100 ppm can enhance the rate of selenium elimination via the bile. Low selenium, high quality, high protein diets reportedly aid in the treatment of chronic selenosis.

CONCLUDING REMARKS AND FUTURE DIRECTIONS

Selenium deficiency and toxicity are problems which have caused extensive financial losses in the livestock industry and have been extensively researched. However, recent research demonstrates that there remains a significant amount of knowledge that needs to be discovered in order to fully understand all of the roles of selenium, especially with regards to reproductive effects. Since it is now known that different chemical forms of selenium can have different physiologic responses, it is now essential that we develop a better understanding of both the beneficial and detrimental effects of different chemical forms of selenium and to understand their relative roles in the toxic effects on reproduction. In this light, it is critical that researchers clearly identify chemical forms of selenium from field cases in order to adequately research the clinical syndromes with the correct chemical form of selenium under controlled conditions. There is also a need to understand the role of the many selenoenzymes in reproductive organs whose roles have not yet been determined.

REFERENCES

Alexander J, Hogberg J, Thomassen Y, Aaseth J (1987) Selenium. In *Handbook on Toxicity of Inorganic Compounds* (Seiler HG, ed.). Marcel Dekker, New York, p. 585.

Amer, MA, St-Laurent GJ, Brisson GJ (1973) Supplemental copper and selenium for calves. Effects upon ceruloplasmin activity and liver copper concentration. *Can J Physiol Pharmacol* **51:** 649.

Ammerman CB, Miller SM (1974) Selenium in ruminant nutrition: a review. *J Dairy Sci* **58:** 1561–76.

Awadeh FT, Rahman A, Kincaid RL, Finley JW (1998) Effect of selenium supplements on the distribution of selenium among serum proteins in cattle. *J Dairy Sci* **81:** 1089–94.

Balogh K, Weber M, Erdelyi M, Mezes M. (2004) Effects of excess selenium supplementation on the glutathione redox system in broiler chickens. *Acta Vet Hung* **52:** 403–11.

Beath OA, Eppson HF, Gilbert CS, Bradley WB (1939) Poisonous plants and livestock poisoning. *Wyo Agr Exp Sta Bull* **231:** 1–104.

Behne D, Hillmert H, Scheid S, Gessner H, Elger W (1988) Evidence for specific target tissues and new biologically important SelP. *Biochim Biophys Acta* **966:** 12–21.

Behne D, Hofer T, Berswordt-Wallrabe R, Elger W (1982) Selenium in the testis of the rat: studies on its regulation and its importance for the organism. *J Nutr* **112:** 1682–7.

Behne D, Weiler H, Kyriakopoulos A (1996) Effects of selenium deficiency on testicular morphology and function in rats. *J Reprod Fertil* **106:** 291–7.

Benavides ST, Mojica FS (1965) *Selenosis*, 2nd edition. Instituto Geografico Augustin Codazzi, Bogota, Columbia.

Boitani C, Puglisi R (2008) Selenium, a key element in spermatogensis and male fertility. In *Molecular Mechanisms in Spermatogenesis* (Cheng CY, ed.). Landes Bioscience and Springer Science Buisness, Austin, Texas, pp. 65–73.

Bopp BA, Sonders RC, Kesterson JW (1982) Metabolic fate of selected selenium compounds in laboratory animals and man. *Drug Metab Rev* **13:** 271–318.

Brown DG, Burk RF (1973) Selenium retention in tissues and sperm of rats fed a torula yeast diet. *J Nutr* **103:** 102–8.

Brown KM, Arthur JR (2001) Selenium, selenoproteins and human health: a review. *Public Health Nutr* **4:** 593–9.

Burk RF, Brown DG, Seely RJ, Scaief CC III (1972) Influence of dietary and injected selenium on whole-body retention, route of excretion, and tissue retention of $^{75}SeO_3^{2-}$ in the rat. *J Nutr* **102:** 1049–55.

Burk RF, Hill KE, Motley AK (2001) Plasma selenium in specific and non-specific forms. *Biofactor* **14:** 107–14.

Caravaggi C, Clark FL, Jackson ARB (1970) Acute selenium toxicity in lambs following intramuscular injection of sodium selenite. *Res Vet Sci* **11:** 146–9.

Casteel SW, Blodgett DJ (2004) Selenium. In *Clinical Veterinary Toxicology* (Plumlee K, ed.). Mosby, pp. 214–7.

Chen X (1986) Selenium and cardiomyopathy (Keshan disease). *Acta Pharmacol Toxicol* **59:** 325–30.

Cohen HJ, Avissar N (1994) Extracellular glutathione peroxidase: a distinct selenoprotein. In *Selenium in Biology and Human Health* (Burk RF, ed.). Springer-Verlag, New York, pp. 79–92.

Combs GF (1997) Selenium and cancer prevention. In *Antioxidants and Disease Prevention* (Garewal HA, ed.). CRC Press, New York, pp. 97–113.

Cousins FB, Cairney IM (1961) Some aspects of selenium metabolism in sheep. *Aust J Agric Res* **12:** 927–33.

Davidson WB, Kennedy DG (1993) Synthesis of [^{75}Se] selenoproteins is greater in selenium-deficient sheep. *J Nutr* **123:** 689–94.

Duthie GG, Wahle KWJ, James WPJ (1989) Oxidants, antioxidants and cardiovascular disease. *Nutr Res Rev* **2:** 51–62.

Echevarria M, Henry PR, Ammerman CB, Rao PV (1988) Effects of time and dietary selenium concentration as sodium selenite on tissue selenium uptake by sheep. *J Anim Sci* **66:** 2299–305.

Eggert RO, Patterson E, Akers WJ, Stokstad ELR (1957) The role of vitamin E and selenium in the nutrition of the pig. *J Anim Sci* **16:** 1037–45.

Ellis RG, Herdt TH, Stowe HD (1997) Physical, hematologic, biochemical, and immunological effects of supranutritional supplementation with dietary selenium in Holstein cows. *Am J Vet Res* **58:** 760–4.

Flohe L, Gunzler WA, Shock HH (1973) Glutathione peroxidase: a selenoenzyme. *FEBS Lett* **32:** 132–4.

Franke KW (1934) A new toxicant occurring naturally in certain samples of plant foodstuffs. I. Results obtained in preliminary feeding trials. *J Nutr* **8:** 597–608.

Franke KW, Moxon AL (1936) A comparison of the minimum fatal doses of selenium, tellurium, arsenic, and vanadium. *J Pharm Exptl Therap* **58:** 454–9.

Freeman JL, Zhang LH, Marcus MA, Fakra S, McGrath SP, Pilon-Smits EA (2006) Spatial imaging, speciation, and quantification of selenium in the hyperaccumulator plants *Astragalus bisulcatus* and *Stanleya pinnata*. *Plant Physiol* **142:** 124–34.

Furchner JE, London JE, Wilson JS (1975) Comparative metabolism of radionuclides in mammals – IX. Retention of ^{75}Se in the mouse, rat, monkey and dog. *Health Physics* **29:** 641–8.

Gasiewicz TA, Smith JC (1978) The metabolism of selenite by intact rat erythrocytes in vitro. *Chem Biol Interact* **21:** 299–313.

Godwin KO, Fraser FJ (1966) Abnormal electrocardiograms, blood pressure changes, and some aspects of the histopathology of selenium deficiency in lambs. *Quart J Exp Physiol* **51:** 94–102.

Goehring TB, Palmer IS, Olson OE, Libal GW, Wahlstorm RC (1984) Effects of seleniferous grains and inorganic selenium on tissue and blood composition of and growth performance of rats and swine. *J Anim Sci* **59:** 725–32.

Grace ND (1994) Selenium. In *Managing Trace Element Deficiencies* (Grace ND, ed.). New Zealand Pastoral Agricultural Research Institute, Simon Print, Palmerston North, New Zealand.

Hamilton SJ (2004) Review of selenium toxicity in the aquatic food chain. *Sci Total Environ* **326:** 1–31.

Hansson E, Jacobsson SO (1966) Uptake of [^{75}Se] selenomethionine in the tissues of the mouse studied by whole-body autoradiography. *Biochim Biophys Acta 28* **115:** 285–93.

Harr JR, Muth OH (1972) Selenium poisoning in domestic animals and its relationship to man. *Clin Toxicol* **5:** 175–86.

Hasegawa T, Okuno T, Nakamuro K, Sayato Y (1996) Identification and metabolism of selenocysteine–glutathione selenenyl sulfide (CySeSG) in small intestine of mice orally exposed to selenocystine. *Arch Toxicol* **71:** 39–44.

Heinz GH, Hoffman DJ (1996) Comparison of the effects of seleno-L-methionine, seleno-Dl-methioine, and selenized yeast on reproduction of mallards. *Environ Pollut* **91:** 169–75.

Heinz GH, Hoffman DJ, Krynitsky AJ, Weller DMG (1987) Reproduction of mallards fed selenium. *Environ Toxicol Chem* **6:** 423–33.

Hidiroglou M, Jenkins KJ (1973) Absorption of ^{75}Se-selenomethionine from the rumen of sheep. *Can J Anim Sci* **53:** 345–7.

Hoffman DJ (2002) Role of selenium toxicity and oxidative stress in aquatic birds. *Aquatic Toxicology* **57:** 11–26.

Hoffman JL (1977) Selenite toxicity, depletion of liver S-adenosylmethionine, and inactivation of methionine adenosyltransferase. *Arch Biochem Biophys* **179:** 136–40.

Hudman JF, Glenn AR (1984) Selenite uptake and incorporation by Selenomonas ruminantium. *Arch Microbiol* **140:** 252–6.

Itoh M, Suzuki KT (1997) Effects of dose on the methylation of selenium to monomethylselenol and trimethyl selenonium ion in rats. *Arch Toxicol* **71:** 461–6.

Jacobsson SO (1966) Excretion of a single dose of selenium in sheep. *Acta Vet Scand* **7:** 226–39.

Jiang S, Robberecht H, Vanden Berghe D (1983) Elimination of selenium compounds by mice through formation of different volatile selenides. *Experientia* **39:** 293–4.

Kajander EO, Harvima RJ, Elonranta TO, Martikainen H, Kantola M, Karenlampi SO, Akerman K (1991) Metabolism, cellular actions, and cytotoxicity of selenomethionine in cultured cells. *Biol Trace Elem Res* **28:** 57–68.

Kaur P, Bansal MP (2005) Effect of selenium-induced oxidative stress on the cell kinetics in testis and reproductive ability of male mice. *Nutrition* **21:** 351–7.

Kaur R, Sharma S, Rampal S (2003) Effects of subchronic selenium toxicosis on lipid peroxidation, glutathione redox cycle, and antioxidant enzymes in calves. *Vet Hum Toxicol* **45:** 190–2.

Kim YY, Mahan DC (2001) Comparative effects of high dietary levels of organic and inorganic selenium on selenium toxicity of growing-finishing pigs. *J Anim Sci* **79:** 942–8.

Kim YY, Mahan DC (2001) Prolonged feeding of high dietary levels of organic and inorganic selenium to gilts from 25 kg BW through one parity. *J Anim Sci* **79:** 956–66.

Kinder LL, Angel CR, Anthony NB (1995) Apparent selenium toxicity in emus (*Dromaius novaehollandiae*). *Avian Dis* **39:** 652–7.

Koenig KM, Rode LM, Cohen RDH, Buckley WT (1997) Effect of diet and chemical form of selenium in sheep. *J Anim Sci* **75:** 817–27.

Koga M, Tanaka H, Yomogida K, Tsuchida J, Uchida K, Kitamura M, Sakoda S, Matsumiya K, Okuyama A, Nishimune Y (1998) Expression of selenoprotein messenger ribonucleic acid in the rat testis. *Biol Reprod* **58:** 261–5.

Kryukov GV, Castellano S, Novoselov SV, Lobanov AV, Zahtab O, Guigo R, Gladyshev VN (2003) Characterization of mammalian selenoproteomes. *Science* **300:** 1439–43.

Lakin HW (1961) Geochemistry of selenium in relation to agriculture. In *Selenium in Agriculture. US Department of Agriculture, Agric. Handb. 2001.* US Government Printing Office, Washington DC.

Langlands JP, Bowles JE, Donald GE, Smith AJ (1986) Selenium excretion in sheep. *Aust J Agric Res* **37:** 201–9.

Latshaw JD, Morishita TY, Sarver CR, Thilsted J (2004) Selenium toxicity in breeding ring-necked pheasants (*Phasianus colchicus*). *Avian Dis* **48:** 935–9.

Lawler TL, Taylor JB, Finley JW, Canton JS (2004) Effects of supranutritional and organically bound selenium on performance, carcass characteristics, and selenium distribution in finishing beef steers. *J Anim Sci* **82:** 1488–93.

Leng L, Boldizarova K, Faix S, Kovac G (2000) The urinary excretion of selenium in sheep treated with a vasopressin analogue. *Vet Res* **31:** 499–505.

Levander OA (1987) Selenium. In *Trace Elements in Human and Animal Nutrition*, 5th edition, vol. 2 (Mertz W, ed.). Academic Press, New York, pp. 209–79.

Mahan DC, Magee PL (1991) Efficacy of dietary sodium selenite and calcium selenite provided in the diet at approved, marginally toxic, and toxic levels to growing swine. *J Anim Sci* **69:** 4722–25.

Mahan DC, Moxon AL (1984) Effect of inorganic selenium supplementation on selenosis in post-weaning swine. *J Anim Sci* **58:** 1216–21.

Marschner H (1995) *Mineral Nutrition of Higher Plants*, 2nd edition. London, Academic Press.

Martin JL (1973) Selenium compounds in nature and medicine. In *Organic Selenium Compounds: Their Chemistry and Biology* (Klayman DL, Gunther WHH, eds.). John Wiley & Sons, New York, pp. 663–91.

McConnell KP, Burton RM, Kute T, Higgins PJ (1979) Selenoproteins from rat testis cytosol. *Biochim Biophys Acta* **588:** 113–19.

McConnell KP, Cho GJ (1967) Active transport of L-selenomethionine in the intestine. *Am J Physiol* **213:** 150–6.

McConnell KP, Roth DM (1964) Passage of selenium across the placenta and also into the milk of the dog. *J Nutr* **84:** 340–4.

McConnell KP, Roth DM (1966) Respiratory excretion of selenium. *Proc Soc Exp Biol Med* **123:** 919–21.

McDowell LR (2003) *Minerals in Animal and Human Nutrition*, 2nd edition. Elsevier Science BV, Amsterdam, The Netherlands.

Miller WT, Williams KT (1940) Minimum lethal dose of selenium as sodium selenite for horses, mules, cattle and swine. *J Agric Res* **60:** 153–73.

Munsell HE, Devaney GM, Kennedy MH (1936) Toxicity of food containing selenium as shown by its effect on the rat, USDA Tech Bull No 534, USDA Washington, DC, 25pp.

Muth OH, Oldfield JE, Remmert LF, Schubert JR (1958) Effects of selenium and Vit. E on white muscle disease. *Science* **128:** 1090–7.

Muth OH, Pendell HW, Watson CR, Oldfield JE, Weswig PH (1967) Uptake and retention of parenterally administered 75Se in ewes on different selenium regimens. *Am J Vet Res* **28:** 1397–406.

Nakamuro K, Nakanishi K, Okuno T, Hasegawa T, Sayato Y (1997) Comparison of methylated selenium metabolites in rats after oral administration of various selenium compounds. *Jpn J Toxicol Environ Health* **43:** 1482–9.

National Research Council (NRC) (1983) *Selenium in Nutrition*, revised ed. Subcommittee on Selenium, Committee on Animal Nutrition, Washington DC.

National Research Council (NRC) (2006) Selenium. In *Mineral Tolerance of Animals*, 2nd edition. National Academies Press, Washington DC, pp. 321–47.

O'Toole D, Raisbeck MF (1995) Pathology of experimentally induced chronic selenosis ("alkali disease") in yearling cattle. *J Vet Diagn Invest* **7:** 364–73.

Oldfield JE (2003) Some recollections of early swine research with selenium and vitamin E. *J Anim Sci* **81:** E145–E148.

Olson, GE, Winfrey VP, Hill KE, Raymond RF (2004) Sequential development of flagellar defects in spermatids and epididymal spermatozoa of selenium-deficient rats. *Reproduction* **127:** 335–42.

Olson GE, Winfrey VP, NagDas SK, Hill KE, Burk RF (2005) Selenoprotein P is required for mouse sperm development. *Biol Rep* **73:** 201–11.

Ort JF, Latshaw JD (1978) The toxic level of sodium selenite in the diet of laying chickens. *J Nutr* **108:** 1114–20.

Oster O, Prellwitz W (1990) The renal excretion of selenium. *Biol Trace Elem Res* **24:** 119–46.

Palmer IS, Fischer DD, Halverson AW, Olson OE (1969) Identification of a major selenium excretory product in rat urine. *Biochim Biophys Acta* **177:** 336–42.

Panter KE, Hartley WJ, James LF, Mayland HF, Stegelmeier BL, Kechele PO (1996) Comparative toxicity of selenium from seleno-DL-methionine, sodium selenate, and *Astragalus bisulcatus* in pigs. *Fundam Appl Toxicol* **32:** 217–23.

Panter KE, James LF, Mayland HF (1995) Reproductive response of ewes fed alfalfa pellets containing sodium selenite or *Astragalus bisulcatus* as a selenium source. *Vet Hum Toxicol* **37:** 30–2.

Patterson EL, Milstrey R, Stokstad ELR (1957) Effect of selenium in preventing exudative diathesis in chicks. *Proc Soc Exp Biol Med* **95:** 617–20.

Peter DW, Whanger PD, Lindsay JP, Buscall DJ (1982) Excretion of selenium, zinc and copper by sheep receiving continuous intraruminal infusions of selenite or selenomethionine. *Proc Nutr Soc* **7:** 178.

Pickering IJ, Wright C, Bubner B, Ellis D, Persans MW, Yu EY, George GN, Prince RC, Salt DE (2003) Chemical form and distribution of selenium and sulfur in the selenium hyperaccumulator *Astragalus bisulcatus*. *Plant Physiol* **131:** 1460–7.

Poley WE, Wilson WO, Moxon AL, Taylor JB (1941) The effect of selenized grains on the rate of growth in chicks. *Poultry Sci* **20:** 171–9.

Poulsen HD, Danielsen V, Nielsen TK, Wolstrup C (1989) Excessive dietary selenium to primiparous sows and their offspring. I. Influence on reproduction and growth. *Acta Vet Scand* **30:** 371–8.

Puls R (1994) *Mineral Levels in Animal Health*, 2nd ed. Diagnostic data. Sherpa International, British Columbia, Canada.

Raisbeck MF (2000) Selenosis. *Vet Clin North Am Food Anim Pract* **16:** 465–80.

Robinson MF, Rea RM, Friend GM, Stewart RDR, Scow PC, Thomson CD (1978) On supplementing the selenium intake of New Zealanders. 2. Prolonged metabolic experiments with daily supplements of selenomethionine, selenite and fish. *Br J Nutr* **39:** 589–95.

Rosenfeld I, Beath OA (1964) *Selenium: Geobotany, Biochemistry, Toxicity, and Nutrition*. Academic Press, New York.

Rotruck JT, Pope AL, Ganther HE, Swanson AB, Hafeman DL, Hoekstra WG (1973) Selenium: biochemical role as a component of glutathione peroxidase. *Science* **179:** 588–90.

Schrauzer GN (1994) Selenium in the maintenance and therapy of HIV-infected patients. *Chem Biol Interact* **91:** 199–205.

Schroeder HA, Mitchener M (1972) Selenium and tellurium in mice. Effects on growth, survival and tumors. *Arch Environ Health* **24:** 66.

Schwarz K, Foltz CM (1957) Selenium as an integral part of Factor 3 against dietary necrotic liver degeneration. *J Am Chem Soc* **78:** 3292.

Serra AB, Serra SD, Fujihara T (1996) Influence of dietary protein on the fractionation of selenium in the rumen of sheep. *Biol Trace Elem Res* **9:** 557–62.

Shalini S, Bansal MP (2005) Role of selenium in regulation of spermatogenesis: involvement of activator protein 1. *Biofactors* **23:** 151–62.

Shalini S, Bansal MP (2007) Dietary selenium deficiency as well as excess supplementation induces multiple defects in mouse epididymal spermatozoa: understanding the role of selenium in male fertility. *Int J Androl* **31:** 438–49.

Shrift A, Virupaksha TK (1965) Seleno-amino acids in selenium-accumulating plants. *Biochim Biophys Acta* **100:** 65–75.

Smith DG, Senger PL, McCutchan JF, Landa CA (1979) Selenium and glutathione peroxidase distribution in bovine semen and selenium-75 retention by the tissues of the reproductive tract in the bull. *Biol Reprod* **20:** 377.

Smith MI, Franke KW, Westfall BB (1936) The selenium problem in relation to public health. A preliminary survey to determine the possibility of selenium intoxication in the rural population living on seleniferous soil. *US Public Health Rept* **51:** 1496–505.

Soda K, Esaki N, Nakamura T, Tanaka H (1987) Selenocysteine β-lyase: an enzymological aspect of mammalian selenocysteine metabolism. In *Selenium in Biology and Medicine, Part A. Proceedings of the Third International Symposium on Selenium in Biology and Medicine*. May 27–June 1, 1984 at Beijing, China. AVI Book Pub by Van Nostrand Reinhold Co., New York, pp. 160–71.

Stowe HD, Herdt TH (1992) Clinical assessment of selenium status of livestock. *J Anim Sci* **70:** 3928–33.

Su D, Novoselov SV, Sun QA, Moustafa Me, Zhou Y, Oko R, Hatfield DL, Gladyshev VN (2005) Mammalian selenoprotein thioredoxin-glutathione reductase: roles in disulfide bond formation and sperm maturation. *J Biol Chem* **280:** 26491–8.

Sunde RA (1994) Intracellular glutathione peroxidases – structure, regulation and function. In: *Selenium in Biology and Human Health* (Burk RF, ed.). Springer-Verlag, New York, pp. 45–78.

Suttle NF, Jones DG (1989) Recent developments in trace element metabolism and function: trace elements, disease resistance and immune responsiveness in ruminants. *J Nutr* **119:** 1055–61.

Swanson CA, Patterson BH, Levander OA, Veillon C, Taylor P, Helzsouer K, McAdam PA, Zech LA (1991) Human (^{74}Se)seleno-methionine metabolism: a kinetic model. *Am J Clin Nutr* **54:** 917–26.

Szeleszczuk P, Karpinska E, Bielecki W, Koroaska G, Borzemaska W (2004) Evaluation of lithium and selenium toxicity for chicken embryos and one day old chicks. *Medycyna-Weterynaryjna* **60:** 492–295.

Thompson JM, Scott ML (1969) Role of selenium in the nutrition of the chick. *J Nutr* **97:** 335–42.

Thomson CD (1998) Selenium speciation in human body fluids. *Analyst* **123:** 827–31.

Thomson CD, Stewart RDH (1974) The metabolism of [^{75}Se] in young women. *Br J Nutr* **32:** 47–57.

Tiwary AK (2004) Differences between inorganic and organic selenium toxicosis in sheep. Masters Thesis, Utah State University, Logan, UT.

Tiwary AK, Panter KE, Stegelmeier BL, James LF, Hall JO (2005) Evaluation of respiratory elimination kinetics of selenium after oral administration in sheep. *Am J Vet Res* **66:** 1–7.

Underwood EJ, Suttle NF (1999) *The Mineral Nutrition of Livestock*, 3rd edition. Wallingford, Oxon, UK.

Ursini F, Heim S, Kiess M, Maiorina M, Roveri A, Wissing J, Flohe L (1999) Dual function of the selenoprotien PHGPx during sperm maturation. *Science* **285:** 1393–6.

Vendeland, SC, Butler JA, Whanger PD (1992) Intestinal absorption of selenite, selenate and selenomethionine in the rat. *J Nutr Biochem* **3:** 359–65.

Vendeland SC, Deagen JT, Butler JA, Whanger PD (1994) Uptake of selenite, selenomethionine and selenate by brush border membrane vesicles isolated from rat small intestine. *Biometals* **7:** 305–12.

Vernie LN, Ginjarr HB, Wilders IT, Bont WS (1978) Amino acid incorporation in a cell-free system derived from rat liver studied with the aid of selenodiglutathione. *Biochem Biophys Acta* **518:** 507–17.

Watanabe T, Endo A (1991) Effects of selenium deficiency on sperm morphology and spermatocyte chromosomes in mice. *Mutat Res* **262:** 93–9.

Whanger PD (2002) Selenocompounds in plants and animals and their biological significance. *J Am Coll Nutr* **21:** 223–32.

Whanger PD, Pedersen ND, Hatfield J, Weswig PH (1976) Absorption of selenite and selenomethionine from ligated digestive tract segments in rats. *Proc Soc Exp Biol Med* **153:** 295.

Whanger PD, Weswig PH, Muth OH (1968) Metabolism of 7 s Se-selenite and v s Se-selenomethionine by rumen microorganisms. *Fed Proc* **27:** 418.

Wolffram S, Grenacher B, Scharrer E (1988) Transport of selenate and sulphate across the intestinal brush-border membrane of pig jejunum by two common mechanisms. *Q J Exp Physiol* **73:** 103–11.

Wright PL, Bell MC (1966) Comparative metabolism of selenium and tellurium in sheep and swine. *Am J Physiol* **211:** 6–10.

Wu AS, Oldfield JE, Shull LR, Cheeke PR (1979) Specific effect of selenium deficiency on rat sperm. *Biol Reprod* **20:** 793–8.

Yaeger MJ, Neiger RD, Holler L, Fraser TL, Hurley DJ, Palmer IS (1998) The effect of subclinical selenium toxicosis on pregnant beef cattle. *J Vet Diagn Invest* **10:** 268–73.

Zeisel SH, Ellis AL, Sun XF, Pomfret EA, Ting BTG, Janghorbani M (1987) Dose–response relations in urinary excretion of trimethylselenonium ion in the rat. *J Nutr* **117:** 1609–14.

Section 8

Pesticides and Other Environmental Contaminants

C H A P T E R

37

Organophosphate and carbamate pesticides

Ramesh C. Gupta, Jitendra K. Malik and Dejan Milatovic

INTRODUCTION

Organophosphates (OP) and carbamates (CM) constitute a large class of synthetic compounds that are used for a variety of purposes, such as: (1) insecticides to protect crops, gardens, homes and offices, (2) agents of warfare, threat and terror, and (3) therapeutic agents in human and veterinary medicine. These compounds are heavily used to protect public health from diseases like malaria, West Nile, Lyme disease and others by controlling vectors such as mosquitoes, ticks, etc. In addition, these pesticides are used in intentional poisonings in humans, and malicious poisonings in animals and wildlife. Currently, OPs and CMs (hereafter referred to as anticholinesterases) are the most commonly used pesticides in agriculture and forestry around the world. This trend is partly due to their lack of residue persistence in the environment and in mammalian species, and also due to the development of lesser resistance in insects compared to the organochlorine pesticides. However, the anticholinesterase (anti-ChE) pesticides lack species selectivity and being extremely toxic chemicals, they pose a serious threat to the environment as well as to the health of human, domestic animal, wildlife and aquatic species. Overexposure of individuals can occur at the sites of production, transportation and end user level, and often result in poisoning (Zwiener and Ginsburg, 1988; Karaliede and Senanayake, 1989; O'Malley, 1997; Eddleston, 2002).

OPs and CMs produce toxicity primarily by virtue of the inhibition of acetylcholinesterase (AChE) enzyme, which terminates the action of the neurotransmitter acetylcholine (ACh) at the synapses in the brain and at the neuromuscular junction (NMJ). Inhibition of AChE results in accumulation of ACh, which overstimulates muscarinic and nicotinic ACh receptors, thereby producing the toxic signs of hypercholinergic preponderance lasting from a few hours to a few days or weeks. While OPs are extremely toxic irreversible AChE inhibitors, CMs are considered relatively less toxic due to their reversible AChE inhibition. Toxicity of these pesticides has been studied in various body organs and systems, including the central nervous system (CNS), skeletal muscles, cardiovascular, respiratory, ocular, endocrine, dermal and immune (Gupta, 2006). The nervous system as a primary target organ for toxicity has been the focus of much attention for more than half a century. Anti-ChE pesticides are known to affect the reproductive system in both males and females. Maternal and/or paternal exposure to these pesticides can adversely influence conception, pregnancy or health of offspring. In mammals, the fetus is often indirectly exposed during gestation via maternal intake of anti-ChE pesticides. Following prenatal exposure, these chemicals cross the placental barrier and produce toxicity in conceptus, as well as in mother and placenta. Anti-ChEs are known to elicit a variety of toxic effects in the embryo and the fetus ranging from biochemical/neurochemical alteration to teratogenesis. During the neonatal period, offspring may be affected by anti-ChE pesticides either by ingesting mother's milk, or by direct exposure to these pesticides. Since the brain is the most sensitive organ for the toxicity of OPs and CMs, *in utero* exposure to these pesticides is likely to affect the developing brain with subsequent dysfunctions later in life (Levin *et al.*, 2001; Timofeeva *et al.*, 2008a,b). This chapter describes the reproductive and developmental toxicity of OP and CM pesticides.

HISTORICAL BACKGROUND

The first OP compound, tetraethyl pyrophosphate, was synthesized in France in 1854 by Phillipe de Clermont. Later, in1932 in Germany, Lange and Kruger synthesized dimethyl and diethyl phosphorofluoridate and observed that inhalation of vapors of either compound produced dimness of vision and choking sensation. These findings led Gerhard Schrader to the exploration of the OP class of compounds, while he was engaged in the development of insecticides for I.G. Farbenindustrie. In the truest sense, this is considered the landmark or birthplace of OP compounds. Parathion was one of the earliest OP pesticides, synthesized by the Schrader group, which is still commonly used throughout the world. Prior to World War II (WWII), the German Defense Ministry shifted the quests of Schrader and his group to synthesize highly toxic OP compounds that could be deployed as nerve agents/gases in chemical warfare, instead of insecticides. They developed diisopropylphosphorofluoridate (DFP), which was not toxic enough to be used as a nerve agent, but too toxic to be used as an insecticide. Even today, DFP is widely used as an experimental or prototype OP compound. Soon after the synthesis of DFP, OPs of the G series (tabun, GA; sarin, GB; and

Reproductive and Developmental Toxicology, Edited by Ramesh C. Gupta
ISBN: 978-0-12-382032-7

soman, GD) were developed, which were considerably more toxic. During WWII and thereafter, OP nerve agents of the V series (VX, Russian VX and Chinese VX) were developed with a much greater toxicity than the G series OP nerve agents.

Since the 1950s, thousands of OPs have been synthesized worldwide for the quest of insecticidal activity with species selective toxicity, i.e. highly toxic to insects and least toxic to non-target mammalian, avian and aquatic species. The advent of malathion fulfilled these expectations and it has been the most popular insecticide worldwide for more than half a century. Even with malathion, many incidents of poisoning still occur. In 1976 in Pakistan, out of 7,500 men who sprayed the pesticide, 2,800 became poisoned and five died from isomalathion that was produced during the storage of formulated malathion. Many such poisoning incidences have been encountered in the past with several other OPs and CMs. Today, more than 100 OPs are on the market for a variety of purposes, but primarily as insecticides.

During the mid-19th century, the first CM compound physostigmine was extracted from the Calabar beans (ordeal poison) of the perennial plant *Physostigma venenosum* commonly found in tropical West Africa. The Calabar beans were used for witchcraft and physostigmine was used for the treatment of glaucoma. Almost a half century later, neostigmine (an aromatic ester of carbamic acid) was synthesized and used in the treatment of myasthenia gravis. During the 1960s and 1970s, dozens of CMs (esters of carbamic acid) were synthesized for pesticidal use. Carbaryl was the first CM to be used as an insecticide. To mimic the structure of ACh, aldicarb was synthesized, which has a toxicity greater than any other compounds of this class. In general, CMs (used as insecticides, herbicides and fungicides) are considered relatively less toxic than OPs, because CMs cause AChE inactivation by carbamylation unlike OPs, which inactivate AChE by phosphorylation. Based on acute toxicity, some of the CM pesticides (aldicarb, carbofuran, oxamyl and methomyl) are extremely toxic. In terms of volume, currently the use of CMs exceeds the use of OPs.

Epidemiological studies suggest that each year approximately one million people are poisoned with anti-ChE pesticides around the world, and several hundred thousand of them die. Pesticide poisoning incidents often occur from intentional, accidental or illegal use, and the number of victims in each incident can vary from a single person to several thousands (Goldman *et al.*, 1990; Gupta, 2006; Satoh, 2006; Varma and Mulay, 2006; Dewan *et al.*, 2008). Survivors of acute or chronic OP poisonings often suffer from delayed effects. Exposure of child-bearing age or pregnant women to these pesticides is inevitable in the farming or greenhouse environment. In many studies, both OPs and CMs have been reported to induce some adverse reproductive effects, but more likely developmental effects. Following *in utero* exposure, consequences can be devastating as these pesticides are known to produce embryotoxicity, fetotoxicity, teratogenesis, and in later life individuals can suffer from chronic diseases, like diabetes, and/or neurodegenerative diseases, such as Alzheimer's or Parkinson's disease (Timofeeva *et al.*, 2008a,b).

TOXICOKINETICS

Even though all OP and CM pesticides share a common property, i.e. AChE inactivation, they differ in their toxicokinetic properties (absorption, distribution, metabolism and excretion, ADME). Toxicokinetics has and will continue to play an important role in assessing OP and CM pesticide dosimetry, biological response and risk in humans exposed to these agents (Timchalk, 2006). Toxicokinetic studies provide important data on the amount of toxicant delivered to a target site as well as species-, age- and gender-specific and dose-dependent differences in biological response. Such studies have been conducted with OP and CM pesticides in multiple species, at various dose levels, and across different routes of exposure to understand how *in vivo* kinetics contributes to the observed toxicological response. Literature substantiates that dose, vehicle, route of administration and species, along with several other factors, can greatly influence the pharmacokinetics/toxicokinetics of a particular AChE inhibitor (Gupta, 1994, 1995; Pelkonen *et al.*, 2006; Eaton *et al.*, 2008; Smith *et al.*, 2009). More importantly, toxicokinetic studies with these pesticides are useful to facilitate extrapolation of dosimetry and biological response from animals to humans, which is required for the assessment of human health risk.

Most of the toxicokinetic studies of OPs and CMs have been conducted in adult laboratory animals (rats, mice, rabbits and guinea pigs). However, there is paucity of data in pregnant animals. It is beyond the scope of this chapter to describe the toxicokinetics of each OP or CM pesticide. Therefore, certain issues related to the toxicokinetics of only selected anti-ChEs are described here in brief.

In occupational and non-occupational poisonings, exposure to these pesticides may occur via oral, inhalation or dermal route. But the majority of studies available in the literature involve the oral route. In general, following oral exposure, these pesticides are rapidly absorbed, widely distributed, metabolized in the liver and eliminated in the urine. Absorption following inhalation is also rapid. Dermal absorption varies depending on the site of application and dose. Compared to many OPs, dermal absorption of chlorpyrifos is low. Pena-Egido *et al.* (1988) reported plasma kinetics of parathion in rabbits after i.v. administration of a dose of 1.5 mg/kg and oral administration of 3 mg/kg. The time course of parathion plasma levels administered i.v. followed a three-compartment kinetic model, whereas following oral administration, the optimum kinetic model proved to be two-compartmental. The process of the absorption of parathion is very rapid with a mean value for the absorption constant (k_a) of $33 \pm 15.41\,h^{-1}$. The slow disposition half-lives for i.v. and oral administration had mean values of 5.08 ± 3.08 and 1.08 ± 0.27 h, respectively. It can be suggested from this study that parathion has wide accessibility and distribution to the different body organs and tissues. Although parathion has a high elimination constant, this process is not limited to distribution. In an earlier study, Braeckman *et al.* (1983) reported toxicokinetics of parathion and methyl parathion in dogs following i.v. and oral administration.

Toxicokinetic studies with dichlorvos revealed that it is rapidly absorbed, distributed and metabolized in both animals and humans (Blair *et al.*, 1975; Nordgren *et al.*, 1980). None of the data indicated that different species handle dichlorvos differently following either oral or inhalation exposure. In such a scenario no specific toxicokinetic adjustments between species are considered necessary. Kinetic considerations relevant to the issue of ChE inhibition itself have been addressed by considering exposure duration as a variable.

Toxicokinetic studies with OPs and CMs in pregnant women or animals are almost non-existent. It is well established that residues of OP and CM pesticides and their metabolites cross the placental barrier with little or no restriction and have been detected in the placenta, fetal cord and in the fetus (Gupta, 1995, 2009). Weitman *et al.* (1983) reported that pregnancy influences parathion disposition and consequently its overall toxicity. In the context of toxicokinetics, understanding metabolism of these pesticides is crucial. For example, OPs of the "thioate" group (malathion, parathion, chlorpyrifos, diazinon, guthion, etc.) are bioactivated primarily in the liver by a biochemical process known as "desulfuration" which then forms their active "oxon" metabolites (malaoxon, paraoxon, chlorpyrifos-oxon, diazoxon, guthoxon, respectively). The oxon metabolites are several times more toxic than their parental compounds, because of their greater potency for AChE inactivation. For example, the acute toxicity of malaoxon is approximately 100 times that of malathion. With a few exceptions, the metabolites of CMs are usually less toxic or non-toxic compared to their parent compounds. The two metabolites of carbofuran (3-hydroxycarbofuran and 3-ketocarbofuran) have a significant impact on the overall toxicity of carbofuran. 3-Hydroxycarbofuran has potency for AChE inhibition equal to carbofuran and plasma elimination $t_{½}$ twice (64 min) that compared to carbofuran (29 min), as it is involved in the enterohepatic circulation. Therefore, in toxicokinetic studies, metabolites should be taken into account for dosimetry, biological response and risk assessment. Due to extensive metabolism of these pesticides, only few metabolites are excreted and detected in the urine, feces, saliva and milk. Detailed information on toxicokinetics and physiologically based pharmacokinetics of OPs and CMs can be found in *Toxicological Profiles* (published by Agency for Toxic Substances and Disease Registry) and elsewhere (Gupta, 1994; Timchalk, 2006; Eaton *et al.*, 2008; Nong *et al.*, 2008; Smith *et al.*, 2009; Voicu *et al.*, 2010).

MECHANISM OF ACTION IN GENERAL TOXICITY

Both OPs and CMs elicit signs of acute intoxication by virtue of AChE inactivation (phosphorylation by OPs and carbamylation by CMs) at the synapses in the brain and at neuromuscular junctions (NMJs). Very recently, Sultatos (2006) and Timchalk (2006) described molecular interactions involved between OPs/CMs and ChEs and the mechanisms by which the enzyme's inhibition takes place. These pesticides have a high affinity for binding to and inhibiting AChE, an enzyme specifically responsible for the destruction of the neurotransmitter ACh. A graphic representation for the comparison of the AChE inhibition dynamics for the interaction of ACh, carbaryl, or chlorpyrifos-oxon with AChE is shown in Figure 37.1. The general rate of bound AChE hydrolysis is ACh > carbaryl > chlorpyrifos-oxon (Timchalk, 2006).

Inhibition of AChE by OPs and CMs leads to excessive ACh accumulation at the synapses and NMJs, which results in overstimulation of muscarinic and nicotinic ACh receptors. Muscarinic receptor-associated effects include salivation, lacrimation, urination, diarrhea (SLUD), in addition to miosis and tracheobronchial secretion. Nicotinic receptor-associated effects include tremors, muscle fasciculations and convulsions (Figure 37.2). Death ensues due to respiratory failure. It is important to mention that the level of AChE activity is low during pregnancy, resulting in higher concentration of ACh and hyperactivity within the nervous system (Gupta, 2009). Compared to OPs, CMs are studied to a lesser extent. Toxicological profiles of the common CM pesticides (aldicarb, carbaryl, carbofuran and propoxur) reports a variety of reversible neurotoxic and neurobehavioral effects in vertebrates, all associated with acute or subacute poisonings (Cranmer, 1986; Gupta and Kadel, 1989, 1991; Gupta, 1994).

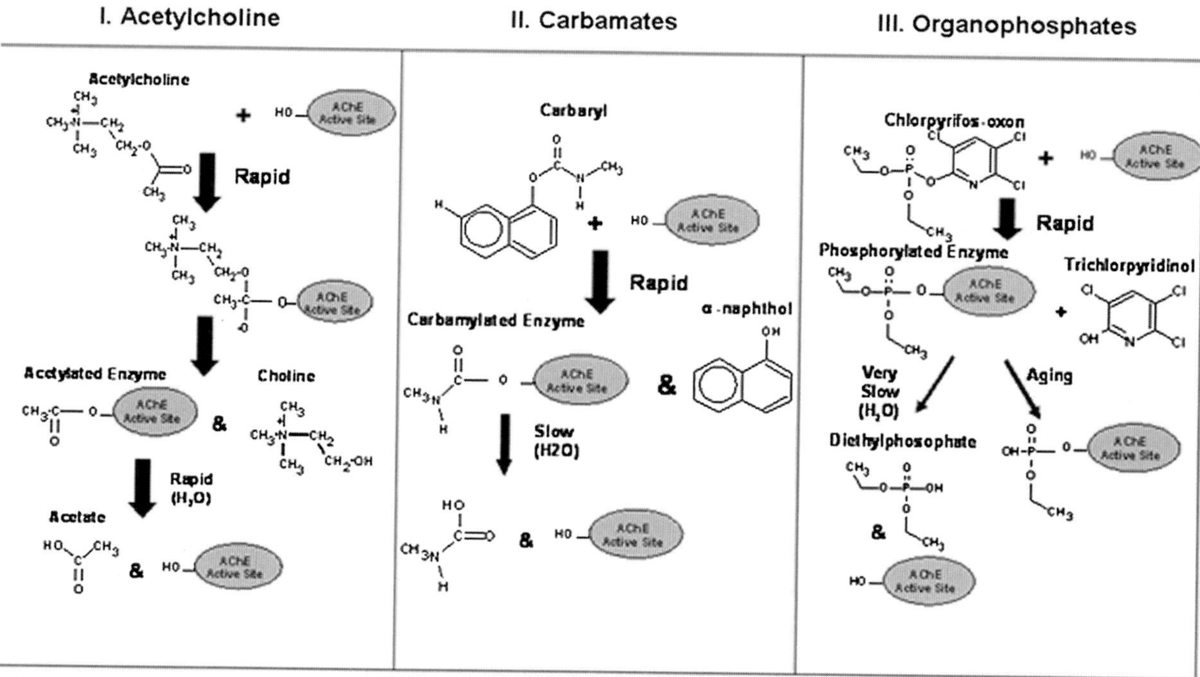

FIGURE 37.1 Interaction of ACh (I), carbaryl (II) and chlorpyrifos-oxon (III) with the active site of AChE (adapted from Timchalk, 2006).

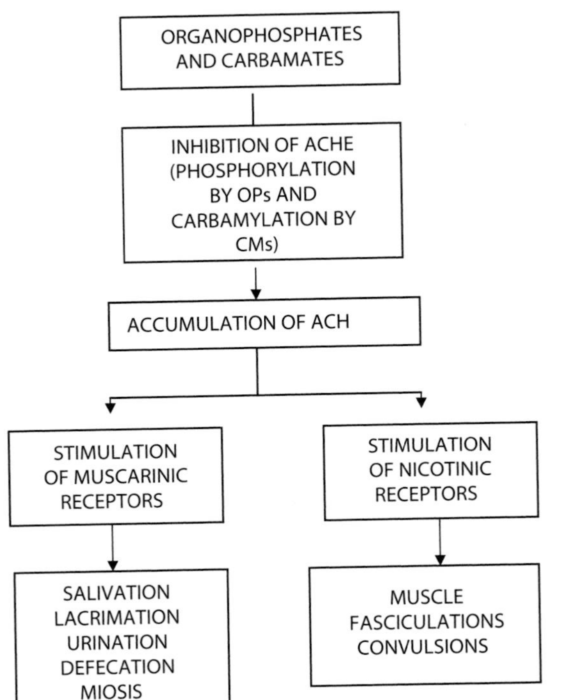

FIGURE 37.2 Sequence of events involved in mechanism of toxicity of OPs and CMs.

It needs to be pointed out that not all OPs or CMs elicit poisoning by the same mechanism (Gupta *et al.*, 1986, 1987; Gupta and Kadel, 1989, 1991; Gupta, 1994; Pope, 1999). Evidence suggests that like some OPs (Katz *et al.*, 1997), CMs interact directly with receptors of the cholinergic system. Physostigmine and related ChE inhibitors displace the muscarinic ACh receptor agonist [^{3}H]-oxotremorine-M from its receptors in rat cortex and brainstem (Van den Beukel *et al.*, 1997; Lockhart *et al.*, 2001). Additional evidence suggests that some of these ChE inhibitors are muscarinic ACh receptor agonists (Volpe *et al.*, 1985; Lockhart *et al.*, 2001). By now, the agonistic, antagonistic, potentiating and inhibitory effects of physostigmine and related ChE inhibitors on nicotinic ACh receptors (nAChRs) have been described. Van den Beukel (1998) described differential effects of CMs and OPs on nicotinic receptors in neuronal cells of different species. In another study, Smulders *et al.* (2003) compared the potencies of CMs on the nAChRs with AChE inhibition in the brain. These authors compared CMs potency on $\alpha 4\beta 4$ nAChRs, and found in the order of fenoxycarb>EPTC (*S*-ethyl *N,N*-dipropylthiocarbamate)>carbaryl, bendiocarb>propoxur>aldicarb, with that of the effects on rat brain AChE, i.e. bendiocarb>propoxur, aldicarb>carbaryl>EPTC, fenoxycarb. It is striking that the more potent interaction with nAChR is seen with the less potent inhibitors of AChE. It appears that nAChRs are additional non-AChE targets for the CM pesticides, and contribute to the toxicity of some CMs.

Both types of pesticides have been shown to perturb cholinergic and non-cholinergic systems in several organs, including brain, skeletal muscles, respiratory and heart (Gupta *et al.*, 2000, 2001a,b, 2007, 2009; Gupta, 2004; Dettbarn *et al.*, 2006; Hilmas *et al.*, 2006; Pope, 2006; Narahashi, 2006; Zoltani et *al.*, 2006; Zaja-Milatovic *et al.*, 2009; Ray *et al.*, 2009). These pesticides are neurotoxicants and the mechanisms involved in neuronal damage appear to be linked with free radical mediated injury and excitotoxicity associated with cholinergic and glutamatergic systems (Figure 37.3). Evidence suggests that many of the pharmacological/toxicological actions of OPs and CMs are much more complex and have no direct relationship to AChE inhibition or ACh accumulation (Milatovic *et al.*, 2005; Dettbarn *et al.*, 2006; Gupta *et al.*, 2007; Saulsbury *et al.*, 2009; Zaja-Milatovic *et al.*, 2009; Gupta and Milatovic, 2010).

MECHANISMS IN REPRODUCTIVE AND DEVELOPMENTAL TOXICITY

In many studies, OPs and CMs have been demonstrated to induce reproductive toxicity, developmental toxicity, endocrine disruption and oxidative stress in both male and female models (Gupta *et al.*, 1984, 1985; Güven *et al.*, 1999; Goad *et al.*, 2004; Qiao *et al.*, 2005; Sikka and Gurbuz, 2006; Verma and Mohanty, 2009). OPs and CMs and their metabolites readily cross the placenta, act on the cholinergic and non-cholinergic components of the developing nervous system and affect vital organs (Gupta *et al.*, 1984, 1985; Gupta, 1995, 2009; Mattsson *et al.*, 2000; Pelkonen *et al.*, 2006). Following prenatal exposure to OPs (chlorpyrifos, dicrotophos, malathion, methyl parathion, quinalphos and several others), significant inhibition of AChE has been demonstrated in maternal and fetal tissues of rats and mice (Bus and Gibson, 1974; Gupta *et al.*, 1985; Srivastava *et al.*, 1992). Similar results have been reported for CMs, including aldicarb, carbaryl, carbofuran and pirimicarb (DeClume and Derache, 1977; Cambon *et al.*, 1979, 1980). It is interesting to note that the sensitivity of cholinesterase inhibition is not different in fetuses or neonates from dams treated perinatally with the OP chlorpyrifos (Mattsson et al., 2000). With some of these pesticides, ChE inhibition has also been observed in the placenta (Gupta, 1995, 2009). These studies suggest AChE inhibition as the primary but not sole biochemical mechanism of toxicity in a developing organism.

Many OPs and CMs are developmental neurotoxicants, and therefore it is of great interest to focus on the effects of anti-ChEs on the developing CNS. It has been reported that multiple neurotransmitter systems are modulated by these pesticides. Developmental exposure to OPs (parathion, methyl parathion, chlorpyrifos, diazinon, etc.) is known to produce persistent modulations in cholinergic and non-cholinergic neurochemicals and receptors (Gupta *et al.*, 1984, 1985; Song *et al.*, 1997; Dam *et al.*, 1998, 1999; Aldridge *et al.*, 2003; Gupta, 2004; Richardson and Chambers, 2005; Slotkin, 2006; Guo-Ross *et al.*, 2007; Slotkin *et al.*, 2009). Interestingly, these effects can be modulated by environmental factors and dietary components.

Without any doubt, ACh is one of the neurotransmitters that provide neurotrophic input, regulating the replication, differentiation and migration of its target cells. But due to AChE inhibition, accumulated ACh and enhanced cholinergic cell signaling appears as a primary mechanism for neurotoxicity (Slotkin, 2006). In a detailed *in vivo* study, Gupta *et al.* (1985) treated pregnant rats with methyl parathion (1 or 1.5 mg/kg/day, p.o.) on GD 6–20, and examined fetal and maternal brains for key cholinergic elements. Exposure to 1 mg/kg/day caused significant but small and transient reductions in maternal and fetal AChE activity, and

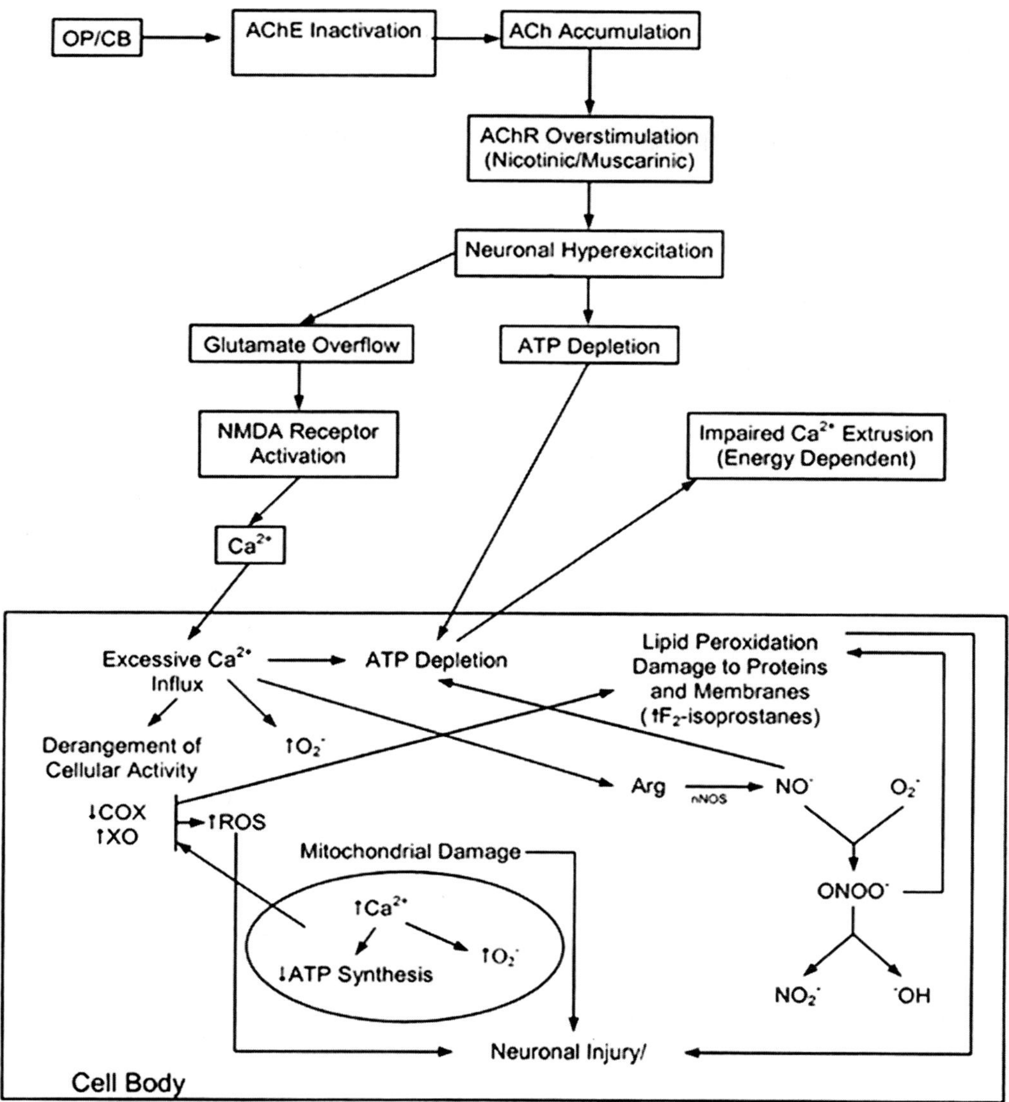

FIGURE 37.3 A schematic diagram showing possible cholinergic and non-cholinergic mechanisms involved in organophosphate (OP)- and carbamate (CM)-induced toxicity.

an increase in maternal but not fetal brain ChAT activity, and a decrease in maternal but not in fetal muscarinic ACh receptors (Tables 37.1 and 37.2). No visible signs of maternal or fetal toxicity were observed. Exposure to 1.5 mg/kg/day, on the other hand, significantly reduced AChE activity and increased ChAT activity in the maternal brain and in all fetal brain regions at various stages during development (Figure 37.4). Interestingly, chronic administration of methyl parathion also increased ChAT activity in frontal cortex and striatum of non-pregnant rats, suggesting that it is not a phenomenon peculiar to pregnancy. Muscarinic ACh receptors (mAChRs) binding sites (B_{max}) were decreased in maternal but not fetal brains. Signs of cholinergic hyperactivity were seen in some of the dams. A slight but significant reduction in maternal weight gain and an increased incidence of fetal resorptions were also observed at 1.5 mg/kg/day. No gross structural abnormalities or change in brain morphology were found in the fetuses. Impairment of behavior (decreased latency for cage emergence, reduction in accommodated locomotor activity and impairment of operant behavior) was found in 2–6-month-old offspring of dams fed methyl parathion at 1 mg/kg/day in peanut butter, but not in offspring of those administered 1.5 mg/kg/day in oil by gavage. The observed differences may have been caused by the differences in method and vehicle of administration, or potential non-linearity in the dose–response for behavioral effects.

From earlier studies it became evident that the mechanisms responsible for OP- or CM- induced embryonic/fetal development and teratogenesis appeared to be different from those involved in general toxicity in adults. Alkylation of nicotinamide adenine dinucleotide (NAD^+) coenzyme by OPs seemed to be the major mechanism involved in the induction of teratogenesis (Schoental, 1977). Other investigators proposed altered levels of RNA, glycogen, sulfated mucopolysaccharides and calcium in the developing bone as the mechanisms (Ho and Gibson, 1972). In another study, Gupta *et al.* (1984) examined the effects of methyl parathion (doses and treatment regimen as described above) on *in vivo*

TABLE 37.1 Effect of methyl parathion (MPTH) on postnatal development of AChE activity in rat brain regions

Brain region	MPTH (mg/kg)	AChE activity at postnatal day				
		1	7	14	21	28
Frontal cortex	1.0	63.8 ± 4.0*	80.2 ± 10.2	98.0 ± 4.1	95.0 ± 3.1	92.9 ± 1.8
	1.5	55.3 ± 6.9*	58.9 ± 6.1*	59.0 ± 4.9*	67.8 ± 5.0*	69.2 ± 4.9*
Brainstem	1.0	82.6 ± 1.6*	73.0 ± 8.3*	83.9 ± 4.9*	87.6 ± 3.4*	97.4 ± 4.3
	1.5	52.4 ± 3.5*	64.4 ± 1.7*	62.8 ± 6.7*	68.5 ± 4.8*	74.8 ± 1.1*
Striatum	1.0	–	–	86.1 ± 4.1*	94.7 ± 3.7	98.0 ± 5.6
	1.5	–	–	58.9 ± 5.1*	65.4 ± 1.4*	70.3 ± 3.1*
Hippocampus	1.0	–	–	99.8 ± 4.5	98.1 ± 3.5	91.4 ± 3.5
	1.5	–	–	52.4 ± 3.7*	67.0 ± 2.2*	80.4 ± 2.1*

Values are expressed as a percentage of control activity and represent the mean ± SEM (n = 5–6 litters)
*Values are significantly different between controls and MPTH-treated rats ($p < 0.05$)
Reproduced from Gupta *et al.* (1985a)

TABLE 37.2 Effect of subchronic exposure to methyl parathion (MPTH) on ChAT and AChE activities and [^{3}H]QNB binding in rat brain cortex on day 19 of gestation

Biochemical parameter	Dose of MPTH (mg/kg)		
	0	1.0	1.5
ChAT activity (nmol ACh synthesized/h/mg protein)	10.03 ± 0.17	13.07 ± 0.74*	15.25 ± 1.00*
AChE activity (% control)	100.0 ± 2.90	79.74 ± 3.73*	40.17 ± 7.50*
[^{3}H]-QNB binding	377 ± 48	270 ± 13*	275 ± 7*
B_{max} (fmol/mg protein)	458 ± 104	397 ± 56	307 ± 70
K_D (pM)			

Values represent the means ± SEM (n = 6–7 litters)
*Significantly different from controls ($p < 0.05$)
Reproduced from Gupta *et al.* (1985a)

protein synthesis in maternal, placental and fetal tissues. Methyl parathion exposures inhibited [^{14}C]valine incorporation into protein in maternal, placental, and fetal tissues. A dose-related inhibition was observed in (free as well as protein-bound pool) maternal brain, viscera, placenta and whole embryo in rats on day 15 and in fetal brain and visceral tissues on day 19. The inhibitory effect of methyl parathion on protein synthesis was greater on day 19 than on day 15 of gestation and was more pronounced in fetal than in maternal tissues. No such studies have been reported for CMs (Figure 37.5).

AChE inhibitors have been shown to disrupt cell replication and differentiation, synaptogenesis and axonogenesis (Lauder and Schambra, 1999; Bigbee *et al.*, 2000; Chang *et al.*, 2006; Sidiropoulou *et al.*, 2009). In recent studies, chlorpyrifos has been shown to disrupt the developing brain during glial proliferation and differentiation (Slotkin, 2006). Garcia *et al.* (2005) reported that chlorpyrifos effects in C6 glioma cells mirrored effects in the intact brain for inhibited DNA synthesis; interfered with adenylyl cyclase signaling; obstructed DNA binding to transcription factors involved in cell differentiation; and enhanced ROS formation. Garcia *et al.* (2005) administered chlorpyrifos to prenatal and neonatal rats and examined the brain for markers of astrocytes, oligodendrocytes and neurons. The findings revealed that males were targeted during postnatal exposures, while females experienced delayed effects following gestational exposure, commensurate with behavioral outcomes. These alterations in glial cell development contribute to chlorpyrifos neurotoxicity, extending vulnerability to myelination, synaptic plasticity and architectural modeling, and continue into adolescence. For further details on developmental toxicity of chlorpyrifos, readers are referred to a recent publication by Eaton *et al.* (2008).

OPs and CMs are known to cause impairment in learning and memory through multiple mechanisms (Gupta *et al.*, 1985; Moser and Padilla, 1998; Eaton *et al.*, 2008). One of those mechanisms appears to be alterations in the cholinergic system, which is known to play a critical role in learning and memory (Bartus *et al.*, 1982; Coyle *et al.*, 1983; Gupta *et al.*, 1985; Pauli and O'Reilly, 2008). Prenatal exposures to methyl parathion have also been shown to inhibit protein synthesis (Gupta *et al.*, 1984), which is normally required for learning and long-term memory (Alkon *et al.*, 2005). Furthermore, an exposure of rats to the CM pesticide carbofuran (Goad *et al.*, 2004) or OP pesticide dimethoate (Varma and Mohanty, 2009) resulted in significant decreases in testosterone levels, which can be linked to impairment in cognition and memory (Choi and Silverman, 2002; Lacreuse *et al.*, 2009). Literature reveals that postnatal exposure of rats to different OPs (chlorpyrifos, diazinon, parathion or methyl parathion) at low doses can have quite different neurotoxic effects and result in different patterns of memory impairment (Levin *et al.*, 2001; Timofeeva *et al.*, 2008a,b; Johnson *et al.*, 2009). Some of these effects can be unrelated to their shared property of ChE inhibition. Furthermore, since these pesticides differ in their patterns of AChE inhibition and recovery, they may differ in inducing impairment in cognition, memory and behavior as well (Gupta *et al.*, 1984, 1985; Moser and Padilla, 1998; Levin *et al.*, 2001; Eaton *et al.*, 2008; Johnson *et al.*, 2009). In a very recent report, Billauer-Haimovitch *et al.* (2009) demonstrated reversal of chlorpyrifos-induced neurobehavioral teratogenicity in mice by either nicotine or neural stem cell transplantation, thereby suggesting novel pharmacologic and stem cell-based therapeutic approaches.

Oxidative stress in developmental neurotoxicity

From *in vivo* and *in vitro* studies, OPs (chlorpyrifos, diazinon, parathion, methyl parathion and many others) have been demonstrated as developmental neurotoxicants (Gupta *et al.*, 1985; Crumpton *et al.*, 2000; Garcia *et al.*, 2005; Giordano *et al.*, 2007). These pesticides have been shown to elicit cell damage through their shared ability to induce AChE inhibition

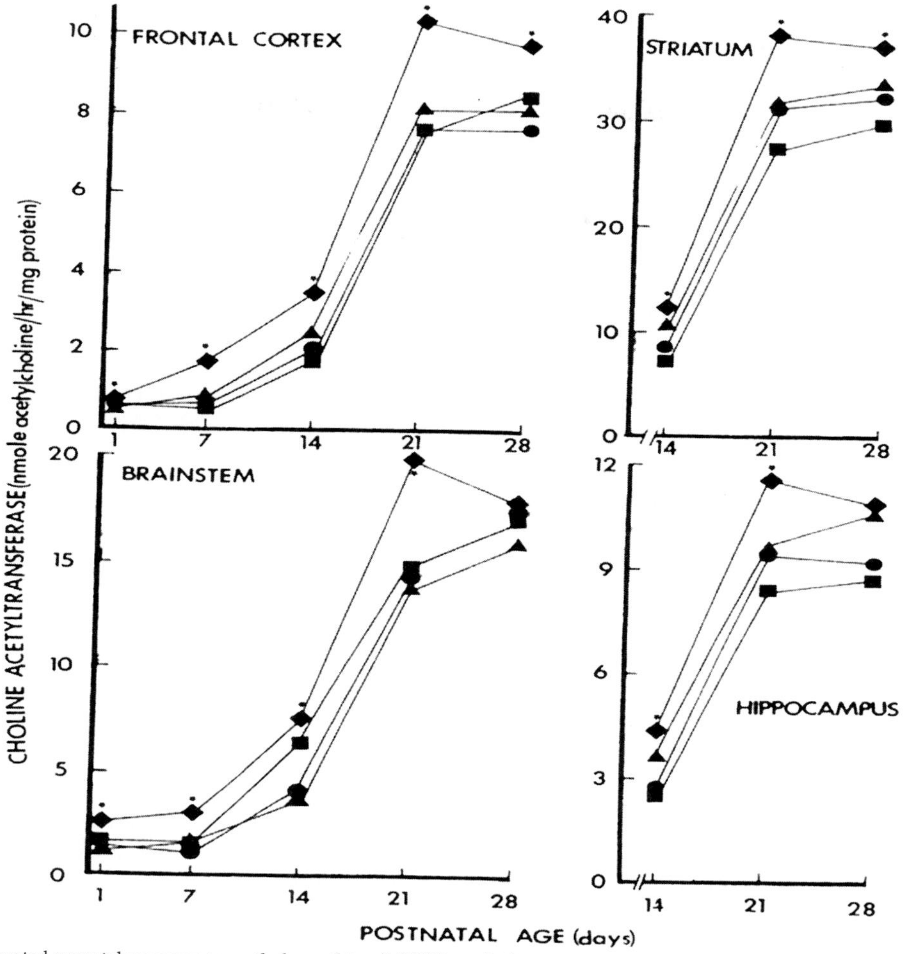

FIGURE 37.4 Effect of repeated prenatal exposure to methyl parathion (MPTH) on choline acetyltransferase (ChAT) activity. Circle, diet control; square, gavage control; triangle, 1.0mg MPTH/kg; diamond, 1.5mg MPTH/kg. Values are expressed nmol ACh synthesized/mg protein/h, and expressed as mean ± SEM (n = 5–6 litters). * = significant difference between values from control rats and MPTH-treated rats ($p < 0.05$). Reproduced from Gupta *et al.* (1985).

and oxidative stress (Gitto *et al.*, 2002; Ranjbar *et al.*, 2002; Gupta, 2004; Gupta *et al.*, 2007; Milatovic *et al.*, 2009; Zaja-Milatovic *et al.*, 2009; Slotkin and Seidler, 2009). The brain is particularly vulnerable to oxidative damage, because it has a high rate of oxygen consumption, and a membrane lipid composition that is enriched in oxidizable polyunsaturated fatty acids (Gupta, 2004). Furthermore, the brain has lower reserves of antioxidants and protective enzymes (Gupta, 2004) and has a higher ratio of neurons to glia, the cells that usually protect neurons from oxidative molecules (Tanaka *et al.*, 1999), while at the same time facing the increased metabolic demand associated with brain growth. The combination of these factors explains why many environmental contaminants elicit oxidative stress within the developing brain (Jett and Navoa, 2000). Most recently, in an *in vitro* study using PC12 cells, Slotkin and Seidler (2009) noted that chlorpyrifos has a greater effect on oxidative stress-related genes in differentiating cells compared with the undifferentiated state. Chlorpyrifos and diazinon showed significant concordance in their effects on glutathione-related genes, but they were negatively correlated for effects on catalase and superoxide dismutase isoforms and had no concordance for effects on ionotropic glutamate receptors. Surprisingly, the correlations were stronger between diazinon and dieldrin than between

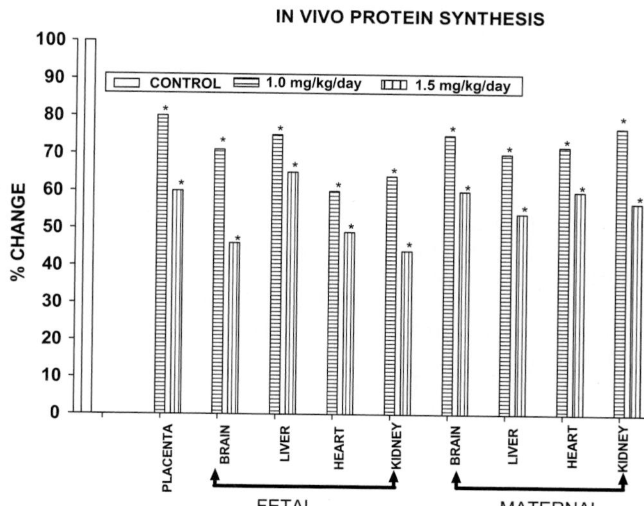

FIGURE 37.5 Effect of repeated prenatal exposure to methyl parathion (MPTH) on *in vivo* protein synthesis in placental, fetal and maternal tissues in rats. Values are means ± SEM (n = 5–6 litters). * = significant difference between values from control rats and MPTH-treated rats ($p < 0.05$). Reproduced from Gupta *et al.* (1984).

chlorpyrifos and diazinon. Therefore, the underlying mechanisms by which different OPs produce disparate neurotoxic outcomes differ from their shared property as ChE inhibitors. Apparently unrelated neurotoxicants may produce similar outcomes because of similar convergence on oxidative stress and excitotoxicity. Furthermore, the combined use of cell cultures and microarrays points to specific endpoints that can distinguish similarities and disparities in the effects of diverse developmental neurotoxicants. In a series of *in vivo* and *in vitro* studies, Slotkin and co-workers demonstrated the involvement of targeting neurotrophic factors, their receptors and signaling pathways in the developmental neurotoxicity of OPs (Slotkin *et al.*, 2008a–d). Thus, multiple cholinergic and non-cholinergic mechanisms may be involved in OPs-/CMs-induced developmental toxicity and teratogenesis.

Endocrine disruption

Chemical toxicants may cause endocrine disruption by influencing the synthesis, secretion, transport, binding or elimination of natural hormones in the body that are responsible for the maintenance of homeostasis, reproduction, development and/or behavior. OPs and CMs can disrupt the endocrine system by interfering with a single or multiple steps. These pesticides can also cause disturbances to the pituitary–adrenal axis or pituitary–testicular axis of the neonate, which may result in persistent endocrine dysfunction in the mature offspring. In a recent study, Verma and Mohanty (2009) reported disruption of the pituitary–testicular axis by demonstrating reduction in the number and size of luteinizing hormone (LH) cells, lowered plasma LH and testosterone levels in the neonates exposed to dimethoate. A drastic reduction in the testosterone level (~70%) was suggestive of a direct toxic impact of dimethoate on the Leydig cells and inhibition of steroidogenesis. It appears that insult to the developing organism is more apt to cause persistent damage than insult to the adult (Spyker, 1975; Goad *et al.*, 2004; Sikka and Gurbuz, 2006; Verma and Mohanty, 2009).

Recently, Kitamura *et al.* (2006) described in detail the endocrine disruption by OP and CM pesticides. Most of the studies in the area of endocrine disruption, and OPs and CMs toxicity, have been done in laboratory animals. The observed effects have included disruption of male and female reproductive functions, such as disruption of normal sexual differentiation, ovarian function, sperm production, pregnancy, etc. In adults, hormones mainly regulate ongoing physiological processes, and as a result they sometimes compensate for or recover from hormonal modulation(s). Endocrine disrupting pesticides have more devastating effects in the fetus and developing organisms than in adults, because they affect gene expression that governs development of organs as well as lifelong hormonal "set points", such as receptor numbers and hormonal production.

Early efforts to identify and characterize environmental endocrine-active chemicals focused on xenoestrogens, which are chemicals capable of interfering with estrogen receptor function (White *et al.*, 1994; Chen *et al.*, 1997; Gaido *et al.*, 1997). Of course, the literature also described environmental chemicals with antiandrogenic activity with research effort to include screening for chemicals capable of interfering with androgen receptor function (Kelce *et al.*, 1995; Maness *et al.*, 1998). Male reproductive tract development *in utero* is one of the most sensitive periods for exposure to antiandrogens. Tamura *et al.* (2001) described antiandrogenic activity in *in vitro* and in Hershberger *in vivo* assays to induce malformations in male rat offspring at lower dosage levels following *in utero* exposure. These authors investigated the interaction of the OP pesticide fenitrothion with the human androgen receptor (AR). Fenitrothion blocked dihydrotestosterone-dependent AR activity in a concentration-dependent and competitive manner in HepG2 human hepatoma liver cells transiently transfected with human AR and an AR-dependent luciferase reporter gene. In order to determine antiandrogenic potential of fenitrothion *in vivo*, Tamura and his colleagues dosed 7-week-old castrated Sprague-Dawley rats once a day for 7 days with testosterone propionate (50 μg/day, s.c.) plus gavage doses of either corn oil vehicle or fenitrothion (15 or 30 mg/kg/day). An additional group of rats was given testosterone propionate and the reference antiandrogen flutamide (50 mg/kg/day). Both fenitrothion and flutamide caused significant decreases in the ventral prostate, seminal vesicle and levator ani plus bulbocavernosus muscles tissue weights. These investigators demonstrated that fenitrothion is a competitive AR antagonist, comparable in potency to flutamide, and more potent than the known environmental antiandrogens linuron and *p,p′*-bis(p-hydroxyphenyl)-1,1-dichloroethylene (*p,p′*-DDE). However, in a detailed study, Okahashi *et al.* (2005) found that fenitrothion had no effects on the reproductive or endocrine systems of the parental animals and F_1 generations, even at toxic doses that markedly suppressed brain ChE activity in parental animals. The results suggested that fenitrothion at levels in the environment is unlikely to cause disruption of human endocrine systems. It is important to mention that testing of some OP pesticides (phoxim, malathion, monocrotophos, dimethoate and opunal) revealed no estrogenic potential using three *in vitro* methods (E-screen assay, estrogen receptor (ER) competitive binding assay and pS2 expression assay) (Chen *et al.*, 2002).

In an acute study, Goad *et al.* (2004) determined the effects of carbofuran (1.5 mg/kg, s.c.) on the levels of endocrine hormones in the serum of male Sprague-Dawley rats. Using chemiluminescent immunoassay, the hormones determined included progesterone, cortisol, estradiol, testosterone, triidothyronine (T3), total thyroxine (total T4) and non-protein-bound thyroxine (free T4). A 24-hour time course revealed significant alterations in hormone levels during 0.5 to 3 hours, with the exception of estradiol at 6 hours. The levels of progesterone, cortisol and estradiol were significantly increased (1279%, 202% and 150%, respectively), while the levels of testosterone were decreased by 88%. No significant change occurred in thyroid hormones (T3, total T4 and free T4) at any interval during the time course study, despite the fact that body temperature was significantly lowered at 1 to 2 hours after carbofuran administration. Carbofuran induced significant hyperglycemia for 3 hours could be due to multiple factors, including elevated levels of corticosterone, catecholamines and possibly glucagon, and depressed levels of insulin, as observed with an acute or subchronic exposure to the OP nerve agent soman (Fletcher *et al.*, 1988; Peoples *et al.*, 1988). Cranmer *et al.* (1978) also reported elevated plasma corticosterone levels in mice exposed to carbofuran or diazinon without a concomitant increase in adrenal steroidogenesis. It can be suggested that anti-ChEs can cause transient endocrine disruption following acute exposure, which may consequently lead to serious reproductive problems following repeated exposures.

TOXICITY

General consideration

Reproductive toxicity is expressed as alterations in sexual behavior and performance, infertility and/or loss of the fetus during pregnancy. Chemical exposure may cause alterations in the male and female reproductive systems. This may include adverse effects to the onset of puberty, gamete production and transport, reproductive cycle normality, sexual behavior, fertility and parturition; and premature reproductive senescence or modifications in other functions that are dependent on the integrity of the reproductive system of both the male and the female (Turner *et al.*, 2002; Sikka and Gurbuz, 2006). Literature abounds showing that exposure of laboratory animals to anti-ChE pesticides prior to or during gestation or lactation can perturb the reproductive system/activity of both males and females. OPs and CMs and their metabolites have been demonstrated to cross the placental barrier and have shown the potential for inducing embryotoxicity, embryolethality, endocrine disruption, fetotoxicity, teratogenicity and behavioral alterations. These effects appear to vary depending upon the particular OP or CM pesticide. In general, embryolethality is encountered more often, and as a result teratogenesis is rarely expressed.

Sensitivity of young vs. adult: is brain the primary target?

In mammals, the fetus can be exposed to pesticides during gestation via maternal intake of pesticides, while the neonate is exposed by ingesting contaminated mother's milk or food and water (NRC, 1993). An incident in Mississippi was an eye-opener, in which exposure to methyl parathion caused severe neurotoxic effects and even death in children, while adults exposed in the same household experienced only mild symptoms (Dean and Pugh, 1984). Since then, many studies have reported that children and young animals are significantly more sensitive than adults to anti-ChE pesticides toxicity (Gupta *et al.*, 1985; Eskenazi *et al.*, 1999; Liu *et al.*, 1999; Slotkin, 2006; Timchalk, 2006; Eaton *et al.*, 2008), and vulnerability often depends on stage of development. The importance of this issue was greatly recognized by the NRC's report, "Pesticides in the Diets of Infants and Children", which led to the passage of the "Food Quality Protection Act". It has been recognized for a long time that children are not just "small adults" but rather "a unique subpopulation that may be particularly vulnerable to chemical insult. In the case of ChE-inhibitors, this could be due to a number of factors, such as: (1) differences in toxicokinetics and toxicodynamics (Ginsberg *et al.*, 2004; Timchalk, 2006), (2) lower levels of AChE (Gupta *et al.*, 1985), (3) polymorphisms that affect cholinesterase and paraoxonase (Costa *et al.*, 2006), (4) immature blood–brain barrier (Adinolfi, 1985), and (5) very low antioxidant capacity (Rice and Barone, 2000; Gupta, 2004, 2009).

In general, the organogenesis period is considered to be the most critical period in terms of susceptibility for developmental neurotoxicity and teratogenesis. The organogenesis period varies from species to species, i.e. GD 7–16 in mouse, GD 20–45 in monkey and GD 20–55 in humans. So, it is important to select the time and duration of exposure in the animal model to match the window of exposure during organogenesis in humans (Slikker, 1994). Further, a brief description of brain development is also considered necessary because the brain is not only the target organ for the toxicity of OPs and CMs, but it is also more sensitive in the developmental (fetal/neonatal) stage than in the adult. The human brain forms over an unusually long period of time compared to other organs, including periods that can be critical for its normal maturation (Eriksson, 1997). While most of the basic structure is laid down before birth, neuron proliferation and migration continue in the postnatal period. In many mammalian species a rapid growth of the brain occurs during perinatal development, the so-called "brain growth spurt". In humans, this period begins during the third trimester of pregnancy and continues throughout the first 2 years of life. In the mouse and rat this period is neonatal, spanning the first 3–4 weeks of life, during which the brain undergoes several fundamental developmental phases, such as maturation of axonal and dendritic outgrowth, establishment of neural connections, synaptogenesis, multiplication of glia cells with accompanying myelinization, and cell, axonal and dendritic death (Kolb and Whishaw, 1989). During the "brain growth spurt", the development of the mammalian brain is associated with numerous biochemical changes that transform the feto-neonatal brain into that of the mature adult. Eriksson (1997) described that low dose exposure in mice to environmental agents, including OPs, during the "brain growth spurt" can lead to irreversible changes in adult brain function. The induction of cholinergic and behavioral disturbances in the adult animal appears to be limited to a short period during neonatal development, around postnatal day 10, and following doses that apparently have no permanent effects when administered to the adult animal. Furthermore, neonatal exposure to a low dose of a neurotoxic agent can lead to an increased susceptibility in adults to an agent having a similar neurotoxic action, resulting in additional behavioral disturbances and learning disabilities.

In humans, the blood–brain barrier (BBB) is not fully developed until the middle of the first year of life. There appears to be great postnatal activity in the development of receptors and transmitter systems, formation of architecture and circuitry, as well as in the production of myelin (Adinolfi, 1985; Rodier, 1995). OPs and CMs can damage the developing brain by interfering with one or more of these developmental processes (Gupta *et al.*, 1985; Gupta, 1995, 2009; Garcia *et al.*, 2005; Slotkin, 2006; Slotkin and Seidler, 2009; Slotkin *et al.*, 2009).

Current literature based on numerous animal studies presents evidence of links between exposure to OPs and suboptimal neurodevelopment (Eskenazi *et al.*, 2004). Many studies have shown that neonatal animals are more sensitive than adults to the toxic effects of chlorpyrifos. Rats exposed to chlorpyrifos during postnatal development showed behavioral changes, ChE inhibition and downregulation of muscarinic ACh receptors in the brain at doses five times lower than doses that would cause similar effects in adults (Moser and Padilla, 1998). It has been suggested that OP exposure may contribute to poorer neurobehavioral functioning in young animals by causing cellular deficits in their developing brains, particularly rich with cholinergic projections (Gupta *et al.*, 1985; Campbell *et al.*, 1997; Eskenazi *et al.*, 2004). Evidence exists that these deficits may result even with lower-level exposure if it occurs during critical periods of brain development (Gupta *et al.*, 1984, 1985; Gupta, 1985, 2009; Eskenazi *et al.*, 2004). Recent studies have also revealed that neonatal exposure to chlorpyrifos produces numerous persistent deficiencies in cholinergic synaptic function, which can continue into adolescence and adulthood (Slotkin *et al.*, 2001; Garcia *et al.*, 2005; Slotkin and Seidler, 2009).

In the context of neurodevelopmental toxicity of OPs and CMs, a brief discussion of brain regional heterogeneity is crucial. The complexity of the brain begins from its very early developmental stage, as it grows into various discrete areas, which are interconnected. From a neurochemical standpoint, growth of only a few brain regions is completed by the time of birth, while for other regions it takes a few months postnatally in laboratory animals and years in humans. Each brain region differs from others not only anatomically but also physiologically and pharmacologically. Until the maturation of the brain, most of the brain regions change drastically in terms of cholinergic and non-cholinergic biochemical/neurochemical determinants. Evidence from experimental animal studies suggests that in OP or CM toxicity, only selected brain regions are involved in initiation and propagation of a cascade of events leading into toxicological signs, including convulsions, seizures and death (Gupta, 2004; Gupta *et al.*, 2007; Zaja-Milatovic *et al.*, 2009). Biochemical/neurochemical determinants differ qualitatively and quantitatively from region to region and in some cases within subregions. In general, the brain areas most affected by AChE inhibitors are the cerebral cortex, brainstem, midbrain, striatum, thalamus/hypothalamus, hippocampus and cerebellum (Gupta, 2004). Each region or subregion in the brain may respond differently to the toxic insult of OPs and CMs. Moreover, the induced neurochemical and histopathological changes may differ: (1) from pesticide to pesticide, (2) acute vs. chronic exposure, (3) low vs. high dose, and (4) developing vs. adult organism.

Effects in males

Anti-ChE pesticides can exert toxicity to the male reproductive system by affecting sperm production and their motion, morphology and function, and by altering sexual behavior and performance. This can result in infertility, erectile dysfunction (ED) and eventually reduced quality of life (Sikka and Gurbuz, 2006). Earl *et al.* (1971) reported testicular atrophy and arrested spermatogenesis in beagles treated with diazinon for 8 months (10 to 20 mg/kg/day, p.o.). Everett (1982) noted decreased sperm production in bulls to which an undetermined amount of chlorpyrifos had been dermally applied. Farag *et al.* (2010) reported that exposure of male mice to chlorpyrifos (15 or 25 mg/kg, p.o.) for 4 weeks before mating with untreated females, resulted in increased dead fetuses, decreased sperm motility and abnormal spermatozoa, in addition to histological changes in brain and skeletal muscles. Krause *et al.* (1976) evaluated the effect of a very commonly used OP pesticide, malathion, on spermatogenesis in juvenile Wistar rats. Rats were sacrificed at various times up to the 50th day of life following two single gavage doses of 40 mg/kg/day of malathion on the 4th and 5th day of life, and the testes were examined. Significant findings included a slight reduction in the number of Sertoli and Leydig cells on the 6th day, reduction of spermatogonia on days 6 and 12 and reduction of spermatocytes on day 18. Mathew *et al.* (1992) showed that doses between 9.4 and 75 mg methyl parathion/kg increased the percentage of abnormal sperm cells in a dose-related manner. In another study, edema, congestion and desquamation of lining cells of the seminiferous epithelium were observed in rats gavaged daily for 12 weeks with 45 mg/kg/day of malathion (Balasubramanian *et al.*, 1987a). The same treatment also lowered the pH of seminal fluid, decreased testicular protein, decreased relative testis weight and decreased activities of testicular lactic dehydrogenase, alkaline phosphatase and acid phosphatase (Balasubramanian *et al.*, 1987b). Wistar rats treated with 390 mg malathion/kg/day for 6 weeks had a reduction in the number of germinal layers in the testes, accumulation of eosinophilic cellular debris in the lumen of the seminiferous tubules and intertubular edema (Piramanayagam and Manohar, 2002). Turner *et al.* (2002) found that OP pesticides can affect weight and morphology of gonads and accessory glands, sperm counts, hormone levels and fertility in rodents. Recently, Okamura *et al.* (2005) treated adult rats with dichlorvos (0, 1, 2 or 4 mg/kg, s.c./day), 6 days a week for 9 weeks, and found AChE inhibition in a dose-dependent manner, and deterioration of sperm motility with higher doses. However, no significant changes were noted in sperm counts, sperm morphology, histopathology of testes and plasma testosterone concentrations. In a series of studies, Narayana *et al.* (2006a–c) demonstrated that methyl parathion exposure during the early postnatal period of male rats induced biochemical and histological alterations in testes and accessory glands, in addition to endocrine disruption.

Very recently, Verma and Mohanty (2009) evaluated the reproductive toxicity of dimethoate at two different stages of postnatal development. The impact of immediate exposure through the mother (gestation and lactation) was assessed at the prepubertal stage of postnatal day (PND) 22. The other assessment was done at PND 63 (age of sexual maturity) to address whether or not the observed adverse effects persist to adulthood. Gonadal inhibition was reflected in the significant reduction of weight and distinct histopathological alteration of testis and epididymis, as well as in decreased sperm counts, which could be linked to the hormonal imbalance caused by dimethoate-induced interference of the reproductive axis. Developmental toxicity was evident, as gestation length and stillbirths were significantly increased, along with a decrease in body weight and anogenital distance of the fetuses. These authors concluded that maternal exposure of dimethoate during gestation and lactation periods adversely affected the pituitary–testicular axis of mouse neonates, which could further cause reproductive dysfunction of young adult mice.

Effects in females

In early studies, Deacon *et al.* (1980) carried out a developmental toxicity study of chlorpyrifos with varying doses (0, 1, 10 or 25 mg/kg/day) on GD 6–15 in mice. Significant increases in skeletal variations were observed in litters exposed to 25 mg/kg/day of chlorpyrifos, a level also causing significant maternal toxicity. Increases were seen in the number of fetuses with delayed ossification of the skull bones (6.8-fold), delayed ossification of the sternebrae (2.1-fold) and unfused sternebrae (4-fold) at the same dosage. For the detailed developmental toxicity of chlorpyrifos, readers are referred to Eaton *et al.* (2008). An increased incidence of supernumerary ribs and reduced fetal body weight gain were observed in the offspring of pregnant mice administered a single oral dose of guthion at 16 and 20 mg/kg, respectively (Kavlock *et al.*, 1985). Repeated exposure of pregnant rats to an oral dose of methyl parathion (1.5 mg/kg/day), a dose that caused frank neurotoxicity, resulted in increased fetal resorptions (Gupta *et al.*, 1984, 1985). Similar exposure of pregnant rats to 1 mg/kg/day of methyl parathion resulted in alterations in some behavioral endpoints in their offspring, evaluated at 2–6 months of age (Gupta *et al.*, 1985), suggesting that *in utero* exposure may lead to persistent behavioral effects. In another study, methyl parathion resulted in an increased incidence of cleft palate in the fetuses as well as fetal deaths (Tanimura *et al.*, 1967). In later studies, decreased ovarian weight gain and inhibition of compensatory ovarian hypertrophy were observed in hemi-ovariectomized rats injected with methyl parathion (5 mg/kg/day, i.p.) for 15 days (Asmathbanu and Kaliwal, 1997; Dhondup and Kaliwal, 1997). A decrease in the number of healthy follicles, no change in the number of atretic follicles, increase in duration of diestrus, decrease in the number of estrus cycles, and decrease in uterine weight were observed in the methyl parathion-treated rats.

In experimental studies, diazinon adversely affected the pups due to impairment of placental transport of nutrients or maternal regulation of fetal growth, or directly via antagonism to cholinergic development of the fetus. In humans, babies born to mothers exposed to OPs such as methyl oxydemeton and mevinphos showed cardiac defects (ventricular and atrial septal defects), stenosis of the pulmonary artery and a patent ductus arteriosus, bilateral optic nerve colobomas, microphthalmia of the left eye, cerebral and cerebellar atrophy and facial anomalies (Ogi and Hamada, 1965; Romero *et al.*, 1989). Many reproductive-developmental studies conducted in rats, mice, rabbits and hamsters showed no teratogenicity following exposure to some OPs, while in some other studies growth retardation and embryotoxicity were observed at maternotoxic doses. However, some OPs have been demonstrated to produce developmental alterations in rats, mice, hamsters and rabbits. In a classical study, Khera (1979) reported polydactyly in fetuses of cats treated with dimethoate (12 mg/kg/day) during the 14th to 22nd day of pregnancy (Figure 37.6).

Interestingly, some impurities present in technical grade OP pesticides are extremely toxic and can induce reproductive and developmental toxicity. *O,O-S*-trimethyl phosphorothioate (*O,O,S*-TMP) is an impurity present in a number of widely used OPs (malathion, phenthoate, acephate and fenitrothion) and it has been recognized as a potent lung toxicant. Koizumi *et al.* (1988) treated pregnant rats orally with *O,O,S*-TMP on GD 20 at 0.5, 2.5, 10 and 40 mg/kg. Neonates from treated dams died within 72 hours after birth in a dose-related manner (100% at 40 mg/kg, 86% at 10 mg/kg, 15% at 2.5 mg/kg and 1% at 0.5 mg/kg). Histopathological examination revealed dose-related proliferation of type II pneumocytes in dams and proliferation of interstitial cells and delayed septal/capillary development in neonates. Even at a dose of 0.5 mg/kg, changes occurred in the pulmonary morphology of dams and neonates. However, no changes were detected in other organs, such as liver, brain, spleen, kidney and adrenal gland of dams or neonates at 40 mg/kg dose. It was concluded that *O,O,S*-TMP caused lung injury in neonates by intrauterine exposure and elicited a lethal response in the neonates. In another study, Koizumi *et al.* (1986) reported increased resorption of embryos (63.2%) in *O,O,S*-TMP (20 mg/kg)-treated pregnant rats (GD8 and GD10). Fetuses from *O,O,S*-TMP treated mothers showed slight growth retardation. Skeletal examination revealed a missing vertebra and delayed ossification.

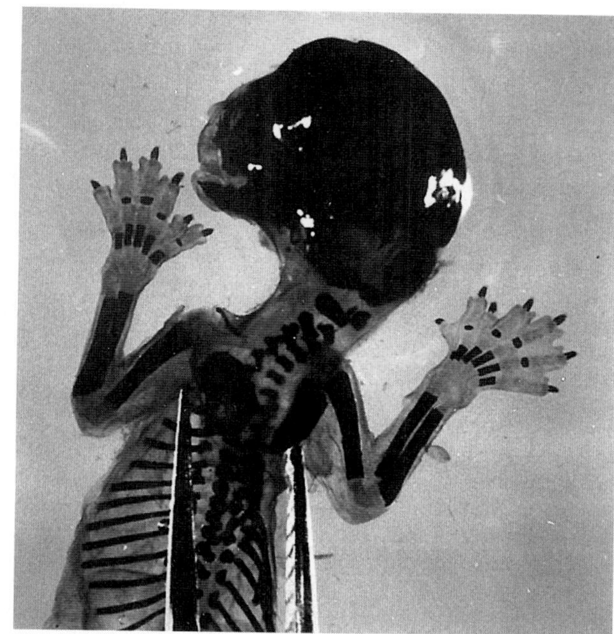

FIGURE 37.6 A cat fetus showing heptadactyly of right and hexadactyly of left forepaw from a cat exposed to dimethoate during 14th to 22nd day of pregnancy. From Khera, 1979.

Literature reveals that among CM pesticides, carbaryl has been studied in detail for its reproductive and developmental toxicity. Just like OPs, CMs have a greater potential for embryolethality and fetotoxicity, which precludes an expression of teratogenicity. A study conducted with carbaryl in beagles showed dystocia due to atonic uterine musculature and evidence of teratogenicity in 21 of a total of 181 pups. Fetal abnormalities included abnormal thoracic fissures with varying degrees of intestinal agenesis and displacement, brachygnathia, ecaudate pups, failure of skeletal formation and superfluous phalanges (Smalley *et al.*, 1968).

Carbaryl exposure during organogenesis produced terata in guinea pigs, but not in hamsters and rabbits (Robens, 1969). Pregnant rats exposed to carbofuran at 1, 2.9, 5.8, 7.7 or 9.7 mg/kg/day (FMC, 1980) or at 1, 3 or 8 mg/kg/day (FMC, 1981a) on GD 6–19 did not show any observable clinical signs of toxicity or adverse effects on pup survival or visceral or skeletal development. In similar experiments, rabbits exposed to carbofuran at 0.12, 0.5 or 2 mg/kg/day by gavage on GD 6–18 showed no developmental effects in the offspring (FMC, 1981b). In later studies, Jayatunga *et al.* (1998a,b) reported detrimental pregnancy outcome in rats.

RISK ASSESSMENT

Risk assessment can be defined as an empirically based process used to determine the probability that adverse effects are associated with exposure to a chemical. The risk assessment process involves four steps: (1) hazard identification, (2) dose–response assessment, (3) exposure assessment, and (4) risk characterization. AChE inhibiting OPs and CMs are economically important classes of pesticides as they are widely used in agriculture and landscape pest control, as well as to protect human health from endemic/pandemic outbreaks of certain diseases by controlling vectors. Although limited use of less hazardous pesticides is generally considered to be economically beneficial and to pose minimal health risks, overuse of the more potent pesticides is an increasing concern among public health officials worldwide. This trend is increasing as insects become more resistant and vector-borne diseases increase. Due to such widespread use, these pesticides pose a potential threat to human health because of unavoidable exposure. Studies suggest that young experimental animals and children are at greater risk of exposure of anti-ChEs and more vulnerable to their harmful effects than adults. Although entire subsets of a population experience reduced levels of neurologic functions, it is more prevalent in the young. It should be addressed that OPs and CMs are neurotoxicants, and therefore endpoints of neurotoxicity and neurobehavioral toxicity should be taken into account for a full spectrum of risk assessment. Since the developing brain is more susceptible than the adult brain to AChE inhibitors, it is important from a regulatory and public health perspective to assess the potential of individual AChE inhibitor to produce damage in children. Thus far, only a few OPs and CMs have been tested for developmental neurotoxicity during the risk assessment process. It is suggested that future studies should determine the dose–responsive effect of OPs and CMs on male and female reproductive tract development following *in utero* exposure. This will be more relevant for risk assessment.

One of the most important goals for the EPA's review of developmental neurotoxicity studies has been the ability to effectively extrapolate data acquired from animal models to humans (Claudio *et al.*, 2000). Virtually all developmental neurotoxicity tests submitted to the EPA are performed in rats. But for some chemicals, rats have different sensitivities than humans. For example, delayed neurotoxicity is observed in OP-exposed humans and chickens, but may not be observed in rats, rabbits and primates (Moretto and Lotti, 2006).

Biomarkers

Various endpoints for the reproductive and developmental toxicity of OPs and CMs are suggested as biomarkers that can be utilized in risk assessment. Biomarkers of exposure to OPs and CMs include residues of OPs and CMs and their metabolites in blood/plasma, urine, amniotic fluid and other body fluids (Bradman *et al.*, 2003; Makris, 2006; Eaton *et al.*, 2008). RBC–AChE inhibition has been identified by the scientific and regulatory communities as the sensitive biomarker of exposure to OPs and CMs because it serves as a sensitive surrogate endpoint for the inhibition of brain cholinesterase (Unni *et al.*, 1994; USEPA, 1993, 2000; WHO-JMPR, 1999). Walker (2000) reported that schizophrenic and depressive reactions with severe memory impairment and difficulties in concentration were observed in a group of workers exposed to these pesticides, and RBC–AChE was used as a biomarker of these effects. AChE inhibition, especially in blood, is therefore still considered one of the most sensitive and reliable biomarkers of exposure and effects of these pesticides. It is important to mention that human blood–AChE inhibition by OPs is no greater than in laboratory animals, suggesting equal sensitivity of AChE inactivation (MacGregor *et al.*, 2005). In recent years, egasyn-β-glucuronidase has gained significant attention for being a sensitive biomarker of OP exposure (Fujikawa *et al.*, 2005). Other biomarkers that can be used in risk assessment include *in vivo* protein synthesis (Gupta et al., 1984), key cholinergic elements (Gupta et al., 1985), endocrine disruption (Kitamura *et al.*, 2006) and leukocytosis (Güven *et al.*, 2005). Anti-ChE pesticides are also known to produce neurotoxicity and neurobehavioral alterations (Bushnell and Moser, 2006; Pope, 2006). Unfortunately, the data needed to estimate the overall magnitude of the problem do not exist.

As mentioned earlier, literature provides the evidence that pesticides exposure may be a contributing factor for neurodegenerative diseases, such as Parkinson's and Alzheimer's disease. If pesticides are risk factors for neurodegenerative diseases, their contribution probably accounts for a minor portion of the total risk. But even minor contributions of this nature, distributed across a large population, provoke a significant public health challenge. According to Weiss (2000) vulnerability to pesticide neurotoxicity is a lifetime issue. For further details on risk assessment and regulatory considerations of OP and CM pesticides, readers are referred to recent publications elsewhere (Lowit, 2006; Makris, 2006).

TREATMENT

OPs and CMs are highly toxic chemicals and present a serious threat to human health. The high mortality ascribed to these pesticides can be due to delayed diagnosis and improper treatment. Development of effective antidotes against OPs and CMs has been a big challenge since the inception of antiChE agents. Currently, atropine sulfate (muscarinic receptor blocker) is indicated in CM poisoning, while atropine sulfate and oximes (AChE reactivators) are indicated in OP poisoning (Eddleston *et al.*, 2002; Marrs and Vale, 2006; Jokanovic, 2009; Milatovic and Jokanovic, 2009). To date, hundreds of oximes have been synthesized and evaluated for their ChE reactivation potency against OPs in *in vitro* and *in vivo* studies, but only five (pralidoxime, trimedoxime, methoxime, obidoxime and HI-6) are commercially marketed. New reactivators are presently under evaluation, and there is a strong possibility for their commercial availability in the near future (Kuca *et al.*, 2009). In a recent report, Stefanovic *et al.* (2006) suggested that the addition of sodium bicarbonate to atropine sulfate improves the protective effects of standard antidotes (atropine and oxime) against OPs. In some studies, an anticonvulsant, diazepam, has proven beneficial in OP poisoning cases. Special care is needed while using these antidotes in pregnancies and the pediatric population.

CONCLUDING REMARKS AND FUTURE DIRECTIONS

OPs and CMs are used worldwide as pesticides in agriculture and public health protection, and in veterinary and human medicine. There is mounting evidence suggesting that these pesticides produce reproductive and developmental toxicity. These compounds can illicit embryotoxicity, fetotoxicity, teratogenesis, endocrine disruption and a variety of biochemical and neurochemical modulations. For both types of pesticides, the brain is the primary target organ, especially during prenatal and neonatal periods, and appears to be much more vulnerable than the adult brain. Exposure to anti-ChE pesticides seems to predispose humans to chronic ailments like diabetes or neurodegenerative diseases like Alzheimer's or Parkinson's disease. Future studies need to be conducted to provide clearer insights into the molecular aspects of developmental and neurobehavioral toxicity.

REFERENCES

Adinolfi M (1985) The development of the human blood–CSF–brain barrier. *Dev Med Child Neurol* **27:** 532–7.

Aldridge JE, Seidler FJ, Meyer A, Thillai I, Slotkin TA (2003) Serotonergic systems targeted by developmental exposure to chlorpyrifos: effects during different critical periods. *Environ Health Perspect* **111:** 1736–43.

Alkon DL, Epstein H, Kuzirian A, Bennett MC, Nelson TJ (2005) Protein synthesis required for long-term memory is induced by PKC activation on days before associative learning. *Proc Natl Acad Sci USA* **102:** 16432–7.

Asmathbanu I, Kaliwal BB (1997) Temporal effect of methyl parathion on ovarian compensatory hypertrophy, follicular dynamics and estrous cycle in hemi-castrated albino rats. *J Basic Clin Physiol Pharmacol* **8:** 237–54.

Balasubramanian K, Ratnakar C, Ananthanarayan PH, *et al.* (1987a) Histopathological changes in the testes of malathion treated albino rats. *Med Sci Res* **15:** 509–10.

Balasubramanian K, Vijayan AP, Ananthanarayan PH, *et al.* (1987b) Effect of malathion on the testes of male albino rats. *Med Sci Res* **15:** 229–30.

Bartus RT, Dean RLI, Beer B, Lippa AS (1982) The cholinergic hypothesis of geriatric memory dysfunction. *Science* **217:** 408–17.

Bigbee JW, Sharma KV, Chan FL, Bogler O (2000) Evidence for the direct role of acetylcholinesterase in neurite outgrowth in primary dorsal root ganglion neurons. *Brain Res* **861:** 354–62.

Billauer-Haimovitch H, Slotkin TA, Dotan S, Langford R, Pinkas A, Yanai J (2009) Reversal of chlorpyrifos neurobehavioral teratogenicity in mice by nicotine administration and neural stem cell transplantation. *Behav Brain Res* **205:** 499–504.

Blair D, Hoadley EC, Hutson DH (1975) The distribution of dichlorvos in the tissues of mammals after its inhalation or intravenous administration. *Toxicol Appl Pharmacol* **31:** 243–53.

Bradman A, Barr DB, Claus Henn BG, Drumheller T, Curry C, Eskenazi B (2003) Measurement of pesticides and other toxicants in amniotic fluid as a potential biomarker of prenatal exposure: a validation study. *Environ Health Perspect* **111:** 1779–82.

Braeckman RA, Audenaert F, Willems JL, Belpaire FM, Bogaert MG (1983) Toxicokinetics of methyl parathion and parathion in the dog after intravenous and oral administration. *Arch Toxicol* **54:** 71–82.

Bus JS, Gibson JE (1974) Bidrin: perinatal toxicity and effects on the development of brain acetylcholinesterase and choline acetyltransferase in mice. *Food Cosmet Toxicol* **12:** 313–22.

Bushnell PJ, Moser VC (2006) Behavioral toxicity of cholinesterase inhibitors. In *Toxicology of Organophosphate and Carbamate Compounds* (Gupta RC, ed.). Academic Press/Elsevier, Amsterdam, pp. 347–60.

Cambon C, DeClume C, Derache R (1979) Effect of the insecticidal carbamate derivatives (carbofuran, pirimicarb, aldicarb) on the activity of acetylcholinesterase in tissues from pregnant rats and fetuses. *Toxicol Appl Pharmacol* **49:** 203–8.

Cambon C, DeClume C, Derache R. (1980) Fetal and maternal rat brain acetylcholinesterase. Isoenzymes changes following insecticidal carbamate derivatives poisoning. *Arch Toxicol* **45:** 257–62.

Campbell CG, Seidler FJ, Slotkin TA (1997) Chlorpyrifos interferes with cell development in rat brain regions. *Brain Res Bull* **43:** 179–89.

Chang P-A, Wu Y-J, Li W, Leng X-F (2006) Effect of carbamate esters on neurite outgrowth in differentiating human SK-N-SH neuroblastoma cells. *Chemico-Biol Interact* **159:** 65–72.

Chen CW, Hurd C, Vorojeikina DP, Arnold SF, Notides AC (1997) Transcriptional activation of the human estrogen receptor by DDT isomers and metabolites in yeast and MCF-7 cells. *Biochem Pharmacol* **53:** 1161–72.

Chen H, Xiao J, Hu G, Zhou J, Xiao H, Wang X (2002) Estrogenicity of organophosphorus and pyrethroid pesticides. *J Toxicol Environ Health Part A* **65:** 1419–35.

Choi J, Silverman I (2002) The relationship between testosterone and route-learning strategies in humans. *Brain Cogn* **50:** 116–20.

Claudio L, Kwa WC, Russell AL, Wallinga D (2000) Testing methods for developmental neurotoxicity of environmental chemicals. Contemporary issue in toxicology. *Toxicol Appl Pharmacol* **164:** 1–14.

Costa LG, Cole TB, Vitalone A, Furlong CE (2006) Paraoxonase polymorphisms and toxicity of organophosphates. In *Toxicology of Organophosphate and Carbamate Compounds* (Gupta RC, ed.). Academic Press/Elsevier, Amsterdam, pp. 247–55.

Coyle JT, Price DL, Delong MR (1983) Alzheimer's disease: a disorder of cortical cholinergic neurons. *Science* **219:** 1184–90.

Cranmer JS, Avery DL, Grady RR, Kitay JI (1978) Postnatal endocrine dysfunction resulting from prenatal exposure to carbofuran, diazinon or chlordane. *J Environ Pathol Toxicol* **2:** 357–69.

Cranmer MF (1986) Carbaryl: a toxicological review and risk analysis. *Neurotoxicology* **7:** 247–28.

Crumpton TL, Seidler FJ, Slotkin TA (2000) Is oxidative stress involved in the developmental neurotoxicity of chlorpyrifos? *Dev Brain Res* **121:** 189–95.

Dam K, Seidler FJ, Slotkin TA (1998) Developmental neurotoxicity of chlorpyrifos: delayed targeting of DNA synthesis after repeated administration. *Develop Brain Res* **108:** 39–45.

Dam K, Garcia SJ, Seidler FJ, Slotkin TA (1999) Neonatal chlorpyrifos exposure alters synaptic development and neuronal activity in cholinergic and catecholaminergic pathways. *Devlop Brain Res* **108:** 9–20.

Deacon MM, Murray JS, Pilney MK, *et al.* (1980) Embryotoxicity and fetotoxicity of orally administered chlorpyrifos in mice. *Toxicol Appl Pharmacol* **54:** 31–40.

Dean A, Pugh J (1984) Organophosphate insecticide poisoning among siblings – Mississippi. *Morbidity Mortality Weekly Report*. October 26, 1984.

DeClume C, Derache R. (1997) Placental passage of an anticholinesterase carbamate on the effectivity of carbaryl insecticide. *Chemosphere* **6:** 141–6.

Dettbarn W-D, Milatovic D, Gupta RC (2006) Oxidative stress in anticholinesterase-induced excitotoxicity. In *Toxicology of Organophosphate and Carbamate Compounds* (Gupta RC, ed.). Academic Press/Elsevier, Amsterdam, pp. 511–32.

Dewan A, Patel AB, Pal R, Jani U, Singel VC, Panchal MD (2008) Mass ethion poisoning with high mortality. *Clin Toxicol* **46:** 85–8.

Dhondup P, Kaliwal, BB (1997) Inhibition of ovarian compensatory hypertrophy by the administration of methyl parathion in hemi-castrated albino rats. *Reprod Toxicol* **11:** 77–84.

Earl FL, Melveger BE, Reinwall JE Jr (1971) Diazinon toxicity-comparative studies in dogs and swine. *Toxicol Appl Pharmacol* **18:** 285–95.

Eaton DL, Daroff RB, Autrup H, Bridges J, Buffler P, Costa LG, Coyle J, McKhann G, Mobley WC, Nadel L, Neubert D, Schulte-Hermann R, Spencer PS (2008) Review of the toxicology of chlorpyrifos with an emphasis on human exposure and neurodevelopment. *Crit Rev Toxicol* **100:** 1–125.

Eddleston M (2002) Patterns and problems of deliberate self-poisoning in the developing world. *Q J Med* **93(11):** 715–31.

Eddleston M, Szinicz L, Eyer P, Buckley N (2002) Oximes in acute organophosphorus pesticide poisoning. *Q J Med* **95(5):** 275–83.

Eriksson P (1997) Developmental neurotoxicity of environmental agents in the neonate. *Neurotoxicology* **18(3):** 719–26.

Eskenazi B, Bradman A, Castorina R (1999) Exposures of children to organophosphate pesticides and their potential adverse health effects. *Environ Health Perspect* **107 (Suppl. 3):** 409–19.

Eskenazi B, Harley K, Bradman A, Weltzien E, Jewell NP, Barr DB, Furlong CE, Holland NT (2004) Association of *in utero* organophosphate pesticide exposure and fetal growth and length of gestation in an agricultural population. *Environ Health Perspect* **112:** 1116–24.

Everett RW (1982) Effect of Dursban 44 on semen output of Holstein bulls. *J Dairy Sci* **65:** 1781–94.

Farag AT, Radwan AH, Sorour F, Okazy AE, El-Agamy E-S, El-Sebae AE (2010) Chlorpyrifos induced reproductive toxicity in male mice. *Reprod Toxicol* **29:** 80–5.

Fletcher HP, Akbar WJ, Peoples RW, Spratto GR (1988) Effect of acute soman on selected endocrine parameters and blood glucose in rats. *Fund Appl Toxicol* **11:** 580–6.

FMC Corp., Agricultural Chemical Group (1980) Pilot teratology study in the rat with carbofuran in the diet. Study no. FMC A-80 443/IRDC 167-116. US EPA accession no. 244389. US EPA Office of Pesticide Programs, Washington DC.

FMC Corp., Agricultural Chemical Group (1981a) Teratology and postnatal study in the rat with carbofuran dietary administration. Study no. FMC A-80 444/IRDC 167-154. US EPA accession no. 244388. US EPA Office of Pesticide Programs, Washington DC.

FMC Corp., Agricultural Chemical Group (1981b) Teratology study in the rabbit with carbofuran. Study no. FMC A-80 452/IRDC 167-156. US EPA accession no. 1245268. US EPA Office of Pesticide Programs, Washington DC.

Fujikawa Y, Satoh T, Suganuma A, Suzuki S, Niikura Y, Yui S, Tamaura Y (2005) Extremely sensitive biomarker of acute organophosphorus insecticide exposure. *Human Exp Toxicol* **24:** 333–6.

Gaido KW, Leonard LS, Lovell S, Gould JC, Babai D, Portier CJ, McDonnell DP (1997) Evaluation of chemicals with endocrine-modulating activity in a yeast-based steroid hormone receptor gene transcription assay. *Toxicol Appl Pharmacol* **143:** 205–12.

Garcia SJ, Seidler FJ, Slotkin TA (2005) Developmental neurotoxicity of chlorpyrifos: targeting glial cells. *Environ Toxicol Pharmacol* **19:** 455–61.

Ginsberg G, Hattis D, Sonawane B (2004) Incorporating pharmacokinetic differences between children and adults in assessing children's risk to environmental toxicants. *Toxicol Appl Pharmacol* **198:** 164–83.

Giordano G, Afsharinejad Z, Guizzetti M, Vitalone A, Kavanagh TJ, Costa LG (2007) Organophosphorus insecticides chlorpyrifos and diazinon and oxidative stress in neuronal cells in a genetic model of glutathione deficiency. *Toxicol Appl Pharmacol* **219:** 181–89.

Gitto E, Reiter RJ, Karbownik M, Tan DX, Gitto P, Barberi S, *et al.* (2002) Causes of oxidative stress in the pre- and perinatal period. *Biol Neonate* **81:**146–57.

Goad RT, Goad JT, Atieh BH, Gupta RC (2004) Carbofuran-induced endocrine disruption in adult male rats. *Toxicol Mech Meth* **14:** 233–9.

Goldman LR, Smith OF, Neutra RR, *et al.* (1990) Pesticide food poisoning from contaminated watermelons in California. *Arch Environ Health* **45:** 229–32.

Guo-Ross SX, Chambers JE, Meek EC, Carr RL (2007) Altered muscarinic acetylcholine receptor subtype binding in neonatal rat brain following exposure to chlorpyrifos or methyl parathion. *Toxicol Sci* **100:** 118–27.

Gupta RC, Thornburg JE, Stedman DB, Welsch F (1984) Effect of subchronic administration of methyl parathion on *in vivo* protein synthesis in pregnant rats and their conceptuses. *Toxicol Appl Pharmacol* **72:** 457–68.

Gupta RC, Rech RH, Lovell KD, Welsch F, Thornburg JE (1985) Brain cholinergic, behavioral and morphological development in rats exposed *in utero* to methyl parathion. *Toxicol Appl Pharmacol* **77:** 405–13.

Gupta RC, Patterson GT, Dettbarn W-D (1986) Mechanisms of toxicity and tolerance to diisopropylphosphorofluoridate at the neuromuscular junction of the rat. *Toxicol Appl Pharmacol* **84:** 541–50.

Gupta RC, Patterson GT, Dettbarn W-D (1987) Biochemical and histochemical alterations following acute soman intoxication in the rat. *Toxicol Appl Pharmacol* **87:** 393–407.

Gupta RC, Kadel WL (1989) Prevention and antagonism of acute carbofuran intoxication by memantine and atropine. *J Toxicol Environ Health* **28:** 111–22.

Gupta RC, Kadel WL (1991) Novel effects of memantine in antagonizing acute aldicarb toxicity: mechanistic and applied considerations. *Drug Dev Res* **24:** 329–41.

Gupta RC (1994) Carbofuran toxicity. *J Toxicol Environ Health* **43:** 383–418.

Gupta RC (1995) Environmental agents and placental toxicity: anticholinesterase and other insecticides. In *Placental Toxicology* (Sastry BVR, ed.). CRC Press, Boca Raton, FL, pp. 257–78.

Gupta RC, Goad JT, Milatovic D, Dettbarn W-D (2000) Cholinergic and noncholinergic brain biomarkers of insecticides exposure and effects. *Hum Exp Toxicol* **19:** 297–308.

Gupta RC, Milatovic D, Dettbarn W-D (2001a) Nitric oxide (NO) modulates high-energy phosphates in rat brain regions with DFP or carbofuran: prevention by PBN or vitamin E. *Arch Toxicol* **75:** 346–56.

Gupta, RC, Milatovic D, Dettbarn W-D (2001b) Protection by antioxidants of DFP- or carbofuran-induced depletion of high-energy phosphates and their metabolites in rat brain regions. *Neurotoxicology* **22:** 217–82.

Gupta RC (2004) Brain regional heterogeneity and toxicological mechanisms of organophosphates and carbamates. *Toxicol Mechan Methods* **14:** 541–50.

Gupta RC (2006) *Toxicology of Organophosphate and Carbamate Compounds* (Gupta RC, ed.). Academic Press/Elsevier, Amsterdam, pp. 1–733.

Gupta RC, Milatovic S, Dettbarn W-D, Aschner M, Milatovic D (2007) Neuronal oxidative injury and dendritic damage induced by carbofuran: protection by memantine. *Toxicol Appl Pharmacol* **219:** 97–105.

Gupta RC (2009) Toxicology of the placenta. In *General and Applied Toxicology*, 3rd edition (Ballantyne B, Marrs TC, Syversen T, eds.). John Wiley & Sons, Ltd, Chichester, pp. 2003–40.

Gupta RC, Dettbarn W-D, Milatovic, D (2009) Skeletal muscle. In *Handbook of Toxicology of Chemical Warfare Agents* (Gupta RC, ed.). Academic Press/Elsevier, Amsterdam, pp. 509–31.

Gupta RC, Milatovic D (2010) Oxidative injury and neurodegeneration by OPs: protection by NMDA receptor antagonists and antioxidants. In *The Neurochemical Consequences of Organophosphate Poisoning in the CNS* (Weissman BA, Raveh L, eds.). Transworld Research Network, Kerala, pp. 19–39.

Güven M, Bayram F, Unlühizraci K, Kelestimur F (1999) Endocrine changes in patients with acute organophosphate poisoning. *Hum Exp Toxicol* **18:** 598–601.

Güven M, Dogukan A, Taskapan H, Cetin M (2005) Leukocytosis as a parameter in management of organophosphate intoxication. *Turk J Med Sci* **30:** 499–500.

Hilmas CJ, Adler M, Baskin SI (2006) Pulmonary toxicity of cholinesterase inhibitors. In *Toxicology of Organophosphate and Carbamate Compounds* (Gupta RC, ed.). Academic Press/Elsevier, Amsterdam, pp. 389–97.

Ho M, Gibson MA (1972) A histochemical study of developing tibiotarsus in malathion-treated chick embryos. *Cab J Zool* **5:** 1293–98.

Jayatunga YNA, Dangalle CD, Ratnasooriya WD (1998a) Hazardous effects of carbofuran on pregnancy outcome of rats. *Med Sci Res* **26:** 33–7.

Jayatunga YNA, Dangalle CD, Ratnasooriya WD (1998a) Effects of mid term exposure to carbofuran on pregnancy outcome of female rats. *Med Sci Res* **26:** 679–83.

Jett DA, Navoa RV (2000) *In vitro* and *in vivo* effects of chlorpyrifos on glutathione peroxidase and catalase in developing rat brain. *Neurotoxicology* **21:** 141–5.

Johnson FO, Chambers JE, Nail CA, Givarungsawat S, Carr RL (2009) Developmental chlorpyrifos and methyl parathion exposure alters Radial Arm Maze performance in juvenile and adult. *Toxicol Sci* **109:** 132–42.

Jokanovic M (2009) Medical treatment of acute poisoning with organophosphate and carbamate pesticides. *Toxicol Lett* **190:** 107–15.

Karaliede L, Senanayake N (1989) Organophosphorus insecticide poisoning. *Bri J Anaesth* **63:** 736–50.

Katz EJ, Kortes VI, Eldefrawi ME, Eldefrawi AT (1997) Chlorpyrifos, parathion, and their oxons bind to and desensitize nicotinic acetylcholine receptor: relevance to their toxicities. *Toxicol Appl Pharmacol* **146:** 227–36.

Kavlock RJ, Chernoff N, Rogers EH (1985) The effect of acute maternal toxicity on fetal development in the mouse. *Teratog Carcinog Mutagen* **5:** 3–13.

Kelce WR, Stone CR, Laws SC, Gray LE, Kemppainen JA, Wilson EM (1995) Persistent DDT metabolite p,p′-DDE is a potent androgen receptor antagonist. *Nature* **375:** 581–5.

Khera KS (1979) Evaluation of dimethoate (Cygon 4E) for teratogenic activity in the cat. *J Environ Pathol Toxicol* **2:** 1283–8.

Kitamura S, Sugihara K, Fugimoto N (2006) Endocrine disruption by organophosphate and carbamate pesticides. In *Toxicology of Organophosphate and Carbamate Compounds* (Gupta RC, ed.). Academic Press/Elsevier, Amsterdam, pp. 481–94.

Kolb B, Whishaw IQ (1989) Plasticity in the neocortex: mechanisms underlying recovery from early brain damage. *Progr Neurobiol* **32:** 235–76.

Koizumi A, Montalbo M, Nguyen O, Hasegawa L, Imamura T (1988) Neonatal death and lung injury in rats caused by intrauterine exposure to *O,O,S*-trimethylphosphorothioate. *Arch Toxicol* **61:** 378–86.

Koizumi A, McCloud L, Imamura T (1986) Increased resorption of embryos in *O,O,S*-trimethylphosphorothioate-treated rats. *Toxicol Lett* **32:** 185–94.

Krause W, Hamm K, Weissmuller J (1976) Damage to spermatogenesis in juvenile rat treated with DDVP and malathion. *Bull Environ Contam Toxicol* **15:** 458–62.

Kuca K, Gupta RC, Musilek K, Jun D, Pohanka M. (2009) *In vitro* identification of novel acetylcholinesterase reactivators. *Toxin Rev* **28**(4): 238–44.

Lauder JM, Schambra UB (1999) Morphogenetic roles of acetylcholine. *Environ Health Perspect* **107 (Suppl. 1):** 65–9.

Lacreuse A, Chiavetta MR, Shirai S-A, Meyer JS, Grow DR (2009) Effects of testosterone on cognition in young adult male rhesus monkeys. *Physiol Behav* **98:** 524–31.

Levin ED, Addy N, Nakajima A, Christopher NC, Seidler FJ, Slotkin TA (2001) Persistent behavioral consequences of neonatal chlorpyrifos exposure. *Develop Brain Res* **130:** 83–9.

Liu J, Olivier K, Pope CN (1999) Comparative neurochemical effects of repeated methyl parathion or chlorpyrifos exposures in neonatal and adult rats. *Toxicol Appl Pharmacol* **158:** 186–96.

Lockhart B, Closier M, Howard K, Steward C, Lestage P (2001) Differential inhibition of [^{3}H]-oxotremorine-M and [^{3}H]-quinuclidinyl benzilate binding to muscarinic receptors in rat brain membranes with acetylcholinesterase inhibitors. *Naunyn-Schmiedeberg's Arch Pharmacol* **363:** 429–38.

Lowit A (2006) Federal regulations and risk assessment of organophosphate and carbamate pesticides. In *Toxicology of Organophosphate and Carbamate Compounds* (Gupta RC, ed.). Academic Press/Elsevier, Amsterdam, pp. 617–32.

MacGregor JA, Plunkett LM, Youngren SH, Manley A, Plunkett JB, Starr TB (2005) Humans appear no more sensitive than laboratory animals to the inhibition of red blood cell cholinesterase by dichlorvos. *Regul Toxicol Pharmacol* **43:** 150–67.

Makris SL (2006) Regulatory considerations in developmental neurotoxicity of organophosphate and carbamate pesticides. In *Toxicology of Organophosphate and Carbamate Compounds* (Gupta RC, ed.). Academic Press/Elsevier, Amsterdam, pp. 633–41.

Maness SC, McDonnell DP, Gaido KW (1998) Inhibition of androgen receptor-dependent transcriptional activity by DDT isomers and methoxychlor in HepG2 human hepatoma cells. *Toxicol Appl Pharmacol* **151:** 135–42.

Marrs TC, Vale JA (2006) Management of organophosphorus pesticide poisoning. In *Toxicology of Organophosphate and Carbamate Compounds* (Gupta RC, ed.). Academic Press/Elsevier, Amsterdam, pp. 617–32.

Mathew G, Vijayalaxmi KK, Rahiman MA (1992) Methyl parathion-induced sperm shape abnormalities in mice. *Mutat Res* **280:** 169–73.

Mattsson JL, Maurissen JPJ, Nolan RJ, Brzak KA (2000) Lack of differential sensitivity to cholinesterase inhibition in fetuses and neonates compared to dams treated perinatally with chlorpyrifos. *Toxicol Sci* **53:** 438–46.

Milatovic D, Gupta RC, Dekundy A, Montine TJ, Dettbarn W-D (2005) Carbofuran-induced oxidative stress in slow and fast skeletal muscles: prevention by memantine and atropine. *Toxicology* **208:** 13–24.

Milatovic D, Jokanovic M (2009) Pyridinium oximes as cholinesterase reactivators in the treatment of poisoning with organophosphorus compounds. In *Handbook of Toxicology of Chemical Warfare Agents* (Gupta RC, ed.). Academic Press/Elsevier, Amsterdam, pp. 985–96.

Milatovic D, Gupta RC, Zaja-Milatovic S, Aschner M (2009) Excitotoxicity, oxidative stress and neuronal injury. In *Handbook of Toxicology of Chemical Warfare Agents* (Gupta RC, ed.). Academic Press/Elsevier, Amsterdam, pp. 633–51.

Moretto A, Lotti M (2006) Peripheral nervous system effects and delayed neuropathy. In *Toxicology of Organophosphate and Carbamate Compounds* (Gupta RC, ed.). Academic Press/Elsevier, Amsterdam, pp. 361–70.

Moser VC, Padilla S (1998) Age and gender-related differences in the time course of behavioral and biochemical effects produced by oral chlorpyrifos in rats. *Toxicol Appl Pharmacol* **149:** 107–19.

Narahashi T (2006) Electrophysiological mechanisms in neurotoxicity of organophosphates and carbamates. In *Toxicology of Organophosphate and Carbamate Compounds* (Gupta RC, ed.). Academic Press/Elsevier, Amsterdam, pp. 339–45.

Narayana K, Prashanthi N, Nayanatara A, Kumar HHC, Abhilash K, Bairy KL (2006a) Neonatal methyl parathion exposure affects the growth and functions of the male reproductive system in the adult rat. *Folia Morphol* **65:** 26–33.

Narayana K, Prashanthi N, Nayanatara A, Bairy KL, D'Souza UJA (2006b) An organophosphate insecticide methyl parathion (*O-O*-dimethyl *O*-4-nitrophenyl phosphorothioate) induces cytotoxic damage and tubular atrophy in the testis despite elevated testosterone level in the rat. *J Toxicol Sci* **31:** 177–89.

Narayana K, Prashanthi N, Nayanatara A, Kumar SG, Kumar HHC, Bairy KL, D'Souza UJA (2006c) A broad spectrum organophosphate pesticide *O-O*-dimethyl *O*-4-nitrophenyl phosphorothioate (methyl parathion) adversely affects the structure and function of male accessory reproductive organs in the rat. *Environ Toxicol Pharmacol* **22:** 315–24.

National Research Council (1993) *Pesticides in the Diets of Infants and Children*. National Academies Press, Washington DC, USA.

Nong A, Tan YM, Krolski ME, Wang J, Lunchick C, Conolly RB, Clewell HJ (2008) Bayesian calibration of a physiologically based pharmacokinetic/pharmacodynamic model of carbaryl cholinesterase inhibition. *J Toxicol Environ Health Part A* **71:** 1363–81.

Nordgren I, Holmsted B, Bentsson E, Finkel Y (1980) Plasma levels of metrifonate and dichlorvos during treatment of schistosomiasis with bilacril. *Am J Trop Med Hyg* **29:** 426–30.

Ogi D, Hamada JA (1965) Case reports on fetal deaths and malformations of extremities probably related to insecticide poisoning: *Jpn Obstet Gynecol Soc* **17:** 569.

Okahashi N, Sano M, Miyata K, Tamano S, Higuchi H, Kamita Y, Seki T (2005) Lack of evidence for endocrine disrupting effects in rats exposed to fenitrothion *in utero* and from weaning to maturation. *Toxicology* **206:** 17–31.

Okamura A, Kamijima M, Shibata E, Ohtani K, Takagi K, Ueyama J, Watanabe Y, Omura M, Wang H, Ichihara G, Kondo T, Nakajima T (2005) A comprehensive evaluation of the testicular toxicity of dichlorvos in Wistar rats. *Toxicology* **213:** 129–37.

O'Malley M (1997) Clinical evaluation of pesticide exposure and poisonings. *Lancet* **349:** 1161–6.

Pauli WM, O'Reilly RC (2008) Attentional control of associative learning – a possible role of the central cholinergic system. *Brain Res* **1202:** 43–53.

Pelkonen O, Vahakangas K, Gupta RC (2006) Placental toxicity of organophosphate and carbamate pesticides. In *Toxicology of Organophosphate and Carbamate Compounds* (Gupta RC, ed.). Academic Press/Elsevier, Amsterdam, pp. 463–79.

Pena-Egido MJ, Rivas-Gonzalo JC, Marino-Hernandez EL (1988) Toxicokinetics of parathion in the rabbit. *Arch Toxicol* **61:** 196–200.

Peoples RW, Spratto GR, Akbar WJ, Fletcher HP (1988) Effect of repeated administration of soman on selected endocrine parameters and blood glucose in rats. *Toxicol Appl Pharmacol* **11:** 587–93.

Piramanayagam S, Manohar BM (2002) Histological changes induced by malathion in rats. *Indian Vet J* **79:** 114–7.

Pope CN (1999) Organophosphorus pesticides: do they all have the same mechanism of toxicity? *J Toxicol Environ Health* **2:** 161–81.

Pope CN (2006) Central nervous system effects and neurotoxicity. In *Toxicology of Organophosphate and Carbamate Compounds* (Gupta RC, ed.). Elsevier/Academic Press, Amsterdam, pp. 511–32.

Qiao D, Seidler FJ, Slotkin TA (2005) Oxidative mechanisms contributing to the developmental neurotoxicity of nicotine and chlorpyrifos. *Toxicol Appl Pharmacol* **206:** 17–26.

Ranjbar A, Pasalar P, Abdollahi M (2002) Induction of oxidative stress and acetylcholinesterase inhibition in organophosphorus pesticide manufacturing workers. *Human Exp Toxicol* **21:** 179–82.

Ray A, Liu J, Karanth S, Gao Y, Brimijoin S, Pope CN (2009) Cholinesterase inhibition and acetylcholine accumulation following intracerebral administration of paraoxon in rats. *Toxicol Appl Pharmacol* **236:** 341–7.

Rice D, Barone S (2000) Critical periods of vulnerability for the developing nervous system: evidence from humans and animal models. *Environ Health Perspect* **108:** S511–S33.

Richardson JR, Chambers JE (2005) Effects of repeated oral postnatal exposure to chlorpyrifos on cholinergic neurochemistry in developing rats. *Toxicol Sci* **84:** 352–9.

Robens JF (1969) Teratologic studies of carbaryl, diazinon, norea, disulfiram and thiram in small laboratory animals. *Toxicol Appl Pharmacol* **15:** 152–63.

Rodier PM (1995) Developing brain as a target of toxicity. *Environ Health Perspect* **10 (Suppl. 6):** 73–6.

Romero P, Barnett PG, Midtling JE (1989) Congenital anomalies associated with maternal exposure to oxydemeton. *Environ Res* **50:** 256.

Saulsbury MD, Heyliger SO, Wang K, Johnson DJ (2009) Chlorpyrifos induces oxidative stress in oligodendrocytes progenitor cells. *Toxicology* **259:** 1–9.

Satoh T (2006) Global epidemiology of organophosphate and carbamate poisonings. In *Toxicology of Organophosphate and Carbamate Compounds* (Gupta RC, ed.). Academic Press/Elsevier, Amsterdam, pp. 89–100.

Schoental R (1977) Depletion of coenzymes at the site of rapidly growing tissues due to alkylation; the biochemical basis of the teratogenic effects of alkylating agents, including organophosphorus and certain other compounds. *Biochem Soc Trans* **5:** 1016–7.

Sidiropoulou E, Sachana M, Flaskos J, Harris W, Hargreaves AJ, Woldehiwet Z (2009) Diazinon oxon affects the differentiation of mouse N2a neuroblastoma cells. *Arch Toxicol* **83:** 373–80.

Sikka SC, Gurbuz N (2006) Reproductive toxicity of organophosphate and carbamate pesticides. In *Toxicology of Organophosphate and Carbamate Compounds* (Gupta RC, ed.). Academic Press/Elsevier, Amsterdam, pp. 447–62.

Slikker, W Jr (1994) Principles of developmental toxicology. *Neurotoxicology* **15:** 11–16.

Slotkin TA (2006) Developmental neurotoxicity of organophosphates: A case study of chlorpyrifos. In *Toxicology of Organophosphate and Carbamate Compounds* (Gupta RC, ed.). Academic Press/Elsevier, Amsterdam, pp. 293–14.

Slotkin TA, Bodwell BE, Levin ED, Seidler FJ (2008a) Neonatal exposure to low doses of diazinon: long-term effects on neural cell development and acetylcholine systems. *Environ Health Perspect* **116:** 340–8.

Slotkin TA, Bodwell BE, Ryde IT, Levin ED, Seidler FJ (2008b) Exposure of neonatal rats to parathion elicits sex-selective impairment of acetylcholine systems in brain regions during adolescence and adulthood. *Environ Health Perspect* **116:** 1308–14.

Slotkin TA, Ryde IT, Levin ED, Seidler FJ (2008c) Developmental neurotoxicity of low-dose diazinon exposure of neonatal rats: effects on serotonin systems in adolescence and adulthood. *Brain Res Bull* **75:** 640–7.

Slotkin TA, Seidler FJ, Fumagalli F (2008d) Targeting of neurotrophic factors, their receptors, and signaling pathways in the developmental neurotoxicity of organophosphates *in vivo* and *in vitro*. *Brain Res Bull* **76:** 424–38.

Slotkin TA, Seidler, FJ (2009) Oxidative and excitatory mechanisms of developmental neurotoxicity: transcriptional profiles for chlorpyrifos, diazinon, dieldrin, and divalent nickel in PC12 cells. *Environ Health Perspect* **117:** 587–96.

Slotkin TA, Wrench N, Ryde IT, Lassiter TL, Levin ED, Seidler FJ (2009) Neonatal parathion exposure disrupts serotonin and dopamine synaptic function in rat brain regions: modulation by a high-fat diet in adulthood. *Neurotoxicol Teratol* **31:** 390–9.

Smalley HE, Curtis JM, Earl FL (1968) Teratogenic action of carbaryl in beagle dogs. *Toxicol Appl Pharmacol* **13:** 392–403.

Smith JN, Campbell JA, Busby-Hjerpe AL, Lee S, Poet TS, Barr DB, Timchalk C (2009) Comparative chlorpyrifos pharmacokinetics via multiple routes of exposure and vehicles of administration in the adult rat. *Toxicology* **261:** 47–58.

Smulders CJGM, Bueters TJH, Van Kleef RGDM, Vijverberg HPM (2003) Selective effects of carbamate pesticides on rat neuronal nicotinic acetylcholine receptors and rat brain acetylcholinesterase. *Toxicol Appl Pharmacol* **193:** 139–46.

Song X, Seidler FJ, Salesh JL, Zhang J, Padilla S, Slotkin TA (1997) Cellular mechanisms for developmental toxicity of chlorpyrifos: targeting the adenylyl cyclase signaling cascade. *Toxicol Appl Pharmacol* **145:** 158–74.

Spyker JM (1975) Assessing the impact of low level chemicals on development: implications over the total lifespan. *Fed Proc* **14:** 1835–44.

Srivastava MK, Raizada RB, Dikshith TS (1992) Fetotoxic response to technical quinalphos in rats. *Vet Hum Toxicol* **34:** 131–3.

Stefanovic D, Antonijevic B, Bokonjic D, Stojiljkovic MP, Milovanovic ZA, Nedeljkovic M (2006) Effect of sodium bicarbonate in rats acutely poisoned with dichlorvos. *Basic Clin Pharmacol Toxicol* **98:** 173–80.

Sultatos LG (2006) Interactions of organophosphorus and carbamate compounds with cholinesterases. In *Toxicology of Organophosphate and Carbamate Compounds* (Gupta RC, ed.). Academic Press/Elsevier, Amsterdam, pp. 209–18.

Tamura H, Maness SC, Reischmann K, Dorman DC, Gray LE, Gaido KW (2001) Androgen receptor antagonism by the organophosphate insecticide fenitrothion. *Toxicol Sci* **60:** 56–62.

Tanaka J, Toku K, Zhang B, Isihara K, Sakanaka M, Maeda N (1999) Astrocytes prevent neuronal death induced by reactive oxygen and nitrogen species. *Glia* **28:** 85–96.

Tanimura T, Katsuya T, Nishimura H (1967) Embryotoxicity of acute exposure to methyl parathion in rats and mice. *Arch Environ Health* **15:** 609–13.

Timchalk C (2006) Physiologically based pharmacokinetic modeling of organophosphorus and carbamate pesticides. In *Toxicology of Organophosphate and Carbamate Compounds* (Gupta RC, ed.). Academic Press/Elsevier, Amsterdam, pp. 103–25.

Timofeeva OA, Roegge CS, Seidler FJ, Slotkin TA, Levin ED (2008a) Persistent cognitive alterations in rats after early postnatal exposure to low doses of the organophosphate pesticide, diazinon. *Neurotoxicol Teratol* **30:** 38–45.

Timofeeva OA, Sanders D, Seeman K, Yang L, Hermanson D, Regenbogen S, *et al.* (2008b) Persistent behavioral alterations in rats neonatally exposed to low doses of the organophosphate pesticide, parathion. *Brain Res Bull* **77:** 404–11.

Turner KJ, Barlow NJ, Struve MF, Wallace DG, Gaido KW, Dorman DC, Foster PMD (2002) Effects of *in utero* exposure to the organophosphate insecticide fenitrothion on androgen-dependent reproductive development in the Crl:CD(SD)BR rat. *Toxicol Sci* **68:** 174–83.

Unni L, Womack C, Hannant M, Becker R (1994) Pharmacokinetics and pharmacodynamics of metrifonate in humans. *Methods Find Exp Clin Pharmacol* **16:** 285–9.

US Environmental Protection Agency (USEPA) (1993) Reference dose (RfD): description and use in health risk assessment. IRIS background document. Office of Health and Environmental Assessment, National Center for Environmental Assessment. Cincinnati, OH.

US Environmental Protection Agency (USEPA) (2000) The use of data on cholinesterase inhibition for risk assessment of organophosphorus and carbamate pesticides. USEPA, Office of Pesticide Programs, Washington DC. Online at: http://www.epa.gov/pesticides/trac/science/cholin.pdf. August 18, 2000.

Van den Beukel I, Dijcks FA, Vanderheijden P, Vaucquelin G, Oortgiesen M (1997) Differential muscarinic receptor binding of acetylcholinesterase inhibitors in rat brain, human brain and Chinese hamster ovary cells expressing human receptors. *J Pharmacol Exp Therap* **281:** 1113–19.

Van den Beukel I, Van Kleef RGDM, Oortgiesen M (1998) Differential effects of physostigmine and organophosphates on nicotinic receptors in neuronal cells of different species. *Neurotoxicology* **19:** 777–88.

Varma DR, Mulay S (2006) The Bhopal accident and methyl isocyanate toxicity. In *Toxicology of Organophosphate and Carbamate Compounds* (Gupta RC, ed.). Academic Press/Elsevier, Amsterdam, pp. 79–88.

Verma R, Mohanty B (2009) Early-life exposure to dimethoate-induced reproductive toxicity: evaluation of effects on pituitary-testicular axis of mice. *Toxicol Sci* **112:** 450–8.

Voicu VA, Thiermanm H, Radulescu FS, Mircioiu C, Miron DS (2010) The toxicokinetics and toxicodynamics of organophosphonates versus the pharmacokinetics and pharmacodynamics of oxime antidotes: biological consequences. *Basic Clin Pharmacol Toxicol* **106:** 73–85.

Volpe LS, Biagioni TM, Marquis JK (1985) *In vitro* modulation of bovine caudate muscarinic receptor number by organophosphates and carbamates. *Toxicol Appl Pharmacol* **78:** 226–34.

Walker W (2000) Neurotoxicity in human beings. *J Lab Clin Med* **136:** 168–80.

Weitman SD, Vodicnik MJ, Lech JJ (1983) Influence of pregnancy on parathion toxicity and disposition. *Toxicol Appl Pharmacol* **71:** 215–24.

Weiss B (2000) Vulnerability to pesticide neurotoxicity is a lifetime issue. *Neurotoxicology* **21:** 67–74.

White R, Jobling S, Hoare SA, Sumpter JP, Parker MG (1994) Environmentally persistent alkylphenolic compounds are estrogenic. *Endocrinology* **135:** 175–82.

World Health Organization Joint Meeting on Pesticide Residues (WHO-JMPR) (1999) FAO/WHO Joint Meeting on Pesticide Residues. Report of the 1998 FAO/WHO Joint Meeting on Pesticide Residues. Food and Agricultural Organization-United Nations. Rome, Italy.

Zaja-Milatovic S, Gupta RC, Aschner M, Milatovic M (2009) Protection of DFP-induced oxidative damage and neurodegeneration by antioxidants and NMDA receptor antagonist. *Toxicol Appl Pharmacol* **240:** 124–31.

Zoltani CK, Thorne GD, Baskin SI (2006) Cardiovascular toxicity of cholinesterase inhibitors. In *Toxicology of Organophosphate and Carbamate Compounds* (Gupta RC, ed.). Academic Press/Elsevier, Amsterdam, pp. 381–8.

Zwiener RJ, Ginsburg CM (1988) Organophosphate and carbamate poisoning in infants and children. *Pediatrics* **81:** 121–6.

C H A P T E R

38

Chlorinated hydrocarbons and pyrethrins/pyrethroids

Jitendra K. Malik, Manoj Aggarwal, Starling Kalpana and Ramesh C. Gupta

INTRODUCTION

Insecticides have been widely used to control noxious insects in agriculture, forestry, horticulture, public health and medicine. Their use in agriculture has contributed to dramatic increases in crop production and in the quantity and variety of the diet. Insecticides have also played a crucial role in limiting the spread of human and animal vector-borne diseases. The chlorinated hydrocarbon insecticides were heavily used after their introduction, but the disadvantages of using compounds that do not readily degrade under environmental conditions soon became apparent. Their acute toxicity is moderate and less than that of organophosphates and carbamates, but chronic exposure may be associated with adverse health effects. Primarily because of ecological considerations, these compounds have been banned in most countries in the past 30 years. Yet, because of their environmental persistence and high lipophilicity, exposure to these compounds continues, most notably through the diet. Dichlorodiphenyltrichloroethane (DDT) and its metabolite 1,1-bis(*p*-chlorophenyl)-2,2-dichloroethylene (DDE) are ubiquitous and can be found in various human tissues throughout the world (Turusov *et al.*, 2002). Moreover, it has been consistently found in follicular fluids and serum of women (Baukloh *et al.*, 1985). It is also known that an isomer of DDT *o,p′*-DDT possesses sex steroid activities which are able to alter the properties and functions of the female reproductive system (Kamrin *et al.*, 1994). Furthermore, some insecticides, such as DDT, are being reintroduced in parts of the world for malaria control; hence, toxicity, especially reproductive and developmental toxicity, induced by chlorinated hydrocarbon insecticides is currently under discussion (Toft *et al.*, 2004; Costa, 2008; Tiemann, 2008).

Environmental accumulation of persistent organic pollutants including chlorinated hydrocarbon insecticides has been suggested as a major cause of reproductive dysfunction in humans and animals (Daston *et al.*, 1997; Campagna *et al.*, 2002). Prolonged exposure to chlorinated hydrocarbon insecticides is associated with reproductive abnormalities in several species and is able to influence the development of oocytes and preimplantation embryos (Walker *et al.*, 2000). Significant diet exposure starts early in postnatal life with breastfeeding, as underscored by the evidence that high levels of chlorinated hydrocarbon insecticides have been detected in breast milk (Lackmann *et al.*, 2004). Recent findings suggest serum concentrations of chlorinated hydrocarbon insecticides change across critical windows of human reproduction, signifying the importance of the sampling time (Bloom *et al.*, 2009).

Pyrethroids (synthetic pyrethrins) are one of the important groups of insecticides. As the usage of many chlorinated hydrocarbons has diminished in many parts of the world, synthetic pyrethroids have often served as replacements. Pyrethroids, broad-spectrum insecticides with low mammalian toxicity and rapid rate of degradation, are used widely as insecticides both in the house and in agriculture, and in medicine for the topical treatment of external parasites (Costa, 2008). For enhancing their insecticidal activity most pyrethrins and many pyrethroids are combined with a synergist, such as piperonyl butoxide, N-octyl-bicycloheptene dicarboximide, sulfoxide, sesamin, sesame oil, sesamolin and isosafrole which may also inhibit microsomal oxidation. Some formulations include additional insecticides, insect repellents, or both, and many contain hydrocarbon solvents (Valentine and Beasley, 1989; Anadon *et al.*, 2009).

A search through the literature shows that most of the previous research on pesticide-induced developmental and reproductive toxicity is focused on organophosphate and chlorinated hydrocarbon insecticides and very little attention was given to the pyrethroids. However, animal studies on pyrethroids such as cypermethrin, deltamethrin and fenvalerate demonstrated insecticide-related reproductive untoward effects both in male and fetal organisms. These studies also showed growth retardation and/or fetal loss due to exposure to pyrethroids to pregnant animals. Recently, pyrethroids have been reported to cause developmental neurotoxicity (Shafer *et al.*, 2005) and interference with the semen quality (Xia *et al.*, 2008) in humans.

HISTORICAL BACKGROUND

The period between 1935 and 1950 was characterized by the development of major classes of pesticides, particularly insecticides. In 1939 Swiss chemist Paul Hermann Mueller

Reproductive and Developmental Toxicology, Edited by Ramesh C. Gupta
ISBN: 978-0-12-382032-7

found that DDT, which had been first synthesized in 1874, acted as a poison on flies, mosquitoes and other insects. DDT was commercialized in 1942 and used extensively and successfully for the control of typhus epidemics and particularly malaria. Together with DDT, other chlorinated hydrocarbon insecticides were developed. In the early 1940s, scientists in England and France recognized the gamma isomer of hexachlorocyclohexane, known as lindane, which had been first synthesized in 1825 by Faraday as a highly potent insecticide. Starting in the mid-1940s several other chlorinated hydrocarbon insecticides were commercialized, including chlordane, heptachlor, aldrin and dieldrin (Costa, 2008).

Pyrethrins were first developed as insecticides from extracts of the flower heads of *Chrysanthemum cinerariaefolium*, whose insecticidal potential was appreciated in ancient China and Persia. There are six compounds that comprise the natural pyrethrins, namely, pyrethrins I and II, cinerins I and II, and jasmolins I and II. However, because pyrethrins were decomposed rapidly by light, synthetic analogs were developed, called pyrethroids, to improve stability, leading to their widespread application as agricultural and industrial insecticides (Elliott *et al.*, 1978; Anadon *et al.*, 2009).

The first generation pyrethroids, developed in the 1960s, include bioallethrin, tetramethrin, resmethrin and bioresmethrin. They are more active than the natural pyrethrum, but are unstable in sunlight. Activity of pyrethrum and first generation pyrethroids is often enhanced by addition of the synergist piperonyl butoxide which is not itself biologically active. By 1974, a second generation of more persistent compounds, notably permethrin, cypermethrin and deltamethrin, was discovered. They are substantially more resistant to degradation by light and air, thus making them suitable for use in agriculture, but they have significantly higher mammalian toxicities. Over the subsequent decades, these were followed by discovery of other compounds such as fenvalerate, lambda-cyhalothrin and beta-cyfluthrin. One of the less desirable characteristics, especially of second generation pyrethroids, is that they can be irritant to the skin and eyes, so special formulations such as capsule suspensions have been developed. Because of high insecticidal potency, relatively low mammalian toxicity, lack of environmental persistence, and low tendency to induce insect resistance of pyrethroids, they have encountered much success in the past 30 years, and now account for more than 25% of the global insecticide market (Elliott *et al.*, 1978; Soderlund *et al.*, 2002; Costa, 2008; Anadon *et al.*, 2009). The intent of this chapter is to describe the reproductive and developmental toxicity of chlorinated hydrocarbon and pyrethrin/pyrethroid insecticides.

TOXICOKINETICS

The characterization of toxicokinetic profiles of insecticides including absorption, distribution, metabolism and excretion is important in evaluating their dosimetry, biological response and risk assessment in human beings exposed to these compounds. Toxicokinetic studies provide pertinent information on the quantity of toxicant delivered to its target site as well as differences in biological response relating to dose, gender, age and species. Toxicokinetic/pharmacokinetic studies of chlorinated hydrocarbon and pyrethroid insecticides have been conducted in a variety of species at various dose levels and following different exposure routes. Several factors including dose, nature of vehicle, route of exposure and species are known to markedly influence the toxicokinetic/pharmacokinetic behavior of an insecticide. Compartmental pharmacokinetic models do not require information on anatomic structure and physiology and cannot predict tissue concentrations whereas physiologically based pharmacokinetic models can predict tissue concentrations of toxicants. The toxicokinetic studies of chlorinated hydrocarbon and pyrethroid insecticides available in literature have been generally conducted in adult laboratory animals and toxicokinetic data of these insecticides are scarce in pregnant animals. It is not the intent of this chapter to give an encyclopedic coverage of the subject but rather to briefly describe certain aspects of toxicokinetics/pharmacokinetics of only selected chlorinated hydrocarbon and pyrethroid insecticides.

Regardless of the route of exposure, insecticides entering the human or animal body undergo chemical or biochemical transformations by various mechanisms. The types of biotransformation a pesticide may undergo in the body are varied and an understanding of the fate of an insecticide in food animals is necessary in determining its selectivity and toxicity. This is an important consideration in view of regular exposure of non-target species to a variety of pesticides which may result due to their universal usage in different fields. Studies relating to metabolism of insecticides in farm animals and birds have been carried out to protect humans from possible deleterious effects of insecticide residues in egg, milk and meat. Residues comprising degradation products alone or in combination with a parent compound may be of toxicological significance.

Due to their high lipid solubility, chlorinated hydrocarbon insecticides can be absorbed orally and topically. Inhalation is not a normal route of exposure as these compounds are not highly volatile. Following absorption, these insecticides are distributed in liver, kidney, brain and adipose tissue. Residues of persistent chlorinated hydrocarbon insecticides follow the well-known kinetics of the food chain which begins in the environment with soil and plants then affects domestic animals and poultry and terminates with the human consumer. Due to their slow rate of biodegradability, persistence, ubiquitous nature and tendency to concentrate in the living organisms, chlorinated hydrocarbon insecticides accumulate in the food chain.

DDT and other diphenyl aliphatic compounds are dechlorinated by cytochrome P450-dependent monooxygenase system. Paradichlorobenzene and other aryl hydrocarbons undergo glucuronidation and sulfation. The cyclodiene insecticides such as endrin undergo epoxidation by mixed function oxidases. Lay *et al.* (1982) reported no significant differences in the pattern of metabolism as a consequence of different doses and/or routes of administration of dieldrin in rats. There are marked differences in the rate of elimination among chlorinated hydrocarbon insecticides. For example, methoxychlor is rapidly eliminated by dechlorination and oxidation as compared to DDT. The metabolites of chlorinated hydrocarbon insecticides may be more toxic than the parent compound (Jaeger *et al.*, 1975; Ensley, 2007a).

The chlorinated hydrocarbon insecticides are excreted via bile into the gastrointestinal tract and consequently may enter the enterohepatic cycle. Since metabolites of chlorinated hydrocarbon insecticides are also lipophilic, they are preferentially taken up by the adipose tissue and are released slowly from the depot site (Sell *et al.*, 1977). The elimination half-lives of the cyclodienes and some diphenyl aliphatic insecticides, such as DDT, may vary from days to years (Council for Agricultural Science and Technology, 1974). The disposition kinetics of chlorinated hydrocarbon insecticides can sometimes be explained by a two-compartment open model with rapid distribution phase and longer elimination phase (Ensley, 2007a).

Cytochrome P450 isoforms involved in the biotransformation of α-endosulfan and β-endosulfan have been recently identified. Studies with human recombinant P450s showed that α-endosulfan metabolism is mediated by CYP2B6, CYP3A4 and CYP3A5 and β-endosulfan is mediated by CYP3A4 and CYP3A5 (Lee *et al.*, 2006). Metabolism of α-endosulfan by human liver microsomes *in vitro* produced only endosulfan sulfate and P450 isoforms CYP3A4 and CYP2B6 are the primary enzymes catalyzing the biotransformation of α-endosulfan (Casabar *et al.*, 2006; Hodgson and Rose, 2008).

In humans, the absorption of cypermethrin across skin is minimal and after dermal application peak excretion rates were not measured until 12–36 h after exposure. These compounds may be sequestered in the skin and then slowly released into the systemic circulation (He *et al.*, 1989). An uptake of permethrin in humans wearing permethrin-impregnated battle dress uniforms has been demonstrated as higher concentrations of urinary insecticide metabolites were detected (Rossbach *et al.*, 2010). Exposure by oral or inhalation routes results in faster systemic exposure (Anadon *et al.*, 1996). An orally ingested dose is absorbed approximately to the extent of 40–60%. Following oral administration of cypermethrin to male volunteers, absorption ranged from 27 to 57% of the given dose and peak excretion rates were observed in the urine between 8 and 24 h after dosing. In adult human males exposed to cyfluthrin at 160 μg/m^3, 93% of the metabolites were excreted in the first 24 h and the peak excretion rates ranged from 0.5 to 3 h (Ensley, 2007b).

Being lipophilic in nature, pyrethroids following absorption distribute to the tissues with high lipid content such as fat and nervous tissue in addition to liver, kidney and milk. Following oral ingestion, pyrethroids and pyrethrins are rapidly hydrolyzed in the gastrointestinal tract and the absorbed compounds are biotransformed by mixed function oxidases and esterases. Biotransformation of pyrethroids results in water soluble metabolites. In general, biotransformation pathways include hydrolysis of the central ester bond, oxidation at several sites and conjugation with glucuronide, sulfate, glucosides or glycine. The ester bond cleavage leads to considerable decrease in toxicity. The rate of hydrolysis of the ester bond is decreased by the presence of the alpha-cyano group present in type II pyrethroids. In these pyrethroids, the cleaved alpha-cyano group leads to rapid conversion of the cyano group to thiocyanate.

Rat and human liver microsomes differ with respect to the biotransformation pathway responsible for the clearance of deltamethrin and esfenvalerate. Rat cytochrome P450 isoforms CYP1A1, CYP2C6, CYP2C11 and CYP3A2 and human P450 isoforms CYP2C8, CYP2C19 and CYP3A5 are capable of metabolizing both pyrethroids. Human CYP2C9 metabolized esfenvalerate but not deltamethrin. Besides liver, an important site of metabolism of pyrethroids is the blood via serum carboxylesterase hydrolysis in rats. The serum of rats contains significant quantities of carboxylesterase but not that of humans. Thus, metabolic elimination of deltamethrin and esfenvalerate in blood may be important to their disposition in rats but not in humans (Godin *et al.*, 2007). In a recent *in vitro* study, it was shown that human cytochrome P450 isoform CYP3A4 is also involved in the metabolism of multiple pyrethroid insecticides (Scollon *et al.*, 2009).

Pyrethroids are excreted as parent compounds and their metabolites primarily by urinary and fecal routes. Their elimination usually follows first order kinetics and most of the administered dose is eliminated during the first 12–24 h after absorption. Dermal and oral bioavailability of pyrethroids in humans is approximately 1 and 36%, respectively. Following oral ingestion, pyrethroids are absorbed mostly from the stomach and due to their lipophilic nature are rapidly distributed in the body. In general, the plasma elimination half-lives of pyrethroids are in hours even after oral administration. The elimination half-life of cyfluthrin is 19–86 min (Ensley, 2007b). Anadon *et al.* (2006) characterized the toxicokinetics of lambda-cyhalothrin after single 20 mg/kg oral and 3 mg/kg intravenous doses in rats. The plasma elimination half-lives were 7.55 and 10.27 h after intravenous and oral administration, respectively. The elimination half-lives for lambda-cyhalothrin were significantly longer for the nerve tissues, including neuromuscular fibers (12–26 and 15–34 h after intravenous and oral doses) than that for plasma. For forecasting pyrethroid dosimetry in young and aged individuals, Tornero-Velez *et al.* (2010) developed maturing rat physiologically based pharmacokinetic model of deltamethrin which allows for updating with age- and chemical-dependent parameters. This model provides a methodology for risk assessors to consider age-specific adjustments to oral reference doses on the basis of differences in pharmacokinetic behavior.

MECHANISM OF ACTION IN GENERAL TOXICITY

Chlorinated hydrocarbon insecticides are classified into three groups: (1) dichlorodiphenylethanes (DDTs) (dichlorodiphenyltrichloroethane, dicofol, methoxychlor and perthane); (2) hexachlorocyclohexanes (benzene hexachloride, chlordane, lindane, mirex and toxaphene); and (3) chlorinated cyclodienes (aldrin, dieldrin, endrin, chlordane, endosulfan and heptachlor). The chemical structures of some chlorinated hydrocarbon insecticides are shown in Figure 38.1.

The mechanism of action of chlorinated hydrocarbon insecticides is not yet fully elucidated. The diphenyl aliphatic chlorinated hydrocarbons such as DDT affect the peripheral nerves and brain by slowing sodium influx and inhibiting potassium outflow resulting in excess intracellular potassium in the neuron which partially depolarizes the cell. The threshold for another action potential is decreased leading to premature depolarization of the neuron (Narahashi, 1987; Ensley, 2007a).

In addition to decreasing action potentials, the chlorinated cyclodiene insecticides may inhibit the post-synaptic binding of γ-aminobutyric acid (GABA) (Lummis *et al.*, 1990; French-Constant, 1993; Hahn, 1998; Carr *et al.*, 1999). The cyclodienes induced hyperactivity of the central nervous system and convulsions can be explained based on their structural resemblance to the GABA receptor antagonist picrotoxin. The cyclodienes act by competitive inhibition of the binding of GABA, an inhibitory neurotransmitter in central

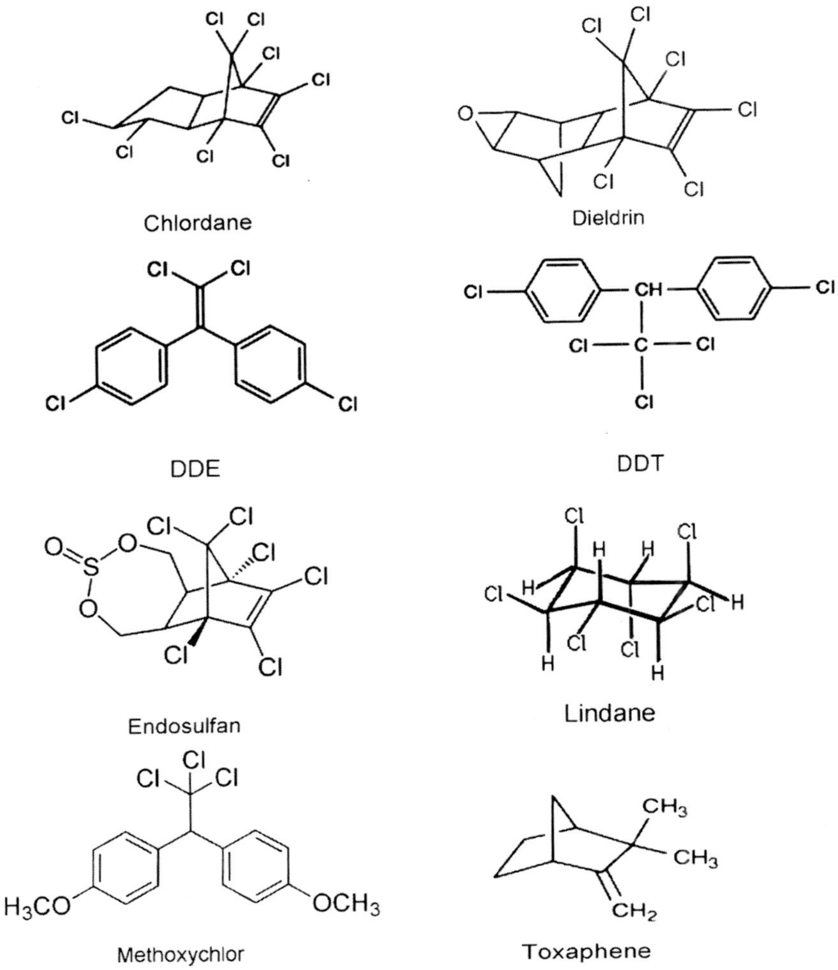

FIGURE 38.1 Structures of selected chlorinated hydrocarbon insecticides.

nervous system of mammals. Both $GABA_A$ and $GABA_B$ receptors play a vital role in mammals. $GABA_A$ receptors present in mammalian synapse are ligand gated chloride ion channels. In the human brain, $GABA_A$ receptor consists of four or five 50–60 kDa glycoprotein subunits, each containing four hydrophobic domains, namely, M_1, M_2, M_3 and M_4. The five M_2 domains are arranged to form a 5.6 Å diameter ion channel. $GABA_B$ receptors present in mammals are coupled to calcium and potassium channels and the action of this neurotransmitter is mediated by G-proteins. Following its release in the synapse, GABA diffuses to the presynaptic terminal of another nerve, where GABA binds to its $GABA_A$ receptors. The binding of GABA to its receptor causes chloride ions to enter the synapse leading to hyperpolarization of the terminal which inhibits the release of other neurotransmitters. Due to such inhibition, postsynaptic stimulation of other nerves by other neurotransmitters such as acetylcholine is reduced. As a consequence of inhibition of GABA, there is no synaptic downregulation and there can be excessive release of other neurotransmitters (Joy, 1976, 1982; Gandolfi *et al.*, 1984; Ensley, 2007a). In the central nervous system, symptoms observed in animals by chlorinated cyclodienes include tremors, convulsions, ataxia and changes in EEG patterns. The central nervous system symptoms could be due either to (1) inhibition of the Na^+/K^+-ATPase or the Ca^{2+}/Mg^{2+}-ATPase activity, which can then interfere with nerve action or release of neurotransmitters, and/or (2) inhibition of the GABA receptor function (Gupta, 2007). In a recent study, Mladenovic *et al.* (2010) presented a nonspecific mechanism involved in lindane-induced seizures. These investigators suggested that lipid peroxidation may contribute to the neurotoxic effects of lindane in early acute intoxication and that behavioral manifestations correlate with lipid peroxidation in the rat brain hippocampus, which is one of the sites for initiation and propagation of seizures.

Pyrethroids are of two types. Type I pyrethroids are those which lack α-cyano moiety and give rise to the tremor syndrome (T syndrome). A few examples of type I are pyrethrin I, allethrin, tetramethrin, resmethrin, cismethrin, phenothrin and permethrin. Type II pyrethroids are those which contain α-cyano moiety and cause the choreoathetosis/salivation (CS) syndrome. A few examples of type II pyrethroids include cyphenothrin, cypermethrin, deltamethrin, fenvalerate, cyfluthrin, cyhalothrin, flucynthrate and esfenvalerate. The chemical structures of some pyrethrin/pyrethroid insecticides are shown in Figure 38.2.

The primary site of action of pyrethroids is the sodium channel of cells but they also affect chloride and calcium channels. Toxicity by pyrethroids results primarily from hyperexcitation of the nervous system. Type II syndrome

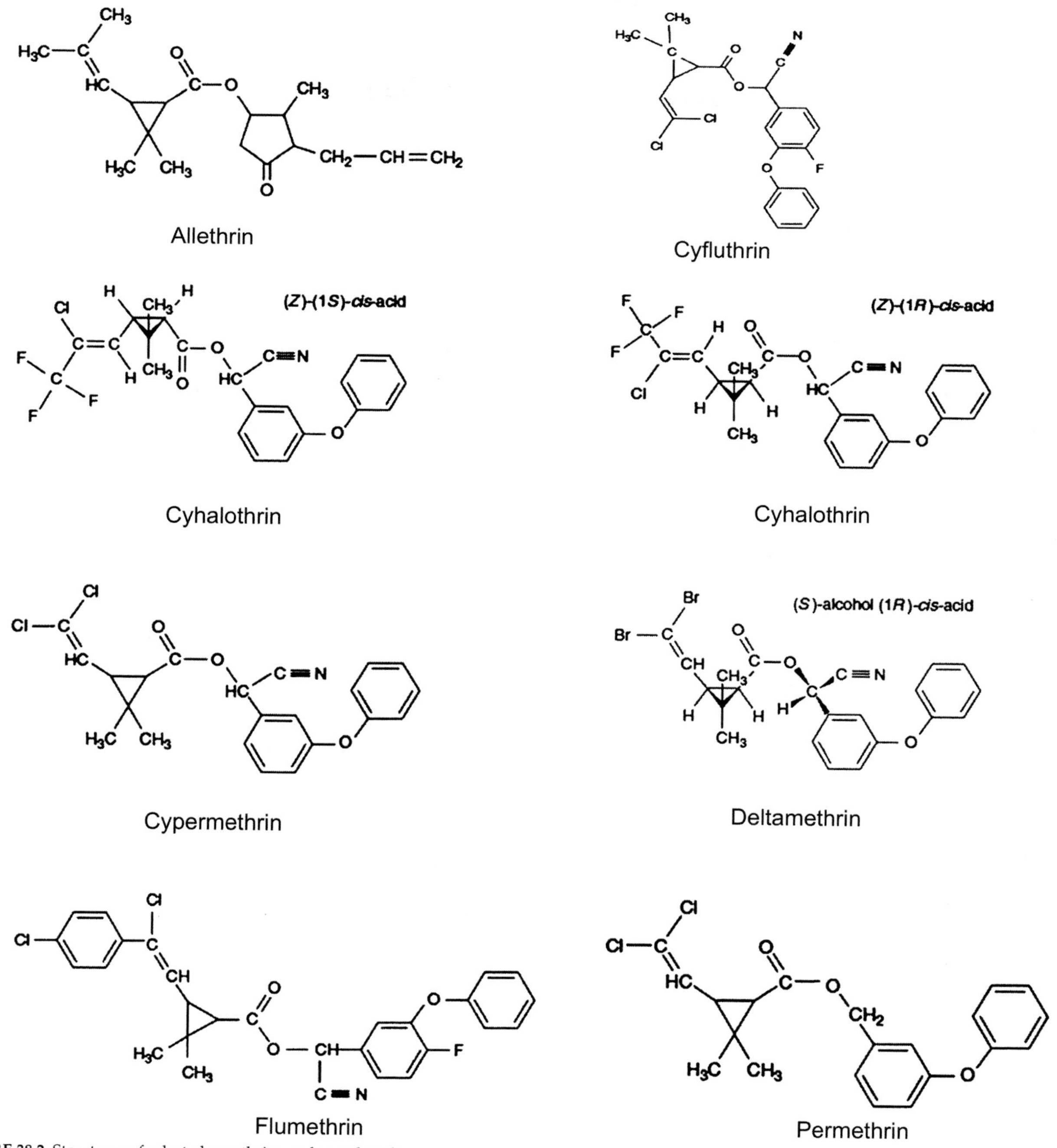

Allethrin

Cyfluthrin

(Z)-(1S)-cis-acid

Cyhalothrin

(Z)-(1R)-cis-acid

Cyhalothrin

Cypermethrin

(S)-alcohol (1R)-cis-acid

Deltamethrin

Flumethrin

Permethrin

FIGURE 38.2 Structures of selected pyrethrins and pyrethroids.

involves primarily an action in the central nervous system, whereas with type I syndrome, peripheral nerves are also involved. Hyperexcitation of the nervous system is caused by repetitive firing and depolarization in nerve axons and synapses. These compounds slow the opening and closing of the sodium channels ultimately leading to the excitation of the cell (Marban *et al.*, 1998). An increase of sodium in the sodium channels results in a cell which is in a stable, hyperexcitable state. The duration of the sodium action potential is much shorter for type I pyrethroids than for type II pyrethroids. While type I pyrethroids result in primarily repetitive charges, cell membrane depolarization is the main mechanism of toxic action exerted by type II pyrethroids. The effect of type I pyrethroids on sodium channels in nerve membranes is similar to those produced by DDT-type insecticides. The direct action of pyrethroids on sensory nerve endings leads to paresthesia as they cause repetitive firing. Pyrethroids must modify less than 1% sodium channels in order to produce neurological signs (Ensley, 2007b; Gupta, 2007).

In addition to sodium channels, pyrethrins also affect the voltage-dependent chloride channels. These channels play a role in controlling cell excitability and are present in the brain, nerve, muscle and salivary gland. Most of the pyrethroids-affected channels are maxi-chloride channel class. These channels are activated by depolarization, possess high conductance, are not dependent on calcium and are activated by protein kinase C phosphorylation. Pyrethroids cause a decrease in the maxi-chloride channel current which results in increase in the excitability of the cell. Type II pyrethroids at high concentrations may also act on GABA-gated chloride channels (Bloomquist *et al.*, 1986; Ensley, 2007b).

There are several factors contributing to the selective toxicity of pyrethroids. Mammals more efficiently detoxify pyrethroids before they reach their target site. They bind less strongly with sodium channels at the mammals' ambient temperature. Furthermore, mammalian sodium channels are at least 1,000 times less sensitive to pyrethroids as compared to sodium channels of insects. The recovery is much faster from depolarization in mammalian sodium channels.

Pyrethroids at high concentrations or hyperactivity beyond the tolerance of the cell will cause depolarization and conduction block. The compounds capable of holding the sodium channel open for the longest period will produce the greatest amount of depolarization. Pyrethroids exhibit marked stereospecificity in their action on sodium channel leading to varying toxicity of different isomers (Soderlund, 1985). Among the two isomers, *cis* isomers are generally more toxic than the *trans* isomers. Depending on the amount of *cis* isomer present, the toxicity of commercial pyrethroid can vary markedly. Permethrin was shown to induce reproductive toxicity in adult mouse due to *cis* isomer and not due to *trans* isomer (Zhang *et al.*, 2008). It has been shown that *1R* and *1S cis* isomers bind non-competitively to another site (Narahashi, 1986). Among *1R* and *1S* isomers, the former are active and the latter are inactive in mammalian species and hence *1S* isomers are non-toxic.

MECHANISMS IN REPRODUCTIVE AND DEVELOPMENTAL TOXICITY

The developing brain is particularly vulnerable to adverse effects of neurotoxic chemicals. It has been documented that the first trimester of pregnancy is critical for the central nervous system and development of neurons. The development of the central nervous system is a sequential and limiting process, the injury being greater the earlier it occurs (Rice and Barone, 2000). The chlorinated hydrocarbon and pyrethroid insecticides may cause neurodevelopmental toxicity and the adverse effects on brain development can be severe and irreversible. Multiple mechanisms may be involved in chlorinated hydrocarbon and pyrethroid insecticides-induced developmental neurotoxicity.

Two possible mechanisms of neurologic damage induced by DDT and/or its metabolites have been suggested. These compounds produce direct effect on motor fibers and on the motor area of the cerebral cortex or act as endocrine disruptors in the hypothalamic–hypophysis–thyroid axis. Neonatal exposure to DDT caused a significant reduction in the density of muscarinic receptors in the cerebral cortex of mice. These receptors are predominantly cholinergic and have a direct involvement in the process of neuronal excitement and inhibition (Eriksson *et al.*, 1992). Another mechanism of action which is probably the most widely accepted for explaining the chronic effect of DDT is disruption of the thyroid system (Takser *et al.*, 2005). DDT alone or its metabolites alter the production of thyroidal hormone and its availability at target tissues, given that the insecticide blocks glucuronidation. Thyroid hormone is known to play a pivotal role in the development of cerebral cortex. This hormone serves as a signal for neuronal differentiation and maturation as well as participates in neuronal migration and proliferation, synaptogenesis and myelinization (Rice and Barone, 2000; Anderson *et al.*, 2003; Lavado-Autric *et al.*, 2003).

Developmental exposure to dieldrin has been shown to alter the dopamine system and increase neurotoxicity in an animal model of Parkinson's disease. The dopamine transporter (DAT) and the vesicular monoamine transporter 2 (VMAT2) play an integral role in maintaining dopamine homeostasis and alteration of their levels during development could result in increased vulnerability of dopamine neurons later in life. Perinatal exposure of mice during gestation and lactation to low levels of dieldrin (0.3, 1 or 3 mg/kg every 3 days), caused a dose-dependent increase in protein and mRNA levels of DAT and VMAT2 in their offspring at 12 weeks of age (Richardson *et al.*, 2006).

Studies of developmental neurotoxicity of pyrethroids have been conducted with rodents as test animals. Several of these experimental animal studies have reported persistent changes in behavior and/or neurochemistry in the animals, but results seem to be somewhat inconsistent. Prenatal or early postnatal exposure to pyrethroids including cypermethrin, fenvalerate and others has been linked with significant neurochemical alterations in neonatal rats (Husain *et al.*, 1991, 1992; Malaviya *et al.*, 1993). Delayed maturation of the cerebral cortex occurs due to alterations in key enzymes of the neurotransmission process such as monoamine oxidase, acetylcholinesterase and Na^+/K^+-ATPase. Prenatal exposure to these compounds significantly delays differential responses in the levels of brain regional polyamines and ontogeny of sensory and motor reflexes in offspring. Other biochemical and neurochemical effects of these insecticides include impairment at the neurotransmitter receptors, including dopaminergic, cholinergic and catecholaminergic (Gupta, 2007, 2009).

Endocrine disruption

As a result of recent research in the growing discipline of endocrine disruption, knowledge has accumulated rapidly about the biological systems that control reproduction, sexual development and fertility, and their vulnerability. Chemicals, so-called endocrine disruptors, may be able to react directly or indirectly with the hormone structure to alter its function, change the pattern of hormone synthesis, or modulate the number of hormone receptors and their affinities for specific molecules. These chemicals even prior to fertilization interfere with gene-controlled signaling systems that control prenatal and postnatal development and function throughout life (Kupfer, 1975; Chapin *et al.*, 1996; Armenti *et al.*, 2008).

The chlorinated hydrocarbon and pyrethroid insecticides may cause endocrine disruption by hindering the ability of cells, tissues and organs to communicate hormonally by influencing the synthesis, transport, binding or elimination of natural hormones in the body which are responsible for the maintenance of homeostasis, reproduction, development and/or behavior. Exposure to endocrine disrupting pesticides may result in a variety of adverse health effects including reduced fertility and fecundity, spontaneous abortion, changes in sex ratio within the offspring of exposed subjects, male and female reproductive tract abnormalities, precocious puberty, polycystic ovary syndrome, neurobehavioral disorders, impaired immune function and cancer (McKinlay *et al.*, 2008). Most of the studies on endocrine disruption caused by chlorinated hydrocarbon and pyrethroid insecticides have been conducted in laboratory animals.

As compared to adults, endocrine disrupting pesticides have more devastating effects in embryo and fetus without a developed blood–brain barrier and with rudimentary DNA repair mechanisms and hepatic detoxifying and metabolizing capabilities. Important organizational events taking place during gonadal and phenotypic sexual differentiation are very sensitive to disruption in normal endocrine milieu. These compounds influence gene expression that controls development of organs and lifelong hormonal set points including number of receptors and production of hormones. In adults, hormones principally regulate ongoing physiological processes and sometimes compensate for or recover from hormonal modulation(s). Early examples of endocrine disruption in wildlife species were the declines in raptor populations due to the bioaccumulation of DDE metabolite of DDT disrupting eggshell formation (Carson, 1962; Vos *et al.*, 2000). The deleterious effects of endocrine disruption in wildlife species can be applied to endocrine disrupting chemical exposures involving human beings.

Endocrine disruption caused by chlorinated hydrocarbon and pyrethroid insecticides encompasses a wide range of mechanisms of action which can ultimately result in deleterious effects in an organism. Aldrin, chlordane, DDT and metabolites, dieldrin, endosulfan, endrin and methoxychlor have been shown to antagonize the action of androgens via binding competitively to their receptors and inhibiting the genetic transcription they induce (Lemaire *et al.*, 2004). DDT and its metabolites also mimic the action of estrogen and promote the proliferation of androgen-sensitive cells. These compounds as well as dieldrin and endosulfan mimic the actions of estrogens indirectly by stimulating the production of their receptors (Tessier and Matsumura, 2001; Tapiero *et al.*, 2002; Bulayeva and Watson, 2004). Additionally, endosulfan acts as a weak aromatase inhibitor (Andersen *et al.*, 2002). Acaricide dicofol inhibits androgen synthesis, increases the synthesis of estrogens and also binds to the estrogen receptor (Okubo *et al.*, 2004; Thibaut and Porte, 2004). Lindane shortens the estrous cycles, lowers luteal progesterone concentrations, increases the blood serum concentrations of insulin and estradiol and decreases thyroxine concentrations (Rawlings *et al.*, 1998; Beard and Rawlings, 1999). Methoxychlor is a strong estrogen mimic which interacts with the pregnane X cellular receptor and also interferes with the synthesis of enzymes responsible for steroid hormone metabolism (Lemaire *et al.*, 2004). Toxaphene increases the proliferation of estrogen-sensitive cells and inhibits corticosterone synthesis in the adrenal cortex (Soto *et al.*, 1994; Cocco, 2002).

Among pyrethroid insecticides, cypermethrin mimics the action of estrogen and its metabolites also have estrogenic effects (Chen *et al.*, 2002; McCarthy *et al.*, 2006). Cyhalothrin decreases the secretion of thyroid hormones (Akhtar *et al.*, 1996) whereas deltamethrin shows weak estrogenic activity (Andersen *et al.*, 2002). Fenvalerate inhibits the proliferation of estrogen-sensitive cells and antagonizes the action of progesterone (Garey and Wolff, 1998; Kim *et al.*, 2004). Permethrin also inhibits the proliferation of estrogen-sensitive cells and in addition its metabolites exert estrogenic effects (Kim *et al.*, 2004; McCarthy *et al.*, 2006). Resmethrin binds weakly to sex hormone binding globulin which is a hormone carrier protein (Eil and Nisula, 1990). Sumithrin increases the proliferation of estrogen-sensitive cells and antagonizes the action of progesterone (Garey and Wolff, 1998; Kim *et al.*, 2004). Tetramethrin exhibits estrogen-antagonistic effects in females only (Kim *et al.*, 2005).

TOXICITY

The acute toxic signs associated with DDT and chlorinated benzene types of insecticides include paresthesia of the tongue, lips and face, apprehension, tremors and convulsions. Stimulation of the central nervous system is the most prominent effect. The toxic signs following chronic exposure to these insecticides include anorexia, loss of weight, mild anemia, tremors, muscular weakness, anxiety, nervous tension and hyperexcitability. The acute signs and symptoms produced by chlorinated cyclodienes include dizziness, nausea, vomiting, myoclonic jerking, motor hyperexcitability and convulsive seizures. The toxic signs after chronic exposure to chlorinated cyclodiene insecticides include headache, dizziness, hyperexcitability, intermittent muscle twitching and myoclonic jerking, loss of consciousness, insomnia, anxiety, irritability, epileptiform convulsions, skin rashes, ataxia, visual difficulty, muscle weakness, tremors of hands, nervousness, irritability and depression. Repeated exposure to dieldrin induces hyperglycemia in animals (Malik *et al.*, 1975). Similar to other chlorinated hydrocarbon insecticides, mirex and kepone cause stimulation of the central nervous system, hepatotoxicity and induction of the mixed-function oxidases.

As compared to other classes of insecticides, the use of synthetic pyrethroids has increased tremendously in the recent times because of their selectively high toxicity to insects and low toxicity to mammals. Type I pyrethroids give rise to the tremor syndrome (T syndrome). The syndrome includes the signs of whole body tremors, incoordination, prostration, tonic–clonic convulsions and death. Type II pyrethroids cause the choreoathetosis/salivation (CS) syndrome. The CS syndrome is characterized by hyperactive behavior, profuse salivation, tremors, motor incoordination and hunch-backed posture (Gupta, 2007).

Many xenobiotics including chlorinated hydrocarbon and pyrethroid insecticides reach the fetus with very little or no restrictions. In general, xenobiotic-metabolizing enzymes present in the placenta protect the fetus from potentially chemical toxicants. Cytochrome P450 systems can also form metabolites that are relatively more toxic than their parent compounds. For example, chlorinated cyclodienes are biotransformed to their epoxides which have a greater potential for fetotoxicity/teratogenicity than their parent compounds. Only a few placental toxicity studies have been conducted with chlorinated hydrocarbon insecticides. In an experimental study, exposure of Swiss mice to lindane at different stages of pregnancy produced various toxicological effects, such as fetotoxicity and reproductive failure (Sircar and Lahiri, 1989). Lindane exposure during early pregnancy (days 1–4) caused total absence of any implantation; during mid-pregnancy (days 6–12) caused total resorptions of fetuses; and during late-pregnancy (days 14–19) caused the death of all pups within 12 h to 5 days after parturition. A decrease in fertility and an increase in resorptions were observed in female rats acutely exposed to 1.8 mg/kg/day. Reduced fertility has also been observed in mice exposed to 8.4 mg/kg/day. A number of animal studies have demonstrated that exposure to heptachlor can result in decreased fertility and pregnancy losses. Impaired fertility was reported in female rats administered via gavage of 0.6 mg/kg/day heptachlor in groundnut oil for 14 days prior to mating (Amita Rani and Krishnakumari, 1995). There are reports that dieldrin produced teratogenic effects, such as supernumerary ribs, with concomitant decrease in ossification centers in fetal hamsters (Chernoff *et al.*, 1975, 1979). In rats, exposure to mirex during pregnancy has been associated with perinatal deaths due to persistent cardiovascular problems, such as first- to third-degree fetal heart blockade (Grabowski, 1983). In addition, mirex causes altered lens growth and cataracts, along with other biochemical, physiological and histological changes (Rogers and Grabowski, 1983).

Exposure of rats to methoxychlor for longer periods resulted in early vaginal opening and first estrus, irregular estrous cycles, reduced pregnancy rate and litter size, and early cessation of estrous cycles (Gray *et al.*, 1989; Chapin *et al.*, 1997). This insecticide affects early ovarian development, folliculogenesis and adult ovarian function.

The transient developmental methoxychlor exposure directly affects the ovary, leading to adult ovarian dysfunction and female infertility. Armenti *et al.* (2008) investigated the effect of transient developmental methoxychlor exposure on adult ovarian dysfunction in rats at environmentally relevant dose (20 μg/kg/day) and high dose (100 mg/kg/day) between 19 days postcoitum and postnatal day (PND) 7. A high dose accelerated pubertal onset and first estrus, reduced litter size and increased irregular cyclicity. The superovulatory response to exogenous gonadotropins in prepubertal females was reduced following exposure to methoxychlor. Rats exposed to a high dose of methoxychlor showed abnormal cycles by 6 months and a decrease in serum progesterone but an increase in luteinizing hormone (LH). Exposure to a high dose of methoxychlor reduced estrogen receptor β whereas anti-Mullerian hormone was upregulated by low and high doses of methoxychlor in preantral and early antral follicles. A high dose of methoxychlor significantly reduced LH receptor expression in large antral follicles and downregulated cytochrome P450 side-chain cleavage.

Lindane produces detrimental effects on reproduction and testes are highly sensitive target organs for this insecticide. It accumulates in rat testes and causes degenerative changes in germinal epithelium and Sertoli cell fragmentation, impairs androgen synthesis in Leydig cells, decreases sperm counts and increases sperm abnormalities (Prasad *et al.*, 1995; Dalsenter *et al.*, 1996; Ronco *et al.*, 2001; Saradha and Mathur, 2006). Recently, Pathak *et al.* (2010) demonstrated association between blood γ-hexachlorocyclohexane levels and women with recurrent miscarriages.

A number of studies have indicated that DDT or its metabolites are associated with significant or suggestive declines in semen quality (Aneck-Hahn, 2007; Perry, 2008; Phillips and Tanphaichitr, 2008). Although results between studies are inconsistent, it has been shown that DDT and/or DDE is positively associated with sperm DNA damage (Bonde *et al.*, 2008; Hauser *et al.*, 2003; Perry, 2008). A few studies have also examined relationships between exposure to DDT/DDE and endocrine-related disorders. An increased risk of diabetes in relation to exposure to DDT/DDE has been reported (Everett *et al.*, 2007; Philibert *et al.*, 2009). Chlorinated hydrocarbon insecticides may also impact thyroid signaling but results obtained from human studies so far have not been consistent. Blood concentrations of DDE have been shown to be associated with increased risk of testicular germ cell tumors (McGlynn *et al.*, 2008) but no such association was evident in another study of adult men (Biggs *et al.*, 2008).

Studies on central nervous system effects in workers chronically exposed to DDT have revealed alterations in the visual-motor and cognitive functions (Misra *et al.*, 1984; Van Wendel de Joode *et al.*, 2001). Findings from two prospective infant cohorts showed an effect between prenatal DDE levels and hyporeflexia at 1 month of age (Rogan *et al.*, 1986) and damage to psychomotor and mental developmental at 13 months of age (Ribas Fitó *et al.*, 2003). In a recent study, Torres-Sanchez *et al.* (2007) examined the prenatal window of exposure to DDE and its effect on psychomotor and mental development during the first year of life in children of mothers who were not occupationally exposed to this compound. Only DDE levels during the first trimester of pregnancy were associated with a significant reduction in psychomotor development index whereas DDE was not associated with mental development index. Thus, a critical window of exposure to DDE *in utero* may be the first trimester of the pregnancy and the target of DDE is psychomotor development. In a follow-up study, these investigators reported that the association between prenatal DDE exposure and neurodevelopment does not persist beyond 12 months of age and the effects seem to be reversible (Torres-Sanchez *et al.*, 2009).

Compared to other classes of insecticides, pyrethroids are not well studied for placental toxicity because they are relatively less toxic to mammalian species. Permethrin at concentrations of 2,000–4,000 ppm showed only a weak to moderate influence on *in utero* fetal development. Female rats dermally exposed to cyhalothrin throughout gestation period had offspring with delayed fur development, delayed ear and eye opening and delayed descent of the testes, but with no change in the age of vaginal opening. In adulthood, however, the sexual behavior of both male and female rats exposed to cyhalothrin prenatally is no different from that of control animals (Gomes *et al.*, 1991a,b). Prenatal exposure of rats to deltamethrin caused increase in early embryonic deaths and fetuses with retarded growth, hyperplasia of the lungs, dilatation of the renal pelvis and increase in placental weight (Abdel-Khalik *et al.*, 1993).

It has been recognized that humans including pregnant women, infants and children are exposed to pyrethroid insecticides (Shafer *et al.*, 2005). Pyrethroids are known to induce neurobehavioral effects in laboratory animals as well as in humans. Although neurotoxicity induced by pyrethroids has been well characterized in adults, little is known about the developmental neurotoxicity of these compounds. The neonatal exposure to pyrethroids may induce developmental toxicity in adults characterized by alterations in behavior, neurohistology, neurochemistry and/or dysmorphology of the central nervous system. Mice exposed to deltamethrin and bioallethrin during PND 10–16 exhibited increased motor activity and changes in cholinergic muscarinic receptor after withdrawal of exposure (Eriksson and Fredriksson, 1991). The effects seem to be linked to exposure during development and are not likely to be associated with residual tissue concentrations of pyrethroids in view of their short half-lives. Pyrethroids have been reported to produce persistent changes in behavior and/or biochemistry, including learning (Moniz *et al.*, 1990), motor activity (observed with deltamethrin only; Husain *et al.*, 1992), sexual behavior (Lazarini *et al.*, 2001), muscarinic acetylcholine receptor binding (Aziz *et al.*, 2001) and permeability of the blood–brain barrier (Gupta *et al.*, 1999).

Type II pyrethroid insecticides fenvalerate and cypermethrin are known to produce steroidogenic alterations in testes and sera of rats leading to impairment of spermatogenesis and the reduction of sperm output and sperm motility (Mani *et al.*, 2002; Manna *et al.*, 2004; Xu *et al.*, 2004). Cypermethrin caused a significant decrease in the number of cell layers of the seminiferous tubules, epididymal and testicular sperm counts and daily sperm production (Elbetieha *et al.*, 2001). The normal development of testes and the maintenance of spermatogenesis are known to be controlled by testosterone. In humans, there is a trend toward a significant positive correlation between abnormal semen analysis and seminal plasma testosterone levels. In infertile men low concentrations of nitric oxide adversely affect sperm quality, probably by decreasing testosterone synthesis and/or secretion (Huang *et al.*, 2006; Carreau *et al.*, 2007). Fenvalerate impaired male reproductive function, increased incidences of sperm abnormalities and caused significant reduction in sperm count, sperm motility and testicular marker enzymes for testosterone biosynthesis (Pati and Bhunya, 1989; Mani *et al.*, 2002; Xu *et al.*, 2004). Cytochrome P450 cholesterol side-chain cleavage enzyme initiates the first step in testosterone biosynthesis in the inner mitochondrial membrane of Leydig cells and the expression of this enzyme was significantly downregulated in testes of permethrin-exposed adult male mouse (Zhang *et al.*, 2008). A recent study showed that exposure of young male mice to cypermethrin (25 mg/kg) by gavage daily from PND 35 to PND 70 caused marked decrease in the levels of serum and testicular testosterone. Cypermethrin was found to alter testosterone synthesis via downregulating the expression of testicular steroidogenic acute regulatory protein and this decreased synthesis of testosterone may be associated with impairment in spermatogenesis in mice (Wang *et al.*, 2010).

Sperm motility is one of the most important parameters examining the fertilizing ability of sperm as its appropriate motility is essential for fertilization of oocytes. Conversely, abnormal sperm motility may adversely impact the ability of sperm to successfully fertilize oocytes. Accordingly, sperm motility following exposure to insecticides has been used as an approach to evaluate their potential reproductive toxicity. Song *et al.* (2008) analyzed motility parameters of rat sperms treated with fenvalerate and cypermethrin with a computer-assisted sperm analysis (CASA) system. CASA is a reproducible method for detecting sperm motility which is one of the highly important parameters in evaluating the fertilizing ability of sperm (Hirano *et al.*, 2001). Sperm suspensions were treated with the pyrethroids at concentrations of 1, 4, 16 and 64 μmol/L for 1, 2 and 4 h. Both fenvalerate and cypermethrin reduced sperm motility in a concentration- and time-dependent manner. Among fenvalerate and cypermethrin, the latter had greater effect on motility patterns, alterations in vigor and progression, and sperm swimming patterns. Both pyrethroids exerted their effects via a direct interaction with sperm, but the underlying exact mechanisms still remain to be elucidated. It has been postulated that reduction in sperm motility following exposure to fenvalerate and cypermethrin might lead to decreased fertility in the affected individuals.

In fenvalerate-exposed workers, the insecticide induced morphologic abnormality, genotoxic defects in spermatozoa and reduction of some sperm motility parameters (Bian *et al.*, 2004; Xia *et al.*, 2004; Tan *et al.*, 2006). Pyrethroid insecticides are also being used in conjunction with organophosphorus insecticides to obtain higher insecticidal effects of pyrethroids on target insects, in particular those that have developed pyrethroid resistance. Higher exposure to such a combination was found to lower sperm concentration in humans (Perry *et al.*, 2007). A study conducted in humans revealed inverse associations between urinary pyrethroid metabolites and sperm concentration, motility and morphology, and a positive relationship between pyrethroid metabolites and sperm DNA damage (Meeker *et al.*, 2008). Recent studies have reported a positive relationship between pyrethroid metabolites and gonadotropins whereas association was inverse with inhibin B and steroid hormones (Han *et al.*, 2008; Meeker *et al.*, 2009).

The development exposure to pyrethroids may influence the dopaminergic system. Deltamethrin and bioallethrin caused an increase in 3,4-dihydroxyphenylacetic acid levels in the adult striatum after developmental exposure (Lazarini *et al.*, 2001; Shafer *et al.*, 2005). In a recent study, Nasuti *et al.* (2007) evaluated the effect of neonatal exposition to two commonly used pyrethroid insecticides permethrin and cypermethrin on dopaminergic system modulation, behavioral changes and oxidative stress in rats. Cypermethrin and permethrin were given orally in doses of 1.49 and 34.05 mg/kg to rats from the 8th to the 15th day of life. Rats exposed to both insecticides exhibited lasting behavioral effects, alterations in monoamine concentrations in the striatum as well as increased oxidative stress. In another study, exposure of both male and female mice to permethrin (parental exposure to 9.8 mg/kg/day or more for 4 weeks before mating) affected development of reflexes, swimming ability and open field activity in offspring (Farag *et al.*, 2006). The deleterious effects of pyrethroids have also been investigated *in vitro* using cell lines. The non-toxic concentration of bifenthrin (10^{-6} M) was shown to inhibit neurite outgrowth in PC12 cells (Tran *et al.*, 2006).

Apoptosis, also known as programmed cell death, is a common process in multicellular organisms. It enables the elimination of single cells or their assemblies when they are damaged or mutated to such an extent that their future existence might be dangerous to the whole organism (Malik *et al.*, 2005). In particular, apoptosis plays an important role during embryogenesis, metamorphosis, endocrine tissue atrophy, tumor regression, wound healing, immune responses and in the growth and maturation of individual organs. Besides playing an important role in fundamental biological processes, programmed cell death is crucial in regulating total cell number. These functions serve to protect human beings and animals from various diseases including cancer. Any disruption in the apoptotic process may lead to unwanted cell survival and can cause development of abnormalities.

Spermatogenesis occurring in seminiferous tubules of the testes is a highly synchronized process. The size of the spermatogenic cell population is controlled by cell proliferation as well as through a dynamic balance with cell death. In recent times, apoptosis has gained much attention. It has been documented that apoptotic degeneration of early spermatogenic cells is the key mechanism limiting the size of the germ cell population in testes of rats (Kerr, 1992). A more recent study conducted to elucidate the mechanism(s) underpinning the gonadal effects of lindane demonstrated that lindane-induced testicular apoptosis in adult rats was mediated via both mitochondria-dependent and Fas-FasL pathways (Saradha *et al.*, 2009).

Repeated exposure of rats to pyrethroid deltamethrin was found to induce testicular apoptosis. The induction of apoptosis by deltamethrin (1 mg/kg/day for 21 days) was evident by characteristic DNA migration patterns (laddering) in testicular tissues of exposed rats. Apoptosis was confined to the basal germ cells, primary and secondary spermatocytes; there was also the appearance of Sertoli cell vacuoles indicating suppression of spermatogenesis. It was suggested that apoptosis is the major mechanism of cell death in the testicular tissues of deltamethrin-exposed animals and this effect was mediated by nitric oxide (El-Gohary *et al.*, 1999).

Nitric oxide is known to play an important role in the regulation of endocrine systems. Endothelial nitric oxide synthase (eNOS) is distributed in human testis, epididymis and vas deferens and is involved in testis pathology suggesting a possible role of nitric oxide in spermatogenesis, sperm maturation and germ cell degeneration (Zini *et al.*, 1996). NOS has also been found in the rat testis and epididymis. Nitric oxide is known to suppress the major regulatory aspects of testicular function, such as testosterone secretion and testicular interstitial fluid formation implicating a pivotal role of nitric oxide in controlling testicular steroidogenesis and in regulation of male fertility and sexual function (Adams *et al.*, 1994; Punta *et al.*, 1996). The pharmacological manipulation of apoptosis by selective NOS inhibitors such as N^G-nitro monomethyl L-arginine hydrochloride (L-NMMA) has been attempted for the control of deltamethrin-induced testicular dysfunction. Administration of L-NMMA (1 mg/kg daily for 21 days, intraperitoneally) to rats 2 h before exposure to deltamethrin (1 mg/kg daily for 21 days, intraperitoneally) was effective in the reduction of the typically testicular apoptotic DNA fragmentation pattern and the associated histopathological changes (El-Gohary *et al.*, 1999).

It has been recognized that reproductive toxicity of chlorinated hydrocarbon and pyrethroid insecticides may be mediated by reactive oxygen species (ROS). The production of ROS is a normal physiological event in various organs including testis. Overproduction of ROS, however, can be detrimental to sperm, being associated with male infertility. The repeated exposure of male rabbits to lambda-cyhalothrin resulted in deterioration of semen quality, decreased testosterone levels and significant increase in concentrations of thiobarbituric acid-reactive substances in seminal plasma (Yousef, 2010). Antioxidants such as vitamin E and curcumin have proven beneficial in ameliorating reproductive toxicity induced by lindane in male rats (Sharma and Singh, 2010) and lambda-cyhalothrin in male rabbits (Yousef, 2010).

RISK ASSESSMENT

The risk assessment process involves four steps, namely, hazard identification, dose–response assessments, exposure estimates and risk characterization. Exposure to pesticides is inherent in most agriculture-related occupations, and studies on pesticides use and pregnancy outcome generally focus on birth defects and the effects on the reproductive system. There is a growing concern about the safety of pesticides and how exposure to these chemicals may affect human health in general and reproductive outcome in particular. Pesticides affecting reproduction may act on selected stages targeting the prenatal stage, the pre-pubertal stage or the adult, resulting in developmental impairments and/or damage to the reproductive organs and/or impaired fertility. The process of reproductive and developmental toxicity testing for regulatory purposes is governed by a framework of guidelines, including screening of single to multi-generation studies, e.g. OECD TG 414, 415, 416, 421, 422 and 426. These guidelines are designed to identify developmental and reproductive effects by examining parental animals and offspring dosed pre- and postnatally to establish a no-observed-adverse-effect level (NOAEL) for the most sensitive effects, thus providing the basis for quantitative assessments. They are more focused on potential adverse human health impacts assessment to the development, reproduction and fertility through the necessary information for identifying potentially sensitive target organ systems, maternal toxicity, embryonic and fetal lethality, morphological anomalies, specific types of malformations, and altered birth weight and growth retardation. While, test guidelines for simultaneous assessment of developmental immunotoxicity, developmental neurotoxicity and endocrine disruption associated with chemical exposure are under current discussion (Iyer, 2001; Cooper, 2009).

It is generally agreed that pesticides will be needed indefinitely and their use will rather expand, in spite of the exploitation of alternative methods of control of pests. A variety of insecticidal chemicals are used widely for agricultural, home, municipal and medical purposes. As insects are becoming more resistant and vector-borne diseases are on the increase, use of insecticides is increasing. Unfortunately, the biological activity of insecticides is not limited just to target species but is also potentially dangerous to other forms of life, including humans because of unavoidable exposure. Among various classes of insecticides, the most problematic chemicals have been the chlorinated hydrocarbon insecticides.

Chlorinated hydrocarbon insecticides persist in the natural environment and may accumulate in body tissues. In view of concern about their potential carcinogenicity and environmental harmfulness, chlorinated hydrocarbon insecticides were banned for most uses in developed nations during the 1970s and 1980s. These insecticides have retained economic relevance in many developing countries where they are still used in agriculture, forestry and public health. As a result of their persistence and ubiquity in the environment, tissue residues of a number of chlorinated hydrocarbon insecticides are found in the general population.

Among chlorinated hydrocarbon insecticides, endosulfan has less environmental persistence and is a contact and stomach insecticide for food and non-food crops. Endosulfan has been shown to cause perturbations in immune responses and induction of apoptosis in developing chicks (Aggarwal *et al.*, 2005, 2008a,b). The risk assessment concerns have been shown that endosulfan exposure during critical development stages (*in utero* or to infants and children) will result in endocrine disruption and subsequent neurotoxicity, developmental or reproductive adverse effects that are irreversible. On the contrary, the data presented in a recent review, after suitable analysis, do not support the case that endosulfan is a developmental or reproductive toxicant or an endocrine disruptor (Silva and Gammon, 2009).

Despite the imposition of a restriction or ban in the industrial nations, the residues of chlorinated hydrocarbon insecticides are still present in eco- and animal systems. In a recent study, Moon *et al.* (2009) assessed the potential human health risks on the dietary intake of chlorinated hydrocarbon pesticides and polychlorinated biphenyls (PCBs) resulting from seafood consumption in South Korea during 2005–2007. Among various age groups studied, infants <2 years of age had the highest dietary exposure to organochlorines. Their study revealed that the intake of PCBs and DDTs by only seafood consumption can cause carcinogenic effects in the human body. Males may have higher cancer risks for all of the organochlorines than females. Children 3–6 years and <2 years showed higher cancer risks compared with adults.

Imposition of new restrictions on the usage of chlorpyrifos and other common organophosphate insecticides has led to the increased availability and usage of synthetic pyrethroid insecticides. Osimitz *et al.* (2009) investigated the effects of exposure of insecticides containing pyrethrins and piperonyl butoxide on humans. Despite their widespread use, these compounds are not likely to cause reactions in people with asthma or allergies and these products can be used with a relatively low risk of adverse effects. The effects produced by endocrine disrupting pesticides in wildlife are valuable indicators of human health risks. Higher damage caused by endocrine disrupting pesticides appears to be during gametogenesis and the early development of the fetus and the effects may be apparent in adulthood which makes it difficult to establish links between endocrine disrupting pesticides and human diseases. Exposure of fetuses and babies to these chemicals is higher because of mobilization of maternal fat reserves during gestation and breastfeeding and infants and children also have high consumption of food in relation to body weight (Tilson, 1998; Anderson and Wolff, 2000; Przyrembel *et al.*, 2000; Waliszewski *et al.*, 2000). Many endocrine disrupting pesticides may produce effects at very much lower levels than those used in standard toxicology tests, which is not taken into account by current regulations and risk assessments. Determination of residues of insecticides may be a greater source of exposure in view of individual behaviors and varying degrees of contamination between individual food items. Incorporation of the most appropriate exposure measures in future study designs is desirable.

Studies have documented a consistent epidemiological linkage between insecticide exposure and the incidence of Parkinson's disease (Semchuk *et al.*, 1992; Butterfield *et al.*, 1993; Gorell *et al.*, 1998). Effects of pyrethroid insecticides on dopaminergic nerve pathways may be a contributing factor in the etiology of environmentally induced Parkinson's disease. It has been pointed out that there is no information on age-dependent toxicity for most pyrethroids. Shafer *et al.* (2005) examined scientific data related to potential for age-dependent and developmental neurotoxicity. It was suggested that for understanding the potential for developmental exposure to cause neurotoxicity, additional well-designed and well-executed developmental neurotoxicity studies of pyrethroids are needed and such studies would be more relevant for risk assessment in future.

Biomarkers

Chlorinated hydrocarbon insecticides can be monitored by testing blood, milk and tissue samples. With the availability of advanced chemical analytical technology and non-invasive sampling protocols, it is now easier to measure chlorinated hydrocarbon insecticides and their metabolites at very low concentrations in humans and animal tissues. Studies dealing with biomonitoring have revealed that insecticides penetrate reproductive tissues and organs of both sexes and this may initiate deleterious effects to their offspring starting before fertilization throughout gestation and lactation. Chlorinated hydrocarbon insecticides and/or their metabolites residues have been found in various human reproductive tissues including amniotic fluid, blood serum, maternal blood, umbilical cord blood, breast milk, colostrum, placenta, semen and urine (Colborn and Carroll, 2007).

Monitoring exposure to pyrethroids is done by testing urine samples for the presence of their metabolites and being a less invasive option is now used in large-scale surveys. The metabolites *trans*-chrysanthemumdicarboxylic acid, *cis*- and *trans*-3-(2,2-dichlorovinyl)-2,2-dimethylcyclopropane carboxylic acid, *cis*-3-(2,2-dibromovinyl)-2,2-dimethylcyclopropane carboxylic acid, 3-phenoxybenzoic acid and 4-fluoro-3-phenoxybenzoic acid in human urine are the relevant biomarkers for an exposure to pyrethrins and pyrethroids (Table 38.1). With the help of the gas chromatographic-high resolution mass spectrometric method a complete assessment of exposure to pyrethroid and pyrethrin insecticides is possible (Leng and Gries, 2005).

TREATMENT

There are no specific antidotes for chlorinated hydrocarbon and pyrethroid insecticide poisonings. In both types of poisonings, general decontamination and supportive treatment are advocated. In chlorinated hydrocarbon insecticide poisoning, benzodiazepine diazepam (0.3 mg/kg intravenously; maximum dose of 10 mg) or long-acting barbiturate phenobarbital (15 mg/kg intravenously; maximum dose of 1.0 g) may be administered intravenously by slow injection. This treatment is given to control insecticide-induced convulsions which may be repeated as necessary (Ecobichon, 2001). In acute dieldrin intoxication, administration of chloral hydrate and magnesium sulfate combination along with atropine and d-tubocurarine was found to be effective in enhancing the survival time in poisoned animals (Malik *et al.*, 1973).

TABLE 38.1 Metabolites of pyrethroids in urine used as biomarkers for an exposure to pyrethroid insecticides

Insecticide	Biomarker
Allethrin	*trans*-Chrysanthemumdicarboxylic acid
Cyfluthrin	4-Fluoro-3-phenoxybenzoic acid; 3-Phenoxybenzoic acid
Cypermethrin	*cis*- and *trans*-3-(2,2-Dichlorovinyl)-2,2-dimethylcyclopropane carboxylic acid; 3-Phenoxybenzoic acid
Deltamethrin	*cis*- and *trans*-3-(2,2-Dichlorovinyl)-2,2-dimethylcyclopropane carboxylic acid; *cis*-3-(2,2-Dibromovinyl)-2,2-dimethylcyclopropane carboxylic acid; 3-Phenoxybenzoic acid
Permethrin	*cis*- and *trans*-3-(2,2-Dichlorovinyl)-2,2-dimethylcyclopropane carboxylic acid; 3-Phenoxybenzoic acid
Phenothrin	*trans*-Chrysanthemumdicarboxylic acid
Pyrethrum	*trans*-Chrysanthemumdicarboxylic acid
Resmethrin	*trans*-Chrysanthemumdicarboxylic acid
Tetramethrin	*trans*-Chrysanthemumdicarboxylic acid

In pyrethroid insecticide poisoning, apart from prevention from further exposure, lavage with vegetable and/or vitamin E cream is used to alleviate dermal paresthesia (Flannigan *et al.*, 1985). Symptomatic treatment includes topical application of steroids for contact dermatitis, decongestants, antihistaminics and steroid nasal spray for rhinitis and inhalation of steroids for asthma (O'Malley, 1997). In particular, in type II pyrethroid poisoning, ivermectin and pentobarbital may be of benefit (Ecobichon, 2001).

CONCLUDING REMARKS AND FUTURE DIRECTIONS

The chlorinated hydrocarbon insecticides were heavily used after their introduction but primarily because of ecological considerations, these compounds have been banned in most countries for the past three decades. These insecticides have retained economic relevance in many developing countries where they are still used in agriculture, forestry and public health. As a result of the persistence and ubiquity in the environment, tissue residues of a number of chlorinated hydrocarbon insecticides are found in general population. As the usage of many chlorinated hydrocarbon insecticides has diminished in many parts of the world, pyrethroid insecticides are used widely in agriculture, forestry, horticulture, public health and medicine. There is an increasing concern that chlorinated hydrocarbon and pyrethroid insecticides produced reproductive and developmental toxicity. Both classes of insecticides cause toxicity to growing embryos, fetuses and elicit a number of biochemical and neurochemical modulations. These compounds can cause endocrine disruption at lower doses and their effects are of notable concern for vulnerable groups such as fetuses, young children and for persons genetically susceptible to the effects of endocrine disruptors. There is evidence suggesting that effects of the pyrethroids on dopaminergic nerve pathways may be a contributory factor in the etiology of environmentally induced Parkinson's disease. More information is needed on the toxicokinetics and exposure to pyrethroids and to appropriately assess the range of internal doses of pyrethroids in humans. Further studies are needed to examine the deleterious effects following simultaneous exposure to these insecticides and other chemicals and to improve our understanding of the molecular aspects of reproductive and neurodevelopmental toxicity.

REFERENCES

Abdel-Khalik MM, Handfy MS, Abdel-Aziz MI (1993) Studies on the teratogenic effects of deltamethrin in rats. *Dtsch Tierarztl Wochenschr* **100:** 142–3.

Adams ML, Meyer ER, Sewing BN, Cicero TJ (1994) Effects of nitric oxide related agents on rat testicular function. *J Pharmacol Exp Ther* **269:** 230–7.

Aggarwal M, Malik JK, Rao GS, Suresh Babu N, Tiwari AK, Dandapat S (2005) Effects of arsenic, endosulfan and their combination on induction of immunotoxicity and apoptosis in broiler chicks. *Toxicol Lett* **158S:** S86.

Aggarwal M, Naraharisetti SB, Dandapat S, Degen GH, Malik JK (2008a) Perturbations in immune responses induced by concurrent subchronic exposure to arsenic and endosulfan. *Toxicology* **251:** 51–60.

Aggarwal M, Naraharisetti SB, Tiwari AK, Degen GH, Malik JK (2008b) Assessment of apoptosis in peripheral blood lymphocytes and splenocytes of chickens simultaneously exposed to arsenite in drinking water and endosulfan in feed. *Toxicol Lett* **180S:** S208.

Akhtar N, Kayani SA, Ahmad MM, Shahab M (1996). Insecticide-induced changes in secretory activity of the thyroid gland in rats. *J Appl Toxicol* **16:** 397–400.

Amita Rani BS, Krishnakumari MK (1995) Prenatal toxicity of heptachlor in albino rats. *Pharmacol Toxicol* **76:** 112–4.

Anadon A, Martinez Larranage MR, Fernandez Cruz ML, Diaz MJ, Fernandez MC, Martinez MA (1996) Toxicokinetics of deltamethrin and its 4'-HO-metabolite in the rat. *Toxicol Appl Pharmacol* **141:** 8–16.

Anadón A, Martínez M, Martínez MA, Díaz MJ, Martínez-Larrañaga MR (2006) Toxicokinetics of lambda-cyhalothrin in rats. *Toxicol Lett* **165:** 47–56.

Anadon A, Martinez-Larranaga MA, Martinez MA (2009) Use and abuse of pyrethrins and synthetic pyrethroids in veterinary medicine. *The Vet J* **182:** 7–20.

Andersen HR, Cook SJ, Waldbillig D (2002) Effects of currently used pesticides in assays for estrogenicity, androgenicity, and aromatase activity in vitro. *Toxicol Appl Pharmacol* **179:** 1–12.

Anderson GW, Schoonover CM, Jones SA (2003) Control of thyroid hormone action in developing rat brain. *Thyroid* **13:** 1039–56.

Anderson H, Wolff MS (2000) Environmental contaminants in human milk. *J Expo Anal Environ Epidemiol* **10:** 755–60.

Aneck-Hahn NH, Schulenburg GW, Bornman MS, Farias P, de Jager C (2007) Impaired semen quality associated with environmental DDT exposure in young men living in a malaria area in the Limpopo Province, South Africa. *J Androl* **28:** 423–34.

Armenti AE, Zama AM, Passantino L, Uzumcu M (2008) Developmental methoxychlor exposure affects multiple reproductive parameters and ovarian folliculogenesis and gene expression in adult rats. *Toxicol Appl Pharmacol* **233:** 286–96.

Aziz MH, Agrawal AK, Adhami VM, Shukla Y, Seth PK (2001) Neurodevelopmental consequences of gestational exposure (GD14–GD20) to low dose deltamethrin in rats. *Neurosci Lett* **300:** 161–5.

Baukloh V, Bohnet HG, Trapp M, Heeschen W, Feichtinger W, Kemeter P (1985) Biocides in human follicular fluid. *Ann NY Acad Sci* **442:** 240–50.

Beard AB, Rawlings NC (1999) Thyroid function and effects on reproduction in ewes exposed to the organochlorine pesticides lindane or pentachlorophenol (PCP) from conception. *J Toxicol Environ Health A* **58:** 509–30.

Bian Q, Xu LC, Wang SL, Xia YK, Tan LF, Chen JF, Song L, Chang HC, Wang XR (2004) Study on the relation between occupational fenvalerate exposure and spermatozoa DNA damage of pesticide factory workers. *Occup Environ Med* **61:** 999–1005.

Biggs ML, Davis MD, Eaton DL, Weiss NS, Barr DB, Doody DR, Fish S, Needham LL, Chen C, Schwartz SM (2008) Serum organochlorine pesticide residues and risk of testicular germ cell carcinoma: a population-based case-control study. *Cancer Epidemiol Biomarkers Prev* **17:** 2012–18.

Bloom MS, Louis GMB, Schisterman EF, Kostyniak PJ, Vena JE (2009) Changes in maternal serum chlorinated pesticide concentrations across critical windows of human reproduction and development. *Environ Res* **109:** 93–100.

Bloomquist JR, Adams PM, Soderlund DM (1986) Inhibition of gamma-aminobutyric acid-stimulated chloride flux in mouse brain vesicles by polychloroalkane and pyrethroid insecticides. *Neurotoxicology* **7:** 11–20.

Bonde JP, Toft G, Rylander L, Rignell-Hydbom A, Giwercman A, Spano M, Manicardi GC, Bizzaro D, Ludwicki JK, Zvyezday V, Bonefeld-Jørgensen EC, Pedersen HS, Jönsson BA, Thulstrup AM (2008) Fertility and markers of male reproductive function in Inuit and European populations spanning large contrasts in blood levels of persistent organochlorines. *Environ Health Perspect* **116:** 269–77.

Bulayeva NN,Watson CS (2004) Xenoestrogen-induced ERK-1 and ERK-2 activation via multiple membrane-initiated signaling pathways. *Environ Health Perspect* **112:** 1481–87.

Butterfield PG, Valanis BG, Spencer PS, Lindeman CA, Nutt JG (1993) Environmental antecedents of young-onset Parkinson's disease. *Neurology* **43:** 1150–8.

Campagna C, Guillemette C, Paradis R, Sirard M, Ayotte P, Bailey JL (2002) An environmentally relevant organochlorine mixture impairs sperm function and embryo development in the porcine model. *Biol Reprod* **67:** 80–7.

Carr RL, Couch TA, Liu J, Coats JR, Chambers JE (1999) The interaction of chlorinated alicyclic insecticides with brain GABA(A) receptors in channel catfish (*Ictalurus punctatus*). *J Toxicol Environ Health A* **56:** 543–53.

Carreau S, Silandre D, Bourguiba S, Hamden K, Said L, Lambard S, Galeraud-Denis I, Delalande C (2007) Estrogens and male reproduction: a new concept. *Braz J Med Biol Res* **40:** 761–8.

Carson R (1962) *Silent Spring*. Penguin Books, London, pp. 317.

Casabar RCT, Wallace AD, Hodgson E, Rose RL (2006) Metabolism of endosulfan-a by human liver microsomes and its utility as a simultaneous in vitro probe for CYP2B6 and CYP3A4. *Drug Metab Dispos* **34:** 1779–85.

Chapin RE, Harris MW, Davis BJ, Ward SM, Wilson RE, Mauney MA, Lockhart AC, Smialowicz RJ, Moser VC, Burka LT, Collins BJ (1997) The effects of perinatal/juvenile methoxychlor exposure on adult rat nervous, immune, and reproductive system function. *Fundam Appl Toxicol* **40:** 138–57.

Chapin RE, Stevens JT, Hughes CL, Kelce WR, Hess RA, Daston GP (1996) Endocrine modulation of reproduction. *Fundam Appl Toxicol* **29:** 1–17.

Chen H, Xiao J, Hu G, Zhou J, Xiao H, Wang X (2002) Estrogenicity of organophosphorus and pyrethroid pesticides. *J Toxicol Environ Health A* **65:** 1419–35.

Chernoff N, Kavlock RJ, Hanisch RC, Whitehouse DA, Gray JA, Gray LE Jr, Sovocool GW (1979) Perinatal toxicity of endrin in rodents. Fetotoxic effects of prenatal exposure in hamsters. *Toxicology* **13:** 155–65.

Chernoff N, Kavlock RJ, Kathrein JR, Dunn JM, Haseman JK (1975) Prenatal effects of dieldrin and photodieldrin in mice and rats. *Toxicol Appl Pharmacol* **31:** 302–8.

Cocco P (2002) On the rumors about the silent spring. Review of the scientific evidence linking occupational and environmental pesticide exposure to endocrine disruption health effects. *Cad Saúde Pública* **18:** 379–402.

Colborn T, Carroll LE (2007) Pesticides, sexual development, reproduction, and fertility: current perspective and future direction. *Hum Ecol Risk Assess* **13:** 1078–110.

Cooper RL (2009) Current developments in reproductive toxicity of pesticides. *Reprod Toxicol* **28:** 180–7.

Costa LG (2008) Toxic effects of pesticides. In *Casarett and Doull's Toxicology. The Basic Science of Poisons* (Klaassen CD, ed.). McGraw-Hill, New York, pp. 883–930.

Council for Agricultural Science and Technology (1974) Aldrin and dieldrin in agriculture. Report No. 34.

Dalsenter PR, Faqi AS, Webb J, Merker HJ, Chahoud I (1996) Reproductive toxicity and tissue concentrations of lindane in adult male rats. *Hum Exp Toxicol* **15:** 406–10.

Daston PG, Gooch JW, Breslin WJ, Shuey DL, Nikiforov AI, Fico TA, Gorsuch JW (1997) Environmental estrogens and reproductive health: a discussion of the human and environmental data. *Reprod Toxicol* **11:** 564–81.

Ecobichon DJ (2001) Toxic effects of pesticides. In *Casarett and Doull's Toxicology. The Basic Science of Poisons* (Klaassen CD, ed.). McGraw-Hill, New York, pp. 763–810.

Eil CC, Nisula BC (1990) The binding properties of pyrethroids to human skin fibroblast androgen receptors and to sex hormone binding globulin. *J Steroid Biochem* **35:** 409–14.

Elbetieha A, Da'as SI, Khamas W, Darmani H (2001) Evaluation of the toxic potentials of cypermethrin pesticide on some reproductive and fertility parameters in the male rats. *Arch Environ Contam Toxicol* **41:** 522–8.

El-Gohary M, Awara WM, Nassar S, Hawas S (1999) Deltamethrin-induced testicular apoptosis in rats: the protective effect of nitric oxide synthase inhibitor. *Toxicology* **132:** 1–8.

Elliott M, Farnham AW, Janes NF, Soderlund DM (1978) Insecticidal activity of the pyrethrins and related compounds: Part XI. Relative potencies of isomeric cyano-substituted 3-phenoxybenzyl esters. *Pestic Sci* **9:** 112–16.

Ensley S (2007a) Organochlorines. In *Veterinary Toxicology: Basic and Clinical Principles* (Gupta RC, ed.). Academic Press/Elsevier, Amsterdam, pp. 489–492.

Ensley S (2007b) Pyrethrins and pyrethroids. In *Veterinary Toxicology: Basic and Clinical Principles* (Gupta RC, ed.). Academic Press/Elsevier, Amsterdam, pp. 494–8.

Eriksson P, Ahlborn J, Fredriksson A (1992) Exposure to DDT during a defined period in neonatal life induces permanent changes in brain muscarinic receptors and behaviour in adult mice. *Brain Res* **582:** 277–81.

Eriksson P, Fredriksson A (1991) Neurotoxic effects of two different pyrethroids, bioallethrin and deltamethrin, on immature and adult mice: changes in behavioral and muscarinic receptor variables. *Toxicol Appl Pharmacol* **108:** 78–85.

Everett CJ, Frithsen IL, Diaz VA, Koopman RJ, Simpson WM Jr, Mainous AG 3rd (2007) Association of a polychlorinated dibenzo-p-dioxin, a polychlorinated biphenyl, and DDT with diabetes in the 1999–2002 National Health and Nutrition Examination Survey. *Environ Res* **103:** 413–18.

Farag AT, Goda NF, Mansee AH, Shaaban NA (2006) Effects of permethrin given before mating on the behavior of F1-generation in mice. *Neurotoxicology* **27:** 421–8.

Flannigan SA, Tucker SB, Key MM, Ross CE, Fairchild EJ 2nd, Grimes BA, Harrist RB (1985) Synthetic pyrethroid insecticides: a dermatological evaluation. *Br J Ind Med* **42:** 363–72.

French-Constant RH (1993) Cloning of a putative GABAA receptor from cyclodiene-resistant *Drosophila*: a case study in the use of insecticide-resistant mutants to isolate neuroreceptors. *Exs* **63:** 210–23.

Gandolfi O, Cheney DL, Hong JS, Costa E (1984) On the neurotoxicity of chlordecone: a role for gamma-aminobutyric acid and serotonin. *Brain Res* **303:** 117–23.

Garey J, Wolff MS (1998) Estrogenic and antiprogestagenic activities of pyrethroid insecticides. *Biochem Biophys Res Commun* **251:** 855–9.

Godin SJ, Crow JA, Scollon EJ, Hughes MF, DeVito MJ, Ross MK (2007) Identification of rat and human cytochrome P450 isoforms and a rat serum esterase that metabolize the pyrethroid insecticides deltamethrin and esfenvalerate. *Drug Metab Dispos* **35:** 1664–71.

Gomes MDS, Bernardi MM, Spinosa HDS (1991a) Pyrethroid insecticides and pregnancy: effect on physical and behavioral development of rats. *Vet Hum Toxicol* **33:** 315–17.

Gomes MDS, Bernardi MM, Spinosa HDS (1991b) Effect of prenatal pyrethroid insecticide exposure on the sexual development of rats. *Vet Hum Toxicol* **33:** 427–8.

Gorell JM, Johnson CC, Rybicki BA, Peterson EL, Richardson RJ (1998) The risk of Parkinson's disease with exposure to pesticides, farming, well water, and rural living. *Neurology* **50:** 1346–50.

Grabowski CT (1983) Persistent cardiovascular problems in newborn rats prenatally exposed to sub-teratogenic doses of the pesticide, mirex. *Dev Toxicol Environ Sci* **11:** 537–40.

Gray Jr LE, Ostby J, Ferrell J, Rehnberg G, Linder R, Cooper R, Goldman J, Slott V, Laskey J (1989) A dose–response analysis of methoxychlor-induced alterations of reproductive development and function in the rat. *Fundam Appl Toxicol* **12:** 92–108.

Gupta A, Agarwal R, Shukla GS (1999) Functional impairment of blood–brain barrier following pesticide exposure during early development in rats. *Hum Exp Toxicol* **18:** 174–9.

Gupta RC (2007) Placental toxicity. In *Veterinary Toxicology: Basic and Clinical Principles* (Gupta RC, ed.). Academic Press/Elsevier, Amsterdam, pp. 245–62.

Gupta RC (2009) Toxicology of the placenta. In *General and Applied Toxicology*, 3rd edition (Ballantyne B, Marrs T, Syversen T, eds.). John Wiley and Sons, West Sussex, UK, pp. 2003–39.

Hahn ME (1998) The aryl hydrocarbon receptor: a comparative perspective. *Comp Biochem Physiol C Pharmacol Toxicol Endocrinol* **121:** 23–53.

Han Y, Xia Y, Han J, Zhou J, Wang S, Zhu P, Zhao R, Jin N, Song L, Wang X (2008) The relationship of 3-PBA pyrethroids metabolite and male reproductive hormones among non-occupational exposure males. *Chemosphere* **72:** 785–90.

Hauser R, Singh NP, Chen Z, Pothier L, Altshul L (2003) Lack of an association between environmental exposure to polychlorinated biphenyls and p,p′-DDE and DNA damage in human sperm measured using the neutral comet assay. *Hum Reprod* **18:** 2525–33.

He FS, Wang SG, Liu LH, Chen SY, Zhang ZW, Sun JX (1989) Clinical manifestations and diagnosis of acute pyrethroid poisoning. *Arch Toxicol* **63:** 54–8.

Hirano Y, Shibahara H, Obara H, Suzuki T, Takamizawa S, Yamaguchi C, Tsunoda H, Sato I (2001) Relationships between sperm motility characteristics assessed by the computer-aided sperm analysis (CASA) and fertilization rates in vitro. *J Assist Reprod Genet* **18:** 213–18.

Hodgson E, Rose RL (2008) Metabolic interactions of agrochemicals in humans. *Pest Manag Sci* **64:** 617–21.

Huang I, Jones J, Khorram O (2006) Human seminal plasma nitric oxide: correlation with sperm morphology and testosterone. *Med Sci Monit* **12:** CR103–CR106.

Husain R, Gupta A, Khanna VK, Seth PK (1991) Neurotoxicological effects of a pyrethroid formulation fenvalerate in rat. *Commun Chem Pathol Pharmacol* **73:** 111–14.

Husain R, Malaviya M, Seth PK, Husain R (1992) Differential responses of regional brain polyamines following in utero exposure to synthetic pyrethroid insecticides: a preliminary report. *Bull Environ Contam Toxicol* **49:** 402–9.

Iyer P (2001) Developmental and reproductive toxicology of pesticides. In *Handbook of Pesticide Toxicology*, Vol. 1, 2nd edition (Krieger R, ed.). Academic Press, San Diego, pp. 375–420.

Jaeger RJ, Conolly RB, Reynolds ES, Murphy SD (1975) Biochemical toxicology of unsaturated halogenated monomers. *Environ Health Perspect* **11:** 121–8.

Joy RM (1976) The alteration by dieldrin of corticol excitability conditioned by sensory stimuli. *Toxicol Appl Pharmacol* **38:** 357–68.

Joy RM (1982) Mode of action of lindane, dieldrin and related insecticides in the central nervous system. *Neurobehav Toxicol Teratol* **4:** 813–23.

Kamrin MA, Carney EW, Chou K, Cummings A, Dostal LA, Harris C, Henck JW, Loch-Caruso R, Miller RK (1994) Female reproductive and developmental toxicology: overview and current approaches. *Toxicol Lett* **74:** 99–119.

Kerr JB (1992) Spontaneous degeneration of germ cells in rat testis: assessment of cell types and frequency during the spermatogenic cycle. *J Reprod Fertil* **95:** 825–30.

Kim IY, Shin JH, Kim HS, Lee SJ, Kang IH, Kim TS, Moon HJ, Choi KS, Moon A, Han SY (2004) Assessing estrogenic activity of pyrethroid insecticides using in vitro combination assays. *J Reprod Dev* **50:** 245–55.

Kim SS, Kwack SJ, Lee RD, Lim KJ, Rhee GS, Seok JH, Kim BH, Won YH, Lee GS, Jeung EB, Lee BM, Park KL (2005) Assessment of estrogenic and androgenic activities of tetramethrin in vitro and in vivo assays. *J Toxicol Environ Health A* **68:** 2277–89.

Kupfer D (1975) Effects of pesticides and related compounds on steroid metabolism and function. *Crit Rev Toxicol* **4:** 83–124.

Lackmann GM, Schaller KH, Angerer J (2004) Organochlorine compounds in breast-fed vs. bottle-fed infants: preliminary results at six weeks of age. *Sci Total Environ* **329:** 289–93.

Lavado-Autric R, Ausó E, García-Velasco JV, Arufe Mdel C, Escobar del Rey F, Berbel P, Morreale de Escobar G (2003) Early maternal hypothyroxinemia alters histogenesis and cerebral cortex cytoarchitecture of the progeny. *J Clin Invest* **111:** 1073–82.

Lay JP, Malik JK, Klein W, Korte F (1982) Effects of dosing and routes of administration on excretion and metabolism of (^{14}C)dieldrin in rats. *Chemosphere* **11:** 1231–42.

Lazarini CA, Florio JC, Lemonica IP, Bernardi MM (2001) Effects of prenatal exposure to deltamethrin on forced swimming behavior, motor activity, and striatal dopamine levels in male and female rats. *Neurotoxicol Teratol* **23:** 665–73.

Lee H-K, Moon J-K, Chang C-H, Choi H, Park H-W, Park B-S, Lee H-S, Hwang E-C, Lee Y-D, Liu K-H, Kim J-H (2006) Stereoselective metabolism of endosulfan by human liver microsomes and human cytochrome P450 isoforms. *Drug Metabol Disp* **34:** 1090–5.

Lemaire G, Terouanne B, Mauvais P, Michel S, Rahmani R (2004) Effect of organochlorine pesticides on human androgen receptor activation in vitro. *Toxicol Appl Pharmacol* **196:** 235–46.

Leng G, Gries W (2005) Simultaneous determination of pyrethroid and pyrethrin metabolites in human urine by gas chromatography-high resolution mass spectrometry *Chromatogr B Analyt Technol Biomed Life Sci* **814:** 285–94.

Lummis SC, Buckingham SD, Rauh JJ, Sattelle DB (1990) Blocking actions of heptachlor at an insect central nervous system GABA receptor. *Proc R Soc Lond B Biol Sci* **240:** 97–106.

Malaviya M, Husain R, Seth PK, Husain R (1993) Perinatal effects of two pyrethroid insecticides on brain neurotransmitter function in the neonate rat. *Vet Hum Toxicol* **35:** 119–22.

Malik JK, Aggarwal M, Rao GS (2005) Induction of apoptosis by metals. In *Role of Toxic Metals in Defence Electronics and Their Safety* (Flora SJS, Vijayaraghavan R, eds.). DRDE, Gwalior, pp. 92–102.

Malik JK, Bahga HS, Sud SC (1973) Evaluation of therapeutic measures in acute dieldrin poisoning in buffalo calves. *Indian J Anim Sci* **43:** 711–14.

Malik JK, Bahga HS, Sud SC (1975) A note on subacute toxicity of dieldrin in buffalo calves. *Indian J Anim Sci* **45:** 499–502.

Mani U, Islam F, Prasad AK, Kumar P, Suresh Kumar V, Maji BK, Dutta KK (2002) Steroidogenic alterations in testes and sera of rats exposed to formulated fenvalerate by inhalation. *Hum Exp Toxicol* **21:** 593–7.

Manna S, Bhattacharyya D, Mandal TK, Das S (2004) Repeated dose toxicity of alpha-cypermethrin in rats. *J Vet Sci* **5:** 241–5.

Marban E, Yamagishi T, Tomaselli GF (1998) Structure and function of voltage-gated sodium channels. *J Physiol* **508:** 647–57.

McCarthy AR, Thomson BM, Shaw IC, Abella AD (2006) Estrogenicity of pyrethroid insecticide metabolites. *J Environ Monit* **8:** 197–202.

McGlynn KA, Quraishi SM, Graubard BI, Weber JP, Rubertone MV, Erickson RL (2008) Persistent organochlorine pesticides and risk of testicular germ cell tumors. *J Natl Cancer Inst* **100:** 663–71.

McKinlay R, Plant JA, Bell JN, Voulvoulis N (2008) Endocrine disrupting pesticides: implications for risk assessment. *Environ Int* **34:** 168–83.

Meeker JD, Barr DB, Hauser R (2009) Pyrethroid insecticide metabolites are associated with serum hormone levels in adult men. *Reprod Toxicol* **27:** 155–60.

Meeker JD, Barr DB, Hauser R (2008) Human semen quality and sperm DNA damage in relation to urinary metabolites of pyrethroid insecticides. *Hum Reprod* **23:** 1932–40.

Misra UK, Nag D, Krishna Murti CR (1984) A study of cognitive functions in DDT sprayers. *Ind Health* **22:** 199–226.

Mladenovic D, Djuric D, Petronijevic N, Radosavljevic T, Radonjic N, Matic D, Hrncic D, Rasic-Markovic A, Vucevic D, Dekanski D, Stanojlovic O (2010) The correlation between lipid peroxidation in different brain regions and the severity of lindane-induced seizures in rats. *Mol Cell Biochem* **333:** 243–50.

Moniz AC, Bernardi MM, Souza-Spinosa HS, Palermo-Neto J (1990) Effects of exposure to a pyrethroid insecticide during lactation on the behavior of infant and adult rats. *Braz J Med Biol Res* **23:** 45–8.

Moon HB, Kim HS, Choi M, Yu J, Choi HG (2009) Human health risk of polychlorinated biphenyls and organochlorine pesticides resulting from seafood consumption in South Korea, 2005–2007. *Food Chem Toxicol* **47:** 1819–25.

Narahashi T (1986) Mechanisms of action of pyrethroids on sodium and calcium channel gating. In *Neuropharmacology of Pesticide Action* (Ford GG, Lunt GG, Reay RC, Usherwood PNR, eds.). Ellis Horwood, Chichester, pp. 36–40.

Narahashi T (1987) Nerve membrane ion channels as the target site of environmental toxicants. *Environ Health Perspect* **71:** 25–9.

Nasuti C, Gabbianelli R, Falcioni ML, Di Stefano A, Sozio P, Cantalamessa F (2007) Dopaminergic system modulation, behavioral changes, and oxidative stress after neonatal administration of pyrethroids. *Toxicology* **229:** 194–205.

O'Malley M (1997) Clinical evaluation of pesticide exposure and poisonings. *Lancet* **349:** 980–1.

Okubo T, Yokoyama Y, Kano K, Soya Y, Kano I (2004) Estimation of estrogenic and antiestrogenic activities of selected pesticides by MCF-7 cell proliferation assay. *Arch Environ Contam Toxicol* **46:** 445–53.

Osimitz TG, Sommers N, Kingston R (2009) Human exposure to insecticide products containing pyrethrins and piperonyl butoxide (2001–2003). *Food Chem Toxicol* **47:** 1406–15.

Pathak R, Mustafa M, Ahmed RS, Tripathi AK, Guleria K, Banerjee BD (2010) Association between recurrent miscarriages and organochlorine pesticide levels. *Clin Biochem* **43:** 131–5.

Pati PC, Bhunya SP (1989) Cytogenetic effects of fenvalerate in mammalian in vivo test system. *Mutat Res* **222:** 149–54.

Perry MJ, Venners SA, Barr DB, Xu X (2007) Environmental pyrethroid and organophosphorus insecticide exposures and sperm concentration. *Reprod Toxicol* **23:** 113–18.

Perry MJ (2008) Effects of environmental and occupational pesticide exposure on human sperm: a systematic review. *Hum Reprod Update* **14:** 233–42.

Philibert A, Schwartz H, Mergler D (2009) An exploratory study of diabetes in a First Nation community with respect to serum concentrations of p, p′-DDE and PCBs and fish consumption. *Int J Environ Res Public Health* **6:** 3179–89.

Phillips KP, Tanphaichitr N (2008) Human exposure to endocrine disrupters and semen quality. *J Toxicol Environ Health B Crit Rev* **11:** 188–220.

Prasad AK, Pant N, Srivastava SC, Kumar R, Srivastava SP (1995) Effect of dermal application of hexachlorocyclohexane (HCH) on male reproductive system of rat. *Hum Exp Toxicol* **14:** 484–8.

Przyrembel H, Heinrich-Hirsch B, Vieth B (2000) Exposition to and health effects of residues in human milk. *Adv Exp Med Biol* **478:** 307–25.

Punta KD, Charreau EH, Pignataro OP (1996) Nitric oxide inhibits Leydig cell steroidogenesis. *Endocrinology* **137:** 5337–43.

Rawlings NC, Cook SJ, Waldbillig D (1998) Effects of the pesticides carbofuran, chlorpyrifos, dimethoate, lindane, triallate, trifluralin, 2,4-D, and pentachlorophenol on the metabolic endocrine and reproductive endocrine system in ewes. *J Toxicol Environ Health A* **54:** 21–36.

Ribas-Fitó N, Cardo E, Sala M, Eulàlia de Muga M, Mazón C, Verdú A, Kogevinas M, Grimalt JO, Sunyer J (2003) Breastfeeding, exposure to organochlorine compounds and neurodevelopment in infants. *Pediatrics* **111:** 580–5.

Rice D, Barone S Jr (2000) Critical periods of vulnerability for the developing nervous system: evidence from humans and animal models. *Environ Health Perspect* **108:** 511–33.

Richardson JR, Caudle WM, Wang M, Dean ED, Pennell KD, Miller GW (2006) Developmental exposure to the pesticide dieldrin alters the dopamine system and increases neurotoxicity in an animal model of Parkinson's disease. *FASEB J* **20:** 1695–97.

Rogan WJ, Gladen BC, McKinney JD, Carreras N, Hardy P, Thullen J, Tinglestad J, Tully M (1986) Neonatal effects of transplacental exposure to PCBs and DDE. *J Pediatr* **109:** 335–41.

Rogers JM, Grabowski CT (1983) Mirex-induced fetal cataracts: lens growth histology and cation balance, and relationship to edema. *Teratology* **27:** 343–9.

Ronco AM, Valdes K, Marcus D, Llanos M (2001) The mechanism for lindane-induced inhibition of steroidogenesis in cultured rat Leydig cells. *Toxicology* **159:** 99–106.

Rossbach B, Appel KE, Mross KG, Letzel S (2010) Uptake of permethrin from impregnated clothing. *Toxicol Lett* **192:** 50–5.

Saradha B, Mathur PP (2006) Induction of oxidative stress by lindane in epididymis of adult male rats. *Environ Toxicol Pharmacol* **22:** 90–6.

Saradha B, Vaithinathan S, Mathur PP (2009) Lindane induces testicular apoptosis in adult Wistar rats through the involvement of Fas-FasL and mitochondria-dependent pathways. *Toxicology* **255:** 131–9.

Scollon EJ, Starr JM, Godin SJ, DeVito MJ, Hughes MF (2009) In vitro metabolism of pyrethroid pesticides by rat and human hepatic microsomes and cytochrome P450 isoforms. *Drug Metab Dispos* **37:** 221–8.

Sell JL, Davison KL, Bristol DW (1977) Depletion of dieldrin from turkeys. *Poult Sci* **56:** 2045–51.

Semchuk KM, Love EJ, Lee RG (1992) Parkinson's disease and exposure to agricultural work and pesticide chemicals. *Neurology* **42:** 1328–35.

Shafer TJ, Meyer DA, Crofton KM (2005) Developmental neurotoxicity of pyrethroid insecticides: critical review and future research needs. *Environ Health Perspect* **113:** 123–36.

Sharma P, Singh R (2010) Protective role of curcumin on lindane induced reproductive toxicity in male Wistar rats. *Bull Environ Contam Toxicol* **84:** 378–84.

Silva MH, Gammon D (2009) An assessment of the developmental, reproductive, and neurotoxicity of endosulfan. *Birth Defects Res B Dev Reprod Toxicol* **86:** 1–28.

Sircar S, Lahiri P (1989) Lindane (gamma-HCH) causes reproductive failure and fetotoxicity in mice. *Toxicology* **59:** 171–7.

Soderlund DM (1985) Pyrethroid–receptor interactions: stereospecific binding and effects on sodium channels in mouse brain preparations. *Neurotoxicology* **6:** 35–46.

Soderlund DM, Clark JM, Sheets LP, Mullin LS, Piccirillo VJ, Sargent D, Stevens JT, Weiner ML (2002) Mechanisms of pyrethroid neurotoxicity: implications for cumulative risk assessment. *Toxicology* **171:** 3–59.

Song L, Wang YB, Sun H, Yuan C, Hong X, Qu JH, Zhou JW, Wang XR (2008) Effects of fenvalerate and cypermethrin on rat sperm motility patterns in vitro as measured by computer-assisted sperm analysis. *J Toxicol Environ Health A* **71:** 325–32.

Soto AM, Chung KL, Sonnenschein C (1994) The pesticides endosulfan, toxaphene, and dieldrin have estrogenic effects on human estrogen-sensitive cells. *Environ Health Perspect* **102:** 380–83.

Takser L, Mergler D, Baldwin M, de Grosbois S, Smargiassi A, Lanfond J (2005) Thyroid hormones in pregnancy in relation to environmental exposure to organochlorine compounds and mercury. *Environ Health Perspect* **113:** 1039–45.

Tan L, Wang S, Ji J, Sun X, Li Y, Wang Q, Chen L (2006) Effects of fenvalerate exposure on semen quality among occupational workers. *Contraception* **73:** 92–6.

Tapiero H, Ba GN, Tew KD (2002) Estrogens and environmental estrogens. *Biomed Pharmacother* **56:** 36–44.

Tessier D, Matsumura F (2001) Increased ErbB-2 tyrosine kinase activity, MAPK phosphorylation, and cell proliferation in the prostate cancer cell line LNCaP following treatment by select pesticides. *Toxicol Sci* **60:** 38–43.

Thibaut R, Porte C (2004) Effects of endocrine disrupters on sex steroid synthesis and metabolism pathways in fish. *J Steroid Biochem Mol Biol* **92:** 485–94.

Tiemann U (2008) In vivo and in vitro effects of the organochlorine pesticides DDT, TCPM, methoxychlor, and lindane on the female reproductive tract of mammals: a review. *Reprod Toxicol* **25:** 316–26.

Tilson HH (1998) Developmental neurotoxicology of endocrine disruptors and pesticides: identification of information gaps and research needs. *Environ Health Perspect* **106:** 807–11.

Toft G, Hagmar L, Giwercman A, Bonde J (2004) Epidemiological evidence on reproductive effects of persistent organochlorines in humans. *Reprod Toxicol* **19:** 5–26.

Tornero-Velez R, Mirfazaelian A, Kim KB, Anand SS, Kim HJ, Haines WT, Bruckner JV, Fisher JW (2010) Evaluation of deltamethrin kinetics and dosimetry in the maturing rat using a PBPK model. *Toxicol Appl Pharmacol* **244:** 208–17.

Torres-Sánchez L, Rothenberg SJ, Schnaas L, Cebrián ME, Osorio E, Del Carmen Hernández M, García-Hernández RM, Del Rio-Garcia C, Wolff MS, López-Carrillo L (2007) In utero p,p′-DDE exposure and infant neurodevelopment: a perinatal cohort in Mexico. *Environ Health Perspect* **115:** 435–39.

Torres-Sánchez L, Schnaas L, Cebrián ME, Del Carmen Hernández M, Valencia EO, Hernandez RMG, López-Carrillo L (2009) Prenatal dichlorodiphenyldichloroethylene (DDE) exposure and neurodevelopment: a follow-up from 12 to 30 months of age. *Neurotoxicology* **30:** 1162–5.

Tran V, Hoffman N, Mofunanaya A, Pryor SC, Ojugbele O, McLaughlin A, Gibson L, Bonventre JA, Flynn K, Weeks BS (2006) Bifenthrin inhibits neurite outgrowth in differentiating PC12 cells. *Med Sci Monit* **12:** BR57–BR62.

Turusov V, Rakitsky V, Tomatis L (2002) Dichlorodiphenyltrichloroethane (DDT): ubiquity, persistence, and risks. *Environ Health Perspect* **110:** 125–8.

Valentine VM, Beasley VR (1989) Pyrethrins and pyrethroids. In *Current Veterinary Therapy X, Small Animal Practice* (Kirk RW, Bonagura JD, eds.). WB Saunders, Philadelphia, pp. 137–40.

Van Wendel de Joode B, Wesseling C, Kromhout H, Monge P, Garcia M, Mergler D (2001) Chronic nervous-system effects of long-term occupational exposure to DDT. *Lancet* **357:** 1014–15.

Vos JG, Dybing E, Greim HA, Ladefoged O, Lambré C, Tarazona JV, Brandt I, Vethaak AD (2000) Health effects of endocrine-disrupting chemicals on wildlife, with special reference to the European situation. *Crit Rev Toxicol* **30:** 71–133.

Waliszewski S, Aguirre AA, Infanzón RM, Siliceo J (2000) Carry-over of persistent organochlorine pesticides through placenta to fetus. *Salud Publica Mex* **42:** 384–90.

Walker SK, Hartwich KM, Robinson JS (2000) Long term effects on offspring of exposure of oocytes and embryos to chemical and physical agents. *Hum Reprod Update* **6:** 564–77.

Wang H, Wang Q, Zhao XF, Liu P, Meng XH, Yu T, Ji YL, Zhang H, Zhang C, Zhang Y, Xu DX (2010) Cypermethrin exposure during puberty disrupts testosterone synthesis via downregulating StAR in mouse testes. *Arch Toxicol* **84:** 53–61.

Xia Y, Bian Q, Xu L, Cheng S, Song L, Liu J, Wu W, Wang S, Wang X (2004) Genotoxic effects on human spermatozoa among pesticide factory workers exposed to fenvalerate. *Toxicology* **203:** 49–60.

Xia Y, Han Y, Wu B, Wang S, Gu A, Lu N, Bo J, Song L, Jin N, Wang X (2008) The relation between urinary metabolite of pyrethroid insecticides and semen quality in humans. *Fertil Steril* **89:** 1743–50.

Xu LC, Zhan, NY, Liu R, Song L, Wang XR (2004) Joint action of phoxim and fenvalerate on reproduction in male rats. *Asian J Androl* **6:** 337–41.

Yousef MI (2010) Vitamin E modulates reproductive toxicity of pyrethroid lambda-cyhalothrin in male rabbits. *Food Chem Toxicol* **48:** 1152–9.

Zhang SY, Ueyama J, Ito Y, Yanagiba Y, Okamura A, Kamijima M, Nakajima T (2008) Permethrin may induce adult male mouse reproductive toxicity due to *cis* isomer not *trans* isomer. *Toxicology* **248:** 136–41.

Zini A, O'Bryan MK, Magid MS, Schlegel PN (1996) Immunohistochemical localization of endothelial nitric oxide synthase in human testis, epididymis, and vas deferens suggests a possible role for nitric oxide in spermatogenesis, sperm maturation, and programmed cell death. *Biol Reprod* **55:** 935–41.

CHAPTER

39

Herbicides and fungicides

P. K. Gupta

INTRODUCTION

Ever since the dawn of civilization, it has been the major task of the human race to engage in a continuous endeavor to improve its living conditions. One of the main tasks in which human beings have been engaged is securing relief from hunger, one of the basic needs. In addition, the control of insects, weeds, fungi and other pests is of utmost importance to our environment (Gupta, 1984). Thus, pesticides occupy a unique position among the synthetic chemicals that humans encounter daily. Among pesticides, herbicides and fungicides have found extensive use in the control of plant diseases and the eradication of unwanted plants (Gupta, 1985a). In fact, these chemicals have significantly reduced the strong competition of weeds with important and essential food crops. Along with improved crop varieties, both herbicides and fungicides have increased crop yields, decreased food costs and enhanced the appearance of food. Without proper controls, however, the residues of these chemicals that remain on foods can create potential health risks (Gupta, 1985b, 1987a).

Before 1910, no legislation existed to ensure the safety of food and feed crops that were sprayed and dusted with pesticides. In 1910, the first pesticide legislation was designed to protect consumers from impure or improperly labeled products. During the 1950s and 1960s, pesticide regulation including herbicides and fungicides evolved to require maximum allowable residue levels of pesticides on foods and to deny registrations for unsafe or ineffective products (Gupta, 1986). In 1961 severe birth defects in infants following thalidomide ingestion by pregnant mothers had a major impact on the field of developmental toxicity. As a result of the thalidomide catastrophe, regulatory agencies in many countries began developing animal testing requirements for evaluating the effects of drugs on pregnancy outcome separately from chronic toxicity studies. Their biochemical mechanisms are complex and less was known about the use of these synthetic chemicals. Subsequent research revealed that long-term, low dose exposure is linked to ill effects, such as immune suppression, hormone disruption, diminished intelligence, reproductive and development abnormalities, decline of bird populations and even cancer (Vettorazzi, 1985; Gupta, 1993). With a few exceptions, most of the newly developed chemicals have a low order of toxicity to mammals (Gupta, 2006b, 2010). Out of these, several have been evaluated for their toxic potential and acceptable daily intake by the WHO/FAO Joint Meeting on Pesticide Residues, and guidelines for pesticide residues have been recommended (Gupta, 2006a). Currently, most of the data available is still derived from experiments performed on laboratory species or *in vitro* models. Great care should be taken when extrapolations to other species or environmental situations are attempted. This chapter describes the reproductive and developmental toxicity of herbicides and fungicides in humans and animals.

HERBICIDES

Herbicides are phytotoxic chemicals used for destroying various weeds or inhibiting their growth. They have variable degrees of specificity. The worldwide use of herbicides is almost 48% of the total pesticide usage. The consumption of herbicides in developing countries is low because weed control is mainly done by hand weeding (Gupta, 2004). Many of the earlier chemicals used as herbicides include sulfuric acid, sodium chlorate, arsenic trioxide, sodium arsenate, petroleum oils, etc. Iron and copper sulfate or sodium borate were generally hard to handle and/or were toxic, relatively non-specific or phytotoxic to the crop/plant, if not applied at the proper time. The biochemical differences in plants make it possible to design herbicides that have a selective toxicity potential against various species of plants (Gupta, 2007). In the past three decades, herbicides have represented the most rapidly growing section of the pesticide industry. Most of the health problems that result from exposure to herbicides are due to their improper use (Gupta and Sanjay, 1988). The classification of herbicides based on chemical nature and common mechanism of action is summarized in Table 39.1.

HISTORICAL BACKGROUND

The first important discovery in the field of selective weed control was the introduction of 2,4-dinitro-o-cresol (DNOC) in France in 1933. This is very toxic to mammals and can cause bilateral cataract in humans. During World War II, considerable effort was directed toward the development of phenoxy

Reproductive and Developmental Toxicology, Edited by Ramesh C. Gupta
ISBN: 978-0-12-382032-7

TABLE 39.1 Classification of herbicides based on chemical nature and common mechanism of action

Classification class	Examples
Phenoxy acid derivatives	2,4-D, 2,4,5-T, dichlorprop or 2,4-DP, 2,4-DB, dalapon, MCPB, MCPA, mecoprop, mecoprop-P, Silvex or fenprop
Bipyridyl derivatives	Paraquat, diquat
Ureas and thioureas (phenyl or substituted ureas)	Chlorbromuron, chlorotoluron, diuron, fenuron, fenuron-tca, fluometuron, flupyrsulfuron, isoproturon, linuron, metobromuron, metoxuron, monolinuron, monuron, monuron-tca, neburon, noruron, siduron, tebuthiuron, thidiazuron
Organic phosphorus/ phosphonomethyl amino acids or inhibitors of aromatic acid biosynthesis	Glyphosate, glufosinate
Protoporphyrinogen oxidase inhibitors (PROTOX) DPE or non-DPE	Nitrofen, oxadiazon, carfentrazone, JV 485 and oxadiargyl
Triazines and triazoles	
Symmetrical triazines	Simazine, atrazine, propazine, cyanazine, ametryn, prometryn, terbutryn, prometon
Asymmetrical triazines	Metribuzin
Subsituted anilines	Alachlor, acetochlor, butachlor[a], metolachlor[a], propachlor
Amides and acetamides	Bensulide[a], dimethenamid-P, propanil
Dinitro compounds	Binapacryl, DNOC, dinoterb, dinoseb
Triazolopyrimidines	Cloransulam-methyl, diclosulam, flumetsulam, metosulam
Imidazolinones	Imazapyr, imazamethabenzmethyl, imazethapyr, imazaquin
Benzoic acids	Chloramben, dicamba, napalm
Carbamate and thiocarbamate compounds	Asulam, chlorpropham, butylate[a], EPTC[a], di-allate, pebulate[a], terbutol, thiobencarb[a], triallatea[a], vernolate[a]
Methyl uracil compounds	Bromacil, terbacil
Polycyclic alkanoic acids	Diclofop, fenoxaprop ethyl, fenthiaprop, fluazifop, haloxyfop
Sulfonylureas	Chlorsulfuron, sulfometuron, metsulfuron methyl, primisulfuron
Dintroaniline	Trifluralin, tridiphane
Nitriles	Ioxynil, bromoxynil

Compiled from Gupta (2007)
[a] = Liquid
DPE = Diphenyl ether
PROTOX = Protoporphyrinogen oxidase inhibitors (DPE or non-DPE)

herbicides, such as 2,4-dichlorophenoxy acetic acid (2,4-D), 2,4,5- trichlorophenoxy acetic acid (2,4,5-T) and derivatives including the acids, salts, amines and esters. These were first available commercially in 1946 (Gupta, 1989). This class of herbicides has been in continuous, extensive and uninterrupted use since 1947 and is the most widely used family of herbicides. Due to potential for contamination of 2,4,5-T with the highly and unwanted by-product 2,3,7,8-tetrachloro dibenzo-*p*-dioxin, this herbicide was removed from commercial use in the USA. Another chemical class of herbicides deserving particular attention is the bipyridyl group, specifically paraquat and diquat. Their herbicidal properties were discovered by ICI in 1955 and bipyridyl became commercially available in 1962 (Smith, 1997). The first urea herbicide, *N,N*-dimethyl-N′ (chlorophenyl)-urea, was introduced in 1952 by Du Pont under the common name of Monouron. Protopyrinogen oxidase (Protox)-inhibiting herbicides have been used since the 1960s and now represent a relatively large and growing segment of the herbicide market. Nitrofen, a diphenyl ether (DPE) herbicide, was the first Protox-inhibiting herbicide to be introduced for commercial use in 1964. This compound was a weak inhibitor of Protox, but was the lead compound of an entire class of structurally related herbicides that were much more active. Subsequently, several DPE herbicides have been successfully commercialized. Substituted aniline, an Alachlor herbicide, was registered and introduced in 1967. Inhibitors of aromatic acid biosynthesis such as glyphosate were developed by Monsanto in 1970. There are other triazine and triazole herbicides which have been extensively used in agriculture in the USA and other parts of the world for more than 40 years (Steven and Summer, 1991). Another class of synthetic chemical compounds called the imidazolinone herbicides was discovered in the 1970s, with the first US patent awarded in 1980 for imazamethabenz-methyl (Hess *et al.*, 2001).

REPRODUCTIVE TOXICITY

Male reproductive toxicity

Male reproduction encompasses a wide range of physiological processes and associated behavior and anatomical structures involved in the production of the next generation and the survival of a given species of mammals (Senger, 2003). Any disturbance(s) in the physiological process will cause production of insufficient numbers of, or defective, sperm, and result in sterile matings. Pathological alterations may be induced in spermatogenic tissue, as well as loss of libido and competence.

There is increasing experimental and anecdotal evidence that exposure of the male to herbicides also affects developmental events in the conceptus. Although the key role principally ends at fertilization, factors relating to both pre-fertilization and peri-fertilization exposure also play a role post-fertilization. Direct effects on sperm are a likely factor in causing such developmental toxicity, but several related phenomena have been suggested as contributing mechanistic factors (Korach, 1998).

The most toxic and best-studied chemical that can lead to male reproductive toxicity is dioxin. Dioxin is the generic name for a broad group of chemical compounds that have a similar structure, common mechanism of action and common spectrum of biochemical and toxicological effects. Examination of functional sequelae of prenatal exposure to dioxin and related compounds such as 2,3,7,8-tetrachlorodibenzo-*p*-dioxin (TCDD) has resulted in key findings over the past several years (TCDD was identified as a toxic contaminant during production of certain herbicides). TCDD has been shown to cause functional developmental toxicity in multiple species, but additional structural abnormalities have been noted that are delayed in their appearance. In TCDD-treated male hamster offspring, delay in puberty and a permanent decrease in the epididymal and ejaculation sperm count have been reported. This may be due to a distruption of hypothalamic or pituitary control of testicular function (Bjerke and Peterson, 1994; Richard *et al.*, 1997).

In another developmental toxicity study with dioxin, at birth and postnatally at day 4, treated pups had a decreased anogenital distance. At adulthood, the weights of the accessory sex organs of the prenatally exposed male offspring were decreased. Both testicular and epididymal sperm counts were permanently low. Reproductive behavior was also altered. The male took longer to mount receptive females, had increased difficulty in achieving intromission and took additional thrusts to achieve ejaculation. These investigators hypothesized that the effects of dioxin might be due to decreased levels of androgens in the pups, a response noted following high doses to adult males. It was postulated that dioxin exposure not only demasculinizes the male offspring, but can also feminize the central nervous system (Charles *et al.*, 1996; Kennepohl and Munro, 2001).

Short-term feeding of diets containing dinoseb in rats caused decreased epididymal sperm counts, atypical epididymal spermatozoa and minimal testicular changes. Reproduction was unaffected and the anomalies were reversible (Linder *et al.*, 1982). Derivatives of phenoxy acid and other herbicides including 2,4-D decreased testes/body weight ratios, accompanied by slight histopathological abnormalities and evidence of atrophy. In dogs, at higher dose, decreased testicular weights were observed. The toxicological significance of these findings is uncertain since the organ weight changes were not accompanied by any corroborative histopathological changes (Charles *et al.*, 1996). A mixture of herbicide formulation Tordon 75D® (a mixture of 2,4-D and picloram) caused small testes, and showed shrunken tubules with germ cell depletion without any recovery. There was no change in the serum concentration of testosterone. The study suggested no involvement of endocrine hormones (Oakes *et al.*, 2002). Another herbicide, isoproturon in male rats, induced pathomorphological changes in various organs. Seminiferous tubules of testes showed degeneration and desquamation of spermatogonial cells and a reduction in the number of mature spermatozoa (Sarkar *et al.*, 1994). Exposure of male mice to amitraz has shown an adverse effect on fertility and the reproductive system of male mice. A significant increase in the total number of resorptions and the number of females with resorptions was observed in females impregnated by the exposed males (Al-Thani *et al.*, 2003). Diuron, although considered to have a very low toxicity in male rats, caused slight testicular damage during reproductive toxicity studies (Fernandes *et al.*, 2007). In another study, the number of fetuses in litters from diuron-treated male rats was slightly smaller, but diuron did not affect fertility and reproductive performance (Glaura *et al.*, 2007).

A reproductive toxicity study of aryloxyphenoxypropionic (haloxyfop-*p*-methyl, quizalofop-*p*-ethyl) and chlorotriazine herbicides in mice indicated significant differences in weight and the organ coefficients of testes (Chen *et al.*, 2007). Recent reports indicated that chlorotoluron and atrazine can perturb male mouse reproductive function. The epithelium of seminiferous tubules was loosely arranged and lacked order, spermatogenic cells were shed and fewer layers formed. Mitochondria in the seminiferous epithelium appeared vacuolated and nuclei were enlarged and irregular. In addition, the number of Sertoli cells was reduced, and part of the tight junction was destroyed. The toxic effects of chlorotoluron were more potent than those of atrazine when administrated separately. Moreover, when administered in combination, the two compounds had synergistic toxic effects (Hong *et al.*, 2008). Dinoseb and DNOC induced spermatotoxicity by disturbing spermogenesis or the maturation process of sperm in the epididymis, and the most probable target cells of spermatotoxicity were thought to be testicular spermatids. Both of these compounds produced infertility in rats (Matsumoto *et al.*, 2008). The testicular seminiferous tubules of rats treated with glyphosate indicated decreased epithelium lengths. The diameters from the tubular lumen were also increased. Besides variations in the epithelium length and the tubular lumen, the total tubular diameter remained unchanged, indicating that the alterations occurred only with the reduction in germinal epithelium (Figure 39.1) (Romano *et al.*, 2010).

Female reproductive toxicity

As has been discussed previously, the female reproductive cycle is a complex process characterized by the distinct phases of gametogenesis and embryogenesis. Therefore, evaluations of reproductive toxicants have been restricted to the measures of ovarian toxicity (i.e., histopathology, oocyte counts and folliculogenesis), effects on fertility or examination of the potential teratogenicity of environmental agents when administered during pregnancy. Published data indicate that exposure to environmental chemicals causes alterations in reproductive behavior and contribute to subfecundity, infertility, pregnancy loss, growth retardation, intrauterine fetal demise, birth defects and ovarian failure. There is clear evidence that a number of environmental toxicants alter female reproductive function through the CNS and, to a lesser extent, the pituitary mechanism (Korach, 1998).

The potential of 2,4-D to cause adverse effects on the ovary has been extensively evaluated in a series of studies in rats and other species of experimental animals. There were decreased ovary/body weight ratios, accompanied by slight histopathological evidence of atrophy in rats. In dogs, at higher doses, decreased ovary weights were observed (Charles *et al.*, 1996). The effects of prenatal exposure to TCDD on the developing reproductive system of female rats and hamsters indicated a delay in vaginal opening and clefting of the external genitalia. This may reflect a lack of appropriate differentiation. Fertility was also decreased in female hamster offspring, likely due to the structural problems or

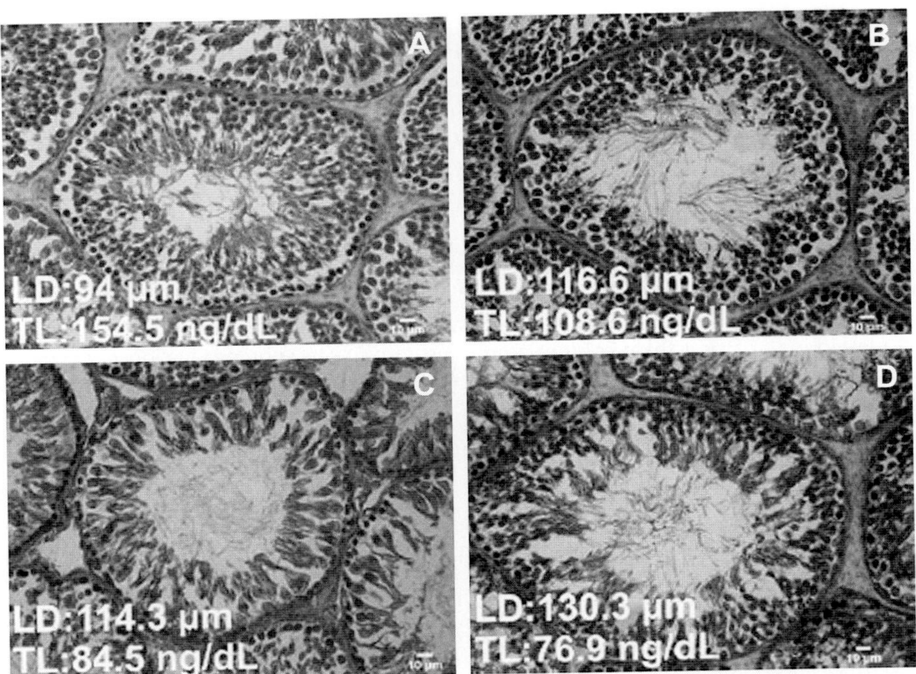

FIGURE 39.1 Effects of the herbicide glyphosate (Roundup) on testicular morphology: control group (a), glyphosate-treated groups at the doses of 5 mg/kg (b), 50 mg/kg (c) or 250 mg/kg (d). All seminiferous tubules of treated groups (b, c, d) presented increase in luminal diameter (LD) and reduction in seminiferous epithelium in relation to control group (a). The testosterone level (TL) is also shown in the picture. RU = Roundup. *Scale bar* = 10 µm. Hematoxilin and eosin stain. From Romano *et al.*, 2010.

the external genitalia (Cooper, 1997). Prenatal exposure to the herbicide nitrofen, a protoporphyrinogen oxidase inhibitor, at 400 mg/d on gestation day (GD) 8/9 or 11/12 induced anomalous development of the para- and mesonephric duct in the hamster. This may result in occasional uterus unicornis, ipsilateral renal agenesis and reduced fertility in treated male progeny. Treatment of female rats with high doses of atrazine disrupted the ovarian cycle and induced repetitive pseudopregnancy (Cooper *et al.*, 1996). From various studies, it has been concluded that herbicides can alter mammalian sex differentiation through unknown mechanisms of toxicity (Gray, 1997). The chemicals that disrupt endocrines are discussed in greater detail later in this chapter.

DEVELOPMENTAL TOXICITY

Experimental studies

A large number of the herbicides that have been tested have shown at least some form of developmental and reproductive toxicity in one or more species of animals. A non-exhaustive list of herbicides that cause developmental toxicity in experimental animals is summarized in Table 39.2.

Phenoxy acid derivatives

Most of the newly developed chemicals have a low order of toxicity to mammals, with the exception of those few that have some adverse effects on the developing embryo. Developmental toxicity associated with exposure to dioxin has been known for almost 40 years. Exposures to herbicides contaminated with TCDD and/or related chemicals resulted in fetal damage in multiple species both in the laboratory and in the wild. For example, lack of reproduction in lake trout in Lake Ontario is well known (EPA, 1993). This chemical, one of 75 known dioxins, was a contaminant of some phenoxy acid derivatives of commonly used herbicides such as 2,4-D and 2,4,5-T. The chemical manufacturer believed that contamination of chemicals during manufacture impart some or all of the developmental toxicity of that chemical in animals and humans.

Initial teratogenic studies were carried out with TCDD and 2,4,5-T in the early 1970s. Several groups of investigators demonstrated that the teratogenic effects of 2,4,5-T in mice and rats from prenatal exposure with low oral doses were due to contamination with TCDD. These consisted of clefting of the secondary palate and hydronephrosis (Courtsey and Moore, 1971). The peak window for sensitivity for induction of cleft palate was GD 11–12. Treatment required higher doses of TCDD. Dosing on GD 13 was less effective and from day 14 on, cleft palate could not be induced by prenatal dioxin exposure. Hydronephrosis was a more sensitive response and could also be brought about following lactation exposure to dioxin; however, this was less efficient than transplacental treatment (Birnbaum, 1998; Boekelheide *et al.*, 1997). Subsequently, several studies confirmed these findings and such abnormalities were also observed in other species of animals. TCDD has also been indicted as an environmental teratogen in the wild bird population (Hoffman *et al.*, 1987). It is known that TCDD suppresses cellular immunity in rodents and alters reproductive functions in the immature rat model through effects on the hypothalamic–pituitary axis as well by direct effects on the ovary (Li *et al.*, 1995).

TABLE 39.2 Non-exhaustive list of herbicides that are known to cause development toxicity in experimental animals

Chemical	Malformations
Atrazine	Disruption of ovarian cycle and induced repetitive pseudopregnancy (rats, at high doses)
Buturon	Cleft palate, increased fetal mortality (mice)
Butiphos	Teratogenic (rabbit)
Chloridazon	Malformations
Chlorpropham	Malformations or other developmental toxicity (mice)
Cynazine	Malformations such as cyclopia and diaphragmatic hernia (rabbits). Skeletal variations in rats
2,4-D*, 2,4,5-T* alone or in combination	Malformations such as cleft palate, hydronephrosis, teratogenic (mice, rats)
Dichlorprop	Teratogenic (mice), affects postnatal behavior (rats)
Dinoseb[a]	Multiple defects (mice, rabbits)
Dinoterb	Skeletal malformations (rats), skeletal, jaw, head and visceral (rabbits)
Linuron	Malformations (rats)
Mecoprop	Malformations (mice)
Monolinuron	Cleft palate (mice)
MCPA	Teratogenic and embryotoxic (rats), teratogenic (mice)
Prometryn	Head, limbs and tail defects (rat)
Propachlor	Slightly teratogenic (rats)
Nitrofen[a]	Malformations (mice, rats, hamsters)
Silvex	Teratogenic (mice)
TCDD*	Malformations/teratogenic (fetotoxicity in chicken, rats, mice, rabbits, guinea pigs, hamsters and monkeys)
Tridiphane	Malformations such as cleft palate (mice), skeletal variations (rats)

Compiled from Gupta (2007)
[a] = Obsolete
*TCDD is a common contaminant of 2,4-D and 2,4,5-T

Experimental studies with multiple animal species have revealed that TCDD exposure during organogenesis resulted in fetotoxicity in chickens, rats, mice, rabbits, guinea pigs, hamsters and monkeys. At dosage levels below those where overt toxicity occurred in the dams, growth retardation was detected in the offspring. Higher levels of exposure were associated with fetal death and resorptions. The compound 2,4,5-T has been tested for teratogenic potential in many studies. Results have not been conclusive largely due to lack of information about the quantity of TCDD present in the manufactured chemical (Sterling, 1971). All studies reported in mice have demonstrated teratogenicity, usually evidenced by cleft palate and sometimes skeletal defects and resorptions. Strain differences in mice were also observed (Gaines *et al.*, 1975). Studies in sheep, rabbits and primates have been negative, even though dioxin contaminants were present in concentrations of 0.05–1 ppm. Several esters of 2,4,5-T have also been found to be teratogenic in rodents. These include the butyl, isooctyl and the propylene glycol butyl ether ester in rodents. 2,4,5-T phenol was not teratogenic in the mouse. Since formulations of 2,4,5-T contained dioxin which increased the toxicity of technical grade herbicides, the safe use of phenoxy herbicides was questioned. This led to a ban from use in the USA (EPA, 1979). Developmental effects of dioxin and the teratogenic potential of 2,4,5-T have been reviewed in greater details by Birnbaum (1998) and Schardein (2000). It seems about one-half of the herbicides that have been tested have been teratogenic in animals. However, a few of them did not cause malformations, but led to other types of developmental abnormalities. For example, pure compounds of phenoxy acid derivatives such as 2,4-D, 2,4,5-T, 2,4-DB {4-(2,4-dichlorophenoxy) butyric acid}, dalapon, dichlorprop or 2,4-DP {2-(2-methyl-4-chlorophenoxy propionic acid}, mecoprop (MCPP) (2-4-chloro-2-methylphenoxy propionic acid), MCPA (2-methyl-4-chlorophenoxyacetic acid) and Silvex {2-(2,4,5-trichlorophenoxy) propionic acid} are not all teratogens.

Out of phenoxy acid derivatives, 2,4-D is the most commonly used herbicide and is one of the best-studied agricultural chemicals. Several multigenerational and developmental animal studies have been conducted to see the potential of 2,4-D to affect reproduction and the developing fetus (Kennepohl and Munro, 2001). The results of the available studies indicate that 2,4-D is not teratogenic and does not affect reproduction, except at maternally toxic doses. 2,4-D does not produce any testicular damage or induce any abnormal reproductive disorders; however, 2,4-D contaminated with TCDD has been reported to have a teratogenic potential in animals. In mice, cleft palate and other classes of developmental toxicity were induced with the chemical in two strains following oral treatment. In mice, up to 70% of fetuses per litter were malformed from oral prenatal treatment. Administration of 2,4-D to hamsters resulted in 22% of the offspring with malformations, most notably fused ribs. The esters of 2,4-D are equally potent teratogens. The butyl and isooctyl esters were teratogenic in two or more species. The isopropyl and methyl esters were active in mice, and the butoxyethanol, diethylamine and dimethylamine esters were all teratogenic in rats. The propylene glycol butyl ether ester had no teratogenic activity in rats. The butoxyethyl ester and isopropylamine and triisopropylamine salts were not teratogenic in the rabbit (Liberacki *et al.*, 1994).

A combination of 2,4-D and 2,4,5-T, popularly known as "Agent Orange" was also teratogenic in mice. In the rat, this combination did not result in malformations, but behavioral effects were seen postnatally in some offspring. A combination of 2,4-D and picloram, given in an unconventional regimen to mice, resulted in malformation and other embryotoxicity only when both preconceptual and gestational exposures were administered (Schardien, 2000).

In general, ureas and thioureas do not cause developmental and reproductive toxicity; however, monolinuron, linuron and buturon are known to cause some teratogenic abnormalities in experimental animals. Linuron produced a high incidence of malformations in rat fetuses when given by gavage, but the chemical had no teratogenic potential in the rabbit under a dietary regimen (Hodge *et al.*, 1968). A related chemical monolinuron caused cleft palate in mice (Matthiaschk and Roll, 1977).

Another herbicide of this class, MCPA, was found to be teratogenic and embryotoxic in rats, and teratogenic in mice. Its ethyl ester was also found to be teratogenic, as it induced cleft palate, ear and renal anomalies at 31% incidence in rats when given at a maternally toxic dose (Yasuda and Maeda, 1972). Mecoprop induced malformations in mice, but when administered prenatally on GD 4, produced only some postnatal behavioral alterations, and no malformations in rats (Buschmann *et al.*, 1986). Silvex is teratogenic in mice and is not teratogenic in rats (Courtsey, 1977).

Bipyridyl derivatives

This chemical class of herbicides includes paraquat and diquat. Paraquat is usually formulated as the dichloride salt (methyl viologen). Paraquat is the most toxic of the commonly used herbicides and its toxicity varies in different species and depending upon the formulation.

The compound is apparently non-teratogenic under standard testing regimens. At high doses injected into pregnant rats and mice on various GD, paraquat caused significant maternal toxicity but did not produce teratogenic effects (Bus and Gibson, 1975). At lower doses, gross soft tissue and slight skeletal anomalies have been reported. In rats, costal cartilage malformtions were reported. Diquat had no effect on fertility, was not teratogenic, and only produced fetotoxicity at doses that were maternally toxic. In the multigenerational study, cataract has been observed in rats given higher doses (Lock and Wilks, 2001).

Ureas and thioureas

The ureas and thioureas (polyureas) are available under different names such as diuron, fluometuron, isoproturon, linuron, buturon, chlorbromuron, chlortoluron, chloroxuron, difenoxuron, fenuron, methiuron, metobromuron, metoxuron, monuron, neburon, parafluron, siduron, tebuthiuron, tetrafluron and thidiazuron. Of these, diuron and fluometuron are most commonly used in the USA, whereas isoproturon is most commonly used in other countries, including India. Ureas have low acute toxicity and do not cause developmental and reproductive toxicity, with the exception of monolinuron, linuron, buturon and tebuthiuron. These chemicals are known to cause some developmental malformations in experimental animals. Linuron produced a high incidence of malformations in rat fetuses when given by gavage, but the chemical had no teratogenic potential in the rabbit under dietary regimen. Monolinuron caused cleft palate in mice (Hodge *et al.*, 1968; Matthiaschk and Roll, 1977). Sarkar and Gupta (1993) have reported minor abnormalities in rat fetuses born to mothers exposed to isoproturon during the period of organogenesis (GD 6–15). In general, cattle are more sensitive to polyurea herbicides than sheep, cats and dogs (Gupta, 2007).

Phosphonomethyl amino acids or inhibitors of aromatic acid biosynthesis

Two organophosphorus compounds, glyphosate (Roundup, Vision) and glufosinate (Basta), are marketed as the isopropyl amine or trimethylsulfonium salts of glyphosate and the ammonium salt of glufosinate. Glyphosate has a low acute oral toxicity in mice and rats and is unlikely to pose acute hazard with normal use. No adverse effects on reproductive or developmental systems have been reported (Farmer, 2001).

Protoporphyrinogen oxidase inhibitors

The protoporphyrinogen oxidase (Protox) inhibitors may be diphenyl ether (DPE) or non-diphenyl ether (non-DPE) herbicides. In 1964, nitrofen was the first Protox-inhibiting herbicide introduced (Reddy *et al.*, 1998). Nitrofen is a developmental toxicant and produces varying results in different species. It produced a high incidence of diaphragmatic hernias and harderian gland alterations in mice following oral treatment, and hydronephrosis and respiratory difficulties in rats. In hamsters, the compound, when administered orally during gestation, resulted in abnormal development of the para- and mesonephric ducts and ureteric bud, which was occasionally accompanied by renal agenesis in female offspring and predominantly left-sided agenesis of vas or epididymis and seminal vesicles in male. It was concluded that the teratogenic activity of nitrofen is mediated by alterations in maternal and fetal thyroid hormone status (Manson *et al.*, 1984; Dayan *et al.*, 2001).

After the first generation of Protox inhibitors (with the exception of oxadiazon), which were based on the DPE, numerous other non-oxygen-bridged compounds (non-DPE Protox inhibitors) with the same site of action (carfentrazone, JV 485 and oxadiargyl) were commercialized. These compounds have little acute toxicity and are unlikely to pose any acute hazard with normal use. The developmental toxicity studies conducted on rats and rabbits indicate that the majority of compounds did not show any reproductive, developmental or teratogenic abnormalites, except at very high doses that elicit maternal toxicity. Development toxicity correlates with Protox accumulation (JMPR, 2004).

Triazines and triazoles

Triazine and triazole herbicides have been used extensively for more than 40 years. These herbicides are inhibitors of photosynthesis and include both the asymmetrical and symmetrical triazines. Examples of symmetrical triazines are chloro-s-triazines (simazine, atrazine, propazine and cyanazine); the thiomethyl-s-triazines (ametryn, prometryn, terbutryn) and the methoxy-s-triazine (prometon). The most commonly used asymmetrical triazine is metribuzin. These herbicides have a low oral toxicity and are unlikely to pose acute hazards with normal use and do not produce developmental toxicity, with the exception of ametryn, metribuzin, atrazine and cyanazine, which may be slightly to moderately hazardous. Atrazine induced no structural malformations in either rats or rabbits. Simazine provided contradictory results of developmental toxicity in different studies carried out in different species using various dose levels (Dilley *et al.*, 1977). Cyanazine is more acutely toxic and resulted in developmental toxicity, presumably because of the presence of cyano moiety (Hodgson and Meyer, 1997). Effects noted at doses that were toxic to the mothers were cyclopia and diaphragmatic hernia in rabbits, and an apparent increase in the incidences of skeletal variations in rats (EPA, 1993).

Substituted anilines

Substituted anilines are used as systemic herbicides. The commonly used herbicides are alachlor, acetochlor, butachlor, metolachlor and propachlor. This class of herbicides is slightly hazardous, except butachlor, which is not likely to pose any hazard. The results from the reproductive and developmental toxicity studies indicate that these herbicides are not reproductive toxicants, development toxicants or teratogens. However, in the rabbit study with butachlor, a slight increase in postimplantation loss and decreased fetal weights were observed at maternally toxic doses. At dietary concentrations, no adverse effects on reproductive performance or pup survival were observed in a study conducted for two successive generations (Wilson and Takei, 1999).

Amides and acetamides

These commonly used herbicides include bensulide, dimethenamid-P and propanil. They are slightly or moderately hazardous with normal use. Dimethenamid is a racemic mixture of the M and P stereoisomers, whereas the P isomer has useful herbicidal activity. Dimethenamid can reduce fetal body weight, but is not teratogenic (Gupta, 2007).

Dinitrophenol compounds

Dinitrophenol herbicides include DNP (2,4-dinitrophenol), DNOC, dinoseb and dinoterb. The dinitro compounds are slightly water-soluble, highly hazardous to animals and may cause developmental toxicity. Dinoseb is known to cause teratogenic effects in several species. The compound when given by gavage to rats at maternally toxic doses reduced fetal body weight and increased the frequency of extra ribs. In rabbits, after dermal exposure, eye defects and neural malformations, accompanied by maternal toxicity, have been reported. With the dinitro compounds, abortions have been reported in sows (Lorgue *et al.*, 1996). The chemical has been banned from use in the USA. Dinoterb, another chemical of the same group, induced skeletal malformations by both oral and dermal administration in the rat, and skeletal, jaw, head and visceral malformations in the rabbit (Schardein, 2000).

Triazolopyrimidine herbicides

Triazolopyrimidine herbicides include cloransulam-methyl, diclosulam, florasulammethyl, flumetsulam and metosulam. The acute oral toxicity of the triazolopyrimidine herbicides is very low. In general, this group of herbicides does not affect reproduction, fetal development or multigenerational reproduction. No evidence of maternal toxicity, embryo-fetotoxicity or teratogenicity has been observed in experimental animals (EPA, 1997a,b; Hanley and Billington *et al.*, 2001).

Imidazolinones

Imidazolinone herbicides include imazapyr, imazethapyr, imazamethabenzmethyl, imazapic, imazamox and imazaquin. These herbicides are relatively non-toxic. Results from the reproductive and developmental toxicity studies indicate that the imidazolinone herbicides are not reproductive toxicants, developmental toxicants or teratogens (Hess *et al.*, 2001).

Benzoic acids

The herbicides in this group include chloramben, dicamba and naptalam. These have a low order of toxicity. In practice, dicamba is often combined with other herbicides. The signs of toxicity with benzoic acid herbicides are similar to those described for the chlorophenoxy acids. Poisoning after normal use has not been reported in domestic animals. The compound did not show any developmental abnormalities in a three-generation study in rats (Harp, 2001).

Carbamates, thiocarbamates and dithiocarbamate compounds

The compounds in this category include derivatives of carbamic acid (asulam, barban, chlorpropham, chlorbufam, karbutilate and phenmedipham), derivatives of thiocarbarnic acid (butylate, cycloate, di-allate, EPTC, molinate and tri-allate) and derivatives of dithiocarbamic acid (metham-sodium). These herbicides have a low to moderate toxicity in rats and do not pose acute hazards. Chlorpropham at high oral doses given during the organogenesis period caused malformations and various types of developmental toxicity (Gupta, 2007).

Dinitroaniline

Tridiphane, a dinitroaniline compound, is a potent developmental toxicant in the mouse, induced cleft palate and other toxicity at maternally toxic doses, but under the same conditions in the rat the compound increased the frequency of minor skeletal variations (Hanley *et al.*, 1987).

Others

There are several other herbicides that may cause various types of developmental and reproductive abnormalities in animals. For example, aminotriazole or amitrole did not induce structural malformations in rats or mice but when administered in the drinking water of rats, it caused fetal thyroid lesions, as it is also an antithyroid agent (Shalette *et al.*, 1963). Butiphos was reported to be teratogenic in the rabbit, but was not in the rat (Mirkhamidova *et al.*, 1981). Chloridazon caused only resorptions in the rat, but caused rib and tail anomalies in hamster fetuses of several litters. Prometryn produced head, limb and tail defects in rat fetuses following daily administration during gestation (Schardein, 2000).

Epidemiological evidence

It is well known that humans are exposed to a variety of chemicals in the home, occupationally and in the environment. Risks to human reproduction and development are quite different depending on the source of exposure. In addition to these types of exposures – herbicide spraying in Vietnam and elsewhere in the 1960s; accidental mixing of a noxious chemical into cattle feed in Michigan (USA), a plant discharge of dioxin in Seveso (Italy) and general chemical dumping into Love Canal (USA), all in the 1970s; an atmospheric release of an industrial poison in Bhopal (India) in the 1980s; and perceived poisoning by chemical warfare agents during the Gulf War in the 1990s – it is no wonder the populace globally is highly concerned about chemical exposure and the hazards they pose (Schardein, 2000). Therefore, several good examples of human developmental toxicants are those that occurred by accident or circumstantial exposure to environmental

TABLE 39.3 Non-exhaustive list of herbicides responsible for reproductive problems/malformations in humans

Chemical	Location	Year	Malformations
Butiphos	Russia	1970s	Aggravated parturition, congenital malformations and stillbirths
2.4-D+2,4,5-T (Agent Orange)	Vietnam	1960s	Miscarriages, stillbirths and congenital malformations
2,4,5-T and dioxin	New Zealand	1970s	Mylomeningocele
Oryzalin	New York	1970s	Miscarriages, stillbirths and heart defects
Picloram	Brazilian state of Para	1984	Miscarriages and malformed fetuses
Silvex	Arizona	1968–1969	Malformations in pets, domestic animals and wildlife, as well as human reproductive toxicity
TCDD	Times Beach (USA)	1970s	Miscarriages and birth defects

chemicals. A non-exhaustive list of herbicides that cause malformations in humans is summarized in Table 39.3.

Epidemiological survey indicated the association of herbicides and birth defects in humans in Vietnam where a mixture of 2,4-D and 2,4,5-T was sprayed. There were an increased number of miscarriages that occurred within 2 months following spraying of dioxin-contaminating herbicides in Vietnam (Laporte, 1977). The EPA banned the use of 2,4,5-T. The major basis for this was a new study linking exposure to dioxin, the unavoidable contaminant of 2,4,5-T and Silvex herbicides, and an increased risk of miscarriages (EPA, 1979). Other herbicides have also been associated with the induction of malformation in humans. Two cases of myelomeningocele from first exposure in women drinking water contaminated with 2,4,5-T from agricultural spraying of their farms in New Zealand has been reported (Sare and Forbes, 1972). A case of encephalocele in the Gulf Islands (Canada) and isolated cases of anencephaly and multiple congenital formations in the child of a woman exposed to Agent Orange at 5 weeks' gestation have also been reported (Lowry and Allen, 1977; Hall *et al.*, 1980). Numerous cases of malformatuions due to the use of Agent Orange and 2,4,5-T have been reported from different parts of the world (Schardein, 2000). Another herbicide to be associated with human birth defects is 2,4-D, where a woman was exposed to the chemical at high doses before conception until the 5th week of her gestation. Her baby had severe mental retardation and multiple congenital defects (Casey and Collie, 1984).

In another survey, occupational contact with butiphos in Russian agricultural workers resulted in aggravated parturition, congenital malformations and stillbirths (Kasymova, 1976). The herbicide oryzalin caused one miscarriage and three cases of heart defects in offspring born to four women whose spouses were exposed to the chemical in a New York manufacturing plant (Dickson, 1979). The herbicide Silvex was involved in a spraying accident in Arizona in 1968–1969. Two families reported malformations in pets, domestic animals and wildlife, as well as human reproductive toxicity (Trost, 1984). In another case, picloram exposure was related to a spate of miscarriages and malformed fetuses which occurred in 1984 in the Brazilian state of Para (Elkington, 1985). However, since that case, no incidences of human developmental toxicity with these chemicals have been reported.

TABLE 39.4 Classification of fungicides based on chemical nature

Chemical class	Examples
Halogenated substituted monocyclic aromatics	Chlorothalonil, tecnazene, dicloran, hexachlorobenzene, quintozene, dinocap, dichlorophen, pentachlorophenol, chloroneb
Chloroalkylthiodicarboximides	Captan, captafol, folpet
Anilinopyrimidines	Mepanipyrim, pyrimethanil, cyprodinil
Carbamic acid derivatives	Ferbam, thiram, ziram, propamocarb, maneb, mancozeb, zineb, nabam, metiram
Benzimidazoles	Benomyl, thiophanate-methyl, carbendazim, fuberidazole
Conazoles	Cyproconazole, diniconazole, etridiazole, hexaconazole, penconazole, triadimefon, azaconazole, triadimenol, bromuconazole, propiconazole, tetraconazole (oil), imazalil
Morpholines	Dodemorph (liquid), fenpropimorph (oil), tridemorph
Amides	Fenhexamid, benalaxyl, metalaxyl, flutolanil, tolyfluanid, dichlofluanid
Others	Thiabendazole, cycloheximide, fludioxonil, dimethomorph, trifloxystrobin, fenpyroximate

FUNGICIDES

Fungicides are used to prevent or eradicate fungal infections from plants or seeds. In agriculture, they are used to protect tubers, fruits and vegetables during storage and are applied directly to ornamental plants, trees, field crops, cereals and turf grasses. Numerous substances with widely varying chemical constituents are used as fungicides (Gupta, 1988). With a few exceptions, most of the newly developed chemicals have a low order of toxicity to mammals. Public concern has focused on their potential to cause reproductive and developmental toxicity in mammals because of their impact on endocrine systems (Gupta, 1987b). The classification of fungicides based on chemical nature is presented in Table 39.4.

HISTORICAL BACKGROUND

The earliest fungicides were inorganic material such as sulfur, lime, copper and mercury compounds. The use of elemental sulfur as a fungicide was recommended as early as 1803. Another compound, hexachlorobenzene (HCB), was extensively used from the 1940s through the 1950s as a fungicidal dressing applied to seed grains. Between 1955 and 1959, an epidemic of poisoning occurred in Turkey. HCB is a highly toxic compound which can lead to severe skin manifestations, including hypersensitivity. Subsequently, many compounds have been developed and used to control fungal diseases in plants, seeds and produce. For example, during the 1940s carbamic acid derivatives such as ethylenebisdithiocarbamates (EBDCs), mancozeb, maneb, metiram, zineb and nabam were developed. Captan, folpet and captafol have been in use for over 50 years. Another compound chlorothalonil, a halogenated benzonitrile fungicide, was first registered for use as an agrochemical in the USA in 1966. The benzimidazole fungicides benomyl and carbendazim have been in use for over 35 years. Recently, anilinopyrimidines, a new class of fungicides (cyprodinil, mepanipyrim and pyrimethanil) has been introduced (Gupta, 2007; Gupta and Agarwal, 2007).

REPRODUCTIVE TOXICITY

Male reproductive toxicity

As has been stated earlier, the potential adverse effects of fungicides on reproductive health have generated much concern. Direct effects on sperm are a likely factor in causing such developmental toxicity, but several related phenomena have been suggested as contributing mechanistic factors (Korach, 1998). During the early stages of testing of benzimidazole fungicides (inhibitors of DNA biosynthesis mitosis) such as benomyl and carbamates, it was observed that high doses by gavage could cause testicular effects, such as decreased sperm count, decreased testicular weights and histopathological changes. Biotransformation studies showed the rapid conversion of benomyl to carbendazim, therefore, other studies were conducted with carbendazim rather than benomyl. Occlusion of the efferent ductules was common following exposure to the fungicide benomyl and its metabolite carbendazim. A single dose of benzimidazole carbamates induced rapid testicular effects, detectable within hours as an increase in testis weight, but having long-term effects that led to testicular atrophy and infertility. At lower doses, direct effects were on the seminiferous epithelium thereby affecting epididymal sperm. Long-term atrophic effects on the testis were more severe after carbendazim than benomyl. The inflammatory response with occluded ductules caused subsequent damage to the ductal epithelium. The rete testis was swollen with compacted sperm and the seminiferous tubules were atrophic with edematous interstitial space. It was further concluded that all the testicular damage and microtubule disruption seen after treatment with benomyl can be explained by the carbendazim released from benomyl rather than benomyl itself (Carter *et al.*, 1987; Ilio and Hess, 1994; Naki and Hess, 1997).

Following long-term exposure, benalaxyl caused liver steatosis and hematological changes in rats and atrophy of seminiferous tubules in dogs. Fungicidal mercury caused Young's syndrome, leading to failure of normal efferent ductule function and infertility. In this syndrome, luminal fluid showed increased viscosity, the epithelium of efferent ductules exhibited an abnormal accumulation of lipid responsible for the decreased flow of fluid through the ductules (Mitchinson *et al.*, 1975; Hendry *et al.*, 1990). Prochloraz feminizes the male offspring after perinatal exposure, therefore leading to diminished fetal steroidogenesis (Vinggaard et al., 2005). It was suggested that prochloraz has multiple mechanisms of action that may influence the demasculinizing and reproductive toxic effects of the compound. Rats, when dosed perinatally, showed mild dysgenesis of the male external genitalia, as well as reduced anogenital distance and retention of nipples in male pups. An increased anogenital distance indicated virilization of female pups. Inhibition of steroidogenesis in male fetuses led to decreased testicular and plasma levels of testosterone and increased levels of progesterone (Laier *et al.*, 2006).

Female reproductive toxicity

The female reproductive system is complex and only a few studies have been conducted which indicate reproductive toxicity. Earlier studies done with benzimidazoles (benomyl, carbendazim) on female reproductive organs indicated an increase in uterine weights. There was no direct or indirect evidence of hormonal activity (Spencer *et al.*, 1996). The effects observed on the oocytes and uterine weight in female rats was direct and was not mediated by endocrine changes. A high dose of carbendazim caused an increased incidence of diffuse proliferation of parafollicular cells of the thyroid in female rats (Jeffay *et al.*, 1996; Spencer *et al.*, 1996). Exposure of blastocysts to various concentrations of mercury or methyl mercuric chloride caused significant inhibition in cell proliferation and protein synthesis of the blastocyst stage embryo (Dwivedi and Iannaccone, 1998). Mancozeb, when administered orally in rats or mice, decreased the number of estrous cycles, duration of proestrus, estrus and metestrus with concomitant significant increase in the duration of diestrus. There was a significant decrease in the number of healthy follicles and a significant increase in the number of atretic follicles. The histologic observation of the ovary revealed the presence of less corpora lutea and the size of the ovary was also reduced. The thyroid weight was increased (Baligar and Kaliwal, 2001). Whether the decreased number of implantations by mancozeb is due to hormonal imbalance or its toxic effects still remains to be seen (Bindali and Kaliwal, 2002).

At high doses, several azole fungicides and other azole compounds are known to affect reproductive organs, fertility and development in several species. These effects may be due to inhibition of sterol 14-alpha-demethylase and/or aromatase. In fact, several azole compounds were shown to inhibit these enzymes *in vitro*, and there is also strong evidence for inhibiting activity *in vivo*. Many azole compounds developed as inhibitors of fungal sterol 14-alpha-demethylase are also inhibitors of mammalian sterol 14-alpha-demethylase and mammalian aromatase with unknown potencies (Zarn *et al.*, 2003). A recent study has shown that fungicides such as propiconazole, myclobutanil and triadimefon adversely affect female rodent reproductive development through inhibition of sterol 14-alpha-demethylase and/or aromatase (Rockett *et al.*, 2006).

DEVELOPMENTAL TOXICITY

Experimental studies

The earlier fungicides such as potassium azide, potassium thiocyanate and titrated or sublimed sulfur, were used during the 19th and early 20th centuries. Elemental sulfur and crude lime sulfur (calcium polysulfide and barium polysulfide) have been used as fungicides in the USA. The

TABLE 39.5 Non-exhaustive list of fungicides that cause development toxicity in experimental animals

Chemical	Malformations
Ammonium salts, manganese and zinc	Multiple defects (rats)
Benomyl	Skeletal malformations, increased mortality (rats), multiple anomalies (mice), small renal papillae but no malformations (rabbits)
Bis(tri-*n*-butyltin) oxide	Cleft palate and development toxicity (rats, mice)
Bitertanol	Tail, palate, jaw, eye defects (rat)
Captafol, folpet	CNS, rib, tail and limb defects (hamsters); no teratogenic effects in other four species
Captan	Multiple defects, CNS and rib (rabbits, hamsters)
Carbendazim	Limb malformations, postnatal behavior alterations, postural reflex, open field behavior (rat)
Conazoles	Variable multiple defects
Cycloheximide[b]	Skeletal defects, dactyly, hydrocephaly or other developmental defects
Dinocap[a]	Multiple malformations, hyprocephaly (rabbit)/experimental teratogen
EBDCs (maneb and zineb metabolite ethylenethiuram monosulfide, and ETU)	Multiple malformations and embryo-fetotoxic effects
Fenpropimorph	Developmental toxicity and malformations
Ferbam	Soft-tissue and skeletal (rats)
Fusilazole	Malformations
Hexachlorobenzene	Variety of defects, renal and palate (hamsters, mice), rib variation and reduced weight (rats)
Mancozeb	Variety of defects
Methyl mercury	Multiple malformations and embryotoxic
Polycarbacin	Embryotoxic, malformations
Probineb	Malformations
Propioconazole	Developmental toxicant
Thiram	Multiple malformations
Triadimenol	Developmental toxicant
Triadimefon	Scapula malformations (rabbits)
Tridemorph	Cleft palate, other malformations and developmental toxicity (rats, mice)

[a] = Withdrawn by manufacturer
[b] = Obsolete
Variable: results need further studies
ETU = Ethylenethiourea
EBDCs = Ethylenebisdithiocarbamates

metallic compounds used as fungicides are protective and preventive. The group of compounds includes mercury, mercuric and mercurous compounds, ethylmercury phosphate, 2-methoxyethylmercury chloride, phenyl mercury chloride and phenylmercury acetate. These are used as seed dressings and treatments for cereals and fodder beets (Gupta, 2007). A large number of fungicides that have been tested have shown at least some form of developmental and reproductive toxicity in one or more species of animals. A non-exhaustive list of fungicides that cause developmental toxicity in experimental animals is summarized in Table 39.5.

Environmental exposure to elemental sulfur does not lead to any reproductive or developmental toxicity in animals or in humans. Ammonium salts, manganese and zinc have been reported to cause multiple defects in experimental animals. Administration of methyl mercury to pregnant mice induced a high incidence of resorptions and dead fetuses, brain and jaw defects, cleft palate and post-behavioral alterations. It has also been shown to be embryotoxic and teratogenic in golden hamsters and mice (Gammon *et al.*, 2001). Another compound, *bis* (tri-*n*-butylin) oxide, induced cleft palate and other developmental toxicity in both mice and rats. Bitertanol, given to rats on single days of gestation, caused tail, palate, jaw and eye defects in their offsprings (Vergieva, 1990).

Halogenated substituted monocyclic aromatics

This class of chemicals includes chlorothalonil, dicloran, HCB, quintozene, PCP, dichlorophen, dinocap, tecnazene and chloroneb. HCB was teratogenic in hamsters and mice (renal and palate malformations) and in rats (increased incidence of 14th rib). HCB was also toxic to developing perinatal animals. The potential to induce developmental toxicity has been investigated in the rat and rabbit. The compound at high doses caused maternal toxicity and postimplantation loss due to early embryonic death. Subsequently, several teratogenic studies conducted with this chemical using different animal species showed variable results (Rogers *et al.*, 1986). HCB induced a variety of defects in the mouse and is a developmental neurotoxicant in the rat (Courtney *et al.*, 1976; Goldey and Tayler, 1992). In 1984, the manufacturer of the fungicide dinocap canceled its use as a fungicide and an acaricide because it caused hydrocephaly in rabbits. In 1986, in developmental studies, dinocap was found to be teratogenic in mice at maternally non-toxic doses, caused cleft palate, exencephaly and extra ribs, as well as reduced fetal weight and increased fetal death. Another compound, chlorothalonil, was not a developmental toxicant (Parsons, 2001).

Chloroalkylthiodicarboximides (phthalimides)

This class of chemicals includes broad spectrum fungicides such as captan, captafol and folpet. They are usually nontoxic to mammals. Folpet induces incidences of diarrhea, vomiting, salivation, reduced food intake and reduced body weight gain. Testes weights are reduced in dogs. Captan, captafol and the ammonium salt of alkyldithiocarbamic acid induced multiple defects in various experimental species. Captan was teratogenic in rabbits and hamsters and induced CNS and rib defects, but was not teratogenic in mice, rats or primates. In the dog, there were variable results. Folpet and captafol in hamsters caused CNS, tail and rib defects following a single oral dose to the mother during gestation but had no teratogenic potential in rats, mice, rabbits and primates (Vondruska *et al.*, 1971; Kennedy *et al.*, 1972; Schardein, 2000).

Anilinopyrimidines

The nilinopyrimidine class of fungicides includes cyprodinil, mepanipyrim and pyrimethanil. In general, anilinopyrimidines are unlikely to present an acute hazard in normal use.

They do not induce adverse effects on developmental systems (Waechter *et al.*, 2001).

Carbamic acid derivatives or dialkyldithiocarbamates (EBDCs)

The carbamic acid class of fungicides includes dithiocarbamates (ferbam, thiram, ziram, propamocarb) and ethylenebisdithiocarbamates (EBDCs) such as maneb, mancozeb, zineb, nabam, metiram, etc. These fungicides alter thyroid hormone levels and/or weights. The reproductive system is generally unaffected by exposure to EBDCs {common metabolite, ethylenethiourea (ETU)}. The developmental toxicity included malformations and embryo-fetotoxic effects at maternally toxic dose levels with EBDCs in rats (Ollinger *et al.*, 2001). Exposure to ETU at the critical stages of pregnancy produced malformations in rats, predominantly those of the CNS. Sensitivity varied with species. Mice and rabbits are less sensitive. The malformations produced by ETU exposure *in vivo* were those expected as a result of thyroid insufficiency. The malformations have been prevented by coadministration of thyroxine (Emmerling, 1978). Guinea pigs and cats did not show any evidence of teratogenic or other developmental toxicity (Khera, 1987).

Different studies conducted on 2-imidazolidinethione, a plant metabolite of fungicide maneb, and other related fungicides such as mancozeb, showed different malformations in different species of experimental animals. Rabbits and mice were resistant to oral doses, whereas cleft palate, tail and digital defects, and anal atresia were observed in hamster embryos (Teramoto *et al.*, 1978). Ethylenethiuram monosulfide, the degradation product of the fungicide maneb, and parent compounds such as zineb and maneb, were teratogenic in rats but not in mice (Vergieva, 1984). Ferbam increased the incidence of soft tissue and skeletal abnormalities in rats but not in mice. Thiram induced cleft palate in one study and developmental toxicity in another study. In hamsters and rabbits, thiram induced multiple malformations including skeletal and tail defects, whereas no such malformations have been reported in rats (Schardein, 2000).

Benzimidazoles

The major benzimidazole fungicides include benomyl, carbendazim and fuberidazole. Benomyl and carbendazim have a low toxicity, whereas fuberidazole has a moderate toxicity. Benomyl, captan, ammonium salt of alkyldithiocarbamic acid and carbendazim all induced multiple defects in various experimental species. The fungicide benomyl produced skeletal malformations and increased mortality in rats and multiple anomalies in mice when given orally during organogenesis. Benomyl was not teratogenic in rats and rabbits (Munley and Hurtt, 1996), whereas teratogenic studies with captan have been variable in animals. Captan was not teratogenic in mice, rats or primates. Some investigators have reported CNS and rib defects, whereas in another study, limb, head and cleft lip have been reported (McLaughlin *et al.*, 1969; Gordon, 2001). In the dog, there were variable results. Carbendazim was teratogenic in rats. High oral doses produced limb malformations, whereas lower doses caused alterations in postnatal behavior, postnatal reflex and open-field behavior (Schardein, 2000).

Conazoles

The conazole class of fungicides includes cyproconazole, diniconazole, triadimefon, triadimenol, propiconazole, imazalil, etc. and has low to moderate acute toxicity. Developmental toxicity indicates increased ovary and testes weights, increased supernumerary lumbar ribs with triadimenol, increased scapula malformations at maternal toxic doses in rabbits after triadimefon. Following long-term exposure, propiconazole causes liver hypertrophy and tumors in mice, uterine lumen dilation in rats and developmental toxicity indicative of reduced pup weight at parentally toxic doses and skeletal variations in laboratory animals (JMPR, 2004).

Morpholines

The class of morpholine fungicides includes dodemorph, fenpropimorph and tridemorph. These compounds are unlikely to cause acute hazards, except tridemorph which is moderately hazardous. Fenpropimorph is a mild irritant to rabbit skin. Tridemorph and fenpropimorph lead to developmental toxicity with an increase in the total number of malformations (JMPR, 2004).

Amides

Commonly used amide fungicides are fenhexamid, benalaxyl, metalaxyl, flutolanil, tolylfluanid and dichlofluanid. These compounds are of low toxicity, with the exception of metalaxyl, which is slightly hazardous. In mice, increased mortality associated with amyloidosis has been observed. Reproductive abnormalities in rats included decreased body weight gain, increased liver weight of pups and delayed ossification of cranial bones. Minor skeletal deviations at maternally toxic levels have been reported in rabbits. Tolylfluanid induced alterations in the levels of thyroid hormones in a number of studies conducted in rats. The compound caused decreased pup viability at maternally toxic doses but was not teratogenic (JMPR, 2002). Another compound, fenhexamid, resulted in delayed ossification in rabbits but was not teratogenic (JMPR, 2005).

Others

The fungicide cycloheximide is extremely toxic and no longer available. Following parenteral administration, cycloheximide has been shown to cause skeletal defects and dactyly in mice. Polycarbacin was embryotoxic and induced malformations. Probineb caused tail and developmental anomalies and flusilazole caused eye, jaw, tongue and palate defects in rat fetuses (Lary and Hood, 1978). Fludioxonil and trifloxystrobin have a low acute toxicity in rats. Following long-term exposure, fludioxonil caused decreased pup weight gains in rats at paternally toxic doses. Trifloxystrobin induced developmental toxicity as evidenced by decreased body weight gain of pups, accompanied by delayed eye opening at parental toxic doses (JMPR, 2004).

TABLE 39.6 Non-exhaustive list of fungicides responsible for reproductive problems/malformations in humans

Chemical	Location	Year	Reproductive abnormalities
Methyl mercury	Japan, New Mexico, Iraq, Sweden, and the USSR	1953 and subsequent years	Disrupts CNS developmental processes in the unborn and infants
Benomyl	England and Wales	1990s	Tetramelia, eye defects, miscarriages, premature delivery and infants with congenital anomalies
Captan and/or with other pesticides	England	1990s	Miscarriages, premature delivery and infants with congenital anomalies
Hexacholorobenzene	Turkey	1955–1957	Stillbirths and neonatal mortality
Zineb		1970s	Reproductive problems

Epidemiological evidence

The epidemiological survey has revealed that exposure to fungicides causes developmental toxicity in humans. A non-exhautive list of fungicides responsible for reproductive problems/malformations in human beings is summarized in Table 39.6.

In the past, the metal mercury was used as a fungicide, but is now banned. Inorganic mercury discharged into rivers, lakes and oceans undergoes microbial conversion to the methyl form of organic mercury by methanogenic bacteria present in the bottom of bodies of water. This form tends to accumulate in the aquatic food chain (Dwivedi and Iannaccone, 1998). In 1953 the waste from a fertilizer manufacturing plant was dumped into Minamata Bay in southern Japan and accumulated in fish that were a staple in the local diet. The effects of methyl mercury poisoning come primarily from epidemic poisonings in Iraq and Japan. In Iraq more than 6,000 individuals were hospitalized and 459 died as a result of methyl mercury poisoning. The Japan and Iraq epidemics have clearly established mercury as an agent that can disrupt developmental processes in the unborn and infant populations. Researchers have also observed a heightened incidence of cerebral palsy in children born to mothers in the Minamata Bay area (Matsumoto *et al.*, 1965). The compound crosses the placenta and has proven to be a potent teratogen. It includes a number of abnormalities, especially of the central nervous system. Methyl mercury was the cause of birth defects and neurological deficits in Minamata disease (Takeuchi, 1966). A large number of a population showed neurological symptoms, microcephaly, cerebral palsy and abnormal dentition from prenatal exposure at 6–8 months of gestation. Subsequently, the exposure of mothers in New Mexico, Iraq, Sweden and the USSR to methyl mercury was through the food chain, and about 150 cases of fetal Minamata disease were reported (Murakami, 1972). Children born to mercury-poisoned mothers were of a smaller, total weight, had decreased brain weights at birth with fewer nerve cells in the cerebral cortex, and experienced an abnormal pattern of neuronal migration. Many of the children that survived the epidemic experienced severe developmental effects throughout their childhood, such as impaired motor and mental function, hearing loss and blindness (Amin-Zaki *et al.*, 1974).

In addition to malformations due to mercury, the fungicide benomyl caused tetramelia in women exposed to the chemical in England. Infants born had anophthalmia or related eye defects. In females exposed to captan, infants with congenital anomalies were increased. Concurrent exposure of captan and benomyl increased the frequency of miscarriages and premature delivery. In another case, a child born from a female engaged in the spraying operation of captan and other pesticides had small size arms and legs (Restrepo *et al.*, 1990; Lappe, 1991).

In Turkey in 1955–1957 reproduction abnormalities due to HCB were reported in pregnant women who had been ingesting 50–200 mg of HCB in flour from treated grains. There were no malformations; however, there were increased stillbirths and neonatal mortality, without any apparent signs of toxicity in the mother (Cam, 1960). In a survey of women occupationally exposed to zineb there was an increased incidence of reproductive problems (Makletsova and Lanivoi, 1981). In another survey the thyroid function of formulators exposed to a combination of pesticides indicated suppression of total T3 and a marginal decrease (7%) in T4 level. Thyroid stimulating hormone (TSH) levels were also elevated by 28%, but the increase was statistically insignificant. There was an increase in the incidence of reproductive abnormalities as compared to unexposed workers (Rupa *et al.*, 1991; Zaidi *et al.*, 2000).

ENDOCRINE DISRUPTION

The ultimate aim of reproduction is birth and it depends upon both male and female reproductive systems. However, the initiation and maintenance of milk production (lactation) for the postparturition of the offspring can also be considered a critical aspect of mammalian reproduction (Evans *et al.*, 2007). In males, normal reproductive function involves interaction of the hypothalamic–pituitary–testis axis and the thyroid gland (Johnson *et al.*, 1997). Chemicals that are toxic to endocrine cells and that deplete germ cells are beyond the scope of this chapter. Chemicals listed in Table 39.7 are representative of those that affect male reproduction through different mechanisms of actions by endocrine disruption.

TCDD is lipophilic, relatively resistant to metabolism and it accumulates in human and animal tissues (Peterson *et al.*, 1993). During pregnancy, and to a greater extent during lactation, a portion of the maternal body burden of these chemicals is transferred to the offspring. The chemical acts as an aryl hydrocarbon receptor agonist (AhR mechanism) and leads to a reduction of prostate growth, cauda epididymus and ejaculated sperm numbers. The mechanism underlying the spectrum of male reproductive effects caused by *in utero* and lactation exposure to TCDD is poorly understood at the molecular level. Although thyroid hormones have historically not been considered a

TABLE 39.7 Non-exhaustive list of herbicides and fungicides with known or suspected endocrine disrupting properties, mechanisms and effects on the male reproductive system in experimental animals

Class of endocrine disruptor	Examples
Reproductive endocrine disruptors	
Antiestrogens (ER-mediated or aromatase inhibition)	TCDD*, downregulates ER and increases estrogen metabolism (mammals, birds and fish), fenarimol, prochloraz, chlorthalonil, glyphosate
Antiandrogens (Ar-mediated or 5 alpha reductase inhibition)	Procymidone, vinclozolin metabolites
Aryl hydrocarbon receptor (AhR) agonists (AhR-mediated)	TCDD (mammals, birds and fish) Dibenzofuran and biphenyl congeners
Toxicants that inhibit hormone production	TCDD (inhibits testosterone synthesis in adult male rats)
Toxicants that alter hormonal status by depleting germ cells	Dibromochloropropane (kills germ cells) (mammals)
Antithyroid endocrine disruptors	
Antithyroid endocrine disruptors	Ethylene thiourea, linuron, TCDD, polychlorinated dibenzofurans, polychlorinated biphenyls, nitrofen (mammals)

Compiled from Richard *et al.* (1997), Derfoul *et al.* (2003), Svechnikov *et al.* (2005), Ankley (2005) and Noriega *et al.* (2005)
ER, estrogen receptor; AhR (Aryl hydrocarbon receptor); Ar = Alpha reductase
*Common contaminant of 2,4-D, 2,4,5-T and Silvex

major factor in male reproduction, recent studies indicate that these hormones are important regulators of testicular development (Mably *et al.*, 1992; Roman *et al.*, 1995). Female pups prenatally exposed to the compound showed moderately decreased levels of plasma T4 at weaning. In certain studies, this led to an increase in TSH levels, which may play an important role in thyrotoxicity of these chemicals (i.e., goiter). In another study, mixtures of Aroclor decreased (80–90%) serum T4 in developing rats. Herbicides such as linuron or decomposition products of ethylenethiourea also produced hypothyroidism. Ethylenethiourea is structurally related to goitrogens such as propylthiouracil (PTU) and produced hypothyroidism by directly impairing T4 production. Maternal ingestion of Aroclor 1254 increased neonatal thyroid weight (Birnbaum, 1998).

Anderson *et al.* (2002) demonstrated that fenarimol caused infertility in male rats by inhibiting aromatization of testosterone to 17 beta estradiol within the brain. Fenarimol acted as an estrogen agonist and an androgen antagonist and, in addition, inhibited aromatase activity in human placental microsomes. Normal aromatization is essential for masculinization of the male rodent CNS and for the development of normal male mating berhavior. Prochloraz significantly inhibited aromatase activity, and chlorothalonil inhibited greater than 50%. One molecular target of the endocrine effects in the placenta may be intracellular calcium homeostasis since estrogenic fungicides change calcium handling by trophoblasts and this effect may be endocrinally controlled (Derfoul *et al.*, 2003). These compounds act through inhibition of CYP450 enzymes involved in steroid metabolism and alter sexual differentiation through antagonism of the androgen receptor(s) (Ankley *et al.*, 2005; Noriega *et al.*, 2005).

The fungicide vinclozolin has been shown to have endocrine-modulating effects in male rat offspring when dams were treated during the last one-third of gestation through postnatal day 3. The anogenital distance was reduced and there were cleft palates, hypospadias and other reproductive malformations (Gray *et al.*, 1994). Procymidone has anti-androgenic properties. Chronic exposure of rats to procymidone had different effects on the pituitary–gonadal axis *in vivo* and on Leydig cell steroidogenesis *ex vivo*. The disruption of hormonal feedback could be due to its anti-androgenic action through activation of endocrine axis, thereby causing hypergonadotropic activation of the testicular steroidogenesis (Svechnikov et al., 2005). No change in plasma testosterone concentrations or in parameters of daily sperm production, sperm reserves in the epididymis, sperm morphology or measured components of male sexual behavior were observed after diuron (Glaura *et al.*, 2007).

The herbicide glyphosate in low non-toxic concentrations caused disruption of the aromatase enzyme in human placental cells *in vitro*. It reduced the aromatase enzyme activity responsible for the synthesis of estrogens (Richard *et al.*, 2005). Recent studies indicate that male reproductive toxicity of glyphosate is due to the inhibition of a StAR protein and an aromatase enzyme, which caused an *in vitro* reduction in testosterone and estradiol synthesis. The study suggested that the commercial formulation of glyphosate (Roundup, Monsanto Co.) is a potent endocrine disruptor *in vivo* which caused disturbances in the reproductive development of rats when the exposure was performed during puberty (Romano *et al.*, 2010).

In females, normal reproductive function involves appropriate interactions of the CNS, anterior pituitary, oviducts, uterus, cervix and ovaries. There are relatively few studies addressing the possibility that these tissues serve as the primary target sites for environmental toxicants. There are several reasons for this lack of information. The majority of in-depth studies evaluating the effects of environmental toxicants on reproductive function have focused on the male. In females, increased concentrations of xenoestrogens may affect ovarian function through the disruption of feedback mechanisms in the hypothalamus–pituitary–gonadal axis (Flaws and Hirshfield, 1997; Bretveld, 2006). Both herbicides and fungicides, like other chemicals, may disrupt all stages of hormonal function of the female reproductive system and, in particular, the ovarian cycle. In many studies, the mechanisms were either not specified or were described for effects of these chemicals on cell culture studies (*in vitro*) and on experimental animal studies (*in vivo*) (Bretveld, 2006). The possible mechanisms of endocrine disruption that provide the first indications of potential effects on the female reproductive system in more general terms are summarized in Table 39.8.

Earlier studies dealing with the mechanism of action had revealed that high doses of TCDD modulate the activity of multiple endocrine systems, including both steroid and peptide hormones in females. TCDD has antiestrogenic action,

TABLE 39.8 Herbicides and fungicides with known or suspected endocrine disrupting properties, mechanisms and effects on the female reproductive system in experimental models

Chemicals	Mechanism(s)	Effects in experimental animals
Alachlor	– binding and activating the estrogen receptor – binding other receptors	unknown
Amitraz	– interference with hormone storage and release	unknown
Atrazine	– interference with hormone synthesis – binding without activating the estrogen receptor – modulation of hormone concentrations	ovarian cycle irregularities
Biphenyl	– binding other receptors	unknown
Chlorophenoxy acids	– interference with overall metabolic rate	unknown
Diaminochlorotriazine	– binding without activating the estrogen receptor	unknown
Fenarimol	– interference with hormone synthesis – binding and activating the estrogen receptor – binding other receptors	impaired fertility
Iprodion	– interference with hormone synthesis	unknown
Ketaconazole	– interference with hormone synthesis	unknown
Linuron	– binding other receptors – unknown	unknown
Mancozeb	– unknown	ovarian cycle irregularities impaired fertility
Pirimicarb	– interference with hormone synthesis	unknown
Prochloraz	– interference with hormone synthesis – binding without activating the estrogen receptor – binding other receptors	unknown
Procymidone	– binding other receptors	unknown
Propamocarb	– interference with hormone synthesis	unknown
Propazine	– interference with hormone synthesis	unknown
Simazine	– interference with hormone synthesis – binding without activating the estrogen receptor	modulation of hormone concentrations
Sodium-N-methyl- dithiocarbamate	– interference with hormone synthesis	ovarian cycle irregularities
TCDD[8]	– hormone receptor activation	unknown
Thiram	– interference with hormone synthesis – interference with hormone storage and release	ovarian cycle irregularities
Triadimefon	– binding and activating the estrogen receptor	unknown
Triadimenol	– binding and activating the estrogen receptor	unknown
Vinclozolin	– binding other receptors	unknown

Compiled from Bretveld *et al.* (2006)
[*]TCDD, a common contaminant of phenoxy acid herbicides

causing a decreased number of estrogen receptors in the immature uterus and breast tissues. Mink are extremely sensitive to dioxin-induced reproductive toxicity. Many of the malformations observed following *in utero* and lactational exposure to TCDD in female rats and hamsters are "estrogen-like" (Birnbaum, 1998). Large doses of Aroclor 1242 or 1254, which have been shown to have estrogenic activity in the rat, failed to induce implantation in the hypophysectomized P_4-primed delayed implanting rat. These weak estrogen-like compounds were perhaps unable to reach the threshold level of estrogenic action required for implantation (Das *et al.*, 1997). Chemicals such as fenarimol, prochloraz and other imidazoles decreased estrogen biosynthesis through CYP450-19 aromatase inhibition *in vitro*, preventing the conversion of androgens to estrogens. Ketaconazole inhibited various enzymes which belong to the CYP450-dependent monooxygenases and also inhibited progesterone synthesis. Atrazine, simazine and propazine (2-chloro-triazine herbicides) induced aromatase activity *in vitro*. The compounds methomyl, pirimicarb, propamocarb and iprodion weakly stimulated aromatase activity, whereas thiram, sodium *N*-methyldithiocarbamate (SMD) and other dithiocarbamates suppressed the dopamine-*beta*-hydroxylase activity leading to a reduced conversion of dopamine to norepinephrine. This has led to changes in hypothalamic catecholamine activity involved in generating the proestrus surge in LH and has stimulated the final stages of ovulation (Goldman *et al.*, 1994; Gray *et al.*, 1999; Anderson *et al.*, 2002). Chlordimeform and amitraz (acaricide) blocked norepinephrine binding to the alpha 2-adrenoreceptors. Norepinephrine is critical for the preovulatory increase in the pulsatile release of GnRH and the subsequent ovulatory surge of LH. Thiram suppressed the proestrus surge of LH and delayed ovulation in the female rat (Stoker *et al.*, 1996, 2001). Atrazine, simazine and diaminochlorotriazine expressed antiestrogenic activity in uteri of female rats without expressing intrinsic estrogenic activity, but the precise mechanism is not known. Vinclozolin and two of its metabolites bind to the androgen receptor and act as androgen receptor antagonists *in vitro* and *in vivo*. Procymidone, linuron and biphenol act as androgen antagonists *in vitro* and/or *in vivo*. The presence of a potent androgen antagonist in a sufficient internal dose may create an overall estrogenic effect. Prochloraz acts as estrogen and androgen antagonist (Kelce *et al.*, 1997; Sohoni and Sumpter, 1998; Ostby *et al.*, 1999; Vinggaard *et al.*, 1999a,b; Lambright *et al.*, 2000; Gray *et al.*, 2001; Anderson *et al.*, 2002). A few other chemicals or their metabolites have been reported to possess estrogenicity *in vivo*, e.g. fenarimol, triadimefon, triadimenol, methiocarb, pentachrophenol, nonylphenol, alachlor and sumithrin. Some of them are weakly estrogenic, but may have additive effects in combination. When mixed together, they may induce estrogenic responses at concentrations lower than those required when each compound is administered alone (Vinggaard *et al.*, 1999a,b; Bretveld, 2006).

The effect of these chemicals on ovarian cycle irregularities include disturbances in the ovarian cycle (e.g., longer cycle, persistent estrus) and ovulation problems (deferred ovulation or anovulation). In most studies, the effects still remain unknown. For example, atrazine, an antagonist of the estradiol receptor, altered estrus cyclicity in rats, caused an extension of the estrus cycle and increased the number of days in estrus. The compounds HCB, mancozeb and 3,3′,4,4′-tetrachloroazoxybenzene decreased the number of estrus cycles and increased the duration of diestrus. Exposure to mancozeb led to a decrease in the number of healthy follicles and an increase in the number of atretic follicles, a decrease in uterine weight as well as the number of implantations. Atrazine in rats caused anovulation. Thiram and sodium *N*-methyldithiocarbamate inhibited ovulation that was related to the suppression of LH secretion. Fenarimol was found to cause a dose-related decrease in fertility in rats. However, in most of the studies it is still unknown whether impaired fertility is due to a hormonal imbalance or is related to other toxic effects of these chemicals (Foster *et al.*, 1995; Baligar and Kaliwal, 2001, 2002; Bindali and Kaliwal, 2002; Pocar *et al.*, 2003; Bretveld *et al.*, 2006).

From the experimental studies, it has been concluded that both herbicides and fungicides can disturb reproduction and developmental processes of both males and females through endocrine signals in organisms indirectly exposed during prenatal or early postnatal life. Such effects during development are permanent and irreversible. They may act through hormone receptors and enhance or diminish the activity normally controlled by endogenous hormones. These chemicals influence virtually every aspect of the mammalian reproductive process by effecting the morphology and physiology of reproductive organs and by causing alterations in sexual behavior (Chaplin *et al.*, 1996).

According to one estimate in 2003, approximately 60 chemicals were identified as endocrine disruptors, exogenous agents that interfere with various aspects of natural hormone physiology. Most of these were identified accidentally rather than as a result of an exhaustive screening process (Pocar *et al.*, 2003). Out of these, 16 chemicals are herbicides and fungicides shown in Table 39.9.

It is likely that the number of chemicals having endocrine disruptor properties has increased. Several chemicals are still under investigation. Although a substantial amount of research has been conducted to associate occupational exposure to herbicides and fungicides (phenoxy herbicides, triazines, glyphosate, thiocarbamates) with fertility problems in men, studies on women are scarce. However, epidemiological studies have revealed that exposure to pesticides has been associated with menstrual cycle disturbances, reduced fertility, prolonged time-to-pregnancy, spontaneous abortion, reduced fecundity, stillbirths and developmental defects, which may or may not be due to disruption of the female hormonal function. Since several phases under endocrine control (e.g., parturition) are different between humans and rodents, direct extrapolation of findings may be difficult (Gupta, 2004; Rescia and Mantovani, 2007).

TABLE 39.9 Common herbicides and fungicides known as or suspected to be endocrine disruptors

Herbicides	Fungicides
2,4-D	Benomyl
2,4,5-T	Hexachlorobenzene
Alachlor	Mancozeb
Amitrole	Maneb
Atrazine	Metriam complex
Metribuzin	Tributyltin
Trifluralin	Zineb
Nitrofen	Ziram

Compiled from Pocar *et al.* (2003)
2,4-D = Dichlorophenoxyacetic acid
2,4,5-T = Trichlorophenoxyacetic acid

CONCLUDING REMARKS AND FUTURE DIRECTIONS

Numerous chemicals including herbicides and fungicides are ubiquitous in the environment. Some of them obviously offer the potential for reproductive and developmental toxicity. Despite their wide use, little attention has been given to their health effects among animal and human populations. During the dynamic process of mammalian development, physiological, functional and morphological changes occur rapidly in spatial and temporal patterns that may influence the potential effects of harmful chemicals in very different ways. Therefore, the determination of cause(s) of reproductive developmemtal and fetotoxicity is extremely complex due to the maternal responses to multiple chemicals, numerous compounding factors and the dynamic changes taking place in the fetus and placenta. The specific cellular pathways activated by these compounds are still unclear. Furthermore, the lack of information on the metabolism and tissue distribution of these chemicals, which greatly depends on species physiology, concentrations and duration of exposure, as well as interactions between single components of the complex mixtures present in the environment, further complicate the conclusions drawn from such studies. In view of developmental toxicity, several herbicides and fungicides have been deregistered or banned in many countries; however, some of them are still in use in other less regulated parts of the world. Some of the synthetic herbicides and fungicides are undergoing re-evaluation because of suspected reproductive and developmental toxicants. However, epidemiological studies clearly indicate that exposure to these chemicals may be associated with menstrual cycle disturbances, reduced fertility, prolonged time-to-pregnancy, spontaneous abortions, stillbirths and developmental defects. In most of these studies, specific information on pesticide exposure and the pathophysiological mechanisms involved is missing. Since most of the data presently available have been derived from experiments performed on laboratory species or *in vitro* models, extrapolations to other species or situations should be done with caution.

REFERENCES

Al-Thani RK, Al-Thani AS, Ahmed E, Darmani H (2003) Assessment of reproductive and fertility effects of amitraz pesticide in male mice. *Toxicol Lett* **138:** 253–60.

Amin-Zaki L, Elhassani S, Majeed MA, Clarkson TW, Doherty RA, Greenwood M (1974) Intrauterine methyl mecury poisoning in Iraq. *Pediatrics* **54:** 587–95.

Anderson HR, Vinggaard AM, Rasmussen TH, Gjermandsen IM, Bonefeld-Jorgensen EC (2002) Effects of currently used pesticides in assays for estrogenicity, androgenicity, and aromatase activity *in vitro*. *Toxicol Appl Pharmacol* **179:** 1–12.

Ankley GT, Kathleen M, Jensen KM, Durhan EJ Makynen EA, Butterworth BC, Kahl MD, Villeneuve DL, Linnum A, Gray LE, Cardon M, Wilson VS (2005) Effects of two fungicides with multiple modes of action on reproductive endocrine function in the fathead minnow (*Pimephales promelas*). *Toxicol Sci* **86:** 300–8.

Baligar PN, Kaliwal BB (2001) Induction of gonadal toxicity to female rats after chronic exposure to mancozeb. *Indl Hlth* **39:** 235–43.

Baligar PN, Kaliwal BB (2002) Reproductive toxicity of carbofuran to the female mice: effects on estrous cycle and follicles. *Indl Hlth* **40:** 345–52.

Bindali BB, Kaliwal BB (2002). Anti-implantation effect of a carbamate fungicide mancozeb in albino mice. *Indl Hlth* **40:** 191–7.

Birnbaum LS (1998) Development effects of dioxins. In *Reproductive and Development Toxicoloy* (Korach KS, ed.). Marcell Dekker, Inc., New York, USA, pp. 87–112.

Bjerke DL, Peterson RE (1994) Reproductive toxicity of 2,3,7,8-tetrachlorodibenzo-*p*-dioxin in male rats: defferent effecs of *in utero* versus lactational exposure. *Toxicol Appl Pharmacol* **127:** 241–9.

Boekelheide K, Robert C, Patricia H, Craig H (1997) *Comprehensive Toxicology: Reproductive and Endocrine Toxicology*, Vol. 10. Pergamon, Elsevier Science, Inc., USA.

Bretveld RW, Thomas C, Scheepers MG, Zielhuis PTJGA, Roeleveld N (2006). Pesticide exposure: the hormonal function of the female reproductive system disrupted. *Reprod Biol Endocrinol* **4:** 30–43.

Bus JS, Gibson JE (1975) Postnatal toxicity of chronically administered paraquat in mice and interactions with oxygen and bromobenzene. *Toxicol Appl Pharmacol* **33:** 461–70.

Buschmann J, Clausing P, Salecki E, Fischer B, Peetz U (1986) Comparative prenatal toxicity of phenoxy herbicides: effects on postnatal development and behavior in rats. *Teratology* **33:** 11A–12A.

Cam C (1960) Une nouvelle dermacose epidemique des enfants. *Ann Dermatol* **87:** 393–7.

Carter SD, Hess RA, Laskey JW (1987) The fungicide methyl 2-benzimidazole carbamate causes infertility in male Sprague-Dawley rats. *Biol. Reprod* **37:** 709–17.

Casey PH, Collie WR (1984) Severe mental retardation and multiple congenital anomalies of uncertain cause after extreme prenatal exposure to 2,4-D. *J Pediatr* **104:** 313–15.

Chaplin RE, Steven JT, Hughes CL, Kelce WR, Hess RA, Daston GP (1996) Endocrine modulation of reproduction. *Fund Appl Toxicol* **29:** 1–27.

Charles JM, Cunny HC, Wilson RD, Bus JS (1996) Comparative subchronic study on 2,4,dichlorophenoxyacetic acid, amine, and ester in rats. *Fundam Appl Toxicol* **33:** 161–5.

Chen RP, Chen T, Yu SY, Gu LJ, Zhang X (2007) Comparison of reproductive toxicity of several herbicides on testes of mice. *Huanjing yu Zhiye Yixue* **24:** 522–3.

Cooper RL (1997) Neuroendocrine control of female reoroduction. In *Comprehensive Toxicology. Reproductive and Endocrine Toxicology*, Vol. 10 (Boekelheide K, Chapin R, Hoyer P, Harris C, eds.). Pergamon, Elsevier Science, Inc., USA, pp. 273–81.

Cooper RL, Stoker TE, Goldman JM, Parish MB, Tyrey L (1996) Effect of atrazine on ovarian function in the rat. *Reprod Toxicol* **10:** 257–64.

Courtney KD, Copeland MF, Robbins A (1976) The effect of pentachoronitrobenzene, hexacholorobenzene, and related compounds on fetal development. *Toxicol Appl Pharmacol* **35:** 239–56.

Courtsey KD (1977) Prenatal effects of herbicides: evaluation by the prenatal development index. *Arch Environ Contam Toxicol* **6:** 33–46.

Courtsey KD, Moore JA (1971) Teratology studies with 2,4,5-trichlorophenoxyacetic acid and 2,3,7,8-tetracholorodibenzo-*p*-dioxin. *Toxicol Appl Pharmacol* **20:** 396–403.

Das SK, Paria BC, Johnson DC, Dey SK (1997) Embryo-uterine interactions during implantation: potential sites of interference by environmental toxins. In *Comprehensive Toxicology. Reproductive and Endocrine Toxicology*, Vol. 10 (Boekelheide K, Chapin R, Hoyer P, Harris C, eds.). Pergamon, Elsevier Science, Inc., USA, pp. 317–27.

Dayan FE, Romagni JG, Duke SO (2001) Protophyrinogen oxidase inhibitors. In *Handbook of Pesticide Toxicology*, 2nd edition, Vol. 2 (Krieger R, ed.). Academic Press, San Diego, pp. 1529–41.

Derfoul A, Lin FJ, Awumey EM, Kolodzeski T, Hall DJ, Tuan RS (2003) Estrogenic endocrine distruptive components interfere with calcium handling and differentiation of human tropoblast cells. *J Cell Biochem* **89:** 755–70.

Dickson D (1979) Herbicide claimed responsible for birth defects. *Nature* **282:** 230.

Dilley JV, Chernoff N, Kay D, Winslow N, Newell W (1977) Inhalation teratology studies of five chemicals in rats. *Toxicol Appl Pharmacol* **41:** 196.

Dwivedi RS, Iannaccone PM (1998) Effects of environmental chemicals on early development. In *Reproductive and Development Toxicology* (Korach KS, ed.). Marcell Dekker, Inc., New York, USA, pp. 11–46.

Elkington J (1985) *The Poisoned Womb: Human Reproduction in a Polluted World.* Penguin Books, Harmondsworth, England.

Emmerling DC (1978) The effects of thyroid hormones on the teratogenic potential of ethylenethioureas in rats. Report from Battelle Laboratories, Columbus, USA.

EPA (1979). Six years spontaneous abortion rates in Oregon areas in relation to forest 2,4,5-T spray practices. Epidemiology Studies Division, US EPA February 1979.

EPA (1993) Interim report on data and methods for assessment of 2,3,7,8-tetrachlorodibenzo-*p*-dioxin risks to aquatic life and associated wildlife. Office of Research and Development, Environmental Research Laboratory at Duluth, MN. EPA /600/R-93/055.

EPA (1997a) Cloransulam-methyl: Pesticide Fact Sheet. OPPTS, 7501 C, USA.

EPA (1997b) Cloransulam-methyl: Pesticide Tolerances. 40 CR 180. *Federal Register* 62 (182). 49158 (Friday, November 20, 1998), USA.

Evans TJ, Constantinescu GM, Ganjam VK (2007) Clinical reproductive anatomy and physiology of the mare. In *Current Veterinary Therapy Large Animal Theriogenology*, 2nd edition (Youhquist RS, Threlfall WR, eds.). Saunders Elsevier, St. Louis, pp. 47–67.

Farmer D (2001) Inhibitors of aromatic acid biosynthesis. In *Handbook of Pesticide Toxicology*, 2nd edition, Vol. 2 (Krieger R, ed.). Academic Press, San Diego, pp. 1667–71.

Fernandes GSA, Arena AC, Fernandez CDB, Mercadante A, Barbisan LF, Kempinas GWG (2007) Reproductive effects in male rats exposed to diuron. *Reprod Toxicol* **23:** 106–12.

Flaws JA, Hirshfield AN (1997) Reproductive, development, and endocine toxicology. In *Comprehensive Toxicology: Reproductive and Endocrine Toxicology*, Vol 10 (Boekelheide K, Chapin R, Hoyer P, Harris C, eds.). Pergamon, Elsevier Science, Inc., USA, pp. 283–91.

Foster WG, McMahon A, Younglai EV, Jarrell JF, Lecavalier P (1995) Alterations in circulating ovarian steroids in hexachlorobenzene exposed monkeys. *Reprod Toxicol* **9:** 541–8.

Gaines IB, Holson JF, Nelson CJ, Schumacher HJ (1975) Analysis of strain differences in sensitivity and reproducibility of results in assessing 2,4,5-T tertogenicity in mice. *Toxicol Appl Pharmacol* **33:** 174–5.

Gammon DW, Moore TB, O'Malley MA (2001) A toxicological assessment of sulfur as a pesticide. In *Handbook of Pesticide Toxicology*, 2nd edition, Vol. 2 (Krieger R, ed.). Academic Press, San Diego, pp. 1781–91.

Glaura SA, Fernandes ACA, Fernandez CDB, Mercadante A, Barbisan LF, Kempinas WG (2007) Reproductive effects in male rats exposed to diuron *Reprod Toxicol* **23:** 106–12.

Goldey ES, Tayler DH (1992) Development neurotoxicity following premating maternal exposure to hexacholorobenzene in rats. *Neurotoxicol Teratol* **14:** 15–21.

Goldman JM, Stoker TE, Cooper RL, McElroy WK, Hein JF (1994) Blockade of ovulation in the rat by the fungicide sodium N-methyldithiocarbamate: relationship between effects on the luteinizing hormone surge and alterations in hypothalamic catecholamines. *Neurotoxicol Teratol* **16:** 257–68.

Gordon EB (2001) Captan and folpet. In *Handbook of Pesticide Toxicology*, 2nd edition, Vol. 2 (Krieger R, ed.). Academic Press, San Diego, pp. 1711–42.

Gray LE (1997) Chemically induced alterations of reproductive development in female mammals. In *Comprehensive Toxicology: Reproductive and Endocrine Toxicology*, Vol. 10 (Boekelheide K, Chapin R, Hoyer P, Harris C, eds.). Pergamon, Elsevier Science, Inc., USA, pp. 329–38.

Gray LE, Ostby J, Furr J, Wolf CJ, Lambright C, Parks L, Veeramachaneni DN, Wilson V, Price M, Hotchkiss A, Orlando E, Guillette L (2001) Effects of environmental antiandrogens on reproductive development in experimental animals. *Hum Reprod Updat* **7:** 248–64.

Gray LE, Ostby JS, Kelce WR (1994) Developmental effects of an environmental antiandrogen; the fungicide vinclozin alters sex differentiation of the male rat. *Toxicol Appl Pharmacol* **129:** 46–52.

Gray LE Jr, Wolf C, Lambright C, Mann P, Price M, Cooper RL, Ostby J (1999) Administration of potentially antiandrogenic pesticides (procymidone, linuron, iprodione, chlozolinate, p,p′-DDE, and ketoconazole) and toxic substances (dibutyl- and diethylhexyl phthalate, PCB 169, and ethane dimethane sulphonate) during sexual differentiation produces diverse profiles of reproductive malformations in the male rat. *Toxicol Ind Health* **15:** 94–118.

Gupta PK (1984) Toxicology of pesticides: a review of the problem. In *Proc Sem Eff Pest Aq Fau* (Agarwal VS, Rana SV, eds.). Jagmander Book Agency, New Delhi, India, pp. 19–36.

Gupta PK (1985a) Pesticides. In *Modern Toxicology: Adverse Effects of Xenobiotics and Other Chemicals*, Vol. 2 (Gupta PK, Salunkhe DK, eds.). Metropolitan Book Co. Pvt Ltd, Delhi, India, pp. 1–60.

Gupta PK (1985b) Rural prosperity vis-à-vis hazards of pesticides. In *Environmental and Natural Resources* (Agarwal VS and Rana SV, eds.). Jagmander Book Agency, New Delhi, India, pp. 43–63.

Gupta PK (1986) *Pesticides in the Indian Environment*. Interprint. New Delhi, India.

Gupta PK (1987a) Environmental pollution of pesticides and associated health hazards. In *Science Development and Environment* (Agarwal VS, Rana SV, eds.). Jagmander Book Agency, New Delhi, India, pp. 47–57.

Gupta PK (1987b) Hazards of pesticides: developed vs developing countries In *Environment and Ecotocicology* (Dalela RC, Sahai VS, Gupta S, eds.). Academy of Environ Science, India, pp. 23–37.

Gupta PK (1988) *Veterinary Toxicology*. Cosmo Publications, New Delhi, India.

Gupta PK (1989) Pesticide production – an overview. In *Soil Pollution and Soil Organisms* (Mishra PC, ed.). Ashish Publishing House, New Delhi, India, pp. 1–16.

Gupta PK (1993) Environmental chemicals: problems associated with xenobiotics in livestock in developing countries. In *Environment Impact of Aquatic and Terrestrial Habbitats* (Agarwal VP, Abidi SAH, Verma GP, eds.). Society of Biosciences, Muzaffarnagar, India, pp. 237–92.

Gupta PK (2004) Pesticide exposure – Indian scene. *Toxicology* **198:** 83–90.

Gupta PK (2006a) WHO/FAO guidelines for cholinesterase-inhibiting pesticide residues in food. In *Toxicology of Organophosphate and Carbamate Compounds* (Gupta RC, ed.). Academic Press/Elsevier, Amsterdam, pp. 643–54.

Gupta PK (2006b) Status of biopesticides – Indian scene. *Toxicol Intl* **13:** 65–73.

Gupta PK (2007) Toxicity of herbicides. In *Veterinary Toxicology: Basic and Clinical Principles* (Gupta RC, ed.). Academic Press/Elsevier, Amsterdam, pp. 567–86.

Gupta PK (2010) Epidemiology of anticholinesterase pesticides: India. In *Anticholinesterase Pesticides: Metabolism, Neurotoxicity, and Epidemiology* (Satoh T, Gupta RC, eds.). John Wiley & Sons, USA.

Gupta PK, Agarwal M (2007) Toxicity of fungicides. In *Veterinary Toxicology: Basic and Clinical Principles* (Gupta RC, ed.). Academic Press/Elsevier, Amsterdam, pp. 587–601.

Gupta PK, Sanjay K (1988) Pesticide residues in India and future strategies for their monitoring. In *Advances in Toxicology* (Gupta PK, Ravi PV, eds.). Jagmander Book Agency, New Delhi, India, pp. 273–314.

Hall JG, Pallister PD, Clarren SK, Beckwith, JB, Wiglesworth, FW, Frazer FC, Cho S, Benke, PJ, Reed SD (1980) Congenital hypothalamic hematoblastoma, hypopituitarism, imperforate anus, and postaxial polydactyly – a new syndrome. Part 1: Clinical, causal and pathogenetic considerations. *Am J Med Genetic* **7:** 47–74.

Hanley TR Jr, Billington R (2001) Toxicology of triazolopyrimidine herbicides. In *Handbook of Pesticide Toxicology*, 2nd edition, Vol. 2 (Krieger R, ed). Academic Press, San Diego, pp. 1653–65.

Hanley TR, John-Greene JA, Hayes WC, Rao KS (1987) Embryotoxicity and fetotoxicity of orally administered tridiphane in mice and rats. *Fund Appl Toxicol* **8:** 179–87.

Harp P (2001) Dicamba. In *Handbook of Pesticide Toxicology*, 2nd edition, Vol. 2 (Krieger R, ed.). Academic Press, San Diego, pp. 1639–40.

Hendry WF, Levison DA, Parkinson MC, Parslow JM, Royle MG (1990) Testicular obstruction: clinicopathological studies. *Ann Royal Coll Surg Engl* **72:** 396–407.

Hess FG, Harris JE, Pendino K, Ponnock K (2001) Imidazolinones. In *Handbook of Pesticide Toxicology*, 2nd edition, Vol. 2 (Krieger R, ed.). Academic Press, San Diego, pp. 1641–52.

Hodge HC, Downs WL, Panner BS, Smith DW, Maynard EA (1968) Oral toxicity and metabolism of diuron (*N*-3,4-dichlorophenyl-*N′*,*N′*-dimethylurea) in rats and dogs. *Food Cosmet Toxicol* **5:** 513–31.

Hodgson E, Meyer SA (1997) Pesticides. In *Comprehensive Toxicology – Hepatic and Gastrointestinal Toxicology*, Vol. 9 (Sipes G, McQueen CA, Gandolfi J, eds.). Pergamon, Elsevier Science, Inc., USA, pp. 369–87.

Hoffman DJ, Rattner BA, Sileo L, Docherty D, Kubick TJ (1987) Embryotoxicity, teratogenicity and aryl hydrocarbon hydroxylase activity in Forster's terns on Green Bay, Lake Michigan. *Environ Res* **42:** 176–84.

Hong Mu , Zhang P, Jian Xu (2008) Testicular toxicity and mechanisms of chlorotoluron compounds in the mouse. *Toxicol Mechan Methods* **18:** 399–403.

Illio KY, Hess RA (1994) Structure and function of the ductuli efferentes: a review. *Microsc Res Tech* **29:** 432–67.

Jeffay S, Libbus B, Barbee R, Perreault S (1996) Acute exposure of female hamsters to carbendazim (mbc) during meiosis results in aneuploid oocytes with subsequent arrest of embryonic cleavage and implantations. *Reprod Toxicol* **10:** 183–9.

JMPR (2002) Pesticide residues in food. Report of the Joint Meeting of the FAO. Panel of Experts on Pesticide Residues in Food and the Environment and a WHO Expert Group on Pesticide Residues. FAO Plant Production and Protection Paper, 176, Rome.

JMPR (2004) Pesticide residues in food. Report of the Joint Meeting of the FAO. Panel of Experts on Pesticide Residues in Food and the Environment and a WHO Expert Group on Pesticide Residues. FAO Plant Production and Protection Paper, 178, Rome.

JMPR (2005) Pesticide residues in food. Report of the Joint Meeting of the FAO Panel of Experts on Pesticide Residues in Food and the Environment and a WHO Expert Group on Pesticide Residues. FAO Plant Production and Protection Paper, 179, Rome.

Johnson L, Welsh TH Jr, Wilker CE (1997) Anatomy and physiology of the male reproductive system and potential targets of toxicants. In *Comprehensive Toxicology: Reproductive and Endocrine Toxicology*, Vol. 10 (Boekelheide K, Chapin R, Hoyer P, Harris C, eds.). Pergamon, Elsevier Science, Inc., USA, pp. 5–61.

Kasymova RA (1976) Experimental and clinical data on the embryonic effect of butiphos. *Probl Gig Organ Zdravookhr Uzb* **5:** 101–3.

Kelce WR, Lambright CR, Gray LE Jr, Roberts KP (1997) Vinclozolin and p, p′-DDE alter androgen-dependent gene expression: *in vivo* confirmation of an androgen receptor-mediated mechanism. *Toxicol Appl Pharmacol* **142:** 192–200.

Kennedy GL, Vondruska JF, Fancher OE, Calandra JC (1972) The teratogenic potential of captan, folpet, and difolatan. *Teratology* **4:** 259–60.

Kennepohl E, Munro IC (2001) Phenoxy herbicides (2,4-D). In *Handbook of Pesticides*, 2nd edition, Vol. 2 (Krieger R, ed.). Academic Press, San Diego, pp. 1623–38.

Khera KS (1987) Ethylenethiourea: a review of teratogenicity and distribution studies and as assessment of reproduction risk. *CRC Cric Rev Toxicol* **18:** 129–39.

Korach KS (ed.) (1998) *Reproductive and Development Toxiology*. Marcell Dekker, Inc., New York, USA, pp. 567–9.

Laier P, Metzdorff SB, Borch J, Hagen ML, Hass U, Christiansen S, Axelstad M, Kledal T, Dalgaard M, McKinnell C, Brokken LJS, Vinggaard AM (2006) Mechanisms of action underlying the antiandrogenic effects of the fungicide prochloraz. *Toxicol Appl Pharmacol* **213:** 160–71.

Lambright C, Ostby J, Bobseine K, Wilson V, Hotchkiss AK, Mann PC, Gray LE Jr (2000) Cellular and molecular mechanisms of action of linuron: an antiandrogenic herbicide that produces reproductive malformations in male rats. *Toxicol Sci* **56:** 389–99.

Laporte JR (1977) Effects of dioxin exposure. *Lancet* **1:** 1049–50.

Lappe M (1991) *Chemical Deception: The Toxic Threat to Health and the Environment*. Sierra Club Books, San Francisco, USA.

Lary JM, Hood RD (1978) Development interactions between cycloheximide and T-locus alleles in the mouse. *Teratology* **17:** 41A.

Li X, Johnson DC, Rozman KK (1995) Reproductive effects of 2,3,7,8-tetrachlorodibenzo-*p*-dioxin (TCDD) in female rats: ovulation, hormonal regulation, and possible mechanism(s). *Toxicol Appl Pharmcol* **133:** 321–7.

Liberacki AB, Zablotny CL, Yano BL, Breslin WJ (1994) Developmental toxicity studies on a series of 2,4,-D salts and esters in rabbits. *Toxicologist* **14:** 162.

Linder RE, Scotti TM, Svendsgaard DJ, McElroy WK, Curley A (1982) Testicular effects of dinoseb in rats. *Arch Environ Contam Toxicol* **11:** 475–85.

Lock EA, Wilks MF (2001) Diquat. In *Handbook of Pesticide Toxicology*, 2nd edition, Vol. 2 (Krieger R, ed.). Academic Press, San Diego, pp. 1605–21.

Lorgue G, Lechenet J, Riviere A (1996) *Clinical Veterinary Toxicology* (English version by MJ Chapman). Blackwell Science, Oxford.

Lowry RB, Allen AB (1977) Herbicides and spina bifida. *Can Med Assoc J* **2:** 117–580.

Mably TA, Bjerke DL, Moore RW, Gendron-Ferzpatrick A, Peterson RE (1992) *In utero* and lactational exposure of male rats to 2,3,7,t-tetrabenzo-*p*-dioxin. 3. Effects of spermatogenesis and reproductive capability. *Toxicol Appl Pharmacol* **114:** 118–26.

Makletsova NY, Lanivoi ID (1981) Status of gynaecological morbidity of women with occupational contact with pesticide zineb. *Pediatr Akush Ginekol* **43:** 60–1.

Manson JM, Brown TJ, Baldwin DM (1984) Teratogenicity of nitrofen (2,4-dinitro-4′-nitrodiphenyl ether) and thyroid function in rat. *Toxicol Appl Pharmacol* **73:** 323–35.

Matsumoto H, Koya G, Takeuchi T (1965) Fetal Minamata disease. *J Neuropathol Exp Neurol* **24:** 563–74.

Matsumoto M, Hirose A, Ema M (2008) Review of testicular toxicity of dinitrophenoli compounds, 2-*sec*-butyl-4,6-dinitrophenol, 4,6-dinitro-*o*-cresol and 2,4-dinitrophenol. *Reprod Toxicol* **26:** 185–90.

Matthiaschk G, Roll R (1977) Studies on the embryotoxicity of monolinuron and buturon in NMBI-mice. *Arch Toxicol (Berl)* **38:** 261–74.

McLaughlin J, Reynolds EF, Lamar JK, Marliac JP (1969) Teratology studies in rabbits with captan, folpet, and thalidomide. *Toxicol Appl Pharmacol* **14:** 641.

Mirkhamidova P, Mirakhmedov AK, Sagatova GA, Isakova AV, Khamidov DK (1981) Effect of butiphos on the structure and function of the liver in rabbit embryos. *Uzb Biol Zh* **5:** 45–7.

Mitchinson MJ, Sherman KP, Stainer-Smith AM (1975) Brown patches in epididymis. *J Path* **115:** 57–62.

Munley SM, Hurtt ME (1996) Development toxicity study of benomyl in rabbits. *Toxicologist* **30:** 192.

Murakami U (1972) The effect of organic mercury on intrauterine life. In *Drugs and Fetal Development* (Kingberg MA, Abramovici A, Chemke J, eds.). Plenum Press, New York, pp. 301–36.

Naki M, Hess RA (1997) Effects of carbendazim (methyl 2-benzimidazole carbamate; mbc) on meiotic spermatocytes and subsequent spermatogenesis in the rat testis. *Anat Rec* **247:** 379–87.

Noriega NC, Ostby J, Lambright C, Wilson VS, Gray LE Jr (2005) Late gestational exposure to the fungicide prochloraz delays the onset of parturition and causes reproductive malformations in male but not female rat offspring. *Biol Reprod* **72:** 1324–35.

Oakes DJ, Webster WS, Brown-Woodman PDC, Ritchie HE (2002) Testicular changes induced by chronic exposure to the herbicide formulation, Tordon 75D® (2,4-dichlorophenoxyacetic acid and picloram) in rats. *Reprod Toxicol* **16:** 281–9.

Ollinger SJ, Arce G, Bui Q, Tobia AJ, Ravenswaay BV (2001) Dialkyldithiocarbamates (EBDCs). In *Handbook of Pesticide Toxicology*, 2nd edition, Vol. 2 (Krieger R, ed.). Academic Press, San Diego, pp. 1759–79.

Ostby J, Kelce WR, Lambright C, Wolf CJ, Mann P, Gray LE Jr (1999) The fungicide procymidone alters sexual differentiation in the male rat by acting as an androgen-receptor antagonist *in vivo* and *in vitro*. *Toxicol Ind Health* **15:** 80–93.

Parsons PP (2001) Mammalian toxicokinetics and toxicity of chlorothalonil. In *Handbook of Pesticide Toxicology*, 2nd edition, Vol. 2 (Krieger R, ed.). Academic Press, San Diego, pp. 1743–57.

Peterson RE, Theobald HM, Kimmel GL (1993) Development and reproductive toxicity of dioxins and related compound: cross species comparisons. *CRC Crit Rev Toxicol* **23:** 283–335.

Pocar P, Brevini TAL, Fischer B, Gandolfi F (2003) The impact of endocrine disruptors on oocyte competence. *Reproduction* **125:** 313–25.

Reddy KN, Dayan FE, Duke SO (1998) QSAR analysis of protoporphyrinogen oxidase inhibitors. In *Comparative QSAR* (Devillers J, ed.). Taylor and Francis, London, pp. 197–234.

Rescia M, Mantovani A (2007) Pesticides as endocrine disrupters: identification of hazards for female reproductive function. In *Reproductive Health and the Environment*, Vol. 22 (Nicolopoulou-Stamati P, Hens L, Howard CV, eds.). Springer, Netherlands, pp. 227–48.

Restrepo M, Minoz N, Day NE, Parra JE, Deromero L, Xuan ND (1990) Prevalence of adverse reproductive outcomes in a population occupationally exposed in Columbia. *Scand J Work Environ* **16:** 232–8.

Richard EP, Paul SC, William RK, Gray LE (1997) Environmental endocrine disruptors. In *Comprehensive Toxicology: Reproductive and Endocrine Toxicology*, Vol. 10 (Boekelheide K, Chapin R, Hoyer P, Harris C, eds.). Pergamon, Elsevier Science, Inc., USA, pp. 181–91.

Richard S, Moslemi S, Sipahutar H, Benachour N, Seralini G (2005) Differential effects of glyphosate and Roundup on human placental cells. *Environ Health Perspect* **113:** 716–20.

Rockett JC, Narotsky MG, Thompson KE, Thillainadarajah I, Blystone CR, Goetz AK, Ren H, Best DS, Murrell RN, Nichols HP, Schmid JE, Wolf DC, Dix DJ (2006) Effect of conazole fungicides on reproductive development in the female rat. *Reprod Toxicol* **22:** 647–58.

Rogers JM, Carver B, Gray JA, Kavlock RJ (1986) Teratogenic effects of fungicide dinovap in the mouse. *Toxicologist* **6:** 91.

Roman BL, Sommer RJ, Shinomiya K, Peterson RE (1995) *In utero* and lactational exposure of the male rat to 2,3,7,8-tetrachlorodibenzo-*p*-dioxin: impaired prostate growth and development without inhibited androgen production. *Toxicol Appl Pharmacol* **134:** 241–50.

Romano RM, Romano MA, Bernardi MM, Furtado PV, Oliveira CA (2010) Prepubertal exposure to commercial formulation of the herbicide glyphosate alters testosterone levels and testicular morphology. *Arch Toxicol* **84:** 309–17.

Rupa DS, Reddy PP, Reddy OS (1991) Reproductive performance in population exposed to pesticides in cotton fields in India. *Environ Res* **44:** 1–7.

Sare WM, Forbes PI (1972) The herbicide 2,4,5-T and its possible dysmorphogenic effects of an agricultural chemical: 2,4,5-T. *New Zealand Med J* **75:** 37–8.

Sarkar SN, Chattopadhya S, Gupta PK (1994) Isoproturon-induced histopathological alterations in rats. *Adv Bios* **13:** 87–94.

Sarkar SN, Gupta PK (1993) Feto-toxic and teratogenic potential of substituted phenylurea herbicide, isoproturon in rats. *Indian J Exp Biol* **31:** 280–2.

Schardein JL (2000) Pesticides. In *Chemically Induced Birth Defects*, 3rd revised and expanded edition. Marcel Dekker, New York, USA, pp. 819–74.

Senger PL (2003) *Pathway to Pregnancy and Parturition*, 2nd edition. Current Conceptions, Inc., Moscow, ID, pp. 1–368.

Shalette MI, Cotes N, Goldsmith ED (1963) Effects of 3-amino-1,2,4-triazole treatment during pregnancy on the development and structure of the thyroid of the fetal rat. *Anat Rec* **145:** 284.

Smith LL (1997) Paraquat. In *Comprehensive Toxicology – Toxicology of the Respiratory System*, Vol. 8 (Sipes IG, McQueen CA, Gandolfi JA, eds.). Pergamon, Elsevier Science, Inc., USA, pp. 581–9.

Sohoni P, Sumpter JP 1998) Several environmental estrogens are also antiandrogens. *J Endocrinol* **158:** 327–39.

Spencer F, Chi L, Zhu M (1996) Effect of benomyl and carbendazim on steroid and molecular mechanisms in uterine decidual growth in rats. *J Appl Toxicol* **16:** 211–4.

Steven JT, Summer DD (1991) Herbicides. In *Handbook of Pesticides Toxicology* (Hayes WJ, Laws ER, eds.). Academic Press, USA, pp. 1317–408.

Sterling TD (1971) Difficulty of evaluating the toxicity and teratogenicity of 2,4,5-T from existing animal experiments. *Science* **174:** 1358–9.

Stoker TE, Cooper RL, Goldman JM, Andrews JE (1996) Characterization of pregnancy outcome following thiram-induced ovulatory delay in the female rat. *Neurotoxicol Teratol* **18:** 277–82.

Stoker TE, Goldman JM, Cooper RL (2001) Delayed ovulation and pregnancy outcome: effect of environmental toxicants on the neuroendocrine control of the ovary. *Environ Toxicol Pharmacol* **9:** 117–29.

Svechnikov K, Supornsilchai V, Strand ML, Wahlgren A, Seidlova-Wuttke D, Wuttke W, Söder O (2005) Influence of long-term dietary administration of procymidone, a fungicide with anti-androgenic effects, or the phytoestrogen genistein to rats on the pituitary–gonadal axis and Leydig cell steroidogenesis. *J Endocrinol* **187:** 117–24.

Takeuchi T (1966) *Minamata Disease: Study Group of Minamata Disease* (Katsuna M, ed.). Kumamato University, Japan, p. 141.

Teramoto S, Shingu A, Keneda M, Saito R (1978) Teratogenicity studies with ethylenethiourea in rats, mice and hamsters. *Congenital Anomal* **18:** 11–17.

Trost C (1984) *Elements of Risk: The Chemical Industry and its Threats to America.* Times Books, New York.

Vergieva T (1984) Experimental study of the teratogenicity and embryotoxicity of endodan. *Probl Khig* 988–95.

Vergieva T (1990) Triazoles teratogenicity in rats. *Teratology* **42:** 27A–28A.

Vettorazzi G (1985) Reproduction toxicity and tertogenicity. In *Modern Toxicology: Basis of Organ and Reproduction Toxicity*, Vol. 1 (Gupta PK, Salunkhe DK, eds.). Metropolitan Book Co. Pvt Ltd, Delhi, India.

Vinggaard AM, Breinholt V, Larsen JC (1999a) Screening of selected pesticides for estrogen receptor activation *in vitro*. *Food Addit Contam* **16:** 533–42.

Vinggaard AM, Joergensen EC, Larsen JC (1999b) Rapid and sensitive reporter gene assays for detection of antiandrogenic and estrogenic effectsof environmental chemicals. *Toxicol Appl Pharmacol* **155:** 150–60.

Vinggaard AM, Christiansen S, Laier P, Poulsen ME, Breinholt V, Jarfelt K, Jacobsen H, Dalgaard M, Nellemann C, Hass U (2005) Perinatal exposure to the fungicide prochloraz feminizes the male rat offspring. *Toxicol Sci* **85:** 886–97.

Vondruska JF, Fancher OF, Calandra JC (1971) An investigation into the teratogenic potential of captan, folpet, and difoltan in nonhuman primates. *Toxicol Appl Pharmacol* **18:** 619–24.

Waechter F, Weber E, Herner T (2001) Cyprodinil: a fungicide of the anilinopyrimidine class. In *Handbook of Pesticide Toxicology,* 2nd edition, Vol. 2 (Krieger R, ed.). Academic Press, Sàn Diego, pp. 1701–10.

Wilson AGE, Takei AS (1999) Summary of toxicology studies with butachlor. *J Pestic Sci* **25:** 75–83.

Yasuda M, Maeda H (1972) Teratogenic effects of 4-chloro-2-methylphenoxyacetic acid ethyl ester (MCPEE) in rats. *Toxicol Appl Pharmacol* **23:** 326–33.

Zaidi SSA, Bhatnagar VK, Gandhi SJ, Shah MP, Kulkarni PK, Sayed SN (2000) Assessment of thyroid functions in pesticide formulators. *Human Exp Toxicol* **19:** 497–500.

Zarn JA, Brüschweiler BJ, Schlatter JR (2003) Azole fungicides affect mammalian steroidogenesis by inhibiting sterol 14 alpha-demethylase and aromatase. *Environ Health Perspect* **111:** 255–61.

CHAPTER

40

Brominated flame retardants

Prasada Rao S. Kodavanti, David T. Szabo, Tammy E. Stoker and Suzanne E. Fenton

INTRODUCTION

Brominated flame retardants (BFRs) belong to a large class of compounds known as organohalogens. BFRs are currently the largest marketed flame retardant group due to their high performance efficiency and low cost. In the commercial market, more than 75 different BFRs are recognized. Some BFRs, such as the polybrominated biphenyls (PBBs), were removed from the market in the early 1970s after an incidental poisoning resulted in the loss of livestock due to the ingestion of PBB-contaminated animal feed, which demonstrated the toxicity of this BFR class (Mercer *et al.*, 1976; Fries, 1985). "Tris-BP" is another BFR that was removed from children's clothing, including pajamas, due to its mutagenic and nephrotoxic effects, (Soderlund *et al.*, 1980). Of the BFRs still on the market, brominated bisphenols, diphenyl ethers and cyclododecanes are three major classes which represent the highest production volumes. These BFRs are used as additive or reactive components in a variety of polymers such as foam, high-impact polystyrene and epoxy resins, which are then used in commercial products such as computers, electronics and electrical equipment, thermal insulation, textiles and furniture foam.

Tetrabromobisphenol A (TBBPA; Figure 40.1) is a reactive BFR in printed circuit boards and is added to several types of polymers. TBBPA is highly lipophilic (log Kow = 4.5) and has low water solubility (0.72 mg/ml). TBBPA has been measured in the air (Zweidinger *et al.*, 1979), soil and sediment (Watanabe *et al.*, 1983), but is generally not found in water samples. Hexabromocyclododecane (HBCD; Figure 40.1) is a non-aromatic brominated cyclic alkane, mainly used as an additive flame retardant in thermoplastic polymers with final applications in styrene resins (National Research Council, 2000). Like other BFRs, HBCD is highly lipophilic, with a log Kow of 5.6 and has low water solubility (0.0034 mg/L) (MacGregor and Nixon, 1997). Studies have shown that HBCD is highly persistent, with a half-life of 3 days in air and 2,025 days in water (Lyman, 1990), and is bioaccumulative with a bioconcentration factor of approximately 18,100 in fathead minnows (Veith and Defoe, 1979). HBCD has been detected in workplace air samples at levels up to 1,400 µg/kg in dust (Leonards *et al.*, 2001). Diet is considered an important source for HBCD exposure (Schecter *et al.*, 2010b), especially for humans consuming large quantities of fish, which reportedly contains relatively high HBCD levels; 1,110 ng/g lipid (Janák *et al.*, 2005; Xian *et al.*, 2007). Besides diet, house dust is probably another important pathway of human exposure, since dust consists of high levels of HBCD (Roosens *et al.*, 2009). Although we discuss some aspects of BFRs in general, the main focus of this chapter will be on polybrominated diphenyl ethers (PBDEs) with some mention of other BFRs where appropriate. We will discuss the developmental and reproductive effects of PBDEs, toxicokinetics, possible mode(s) of action and structural similarities with polychlorinated biphenyls (PCBs).

PBDEs constitute an important group of flame retardants. They are added to consumer products to either prevent the products from catching fire or delay the ignition process if exposed to flame or heat. PBDEs are added to plastics, upholstery, fabrics and foams and in common products such as computers, television sets, mobile phones, furniture and carpet pads. Nearly 90% of electrical and electronic appliances contain PBDEs and Bromine Science and Environmental Forum (BSEF) claims that adding flame retardants gives 15 times greater escape time in case of a fire (BSEF, 2010). Polybrominated dioxins (PBDDs)/dibenzofurans (PBDFs) have toxicological profiles similar to those of their chlorinated homologs (Birnbaum *et al.*, 2003), but more toxic than PBDEs, and are formed during heating or incineration of PBBs and PBDEs. Low levels of PBDDs/PBDFs detected in environmental samples suggest relatively lower exposure of these compounds to biota (fish) and humans when compared to PBDEs. Although PBDEs are ubiquitous, they are primarily considered as indoor pollutants based on human exposure scenaries. They leach into the environment when household wastes decompose in landfills or are incompletely incinerated. Human health concerns stem from the fact that PBDEs are persistent, bioaccumulative and chemically related to PCBs (Figure 40.1). PBDE concentrations are rapidly increasing in the global environment and in human blood, breast milk, liver, as well as other lipophilic tissues. However, in defined areas like the European Union, environmental PBDEs are leveling off or declining due to regulation on these compounds (Law *et al.*, 2006b). Although these chemicals are ubiquitous in the environment and bioaccumulate in wildlife and humans, information on their potential toxic effects are now accruing (Kodavanti, 2005; Stoker et al., 2005; Costa *et al.*, 2008; Lorber, 2008; Szabo *et al.*, 2009; Kodavanti *et al.*, 2010).

Similar to PCBs, PBDEs are synthetic chemicals manufactured in large quantities. They are comprised of two

Reproductive and Developmental Toxicology, Edited by Ramesh C. Gupta
ISBN: 978-0-12-382032-7

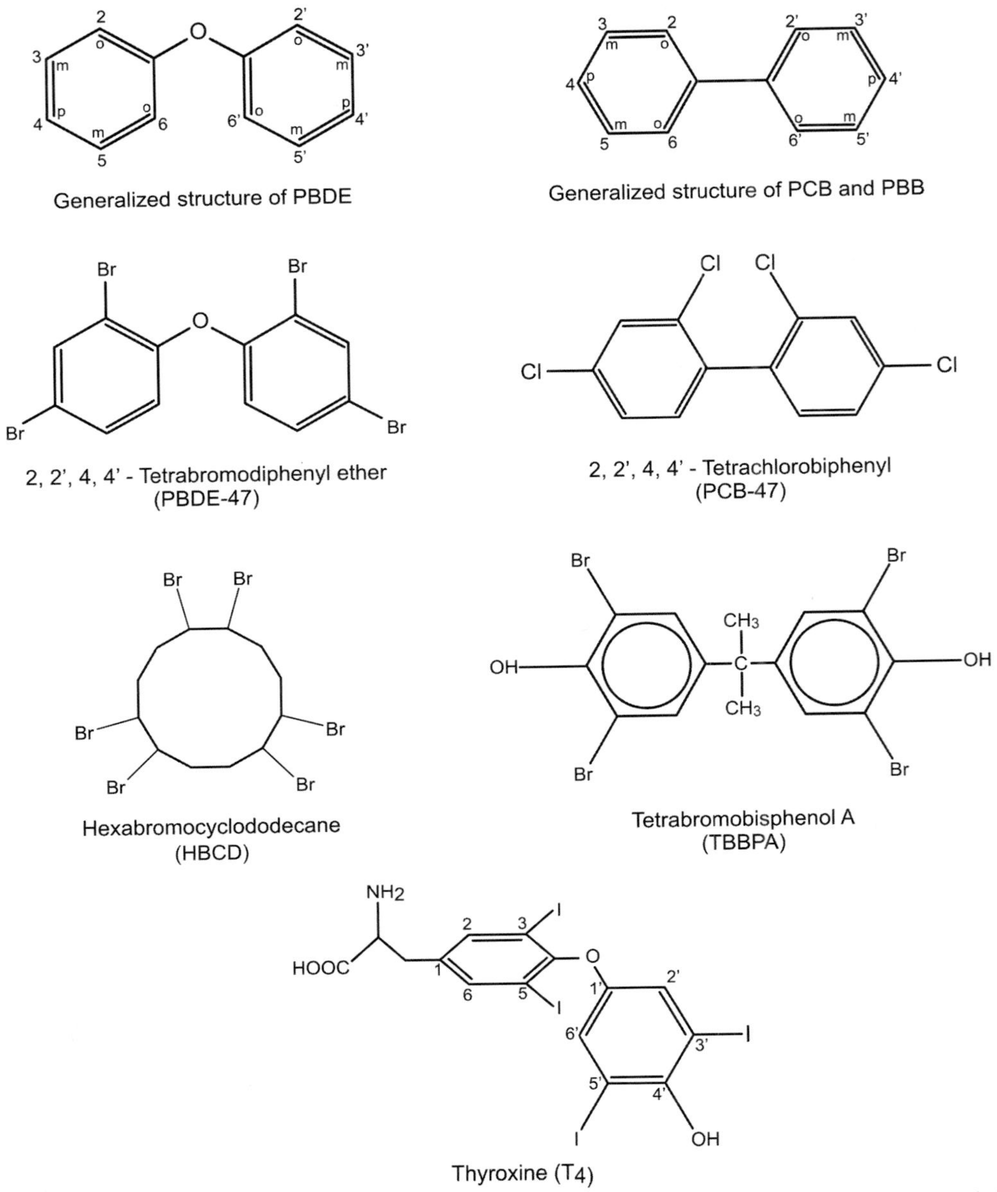

Generalized structure of PBDE

Generalized structure of PCB and PBB

2, 2', 4, 4' - Tetrabromodiphenyl ether (PBDE-47)

2, 2', 4, 4' - Tetrachlorobiphenyl (PCB-47)

Hexabromocyclododecane (HBCD)

Tetrabromobisphenol A (TBBPA)

Thyroxine (T4)

FIGURE 40.1 Chemical structures of selected brominated flame retardants along with thyroxine (T_4) and a representative structure of polychlorinated biphenyls (PCBs). Core structures as well as predominant congeners with similar position and number of halogens for PCBs and PBDEs are shown to highlight the structural similarities between these two groups of chemicals. The letters (o), (m) and (p) indicate ortho, meta and para substitutions for chlorines or bromines. The numbers indicate position of halogens.

phenyl rings linked by oxygen (thus the designation as "ether"; Figure 40.1). PBDEs are quite resistant to physical, chemical and biological degradation. Compared to chlorine atoms, bromine atoms are a better leaving group rendering PBDEs susceptible to various types of degradation and metabolism more readily than PCBs. The exact identity and pattern of various congeners in numerous commercial mixtures depends on the manufacturer and the specific product. Among these, the commercial "penta" mixture generally consists of PBDE congeners 99 (pentaBDE) and 47 (tetraBDE) as the major constituents, which make up about 70% of the mixture (Huber and Ballschmitter, 2001). PBDE congener 100 (pentaBDE) is present at less than 10%, with PBDE congeners 153 and 154 (hexaBDEs) at less than 5% each. The commercial "octa" mixture is 10–12% hexaBDE, 43–44% heptaBDE, 31–35% octaBDE, 9–11% nonaBDE and 0–1% decaBDE. The "deca" commercial mixture consists of 98% decaBDE, with a small percentage of nonaBDEs (WHO, 1994; La Guardia *et al.*, 2006). Trace analysis of these commercial mixtures for other brominated contaminants revealed the presence of PBBs and PBDFs, but not PBDDs at levels above the limit of detection (Hanari *et al.*, 2006). It is known that PBDEs, upon pyrolysis at 900°C, release PBDFs and PBDDs and the amount of these contaminants depends on the conditions of pyrolysis (Buser, 1986; Thoma *et al.*, 1986).

ENVIRONMENTAL CONTAMINATION AND HUMAN EXPOSURE

PBDE residues have been detected in indoor air, house dust and foods. PBDE exposure to humans may be possible via multiple sources (air, water, food and dust). Recent lifestyle exposure analysis studies found that PBDE-47, PBDE-99 and PBDE-209 were present in highest concentrations and that US samples were approximately 50 times higher than samples from Germany (Sjodin *et al.*, 2008). The median total PBDE levels in the US dust were more than 10 times higher than the median German levels (Schecter *et al.*, 2009). High concentrations of PBDEs are also found in sewage sludge, with levels in the USA running 10- to 100-fold higher than those in Europe. Over half of the sewage sludge produced annually in the USA is applied to land as fertilizer (US EPA, 1999). Thus, application of sewage sludge may represent a source of exposure to humans and wildlife through direct contact or uptake by plants. A survey of US foods showed that PBDE levels were highest in fish (median: 1,725 pg/g), followed by meat (283 pg/g), and lowest in dairy products (31.5 pg/g) (Schecter *et al.*, 2004). Significant levels of PBDEs may be found in outdoor air, even at rural locations. PBDE concentrations in indoor measures were 15–20 times higher than in outdoor air (Butt *et al.*, 2004).

Lipophilic chemicals in milk have been heavily studied, as they bioaccumulate, have a long-half-life in humans and have been detected for decades, based on their persistence. Like the well-studied persistent organic pollutants (dioxins, furans, PCBs and persistent organochlorine pesticides), PBDEs have been measured in milk and other biological matrices. Because most mammals receive milk from their mother as the primary nutritional source for the first weeks of their life, PBDEs in milk are a critical consideration when evaluating potential developmental exposures to these chemicals. Breast milk has a complex make-up; human milk is composed primarily of lipids (~2–4%), proteins (~1%), lipoproteins, immune factors, lactose and water (LaKind *et al.*, 2009). Rodents differ slightly in that the fat and protein percentages can vary from 4–12% and 8% in rats to 17–26% and 11% in mice, respectively (Godbole *et al.*, 1981; Görs *et al.*, 2009). The percentage of milk fat is highest early in lactation regardless of species.

PBDEs were first reported in breast milk 12 years ago (Meironyté-Guvenius *et al.*, 1999). PBDEs have increased in concentration in breast milk from the 1970s through the 1990s, leading to the 2004 ban on penta- and octa-congeners in Europe. The USA is the country reporting some of the highest PBDE breast milk levels in the world and is regulating the use of the PBDE congeners on a state-by-state basis. However, the sole US manufacturer of penta- and octaBDE mixtures voluntarily ceased production in 2004. The USEPA further used SNUR (significant new use rule) to prevent new production in 2007. The BSEF (2010) reports that its member companies voluntarily phased out the production and use of penta- and octaBDEs in 2004, and of decaBDE by 2012 in cooperation with the USEPA. To date, 10 states have adopted legislation banning penta- and octaBDE (CA, HI, IL, ME, MA, MI, NY, OR, RI, WA) with three of those also enacting limited bans on decaBDE (ME, OR, WA), and one state has banned decaBDE (VT).

In studies measuring PBDEs in humans, the median PBDE concentration in a Texas study was 34 ng/g lipid, with a range of 6–419 ng/g (Schecter *et al.*, 2003). In a US study conducted in Massachusetts, PBDE levels in breast milk ranged from 0.06 to 1,910 ng/g lipid weight for various PBDE congeners (Johnson-Restrepo *et al.*, 2007). In other studies, the median for breast milk levels was 58 ng/g, with a range of 9.5–1,078 ng/g lipid. There are several studies that have evaluated the partitioning of tri-hepta PBDEs in human milk vs. serum (Schecter *et al.*, 2003, 2010a; LaKind *et al.*, 2009) and all of them reported milk to serum ratios in excess of 1.0, indicating the accumulation or preferential storage of the compounds in milk fat. Of the PBDEs at highest concentration (47, 99, 100, 153), only 153 approached a milk:serum ratio of 1.0 (Schecter *et al.*, 2010a). In those studies, the mean sum PBDE concentrations ranged from 74 to 96 ng/g lipid in breast milk. Although PBDEs were found at significant levels in breast milk, their concentration did not decrease or depurate over the period of lactation (LaKind *et al.*, 2009; Daniels *et al.*, 2010). From those data, it appears that milk can be a significant source of PBDE exposure for the developing child or rodent. This exposure source may explain why Australian toddlers (2.6–3 years old) exhibited five-fold higher and infants (0–0.5 years old) 50% higher serum PBDE levels than adults (Toms *et al.*, 2009).

Levels of PBDEs in human tissues, specifically blood, milk and fat, have increased exponentially since the 1970s in several countries, including the USA, Canada and Sweden (Schecter *et al.*, 2005). The EU has decreased PBDE use by two-thirds in recent years. Currently in Sweden, breast milk levels are decreasing, presumably as a result of a decrease in the use of PBDE-containing products. Levels of PBDEs among individuals in North America, as measured in blood, breast milk or adipose tissue, are 10–70 times higher than in Europe or Japan (Schecter *et al.*, 2005). Elevated levels of PBDEs in North America were attributed to the higher use of the pentaBDE mixture when compared to the rest of the world. Like other lipophilic compounds, PBDEs readily cross the placenta into the fetus. This provides the opportunity for PBDEs to interfere with human developmental processes, producing adverse effects in not only the infant, but, due to the bioaccumulative nature of the compounds, the adolescent too.

EFFECTS ON HUMAN HEALTH

Epidemiological studies on the health effects of PBDE exposure are few in number, but rapidly increasing. This is largely due to recent findings that PBDEs are persistent organic pollutants. An initial report from Denmark in 2007 (Main *et al.*, 2007) showed that increased PBDE levels in breast milk are positively associated with congenital cryptorchidism. Later studies indicated elevated serum thyroid stimulating hormone (TSH) levels with increased serum PBDE levels in Chinese workers from an E-waste dismantling site (Yuan *et al.*, 2008), an association of prenatal PCB and PBDE exposures with decreased total and free thyroxine (T_4) levels in infants born by spontaneous delivery (Herbstman *et al.*, 2008), and a strong inverse association of dust PBDE concentrations with serum luteinizing hormone and follicle stimulating hormone (Meeker *et al.*, 2009). Recent studies indicate association of PBDEs with longer time to pregnancy in women (Harley *et al.*, 2010) and reduced development of children at school age that included psychomotor development index and full scale IQ performance (Roze *et al.*, 2009; Herbstman *et al.*, 2010).

The ubiquitous nature of PBDEs allows for many routes of human exposure, although ingestion seems to be the primary exposure route. Several studies have documented significant PBDE levels in oils and fats, fish and shellfish, meat and meat products, and eggs, corresponding to a dietary intake ranging from 26 to 150 ng/day (Darnerud *et al.*, 2001; Huwe *et al.*, 2002; Ohta *et al.*, 2002; Bocio *et al.*, 2003; Schecter *et al.*, 2006; Wu *et al.*, 2007). Additionally, indoor environmental exposure has been implicated in human PBDE intake. High PBDE levels in indoor air, airborne particles and house dust have been discovered in all parts of the world. One study determined the adult daily exposure dose of PBDE due to inhalation, incidental oral ingestion and dermal absorption of house dust to be 0.14, 1.3 and 0.34 ng/kg/day, respectively (Johnson-Restrepo and Kannan, 2009). In infants, the major route of PBDE exposure seems to be maternal transfer and breast milk consumption, but could also result from toddlers and crawling infants acquiring hand to mouth exposures in the home. Alarmingly, Johnson-Restrepo and Kannan (2009) determined that the infant daily exposure dose of PBDE due to inhalation, incidental oral ingestion and dermal absorption of house dust was significantly higher than that of the adult, measuring 0.60, 6.7 and 0.77 ng/kg/day, respectively. As stated earlier, breast milk can contain substantial PBDEs; the serum samples of infants aged 0–4 years contained significantly higher PBDE concentrations as compared to children 5–15 years of age (Toms *et al.*, 2009). These levels of PBDE in pregnant mothers and their breast milk may pose a developmental toxicity risk for developing fetuses and neonates. But, it must be noted that there are numerous benefits to breastfeeding, both to the mother and child, so women would need to weigh the benefit to risk ratio.

The median value in breast milk is about 10 times higher for PCBs than for current concentrations of PBDEs; however, the concentration ranges do overlap. The current doubling time for levels of PBDEs in milk in North America is as short as 2.6 years. Assuming that the current exponential increase continues, doubling times will continue to decrease. In such an event, levels that are known to produce developmental neurotoxicity would be reached in fewer than 10 years. It is also important to remember that a no adverse effect level (NOAEL) for PCBs has not been determined. Therefore, it is not known whether current concentrations of PBDEs in the environment are producing adverse effects, assuming that PBDEs have effects at approximately the same concentrations as PCBs. In addition, it is likely that the effects of PCBs and PBDEs are additive, at least for neurotoxicity. Therefore, the levels of PBDEs currently in the environment may well be producing adverse effects.

Although the US federal government has not banned penta- or octaBDE mixtures, they have been voluntarily withdrawn by the US manufacturers and state governments are taking actions independently. This withdrawal should result in at least a decreasing rate of the doubling time. Since the vast majority of the PBDEs currently in use are the decaBDE mixture, it is expected that its metabolic products will make up an increasingly important fraction of the lower brominated PBDE concentrations in the human body, if production does not cease. It is not possible to estimate, based on current information, how quickly decaBDE and its products would increase in the environment.

HEALTH EFFECTS IN ANIMALS AND WILDLIFE

Since PBDEs are a class of chemicals that are mostly used indoor, data on their effects on wildlife is limited. Few studies indicate that PBDE exposure at environmentally relevant concentrations increases nestling growth (Fernie *et al.*, 2006) and causes changes in reproductive courtship behaviors in adult American kestrels (Fernie *et al.*, 2008). However, a number of studies of laboratory animals have indicated that commercial PBDE mixtures as well as individual PBDE congeners that compose them affect the nervous, endocrine, reproductive and immune systems.

Developmental effects

With regard to neurotoxic effects, several studies indicated that HBCD and PBDEs cause permanent aberrations in spontaneous behavior and habituation capability in mice after a single exposure at postnatal day (PND) 10 (a period of rapid brain growth development). In fact, the pattern of effect was similar for PBDE congeners 47, 99, 153, 183 (a heptaBDE), 203 (octaBDE), 206 (nonaBDE) and 209 (decaBDE) (Eriksson *et al.*, 2001, 2002; Viberg *et al.*, 2003a,b, 2004). It is interesting to note that the effects seen on this behavioral paradigm with PBDEs are identical to those produced by PCBs (Eriksson and Fredriksson, 1996). PBDEs are neurotoxic in various *in vitro* assays (Kodavanti and Derr-Yellin, 2002; Mariussen and Fonnum, 2003, 2006; Kodavanti *et al.*, 2005), suggesting possible mechanisms of PBDE-induced toxicity. Neural defects in fish larvae following embryonic exposure to 2,2′4,4′-tetrabromodiphenyl ether (PBDE-47) have also been reported (Lema *et al.*, 2007).

Mice exposed to a single dose of PBDE-47 on PND 10 demonstrated delayed ontogeny of neuromotor function and hyperactivity when they attained adult age without any alterations in circulating thyroid hormone (TH) levels (Gee and Moser, 2008; Gee *et al.*, 2008). These studies are in agreement with previous reports on PBDE-99 where hyperactivity was observed in CD-1 Swiss mice following developmental exposure, in the absence of significant changes in circulating TH levels when assessed at PND 22 (Branchi *et al.*, 2005). Other studies showed developmental delays in the acquisition of the palpebral reflex following neonatal exposure to PBDE-209 along with changes in circulating T4 levels (Rice *et al.*, 2007). Because of these differential reports, the role of hypothyroxinemia in the behavioral effects of PBDEs is unclear. Kuriyama *et al.* (2005) indicated that gestational exposure of pregnant rats to low doses of PBDE-99 caused hyperactivity in the offspring, an effect that extended into adulthood. Similarly, Branchi *et al.* (2002, 2003, 2004) reported that prolonged developmental exposure to PBDE-99 affected sensory-motor development, as indicated by a delay in screen climbing response, and spontaneous behavior, as indicated by hyperactivity and impaired habituation in mice. During developmental exposure in rats, increased locomotor activity was observed by PBDE-47 (Suvorov *et al.*, 2009) while Cheng *et al.* (2009) reported a delayed appearance of cliff drop and negative geotaxis reflexes by PBDE-99.

Recent studies indicate that DE-71, a commercial pentabrominated mixture, when administered during development did not alter maternal or male body weights. However, female offspring were smaller compared to controls between PND 35–60. DE-71 exposure also accumulated PBDE congeners in various tissues including the brain suggesting that PBDEs can cross the blood–placenta and blood–brain barriers. Furthermore, this can cause subtle changes in neurobehavior and dramatic changes in circulating thyroid hormone levels, as well as changes in both male and female reproductive endpoints (Kodavanti *et al.*, 2010).

There is evidence that PBDEs affect the cholinergic neurotransmitter system (Viberg *et al.*, 2003a,b), which is involved in memory and motor function, among others. The effects of several PBDE congeners have been compared to PCBs for their ability to affect intracellular signaling in a cerebellar (brain) culture system (Kodavanti and Ward, 2005; Kodavanti *et al.*, 2005). The Ca/protein kinase C signaling pathways are proposed mechanisms of neurotoxicity for a number of chemicals, including PCBs and PBDEs. The order of potency for their effects on intracellular signaling was DE-71 (a commercial mixture of tetra-, penta- and hexaBDEs) > 47 > 100 > 99. On a molar basis, DE-71 was equipotent with Aroclor 1254; the most widely used commercial PCB mixture. A Swedish study found that PBDE-99 and PCB-52 produced effects on behavior when given together but not at the same dose given alone (Eriksson *et al.*, 2006). These results suggest that there may be little difference in neurotoxic potency between PBDEs and PCBs for neurotoxicity, and that effects of PCBs and PBDEs are additive. This implies that body burdens of PCBs and PBDEs in humans may need to be added when assessing risk.

PBDEs also affect the TH system both *in vivo* and *in vitro*. *In vivo* studies show reductions in serum T_4 levels following exposure to PBDEs, after both acute and subacute exposure (Fowles *et al.*, 1994) and after developmental exposure (Hallgren *et al.*, 2001; Richardson *et al.*, 2008; Kodavanti *et al.*, 2010). Hallgren *et al.* (2001) showed that PCBs are more potent compounds in reducing circulating T_4 levels than PBDEs. Interaction studies with human transthyretin (TTR) showed that PBDEs have to undergo metabolic activation before the compounds are able to competitively inhibit the binding of T_4 (Meerts *et al.*, 2000; Hamers *et al.*, 2006). This interaction between PBDEs and TTR, however, appears to vary with species, since several PBDE congeners (BDE-47, BDE-99) bind the piscine form of TTR with high affinity (Morgado *et al.*, 2007). These species differences in PBDE interaction with TTR are likely due to differences in the structural properties of mammalian and piscine TTRs (Eneqvist *et al.*, 2004). Zhou *et al.* (2001) concluded that short-term exposure to some commercial PBDE mixtures interferes with the TH system via upregulation of uridine diphosphate glucuronyl transferases (UGTs). Richardson *et al.* (2008) indicated that the decreases in circulating T_4 levels by PBDE-47 exposure might involve other mechanisms although there was induction of hepatic UGTs. However, several other reports indicated good correlation between the degree of TH reduction by PCBs and PBDEs with a decrease in the *ex vivo* binding of ^{125}I-T_4 to TTR and lack of correlation with UGT induction (Hallgren *et al.*, 2001; Hallgren and Darnerud, 2002). Further studies indicated that decabromodiphenyl ether (PBDE-209) decreased serum triiodothyronine (T_3) levels, but not T_4 levels in the absence of any induction of UGTs (Tseng *et al.*, 2008). These studies with PBDEs are in agreement with the reports on PCBs and support the conclusion that UGTs may not play a significant role in decreasing circulating TH levels by these groups of chemicals. Displacement of T_4 and binding of PCBs or PBDEs with the TTR transport protein might be a critical event in decreasing circulating TH levels.

Szabo *et al.* (2009) conducted extensive studies on different mechanisms involved in TH disruption after exposure to a PBDE mixture. Developmental exposure to the DE-71 commercial mixture resulted in significant increases in hepatic cytochrome P450 enzyme activities and gene expression, and decreases in hepatic deiodinase I (D1) activity and gene expression. The results from this study indicated that deiodination, active transport and sulfation, in addition to glucuronidation, may be involved in the disruption of TH homeostasis due to perinatal exposure to the commercial PBDE mixture, DE-71 (Szabo *et al.*, 2009; Figure 40.2). In addition to the effects on circulating TH levels, PBDEs also interfere with TH receptor (TR)-mediated TH signaling. Schriks *et al.* (2007) reported that hydroxyl-PBDEs increased T_3-induced TRα-activation, but not T_3-induced TRβ-activation while 2,2′,3,3′,4,4′,5,5′,6-brominated diphenyl ether (PBDE-206) was antagonistic on both TRs. Lema *et al.* (2008) recently reported depressed plasma T_4 levels in flathead minnows exposed to PBDE-47 and this was accompanied by elevated mRNA levels for TSH-β in the pituitary. PBDE-47 exposure also elevated transcription of TRα in the brain of females and decreased mRNA levels for TRβ in the brain of both sexes of fathead minnows (Lema *et al.*, 2008). The PBDE effects on TR would have physiological implications such as alterations in the development of neuronal cells as reported by Schreiber *et al.* (2010).

Based on the literature, the possible mechanism(s) of disruption of TH by exposure to PBDEs are shown in Figure 40.2. PBDE congeners as well as the contaminants such as PBDD/PBDF enter circulation through gastric absorption. T_4 is synthesized and released into circulation by the thyroid gland. In circulation, PBDEs displace T_4 from serum binding proteins such as TTR. The reductions in circulating T_4 levels increase TSH production via reduced negative feedback on the hypothalamic–pituitary axis (Lema *et al.*, 2008), which induces increased synthesis and secretion of T_4 by the thyroid gland. PBDEs bound to TTR along with T_4 will reach target organs including the brain to elicit their effects. The resulting free T_4 released from TTR will be subjected to hepatic metabolism and elimination. In the liver, PBDEs activate nuclear receptors initiating transcription of xenobiotic metabolizing enzymes (XMEs) for T_4 elimination. XMEs consequently conjugate T_4 by phase II enzymes, UGT and sulfotransferease (SULT). Deiodinase 1 (D1) can deiodinate T_4 to its metabolites (T_3 or rT_3). Influx transporters (Oatp1a4) further increase the T_4 uptake for metabolism. Efflux transporters eliminate T_4 or its conjugates from hepatocytes either into the serum (Mrp3) or the bile (Mrp2). Thus, TH disruption by PBDEs involve multiple mechanisms including phase II glucoronidation and sulfation, TTR displacement, decreased hepatic deiodinase I activity and increases in hepatic transporter phase III elimination.

The immune effects of some PBDEs have also been studied indicating that some congeners are immunotoxic (similar to PCBs). DE-71 produced a suppression of the ability to mount an immune response in adult mice following subchronic exposure (Fowles *et al.*, 1994). Decreased number of splenocytes and decreased production of IgG antibodies in response to a challenge were observed following administration of Bromkal 70-5DE (a commercial mixture of penta- and hexaBDE) or BDE-47 in rats and/or mice (Darnerud and Thuvander, 1999). PCBs had similar effects in this study. The immunosuppressive potential of tetra-, penta- or hexaBDEs was assessed in adult mice (Howie *et al.*, 1990). All congeners suppressed the splenic plaque-forming cell response, with

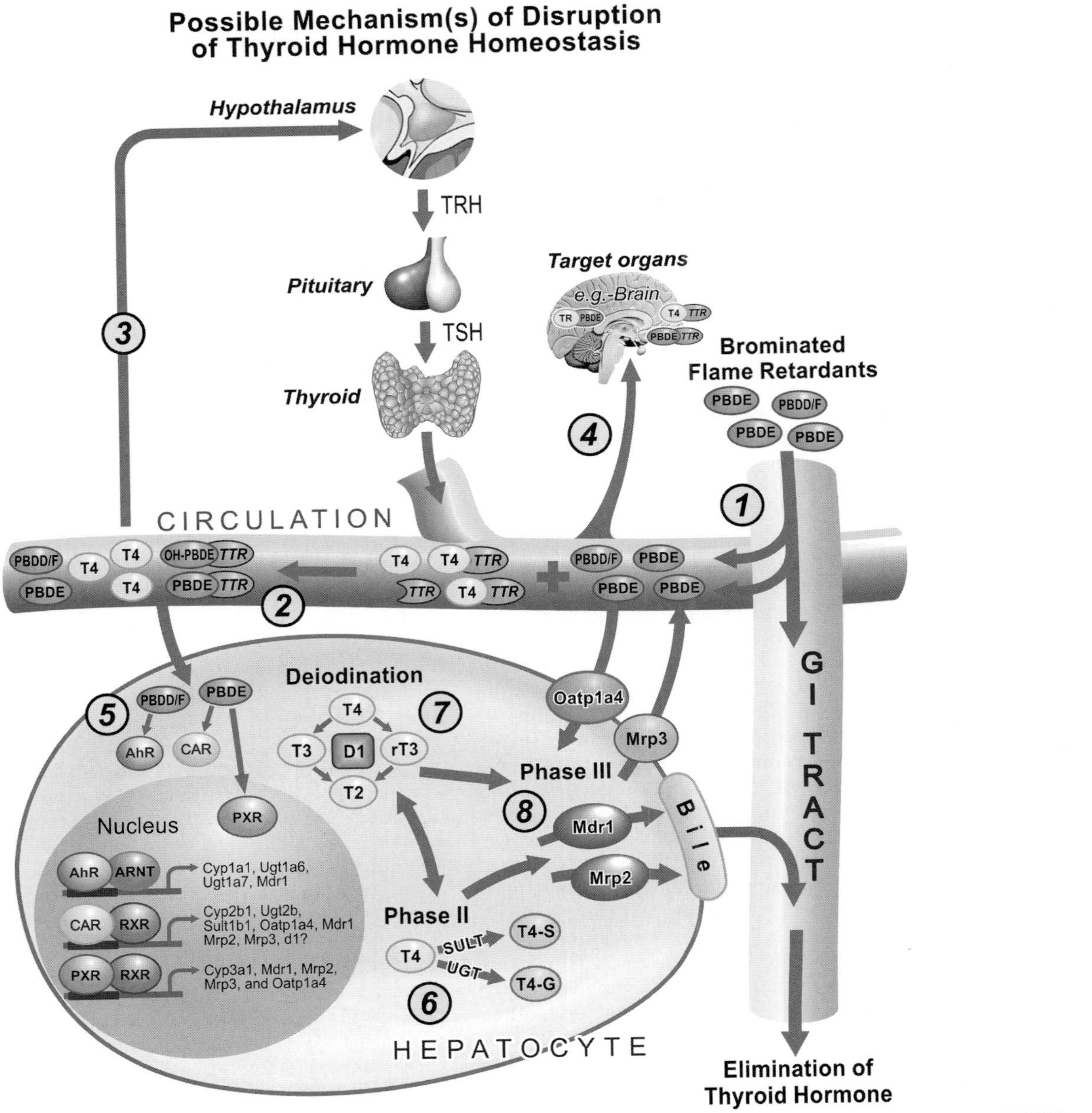

FIGURE 40.2 Possible mechanism(s) of disruption of thyroid hormone homeostasis following developmental exposure to commercial PBDE mixtures. (1) PBDEs as well as PBDD/Fs enter the circulation from gastrointestinal (GI) tract. (2) PBDEs in the parent or hydroxylated form can displace thyroxine (T_4) from serum binding proteins such as transthyretin (TTR). The resulting free T_4 will be subjected to hepatic metabolism and elimination. (3) Reduced circulating T_4 levels trigger the hypothalamic–pituitary axis to synthesize and secrete more T_4 by thyroid. (4) PBDEs bound to TTR along with T_4 will reach target organs including brain, where it can bind to thyroid hormone receptor to elicit a biological/toxicological effect. (5) PBDEs and PBDD/Fs activate nuclear receptors in hepatocytes initiating transcription of xenobiotic metabolizing enzymes (XMEs) for T_4 elimination. (6) XMEs consequently conjugate T_4 by phase II enzymes, uridine diphosphate glucuronyl transferase (UGT) and sulfotransferase (SULT). (7) Deiodinase 1 (D1) deiodinates T_4 to its metabolites. (8) Influx transporters (Oatp1a4) further increase the T_4 uptake for metabolism. Efflux transporters eliminate T_4 or its conjugates from hepatocytes into either the serum (Mrp3) or the bile (Mrp2). (Adapted from Szabo *et al.*, 2009; Kodavanti and Curras-Collazo, 2010.) Please refer to color plate section.

potencies varying among congeners. In an *in vitro* study in human lymphocytes (Fernlöf *et al.*, 1997), neither PCBs nor PBDEs had an effect on cell proliferation. In contrast, it is well established that PCBs are immunotoxic *in vivo* in humans. The negative results of the *in vitro* study are presumably the result of the fact that PCBs (and perhaps PBDEs) exert their effect through an indirect mechanism.

With regard to carcinogenic potential, only decaBDE has been assessed for carcinogenicity in a chronic bioassay, conducted on rats and mice by the US National Toxicology Program in 1986. In mice, non-significant increases in combined hepatocellular adenomas and carcinomas were observed at 3,200 or 6,650 mg/kg body weight/day in males, and in combined thyroid follicular cell adenomas and carcinomas in both sexes. In rats, females were dosed with 1,200 or 2,550 mg/kg body weight/day and males with 1,120 or 2,240 mg/kg body weight/day for 103 weeks. A significant dose-dependent increase in the incidence of adenomas of the liver was observed in both sexes, and there was a significant dose-dependent increase in acinar cell adenoma in males.

TABLE 40.1 Effects of PBDE on male reproductive end points

PBDE	Doses (mg/kg)*	Dose length	Strain	Effects	Reference
BDE-209	5, 40, 320	GD 6–18	SD rat	No effects on testosterone or androgen-dependent tissue weights	Kim *et al.*, 2009
PBDE-99	60, 300 μg/kg	GD 6	Wistar rat	↓ sperm counts (60, 300), ↓ ejaculation, ↓ relative testes, epididymal weights	Kuriyama *et al.*, 2005
PBDE-99	1, 10	GD 10–18	LE rats	↓ Testosterone at PND 21/160 ↓ AGD (10), ↑ sweet preference (1, 10)	Lilienthal *et al.*, 2006
DE-71	1.7, 10.2, 30.6	GD 6–PND 21	Wistar rat	Delay in PPS (30.6)	Kodavanti *et al.*, 2010
DE-71	60, 120	PND 23–53	Wistar rat	Delay in PPS of 4 and 5 days	Stoker *et al.*, 2005
DE-71	30–240	PND 53–61	Wistar rat	↓ VP (30–240), ↓ SV (60–240), ↓ CG (120, 240), ↓ LABC AND GP (240) weights	Stoker *et al.*, 2005
DE-71	3, 30, 60	PND 23–53	Wistar rat	Delay in PPS (30, 60)	Stoker *et al.*, 2004
PBDE-209	10, 100, 500, 1,500	PND 21–71	CD-1 mice	Reduces sperm lateral head displacement, ↓ sperm mitochondrial membrane potential, generated H_2O_2 (500, 1,500)	Tseng *et al.*, 2006
pentaBDE	0.27, 0.82, 2.47, 7.4, 22.2, 66.7, 200	PND 56–84	Wistar rat	Dose-dependent ↓ epididymis, SV, prostate weights, ↑ sperm head deformities	van der Ven *et al.*, 2008
decaBDE	1.9, 3.8,7.5, 5, 30, 60	PND 56–84	Wistar rat	Dose-dependent ↓ epididymis weights, Dose-dependent ↑ SV weights	van der Venet *et al.*, 2008

*Unless noted otherwise
Doses were administered orally in all studies
GD – gestational day, PND – postnatal day, PPS – preputial separation, VP – ventral prostate, SV – seminal vesicle, CG – cowpers gland

The US EPA classifies decaBDE as a possible human carcinogen. Several studies, involving emerging BFRs and specific PBDE congeners 47, 99 and 153, are currently under way at the NTP to assess their effects on carcinogenicity, neurotoxicity and reproductive toxicity.

Male reproductive effects

Until recently, very little was known about the effects of brominated flame retardants on male reproductive development or function. With increasing concentrations being detected in the environment and in tissue/milk samples of humans and animals (Rayne *et al.*, 2003; Schecter *et al.*, 2005; Frederiksen *et al.*, 2009), the ability of the PBDEs to act as endocrine disruptors or reproductive toxicants has raised new concerns about the possible effects on human reproductive and nervous system development. Several *in vivo* studies have more recently examined the effects of PBDEs on male reproductive outcomes in rodents (summarized in Table 40.1) and on steroid receptors, synthesis and clearance in cell-based assays.

In vivo *studies in rodents*

The earliest studies in rodents demonstrated that male rats treated peripubertally with oral exposure to DE-71 displayed a significant delay in puberty at 30, 60 and 120 mg/kg by 2, 3.5 and 5 days, respectively (Stoker *et al.*, 2004, 2005). In addition to the delay in preputial separation, a marker of pubertal progression, the weight of certain androgen-dependent tissues including the ventral prostate and seminal vesicles were decreased. The later study was primarily designed to evaluate changes in steroid hormones/androgen receptor (AR) function following DE-71 exposure. In that study, it was discovered that the DE-71 mixture as well as the predominant congeners present in the PBDE mixture were AR antagonists, both *in vivo* and *in vitro*, which confirmed their anti-androgenic activity (Stoker *et al.*, 2005).

A number of other studies have since shown that adult exposures to BFRs can also disrupt androgen homeostasis and thereby alter the function of male reproductive organs. For example, adult male rats exposed to DE-71 displayed decreased epididymal, seminal vesicle and prostate weights, sperm head deformities, perturbations in circulating LH and testosterone levels, and altered activity of enzymes important for xenobiotic metabolism and steroidogenesis (van der Ven *et al.*, 2008; Stoker *et al.*, 2005). Stoker *et al.* (2005) also tested DE-71 in a Hershberger assay to confirm changes observed on pubertal onset and the effects observed *in vitro* on AR antagonism. This assay uses castrated male rats to determine competition for androgen-induced growth using a co-treatment of the compound and testosterone proprionate (a synthetic androgen). In this study, the ventral prostate and seminal vesicle weights were suppressed in a dose–response fashion including lower dosage groups (30 mg/kg) and were the most sensitive (compared to the other androgen-dependent tissues) to the anti-androgenic effects of DE-71 (see Table 40.1).

In another study, TBBPA exposure in adult male rats also resulted in an increase of gonad weights in F_1 males with accompanying effects on circulating testosterone secretion. In addition, BDE-209 and DE-71 exposure caused a decrease in male accessory reproductive organs and induction of androgen synthesis in female adrenals (van der Ven *et al.*, 2007). Tseng *et al.* (2006) did not find effects on sperm count or function at high concentrations of PBDE-209 (500-1,500 mg/kg/day from PND 21 to 70), but they did find indications of oxidative stress in sperm.

Recently, gestational exposures to BFRs were also evaluated to examine effects on the reproductive development of the male rat offspring. It was important to determine if AR inhibitors would demasculinize/feminize male rat offspring following a gestational and/or neonatal exposure scenario, as other anti-androgenic compounds have been shown to have these effects (Hotchkiss *et al.*, 2002, 2003; Gray *et al.*, 2004). Some work has been conducted on individual congeners following gestational exposures; evaluating effects on reproductive outcomes in the fetus. For example, Kuriyama *et al.* (2005) showed a decrease in spermiogenesis in the male offspring of dams exposed to a single low dose of 60 or 300 μg/kg of PBDE-99 on GD 6 (Table 40.1). Another study also found that a PBDE-99 oral exposure from GD 10–18 (1 or 10 mg/kg) reduced anogenital distance in male offspring (10 mg/kg) and resulted in decreased serum testosterone at weaning and PND 160 (Lilienthal *et al.*, 2006). In the same study, they also found an increase in sweet preference in the male offspring of both dose groups, which indicates a feminization of sexually dimorphic behavior (Hany *et al.*, 1999). Another study evaluated the effects of an orally dosed gestational exposure to decabromodiphenyl ether (PBDE-209) at doses of 5 to 320 mg/kg, but found no effects on testosterone- or androgen-dependent tissue weights on PND 42 (Kim *et al.*, 2009). Since SD male rats historically are not reproductively mature at PND 42 when the average PPS occurs, this time point may not have been the best time to measure testosterone or weigh the androgen-dependent tissues (Stoker *et al.*, 2000).

In a more recent study, Long Evans rat dams were dosed from GD 6 to weaning with 0, 1.6, 10.4 and 30.6 mg/kg of DE-71 by oral gavage (Kodavanti *et al.*, 2010) and the male offspring were evaluated for effects on reproductive developmental endpoints. There were no significant differences in the anogenital distance of the male offspring on PND 7 in any of the DE-71 dose groups as compared to the controls. In addition, this DE-71 exposure to the dam from pregnancy through PND 22 dose-dependently delayed the age of onset of preputial separation (PPS) by 1.0 and 1.8 days in the 10.2 and 30.6 mg/kg dose groups, respectively. However, only the 1.8 day delay in the high dose group was statistically different as compared to the control males. There was no significant difference in body weight at the time of puberty (PND 40 to 45), so the delay in PPS did not appear to be the result of altered body weight. There were no differences in the PND 60 weights of the seminal vesicles, epididymis, testis or ventral prostate. Although there appeared to be a decrease in the mean serum testosterone concentration at the highest dose, there was no statistical difference between the control mean and any of the DE-71 dose groups.

The observation of a delay in preputial separation in the male offspring in this recent study indicates that there is a decreased response to the circulating androgens or a suppression of androgen function. As mentioned, DE-71 was shown to be anti-androgenic in several *in vivo* and *in vitro* assays (Stoker *et al.*, 2004), and certain congeners inhibit the binding of androgens to the receptor. PBDE-100 was the most potent androgen receptor antagonist, and was determined to be a competitive AR antagonist, with an inhibition constant of 1 μM. This single congener is present in the mixture and does not appear to decrease in concentration over time of lactation. Since earlier studies had shown that DE-71 can delay the onset of preputial separation in the Wistar rat when administered during the peri-pubertal period (Stoker *et al.*, 2004), it is not surprising that a dose of 30 mg/kg to the lactating dam would lead to an accumulation of DE-71 in circulation and result in a 2 day delay in PPS. Although reproductive tract development was impaired in the previous study following a direct 30 day exposure from PND 23 to PND 53, we hypothesize that the DE-71 concentrations in this study were not high enough beyond puberty to prevent normal development of these androgen-dependent tissues.

In vitro studies examining effects on steroid binding, synthesis and clearance

Effects on AR binding

Because many of the *in vivo* rat studies with PBDEs demonstrated delays in pubertal progression and altered androgen-dependent tissue weights, Stoker *et al.* (2005) evaluated the five congeners of DE-71 and found that several of them showed anti-androgenicity in several *in vitro* systems. DE-71, BDE-47, BDE-99, BDE-100 and BDE-154 inhibited the binding of [^{3}H]R1881 (methyltrienolone 17 beta-hydroxy-17 alpha-methyl-estra-4,9,11-trien-3-one, AR agonist) to the cytosolic AR in a rat cytosol AR binding assay (Figure 40.3A). BDE-154 did not inhibit the binding of [^{3}H]R1881 beyond 40%, while BDE-99 and BDE-47 did display an IC_{50} of approximately 33 μM and 16.7 μ M. DE-71 and the congener BDE-100 displayed the most effective inhibition of the ligand for the receptor, shown by the most inhibition at lower concentrations (80% and 98% at 33 μM concentrations) and IC_{50}s of 5 μM and 3 μM, respectively. While the relative binding affinity curves for these compounds suggest that all compounds are competing with [^{3}H]R1881 for binding to the AR, this was confirmed by using fixed concentrations of BDE-100 against increasing concentrations of [^{3}H]R1881 for K_i determination (Figure 40.3B). The pattern of inhibition shown in the double-reciprocal plot indicates that BDE-100 is a true competitive inhibitor of [^{3}H]R1881 binding to the AR, in that concentrations of BDE-100 form a pattern of lines which intersect on the ordinate (Siegel, 1975). The linear slope replot confirmed that the *in vitro* mechanism is competitive inhibition and the calculated K_i for BDE-100 is 1 μM (Figure 40.3C).

Stoker *et al.* (2005) also evaluated the DE-71 commercial mixture and its individual congeners in the MDA-kb2 cell line (transfected with a human androgen receptor-hAR) to examine the anti-androgenic activity of the compounds by measuring gene expression. DE-71, BDE-47 and BDE-100 inhibited DHT-induced hAR transcriptional activation in a concentration-dependent manner (Figure 40.3D). The log-transformed data, which corrected for heterogeneity of variance, showed a decrease of DHT activity by 50% in the 5 μM concentration of DE-71, BDE-47 and BDE-100. The other three congeners, BDE-99, 153 and 154, did not inhibit DHT-induced transcription. The results of a lactose dehyrogenase assay confirmed that no cytotoxicity was observed in this study.

Other studies have recently evaluated other sets of PBDEs and flame retardants for androgenic or anti-androgenic activity. For example, in a large *in vitro* screen, AR-antagonistic potencies have been found for 18 out of 27 BFRs (Hamers *et al.*, 2006). They found that both BDE-19 and BDE-100 have a higher anti-androgenic activity than the prostate therapeutic drug flutamide (IC_{50} 60 and 100 nM, respectively; Hamers *et al.* 2006). This was also shown when Kojima *et al.* (2009) tested 12 PBDEs including metabolites and found AR antagonistic activity in several, with 4′-HO-BDE-17 showing the most potent activity followed by BDE-100. Quantitative structure–activity relationship models based on androgen antagonism also suggest that lower brominated BDEs with bromine substitutions in the *ortho*-positions and bromine-free *meta*- and *para*-positions have the highest potencies (Harju *et al.*, 2007; Kojima *et al.*, 2009).

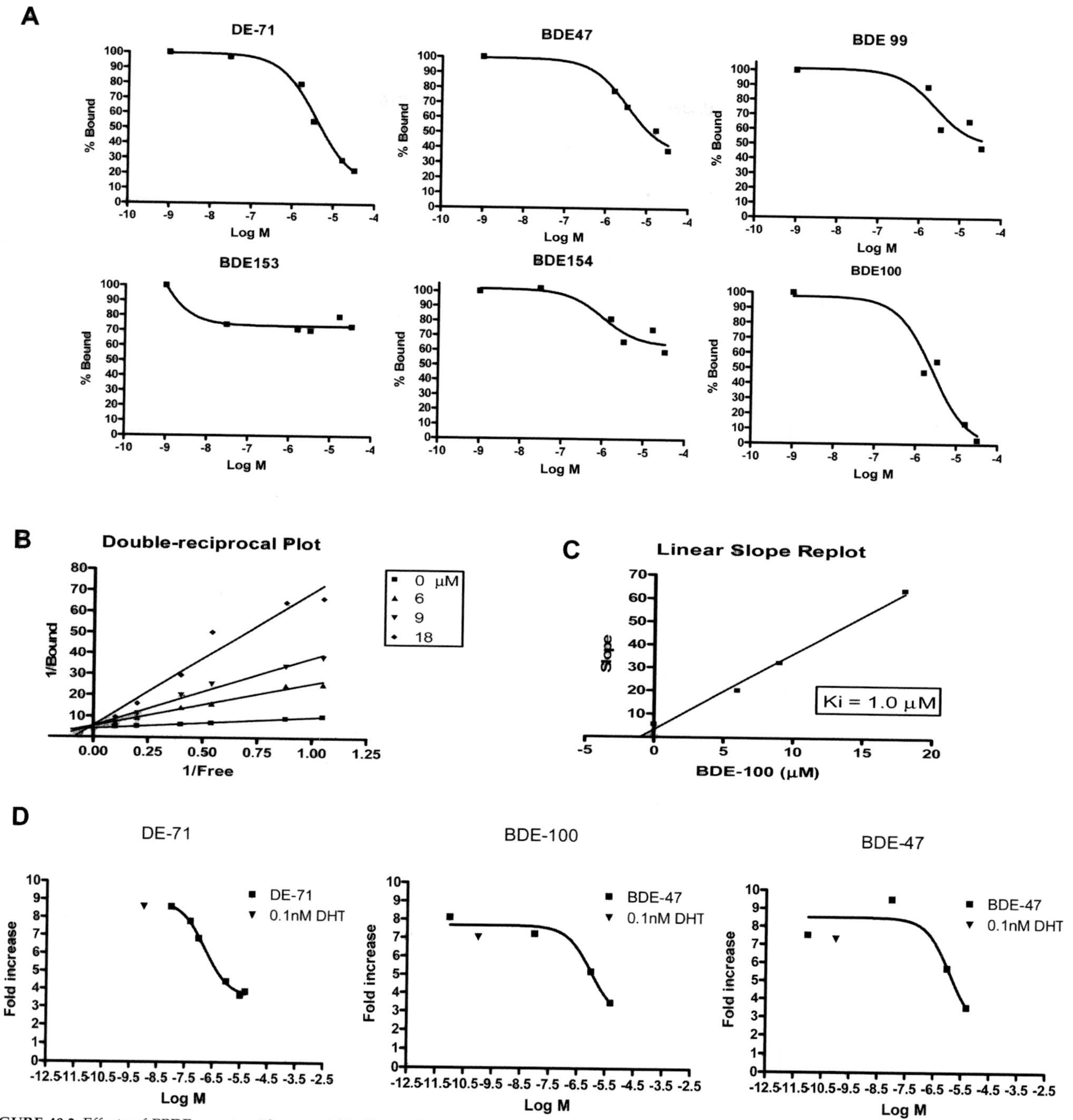

FIGURE 40.3 Effects of PBDEs on steroid receptor binding and activation. (A) DE-71 and individual congeners inhibition of [^{3}H] R1881 binding in the rat VP cytosol assay. 1.0 nM [^{3}H] R1881 was competed against varying concentrations of PBDEs overnight at 4°C. Data are presented as % [^{3}H] R1881 Bound. (B) Double-reciprocal analysis of the competitive inhibition of [^{3}H] R1881 specific binding to rat VP cytosolic AR by increasing BDE-100 concentrations (0, 6, 9 or 18 μM). ($n=2$ replicates with duplicate tubes/replicate.) (C) The slope replot analysis ($K_i = 1$ μM) of BDE-100 illustrating that the slope of the double-reciprocal plots vary linearly with increasing inhibitor concentrations. (D) Using the MDA-kb2 stable human AR/luciferase cell line, 0.1 nM DHT was competed against varying concentrations of DE-71, BDE-47 and BDE-100 overnight at 37°C. Hydroxyflutamide at 1 μM is also shown as a positive control in this assay. Data are presented as fold induction of luciferase activity over media control. ($n=3$ replicates with four wells/replicate.) (Reproduced from Stoker *et al.*, 2005, with permission from Elsevier.)

In contrast to the anti-androgenic potential of some flame retardants, BCH (1,2-dibromo-4-(1,2,-dibromoethyl)-cyclohexane), a BFR used in construction material, plastic parts of appliances and electric cable coating, was shown to be an androgen agonist (Larsson *et al.*, 2006). BCH binds to the AR and induces luciferase activity in human hepatocellular liver carcinoma cells transiently transfected with the human AR and a luciferase reporter gene at low μM concentrations. Further, their modeling of binding studies of the AR showed that BCH preferentially located to the ligand pocket (Larsson *et al.*, 2006). However, an *in vivo* study will need to be performed in a rodent model to assess the relevant exposures to humans.

Effects on steroidogenesis

In addition to studies showing effects of BFRs on the androgen receptor, other *in vitro* studies indicate that altered steroidogenesis may be involved in some of the anti-androgenic effects observed *in vivo*. Several cytochrome P450 (CYP) enzymes are responsible for the highly specific reactions in the steroid biosynthesis pathway and have been shown to be potential targets for endocrine disruption. These steroidogenic enzymes are responsible for the biosynthesis of various steroid hormones, including glucocorticoids, mineralocorticoids, progestins and sex hormones (estrogens and androgens). Androgens and subsequently estrogens are ultimately synthesized from cholesterol via the formation of pregnenolone, 17-alpha-hydroxypregnenolone and dehydroepiandrosterone (DHEA), the latter two synthesized by CYP17. Androgens may subsequently be converted to estrogens by the enzyme aromatase (CYP19). Also, both of these enzymes (CYP17 and CYP19) catalyze key steps in the production of sex hormones in humans.

Some PBDEs and their metabolites have been shown to induce or inhibit steroidogenic enzymes important in the conversion of testosterone to estradiol (aromatase, CYP19) and in the biosynthesis of the weak androgens DHEA and androstenedione in the adrenals, as well as testosterone in the testes (CYP17). Studies conducted in the H295R adrenocortical carcinoma cell line have shown that some of the hydroxylated and methoxylated PBDE metabolites are able to inhibit CYP19 at low μM concentrations, while 2,4,6-tribromophenol (2,4,6-TBP) induces this enzyme (Canton *et al.*, 2005). In addition, using human placental microsomes, they found that the 11 hydroxylated BDEs all inhibit placental aromatase activity with IC_{50}s in the μM range. They also showed in the H295R cells that hydroxylated metabolites of BDEs inhibit CYP17, but some of these metabolites showed cytotoxicity at high concentrations confounding the observed effect (Canton *et al.*, 2006). Only BDE-183, 6-OH-BDE-99 and 2-OH-BDE-47 inhibited CYP17 without displaying cytotoxicity. In another study, Ding *et al.* (2007) showed that 2,4,6-TBP suppressed CYP17 mRNA expression.

Effects on steroid metabolism

It has also been shown that the induction of the pregnane X receptor (PXR, called steroid X receptor) and the constitutive androstane receptor (CAR) affect the homeostasis of endogenous substances including steroids. Pacymiak *et al.* (2007) have studied the role of PXR in BFR-related effects and showed that BDE-47, 99 and 209 activated PXR. Others have also shown similar effects with HBCD and BDE-47, 99 and 153 (Sanders *et al.*, 2005; Germer *et al.*, 2006; Wahl *et al.*, 2007). Therefore, it is possible that some of the effects observed previously *in vivo* may also involve changes to the CAR/PXR signaling pathways.

Female reproductive effects

PBDEs have been reported to have a variety of female reproductive effects in animal models for human disease, but to date there is only one report of this family of compounds potentially impacting human reproduction. Harley and coworkers (Harley *et al.*, 2010) collected blood at around 26 weeks of pregnancy from 223 women in the CHAMACOS study and found a strong 40–50% decrease in the odds of becoming pregnant with each 10-fold increase in serum concentrations of BDE-100 or 153. There was also a 30% decrease in the odds of becoming pregnant each month with each 10-fold increase in serum BDE-47, 99, 100 and 153, when considered together. The only other epidemiological study addressing human developmental concerns was in Taiwan (Chao *et al.*, 2007). That study reported that increased PBDEs in milk was related to altered birth weight and length, infant chest circumference and the length of the mother's menstrual cycle.

Using rodent models, other effects of PBDEs on female reproductive outcomes have been delineated. Following exposure to the DE-71 mixture under the EDSP Pubertal Protocol (oral dosing from PND 22 to 41; Laws *et al.*, 2000), female Wistar rats demonstrated a 1.8 day delay in the onset of puberty (60 mg/kg), decreased serum T_4 (30 mg/kg), increased liver size and induction of hepatic enzymes (30 mg/kg), without effects on body weight (Stoker *et al.*, 2004). The only other DE-71 study to report effects on female pubertal indices (Kodavanti *et al.*, 2010) demonstrated significantly delayed mammary gland development in Long Evans rat offspring exposed to DE-71 (orally, 10.2 and 30.6 mg/kg) from GD 6 to PND 21 (Figure 40.4). The mammary effects were evident on PND 21, nearly 2 weeks earlier than vaginal opening (VO), using a mammary gland whole mount approach. Another study, exposing pregnant rats to DE-71 (60 μg/kg) from GD 1.5 through PND 20 did not evaluate pubertal indices in F_1 offspring and found no effects of treatment on reproductive endpoints (LaVoie *et al.*, 2008).

In an adult ovariectomized mouse assay comparing the effects of DE-71 in C57Bl/6 and Balb/C strains, there was a strain-dependent effect on the uterus, with increased uterine epithelial height and vaginal epithelial thickness in the Balb/C given 50 mg/kg DE-71 subcutaneously for 34 days. Little effect was seen after a 3 day subcutaneous exposure and no effects were seen when DE-71 was administered orally up to 300 mg/kg (Mercado-Feliciano and Bigsby, 2008). These authors also reported DE-71-induced proliferation of MCF-7 cells, which was blocked by the estradiol antagonist ICI 182 780. They demonstrated significant DE-71 dose-dependent inhibition of estradiol-induced proliferation at 1, 5 and 10 μM.

Many other studies have evaluated individual congeners for their effects on female reproductive endpoints, and have utilized either a gestational or gestational and lactational window of exposure. The developmental effects of BDE-99 were evaluated by Talsness *et al.* (2005). In that study, 0.06 or 0.3 mg/kg PBDE-99 was administered by gavage to Wistar rats on GD 6. At approximately 5 months of age, female F_1 offspring from each group were mated with untreated males to evaluate fertility. Pregnancy rate, total implantation sites, mean implantation sites per gravid dam, total live fetuses per dam, resorption rate and percentage of dams with resorptions in the F_1 females were similar to controls at both doses of BDE-99. Increased mean fetal weights at 0.06 mg/kg BDE-99, but not at 0.3 mg/kg BDE-99, were reported. Follicle counts were performed in the F_1 females and although there was no difference seen, evaluation by electron or light microscopy of the ovary, uterus and vagina of 90 day old F_1 female offspring detected ultrastructural changes in the ovaries and hyperplastic vacuolar degeneration of the vaginal epithelium in both BDE-99 exposed groups. Long Evans rats were also administered BDE-99 (s.c., 1 and 10 mg/kg) from GD 10 to 18 (Ceccatelli *et al.*, 2006). Anogenital distance, VO and uterine weight were unchanged compared to controls, although

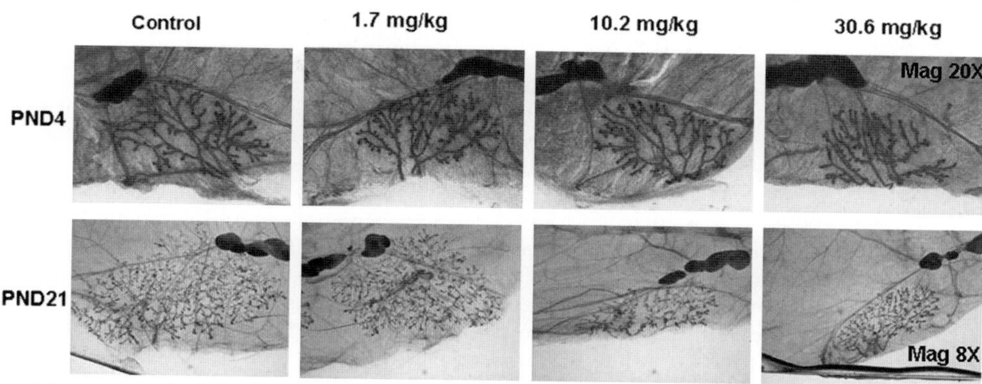

FIGURE 40.4 Prepubertal mammary gland development in female pups at PND 4 and PND 21 following developmental exposure to DE-71. Significant developmental delays were observed at PND 21 at 10.2 and 30.6 mg/kg DE-71. Magnifications differ between PND 4 and 21 and are noted. (Reproduced from Kodavanti *et al.*, 2010, with permission from Oxford University Press.)

BDE-99 demonstrated a positive trend for delayed VO. Ovarian weight and ovarian weight relative to body weight were significantly increased at the highest dose. Adult uterine progesterone receptor expression was decreased compared to controls, at both doses evaluated. Uterine ER-β and IGF-I gene expression were upregulated at the lower dose. A near repeat of this study by another research lab (Lilienthal *et al.*, 2006), using the same strain, route of administration and doses of BDE-99 found significantly smaller thyroid weights in 21-day-old female pups, a significant delay in VO (high dose) and decreased primordial (low dose) and secondary (high dose) follicle counts. Although both of the studies saw a response in delayed VO in the high dose group, the timing of VO in the two studies was quite different; control and high dose VO occurred on PND 33.7 and 34.0 (Lilienthal *et al.*, 2006) vs. 39.6 and 40.9 (Ceccatelli *et al.*, 2006), respectively. Different Long Evans distributors were utilized (Denmark and France).

Talsness *et al.* (2008) also evaluated the effects of an oral GD 6 exposure to BDE-47 (140 or 700 μg/kg) for effects in the female offspring. They found a significant decrease in ovarian weight at the lower dose, decreased secondary follicle counts at both BDE levels, and decreased tertiary follicles and serum estradiol concentrations at the higher dose. Persistent effects on the thyroid gland were also observed. The females were mated with unexposed males and no changes in reproductive indices were observed (Talsness *et al.*, 2008). Preliminary data in Wistar rats gavaged with 20 mg/kg of BDE-47 or 5 mg/kg 6-OH-BDE-47 from GD 10 to 16 did not exhibit any effect on female offspring growth, timing of vaginal opening or estrous cycle length as adults (Buitenhuis *et al.*, 2004). In another study, Wistar rats were given intravenous BDE-47 at 0.2 mg/kg from GD 15 to PND 20, every 5th day (Suvorov *et al.*, 2009), and found no changes in fur development, incisor eruption, eye opening or VO in the female offspring.

Some of the most recent concerns regarding the potential for adverse effects of TBBPA focus on the possibility that it may act as an endocrine disruptor. The structural similarity of TBBPA to bisphenol A, a known weak environmental estrogen, has suggested that this chemical might have the ability to bind to the estrogen receptor and disrupt signaling. TBBPA has been shown to induce malformations in zebrafish embryos at concentrations of 1.5 μM, and at 6 μM caused a failure to hatch (Kuiper *et al.*, 2007). Meerts *et al.* (2001) examined the estrogenic potency of TBBPA and related compounds in the T47D human breast cancer cell line, as well as cells stably transfected with ER-α and ER-β luciferase-linked constructs to evaluate estrogen receptor-dependent activation and gene expression. TBBPA had little estrogenic effect, but lower brominated bisphenols demonstrated the highest estrogenic potencies (Meerts *et al.*, 2001). Their results indicated that several BDE congeners, but especially the OH-BDE and brominated BPA analogs, are ER agonists. Furthermore, hydroxylated TBBPA metabolites have been shown to inhibit estrogen sulfotransferase activity *in vitro* (Kester *et al.*, 2002). If such an inhibition were to occur *in vivo*, it could result in elevated levels of circulating estrogens because sulfation is a major elimination pathway for endogenous estrogenic hormones.

In summary, although the rodent studies have not repeatably shown the same effects in female offspring (likely due to differences in dose, rat strain, various end targets evaluated, etc.), they have consistently demonstrated effects of the PBDEs on steroid-responsive target tissues (uterus, mammary gland and ovary), as well as altered steroid and steroid receptor gene expression. *In vitro* culture studies confirm that steroid receptor activation or steroidogenesis appears to be targets for BDE-related effects. In fact, cultures of porcine theca and granulosa cells exposed to a range (0.05 to 50 ng/ml) of BDE congeners (47, 99, 100 and 209) produced increased progesterone secretion, as well as other irreversible effects on estradiol and testosterone secretion (Karpeta and Gregoraszcuk, 2010).

Rats may not be the most sensitive species of animal in which to test the PBDEs. Complete reproductive failure has been reported in mink fed 2.5 ppm DE-71 in the diet (Zhang *et al.*, 2009). Also, at 0.5 ppm in the diet, males and females displayed increased liver size and reduced tT_3, and females exhibited increased tT_4. This species seems highly sensitive to the effects of PBDEs, and are known to have a greater capacity than rodents to biotransform BDE-99.

TOXICOKINETICS AND METABOLITES

With regard to toxicokinetics, we have discussed all three groups of predominant BFRs.

TBBPA

Despite generally low concentrations of TBBPA in the US and European diet, it is still considered the major pathway of exposure to the general population (EU-Report, 2005). The low systemic bioavailability of TBBPA results in low blood levels of parent and metabolites. Because of this, TBBPA is thought to have a low potential for toxic effects after administration of high doses in rodents. In repeated exposure studies the NOAEL was relatively high (>1,000 mg/kg body weight; EU-Report, 2005). Parent TBBPA and its derived metabolites were detected in bile, and excreted predominantly in feces; however, metabolites were only found in the urine. The metabolites identified in the bile of rats were TBBPA-glucuronide, a diglucuronide, and a mixed glucuronide-sulfate (Hakk *et al.*, 2000). After only intravenous (i.v.) injection in rats, TBBPA was also rapidly cleared where the majority of an i.v. dose was also recovered in the feces (Kuester *et al.*, 2007). It is suspected that biliary elimination rates of TBBPA may differ between rats and humans. Results obtained from kinetic studies in rodents and humans suggest low absorption of TBBPA from the gastrointestinal tract along with rapid metabolism (Schauer *et al.*, 2006; Kuester *et al.*, 2007). These results further support that TBBPA has a low potential for bioaccumulation in mammals. In summary, systemic levels of TBBPA are low most likely due to efficient hepatic metabolism and biliary elimination of its conjugated metabolities.

HBCD

Information on the toxicokinetics of HBCD is limited. The current literature has been dominated with studies focusing on the commercially available HBCD mixture via oral and dermal routes of exposure. HBCD is reported to be absorbed from the gastrointestinal tract and it is hypothesized that food and dust intake is the largest source of human exposure to HBCD. Unfortunately, most toxicokinetic and toxicity studies have been compromised as animals were administered HBCD suspensions in oil. Undissolved particles of HBCD in oil as well as absorption to glass results in decreased administration and decreased internal absorption. These factors create further uncertainties when comparing dose and effects across studies.

There are three main diastereoisomers in the commercial HBCD mixture, denoted as alpha (α), beta (β) and gamma (γ) with the γ-diastereoisomer predominating (>70%) (Heeb *et al.*, 2005). High concentrations of HBCD in some top predators indicate persistence and biomagnification of HBCD. Most of the early studies of HBCD did not examine individual diastereoisomers but only the commercial mixture. Recent studies have shown that there is a predominance of α-HBCD in biota (Law *et al.*, 2006a) and that individual diastereomers have different physical and chemical properties. As continued biological, physical and chemical differences of the HBCD diastereomers are uncovered, there is a growing need to understand the individual diastereomers that make up the commercial mixture.

A study by Szabo *et al.* (2010) was conducted to characterize absorption, distribution, metabolism and excretion parameters of the major HBCD diastereomer, γ-HBCD, with respect to dose and time following a single acute oral exposure and a 10 day repeated exposure in adult female C57BL/6 mice. γ-[^{14}C]HBCD was purified from the commercial mixture, dissolved properly and completely in corn oil and orally administered. Results suggest that 85% of the administered dose (3 mg/kg) was absorbed after oral exposure. Disposition was dose-independent after a single exposure to 3, 10, 30 and 100 mg/kg of γ-HBCD and disposition did not significantly change after 10 days of exposure. Liver was the major depot (<0.3% of dose) 4 days after treatment followed by blood, fat and brain; however, less than 1% of the dose remained in the tissues by 4 days. γ-HBCD was rapidly metabolized and eliminated in the urine (30%) and feces (55%) by day 4. For the first time, *in vivo* stereoisomerization was observed of the γ-HBCD diastereoisomer to the β-HBCD diastereoisomer in liver and brain tissues, and to the α- and β-HBCD diastereoisomer in fat and feces (Figure 40.5). Polar metabolites in the blood and urine were a major factor in determining the initial whole-body half-life (1 day) after a single oral exposure. Elimination, both whole-body and from individual tissues, was biphasic. Initial half-lives were approximately 1 day, whereas terminal half-lives were up to 4 days, suggesting limited potential for γ-diastereoisomer bioaccumulation. This first complete *in vivo* report on the toxicokinetics of γ-HBCD indicated that two factors may be responsible for the shift observed from the predominance of γ-HBCD in the commercial mixture and environment relative to α-HBCD in biota. First, γ-HBCD was observed to be rapidly metabolized and eliminated. Second, *in vivo* stereoisomerization of γ-HBCD to α- and β- occurred (Figure 40.5). Szabo *et al.* (2010) concluded that the biological persistence of γ-HBCD in mice was low and may explain low levels of γ-HBCD in biota. This ADME data would support the Szabo *et al.* (2010) hypothesis that metabolism and stereoisomerization, in addition to differential exposure, play a role in the observed stereoisomer profiles in biota. The toxicokinetic behavior reported has important implications for the extrapolation of toxicological studies of the commercial HBCD mixture to the assessment of risk.

A few studies (although flawed with improper dosing solution as mentioned above) have been conducted using the commercial HBCD mixture. In experimental studies, the HBCD commercial mixture was found to be deposited in several organs after oral administration, with accumulation in adipose tissue. Several (unidentified) metabolites are also shown in experimental studies (Yu and Atallah, 1980). HBCD partitions to adipose tissue at higher concentrations in females and this was observed in a rat 90 day study (Chengelis, 2001). This has been suggested to be possibly due to a faster elimination in male compared to female rats (Yu and Atallah, 1980). The excreted HBCD in that study, both in the feces and in the urine, was most likely completely metabolized, indicating complete absorption of the orally dosed compound which was similarly seen with γ-HBCD (Szabo *et al.*, 2010). Another study by Arita *et al.* (1983) exposed rats to the commercial HBCD mixture (Pyroguard SR-103; Daiichi Kogyo Seiyaku K.K.) with a suspension of 500 mg/kg HBCD administered for 5 days. No urinary excretion of parent HBCD was reported (only an unknown metabolite) and the cumulative fecal excretion of HBCD was 32–35%. Considering the high dose (500 mg/kg) and the use of a particle suspension, the degree of gastrointestinal tract absorption is questioned. Whether the presence of HBCD or its bioaccumulation seen here was due to alpha, beta or gamma remained unknown.

A dermal *in vitro* study on human skin has been performed according to OECD Test Guideline 428 in order to assess the

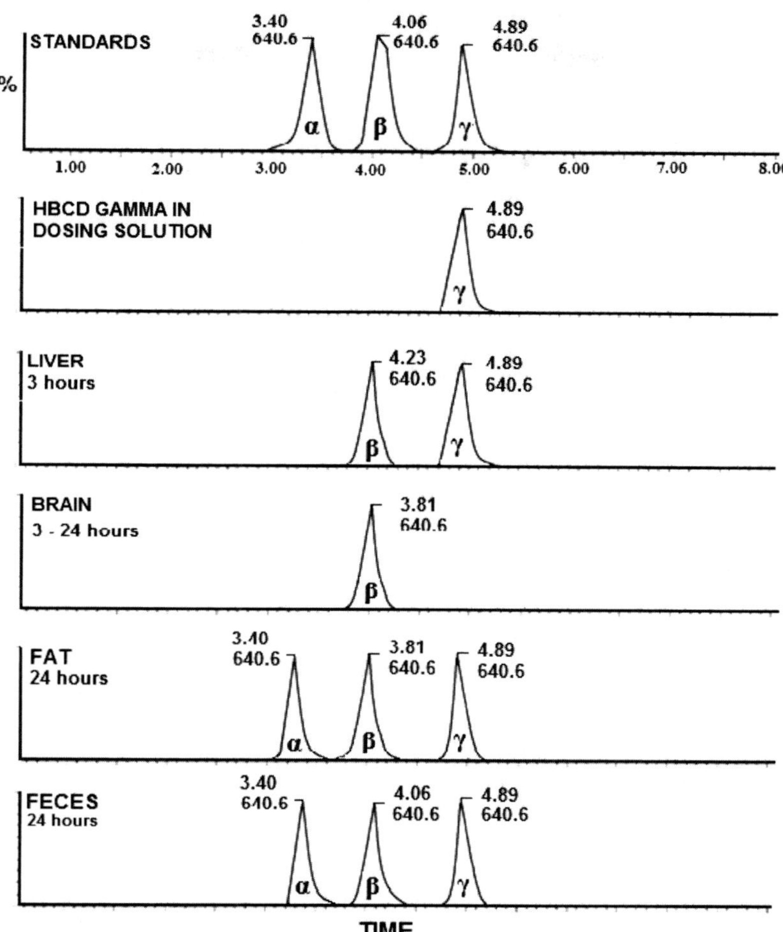

FIGURE 40.5 Evidence of *in vivo* stereoisomerization of γ-HBCD: LC-MS chromatograms of tissues and excreta after oral administration of γ-HBCD in mice. ^{14}C derived radioactivity was determined based on retention time and molecular weight using LC/MS. Chromatograms of α-HBCD, β- and γ- standards, liver and feces peaks from TLC were analyzed after mice were orally exposed to the diastereomer γ-HBCD. Standards are a representative sample and retention times varied slightly from day to day. To conserve low levels of radioactivity, fat as well as brain tissue were pooled and Gel Permeation Chromatography (GPC) was used prior to LC/MS analysis. This demonstrates that γ-HBCD can undergo *in vivo* stereoisomerization to form α-HBCD and β-HBCD diastereomers and the presence of the stereoisomers are tissue and matrix specific. (Adapted from Szabo *et al.*, 2010.)

rate and extent of HBCD absorption (Roper, 2005). Samples of human breast skin were obtained from seven patients, 19–68 years old. ^{14}C-HBCD commercial product was mixed in acetone by inversion until the mixture was dissolved. Five consecutive 6 µl aliquots were applied to the skin for a total of 640 µg ^{14}C-HBCD of the dose solution. These samples were analyzed by combustion/liquid scintillation counting. The corrected total mass of ^{14}C-HBCD applied to the skin was calculated to be 607 µg. The results are based on nine samples of skin obtained from six different donors. Receptor fluid was collected in hourly fractions for 0–8 hours and then every 2 hours for 8–24 hours post dose and mixed with liquid scintillation fluid and counted. The underside of the skin was washed with receptor fluid and was analyzed by scintillation counting. The stratum corneum was removed with 20 successive tape strips. The first five strips were pooled and analyzed together. There were two steady-state fluxes observed in the study, the first from 0 to 6 hours and the second from 6 to 24 hours. Considering the solubility of HBCD in water is low (2.1, 14.7 and 48.8 µg/l for γ-, β- and α-HBCD, respectively) it was not surprising to see the amount of HBCD found in the receptor fluid close to the solubility of gamma-HBCD in water. The authors concluded that the total dermal absorption was estimated to be 4% of the applied dose.

PBDE

Current data on the toxicokinetics of PBDEs have focused on an oral or dermal route of exposure with very little information via other routes, since these routes appear to be the most relevant for environmental or indoor exposure. There are significant differences in the toxicokinetic behavior between individual PBDE congeners and mixtures. These differences in adsorption, distribution, metabolism and excretion (ADME) depend on the test animal species used and the degree of bromination of the administered compound. As the number of bromine atoms increases from four bromines to 10 bromines (tetraBDE to decaBDE), there are decreases in oral absorption which lead to shortened half-lives and increased elimination in both the urine and feces.

Higher brominated PBDE congeners

Decabromodiphenyl ether (decaBDE or PBDE-209) is the fully brominated PBDE congener containing 10 bromine atoms and is not absorbed well by either humans or animals. It is believed that the low amounts of decaBDE absorbed can be metabolized (ATSDR, 2004). This has been seen in rats where decaBDE is poorly absorbed with greater than 90% of the dose excreted within 48 hours (Morck *et al.*, 2003). However, once absorbed and in the body, decaBDE may be excreted (as parent) or eliminated (as metabolites), mainly in the feces and to a lesser extent in the urine within a few days (ATSDR, 2004). Workers occupationally exposed to decaBDEs have shown half-lives around 15 days (Thuresson *et al.*, 2006) which is considerably shorter than other lower brominated BDE congeners. DecaBDE has been found in the blood and breast milk of humans in the general population, but at lower levels than other PBDE congeners (Lorber, 2008).

Debromination of PBDE congeners

Debromination of decaBDE leads to formation of lower brominated congeners. Debromination has been postulated to be another possible source of lower brominated PBDE congeners in the environment (Riess *et al.*, 2000, Sorderstrom *et al.*, 2004; Huwe and Smith, 2007). The loss of bromines has shown to occur through *in vivo* metabolism, microbacteria, thermal conversion and photodegradation. Evidence that decaBDE undergoes *in vivo* metabolic debromination have been observed in several species including fish (Holbrook, 2006), birds (van den Steen *et al.*, 2007), cows (Kierkegaard *et al.*, 2007) and rats (Huwe *et al.*, 2007). The major debromination products were hepta- to nonaPBDEs for fish, birds and cows, and octa- and nonaPBDEs for rats. Evidence that microorganisms can debrominate higher BDE congeners to lower congeners has been observed with anaerobic bacteria from soils and sediments (Lee and He, 2010). Thermal debromination reactions of PBDEs are enhanced at temperatures above 500°C (Weber and Kuch, 2003). PBDEs can also be directly converted to PBDD/PBDF within thermal systems (Weber and Kuch, 2003). The kinetics of the thermal conversion of PBDEs to PBDDs and PBDFs appears to be more favorable for the lower-brominated diphenyl ethers than for decaBDE (Weber and Kuch, 2003). Photolytic debromination of BDE-28, BDE-47, BDE-99, BDE-100, BDE-153 and BDE-183 has been observed following pseudo-first-order kinetics (Fang *et al.*, 2008). Higher brominated PBDE congeners degrade at a faster rate than lower brominated congeners where reductive debromination was the main mechanism during photolysis forming lower brominated PBDE congeners.

Lower brominated PBDE congeners

Lower brominated PBDEs, in contrast to decaBDE, are more readily absorbed and persist in the body for many years, since they are mainly stored in body fat. Lower brominated congeners such as the tetraBDE (BDE-47) and the pentaBDE (BDE-99) are well absorbed and highly distributed to lipophilic tissues, such as adipose, skin and liver (Orn and Klasson-Wehler, 1998; Hakk *et al.*, 2002; Staskal *et al.*, 2005). In rats, tetra- and pentaBDEs are metabolized and eliminated slowly (Hakk *et al.*, 2002) while in mice, PBDE-47 is also well absorbed and distributed, but its elimination is rapid (Staskal *et al.*, 2005). Uptake efficiencies of BDE-47, BDE-99 and BDE-153 by pike fed trout injected with the congeners were 90%, 62% and 40%, respectively (Burreau *et al.*, 1997). Von Meyerinck *et al.* (1990) tested the components of a commercial pentaBDE product, Bromkal 70 and concluded that the degree of bromination directly influences the rate of elimination. In another rat-feeding study, Huwe *et al.* (2007) reported the retention of the BDE congeners in tissues decreased from 40–50% for BDE-47, 99 and 100 to 25–30% for BDE-153 and 154.

PBDE metabolites

Hydoxylated PBDE metabolites are a concern as they outcompete thyroxine for serum binding proteins. This increases total body burden of the administered compound and prolongs exposure and possible delivery to target tissues. This binding has been hypothesized as a mode of action in the displacement, increased metabolism and elimination of thyroid hormones (Szabo *et al.*, 2009). Hydroxylated and/or methoxylated PBDE congeners have been detected in several species including Baltic salmon, herring, ringed seal, gray seal, rats and humans (Asplund *et al.*, 1997, 1999; Haglund *et al.*, 1997; Kierkegaard *et al.*, 1999; Hakk *et al.*, 2002; Athanasiadou *et al.*, 2008). BDE-99 and BDE-100 have been found to be metabolized to OH-pentaBDE and OH-tetraBDE in the rat (Hakk *et al.*, 2002, 2006). Hydroxylated metabolites have been reported to be retained in mouse plasma after exposure to a commercial pentaBDE product (Qiu *et al.*, 2007). OH-BDEs have been detected and identified as metabolites of BDE-47, 99, 100 and 153 in urine and feces from female mice (Chen *et al.*, 2006; Staskal *et al.*, 2006).

PBDE mixture studies

Studies on lower brominated BDE commercial mixtures (pentaBDE and octaBDE commercial mixtures) show similar pharmacokinetic behaviors as individual lower brominated congeners. Huwe *et al.* (2007) exposed rats to environmental levels (2.9 ppb) of the commercial PBDE mixture Great Lakes DE-71 in peanut oil for 21 days via a feeding study. BDE-47 and 99 were the two congeners present at the highest levels in the dose, liver, carcass and feces. Because the congener pattern of the five major PBDEs remained similar in the dose, carcass and feces of the rats, they concluded that there were no significant differences between the bioavailability and accumulation of the major brominated congeners investigated in this study. A comparable study was conducted by Huwe *et al.* (2002) where male Sprague-Dawley rats were fed 33 ng/day/animal of the octaBDE commercial mixture, DE-79, in peanut oil for 21 days. While BDE-183 was the dominant congener detected in the administered dosing solution, feces, liver and carcass, BDE-153 bioaccumulated to the highest degree, with >60% of the dose remaining in the tissues. The authors concluded that bioaccumulation was inversely related to the degree of bromination for hexa- to octaBDEs and that some of the higher PBDE congeners were metabolized, since total recovery was <60%. Based on these two studies, on average, after 21 days of exposure, 0.7% of a commercial pentaBDE dose remained in the liver and 43% remained in the carcass. Furthermore, 1% of commercial octaBDE dose remained in the liver and 34% remained in the carcass. A study by Szabo *et al.* (2009) demonstrated that after oral administration of DE-71 to pregnant Long Evans rats, the effects of the BDE mixture causes hypothyroidism in offspring, including hepatic effects in the male offspring at postnatal day ages 4 and 22. Once the pups were weaned, gene expression levels and enzyme activities went back to basal levels at postnatal age 60. This study suggested that the PBDE congeners could cross the placenta (*in utero* exposure) and pass through the breast milk (lactational transference).

There have been a few studies that have measured PBDEs after dermal exposure. Hughes *et al.* (2001) examined dermal absorption after exposure to decaBDE. This *in vitro* system used skin from the adult hairless female mouse which was removed and mounted in flow-through diffusion cells. The percent of the administered dose detected in the skin after 1 day was low and ranged from 2 to 20%. Staskal *et al.* (2005) conducted an *in vivo* study in mice to measure dermal absorption of BDE-47. Approximately 62% of the administered dose was absorbed over a 5 day period. The dermal absorption of BDE-47 was also examined by Roper *et al.* (2006) using rat and human skin *in vitro*. The total absorbed dose in human and rat skin after 24 hours was 3.1% and 17.9%, respectively (Roper *et al.*, 2006) demonstrating that rat skin was more permeable than human skin to BDE-47.

CONCLUDING REMARKS AND FUTURE DIRECTIONS

Brominated flame retardants belong to a large group of organohalogen chemicals. They can be highly persistent, bioaccumulative and cause adverse effects in humans and wildlife. Although some BFRs are banned or voluntarily withdrawn from usage by the manufacturer, emerging and existing BFRs continue to be used in industrialized countries. Because of the widespread use and large quantities of these chemicals in consumer products and household items, indoor contamination is proposed to be a significant source of human exposure. Other exposure routes are oral – both via breast milk, fat-containing foods, hand to mouth activity, etc.

Recent epidemiological studies clearly indicated that BFRs affect human health. The human health effects include cryptorchidism, alterations in thyroid hormone homeostasis, reproductive effects and reduced development of children at school age that include psychomotor development index and IQ performance. Studies have also indicated that the infant daily exposure dose of PBDEs due to inhalation, accidental oral ingestion and dermal absorption of house dust was significantly higher than that of the adults. Many rodent studies have confirmed that developmental exposure to these compounds should be limited. Studies in rodents indicated that several BFRs are developmental neurotoxicants affecting the nervous system growth and function. Several studies have also confirmed that the brominated flame retardants are indeed endocrine disruptors, with the potential to disrupt male and female reproductive development and adult reproductive function by having anti-androgenic actions (males) and by altering steroidogenic activities. This has been demonstrated in several *in vivo* studies using rodent models and by *in vitro* systems to determine effects on receptor binding (AR, CAR and PXR) and on steroidogenesis. These potential modes of action may also be relevant to humans. This is incredibly important to consider as there have been several reports of adverse health consequences associated with increased PBDE exposure in humans in the last few years (Meeker *et al.*, 2009; Roze *et al.*, 2009; Harley *et al.*, 2010; Herbstman *et al.*, 2010). Further research is needed to determine the long-term adverse consequences of exposures to the BFR described herein as well as a number of emerging replacement chemicals coming onto the market, since these compounds are known to bioaccumulate and can be transplacentally and lactationally transferred.

ACKNOWLEDGMENTS

The authors thank Mr. Jonathan Besas for collection of relevant literature, Mr. John Havel for excellent graphic assistance, Drs. Linda Birnbaum and June Dunnick of National Institute of Environmental Health Sciences, Research Triangle Park, NC, and Drs. Heldur Hakk and Janice Huwe of US Department of Agriculture, Fargo, ND, for constructive review of this chapter. The contents of this chapter has been reviewed by the National Institute of Environmental Health Sciences and the National Health and Environmental Effects Research Laboratory of the US Environmental Protection Agency, and approved for publication. Approval does not signify that the contents necessarily reflect the views and policies of the Institute or Agency, nor does mention of trade names or commercial products constitute endorsement or recommendation for use.

REFERENCES

Agency for Toxic Substances and Disease Registry (2004) Toxicological Profile for Polybrominated Biphenyls and Polybrominated Diphenyl Ethers (PBBs and PBDEs). Atlanta, GA: US Department of Health and Human Services, Public Health Service, September 2004.

Arita R, Miyazaki K, Mure S (1983) Metabolic test of hexabromocyclododecane. Test on chemical substances used in household items. Studies on pharmacodynamics of hexabromocyclododecane. Department of Pharmacy, Hokkaido University Hospital (unpublished report).

Asplund L, Athanasiadou M, Eriksson U, Sjodin A, Borjeson H, Bergman A (1997) Mass spectrometric screening for organohalogen substances (OHs) in blood plasma from Baltic salmon (*Salmo salar*). *Organohalogen Comp* **33:** 355–9.

Asplund L, Athanasiadou M, Sjodin A, Bergman A, Borjeson H (1999) Organohalogen substances in muscle, egg and blood from healthy Baltic salmon (*Salmo salar*) and Baltic salmon affected by the M74 syndrome. *Ambio* **28:** 67–76.

Athanasiadou M, Cuadra SN, Marsh G, Bergman Å, Jakobsson K (2008) Polybrominated diphenyl ethers (PBDEs) and bioaccumulative hydroxylated PBDE metabolites in young humans from Managua, Nicaragua. *Environ Health Perspect* **116:** 400–8.

Birnbaum LS, Staskal DF, Diliberto JJ (2003) Health effects of polybrominated dibenzo-p-dioxins (PBDDs) and dibenzofurans (PBDFs). *Environ Int* **29:** 855–60.

Bocio A, Llobet JM, Domingo JL, Corbella J, Teixido A, Casas C (2003) Polybrominated diphenyl ethers (PBDEs) in foodstuffs: human exposure through the diet. *J Agric Food Chem* **51:** 3191–5.

Branchi I, Alleva E, Costa JG (2002) Effects of perinatal exposure to a polybrominated diphenyl ether (PBDE 99) on mouse neurobehavioral development. *Neurotoxicology* **23:** 375–84.

Branchi I, Capone F, Alleva E, Costa LG (2003) Polybrominated diphenyl ethers: neurobehavioral effects following developmental exposure. *Neurotoxicology* **24:** 449–62.

Branchi I, Capone F, Vitalone A, Madia F, Santucci D, Alleva E, Costa LG (2005) Early developmental exposure to BDE 99 or Aroclor 1254 affects neurobehavioural profile: interference from the administration route. *Neurotoxicology* **26:** 183–92.

BSEF. Bromine Science and Environmental Forum. Legislation on BFRs in North America. http://www.bsef.com/regulation/north-america/ Accessed June 21, 2010.

Buitenhuis C, Cenijn PC, Lilienthal H, Malmberg T, Bergman Å, Gutleb AC, Legler J, Brouwer A (2004) Effects of prenatal exposure to hydoxylated PCB metabolites and some brominated flame retardants on the development of rats. *Organohalogen Compounds* **66:** 3586.

Burreau S, Axelman J, Broman D, Jakobsson E (1997) Dietary uptake in pike (*Esox lucius*) of some polychlorinated biphenyls, polychlorinated naphthalenes and polybrominated diphenyl ethers administered in natural diet. *Environ Toxicol Chem* **16:** 2508–13.

Buser HR (1986) Polybrominated dibenzofurans and dibenzo-p-dioxins: thermal reaction products of polybrominated diphenyl ether flame retardants. *Environ Sci Technol* **20:** 404–8.

Butt CM, Diamond ML, Truong J, Ikonomou MG, ter Schure AF (2004) Spatial distribution of polybrominated diphenyl ethers in southern Ontario as measured in indoor and outdoor window organic films. *Environ Sci Technol* **38:** 724–31.

Canton RF, Sanderson JT, Letcher RJ, Bergman A, van den Berg M (2005) Inhibition and induction of aromatase (CYP19) activity by brominated flame retardants in H295R human adrenocortical carcinoma cells. *Toxicol Sci* **88:** 147–55.

Canton RF, Sanderson JT, Nijmejer S, Bergman A, Letcher RJ, van den Berg M (2006) *In vitro* effects of brominated flame retardants and metabolites on CYP17 catalytic activity: a novel mechanism of action? *Toxicol Appl Pharmacol* **227:** 68–75.

Ceccatelli R, Faass O, Schlumpf M, Lichtensteiger W (2006) Gene expression and estrogen sensitivity in rat uterus after developmental exposure to the polybrominated diphenylether PBDE 99 and PCB. *Toxicology* **220:** 104–16.

Chao H-R, Wang S-L, Lee W-J, Wang Y-F, Papke O (2007) Levels of polybrominated diphenyl ethers (PBDEs) in breast milk from central Taiwan and their relationship to infant birth outcome and maternal menstruation effects. *Environ Intl* **33:** 239–45.

Chen LJ, Lebetkin EH, Sanders JM, Burka LT (2006). Metabolism and disposition of 2,2′,4,4′,5-pentabromodiphenyl ether (BDE99) following a single or repeated administration to rats or mice. *Xenobiotica* **36:** 515–34.

Cheng J, Gu J, Ma J, Chen X, Zhang M, Wang W (2009) Neurobehavioural effects, redox responses and tissue distribution in rat offspring developmental exposure to BDE-99. *Chemosphere* **75:** 963–8.

Chengelis CP (2001) A 90-Day Oral (Gavage) Toxicity Study of HBCD in Rats. WIL Research Laboratories, Ashland, OH.

Costa LG, Giordano G, Tagliaferri S, Caglieri A, Mutti A (2008) Polybrominated diphenyl ether (PBDE) flame retardants: environmental contamination, human body burden and potential adverse health effects. *Acta Biomed* **79:** 172–83.

Daniels JL, Pan I-J, Jones R, Anderson S, Patterson DG Jr, Needham LL, Sjodin A (2010) Individual characteristics associated with PBDE levels in US human milk samples. *Environ Health Perspect* **118:** 155–60.

Darnerud PO, Eriksen GS, Johannesson T, Larsen PB, Viluksela M (2001) Polybrominated diphenyl ethers: occurrence, dietary exposure, and toxicology. *Environ Health Perspect* **109:** 49–68.

Darnerud PO, Thuvander A (1999) Effects of polybrominated diphenyl ether (PBDE) and polychlorinated biphenyl (PCB) on some immunological parameters after oral exposure in rats and mice. *Toxicol Environ Chem* **70:** 229–42.

Ding L, Murphy MB, He Y, Yeung LW, Wang J, Zhou B, Lam PK, Wu RS, Giesy JP (2007) Effects of brominated flame retardants and brominated dioxins on steroidogenesis in H295R human adrenocortical carcinoma cell line. *Environ Toxicol Chem* **26:** 764–72.

Eneqvist T, Lundberg E, Karlsson A, Huang S, Santos CR, Power DM, Sauer-Eriksson AE (2004) High resolution crystal structures of piscine transthyretin reveal different binding modes for triiodothyronine and thyroxine. *J Biol Chem* **279:** 26411–16.

Eriksson P, Fischer C, Fredriksson A (2006) Polybrominated diphenyl ethers, a group of brominated flame retardants, can interact with polychlorinated biphenyls in enhancing developmental neurobehavioral defects. *Toxicol Sci* **94:** 302–309.

Eriksson P, Fredriksson A (1996) Developmental neurotoxicity of four ortho-substituted polychlorinated biphenyls in the neonatal mouse. *Environ Toxicol Pharmacol* **1:** 155–65.

Eriksson P, Jakobsson E, Fredriksson A (2001) Brominated flame retardants: a novel class of developmental neurotoxicants in our environment? *Environ Health Perspect* **109:** 903–8.

Eriksson P, Viberg H, Jakobsson E, Orn U, Fredriksson A (2002) A brominated flame retardant, 2,2′,4,4′,5-pentabromodiphenyl ether: uptake, retention, and induction of neurobehavioral alterations in mice during a critical phase of neonatal brain development. *Toxicol Sci* **67:** 98–103.

EU-Report (2005) European Union Risk Assessment Report on 2,2#,6,6#-tetrabromo-4,4#-isopropylene diphenol (tetrabromobisphenol-A). CAS No. 79-94-7, EINECS No. 201-36-9, European Chemicals Bureau, Ispra, Italy.

Fang L, Huang J, Yu G, Wang L (2008) Photochemical degradation of six polybrominated diphenyl ether congeners under ultraviolet irradiation in hexane. *Chemosphere* **71:** 258–67.

Fernie KJ, Shutt JL, Letcher RJ, Ritchie JI, Sullivan K, Bird DM (2008) Changes in reproductive courtship behaviors of adult American kestrels (*Falco sparverius*) exposed to environmentally relevant levels of the polybrominated diphenyl ether mixture, DE-71. *Toxicol Sci* **102:** 171–8.

Fernie KJ, Shutt JL, Ritchie IJ, Letcher RJ, Drouillard K, Bird DM (2006) Changes in the growth, but not the survival, of American kestrels (*Falco sparverius*) exposed to environmentally relevant polybrominated diphenyl ethers. *J Toxicol Environ Health A* **69:** 1541–54.

Fernlöf G, Gadhasson I, Pödra K, Darnerud PO, Thuvander A (1997) Lack of effects of some individual polybrominated diphenyl ether (PBDE) and polychlorinated biphenyl (PCB) on human lymphocyte functions in vitro. *Toxicol Lett* **90:** 189–97.

Fowles JR, Fairbrother A, Baecher-Steppan L, Kerkvliet NI (1994) Immunologic and endocrine effects of the flame-retardant pentabromodiphenyl ether (DE-71) in C57BL/6J mice. *Toxicology* **86:** 49–61.

Frederiksen M, Vorkamp K, Thomsen M, Knudsen LE (2009) Human internal and external exposures to PBDEs – a review of levels and sources. *Int J Hyg Environ Health* **212:** 109–34.

Fries GF (1985) Bioavailability of soil-borne polybrominated biphenyls ingested by farm animals. *J Toxicol Environ Health* **16:** 565–79.

Gee JR, Hedge JM, Moser VC (2008) Lack of alterations in thyroid hormones following exposure to polybrominated diphenyl ether 47 during a period of rapid brain development in mice. *Drug Chem Toxicol* **31:** 245–54.

Gee JR, Moser VC (2008) Acute exposure to brominated diphenyl ether 47 delays neuromotor ontogeny and alters motor activity in mice. *Neurotoxicol Teratol* **30:** 79–87.

Germer S, Piersma AH, van der Ven L, Kamyschnikow A, Fery Y, Schmitz HJ, Schrenk D (2006) Subacute effects of the brominated flame retardants hexabromocyclododecane and tetrabromobisphenol A on hepatic cytochrome P450 levels in rats. *Toxicology* **218:** 229–36.

Godbole VY, Grundleger ML, Pasquine TA, Thenen SW (1981) Composition of rat milk from day 5 to 20 of lactation and milk intake of lean and preobese Zucker pups. *J Nutr* **111:** 480–7.

Görs S, Kucia M, Langhammer M, Junghans P, Metges CC (2009) Milk composition in mice – methodological aspects and effects of mouse strain and lactation day. *J Dairy Sci* **92:** 632–7.

Gray LE Jr, Wilson V, Noriega N, Lambright C, Furr J, Stoker TE, Laws SC, Goldman J, Cooper RL, Foster PM (2004) Use of the laboratory rat as a model in endocrine disruptor screening and testing. *ILAR J* **45:** 425–37.

Haglund PS, Zook DR, Buser H and Hu J (1997) Identification and quantification of polybrominated diphenyl ethers and methoxy-polybrominated diphenyl ethers in baltic biota. *Environ Sci Technol* **31:** 3281–7.

Hakk H, Huwe J, Low M, Rutherford D, Larsen G (2006) Tissue disposition, excretion and metabolism of 2,2′,4,4′,6-penta-bromodiphenyl ether (BDE-100) in male Sprague-Dawley rats. *Xenobiotica* **36:** 79–94.

Hakk H, Larsen G, Bergman A, Orn U (2000) Metabolism, excretion and distribution of the flame retardant tetrabromobisphenol A in conventional and bile-duct cannulated rats. *Xenobiotica* **30:** 881–90.

Hakk H, Larsen G, Klasson-Wehler E (2002) Tissue disposition, excretion and metabolism of 2,2′,4,4′,5-pentabromodiphenyl ether (BDE-99) in the male Sprague-Dawley rat. *Xenobiotica* **32:** 369–82.

Hallgren S, Darnerud PO (2002) Polybrominated diphenyl ethers (PBDEs), polychlorinated biphneyls (PCBs) and chlorinated paraffins (CPs) in rats – testing interactions and mechanisms for thyroid hormone effects. *Toxicology* **177:** 227–43.

Hallgren S, Sinjari T, Hakansson H, Darnerud HO (2001) Effects of polybrominated diphenyl ethers (PBDEs) and polychlorinated biphenyls (PCBs) on thyroid hormone and vitamin A levels in rats and mice. *Arch Toxicol* **75:** 200–208.

Hamers T, Kamstra JH, Sonneveld E, Murk AJ, Kester MH, Andersson PL, Legler J, Brouwer A (2006) In vitro profiling of the endocrine-disrupting potency of brominated flame retardants. *Toxicol Sci* **92:** 157–73.

Hanari N, Kannan K, Miyake Y, Okazawa T, Kodavanti PRS, Aldous KM, Yamashita N (2006) Occurrence of polybrominated biphenyls, polybrominated dibenzo-p-dioxins, and polybrominated dibenzofurans as impurities in commercial polybrominated diphenyl ether mixtures. *Environ Sci Technol* **40:** 4400–5.

Hany J, Lilienthal H, Sarasin A, Roth-Härer A, Fastabend A, Dunemann L, Lichtensteiger W, Winneke G (1999) Developmental exposure of rats to a reconstituted PCB mixture or Aroclor 1254: effects on organ weights, aromatase activity, sex hormone levels, and sweet preference levels. *Toxicol Appl Pharmacol* **158:** 231–43.

Harju M, Hamers T, Kamstra JH, Sonneveld E, Boon JP, Tyskind M, Andersson PL (2007) Quantitative structure–activity relationship modeling on in vitro endocrine effects and metabolic stability involving 26 selected brominated flame retardants. *Environ Toxicol Chem* **26:** 816–26.

Harley KG, Marks AR, Chevrier J, Bradman A, Sjödin A, Eskenazi B (2010) PBDE concentrations in women's serum and fecundability. *Environ Health Perspect* **118:** 699–704.

Heeb NV, Schweizer WB, Kohler M, Gerecke AC (2005) Structure elucidation of hexabromocyclododecanes – a class of compounds with a complex stereochemistry. *Chemosphere* **61:** 65–73.

Herbstman JB, Sjodin A, Apelberg BJ, Witter FR, Halden RU, Patterson DG, Panny SR, Needham LL, Goldman LR (2008) Birth delivery mode modifies the associations between prenatal polychlorinated biphenyl (PCB) and polybrominated diphenyl ether (PBDE) and neonatal thyroid hormone levels. *Environ Health Perspect* **116:** 1376–82.

Herbstman JB, Sjodin A, Lederman SA, Jones RS, Rauh V, Needham LL, Tang D, Niedzwiecki M, Wang RY, Perera F (2010) Prenatal exposure to PBDEs and neurodevelopment. *Environ Health Perspect* (Epub ahead of print).

Holbrook RD (2006) In vivo and in vitro debromination of decabromodiphenyl ether (BDE 209) by juvenile rainbow trout and common carp. *Environ Sci Technol* **40:** 4653–8.

Hotchkiss AK, Ostby JS, Vandenburgh JG, Gray LE Jr (2002) Androgens and environmental antiandrogens affect reproductive development and play behavior in the Sprague-Dawley rat. *Environ Health Perspect* **110:** 435–9.

Hotchkiss AK, Ostby JS, Vandenburgh JG, Gray LE Jr (2003) An environmental antiandrogen, vinclozolin, alters the organization of play behavior. *Physiol Behav* **79(2):** 151–6.

Howie L, Dickerson R, Davis D, Safe S (1990) Immunosuppressive and monooxygenase induction activities of polychlorinated diphenyl ether congeners in C57BL/6N mice: quantitative structure–activity relationships. *Toxicol Appl Pharmacol* **105:** 254–63.

Huber S, Ballschmiter K (2001) Characterisation of five technical mixtures of brominated flame retardants. *Fersenius J Anal Chem* **371:** 882–90.

Hughes M, Edwards BC, Mitchell CT, Bhooshan B (2001) In vitro dermal absorption of flame retardant chemicals. *Food Chem Toxicol* **39:** 1263–70.

Huwe JK, Hakk H, Lozentzsen M (2002) A mass balance feeding study of a commercial octabromo diphenyl ether mixture in rats. *Organohalogen Compounds* **58:** 229–32.

Huwe JK, Hakk H, Lorentzsen M (2007) Bioavailability and mass balance studies of a commercial pentabromodiphenyl ether mixture in male Sprague-Dawley rats. *Chemosphere* **66:** 259–66.

Huwe JK, Smith DJ (2007) Accumulation, whole-body depletion, and debromination of decabromodiphenyl ether in male Sprague-Dawley rats following dietary exposure. *Environ Sci Technol* **41:** 2371–7.

Janák K, Covaci A, Voorspoels S, Becher G (2005) Hexabromocyclododecane in marine species from the Western Scheldt Estuary: diastereoisomer- and enantiomer-specific accumulation. *Environ Sci Technol* **39:** 1987–94.

Johnson-Restrepo B, Addink R, Wong C, Arcaro K, Krishnan K (2007) Polybrominated diphenyl ethers and organochlorine pesticides in human breast milk from Massachusetts, USA. *J Environ Monit* **9:** 1205–12.

Johnson-Restrepo B, Kannan K (2009) An assessment of sources and pathways of human exposure to polybrominated diphenyl ethers in the United States. *Chemosphere* **76:** 542–8.

Karpeta A, Gregoraszczuk E (2010) Mixture of dominant PBDE congeners (BDE-47, -99, -100 and -209) at levels noted in human blood dramatically enhances progesterone secretion by ovarian follicles. *Endocr Regul* **44:** 49–55.

Kester MH, Bulduk S, van Toor H, Tibboel D, Meinl W, Glatt H, Falany CN, Coughtrie MW, Schuur AG, Brouwer A, Visser TJ (2002) Potent inhibition of estrogen sulfotransferase by hydroxylated metabolites of polyhalogenated aromatic hydrocarbons reveals alternative mechanism for estrogenic activity of endocrine disrupters. *J Clin Endocrinol Metab* **87:** 1142–50.

Kierkegaard A, Asplund L, de Wit CA, *et al.* (2007) Fate of higher brominated PBDEs in lactating cows. *Environ Sci Technol* **41(2):** 417–23.

Kierkegaard A, Balk L, Tjarnlund U, de Wit C, Jansson B (1999) Dietary uptake and effects of decabromodiphenyl ether in the rainbow trout (*Oncorhynchus mykiss*). *Environ Sci Technol* **33:** 1613–17.

Kim TH, Lee YJ, Lee E *et al.* (2009) Effects of gestational exposure to decabromodiphenyl ether on reproductive parameters, thyroid hormone levels, and neuronal development in Sprague-Dawley rats offspring. *J Toxicol Environ Health, Part A* **72:** 1296–303.

Kodavanti PRS (2005) Neurotoxicity of persistent organic pollutants: possible mode(s) of action and further considerations. *Dose Response* **3:** 273–5.

Kodavanti PRS, Coburn CG, Moser VC, MacPhail RC, Fenton SE, Stoker TE, Rayner JL, Kannan K, Birnbaum LS (2010) Developmental exposure to a commercial PBDE mixture, DE-71: neurobehavioral, hormonal, and reproductive effects. *Toxicol Sci* **116:** 297–312.

Kodavanti PRS, Curras-Collazo MC (2010) Neuroendocrine actions of organohalogens: thyroid hormones, arginine vasopressin, and neuroplasticity. *Front Neuroendocrinology* **31:** 479–96.

Kodavanti PRS, Derr-Yellin EC (2002) Differential effects of polybrominated diphenyl ethers and polychlorinated biphenyls on [3H]arachidonic acid release in rat cerebellar granule neurons. *Toxicol Sci* **68:** 451–7.

Kodavanti PRS, Ward TR (2005) Differential effects of commercial polybrominated diphenyl ether and polychlorinated biphenyl mixture on intracellular signaling in rat brain *in vitro*. *Toxicol Sci* **85:** 952–2.

Kodavanti PRS, Ward TR, Ludewig G, Robertson LW, Birnbaum LS (2005) Polybrominated diphenyl ether (PBDE) effects in rat neuron cultures: ^{14}C-PBDE accumulation, biological effects, and structure–activity relationships. *Toxicol Sci* **88:** 181–92.

Kojima H, Takeuchi S, Uramaru N, Kazumi S, Yoshida T, Kitamura S (2009) Nuclear hormone receptor activity of polybrominated diphenyl ethers and their hydroxylated and methoxylated metabolites in transactivation assays using Chinese hamster ovary cells. *Environ Health Perspect* **117:** 1210–18.

Kuester RK, Solyom AM, Rodriguez VP, Sipes IG (2007) The effects of dose, route, and repeated dosing on the disposition and kinetics of tetrabromobisphenol A in male F-344 rats. *Toxicol Sci* **96:** 237–45.

Kuiper RV, van den Brandhof EJ, Leonards PEG, van der Ven LTM, Wester PW, Vos JG (2007) Toxicity of tetrabromobisphenol A (TBBPA) in zebrafish (*Danio rerio*) in a partial life-cycle. *Arch Toxicol* **81:** 1–9.

Kuriyama SN, Talsness CE, Grote K, Chahoud I (2005) Developmental exposure to low-dose PBED-99: effects on male fertility and neurobehavior in rat offspring. *Environ Health Perspect* **113(2):** 149–54.

La Guardia M, Hale RC, Harvey E (2006) Detailed polybrominated diphenyl ether (PBDE) congener composition of the widely used penta-, octa-, and deca-PBDE technical flame-retardant mixtures. *Environ Sci Technol* **40:** 6247–54.

LaKind, JS, Berlin CM, Sjodin A, Turner W, Wang RY, Needham LL, Paul IM, Stokes JL, Naiman DQ, Patterson DG Jr (2009) Do human milk concentrations of persistent organic chemicals really decline during lactation? Chemical concentrations during lactation and milk/serum partitioning. *Environ Health Perspect* **117:** 1625–31.

Larsson A, Eriksson LA, Andersson RL, Evarson P, Olssom PE (2006) Identification of the brominated flame retardant 1,2-dibromo-4-(1,2-dibromoethyl-cyclohexane as an androgen agonist. *J Med Chem* **49:** 7366–72.

LaVoie HA, Hui YY, McCoy GL, Blake CA (2008) Perinatal exposure to low dose DE-71 affects thyroid and gonadal endpoints. *Biol Reprod (Suppl)* **78:** 116.

Law K, Palace VP, Halldorson T, Danell R, Wautier K, Evans B, Alaee M, Marvin C, Tomy GT (2006a) Dietary accumulation of hexabromocyclododecane diastereoisomers in juvenile rainbow trout (*Oncorhynchus mykiss*). I: Bioaccumulation parameters and evidence of bioisomerization. *Environ Toxicol Chem* **25:** 1757–61.

Law RJ, Allchin CR, de Boer J, Covaci A, Herzke D, Lepom P, Morris S, Tronczynski J, de wit CA (2006b) Levels and trends of brominated flame retardants in the European environment. *Chemosphere* **64:** 187–208.

Laws SC, Ferrell JM, Stoker TE, Schmid J, Cooper RL (2000) The effects of atrazine on female Wistar rats: an evaluation of the protocol for assessing pubertal development and thyroid function. *Toxicol Sci* **58:** 366–76.

Lee LK, He J (2010) Reductive debromination of polybrominated diphenyl ethers by anaerobic bacteria from soils and sediments. *Appl Environ Microbiol* **76:** 792–802.

Lema SC, Dickey JT, Schultz IR, Swanson P (2008) Dietary exposure to 2,2′,4,4′-tetrabromodiphenyl ether (PBDE 47) alters thyroid status and thyroid hormone-regulated gene transcription in the pituitary and brain. *Environ Health Perspect* **116:** 1694–9.

Lema SC, Schultz IR, Scholz NL, Incardona JP, Swanson P (2007) Neural defects and cardiac arrhythmia in fish larvae following embryonic exposure to 2,2′,4,4′-tetrabromodiphenyl ether (PBDE 47). *Aquat Toxicol* **82:** 296–307.

Leonards PEG, Santillo D, Brigden K, van der Veen I, Hesselingen J (2001) Brominated flame retardants in office dust samples [Abstract]. Presented at the Second International Workshop on Brominated Flame Retardants, May 14–16, 2001, Stockholm, Sweden.

Lilienthal H, Hack A, Roth-Harer A, Wichert Grande S, Talsness CE (2006) Effects of developmental exposure to 2,2′,4,4′,5-pentabromodiphenyl ether (PBDE-99) on sex steroids, sexual development, and sexually dimorphic behavior in rats. *Environ Health Perspect* **114:** 194–201.

Lorber M (2008) Exposure of Americans to polybrominated diphenyl ethers. *J Expo Sci Environ Epidemiol* **18(1):** 2–19.

Lyman WJ (1990) *Handbook of Chemical Property Estimation Methods*. Washington, DC, American Chemical Society.

MacGregor JA, Nixon WB (1997) Hexabromocyclododecane (HBCD): Determination of n-Octanol/Water Partition Coefficient. Wildlife International Ltd 439C-104, Arlington, VA: Brominated Flame Retardant Industry Panel, Chemical Manufacturers Association.

Main KM, Kiviranta H, Virtanen HE, Sundqvist E, Tuomisto JT, Tuomisto J, Vartiainen T, Skakkebaek NE, Toppari J (2007) Flame retardants in placenta and breast milk and cryptorchidism in newborn boys. *Environ Health Perspect* **115:** 1519–26.

Mariussen E, Fonnum F (2003) The effect of brominated flame retardants on neurotransmitter uptake into rat brain synaptosomes and vesicles. *Neurochem Int* **43:** 533–42.

Mariussen E, Fonnum F (2006) Neurochemical targets and behavioral effects of organohalogen compounds; an update. *Crit Rev Toxicol* **36:** 253–89.

Meeker JD, Johnson PI, Camann D, Hauser R (2009) Polybrominated diphenyl ether (PBDE) concentrations in house dust are related to hormone levels in men. *Sci Total Environ* **407:** 3425–9.

Meerts IATM, Assink Y, Cenijn PH, van den Berg JHJ, Weijers BM, Bergman A, Koeman JH, Brouwer A (2000) Placental transfer of a hydroxylated polychlorinated biphenyl and effects on fetal and maternal thyroid hormone homeostasis in the rat. *Toxicol Sci* **68:** 361–71.

Meerts IATM, Letcher RJ, Hoving S, Marsh G, Bergman A, Lemmen JG, van der Burg B, Brouwer A (2001) *In vitro* estrogenicity of polybrominated diphenyl ethers, hydroxylated PBDEs, and polybrominated bisphenol A compounds. *Environ Health Perspect* **109:** 399–407.

Meironyte-Guvenius DM, Noren K, Bergman A (1999) Analysis of polybrominated diphenyl ethers in Swedish human milk. A time related trend study, 1972–1997. *J Toxicol Environ Health A* **58:** 329–41.

Mercado-Feliciano M, Bigsby RM (2008) The polybrominated diphenyl ether mixture DE-71 is mildly estrogenic. *Environ Health Perspect* **116:** 605–11.

Mercer HD, Teske RJ, Condon A (1976) Herd health status of animals exposed to polybrominated biphenyls (PBB). *J Toxicol Environ Health* **2:** 335–49.

Morck A, Hakk H, Orn U, Wehler EK (2003) Decabromodiphenyl ether in the rat: absorption, distribution, metabolism and excretion. *Drug Metab Disp* **31:** 900–7.

Morgado I, Hamers T, Van der Ven L, Powers DM (2007) Disruption of thyroid hormone binding to sea bream recombinant transthyretin by ioxinyl and polybrominated diphenyl ethers. *Chemosphere* **69:** 155–63.

National Research Council (2000) Hexabromocyclododecane. In *Toxicological Risks of Selected Flame-Retardant Chemicals*. Washington DC, National Academy Press, pp. 53–71. Available: http://www.nap.edu/books/0309070473/html/ (accessed November 10, 2003).

Ohta S, Ishizuka D, Nishimura H, Nakao T, Aozasa O, Shimidzu Y, Ochiai F, Kida T, Nishi M, Miyata H (2002) Comparison of polybrominated diphenyl ethers in fish, vegetables, and meats and levels in human milk of nursing women in Japan. *Chemosphere* **46:** 689–96.

Orn U, Klasson-Wehler E (1998) Metabolism of 2,2′,4,4′-tetrabromodiphenyl ether in rat and mouse. *Xenobiotica* **28:** 199–211.

Pacymiak EK, Cheng X, Cunningham ML, Crofton K, Klaassen CD, Guo GL (2007) The flame retardants polybrominated diphenyl ethers are pregnane X receptor activators. *Toxicol Sci* **97:** 94–102.

Qiu X, Mercado-Feliciano M, Rigsby RM, Hites RA (2007) Measurement of polybrominated diphenyl ethers and metabolites in mouse plasma after exposure to a commercial pentabromo diphenyl ether mixture. *Environ Health Perspect* **115:** 1052–8.

Rayne S, Ikonomou MG, Antcliffe B (2003) Rapidly increasing polybrominated diphenyl ether concentrations in the Columbia River system from 1992 to 2000. *Environ Sci Technol* **37:** 2847–54.

Rice DC, Reeve EA, Herlihy A, Zoeller RT, Thompson WD, Markowski VP (2007) Developmental delays and locomotor activity in the C57BL6/J mouse following neonatal exposure to the fully brominated PBDE, decabromodiphenyl ether. *Neurotoxicol Teratol* **29:** 511–20.

Richardson VM, Staskal DF, Ross DG, Diliberto JJ, DeVito MJ, Birnbaum LS (2008) Possible mechanisms of thyroid hormone disruption in mice by BDE 47, a major polybrominated diphenyl ether congener. *Toxicol Appl Pharmacol* **226:** 244–50.

Riess M, Ernst T, Popp R, Muller B, Thoma H, Vierle O, Wolf M, van Eldik R (2000) Analysis of flame retarded polymers and recycling materials. *Chemosphere* **40:** 937–41

Roosens L, Abdallah MA, Harrad S, Neels H, Covaci A (2009) Exposure to hexabromocyclododecanes (HBCDs) via dust ingestion, but not diet, correlates with concentrations in human serum: preliminary results. *Environ Health Perspec* **117:** 1707–12.

Roper CS (2005) The in vitro percutaneous absorption of radiolabelled hexabromocyclododecane (HBCD) through human skin. *Organohalogen Compounds* **58:** 36.

Roper CS, Simpson AG, Madden S, Serex TL, Biesemeier JA (2006) Absorption of [^{14}C]-tetrabromodiphenyl ether (TeBDE) through human and rat skin *in vitro*. *Drug Chem Toxicol* **29:** 289–301.

Roze E, Meijer L, Bakker A, Van Braeckel KNJA, Sauer PJJ, Bos AF (2009) Prenatal exposure to organohalogens, including brominated flame retardants, influences motor, cognitive, and behavioral performance at school age. *Environ Health Perspect* **117:** 1953–8.

Sanders JM, Burka LT, Smith CS, Black W, James R, Cunningham ML (2005) Differential expression of CYP1A, 2B and 3A genes in the F344 rat following exposure to polybrominated diphenyl ether mixture or individual components. *Toxicol Sci* **88:** 127–33.

Schauer UM, Volkel W, Dekant W (2006) Toxicokinetics of tetrabromobisphenol a in humans and rats after oral administration. *Toxicol Sci* **91:** 49–58.

Schecter A, Colacino J, Sjodin A, Needham L, Birnbaum LS (2010a) Partitioning of polybrominated diphenyl ethers (PBDEs) in serum and milk from the same mothers. *Chemosphere* **78:** 1279–84.

Schecter A, Haffner D, Colacino J, Patel K, Päpke O, Opel M, Birnbaum L (2010b) Polybrominated diphenyl ethers (PBDEs) and hexabromocyclodecane (HBCD) in composite U.S. food samples. *Environ Health Perspect* **118:** 357–62.

Schecter A, Papke O, Harris TR, Tung KC, Musumba A, Olson J, Birnbaum L (2006) Polybrominated diphenyl ether (PBDE) levels in an expanded market basket survey of U.S. food and estimated PBDE dietary intake by age and sex. *Environ Health Perspect* **114:** 1515–20.

Schecter A, Papke O, Tung KC, Joseph J, Harris TR, Dahlgren J (2005) Polybrominated diphenyl ether flame retardants in the U.S. population: current levels, temporal trends, and comparison with dioxins, debenzofurans, and polychlorinated biphenyls. *J Occup Environ Med* **47:** 199–211.

Schecter A, Papke O, Tung KC, Staskal D, Birnbaum L (2004) Polybrominated diphenyl ethers contamination of United States food. *Environ Sci Technol* **38:** 5306–11.

Schecter A, Pavuk M, Papke O, Ryan JJ, Birnbaum L, Rosen R (2003) Polybrominated diphenyl ethers (PBDEs) in U.S. mothers' milk. *Environ Health Perspect* **111:** 1723–9.

Schecter A, Shan N, Colacino JA, Brummitt SI, Ramakrishnan V, Robert Harris T, Papke O (2009) PBDEs in US and German clothes dryer lint: a potential source of indoor contamination and exposure. *Chemosphere* **75:** 623–8.

Schreiber T, Gassmann K, Gotz C, Hubenthal U, Moors M, Krause G, Merk HF, Nguyen N-H, Scanlan TS, Abel J, Rose CR, Fritsche E (2010) Polybrominated diphenyl ethers induce developmental neurotoxicity in a human in vitro model: evidence for endocrine disruption. *Environ Health Perspect* **118:** 572–8.

Schriks M, Roessig JM, Murk AJ, Furlow JD (2007) Thyroid hormone receptor isoform selectivity of thyroid hormone disrupting compounds quantified with an in vitro reporter gene assay. *Environ Toxicol Pharmacol* **23:** 302–7.

Siegel JH (1975) Simple inhibition systems. In *Enzyme Kinetics: Behavior and Analysis of Rapid Equilibrium and Steady-state Enzyme Systems*. John and Sons, New York, pp. 100–160.

Sjodin A, Papke O, McGahee E, Focant JF, Jones RS, Pless-Mulloli T, Toms LM, Herrmann T, Muller J, Needham LL, Patterson DG Jr (2008) Concentrations of polybrominated diphenyl ethers (PBDEs) in household dust from various countries. *Chemosphere* **73 (1 Suppl.):** S131–6.

Soderlund E, Dybing E, Nelson SD (1980) Nephrotoxicity and hepatotoxicity of tris(2,3-dibromopropyl)phosphate in the rat. *Toxicol Appl Pharmacol* **56:** 171–81.

Söderström G, Sellström U, de Wit CA, Tysklind M (2004) Photolytic debromination of decabromodiphenyl ether (DeBDE). *Environ Sci Technol* **38:** 127–32.

Staskal DF, Diliberto JJ, DeVito MJ, Birnbaum LS (2005) Toxicokinetics of BDE 47 in female mice: effect of dose, route of exposure, and time. *Toxicol Sci* **83:** 215–23.

Staskal DF, Hakk H, Bauer D, Diliberto JJ, Birnbaum LS (2006) Toxicokinetics of polybrominated diphenyl ether congeners 47, 99, 100, and 153 in mice. *Toxicol Sci* **94:** 28–37.

Stoker TE, Cooper RL, Lambright CS, Furr J, Wilson V, Gray LE (2005) In vivo and in vitro anti-androgenic effects of DE-71, A commercial polybrominated diphenyl ether (PBDE) Mixture. *Toxicol Appl Pharmacol* **207(1):** 78–88.

Stoker TE, Laws SL, Crofton KM, Hedge JM, Ferrell JM, Cooper RL (2004) Assessment of DE-71, a commercial polybrominated diphenyl ether (PBDE) mixture, in the EDSP male and female pubertal protocols. *Toxicol Sci* **78:** 144–55.

Stoker TE, Parks LG, Gray LE, Cooper RL (2000) Endocrine-disrupting chemicals: prepubertal exposures and effects on sexual maturation and thyroid function in the male rat. A focus on the EDSTAC recommendations. *Crit Rev Toxicol* **30(2):** 197–252.

Suvorov A, Battista M-C, Takser L (2009) Perinatal exposure to low-dose 2,2′,4,4′-tetrabromodiphenyl ether affects growth in rat offspring: what is the role of IGF-1? *Toxicology* **260:** 126–31.

Szabo DT, Diliberto JJ, Hakk H, Huwe J, Birnbaum LS (2010) Toxicokinetics of the flame retardant hexabromocyclododecane gamma: effect of dose, timing, route, repeated exposure and metabolism. *Toxicol Sci.* **117:** 282–93.

Szabo DT, Richardson VM, Ross DG, Diliberto JJ, Kodavanti PRS, Birnbaum LS (2009). Effects of perinatal PBDE exposure on hepatic phase I, phase II, phase III, and deiodinase 1 gene expression involved in thyroid hormone metabolism in male rat pups. *Toxicological Sciences* **107:** 27–39.

Talsness CE, Kuriyama SN, Sterner-Kock A, Schnitker P, Grande SW, Shakibaei M, Andrade A, Grote K, Chadoud I (2008) In utero and lactational exposures to low doses of polybrominated diphenyl ether-47 alter the reproductive system and thyroid gland of female rat offspring. *Environ Health Perspect* **116:** 308–14.

Talsness CE, Shakibaei M, Kuriyama SN, Grande SW, Sterner-Kock A, Schnitker P, de Souza C, Grote K, Chahoud I (2005) Ultrastructural changes observed in rat ovaries following in utero and lactational exposure to low doses of a polybrominated flame retardant. *Toxicol Lett* **157:** 189–202.

Thoma H, Rist S, Hauschulz G, Hutzinger O (1986) Polybrominated dibenzodioxins and -furans from the pyrolysis of some flame retardants. *Chemosphere* **15:** 649–52.

Thuresson K, Höglund P, Hagmar L, Sjödin A, Bergman A, Jakobsson K (2006) Apparent half-lives of hepta- to decabrominated diphenyl ethers in human serum as determined in occupationally exposed workers. *Environ Health Perspect* **114(2):** 176–81.

Toms L-ML, Sjodin A, Harden F, Hobson P, Jones R, Edenfield E, Mueller JF (2009) Serum polybrominated diphenyl ethers (PBDEs) in pooled serum are higher in children (2–5 years of age) than in infants and adults. *Environ Health Perspect* **117:** 1461–5.

Tseng LH, Lee CW, Pan MH, Tsai SS, Li MH, Chen JR, Lay JJ, Hsu RC (2006) Postnatal exposure of the male mouse to 2,2′, 3,3′, 4,4′, 5,5′, 6,6′-decabrominated diphenyl ether: decreased epididymal sperm functions without alterations in DNA content and histology in testis. *Toxicology* **224:** 33–43.

Tseng LH, Li MH, Tsai SS, Lee CW, Pan MH, Yao WJ, Hsu PC (2008) Developmental exposure to decabromodiphenyl ether (PBDE 209): effects on thyroid hormone and hepatic enzyme activity in male mouse offspring. *Chemosphere* **70:** 640–7.

US Environmental Protection Agency (1999) *Biosolids Generation, Use and Disposal in the United States*. EPA530-R-99-009, Washington, DC: Environmental Protection Agency.

Van den Steen E, Covaci A, Jaspers VL, *et al.* (2007) Accumulation, tissue-specific distribution and debromination of decabromodiphenyl ether (BDE 209) in European starlings (*Sturnus vulgaris*). *Environ Pollut* **148(2):** 648–53.

Van der Ven LTM, van de Kuil T, Hamers T, Leonards REG, Visser TJ, Canton RF, Lilienthal H, Verhoef A, Peirsma AH (2007) Endocrine modulating activity of some brominated flame retardants in rats. In Fourth International BFR Workshop, Amsterdam, The Netherlands, April 24–27. http://www.bfr2007.com/

Van der Ven LT, van de Kuil T, Verhoef A, Leonards PE, Slob W, Canton RF, Germer S, Hamers T, Visser TJ, Litens S, Hakansson H, Fery Y, Schrenk D, van den Berg M, Piersma AH, Vos JG (2008) A 28-day oral dose toxicity study enhanced to detect endocrine effects of a purified technical pentabromodiphenyl ether (pentaBDE) mixture in Wistar rats. *Toxicology* **245(12):** 109–22.

Veith GD, Defoe DL (1979) Measuring and estimating the bioconcentration factor of chemicals in fish. *J Fish Res Board Canada* **36:** 1040–8.

Viberg H, Fredriksson A, Eriksson P (2003a) Neonatal exposure to polybrominated diphenyl ether (PBDE 153) disrupts spontaneous behaviour, impairs learning and memory, and decreases hippocampal cholinergic receptors in adult mice. *Toxicol Appl Pharmacol* **192:** 95–106.

Viberg H, Fredriksson A, Jakobsson E, Orn U, Eriksson P (2003b) Neurobehavioral derangements in adult mice receiving decabrominated diphenyl ether (PBDE 209) during a defined period of neonatal brain development. *Toxicol Sci* **76:** 112–20.

Viberg H, Fredriksson A, Eriksson P (2004) Neonatal exposure to the brominated flame retardant, 2, 2′, 4, 4′, 5-pentabromodiphenyl ether, decreases cholinergic nicotinicreceptors in hippocampus and affects spontaneous behaviour in the adult mouse. *Environ Toxicol Pharmacol* **17:** 61–5.

Von Meyerinck L, Hufnagel B, Schmoldt A, Benthe HF (1990) Induction of rat liver microsomal cytochrome P-450 by the pentabromodiphenyl ether Bromkal 70 and half lives of its components in the adipose tissue. *Toxicology* **61:** 259–74.

Wahl M, Weiss C, Kuch B, Strack S (2007) BDE-47 batch containing traces of brominated dibenzofurans alters cell cycle regulation in vitro. In Fourth International BFR Workshop. Amsterdam, The Netherlands. April 24–27. <http://www.bfr2007.com/>

Watanabe I, Kashimoto T, Tatsukawa R (1983) The flame retardant tetrabromobisphenol A and its metabolite found in river and marine sediments in Japan. *Chemosphere* **12:** 1533–9.

Weber R, Kuch B (2003) Relevance of BFRs and thermal conditions on the formation pathways of brominated and brominated-chlorinated dibenzodioxins and dibenzofurans. *Environ Int* **29:** 699–710.

World Health Organization (1994) Environmental Health Criteria: Brominated Diphenyl Ethers, Vol. 162, World Health Organization, Geneva, Switzerland.

Wu N, Herrmann T, Paepke O, Tickner J, Hale R, Harvey E, La Guardia M, McClean MD, Webster TF (2007) Human exposure to PBDEs: Association of PBDE body burdens with food consumption and house dust concentrations. *Environ Sci Toxicol* **41:** 1584–9.

Xian Q, Ramu K, Isobe T, Sudaryanto A, Liu X, Gao Z, Takahashi S, Yu H, Tanabe S (2007) Levels and body distribution of polybrominated diphenyl ethers (PBDEs) and hexabromocyclododecanes (HBCDs) in freshwater fishes from the Yangtze River, China. *Chemosphere* **71:** 268–76.

Yu CC, Atallah YH (1980) Pharmacokinetics of HBCD in rats, pp. 24. Vesichol Chemical Corporation (unpublished report).

Yuan J, Chen L, Chen D, Guo H, Bi X, Ju Y, Jiang P, Shi J, Yu Z, Yang J, Li L, Jiang Q, Sheng G, Fu J, Wu T, Chen X (2008) Elevated serum polybrominated diphenyl ethers and thyroid stimulating hormone associated with lymphocytic micronuclei in Chinese workers from an E-waste dismantling site. *Environ Sci Technol* **42:** 2195–200.

Zhang S, Bursian SJ, Martin PA, Chan HM, Tomy G, Palace VP, Mayne GJ, Martin JW (2009) Reproductive and developmental toxicity of a pentabrominated diphenyl ether mixture, DE-71, to ranch mink (*Mustela vison*) and hazard assessment for wild mink in the Great Lakes region. *Toxicol Sci* **110:** 107–16.

Zhou T, Ross DG, DeVito MJ, Crofton KM (2001) Effects of short-term in vivo exposure to polybrominated diphenyl ethers on thyroid hormones and hepatic enzyme activities in weanling rats. *Toxicol Sci* **61:** 76–82.

Zweidinger RA, Cooper SD, Erickson MD, Michael LC, Pellizzair ED (1979) Sampling and analysis for semi volatile brominated organics in ambient air. In *Monitoring Toxic Substances* (Schuetzle D, ed.). ACS Symposium Series, Vol. 94. Washington, DC, American Chemical Society, pp. 217–31.

CHAPTER

41

Polychlorinated biphenyls, polychlorinated dibenzo-*p*-dioxins and polychlorinated dibenzofurans

Steven J. Bursian, John L. Newsted and Matthew J. Zwiernik

INTRODUCTION

Polychlorinated biphenyls (PCBs), polybrominated biphenyls (PBBs), polychlorinated dibenzo-*p*-dioxins (PCDDs) and polychlorinated dibenzofurans (PCDFs) form a large group of compounds, the polyhalogenated aromatic hydrocarbons or PHAHs, which are structurally related and are environmentally and biologically persistent (Safe, 1990, 1998; Van den Berg *et al.*, 1994; Fries, 1995; Huwe, 2002; Mandal, 2005; Schecter *et al.*, 2006).

Polychlorinated biphenyls and PBBs were produced commercially for a variety of applications while the PCDDs and PCDFs occur as by-products of industrial and natural processes. The structurally similar PCBs and PBBs are formed by substituting chlorine or bromine, respectively, for hydrogen on the biphenyl molecule that consists of two benzene rings (Figure 41.1). Theoretically, there are 209 possible PCB and PBB congeners considering the five chlorine or bromine binding sites on each ring. Each congener has been assigned a unique number from 1 to 209 in accordance with the rules of the International Union of Pure and Applied Chemistry (IUPAC). Commercial PCB and PBB products were mixtures of congeners that differed with respect to the extent and positions of chlorination or bromination. Polychlorinated dibenzo-*p*-dioxins are composed of two benzene rings connected by two oxygen atoms and contain four to eight chlorines, for a total of 75 congeners (Figure 41.1). Polychlorinated dibenzofurans are also composed of two benzene rings. The rings have one oxygen molecule between them and have four chlorine binding sites available on each ring (Figure 41.1). There are 135 different PCDF congeners (DiCarlo *et al.*, 1978; Safe, 1990, 1998; Fries, 1995: Headrick *et al.*, 1999; Huwe, 2002; Mandal, 2005; Schecter *et al.*, 2006).

Certain approximate stereoisomers in this group, often referred to collectively as dioxins and dioxin-like compounds (DLCs), induce a common suite of effects and have a common mechanism of action mediated by binding of the PHAH ligand to a specific high-affinity cellular protein. This group of dioxins and DLCs includes seven PCDD congeners, 10 PCDF congeners and 12 PCB congeners. While the PBB congeners analogous to the 12 PCB congeners could also be considered dioxin-like chemicals, the relatively short commercial lifespan and restricted environmental distribution of PBBs generally precludes them from consideration. The prototype for the dioxins is 2,3,7,8-tetrachlorodibenzo-*p*-dioxin or 2,3,7,8-TCDD. Toxicity and persistence of the PHAHs are determined by structure, with lateral substitutions on the ring resulting in the highest degree of toxicity. For the PCDDs and PCDFs, congeners with chlorines in the 2, 3, 7 and 8 positions fall into this category. The 2,3,7,8-TCDD-like PCB congeners are the non-ortho- and mono-ortho-substituted compounds with no chlorines or no more than one chlorine (or bromine) on the 2, 2′, 6 or 6′ position (Safe, 1990; Fries, 1995; Headrick, 1999; Huwe, 2002; Mandal, 2005; Schecter *et al.*, 2006).

Mechanistic studies indicate that the toxic and biochemical effects associated with exposure to 2,3,7,8-TCDD and its approximate stereoisomers are mediated by initial binding of the chemical to the cytosolic aryl hydrocarbon receptor (AhR) present in target tissues and organs. There is a correlation between the AhR binding affinity of these chemicals and their structure–toxicity relationships, which supports the idea that the Ah receptor is involved in the mediation of responses induced by the 2,3,7,8-TCCD-like PCDD, PCDF and PCB congeners (Okey *et al.*, 1994; Hahn, 1998, 2002; Safe, 1998; Denison *et al.*, 2002; Denison and Nagy, 2003; Mandal, 2005).

The common mechanism of action of 2,3,7,8-TCDD and related compounds allows for use of the toxic equivalency factor (TEF) approach to estimate the 2,3,7,8-TCDD-like toxicity of complex mixtures containing chemicals that resemble 2,3,7,8-TCDD. The TEF value for a 2,3,7,8-TCDD-like congener is defined as the potency of the individual congener relative to 2,3,7,8-TCDD. Using the TEF concept, 2,3,7,8-TCDD toxic equivalents (TEQ), which is the sum of the product of the concentration of each congener and its respective TEF, can be calculated for any complex mixture containing

Reproductive and Developmental Toxicology, Edited by Ramesh C. Gupta
ISBN: 978-0-12-382032-7

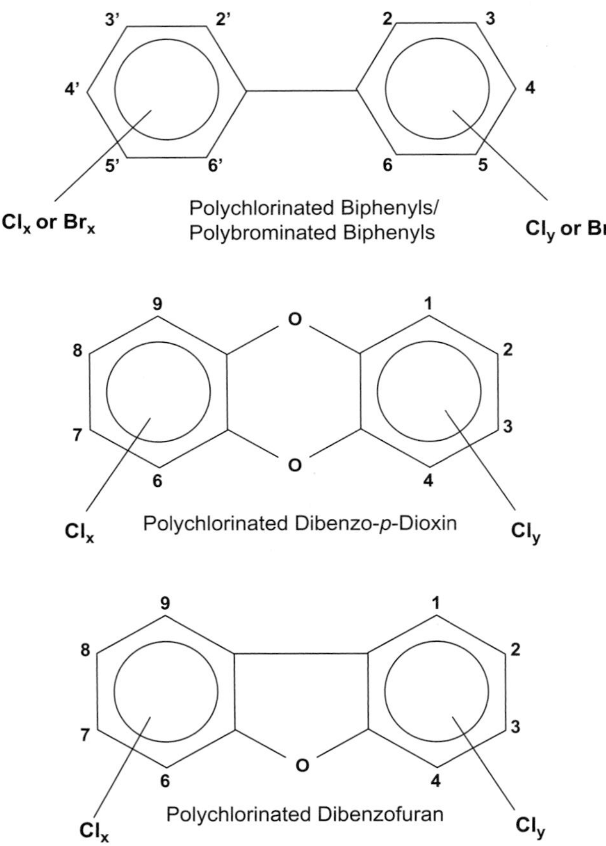

FIGURE 41.1 Structures and numbering of generic polychlorinated/polybrominated biphenyl (PCB/PBB), polychlorinated dibenzo-*p*-dioxin and polychlorinated dibenzofuran molecules.

2,3,7,8-TCDD-like chemicals to provide an estimation of the total 2,3,7,8-TCDD-like toxicity (Safe, 1998; Huwe, 2002).

The PCDDs, PCDFs and PCBs are widely distributed into the global environment and, due to long-range transport, can be very resistant to environmental degradation and metabolism. As a result, they readily accumulate in the food chain with the greatest tissue concentrations being found in species at the higher trophic levels. Residues have been detected in a variety of animal species, including humans (Van den Berg *et al.*, 1994; Safe, 1998). In some situations, the environmental concentrations of these contaminants are such that there is a health risk to animals and humans. Because of this risk, there continues to be an effort on the part of state, federal and international regulatory agencies to minimize exposure to this significant class of environmental contaminants.

HISTORICAL BACKGROUND

Sources of PCBs, PCDDs, PCDFs and PBBs

PCBs

Polychlorinated biphenyls were first synthesized by Schmidt and Schultz in 1881. Commercial production of PCBs for a variety of uses began in the USA in 1929 until 1977, primarily by the Monsanto Corporation (Kimbrough, 1987, 1995; Tanabe, 1988; Headrick *et al.*, 1999). They were used in closed use systems in electrical transformers, capacitors and heat transfer and hydraulic systems. For a period of time, PCBs also had a large number of open-ended applications. They were used in paints, polymers and adhesives, as lubricants, plasticizers, fire retardants and immersion oils, vehicles for pesticide application and as agents for the suspension of pigments in carbonless copy paper (Safe, 1990; Headrick *et al.*, 1999). The PCB products that were manufactured by Monsanto in the USA had the trade name Aroclor followed by four digits that identified the particular mixture. The first two digits referred to the 12 carbon atoms of the biphenyl molecule and the last two digits referred to the percent of chlorine in the mixture, by weight. Aroclors 1221, 1232, 1242, 1254 and 1260 were the commercial PCB products that were produced by Monsanto, containing 21, 32, 42, 54 and 60% chlorine by weight, respectively. Similar commercial PCB mixtures were produced by other manufacturers worldwide including the Clophens (Bayer, Germany), Pheoclors and Pyralenes (Prodelec, France), Fenclors (Caffro, Italy) and Kanechlors (Kanegafuchi, Japan) (Kimbrough, 1987, 1995; Safe, 1994).

The physical and chemical properties of PCBs, such as high stability, inertness and dielectric properties, which were advantageous for many industrial purposes, led to the international use of PCBs in large quantities (Tanabe, 1988). For example, the estimated cumulative production of PCBs in the USA between 1930 and 1975 was 700,000 tons and 1.2 million tons were estimated to have been produced worldwide. Domestic sales of PCBs in the USA during this time period totaled 627,000 tons (Kimbrough 1987, 1995; Tanabe, 1988). As a result of widespread use, PCBs were identified in environmental media and biota as early as the 1960s. After the discovery of their widespread environmental contamination in the 1970s, PCB production decreased and eventually ceased (Tanabe, 1988). In 1971, Monsanto voluntarily stopped production of PCBs for open-ended uses and subsequently only the lower chlorinated biphenyls were produced (Aroclor 1242 and 1016). In 1977, Monsanto ceased production entirely (Kimbrough, 1987, 1995).

Although PCBs are no longer used commercially because of their persistence, they are still present in the environment. About 31% (370,000 tons) of all the PCBs produced is present in the global environment. It is estimated that 780,000 tons are still in use in older electric equipment and other products, deposited in landfills and dumps or in storage (Tanabe, 1988).

PCDDs and PCDFs

Polychlorinated dibenzo-*p*-dioxins and PCDFs are by-products that are formed during the synthesis of certain industrial halogenated aromatic chemicals, by-products from other commercial processes and by-products of combustion (Safe, 1990). Some of the important industrial sources of PCDDs and PCDFs have included their formation as by-products in the production of PCBs, chlorinated phenols and chlorinated phenol-derived chemicals, hexachorobenzene, technical hexachlorocyclohexanes and chlorides of iron, aluminum and copper. PCDDs and PCDFs have also been identified in effluents, wastes and pulp samples from the pulp and paper industry and in finished paper products. Emissions from municipal and hazardous waste incinerators as well as home heating systems that use wood and coal, diesel engines, forest and grass fires and agricultural and backyard burning contain PCDDs and PCDFs. Another contribution might come from naturally formed PCDDs and PCDFs, which have been detected in deep soils and clays from the southern USA and Germany (Safe, 1990; Huwe, 2002).

The US Environmental Protection Agency (EPA) estimated that annual emissions of PCDDs and PCDFs decreased from 13.5 to 2.8 kg TEQ/year between 1987 and 1995. This was due primarily to improvements in incinerator performance and removal of incinerators that could not meet emission standards. Other regulations, including bans or restrictions on the production and use of chemicals such as the wood preservative pentachlorophenol (PCP), the phase-out of leaded gasoline that contained halogenated additives and the elimination of chlorine bleaching in the pulp industry also contributed to reducing concentrations of PCDDs and PCDFs (Huwe, 2002).

PBBs

Polybrominated biphenyls were manufactured for use as flame retardants in industrial and consumer products (Damstra *et al.*, 1982). It is estimated that approximately 13 million pounds were produced in the USA from 1970 to 1976 and used by more than 130 companies for incorporation into plastic products that included business machine housings, radios, televisions, thermostats, electric shavers, hand tools and various automotive parts (DiCarlo *et al.*, 1978; Headrick *et al.*, 1999). Three commercial PBB products were manufactured in the USA: hexabromobiphenyl, octabromobiphenyl and decabromobiphenyl (DiCarlo *et al.*, 1978; Hardy, 2000). Hexabromobiphenyl was the predominant product with approximately 11.8 million pounds being produced solely by Michigan Chemical Company. Over 98% of the hexabromobiphenyl was produced as FireMaster BP-6 with the remainder being produced as FireMaster FF-1 (Hesse and Powers, 1978) after addition of an anti-caking agent to FireMaster BP-6. Michigan Chemical Company stopped production of their PBB products in 1974 (DiCarlo *et al.*, 1978). White Chemical Company and Hexcel Corporation manufactured octa- and decabromobiphenyl in the USA until 1979 (IARC, 1986). Production of decabromobiphenyl was discontinued in Great Britain in 1977 and Germany stopped production of brominated biphenyls in 1985. In 2000, France discontinued the remaining commercial production of PBBs (Hardy, 2000).

While FireMaster BP-6 was sold as a hexabromobiphenyl, it consisted of 18 different congeners, some of which were tetra-, penta-, hepta- and octabromobiphenyls. The predominant hexabromobiphenyl was 2,4,5,2′,4′,5′-hexabromobiphenyl. Commercial octabromobiphenyl contained at least four congeners; a heptabromobiphenyl, isomeric octabromobiphenyls and a nonabromobiphenyl, which constituted the majority of the mixture. Commercial decabromobiphenyl was over 95% decabromobiphenyl with the remainder being a nonabromobiphenyl and an octabromobiphenyl (DiCarlo *et al.*, 1978).

Environmental fate of PCBs, PCDDs, PCDFs and PBBs

The release of PCBs into the environment primarily has been the result of leaks, spills and improper disposal. As stated earlier, it is estimated that approximately 370,000 tons of PCBs are present in the global environment (Tanabe, 1988). The volatility of PCBs allows their evaporation from water surfaces and movement through the atmosphere, resulting in widespread environmental dispersal (Headrick *et al.*, 1999). Polychlorinated dibenzo-*p*-dioxins and PCDFs are released into the atmosphere primarily by combustion sources and by evaporation from PCDD/PCDF-containing soils and water. Similar to PCBs, the PCDDs and PCDFs can be transported long distances by winds, contributing both to general background concentrations and contamination of remote areas far from the original source. Polychlorinated biphenyls, PCDDs and PCDFs are removed from the atmosphere by physical processes such as wet and dry deposition and vapor uptake and are deposited on soils, surface waters and plant surfaces. Most of the PCBs, PCDDs and PCDFs that are deposited on surface waters sorb onto suspended sediments. Once bound to soil and sediment, these chemicals generally remain fixed except for bulk transport due to soil erosion, flooding and dredging (Dickson and Buzik, 1993). Ingestion of these compounds by animals results in their preferential bioaccumulation and biomagnification in higher trophic levels of the food chain (Safe, 1994).

Because PBBs were manufactured for a relatively short time and because of their restricted use, they are not considered to be a significant environmental contaminant with the exception of specific locations in Michigan related to production and disposal. Environmental losses of PBBs from manufacturing sites were estimated to be 0.11% into the atmosphere as particulate matter, negligible losses to storm sewers and 5% as solid waste to landfills. Soil samples collected from the loading and bagging area of the Michigan Chemical Company plant manufacturing FireMaster BP-6 and FF-1 contained 3,500 and 2,500 ppm (mg/kg) PBBs, respectively (DiCarlo *et al.*, 1977). Like PCBs, PCDDs and PCDFs, PBBs are very stable compounds and persist in the environment. Studies have indicated that PBBs have a high affinity for soil and undergo very little degradation and translocation into vegetation (Fries, 1985). Like PCBs, PCDDs and PCDFs, the PBBs are very lipophilic and have the potential to bioaccumulate and biomagnify in the food chain (Damstra *et al.*, 1982).

It is important to remember that the commercial PCB products and PCBs, PCDDs and PCDFs in environmental extracts are complex mixtures of congeners. Because of various physical and biological processes, the composition of the commercial PCB mixture and an environmental PCB/PCDD/PCDF mixture may vary significantly from one another. Thus, the impacts of PCBs, PCDDs and PCDFs on the environment and biota are due to the individual components of these mixtures, their additive and/or non-additive (synergistic/antagonistic) interactions with themselves and other classes of pollutants (Safe, 1994).

Exposure to PCBs, PCDDs, PCDFs and PBBs

PCBs, PCDDs and PCDFs

There are a number of ways by which animals can be and have been exposed to PCBs, PCDDs/PCDFs and PBBs. Some of the scenarios described involve ingestion of low concentrations of these chemicals through consumption of environmentally contaminated feed or feed components while other scenarios involve accidental incorporation of the chemical into the feed resulting in exposure to relatively high concentrations of the contaminant. Usually, food animal exposures to PCBs, PCDDs and PCDFs occur below concentrations resulting in acute toxicity. Clinical signs are not evident and there often is not a noticeable economic impact on the health of the animal, although there may be detectable contamination of food products such as milk, meat and eggs (Headrick *et al.*, 1999).

During the 1940s and 1950s, silos constructed with concrete were sealed with a PCB-containing paint, which eventually peeled off from the walls resulting in contaminated silage. Dairy and beef cattle were exposed to the paint in the feed resulting in accumulation of PCBs in adipose tissue. As a result, food products such as milk and meat contained detectable concentrations of PCBs. Examples of other exposure incidents resulting in PCB residues in food animals were summarized by Headrick *et al.* (1999). These include consumption of tar paper by veal calves, consumption of fish viscera by swine, pullet consumption of feed containing PCB-contaminated fat added during processing, exposure of chickens to ceiling insulation and fiberglass insulation that contained PCBs and treatment of boars with a topical pesticide containing PCB-contaminated oil. In 1979, a spare electrical transformer in a Montana hog slaughter plant was damaged allowing PCBs to leak into the plant's drainage system. The PCBs and animal wastes were processed into grease and animal feed, which was distributed and subsequently fed to hogs, beef cattle, dairy cattle, chickens and mink in 19 states in the USA and in Canada and Japan before the contamination was detected. Ultimately, 800,000 chickens, nearly 4,000,000 eggs, 4,000 hogs, 74,000 bakery items, 800,000 pounds of animal feeds and 1,200,000 pounds of grease were destroyed with an estimated cost of recalls and destroyed products amounting to over $2 million (Headrick *et al.*, 1999).

Michigan PBB incident

The most extensive exposure of food animals and humans to PBBs occurred in Michigan in the mid-1970s. In 1970, the Michigan Chemical Company began to manufacture PBBs under the trade name of FireMaster BP-6 in St. Louis, MI (Fries, 1985). FireMaster BP-6 was a mixture of PBB congeners containing two to eight bromines. The major constituents of FireMaster BP-6 were 2,2′,4,4′,5,5′-hexabromobiphenyl (56%) and 2,2′,3,4,4′,5,5′-heptabromobiphenyl (27%) (Damstra *et al.*, 1982). In 1972, the company changed the formulation of the retardant by grinding BP-6 and adding 2% calcium silicate as an anti-caking agent. This new formulation, now called FireMaster FF-1, was a white powder as opposed to brown flakes, which was the appearance of BP-6 (Fries, 1985).

In May 1973, 650 pounds of FF-1 were mistakenly included in a shipment of feed-grade magnesium oxide to a feed mill in Climax, MI. Michigan Chemical Company, in addition to producing FireMaster FF-1, also produced the magnesium oxide product, which had an appearance identical to FireMaster FF-1 and was sold under the trade name NutriMaster. Normally the two products were packaged in paper bags with unique color codes. However, during a paper shortage, both FireMaster and NutriMaster were packaged in plain brown bags differentiated only by the product names stenciled on the bags. Both products were stored in the same warehouse (Dunckel, 1975; Fries, 1985).

A portion of the magnesium oxide that was shipped to the Climax feed mill was used to mix feeds primarily for dairy cattle at that location, which were subsequently shipped to area farms or other retail units. The remaining magnesium oxide was shipped to other mills within the state and used in feeds mixed at those locations. Feeds that were not formulated to contain magnesium oxide also became contaminated because of carryover from the contaminated feed-mixing equipment (Fries, 1985). In total, 101 feed mills were affected (Dunckel, 1975).

Most of the high-level exposures occurred during the fall of 1973 before sale of the initial batch of feed was stopped in December 1973 because of dairy producer complaints of animal health problems. Three initial feed preparations containing different concentrations of PBBs were Feed No. 405, which had 2.4 μg/g(ppm) PBBs, No. 410 having 1,790 ppm PBBs and No. 407, which contained 4,300 ppm PBBs. The highest feed concentration reported was 13,500 ppm PBBs (DiCarlo *et al.*, 1978; Damstra *et al.*, 1982). Low-level contamination of feed continued beyond the chance identification of PBBs as the contaminant in April 1974 because of their persistence. In 1974, 68% of 1,770 feed samples collected in Michigan contained PBB residues. Resampling in 1975 indicated that 6% of 1,208 feed samples were contaminated and in 1976, only 0.3% of 663 samples contained PBBs (DiCarlo *et al.*, 1978). Shortly after PBBs were identified as the feed contaminant, the US Food and Drug Administration (FDA) set a temporary guideline of 1 ppm PBBs in milk fat, meat and poultry, 0.1 ppm in whole eggs and 0.3 ppm in animal feeds. The Michigan Department of Agriculture started to identify and quarantine all dairy herds with PBB concentrations in excess of 5 ppm. Because of the long half-life of PBBs, the decision was made to depopulate affected farms and to dispose of the animals at a burial site in northern Michigan. Initially, 9,400 head of cattle, 2,000 swine, 400 sheep and 2,000,000 chickens were buried in addition to 865 tons of feed and animal by-products such as cheese, butter, dry milk products and eggs (DiCarlo *et al.*, 1978; Damstra *et al.*, 1982; Fries, 1985, Headrick *et al.*, 1999). In October 1974, the FDA lowered the guidelines for PBBs in milk and meat from 1 ppm to 0.3 ppm, which resulted in disposal of 20,000 additional head of cattle as well as 3,900 swine and 1,100 sheep (Damstra *et al.*, 1982). In total, 507 farms were affected (Dunckel, 1975). In response to increasing concerns about the effects of PBBs on human and animal health, the Michigan legislature lowered the PBB tolerance to 0.02 ppm in body fat of all dairy cattle offered for slaughter in 1977. A small number of dairy producers who had repopulated after the initial quarantine in 1974 continued to have violative cattle because of residual contamination on their facilities, although this number was less than 2% of all culled cows. Over the next five years, the number of violative cattle diminished rapidly as they approached the end of production.

A potential environmental source of exposure to animals on contaminated farms was the soil, if animals had direct access to the contaminated soil. Four years after the initial PBB contamination incident, there were several farms in Michigan that exceeded the 20 ng/g(ppb) tolerance for PBBs in fat of culled cows even though farmers had depopulated, cleaned up the premises and repopulated with clean animals. The major route of animal exposure was through soil consumption because crops grown on contaminated soils did not accumulate PBBs (Fries, 1985). Major sources of PBBs on the farms were soils of fields on which manure had been spread and soil of unpaved exercise lots where feces were deposited and feed was spilled. It was shown that all of the problem farms were using unpaved lots that had been used in 1974 for some part of their production system and that ingestion of soil from unpaved lots was the major route of PBB exposure causing animal contamination on problem farms (Fries, 1995).

For livestock, atmospheric deposition of PCDDs and PCDFs onto forage and soils is assumed to be the major source of exposure (Huwe, 2002). Extensive field studies in contaminated areas have demonstrated a positive correlation between PCDD and PCDF concentrations in animals and their soil contact (Van den Berg *et al.*, 1994). The relative importance of soil depends upon the species of animal and the management system. Ruminants are expected to be more vulnerable to PCDD and PCDF exposure than poultry and swine because of their grazing activities. The use of pasture is of particular importance because consumption of contaminated plants is additive to soil ingestion of PCDDs and PCDFs. Volatilization of PCDDs and PCDFs from soil and deposition on plants is an important pathway of animal exposure when forage is abundant. However, that soil may be more important when grazing is sparse. The soil ingestion pathway is not limited to grazing animals. Cattle confined to unpaved lots consume small amounts of soil that can lead to product residues. Although most poultry and pork production is conducted in confined operations, the soil ingestion pathway of exposure may be important when these species have access to contaminated soil (Fries, 1995).

In addition to exposure to PCDDs and PCDFs through consumption of contaminated soil and/or forage, a number of other incidents of animal exposure to these compounds have been reported. The first known exposure to PCDDs occurred in the late 1950s. "Chick edema disease", as the condition was initially called, resulted from consumption of feed containing fat contaminated with a number of PCDD congeners originating from the production of PCP. In 1975, several horses died in Missouri as a result of exposure to TCDD-contaminated waste oil that was used for dust control on horse tracks. The oil contained waste from a hexachlorophene manufacturing plant and it had also been used for dust control on the unpaved streets of Times Beach. The high concentrations of TCDD in the residential soils led to purchase and evacuation of the town by the US government (Fries, 1995). In a geographical survey, high concentrations of TEQs in cattle were strongly correlated to PCP-treated wood used for fence posts and feed bunks at several beef cattle operations across 13 states in the USA. Although the use of PCP was restricted in the 1980s, PCP was used heavily on farms as a wood preservative in the late 1970s (Huwe, 2002). In an EPA survey of poultry, two chicken samples were found with PCDD concentrations considerably above background. The origin of this contamination was ball clay, which had been added as an anti-caking agent to soy meal in the feed. This same contaminated feed was also used by the catfish industry and resulted in high TEQ concentrations in catfish from Arkansas (Huwe, 2002).

Several dioxin contamination incidents have occurred in Europe. In 1998, during routine monitoring, dairy products were identified that had dioxin concentrations that were two to four times higher than background concentrations. The source of the contamination was traced to citrus pulp used as a cattle feed component. The citrus pulp and contaminated feeds were immediately removed from the market. In another incident, PCB/PCDD/PCDF-contaminated oil was added to recycled fat used as an additive in animal feeds. The affected feeds contaminated Belgian poultry, dairy and meat and were discovered only after toxic effects characteristic of "chick edema disease" were seen in chickens. Animals and products were quarantined, recalled and eventually destroyed.. The incident led to international recalls and bans against Belgian products (Van Larebeke *et al.*, 2001; Bernard *et al.*, 2002; Huwe, 2002).

Differential toxicity

Comparison of the relative toxicity of PCDDs, PCDFs and PCBs as three separate classes suggests that the dioxins are more toxic than the furans, which in turn are more toxic than the PCBs. It was concluded that PBBs are slightly more toxic than their chlorinated counterparts (McConnell, 1985). Studies also suggest that the toxicity of commercial PCB formulations increases with increasing chlorine content (Aroclor 1221 <1232<1242<1248<1254), but highly chlorinated Aroclors 1260, 1262 and 1268 are less toxic than Aroclor 1254 (Tanabe, 1988).

2,3,7,8-Tetrachlorodibenzo-*p*-dioxin binds with the greatest affinity to the AhR and is the most potent isomer in terms of toxicity. Polychlorinated dibenzo-*p*-dioxins and PCDFs substituted with chlorines in at least three of the four lateral positions (2,3,7 and 8; Figure 41.1) bind most strongly to the AhR. If chlorines are removed from these lateral positions or if chlorines are added to the non-lateral positions (1,4,6,9; Figure 41.1), binding affinities decrease markedly, as do toxicities. There are seven 2,3,7,8-substituted PCDDs (2,3,7,8-TCDD, 1,2,3,7,8-pentaCDD, 1,2,3,4,7,8-hexaCDD, 1,2,3,6,7,8-hexaCDD, 1,2,3,7,8,9-hexaCDD, 1,2,3,4,6,7,8-heptaCDD and octa-CDD) and 10 2,3,7,8-substituted PCDFs (2,3,7,8-TCDF, 1,2,3,7,8-pentaCDF, 2,3,4,7,8-pentaCDF, 1,2,3,4,7,8-hexaCDF, 1,2,3,6,7,8-hexaCDF, 1,2,3,7,8,9-hexaCDF, 2,3,4,6,7,8-hexa CDF, 1,2,3,4,6,7,8-heptaCDF, 1,2,3,4,6,7,8-heptaCDF and octaCDF) that induce 2,3,7,8-TCDD-like toxicity. There are 209 theoretically possible PCB congeners having different toxic and biologic responses. The most toxic PCB congeners have four or more chlorine atoms at both the para (4,4′) and meta positions (3,3′,5,5′; Figure 41.1) in the biphenyl rings, but no chlorine atoms in the ortho positions (2,2′,6,6′; Figure 41.1). Of the 209 PCB congeners, four PCB congeners (3,3′,4,4′-tetraCB (IUPAC 77), 3,4,4′,5-tetraCB (IUPAC 81), 3,3′,4,4′,5-pentaCB (IUPAC 126)and 3,3′,4,4′,5,5′-hexaCB (IUPAC 169)) are approximate stereoisomers of the highly toxic 2,3,7,8-TCDD and thus bind to the AhR and elicit toxic and biologic responses typical of TCDD, although at higher doses. These four congeners are considered to be coplanar because both rings of the biphenyl molecule lie in the same plane, which enables binding to the AhR (Tanabe, 1988). There are eight PCB congeners with chlorine substitution in one of the ortho positions (2,2′,6,6′). These congeners may have partial coplanarity and thus exhibit lower competitive binding affinities for the AhR and lower toxic potency. The mono-ortho PCB congeners are 2,3,3′,4,4′-pentaCB (IUPAC 105), 2,3,4,4′,5-pentaCB (IUPAC 114), 2,3′,4,4′,5-pentaCB (IUPAC 118), 2′,3,4,4′,5-pentaCB (IUPAC 123), 2,3,3′,4,4′,5-hexaCB (IUPAC 156), 2,3,3′,4,4′,5-hexaCB (IUPAC 157), 2,3′,4,4′,5,5′-hexaCB (IUPAC 167) and 2,3,3′,4,4′,5,5′-heptaCB (IUPAC 189) (Poland and Knutson, 1982; Tanabe, 1988; Safe, 1990, 1998; Giesy and Kannan, 1998; Huwe, 2002; Whyte *et al.*, 2004).

Toxic equivalency factors

The relationship between the structure of individual PCDD, PCDF and PCB congeners and their toxicity is the basis of toxicity equivalency factors (TEFs) and the toxic equivalency (TEQ) approach. The TEQ approach is used to determine the toxic potency of complex mixtures of PCDDs, PCDFs and PCBs found in the environment. Assuming a similar mechanism of action (binding to the AhR), the potency of each chemical in a mixture to cause a particular toxic or biological effect can be expressed as a fraction of the potency of 2,3,7,8-TCDD to cause the same effect. Thus, the TEF is a ratio of EC_{50} (2,3,7,8-TCDD-like chemical)/EC_{50} (2,3,7,8-TCDD). 2,3,7,8-Tetrachlorodibenzo-*p*-dioxin has been assigned a TEF value of 1.0. Based on a variety of biological endpoints, relative potency factors (RPFs) are assigned to the different 2,3,7,8-TCDD-like congeners. All RPFs for an individual congener are evaluated to derive a consensus value (the TEF) that describes an order-of-magnitude potency for that congener. The toxic potency of a mixture of PCDDs, PCDFs and/or PCBs is estimated by multiplying the concentrations of individual congeners by their respective TEFs and summing the products to yield a total TEQ. The total TEQ expresses the toxicity as if the mixture were pure 2,3,7,8-TCDD (Dickson and Buzik, 1993; Safe, 1990, 1998; Fries, 1995; Van den Berg *et al.*, 1998, 2006; Whyte *et al.*, 2004, Schecter *et al.*, 2006). Several assumptions are made when using the TEF approach: (1) the effects of individual PCDDs, PCDFs and/or PCBs in a mixture are additive; (2) only tissue and environmentally persistent organochlorine compounds have been assigned TEFs; (3) all of these compounds bind to the Ah receptor and elicit receptor-mediated biochemical and toxic responses (Safe, 1998). The TEQ approach and current values (Table 41.1) have been adopted internationally as the most appropriate way to estimate the potential health risk of mixtures of 2,3,7,8-TCDD-like chemicals (Schecter *et al.*, 2006).

Table 41.2 illustrates how the TEF approach can be used. The table presents the concentrations of various PCDD, PCDF and PCB congeners found in fish collected downstream from the abandoned site of a manufacturing facility that used PCBs. By multiplying the congener concentration detected in the fish by the appropriate TEF value, the quantity of the 2,3,7,8-TCDD-like toxicity contributed by each congener can be determined. In the example given, the PCDDs contribute 0.8 pg TEQ/g, the PCDFs contribute 3.8 pg TEQs/g and the non-ortho PCBs contribute 41 pg TEQs/g or over 90% of the 2,3,7,8-TCDD-like activity in the fish sample. While the relative toxicities of the mono-ortho PCB congeners are relatively low, as indicated by their TEF values, their high concentrations in the fish allow them to contribute a measurable quantity of 2,3,7,8-TCDD-like activity.

TABLE 41.1 Summary of World Health Organization (WHO) 2005 Toxic Equivalency Factor (TEF) values for mammals[1]

Compound	WHO 2005 TEF
Chlorinated dibenzo-p-dioxins	
2,3,7,8-TCDD	1
1,2,3,7,8-PeCDD	1
1,2,3,4,7,8-HxCDD	0.1
1,2,3,6,7,8-HxCDD	0.1
1,2,3,7,8,9-HxCDD	0.1
1,2,3,4,6,7,8-HpCDD	0.01
OCDD	0.0003
Chlorinated dibenzofurans	
2,3,7,8-TCDF	0.1
1,2,3,7,8-PeCDF	0.03
2,3,4,7,8-PeCDF	0.3
1,2,3,4,7,8-HxCDF	0.1
1,2,3,6,7,8-HxCDF	0.1
1,2,3,7,8,9-HxCDF	0.1
2,3,4,6,7,8-HxCDF	0.1
1,2,3,4,6,7,8-HpCDF	0.01
1,2,3,6,7,8,9-HpCDF	0.01
OCDF	0.0003
Non-ortho-substituted PCBs	
3,3′,4,4′-tetraCB (PCB 77)	0.0001
3,4,4′,5-tetraCB (PCB 81)	0.0003
3,3′,4,4′,5-pentaCB (PCB 126)	0.1
3,3′,4,4′,5,5′-hexaCB (PCB 169)	0.03
Mono-ortho-substituted PCBs	
2,3,3′,4,4′-pentaCB (PCB 105)	0.00003
2,3,4,4′,5-pentaCB (PCB 114)	0.00003
2,3′,4,4′,5-pentaCB (PCB 118)	0.00003
2′,3,4,4′,5-pentaCB (PCB 123)	0.00003
2,3,3′,4,4′,5-hexaCB (PCB 156)	0.00003
2,3,3′,4,4′,5′-hexaCB (PCB 157)	0.00003
2,3′,4,4′,5,5′-hexaCB (PCB 167)	0.00003
2,3,3′,4,4′,5,5′-heptaCB (PCB 189)	0.00003

[1]Van den Berg *et al.* (2006)

TOXICOKINETICS

PCBs and PBBs

Because commercial PCB and PBB products are mixtures of individual congeners that differ in the number and position of chlorine or bromine atoms and thus differ in terms of their biological activities, it is difficult to accurately assess their absorption, distribution, metabolism and elimination. A number of experiments have been conducted with a variety of species including cows, pigs, rats and birds on the absorption, distribution, metabolism and elimination of the commercial PBB mixture, FireMaster BP-6, which have been summarized in an extensive review by Fries (1985). Because of the similarities between PCBs and PBBs, information pertaining to one can generally be applied to the other.

In general, PBBs are rapidly and extensively absorbed, with absorption being inversely dependent on the number of bromine atoms (Damstra *et al.*, 1982; Fries, 1985). For example, less than 10% of a dose of C^{14}-labeled 2,2′,4,4′,5,5′-hexabromobiphenyl was eliminated in rats (Matthews *et al.*, 1977; Fries, 1985) indicating almost complete absorption compared to 62% fecal elimination of C^{14}-labeled octobromobiphenyl 24 hours after dosing suggesting incomplete absorption (Norris *et al.*, 1975; Fries, 1985).

PBBs are widely distributed throughout the body of all species studied. Initial concentrations are generally greatest in the liver and adipose tissue (Damstra *et al.*, 1982; Fries, 1985) with highest equilibrium concentrations on a wet tissue basis being adipose tissue (Miceli and Marks, 1981; Damstra *et al.*, 1982; Fries, 1985). Concentrations of PBBs in muscle and organ tissues are usually an order of magnitude lower (Fries, 1985) compared to adipose tissue. Generally, differences in

TABLE 41.2 Concentrations of polychlorinated dibenxo-*p*-dioxin (PCDD), polychlorinated dibenzofuran (PCDF) and polychlorinated biphenyl (PCB) congeners and toxic equivalents (TEQ) in fish collected downstream from a contaminated industrial site

Compound	TEF	Congener and (TEQ) concentration (pg/g)
PCDDs		
2,3,7,8-TCDD	1.00000	0.5 (0.5)
1,2,3,7,8-PeCDD	1.00000	0.3 (0.3)
TEQ from PCDDs		0.8
% total TEQ		1.8
PCDFs		
2,3,7,8-TCDF	0.10000	3.0 (0.3)
2,3,4,7,8-PeCDF	0.30000	4.6 (1.4)
TEQ from PCDFs		1.7
% total TEQ		3.8
Non-ortho PCBs		
#126	0.10000	410 (41.0)
TEQ from non-ortho PCBs		41.0
% total TEQ		90.5
Mono-ortho PCBs		
#123	0.00003	38,000 (1.1)
#156	0.00003	23,000 (0.7)
TEQ from mono-ortho PCBs		1.8
% total TEQ		4.0
Grand total TEQ (pg/g wet weight)		45.3

concentration between tissues can be attributed, at least in part, to variations in fat content of the tissues.

Individual PBB congeners in FireMaster BP-6 undergo hydroxylation by metabolic routes that are similar for the related PCBs with the rate of metabolism being determined primarily by the position of bromine atoms on the ring and secondarily by the bromine content of the molecule (Damstra *et al.*, 1982). *In vivo* studies suggest that, like PCBs, metabolism can occur if there are two adjacent unbrominated positions (Matthews *et al.*, 1978; Fries, 1985), although no studies indicated significant metabolism of congeners comprising the commercial PBB mixture (Fries *et al.*, 1976).

Elimination of individual PBB congeners occurs at different rates with those congeners that are more slowly removed becoming more concentrated in tissues relative to those congeners that are more rapidly eliminated. The predominant congener in FireMaster BP-6, 2,2′4,4′,5,5′-hexabromobiphenyl, is the most persistent congener in the various species studied (Damstra *et al.*, 1982). PBBs are eliminated primarily by biliary excretion into the feces, but fecal concentrations are low compared to whole-body concentrations (Damstra *et al.*, 1982; Fries, 1985). For example, less than 7% of an intravenous dose of 2,2′,4,4′,5,5′-hexabromobiphenyl was eliminated by rats over a 42-day period (Matthews *et al.*, 1977; Fries, 1985) and rhesus monkeys excreted on a daily basis approximately 0.5% of a single dose of the same congener from 10 to 42 days post-dosing (Rozman *et al.*, 1982; Fries, 1985).

Placental transfer of PBBs occurs to some extent, but the concentrations in fetal or offspring tissues are relatively small compared to concentrations in maternal tissues. Transfer of PBBs to the offspring during nursing results in much greater whole-body concentrations compared to PBB transfer during gestation. For example, pigs from sows that were fed PBBs during gestation and lactation had a five-fold increase in body burden during the 4-week lactation period with residues accumulated during lactation accounting for 95% of the total body burden (Werner and Sleight, 1981; Fries, 1985).

As suggested above, milk is the major route of elimination of PBBs for lactating mammals, although in the case of females nursing their young, the contaminant is simply transferred from one animal to another. Concentrations of PBBs in milk fat generally exceed dietary concentrations, with bovine milk fat concentrations exceeding dietary concentrations by three- to four-fold (Fries and Marrow, 1975; Willett and Irving, 1976; Damstra *et al.*, 1982; Fries, 1985).

The egg is a major route of elimination for egg-laying birds with concentrations in chicken or Japanese quail eggs being 1 to 1.5 times that of dietary concentrations (Babish *et al.*, 1975; Fries *et al.*, 1976; Polin and Ringer, 1978a; Damstra *et al.*, 1982; Fries, 1985). Elimination of PBBs via the egg can account for as much as 50% of the daily dose if there is no deleterious effect on egg production (Fries *et al.*, 1976).

Dairy cows at different stages of production were administered daily doses of FireMaster BP-6 ranging from 0.25 mg to 25 g for periods ranging from 1 to 202 days. Penta-, hexa- and heptabromobiphenyls in the commercial mixture were absorbed through the gastrointestinal tract and were detected in the plasma after 4 hours and reached steady-state concentrations after 15 days. The concentration of PBBs in tissues was, in general, correlated with the lipid content of the particular tissue with exception of the liver, which contained relatively high concentrations of PBBs in relation to its lipid content. Fecal elimination was the predominant route of excretion in non-lactating cows, while milk fat was the major route of elimination in those animals that were lactating. Concentrations of PBBs in milk were approximately three times those in feces. The half-life of PBBs being excreted via lactation was 28 days (Willett and Durst, 1978; Damstra *et al.*, 1982).

Chickens fed FireMaster FF-1 for 5 weeks accumulated PBB residues at average ratios of tissue PBBs:diet PBBs of 3:1 for adipose tissue, 1.5:1 for whole egg, 0.8:1 for liver and 0.008:1 for muscle (Polin and Ringer, 1978a,b). The distribution of a chicken's daily intake of PBBs on reaching a steady state was estimated to be: excreta – 11%; eggs – 58%; adipose – 10%; muscle – 12%; liver – 2%; unknown – 7% (Ringer and Polin, 1977). A second chicken study demonstrated that after 63 days of consuming a diet containing PBBs, body fat concentrations were approximately four times greater than dietary concentrations (Fries *et al.*, 1976; Damstra *et al.*, 1982).

The concentrations of PBBs in adipose tissue of mink fed various concentrations of FireMaster FF-1 were about 60 times higher than dietary concentrations (Aulerich and Ringer, 1979).

The kinetics of some individual PBB congeners has been studied. Rats orally administered ^{14}C-labeled 2,2′,4,4′,5,5′-hexabromobiphenyl at doses up to 30 mg/kg over 4 days absorbed at least 90% of the congener. Twenty-four hours after the last dose, 40% of the radioactivity was measured in the muscle, 10% in the liver and 25% in the adipose tissue. After 7 days, adipose tissue contained 60% of the radioactivity while the liver and muscle contained 2% and 7%, respectively. Very little of the congener was metabolized and eliminated. It was estimated that less than 10% of the total dose would undergo fecal excretion (Matthews *et al.*, 1977; DiCarlo *et al.*, 1978). An octabromobiphenyl mixture consisting of hepta-, octa-, nona- and decabromobiphenyls that comprised approximately 11% of FireMaster BP-6 was fed to rats at a dietary concentration of

1,000 ppm for 4 weeks. Bromine concentrations in the adipose tissue of these animals were approximately 600 times greater than bromine concentrations in the adipose tissue of untreated rats. Adipose tissue concentrations of bromine increased to 800 times greater than concentrations in untreated animals 18 weeks after the treated animals had been placed on clean feed. These results indicated that the octabromobiphenyl mixture was resistant to metabolism and elimination (Lee *et al.*, 1975; Damstra *et al.*, 1982)

PBBs can have a relatively long biological half-life in animals. Data suggested that only 10% of the total dose of 2,2′4,4′5,5′-hexabromobiphenyl would be eliminated during the lifetime of a rat (Matthews *et al.*, 1977; DiCarlo *et al.*, 1978). Rats receiving a single dose of C^{14}-octabromobiphenyl had biphasic fecal excretion with the initial half-life being less than 24 hours and second phase half-life being greater than 16 days (Norris *et al.*, 1975; DiCarlo *et al.*, 1978). Studies with cows suggested biphasic elimination of PBBs via the milk with an initial half-life of 11 days and a second half-life of 58 days (Fries and Marrow, 1975; Gutenmann and Lisk, 1975; DiCarlo *et al.*, 1978). In cases where observation periods were long, a biological half-life of 180 days was estimated for lactating cows (Fries, 1985). It was estimated that the concentration of FireMaster BP-6 in bovine milk fat would decrease from approximately 300 ppm to 0.3 ppm in 120 weeks (Detering *et al.*, 1975; DiCarlo *et al.*, 1978). A half-life of 17 days was calculated for FireMaster FF-1 in the eggs of chickens fed a diet containing the commercial mixture. Half-lives of 17 days and 31 days were calculated for muscle and liver, respectively, and the concentration of PBBs in adipose tissue was essentially unchanged after 56 days (Ringer and Polin, 1977; Polin and Ringer, 1978b). It was estimated that a chicken exposed to 1 ppm PBB in the feed for at least 10 days (the minimum time required to attain a steady-state concentration in the contents of a whole egg) would require 87 days of feeding uncontaminated feed to reach a concentration of 0.05 ppm in the whole egg (Ringer and Polin, 1977). The half-life of hexabromobiphenyl was 28 days and that of heptabromobiphenyl was 20 days in chicken eggs (Fries *et al.*, 1976; DiCarlo *et al.*, 1978).

PCDDs and PCDFs

The absorption, distribution, metabolism and elimination of PCDDs and PCDFs have been extensively reviewed by Van den Berg and associates (1994). Absorption from the gastrointestinal tract of mammals is effective and can exceed 75% of the dose for the lower chlorinated congeners. With increasing molecular size, absorption from the intestines is greatly reduced, which is most apparent for the hepta- and octachlorinated congeners. The liver and adipose tissue are the major storage sites of PCDDs and PCDFs for most mammalian and avian species. The biotransformation of PCDDs and PCDFs depends on the number and position of the chlorine atoms on the molecule. Metabolic reactions include oxidation and reductive dechlorination as well as breakage of the oxygen bonds. Sulfur containing metabolites have also been identified. In general, the urinary and biliary elimination of 2,3,7,8-substituted congeners depends on the metabolism of these compounds. Whole-body half-lives of the group of 2,3,7,8-substituted congeners in rodents range from a few to more than 100 days.

The absorption of PCDDs and PCDFs from the gastrointestinal tract has been studied for a number of individual congers. The extent of absorption of 2,3,7,8-TCDD or related compounds is variable, depending on the vehicle and the substitution pattern of the congener. There appear to be no differences between species in terms of absorption of these compounds through the gastrointestinal tract. There are indications that passage across the intestinal wall is predominately limited by molecular size and solubility with the influence of these two parameters being most significant for hepta- and octachlorinated congeners, which exhibit decreased absorption. Studies with rats, mice, hamsters, guinea pigs, cows and chickens, in general, indicate that 2,3,7,8-tetra- and pentachlorinated congeners are well absorbed from the gastrointestinal tract (50 to 90%), and OCCD is absorbed only to a limited extent (2 to 15%) (Pohjanvirta and Tuomisto, 1994; Van den Berg *et al.*, 1994).

The tissue distribution of PCDDs and PCDFs has been extensively studied in laboratory experiments using rodents and non-human primates. Upon absorption, 2,3,7,8-substituted PCDDs and PCDFs are bound to chylomicrons, lipoproteins and other serum proteins and transported throughout the circulatory system. The liver and adipose tissue are the major storage sites of PCDDs and PCDFs for most mammalian and avian species, whereas, depending on species, the skin and adrenals can also act as primary sites for deposition. Several studies with rats, mice, hamsters, guinea pigs and monkeys indicated that the 2,3,7,8-substituted PCDDs and PCDFs are the predominant congeners retained in tissues and body fluids. In rats and mice, most of the 2,3,7,8-substituted penta- to octachlorinated congeners are retained in the liver at higher concentrations than 2,3,7,8-TCDD and TCDF. In the hamster, the adrenal glands also appear to be a major storage site in addition to the liver and adipose tissue. Recent studies suggest that the tissue distribution of 2,3,7,8-TCDD and related compounds is dose dependent in that as the dose increases, so does the liver:adipose distribution ratio. In the liver, 2,3,7,8-TCDD induces both cytochromes CYP1A1 and CYP1A2. Induced CYP1A2, in turn, appears to be a crucial binding species for 2,3,7,8-TCDD and related compounds in rodents. The hepatocellular binding of 2,3,7,8-TCDD to CYP1A1 is so strong that only a very limited amount will be released back into the circulation. Placental transfer of 2,3,7,8-substituted PCDDs and PCDFs was found to be strongly dependent on molecular size with 2,3,7,8-TCDD being retained to the greatest extent in the fetus. In a number of mammalian species, the transfer of PCDDs and PCDFs from the mother to the offspring via lactation is quantitatively more important than transport to the fetus across the placenta. Excretion via lactation generally decreases as chlorine content increases, being most pronounced for the hepta- and octachlorinated congeners (Pohjanvirta and Tuomisto, 1994; Van den Berg *et al.*, 1994).

As in mammals, the liver and adipose tissue of avian species are the major sites for storage and accumulation of 2,3,7,8-substitiuted PCDDs and PCDFs. Hepatic deposition of 2,3,7,8-substituted PCDDs and PCDFs appeared to increase with increasing chlorination, resulting in a limited transfer of the more highly chlorinated congeners to the egg (Van den Berg *et al.*, 1994).

Metabolism of 2,3,7,8-TCDD and related compounds is necessary for urinary and biliary elimination, thus playing a major role in regulating the rate of excretion of these compounds. In rats, metabolic reactions include oxidation, preferably in the lateral positions, and reductive dechlorination as well as oxygen bridge cleavage of the diphenyl ether in 2,3,7,8-substituted PCDDs. As with lower chlorinated PCDDs, oxidation of PCDFs preferably occurs on the 2 and 3 positions. Metabolism of 2,3,7,8-TCDF results in a number of metabolites containing one and two hydroxyl groups. However, in contrast to 2,3,7,8-TCDD, there was no cleavage of the oxygen bridge. In the 2,3,7,8-substituted PCDF molecule, the 4 and 6 positions are more susceptible to metabolic attack than the 1 and 9 positions. As a result, PCDFs with chlorines in the 4 and 6 positions are highly persistent in biota (Van den Burg *et al.*, 1994). Metabolism of PCDDs and PCDFs is generally thought to be a detoxification process, thus toxicity is attributable to the unchanged parent compound (Pohjanvirta and Tuomisto, 1994).

The induction of CYP1A1 and CYP1A2 enzyme activities by 2,3,7,8-substituted PCDDs and PCDFs has been shown to be one of the most sensitive parameters for biological activity of these compounds. The enzymes most studied are the CYP1A1-dependent ethoxyresorufin-*O*-deethylase (EROD) and aryl hydrocarbon hydroxylase (AHH). In addition, 2,3,7,8-substituted PCDDs and PCDFs also induce Phase II enzymes (Van den Berg *et al.*, 1994).

In mammals, the liver and adipose tissue are the major compartments for the deposition of PCDDs and PCDFs. The elimination of polar metabolites of 2,3,7,8-substituted PCDDs and PCDFs occurs predominantly via the bile and feces, with urinary excretion playing a minor role. However, urinary elimination plays an important role in the hamster. In rats, the whole-body half-lives of PCDDs and PCDFs range from 17 to 31 days, depending on the dose and strain of rat used, while in hamsters and mice, the whole-body half-lives range from 11 to 15 days and 11 to 24 days, respectively. In rats, it was shown that lactation can reduce the half-life of these compounds while egg-laying can reduce the half-life in avian species. In lactating cows, mean half-lives ranged from 40 to 50 days for tetra- to heptaCDDs and CDFs. 2,3,7,8-Tetrachlorodibenzofuran is eliminated more rapidly than 2,3,7,8-TCDD, having a whole-body half-life of 2 days. The rapid elimination of 2,3,7,8-TCDF is thought to be due to its rapid metabolism. In contrast, 2,3,4,7,8-pentaCDF is eliminated very slowly in the rat, with a whole-body half-life of 64 days. The slow elimination rate is probably due to tight binding of this congener by CYP1A2, in addition to limited metabolism. As chlorine content increases, the rate of elimination of PCDDs and PCDFs decreases (Pohjanvirta and Tuomisto, 1994; Van den Berg *et al.*, 1994).

Interspecies differences in toxicity can only be partly explained by differences in toxicokinetics. The hamster is the species most resistant to the acute toxicity of 2,3,7,8-TCDD. Although the elimination rate of 2,3,7,8-TCDD is two- to three-fold greater in the hamster than the rat and mouse, this does not explain entirely the 10- to 100-fold difference in acute toxicity between the hamster and other rodent species. The guinea pig is most sensitive to the acute effects of 2,3,7,8-TCDD and it is the species with the slowest metabolism and elimination of 2,3,7,8-TCDD, suggesting that toxicokinetics in part explains the unique sensitivity of the guinea pig to the acute toxicity of 2,3,7,8-TCDD and 2,3,7,8-TCDF (Van den Berg *et al.*, 1994).

MECHANISM OF ACTION

The AhR is a ligand-activated transcription factor that is involved in the regulation of a number of genes, including those for enzymes that play a role in the metabolism of xenobiotics as well as genes involved in cell growth regulation and differentiation (Okey *et al.*, 1994; Safe, 1994; Hahn, 1998, 2002; Denison *et al.*, 2002; Denison and Nagy, 2003; Mandal, 2005). The AhR plays an important role in the altered gene expression and species- and tissue-specific toxicity resulting from exposure to specific PCB congeners and PCDD and PCDF isomers. It is now well established that the majority of the toxic effects attributed to 2,3,7,8-TCDD and 2,3,7,8-TCDD-like chemicals require activation of the AhR. The toxicity of individual isomers and congeners is closely related to the affinity with which these compounds bind to the AhR with the most toxic compounds being those that bind with the greatest affinity (Okey *et al.*, 1994). There are large species and strain differences in sensitivity to 2,3,7,8-TCDD and related chemicals. Mouse and rat strain differences in sensitivity to 2,3,7,8-TCDD can be partially explained by differences in the ligand-binding affinity of their polymorphic AhR variants. A recent study in birds indicated that species differences in sensitivity to 2,3,7,8-TCDD and related chemicals could be due, at least in part, to differences in amino acid composition of the ligand-binding domain of the AhR (Karchner *et al.*, 2006). However, differences in AhR concentration or binding affinity do not fully explain the differences in species susceptibility to 2,3,7,8-TCDD and 2,3,7,8-TCDD-like chemicals (Denison *et al.*, 1986).

The AhR is a basic helix-loop-helix (bHLH) and Per-Arnt-Sim (PAS)-containing transcription factor (Denison *et al.*, 2002; Denison and Nagy, 2003). In the absence of a ligand, AhR occurs as a soluble multiprotein complex in the cytosol of the cell. The chaperone proteins are two molecules of hsp90 (a heat shock protein of 90 kDa), the X-associated protein 2 (XAP2) and p23 (a co-chaperone protein of 23 kDa). When 2,3,7,8-TCDD or another ligand diffuses across the plasma membrane and binds to the AhR, the ligand AhR complex undergoes a conformational change that exposes a nuclear localization sequence or NLS (Figure 41.2). The complex translocates into the nucleus of the cell and the chaperone proteins dissociate from the complex. The AhR–ligand then binds to the bHLH-PAS nuclear protein, AhR nuclear translocator or Arnt. The formation of this heterodimer initiates conversion of the complex into a form that binds to DNA with high affinity on a specific recognition site called the dioxin responsive element or DRE. Binding of the ligand–AhR–Arnt complex to the DRE stimulates transcription of genes encoding ctyochrome P450 enzymes in the CYP1A1 subfamily and other AhR-responsive genes that are located upstream of the DRE (Denison *et al.*, 2002; Denison and Nagy, 2003). Continuous and inappropriate modulation of gene expression is thought to be responsible for a series of biochemical, cellular and tissue changes that result in toxicity characteristic of 2,3,7,8-TCDD and related compounds (Denison and Heath-Pagliuso, 1998; Mandal, 2005).

TOXICITY

General considerations

Exposure to PBBs, PCBs, PCDDs and PCDFs has been linked with a broad spectrum of effects, both *in vivo* and *in vitro*, which vary depending on method/age of exposure, sex of the individual and dose/duration of exposure (Steinberg *et al.*, 2008). Fetal and early developmental exposures to these

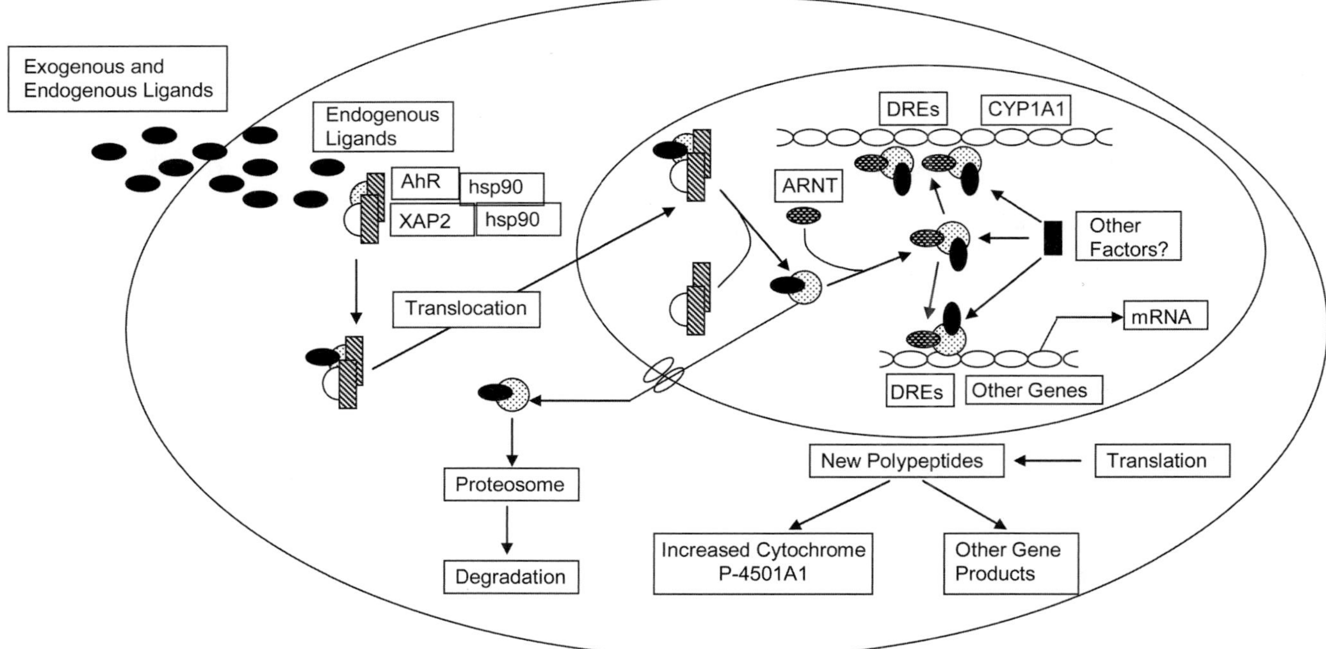

FIGURE 41.2 The proposed molecular mechanism of action of 2,3,7,8-tetrachorinated dibenzo-*p*-dioxin (TCDD) and TCDD-like chemicals. See text for details.

chemicals are particularly devastating, and can have different outcomes from adult exposure (Crews *et al.*, 2000). As stated by Steinberg *et al.* (2008), latent effects of early exposures include, but are not limited to, depressed circulating thyroid hormone and abnormal thyroid cytology (Porterfield, 1994; Goldey *et al.*, 1995; Morse *et al.*, 1996a; Chauhan *et al.*, 2000; Bansal *et al.*, 2005), developmental effects of the heart, palate and kidney (Foster *et al.*, 2010), delayed cognitive development (Chen *et al.*, 1992; Jacobson and Jacobson, 1997), altered sensory and motor abilities (Bowman *et al.*, 1981; Laskey *et al.*, 2002; Roegge *et al.*, 2004), reproductive impairment (Sager and Girard, 1994; Arnold *et al.*, 1995; Meerts *et al.*, 2004; Yang *et al.*, 2005) and compromised neural function (Morse *et al.*, 1996b; Provost *et al.*, 1999; Donahue *et al.*, 2004; Seegal *et al.*, 2005).

Significant differences in toxic effects will result depending upon when exposure occurs during gestation (Miller *et al.*, 2004). For example, in the mouse, gestational development begins with fertilization, cleavage and blastulation that occur in the oviduct between gestation day (GD) 0 and GD 5. Between GD 5 and 10, the ectoderm, mesoderm and endoderm are formed and early organogenesis is initiated. At GD 9, the heart begins to beat, the neuropore closes and organogenesis continues through GD 15. Primordial germ cells enter the genital ridges at GD 11 and sexual differentiation of the gonads occurs at GD 12.5. Further fetal growth and development and bone formation occur from GD 14 through GD 19. Exposure to chemicals prior to GD 12 will have a significant effect on organogenesis and sex-appropriate differentiation of the gonads. Exposures that occur after GD 14 will predominantly affect the overall growth of the fetus because the organ systems have essentially developed prior to this point.

Many environmental contaminants may mediate their effects by receptor binding, modulation of hormone-regulated mechanisms or direct toxic effects. 2,3,7,8-TCDD and related compounds such as the non-ortho PCBs are considered to be antiestrogenic while ortho-substituted PCBs have estrogenic properties (Pflieger-Bruss and Schill, 2000; Pflieger-Bruss *et al.*, 2004).

PBBs

Toxicological assessment of FireMaster FF-1 is complicated by the fact that the commercial product is a mixture of individual congeners of differing toxicities. In addition, the commercial mixture also contained traces of brominated naphthalenes as impurities with their own toxicity. As with many chemicals, the type and severity of effects are influenced by species, age, duration of exposure and dose. None of the effects caused by PBBs are unique to this particular group of brominated congeners, but they are characteristic of polyhalogenated hydrocarbons including PBBs, PCBs, PCDDs and PCDFs.

A number of studies have demonstrated PBB-induced reproductive effects in a variety of species. Exposure of poultry to deleterious concentrations of PBBs resulted in an initial decrease in feed consumption accompanied by a decrease in egg production. At sufficiently high concentrations, there was a dose-related decrease in egg hatchability with embryo mortality occurring late in incubation (Fries, 1985). Dietary concentrations of FireMaster FF-1 greater than 30 ppm resulted in a significant decrease in egg production of chickens, which returned to control values from 2 to 6 weeks after withdrawal of the contaminated feed. Concentrations above 30 ppm also had an adverse effect on hatchability and subsequent survivability of chicks (Ringer and Polin, 1977; Polin and Ringer, 1978a). Edema of the abdominal and cervical regions of the chicken embryos and hatchlings was the prevalent pathological condition observed and was the only effect that had an increased incidence compared to the incidence of abnormalities observed in controls (Ringer and Polin, 1977; Polin and Ringer, 1978b). A dietary PBB concentration of 20 ppm had no effect on egg production and hatchability in Japanese quail, but 100 ppm resulted in a significant decrease in both parameters (Babish *et al.*, 1975). Rats administered FireMaster BP-6 at doses of 5 or 25 mg/kg body weight every other day for 14 days had a reduced number of implantation sites compared to controls at both doses and increased resorptions and fetal deaths at the higher dose (Beaudoin, 1977; Damstra *et al.*, 1982). Single doses of 400 and 800 mg/kg body weight caused a decrease in rat fetal weights at term as well as an increased incidence of cleft palate and diaphragmatic hernia. Pregnant rats fed diets containing 100 and 1,000 ppm FireMaster BP-6 experienced increased fetal mortality and fetal weights were reduced at term (Corbett *et al.*, 1975, 1978; Damstra *et al.*, 1982). Mice exposed to 200 ppm dietary PBBs on GD 4 through GD 16 had an increase in fetal deaths and resorptions as well as reduced fetal weights at term (Preache *et al.*, 1976; Damstra *et al.*, 1982). Exencephaly and cleft palate were observed in offspring of mice fed FireMaster BP-6 at concentrations up to 1,000 ppm (Corbett *et al.*, 1975, 1978; DiCarlo *et al.*, 1978). The predominant congener in FireMaster BP-6, 2,2′,4,4′,5,5′-hexabromobiphenyl, did not cause any effects in offspring when administered to pregnant mice at a dose of 40 mg/kg body weight on gestation days 10 through 16 (Damstra *et al.*, 1982). Pigs that were fed diets containing up to 200 ppm PPBs during gestation had normal young but as the offspring nursed, there was 50% mortality in those receiving 200 ppm via lactation and significant growth depression in offspring consuming 100 ppm in the milk (Werner and Sleight, 1981; Fries, 1985). Rhesus monkeys fed diets containing 0.3 ppm FireMaster FF-1 for 7 months prior to breeding had prolonged menstrual cycles and decreased progesterone concentrations. Offspring had depressed birth weights and growth rates through 16 weeks of age (Allen and Lambrecht, 1978; Damstra *et al.*, 1982). Mink were fed diets containing FireMaster FF-1 at concentrations ranging from 1.0 to 15.6 ppm, a diet containing contaminated chicken that provided a PBB concentration of 1.5 ppm or a diet containing contaminated beef that provided a PBB concentration of 12.0 ppm for up to 10 months. Adults experienced increased mortality at dietary concentrations of 6.25 ppm or greater. There was also a significant decrease in litter size, birth weights and kit survivability through 4 weeks of age at dietary concentrations from 1.0 to 2.5 ppm and greater. Results indicated that the PBB-contaminated poultry and beef were more toxic than the commercial mixture. A concentration lethal to 50% of the population (LC_{50}) for FireMaster FF-1 was estimated to be 4 ppm when fed for over 300 days. This study indicated that PBBs were not as fetotoxic as two commercial PCB mixtures (Aroclors 1242 and 1254) but were lethal to adults at a lower dietary concentration (Aulerich and Ringer, 1979).

PCBs, PCDDs and PCDFs

General effects

The toxic and biochemical effects of various commercial PCB mixtures have been studied in various laboratory animals, fish and wildlife species and have been summarized by Safe (1994). Commercial PCBs cause a broad spectrum of toxic responses that are dependent on several factors including the chlorine content and purity of the commercial mixture, the route and duration of exposure as well as on the age, sex, species and strain of animal. The majority of effects caused by commercial PCB mixtures are the same as those induced by 2,3,7,8-TCDD because the responses caused by commercial PCB mixtures are due, in part, to the individual non-ortho coplanar and mono-ortho coplanar PCBs present in these mixtures that act as AhR agonists. Because some of the mono-ortho coplanar PCBs are present in relatively high concentrations in commercial mixtures and environmental extracts, this class of PCBs may contribute significantly to the 2,3,7,8-TCDD-like activity of PCB mixtures (Safe, 1994).

There are a number of reports that describe the common effects induced by 2,3,7,8-TCDD and related PCDDs, PCDFs and PCBs. The only major difference in these compounds is their relative toxic potencies. These effects are thought to be mediated by initial binding to the AhR and are dependent on dose, age, sex, species and strain of animal. In most cases, if a given species is more sensitive to a given class of compound (for example, PCBs), this species will also be sensitive to the other classes (PCDDs, PCDFs, PBBs). It has also been observed that in most instances young animals are more sensitive than adults and females more sensitive than males. Generally speaking, chickens, guinea pigs and mink are the most sensitive species of animals to the toxic effects induced by 2,3,7,8-TCDD and 2,3,7,8-TCDD-like chemicals. In contrast, hamsters and amphibians appear to be fairly resistant to the toxic effects. The effects include acute lethality, wasting syndrome, thymic and splenic atrophy, impairment of immune responses, hepatotoxicity and porphyria, chloracne and related dermal lesions, tissue-specific hypo- and hyperplastic responses, disruption of multiple endocrine pathways, carcinogenesis, teratogenicity and reproductive toxicity (Poland and Knutson, 1982; McConnell, 1985; Safe, 1986, 1990, 1998; Dickson and Buzik, 1993; Fries, 1995, Schecter *et al.*, 2006).

Female reproductive effects

2,3,7,8-TCDD and approximate stereoisomers have been shown to affect female reproductive endpoints in a variety of animal studies. Among the effects reported are a decrease in the number of females mated in rats, mink and monkeys, fewer completed pregnancies in rats, mink and monkeys, lower maternal weight gain during pregnancy in rats, rabbits and monkeys, decreased litter size in rats, rabbits, mink and swine, effects on female gonads in guinea pigs and mice and altered estrous and menstrual cycles in mice, rats and monkeys. Decreased egg production and hatchability occur in a number of avian species. Numerous studies have indicated that 2,3,7,8-TCDD and related chemicals are anti-estrogenic presumably due to increased metabolism of estrogen and a decreased number of estrogen receptors. One manifestation of the anti-estrogenic effect is the 2,3,7,8-TCDD-induced decrease in uterine weight in rats. Occasionally, some signs of ovarian dysfunction such as anovulation and suppression of the estrous cycle have been reported (Golub *et al.*, 1991; Peterson *et al.*, 1993; Safe, 1994). Specific topics are addressed below.

Sexual development

Den Hond *et al.* (2002) reported that fewer adolescent females living near two waste incinerators in Flanders, Belgium, had achieved the adult stage of breast development compared to youth living in the control area. There was a negative association between serum concentrations of 2,3,7,8-TCDD-like chemicals and breast development.

Fecundity

Buck *et al.* (2000) reported that consumption of PCB-contaminated fish from Lake Ontario by women of reproductive age was associated with a reduction in fecundity. Specifically, women who consumed fish for 3 to 6 years or who reported recent consumption of at least one monthly fish meal were approximately 25% less likely to become pregnant per cycle than women who did not consume fish. Mendola *et al.* (1997) reported a significant reduction in menstrual cycle length associated with consumption of PCB-contaminated sport fish from Lake Ontario raising concern about the effect(s) of environmental aquatic contaminants on female fecundity. Abnormal menstrual bleeding was reported to be higher among women exposed to PCBs and PCDFs as a result of consumption of contaminated rice oil in Yucheng, Taiwan, between 1978 and 1979 in comparison to controls (Yu *et al.*, 2000). Chao *et al.* (2007) assessed placental concentrations of TEQ contributed by PCDDs/PCDFs ($TEQ_{PCDD/PCDF}$) and PCBs (TEQ_{PCB}) and irregular menstrual cyclicity in Taiwanese mothers. Results indicated that placental $TEQ_{PCDD/PCDF}$ concentrations were greater in women with an irregular menstrual cycle compared to women with a regular cycle and TEQ_{PCB} were greater in women with menstrual cycles longer than 33 days compared to women with cycles with a duration less than 33 days. Yang *et al.* (2008) recently reported prolonged time to pregnancy and reduced fertility in women exposed *in utero* to PCBs and PCDFs during the Yucheng incident.

Embryotoxicity

Oral administration of Aroclor 1260 to female rabbits (4 mg/kg body weight for 14 weeks) resulted in a significant accumulation of PCBs in 6-day-old blastocysts and increased preimplantation embryo mortality (Seiler *et al.*, 1994). Lindenau and Fischer (1996) assessed the direct toxicity of Aroclor 1260 on preimplantation rabbit embryos by *in vitro* culture. One-day-old cleavage stages and 3-day-old rabbit morulae exposed to 5.0 or 50 μg Aroclor 1,260/ml culture medium for 24 hours displayed dose-related developmental arrest or degeneration of embryos.

Endometriosis

Endometriosis is a common gynecological disorder affecting at least 5 to 10% of the reproductive age women in the USA and is characterized by the presence of endometrial glands and stroma outside the uterus (Bruner-Tran and Osteen, 2010). Rier *et al.* (1993) were the first to report an association between chronic exposure to 2,3,7,8-TCDD-like chemicals and endometrosis in rhesus monkeys. This finding prompted epidemiological studies that attempted to correlate the body burden of 2,3,7,8-TCDD and PCBs and the incidence of endometriosis in humans. In a review of the relation between exposure to 2,3,7,8-TCDD-like chemicals and the incidence of endometriosis in humans, Bruner-Tran and Osteen (2010) state that these studies do not come to consistent conclusions. An association between endometriosis and 2,3,7,8-TCDD was observed in a case–control study conducted in Israel (Mayani *et al.*, 1997). In a Belgian case–control study carried out on 42 infertile endometriosis cases and 27 mechanical infertile controls, no significant association was demonstrated between exposure to 2,3,7,8-TCDD-like compounds and the occurrence of endometriosis (Pauwels *et al.*, 2001). In a study carried out on a large group of women exposed to 2,3,7,8-TCDD in Seveso, Italy, a two-fold non-significant risk for endometriosis was observed among women with 2,3,7,8-TCDD concentrations equal to or greater than 100 ng/l (parts per trillion or ppt) but there was no evidence of a dose–response relationship (Eskenazi *et al.*, 2002). De Felip *et al.* (2004) reported no significant differences in body burdens of 2,3,7,8-TCDD-like chemicals in Belgium and Italian women with and without endometriosis, despite the observation that the incidence and severity of endometriosis as well as exposure to 2,3,7,8-TCDD-like chemicals in Belgium is greater compared to other industrialized countries.

Ovary

The ovary is responsible for oocyte and follicle development as well as synthesis of steroid hormones. Thus, chemicals affecting the ovary may affect fertility, menstrual/estrous cyclicity and timing of puberty and menopause. Because the ovary is composed of multiple cell types and follicles are in different stages of development, it can be difficult to identify those cell types that may be targeted by a specific toxicant (Miller *et al.*, 2004).

Synthesis of the ovarian steroid hormones estrogen and progesterone is regulated by follicle stimulating hormone (FSH) and luteinizing hormone (LH), which in turn are synthesized and released from the anterior pituitary in response to gonadotropin-releasing hormone (GnRH), which is released from the hypothalamus. As a result, hormonal regulation of follicular growth and ovulation is regulated by the neuroendocrine system acting on the ovary. Ovarian toxicity can thus result from direct action of the toxicant on the ovary or indirectly through modulation of the neuroendocrine system.

2,3,7,8-Tetrachlorodibenzo-*p*-dioxin-induced ovarian toxicity appears to be strain dependent. Long-Evans rats exposed to 1 μg 2,3,7,8-TCDD/kg body weight on GD 8 had reduced ovarian weight, a decline in fertility and persistent vaginal estrous, which can lead to infertility. Exposure to 0.8 μg 2,3,7,8-TCDD/kg body weight on GD 15 resulted in fewer functional effects compared to exposure on GD 8 (Gray and Otsby, 1995; Gray *et al.*, 1997). In Sprague-Dawley rats, exposure to 2,3,7,8-TCDD on GD 15 resulted in a decrease in the number of days spent in estrous (1 μg/kg body weight) and a decrease in or elimination of ovulation (2.5 μg/kg body weight) (Salisbury and Marcinkiewicz, 2002). The non-ortho PCB congener 3,3′,4,4′-tetrachlorobiphenyl (IUPAC 77) resulted in a reduction in germ cells and follicles of all stages in the ovaries of C57B1/6 mice on postnatal day (PND) 28 when injected on GD 13 (Ronnback, 1991). Salisbury and Marcinkiewicz (2002) reported that a single dose of 1 or 10 μg 2,3,4,7,8-pentachlorodibenzofuran/kg body weight injected on GD 15 caused periods of diestrus and corresponding irregular cyclicity. Additionally, ovulation rates were reduced (1 μg/kg body weight) or ovulation was eliminated entirely (10 μg/kg body weight). Miller *et al.* (2004), in evaluating the previous studies, summarized a number of possible mechanisms of action for the 2,3,7,8-TCDD-like chemicals that included alteration of steroidogenic and transcriptional pathways due to binding of the ligand to the ovarian AhR, reduction of the responsiveness of the developing follicle to gonadotropins and blocking of the LH surge needed to induce ovulation.

Gandolfi *et al.* (2002) reviewed literature related to the effects of various endocrine disrupters including PCBs on ovarian function and embryonic development. In general, published data indicate that PCBs (single congeners or commercial mixtures) disrupt mammalian oocyte maturation even at very low concentrations, acting through different cellular and molecular mechanisms. However, they state that it is unclear which specific cellular pathway(s) these compounds activate.

Placenta

The placenta, a highly vascularized tissue that develops during early gestation, is involved in the circulation of blood, oxygen, glucose and nutrients between the mother and fetus. The placenta synthesizes estrogen and progesterone as well as other hormones associated with pregnancy. Exposure to toxicants during pregnancy can comprise placental development and function as well as alter hormonal signaling that is critical for *in utero* development of the fetus (Miller *et al.*, 2004).

It has been suggested that *in utero* exposure to 2,3,7,8-TCDD results in placental hypoxia. The hypoxic response to 2,3,7,8-TCDD is thought to be the ultimate cause of death in Holtzman rats exposed to 1.6 μg/kg body weight on GD 15 (Ishimura *et al.*, 2002a). Additionally, placental exposure to 2,3,7,8-TCDD may interfere with glucose kinetics in that tissue. Because glucose transport from the mother to the fetus is facilitated by the placenta and because the placenta itself utilizes glucose, disruption of glucose kinetics could lead to an increase in fetal deaths in late pregnancy as suggested by Ishimura *et al.* (2002b) who administered a single 1.6 μg/kg body weight dose to Holtzman rats on GD 15.

Uterus, vagina and cervix

The ability of a female to maintain pregnancy can be compromised by structural abnormalities in the uterus, vagina and cervix. A number of studies have been conducted that examined the effects of 2,3,7,8-TCDD and related compounds on external genitalia of rats as summarized by Miller *et al.* (2004). Gray and Otsby (1995) reported a decline in fertility in female offspring of Long-Evans rats administered a single dose of 1 μg 2,3,7,8-TCDD/kg body weight on GD 8 due to an increase in endometrial hyperplasia. When an identical dose of 2,3,7,8-TCDD was administered on GD 15, female progeny of Long-Evans and Holtzman rats had a delay in puberty due to phallic clefting and the presence of a vaginal thread with the effect being more prominent in the latter strain. Gray *et al.* (1997) reported that there was a dose-related increase in the incidence of these effects in female offspring of Long-Evans rats injected with single doses of 2,3,7,8-TCDD ranging from 0.2 to 1.0 μg/kg body weight. Wolf *et al.* (1999) reported delayed vaginal opening, reduced fertility and increased incidence of cleft phallus in hamsters, although at a dose that was greater than the effective dose in rats. Vaginal threads were not apparent in hamsters.

Mammary gland

As a source of nourishment for perinatal mammalian offspring, the mammary gland is an important part of the female reproductive system. While the majority of development of the gland occurs in adult females during pregnancy, the organ is formed during embryonic development (Miller *et al.*, 2004). Fenton *et al.* (2002) and Fenton (2006) describe the development of the rodent mammary gland. The mammary epithelial bud is formed by GD 12 to GD 14 followed by a short period of inactivity. At GD 16 to GD 17, the epithelial bud begins to migrate and fill the stromal portion of the gland. At parturition, the ductal tree is formed, consisting of several ducts and lateral branches from each primary duct. The time period between parturition and puberty is characterized by slow growth of the gland as the fat pad and epithelium from the nipple extend backward. During puberty, growth of the gland is exponential with rapid development of terminal end buds at the ends of the lateral ductal branches. This phase is then followed by a period whereby terminal end buds are replaced by terminal ducts and small lobules. Exposure to toxicants during gestation can directly affect the development of the mammary gland and influence the ability of the female to adequately nurse her young (Miller *et al.*, 2004).

Fenton *et al.* (2002) reported that *in utero* and lactational exposure of Long-Evans rats to 2,3,7,8-TCDD (1 μg/kg body weight) on GD 15 delayed maturation of the mammary gland and could increase the incidence of breast cancer due to increased susceptibility of the gland to carcinogens. Exposure to 2,3,7,8-TCDD on GD 20 had no effect on the mammary gland. When 2,3,7,8-TCDD-exposed female rat offspring were bred and subsequently raised their offspring, the mammary glands of the second-generation females were smaller compared to control females. Brown *et al.* (1998) treated Sprague-Dawley rats prenatally with 1 μg 2,3,7,8-TCDD/kg body weight, which resulted in more terminal end buds and less lobules II at PND 50 compared to controls. Because terminal end buds are less mature than lobules, they are more susceptible to chemical carcinogens. Brown *et al.* (1998) demonstrated that rats exposed to 2,3,7,8-TCDD prenatally had twice as many mammary adenocarcinomas as a result of subsequent exposure to dimethylbenzanthracene compared to rats treated with dimethylbenzanthracene only. Exposure to non-ortho PCB congeners results in similar effects. Sprague-Dawley rats exposed prenatally to IUPAC 126 at a dose of 0.25 μg/kg body weight resulted in an increase in the number of terminal end buds and a decrease in alveolar buds and lobules, which in turn was associated with an increase incidence of postnatal dimethylbenzanthracene-induced mammary carcinomas (Muto *et al.*, 2002). Exposure to 2,3,7,8-TCDD-like chemicals during the time of puberty can also influence mammary gland development. Brown and Lamartiniere (1995) reported that when 2,3,7,8-TCDD (2.5 μg/kg body weight) was administered to rats on PND 25, 27, 29 and 31, there was an inhibition of mammary epithelial outgrowth and fewer terminal end buds on PND 32 compared to controls.

Another critical time of mammary gland development that can be affected by exposure to 2,3,7,8-TCDD-like chemicals is during pregnancy as the gland prepares for lactation

(Fenton, 2006). Vorderstrasse *et al.* (2004) reported that pregnant C57B1/6 mice exposed to 5 μg 2,3,7,8-TCDD/kg body weight on days GD 0, 7 and 14 and assessed for mammary gland effects on GD 9, 12 and 17 as well as on the day of parturition, had stunted gland growth, decreased branching and poor formation of lobular alveolar structures. In addition, expression of a specific milk protein in the gland was suppressed and all pups born to 2,3,7,8-TCDD-treated dams died within 24 hours of birth.

Male reproductive effects

2,3,7,8-Tetrachlorodibenzo-*p*-dioxin and related compounds decrease testis and accessory sex organ weight, cause abnormal testicular morphology, decrease spermatogenesis and reduce fertility when given to adult animals in doses sufficient to reduce feed intake and/or body weight. Some of these effects have been reported in chickens, rhesus monkeys, rats, guinea pigs and mice treated with overtly toxic doses of 2,3,7,8-TCDD or 2,3,78-TCDD-like chemicals. 2,3,7,8-Tetrachlorodibenzo-*p*-dioxin effects on spermatogenesis are characterized by loss of germ cells, the appearance of degenerating spermatocytes and mature spermataozoa within the lumens of seminiferous tubules and a reduction in the number of tubules containing mature spermatozoa. Effects of 2,3,7,8-TCDD on the male reproductive system are thought to be due in part to an androgen deficiency. The deficiency in rats is caused by decreased plasma testosterone and dihydrotestosterone (DHT) concentrations and unchanged plasma clearance of androgens and LH (Dickson and Buzik, 1993; Peterson *et al.*, 1993; Safe, 1994). Pflieger-Bruss *et al.* (2004) provide a review of the effects of various endocrine-disrupting chemicals, including PCBs/PCDDs/PCDFs, on the male reproductive system. Specific topics are addressed below.

Sexual development

Aoki (2001) summarized effects in humans exposed to PCBs and PCDFs in contaminated rice oil resulting in Yusho disease (Japan) and Yucheng disease (Taiwan). Sexual development of Yucheng boys was delayed and was thought to be due to altered hormonal status caused by PCBs and related congeners (Guo *et al.*, 1995). Den Hond *et al.* (2002) reported that fewer adolescent males living near two waste incinerators had achieved adult stages of genital development and pubic hair growth compared to youth living in the control area and that there was an negative association between serum concentrations of IUPAC 153 and genital development.

Sperm

Epidemiological studies have indicated variable effects of potential PCB/PCDD/PCDF exposure on semen quality and sperm counts. Guo *et al.* (2000) reported that sperm collected from males exposed prenatally to PCBs and PCDFs as a result of consumption of contaminated rice oil in Yucheng, Taiwan, between 1978 and 1979 was characterized by abnormal morphology, reduced motility and reduced capacity to penetrate hamster oocytes. Hsu *et al.* (2003a) reported a higher percentage of oligospermia, abnormal sperm morphology and reduced sperm binding capability and penetration in the same cohort. Decreases in sperm concentration and sperm motility (Van Waeleghem *et al.*, 1996) and total sperm count (Comhaire *et al.*, 2007) were reported in males exposed to 2,3,7,8-TCDD in Belgium. Mocarelli *et al.* (2008) reported that men exposed to 2,3,7,8-TCDD during the 1976 Seveso incident prior to puberty had reduced sperm count and motility as adults, while males exposed during adolescence exhibited increased sperm counts and motility. White and Birnbaum (2009) point out that these effects occurred at a concentration (less than 69 ppt in serum lipid in 1976) that is within an order of magnitude of present mean concentrations (15 ppt on a serum lipid basis).

Foster *et al.* (2010) state that of the reproductive/developmental effects of 2,3,7,8-TCDD, decreased sperm counts are considered to be the most sensitive outcome. A single exposure of rats to 0.064 μg 2,3,7,8-TCDD/kg body weight on GD 15 resulted in a significant decrease (36%) in epididymal sperm counts (Mably *et al.*, 1992). The World Health Organization (WHO) used this endpoint in establishing a tolerable daily intake for 2,3,7,8-TCDD of approximately 2 pg/kg body weight/day (Foster *et al.*, 2010). However, results of recent studies generally have not indicated an effect of *in utero* exposure to 2,3,7,8-TCDD on epididymal sperm counts. Foster *et al.* (2010) propose that the primary effect of 2,3,7,8-TCDD in relation to reduced sperm counts are due to developmental abnormalities of the male reproductive tract and epididymal structure and/or function.

In a review on 2,3,7,8-TCDD-induced changes in epididymal sperm count and spermatogenesis, Foster *et al.* (2010) demonstrated that developmental exposure to 2,3,7,8-TCDD has been consistently linked with decreased cauda epididymal and ejaculatory sperm counts in different rodent species, although doses at which the effects occur vary. They further state that the evidence linking *in utero* 2,3,7,8-TCDD exposure and spermatogenesis is less convincing and that effects of 2,3,7,8-TCDD on androgen signaling, reproductive organ weights and sperm transit through the epididymides may better account for the decrease in epididymal sperm counts.

There are studies that have examined the functional effects of exposure to commercial PCB mixtures in male rodents. Fielden *et al.* (2001) state that the effects of developmental exposure to PCBs on testis weight and fertility in laboratory rodents depend on the test congener or mixture, the dosage, the developmental stage during exposure, and the age of the animal at the time of examination, as well as species and strain. For example, Sager and associates (1983, 1987, 1994) reported that male Holtzman rats exposed to Aroclor 1254 from birth to 9 days of age had decreased fertility at 18 weeks of age and increased testis weight at 23 weeks of age. Epididymal sperm count and sperm morphology and motility were not adversely affected, but there was a decline in the ability of sperm to fertilize eggs. Cooke *et al.* (1996) demonstrated that neonatal exposure (from birth to day 25 of age) of Sprague-Dawley rats to Aroclor 1254 and Aroclor 1242 increased testis weight and daily sperm production at 19 weeks of age that were attributed to PCB-induced hypothyroidism. In contrast to the reduced fertility of Aroclor 1254-exposed pups reported by Sager and associates (1983, 1987, 1991), all Aroclor 1242-treated male pups bred successfully. Fielden *et al.* (2001) conducted a study to determine if gestational and lactational exposure of B6D2F1 mice to Aroclor 1242 could induce alterations in organ development and sperm quality and fertility in young adult (16 weeks of age) male offspring and to determine if the effects persisted into middle age (45 weeks of age). They reported no increase in testes size and epididymal sperm count at either age. However, *in vitro* sperm fertilizing ability was significantly decreased at both 16 and 45 weeks of age, suggesting that fertility in the adult mouse is susceptible to developmental exposure to Aroclor 1242 and that it is independent of testis weight or epididymal sperm count.

Hsu *et al.* (2003a,b) examined the effects of two ortho-substituted PCB congeners on sperm function and hormone concentrations in male rats. Male Sprague-Dawley rats were administered a single dose (9.6 or 96 mg/kg body weight) of 2,2′,3,3′4,6′-hexachlorobiphenyl (IUPAC 132) or 2,2′,3,4′5′,6-hexachlorobiphenyl (IUPAC 149) at 21 days of age and assessed at 16 weeks of age. Exposure to 96 mg IUPAC 132 or IUPAC 149/kg body weight resulted in decreased sperm motility, velocity and the ability of sperm to penetrate oocytes. Hsu *et al.* (2007) reported that prenatal exposure to IUPAC 132 (1 or 10 mg/kg body weight) resulted in a decrease in cauda epididymal weight, epididymal sperm count and motile epididymal sperm count in adult offspring. Kuriyama and Chahoud (2004) administered a single dose of 375 μg 2,3′,4,4′,5-pentachlorobiphenyl (IUPAC 118)/kg body weight to female Sprague-Dawley rats on GD 6. When male offspring were assessed on PND 170, effects on reproductive organs were observed in PCB-exposed animals that included smaller testes, epididymides and seminal vesicles (absolute and relative weights). Decreases in sperm and spermatid numbers and impairment of daily sperm production were also observed, although there was no effect on fertility. Oskam *et al.* (2005) administered the non-ortho PCB congener IUPAC 126 (49 ng/kg body weight/day) or the ortho-substituted IUPAC 153 (98 ng/kg body weight/day) to female goats from GD 60 until parturition at approximately GD 150. Lactational exposure of offspring continued until PND 40. Male offspring treated with IUPAC 153 had testes with a lesser diameter in comparison to the control group. There were no significant differences in plasma FSH concentrations but IUPAC 153-treated males differed significantly from the control group with respect to plasma LH and testosterone concentrations, whereas IUPAC 126-treated goats differed from the controls only in plasma testosterone concentrations. Neither the IUPAC 126 nor the IUPAC 153 group differed from the controls with respect to the conventional sperm parameters or testis histology. The authors concluded that IUPAC 153 was able to induce alterations in reproductive endpoints related to the hypothalamic–pituitary–axis as well as to the testis.

Developmental effects

Exposure to 2,3,7,8-TCDD during pregnancy causes prenatal mortality in the mouse, rat, guinea pig, hamster, rabbit, mink and monkey. The time period during which exposure of the embryo/fetus to 2,3,7,8-TCDD occurs is just as important as the dose of 2,3,7,8-TCDD administered in terms of prenatal mortality. In most laboratory mammals, gestational exposure to 2,3,7,8-TCDD produces a characteristic pattern of fetotoxic responses that consist of thymic hypoplasia, subcutaneous edema, decreased fetal growth and prenatal mortality. In addition to these common fetotoxic effects, there are other effects of 2,3,7,8-TCDD that are highly species specific. Such effects include cleft palate formation in the mouse and intestinal hemorrhage in the rat. In the mouse, hydronephrosis is the sensitive sign of prenatal toxicity, followed by cleft palate formation and atrophy of the thymus at higher doses, and by subcutaneous edema and mortality at maternally toxic doses. In the rat, 2,3,7,8-TCDD prenatal toxicity is characterized by intestinal hemorrhage, subcutaneous edema, decreased fetal growth and mortality. Structural abnormalities occur in the rat only at relatively large doses. In the hamster fetus, hydronephrosis and renal congestion are the most sensitive effects, followed by subcutaneous edema and mortality. In the rabbit, an increased incidence of extra ribs and prenatal mortality is found, whereas in the guinea pig and rhesus monkey, prenatal mortality is seen (Dickson and Buzik, 1993; Peterson *et al.*, 1993).

Avian embryos are more sensitive to 2,3,7,8-TCDD toxicity compared to mammals based on LD_{50} values. Among bird species, most of the developmental toxicity research has been done on the chicken, which is considered to be the most sensitive avian species to 2,3,7,8-TCDD-like chemicals. Injection of 2,3,7,8-TCDD or its approximate stereoisomers into fertilized chicken eggs causes a toxicity syndrome in the embryo characterized by pericardial and subcutaneous edema, liver lesions, inhibition of lymphoid development in the thymus and bursa of Fabricius, microophthalmia, beak deformities, cardiovascular malformations and mortality. Clinical signs in turkey embryos include microophthalmia, beak deformities and embryo mortality, but not liver lesions, edema or thymic hypoplasia while ring-necked pheasant embryos experienced only mortality. Thus, the clinical signs of toxicity of 2,3,7,8-TCDD and its approximate stereoisomers are species dependent with embryo mortality being the only common effect (Peterson *et al.*, 1993).

Cardiac effects

The developing cardiovascular system is a sensitive target of many environmental pollutants, including 2,3,7,8-TCDD and 2,3,7,8-TCDD-like chemicals. Kopf and Walker (2009) reviewed studies of the effects of 2,3,7,8-TCDD and 2,3,7,8-TCDD-like PCBs on the developing heart. These studies have shown that fish, avian and mammalian embryos exhibit cardiovascular structural changes and functional deficits, although the specific characteristics vary with species. Fish models typically exhibit reduced blood flow, altered heart looping and reduced heart size and contraction rate. The chick embryo exhibits extensive cardiac dilation, thinner ventricle walls and reduced responsiveness to chronotropic stimuli, while the mouse embryo exhibits reduced heart size. In all of the models, the 2,3,7,8-TCDD-induced cardioteratogenicity is associated with increases in cardiovascular apoptosis and decreases in cardiocyte proliferation. While the cardioteratogenicity in fish and avian species is associated with overt morbidity and mortality, this is not the case for the mouse embryo. However, murine offspring exposed during development to 2,3,7,8-TCDD exhibit cardiac hypertrophy and an increased sensitivity to a second cardiovascular insult in adulthood. Thus, although the mammalian embryo is less sensitive to cardiovascular defects induced by 2,3,7,8-TCDD and 2,3,7,8-TCDD-like compounds, developmental exposure increases the risk of cardiovascular disease later in life. The impact of developmental exposure to 2,3,7,8-TCDD-like chemicals on human cardiovascular disease susceptibility is not known. However, recent animal studies confirmed human epidemiology studies that exposure to 2,3,7,8-TCDD in adulthood is associated with hypertension and cardiovascular disease (Kopf and Walker, 2009).

Studies characterizing the developmental cardiovascular toxicity of 2,3,7,8-TCDD in mammalian species have focused on mice. Since fetal exposure to 2,3,7,8-TCDD in mice does not cause overt toxicity and mortality when exposure occurs after the fusion of the palate, studies assessing the developmental effects of 2,3,7,8-TCDD on the heart have conducted exposures on GD 14.5, a developmental window of cardiomyocyte proliferation (Kopf and Walker, 2009). Fetal heart-to-body weight ratio is decreased on GD 17.5, with a reduction in myocyte proliferation. This decreased heart-to-body weight ratio persisted with a trend in PND 7 pups. However, PND 21 pups from 2,3,7,8-TCDD-treated litters exhibited a significant increase in heart-to-body weight ratios, which was associated with an increase in atrial natriuretic factor (ANF) mRNA expression (Thackaberry *et al.*, 2005). Atrial natriuretic factor is an indicator of cardiac stress and hypertrophy (Kopf and Walker, 2009). In addition, basal heart rate is decreased in 2,3,7,8-TCDD-exposed mice on PND21 (Thackaberry *et al.*, 2005). Expression of extracellular matrix remodeling genes and cardiac hypertrophy genes were dysregulated in both fetal (GD 17.5) and adult (3 months) hearts, suggestive of cardiac remodeling that persists into adulthood. Additionally, adult mice exposed to 2,3,7,8-TCDD *in utero* had increased left ventricle weight, mild hydronephrosis in the kidney and decreased plasma volume (Aragon *et al.*, 2008).

Thyroid effects

Thyroid hormone homeostasis plays an important role in vertebrate metabolism, growth and development. Thyroid hormones are also necessary for normal brain development in the human fetus and newborn infant, since deficits in pregnant women result in neurological disorders accompanied by severe cognitive and/or mental deficits in their offspring. The thyroid system operates in basically the same way in all vertebrates including humans. The thyroid gland produces predominantly thyroxine (T4), which is transported to target tissues by the serum transport proteins, transthyretin (TTR), thyroxine-binding globulin (TBG) and albumins (Kashiwagi *et al.*, 2009).

Polychlorinated biphenyls are structurally similar to the thyroid hormones and have been documented to disrupt normal thyroid function in laboratory animals (Brouwer *et al.*, 1998). Exposure to PCBs and related compounds causes a reduction in thyroid hormones in developing and adult animals although PCBs do not seem to adversely affect thyroid stimulating hormone (TSH) activity. For example, no effects on TSH were seen when developing rats were exposed to Aroclor 1254 *in utero*, in spite of changes in plasma total and free T4 concentrations, triidothyronine (T3) concentrations and deiodinase activity (Morse *et al.*, 1996a).

The following mechanisms have been summarized by Kashiwagi *et al.* (2009) to explain how PCBs alter thyroid function. PCBs and related compounds are structurally similar to thyroid hormones and therefore bind to TTR or thyroid hormone receptors to act as either a thyroid hormone agonist or antagonist. 2,3,7,8-Tetrachlorodibenzo-*p*-dioxin-like PCBs act through the AhR. These PCBs can bind to the AhR and induce hepatic uridine diphosphate glucuronyl transferases (UDPGTs), leading to biliary excretion and elimination of T4.

Dentition effects

Dental deformities and periodontal diseases have been documented in humans exposed to PCBs and related chemicals. A case report of a 12-year-old Japanese girl with Yusho poisoning determined that her periodontal disease and alveolar bone resorption were caused by the consumption of contaminated rice bran oil at 6 years of age (Shimizu *et al.*, 1992). Wang *et al.* (2003) demonstrated a dose–response relationship between perinatal PCBs and PCDF exposure and dental defects in Yucheng children. The developmental defects were directly impacted by the maternal serum concentrations of contaminants and were apparent when total PCB concentrations were less than 10 μg/l (parts per billion or ppb). In a 14-year follow-up study of Yucheng victims, focusing on people exposed as children rather than *in utero* or via breast milk, gum pigmentation, gum swelling and broken teeth were prevalent (Guo *et al.*, 1999). Similarly, a Finnish study of children (Alaluusua *et al.*, 1999) determined that hypomineralized enamel defects of molar teeth could be the best available biomarker for 2,3,7,8-TCDD exposure, since the defects were present after low exposure through breast milk. Continued research in Finland supplied further evidence of the relationship between PCDDs and PCDFs and dental defects in children. Women living along the heavily polluted Kymijoki River, which eventually empties into the Gulf of Finland (part of the Baltic Sea), had breast milk international TEQ between 10.9 and 13.4 pg/g fat. The duration of breastfeeding was positively correlated with prevalence of dental defects in children (Holtta *et al.*, 2001). The effects of long-term exposure to PCBs on developmental dental defects were also examined in children from Slovakia demonstrating a dose–response relationship between PCB exposure and developmental enamel defects of permanent teeth in children (Jan *et al.*, 2007).

Hydronephrosis and cleft palate

The teratogenic responses induced by 2,3,7,8-TCDD-like chemicals are species and strain specific. The induction of terata is one of the most sensitive indicators of 2,3,7,8-TCDD toxicity in mice, as hydronephrosis and cleft palate are induced at doses below those resulting in either maternal or embryo/fetal toxicity (Couture *et al.*, 1990). Indices of maternal and embryo/fetal toxicity classically reported for 2,3,7,8-TCDD-exposed mice include increased maternal mortality, overt clinical signs of maternal toxicity, decreased maternal weight gain, increased maternal liver-to-body weight ratios, increased fetal mortality and decreased fetal weight (Courtney and Moore, 1971; Neubert and Dillman, 1972; Courtney, 1976). In susceptible strains of mice, such as the C57BL strain, the teratogenic response is tissue specific in that only the kidney, secondary palate and thymus show alterations. Hydronephrosis is induced in the absence of palatal clefting; thus, the urinary tract is more sensitive to 2,3,7,8-TCDD than is the secondary palate (Moore *et al.*, 1973; Birnbaum *et al.*, 1989; Couture *et al.*, 1990). In addition, while palatal sensitivity to 2,3,7,8-TCDD increases with gestational age at days 6–12 in the C57BLl 6N mouse, the urinary tract appears to be equally sensitive throughout the major period of organogenesis (Couture *et al.*, 1990).

The mechanism by which 2,3,7,8-TCDD induces hydronephrosis has been examined in C57BL/6N mice and has been found to be a consequence of increased proliferation of the ureteric epithelial cells (Abbott *et al.*, 1987). Hyperplasia of the epithelial lining of the ureter results in occlusion of the lumen and restriction of urine outflow. The end result is the development of hydroureter and hydronephrosis. The hyperplastic response induced in the ureter was found to correlate with increased ureteric epithelial expression of EGF receptors (Abbott and Birnbaum, 1990).

Cleft palate in mice has been studied extensively (Abbott and Birnbaum, 1991; Abbott *et al.*, 1992; Moriguchi *et al.*, 2003). In order to form a barrier between the oral and nasal cavities, two opposing palatal shelves normally meet and fuse. The opposing medial edges consist of an outer layer of continuously shed periderm that overlays a layer of basal cells resting on basal lamina. Before fusion, the lamina disappears, basal cells of the apposing medial seam lose epithelial characteristics, extend filopodia into the adjacent connective tissue and gain fibroblast-like features (epithelial to mesenchyme transformation). In this way a single fused tissue is formed. 2,3,7,8-Tetrachlorodibenzo-*p*-dioxin-exposed murine palatal shelves grow and make contact, but the subsequent process of epithelial-to-mesenchyme transformation does not occur. Therefore, a cleft is formed as the palatal shelves continue to grow without fusing (Bock and Kohle, 2006). Human embryonic palatal shelves are similarly affected, but at a much higher 2,3,7,8-TCDD concentration (Abbott and Birnbaum, 1991). The observation that humans are less sensitive than mice is supported by studies with AhR-transgenic "humanized" mice (Moriguchi *et al.*, 2003).

Behavioral effects

In humans as well as wildlife, laboratory along with epidemiological studies have shown that exposure to 2,3,7,8-TCDD-like compounds can impair cognitive functions, motor development as well as gender-related behavior (Schantz *et al.*, 2003). Furthermore, these studies have indicated that the behavioral effects associated with PCB exposure appear to be species independent and that the most susceptible period of exposure is during development and nursing. In children of mothers who consumed contaminated rice oil in Japan (Yusho) and Taiwan (Yucheng), developmental and cognitive dysfunctions were observed that were associated with exposure to complex mixtures of 2,3,7,8-TCDD-like chemicals including PCBs, PCDFs and polychlorinated quarterphenyls (PCQs) in the rice (Hsu *et al.*, 1985; Chen *et al.*, 1994). In some patients, exposure to these compounds resulted in several peripheral nervous system symptoms that included decreased nerve conduction velocity, numbness and weakness in limbs as well as central nervous system signs that included tiredness and respiratory disturbances (Fonnum and Mariussen, 2009). Children exposed prenatally and/or through breastfeeding to PCBs displayed clinical signs including delayed motor development, defects in short-term memory and lower scores on intelligence quotient tests (Rogan *et al.*, 1988; Tilson *et al.*, 1990). In several studies conducted in Michigan and North Carolina, there were correlations between the PCB exposure levels in mothers who consumed fish contaminated with PCBs and impairment of their children in terms of behavioral test performance and display of fine motor skills (Fein *et al.*, 1984; Jacobson and Jacobson, 1996; Stewart *et al.*, 2000). However, unlike their children, the mothers exhibited no effects of the exposure. Similar signs have been observed in children exposed to PCBs in the Faroe Islands, Germany and the Netherlands where in nearly all cases there was a negative correlation between PCB exposure and cognition in children (Schantz *et al.*, 2003). In a more recent study on 9-year-old boys, it was estimated that for each 1 ng PCB/g increase in placental tissue, full-scale IQ dropped by three points and verbal IQ dropped by four points (Stewart *et al.*, 2008; Fonnum and Mariussen, 2009). Moreover, even when the authors controlled for potential confounders such as prenatal exposure to methyl mercury, DDT and lead, this association was still statistically significant.

In humans, most studies of PCB exposure on behavior and cognitive function have focused on young children, but the effects can also be observed in adolescents and adults with adverse effects being memory impairment and decreased motor activity (Schantz and Widholm, 2001; Newman *et al.*, 2006). Animal studies have also demonstrated this phenomenon. In female rats, exposure to ortho-substituted PCB congeners (IUPAC 28, 118 or 153) during gestation and lactation resulted in spatial learning deficits but not mnemonic deficits in adulthood, indicating that the effects could be delayed or persist from an earlier exposure (Chen and Hsu, 1994; Schantz *et al.*, 1995). In a study relevant to humans, monkeys exposed to a PCB mixture (7.5 μg/kg body weight/day) from birth to 20 weeks of age had deficits on a spatial delay alteration task, and displayed perseverative behavior and the inability to inhibit inappropriate responding when tested between 2.5 and 5 years of age (Rice, 1999).

Several epidemiological studies have indicated that exposure to PCBs can contribute to hyperactivity and may contribute to the prevalence of attention deficit hyperactivity disorder (ADHD) in humans (Bowman *et al.*, 1981; Rice, 2000; Hardell *et al.*, 2002). Exposure to PCBs during brain development has been shown to increase activity levels in rats and mice indicating that PCB exposure could potentially lead to ADHD-like symptoms (Tilson and Cabe, 1979; Eriksson, 1991; Eriksson and Fredriksson, 1996, 1998; Berger *et al.*, 2001; Branchi *et al.*, 2005).

Exposure to PCBs and other 2,3,7,8-TCDD-like compounds has also been shown to alter the pubertal transition to adult in humans and animals (Sisk and Foster, 2004; Dickerson and Gore, 2007). Exposure to PCBs can result in precocious puberty, delayed puberty or no change in timing of puberty depending on the PCB congener and sex of the animal. In female rats, exposure to IUPAC 126 during embryonic development can result in a delay of the onset of female puberty while onset of puberty is unaffected in males (Faqi *et al.*, 1998; Shirota *et al.*, 2006). However, while IUPAC 126 did not affect the onset of puberty in male rats, demasculinization of the anogenital distance (AGD) was observed. In male rats, gestational exposure to Aroclor 1254 delayed the onset of puberty and early postnatal exposure did not, while in female rats, pubertal onset was delayed by both gestational and postnatal exposures (Sager and Girard, 1994). In contrast, in female rats exposed postnatally to Aroclor 1221 (1 mg/kg body weight), the onset of puberty was advanced (Gellert, 1978; Salama *et al.*, 2003). While the reason for contrasting responses in female rats exposed to the two Aroclor mixtures is unknown, it may be due to differences in PCB congener composition. Aroclor 1254 has a greater proportion of highly chlorinated, 2,3,7,8-TCDD-like congeners that have a greater affinity for the AhR, while Aroclor 1221 has a greater proportion of lower chlorinated congeners that have much lesser AhR affinities.

Exposure to PCBs during early development consistently has been shown to affect female reproductive behavior and cycles. In rats, embryonic exposure to IUPAC 47 (20 mg/kg body weight) or IUPAC 77 (0.25 mg/kg body weight) reduced adult female-typical sexual behavior that included sexual receptivity and lordosis behavior (Wang *et al.*, 2002). Similar findings were also reported for female rats treated with Aroclor 1221 or Aroclor 1254 during embryonic (Chung and Clemens, 1999) or early postnatal (Chung *et al.*, 2001) development. Moreover, prenatal exposure of adult rats to Aroclor 1221 resulted in the diminution of several sexual behavior parameters including impaired paced mating behaviors that exhibited an inverted-U or U-shaped dose–response curve that has been associated with the effects of endocrine disrupting chemicals on physiological and endocrine endpoints (Gore *et al.*, 2006; Steinberg *et al.*, 2007). In male rats, exposure to 2,3,7,8-TCDD-like compounds has also been shown to alter sexual behavior. For instance, acute gestational exposure to IUPAC 126 decreases the number of mounts with intromissions (Faqi *et al.*, 1998). Reduced adult male reproductive behavior, fertility and weight of reproductive organs have been observed in male rats exposed to Aroclor 1254 (Sager, 1983). Overall, these studies indicate that both 2,3,7,8-TCDD-like and non-2,3,7,8-TCDD-like compounds have the potential to alter behavior through a variety of modes of action.

Neurochemical effects

Laboratory studies with animals and epidemiological studies with humans have provided extensive evidence for an association between exposure to 2,3,7,8-TCDD-like chemicals and adverse effects on behavior and cognition; however, linkages of these changes to alterations in specific nervous tissue are still a significant challenge for toxicologists. In part, this difficulty is due to these compounds acting on a range of neurochemical and neuroendocrine targets that can vary in their significance depending on the exact nature of the chemical, species, gender and age. Targets that are most likely to be affected by these chemicals are neurotransmitter processes and systems including neurotransmitter transport and receptors, calcium homeostasis and oxidative stress (Fonnum and Mariussen, 2009). Additional effects further downstream of the initial interaction with neurotransmitter systems include the activation or inhibition of a variety of signal transduction enzymes including nitric oxide synthase (NOS) and protein kinase C (PKC) as well as alterations in Ca^{2+} homeostasis and synaptic plasticity (Smith *et al.*, 2002).

Numerous studies have shown that ortho-substituted PCBs can alter dopamine (DA) concentrations and turnover in the brain (Seegel, 1996; Giesy and Kannan, 1998; Mariussen and Fonnum, 2006). This PCB-related decrease in brain DA concentrations also appears to be dependent on whether an animal is exposed during development or as an adult. In adult pig-tailed macaques (*Macaca nemestrina*) exposed to Aroclor 1016 or Aroclor 1260 at doses of 0.8, 1.6 or 3.2 mg/kg body weight/day for 20 weeks, significant reductions in DA concentrations were observed in certain regions of the brain where DA synthesis occurs (Seegal, 1996; Seegal *et al.*, 2002). In contrast, offspring of rats exposed up to 25 mg/kg body weight/day of Aroclor 1016 exhibited an increase in brain DA concentrations (Seegal, 1994). In rats exposed to non-ortho PCBs at doses ranging from 1 μg/kg body weight/day to 1 mg/kg body weight/day from GD 6 through weaning, DA concentrations were elevated in the prefrontal cortex whereas rats exposed to 20 mg/kg body weight/day of ortho-substituted PCBs during the same developmental period exhibited a decrease in brain DA concentrations (Seegal *et al.*, 2002, 2005). This finding is not unique to DA in that brain concentrations of other biogenic amines such as norepinephrine and serotonin also exhibit a similar pattern in rats exposed to different PCB congeners (Chishti *et al.*, 1996; Messeri *et al.*, 1997; Lee and Opanashuk, 2004). The congener-specific effect has also been observed *in vitro*. In pheochromocytoma (PC12) cells, exposure to Aroclor 1254 reduced DA activity (Greene and Rein, 1977; Seegal *et al.*, 1989). In studies designed to characterize the relationship between the structure of individual PCB congeners and their ability to alter PC12 cellular DA content, di-ortho- through tetra-ortho-substituted congeners were the most potent, whereas non-ortho PCB congeners were ineffective (Shain *et al.*, 1991). Moreover, chlorination in a meta-position decreased the potency of ortho-substituted congeners, but meta-substitution had little effect on congeners with both ortho- and para-substitutions. These results support the hypothesis that PCB congeners predicted to have little 2,3,7,8-TCDD-like activity decreased DA concentrations in the nervous system and that neurotoxicity might be due to a mechanism independent of AhR activation.

Recently, studies have shown that PCBs can adversely affect neurotransporter systems including the inhibition of the vesicular monoamine transporter (VMAT) in synaptic vesicles and the plasma membrane DA transporter (DAT) in synaptosomes (Mariussen and Fonnum, 2001a,b; Mariussen *et al.*, 2001). The VMAT is a common transporter for biogenic amines and is an analog of the so-called multidrug transporter that can transport potential cytotoxic components out of cells (Peter *et al.*, 1995; Yelin and Shuldiner, 1995). It is suggested that the neurodegenerative effects of other VMAT inhibitors such as amphetamines are due to the redistribution of DA to the cytoplasm resulting in an outflow of vesicular DA, generation of oxidative stress and impairment of intraneuronal metabolism followed by a depletion of intracellular DA concentrations (Gainetdinov and Caron, 2003). Ortho-substituted PCBs can also inhibit plasma membrane DA transport and this reduction in DAT is correlated with reductions in DA concentrations (Gainetdinov and Caron, 2003). Another factor related to the alteration of DA concentrations is the imbalance between VMAT and DAT inhibition. Strong inhibition of brain VMAT compared to DAT can increase the susceptibility to DA-induced neurotoxicity (Miller *et al.*, 1999). Results from PCB structure–activity studies have indicated that inhibition of the plasma membrane uptake of DA is mainly due to lower chlorinated ortho-substituted PCBs while the inhibition of vesicular uptake is theoretically possible by all ortho-substituted PCBs, independent of chlorination (Mariussen and Fonnum, 2006; Maurissen and Fonnum, 2001a,b). This hypothesis is supported by the results of Seegal *et al.* (2002) where adult male rats were exposed to 25 mg Aroclor 1254/kg body weight/day and brain DA concentrations were evaluated for 8 weeks. Rat brain DA concentrations increased after 3 days of exposure followed by a sustained decrease in extracellular DA that may have been due to an acute extracellular overflow of DA due to DAT inhibition followed by a reduction in DA due to inhibition of VMAT and reduced DA synthesis. In rat synaptosomes exposed to different PCB congeners and mixtures, reductions in synaptosomal DA concentrations were thought to be due to VMAT inhibition (Bemis and Seegal, 2004). Richardson and Miller (2004) fed rats a single dose of Aroclor 1260 or Aroclor 1016 (500 mg/kg body weight) and reported that the expression of DAT was primarily reduced by Aroclor 1016 while VMAT was primarily reduced by the Aroclor 1260 mixture. PCBs and similar compounds can also alter DA concentrations in the brain by inhibiting its synthesis. It has been proposed that PCBs (greater than 50 μM) can inhibit tyrosine hydroxylase (TH), the rate-limiting enzyme involved in the catalysis of the DA precursor L-DOPA from tyrosine (Seegal *et al.*, 1991; Schwartz, 1991).

Other neurotransmitters that may be involved in PCB-induced alterations in behavior such as changes in cognitive function and hyperactivity include the cholinergic neurotransmitter system (Eriksson and Norberg, 1986; Eriksson, 1997). Findings from these studies indicated that PCB exposure resulted in increased concentrations of brain muscarinic receptors and a reduction in nicotine receptors in the hippocampus but not the cerebral cortex (Eriksson *et al.*, 1991; Eriksson and Fredriksson, 1998). Other neurotransmitter systems altered by PCB exposure include a reduction in N-methyl-D-aspartic acid (NMDA) receptor binding sites in the visual cortex of developmentally exposed rats (Altmann *et al.*, 2001). Results from other studies support the concept that PCBs can also influence the glutamatergic, GABAergic and dopaminergic systems (Myhrer, 2003). PCBs have been shown to be weak inhibitors of vesicular glutamate and GABA uptake (Mariussen *et al.*, 1999) where relatively low concentrations (less than 4 μM) of ortho-substituted PCBs (less than five chlorines) inhibited both glutamine and GABA uptake into synaptosomes while ortho-substituted PCBs containing more than five chlorines at low concentrations (5 μM) inhibit glutamate and GABA uptake by about 40% (Mariussen and Fonnum, 2001b). Thus, PCB-mediated reduction in the uptake of glutamate and GABA could possibly result in increased extracellar concentrations and lead to excitotoxicity and neurotoxic consequences.

Investigations of the effects of various PCB congeners on Ca^{2+} homeostasis and PKC translocation in cerebellar granule cells indicate a similar structure–activity relationship in that the ortho-substituted PCBs have potential to alter Ca^{2+} homeostasis in the brain, while the AhR-active congeners were reported to be inactive (Kodavanti *et al.*, 1998). Disruption of Ca^{2+} homeostatic processes by PCBs can result in various adverse effects including the production of reactive oxygen species (ROS), altered neurotransmitter release, activated phosphokinase, phosphatase, phospholipase and protease activity, enhanced apoptotic processes, alteration of other Ca^{2+}-dependent enzyme activities including NOS, and long-term potentiation (LTP) and synaptic plasticity (Mariussen and Fonnum, 2006). In general, exposure to PCBs results in an influx of extracellular Ca^{2+} from a variety of sources and routes. Routes of extracellular Ca^{2+} into cells include entry via L-type voltage-sensitive Ca^{2+} channels, release of Ca^{2+} from inositol triphosphate (IP3)-sensitive Ca^{2+} stores in the endoplasmic reticulum (ER), influx of Ca^{2+} from store-operated Ca channels and glutamate receptors channels (Inglefield *et al.*, 2001). Ryanodine receptors, which regulate Ca^{2+} release from the ER, may also be involved in PCB-altered Ca^{2+} homeostasis. Wong *et al.* (1997) reported that exposure to ortho-substituted PCBs enhanced ryanodine binding in membrane preparations from rat brain hippocampus, cerebellum and cortex and induced a ryanodine-sensitive Ca^{2+} mobilization in cortex preparations. Schantz *et al.* (1997) reported decreased ryanodine-specific binding in the hippocampus and an increase in binding in the cerebral cortex in offspring of rats exposed to IUPAC 95. Another study has also indicated an ortho-substituted PCB-mediated effect on ryanodine receptors was associated with an increase in apoptosis in rat hippocampal neurons (Howard *et al.*, 2003).

Protein kinase C has been shown to have an important role in PCB-induced toxicity (Kodavanti *et al.*, 1998). In mammals, there are at least 12 different isoforms of PKC and they influence a range of activities including modulation of neurotransmitter release, synaptic plasticity and long-term potentiation, apoptotic processes and neurological diseases (Sweatt, 1999; Way *et al.*, 2000; Battaini, 2001). Studies have shown that PCBs increase PKC translocation and affect the inositol phosphate binding and accumulation in cerebellar granule cells *in vitro* (Kodavanti *et al.*, 1994; Shafer *et al.*, 1996) and that the phenomenon is enantiomer selective (Lehmler *et al.*, 2005). While the exact mechanism for these effects is not yet known, it is believed that extracellular calcium is necessary. However, Yang and Kodavanti (2001) have shown that ortho-substituted PCBs induce translocation of the calcium-dependent isoform of PKC-α as well as the calcium-independent isoform PKC-ε. In a later study with rats exposed to 6 mg Aroclor 1254/kg body weight/day from GD 6 to PND 21, three different isoforms of PKC (-α, -ε, -γ) in subcellular fractions of brain preparations were altered (Yang *et al.*, 2003). PCBs have been suggested to inhibit brain NOS activity (Kang *et al.*, 2002; Yun *et al.*, 2005). Glutamate receptors and calcium/calmodulin have been shown to regulate NOS activity (Moncada *et al.*, 1991). NOS is involved in long-term potentiation and is implicated in oxidative injury (Sweatt, 1999). Thus, inhibition of NOS could influence the generation of LTP and therefore learning and memory deficits. In rats exposed to Aroclor 1254, extracellular dopamine concentrations in the striatum were decreased while there was an increase in the expression of phosphorylated NOS (Yun *et al.*, 2005). These effects were attenuated by prior treatment with α-tocopherol, an antioxidant with membrane stabilization properties. However, the exact nature of NOS effects on dopaminergic systems in PCB-exposed animals is still under investigation.

TREATMENT

The PBB incident in Michigan that resulted in the contamination and subsequent disposal of thousands of animals because of long biological half-lives of these compounds and millions of pounds of contaminated food products prompted investigation of ways to enhance elimination of persistent polyhalogenated aromatic hydrocarbons. Strategies reported in Fries (1985) included activated charcoal in rats and cows (Cook *et al.*, 1978; McConnell *et al.*, 1980), mineral oil in rats and monkeys (Kimbrough *et al.*, 1980; Rozman *et al.*, 1982), high fiber diets in rats (Kimbrough *et al.*, 1980), phenobarbital in cows (Cook *et al.*, 1978) and colestipol, mineral oil, propylene glycol or petroleum jelly with and without restricted feeding in chickens (Polin and Ringer, 1978a,b). In general, none of these elimination enhancement strategies proved to be effective despite the fact that they were employed for periods of 3 to 6 months (Fries, 1985). More recently, studies have been conducted that have examined different strategies to increase clearance of 2,3,7,8-TCDD from animals. Rats fed clenbuterol-supplemented feed for 10 days after exposure to 2,3,7,8-TCDD had 30% less fat than control rats and a 30% decrease in the 2,3,7,8-TCDD body burden. In other studies, rats and mice fed dietary fiber, chlorophyll or an insoluble evacuation substance (chlorophyllin-chitosan) significantly increased excretion of PCDDs and PCDFs and reduced the TEQ body burden (Huwe, 2002).

As suggested above, once animals have been contaminated with the persistent polyhalogenated aromatic hydrocarbons, there are currently no practical methods available to quickly reduce body burdens. Therefore, in a contamination incident, products are removed from the market and animals may have to be destroyed. A common strategy to reduce concentrations of contaminants in exposed animals is to provide the animal with uncontaminated feed and withhold products from the market until concentrations of the contaminant have decreased to an acceptable level. In the case of the persistent PCBs, PBBs, PCDDs, long half-lives in the animals require long withdrawal periods. Estimates of the half-lives of PCBs/PCDDs/PCDFs in milk range from 40 to 190 days. In beef cattle adipose tissue, half-lives are in the range of 100 to 200 days. The half-lives of 2,3,7,8-TCDD-like chemicals in adipose tissue and eggs of chickens range from 25 to 60 days. Depuration is the only way to reduce body burdens, but may be uneconomical in many situations because of the length of time required (Huwe, 2002).

At present, the best way to reduce concentrations of 2,3,7,8-TCDD-like chemicals in livestock is to minimize exposure. In general, the substitution of plant meals for animal and fish meals may prove to be effective in lowering intake of 2,3,7,8-TCDD-like chemicals intake in livestock and aquaculture (Huwe, 2002).

CONCLUDING REMARKS AND FUTURE DIRECTIONS

The PHAHs, which include PCBs, PBBs, PCDDs and PCDFs, are environmentally persistent, lipophilic compounds that have a tendency to bioaccumulate and biomagnify at the higher levels of the food chain. Concentrations of these chemicals have been detected in remote areas of the world and in a variety of animal species, including humans. While certain congeners and isomers can pose a very serious threat to the health of animals and humans, exposure situations are generally such that risks of health effects are generally low. The most significant problem for those involved in producing a safe food supply is contamination of food products beginning at the animal. Additionally, there are areas of the environment that are heavily contaminated by these chemicals because of past industrial activities. Animals and humans residing in or near contaminated locations certainly are at risk of serious health effects. In those situations, efforts must continue to eliminate or reduce exposure to these very persistent and toxic chemicals.

REFERENCES

Abbott BD, Birnbaum LS (1990) Effects of TCDD on embryonic ureteric epithelial EGF receptor expression and cell proliferation. *Teratology* **41:** 71–84.

Abbott BD, Birnbaum LS (1991) TCDD exposure of human palatal shelves in organ culture alters the differentiation of medial epithelial cells. *Teratology* **43:** 119–32.

Abbott BD, Birnbaum LS, Pratt RM (1987) TCDD-induced hyperplasia of the ureteral epithelium produces hydronephrosis in murine species. *Teratology* **35:** 329–34.

Abbott BD, Harris MW, Birnbaum LS (1992) Comparisons of the effects of TCDD and hydrocortisone on growth factor expression provide insight into their interaction in the embryonic mouse palate. *Teratology* **45:** 35–53.

Alaluusua S, Lukinmaa PL, Torppa J, Tuomisto J, Vartiainen T (1999) Developing teeth as biomarker of dioxin exposure. *Lancet* **353:** 206.

Allen JR, Lambrecht L (1978) Response of rhesus monkeys to polybrominated biphenyls. *Toxicol Appl Pharmacol* **45:** 340–1.

Altmann L, Mundy WR, Ward TR, Fastabend A, Lilienthal H (2001) Developmental exposure of rats to a reconstituted PCB mixture or Aroclor 1254: effects on long-term potentiation and [H-3]MK-801 binding in occipital cortex and hippocampus. *Toxicol Sci* **61:** 321–30.

Aoki Y (2001) Polychlorinated biphenyls, polychlorinated dibenzo-*p*-dioxins, and polychlorinated dibenzofurans as endocrine disrupters – what have we learned from Yusho disease. *Environ Res* **86:** 2–11.

Aragon AC, Kopf PG, Campen MJ, Huwe JK, Walker MK (2008) In utero and lactational 2,3,7,8-tetrachlorodibenzo-p-dioxin exposure: effects on fetal and adult cardiac gene expression and adult cardiac and renal morphology. *Toxicol Sci* **101:** 321–30.

Arnold DL, Bryce F, McGuire PF, Stapley R, Tanner JR, Wrenshall E, Mes J, Fernie S, Tryphonas H, Hayward S, Malcolm S (1995) Toxicological consequences of Aroclor 1254 ingestion by female rhesus (*Macaca mulatta*) monkeys. Part 2. Reproduction and infant findings. *Food Chem Toxicol* **33:** 457–74.

Aulerich RJ, Ringer RK (1979) Toxic effects of dietary polybrominated biphenyls on mink. *Arch Environ Contam Toxicol* **8:** 487–98.

Babish JG, Gutenmann WH, Stoewsand GS (1975) Polybrominated biphenyls: tissue distribution and effect on hepatic microsomal enzymes in Japanese quail. *J Agric Food Chem* **23:** 879–82.

Bansal R, You SH, Herzig CT, Zoeller RT (2005) Maternal thyroid hormone increases HES expression in the fetal rat brain: an effect mimicked by exposure to a mixture of polychlorinated biphenyls (PCBs). *Dev Brain Res* **156:** 13–22.

Battaini F (2001) Protein kinase C isoforms as therapeutic targets in nervous system disease states. *Pharmacol Res* **44:** 353–61.

Beaudoin AR (1977) Teratogenicity of polybrominated biphenyls in rats. *Environ Res* **14:** 81–6.

Bemis JC, Seegal RF (2004) PCB-induced inhibition of the vesicular monoamine transporter predicts reductions in synaptosomal dopamine content. *Toxicol Sci* **80:** 288–95.

Berger DF, Lombardo JP, Jeffers PM, Hunt AE, Bush B, Case A, Quimby F (2001) Hyperactivity and impulsiveness in rats fed diets supplemented with either Aroclor 1248 or PCB-contaminated St. Lawrence River fish. *Behav Brain Res* **126:** 1–11.

Bernard A, Broeckaert F, De Poorter G, De Cock A, Hermans C, Saegerman C, Houins G (2002) The Belgian PCB/dioxin incident: analysis of the food chain contamination and health risk evaluation. *Environ Res* **88A:** 1–18.

Birnbaum LS, Harris MW, Stocking LM, Clark AM, Morrissey RE (1989) Retinoic acid and 2,3,7,8-tetrachlorodibenzo-p-dioxin (TCDD) selectively enhance teratogenesis in C57BLi6N mice. *Toxicol Appl Pharmacol* **98:** 487–500.

Bock KW, Kohle C (2006) Ah receptor: dioxin-mediated toxic responses as hints to deregulated physiologic functions. *Biochem Pharmacol* **72:** 393–404.

Bowman RE, Heironimus MP, Barsotti DA (1981) Locomotor hyperactivity in PCB-exposed rhesus monkeys. *Neurotoxicology* **2:** 251–68.

Branchi I, Capone F, Vitalone A, Madia F, Santucci D, Alleva E, Costa LG (2005) Early developmental exposure to BDE 99 or Aroclor 1254 affects neurobehavioural profile: interference from the administration route. *Neurotoxicology* **26:** 183–92.

Brouwer A, Morse DC, Lans MC, Schuur AG, Murk AJ, Klosson-Wehler E, Bergman Å, Visser T J (1998) Interactions of persistent environmental organohalogens with the thyroid hormone system: mechanisms and possible consequences for animal and human health. *Toxicol Ind Health* **14:** 59–84.

Brown NM, Lamartiniere CA (1995) Xenoestrogens alter mammary gland differentiation and cell proliferation in the rat. *Environ Health Perspect* **103:** 708–13.

Brown NM, Manzolillo PA, Zhang JX, Wang J, Lamartiniere CA (1998) Prenatal TCDD and predisposition to mammary cancer in the rat. *Carcinogenesis* **19:** 1623–9.

Bruner-Tran KL, Osteen KG (2010) Dioxin-like PCBs and endometriosis. *Systems Biol Reprod Med* **56:** 132–46.

Buck GM, Vena JE, Schisterman EF, Dmochowski J, Mendola P, Sever LE, Fitzgerald E, Kostyniak P, Greizerstein H, Olson J (2000) Parental consumption of contaminated sport fish from Lake Ontario and predicted fecundability. *Epidemiology* **11:** 388–93.

Chao HR, Wang SL, Lin LY, Lee WJ, Papke O (2007) Placental transfer of polychlorinated-*p*-dioxins, dibenzofurans, and biphenyls in Taiwanese mothers in relation to menstrual cycle characteristics. *Food and Chem Toxicol* **45:** 259–65.

Chauhan KR, Kodavanti PR, McKinney JD (2000) Assessing the role of ortho-substitution on polychlorinated biphenyl binding to transthyretin, a thyroxine transport protein. *Toxicol Appl Pharmacol* **162:** 10–21.

Chen YC, Guo YL, Hsu CC (1992) Cognitive development of children prenatally exposed to polychlorinated biphenyls (Yu-Cheng children) and their siblings. *J Formos Med Assoc* **91:** 704–7.

Chen YC, Yu M, Rogan WJ, Gladen BC, Hsu CC (1994) A 6-year follow-up of behavior and activity disorders in the Taiwan Yu-Cheng children. *Am J Public Health* **84:** 415–21.

Chen YJ, Hsu CC (1994) Effects of prenatal exposure to PCBs on the neurological function of children: a neuropsychological and neurophysiological study. *Dev Med Child Neurol* **36:** 312–20.

Chishti MA, Fisher JP, Seegal RF (1996) Aroclors 1254 and 1260 reduce dopamine concentrations in rat striatal slices. *Neurotoxicology* **17:** 653–60.

Chung YW, Clemens LG (1999) Effects of perinatal exposure to polychlorinated biphenyls on the development on female sexual behavior. *Bull Environ Contam Toxicol* **62:** 664–70.

Chung YW, Nunez AA, Clemens LG (2001) Effects of neonatal polychlorinated biphenyl exposure on female sexual behavior. *Physiol Behav* **74:** 363–70.

Comhaire FH, Mahmoud AM, Schoonjans F (2007) Sperm quality, birth rates, and the environment in Flanders (Belgium). *Reprod Toxicol* **23:** 133–7.

Cook RM, Prewitt LR, Fries GF (1978) Effects of activated carbon, phenobarbital, and vitamins A, D, and E on polybrominated biphenyl excretion in cows. *J Dairy Sci* **61:** 414–9.

Cooke PS, Zhao YD, Hansen LG (1996) Neonatal polychlorinated biphenyl treatment increases adult testis size and sperm production in the rat. *Toxicol Appl Pharmacol* **136:** 112–7.

Corbett TH, Beaudoin AR, Cornell RG, Anver MR, Schumacher R, Endres J, Szwambowska M (1975) Toxicity of polybrominated biphenyls (Firemaster BP-6) in rodents. *Environ Res* **10:** 390–6.

Corbett TH, Simmons JL, Kawanishi H, and Endres JL (1978) EM changes and other toxic effects of FireMaster BP-6® (polybrominated biphenyls) in the mouse. *Environ Health Perspect* **23:** 275–81.

Courtney KD (1976) Mouse teratology studies with chlorodibenzo-p-dioxins. *Bull Environ Contam Toxicol* **16:** 674–81.

Courtney KD, Moore JA (1971) Teratology studies with 2,4,5-T and 2,3,7,8 TCDD. *Toxicol Appl Pharmacol* **20:** 396–403.

Couture LA, Abbott BD, Birnbaum LS (1990) A critical review of the developmental toxicity and teratogenicity of 2,3,7,8-tetrachlorodibenzo-*p*-dioxin: recent advances toward understanding the mechanism. *Teratology* **42:** 619–27.

Crews D, Willingham E, Skipper JK (2000) Endocrine disruptors: present issues, future directions. *Q Rev Biol* **75:** 243–60.

Damstra T, Jurgelski, Jr W, Posner HS, Vouk VB, Bernheim NJ, Guthrie J, Luster M, Falk HL (1982) Toxicity of polybrominated biphenyls in domestic and laboratory animals. *Environ Health Perspect* **44:** 1765–188.

De Felip E, Porpora MG, di Domenico A, Ingelido AM, Cardelli M, Cosmi EV, Donnex J (2004) Dioxin-like compounds and endometriosis: a study on Italian and Belgium women of reproductive age. *Toxicol Lett* **150:** 203–9.

Den Hond E, Roels HA, Hoppenbrouwers K, Nawrot T, Thijs L, Vandermeulen C, Winneke G, Vanderschueren D, Staessen JA (2002) Sexual maturation in relation to polychlorinated aromatic hydrocarbons: Sharpe and Skakkebaek's hypothesis revisted. *Environ Health Perspect* **110:** 771–6.

Denison MS, Heath-Pagliuso S (1998) The Ah receptor: a regulator of the biochemical and toxicological actions of structurally diverse chemicals. *Bull Environ Contam Toxicol* **61:** 557–68.

Denison MS, Nagy SR (2003) Activation of the aryl hydrocarbon receptor by structurally diverse exogenous and endogenous chemicals. *Annu Rev Pharmacol Toxicol* **43:** 309–34.

Denison MS, Pandini A, Nagy SR, Baldwin EP, Bonati L (2002) Ligand binding and activation of the Ah receptor. *Chem-Biol Interact* **141:** 3–24.

Denison MS, Vella LM, Okey AB (1986) Structure and function of the Ah receptor for 2,3,7,8-tetrachlorodibenzo-*p*-dioxin: species differences in molecular properties of the receptor from mouse and rat hepatic cytosol. *J Biol Chem* **261:** 3987–95.

Detering CN, Prewitt LR, Cook RM, Fries GF (1975) Placental transfer of polybrominated biphenyls by Holstein cows. *J Dairy Sci* **58:** 764–5.

DiCarlo FJ, Seifter J, DeCarlo VJ (1978) Assessment of the hazards of polybrominated biphenyls. *Environ Health Perspect* **23:** 351–65.

Dickerson SM, Gore AC (2007) Estrogenic environmental endocrine-disrupting chemical effects on reproductive neuroendocrine function and dysfunction across the life cycle. *Rev Endocr Metab Disord* **8:** 143–59.

Dickson LC, Buzik, SC (1993) Health risks of "dioxins": a review of environmental and toxicological considerations. *Vet Hum Toxicol* **35:** 68–77.

Donahue DA, Dougherty EJ, Meserve LA (2004) Influence of a combination of two tetrachlorobiphenyl congeners (PCB 47; PCB 77) on thyroid status, choline acetyltransferase (ChAT) activity, and short- and long-term memory in 30-day-old Sprague-Dawley rats. *Toxicology* **203:** 99–107.

Dunckel AE (1975) An updating on the polybrominated biphenyl disaster in Michigan. *J Am Vet Med Assoc* **167:** 838–41.

Eriksson P (1997) Developmental neurotoxicity of environmental agents in the neonate. *Neurotoxicology* **18:** 719–26.

Eriksson P, Fredriksson A (1996) Developmental neurotoxicity of four ortho-substituted polychlorinated biphenyls in the neonatal mouse. *Environ Toxicol Pharmacol* **1:** 155–65.

Eriksson P, Fredriksson A (1998) Neurotoxic effects in adult mice neonatally exposed to 3,3′,4,4′,5-pentachlorobiphenyl or 2,3,3′,4,4′-pentachlorobiphenyl. Changes in brain nicotinic receptors and behaviour. *Environ Toxicol Pharmacol* **5:** 17–27.

Eriksson P, Norberg A (1986) The effects of DDT, DDOH-palmitic acid and a chlorinated paraffin on muscarinic receptors and the sodium-dependent chloline uptake in the central nervous system of immature mice. *Toxicol Appl Pharmacol* **85:** 112–27.

Eriksson P, Lundkvist U, Fredriksson A (1991) Neonatal exposure to 3,3′,4,4′-tetrachlorobiphenyl: changes in spontaneous behavior and cholinergic muscarinic receptors in the adult mouse. *Toxicology* **69:** 27–34.

Eskenazi B, Mocarelli P, Warner M, Samuels S, Vercellini P, Olive D, Needham LL, Patterson DG, Brambilla P, Gavoni N, Casalini S, Panazza S, Turner W, Gerthoux PM (2002) Serum dioxin concentrations and endometriosis: a cohort study in Seveso, Italy. *Environ Health Perspect* **110:** 629–34.

Faqi AS, Dalsenter PR, Merker HJ, Chahoud I (1998) Effects on developmental landmarks and reproductive capability of 3,3′,4,4′-tetrachlorobiphenyl and 3,3′,4,4′,5-pentachlorobiphenyl in offspring of rats exposed during pregnancy. *Hum Exp Toxicol* **17:** 365–72.

Fein GG, Jacobson JL, Jacobson SW, Schwartz PM, Dowler JK (1984) Prenatal exposure to polychlorinated biphenyls – effects on birth size and gestational age. *J Pediatr* **105:** 315–20.

Fenton SE (2006) Endocrine-disrupting compounds and mammary gland development: early exposure and later life consequences. *Endocrinology* **147:** S18–S24.

Fenton SE, Hamm JT, Birnbaum LS, Youngblood GL (2002) Persistent abnormalities in the rat mammary gland following gestational and lactational exposure to 2,3,7,8-tetrachlorodibenzo-*p*-dioxin (TCDD). *Toxicol Sci* **67:** 63–74.

Fielden MR, Halgren RL, Tashiro CHM, Yeo BR, Chittim B, Chou K, Zacharewski TR (2001) Effects of gestational and lactational exposure to Aroclor 1242 on sperm quality and in vitro fertility in early adult and middle-aged mice. *Reprod Toxicol* **15:** 281–92.

Fonnum F, Mariussen E (2009) Mechanisms involved in the neurotoxic effects of environmental toxicants such as polychlorinated biphenyls and brominated flame retardants. *J Neurochem* **111:** 1327–47.

Foster WG, Maharaj-Briceno S, Cyr DG (2010) Dioxin-induced changes in epididymal sperm count and spermatogenesis. *Environ Health Perspect* **118:** 458–64.

Fries G (1995) A review of the significance of animal food products as potential pathways of human exposure to dioxins. *J Anim Sci* **73:** 1639–50.

Fries GF (1985) The PBB episode in Michigan: an overall appraisal. *Crit Rev Toxicol* **16:** 105–56.

Fries GF, Marrow GS (1975) Excretion of polybrominated biphenyls into the milk of cows. *J Dairy Sci* **58:** 947–75.

Fries GF, Cecil HC, Bitman J, Lillie RJ (1976) Retention and excretion of polybrominated biphenyls by hens. *Bull Environ Contam Toxicol* **15:** 278–82.

Gainetdinov RR, Caron MG (2003) Monoamine transporters: from genes to behavior. *Annu Rev Pharmacol Toxicol* **43:** 261–84.

Gandolfi F, Pocar P, Brevini TAL, Fischer B (2002) Impact of endocrine disrupters on ovarian function and embryonic development. *Domest Anim Endocrinol* **23:** 189–201.

Gellert RJ (1978) Uterotrophic activity of polychlorinated biphenyls (PCB) and induction of precocious reproductive aging in neonatally treated female rats. *Environ Res* **16:** 123–30.

Giesy JP, Kannan K (1998) Dioxin-like and non-dioxin-like toxic effects of polychlorinated biphenyls (PCBs): implications for risk assessment. *Crit Rev Toxicol* **28:** 511–69.

Goldey ES, Kehn LS, Lau C, Rehnberg GL, Crofton KM (1995) Developmental exposure to polychlorinated biphenyls (Aroclor 1254) reduces circulating thyroid hormone concentrations and causes hearing deficits in rats. *Toxicol Appl Pharmacol* **135:** 77–88.

Golub MS, Donald JM, Reyes, JA (1991) Reproductive toxicity of commercial PCB mixtures: LOAELs and NOAELs from animal studies. *Environ Health Perspect* **94:** 245–53.

Gore AC, Heindel JJ, Zoeller RT (2006) Endocrine disruption for endocrinologists (and others). *Endocrinology* **147:** S1–S3.

Gray LE Jr, Otsby JS (1995) In utero 2,3,7,8-tetrachlorodibenzo-*p*-dioxin (TCDD) alters reproductive morphology and function in female rat offspring. *Toxicol Appl Pharmacol* **133:** 285–94.

Gray LE Jr, Wolf C, Mann P, Otsby JS (1997) In utero exposure to low doses of 2,3,7,8-tetrachlorodibenzo-*p*-dioxin alters reproductive development of female Long Evans hooded rat offspring. *Toxicol Appl Pharmacol* **146:** 237–44.

Greene LA, Rein G (1977) Release, storage and uptake of catecholamines by a clonal cell line of nerve growth factors (NGF) responsive pheochromocytoma cells. *Brain Res* **129:** 247–56.

Guo YL, Hsu PC, Hsu CC, Lambert GH (2000) Semen quality after prenatal exposure to polychlorinated biphenyls and polychlorinated dibenzofurans. *Lancet* **356:** 1240–1.

Guo Y, Lambert GH, Hsu CC (1995) Growth abnormalities in the population exposed in utero and early postnatally to polychlorinated biphenyls and dibenzofurans. *Environ Health Perspect* **103:** 117–22.

Guo YL, Yu ML, Hsu CC, Rogan WJ (1999) Chloracne, goiter, arthritis, and anemia after polychlorinated biphenyl poisoning: 14-year follow-up of the Taiwan Yucheng cohort. *Environ Health Persp* **107:** 715–9.

Gutenmann WH, Lisk DJ (1975) Tissue storage and excretion in milk of polybrominated biphenyls in ruminants. *J Agric Food Chem* **23:** 1005–7.

Hahn ME (1998) The aryl hydrocarbon receptor: a comparative perspective. *Comp Biochem Physiol* **121C:** 23–53.

Hahn ME (2002) Aryl hydrocarbon receptors: diversity and evolution. *Chem-Biol Interact* **141:** 131–60.

Hardell L, Lindstrom G, Van Bavel B (2002) Is DDT exposure during fetal period and breast-feeding associated with neurological impairment? *Environ Res* **88:** 141–4.

Hardy ML (2000) The toxicity of the commercial polybrominated diphenyl oxide flame retardants: DBDPO, OBDPO, PeBDPO. *Organohalogen Compounds* **47:** 41–4.

Headrick ML, Hollinger K, Lovell RA, Matheson JC (1999) PBBs, PCBs, and dioxins in food animals, their public health implications. *Vet Clin North America: Food Anim Pract* **15:** 109–31.

Hesse JL, Powers RA (1978) Polybrominated biphenyl (PBB) contamination of the Pine River, Gratiot and Midland Counties, Michigan. *Environ Health Perspect* **23:** 19–25.

Holtta P, Kiviranta H, Leppaniemi A, Vartiainen T, Lukinmaa PL, Alaluusua S (2001) Developmental dental defects in children who reside by a river polluted by dioxins and furans. *Arch Environ Health* **56:** 522–8.

Howard AS, Fitzpatrick R, Pessah I, Kostyniak P, Lein PJ (2003) Polychlorinated biphenyls induce caspase-dependent cell death in cultured embryonic rat hippocampal but not cortical neurons via activation of the ryanodine receptor. *Toxicol Appl Pharmacol* **190:** 72–86.

Hsu PC, Huang W, Yao WJ, Wu MH, Guo YL, Lambert GH (2003a) Sperm changes in men exposed to polychlorinated biphenyls and dibenzofurans. *J Amer Med Assoc* **289:** 2943–4.

Hsu PC, Li MH, Guo YL (2003b) Postnatal exposure of 2,2′,3,3′,4,6′-hexachlorobiphenyl and 2,2′,3,4′,5′,6-hexachlorobiphenyl on sperm function and hormone levels in adult rats. *Toxicology* **187:** 117–26.

Hsu PC, Pan MH, Li LA, Chen CJ, Tsai SS, Guo YL (2007) Exposure in *utero* to 2,2′,3,3′,4,6′-hexachlorobiphenyl (PCB 132) impairs sperm function and alters testicular apoptosis-related gene expression in rat offspring. *Toxicol Appl Pharmacol* **221:** 68–75.

Hsu ST, Ma CI, Hsu SK, Wu SS, Hsu NH, Yeh CC, Wu SB (1985) Discovery and epidemiology of PCB poisoning in Taiwan: a four-year follow-up. *Environ Health Perspect* **59:** 5–10.

Huwe JK (2002) Dioxins in food: a modern agricultural perspective. *J Agric Food Chem* **50:** 1739–50.

Inglefield JR, Mundy WR, Shafer TJ (2001) Inositol 2,4,5-triphosphate receptor-sensitive Ca^{2+} release, store-operated Ca^{2+} entry, and cAMP responsive element binding protein phosphorylation in developing cortical cells following exposure to polychlorinated biphenyls. *J Pharmacol Exp Ther* **297:** 762–73.

International Agency for Research on Cancer (IARC) (1986) IARC monographs of the evaluation of carcinogenic risks to humans. Volume 41: Some halogenated hydrocarbons and pesticide exposures. World Health Organization, Lyon, France, 261–92.

Ishimura R, Ohsako S, Kawakami T, Sakaue M, Aoki Y, Tohyama C (2002a) Altered protein profile and possible hypoxia in the placenta of 2,3,7,8-tetrachlorodibenzo-*p*-dioxin-exposed rats. *Toxicol Appl Pharmacol* **185:** 197–206.

Ishimura R, Ohsako S, Miyabara Y, Sakaue M, Kawakami T, Aoki Y, Yonemoto J, Tohyama C (2002b) Increased glycogen content and glucose transporter 3 mRNA levels in the placenta of Holtzman rats after exposure to 2,3,7,8-tetrachlorodibenzo-*p*-dioxin. *Toxicol Appl Pharmacol* **178:** 161–71.

Jacobson JL, Jacobson SW (1996) Dose–response in perinatal exposure to polychlorinated biphenyls (PCBs): the Michigan and North Carolina cohort studies. *Toxicol Ind Health* **12:** 435–45.

Jacobson JL, Jacobson SW (1997) Evidence for PCBs as neurodevelopmental toxicants in humans. *Neurotoxicology* **18:** 415–24.

Jan JJ, Sovcikova A, Kocan L, Wsolova L, Trnovec T (2007) Developmental dental defects in children exposed to PCBs in eastern Slovakia. *Chemosphere* **67:** S350–S354.

Kang JH, Jeong W, Park Y, Lee SY, Chung MW, Lim HK, Park IS, Choi KH, Chung SY, Kim DS, Park CS, Hwang O, Kim J (2002) Aroclor 1254-induced cytotoxicity in catecholaminergic CATH.a cells related to the inhibition of NO production. *Toxicology* **177:** 157–66.

Karchner SI, Franks DG, Kennedy SW, Hahn ME (2006) The molecular basis for differential dioxin sensitivity in birds: role of the aryl hydrocarbon receptor. *Proc Natl Acad Sci USA* **103:** 6252–7.

Kashiwagi K, Furuno N, Kitamura S, Ohta S, Sugihara K, Utsumi K, Hanada H, Taniguchi K, Suzuki K, Kashiwagi A (2009) Disruption of thyroid hormone function by environmental pollutants. *J Health Sci* **55:** 147–60.

Kimbrough RD (1987) Human health effects of polychlorinated biphenyls (PCBs) and polybrominated biphenyls (PBBs). *Ann Rev Pharmacol Toxicol* **27:** 87–111.

Kimbrough RD (1995) Polychlorinated biphenyls (PCBs) and human health: an update. *Crit Rev Toxicol* **25:** 133–63.

Kimbrough RD, Korver MP, Burse VW, Groce DF (1980) The effect of different diets or mineral oil on liver pathology and polybrominated biphenyl concentration in tissues. *Toxicol Appl Pharmacol* **52:** 442–53.

Kodavanti PRS, Derr-Yellin EC, Mundy WR, Shafer TJ, Herr DW, Barone S, Choksi NY, MacPhail RC, Tilson HA (1998) Repeated exposure of adult rats to Aroclor 1254 causes brain region-specific changes in intracellular Ca^{2+} buffering and protein kinase C activity in the absence of changes in tyrosine hydroxylase. *Toxicol Appl Pharmacol* **153:** 186–98.

Kodavanti PRS, Shafer TJ, Ward TR, Mundy WR, Freudenrich T, Harry GJ, Tilson HA (1994) Differential effects of polychlorinated biphenyl congeners on phosphoinositide hydrolysis and protein kinase C translocation in rat cerebellar granule cells. *Brain Res* **662:** 75–82.

Kopf PG, Walker MK (2009) Overview of developmental heart defects by dioxins, PCBs, and pesticides. *J Environ Sci Health Part C* **27:** 276–85.

Kuriyama SN, Chahoud I (2004) In utero exposure to low dose 2,3′,4,4′,5-pentachlorobiphenyl (PCB 118) impairs male fertility and alters neurobehavior in rat offspring. *Toxicology* **202:** 185–97.

Lasky RE, Widholm JJ, Crofton KM, Schantz SL (2002) Perinatal exposure to Aroclor 1254 impairs distortion product otoacoustic emissions (DPOAEs) in rats. *Toxicol Sci* **68:** 458–64.

Lee DW, Opanashuk LA (2004) Polychlorinated biphenyl mixture Aroclor 1254-induced oxidative stress plays a role in dopaminergic cell injury. *Neurotoxicology* **25:** 925–39.

Lee KP, Herbert RR, Sherman H, Aftosmis JG, Waritz RS (1975) Bromine tissue residue and hepatotoxic effects of octabromobiphenyl in rats. *Toxicol Appl Pharmacol* **34:** 115–27.

Lehmler HJ, Robertson LW, Garrison AW, Kodavanti PRS (2005) Effects of PCB 84 enantiomers on [^{3}H]-phorbol ester binding in rat cerebellar granule cells and $^{45}Ca^{2+}$-uptake in rat cerebellum. *Toxicol Lett* **156:** 391–400.

Lindenau A, Fischer B (1996) Embryotoxicity of polychlorinated biphenyls (PCBs) for preimplantation embryos. *Reprod Toxicol* **10:** 227–30.

Mably TA, Bjerke DL, Moore RW, Gendron-Fitzpatrick A, Peterson RE (1992) In utero and lactational exposure of male rats to 2,3,7,8-tetrachlorodibenzo-*p*-dioxin. 3. Effects on spermatogenesis and reproductive capability *Toxicol Appl Pharmacol* **114:** 118–26.

Mandal PK (2005) Dioxin: a review of its environmental effects and its aryl hydrocarbon receptor biology. *J Comp Physiol B* **175:** 221–30.

Mariussen E, Fonnum F (2001a) The effect of polychlorinated biphenyls on the high affinity uptake of the neurotransmitters, dopamine, serotonin, glutamate and GABA, into rat brain synaptosomes. *Toxicology* **159:** 11–21.

Mariussen E, Fonnum F (2001b) The effects of polychlorinated biphenyls at the neurotransmitter receptor level of the brain. *Organohalogen Compounds* **53:** 190–3.

Mariussen E, Fonnum F (2006) Neurochemical targets and behavioral effects of organohalogen compounds: an update. *Crit Rev Toxicol* **36:** 253–89.

Mariussen E, Andersen JM, Fonnum F (1999) The effect of polychlorinated biphenyls on the uptake of dopamine and other neurotransmitters into rat brain synaptic vesicles. *Toxicol Appl Pharmacol* **161:** 274–82.

Mariussen E, Anderssson PL, Tysklind M, Fonnum F (2001) Effect of polychlorinated biphenyls on the uptake of dopamine into rat brain synaptic vesicles: a structure–activity study. *Toxicol Appl Pharmacol* **175:** 176–83.

Matthews HB, Fries G, Gardner A, Garthoff L, Goldstein J, Ku Y, Moore J (1978) Metabolism and biochemical toxicity of PCBs and PBBs. *Environ Health Perspect* **24:** 147–55.

Matthews HB, Kato S, Morales NM, Tuey DB (1977) Distribution and excretion of 2,4,5,2′,4′,5′-hexabromobiphenyl, the major component of Firemaster BP-6®. *J Toxicol Environ Health* **3:** 599–605.

Mayani A, Barel S, Soback S, Almagor M (1997) Dioxin concentrations in women with endometriosis. *Hum Reprod* **12:** 373–5.

McConnell EE (1985) Comparative toxicity of PCBs and related compounds in various species of animals. *Environ Health Perspect* **60:** 29–33.

McConnell EE, Harris MW, Moore JA (1980) Studies on the use of activated charcoal and cholestyramine for reducing the body burden of polybrominated biphenyls. *Drug Chem Toxicol* **3:** 277–92.

Meerts IA, Hoving S, van den Berg JH, Weijers BM, Swarts HJ, van der Beek EM, Bergman A, Koeman JH, Brouwer A (2004) Effects of in utero exposure to 4-hydroxy-2,3,3′,4′,5-pentachlorobiphenyl (4-OH-CB107) on developmental landmarks, steroid hormone levels, and female estrous cyclicity in rats. *Toxicol Sci* **82:** 259–67.

Mendola P, Buck GM, Sever LE, Zielezny M, Vena JE (1997) Consumption of PCB-contaminated freshwater fish and shortened menstrual cycle length. *Am J Epidemiol* **146:** 955–60.

Messeri MD, Bickmeyer U., Weinsberg F, Wiegand H (1997) Congener specific effects by polychlorinated biphenyls on catecholamine content and release in chromaffin cells. *Arch Toxicol* **71:** 416–21.

Miceli JN, Marks BH (1981) Tissue distribution and elimination kinetics of polybrominated biphenyls (PBB) from rat tissue. *Toxicol Lett* **9:** 315–20.

Miller GW, Gainetdinov RR, Levy AI, Caron MG (1999) Dopamine transporters and neuronal injury. *Trends Pharmacol Sci* **20:** 424–9.

Miller KP, Borgeest C, Greenfeld C, Tomic D, Flaws JA (2004) In utero effects of chemicals on reproductive tissues in females. *Toxicol Appl Pharmacol* **198:** 111–31.

Mocarelli P, Gerthoux PM, Patterson DG, Milani S, Limonta G, Bertona M, Signorini S, Tramacere P, Colombo L, Crespi C, Brambilla P, Sarto C, Carreri V, Sampson EJ, Turner WE, Needham LL (2008) Dietary exposure, from infancy through puberty, produces endocrine disruption and affects human semen quality. *Environ Health Perspect* **116:** 70–7.

Moncada S, Palmer RM, Higgs EA (1991) Nitric oxide: physiology, pathophysiology, and pharmacology. *Pharmacol Rev* **43:** 109–42.

Moore JA, Gupta BN, Zinkl JG, Vos JG (1973) Postnatal effects of maternal exposure to 2,3,7,8-tetrachlorodibenzo-p-dioxin (TCDD). *Environ Health Perspect* **5:** 81–5.

Moriguchi T, Motohashi H, Hosaya T, Nakajima O, Takahashi S, Ohsako S, Aoki Y, Nishimura N, Tohyama C, Fujii-Kurlyama Y, Yamamoto M (2003) Distinct responses to dioxin in an aryl hydrocarbon receptor (AhR)-humanized mouse. *Proc Natl Acad Sci USA* **100:** 5652–7.

Morse DC, Seegal RF, Borsch KO, Brouwer A (1996b) Long-term alterations in regional brain serotonin metabolism following maternal polychlorinated biphenyl exposure in the rat. *Neurotoxicology* **17:** 631–8.

Morse DC, Wehler EK, Wesseling W, Koeman JH, Brouwer A (1996a) Alterations in rat brain thyroid hormone status following pre- and postnatal exposure to polychlorinated biphenyls (Aroclor 1254). *Toxicol Appl Pharmacol* **136:** 269–79.

Muto T, Wakui S, Imano N, Nakaaki K, Takahashi H, Hano H, Furusato M, Masaoka T (2002) Mammary gland differentiation in female rats after prenatal exposure to 3,3′,4,4′,5-pentachlorobiphenyl. *Toxicology* **177:** 197–205.

Myhrer T (2003) Neurotransmitter systems involved in learning and memory in the rat: a meta-analysis based on studies of four behavioral tasks. *Brain Res* **41:** 268–87.

Neubert D, Dillman I (1972) Embryotoxic effects in mice treated with 2,4,5-trichlorophenoxyacetic acid and 2,3,7,8-tetrachlorodibenzo-p-dioxin. *Arch Pharmacol* **272:** 243–64.

Newman J, Aucompaugh AG, Schell LM, Denham M, DeCaprio AP, Gallo MV, Ravenscroft J, Kao CC, Hanover MR, David D, Jacobs AM, Tarbell AM, Worswick P (2006) PCBs and cognitive functioning of Mohawk adolescents. *Neurotox Teratology* **28:** 439–45.

Norris JM, Kociba RJ, Schwetz BA, Rose JQ, Humiston CG, Jewett GL, Gehring PJ, Mailhes JB (1975) Toxicology of octabromobiphenyl and decabromobiphenyl oxide. *Environ Health Perspect* **11:** 153–61.

Okey AB, Riddick DS, Harper PA (1994) The Ah receptor: mediator of the toxicity of 2,3,7,8-tetrachlorodibenzo-*p*-dioxin (TCDD) and related compounds. *Toxicol Lett* **70:** 1–22.

Oskam IC, Lyche JL, Krogenates A, Thomassen R, Skaare JU, Wiger R, Dahl E, Sweeney T, Stien A, Ropstad E (2005) Effects of long-term maternal exposure to low doses of PCB 126 and PCB 153 on the reproductive system and related hormones of young male goats. *Reproduction* **130:** 731–42.

Pauwels A, Schepens PJC, D'Hooghe T, Delbeke L, Dhont M, Brouwer A, Weyler J (2001) The risk of endometriosis and exposure to dioxins and polychlorinated biphenyls: a case–control study of infertile women. *Hum Reprod* **16:** 2050–5.

Peter D, Liu YJ, Sternini C, Degiorgio R, Brecha N, Edwards RH (1995) Differential expression of 2 vesicular monoamine transporters. *J Neurosci* **15:** 6179–88.

Peterson RE, Theobald HM, Kimmel GL (1993) Developmental and reproductive toxicity of dioxins and related compounds: cross-species comparisons. *Crit Rev Toxicol* **23:** 283–335.

Pflieger-Bruss S, Schill WB (2000) Effects of chlorinated hydrocarbons on sperm function in vitro. *Andrologia* **32:** 311–5.

Pflieger-Bruss S, Schuppe HC, Schill WB (2004) The male reproductive system and its susceptibility to endocrine disrupting chemicals. *Andrologia* **36:** 337–45.

Pohjanvirta R, Tuomisto J (1994) Short-term toxicity of 2,3,7,8-tetrachlorodibenzo-*p*-dioxin in laboratory animals: effects, mechanisms, and animal models. *Pharmacol Rev* **46:** 483–549.

Poland A, Knutson JC (1982) 2,3,7,8-Tetrachlorodibenzo-*p*-dioxin and related halogenated aromatic hydrocarbons: examination of the mechanism of toxicity. *Ann Rev Pharmacol Toxicol* **22:** 517–54.

Polin D, Ringer RK (1978a) PBB fed to adult female chickens: its effect on egg production, viability of offspring, and residues in tissues and eggs. *Environ Health Perspect* **23:** 283–90.

Polin D, Ringer RK (1978b) Polybrominated biphenyls in chicken eggs vs. hatchability. *Proc Soc Exp Biol Med* **159:** 131–5.

Porterfield SP (1994) Vulnerability of the developing brain to thyroid abnormalities: environmental insults to the thyroid system. *Environ Health Perspect* **102:** 125–30.

Preache MM, Cagan SJ, Gibson JE (1976) Perinatal toxicity in mice following dietary exposure to polybrominated biphenyls. *Toxicol Appl Pharmacol* **37:** 171.

Provost TL, Juarez de Ku LM, Zender C, Meserve LA (1999) Dose- and age-dependent alterations in choline acetyltransferase (ChAT) activity, learning and memory, and thyroid hormones in 15- and 30-day old rats exposed to 1.25 or 12.5 ppm polychlorinated biphenyl (PCB) beginning at conception. *Prog Neuropsychopharmacol Biol Psychiatry* **23:** 915–28.

Rice DC (1999) Behavioral impairment produced by low-level postnatal PCB exposure in monkeys. *Environ Res* **80:** S113–S121.

Rice DC (2000) Parallels between attention deficit hyperactivity disorder and behavioral deficits produced by neurotoxic exposure in monkeys. *Environ Health Perspect* **108:** 405–8.

Richardson JR, Miller GE (2004) Acute exposure to Aroclor 1016 or 1260 differentially affects dopamine transporter and vesicular monoamine transporter 2 levels. *Toxicol Lett* **148:** 29–40.

Rier SE, Martin DC, Bowman RE, Dmowski WP, Becker JL (1993) Endometriosis in rhesus monkeys (*Macaca mulatta*) following chronic exposure to 2,3,7,8-tetrachlorodibenzo-*p*-dioxin. *Fundam Appl Toxicol* **21:** 433–41.

Ringer RK, Polin D (1977) The biological effects of polybrominated biphenyls in avian species. *Fed Proc* **36:** 1894–8.

Roegge CS, Wang VC, Powers BE, Klintsova AY, Villareal S, Greenough WT, Schantz SL (2004) Motor impairment in rats exposed to PCBs and methylmercury during early development. *Toxicol Sci* **77:** 315–24.

Rogan WJ, Gladen BC, Hung KL, Koong SL, Shih LY, Taylor JS, Wu YC, Yang D, Ragan NB, Hsu CC (1988) Congenital poisoning by polychlorinated biphenyls and their contaminants in Taiwan. *Science* **241:** 334–6.

Ronnback C (1991) Effects of 3,3′4,4′-tetrachlorobiphenyl on ovaries of foetal mice. *Pharmacol Toxicol* **68:** 340–5.

Rozman KK, Rozman TA, Williams J, Greim HA (1982) Effects of mineral oil and/or cholestryamine in the diet on biliary and intestinal elimination of 2,2′,4,4′,5,5′-hexachlorobiphenyl in the rhesus monkey. *J Toxicol Environ Health* **9:** 611–8.

Safe S (1986) Comparative toxicology and mechanism of action of polychlorinated dibenzo-*p*-dioxins and dibenzofurans. *Annu Rev Pharmacol Toxicol* **26:** 371–99.

Safe S (1990) Polychlorinated biphenyls (PCBs), dibenzo-p-dioxins (PCDDs), dibenzofurans (PCDFs), and related compounds: environmental and mechanistic considerations which support the development of toxic equivalency factors (TEFs). *Crit Rev Toxicol* **21:** 51–88.

Safe S (1994) Polychlorinated biphenyls (PCBs): environmental impact, biochemical and toxic responses, and implications for risk assessment. *Crit Rev Toxicol* **24:** 87–149.

Safe S (1998) Development validation and problems with the toxic equivalency factor approach for risk assessment of dioxins and related compounds. *J Anim Sci* **76:** 134–41.

Sager D, Girard D, Nelson D (1991) Early postnatal exposure to PCBs: sperm function in rats. *Environ Toxicol Chem* **10:** 717–46.

Sager DB (1983) Effect of postnatal exposure to polychlorinated biphenyls on adult male reproductive function. *Environ Res* **31:** 76–94.

Sager DB, Girard DM (1994) Long-term effects on reproductive parameters in female rats after translactational exposure to PCBs. *Environ Res* **66:** 52–76.

Sager DB, Shih-Schroeder W, Girard D (1987) Effect of early postnatal exposure to polychlorinated biphenyls (PCBs) on fertility in male rats. *Bull Environ Contam Toxicol* **38:** 946–53.

Salama J, Chakraborty TR, Ng L, Gore AC (2003) Effects of polychlorinated biphenyls on estrogen receptor-beta expression in the anteroventral periventricular nucleus. *Environ Health Perspect* **111:** 1278–82.

Salisbury TB, Marcinkiewicz JL (2002) In utero and lactational exposure to 2,3,7,8-tetrachlorodibenzo-*p*-dioxin and 2,3,4,7,8-pentachlorodibenzofuran reduces growth and disrupts reproductive parameters in female rats. *Biol Reprod* **66:** 1621–6.

Schantz SL, Moshtaghian J, Ness DK (1995) Spatial learning deficits in adult rats exposed to ortho-substituted PCB congeners during gestation and lactation. *Fundam Appl Toxicol* **26:** 117–26.

Schantz SL, Seo BW, Wong PW, Pessah IN (1997) Long-term effects on developmental exposure to 2,2,3,5,6-pentachlorobiphenyl (PCB95) on locomotor activity, spatial learning and memory and brain ryanodine binding. *Neurotoxicology* **18:** 457–67.

Schantz SL, Widhom JJ (2001) Cognitive effects of endocrine-disrupting chemicals in animals. *Environ Health Perspect* **109:** 1197–206.

Schantz SL, Widholm JJ, Rice DC (2003) Effects of PCB exposure on neuropsychological function in children. *Environ Health Perspect* **111:** 357–76.

Schecter A, Birnbaum L, Ryan JJ, Constable JD (2006) Dioxins: an overview. *Environ Res* **101:** 419–28.

Schwartz JH (1991) Chemical messengers: small molecules and peptides. In *Principles of Neural Sciences* (Kandell ER, Schwartz JH, Jessel TM, eds.). Appleton and Lange, East Norwalk, Connecticut, pp. 213–24.

Seegal RF (1994) The neurochemical effects of PCB exposure are age-dependent. *Arch Toxicol* **16:** 128–37.

Seegal RF (1996) Epidemiological and laboratory evidence of PCB-induced neurotoxicity. *Crit Rev Toxicol* **26:** 709–37.

Seegal RF, Brosch KO, Bush B, Ritz M, Shain W (1989) Effects of Aroclor 1254 on dopamine and norepinephrine concentrations in pheochromocytoma (PC-12) cells. *Neurotoxicology* **10:** 757–68.

Seegal RF, Brosch KO, Okoniewski RJ (2005) Coplanar PCB congeners increase uterine weight and frontal cortical dopamine in the developing rat: implications for developmental neurotoxicity. *Toxicol Sci* **86:** 125–31.

Seegal RF, Bush B, Shain W (1991) Neurotoxicology of ortho-substituted polychlorinated byphenyls. *Chemosphere* **23:** 1941–9.

Seegal RF, Okoniewski RJ, Brosch KO, Bemis JC (2002) Polychlorinated biphenyls alter extraneuronal but not tissue dopamine concentrations in adult rat striatum: an in vivo microdialysis study. *Environ Health Perspect* **110:** 1113–7.

Seiler P, Fischer B, Lindenau A, Beier HM (1994) Effects of persistent chlorinated hydrocarbons on fertility and embryonic development in the rabbit. *Hum Reprod* **9:** 1920–6.

Shafer TJ, Mundy, WR, Tilson HA, Kodavanti PRS (1996) Disruption of inositol phosphate accumulation in cerebellular granule cells by polychlorinated biphenyls: a consequence of altered Ca^{2+} homeostasis. *Toxicol Appl Pharmacol* **141:** 448–55.

Shain W, Bush B, Seegal R (1991) Neurotoxicology of ortho-substituted polychlorinated biphenyls: structure–activity relationships of individual congeners. *Toxicol Appl Pharmacol* **111:** 33–45.

Shimizu K, Nakata S, Murakami T, Tamari K, Takahama Y, Akamine A, Aono M (1992) Long-term occlusal guidance of a severely intoxicated patient with *yusho* (PCB poisoning): a case report. *Am J Orthodon Dentofac* **101:** 393–402.

Shirota M, Mukai M, Sakurada Y, Doyama A, Inoue K, Haishima A, Akohori F, Shirota K (2006) Effects of vertically transferred 3,3′,4,4′,5-pentachlorobiphenyl (PCB126) on the reproductive development of female rats. *J Reprod Dev* **52:** 751–61.

Sisk CL, Foster DL (2004) The neural basis of puberty and adolescence. *Nat Neurosci* **7:** 1040–7.

Smith JW, Evans AT, Costallm B, Smythe JW (2002) Thyroid hormones, brain function and cognition: a brief review. *Neurosci Biobehav Rev* **26:** 45–60.

Steinberg RM., Juenger TE, Gore AC (2007) The effects of prenatal PCBs on adult female paced mating reproductive behaviors in rats. *Horm Behav* **51:** 364–72.

Steinberg RM, Walker DM, Juenger TE, Woller MJ, Gore AC (2008) Effects of perinatal polychlorinated biphenyls on adult female rat reproduction: development, reproductive physiology, and second generational effects. *Biol Reprod* **78:** 1091–101.

Stewart P, Pagano J, Sargent D, Darvill T, Lonky E, Reihman J (2000) Effects of Great Lakes fish consumption on brain PCB pattern, concentration, and progressive-ratio performance. *Environ Res* **82:** 18–32.

Stewart PW, Lonky E, Reiman J, Pagano J, Gump BB, Darvill T (2008) The relationship between prenatal PCB exposure and intelligence (IQ) in 9 year old children. *Environ Health Perspect* **116:** 1416–22.

Sweatt JD (1999) Toward a molecular explanation for long term potentiation. *Learn Mem* **6:** 399–416.

Tanabe S (1988) PCB problems in the future: foresight from current knowledge. *Environ Pollut* **50:** 5–28.

Thackaberry EA, Nunez BA, Ivnitski-Steele ID, Friggins M, Walker MK (2005) Effect of 2,3,7,8-tetrachlorodibenzo-p-dioxin on murine heart development: alteration in fetal and postnatal cardiac growth, and postnatal cardiac chronotropy. *Toxicol Sci* **88:** 242–9.

Tilson HA, Cabe PA (1979) Studies on the neurobehavioral effects of polychlorinated biphenyls in rats. *Ann NY Acad Sci* **320:** 325–36.

Tilson HA, Jacobson JL, Rogan WJ (1990) Polychlorinated biphenyls and the developing nervous-system. Cross-species comparisons. *Neurotoxicol Teratol* **12:** 239–48.

Van den Berg M, Birnbaum L, Bosveld AT, Brunstrom B, Cook P, Feeley M, Giesy JP, Hanberg A, Hasegawa R, Kennedy SW, Kubiak T, Larsen JC, van Leeuwen FX, Liem AK, Nolt C, Peterson RE, Poellinger L, Safe S, Schrenk D, Tillitt D, Tysklind M, Younes M, Woern F, Zacharewski T (1998) Toxic equivalency factors (TEFs) for PCBs, PCDDs, PCDFs for humans and wildlife. *Environ Health Perspect* **106:** 775–92.

Van den Berg M, Birnbaum LS, Denison M, DeVito M, Farland W, Feeley M, Fiedler H, Hakansson H, Hanberg A, Haws L, Rose M, Safe S, Schrenk D, Tohyama C, Tritscher A, Tuomisto J, Tysklind M, Walker N, Peterson RE (2006) The 2005 World Health Organization re-evaluation of human and mammalian toxic equivalency factors for dioxins and dioxin-like compounds. *Toxicol Sci* **93:** 223–41.

Van den Berg M, De Jongh J, Poiger H, Olson JR (1994) The toxicokinetics and metabolism of polychlorinated dibenzo-*p*-dioxins (PCDDs) and dibenzofuran (PCDFs) and their relevance for toxicity. *Crit Rev Toxicol* **24:** 1–74.

Van Larebeke N, Hens L, Schepens P, Covaci A, Baeyens J, Everaert K, Bernheim JL (2001) The Belgian PCB and dioxin incident of January–June 1999: exposure data and potential impact on health. *Environ Health Perspect* **109:** 265–73.

Van Waeleghem K, De Clercq N, Vermeulen L, Schoonjans F, Comhaire F (1996) Deterioration of sperm quality in young healthy Belgium men. *Hum Reprod* **11:** 325–9.

Vorderstrasse BA, Fenton SE, Bohn AA, Cundiff JA, Lawrence BP (2004) A novel effect of dioxin: exposure during pregnancy severely impairs mammary gland differentiation. *Toxicol Sci* **78:** 248–57.

Wang SL, Chen TT, Hsu JF, Hsu CC, Chang LW, Ryan JJ, Guo YLL, Lambert GH (2003) Neonatal and childhood teeth in relation to perinatal exposure to polychlorinated biphenyls and dibenzofurans: observations of the Yucheng children in Taiwan. *Environ Res* **93:** 131–7.

Wang XQ, Fang J, Nunez AA, Clemens LG (2002) Developmental exposure to polychlorinated biphenyls affects behavior of rats. *Physiol Behav* **75:** 689–96.

Way KJ, Chou E, King GL (2000) Indentification of PKC-isoform-specific biological actions using pharmacological approaches. *Trends Pharmacol Sci* **21:** 181–7.

Werner PR, Sleight SD (1981) Toxicosis in sows and their pigs caused by feeding rations containing polybromonated biphenyls to sows during pregnancy and lactation. *Amer J Vet Res* **42:** 183–9.

White SS, Birnbaum LS (2009) An overview of the effects of dioxins and dioxin-like compounds on vertebrates, as documented in human and ecological epidemiology. *J Environ Sci Health Part C* **27:** 197–211.

Whyte JJ, Schmitt CJ, Tillitt DE (2004) The H4IIE cell bioassay as an indicator of dioxin-like chemicals in wildlife and the environment. *Crit Rev Toxicol* **34:** 1–83.

Willett LB, Durst HI (1978) Effects of PBBs on cattle. IV. Distribution and clearance of components of FireMaster BP-6®. *Environ Health Perspect* **23:** 67–74.

Willett LB, Irving HA (1976) Distribution and clearance of polybrominated biphenyls in cows and calves. *J Dairy Sci* **59:** 1429–39.

Wolf CJ, Otsby JS, Gray LE Jr (1999) Gestational exposure to 2,3,7,8-tetrachlorodibenzo-*p*-dioxin (TCDD) severely alters reproductive function of female hamster offspring. *Toxicol Sci* **51:** 259–64.

Wong PW, Brackney WR, Pessah IN (1997) Ortho-substituted polychlorinated biphenyls alter microsomal calcium transport by direct interaction with ryanodine receptors of mammalian brain. *J Biol Chem* **272:** 15145–53.

Yang CH, Wang YJ, Chen PC, Tsai SJ, Guo YL (2008) Exposure to a mixture of polychlorinated biphenyls and polychlorinated dibenzofurans resulted in a prolonged time to pregnancy in women. *Environ Health Perspect* **116:** 599–604.

Yang CY, Yu ML, Guo HR, Lai TJ, Hsu CC, Lambert G, Guo YL (2005) The endocrine and reproductive function of the female Yucheng adolescents prenatally exposed to PCBs/PCDFs. *Chemosphere* **61:** 355–60.

Yang JH, Kodavanti PRS (2001) Possible molecular targets of halogenated aromatic hydrocarbons in neuronal cells. *Biochem Biophys Res Commun* **280:** 1372–7.

Yang JH, Derr-Yellin EC, Kodavanti PRS (2003) Alterations in brain protein kinase C isoforms following developmental exposure to polychlorinated biphenyl mixture. *Mol Brain Res* **111:** 123–35.

Yelin R, Shuldiner S (1995) The pharmacological profile of the vesicular monoamine transporter resembles that of multidrug transporters. *FEBS Lett* **377:** 201–7.

Yu ML, Guo YLL, Hsu CC, Rogan WJ (2000) Menstruation and reproduction in women with polychlorinated biphenyl (PCB) poisoning: long-term follow-up interviews of the women from the Taiwan Yucheng cohort. *Int J Epidemiol* **29:** 672–7.

Yun JS, Na HK, Park KS, Lee YH, Kim EY, Lee SY, Kim JI, Kang JH, Kim DS, Choi KH (2005) Protective effects of vitamin E on endocrine disruptors, PCB-induced dopaminergic neurotoxicity. *Toxicology* **216:** 140–6.

C H A P T E R

42

Developmental dioxin exposure and endometriosis

Tultul Nayyar, Kaylon L. Bruner-Tran and Kevin G. Osteen

INTRODUCTION

Humans are exposed to an astonishing array of natural and synthetic chemicals that have the potential to negatively affect our overall health. Importantly, many toxicants are persistent, with long half-lives; thus these agents accumulate within our bodies and have the capacity to be transferred to the developing fetus during pregnancy. Indeed, a recent analysis of human umbilical cord blood by the Environmental Working Group revealed the presence of 287 different chemicals (EWG, 2005) and although not every child was exposed to all toxicants analyzed, no child was without some exposure. While it is difficult to accurately ascertain the combinatorial effects of these numerous chemicals, developmental exposure to various individual toxicants has been clearly linked to alterations in adult reproductive tract function (Anway and Skinner, 2006, 2008; Heindel, 2006; Skinner, 2007; Bruner-Tran and Osteen, in press).

Among multiple environmental toxicants of human health concern, TCDD (2,3,7,8-tetrachlorodibenzo-*p*-dioxin or commonly, dioxin (throughout this chapter "TCDD" refers to the specific dioxin 2,3,7,8-tetrachlorodibenzo-*p*-dioxin; while the term "dioxin" will refer to the family of toxicants to which TCDD belongs), is a ubiquitous chemical and known endocrine disruptor. While TCDD is noted to be perhaps the most highly toxic contaminant ever manufactured (Jacobson-Dickman and Lee, 2009), other toxicants can exhibit similar dioxin-like biological activity and likely work collectively to disrupt reproductive tract function. As with most environmental toxicants, humans and other animals are particularly sensitive to TCDD exposure during the time of development (Birnbaum, 1994). However, since prospective developmental toxicology studies cannot be conducted in humans, it is necessary to utilize appropriate animal models to ascertain the potential risk of early life exposure to the development of adult disease. Within our group, we were interested in examining the impact of developmental TCDD exposure on physiologic processes which might impact adult risk of endometriosis.

Endometriosis, characterized as the growth of endometrial tissue outside the uterus, is a persistent, estrogen-dependent gynecological disorder frequently associated with pain and infertility. It is a common condition, estimated to affect 10–15% of all reproductive age women and up to 40% of infertile women in the USA (Giudice and Kao, 2004). Transfer of endometrial tissue to the peritoneal cavity via retrograde menstruation is considered the primary *mechanical* risk factor for development of endometriosis; however, since most menstruating women experience some degree of retrograde menstruation additional factors must contribute to determining whether or not an individual will actually develop this disease (Sampson, 1927; Bulun, 2009). For example, under normal circumstances, cells within refluxed menstrual tissue are terminally differentiated and apoptotic; thus these cells are rapidly cleared by the innate immune system. In women with endometriosis, it is suspected that cells within the menses are not apoptotic; furthermore, these cells are capable of evading immune detection, perhaps due to alterations in immune surveillance within the peritoneal cavity (Dmowski and Braun, 2004). In addition to immunological alterations, women with endometriosis have been found to exhibit endocrine system alterations which also likely contribute to the development of endometriosis. More recently, a potential role for exposure to endocrine disrupting environmental toxicants such as TCDD has emerged as an additional factor which may contribute to the incidence of endometriosis since this toxicant is capable of disrupting the normal regulation of both the endocrine and immune systems (Gregoraszczuk *et al.*, 2001; Bruner-Tran *et al.*, 2010).

Numerous epidemiologic studies have attempted to link a woman's adult body burden of TCDD and/or similar toxicants to the diagnosis of endometriosis; however, as will be discussed below, no clear consensus has emerged. Thus, defining the precise role(s) that environmental TCDD exposure plays in this or any other disease within a human population will require a better understanding of how this toxicant disrupts specific biological processes. Furthermore, since humans and other animals are most sensitive to endocrine disrupting toxicants during development, animal models allowing for experimental, early life exposure to TCDD, in addition to adult human exposure studies, will be necessary to fully understand the role of environmental toxicants in the

Reproductive and Developmental Toxicology, Edited by Ramesh C. Gupta
ISBN: 978-0-12-382032-7

natural history of endometriosis. To this end, it is important to note that several recent animal studies have suggested that developmental exposure to environmental toxicants may not only negatively affect an individual's reproductive health but also impact the reproductive capacity of future generations (Guerrero-Bosagna and Skinner, 2009 for review; Bruner-Tran and Osteen, in press). In this chapter, we will discuss some of the potential mechanisms by which TCDD may promote the development of endometriosis, including a discussion on accumulating data derived from animal studies suggesting that the development of endometriosis may reflect the consequences of an early life exposure to environmental toxicants with dioxin-like activity.

TOXICOKINETICS AND RISK ASSESSMENT

The dioxin family of environmental contaminants includes polychlorinated dibenzodioxins (PCDDs) (Rier and Foster, 2002), polychlorinated dibenzofurans (PCDFs) and co-planar and mono-ortho-substituted polychlorinated biphenyls (PCBs) which are structurally similar to PCDDs and PCDFs (Van den Berg *et al.*, 1994; Safe, 1994). Among the numerous environmental toxicants which comprise the dioxin family, TCDD (Figure 42.1) is considered the most toxic, and has been shown to be a prototypical disruptor of steroid receptor levels as well as steroid metabolism and serum transport (Heimler *et al.*, 1998; Morán *et al.*, 2003; Pocar *et al.*, 2005). The biological effects of TCDD in responsive cells are mediated through high affinity binding to the arylhydrocarbon receptor (AhR), an orphan nuclear receptor, which subsequently forms an activated heterodimer complex with a structurally related nuclear transport protein (ARNT; Whitlock *et al.*, 1999). This activated complex can bind to specific DNA enhancer sequences known as dioxin response elements (DREs) in order to affect the expression of specific genes (Whitlock *et al.*, 1997; Schrenk, 1998). Dioxin-like PCBs, also known as the co-planar PCBs, bind the AhR and thus are capable of producing dioxin-like effects including altering endocrine status in humans (Koopman-Esseboom *et al.*, 1994; Aoki, 2001). However, little data exist regarding human exposure to dioxin-like PCBs and the development of endometriosis (for review, see Anger and Foster, 2008; Bruner-Tran and Osteen, 2010), thus these agents will not be discussed in detail.

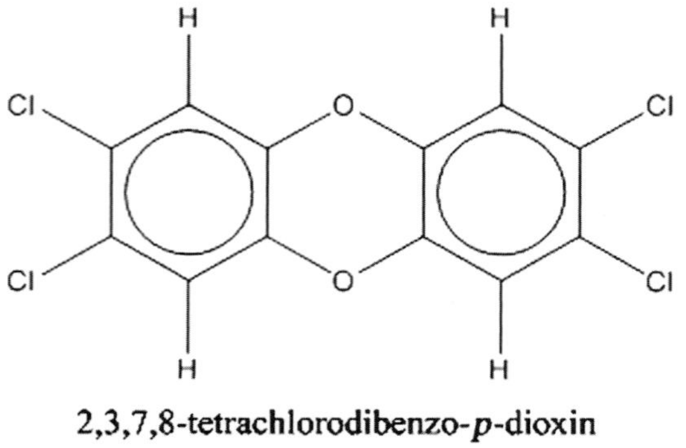

FIGURE 42.1 Chemical structure of 2,3,7,8-tetrachlorodibenzo-*p*-dioxin.

Although TCDD was introduced to our environment largely as an unwanted by-product of manufacturing processes and incineration (Zook and Rappe, 1994), PCBs with dioxin-like activity have widespread commercial application and were heavily manufactured until being prohibited in the USA in 1979; a worldwide ban followed a few years later. These organochlorides are extremely resistant to degradation and, due to their lipophilic nature, bioaccumulate and biomagnify within the food chain (Birnbaum, 1994). Although environmental contamination with these toxicants appears to be declining, their resistance to environmental and biologic degradation results in a significant degree of bioaccumulation. Furthermore, once formed, TCDD disperses throughout the atmosphere, soil and water, affecting populations distant from the original point of production, although the level of exposure and contamination varies between countries (Bruner-Tran *et al.*, 2010 for review). Among human and animal populations, ingestion of contaminated food is the primary source of dioxin and PCB exposure (Schecter *et al.*, 2002; Harrad *et al.*, 2003; Pompa *et al.*, 2003), and thus, consumption of contaminated food over a lifetime would likely lead to very high body burdens of these toxicants (Van der Molen *et al.*, 1996) since the lipophilic nature of dioxins limits their excretion in urine and promotes accumulation in adipose tissues (Domingo and Boccio, 2007).

Accurately linking an external toxicant exposure to the internal dosimetry that may be associated with the observed effects requires determination of internal effective concentrations, i.e., the concentration within the target tissues where toxic effects arise (Safe, 1990). Internal dosimetry depends on the toxicokinetics of the substance that are governed by its absorption, distribution, metabolism and excretion (ADME). Further complicating the ability to accurately assess the impact of an *individual* toxicant exposure to any disease or outcome is the fact that humans are exposed to *mixtures* of synthetic and natural toxicants. Therefore, the World Health Organization (WHO) developed a weighted scheme to determine the toxicity of mixtures of TCDD and dioxin-like compounds. Total exposure to mixtures of dioxins can be assessed by calculating the toxic equivalents (TEQ). A toxic equivalency factor (TEF) is assigned to each dioxin-like chemical based on its potency compared to TCDD. The TEQ is the sum of the magnitude of exposure for each constituent dioxin multiplied by its respective TEF (Safe, 1990). The use of the TEQ is appropriate for PCDDs and PCDFs where TCDD alone or a mixture with an equivalent TEQ produces similar biologic effects (DeVito *et al.*, 1995).

In humans, dioxins are metabolized slowly, as evidenced by the estimated TCDD half-life of 5.8 to 14.1 years (Michalek *et al.*, 1996; Wolfe *et al.*, 1994). Residents of the USA have an average dioxin concentration of approximately 5 ppt in their adipose tissue alone (Orban *et al.*, 1994). Human exposure is frequently assessed by measuring the concentrations of dioxins in the lipid fraction of the blood, which typically is 36 to 58 ppt TEQ in adults. Additionally, dioxins can be transferred from the mother to the fetus via the placenta during pregnancy, and from the mother to the child via the breast milk when nursing. Based on analysis of breast milk, infants have a daily exposure of approximately 70 pg TEQ/kg/day, which exceeds average adult daily exposures by an order of magnitude (Pohl, 1996).

TCDD is a known endocrine disruptor (Mandal, 2005) and thus the initial association of this toxicant with the potential development of endometriosis in a primate colony resulted in a great deal of both scientific interest and public concern (Rier, 1993). Certainly, exposure of humans to high levels of dioxin is known to increase the incidence of both spontaneous abortion and congenital malformations in surviving offspring (Sever *et al.*, 1997; Le and Johansson, 2001). Nevertheless, most human populations are exposed to "background" levels of TCDD and other toxicants, the impact of which is less clear. In this regard, experimental animal models can enhance the understanding of the effects of low-level TCDD exposure, particularly when accumulating evidence suggests that humans respond similarly to animals. Although there are species-specific differences in pharmacokinetics, experimental animal models demonstrate AhR-dependent health effects similar to those found in exposed human populations (DeVito *et al.*, 1995). Integration of all available information describing the toxicokinetics, biochemistry and health effects of dioxins in both human studies and animal models are used to develop mechanistic models for risk assessment. This approach is used to infer human responses by comparing human and animal *in vitro* data with the *in vivo* effects in animals. However, the doses used in animal models do not always reflect the levels of human exposure due to differences in sensitivity and metabolism; nevertheless, it is possible to mimic body burdens between species (DeVito *et al.*, 1995).

Several alternative dose metrics are used for quantitative comparisons of TCDD response between species. Among them are intake, tissue concentration, body burden and total cumulative dose. Intake of dioxins is usually expressed as average daily dose (picograms/kilogram/day) and this is the most convenient method of measuring exposures in animal models. In humans, average daily dose can be estimated by measuring levels in foodstuffs and monitoring consumption. However, tissue concentrations and body burden more closely estimate individual internal dose than estimations made via monitoring intake. Finally, accuracy of TCDD exposures expressed as body burdens can be enhanced by correcting for the proportion of the body mass consisting of lipids, usually 22% in humans (DeVito *et al.*, 1995).

TCDD AND ENDOMETRIOSIS

Although animal and human research has suggested that exposure to environmental agents may adversely affect the development and function of the reproductive system (reviewed by Miller *et al.*, 2004), the association of toxicants with the development of endometriosis remains unclear. In 1993, Rier *et al.* reported a dose–response relationship between TCDD levels (5 and 25 ppt) in feed and the incidence and severity of endometriosis in adult rhesus monkeys, diagnosed several years after dosing ceased. These investigators found that disease was present in 71 and 86% of animals in the 5 and 25 ppt groups, respectively, both of which were significantly different from the percentage of animals exhibiting disease in the control group (33%, $p<0.05$). Although chronic administration of 5 ng TCDD per kg of diet was shown to represent the lowest dose observed to elicit an adverse affect resulting in endometriosis in the female rhesus monkey, there are numerous concerns with the study of Rier *et al.* (1993) mainly due to the small sample sizes and statistical analysis (Guo, 2004). However, in a separate primate study, Yang *et al.* (2000) were able to demonstrate a dose-related divergence in the growth response of endometrial implants to TCDD: the implants in the high dose group were significantly larger than those of controls, while the implants in the medium and low dose groups were either not different, or significantly smaller relative to controls.

Among human studies, numerous investigators have attempted to link adult body burden of TCDD and dioxin-like PCBs in women to the presence or absence of endometriosis (see Bruner-Tran and Osteen, 2010 for review). An Israeli study (Mayani, 1997) reported low levels of TCDD in eight of the 44 cases (18%; range = 0.7–1.2 ppt) but in only one of the 35 (2%) controls (0.4 ppt), yielding a non-significant odds ratio (OR) of 7.6. Using the CALUX assay, a Belgian study (Pauwels *et al.*, 2001) reported a high TEQ (>100 pg/g) in six of 42 cases (14%) but in only one of 27 controls (4%), for a non-significant crude OR of 4.3 (95% confidence interval (CI) = 0.49–43.6). Studies in the USA (Boyd *et al.*, 1995) and Canada (Boyd *et al.*, 1995; Lebel *et al.*, 1998) have found no association between human levels of selected environmental chemicals and the prevalence of endometriosis. The US study measured TCDD and 21 other PCDDs, PCDFs and PCB congeners, but had a small sample size (15 cases and geographically matched controls). However, the Canadian study (86 cases and 70 controls) found no differences between levels in cases and controls when measuring 14 non-coplanar and co-planar PCB congeners and 11 chlorinated pesticides. None of the above studies specifically measured the dioxin-like PCB congeners also found to be related to endometriosis in a follow-up study by Rier *et al.* (2001), who originally reported this disease in TCDD-exposed rhesus monkeys (Rier *et al.*, 1993). In general, small sample size and/or a failure to evaluate exposure to TCDD or other dioxin-like compounds limited most of these endometriosis-related studies. Among the most important investigations related to human exposure to TCDD, Eskenazi *et al.* (2002) conducted a population-based historical cohort study 20 years after the 1976 factory explosion in Seveso, Italy. This accident resulted in the highest known population exposure to TCDD. Of those exposed, 601 female residents of the Seveso area who were ≤30 years old in 1976 with adequate stored sera participated in the study. Endometriosis disease status was defined by pelvic surgery, transvaginal ultrasound, pelvic examination and patient history of infertility and/or pelvic pain. "Cases" included women who had surgically confirmed disease or ultrasound findings consistent with endometriosis. "Non-diseased" women had surgery with no evidence of endometriosis or any signs or symptoms while other women had uncertain status. To assess TCDD exposure, individual levels of TCDD were measured in stored sera that had been collected soon after the accident. The study identified 19 women with endometriosis and 277 disease-free women. The relative risk ratios (RRRs) for women with serum TCDD levels of 20.1–100 ppt and >100 ppt were 1.2 (90% CI = 0.3–4.5) and 2.1 (90% CI = 0.5–8.0), respectively, relative to women with TCDD levels ≤20 ppt. Tests for trends using the above exposure categories were non-significant. Nevertheless, Eskenazi and colleagues reported a doubled, though non-significant, risk for endometriosis among women with serum TCDD levels of 100 ppt or higher. As noted by the investigators, unavoidable disease misclassification in a population-based study may have led to an underestimate of the true risk of endometriosis. In yet another study, increased levels of dioxin-like compounds were found in the serum of women with peritoneal endometriosis and deep endometriotic (adenomyotic) nodules (Heilier *et al.*, 2005). Thus, while the human data are enticing, they remain equivocal despite the numerous animal studies which provide support for a dioxin–endometriosis link (Osteen *et al.*, 1997; Bruner-Tran *et al.*, 1999; Koninckx, 1999; Kogevinas, 2001; Birnbaum and Cummings, 2002; Rier *et al.*, 2002). In light of these confounding observations, it would appear that attempting to link *adult* body burden to the presence or absence of concurrent disease will remain a difficult and perhaps flawed approach. As stated earlier, humans and animals are most sensitive to toxicant exposure during development; therefore understanding the mechanism(s) behind environmental toxicant disruption of organ systems at each stage of life (*in utero* through adulthood) is necessary to develop more precise risk assessments.

POTENTIAL MECHANISMS OF TCDD ACTION AND THE DEVELOPMENT OF ENDOMETRIOSIS

TCDD influences numerous biological systems which could potentially affect a woman's risk for developing endometriosis. For example, TCDD is known to alter the development of the immune system, inhibit T lymphocytes and cytokine production and decrease natural killer cell activity. This toxicant can also alter the impact of steroid action in the reproductive tract, affecting both estrogen and progesterone action (Bruner-Tran *et al.*, 1999; Ohtake *et al.*, 2003). However, since the development of endometriosis is restricted to menstruating species, the search for toxicant-mediated mechanisms must include the potential for disruption of normal endometrial function related to menstruation. In this regard, both *in vivo* and *in vitro* studies have shown that women with endometriosis exhibit a decreased endometrial sensitivity to progesterone that increases the expression of matrix degrading enzymes prior to menstruation (Bruner-Tran *et al.*, 2002). Given the anti-inflammatory effects of progesterone (Tibbetts *et al.*, 1999; Majewski and Hansen, 2002; Mendelson and Hardy, 2006), reduced sensitivity to this steroid could contribute to the pathophysiology of endometriosis by disrupting immune function related to menstruation. During the secretory phase of each menstrual cycle, immune cells actively migrate into the human endometrium and organize themselves into distinct clusters prior to endometrial breakdown to assist in this process (Yeaman *et al.*, 2001). Thus, although the biology of the endometrium in menstruating species is complex, exposure to environmental toxicants capable of disrupting progesterone action could dramatically affect the process of menstruation. Prior to menstruation, progesterone acts to promote endometrial stability by inducing endometrial differentiation (Osteen *et al.*, 2003) and suppressing the ability of locally produced proinflammatory cytokines to stimulate matrix degrading enzymes (Keller *et al.*, 2000). Thus, an important action of progesterone prior to menstruation is to prevent endometrial cell reactivity to locally produced chemokines and cytokines that normally trigger tissue breakdown and bleeding (Bruner-Tran *et al.*, 2008). Perhaps due to the occurrence of endometriosis only in primates and humans, the impact of TCDD on specific elements of cell behavior in the reproductive tract has not been extensively studied. Nevertheless, experimental studies using human endometrial cell cultures have shown that TCDD induces a time dependent loss of progesterone receptor expression, disrupting normal cell–cell communication ultimately leading to a concomitant resistance to progesterone-mediated suppression of matrix degrading enzymes (Igarashi *et al.*, 2005). Thus, through these and other mechanisms, TCDD exposure may act to predispose women to the development of endometriosis (Birnbaum and Cummings, 2002; Rier and Foster, 2002) (Figure 42.2). Specifically, it appears plausible that by altering steroid action, TCDD acts to disrupt production of various cytokines and growth factors, alters remodeling of endometrial tissue via the matrix degrading enzymes and promotes a hyperinflammatory tissue phenotype prior to menstruation. Nevertheless, epidemiologic studies published to date have failed to conclusively link an increased body burden of TCDD to the incidence of endometriosis, leading our group and others to pursue the possible relevance of an early life toxicant exposure on the development of adult disease. As discussed below, an individual's exposure to TCDD during different periods of reproductive tract development may ultimately determine the extent of the impact of this toxicant on development of adult reproductive tract diseases, including endometriosis (Nayyar *et al.*, 2007).

DEVELOPMENTAL TCDD EXPOSURE AND THE ENDOMETRIOSIS PHENOTYPE

Until recently, a critical factor often overlooked in the study of environmental toxicants is the relative risk that exposures may play at different stages of life. In particular, a concept known as developmental origins of human disease (DOHaD) has emerged that requires that we begin to examine the potential role of fetal/neonatal programming on adult susceptibility to disease. Since human and animal exposures actually begin *in utero,* when toxicant sensitivity is greatest, developing a clearer understanding of the potential effects of TCDD and other environmental contaminants will require examining the impact of early life exposure. The necessary prospective experimental studies of early life exposures are not possible in humans; therefore, we developed a murine pregnancy model in order to examine whether developmental exposure to TCDD impacts the sensitivity of the reproductive tract to future toxicant exposures.

Specifically, a murine model was developed in which offspring were exposed at one or more developmental timepoints (*in utero,* prepubertal and pubertal) in order to examine the impact of TCDD exposure on the adult uterine phenotype (Nayyar *et al.*, 2007). Interestingly, we found that female mice exposed to TCDD *in utero*, and again during the development of reproductive potential, demonstrate a progressive loss of uterine progesterone receptor expression. Significantly, our studies indicate that the adult uterine phenotype of toxicant-exposed mice is markedly similar to the endometrial phenotype that is found in women with endometriosis (Nayyar *et al.*, 2007). These findings support the possibility that exposure of children to TCDD during critical periods (i.e., *in utero* development, perinatally or as young adults) could play a cumulative role in disrupting adult endometrial function, potentially predisposing some women to the development of endometriosis. Further, since developmental exposure to TCDD leads to reduced uterine sensitivity to progesterone

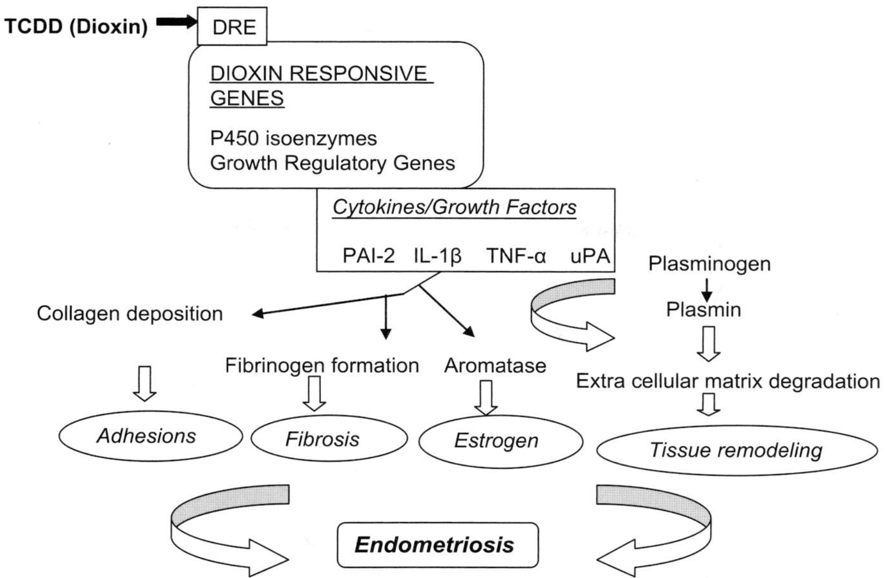

FIGURE 42.2 DREs within target genes affect tissue response at multiple levels, including altered expression of cytokines and growth factors as well as cytochrome P450. Dioxins initially bind with the intracellular AhR and move from the cytoplasm to the nucleus through ARNT which acts as a signal transducer and transcription factor for target genes. Tumor necrosis factor-α (TNF-α) and interleukin-1β (IL-1β) stimulate collagen deposition and fibrinogen formation which might account for the fibrosis and adhesions observed in endometriosis. Urokinase plasminogen activator (uPA) activates plasminogen to plasmin, and modulates extracellular matrix (ECM) degradation. Enhancement of aromatase activity leads to localized estrogen production and thus could further contribute to endometriosis formation.

in adult female animals, suggesting that reproductive success also may be compromised in toxicant-exposed animals (Bruner-Tran and Osteen, in press).

We have recently extended our murine model of developmental toxicant exposure in order to determine if the TCDD-mediated loss of progesterone responsiveness affected fertility and whether the observed effects could be transmitted to subsequent generations of exposed dams (Bruner-Tran *et al.*, 2010; Bruner-Tran and Osteen, in press). To this end, we exposed pregnant mice (F_0 generation) to TCDD on gestation day 15.5 (E15.5) and followed the reproductive success of offspring (the F_1 generation) in the presence and absence of additional exposures. Importantly, TCDD exposure of a pregnant animal also results in exposure of the F_1 generation as germ cells present in the F_2 animal are present at E15.5 (see Figure 42.3). In this study, 44% of mice exposed to TCDD only once (*in utero*) and 66% of mice exposed both *in utero* and at 4 weeks of age (prepuberty) demonstrated an ability to achieve pregnancy. Surviving offspring of mice which were able to achieve pregnancy were also mated and examined. Although the rate of fertility increased in successive generations, infertility was still observed in the F_4 generation, the last generation examined in this study (Bruner-Tran and Osteen, in press).

FUTURE DIRECTIONS

One plausible mechanism by which early life toxicant exposure leads to the development of adult disease is via altered fetal programming through epigenetic modifications. Epigenetic marking of DNA, via methylation of cytosine, is an important mechanism by which a gene can be turned off during development. Although these marks are not necessarily

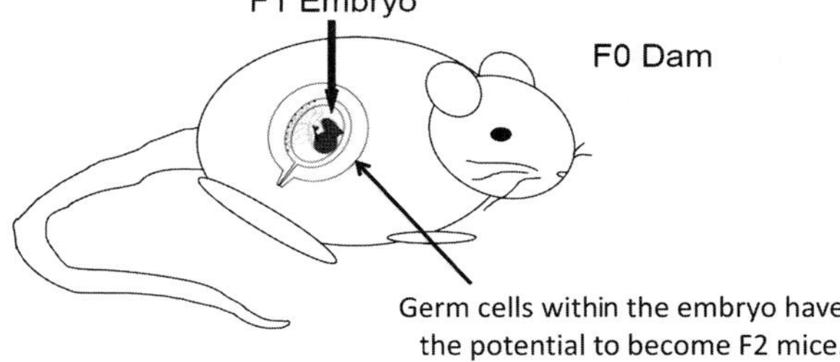

FIGURE 42.3 Schematic depicting the F_0 pregnant mouse which is exposed to 10 ug/kg TCDD by gavage. Pups *in utero* will become the F_1 generations, while F_1 germ cells will ultimately become F_2 mice.

permanent, they are stable and inheritable (Morgan *et al.*, 2005). During development, many cells undergo epigenetic reprogramming which involves the replacement of current marks with new ones and ultimately results in cellular differentiation along a particular path. Differentiated cells do not normally undergo reprogramming, but diseases associated with dedifferentiation (i.e., cancer) are frequently associated with changes in methylation patterns (Morgan *et al.*, 2005). Exposure to TCDD has been found to induce changes in expression of a number of progesterone-responsive genes via epigenetic alterations (for example, Ray and Swanson, 2004).

Recently, epigenetic alterations, including hypermethylation of the progesterone receptor gene, have been described in eutopic and ectopic tissues from women with endometriosis (Wu *et al.*, 2006). Hypermethylation of the progesterone receptor would likely lead to reduced protein expression, thereby inducing a reduced endometrial responsiveness to progesterone, which has been identified in women with endometriosis (Osteen *et al.*, 2005). Future studies are crucial for determining if epigenetic modification of the progesterone receptor gene could provide the missing link between developmental exposure to TCDD and the risk for the development of endometriosis.

REFERENCES

Anger DL, Foster WG (2008) The link between environmental toxicant exposure and endometriosis. *Frontiers Biosci* **13:** 1578–93.

Anway MD, Skinner MK (2006) Epigenetic transgenerational actions of endocrine disruptors. *Endocrinology* Epub; **47 (6 Suppl.):** S43–S9.

Anway MD, Skinner MK (2008) Epigenetic programming of the germ line: effects of endocrine disruptors on the development of transgenerational disease. *Reprod Biomed Online* **16:** 23–5.

Aoki Y (2001) Polychlorinated biphenyls, polychlorinated dibenzo-p-dioxins, and polychlorinated dibenzofurans as endocrine disrupters – what we have learned from Yusho disease. *Environ Res* **86:** 2–11.

Birnbaum LS (1994) The mechanism of dioxin toxicity: relationship to risk assessment. *Environ Health Perspect* **102 (Suppl. 9):** 157–67.

Birnbaum LS, Cummings AM (2002) Dioxins and endometriosis: a plausible hypothesis. *Environ Health Perspect* **110(1):** 15–21.

Boyd JCG, Walmer D, Patterson D, Needham L, Lucier G (1995) Endometriosis and the environment: biomarkers of toxin exposure. [Abstract] Presented at Endometriosis 2000 conference, May 15, 1995. Bethesda, MD.

Bruner-Tran KL, Ding T, Osteen KG (2010) Dioxin and endometrial progesterone resistance. *Semin Reprod Med* **28:** 59–68.

Bruner-Tran KL, Eisenberg E, Yeaman GR, Anderson TA, McBean J, Osteen KG (2002) Steroid and cytokine regulation of matrix metalloproteinase expression in endometriosis and the establishment of experimental endometriosis in nude mice. *J Clin Endocrinol Metab* **87(10):** 4782–91.

Bruner-Tran KL, Osteen KG (2010) Dioxin-like PCBs and endometriosis. *Systems Biol Reprod Med* **56(2):** 132–46.

Bruner-Tran KL, Osteen KG (in press) Developmental eExposure to TCDD reduces fertility and negatively affects pregnancy outcomes across multiple generations. *Reprod Toxicol.*

Bruner-Tran KL, Rier SE, Eisenberg E, Osteen KG (1999) The potential role of environmental toxins in the pathophysiology of endometriosis. *Gynecologic Obstetric Invest* **48 (Suppl. 1):** 45–56.

Bruner-Tran KL, Yeaman GR, Crispens MA, Igarashi TM, Osteen KG (2008) Dioxin may promote inflammation-related development of endometriosis. *Fertil Steril* **89 (5 Suppl.):** 1287–98.

Bulun SE (2009) Endometriosis. *New Eng J Med* **360(3):** 268–79.

DeVito MJ, Birnbaum LS, Farland WH, Gasiewicz TA (1995) Comparisons of estimated human body burdens of dioxinlike chemicals and TCDD body burdens in experimentally exposed animals. *Environ Health Perspect* **103(9):** 820–31.

Dmowski PW, Braun DP (2004) Immunology of endometriosis. Best practice and research. *Clin Obstet Gynaecol* **18:** 245–63.

Domingo JL, Bocio A (2007) Levels of PCDD/PCDFs and PCBs in edible marine species and human intake: a literature review. *Environ Intern* **33(3):** 397–405.

Environmental Working Group (2005) Body burden – the pollution in newborns: a benchmark investigation of industrial chemicals, pollutants and pesticides in umbilical cord blood. [Internet] July 14, 2005 (cited May 6, 2010) Available from: http://www.ewg.org/reports/bodyburden2/execsumm.php

Eskenazi B, Mocarelli P, Warner M, Samuels S, Vercellini P, Olive D, Needham LL, Patterson DG, Brambilla P, Gavoni N, Casalini S, Panazza S, Turner W, Gerthoux PM (2002) Serum dioxin concentrations and endometriosis: a cohort study in Seveso, Italy. *Environ Health Perspect* **110(7):** 629–34.

Giudice LC, Kao LC (2004) Endometriosis. *Lancet* **364(9447):** 1789–99.

Gregoraszczuk EL, Zabielny E, Ochwat D (2001) Aryl hydrocarbon receptor (AhR)-linked inhibition of luteal cell progesterone secretion in 2,3,7,8-tetrachlorodibenzo-p-dioxin treated cells. *J Physiol Pharmacol* **52:** 303–11.

Guerrero-Bosagna CM, Skinner MK (2009) Epigenetic transgenerational effects of endocrine disruptors on male reproduction. *Seminars Reprod Med* **27(5):** 403–8.

Guo SW (2004) The link between exposure to dioxin and endometriosis: a critical reappraisal of primate data. *Gynecologic Obstetric Invest* **57:** 157–73.

Harrad S, Wang Y, Sandaradura S, Leeds A (2003) Human dietary intake and excretion of dioxin-like compounds. *J Environ Monit* **5:** 224–8.

Heilier JF, Nackers F, Verougstraete V, Tonglet R, Lison D, Donnez J (2005) Increased dioxin-like compounds in the serum of women with peritoneal endometriosis and deep endometriotic (adenomyotic) nodules. *Fertil Steril* **84(2):** 305–12.

Heimler I, Rawlins RG, Owen H, Hutz RJ (1998) Dioxin perturbs, in a dose- and time-dependent fashion, steroid secretion, and induces apoptosis of human luteinized granulosa cells. *Endocrinology* **139:** 4373–9.

Heindel JJ (2006) Role of exposure to environmental chemicals in the developmental basis of reproductive disease and dysfunction. *Semin Reprod Med* **24:** 168–77.

Igarashi TM, Bruner-Tran KL, Yeaman GR, Lessey BA, Edwards DP, Eisenberg E, Osteen KG (2005) Reduced expression of progesterone receptor-B in the endometrium of women with endometriosis and in cocultures of endometrial cells exposed to 2,3,7,8-tetrachlorodibenzo-*p*-dioxin. *Fertil Steril* **84:** 67–74.

Jacobson-Dickman E, Lee MM (2009) The influence of endocrine disruptors on pubertal timing. *Curr Opin Endocrinol Diabetes Obesity* **16:** 25–30.

Keller NR, Sierra-Rivera E, Eisenberg E, Osteen KG (2000) Progesterone exposure prevents matrix metalloproteinase-3 (MMP-3) stimulation by interleukin-1a in human endometrial stromal cells. *J Clin Endocrinol Metab* **85:** 1611–9.

Kogevinas M (2001) Human health effects of dioxins: cancer, reproductive and endocrine system effects. *Human Reprod* update **7(3):** 331–9.

Koninckx PR (1999) The physiopathology of endometriosis: pollution and dioxin. *Gynecologic Obstetric Invest* **47 (Suppl. 1):** 47–9; discussion 50.

Koopman-Esseboom C, Morse DC, Weisglas-Kuperus N, Lutkeschipholt IJ, Van der Paauw CG, Tuinstra LG, Brouwer A, Sauer PJ (1994) Effects of dioxins and polychlorinated biphenyls on thyroid hormone status of pregnant women and their infants. *Pediatric Res* **36:** 468–73.

Le TN, Johansson A (2001) Impact of chemical warfare with agent orange on women's reproductive lives in Vietnam: a pilot study. *Reprod Health Matters* **9:** 156–64.

Lebel G, Dodin S, Avotte P, Marcoux S, Ferron LA, Dewailly E (1998) Organochlorine exposure and the risk of endometriosis. *Fertil Steril* **69(2):** 221–8.

Majewski AC, Hansen PJ (2002) Progesterone inhibits rejection of xenogeneic transplants in the sheep uterus. *Hormone Res* **58:** 128–35.

Mandal PK (2005) Dioxin: a review of its environmental effects and its aryl hydrocarbon receptor biology. *J Comp Physiol B* **175:** 221–30.

Mayani A, Barel S, Soback S, Almagor M (1997) Dioxin concentrations in women with endometriosis. *Human Reprod* **12(2):** 373–5.

Mendelson CR, Hardy DB (2006) Role of the progesterone receptor (PR) in the regulation of inflammatory response pathways and aromatase in the breast. *J Steroid Biochem Mol Biol* **102:** 241–9.

Michalek JE, Pirkle JL, Caudill SP, Tripathi RC, Patterson DG Jr, Needham LL (1996) Pharmacokinetics of TCDD in veterans of Operation Ranch Hand: 10-year follow-up. *J Toxicol and Environ Health* **47(3):** 209–20.

Miller KP, Borgeest C, Greenfeld C, Tomic D, Flaws JA (2004) In utero effects of chemicals on reproductive tissues in females. *Toxicol Appl Pharmacol* **198:** 111–31.

Morán FM, VandeVoort CA, Overstreet JW, Lasley BL, Conley AJ (2003) Molecular target of endocrine disruption in human luteinizing granulosa cells by 2,3,7,8-tetrachlorodibenzo-p-dioxin: inhibition of estradiol secretion due to decreased 17a-hydroxylase/17,20-lyase cytochrome P450 expression. *Endocrinology* **144(2):** 467–73.

Morgan HD, Santos F, Green K, Dean W, Reik W (2005) Epigenetic reprogramming in mammals. *Human Mol Gen* **14 Spec. No. 1:** R47–R58.

Nayyar T, Bruner-Tran KL, Piestrzeniewicz-Ulanska D, Osteen KG (2007) Developmental exposure of mice to TCDD elicits a similar uterine phenotype in adult animals as observed in women with endometriosis. *Reprod Toxicol* **23(3):** 326–36.

Ohtake F, Takeyama K, Matsumoto T, Kitagawa H, Yamamoto Y, Nohara K, Tohyama C, Krust A, Mimura J, Chambon P, Yanagisawa J, Fujii-Kuriyama Y, Kato S (2003) Modulation of oestrogen receptor signalling by association with the activated dioxin receptor. *Nature* **423(6939):** 545–50.

Osteen KG, Sierra-Rivera E (1997) Does disruption of immune and endocrine systems by environmental toxins contribute to development of endometriosis? *Semin Reprod Endocrinol* **15(3):** 301–8.

Osteen KG, Bruner-Tran KL, Eisenberg E (2005) Reduced progesterone action during endometrial maturation: a potential risk factor for the development of endometriosis. *Fertil Steril* **83(3):** 529–37.

Osteen KG, Igarashi TM, Bruner-Tran KL (2003) Progesterone action in the human endometrium: induction of a unique tissue environment which limits matrix metalloproteinase (MMP) expression. *Frontiers Biosci* **8:** d78–86.

Pauwels A, Schepens PJ, D'Hooghe T, Delbeke L, Dhont M, Brouwer, A, Weyler J (2001) The risk of endometriosis and exposure to dioxins and polychlorinated biphenyls: a case–control study of infertile women. *Human Reprod* **16(10):** 2050–5.

Pocar P, Fischer B, Klonisch T, Hombach-Klonisch S (2005) Molecular interactions of the aryl hydrocarbon receptor and its biological and toxicological relevance for reproduction. *Reproduction* **129(4):** 379–89.

Pohl HR, Hibbs BF (1996) Breast-feeding exposure of infants to environmental contaminants – a public health risk assessment viewpoint: chlorinated dibenzodioxins and chlorinated dibenzofurans. *Toxicol Indust Health* **12(5):** 593–611.

Pompa G, Caloni F, Fracchiolla ML (2003) Dioxin and PCB contamination of fish and shellfish: assessment of human exposure. Review of the international situation. *Vet Res Comm* **27 (Suppl. 1):** 159–67.

Ray SS, Swanson HI (2004) Dioxin-induced immortalization of normal human keratinocytes and silencing of p53 and p16INK4a. *J Biol Chem* **279(26):** 27187–93.

Rier S, Foster WG (2002) Environmental dioxins and endometriosis. *Toxicol Sci* **70(2):** 161–70.

Rier S, Bowman R, Dmowski W, Becker J (1993) Endometriosis in rhesus monkeys (Macaca mulatta) following chronic exposure to 2,3,7,8-tetrachlorodibenzo-pdioxin. *Fund Appl Toxicol* **21:** 433–41.

Safe SH (1994) Polychlorinated biphenyls (PCBs): environmental impact, biochemical and toxic responses, and implications for risk assessment. *Crit Rev Toxicol* **24(2):** 87–149.

Safe SH (1990) Polychlorinated biphenyls (PCBs), dibenzo-p-dioxins (PCDDs), dibenzofurans (PCDFs), and related compounds: environmental and mechanistic considerations which support the development of toxic equivalency factors (TEFs). *Crit Rev Toxicol* **21(1):** 51–88.

Sampson JA (1927) Peritoneal endometriosis due to menstrual dissemination of endometrial tissues into the peritoneal cavity. *Am J Obstet Gynecol* **14:** 422–69.

Schecter A, Wallace D, Pavuk M, Piskac A, Papke O (2002) Dioxins in commercial United States baby food. *J Toxicol Environ Health. Part A* **65:** 1937–43.

Schrenk D (1998) Impact of dioxin-type induction of drug metabolizing enzymes on the metabolism of endo- and xenobiotics. *Biochem Pharmacol* **55(8):** 1155–62.

Sever LE, Arbuckle TE, Sweeney A (1997) Reproductive and developmental effects of occupational pesticide exposure: the epidemiologic evidence. *J Occup Med* **12:** 305–25.

Skinner MK (2007) Endocrine disruptors and epigenetic transgenerational disease etiology. *Pediatric Res* **61(5 Pt 2):** 48R–50.

Tibbetts TA, Conneely OM, O'Malley BW (1999) Progesterone via its receptor antagonizes the proinflammatory activity of estrogen in the mouse uterus. *Biol Reprod* **60:** 1158–65.

Van den Berg M, De Jongh J, Poiger H, Olson JR (1994) The toxicokinetics and metabolism of polychlorinated dibenzo-p-dioxins (PCDDs) and dibenzofurans (PCDFs) and their relevance for toxicity. *Crit Rev Toxicol* **24(1):** 1–74.

Van der Molen GW, Kooijman SA, Slob W (1996) A generic toxicokinetic model for persistent lipophilic compounds in humans: an application to TCDD. *Fund Appl Toxicol* **31(1):** 83–94.

Whitlock JP Jr (1999) Induction of cytochrome P4501A1. *Annu Rev Pharmacol Toxicol* **39:** 103–25.

Whitlock JP Jr, Chichester CH, Bedgood RM, Okino ST, Ko HP, Ma Q, Dong L, Li H, Clarke-Katzenberg R (1997) Induction of drug-metabolizing enzymes by dioxin. *Drug Metab Rev* **29(4):** 1107–27.

Wolfe WH, Michalek JE, Miner JC, Pirkle JL, Caudill SP, PattersonDG Jr, Needham LL (1994) Determinants of TCDD half-life in veterans of operation ranch hand. *J Toxicol Environ Health* **41(4):** 481–8.

Wu Y, Strawn E, Basir Z, Halverson G, Guo SW (2006) Promoter hypermethylation of progesterone receptor isoform B (PR-B) in endometriosis. *Epigenetics* **1(2):** 106–11.

Yang JZ, Agarwal SK, Foster WG (2000) Subchronic exposure to 2,3,7,8-tetrachlorodibenzo-*p*-dioxin modulates the pathophysiology of endometriosis in the cynomolgus monkey. *Toxicol Sci* **56(2):** 374–81.

Yeaman GR, Collins JE, Fanger MW, Wira CR, Lydyard PM (2001) CD8+ T cells in human uterine endometrial lymphoid aggregates: evidence for accumulation of cells by trafficking. *Immunology* **102:** 434–40.

Zook D, Rappe C (1994) Environmental sources, distribution and fate of polychlorinated dibenzodioxins, dibenzofurans, and related organochlorines. In *Dioxins and Health* (Schecter A, ed.). Plenum Press, New York, pp. 79–113.

C H A P T E R

43

Reproductive toxicity of polycyclic aromatic hydrocarbons: occupational relevance

Aramandla Ramesh and Anthony E. Archibong

INTRODUCTION

Polycyclic aromatic hydrocarbons (PAHs) constitute a large generic group of organic compounds with two or more fused aromatic rings. They are semi-volatile, lipophilic, high molecular weight compounds that are products of combustion and can accumulate in crops via absorption from contaminated soils. Polycyclic aromatic hydrocarbons are formed mainly as a result of pyrolytic processes, especially the incomplete combustion of organic materials during industrial and other human activities, such as processing of coal and crude oil, combustion of natural gas for cooking and home heating. Other human activities that result in B(a)P emission include the combustion of refuse, vehicle traffic, cooking and tobacco smoking, as well as in natural processes such as carbonization. There are several hundred PAHs; the best known prototype being benzo(a)pyrene (B(a)P).

Exclusive sources for B(a)P contamination of the environment and exposure to humans include industrial and automobile emissions, hazardous waste sites, cigarette smoke, biomass burning, municipal incinerators, volcanic eruptions, home heating and consumption of charcoal broiled and smoked foods (ATSDR, 1995; IPCS, 1998). Both food ingestion and inhalation represent major routes of PAH exposure for distinct segments of the general population (Butler *et al.*, 1993; Van Rooij *et al.*, 1994). Vulnerable organs such as the gonads are exposed directly to inhaled B(a)P without undergoing "first pass effect" through the liver for metabolism and detoxification. However, the reverse is true for orally administered B(a)P. Regardless of the route of exposure (inhalation or oral) B(a)P elicits toxic effects on the functional development of the testis and ovary.

HISTORICAL BACKGROUND

Several reports (reviewed in Toppari *et al.*, 1996; Moline *et al.*, 2000; Schettler *et al.*, 2000) suggest that human health globally is adversely influenced by exposure to toxic chemicals that act as endocrine disruptors. One of the environmental/occupational reproductive endocrine disruptors is benzo(a)pyrene (B(a)P), a prototypical member of the PAH family of compounds (Charles *et al.*, 2000; Archibong *et al.*, 2002; Inyang *et al.*, 2003; Kim *et al.*, 2004). Several PAHs are associated with testicular toxicity and numerous studies have documented that B(a)P and cigarette smoking, a source of B(a)P, are associated with reduced semen quality (Zinaman *et al.*, 2000; Kunzle *et al.*, 2003). Also, Huang *et al.* (2008) demonstrated that inhalation of motorcycle exhaust (ME) fumes, another source of B(a)P, by adult male Wister rats significantly reduced circulating testosterone concentrations, testis weight, spermatid numbers and stored sperm density compared with controls. Their data also indicated that ME caused histopathological changes such as testicular spermatocytic necrosis, seminiferous tubule atrophy and formation of clusters of pyknotic and necrotic stored spermatozoa. Caging of ME-exposed male rats with unexposed females for the purpose of mating resulted in decreased male mating index, female fertility index and an increase in implantation site losses. The adverse effect of B(a)P on male fertility indices was confirmed when adult male rats were exposed to B(a)P via inhalation. Specifically, a subacute exposure (10 days) of adult F-344 male rats via inhalation to B(a)P (75 μg B(a)P/cm^3) caused a significant reduction in stored sperm motility and circulating testosterone concentrations (Inyang *et al.*, 2003). Furthermore, a subchronic exposure of adult F-344 male rats to this PAH significantly reduced testis weight, spermatid numbers, stored sperm density, progressive motility, spermatozoa with normal morphology, intratesticular testosterone concentrations and circulating testosterone (Archibong *et al.*, 2008; Ramesh *et al.*, 2008).

Endocrine disrupting chemicals may have very specific effects on the cells within the ovary and because of the intense interdependency of cells in this organ, cause a disruption in normal folliculogenesis, ovulatory process, fertilization and subsequent embryo development. One of the endocrine disrupting compounds is benzo(a)pyrene (B(a)P). Polycyclic aromatic hydrocarbons including B(a)P have steric resemblance to steroid molecules (Santodonato, 1997) and have been demonstrated to have both estrogenic and antiestrogenic activities (Pasqualini *et al.*, 1990; Chaloupka *et al.*,

Reproductive and Developmental Toxicology, Edited by Ramesh C. Gupta
ISBN: 978-0-12-382032-7

1992; Santodonato, 1997; Charles *et al.*, 2000). These findings suggest that PAHs can influence reproductive efficiency in exposed subjects. Our studies (Archibong *et al.*, 2002; Inyang *et al.*, 2003; Archibong *et al.*, 2008; Ramesh *et al.*, 2008) indicate that fertility is perturbed in rats subjected via inhalation, to subacute and subchronic B(a)P exposures. Taken together, exposures to PAHs contribute significantly to both male and female infertility and the aforementioned studies set the stage for ongoing mechanism-based investigations by our research group and several others in this area.

PHARMACOKINETICS/ TOXICOKINETICS

In addition to biotransformation of B(a)P to reactive metabolites, another key factor of contention is the dose of B(a)P administered, as it plays an important role in the toxicity and risk associated with this chemical. In the context of toxicity, the external or administered dose is not the most appropriate one to consider in terms of functional importance at the cellular or molecular level. Of importance is the amount that actually reaches the target site where adverse effects occur designated as "internal dose" and represent only a fraction of the "delivered" or "external dose" (Paustenbach, 2000). The internal dose, also referred to as the "absorbed" or "bioavailable dose", is estimated by toxicokinetic parameters (Hrudey *et al.*, 1996).

Toxicokinetics is a term used to quantitatively define pharmacokinetic parameters in the context of toxicity. The pharmacokinetic parameters of toxicants aid in the interpretation of toxicology data and risk assessment (Wier, 2006). Pharmacokinetics of PAHs is inextricably linked to processes such as absorption, distribution, metabolism and elimination of these compounds.

The pharmacokinetic (PK) behavior of PAHs in animal models has been investigated (Moir *et al.*, 1998; Ramesh *et al.*, 2001; Uno *et al.*, 2006; Walker *et al.*, 2007; Harris *et al.*, 2008) from the standpoint of toxicity to somatic tissues. These studies were equivocal in the agreement that pharmacokinetic properties of B(a)P favor a greater residence time for this lipophilic toxicant in target tissues. Therefore, the likelihood of B(a)P and/or its metabolites residing in steroidogenic tissues such as testis or ovary pose a greater threat to the reproductive health of the mammalian species in general. Unfortunately, there is a dearth of information in PAH pharmacokinetics from the standpoint of toxicity to the reproductive system. The available literature focuses mostly on temporal disposition kinetics of B(a)P (Ramesh *et al.*, 2001, 2010) and fluoranthene (Walker *et al.*, 2007) in male reproductive tissues subsequent to acute exposures. Pharmacokinetic studies for PAHs are warranted in both genders of animal models in different age groups that correspond to adolescence, puberty, adult and senile age groups in humans. Towards this end, there is a need to employ physiologically based pharmacokinetic (PBPK) models. These models provide a reliable estimate of toxicant uptake and disposition (Wier, 2006) as they take into consideration several anatomical, physiological, biochemical and physicochemical parameters to assess the fate of ingested/inhaled PAH compound. While PBPK models have been constructed for various reproductive toxicants, a paucity of information exists for PAHs in this area, which qualifies for immediate data needs.

MECHANISM OF ACTION

Benzo(a)pyrene and other PAHs are toxic to tissues and organs after biotransformation to reactive intermediates. The first step in the action of PAHs is interaction with a cellular protein known as the aryl hydrocarbon receptor (Ah) receptor (reviewed in Birnbaum, 1994). The Ah receptor, so named because it was first associated with the enzyme induction by aryl hydrocarbons is a member of the basic helix–loop–helix family of regulatory proteins (Swanson and Bransfield, 1993). It is the first member of this family known to be ligand activated. It is normally present in the cell complexed to heat shock protein 90 as well as additional proteins. Upon binding of PAHs, the ligand-binding subunit undergoes a conformational change leading to disassociation of the complex and release of the other proteins. The ligand-bound Ah receptor then associates with its heterodimeric partner, aryl hydrocarbon nuclear translocase (ARNT). Aryl hydrocarbon nuclear translocase is another basic helix–loop–helix protein that has significant sequence similarity to the Ah receptor (Reyes *et al.*, 1992). A family of ARNT-like proteins that dimerize with the Ah receptor and the ligand-bound heterodimer then bind to a specific DNA sequence, functioning as a transcriptional heterodimer (Whitlock, 1993). Additional proteins may also play a role in the activation function of the Ah receptor. Functional xenobiotic response elements (XREs) have been found in the regulatory region of several genes involved in biotransformation such as CYP1A1, CYP1A2, CYP1B1, glutathione-S-transferase, menadione reductase, uridine diphosphoglucuronylsyl transferase and aldehyde dehydrogenase. In the gonads, the transcription of CYP1B1 results in the generation of intermediates, the most notable reactive forms being diol epoxides and quinones. In addition, XREs have been detected in the genes of several cytokines, growth factors and steroid receptors (White and Gasiewicz, 1993).

Both the Ah receptor and ARNT are present in the embryo. Using *in situ* hybridization to detect mRNA and immunohistochemical staining to recognize the presence of expressed protein, Abbott and coworkers demonstrated tissue-specific localization of both the Ah receptor (Abbott *et al.*, 1994) and ARNT (Abbott and Probst, 1995) in mouse embryo from gestation days (GDs) 10–16. The presence of both proteins is developmentally regulated, being specific for cell type, organ/tissue and developmental stage. The expression of these heterodimeric partners is generally coordinated. High levels of ARNT, which decrease toward the end of organogenesis, are expressed in the developing brain and heart. Low levels are present in the liver on GD 10, which then increase to represent the highest levels in the fetus by GD 16. A similar pattern is present in the bone. Low-to-moderate levels are present in kidney, muscle and lung by the end of organogenesis, whereas high levels appear in the skin and the adrenal glands by GD 16. Non-coordinate expression of the Ah receptor and ARNT occurs in the adrenal glands with levels of ARNT being much higher than Ah receptor. The Ah receptor is also present in the renal tubules and differentiating glomeruli, whereas ARNT is present in the developing collecting ducts and ureter. Expression in other organs appears after GD 13 and increase with gestational age. In the developing human palate, co-staining studies by Abbott *et al.* (1994) demonstrated that most cells that express Ah receptor also express ARNT and vice versa; however, some cells express only one of the two proteins. Their data also indicated that the developmental regulation of Ah receptor and ARNT did not only occur at the levels of the tissue and organ, but included subcellular localization. Furthermore, in neural tissue and bone, both proteins were predominantly nuclear throughout organogenesis. In contrast, these proteins were both nuclear and cytoplasmic in muscle and skin. In the adrenals, the Ah receptor was strongly nuclear and ARNT was highly cytoplasmic. They also observed that liver Ah receptor and ARNT were both nuclear and cytoplasmic on GD 10, but by GD 16 both had become strongly nuclear.

Other investigators have detected the presence of the Ah receptor and/or ARNT earlier in development. Peters and Wiley (1995) used RT-PCR to determine whether the Ah receptor is expressed during murine preimplantation embryo development. Their results suggest that mouse embryo transcribes, rather than maternally inherits, Ah receptor mRNA. They first detected Ah receptor mRNA at the compacted eight cell stage, suggesting that the Ah receptor begins to function in preimplantation embryos that are well into the eight cell stage. Aryl hydrocarbon receptor protein was detected in the blastocyst. As observed in other biological systems where Ah receptor functions during proliferation and differentiation, this receptor plays a major role in the differentiation of the trophectoderm as well as influences embryonic growth by enhancing cell proliferation. At the end of organogenesis, levels of Ah receptor mRNA are low compared to those for ARNT (Carver *et al.*, 1994). However, in human placenta at term, Ah receptor levels are high compared to those found in most adult tissues (Dolwick *et al.*, 1993). The critical importance of this signal transduction system in normal development is supported by the decreased viability and immune deficiencies of transgenic mice in which Ah receptor gene has been knocked out (Fernandez-Salguero *et al.*, 1995).

Although the direct transcriptional activation of the Ah receptor is well demonstrated, recent studies suggest that the Ah receptor has an alternative mode of action involving the direct activation of second messenger systems. Phosphorylation of tyrosine residues has been shown to be a rapid and sensitive response to dioxin exposure both *in vivo* and *in vitro*. Activation of cellular-sarcoma (c-src) gene and the epidermal growth factor (EGF) receptor have been documented. Analogous to the steroid hormone receptors, which have non-nuclear functions, both Birnbaum (1994, 1996) and Matsumura (1994) have suggest that additional proteins present in the multimeric protein complex present in the absence of ligand may be tyrosine kinases or proteins involved in the activation of tyrosine kinases. Upon binding to dioxin, these proteins are released from the Ah receptor complex and from its inhibitory control. A negative role has been shown for other helix–loop–helix proteins such as inhibitor of DNA binding (Id) which blocks the transcriptional activation function of NF-kappa (Beg *et al.*, 1995).

TOXICITY

Effect of benzo(a)pyrene on female reproduction

The receptor-mediated action of B(a)P and many other functional analogs between the steroid receptors and the Ah receptor (AhR) has led to the classification of B(a)P and other PAHs as potential environmental hormones (Safe, 2001). In testimony, B(a)P affects the serum concentrations of progesterone, androgens, estrogens, prolactin and indirectly on LH (Archibong *et al.*, 2002; Inyang *et al.*, 2003; Ramesh *et al.*, 2008). Furthermore, this PAH has been shown to affect growth factors such as insulin-like growth factor (IGF) EGF, transforming growth factor (TGF) and retinoic acid (Rodríguez-Fragoso *et al.*, 2009; Song and Xu, 2009), the receptors to which are either up- or downregulated in response to B(a)P exposure. Similar to any hormone or growth factor, the response to B(a)P exposure is tissue specific and the intensity of damage is dependent on the interactive action of multiple regulatory molecules in the affected tissue(s). Hence, the understanding that B(a)P can alter multiple endocrine and growth factor pathways makes it comprehendible that PAHs function as potent endocrine and growth disruptors, altering both proliferation and differentiation.

Polycyclic aromatic hydrocarbons including B(a)P are typically activated by phase I (oxidation-reduction) enzymes to reactive intermediates that bind covalently to nucleic acids and proteins; however, PAHs are detoxified by both phase I and phase II (conjugation) enzymes. Polycyclic aromatic hydrocarbons affect the expression of many other genes by way of both AhR-dependent and AhR-independent mechanisms (Ryu *et al.*, 1996; Nebert *et al.*, 2000, 2004; Puga *et al.*, 2000; Miller and Ramos, 2001). The expression of CYP1A1 is constitutively absent but is markedly induced in a large number of tissues after induction by PAHs (Nebert *et al.*, 2004). In contrast, substantial levels of basal CYP1A2 activity occur in mammalian liver. The human and rodent CYP1A2 gene is inducible by PAHs in liver, gastrointestinal tract, pancreas, brain and lung (Sesardic *et al.*, 1990; Farin and Omiecinski, 1993; Foster *et al.*, 1993; Dey *et al.*, 1999; Tatemichi *et al.*, 1999; Wei *et al.*, 2001). However, CYP1B1 has a high basal activity in such tissues as adrenal cortex, ovary, testis, uterus, prostate and mammary gland, gastrointestinal tract and immune cells (Guengerich *et al.*, 2003; Galvan *et al.*, 2005). Constitutive CYP1B1 is extremely low in liver and gastrointestinal tract but is detectable after PAH treatment (Buesen *et al.*, 2002; Zhang *et al.*, 2003). Hence, the metabolism of PAHs by CYP1B1 in steroidogenic and reproductive tissues is detrimental to hormonally regulate developmental events such as male and female gamete production, their ability to interact and the development of generated embryo to a viable young.

Although there is little evidence that B(a)P or and its related isosteromers are directly mutagenic, exposures can lead to secondary genotoxicity. Polycyclic aromatic hydrocarbons are clearly immunotoxic in several species, affecting both T- and B-cell responses. Several studies have shown that PAHs are neurotoxic, causing both central and peripheral effects as well as affecting learning and memory. The liver, gastrointestinal and genitourinary tracts and cardiovascular system have all been shown to be targets for PAHs' adverse effects. Polycyclic aromatic hydrocarbons have also been shown to be both developmental and reproductive toxicants in multiple species. Both structural and functional defects have been noted, as well as altered fertility.

Overview of developmental effects of benzo(a)pyrene

Developmental toxicity associated with exposure to B(a)P has been a target of intense recent research. We now know that the lack of reproduction in teleost fish has been caused by the presence of B(a)P in their habitat (Cheshenko *et al.*, 2008). According to these investigators, two cyp19 genes are present in most teleosts, cyp19a and cyp19b, primarily expressed in the ovary and brain, respectively. Both aromatase CYP19 isoforms are involved in the sexual differentiation and regulation of the reproductive cycle and male reproductive behavior in diverse teleost species. Alteration of aromatase CYP19 expression and/or activity, be it upregulation or downregulation, may lead to diverse disturbances of the above-mentioned processes.

Polycyclic hydrocarbons have toxic effects on mammalian embryonic development. Pregnant mice or rats treated during early or middle gestation with B(a)P, 3-methylcholanthrene or 7,12-dimethylbenzo(a)anthracene show significant increases in embryolethality and resorption; surviving fetuses have a greater incidence of malformation (reviewed in Galloway *et al.*, 1980). Exposure during late gestation substantially increases the incidence of tumors in the progeny (Urso and Gengozian, 1980). A demonstrated correlation between embryotoxicity and genetic capacity for B(a)P metabolism (Galloway *et al.*, 1980) suggests that embryo damage involves the metabolism of B(a)P to chemically active form(s). The adverse effects of B(a)P in cigarette smoke on human health is well documented. Cigarette smoking during pregnancy is associated with an increased risk of a number of adverse obstetric and fetal outcomes including spontaneous miscarriage, placenta previa, premature rupture of the membranes, preterm birth and low birth weight (Shiverick and Salafia, 1999; Andres and Day, 2000). Furthermore there is a significant association between smoking and reduced fertility among female smokers (Zenzes, 2000; Lintsen *et al.*, 2005; Soares *et al.*, 2007). Therefore it is generally accepted that women who smoke should be counseled to desist from the practice prior to attempting pregnancy. Smoking by men and passive and active smoking by women are associated with a longer time to pregnancy (TTP; Hull *et al.*, 2000). These authors reported that smoking 20 cigarettes per day by either partner was associated with longer TTP. Little evidence of any trend was seen with smoking from one to 14 cigarettes per day.

Effect of benzo(a)pyrene on follicular growth

The AhR is abundantly expressed in oocytes (Robles *et al.*, 2000) and can be triggered by a number of chemicals including B(a)P. Upon ligand binding, the AhR translocates to the nucleus and interacts with genes that contain a common nucleotide sequence (known as the AhR response element) resulting in altered expression of AhR regulated genes (Matikainen *et al.*, 2001). Oocytes in fetal mouse ovaries undergo apoptosis in an AhR-dependent fashion following PAH exposure (Matikainen *et al.*, 2001). A similar response to PAHs has been shown in primordial follicles from human ovarian tissue (Matikainen *et al.* 2002). The ovotoxicity of B(a)P may not be limited to humans in that a similar observation has been made in rodents. The 7,12-dimethylbenz(a) anthracene (DMBA), 3-methylcholanthrene (3-MC) and B(a)P destroy oocytes in small ovarian follicles of rats and mice within 14 days following a single injection of the aforementioned PAHs (Mattison, 1979). Under these conditions, mice were more susceptible to PAH-induced ovotoxicity than rats with DMBA being the most toxic to primordial follicles followed by 3-MC and then B(a)P (Mattison and Thorgeirsson, 1979) in a dose-dependent manner. Similarly, the aforementioned PAHs also cause follicular toxicity in F-344 rats and B6 mice (Borman *et al.*, 2000). Using an isolated rat follicle culture assay, Neal *et al.* (2007) also have demonstrated that B(a)P inhibits follicular growth. Daily oral exposure of mice between GD 7 and 16 to high doses of BaP (40 and 160 mg/kg) also caused complete sterility in the female offspring (Mackenzie and Angevine, 1985). Furthermore, pregnant mice exposed to a lower dose of B(a)P (10 mg/kg) gave birth to offspring with severely compromised fertility.

In general, PAHs are not directly ovotoxic. They require metabolic biotransformation to reactive metabolites. Ovarian enzymes involved in the biotransformation of PAHs (CYP1B1, AHH and epoxide hydrolase) have been identified in the mice, rats and primates (Hoyer, 2004; Harris *et al.*, 2009). Consequently, oocyte destruction by PAHs may be preceded by the distribution of the parent compound to the ovary where PAH transformation enzymes metabolize the compounds to reactive intermediates (Mattison, 1983; Smith *et al.*, 2007; Harris *et al.*, 2009). These reactive intermediates are capable of covalent binding to macromolecules such as DNA, RNA and proteins (Ramesh *et al.*, 2010).

Activated AhR has been reported to regulate female gametogenesis through Bax gene (a proapoptotic member of the Bcl-2 family of cell death regulators; Oltvai *et al.*, 1993)-mediated transcription in germ cells (Pru and Tilly, 2001). Reactive metabolites of PAHs such as 9,10-DMBA were found to induce expression of Bax gene and apoptosis in oocytes of prenatal (Matikainen *et al.*, 2001) and neonatal (Matikainen *et al.*, 2002) mouse ovaries. Hence it can be surmised that BaP-induced AhR contributes to apoptosis of oocytes and consequently the ovulation of fewer mature ova.

Perhaps the destruction of oocytes by B(a)P reactive metabolites results from the inability of granulosa cells to support oocyte maturation due to the inhibition of aromatase activity in these cells. Dong *et al.* (2008) have demonstrated that B(a)P inhibits aromatase expression and consequently the inhibition of the conversion of androgens to E2. The normal maturation of oocytes is dependent on the ability of follicular granulosa cells to progressively produce E2, failing which oocytes become atretic.

Effect of benzo(a)pyrene on fetal survival

Transplacental exposures of fetuses to PAHs affect fetal development and pregnancy outcomes in both laboratory animals and humans. Huel *et al.* (1993) reported an association between the PAH-induced human placental aryl hydrocarbon hydroxylase induction and threatened preterm delivery. Metabolites of PAHs were implicated as abortifacient agents by these authors. Furthermore, the molecular epidemiologic studies of Perera *et al.* (1998) and Sram *et al.* (1999) suggest that some environmental PAHs significantly affected birth outcomes in Poland and the Czech Republic. A recent study reported chromosomal aberrations in Czech mothers exposed to PAHs through inhalation and also in their newborns (Rossnerova *et al.*, 2010). Our findings (Archibong *et al.*, 2002) indicate that B(a)P affects fetal survival, intrauterine growth and pregnancy-related hormones. In this study, pregnancy and number of conceptuses *in utero* were established in time-pregnant rats via midventral laparotomy on GD 8. Confirmed pregnant rats were divided into three groups based on the number of conceptuses in the uterus. The groups consisted of animals that had 4–6, 7–9 and more than 9 conceptuses *in utero*. Rats in each group were then assigned randomly to treatment groups and two control groups. Treatment consisted of subacute exposure of rats to 25, 75 and 100 µg B(a)P/m^3 via nose-only inhalation, 4 h daily for 10 days (GD 11–20). Control animals were either sham exposed to carbon black (CB), to control for the inert carrier of B(a)P, or served as unexposed control (UNC). Blood samples were collected on GD 15 and 17 via orbital sinus veini-puncture, plasma harvested and assayed for estrogen, progesterone and prolactin. Prolactin concentration was taken as an indirect measure of decidual luteotropin activity. Percentage fetal survival was calculated by dividing the total number of pups by the number of implantation sites determined on GD 8 times 100. Individual pup weight (g) and crown–rump length (mm) per litter per treatment were determined on postnatal day (PND) 4 (PND 0 = day of parturition). Exposure of pregnant rats to increasing exposure concentrations of B(a)P indicated above caused decreased fetal survival rates in a dose-dependent manner (Table 43.1). Mean pup weights were similar among litters in both control groups and the group exposed to B(a)P 25 µg/m^3. Exposure to 75 and 100 µg B(a)P/m^3 resulted in a decrease in mean pup weight (Table 43.1). There was no difference in pup weights between the two high dose groups. Crown–rump length did not differ among groups (Table 43.1). Furthermore, exposure of pregnant rats to inhaled B(a)P caused a decrease in plasma progesterone, estradiol and prolactin in rats exposed to 75 µg B(a)P/m^3 and above on GD 17 (because the reproductive characteristics between pregnant rats exposed to 75 and 100 µg B(a)P/m^3 did not differ, endocrine data for rats exposed to 75 µg B(a)P/m^3 are represented herein; Figures 43.1–43.3). Even though our study did not identify any teratogenic effect of B(a)P on rat neonates, Sanyal and Li (2007) demonstrated damage to the vasculature of the placentae and within the cranium of fetuses of rats treated intraperitoneally with high doses of B(a)P. Studies conducted by

TABLE 43.1 Pregnancy outcome (mean ± SEM, $n = 10$ dams per treatment) in F-344 rats exposed to benzo(a)pyrene through inhalation (Archibong *et al.*, 2002)

	Treatment				
	Controls		Benzo(a)pyrene (µg/m^3)		
Outcome parameter	Unexposed	Carbon black	25	75	100
Implantation sites (n)	8.6 ± 0.2	8.8 ± 0.1	8.8 ± 0.5	9.0 ± 0.2	8.8 ± 0.1
Pups per litter (n)	8.5 ± 0.2^a	8.7 ± 0.2^a	7.4 ± 0.5^b	4.2 ± 0.1^c	3.0 ± 0.2^c
Survival (litter %)	98.9 ± 1.1^a	96.7 ± 1.7^a	78.3 ± 4.1^b	38.0 ± 2.1^c	33.8 ± 1.3^d
Pup weight (g per litter)	10.6 ± 0.1^a	8.8 ± 0.1^a	10.5 ± 0.2^a	9.1 ± 0.2^b	8.9 ± 0.1^b
Crown–rump length (mm per litter)	29.4 ± 0.6	29.3 ± 0.5	28.0 ± 0.6	27.3 ± 0.7	27.9 ± 0.7

Entries within rows with different letters (a–d) are different from one another at $P \leq 0.05$ by one-tailed post-hoc t-testing following ANOVA

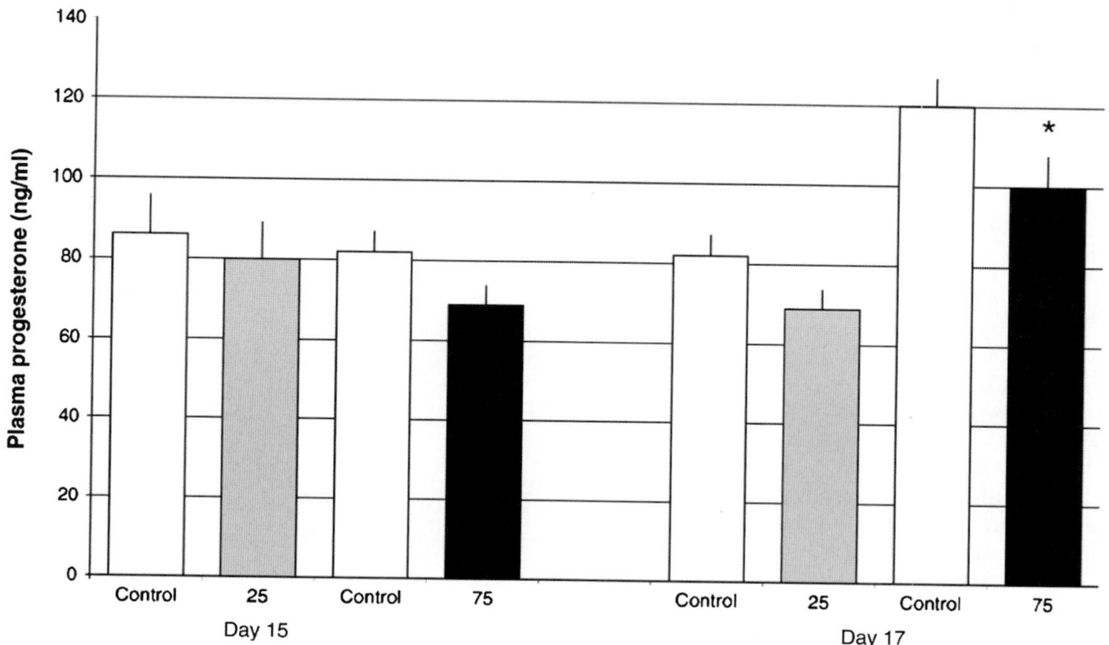

FIGURE 43.1 Plasma progesterone (mean ± SEM) in untreated controls and animals exposed to 25 or 75 µg B(a)P/m^3 from gestation days 8 through 17 (Archibong *et al.*, 2002). Control group is shown immediately to the left of its respective B(a)P-exposed group. (*) $P < 0.05$ compared to respective control. $n = 10$ per group.

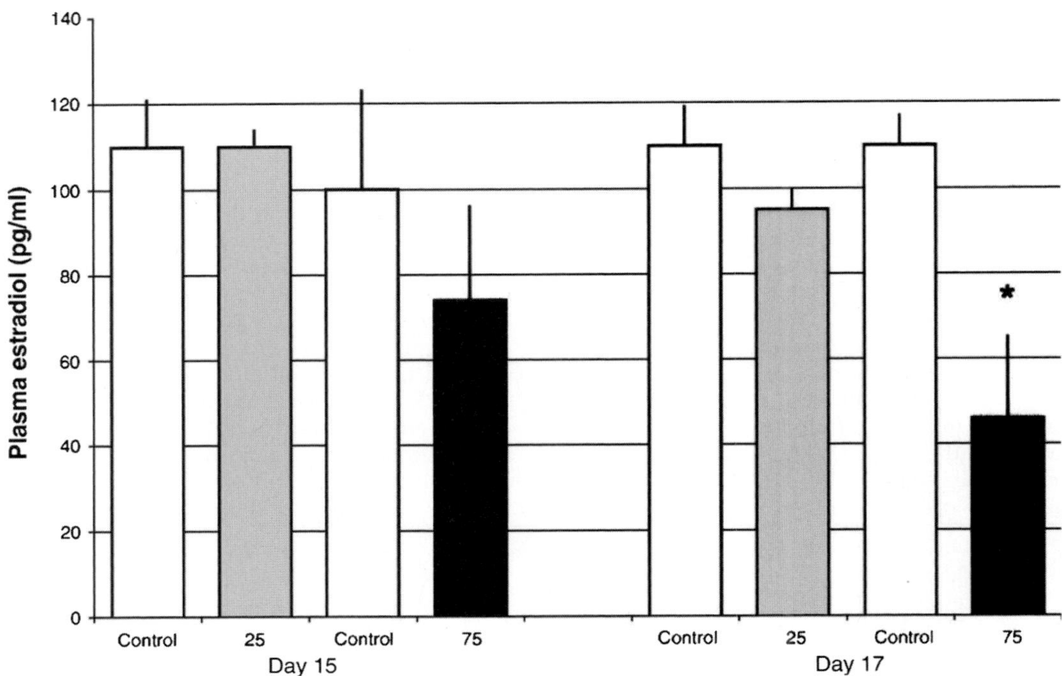

FIGURE 43.2 Plasma estradiol-17β (mean ± SEM) in untreated controls and animals exposed to 25 or 75 μg B(a)P/m^3 from gestation days 8 through 17 (Archibong *et al.*, 2002). Control group is shown immediately to the left of its respective B(a)P-exposed group. (*) $P < 0.05$ compared to respective control. $n = 10$ per group.

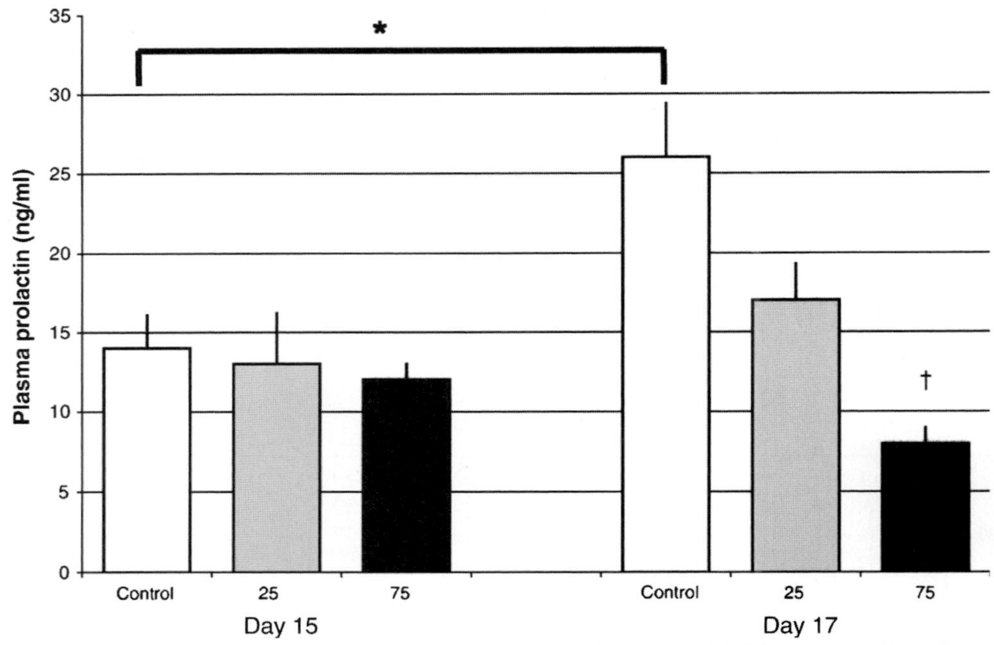

FIGURE 43.3 Plasma prolactin (mean ± SEM) in untreated controls and animals exposed to 25 or 75 μg B(a)P/m^3 from gestation days 8 through 17 (Archibong *et al.*, 2002). Plasma prolactin was taken as an indirect measure of decidual luteotropin. (*) $P < 0.05$ GD 15 vs. GD 17 controls. (†) $P < 0.05$ compared to respective control. $n = 10$ per group.

Detmar *et al.* (2006) also have shown that chronic exposure of mice to PAHs prior to conception resulted in a greater number of resorptions. The foregone data have led these authors to conclude that exposure of embryos at early stages of development to PAHs reduces the allocation of cells to embryonic and placental lineage by inducing the proapoptotic gene, Bax, and therefore reducing the ability of embryos to develop.

Effect of benzo(a)pyrene-induced reduction in estrogen synthesis on puberty, reproductive tract function and menopause

The sexual maturation and growth of the female (vagina, uterus, oviduct, secondary sexual characteristics, breast stromal and ductal development, accelerated bone growth phase and closure of the epiphysis of long bones, growth of ancillary hair and pubic hair, alteration of body fat to produce typical female contours, pigmentation nipples, areolae and the genital area) are under estrogen regulation. Hence a B(a)P-induced reduction of estrogen secretion at puberty when sexual maturation and growth are expected to occur could delay these processes. Furthermore, in addition to the growth effects estrogen has on the uterine and oviductal musculature, it plays a major role in the development of the endometrial lining. Consequently, B(a)P-induced reduction in estrogen secretion can compromise the ability of the uterus (Khorram *et al.*, 2010) and oviduct to facilitate spermatozoa and mature ovum transport to the site of fertilization (oviduct) and subsequent implantation in the uterus (Cooper and Moley, 2008). Because of the near universally accepted theory that oocytes are endowed as a fixed and non-renewing stockpile at birth (Zuckerman and Baker, 1977), pathologic destruction of oocytes has been viewed as irreversible. This being the case, the destruction of oocytes by B(a)P (Mattison *et al.*, 1980) especially via cigarette smoke can lead to early age at menopause with the attendant vasomotor reflexes and vaginal dryness and atrophy due the absence of follicular estrogen production.

Published reports suggest that PAHs interact with the ER α and β signaling pathways in a variety of test systems (Tran *et al.*, 1996; Arcaro *et al.*, 1999; Fertuck *et al.*, 2001) interfering with estrogen signaling in important reproductive processes. Exposure to PAHs has been shown to suppress estrogen response element-controlled gene expression, increase estradiol metabolism and downregulate ERα levels (reviewed in Safe, 2001).

Using fish tissues, *in vitro* studies conducted by Rochas-Montiero *et al.* (2000) revealed that at 15 μM concentration, PAHs such as B(a)P, phenanthrene and chrysene inhibited androstenedione secretion by 50% and E_2 synthesis from 10 to 40%. Furthermore, these authors also observed a significant reduction in the concentrations of conjugated E_2 metabolites in conditioned media, clearly indicating that PAH action in ovary is mediated mainly by the inhibition of steroidogenic enzymes. It is noteworthy that B(a)P's action on the steroidogenic activities in the ovary is not limited to inhibition of estrogen production. It also enhances the clearance of circulating estrogens. Induction of CYP1A1 in porcine ovarian granulosa cells by 3-MC indicates that PAHs may decrease plasma estrogens by enhancing their clearance, through CYP1A1 induction (Leighton *et al.*, 1995). The P450 isoforms CYP1A1, CYP1A2 and CYP1B1 are involved in PAH biotransformation (reviewed in Ramesh *et al.*, 2004a). Induction of P450s by PAHs also may lead to an increased metabolism of estrogens as the same P450 isoforms are involved in estrogen catabolism. For example, estrogens are metabolized by CYP1A1, CYP1B1, CYP3A4 and CYP3A7 to catechol estrogens. The catechols undergo metabolic redox cycling to generate free radicals such as reactive quinone/semiquinone intermediates (reviewed in Jefcoate *et al.*, 2000). These metabolic intermediates initiate toxicity. Therefore, it can be concluded that the repression of estrogen biosynthesis and enhanced metabolism of E_2 by B(a)P can result in the reduction of the circulating concentrations of this ovarian steroid below physiological threshold essential for maintaining bone and reproductive health.

Even though the toxicity of B(a)P on various organ systems has been established, not much information is available on their effects on the bone. It was reported that in exposed animals, B(a)P and DMBA were bioavailable in the bone marrow and induced cytotoxicity (Page *et al.*, 2004; Galvan *et al.*, 2005). The PAH compound 3-MC was reported to inhibit the proliferation and differentiation of osteoblasts (Naruse *et al.*, 2002). Investigations by Naruse *et al.* (2004) also revealed that 3-MC affects osteoclast supporting cells. Consistent with the findings of Naruse *et al.* (2002, 2004), Voronov *et al.* (2005) observed that B(a)P inhibits rabbit osteoclast differentiation. Using *in vitro* systems, Tsai *et al.* (2004) reported that B(a)P induces osteoblast proliferation through estrogen receptor-related cyclooxygenase-2 (COX-2) mechanisms.

To date, only two studies document an association between bone damage and PAH exposure *in vivo*. Exposure to 3-MC was found to cause a delay in the ossification of the forelimb, hindlimb, cervical and thoracic vertebrae in fetal mice (Naruse *et al.*, 2002). Also, exposure to B(a)P resulted in a loss of bone mass and bone strength in ovariectomized adult rats (Lee *et al.*, 2002). Thus, there is a clear data gap in the knowledge regarding the mechanisms of bone damage caused by PAHs in an *in vivo* model.

Effect of benzo(a)pyrene on male reproduction/fertility

The hazardous effects of B(a)P on human male reproduction have been extrapolated from sources that contain other contaminants that can adversely alter male fertility (Table 43.2). The commonest source of environmental B(a)P exposure is cigarette smoke because non-smokers can be exposed indirectly via side stream exposure. Experimental studies show that whole animal exposure to cigarette smoke or exposure of human spermatozoa to cotinine (the metabolite of a component of cigarette smoke, nicotine) *in vitro* can decrease the percentage of motile and viable spermatozoa and the ability

TABLE 43.2 Environmental sources of B(a)P and consequence on male fertility

Source of B(a)P	Effects	References
Cigarette smoke	Sperm count among smokers average about 13–17% lower than non-smokers	Vine *et al.* (1994)
Cigarette smoke	Smoking cessation improved sperm counts 50–800%, suggesting that toxic chemicals in the smoke are responsible and any reduction in sperm count is reversible	Vine *et al.* (1994)
Cigarette smoke	Cigarette smoking significantly decreases seminal plasma ascorbic acid sperm count, motility and normal morphology vs. their control counterparts	Mostafa *et al.* (2006)
Coke oven industry	Male coke oven workers have an increase in sperm morphological abnormalities (32.3%) vs. controls (14.6%), thereby suggesting a mutagenic effect	Hsu *et al.* (2006)
Diesel polluted air	Diesel fumes decrease motility and sperm counts in exposed men	Guven *et al.* (2008)

of these male gametes to penetrate the mature ova (Kapawa *et al.*, 2004; Sofikitis *et al.*, 2008). It is very difficult to isolate the effect of B(a)P in cigarette smoke from other hazardous chemicals in this source of B(a)P on male fertility inasmuch as cigarette smoke contains approximately 4,000 toxic chemicals including nicotine, nitroso compounds, aromatic amines, protein pyrolysates and polycyclic aromatic hydrocarbons (PAHs; Lodovici *et al.*, 2004). Only a few of these have been studied for their effects on the male reproductive system (Zenzes, 2000). Exposure of adult male rats to subacute (10 consecutive days) oral B(a)P (50 mg/kg/day) causes a reduction in testis weight, and an induction of pyknosis and necrobiotic changes as well as chromatolysis in the nuclei of spermatocytes (Arafa *et al.*, 2009). Under this regimen of exposure, epididymal function deteriorates as exemplified by decreases in cauda epididymal (stored) sperm density and motility (Arafa *et al.*, 2009).

Exposure of Wistar rats to oral B(a)P for 14, 28 and 90 days resulted in a reduction in sperm density, viability and percentage of motile spermatozoa (Paltanaviciene *et al.*, 2006). Subchronic exposure of F-344 rats to oral doses of 15, 30 and 60 μg PAH-loaded airborne particulates/L caused a significant reduction in daily sperm production and sperm motility (Jeng and Yu, 2008). Similarly, Sprague-Dawley rats exposed orally for 30 days to organic extracts of river water heavily contaminated by PAHs, at doses of 2, 16 and 80 L/kg body weight had pathological damage to testicular tissue, followed concomitantly by decreased testosterone concentrations and the production of abnormal morphologic forms of spermatozoa (Cao *et al.*, 2009). Furthermore, exposure of adult F-344 rats to inhaled B(a)P at an exposure concentration of 75 μg/cm^3, which is within the legally enforceable limit of 100 μg/m^3 recommended by the OSHA, alters fertility indices in the exposed animals (Inyang *et al.*, 2003). Even though testis weight and stored sperm density were not affected by subacute inhaled B(a)P, testosterone synthesis and release and the ability of the epididymis to impart motility to spermatozoa (based on reduced stored sperm progressive motility) were impaired (Inyang *et al.*, 2003). However, exposure of adult F-344 male rats to subchronic (60 days) B(a)P via inhalation at the exposure concentration used in the study by Inyang *et al.* (2003) revealed that whatever adverse effect B(a)P has on fertility is not mediated by lack of thrift based on similar trend of weekly weight gain (Ramesh *et al.*, 2008; Figure 43.4). This subchronic exposure of rats to B(a)P significantly altered some testis morphometric data (Table 43.3). According to data generated by Ramesh *et al.* (2008) inhaled B(a)P reduced testis weight by approximately 34% compared with controls. In this study, B(a)P did not affect seminiferous tubular diameter and percentage of these tubules exhibiting elongated spermatids. It was further observed (Ramesh *et al.*, 2008) that inhaled B(a)P significantly reduced total seminiferous tubular volume, total weight of seminiferous tubules and total seminiferous tubular length per paired testes compared with those of their control counterparts. Other morphometric data reduced by B(a)P include total volume and total weight of interstitium (approximately 12% reduction) per paired testes compared with those of rats in the control group (Ramesh *et al.*, 2008). Some of the pathological changes imposed by B(a)P on the testis are depicted in the photomicrographs of B(a)P and control hematoxylin–eosin-stained testis histologies (Figure 43.5).

Present in the testis, lung and liver tissues are inducible and constitutive enzymes CYP1A1 and CYP1B1, necessary

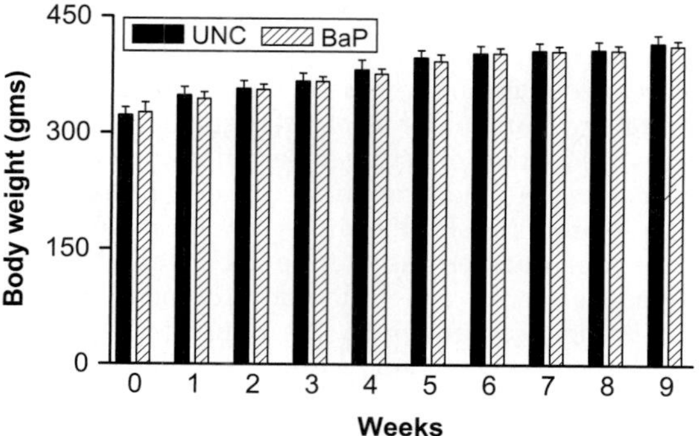

FIGURE 43.4 Weekly weight profile of control and B(a)P-exposed male rats. From Ramesh *et al.*, 2008.

TABLE 43.3 Morphometric analysis of testicular parameters in rats inhalationally exposed to 75 μg B(a)P/m^3 B(a)P

Parameter	Control	B(a)P exposed
Testis weight (g/paired testis)	3.0 ± 0.16	2.0 ± 0.11*1
Tubule diameter (μm)	250 ± 8.5	230 ± 8.2*2
Tubules with elongated spermatids (%)	99 ± 1.0	99 ± 1.0
Tubular volume (×10^9 μm^3)	2.0 ± 0.7	1.6 ± 0.004*3
Total weight of tubules (g)	2.20 ± 0.7	1.6 ± 0.004
Total tubular length (μm)	55 ± 1.0	33 ± 1.0*5
Total volume of interstitium per paired testis (μm^3)	0.43 ± 0.01	0.38 ± 0.01
Total weight of interstitium per paired testis (g)	0.45 ± 0.01	0.37 ± 0.01*4

*1 $p < 0.025$
*2 $p < 0.09$
*3 $p < 0.002$
*4 $p < 0.05$
*5 $p < 0.01$

for the metabolism of B(a)P to reactive metabolites. Ramesh *et al.* (2008) indicated that inhaled B(a)P elevates the concentrations of B(a)P reactive metabolites of toxicological interest ([7,8-dihydrodiol; precursor for 7,8-diol 9,10-epoxide] and 3,6-dione) in testicular, liver and lung tissues relative to the aforementioned tissues recovered from control rats. Furthermore, aryl hydrocarbon hydroxylase (AHH, a marker for CYP1A1 and CYP1B1 enzymatic activity (Ou and Ramos, 1992)) activity increases in testicular, liver and lung tissues recovered from B(a)P-exposed rats compared with that measured in corresponding tissues from control rats (Table 43.3). These metabolizing enzymes are aryl hydrocarbon receptor (AhR) and the AhR nuclear translocator (ARNT) complex regulated (Nebert *et al.*, 2000). A recent study by Deb *et al.* (2010) reported that B(a)P failed to induce CYP1B1 expression at oral doses of 10, 25, 50, 100 or 200 mg/kg body weight. Whether AhR expression protein blocks the induction of CYP1B1 by B(a)P or whether hormonal pathway supersedes AhR pathway in the regulation of testicular CYP1B1 in the B(a)P-exposed animals mentioned above is open for speculation. The aforementioned B(a)P reactive metabolites ultimately produce reactive oxygen species (ROS; Senft *et al.*, 2002) enough to overwhelm the antioxidant defense system. Hence the reduction in testicular lactate dehydrogenase (LDH-X), superoxide dismutase (SOD) and glutathione-S-transferase (GST) activity as well

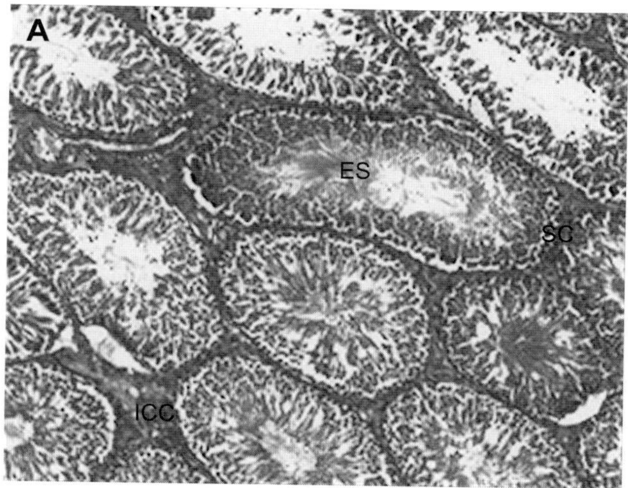

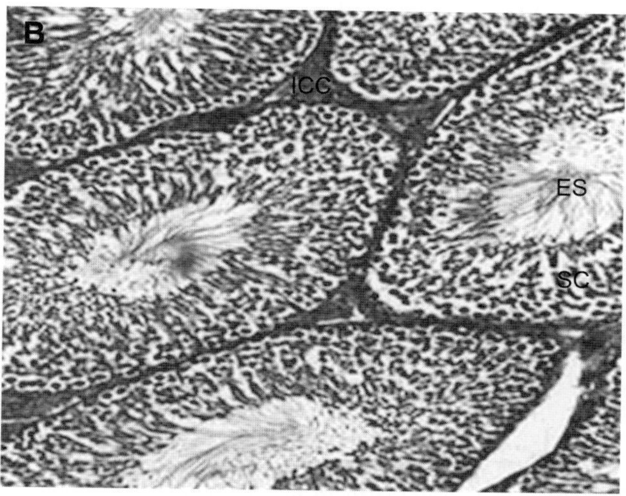

FIGURE 43.5 Photomicrographs of testes histologies from (A) unexposed control F-344 rat; (B) F-344 rat exposed to subchronic concentration of 75 μg benzo(a)pyrene/m^3 (Ramesh *et al.*, 2008). Magnification bar = 250 μm; ICC = interstitial cell compartment; ES = elongated spermatids; SC = Sertoli cells. Though the seminiferous tubules appear qualitatively similar, the size of tubular lumens and length decreased in B(a)P-exposed rats, compared with controls. This indicates a reduction in spermatogenic activity and loss of fluid in the seminiferous tubules due to decreased testosterone production, thus the decreased testis size.

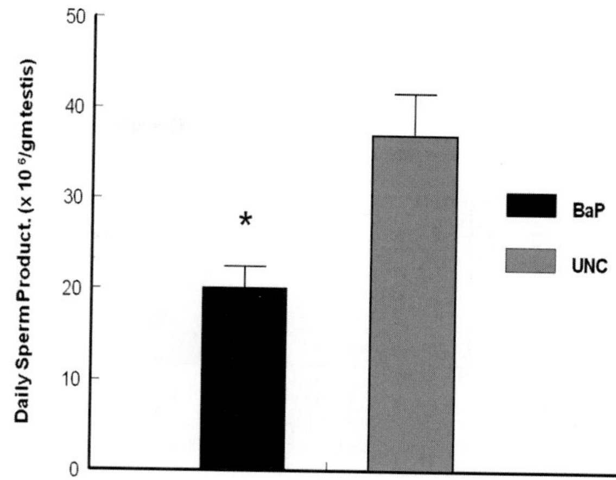

FIGURE 43.6 Effect of inhaled B(a)P on daily sperm production per gram of testis in F-344 male rats exposed to subchronic exposure concentrations of 75 μg B(a)P/m^3 (Archibong *et al.*, 2008); $n = 10$ per treatment or control group. Results are expressed as mean ± SE (UNC = unexposed control; B(a)P = B(a)P-inhaled rats. Asterisks indicate a significant difference from controls ($P < 0.05$).

TABLE 43.4 Sperm characteristics in rats inhalationally exposed to 75 μg B(a)P/m^3 B(a)P (Ramesh *et al.*, 2008)

Characteristic	Control	B(a)P treated
Sperm progressive motility (%)	85 ± 5.0	23 ± 2.0*1
Density of stored spermatozoa (×10^6)	81 ± 4.0	25 ± 6.0*1
Morphologically normal sperm (%)	67 ± 4.0	13 ± 3.9*2
Decapitated spermatozoa (%)	7.2 ± 2.3	60 ± 11*3
Sperm with abnormal tail (%)	26 ± 3.0	28 ± 7.0

*1 $p < 0.05$
*2 $p < 0.001$
*3 $p < 0.01$

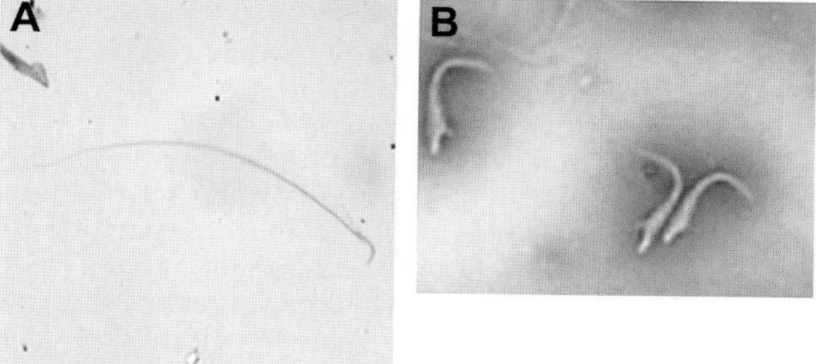

FIGURE 43.7 Photomicrograph showing (A) a normal spermatozoan taken from unexposed F-344 rat; (B) spermatozoa with decapitated heads taken from an F-344 rat exposed to subchronic exposure concentration of 75 μg benzo(a) pyrene/m^3. From Ramesh *et al.*, 2008.

as intratesticular reduced glutathione (GSH) accompanied by increased testicular malondialdehyde (MDA) contents (Arafa *et al.*, 2009).

Benzo(a)pyrene-exposed animals produce fewer intratesticular spermatozoa (Figure 43.6), percentage of progressively motile stored spermatozoa, stored sperm density and morphologically normal spermatozoa than their control counterparts (Archibong *et al.*, 2008; Ramesh *et al.*, 2008; Table 43.4). Mostly, the prevalent abnormal morphologic form of spermatozoa present in the cauda epididymides of rats exposed to B(a)P compared with those of control rats (Table 43.4) is decapitated spermatozoa (Figure 43.7).

Fertility indices described above and the functioning of the male reproductive system in general are regulated by testosterone whose synthesis and release by the testis is repressed by B(a)P (Figure 43.8). The mechanism by which B(a)P perturbs testosterone synthesis and release is linked to ROS-induced oxidative aging of the Leydig cells (Mandal *et al.*, 2001; Senft *et al.*, 2002). Data generated by Peltola *et al.* (1996) indicate that ROS can damage critical components of the steroidogenic pathway in the Leydig cells, including steroidogenic acute regulatory (StAR) protein (Diemer *et al.*, 2003) and consequently the repression of testosterone synthesis. It is apparent from the data generated by Ramesh *et al.* (2008) and Archibong *et al.* (2008) that B(a)P-induced

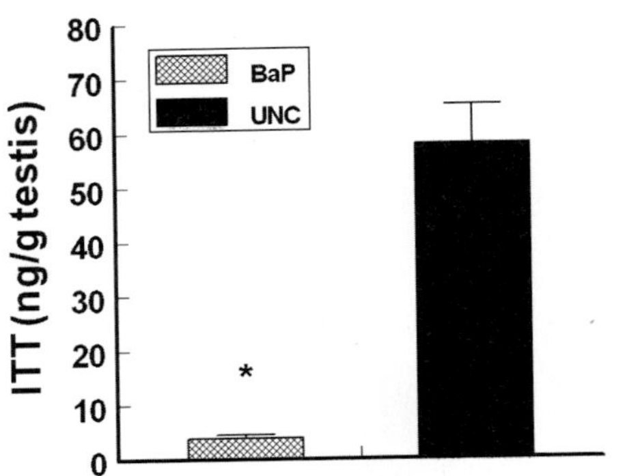

FIGURE 43.8 Effect of inhaled B(a)P on intratesticular testosterone concentrations in F-344 male rats exposed to subchronic exposure concentrations of 75 µg BaP/m^3; $n=10$ per treatment or control group (Archibong *et al.*, 2008). Results are expressed as mean ± SE (UNC = unexposed control; BaP = B(a) P-inhaled rats. Asterisks indicate a significant difference from controls ($P<0.05$).

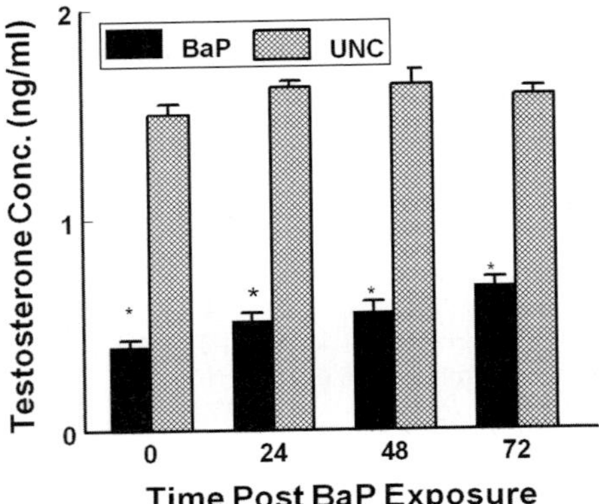

FIGURE 43.9 Effect of inhaled B(a)P on plasma testosterone concentrations in F-344 male rats exposed to subchronic exposure concentrations of 75 µg B(a) P/m^3; $n=10$ per treatment or control group (Archibong *et al.*, 2008). Results are expressed as mean ± SE (UNC = unexposed control; BaP = B(a)P-inhaled rats). Asterisks indicate a significant difference from controls ($P<0.05$).

reduction in testosterone secretion is not based on a direct effect of this PAH on the anterior pituitary. Data from these studies indicate that B(a)P exposure significantly reduced plasma testosterone concentrations on the last day of exposures (day 60) and at 24, 48 and 72 hours later compared with controls (Figure 43.9). However, LH concentrations in plasma samples of B(a)P-exposed rats were significantly elevated throughout the above-mentioned four time periods studied compared with controls.

Spermatogenesis in an adult mammal is regulated and maintained by testosterone, the reduction of which could decrease spermatogenesis. We observed a significant reduction in daily sperm production (DSP) per gram of testicular tissue in B(a)P-exposed rats compared with their control counterparts (Archibong *et al.*, 2008), probably due to B(a) P-induced reduction in intratesticular testosterone secretion and/or dysfunction of exposed Sertoli cells. Raychoudhury and Kubinski (2003) reported that *in vitro* exposure of isolated rat Sertoli cells to B(a)P resulted in cellular changes characteristic of apoptosis. Sertoli cells initiate, support, maintain and regulate spermatogenesis in mammals by (1) providing a structural and functional barrier that regulates the movement of extratubular blood-borne components into the seminiferous tubular environment; (2) synthesizing and secreting various nutrients utilized by developing germ cells; and (3) synthesizing and secreting paracrine mediators proposed to be involved in the regulation of spermatogenesis (Ku and Chapin, 1993). Thus, the reduced DSP per gram testis observed in our study (Archibong *et al.*, 2008) may have been due to reduced spermatogenesis resulting from B(a) P-induced reduction in ITT (Archibong *et al.*, 2008) and/or DNA damage and apoptosis in Sertoli cells (Revel *et al.*, 2001; Raychoudhury and Kubinski, 2003). The consequences of B(a)P-induced reduction in testosterone secretion, apart from the reduction in spermatogenesis, include perturbation of epididymal sperm maturation, compromised functions of the prostate gland, seminal vesicles, bulbo-urethral gland and erectile dysfunction.

Ejaculated spermatozoa have to undergo further maturational changes in the female reproductive tract; a dictum referred to as "capacitation" and characterized by hyperactive patterns of motility. The failure of mature spermatozoa to capacitate normally results in failed fertilization of mature ova. Benzo(a)pyrene has been reported to affect important motion characteristics of spermatozoa such as hyperactivation as well as premature acrosome reaction (Mukhopadhyay *et al.*, 2010) in human sperm samples, which caregivers are to be aware of when counseling occupationally exposed workers suffering from idiopathic male infertility. A correlation between urinary concentrations of PAH metabolites and increased idiopathic male infertility was reported by Xia *et al.* (2009). The presence of AhR and ARNT in spermatozoa (Khorram *et al.*, 2004) suggest that exposure to PAHs stimulate the AhR that in turn increase the metabolism of PAHs to reactive metabolites that can influence sperm function. Microarray analysis and Q-PCR studies also have shown that mRNA of CYP1A1 and CYP1B1 are detectable in spermatozoa (Linschooten *et al.*, 2009) confirming the ability of germ cells to produce these CYP enzymes to metabolize environmental toxicants such as PAHs.

Polycyclic aromatic hydrocarbon-induced DNA damage in reproductive tissues

One of the mechanisms through which PAHs cause toxicity/cancer is through binding with nucleophilic sites of cellular macromolecules such as proteins, and nucleic acids (Ramesh and Knuckles, 2006) interfere with the organ function and as a consequence cause reproductive failure. Deoxyribonucleic acid damage occurring in target reproductive tissues can be of value as a biomarker of PAH exposure. Bulky PAH-DNA adducts serve as biomarkers of biologically effective dose of PAH exposure whose persistence is dependent on metabolism and DNA repair factors (Perera and Weinstein, 2000). On the other hand, oxidative DNA lesions induced by PAHs can also be used as biomarkers of effect; however, these biomarkers are not specific and are likely to be influenced by endogenous and exogenous factors (Mangal *et al.*, 2009; Tarantini *et al.*, 2009).

Polyaromatic hydrocarbons have been known to cause DNA damage both in laboratory animals and humans. Benzo(a)pyrene causes DNA adduct formation in exposed spermatozoa and testicular tissues of mice and rats, respectively (Revel *et al.*, 2001; Ramesh *et al.*, 2004b). A recent study by Verhofstad *et al.* (2010) indicates that a single oral exposure to 13 mg B(a)P/kg body weight causes DNA adducts to persist up to 42 days in spermatozoa and other testicular tissues of mice post-B(a)P exposure. The adduct persistence was found to be remarkably high in DNA repair deficient mice (xpc (-1-)) compared to their wild-type counterparts.

In addition to laboratory animal studies, human studies also yielded interesting results. Zenzes and coworkers (1999a) were the first team to report B(a)P-DNA adducts in the spermatozoa of smokers. This team (Zenzes *et al.*, 1999b) also detected B(a)P-DNA adducts in preimplantation embryos derived from the fertilization of a non-smoker's mature ova with spermatozoa from a smoking father. These studies bring forth an interesting argument that developmental problems found in children are male mediated. Subsequent studies stress that paternal transmission of DNA modified upon exposure to chemical carcinogens will have profound multigenerational effects. In *in vitro* studies, B(a)P has been shown to cause DNA strand breaks in human spermatozoa (Russo *et al.*, 2006). Polyaromatic hydrocarbon-DNA adduct concentrations in human spermatozoa were used as a biomarker for DNA damage. Samples collected from an infertility clinic in Italy revealed a significant relationship between PAH-DNA adduct concentrations in spermatozoa and occupational exposure to PAHs (Gaspari *et al.*, 2003). Hsu *et al.* (2006) reported a relationship between PAH exposure and sperm DNA damage in coke oven workers. The small sample size notwithstanding, these studies indicate the possibility that PAHs may impact the integrity of DNA in spermatozoa. Similarly, Singh *et al.* (2007) documented oxidative damage to DNA and DNA adducts in blood samples of people exposed to PAHs through inhalation of polluted air. Sperm samples collected from infertile men showed a correlation between PAH exposure (assessed by urinary PAH metabolites) and sperm DNA damage (Ji *et al.*, 2010). Interestingly, some of these patients who were presumed to have been exposed to PAHs also showed a polymorphism in the X-ray repair cross complementing group 1 (XRCC1) gene involved in base excision repair of DNA. The combined effect of XRCC1 polymorphisms and PAH exposure seem to exacerbate the damage to DNA of spermatozoa in these patients. In this context, it is imperative to mention the studies conducted earlier in the Czech Republic wherein men exposed to polluted air rich in PAHs showed abnormal chromatin/fragmented DNA in spermatozoa (Rubes *et al.*, 2007). These men were found to carry a homozygous null glutathione-S-transferase 1 (GSTM1) gene. Also, a statistically significant relationship was observed between GSTM1 null genotype and increased DNA fragmentation index in these individuals. Studies conducted by Paracchini *et al.* (2005) on infertile men in Italy also exhibited the same trend observed by Rubes *et al.* (2007) with regard to GSTM1 deficiency. The GSTM1 deletions in these men showed a significant increase in PAH-DNA adduct concentrations in spermatozoa. The above-mentioned studies document key pieces of evidence for the presence of gene–environment interaction in PAH-induced toxicity of the male reproductive system.

Some studies (Linschooten *et al.*, 2009) advocate using mRNA profiles of spermatozoa as indicators of the processes that may have occurred in the testis after exposure to environmental toxicants. Since mRNA along with DNA in spermatozoa is transferred to oocytes during fertilization (Ostermeier *et al.*, 2004), it has a high potential to play a key role during embryogenesis (Krawetz, 2005). These studies highlight the possibility of using gene expression profiles in spermatozoa to unravel gene–environment interactions in relation to male infertility.

Although information available on B(a)P-induced DNA damage in the ovary has not received as much attention as the testis, their protracted residence in ovaries from the standpoint of damage to gametes cannot be overlooked. Ramesh *et al.* (2010) studied the persistence of B(a)P-DNA adducts in ovary of F-344 rats 1, 7, 14, 21 and 28 days post-exposure to a single acute oral dose of 5 mg of B(a)P/kg body weight. The B(a)P-DNA adducts concentrations in this reproductive organ showed an insignificant decline from day 1 to day 7 and showed a gradual decline thereafter until 28 days (Figure 43.10). Carrier lipoproteins were demonstrated to react with B(a)P and sequester this toxicant in blood at high doses (Grova *et al.*, 2009). The sequestered B(a)P was found to be redistributed and repartitioned into target tissues, altering the bioavailability of this chemical. Our supposition is that a slow release of B(a)P from lipid-rich tissues may have taken place followed by an uptake by the ovary. Ramesh *et al.* (2010) also observed a concordance between B(a)P reactive metabolite concentrations and adduct concentrations.

The connection between B(a)P metabolism and adduct formation is revealed by the studies of Buters *et al.* (2003). These authors administered 20 μg/day of dimethylbenz(a) anthracene to wild-type and CYP1B1 null mice. Wild-type mice had more hyperplasias and DMBA-DNA adducts in ovary than the CYP1B1-null mice. It is well established that CYP1B1 is the predominant PAH biotransformation enzyme in the reproductive organs (Guengerich *et al.*, 2003). Quite naturally, the wild-type mice are more likely to develop ovarian tumors as this enzyme metabolizes DMBA to carcinogenic metabolites.

Taken together, the findings of Buters *et al.* (2003) and Ramesh *et al.* (2010) indicate that the bioavailability of reactive metabolites determines the extent of their binding to DNA and consequently the formation and persistence of adducts. The latter statement is in agreement with the observation that tissue DNA acts as the internal trapping agent for reactive metabolites (Ginsberg and Atherholt, 1989; Garg *et al.*, 1993) produced in post-exposure liver and reproductive organs. Such delayed clearance of B(a)P metabolites

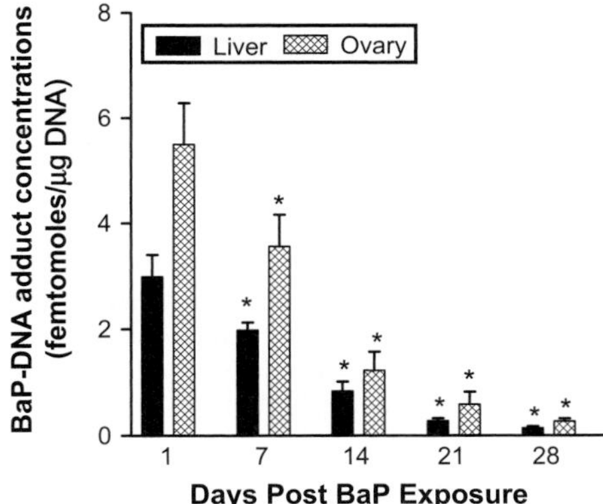

FIGURE 43.10 Time-course distribution (persistence) of B(a)P-DNA adducts in ovaries and liver of F-344 rats that received B(a)P via oral gavage (Ramesh *et al.*, 2010). Asterisks denote statistical significance ($p<0.05$) in B(a)P-DNA adduct concentrations at various post-exposure time-points in ovary or liver compared to day 1 post-exposure time-point. DNA was extracted from these samples, B(a)P-derived adducts were ^{32}P post-labeled, and TLC was performed as described in the materials and methods section. Films were exposed for 24 hours at −80ºC. Values represent mean ± SE ($n=6$). Asterisks denote statistical significance ($p<0.05$) at the respective time-point compared to day 1 post-exposure.

and DNA adducts (60 day persistence post-B(a)P exposures) from extrahepatic tissues were also recorded in AhR wild-type mice treated orally with a single dose of 100 mg/kg B(a)P (Sagredo *et al.*, 2009). A single oral dose of 10 mg/kg B(a)P generated B(a)P-DNA adduct concentrations in extrahepatic tissues of Lewis rats that were sustainable for 20 days post-exposure (Godschalk *et al.*, 2000).

If a single acute exposure to a high dose of B(a)P could sustain reactive metabolites and adducts up to a month after exposure (Ramesh *et al.*, 2010), the likelihood of the damage caused in subacute (short-term) and subchronic (long-term) exposures in human is of concern from the standpoint of toxicity and carcinogenesis. Evidence subscribing to this viewpoint is furnished by the studies of Zenzes *et al.* (1998) who reported the presence of B(a)P-DNA adducts in granulosa cells and oocytes of female cigarette smokers. Cigarette smoke is a rich source of PAHs that puts these women at an increased risk as transmission of altered DNA to preimplantation embryos increases the likelihood of contributing to childhood cancers.

Human ovarian tissue samples collected from hospitals also showed the presence of B(a)P-DNA adducts (Shamsuddin and Gan, 1988), an indication that mature ova from the sample donors could carry defective genes that may or may not express themselves during intra-uterine residence but could do so postpartum. Besides the ovary, B(a)P metabolites have also been reported to exert an inhibitory effect on human cervical cells by enhancing cell death (Rorke *et al.*, 1998) and B(a)P-DNA adduct formation (Melikian *et al.*, 1999).

CONCLUDING REMARKS AND FUTURE DIRECTIONS

This chapter raises the awareness that exposure to B(a)P contributes to the declining fertility in men and women due to declining sperm production and altered endocrine regulated events that lead to gamete maturation. The adverse effects of this endocrine disruptor on reproduction will not abate inasmuch as exposures of men and women to this xenobiotic continue. It is important, therefore, for healthcare givers to advise patients during infertility counseling sessions, to curtail exposures to B(a)P in order to reduce the risk to infertility, should the patients fall within the "at risk" category for B(a)P exposure. This "at risk" category includes smokers; workers in coke oven, coal tar, distillery, iron foundry, aluminum, bitumen, creosote and carbon electrode manufacturing industries and thermo-electric power plants; roofers; ship builders; painters; fire fighters; auto and aircraft mechanics; incineration plant workers; restaurant cooks; and individuals that live near hazardous waste sites.

REFERENCES

Abbott BD, Probst MR (1995) Developmental expression of two members of a new class of transcription factors: II. Expression of aryl hydrocarbon receptor nuclear translocator in the C57BL/6N mouse embryo. *Dev Dyn* **204:** 144–55.

Abbott BD, Probst MR, Perdew GH (1994) Immunohistochemical double-staining for Ah receptor and ARNT in human embryonic palatal shelves. *Teratology* **50:** 361–6.

Andres RL, Day MC (2000) Perinatal complications associated with maternal tobacco use. *Semin Neonatol* **5:** 231–41.

Arafa HMM, Aly HAA, Abd-Elloah MF, El-Refaey HM (2009) Hesperidin attenuates benzo[α]pyrene-induced testicular toxicity in rats via regulation of oxidant/antioxidant balance. *Toxicol Ind Hlth* **25:** 417–27.

Arcaro KF, O'Keefe PW, Yang Y, Clayton W, Gierthy JF (1999) Antiestrogenicity of environmental polycyclic aromatic hydrocarbons in human breast cancer cells. *Toxicology* **133:** 115–27.

Archibong AE, Inyang F, Ramesh A, Greenwood M, Nayyar T, Kopsombut P, Hood DB, Nyanda AM (2002) Alteration of pregnancy related hormones and fetal survival in F-344 rats exposed by inhalation to benzo(a)pyrene. *Reprod Toxicol* **16:** 801–8.

Archibong AE, Ramesh A, Niaz MS, Brooks CM, Roberson SI, Lunstra DD (2008) Effects of benzo(a)pyrene on intratesticular function in F-344 rats. *Int J Environ Res Public Health* **5:** 32–40.

ATSDR (1995) Toxicological profile for polycyclic aromatic hydrocarbons (PAHs). Agency for Toxic Substances and Disease Registry, US Department of Health and Human Services, US Public Health Service, Atlanta, GA, 271 pp.

Beg AA, Sha WC, Bronson RT, Ghosh S, Baltimore D (1995) Embryonic lethality and liver degeneration in mice lacking the RelA component of NF-kappa B. *Nature* **376:** 167–70.

Birnbaum LS (1994) The mechanism of dioxin toxicity: relationship to risk assessment. *Environ Health Perspect* **102:** 157–67.

Birnbaum LS (1996) Developmental effects of dioxins and related endocrine disrupting chemicals. *Toxicol Lett* **83:** 743–50.

Borman SM, Christian PJ, Sipes IG, Hoyer PB (2000) Ovotoxicity in female Fischer rats and B6 mice induced by low-dose exposure to three polycyclic aromatic hydrocarbons: comparison through calculation of an ovotoxic index. *Toxicol Appl Pharmacol* **167:** 191–8.

Buesen R, Mock M, Seidel A, Jacob J, Lampen A (2002) Interaction between metabolism and transport of benzo[a]pyrene and its metabolites in enterocytes. *Toxicol Appl Pharmacol* **183:** 168–78.

Buters J, Quintanilla-Martinez L, Schober W, Soballa VJ, Hintermair J, Wolff T, Gonzalez FJ, Greim H (2003) CYP1B1 determines susceptibility to low doses of 7,12-dimethylbenz(a)anthracene-induced ovarian cancers. *Carcinogenesis* **24:** 327–34.

Butler JP, Post GB, Lioy PJ, Waldman JM, Greenberg A (1993) Assessment of carcinogenic risk from personal exposure to benzo(a)pyrene in the total human environmental exposure study (THEES). *J Air Waste Manage Assoc* **43:** 970–7.

Cao B, Ren Q, Cui Z, Li P, Cao J (2009) Evaluation of reproductive toxicity in rats caused by inorganic extracts of Jiangling river water of Chonging, China. *Environ Toxicol Pharmacol* **27:** 357–65.

Carver LA, Hogenesch JB, Bradfield CA (1994) Tissue specific expression of the rat Ah-receptor and ARNT mRNAs. *Nucleic Acids Res* **22:** 3038–44.

Chaloupka K, Krishnan V, Safe S (1992) Polynuclear aromatic hydrocarbon carcinogens as antiestrogens in MCF-7 human breast cancer cells: role of the Ah receptor. *Carcinogenesis* **13:** 2233–9.

Charles GD, Bartels MJ, Zacharewski TR, Gollapudi BB, Freshour NL, Carney EW (2000) Activity of benzo(a)pyrene and its hydroxylated metabolite in an estrogen receptor-α reporter gene assay. *Tox Sci* **55:** 320–6.

Cheshenko K, Pakdel F, Segner H, Kah O, Eggen RI (2008) Interference of endocrine disrupting chemicals with aromatase CYP19 expression or activity, and consequences for reproduction of teleost fish. *Gen Comp Endocrinol* **155:** 31–62.

Cooper AR, Moley KH (2008) Maternal tobacco use and its preimplantation effects on fertility: more reasons to stop smoking. *Semin Reprod Med* **26:** 204–12.

Deb S, Kawai M, Chang TKH, Bandiera SM (2010) Effect of aryl hydrocarbon receptor agonists on CYP1B1 expression in rat testis and Leydig cells. *Xenobiotica*. In press.

Detmar J, Rabaglino T, Taniuchi Y, Oh J, Acton BM, Benito A, Nunez G, Jurisicova A (2006) Embryonic loss due to exposure to polycyclic aromatic hydrocarbons is mediated by Bax. *Apoptosis* **11:** 1413–25.

Dey A, Jones JE, Nebert DW (1999) Tissue- and cell type-specific expression of cytochrome P450 1A1 and cytochrome P450 1A2 mRNA in the mouse localized by in situ hybridization. *Biochem Pharmacol* **58:** 525–37.

Diemer T, Allen JA, Hales KH, Hales DB (2003) Reactive oxygen disrupts mitochondria in MA-10 tumor Leydig cells and inhibits steroidogenic acute regulatory (StAR) protein and steroidogenesis. *Endocrinology* **144:** 2882–91.

Dolwick KM, Schmidt JV, Carver LA, Swanson HI, Bradfield CA (1993) Cloning and expression of a human Ah receptor cDNA. *Mol Pharmacol* **44:** 911–17.

Dong W, Wang L, Thornton C, Scheffler BE, Willett KL (2008) Benzo(a)pyrene decreases brain and ovarian aromatase mRNA expression in *Fundulus heteroclitus*. *Aquat Toxicol* **88:** 289–300.

Farin FM, Omiecinski CJ (1993) Regiospecific expression of cytochromes P-450 and microsomal epoxide hydrolase in human brain tissue. *J Toxicol Environ Health* **40:** 317–35.

Fernandez-Salguero P, Pineau T, Hilbert DM, McPhail T, Lee SS, Kimura S, Nebert DW, Rudikoff S, Ward JM, Gonzalez FJ (1995) Immune system impairment and hepatic fibrosis in mice lacking the dioxin-binding Ah receptor. *Science* **268:** 722–6.

Fertuck KC, Matthews JB, Zacharewski TR (2001) Hydroxylated benzo(a) pyrene metabolites are responsible for in vitro estrogen receptor-mediated gene expression induced by benzo(a)pyrene, but do not elicit uterotrophic effects in vivo. *Toxicol Sci* **59:** 231–40.

Foster JR, Idle JR, Hardwick JP, Bars R, Scott P, Braganza JM (1993) Induction of drug-metabolizing enzymes in human pancreatic cancer and chronic pancreatitis. *J Pathol* **169:** 457–63.

Galloway SM, Perr PE, Meneses J, Nebert DW, Pedersen RA (1980) Cultured mouse embryos metabolize benzo[a]pyrene during early gestation: genetic differences detectable by sister chromatid exchange. *Proc Natl Acad Sci USA* **77:** 3524–8.

Galvan N, Teske DE, Zhou G, Moorthy B, MacWilliams PS, Czuprynski CJ, Jefcoate CR (2005) Induction of CYP1A1 and CYP1B1 in liver and lung by benzo(a)pyrene and 7,12-dimethylbenz(a)anthracene do not affect distribution of polycyclic hydrocarbons to target tissue: role of AhR and CYP1B1 in bone marrow cytotoxicity. *Toxicol Appl Pharmacol* **202:** 244–57.

Garg A, Beach AC, Gupta RC (1993) Interception of reactive, DNA adduct-forming metabolites present in rodent serum following carcinogen exposure: implications in biomonitoring. *Teratog Carcinog Mutagen* **13:** 151–66.

Gaspari L, Chang SS, Santella RM, Garte S, Pedotti P, Taioli E (2003) Polycyclic aromatic hydrocarbon-DNA adducts in human sperm as a marker of DNA damage and infertility. *Mutat Res* **535:** 155–60.

Ginsberg GL, Atherholt TB (1989) Transport of DNA-adducting metabolites in mouse serum following benzo[a]pyrene administration. *Carcinogenesis* **10:** 673–9.

Godschalk RWL, Moonen EJC, Schilderman PAEL, Broekmans WMR, Kleinjans JCS, van Schooten FJ (2000) Exposure-route-dependent DNA adduct formation by polycyclic aromatic hydrocarbons. *Carcinogenesis* **1:** 87–92.

Grova N, Prodhomme EJF, Schellenberger MT, Farinelle S, Muller CP (2009) Modulation of carcinogen bioavailability by immunization with benzo(a) pyrene-conjugate vaccines. *Vaccine* **27:** 4142–51.

Guengerich FP, Chun YJ, Kim D, Gillam EM, Shimada T (2003) Cytochrome P450 1B1: a target for inhibition in anticarcinogenesis strategies. *Mutat Res* **523–524:** 173–82.

Guven A, Kayikci A, Cam K, Arbak P, Balbay O, Cam M (2008) Alterations in semen parameters of toll collectors working at motorways: does diesel exposure induce detrimental effects on semen? *Andrologia* **40:** 346–51.

Harris DL, Hood DB, Ramesh A (2008) Vehicle-dependent disposition of fluoranthene in Fisher-344 rats. *Int J Environ Res Public Health* **5:** 41–8.

Harris DL, Huderson AC, Niaz MS, Ford JJ, Archibong AE, Ramesh A (2009) Comparative metabolism of benzo(a)pyrene by ovarian microsomes of various species. *Environ Toxicol* **24:** 603–9.

Hoyer P (2004) *Ovarian Toxicology*. Informa Healthcare, New York, 248 pp.

Hrudey SE, Chen W, Rousseaux CG (1996) *Bioavailability in Environmental Risk Assessment*. CRC Press Inc., Boca Raton, Florida, 294 pp.

Hsu PC, Chen IY, Pan CH, Wu KY, Pan MH, Chen JR, Chen CJ, Chang-Chien GP, Hsu CH, Liu CS, Wu MT (2006) Sperm DNA damage correlates with polycyclic aromatic hydrocarbon biomarker in coke-oven workers. *Int Arch Occup Environ Health* **79:** 349–56.

Huang JY, Liao JW, Liu YC, Lu SY, Chou CP, Chan WH, Chen SU, Ueng TH (2008) Motorcycle exhaust induces reproductive toxicity and testicular interleukin-6 in male rats. *Toxic Sci* **103:** 137–48.

Huel G, Godin J, Frery N, Girard F, Moreau T, Nessmann C, Blot P (1993) Arylhydrocarbon hydroxylase activity in human placenta and threatened preterm delivery. *J Expo Anal Environ Epidemiol* **3 (Suppl. 1):** 187–99.

Hull MG, North K, Taylor HM, Farrow A, Ford CW (2000) Delayed conception and active and passive smoking. *Fertil Steril* **74:** 725–33.

Inyang F, Ramesh A, Kopsombut P, Niaz MS, Hood DB, Nyanda AM, Archibong AE (2003) Disruption of testicular steroidogenesis and epididymal function by inhaled benzo(a)pyrene. *Reprod Toxicol* **17:** 527–37.

IPCS (1998) Environmental Health Criteria 202: selected non-heterocyclic polycyclic aromatic hydrocarbons. International Programme on Chemical Safety, World Health Organization, Lyon, France.

Jefcoate CR, Liehr JG, Santen RJ, Sutter TR, Yager JD, Yue W, Santner SJ, Tekmal R, Demers L, Pauley R, Naftolin F, Mor G, Berstein L (2000) Tissue-specific synthesis and oxidative metabolism of estrogens. *J Natl Cancer Inst Monogr* **27:** 95–112.

Jeng HA, Yu L (2008) Alteration of sperm quality and hormone levels by polycyclic aromatic hydrocarbons on airborne particulate particles. *J Environ Sci Health A Tox Hazard Subst Environ Eng* **43:** 675–81.

Ji G, Gu A, Zhu P, Xia Y, Zhou Y, Hu F, Song L, Wang S, Wang X (2010) Joint effects of XRCC1 polymorphisms and polycyclic aromatic hydrocarbons exposure on sperm DNA damage and male infertility. *Tox Sci*. In press.

Kapawa A, Giannakis D, Tsoukanelis K, Kanakas N, Baltogiannis D, Agapitos E, Loutradis D, Miyagawa I, Sofikitis N (2004) Effects of paternal cigarette smoking on testicular function, sperm fertilizing capacity, embryonic development, and blastocyst capacity for implantation in rats. *Andrologia* **36:** 57–68.

Khorram O, Garthwaite M, Jones J, Golos T (2004) Expression of aryl hydrocarbon receptor (AHR) and aryl hydrocarbon receptor nuclear translocator (ARNT) mRNA expression in human spermatozoa. *Med Sci Monit* **10:** 135–8.

Khorram O, Han G, Magee T (2010) Cigarette smoke inhibits endometrial epithelial cell proliferation through a nitric oxide-mediated pathway. *Fertil Steril* **93:** 257–63.

Kim J-C, Kim S-H, Shin D-H, Ahn T-H, Kim H-C, Kim Y-B, Jiang C-Z, Han J, Chung M-K (2004) Effects of prenatal exposure to the environmental pollutant 2-bromopropane on embryo-fetal development in rats. *Toxicology* **196:** 77–86.

Krawetz SA (2005) Paternal contribution: new insights and future challenges. *Nat Rev Genet* **6:** 633–42.

Ku WW, Chapin RE (1993) Preparation and use of Sertoli cell-enriched cultures from 18-day-old rat. In *Male Reproductive Toxicology, Methods in Toxicology*, Vol. 3 (Chapin RE, Heindel JJ, eds.). Academic Press, San Diego, pp. 210–29.

Künzle R, Mueller MD, Hänggi W, Birkhäuser MH, Drescher H, Bersinger NA (2003) Semen quality of male smokers and nonsmokers in infertile couples *Fertil Steril* **79:** 287–91.

Lee LL, Lee JSC, Waldman SD, Casper RF, Grynpas MD (2002) Polycyclic aromatic hydrocarbons present in cigarette smoke cause bone loss in an ovariectomized rat model. *Bone* **30:** 917–23.

Leighton JK, Canning S, Guthrie HD, Hammond JM (1995) Expression of cytochrome P450 1A1, and estrogen hydroxylase in ovarian granulose cells is developmentally regulated. *J Steroid Biochem Mol Biol* **52:** 351–6.

Linschooten JO, van Schooten FJ, Baumgartner A, Cemeli E, vanDelft J, Anderson D, Godschalk RWL (2009) Use of spermatozoa mRNA profiles to study gene-environment interactions in human germ cells. *Mutat Res* **667:** 70–6.

Lintsen AME, Pasker-de Jong PCM, de Boer EJ, Burger CW, Jansen CAM, Braat DDM, van Leeuwen FE (2005) Effects of subfertility cause, smoking and body weight on the success rate of IVF. *Hum Reprod* **20:** 1867–75.

Lodovici M, Akpan V, Evangelisti C, Dolara P (2004) Sidestream tobacco smoke as the main predictor of exposure to polycyclic aromatic hydrocarbons. *J Appl Toxicol* **24:** 277–81.

Mackenzie KM, Angevine DM (1981) Infertility in mice exposed in utero to benzo(a)-pyrene. *Biol Reprod* **24:** 183–91.

Mandal PK, McDaniel LR, Prough RA, Clark BJ (2001) 7, 12-Dimethylbenz(a) anthracene inhibition of steroid production in MA-10 mouse Leydig tumor cells is not directly linked to induction of CYP1B1. *Toxicol Appl Pharmacol* **175:** 200–8.

Mangal D, Vudathala D, Park JH, Lee SH, Penning TM, Blair IA (2009) Analysis of 7,8-dihydro-8-oxo-2′-deoxyguanosine in cellular DNA during oxidative stress. *Chem Res Toxicol* **22:** 788–97.

Matikainen T, Perez GI, Jurisicona A, Pru JK, Schlezinger JJ, Ryu H-Y, Laine J, Sakai T, Korsmeyer SJ, Casper RF, Sherr DH, Tilly JL (2001) Aromatic hydrocarbon receptor-driven Bax gene expression is required for premature ovarian failure caused by biohazardous environmental chemicals. *Nature Genetics* **28:** 355–60.

Matikainen TM, Moriyama T, Morita Y, Perez GI, Korsmeyer SJ, Sherr DH, Tilly JL (2002) Ligand activation of the aromatic hydrocarbon receptor transcription factor drives Bax-dependent apoptosis in developing fetal ovarian germ cells. *Endocrinology* **143:** 615–20.

Matsumura F (1994) How important is the protein phosphorylation pathway in the toxic expression of dioxin-type chemicals? *Biochem Pharmacol* **48:** 215–24.

Mattison DR (1979) Difference in sensitivity of rat and mouse primordial oocytes to destruction by polycyclic aromatic hydrocarbons. *Chem Biol Interact* **28:** 133–7.

Mattison DR (1983) The mechanism of action of reproductive toxins. *Am J Ind Med* **4:** 65–79.

Mattison DR, Thorgeirsson SS (1979) Ovarian aryl hydrocarbon hydroxylase activity and primordial oocyte toxicity of polycyclic aromatic hydrocarbons in mice. *Cancer Res* **39:** 3471–5.

Mattison DR, White NB, Nightingale MR (1980) The effect of benzo(a)pyrene on fertility, primordial oocyte number, and ovarian response to pregnant mare's serum gonadotropin. *Pediatr Pharmacol* **1:** 143–51.

Melikian AA, Sun P, Prokopczyk B, ElBayoumy K, Hoffman D, Wang X, Waggoner S (1999) Identification of benzo(a)pyrene metabolites in cervical mucus and DNA adducts in cervical tissues in humans by gas chromatography-mass spectrometry. *Cancer Lett* **146:** 127–34.

Miller KP, Ramos KS (2001) Impact of cellular metabolism on the biological effects of benzo(a)pyrene and related hydrocarbons. *Drug Metab Rev* **33:** 1–35.

Moir D, Viau A, Chu I, Withey J, McMullen E (1998) Pharmacokinetics of benzo[a]pyrene in the rat. *J Toxicol Environ Health A* **53:** 507–30.

Moline JM, Golden A, Bar-Chama N, Smith E, Rauch M, Chapin R, Perreault S, Schrader S, Suk W, Landrigan P (2000) Exposure to hazardous substances and male reproductive health: a research framework. *Environ Hlth Perspect* **108:** 803–13.

Mostafa T, Tawadrous G, Roaia MM, Amer MK, Kader RA, Aziz A (2006) Effect of smoking on seminal plasma ascorbic acid in infertile and fertile males. *Andrologia* **38:** 221–4.

Mukhopadhyay D, Nandi P, Varghese AC, Gutgutia R, Banerjee S, Bhattacharyya AK (2010) The in vitro effect of benzo(a)pyrene on human sperm hyperactivation and acrosome reaction. *Fertil Steril*. In press.

Naruse M, Ishihara Y, Miyagawa-Tomita S, Koyama A, Hagiwara H (2002) 3-methylcholanthrene, which binds to the arylhydrocarbon receptor, inhibits proliferation and differentiation of osteoblasts in vitro and ossification in vivo. *Endocrinology* **143:** 3575–81.

Naruse M, Otsuka E, Naruse M, Ishihara Y, Miyagawa-Tomita S, Hagiwara H (2004) Inhibition of osteoclast formation by 3-methylcholanthrene, a ligand for arylhydrocarbon receptor: suppression of osteoclast differentiation factor in osteogenic cells. *Biochem Pharmacol* **67:** 119–27.

Neal MS, Zhu J, Holloway AC, Foster WG (2007) Follicle growth is inhibited by benzo(a)pyrene, at concentrations representative of human exposure, in an isolated rat follicle culture assay. *Hum Reprod* **22:** 961–7.

Nebert DW, Dalton TP, Okey AB, Gonzalez FJ (2004) Role of aryl hydrocarbon receptor-mediated induction of the CYP1 enzymes in environmental toxicity and cancer. *J Biol Chem* **279:** 23847–50.

Nebert DW, Roe AL, Dieter MZ, Solis WA, Yang Y, Dalton TP (2000) Role of the aromatic hydrocarbon receptor and [Ah] gene battery in the oxidative stress response, cell cycle control and apoptosis. *Biochem Pharmacol* **59:** 65–85.

Oltvai ZN, Milliman CL, Korsmeyer SJ (1993) Bcl-2 heterodimerizes in vivo with a conserved homolog, Bax, that accelerates programmed cell death. *Cell* **74:** 609–19.

Ostermeier GC, Miller D, Huntriss JD, Diamond MP, Krawetz SA (2004) Reproductive biology: delivering spermatozoan RNA to the oocyte. *Nature* **429:** 154.

Ou X, Ramos KS (1992) Modulation of aortic protein phosphorylation by benzo(a)pyrene: implications in PAH-induced atherogenesis. *Biochem Toxicol* **7:** 147–54.

Page TJ, MacWilliams PS, Suresh M, Jefcoate CR, Czuprynski CJ (2004) 7–12 dimethylbenz[a]anthracene-induced bone marrow hypocellularity is dependent on signaling through both the TNFR and PKR. *Toxicol Appl Pharmacol* **198:** 21–8.

Paltaviciene A, Zabulyte D, Kalibatas J (2009) Combined effect of cadmium, benzo(a)pyrene and pyrene on the Wistar male rats reproductive system. *Trace Elem Electro* **23:** 251–7.

Paracchini V, Chang S-S, Santella RM, Garte S, Pedotti P, Taioli E (2005) GSTM1 deletion modifies the levels of polycyclic aromatic hydrocarbon-DNA adducts in human sperm. *Mutat Res* **586:** 97–101.

Pasqualini C, Sarrieau A, Dussaillant M, Corbani M, Bojda-Diolez F, Rostène W, Kerdelhué B (1990) Estrogen-like effects of 7,12-dimethylbenz(a)anthracene on the female rat hypothalamo-pituitary axis. *J Steroid Biochem* **36:** 485–91.

Paustenbach DJ (2000) The practice of exposure assessment. A state of the art review. *J Toxicol Environ Health B* **3:** 179–291.

Peltola V, Huhtaniemi I, Metsa-Ketela T, Ahotupa M (1996) Induction of lipid peroxidation during steroidogenesis in the rat testis. *Endocrinology* **137:** 105–12.

Perera FP, Weinstein IB (2000) Molecular epidemiology: recent advances and future directions. *Carcinogenesis* **21:** 517–24.

Perera FP, Whyatt RM, Jedrychowski W, Rauh V, Manchester D, Santella RM, Ottoman R (1998) Adverse reproductive outcomes from exposure to environmental polycyclic aromatic hydrocarbons on birth outcomes in Poland. *Am J Epidemiol* **147:** 309–14.

Peters JM, Wiley LM (1995) Evidence that murine preimplantation embryos express aryl hydrocarbon receptor. *Toxicol Appl Pharmacol* **134:** 214–21.

Pru JK, Tilly JL (2001) Programmed cell death in the ovary: insights and future prospects using genetic technologies. *Mol Endocrinol* **15:** 845–53.

Puga A, Maier A, Medvedovic M (2000) The transcriptional signature of dioxin in human hepatoma HepG2 cells. *Biochem Pharmacol* **60:** 1129–42.

Ramesh A, Knuckles ME (2006) Dose-dependent benzo(a)pyrene [B(a)P]-DNA adduct levels and persistence in F-344 rats following subchronic dietary exposure to B(a)P. *Cancer Lett* **240:** 268–78.

Ramesh A, Archibong AE, Niaz MS (2010) Ovarian susceptibility to benzo(a) pyrene: tissue burden of metabolites and DNA adducts in F-344 rats. *J Toxicol Environ Hlth B*. In press.

Ramesh A, Inyang F, Hood DB, Archibong AE, Knuckles ME, Nyanda AM (2001) Metabolism, bioavailability, and toxicokinetics of benzo(a)pyrene in F344 rats following oral administration. *Exp Toxic Pathol* **53:** 275–90.

Ramesh A, Inyang F, Knuckles ME (2004b) Modulation of adult rat benzo(a) pyrene metabolism and DNA adduct formation by neonatal diethylstilbestrol exposure. *Exp Toxic Pathol* **56:** 129–38.

Ramesh A, Inyang F, Lunstra DD, Niaz MS, Kopsombut P, Jones KM, Hood DB, Hills ER, Archibong AE (2008) Alteration of fertility endpoints in adult male F-344 rats by subchronic exposure to inhaled benzo(a)pyrene. *Exp Toxic Pathol* **60:** 269–80.

Ramesh A, Walker SA, Hood DB, Guillén MD, Schneider K, Weyand EH (2004a) Bioavailability and risk assessment of orally ingested polycyclic aromatic hydrocarbons. *Int J Toxicol* **23:** 301–33.

Raychoudhury SS, Kubinski D (2003) Polycyclic aromatic hydrocarbon induced cytotoxicity in cultured rat sertoli cells involves differential apoptotic response. *Environ Hlth Perspect* **111:** 33–8.

Revel A, Raanani H, Younglai E, Xu J, Han R, Savouret JF, Casper RF (2001) Resveratrol, a natural arylhydrocarbon receptor antagonist, protects sperm from DNA damage and apoptosis caused by benzo(a)pyrene. *Rep Toxicol* **15:** 479–86.

Reyes H, Reisz-Porszsz S, Hankinson O (1992). Identification of the Ah receptor nuclear translocator protein (Arnt) as a component of the DNA binding form of the Ah receptor. *Science* **256:** 1193–5.

Robles R, Morita Y, Mann KK, Perez GI, Yang S, Matikainen T, Sherr DH, Tilly JL (2000) The aryl hydrocarbon receptor, a basic helix–loop–helix transcription factor of the PAS gene family, is required for normal ovarian germ cell dynamics in the mouse. *Endocrinology* **141:** 450–3.

Rochas-Monteiro PR, Reis-Henriques MA, Coimbra J (2000) Polycyclic aromatic hydrocarbons inhibit in vitro ovarian steroidogenesis in the flounder (*Platichthys flesus* L.). *Aquat Toxicol* **48:** 549–59.

Rodríguez-Fragoso L, Melendez K, Hudson LG, Lauer FT, Burchiel SW (2009) EGF-receptor phosphorylation and downstream signaling are activated by benzo[a]pyrene 3,6-quinone and benzo[a]pyrene 1,6-quinone in human mammary epithelial cells. *Toxicol Appl Pharmacol* **235:** 321–8.

Rorke EA, Sizemore N, Mukhtar H, Couch LH., Howard PC (1998) Polycyclic aromatic hydrocarbons enhance terminal cell death of human ectocervical cells. *Int J Oncol* **13:** 557–63.

Rossnerova A, Balascak I, Rossner P Jr, Sram RJ (2010) Frequency of chromosomal aberrations in Prague mothers and their newborns. *Mutat Res*. In press.

Rubes J, Selevan SG, Sram RJ, Evenson DP, Perreault SD (2007) GSTM1 genotype influences the susceptibility of men to sperm DNA damage associated with exposure to air pollution. *Mutat Res* **625:** 20–8.

Russo A, Troncoso N, Sanchez F, Garbarino JA, Vanella A (2006) Propolis protects human spermatozoa from DNA damage caused by benzo(a)pyrene and exogenous reactive oxygen species. *Life Sci* **78:** 1401–6.

Ryu DY, Levi PE, Fernandez-Salguero P, Gonzalez FJ, Hodgson E (1996) Piperonyl butoxide and acenaphthylene induce cytochrome P450 1A2 and 1B1 mRNA in aromatic hydrocarbon-responsive receptor knock-out mouse liver. *Mol Pharmacol* **50**: 443–6.

Safe S (2001) Molecular biology of the Ah receptor and its role in carcinogenesis. *Toxicol Lett* **120:** 1–7.

Sagredo C, Mollerup S, Cole KJ, Phillips DH, Uppstad H, Øvrebø S (2009) Biotransformation of benzo(a)pyrene in Ahr knockout mice is dependent on time and route of exposure. *Chem Res Toxicol* **22:** 584–91.

Santodonato J (1997) Review of the estrogenic and antiestrogenic activity of polycyclic aromatic hydrocarbons: relationship to carcinogenicity. *Chemosphere* **34:** 835–48.

Sanyal MK, Li YL (2007) Deleterious effects of polynuclear aromatic hydrocarbon on blood vascular system of the rat fetus. *Birth Defects Res B Dev Reprod Toxicol* **80:** 367–73.

Schettler T, Stein J, Reich F, Valenti M (2000) In harm's way: toxic threats to child development. Greater Boston Physicians for Social Responsibility.

Senft AP, Dalton TP, Nebert DW, Genter MB, Puga A, Hutchinson RJ, Kerzee JK, Uno S, Shertzer HG (2002) Mitochondrial reactive oxygen production is dependent on the aromatic hydrocarbon receptor. *Free Radic Biol Med* **33:** 1268–78.

Sesardic D, Pasanen M, Pelkonen O, Boobis AR (1990) Differential expression and regulation of members of the cytochrome P450 IA gene subfamily in human tissues. *Carcinogenesis* **11**: 1183–8.

Shamsuddin AK, Gan R (1988). Immunocytochemical localization of benzo(a) pyrene-DNA adducts in human tissue. *Hum Pathol* **19:** 309–15.

Shiverick KT, Salafia C (1999) Cigarette smoking and pregnancy. I: Ovarian, uterine and placental effects. *Placenta* **20:** 265–72.

Singh R, Sram RJ, Binkova B, Kalina I, Popov TA, Georgieva T, Garte S, Taioli E, Farmer PB (2007) The relationship between biomarkers of oxidative DNA damage, polycyclic aromatic hydrocarbon-DNA adducts, antioxidant status and genetic susceptibility following exposure to environmental air pollution in humans. *Mutat Res* **620:** 83–92.

Smith TL, Merry ST, Harris DL, Ford J, Ike J, Archibong AE, Ramesh A (2007) Species-specific testicular and hepatic microsomal metabolism of benzo(a) pyrene, a ubiquitous toxicant and endocrine disruptor. *Toxicol in Vitro* **4:** 753–8.

Soares SR, Simon C, Remohí J, Pellicer A (2007) Cigarette smoking affects uterine receptiveness. *Hum Reprod* **22:** 543–7.

Sofikitis N, Giotitsas N, Tsounapi P, Baltogiannis D, Giannakis D, Pardalidis NJ (2008) Hormonal regulation of spermatogenesis and spermiogenesis. *Steroid Biochem Mol Biol* **109:** 323–30.

Song S, Xu X-C (2009) Effect of benzo[a]pyrene diol epoxide on expression of retinoic acid receptor-β in immortalized esophageal epithelial cells and esophageal cancer cells. *Biochem Biophys Res Commun* **281:** 872–7.

Sram RJ, Binkova B, Rössner P, Rubeš J, Topinka J, Dejmek J (1999) Adverse reproductive outcomes from exposure to environmental mutagens. *Mutat Res* **428:** 203–15.

Swanson HI, Bradfield CA (1993) The AH-receptor: genetics, structure and function. *Pharmacogenetics* **3:** 213–320.

Tarantini A, Maitre A, Lefebvre E, Marques M, Marie C, Ravanat JL, Douki T (2009) Relative contribution of DNA strand breaks and DNA adducts to the genotoxicity of benzo(a)pyrene as a pure compound and in complex mixtures. *Mutat Res* **671:** 67–75.

Tatemichi M, Nomura S, Ogura T, Sone H, Nagata H, Esum H (1999) Mutagenic activation of environmental carcinogens by microsomes of gastric mucosa with intestinal metaplasia. *Cancer Res* **59**: 3893–8.

Toppari J, Larsen JC, Christiansen P, Giwercman A, Grandjean P, Guillette LJ Jr, Jegou B, Jensen TK, Jouannet P, Keiding N, Leffers H, McLachlan JA, Meyer O, Muller J, Rajpert-DeMeyts E, Scheike, T, Sharpe R, Sumpter J, Skakkebaek NE (1996) Male reproductive health and environmental xenoestrogens. *Environ Health Perspect* **104 (Suppl. 4):** 741–803.

Tran DQ, Ide CF, McLachlan JA, Arnold SF (1996) The anti-estrogenic activity of selected polynuclear aromatic hydrocarbons in yeast expressing human estrogen receptor. *Biochem Biophys Res Commun* **229:** 101–8.

Tsai KS, Yang RS, Liu SH (2004) Benzo(a)pyrene regulates osteoblast proliferation through an estrogen receptor-related cyclooxygenase-2 pathway. *Chem Res Toxicol* **17:** 679–84.

Uno S, Dalton TP, Gragin N, Curran CP, Derkenne S, Miller ML, Shertzer HG, Gonzalez FJ, Nebert DW (2006) Oral benzo(a)pyrene in CYP1 knockout mouse lines: CYP1A1 important in detoxication, CYP1B1 metabolism required for immune damage independent of total body burden and clearance rate. *Mol Pharmacol* **69:** 1103–14.

Urso P, Gengozian N (1980) Depressed humoral immunity and increased tumor incidence in mice following *in utero* exposure to benzo[*a*]pyrene. *J Toxicol Environ Hlth, Part A* **6:** 569–76.

Van Rooij JG, Veeger MM, Bodelier-Bade MM, Scheepers PT, Jongeneelen FJ (1994) Smoking and dietary intake of polycyclic aromatic hydrocarbons as sources of interindividual variability in the baseline excretion of 1-hydroxypyrene in urine. *Int Arch Occup Environ Health* **66:** 55–65.

Verhofstad N, van Oostrom CTM, van Benthem J, van Schooten FJ, van Steeg H, Godschalk RWL (2010) DNA adduct kinetics in reproductive tissues of DNA repair proficient and deficient male mice after oral exposure to benzo(a)pyrene. *Environ Mol Mutagen* **51:** 123–59.

Vine MF, Margolin BH, Morrison HI, Hulka BS (1994) Cigarette smoking and sperm density: a meta-analysis. *Fertil Steril* **61:** 35–43.

Voronov I, Heersche JNM, Casper RF, Tenenbaum HC, Manolson MF (2005) Inhibition of osteoclast differentiation by polycyclic aryl hydrocarbons is dependent on cell density and RANKL concentration. *Biochem Pharmacol* **70:** 300–7.

Walker SA, Addai AB, Mathis M, Ramesh A (2007) Effect of dietary fat on metabolism and DNA adduct formation after acute oral exposure of F-344 rats to fluoranthene. *J Nutr Biochem* **18:** 236–49.

White TEK, Gasiewicz TA (1993) The human estrogen receptor structural gene contains a DNA sequence that binds activated mouse and human Ah receptors: a possible mechanism of estrogen receptor regulation by 2,3,7,8-tetrachlorodibenzo-p-dioxin. *Biochem Biophys Res Commun* **193:** 956–62.

Whitlock Jr JP (1993) Mechanistic aspects of dioxin action. *Chem Res Toxicol* **6:** 754–63.

Wei C, Caccavale RJ, Kehoe JJ, Thomas PE, Iba MM (2001) CYP1A2 is expressed along with CYP1A1 in the human lung. *Cancer Lett* **171**: 113–20.

Wier PJ (2006) Use of toxicokinetics in developmental and reproductive toxicology. In *Developmental and Reproductive Toxicology* (Hood RD, eds.). Taylor and Francis Group, Boca Raton, Florida, pp. 571–97.

Xia Y, Zhu P, Han Y, Lu C, Wang S, Gu A, Fu G, Zhao R, Song L, Wang X (2009) Urinary metabolites of polycyclic aromatic hydrocarbons in relation to idiopathic male infertility. *Human Reproduction* **1:** 1–8.

Zenzes MT (2000) Smoking and reproduction: gene damage to human gametes and embryos. *Hum Reprod Update* **6:** 122–31.

Zenzes MT, Bielecki R, Reed TE (1999) Detection of benzo(a)pyrene diol epoxide-DNA adducts in sperm of men exposed to cigarette smoke. *Fertil Steril* **72:** 330–5.

Zenzes MT, Puy LA, Bielecki R (1998) Immunodetection of benzo(a)pyrene adducts in ovarian cells of women exposed to cigarette smoke. *Mol Hum Reprod* **4:** 159–65.

Zhang QY, Dunbar D, Kaminsky LS (2003) Characterization of mouse small intestinal cytochrome P450 expression. *Drug Metab Dispos* **31**: 1346–51.

Zinaman MJ, Brown CC, Selevan SG, Clegg ED (2000) Semen quality and human fertility: a prospective study with healthy couples. *J Androl* **21:** 145–53.

Zuckerman S, Baker TG (1977) The development of the ovary and the process of oogenesis. In *The Ovary* (Zuckerman S, Weir BJ, eds.). Academic Press, New York, pp. 41–67.

C H A P T E R

44

Developmental toxicity of polycyclic aromatic hydrocarbons

Darryl B. Hood, Aramandla Ramesh, Sanika Chirwa, Habibeh Khoshbouei and Anthony E. Archibong

INTRODUCTION

Recent studies have documented the unique vulnerability within the context of gene x environment interactions of young children that were exposed *in utero* to PAHs (Wang *et al.*, 2010). Paradoxically, while this is true, it remains a fact that very little is known about the extent to which environmental pollutants contribute to the overall neurodevelopmental disease burden of children in America. The most serious diseases confronting children in the USA are chronic, disabling illnesses that place an enormous burden on our healthcare resources. These diseases include asthma, leukemia and other childhood cancers, and neurobehavioral disorders such as learning disabilities, cognitive delay, autism, mental retardation and attention deficit hyperactivity disorder. Children continue to be especially vulnerable and susceptible to the thousands of high volume chemicals that contaminate our air, water and food. Children receive proportionately larger doses of chemical toxicants than adults, and these exposures occur at a time when children's organs and tissues are rapidly growing and developing.

The group of researchers led by Frederica Perera and Phil Landrigan, located in New York City (Columbia University and at Mount Sinai School of Medicine), have recently estimated the contribution of environmental pollutants to the incidence, mortality and costs of four categories of childhood diseases: lead poisoning, asthma, cancer and neurobehavioral disorders. The fraction of each disease that was attributable to environmental exposures, the prevalence of these diseases and the size of the population at risk was calculated and is shown in Figure 44.1. Based on these factors, these researchers have estimated that the annual costs associated with environmental exposure-related illness in American children are approximately \$54.9 billion. Of this amount, \$43.4 billion is due to lead poisoning, \$2.0 billion to asthma, \$0.3 billion to childhood cancer and \$9.2 billion to neurobehavioral disorders (Landrigan *et al.*, 2002).

PHARMACOKINETICS/ TOXICOKINETICS

Though studies have been conducted on the pharmacokinetic (PK) behavior of PAHs in adult animals (Foth *et al.*, 1988; Withey *et al.*, 1994; Moir *et al.*, 1998; Ramesh *et al.*, 2001a,b; Uno *et al.*, 2006; Walker *et al.*, 2007; Harris *et al.*, 2008), PK studies of PAHs in developing offspring are non-existent. Animal studies utilizing the susceptibility–exposure paradigm have documented deficits in cortical neuronal activity from adult offspring that were exposed *in utero* to B(a)P (McCallister *et al.*, 2008). These data pose the question as to whether sufficient amounts of the maternal B(a)P dose are bioavailable in offspring so as to cause the observed neurotoxicity. Within the context of neurotoxicity, the administered dose is not the most appropriate one to consider in terms of functional importance at the cellular or molecular level. The amount that actually reaches the target site where the adverse effect occurs is called as the "internal dose" and may represent only a fraction of the "delivered dose" (Paustenbach, 2000). The "internal dose" or "bioavailable dose" is estimated by toxicokinetic parameters (Hrudey *et al.*, 1996).

Toxicokinetics is a quantitative definition of pharmacokinetic parameters in the context of neurotoxicity. The pharmacokinetic parameters of toxicants help us in the interpretation of toxicology data and risk assessment (Wier, 2000). The pharmacokinetics of PAHs is inextricably linked to processes such as absorption, distribution, metabolism and elimination (ADME) of these compounds. Since biotransformation and ADME of PAHs are beyond the scope of this chapter, we are not presenting that information here. Interested readers may refer to the works of Shimada *et al.* (2001, 2003) and Ramesh *et al.* (2004) for a comprehensive perspective. One aspect that may limit the ability to pursue PK studies in offspring is the fact that collection of fetal blood/tissue requires terminal surgeries on multiple days of gestation. In order to obtain robust and statistically reliable data, several dams/fetuses must be sacrificed, which raises ethical questions from an animal welfare standpoint. Hence, developmental PBPK models

Reproductive and Developmental Toxicology, Edited by Ramesh C. Gupta
ISBN: 978-0-12-382032-7

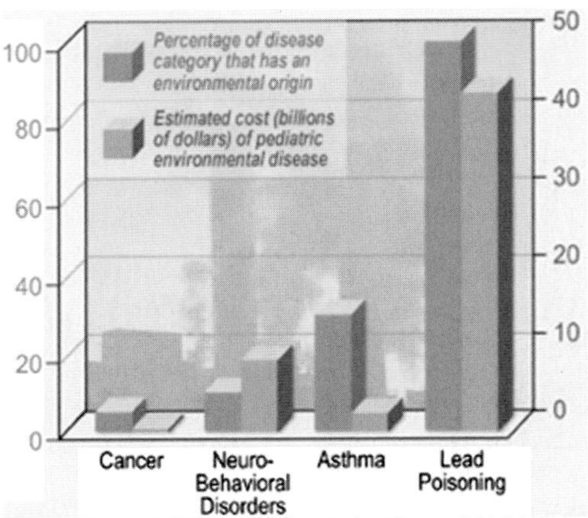

FIGURE 44.1 Estimated cost and percent of pediatric disease attributable to environmental pollutants. (Adapted from Landrigan *et al.*, 2002).

have been advocated to model toxicant uptake and disposition (Wier, 2000) during fetal neurogenesis and organogenesis processes. These models take into consideration several anatomical, physiological, biochemical and physicochemical parameters to assess the fate of ingested/inhaled toxicants and minimize the use of experimental animals.

A report by Neubert and Tapken (1988) was the first systematically conducted study that documents oral disposition of B(a)P to embryos and fetuses. This study used a single dose of 12 mg/kg. There were no other studies in this area until Hood and co-workers conducted a series of carefully planned experiments to reveal the prenatal disposition of B(a)P and its metabolites in rats exposed via both inhalation and oral exposures (Hood *et al.*, 2000; Wu *et al.*, 2003; Brown *et al.*, 2007; McCallister *et al.*, 2008). In lieu of the toxicokinetic data, plasma and tissue disposition data of B(a)P and metabolites generated by Hood and co-workers are considered as an approximate measure of the "internal or bioavailable dose" for the purposes of the discussion here.

The time course of total B(a)P metabolite concentrations in cerebral cortex, hippocampus and liver in offspring pups born from dams that were exposed to 25 μg/kg B(a)P and 150 μg/kg B(a)P is shown in Figure 44.2. The data reveal an approximate three-fold increase on postnatal day (PND) 2 in total B(a)P metabolite disposition to cerebral cortex, hippocampus and liver as the gestational dosing regimen is increased from 25 μg/kg B(a)P to 150 μg/kg B(a)P in preweaning offspring pups. No detectable levels of metabolites were found in the vehicle-exposed control offspring.

Figure 44.3 is a presentation of the total B(a)P metabolite load per gram of tissue in brain. Additionally, Figure 44.4 presents the qualitative distribution of metabolites in brain regions and is very important to the outcome of toxicity. The qualitative distribution of hippocampal and hepatic B(a)P metabolites is also presented as Figure 44.4. The concentrations of B(a)P diol metabolites (4, 5; 7, 8 and 9, 10 diols) were high up to PND 10, whereas the hydroxy metabolites (3- and 9-OH) constituted higher percentages at PND 15 and 20. The differences between these two metabolite groups at each of the time points (PND) monitored were statistically significant ($p < 0.05$ ANOVA with Tukeys post hoc). The formation of diols during this early period of development is interesting in that the diols can be converted further into dihydrodiol epoxides. From a toxicity standpoint, the dihydrodiol

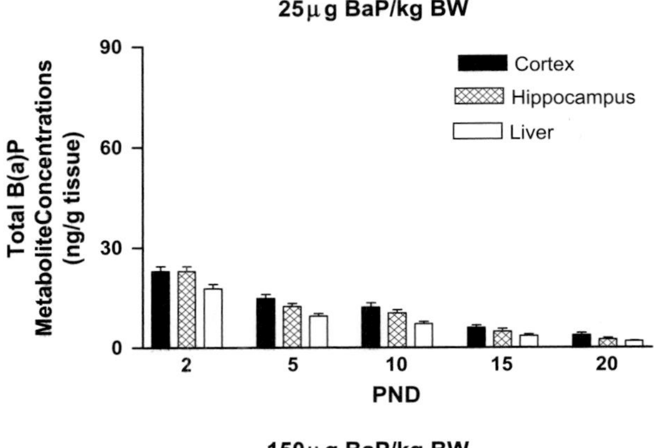

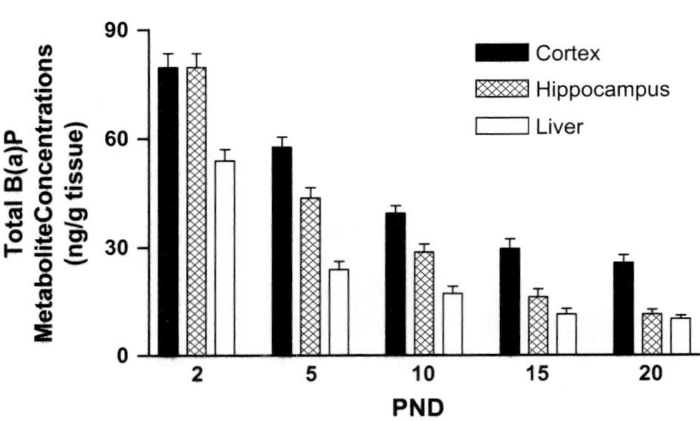

FIGURE 44.2 Time-course distribution of bioavailable B(a)P metabolites in cerebral cortex, hippocampus and liver of offspring (Brown *et al.*, 2007). Timed-pregnant dams received (A) 25 mg or (B) 150 mg B(a)P/kg body weight via gavage on GD 14–17. Offspring pups were sacrificed on PND 2, 5, 10, 15 and 20 and metabolite levels were determined as outlined in the methods and materials section. Values represent mean ± SEM.

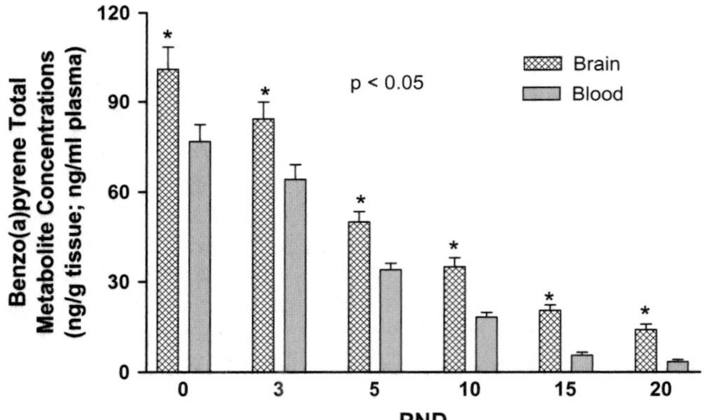

FIGURE 44.3 Time-course distribution of bioavailable B(a)P total metabolites in brain tissues and blood (McCallister *et al.*, 2008). Timed-pregnant dams received 300 μg B(a)P/kg body weight via gavage on GD 14–17. Offspring pups were sacrificed on PND 0, 3, 5, 10, 15 and 20 and metabolite levels were determined as outlined in the text. The detection limit (evaluated by a minimum signal to noise ratio of 3) of B(a)P metabolites by HPLC was approximately 300 fg/total sample on column. Values represent mean ± SEM. Owing to the limited volume of blood that could be obtained at PND 0 and PND 5, whole blood was used in lieu of plasma, whereas plasma was used for the remaining time-points for metabolite analysis. Values are mean ± SEM with $^*p < 0.05$ for $n = 3$ litters for control and $n = 3$ litters for B(a)P-exposed cerebrocortical brain tissue for metabolite concentrations in brain tissues as compared to plasma. The asterisks denote statistical significance.

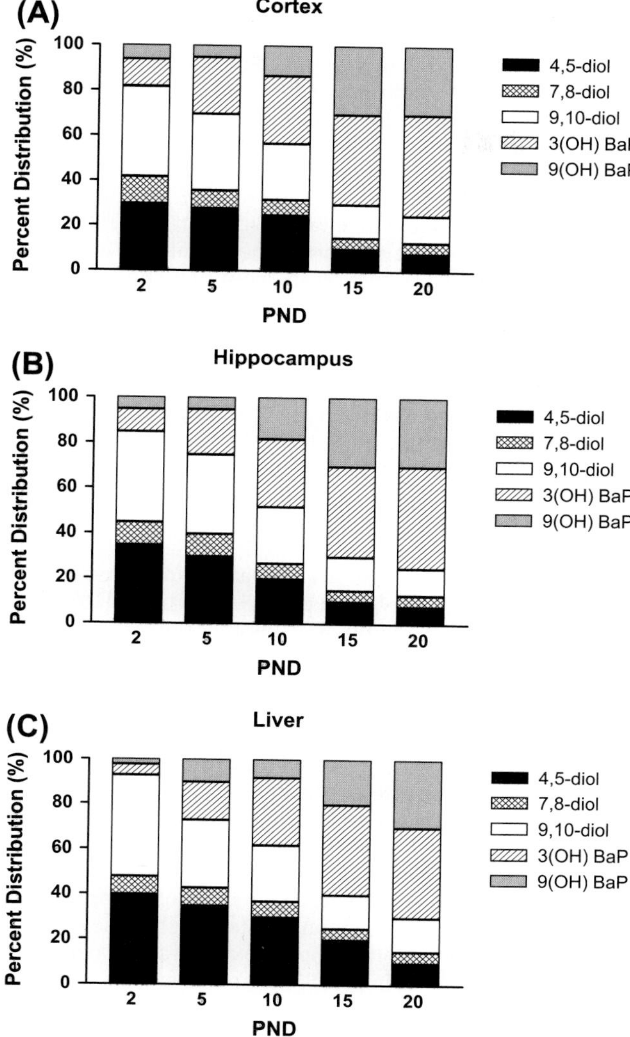

FIGURE 44.4 Percentage distribution of B(a)P metabolites in offspring; (A) cerebral cortex, (B) hippocampus and (C) liver (Brown *et al.*, 2007). Timed pregnant dams were dosed with 25 mg B(a)P/kg body weight. Offspring pups were sacrificed on PND 2, 5, 10, 15 and 20 and metabolite concentrations were determined and authenticated using standards obtained from the NCI as outlined in Ramesh *et al.* (2001).

epoxides are important as they are very reactive to nucleophilic attack by cellular macromolecular nucleophiles. The distribution profile of B(a)P metabolites among the hepatic and brain tissues were similar, which is consistent with the oral route of exposure where the metabolic processing of B(a)P by liver is reflected in the distribution of metabolites in extrahepatic tissues. It is readily apparent from analysis of the time course disposition profiles at both doses that the percent distribution of the 7,8-dihydrodiol metabolite concentrates in the hippocampus during the pre-weaning testing period.

The formation and accumulation of the 7,8-diol during this early postnatal period during the time when synapses are developing for the first time is interesting in that this diol can be converted further into B(a)P dihydrodiol epoxide (BPDE) (McCallister *et al.*, 2008). The covalent interaction of BPDE with nucleophilic centers in cellular macromolecules, such as DNA and protein, is also a critical event in the initiation of toxicity. The subacute exposure of pregnant dams to B(a)P may have contributed to an increased production of BPDE from 7,8-diol and an elevated uptake of BPDE by neurons. The lipophilicity of BPDE has been reported to allow partitioning across membranes to reach all cellular compartments (Reed and Jones, 1996). The modification of cellular macromolecules or alteration of cellular signaling events by this B(a)P derivative may be a critical determinant in the resulting neurotoxic response. The predominance of 3-hydroxy metabolites at PND 15 and PND 20 indicate that the mechanism of detoxification may be more prominent at later stages of development. As toxification overrides the detoxification processes during the critical period of synaptogenesis, the preferential disposition of B(a)P 7,8-diol to brain tissues and its bioavailability provide sufficient evidence to implicate this metabolite as a potential causative agent of the observed neurotoxicity.

Our findings on the disposition of B(a)P/metabolites in blood and whole brain tissue from offspring suggest that *in utero* exposure to B(a)P results in accumulation of metabolites, which persist in offspring tissue up to PND 20. The findings from this study corroborated earlier findings (Wu *et al.*, 2003; Brown *et al.*, 2007) demonstrating transplacental disposition of metabolites from dam to fetus during gestation and subsequent persistence in tissues throughout the pre-weaning period. Lactational transfer of B(a)P from mother to the newborn has been reported for rats (Yoshiko *et al.*, 2004), ruminants (Lapole *et al.*, 2007) and humans (Zanieri *et al.*, 2007). Thus, developing rat pups will not only have a constant infusion of B(a)P *in utero* (via placental transfer; Sanyal and Li, 2007) but also during the neonatal pre-weaning period (lactational transfer; cited above). In addition to transplacental transfer of maternal metabolites, fetal metabolic conversion of B(a)P transferred through the placenta (Kihlström, 1986; Withey *et al.*, 1993) may also contribute to the global B(a)P metabolite pool in offspring pups. The bioavailable reactive metabolites of B(a)P such as the B(a)P 7,8-diol 9,10-epoxide in neuronal tissues may also contribute to the total *in utero* oxidative milieu and potentiate the formation of F_2-isoprostanes to result in deficits in cortical neuronal activity phenotypes.

The pharmacokinetic properties of B(a)P favor a greater residence time for this toxicant in target tissues. Studies conducted in F-344 rats from our group (Ramesh *et al.*, 2001b) and those of others in Sprague–Dawley rats (Moir *et al.*, 1998) have documented that the half-life of B(a)P subsequent to a single exposure is 10 h. Hence, there may be greater tissue accumulation of B(a)P metabolites due to the subacute dosing regimen (since dosing would occur again before all the compound has cleared), and that lactational transfer may be occurring since the parent compound and metabolites are found in the pups well after dosing has ended. These studies did not determine the half-life in either the dams or offspring and the repeated dosing regimen and lactational transfer make it difficult to do so or even to speculate about this (Figure 44.5).

MECHANISM OF ACTION

The model presented in Figure 44.6 is supported by our studies in control $Cpr^{lox/lox}$ and B(a)P-exposed $Cpr^{lox/lox}$ offspring. Since the production of metabolites of parent B(a)P in offspring is a physiological marker of exposure *in utero*, our recent work has utilized mice that do not express the

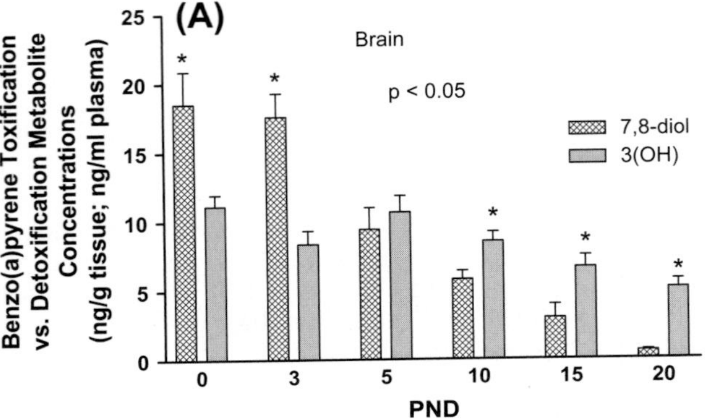

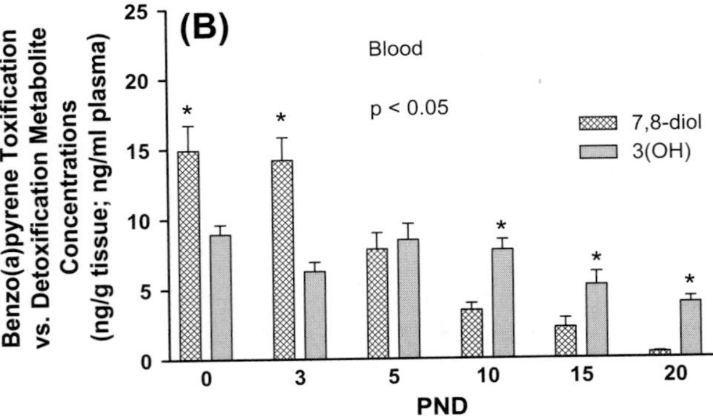

FIGURE 44.5 Time-course distribution of B(a)P metabolites representative of toxification (B(a)P 7,8-diol) and detoxification (3-OH B(a)P) processes in (A) brain tissues and (B) plasma (McCallister *et al.*, 2008). Timed-pregnant dams received 300 mg B(a)P/kg body weight via gavage on GD 14–17. Offspring pups were sacrificed on PND 0, 3, 5, 10, 15 and 20 and metabolite levels were determined by reverse phase HPLC with fluorescence detection. Values represent mean ± SEM. Owing to the limited volume of blood that could be obtained at PND 0 and 5, whole blood was used in lieu of plasma, whereas plasma was used for the remaining time points for metabolite analysis. Values are mean ± SEM with $*p < 0.05$ for $n = 3$ litters for control and $n = 3$ litters for B(a)P-exposed cerebrocortical brain tissue for metabolite concentrations in brain tissues as compared to plasma. The asterisks denote statistical significance.

NADPH reductase associated with cortical CYP450 1B1. We are using these *Cpr*-null mice to test our hypotheses because such null mice no longer possess the ability to produce B(a)P metabolites. Further, these mice will allow us to determine the extent to which oxidative metabolites of B(a)P are responsible for any observed neurodevelopmental defects. So far, data with $Cpr^{lox/lox}$ offspring is suggestive of a mechanism that requires Sp4 protein and target gene expression during the early postnatal period which is critical for establishment of strong glutamatergic circuits and synapses. Sp4 target gene NR2A (NMDA-NR2A receptor subunit) expression facilitates in establishing glutamatergic currents that are key to enhancing the strength of synaptic connections. Temporal Sp4-mediated target gene expression is key for NR2A-driven neuronal activity during the period from P 7 to P 15 in $Cpr^{lox/lox}$ offspring to give a normal behavioral phenotype. Data with B(a)P-exposed $Cpr^{lox/lox}$ offspring suggest that this process is dysregulated as a result of *in utero* exposure. $Cpr^{lox/lox}$ mice exposed to B(a)P aerosol from E 14 to E 17 give birth to offspring on E 20. B(a)P-exposed $Cpr^{lox/lox}$ offspring demonstrate a premature peak of Sp4 expression and altered target gene expression (NR2A receptor subunit). The resulting NMDA receptor containing NR2A subunit is predicted to exhibit altered NR2A-driven neuronal activity that manifest as a behavioral deficit phenotype.

For instance, recent mechanistic studies from our group have demonstrated that normal function of the somatic sensory cortex is impaired for at least 4 months after birth as a result of *in utero* B(a)P exposure. The suppression of evoked cortical neuronal activity was found to correlate with alterations in NMDA-receptor subunit expression. The physiological deficit was shown to be characterized by robust reductions in sensory stimulus-evoked cortical neuronal activity (Figure 44.7). The persistent reduction in the initial shorter latency epochs (3–10 msec) from *in utero* B(a)P-exposed offspring was found to be similar to what has been previously observed in 2,3,7,8-tetrachloro-dibenzo-p-dioxin (TCDD)-exposed offspring (Hood *et al.*, 2006). In normal and control animals, this shorter latency response is almost completely dependent on glutamatergic receptors (Armstrong-James *et al.*, 1993) localized in thalamocortical synapses in cortical layer IV. The latter part of the short latency (11–20 msec) response depends largely on the NMDA type glutamate receptors subunit expression (Armstrong-James *et al.*, 1993; Rema *et al.*, 1998). Thus, the suppression of these early latency responses in B(a)P-exposed offspring predicts a perturbation of NMDA receptor subunit function, and possibly of other types of glutamate receptors.

Prenatal B(a)P exposure produces many of its long lasting effects by adding to cortically based sensory deprivation caused by B(a)P exposure-induced suppression of glutamate receptor subunit expression during the early postnatal period. When the reported results from low input activity are compared with similar effects of prenatal B(a)P exposure, it raises the possibility that B(a)P produces a "central" deprivation by reducing cortical activity below the levels needed for normal experience-dependent maturation of synaptic function. Mechanistically, it remains plausible that the delay in the observed response onset could be due to slow conduction and sluggish synapses in the (S1) primary sensory cortex circuit pathway. It remains a possibility that both the magnitude of response and latency could be affected via trigeminal or thalamic relay neurons in the S1 pathway.

Our group, using patch-clamp electrophysiology, demonstrated a voltage-dependent decrease in inward current of rat cortical neurons exposed to 25 nM B(a)P (unpublished data). The studies have also recently been extended to neurons derived from $Cpr^{lox/lox}$ offspring exposed *in utero* to B(a)P aerosol. The current–voltage relationship and the average reversal potential ($E_{rev} = 1.6$ mV) found in these studies are in agreement with findings by Li *et al.* (Li *et al.*, 2004). The values for E_{rev} found in the studies from the Hood laboratory and that of Li *et al.* are close to the equilibrium potential for a nonspecific cation channel such as NMDA.

Several laboratories have shown that environmental toxicant exposure, in general, has differential effects on specialized subunits of glutamate receptors (Guilarte and McGlothan, 1998; Nihei and Guilarte, 1999; Chen *et al.*, 2004; Wormley *et al.*, 2004b; Hood *et al.*, 2006; Grova *et al.*, 2007). The novel results reported by McCallister *et al.* (2008) demonstrated for the first time that *in utero* exposure to B(a)P degrades the function of the somatic sensory cortex in a distinctive and quantifiable manner as assessed in offspring progeny. The findings were novel due to the fact that the circuit that was used as a model to assess the effects of prenatal B(a)P exposure in offspring had not been previously utilized in this manner. The physiological deficits reported then are now supported

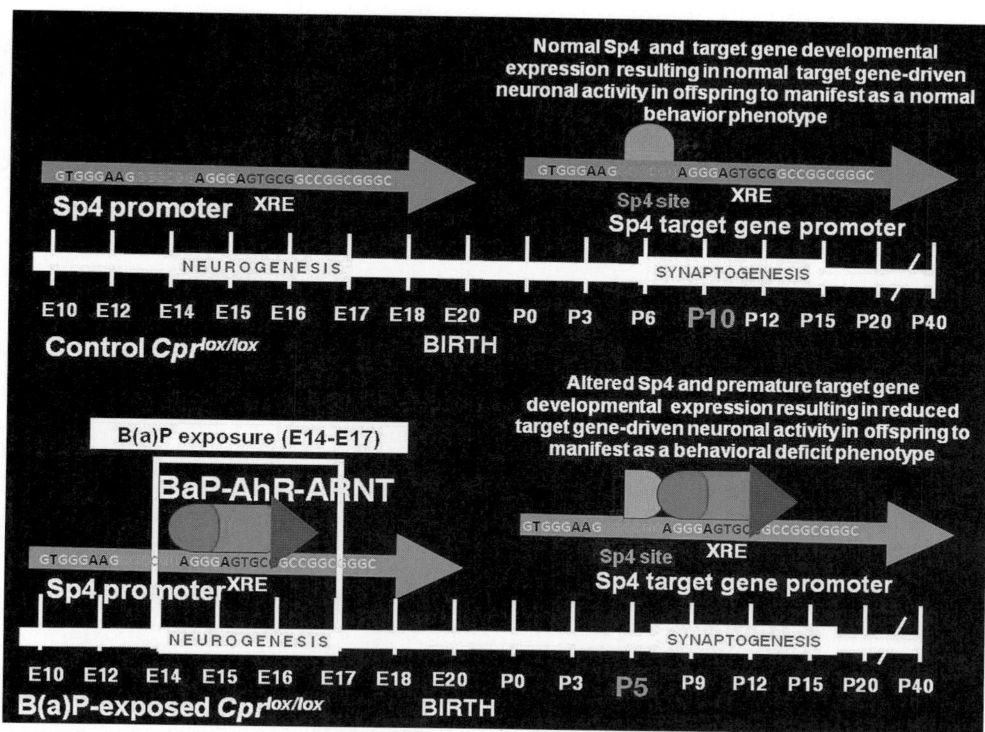

FIGURE 44.6 Proposed signaling subsequent to *in utero* B(a)P exposure. *Top panel*: normal homeostasis; normal temporal activation of Sp4 expression and of its target genes during embryonic development in timed-pregnant control $Cpr^{lox/lox}$ mice is depicted from E 10 to 20 (birth). During the early postnatal period, target gene expression is necessary for the establishment of glutamatergic (NMDA) circuits and synapses. Sp4 target genes facilitate in establishing glutamatergic currents that are key to enhancing the strength of synaptic connections. Temporal Sp4 and target gene expression is key to glutamatergic-driven neuronal activity during the period from P 7 to 15 in $Cpr^{lox/lox}$ offspring to give a normal behavioral phenotype. *Bottom panel*: dysregulated homeostasis; $Cpr^{lox/lox}$ mice exposed to B(a)P aerosol from E14 to 17 give birth to offspring on E 20. B(a)P-exposed $Cpr^{lox/lox}$ offspring demonstrate a premature peak of Sp4 expression and altered target gene expression. The resulting target gene subunit is predicted to exhibit altered glutamatergic-driven neuronal activity that manifests as a behavioral deficit phenotype. Please refer to color plate section.

by additional data demonstrating alterations in glutamatergic receptor subunit levels (Sheng *et al.*, 2010). These new data corroborate earlier observations reported by our group (Brown *et al.*, 2007). The implications of these reports are that *in utero* B(a)P exposure-induced effects in offspring occur at a time when excitatory synapses are being formed for the first time in the somatosensory cortex. The results suggest that *in utero* exposure to B(a)P results in diminished expression of certain NMDA receptor subunits that manifest as later life deficits in cortical neuronal activity in the offspring. These findings have led to a strong prediction that *in utero* exposure to B(a)P at a time when synapses are first formed and adjusted in strength by activity in the sensory pathways will produce a strong negative effect on brain function in offspring progeny to result in robust behavioral deficits.

PRENATAL B(a)P EXPOSURE-INDUCED MODULATION OF HIPPOCAMPAL LONG-TERM POTENTIATION

As the preceding section illustrates, there is growing recognition that PAHs, such as B(a)P, exert a wide range of effects on the developing brain that may result in altered patterns in neuroendocrine function and behavior in adulthood, including cognitive function (MacLusky *et al.*, 1998). In particular, B(a)P has been associated with several behavioral deficits including decreased motor activity, neuromuscular, physiological and autonomic abnormalities and decreased responsiveness to sensory stimuli (Saunders *et al.*, 2002). In humans, coke-production plant workers in Poland developed varying degrees of neurotic syndrome with vegetative dysregulation, and short-term memory loss (Majchrzak *et al.*, 1990). Similarly neurological symptoms were reported from a community that was chronically exposed to B(a)P and other PAHs dumped at contaminated sites around the USA from the 1960s until the mid-1970s (Dahlgren *et al.*, 2003; Wormley *et al.*, 2004a,b). Consistent with this finding are reports that children born in years of maximal air pollution in the former Czech Republic showed poor neurobehavioral performance (Otto *et al.*, 1997). Studies in animal models further reveal that the neurotoxic effects of PAHs extend to the gestation period as well. Thus, pregnant mice treated with PAHs produced offspring with a high incidence of brain tumors (Rice *et al.*, 1978). Also, malignant transformations of fetal mouse brain cells were observed subsequent to *in vitro* B(a)P exposure (Markovits *et al.*, 1979). Microinjections of diesel exhaust fraction (rich in PAHs) in rat hippocampus and striatum caused neuronal lesions (Andersson *et al.*, 1998). *In utero* exposure to toxic chemicals caused functional alterations in nervous system functioning resulting in developmental disorders or behavioral impairments in higher mammals (Sram *et al.*, 1999). All of these results suggest that a likely long-term effect of prenatal exposure to these environmental contaminants is to interfere with the development of higher cognitive functions (i.e., thinking, communication, memory, etc.). We tested this idea by examining how *in utero* exposure to B(a)P affected

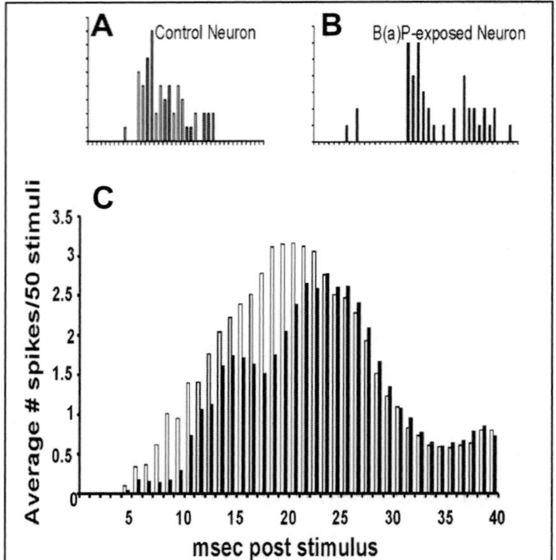

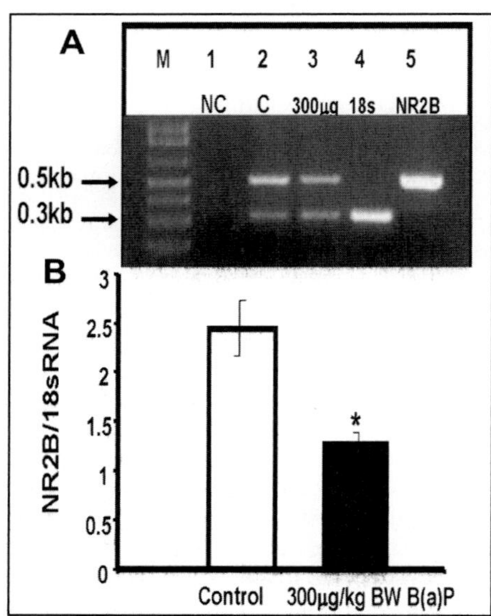

FIGURE 44.7 *Top panel*: post-stimulus time histograms illustrate the deficit in short latency responses to whisker stimulation by S1 cortical neurons. Panels A and B show responses to a single round of 50 whisker stimulations from control and B(a)P-exposed neurons, respectively. Panel C shows comparison of average responses from all control versus all B(a)P-exposed neurons recorded. *Bottom panel*: control and B(a)P-exposed offspring cerebrocortical NR2B mRNA expression on PND 100. Panel A shows a representative agarose gel electrophoresis result from semi-quantitative RT-PCR analysis. The upper band is the NR2B (534 bp) subunit and the lower band is the internal control, 18sRNA (324 bp). M represents the DNA marker: (lane 1) negative control; offspring control cerebrocortical template cDNA minus NR2B primers; (lane 2) positive control; offspring control cerebrocortical template cDNA with NR2B+ 18sRNA primers; (lane 3) 300 mg/kg BW B(a)P-exposed offspring cerebrocortical template cDNA with NR2B+18sRNA primers; (lane 4) control cerebrocortical template cDNA+18sRNA primers; (lane 5) control cerebrocortical template cDNA+NR2B primers. Panel B displays a histogram of the densitometric quantitation of the relative expression of NR2B to internal 18sRNA control quantified from the ratios in lane 2 (white bar – control) and lane 3 (black bar – 300 µg/kg body weight B(a)P-exposed offspring) from panel A. *$p < 0.05$ vs. control in the PND 100 samples.

neural networks in the hippocampus that are critical for memory formation in F_1 offspring (Wormley *et al.*, 2004a,b).

To study memory at the cellular level, most investigators use well-defined animal models that measure activity-induced changes in synaptic strength, termed long-term potentiation (LTP) and long-term depression (LTD). Specifically, LTP is an enduring enhancement in synaptic efficacy following activity-induced modifications of specific inputs (Bliss and Collingridge, 1993). This phenomenon is widely accepted as a cellular model for learning and memory. LTP is taken to reflect synaptic enhancement due to molecular and structural "remodeling" of synapses (Engert and Bonhoeffer, 1999; Maletic-Savatic *et al.*, 1999). Like memory, LTP occurs in two temporally distinct phases; early-LTP depends on modification of preexisting proteins and lasts only 1–2 hours, whereas late-LTP requires transcription and synthesis of new proteins and lasts for hours to days (Duffy *et al.*, 1981; Frey *et al.*, 1993; Frey and Morris, 1998; Lynch, 2004; Chirwa *et al.*, 2005). Thus, studying LTP in the rodent hippocampus offers unique capabilities for assessing alterations in mneumonic functions as a consequence of exposure to B(a)P *in utero*. Other investigators have utilized the LTP model to link exposure to environmental contaminants to alterations in the characteristics of LTP in the hippocampus (Gilbert and Crofton, 1999; Gilbert *et al.*, 2000) and visual cortex (Altmann *et al.*, 2001). In the latter study, a PCB mixture reconstituted according to the pattern found in human breast milk altered LTP in the occipital cortex of offspring. The exposure began 50 days prior to mating and continued through parturition. The effect shown was persistent, affecting cortical LTP of the adult animals, even though they were not exposed to PCBs after weaning. The former reported that maternal exposure to the commercial mixture A1254 reduced LTP in the hippocampal dentate gyrus of adult offspring.

In an effort to further understand the neurotoxic impact of B(a)P on memory functions, we modified the LTP model to investigate the effects of a B(a)P aerosol on LTP (Wormley *et al.*, 2004a,b). Briefly, timed pregnant Fisher (F-344) dams were randomized into control and B(a)P groups. On embryonic day (ED) 14, timed-pregnant dams were placed in nose-only inhalation chambers to receive B(a)P: carbon black aerosol (100 µg/m^3) for 4 hours per day on ED 14–17. After birth, F_1 generation pups were anesthetized and prepared for evoked field recordings from the hippocampus. Rats were anesthetized with urethane (1,500 mg/kg i.p.) and secured in a stereotaxic unit. Small access holes (1–2 mm diameter) were made in the skull for placement of a bipolar tungsten-stimulating electrode in the left entorhinal cortex (in mm: 4 lateral and 7.2 posterior to bregma; 2.2 ventral from surface of skull). A similar bipolar electrode was positioned in the left dentate gyrus region (in mm: 2 lateral and 3.5 posterior to bregma; 3.5 ventral from surface of skull) to record evoked electrical field potentials. Then the entorhinal region was stimulated at low frequency to elicit population spikes in the dentate gyrus (Figure 44.8). Once stable population spikes were verified in the dentate gyrus, stimulus input and response output (I–O) curves were plotted and used to select stimulus parameters evoking 60–80% of "plateau" population spikes. Then twin pulses were applied at 50 msec intervals (4–6 consecutive sweeps) to check for paired-pulse facilitation; this stimulation was followed by return to single-pulse low frequency test stimulation. After ~30 minutes of recording stable baseline population spikes, a high frequency train (100 Hz for 1 sec, 3 trains at 5 sec intervals) was applied to the entorhinal cortex.

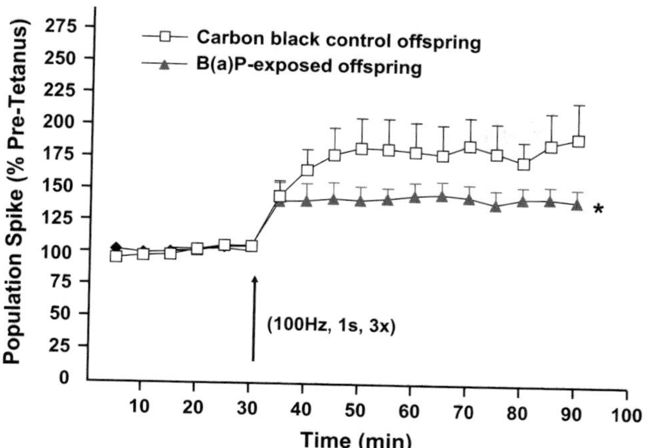

FIGURE 44.8 Long-term potentiation across the perforant paths and granule cell synapses in the dentate gyrus in the F_1 generation *in vivo*. Tetanic stimulation (100 Hz for 1 sec, 3 trains at 5 sec intervals) was applied to the entorhinal cortex after 30 min of baseline recording (arrow). Robust LTP was produced in the unexposed, control rats, whereas only a "weak" LTP was evident in the B(a)P group.

This was followed by resumption of low frequency test stimulation that was continued for 60 min. At the end of this post-tetanic period, the following parameters were re-examined; I–O curves, onset latencies (i.e., time from start of stimulus artifact to peak negativity of population spike), population spike amplitude and paired-pulse facilitation. The features extracted from the evoked field potentials included the population spike amplitude and onset latency. Paired-pulse facilitation was calculated by taking the ratio of the amplitude of the second population spike relative to the first population spike in each evoked pair. The criterion for synaptic potentiation was an enduring enhancement of evoked population spikes that were statistically different from pre-tetanus responses. We found that all recordings exhibited paired-pulse facilitation when tested with twin pulses at inter-pulse intervals of 50 msec; however, the magnitude of the facilitation tended to be less in offspring exposed to B(a)P *in utero*. After a period of conditioning tetanic stimuli, very robust LTP was found in rats in the control group (pre-tetanus population spike amplitude, 101.92±2.23%; 60 min post-tetanic stimulation 188.73±27.88%%; $n=9$). The synaptic potentiation of the control group was associated with a decrease in population spike onset latency as well as a leftward shift in input–output plots. In contrast, rats obtained from pregnant dams exposed to B(a)P seemed to develop a "weak" but enduring potentiation (pre-tetanus population spike amplitude, 102.34±1.34%; 60 min post-tetanic stimulation 139.07±9.51%; $n=5$; Figure 44.8). Taken together, the data showed that prenatal exposure to B(a)P decreased the capacity for synaptic plasticity in the F_1 generation. The full report of our investigation has been published elsewhere (Wormley *et al.*, 2004a,b).

Our study did not reveal the exact mechanisms that accounted for the apparent reduction of LTP after prenatal exposure to B(a)P. However, the observed attenuation of LTP appeared to rule out certain factors. First, the magnitudes of evoked population spikes during pre-tetanic synaptic transmission (i.e., low frequency stimulation) were similar in the treatment groups. Moreover, there were no detectable differences in the basic features of the synaptically evoked population spikes prior to tetanic stimulation. Thus, failure to produce LTP in the experimental groups could not be ascribed to differences in the baseline responses among the animal groups. Second, a concern particularly associated with conducting hippocampal recordings *in vivo* relates to the distinction between synaptically activated population spikes (i.e., orthodromic activation) vs. non-synaptically activated spikes (i.e., antidromic activation). This is a key consideration since antidromic population spikes do not develop LTP (Schwartzkroin and Wester, 1975). However, this seemed unlikely because the axons of granule cells, the mossy fibers, do not project to the entorhinal region. Moreover, our experiments exhibited paired-pulse facilitation. This phenomenon is indicative of presynaptic involvement in facilitation at the inter-pulse intervals utilized in our study (Katz and Miledi, 1968; McNaughton, 1980; Thompson, 2000). Given these considerations it was very likely that the evoked field potentials were synaptically activated population spikes produced by orthodromic stimulation. Third, it was unlikely that our prenatal treatment methods produced trauma that may have contributed to the observed reduction in success rates to induce robust LTP. Both experimental and control animals underwent similar handling and processing. The methods used to administer B(a)P are well established and proven effective (Ramesh *et al.*, 2001a,b). The animals recovered well from these procedures. Hence, we concluded that inhibition of LTP in the F_1 progeny was a consequence of prenatal B(a)P exposure.

Our study and those of others clearly showcase the utility of the LTP model for examining the consequences of environmental toxins such as B(a)P on neural processes thought to undergird memory functions. Several key insights become evident and these open up areas for further investigation. Although paired-pulse facilitation had been obtained in all animal groups, it was more robust in the control group relative to the experimental groups. To the extent that paired-pulse facilitation provides insights on presynaptic mobilization of transmitter release, we predict that exposure to B(a)P exerted their deleterious effects in part through presynaptic exocytotic failure. It could also reflect dysregulation of postsynaptic receptor functions. The induction of LTP is dependent on coincident "suprathreshold" depolarization of both presynaptic and postsynaptic regions (Malinow and Miller, 1986). In this regard, converging inputs partly exhibit cooperativity that facilitates adequate depolarization of synapses being conditioned (Lee, 1983). Thus, it could be that optimal cooperativity was not achieved in the treatment groups, using the high frequency conditioning protocol of our study. That is, the timing of synaptic activation could be altered. B(a)P may alter axonal properties making them less able to support high frequency conduction of action potentials. Mammalian development undergoes a myriad of complex processes, which serve to maintain homeostasis *per se* within the embryo and fetus. Prenatal exposure to environmental contaminants may cause a collapse in one of these critical processes, resulting in malformations and physiological dysfunction.

NMDA-type glutamate receptors are highly permeable to calcium (Ca^{2+}) and play an important role in the regulation of activity-dependent neuroplasticity and excitotoxicity, which underlie many physiological and pathological processes including learning and memory, ethanol sensitivity, epilepsy, neuronal death and mental disorders (Collingridge, 1987; Dingledine *et al.*, 1999). The NMDAR is involved in neuronal differentiation, migration, synapse formation and axonal outgrowth patterns during the development of the central nervous system (Balazs *et al.*, 1988; Komuro *et al.*, 1993; Dingledine *et al.*, 1999; Dahlgren *et al.*, 2003). Thus, modulation of this receptor may lead to sustainable alterations in functional synaptic maturation and plasticity. In our susceptibility–exposure paradigm, B(a)P was administered during the developmental period of neurogenesis and its metabolites are present during synaptogenesis when neurons are very sensitive to specific disturbances in their synaptic environment. During this period, abnormalities in NMDA receptor profiles may have occurred as a consequence of B(a)P exposure. Resolving this possibility will require further investigations. It will also be important to correlate histological data about cell morphology and densities with electrical recordings. These experiments should include an ultrastructural examination of axons and synaptic structures to determine whether pre- or postsynaptic elements are altered by B(a)P exposure during development. In addition, there is a need to tie residual levels of B(a)P metabolites with behavioral phenotypes and reconcile their relationship to changes in LTP in the offspring. In summary, *in utero* exposure to B(a)P appears to produce significant reductions in synaptic modification after the fetus is born and mature. The results from our *in vivo* experiments taken together with those of other investigators correlate well with behavioral studies in animals and humans which have reported deficits in learning and memory tasks produced by *in utero* exposure to halogenated aromatic hydrocarbons and their mixtures; these deficits appear to persist through adulthood long after the end of exposure (Gilbert *et al.*, 2000).

BENZO(a)PYRENE AND NEURAL CONTROL OF MALE SEXUAL BEHAVIOR

In mammals, sexual differentiation is characterized by three sequential events: the establishment of genetic sex at fertilization, gonadal development and differentiation, and finally the development of the proper sexual phenotype. In both sexes, early gonadal development is characterized by the migration of extra embryonically derived primordial germ cells into the surface epithelium and underlying mesenchyme of the mesonephros and the appearance of the sexually indifferent gonad or genital ridge. Several genes are now known to have definitive roles in gonadal development and sex differentiation; they include steroidogenic factor1 (*SF1*; Luo *et al.*, 1994), the testis-determining gene (*SRY*; Koopman *et al.*, 1991), Wilms' tumor antigen (*WT1*; Kreidberg *et al.*, 1993) and Müllerian inhibiting substance (*MIS*; Matzuk *et al.*, 1995; Mishina *et al.*, 1996). To date, the earliest known marker of gonadal development is the orphan nuclear receptor *SF-1* whose transcripts first appear in the urogenital ridge of ED 9 mouse embryos (Ikeda *et al.*, 1994). In genotypic XY males, the indifferent gonad is directed away from ovarian development and towards testicular differentiation through the action of the testis-determining gene, *SRY*, which is present on the Y chromosome (Gubbay *et al.*, 1990; Sinclair *et al.*, 1990). In the mouse, fetal *Sry* expression is limited to the period of sex differentiation (ED 10.5–12.5) and is thought to act solely in the supporting cell lineage (Palmer and Burgoyne, 1991), triggering them to differentiate into Sertoli cells and organize into testicular cords (Koopman *et al.*, 1990; Palmer and Burgoyne, 1991). Testicular cord formation is then believed to induce the remaining gonadal cell types, Leydig cells included, to follow the male differentiation pathway (Byskov and Hoyer, 1994). Gonadal steroids, especially testosterone, are important modulators of sexual behavior in adult male mammals (Robbins, 1996). Fetal testis has the capacity to synthesize and release testosterone at a critical species-specific stage of development. In the male human fetus, this occurs between the 18th and 19th week of gestation (Huhtaniemi *et al.*, 1997) while in the rat and pig the fetal testes produce testosterone maximally at gestation day 20 (Parks *et al.*, 2000) and between the 34th and 39th day of gestation (Evans and Sack, 1973), respectively.

The exposure of hypothalamus of male fetuses *in utero* during late gestation or male pups during early neonatal development to testosterone results in sexual dimorphism of the central nervous system (CNS), due to testosterone aromatization in the brain to estrogen (Swaab and Fliers, 1985; Dőrner, 1988; Swaab and Hofman, 1988; Swaab *et al.*, 1992; Pilgrim and Reisert, 1992; Gorski, 1991). Prenatal and perinatal estrogen action in the brain is believed to be responsible for the establishment of a male brain (MacLusky and Naftolin, 1981). Interestingly, the brain of the male rat is exposed to higher concentrations of estradiol-17β (E_2) than the brain of its female counterpart, inasmuch as the ovaries synthesize and release less E_2 than testes during this stage of development. Hence, E_2 is produced in the male by the conversion of testosterone produced by the fetal or early postnatal testis. On the contrary, estrogen concentrations are reduced in the female fetus by the binding of these steroids' alpha-fetoprotein (Baum *et al.*, 1991). Consequently, sexual dimorphism of hypothalamic structures develops in rodents, a mechanism that seems to be operative for the establishment of differences in hypothalamic structures between men and women (Meyer-Bahlburg, 1984; Dörner, 1988; LeVay, 1991; Collaer and Hines, 1995).

The inability of the fetal testis to produce enough testosterone at the critical stage of development can nullify dimorphism, a phenomenon that B(a)P exposure can impose. We have demonstrated that the exposures to B(a)P repress testicular testosterone synthesis and release (Inyang *et al.*, 2003; Ramesh *et al.*, 2008; Archibong *et al.*, 2008). Plasma testosterone concentrations were consistently reduced even after 72 hours of post-B(a)P exposures compared with their counterparts in the unexposed control group. However, the reduction in plasma testosterone concentrations by B(a)P exposure is not solely attributable to enhanced phase II metabolism of this steroid by the liver. Rather, most of the reduction in plasma testosterone is contributed to by the repression of intra-testicular synthesis of testosterone. It has been established that maternal exposure to B(a)P, results in an accumulation of a metabolite-rich fraction of this PAH in the fetal compartment (McCabe and Flynn,1990), which could result in the perturbation of testosterone synthesis by the fetal testis.

The role of sex steroids and of testosterone aromatization in the determination of the imprinting of sexual behavior has been considered of primary importance for the determination of both adult sexual orientation and sexual behavior in both animals and humans (Meyer-Bahlburg, 1984; Dörner, 1988; Collaer and Hines, 1995; Byne and Parsons, 1993). A possible role for prenatal hormonal exposure in sexual orientation was suggested (Gorski, 1991; Swaab *et al.*, 2003) on the basis of some differences in hypothalamic structures found between heterosexual and homosexual men (LeVay, 1991; Swaab *et al.*, 2003). In particular, prenatal androgen deficiency and the lack of its estrogenic metabolites were suggested to be responsible for male homosexuality (Gorski, 1991; Morris *et al.*, 2004). The hypothesis of a possible role of sex steroids on the imprinting related to sexuality and sexual orientation considered the prenatal action of sex steroids on the development of some hypothalamic structures as the prerequisite for sexual orientation in adulthood. In particular, it has been supposed that the sexual differentiation of the brain takes place when the peak of testosterone secretion from the testis during fetal life occurs (Baum *et al.*, 1991). According to these findings, the intrinsic pattern of mammalian brain development is retained to be female, and it was suggested that the production of androgens by the male fetus is needed for the development of a male brain and that, paradoxically, the aromatization of androgens to estrogens is the mechanism by which brain differentiation is achieved (Pilgrim and Reisert, 1992). It can then be argued that the B(a)P perturbation of testosterone secretion by the fetal testis may not be the only mechanism by which *in utero* exposure to B(a)P can potentially alter adult male sexual behavior. Dong *et al.* (2008) have demonstrated that B(a)P inhibits aromatase expression in the pituitary and hypothalamus of fundulus. Therefore it is conceivable that *in utero* exposure of the male fetus to B(a)P can act to alter adult male sexual behavior by reducing the secretion of aromatizable testosterone by the fetal testis and inhibiting hypothalamus aromatase enzyme secretion necessary for the conversion of testosterone to estrogen. In fact it is believed that estrogens bring about permanent changes in the organization of certain neural circuits as a prerequisite for the sex-specific regulation of reproductive and sexual behavior (MacLusky and Naftolin, 1981; Pilgrim and Reisert, 1992). Decreased testosterone levels similar to that observed in our research (Archibong *et al.*, 2008; Ramesh *et al.*, 2008) may have implications on successful mating of females by B(a)P-exposed male rats (Karabelyos and Csaba, 1996). Taken together, the lack of estrogen action on the developing brain, in males, is believed to be related to both dimorphism of hypothalamic structures and future sexual orientation (Gorski, 1991; LeVay, 1991; Swaab *et al.*, 2003; Morris *et al.*, 2004).

ROLE OF B(a)P IMPRINTING IN NEONATAL DEVELOPMENT

In the context of developmental toxicity of B(a)P, hormonal imprinting deserves mention. Hormonal imprinting is a phenomenon that takes place when the receptors mature and reach their maximal binding capacity thereby orchestrating the cell's hormone production and different functions that solely rely on receptors and hormones. In most mammals, hormonal imprinting takes place perinatally and controls the receptor–signal–transduction systems and hormone synthesis for life. Many environmental toxicants are able to bind to receptors, provoke faulty imprinting in the critical periods of development resulting in life-long morphological, biochemical, functional or behavioral consequences (Csaba, 2008). Benzo(a)pyrene is one such environmental toxicant and a known endocrine disruptor (Archibong *et al.*, 2002, 2008; Inyang *et al.*, 2003; Ramesh *et al.*, 2008).

Benzo(a)pyrene has been reported to misimprint thymic glucocorticoid receptors regardless of the stage of life, severely curtailing their binding capacity (Csaba and Inczefi-Gonda, 1984). This toxicant has also been demonstrated to influence uterine receptor binding capacity (Csaba and Inczefi-Gonda, 1993) and sexual behavior of rats (Csaba *et al.*, 1993) after neonatal imprinting. What is more interesting and disturbing is the report that neonatal B(a)P treatment has also a transgenerational effect (Csaba and Inczefi-Gonda, 1998). This report documented that the receptor binding capacity of thymic glucocorticoid receptors was sex dependent. While the receptor density in males was reduced up to the F_2 generation, in females this reduction was observed only in the F_1 generation of treated animals.

Furthermore, Tekes *et al.* (2007) have shown that a single intramuscular treatment with 20 μg/kg B(a)P to a newborn male rat (24 h postpartum) resulted in a significant increase in serotonin levels in striatum, but a significant decrease in brainstem, cortex and hippocampus of adult (12-week-old) rats. These studies also beg answers for the questions whether the imprinting effects of B(a)P are direct (at the receptor level) or indirect, caused as a consequence of receptorial defects. Since many functional/regulatory connections are known to exist between steroid hormones and serotonin synthesis (Tekes *et al.*, 2007), further studies are warranted to elucidate the transgenerational imprinting mechanism with regard to environmental toxicants such as PAHs, which are established neurotoxicants and endocrine disruptors.

RISK-COMMUNICATION CORRELATES OF ENVIRONMENTAL EXPOSURE TO PAHs

As mentioned earlier, the principal environmental contaminants arising from combustion processes such as those from coal-fired electrical plant emissions are PAHs. Industrial environmental polluters typically attempt to locate their facilities in areas that are disproportionately comprised of minority populations (NEJAC, 2004). The environmental exposures of historical concern to such *environmental justice communities* come from wood and paper processing plants that are involved in processing creosote (a compound that, when heated, produces high levels of PAHs). Prior to 1975, there were over 250 former wood and paper processing plants operating throughout the USA that were primarily located in minority neighborhoods (Dahlgren *et al.*, 2003)

As discussed earlier, exposure to the prototypical PAH, B(a)P occurs primarily through the inhalation of particulates in the air, which are produced and emitted into the environment as a result of industrial production activities (Choi *et al.*, 2008). Illustrative of this fact is the recent coal-ash release disaster incident from a coal-fired electric power plant known as the Kingston Fossil Plant (KIF) in Harriman, Tennessee, as an example of two types of emissions that pose threats to communities. This plant is located at the confluence of the Emory and Clinch Rivers on Watts Bar Reservoir near Kingston, Tennessee. The Kingston Fossil Plant is one of the Tennessee Valley Authority (TVA)'s larger fossil plants. It generates 10 billion kilowatt-hours of electricity a year, enough to supply the needs of about 670,000 homes in the Tennessee Valley. The construction for this plant began in 1951 and was completed in 1955. The Kingston Fossil Plant has nine coal-fired generating units. The net dependable generating capacity at the Kingston Fossil Plant is 1,456 megawatts and this plant produces fossil fuel emissions from the combustion of 14,000 tons/day of coal. This represents the most significant pathway for exposure to PAHs but not the only exposure pathway (Hines, 2007).

On Monday, December 22, 2008, a coal-ash spill occurred at this plant allowing a large amount of coal ash to escape into the adjacent waters of the Emory River. This coal ash, a by-product of a coal-fired power plant, is stored in containment areas. Failure of the dredge cell dike was responsible for causing about 60 acres of coal ash in the 84-acre containment area to be displaced and released into the environment (river and air). At the time of this accident, the area contained about 9.4 million cubic yards of coal ash. The coal ash that was released into the surrounding environment originated from the coal burned in boilers for electrical power production. This then represents a second pathway for exposure to nearby community residents. This is but the most recent example of the potential that exists for communities to be exposed from "industrial sources of pollution".

Technology now exists that can largely mitigate these potential effects and air-pollution control devices can greatly influence emissions from waste-incineration facilities. For example, airborne particles can be controlled with electrostatic precipitators, fabric filters or wet scrubbers. Hydrochloric acid, sulfur dioxide, dioxins and heavy metals can be controlled with wet scrubbers, spray-dryer absorbers or dry-sorbent injection and fabric filters. Oxides of nitrogen can be controlled, in part, by combustion-process modification and ammonia or urea injection through selective catalytic or non-catalytic reduction. Concentrations of dioxins and mercury can be reduced substantially by passing the cooled flue gas through a carbon sorbent bed or by injecting activated carbon into the flue gas.

With current technology, waste incinerators can be designed and operated to produce nearly complete combustion of the combustible portion of waste and to emit low amounts of the pollutants of concern under normal operating conditions. Additionally, well-trained employees can help ensure that an incinerator is operated to its maximal combustion efficiency and that the emission-control devices are operated optimally for pollutant capture or neutralization. However, for all types of incinerators, there is a need to be alert to off-normal (upset) conditions that might result in short-term emissions greater than those usually represented by typical operating conditions or by annual national averages. Such upset conditions usually occur during incinerator startup or shutdown or when the composition of the waste being burned changes sharply. Upset conditions can also be caused by malfunctioning equipment, operator error, poor management of the incineration process or inadequate maintenance. The integrated gasification combined cycle (IGCC) power plants are equipped with the best available technology to greatly reduce pollutant emissions. This technology, however, was not considered in the case that we present below.

Recently published human epidemiological evidence demonstrates that unintended prenatal exposure of the fetus to PAHs adversely affects fetal development resulting in low birth weight and reduced head circumference which can manifest as neurobehavioral deficits in the early years of childhood (Hack *et al.*, 1999; Perera *et al.*, 2003; Landrigan *et al.*, 2004; Jedrychowski *et al.*, 2009). Neurobehavioral deficits in the children of PAH-exposed mothers have been quantified as low scores on selective types of cognitive and neuromotor instruments (Perera *et al.*, 2006). Recently, studies characterizing PAH-exposed cohorts have been published, providing further evidence that prenatal exposure to environmentally relevant levels of PAH adversely affects childhood development and intelligence quotient as assessed by the mental development index on the Bayley Scales of Infant Development (BSID-II) and Wechsler Intelligence Quotient, respectively (Dayal *et al.*, 1995).

Negative outcomes in environmental justice communities (a community that is disproportionately affected by environmental hazards and that, consequently, suffers from health and/or environmental problems associated with those hazards) with respect to exposure to polycyclic aromatic hydrocarbons in the USA include the reporting of neurological symptoms from a community that was chronically exposed to B(a)P, benz(a)anthracene, chrysene, naphthalene, fluorine and pyrene, all of which were dumped at a site in Texas from the mid-1960s through the mid-1970s (Dahlgren *et al.*, 2003). Similarly, residents in close proximity to a combustion Superfund site in Louisiana were reported to have displayed neurophysiological and neuropsychological impairments. Additionally, paternal occupational exposure to polycyclic aromatic hydrocarbons has been shown to be associated with an increased risk of neuroectodermal tumors in children from Italy, France and Spain (Cordier *et al.*, 1997). Further, an association between paternal exposure to creosote (rich in PAHs) and diagnosed cases of neuroblastoma in children has been reported. Earlier work has also demonstrated that *in utero* exposure to environmental toxicants produces functional alterations in nervous system functioning resulting in various forms of developmental disorders or behavioral impairments in higher mammals (Kerr *et al.*, 2000).

Since 2000, approximately 151 coal-fired power plants have been proposed, 10 of which are operational today (NETL, 2007). In 2006, the city of Perry, Florida (FL), which is located in Taylor County, was targeted for the construction of a coal-fired electrical power plant by the Taylor Energy Center (TEC) consortium of the Florida Municipal Power Agency, the Jacksonville Electric Authority (JEA), the City of Tallahassee and the Reedy Creek Improvement District (Walt Disney World). This was cause for significant concern because Perry is recognized as an *environmental justice community* (Brulle and Pellow, 2006).

The designation of this community as an environmental justice community is, in part, the result of the presence of the Buckeye Florida Limited Partnership (LP) pulp and paper mill. This industrial environmental pollution is close to the city of Perry, on the Fenholloway River near the Gulf Coast. The paper mill discharges up to 50,000,000 gallons per day and approximately 157,649,588 gallons per year (≈440,000 metric tons per year) of treated industrial effluent (Ferguson, 1995; Andrew, 2006). The treated industrial effluent is a by-product of the dissolving pulp, cellulose fiber extraction and kraft bleach processes that employ the use of dangerous chemical toxicants such as chlorine, polychlorophenols, hypochlorite, sodium hydroxide and chlorine dioxide. This particular pulp and paper mill, originally owned by Procter and Gamble, opened in 1954. Amid concerns voiced by local and federal authorities that the Fenholloway River was contaminated with dioxin, residents filed a lawsuit against Procter and Gamble. Allegations ranged from "property damage to contaminated well-drawn drinking water that smelled like rotten eggs". The managing authorities at the pulp and paper mill attempted to downplay the dangers of human exposure to dioxin and finally sold the mill in 1992 (Andrew, 2005).

The current health status of the residents of Taylor County, FL, is further cause for concern. Taylor County ranks in the fourth quartile (least favorable) in age-adjusted rates of the following: (1) lung cancer deaths; (2) lung cancer incidence; (3) chronic lower respiratory disease (CLRD) hospitalizations; (4) stroke deaths; (5) stroke hospitalizations; (6) heart failure deaths; (7) congestive heart failure hospitalizations; (8) diabetes deaths; and (9) diabetes hospitalizations. All of these disproportionately adverse health outcomes are associated with and/or exacerbated by particulate air pollution (from contaminants such as PAHs, mercury, sulfur dioxide, nitrogen oxides, particulate matter, lead and carbon dioxide) emitted by coal-fired power plants (Meij and Winkel, 2006; Goldberg *et al.*, 2006; Bai *et al.*, 2007; Joubert *et al.*, 2007; Kampa and Castanas, 2010).

The socio-demographic status of Taylor County is also an important area of concern. Taylor County ranks in the fourth quartile in median income, unemployment and population over 25 without a high school diploma or the equivalent. Taylor County also ranks in the third quartile for residents with a household income 100% below the poverty level (CHARTS, 2007a-e). When the TEC proposed its new coal-fired electrical power plant, residents of Perry and other concerned persons complained that "TEC" more accurately stood for the "Taylor Emphysema Center", that the Taylor County Commission was unfairly dismissing their health and environmental concerns, and that only a small group of individuals were making the decisions in Taylor County. One concerned Perry resident and a member of Taylor Residents United for the Environment (TRUE) requested that the Taylor County Development Authority (TCDA) conduct a health impact assessment (HIA) which would incorporate a cumulative chemical assessment. That request was summarily denied.

In order for the community to fully appreciate the potential hazards associated with the establishment of this coal-fired electrical power plant, it was necessary to conduct research in a number of areas. It is well known that the electrical power plant siting and permitting process is tedious, and both the average layperson as well as the community health professional may find the process extremely difficult to navigate. A preexisting partnership between Florida Agricultural and Mechanical University (FAMU), WildLaw (a non-profit environmental law firm) and the community-based organization TRUE facilitated the bridging of this gap. At the time, no community coalition existed that was capable of fighting against the proposed coal-fired electrical power plant.

Through a grant funded by the Agency for Toxic Substances and Disease Registry/Association of Minority Professional Health Schools (ATSDR/AMPHS Grant # U50/ATU473408-03) in response to these needs, the Taylor County No Coal Coalition (TCNCC) was created. Subsequently, a clear and concise, step-by-step blueprint was created. The blueprint outlined the electrical power plant siting process and detailed as to how an affected community could organize so as to effectively prevent the siting of coal-fired electrical power plants through initiation of a risk-communication/public participation/community involvement campaign. The universal blueprint is based on the experiences of the TCNCC in Taylor County, FL (Stokes *et al.*, 2010). The framework that is provided in Stokes *et al.* (2010) will enable other communities to use a similar approach in assembling information highlighting the dangers associated with coal-fired electrical power plants relative to the potential negative impacts on human health as well as upon the environment. The final outcome of this risk communication process resulted in the withdrawal of the application during the permitting process by the energy consortium. Proactive measures such as these serve to decrease the potential adverse health effects associated with exposure to airborne PAHs in communities that are disproportionately exposed to environmental pollutants.

CONCLUDING REMARKS AND FUTURE DIRECTIONS

Our susceptibility–exposure paradigm remains an excellent model that will continue to be utilized in future studies to unravel the basic, molecular level mechanisms that are causative for the observed neurotoxicity resulting from "*in utero*" exposure to PAHs. The specific class of airborne environmental pollutants will continue to be surveyed due to their propensity to be released as emissions from environmental polluters throughout the USA that are located in areas that are disproportionately comprised of minority populations (Fla. Stats, 2007a,b). Future studies in this area should be focused on testing hypotheses to determine the specific mechanistic associations between environmental pollutant-induced insults to the normal process of cortical neurogenesis (E 14–17) and how this influences experience-dependent gene expression during the postnatal period when synapses are forming for the first time (PND 7–14). To date, data from the use of our susceptibility–exposure paradigm suggests that deleterious exposures during this peak period for cortical neurogenesis and synaptogenesis is detrimental and contributory to the specific PAH exposure-induced cognitive deficit phenotype found in children born to African American women that were exposed to PAHs early in their pregnancy described by Perera *et al.* (2009) and Wang *et al.* (2010). Negative environmental exposures such as these that occur "*in utero*" can be predicted to produce defects in activity and experience-dependent gene expression which may contribute to deficits in mental development index scores and intelligence quotients in specific subsets of susceptible and vulnerable children exposed to environmental levels of PAHs *in utero*.

ACKNOWLEDGMENTS

The work conducted and referred to in this chapter was supported, in part, by NIH grants S11ES014156, U50NS041071 and R56ES017448 to DBH, R01ES007462 to XD, R01CA142845-01A1 to AR and a grant from the Simons Foundation Autism Research Initiative to DBH. Institutional grants G12RRO3032, S06GM08037 and T32MH065782 (MMC-VU Alliance for Research Training in Neuroscience) also supported this work.

REFERENCES

Altmann L, Mundy WR, Ward TR, Fastabend A, Lilienthal H (2001) Developmental exposure of rats to a reconstituted PCB mixture or aroclor 1254: effects on long-term potentiation and (3H)MK-801 binding in occipital cortex and hippocampus. *Tox Sci* **61:** 321–30.

Andersson H, Lindqvist E, Westerholm R, Gragg K, Almen J, Olson L (1998) Neurotoxic effects of fractionated diesel exhausts following microinjections in rat hippocampus and striatum. *Environ Res* **76:** 41–51.

Andrew SA (2005) Fenholloway River Evaluation Initiative: collaborative problem-solving within the permit system. In *Adaptive Governance and Water Conflict: New Institutions for Collaborative Planning* (Scholz JT, Stiftel B, eds.). Resources for the Future, Washington DC, p. 41.

Archibong AE, Inyang F, Ramesh A, Greenwood M, Nayyar T, Kopsombut P, Hood DB, Nyanda AM (2002) Alteration of pregnancy related hormones and fetal survival in F-344 rats exposed by inhalation to benzo(a)pyrene. *Reprod Toxicol* **16(6):** 801–8.

Archibong AE, Ramesh A, Niaz MS, Brooks CM, Roberson SI, Lunstra DD (2008). Effects of benzo(a)pyrene on intra-testicular function in F-344 rats. *Int J Environ Res Public Health* **5:** 32–40.

Armstrong-James M, Welker E, Callahan CA (1993) The contribution of NMDA and non-NMDA receptors to fast and slow transmission of sensory information in the rat S-I barrel cortex. *J Neurosci* **13:** 2149–60.

Bai N, Khazaei M, van Eeden SF, *et al.* (2007) The pharmacology of particulate matter air pollution-induced cardiovascular dysfunction. *Pharmacol Therapeut* **113:** 16–29.

Balazs R, Jorgensen OS, Hack N (1988) N-methyl-D-aspartate promotes the survival of cerebellar granule cells in culture. *Neuroscience* **27:** 437–51.

Baum MJ, Woutersen JA, Slob AK (1991) Sex difference in whole-body androgen content in rats on fetal days 18 and 19 without evidence that androgen passes from males to females. *Biol Reprod* **44:** 747–51.

Bliss TV, Collingridge GL (1993) A synaptic model of memory: long-term potentiation in the hippocampus. *Nature* **361:** 31–9.

Brown LA, Khoshbouei H, Goodwin SJ, Irvin-Wilson C, Ramesh A, Sheng L, McCallister M, Jiang GT, Aschner M, Hood DB (2007) Downregulation of early ionotrophic glutamate receptor subunit developmental expression as a mechanism for observed plasticity deficits following gestational exposure to benzo(a)pyrene. *Neurotoxicology* **28:** 965–78.

Brulle RJ, Pellow DN (2006) Environmental justice: human health and environmental inequalities. *Ann Rev Public Hlth* **27:** 103–24.

Byne W, Parsons B (1993). Human sexual orientation: the biologic theories reappraised. *Arch Gen Psychiatry* **50:** 228–39.

Byskov AG, Hoyer PE (1994) Embryology of mammalian gonads and ducts. In *The Physiology of Reproduction* (Knobil E, Neill JD, ed.). Raven Press, New York, pp. 487–540.

CHARTS (Florida Community Health Assessment Research Tool Set) (2007a) Taylor county chronic disease profile. Tallahassee, Florida. Available at http://www.floridacharts.com/charts/DisplayHTML.aspx?ReportType=1346&County=62&year=2006.

CHARTS (Florida Community Health Assessment Research Tool Set) (2007b). Median household income (in dollars). Tallahassee, Florida. Available at http://www.floridacharts.com/charts/DisplayHTML.aspx?ReportType=1344&Sid=jsct3145vwv5zr45inwu323c3&IndCode=0600000293.

CHARTS (Florida Community Health Assessment Research Tool Set) (2007c). Unemployment rate. Tallahassee, Florida. Available at http://www.floridacharts.com/charts/DisPlayHTML.aspx?Sid=jsct3145vwv5zr45inwu323c8&ReportType=17.

CHARTS (Florida Community Health Assessment Research Tool Set) (2007d) Percentage of population 25 years and over with no high school diploma. Tallahassee, Florida. Available at http://www.floridacharts.com/charts/DisplayHTML.aspx?ReportType=1344&Sid=jsct3145vwv5zr45inwu323c4&IndCode=0600000402.

CHARTS (Florida Community Health Assessment Research Tool Set) (2007e) Percentage of total population below poverty level. Tallahassee, Florida, 2007. Available at http://www.floridacharts.com/charts/DisplayHTML.aspx?ReportType=1344&Sid=jsct3145vwv5zr45inwu323c5&IndCode=0600000294.

Chen PE, Johnston AR, Mok MH, Schoepfer R, Wyllie DJ (2004) Influence of a threonine residue in the S2 ligand binding domain in determining agonist potency and deactivation rate of recombinant NR1a/NR2D NMDA receptors. *J Physiol* **558(Pt 1):** 45–58.

Choi H, Rauh V, Garfinkel R, Tu Y, Perera FP (2008) Prenatal exposure to airborne polycyclic aromatic hydrocarbons and risk of intrauterine growth restriction. *Environ Health Perspect* **116:** 658–65.

Chirwa S, Aduonum A, Pizarro J, Reasor J, Kawai Y, Gonzalez M, McAdory BS, Onaivi E, Barea-Rodriguez EJ (2005) Dopaminergic DA1 signaling couples growth-associated protein-43 and long-term potentiation in guinea pig hippocampus. *Brain Res Bull* **64(5):** 433–40.

Collaer ML, Hines M (1995) Human behavioral sex differences: a role for gonadal hormones during early development? *Psychological Bulletin* **118:** 55–107.

Collingridge G (1987) Synaptic response level. The role of NMDA receptors in learning and memory. *Nature* **330:** 604–5.

Cordier S, Lefeuvre B, Filippini G, Peris-Bonet R, Farinotti M, Lovicu G, Mandereau L (1997) Parental occupation, occupational exposure to solvents and polycyclic aromatic hydrocarbons and risk of childhood brain tumors (Italy, France, Spain). *Cancer Causes Control* **8:** 688–97.

Csaba G (2008) Hormonal imprinting: phylogeny, ontogeny, diseases and possible role in present-day human evolution. *Cell Biochem Funct* **26:** 1–10.

Csaba G, Inczefi-Gonda Á (1984) Effect of benzo(a)pyrene treatment of neonatal and growing rats on steroid receptor binding capacity in adulthood. *Gen Pharmacol* **15:** 557–8.

Csaba G, Inczefi-Gonda Á (1993) Uterus estrogen receptors binding capacity is reduced in rat if exposed by benzo(a)pyrene neonatally. *J Develop Physiol* **19:** 217–19.

Csaba G, Inczefi-Gonda Á (1998) Transgenerational effect of a single neonatal benzo(a)pyrene treatment on the glucocorticoid receptor of the rat thymus. *Hum Exp Toxicol* **17:** 88–92.

Csaba G, Karabélyos C, Dalló J (1993) Fetal and neonatal action of a polycyclic hydrocarbon (benzpyrene) or a synthetic steroid hormone (allylestrenol) as reflected by the sexual behaviour of adult rats. *J Dev Physiol* **19(2):** 67–70.

Dahlgren J, Warshaw R, Thornton J, Anderson-Mahoney CP, Takhar H (2003) Health effects on nearby residents of a wood treatment plant. *Environ Res* **92:** 92–8.

Dayal H, Gupta S, Trieff N, Maierson D, Reich D (1995) Symptom clusters in a community with chronic exposure to chemicals in two superfund sites. *Arch Environ Health* **50:** 108–11.

Dingledine R, Borges K, Bowie D, Traynelis SF (1999) The glutamate receptor ion channels. *Pharmacol Rev* **51:** 7–61.

Dong W, Wang L, Thornton C, Scheffler BE, Willett L (2008) Benzo(a)pyrene decreases brain and ovarian aromatase mRNA expression in Fundulus heteroclitus. *Aquat Toxicol* **88:** 289–300.

Dörner G (1988) Neuroendocrine response to estrogen and brain differentiation in heterosexuals, homosexuals, and transsexuals. *Arch Sex Behav* **17:** 57–75.

Duffy C, Teyler TJ, Shashoua VE (1981) Long-term potentiation in the hippocampal slice: evidence for stimulated secretion of newly synthesized proteins. *Science* **212:** 1148–51.

Engert F, Bonhoeffer T (1999) Dendritic spine changes associated with hippocampal long-term synaptic plasticity. *Nature* **399:** 66–70.

Evans HE, Sack WO (1973) Prenatal development of domestic and laboratory mammals: growth curves, external features and selected references. *Anat Histol Embryol* **2:** 11–45.

Ferguson KH (1995) Buckeye's foley mill solves effluent issue with government cooperation. *Pulp & Paper* **69:** 133–5.

Fla. Stats. (2007a) Public notice. §403.5115.

Fla. Stats. (2007b) Preliminary statements of issues, reports, project analyses, and studies. §403.507.

Foth H, Kahl R, Kahl GF (1988) Pharmacokinetics of low doses of benzo[a]pyrene in the rat. *Food Chem Toxicol* **26:** 45–51.

Frey U, Huang YY, Kandel ER (1993) Effects of cAMP simulate a late stage of LTP in hippocampal CA1 neurons. *Science* **260:** 1661–4.

Frey U, Morris RG (1998) Synaptic tagging: implications for late maintenance of hippocampal long-term potentiation. *Trends Neurosci* **21:** 181–8.

Gilbert ME, Crofton KM (1999) Developmental exposure to a commercial PCB mixture (Aroclor 1254) produces a persistent impairment in long-term potentiation in the rat dentate gyrus in vivo. *Brain Res* **850:** 87–95.

Gilbert ME, Mundy W R, Crofton KM (2000) Spatial learning and long-term potentiation in the dentate gyrus of the hippocampus in animals developmentally exposed to Aroclor 1254. *Toxicol Sci* **57:** 102–11.

Goldberg MS, Burnett RT, Yale JF, Valois MF, Brook JR (2006) Associations between ambient air pollution and daily mortality among persons with diabetes and cardiovascular disease. *Environ Res* **100:** 255–67.

Gorski RA (1991) Sexual differentiation of the endocrine brain and its control. In *Brain Endocrinology* (Motta M, ed.). Raven Press, New York, pp. 71–104.

Grova N, Valley A, Turner JD, Morel A, Muller C, Schroeder H (2007) Modulation of behavior and NMDA-R1 gene mRNA expression in adult female mice after subacute administration of benzo(a)pyrene. *Neurotoxicology* **28:** 630–6.

Gubbay J, Collignon J, Koopman P, Capel B, Economou A, Munsterberg A, Vivian N, Goodfellow P, Lovell-Badge R (1990) A gene mapping to the sex-determining region of the mouse Y chromosome is a member of a novel family of embryonically expressed genes. *Nature* **346:** 245–50.

Guilarte TR, McGlothan JL (1998) Hippocampal NMDA receptor mRNA undergoes subunit specific changes during developmental lead exposure. [Internet]. *Brain Res* 790(1-2): 98–107

Hack M, Breslau N, Weissman B, Aram D, Klein N, Borawski E (1991) Effect of very low birth weight and subnormal head size on cognitive abilities at school age. *N Engl J Med* **325(4):** 231–7.

Harris DL, Hood DB, Ramesh A (2008) Vehicle-dependent disposition of fluoranthene in Fisher-344 rats. *Int J Environ Res Public Health* **5:** 41–8.

Hines R (2007) Race, environmental justice, and interest group mobilizations: hazardous waste and the case of Sumter County, Alabama. *The Western Journal of Black Studies* **3:** 50–7.

Hood DB, Nayyar T, Ramesh A, Greenwood M, Inyang F (2000) Modulation in the developmental expression profile of SP1 subsequent to transplacental exposure of fetal rats to desorbed benzo(a)pyrene following maternal inhalation. *Inhalat Toxicol* **12:** 511–35.

Hood DB, Woods L, Brown LA and Ebner FF (2006) Gestational 2,3,7,8-tetrachlorodibenzo-p-dioxin exposure effects on sensory cortex function. *Neurotoxicology* **27:** 1032–42.

Hrudey SE, Chen W, Rousseaux CG (1996) *Bioavailability in Environmental Risk Assessment*. CRC Press Inc., Boca Raton, Florida, 294 pp.

Huhtaniemi IT, Korenbrot CC, Jaffe RB (1977) hCG binding and stimulation of testosterone biosynthesis in the human fetal testis. *J Clin Endocrinol Metab* **44:** 963–7.

Ikeda Y, Shen WH, Ingraham HA., Parker KL (1994) Developmental expression of mouse steroidogenic factor-1, an essential regulator of the steroid hydroxylases. *Mol Endocrinol* **8:** 654–62.

Inyang F, Ramesh A, Kopsombut P, Niaz MS, Hood DB, Nyanda AM, Archibong AE (2003) Disruption of testicular steroidogenesis and epididymal function by inhaled benzo(a)pyrene. *Reprod Toxicol* **17:** 527–37.

Jedrychowski W, Perera FP, Jankowski J, Mrozek-Budzyn D, Mroz E, Flak E, Edwards S, Skarupa A, Lisowska-Miszczyk I (2009) Very low prenatal exposure to lead and mental development of children in infancy and early childhood: Krakow prospective cohort study. *Neuroepidemiology* **32:** 270–8.

Joubert J, Cumming TB, McLean AJ (2007) Diversity of risk factors for stroke: the putative roles and mechanisms of depression and air pollution. *J Neurol Sci* **62:** 71–6.

Kampa M, Castanas E Human health effects of air pollution. *Environ Pollut*. In press.

Karabelyos CS, Csaba G (1996) Benzo(a)pyrene treatment decreases the sexual activity of adult rats. What is reversed in neonatally allystrenol-treated animals? *Acta Physiol Hung* **84:** 131–7.

Katz B, Miledi R (1968) The role of calcium in neuromuscular facilitation. *J Physiol* **195:** 481–92.

Kerr MA, Nasca PC, Mundt KA, Michalek AM, Baptiste MS, Mahoney MC (2000) Parental occupational exposures and risk of neuroblastoma: a case control study (United States). *Cancer Causes Control* **11:** 635–43.

Kihlström I (1986) Placental transfer of benzo(a)pyrene and its hydrophilic metabolites in the guinea pig. *Acta Pharmacol Toxicol* **58:** 272–6.

Komuro H, Rakic P (1993) Modulation of neuronal migration by NMDA receptors. *Science* **260:** 95–7.

Koopman P, Gubbay J, Vivian N, Goodfellow P, Lovell-Badge R (1991) Male development of chromosomally female mice transgenic for Sry. *Nature* **351:** 117–21.

Koopman P, Munsterberg A, Capel B, Vivian N, Lovell-Badge R (1990) Expression of a candidate sex-determining gene during mouse testis differentiation. *Nature* **348:** 450–2.

Kreidberg JA, Sariola H, Loring JM, Maeda M, Pelletier J, Housman D, Jaenisch R (1993) WT-1 is required for early kidney development. *Cell* **74:** 679–91.

Landrigan PJ, Kimmel CA, Correa A, Eskenazi B (2004) Children's health and the environment: public health issues and challenges for risk assessment. *Environ Health Perspect* **112:** 257–65.

Landrigan PJ, Schechter CB, Lipton JM, Fahs MC, Schwartz J (2002) Environmental pollutants and disease in American children: estimates of morbidity, mortality, and costs for lead poisoning, asthma, cancer, and developmental disabilities. *Environ Health Perspect* **110(7):** 721–8.

Lapole D, Rychen G, Grova N, Monteau F, LeBizec B, Feidt C (2007) Milk and urine excretion of polycyclic aromatic hydrocarbons and their hydroxylated metabolites after a single oral administration in ruminants. *J Dairy Sci* **90:** 2624–9.

Lee KS (1983) Cooperativity among afferents for the induction of long-term potentiation in the CA1 region of the hippocampus. *J Neurosci* **3:** 1369–72.

LeVay S (1991) A difference in hypothalamic structure between heterosexual and homosexual men. *Science* **253:** 1034–7.

Li J, McRoberts JA, Nie J, Ennes HS, Mayer EA (2004) Electrophysiological characterization of N-methyl-D-aspartate receptors in rat dorsal root ganglia neurons. *Pain* **109:** 443–52.

Luo X, Ikeda Y, Parker KL (1994) A cell-specific nuclear receptor is essential for adrenal and gonadal development and sexual differentiation. *Cell* **77:** 481–90.

Lynch MA (2004) Long-term potentiation and memory. *Physiol Rev* **84:** 87–136.

MacLusky NJ, Brown TJ, Schantz S, Seo BW, Peterson RE (1998) Hormonal interactions in the effects of halogenated aromatic hydrocarbons on the developing brain. *Toxicol Ind Health* **14:** 185–208.

MacLusky NJ, Naftolin F (1981) Sexual differentiation of the central nervous system. *Science* **211:** 1294–303.

Majchrzak R, Sroczynski J, Chelmecka E (1990) Evaluation of the nervous system in workers in the furnace and coal divisions of the coke-producing plants. *Med Pr* **41:** 108–13.

Maletic-Savatic M, Malinow R, Svoboda K (1999) Rapid dendritic morphogenesis in CA1 hippocampal dendrites induced by synaptic activity. *Science* **283:** 1923–7.

Malinow R, Miller JP (1986) Postsynaptic hyperpolarization during conditioning reversibly blocks induction of long-term potentiation. *Nature* **320:** 529–30.

Markovits P, Maunoury R, Tripier MF, Coulomb B, Levy S, Papadopoulo D, Vedrenne C, Benda P (1979) Normal and benzo(a)pyrene-transformed fetal mouse brain cell. I. Tumorigenicity and immunochemical detection of glial fibrillary acidic protein. *Acta Neuropathol (Berl)* **47:** 197–203.

Matzuk MM, Finegold MJ, Mishina Y, Bradley A, Behringer RR (1995) Synergistic effects of inhibins and Müllerian-inhibiting substance on testicular tumorigenesis. *Mol Endocrinol* **9:** 1337–45.

McCabe DP, Flynn EJ (1990) Deposition of low dose benzo(a)pyrene into fetal tissue: influence of protein binding. *Dev Pharmacol Toxicol* **41:** 85–95.

McCallister NM, Maguire M, Ramesh A, Aimin Q, Liu S, Khoshbouei H, Aschner M, Ebner FF, Hood DB (2008) Prenatal exposure to benzo(a) pyrene impairs later-life cortical neuronal function. *Neurotoxicology* **29:** 846–54.

McNaughton BL (1980) Evidence for two physiologically distinct perforant pathways to the fascia dentata. *Brain Res* **199:** 1–19.

Meij R, te Winkel H The emissions of heavy metals and persistent organic pollutants from modern coal-fired power stations. *Atmos Environ*. In press.

Meyer-Bahlburg HF (1984) Psychoendocrine research on sexual orientation: current status and future options. *Progr Brain Res* **61:** 375–98.

Mishina Y, Rey R, Finegold MJ, Matzuk MM, Josso N, Cate RL, Behringer RR (1996) Genetic analysis of the Müllerian inhibiting substance signal transduction pathway in mammalian sexual differentiation. *Genes Dev* **10:** 2577–87.

Moir D, Viau A, Chu I, Withey J, McMullen E (1998) Pharmacokinetics of benzo[a]pyrene in the rat. *J Toxicol Environ Health A* **53:** 507–30.

Morris JA, Gobrogge KL, Jordan CL, Breedlove SM (2004) Brain aromatase: dyed-in-the-wool homosexuality. *Endocrinology* **145:** 475–7.

National Energy Technology Laboratory (NETL) (2007) Tracking new coal-fired powered plants: coal's resurgence in electric power generation. Available at http://cmnow.org/NETLNewCoal5.2007.pdf

National Environmental Justice Advisory Council (NEJAC) (2004) *Ensuring Risk Reduction in Communities with Multiple Stressors: Environmental Justice and Cumulative Risks/Impacts*. Washington, DC: United States Environmental Protection Agency.

Neubert D, Tapken S (1988) Transfer of benzo(a)pyrene into mouse embryos and fetuses. *Arch Toxicol* **62:** 236–9.

Nihei MK, Guilarte TR (1999) NMDAR-2A subunit protein expression is reduced in the hippocampus of rats exposed to Pb2+ during development. *Brain Res Mol Brain Res* **66(1-2):** 42–9.

Otto D, Skalik I, Bahboli R, Hudnell K, Sram R (1997) Neurobehavioral performance of Czech school children born in years of maximal air pollution. *Neurotoxicology* **18:** 903.

Palmer SJ, Burgoyne PS (1991) In situ analysis of fetal, prepubertal and adult XX-XY chimaeric mouse testes: Sertoli cells are predominantly, but not exclusively, XY. *Development* **112:** 265–8.

Parks LG, Joe S, Ostby JS, Christy R, Lambright CR, Barbara D, Abbott BD, Klinefelter GR, Norman J, Barlow NJ, Gray Jr LE (2000) The plasticizer diethylhexyl phthalate induces malformations by decreasing fetal testosterone synthesis during sexual differentiation in the male rat. *Toxic Sci* **58:** 339–49.

Paustenbach DJ (2000) The practice of exposure assessment. A state of the art review. *J Toxicol Environ Health B* **3:** 179–291.

Perera FP, Li Z, Whyatt R, Hoepner L, Wang S, Camann D, Rauh V (2009) Prenatal airborne polycyclic aromatic hydrocarbon exposure and child IQ at age 5 years. *Pediatrics* **124:** 195–202.

Perera FP, Rauh V, Tsai WY, Kinney P, Camann D, Barr D, Bernert T, Garfinkel R, Tu YH, Diaz D, Dietrich J, Whyatt RM (2003) Effects of transplacental exposure to environmental pollutants on birth outcomes in a multiethnic population. *Environ Health Perspect* **111:** 201–5.

Perera FP, Rauh V, Whyatt RM, Tsai WY, Tang D, Diaz D, Hoepner L, Barr D, Tu YH, Camann D, Kinney P (2006) Effect of prenatal exposure to airborne polycyclic aromatic hydrocarbons on neurodevelopment in the first 3 years of life among inner-city children. *Environ Health Perspect* **114:** 1287–92.

Pilgrim C, Reisert J (1992) Differences between male and female brains – developmental mechanisms and implications. *Horm Metab Res* **24:** 353–59.

Ramesh A, Greenwood M, Inyang F, Hood DB (2001a) Toxicokinetics of inhaled benzo(a)pyrene: plasma and lung bioavailability. *Inhal Toxicol* **13:** 533–55.

Ramesh A, Inyang F, Hood DB, Archibong AE, Knuckles ME, Nyanda AM (2001b) Metabolism, bioavailability, and toxicokinetics of benzo(a) pyrene in F-344 rats following oral administration. *Exp Toxicol Pathol* **53:** 275–90.

Ramesh A, Inyang,F, Lunstra DD, Niaz MS, Greenwood M, Kopsombut PM, Jones KM, Hood DB, Hills ER, Archibong AE (2008) Alteration of fertility endpoints in adult male F-344 rats by subchronic exposure to inhaled benzo(a)pyrene. *Exp Toxicol Pathol* **60:** 269–80.

Ramesh A, Walker SA, Hood DB, Guillen MD, Schneider H, Weyand EH (2004) Bioavailability and risk assessment of orally ingested polycyclic aromatic hydrocarbons. *Int J Toxicol* **23:** 301–33.

Reed GA, Jones BC (1996) Enhancement of benzo[a]pyrene diol epoxide mutagenicity by sulfite in a mammalian test system. *Carcinogenesis* **17:** 1063–8.

Rema V, Armstrong-James M, Ebner FF (1998) Experience-dependent plasticity of adult rat S1 cortex requires local NMDA receptor activation. *J Neurosci* **18:** 10196–206.

Rice JM, Joshi SR, Shenefelt RE, Wenk ML (1978) Transplacental carcinogenic activity of 7, 12-dimethylbenz[a]anthracene. In *Carcinogenesis – A Comprehensive Survey*, Vol. 3 (Freudenthal RI, Jones PW, ed.). Raven Press, New York, pp. 413–22.

Robbins A (1996) Androgens and male sexual behavior. *Trends Endocrinol Metab* **7:** 345–50.

Sanyal MK, Li YL (2007) Deleterious effects of polynuclear aromatic hydrocarbon on blood vascular system of the rat fetus. *Birth Defects B Dev Reprod Toxicol* **80:** 367–73.

Saunders CR, Ramesh A, Shockley DC (2002) Modulation of neurotoxic behavior in F-344 rats by temporal disposition of benzo(a)pyrene. *Toxicol Lett* **129:** 33–45.

Schwartzkroin PA, Wester K (1975) Long-lasting facilitation of a synaptic potential following tetanization in the in vitro hippocampal slice. *Brain Res* **89:** 107–19.

Sheng L, Ding X, Maguire M, Ferguson, M, Rhoades R, Ramesh A, Aimin Q, Aschner M, Campbell D, Levitt P and Hood DB (2010) Prenatal polycyclic aromatic hydrocarbon exposure leads to behavioral deficits and reduced expression of the autism risk gene, Met receptor tyrosine kinase. *Environ Health Perspect*. In press.

Shimada T, Oda Y, Gillam EM, Guengerich FP, Inoue K (2001) Metabolic activation of polycyclic aromatic hydrocarbons and other procarcinogens by cytochromes P450 1A1 and P450 1B1 allelic variants and other human cytochromes P450 in *Salmonella typhimurium* NM2009. *Drug Metab Dispos* **29:** 1176–82.

Shimada T, Sugie A, Yamada T, Kawazoe H, Hashimoto M, Azuma E, Nakajima T, Inoue K, Oda Y (2003) Dose–response studies on the induction of liver cytochromes P4501A1 and 1B1 by polycyclic aromatic hydrocarbons in arylhydrocarbon-responsive C57BL/6J mice. *Xenobiotica* **33:** 957–71.

Sinclair, AH, Berta P, Palmer MS, Hawkins JR, Griffiths BL, Smith MJ, Foster JW, Frischauf AM, Lovell-Badge R, Goodfellow PN (1990) A gene from the human sex-determining region encodes a protein with homology to a conserved DNA-binding motif. *Nature* **346:** 240–4.

Sram RJ, Binkova B, Rossner P, Rubes J, Topinka J, Dejmek J (1999) Adverse reproductive outcomes from exposure to environmental mutagens. *Mutat Res* **428:** 203–15.

Stokes SC, Hood DB, Zokovitch J, Close FT (2010) Blueprint for preventing environmental injustice. *J Health Care Poor Underserved* **21:** 35–52.

Swaab D, Gooren LJG, Hofman MA (1992) Gender and sexual orientation in relation to hypothalamic structures. *Horm Res* **38:** 51–61.

Swaab DF, Fliers E (1985) A sexually dimorphic nucleus in the human brain. *Science* **228:** 1112–5.

Swaab DF, Hofman MA (1988) Sexual differentiation of the human hypothalamus: ontogeny of the sexually dimorphic nucleus of the preoptic area. *Dev Brain Res* **44:** 314–18.

Swaab DF, Wilson CJC, Frank PMK (2003) Sex differences in the hypothalamus in the different stages of human life. *Neurobiol Aging* **24:** 1–16.

Tekes K, Tóthfalusi L, Hantos M, Csaba G (2007) Effect of neonatal benzo(a) pyrene imprinting on the brain serotonin content and nocistatin level in adult male rats. *Acta Physiol Hung* **94:** 183–9.

Thompson AM (2000) Facilitation, augmentation, and potentiation at central synapses. *Trends in Neurosci* **23:** 305–12.

Uno S, Dalton TP, Gragin N, Curran CP, Derkenne S, Miller ML, Shertzer HG, Gonzalez FJ, Nebert DW (2006) Oral benzo(a)pyrene in CYP1 knockout mouse lines: CYP1A1 important in detoxication, CYP1B1 metabolism required for immune damage independent of total body burden and clearance rate. *Mol Pharmacol* **69:** 1103–14.

Walker SA, Addai AB, Mathis M, Ramesh A (2007) Effect of dietary fat on metabolism and DNA adduct formation after acute oral exposure of F-344 rats to fluoranthene. *J Nutr Biochem* **18:** 236–49.

Wang S, Chanock S, Tang D, Li Z, Edwards S, Jedrychowski W, Perera FP (2010) Effect of gene–environment interactions on mental development in African American, Dominican, and Caucasian mothers and newborns. *Ann Hum Genet* **74:** 46–56.

Wier PJ (2000) Use of toxicokinetics in developmental and reproductive toxicology. In *Developmental and Reproductive Toxicology* (Hood RD, ed). Taylor and Francis, Boca Raton, Florida, pp. 571–97.

Withey JR, Burnett R, Law FC, Abedini S, Endrenyi L (1994) Pharmacokinetics of inhaled pyrene in rats. *J Toxicol Environ Health* **43:** 103–16.

Withey JR, Shedden J, Law FC, Abedini S (1993) Distribution of benzo[a] pyrene in pregnant rats following inhalation exposure and a comparison with similar data obtained with pyrene. *J Appl Toxicol* **13:** 193–202.

Wormley DD, Chirwa S, Nayyar T, Wu J, Johnson S, Brown LA, Harries E, Hood DB (2004a) Inhaled benzo(a)pyrene impairs long-term potentiation in the F1 generation rat dentate gyrus. *Cell Mol Biol* **50:** 715–21.

Wormley DD, Ramesh A, Hood DB (2004b) Environmental contaminant-mixture effects on CNS development, plasticity and behavior. *Toxicol Appl Pharmacol* **197:** 49–65.

Wu J, Ramesh A, Nayyar T, Hood DB (2003) Assessment of metabolites and Ahr and CYP1A1 mRNA expression subsequent to prenatal exposure to inhaled benzo(a)pyrene. *Int J Devl Neuroscience* **21:** 333–46.

Yoshiko T, Nobue W, Masanobu O, Akira T, Ryoichi K, Kazuichi H (2004) Transfer of polycyclic aromatic hydrocarbons to fetuses and breast milk of rats exposed to diesel exhaust. *J Health Sci* **50:** 497–502.

Zanieri L, Galvan P, Checchini L, Cincinelli A, Lepri L, Donzelli GP, Del Bubba M (2007) Polycyclic aromatic hydrocarbons (PAHs) in human milk from Italian women: influence of cigarette smoke and residential area. *Chemosphere* **67:** 1265–74.

CHAPTER

45

Ethylene glycol

Edward W. Carney

INTRODUCTION

Ethylene glycol (EG) is a major industrial chemical perhaps best known as the compound poured into automobile radiators and sprayed onto airplane wings to help keep both from freezing in the winter. This very small molecule (molecular weight, 62.07; Table 45.1) has a very large number of uses, with total US production typically exceeding 5 billion pounds annually. While a great deal of the EG produced each year is used in antifreeze and deicing fluids, its largest use is in the production of polyester fibers and films and polyethylene terephthalate (PET) plastics. EG also is found in paints, hydraulic fluids, surfactants, emulsifiers and heat transfer fluids (NTP-CERHR, 2004). Consistent with these uses, skin contact is the primary route of potential human exposure, followed by inhalation of EG aerosols or vapors. Oral exposure is not typical, and generally is restricted to either accidental ingestion of EG-containing products or intentional misuse (e.g., suicide).

This chapter describes the reproductive and developmental toxicology of EG, with greater emphasis being placed on the latter, commensurate with the scientific literature on these topics. Also, EG serves as an excellent case study to illustrate certain fundamental principles in developmental toxicology. First and foremost, as is true for any toxicity, EG exemplifies the conditional nature of developmental toxicity. To paraphrase "Karnofsky's law" (Karnofsky, 1965; Schardein, 1985), "...a teratogenic response depends upon the administration of a particular treatment to a susceptible species during a susceptible stage of development". For EG, the most effective way to induce a teratogenic response is high dose/high dose-rate administration by the oral route. The susceptible species are primarily rats and mice, and the susceptible stage of development is the embryonic period, particularly during development of the axial skeleton and craniofacial structures. EG also provides an excellent example of how *in vivo* developmental toxicity studies, toxicokinetics and *in vitro* methods can be integrated to understand mode-of-action (MOA) and to define specific internal dose metrics delineating safe vs. unsafe exposures in humans.

TABLE 45.1 Characteristics and physicochemical properties of ethylene glycol

Chemical formula	HO–CH_2–CH_2–OH
Molecular weight	62.01
CAS no.	107-21-1
Freezing point	−13.4
Boiling point	197.4
Vapor pressure	0.092 mm Hg @ 25 °C
Saturated vapor conc.	400 mg/m^3 (158 ppm) @ 25°C

Reviewed in Carney (1994)

HISTORICAL BACKGROUND

EG has been studied since the 1930s when it was first found to cause acute renal toxicity in humans and domestic animals. Following oral consumption of large quantities of EG (typically >100 ml in humans), signs of acute toxicity are usually noted within 1 hour and involve central nervous system depression attributable to the solvent-type effects of parent EG (Jacobsen and McMartin, 1986). More debilitating effects of EG only come about 12–24 hours later following biotransformation of EG to more toxic metabolites. Most of these metabolites are weak acids, among them glycolic acid (GA), and at high concentrations they induce a metabolic acidosis and associated cardiopulmonary changes. In the third and final stage of acute toxicity, renal toxicity ensues anywhere from 1 to 3 days post-exposure and is a consequence of both metabolic acidosis as well as formation of the terminal metabolite, oxalic acid. Oxalic acid combines with calcium and precipitates to form needle-shaped crystals which damage the renal tubular epithelium.

Over the years, a robust database has been developed, covering the major subdisciplines of toxicology, including reproductive and developmental toxicity. Developmental toxicology has been particularly interesting, as initial assessments conducted in the 1980s revealed teratogenic effects, sparking a long series of research studies aimed at understanding the MOA and applying it to improve the scientific basis of human risk assessments for EG. A great deal has since been learned about the toxicokinetics of EG in both non-pregnant and pregnant animals, including rats and rabbits, and a physiologically based pharmacokinetic model (PBPK) has been developed to extrapolate internal dose to the human (Corley *et al.*, 2005a,b).

Reproductive and Developmental Toxicology, Edited by Ramesh C. Gupta
ISBN: 978-0-12-382032-7

DEVELOPMENTAL TOXICITY

Gavage studies

It was not until five decades after the discovery of EG's acute renal toxicity that studies were conducted to evaluate EG's potential to harm the developing fetus. Initial studies utilized the gavage route in rats and mice, and employed dose levels well in excess of 1,000 mg/kg/day (Table 45.2). In one of the first of these studies, dose levels of 0, 750, 1,500 or 3,000 mg/kg/day EG were given to CD-1 mice by gavage on gestation day (GD) 6–15 (Price *et al.*, 1985). Decreased fetal body weights and increased fetal malformations were noted at all dose levels, accompanied by maternal toxicity at the middle and high dose levels. This study revealed what turned out to be a signature profile of EG-induced axial skeleton malformations involving fused, extra or misshapen vertebrae and ribs. A similar profile of toxicity was observed in a companion study in which EG doses of 0, 1250, 2,500 or 5,000 mg/kg/day were given to CD rats on GD 6–15. In both studies, increases in craniofacial malformations (e.g., cleft palate) were noted at the highest dose levels.

Additional gavage studies in mice and rats were conducted so that no-observable-effect-levels (NOELs) for maternal and developmental toxicity could be identified for use in risk assessment and regulation (Neeper-Bradley *et al.*, 1995). CD-1 mice were gavaged with 0, 50, 150, 500 or 1,500 mg/kg/day of EG on GD 6–15, while CD rats similarly received 0, 150, 500, 1,000 or 2,500 mg/kg/day. In mice, 1,500 mg/kg/day caused decreases in fetal body weights as well as increases in the incidence of axial skeletal malformations, including fused or extra ribs, fused thoracic or lumbar vertebral arches, as well as some minor skeletal variations (poorly ossified thoracic or lumbar vertebral centra). At 500 mg/kg/day, the only developmental effect was an increase in the extra 14th rib, which is a relatively common skeletal variation in mice. There was no significant maternal toxicity at any dose level, and no developmental effects at 150 or 50 mg/kg/day. Thus, the NOEL for developmental toxicity in mice was considered to be 150 mg/kg/day, although in this author's opinion, 500 mg/kg/day can be considered a no-observable-*adverse*-effect-level (NOAEL) in mice. In rats, axial skeletal defects and reduced fetal body weights were noted at dose levels of 1,000 and 2,500 mg/kg/day, while maternal toxicity was detected only at 2,500 mg/kg/day. Therefore, the NOELs for developmental and maternal toxicity in rats were 500 and 1,000 mg/kg/day, respectively.

In contrast to rats and mice, EG was not developmentally toxic in the rabbit, as shown in a study of New Zealand white rabbits given 0, 100, 500, 1,000 or 2,000 mg/kg/day of EG by gavage on GD 6–19 (Tyl *et al.*, 1993). Although the top dose induced severe maternal toxicity (42% maternal mortality), there was no evidence of developmental toxicity in the fetuses from surviving does at this dose level. Lower dose levels produced no maternal or developmental toxicity.

TABLE 45.2 Summary of key regulatory guideline developmental toxicity studies in rats, mice and rabbits

Route	Species/strain	Dose levels (mg/kg/day)	Maternal toxicity	Developmental toxicity: ↓ Fetal body weight	Developmental toxicity: Skeletal malformations	Developmental toxicity: Craniofacial malformations	Ref.
Gavage	Rat/CD	150	–	–	–	–	Neeper-Bradley *et al.* (1995)
		500	–	–	–	–	
		1,000	–	X	X	–	
		2,500	X	X	X	X	
Gavage	Mouse/CD-1	50	–	–	–	–	Neeper-Bradley *et al.* (1995)
		150	–	–	–	–	
		500	–	–	–	–	
		1,500	–	X	X		
Gavage	Rabbit/NZW	100	–	–	–	–	Tyl *et al.* (1993)
		500	–	–	–	–	
		1,000	–	–	–	–	
		2,000	X	–	–	–	
Diet	Rat/F344	40	–	–	–	–	Maronpot *et al.* (1983)
		200	–	–	–	–	
		1,000	–	–	–	–	
Inhal. (whole body)	Rat/CD	150 mg/m^3	–	–	–	–	Tyl *et al.* (1995)
		1,000 mg/m^3	–	–	–	–	
		2,500 mg/m^3	X	–	–	–	
Inhal. (nose only)	Mouse/CD-1	500 mg/m^3	–	–	–	–	Tyl *et al.* (1995)
		1,000 mg/m^3	X	–	–	–	
		2,500 mg/m^3	X	X	X	–	
Dermal	Mouse/CD-1	404	–	–	–	–	Tyl *et al.* (1995)
		1,677	–	–	–	–	
		3,549	–	–	–	–	

Other routes of exposure

EG also was evaluated in developmental toxicity studies utilizing dietary, whole-body inhalation, nose-only inhalation and dermal routes of exposure. These routes of exposure are characterized by slower, non-bolus dose-rates relative to gavage dosing, and all show a much lower propensity to induce developmental toxicity. For example, there was no evidence of developmental toxicity in a feeding study in rats using dose levels as high as 1,000 mg/kg/day (Maronpot *et al.*, 1983). The only developmental effects seen in a mouse dermal study occurred at the high dose level of 3,549 mg/kg/day and consisted of increases in two very minor skeletal variations (delayed ossification of phalanges and skull), with no evidence of teratogenicity. Inhalation studies on EG exhibited developmental toxicity only at very high aerosol concentrations which were several-fold above the saturated vapor concentration (Tyl *et al.*, 1995a,b,c). These studies were confounded by deposition of large quantities of EG on the fur of the animals. EG has a sweet taste that animals find palatable, which appears to have led to oral ingestion of significant quantities. As much as 1,000 mg/kg/day of EG in the whole-body inhalation studies and up to 330 mg/kg/day of EG in the nose-only study were potentially available for oral ingestion.

Postnatal effects and reversibility

The effects of *in utero* exposure to EG on postnatal development have also been examined. At very high dose levels (>2,000 mg/kg/day via gavage), pup mortality increased and pup weight gain decreased, while kidney weights decreased through postnatal day 63 in pups from dams given 1,250 mg/kg/day (Price *et al.*, 1988). Despite the high dose and associated systemic toxicity, there were no effects of treatment on any developmental landmarks such as incisor eruption, testes descent or vaginal opening, or on any neurodevelopmental endpoints, such as wire-grasping skills (forelimb and hindlimb grip).

The persistence of skeletal effects induced by high dose *in utero* exposure (GD 6–15) to EG was examined in rat pups at 1, 4, 14, 21 and 63 days of age. Although skeletal effects characteristic of EG exposure were noted during early postnatal development, their incidence steadily decreased with age, such that by postnatal day 63 there was no detectable difference between pups from EG-treated and control dams. The apparent reversibility of these skeletal malformations is remarkable given the severity of some of them (e.g., fused ribs, extra ribs). However, recent research has revealed an extensive capacity of the developing skeleton to remodel postnatally (Carney and Kimmel, 2007; Macsai *et al.*, 2008).

REPRODUCTIVE TOXICITY

EG has been evaluated in detail by the US National Toxicology Program's Center for the Evaluation of Risks to Human Reproduction and is considered to have a low potential for reproductive effects at exposures of relevance to humans. Any effects seen were generally limited to dose levels in excess of 1,000 mg/kg/day (NTP-CERHR, 2004). For example, EG was administered via drinking water in a mouse continuous breeding study in which breeding pairs were continually co-housed for 14 weeks and reproductive performance was assessed. Dose levels were 0, 400, 800 and 1,600 mg/kg/day. Most of the F_1 litters were retained until young adults and then mated to produce an F_2 generation. Effects were limited to a slight decrease in the number of F_1 offspring produced by the high dose level breeding pairs (10.2 pups/litter) relative to controls (10.8 pups/litter), but there were no such decreases in those F_1 animals which were then mated to produce F_2 litters. There were no reproductive effects resulting from continuous exposure to the other doses, 400 and 800 mg/kg/day.

Fisher 344 rats were continuously exposed via diet for three generations at dose levels of 0, 40, 200 or 1,000 mg/kg/day (DePass *et al.*, 1986). Although mild renal toxicity was noted at the high dose level, there were no effects on reproductive performance, pup survival or pup growth at any dose level. This study also was combined with a dominant lethal assay; there were no adverse effects observed at any dose level in that assay.

TOXICOKINETICS

Absorption

The absorption of EG shows marked route-dependent differences which have a major impact on toxicity. In all species studied, absorption of EG administered by oral gavage is rapid and shows nearly 100% bioavailability (Frantz *et al.*, 1996a; Gessner *et al.*, 1961; Jacobsen *et al.*, 1984; Pottenger *et al.*, 2001). Peak blood EG levels are reached within 1 hour of gavage exposure in rats, mice and rabbits. Oral absorption rates in humans are difficult to define precisely because most clinical cases do not present until several hours after exposure. Nonetheless, the available data are consistent with rapid and complete oral absorption in humans (Jacobsen *et al.*, 1984).

In contrast to oral exposure, dermal absorption is extremely slow and incomplete. Rats and mice were exposed to neat EG or a 50% aqueous EG solution for 6 hours, followed by wash-off and subsequent sampling of blood and urine for up to 96 hours (Frantz *et al.*, 1996a,b,c). The half-life for absorption in rats was 4.5 hours, which is over 20 times slower than oral gavage. *In vitro* studies with human cadaver skin also report a slow rate of dermal absorption (Saghir *et al.*, 2010; Sun *et al.*, 1995).

A study which evaluated absorption via inhalation of EG vapors and aerosols in rats reported that 60% of the inhaled dose was deposited in the nasal cavity, with 75–80% of the initial body burden found systemically (Marshall and Cheng, 1983). Absorption data on humans exposed to EG vapors and aerosols are inconclusive. However, human blood:air partition coefficients measured *in vitro* for EG were very high (>17,542), suggesting rapid absorption (Corley *et al.*, 2005a,b).

Distribution

Consistent with other low molecular weight alcohols, unchanged EG is extensively and uniformly distributed throughout the body, following total body water. However, distribution of certain key metabolites shows some unique features during pregnancy, as will be discussed later.

Metabolism

The metabolism of EG (Figure 45.1) has been described in numerous studies and reviews and follows the same pathways in all species examined (Carney, 1994; Frantz *et al.*, 1996a,b,c; Jacobsen *et al.*, 1984, 1988; Jacobsen and McMartin, 1986). The initial step in the metabolic pathway consists of oxidation of EG to glycoaldehyde, which is extremely labile and undergoes nearly instantaneous conversion to glycolic acid (GA). Biotransformation of EG to GA occurs primarily in the liver through the alcohol dehydrogenase/aldehyde dehydrogenase (ADH/ALDH) complex. GA is subsequently oxidized to glyoxylic acid, followed by formation of the terminal metabolites, oxalic acid and CO_2.

The conversion of GA to glyoxylic acid is of critical importance in the toxicity of EG as this is the key rate-limiting step in the EG metabolic pathway. While at low doses GA is readily oxidized to downstream metabolites leading ultimately to CO_2, at high doses and/or high dose-rates, a shift to non-linear kinetics occurs as the rate of GA formation exceeds that of further GA metabolism. An intravenous bolus study in male rats (Marshall, 1982) indicated that this dose-dependent shift occurs at dose levels between 200 and 1,000 mg/kg (Figure 45.2). As will be discussed later (see Mode of Action), research has identified this shift in GA kinetics as a required step in the progression toward developmental toxicity. As a result of this kinetic shift, peak blood GA levels rose disproportionately and reached a range of 4.1–4.8 mM following a 1,000 mg/kg dose in female rats (Pottenger *et al.*, 2001; Carney *et al.*, 2010). In poisoning cases, blood GA concentrations as high as 29 mM have been reported (Jacobsen *et al.*, 1984). In contrast, dermal exposures of up to 1,000 mg/kg in rats showed no such shift in metabolism, with the majority of the EG dose being eliminated as CO_2 (Frantz *et al.*, 1996a,b,c).

The terminal metabolite, oxalic acid, is mainly of significance for renal toxicity, as it can come out of solution during concentration in the renal tubule and form calcium oxalate crystals (Corley *et al.*, 2005a,b). Unlike GA, which is highly soluble in water, the solubility of oxalic acid is low. These crystals are readily apparent during microscopic analysis of urine and kidney sections and are a diagnostic hallmark of EG intoxication. While calcium oxalate crystals have also been reported in the chorioallantoic placenta of pregnant rats exposed to EG, the doses employed were extremely high (Khera, 1991) such that oxalate is not considered to be a significant factor in the developmental toxicity of EG.

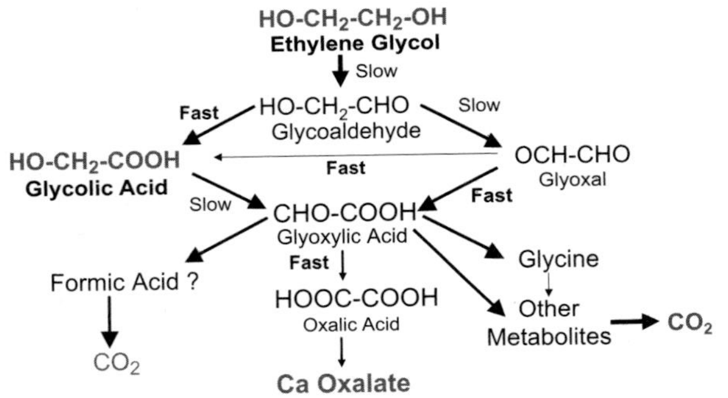

FIGURE 45.1 Metabolism of ethylene glycol. (Reprinted with permission from Corley *et al.*, 2005.)

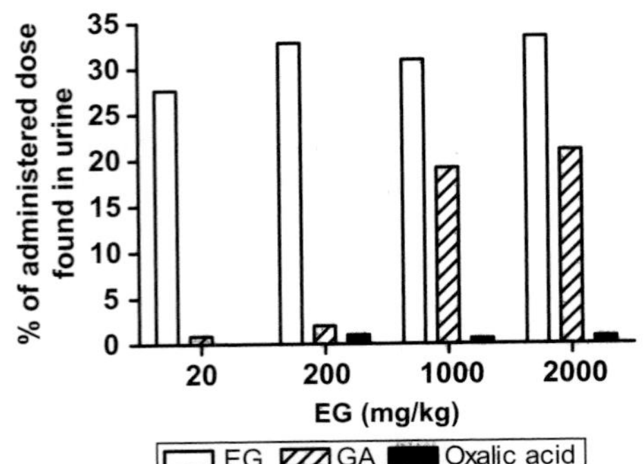

FIGURE 45.2 Dose-dependent urinary excretion of unchanged ethylene glycol (EG) and certain metabolites (glycolic acid, GA) following various intravenous doses of EG in male rats. Levels of glycoaldehyde and glyoxylic acid were below the limit of detection. (Based on Marshall, 1982.)

Elimination

Unchanged EG is rapidly eliminated in the urine, with half-lives of 1–3 h in rats (Frantz *et al.*, 1996a,b,c), 1–2 h in rabbits (Carney *et al.*, 2008) and 2.5–8.4 h in humans (Jacobsen *et al.*, 1988). In a radiotracer study with male rats, unchanged EG eliminated in the urine generally represented about one-third of the total EG dose administered (Frantz *et al.*, 1996a,b,c).

Elimination of GA and other metabolites varies as a function of GA's dose-dependent metabolism. At non-saturating doses, metabolites are almost completely oxidized to CO_2 which is eliminated through the respiratory tract, with a relatively small proportion of intermediary metabolites appearing in urine. Conversely, at high doses which saturate metabolism, the percentage of dose eliminated as expired CO_2 decreases with a commensurate increase in the percentage of metabolites (mainly GA) eliminated in the urine (Frantz *et al.*, 1996a,b,c). Consistent with the dose-dependent saturation of GA metabolism following oral exposure, very little GA is found in urine following a low (10 mg/kg) dose of EG, whereas GA accounted for 37.5% of total urinary elimination. In contrast, no evidence of a shift in urinary elimination was seen following dermal exposure, which is explained by the low rate of dermal absorption, thus precluding the achievement of saturating concentrations of GA.

Toxicokinetics in pregnancy

Pregnancy appears to have essentially no effect on the toxicokinetic profile of EG, GA or oxalic acid in maternal blood based on a study in which jugular vein-cannulated, female non-pregnant or pregnant CD rats were administered ^{13}C-labeled EG on GD 10 by gavage at dose levels of 10 or 2,500 mg/kg (Pottenger *et al.*, 2001). In addition, evaluation of toxicokinetics in pregnant rats given 10, 150, 500, 1,000 or 2,500 mg/kg EG revealed similar dose-dependent GA kinetics as reported previously for non-pregnant rats (Marshall, 1982; Frantz *et al.*, 1996a,b,c). Oxalic acid was a very minor metabolite in both blood and urine at all dose levels in pregnant rats.

The lack of an effect of pregnancy on EG toxicokinetics is consistent with the fact that EG metabolism is mainly carried out in maternal liver by ADH/ALDH. Both human and rat chorioallantoic placenta show little ADH/ALDH activity (Sjoblom *et al.*, 1978; Pares *et al.*, 1984). Postnatally, hepatic ADH activity increases slowly in humans with adult levels of activity not reached until 5 years of age (Pikkarainen and Raiha, 1967), while in rats, ADH activity increases rapidly after birth and is close to adult activity levels by 7 weeks of age (Sjoblom *et al.*, 1978)

While pregnancy does not appear to affect the kinetics of EG, GA or oxalic acid in blood, there are some unique considerations with respect to disposition of GA to the conceptus that are important in developmental toxicity. In particular, GA distribution to the conceptus shows marked differences between rats and rabbits, and the understanding of the factors regulating these differences have implications for assessing potential risk from EG exposure during human pregnancy.

In rats, GA becomes concentrated in the mid-gestation (GD 10–12) embryo, as well as in the exocoelomic fluid contained within the visceral yolk sac placenta, to levels which are ~2-fold higher than corresponding maternal blood levels (Figure 45.3). The higher levels of GA in rat embryo and exocoelomic fluid appear to be due to a phenomenon called ion-trapping (Nau and Scott, 1986; Scott and Nau, 1987; Srivastava *et al.*, 1991; Carney *et al.*, 2004). Early in development, the pH of mouse and rat embryos, as well as the exocoelomic fluid, is 0.2–0.4 pH units higher than that of maternal plasma. The unionized fraction of weak acids such as GA cross into the exocoelomic fluid and/or embryonic cells, become ionized due to the higher pH of those environments, and thus are unable to diffuse back out. Weak acid ion-trapping in organogenesis stage rodent embryos has been documented for a number of compounds, including methoxyacetic acid, valproic acid, butyric acid, propionic acid and glycolic acid. In fact, during fetal stages of development, the direction of the pH gradient is opposite that of early development, driving a reversal in the partitioning of many weak acid or weak base compounds. It should also be noted that ion trapping is only significant for compounds with low protein binding, as only the free fraction is available for exchange. GA protein binding is relatively low (<25%) in humans, rats and rabbits (Corley *et al.*, 2005a,b).

In rabbits, the yolk sac cavity fluid that surrounds the GD 9–12 embryo is acidic with respect to maternal blood; thus, the pH gradient is in the opposite direction to that of rats (Carney *et al.*, 2008). Consistent with pH-mediated distribution, peak embryonic GA levels in the rabbit embryo and yolk sac cavity fluid were only 30% of maximal maternal blood GA. In humans, measurement of acid–base status in the first trimester of pregnancy has been accomplished via ultrasound-guided sampling in women undergoing elective termination of pregnancy (Jauniaux *et al.*, 1994). The pH of the conceptus fluid surrounding the embryos (called coelomic fluid) is 0.2 pH units lower than that of maternal blood. Therefore, if embryonic dosimetry was based solely on these pH gradients, one would expect GA concentration in the human embryo to be about half that of maternal blood, which contrasts with the opposite situation in the rat.

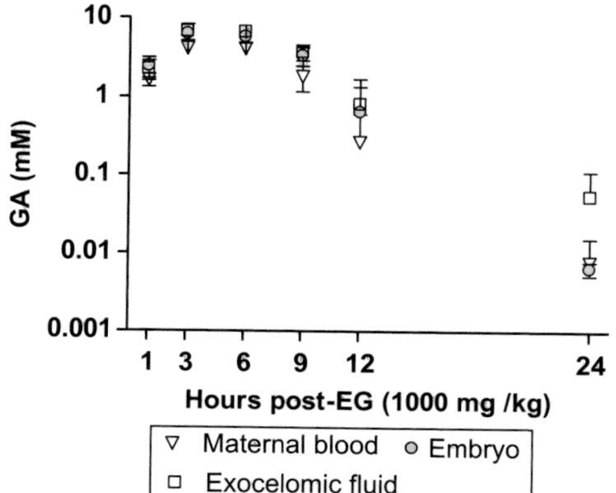

FIGURE 45.3 Pharmacokinetic time-course of glycolic acid (GA) in rat maternal blood, exocoelomic fluid and embryo following gavage dose of 1,000 mg/kg EG on GD 11. Note higher concentrations of GA in embryo and exocoelomic fluid relative to maternal blood. (Based on Carney *et al.*, 2010.)

MECHANISM OF ACTION

Identification of proximate toxicant

One of the first steps in any mode-of-action (MOA) investigation is to discern whether the toxic effect of interest is due to the parent molecule itself or to one or more of its metabolites. For EG, the whole embryo culture model was extremely useful in addressing this question as the cultures contain no significant ADH/ALDH metabolizing capability of their own, thus enabling the evaluation of the effects of specific metabolites directly on the developing conceptus (Sjoblom *et al.*, 1978). Whole embryo culture starts with the explantation from the uterus of postimplantation rodent embryos intact within the visceral yolk sac placenta, amnion and other extraembryonic tissues (Cockroft, 1990). The conceptuses are then grown in a rotating bottle culture apparatus for up to 48 hours, during which time they undergo extensive development. In two independent rat whole embryo culture studies, parent EG was tested at extremely high concentrations and was found to have little effect on embryo development *in vitro* (Carney *et al.*, 1996; Klug *et al.*, 2001). Interestingly, high concentrations of a low molecular weight compound such as EG generate extremely high osmotic pressures in the culture media (up to 418 mOsmol/kg H_2O vs. 299 for control media in the Carney *et al.* experiment). The lack of effects of EG in whole embryo culture suggests that the visceral yolk sac placenta is able to maintain homeostasis in the face of significant hyperosmotic challenge.

In parallel to the central role of EG's metabolites in acute and systemic toxicity, it was also logical to consider one of these metabolites as the potential proximate toxicant. The GA metabolite specifically was suggested based on the observation that the dose levels at which GA kinetics shift from linear to non-linear kinetics just slightly precede the LOEL for developmental toxicity.

The developmental toxicity of GA was evaluated in CD rats given 0, 75, 150, 300 or 600 mg/kg/day by gavage to rats on GD 7–21, as well as in rat whole embryo culture studies which examined the direct effects of GA and several other metabolites (Carney *et al.*, 1999, 1996; Munley *et al.*, 1999; Klug *et al.*, 2001). *In vivo*, maternal GA exposure (>300 mg/kg/day) caused the same signature of fetal axial skeletal effects as caused by EG. *In vitro*, GA affected the developing somites, which are the anlagen for the axial skeleton, and the maxillary process, which eventually develops into the upper jaw and palate, corresponding with the cleft palate observed following very high doses of EG *in vivo*. Furthermore, the concentrations of GA in whole embryo culture at teratogenic doses (6 mM) corresponded closely with the levels of GA found in the rat conceptus following a teratogenic dose of EG *in vivo*. In contrast, all of the other metabolites tested (i.e., glycoaldehyde, glyoxylic acid, oxalic acid) only affected rat embryo development at concentrations which were much higher than those occurring *in vivo*. Based on this weight of evidence, it is now well accepted that GA is the proximate toxicant in the developmental toxicity of EG (NTP-CERHR, 2004).

Role of metabolic acidosis

The identification of GA as the proximate toxicant raised interesting questions about its MOA. GA is an acidic metabolite (pK_a 3.83), and is the major contributor to the metabolic acidosis seen following acutely toxic exposures to EG (Clay and Murphy, 1977; Jacobsen *et al.*, 1984). This fact led to early exploration of the hypothesis that maternal metabolic acidosis was the mode of action for EG glycol developmental toxicity. This was first explored in an *in vivo* study in which 3.3g/kg of EG was given via subcutaneous injection to GD 11 rats, either with or without co-administration of sodium bicarbonate to neutralize the acidosis which occurred with EG alone (Khera, 1991). Consistent with earlier studies, high dose bolus administration of EG caused a high (85%) incidence of skeletal defects. However, the incidence of skeletal defects was considerably reduced (55%), but not eliminated, with co-administration of sodium bicarbonate. Although this study indicated that metabolic acidosis contributed to developmental toxicity following high dose administration of EG, the lack of complete amelioration and the use of a single high dose level precluded determination of whether the induction of metabolic acidosis was required in EG's mode of action for developmental effects.

To address this question further, a novel *in vivo* study was conducted in which equimolar doses (8.5mM/kg/day) of either GA (free acid form) or sodium glycolate at neutral pH were given to pregnant rats on GD 6–15 to compare their effects on acid–base balance, toxicokinetic parameters, and embryo/fetal development. Both treatments resulted in very similar kinetics for total glycolate in maternal blood, but free GA caused metabolic acidosis whereas sodium glycolate did not. Free GA caused reductions in fetal body weights and the signature profile of axial skeletal defects characteristic of EG. In the sodium glycolate group, the incidence of skeletal malformations was lower than in the free GA group, but nonetheless, there still remained treatment-related decreases in fetal body weight, increases in the incidence of hemivertebrae and missing ribs, and increases in three minor skeletal variations, despite lack of any metabolic acidosis.

These *in vivo* results were consistent with rat whole embryo culture data showing that free GA (pH6.7) and sodium glycolate at (pH7.4) caused similar rates of morphological defects. Taken together, these results demonstrated that developmental toxicity is due specifically to GA, rather than a secondary result of acidosis. The identification of GA as the true proximate toxicant then set the stage for determination of a threshold for developmental toxicity based on the internal dosimetry of GA.

Linking developmental toxicity and kinetics

The fact that GA kinetics exhibit saturation at dose levels just below those associated with developmental toxicity suggested that the relevant internal dose metric for defining a threshold was *peak* GA in maternal blood or embryo. As summarized in Table 45.3, peak maternal blood GA values at the NOEL (500mg/kg/day) and LOEL (1,000mg/kg/day) for developmental toxicity in rats were 1.7 and 4.1–4.8mM, respectively (Pottenger *et al.*, 2001; Carney, 2010), while whole embryo culture studies indicated a no-effect concentration of 3mM and a lowest-effect concentration of 6mM GA (Carney *et al.*, 1996; Klug *et al.*, 2001). The higher values in whole embryo culture are in line with the ~2-fold concentration of GA in the embryo compared to the maternal blood (Carney *et al.*, 2008). By linking these toxicokinetic and whole embryo culture values back to the *in vivo* developmental toxicity NOEL and LOEL (Table 45.3), threshold values of 2mM GA in maternal blood and 4mM GA in embryo were proposed.

To test the validity of these proposed threshold values, a study was done to compare equivalent doses of EG given as a bolus (fast dose-rate) vs. as a slow continuous infusion (slow dose-rate) for their impact on kinetics and developmental outcome (Carney, 2010). This was accomplished by administering subcutaneous (SC) bolus injections of 0, 1,000 or 2,000mg/kg/day of EG on gestation day (GD) 6–15 once daily to pregnant CD rats, while three corresponding groups were given the same daily doses as continuous SC infusions administered via an implantable pump from GD 6 to 15. As expected, the fast dose-rate groups had peak maternal blood GA levels in excess of the putative 2mM threshold and the fetuses from these dams showed significant increases in skeletal malformations and variations. In the slow dose-rate groups, GA levels remained below the putative threshold and there was no increase in the incidence of skeletal defects. Supporting the validity of the 2mM maternal blood threshold, blood GA in the 2,000mg/kg/day slow dose-rate group was maintained just barely below the 2mM threshold (range of 0.7–1.1mM) from the initiation of infusion on GD 6 until its termination on GD 15, yet the fetuses from these dams exhibited no effects of treatment.

Species-specific GA kinetics and developmental toxicity

As mentioned previously, EG is not developmentally toxic in the rabbit (Tyl *et al.*, 1993). An understanding of the mechanisms behind this discordance between species may aid in

TABLE 45.3 Correlations across developmental toxicity and toxicokinetics in rats to establish a threshold for induction of developmental effects based on internal dose

	In vivo dose	Peak GA (maternal blood)	Peak GA (embryo)	GA concentration in whole embryo culture
No-effect dose	500 mg/kg/day	1.7 mM	No data	3 mM
Low-effect dose	1,000 mg/kg/day	4.1–4.8 mM	6.3 mM	6 mM

References: Carney *et al.* (1996); Klug *et al.* (2001); Pottenger *et al.* (2001); Carney (2010)

the understanding of the relevance of EG developmental toxicity to humans. In other words, which is a better predictor of EG's effects in humans – the rat or the rabbit? To address this question further, a toxicokinetic study of EG and GA in rabbit maternal and conceptus tissues following dosing on GD 9 was conducted (Carney *et al.*, 2008) and the data compared to the previously discussed toxicokinetic data in pregnant rats (Carney *et al.*, 2010; Pottenger *et al.*, 2001; Slikker *et al.*, 2004). The rabbit toxicokinetic study demonstrated a 10-fold lower concentration of GA in the embryo following administration of 1,000 mg/kg of EG relative to the pregnant rats given equivalent doses of EG at an equivalent stage of gestation (Figure 45.4). This interspecies difference was not explained by differences in absorption of EG, elimination of EG or GA, or GA protein binding, all of which were similar in rats and rabbits. Instead, the lower tissue levels of GA in the rabbit embryo appeared to be due to a combination of slower rates of GA formation and decreased disposition of GA from the maternal circulation to the rabbit embryo. Maximum concentrations of GA in rabbit maternal blood were slightly less than half those of rats given an identical dose of EG. The *in vivo* differences in GA kinetics in maternal blood were consistent with an *in vitro* liver slice metabolism study showing that rabbits metabolize EG to GA at a slower rate than rats (Booth *et al.*, 2004).

Compounding the species differences in maternal metabolism was a clear difference in disposition of GA to the embryo and conceptus fluids. Whereas rat embryos concentrate GA by ~2-fold over maternal blood levels, peak GA concentrations in the rabbit embryo were only 0.3 times those of peak maternal blood levels. As described previously, this concentration of GA in the rat is likely due to ion-trapping driven by a pH gradient between maternal blood and the exocoelomic fluid contained within the rat visceral yolk sac which encloses the rat embryo (Carney *et al.*, 2004; Jollie, 1990). Concentration is also favored by the small volume of conceptus fluid in rat, which is conducive to rapid equilibrium between maternal blood, exocoelomic fluid and embryo. In contrast, the volume of fluid surrounding the rabbit embryo is quite large relative to the size of the embryo. Also, pH gradients between maternal blood and conceptus fluids of rabbits are in the opposite direction to those of rats (see Carney *et al.*, 2004 for a detailed discussion), thus favoring retention of GA in maternal blood.

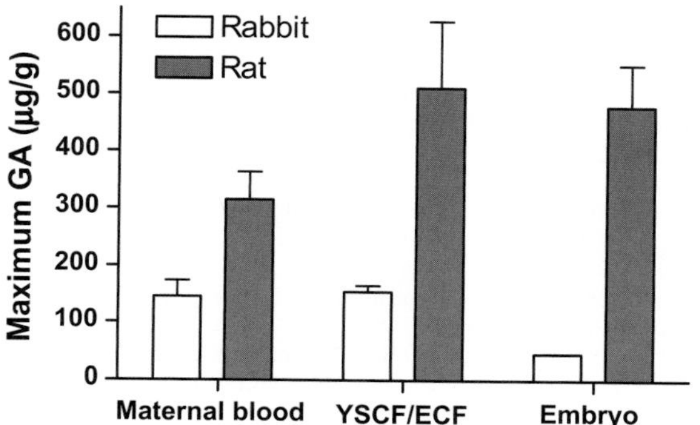

FIGURE 45.4 Comparison of peak glycolic acid (GA) in maternal blood, embryo and conceptus fluids of GD 9 rabbits and GD 11 rats given 1,000 mg/kg via gavage. YSCF = yolk sac cavity fluid of the rabbit; ECF = exocoelomic fluid of the rat. (From Carney *et al.*, 2008.)

Implications for humans

In humans it appears that metabolism of EG as well as disposition of GA to the embryo are likely to be more similar to rabbits than rats. This is based on *in vitro* metabolism studies which indicated a slower rate of GA formation in humans than in rats (Booth *et al.*, 2004). This conclusion is also supported by estimates developed using validated PBPK models for EG in rats and humans (Corley *et al.*, 2005a,b). For example, the PBPK model predicted blood GA to be 7-to 8-fold lower in humans than in rats following inhalation exposure concentrations ranging from 3 to 1,000 mg/m^3 (Corley *et al.*, 2005a,b). For the oral route, the PBPK model predicted that a 58 kg human female would need to consume a bolus dose in excess of 20 g EG to achieve a blood concentration of 2 mM GA.

As described in a review paper comparing toxicant disposition in early pregnancy, the first trimester human conceptus possesses several characteristics that bear similarity to the rabbit, but which fundamentally differ from the rat (Carney *et al.*, 2004). Human coelomic fluid is similar to the rabbit yolk sac cavity fluid in that it directly bathes the embryo and its volume is very large relative to the embryo. Interestingly, the pH gradient between human maternal blood and the coelomic fluid is similar to that of the rabbit, but opposite that of rats and mice (Jauniaux *et al.*, 1994). Predictions of GA partitioning based on pH indicate that GA levels in the human conceptus would be approximately 0.5× those of maternal blood, similar to the 0.3× factor observed in the rabbit.

RISK ASSESSMENT

Model of EG developmental toxicity

By using an integrated approach which combined animal developmental toxicity studies, whole embryo culture experiments and an extensive array of toxicokinetic data, a strong body of evidence was compiled to implicate GA as the proximate toxicant. Furthermore, studies in rats supported a proposed threshold of at least 2 mM GA in maternal blood (4 mM in conceptus) which must be exceeded in order to induce developmental effects. Achievement of such high internal concentrations of GA is favored by some specific conditions, namely: high dose, route characterized by rapid absorption (e.g., oral) and/or high dose-rate (Figure 45.5). These three variables converge to bring about very high blood levels of EG, which is readily metabolized to GA. The resulting

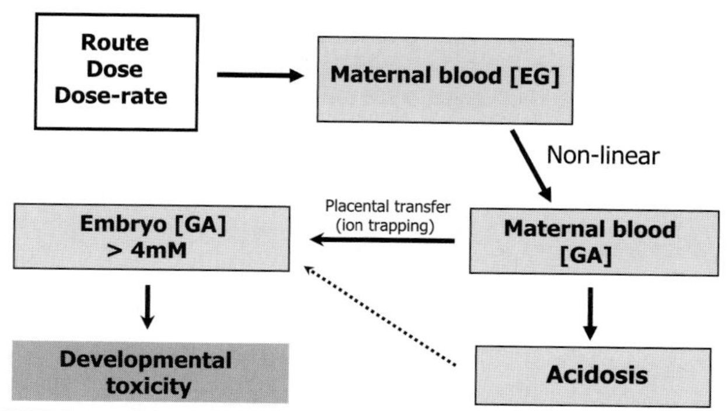

FIGURE 45.5 Schematic depiction of the MOA for EG-induced developmental toxicity in rodents.

high GA levels saturate the metabolism of GA to glyoxylic acid, such that GA production exceeds the rate of its further metabolism, resulting in a disproportionate or non-linear increase in blood GA concentrations. In species such as the rat and mouse, which concentrate weak acids within the conceptus, exposure of the embryo to GA is further increased, whereas in species such as the rabbit, GA is poorly distributed to the conceptus and embryonic GA levels are less than those of maternal blood. Given similarities in conceptus fluid volumes and pH gradients, GA disposition in the human is more likely to mirror the rabbit.

Risk to humans

Based on this understanding, it is clear that EG developmental toxicity requires very specific exposure conditions that are unlikely to occur under normal handling and use circumstances in humans. Typical exposures to EG involve doses much lower than those tested in animal studies; the principal route of exposure is dermal and, secondarily, inhalation and exposures tend to be spread over time rather than as a bolus with a high dose-rate. Under these conditions, GA should be readily metabolized with no shift to non-linear kinetics.

In addition, comparative toxicokinetics indicate that rodents form GA more quickly than other species, including the human, and appear to be unique in their propensity to concentrate GA within the conceptus. Thus, for a given exposure to EG, GA blood and tissue levels would be expected to be significantly lower in humans than in rats. Taken together, research on EG suggests there is negligible concern for developmental or reproductive toxicity in humans exposed to EG, which is in fact the conclusion drawn in a rigorous assessment of EG conducted by the National Toxicology Program's Center for the Evaluation of Risks to Human Reproduction (NTP-CERHR, 2004).

CONCLUDING REMARKS AND FUTURE DIRECTIONS

The "EG story" is the tale of a chemical identified over 25 years ago as having teratogenic potential in high dose animal studies, and an ensuing research journey which ultimately determined that EG-induced teratogenicity requires unique exposure circumstances which are highly unlikely to occur in human populations.

Beyond the specific implications for risk assessments on this high production volume chemical, the EG story illustrates a number of fundamental principles which are of much broader applicability. First and foremost, it is an excellent example of Karnofsky's law (Karnofsky, 1965), which reminds us that all chemical agents are potential teratogens under certain conditions. Indeed, the research on EG focused on definition of those conditions which differentiate safe vs. unsafe exposures to EG. In the case of EG, dose, dose-rate and route of exposure are the key determinants of developmental toxicity. This is likely to be true for a large number of other chemical agents as well.

Research on EG also led to new understanding of species differences in maternal and placental transfer physiology during early pregnancy, and how maternal blood levels are not always reliable predictors of exposure to the embryo. The research also shed light on the fundamental biology of the pregnant rabbit model, about which, despite its many decades of use in developmental toxicity testing, little had been known concerning factors such as the rabbit yolk sac or mechanisms of toxicant disposition to the embryo.

Finally, the lessons taught by the EG story have broader implications for the practice of developmental toxicity testing. Regulatory guidelines for prenatal developmental toxicity studies traditionally have required testing at maximally tolerated doses, with gavage as the default route of exposure. In fact, this practice was what led to the initial identification of EG's teratogenicity, and what required years of subsequent research which ultimately showed that these effects were not relevant to typical human exposures. In recent years, we are seeing a gradual trend away from these high dose and high dose-rate exposures, and instead a move toward dosing which better reflects human exposure characteristics. To support this approach, it will be necessary to incorporate more toxicokinetic measures into standardized testing, such as internal dose metrics, as well as to improve methods for estimating human exposures. Hopefully testing approaches have evolved such that a 20-year research program to prove that high dose effects are not relevant to humans will be a relic of the past.

ACKNOWLEDGMENT

The author thanks Dr. Lynn Pottenger (The Dow Chemical Company) for critical review of the manuscript.

REFERENCES

Booth ED, Dofferhoff O, Boogaard PJ, Watson WP (2004) Comparison of the metabolism of ethylene glycol and glycolic acid in vitro by precision-cut tissue slices from female rat, rabbit and human liver. *Xenobiotica* **34:** 31–48.

Carney EW (1994) An integrated perspective on the developmental toxicity of ethylene glycol. *Reprod Toxicol* **8:** 99–113.

Carney EW, Freshour NL, Dittenber DA, Dryzga MD (1999) Ethylene glycol developmental toxicity: unraveling the roles of glycolic acid and metabolic acidosis. *Toxicol Sci* **50:** 117–26.

Carney EW, Kimmel CA (2007) Interpretation of skeletal variations for human risk assessment: delayed ossification and wavy ribs. *Birth Defects Res B Dev Reprod Toxicol* **80:** 473–96.

Carney EW, Liberacki AB, Bartels MJ, Breslin WJ (1996) Identification of proximate toxicant for ethylene glycol developmental toxicity using rat whole embryo culture. *Teratology* **53:** 38–46.

Carney EW, Scialli AR, Watson RE, DeSesso JM (2004) Mechanisms regulating toxicant disposition to the embryo during early pregnancy: an interspecies comparison. *Birth Defects Res C Embryo Today* **72:** 345–60.

Carney EW, Tornesi B, Liberacki AB, Markham DA, Weitz DD, Luders TM, Studniski KG, Blessing JC, Gies RA, Corley RA (2010) The impact of dose-rate on ethylene glycol developmental toxicity and pharmacokinetics in pregnant CD rats. *Toxicol Sci* (in press).

Carney EW, Tornesi B, Markham DA, Rasoulpour RJ, Moore N (2008) Species-specificity of ethylene glycol-induced developmental toxicity: toxicokinetic and whole embryo culture studies in the rabbit. *Birth Defects Res B Dev Reprod Toxicol* **83:** 573–81.

Clay KL, Murphy RC (1977) On the metabolic acidosis of ethylene glycol intoxication. *Toxicol Appl Pharmacol* **39:** 39–49.

Cockroft DL (1990) Dissection and culture of postimplantation embryos. In *Postimplantation Embryos: A Practical Approach* (Copp AJ, Cockroft DL, eds.). New York, Oxford University Press, pp. 15–40.

Corley RA, Bartels MJ, Carney EW, Weitz KK, Soelberg JJ, Gies RA, Thrall KD (2005a) Development of a physiologically based pharmacokinetic model for ethylene glycol and its metabolite, glycolic acid, in rats and humans. *Toxicol Sci* **85:** 476–90.

Corley RA, Meek ME, Carney EW (2005b) Mode of action: oxalate crystal-induced renal tubule degeneration and glycolic acid-induced dysmorphogenesis – renal and developmental effects of ethylene glycol. *Crit Rev Toxicol* **35:** 691–702.

DePass LR, Woodside MD, Maronpot RR, Weil CS (1986) Three-generation reproduction and dominant lethal mutagenesis studies of ethylene glycol in the rat. *Fundam Appl Toxicol* **7:** 566–72.

Frantz SW, Beskitt JL, Grosse CM, Tallant MJ, Dietz FK, Ballantyne B (1996a) Pharmacokinetics of ethylene glycol. I. Plasma disposition after single intravenous, peroral, or percutaneous doses in female Sprague-Dawley rats and CD-1 mice. *Drug Metab Dispos* **24:** 911–21.

Frantz SW, Beskitt JL, Grosse CM, Tallant MJ, Dietz FK, Ballantyne B (1996b) Pharmacokinetics of ethylene glycol. II. Tissue distribution, dose-dependent elimination, and identification of urinary metabolites following single intravenous, peroral or percutaneous doses in female Sprague-Dawley rats and CD-1 mice. *Xenobiotica* **26:** 1195–220.

Frantz SW, Beskitt JL, Tallant MJ, Zourelias LA, Ballantyne B (1996c) Pharmacokinetics of ethylene glycol. III. Plasma disposition and metabolic fate after single increasing intravenous, peroral, or percutaneous doses in the male Sprague-Dawley rat. *Xenobiotica* **26:** 515–39.

Gessner PK, Parke DV, Williams RT (1961) Studies in detoxication. 86. The metabolism of 14C-labelled ethylene glycol. *Biochem J* **79:** 482–9.

Jacobsen D, Hewlett TP, Webb R, Brown ST, Ordinario AT, McMartin KE (1988) Ethylene glycol intoxication: evaluation of kinetics and crystalluria. *Am J Med* **84:** 145–52.

Jacobsen D, McMartin KE (1986) Methanol and ethylene glycol poisonings. Mechanism of toxicity, clinical course, diagnosis and treatment. *Med Toxicol* **1:** 309–34.

Jacobsen D, Ovrebo S, Ostborg J, Sejersted OM (1984) Glycolate causes the acidosis in ethylene glycol poisoning and is effectively removed by hemodialysis. *Acta Med Scand* **216:** 409–16.

Jauniaux E, Jurkovic D, Gulbis B, Collins WP, Zaidi J, Campbell S (1994) Investigation of the acid–base balance of coelomic and amniotic fluids in early human pregnancy. *Am J Obstet Gynecol* **170:** 1365–9.

Jollie WP (1990) Development, morphology, and function of the yolk-sac placenta of laboratory rodents. *Teratology* **41:** 361–81.

Karnofsky DA (1965) Drugs as teratogens in animals and man. *Annu Rev Pharmacol* **10:** 447–72.

Khera KS (1991) Chemically induced alterations in maternal homeostasis and histology of conceptus: their etiologic significance in rat fetal anomalies. *Teratology* **44:** 259–97.

Klug S, Merker HJ, Jackh R (2001) Effects of ethylene glycol and metabolites on in vitro development of rat embryos during organogenesis. *Toxicol in Vitro* **15:** 635–42.

Macsai CE, Foster BK, Xian CJ (2008) Roles of Wnt signalling in bone growth, remodelling, skeletal disorders and fracture repair. *J Cell Physiol* **215:** 578–87.

Maronpot RR, Zelenak JP, Weaver EV, Smith NJ (1983) Teratogenicity study of ethylene glycol in rats. *Drug Chem Toxicol* **6:** 579–94.

Marshall TC (1982) Dose-dependent disposition of ethylene glycol in the rat after intravenous administration. *J Toxicol Environ Health* **10:** 397–409.

Marshall TC, Cheng YS (1983) Deposition and fate of inhaled ethylene glycol vapor and condensation aerosol in the rat. *Fundam Appl Toxicol* **3:** 175–81.

Munley SM, Kennedy GL, Hurtt ME (1999) Developmental toxicity study of glycolic acid in rats. *Drug Chem Toxicol* **22:** 569–82.

Nau H, Scott WJ Jr (1986) Weak acids may act as teratogens by accumulating in the basic milieu of the early mammalian embryo. *Nature* **323:** 276–8.

Neeper-Bradley TL, Tyl RW, Fisher LC, Kubena MF, Vrbanic MA, Losco PE (1995) Determination of a no-observed-effect level for developmental toxicity of ethylene glycol administered by gavage to CD rats and CD-1 mice. *Fundam Appl Toxicol* **27:** 121–30.

NTP-CERHR (2004) NTP-CERHR Expert Panel report on the reproductive and developmental toxicity of ethylene glycol. *Reprod Toxicol* **18:** 457–532.

Pares X, Farres J, Vallee BL (1984) Organ specific alcohol metabolism: placental chi-ADH. *Biochem Biophys Res Commun* **119:** 1047–55.

Pikkarainen PH, Raiha NC (1967) Development of alcohol dehydrogenase activity in the human liver. *Pediatr Res* **1:** 165–8.

Pottenger LH, Carney EW, Bartels MJ (2001) Dose-dependent nonlinear pharmacokinetics of ethylene glycol metabolites in pregnant (GD 10) and non-pregnant Sprague-Dawley rats following oral administration of ethylene glycol. *Toxicol Sci* **62:** 10–19.

Price CJ, George JD, Marr MC, Kimmel CA, Schwetz BA, Morrissey RE (1988) Developmental toxicity evaluation of ethylene glycol (CAS 107-21-1) in CD rats. Report of the National Toxicology Program.

Price CJ, Kimmel CA, Tyl RW, Marr MC (1985) The developmental toxicity of ethylene glycol in rats and mice. *Toxicol Appl Pharmacol* **81:** 113–27.

Saghir SA, Bartels MJ, Snellings WM (2010) Dermal penetration of ethylene glycol through human skin in vitro. *Int J Toxicol* **29:** 268–76.

Schardein JL (1985) *Chemically Induced Birth Defects*. New York, Marcel Dekker, Inc. pp. 879.

Scott WJ Jr, Nau H (1987) Accumulation of weak acids in the young mammalian embryo. In *Pharmacokinetics in Teratogenesis* (Nau H, Scott WJ Jr, ed.). Boca Raton, CRC Press, Inc. pp. 71–7.

Sjoblom M, Pilstrom L, Morland J (1978) Activity of alcohol dehydrogenase and acetaldehyde dehydrogenases in the liver and placenta during the development of the rat. *Enzyme* **23:** 108–15.

Slikker W Jr, Andersen ME, Bogdanffy MS, Bus JS, Cohen SD, Conolly RB, David RM, Doerrer NG, Dorman DC, Gaylor DW, Hattis D, Rogers JM, Setzer RW, Swenberg JA, Wallace K (2004) Dose-dependent transitions in mechanisms of toxicity: case studies. *Toxicol Appl Pharmacol* **201:** 226–94.

Srivastava M, Collins MD, Scott WJ Jr, Wittfoht W, Nau H (1991) Transplacental distribution of weak acids in mice: accumulation in compartments of high pH. *Teratology* **43:** 325–9.

Sun J, Frantz SW, Beskitt JL (1995) In vitro skin penetration of ethylene glycol using excised skin from mice and humans. *J Toxicol Cutan Ocular Toxicol* **14:** 273–86.

Tyl RW, Ballantyne B, Fisher LC, Fait DL, Dodd DE, Klonne DR, Pritts IM, Losco PE (1995a) Evaluation of the developmental toxicity of ethylene glycol aerosol in CD-1 mice by nose-only exposure. *Fundam Appl Toxicol* **27:** 49–62.

Tyl RW, Ballantyne B, Fisher LC, Fait DL, Savine TA, Dodd DE, Klonne DR, Pritts IM (1995b) Evaluation of the developmental toxicity of ethylene glycol aerosol in the CD rat and CD-1 mouse by whole-body exposure. *Fundam Appl Toxicol* **24:** 57–75.

Tyl RW, Fisher LC, Kubena MF, Vrbanic MA, Losco PE (1995c) Assessment of the developmental toxicity of ethylene glycol applied cutaneously to CD-1 mice. *Fundam Appl Toxicol* **27:** 155–66.

Tyl RW, Price CJ, Marr MC, Myers CB, Seely JC, Heindel JJ, Schwetz BA (1993) Developmental toxicity evaluation of ethylene glycol by gavage in New Zealand white rabbits. *Fundam Appl Toxicol* **20:** 402–12.

C H A P T E R

46

Methyl *tert*-butyl ether

Dongmei Li and Xiaodong Han

INTRODUCTION

Methyl *tert*-butyl ether (MTBE) is a kind of oxygenate used as a fuel additive in gasoline. It enables fuel to burn more efficiently and helps prevent engine knocking by raising the oxygen content of gasoline and increasing its octane rating. Aside from its use as an oxygenate, MTBE is also used therapeutically for dissolving gallstones in humans (Hellstern *et al.*, 1998). MTBE is the main component of ether oxygenates; and as such MTBE production all over the world is in a considerable volume. For example, in 1999, the estimated production capacity of MTBE in the USA was over 200,000 barrels per day. As of 2010, the global production capacity of MTBE is estimated to be approximately 18 million metric tons annually. Thus, the potential exposure of humans to MTBE should be monitored.

In 1979, small amounts of MTBE began to be used in gasoline in order to replace tetra-ethyl lead in the USA. MTBE has more favorable qualities than other oxygenates, such as its low sulfur content, boiling point, blending vapor pressure and high octane number. It is also inexpensive. In 1990, the Clean Air Act Amendments was passed by the US Congress, which mandated the use of oxygenated fuels in some areas without having to meet the National Ambient Air Quality Standards during winter. Since 1992, MTBE volumes in some gasoline blends reached 15% to fulfill oxygenate requirements. However, due to its high solubility in water, once fuels leak from underground storage tanks, MTBE rapidly moves into surface or groundwater at a rate faster than any of the other components in the fuel. In 1996, 50% of public water suppliers were obliged to close because high levels of MTBE were detected in the water wells of Santa Monica, and MTBE contamination began to arouse public concern. US findings subsequently found that tens of thousands of contaminated water wells were distributed across the country. Since 1999, MTBE began to be phased out in California and other locations. The federal requirement for oxygen content in reformulated gasoline has been modified in the Energy Policy Act of 2005, and as of 2010, MTBE will be completely banned in the USA. Due to these reasons, the US production of MTBE has declined. For other countries, however, MTBE will continue to be a major component of clean gasoline.

Recently, McGregor *et al.* (2006) described metabolic pathways of MTBE in detail. Metabolic studies have found that CYP2A6 is the major enzyme involved in the initial oxidation of MTBE into *tert*-butyl alcohol (TBA) and formaldehyde in liver microsomes (Hutcheon *et al.*, 1996; Hong *et al.*, 1997a,b, 2001; Bernauer *et al.*, 1998; Amberg *et al.*, 1999; Gal *et al.*, 2001). TBA may be further converted into 2-methyl-1,2-propanediol and 2-hydroxyisobutyrate, both of which are the major metabolites of MTBE detected in rat and human urine (Hutcheon *et al.*, 1996; Bernauer *et al.*, 1998; Amberg *et al.*, 1999). There is similar biotransformation in terms of quality and quantity between rats and humans, and no gender differences have been found in either species (Amberg *et al.*, 1999).

The toxicity, human health hazards and toxicokinetics of MTBE have been described in detail in several publications (Hutcheon *et al.*, 1996; Ahmed, 2001; McGregor *et al.*, 2006; Phillips *et al.*, 2008). In recent years, incidents of reproductive diseases, especially in males, such as testicular cancer, cryptorchidism and hypospadias, have increased (Chilvers *et al.*, 1984; Matlai and Beral, 1985; Adami *et al.*, 1994; Forman and Moller, 1994; Toppari *et al.*, 1996; Paulozzi *et al.*, 1997), and semen quality and quantity have declined (Carlsen *et al.*, 1992; Swan *et al.*, 1997; Andersen *et al.*, 2000). The use of environmental chemicals has been regarded as an important consideration in determining possible reproductive and developmental toxicity. Although the use of MTBE had been banned in the USA, water supplies used for drinking, bathing, cooking and recreation may still be contaminated with MTBE (Davis and Farland, 2001).

This chapter describes the reproductive and developmental toxicity of MTBE in different species, including rodents, rabbits and aquatic organisms, since the human toxicity data are limited.

REPRODUCTIVE TOXICITY

Male reproductive toxicity

In *in vivo* studies, no significant effects, such as on relative testicular weight and testicular histology, were reported in subchronic studies on male rats or mice exposed to MBTE by inhalation. In subchronic studies by gavage, the relative testicular weights of male Sprague–Dawley rats decreased

Reproductive and Developmental Toxicology, Edited by Ramesh C. Gupta
ISBN: 978-0-12-382032-7

significantly after exposure to 400, 800 and 1,500 mg/kg body weight MTBE for 14 days. In addition, their testicular histology changed significantly only at 1,500 mg/kg body weight MTBE after treatment for 28 days (Li *et al.*, 2009a). The relative testicular weights of these rats also increased significantly only following oral administration of 1,500 mg/kg body weight MTBE for 28 days (Williams *et al.*, 2000a). No testicular histology or changes in relative testicular weight were found in CD-1, B6C3F1 or BALB/c mice exposed to MTBE or TBA (Chun *et al.*, 1992; NTP, 1995; de Peyster *et al.*, 2008), and no significant testicular histology changes related to treatment were reported in F344 rats treated via drinking water with TBA after 2 years' exposure (NTP, 1995). However, interstitial cell hyperplasia was reported to occur in both an inhalation study of F344 rats exposed to MTBE for 2 years (Chun *et al.*, 1992) and in a gavage study of Sprague–Dawley rats (Belpoggi *et al.*, 1998).

In vitro studies have found that only high concentrations (≥50 mM and ≥5 mM) of MTBE have direct toxic effects on Sertoli cells and mixed adult spermatogenic cells in the testes (Li *et al.*, 2007, 2009b). DNA damaged by oxidative stress may be one of the mechanisms that induce the toxicity of MTBE (Li *et al.*, 2009b). No studies on the effects of MBTE on Leydig cells *in vitro* have been reported.

Female reproductive toxicity

After female B6C3F1 mice were exposed to 8,000 ppm MTBE vapor for either 3 or 21 days or 4 or 8 months, their body weight gain and ovary and uterine weights significantly decreased, and the number of uterine glands and epithelial layers in their cervix and vagina also decreased (Moser *et al.*, 1998). Similarly, MTBE-exposed mice showed a dose-dependent decrease in the incidence of uterine endometrial cystic hyperplasia compared with air-exposed controls (Burleigh-Flayer *et al.*, 1991). In an *in vivo* study where female Simonson albino rats were exposed to 0.3% MTBE in their drinking water for 2 weeks preceding oocytes recovery, female rats exposed to MTBE were found to have lower weight gains than the controls, but MTBE appeared to have no effects on either the percentage of ovulating females or the number of oocytes produced per ovulating female (Berger and Horner, 2003). No adverse effects on reproductive parameters were reported for female F344/N rats or female B6C3F1 mice exposed to TBA at concentrations of 450, 900, 1,750, 3,500 and 7,000 ppm 6 hours per day and 5 days per week for 12 exposure days, and at concentrations of 0, 135, 270, 540, 1,080 and 2,100 ppm 6 hours per day and 5 days per week for 13 weeks via whole-body inhalation (Mahler, 1997).

Reproductive dysfunction in aquatic organisms

MTBE has been tested for its effects on the reproduction of aquatic organisms (Moreels *et al.*, 2006a). In a long-term exposure study of adult zebrafish (*Danio rerio*) to environmentally relevant concentrations of MTBE in flow-through systems, exposure to as low as 0.11 mg/L of MTBE over 3 weeks led to a significant increase in vitellogenin concentrations in male fish. These results indicate that MTBE possesses estrogenic activity at environmentally relevant concentrations. Fecundity, fertilization or hatch rate were not affected significantly in the 8-week exposure period at effective concentrations, ranging from 0.44 to 220 mg/L, but sperm motility was significantly affected. The spermatozoa of all MTBE-exposure groups showed a significantly lower straight-line velocity and lower average path velocity. This suggests that chronic exposure to MTBE in the environment at relevant low concentrations affected fish sperm motility (Moreels *et al.*, 2006a).

Tumor incidence of endocrine-sensitive tissues

After treatment with MTBE by inhalation and gavage, the incidence of testicular Leydig cell tumors in Sprague–Dawley and Fisher 344 rats increased, and the incidence of tumors in the mammary, adrenal and pituitary glands in female Sprague–Dawley rats decreased (Burleigh-Flayer *et al.*, 1991; Chun *et al.*, 1992; Belpoggi *et al.*, 1995). These indicate that the disturbance of endocrine effects is a potential mechanism of MTBE, thus resulting in modifications of the rodent tumor profile of endocrine-sensitive organ systems.

In male rats, related studies on the mechanisms of Leydig cell carcinogenesis induced by MTBE chronic disruption in normal hypothalamic–pituitary–gonadal and/or liver functions have been reported. The mean serum testosterone levels of control rats showed decreases of 27% and 57% 4–5 h after treatment with 1,500 and 1,000 mg/kg MTBE, respectively. A slight dose-related reduction in testosterone level was observed 14 days later. However, the group testosterone levels were not statistically different 28 days after treatment (de Peyster *et al.*, 2003). In contrast, mild hormonal level changes occurred in Sprague–Dawley rats orally administered with high MTBE doses for 15 or 28 days (Williams *et al.*, 2000a; Li *et al.*, 2008). Serum testosterone levels were decreased in rats treated for 15 days but not 28 days, and increased luteinizing hormone (LH) and follicle stimulating hormone (FSH) levels were commonly observed following exposure to chemicals for 15 days (Li *et al.*, 2008). *In vitro*, isolated rat, Leydig cell cultures exposed to 50 mM and 100 mM MTBE and TBA, respectively, for 3 h with and without stimulation by human chorionic gonadotropin (hCG) showed testosterone secretion reductions by at least 50% as compared to the RPMI vehicle control (de Peyster *et al.*, 2003). Hepatic microsomal cytochrome P450 (CYP), such as CYP2B1/2 CYP1A1/2, CYP2A1 and CYP2E1, increased in 15 day-treated and 28 day-treated rats orally administered with 1,500 mg MTBE/kg/day, indicating that the decrease in serum testosterone with MTBE may be the result of enhanced testosterone metabolism and subsequent clearance (Williams *et al.*, 2000b).

Although the incidence of Leydig cell tumors has been reported in both Fischer 344 rats by inhalation and in Sprague-Dawley rats by gavage (Bird *et al.*, 1997; Belpoggi *et al.*, 1997), there are still questions that to need to be answered. Increases in luteinizing hormone (LH) to overstimulate Leydig cells chronically and result in Leydig cell hyperplasia and neoplasia may be one of the mechanisms of rat Leydig cell carcinogens. The recovery of testosterone levels after 4 weeks may have been due to self-induction of MTBE metabolism and a compensatory rise in (LH). At only 2 weeks, however, circulating LH showed an increase, while no increase was observed at 4 weeks post-treatment with MTBE (Li *et al.*, 2008). Peroxisome proliferation was regarded as another possible mechanism of Leydig cell tumor induction by MTBE, but no such proliferation has yet been demonstrated (de Peyster *et al.*, 2003).

There are significant species differences in terms of Leydig cell physiology between rats and humans, as demonstrated by McGregor (2006): (1) there is a 13-fold lower density of LH receptors in the Leydig cells of humans compared with those of rats; (2) human Leydig cells respond to human chorionic gonadotropin (a hormone equivalent to LH by hypertrophy), whereas rat Leydig cells only respond by hyperplasia; and (3) human or mouse Leydig cells do not contain gonadotropin-releasing hormone (GnRH) receptors, but they are present in rats. Therefore, the mouse model is a closer approximation to human disease than the rat model, although differences in Leydig cell physiology still exist between humans and mice. In addition, the incidence of Leydig-cell tumors in humans is very low, a factor that makes their study particularly difficult. No increases in the incidence of any type of testicular tumor have been demonstrated in mouse studies with MTBE, TBA or methanol, so confirming that MTBE-induced Leydig cell tumors in human is difficult. Therefore, the American Conference of Governmental Industrial Hygienists classified MTBE as a "confirmed animal carcinogen with unknown relevance to humans" (group A3) (ACGIH, 2005).

In female Sprague–Dawley rats, the incidence of tumors in estrogen-sensitive tissues, such as the mammary, adrenal and pituitary glands, decreased, while in CD-1 mice, these estrogen-sensitive tissues appeared indicative of estrogen antagonism after MTBE exposure (Moser *et al.*, 1998). Based on these findings of MTBE-induced endocrine effects in female rodents, MTBE is suggested to be anti-estrogen. Neither serum estrogen levels nor the location or intensity of estrogen receptor immunoreactivity in the uterus, cervix and vagina, however, appeared to be altered after MTBE exposure in CD-1 mice. The binding of $[^3H]$-17β-estradiol to estrogen receptors (ERs) was not inhibited by MTBE, TBA or formaldehyde. In addition, transiently infected HepG2 cells exposed to MTBE showed that binding of the ER to the response element in DNA was not altered, and the interaction of estradiol with ER was not antagonized (Moser *et al.*, 1998). Therefore, although MTBE exposure can cause multiple changes in estrogen-sensitive tissues and cellular responses, these effects were not mediated through ER.

DEVELOPMENTAL TOXICITY

In a study on the effect of MTBE (up to 100 mg/L) and TBA (up to 1,400 mg/L) on the hatch rate and larval development of African catfish (*Clarias gariepinus*), exposure to doses of MTBE higher than 50 mg/L was found to result in deformed eyes, mouthparts and spinal cords, and increased larval mortality. TBA also induced a decline in hatch rate (Moreels *et al.*, 2006b). In mice, rats and rabbits, no significant reproductive and developmental toxicity or teratogenic responses were reported after MTBE exposure (Conaway *et al.*, 1985; Biles *et al.*, 1987; Bevan *et al.*, 1997a,b). In a single generation reproduction study, prior to mating, male and female rats were exposed to target concentrations of MTBE of 300, 1,300 and 3,400 ppm 6 hours/day and 5 days/week for 12 and 3 weeks, respectively (Biles *et al.*, 1987). The results showed that MTBE did not induce significant or specific toxicity to reproduction in Sprague–Dawley rats. In a two-generation study, the effects of MTBE exposure on reproductive functions were evaluated (Bevan *et al.*, 1997a). Sprague–Dawley rats were exposed to either 0, 400, 3,000 or 8,000 ppm MTBE 6 h/day for 10 weeks prior to mating, throughout mating and gestation, and then from day 5 of lactation. F_1 rats were exposed to the same doses of MTBE for 4 weeks. The data revealed that reproduction was not affected even after exposure to MTBE vapors of up to 8,000 ppm. Parental toxicity resulted from prolonged exposure to 3,000 and 8,000 ppm MTBE vapors. Adult animals exposed to 3,000 and 8,000 ppm MTBE showed adverse clinical signs indicative of central nervous system depression, such as hypoactivity and lack of startle reflex. At 8,000 ppm, these same effects were more severe and were even accompanied by reduced body weights. Liver weights increased in both sexes of F_1 generation rats in the 8,000 and 3,000 ppm groups, but no histological differences were observed in their reproductive organs. In addition, none of the parameters measured in the study suggested treatment-related reproductive effects. The only remarkable changes observed were lowered body weights in both generations of pups at 3,000 and 8,000 ppm, and a significant increase in dead F_2 pups in the 8,000 ppm group on postnatal day 4. Thus, no reproductive toxicity was found in two generations of Sprague–Dawley rats exposed to MTBE vapors even in the presence of parental toxicity at concentrations of 3,000 and 8,000 ppm.

Four developmental studies on rodents and New Zealand white rabbits exposed to MTBE by inhalation have been performed (Conaway *et al.*, 1985; Bevan *et al.*, 1997b). In a study conducted by Conaway *et al.* (1985), mated Sprague–Dawley rats and CD-1 mice were exposed for 6 h/day to target concentrations of 0, 250, 1,000 and 2,500 ppm MTBE during organogenesis. In another study, CD-1 mice and New Zealand white rabbits were exposed to up to 8,000 ppm MTBE vapor by inhalation for 6 h/day on gestation days 6–15 and 6–18, respectively (Bevan *et al.*, 1997b). In these studies, maternal and developmental toxicity occurred only at MTBE concentrations of 4,000 and 8,000 ppm. In mice (Bevan *et al.*, 1997b), maternal body weight, body weight gain and food consumption were significantly reduced at 8,000 ppm during the exposure period. Treatment-related clinical signs, such as hypoactivity and ataxia, were observed at 4,000 and 8,000 ppm. The inhalation exposure of mice clearly resulted in fetotoxic effects, such as reduced body weights and reduced ossification in fetal skeletal districts. In particular, a significantly increased incidence of cleft palates was found in fetuses, but this developmental toxicity was observed only at maternally toxic doses (Bevan *et al.*, 1997b). Postimplantation deaths significantly increased, and live male fetuses significantly decreased at 8,000 ppm MTBE exposure. Fetal body weights per litter were also reduced at 4,000 and 8,000 ppm. Markedly elevated corticosterone concentrations have been previously shown to occur in female Fischer 344 rats and CD-1 mice exposed to 8,000 ppm MTBE (Dodd and Kintigh, 1989). Therefore, maternal stress is considered to play an important role in the formation of cleft palates (Barlow *et al.*, 1975). In addition, a slight increase in fetal resorption was observed, but this was not associated with the treatment itself (Conaway *et al.*, 1985). Developmental studies on rats and rabbits showed no evidence of treatment-related teratogenicity, except that exposure to 8,000 ppm MTBE reduced body weight gain and food consumption in adult rabbits, and resulted in transient reduction in food consumption in adult rats. For rats and rabbits, no remarkable adverse maternal effects were observed.

CONCLUDING REMARKS AND FUTURE DIRECTIONS

In conclusion, in both reproductive and developmental studies of rodents and rabbits with MTBE exposure, no-observed-adverse-effect level (NOAEL) for reproduction and developmental toxicity was at least 1,000 ppm in rodents or rabbits, much higher than the current non-occupational exposure dose (1 ppm). Whether or not the results found in rats or mice are indicative of human responses in terms of health risks associated with MTBE exposure is not currently known. The mouse model seems to be more appropriate to compare with humans than the rat model, but no significant effects to mouse testes or other reproductive organs have been induced by MTBE. Therefore, MTBE unlikely poses human reproductive or developmental hazards.

REFERENCES

Adami HO, Bergstrom R, Mohner M, Zatonski W, Storm H, Ekbom A, Tretli S, Teppo L, Ziegler H, Rahu M, Gurevicius R, Stengrevics A (1994) Testicular cancer in nine northern European countries. *Int J Cancer* **59:** 33–8.

Ahmed FE (2001) Toxicology and human health effects following exposure to oxygenated or reformulated gasoline. *Toxicol Lett* **123:** 89–113.

Amberg A, Rosner E, Dekant W (1999) Biotransformation and kinetics of excretion of methyl-*tert*-butyl ether in rats and humans. *Toxicol Sci* **51:** 1–8.

American Conference of Governmental Industrial Hygienists (ACGIH) (2005) TLVs and BEIs based on the documentation of the threshold limit values for chemical substances and physical agents and biological indices. Cincinnati, USA, ACGIH.

Andersen AG, Jensen TK, Carlsen E, Jorgensen N, Andersson AM, Krarup T, Keiding N, Skakkebaek NE (2000) High frequency of sub-optimal semen quality in an unselected population of young men. *Hum Reprod* **15:** 366–72.

Barlow SM, McElhatton PR, Sullivan FM (1975) The relation between maternal restraint and food deprivation, plasma corticosterone, and induction of cleft palate in the offspring of mice. *Teratology* **12:** 97–103.

Belpoggi F, Soffritti M, Maltoni C (1995) Methyl-*tertiary*butyl ether (MTBE) – a gasoline additive – causes testicular and lymphohematopoietic cancers in rats. *Toxicol Ind Health* **11:** 119–49.

Belpoggi F, Soffritti M, Filipinni F, Maltoni C (1997) Results of long-term experimental studies on the carcinogenicity of methyl *tert*-butyl ether. *Ann NY Acad Sci* **837:** 77–95.

Belpoggi F, Soffritti M, Maltoni C (1998) Pathological characterization of testicular tumours and lymphomas–leukaemias, and of their precursors observed in Sprague-Dawley rats exposed to methyl *tertiary*-butyl-ether (MTBE). *Eur J Oncol* **3:** 201–6.

Berger T, Horner CM (2003) In vivo exposure of female rats to toxicants may affect oocyte quality. *Reproductive Toxicology* **17:** 273–81.

Bernauer U, Amberg A, Scheutzow D, Dekant W (1998) Biotransformation of 12C- and 2-13C-labeled methyl *tert*-butyl ether, ethyl *tert*-butyl ether, and *tert*-butyl alcohol in rats: identification of metabolites in urine by 13C nuclear magnetic resonance and gas chromatography/mass spectrometry. *Chem Res Toxicol* **11:** 651–8.

Bevan C, Neeper-Bradley TL, Tyl RW, Fisher LC, Panson RD, Kneiss JJ, Andrews LS (1997a) Two-generation reproductive toxicity study of methyl tertiary-butyl ether (MTBE) in rats. *J Appl Toxicol* **17 (Suppl. 1):** S13–S19.

Bevan C, Tyl RW, Neeper-Bradley TL, Fischer LC, Panson RD, Douglas JF, Andrews LS (1997b) Developmental toxicity evaluation of methyl *tertiary* butyl ether (MTBE) by inhalation in mice and rabbits. *J Appl Toxicol* **17 (Suppl. 1):** S21–S29.

Biles RW, Schroeder RE, Holdworth CE (1987) Methyl *tertiary* butyl ether inhalation in rats: single generation reproduction study. *Tox Ind Health* **3:** 519–34.

Bird MG, Burleigh-Flayer H, Chun JS, Douglas JF, Kneiss JJ, Andrews LS (1997) Oncogenicity study of inhaled methyl *tertiary*-butyl ether (MTBE) in CD-1 mice and F-344 rats. *J Appl Toxicol* **17:** S45–S55.

Burleigh-Flayer HD, Doss DE, Bird MG, Ridlon SA (1991) *Oncogematy Study of Inhaled Methyl Tertiary Butyl Ether (MTBE) in CD-I Mouse. Methyl Tertiary Butyl Ether (MTBE): Health Effects Testing Program under EPA Consent Order.* MTBE Task Force, Oxygenated Fuels Association, Washington DC.

Carlsen E, Giwercman A, Keiding N, Skakkebaek NE (1992) Evidence for decreasing quality of semen during past 50 years. *Brit Med J* **305:** 609–13.

Chilvers C, Pike MC, Forman D, Fogelman K, Wadsworth ME (1984) Apparent doubling of frequency of undescended testis in England and Wales in 1962–81. *Lancet* **2:** 330–2.

Chun JS, Burleigh-Flayer HD, Kintigh WJ (1992) Methyl tertiary butyl ether: vapor inhalation oncogenicity study in Fischer 344 rats. Export, PA, Bushy Run Research Center.

Conaway CC, Schroeder RE, Snyder NK (1985) Teratology evaluation of methyl *tertiary* butyl ether in rats and mice. *J Toxicol Environ Health* **66:** 797–809.

Davis MJ, Farland WH (2001) The paradoxes of MTBE. *Tox Sci* **61:** 211–17.

de Peyster A, MacLean KJ, Stephens BA, Ahern LD, Westover CM, Rozenshteyn D (2003) Subchronic studies in Sprague-Dawley rats to investigate mechanisms of MTBE-induced Leydig cell cancer. *Toxicol Sci* **72:** 31–42.

de Peyster A, Rodriguez Y, Shuto R, Goldberg B, Gonzales F, Pu X, Klaunig JE (2008) Effect of oral methyl-*t*-butyl ether (MTBE) on the male mouse reproductive tract and oxidative stress in liver. *Reprod Toxicol* **26:** 246–53.

Dodd DE, Kintigh WJ (1989) Methyl tertiary butyl ether (MTBE): repeated (13-week) vapor inhalation study in rats with neurotoxicity evaluation. Unpublished study, Union Carbide, Bushy Run Research Center for MTBE Committee, TSCATS 403189, EPA/OTS # FYI-OTS-0889-0689.

Forman D, Moller H (1994) Testicular cancer. *Cancer Surv* **19–20:** 323–41.

Gal AL, Dreáno Y, Gervasi PG, Berthou FO (2001) Human cytochrome P450 2A6 is the major enzyme involved in the metabolism of three alkoxyethers used as oxyfuels. *Toxicol Lett* **124:** 47–58.

Hellstern A, Leuschner U, Benjaminov A, Ackermann H, Heine T, Festi D, Orsini M, Roda E, Northfield TC, Jazrawi R, Kurtz W, Schmeck-Lindenau HJ, Stumpf J, Eidsvoll BE, Aadland E, Lux G, Boehnke E, Wurbs D, Delhaye M, Cremer M, Sinn I, Horing E, Gaisberg UV, Neubrand M, Sauerbruch T, Salamon V, Swobodnik W, Sanden HV, Schmitt W, Käser T, Schomerus H, Wechsler JG, Janowitz P, Lohmann J, Porst H, Attili AF, Bartels E, Arnold W, Strohm WD, Paul F (1998) Dissolution of gallbladder stones with methyl tert-butyl ether and stone recurrence. *Dig Dis Sci* **43:** 911–20.

Hong J-Y, Yang CS, Lee M, Wang Y-Y, Huang W, Tan Y, Pattern CJ, Bondoc Y (1997a) Role of cytochrome-P450 in the metabolism of methyl *tert*-butyl ether in human livers. *Arch Toxicol* **71:** 266–9.

Hong J-Y, Wang YY, Bondoc FY, Yang CS, Lee M, Huang WQ (1997b) Rat olfactory mucosa displays a high activity in metabolizing methyl *tert*-butyl ether and other gasoline ethers. *Fundam Appl Toxicol* **40:** 205–10.

Hong J-Y, Wang Y-Y, Mohr SN, Bondoc FY, Deng C (2001) Human cytochrome P450 isozymes in metabolism and health effects of gasoline ethers. *Health Effects Institute Research Report* **102:** 7–27.

Hutcheon DE, Arnold JD, ten Hove W, Boyle J III (1996) Disposition, metabolism, and toxicity of methyl tertiary butyl ether, an oxygenate for reformulated gasoline. *J Toxicol Environ Health* **47:** 453–64.

Li D, Yuan C, Gong Y, Huang Y, Han X (2008) The effects of methyl tert-butyl ether (MTBE) on the male rat reproductive system. *Food Chem Toxicol* **46:** 2402–8.

Li D, Gong Y, Yuan C, Huang Y, Han X (2009a) Effects of subchronic methyl *tert*-butyl ether exposure on male Sprague–Dawley rats. *Toxicol Indust Health* **25:** 15–23.

Li D, Liu Q, Gong Y, Huang Y, Han X (2009b) Cytotoxicity and oxidative stress study in cultured rat Sertoli cells with methyl *tert*-butyl ether (MTBE) exposure. *Reprod Toxicol* **27:** 170–6.

Li D, Yin D, Han X (2007) Methyl *tert*-butyl ether (MTBE)-induced cytotoxicity and oxidative stress in isolated rat spermatogenic cells. *J Appl Toxicol* **1:** 10–7.

Matlai P, Beral V (1985) Trends in congenital malformations of external genitalia. *Lancet* **1:** 108.

Mahler J (1997) NTP technical report on toxicity studies of t-butyl alcohol (CAS No. 75-65-0). Administered by inhalation to F344/N rats and B6C3F1 mice. *Toxic Rep Ser* **53:** 1–56, A1–D9.

McGregor D (2006) Methyl tertiary-butyl ether: studies for potential human health hazards. *Crit Rev Toxicol* **36:** 319–58.

Moreels D, Cauwenberghe KV, Debaere B, Rurangwa E, Vromant N, Bastiaens L, Diels L, Springael D, Merckx R, Ollevier F (2006a) Long-term exposure to environmentally relevant doses of methyl-tert-butyl ether causes significant reproductive dysfunction in the zebra fish (*Danio Rerio*). *Environ Toxicol Chem* **25:** 2388–93.

Moreels D, Lodewijks P, Zegers H, Rurangwa E, Vromant N, Bastiaens L, Diels L, Springael D, Merckx R, Ollevier F (2006b) Effect of short-term exposure to methyl-*tert*-butyl ether and *tert*-butyl alcohol on the hatch rate and development of the African catfish, *Clarias gariepinus*. *Environ Toxicol Chem* **25:** 514–9.

Moser GJ, Wolf DC, Sar M, Gaido KW, Janszen D, Goldsworthy TL (1998) Methyl tertiary butyl ether-induced endocrine alterations in mice are not mediated through the estrogen receptor. *Toxicol Sci* **41:** 77–87.

National Toxicology Program (1995) Toxicology and carcinogenesis studies of *tert*-butyl alcohol in F344/N rats and B6C3F1 mice (Tech. Rep. Ser. No. 436; NIH Publ. No. 95-3167). Research Triangle Park, NC, NTP.

Paulozzi LJ, Erickson JD, Jackson RJ (1997) Hypospadias trends in two US surveillance systems. *Pediatrics* **100:** 831–4.

Phillips S, Palmer RB, Brody A (2008) Epidemiology, toxicokinetics, and health effects of methyl *tert*-butyl ether (MTBE). *J Med Toxicol* **4:** 115–26.

Swan SH, Elkin EP, Fenster L (1997) Have sperm densities declined? A reanalysis of global trend data. *Environ Health Perspect* **105:** 1228–32.

Toppari J, Larsen JC, Christiansen P, Giwercman A, Grandjean P, Guillette Jr LJ, Jegou B, Jensen TK, Jouannet P, Keiding N, Leffers H, McLachlan JA, Meyer O, Muller J, Rajpert-De Meyts E, Scheike T, Sharpe R, Sumpter J, Skakkebaek NE (1996) Male reproductive health and environmental xenoestrogens. *Environ Health Perspect* **104 (Suppl. 4):** 741–803.

Williams TM, Cattley RC, Borghoff SJ (2000a) Alterations in endocrine responses in male Sprague–Dawley rats following oral administration of methyl *tert*-butyl ether. *Toxicol Sci* **54:** 168–76.

Williams TM, Borghoff SJ (2000b) Induction of testosterone biotransformation enzymes following oral administration of methyl *tert*-butyl ether to male Sprague–Dawley rats. *Toxicol Sci* **57:** 147–55.

C H A P T E R

47

Perfluorooctane sulfonate (PFOS) and perfluorooctanoic acid (PFOA)

Henrik Viberg and Per Eriksson

INTRODUCTION

Perfluorinated compounds (PFCs) comprise a large group of chemicals that have been produced for about 50 years. PFCs are fully fluorinated chemicals, which are synthetic with unique properties and have been recognized as a class of emerging, persistent contaminants. Carbon–fluorine bonds are among the strongest in organic chemistry. This stability makes these compounds practically non-biodegradable and persistent in the environment (Key *et al.*, 1997, 1998).

Perfluorinated sulfonates, such as perfluorooctane sulfonate (PFOS), and perfluorinated carboxylates (PFCAs), such as perfluorooctanoic acid (PFOA) (Figure 47.1), are not reactive, resist hydrolysis and photolysis, and are not easily degraded in biological systems (Kissa, 2001), making them persistent in the environment. The fluorocarbon part is hydrophobic, lipophilic and hence non-polar, while the "tail" sections of the molecules add polarity since they are hydrophilic and lipophobic (for detailed characteristics see Table 47.1). Both PFOS and PFOA are fluorosurfactans that can drastically lower the surface tension of water. These chemicals are produced for numerous applications in industrial processes and are used to make consumer products, such as water-, oil- and stain-resistant coatings for clothing fabrics, leather and carpets, and oil-resistant coatings for paper products for food contact. They are also used in surfactants, photographic emulsifier, aviation hydraulic fluids, fire-fighting foams, floor polishes and insecticide formulations (Renner, 2001; Seacat *et al.*, 2002). During the last two decades several reports have surfaced concerning toxicity of PFOS and PFOA in both humans and wildlife. This chapter describes reproductive and developmental toxicity of PFOS and PFOA.

HISTORICAL BACKGROUND

In the 1940s the company 3M began producing fluorinated compounds by electrochemical fluorination, first PFOA in 1947 (3MCompany, 1995) and then PFOS-based compounds in 1949 (3MCompany, 1999). It has been clear for several years that these fluorinated compounds can induce toxicological effects in animals, since DuPont knew already in 1961 that PFOA induced liver anomalies (hepatomegaly) in mice. Not that much later, in 1968, organofluorine content was discovered in human blood serum, but it was not until 1976 before it was clear that this came from PFOS, PFOA and other related compounds (Taves, 1968; Shen and Taves, 1974; Lau *et al.*, 2004). During the 1990s researchers have been interested in monitoring the concentrations and studying the possible toxicological effects of these compounds and in 1999 the United States Environmental Protection Agency (US EPA) started to investigate perfluorinated compounds as a result of 3M's detection of PFOS in blood from global blood banks in 1997 and receiving data on the global distribution and toxicity of PFOS (Kennedy *et al.*, 2004). Since then 3M has phased out their production in the USA, but other companies inside and outside the USA are still producing these perfluorinated compounds, which contribute to the continuing spread of these compounds. In recent years a lot of interest has been focused on the negative effects of these compounds, both environmentally and physiologically. The reproductive and developmental toxicity of these compounds are discussed in this chapter.

Exposure situation

Environment

In the early 2000s, it was established that PFOS, which is also the stable and extremely persistent end-product of degradation of various sulfonated fluorochemicals, is universally present and bioaccumulating (Giesy and Kannan, 2001; Kannan *et al.*, 2001). Both abiotic matrices, like air, lakes and rivers (Nakayama *et al.*, 2005; Loos *et al.*, 2009), and biotic matrices have been shown to contain significant concentrations of these compounds, and several wildlife species from all over the world have been shown to be exposed to PFOS and PFOA. Furthermore these compounds are also known to biomagnify in the food chain, which, together with their high persistency, make them a possible threat to wildlife species,

Reproductive and Developmental Toxicology, Edited by Ramesh C. Gupta
ISBN: 978-0-12-382032-7

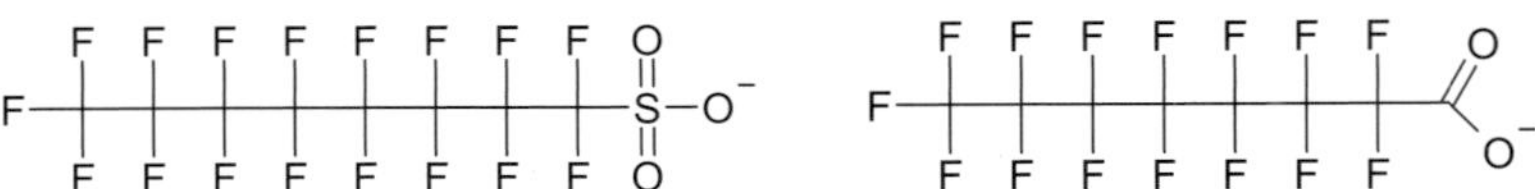

FIGURE 47.1 The structure formula of PFOS (left) and PFOA (right).

e.g., top predators (Hekster *et al.*, 2003; Kannan *et al.*, 2005). Despite the distant location away from human activities and sources, polar bears contain PFOS and PFOA indicating global distribution patterns of perfluorinated compounds, similar to those of other organohalogen compounds (OHC). Furthermore it is clear that exposure has increased drastically during the last 20 years and concentrations are now higher than for several other persistent organic pollutants with known negative health effects (Smithwick *et al.*, 2005; Dietz *et al.*, 2008).

TABLE 47.1 Chemical and physical properties of PFOS and PFOA

CAS number	1763-23-1	335-67-1
Molecular formula	$C_8HF_{17}O_3S$	$C_8HF_{15}O_2$
Molar mass	500.13 g/mol	414.07 g/mol
Appearance	white powder	colorless liquid
Density	1.25 g/cm^3	1.8 g/cm^3
Melting point	90°C	40–50°C
Boiling point	258–260°C	189–192°C
Solubility in water	519 mg/L at 20°C	soluble, 9.5 g/L
Solubility in other solvents	polar organic solvents	polar organic solvents
Acidity (p*K*a)	–	2–3

Human

Exposure to PFOS and PFOA is not only an environmental problem, but also well documented in humans. The major route of exposure seems to be via food and drinking water (Tittlemier *et al.*, 2007; Trudel *et al.*, 2008; Nolan *et al.*, 2010), resulting in chronic long-term exposure. PFOS and PFOA are found in a variety of different food products, and concentrations tend to be highest in meats, fish/shellfish and dairy products (Tittlemier *et al.*, 2007; Ericson *et al.*, 2008; Trudel *et al.*, 2008). The estimated daily intake from food varies a lot depending on the study (see Table 47.2). Of great concern though is that younger individuals, toddlers and newborns experience higher exposure through higher daily intake.

The indoor environment also contains PFOS and PFOA (Moriwaki *et al.*, 2003; Strynar and Lindstrom, 2008; Bjorklund *et al.*, 2009). Generally newer buildings have higher levels of PFOS and PFOA and there is a high correlation between the degree of carpeting and high dust concentrations (Kubwabo *et al.*, 2005). Since PFOS and PFOA are found in indoor air and dust, both inhalation and ingestion can be of importance in all humans ranging from newborns and toddlers to adults.

People from several different countries have been studied (see Table 47.3) as well as people of both genders and of different ages. Generally it can be said that human levels of PFOS are higher than levels of PFOA and the levels of both compounds have increased over time. Males have higher levels than females and older people have higher levels than younger people, with the exception of newborns and toddlers who can have very high levels (Harada *et al.*, 2004, 2005a; Kärrman *et al.*, 2007, 2009; Ericson *et al.*, 2007; Toms *et al.*, 2009). In addition, educational status seems to be positively correlated with higher levels of PFOS and PFOA (Calafat *et al.*, 2007a; Fromme *et al.*, 2009; Vestergren and Cousins, 2009).

Employees in fluorochemical manufacturing industries and people living in areas close to production sites (Fromme *et al.*, 2009) are showing significantly higher serum concentrations of PFOS and PFOA, where concentrations can be several orders of magnitude higher. Blood samples from retired workers have also shown that the serum concentrations of PFOS and PFOA are still very high up to 5 years after retirement, indicating that in humans PFOS and PFOA have long half-lives, contributing to the long-term exposure situation from these compounds (Olsen *et al.*, 2003a,b, 2007; Ehresman *et al.*, 2007).

TABLE 47.2 Estimated daily intake doses of PFOS and PFOA from the diet

Country	Year	PFOS(ng/ kg_{bw}/day)	PFOA(ng/ kg_{bw}/day)	Study
Canada	1992–2004	1.77	1.13	Tittlemier *et al.* (2007)
North America	1999–2007	7–219	0.4–128	Trudel *et al.* (2008)
Spain	2006	1.07	<LOD	Ericson *et al.* (2008)
UK	2004	100	70	UK Food Standards Agency (2007)
Europe	1999–2007	3–216	0.7–114	Trudel *et al.* (2008)
Japan	2004	1.47	1.28	Karrman *et al.* (2009)

TABLE 47.3 Levels of PFOS and PFOA in humans from different countries mean or median concentrations

Country	Year	Median PFOS (μg/l)	Median PFOA (μg/l)	Study
Australia	2002–2003	20.8	7.6	Kärrman *et al.* (2006)
	2006–2207	15.2	6.4	Toms *et al.* (2009)
Brazil	2003	13.5	<20	Kannan *et al.* (2004)
Belgium	1998–2000	16.8	5.0	Kannan *et al.* (2004)
Colombia	2003	8.5	6.2	Kannan *et al.* (2004)
India	2000	1.7	3.5	Kannan *et al.* (2004)
Italy	2001	4.3	<3	Kannan *et al.* (2004)
Japan	2002	14.1	<6.8	Kannan *et al.* (2004)
	2003–2004	28.7	12.74	Harada *et al.* (2005a, 2007)
Korea	2003	27.1	35.5	Kannan *et al.* (2004)
Malaysia	2004	13.2	<10	Kannan *et al.* (2004)
Peru	2003	0.7	0.1	Calafat *et al.* (2006)
Poland	2003	55.4	20.5	Kannan *et al.* (2004)
Spain	2006	7.6	1.8	Ericson *et al.* (2007)
USA	2003–2004	41.2	7.8	Calafat *et al.* (2007b)
Vietnam	2005	3.2	1.6	Rylander *et al.* (2009)

From the fertilization of the egg, through gestation and during the first years after birth, a continuous development is going on and disturbances during susceptible periods can induce many different types of negative alterations in the organism. Knowledge about the exposure situation in fetuses, newborns and toddlers, since transfer of xenobiotics occur from the mother to the fetus through the umbilical cord, via mother's milk to the newborn and via direct inhalation and ingestion to the newborn and toddler is therefore important in order to predict toxic effects. The concentrations of PFOS and PFOA are significantly higher in maternal serum (4.9–18.1 and 0.5–2.6 μg/L, respectively) than in umbilical cord serum (1.6–7.3 and 1.6–3.4 μg/L, respectively) (Inoue *et al.*, 2004; Apelberg *et al.*, 2007a; Midasch *et al.*, 2007; Monroy *et al.*, 2008), but in umbilical cord serum the difference between PFOS and PFOA concentrations is not as pronounced, which means that PFOA, but not PFOS, crosses the placental barrier obviously unhindered (Midasch *et al.*, 2007).

Newborns, toddlers and children are the most exposed part of the population, on a body weight basis, since they tend to inhale and ingest more than the adult population (Trudel *et al.*, 2008). When comparing the serum concentrations of PFOS and PFOA between adults from the general population and children the picture is not uniform, sometimes concentrations are higher in children and sometimes the same as in the adult population (Olsen *et al.*, 2004; Holzer *et al.*, 2008; Toms *et al.*, 2009; Wilhelm *et al.*, 2009). However, this discrepancy might be related to the fact that different studies measure children of different age.

It is a well-known fact that many environmental pollutants end up in the mother's milk exposing the nursing neonate to a cocktail of chemicals, including PFOS and PFOA (So *et al.*, 2006; Karrman *et al.*, 2007; Tao *et al.*, 2008a, b; Völkel *et al.*, 2008). The concentrations of PFOS and PFOA in breast milk are highest in the USA and it is also seen that mother's nursing for the first time have higher concentrations in their milk compared to mothers who have previously nursed (Tao *et al.*, 2008a). Estimated average daily intake of PFOS (for example, 11.8 ± 10.6 ng/kg body weight/day) and PFOA (for example, 9.6 ± 4.9 ng/kg body weight/day) by infants, via breastfeeding, is considerably higher than the estimated adult dietary intakes (Tao *et al.*, 2008b).

TOXICOKINETICS

The toxicokinetics and pharmacokinetic properties of PFOS and PFOA have been well characterized. Generally, both compounds are well absorbed and undergo extensive uptake from the enterohepatic circulation, but are poorly excreted and are not known to be metabolized (Johnson *et al.*, 1984; Harada *et al.*, 2005a). For example, after a single oral dose of PFOS, at least 95% is systemically absorbed after 24 h (Johnson *et al.*, 1979). Both PFOS and PFOA are distributed mainly to the serum, kidney and liver, and not to more lipid-rich tissues and liver concentrations are several times higher than serum concentrations (Johnson and Ober, 1979; Seacat *et al.*, 2002, 2003). The distribution is suggested to be mainly extracellular, since the volume of distribution at steady state of PFOS is approximately 200 ml/kg in the cynomolgus monkey. Both PFOS and PFOA are binding to several types of proteins in serum, e.g., β-lipoproteins, albumin and liver fatty acid-binding protein (L-FABP) (Lau *et al.*, 2007). PFOS is distributed to the brain, but the concentrations in the brain are considerably lower than in other tissues, but can increase gradually with time after exposure (Sato *et al.*, 2009). PFOS can also be detected in the brain in offspring of dams treated with PFOS during the gestational period (Chang *et al.*, 2009). The distribution pattern of PFOS also changes with age and there are also gender differences in the distribution, which increase with increasing age (Liu *et al.*, 2009a). In humans, there are detectable levels of PFOS and PFOA in umbilical cord blood, indicating that these chemicals cross the placenta. Although PFOS concentrations are higher than PFOA concentrations in maternal serum, the difference between PFOS and PFOA concentrations in umbilical cord serum is not as pronounced, suggesting that PFOA, but not PFOS, crosses the placental barrier obviously unhindered (Midasch *et al.*, 2007). PFOS is found in maternal milk of both animals and humans (Kuklenyik *et al.*, 2004). In general, the rate of elimination of perfluorinated compounds is enhanced with decreasing carbon chain length, and the elimination half-life of PFOA is shorter than that of PFOS, but the rate of elimination varies considerably between species and genders. The elimination of PFOS, shown by the half-life, in rat is 100 days, compared to 5.4 years in human (Olsen *et al.*, 2007) and the elimination half-life of PFOA in adult female rats is 2–4 h, but is 4–6 days in adult male rats. The elimination is not always faster in females; in mice and rabbits gender differences are absent and in hamsters the excretion is faster in males than in females. For instance, male hamsters excrete PFOA more rapidly than female hamsters (Butenhoff *et al.*, 2004; Hundley *et al.*, 2006; Lau *et al.*, 2007; Tan *et al.*, 2008). In humans there are no known differences in elimination of PFOS and PFOA between men and women. The elimination half-lives of PFOS and PFOA in several species are summarized in Table 47.4.

The reason for species and gender differences in elimination of PFOA is not fully understood, but researchers believe that sex hormones are involved, since the elimination of PFOA in rats is upregulated by estradiol in male rats (Ylinen *et al.*, 1989) and downregulated by testosterone in both female and castrated male rats (Vanden Heuvel *et al.*, 1992; Kudo *et al.*, 2001, 2002). Some of these differences develop during the period of sexual maturation and several transporter proteins in the kidney are expressed differentially in male and female adult rats, probably contributing to the excretion differences (Buist *et al.*, 2002; Buist and Klaassen, 2004). These transport proteins are thus rate limiting for excretion since the renal resorption process can be saturable (Olsen *et al.*, 2007).

TABLE 47.4 Elimination (T1/2) of PFOS and PFOA in plasma/serum

Species	PFOS	PFOA	References
Mouse		19 days	Lau *et al.* (2007)
Rat	100 days	4–6 days	Lau *et al.* (2007)
Rabbit		5.5 h	Hundley *et al.* (2006)
Dog		20–30 days	Hanhijarvi *et al.* (1982)
Monkey	150 days	21 days	Butenhoff *et al.* (2004); Andersen *et al.* (2006); Lau *et al.* (2007)
Human	5.4 years	3.8 years	Olsen *et al.* (2005); Lau *et al.* (2007)

MECHANISM OF ACTION

The physico-chemical characteristics of PFOS and PFOA are the determinants of the toxicokinetics of the compounds and this in turn is important for the mechanism of action of the compounds. Since the gross and microscopical physiology is very variable throughout the body several different mechanisms of action can be involved, such as oxidative stress, apoptosis and alterations in the function of calcium channels, but this chapter is focused on the three most studied mechanisms, namely peroxisome proliferator-activated receptors (PPAR), thyroid hormone system and fatty acid homeostasis.

Peroxisome proliferator-activated receptor (PPAR)

One well-characterized mechanism of action is the influence of PFOS and PFOA on the PPAR. PPARs are a group of nuclear receptor proteins that function as transcription factors regulating the expression of genes. PPARs play essential roles in the regulation of cellular differentiation, development, metabolism (carbohydrate, lipid, protein) and hence are important in reproduction and development.

PFOS and PFOA exposure of rodents, during gestation, results in an array of toxic effects, such as developmental delay, growth deficits and neonatal deaths. PFOS and PFOA can cause acute hepatic peroxisome proliferation in rats (Berthiaume and Wallace, 2002) and PPAR is also known to modify lipid and lipoprotein metabolism (Li and Glass, 2004). It has also been known since the 1990s that PFOA exposure could also modify lipid and lipoprotein metabolism (Haughom and Spydevold, 1992). Together these findings led to the suspicions that the mechanism of action of PFOS and PFOA could be connected to the PPARs. Studies in cell cultures from human, mouse and rat showed that PPARalpha could be activated by PFOA and PFOS. PPARbeta was less sensitive to the agents tested, with only PFOA affecting the mouse receptor. PFOA and PFOS can also activate human, mouse and rat PPARgamma, although the maximum induction of PPARgamma was low, suggesting that PFOA and PFOS are partial agonists of this receptor. Today there is support that PPARalpha is the most likely target of PFOA and PFOS, although PPARgamma is also activated to some extent (Vanden Heuvel *et al.*, 2006; Takacs and Abbott, 2007; Wolf *et al.*, 2008).

These *in vitro* studies have more recently been supported by *in vivo* studies, where full-term fetuses from pregnant mice, orally dosed with different doses of PFOA, had altered gene expression in genes related to fatty acid catabolism in both the fetal liver (748–1,465 genes depending on the dose) and lung (44–336 genes depending on the dose). In the fetal liver, the effects of PFOA were robust, and also included genes associated with lipid transport, ketogenesis, glucose metabolism, lipoprotein metabolism, cholesterol biosynthesis, steroid metabolism, bile acid biosynthesis, phospholipid metabolism, retinol metabolism, proteosome activation and inflammation (Rosen *et al.*, 2007). It has also been reported that pups from PPARalpha knockout mice, exposed to PFOA during gestation, had higher survival rates and did not experience delayed eye opening and deficits in postnatal weight gain as the wild-type animals did, meaning that PPARalpha was required for PFOA-induced postnatal lethality. The expression of one copy of the gene was sufficient to mediate this effect (Abbott *et al.*, 2007).

PFOS induces the same type of developmental effects as PFOA and when looking at gene transcripts from rat pups of dams exposed to PFOS during gestation, changes in hepatic metabolic status are also seen, where 225 transcripts increased and 220 decreased. PPARalpha transcript itself was not affected, but there was an increase in expression of gene transcripts associated with hepatic peroxisomal proliferation as well as those responsible for fatty acid activation, transport and oxidation pathways (both mitochondrial and peroxisomal) (Bjork *et al.*, 2008). A similar picture is seen in mice where PFOS and PFOA induce the same type of alterations in the expression of gene transcripts (Rosen *et al.*, 2009). On the other hand, contradicting reports about the mechanism of action of developmental PFOS toxicity have recently been presented. The developmental effects of PFOS may be independent of PPARalpha activation as wild-type mice and PPARalpha knockout mice responded in the same way to PFOS exposure during the last days of gestation (gestational days 15–19), showing reduced neonatal survival, delayed eye-opening and increased liver weights (Abbott *et al.*, 2009). The closest thing to a mechanistic explanation of the PPAR changes came when measuring mitochondrial respiration and membrane potential in energized rat liver mitochondria. However, this discrepancy might be dose dependent, since sufficiently high concentrations of PFOA and PFOS caused a slight increase in the intrinsic proton leak of the mitochondrial inner membrane, which resembled a surfactant-like change in membrane fluidity. The uncoupling action of these compounds in mitochondria may be critical to the mechanism by which these compounds interfere with mitochondrial metabolism to induce peroxisome proliferation *in vivo* (Starkov and Wallace, 2002).

Thyroid hormone system

The importance of thyroid hormones for normal development and maturation is well established and several other persistent organic pollutants are affecting the thyroid hormone system, therefore it came as no surprise when it first was shown that the reproductive and developmental toxicity of PFOS and PFOA could be a result of this type of mechanism of action. The thyroid hormone system in the fetus develops late and the fetus relies on the maternal thyroid hormone system until just before birth, which means that the maternal thyroid hormone system is of biggest interest prenatally and around birth, and postnatally the interest shifts to that of the offspring, when also the hypothalamic–pituitary–thyroid axis develops and gains normal function (Dussault and Labrie, 1975).

Zebrafish (a new model organism to study reproductive toxicity) exposed to low PFOS concentrations (0-400 μg/L), the expression of several genes in the hypothalamic–pituitary–thyroid system, were affected 15 days post-fertilization. Genes corresponding to synthesis, regulation and action of thyroid hormones were altered, such as corticotropin-releasing factor, thyroid-stimulating hormone, thyroid peroxidase, transthyretin and thyroid receptor alpha and beta. Triiodothyronine (T3) levels were significantly increased indicating a disrupted thyroid hormone status after PFOS exposure in developing fish (Shi *et al.*, 2009).

Repeated long-term PFOS exposure has been studied in several species, for example rat, mouse and monkey. In the adult monkeys thyroid stimulating hormone (TSH) increased (approximately twice control) and total triiodothyronine (T3) decreased, accompanied by lower concentrations of free T3 (Seacat *et al.*, 2002). Female rats exposed to different doses of PFOS during gestation had reduced serum thyroxin (T4) and T3 as early as one week after chemical exposure, although no feedback response of TSH was observed. This reduction in T4 is also seen in pregnant mice (Thibodeaux *et al.*, 2003; Chang *et al.*, 2008). These effects in adult animals were compared with effects in pups after maternal exposure. In rat pups hypothyroxinemia was detected as early as on postnatal day 2. Both total T4 and free T4 concentrations in serum were reduced, and this reduction in free T4 persisted into adolescence, while the levels of total T4 appeared to be recovered by the age of weanling. T3 and TSH in the pups were not affected by the maternal PFOS exposure during gestation. In mice the serum thyroxin level was reduced. This shows that gestational exposure to PFOS can alter the thyroid hormone system in both rats and mice during development, which in turn may be one of the mechanisms of action behind the reproductive and developmental toxicity of PFOS (Lau *et al.*, 2003; Chang *et al.*, 2009). These effects have been confirmed in other studies where PFOS-exposed dams had significant reductions in total T3 and total T4, while the TSH concentrations were unchanged. In pups from the PFOS-treated dams significant reductions in free T4 and total T4, down to immeasurable levels, were observed, which also confirm earlier studies (Luebker *et al.*, 2005). Due to the lack of effects on TSH it is concluded that PFOS does not induce a hypothyroid state, since the diagnosis of primary hypothyroidism is based on reduced serum-free T4 and consequent compensatory elevation of TSH. The inherent property of PFOS to induce changes in the thyroid hormone system, secondarily giving rise to reproductive and developmental toxicity, is apparently dose related, meaning that the effects are bigger or worse the higher the dose.

There is little knowledge about PFOA and its effects on the thyroid hormone system, but it has been seen in male workers from production sites that PFOA serum concentrations have a negative association with free T4 and positive association with T3 (Olsen and Zobel, 2007). In animal studies, PFOA-exposed rats had perturbations in genes related to thyroid hormone metabolism and these perturbations were matched by serum thyroid hormone depletion *in vivo* (Martin *et al.*, 2007). In addition it has been seen in cDNA microarrays in fish (rare minnows, *Gobiocypris rarus*) that subchronic exposure to PFOA inhibits genes responsible for thyroid hormone biosynthesis (Wei *et al.*, 2008), but data on reproductive and developmental toxicity of PFOA is basically non-existent.

Fatty acid homeostasis

Yet another possible type of mechanism of action of PFOS and PFOA is changes in the fatty acid homeostasis. In some cases the changes in fatty acid homeostasis, from PFOA exposure, are suggested to be attributed to effects in PPAR, but there are suggestions that mechanisms other than PPAR can be involved (Rosen *et al.*, 2008b).

The first reports about PFOS and PFOA altering important factors in the fatty acid homeostasis came in 1992, when researchers discovered that dietary exposure of rats with PFOS and PFOA resulted in rapid and pronounced reduction in both cholesterol and triacylglycerols in serum and the following was reported: (1) concentration of liver triacylglycerols was increased by about 300% by PFOS; (2) free cholesterol was increased by both perfluorocompounds and PFOS reduced cholesteryl ester to 50%; (3) in hepatocytes from fed rats, both PFOS and PFOA resulted in reduced cholesterol synthesis from acetate, pyruvate and hydroxymethyl glutarate; (4) the oxidation of palmitate, one of the most common saturated fatty acids found in animals and the first fatty acid produced during lipogenesis (fatty acid synthesis) and from which longer fatty acids can be produced, was also increased by PFOS and PFOA exposure; (5) PFOS and PFOA caused some reduction in fatty acid synthesis; (6) the activity of liver HMG-CoA reductase was reduced to 50% and lower activity of acyl-CoA was seen after both PFOS and PFOA treatment. All these changes led to the conclusion that the hypoliponic effect of PFOS and PFOA may be mediated via a common mechanism, namely impaired production of lipoprotein particles due to reduced synthesis and esterification of cholesterol together with enhanced oxidation of fatty acids in the liver (Haughom and Spydevold, 1992). Since then several studies have confirmed these effects in adult animals and also shown that PFOA can alter the fatty acid homeostasis (Martin *et al.*, 2007).

In studies where pregnant rats were exposed to PFOS during the whole gestational period, several genes associated with fetal hepatic fatty acid biosynthesis increased significantly. Among the genes with increased expression were acyl-CoA carboxylase (Acac), coding for the rate-limiting enzyme in fatty acid biosynthesis, and fatty acid synthase (Fas), fatty acid CoA ligase 5 (Facl5), fatty acid elongase 1 and 2 (rELO1, 2), stearoyl-coenzyme A desaturase 1 (Scd1) and sterol regulatory element binding factor 1 (Srebf1), a key nuclear transcription factor controlling expression of fatty acid and cholesterol synthesis genes (Bjork *et al.*, 2008). When pregnant mice and rats were exposed to PFOA during the gestational period, the expression of genes related to fatty acid catabolism was altered in both the fetal liver and lung and also included genes associated with lipid transport, ketogenesis, glucose metabolism, lipoprotein metabolism, cholesterol biosynthesis, steroid metabolism, bile acid biosynthesis, phospholipid metabolism, retinol metabolism, proteosome activation and inflammation. In mice, all together 127 genes related to lipid homeostasis were altered in fetal liver and 18 genes related to lipid homeostasis were altered in lung (Rosen *et al.*, 2007, 2008a).

Cell communication

Inter- and intracellular communication is vital for biological processes to work properly and disturbances in this communication can be disastrous for a tissue or the whole organism. Gap junctional intercellular communication (GJIC) is the major pathway of intercellular signal transduction, and is thus important for normal cell growth and function. In cell lines from rat liver (WB-F344) and dolphin kidney (CDK) as well as in intact Sprague-Dawley rats, exposed to different doses of PFOS (3.1, 6.25, 12.5, 50, 100 and 160 μM for cell lines and 5 mg PFOS/kg body weight/day for 3 days or 3 weeks in rats), inhibition of GJIC was seen in a dose-dependent fashion and this inhibition occurred rapidly and was reversible. Since the results from the two cell lines and the *in vivo* exposure are comparable these inhibitory effects on GJIC are neither species nor tissue specific and can occur both *in vitro* and *in vivo* making them reliable as a possible mechanism of action of PFOS (Hu *et al.*, 2002). Furthermore, other studies have shown that PFOS and PFOA alter the structure and organization of lipid membranes. The presence of PFOS or PFOA leads to the formation of a more fluidic lipid layer at the air/water interface and PFOS also penetrates slowly into already preformed lipid layers, leading to a change of their properties with time (Matyszewska *et al.*, 2007). Changes of membrane properties are likely to affect cell communications and maybe also effects on ion channels can be part of this mechanism of action. Both PFOS and PFOA altered the activation and inactivation kinetics of calcium currents in myocytes from guinea-pig and increased the voltage-activated peak amplitude. PFOA showed less potent effects. These shifts of the activation and inactivation curves are due to changes in the actual membrane potentials induced by insertion of PFOS or PFOA into the outer layer of the cell membrane. Incorporation of PFOS or PFOA into the outer monolayer of the cell membrane should increase the fixed negative charge, thereby rendering the actual transmembrane potential less negative, and resulting in shifts of both the activation and inactivation kinetics. The concentrations used to these membrane characteristics are actually lower than seen in samples from occupational exposure, making effects on membranes and/or calcium channels a realistic toxicological target for PFOS and PFOA (Harada *et al.*, 2005b).

TOXICITY

PPAR, the thyroid hormone system and fatty acid homeostasis may be the three most studied and likely mechanisms of action, but what do all the different mechanisms of action lead to, and what are the toxicological responses to PFOS and PFOA exposure during reproduction and development? Many different endpoints have been studied in both human and experimental animals and still many questions are unanswered and need explanation, therefore here we are going to discuss the most important ones in human and in experimental animals.

Human studies

It is always hard to study toxicological effects in humans especially when it comes to reproductive and developmental effects. Despite that, a lot of effort has been put into epidemiological studies to investigate if there are connections or correlations between levels/concentrations of PFOS and/or PFOA in maternal serum, umbilical cord serum and birth weight, size and other markers of development in humans. In 2007, reports came from Maryland, USA, that both PFOS and PFOA concentrations in umbilical cord serum were negatively associated with birth weight, ponderal index (a measure of leanness of a person, calculated as a relationship between mass and height) and head circumference. This correlation was seen despite the relatively low cord serum concentrations (Apelberg *et al.*, 2007b). When studying women and their infants both PFOS (Stein *et al.*, 2009) and PFOA levels (Fei *et al.*, 2007) are inversely associated with birth weight, and for PFOS this risk showed a dose–response gradient. When looking at maternal concentrations of PFOS and PFOA in relation to motor and mental developmental in children, it can be seen that children from mothers with high PFOS concentrations are slightly delayed in time of sitting without support (Fei *et al.*, 2008a) and also self-reported birth defects were associated with high PFOA exposures (Stein *et al.*, 2009). From the same studies it was evaluated whether PFOS and PFOA could reduce organ growth. The following findings were made: (1) maternal PFOA levels in early pregnancy were associated with smaller abdominal circumference and birth length; (2) for each ng/ml increase in PFOA, birth length decreased by 0.069 cm (95% confidence interval: 0.024, 0.113) and abdominal circumference decreased by 0.059 cm (95% confidence interval: 0.012, 0.106); (3) maternal PFOS levels were not associated with changes in any of the five fetal growth indicators. These findings suggest that fetal exposure to PFOA but not PFOS during organ development may affect the growth of organs and the skeleton (Fei *et al.*, 2008b). Preeclampsia, a condition in pregnancy characterized by abrupt hypertension (a sharp rise in blood pressure), albuminuria (leakage of large amounts of the protein albumin into the urine) and edema (swelling) of the hands, feet and face, were weakly associated with PFOA and PFOS exposures (Stein *et al.*, 2009).

In addition to the effects seen in pregnant mothers and their fetuses/newborns other types of effects on reproduction have been discovered in both adult females and males. First, high levels of PFOS and PFOA in females were related to longer time to pregnancy, which can be interpreted as reduced fecundity (Fei *et al.*, 2009). Second, human testicular function has been investigated in relation to PFOS and PFOA and a reduction of the number of normal spermatozoa per ejaculate was seen in men with high combined levels of PFOS and PFOA. These men also had lower sperm concentration, total sperm count and altered concentrations of testosterone, estradiol, sex hormone binding globulin (SHBG), luteinizing hormone (LH), follicle-stimulating hormone (FSH) and inhibin B (Joensen *et al.*, 2009). Clearly, high serum concentrations of PFOS and PFOA can affect both female and male fecundity.

Animal studies

Although there have been few studies on humans it is obvious that PFOS and PFOA have toxic effects in humans despite the limited methods of measuring both exposure and effects. In animal studies there are a vast number of different experimental methods that can measure a variety of endpoints from several different exposure paradigms, with different doses, in several different species. Results generated from animal studies can be used to extrapolate and predict human toxicity. Generally, it can be said that PFOS and PFOA toxicity have been studied in all types of animals including fish, birds and mammals, and it has been seen that different toxicological effects and the vast majority of reproductive and developmental toxicology studies with PFOS and PFOA are done in rats and mice.

General reproductive and developmental toxicity

Most of the knowledge concerning PFOS and PFOA reproductive and developmental toxicity comes from *in utero* exposure, where the dam has been exposed during parts of or the whole gestational period. Exposure of mice and rats exposed to different doses of PFOS (1–20 mg/kg body weight/day and 1–10 mg/kg body weight/day, respectively) during the whole gestational period (gestational day 1–17 and 2–20, respectively) causes toxic effects in both the dams, fetuses and newborn pups. Maternal weight gain in both mice and rats can be suppressed by PFOS in a dose-dependent manner, likely attributed to reduced food and water intake, and as discussed previously in this chapter effects on the thyroid hormone system and fatty acid homeostasis can be seen in the dams. The reduced food and water intake is probably mediated via the activation of hypothalamic urocortin 2 and corticotropin-releasing factor type 2 receptor, together with the suppression of gastroduodenal motor activity (Asakawa *et al.*, 2007). In rat small deficits in fetal weight were noted and a host of birth defects, including cleft palate, anasarca, ventricular septal defect and enlargement of the right atrium, were seen in both rats and mice, primarily after the highest exposures (Thibodeaux *et al.*, 2003). Pups born alive from exposed mice and rats initially appear to be active, but within the first 30–60 minutes pups from the highest dosage groups become pale, inactive and moribund and all died soon afterward. These effects were dose–response related because the lower the PFOS dose, the more pups survived. Small but significant and persistent growth lags were also seen in surviving rat and mouse pups exposed to PFOS prenatally, and slight delays in eye-opening were noted. These effects in newborn pups were accompanied by changes in the thyroid hormone system (see the section on mechanisms of action). This indicates that *in utero* exposure to PFOS severely compromises postnatal survival of neonatal rats and mice, and causes delays in growth and development in the surviving rat pups (Lau *et al.*, 2003). Lower doses (0.8–2.0 mg/kg body weight/day) decreased gestational length and decreased viability up to postnatal day 5 and the decreased gestational length and decreased viability were positively correlated. This suggested that late-stage fetal development may be affected in pups exposed to PFOS *in utero* and may contribute to the observed mortality (Luebker *et al.*, 2005).

PFOA exposure (1–40 mg/kg body weight/day) of mice during the gestational period (GD 1–17) produce dose-dependent fetal resorption, and all exposed to the highest dose resorbed the whole litter. The percent of live fetuses was lower only in the 20 mg/kg group (74 vs. 94% in controls), and fetal weight was also significantly lower in this group. In the 10 and 20 mg/kg groups the incidence of live birth and postnatal survival was lowered by PFOA compared to controls. Dose-dependent growth deficits, such as enlarged fontanel and reduced ossification of sternebrae, caudal vertebrae, metacarpals, metatarsals, phalanges, calvaria, supraoccipital and hyoid, plus minor tail and limb defects and microcardia, were detected in all PFOA-treated litters above 1 mg/kg group. Just as with PFOS treatment, PFOA treatment resulted in delayed eye-opening (2–3 days) in pups from dams exposed to 5 mg/kg and higher doses. In these offspring an accelerated sexual maturation was observed in males, manifested as earlier prepuce separation, but no difference in sexual maturation was seen in females (Lau *et al.*, 2006).

Looking at the timing of PFOS and PFOA exposure it is clear the severity of effects of *in utero* exposure differ with the timing of exposure. Rats exposed to 25 mg PFOS/kg body weight/day on gestational days (GD) 2–5, 6–9 and 10–13 had pups with reduced weights. This decrease in weights occurred after exposure during the embryonic period. Another effect seen when PFOS exposure occurred during the fetal period, GD 14–17 or 17–20, was that neonatal survival decreased in groups dosed later during gestation, approaching 100% with dosing on GD 17–20. The majority of deaths occurred within the first 24 hours, but continued up to postnatal day 4. Following a 2-day treatment on GD 19–20, PFOS groups experienced significant pup mortality by PND 1 and continuing through PND 5, when survival was 98, 66 and 3% for the 0, 25 and 50 mg/kg groups, respectively, and this type of treatment reduced pup weight in surviving litters (Grasty *et al.*, 2003). An attempt has also been made in a study to segregate the contributions of gestational and lactational exposures to PFOA and consider the impact of restricting PFOA exposure to specific gestational periods. Generally, the longer and the earlier the PFOA exposure is, during the gestational period, the more severe the effects become and if this is a function of higher total dose or if there is a more developmentally sensitive period is not known. Furthermore, the early postnatal developmental effects of PFOA are due to gestational exposure rather than lactational exposure and these effects include increased incidence of whole litter loss, reduced birth weights, developmental delay in eye-opening and hair growth (Wolf *et al.*, 2007).

Liver toxicity

One characteristic that seem to be shared by PFOS and PFOA is an ability to cause hepatomegaly and, in some cases, hepatotoxicity, in rodents and primates, including an increased incidence of hepatocellular adenoma in rats. Many PPARalfa agonists, like PFOA, induce low incidences of tumors of the rat liver, pancreas and testis. These compounds are non-genotoxic and produce these tumors by a non-DNA reactive mode-of-action involving binding to and stimulation of PPARalfa, leading to increased cell proliferation and, ultimately, low incidences of tumors. The administration of PFOA to rats also leads to hepatomegaly and can result in reduced weight gain or actual weight loss, presumably via the increased oxidation of fat. PFOA exposure can also lead to changes in the expression of genes involved in xenobiotic metabolism, including both phase I and phase II genes. The mechanism of action behind the liver toxicity of PFOS and PFOA has been attributable to all of the topics discussed above, but general consensus is that PPARalfa is the most important or dominating mechanism of action.

Pulmonary toxicity

One of the more pronounced effects of prenatal PFOS exposure in rodents is neonatal mortality occurring during the first postnatal week. Pups born alive, but affected, have difficulties breathing accompanied by pale lungs that did not expand fully on perfusion. Gross dissection and histological examination of lungs have revealed differences in maturation between exposed and non-exposed animals on PND 0. In lungs of PFOS-exposed newborns (25 or 50 mg/kg body weight/day) alveolar walls were thicker compared to controls. The ratio of solid tissue: small airway was increased and these morphometric changes in lungs of PFOS exposed neonates were suggestive of immaturity. Therefore exposure to PFOS late in gestation is sufficient to induce 100% pup mortality suggesting that inhibition of lung maturation may be involved (Grasty *et al.*, 2003, 2005).

Neurotoxicity

Usually, in order to exert an effect a compound has to be present in the target organ. In the section about the toxicokinetics of PFOS and PFOA it was described that both compounds can reach the brain, both during development and in adults, which indicates that neurotoxic effects may arise. There are several known neurotoxic effects of PFOS and PFOA and here we will look into some of them.

In utero exposure to 3 mg PFOS/kg body weight/day, during the gestational period, in rats resulted in decreased activity of choline acethyltransferase in prefrontal cortex at different postnatal ages (Lau *et al.*, 2003). Choline acetyltransferase (ChAT), a very important enzyme in the cholinergic system of mammals, is involved in the recycling of the neurotransmitter acethylcholine by joining of acetyl-CoA and choline to reform acethylcholine. The cholinergic system is involved in many physiological functions, including cognitive capacity. However, despite the decrease of ChAT the development of learning in these animals was not affected by the *in utero* exposure to PFOS. PFOS exposure in mice during the gestational period (6 mg/kg body weight/day) delayed a couple of landmarks of neuromotor maturation, such as decreased resistance to backward pull on postnatal days 10 and 11 and decreased climb ability and forelimb strength on postnatal day 11. These effects were transient and not seen later during the postnatal period and also here no effects were seen on the development of learning (Fuentes *et al.*, 2007). In a more recent study dams were exposed to different doses (0.1, 0.3 and 1.0 mg/kg body weight/day) of PFOS from gestational day 0 through postnatal day 20. PFOS treatments had no effect during the postnatal period when looking at the auditory startle response and learning and memory in a swim maze. However, locomotor activity increased in PFOS-treated animals (0.3 and 1.0 mg/kg body weight/day) on postnatal day 17, which ultimately leads to the inability of the animals to habituate to the novel test environment (Butenhoff *et al.*, 2009).

Increase in locomotor activity and inability to habituate to a novel home environment had earlier been seen in adult mice exposed only to one single oral dose of PFOS (0.75 and 11.3 mg/kg body weight) or PFOA (0.58 and 8.7 mg/kg body weight) on postnatal day 10, during the postnatal brain development, known as the brain growth spurt. Here the spontaneous behavior, locomotion (horizontal movement), rearing (vertical movement) and total activity were measured for an hour. In the beginning of the 60-minute test period the activity was decreased in animals exposed to the highest PFOS or PFOA dose, but in the end these animals had not habituated to the novel environment and the activity was higher than in the control animals. This type of behavior was observed in both 2- and 4-month-old animals (Figure 47.2) and these behavioral effects were persistent and actually worsen with age. A third perfluorinated compound, PFDA (perfluorodecanoic acid), had no effects on adult behavior. The spontaneous behavior tested here also measures the cognitive function and in earlier studies it had been seen that neonatal exposure to other environmental pollutants, like PBDEs and PCBs, can affect the cholinergic system and when these PFOS- and PFOA-exposed animals were challenged with an injection of nicotine, as adults, they had developed an increased susceptibility of the cholinergic system. They became hypoactive, meaning that locomotion, rearing and total activity decreased compared to the controls that become hyperactive by the nicotine injection.

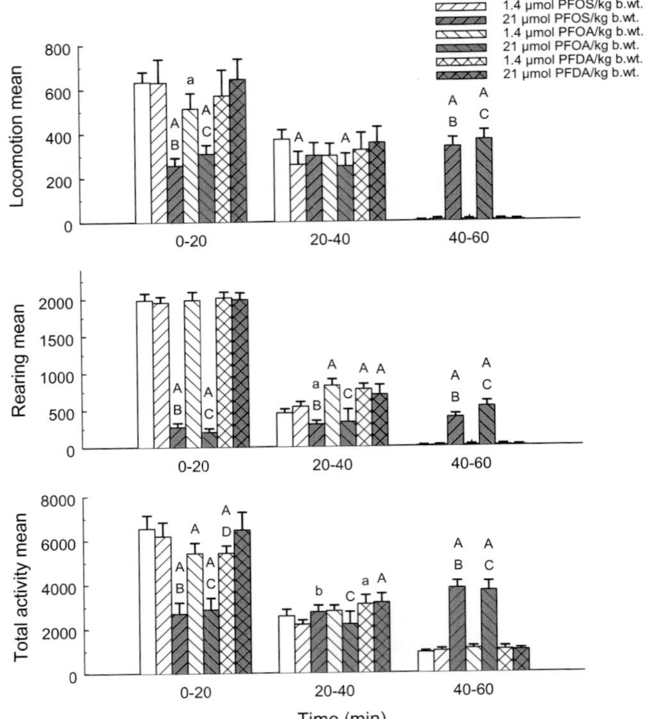

FIGURE 47.2 Spontaneous behavior of 4-month-old NMRI male mice exposed to a single-oral dose of either 10 ml/kg body weight of the 20% fat emulsion vehicle, 1.4 or 21 µmol/kg body weight of PFOS (0.75 or 11.3 mg/kg body weight), PFOA (0.58 or 8.70 mg/kg body weight) or PFDA (0.72 or 10.8 mg/kg body weight), at the age of 10 days. Statistical differences are indicated as (A) significantly different vs. controls $P<0.01$; (a) significantly different vs. controls $P<0.05$; (B) significantly different vs. 1.4 µmol PFOS/kg body weight $P<0.01$; (b) significantly different vs. 1.4 µmol PFOS/kg body weight $P<0.05$; (C) significantly different vs. 1.4 µmol PFOA/kg body weight $P<0.01$; (c) significantly different vs. 1.4 µmol PFOA/kg body weight $P<0.05$. Bar height represents mean value ± SD.

This means that PFOS and PFOA can cause alterations in the developing cholinergic system, which could be one of the possible mechanisms behind the adult behavioral disturbances (Johansson *et al.*, 2008). To further look into the mechanisms behind the adult functional changes, neonatal animals were exposed to PFOS or PFOA on postnatal day 10 and sacrificed 24 hours later. Proteins important for normal brain development, axonal growth and synaptogenesis were analyzed and interesting results were seen. Both PFOS and PFOA exposure led to increases in the four proteins CaMKII (Ca^{2+} calmodulin-dependent protein kinase II), GAP-43 (growth-associated protein 43), synaptophysin and tau in hippocampus, and in cortex the levels of synaptophysin and tau were elevated (Figure 47.3). Because hippocampus and cortex are directly involved in behavioral and cognitive processes such as learning and memory, changes in these proteins during the brain growth spurt may lead to adult functional alterations (Johansson *et al.*, 2009). The effects on these proteins by PFOS and PFOA are supported by changes in the gene expression of calcium-dependent signaling molecules in rat hippocampus after perinatal PFOS exposure. The expression of calcium-related signaling molecules, which are critical to the function of the central nervous system, such as N-methyl-D-aspartate receptor subtype-2B, calmodulin, Ca(2+)/calmodulin-dependent kinase II alpha and cAMP-response element-binding, were

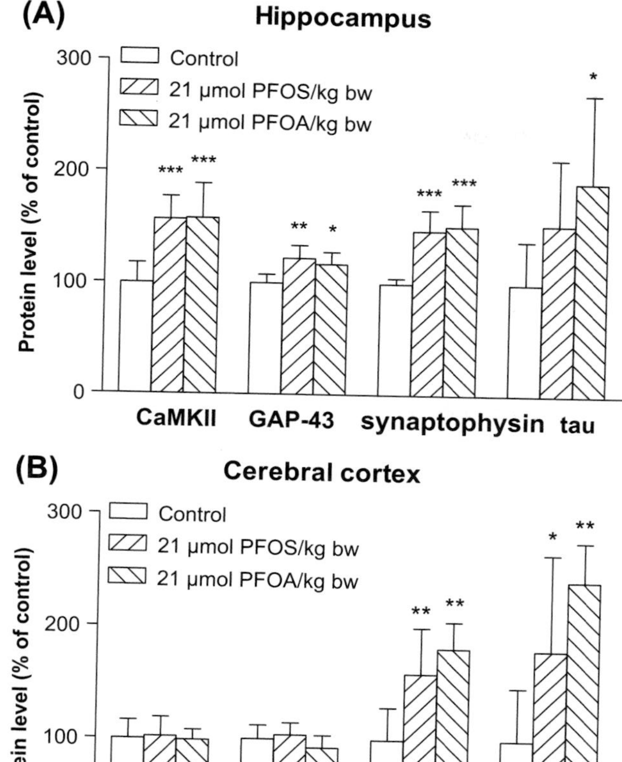

FIGURE 47.3 Protein levels of CaMKII, GAP-43, synaptophysin and tau in (A) hippocampus and (B) cerebral cortex of animals exposed to 21 μmol PFOS or PFOA/kg body weight on postnatal day 10 and sacrificed 24 hours later. The data were analyzed with a one-way ANOVA and Newman-Keuls post hoc test. Statistical differences are indicated by (***) significantly different vs. control, $P<0.001$; (**) significantly different vs. control, $P<0.01$; (*) significantly different vs. control, $P<0.05$. The height of the bars represents the mean value ± SD.

increased in the PFOS exposure group on postnatal day 1 (PND 1). In some cases these changes lasted for short periods in postnatal life, but only calmodulin and as N-methyl-D-aspartate receptor subtype-2B were still reduced on postnatal day 35 (Liu *et al.*, 2009b). Also, results from *in vitro* studies with PC12 cells, a neuronotypic cell line used to characterize neurotoxicity, show that PFOS can affect the differentiation of developing neurons by reducing DNA synthesis in undifferentiated PC12 cells and promoting differentiation of the PC12 cells into the acethylcholine neurotransmitter phenotype at the expense of the dopamine neurotransmitter phenotype. PFOA had little or no effect on phenotypic specification (Slotkin *et al.*, 2008). When comparing the doses used and the duration of the exposure, it seems as though the developing central nervous system is the most susceptible part of the organism.

RISK ASSESSMENT

As we have seen, PFOS and PFOA can affect many different organisms and several different types of endpoints at different stages of an organism's lifecycle. But as we also have seen, the studies are very diverse and the exposures and doses are not the same. How do we interpret all these studies? One attempt has been made to create a scaling system for perfluorinated compounds, including PFOS and PFOA, analogous to the toxic equivalency factor (TEF) system used for polychlorinated biphenyls, polychlorinated dibenzo-p-dioxins and polychlorinated dibenzofurans, but it was impossible to identify a scaling system that gave values consistently within an order of magnitude for the same compounds (Scialli *et al.*, 2007). Instead, risk assessors and other governmental authorities have used the present knowledge for risk assessment and legislation and the situation differs between different countries in the world.

In the European Union a directive (2006/122/EG) to limit the use of PFOS and PFOS-related compounds came into force on June 27, 2008. This directive means a ban against PFOS and compounds that can be degraded to PFOS in chemical products and merchandise. In reality, almost all the remaining use is excepted from the ban, such as:

- use of remaining PFOS-based stocks of fire-fighting foams;
- aviation hydraulic fluids;
- critical applications in the photographic sector; and
- critical applications in photolithography and semiconductors.

Fire-fighting foam containing PFOS, for example, is allowed until June 2011. Furthermore, the directive includes the possibility to discontinue the exceptions and also to start to investigate a limitation of the use of PFOA and other compounds that can be degraded to PFOS.

In North America there are different regulations compared to Europe and there are also differences between the USA and Canada. The USA, through the Environmental Protection Agency, have joined a global PFOA Stewardship program where companies commit to drastically decrease the content of PFOA and PFOA-related compounds in products and in emissions from production, i.e. 95% until 2010 and a total elimination until 2015 (Reneman *et al.*, 2001). Canada banned import and production of four fluoro-telomere-based compounds in 2004 for a period of two years, but has since proposed prohibition on manufacture, use, sale, offer for sale and import of PFOS, its salts and its precursors, and products or formulations containing PFOS, its salts and its precursors.

On an international note it can also be said that the Swedish Chemicals Agency (KemI) has nominated PFOS as a POP candidate (persistent organic pollutant) in the United Nations LRTAP convention (long-range transboundary air pollution) and in the Stockholm convention, in hope of reaching a global ban.

CONCLUDING REMARKS AND FUTURE DIRECTIONS

As been discussed above, different countries have chosen different ways of regulation and legislation. In order to gather new valuable information for further understanding and risk assessment, there are a couple of crucial aspects to focus on. First, it is important to further evaluate the exposure situation to understand both the magnitude of the exposure and if certain demographic groups are at higher risk of exposure. The most recent findings suggest that infants and toddlers are at high risk due to the combined exposure from lactation, dust and particle ingestion and inhalation. Furthermore it is important to characterize vulnerable and sensitive periods during the organism's life-course, as well as the most vulnerable and sensitive endpoints of toxicity. According to what is known at the moment it looks as though neurotoxicological endpoints, including behavior and molecular disturbances in the brain, are very sensitive and are induced at the lowest doses, compared to induction of toxicity in other organs or systems, especially when looking at exposure during the neonatal period, a period also coinciding with the highest exposure in the general population.

Finally, there is no doubt that PFOS and PFOA can induce reproductive and developmental toxic effects in various organs and tissues. Reality, though, is much more complicated than exposure to one single compound at the time. We are constantly exposed to a cocktail of chemicals, both compounds which we administer voluntarily and compounds entering our bodies involuntarily. Therefore, effects of PFOS and PFOA in combination and/or in combination with other xenobiotics need to be investigated. At the moment two known cases of interaction effects have been seen. In cell cultures from chicken embryo primary hepatocytes co-exposure to PFOS plus TCDD and co-exposure to PFOA and TCDD induced cytochrome P450 mRNA compared with exposure to TCDD, PFOS and PFOA alone (Watanabe *et al.*, 2009) showing that combined exposures can induce effects that PFOS or PFOA alone cannot. Furthermore, combined exposure to low doses of PFOA and the polybrominated diphenyl ether PBDE 209, during the neonatal period, can interact and exacerbate adult functional neurobehavioral effects, compared to the single compounds alone (Johansson, 2009).

REFERENCES

3MCompany (1995) 3M The leader in electrofluorination. In *Technical Bulletin* (3MCompany, ed.). St. Paul, MN, USA.

3MCompany (1999) The science of organic fluorochemistry. AR226-0547.

Abbott BD, Wolf CJ, Das KP, Zehr RD, Schmid JE, Lindstrom AB, Strynar MJ, Lau C (2009) Developmental toxicity of perfluorooctane sulfonate (PFOS) is not dependent on expression of peroxisome proliferator activated receptor-alpha (PPAR alpha) in the mouse. *Repro Toxicol* **27:** 258–65.

Abbott BD, Wolf CJ, Schmid JE, Das KP, Zehr RD, Helfant L, Nakayama S, Lindstrom AB, Strynar MJ, Lau C (2007) Perfluorooctanoic acid induced developmental toxicity in the mouse is dependent on expression of peroxisome proliferator activated receptor-alpha. *Toxicol Sci* **98:** 571–81.

Andersen ME, Clewell HJ 3rd, Tan YM, Butenhoff JL, Olsen GW (2006) Pharmacokinetic modeling of saturable, renal resorption of perfluoroalkylacids in monkeys – probing the determinants of long plasma half-lives. *Toxicology* **227:** 156–64.

Apelberg BJ, Goldman LR, Calafat AM, Herbstman JB, Kuklenyik Z, Heidler J, Needham LL, Halden RU, Witter FR (2007a) Determinants of fetal exposure to polyfluoroalkyl compounds in Baltimore, Maryland. *Environ Sci Techn* **41:** 3891–7.

Apelberg BJ, Witter FR, Herbstman JB, Calafat AM, Halden RU, Needham LL, Goldman LR (2007b) Cord serum concentrations of perfluorooctane sulfonate (PFOS) and perfluorooctanoate (PFOA) in relation to weight and size at birth. *Environ Health Perp* **115:** 1670–6.

Asakawa A, Toyoshima M, Fujimiya M, Harada K, Ataka K, Inoue K, Koizumi A (2007) Perfluorooctane sulfonate influences feeding behavior and gut motility via the hypothalamus. *Int J Mol Med* **19:** 733–9.

Berthiaume J, Wallace KB (2002) Perfluorooctanoate, perflourooctanesulfonate, and N-ethyl perfluorooctanesulfonamido ethanol; peroxisome proliferation and mitochondrial biogenesis. *Toxicol Lett* **129:** 23–32.

Bjork JA, Lau C, Chang SC, Butenhoff JL, Wallace KB (2008) Perfluorooctane sulfonate-induced changes in fetal rat liver gene expression. *Toxicology* **251:** 8–20.

Bjorklund JA, Thuresson K, De Wit CA (2009) Perfluoroalkyl compounds (PFCs) in indoor dust: concentrations, human exposure estimates, and sources. *Environ Sci Techn* **43:** 2276–81.

Buist SC, Cherrington NJ, Choudhuri S, Hartley DP, Klaassen CD (2002) Gender-specific and developmental influences on the expression of rat organic anion transporters. *J Pharmacol Exp Ther* **301:** 145–51.

Buist SC, Klaassen CD (2004) Rat and mouse differences in gender-predominant expression of organic anion transporter (Oat1-3; Slc22a6-8) mRNA levels. *Drug Metab Dispos* **32:** 620–5.

Butenhoff JL, Ehresman DJ, Chang SC, Parker GA, Stump DG (2009) Gestational and lactational exposure to potassium perfluorooctanesulfonate (K+PFOS) in rats: developmental neurotoxicity. *Repro Toxicol* **27:** 319–30.

Butenhoff JL, Kennedy GL Jr, Hinderliter PM, Lieder PH, Jung R, Hansen KJ, Gorman GS, Noker PE, Thomford PJ (2004) Pharmacokinetics of perfluorooctanoate in cynomolgus monkeys. *Toxicol Sci* **82:** 394–406.

Calafat AM, Kuklenyik Z, Reidy JA, Caudill SP, Tully JS, Needham LL (2007a) Serum concentrations of 11 polyfluoroalkyl compounds in the U.S. population: data from the national health and nutrition examination survey (NHANES). *Environ Sci Techn* **41:** 2237–42.

Calafat AM, Needham LL, Kuklenyik Z, Reidy JA, Tully JS, Aguilar-Villalobos M, Naeher LP (2006) Perfluorinated chemicals in selected residents of the American continent. *Chemosphere* **63:** 490–6.

Calafat AM, Wong LY, Kuklenyik Z, Reidy JA, Needham LL (2007b) Polyfluoroalkyl chemicals in the U.S. population: data from the National Health and Nutrition Examination Survey (NHANES) 2003–2004 and comparisons with NHANES 1999–2000. *Environ Health Pers* **115:** 1596–602.

Chang SC, Ehresman DJ, Bjork JA, Wallace KB, Parker GA, Stump DG, Butenhoff JL (2009) Gestational and lactational exposure to potassium perfluorooctanesulfonate (K+PFOS) in rats: toxicokinetics, thyroid hormone status, and related gene expression. *Repro Toxicol* **27:** 387–99.

Chang SC, Thibodeaux JR, Eastvold ML, Ehresman, DJ, Bjork JA, Froehlich JW, Lau C, Singh RJ, Wallace KB, Butenhoff JL (2008) Thyroid hormone status and pituitary function in adult rats given oral doses of perfluorooctanesulfonate (PFOS). *Toxicology* **243:** 330–9.

Dietz R, Bossi R, Riget FF, Sonne C, Born EW (2008) Increasing perfluoroalkyl contaminants in east Greenland polar bears (Ursus maritimus): a new toxic threat to the Arctic bears. *Environ Sci Technol* **42:** 2701–7.

Dussault JH, Labrie F (1975) Development of the hypothalamic–pituitary–thyroid axis in the neonatal rat. *Endocrinology* **97:** 1321–4.

Ehresman DJ, Froehlich JW, Olsen GW, Chang SC, Butenhoff JL (2007) Comparison of human whole blood, plasma, and serum matrices for the determination of perfluorooctanesulfonate (PFOS), perfluorooctanoate (PFOA), and other fluorochemicals. *Environ Res* **103:** 176–84.

Ericson I, Gomez M, Nadal M, van Bavel B, Lindstrom G, Domingo JL (2007) Perfluorinated chemicals in blood of residents in Catalonia (Spain) in relation to age and gender: a pilot study. *Environ Int* **33:** 616–23.

Ericson I, Marti-Cid R, Nadal M, Van Bavel B, Lindstrom G, Domingo JL (2008) Human exposure to perfluorinated chemicals through the diet: intake of perfluorinated compounds in foods from the Catalan (Spain) market. *J Agr Food Chem* **56:** 1787–94.

Fei C, McLaughlin JK, Lipworth L, Olsen J (2008a) Prenatal exposure to perfluorooctanoate (PFOA) and perfluorooctanesulfonate (PFOS) and maternally reported developmental milestones in infancy. *Environ Health Persp* **116:** 1391–5.

Fei C, McLaughlin JK, Lipworth L, Olsen J (2009) Maternal levels of perfluorinated chemicals and subfecundity. *Human Repro* **24:** 1200–5.

Fei C, McLaughlin JK, Tarone RE, Olsen J (2007) Perfluorinated chemicals and fetal growth: a study within the Danish National Birth Cohort. *Environ Health Persp* **115:** 1677–82.

Fei C, McLaughlin JK, Tarone RE, Olsen J (2008b) Fetal growth indicators and perfluorinated chemicals: a study in the Danish National Birth Cohort. *Am J Epidemiol* **168:** 66–72.

Fromme H, Tittlemier SA, Volkel W, Wilhelm M, Twardella D (2009) Perfluorinated compounds – exposure assessment for the general population in Western countries. *Int J Hyg Environ Health* **212:** 239–70.

Fuentes S, Colomina MT, Vicens P, Franco-Pons N, Domingo JL (2007) Concurrent exposure to perfluorooctane sulfonate and restraint stress during pregnancy in mice: effects on postnatal development and behavior of the offspring. *Toxicol Sci* **98:** 589–98.

Giesy JP, Kannan K (2001) Global distribution of perfluorooctane sulfonate in wildlife. *Environ Sci Technol* **35:** 1339–42.

Grasty RC, Bjork JA, Wallace KB, Wolf DC, Lau CS, Rogers JM (2005) Effects of prenatal perfluorooctane sulfonate (PFOS) exposure on lung maturation in the perinatal rat. *Birth Defects Research* **74:** 405–16.

Grasty RC, Wolf DC, Grey BE, Lau CS, Rogers JM (2003) Prenatal window of susceptibility to perfluorooctane sulfonate-induced neonatal mortality in the Sprague-Dawley rat. *Birth Defects Res* **68:** 465–71.

Hanhijarvi H, Ophaug RH, Singer L (1982) The sex-related difference in perfluorooctanoate excretion in the rat. *Proc Soc Exp Biol Med* **171:** 50–5.

Harada K, Inoue K, Morikawa A, Yoshinaga T, Saito N, Koizumi A (2005a) Renal clearance of perfluorooctane sulfonate and perfluorooctanoate in humans and their species-specific excretion. *Environ Res* **99:** 253–61.

Harada K, Koizumi A, Saito N, Inoue K, Yoshinaga T, Date C, Fujii S, Hachiya N, Hirosawa I, Koda S, Kusaka Y, Murata K, Omae K, Shimbo S, Takenaka K, Takeshita T, Todoriki H, Wada Y, Watanabe T, Ikeda M (2007) Historical and geographical aspects of the increasing perfluorooctanoate and perfluorooctane sulfonate contamination in human serum in Japan. *Chemosphere* **66:** 293–301.

Harada K, Saito N, Inoue K, Yoshinaga T, Watanabe T, Sasaki S, Kamiyama S, Koizumi A (2004) The influence of time, sex and geographic factors on levels of perfluorooctane sulfonate and perfluorooctanoate in human serum over the last 25 years. *J Occup Health* **46:** 141–7.

Harada K, Xu F, Ono K, Iijima T, Koizumi A (2005b) Effects of PFOS and PFOA on L-type Ca2+ currents in guinea-pig ventricular myocytes. *Biochem Biophys Res Comm* **329:** 487–94.

Haughom B, Spydevold Ø (1992) The mechanism underlying the hypolipemic effect of perfluorooctanoic acid (PFOA), perfluorooctane sulphonic acid (PFOSA) and clofibric acid. *Biochim et Biophys Acta (BBA) – Lipids and Lipid Metabol* **1128:** 65–72.

Hekster FM, Laane RW, de Voogt P (2003) Environmental and toxicity effects of perfluoroalkylated substances. *Rev Environ Contam Toxicol* **179:** 99–121.

Holzer J, Midasch O, Rauchfuss K, Kraft M, Reupert R, Angerer J, Kleeschulte P, Marschall N, Wilhelm M (2008) Biomonitoring of perfluorinated compounds in children and adults exposed to perfluorooctanoate-contaminated drinking water. *Environ Health Persp* **116:** 651–7.

Hu W, Jones PD, Upham BL, Trosko JE, Lau C, Giesy JP (2002) Inhibition of gap junctional intercellular communication by perfluorinated compounds in rat liver and dolphin kidney epithelial cell lines in vitro and Sprague-Dawley rats in vivo. *Toxicol Sci* **68:** 429–36.

Hundley SG, Sarrif AM, Kennedy GL (2006) Absorption, distribution, and excretion of ammonium perfluorooctanoate (APFO) after oral administration to various species. *Drug Chem Toxicol* **29:** 137–45.

Inoue K, Okada F, Ito R, Kato S, Sasaki S, Nakajima S, Uno A, Saijo Y, Sata F, Yoshimura Y, Kishi R, Nakazawa H (2004) Perfluorooctane sulfonate (PFOS) and related perfluorinated compounds in human maternal and cord blood samples: assessment of PFOS exposure in a susceptible population during pregnancy. *Environ Health Persp* **112:** 1204–7.

Joensen UN, Bossi R, Leffers H, Jensen AA, Skakkebaek NE, Jorgensen N (2009) Do perfluoroalkyl compounds impair human semen quality? *Environ Health Persp* **117:** 923–7.

Johansson N (2009) Neonatal exposure to highly brominated diphenyl ethers and perfluorinated compoounds. Developmental dependent toxicity and interaction. Acta Univ. Ups., Comprehensive Summaries of Uppsala Dissertations from the Faculty of Science and Technology. In *Environmental Toxicology*, pp. 67. Uppsala University, Uppsala.

Johansson N, Eriksson P, Viberg H (2009) Neonatal exposure to PFOS and PFOA in mice results in changes in proteins which are important for neuronal growth and synaptogenesis in the developing brain. *Toxicol Sci* **108:** 412–8.

Johansson N, Fredriksson A, Eriksson P (2008) Neonatal exposure to perfluorooctane sulfonate (PFOS) and perfluorooctanoic acid (PFOA) causes neurobehavioural defects in adult mice. *Neurotoxicology* **29:** 160–9.

Johnson JD, Gibson SJ, Ober RE (1979) Extent and route of excretion and tissue distribution of total carbon-14 in rats after a single intravenous dose of FC-95-14C. Project No. 8900310200. Riker Laboratories, Inc., St. Paul, MN. USEPA Docket No. 8(e) HQ-1180-00374.

Johnson JD, Gibson SJ, Ober RE (1984) Cholestyramine-enhanced fecal elimination of carbon-14 in rats after administration of ammonium [14C]perfluorooctanoate or potassium [14C]perfluorooctanesulfonate. *Fund Appl Toxicol* **4:** 972–6.

Johnson JD, Ober RE (1979) Absorption of FC-95-14C in rats after a single oral dose. Project No. 8900310200, Riker Laboratories, Inc., St. Paul, MN (US EPA Docket No. 8(e)HQ-1180-00374).

Kannan K, Corsolini S, Falandysz J, Fillmann G, Kumar KS, Loganathan BG, Mohd MA, Olivero J, Van Wouwe N, Yang JH, Aldoust KM (2004) Perfluorooctanesulfonate and related fluorochemicals in human blood from several countries. *Environ Sci Technol* **38:** 4489–95.

Kannan K, Koistinen J, Beckmen K, Evans T, Gorzelany JF, Hansen KJ, Jones PD, Helle E, Nyman M, Giesy JP (2001) Accumulation of perfluorooctane sulfonate in marine mammals. *Environ Sci Technol* **35:** 1593–8.

Kannan K, Tao L, Sinclair E, Pastva SD, Jude DJ, Giesy JP (2005) Perfluorinated compounds in aquatic organisms at various trophic levels in a Great Lakes food chain. *Arch Environ Conta Toxicol* **48:** 559–66.

Karrman A, Ericson I, van Bavel B, Darnerud PO, Aune M, Glynn A, Lignell S, Lindstrom G (2007) Exposure of perfluorinated chemicals through lactation: levels of matched human milk and serum and a temporal trend, 1996–2004, in Sweden. *Environ Health Persp* **115:** 226–30.

Karrman A, Harada KH, Inoue K, Takasuga T, Ohi E, Koizumi A (2009) Relationship between dietary exposure and serum perfluorochemical (PFC) levels – a case study. *Environ Int* **35:** 712–7.

Kärrman A, Mueller JF, van Bavel B, Harden F, Toms LM, Lindstrom G (2006) Levels of 12 perfluorinated chemicals in pooled Australian serum, collected 2002–2003, in relation to age, gender, and region. *Environ Sci Technol* **40:** 3742–8.

Kennedy GL Jr, Butenhoff JL, Olsen GW, O'Connor JC, Seacat AM, Perkins RG, Biegel LB, Murphy SR, Farrar DG (2004) The toxicology of perfluorooctanoate. *Crit Rev Toxicol* **34:** 351–84.

Key BD, Howell RD, Criddle CS (1998) Defluorination of organofluorine sulfur compounds by Pseudomonas sp. strain D2. *Environ Sci Technol* **32:** 2283–7.

Key BD., Howell RD, Criddle CS (1997) Fluorinated organics in the biosphere. *Environ Sci Technol* **31:** 2445–54.

Kissa E (2001) *Fluorinated Surfactants and Repellents*, 2nd edition. Mercel Dekker, New York, USA.

Kubwabo C, Stewart B, Zhu J, Marro L (2005) Occurrence of perfluorosulfonates and other perfluorochemicals in dust from selected homes in the city of Ottawa, Canada. *J Environ Monit* **7:** 1074–8.

Kudo N, Katakura M, Sato Y, Kawashima Y (2002) Sex hormone-regulated renal transport of perfluorooctanoic acid. *Chem Biol Interact* **139:** 301–16.

Kudo N, Suzuki E, Katakura M, Ohmori K, Noshiro R, Kawashima Y (2001) Comparison of the elimination between perfluorinated fatty acids with different carbon chain length in rats. *Chem Biol Interact* **134:** 203–16.

Kuklenyik Z, Reich JA, Tully JS, Needham LL, Calafat AM (2004) Automated solid-phase extraction and measurement of perfluorinated organic acids and amides in human serum and milk. *Environ Sci Technol* **38:** 3698–704.

Lau C, Anitole K, Hodes C, Lai D, Pfahles-Hutchens A, Seed J (2007) Perfluoroalkyl acids: a review of monitoring and toxicological findings. *Toxicol Sci* **99:** 366–94.

Lau C, Butenhoff JL, Rogers JM (2004) The developmental toxicity of perfluoroalkyl acids and their derivatives. *Toxicol Appl Pharmacol* **198:** 231–41.

Lau C, Thibodeaux JR, Hanson RG, Rogers JM, Grey BE, Stanton ME, Butenhoff JL, Stevenson LA (2003) Exposure to perfluorooctane sulfonate during pregnancy in rat and mouse. II: Postnatal evaluation. *Toxicol Sci* **74:** 382–92.

Lau C., Thibodeaux JR, Hanson RG, Narotsky MG, Rogers JM, Lindstrom AB, Strynar MJ (2006) Effects of perfluorooctanoic acid exposure during pregnancy in the mouse. *Toxicol Sci* **90:** 510–8.

Li AC, Glass CK (2004) PPAR- and LXR-dependent pathways controlling lipid metabolism and the development of atherosclerosis. *J Lipid Res* **45:** 2161–73.

Liu L, Liu W, Song J, Yu H, Jin Y, Oami K, Sato I, Saito N, Tsuda S (2009a) A comparative study on oxidative damage and distributions of perfluorooctane sulfonate (PFOS) in mice at different postnatal developmental stages. *Toxicol Sci* **34:** 245–54.

Liu X, Liu W, Jin Y, Yu W, Wang F, Liu L (2010) Effect of gestational and lactational exposure to perfluorooctanesulfonate on calcium-dependent signaling molecules gene expression in rats' hippocampus. *Arch Toxicol* **84:** 71–9.

Loos R, Gawlik BM, Locoro G, Rimaviciute E., Contini S, Bidoglio G (2009) EU-wide survey of polar organic persistent pollutants in European river waters. *Environ Pollut* **157:** 561–8.

Luebker DJ, York RG, Hansen KJ, Moore JA, Butenhoff JL (2005) Neonatal mortality from in utero exposure to perfluorooctanesulfonate (PFOS) in Sprague-Dawley rats: dose–response, and biochemical and pharamacokinetic parameters. *Toxicology* **215:** 149–69.

Martin MT, Brennan RJ, Hu W, Ayanoglu E, Lau C, Ren H, Wood CR, Corton JC, Kavlock RJ, Dix DJ (2007) Toxicogenomic study of triazole fungicides and perfluoroalkyl acids in rat livers predicts toxicity and categorizes chemicals based on mechanisms of toxicity. *Toxicol Sci* **97:** 595–613.

Matyszewska D, Tappura K, Oradd G, Bilewicz R (2007) Influence of perfluorinated compounds on the properties of model lipid membranes. *J Phys Chem B* **111:** 9908–18.

Midasch O, Drexler H, Hart N, Beckmann MW, Angerer J (2007) Transplacental exposure of neonates to perfluorooctanesulfonate and perfluorooctanoate: a pilot study. *Int Arch Occup Environ Health* **80:** 643–8.

Monroy R, Morrison K, Teo K, Atkinson S, Kubwabo C, Stewart B, Foster WG (2008) Serum levels of perfluoroalkyl compounds in human maternal and umbilical cord blood samples. *Environ Res* **108:** 56–62.

Moriwaki H, Takatah Y, Arakawa R (2003) Concentrations of perfluorooctane sulfonate (PFOS) and perfluorooctanoic acid (PFOA) in vacuum cleaner dust collected in Japanese homes. *J Environ Monit* **5:** 753–7.

Nakayama S, Harada K, Inoue K, Sasaki K, Seery B, Saito N, Koizumi A (2005) Distributions of perfluorooctanoic acid (PFOA) and perfluorooctane sulfonate (PFOS) in Japan and their toxicities. *Environ Sci* **12:** 293–313.

Nolan LA, Nolan JM, Shofer FS, Rodway NV, Emmett EA (2010) Congenital anomalies, labor/delivery complications, maternal risk factors and their relationship with perfluorooctanoic acid (PFOA)-contaminated public drinking water. *Repro Toxicol* **29:** 147–55.

Olsen GW, Burris JM, Ehresman DJ, Froehlich JW, Seacat AM, Butenhoff JL, Zobel LR (2007) Half-life of serum elimination of perfluorooctanesulfonate ,perfluorohexanesulfonate, and perfluorooctanoate in retired fluorochemical production workers. *Environ Health Persp* **115:** 1298–305.

Olsen GW, Church TR, Hansen KJ, Burris JM, Butenhoff JL, Mandel JH, Zobel LR (2004) Quantitative evaluation of perfluorooctanesulfonate (PFOS) and other fluorochemicals in the serum of children. *J Child Health* **2:** 53–76.

Olsen GW, Hansen KJ, Stevenson LA, Burris JM, Mandel JH (2003a) Human donor liver and serum concentrations of perfluorooctanesulfonate and other perfluorochemicals. *Environ Sci Toxicol* **37:** 888–91.

Olsen GW, Huang HY, Helzlsouer KJ, Hansen KJ, Butenhoff JL, Mandel JH (2005) Historical comparison of perfluorooctanesulfonate, perfluorooctanoate, and other fluorochemicals in human blood. *Environ Health Persp* **113:** 539–45.

Olsen GW, Logan PW, Hansen KJ, Simpson CA, Burris JM, Burlew MM, Vorarath PP, Venkateswarlu P, Schumpert JC, Mandel JH (2003b) An occupational exposure assessment of a perfluorooctanesulfonyl fluoride production site: biomonitoring. *AIHA J (Fairfax, Va)* **64:** 651–9.

Olsen GW, Zobel LR (2007) Assessment of lipid, hepatic, and thyroid parameters with serum perfluorooctanoate (PFOA) concentrations in fluorochemical production workers. *Intern Arch Occup Environ Health* **81:** 231–46.

Reneman L, Majoie CB, Habraken JB, den Heeten GJ (2001) Effects of ecstasy (MDMA) on the brain in abstinent users: initial observations with diffusion and perfusion MR imaging. *Radiology* **220:** 611–7.

Renner R (2001) Growing concern over perfluorinated chemicals. *Environ Sci Technol* **35:** 154A–60.

Rosen MB, Abbott BD, Wolf DC, Corton JC, Wood CR, Schmid JE, Das KP, Zehr RD, Blair ET, Lau C (2008a) Gene profiling in the livers of wild-type and PPARalpha-null mice exposed to perfluorooctanoic acid. *Toxicologic Pathol* **36:** 592–607.

Rosen MB, Lee JS, Ren H, Vallanat B, Liu J, Waalkes MP, Abbott BD, Lau C, Corton JC (2008b) Toxicogenomic dissection of the perfluorooctanoic acid transcript profile in mouse liver: evidence for the involvement of nuclear receptors PPAR alpha and CAR. *Toxicol Sci* **103:** 46–56.

Rosen MB, Schmid JE, Das KP, Wood CR, Zehr RD, Lau C (2009) Gene expression profiling in the liver and lung of perfluorooctane sulfonate-exposed mouse fetuses: comparison to changes induced by exposure to perfluorooctanoic acid. *Repro Toxicol* **27:** 278–88.

Rosen MB, Thibodeaux JR, Wood CR, Zehr RD, Schmid JE, Lau C (2007) Gene expression profiling in the lung and liver of PFOA-exposed mouse fetuses. *Toxicology* **239:** 15–33.

Rylander C, Phi DT, Odland JO, Sandanger TM (2009) Perfluorinated compounds in delivering women from south central Vietnam. *J Environ Monit* **11:** 2002–8.

Sato I, Kawamoto K, Nishikawa Y, Tsuda S, Yoshida M, Yaegashi K, Saito N, Liu W, Jin Y (2009) Neurotoxicity of perfluorooctane sulfonate (PFOS) in rats and mice after single oral exposure. *Toxicol Sci* **34:** 569–74.

Scialli AR, Iannucci A, Turim J (2007) Combining perfluoroalkane acid exposure levels for risk assessment. *Regul Toxicol Pharmacol* **49:** 195–202.

Seacat AM, Thomford PJ, Hansen KJ, Clemen LA, Eldridge SR, Elcombe CR, Butenhoff JL (2003) Sub-chronic dietary toxicity of potassium perfluorooctanesulfonate in rats. *Toxicology* **183:** 117–31.

Seacat AM, Thomford PJ, Hansen KJ, Olsen GW, Case MT, Butenhoff JL (2002) Subchronic toxicity studies on perfluorooctanesulfonate potassium salt in cynomolgus monkeys. *Toxicol Sci* **68:** 249–64.

Shen YW, Taves DR (1974) Fluoride concentrations in the human placenta and maternal and cord blood. *Am J Obstet Gynecol* **119:** 205–7.

Shi X, Liu C, Wu G, Zhou B (2009) Waterborne exposure to PFOS causes disruption of the hypothalamus–pituitary–thyroid axis in zebrafish larvae. *Chemosphere* **77:** 1010–8.

Slotkin TA, MacKillop EA, Melnick RL, Thayer KA, Seidler FJ (2008) Developmental neurotoxicity of perfluorinated chemicals modeled in vitro. *Environ Health Persp* **116**, 716–22.

Smithwick M, Muir DC., Mabury SA, Solomon KR, Martin JW, Sonne C, Born EW, Letcher R. J, Dietz R (2005) Perflouroalkyl contaminants in liver tissue from East Greenland polar bears (Ursus maritimus). *Environ Toxicol Chem/ SETAC* **24:** 981–6.

So MK, Yamashita N, Taniyasu S, Jiang Q, Giesy JP, Chen K, Lam PK (2006) Health risks in infants associated with exposure to perfluorinated compounds in human breast milk from Zhoushan, China. *Environ Sci Techn* **40:** 2924–9.

Starkov AA, Wallace KB (2002) Structural determinants of fluorochemical-induced mitochondrial dysfunction. *Toxicol Sci* **66:** 244–52.

Stein CR, Savitz DA, Dougan M (2009) Serum levels of perfluorooctanoic acid and perfluorooctane sulfonate and pregnancy outcome. *Am J Epidemiol* **170:** 837–46.

Strynar MJ, Lindstrom AB (2008) Perfluorinated compounds in house dust from Ohio and North Carolina, USA. *Environ Sci Technol* **42:** 3751–6.

Takacs ML, Abbott BD (2007) Activation of mouse and human peroxisome proliferator-activated receptors (alpha, beta/delta, gamma) by perfluorooctanoic acid and perfluorooctane sulfonate. *Toxicol Sci* **95:** 108–17.

Tan YM, Clewell HJ 3rd, Andersen ME (2008) Time dependencies in perfluorooctylacids disposition in rat and monkeys: a kinetic analysis. *Toxicol Lett* **177**, 38–47.

Tao L, Kannan K, Wong CM, Arcaro KF, Butenhoff JL (2008a) Perfluorinated compounds in human milk from Massachusetts, U.S.A. *Environ Sci Technol* **42:** 3096–101.

Tao L, Ma J, Kunisue T, Libelo EL, Tanabe S, Kannan K (2008b) Perfluorinated compounds in human breast milk from several Asian countries, and in infant formula and dairy milk from the United States. *Environ Sci Technol* **42:** 8597–602.

Taves DR (1968) Evidence that there are two forms of fluoride in human serum. *Nature* **217:** 1050–1.

Thibodeaux JR, Hanson RG, Rogers, JM, Grey BE, Barbee BD, Richards JH, Butenhoff JL, Stevenson LA, Lau C (2003) Exposure to perfluorooctane sulfonate during pregnancy in rat and mouse. I: maternal and prenatal evaluations. *Toxicol Sci* **74**, 369–81.

Tittlemier SA, Pepper K, Seymour C, Moisey J, Bronson R, Cao XL, Dabeka RW (2007) Dietary exposure of Canadians to perfluorinated carboxylates and perfluorooctane sulfonate via consumption of meat, fish, fast foods, and food items prepared in their packaging. *J Agr Food Chem* **55:** 3203–10.

Toms LM, Calafat AM, Kato K, Thompson J, Harden F, Hobson P, Sjodin A, Mueller JF (2009) Polyfluoroalkyl chemicals in pooled blood serum from infants, children, and adults in Australia. *Environ Sci Technol* **43:** 4194–9.

Trudel D, Horowitz L, Wormuth M, Scheringer M, Cousins IT, Hungerbuhler K (2008) Estimating consumer exposure to PFOS and PFOA. *Risk Anal* **28:** 251–69.

Vanden Heuvel JP, Davis JW 2nd, Sommers R, Peterson RE (1992) Renal excretion of perfluorooctanoic acid in male rats: inhibitory effect of testosterone. *J Biochem Toxicol* **7:** 31–6.

Vanden Heuvel JP, Thompson JT, Frame SR, Gillies PJ (2006) Differential activation of nuclear receptors by perfluorinated fatty acid analogs and natural fatty acids: a comparison of human, mouse, and rat peroxisome proliferator-activated receptor-alpha, -beta, and -gamma, liver X receptor-beta, and retinoid X receptor-alpha. *Toxicol Sci* **92:** 476–89.

Vestergren R, Cousins IT (2009) Tracking the pathways of human exposure to perfluorocarboxylates. *Environ Sci Technol* **43:** 5565–75.

Völkel W, Genzel-Boroviczeny O, Demmelmair H, Gebauer C, Koletzko B, Twardella D, Raab U, Fromme H (2008) Perfluorooctane sulphonate (PFOS) and perfluorooctanoic acid (PFOA) in human breast milk: results of a pilot study. *Int J Hyg Environ Health* **211:** 440–6.

Watanabe MX, Jones SP, Iwata H, Kim EY, Kennedy SW (2009) Effects of co-exposure to 2,3,7,8-tetrachlorodibenzo-p-dioxin and perfluorooctane sulfonate or perfluorooctanoic acid on expression of cytochrome P450 isoforms in chicken (Gallus gallus) embryo hepatocyte cultures. *Comp Biochem Physiol C Toxicol Pharmacol* **149:** 605–12.

Wei Y, Liu Y, Wang J, Tao Y, Dai J (2008) Toxicogenomic analysis of the hepatic effects of perfluorooctanoic acid on rare minnows (Gobiocypris rarus). *Toxicol Appl Pharmacol* **226:** 285–97.

Wilhelm M, Angerer J, Fromme H, Holzer J (2009) Contribution to the evaluation of reference values for PFOA and PFOS in plasma of children and adults from Germany. *Int J Hyg Environ Health* **212:** 56–60.

Wolf CJ, Fenton SE, Schmid JE, Calafat AM, Kuklenyik Z, Bryant XA, Thibodeaux J, Das KP, White SS, Lau CS, Abbott BD (2007) Developmental toxicity of perfluorooctanoic acid in the CD-1 mouse after cross-foster and restricted gestational exposures. *Toxicol Sci* **95:** 462–73.

Wolf CJ, Takacs ML, Schmid JE, Lau C, Abbott BD (2008) Activation of mouse and human peroxisome proliferator-activated receptor alpha by perfluoroalkyl acids of different functional groups and chain lengths. *Toxicol Sci* **106:** 162–71.

Ylinen M, Hanhijarvi H, Jaakonaho J, Peura P (1989) Stimulation by oestradiol of the urinary excretion of perfluorooctanoic acid in the male rat. *Pharmacol Toxicol* **65:** 274–7.

C H A P T E R

48

Phthalates

Jan L. Lyche

INTRODUCTION

Advances in materials sciences and engineering during the last decades have led to a widespread use of phthalates (phthalic acid esters) in a wide range of industrial products. Phthalates are used as plasticizers that impart flexibility and durability to polyvinylchloride (PVC) products. They are also used in solvents, lubricating oils, fixatives and as detergents in personal care products. When incorporated into PVC, phthalates are not covalently bound and are therefore easily released to the surroundings, leading to contamination of the external environment. Phthalates are detected in several media including food, water, house dust and air, thereby exposing animals and humans.

Phthalates were first introduced as a plasticizer in the 1920s and quickly replaced the volatile and odorous camphor. In 1931 polyvinyl chloride became commercially available and the development of di-2-ethylhexyl phthalate led the boom of the plasticizer PVC industry starting from the 1950s. Between 1970 and 2006 worldwide production grew from 1.8 to 4.3 million tons (Habert *et al.*, 2009). In 2006 di-isononyl phthalate (DINP) had the highest production volume, followed by di-isodecyl phthalate (DIDP) and di(2-ethylhexyl) phthalate (DEHP), then butyl benzyl phthalate (BBP), dibutyl phthalate (DBP), di-*n*-octyl phthalate (DnOP) and di-isobutyl phthalate (DIBP).

Because of widespread use, ubiquitous and constant environmental presence, exposure to humans, domestic animals and wildlife is virtually unavoidable. In the general population the major source of human exposure is through ingestion of contaminated food and water. Other significant sources are inhalation of indoor air and dermal uptake via cosmetics (Kavlock *et al.*, 2006; Koo and Lee, 2007). Humans are also exposed to high doses of phthalates from medical devices during medical procedures such as blood transfusions and hemodialysis (Calafat *et al.*, 2004). Furthermore, increased human exposure is documented in patients treated with pharmaceuticals where phthalates are incorporated in the coatings. The widespread exposure of the general population is documented in several recent monitoring studies in the USA and Europe (Koch and Calafat, 2009). Phthalate esters and their metabolites are detected in human urine (Koch *et al.*, 2006), breast milk (Lottrup *et al.*, 2006; Main *et al.*, 2006; Zhu *et al.*, 2006), and amniotic fluid (Silva *et al.*, 2004a,b). Furthermore, phthalates are also able to cross the placenta, and fetal exposure is closely correlated with maternal exposure (Latini *et al.*, 2003a).

Phthalate esters are suggested to have endocrine disrupting properties (Latini, 2005) and exposures to high concentrations were shown to induce fetal death, cancer, malformations, liver and kidney injury and reproductive toxicity in animals (Lovekamp-Swan and Davis, 2003; Hauser and Calafat, 2005; Latini *et al.*, 2006). Furthermore, phthalates are well-known antiandrogens in experimental animals, with perinatal exposure as the apparently most sensitive life stage. Reduced testosterone and adverse male reproductive system development are extensively documented in rodents and the adverse effects observed in animals raise concerns as to whether phthalates represent a potential health risk to humans (Kavlock *et al.*, 2006). The observed high sensitivity of the prenatal developmental stage for endocrine disruption has led to the postulation that increased incidence of human reproductive deficits may be produced by exposure to environmental chemicals during fetal and/or pre-pubertal life (Sharp and Skakkebaek, 2008). Reports have been published which also associate exposure to phthalates with increasing incidence of other human diseases such as obesity, insulin resistance and type 2 diabetes, asthma and allergies and neurological disorders such as ADHD and autism.

Even though association between adverse human health effects and exposure to phthalates has been reported, no clear cause–effect relationships are presently documented. However, based on the animal data, the Environment Directorate-General of the European Commission categorized DEHP, DBP and BBP as "reproductive-toxic". DEHP and DBP are also anticipated to be a human carcinogen. Therefore the use of the phthalates DEHP, DBP and BBP is forbidden in toys, cosmetics and food contact materials. The use of DINP, DIDP and DNOP (di-*n*-octylphthalate) is also forbidden for toys and baby clothes.

EXPOSURE

Phthalates are diesters of 1,2-benzenedicarboxylic acid (phthalic acid) containing a benzene ring with two ester functional groups (Figure 48.1). The water solubility is low and

Reproductive and Developmental Toxicology, Edited by Ramesh C. Gupta
ISBN: 978-0-12-382032-7

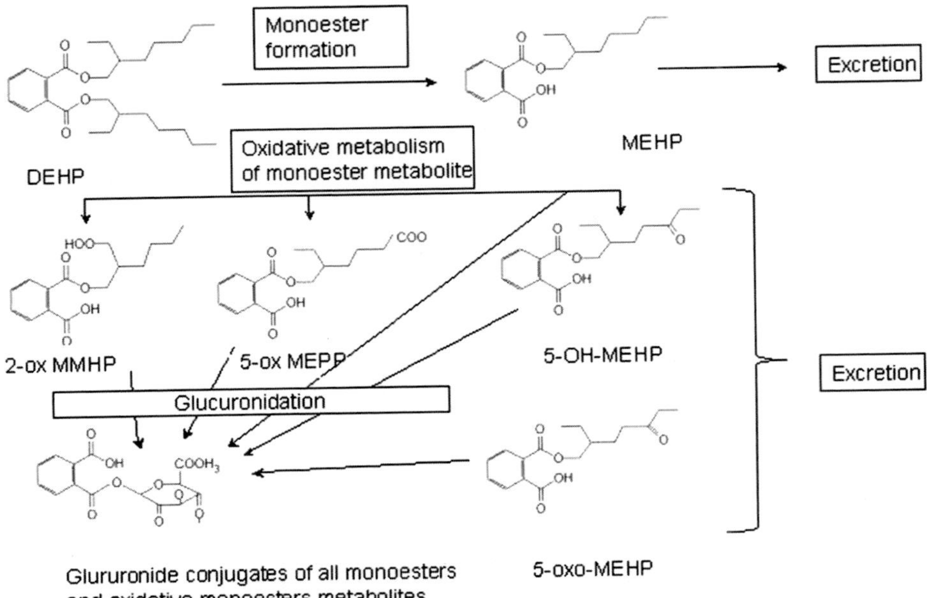

FIGURE 48.1 DEHP and metabolites used to estimate DEHP exposure.

decreases with increasing length of the side chain (the alcohol moiety) or with higher molecular weight (MW). As a consequence, low molecular weight phthalates with short alkyl groups such as DMP and DBP are more water soluble whereas the long-chained phthalates are poorly soluble. Volatility at standard temperature is low, particularly for long-chain phthalates such as DEHP and BBP (Rusyn *et al.*, 2006). Uses of the various phthalates mainly depend on their molecular weight (MW). Higher MW DEHP, DiNP, and DiDP are used in construction materials and numerous PVC products including clothing (footwear, raincoats), flooring and wall coverings, food packaging, children's products (toys, grip bumpers), and medical devices. Manufacturers use low MW phthalates such as di-methyl phthalate (DMP), di-ethyl phthalate (DEP) and DBP as solvents in personal care products (perfumes, lotions, cosmetics), insecticides, lacquers and in coatings including those used to provide timed releases in some pharmaceuticals. They are also used in PVC (Heudorf *et al.*, 2007).

Humans are exposed to phthalates through ingestion, inhalation and dermal contact. For the general population the major route of exposure for most phthalates is ingestion of food and water. Infants and young children (0.5–4 years of age) consume more calories per kg body weight and consume relatively more fatty foods compared to adults. The estimated total dietary DEHP intake is highest in children followed by adolescents younger than 19 years of age. In addition to dietary exposure, oral intake of phthalates also occurs when children mouth, suck or chew on toys containing phthalates (Bouma and Schakel, 2002). As a consequence, the European Union (EU) banned the use of DEHP, DBP, BBP and DiDP in children's toys and child-care items for children below 3 years of age in 1999 (EU Decision, 1999), and in 2005 the EU prohibited DEHP from all toys and child-care products (EU Directive, 2005). In the USA it is still permitted to use DiNP in toys and it was shown that children receive considerable levels of DiNP as a result of mouthing activities (Kavlock *et al.*, 2002).

Humans may also be exposed orally to phthalates incorporated in the coatings of commonly used pharmaceuticals.

TABLE 48.1 Concentrations of DEHP in various environmental matrices (Clark *et al.*, 2003b)

Matrix	Mean	Range
Drinking water (μg/L)	0.55	0.16–170
Sediments (μg/g)	1.4	0.0003–218
Soil (μg/g)	0.03	0.03–1280
Outdoor air (ng/m^3)	5	<0.4–65
Indoor air (ng/m^3)	109	20–240
Dust (g/kg)	3.24	2.38–4.1
Wastewater (μg/L)	27	0.01–4400
Sludge (g/kg)	0.3	0.0004–58.3

Herbal preparations and nutritional supplements, including some intended for use during pregnancy, may also contain phthalates in the formulation (Schettler, 2006).

Phthalates may permeate into humans via inhalation of indoor air in rooms with large surfaces of PVC-containing products (Table 48.1). The most common phthalate found indoors is DEHP. Other phthalates detected in indoor air include butyl benzyl phthalate (BBzP) di-*n*-butyl phthalate (DnBP), di-isobutyl phthalate (DiBP) and DEP (Bornehag and Nanberg, 2010). Concentrations of DEHP in indoor air in Japan were reported to be up to 1,000-fold higher than outdoor air concentrations (Otake *et al.*, 2004). In Germany higher levels of DEHP were detected in kindergartens compared to apartments (Fromme *et al.*, 2004). In Sweden significantly higher DEHP levels in dust were found in homes of children with doctor-diagnosed asthma (Bornehag *et al.*, 2004). This exposure route is suggested to be of limited importance for adults.

Dermal exposure may also be important routes of exposures to phthalates such as DBP, which are used in many cosmetics including perfume, hair gels, hair sprays, body lotion, deodorant and nail polish (Koch *et al.*, 2003a; Koo and Lee, 2007). In the USA, the urinary levels of DBP

TABLE 48.2 The levels of urinary DEHP metabolites measured in patients undergoing medical treatments

Intervention	Exposure	References
Infants undergoing multiple medical procedures	6 mg/kg bw/day	Silva *et al.* (2004b); Koch *et al.* (2006)
Parenteral nutrition to preterm neonates	20 mg/day	Loff *et al.* (2000, 2002); Subotic *et al.* (2007)
Blood transfusion in adults	>4 mg/kg bw/day	FDA (2004)
Blood transfusion in premature infants	20–fold increase	Calafat *et al.* (2004)
Kidney dialysis patients	0.8 mg/kg bw/treatment	Dine *et al.* (2000)

TABLE 48.3 Markers of DEHP exposure measured in a variety of matrices to assess exposure to DEHP

Marker	Marker type	Matrices	References
DEHP	Parent diester	Environmental samples, serum	McKee (2004)
MEHP	Monoester metabolite	Serum, urine, amniotic fluid, saliva, breast milk	Silva *et al.* (2004) Calafat *et al.* (2004) Kato *et al.* (2004) Silva *et al.* (2005)
5-OH-MEHP	Oxidized monoester metabolite	Serum, urine, amniotic fluid, saliva, breast milk	Kato *et al.* (2004) Silva *et al.* (2005) Barr *et al.* (2003)
5-oxo-MEHP	Oxidized monoester metabolite	Serum, urine, amniotic fluid, saliva, breast milk	Kato *et al.* (2004) Silva *et al.* (2005) Barr et *al.* (2003)
2-cx-MEHP	Oxidized monoester metabolite	Serum, urine, amniotic fluid, saliva, breast milk	Koch *et al.* (2005a,b) Preuss *et al.* (2005)
5-cx-MEHP	Oxidized monoester metabolite	Serum, urine, amniotic fluid, saliva, breast milk	Koch *et al.* (2005a) Preuss *et al.* (2005)

metabolites are significantly higher in women of reproductive age (20–40 years) compared with concentrations in males or other age groups (Blount *et al.*, 2000) probably originating from beauty products containing DBP (Lowekamp-Swan and Davis, 2003). It may be difficult for people to avoid exposure from cosmetic products even though they are subjected to strict labeling requirements. In one study, 72 products, purchased directly from stores, were analyzed for their phthalate ester content. Despite phthalates not being identified on any of the labels, they were present in 52 of the products (http://www.environmentalhealth.ca/fall02pretty.html). Baby-care products represent a dermal route of phthalate exposure with relevance for infants, as exposure to lotions, powder and shampoo was associated with increased levels of metabolites in infant urine (Sathyanarayana *et al.*, 2008).

Neonates may be exposed to high doses during blood transfusions and other life-saving procedures (Table 48.2) because medical devices for administration of medicines or nutrients may contain high levels of DEHP (20–40%) resulting in MEHP concentrations several orders of magnitude higher than the general population (Center for Devices and Radiological Health, 2001). In addition, adults are exposed to DEHP doses in excess of the TDI when receiving blood transfusions or during kidney dialysis (Dine *et al.*, 2000; Buchta *et al.*, 2003, 2005; Koch *et al.*, 2005b).

Exposure assessment

Historically, exposure assessment relied on concentrations found in environmental samples and food. In order to estimate internal levels based on external exposures, not only do phthalate levels in water and different food products need to be known, but also ingestion and inhalation rates are required. In contrast, human biomonitoring assesses exposure by measuring the chemicals in blood or urine (Table 48.3). This method allows the assessment of human exposure without knowing external exposure. Biomonitoring can be used to compare exposure levels in the general populations with specific subpopulations.

For risk assessment biomonitoring/biomarker of exposure measurements are used to determine the exposure level, which can be compared with toxicological data obtained from previous research. During the last two decades urinary concentrations of phthalates have been measured as part of biomonitoring studies and used to determine exposure levels of the general population around the world (Koch and Calafat, 2009). This data demonstrated that exposure to DEHP from food consumption was in the range of the tolerable daily intake (TDI) and at least some individuals exceed TDI values on single occasions (Fromme *et al.*, 2007c) suggesting that background exposure may represent a health risk for the general population.

Exposure assessment is also a vital component in environmental epidemiologic studies. Inadequate exposure estimation can lead to exposure misclassification which in turn leads to wrong conclusions regarding associations between exposure and outcome. Because phthalates have short biological half-lives and are quickly excreted from the body, it may be difficult to determine exposure over time by measuring a person's exposure at a single time point. However, Hauser *et al.* (2004) documented high day-to-day and month-to-month variability in phthalate concentrations, but still the authors showed that a single measurement may adequately predict average concentrations over a 3-month period for low molecular weight phthalates. Because single urinary measures are less predictive for high molecular weight phthalates it is suggested that a measurement of a second urine sample after 30 days be taken (Hauser *et al.*, 2004).

The selection of the proper biomarker which reflects the actual internal exposure is dependent of the individual phthalate. In a first rapid step, phthalate diesters are cleaved to the respective hydrolytic monoesters when passing biological membranes into the body, followed by a second step with formation of oxidative metabolites. In a third step this metabolite can be conjugated with glucuronic acid and finally excreted (Koch and Calafat, 2009). The rapid transformation of the intact diester to the hydrolytic monoester indicates that the levels would be very low, rather transient or artefacts of analytical background contamination suggesting the diesters as improper biomarkers of exposure (Koch and Calafat, 2009).

Because the low molecular weight phthalates are more water soluble they are mostly excreted as the primary metabolites (hydrolytic monoesters) while more lipophilic high molecular weight phthalates need to be transformed to the secondary oxidative metabolites to increase water solubility so they can be metabolized via urine. Therefore, using the hydrolytic primary metabolites may underestimate the internal exposure of high molecular weight phthalates. For example, approximately 70% of an oral dose of DBP (low molecular weight phthalate) while only 10% of DEHP and 2% of DiNP (high molecular weight phthalates) are excreted in urine as the primary hydrolytic monoester (Koch and Calafat, 2009). Therefore, the proper biomarker should be chosen based on the individual phthalate to be studied.

Exposure estimates based on DEHP levels in environmental samples and food

Based on elaborate exposure assessments it was estimated that more than 90% of the DEHP intake in adult humans is from food (Clark *et al.*, 2003a, b; Wormuth *et al.*, 2006), whereas food intake accounts only for 44 and 60% for formula-fed and breast-fed infants, respectively (Clark *et al.*, 2003a, b). DEHP concentrations were reported for a great variety of environmental and food matrices (Table 48.4). Food ingested by adults from Denmark was calculated to contain less than 0.19 μg/g DEHP resulting in a minimum and maximum daily intake of 2.7 and 4.3 μg/kg body weight (Petersen and Breindahl, 2000). A more recent estimation based on concentrations in German diets gave comparable results with a range from 1 to 4.2 μg/kg body weight/day (Fromme *et al.*, 2007b), which is less than 10% of the TDI of 50 μg/kg body weight/day. In Japan daily intake up to 11.8 μg DEHP/g was estimated which was attributed to DEHP in the wrappings of pre-packaged meals (Tsumura *et al.*, 2001a). Heating of food in a microwave while in contact with PVC significantly elevated phthalate concentrations in packed lunch preparations, increasing the intake to 92% of TDI (Chen *et al.*, 2008) while a positive correlation was found between packing date and DEHP concentrations in curry paste (Kueseng *et al.*, 2007). Tsumara *et al.* (2001b) found high levels of DEHP originating from disposable gloves used in the preparation of the food. Regulation of these type of gloves by the Japanese Ministry of Health, Labour and Welfare reduced the estimated daily intake from 7.4 to 2.3 μg/kg/day after the regulation was instituted (Tsumura *et al.*, 2003).

Although human DEHP exposure starts *in utero* as shown by placental transfer (Shea, 2003; Latini *et al.*, 2003b), it was suggested that exposure via breast milk to newborns is markedly higher (Calafat *et al.*, 2004; Main *et al.*, 2006). Babies are also exposed via infant formula containing DEHP (Petersen and Breindahl, 2000), and it was calculated that the infants receive comparable doses via formula and breast milk (Clark *et al.*, 2003a; Latini *et al.*, 2004). The calculated postnatal exposures are well below the European Commission TDI and US EPA oral reference dose (RfD) (Table 48.5).

Exposure estimates based on biomarkers

The predictive value of a single urine measurement in characterizing exposures to DEHP as high, medium or low over the course of 3 months was highest for the secondary metabolites and lowest for MEHP (Hauser *et al.*, 2004). Urinary levels for 5-OH-MEHP and 5-oxo-MEHP were 10-fold higher than MEHP levels (Kato *et al.*, 2004) and the sum of 5-OH-MEHP, 5-oxo-MEHP, 5-cx-MEPP and 2-cx-MMHP represents about 70% of the DEHP excretion compared to only 6% excreted as MEHP (Koch *et al.*, 2006) indicating that DEHP metabolites in urine provide a more reliable estimate of the DEHP exposure (Barr *et al.*, 2003; Koch *et al.*, 2003b, 2005a; Weuve *et al.*, 2006).

TABLE 48.4 Selected food concentrations of DEHP (μg/g)

Food	Mean	Range	References
Baby food	0.12	0.01–0.6	Clark *et al.* (2003a)
Breast milk	0.062	0.01–0.6	Clark *et al.* (2003a)
Cereals	0.05	0.02–1.7	Clark *et al.* (2003a)
Cream		0.2–2.7	Sharman *et al.* (1994)
Dairy (not milk)	0.96	0.059–16.8	Clark *et al.* (2003a)
Egg	0.12	<0.01–0.6	Clark *et al.* (2003a)
Fats and oils	2.4	0.7–11.9	Clark *et al.* (2003a)
Infant formula	0.12	<0.012–0.98	Clark *et al.* (2003a)
Meat	0.05	<0.1–0.8	Clark *et al.* (2003a)
Milk (cow)	0.035	<0.05–1.4	Clark *et al.* (2003a)
Milk (human)	0.22	0.16–0.4	Zhu *et al.* (2006)
Poultry	0.9	0.05–2.6	Clark *et al.* (2003a)
Vegetables	0.048	0.0098–2.2	Clark *et al.* (2003a)

TABLE 48.5 Exposure estimates based on DEHP concentration in environmental samples and in (A) food and on urinary metabolites (B)

	Life stage	DEHP intakeμg/kg/bw/day	References
A: Concentration in food			
USA	20–70 years	8.2	Clark *et al.* (2003a)
Denmark	adults	2.7–4.3	Petersen and Breindahl (2000)
Germany	14–60 years	2.5–4.3	Fromme *et al.* (2007b)
USA	12–19 years	10.0	Clark *et al.* (2003a)
USA	5–11 years	18.9	Clark *et al.* (2003a)
USA	USA	25,8	Clark *et al.* (2003a)
USA formula fed	0–6 months	5.0	Clark *et al.* (2003a)
USA breast feed	0–6 months	7.3	Clark *et al.* (2003a)
UK formula feed	(0–3 months) (3–12 months)	(13.0) (8.0)	Latini *et al.* (2004)
UK breast feed	(0–3 months) (3–12 months)	(21.0) (8.0)	Latini *et al.* (2004)
B: Urinary metabolites			
USA	20–60 years	0.7–3.6	Wittassek *et al.* (2007)
Germany	14–60 years	2.2–7.7	Fromme *et al.* (2007)
German students	20–29 years	2.7–6.4	Wittassek *et al.* (2007)
German children	2–14 years	4.3–15.2	Wittassek *et al.* (2007)
USA pregnant women	20–40 years	1.32–9.32	Fromme *et al.* (2007b)
USA medical exposure	neonates	130–6,000	Calafat *et al.* (2004)

The ratio of oxidative metabolites to monoester metabolites changes almost linearly with age group but not with gender or ethnicity with children aged 6–11 years producing a larger fraction of oxidative metabolites than adolescents or adults (Silva *et al.*, 2004a, b; Fromme *et al.*, 2007a). Koch *et al.* (2003a, b) determined a median DEHP intake of 13.8 μg/kg/day based on urinary oxidative metabolites of DEHP, 5OH-MEHP and 5oxo-MEHP, in male and female Germans ($n = 85$; aged 18–40). Twelve percent of subjects exceeded the TDI of the EU-CSTEE (50 μg/kg/day) and 31% of the subjects exceeded the US EPA oral RfD of (20 μg/kg/day).

Fromme *et al.* (2007b) compared the daily DEHP intake based on concentration in food and on urinary metabolites in the same study subjects and found almost equal estimates independent of quantification method, confirming food as the major source of DEHP exposure (Table 48.5). However, in the same study, daily DnBP and DiBP intake estimated from levels in food was lower than TDI calculated by the biomonitoring approach suggesting that sources other than food contribute to human phthalates body burden. In a retrospective human biomonitoring study, Wittassek *et al.* (2007) extrapolated the daily parent phthalate exposure in Germany based on the levels of urinary metabolites in samples collected between 1988 and 2003, and found comparable exposure doses as for studies using external doses to assess the daily intake (Table 48.5). In the same study a downward temporal trend of 40% in the levels of DEHP and DnBP from 1996 to 2003 was observed.

TOXICOKINETICS

Absorption

No human *in vivo* dermal absorption studies are available. However, *in vitro* comparison of absorption of phthalate esters through rat and human skin showed that phthalates were absorbed faster through rat skin (Scott *et al.*, 1987). Nevertheless dermal absorption in rodents is relatively slow (Elsisi *et al.*, 1989), but once absorbed phthalates are distributed in the same manner as orally administered compounds. In guinea-pigs only 3 and 21% of the applied dermal dose was absorbed and excreted after 1 and 7 days, respectively (Ng *et al.*, 1992). There is no study available on absorption of inhaled phthalates in humans. However, indirect evidence for absorption via the lungs was observed in infants ventilated with PVC respiratory tubes, and in workers occupationally exposed to phthalates. In infants and workers significantly higher levels of MEHP and secondary metabolites were detected in urine suggesting that intake via the inhalation route occurs (Kavlock *et al.*, 2002; Pan *et al.*, 2006). Furthermore, radiolabeled DEHP was rapidly absorbed in rats exposed via inhalation (General Motors, 1982).

Phthalates are absorbed from rat intestine in a wide concentration-dependent range, mainly in the form of monoesters, due to rapid hydrolysis by gut lipases. DEHP was not detected in urine of any of the species studied, but was found in feces in amounts inversely related to the degree of metabolites in urine (Kavlock *et al.*, 2002) suggesting little absorption of the parent compounds from the gastrointestinal tract. More than 90% of DBP and 40–50% of DEHP incorporated in feed were detected in urine following oral administration to rodents, indicating that phthalates in food are well absorbed (Kluwe, 1982). Koch *et al.* (2006) estimated oral absorption rate for DEHP in a healthy Caucasian male volunteer by measuring the levels of metabolites in urine. After 24 h 67% of the dose was excreted in urine followed by an additional 3.8% on the second day, indicating that the majority of the ingested DHEP is systemically absorbed and excreted in urine in humans.

Distribution

Once absorbed, phthalates and their metabolites are distributed throughout the body in all tissues (Table 48.3). Several studies of DEHP distribution in different species indicate highest concentrations in liver and kidneys. In addition, in humans, phthalates are also detected in seminal fluid, amniotic fluid, breast milk, saliva and placenta (Koch *et al.*, 2003a,b; Calafat *et al.*, 2004; Silva *et al.*, 2004a,b, 2005; Mortensen *et al.*, 2005). No significant cumulative accumulation in tissues was noted with less than 1% of the dose retained a few days after administration (Kavlock *et al.*, 2002). In mice, however, Tomita *et al.* (1986) found specific sequestration in pancreas.

Phthalates are transported to the fetus via the placenta, indicating that exposure to these chemicals occurs during intrauterine life (Latini *et al.*, 2003b, 2006; Mose *et al.*, 2007), and fetal phthalate levels correlate with maternal concentrations. In addition, phthalates were also detected in human breast milk, which is the major source of nutrition for infants (Mortensen *et al.*, 2005; Zhu *et al.*, 2006). Transfer of phthalates to the fetus via the placenta and the newborn via breast milk was also documented in rodents (Srivastava *et al.*, 1989).

Biotransformation and excretion

Following oral ingestion, diester phthalates undergo a rapid cleavage into their monoester metabolites by non-specific esterases and lipases in the gastrointestinal tract. Human neonates have lower levels of pancreatic lipase compared to adults suggesting a reduced metabolic capacity in babies. Following absorption, the monoesters are further metabolized by various oxidation and hydroxylation reactions resulting in secondary metabolites, which are excreted via urine or conjugated to glucuronic acid before excretion (Table 48.1). In children, the glucuronidation pathways are not fully mature until they are 3 months old, suggesting that this important clearance mechanism is not fully available to neonates and young infants, which may increase the internal doses of toxic metabolites (Cresteil, 1998).

In a human study, two male volunteers received DEHP and approximately 13% of the dose was excreted in urine within 24 hours when only the levels of MEHP were analyzed (Schmid and Schlatter, 1985). In contrast, when the secondary metabolites (5OH-MEHP), mono(2-ethyl-5-oxohexyl)phthalate (5oxo-MEHP), mono(2-ethyl-5-carboxypentyl)phthalate (5cx-MEPP) and mono[2-(carboxymethyl)hexyl]phthalate (2cx-MMHP) were included as markers of exposure, around 70% of the administered dose was detected in urine of a male volunteer indicating that the previous focus on only monoesters may significantly underestimate the level of exposure (Koch *et al.*, 2003b, 2006; Fromme *et al.*, 2007b).

As discussed above, the low molecular weight phthalates, including among others DEP and DBP, appear to be less transformed to the oxidative secondary metabolites indicated by the observation that 70% of an oral dose of DBP (four carbons in the alkyl chain) is excreted in the urine as the primary monoester (Anderson *et al.*, 2001). In contrast, for the high molecular weight phthalate DiNP with 10 carbon atoms in the alkyl chain, no significant levels of the hydrolytic monoester are excreted in urine (Koch and Calafat, 2009) suggesting that the monoesters are inadequate as biomarkers of exposure for high molecular weight phthalates. For risk assessment and epidemiologic studies recent research has focused on identifying and characterization of suitable oxidative metabolites (Koch and Calafat, 2009).

MECHANISM OF ACTION

There is substantial evidence available which shows that the C4–C6 phthalates, DBP, BBP and DEHP, produce similar alterations in male reproductive tract functions, and it was therefore suggested that there may be a similar mode of action. The underlying mechanisms of these effects are not clear but have been the focus of numerous investigations. Initial mechanistic studies focused on phthalates acting as environmental estrogens or antiandrogens. However, by using estrogenic and androgenic screening assays it was demonstrated that only the unmetabolized phthalates are able to bind to steroid receptors whereas the monoesters which are absorbed exert little or no affinity for ER and AR, indicating a lack of receptor-mediated effects under *in vivo* condition (David, 2006).

A key mechanistic step for phthalate toxicity is formation of the monoester prior to absorption from GIT. *In vitro* studies with cultured testicular cells showed that MEHP is a more potent testicular toxicant compared to DEHP. Another important concept for phthalate toxicity is that the modes of action appear to depend upon developmental timing and dosing. During rodent development, two sets of Leydig cells, which are the predominant testosterone producing cells in males, develop successively. The first set, fetal Leydig cells, differentiate into fully competent steroidogeneic cells at gestation day 12 in rats (Huhtaniemi and Pelliniemi, 1992). Testosterone and INSL3 produced by these cells are critical for normal male secondary differentiation (Huhtaniemi and Pelliniemi, 1992). Fetal Leydig cells remain in the rodent testis until after birth followed by a substitution by adult Leydig cells which start to appear at postnatal day 11. In humans, fetal Leydig cells differentiate around week 8 of intrauterine life and persist at least for a few months after birth. At the beginning of the pubertal period, or following choriogonadotropin hormone (hCG) administration during childhood, cells of mesenchymal origin start to proliferate and differentiate into adult-type Leydig cells (Codesal *et al.*, 1990; Ariyaratne *et al.*, 2000; Habert *et al.*, 2001). Exposures of fetal vs. adult Leydig cells are proposed to produce different adverse effects. For example, phthalates were found to induce aggregation of fetal Leydig cells (Mylchreest *et al.*, 2000; Barlow *et al.*, 2004; Ge *et al.*, 2007), whereas such an effect was not observed in adult Leydig cells (Dostal *et al.*, 1988; Parks *et al.*, 2000; Ge *et al.*, 2007). Furthermore, when exposed to high doses, phthalates inhibit testosterone production in both fetal and adult Leydig cells. In contrast, low doses of phthalates increase the number of adult Leydig cells and enhance testosterone production leading to advanced onset of puberty, whereas high doses reduce testosterone synthesis and delay puberty (Ge *et al.*, 2007). No such biphasic pattern was documented in fetal Leydig cells. An explanation for these contradictory results may be that DEHP interferes with different mechanisms during different life stages (e.g., fetal life vs. adulthood). This phenomenon, that effects do not increase monotonically with dosage, is frequently noted in toxicological and pharmacological studies (Calabrese and Baldwin, 2003; Kohn and Melnick, 2007).

The mode of action underlying phthalate toxicity on Leydig cells remains unclear. However, it was proposed that peroxisome proliferator-activated receptors (PPAR) may be involved in testicular toxicity following phthalate exposure because many phthalate monoesters including MEHP and MDP were found to induce PPAR *in vitro* (Hurst and Waxmann, 2003; Corton and Lapinskas, 2005; Ge *et al.*, 2007) and that these receptors may be expressed differently in Leydig cells and other testicular cells at different life stages. The PPAR family contains three subtypes, PPARα, PPARβ and PPARγ, encoded by different genes, and the activation of PPAR regulates genes which are generally involved in metabolism, cell growth and stress responses (Lemberger *et al.*, 1996). In rats, Schultz *et al.* (1999) showed that both PPARα and PPARγ are strongly expressed in fetal Leydig cells whereas only PPARα is expressed in Leydig cells of adult rats. Although apparently not expressed in adult Leydig cells, testis homeogenates from juvenile male rats exposed from week 4 to 8 of age to DEHP demonstrated a concentration-dependent increase in PPARγ protein, indicating that other testicular cells may contain PPARγ. Further, in the same study, the levels of RXRalpha and several apoptotic proteins were also upregulated in testes suggesting that DEHP exposure may induce the expression of apoptosis-related proteins in testes through induction of PPARγ (Ryu *et al.*, 2007a). Juvenile exposure to DBP was also found to raise the expression of the PPARγ gene in testes of Sprague-Dawley rats (Ryu *et al.*, 2007b). A possible involvement of PPAR in male reproductive toxicity is supported by the observation that DEHP exposure did not affect testosterone production in PPARα-null mice to the same extent as in wild-type mice (Corton and Lapinskas, 2005). Maloney and Waxman (1999) also showed that MEHP activates human PPARα and PPARγ in COS-1 cells. However, there are no clear data to support or reject the suggested involvement of PPARs in the dysgenesis of the male reproductive tract following fetal exposure (David, 2006).

DEHP or DBP was also found to dysregulate genes involved in cholesterol transport across mitochondrial membrane and steroidogenic enzyme activities in Leydig cells with subsequent decrease in testicular testosterone production, which may adversely affect the differentiation of androgen-dependent tissues (Akingbemi *et al.*, 2001; Shultz *et al.*, 2001; Barlow *et al.*, 2003). Ryu *et al.* (2007b) exposed juvenile Sprague-Dawley rats to DBP for 30 days and observed that genes involved in steroidogenensis (SR-B1, StAr, P450$_{scc}$, CYP17, CYP19) were expressed differently compared to control.

Reduced testosterone levels were also observed in male rats exposed prenatally to 50 mg/kg DBP (Lehmann *et al.*, 2004) and 10 mg/kg DEHP (Akingbemi *et al.*, 2001). Howdeshell *et al.* (2008) exposed fetal rats to a mixture of phthalates containing DEHP, BBP, DBP and di-isobutyl (DiBP) and co-administration of these phthalates reduced testosterone production in a dose additive fashion. Evidence indicated that the individual phthalates induce cumulative, dose additive effects on fetal testosterone production when administered as a mixture due to the similar mechanisms of action. Furthermore, Borch *et al.* (2006) showed that DiBP exerted similar effects as DEHP, DBP and DiNP on rat fetal testicular testosterone production and testicular histopathology following exposure *in utero*. The proteins StAR and P450scc involved in steroid synthesis in testes were also decreased by DiBP as shown for other phthalates. These findings contradict the conclusion in an EFSA (2005b) report which stated that no group-TDI could be allocated for phthalates because different mechanisms are involved.

Elevation of glucocorticoid has been associated with suppression of reproductive functions, obesity and type 2 diabetes. Glucocorticoids are controlled by 11β-hydroxysteroid dehydrogenase (11β-HSD) which catalyzes conversion of active cortisol to inert steroids. Using human and rat kidney microsomes and murine gonadotrope LβT2 cells, it was demonstrated that MEHP, di-*n*-butyl-phthalate (DBP), dipropyl phthalate (DPrP) and di-cyclohexyl phthalate (DCHP) downregulated 11β-HSD leading to increased cortisol concentration (Hong *et al.*, 2009). Downregulation of 11β-HSD in Leydig cells accompanied by increased cortisol is shown to inhibit Leydig cell testosterone production (Hu *et al.*, 2008), suggesting a new mechanism for testicular toxicity induced by phthalates.

In addition to the adverse effects of androgens on steroidogenesis, phthalates were also found to reduce the expression of insulin-like factor 3 (insl3) gene (Wilson *et al.*, 2004; McKinnell *et al.*, 2005, Ryu *et al.*, 2007b). The insl3 protein is involved in the initial stages of testicular descent and together with androgens controls normal testicular descent into the scrotum, while failure of this process results in cryptorchidism (Sharpe, 2006). Decreased insl3 expression observed after fetal exposure to DEHP, DBP and BBP may be related to increased incidence of cryptorchidism (David, 2006). Knockouts of this gene in mice show complete cryptorchidism (Nef and Parada, 2000).

The observation that phthalate exposure reduces Sertoli cell proliferation and triggers formation of multinucleated gonocytes may be an indirect effect due to reduced androgen production by Leydig cells (David, 2006). However, direct effects of phthalates on Sertoli cells have also been proposed. DEHP exposure of neonatal Sertoli cells decreased the cell cycle gene cyclin D2 and reduced proliferation. Furthermore, Kang *et al.* (2002) demonstrated that DEHP (500 microM) inhibited apoptosis in TM5 Sertoli cells, preceded by the downregulation of gap junctional intercellular communication. Sertoli cell communication is essential for proliferation of gonocytes, and a reduction of Sertoli cells may result in dysgenesis of gonocytes (David, 2006) similar to changes observed when rats are exposed to phthalates (Mylchreest *et al.*, 2002; Barlow *et al.*, 2003; Fisher *et al.*, 2003).

DNA methylation controls gene expression and epigenetic modulation of DNA, which may represent an important newly discovered mechanism for endocrine disruption of gene expression during development leading to permanent effects (Gore, 2008). Treatment of MCF7 cells with BBP or DBP at 10^{-5} M led to the demethylation of ERalpha promoter-associated CpG islands suggesting that phthalates may disrupt endocrine function by epigenetic mechanisms (Kang and Lee, 2005).

Mechanisms of action in females

As primary effects of phthalates on female rats appear to be associated with reduction in plasma estradiol concentrations, different phthalates were tested for their effects on estradiol levels. To study whether reduced production and/or increased metabolism contributed to the lower estradiol levels, the concentrations of estradiol and estrone, the primary metabolite, were determined and both DEHP and DBP decreased the estradiol to estrone ratio indicative of an increased estrogen metabolism following exposure to these compounds (Lovekamp-Swan and Davis, 2003). In contrast, MEHP, the active metabolite of DEHP, was the only phthalate monoester that significantly decreased estradiol production in rat granulosa cells *in vitro* suggesting that DEHP lowered estradiol levels by interfering with both production and metabolism whereas DBP affected only the metabolic pathway.

Mechanistic studies with primary rat granulosa cell cultures demonstrated that DEHP decreased estradiol production by reducing the levels of aromatase, the enzyme that converts testosterone to estradiol (Lovekamp and Davis, 2001). This dysregulation of aromatase may be due to DEHP-induced activation of PPARα and PPARγ in rat granulosa cells. By comparing known PPAR ligands with DEHP, Lovekamp and Davis (2001) showed that phthalates inhibit aromatase expression and activity in rat granulosa cells in the same manner. By activating PPARγ, DEHP disrupted the critical timing and growth of the ovarian follicle. Sufficient estradiol production prior to ovulation is thus critical for induction of the ovulatory LH surge. After ovulation aromatase activity is rapidly decreased both by increased degradation of mRNA and inhibition of transcription (Fitzpatrick *et al.*, 1997). PPARγ activation also diminishes the activation of the aromatase gene and increases the turnover of mRNA (Mu *et al.*, 2001). This is probably part of the normal program involved in LH-induced luteinization. Consequently, DEHP triggers granulosa cell differentiation without ovulation by activation of PPARγ (Lovekamp-Swan and Davis, 2003). Based on this information from studies in rats it is likely that DEHP also affects human female reproductive function since (1) PPARγ is expressed in human and rodent ovaries and (2) DEHP stimulates transcriptional activity of both human and rodent PPARγ (Lovekamp-Swan and Davis, 2003).

TOXICITY

In animal studies phthalates produced a variety of adverse effects including liver tumors in rats and mice as well as Leydig cell and pancreatic cell tumors in rats (Kavlock *et al.*, 2006). Based on those observations the US Environmental Protection Agency (EPA) classified the risk for DEHP carcinogenicity as B2 (probable human carcinogen) in 1993. However, in 2000, the International Agency for Research on Cancer (IARC) downgraded the level of potential health risks of DEHP from 2B (possibly carcinogenic to humans) to 3 (not classifiable as to carcinogenicity to humans) based on an expert panel's acceptance that DEHP induces liver tumors in rodents by a mechanism dependent on PPARα activation that is not relevant in humans (Guyton *et al.*, 2009). This decision has been variously argued by several scientists based on the lack of experimental studies that support the PPARα hypothesis to dismiss the human relevance of effects observed in laboratory animals (Guyton *et al.*, 2009). Furthermore, two recent studies showed that DEHP induces liver tumors in PPARα knockout mice suggesting that DEHP may produce liver tumors by alternative mechanisms (Ito *et al.*, 2007). Based on those uncertainties, in contrast to IARC's classification, the Japan Society for Occupational Health has maintained the 2B class of DEHP carcinogenicity because of the obvious rodent carcinogenicity (Japan Society for Occupational Health 2007, http://joh.med.uoeh-u.ac.jp/oel/index.html).

More recently phthalates have attracted special attention because of their possible endocrine disrupting potential that may disrupt biological functions including sexual development and reproductive functions in adults. The first finding of phthalate induced reproductive toxicity were testicular injury in experimental animals (Schaffer *et al.*, 1945). Later male reproductive and developmental effects that are observed in animal models include pathological changes in testes and male reproductive accessory glands, hypospadias, cryptorchidism, retention of nipples, reduced ano-genital distance (AGD) and reduced sperm production. These postnatal changes were preceded by an impairment of fetal Leydig cell function associated with reduced testosterone production (Mylchreest *et al.*, 2000; Parks *et al.*, 2000; Fisher *et al.*, 2003; Foster, 2006; Latini *et al.*, 2006; Sharpe, 2006) and insulin-like factor 3 (insl3) mRNA levels (Wilson *et al.*, 2004). Furthermore, fetal exposure to DBP also resulted in testicular Leydig cell adenomas in adult life (Mylchreest *et al.*, 2000; Barlow and Foster, 2003; Barlow *et al.*, 2003). At present the general consensus is that DEHP, DBP, BBP and DINP have potential to disrupt normal development and reproduction (Fabjan *et al.*, 2006). However, other phthalates need further evaluation before definite conclusions can be drawn with respect to their developmental and reproductive toxicity (Fabjan *et al.*, 2006).

The adverse effects induced by phthalates depend upon the dose and timing. Previous standard teratology studies in rats using exposure on gestation day (GD) 6–15 were only able to demonstrate effects following exposure to high doses (Ema *et al.*, 1993; Hellwig *et al.*, 1997; Waterman *et al.*, 1999). However, those studies did not expose pregnant dams during the period when the reproductive system differentiates (GD 12–20). More recent studies showed that all of the adverse responses on reproductive development were induced at lower doses when exposure occurred in late gestation (Mylchereest *et al.*, 2000; Gray *et al.*, 2000; Foster *et al.*, 2001, 2006; Tyl *et al.*, 2004; Ryu *et al.*, 2007a). The most frequently investigated phthalates are DEHP, DBP and BBP and they were found to produce almost identical responses with a relative toxic potency of DEHP > DBP > BBP (Foster, 2005). However, despite limited data regarding the reproductive toxic potential of other phthalates, there are reports suggesting that other phthalates such as di-*n*-hexyl phthalate (DnHP), di-isobutyl phthalate (DiBP) and di-isononyl phthalate (DiNP) may also induce reproductive toxicity (Fabjan *et al.*, 2006; Borch *et al.*, 2006; Howdeshell *et al.*, 2006).

The effects observed in rodent studies resemble testicular dysgenesis syndrome (TDS) in humans (Sharpe and Skakkebaek, 2008). TDS represents a number of reproductive disorders in humans, hypothesized to be induced by exposure to endocrine disruptive chemicals during development. This syndrome was proposed to explain the reported increase in male reproductive deficits such as decline in sperm count, elevated incidence of testicular and prostate cancers and higher incidence of cryptorchidism and hypospadias (Sharpe and Skakkebaek, 2008). Although the present data suggest a link between phthalate exposure and adverse human reproductive health effects, the evidence is too limited to establish cause–effect relationships between human exposure and these effects. However, the attempt to relate toxic events during fetal and neonatal life to subsequent adult diseases is an exceedingly difficult challenge for epidemiology (Foster, 2005; Latini, 2006; Skakkebaek *et al.*, 2006; Matsumoto *et al.*, 2008).

Although far less investigated, there are reports that suggest that phthalates may adversely affect other functions and systems such as thyroid signaling, immune functions, metabolic homeostasis, behavior and neuronal development and functioning (Román, 2007; Stahlhut *et al.*, 2007; Jaakkola and Knight, 2008; Meeker *et al.*, 2009; Bornehag and Nanberg, 2010). Due to the observation that low testosterone in adult males is associated with obesity and increased risk of type 2 diabetes it has also been suggested that phthalates may represent one of the etiologic factors for the increased prevalence of these diseases reported in developed countries (Stahlhut *et al.*, 2007; Latini *et al.*, 2009).

Male human studies

In humans a few studies are available assessing the association between developmental phthalate exposure and adult male reproductive and developmental endpoints such as hormone levels, adverse semen parameters, time to pregnancy and infertility diagnosis (Table 48.6). Various studies suggested a possible association between phthalate exposure and disturbance of normal sperm function (Matsumoto *et al.*, 2008) such as fewer motile sperm (Jönsson *et al.*, 2005), low sperm concentration and motility (Hauser *et al.*, 2006), sperm malformations (Rozati *et al.*, 2002; Zhang *et al.*, 2006) and increased DNA damage (Rozati *et al.*, 2002; Hauser *et al.*, 2007).

Two studies reported an association between DEP exposure and increased DNA damage in sperm (Duty *et al.*, 2003; Hauser, 2008). Urinary MEP levels have also been associated with enlarged testes, fewer motile sperm and lower serum luteinizing hormone (LH) levels (Hauser *et al.*, 2005; Jönsson *et al.*, 2005). Interestingly, no adverse effects of DEP exposure have thus far been noted in animal studies.

Significant dose–response relationships were found between DBP exposure and low sperm concentration and motility in male partners of subfertile couples, whereas in this study no relationships were observed between DEP and DEHP and semen quality (Hauser *et al.*, 2006). In another study both DBP and DEHP were associated with lower plasma testosterone levels in occupationally exposed workers (Pan *et al.*, 2006). DEHP was also correlated with increased DNA damage in a group of men exposed to doses comparable to those reported for the US general population, suggesting that exposure to DEHP may affect the population distribution of sperm DNA damage (Hauser *et al.*, 2007). Higher levels of total phthalates (DMP, DEP, DBP, BBP, DOP, DEHP) were found in a group of infertile men compared to controls (Rozati *et al.*, 2002). In this group, a significant correlation was found between sum phthalates and normal sperm morphology and percent single stranded DNA in the sperm (Rozati *et al.*, 2002). In a study of phthalate concentration in breast milk, significant negative correlation was observed between DBP and free testosterone, positive correlation between DEP, DMP, DBP and DiNP and LH and between DEP and DBP and sex hormone binding globulin (Main *et al.*, 2006).

Female human studies

In females data are limited to a few studies. Two studies suggested a possible association between phthalates and endometriosis (Cobellis *et al.*, 2003; Reddy *et al.*, 2006). In the first study higher plasma concentrations of DEHP and MEHP were found in women with endometriosis (study group) compared to controls. In the second study higher levels of DBP, BBP, DOP and DEHP were detected in the study group. Latini *et al.* (2003b) found an association between cord blood concentrations of DEHP and a lower gestational age, and it was suggested that the increased number of premature babies might be due to induction of intrauterine inflammation by DEHP. Disturbance of immune functions may also trigger the development of endometriosis (Matsumoto *et al.*, 2008). In Puerto Rico, premature breast development was associated with high blood levels of DMP, DEP, DBP and DEHP (Colón *et al.*, 2000). These results were challenged by McKee (2004) because the levels detected were unusually high and may reflect contamination of the samples during analysis, and because no such effects are observed in animal studies. Recently, Meeker *et al.* (2009) found significant association between phthalate exposure (DEHP, DBP, DOP, BBzP) and increased risk for preterm birth among a group of Mexican women.

Human infant studies

Anogenital distance (AGD) is a commonly used endpoint for hormonally regulated sex differentiation in rodents. AGD in male rats is normally twice that in females, and a similar sex difference occurs in humans (Salazar-Martinez *et al.*, 2004). A negative association between anogenital index (AGI; AGD/weight) in boys of 2–36 months of age and the levels of MEP, MBP, MBzP and MiBP detected in their mothers' urine was reported (Swan *et al.*, 2005). Furthermore, in a recent study, Huang *et al.* (2009) found negative correlations between AGI in newborns and levels of MEHP and MBP in amniotic fluid. Main *et al.* (2006) found no association between phthalate exposure via breast milk and testicular descent. However, in the same study, positive correlations were noted between (1) DEP and DBP and sex hormone binding protein, (2) DBP and the ratio of LH/free testosterone, and (3) negative correlation

TABLE 48.6 Male reproductive effects in human populations

Compounds	Study subjects	Significant associated effects	References
MEP	$n = 168$	DNA damage in sperm	Duty *et al.* (2003)
	$n = 234$	↑large testis ↓sperm motility, ↓LH 113 mg/kg bw/day	Jönsson *et al.* (2005)
	$n = 379$	↑DNA damage in sperm	Hauser *et al.* (2007)
DBP	$n = 37$	↓semen volume	Zhang *et al.* (2006)
MBP	$n = 168$	↓sperm concentration, ↓sperm motility	Duty *et al.* (2003)
	$n = 463$	↓sperm concentration, ↓sperm motility	Hauser *et al.* (2006)
	$n = 74$	↓plasma free testosterone	Pan *et al.* (2006)
DEHP	$n = 37$	↓semen volume, ↑rate of sperm malformation	Zhang *et al.* (2006)
MEHP	$n = 187$	↓straight-line velocity and curvilinear velocity of sperm	Duty *et al.* (2004)
	$n = 74$	↓plasma free testosterone	Pan *et al.* (2006)
	$n = 379$	↑sperm DNA damage	Hauser *et al.* (2007)
Sum phthalates	$n = 21$	↓sperm normal morphology, ↑percent of single-stranded DNA in sperm	Rozati *et al.* (2002)

↓ = decrease, ↑ = increase

between DBP and free testosterone (Main *et al.*, 2006). The study did not analyze the secondary metabolites. Furthermore, the samples might have been contaminated because they used breast pumps containing phthalates. Although these studies suggest a possible association between exposures to phthalates and adverse effects in humans, no effects were observed in adolescents exposed as neonates to high levels of DEHP from medical devices (Rais-Bahrami *et al.*, 2004). However, in this study, controls were not included, the levels of phthalates were not measured and the small size of the study group limits the power to elucidate statistical significance (Kavlock *et al.*, 2006).

Animal studies

The existing human data are insufficient to evaluate the reproductive effects of phthalate exposure in humans. In animals, however, there are strong indications that phthalates have the potential to adversely affect normal development and disrupt reproductive functions (Kavlock *et al.*, 2006). In a number of studies reproductive and endocrine endpoints were investigated in rodents exposed during development (Table 48.7).

Some studies used multiple doses giving the opportunity to establish dose–response relationships. The remaining investigations are single dose studies focusing on modes of action for developmental reproductive toxicity. In one study Sprague-Dawley rats were orally dosed with DEHP at 0, 375, 750 or 1,500 mg/kg body weight/day from GD 3 to PND 21 and endpoints related to sexual development were studied through puberty and adulthood in male and female offspring. The two highest doses reduced the prenatal maternal weight gain. In the high dose group the number of pups was reduced and the postnatal mortality was increased at the two highest dose levels. However, at all doses increased aerolae or nipple sizes in the male offspring were observed and this effect was persistent until adulthood. Furthermore, a range of male accessory reproductive organ developmental effects was observed at the two highest doses and the changes also persisted until adulthood. Although not statistically significant, similar effects were also found at the lowest dose levels and these findings were regarded as biologically significant because of the rarity of such effects. In the female offspring no effects were associated with the DEHP treatment. Because effects were observed in all treatment groups the study could not identify a no-observable-adverse-effect level (NOAEL) but a lowest-observable-adverse-effect level (LOAEL) at 375 mg/kg body weight/day was identified based on a significant decrease in anterior prostate weight and an increase in permanent nipple retention (Moore *et al.*, 2001). Retained nipples were also found in Wistar rats orally treated with 1,088 mg/kg body weight/day DEHP during gestation and lactation. In the same study, focal tubular atrophy was shown at all doses giving an LOAEL at 113 mg/kg body weight/day for reproductive toxicity. At this dose no systemic toxicity was observed (Schilling *et al.*, 2001). In another study using Sprague-Dawley rats, exposure to 100–500 mg/kg body weight DEHP reduced Sertoli cell proliferation and increased the number of large gonocytes containing 2–4 nuclei in their pups in a dose-dependent manner (Li *et al.*, 2000). Increased levels of multinucleated germ cells at ≥125 mg/kg body weight/day and interstitial hyperplasia at 250 or 500 mg/kg body weight/day were also observed in offspring of rats exposed orally to DEHP from GD 7 to 18 (Shirota *et al.*, 2005).

Cammack *et al.* (2003) studied reproductive development of Sprague-Dawley rats exposed i.v. or orally for 3 weeks postnatally to multiple doses of DEHP. Depletion of germinal tubule and decreased seminiferous tubule diameter were observed in the groups treated with 300 or 600 mg/kg body weight by both exposure routes. Furthermore, decreased seminiferous tubule diameter persisted until adult life in the groups receiving ≥300 mg/kg body weight DEHP. Reproductive effects of DEHP exposure in feed were investigated in a comprehensive multiple dose multigenerational breeding study in Sprague-Dawley rats sponsored by the US National Toxicology Programme (NTP). Adverse reproductive effects such as seminiferous tubuli atrophy, decrease in pregnancy index, number of litters per pair, male reproductive organ weights, sperm counts and sperm motility were observed in all generations. The NTP-CEHR reviewed the data from this study, and based on the occurrence of small reproductive organ weights in F_1 and F_2 generation the panel considered 14–23 mg/kg body weight/day to be the LOAEL giving an NOAEL of 3–5 mg/kg body weight/day (Kavlock *et al.*, 2006).

TABLE 48.7 Summary of male reproductive toxicity data from studies in rats

Species and dosing	Most sensitive outcome	Effect level	References
Sprague-Dawley: DEHP orally at 0, 375, 750, 1,500 mg/kg bw/day. GD 3–PND 21	Increased aerolae or nipples sizes in the male offspring	LOAEL 375 mg/kg bw/day	Moore *et al.* (2001)
Wistar rats: DEHP orally at 0, 113, 340, 1,088 mg/kg bw/day Gestation and lactation	Focal tubular atrophy	LOAEL 113 mg/kg bw/day	Schilling *et al.* (2001)
Sprague-Dawley: DEHP orally at 0, 100, 250, 500 mg/kg bw/day. GD 7–18	Reduced Sertoli cell proliferation. Increased large gonocytes with 2–4 nuclei	LOAEL 100 mg/kg bw/day	Shirota *et al.* (2005)
Sprague-Dawley: DEHP orally at 0, 150, 300, 600 mg/kg bw/day. PND 0–21	Persistent decreased seminiferous tubule diameter until adulthood	LOAEL 300 mg/kg bw/day	Cammack *et al.* (2003)
Sprague-Dawley; DEHP orally at 1.5, 10, 30, 100, 300, 1,000, 7,500 or 10,000 ppm. Continously 3 generations	F_2 percent mobile sperm	NOAEL 100 ppm (3–5 mg/kg bw/day)	Kavlock *et al.* (2006)
Rat, Long-Evans: DEHP orally at 0, 1, 10, 100 or 200 mg/kg bw/day 14 or 28 days	Decreased 17α-hydroxylase in testis, altered *ex vivo* Leydig cell testosterone synthesis	NOAEL 1 mg/kg bw/day	Akingbemi *et al.* (2004)
Sprague-Dawley: DBP injected s.c. PND 5–14	Reduced weights of testes and accessory glands. Affected tubules	20 mg/animal	Kim *et al.* (2004)

Long-Evans rats orally dosed with DEHP from postnatal day (PND) 21 (weaning) to PND 120 showed no signs of overt toxicity. However, exposure to a dose as low as 10 mg/kg body weight/day reduced Leydig cell testosterone production *ex vivo*, increased serum LH, testosterone and 17 β-estradiol and led to Leydig cell hypoplasia, suggesting an NOAEL of 1 mg/kg body weight/day (Akingbemi *et al.*, 2004). The increased steroid levels were probably produced by increased number of Leydig cells and chronically increased LH levels induced by DEHP exposure. The rise in testosterone levels found in this study contrasts with the decrease in testosterone amounts observed in studies where exposure to DEHP occurred prenatally.

In a multi-dose study, rats were injected subcutaneously from PND 5 to PND 14 with corn oil (control) or DBP (5, 10 or 20 mg/animal). DBP exposure (20 mg/animal) significantly reduced the weights of testes and accessory sex organs in the same manner as DEHP. These adverse effects persisted through puberty at PND 42. Histomorphological examination showed mild diffuse Leydig cell hyperplasia in the interstitium of severely affected tubules on PND 31. Furthermore, DBP (20 mg/animal) significantly decreased the expression of androgen receptor (AR), whereas estrogen receptor (ER) expression and steroidogenic factor 1 (SF-1) expression were increased in a dose-dependent manner on PND 31 in the rat testes (Kim *et al.*, 2004).

Effects observed in single dose studies are similar to those found in the multiple dose level studies. For example, treatment of dams with a single dose of DEHP at 750 mg/kg body weight in late gestation or early lactation decreased testicular weights and increased testicular lesions in the offspring. Additional effects observed in male rats exposed to a single dose of DEHP at 750 mg/kg body weight included retained nipples, reduced AGD, lack of testicular descent, agenesis of accessory reproductive organs and incomplete preputial separation (Gray *et al.*, 2000; Parks *et al.*, 2000; Borch *et al.*, 2004). In a 65-week oral toxicity study in marmosets, DEHP was administered from prior to puberty until young adulthood. Although a dose-dependent delay in the onset of puberty was found in males, no testicular toxicity was observed at the highest dose level (2,500 mg/kg body weight/day) suggesting that male marmosets are less sensitive compared to rodents. These conflicting results may be explained by a lower absorption of DEHP from the intestine in marmosets (Tomonari *et al.*, 2006).

Female animal studies

Although less studied, phthalates were also reported to induce adverse reproductive effects in females (Table 48.8). In the 65-week oral DEHP toxicity study in marmosets (Tomonari *et al.*, 2006), DEHP at ≥500 mg/kg body weight/day elevated serum estradiol levels, advanced the onset of puberty and increased ovarian and uterine weights. In the same study no differences were observed in weights of the male accessory sex organs. In female rats gestational and lactational exposure to DBP induced uterine malformations and reduced fecundity at the same doses (500 or 750 mg/kg/day), which produced malformations in males (Mylcherest *et al.*, 1998). In a multiple dose, two-generation reproductive study in rats, DEHP exposure reduced the weight and weight gain in F_2 pups in the high dose group (1,088 mg/kg body weight/day; Schilling *et al.*, 2001). Furthermore, in the high dose females deficits in growing follicles and corpora lutea were noted. Exposure of adult Sprague-Dawley rats with 2 g/kg DEHP decreased serum estradiol levels, prolonged estrus cycles and there was an absence of ovulation. Missing ovulation led to an absence of the development of corpora lutea and follicles became cystic. Histological analysis of the preovulatory follicles showed significantly smaller granulosa cells in the DEHP-exposed rats (Davis *et al.*, 1994). Perinatal exposure to DEHP at 5, 15, 45, 135 or 405 mg/kg body weight/day was studied by Grande *et al.* (2006, 2007). There was delayed puberty at 15 mg/kg body weight/day in female Wistar rats in addition to inducing a significant increase in tertiary atretic follicles in adult female offspring exposed to 405 mg/kg body weight/day. An NOAEL of 5 mg/kg body weight/day was estimated for female reproductive toxicity (Grande *et al.*, 2006, 2007).

Developmental effects in other organs and systems

Normal thyroid hormone function was shown to be important for reproductive system development and function in both males and females (Poppe *et al.*, 2007). Furthermore, deficiency of thyroid hormones during critical periods of brain development both pre- and postnatally is a well-recognized etiologic factor for brain damage leading to various neurologic disorders (Román, 2007) Serum thyroid hormone (TH) and thyroid stimulating hormone (TSH) levels were

TABLE 48.8 Summary of female reproductive toxicity data from animal studies

Species and dosing	Most sensitive outcome	Effect level	References
Marmosets: DEHP orally at 0, 100, 500 or 2,500 mg/kg daily 3–18 months	Increased serum estradiol levels, advanced onset of puberty, increased ovarian and uterine weights	NOAEL 250 mg/kg bw/day	Tomonari *et al.* (2006)
Sprague-Dawley: DBP orally at 0, 250, 500 or 750 mg/kg/day. GD 3–PND 21	Uterine malformations, reduced fecundity	NOAEL 100 mg/kg bw/day	Mylcherest *et al.* (1998)
Wistar rats: DEHP orally at 0, 113, 340, 1,088 mg/kg bw/day Gestation and lactation	Deficits in growing follicles and corpora lutea	NOAEL 340 mg/kg bw/day	Schilling *et al.* (2001)
Sprague–Dawley: Adults DEHP orally at 2 g/kg DEHP for 12 days	Decreased estradiol, prolonged estrus cycles, significantly smaller granulosa cells	LOAEL 2,000 mg/kg bw/day	Davis *et al.* (1994)
Wistar rats: DEHP orally at 5, 15, 45, 135 and 405 mg/kg bw/day. GD 3–PND 21	Delayed puberty	NOAEL 5 mg/kg bw/day	Grande *et al.* (2006, 2007)

inversely correlated with urinary MEHP concentrations comparable with levels reported for the general US population (Meeker *et al.*, 2007, 2009). In Taiwanese pregnant women, urinary MBP levels showed significant negative associations with thyroxine and free thyroxine (Huang *et al.*, 2009). In animal studies, rats receiving diets with added DEHP had lower plasma thyroxin (T4) concentrations compared with controls (Hinton *et al.*, 1986; Poon *et al.*, 1997; Howarth *et al.*, 2001). A dose-dependent inverse association between DBP and both triiodothyronine (T3) and T4 has also been reported in male rats (O'Connor *et al.*, 2002). Furthermore, in a recent *in vitro* study the TH disrupting potential of various phthalates was determined by the effect on the TH-dependent rat pituitary GH3 cell proliferation (T-screen) and BBP, DBP, DOP, DIDP, DINP and DEHP was shown to significantly affect the GH3 cell proliferation (Ghisari and Bonefeld-Jorgensen, 2009). Association between severe hypothyroxemia and neurological disorders such as reduced IQ and motor deficiency is well described (Ohara *et al.*, 2004). However, even mild subclinical maternal hypothyroxemia has been documented to affect fetal neurodevelopment (Haddow *et al.*, 1999; Pop *et al.*, 1999). Engel *et al.* (2009) reported significant association between prenatal exposure and performance on the Neonatal Behavior Assessment Scale in a multiethnic cohort from New York. Based on the reported effect of phthalates on thyroxin function, the authors suggested maternal hypothyroxemia as a possible mechanism for the observed effect. Another study reported association between DEHP and attention-deficit/hyperactivity disorder (ADHD) in school-age children (Kim *et al.*, 2009a). Associations between phthalates and hyperactivity are also reported in animal studies (Ishido *et al.*, 2004). Furthermore, behaviors of young rats were more seriously affected when exposure occurred during differentiation and synaptogenesis compared to later life stages suggesting that the level of vulnerability of the developing brain is dependent on the life stage at which the exposure occurs (Kim *et al.*, 2009a). Many studies have documented an association between the midbrain dopaminergic system and the pathogenesis for ADHD. Tyrosine hydroxylase, the rate-limiting enzyme of dopamine production, was downregulated in midbrain dopaminergic nuclei in mice exposed to doses of DEHP below the NOAEL (Tanida *et al.*, 2009). Decreased tyrosine hydroxylase expression was also observed in rats exposed to dicyclohexylphthalate (DCHP). Furthermore, microarray data revealed that DEHP and DBP changed the gene expression of other genes, dopamine receptor D4 (DRD4) and dopamine transporter in the midbrain of rats (Masuo *et al.*, 2004). Modulation of DRD4 and dopamine transporter can lead to changes in extracellular dopamine and neuronal dopamine sensitivity resulting in hyperactivity and impulsivity in rats. Accordingly, overexpression of dopamine transporter was one of the consistent findings in ADHD children (Dougherty *et al.*, 1999; Kim *et al.*, 2009b). Because thyroid hormones play crucial roles in brain development of both humans and experimental animals and since phthalates are suggested to affect thyroid functions it is likely that prenatal modulation of dopamine production and sensitivity may be due to disruption of thyroid hormone signaling. Thus, the reduced levels of tyrosine hydroxylase in midbrain dopaminergic nuclei observed in rodents exposed to phthalates may be caused by disruption of thyroid hormone-dependent gene expression (Tanida *et al.*, 2009).

Because of the documented antiandrogenic effects of certain phthalates in animal models and the suggestive results from human epidemiological studies, it has been questioned whether low testosterone in adult males may be associated with an increased prevalence of obesity and type 2 diabetes (Ding *et al.*, 2006). Stahlhut *et al.* (2007) compared urinary phthalate metabolites with increased waist circumference and insulin resistance in adult American men and found significant positive correlation between those parameters. Based on their results, it was suggested that phthalates might contribute to the ongoing increase in prevalence of obesity, insulin resistance and related clinical disorders (metabolic syndrome) observed in US humans via endocrine disruptive mechanisms. In rats, prenatal exposure to DiBP reduced plasma protein levels of insulin in male and female offspring and plasma testosterone and liver and testis mRNA levels of PPARα in males (Boberg *et al.*, 2008). The recent environmental obesogen hypothesis suggests that environmental chemicals may contribute to the development of obesity and metabolic disorders such as type 2 diabetes by chemical interaction with nuclear receptors including steroid receptors, retionid x-receptor (RXR) and PPARs (Newbold *et al.*, 2007). Furthermore, reduced leptin levels in gestation lead to adiposity in adult offspring (Vickers, 2007). The existing human and animal data provide preliminary evidence of a potential contributing role of phthalates in the increasing prevalence of obesity diabetes and related clinical condition, but additional studies are needed (Meeker *et al.*, 2009).

Exposure to phthalates during fetal and neonatal life may also affect the normal development of the immune system leading to immune system disorders such as asthma and allergies. In Oslo, Norway, indoor PVC surface materials in the home were associated with increased risk of bronchial obstruction in small children (Jaakkola and Knight, 2008). In Swedish children (aged 3–8 years), significantly higher concentrations of DEHP and butyl benzyl phthalate (BBzP) were associated with eczematous and asthmatic symptoms (Bornehag *et al.*, 2004). Similar effects were observed in Bulgarian children where high levels of DEHP were associated with increased asthma/wheezing in a dose-dependent manner (Kolarik *et al.*, 2008). These studies are of cross-sectional design that reduces the possibility of conclusive results. However, positive association between PVC flooring and increased incidence of asthma was found in a Swedish study with longitudinal design (Larsson *et al.*, 2009). Other shortcomings in these studies include that none of the studies focus on early-life exposure and that PVC materials instead of phthalates were used as exposure data (Bornehag and Nanberg, 2010).

Animal studies using mice models demonstrated that DEHP as well as DiNP, DnBP and DnOP at low doses administered subcutaneously (s.c.) or by intraperitoneal injection and in long-term inhalation protocols produced Th2 response with induction of IgE and IgG1 (Larsen *et al.*, 2001, 2007; Lee *et al.*, 2004). Furthermore, increased lymphocyte-dependent production of Th2 cytokines including IL-4, IL-5 and IL-10 following DEHP exposure was also shown in mice (Larsen *et al.*, 2001, 2007; Lee *et al.*, 2004). In contrast topical application or s.c. injection of high doses of DEHP did not induce IgE and IgG1 (Kimber and Dearman, 2010). Even though the individual studies differ in several critical aspects such as strain, antigen, method for sensitization, route of administration, time of exposure and doses of the phthalates studied, the overall picture of the results suggests that several phthalates affect Th2 differentiation and Th2 promoted antigen production of IgG1 and IgE (Bornehag and Nanberg, 2010).

MIXTURE EXPOSURES

There is widespread recognition that humans, fish and wildlife are simultaneously exposed to multiple phthalates as well as other contaminants on a continuous basis. The chemicals frequently detected in biological samples include pesticides, industrial chemicals, pharmaceuticals and hormones. To date, risk assessments are typically conducted on a chemical-by-chemical basis and regulatory efforts have not accounted for realistic environmental exposure to mixture of phthalates and other contaminants. However, recent studies have documented that individual phthalates induce cumulative, dose additive effects by the same mechanism of action when administered as a mixture (Borch *et al.*, 2006; Howdeshell *et al.*, 2008). These findings contradict the conclusion in an EFSA (2005b) report which stated that no group-TDI could be allocated for phthalates because different mechanisms are involved. Furthermore, exposure to phthalates in combination with other groups of chemicals including phenols, dioxins, pesticides and pharmaceuticals are reported to induce antagonistic, additive or synergistic effects depending on the different combinations (Christiansen *et al.*, 2009; Ghisari and Bonefeld-Jorgensen, 2009; Tanida *et al.*, 2009). These results indicate that compounds that act by different modes of action interact when present in combination. The results also suggest that a modification of the approach for cumulative risk assessments should be considered, from one based upon "common mechanism of toxicity" to one that includes the cumulative assessment of chemicals that disrupt development of the same tissues or biological systems resulting in a target organ- and timing-based approach rather than on a narrow mechanism of toxicity. The cumulative risk assessment could then potentially include all chemicals that target one system during the same critical developmental period (Rider *et al.*, 2009).

RISK ASSESSMENT AND PHTHALATE ACTION PLANS

The five main phthalate plasticizers, DINP, DIDP, DEHP, BBP and DBP, have all undergone comprehensive European Union Risk Assessments conducted under European Union Regulation 793/93, by the Scientific Committee on Toxicity, Ecotoxicity and the Environment (http://www.phthalates.com/RAs)

The risk assessments stated that di-isononyl phthalate (DINP) and di-isodecyl phthalate (DIDP) pose no risk to either human health or the environment from any current use. However, in Europe, based on the precautionary principle, DINP can no longer be used in toys and child-care items that can be put in the mouth even though the EU scientific risk assessment concluded that its use in toys does not pose a risk to human health or the environment. DIDP, however, is still allowed in toys and child-care items.

For BBP, the conclusion of the assessment of the risks to human health is that there is at present no need for further information and/or testing or for risk reduction measures beyond those which are being applied. It is further concluded that there is a need for better information to adequately characterize the risks to aquatic ecosystem and terrestrial ecosystems. For example, a long-term fish study on reproductive and endocrine effects was mentioned as a specific requirement.

The assessment of the risks of DBP exposure to humans and aquatic and terrestrial ecosystems stated that there is no need for further information or testing or risk reduction measures beyond those which are being applied already. However, for workers more information is required because of concerns for general systemic toxicity as a consequence of repeated dermal exposure arising from aerosol forming activities and adverse local effects in the respiratory tract as a consequence of repeated inhalation exposure in all occupational exposure scenarios.

The risk assessment demonstrates that DEHP poses no risk to the general population and that no further measures need to be taken to manage the substance in any of its key end-use applications. The areas of possible risk identified in the assessment relate to the use of DEHP in children's toys and DEHP is no longer permitted in toys and child-care articles in the EU. Some localized environmental exposures near to factories are documented and the European Union has initiated measures relating to emission controls from converters' plants. An EU Scientific Review was requested to determine whether there may be any risk from the use of DEHP in certain medical applications (children and neonates undergoing long-term blood transfusion and adults undergoing long-term hemodialysis). In February 2008, the EU Scientific Committee on Emerging and Newly Identified Health Risks (SCENIHR) published an Opinion in which they said there is reason for some concern for prematurely born male neonates although follow-up studies after high DEHP exposures in neonates do not indicate there is an effect of DEHP on the development of the human male reproductive system.

In an EU risk assessment on cumulative effects of mixtures of phthalates it was concluded that no group-TDI could be allocated for phthalates because different mechanisms are involved (EFSA, 2005b). This conclusion contradicts recent data which show that different phthalates exert toxicity in a dose-additive fashion by the same mode of actions.

A major concern regarding the risk assessments conducted by the EU is that experimental and epidemiological data published after 2000 are not considered. Furthermore, at present the EU has not initiated any specific action plan on phthalates (http://www.phthalates.com/RAs).

In a review on DEHP in 2006, the National Toxicology Program, Centre for the Evaluation of Risks to Human Reproduction (NTP-CERHR) expressed a reduced level of concern for the effects of DEHP on male offspring exposed to general population levels during pregnancy and lactation due to greater confidence in exposure levels in humans and in effect levels in experimental animals. The expert panel underlines that it has concern for possible effects on male children of women undergoing medical treatment during pregnancy and lactation leading to additional exposure to DEHP during development (Kavlock *et al.*, 2006). In 2002, the NTP concluded in its review on the potential human impact of DBP exposure that, "Based upon recent estimated DBP exposures among women of reproductive age, the NTP has some concern for DBP causing adverse effects to human development, particularly development of the reproductive system."

A major concern regarding the risk assessments conducted by the EU is that experimental and epidemiological data published after 2000 are not considered. Furthermore, at present the EU has not initiated any specific action plan on phthalates. In contrast the US Environmental Protection Agency (EPA) recently published their phthalates management plan that includes eight phthalates (DIBP, DINP, DIDP, BBP, DBP, DEHP, DnPP, DnOP). In developing this plan, the EPA considered the toxicity of phthalates, their prevalence in the environment and their widespread use and human exposure (www.epa.gov/oppt/.../pubs/actionplans/phthalates.html).

The EPA is concerned about phthalates because of their toxicity and the evidence of pervasive human and environmental exposure to them. Thus, the EPA intends to initiate action to address the manufacturing, processing, distribution in commerce and use of these eight phthalates. The EPA intends to take action as part of a coordinated approach with the Consumer Product Safety Commission (CPSC) and the Food and Drug Administration (FDA).

Because of the reported cumulative effects of mixtures the EPA has scheduled a major cumulative hazard assessment conduced by the CPSC with planned date of completion in 2012.

Because of the reported adverse effects observed in test animals the Consumer Product Safety Improvement Act of 2008 (CPSIA) banned the use of six phthalates in toys and child-care items at concentrations greater than 0.1%: DEHP, DBP, BBP, DINP, DIDP and DnOP. The Food and Drug Administration (FDA) regulates phthalates in food contact substances (such as plastic wrap), cosmetics, pharmaceuticals and medical devices. The FDA announced in June 2008 that it was reviewing available use and toxicology information associated with phthalate exposure from FDA regulated products to better characterize any potential risk from these uses.

CONCLUDING REMARKS AND FUTURE DIRECTIONS

The widespread use of phthalates in consumer products leads to ubiquitous exposure of humans to these compounds from fetal life to adulthood. At present, exposure data are inconsistent because of the different methods used to assess exposure levels. Oxidized metabolites of DEHP were recently recognized as the major urinary metabolites in humans, suggesting an underestimation of exposure when using only the primary metabolite MEHP as a biomarker of DEHP exposure. Furthermore, there are little data available on human TK and metabolism of other phthalates.

Estimated DEHP concentrations in the general population were found to be highest in children and decreased with age. The human levels approximate currently accepted TDI (EFSA, 2005a) suggesting that at least in some individuals TDI are exceeded (Fromme *et al.*, 2007c). However, DEHP concentrations measured in neonates receiving medical treatments are several orders of magnitude higher than in the general population. Thus, neonates constitute a population at particular risk. Other groups, which may be exposed to high levels, are occupationally exposed workers, adults undergoing medical treatments with medical devices or pharmaceutical drugs containing phthalates.

The current human toxicological data are insufficient to evaluate the prenatal and childhood effects following phthalate exposure. Animal data are, however, sufficient to conclude that DEHP, DBP and BBP are potential reproductive toxicants in rats. The critical period for effects on male reproductive development appears to be late gestation and into the immediate postnatal period. Although most of the animal studies focused on male toxicity there are both human and animal data available, which indicate that exposure to phthalates may also affect female reproductive functions.

Recent data demonstrated that individual phthalates with a similar mechanism of action elicit cumulative, dose-additive effects on fetal testosterone production and testicular histopathology when administered as a mixture (Howdeshell *et al.*, 2008). These findings emphasize the need for testing combinations of phthalates to better assess the health risks of known human exposure to multiple sources of these chemicals. Additional TK and toxicodynamic (TD) data on less well-studied phthalates are needed. Further, new endpoints need to be included in the study of putative phthalate toxicity on humans.

Due to the fact that there are substantial gaps in knowledge in both phthalate levels of exposure and consequent health effects in humans, additional research is warranted.

1. It is of key importance to improve the knowledge of human TK and toxicity, specifically during pregnancy and the nursing period, because *in utero* and early postnatal exposure appears to be the most vulnerable period during development.
2. Well-designed follow-up studies of reproductive system development and functions in the most heavily exposed and most vulnerable human populations may address the question of whether phthalates produce adverse human reproductive effects. Reproductive developmental toxicity is well studied in male animals. However, data on female reproductive toxicity are scarce and need further research. Further *in vitro* and *in vivo* studies are also warranted to improve the understanding of the modes of action of phthalates in humans.
3. Most studies focused on adverse reproductive and developmental effects associated with exposure to single phthalates. However, because humans are exposed to mixtures of phthalates both concurrently and sequentially, and available experimental evidence suggests that mixtures of phthalates may induce endocrine disruption in a cumulative fashion, it is necessary to initiate studies which focus on mixture effects.
4. Phthalates with shorter and longer C backbones may need further evaluation before definite conclusions are drawn correlating physicochemical properties to toxicity.
5. It is also important to identify the most reliable biomarkers of exposure and the biologic media best suited for biomarker analysis. Phthalates occur as mixtures in nature and it needs to be considered whether a summary of the different phthalates and their metabolites might be a more appropriate measurement for biomarkers of exposure.
6. Focus should be extended to endpoints other than reproductive toxicity.

REFERENCES

Akingbemi BT, Sottas CM, Koulova AI, Klinefelter GR, Hardy MP (2004) Inhibition of testicular steroidogenesis by the xenoestrogen bisphenol A is associated with reduced pituitary luteinizing hormone secretion and decreased steroidogenic enzyme gene expression in rat Leydig cells. *Endocrinology* **145:** 592–603.

Akingbemi BT, Youker RT, Sottas CM, Ge R, Katz E, Klinefelter GR, Zirkin BR, Hardy MP (2001) Modulation of rat Leydig cell steroidogenic function by di(2-ethylhexyl)phthalate. *Biol Reprod* **65:** 1252–9.

Anderson WA, Castle L, Scotter MJ, Massey RC, Springall C (2001) A biomarker approach to measuring human dietary exposure to certain thalate diesters. *Food Addit Contam* **18:** 1068–74.

Ariyaratne HB, Chamindrani Mendis-Handagama S (2000) Changes in the testis interstitium of Sprague Dawley rats from birth to sexual maturity. *Biol Reprod* **62:** 680–90.

Barlow NJ, Foster PM (2003) Pathogenesis of male reproductive tract lesions from gestation through adulthood following in utero exposure to di(n-butyl) phthalate. *Toxicol Pathol* **31:** 397–410.

Barlow NJ, McIntyre BS, Foster PM (2004) Male reproductive tract lesions at 6, 12, and 18 months of age following in utero exposure to di(n-butyl) phthalate. *Toxicol Pathol* **32:** 79–90.

Barlow NJ, Phillips SL, Wallace DG, Sar M, Gaido KW, Foster PM (2003) Quantitative changes in gene expression in fetal rat testes following exposure to di(n-butyl) phthalate. *Toxicol Sci* **73:** 431–4.

Barr DB, Silva MJ, Kato K, Reidy JA, Malek NA, Hurtz D, Sadowski M, Needham LL, Calafat AM (2003) Assessing human exposure to phthalates using monoesters and their oxidized metabolites as biomarkers. *Environ Health Perspect* **111:** 1148–51.

Blount BC, Silva MJ, Caudill SP, Needham LL, Pirkle JL, Sampson EJ, Lucier GW, Jackson RJ, Brock JW (2000) Levels of seven urinary phthalate metabolites in a human reference population. *Environ Health Perspect* **108:** 979–82.

Boberg J, Metzdorff S, Wortziger R, Axelstad M, Brokken L, Vinggaard AM, Dalgaard M, Nellemann C (2008) Impact of diisobutyl phthalate and other PPAR agonists on steroidogenesis and plasma insulin and leptin levels in fetal rats. *Toxicology* **250:** 75–81.

Borch J, Axelstad M, Vinggaard AM, Dalgaard M (2006) Diisobutyl phthalate has comparable anti-androgenic effects to di-n-butyl phthalate in fetal rat testis. *Toxicol Lett* **163:** 183–90.

Borch J, Ladefoged O, Hass U, Vinggaard AM (2004) Steroidogenesis in fetal male rats is reduced by DEHP and DINP, but endocrine effects of DEHP are not modulated by DEHA in fetal, prepubertal and adult male rats. *Reprod Toxicol* **18:** 53–61.

Bornehag CG, Nanberg E (2010) Phthalate exposure and asthma in children. *Int J Androl.* Epub ahead of print.

Bornehag CG, Sundell J, Weschler CJ, Sigsgaard T, Lundgren B, Hasselgren M, Hägerhed-Engelman L (2004) The association between asthma and allergic symptoms in children and phthalates in house dust: a nested case-control study. *Environ Health Perspect* **112:** 1393–7.

Bouma K, Schakel DJ (2002) Migration of phthalates from PVC toys into saliva simulant by dynamic extraction. *Food Addit Contam* **19:** 602–10.

Buchta C, Bittner C, Heinzl H, Hocker P, Macher M, Mayerhofer M, Schmid R, Seger C, Dettke M (2005) Transfusion-related exposure to the plasticizer di(2-ethylhexyl)phthalate in patients receiving platelet pheresis concentrates. *Transfusion* **45:** 798–802.

Buchta C, Bittner C, Hocker P, Macher M, Schmid R, Seger C, Dettke M (2003) Donor exposure to the plasticizer di(2-ethylhexyl)phthalate during plateletpheresis. *Transfusion* **43:** 1115–20.

Calabrese EJ, Baldwin LA (2003) The hormetic dose–response model is more common than the threshold model in toxicology. *Toxicol Sci* **71:** 246–50.

Calafat AM, Needham LL, Silva MJ, Lambert G (2004) Exposure to di-(2-ethylhexyl) phthalate among premature neonates in a neonatal intensive care unit. *Pediatrics* **113:** 429–34.

Cammack JN, White RD, Gordon D, Gass J, Hecker L, Conine D, Bruen US, Friedman M, Echols C, Yeh TY, Wilson DM (2003) Evaluation of reproductive development following intravenous and oral exposure to DEHP in male neonatal rats. *Int J Toxicol* **22:** 159–74.

Center for Devices and Radiological Health (2001) Device Advice. US Food and Drug Administration. http://www.fda.gov/downloads/MedicalDevices/DeviceRegulationandGuidance.

Chen M-L, Chen J-S, Tang C-L, Mao I-F (2008) The internal exposure of Taiwanese to phthalate – an evidence of intensive use of plastic materials. *Environ Int* **34:** 79–85.

Christiansen S, Scholze M, Dalgaard M, Vinggaard AM, Axelstad M, Kortenkamp A, Hass U (2009) Synergistic disruption of external male sex organ development by a mixture of four antiandrogens. *Environ Health Perspect* **117:** 1839–46.

Clark K, Cousins IT, Mackay D (2003a) Assessment of critical exposure pathways. In The *Handbook of Environmental Chemistry* (Staples CA, ed.). New York, Springer-Verlag, pp. 227–62.

Clark K, Cousins IT, Mackay D, Yamada K (2003b) Observed concentrations in the environment. In *The Handbook of Environmental Chemistry* (Staples CA, ed.). New York, Springer-Verlag, pp. 125–77.

Cobellis L, Latini G, De Felice C, Razzi S, Paris I, Ruggieri F, Mazzeo P, Petraglia F (2003) High plasma concentrations of di-(2-ethylhexyl)-phthalate in women with endometriosis. *Human Reprod* **18:** 1512–15.

Codesal J, Regadera J, Nistal M, Regadera-Sejas J, Paniagua R (1990) Involution of human fetal Leydig cells. An immunohistochemical, ultrastructural and quantitative study. *J Anat* **172:** 103–14.

Colón I, Caro D, Bourdony CJ, Rosario O (2000) Identification of phthalate esters in the serum of young Puerto Rican girls with premature breast development. *Environ Health Perspect* **108:** 895–900.

Corton JC, Lapinskas PJ (2005) Peroxisome proliferator-activated receptors: mediators of phthalate ester-induced effects in the male reproductive tract? *Toxicol Sci* **83:** 4–17.

Cresteil T (1998) Onset of xenobiotic metabolism in children: toxicological implications. *Food Addit Contam* **15 (Suppl):** 45–51.

David RM (2006) Proposed mode of action for in utero effects of some phthalate esters on the developing male reproductive tract. *Toxicol Pathol* **34:** 209–19.

Davis BJ, Maronpot RR, Heindel JJ (1994) Di-(2-ethylhexyl) phthalate suppresses estradiol and ovulation in cycling rats. *Toxicol Appl Pharmacol* **128:** 216–23.

Dine T, Luyckx M, Gressier B, Brunet C, Souhait J, Nogarede S, *et al.* (2000) A pharmacokinetic interpretation of increasing concentrations of DEHP in haemodialysed patients. *Med Eng Phys* **22:** 157–65.

Ding EL, Song Y, Malik VS, Liu S (2006) Sex differences of endogenous sex hormones and risk of type 2 diabetes: a systematic review and meta-analysis. *JAMA* **295:** 1288–99.

Dostal LA, Chapin RE, Stefanski SA, Harris MW, Schwetz BA (1988) Testicular toxicity and reduced Sertoli cell numbers in neonatal rats by di(2-ethylhexyl)phthalate and the recovery of fertility as adults. *Toxicol Appl Pharmacol* **95:** 104–21.

Dougherty DD, Bonab AA, Spencer TJ, Rauch SL, Madras BK, Fischman AJ (1999) Dopamine transporter density in patients with attention deficit hyperactivity disorder. *Lancet* **354:** 2132–3.

Duty SM, Singh NP, Silva MJ, Barr DB, Brock JW, Ryan L, Herrick RF, Christiani DC, Hauser R (2003) The relationship between environmental exposures to phthalates and DNA damage in human sperm using the neutral comet assay. *Environ Health Perspect* **111:** 1164–9

EFSA (2005a) Opinion of the Scientific Panel on Food Additives, Flavourings, Processing Aids and Materials in Contact with Food (AFC) on a request from the Commission related to Bis(2-ethylhexyl)phthalate (DEHP) for use in food contact materials. *The EFSA Journal* **243:** 1–20.

EFSA (2005b) Statement of the Scientific Panel on Food Additives, Flavourings, Processing Aids and Materials in Contact with Food on a request from the Commission on the Possibility of Allocating a Group-TDI for Butylbenzylphthalate (BBP), di-Butylphthalate (DBP), Bis(2-ethylhexyl) phthalate (DEHP), di-Isononylphthalate (DINP) and di-Isodecylphthalate (DIDP). http://www.efsa.europa.eu/EFSA/Statement/phthalategroup_minutes_statement1,0.pdf

Elsisi AE, Carter DE, Sipes IG (1989) Dermal absorption of phthalate diesters in rats. *Fundam Appl Toxicol* **12:** 70–7.

Ema M, Itami T, Kawasaki H (1993) Teratogenic phase specificity of butyl benzyl phthalate in rats. *Toxicology* **79:** 11–19.

Engel SM, Zhu C, Berkowitz GS, Calafat AM, Silva MJ, Miodovnik A, Wolff MS (2009) Prenatal phthalate exposure and performance on the Neonatal Behavioral Assessment Scale in a multiethnic birth cohort. *Neurotoxicology* **30:** 522–8.

EU Decision 198/815/EC of December 7 (1999) *Official Journal of the European Communities* (OJCE) L 315 of December 9, 1999.

EU Directive 2005/84/EC of the European Parliament and of the Council of December 14, 2005.

Fabjan E, Hulzebos E, Mennes W, Piersma AH (2006) A category approach for reproductive effects of phthalates. *Crit Rev Toxicol* **36:** 695–726.

FDA (2004) Safety assessment of di(2-ethylhexyl)phthalate (DEHP) released from PVC medical devices. *Govt. Reports Announcements & Index*, p. 21.

Fisher JS, Macpherson S, Marchetti N, Sharpe RM (2003) Human "testicular dysgenesis syndrome": a possible model using in-utero exposure of the rat to dibutyl phthalate. *Human Reprod* **18:** 1383–94.

Fitzpatrick SL, Carlone DL, Robker RL, Richards JS (1997) Expression of aromatase in the ovary: down-regulation of mRNA by the ovulatory luteinizing hormone surge. *Steroids* **62:** 197–206.

Foster PM, Mylchreest E, Gaido KW, Sar M (2001) Effects of phthalate esters on the developing reproductive tract of male rats. *Human Reprod* **7(3):** 231–5.

Foster PM (2005) Mode of action: impaired fetal Leydig cell function – effects on male reproductive development produced by certain phthalate esters. *Crit Rev Toxicol* **35:** 713–19.

Foster PM (2006) Disruption of reproductive development in male rat offspring following in utero exposure to phthalate esters. *Int J Androl* **29:** 140–7; discussion 181–5.

Fromme H, Albrecht M, Angerer J, Drexler H, Gruber L, Schlummer M, Parlar H, Körner W, Wanner A, Heitmann D, Roscher E, Bolte G (2007b) Integrated exposure assessment survey (INES) exposure to persistent and bioaccumulative chemicals in Bavaria, Germany. *Int J Hyg Environ Health* **210:** 345–9.

Fromme H, Bolte G, Koch HM, Angerer J, Boehmer S, Drexler H, Mayer R, Liebl B (2007a) Occurrence and daily variation of phthalate metabolites in the urine of an adult population. *Int J Hyg Environ Health* **210:** 21–33.

Fromme H, Gruber L, Schlummer M, Wolz G, Böhmer S, Angerer J, Mayer R, Liebl B, Bolte G (2007c) Intake of phthalates and di(2-ethylhexyl)adipate: results of the integrated exposure assessment survey based on duplicate diet samples and biomonitoring data. *Environ Int* **33:** 1012–20.

Fromme H, Lahrz T, Piloty M, Gebhart H, Oddoy A, Ruden H (2004) Occurrence of phthalates and musk fragrances indoor air and dust from apartments and kindergartens in Berlin (Germany). *Indoor Air* **14:** 188–95.

Ge RS, Chen GR, Dong Q, Akingbemi B, Sottas CM, Santos M, Sealfon SC, Bernard DJ, Hardy MP (2007) Biphasic effects of postnatal exposure to diethylhexylphthalate on the timing of puberty in male rats. *J Androl* **28:** 513–20.

General Motors (1982) Disposition of di(2-ethylhexyl) phthalate following inhalation and peroral exposure in rats. TSCATS: PTS0530339, Doc. I.D.: 86-910000683: General Motors Corp.

Ghisari M, Bonefeld-Jorgensen EC (2009) Effects of plasticizers and their mixtures on estrogen receptor and thyroid hormone functions. *Toxicol Lett* **189:** 67–77.

Gore AC (2008) Developmental programming and endocrine disruptor effects on reproductive neuroendocrine systems. *Front Neuroendocrinol* **29:** 358–74.

Grande SW, Andrade AJ, Talsness CE, Grote K, Chahoud I (2006) A dose–response study following in utero and lactational exposure to di(2-ethylhexyl)phthalate: effects on female rat reproductive development. *Toxicol Sci* **91:** 247–54.

Grande SW, Andrade AJ, Talsness CE, Grote K, Golombiewski A, Sterner-Kock A, Chahoud I (2007) A dose–response study following in utero and lactational exposure to di-(2-ethylhexyl) phthalate (DEHP): reproductive effects on adult female offspring rats. *Toxicology* **229:** 114–22.

Gray LE Jr, Ostby J, Furr J, Price M, Veeramachaneni DN, Parks L (2000) Perinatal exposure to the phthalates DEHP, BBP, and DINP, but not DEP, DMP, or DOTP, alters sexual differentiation of the male rat. *Toxicol Sci* **58:** 350–65.

Guyton KZ, Chiu WA, Bateson TF, Jinot J, Scott CS, Brown RC, Caldwell JC (2009) A reexamination of the PPAR-alpha activation mode of action as a basis for assessing human cancer risks of environmental contaminants. *Environ Health Perspect* **117:** 1664–72.

Habert R, Lejeune H, Saez JM (2001) Origin, differentiation and regulation of fetal and adult Leydig cells. *Mol Cell Endocrinol* **179:** 47–74.

Habert R, Muczynski V, Lehraiki A, Lambrot R, Lécureuil C, Levacher C, Coffigny H, Pairault C, Moison D, Frydman R, Rouiller-Fabre V (2009) Adverse effects of endocrine disruptors on the foetal testis development: focus on the phthalates. *Folia Histochem Cytobiol* **47:** 67–74.

Haddow JE, Palomaki GE, Allan WC, Williams JR, Knight GJ, Gagnon J (1999) Maternal thyroid deficiency during pregnancy and subsequent neuropsychological development of the child. *N Engl J Med* **341:** 549–55.

Hauser R (2008) Urinary phthalate metabolites and semen quality: a review of a potential biomarker of susceptibility. *Int J Androl* **31:** 112–17.

Hauser R, Calafat AM (2005) Phthalates and human health. *Occup Environ Med* **62:** 806–18.

Hauser R, Meeker JD, Duty S, Silva MJ, Calafat AM (2006) Altered semen quality in relation to urinary concentrations of phthalate monoester and oxidative metabolites. *Epidemiology* **17:** 682–91.

Hauser R, Meeker JD, Singh NP, Silva MJ, Ryan L, Duty S, Calafat AM (2007) DNA damage in human sperm is related to urinary levels of phthalate monoester and oxidative metabolites. *Human Reprod* **22:** 688–95.

Hauser R, Williams P, Altshul L, Calafat AM (2005) Evidence of interaction between polychlorinated biphenyls and phthalates in relation to human sperm motility. *Environ Health Perspect* **113:** 425–30.

Hauser R, Meeker JD, Park S, Silva MJ, Calafat AM (2004) Temporal variability of urinary phthalate metabolite levels in men of reproductive age. *Environ Health Perspect* **112:** 1734–40.

Hellwig J, Freudenberger H, Jäckh R (1997) Differential prenatal toxicity of branched phthalate esters in rats. *Food Chem Toxicol* **35:** 501–12.

Heudorf U, Mersch-Sundermann V, Angerer J (2007) Phthalates: toxicology and exposure. *Int J Hyg Environ Health* **210:** 623–34.

Hinton RH, Mitchell FE, Mann A, Chescoe D, Price SC, Nunn A, Grasso P, Bridges JW (1986) Effects of phthalic acid esters on the liver and thyroid. *Environ Health Perspect* **70:** 195–210.

Hong D, Li XW, Lian QQ, Lamba P, Bernard DJ, Hardy DO, Chen HX, Ge RS (2009) Mono-(2-ethylhexyl) phthalate (MEHP) regulates glucocorticoid metabolism through 11beta-hydroxysteroid dehydrogenase 2 in murine gonadotrope cells. *Biochem Biophys Res Commun* **389:** 305–9.

Howarth JA, Price SC, Dobrota M, Kentish PA, Hinton RH (2001) Effects on male rats of di-(2-ethylhexyl) phthalate and di-n-hexylphthalate administered alone or in combination. *Toxicol Lett* **121:** 35–43.

Howdeshell KL, Wilson VS, Furr J, Lambright CR, Rider CV, Blystone CR, Hotchkiss AK, Gray LE Jr (2008) A mixture of five phthalate esters inhibits fetal testicular testosterone production in the Sprague-Dawley rat in a cumulative, dose-additive manner. *Toxicol Sci* **105:** 153–65.

Hu GX, Lin H, Sottas CM, Morris DJ, Hardy MP, Ge RS (2008) Inhibition of 11beta-hydroxysteroid dehydrogenase enzymatic activities by glycyrrhetinic acid in vivo supports direct glucocorticoid-mediated suppression of steroidogenesis in Leydig cells. *J Androl* **29:** 345–51.

Huang PC, Kuo PL, Chou YY, Lin SJ, Lee CC (2009) Association between prenatal exposure to phthalates and the health of newborns. *Environ Int* **35:** 14–20.

Huhtaniemi I, Pelliniemi LJ (1992) Fetal Leydig cells: cellular origin, morphology, life span, and special functional features. *Proc Soc Exp Biol Med* **201:** 125–40.

Hurst CH, Waxman DJ (2003) Activation of PPARalpha and PPARgamma by environmental phthalate monoesters. *Toxicol Sci* **74:** 297–308.

Ishido M, Masuo Y, Sayato-Suzuki J, Oka S, Niki E, Morita M (2004) Dicyclohexylphthalate causes hyperactivity in the rat concomitantly with impairment of tyrosine hydroxylase immunoreactivity. *J Neurochem* **91:** 69–76.

Ito Y, Yamanoshita O, Asaeda N, Tagawa Y, Lee CH, Aoyama T, Ichihara G, Furuhashi K, Kamijima M, Gonzalez FJ, Nakajima T (2007) Di(2-ethylhexyl)phthalate induces hepatic tumorigenesis through a peroxisome proliferator-activated receptor alpha-independent pathway. *J Occup Health* **49:** 172–82.

Jaakkola JJ, Knight TL (2008) The role of exposure to phthalates from polyvinyl chloride products in the development of asthma and allergies: a systematic review and meta-analysis. *Environ Health Perspect* **116:** 845–53.

Jönsson BA, Richthoff J, Rylander L, Giwercman A, Hagmar L (2005) Urinary phthalate metabolites and biomarkers of reproductive function in young men. *Epidemiology* **16:** 487–93.

Kang KS, Lee YS, Kim HS, Kim SH (2002) DI-(2-ethylhexyl) phthalate-induced cell proliferation is involved in the inhibition of gap junctional intercellular communication and blockage of apoptosis in mouse Sertoli cells. *J Toxicol Environ Health A* **65:** 447–59.

Kang SC, Lee BM (2005) DNA methylation of estrogen receptor alpha gene by phthalates. *J Toxicol Environ Health A* **68:** 1995–2003.

Kato K, Silva MJ, Reidy JA, Hurtz D 3rd, Malek NA, Needham LL, Nakazawa H, Barr DB, Calafat AM (2004) Mono(2-ethyl-5-hydroxyhexyl) phthalate and mono-(2-ethyl-5-oxohexyl) phthalate as biomarkers for human exposure assessment to di-(2-ethylhexyl) phthalate. *Environ Health Perspect* **112:** 327–30.

Kavlock R, Barr D, Boekelheide K, Breslin W, Breysse P, Chapin R, Gaido K, Hodgson E, Marcus M, Shea K, Williams P (2006) NTP-CERHR Expert Panel update on the reproductive and developmental toxicity of di(2-ethylhexyl) phthalate. *Reprod Toxicol* **22:** 291–399.

Kavlock R, Boekelheide K, Chapin R, Cunningham M, Faustman E, Foster P, Golub M, Henderson R, Hinberg I, Little R, Seed J, Shea K, Tabacoba S, Tyl R, Williams P, Zacharewski T (2002) NTP Center for the evaluation of risks to human reproduction; phthalates expert panel report on the reproductive and developmental toxicity of di(2-ethylhexyl)phthalate. *Reprod Toxicol* **16:** 529–653.

Kim B, Koo MS, Jun JY, Park IH, Oh DY, Cheon KA (2009b) Association between dopamine D4 receptor gene polymorphism and scores on a continuous performance test in Korean children with attention deficit hyperactivity disorder. *Psychiatry Investig* **6:** 216–21.

Kim BN, Cho SC, Kim Y, Shin MS, Yoo HJ, Kim JW, Yang YH, Kim HW, Bhang SY, Hong YC (2009a) Phthalates exposure and attention deficit/hyperactivity disorder in school-age children. *Biol Psychiatry* **66:** 958–63.

Kim HS, Kim TS, Shin JH, Moon HJ, Kang IH, Kim IY, Oh JY, Han SY (2004) Neonatal exposure to di(n-butyl) phthalate (DBP) alters male reproductive-tract development. *J Toxicol Environ Health A* **67:** 2045–60.

Kimber I, Dearman RJ (2010) An assessment of the ability of phthalates to influence immune and allergic responses. *Toxicology* **271:** 73–82.

Kluwe WM (1982) Overview of phthalate ester pharmacokinetics in mammalian species. *Environ Health Perspect* **45:** 3–9.

Koch HM, Bolt HM, Preuss R, Angerer J (2005a) New metabolites of di(2-ethylhexyl)phthalate (DEHP) in human urine and serum after single oral doses of deuterium-labelled DEHP. *Arch Toxicol* **79:** 367–76.

Koch HM, Bolt HM, Preuss R, Eckstein R, Weisbach V, Angerer J (2005b) Intravenous exposure to di-(2ethylhexyl)phthalate (DEHP): metabolites of DEHP in urine after a voluntary platelet donation. *Arch Toxicol* **79:** 689–93.

Koch HM, Calafat AM (2009) Human body burdens of chemicals used in plastic manufacture. *Philos Trans R Soc Lond B Biol Sci* **364:** 2063–78.

Koch HM, Drexler H, Angerer J (2003a) An estimation of the daily intake of di(2-ethylhexyl)phthalate (DEHP) and other phthalates in the general population. *Int J Hyg Environ Health* **206:** 77–83.

Koch HM, Preuss R, Angerer J (2006) Di(2-ethylhexyl)phthalate (DEHP): human metabolism and internal exposure – an update and latest results. *Int J Androl* **29:** 155–65.

Koch HM, Rossbach B, Drexler H, Angerer J (2003b) Internal exposure of the general population to DEHP and other phthalates – determination of secondary and primary phthalate monoester metabolites in urine. *Environ Res* **93:** 177–85.

Kohn MC, Melnick RL (2007) Biochemical origins of the non-monotonic receptor-mediated dose–response. *J Mol Endocrinol* **29:** 113–23.

Kolarik B, Naydenov K, Larsson M, Bornehag CG, Sundell J (2008) The association between phthalates in dust and allergic diseases among Bulgarian children. *Environ Health Perspect* **116:** 98–103.

Koo HJ, Lee BM (2007) Toxicokinetic relationships between di-(2-ethylhexyl)-phthalate (DEHP) and mono(2-ethylhexyl)-phthalate in rats. *J Toxicol Environ Health* **70:** 383–7.

Kueseng P, Thavarungkul P, Kanatharana P (2007) Trace phthalate and adipate esters contaminated in packaged food. *J Environ Sci Health B* **42:** 569–76.

Larsen ST, Hansen JS, Hansen EW, Clausen PA, Nielsen GD (2007) Airway inflammation and adjuvant effect after repeated airborne exposures to di-(2-ethylhexyl)phthalate and ovalbumin in BALB/c mice. *Toxicology* **235:** 119–29.

Larsen ST, Lund RM, Nielsen GD, Thygesen P, Poulsen OM (2001) Di-(2-ethylhexyl) phthalate possesses an adjuvant effect in a subcutaneous injection model with BALB/c mice. *Toxicol Lett* **125:** 11–18.

Larsson M, Weiss B, Janson S, Sundell J, Bornehag CG (2009) Associations between indoor environmental factors and parental-reported autistic spectrum disorders in children 6–8 years of age. *Neurotoxicology* **30:** 822–31.

Latini G (2005) Monitoring phthalate exposure in humans. *Clin Chim Acta* **361:** 20–9.

Latini G, De Felice C, Del Vecchio A, Presta G, De Mitri B, Ruggieri F, Mazzeo P (2003a) Lactational exposure to di-(2-ethylhexyl)-phthalate. *Pediatr Res* **54:** 56A.

Latini G, De Felice C, Presta G, Del Vecchio A, Paris I, Ruggieri F, Mazzeo P (2003b) In utero exposure to di-(2-ethylhexyl) phthalate and duration of human pregnancy. *Environ Health Perspect* **111:** 1783–5.

Latini G, De Felice C, Verrotti A (2004) Plasticizers, infant nutrition and reproductive health. *Reprod Toxicol* **19:** 27–33.

Latini G, Del Vecchio A, Massaro M, Verrotti A, De Felice C (2006) In utero exposure to phthalates and fetal development. *Curr Med Chem* **13:** 2527–34.

Latini G, Marcovecchio ML, Del Vecchio A, Gallo F, Bertino E, Chiarelli F (2009) Influence of environment on insulin sensitivity. *Environ Int* **35:** 987–93.

Lee MH, Park J, Chung SW, Kang BY, Kim SH, Kim TS (2004) Enhancement of interleukin-4 production in activated CD4+ T cells by diphthalate plasticizers via increased NF-AT binding activity. *Int Arch Allergy Immunol* **134:** 213–22.

Lehmann KP, Phillips S, Sar M, Foster PM, Gaido KW (2004) Dose-dependent alterations in gene expression and testosterone synthesis in the fetal testes of male rats exposed to di (n-butyl) phthalate. *Toxicol Sci* **81:** 1–2.

Lemberger T, Braissant O, Juge-Aubry C, Keller H, Saladin R, Staels B, Auwerx J, Burger AG, Meier CA, Wahli W (1996) PPAR tissue distribution and interactions with other hormone-signaling pathways. *Ann NY Acad Sci* **804:** 231–51.

Li LH, Jester WF Jr, Laslett AL, Orth JM (2000) A single dose of di-(2-ethylhexyl) phthalate in neonatal rats alters gonocytes, reduces Sertoli cell proliferation, and decreases cyclin D2 expression. *Toxicol Appl Pharmacol* **166:** 222–9.

Loff S, Kabs F, Witt K, Sartoris J, Mandl B, Niessen KH, Waag KL (2000) Polyvinylchloride infusion lines expose infants to large amounts of toxic plasticizers. *J Pediatr Surg* **35:** 1775–81.

Lottrup G, Andersson AM, Leffers H, Mortensen GK, Toppari J, Skakkebaek NE, Main KM (2006) Possible impact of phthalates on infant reproductive health. *Int J Androl* **29:** 172–80; discussion 181–5.

Lovekamp TN, Davis BJ (2001) Mono-(2-ethylhexyl) phthalate suppresses aromatase transcript levels and estradiol production in cultured rat granulosa cells. *Toxicol Appl Pharmacol* **172:** 217–24.

Lovekamp-Swan T, Davis BJ (2003) Mechanisms of phthalate ester toxicity in the female reproductive system. *Environ Health Perspect* **111:** 139–45.

Main KM, Mortensen GK, Kaleva MM, Boisen KA, Damgaard IN, Chellakooty M, Schmidt IM, Suomi AM, Virtanen HE, Petersen DV, Andersson AM, Toppari J, Skakkebaek NE (2006) Human breast milk contamination with phthalates and alterations of endogenous reproductive hormones in three months old infants. *Environ Health Perspect* **114:** 270–6.

Maloney EK, Waxman DJ (1999) trans-Activation of PPARalpha and PPARgamma by structurally diverse environmental chemicals. *Toxicol Appl Pharmacol* **161:** 209–18.

Masuo Y, Morita M, Oka S, Ishido M (2004) Motor hyperactivity caused by a deficit in dopaminergic neurons and the effects of endocrine disruptors: a study inspired by the physiological roles of PACAP in the brain. *Regul Pept* **123**: 225–34.

Matsumoto M, Hirata-Koizumi M, Ema M (2008) Potential adverse effects of phthalic acid esters on human health: a review of recent studies on reproduction. *Reg Toxicol Pharmacol* **50:** 37–49.

McKee RH (2004) Phthalate exposure and early thelarche. *Environ Health Perspect* **112:** A541–A543.

McKinnell C, Sharpe RM, Mahood K, Hallmark N, Scott H, Ivell R, Staub C, Jégou B, Haag F, Koch-Nolte F, Hartung S (2005) Expression of insulin-like factor 3 protein in the rat testis during fetal and postnatal development and in relation to cryptorchidism induced by in utero exposure to di (n-Butyl) phthalate. *Endocrinology* **146:** 4536–44.

Meeker JD, Calafat AM, Hauser R (2007) Di(2-ethylhexyl) phthalate metabolites may alter thyroid hormone levels in men. *Environ Health Perspect* **115:** 1029–34.

Meeker JD, Sathyanarayana S, Swan SH (2009) Phthalates and other additives in plastics: human exposure and associated health outcomes. *Philos Trans R Soc Lond B Biol Sci* **364:** 2097–113.

Moore RW, Rudy TA, Lin TM, Ko K, Peterson RE (2001) Abnormalities of sexual development in male rats with in utero and lactational exposure to the antiandrogenic plasticizer di(2-ethylhexyl) phthalate. *Environ Health Perspect* **109:** 229–37.

Mortensen GK, Main KM, Andersson AM, Leffers H, Skakkebaek NE (2005) Determination of phthalate monoesters in human milk, consumer milk, and infant formula by tandem mass spectrometry (LC-MS-MS). *Anal Bioanal Chem* **382:** 1084–92.

Mose T, Knudsen LE, Hedegaard M, Mortensen GK (2007) Transplacental transfer of monomethyl phthalate and mono(2-ethylhexyl) phthalate in a human placenta perfusion system. *Int J Toxicol* **26:** 221–9.

Mu YM, Yanase T, Nishi Y, Takayanagi R, Goto K, Nawata H (2001) Combined treatment with specific ligands for PPARgamma:RXR nuclear receptor system markedly inhibits the expression of cytochrome P450arom in human granulosa cancer cells. *Mol Cell Endocrinol* **181:** 239–48.

Mylchreest E, Cattley RC, Foster PM (1998) Male reproductive tract malformations in rats following gestational and lactational exposure to di(n-butyl) phthalate: an antiandrogenic mechanism? *Toxicol Sci* **43:** 47–60.

Mylchreest E, Wallace DG, Cattley RC, Foster PM (2000) Dose-dependent alterations in androgen-regulated male reproductive development in rats exposed to di(n-butyl) phthalate during late gestation. *Toxicol Sci* **55:** 143–51.

Mylchreest E, Sar M, Wallace DG, Foster PM (2002) Fetal testosterone insufficiency and abnormal proliferation of Leydig cells and gonocytes in rats exposed to di(n-butyl) phthalate. *Reprod Toxicol* **16:** 19–28.

Nef S, Parada LF (2000) Hormones in male sexual development. *Genes Dev* **14:** 3075–86.

Newbold RR, Padilla-Banks E, Snyder RJ, Phillips TM, Jefferson WN (2007) Developmental exposure to endocrine disruptors and the obesity epidemic. *Reprod Toxicol* **23:** 290–6.

Ng KM, Chu I, Bronaugh RL, Franklin CA, Somers DA (1992) Percutaneous absorption and metabolism of pyrene, benzo[a]pyrene, and di(2-ethylhexyl) phthalate: comparison of in vitro and in vivo results in the hairless guinea pig. *Toxicol Appl Pharmacol* **115:** 216–23.

O'Connor JC, Frame SR, Ladics GS (2002) Evaluation of a 15-day screening assay using intact male rats for identifying anti-androgens. *Toxicol Sci* **69:** 92–108.

Ohara N, Tsujino T, Maruo T (2004) The role of thyroid hormone in trophoblast function, early pregnancy maintenance, and fetal neurodevelopment. J Obstet Gynaecol Can **26:** 982–90.

Otake T, Yoshinaga J, Yanagisawa Y (2004) Exposure to phthalate esters from indoor environment. *J Exp Anal Environ Epidemiol* **14:** 524–8.

Pan G, Hanaoka T, Yoshimura M, Zhang S, Wang P, Tsukino H, Inoue K, Nakazawa H, Tsugane S, Takahasho K (2006) Decreased serum free testosterone in workers exposed to high levels of di-*n*-butyl phthalate (DBP) and di-2-ethylhexyl phthalate (DEHP): a cross section study in China. *Environ Health Perspect* **114:** 1643–8.

Parks LG, Ostby JS, Lambright CR, Abbott BD, Klinefelter GR, Barlow NJ, Gray LE Jr (2000) The plasticizer diethylhexyl phthalate induces malformations by decreasing fetal testosterone synthesis during sexual differentiation in the male rat. *Toxicol Sci* **58:** 339–49.

Petersen JH, Breindahl T (2000) Plasticizers in total diet samples, baby food and infant formulae. *Food Additiv Contam* **17:** 133–41.

Poon R, Lecavalier P, Mueller R, Valli VE, Procter BG, Chu I (1997) Subchronic oral toxicity of di-n-octyl phthalate and di(2-ethyl-hexyl) phthalate in the rat. *Food Chem Toxicol* **35:** 225–39.

Pop VJ, Kuijpens JL, van Baar AL, Verkerk G, van Son MM,de Vijlder JJ, Vulsma T, Wiersinga WM, Drexhage HA, Vader HL (1999) Low maternal free thyroxine concentrations during early pregnancy are associated with impaired psychomotor development in infancy. *Clin Endocrinol (Oxf)* **50:** 149–55.

Poppe K, Velkeniers B, Glinoer D (2007) Thyroid disease and female reproduction. *Clin Endocrinol* **66:** 309–21.

Preuss R, Koch HM, Angerer J (2005) Biological monitoring of the five major metabolites of di-(2-ethylhexyl)phthalate (DEHP) in human urine using column-switching liquid chromatography-tandem mass spectrometry. *J Chromatogr B Anal Technol Biomed Life Sci* **816:** 269–80.

Rais-Bahrami K, Nunez S, Revenis ME, Luban LC, Short BL (2004) Adolescents exposed to DEHP in plastic tubing as neonates: research briefs. *Pediatr Nurs* **30:** 406–33.

Reddy BS, Rozati R, Reddy BV, Raman NV (2006) Association of phthalate esters with endometriosis in Indian women. *BJOG* **113:** 515–20.

Rider CV, Wilson VS, Howdeshell KL, Hotchkiss AK, Furr JR, Lambright CR, Gray LE Jr (2009) Cumulative effects of in utero administration of mixtures of "antiandrogens" on male rat reproductive development. *Toxicol Pathol* **37:** 100–13.

Román GC (2007) Autism: transient in utero hypothyroxinemia related to maternal flavonoid ingestion during pregnancy and to other environmental antithyroid agents. *J Neurol Sci* **262:** 15–26.

Rozati R, Reddy PP, Reddanna P, Mujtaba R (2002) Role of environmental estrogens in the deterioration of male factor fertility. *Fertil Steril* **78:** 1187–94.

Rusyn I, Peters JM, Cunningham ML (2006) Modes of action and species-specific effects of di-(2-ethylhexyl)phthalate in the liver. *Crit Rev Toxicol* **36:** 459–79.

Ryu JY, Lee BM, Kacew S, Kim HS (2007b) Identification of differentially expressed genes in the testis of Sprague-Dawley rats treated with di(n-butyl) phthalate. *Toxicology* **234:** 103–12.

Ryu JY, Whang J, Park H, Im JY, Kim J, Ahn MY, Lee J, Kim HS, Lee BM, Yoo SD, Kwack SJ, Oh JH, Park KL, Han SY, Kim SH (2007a) Di(2-ethylhexyl) phthalate induces apoptosis through peroxisome proliferators-activated receptor-gamma and ERK 1/2 activation in testis of Sprague-Dawley rats. *J Toxicol Environ Health A* **70:** 1296–303.

Salazar-Martinez E, Romano-Riquer P, Yanez-Marquez E, Longnecker MP, Hernandez-Avila M (2004) Anogenital distance in human male and female newborns: a descriptive, cross-sectional study. *Environ Health* **3:** 8.

Sathyanarayana S, Karr CJ, Lozano P, Brown E, Calafat AM, Liu F, Swan SH (2008) Baby care products: possible sources of infant phthalate exposure. *Pediatrics* **121:** 260–8.

Schaffer C, Carpenter C, Smyth H Jr (1945) Acute and subacute toxicity of di(2-ethylhexyl)phthalate with note upon its metabolism. *J Ind Hyg Toxicol* **27:** 130–5.

Schettler T (2006) Human exposure to phthalates via consumer products. *Int J Androl* **29:** 134–9; discussion 181–5.

Schilling K, Gembardt C, Hellwig J (2001) Di-2-ethylhexyl phthalate-two generation reproduction toxicity study in Wistar rats, continous dietary administration, Germany: BASF Atiengesellchaft.

Schmid P, Schlatter C (1985) Excretion and metabolism of di(2-ethylhexyl) phthalate in man. *Xenobiotica* **15:** 251–6.

Schultz R, Yan W, Toppari J, Völkl A, Gustafsson JA, Pelto-Huikko M (1999) Expression of peroxisome proliferator-activated receptor alpha messenger ribonucleic acid and protein in human and rat testis. *Endocrinology* **140:** 2968–75.

Scott RC, Dugard PH, Ramsey JD, Rhodes C (1987) In vitro absorption of some o-phthalate diesters through human and rat skin. *Environ Health Perspect* **74:** 223–7.

Sharman M, Read WA, Castle L, Gilbert J (1994) Levels of di-(2-ethylhexyl) phthalate and total phthalate esters in milk, cream, butter and cheese. *Food Add Contam* **11:** 375–85.

Sharpe RM (2006) Pathways of endocrine disruption during male sexual differentiation and masculinization. *Best Pract Res Clin Endocrinol Metab* **20:** 91–110.

Sharpe RM, Skakkebaek NE (2008) Testicular dysgenesis syndrome: mechanistic insights and potential new downstream effects. *Fertil Steril* **89(2 Suppl.):** 33–8.

Shea KM; American Academy of Pediatrics Committee on Environmental Health (2003) Pediatric exposure and potential toxicity of phthalate plasticizers. *Pediatrics* **111:** 1467–74.

Shirota M, Saito Y, Imai K, Horiuchi S, Yoshimura S, Sato M, Nagao T, Ono H, Katoh M (2005) Influence of di-(2-ethylhexyl)phthalate on fetal testicular development by oral administration to pregnant rats. *J Toxicol Sci* **30:** 175–94.

Shultz VD, Phillips S, Sar M, Foster PM, Gaido KW (2001) Altered gene profiles in fetal rat testes after *in utero* exposure to di(n-butyl) phthalate. *Toxicol Sci* **64:** 233–42.

Silva MJ, Barr DB, Reidy JA, Malek NA, Hodge CC, Caudill SP, Brock JW, Needham LL, Calafat AM (2004a) Urinary levels of seven phthalate metabolites in the U.S. population from the National Health and Nutrition Examination Survey (NHANES) 1999–2000. *Environ Health Perspect* **112:** 331–8.

Silva MJ, Reidy JA, Herbert AR, Preau JL, Needham LL, Calafat AM (2004b) Detection of phthalate metabolites in human amniotic fluid. *Bull Environ Contam Toxicol* **72:** 1226–31.

Silva MJ, Reidy JA, Samandar E, Herbert AR, Needham LL, Calafat AM (2005) Detection of phthalate metabolites in human saliva. *Arch Toxicol* **79:** 647–52.

Skakkebaek NE, Jørgensen N, Main KM, Rajpert-De Meyts E, Leffers H, Andersson AM, Juul A, Carlsen E, Mortensen GK, Jensen TK, Toppari J (2006) Is human fecundity declining? *Int J Androl* **29:** 2–11.

Srivastava S, Awasthi VK, Srivastava SP, Seth PK (1989) Biochemical alterations in rat fetal liver following in utero exposure to di(2-ethylhexyl) phthalate (DEHP). *Indian J Exp Biol* **27:** 885–8.

Stahlhut RW, van Wijngaarden E, Dye TD, Cook S, Swan SH (2007) Concentrations of urinary phthalate metabolites are associated with increased waist circumference and insulin resistance in adult U.S. males. *Environ Health Perspect* **115(6):** 876–82.

Subotic U, Hannmann T, Kiss M, Brade J, Breitkopf K, Loff S (2007) Extraction of the plasticizers diethylhexylphthalate and polyadipate from polyvinylchloride nasogastric tubes through gastric juice and feeding solution. *J Ped Gastroenter Nutr* **44:** 71–6.

Swan SH, Main KM, Liu F, Stewart SL, Kruse RL, Calafat AM, Mao CS, Redmon JB, Ternand CL, Sullivan S, Teague JL, Study for the Future of Families Research Team (2005) Decrease in anogenital distance among male infants with prenatal phthalate exposure. *Environ Health Perspect* **113:** 1056–61.

Tanida T, Warita K, Ishihara K, Fukui S, Mitsuhashi T, Sugawara T, Tabuchi Y, Nanmori T, Qi WM, Inamoto T, Yokoyama T, Kitagawa H, Hoshi N (2009) Fetal and neonatal exposure to three typical environmental chemicals with different mechanisms of action: mixed exposure to phenol, phthalate, and dioxin cancels the effects of sole exposure on mouse midbrain dopaminergic nuclei. *Toxicol Lett* **189:** 40–7.

Tomita I, Nakamura Y, Yagi Y, Tutikawa K (1986) Fetotoxic effects of mono-2-ethylhexyl phthalate (MEHP) in mice. *Environ Health Perspect* **65:** 249–54.

Tomonari Y, Kurata Y, David RM, Gans G, Kawasuso T, Katoh M (2006) Effect of di(2-ethylhexyl) phthalate (DEHP) on genital organs from juvenile common marmosets: I. Morphological and biochemical investigation in 65-week toxicity study. *J Toxicol Environ Health A* **69:** 1651–72.

Tsumura Y, Ishimitsu S, Kaihara A, Yoshii K, Nakamura Y, Tonogai Y (2001a) Di(2-ethylhexyl) phthalate contamination of retail packed lunches caused by PVC gloves used in the preparation of foods. *Food Additiv Contam* **18:** 569–79.

Tsumura Y, Ishimitsu S, Saito I, Sakai, H., Kobayashi Y, Tonogai Y (2001b) Eleven phthalate esters and di(2-ethylhexyl) adipate in one-week duplicate diet samples obtained from hospitals and their estimated daily intake. *Food Additiv Contam* **18:** 449–60.

Tsumura Y, Ishimitsu S, Saito I, Sakai H, Tsuchida Y, Tonogai Y (2003) Estimated daily intake of plasticizers in 1-week duplicate diet samples following regulation of DEHP-containing PVC gloves in Japan. *Food Additiv Contam* **20:** 317–24.

Tyl RW, Myers CB, Marr MC, Fail PA, Seely JC, Brine DR, Barter RA, Butala JH (2004) Reproductive toxicity evaluation of dietary butyl benzyl phthalate (BBP) in rats. *Reprod Toxicol* **18:** 241–64.

Vickers MH (2007) Developmental programming and adult obesity: the role of leptin. *Curr Opin Endocrinol Diabetes Obes* **14:** 17–22.

Waterman SJ, Ambroso JL, Keller LH, Trimmer GW, Nikiforov AI, Harris SB (1999) Developmental toxicity of di-isodecyl and di-isononyl phthalates in rats. *Reprod Toxicol* **13:** 131–6.

Weuve J, Sánchez BN, Calafat AM, Schettler T, Green RA, Hu H, Hauser R (2006) Exposure to phthalates in neonatal intensive care unit infants: urinary concentrations of monoesters and oxidative metabolites. *Environ Health Perspect* **114:** 1424–31.

Wilson VS, Lambright C, Furr J, Ostby J, Wood C, Held G, Gray LE Jr (2004) Phthalate ester-induced gubernacular lesions are associated with reduced insl3 gene expression in the fetal rat testis. *Toxicol Lett* **146:** 207–15.

Wittassek M, Wiesmüller GA, Koch HM, Eckert R, Dobler L, Müller J, Angerer J, Schlütter C (2007) Internal phthalate exposure over the last two decades – a retrospective human biomonitoring study. *Int J Hyg Environ-Health* **210:** 319–33.

Wormuth M, Scheringer M, Vollenweider M, Hungerbühler K (2006) What are the sources of exposure to eight frequently used phthalic esters in Europeans? *Risk Anal* **26:** 803–24.

Zhang YH, Zheng LX, Chen BH (2006) Phthalate exposure and human semen quality in Shanghai: a cross-sectional study. *Biomed Environ Sci* **19:** 205–9.

Zhu J, Phillips SP, Feng YL, Yang X (2006) Phthalate esters in human milk: concentration variations over 6-month postpartum time. *Environ Sci Technol* **40:** 5276–81.

CHAPTER

49

Organotins (tributyltin and triphenyltin)

John D. Doherty and William A. Irwin

Disclaimer. This chapter was prepared to stimulate interest in and discussion of the toxicity issues related to organotins and no references to regulatory policy are implied. The opinions expressed in this review are the opinions of the authors and do not represent the views and/or policy of the United States Environmental Protection Agency.

INTRODUCTION

Organotins (OTs) are a family of chemicals that vary widely in their toxicity. The family includes potent neurotoxicants and immunotoxicants and some OTs have characteristics of reproductive and developmental toxicants. From an environmental toxicological perspective, the two most widely studied OTs are tributyltin (TBT)[1] and triphenyltin (TPhT). For many years TBT was used to control fouling of boat bottoms by mollusks, as a wood preservative and general biocide and TPhT has many applications as a fungicide, acaricide and insecticide. OTs also have uses as stabilizers in plastics, rubber and other materials. The use of OTs has resulted in contamination of waterways and it is generally recognized that water contaminated with certain OTs is correlated with imposex or the formation of male sex organs in females especially in gastropods (Horiguchi *et al.*, 1997; Gagné *et al.*, 2003). Alterations in endocrine function or disruption have been established in the process of masculinization of female mollusks (Siah *et al.*, 2003; Iguchi *et al.*, 2007) and fish species (McAllister and Kime, 2003; Shimasaki *et al.*, 2003). Although the effects of the OTs in aquatic species are better established, the potential for OTs to affect the mammalian endocrine systems and reproduction and development is less well characterized. TBT (Dobson, 1990; Benson, 1997) and TPhT (Sekizawa, 1999) are currently regulated on their immunotoxicity potential but effects on reproduction and development occur at higher doses than effects observed for other endpoints in the studies submitted to support the registration of these chemicals as pesticides. This chapter provides the latest information on TBT's and TPhT's ability to affect the reproductive organs and developmental toxicity in mammals, and includes detailed studies reporting alterations in hormonal levels *in vivo*, inhibition of enzymes in steroidogenesis and the interactions with nuclear receptors. The role of the mitochondria as a target is discussed to correlate these findings with a proposed common mechanism of action for TBT and TPhT toxicity.

HISTORICAL BACKGROUND

The subject of OTs and reproduction and development in mammals has been reviewed (Ema and Hirose, 2006). It is generally accepted that the predominant effects of both TBT and TPhT in male rats include degeneration of the testis and other male structures, including the prostate as well as decreased spermatogenesis. In female rats, TBT and TPhT have been shown to reduce fertility by interfering with decidualization and preventing implantation, an effect that is reversed by progesterone. TBT and TPhT inhibit aromatase, the enzyme responsible for converting androgens to estrogens. The evidence that aromatase, or some aspect of steroidogenesis, is involved in the formation of imposex in female mollusks is supported because the specific inhibitor of aromatase (atamestane) mimics TBT in the formation of imposex and adding steroids to the water reverses TBT-induced imposex, as does adding an antiandrogen agent cyproterone acetate (Bettin *et al.*, 1996). Male and female sexual development and successful implantation in mammals are dependent on hormones. The possibility that TPhT is an endocrine disruptor in mammals has been discussed previously (Golub and Doherty, 2004). Aromatase inhibition does not seem to be the sole mode of action of TBT and TPHT (Grun and Blumberg, 2006; Iguchi *et al.*, 2008; Nakanishi, 2008). These reviews discuss that TBT and TPhT are agonists at nanomolar (nM) concentrations for the retinoid X (RXR) and/or the peroxisome proliferator-activated nuclear receptors (PPARγ) that are intricately involved with steroid hormone production and related cellular alterations. The broader interpretation of these reviews is that the OTs may act, in part, through activation of the nuclear receptors in concert with aromatase inhibition and that other cellular

[1]TBT is currently registered in the USA as the oxide, maleate and benzoate compounds and use is restricted to minimize human exposure. TPhT is registered as the hydroxide form and has current uses as a fungicide, acaricide and insecticide and has tolerances for several food items.

Reproductive and Developmental Toxicology, Edited by Ramesh C. Gupta
ISBN: 978-0-12-382032-7

physiological/biochemical processes play a role in toxicological outcomes. It has been known for many years that some OTs affect basic mitochondrial functions (Aldrich *et al.*, 1977; Kass *et al.*, 1999) and that these effects may contribute to the toxicity OTs (Golub and Doherty, 2004).

CHEMISTRY, METABOLISM AND PHARMACOKINETICS OF OTs

An understanding of the toxicity of OTs requires an understanding of their chemistry, metabolism and pharmacokinetics in the body. This section describes certain aspects of the OTs that we took into account to develop a new proposed model for OT mechanism of action.

Multiple chemical forms of OTs

In commercial OT products, the organically substituted tin is commonly associated with anions such as halides, acetate, hydroxide, oxide, benzoate, hydride, maleate or methacrylate. In water, the halide and acetate forms of TPhT are hydrolyzed to the hydroxide form that has a water solubility of only 2.7 μM which must be considered in experimental result analysis. TPhT is hydrophobic, with a log K_{OW} of 3.43, and the hydrophobicity is an important aspect of the proposed model for OTs' mechanism of action. In some cases the anion has two OTs associated with it as in *bis*-tributylin. OTs commonly occur in the tri-substituted form, but di- and mono- variations have some commercial uses and occur often resulting from metabolism from the tri-substituted forms. For the sake of simplicity in this chapter, the anion form of TBT or TPhT is not mentioned since the focus of this chapter is to examine the evidence that organotin moiety of TBT or TPhT causes the observed adverse effect. It should not be implied that all anionic forms of the OTs will have exactly the same potential toxicity.

Organotin chemistry

Tin belongs to Group 14 elements, whose bonding type to other molecules depends on the radius of the atom. The larger the radius, the more likely the compound will have ionic bonding. Carbon has the smallest radius and therefore has almost entirely covalent bonding, while tin has a much larger atomic radius, thus its bonding has been described as the "ionic covalent" type. For example, one form of organotin, tributyltin hydride, is sometimes called TBTH cation and a model by Aldridge also depicts OTs with a positive charge (Aldridge *et al.*, 1977). Triethyltin (TET) has been classified as an anionophore, supporting its cationic nature (Davidoff *et al.*, 1978). It is possible that TBT and TPhT are also anionophores. OTs can form free radicals and are commonly utilized in organic synthesis due to this reactivity. These characteristics of organotin chemistry may also explain some of their adverse effects.

Tissue retention and lactational transfer

Some aspects of the pharmacokinetics of OTs (Appel, 2004) that are considered important to reproductive and developmental toxicity are described in this paragraph. OTs do not seem to have a specific affinity for male or female reproductive organs. The kidney and liver (oxidative tissues) have been shown to have the highest levels of TBT or TPhT concentration in rats following oral dosing. The testis also may accumulate some TPhT since content in the testis was increased following repeat dosing but only by a slightly higher factor than for the kidney. Exposure to TBT on gestation day 8 until weaning demonstrated that suckling rat pups had negligible levels of either TBT or dibutyltin (DBT) in their stomachs indicating that lactational transfer of TBT is insignificant (Cooke *et al.*, 2004). Another comprehensive study (Cooke *et al.*, 2008) assessed the tissue distribution and speciation of TBT and its metabolites in rat dams, fetuses and neonates. In this study, rat dams were dosed orally with TBT on gestation day 8 through lactation day 20. The tissues from both the dam and fetuses were harvested at gestation day 20 and PND 6 and 12 for the pups, and analyzed for TBT and its metabolites. It was concluded that TBT crosses the placenta, but that exposure via lactation was limited because of the low level of TBT in the milk of the dams. The GD 20 fetuses generally had the highest concentration in the liver and brains and these levels were about 50% less than the corresponding levels in the dams. The TBT level declined during weaning but DBT in the weanlings tended to increase, probably by conversion from TBT. Several studies by Ema and his colleagues (Ema and Hirose, 2006) were conducted with DBT, assuming it is the more active form for inducing reproductive effects. There was no detectable TPhT or its metabolites in rat milk following an acute dose. After 10 days of dosing with 4 mg/kg, mean concentrations of total TPhT in rat milk were 0.10 ± 0.03 μg/mL 6 hours post-dose. The residues in milk were below the limits of detection within 5 days of cessation of treatment (Taylor *et al.*, 2003). TBT crosses the blood–brain barrier and based on some indirect behavioral studies TPhT is also thought to cross the blood–brain barrier (Appel, 2004).

Organotin bioaccumulation in cells

Pharmacokinetics is important to understand the toxicity and mechanisms of the OTs and this section describes how both the hydrophobicity and charge are important determinants of distribution of OTs within cells. Electron micrographs of tissue have revealed organotin compound precipitation inside the mitochondria, with similarity to Nernst cationic dyes like JC-1, which also accumulate in the mitochondria and form aggregates (Cima *et al.*, 1996). The Nernst equation, for which Walter Nernst won the Nobel Prize in 1920, describes how ion gradients form electrical potentials. The Nernst equation also predicts how charged molecules can be partitioned across membranes by membrane potentials and this phenomenon is commonly utilized to measure membrane potentials in cells by employing organic cation dyes (Figure 49.1).

TPhT has a striking structural similarity to tetraphenyl phosphonium, a membrane potential probe with almost ideal Nernst properties (i.e., accumulation closely agrees with Nernst equation predictions). The Nernst equation states that hydrophobic cations are concentrated by a factor of 10 for each 61.5 mV of membrane potential. The plasma membrane typically has a membrane potential of 60–70 mV, while the mitochondria typically have a membrane potential of 180–220 mV. These data suggest that organotin cations could be concentrated by a factor of 10 into the cytosol and by another factor of 1,000 into the mitochondria. Overall,

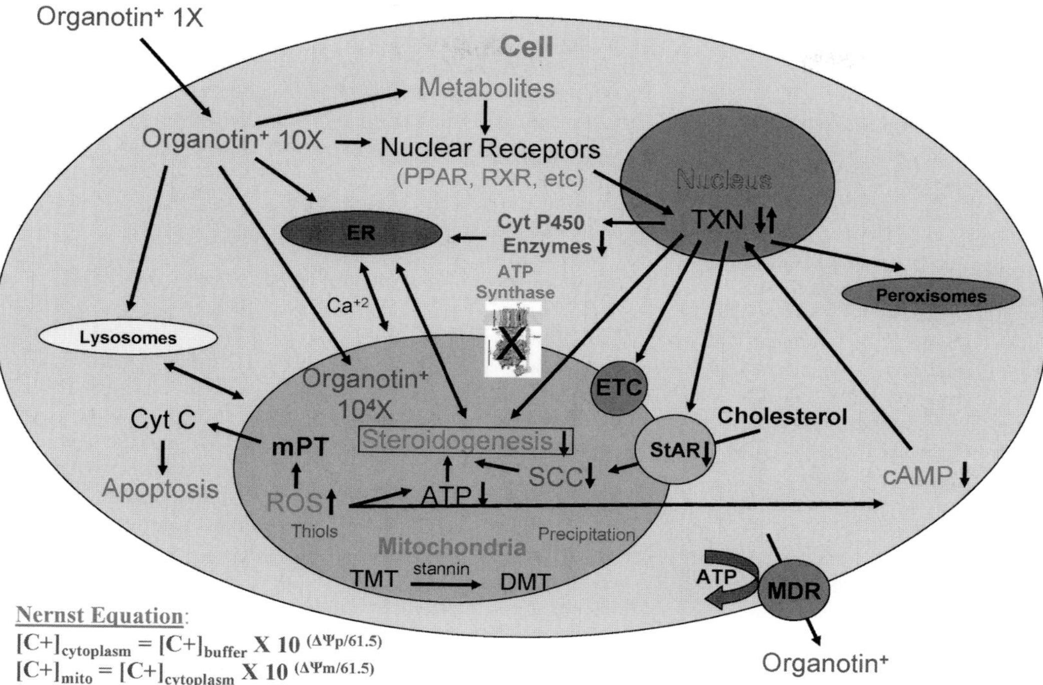

FIGURE 49.1 Organotin integrative model of toxicity. Organotins and their metabolites have effects on cells at multiple levels, including nuclear receptors, gene transcription, enzyme inhibition, free radical production, ATP generation, steroid production and apoptosis. Organotin cations can be bio-accumulated into the cells according to the Nernst equation, by a factor of 10 into the cytosol and by a factor of 10,000 into the mitochondria. Abbreviations: Cyt C – cytochrome C; SCC – side chain cleavage enzyme or desmolase; ROS – reactive oxygen species; ATP – adenosine triphosphate; TXN – transcription; mPT – mitochondrial permeability transition (swelling); ETC – electron transport chain; StAR – steroid hormone acute regulatory protein; Cyt P450 – cytochrome P450 enzymes; cAMP – cyclic adenosine monophosphate; TMT – trimethyltin; DMT– dimethyltin; $\Delta\Psi_p$ – plasma membrane potential in mV; $\Delta\Psi_m$ – mitochondrial potential; ER – endoplasmic reticulum; MDR – multi-drug resistance xenobiotic pumps. Please refer to color plate section.

OTs could be concentrated by several orders of magnitude into the mitochondria relative to extracellular concentrations and this might explain their high bioaccumulation not predicted by hydrophobicity alone. Even if only a few percent of organotin compounds exist in the ionic bonding state in the extracellular space as more organotin cation is taken up by the cells from the extracellular space, the extracellular equilibrium would shift to the ionic cation form by Le Chatelier's principle. Thus, a considerable amount of organotin cation could be taken up by cells and mitochondria by the Nernst effect. Curiously, several studies have shown that hydrophobic TPhT does not predominantly concentrate in the fatty tissues (Sekizawa, 1999). Rather TPhT concentrates in mitochondrial-rich tissues such as liver, kidney and muscle, suggesting a completely different model of bioaccumulation and tissue persistence (Berge *et al.*, 2004) such as through a Nernst principle model. Also, inhibition of specific cytochrome (cyt) P450 enzymes by TBT is much more pronounced in intact cells vs. isolated organelles, suggesting that the intact cells bioconcentrate TBT to inhibit enzymes more extensively (Yamazaki *et al.*, 2005), Eventually, the Nernst accumulation model may be able to explain multiple discrepancies in the data related to why EC_{50} at both the nM and μM levels of OTs *in vitro* can have such profound effects on cells *in vivo* since their effective concentrations within the cells organelles may be much higher than external levels. Thus, the charge as well as the hydrophobic nature of the OTs may be important to their toxicity.

TOXICITY

General toxicity

The effects of the OTs on reproduction or development need to be considered in the context of overall toxicity. A brief description of other aspects of the potential toxicity of the TBT and TPhT helps to understand models that may be developed for defining the mechanism of toxic action of these OTs.

Systemic toxicity

Inorganic tin is poorly absorbed (i.e., <3%) from the gastrointestinal tract and is relatively non-toxic but can cause acute gastroenteritis. Inclusion of organic substituents on elemental tin results in severe systemic toxicity depending upon the substitution. Many *in vivo* toxicity studies exist, both those described in the literature and studies conducted to support regulatory purposes. In these studies, systemic toxicity of TPhT and TBT is noted at doses starting above 1–5 mg/kg oral dosing, depending upon species, strain, chemical form and vehicle. Body weight decreases commonly occur in toxicity studies at higher doses and may be related to non-specific toxicity. Hepatic alterations are also observed and may be related to increased metabolism of xenobiotics. But since OTs are cytotoxic and potentially affect many enzyme systems, direct toxicity to the liver may also be occurring. Effects on the spleen and thymus may relate to more specific effects on the immune system.

Neurotoxicity and immunotoxicity

The relative specificity of the OTs with regard to nervous and immune systems was described previously (Snoeji *et al.*, 1987) where it was concluded that "the lower trialkyltins (TMTC, TETC) are essentially neurotoxic, the intermediate trialkyltins (TPTC, tripropyl tin chloride, TBTC) and triphenyltin are primarily immunotoxic, and the higher homologs (THTC (trihexyltin chloride), TOTC (trioctyltin chloride)) are only slightly toxic or not toxic at all". This paper also concluded that atrophy of the thymus was considered to be the predominant effect of the intermediate trialkyltins associated with immunotoxicity. A recent report demonstrated that the anti-proliferative effects of TBT and TPhT, rather than apoptosis, are the cause of thymic atrophy (Ueno *et al.*, 2009). The low molecular weight alkyl tins, trimethyltin (TMT) and triethyltin (TET), are well-known potent neurotoxins and are often used as positive controls to establish the reliability of testing laboratories to detect specific responses to a given chemical (Moser, 1996). Although both have short chain alkyl substitute groups, there are significant differences in their neurotoxicity. TMT damages neurons and gray matter (Krinke, 2000a) while TET damages white matter (Krinke, 2000b). Any reproductive and developmental effects that occur from exposure to TMT or TET may be secondary effects of their neurotoxicity as opposed to the TBT and TPhT toxicity pathways. It has been reported that mitochondrial stannin, a protein which is responsible for TMT toxicity (Reese *et al.*, 2005) and a role for stannin in TBT and TPhT toxicity, is possible and under investigation.

Teratogenicity

The Ema and Hirose review (2006) described the results of several studies to assess the developmental effects in offspring assessed at parturition in teratology studies (dosing during gestation and examination of fetuses). These studies demonstrate that at doses that are usually maternally toxic, a variety of visceral and skeletal fetal alterations and malformations may result. These effects are recognized but this chapter focuses on effects on the reproductive tract and developmental effects that may persist to adulthood.

Carcinogenicity

The pesticides fenbutyltin (FenBT) and tricyclohexyltin (TCHT) are not considered carcinogens. The carcinogenicity classification of TBT is confounded because of the high spontaneous rates of benign pituitary tumors, pheochromocytomas and parathyroid tumors in rats; however, there were no increases in tumors in the mouse study deemed to be treatment related. TPhT was determined to be associated with increases in pituitary gland adenomas in females and Leydig cell tumors in rats and liver adenomas and/or carcinomas in mice. The relevance of these increases was considered not significant by the WHO (Sekizawa, 1999) but the WHO report mentioned that the Leydig cell tumors may be a result of hormonal effects. Neither TBT nor TPhT are considered genotoxic or mutagenic.

Reproductive and developmental toxicity

As noted in the introduction section, the purpose of this chapter is to describe the science surrounding the ability of the OTs to cause reproductive and developmental effects and to integrate this information into a comprehensive model for the mechanisms of action for OTs for the reproductive and developmental effects. This section will summarize what is known about the ability of the OTs to disrupt the reproductive function and development.

Effects on the male reproductive system

The effects of TPhT on male adult rats were reported as early as 1968 (Pate and Hayes, 1968). Ema and Hirose (2006) concluded that TPhT when dosed to adult rodents at levels causing weight loss decreased male fertility due to degenerative changes in testicular tissue. TBT caused decreases in the weight of testis, epididymis and ventral prostate and spermatid and sperm counts in male offspring resulting from continuous dosing in a two generation rat reproduction study (Omura *et al.*, 2001). The fertility rate for males in this study was, however, unaffected in the F_1 generation. Table 49.1 lists some more recent studies reinforcing the conclusions of Ema and Hirose, demonstrating the effects of TBT and TPhT in males as a result of dosing at different life stages (fetal, neonatal, pubertal and adult). Recent studies (Yu *et al.*, 2003; Grote *et al.*, 2004; Reddy *et al.*, 2006; Barthelemy *et al.*, 2007; Kishta *et al.*, 2007; Chen *et al.*, 2008) confirm the earlier observations that exposure to pubertal and adult male rats results in decreased testis and prostate weights. Of particular note is that gestational exposure in rats results in increased lipid droplets in Sertoli cells (Kishta *et al.*, 2007). Similar alterations in fat were noted in mice exposed *in utero* where increased epididymal adipose mass was seen when assessed at postnatal day (PND) 70 (Grun *et al.*, 2006). Ectopic adipocytes near gonads were also seen in exposed tadpoles when assessed as mature adult frogs (Grun *et al.*, 2006). As will be discussed later, the increased adipose mass in the epididymides in mice and adipocytes near the gonads in frogs suggest interaction with nuclear receptors leading to these effects. Increase in adipose tissue without increases in organism weight suggests alterations in tissue differentiation, an important component in development and some disease states. Additional support for effects persisting into adulthood in males following gestational and/or early postnatal exposure to TPhT included reduced body weight and reduced weights of the testis, prostate and epididymides, when assessed at PND 64–65 (Grote *et al.*, 2009). TBT also demonstrated delayed preputial separation (Grote *et al.*, 2004). The persistent effect of TBT in the prostate of rats was further analyzed (Barthelemy *et al.*, 2007) and it was demonstrated that following gestational exposure, the decreased prostate weight was associated with permanent developmental alterations in the expression and distribution of adhesion and tight junctional proteins on PND 91.

Effects in females

TPhT caused implantation loss at low doses which was correlated with an effect on decidualization in rodents which in turn correlated with a reduction in progesterone (Ema and Hirose, 2006). Similarly, TBT caused implantation loss, altered

TABLE 49.1 Examples of organotin effects on the male reproductive parameters following dosing to adults or to male offspring with gestational and/or early postnatal exposure

Reference	Chemical	Dosing/Species	Results
Continuous exposure in reproduction study			
Omura *et al.* (2001)	TBT	Continuous in reproduction study in rats	Decreased testis, ventral prostate and epididymis weights, homogenization-resistant sperm and sperm count; vacuolization of seminiferous epithelium, spermatid retention, and delayed spermiation, but no effect on fertility.
Pubertal (post-weaning) and adult male exposure			
Chen *et al.* (2008)	TBT	Puberty in mice	↓Gonadotrophic index ↓Spermatogenesis
Grote *et al.* (2004)	TBT	PND 23 to 53 in rats	Delay in preputial separation ↓Reproductive organ weights
Grote *et al.* (2004)	TPhT	PND 23 to 53 in rats	No effect on preputial separation ↓ Male reproductive organ weights
Yu *et al.* (2003)	TBT	PND 35 to 45 in rats	↓Homogenization-resistant sperm counts, caudal epididymal sperm count, motion kinetic parameters
Reddy *et al.* (2006)	TPhT and FenBT	Adults (i.p.) in mice	↓Sperm count, motility, viability and function (HOS coiling)
Male offspring following gestational/lactational exposure			
Kishta *et al.* (2007)	TBT	GD 0–19 or 8–19 in rats	↑Lipid droplets in Sertoli cells, electron microscopy revealed abnormally dilated endoplasmic reticulum in Sertoli cells and gonocytes, reduced gap junction connexin protein
Sarpa *et al.* (2007)	TPhT	GD 6–17 in mice	Malpositioned testis
Barthelemy *et al.* (2007)	TBT	GD 0–19 in rats	Decreased prostate weight. Permanent alterations in the expression and distribution of adhesion and tight junctional proteins (PND 91)
Makita *et al.* (2004)	TBT	GD 1–PND 21 – rats	Suppressed growth and delayed eye-opening and physical condition; prostate weight (PND 42), interaction with DDE
Grote *et al.* (2009)	TPhT	GD 6–PND 21	Delayed preputial separation, reproductive organ weights (testis, epididymides prostate), body weight, testosterone level (PND 64–5)
Grun *et al.* (2006b)	TBT	GD 12–18	Epididymal adipose mass 20% greater than control. Body weight not increased (PND 70)
Asakawa (2009)	TBT	G/L – rats	↓Total locomotion and distance, wall rearing, thymus weight (PND 105)
Delgado *et al.* (2009)	TPhT	G – mice	Less resistance to *P. yoelii* (PND 50)

GD – Gestation day; PND – Postnatal day; L – lactation

decidualization and a reduction in progesterone. An important series of papers demonstrated that progesterone administration was shown to protect against the TBT effects of inducing implantation loss (Ema and Hirose, 2006). The female responses in a dietary reproductive study (Ogata *et al.*, 2001) where rats were exposed through two generations demonstrated several effects (Table 49.2), such as an increased ano-genital distance in females that suggests masculinization. However, similar to the report in males (Omura *et al.*, 2001) from this same study, the fertility index was not affected. The possibility of biphasic effects on female development was raised by the demonstration that 2mg/kg TPhT (Grote *et al.*, 2006a, 2009) showed advanced vaginal opening but the higher dose of 6mg/kg showed delayed vaginal opening when pubertal rats were dosed (Grote *et al.*, 2006a). Another study from this same laboratory (Waterman *et al.*, 2008) reports that daily exposure of 2 or 6mg/kg TPhT to pubertal or adult rats did not result in histological changes in the oviduct, uterus, vagina and "mamma" but increased the number of follicle cells in tertiary and preovulatory follicles at a dose of 6mg/kg, suggesting hormonal interference. The 6mg/kg dose was also systemically toxic to rats. Of particular interest are two more recent reports (Ema *et al.*, 2007, 2009) on studies with monkeys, where DBT (7.5mg/kg) was demonstrated to be embryolethal but did not have obvious effects in the surviving fetuses. The studies with monkeys unfortunately did not include an assessment of circulating hormone levels in the mothers or a detailed histological assessment of the reproductive organs in either the mothers or the fetuses.

Developmental effects on behavior, learning and memory

The issue of fetal and/or neonatal exposure resulting in altered behavioral parameters in adults, including effects on learning and memory, is of concern for metals as well as other chemicals. An earlier study demonstrated that prenatal exposure on days 7–15 of gestation to TPhT resulted in adverse effects on behavior and conditioned learning in the pups (Lehotzky *et al.*, 1982a,b) and a claim that spontaneous motor activity was increased and conditioned avoidance was acquired more rapidly. Decreased locomotor and wall and center rearing in rats (assessed 15 weeks after administration

TABLE 49.2 Examples of organotin effects on the female reproductive parameters, including dosing during gestation or otherwise, or to female offspring with gestational and/or early postnatal exposure

Reference	Chemical	Dosing/Species	Results
Continuous exposure in reproduction study			
Ogata *et al.* (2001)	TBT	Continuous in reproduction study in rats	Number and body weight of pups percent of live pups decreased. Delay in vaginal opening, eye-opening impaired estrus cyclicity, increase in ano-genital distance to suggest masculinization effect
Pubertal and adult female exposure			
Grote *et al.* (2006a)	TPhT	PND 23 to 33 or to first estrus in rats	Delay in vaginal opening at 6 mg/k but advanced opening at 2 mg/kg ↑Ovarian weight
Waterman *et al.* (2008)	TPhT	PND 23 – first estrus in rats	No histological changes in oviduct, uterus, vagina and mamma but increase in number of all follicle stages and reduction in diameter of tertiary follicles and increase in atretic follicles. Also decrease in number of apoptic cells in the thymus
Exposure during gestation			
Ema *et al.* (2007)	DBT	Several windows of gestation in monkeys	Embryolethality but not teratogenic
Sarpa *et al.* (2007)	TPhT	G 6–17 in mice	Enhanced embryolethality, lower fetal weight, malpositioned uteri
Kishta *et al.* (2007)	TBT	G 0–19 or 8–19 in rats	↓Germ cells in fetuses
Grote *et al.* (2009)	TPhT	G/L – rats	Precocious vaginal opening

of TBT) were also reported in a more current study (Asakawa *et al.*, 2009). Another attempt to assess learning and development in rat pups from dams exposed to 4 or 8 mg/kg of TPhT on days 6 to day 20 of gestation (Miyake *et al.*, 1991) reported that the Sidman avoidance test revealed that the avoidance rate was reduced in females at both TPhT doses. The authors concluded that the gestational TPhT exposure affects the "learning acquisition of rats". Unfortunately the data tables for this study are not available for analysis. Gestational exposure to TBT to rats (at dose levels reported not to affect maternal toxicity) resulted in delayed acquisition in the radial arm maze and a potentiation of d-amphetamine-induced hyperactivity (Gardland *et al.*, 1991). Conversely, a developmental neurotoxicity study in rats with TPhT (Myers *et al.*, 2003), conducted according to current guidelines for submission of data to support product registration, did not demonstrate adverse effects on motor activity or on learning and memory in either the weanlings or the adults. Thus, whether learning and memory in adults can be affected following gestational exposure to OTs remains an area for future investigations.

Developmental effect on the immune system

The issue of whether or not *in utero* exposure to OTs can result in impaired development of the immune system was investigated recently in an experiment where TPhT was administered to pregnant mice on days 6–17 of gestation (Delgado *et al.*, 2008). On PND 50, the pups were challenged with *Plasmodium yoelii* (a commonly used model to test for resistance to malaria). At maternal dosing of ≥15 mg/kg "a shorter latency to peak parasiternia and a reduced malaria-induced spleen enlargement were observed" implying that gestational treatment with TPhT interfered with the response to infection in adulthood. Thus, a developmental effect of TPhT was demonstrated, although a relatively high dose was needed.

MECHANISM OF ACTION

Mechanisms in effects on hormones, steroidogenesis and nuclear receptors

The previous section presented an overview of reports on anatomical alterations, particularly in the sex organs that occur following exposure to OTs and identified alterations persisting to adulthood, including behavioral and immunological, following *in utero* or early postnatal exposure. This section describes reports on the effects TBT and TPhT on circulating hormone levels, enzymes involved in steroidogenesis, nuclear receptors and alterations in mRNA resulting from exposure in an attempt to understand the mechanisms that may be involved in the effects of TBT or TPhT on the reproductive and developmental outcomes.

Alterations in circulating hormones

As potential hormone disruptors, TBT and TPhT might be expected to alter circulating hormone levels leading to the alterations in male and female reproductive and/or developmental effects mentioned above or the otherwise damaged organs may affect hormone levels. Table 49.3 demonstrates that circulating levels for several hormones are altered following administration of TBT or TPhT. Progesterone levels were decreased consistently in several studies investigating the cause of implantation loss (Ema and Hirose, 2006). More recent studies confirm alterations in progesterone (Grote *et al.*, 2006b, 2009) in rats. Testosterone was decreased in several studies (Grote *et al.*, 2004, 2009; Reddy *et al.*, 2006; Chen *et al.*, 2008; Kim *et al.*, 2008) following gavage dosing. However, in the reproduction study (Omura *et al.*, 2001) with continuous dietary dosing it was elevated. Gavage administration

TABLE 49.3 Representative reports demonstrating alterations in circulating hormone levels

Hormone	Dosing	Effect	Reference
Progesterone	• TPhT, DPhT, TBT, DBT all on days 0–3 or 4–7 in pseudopregnant or pregnant rat	• Decreased	• Ema *et al.* (2006)
	• DBT on days GD 0–3 or 4–7	• Decreased	• Ema *et al.* (2007)
	• TPhT: 2 and 6 mg/kg in rats PND 23 to 33 or first estrus	• ↓Slight (ns) decrease at PND 33, ~42–46% decrease at PND 53	• Grote *et al.* (2006a)
	• TPhT: 2 mg/kg in rats until weaning or termination	• No effect	• Grote *et al.* (2009)
Estradiol	• TBT: 100 mg/kg acute dose to 3-week-old mice testis	• ↓~22% (ns)	• Kim *et al.* (2008)
	• TPhT: Both 2 and 6 mg/kg in rats at PND 33 or 53 (first estrus)	• ↑(33%, ns at 2 mg; and ~50% $p < 0.05$) at 6 mg at first estrus	• Grote *et al.* (2006a)
	• TPhT: 2 mg/kg in rats until weaning or termination	• No effect	• Grote *et al.* (2009)
17β estradiol	• DBT: 30.4 mg/kg on days 0–3 or 4–7 of gestation in mice	• ↑~9–fold following days 4–7 but no or little effect following days 0–3	• Ema *et al.* (2007)
	• TBT: Up to 50 μg/kg each third day for 30 days in mice	• ↓34%	• Chen *et al.* (2008)
	• TBT: Reproduction study – male rats	• ↓45% in both generations	• Omura *et al.* (2001)
	• TBT: Reproduction study – female rats	• No effect	• Ogata *et al.* (2001)
Testosterone	• TBT: 100 mg/kg acute dose to 3-week-old mice	• ↓78%	• Kim *et al.* (2008)
	• TBT: 15 mg/kg PND 23–53 in rats	• ↓~70% (based on medium)	• Grote *et al.* (2004)
	• TPhT: 2, 6 or 12 mg/kg PND 23–53 in rats	• ↓~27, 55 or 87% (based on medium)	• Grote *et al.* (2004)
	• TBT: 2 mg/kg to weaning or adult in rats	• No effect in weaning but decrease in adults	• Grote *et al.* (2009)
	• TBT: Up to 50 μg/kg each third day for 30 days in adult mice	• Not altered	• Chen *et al.* (2008)
	• TPhT or FenBT: 10 or 25 μg/kg (i.p.) on first, third and fifth day in adult mice	• ↓~30 and 60% for both chemicals	• Reddy *et al.* (2006)
	• TBT: Reproduction study – male rats	• ↑~88% in F_1 and 44% in F_2	• Omura *et al.* (2001)
	• TBT: Reproduction study – female rats	• No effect	• Ogata *et al.* (2001)
Follicular stimulating hormone	• TPhT or fenbutatin: 10 or 25 μg/kg on first, third and fifth day in adult mice	• ↑~63–70% and 146–159% for both chemicals	• Reddy *et al.* (2006)
Luteinizing hormone	• TPhT or FenBT: 10 or 25 μg/kg on first, third and fifth day in adult mice	• ↑~200% to 444 – 640% for both chemicals	• Reddy *et al.* (2006)
	• TPhT: 6 mg/kg in rats	• ↑~doubled	• Grote *et al.* (2004)
	• TBT in a rat reproduction study	• ↑58% in F_2 generation	• Omura *et al.* (2001)
Thyroid	• TBT: 10 or 20 mg/kg during gestation or PND 8–19 in rats	• ↓Thyroxine and triiodothyronine (nearly obliterated at 20 mg/kg) during gestation but only thyroxine reduced following GD 8–19	• Adeeko *et al.* (2003)
	• TBT: 2.5 mg/kg for 90 days in rats	• ↓T4 ~27% ($p < 0.01$)	• Cooke *et al.* (2004)
	• TPhT: 3 or 30 ppm in a quail reproduction study	• ↓18 and 29% in both males and females	• Grote *et al.* (2006)
	• TBT: 1, 10 or 100 ng/L in water in fish	• ↓T3 (about 7% for 1 and 10 and 21% for 100 ng/L) and T4 (about 5, 11 and 25% for 1, 10 and 100 ng/L)	• Zhang *et al.* (2009)
In vitro: Cortisone and androstenedione	• 10–100 nM in bovine adrenal cultures	• Suppresses secretion	• Yamazaki *et al.* (2005)

may result in much higher C_{max} values with resulting differences in effects relative to dietary dosing. Several other steroid hormones are listed in Table 49.3 as being affected by TBT and/or TPhT and alterations in these hormones may be related to the same mechanisms that cause alterations in testosterone and progesterone.

There are several studies which demonstrate that circulating T3 and T4 thyroid hormones are reduced in rats (Adeeko *et al.*, 2008, Cooke *et al.*, 2004), quail (Grote *et al.*, 2006a) and fish (Zhang *et al.*, 2009) in such a manner that some investigators suggested that altered thyroid function is responsible for some aspects of the reproductive effects of TBT or TPHT.

TABLE 49.4 Examples of organotin effects on enzymes in steroid hormone metabolism

Target	Function	Chemical and effects	References
Aromatase (smooth endoplastic reticulum)	Formation of estrogens from androgens (testosterone to estradiol)	• Both TBT and TPhT lower doses *induce* aromatase activity in human placental choriocarcinoma cells • TBT and TPhT inhibit aromatase • 6 mg/kg TPhT daily for 30 days ovary enzyme inhibited *only* about ~37% • Comparisons of organotins as inhibitors on human aromatase. TBT and DBT but not MBT or monooctyltins effective competitive inhibitors. K_i for TBT = 37 to 65 μM in cellular extracts • IC_{50} = 1.5 μM for TPhT in human tissues • 1 and 3 nM TBT induces activity in JEG-3 cells	• Nakanishi *et al.* (2002) • Saitoh *et al.* (2001) • Grote *et al.* (2006a) • Cooke (2002) • Lo *et al.* (2003) • Laville (2006)
17β-Hydroxysteroid dehydrogenase (17β-HSD, smooth endoplastic reticulum)	Converts estrone to estradiol; androstenedione to testosterone	• ↓Testicular activity *in vivo* • ↑Activity in human choriocarcinoma JAr cells • TPhT IC_{50} = 2.6 μM; TBT less effective for cellular extracts • TPhT IC_{50} = 4.3 for type 3 and 10.5 for type 1 μM • Not inhibited by TBT in rat testis	• Reddy *et al.* (2006) • Nakanishi *et al.* (2006) • Ohno *et al.* (2005) • Lo *et al.* (2003) • McVey and Cooke (2003)
17α-Hydroxylase/C17-20 lyase (smooth endoplastic reticulum)	Converts pregnenolone to 17-pregnonolone	• IC_{50} = 117 μM TPhT • IC_{50} ~59 μM for TBT	• Ohno *et al.* (2005) • McVey and Cooke (2003)
3β-Hydroxysteroid dehydrogenase (3β-HSD, smooth endoplastic reticulum)	Δ^4–Δ^5 isomerase converts pregnenolone to progesterone	• ↓Testicular activity *in vivo* TPhT, FenBT • TPhT IC_{50} = 4.0 μM (in LNCaP cells) • 12 μM TBT almost total inhibition • No inhibition at <10 μM TBT	• Reddy *et al.* (2006) • Lo *et al.* (2007) • McVey and Cooke (2003) • Yamasaki *et al.* (2005)
11β-Hydroxysteroid dehydrogenase type 2 (mitochondrial)	Converts active 11-hydroxy corticoids deoxycortisol to inactive 11-ketoglucocorticoids	• TBT, DBT, TPhT, DPhT inhibit with IC_{50}s in the 500 nM to 3 μM range. (Relates to thymus involution and placenta functions)	• Atanasov *et al.* (2005)
5α-Reductase (smooth endoplastic reticulum)	Converts testosterone to dihydrotestosterone	• IC_{50} for DBT, TBT and TPhT in range of 2.7 to 11.2μM. MBT no effect in human LNCaP cells. Reversal by dithiothreitol • IC_{50} = 0.95 μM for human enzyme • IC_{50} =19.9 μM for TBT for type 1 (human brain); IC_{50} = 10.8 μM for type 2 (human prostate)	• Lo *et al.* (2007) • Lo *et al.* (2003) • Doering *et al.* (2002)

Inhibition of enzymes in hormone metabolism

Since alterations in progesterone and testosterone as well as several other steroids are reported as resulting from exposure to TBT and/or TPhT investigations into the inhibition of enzymes involved in their synthesis/degradation may help to determine the cause of these alterations. Reports demonstrating inhibition of enzymes involved in the metabolism of steroid hormones are shown in Table 49.4. Aromatase is inhibited by TBT and TPhT but the concentrations necessary are in the μM range in cellular extracts (Cooke, 2002) and at nM levels in intact cells (Lo *et al.*, 2003). Lower concentrations have been demonstrated to increase production of aromatase (Nakanishi *et al.*, 2002) in cell cultures. Attempts to demonstrate inhibition of aromatase *in vivo* have produced mixed results (Grote *et al.*, 2006a).

In a series *in vitro* papers it was first reported that TBT or DBT (30–300 nM) and TPhT (10–300 nM) "powerfully suppressed human chorionic gonadotropin- and 8-bromo-cAMP-stimulated testosterone production in intact pig Leydig cells at relatively low concentrations that were not cytotoxic" (Nakajima *et al.*, 2003). This study was followed by investigations on the activity and inhibition of enzymes involved in testosterone production (Ohno *et al.*, 2005). TPhT inhibited 17β-hydroxysteroid dehydrogenase (17-β-HSD, IC_{50} 2.6 = μM) and cytochrome P450 17α-hydroxylase/C(17α-HSD, IC_{50} = 117 μM) in cellular extracts. Inhibition of these enzymes would explain the decreases in testosterone

TABLE 49.5 Representative examples of the interaction of organotins with nuclear receptors *in vitro*

Receptor	Source	Chemical and effect	Reference
Peroxisome proliferator-activated receptor γ (PPARγ)	• Human cell high throughput assay • Human JEG-3 cell line	• TPhT – EC_{50} = 95 nM strong agonist effect TBT – lesser effect • TPhT K_d = 66.6 ± 5.2 nM, TPhT, TBT, but not DBT competitively block rosi	• Kanayama *et al.* (2005) • Hiromori *et al.* (2009)
	• GAL4 • JEG-3 human choriocarcinoma cells	• TBT EC_{50} 20 nM TPhT EC_{50} 20 nM • Directly bind and have high affinity for transcriptional activity	• Grun and Blumberg (2006) • Nakanishi *et al.* (2005)
Retinoid X receptor (RXRα)	• Human cell high throughput assay • GAL4	• TBT – strong agonist EC_{50} = 74 nM TPhT – weaker effect • TBT 3–8 nM EC_{50} DBT 3,000 nM EC_{50} TPhT 2–10 nM EC_{50}	• Kanayama *et al.* (2005) • Grun and Blumberg (2006)
RXR and PPAR	• HGELN human cell lines	• TBT activates all three RXR/PPARα, γ and δ heterodimers	• le Maire *et al.* (2009)
Glucocorticoid receptor	• HEK-293 cells	• DBT (but not other organotins) at nM levels *inhibits* ligand binding	• Gumy *et al.* (2008)

but rather high concentrations are needed. In contrast, side chain cleavage by cytochrome P450 and 3β-HSD/*delta*(4)-*delta*(5) isomerase were even less inhibited in isolated enzymes. From a mechanistic perspective, OTs have an affinity for di-thiol enzymes and the inhibitory effect of TPhT on microsomal 17β-HSD activity was eliminated by pretreatment with thiol protective agents such as dithiothreitol or dithioerythritol (Lo *et al.*, 2003). Testosterone production from androstendione in intact pig Leydig cells was inhibited at only 30 nM of TPhT and 100 nM TBT and the authors (Ohno *et al.*, 2005) indicated that inhibition of 17β-HSD activity in the cell culture blocked the conversion, with estimated *in vivo* IC_{50}s at 48 and 114 nM for TPhT and TBT, respectively.

In general, some of the enzymes involved in steroid hormone synthesis may have IC_{50}s in the sub-μM range, depending on whether the experiments were done in intact cells or with cellular extracts. However, other enzyme systems may also be inhibited in the same range including plasma membrane and mitochondrial enzymes. These concentrations approach levels that cause apoptosis. A caveat to the IC_{50}s based on *in vitro* studies is that the most active form of TBT or TPhT *in vivo* may accumulate to high concentration within the cell and the IC_{50}s based on *in vitro* cellular extracts may be misleading relative to intact viable cells. Overall direct inhibition of steroid metabolizing enzymes as a primary critical target for the mechanism(s) that result in expression of toxicity to reproductive organs and postnatal development in rats and mice cannot be ruled out as *contributing* to the overall toxicity of TBT or TPhT.

Affinity of TBT and TPhT for nuclear receptors

Demonstrating that the OTs affect the receptors for hormones may explain some of their actions on reproduction and development such as altered hormone levels as well as other aspects of OT toxicity such as immunotoxicity. Nuclear receptors are the intracellular receptors for the various steroids and thyroid hormones. Environmental pollutants that are either agonists or antagonists for nuclear receptors can potentially induce or prevent the same intracellular events that are initiated by the natural hormones potentially leading to many consequences. As indicated in Table 49.5 recent reports demonstrate that TBT and/or TPhT are agonists for the nuclear receptors PPAR and RXR families and in most cases the effective doses are in the nM range. In a high throughput screening study (Kanayama *et al.*, 2005), where 40 suspected environmental endocrine disruptors were assessed, TPhT was demonstrated to have an affinity nearly as strong as the specific agonist rosiglitazone (rosi) for the PPARγ receptor, and TBT showed a strong agonist effect for the RXRα receptor also nearly equivalent to the specific agonist 9-*cis*-retinoic acid. Of the 40 suspect environmental endocrine disruptors assessed (Kanayama *et al.*, 2005), TBT and TPhT were among the most effective as agonists. The same paper also demonstrated that activation of events downstream from the nuclear receptors such as transcriptional activity through activation of the PPARγ and RXRα were induced (Table 49.6). Both the agonist effects and transcriptional effects (Table 49.6) were statistically significant starting at 10 nM. Cellular lipid accumulation induced by TBT and TPhT was similar to cellular lipid accumulation induced by rosi. Although TPhT and TBT demonstrated contrasting strong affinities for the PPARγ and RXRα nuclear receptors, respectively (Kanayama *et al.*, 2005), the affinities were similar in another study (Grun *et al.*, 2006) suggesting molecular specificity for these receptors may depend on the cell lines tested. Addition of the RXR ligand 9-*cis*-retinoic acid has been reported to induce imposex in gastropods mimicking TBT (Nishikawa *et al.*, 2004), supporting RXR signaling in this effect. It was reported (Grun *et al.*, 2006) that DBT has much lower affinity for the RXR receptor than TBT. DBT, however, while not affecting these nuclear receptors, still effectively causes the same reproductive effects in female rats (Ema and Hirose, 2006) suggesting that these nuclear receptors may not be involved in the reproductive effects of TBT or TPhT in female rats and other mechanisms are possible. DBT was not evaluated in the high throughput study (Kanayama *et al.*, 2005). As indicated in Table 49.5, other investigators also report strong affinities of the OTs for other hormone receptors. In particular, the glucocorticoid receptor is disrupted by DBT (Gumy *et al.*, 2008) but not other OTs. There are several papers describing the molecular interactions of the OTs with the hormone receptors (Gumy *et al.*, 2008; Hiromori *et al.*, 2009; le Maire *et al.*, 2009).

TABLE 49.6 Examples of organotin alterations in mRNA and gene expression or levels

Chemical	Dosing/Species/System	Results	Reference
In vivo			
TBT	Gestation – rats	Genes related to cell adhesion and cell polarity, E-caderthrin mRNA affected by (2.5 to 20 mg/kg)	Barthelemy *et al.* (2007)
TBT	Gestation – rats	40 out of 1,176 genes in testis upregulated 8 genes downregulated in ovary by 20 mg/kg	Kishta *et al.* (2007)
TBT	3-week-old males	17α-hydroxylase ($P450_{17}\alpha$, desmolase) 3β-hydroxysteroid dehydrogenase (3β-HSD) 17β-hydroxysteroid dehydrogenase (17β-HSD) mRNAs all *down*regulated.	Kim *et al.* (2008)
TBT	Salmon	↓Transcription StAR and desmolase (rate limiting steps in steroidogenesis)	Pavilkova *et al.* (2010)
In vitro			
Several	Different cell lines	Increases mRNA for human chorionic gonadotropin and aromatase in human choriocarcinoma cells but decreases aromatase expression in ovarian granulosa cell lines	Nakanishi *et al.* (2006)
TBT/TPhT	Human granulose-like tumor cell line	Decreases mRNA for aromatase.	Saitoh *et al.* (2001)
TPhT TBT	3T3 L1 cells	Induction of adipocyte differentiation marker genes, induction of mRNA for aP2 at 30 or 100 nM	Kanayama *et al.* (2005)
TBT	Rat thymocytes	Many transcriptional effects related to apoptotic processes – some increases and some decreases	Baken *et al.* (2007)
TBT	Human bone marrow cells	TBT increases adipocyte differentiation marker (aP2), PPARγ (but not RXR) mRNA, other factors decreased	Carfi *et al.* (2008)
TBT	JEG-3 human choriocarcinoma	↑mRNA for CPY19 for aromatase *induced* at 1–3 nM TBT	Laville *et al.* (2006)
TBT	PC 12 line	↓mRNA for tyrosine hydroxylase with ↓in enzyme activity and L-dopa at 0.1 μM TBT but no cytotoxicity	Kim *et al.* (2007)
TBT	Rat cortical neurons	↓GLuR2 NR1, NR2A, GluR1 and GluR2 expression. ↑NR2B, GluR3 and GluR4 all at 20 nM. TBT treated cells had increased Ca influx with GluR2 decreased expression	Nakatsu *et al.* (2009)
TBT	Bovine adrenal cell cultures	↓mRNA for p450 for 17α, 3β, 11β hydroxysteroid dehydrogenase, c21, and StAR	Yamazaki *et al.* (2005)
DBT	HEK-293 cells	↓Transcriptional activity of the glucocorticoid receptor by DBT	Gumy *et al.* (2008)

Alterations in mRNA and genes

OTs acting on nuclear receptors may affect mRNA levels. Genomic approaches toward understanding the possible modes of alterations induced by the OTs have been reported recently as shown in Table 49.6. As seen in Table 49.6, the mRNA expression is affected as indicated by upregulated/downregulated activity in response to TBT, DBT and/or TPhT treatment. There does not seem to be a consistency with effects on mRNA for aromatase since in some cell lines there is an increase (Nakanishi *et al.*, 2006) and another a decrease in messenger levels (Nakanishi *et al.*, 2006; Saitoh *et al.*, 2001). The differences between primary cells and tumor cell lines biochemistry could be a possible explanation. Alterations on the mRNA for some of the proteins involved in steroid metabolism and/or function may be downregulated to help explain the decreases in testosterone (Kim *et al.*, 2008). Importantly, increases in mRNA levels do not necessarily result in an increase in protein levels or enzyme activity, due to other effects on protein translation or inhibition of the enzyme. However, decreases in mRNA levels typically do result in a decrease in protein levels and enzyme activity, since proteins have a turnover and a definite lifetime in the cell.

DBT, but not other OTs, inhibits ligand binding to the glucocorticoid receptor and inhibits transcriptional activity (Gumy *et al.*, 2008). It is not obvious how to correlate the alterations in glucocorticoids by DBT with the known effects of DBT on reproduction and development when TBT and TPhT are not effective at this time.

Mechanisms – models

Significance of the effects of the TBT and TPhT on nuclear receptors

Probably the most intriguing current hypothesis for the role of OTs as endocrine disruptors concerns their potential affinity for nuclear receptors particularly for the PPAR and RXR family (Grun and Blumberg, 2007; Iguchi *et al.*, 2008; Nakanishi, 2008). The nuclear receptor hypothesis is that, as nuclear receptor agonists, the OTs shift the cellular metabolism from fat oxidation to favor fat generation and thus are adipogenic and ultimately obesogens. According to a recent review (Iguchi *et al.*, 2008) "TBT represents the first example of an environmental endocrine disruptor that promotes adverse effects from gastropods to mammals. Prenatal (TBT) and early postnatal exposures (oestrogens) stand as strong examples of endocrine disrupting compounds that permanently alter the developing programming." Support for this conclusion is the affinity of the OTs for nuclear receptors that may result in promotion of the genes that increase fatty acid storage and inhibit expression of genes that induce lipolysis. Table 49.1 includes a report that prenatal exposure of mice to TBT resulted in increased epididymal fat pad (~20%) at week 10 whereas the body weight was either not affected or slightly decreased (Grun *et al.*, 2006), meaning that total body mass may not differ following OT exposure but the fat composition does. Another example mentioned previously is that adult frogs, exposed as tadpoles to TBT, also have increased fat near their gonads. If TBT and/or TPhT are obesogens as a result of *in utero* exposure as the authors claim, this would certainly indicate a developmental effect of these OTs. Mitochondria are the location for both fatty acid synthesis and oxidation, thus they are important organelles for models involving obesogenesis. TBT potently inhibits the mitochondrial inner membrane anion channel (IMAC) which is involved in some fatty acid transport (Powers and Beavis, 1991). Inhibition of fatty acid matrix transport by default causes inhibition of fatty acid oxidation, thus fatty acids accumulate to cause obesity. Even more recent reports demonstrate that TBT and TPhT at nM levels have been linked to bone loss and adipogenesis via PPAR nuclear receptor signaling, clearly important steps in animal development (Haas *et al.*, 2010; Yanik *et al.*, 2010). These authors suggest that the OTs can cause a differentiation of tissue from one form to adipose tissue, explaining the apparent paradox with regard to absence of weight gain but increase of lipid (Haas *et al.*, 2010; Yanik *et al.*, 2010).

Interestingly, one report (Inadera and Shimomura, 2005), maintained that co-treatment with a PPARγ antagonist did not inhibit the effect of TBT and neither did addition of dihydroxy-testosterone or 17β estradiol induce the same effect on adipocyte differentiation marker (aP2) expression. The authors suggested that the effect of TBT on accumulation of adipose tissue was not via sex steroids or PPAR signaling. The adipogenic effects reported in adults following *in utero* exposure to OTs would be a developmental effect. However, most studies with TBT and TPhT demonstrate weight loss especially at the higher doses and a weight increase that might accompany an adipogenic effect is not a characteristic at lower doses where competing toxicity should be minimal.

More complex are the interactions of TBT and TPhT with the nuclear receptors in relation to causing the predominant effects on the testis, other male reproductive glands and implantation loss as well as developmental effects persisting to adulthood, which are the main focus of this review. Additional experimentation is needed to elucidate the chain of events from the initial interaction with the nuclear receptors to the known outcomes on these parameters in animal models. The reactions within the chain of events following the action of TBT or TPhT on the nuclear receptors may require that some of the other enzymes or physiological functions be affected before the ultimate expression of the toxic response on reproductive and developmental parameters. The identification of enzymes and physiological functions needs to be demonstrated and their contributions of these factors need to be established. It is intriguing that while TBT and TPhT do not always have the same affinities for both the PPAR and RXR they both cause similar responses in male and female rats. In this regard, one issue is that DBT that was used in many of Ema's studies did not have comparable affinity for the RXR receptor that TBT demonstrated (Table 49.6). However, DBT has high affinity for the glucocorticoid receptor whereas other OTs do not.

The mitochondria as a target for OTs

The mitochondria are a clear target for drug and chemical toxicity, with bioaccumulation by the Nernst model as a proven contributing factor in some cases such as MPP+ or rhodamine derivative toxicity (Wallace and Starkov, 2000). With regards to the known effects of TBT and TPhT in rodents, it has been stated that "implantation efficiency correlates with mitochondrial activity (health)" (Wilding *et al.*, 2001). Many aspects of both OT chemistry and toxicological outcomes suggest that the mitochondria are a target for some of the OTs. Once inside the mitochondria, the organotin compounds potentially have profound effects on several mitochondrial processes, including inhibition of the ATP synthase, induction of cytochrome C release, decrease of membrane potential, caspase activation and apoptosis stimulation, with TBT generally having more adverse effects than DBT (Tomiyama *et al.*, 2009). *In vivo*, TBT has been shown to downregulate mouse testis desmolase, reduce testosterone levels, plus induce apoptosis in testis germ cells, important mitochondrial-modulated events affecting steroid production and the resulting organism development (Kim *et al.*, 2008). Sperm and oocytes are particularly rich in mitochondria, which may predispose those tissues to enhanced effects of TBT or TPhT. The rate-limiting steps of all steroid and glucocorticoid synthesis are located in the mitochondria, from the import of cholesterol by the steroid acute regulatory protein (StAR) transporter to its cleavage to pregnenolone by desmolase (cyt P450 11A1). The flow diagram for steroid, glucocorticoid and mineralocorticoid hormone synthesis is depicted in Figure 49.2. Other important mitochondrial hormone steps are the synthesis of cortisol, corticosterone and aldosterone, plus the initial committed step in bile salt synthesis. These latter hormones have a role in stress responses and bile salts are involved in digestion of lipids, plus the excretion of xenobiotics. The effects of TBT and TPhT on implantation loss have been demonstrated to be reversed by the addition of progesterone, suggesting an early step in steroid synthesis is affected before progesterone synthesis (i.e., 3β HSD, desmolase or StAR). In salmon fed a single dose of only 0.1 mg/kg TBT (Pavlikova *et al.*, 2010), StAR and demolase transcription was still depressed by 75%; 3 days later with significant elevations of PPARγ and PXR nuclear receptors, all mitochondrial events were mediated via cAMP. A retinoic acid receptor binding element has been identified in the StAR gene promoter element in bass fish, meaning that OTs that may have an affinity for this receptor may affect the function of StAR at this step. TBT has been shown to modulate key events in hormone synthesis at the mitochondrial level based on studies with bovine adrenal cultures (Yamazaki *et al.*, 2005). These include decreasing StAR gene transcription in the nucleus, and suppressing cortisol secretion while increasing levels of hydroxyprogesterone and deoxycortisol. These data strongly suggest that TBT is modulating hormone synthesis via transcriptional downregulation at two key mitochondrial steps: cholesterol transport and 11B-hydroxylase. The 11B-hydroxylase enzyme level was significantly reduced at very low levels of 1 nM TBT, while PXR signaling has been

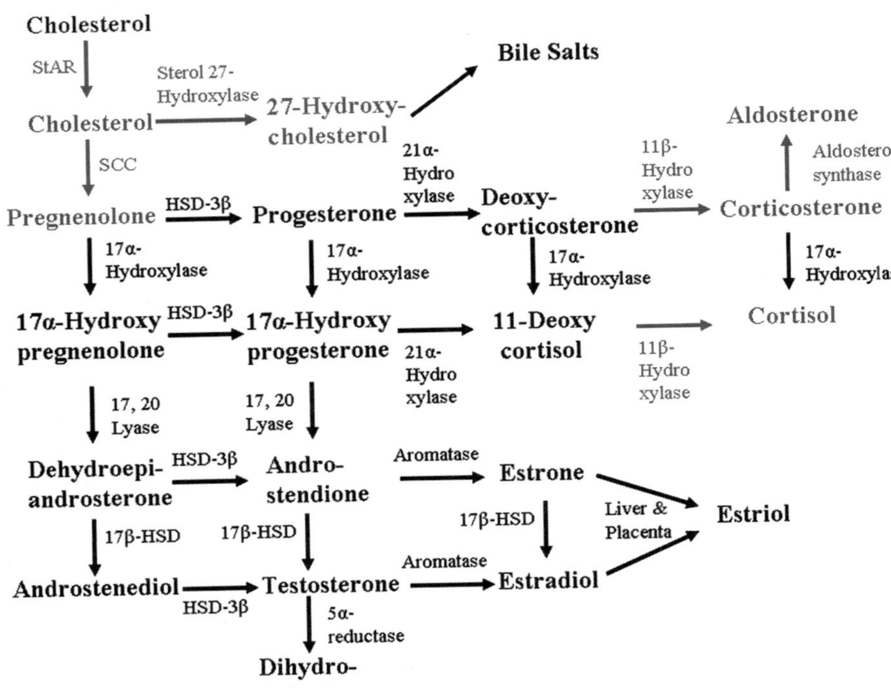

FIGURE 49.2 Steroid, glucocorticoid and mineralocorticoid synthesis pathways. Endoplasmic reticulum products and enzymes are listed in black text and arrows. Mitochondrial products and enzymes are depicted in gray text and arrows. The rate-limiting step in steroid synthesis is cholesterol transport into the mitochondria by StAR. Abbreviations: 17β-HSD – 17 beta hydroxysteroid dehydrogenase; StAR – steroidogenic acute regulatory protein; SCC – side chain cleavage enzyme, desmolase, P450 11A1; HSD-3β – 3 beta hydroxysteroid dehydrogenase.

correlated to 11B-hydroxylase expression. The same study also showed that mitochondrial desmolase was inhibited at a 10,000 times lower dose in intact primary bovine adrenal cells than cellular extracts (i.e., 10^{-7}M vs. 10^{-3}M in 1 hour), in precise agreement with the Nernst equation predictions. Similarly, comparing the results for aromatase activity in Table 49.4, the OT concentrations for inhibition were three orders of magnitude lower in intact cells (Lo *et al.*, 2003) relative to cellular extracts (Cooke, 2002), also supporting the Nernst bioaccumulation model. Cells normally exclude xenobiotics via drug efflux pumps (multi-drug resistance pumps, MDRs). Typically, much higher concentrations of compounds are required for inhibition of cytosolic enzymes in intact cells vs. cell extracts, unless a bioaccumulation phenomenon is occurring. Klaassen's group demonstrated that MDR pump levels may also be regulated by hormones and through nuclear receptors such as PXR and PPAR (Maher *et al.*, 2005), so OTs may induce feedback control on their cytosolic concentrations. Bioaccumulation of OTs via the Nernst model with subsequent MDR pump efflux would cause futile cellular ATP hydrolysis by these mechanisms, thus resulting in deviations of the OTs from ideal Nernst properties. The nuclear receptor NR4A1 has been shown to modulate the rate-limiting steps of hormone synthesis at mitochondrial StAR protein expression and mitochondrial desmolase, as well as Cyp17 and HSD-3B2 enzymes. Similarly, TCDD is known to bind to nuclear receptors and modulate vital mitochondrial electron transport protein levels such as complexes I, III, IV and V (Forgacs *et al.*, 2010). TPhT is metabolized to benzene and phenols, and these metabolites, like TCDD, are potential endocrine disruptors and have been shown to activate the aryl hydrocarbon nuclear receptors in bone marrow cells (Hirabayashi and Inoue, 2010) and may have affinity for the nuclear receptors and effects on mitochondrial functions. It is important to note that the mitochondria typically supply 90% of cellular energy for enzyme synthesis and biomolecular transport. Mitochondrial pathology due to chemical toxicity can suppress normal housekeeping roles of the cell such as hormone production and induce necrosis or apoptosis pathways. Some OTs can inhibit the ATP synthase, and other inhibitors of this complex, such as oligomycin, have been shown to potently sensitize skeletal muscle and other tissues to other stressors or disease states (Irwin *et al.*, 2003). Some OTs can inhibit mitochondrial substrate transporters, such as for a key oxidative substrate such as pyruvate (Skilleter, 1975).

An important proposed component of the model for the ability of OTs to cause toxicity outcomes, including reproduction and development, is their activation of nuclear receptors or free radical production. As indicated above, OTs have been shown to modulate mitochondria and steroidogenesis but other cellular functions and signaling pathways are also affected by the free radical property of the OTs. This section links several of these signaling pathways together for a more integrative approach to OT toxicity. There are many biochemical reactions within the mitochondria that could be targets for OT action on nuclear receptors. Peroxisomal and mitochondrial proliferation is both modulated by dynamin-like protein signaling. The peroxisomes and mitochondria are the major cellular locations of reactive oxygen species (ROS) generation when they are stressed and increased ROS generation has been shown to downregulate steroid production via cAMP control of StAR transporter gene transcription in the nucleus. StAR is a critical rate limiting step in the transport of cholesterol into cells for further metabolism to steroid hormones. Superoxide dismutase mimetics, which scavenge superoxide-free radicals, partially restore progesterone production supporting this ROS mechanism (Shi et *al.*, 2010). Conversely, overexpression of StAR in macrophages upregulates mitochondrial sterol 27-hydroxylase (CYP27A1) via the PPARγ receptor, a competing pathway, for bile salt synthesis from cholesterol, while inhibiting apoptosis. Nuclear receptors may also have a role in the expression of cholesterol efflux transporters, which provide feedback control for hormone and bile synthesis (Ning *et al.*, 2009). Conversely, TBT has been shown to modulate PPAR gamma, which can control StAR expression (also modulated by other nuclear receptors).

The interaction of the OTs with the energy functions of the mitochondria and other organelles, and eventual apoptosis, needs to be considered. OTs have long been known to affect basic mitochondrial functions such as ATP productions (Aldridge *et al.*, 1977). TBT has been shown to inhibit the lysosomal V-ATPases proton pumps with an IC_{50} value of 200 nM (Akiyama *et al.*, 2008). TMT and TBT can induce autophagy of mitochondria by the lysosomes, which also contain cathepsins involved in cell death pathways (Bouldin *et al.*, 1981). TBT inhibits SERCA calcium pumps in the endoplasmic reticulum, raising cytosolic Ca^{++} levels which can lead to cell pathology via mitochondrial mechanisms (Kass and Orrenius, 1999). Some OTs increase mitochondrial Ca^{++} uptake which often causes mitopathology, such as mitochondrial swelling (permeability transition, mPT). Mitochondrial swelling is modulated by dithiol agents. Some dithiol agents (i.e., DTT and DTE) protect against OT enzyme inhibition and may also protect against mitochondrial swelling by OTs. TBT at 2 μM levels induces rapid loss of membrane potential and cytochrome C release in lymphocytes (Stridh *et al.*, 1998). TBT at 300 nM for 1 hour significantly lowers granzyme and perforin levels in natural killer cells, partially through a cAMP response element binding protein mechanism (Thomas *et al.*, 2004). TBT can both induce B cell calcium-mediated mitochondrial apoptosis and alter their development/differentiation in the bone marrow. Both of these effects are altering immune responses in cell models that parallel *in vivo* responses currently utilized to regulate TBT and TPhT.

A comprehensive model integrating the effects of OTs on cells as described above is illustrated in Figure 49.1. Overall, based on the available data, there may not be a single mechanism for the mode of action of TBT and TPhT to cause *all* of their adverse effects including those on reproduction and development in mammals. It appears that several enzyme systems and other parameters such as nuclear receptors are affected in the nM and approaching the μM range. The mitochondria are a main focus for these effects but also included are effects on the peroxisomes, lysosomes and endoplasmic reticulum. The relative contribution of each factor may be the determinant of the expression of differential toxicity. The relative toxicity of OTs to specific tissues could be determined by multiple factors such as compound uptake magnitude, xenobiotic multi-drug resistance pumps (i.e., MDR), specific receptors or signaling pathways, tissue-specific metabolism, protein binding, inhibition of tissue regeneration, etc.

CONCLUDING REMARKS AND FUTURE DIRECTIONS

This chapter was intended to serve as an introduction to the many aspects of the reproductive and developmental toxicity of TBT and TPhT in mammals, as much as to stimulate interest and discussion in possible mechanisms for their action. The authors regret that more inclusive descriptions of some of the papers cited were not more fully described and that some important papers may not be cited in the space allowed. Overall, this chapter should convey that it is established that TBT and TPhT affect the reproductive structures in laboratory rats and/or mice based on experimental data from several laboratories and each gender is affected. Not only are adult animals affected by direct administration, there is evidence that gestational exposure potentially results in persistent developmental differences seen as the animals mature to adults. The OTs have multiple effects on mammals including immunotoxicity and neurotoxicity. Additional research is needed to distinguish any highly specific effects on the reproductive systems and development at lower doses than effects occur on any other system, such as the immune system. In rodents and other species, the role for OTs as endocrine disruptors is becoming established. This chapter should convey that the TBT and TPhT could be endocrine disruptors through their direct effects on nuclear receptors, by regulating genes for enzymes and receptors involved in steroidogenesis, as direct inhibitors of enzymes involved in hormone metabolism or through their effects on basic mitochondrial functions such as energy production and molecular transport. However, so far the reports on TBT and TPhT as mammalian endocrine disruptors focus more on possible adipogenic or immunotoxic effects through their action on nuclear receptors. Less focus was placed on trying to explain precisely how TBT and/or TPhT acting as agonists for nuclear receptors are related to the several adverse effects on male/female reproductive organs and the developmental effects seen in adults following *in utero* exposure. Although a role as endocrine disruptors for the OTs is developing in animal models, other systems that are affected by TBT and/or TPhT at nearly the same dose *in vivo* or concentration *in vitro* may also contribute to the potential toxicity of the OTs. In order to better establish a role for TBT and TPhT as endocrine disruptors in mammals, additional data on all circulating hormones (including the cholesterol precursor levels) in the same model would be very informative. Establishing the relationship of altered hormone levels to the known effects of TBT and TPhT on the male and female reproductive structures, as well as developmental effects from *in utero* that persist to adulthood, would be an important pathway for additional research. One example of a developmental effect that needs to be explained is the increased sensitivity to infections in adults following *in utero* exposure. Many important papers come from laboratories that attempt to address the mechanisms for immunotoxicity and the results of these studies may yield important clues as to the mechanism for the initial effects on the reproductive tracts and on offspring development. This chapter focused on the mitochondria and their many functions for energy production, and roles in steroidogenesis seem to be a promising target for explaining the toxicity outcomes of TBT and TPhT. Elucidating the steps between effects in the mitochondria or other organelles and the expression of toxicity remain to be precisely established. Initial Nernst model results are very promising. However, further experiments are needed to fully validate the Nernst model in more tissues affected by OTs. Side-by-side comparisons of the inhibition of critical enzyme IC_{50} values in cellular extracts vs. intact cells needs to be performed from the same tissue with and without MDR pump inhibitors (i.e., cyclosporin A) to consider the effects of these xenobiotic pumps on experimental results. If an important target of OTs are the mitochondria, which are present in all oxidative cells, pharmacokinetic and pharmacodynamic data are needed to better explain why the male and female reproductive structures and fetal development may preferentially be affected. Lastly, once the pathways between the biochemical events leading to the expression of toxicity are established, experiments in animal models could be done to develop antidotal treatment. Examples may include use of thiols to prevent inhibition and hormonal therapies to address the outcomes from exposure.

ACKNOWLEDGMENT

The authors gratefully acknowledge Dr. Tina Levine and Dr. Jack Fowle for their critical review of the drafts of this manuscript and their many helpful suggestions.

REFERENCES

Adeeko A, Li D, Forsyth DS, Casey V, Cooke GM, Barthelemy J, Cyr DG, Trasler JM, Robaire B, Hales BF (2003) Effects of *in utero* tributyltin chloride exposure in the rat on pregnancy outcome. *Toxicol Sci* **74:** 407–15.

Akiyama K, Chardwiriyapreecha S, Chahomchuen T, Sugimoto N, Sekito T, Nishimoto S, Sugahara T, Kakinuma Y (2008) Vacuolar-type H^+-translocating ATPase is the target of tributyltin chloride. In *Interdisciplinary Studies on Environmental Chemistry – Biological Responses to Chemical Pollutants* (Murakami Y, Nakayama K, Kitamura S-I, Iwata H, Tanabe S, eds.). TERRAPUB, pp. 241–9.

Aldridge WN, Street BW, Skilleter DN (1977) Halide-dependent and halide independent effects of triorganotin and triorganolead compounds on mitochondrial functions. *Biochem J* **168:** 353–64.

Appel KE (2004) Organotin compounds: toxicokinetic aspects. *Drug Metabolism Reviews* **36:** 763–86.

Asakawa H, Tsunoda M, Kaido T, Hosokawa M, Sugaya C, Inoue Y, Kudo Y, Satoh T, Katagiri H, Akita H, Saji M, Wakasa M, Negishi T, Tashiro T, Aizawa Y (2009) Enhanced inhibitory effects of TBT chloride on the development of F1 rats. *Arch Environ Contam Toxicol* (electronic publication).

Atanasov AG, Nashev LG, Tam S, Baker ME, Odermatt A (2005) Organotins disrupt the 11β-hydroxysteroid dehydrogenase type 2-dependent local inactivation of glucocorticoids. *Environ Health Perspect* **113:** 1600–6.

Baken KA, Arkusz J, Pennings JLA, Vandebriel RJ, van Loveren H (2007) *In vitro* immunotoxicity of bis(tri-*n*-butyltin)oxide (TBTO) studied by toxicogenomics. *Toxicology* **237:** 35–48.

Barthelemy J, Adeeko A, Robaire B, Cyr DG (2007) *In utero* exposure to tributyltin alters the expression of E-cadherin and localization of claudin-1 in intercellular junctions of the rat ventral prostate. *Mol Repro Dev* **74:** 455–67.

Benson (1997) Toxicological Review Trobutyltin Oxide (CAS No. 56-35-9) In Support of Summary Information on the Integrated Risk Information System (IRIS).

Berge JA, Brevik EM, Bjorge A, Folsvik N, Gabrielsen GW, Wolkers H (2004) Organotins in marine mammals and seabirds from Norwegian territory. *J Environ Monit* **6:** 108–12.

Bettin C, Oehlmann J, Stroben E (1996) TBT-induced imposex in marine neogastropods is mediated by an increasing androgen level. *Hegolander Meeresuntersuchungen* **50:** 299–317.

Bouldin TW, Goines ND, Bagnell RC, Kingman MR (1981) Pathogenesis of trimethyltin neuronal toxicity. Ultrasound and cytochemical observations. *Am J Pathol* **104:** 237–49.

Carfi M, Croera C, Ferrario D, Campi V, Bowe G, Pieters R, Gribaldo L (2008) TBTC induces adipocyte differentiation in human bone marrow long term culture. *Toxicology* **249:** 11–18.

Chen Y, Zou Z, Chen S, Yan F, Chen Y, Yang Z, Wang C (2008) Reduction of spermatogenesis in mice after tributyltin administration. *Toxicology* **251:** 21–7.

Cima F, Ballerin L, Bressa G, Martinucci G, Burighel P (1996) Toxicity of organotin compounds on embryos of a marine invertebrate *(Styela plicata: tunicata). Ecotoxicol Environ Saf* **35:** 174–82.

Cooke GM (2002) Effect of organotins on human aromatase activity *in vitro*. *Toxicol Lett* **126:** 121–30.

Cooke GM, Forsyth DS, Bondy GS, Tachon R, Tague B, Caody Y (2008) Organotin speciation and tissue distribution in rat dams, fetuses and neonates following oral administration of tributyltin chloride. *J Toxicol Environ Health Part A* **71:** 384–95.

Cooke GM, Tryphonas H, Pulido O, Caldwell D, Bondy GS, Forsyth D (2004) Oral (gavage) *in utero* and postnatal exposure of Sprague-Dawley rats to low doses of tributyltin chloride. Part 1. Toxicology, histopathology and clinical chemistry. *Food Chem Toxicol* **42:** 211–20.

Davidoff F, Bertolini D, Haas D (1978) Enhancement of the mitochondrial Ca2+ uptake rate by phenethylbiguanide and other organic cations with hypoglycemic activity. *Diabetes* **27:** 757–65.

Delgado, IF, Vianna, VG, Sarpa M, Paumgartten FJR (2008) Postnatal development and resistance to *Plasmodium yoelii* infection of mice prenatally exposed to triphenyltin hydroxide. *Environ Toxicol* **24:** 629–35.

Dobson S (1990). Environmental Health Criteria 116. Tributyltin Compounds. Geneva, WHO.

Doering DD, Steckelbroeck S, Doering T, Klingmuller D (2002) Effects of butyltins on human 5alpha-reductase type 1 and type 2 activity. *Steroids* **67:** 859–67.

Ema M, Arima A, Fukunishi K, Matsumoto M, Hirata-Koizumi, M, Hirose A, Ihara T (2009) Developmental toxicity of dibutyltin dichloride given on three consecutive days during organogenesis in cynomolgus monkeys. *Drug Chem Toxicol* **32:** 150–7.

Ema M, Fukunishi K, Matsumoto M, Hirose A, Kamata E, Ihara T (2007) Developmental toxicity of dibutyltin dichloride in cynomolgus monkeys. *Reprod Toxicol* **23:** 12–19.

Ema M, Hirose A (2006) Reproductive and developmental toxicity of organotin compounds. In *Metals, Fertility, and Reproductive Toxicity* (Golub M, ed.). Taylor and Francis, pp. 24–64.

Forgacs A, Burgoon LD, Lynn SG, LaPres JJ, Zacharewski TR (2010) TCDD-mediated gene expression profiling of nuclear encoded mitochondrial genes involved in oxidative phosphorylation. Abstract No. 84 Annual Meeting of the Society of Toxicology, Salt Lake City, Utah.

Gagné F, Blaise C, Pellerin J, Pelletier E, Douville M, Gauthier-Clers S, Vigino L (2003) Sex alteration in soft-shell clams (*Mya arenaria*) in an intertidal zone of the Saint Lawrence river (Quebec, Canada). *Comp Biochem Physiol C Toxicol Pharmacol* **134:** 189–198.

Gardland AT, Archer T, Danielsson K, Frederiksson A, Lindquist NG, Lindstrom H, Luthman J (1991) Effects of prenatal exposure to tributyltin and trihexyltin in behavior in rats. *Neurotoxicol Teratol* **13:** 99–105.

Golub M, Doherty JD (2004) Triphenyltin as a potential human endocrine disruptor. *J Toxicol Environ Health Part B* **7:** 281–95.

Grote K, Anderson JM, Andrade AJM, Grande SW, Kuriyama SN, Talsness CE, Appel KE, Chahoud I (2006a) Effects of peripubertal exposure to triphenyltin on female sexual development of the rat. *Toxicology* **222:** 17–34.

Grote K, Hobler C, Andrade AJM, Grande SW, Gericke C, Talsness CE, Appel KE, Chahoud I (2009) Sex differences in effects on sexual development in rat offspring after pre- and postnatal exposure to triphenyltin chloride. *Toxicology* **260:** 53–9.

Grote K, Niemann L, Gericke C, Selzman B, Chahoud I (2006b) Effects of fentin hydroxide on reproduction of the Japanese quail (*Coturnix coturnix japonica*). *Environ Res* **101:** 81–8.

Grote K, Stahschmidt B, Talsness CE, Gericke C, Appel KE, Chahoud I (2004) Effects of organotin compounds on pubertal male rats. *Toxicology* **202:** 145–58.

Grun F, Blumberg B (2006) Environmental obesogens: organotins and endocrine disruption via nuclear receptor signaling. *Endocrinology* **147:** 550–5.

Grun F, Blumberg B (2007) Perturbed nuclear receptor signaling by environmental obesogens as emerging factors in the obesity crisis. *Rev Endocr Metab Disord* **8:** 161–71.

Grun F, Watanabe H, Zamanian Z, Maeda L, Arima K, Cubacha R, Gardiner DM, Kanno J, Iguchi T, Blumberg B (2006) Endocrine-disrupting organotin compounds are potent inducers of adiopgenesis in vertebrates. *Mol Endocrinol* **20:** 2141–55.

Gumy C, Chandsawangbhuwana C, Dzyakanchuk AA, Kratschmar D, Baker ME Odermatt A (2008) Dibutyltin disrupts glucorcorticoid receptor function and impairs glucorcorticoid-induced suppression of cytokine production. *Plos ONE* **3:** e3545:1–11.

Haas AR, Yanik SC, Sherr DH, Gerstenfeld LC, Schlezinger JJ (2010) Tributyltin: B cell toxicant and bone marrow microenvironment modulator. Presented at the 49th Annual Meeting of the Society of Toxicology, Salt Lake City. Utah, Abstract # 1549.

Hirabayashi Y, Inoue T (2010) Benzene-induced bone-marrow toxicity: a hematopoietic stem-cell.specific, aryl hydrocarbon receptor-mediated adverse effect. *Chem Biol Interact* **184:** 252–8.

Hiromori, Y, Nishikawa J-I, Yoshida I, Nagase H, Nakanishi T (2009) Structure-dependent activation of peroxisome proliferators-activated receptor

(PPAR) γ by organotin compounds. *Chemico-Biological Interactions* **180:** 238–44.

Horiguchi T, Shiraishi H, Shimizu M, Morita M (1997) Effects of triphenyltin chloride and five other organotin compounds on the development of imposex in the rock shell *Thais clavigera*. *Environ Pollut* **95:** 85–91.

Iguchi T, Katsu Y, Horiguchi T, Watanabe H, Blumberg B, Ohta Y (2007) Endocrine disrupting organotin compounds are potent inducers of imposex in gastropods and adiopgenesis in vertebrates. *Mol Cell Toxicol* **3:** 1–10.

Iguchi T, Watanabe H, Ohta Y, Blumberg B (2008) Developmental effects: oestrogen-induced vaginal changes and organotin-induced adipogenesis. *Int J Androl* **31:** 263–8.

Inadera H, Shimomura A (2005) Environmental chemical tributyltin augurnents adipocyte differentiation. *Toxicol Letters* **159:** 226–34.

Irwin W, Bergamin N, Sabatelli P, Merlini L, Megighian A, Reggiani C, Braghetta P, Columbaro M, Volpin D, Bressan GM, Bernardi P, Bonaldo P (2003) Mitochondrial dysfunction and apoptosis in myopathic mice with collagen VI deficiency. *Nature Genetics* **35:** 367–71.

Kanayama T, Kobayashi N, Mamiya S, Nakanishi T, Nishikawa J-I (2005) Organotin compounds promote adipocyte differentiation as agonists of the peroxisome proliferation-activated receptor gamma/retinoid X receptor pathway. *Mol Pharmacol* **67:** 766–74.

Kass GEN, Orrenius S (1999) Calcium signaling and cytotoxicity. *Environ Hlth Perspect* **107:** 25–35.

Kim S-K, Kim JH, Han JH, Yoon Y-D (2008) Inhibitory effect of tributyltin on expression of steroidogenic enzymes in mouse testis. *Internatl J Toxicol* **27:** 175–82.

Kim YM, Lee JJ, Park SK, Lim SC, Hwang BY, Lee CK, Lee MK (2007) Effects of tributyltin acetate on dopamine biosynthesis and L-DOPA-induced cytotoxicity in PC12 cells. *Arch Pharm Res* **30:** 858–65.

Kishta, O, Adeeko A, Li D, Luu T, Brawer JR, Morales C, Hermo L, Robaire B, Hales BF, Barthlemy J, Cyr DG, Trasler JM (2007) *In utero* exposure to tributyltin chloride differentially alters male and female gonad morphology and gene expression profiles in the Sprague-Dawley rat. *Reprod Toxicol* **23:** 1–11.

Krinke G (2000a) Trimethyltin. In *Experimental and Clinical Neurotoxicology*, 2nd edition (Spencer PS, Schaumburg HH, eds.). Oxford, Oxford University Press, pp. 1211–14.

Krinke G (2000b) Trimethyltin. In *Experimental and Clinical Neurotoxicology*, 2nd edition (Spencer PS, Schaumburg HH, eds.). Oxford, Oxford University Press, pp. 1206–8.

Laville N, Balaguer P, Brion F, Hinfray N, Casellas C, Porcher J-M, Ait-Aissa S (2006) Modulation of aromatase activity and mRNA by various selected pesticides in the human choriocarcinoma JEG-3 cell line. *Toxicology* **228:** 98–108.

Lehotzky K, Szeberenyi JM, Gonda Z, Horkay F Kiss A (1982a) Effects of prenatal triphenyl-tin exposure on the development and behavior and conditioned learning in rat pups. *Neurobehav Toxicol Teratol* **4:** 247–50.

Lehotzky K, Szeberenyi JM, Horkay F Kiss A (1982b) The neurotoxicity of organotins: behavioral changes in rats. *Acta Biol Acad Sci Hung* **33:** 15–22.

le Maire A, Grimaldi M, Roecklin D, Dagnino S, Vivat-Hannah V, Balaguer P, Bourguet W (2009) Activation of RXR-PPAR heterodimers by organotins. *EMBO Rep* **10:** 367–73.

Lo S, Allera A, Albers P, Heimbrecht J, Jantzen E, Klingmuller, D, Steckelbroeck S (2003) Dithioerythritol (DTE) prevents inhibitory effects of triphenyltin (TPT) on the key enzymes of the human sex steroid hormone metabolism. *J Steroid Biochem Mol Biol* **84:** 569–76.

Maher JM, Cheng X, Slitt AL, Dieter MZ, Klassen CD (2005) Induction of the multidrug resistance-associated protein family of transporters by chemical activators of receptor-mediated pathways in mouse liver. *Drug Metab Dispos* **33:** 956–62.

Makita Y, Omura M, Ogata R (2004) Effects of perinatal simultaneous exposure to tributyltin (TBT) and *p,p'*-DDE (1,1-dichloro-2,2-bis(*p*-chlorophenyl)ethylene) on male offspring of Wistar rats. *J Toxicol Environ Health Part A* **67:** 385–95.

McAllister BG, Kime DE (2003) Early life exposure to environmental levels of aromatase inhibitor tributyltin causes masculinization and irreversible sperm damage in zebrafish (*Danio rerio*). *Aquat Toxicol* **65:** 309–16.

McVey MJ, Cooke GM (2003) Inhibition of rat testis microsomal 3β-hydroxysteroid dehydrogenase activity by tributyltin. *J Steroid Biochem Mol Biol* **86:** 99–105.

Miyake K, Misawa T, Shigata S (1991) The effects of prenatal triphenyltin exposure on learning and development in the rat. *Nippon Eiseigaku Zasshi* **46:** 769–76.

Moser VC (1996) Rat strain- and gender-related differences in neurobehavioral screening: acute trimethyltin neurotoxicity. *J Toxicol Environ Health* **47:** 567–86.

Myers D (2003) TPTH: Developmental neurotoxicity study in the CD rat by oral administration. Huntingdon Life Sciences Project Id No.: LDA/038/032055. Submitted to the USEPA in support of product registration. MRID No.: 46055701.

Nakajima Y, Sato G, Ohno S, Nakajin S (2003) Organotin compounds suppress testosterone production in Leydig cells from neonatal pig testis. *J Health Sci* **49:** 514–19.

Nakanishi T (2008) Endocrine disruption induced by organotin compounds: organotins function as a powerful agonist for nuclear receptors rather than an aromatase inhibitor. *J Toxicol Sci* **33:** 269–76.

Nakanishi T, Hiromori Y, Yokoyama H, Koyanagi M, Itoh, N, Nishikawa J, Tanaka K (2006) Organotin compounds enhance 17β-hydroxysteroid dehydrogenase type I activity in human choriocarcinoma JAR cells: potential promotion of 17β-estradiol biosynthesis in human placenta. *Biochem Pharmacol* **71:** 1349–57.

Nakanishi T, Kohroki J, Suzuki S, Ishizaki J, Hiromori Y, Takasuga S, Itoh N, Watanabe Y, Utoguchi N, Tanaka K (2002) Trialkyltin compounds enhance human CG secretion and aromatase activity in human placental choriocarcinoma cells. *J Clin Endocrinol Metab* **87:** 2830–7.

Nakatsu Y, Kotake Y, Takshita T, Ohta S (2009) Long-term exposure to endogenous levels of tributyltin decreases GluR2 expression and increases neuronal vulnerability to glutamate. *Toxicol Appl Pharmacol* **240:** 292–8.

Ning Y, Bai Q, Lu H, Li X, Pandak WM, Zhao F, Chen S, Ren S, Yin L (2009) Overexpression of mitochondrial cholesterol delivery protein, StAR, decreases intracellular lipids and inflammatory factors secretion in macrophages. *Atheroscelosis* **204:** 114–20.

Nishikawa J, Mamiya S, Kanayama T, Nishikawa T, Shiraishi F, Horiguchi T (2004) Involvement of the retinoid X receptor in the development of imposex caused by organotins in gastropods. *Environ Sci Technol* **38:** 6271–6.

Ogata R, Omura M, Kubo K, Oshima Y, Aou S, Inoue N (2001) Two-generation reproductive toxicity study of tribytyltin chloride in rats. *J Toxicol Environ Hlth Part A* **63:** 127–44.

Ohno S, Nakajima Y, Nakajin S (2005) Triphenyltin and tributyltin inhibit pig testicular 17β-hydroxysteroid dehydrogenase activity and suppress testicular testosterone biosynthesis. *Steroids* **70:** 645–51.

Omura M, Ogata R, Kubo K, Shimasaki Y, Aou S, Oshima Y, Tanaka A, Hirata M, Makita Y, Inoue N (2001) Two-generation reproduction toxicity study of tributyltin chloride in rats. *Toxicol Sci* **64:** 224–32.

Pate BD, Hayes RL (1968) Histological studies in rats treated with certain insect chemosterilants. *J Econ Entomol* **61:** 32–4.

Pavilkova N, Kortner TM, Arukwe A (2010) Modulation of acute steroidogenesis, peroxisome proliferator-activated receptors and CYP3A/PXR in salmon interregnal tissues by tributyltin and the second messenger activator, forskolin. *Chemico-Biological Interactions* (published online).

Powers MF, Beavis AD (1991) Triorganotins inhibit the mitochondrial inner membrane anion channel. *J Biol Chem* **226:** 17250–6.

Reddy PS, Pushpalatha T, Reddy PS (2006) Reduction of spermatogenesis and steroidogenesis in mice after fentin and fenbutatin administration. *Toxicol Letters* **166:** 53–9.

Reese BE, Davidson C, Billingsley ML, Yun J (2005) Protein kinase C epsilon regulated tumor necrosis factor-alpha-induced stannin gene expression. *J Pharmacol Exp Ther* **314:** 61–9.

Saitoh M, Yanase T, Morinaga H, Tanabe M, Mu YM, Nishi Y, Nomura M, Okabe T, Goto K, Takayanagi R, Nawata H (2001) Tributyltin or triphenyltin inhibits aromatase activity in the human granulose-like tumor cell line KGN. *Biochem Biophys Res Commun* **289:** 198–204.

Sarpa M, De-Carvalho RR, Delgado IF, Paumgartten FJR (2007) Developmental toxicity to triphenyltin hydroxide in mice. *Reg Toxicol Pharmacol* **49:** 43–52.

Sekizawa J (1999) Triphenyltin Compounds. Concise International Chemical Assessment Document 13. INCHEM, World Health Organization.

Shi Z, Feng Y, Wang J, Zhang H, Ding L, Dai J (2010) Perfluorododecanoic acid-induced steroidogenic inhibition is associated with steroidogenic acute regulatory protein and reactive oxygen species in cAMP-stimulated Leydig cells. *Toxicol Sci* **114:** 285–94.

Shimasaki Y, Kitano T, Oshima Y, Inoue S, Imada N, Honjo T (2003) Trybutylin causes masculinization in fish. *Environ Toxicol Chem* **22:** 141–4.

Siah A, Pellerin J, Amiard J-C, Pelletier E, Viglino L (2003) Delayed gametogenesis and progesterone levels in soft-shell clams (*Mya arenaria*) in relation to *in situ* contamination to organotins and heavy metals in the St. Lawrence River (Canada). *Comp Biochem and Physiol Part C* **135:** 145–56.

Skilleter DN (1975) The decrease of mitochondrial substrate uptake caused by trialklytin and trialklylead compounds in chloride media and its relevance to inhibition of oxidative phosphorylation. *Biochem J* **146:** 465–71.

Snoeji NJ, Penniks AH, Seinen W (1987) Biological activity of organotin compounds – an overview. *Environ Res* **44:** 3335–53.

Stridh H, Kimland M, Jones DP, Orrenius S, Hampton MB (1998) Cytochrome c release and caspase activation in hydrogen peroxide- and tributyltin-induced apoptosis. *FEBS Lett* **429:** 351–5.

Taylor LM, Hackett AM, Cordon C, Button SG (2003) Triphenyltin Hydroxide (TPTH) Milk Secretion Study following single and repeated oral doses to the rat. Huntingdon Life Science, Study No. LDA/036. Submitted in support of product registration.

Thomas LD, Shah H, Green SA, Bankhurst AD, Whalen MM (2004) Tributyltin exposure causes decreased granzyme B and perforin levels in human natural killer cells. *Toxicology* **200:** 221–33.

Tomiyama K, Yamaguchi A, Kuriyama T, Arakawa Y (2009) Analysis of mechanisms of cell death of T-lymphocytes induced by organotin agents. *J Immunotoxicol* **6:** 184–93.

Uneo S, Kashimoto T, Susa N, Asai T, Kawaguchi S, Takeda-Homma S, Terada Y, Sugiyama M (2009) Reductions in peripheral lymphocytes and thymus atrophy induced by organotin compounds *in vivo*. *J Vet Med Sci* **7:** 1041–8.

Wallace KB, Starkov AA (2000) Mitochondrial targets of drug toxicity. *Ann Rev Pharmacol Toxicol* **40:** 353–88.

Waterman B, Grote K, Gnass K, Kolodzey H, Thomsen A, Appel KE, Candia-Carnevali D, Schule-Oehlmann U (2008) Histological alterations in ovaries of pubertal female rats induced by triphenyltin. *Exptl Toxicol Pathol* **60:** 313–21.

Wilding M, Dale B, Marino M, di Matteo L, Alviggi C, Pisaturo ML, Lombardi L, De Placido G (2001) Mitochondria aggregation patterns and activity in human oocytes and preimplantation embryos. *Human Reprod* **16:** 909–17.

Yamazaki T, Shimodaira M, Kuwahara H, Wakatsuki H, Horichi H, Matsuda H, Kominami S (2005) Tributyltin disturbs bovine adrenal steroidogenesis by two modes of action. *Steroids* **70:** 913–21.

Yanik S, Sherr DH, Schlezinger JJ (2010) Organotin-mediated PPARγ activation and adipocyte differentiation in bone marrow stromal cells. Presented at the 49th Annual Meeting of the Society of Toxicology, Salt Lake City. Utah, Abstract # 1551.

Yu WJ, Lee BJ, Nam SY, Kim YC, Lee YS, Yun YW (2003) Spermatogenic disorders in adult rats exposed to tributyltin chloride during puberty. *J Vet Med Sci* **65:** 1331–5.

Zhang J, Zuo Z, Hem C, Wu D, Chen Y, Wang C (2009) Inhibition of thyroidal status related to depression of testicular development to *Sebastiscus marmoratus* exposed to tributyltin. *Aquatic Toxicol* **94:** 62–7.

C H A P T E R

50

Bisphenol A

Patrick Allard and Monica P. Colaiácovo

INTRODUCTION

Our perception and understanding of plastics and plasticizers have been greatly reshaped by the last two decades of research. Informed by novel and sometimes serendipitous findings, we have slowly moved from considering them as inert materials to being an integral part of our chemical landscape and able to elicit a vast array of biological responses. From phthalate esters to nonyl-phenol and Bisphenol A, both the number and, most importantly, the prevalence of compounds that are found in plastics with adverse biological effects are staggering.

4,4′-Dihydroxy-2,2-diphenylpropane or Bisphenol A (BPA) is certainly one of the most common chemicals produced by the plastics industry. It is an organic compound consisting of two phenolic rings connected by a single carbon carrying two methyl groups (Figure 50.1). BPA is the major monomer used in the manufacturing of polycarbonate (approximately 75% of BPA used) and epoxy resins (approximately 20%), and it is also found as an additive in polyvinyl chloride (PVC). Polycarbonate is classically synthesized by the polymerization of BPA monomers in reaction with carbonyl dichloride (phosgene). BPA is easy to manufacture and is also lightweight, clear and highly durable. Due to its remarkable properties, BPA in its polycarbonate form is found in a plethora of common products such as water, milk and baby bottles, eyeglass lenses, sport protective equipment and compact discs, as well as in medical and dental devices (NTP-CERHR, 2008). As epoxy resin, BPA is mainly used to line the inside of food cans and protect them from their content. Thus, BPA is ubiquitously present in our surroundings and is found in close proximity to food and drinks.

This chapter presents a comprehensive examination of the literature on Bisphenol A (BPA), from its invention to the current debate regarding its low dose effects. The chapter also discusses the recent advances in our understanding of its metabolism, its molecular action and the mechanisms underlying its reproductive and developmental effects.

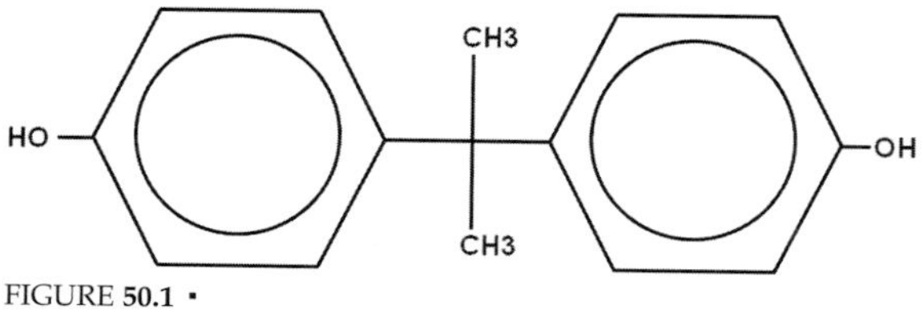

HO — [benzene ring] — C(CH_3)(CH_3) — [benzene ring] — OH

FIGURE **50.1** ·

HISTORICAL BACKGROUND

BPA was first reported by the Russian chemist Aleksandr Dianin in 1891 and synthesized in 1905 by Theodor Zincke from Marburg University, Germany. BPA was created by the reaction of phenol with acetone following a 2 to 1 ratio in the presence of an acid catalyst leaving water as the sole by-product.

The usefulness of BPA became evident by the middle of the 20th century. Although polycarbonates had been produced in the laboratory since the late 19th century, it was not until 1953 that polycarbonates were efficiently synthesized by reacting Bisphenol A with phosgene as discovered by Bayer chemist Dr. Hermann Schnell. The new material was patented in October 1953 under the name of Makrolon and polycarbonate production was rapidly expanded to reach industrial levels by the summer of 1960 (bayermaterialscience.com).

Nowadays, industrial synthesis of BPA still follows Zincke's reaction. It is one of the largest high volume chemicals in the world with a global production of approximately 6 billion pounds (3 million tons) as of 2004, of which approximately 1 million pounds are produced in the USA alone (NTP-CERHR, 2008). The rate of production of BPA has increased significantly throughout the years, growing from a global production of 16 million pounds in the early 1990s to an estimated production capacity of about 10 billion pounds in 2008. Although BPA production has been described as steadily increasing by 6 to 7% every year, it is unclear how the negative press and consumer pressure regarding BPA have affected the demand and, therefore, its production level. The leading manufacturers of BPA in the world are BASF, Bayer Material Science, Dow Chemicals, Hexion Specialty Chemicals, SABIC Innovative Plastics, Shell and Sunoco chemicals.

A biological activity for BPA was first reported in 1936, when Dodds and Lawson analyzed the estrogenic properties of a variety of compounds, including BPA, by injecting them at a dose of 100 mg in ovariectomized rats and monitoring the induction of an estrus (Dodds and Lawson, 1936, 1938).

Reproductive and Developmental Toxicology, Edited by Ramesh C. Gupta
ISBN: 978-0-12-382032-7

These results were repeated and confirmed in 1944 by Reid and Wilson (Reid and Wilson, 1944). In 1993 came the first report of BPA leaching, a major concern in BPA exposure and safety, from polycarbonate flasks following autoclaving (Krishnan et al., 1993). While investigating the synthesis of estrogens in yeast, Krishan and colleagues found that BPA, inadvertently released into the media from the flasks, binds the mammalian estrogen receptor, although less potently than estradiol. In further experiments, the authors also showed that BPA could elicit an estrogenic response in a well-established estrogen responsive cell line (MCF-7) at nanomolar concentrations (Krishnan et al., 1993). This was highly reminiscent of the serendipitous discovery by Soto and colleagues of the estrogenic properties of nonyl-phenol released from polystyrene 2 years earlier (Soto et al., 1991). These experiments led to extensive research on the exposure and effects of BPA in model organisms and humans, which will be discussed in the following sections.

PHARMACOKINETICS/ TOXICOKINETICS

BPA is present in a plethora of products used daily, including baby bottles, water bottles, various consumer plastics, tubings, paper, cardboard, soda cans, food cans and dental sealants (Vandenberg *et al.*, 2007). As BPA is mostly used for the packaging of food and drinks, it is thought that ingestion is the main source of human exposure to BPA. It is worth noting, however, that BPA is detectable in indoor air and dust and therefore might also be inhaled (Rudel *et al.*, 2003; Wilson *et al.*, 2003). It is estimated from urine sample analysis that the daily human intake of BPA ranges from 0 to approximately 2 μg/kg/day (Wilson *et al.*, 2007; Wolff *et al.*, 2007).

Most toxicokinetic data stems from the study of animal models, usually rodents. Following a single intravenous administration of BPA at 10 mg/kg to rats, BPA was rapidly detectable in a variety of adult and fetal tissues. Maximum BPA levels were reached within half an hour following administration, with levels ranging from 2 μg/g to approximately 10 μg/g depending on the organ tested. The liver, kidney and uterus tended to have higher BPA levels than the placenta, fetal liver and total fetal tissue. These results, however, pointed to a rapid transfer of BPA across the placental barrier (Moors *et al.*, 2006).

Several studies have examined the toxicokinetics of BPA in rats using both a low and a high dose of BPA while also comparing two distinct routes of exposure (oral vs. i.v.). The kinetics differed between the two routes of exposure with maximal concentration (15 μg/ml) of BPA being reached within minutes of i.v. administration at 10 mg/kg, and decreasing rapidly to 700 ng/ml. In contrast, whereas gavage at a similar concentration led to a rapid detection of BPA in serum, the maximum concentration (30 to 40 ng/ml) was only reached within several hours irrespective of the dose (10 or 100 mg/kg). Regardless of the route of exposure, BPA serum levels were undetectable 48 hours after administration (Upmeier *et al.*, 2000). A difference in the amount of bioavailable BPA based on the route of administration was also noted in another study with serum levels of BPA being markedly lower in oral compared to subcutaneous or i.v. treated rats irrespective of the dose (Pottenger *et al.*, 2000).

There are currently no data available on the toxicokinetics of BPA in humans that would take into account the fetus. Therefore, a physiological model that incorporates such parameters as blood flow and organ volume in the fetus was built using the mouse data (Mielke and Gundert-Remy, 2009). The experiments showed that total BPA concentration peaks in the blood and liver at 0.4 mg/L and 12 mg/L, respectively, within an hour of a single oral dose of BPA at 1 mg/kg. BPA is then rapidly, albeit not completely, cleared to reach a low steady-state level. In contrast, according to this model and supported by the mouse data, the fetus accumulates BPA with total BPA concentration reaching approximately 0.004 mg/L, 10 hours after BPA administration. Consistent with these results, another human toxicokinetic model also predicts a three-fold higher concentration of BPA in the blood of newborns due to incomplete development of their glucuronation system (see below) (Mielke and Gundert-Remy, 2009).

The two main metabolites of BPA are, in increasing order of importance, its sulfated and glucuronidated forms. The sulfation dramatically lowers BPA uptake and possibly its activity at the estrogen receptor, while an unequivocal decrease in ER activation by BPA has been observed when it is glucuronidated (Snyder *et al.*, 2000; Shimizu *et al.*, 2002; Stowell *et al.*, 2006). However, one major concern regarding the toxicokinetics of BPA is that fetuses and neonates have a lower ability to glucuronidate BPA. Administration of low doses of BPA (35 or 395 μg/kg) to mice was performed comparing two different routes of exposure, subcutaneous and oral, and radiolabeled BPA was measured for 24 hours in the blood of neonates. Interestingly, there was only minimal clearing of BPA within the 24 hour window showing that BPA remains largely non-metabolized in neonate mice (Taylor *et al.*, 2008). An age dependency in the modification of BPA was also observed in rats comparing neonates with adults (Domoradzki *et al.*, 2004). In adults, modified (conjugated) BPA is rapidly excreted and is the main form of BPA detected in milk, bile and urine (Pottenger *et al.*, 2000; Snyder *et al.*, 2000; Kurebayashi *et al.*, 2003), while non-conjugated BPA is the main form found in feces (Pottenger *et al.*, 2000). Differences in the mode of excretion of BPA between species were also noted, with rats relying more heavily on enterohepatic clearing of BPA while renal elimination is thought to be the main route for primates and humans (Tominaga *et al.*, 2006).

By comparing the toxicokinetics of BPA in three different animal species – rats, cynomolgus monkeys and chimpanzees – Tominaga and colleagues drew a comprehensive picture of the kinetics of BPA with likely better relevance to humans (Tominaga *et al.*, 2006). Eight hours after oral and subcutaneous administration of two doses of BPA (10 mg/kg or 100 mg/kg), monkeys and chimpanzees showed a higher serum level of BPA compared to rats, although after 24 hours the trend was reversed for the oral groups (rats showed higher serum levels than the two other groups). The total number of BPA metabolites detectable within 24 hours following administration was also higher in monkeys and chimpanzees than in rats (Tominaga *et al.*, 2006). The terminal elimination half-life was also higher in rats than in the other animals suggesting that human serum clearing might be lower than predicted by rodent models, thus highlighting the difficulty in translating results obtained in rodents to humans.

There is little human data on the toxicokinetics of BPA. Völkel and colleagues administered a single low oral dose of BPA (5 mg) to adults. This resulted in a total serum peak of BPA at around 1.5 hours and a complete recovery of the administered BPA through the urine within 30 hours for both males and females. The terminal half-life of BPA in the blood was estimated to be 5.4 hours. In this study, only the glucuronidated form of BPA was detected in both blood and urine samples (Volkel *et al.*, 2002).

Taken together, these studies point to the need for additional analyses performed in various model species, and if possible more human data, in order to establish the fetal toxicokinetics of BPA and its accumulation in various fetal organs during critical windows of development.

MECHANISM OF ACTION

BPA has been viewed historically as a weak environmental estrogen based on its binding affinity to classical estrogen receptors (ER) when compared to a canonical estrogen such estradiol. Recent research, however, has uncovered a pleiotropy in the mechanism of action of BPA. First, BPA should be considered a selective estrogen receptor modulator, or SERM, as its action as either an estrogen agonist or antagonist is tissue dependent. Second, BPA can elicit an estrogenic cellular response at low concentrations and with potency equivalent to that of estradiol. Finally, BPA elicits biological effects through other receptors and pathways that are non-ER related. These different modes of action of BPA are explored below.

Bisphenol A and the estrogen receptors

Many of the biological responses described for BPA are attributed to its association with both classical and non-classical estrogen receptors. BPA can bind both mammalian ERα and ERβ (Kuiper *et al.*, 1997; Pennie *et al.*, 1998; Hiroi *et al.*, 1999), although its relative binding affinity seems to be between six to ten times higher for ERβ than for ERα (Routledge *et al.*, 2000). This results in estrogen receptor element (ERE) mediated transcriptional activation (Pennie *et al.*, 1998). In these experiments, BPA was shown to associate with the ERs with much lower affinity than estradiol, with approximately 2,000-fold less affinity for ERα and 300-fold less for ERβ (Kuiper *et al.*, 1997). The IC_{50} (concentration of a compound able to decrease ligand binding to a receptor by 50%) of BPA for the two ERs is estimated to be in the micromolar range: 1–8 μM (Kuiper *et al.*, 1998; Kim *et al.*, 2001; Matthews *et al.*, 2001). BPA is not only a partial agonist of both ERα and ERβ (Barkhem *et al.*, 1998; Gould *et al.*, 1998), but as highlighted by a series of *in vitro* experiments, it also interacts with ERα in a way clearly distinct from estradiol, partial agonists like 4OH-tamoxifen or the pure antagonist ICI182780 (Gould *et al.*, 1998).

ERα and ERβ both contain a ligand-dependent transactivation domain termed AF2 that activates transcription of downstream target genes by the recruitment of transcriptional co-factors such as SRC-1 and TIF2 (Berry *et al.*, 1990; Voegel *et al.*, 1996; Henttu *et al.*, 1997). The association of BPA to the ligand-binding domain of ERα and ERβ significantly increases the recruitment of both SRC-1 and TIF2, although the BPA-mediated recruitment of TIF2 is 500-fold higher for ERβ than for ERα (Routledge *et al.*, 2000).

While the affinity of BPA for classical ERs is low, it can bind with high affinity to ERRγ. ERRγ is an orphan nuclear receptor of the ERR (estrogen receptor-related) family and is therefore related to ERα and ERβ (Giguere, 2002). Although the receptors share sequence homology, estradiol does not associate with ERRγ (Takayanagi *et al.*, 2006). By both crystallography structure analysis and computer modeling, BPA has been shown to fit in the ligand-binding domain of ERRγ while preserving its constitutive activity (Matsushima *et al.*, 2007; Nose and Shimohigashi, 2008). The IC_{50} for the interaction of BPA with the ERRγ ligand-binding domain is around 10 nM (Takayanagi *et al.*, 2006; Okada *et al.*, 2008), thus much lower than the corresponding values for ERα and ERβ, and similar to the IC_{50} of 4OH-tamoxifen, a very strong inverse agonist of ERRγ (Coward *et al.*, 2001). The significance of BPA binding to ERRγ is unclear, but it should be noted that ERRs associate with the EREs and share similar transcriptional targets as ERα (Vanacker *et al.*, 1999). Moreover, heterodimerization of ERRγ with ERα suppresses the transcriptional activity of both receptors (Huppunen and Aarnisalo, 2004). Taken together, these results suggest that BPA, via its interaction with ERRγ, can also interfere with classical ER signaling.

BPA and the androgen and thyroid hormone receptors

BPA binds the androgen receptor (AR) with an IC_{50} in the micromolar range, between 0.7 and 10 μM, when compared to 5α-dihydrotestosterone (DHT) or a synthetic reference androgen R1881 (Paris *et al.*, 2002; Lee *et al.*, 2003; Xu *et al.*, 2005; Sun *et al.*, 2006). Furthermore, BPA displays an antagonistic activity at the AR (Xu *et al.*, 2005) by partially and noncompetitively preventing DHT from binding the AR (Lee *et al.*, 2003).

BPA shares structural similarity with triiodothyronine, also known as T3, the more active form of the thyroid hormone. Similarly to its action at the AR, BPA exhibits a weak antagonistic activity towards the thyroid hormone receptors (TRs) with an IC_{50} around 16 μM (Sun *et al.*, 2009). Consistent with these results, BPA in the micromolar range inhibits the transcriptional activity of T3 through both TRα and Trβ, although it inhibits TRβ activity more efficiently than that of TRα (Moriyama *et al.*, 2002; Zoeller *et al.*, 2005; Iwamuro *et al.*, 2006). This antagonist effect of BPA on the TRs can be at least partially explained by the ability of BPA to enhance the interaction of N-CoR, a negative co-regulator of TR transcriptional activity, with the TRs (Moriyama *et al.*, 2002).

Although the IC_{50} of BPA on the androgen and thyroid hormone receptors seems to be weak, it is interesting to note that *in vivo* effects mediated by both receptor types have been demonstrated at low levels of BPA. The mechanistic evidence is discussed in the next section.

Rapid, non-genomic response

The action of estrogens like estradiol is also mediated by non-ER-dependent pathways such as the binding and activation of the endoplasmic reticulum associated G protein coupled receptor GPR30 (Revankar *et al.*, 2005). Estradiol elicits two effects upon binding to GPR30: the mobilization of intracellular calcium and the activation of PI3K signaling (Revankar *et al.*, 2005). BPA binds GPR30 with an IC_{50} of 630 nM at levels approximately 35 times lower than that of estradiol (Thomas and Dong, 2006). This association leads to an increase in cAMP levels. Thus, as pathways downstream of GPR30 include ERK, PI3K, calcium mobilization and cAMP production (Prossnitz *et al.*, 2008), BPA may trigger activation of multiple rapid pathways.

Another example of the rapid action of BPA is in pancreatic cells where BPA exposure results in the modulation of intracellular calcium concentration at levels similar to that of estradiol (Nadal *et al.*, 2000). In beta cells, BPA binds to a membrane-associated catecholaminergic receptor leading to the calcium-dependent activation of the transcription factor CREB (Ropero *et al.*, 2006; Bouskine *et al.*, 2009). In alpha cells, however, BPA associates with a membrane-bound G coupled receptor and its action is mediated by a cGMP/PKG-dependent mechanism (Alonso-Magdalena *et al.*, 2005). Importantly, in both cell types, the effects of BPA were comparable to that of estradiol at similar concentrations.

In the nervous system, a single low dose of BPA (10^{-12} to 10^{-10} M) is sufficient to rapidly activate ERK signaling. Specifically, this activation is observed within six minutes of direct injection of BPA into the cerebellar cortex of rats and is similar in nature to the response observed with estradiol at the same concentration (Zsarnovszky *et al.*, 2005). Interestingly, in this context, co-administration of BPA at low concentration inhibits the estradiol response. In the PC12 neuronal cell line, a low dose of BPA also elicited a rapid response resulting in the inhibition of dopamine efflux within 15 minutes of exposure. This was consistent with the relocalization of the membrane-associated ERs and the dopamine transporter away from the membrane (Alyea and Watson, 2009).

Action of BPA at the DNA level

An intriguing mechanism for the action of BPA involves its potential direct action on the DNA to alter gene expression. BPA has been shown to be oxidized into bisphenol-o-quinone which can then covalently bind deoxyguanosine to form DNA adducts both *in vitro* and *in vivo* (Atkinson and Roy, 1995; Edmonds *et al.*, 2004). The presence of adducts in mice following ingestion of water containing BPA was detected in at least two tissues, the liver and the mammary glands (Izzotti *et al.*, 2009). Although these results suggest a direct role of BPA in causing DNA injuries, some DNA damage can also be mediated by BPA action at the ER. Indeed, in a comet assay performed in MCF-7 cells, BPA was shown to induce DNA damage, although at concentrations 1,000-fold higher than estradiol. This effect could be blocked by co-exposure with the ER antagonist ICI182780 (Iso *et al.*, 2006).

Although the mechanism of BPA effects on the epigenome is unknown, it is now clear that BPA exposure dramatically alters patterns of methylation at genome-wide levels (Yaoi *et al.*, 2008). The effect of BPA seems to be locus specific as both induced methylation and demethylation are detected following exposure (Yaoi *et al.*, 2008). Demethylation in particular has resulted in potentially drastic outcomes, including changes in coat color by BPA-mediated hypomethylation of the *Agouti* locus (Dolinoy *et al.*, 2007) and an upregulation of the hox gene Hoxa10 by induced hypomethylation of its promoter element in the uterus (Bromer *et al.*, 2010). This hypomethylation of Hoxa10 increases the accessibility of its ERE to ERα, once again suggesting an interplay between BPA and ER signaling.

Although a study by Tyl and colleagues failed to detect an effect of BPA on several reproductive endpoints for multiple generations (Tyl *et al.*, 2008), an action of BPA on DNA methylation suggests the possibility of transgenerational effects which should be carefully studied. Furthermore, a better understanding of the non-genomic action of BPA is of particular importance as BPA is thought to be cleared within a few minutes to hours from the blood and rapidly excreted through urine in humans, suggesting that the rapid action of BPA might be an important component of the effects of BPA in humans.

REPRODUCTIVE AND DEVELOPMENTAL TOXICITY

The study of the effects of BPA on development and reproduction has produced a wealth of data on these two topics. In reviewing the research, it is important to keep in mind the model organism used (most commonly mice or rats), the sensitivity of the strain as well as the dose and the route of exposure chosen. When either the developmental endpoints or the fetal basis of adult disease are assayed, it is important to determine the critical window of development for these endpoints in order to inform human risk assessment. In this section, we will explore the various developmental and reproductive processes disrupted by BPA based mainly on rodent models of BPA exposure. The studies and reported effects of BPA mentioned in this section are summarized in Table 50.1.

Mammary gland

The mammary gland is a tissue that sees extensive remodeling starting from puberty and continuing throughout the reproductive life of an individual. The changes in tissue architecture are exquisitely sensitive to circulating hormones such as estradiol and progesterone, and as such vary during both the estrous cycle and pregnancy (Soto *et al.*, 2008). Morphogenetic processes that are hormone dependent include the formation of terminal end buds (TEB), invasion of the fat pad at puberty and branching of the ducts (Soto *et al.*, 2008).

BPA can significantly delay the morphogenesis of the mammary gland at critical windows for development of this structure. First, mouse embryonic exposure to BPA (embryonic day 8 to 18) increases the growth of ducts and the maturation of the fat pads while delaying lumen formation at E 18 (Vandenberg *et al.*, 2007). Second, perinatal exposure to BPA by osmotic pump in mice, even at low doses, leads to a significant increase in the number of TEBs, a decrease in apoptosis and an increase in progesterone-mediated side branching in peripubertal mice (Markey *et al.*, 2001; Munoz-de-Toro *et al.*, 2005). This suggests that early BPA exposure can sensitize the mammary tissue to the action of hormones later in life. Consistent with this idea, the authors noticed an increased sensitivity to estradiol (Munoz-de-Toro *et al.*, 2005; Wadia *et al.*, 2007) and an increased expression of both ERα, the main estrogen receptor in the mammary gland, and the progesterone receptor (Munoz-de-Toro *et al.*, 2005).

The changes in mammary gland architecture observed following BPA administration were associated with a higher propensity to develop pre-cancerous and cancerous lesions. Exposure of rats in utero to a range of BPA doses resulted in the appearance of ductal hyperplasias and carcinoma in situ later in life, at postnatal days 50 and 95 (Murray et al.,

TABLE 50.1 Summary of studies cited in this chapter

Topic	Article cited	Species/ strain	Route	Dose per day	Time of exposure	Reported effects mentioned in this chapter
Mammary gland	Durando *et al.*, 2007	Rat/Wistar	Osmotic pump	25 μg/kg	E 8-E 23	Increased duct hyperplasia at PND 110 and 180 Increased tumor and tumor multiplicity at PND 50 when co-exposed to NMU
	Munoz-de-Toro *et al.*, 2005	Mouse/CD-1	Osmotic pump	25 ng/kg 250 ng/kg	E 9-PND 4	Increase in terminal end buds (TEBs) at PND 30 Decreased apoptosis at PND 30 Increased lateral branching at 4 months for 25 ng/kg
	Murray *et al.*, 2007	Rat/Wistar	Osmotic pump	2.5, 25, 250, 1,000 μg/kg	E 9-PND 1	Increased duct hyperplasia at PND 50 (all doses) Increased duct hyperplasia at PND 95 (lowest dose)
	Wadia *et al.*, 2007	Mouse/CD-1 and C57Bl6	Osmotic pump	250 ng/kg	E 8-PND 2	Increased sensitivity to estradiol Increased number of TEBs at PND 35
Male reproduction	Herath *et al.*, 2004	Rat/Wistar	Subcutaneous	3 mg/kg	PND 50–85	Increased ventral prostate weight
	Ramos *et al.*, 2001	Rat/Wistar	Osmotic pump	25 μg/kg 250 μg/kg	E 8–birth	Decreased androgen receptor (AR)-positive cells in periductal stroma in ventral prostate at PND 30
	Richter *et al.*, 2007	Mouse/CD-1	Cell culture	0–100,000 nM	4 days	Increase in AR expression
	Timms *et al.*, 2005	Mouse/CD-1	Oral	10 μg/kg	E 14–18	Increase in epithelial cell proliferation at E 19 Increase in number and size of ducts at E 19
	Ho *et al.*, 2006	Rat/Sprague-Dawley	Subcutaneous	10 μg/kg	PND 1, 3 and 5	Increased susceptibility to prostate neoplastic lesions at PND 200
	Ashby *et al.*, 2003	Rat/Sprague-Dawley	Oral	20 μg/kg–200 mg/kg	PND 91–97	No effect on testis weight at PND 125
	Kato *et al.*, 2006	Rat/Sprague-Dawley	Subcutaneous	0.002–97 mg/kg	PND 1–10	No effect on testis weight at either PND 35 or 150
	Takahashi and Oishi, 2003	Mouse, Rat/ CD-1, SD	Subcutaneous Intraperitoneal	200 and 400 mg/kg	4 and 8 weeks	Decreased testis, epididymis and prostate weight
	Chitra *et al.*, 2003	Rat/Wistar	Oral	0.2, 2 and 20 μg/kg	PND 45–90	Decreased testis and epididymis weight Increased ventral prostate weight
	Kabuto *et al.*, 2004	Mouse/ICR	Oral	5–10 μg/mL	E 1–PND 28	Decreased testis weight at PND 28
	Fiorini *et al.*, 2004	Rat/Wistar SerW3 cell line	Cell culture	45 μM	24 hours	Decreased Connexin 43 protein levels
	Salian *et al.*, 2009	Rat/ Holtzman	Subcutaneous	100–1,600 μg/kg	PND 1–5	Decreased Connexin 43 immunostaining at PND 45 and 90
	Akingbemi *et al.*, 2004	Rat/Long-Evans	Oral	2.4 μg/kg	PND 21–35	Decreased testosterone production at PND 35
	Nakamura *et al.*, 2010	Rat/Wistar	Subcutaneous	57.1 and 114.2 mg/kg	PND 28–70	Decreased testosterone production at PND 70
	Takao *et al.*, 1999	Mouse/ C57Bl6	Oral	50 μg/ml	PND 35–63 and 91	Decreased testosterone production at PND 63 and 91

(Continued)

TABLE 50.1—*cont'd*

Topic	Article cited	Species/ strain	Route	Dose per day	Time of exposure	Reported effects mentioned in this chapter
	Toyama *et al.*, 2004	Mouse, Rat/ ICR, Wistar	Subcutaneous	20 and 200 μg/ kg	6 days at 3, 4 month	Malformed spermatids after a 6-day treatment
Female reproduction	Rubin *et al.*, 2001	Rat/Sprague-Dawley	Oral	0.1 and 1.2 mg/kg	E 6–PND 21	Lower plasma LH levels in cycling adults
	Fernandez *et al.*, 2009	Rat/Sprague-Dawley	Subcutaneous	25–62 mg/kg	PND 1–10	Decreased LH release from GnRH at PND 13 Increased GnRH pulsatility at PND 13
	Savabiesfahani *et al.*, 2006	Sheep/Suffolk	Subcutaneous	5 mg/kg	E 30–90	Lower LH surge amplitude in cycling adults
	Adewale *et al.*, 2009	Rat/Long-Evans	Subcutaneous	50 μg/kg 50 mg/kg	PND 1–4	Early onset of puberty at 50 μg/kg Abnormal cycle for both doses PND 50–105
	Honma *et al.*, 2002	Mouse/ICR	Subcutaneous	20 μg/kg	E 11–17	Early onset of puberty
	Howdeshell *et al.*, 1999	Mouse/CF-1	Oral	2.4 μg/kg	E 11–17	Early onset of puberty
	Nikaido *et al.*, 2004	Mouse/CD-1	Subcutaneous	0.5 and 10 mg/kg	E 15–E 18	Early onset of puberty
	Markey *et al.*, 2005	Mouse/CD-1	Osmotic pump	250 ng/kg	E 9–PND 4	Increased proliferation of uterine epithelium at PND 90
	Suzuki *et al.*, 2002	Mouse/ICR	Subcutaneous	150 μg/pup	PND 1–5	Vaginal stratification at PND 40 and 90
	Kato *et al.*, 2003	Rat/Sprague-Dawley	Subcutaneous	13.2 mg/kg	PND 1–10	Persistent cornification in adults
	Newbold *et al.*, 2009	Mouse/CD-1	Subcutaneous	0.1–1,000 μg/ kg	E 9–16	Presence of cancerous lesions in the ovary, oviduct and vagina at 16–18 months
	Steinmetz *et al.*, 1998	Rat/Sprague-Dawley, F344	Pellet implantation	0.3 mg/kg	3 days at PND 70	Induced cell proliferation in uterus and vagina at PND 74
	Fernández *et al.*, 2010	Rat/Sprague-Dawley	Subcutaneous	25–62 mg/kg	PND 1–10	Presence of ovarian cysts, infertility at 4–5 months
	Newbold *et al.*, 2007	Mouse/CD-1	Subcutaneous	10–1,000 μg/ kg	PND 1–5	Presence of ovarian cysts and cancerous lesions in ovary, oviduct and uterus at 18 months
	Hunt *et al.*, 2003	Mouse	Oral	20 μg/kg	PND 20–28	Altered meiotic progression, aneuploidy in adults
	Susiarjo *et al.*, 2007	Mouse/ C57Bl6	Pellet implantation	20 μg/kg	E 11–18	Altered meiotic progression at E 18.5 Aneuploidy at 4–5 weeks
	Mlynarcikova *et al.*, 2009	Porcine	Cell culture	100 μM	44 hours	Altered meiotic progression
Brain and behavior	Kubo *et al.*, 2001	Rat/Wistar	Oral	1.5 mg/kg	E 1–PND 21	Elimination of sexual dimorphism of locus coeruleus and avoidance memory at 20 weeks
	Kubo *et al.*, 2003	Rat/Wistar	Oral	30 and 300 μg/ kg	E 1–PND 21	Elimination of sexual dimorphism of locus coeruleus at 14 weeks Elimination of sex differences in open-field test at 6 weeks

TABLE 50.1—*cont'd*

Topic	Article cited	Species/ strain	Route	Dose per day	Time of exposure	Reported effects mentioned in this chapter
Brain and behavior	Patisaul *et al.*, 2006	Rat/Sprague-Dawley	Subcutaneous	~100 mg/kg	PND 1–4	Elimination of sex differences in TH expression in the AVPV nucleus
	Rubin *et al.*, 2006	Mouse/CD-1	Osmotic pump	25 and 250 ng/kg	E 8–PND 16	Elimination of sex differences in TH expression in the AVPV nucleus 22–24 days Elimination of sex differences in open-field test at 6–9 weeks
	Miyatake *et al.*, 2006	Mouse/ICR	Oral	3 μg/kg 200 mg/kh	E 1–PND 21	Increased dopamine-dependent rewarding effect at 7 weeks
	Zhou *et al.*, 2009	Rat/Sprague-Dawley	Subcutaneous	20 μg/kg	E 8–PND 21	Impairs LTP and LTD at PND 21–32
	Miyagawa *et al.*, 2007	Mouse/ C57Bl6	Oral	30 ng/g, 2 mg/g diet	E 1–PND 21	Memory impairment, decrease in Ach production in 7–11 week old males
	Farabollini *et al.*, 2002	Rat/Sprague-Dawley	Oral	40 μg/kg	E 1–PND 21	Increased frequency of lordosis in females at PND 100 Increased intromission latency in prenatal treatment of males at PND 100
	Della Seta *et al.*, 2005	Rat/Sprague-Dawley	Oral	40 μg/kg	E 1–PND 21	Decreased maternal behavior
	Palanza *et al.*, 2002	Mouse/CD-1	Oral	10 μg/kg	E 14–18	Decreased maternal behavior
	Ryan and Vandenbergh, 2006	Mouse/ C57Bl6	Oral	2 and 200 μg/ kg	E 1–PND 21	No effect on spatial memory in adults
	Gioiosa *et al.*, 2007	Mouse/CD-1	Oral	10 μg/kg	E 11–PND 8	Elimination of sex differences in exploratory behavior at PND 30 and PND 70
	Palanza *et al.*, 2008	Mouse/CD-1	Oral	10 μg/kg	E 11–18 E 11–PND 7	Elimination of sex differences in novelty (PND 28–30) and exploratory behavior (adults)
Thyroid function	Zoeller *et al.*, 2005	Rat/Sprague-Dawley	Oral	1–50 mg/kg	E 6–lactation	Increased total serum T_4 at PND 15
	Heimeier *et al.*, 2009	*Xenopus laevis*	Mixed in tank water	10 μM	4 days	Delay in metamorphosis
	Ramakrishnan and Wayne, 2008	Medaka fish	Mixed in tank water	200 μg/l	E 1–3	Acceleration of embryonic development
Adipogenesis	Rubin *et al.*, 2001	Rat / Sprague-Dawley	Oral	0.1 and 1.2 mg/kg	E 6–PND 21	Increase in body weight at PND 4–PND 110
	Masuno *et al.*, 2005	3T3-L1 cell line	Cell culture	80 μM	6 days	Accelerated differentiation into adipocytes, accumulation of triglycerides
	Sargis *et al.*, 2009	3T3-L1 cell line	Cell culture	10–100 nM	3 days	Accelerated differentiation into adipocytes, accumulation of triglycerides

(Continued)

TABLE 50.1 *cont'd*

Topic	Article cited	Species/ strain	Route	Dose per day	Time of exposure	Reported effects mentioned in this chapter
	Masuno *et al.*, 2002	3T3-L1 cell line	Cell culture	20 μg/ml	2 days	Accelerated differentiation into adipocytes, accumulation of triglycerides
	Hugo *et al.*, 2008	Adipose tissue explant	Cell culture	0.1 and 1 nM	6 hours	Suppression of adiponectine release
	Phrakonkham *et al.*, 2008	3T3–L1 cell line	Cell culture	80 μM	2 days	Increased leptin mRNA levels
	Somm *et al.*, 2009	Rat/Sprague-Dawley	Oral	70 μg/kg	E 6–PND 21	Increase weight in females at PND 1 and 21 Adipocyte hypertrophy and increased expression of lipogenic genes at PND 21

E: embryonic day (plug day = day1); PND: postnatal day (birth = day 1)

2007). The proportion of hyperplastic ducts and neoplastic lesions can be further increased by the injection of N-nitroso-N-methylurea (NMU), a carcinogenic compound used at subcarcinogenic levels in this study (Durando *et al.*, 2007).

These results therefore suggest that exposure to BPA early in life predisposes the mammary tissue to respond abnormally to both hormonal signaling and the development of neoplastic lesions later in life.

Male reproductive system

Prostate

Administering BPA affects the histoarchitecture of the adult prostate. It increases the size of both the ventral prostate gland in adults (Herath *et al.*, 2004) and the ratio of fibroblastic to smooth muscle when given prenatally (Ramos *et al.*, 2001). These changes are accompanied by a downregulation in the expression of the androgen receptor (AR) (Ramos *et al.*, 2001), although an upregulation of the AR following BPA exposure at low dose has also been reported (Richter *et al.*, 2007). Low doses of BPA can also impair the development of the embryonic prostate. Specifically, BPA exposure increases the total number of prostate gland ducts and also their volume (Timms *et al.*, 2005). The increase in the size of the ducts is likely due to an increase in cell proliferation as revealed by PCNA staining (Timms *et al.*, 2005).

Similarly to the mammary gland, exposure to low levels of Bisphenol A early in life can predispose to the development of neoplastic lesions in the prostate. Specifically, intraepithelial prostatic neoplasia develops when older rats that were exposed to BPA shortly after birth are subjected to continuous exposure to estrogen and testosterone as adults (Ho *et al.*, 2006).

Testis and sperm production

There is ambiguity regarding whether administering BPA to adult males can affect the testis, with several authors reporting no effect on weight or size (Ashby *et al.*, 2003; Kato *et al.*, 2006) unless BPA is administered at high doses (Takahashi and Oishi, 2003). However, it appears that embryonic and perinatal BPA exposures do lead to a reduction in testis size in mice and rats (Chitra *et al.*, 2003; Kabuto *et al.*, 2004). For example, low doses of BPA administered to mice via their water throughout embryonic life until weaning lead to a significant 18% decrease in testis weight (Kabuto *et al.*, 2004).

Within the testis, one of the targets of BPA seems to be the Sertoli cells, where expression of Connexin 43, a major gap junction component of Sertoli cells that plays a crucial role during spermatogenesis (Brehm *et al.*, 2007; Sridharan *et al.*, 2007), is greatly downregulated following BPA exposure in rats (Fiorini *et al.*, 2004; Salian *et al.*, 2009). The number of Leydig cells and the expression of steroidogenesis genes crucial for testosterone production are also affected by BPA leading to a decrease in the production of the male hormone (Takao *et al.*, 1999; Akingbemi *et al.*, 2004; Nakamura *et al.*, 2010). These testicular defects are the likely cause of the decreased epididymal sperm count and mobility observed following BPA administration (Chitra *et al.*, 2003). The spermatids were also affected with severe deformation of both the nuclei and the acrosomal compartment (Toyama *et al.*, 2004).

Finally, the action of BPA on the testis and other male reproductive organs could account for the decrease in fertility (i.e., the smaller litter size) observed when males exposed perinatally to low BPA doses are mated with non-exposed females (Salian *et al.*, 2009).

Female reproductive system

Effects on the pituitary–gonadal axis, puberty and estrous cycle

One mechanism of BPA-induced effect on reproduction is via disruption of the pituitary–gonadal axis, thus altering the normal estrous cycle. In BPA-treated rats, plasma LH levels are lower than control (Rubin *et al.*, 2001) and LH release in response to GnRH is dampened, while an increase in the number of pulses is observed (Fernandez *et al.*, 2009). A dampening of LH surge amplitude was also observed in ewes treated with BPA (Savabieasfahani *et al.*, 2006). This could be explained by an inability to either upregulate or sustain the activity of downstream effectors such as IP3 and phosphorylated ERK1/2, respectively (Fernandez *et al.*, 2009).

The onset of puberty in rodents can be assessed by the timing of vaginal opening which was significantly lowered both in BPA-exposed rats and mice compared to control (Howdeshell et *al.*, 1999; Honma *et al.*, 2002; Nikaido *et al.*, 2004; Adewale *et al.*, 2009; Fernandez *et al.*, 2009). The estrous cycle was also perturbed with significantly more days spent in estrus vs. either diestrus or proestrus for rats exposed at low doses (Fernandez *et al.*, 2009), or diestrus for mice exposed to mid-to-high doses (Nikaido *et al.*, 2004). In rats, neonatal exposure to BPA ultimately leads to acyclicity (Adewale *et al.*, 2009).

Oviduct, uterus and vagina

BPA exposure can cause dramatic alteration of the tissue architecture and proliferative characteristics of the female genital tract. First, BPA causes malformation of the uterus in both mouse and rat models. Prenatal exposure to low levels of BPA leads to increased proliferation of the uterine lining with stratification of its epithelium (Suzuki *et al.*, 2002; Markey *et al.*, 2005). The vaginal epithelium is also affected, showing a persistent cornification (keratinization) in both species (Kato *et al.*, 2003; Nikaido *et al.*, 2004). These changes in tissue architecture are associated with abnormal proliferation and the appearance of pre-cancerous and cancerous lesions in the oviduct, uterus and vagina (Steinmetz *et al.*, 1998; Newbold *et al.*, 2007, 2009).

Ovary and oocytes

Ovarian morphology is affected by exposure to BPA. In rats exposed to BPA neonatally by subcutaneous injection, the number of corpus lutei and antral follicles is decreased in the ovaries, while an increase in the number of atretic follicles and in follicles resembling cystic follicles are observed (Kato *et al.*, 2003; Newbold *et al.*, 2007; Adewale *et al.*, 2009; Fernandez *et al.*, 2010). Instances of polyovular follicles are also detected (Suzuki *et al.*, 2002). Consistent with these observations in animal models, higher serum BPA levels are found in women with polycystic ovaries (Takeuchi *et al.*, 2004).

Oocyte development is also affected by BPA exposure. In two important studies, Hunt and colleagues showed that exposure to BPA, either during adulthood or *in utero,* alters proper meiotic progression (Hunt *et al.*, 2003; Susiarjo *et al.*, 2007). BPA exposure *in utero,* spanning the embryonic stages when the first step of meiosis (prophase I) unravels, causes the appearance of end-to-end chromosome associations as well as an increase in recombination (Susiarjo *et al.*, 2007). These defects likely result in the increased rate of aneuploidy observed in unfertilized eggs and embryos at adulthood (Susiarjo *et al.*, 2007). Exposure in reproducing adult females, on the other hand, leads to a failure of chromosomes to align properly at the metaphase plate (congression failure), during meiosis I and II, therefore also resulting in aneuploidy (Hunt *et al.*, 2003). Consistent with these results, the ability of porcine oocytes to progress through meiosis I and II is significantly lowered compared to controls (Mlynarcikova *et al.*, 2009).

Brain and behavior

Administering BPA even at a low dose can erase and sometimes even reverse sexually dimorphic differences in the brain. Kubo and colleagues examined the effect of administering BPA to rats at a low oral dose prenatally until weaning age on a sexually dimorphic nucleus: the locus coeruleus (LC), a brainstem nucleus involved in fear and panic response (Kubo *et al.*, 2001, 2003). The LC size difference under control conditions (female LC>male LC) was effectively reversed when exposed to BPA (male LC>female LC) (Kubo *et al.*, 2003). In mice, exposure to even very low doses during the same developmental window affected another region, the periventricular preoptic area which is implicated in the control of estrous cyclicity and characterized by a differential number of tyrosine hydroxylase (TH) neurons (more in females than in males) (Patisaul *et al.*, 2006; Rubin *et al.*, 2006). BPA exposure erased the difference between sexes by specifically reducing the number of TH-positive neurons in females while males were unaffected (Patisaul *et al.*, 2006; Rubin *et al.*, 2006).

BPA exposure can alter the expression or effect of several neurotransmitters. For example, pre- and neonatal exposure to BPA in mice leads to an enhancement of the dopamine-dependent rewarding effect which correlates with an increased dopamine response of neurons and astrocytes *in vitro* (Miyatake *et al.*, 2006). Consistent with these results, the dopaminergic-mediated effect of BPA on hyperlocomotion can be efficiently blocked by using a dopamine 1 receptor specific inhibitor (Zhou *et al.*, 2009). BPA also causes a severe decrease in production of acetylcholine in the hippocampus possibly causing memory impairment (Miyagawa *et al.*, 2007).

BPA appears to have opposing effects on male and female rats in terms of sexual behavior. While in males BPA decreased overall performance by increasing the latency of intromission; in females, BPA increased their sexual receptivity as measured by lordosis behavior (Farabollini *et al.*, 2002).

Maternal behavior in both mice and rats is also affected by exposure to BPA. A decrease in maternal behavior, as judged by time spent nursing, was observed in females exposed to BPA at very low oral doses either prenatally or as adults (Palanza *et al.*, 2002; Della Seta *et al.*, 2005).

While BPA does not seem to affect spatial memory in mice (Ryan and Vandenbergh, 2006), BPA has been shown to negatively impact memory in tests measuring avoidance behavior (Miyagawa *et al.*, 2007). The analysis of both male and female rats revealed that BPA erases the sexually dimorphic behavior in avoidance memory (Kubo *et al.*, 2001). In open field tests, BPA could erase male/female differences in mice (Rubin *et al.*, 2006; Gioiosa *et al.*, 2007; Palanza *et al.*, 2008) and could even revert sex differences in rats, with males acting more like females (Kubo *et al.*, 2001, 2003).

Interference with thyroid hormone function

Physiological levels of BPA efficiently downregulate thyroid hormone target genes *in vitro* by recruiting transcriptional corepressors to the thyroid hormone receptor as shown in mammalian two-hybrid experiments (Moriyama *et al.*, 2002). Studies in rodents suggest that BPA acts specifically on the beta-TR, which mediates the downstream negative effect of TH on the pituitary (Zoeller *et al.*, 2005). In *Xenopus laevis*, BPA inhibits thyroid-mediated processes such as metamorphosis. Interestingly, microarray analysis revealed that most T3 responsive genes are inhibited by BPA exposure confirming the antagonistic action of BPA on the TR (Heimeier *et al.*, 2009). Just like its action on the ER, the action of BPA as either an agonist or antagonist can be context dependent. For example, in medaka fish, BPA accelerates the development of the embryos and advances sexual maturation in a process that can be blocked by a TR-specific antagonist (Ramakrishnan and Wayne, 2008).

Adipogenesis

The study of environmental toxicants able to promote fat accumulation, coined "obesogens", is of growing interest as they may contribute to the worldwide obesity epidemic. BPA belongs to the list of compounds having this property as the rodent models have shown that BPA exposure correlates with weight gain (Rubin *et al.*, 2001; Rubin and Soto, 2009).

Several mechanisms can help explain the effect of BPA on body weight increase. Using a mouse pre-adipocyte cell line that can be differentiated into mature adipocytes, Masuno and others have shown that BPA, as well as BPA in combination with insulin, working through the activation of PI-3 kinase, can dramatically push the fibroblastic cells into an adipocyte differentiation pathway leading to high accumulation of triglycerides and lipoprotein lipase (Masuno *et al.*, 2002, 2005; Sargis *et al.*, 2009).

A possibly related mechanism leading to triglyceride accumulation is the decreased production of the hormone adiponectin from all human adipous tissue tested when exposed to very low levels (below the nanomolar range) of BPA in either cell or explant culture settings (Hugo *et al.*, 2008). Conversely, the expression of leptin, as well as of several enzymes and transcription factors involved in adipogenesis, is upregulated by BPA exposure both *in vivo* and *in vitro* (Phrakonkham *et al.*, 2008; Somm *et al.*, 2009). Taken together, the altered expression and activity of these important mediators of fat metabolism could explain the increase in weight following BPA exposure in rodent models. These results also suggest that along with other obesogens, low but environmentally relevant levels of BPA may contribute to the human obesity phenomenon.

Collectively, these mechanistic insights on the effect of BPA *in vivo* highlight two important features shared between BPA and other toxicants. First, BPA can act at distinct critical windows of development. In terms of meiotic endpoint, for example, exposure to BPA early during fetal life, when meiotic prophase I is under way, significantly impacts the progression through this specific phase of meiosis (Susiarjo *et al.*, 2007). Second, exposure early on in life can cause irremediable changes in tissue architecture or cellular response, rendering specific tissues more prone to the development of particular diseases. This is exemplified by the fetal exposure to BPA and the development of mammary hyperplasia and predisposition to tumors (Durando *et al.*, 2007; Murray *et al.*, 2007). Thus, the determination of the critical windows of development for various endpoints that are affected by BPA is of prime importance for human risk assessment.

RISK ASSESSMENT

While the list of adverse effects attributed to BPA is extensive, the risk associated with BPA exposure to humans is a source of seemingly endless debate (for examples, see vom Saal and Hughes, 2005; Politch, 2006). Although a definite causal relationship between BPA and human disease has yet to be established, several points of concern should be raised.

BPA is present in food and beverage containers used in everyday life. The amount of BPA leaching out of food cans has been estimated to reach up to approximately 20 μg per can (Kang *et al.*, 2003; Vandenberg *et al.*, 2007). As a consequence of its prevalence in our daily environment, BPA is detectable in the urine and serum of over 90% of the population, with urinary levels averaging about 1 to 3 ng/ml (Vandenberg *et al.*, 2007; Calafat *et al.*, 2008) and is also detectable in other fluids such as breast milk, semen and amniotic fluid (Vandenberg *et al.*, 2007). Analysis of the 2003-4 National Health and Nutrition Examination Survey (NHANES) data highlighted the higher urinary levels of BPA in the younger population (layer of the population within reproductive age) as well as a positive correlation between urinary BPA and body mass index (Lang *et al.*, 2008).

BPA accumulates in the placental unit (Schonfelder *et al.*, 2002) and can also cross the placental barrier (Balakrishnan *et al.*, 2010). It is therefore detectable in the fetal serum (Schonfelder *et al.*, 2002). Maternal BPA serum levels ranged from 0.3 to 18.9 ng/ml, fetal levels from 0.2 ng/ml to 9.2 ng/ml while placental levels ranged from 1.0 ng/g to a maximum of 104.9 ng/g (Schonfelder *et al.*, 2002). These results demonstrate fetal exposure to BPA and suggest that BPA is present throughout embryonic and fetal life.

Association studies have suggested several effects of BPA on human health. Elevated urinary BPA levels are correlated with a higher incidence of cardiovascular diseases as well as diabetes (Lang *et al.*, 2008). There is also association between higher BPA levels in maternal serum and amniotic fluid with abnormal karyotypes stemming from the increased presence of trisomy 13, 18 and 21 (Yamada *et al.*, 2002). Consistent with these findings, higher BPA levels were also associated with abnormal karyotypes and an increased incidence of miscarriages (Sugiura-Ogasawara *et al.*, 2005). Occupational studies have also suggested a link between high BPA exposure and sexual dysfunction in males including a diminished sexual drive, erectile and ejaculation difficulties and decreased sexual satisfaction (Li *et al.*, 2010).

Finally, although a few studies have reported no effect of BPA on a multitude of endpoints including behavior, puberty, fertility and anatomy (Tyl *et al.*, 2008; Ryan *et al.*, 2010), there are indications that in rodent models, BPA can act *in vitro*, and in some instances *in vivo*, at concentrations similar to and sometimes below that of human exposure (for reviews see Welshons *et al.*, 2006; Richter *et al.*, 2007; Wetherill *et al.*, 2007). These studies thus raise concerns regarding the effects of BPA on human health especially considering fetal exposure to BPA.

CONCLUDING REMARKS AND FUTURE DIRECTIONS

The research in the field of BPA and its effects *in vivo* is accompanied by a certain degree of controversy, with some even calling for an end to the concerns over BPA (Sharpe, 2010). Research on BPA might appear as distracting and diverting funds that should be available to the study of the many compounds that are released into the environment every year. However, the last decade of research on the effect of BPA has uncovered a plethora of mechanisms (various hormones receptors, non-genomic action, DNA methylation) as well as of endpoints (reproduction, CNS, behavior, adipogenesis) that are affected by exposure to BPA. Through extensive investigation, we now have a deeper understanding of the mechanism of action of not only BPA but also other plastics, plasticizers and endocrine disruptors, and a clearer vision of both what to look for and where when assessing the biological effects of toxicants.

REFERENCES

Adewale HB, Jefferson WN, Newbold RR, Patisaul HB (2009) Neonatal bisphenol-A exposure alters rat reproductive development and ovarian morphology without impairing activation of gonadotropin-releasing hormone neurons. *Biol Reprod* **81(4):** 690–9.

Akingbemi BT, Sottas CM, Koulova AI, Klinefelter GR, Hardy MP (2004) Inhibition of testicular steroidogenesis by the xenoestrogen bisphenol A is associated with reduced pituitary luteinizing hormone secretion and decreased steroidogenic enzyme gene expression in rat Leydig cells. *Endocrinology* **145(2):** 592–603.

Alonso-Magdalena P, Laribi O, Ropero AB, E. Fuentes, Ripoll C, Soria B, Nadal A (2005) Low doses of bisphenol A and diethylstilbestrol impair Ca2+ signals in pancreatic alpha-cells through a nonclassical membrane estrogen receptor within intact islets of Langerhans. *Environ Health Perspect* **113(8):** 969–77.

Alyea RA, Watson CS (2009) Differential regulation of dopamine transporter function and location by low concentrations of environmental estrogens and 17beta-estradiol. *Environ Health Perspect* **117(5):** 778–83.

Ashby J, Tinwell H, Lefevre PA, Joiner R, Haseman J (2003) The effect on sperm production in adult Sprague-Dawley rats exposed by gavage to bisphenol A between postnatal days 91–97. *Toxicol Sci* **74(1):** 129–38.

Atkinson A, Roy D (1995) In vivo DNA adduct formation by bisphenol A. *Environ Mol Mutagen* **26(1):** 60–6.

Balakrishnan B, Henare K, Thorstensen EB, Ponnampalam AP, Mitchell MD (2010) Transfer of bisphenol A across the human placenta. *Am J Obstet Gynecol* **202(4):** 393. e1–7.

Barkhem T, Carlsson B, Nilsson Y, Enmark E, Gustafsson J, Nilsson S (1998) Differential response of estrogen receptor alpha and estrogen receptor beta to partial estrogen agonists/antagonists. *Mol Pharmacol* **54(1):** 105–12.

Berry M, Metzger D, Chambon P (1990) Role of the two activating domains of the oestrogen receptor in the cell-type and promoter-context dependent agonistic activity of the anti-oestrogen 4-hydroxytamoxifen. *EMBO J* **9(9):** 2811–8.

Bouskine A, Nebout M, Brucker-Davis F, Benahmed M, Fenichel P (2009) Low doses of bisphenol A promote human seminoma cell proliferation by activating PKA and PKG via a membrane G-protein-coupled estrogen receptor. *Environ Health Perspect* **117(7):** 1053–8.

Brehm R, Zeiler M, Ruttinger C, Herde K, Kibschull M, Winterhager E, Willecke K, Guillou F, Lecureuil C, Steger K, Konrad L, Biermann K, Failing K, Bergmann M (2007) A Sertoli cell-specific knockout of connexin43 prevents initiation of spermatogenesis. *Am J Pathol* **171(1):** 19–31.

Bromer JG, Zhou Y, Taylor MB, Doherty L, Taylor HS (2010) Bisphenol-A exposure in utero leads to epigenetic alterations in the developmental programming of uterine estrogen response. *FASEB J* **24(7):** 2273–90.

Calafat AM, Ye X, Wong LY, Reidy JA, Needham LL (2008) Exposure of the U.S. population to bisphenol A and 4-tertiary-octylphenol: 2003–2004. *Environ Health Perspect* **116(1):** 39–44.

Chitra KC, Latchoumycandane C, Mathur PP (2003) Induction of oxidative stress by bisphenol A in the epididymal sperm of rats. *Toxicology* **185(1–2):** 119–27.

Coward P, Lee D, Hull MV, Lehmann JM (2001) 4-Hydroxytamoxifen binds to and deactivates the estrogen-related receptor gamma. *Proc Natl Acad Sci USA* **98(15):** 8880–4.

Della Seta D, Minder I, Dessi-Fulgheri F, Farabollini F (2005) Bisphenol-A exposure during pregnancy and lactation affects maternal behavior in rats. *Brain Res Bull* **65(3):** 255–60.

Dodds EC, Lawson W (1936) Synthetic estrogenic agents without the phenanthrene nucleus. *Nature* **137(3476):** 996.

Dodds EC, Lawson W (1938) Molecular structure in relation to oestrogenic activity. Compounds without a phenanthrene nucleus. *Proc R Soc Lond. Series B, Biological Sciences* **125**(839 (April 27, 1938)): 222–32.

Dolinoy DC, Huang D, Jirtle RL (2007) Maternal nutrient supplementation counteracts bisphenol A-induced DNA hypomethylation in early development. *Proc Natl Acad Sci USA* **104(32):** 13056–61.

Domoradzki JY, Thornton CM, Pottenger LH, Hansen SC, Card TL, Markham DA, Dryzga MD, Shiotsuka RN, Waechter JM Jr (2004) Age and dose dependency of the pharmacokinetics and metabolism of bisphenol A in neonatal Sprague-Dawley rats following oral administration. *Toxicol Sci* **77(2):** 230–42.

Durando M, Kass L, Piva J, Sonnenschein C, Soto AM, Luque EH, Munoz-de-Toro M (2007) Prenatal bisphenol A exposure induces preneoplastic lesions in the mammary gland in Wistar rats. *Environ Health Perspect* **115(1):** 80–6.

Edmonds JS, Nomachi M, Terasaki M, Morita M, Skelton BW, White AH (2004) The reaction of bisphenol A 3,4-quinone with DNA. *Biochem Biophys Res Commun* **319(2):** 556–61.

Farabollini F, Porrini S, Della Seta D, Bianchi F, Dessi-Fulgheri F (2002) Effects of perinatal exposure to bisphenol A on sociosexual behavior of female and male rats. *Environ Health Perspect* **110 (Suppl. 3):** 409–14.

Fernández M, Bianchi M, V. Lux-Lantos V, Libertun C (2009) Neonatal exposure to bisphenol a alters reproductive parameters and gonadotropin releasing hormone signaling in female rats. *Environ Health Perspect* **117(5):** 757–62.

Fernández MO, Bourguignon N, Lux-Lantos V, Libertun C (2010) Neonatal exposure to bisphenol A and reproductive and endocrine alterations resembling the polycystic ovarian syndrome in adult rats. *Environ Health Perspect* **119(9):** 1217–22.

Fiorini C, Tilloy-Ellul A, Chevalier S, Charuel C, Pointis G (2004) Sertoli cell junctional proteins as early targets for different classes of reproductive toxicants. *Reprod Toxicol* **18(3):** 413–21.

Giguere V (2002) To ERR in the estrogen pathway. *Trends Endocrinol Metab* **13(5):** 220–5.

Gioiosa L, Fissore E, Ghirardelli G, Parmigiani S, Palanza P (2007) Developmental exposure to low-dose estrogenic endocrine disruptors alters sex differences in exploration and emotional responses in mice. *Horm Behav* **52(3):** 307–16.

Gould JC, Leonard LS, Maness SC, Wagner BL, Conner K, Zacharewski T, Safe S, McDonnell DP, Gaido KW (1998) Bisphenol A interacts with the estrogen receptor alpha in a distinct manner from estradiol. *Mol Cell Endocrinol* **142(1–2):** 203–14.

Heimeier RA, Das B, Buchholz DR, Shi YB (2009) The xenoestrogen bisphenol A inhibits postembryonic vertebrate development by antagonizing gene regulation by thyroid hormone. *Endocrinology* **150(6):** 2964–73.

Henttu PM, Kalkhoven E, Parker MG (1997) AF-2 activity and recruitment of steroid receptor coactivator 1 to the estrogen receptor depend on a lysine residue conserved in nuclear receptors. *Mol Cell Biol* **17(4):** 1832–9.

Herath CB, Jin W, Watanabe G, Arai K, Suzuki AK, Taya K (2004) Adverse effects of environmental toxicants, octylphenol and bisphenol A, on male reproductive functions in pubertal rats. *Endocrine* **25(2):** 163–72.

Hiroi H, Tsutsumi O, Momoeda M, Takai Y, Osuga Y, Taketani Y (1999) Differential interactions of bisphenol A and 17beta-estradiol with estrogen receptor alpha (ERalpha) and ERbeta. *Endocr J* **46(6):** 773–8.

Ho SM, Tang WY, Belmonte de Frausto J, Prins GS (2006) Developmental exposure to estradiol and bisphenol A increases susceptibility to prostate carcinogenesis and epigenetically regulates phosphodiesterase type 4 variant 4. *Cancer Res* **66(11):** 5624–32.

Honma S, Suzuki A, Buchanan DL, Katsu Y, Watanabe H, Iguchi T (2002) Low dose effect of in utero exposure to bisphenol A and diethylstilbestrol on female mouse reproduction. *Reprod Toxicol* **16(2):** 117–22.

Howdeshell KL, Hotchkiss AK, Thayer KA, Vandenbergh JG, vom Saal, FS (1999) Exposure to bisphenol A advances puberty. *Nature* **401(6755):** 763–4.

Hugo ER, Brandebourg TD, Woo JG, Loftus J, Alexander JW, Ben-Jonathan N (2008) Bisphenol A at environmentally relevant doses inhibits adiponectin release from human adipose tissue explants and adipocytes. *Environ Health Perspect* **116(12):** 1642–7.

Hunt PA, Koehler KE, Susiarjo M, Hodges CA, Ilagan A, Voigt RC, Thomas S, Thomas BF, Hassold TJ (2003) Bisphenol a exposure causes meiotic aneuploidy in the female mouse. *Curr Biol* **13(7):** 546–53.

Huppunen J, Aarnisalo P (2004) Dimerization modulates the activity of the orphan nuclear receptor ERRgamma. *Biochem Biophys Res Commun* **314(4):** 964–70.

Iso T, Watanabe T, Iwamoto T, Shimamoto A, Furuichi Y (2006) DNA damage caused by bisphenol A and estradiol through estrogenic activity. *Biol Pharm Bull* **29(2):** 206–10.

Iwamuro S, Yamada M, Kato M, Kikuyama S (2006) Effects of bisphenol A on thyroid hormone-dependent up-regulation of thyroid hormone receptor alpha and beta and down-regulation of retinoid X receptor gamma in Xenopus tail culture. *Life Sci* **79(23):** 2165–71.

Izzotti A, Kanitz S, D'Agostini F, Camoirano A, De Flora S (2009) Formation of adducts by bisphenol A, an endocrine disruptor, in DNA in vitro and in liver and mammary tissue of mice. *Mutat Res* **679(1–2):** 28–32.

Kabuto H, Amakawa M, Shishibori T (2004) Exposure to bisphenol A during embryonic/fetal life and infancy increases oxidative injury and causes underdevelopment of the brain and testis in mice. *Life Sci* **74(24):** 2931–40.

Kang JH, Kito K, Kondo F (2003) Factors influencing the migration of bisphenol A from cans. *J Food Prot* **66(8):** 1444–7.

Kato H, Furuhashi T, Tanaka M, Katsu Y, Watanabe H, Ohta Y, Iguchi T (2006) Effects of bisphenol A given neonatally on reproductive functions of male rats. *Reprod Toxicol* **22(1):** 20–9.

Kato H, Ota T, Furuhashi T, Ohta Y, Iguchi T (2003) Changes in reproductive organs of female rats treated with bisphenol A during the neonatal period. *Reprod Toxicol* **17(3):** 283–8.

Kim HS, Han SY, Yoo SD, Lee BM, Park KL (2001) Potential estrogenic effects of bisphenol-A estimated by in vitro and in vivo combination assays. *J Toxicol Sci* **26(3):** 111–18.

Krishnan AV, Stathis P, Permuth SF, Tokes L, Feldman D (1993) Bisphenol-A: an estrogenic substance is released from polycarbonate flasks during autoclaving. *Endocrinology* **132(6):** 2279–86.

Kubo K, Arai O, Ogata R, Omura M, Hori T, Aou S (2001) Exposure to bisphenol A during the fetal and suckling periods disrupts sexual differentiation of the locus coeruleus and of behavior in the rat. *Neurosci Lett* **304(1–2):** 73–6.

Kubo K, Arai O, Omura M, Watanabe R, Ogata R, Aou S (2003) Low dose effects of bisphenol A on sexual differentiation of the brain and behavior in rats. *Neurosci Res* **45(3):** 345–56.

Kuiper GG, Carlsson B, Grandien K, Enmark E, Haggblad J, Nilsson S, Gustafsson JA (1997) Comparison of the ligand binding specificity and transcript tissue distribution of estrogen receptors alpha and beta. *Endocrinology* **138(3):** 863–70.

Kuiper GG, Lemmen JG, Carlsson B, Corton JC, Safe SH, van der Saag PT, van der Burg B, Gustafsson JA (1998). Interaction of estrogenic chemicals and phytoestrogens with estrogen receptor beta. *Endocrinology* **139(10):** 4252–63.

Kurebayashi H, Betsui H, Ohno Y (2003) Disposition of a low dose of 14C-bisphenol A in male rats and its main biliary excretion as BPA glucuronide. *Toxicol Sci* **73(1):** 17–25.

Lang IA, Galloway TS, Scarlett A, Henley WE, Depledge M, Wallace RB, Melzer D (2008) Association of urinary bisphenol A concentration with medical disorders and laboratory abnormalities in adults. *JAMA* **300(11):** 1303–10.

Lee HJ, Chattopadhyay S, Gong EY, Ahn RS, Lee K (2003) Antiandrogenic effects of bisphenol A and nonylphenol on the function of androgen receptor. *Toxicol Sci* **75(1):** 40–6.

Li D, Zhou Z, Qing D, He Y, Wu T, Miao M, Wang J, Weng X, Ferber JR, Herrinton LJ, Zhu Q, Gao E, Checkoway H, Yuan W (2010) Occupational exposure to bisphenol-A (BPA) and the risk of self-reported male sexual dysfunction. *Hum Reprod* **25(2):** 519–27.

Markey CM, Luque EH, Munoz De Toro M, Sonnenschein C, Soto AM (2001) In utero exposure to bisphenol A alters the development and tissue organization of the mouse mammary gland. *Biol Reprod* **65(4):** 1215–23.

Markey CM, Wadia PR, Rubin BS, Sonnenschein C, Soto AM (2005) Long-term effects of fetal exposure to low doses of the xenoestrogen bisphenol-A in the female mouse genital tract. *Biol Reprod* **72(6):** 1344–51.

Masuno H, Iwanami J, Kidani T, Sakayama K, Honda K (2005) Bisphenol a accelerates terminal differentiation of 3T3-L1 cells into adipocytes through the phosphatidylinositol 3-kinase pathway. *Toxicol Sci* **84(2):** 319–27.

Masuno H, Kidani T, Sekiya K, Sakayama K, Shiosaka T, Yamamoto H, Honda K (2002) Bisphenol A in combination with insulin can accelerate the conversion of 3T3-L1 fibroblasts to adipocytes. *J Lipid Res* **43(5):** 676–84.

Matsushima A, Kakuta Y, Teramoto T, Koshiba T, Liu X, Okada H, Tokunaga T, Kawabata S, Kimura M, Shimohigashi Y (2007) Structural evidence for endocrine disruptor bisphenol A binding to human nuclear receptor ERR gamma. *J Biochem* **142(4):** 517–24.

Matthews JB, Twomey K, Zacharewski TR (2001) In vitro and in vivo interactions of bisphenol A and its metabolite, bisphenol A glucuronide, with estrogen receptors alpha and beta. *Chem Res Toxicol* **14(2):** 149–57.

Mielke H, Gundert-Remy U (2009) Bisphenol A levels in blood depend on age and exposure. *Toxicol Lett* **190(1):** 32–40.

Miyagawa K, Narita M, Akama H, Suzuki T (2007) Memory impairment associated with a dysfunction of the hippocampal cholinergic system induced by prenatal and neonatal exposures to bisphenol-A. *Neurosci Lett* **418(3):** 236–41.

Miyatake M, Miyagawa K, Mizuo K, Narita M, Suzuki T (2006) Dynamic changes in dopaminergic neurotransmission induced by a low concentration of bisphenol-A in neurones and astrocytes. *J Neuroendocrinol* **18(6):** 434–44.

Mlynarcikova A, Nagyova E, Fickova M, Scsukova S (2009) Effects of selected endocrine disruptors on meiotic maturation, cumulus expansion, synthesis of hyaluronan and progesterone by porcine oocyte-cumulus complexes. *Toxicol in Vitro* **23(3):** 371–7.

Moors S, Diel P, Degen GH (2006) Toxicokinetics of bisphenol A in pregnant DA/Han rats after single i.v. application. *Arch Toxicol* **80(10):** 647–55.

Moriyama K, Tagami T, Akamizu T, Usui T, Saijo M, Kanamoto N, Hataya Y, Shimatsu A, Kuzuya H, Nakao K (2002) Thyroid hormone action is disrupted by bisphenol A as an antagonist. *J Clin Endocrinol Metab* **87(11):** 5185–90.

Munoz-de-Toro M, Markey CM, Wadia PR, Luque EH, Rubin BS, Sonnenschein C, Soto AM (2005) Perinatal exposure to bisphenol-A alters peripubertal mammary gland development in mice. *Endocrinology* **146(9):** 4138–47.

Murray TJ, Maffini MV, Ucci AA, Sonnenschein C, Soto AM (2007) Induction of mammary gland ductal hyperplasias and carcinoma in situ following fetal bisphenol A exposure. *Reprod Toxicol* **23(3):** 383–90.

Nadal A, Ropero AB, Laribi O, Maillet M, Fuentes E, Soria B (2000) Nongenomic actions of estrogens and xenoestrogens by binding at a plasma membrane receptor unrelated to estrogen receptor alpha and estrogen receptor beta. *Proc Natl Acad Sci USA* **97(21):** 11603–8.

Nakamura D, Yanagiba Y, Duan Z, Ito Y, Okamura A, Asaeda N, Tagawa Y, Li C, Taya K, Zhang SY, Naito H, Ramdhan DH, Kamijima M, Nakajima T (2010) Bisphenol A may cause testosterone reduction by adversely affecting both testis and pituitary systems similar to estradiol. *Toxicol Lett* **194(1–2):** 16–25.

Newbold RR, Jefferson WN, Padilla-Banks E (2007) Long-term adverse effects of neonatal exposure to bisphenol A on the murine female reproductive tract. *Reprod Toxicol* **24(2):** 253–8.

Newbold RR, Jefferson WN, Padilla-Banks E (2009) Prenatal exposure to bisphenol A at environmentally relevant doses adversely affects the murine female reproductive tract later in life. *Environ Health Perspect* **117(6):** 879–85.

Nikaido Y, Yoshizawa K, Danbara N, Tsujita-Kyutoku M, Yuri T, Uehara N, Tsubura A (2004) Effects of maternal xenoestrogen exposure on development of the reproductive tract and mammary gland in female CD-1 mouse offspring. *Reprod Toxicol* **18(6):** 803–11.

Nose T, Shimohigashi Y (2008) A docking modelling rationally predicts strong binding of bisphenol A to estrogen-related receptor gamma. *Protein Pept Lett* **15(3):** 290–6.

NTP-CERHR (2008) NTP-CERHR Monograph on the Potential Human Reproductive and Developmental Effects of Bisphenol A. NTP CERHR MON(22): i–III1.

Okada H, Tokunaga T, Liu X, Takayanagi S, Matsushima A, Shimohigashi Y (2008) Direct evidence revealing structural elements essential for the high binding ability of bisphenol A to human estrogen-related receptor-gamma. *Environ Health Perspect* **116(1):** 32–8.

Palanza P, Gioiosa L, vom Saal FS, Parmigiani S (2008) Effects of developmental exposure to bisphenol A on brain and behavior in mice. *Environ Res* **108(2):** 150–7.

Palanza PL, Howdeshell KL, Parmigiani S, vom Saal FS (2002) Exposure to a low dose of bisphenol A during fetal life or in adulthood alters maternal behavior in mice. *Environ Health Perspect* **110 (Suppl. 3):** 415–22.

Paris F, Balaguer P, Terouanne B, Servant N, Lacoste C, Cravedi JP, Nicolas JC, Sultan C (2002) Phenylphenols, biphenols, bisphenol-A and 4-tert-octylphenol exhibit alpha and beta estrogen activities and antiandrogen activity in reporter cell lines. *Mol Cell Endocrinol* **193(1–2):** 43–9.

Patisaul HB, Fortino AE, Polston EK (2006) Neonatal genistein or bisphenol-A exposure alters sexual differentiation of the AVPV. *Neurotoxicol Teratol* **28(1):** 111–18.

Pennie WD, Aldridge TC, Brooks AN (1998) Differential activation by xenoestrogens of ER alpha and ER beta when linked to different response elements. *J Endocrinol* **158(3):** R11–R14.

Phrakonkham P, Viengchareun S, Belloir C, Lombes M, Artur Y, Canivenc-Lavier MC (2008) Dietary xenoestrogens differentially impair 3T3-L1 preadipocyte differentiation and persistently affect leptin synthesis. *J Steroid Biochem Mol Biol* **110(1–2):** 95–103.

Politch JA (2006) Bisphenol A and risk assessment. *Environ Health Perspect* **114(1):** A16; author reply A16–A17.

Pottenger LH, Domoradzki JY, Markham DA, Hansen SC, Cagen SZ, Waechter JM Jr (2000) The relative bioavailability and metabolism of bisphenol A in rats is dependent upon the route of administration. *Toxicol Sci* **54(1):** 3–18.

Prossnitz ER, Oprea TI, Sklar LA, Arterburn JB (2008) The ins and outs of GPR30: a transmembrane estrogen receptor. *J Steroid Biochem Mol Biol* **109(3–5):** 350–3.

Ramakrishnan S, Wayne NL (2008) Impact of bisphenol-A on early embryonic development and reproductive maturation. *Reprod Toxicol* **25(2):** 177–83.

Ramos JG, Varayoud J, Sonnenschein C, Soto AM, Munoz De Toro M, Luque EH (2001) Prenatal exposure to low doses of bisphenol A alters the periductal stroma and glandular cell function in the rat ventral prostate. *Biol Reprod* **65(4):** 1271–7.

Reid EE, Wilson E (1944) The relation of estrogenic activity to structure in some 4,4′-dihydroxydiphenylmethanes. *J Am Chem Soc* **66(6):** 967–9.

Revankar CM, Cimino DF, Sklar LA, Arterburn JB, Prossnitz ER (2005) A transmembrane intracellular estrogen receptor mediates rapid cell signaling. *Science* **307(5715):** 1625–30.

Richter CA, Taylor JA, Ruhlen RL, Welshons WV, Vom Saal FS (2007) Estradiol and Bisphenol A stimulate androgen receptor and estrogen receptor gene expression in fetal mouse prostate mesenchyme cells. *Environ Health Perspect* **115(6):** 902–8.

Ropero AB, Alonso-Magdalena P, Ripoll C, Fuentes E, Nadal A (2006) Rapid endocrine disruption: environmental estrogen actions triggered outside the nucleus. *J Steroid Biochem Mol Biol* **102(1–5):** 163–9.

Routledge EJ, White R, Parker MG, Sumpter JP (2000) Differential effects of xenoestrogens on coactivator recruitment by estrogen receptor (ER) alpha and ERbeta. *J Biol Chem* **275(46):** 35986–93.

Rubin BS, Lenkowski JR, Schaeberle CM, Vandenberg LN, Ronsheim PM, Soto AM (2006) Evidence of altered brain sexual differentiation in mice exposed perinatally to low, environmentally relevant levels of bisphenol A. *Endocrinology* **147(8):** 3681–91.

Rubin BS, Murray MK, Damassa DA, King JC, Soto AM (2001) Perinatal exposure to low doses of bisphenol A affects body weight, patterns of estrous cyclicity, and plasma LH levels. *Environ Health Perspect* **109(7):** 675–80.

Rubin BS, Soto AM (2009) Bisphenol A: perinatal exposure and body weight. *Mol Cell Endocrinol* **304(1–2):** 55–62.

Rudel RA, Camann DE, Spengler JD, Korn LR, Brody JG (2003) Phthalates, alkylphenols, pesticides, polybrominated diphenyl ethers, and other endocrine-disrupting compounds in indoor air and dust. *Environ Sci Technol* **37(20):** 4543–53.

Ryan BC, Hotchkiss AK, Crofton KM, Gray LE Jr (2010) In utero and lactational exposure to bisphenol A, in contrast to ethinyl estradiol, does not alter sexually dimorphic behavior, puberty, fertility, and anatomy of female LE rats. *Toxicol Sci* **114(1):** 133–48.

Ryan BC, Vandenbergh JG (2006) Developmental exposure to environmental estrogens alters anxiety and spatial memory in female mice. *Horm Behav* **50(1):** 85–93.

Salian S, Doshi T, Vanage G (2009) Neonatal exposure of male rats to Bisphenol A impairs fertility and expression of sertoli cell junctional proteins in the testis. *Toxicology* **265(1–2):** 56–67.

Sargis RM, Johnson DN, Choudhury RA, Brady MJ (2009) Environmental endocrine disruptors promote adipogenesis in the 3T3-L1 cell line through glucocorticoid receptor activation. *Obesity (Silver Spring)* **18(7):** 1293–9.

Savabieasfahani M, Kannan K, Astapova O, Evans NP, Padmanabhan V (2006) Developmental programming: differential effects of prenatal exposure to bisphenol-A or methoxychlor on reproductive function. *Endocrinology* **147(12):** 5956–66.

Schonfelder G, Wittfoht W, Hopp H, Talsness CE, Paul M, Chahoud I (2002) Parent bisphenol A accumulation in the human maternal-fetal-placental unit. *Environ Health Perspect* **110(11):** A703–A707.

Sharpe RM (2010) Is it time to end concerns over the estrogenic effects of bisphenol A? *Toxicol Sci* **114(1):** 1–4.

Shimizu M, Ohta K, Matsumoto Y, Fukuoka M, Ohno Y, Ozawa S (2002) Sulfation of bisphenol A abolished its estrogenicity based on proliferation and gene expression in human breast cancer MCF-7 cells. *Toxicol in Vitro* **16(5):** 549–56.

Snyder RW, Maness SC, Gaido KW, Welsch F, Sumner SC, Fennell TR (2000) Metabolism and disposition of bisphenol A in female rats. *Toxicol Appl Pharmacol* **168(3):** 225–34.

Somm E, Schwitzgebel VM, Toulotte A, Cederroth CR, Combescure C, Nef S, Aubert ML, Huppi PS (2009) Perinatal exposure to bisphenol A alters early adipogenesis in the rat. *Environ Health Perspect* **117(10):** 1549–55.

Soto AM, Justicia H, Wray JW, Sonnenschein C (1991) p-Nonyl-phenol: an estrogenic xenobiotic released from "modified" polystyrene. *Environ Health Perspect* **92:** 167–73.

Soto AM, Vandenberg LN, Maffini MV, Sonnenschein C (2008) Does breast cancer start in the womb? *Basic Clin Pharmacol Toxicol* **102(2):** 125–33.

Sridharan S, Simon L, Meling DD, Cyr DG, Gutstein DE, Fishman GI, Guillou F, Cooke PS (2007) Proliferation of adult sertoli cells following conditional knockout of the Gap junctional protein GJA1 (connexin 43) in mice. *Biol Reprod* **76(5):** 804–12.

Steinmetz R, Mitchner NA, Grant A, Allen DL, Bigsby RM, Ben-Jonathan N (1998) The xenoestrogen bisphenol A induces growth, differentiation, and c-fos gene expression in the female reproductive tract. *Endocrinology* **139(6):** 2741–7.

Stowell CL, Barvian KK, Young PC, Bigsby RM, Verdugo DE, Bertozzi CR, Widlanski TS (2006) A role for sulfation–desulfation in the uptake of bisphenol A into breast tumor cells. *Chem Biol* **13(8):** 891–7.

Sugiura-Ogasawara M, Ozaki Y, Sonta S, Makino T, Suzumori K (2005) Exposure to bisphenol A is associated with recurrent miscarriage. *Hum Reprod* **20(8):** 2325–9.

Sun H, Shen OX, Wang XR, Zhou L, Zhen SQ, Chen XD (2009) Anti-thyroid hormone activity of bisphenol A, tetrabromobisphenol A and tetrachlorobisphenol A in an improved reporter gene assay. *Toxicol in Vitro* **23(5):** 950–4.

Sun H, Xu LC, Chen JF, Song L, Wang XR (2006) Effect of bisphenol A, tetrachlorobisphenol A and pentachlorophenol on the transcriptional activities of androgen receptor-mediated reporter gene. *Food Chem Toxicol* **44(11):** 1916–21.

Susiarjo M, Hassold TJ, Freeman E, Hunt PA (2007) Bisphenol A exposure in utero disrupts early oogenesis in the mouse. *PLoS Genet* **3(1):** e5.

Suzuki A, Sugihara A, Uchida K, Sato T, Ohta Y, Katsu Y, Watanabe H, Iguchi T (2002) Developmental effects of perinatal exposure to bisphenol-A and diethylstilbestrol on reproductive organs in female mice. *Reprod Toxicol* **16(2):** 107–16.

Takahashi O, Oishi S (2003) Testicular toxicity of dietarily or parenterally administered bisphenol A in rats and mice. *Food Chem Toxicol* **41(7):** 1035–44.

Takao T, Nanamiya W, Nagano I, Asaba K, Kawabata K, Hashimoto K (1999) Exposure with the environmental estrogen bisphenol A disrupts the male reproductive tract in young mice. *Life Sci* **65(22):** 2351–7.

Takayanagi S, Tokunaga T, Liu X, Okada H, Matsushima A, Shimohigashi Y (2006) Endocrine disruptor bisphenol A strongly binds to human estrogen-related receptor gamma (ERRgamma) with high constitutive activity. *Toxicol Lett* **167(2):** 95–105.

Takeuchi T, Tsutsumi O, Ikezuki Y, Takai Y, Taketani Y (2004) Positive relationship between androgen and the endocrine disruptor, bisphenol A, in normal women and women with ovarian dysfunction. *Endocr J* **51(2):** 165–9.

Taylor JA, Welshons WV, Vom Saal FS (2008) No effect of route of exposure (oral; subcutaneous injection) on plasma bisphenol A throughout 24h after administration in neonatal female mice. *Reprod Toxicol* **25(2):** 169–76.

Thomas P, Dong J (2006) Binding and activation of the seven-transmembrane estrogen receptor GPR30 by environmental estrogens: a potential novel mechanism of endocrine disruption. *J Steroid Biochem Mol Biol* **102(1–5):** 175–9.

Timms BG, Howdeshell KL, Barton L, Bradley S, Richter CA, vom Saal FS (2005) Estrogenic chemicals in plastic and oral contraceptives disrupt development of the fetal mouse prostate and urethra. *Proc Natl Acad Sci USA* **102(19):** 7014–19.

Tominaga T, Negishi T, Hirooka H, Miyachi A, Inoue A, Hayasaka I, Yoshikawa Y (2006) Toxicokinetics of bisphenol A in rats, monkeys and chimpanzees by the LC-MS/MS method. *Toxicology* **226(2–3):** 208–17.

Toyama Y, Suzuki-Toyota F, Maekawa M, Ito C, Toshimori K (2004) Adverse effects of bisphenol A to spermiogenesis in mice and rats. *Arch Histol Cytol* **67(4):** 373–81.

Tyl RW, Myers CB, Marr MC, Sloan CS, Castillo NP, Veselica MM, Seely JC, Dimond SS, Van Miller JP, Shiotsuka RN, Beyer D, Hentges SG, Waechter JM Jr (2008) Two-generation reproductive toxicity study of dietary bisphenol A in CD-1 (Swiss) mice. *Toxicol Sci* **104(2):** 362–84.

Upmeier A, Degen GH, Diel P, Michna H, Bolt HM (2000) Toxicokinetics of bisphenol A in female DA/Han rats after a single i.v. and oral administration. *Arch Toxicol* **74(8):** 431–6.

Vanacker JM, Pettersson K, Gustafsson JA, Laudet V (1999) Transcriptional targets shared by estrogen receptor-related receptors (ERRs) and estrogen receptor (ER) alpha, but not by ERbeta. *EMBO J* **18(15):** 4270–9.

Vandenberg LN, Hauser R, Marcus M, Olea N, Welshons WV (2007) Human exposure to bisphenol A (BPA). *Reprod Toxicol* **24(2):** 139–77.

Voegel JJ, Heine MJ, Zechel C, Chambon P, Gronemeyer H (1996) TIF2, a 160 kDa transcriptional mediator for the ligand-dependent activation function AF-2 of nuclear receptors. *EMBO J* **15(14):** 3667–75.

Volkel W., Colnot T, Csanady GA, Filser JG, Dekant W (2002) Metabolism and kinetics of bisphenol A in humans at low doses following oral administration. *Chem Res Toxicol* **15(10):** 1281–7.

vom Saal FS, Hughes C (2005) An extensive new literature concerning low-dose effects of bisphenol A shows the need for a new risk assessment. *Environ Health Perspect* **113(8):** 926–33.

Wadia PR, Vandenberg LN, Schaeberle CM, Rubin BS, Sonnenschein C, Soto AM (2007) Perinatal bisphenol A exposure increases estrogen sensitivity of the mammary gland in diverse mouse strains. *Environ Health Perspect* **115(4):** 592–8.

Welshons WV, Nagel SC, vom Saal FS (2006) Large effects from small exposures. III. Endocrine mechanisms mediating effects of bisphenol A at levels of human exposure. *Endocrinology* **147 (6 Suppl.):** S56–S69.

Wetherill YB, Akingbemi BT, Kanno J, McLachlan JA, Nadal A, Sonnenschein C, Watson CS, Zoeller RT, Belcher SM (2007). In vitro molecular mechanisms of bisphenol A action. *Reprod Toxicol* **24(2):** 178–98.

Wilson NK, Chuang JC, Lyu C, Menton R, Morgan MK (2003) Aggregate exposures of nine preschool children to persistent organic pollutants at day care and at home. *J Expo Anal Environ Epidemiol* **13(3):** 187–202.

Wilson NK, Chuang JC, Morgan MK, Lordo RA, Sheldon LS (2007) An observational study of the potential exposures of preschool children to pentachlorophenol, bisphenol-A, and nonylphenol at home and daycare. *Environ Res* **103(1):** 9–20.

Wolff MS, Teitelbaum SL, Windham G, Pinney SM, Britton JA, Chelimo C, Godbold J, Biro F, Kushi LH, Pfeiffer CM, Calafat AM (2007) Pilot study of urinary biomarkers of phytoestrogens, phthalates, and phenols in girls. *Environ Health Perspect* **115(1):** 116–21.

Xu LC, Sun H, Chen JF, Bian Q, Qian J, Song L, Wang XR (2005) Evaluation of androgen receptor transcriptional activities of bisphenol A, octylphenol and nonylphenol in vitro. *Toxicology* **216(2–3):** 197–203.

Yamada H, Furuta I, Kato EH, Kataoka S, Usuki Y, Kobashi G, Sata F, Kishi R, Fujimoto S (2002) Maternal serum and amniotic fluid bisphenol A concentrations in the early second trimester. *Reprod Toxicol* **16(6):** 735–9.

Yaoi T, Itoh K, Nakamura K, Ogi H, Fujiwara Y, Fushiki S (2008) Genome-wide analysis of epigenomic alterations in fetal mouse forebrain after exposure to low doses of bisphenol A. *Biochem Biophys Res Commun* **376(3):** 563–7.

Zhou R, Zhang Z, Zhu Y, Chen L, Sokabe M (2009) Deficits in development of synaptic plasticity in rat dorsal striatum following prenatal and neonatal exposure to low-dose bisphenol A. *Neuroscience* **159(1):** 161–71.

Zoeller RT, Bansal R, Parris C (2005) Bisphenol-A, an environmental contaminant that acts as a thyroid hormone receptor antagonist in vitro, increases serum thyroxine, and alters RC3/neurogranin expression in the developing rat brain. *Endocrinology* **146(2):** 607–12.

Zsarnovszky A, Le HH, Wang HS, Belcher SM (2005) Ontogeny of rapid estrogen-mediated extracellular signal-regulated kinase signaling in the rat cerebellar cortex: potent nongenomic agonist and endocrine disrupting activity of the xenoestrogen bisphenol A. *Endocrinology* **146(12):** 5388–96.

Section 9

Phytotoxicants

C H A P T E R

51

Toxic plants

Kip E. Panter, Kevin D. Welch and Dale R. Gardner

INTRODUCTION

Investigations of reproductive dysfunction, especially infertility, abortions and teratogenesis, should focus on a thorough examination of animal condition, general health status, management practices and infectious agents while potential toxicants are sought. This requires a systematic approach including individual animal and herd/flock health history, veterinary examination of individual animals, testing of animal tissues including hair, blood, urine, feces, selected organs, gross and pathological/histological postmortem examination, and toxicological screening of samples of feed and/or tissue. In livestock production systems, these investigations are often limited by economic constraints and the extent or battery of tests must be determined between the client, veterinarian and diagnostician.

As synthetic chemicals (anthropogenic) increase in number and prevalence of use, it is not uncommon for farmers or ranchers to immediately suspect a xenobiotic as the cause of reproductive dysfunction or birth defects in livestock. However, reproductive dysfunction may result from any number of other potential causes, including poisonous plants (Table 51.1). The influence of natural toxicants or anthropogenic compounds on animal reproduction may be significant in its economic impact and the subject requires much more research and further experimental substantiation. Most information on livestock comes from field investigations or case reports and the link between the suspected toxicant and the observed reproductive failure (diagnosis) is often by association, and sometimes a weak association at best. Undoubtedly, many cases of toxicant-induced reproductive failure in livestock operations go undiagnosed, unrecognized or unreported. Additionally, poor management practices and lack of experience or understanding may confound the diagnosis. Other factors including stress, nutritional status, genetic variability, disease conditions, etc., make diagnosis of toxicant-induced reproductive failure more difficult.

Reproductive success is dependent on a large number of carefully orchestrated biological events that must occur in a specifically timed sequence. The interference with one or more of these sequences or events may result in total reproductive failure or a more subtle reduction in reproductive potential. Many factors must be considered when reproductive failure occurs such as livestock species implicated, season of the year and animal/plant relationships. Nutritional status and environmental factors (weather, cold, storms, season of the year, etc.) also influence diet selection if toxic plants are present in pastures, which ultimately may impact reproductive success. For example, if plants containing phytoestrogens are grazed by sheep during the seasonal anestrus period very few if any effects may be recognized, whereas if the phytoestrogens are ingested during the breeding season the subsequent reproductive failures are often economically devastating. The specific effects of phytoestrogens on reproduction will be discussed in a separate chapter.

This chapter describes literature on poisonous plants that impact reproduction and embryo–fetal development in livestock species. This chapter is not intended to be all inclusive and other phytochemical causes of reproductive dysfunction will be covered in more detail in other chapters found within this book.

LOCOWEEDS, *ASTRAGALUS* AND *OXYTROPIS* SPP.

Locoweeds, species of *Oxytropis* and *Astragalus* genera containing the indolizidine alkaloid toxin swainsonine (Figure 51.1; Molyneux and James, 1982; Molyneux *et al.*, 1991), reduce reproductive performance in livestock (Panter *et al.*, 1999b). Most aspects of reproduction are affected, including mating behavior, libido and spermatogenesis in males, estrus behavior and conception in females, fetal growth and development, reproductive maturity at puberty and neonatal/maternal behavior. While extensive research has been done to characterize and describe the histological changes, we have just scratched the surface of understanding the magnitude of the physiological problems, the mechanisms of reproductive dysfunction and the management strategies needed to prevent losses.

Once animals begin to graze locoweed, nearly immediate measurable increases in serum swainsonine with concomitant decreases in α-mannosidase occur (Figure 51.2; Stegelmeier *et al.*, 1995a,b). While these measurable changes are diagnostic for locoweed ingestion, the rapid clearance of swainsonine from serum ($t_{(1/2)} \approx 20\,h$) and accompanying

Reproductive and Developmental Toxicology, Edited by Ramesh C. Gupta
ISBN: 978-0-12-382032-7

TABLE 51.1 Teratogenic plants

Plant	Toxicant	Effects	Species and stage of development
Veratrum californicum (skunk cabbage, false hellebore)	Steroidal alkaloids, cyclopamine, jervine, cycloposine	Cyclopia, cleft palate, limb defects, tracheal stenosis and embryonic death	Cattle, goats, sheep; day 14 cyclopia, days 28–31 limb reductions; days 31–33 tracheal stenosis (sheep)
Veratrum eschscholtizi	Unknown, possibly same as above	Cyclopia	Horses
Veratrum album	Same as above	Cyclopia	Llamas and alpacas
Oxytropis/Astragalus	Swainsonine, swainsonine *N*-oxide	Bowed limbs, embryo or fetal death	Sheep, cattle, horses and most stages of pregnancy
Lupinus spp. *L. caudatus* *L. sericeus* *L. nootkatensis* *L. laxiflorus* *L. sulphureus*	Quinolizidine alkaloid Anagyrine	Cleft palate, contracture-type skeletal defects	Cattle, 40–100 days' gestation (cleft palate only 40–50 days' gestation)
L. formosus *L. arbustus* *L. argenteus*	Piperidine alkaloid Ammodendrine	Cleft palate, contracture-type skeletal defects	Cattle, 40–100 (cleft palate only 40–50); sheep and goats, 30–60 (cleft palate only 35–41)
Nicotiana tabacum *N. glauca*	Anabasine	Cleft palate, contracture-type skeletal defects	Pigs, 30–60 (cleft palate only 30–40); cattle, 40–100 (cleft palate only 40–50); sheep and goats, 30–60 (cleft palate only 35–41)
Conium maculatum (poison-hemlock)	Coniine and g-coniceine	Cleft palate, contracture-type skeletal defects	Same as above
Prunus serotina (wild black cherry)	Cyanogenic compounds suspected	Cleft palate, contracture-type skeletal defects	Pigs
Datura stramonium (jimsonweed)	Unknown, possibly alkaloids	Cleft palate, contracture-type skeletal defects	Pigs

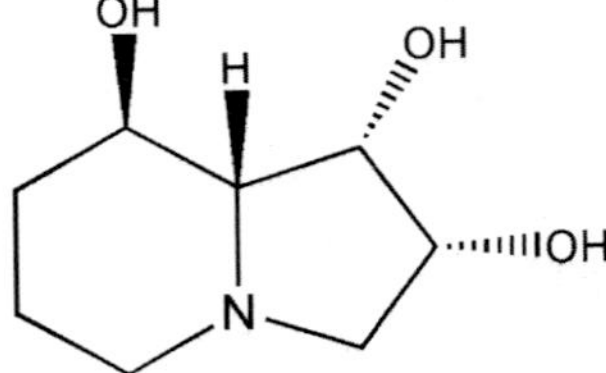

FIGURE 51.1 The locoweed toxin swainsonine, an indolizidine alkaloid.

rapid recovery of α-mannosidase ($t_{(1/2)} \approx 65$ h) limits serum analysis of these parameters as a reliable test for past or long-term locoweed exposure (Stegelmeier *et al.*, 1995a). Currently, diagnosis of locoweed poisoning relies on history of locoweed ingestion, behavioral changes, loss of condition, and, in terminal cases, histological evidence of neurovisceral vacuolation. Histological lesions induced by locoweed and pure swainsonine (James *et al.*, 1991; Panter *et al.*, 1999b) have been compared and are the same. Lesions appear to develop in a threshold-like fashion over time (Van Kampen and James, 1969, 1970; James *et al.*, 1970a,b; Stegelmeier *et al.*, 1999a,b) and animal tissues (such as liver and kidney) that accumulate high swainsonine concentrations develop lesions more rapidly than other organ systems (Stegelmeier *et al.*, 1998). Even though α-mannosidase activity in serum recovers quickly, tissue repair and return to normal organ function occur much more slowly (Stegelmeier *et al.*, 1999a), which is especially true for reproductive function.

Effects on female reproduction

Locoweeds affect almost every aspect of reproduction in the female, such as estrus behavior, estrous cycle length, ovarian function, conception, embryonic and fetal viability, and maternal/infant bonding (Hartley and James, 1975; Panter *et al.*, 1987, 1999b; Pfister *et al.*, 1993, 2006; Panter and Stegelmeier 2000).

Locoweed fed to cattle and sheep at various times and dosages temporarily altered ovarian function, increased estrous cycle length, altered breeding behavior and reduced conception rates (Panter *et al.*, 1999c). Experimental feeding trials with locoweeds (*A. mollissimus, A. lentiginosus* and *O. sericea*) in cycling ewes demonstrated that feeding locoweed free choice as 10–15% of their diet for 20 days altered the estrous cycle, delayed and shortened estrus behavior, decreased conception rates and the number and quality of viable embryos collected from gonadotropin-induced superovulated ewes was significantly reduced.

While only a few abnormal morula-stage embryos were collected from ewes after 30 days of feeding locoweed, *in vitro* data using bovine oocytes demonstrated that swainsonine added to culture media at different concentrations (up to 6.4 μg/mL) did not directly interfere with bovine oocyte maturation (IVM), *in vitro* fertilization (IVF) or embryo growth and development (Wang *et al.*, 1999). Furthermore, pregnancy rates were not different from controls when these swainsonine-cultured (IVM/IVF/IVC) bovine embryos were transferred to recipient heifers. This research suggests that the negative effects that locoweed has on early embryo viability and development *in vivo* are not from direct effects of swainsonine on the oocyte or the preimplantation embryo.

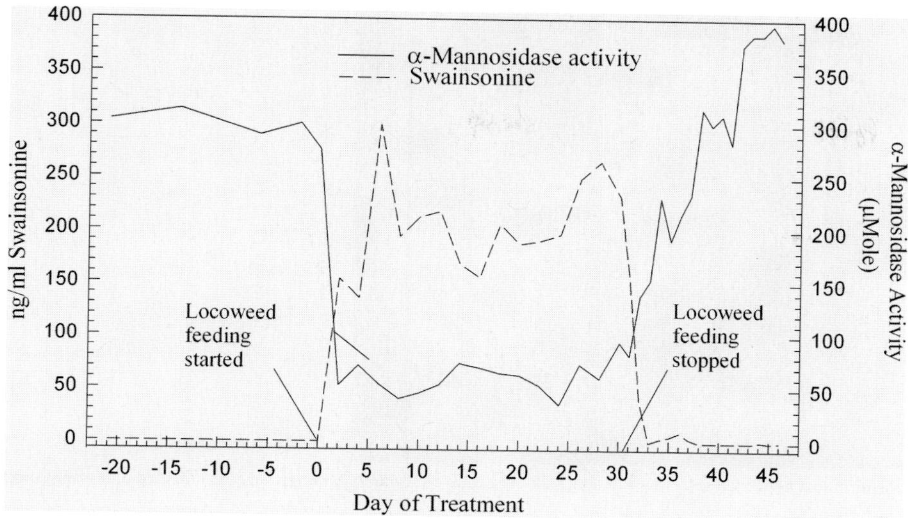

FIGURE 51.2 Average serum swainsonine increase and associated decline in alpha mannosidase as measured in four cows fed *Oxytropis sericea*.

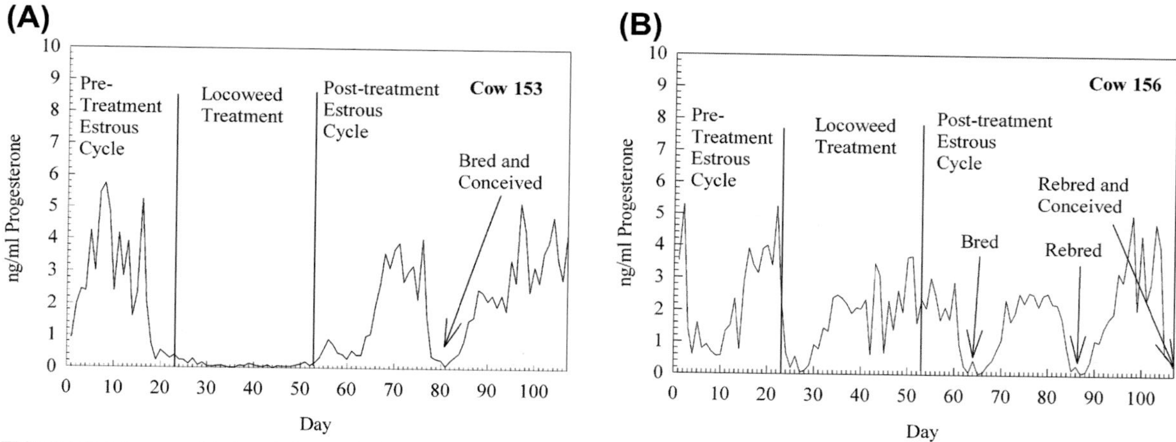

FIGURE 51.3 Locoweed-induced changes in the estrous cycle of cows fed *Oxytropis sericea*. Note the extended follicular (A) and luteal (B) phases and associated repeat breeding.

Therefore, the oocyte/preimplantation embryo effects are apparently secondary and result from effects on other facets of reproduction such as the maternal pituitary/hypothalamic axis where glycoprotein gonadotropins are produced and released, or at the ovarian/utero interface, or the utero/placental interaction once pregnancy recognition is established.

Mature cycling cows fed *Oxytropis sericea* at 20% of their diet for 30 days showed moderate clinical signs of toxicity. However, the estrous cycle length was increased during locoweed feeding and breeding and conception was delayed (Figure 51.3). After locoweed feeding stopped, normal estrous cycles returned relatively soon and while breeding behavior appeared normal, conception was delayed in some cows (repeat breeders) for up to three estrous cycles. In another study, cycling heifers fed *O. sericea* at three dosages of swainsonine (0.25, 0.75 and 2.25 mg/kg/day) showed ovarian dysfunction in a dose-dependent pattern. Heifers receiving the highest dose for 45 days had cystic ovaries within 20 days after locoweed feeding started. Scanning of these ovaries by ultrasound suggested that both the luteal phase (luteal cysts) and follicular phase (follicular cysts) were prolonged and persisted throughout the feeding period (Figure 51.4; Panter unpublished data). Forty-five days after locoweed feeding was stopped, heifers were necropsied and ovaries had returned to normal. Further studies are needed to fully characterize and define the effects of locoweed on ovarian function in cattle and sheep.

While gross and microscopic lesions in the dam may begin to resolve quickly after locoweed ingestion ceases, fetal effects may be prolonged as a result of abnormal placentation (Hafez *et al.*, 2007) and severe enough to result in fetal–embryo death and resorption or abortion, birth of small weak offspring or reduced maternal/infant bonding and impaired nursing ability of the neonate (Panter *et al.*, 1987, 1992b; Pfister *et al.*, 2006). Locoweed ingestion during gestation days 100–130 disrupted normal maternal infant bonding compared to control ewe–lamb pairs (Pfister *et al.*, 2006). Lambs from mothers ingesting locoweed failed to suckle within 2 hours after birth, were slower to stand, and were less vigorous than control lambs. Maternal ingestion of locoweed also disrupted the learning ability of neonatal lambs. Swainsonine is also excreted in the milk and can result in further intoxication of nursing offspring or exacerbate intoxication when offspring begin to graze locoweeds and continue to nurse their locoweed-grazing mothers (James and Hartley, 1977; Panter and James, 1990).

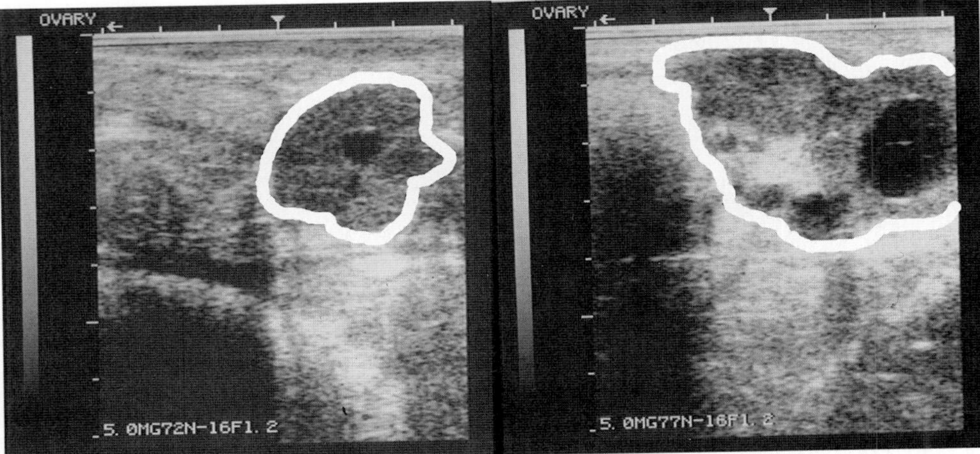

FIGURE 51.4 Cystic ovary (*right*) as observed by ultrasound in a heifer fed locoweed compared to a normal ovary (*left*). Note the large fluid-filled area suggesting a follicular cyst.

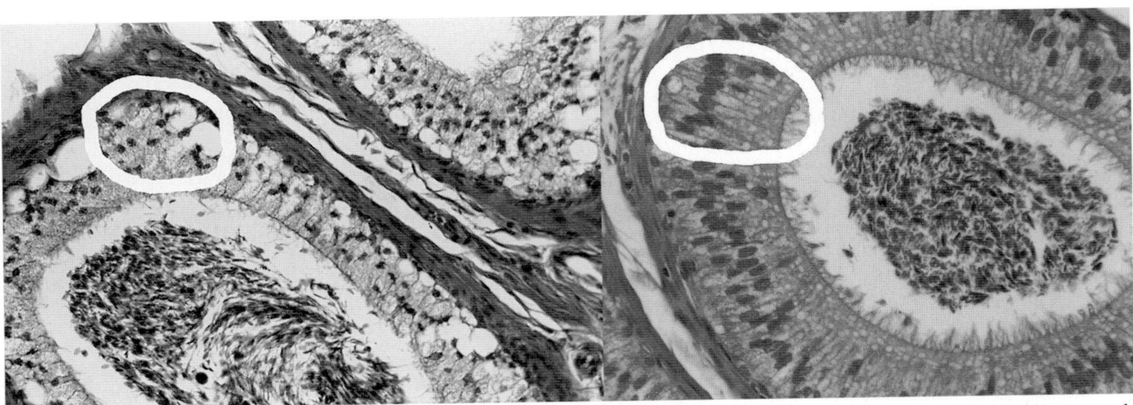

FIGURE 51.5 Seminiferous tubules from a loco-fed (*left*) ram showing foamy vacuolation and reduced spermatogenesis (*circle*) compared to a control (*right*) where normal spermatocytogenesis is observed in the seminiferous epithelium (*circle*).

Effects on male reproduction

Locoweed ingestion by males is equally detrimental to male reproductive functions as it is to female reproduction. However, because of the latent period of spermatogenesis and the importance of a single male in reproductive performance in a herd/flock of females, the outcome may be multiplied or exacerbated. Panter *et al.* (1989) reported induced transient degenerative changes in the seminiferous, epididymal and vas deferens epithelium after feeding locoweed to yearling rams for 70 days. Clinically, there were changes in behavior, reduced libido and loss of body condition. Grossly, there were no observed changes in testicular circumference or gross tissue appearance, but histologically there was foamy cytoplasmic vacuolation in the epithelium of the seminiferous tubules, epididymis and vas deferens and reduced spermatozoa production (Figure 51.5). Semen contained significantly more abnormal spermatozoa, including retained peri-nuclear cytoplasmic droplets, detached tails, kinked tails and marked decreases in motility (Panter *et al.*, 1989). Testicular lesions were transient and spermatogenesis resumed, and by 70 days after locoweed feeding had ended, semen quality appeared relatively normal.

Recent feeding trials in 2-year-old rams demonstrated that changes in breeding behavior occurred within 30 days after locoweed feeding started. Exposure of these rams to ewes in estrus often precipitated uncontrolled muscular tremors, proprioceptive deficits and anxiousness (Panter, unpublished data). Even though these rams had no microscopic changes in semen quality, motility or metabolism at this time, there was a reduction in conception rates when these rams were bred to control ewes (Panter, unpublished data). After 60 days of feeding locoweed, there were severe neurological deficits and microscopic changes in spermatozoa morphology and motility but sperm cell metabolic activity, as measured by reazurin red dye reduction assays, was still not significantly reduced (Wang *et al.*, 1998). Spermatogenesis and spermatozoa defects resolved by 60 to 90 days after locoweed feeding stopped, but five of seven rams continued to lose weight (wasting) and neurologic deficits intensified until they were euthanized. This suggests that permanent neurological deficits may preclude salvaging locoweed affected animals.

Ortiz *et al.* (1997) reported several delayed effects of feeding *Oxytropis sericea* to breeding age ram for 35 days. Thirty-five days after locoweed feeding stopped, they found reduced sperm motility and decreased scrotal circumference in all treated rams. There was also a reduced testosterone response to GnRH challenge, suggesting that locoweed affected testicular function in these rams. This delayed effect is expected as the cycle of spermatogenesis in sheep is about 60 to 70 days

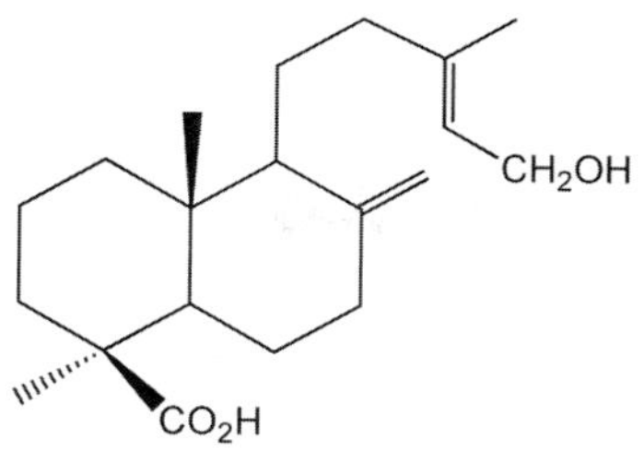

Isocupressic Acid

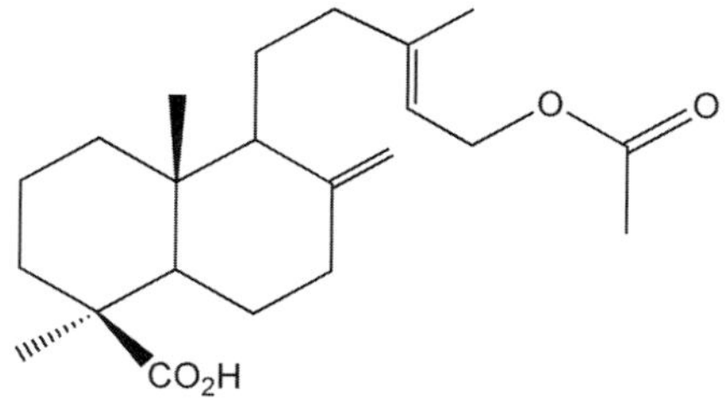

Acetylisocupressic acid

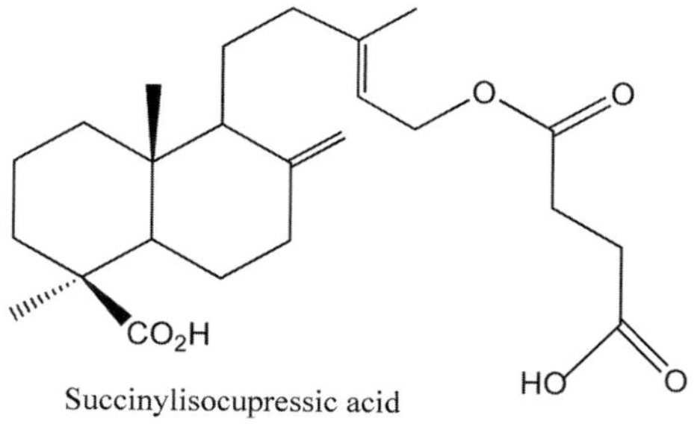

Succinylisocupressic acid

FIGURE 51.6 Isocupressic acid (ICA), the abortifacient compound in Ponderosa pine needles and two ICA derivatives, succinyl and acetyl ICA.

and Panter *et al.* (1989) demonstrated an increase in spermatozoa abnormalities 60 to 70 days after continuous locoweed feeding.

While research and field observations have demonstrated that locoweed affects almost every aspect of reproduction in livestock, several questions still remain unanswered. How long and how much locoweed can livestock eat before reproduction declines? What functions are affected first? When are reproductive effects irreversible? What are the modes of action? How long does it take for reproductive function to return to normal once locoweed ingestion stops? Answers to these fundamental questions will aid in management decisions to improve reproductive performance and allow better utilization of locoweed-infested ranges.

PINE NEEDLE ABORTION, PONDEROSA PINE AND RELATED SPECIES

Ponderosa pine needles (PN) induce abortion in cattle and bison when eaten, primarily during the last trimester of gestation (James *et al.*, 1989; Short *et al.*, 1992; Panter *et al.*, 1992a). Isocupressic acid (ICA), a labdane resin acid, and two ICA derivatives were identified as the abortifacient toxins (James *et al.*, 1994; Gardner *et al.*, 1994, 1997; Figure 51.6). Oral and intravenous (i.v.) administration of ICA induced abortions in a dose-dependent manner with the higher doses inducing abortion in a shorter period of time. Acetyl and succinyl ICA derivatives, naturally present in PN, were also abortifacient when administered orally (Gardner *et al.*, 1996). However, the acetyl and succinyl ICA derivatives were not active when administered i.v. suggesting that intra-ruminal hydrolysis to ICA is important and inclusion of these two compounds in the total resin acid analysis is essential when evaluating relative risk of PN populations to induce abortions as both compounds are hydrolyzed in the rumen to ICA (Gardner *et al.*, 1999). Isocupressic acid metabolites include imbricatoloic acid, agathic acid, dihydroagathic acid, and tetrahydroagathic acid (Figure 51.7). Recently, Utah juniper bark, rich in agathic acid, was demonstrated to induce abortion in later term pregnant cattle thus implicating agathic acid as an abortifacient component of pine needles (Gardner *et al.*, 2010). The relative abortifacient activity of the remaining metabolites compared to ICA is still unknown but remains a main focus of our current research at the Poisonous Plant Research Lab. Ponderosa pine needles are not abortifacient in goats or sheep; ICA was not abortifacient in goats when administered orally or i.v. and ICA metabolites, similar to those detected in cow serum, were detected in goat serum (Gardner, unpublished data).

Serum samples taken from cows 15 minutes after i.v. infusion with ICA revealed that serum ICA disappearance is very rapid, as only residual amounts of ICA were detected (Gardner *et al.*, 1999). Metabolism studies using homogenates of bovine liver determined that ICA is rapidly metabolized to agathic acid and dihydroagathic acid with a $t_{1/2}$ of 15 minutes (Gardner *et al.*, 1999). Similar metabolism occurred in goat, sheep, pig, guinea-pig and rat liver homogenates although the guinea-pig and rat livers were less efficient. Metabolism occurred in the cystolic fraction of the liver homogenate and not in the microsomal fraction.

Thirty-six other tree and shrub species from throughout the western and southern states were analyzed for ICA (Gardner *et al.*, 1998a; Gardner and James, 1999; Table 51.2). Significant levels (>0.5% dry weight) were detected in *Pinus jefferyi* (Jeffrey pine), *P. contorta* (lodgepole pine), *Juniperus scopulorum* (Rocky Mountain juniper), *J. communis* (common juniper) and *Cupressus macrocarpa* (Monterey cypress) from New Zealand and Australia. Similar to Utah juniper (*J. osteosperma*), the bark from western juniper (*J. occidentalis*) contains high concentrations of agathic acid and imbricatoloic acid with very little ICA. Recently, we have found that the bark from western juniper will also induce abortions in cattle (unpublished observations). Abortions were induced when lodgepole pine and common juniper containing 0.7 and 2.5% ICA, respectively, were experimentally fed to pregnant cows, inducing abortions in 9 and 3.5 days, respectively (Gardner *et al.*, 1998a). This research confirmed field reports of

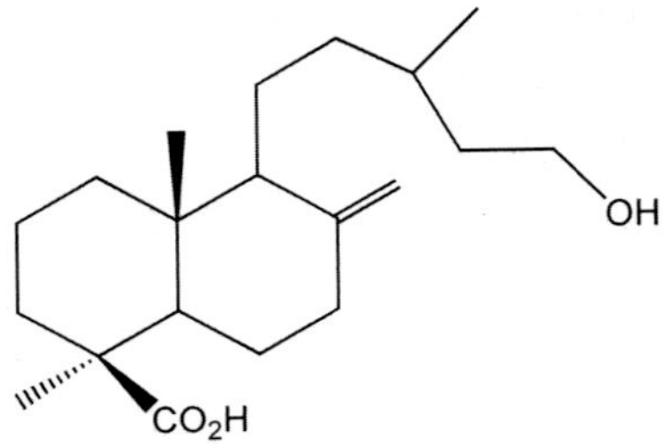

Imbricatoloic acid

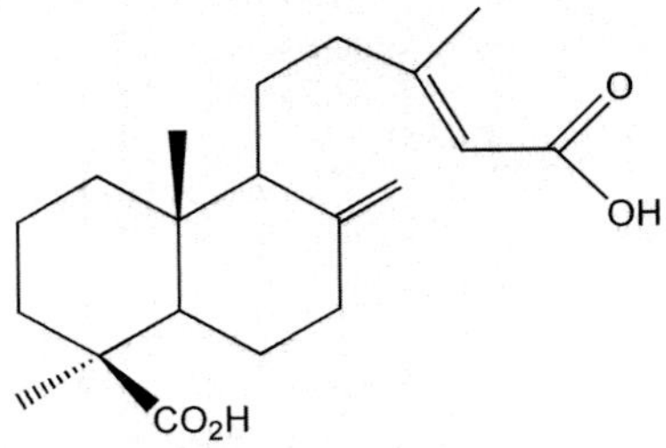

Agathic acid

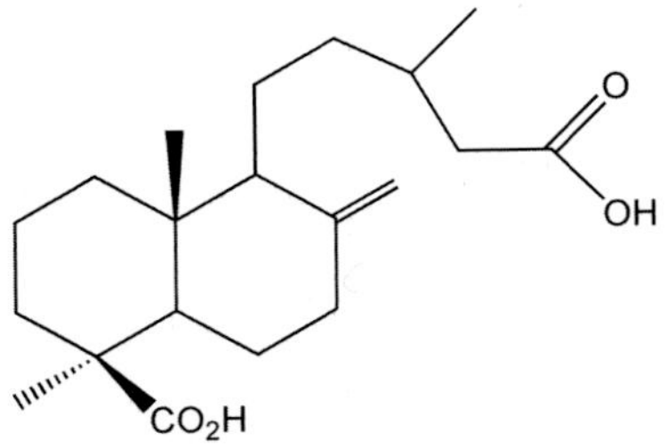

Dihydroagathic acid

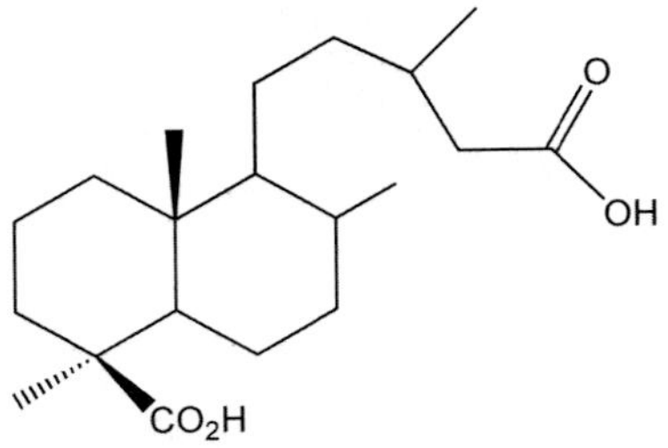

Tetrahydroagathic acid

FIGURE 51.7 Other labdane resin acids found in pine species and suspected to have abortifacient activity.

TABLE 51.2 Concentration of isocupressic acid (ICA) and related metabolic compounds from selected species and locations

Species	Common name	Location	Concentration (% DW)
Abies concolor	White fir	Arizona	n.d.[a]
		California	n.d.
		Colorado	0.04
		Utah	n.d.
Abies grandis	Grand fir	Idaho	n.d.
		Oregon	n.d.
Abies lasiocarpa	Subalpine fir	Oregon	n.d.
		Colorado	n.d.
		Idaho	0.04
		Utah	n.d.
Abies magnifica	Red fir	California	0.05
Cupressus macrocarpa	Monterey cypress	California	n.d.–0.06
		New Zealand	0.89–1.24
Cupressus X ovensii	Ovens cypress	New Zealand	0.81
Juniperus californica	California juniper	California	0.93 needles 0.05 bark
Juniperus communis	Mountain common juniper	Colorado	2.05–2.88
		Utah	1.50–5.0
Juniperus monosperma	One seed juniper	Arizona	0.14
		New Mexico	n.d.
Juniperus occidentalis	Western juniper	Oregon	0.10 Imbricatoloic acid = 1.0
		California	0.10 Imbricatoloic acid = 1.0 stems = 1.83 total labdane acids
Juniperus osteosperma	Utah juniper	Utah	n.d.
		Nevada	0.07
		Arizona	n.d.
		Colorado	n.d.
		Utah	Agathic acid = 1.50
Juniperus scopulorum	Rocky mountain juniper	Utah	0.84
		New Mexico	0.33
		Arizona	0.42
Juniperus virginiana	Eastern red cedar	Nebraska	Needles, low bark, <0.10–high
Larix occidentalis	Western larch	Oregon	n.d.

TABLE 51.2 Concentration of isocupressic acid (ICA) and related metabolic compounds from selected species and locations *(Cont'd)*

Species	Common name	Location	Concentration (% DW)
Libocedrus decurrens	Incense cedar	Oregon	0.07
Picea engelmannii	Engelmann spruce	California	0.27
		Colorado	n.d.
		Idaho	0.04
		Montana	0.31
		Oregon	n.d.
		Utah	n.d.
Picea pungens	Colorado blue spruce	Utah	0.17
		Colorado	n.d.
Pinus aristata	Bristle cone pine	Colorado	0.01–0.05
Pinus arizonica	Arizona pine	California	n.d.
		Arizona	n.d.
Pinus contorta	Lodgepole pine	Oregon	0.28
		Idaho	0.11
		Colorado	0.29–0.47
		Utah	0.66
		Canada (BC)	0.45
Pinus densiflora	Japanese red pine	Korea	n.d.
Pinus echinata	Short leaf pine	Arkansas	n.d.
Pinus edulis	Pinyon pine	Arizona	n.d.
		Colorado	0.12
		New Mexico	0.10
		Utah	0.45
Pinus elliottii	Slash pine	Arkansas	n.d.
Pinus flexilis	Limber pine	Colorado	n.d.–0.06
		Utah	n.d.
Pinus halepensis	Aleppo pine	California	n.d.
Pinus jeffreyi	Jeffrey pine	California	0.04–0.54
Pinus koraiensis	Korean pine	Utah	Positive
		Korea	0.02
Pinus monophylla	Single-leaf pinyon	Nevada	0.32
Pinus montezumae	Montezuma pine	California	n.d.
Pinus palustris	Long-leaf pine	Arkansas	n.d.
Pinus patula	Patula pine	South Africa	<0.10
Pinus ponderosa	Ponderosa pine	Oregon	0.74–1.30
		Arizona	0.49
		California	0.08–1.35
		Utah	0.51
		Colorado	0.49–0.58
		South Dakota	0.10–1.30
		Wyoming	0.58–1.11
		Germany	0.62
Pinus radiata	Radiata pine	New Zealand	n.d.–0.26
Pinus strobus	White pine		n.d.
Pinus taeda	Loblolly pine	Arizona	n.d.
		Arkansas	n.d.
Pseudotsuga menziesii	Douglas fir	Utah	0.04
		Colorado	0.05
		California	n.d.
		Idaho	n.d.
		Arizona	n.d.
		Oregon	n.d
Thuja plicata	Western red cedar	Arizona	0.42
		New Mexico	0.33
		Utah	0.84
		Germany	n.d.
Tsuga mertensiana	Mountain hemlock	Oregon	n.d.

[a]n.d. = not detected (<0.01%)

lodgepole pine needle abortion in British Columbia, Canada (France, personal communication). Monterey cypress is known to cause abortions in cattle in New Zealand and southern Australia and contained ICA levels of 0.89 to 1.24%. Similar labdane resin acids are present in broom snakeweed, but the putative abortifacient and toxic components have not been fully elucidated.

Occasional toxicoses from PN have been reported in field cases but are rare and have only occurred in pregnant cattle. No toxicity has been demonstrated from ICA or ICA derivatives; however, the abietane-type resin acids present in PN, and found in high concentrations in the new growth tips, were shown to be toxic and abortifacient at high doses when administered orally to cattle and toxic in goats and hamsters, causing nephrosis, edema of the central nervous system, myonecrosis and gastroenteritis (Stegelmeier *et al.*, 1996). While we believe these abietane-type resin acids may contribute to the occasional toxicoses reported in the field, we do not believe they contribute to the abortions. Most cow losses in the field are associated with difficult parturition or post-abortion toxemia due to retained fetal membranes.

Cattle readily graze PN (both PN litter on the ground and green needles from trees), especially during the winter months in the western USA. PN consumption increases during cold weather, with increased snow depth, and when other forage is limited (Pfister *et al.*, 1998; Cook *et al.*, 2010). Cattle are easily averted to green PN using an emetic (lithium chloride) paired with PN consumption, but these aversions may be extinguished if cattle are offered dry needles intermingled with dormant grasses.

Currently, recommendations to remove pregnant cattle in the last trimester of pregnancy from Ponderosa pine-infested pastures or to erect fencing around pine trees are the only preventive measures to ensure no losses from grazing pine needles. Current and future research centers on metabolism of the abortifacient labdanes, mechanism of action of the induced parturition, and treatment of premature calves and retained fetal membranes to ultimately reduce losses for livestock producers. Calves born after 260 days' gestation have a good prognosis for survival if given colostrum and supplemented for a few days until lactation in the dam improves.

BROOM SNAKEWEED

Broom snakeweed causes significant losses to cattle, sheep and goat producers in Texas and New Mexico from abortions and associated effects including toxicoses (McGinty, 1985). There are minor similarities to the abortions observed from Ponderosa pine needles; however, pine needles do not affect sheep and goats.

There are two major species of snakeweeds, *Gutierrezia sarothrae* (broom snakeweed, perennial snakeweed or turpentine weed) and *G. microcephala* (threadleaf broomweed). The snakeweeds are widely distributed in the western USA, Mexico and Canada. They extend from central Texas to California and from Saskatchewan, Canada, to northern Mexico (Lane, 1985). Threadleaf snakeweed often grows intermixed with broom snakeweed but is restricted to the southwestern desert regions of the USA and northern Mexico. Snakeweeds are widespread and invade depleted or disturbed rangeland. They are allelopathic and compete with other forages, often dominating the landscape. Their invading properties have resulted in their rapid movement into the dryer areas of the west.

Snakeweeds are short-lived perennial shrubs ranging from 15 to 60 cm tall. The leaves are narrow (3 to 6 mm wide) and 2 to 4 cm long. The flowers are yellow, in numerous clusters with three flowers per head in *G. sarothrae* and one or two per head in *G. microcephala*. The flowers are a distinguishing morphological characteristic between the two species (McDaniel and Loomis, 1985). The average lifespan of snakeweed is about 2.5 years (Parker, 1982). Seedlings are sensitive to soil moisture, competition from other plants and most die within the first year. However, snakeweeds rapidly increase in heavily overgrazed, burned or disturbed sites and during and following drought. Snakeweed seeds germinate when favorable precipitation resumes and it rapidly increases as a result of reduced competition (Parker, 1982). Snakeweeds grow on shallow sandy loam to loam with limestone bedrock underneath. They grow among open grassland communities as well as intermixed among sagebrush and mesquite shrub-dominated communities.

Snakeweeds are invasive and frequently dominate the landscape causing large economic losses through decreased carrying capacity and reduced rangeland utilization. Broom snakeweed is an aggressive invader and thrives following environmental disturbances in semi-arid rangelands of the west. Overgrazing, fires or major drought provide opportunities for snakeweeds to invade and dominate plant communities (Thacker *et al.*, 2008). Seeding with cool-season grasses following these disturbances or after herbicide control of snakeweeds is effective in suppressing reinvasion of snakeweeds and proved to be successful in experimental plots (Ralphs, 2009; Thacker *et al.*, 2009). In targeted grazing experiments where cattle were forced to deplete heavy stands of snakeweed, successful suppression of the snakeweed occurred and where stands of crested wheat grass were established, grass seedling response was improved and crested wheat grass stands were unaffected or somewhat improved following the target-grazing experiment (Ralphs and Banks, 2009). However, this approach requires further experimental substantiation over broader regions and under different environmental conditions.

The snakeweeds are toxic and abortifacient to cattle, sheep and goats. Abortions and retained fetal membranes in cattle are the most serious problems. In 1985, McGinty estimated losses in excess of $15 million annually to the cattle industry in Texas alone and over $30 million when losses in New Mexico and Arizona were included. This does not account for indirect losses such as loss of usable forage, management changes, increased calving intervals or added veterinary care.

The abortion has limited similarities to that of Ponderosa pine needles, i.e. there may be signs of impending parturition such as vulvar swelling, mucous and blood discharge, premature udder development and birth of small weak offspring. Retained fetal membranes are common and toxemia and death may occur. However, differences include: cattle are generally in poorer condition on broom snakeweed ranges compared to the pine pastures in the west; broom snakeweeds appear to possess a broader range of toxic terpenes than pine needles; snakeweeds are toxic and abortifacient to sheep and goats as well as cattle (Dollahite and Allen, 1959) whereas pine needles are only abortifacient in cattle and bison. Clinical signs of snakeweed toxicoses include anorexia, nasal discharge, crusted and sloughing skin on the muzzle, diarrhea followed by constipation. Dollahite *et al.* (1962) demonstrated that death in sheep, steers and goats occurred after ingestion of 3.6 kg, 10.9 kg and 5 kg of green snakeweed over 5, 3 and 14 days, respectively. Recent research suggests livestock usually do not eat snakeweeds if adequate forage is available; however, they will graze considerable amounts when other forage is depleted (Ralphs and Banks, 2009).

In rats, snakeweed at 12.5 and 25% of their diet impaired male and female reproduction, causing increased embryonic mortality in females and increased numbers of abnormal sperm in males (Flores-Rodriguez *et al.*, 1989; Edrington *et al.*, 1993). Aside from the abortifacient effects in ewes and heifers other reproductive effects are inconclusive and appear to not be as severe as those described for rats.

Broom snakeweed is reported to vary in toxicity at different phenological stages and soil sites where growing. It is more toxic when rapidly growing as in early spring. Snakeweeds growing on sandy soils are believed to be more toxic than when growing on limestone soils (Dollahite and Anthony, 1957) but this has not been fully substantiated. The abortifacient and toxic elements in broom snakeweed have not been identified although saponins extracted from broom snakeweed induced death and abortion when injected intravenously in cows, goats and rabbits. A non-toxic, pharmaceutical-grade saponin produced abortion and death in pregnant rabbits (Dollahite *et al.*, 1962). Molyneux *et al.* (1980) identified some major monoterpenes and sesquiterpenes in the essential oil fraction of snakeweed and these included alpha-pinene, myrcene, linalaol, *cis*-verbenol, *trans*-verbenol, verbenone, geraniol, caryophyllene and gamma-humulene. More recently, surface extractions of leaves and stems of *G. sarothrae* produced a resinous exudate amounting to approximately 10% of the dry plant weight. Gas chromatography-mass spectroscopy (GC-MS) analysis revealed numerous diterpene acids most of which have not been identified (Roitman *et al.*, 1994). There was a large difference in chemical composition of the extracts between plant collections apparently due to soil type thus supporting the previous reports from sandy soils vs. limestone soils.

POISONOUS PLANTS THAT AFFECT EMBRYO AND FETAL HEALTH

Lupines, poison-hemlock and *Nicotiana glauca*

Lupines, poison-hemlock (*Conium maculatum*) and *Nicotiana* spp. (*Nicotiana tabacum*; *N. glauca*) will be discussed together as the congenital malformations (skeletal contractures and cleft palates) are the same as is the mechanism of action (Panter *et al.*, 1990). The teratogenic effects of lupines are primarily a problem in cattle, whereas poison-hemlock is reported to cause field cases of skeletal defects in cattle, horses and pigs and *Nicotiana tabacum* has caused outbreaks of malformations in piglets born to pasture-grazed pregnant sows. While *N. glauca* has caused death losses in livestock it has not been reported as a cause of malformations in livestock in field cases. It is a rich source of the teratogenic alkaloid anabasine which is used in our laboratory for basic research and facilitates use of a congenital goat cleft palate model for biomedical research (Weinzweig *et al.*, 1999). Lupines contain quinolizidine and piperidine alkaloids, and poison-hemlock as well as *Nicotiana glauca* contains piperidine alkaloids while *N. tabacum* contains pyridine and piperidine alkaloids. Piperidine and quinolizidine alkaloids are widely distributed in nature and most possess a certain level of toxicity. Some are teratogenic, depending on structural characteristics which are now substantially understood.

Lupine toxicity

Stockmen have long recognized the toxicity of lupines, especially in late summer and fall when the pods and seeds are present. The clinical signs of poisoning begin with nervousness, depression, grinding of the teeth, frothing around the mouth, relaxation of the nictitating membrane of the eye, frequent urination and defecation and lethargy (Panter *et al.*, 1999a). These progress to muscular weakness and fasciculations, ataxia, collapse, sternal recumbency leading to lateral recumbency, respiratory failure and death. Signs may appear as early as 1 hour after ingestion and progressively get worse over the course of 24 to 48 hours even if further ingestion does not occur. Generally, if death does not occur within this timeframe, the animal recovers completely. Because of their foraging behavior and preference for forbs, sheep are more likely to die from acute lupine poisoning than cattle.

More than 150 quinolizidine alkaloids have been structurally identified from the Leguminosae family including *Lupinus, Laburnum, Cytisus, Thermopsis* and *Sophora* (Schmeller *et al.*, 1994; Wink *et al.*, 1995). Quinolizidine alkaloids occur naturally as *N*-oxides as well as free bases, but very little research has been done on the toxicity or teratogenicity of the *N*-oxides. However, the *N*-oxides of pyrrolizidine alkaloids are reduced to the corresponding free bases in the rumen, and it seems likely that quinolizidine alkaloids could undergo a similar conversion (Molyneux, personal communication).

Eighteen western American lupine species have been shown to contain the teratogen anagyrine (Figure 51.8) and 14 of these contain a sufficient concentration of anagyrine to be a risk for causing teratogenesis (Davis and Stout, 1986). Lupine alkaloids are produced by leaf chloroplasts and are translocated via the phloem and stored in epidermal cells and in seeds (Wink and Carey, 1994). Little is known about individual alkaloid toxicity; however, 14 alkaloids isolated from *Lupinus albus*, *L. mutabilis* and *Anagyris foetida* were analyzed for their affinity to nicotinic and/or muscarinic acetylcholine receptors (Schmeller *et al.*, 1994). Of the 14 compounds tested, the α-pyridones (*N*-methyl cytisine and cytisine) showed the highest affinities at the nicotinic receptor (IC_{50} of 0.05 and 0.14 μM for nicotinic vs. 417 and 400 μM for muscarinic receptors, respectively), while several quinolizidine alkaloid types including the teratogen anagyrine (IC_{50} 132 μM at muscarinic receptor vs. 2,096 μM at the nicotinic receptor) were more active at the muscarinic receptor. If one compares binding affinities of the teratogen anagyrine for nicotinic vs. muscarinic receptors, there is 16 times greater binding affinity to muscarinic receptors. Information about the maternal or fetal mechanism of toxicity or teratogenicity of anagyrine can perhaps be implied from this comparison.

Piperidine and quinolizidine alkaloid content as well as individual proportions vary in plants depending on environmental conditions, season of the year and stage of plant growth (Wink and Carey, 1994). Typically, alkaloid content is highest during early growth stages, decreases through the flower stage and increases in the seeds and pods. This knowledge has been used in management strategies to reduce losses to cattle producers.

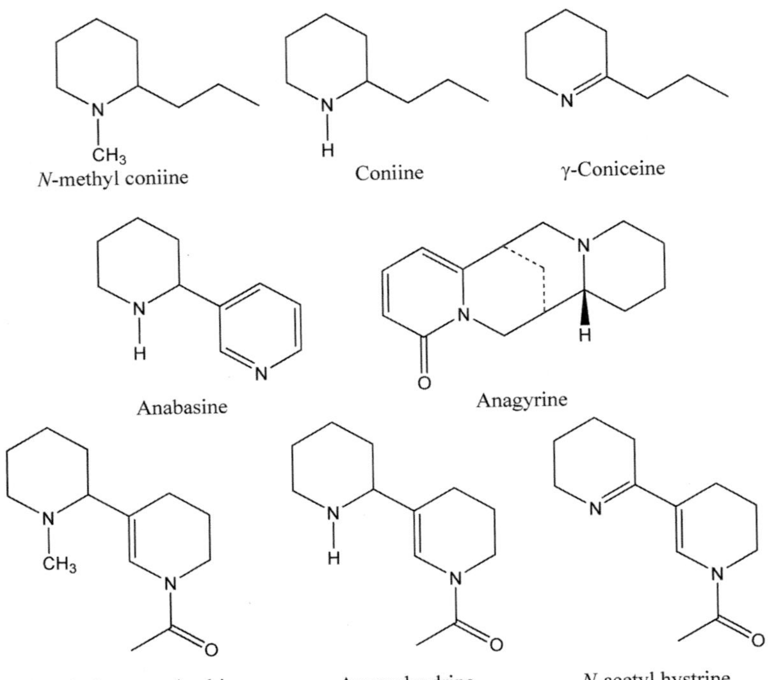

N-methyl coniine Coniine γ-Coniceine

Anabasine Anagyrine

N-methyl ammondendrine Ammodendrine *N*-acetyl hystrine

FIGURE 51.8 Teratogenic alkaloids from *Lupinus*, *Conium* and *Nicotiana* spp. that cause crooked calf disease and associated birth defects.

Alkaloid profiles vary considerably within and between lupine species (Wink and Carey, 1994). Season, environment and location influence alkaloid profile and concentration in a given species of lupine. Site differences in alkaloid levels have been described and are substantial. Total alkaloid content decreases as elevation increases and was shown to be six times higher in plants at 2,700 m vs. plants collected at 3,500 m. This phenomenon persists even when seedlings from the highest and lowest elevations were grown under identical greenhouse conditions, suggesting genetic differences as plants adapt to elevation changes. Generally, alkaloid content is highest in young plants and in mature seeds. For many lupines, the time and degree of seeding varies from year to year. Most direct death losses have occurred under conditions in which animals consume large amounts of pods or toxic plants in a brief period. This is especially true in sheep and happens when livestock are driven through an area of heavy lupine growth, unloaded into such an area, trailed through an area where the grass is covered by snow exposing lupine only, or when animals are forced to eat the plants due to overgrazing (Chestnut and Wilcox, 1901). Most poisonings occur in the late summer or early fall because seed pods are present and lupine remains green after other forage has matured or dried. Most calf losses occur because of teratogenic effects resulting from their mothers grazing lupine plants or pods during susceptible stages of pregnancy.

Some species of lupines are readily grazed by livestock and are acceptable forage under certain range conditions. Grazing of highly toxic species usually occurs because of unusual circumstances. A recent report described the death of 10 yearling stocker calves after grazing *Lupinus argenteus* containing predominantly the piperidine alkaloids ammodendrine and *N*-methyl ammodendrine (Panter *et al.*, 2001). This was an unusual case of piperidine alkaloid-containing lupine toxicosis and was thought to have resulted from overgrazing of the pasture, thus forcing the calves to begin eating lupine plants. Simply moving the calves a few days earlier to fresh pastures would have prevented the loss.

Lupines are responsible for a condition in cattle referred to as "crooked calf syndrome" wherein pregnant cattle grazing lupines containing either the quinolizidine alkaloid anagyrine or piperidine alkaloids of which ammodendrine, *N*-methyl ammodendrine and *N*-acetyl hystrine are the most likely piperidine alkaloid teratogens (Figure 51.8; Panter *et al.*, 1999a). Subsequently, calves may be born with multiple skeletal contracture malformations and/or cleft palate, depending on the stage of pregnancy when the dam grazes the lupines. Not all lupines are teratogenic but all wild lupines contain alkaloids that possess toxicity and some contain the teratogens. While lupines have historically caused large death losses in sheep, the most common losses in the last 50 years have been from the lupine-induced "crooked calf syndrome". While huge death losses were reported in sheep in the early 1900s, the teratogenic effects (crooked calf syndrome; Figure 51.9) are responsible for most recent losses associated with lupine. In more recent times large calf losses from congenital birth defects have been recorded in Oregon, Idaho, Montana and Washington (Panter, unpublished data). In 1992, 56% of the calves from a single herd of cows in Oregon were affected with lupine-induced skeletal malformations and many were euthanized (Panter *et al.*, 1997). In the spring of 1997 over 4,000 calves in Adams County, Washington, were deformed and many of those had to be humanely euthanized. In 2008 one ranch in eastern Washington State reported a 28% incidence of crooked calf syndrome. Similar reports have been recently reported in Montana, Oregon and British Columbia, including one anecdotal report from British Columbia of bison calves being born with classical lupine-type skeletal contractures.

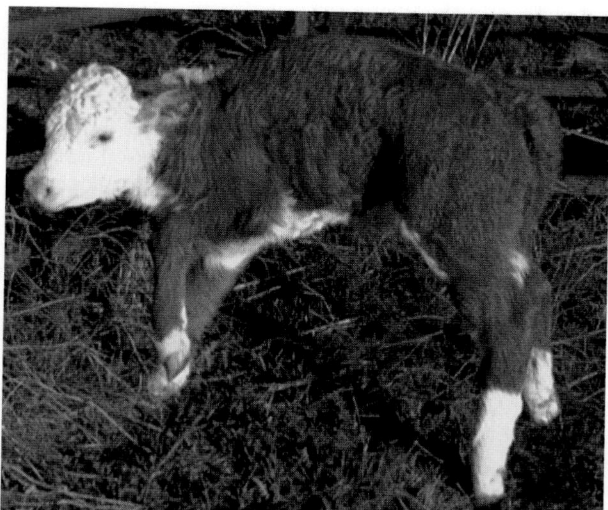

FIGURE 51.9 Crooked calf induced by maternal ingestion of lupines during gestation days 50–70. The left front leg is unable to extend and is rotated laterally.

Poison-hemlock (*Conium maculatum*) toxicoses

Poison-hemlock (*Conium maculatum*) has interesting historic significance as the "hemlock tea" used for execution in ancient Greece and the decoction used to put the philosopher Socrates to death (Daugherty, 1995). Toxicoses in livestock frequently occur and field reports of teratogenic effects in cattle and pigs have been reported (Edmonds *et al.*, 1972; Panter *et al.*, 1985a,b, 1999a). Poison-hemlock contains at least five piperidine alkaloids, all of which are believed to contribute to the toxicity. Coniine and γ-coniceine (Figure 51.8) predominate and are believed also to contribute to the teratogenic effects. The teratogenic effects are the same as those induced in cattle by lupines, i.e. cleft palate and multiple congenital skeletal contractures (MCC).

Clinical signs of poisoning include early signs of nervousness, occlusion of the eyes by the nictitating membrane (most pronounced in pigs and occasionally seen in cows, sheep and goats) progressing quickly through a pattern of nervous system stimulation with peripheral and local effects including frequent urination and defecation, dilated pupils, trembling, incoordination and excessive salivation. The stimulation soon progresses to depression resulting in relaxation, recumbency and eventually death from respiratory paralysis if the dosage is high enough. Cattle, pigs, goats, elk, wild geese and domestic turkeys have demonstrated a preference for *Conium* plant once they have acquired a taste for it (Copithorne, 1937; Macdonald, 1937; Edmonds *et al.*, 1972; Jessup *et al.*, 1986; Frank and Reed, 1990).

Coniine, γ-coniceine and *N*-methyl coniine are the principal alkaloids in *Conium* with relative concentration depending on the stage of plant growth. Gamma-coniceine is a metabolic precursor of coniine and *N*-methyl coniine; it is at highest concentration in early plant growth shifting to coniine and *N*-methyl coniine as the plant matures (Leete and Olson, 1972; Keeler and Balls, 1978). Coniine, γ-coniceine and *N*-methyl coniine have been shown to be toxic and teratogenic (Keeler *et al.*, 1980). Structural differences impart significant differences in toxicity (γ-coniceine>coniine>*N*-methyl coniine; Figure 51.8), but teratogenic potency is unknown although we believe it is related to toxicity (Panter *et al.*, 1999a).

Nicotiana spp.

While *Nicotiana glauca* has not been associated with field cases of teratogenesis in livestock, there have been reported cases of toxicoses (Plumlee *et al.*, 1993). The domesticated relative, *N. tabacum*, caused epidemic proportion outbreaks of malformations in newborn pigs in the late 1960s in Kentucky after tobacco stalks were fed to pregnant sows (Menges *et al.*, 1970). Experimentally, *N. glauca* is teratogenic in cattle, pigs, sheep, as well as goats and was used to establish that anabasine was the teratogenic alkaloid in *N. tabacum* (Keeler *et al.*, 1981, 1984; Panter and Keeler, 1992). *Nicotiana glauca* is primarily used as a rich source of anabasine (a potent teratogen). Similarly, the goat has been established as a model to study the mechanism of action of teratogenic piperidine alkaloids and the induction of cleft palate for both animal and human studies (Panter and Keeler, 1992; Panter *et al.*, 2000; Weinzweig *et al.*, 2008). These malformations were of the same type as those in lupine-induced crooked calf disease.

Nicotiana glauca contains primarily one piperidine alkaloid (anabasine; Figure 51.8) whereas *N. tabacum* contains several pyridine alkaloids (nicotine-like) as major constituents and some piperidine alkaloids as minor constituents. Clinical signs of *N. glauca* poisoning are similar to those described for poison hemlock and include early signs of nervousness, initial stimulation then depression, occlusion of the eyes by the nictitating membrane (most pronounced in pigs and occasionally seen in cows, sheep and goats) progressing quickly through a pattern of nervous system stimulation with peripheral and local effects including frequent urination and defecation, dilated pupils, trembling, incoordination and excessive salivation. The stimulation soon progresses to depression resulting in relaxation, recumbency and eventually death from respiratory paralysis if the dosage is high enough (Panter *et al.*, 1999a). Clinical signs of *N. tabacum* poisoning have similarities to that of *N. glauca*.

Teratogenicity of lupines, poison-hemlock and *Nicotiana glauca*

The teratogenic effects of *Lupinus*, *Conium* and *Nicotiana* spp. are discussed together as the malformations induced are the same, and the mechanism of action is believed to be common among the three genera and similar in susceptible livestock species (Panter *et al.*, 1999a). Current research at the Poisonous Plant Research Laboratory includes defining the specific teratogenic periods of gestation (Table 51.3), differences in susceptibility among livestock species, alkaloid structure–activity relationships, mechanisms of action and management strategies to reduce losses. A goat model using ground *Nicotiana glauca* and extracts therefrom was established to study the mechanism of action of the cleft palate and MCC (Panter *et al.*, 1990). Subsequently, this model has recently been characterized to study the etiology of cleft palate formation in humans and to develop new tools and procedures for treatment of cleft palate in children (Weinzweig *et al.*, 1999).

Susceptible periods of gestation

The periods of gestation when the fetus is susceptible to these plant teratogens have been defined in cattle, sheep, goats and swine (Table 51.3; Shupe *et al.*, 1967; Panter *et al.*, 1985a,b, 1997,

TABLE 51.3 Susceptible periods of gestation for alkaloid-induced cleft palate and multiple skeletal contractures (MCC) in cattle, sheep, goats, and swine

Defect	Cattle	Sheep	Goats	Swine
Cleft palate	40–50	35–41	35–41	30–40
MCC[a]		30–60	30–60	
	40–70			40–53
	40–100			50–63
				30–60

[a] MCC – multiple congenital contractures – include arthrogryposis, scoliosis, kyphosis and torticollis. Rib cage anomalies and asymmetry of the head also occur

1999a; Panter and Keeler, 1992). In swine, cleft palate only occurred when *Conium* was fed during days 30–41 of gestation (Panter *et al.*, 1985b). Skeletal defects, predominantly the forelimbs, spine and neck without cleft palate, were induced when pregnant sows were fed *Conium* during gestation days 40–53 (Panter *et al.*, 1985a). When feeding of *Conium* included days 50–63, rear limbs were affected also. When the *Conium* feeding period included days 30–60, all combinations of the defects described occurred. In sheep and goats, the teratogenic insult period is similar to pigs and includes days 30–60 (Keeler and Crowe, 1984; Panter *et al.*, 1990). In goats, a narrow period for cleft palate induction only was defined to include days 35–41 (Panter and Keeler, 1992). The cleft palate-induction period in cattle was recently defined from 40 to 50 days (Panter *et al.*, 1998). The critical gestational period for exposure in cattle is 40–70 days with susceptible periods extending to 100 days (Shupe *et al.*, 1967; Panter *et al.*, 1997). The severity and type of the malformations are dependent on alkaloid dosage ingested, the stage of pregnancy when the plants are eaten, and the length of time ingestion takes place.

Livestock species differences

The syndrome known as crooked calf disease (Figure 51.9) associated with lupine ingestion was first reported in the late 1950s and included various skeletal contracture-type birth defects and occasionally cleft palate (Palotay, 1959; Wagnon, 1960; Shupe *et al.*, 1967; Panter *et al.*, 1997, 2009). Through epidemiologic evidence and chemical comparison of teratogenic and non-teratogenic lupines, the quinolizidine alkaloid anagyrine was determined to be the teratogen (Keeler, 1976; Figure 51.8). A second teratogen, a piperidine alkaloid called ammodendrine, was found in *Lupinus formosus* to induce the same type of skeletal birth defects (Keeler and Panter, 1989; Panter *et al.*, 1994, 1998; Gardner *et al.*, 1998b; Figure 51.8). Further research determined that the anagyrine-containing lupines only caused birth defects in cattle and did not affect sheep or goats. No breed predilection or genetic susceptibility in cattle to the lupine-induced condition has been determined. The piperidine-containing lupine *L. formosus* caused birth defects experimentally in cattle and goats (Keeler and Panter, 1989; Panter *et al.*, 1994). This led to speculation about possible metabolism or absorption differences between cattle and small ruminants. Keeler and Panter (1989) hypothesized that the cow might metabolize the quinolizidine alkaloid anagyrine to a complex piperidine, meeting the structural characteristics determined for the simple teratogenic piperidine alkaloids in poison-hemlock (Keeler and Balls, 1978). This was supported by feeding trials with other piperidine alkaloid-containing plants, extracts and pure compounds. Even though comparative studies support the hypothesis that the cow may convert the quinolizidine alkaloid anagyrine to a complex piperidine by ruminal metabolism, recent evidence reporting the absorption and elimination patterns of many of the quinolizidine alkaloids, including anagyrine, in cattle, sheep and goats does not support this theory. Further research on this is currently ongoing at the Poisonous Plant Research Laboratory in Logan, Utah.

Structure–activity relationship

Keeler and Balls (1978) fed commercially available structural analogs of coniine to pregnant cows to compare structural relationships to teratogenic effects. Results suggested that the piperidine alkaloids must meet certain structural criteria to be teratogenic. Based on these data, Keeler and Balls (1978) speculated that the piperidine alkaloids with either a saturated ring or a single double bond and a side chain of at least three carbon atoms in length adjacent to the nitrogen atom might be considered potential teratogens. Note that the piperidine alkaloids in Figure 51.8 meet these criteria. Additionally, those alkaloids with a double bond adjacent to the nitrogen atom are more toxic than either the saturated or *N*-methyl derivatives. Relative toxicity of known teratogenic piperidine alkaloids using a mouse bioassay is: anabaseine > anabasine > gamma coniceine > coniine > *N*-methyl anabasine > *N*-methyl coniine > *N*-acetyl hystrine > *N*-methyl ammodendrine > ammodendrine (Panter *et al.*, 1999a).

Mechanism of action

The proposed mechanism of action for lupine, poison-hemlock and *N. glauca*-induced contracture defects and cleft palate is through a chemically induced reduction in fetal movement much as one would expect with a sedative, neuromuscular blocking agent, or anesthetic (Panter *et al.*, 1990). The speculated mechanism of action was supported by experiments using radio ultrasound where a direct relationship between reduced fetal activity and severity of contracture-type skeletal defects and cleft palate in sheep and goats was recorded. Further research suggests that this inhibition of fetal movement must be over a protracted period of time during specific stages of gestation. For example, fresh *Conium* plant was fed to pregnant sheep and goats during gestation days 30–60 and fetal movement monitored at 45, 50 and 60 days' gestation over a 12-hour period after dosing. *Conium* plant inhibited fetal movement for 5 to 9 hours after gavage, but by 12 hours fetal movement was similar to that of controls. The lambs and kids had no cleft palates and only slight to moderate carpal flexure (buck knees), which spontaneously resolved a few weeks after birth. On the other hand, *Conium* seed (with higher teratogen concentration) or *N. glauca* inhibited fetal movement during the entire 12-hour period between dosages (two times daily) over the treatment period of 30 to 60 days. Severe limb, spine and neck defects and cleft palate occurred (Panter *et al.*, 1990).

Further ultrasonographic studies showed that strong fetal movement becomes evident in the untreated goat at about day 35 gestation and these first movements are intermittent extension/flexure-type of the fetal head and neck. The heads

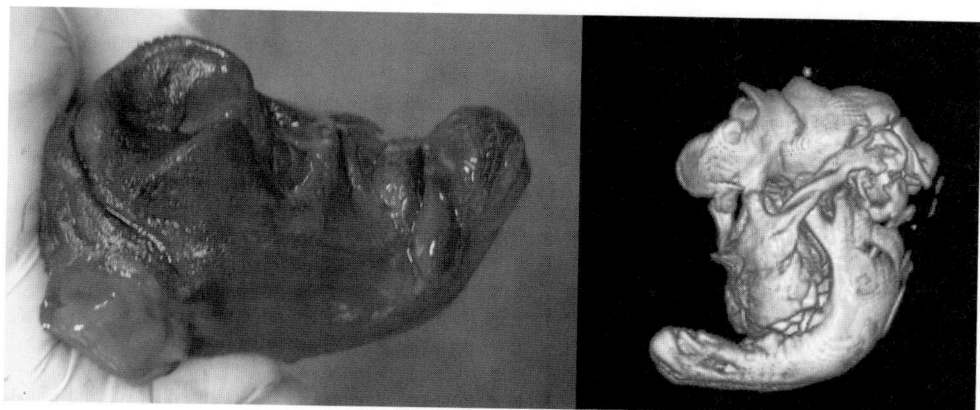

FIGURE 51.10 Congenital cyclopia caused by maternal ingestion of *Veratrum californicum* on gestation day 13 or 14.

of fetuses under the influence of anabasine from 35 to 41 days' gestation remained tightly flexed against the sternum and no movement was seen. Subsequently, the newborn goats had cleft palate but no other defects. Panter and Keeler (1992) suggested that these cleft palates were caused by mechanical interference by the tongue between palate shelves during programmed palate closure time (day 38 in goats; between days 40 and 50 in cows).

In addition to the ultrasonographic studies, which provide direct evidence of reduced fetal movement, the nature of some of the defects in offspring from cows gavaged *L. formosus* and in goats gavaged *Conium* seed or *N. glauca* offers other evidence of the importance of lack of fetal movement in normal development. These defects included depressions in the rib cage, legs or spinal column suggesting a mechanical impact from pressure of a sibling or the head turned back on the rib cage. Based on ultrasonographic studies, the action of teratogens appears to be directly on the fetus (inhibited fetal movement) rather than via maternal toxicity, because fetal movement inhibition persists between doses for a much greater duration than do signs of overt toxicity in the dam (Panter *et al.*, 1990). Furthermore, manual manipulation of the fetus and ultrasound observation during feeding trials revealed that there was adequate space in the uterus for normal body movement, yet the fetus remained totally immobile.

Even though research at the Poisonous Plant Research Lab has been limited to the three genera mentioned above, there are others that contain piperidine and quinolizidine alkaloids structurally similar to what we would expect to be both toxic and teratogenic. These include species in the following genera: *Genista, Prosopis, Lobelia, Cytisus, Sophora, Pinus, Punica, Duboisia, Sedum, Withania, Carica, Hydrangea, Dichroa, Cassia, Ammondendron, Liparia, Colidium* and others (Keeler and Crowe, 1984). Many plant species or varieties from these genera may be included in animal and human diets; however, toxicity and teratogenicity are a matter of dose, rate of ingestion, and alkaloid level and composition in the plant.

Prevention and treatment

Prevention of poisoning and birth defects induced by lupines, poison-hemlock and *Nicotiana* spp. can be accomplished by using a combination of management techniques: (1) coordinating grazing times to avoid the most toxic stage of plant growth such as early growth and seed pod stage for lupine and early growth and green seed stage for *Conium;* (2) changing time of breeding, either advancing or delaying or changing from spring to fall calving, thereby avoiding the most susceptible period of gestation; (3) reducing plant population through herbicide treatment; (4) managing grazing to maximize grass coverage; and (5) intermittent grazing, allowing short duration grazing of lupine pastures with frequent rotation when cows are first observed grazing lupine plants. The risk is reduced when lupine is in flower or post-seed stage and when poison-hemlock has matured.

VERATRUM SPP. (SKUNK CABBAGE, FALSE HELLEBORE)

Veratrum belongs to the Liliaceae (lily) family and is comprised of at least five species in North America. During the mid-20th century, up to 25% of pregnant ewes that grazed on pastures infested with *Veratrum californicum* in the mountains of central Idaho gave birth to lambs with serious craniofacial malformation (James, 1999). The gross malformations ranged from a series of lethal craniofacial defects including synophthalmia (congenital cyclops) to less severe deformities of the upper and lower jaws (Binns *et al.*, 1965; Welch *et al.*, 2009; Figure 51.10). The Basque shepherds called the lambs "chatto", which translates as "monkey faced" lamb syndrome. While losses from *Veratrum* have long been reduced or eliminated on these ranges because of the research and recommended management changes, alkaloid teratogens, isolated and identified at the Poisonous Plant Research Lab and now used as molecular probes, have opened a new frontier for human biomedical research (Gaffield and Keeler, 1996; James *et al.*, 2004; Scales and Sauvage, 2009).

Veratrum californicum grows primarily in the high mountain ranges of the western USA (Kingsbury, 1964; Knight and Walter, 2001). *Veratrum viride* is the most widespread species and grows in the northwestern USA north through western Canada into Alaska and is also widespread in the northeastern USA; *V. insolitum* grows in a relatively small region of northwestern California and southwestern Oregon; *V. parviflorum* grows in the central southeastern states; and *V. woodii* grows from Ohio to Missouri, Oklahoma and Arkansas. Two other species have been reported to cause poisoning in other countries, *V. japonicum* in Korea and *V. album* in Europe. Common names include western false hellebore, hellebore, skunk cabbage, corn lily, Indian poke, wolfsbane, etc. Caution should be used with common names as they may be used interchangeably within these genera but also in unrelated genera. For example, the name hellebore is also used for the genus *Helleborus* in the buttercup family.

Most *Veratrum* spp. are found in similar habitats of moist, open alpine meadows or open woodlands, marshes, along waterways, in swamps or bogs, and along lake edges in high mountain ranges (Kingsbury, 1964; Burrows and Tyrl, 2001). Most species grow at higher elevations. All species are similar with course, erect plants about 4–8 feet tall, with short perennial rootstalks. The leaves are smooth, alternate, parallel veined, broadly oval to lanceolate, up to 1 foot long, 6 inches wide, in three ranks and sheathed at the base. The inflorescence is a panicle, the lower ones often staminate and the upper ones perfect. The flowers of *V. viride* are distinctly green and the fruit is three chambered with several seeds.

Over 50 complex steroidal alkaloids have been identified from the *Veratrum* spp. (Keeler, 1978, 1984; Brown and Keeler, 1978; Keeler *et al.*, 1993; Gaffield and Keeler, 1996). Five classes of steroidal alkaloids have been characterized: veratrines, cevanines, jervanines, solanidines and cholestanes. The veratrines and cevanines are of considerable interest in toxicology as they are neurological toxins and hypotensive agents that bind to sodium channels delaying closure and causing cardio-toxic and respiratory effects (Nanasi *et al.*, 1990). The cevanine alkaloids are also found in *Zigadenus* spp., also members of the lily family. The jervanines are most significant in the teratogenic effects, the most notable of which were named cyclopamine and jervine (Keeler, 1978; Figure 51.11) both potent inducers of the congenital cyclopia ("monkey-faced lamb syndrome" reported in many flocks of sheep in the late 1950s in central Idaho; Binns *et al.*, 1965). This cyclopic defect is induced in the sheep embryo during the blastocyst stage of development when the pregnant mother ingests the plant during the 14th day of gestation. Other defects such as limb defects and tracheal stenosis occur when maternal ingestion includes days 28–33 of gestation (Keeler *et al.*, 1985; Keeler and Stuart, 1987; Keeler, 1990). The solanidine alkaloids are also found in many *Solanum* spp., and are toxic and teratogenic. The cholestanes, other alkaloids found in the plant, have been used as hypotensive drugs but are much less likely to induce the birth defects. Structure–activity relationship is a very important key for potency to produce birth defects (Keeler *et al.*, 1993; Gaffield and Keeler, 1994). It is now known that this structure–activity relationship is key in the mechanism of action which is the inhibition of the sonic hedgehog signaling pathway (Gaffield and Keeler, 1996). This sonic hedgehog gene pathway and the subsequent downstream regulation of gene expression have now been implicated in numerous cancers, birth defects and other anomalies. The toxin, cyclopamine, has become a significant tool in the study of the very complex sonic hedgehog pathway and cyclopamine derivatives such as IPI-926 have shown great promise in phase 1 clinical trials for cancer treatments (Olive *et al.*, 2009; Scales and Sauvage, 2009).

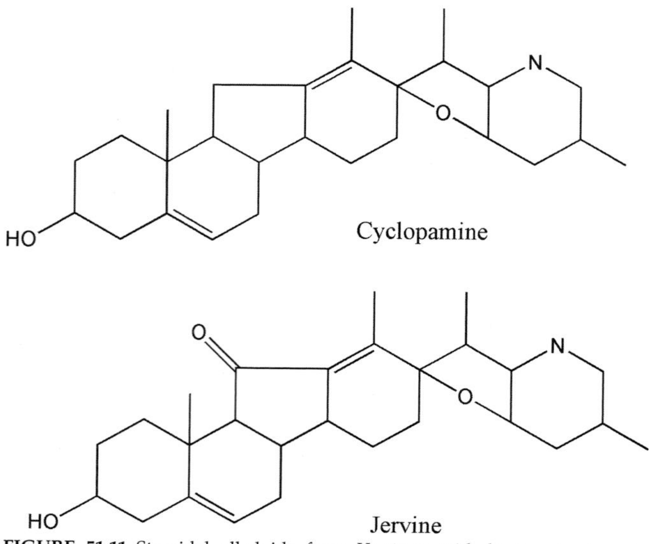

Clinical signs of poisoning in animals are most likely caused by neurotoxic cevanine alkaloids present in most species of *Veratrum*. Typical signs begin with excess salivation with froth around the mouth, slobbering and vomiting progressing to ataxia, collapse and death.

Control of *Veratrum* is relatively easy with herbicides such as broad-leaf herbicides and long-term control has been demonstrated (Williams, 1991). The teratogenic effects of *Veratrum* can be avoided by keeping sheep and other livestock species off pastures containing the plants during the first trimester of pregnancy. Observation of toxicoses in the field is rare unless herders move the animals shortly after exposure. The neurological signs, which are likely produced by the cevanine alkaloids, can be treated with atropine to improve the cardiovascular output. Activated charcoal to adsorb toxins and administration of picrotoxin to improve respiration have been recommended (Burrows and Tyrl, 2001).

HO N O Cyclopamine

HO O N O Jervine

FIGURE 51.11 Steroidal alkaloids from *Veratrum* with known teratogenic potency.

OTHER PLANT SPECIES WITH SUSPECTED TERATOGENIC ACTIVITY

Numerous other plants are suspected to be teratogenic but lack sufficient experimental work to be conclusive. Plants containing cyanogenic glycosides have been reported to induce contracture skeletal defects in pigs and horses when ingested by pregnant dams (Table 51.1). Wild black cherry was implicated in pig contracture deformities (Selby *et al.*, 1971) and sorghum was suggested as a cause of contracted foal syndrome. Jimson weed (Table 51.1) was believed to be the cause of an outbreak of skeletal deformities in pigs; however, experimental feeding trials failed to confirm this (Keeler, 1981). Research evidence and suggested mechanisms of action are inconclusive and further experimentation is needed.

CONCLUDING REMARKS AND FUTURE DIRECTIONS

Reproductive success is the single most important economic multiplier for livestock producers in the USA. Compared to carcass and growth traits, reproductive performance is considered to be 5 and 10 times more significant, respectively.

It must be kept in mind that if reproduction fails, the other values have little relevance. Reproductive performance not only relates to an animal's ability to produce offspring, but to produce it at a proper time interval and provide proper neonatal care and nutrition. The recognition that poisonous plants may have a major impact on reproductive performance is relatively new and not fully realized. Effects on spermatogenesis, oogenesis, libido, fertilization, placentation, embryo–fetal survival, development (birth defects) and growth, postpartum intervals, and neonatal survival and development are all factors affected by poisonous plants.

The following basic concepts will reduce risk of poisonous plants losses:

1. Recognize the plants on your range or pastures or seek appropriate help from extension, university or federal agencies and know the potential hazards of grazing where poisonous plants grow. Know the conditions under which poisoning may occur.
2. Avoid introducing naive animals into unfamiliar pastures or ranges where poisonous plants grow.
3. Do not introduce animals into poisonous plant-infested ranges before adequate quality feed is available. Many toxic plants emerge before grasses are adequate for grazing.
4. Do not discard grass, shrubs or tree clippings where livestock have access, e.g. yew clippings are a common cause of poisoning in cattle and horses.
5. Provide free choice access to fresh water and trace mineral salt.
6. Do not overstock or overgraze pastures.
7. Avoid bedding, lambing/calving, watering, salting or unloading hungry animals near poisonous plant populations.
8. Avoid excess stress to affected animals, especially when animals may be showing clinical effects.
9. Control poisonous plants if economically feasible, either through hand grubbing, mechanical clipping or herbicide treatment.

REFERENCES

Binns W, Shupe JL, Keeler RF, James LF (1965) Chronologic evaluation of teratogenicity in sheep fed *Veratrum californicum*. *J Am Vet Med Assoc* **147:** 839–42.

Brown D, Keeler RF (1978) Structure–activity relation of steroid teratogens. 3. Solanidan epimers. *J Agric Food Chem* **26:** 566–9.

Burrows GE, Tyrl RJ (2001) *Toxic Plants of North America*. Iowa State University Press, Ames, Iowa.

Chestnut VK, Wilcox EV (1901) The stock-poisoning plants of Montana: a preliminary report. *US Dept of Agric Bull No.* **26:** 100–10 Washington DC.

Cook D, Gardner DR, Pfister JA, Panter KE, Stegelmeier BL, Lee ST, Welch KD, Green BT, Davis TZ (2010) Differences in Ponderosa pine isocupressic acid concentrations across space and time. *Rangelands* **32(3):** 14-17.

Copithorne B (1937) Suspected poisonings of goats by Hemlock (*Conium maculatum*). *Vet Record* **49:** 1018–9.

Daugherty CG (1995) The death of Socrates and the toxicology of hemlock. *J Med Biography* **3:** 178–82.

Davis AM, Stout DM (1986) Anagyrine in western American lupines. *J Range Manage* **39:** 29–30.

Dollahite JW, Allen TJ (1959) Feeding perennial broomweed to cattle, sheep, goats, rabbits, guinea pigs, and chickens. *Tex Agric Exp Stn Prog Rpt* **2105**.

Dollahite JW, Anthony WV (1957) Poisoning of cattle with *Gutierrezia microcephala*, a perennial broomweed. *J Am Vet Med Assoc* **130:** 525–30.

Dollahite JW, Shaver T, Camp BJ (1962) Injected saponins as abortifacients. *J Amer Vet Res* **23:** 1261–3.

Edmonds LD, Shelby LA, Case AA (1972) Poisoning and congenital malformations associated with consumption of poison hemlock by sows. *J Am Vet Med Assoc* **160:** 1319–24.

Edrington TS, Flores-Rodriguez GI, Smith GS, Hallford DM (1993) Effect of ingested snakeweed (*Gutierrezia microcephala*) foliage on reproduction, semen quality, and serum clinical profiles of male rats. *J Anim Sci* **71:** 1520–5.

Flores-Rodriguez GI, Smith GS, McDaniel KC (1989) Effects of ingested snakeweed (*Gutierrezia microcephala*) herbage on reproduction, serum progesterone, and blood constituents of female albino rats. *Proc West Sect Am Soc Anim Sci* **40:** 217–21.

Frank AA, Reed WM (1990) Comparative toxicity of coniine, an alkaloid of *Conium maculatum* (poison hemlock), in chickens, quails, and turkeys. *Avian Diseases* **31(2):** 433–7.

Gaffield W, Keeler RF (1994) Structure–activity relations of teratogenic natural products. *Pure Appl Chem* **66:** 2407–10.

Gaffield W, Keeler RF (1996) Steroidal alkaloid teratogens: molecular probes for investigation of craniofacial malformation. *J Toxicol Toxin Rev* **15:** 303–26.

Gardner DR, James LF (1999) Pine needle abortion in cattle: analysis of isocupressic acid in North American gymnosperms. *Phytochem Anal* **10(3):** 132–6.

Gardner DR, Molyneux RJ, James LF, Panter KE, Stegelmeier BL (1994) Ponderosa pine needle-induced abortion in beef cattle: identification of isocupressic acid as the principal active compound. *J Ag Food Chem* **42(3):** 756–61.

Gardner DR, Panter KE, James LF (1999) Pine needle abortion in cattle: metabolism of isocupressic acid. *J Ag Food Chem* **47(7):** 2891–97.

Gardner DR, Panter KE, James LF, Stegelmeier BL (1998a) Abortifacient effects of lodgepole pine (*Pinus contorta)* and common juniper (*Juniperus communis*) on cattle. *Vet Human Toxicol* **40(5):** 260–3.

Gardner DR, Panter KE, Molyneux RJ (1998b) Teratogenic and fetotoxic effects of two piperidine alkaloid-containing lupines (*L. formosus* and *L. arbustus*) in cows. *J Natural Toxins* **7(2):** 131–40.

Gardner DR, Panter KE, Molyneux RJ, James LF, Stegelmeier BL (1996) Abortifacient activity in beef cattle of acetyl- and succinyl-isocupressic acid from ponderosa pine. *J Ag Food Chem* **44(10):** 3257–61.

Gardner DR, Panter KE, Molyneux RJ, James LF, Stegelmeier BL, Pfister JA (1997) Isocupressic acid and related diterpene acids from *Pinus ponderosa* as abortifacient compounds in cattle. *J Nat Toxins* **6:** 1–10.

Gardner DR, Panter KE, Stegelmeier BL (2010) Implication of agathic acid from Utah juniper bark as an abortifacient compound in cattle. *J Appl Toxicol* **30:** 115–9.

Hafez SA, Caceci T, Freeman LE, Panter KE (2007) Angiogenesis in the caprine caruncles in non-pregnant and pregnant normal and swainsonine treated does. *Anatom Rec* **90:** 761–9.

Hartley WJ, James LF (1975) Fetal and maternal lesions in pregnant ewes ingesting locoweed (*Astragalus lentiginosus*). *Amer J Vet Res* **36:** 825–6.

James LF (1999) Teratological research at the USDA-ARS Poisonous Plant Research Laboratory. *J Nat Toxin* **8:** 63–80.

James LF, Hartley WJ (1977) Effects of milk from animals fed locoweed in kittens, calves and lambs. *Amer J Vet Res* **38:** 1263–5.

James LF, Molyneux RJ, Panter KE, Gardner DR, Stegelmeier BL (1994) Effect of feeding Ponderosa pine needle extracts and their residues to pregnant cattle. *Cornell Vet* **84(1):** 33–9.

James LF, Panter KE, Broquist HP, Hartley WJ (1991) Swainsonine-induced high mountain disease in calves. *Vet Human Toxicol* **33:** 217–19.

James LF, Panter KE, Gaffield W, Molyneux RJ (2004) Biomedical applications of poisonous plant research. *J Agric Food Chem* **52:** 3211–30.

James LF, Short RE, Panter KE, Molyneux RJ, Stuart LD, Bellows RA (1989) Pine needle abortion in cattle: a review and report of 1973–84 research. *Cornell Vet* **79:** 39–52.

James LF, Van Kampen KR, Hartley WJ (1970a) Comparative pathology of *Astragalus* (locoweed) and *Swainsona* poisoning in sheep. *Pathol Vet* **7:** 116–25.

James LF, Van Kampen KR, Johnson AE (1970b) Physiopathologic changes in locoweed poisoning in livestock. *Amer J Vet Res* **31:** 663–72.

Jessup DA, Boermans HJ, Kock ND (1986) Toxicosis in tule elk caused by ingestion of poison hemlock. *J Am Vet Med Assoc* **189:** 1173–5.

Keeler RF (1976) Lupin alkaloids from teratogenic and nonteratogenic lupins. III. Identification of anagyrine as the probable teratogen by feeding trials. *J Toxicol Environ Health* **1:** 887–9.

Keeler RF (1978) Cyclopamine and related steroidal alkaloid teratogens: their occurrence, structural relationship, and biologic effects. *Lipids* **13:** 708–15.

Keeler RF (1981) Absence of arthrogryposis in newborn Hampshire pigs from sows ingesting toxic levels of jimsonweed during gestation. *Vet Human Toxicol* **23:** 413–15.

Keeler RF (1984) Teratogens in plants. *J Anim Sci* **58:** 1029–39.

Keeler RF (1990) Early embryonic death in lambs induced by *Veratrum californicum*. *Cornell Vet* **80:** 203–7.

Keeler RF, Balls LD (1978) Teratogenic effects in cattle of *Conium maculatum* and *Conium* alkaloids and analogs. *Clin Toxicol* **12:** 49–64.

Keeler RF, Balls LD, Panter KE (1981) Teratogenic effects of *Nicotiana glauca* and concentration of anabasine, the suspect teratogen in plant parts. *Cornell Vet* **71:** 47–53.

Keeler RF, Balls LD, Shupe JL, Crowe MW (1980) Teratogenicity and toxicity of coniine in cows, ewes and mares. *Cornell Vet* **70:** 19–26.

Keeler RF, Crowe MW (1984) Teratogenicity and toxicity of wild tree tobacco, *Nicotiana glauca* in sheep. *Cornell Vet* **74:** 50–9.

Keeler RF, Crowe MW, Lambert EA (1984) Teratogenicity in swine of the tobacco alkaloid anabasine isolated from *Nicotiana glauca*. *Teratology* **30:** 61–9.

Keeler RF, Gaffield W, Panter KE (1993) Natural products and congenital malformations: structure–activity relationships. In *Dietary Factors and Birth Defects* (Sharma RP, ed.). Pacific Division, San Francisco, CA.

Keeler RF, Panter KE (1989) Piperidine alkaloid composition and relation to crooked calf disease-inducing potential of *Lupinus formosus*. *Teratology* **40:** 423–32.

Keeler RF, Stuart LD (1987) The nature of congenital limb defects induced in lambs by maternal ingestion of *Veratrum californicum*. *Clin Toxicol* **25:** 273–86.

Keeler RF, Young S, Smart R (1985) Congenital tracheal stenosis in lambs induced by maternal ingestion of *Veratrum californicum*. *Teratology* **31:** 83–8.

Kingsbury JM (1964) *Poisonous Plants of the United States and Canada*. Prentice-Hall Inc., Englewood Cliffs, NJ.

Knight AP, Walter RG (2001) *A Guide to Plant Poisoning of Animals in North America*. Teton New Media, Jackson, WY.

Lane M (1985) Taxonomy of *Gutierrezia* Lag (Compositeae: Astereae) in North America. *Systemic Botany* **10(1):** 7–28.

Leete E, Olson JO (1972) Biosynthesis and metabolism of the hemlock alkaloids. *J Am Chem Soc* **94(15):** 5472–7.

MacDonald H (1937) Hemlock poisoning in horses. *Vet Rec* **49:** 1211–12.

McDaniel KC, Loomis LE (1985) Livestock poisoning by perennial snakeweeds. *Weeds Today* **16(1):** 9–11.

McGinty A (1985) Survey suggests broomweed costs far more than previously thought. *Livestock Weekly* September 5–6.

Menges RW, Selby LA, Marienfed CJ, Aue WA, Greer DL (1970) A tobacco related epidemic of congenital limb deformities in swine. *Environ Res* **3:** 285.

Molyneux RJ, James LF (1982) Loco intoxication: indolizidine alkaloids of spotted locoweed (*Astragalus lentiginosus*). *Science* **216:** 190–1.

Molyneux RJ, James LF, Panter KE, Ralphs MH (1991) Analysis and distribution of swainsonine and related polyhydroxyindolizidine alkaloids by thin layer of chromatography. *Phytochem Anal* **2:** 125–9.

Molyneux RJ, Stevens KL, James LF (1980) Chemistry of toxic range plants: volatile constituents of broomweed (*Gutierrezia sarothrae*). *J Agric Food Chem* **28:** 1332–3.

Nanasi PP, Kiss T, Danko M, Lathrop DA (1990) Differenct actions of aconitine and veratrum alkaloids on frog skeletal muscle. *Gen Pharmacol* **21:** 863–8.

Olive KP, Jacobetz MA, Davidson CJ, Gopinathan A, McIntyre D, *et al.* (2009) Inhibition of hedgehog signaling enhances delivery of chemotherapy in a mouse model of pancreatic cancer. *Science* **324(5933):** 1457–61.

Ortiz AR, Hallford DM, Galyean ML, Schneider FA, Kridli RT (1997) Effects of locoweed (*Oxytropis sericea*) on growth, reproduction, and serum hormone profiles in young rams. *J Anim Sci* **75:** 3229–34.

Palotay JL (1959) Crooked calves. *Western Vet* **6:** 16–20.

Panter KE, Bunch TD, James LF, Sisson DV (1987) Ultrasonographic imaging to monitor fetal and placental developments in ewes fed locoweed (*Astragalus lentiginosus*). *Amer J Vet Res* **48:** 686–90.

Panter KE, Bunch TD, Keeler RF, Sisson DV, Callan RJ (1990) Multiple congenital contractures (MCC) and cleft palate induced in goats by ingestion of piperidine alkaloid-containing plants: reduction in fetal movement as the probable cause. *Clin Toxicol* **28:** 69–83.

Panter KE, Gardner DR, Gay CC, James LF, Mills R, Gay JM, Baldwin TJ (1997) Observations of *Lupinus sulphureus*-induced "crooked calf disease". *J Range Manage* **50:** 587–92.

Panter KE, Gardner DR, Molyneux RJ (1994) Comparison of toxic and teratogenic effects of *Lupinus formosus*, *L. arbustus* and *L. caudatus* in goats. *J Nat Toxins* **3(2):** 83–93.

Panter KE, Gardner DR, Molyneux RJ (1998) Teratogenic and fetotoxic effects of two piperidine alkaloid-containing lupines (*L. formosus and L. arbustus*) in cows. *J Nat Toxins* **7(2):** 131–40.

Panter KE, James LF (1990) Natural plant toxicants in milk: a review. *J Anim Sci* **68:** 892–904.

Panter KE, James LF, Gardner DR (1999a) Lupine, poison-hemlock, and *Nicotiana* spp.: toxicity and teratogenicity in livestock. *J Nat Toxins* **8(1):** 117–34.

Panter KE, James LF, Hartley HJ (1989) Transient testicular degeneration in rams fed locoweed (*Astragalus lentiginosus*). *Vet Human Toxicol* **31:** 42–6.

Panter KE, James LF, Molyneux RJ (1992a) Ponderosa pine needle-induced parturition in cattle. *J Anim Sci* **70:** 1604–8.

Panter KE, James LF, Stegelmeier BL, Ralphs MH, Pfister JA (1999b) Locoweeds: effects on reproduction in livestock. *J Nat Toxins* **8(1):** 53–62.

Panter KE, Keeler RF (1992) Induction of cleft palate in goats by *Nicotiana glauca* during a narrow gestational period and the relation to reduction in fetal movement. *J Nat Toxins* **1:** 25–32.

Panter KE, Keeler RF, Buck WB (1985a) Congenital skeletal malformations induced by maternal ingestion of *Conium maculatum* (poison hemlock) in newborn pigs. *Am J Vet Res* **46:** 2064–6.

Panter KE, Keeler RF, Buck WB (1985b) Induction of cleft palate in newborn pigs by maternal ingestion of poison-hemlock (*Conium maculatum*). *Am J Vet Res* **46:** 1368–71.

Panter KE, Keeler RF, James LF, Bunch TD (1992b) Impact of plant toxins on fetal and neonatal development. *J Range Manage* **45:** 52–7.

Panter KE, Mayland HF, Gardner DR, Shewmaker G (2001) Beef cattle losses after grazing *Lupinus argenteus* (silvery lupine). *Vet Human Toxicology* **43(5):** 279–82.

Panter KE, Motteram E, Cook D, Lee ST, Ralphs MH, Platt TE, Gay CC (2009) Crooked calf syndrome: managing lupines on rangelands of the Channel Scablands of east central Washington State. *Rangelands* **31(1):** 10–15.

Panter KE, Ralphs MH, James LF, Stegelmeier BL (1999c) Effects of locoweed (*Oxytropis sericea*) on reproduction in cows with a known history of locoweed consumption. *Vet Human Toxicol* **41(5):** 282–6.

Panter KE, Stegelmeier BL (2000) Reproductive toxicoses of food animals. *Vet Clin North Am: Food Anim Pract* **16(3):** 531–44.

Panter KE, Weinzweig J, Gardner DR, Stegelmeier BL, James LF (2000) Comparison of cleft palate induction by *Nicotiana glauca* in fetal goats and sheep. *Teratology* **61(3):** 203–10.

Parker MA (1982) Association with mature plants protects seedlings from predation in an arid grassland shrub (*Gutierrezia microcephala*). *Oecologia* **53:** 276–80.

Pfister JA, Astorga JB, Panter KE, Molyneux RJ (1993) Maternal locoweed exposure *in utero* and as a neonate does not disrupt taste aversion learning in lambs. *Appl Anim Behav* **36:** 159–67.

Pfister JA, Astorga JB, Panter KE, Stegelmeier BL, Molyneux RJ (2006) Maternal ingestion of locoweed III. Effects on lamb behavior at birth. *Small Rumin Res* **65:** 70–8.

Pfister JA, Panter KE, Gardner DR (1998) Pine needle consumption by cattle during the winter in South Dakota. *J Range Manage* **51:** 551–6.

Plumlee KH, Holstege DM, Blanchard PC, Fiser KM, Galey FD (1993) *Nicotiana glauca* toxicosis of cattle. *J Vet Diagn Invest* **5:** 498–9.

Ralphs MH (2009) Response of broom snakeweed (*Gutierrezia sarothrae*) and cool-season grasses to defoliation. *Invasive Plant Sci Manage* **2:** 28–35.

Ralphs MH, Banks JE (2009) Cattle grazing as a biological control for broom snakeweed: vegetation response. *Range Eco Manage* **62(1):** 38–43.

Roitman JN, James LF, Panter KE (1994) Constituents of broom snakeweed (*Gutierrezia sarothrae*), an abortifacient rangeland plant. In *Plant Associated Toxins: Agricultural, Phytochemical and Ecological Aspects* (Colegate SM, Dorling PR, eds.). CAB International, Wallingford, Oxon OX 109de, United Kingdom, pp. 345–50.

Scales SJ, Sauvage FJ (2009) Mechanisms of hedgehog pathway activation in cancer and implications for therapy. *Trends Pharm Sci* **30(6):** 303–12.

Schmeller T, Sauerwein M, Sporer F, Wink M, Muller WE (1994) Binding of quinolizidine alkaloids to nicotinic and muscarinic acetylcholine receptors. *J Nat Prod* **57:** 1316–9.

Selby LA, Manges RW, Houser EC, Flatt RE, Case AA (1971) Outbreak of swine malformations association with the black cherry, *Prunus serotina*. *Arch Environ Health* **22:** 496–501.

Short RE, James LF, Panter KE, Staigmiller RB, Bellows RA, Malcolm J, Ford SP (1992) Effects of feeding ponderosa pine needles during pregnancy: comparative studies with bison, cattle, goats, and sheep. *J Anim Sci* **70:** 3498–504.

Shupe JL, Binns W, James LF, Keeler RF (1967) Lupine, a cause of crooked calf disease. *J Am Vet Med Assoc* **151:** 198–203.

Stegelmeier BL, Gardner DR, James LF, Panter KE, Molyneux RJ (1996) The toxic and abortifacient effects of Ponderosa pine. *Vet Pathol* **33:** 22–8.

Stegelmeier BL, James LF, Panter KE, Gardner DR, Pfister JA, Ralphs MH, Molyneux RJ (1999a) Dose response of sheep poisoned with locoweed (*Oxytropis sericea*). *J Vet Diagn Investigation* **11:** 446–54.

Stegelmeier BL, James LF, Panter KE, Gardner DR, Ralphs MH, Pfister JA (1998) Tissue swainsonine clearance in sheep chronically poisoned with locoweed (*Oxytropis sericea*). *J Anim Sci* **76:** 1140–4.

Stegelmeier BL, James LF, Panter, KE, Molyneux RJ (1995a) Serum swainsonine concentration and α-mannosidase activity in cattle and sheep ingesting *Oxytropis sericea* and *Astragalus lentiginosus* (locoweeds). *Am J Vet Res* **56:** 149–54.

Stegelmeier BL, James LF, Panter KE, Ralphs MH, Gardner DR, Molyneux RJ, Pfister JA (1999b) The pathogenesis and toxicokinetics of locoweed (*Astragalus* and *Oxytropis* spp.) poisoning in livestock. *J Nat Toxins* **8:** 35–45.

Stegelmeier BL, Molyneux RJ, Elbein AD, James LF (1995b) The comparative pathology of locoweed, swainsonine, and castanospermine in rats. *Vet Pathol* **32:** 289–98.

Thacker ET, Ralphs MH, Call CA, Benson B, Green S (2008) Invasion of broom snakeweed (*Gutierrezia sarothrae*) following evaluating change in a state-and-transition model. *Range Eco Manage* **61:** 263–8.

Thacker E, Ralphs MH, Monaco TA (2009) Seeding cool-season grasses to suppress broom snakeweed (*Gutierrezia sarothrae*) downy brome (*Bromus tectorum*), and weedy forbs. *Invasive Plant Sci Manage* **2:** 237–46.

Van Kampen KR, James LF (1969) Pathology of locoweed poisoning in sheep. *Pathol Vet* **6:** 413–23.

Van Kampen KR, James LF (1970) Pathology of locoweed (*Astragalus lentiginosus*) poisoning in sheep, sequential development of cytoplasmic vacuolation in tissues. *Pathol Vet* **7:** 503–8.

Wagnon KA (1960) Lupine poisoning as a possible factor in congenital deformities in cattle. *J Range Manage* **13:** 89–91.

Wang S, Holyoak GR, Panter KE, Liu G, Evans RC, Bunch TD (1998) Resazurin reduction assay for ram sperm metabolic activity measured by spectrophotometry. *Proc Soc Exp Biol Med* **217:** 197–202.

Wang S, Panter KE, Holyoak GR, Molyneux RJ, Liu G, Evans RC, Bunch TD (1999) Embryo development and viability of bovine preplacentation embryos treated with swainsonine in vitro. *Anim Repro Sci* **56:** 19–29.

Weinzweig J, Panter KE, Pantaloni M, Spangenberger A, Harper JS, Lui F, Gardner D, Wierenga TL, Edstrom LE (1999) The fetal cleft palate: I. Characterization of a congenital model. *Plastic Reconstruct Surg* **103:** 419–28.

Weinzweig J, Panter KE, Patel J, Smith DM, Spangenberger A, Freeman MB (2008) The fetal cleft palate: V. Elucidation of the mechanism of palatal clefting in the congenital caprine model. *Plast Reconstr Surg* **121(4):** 1328–34.

Welch KD, Panter KE, Lee ST, Gardner DR, Stegelmeier BL, Cook D (2009) Cyclopamine-induced synophthalmia in sheep: defining a critical window and toxicokinetic evaluation. *J Appl Toxicol* **29:** 414–21.

Williams MC (1991) Twenty year control of California false hellebore. *Weed Technol* **5:** 40–2.

Wink M, Carey DB (1994) Variability of quinolizidine alkaloid profiles of *Lupinus argenteus* (Fabaceae) from North America. *Biochem Systematics Ecol* **22:** 663–9.

Wink M, Meibner C, Witte L (1995) Patterns of quinolizidine alkaloids in 56 species of the genus *Lupinus*. *Phytochemistry* **38:** 139–53.

C H A P T E R

52

Phytoestrogens

Michelle Mostrom and Timothy J. Evans

INTRODUCTION

Phytoestrogens are non-steroidal, natural plant compounds that are structurally or functionally similar to mammalian estrogens, particularly 17β-estradiol (Figure 52.1). Typically, phytoestrogens or their active metabolites exert their estrogenic effect on the central nervous system and on the reproductive system of males and females, inducing estrus and stimulating growth of the genital tract and mammary glands in females. The classic test for estrogenicity of compounds is proliferation of the female reproductive tract. Phytoestrogens may bind to estrogen receptors, mimicking the conformational structure of estradiol (Kuiper *et al.*, 1997, 1998), and act as agonists, partial agonists or antagonists inducing estrogen-responsive gene products and may exert metabolic effects not related to estrogen receptors. A large volume of literature has been published on phytoestrogens, both for beneficial effects in reducing atherosclerosis, osteoporosis, angiogenesis, diabetes and vasomotor effects (hot flushes) at menopause, and acting as antioxidants, antineoplastics, anti-inflammatories and probiotics and for adverse effects causing infertility in livestock and possible impaired reproductive processes in humans. The focus of this chapter will be on the most extensively studied phytoestrogens found in legumes and beans, such as the isoflavones and coumestans, which affect reproduction.

Phytoestrogens are polyphenolic compounds that can be divided into several broad categories (Table 52.1). Many phytoestrogens are grouped into flavonoids and isoflavonoids, including the isoflavones compounds found in soybeans (*Glycine max* L.), red clover (*Trifolium pretense* L.) and white clover (*Trifolium repens* L.): daidzein, genistein, formononetin, biochanin A and glycitein. The isoflavone content of red clover, normal concentrations between 0.5 to 2.5% of dry matter, can be 2 to 10 times that found in soybeans, which are the more common source of isoflavones in food. An excellent database for foods and flavanoid contents can be found online at the US Department of Agriculture (www.ars.usda.gov). Hops and beer may contain a very potent phytoestrogen, the flavanone 8-prenylnaringenin. β-sitosterol is one of several plant sterols widely distributed in the plant kingdom, with a chemical structure similar to cholesterol. It is found in corn, soybeans, avocados, pistachios, pecans, almonds and saw palmetto. Coumestrol is a potent estrogenic phytoestrogen in the coumestan group. Coumestrol may be found in alfalfa (*Medicago sativa* L.), white clover, spinach and soybean sprouts. The stilbenes, such as trans-resveratrol, are found in red wine (grape skin) and peanuts. Lignans are compounds found in plant cell walls and fiber-rich foods, seeds (flax and sesame seeds), berries, cereals, nuts and fruits. Typically, a mixture of phytoestrogens can be found in plants and processed food. This chapter will not include the estrogenic *Fusarium* spp. mycotoxins, zearalenone, zearalanols and zearalenols, which are resorcyclic acid lactones produced as secondary fungal metabolites in plants and grasses. This review is not all-inclusive and given the limited scope of this chapter, the reader is referred to recent review articles on phytoestrogens related to mechanistic effects (Rosselli *et al.*, 2000), physiology (Kurzer and Xu, 1997; Tham *et al.*, 1998; Benassayag *et al.*, 2002; Patisaul and Jefferson, 2010; Pilšaková *et al.*, 2010), and reproductive functions (Whitten and Patisaul, 2001; Dusza *et al.*, 2006; Cederroth *et al.*, 2009; Baber, 2010).

HISTORICAL BACKGROUND

Over 50 years ago in Australia, a syndrome of temporary or permanent infertility occurred in female sheep grazing subterranean clover (*Trifolium subterraneum* L.) containing high concentrations of isoflavone phytoestrogens,

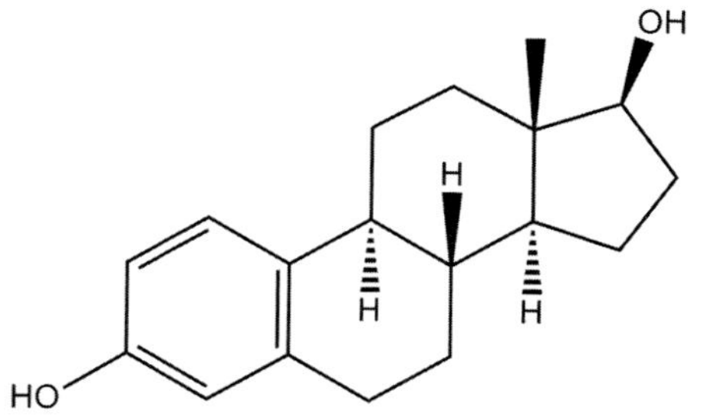

OH H H H HO

17BETA-ESTRADIOL

(8*R*,9*S*,13*S*,14*S*,17*S*)-13-methyl-7,8,9,11,12,13,14,15,16,17-decahydro-6*H*-cyclopenta[*a*]phenanthrene-3,17-diol

FIGURE 52.1 Chemical structure of the estrogen found in animals or 17β-estradiol.

Reproductive and Developmental Toxicology, Edited by Ramesh C. Gupta
ISBN: 978-0-12-382032-7

TABLE 52.1 Categories of phytoestrogens and selected compounds (adapted from Patisaul and Jefferson, 2010)

Category	Phytoestrogen examples	Dietary sources	Basic chemical structure
Isoflavones	Daidzein Genistein Fomononetin Biochanin A Glycitein	Clovers (red and white) Soybeans Beans Split peas	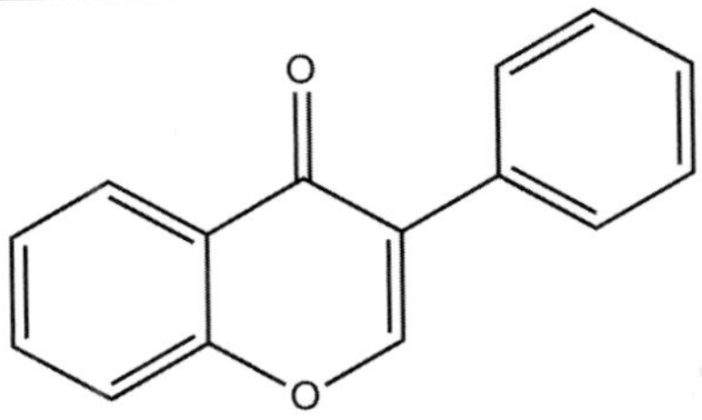 ISOFLAVONE
Flavanones	Naringenin	Hops (8-prenylnaringenin) Apples, red onions	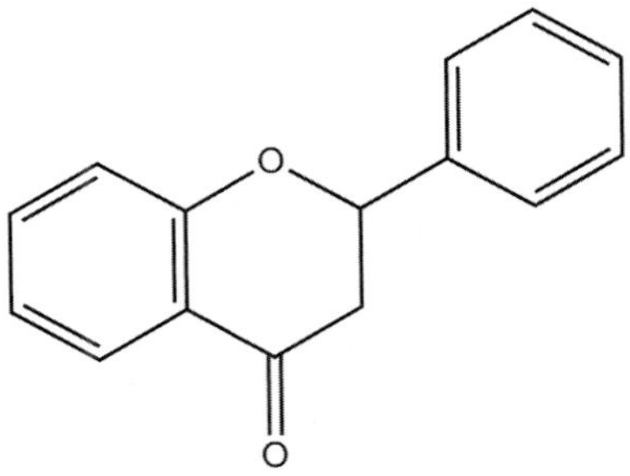 FLAVANONE
Flavonoids	Apigenin Luteolin	Parsley Capsicum pepper Alfalfa	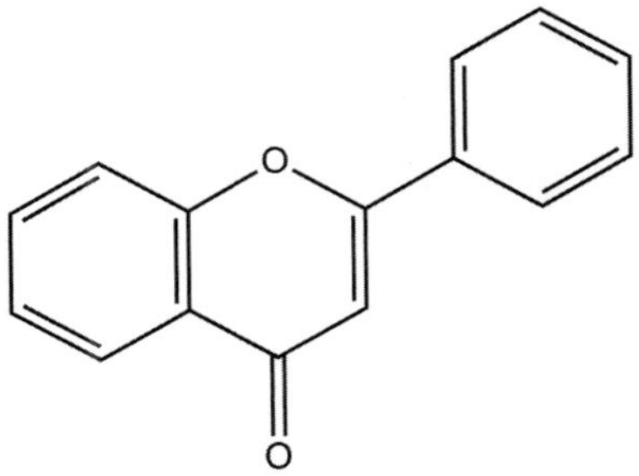 FLAVONE
	Quercetin Kaempferol	Tomatoes Broccoli Apples Onions	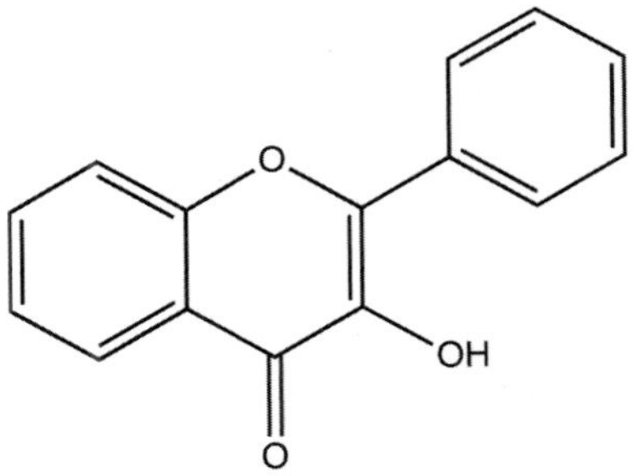 FLAVONOL
Plant sterols	B-sitosterol	Corn Soybeans Sugar beet forage Saw palmetto (*Serenoa repens*) Avocados Pistachios and almonds Wood	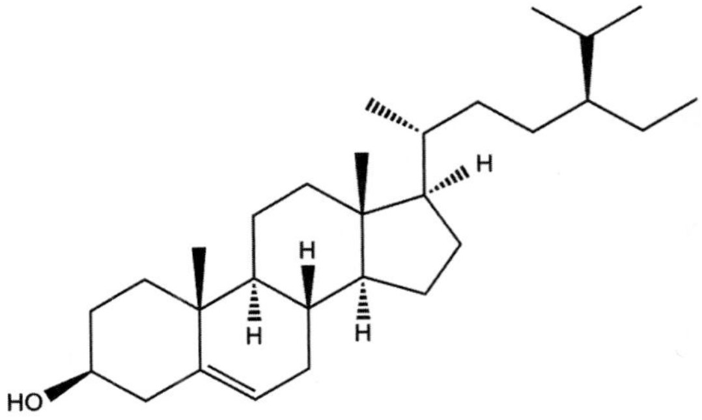 BETA-SITOSTEROL

TABLE 52.1 Categories of phytoestrogens and selected compounds (adapted from Patisaul and Jefferson, 2010) — *Cont'd*

Category	Phytoestrogen examples	Dietary sources	Basic chemical structure
Coumestans	Coumestrol	Legumes (alfalfa, clover) Spinach Split peas, lima beans Soy bean sprouts	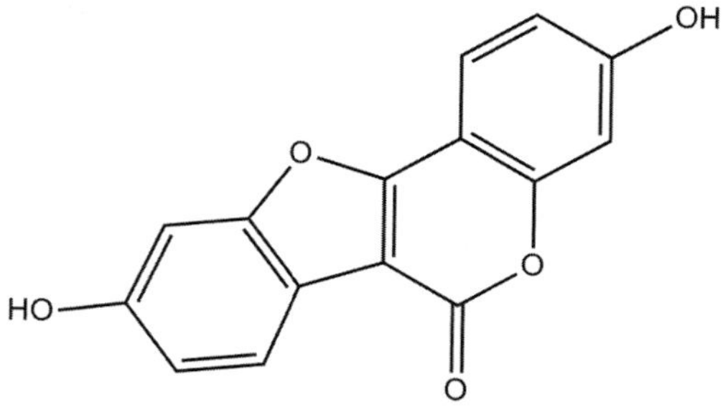 OH, O, O, HO, O COUMESTROL
Stilbenes	Trans-resveratrol (trans-3,5, 4′-trihydroxystilbene)	Grape skin (red wine) peanuts	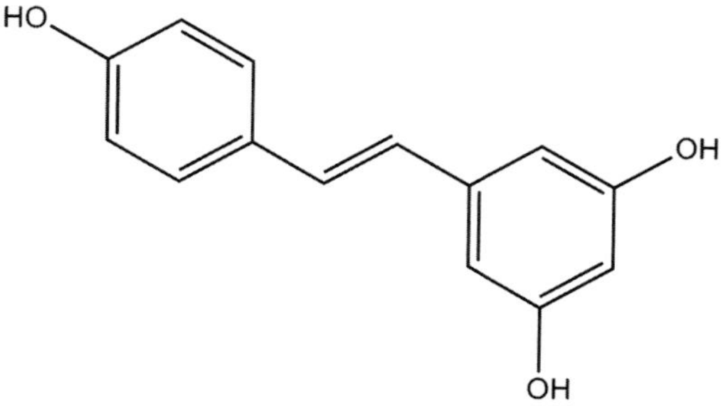 HO, OH, OH RESVERATROL
Lignans	Secoisolariciresinol, matairesinol	Flaxseed (linseed) Squash, pumpkin seeds Tea (black and green) Sunflower seeds Strawberries Cranberries Brans	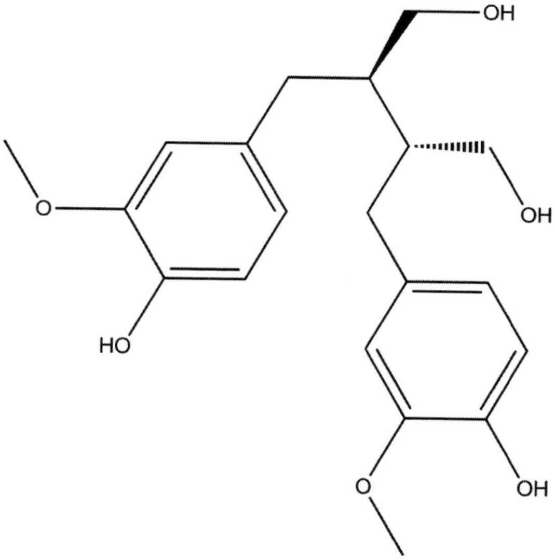 OH, OH, O, HO, O, OH SECOISOLARICIRESINOL

particularly formononetin (Adams, 1995). Temporary infertility was related to direct effects of phytoestrogen on the ovarian follicle decreasing ovulation and increasing embryo mortality and associated with abnormalities of ovum transport and uterine function. Prolonged exposure to growing, green subterranean clover caused permanent infertility in ewes that was related to morphological changes in the cervix, including thick, fused cervical folds and the appearance of cystic tubular glands, and in the uterus with the development of cystic uterine glands and mild endometritis. The cervical mucus became watery and lost viscoelasticity, allowing loss of spermatozoa from the cervix and reducing the chances of conception. External genitalia of some ewes underwent masculinization, with fusion of the vulvar lips at the lower commissure and hypertrophy of the clitoris. The permanent changes in cervical structure were analogous to the organizational effects of estrogen reported in mice treated with estrogen neonatally and in women exposed to diethylstilbestrol during fetal development. Cattle apparently are not permanently affected by phytoestrogens. Elevated concentrations of coumestrol >25 to 30 ppm dry weight basis, or lower concentrations when feedstuffs fed at high proportions of a ration to dairy cows, can cause ovarian dysfunction, early embryonic deaths and repeat breeding (Mostrom, 2010).

Historically, Asian populations had lower rates of breast and prostate cancer, vascular disease, menopausal symptoms and diabetes, as compared to Western populations. Medical and epidemiology studies focused on the use of soy in Asian diets and beneficial effects of phytoestrogens related to preventing cancer, atherosclerosis and osteoporosis. While most individuals are aware of soy in soy milk, tofu and tempeh, soy may be found in over 50% of processed foods because it is cholesterol free, high in fiber and a good vegetable protein. The potential health benefits and adverse effects of phytoestrogens in humans and animals related to reproduction will be discussed.

TABLE 52.2 Typical phytoestrogen concentrations in plants used for livestock forage and soy food (Franke *et al.*, 1995; Saloniemi *et al.*, 1995)

Plant	Phytoestrogen	Concentration (mg/kg or ppm dry weight)
Alfalfa	Coumestrol	25 to 65[a]
Red clover	Formononetin and biochanin A	3,000 to 15,000[b]
		300 to 1,500
	Genistein	<300
	Daidzein	
White clover	Isoflavonoids	100 to 600
	Coumestrol	<10
Soy foods	Daidzein and genistein	~1,000 to 3,500

[a]Concentrations from 18 to >180 mg/kg coumestrol have been associated with infertility in cattle (Mostrom, 2010)

[b]Concentrations >500 to 750 mg/kg have been associated with infertility in cattle (Mostrom, 2010)

PHARMACOKINETICS/ TOXICOKINETICS

Plant impact

The concentration of phytoestrogens in plant material varies widely. In addition to participating in plant defense, these compounds play a role in attraction of pollinators and seed dispersing organisms. Phytoestrogens are not translocated within the vascular pathways of a plant, but are synthesized and degraded in localized areas that vary with the specific tissue. Coumestrol concentrations were found in higher concentrations near the top segment of the alfalfa plant canopy, as compared to the lower part of the plant (Seguin *et al.*, 2004). A number of factors affect production of phytoestrogens. Plant fungal infections, animal predation or insect invasions may increase phytoestrogen production. The growing conditions, in particular temperature and rainfall, can dramatically affect phytoestrogen concentrations in legumes. In cool, wet spring and fall temperatures, legumes may contain high concentrations of phytoestrogens (isoflavones and coumestrol). Generally, the concentrations of phytoestrogens decrease with successive cuttings of legumes in a season, with coumestrol at higher concentration in early and late maturity of the alfalfa crop. Seguin and Zheng (2006) reported that coumestrol concentrations in alfalfa were lower in harvests of seeding than of the post-seeding years, with choice of cultivar having little impact. Fresh herbage tends to have higher concentrations of phytoestrogens than silage or hay (Sivesind and Seguin, 2005). These authors reported that the red clover cultivar "Start" was consistently low in detectable isoflavones during multi-year and multi-site trials. Very high concentrations of phytoestrogens have been detected in alfalfa silages and grass haylages fed to dairy cattle causing infertility and estrogenic clinical signs. Lundh (1995) estimated the daily consumption of phytoestrogens by dairy cows on red clover forage at 50 to 100 grams. Elevated concentrations of coumestrol may also be found in alfalfa cubes, alfalfa extracts and powders, which can be incorporated into nutraceuticals or livestock and pet feeds. Table 52.2 lists typical concentrations of phytoestrogens in legume feeds and soy food.

In soy foods, boiling, milling or processing of the commodity does not appear to destroy daidzein or genistein, but roasting soybeans can reduce these isoflavones by 15% (Franke *et al.*, 1995). Three estrogenic isoflavones, daidzein, genistein and glycitein, were found in soy foods in four chemical forms: aglycone, glucoside, acetylglucoside and malonylglucoside. Fermentation and processing of soy foods increased the aglycone and glycoside forms of the isoflavone, respectively. Soy processing appears to influence isoflavone bioavailability; the unconjugated isoflavones in fermented soy food may be more bioavailable than glucosides. The total isoflavone content of raw soy beans has a wide range from 18 to greater than 500 mg/100 g. People consuming traditional Asian diets may have isoflavone consumption as high as 50 mg/kg body weight/day; whereas in the USA, the typical intake of isoflavones on a "Western" diet is about 1 to 3 mg/day (Mortensen *et al.*, 2009). This translates to blood genistein concentrations of 25 ng/mL for Asian women and less than 2 ng/mL for US women. Using data from various morphologic endpoints in reproductive tissue, effects on hormonal secretion and the hypothalamic–pituitary–gonadal axis, Whitten and Patisaul (2001) estimated that phytoestrogens are biologically active in humans at dietary doses of 0.4 to 10 mg/kg/day, which is similar to daily intakes estimated for adults on soy-rich Asian diets.

Animal and human biotransformation

Similar to any drug or toxin, the dose or intake of phytoestrogens is not equivalent to the dose at the active site or receptor in tissue. Dietary phytoestrogens undergo the processes of absorption in the gastrointestinal tract (GIT), biotransformation, distribution and excretion in urine, bile, feces and milk. Effects of phytoestrogens may vary with the individual phytoestrogen, species exposed, sex, the route, and dose and duration of exposure, particularly the timing during reproductive development and cycling. Most of the phytoestrogens occur in plants as biologically inactive glycoside conjugates with glucose or carbohydrate moieties. Plant glycosides can be hydrolyzed by plant enzymes or after plant consumption the glycosides are hydrolyzed and further demethylated in the acidic gut or rumen by microbes and the heterocyclic phenols (aglycones) are free in the gastrointestinal tract. The gut flora may become adapted to the diet over a matter of days and expand their populations for enhanced metabolism. Microbial metabolism of isoflavones can vary

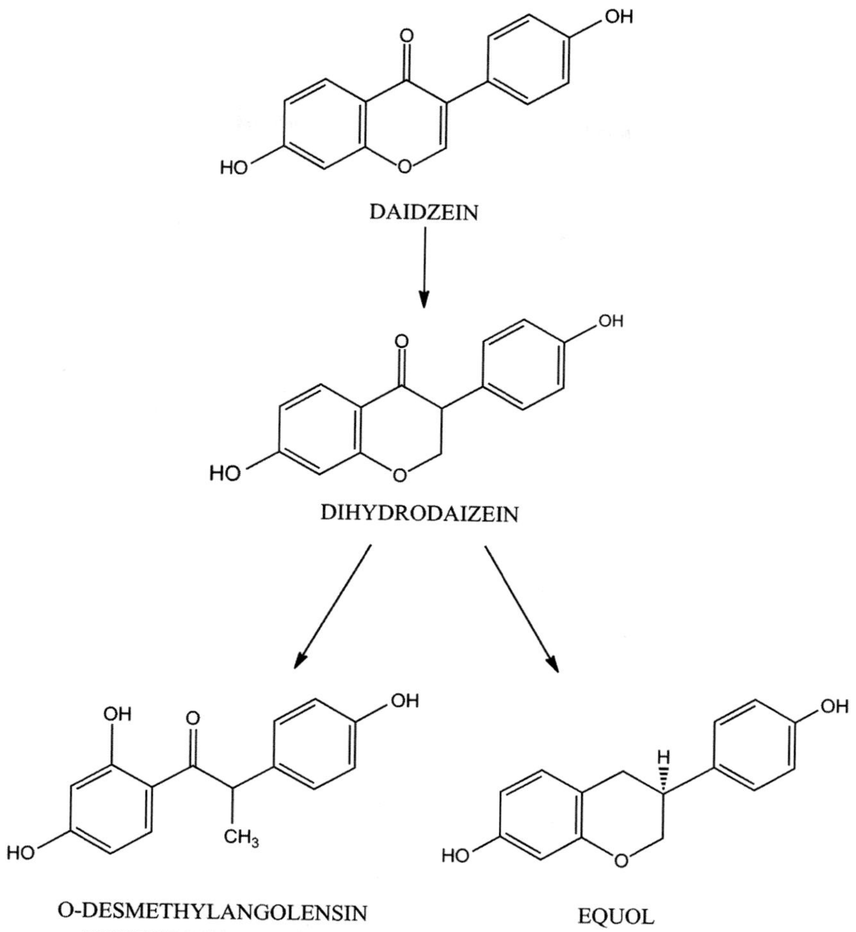

DAIDZEIN

DIHYDRODAIZEIN

O-DESMETHYLANGOLENSIN

EQUOL

FIGURE 52.2 Schematic diagram of human metabolism of the isoflavone daidzein.

greatly between individuals. Isoflavone absorption and bioavailability in humans varies with intestinal microbial population, gut transit time, fecal digestion rates and fiber content in the diet (Neilsen and Williamson, 2007). Some literature suggests that the absorption of isoflavone glucoside and aglucones is similar in humans and unaffected by background diet or food source (Xu *et al.*, 2000).

Several factors appear to influence the metabolism of daidzein to equol in humans, including: diet, gut physiology and individual genetics. In humans, 30 to 50% of the population have microbes capable of metabolism of daidzein to equol, an active estrogenic compound, and 80 to 90% of the population have bacteria that break down daidzein to *O*-desmethylangolensin (Figure 52.2) (Lampe, 2009). The catabolism of genistein by human gut bacteria is eventually to 6′-hydroxy-*O*-DMA (Figure 52.3).

In ruminants, a majority of the metabolic transformations of phytoestrogens occur in the rumen by microbial action. Complete metabolic pathways have not been defined (Lundh, 1995). Basically, in ruminants, biochanin A is demethylated to genistein and via ring cleavage to para-ethyl phenol and organic acids (Figure 52.4). Para-ethyl phenol is considered a non-estrogenic compound. Formononetin is primarily demethylated to daidzein and further metabolized via hydrogenation and ring fission to equol (Figure 52.5). Formononetin can also undergo reduction to *O*-methyl equol or can be metabolized to *O*-desmethylangolensin. In ruminants, daily consumption of phytoestrogens in the diet can lead to adaption and a larger population of rumen microbes capable of phytoestrogen metabolism. Therefore, estrogenic activity of biochanin A and genistein in ruminants is limited to a few initial days of exposure when the unadapted rumen microbes have slower metabolism to non-estrogenic metabolites para-ethylphenol and phenolic acid. With the ingestion of formononetin and daidzein, metabolism may lead to compounds with less or greater estrogenic activity (equol).

Enterodiol and enterolactone are the active, estrogenic mammalian lignans formed by microbes in the human intestinal tract from plant lignans matairesinol and secoisolariciresinol and their glycosides (Wang, 2002) (Figure 52.6).

Only the unconjugated forms (aglycones) and active metabolites appear to exert estrogen-like activity in animals. Most hydrolyzed phytoestrogens are conjugated by glucuronic acid (a minor fraction is conjugated with sulfate) in the gut epithelium, which is a major mechanism for detoxification of phytoestrogens. A small portion of the free, hydrolyzed compounds is absorbed through the gut or rumen mucosa and reaches the blood circulation unconjugated. Absorption of phytoestrogens is fairly rapid; in cattle, formononetin and daidzein (free and conjugated) reached a maximum level in plasma within 1 hour after feeding (Lundh, 1995), and in humans, peak serum resveratrol occurred 30 minutes after consumption. The unconjugated phytoestrogens reaching the circulation are conjugated by

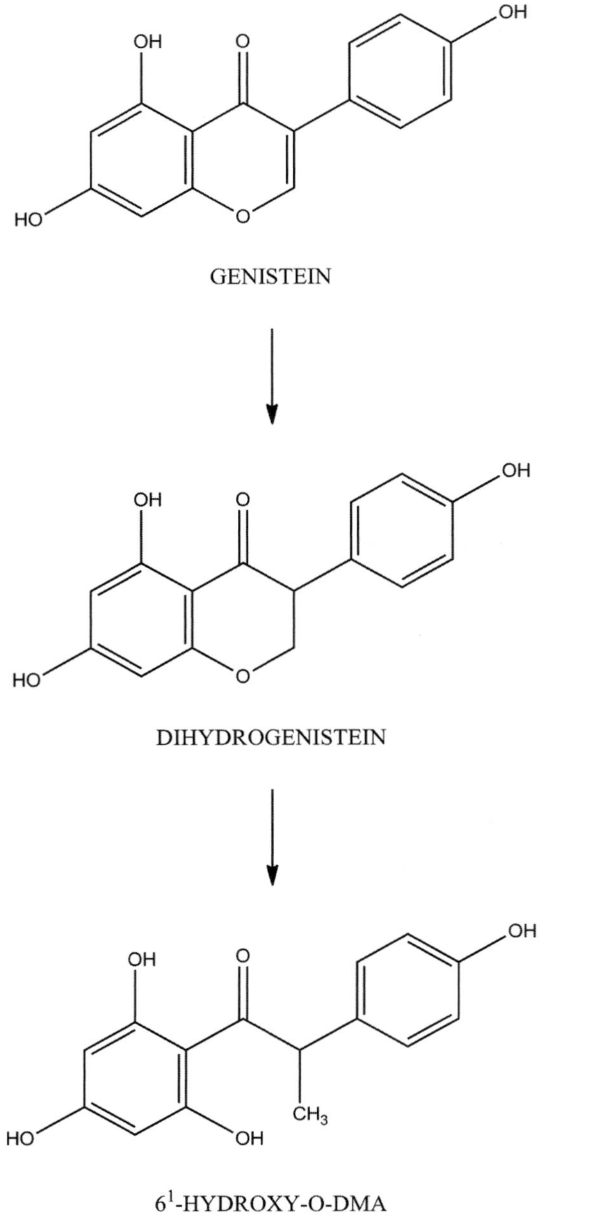

FIGURE 52.3 Schematic diagram of human metabolism of the isoflavone genistein.

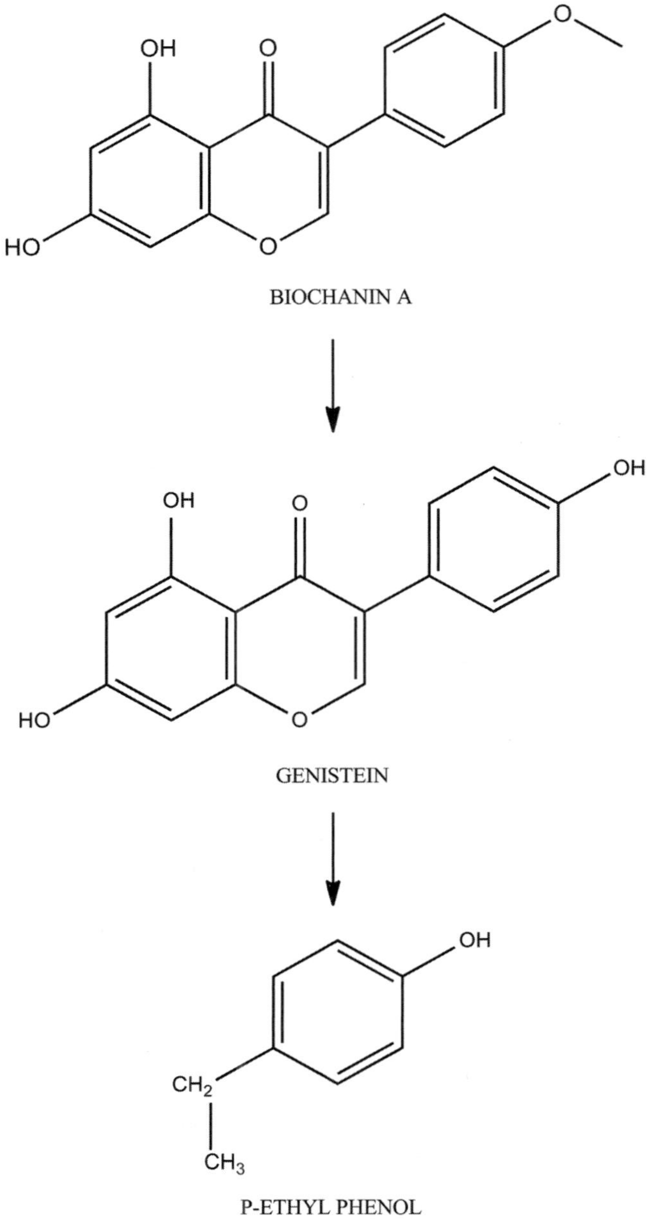

FIGURE 52.4 Schematic diagram of human metabolism of plant lignans.

the liver (hepatic UDP-glucuronosyltransferases and sulfotransferases) and other tissues, perhaps kidney. Glucuronide conjugated compounds and free phytoestrogens circulate through the body. Mammalian lignans and isoflavones can be detected in serum, bile and urine following phytoestrogen consumption. Like endogenous estrogens, these conjugated phytoestrogens undergo enterohepatic circulation. The metabolism of coumestrol has not been characterized.

Conjugated equol in the plasma of cattle or sheep is about 95 to 99% of total equol; whereas in pigs about 50 to 70% of total equol is conjugated (Lundh, 1995). The estrogenic effects are related to free compounds and active metabolites, such as equol, which is suggested to have 0.061% of the potency as 17β-estradiol (Markiewicz *et al.*, 1993). Equol was considered the primary chemical responsible for infertility in sheep consuming isoflavones in subterranean clover. Ingestion of high concentrations of red clover silage by ruminants can lead to extremely high concentrations of unconjugated equol in plasma and potency 100 times higher than the 17β-estradiol activity during estrus. Following consumption of mixed red clover-grass silage, the concentration of free equol was about 10 times greater in bovine plasma, as compared with ovine plasma, which suggested that the differences in isoflavone sensitivity between cattle and sheep was not caused by differences in metabolism or detoxification of formononetin and daidzein (Lundh *et al.*, 1990).

Little data are available on tissue distribution of phytoestrogens in humans. Following an intravenous injection of daidzein in rats (40 mg/kg body weight), daidzein was detected at high concentrations in plasma, liver, lung and kidney, and at lower concentrations in spleen, heart and skeletal muscle (Yueh and Chu, 1977). Isoflavones can be detected in breast tissue of premenopausal women and in prostate

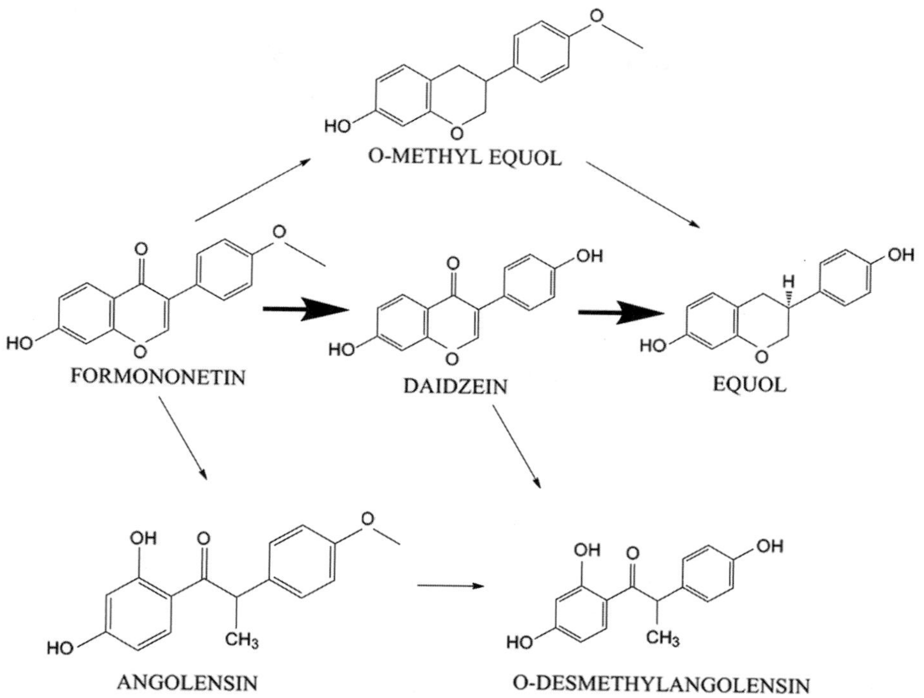

O-METHYL EQUOL
FORMONONETIN
DAIDZEIN
EQUOL
ANGOLENSIN
O-DESMETHYLANGOLENSIN

FIGURE 52.5 Schematic of rumen metabolism of biochanin A to genistein (Cox and Davies, 1988).

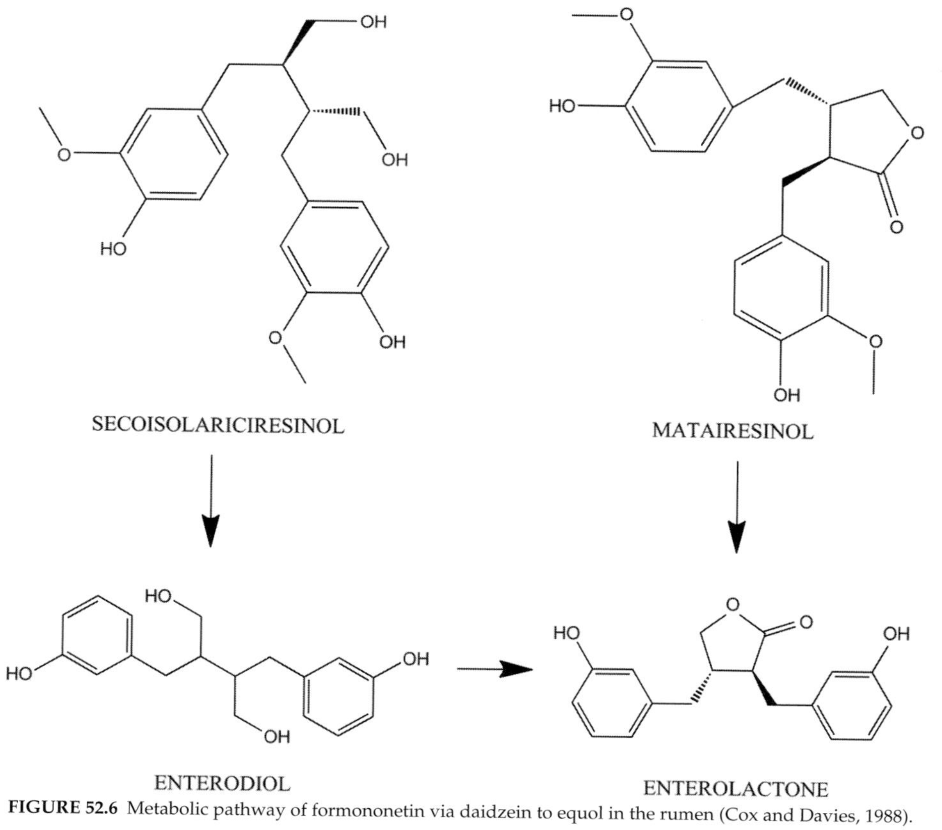

SECOISOLARICIRESINOL
MATAIRESINOL
ENTERODIOL
ENTEROLACTONE

FIGURE 52.6 Metabolic pathway of formononetin via daidzein to equol in the rumen (Cox and Davies, 1988).

glands of men (reviewed by Manach *et al.*, 2005). Conjugated and free metabolites are excreted in urine. Humans exhibit highly variable metabolic capacity for isoflavones. Daidzein and genistein parent compounds have a shorter half-life in urine, as compared with the isoflavone metabolites, equol and O-desmethylangolensin (Kelly *et al.*, 1995). A variable amount of phytoestrogens are excreted into bile and feces; for example, a greater fraction of genistein is eliminated in bile and feces, as compared with daidzein in rats (Manach *et al.*, 2005).

Tissue distribution of isoflavones was determined in two lactating ewes after being fed red clover silage for one month (Urpi-Sarda *et al.*, 2008). The fermented silage contained only aglycones and provided a daily intake of about 157 mg/kg body weight of isoflavones, with an average of 82 mg/kg body weight formononetin, 65 mg/kg body weight biochanin A, 7 mg/kg body weight genistein and 3 mg/kg body weight daidzein. The major compounds recovered in tissues were equol, generally in the largest concentration, and daidzein as glucuronides. The highest concentrations of equol and daidzein were found in the kidney at 10-fold higher concentrations than other tissues. Decreasing concentrations were found in liver, plasma, aorta, suprarenal glands, uterus, thyroid and mammary gland. Lower isoflavone concentrations were detected in lung, pituitary gland, thymus, heart, muscle, olfactory lobe of brain, cerebellum and cerebral hemisphere. The penetration into the brain was very limited. Interestingly, isoflavones were found in the thyroid. Red clover silage ingestion has been documented to stimulate thyroid hormone secretion (total and free triiodothyronine) and increase thyroid follicle size and the ERα immune-reactivity of thyroid glands in ovariectomized ewes (Madej *et al.*, 2002). The two major isoflavones found in red clover, formononetin and biochanin A were not recovered in tissues, which is consistent with extensive rumen metabolism of methylated isoflavones.

Phytoestrogens are excreted in milk, with animal diet playing a major role in detectable concentrations. Data indicate that animal feeds, for example soy meals, clovers and grass/alfalfa feedstuffs, may influence milk phytoestrogen content. In a dairy cow ration of mixed red clover-grass silage, formononetin (0.3 to 0.5%) and biochanin A (0.2%) were the predominant isoflavones. Dairy cows fed a mixed red clover silage produced milk with high concentrations of equol (272 and 364 μg/L or parts per billion, ppb) and enterolactone (21 and 27 μg/L), metabolites of formononetin and the plant lignans (secoisolariciresinol and matairesinol), respectively (Steinshamn *et al.*, 2008). Higher equol concentrations were determined in milk from cows on red-clover silage as compared with white clover silage. Skimmed milk originating from organically managed Finnish diary operations contained higher concentrations of isoflavonoids, with equol concentrations at 411 ± 65 μg/L, than conventionally managed dairy operations (Hoikkala *et al.*, 2007). The presence of equol and enterolactone at elevated concentrations in dairy milk, from 14.1 to 293 μg/L and 14.3 to 94 μg/L, respectively, may be a health concern for children (Antignac *et al.*, 2004). Trace concentrations of methoxylated formononetin and biochanin A and hydroxylated daidzein and genistein (0.1 to 5.0 μg/L) were detected in bovine milk. These authors found phytoestrogen concentrations in skimmed and full cream milk were similar, indicating that phytoestrogens are not very lipophilic compounds. For comparison purposes, the total isoflavone content of soy milk has been reported at 6 to 10 mg aglucone equivalents/100 g of wet weight (Chan *et al.*, 2009).

A major focus of concern is phytoestrogen exposure of infants consuming soy-based formulas for months and its potential health effects. For infants fed only soy-based formulas, the range of isoflavone consumption was 6 to 9 mg/kg per day, which could result in infant plasma concentrations of isoflavones up to 1,000 to 1,455 ng/mL (reviewed by Patisaul and Jefferson, 2010). In contrast, infants fed cow's milk formula or human breast milk had isoflavones concentrations of 9.4 and 4.7 ng/mL, respectively. The exposure of the Asian and "Western" populations to soy is quite opposite. Infants in Asia are generally breast fed and then consume high soy diets throughout their lifespan; whereas, approximately 20 to 25% of infants in the "Western" culture consume soy-based formulations for months and then are switched to low soy exposure throughout their lifespan. Additional dietary foods probably have a role in estrogenic effects in populations, with the Asian population consuming more fish and Western cultures more red meat and higher fatty foods.

MECHANISMS OF ACTION

Phytoestrogens have been reported to affect physiological responses related to reproduction through numerous mechanisms (Table 52.3). Phytoestrogens are considered weak estrogens, with an activity on the order of 10^{-2} to 10^{-3} of 17β-estradiol, but may be present in the body at concentrations 100-fold higher than endogenous estrogens (Adlercreutz and Mazur, 1997). Reproduction is under hormonal regulation and abnormalities in the dynamics of hormone production, metabolism, target molecule binding and elimination can lead to alterations in the structure and/or function of the reproductive system. Estrogens influence cell growth and differentiation of both female and male reproductive tissue. They regulate the ovaries and testes, uterus, vagina, mammary glands, epididymis and prostate gland. A number of phytoestrogens have been shown to stimulate uterine growth in laboratory and farm animals. However, not all mouse strains were susceptible to isoflavone-induced uterine hypertrophy, the Swiss albino CD-1 mouse and ICR mouse showed no or only a slight response, respectively, which may be related to metabolism (reviewed by Kurzer and Xu, 1997). Additionally, the isoflavone genistein has been demonstrated to inhibit important pathways for cellular growth and proliferation in multiple tissues.

Estrogen receptors

Estrogens play an important role in physiological functions via a genomic mechanism. Phytoestrogens can mediate their effects by diffusing through the cell membrane and binding

TABLE 52.3 Several proposed mechanisms of phytoestrogens' actions on reproduction and development

Genomic effects through binding to estrogen receptors α and β causing endocrine disruption
Non-genomic effects through binding to steroid membrane receptors
Affect metabolism through inhibition of enzymes in steroidogenesis (3β- and 17β-hydroxysteroid dehydrogenase, aromatase, 5α-reductase, 17β-hydroxysteroid oxidoreductase Type 1)
Stimulation of sex hormone-binding globulin (SHBG)
Inhibition of protein tyrosine kinase involved with signal transduction and cell proliferation
Inhibition of DNA topoisomerases I and II required for DNA replication
Inhibit matrix metalloproteinase 9 (MMP9) involved in cell growth
Downregulate expression of vascular endothelial growth factor (VEGF) involved with growth factor genes and angiogenesis
Inhibit prostaglandin synthesis via lipoxygenase or cyclo-oxygenase-2 and exert antioxidant activity

to specific estrogen receptors (ERs) in the target cell. After binding, the phytoestrogens do not act like typical estrogen agonists, but act more like selective estrogen receptor modulators (SERMS) that have differential actions as agonists or antagonists in different tissues potentially causing endocrine disruption. The differential action occurs partly from ER ligand conformational changes and the influence of co-regulator proteins (reviewed by Patisaul and Jefferson, 2010). Following phytoestrogen–receptor complex conformation changes, the complex translocates to the nucleus. Within the nucleus, the complex binds to selective regions of the DNA, the estrogen response element (ERE), and stimulates or inhibits specific genes that may result in the production of messenger RNA and subsequently new specific proteins. Numerous studies have focused on the direct effects of phytoestrogen receptor binding *in vitro*. Binding affinities to the ERs, whose subtypes are ERα and ERβ, vary greatly with phytoestrogens and the various cell lines used in studies and chosen endpoints of estrogenic potency (Kuiper *et al.*, 1997, 1998). The most potent activator of binding to ERs was the endogenous hormone 17β-estradiol, as compared with any phytoestrogen tested. Daidzein, genistein, coumestrol, equol and *O*-desmethylangolensin apparently bind to estrogen receptors from sheep uterine cytosol, suggesting estrogenic effects. Formononetin at physiological concentrations did not bind to the estrogen receptor, but can be metabolized to daidzein and eventually to equol, both of which have estrogenic properties (Kuiper *et al.*, 1998). Daidzein preferentially activated binding of ERβ, but with metabolism of daidzein to equol both ERβ and ERα can be activated (Kostelac *et al.*, 2003). Phytoestrogens appear to have a predilection for greater affinity to ERβ. Studies have shown that coumestrol has a two-fold higher affinity for ERβ than for ERα and genistein has a pronounced affinity (30-fold) for ERβ (Kuiper *et al.*, 1997).

While coumestrol may bind to both ERα and ERβ, it is an atypical estrogen because it does not stimulate uterine cellular hyperplasia. Coumestrol significantly increased uterine wet and dry weights in ovariectomized rats, but did not stimulate cytosolic ER depletion or nuclear ER accumulation (Markaverich *et al.*, 1995). These findings suggest that the estrogenic effects of coumestrol may be mediated by increased sensitivity of the tissue to endogenous estradiol. An anti-estrogenic effect of phytoestrogens has been proposed when high concentrations of phytoestrogens compete with endogenous estrogens and bind the estrogen receptor, which blocks endogenous estrogen actions and reduces cellular growth (Rosselli *et al.*, 2000).

Differential expression of ERs has been reported in tissues and several physiological roles have been associated with the ER subtypes (Table 52.4). Both subtypes have been found in blood vessels and in breast, uterus and ovaries of women, but the proportions of α and β subtypes appear to vary with estrogen target tissues, physiological and pathological status, and age of the individual. Each of these two ERs may influence the function of the other, creating a complex process of estrogenic effects in tissues where both subtypes are co-expressed (Benassayag *et al.*, 2002). The resulting changes in physiological functions can be difficult to interpret.

Estradiol can bind with high affinity to plasma membrane forms of steroid receptors and may mediate non-genomic actions with a variety of short-term estrogen effects (Pietras and Szego, 1975; Swego, 1984). Estradiol has been shown to induce rapid changes in intracellular calcium concentrations/flux, potassium conductance and cyclic AMP levels (reviewed by Rosselli *et al.*, 2000). The direct effects of phytoestrogens and membrane estrogen receptors have not been fully defined. Resveratrol, a stilbene phytoestrogen found in red wine, apparently binds to and increases the transcriptional activity of estrogen receptors α and β. Klinge and co-workers (2005) reported that resveratrol, at nanomolar concentrations achieved by reasonable red wine consumption, can activate membrane-initiated (non-genomic) estrogen receptor signaling in endothelial cells that activate mitogen-activated protein kinases (MAPK) involved in signaling pathways and endothelial nitric oxide synthase. Resveratrol increased nitric oxide levels in human umbilical vein endothelial cells after short-term exposure, suggesting to the authors a potential cardioprotective effect.

Impact on steroidogenesis

Certain phytoestrogens may alter key steroidal enzymes in tissues, although most studies have occurred with *in vitro* cell lines or in purified microsomal or enzyme preparation (Lacey *et al.*, 2005). Phytoestrogens may interfere with the synthesis or metabolism of steroid hormones, such as cytochrome P450arom (aromatase), an enzyme that can catalyze the conversion of testosterone to 17β-estradiol and Δ4-androstenedial to estrone. The enzyme aromatase has a critical role in the ovary (important for premenopausal women) and peripheral tissues, which are sites for estradiol synthesis in postmenopausal women and men. Using an *in vitro* assay with human breast cancer MCF-7 cells, Almstrup and co-workers (2002) reported that phytoestrogens, but not genistein, were aromatase inhibitors at low concentrations, <1 μM, but at higher concentrations of >1 μM were estrogenic. The aromatase inhibition at low doses of phytoestrogens may provide antiestrogenic properties that play a role in protection against breast cancer.

TABLE 52.4 Estrogen receptor α and β proposed actions and distribution[a] (based on Kuiper *et al.*, 1998, 1997; Patisaul and Jefferson, 2010)

ERα and ERβ function in:	Normal ovarian follicular development
	Vascular endothelial cells
	Myocardial cells
	Smooth muscle cells
	Breast cells
ERα associated with:	Bone maturation in males and females
	Important role maintaining follicle stimulating hormone and luteinizing hormone in blood
	More predominant is kidney, adrenal, non-pregnant human myometrium
ERβ associated with:	Bone maintenance
	Frontal lobe mediated memory and learning
	Coumestrol and genistein bind with higher estrogenic potential
	Equol has modest affinity for binding
	More predominant in human brain, thymus, bladder, ovarian granulosa cells, testis Sertoli and germ cells, lung, bone and pregnant term human myometrium

[a]Distribution of estrogen receptors in tissues can change over a lifespan and is sexually dimorphic

Phytoestrogens may decrease endogenous estrogen concentrations through effects on the sex (or serum) hormone binding globulin (SHBG). This binding protein has specific affinity for estrogens and androgens. Minor changes in the amount or availability of SHBG, caused by phytoestrogens, may change the free fraction of endogenous hormones in circulation, either locally or systemically. The phytoestrogen enterolactone (1 to 10 μM) stimulated sex hormone binding globulin *in vitro* with HepG2 cells (Adlercreutz *et al.*, 1992). Equol, genistein, daidzein, enterolactone and enterodiol appear to exert a dose-dependent inhibitory effect on binding of steroids to SHBG, displacing 17β-estradiol or testosterone (Benassayag *et al.*, 2002). Additional mechanisms of action may affect steroid hormones. Coumestrol and, to a lesser degree, genistein have been shown to inhibit the enzyme 17β-hydroxysteroid oxidoreductase Type 1, which converts [3H]-estrone to [3H]-estradiol in a dose-dependent manner (Mäkelä *et al.*, 1995). Phytoestrogens have been reported to inhibit 17β-hydroxysteroid dehydrogenase, converting androstenedione to testosterone, and 5α-reductase, converting testosterone to the more potent di-hydrotestosterone using *in vitro* studies (reviewed by Whitten and Patisaul, 2001). Biochanin A displayed dose-dependent inhibition of 3β-hydroxysteroid dehydrogenase, an enzyme which catalyzes the conversion of pregnenolone to progesterone and androstenediol to testosterone, in primary cultures of human granulose–luteal cells (Lacey *et al.*, 2005).

Angiogenesis is essential for ovarian follicle development and for tumor growth, invasion and metastasis. Several studies have reported that phytoestrogens inhibited vascular endothelial growth factor or VEGF-induced endothelial cell functions and signaling pathways. The flavonoid quercetin at 5 and 50 μg/mL (concentrations higher than physiological range) inhibited VEGF production by porcine granulosa cells *in vitro* (Santini *et al.*, 2009). The authors determined that quercetin inhibited steroidogenesis, specifically progesterone production, but not granulosa cell growth.

Genistein has been reported to inhibit ethoxyresorufin-O-deethylase (EROD) activity, part of the enzyme cytochrome P450 family (CYP1A) that is critical in the metabolism of 17β-estradiol to hydroxylated estrogen, in mammalian cell culture lines (Shon *et al.*, 2006). Additionally, ornithine decarboxylase activity, a critical enzyme in polyamine biosynthesis and normal cell growth and proliferation, was markedly reduced after genistein treatment of MCF-7 breast cancer cells, suggesting that genistein might be of therapeutic value in preventing human breast cancer.

Altered signal transduction and cell proliferation

Genistein may alter cell growth at several signal transduction pathways. Genistein can (1) inhibit protein tyrosine kinase activity, (2) downregulate epidermal growth factor (EGF) receptor autophophorylation, which phosphorylates tyrosyl residues of membrane-bound receptors (Akiyama *et al.*, 1987), and (3) downregulate mitogen-activated protein kinase (MAPK) activity and mitogen proliferation in human aortic smooth muscle cells (Dubey *et al.*, 1999). Inhibition of protein tyrosine kinases and MAPK by isoflavones may play a role in improving heart function. Genistein can inhibit DNA replication enzymes associated with cancer growth, including DNA topoisomerases I and II (required for DNA replication) and matrix metalloproteinase 9 (MM9P – a matrix enzyme that can degrade a number of structural components) (Kurzer and Xu, 1997). While inhibition of these pathways may lead to inhibited cell growth and a protective effect, a number of phytoestrogens, including coumestrol, genistein, biochanin A, daidzein and enterolactone, can stimulate cellular proliferation of the estrogen-dependent MCF-7 human breast cancer cells at concentrations below 1 to 10 μM (reviewed by Kurzer and Xu, 1997). The influence of genistein on cells *in vitro* appears to be biphasic in nature, inducing cell growth of MCF-7 cells at low concentrations and inhibiting cell growth at higher concentrations (reviewed by Rosselli *et al.*, 2000). Genistein, which shows a high affinity to ER, has been shown to inhibit growth in both ER-positive and ER-negative cell lines *in vitro*.

The antioxidant activity of phytoestrogens has been reported both *in vitro* and *in vivo*. Isoflavones inhibit lipoxygenase action and prevent sheep erythrocyte hemolysis *in vitro* and inhibit production of hydrogen peroxide in HL60 cells (reviewed by Benassayag *et al.*, 2002). Inhibition of lipoxygenase and possibly cyclo-oxygenase may modulate production of prostaglandins and leukotrienes involved in inflammation, carcinogenesis and reproduction.

ADVERSE HEALTH EFFECTS

Developmental effects

The effects of pre- and neonatal exposure to phytoestrogens on development in laboratory animals have been studied, with variable effects observed (Table 52.5). The impact of phytoestrogens on human development is not clear. Pre- and neonatal treatment of rodents with phytoestrogens has resulted in altered prepubertal or adult morphology and possible function in the uterus, vagina, ovary, breast, pituitary and hypothalamus (Whitten and Patisaul, 2001). *In utero* exposure to several estrogens, including genistein, downregulated the expression of several testicular genes in the rat and mouse (Phillips and Tanphaichitr, 2008). Both male and female rat offspring from dams treated with high levels of genistein, 5,000 μg, had shorter anogenital distances at birth and females in this treatment group had a later onset of vaginal opening or puberty (Levy *et al.*, 1995). High levels of dietary coumestrol (100 mg/kg) fed to weanling female rats on days 21 to 24 or 22 to 60 caused earlier vaginal opening and irregular vaginal cycles (Whitten and Naftolin, 1992). Coumestrol treatment of neonatal female rats, given a 100 μM dose, resulted in premature uterine gland development and increased uterine weights on postnatal days 1 to 5, and at later ages, the uterine weights and ER levels were reduced; however, if coumestrol was administered on postnatal days 10 to 14, the uterine gland growth was inhibited (Benassayag *et al.*, 2002).

Female neonatal rats given a subcutaneous injection of 10 μg of genistein showed an increased pituitary response to gonadotropin releasing hormone, with higher genistein doses causing a decreased luteinizing hormone secretion on postnatal days 1 to 10 (Faber and Hughes, 1993). The effects of the higher doses were similar to the typical effects of estrogens in masculinizing the brain and decreasing pituitary response. Oral exposure of female CD-1 mice to genistein, the glycosylated form of genistein found in soy-based infant formulas, treated on postnatal days 1 to 5, caused estrogenic responses

TABLE 52.5 Selected reproductive effects associated with phytoestrogen exposure in laboratory animals

Reduced the frequency of the gondadotropin releasing hormone pulse generator
Inhibited luteinizing hormone at the pituitary level
Delayed fertilization (2 to 4 cell stage)
Abnormal oviduct environment
Failure of implantation development
Irregular estrous cycling
Increased incidence of multioocyte follicles
Decreased acrosomal reaction and zona–pellucida–spermatozoa binding

including altered ovarian differentiation (multioocyte follicles) and delayed vaginal opening and, subsequently in the adult mouse, abnormal estrous cycles, decreased fertility and delayed parturition (Jefferson *et al.*, 2009a). The authors noted that the glucoside forms of isoflavones were quickly hydrolyzed to produce the aglycone forms and subsequently absorbed. The glycosylated form can be passively transported across the intestinal membrane and enter circulation by the sodium-dependent glucose transporter, unlike passive diffusion by the aglycone form. Major contributions to infertility in genistein-treated neonatal mice were determined to be (1) delay in fertilization by an undetermined mechanism that could lead to altered developmental timing (lack of development between the two- and four-cell stage), (2) adverse oviductal environment because more than half of the embryos were lost in early embryo development, and (3) the reproductive tract (uterus not responsive to hormonal cues) was not capable of sustaining pregnancy (Jefferson *et al.*, 2009b).

Estrogen receptors are located in numerous areas of the brain and phytoestrogens can have extensive effects. The paraventricular nucleus of the hypothalamus (PVN) is a region coordinating reproductive, social and stress behaviors that primarily express ERβ (reviewed by Patisaul and Jefferson, 2010). ERβ is expressed at higher levels than ERα in the basal forebrain, hippocampus and cerebral cortex (areas important for memory) in the adult. Notably, ERα is primarily expressed in the ventromedial nucleus (VMN) of the brain, which along with the PVN nucleus is important for initiation and regulation of sexual behavior. The authors observed that the PVN is the main site for oxytocin production, involved with social behavior and facilitation of sexual behavior. Estrogen binding to ERβ may stimulate oxytocin production from the PVN, which subsequently binds to the oxytocin receptor in the VMN, a nucleus involved in mediating the lordosis response in females. Upregulation of oxytocin receptors involves binding to ERα.

The central nervous system–gonadal axis and male sexual behavior of the rat appear to be sensitive to phytoestrogens in the rat (Santti *et al.*, 1998). Altering the isoflavone dietary concentrations significantly affected both the sexually dimorphic nucleus of the preoptic area and the anteroventral periventricular nucleus in the brain of rodents (Lephart *et al.*, 2005). When rodents were changed from a phytoestrogen-rich to a phytoestrogen-free diet the volume of nucleus of the preoptic area was decreased in males and relatively unchanged in females; conversely on a phytoestrogen-rich diet, the volume of the anteroventral periventricular nucleus was larger in females as compared with males or with females on the phytoestrogen-free diet.

Phytoestrogens may be incorporated as an alternative protein source for aquatic nutrition and have been found in discharged kraft mill effluent and sewage treatment plant effluents, with low concentrations of genistein detected that could impact fish populations. Phytoestrogens may alter sex differentiation in early development, causing a paradoxical sex reversal with increased male phenotypic sex resulting from the administration of an estrogen mimic in the diet. Increased concentrations of genistein, from 0 to 8 mg/g in the diet, fed chronically to sexually undifferentiated channel catfish (*Ictalurus punctatus*), altered gonadal sex differentiation with increasing proportions of intersex fish and phenotypically male individuals (Green and Kelly, 2009).

Preliminary evidence indicates that soy infant formulas may exert estrogenic activity in the developing human reproductive tract. Phytoestrogens can cross the placenta and are capable of crossing the blood–brain barrier to a limited extent. The human myometrium primarily expresses ERβ in late pregnancy and could be a target for genistein, which preferentially binds to this receptor subtype. A pilot study of female infants fed soy formula, cow milk formula and breast milk revealed that soy milk fed infants had re-estrogenization of vaginal cells at 6 months of age (Bernbaum *et al.*, 2008). However, an expert panel report from the National Toxicology Program (NTP) and the National Institute of Environmental Health Sciences concluded in 2006 that there were insufficient human or experimental animal data published to permit determination of the toxicity of soy infant formula on development or reproduction (Rozman *et al.*, 2006).

Hormones and menstrual cycles

Phytoestrogen effects on the adult hypothalamic–pituitary–gonadal axis after adult exposures indicate the potential for suppression. Data from studies in ovariectomized rodent and humans suggest that ingestion of isoflavone-rich soy food may suppress circulating estrogen and progesterone concentrations and can attenuate the preovulatory surge of luteinizing hormone (LH) and follicle stimulating hormone (FSH) (Patisaul and Jefferson, 2010). Several studies have been reported on the effects of soy isoflavones in premenopausal women. In a limited study during one menstrual cycle in six premenopausal women given 45 mg of isoflavones daily, the follicular phase length was increased and delayed menstruation (Cassidy *et al.*, 1994). Follicular estradiol concentrations were increased and mid-cycle surges of luteinizing hormone and follicle stimulating hormone were significantly suppressed. One case report in three women described adverse effects of abnormal uterine bleeding, leiomyomas and endometriosis related to high intakes of soy products; all of the women improved after withdrawal of soy from their diet (Chandrareddy *et al.*, 2008). Studies evaluating phytoestrogens treating symptoms of menopause, particularly vasomotor symptoms of hot flushes and night sweats, have produced inconclusive results, with a large placebo effect noted in many studies.

Infertility

Phytoestrogens have the capability to affect reproduction at many levels, from the hypothalamic–pituitary level to local levels of the ovary and uterus, and testis and prostate gland.

In laboratory animals, intravenous infusion of coumestrol, but not genistein, affected control of luteinizing hormone secretion at both the pituitary and hypothalamic levels. At the pituitary level coumestrol inhibited gonadotropin releasing hormone – luteinizing hormone release *in vivo* and at the hypothalamic level, coumestrol reduced the frequency of the gondadotropin releasing hormone pulse generator (McGarvey *et al.*, 2001). The inhibitory effects of coumestrol on luteinizing hormone at the pituitary level occurred via an estrogen receptor-mediated process. Additional evidence that phytoestrogens immediately affect pituitary responsiveness was found in ewes when genistein was administered directly into the central nervous system (Romanowicz *et al.*, 2004). Lower plasma luteinizing hormone concentrations were detected in ovariectomized ewes infused intracerebroventricularly for 6 hours with two different levels of genistein at 1 μg/100 μL/hour and 10 μg/100 μL/hour. In addition, the plasma prolactin concentrations were significantly higher in treated ewes, as compared with the control ewes. Estrogen has been shown to be a potent stimulator of prolactin release in the pituitary lactotropes.

Initial cases of temporary and permanent infertility in animals related to phytoestrogens occurred in sheep ingesting subterranean clover in Australia (Adams, 1995). Red clover, a popular over-the-counter nutraceutical and livestock forage supplement, caused adverse effects in reproductive organs of ovariectomized sheep with increased teat length (a relatively sensitive parameter), mammary gland development and milky fluid secretions (galactorrhea) from the teats. Nwannenna and co-workers (1995) described clinical effects of edema and mucous discharge from the vulva, fluid accumulation in the uterus, elongated teats and the presence of milky fluid in the mammary glands in ovariectomized heifers fed 20 kg of 100% red clover silage (daily intake of 35 g phytoestrogens, primarily formononetin and biochanin A) per day for 14 days. The magnitude of the pituitary response to gonadotropin-releasing hormone injections was diminished with low luteinizing hormone release. The authors noted that the abnormal mounting behavior in one of the heifers was similar to the sexual behavior of cattle treated with estradiol.

Cattle seem to be less sensitive than sheep to clover forage, with temporary estrogenic signs and infertility occurring following ingestion of clover or alfalfa forages; although coumestrol is thought to have a cumulative type of effect. Concentrations of coumestrol of about 25 mg/kg (dry matter) in forage may have adverse effects on reproduction in livestock and reduce fertility (Saloniemi *et al.*, 1995). Whereas, dietary coumestrol concentrations of 50 mg/kg provided for over 180 hours induced uterine enlargement in rats (Whitten *et al.*, 1992). There is marked variability in the effects of phytoestrogens for different species. High concentrations of daidzein and genistein from soybeans in captive cheetah diets, with an approximate consumption of 50 mg isoflavones/day, may have been a major contributor to the decreased fertility and the veno-occlusive liver disease in the cheetah population (Setchell *et al.*, 1987).

Physiology, particularly the stage of pregnancy or cycling, appears to influence the concentrations of isoflavones (daidzein and genistein) in the plasma of heifers fed 2.5 kg soybeans (Woclawek-Potocka *et al.*, 2008). Pregnancy influenced the kinetics of the isoflavones; plasma concentrations of daidzein and genistein were significantly higher in cycling heifers than in early- or late-pregnant heifers. In addition, heifers at 2 months pregnant had higher concentrations of the active metabolite equol, as compared to heifers at 8 months pregnant or heifers at the mid-luteal phase of the estrous cycle. Piotrowska and co-workers (2006) found elevated concentrations of equol and para-ethylphenol in corpus luteal tissue and plasma of cows fed a soy diet (2.5 kg soybean/animal/day), as compared with a standard diet. These data suggest that cows may be continuously exposed to active phytoestrogens metabolites that can affect the reproductive tract. Metabolites of isoflavones phytoestrogens, for example equol, appear to disturb bovine corpus luteum function *in vitro* by inhibiting luteinized hormone (needed for a pre-ovulatory surge) and prostaglandin stimulated progesterone secretion.

Uterine endometrial release of prostaglandin F2α is under regulation by oxytocin, progesterone (P4) and estradiol (E2) in ruminants and causes luteolysis and regression of the corpus luteum. In cattle and sheep, an increase in oxytocin receptors on endometrial epithelial cells is a primary initiator of luteolysis (Goff, 2004). Oxytocin has a functional role in the regulation of ovarian function in ruminants. Mlynarczuk and co-workers (2009) determined that coumestrol, daidzein and genistein stimulated the expression of several genes that are responsible for synthesis of the oxytocin precursor, neurophysin-I/OT, and post-translation synthesis of oxytocin, peptidyl-glycine-α-amidating monooxygenase or PGA, in granulosa and luteal cells in cattle. These phytoestrogens stimulated the secretion of oxytocin stored in bovine ovarian follicles and corpora lutea, which in cattle may result in premature luteolysis and the formation of persistent corpus luteum.

Higher concentrations of active estrogenic metabolites, i.e. equol, in early pregnancy could lead to increased insemination rates (number of breedings) and decreased number of successful pregnancies in cattle fed soybeans at 2.5 kg/head/day (Woclawek-Potocka *et al.*, 2005a,b). The concentrations of a metabolite of prostaglandin $PGF_2\alpha$ or PGFM were significantly higher in the soybean-fed cattle plasma through the first 21 days after ovulation and artificial insemination; the high concentrations of PGFM were correlated with isoflavone metabolites in the plasma. The authors concluded that the soy-derived phytoestrogens and their metabolites disrupt reproduction and uterine function by modulating the ratio of $PGF_2\alpha$ to PGE_2, which leads to elevated, non-physiological production of luteolytic $PGF_2\alpha$ by the bovine endometrium during the estrous cycle and early pregnancy in cattle. In ruminants, $PGF_2\alpha$ is the major luteolytic agent while PGE2 is considered luteoprotective with anti-luteolytic properties; the ratio of $PGF_2\alpha$ to PGE_2 is important for the development and maintenance of the corpus luteum and establishment of pregnancy.

A majority of the reports on adverse effects on reproduction from phytoestrogens involve isoflavone or coumestrol exposure. One report focused on the effect of plant sterols in cattle reproduction. Elghamry and co-workers (1971) identified β-sitosterol as one of possibly several active estrogenic compounds in sugar beet silage, which when fed at relatively high levels to cows decreased fertility and ovulations and caused cystic ovaries. These reported effects are consistent with reproductive problems in cattle, sheep and horses reported by veterinary practitioners, which include lack of dominant follicles, repeat inseminations or services, early embryonic death and occasionally mammary gland hypertrophy and secretions in the glands. The clinical findings in livestock are supported by the clinical signs of infertility in mice treated with genistein (Jefferson *et al.*, 2009a,b), described earlier under developmental effects.

Male infertility

There are a limited number of adverse effect reports of phytoestrogens on male reproductive function. In a review on soy and male reproductive function, Cederroth *et al.* (2009) stated that overall there are some indications that phytoestrogens may alter reproductive hormones, spermatogenesis, sperm capacitation and fertility. However, there is lack of consistency in human and animal studies examining these effects. Adult male mice fed a soy-rich diet from conception to adulthood exhibited normal male behavior and were fertile, but with a 25% reduction in epididymal sperm counts and a 21% reduction in litter size (Cederroth *et al.*, 2010). Irrigated red clover, containing higher estrogenic activity than non-irrigated clover, was fed with non-irrigated red clover in diets to Japanese quail chicks for 2 weeks (Rochester *et al.*, 2009). Both irrigated and non-irrigated red clover reduced chick growth as compared with control chicks, but irrigated red clover reduced both absolute and relative testes and ovary weights and increased the relative oviduct weights, suggesting isoflavones affect avian reproductive development. Bilgoraj ganders were fed diets containing high concentrations of phytoestrogens (about 140 µg/g of diet) from soy and alfalfa meal during growth, photorefractoriness and laying periods (reviewed by Dusza *et al.*, 2006). Semen samples analyzed from phytoestrogen-fed ganders had decreased volume of ejaculates and increased number of abnormal spermatozoa, but fertility of eggs and percentage of normal hatching were not different in males and females fed the control and phytoestrogen diets during the breeding season.

Male goat kids fed a conventional diet supplement with red clover isoflavones (60% biochanin A), at approximately 3 to 4 mg/kg/day for 3 months, exhibited a rise in plasma-free and total triiodothyronine (T_3) followed by a significant increase in plasma testosterone concentrations during puberty, as compared with control goats (Gunnarsson *et al.*, 2009). The increased concentration of T_3 has a direct effect on pubertal Leydig cell steroidogenesis leading to increased testosterone. In an *in vitro* experiment with pubertal rat Leydig cells, Maran and co-workers (2000) reported that T_3 can modulate luteinizing hormone-mediated secretion of testosterone and estradiol in a dose-dependent manner. Other studies have found that isoflavones do not affect thyroid hormones. A possible explanation is type of isoflavones used in the study diets; biochanin A (found in red clover) is considered an efficient aromatase inhibitor, while genistein, found in soy protein, does not inhibit aromatase and has a higher affinity for ER binding.

Phytoestrogens have been evaluated with normal sperm to determine altered cell signaling through inhibition of tyrosine kinase. Protein tyrosine kinase is believed to have a major role in sperm function in the human and other animals through phosphorylation of tyrosine proteins on the spermatozoa and subsequent capacitation, followed by the zona pellucida-induced acrosomal reaction and penetration of the zona pellucida-intact oocytes (Pukazhenthi *et al.*, 1998). Utilizing *in vitro* genistein exposure and cat spermatozoa, no effect was detected in sperm motility, but genistein inhibited the zona pellucida induced acrosome reaction and reduced sperm penetration into the inner zona pellucida. Menzel and co-workers (2007) reported similar findings in cryopreserved bovine spermatozoa incubated with a range of genistein concentrations, from 0.74 µmol/L to 7.4 µmol/L. Genistein did not affect tyrosine phosphorylation in cryopreserved spermatozoa, but inhibited the progesterone and ZP3-6 peptide-induced acrosomal exocytotic event or reaction and decreased sperm–zona pellucida binding, probably by a process independent of protein tyrosine kinase inhibition.

Data from castrated rats treated with 5α-dihydrotestosterone (DHT) and equol showed that equol bound and sequestered DHT from the androgen receptor resulted in increased plasma concentrations of DHT (Lund *et al.*, 2004). The authors reported that equol administration to intact male rats somewhat blocked the negative feedback effects of DHT on pituitary luteinizing hormone regulation increasing circulating luteinizing hormone levels and reducing ventral prostate and epididymal weights, acting as an anti-androgen. Tan and co-workers (2006) used seven marmoset monkey twins to evaluate potential adverse effects of feeding human male infants with soy milk formula. Male co-twin marmoset monkeys were fed soy milk formula from age 4 to 5 days for approximately 5 to 6 weeks, which resulted in normal body weights, penis length and fertility; however, the soy-fed monkeys had significantly increased testis weights and Sertoli and Leydig cell numbers per testis. Additional studies are needed regarding the influence of phytoestrogens, particularly soy milk formula feed to infants, on male development and subsequent adult male reproductive and endocrine functions.

RISK ASSESSMENT

Humans are exposed to diets that may contain a wide variety of chemicals, both natural and synthetic, with estrogenic activity. Asian populations have consumed high levels of isoflavones from soy for generations without apparent negative impact on reproduction and development and with the beneficial effects of lower rates of breast and prostate cancer and lower rates of osteoporosis and cardiovascular diseases. Van Meeuwen and co-workers (2007) evaluated potential interactions of a combination of phytoestrogens (genistein, coumestrol, naringenin, catechins, epicatechins and quercetin) similar to levels found in the human diet given to juvenile rats in subcutaneous doses for 3 successive days. The combination of phytoestrogens was uterotrophic in the pubertal rats and acted additively with exogenous 17β-estradiol. However, the dose used was orders of magnitude higher than the regular human diet. Reviews of studies evaluating soy infant formula fed to infants have not identified major risk endpoints in human development or reproduction.

Phytoestrogens may result in marked adverse effects on reproduction in livestock. That risk has been recognized for years in livestock, particularly in sheep and cattle production. With regard to sheep grazing subterranean clover in Australia, temporary and permanent fertility are recognized reproductive conditions. The occurrence of adverse reproductive effects from clover or alfalfa forage consumption in livestock cannot be reliably predicted, nor can most of the factors affecting enhanced phytoestrogen concentration be controlled (e.g., weather, insect or fungal invasion). Elevated phytoestrogen concentrations in soy beans and forages can be analyzed in rations and producers can mitigate most of the adverse effects by diluting or eliminating the forage from the ration.

In subchronic and chronic studies of oral genistein dosing in beagle dogs, the no-observed-adverse-effect level (NOAEL) was considered to be >500 mg/kg/day for the 4-week and 52-week studies (McClain *et al.*, 2005). The primary effects reported were in reproductive organs and included: (1) increased uterine weights in female dogs in the 4-week study; (2) atrophy of the testes and prostate gland and absent spermatozoa in the epididymis in males in the 52-week study; and (3) small decreases in ovarian weights in female dogs in the 52-week study. The no-observed-effect level (NOEL) was considered to be 150 mg/kg/day for the 4-week study and 50 mg/kg/day for the 52-week study. A 4-week recovery period, after the 52-week study at 500 mg/kg/day of genistein, resulted in no observed changes in the dogs. To assess teratogenic and fetal toxic potential of genistein in rats, McClain and co-workers (2007) conducted several *in vivo* embryo–fetal developmental safety studies using genistein by gavage, dosages of 0 to 1,000 mg/kg/day from days 6 to 20 of gestation, and dietary admix, dosages of 0 to 500 mg/kg/day from days 5 to 21 of gestation, and an *in vitro* rat whole embryo culture assay (preliminary screen) using genistein from 1 to 100 µg/mL. *In vitro* genistein exposure in the embryo culture at ≥10 µg/mL resulted in anomalies that were not predictive of *in vivo* findings. A slight maternal toxicity was reported at 1,000 mg genistein/kg/day by gavage doses and included decreased maternal body weights and food consumption with adverse effects in pups reported as increased pup mortality and reduced pup body weights and milk uptake. No external malformations were noted in pups, with minor visceral and skeletal variations observed at the high dose. At the high dietary admix dose of 500 mg/kg/day, maternal body weight and feed consumption were reduced and the incidence of fetal resorptions increased with a corresponding decrease in the number of live fetuses per dam. Fetal body weights were reduced, but no treatment-related teratogenic effects were detected during external, visceral and skeletal examinations of fetuses or in bodyweight normalized anogenital distance. The authors concluded that on the basis of the definitive prenatal developmental safety study (oral dietary admix exposure), the NOAEL for maternal toxicity and adverse effect on embryonic development was considered to be 100 mg genistein/kg/day when given orally by dietary admix.

TREATMENT

The focus of phytoestrogens is on both beneficial and adverse effects. Regarding the adverse impact of phytoestrogens on livestock fertility, the current recommendation is either to delete or dilute the estrogenic component of the diet. Typically, the problems with fertility (irregular cycling) or mammary gland hypertrophy in cattle or horses are related to using specific cuttings of alfalfa or clover forages. Forages and soybeans can be analyzed for isoflavones and coumestrol concentrations and non-detectable or low phytoestrogen feeds can be substituted into rations. A washout period of several weeks (4 to 6+ weeks) will usually result in a return to normal reproductive cycling. The current phytoestrogen data in humans does not substantiate any treatment recommendations for humans.

CONCLUDING REMARKS AND FUTURE DIRECTIONS

Because of the variability in multiple parameters of exposure (dose, timing, duration of exposure) of numerous phytoestrogens to experimental animals and humans, there are not adequate data to determine the developmental and reproductive toxicity of soy infant formula in humans. A potential increased risk of premature breast development in young girls (<2 years) fed soy infant formula was identified by the NTP-CERHR report (Rozman *et al.*, 2006). Large, long-term studies of human infant exposure to isoflavones using soy formula with defined exposure parameters and endpoints that evaluate reproductive endpoints (age of puberty, premature breast development, early onset of menopause, endometriosis and reproductive carcinogenesis) and neurobehavioral development of females and males could assist evaluating phytoestrogen impact on reproduction. Laboratory animal experiments using models with similar pharmaco- and toxicokinetic pathways of humans for appropriate extrapolation to the human neonate and dosing with realistic phytoestrogen concentrations for dose–response relationships are necessary to evaluate developmental and reproductive endpoints. A primary focus of laboratory and livestock research should focus on the dose–response relationship of phytoestrogens (particularly isoflavones and coumestrol) on ovarian follicular development, ovarian follicle counts and ovarian failure. The dose–response relationship for isoflavones and coumestrol in forages and potential for adverse effects of ovarian dysfunction and early embryonic death in livestock, particularly in dairy, needs to be determined. Further research is necessary into the mechanisms that underlie the impact, detrimental or beneficial, of phytoestrogens on reproductive processes in humans and farm animals.

REFERENCES

Adams NR (1995) Organizational and activational effects of phytoestrogens on the reproductive tract of the ewe. *Proc Soc Exp Biol Med* **208:** 87–91.

Adlercreutz H, Mazur W (1997) Phyto-oestrogens and western diseases. *Ann Med* **29:** 95–120.

Adlercreutz H, Mousavi Y, Clark J, Höckersted K, Hämäläinen EK, Wähälä K, Mäkelä T, Hase T (1992) Dietary phytoestrogens and cancer: *in vitro* and *in vivo* studies. *J Steroid Biochem Mol Biol* **41:** 331–7.

Akiyama T, Ishida J, Nakagawa S, Ogawara H, Watanabe S-I, Itoh N, Shibuya M, Fukamai Y (1987) Genistein, a specific inhibitor of tyrosine-specific protein kinases. *J Biol Chem* **262:** 5592–5.

Almstrup K, Fernández MF, Petersen J, Olea N, Skakkebæk NE, Leffers H (2002) Dual effects of phytoestrogens result in U-shaped dose–response curves. *Environ Health Perspect* **110:** 743–8.

Antignac J-P, Cariou R, LeBizec R, André F (2004) New data regarding phytoestrogens content in bovine milk. *Food Chem* **87:** 275–81.

Baber R (2010) Phytoestrogens and post reproductive health. *Maturitas.* DOI:10.1016/jmaturitas.2010.03.023.

Benassayag C, Perrot-Applanat M, Ferre F (2002) Phytoestrogens as modulators of steroid action in target cells. *J Chromatogr B* **777:** 233–48.

Bernbaum JC, Umbach DM, Ragan NB, Ballard JL, Archer JI, Schmidt-Davis H, Rogan WJ (2008) Pilot studies of estrogen-related physical findings in infant. *Environ Health Perspect* **116:** 416–20.

Cassidy A, Bingham S, Setchell KDR (1994) Biological effects of a diet of soy protein rich in isoflavones on the menstrual cycle of premenopausal women. *Am J Clin Nutr* **60:** 333–40.

Cederroth C, Zimmermann C, Beny J-L, Schaad O, Combepine C, Descombes P, Doerge D, Pralong FP, Vassalli J-D, Nef S (2010) Potential detrimental effects of a phytoestrogen-rich diet on male fertility in mice. *Mol Cell Endrocrinol* **321:** 152–60.

Cederroth CR, Auger J, Zimmermann C, Eustache F, Nef S (2009) Soy, phyto-oestrogens and male reproductive function: a review. *Int J Androl* **33:** 304–16.

Chan SG, Murphy PA, Ho SC, Kreiger N, Darlington G, So EKF, Chong PYY (2009) Isoflavonoid content of Hong Kong Soy Foods. *J Agric Food Chem* **57:** 5386–90.

Chandrareddy A, Muneyyirci-Delale O, McFarlane SI, Murad OM (2008) Adverse effects of phytoestrogens on reproductive health: a report of three cases. *Compl Therap Clin Pract* **14:** 132–5.

Cox RI, Davies LH (1988) Modification of pasture oestrogens in the gastrointestinal tract of ruminants. *Proc Nutr Soc Aust* **13:** 61–7.

Dubey RK, Gillespie DG, Imthurn B (1999) Phytoestrogens inhibit growth and MAP kinase activity in human aortic smooth muscle cells. *Hypertension* **33:** 177–82.

Dusza L, Ciereszko R, Skarzyńki DJ, Nogowski L, Opalka M, Kamińska B, Nynca A, Kraszewska O, Slomczńska M, Woclawek-Potocka I, Korzekwz A, Pruszńska-Oszmalek E, Szkudelska K (2006) Mechanism of phytoestrogen action in reproductive processes of mammals and birds. *Repro Biol* **6 (Suppl. 1):** 151–74.

Elghamry ME, Grunert E, Aehnelt E (1971) An active principle responsible for estrogenicity in the leaves of *Beta vulgaris*. *Planta Med* **19:** 208–14.

Faber KA, Hughes CL Jr (1993) Dose–response characteristics of neonatal exposure to genistein on pituitary responsiveness to gonadotropin releasing hormone and volume of the sexually dimorphic nucleus of the preoptic area (SDN-POA) in postpubertal castrated female rats. *Repro Toxicol* **7:** 35–9.

Franke AA, Custer LJ, Cerna CM, Narala K (1995) Rapid HPLC analysis of dietary phytoestrogens from legumes and from human urine. *Proc Soc Exp Biol Med* **208:** 18–26.

Goff AK (2004) Steroid hormone modulation of prostaglandin secretion in the ruminant endometrium during the estrous cycle. *Biol Reprod* **71:** 11–16.

Green CC, Kelly AM (2009) Effects of the estrogen mimic genistein as a dietary component on sex differentiation and ethoxyresorufin-O-deethylase (EROD) activity in channel catfish (*Ictalurus punctatus*). *Fish Physiol Biochem* **35:** 377–84.

Gunnarsson D, Selstam G, Ridderstråle Y, Holm L, Ekstedt E, Madej A (2009) Effects of dietary phytoestrogens on plasma testosterone and triiodothyronine (T_3) levels in male goat kids. *Acta Vet Scand* **51:** 51. DOI:10.1186/1751-0147-51-51.

Hoikkala A, Mustonen E, Saastamoinen I, Joekla T, Taponen J, Saloniemi H, Wähälä K (2007) High levels of equol in organic skimmed Finnish cow milk. *Mol Nutr Food Res* **51:** 782–6.

Jefferson WN, Doerge D, Padilla-Banks E, Woodling KA, Kissling GE, Newbold R (2009a) Oral exposure to genistin, the glycosylated form of genistein, during neonatal life adversely affects the female reproductive system. *Environ Health Perspect* **117:** 1883–9.

Jefferson WN, Padilla-Banks E, Goulding EH, Lao S-P, Newbold RR, Williams CJ (2009b) Neonatal exposure to genistein disrupts ability of female mouse reproductive tract to support preimplantation embryo development and implantation. *Biol Reprod* **80:** 425–31.

Kelly GE, Joannou GE, Reeder AY, Nelson C, Waring MA (1995) The variable metabolic response to dietary isoflavones in humans. *Proc Soc Exp Biol Med* **208:** 40–3.

Klinge CM, Blankenship KA, Risinger KE, Bhatnagar S, Noisin EL, Sumanasekera WK, Zhao L, Brey DM, Keynton RS (2005) Reseveratrol and estradiol rapidly activate MAPK signaling through estrogen receptors α and β in endothelial cells. *J Biol Chem* **280:** 7460–8.

Kostelac D, Rechkemmer G, Briviba K (2003) Phytoestrogens modulate binding response of estrogen receptors alpha and beta to the estrogen response element. *J Agric Food Chem* **51:** 7632–5.

Kuiper GG, Carlsson B, Grandien K, Enmark E, Haggblad J, Nilsson S, Gustafsson J-A (1997) Comparison of the ligand binding specificity and transcript tissue distribution of estrogen receptors alpha and beta. *Endocrinology* **138:** 863–70.

Kuiper GG, Lemmen JG, Carlsson B Corton JC, Safe SH, van der Saag PT, van der Burg B, Gustafsson J-A (1998) Interaction of estrogenic chemicals and phytoestrogens with estrogen receptor β. *Endocrinology* **139:** 4252–63.

Kurzer MS, Xu X (1997) Dietary phytoestrogens. *Annu Rev Nutr* **17:** 353–81.

Lacey M, Bohday J, Fonseka SMR, Ullah AI, Whitehead SA (2005) Dose–response effects of phytoestrogens on the activity and expression of 3 β-hydroxysteroid dehydrogenase and aromatase in human granulosa-luteal cells. *J Steroid Biochem Mol Biol* **96:** 279–86.

Lampe JW (2009) Is equol the key to the efficacy of soy foods? *Am J Clin Nutr* **89:** 1664S–7S.

Lephart ED, Setchell KD, Lund TD (2005) Phytoestrogens: hormonal action and brain plasticity. *Brain Res Bull* **65:** 193–8.

Levy JR, Faber KA, Ayyash L, Hughrs CL Jr (1995) The effect of prenatal exposure to the phytoestrogen genistein on sexual differentiation in rats. *Proc Soc Exp Biol Med* **208:** 60–6.

Lund TD, Munson DJ, Haldy ME, Setchell KDR, Lephart ED, Handa RJ (2004) Equol is a novel anti-androgen that inhibits prostate growth and hormone feedback. *Biol Reprod* **70:** 1188–95.

Lundh T (1995) Metabolism of estrogenic isoflavones in domestic animals. *Proc Soc Exp Biol Med* **208:** 33–9.

Lundh T, Pettersson HI, Martinsson KA (1990) Comparative levels of free and conjugated plant estrogens in blood plasma of sheep and cattle fed estrogenic silage. *J Agic Food Chem* **38:** 1530–4.

Madej A, Persson E, Lundh T, Ridderstråle Y (2002) Thyroid gland function in ovariectomized ewes exposed to phytoestrogens. *J Chromatogr B* **777:** 281–7.

Mäkelä S, Poutanen M, Lehtimäki J, Kostian ML, Santti R, Vihko R (1995) Estrogen-specific 17beta-hydroxysteroid oxidoreductase type 1 (E.C.1.1.1.62) as a possible target for the action of phytoestrogens. *Proc Soc Exp Biol Med* **208:** 51–9.

Manach C, Williamson G, Morand C, Scalbert A, Rémésy (2005) Bioavailability and bioefficacy of polyphenols in humans. I. Review of 97 bioavailability studies. *Am J Clin Nutr* **81 (Suppl.):** 230S–42S.

Maran RRM, Arunakaran J, Aruldhas MM (2000) T_3 directly stimulate basal and modulates LH induced testosterone and oestradiol production by rat Leydig cells *in vitro*. *Endocr J* **47:** 417–28.

Markaverich BM, Webb B, Densvore CL, Gregory RR (1995) Effects of coumestrol on estrogen receptor function and uterine growth in ovariectomized rats. *Environ Health Perspect* **103:** 574–81.

Markiewicz L, Garey J, Adlercreutz H, Gurpide E (1993) *In vitro* bioassay of non-steroidal phytoestrogens. *J Steroid Biochem Mol Biol* **45:** 399–405.

McClain RM, Wolz E, Davidovich A, Pfannkuch F, Bausch J (2005) Subchronic and chronic safety studies with genistein in dogs. *Food Chem Toxicol* **43:** 1461–82.

McClain RM, Wolz E, Davidovich A, Edwards J, Bausch J (2007) Reproductive safety studies with genistein in rats. *Food Chem Toxicol* **45:** 1319–32.

McGarvey C, Cates PS, Brooks N, Swanson IA, Milligan SR, Coen CW, O'Byrne KT (2001) Phytoestrogens and gonadotropin-releasing hormone pulse generator activity and pituitary luteinizing hormone release in the rat. *Endocrinology* **142:** 1202–8.

Menzel VA, Hinsch E, Hägele W, Hinsch K-D (2007) Effect of genistein on acrosome reaction and zona pellucid binding independent of protein tyrosine kinase inhibition in bull. *Asian J Androl* **9:** 650–8.

Mlynarczuk J, Wrobel MH, Kotwica J (2009) The adverse effect of phytoestrogens on the synthesis and secretion of ovarian oxytocin in cattle. *Reprod Dom Anim.* doi: 10.1111/j.1439–0531.2009.01529.x.

Mortensen A, Kulling SE, Schwartz H, Rowland I, Ruefer CE, Rimbach G, Cassidy A, Magee P, Millar J, Hall WL, Kramer Birkved F, Sorensen IK, Sontag F (2009) Analytical and compositional aspects of isoflavones in flood and their biological effects. *Mol Nutr Food Res* **53 (Suppl. 2):** S266–S309.

Mostrom, MS (2010) Unpublished observations. NDSU – Veterinary Diagnostic Laboratory, Fargo, North Dakota.

Neilsen IL, Williamson G (2007) Review of the factors affecting bioavailability of soy isoflavones in humans. *Nutr Cancer* **57:** 1–10.

Nwannenna AI, Lundh T, Madej A, Fredriksson G, Björnhag G (1995) Clinical changes in ovariectomized ewes exposed to phytoestrogens and 17β-estradiol implants. *Proc Soc Exp Biol Med* **208:** 92–7.

Patisaul HB, Jefferson W (2010) The pros and cons of phytoestrogens. *Front. Neuroendocrinol.* DOI:10.1016/j.yfrne.2010.03.003.

Phillips KP, Tanphaichitr N (2008) Human exposure to endocrine disrupters and semen quality. *J Toxicol Environ Health B* **11:** 188–220.

Pietras RJ, Szego CM (1975) Endometrial cell calcium and oestradiol action. *Nature* **253:** 357–9.

Pilšáková L, Riečanský I, Jagla F (2010) The physiological actions of isoflavone phytoestrogens. *Physiol Rev*. Epub ahead of press.

Piotrowska K, Woclawek-Potocka I, Bah MM, Piskula M, Pilawski W, Bober A, Skarzynski DJ (2006) Phytoestrogens and their metabolites inhibit the sensitivity of the bovine corpus luteum on luteotropic factors. *J Reprod Dev* **52:** 33–41.

Pukazhenthi BS, Wildt DE, Ottinger MA, Howard J (1998) Inhibition of domestic cat spermatozoa acrosome reaction and zona pellucid penetration by tyrosine kinase inhibitors. *Mol Repro Dev* **49:** 48–57.

Rochester JR, Klasing KC, Stevenson L, Denison MS, Berry W, Millam JR (2009) Dietary red clover (*Trifolium pretense*) induces oviduct growth and decreases ovary and testes growth in Japanese quail chicks. *Reprod Toxicol* **27:** 63–71.

Romanowicz K, Misztal T, Barcikowski (2004) Genistein, a phytoestrogen, effectively modulated luteinizined hormone and prolactin secretion in ovariectomized ewes during seasonal anestrus. *Neuroendorinology* **79:** 73–81.

Rosselli M, Reinhart K, Imthurn B, Keller PJ, Dubey RK (2000) Cellular and biochemical mechanisms by which environmental oestrogens influence reproductive function. *Hum Reprod Update* **6:** 332–50.

Rozman KK, Bhatia J, Calafat AM, Chambers C, Culty M, Etzel RA, Flaws JA, Hansen DK, Hoyer PB, Jeffery EH, Kesner JS, Marty S, Thomas JA, Umbach D (2006) NTP-CERHR expert panel report on the reproductive and developmental toxicity of soy formula. *Birth Defects Res (Part B)* **77:** 280–397.

Saloniemi H, Wähälä K, Nykänen-Kurki P, Kallela K, Saastamoinen I (1995) Phytoestrogen content and estrogenic effect of legume fodder. *Proc Soc Exp Biol Med* **208:** 13–17.

Santini SE, Basini GB, Bussolati S, Grasselli F (2009) The phytoestrogen quercetin impairs steroidogenesis and angiogenesis in swine granulosa cells in vitro. *J Biomed Biotech* DOI:10.1155/2009/419891.

Santti R, Mäkelä S, Strauss L, Korkman J, Kostian M–L (1998) Phytoestrogens: potential endocrine disruptors in males. *Toxicol Ind Health* **14:** 223–37.

Seguin P, Zheng W (2006) Phytoestrogen content of alfalfa cultivars grown in eastern Canada. *J Sci Food Agric* **86:** 765–71.

Seguin P, Zheng W, Souleimanov A (2004) Alfalfa phytoestrogen content: impact of plant maturity and herbage components. *J Agron Crop Sci* **190:** 211–17.

Setchell KDR, Gosselin SJ, Welsh MB, Johnston JO, Balistreri WF, Kramer LW, Dresser BL, Tarr MJ (1987) Dietary estrogens – a probable cause of infertility and liver disease in captive cheetahs. *Gastroenterology* **93:** 225–33.

Shon YH, Park SD, Nam KS (2006) Effective chemopreventive activity of genistein against human breast cancer cells. *J Biochem Mol Biol* **39:** 448–51.

Sivesind E, Seguin P (2005) Effects of the environment, cultivar, maturity, and preservation method on red clover isoflavone concentration. *J Agric Food Chem* **53:** 6397–402.

Steinshamn H, Purup S, Thuen D, Hansen-Møller J (2008) Effects of clover-grass silages and concentrate supplementation on the content of phytoestrogens in dairy cow milk. *J Dairy Sci* **91:** 2715–25.

Swego CM (1984) Mechanisms of hormone action: parallels in receptor-mediated signal propagation for steroid peptide effectors. *Life Sci* **35:** 2381–96.

Tan KA, Walker M, Morris K, Greig I, Mason JI, Sharpe RM (2006) Infant feeding with soy formula milk: effect in puberty progression, reproductive function and testicular cell numbers in marmoset monkeys in adulthood. *Human Reprod* **21:** 896–904.

Tham DM, Gardner CD, Haskell WI (1998) Potential health benefits of dietary phytoestrogens: a review of the clinical, epidemiological, and mechanistic evidence. *J Clin Endodrinol Metab* **83:** 2223–35.

Urpi-Sarda M, Morand C, Besson C, Kraft G, Viala D, Scalbert A, Besle J-M, Manach C (2008) Tissue distribution if isoflavones in ewes after consumption of red clover silage. *Arch Biochem Biophys* **476:** 205–10.

Van Meeuwen JA, Dan den Berg M, Sanderson JT, Verhoef A, Piersma AH (2007) Estrogenic effects of mixtures of phyto- and synthetic chemicals on uterine growth of prepubertal rats. *Toxicol Lett* **170:** 165–76.

Wang L-Q (2002) Mammalian phytoestrogens: enerodiol and enterolactone. *J Chromatog B* **777:** 289–309.

Whitten PL, Naftolin F (1992) Effects of a phytoestrogen diet on estrogen-dependent reproductive processes in immature female rats. *Steroids* **57:** 56–61.

Whitten PL, Patisaul HB (2001) Cross-species and interassay comparisons of phytoestrogen action. *Environ Health Perspect* **109 (Suppl. 1):** 5–20.

Whitten PL, Russell E, Naftolin F (1992) Effects of a normal human concentration phytoestrogen diet on rat uterine growth. *Steroids* **57:** 98–106.

Woclawek-Potocka I, Bah M, Korzekwa A, Piskula M, Wiczkowski W, Depta A, Skarzynski D (2005a) Soybean-derived phytoestrogens regulate prostaglandin secretion in endometrium during cattle estrous cycle and early pregnancy. *Exp Biol Med* **230:** 189–99.

Woclawek-Potocka I, Acosta TJ, Korzekwa A, Bah MM, Shibaya M, Okuda K, Skarzynski D (2005b) Phytoestrogens modulate prostaglandins production in bovine endometrium: cell type specificity and intracellular mechanism. *Exp Biol Med* **230:** 326–33.

Woclawek-Potocka I, Piskula MK, Bah MM, Siemieniuch MJ, Korzekwa A, Brzezicka E, Skarzynski D (2008) Concentrations of isoflavones and their metabolites in the blood of pregnant and non-pregnant heifers fed soy bean. *J Reprod Dev* **54:** 358–63.

Xu X, Wang H-J, Murphy PA, Hendrich S (2000) Neither background diet nor type of soy food affects short-term isoflavone bioavailability in women. *J Nutr* **130:** 798–901.

Yueh TL, Chu HY (1977) The metabolic fate of daidzein. *Sci Sin* **20:** 513–22.

Section 10

Biotoxins

CHAPTER

53

Fumonisins

Kenneth A. Voss, Ronald T. Riley and Janee Gelineau-van Waes

INTRODUCTION

The discovery of the fumonisins (Gelderblom *et al.*, 1988) was a major breakthrough ending the search to identify the mycotoxin(s) causing the animal diseases associated with maize or feeds contaminated with *Fusarium verticillioides* (formerly *F. moniliforme* Sheldon) or *F. proliferatum* (Marasas, 2001). These two species are the most significant fumonisin producers although other *Fusarium* (Bolger *et al.*, 2001) and at least one *Aspergillus* species (*A. niger*) (Månsson *et al.*, 2010) produce minor amounts. Over 28 fumonisins were identified by 2002 (Rheeder *et al.*, 2002). New stereoisomers such as *epi*-FB_3 and *epi*-FB_4 (Gelderblom *et al.*, 2007) and novel congeners such as fumonisin B_6 (Månsson *et al.*, 2010) continue to be discovered and structural confirmation of more is likely (Bartók *et al.*, 2010). Fumonisin B_1 (FB_1) (Figure 53.1) is the predominant isomer and usually accounts for 60% or more of the fumonisins in maize. FB_2 and FB_3 occur in lower amounts with FB_2 being the more prevalent; however, a small number of fungal isolates produce predominantly FB_2 or FB_3 and little to no FB_1 (Riley *et al.*, 1997; Voss *et al.*, 1998; Månsson *et al.*, 2010). Fumonisins have been proven to cause animal diseases including liver and kidney toxicity (Bolger *et al.*, 2001; Voss *et al.*, 2001, 2007) and carcinogenicity in rodents (Gelderblom *et al.*, 1991; Howard *et al.*, 2001) and there is evidence that they pose a health risk for humans under some circumstances.

PHARMACOKINETICS/ TOXICOKINETICS

The bioavailability, distribution and toxicokinetics of fumonisins have been studied in multiple species including laboratory rodents and primates, swine, ruminants and poultry (reviewed by Bolger *et al.*, 2001). Absorption is low and only small amounts accumulate in tissues as illustrated by the findings of Martinez-Larranaga *et al.* (1999). Gastrointestinal absorption was poor and absorbed FB_1 was quickly eliminated from the blood. Minor amounts accumulated in liver and kidneys while only negligible amounts were found in other tissues. T_{max} after oral dosing with 10 mg/kg body weight = 1.02 hour, C_{max} = 0.18 μg/mL, and bioavailability was only about 3.5% of the dose. Elimination from plasma was consistent with a two-compartment open model with an elimination $T_{1/2}$ = 3.2 hours. As in other studies (cited by Martinez-Larranga *et al.*, 1999; Bolger *et al.*, 2001; Voss *et al.*, 2001) FB_1 distributed to liver and, to a greater extent, to kidney. The area under the concentration–time curve (AUC) ratios for liver/plasma and kidney/plasma were 2.0 and 29.9, respectively, and distribution fitted a one-compartment open model. Elimination from liver was more rapid than from kidney: their respective $T_{1/2}$ of elimination was about 4.1 and 7.1 hours.

When diets containing FB_1, FB_2 and FB_3 in the ratio of 1.0:0.45:0.10 (equal to 65, 29 and 7% of the total) were fed to rats, little (≤4% of total recovered fumonisins) FB_2 or FB_3 was found in liver or kidney after 10 days (Riley and Voss, 2006). FB_1 was therefore most readily absorbed, most readily retained in target tissues, most slowly eliminated or accumulated due to some combination of these possibilities. In any event, the significantly higher accumulation of FB_1 in the rat kidney likely contributes to its enhanced sensitivity to fumonisins relative to liver.

MECHANISM OF ACTION

The chemical structure of the fumonisins strongly resembles that of the sphingoid bases sphinganine (Sa) and sphingosine (So). There is no evidence to date that fumonisins undergo Phase I or Phase II hepatic metabolism. Fumonisins having a primary amino group at the C2 position competitively inhibit *de novo* ceramide (*N*-acyl sphingosine) biosynthesis (Wang *et al.*, 1999; Gelineau-van Waes *et al.*, 2009) by competitively binding to ceramide synthase and preventing CoA-dependent acylation of Sa. Consequently, the tissue concentration of Sa increases quickly and dramatically (Figure 53.2). Concentrations of the downstream metabolite sphinganine-1-phosphate (Sa 1-P) also increase. Sphingosine (So) originates during the metabolic turnover of ceramide. It differs structurally from Sa only by the presence of a *trans* 3,4 double bond in the fatty acyl chain (the double bond is

Reproductive and Developmental Toxicology, Edited by Ramesh C. Gupta
ISBN: 978-0-12-382032-7

FIGURE 53.1 The chemical structure of fumonisin B_1 (FB_1), the most common and most thoroughly studied fumonisin. Other fumonisins differ from FB_1 in the number of -OH groups at C3 and C5 (fumonisins B), addition of R groups to the amine function (fumonisins A, P and others), loss of one or both of the tricaballylic acid groups at C14 or C15 (fully or partially hydrolyzed fumonisins) or loss of the C1 methyl group (fumonisins C).

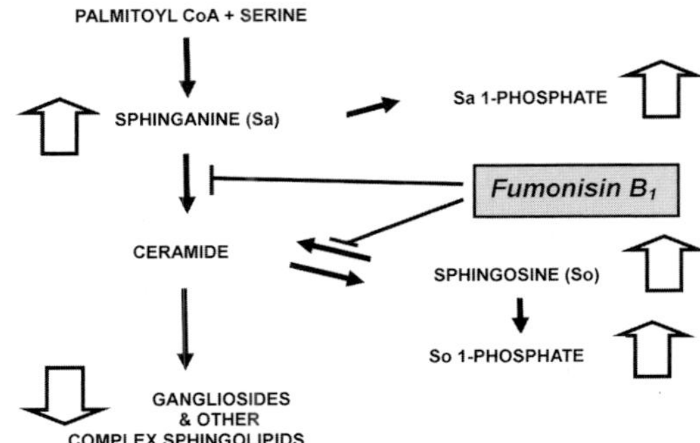

FIGURE 53.2 Simplified schematic of the *de novo* sphingolipid biosynthetic pathway showing the competitive inhibition of ceramide synthase by fumonisin B_1. The consequential increases in sphingoid bases and their 1-phosphate metabolites and decreases in complex sphingolipids are shown by the arrows.

inserted during *de novo* ceramide biosynthesis after condensation of Sa and fatty acyl-CoA). Like Sa, So is acylated by ceramide synthase and accumulates in tissues as a result of ceramide synthase inhibition, although to a lesser extent than Sa. Sphingosine 1-phosphate (So 1-P) concentrations also increase. In addition to sphingoid base and sphingoid base metabolite accumulations, complex sphingolipids downstream of ceramide decrease due to ceramide synthase inhibition. Accumulation of Sa, So and their 1-phosphates in tissues, blood or urine are useful biomarkers of fumonisin exposure and a close correlation between increased sphingoid base concentrations, especially those of Sa, and toxicity have been repeatedly shown in experiments in laboratory animals, horses, swine and other species (Riley and Voss, 2006; Gelineau-van Waes *et al.*, 2009; Eaton *et al.*, in press). These effects decrease rapidly after cessation of exposure and the decreases precede reversal of microscopic indications of tissue damage. The intermediate intracellular or extracellular signaling events linking ceramide synthase inhibition (initial event) and overt toxicity (outcome) in target tissues are not fully understood. Tissue-, strain- and species-related differences likely involve multiple processes including one or more of the following: efficiency of kinases in target tissues to metabolize accumulated Sa or So; ability of tissues to metabolize sphingoid base 1-phoshates to aldehydes, phosphoethanolamine or back to Sa or So by dephosphorylation; ability of cells to eliminate sphingoid bases or metabolites; induction or activation of pro-apoptotic and pro-mitotic cytokines; upregulation of cyclins or other cell cycle modulators; direct or indirect induction of nitric oxide; blockage of cardiac L-type calcium channels by accumulated So; inappropriate intracellular signaling by accumulated So 1-P; binding of accumulated So (or Sa) 1-P to membrane-bound G-protein coupled sphingosine 1-phosphate receptors; altered fatty acid composition of cell membranes; or disruption of membrane lipid raft function as a result of complex sphingolipid depletion. These processes are discussed in Burger *et al.* (2007), Eaton *et al.* (in press), Gelineau-van Waes *et al.* (2009) and Riley and Voss (2006). Mechanistic considerations relevant to reproductive toxicity are discussed below.

Two recent developments are likely to impact understanding of fumonisin-related toxicity. First, at least six ceramide synthases have been identified (designated CerS1–Cer6) (Levy and Futerman, 2010) and one of these, CerS1, appears resistant to the inhibitory effects of fumonisins when overexpressed. (Venkataraman *et al.*, 2002). Upregulation of CerS1 under some circumstances could serve as an adaptive mechanism to offset ceramide depletion. Second, accumulation of 1-deoxysphinganine (1-dSa) and depletion of complex sphingolipids containing 1dSa have been demonstrated in the livers of mice following short-term parenteral (Voss *et al.*, 2009) or long-term dietary (Zitomer *et al.*, 2009) FB_1 exposure. The role of 1-dSa and 1-dSa complex sphingolipids remains to be determined but it is possible that they contribute to the variable species, sex and target organ sensitivities to fumonisins.

SYSTEMIC TOXICITY

Equine leukoencephalomalacia

Horses are the most sensitive species to fumonisins and reviews of the topic are available in Haschek *et al.* (2002) and Voss *et al.* (2007). Classically, horses ingesting contaminated feed develop a syndrome referred to as equine leukoencephalomalacia (ELEM). Symptoms reflect neurologic injury and include ataxia, head pressing, paralysis of the lips and tongue and convulsions. They appear acutely and progress rapidly, and the mortality rate is near 100%. At necropsy, one or more foci of hemorrhagic liquefactive necrosis are characteristically present in the white matter of the brain, predominantly in the cerebrum.

A hepatotoxic syndrome also occurs in horses. Icterus, elevated concentrations of serum bilirubin and liver enzymes, oral petechia, and swelling of the face and head may occur. Necropsy usually reveals a small, firm liver and, upon microscopic examination, centrilobular necrosis and periportal fibrosis are typical. Neurotoxic signs may also develop before death.

FB_1 was proven to cause ELEM (Marasas *et al.*, 1988) when liver and brain lesions were induced by repeated injection of 125 μg/kg body weight FB_1. ELEM was also unequivocally induced by giving repeated oral doses of 1 to 4 mg/kg body weight FB_1 to two horses over a span of 29 to 33 days (Kellerman *et al.*, 1990).

FB_1 is also cardiotoxic to horses (Smith *et al.*, 2002). Decreased heart rates, decreased cardiac contractility and increased systemic vascular resistance were found after exposure to 0.2 mg/kg body weight FB_1 administered intravenously. Repeated daily doses of 0.01 mg/kg body weight FB_1 over 28 days caused no cardiovascular impairment but did affect sphingolipid profiles of cardiac tissues (Foreman *et al.*, 2004).

Porcine pulmonary edema

Like ELEM, porcine pulmonary edema (PPE) is associated with the consumption of moldy feed. Outbreaks are sporadic, can be extensive and can sometimes involve thousands of animals (Haschek *et al.*, 2002). Death is due to pulmonary edema and hydrothorax. The causative role of FB_1 was shown when 0.4 mg/kg body weight per day for 4 days induced the characteristic pulmonary lesions (Harrison *et al.*, 1990). Liver lesions similar to those found in exposed rodents (see below) also occur and pancreatic necrosis has also been found in exposed swine by some investigators (Haschek *et al.*, 2002). The underlying pathophysiological mechanism of PPE is not resolved but likely involves left-sided cardiac insufficiency (Constable *et al.*, 2003). FB_1 increases Sa and So concentrations in the heart and the increased So (and/or Sa) in turn appears to inhibit L-type calcium channels that are critical for myocardial contractility. So 1-P might also alter vascular tension.

Other

Poultry and ruminants are less sensitive than horses or swine (Bolger *et al.*, 2001; Haschek *et al.*, 2002; Voss *et al.*, 2007). Effects include disrupted sphingolipid metabolism, compromised immunity or kidney or liver lesions.

Rodents and rabbits

The systemic toxicity of FB_1 and fumonisins in fungal culture materials in laboratory animals including rats, mice, rabbits and non-human primates have been extensively studied and detailed reviews are available (Bolger *et al.*, 2001; Voss *et al.*, 2001). In summary, the liver or kidneys or both are target organs in all species tested. Fumonisins initially cause apoptosis of renal epithelial cells in the proximal tubules of the outer medulla and in hepatocytes. FB_1 is a liver (hepatocellular carcinoma) and kidney (renal tubule carcinoma, including sarcomatous forms) carcinogen in rodents at dietary concentrations 50 ppm or greater (Gelderblom *et al.*, 1991; Howard *et al.*, 2001).

REPRODUCTIVE AND DEVELOPMENTAL TOXICITY

Interest in the potential adverse effects of fumonisins on reproduction and development began shortly after their discovery. Overall, the effects induced by fungal culture materials or purified mycotoxin are in good agreement, suggesting that fumonisins, especially FB_1, are responsible for the reproductive effects of *F. verticillioides*.

Early investigations

In ovo *and* in vitro *studies*

Javed *et al.* (1993) inoculated eggs with 0, 1, 10 or 100 μM FB_1 or an extract of *F. proliferatum* culture material providing 20 μM FB_1 and 4 μM FB_2 on days 1 or 10 of the 21-day incubation period. Dose-related mortality rose to 100 and 90% in embryos of eggs inoculated with FB_1 on days 1 and 10, respectively. Mortality rates in chicks given the culture material extract were 90 (day 10 inoculation) to 100% (day 1 inoculation) and both FB_1 and culture material extract caused anomalies described as enlarged heads with or without hydrocephalus. Decreased body size was also found in embryos exposed to 1 μM FB_1 on day 1, as were beak enlargement and neck elongation in this and other groups treated on day 1. Overall, embryos from the mid- and high dose groups exhibited delayed development.

Other treatment-related findings included incompletely closed umbilicus, hemorrhagic membranes or yolk sac, discoloration of the feathers, softening of beaks and toenails, weakness, thickened cartilaginous plates in the beak and jaw, hepatocyte necrosis, fragmented myocardial fibers and sloughing of epithelial cells in the renal tubules. Some findings were most prominent at the lower doses while others were seen at the higher doses, indicating that FB_1 stimulated embryo development at low doses but impaired development at high doses. While these findings showed that experimental *in ovo* exposure adversely affects embryo survival and development, the demonstrated absence of carryover into eggs of FB_1-exposed hens (Vudathula *et al.*, 1994) nonetheless indicates that fumonisins do not pose a significant threat to chick development "in the field".

FB_1 retarded the growth of cultured rat embryos exposed to ≥0.28 μM FB_1 for 45 hours beginning embryonic day 9.5 (E 9.5) (Flynn *et al.*, 1996). The percentage of abnormal embryos increased at doses ≥0.7 μM FB_1 and reached 100% at 1.4 to 56 μM. The abnormalities presented no consistent or "distinct" pattern and were therefore likely a consequence of generalized growth and developmental retardation. Simultaneous exposure to *N*-acetylsphinganine or the complex sphingolipid ganglioside GM1 did not protect the embryos, suggesting that the mechanism of growth retardation was not sphingolipid dependent. Embryos similarly exposed to hydrolyzed FB_1 (HFB_1), which is found in alkaline cooked foods, showed significant effects on growth only at 56 μM FB_1 equivalents. Developmental abnormalities were found at ≥2.8 μM FB_1 equivalents and, like those induced by FB_1; they were attributed to general retardation of growth and development. Higher doses of HFB_1 did induce neural tube defects (NTDs) in cultured rat embryos (Flynn *et al.*, 1997) as discussed below.

In vivo experiments

Results of experiments using Syrian hamsters suggested that fumonisins were fetotoxic at doses that did not elicit maternal toxicity. Increased fetal deaths were found in the litters of dams given oral doses of 12 or 18 mg/kg body weight FB_1 on E 8 and E 9 (Floss *et al.*, 1994a). No significant differences in weight or size of offspring were found but the incidence of malformed fetuses was higher in the 18 mg/kg body weight FB_1 group. Malformations included hooked or crooked tail (13% affected), absence of middle digits (18%) and cleft palate (3%). Mild histological changes were also found in the maternal livers (Floss *et al.*, 1994a,b).

When pregnant Syrian hamsters were given 0, 8.7, 10.4, 12.5, 15 or 18 mg/kg body weight FB_1 by gavage on E 8 through E 12 (Penner *et al.*, 1998), the number of litters with live fetuses (3 to 4) and the average number of live fetuses/litter (2.5 to 2.9) were significantly reduced at the two highest doses compared the other groups (9 to 10 litters with live fetuses; 10.6 to 14.5 fetuses/litter). There were also dose-dependent trends toward decreased fetal body weight and crown-to-rump length. Skeletal findings were attributed to delayed development and included poorly ossified hyoid and pelvic bones or sternabrae, enhanced prognathism (protrusion of lower jaw) and small or missing incisors. The percent of affected fetuses increased in a dose-dependent manner and reached 100% in the high dose group. As in other hamster studies (Floss *et al.*, 1994a), maternal toxicity was not apparent by measuring serum aminotransaminase activity or bilirubin concentration or by microscopic examination of maternal tissues. While the findings suggest that fetal effects occurred independently of maternal toxicity, it is significant that the latter was likely underestimated because maternal sphingolipids were not evaluated.

The results of the earliest reproductive studies in rats also suggested maternal toxicity was not a prerequisite for embryotoxicity. Delayed or incomplete ossification of sternebrae and vertebral bodies was found in the fetuses of Fischer 344 dams given 30 or 60 mg/kg body weight FB_1 by gavage on E 8 through E 12 (Lebepe-Mazur *et al.*, 1995). Weights of high dose fetuses were decreased about 20%. Maternal weight gain was unaffected but histopathology, serum chemistry or sphingolipid profiles of FB_1-exposed dams were not included during assessment of maternal toxicity.

More detailed evaluations of maternal toxicity were undertaken (Collins *et al.*, 1998a,b) when pregnant Fischer 344 rats were orally dosed with 1.88 to 15 mg/kg body weight FB_1 on E 3 through E 16 (Collins *et al.*, 1998a). No dose-related skeletal or soft tissue abnormalities were found. Mean weight (3.3 g) and crown-to-rump length (3.7 cm) of high dose female fetuses were minimally but significantly ($p < 0.05$) decreased: the respective control values were 3.4 g and 3.8 cm. No external anomalies or developmental variations were found in the fetuses that could be attributed to FB_1 and there were no specific skeletal variations that could be considered dose dependent. However, the average number of litters with fetuses (≥1.6) having two or more variations was increased (controls = 0.8) at ≥3.75 mg/kg body weight and the number of litters/group having fetuses exhibiting two or more variations increased at 3.75 (15) and 15 (14) mg/kg body weight (controls = 8).

When the dosing regimen was modified so that the dams were given 6.25 to 50 mg/kg body weight FB_1 (Collins *et al.*, 1998a,b), both maternal and fetal toxicity were induced at the high dose. Dose-related trends toward lower feed consumptions and reduced weight gains were found in dams given ≥12.5 mg/kg body weight. Liver and kidney lesions typical of those caused by FB_1 were found in dams dosed with ≥25 and ≥6.25 mg/kg body weight, respectively, and dose-dependent increases in maternal sphinganine to sphingosine ratios were found in kidney at ≥6.25, in liver at ≥12.5, and in serum at ≥25 mg/kg body weight FB_1.

The number of viable fetuses per litter (12.0) (control value = 14.0) was slightly but significantly ($p < 0.05$) reduced at 50 mg/kg body weight and, conversely, dead fetuses per litter were significantly increased at 25 (5.7%) and 50 mg/kg body weight (23.1%) compared to the controls (5.5%). Fetal weights and length were significantly reduced at 50 mg/kg body weight FB_1 and the percentage of fetuses/litter exhibiting two or three variations increased significantly at 25 and 50 mg/kg body weight. Together, these findings (Collins *et al.*, 1998a,b) indicated that FB_1 was not teratogenic and that developmental variations induced by the mycotoxin were mediated by maternal toxicity.

Findings in mice corroborated this interpretation (Reddy *et al.*, 1996). Pregnant CD1 mice were given 0, 12.5, 5, 25, 50 or 100 mg/kg body weight FB_1 orally by gavage on E 7–15. More resorptions (percent of total implants), averaging ≥10.0%, were found at ≥25 mg/kg body weight (control and low dose litters averaged ≤2.6%) and reached a maximum of 95.8% at the high dose. Conversely, the number of live fetuses/litter was reduced so that the survival rate, as a percentage of total implants, was only 4.2 at the high dose. In contrast to the control group, 59.2 to 100% (high dose) of the fetuses in the 25, 50 or 100 mg/kg body weight groups exhibited hydrocephalus. All litters in these groups were affected and the severity of the condition increased with increasing dose. No other developmental effects were found.

FB_1 induced maternal toxicity at ≥25 mg/kg body weight. Findings included ascites, increased plasma alanine aminotransferase and microscopic liver lesions. The latter increased in severity with increasing dose, and included hepatocyte apoptosis, cytoplasmic basophilia, increased mitoses and increased nucleus size. The ratio of sphinganine/sphingosine (Sa/So) in maternal liver was elevated at ≥25 mg/kg body weight FB_1. Sa/So of the fetal livers were, in contrast, unaffected, suggesting that FB_1 either did not cross the placenta or that sphingoid base elevations, if they had occurred, were reversed within 3 days after the last dose.

When FB_1 was given to New Zealand white rabbits by gavage at 0, 0.1, 0.5 or 1.0 mg/kg body weight on E 3 through E 19 (LaBorde *et al.*, 1997), it caused maternal mortality and disrupted maternal sphingolipid metabolism at ≥0.5 mg/kg body weight. However, there were no differences in maternal body weight or weight gain among surviving dams and no differences in the number of non-viable fetuses or number of fetal malformations were found among the groups. While not teratogenic, FB_1 was fetotoxic as shown by the significantly reduced fetal body, kidney and liver weights found at the two highest doses. No evidence of disrupted sphingolipid metabolism was found in the fetuses, which were examined one day following the final dose. Fetal effects were considered secondary to maternal toxicity.

FUMONISINS AND NEURAL TUBE DEFECTS (NTDs)

Background

NTDs are relatively common birth defects resulting from a failure of the neural tube to fuse properly. Depending upon whether the brain or spinal cord is affected, the morphological presentation varies from *spina bifida occulta* to the more severe conditions that are incompatible with life. These include myelomeningiocele (externalization of the meningeal membranes and spinal cord), exencephaly, anencephaly and craniorhachischisis (external exposure of the brain and spinal cord). Neural tube closure in humans occurs within the first month of gestation, often before women are aware that they are pregnant. The etiology of NTDs is poorly understood, but is a multifactorial phenomenon involving complex genetic, nutritional and environmental interactions (Gelineau-van Waes *et al.*, 2009). Among the nutritional factors that influence fetal development, adequate maternal folate appears to have a crucial role in protecting the fetus from exogenous teratogens. Diets that include large amounts of maize as a staple are likely to be folate-deficient because maize naturally contains low amounts of this vitamin (Burton *et al.*, 2008). Deficiency is compounded in regions including Mexico and Central America where alkaline cooking, or nixtamalization, of maize is common (Palencia *et al.*, 2003) because the practice further reduces the amounts of folate and other vitamins (Cárdenas *et al.*, 2001; Burton *et al.*, 2008).

Folate is an essential vitamin. Nutritional deficiencies or genetic variations impacting its homeostasis can lead to an insufficient transfer of folate to a developing fetus, thereby adversely affecting embryogenesis (Piedrahita *et al.*, 1999; Tang and Finnell, 2003; Spiegelstein *et al.*, 2004). Folate's structure includes a pteridine ring attached to a para-aminobenzoic acid side chain. In its reduced form, tetrahydrofolate (THF), folate is an important co-factor in single-carbon transfer reactions and, accordingly, folate is required for incorporating single carbon groups into purine nucleotides or for methylating deoxyuridylate to thymidylate for DNA biosynthesis. Vitamin B_{12} (cobalamin) is another essential vitamin and its metabolism is interdependent with that of folate. Cobalamin is a co-enzyme for methionine synthase, which is involved in the THF-dependent methylation of homocysteine to methionine (Stipanuk, 2004). Cobalamin deficiency might therefore "trap" THF to produce a functional folate deficiency (Shane and Stokstad, 1985).

Human clinical and epidemiological studies have shown an association between maternal use of folic acid supplements or multivitamins with folic acid during early pregnancy and reduced risk for some congenital malformations in offspring, including reductions in the occurrence (Itikala *et al.*, 2001) and recurrence (MRC, 1991) of pregnancies having an NTD outcome. Others found a 50% decrease in NTD incidence with folic acid supplementation in Mexico (Martinez de Villarreal *et al.*, 2002), where dietary fumonisin exposure is likely. The mechanism underlying these beneficial effects is elusive and the mothers of babies born with NTD usually have normal folate levels (Yates *et al.*, 1987). This means that folate deficiency alone does not explain how NTDs arise and reinforces the concept that a combination of genetic, environmental (possibly including fumonisins) or dietary factors influences folate uptake, metabolism or utilization by developing embryos.

A potential link connecting fumonisins, folate metabolism and, by implication, NTDs was first provided by Stevens and Tang (1997) who found that fumonisins depleted glycosphingolipids and inhibited folate uptake *in vitro*. The high affinity folate receptor (murine Folr1; human FRα) is a GPI-anchored protein that associates with detergent-insoluble "lipid rafts" in membranes (Figure 53.3). The lipid rafts are rich in cholesterol and sphingolipids (Elortza *et al.*, 2003). Depletion of cellular cholesterol impaired the uptake of 5-methyltetrahydrofolate into cells (Chang *et al.*, 1992), thus suggesting that lipid rafts have a role in regulating the function of the GPI-anchored folate receptor.

Gangliosides are complex sphingolipids that are found in lipid rafts in which GPI-anchored proteins cluster (Watanabe *et al.*, 2002). Ganglioside GM1 is highly expressed in the developing central nervous system (Silani *et al.*, 1993), and it may be critical for coordinating the protein–lipid interactions and signaling involved in neural tube closure. The GPI-anchored Folr1 co-localizes with GM1 in lipid rafts and has been isolated from lipid rafts that are enriched in signaling molecules such as kinase/phosphatases and heterotrimeric G proteins. It is therefore possible that the folate binding

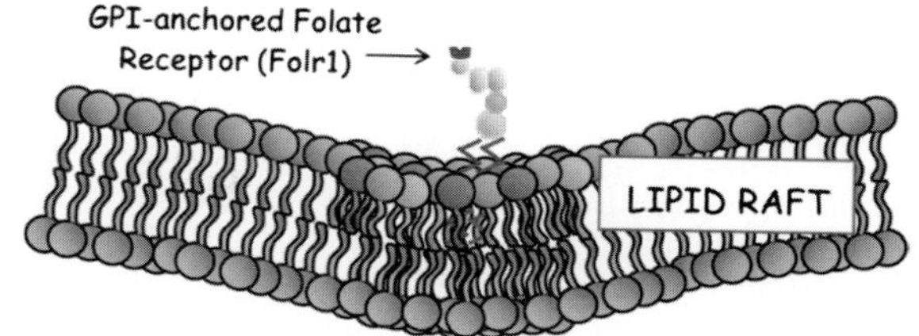

FIGURE 53.3 Murine folate binding protein 1 (Folr1) is homologous to the human folate receptor *alpha* (FRα). The glycosylphosphatidylinositol (GPI)-anchored Folr1 internalizes folate and is found in sphingolipid-enriched "lipid rafts" in the plasma membrane. Lipid rafts also coordinate protein–protein interactions involved in initiating signal transduction cascades and intracellular signaling.

protein is involved in signaling pathways for cell survival, proliferation or cytoskeleton activation that are necessary for normal neural tube closure (Miotti *et al.*, 2000; Elortza *et al.*, 2003; Foster *et al.*, 2003).

Epidemiological observations

The average NTD incidence in the general population of the USA is ≤3 per 10,000 live births but can be over 100 per 10,000 in some areas worldwide where maize is a diet staple (Marasas *et al.*, 2004). The epidemiological evidence that fumonisins increase NTD risk has been reviewed elsewhere (Marasas *et al.*, 2004; Gelineau-van Waes *et al.*, 2009). Briefly, the number of NTD-affected pregnancies doubled among Mexican-American women in the Texas–Mexico border region in 1990–1991, increasing from its average rate of about 15/10,000 to about 27/10,000 live births. An increase in ELEM cases and higher than usual fumonisin concentrations in locally grown maize were also noted in the same area. These observations pointed to the possibility that eating foods prepared from locally grown maize contributed to the "spike" in NTD-affected pregnancies. Other potential risk factors that could act alone or together with fumonisins were also identified. These included hyperthermia, diarrhea and stress (references cited in Voss *et al.*, 2006).

Further evidence was provided by a retrospective population-based case controlled study of the Texas–Mexico border region (Missmer *et al.*, 2006). The results suggested that there was an association between tortilla consumption in the first trimester of pregnancy and increased risk of a pregnancy ending with an NTD outcome. The dose–response followed an inverted U-shape, that is, the association with NTD increased as the number of tortillas eaten rose to 301 to 400 and diminished as consumption increased further. Fumonisin concentrations in the tortillas averaged 0.23 ppm and ranged from 0 to 1.69 ppm. Estimation of fumonisin exposure from tortilla consumption and fumonisin concentration data again revealed an inverted U-shaped response: the highest number of NTD cases was found in women exposed to 0.15 to 0.65 μg/kg body weight FB_1 per day. Finally, an association between NTD and postpartum maternal serum Sa/So ratios was also reported and the dose–response again followed the same inverted U-shaped pattern. Altogether, the findings inferred that NTD risk becomes greater as tortilla consumption (and fumonisin exposure) during the first trimester of pregnancy increases up to a critical point and then decreases due to increasing fetal death. An association between the frequency and amount of FB_1 detected in human urine and tortilla consumption has been independently reported (Gong *et al.*, 2008).

The retrospective nature of the study by Missmer *et al.* (2006) and other considerations require that the aforementioned interpretation be considered provisional. First, the analytical results might not have accurately reflected fumonisin concentrations in the tortillas at the time of consumption. This is especially important because the median exposures in women experiencing both NTD and normal pregnancy outcomes were below the provisional maximum tolerated daily intake of 2 μg/kg body weight (Bolger *et al.*, 2001), Second, little is known about how fumonisins affect sphingolipid metabolism or other biochemical or physiological processes in humans. Efforts to correlate serum or urine sphinganine concentrations or sphingoid base ratios with fumonisin exposures or disease outcomes have been largely unsuccessful (van der Westhuizen *et al.*, 2010). Elevated serum or tissue sphingoid base concentrations in animals are readily reversible upon cessation of exposure (Riley *et al.*, 1997; Voss *et al.* 1998, 2009; Enongene *et al.*, 2002), although elevated concentrations can persist if low-level (relative to the original exposure) fumonisin exposure continues (Wang *et al.*, 1999). This suggests that, unless exposures had remained constant over time, it cannot be concluded that the results of the retrospective epidemiological study correspond to the women's serum sphingoid base status during the time of neural tube closure. Additional studies to determine how fumonisins affect sphingoid bases in humans are a critical need.

In vitro induction of NTDs in mice

Cultured mouse embryos (harvested on E 9) were exposed long term (26 hours) or short term (2 hours) to FB_1 alone or in combination with folinic acid (Sadler *et al.*, 2002). In the long-term experiment, NTDs (exencephaly) were induced at ≥2 μM FB_1 and the incidence increased from 10% of treated embryos at 2 μM to 48% at 100 μM, the highest dose tested. No NTDs were induced at 1 μM; however, growth retardation was found at this and all higher doses. Hypoplasia of the frontonasal prominence was evident at all doses. Supplementation of the culture medium with 1 mM folinic acid partially reversed NTD induction: the percent of NTD-affected embryos dropped from 25 to 9 at 25 μM FB_1, from 27 to 8 at 50 μM FB_1 and from 48 to14 at 100 μM FB_1. Sa/So ratios of the embryos also increased at ≥25 μM FB_1. The ratio was unaffected by co-exposure to folinic acid.

Short-term exposure to 50 μM FB_1 caused NTDs in 67% of the fetuses, facial hypoplasia in 83%, and retarded growth. Folinic acid supplementation again lowered the incidence of embryos exhibiting NTDs (34%) or facial hypoplasia (43%). The results suggested that *in utero* exposure to FB_1 caused growth retardation and developmental abnormalities and further demonstrated that FB_1 inhibits folate uptake or utilization.

In vivo induction of NTDs

In vivo induction of NTDs by FB_1 was first reported by Gelineau-van Waes *et al.* (2005). Inbred LM/Bc mice were given intraperitoneal injections of 0, 5, 10, 15 or 20 mg/kg FB_1 on E 7.5 and E 8.5. As a result, the mean number of litters with at least one NTD-affected fetus rose from four at 5 mg/kg body weight to seven at 10 mg/kg body weight and to 10 at the two highest doses (Figures 53.4 and 53.5). The incidence of NTD-affected fetuses increased similarly from 5% at the lowest dose to 79% at the highest. Histological and ultrastructural evaluation of exencephalic embryos (ED 10.5) revealed that elevation of the neural folds had not occurred normally.

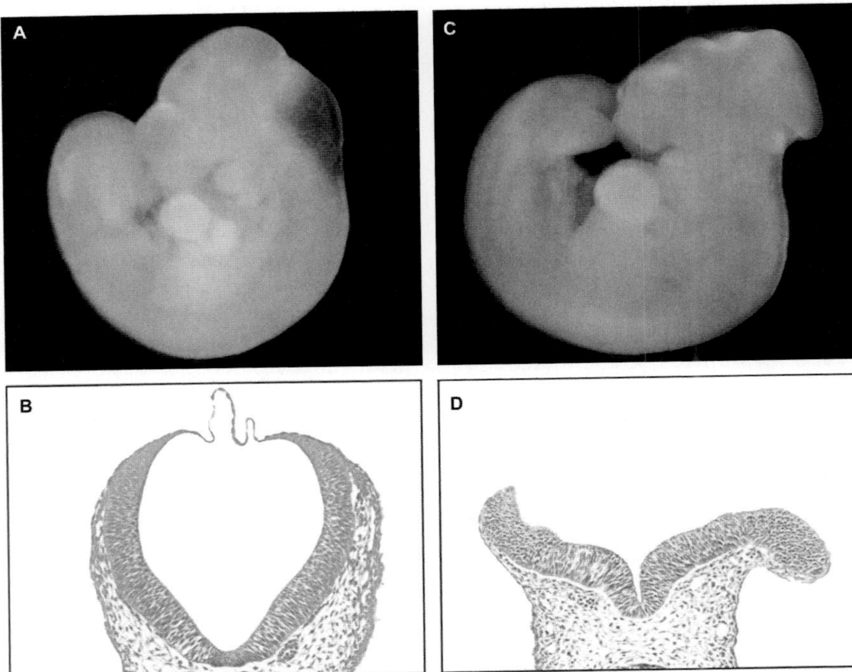

FIGURE 53.4 Gross appearance of normal (A) and exencephalic (C) LM/Bc fetuses, illustrating neural tube defect (NTD) induction effect of fumonisin B_1 when given to the dams on E 7.5 and E 8.5. Microscopic appearance of closed (B, normal fetus) and open neural tubes (D, exencephalic fetus) are also shown.

Administration of 50 mg/kg body weight folic acid (intraperitoneal injection) on E 0.5 through E 9.5 reduced the incidence of NTDs caused by 20 mg/kg body weight FB_1 from 79 to 50% (Figure 53.6). When 20 mg/kg FB_1 was given to dams that were also treated with the ganglioside GM1 (10 mg/kg body weight given by intraperitoneal injection on E 6.5 through E 9.5), only 5% of the fetuses had NTDs (Figure 53.6). Immunohistochemical studies demonstrated the co-localization of the GPI-anchored folate binding protein and GM1 in the neuroepithelium and yolk sac membranes as well as depletion of the folate binding protein in mice exposed to FB_1.

Two likely explanations for the differing results of the experiments in LM/Bc (Gelineau-van Waes *et al.*, 2005) and CD1 mice (Reddy *et al.*, 1996) were the significant differences in the exposure regimens, including both the dose level and route of administration, and possible genetic–physiological differences between the LM/Bc and CD1 mouse strains. The latter possibility was tested by giving 0 (vehicle controls), 15, 30 or 45 mg/kg body weight FB_1 by intraperitoneal injection to pregnant CD1 mice on ED 7 and ED 8 (Voss *et al.*, 2007). Additional groups were given 0, 10, 23, 45 or 100 mg/kg body weight FB_1 in a second trial. Maternal body weights, corpora lutea counts and total implant counts were not adversely affected. There are no statistically significant effects on resorption or live fetus counts in the first series of doses (15 to 45 mg/kg body weight FB_1) although the number of resorptions/dam at 45 mg/kg body weight was increased three-fold (2.4; control value = 0.8). Furthermore, the number of live fetuses/dam was 22 to 36% lower at 45 mg/kg body weight than in the other groups: average live fetus counts were 11.2, 12.3, 13.6 and 8.7 at 0, 15, 30 and 45 mg/kg body weight, respectively. Average weights of the (live) high dose fetuses were also reduced by about 15%. NTDs (exencephaly) occurred in one of nine low dose and four of 10 high dose litters (Figure 53.5). The incidences of NTD per affected low and high dose litter were 10 and 16%, respectively.

Fetotoxicity and a dose-related increase in NTDs (Figure 53.5) were also induced by FB_1 in the second dosing series. Average resorption counts/dam increased from 0.83 in the vehicle control group, to 3.0 at 45 mg/kg body weight (not significantly different from the controls) to 8.0 at 100 mg/kg body weight (significantly different, $p < 0.05$, from groups given ≤23 mg/kg body weight). Conversely, the average number of live fetuses/litter (6.2) at 100 mg/kg body weight was significantly lower than in the other groups (10.4 to 11.8). No NTDs were found in the vehicle controls but at least one litter in each of the treated groups had one or more NTD-positive fetuses. Both the number of affected litters and the incidence of exencephalic fetuses in affected litters increased in a dose-dependent manner. The percentages of affected litters were: 8, 17, 36 and 55% at the respective doses of 10, 23, 45 and 100 mg/kg body weight FB_1 (Figure 53.5). The respective percentages of NTD-positive fetuses per affected litter were 8, 23, 15 and 41%. Results from the two trials were consistent as shown by the similar percentages of NTD-affected litters (36–40%) and fetuses (15–16%) found at 45 mg/kg body weight. NTD induction in mice using the intraperitoneal dosing protocol (Gelineau-van Waes *et al.*, 2005) is therefore not limited to the LM/Bc strain, although the latter is clearly more sensitive than CD1 mice (Figure 53.5).

While the studies of Gelineau-van Waes *et al.* (2005), Sadler *et al.* (2002) and Voss *et al.* (2007) demonstrated the ability of FB_1 to cause NTDs in mice, the relevance of these findings to humans is uncertain because of the dosing route, the relatively high exposure levels as well as *in vivo* evidence indicating that fumonisins do not cross the placental barrier of rats, mice and rabbits (Reddy *et al.*, 1996; Voss *et al.*, 1996; LaBorde *et al.*, 1997; Collins *et al.*, 1998a,b) after oral exposure. Intraperitoneal injection of 5 mg/kg body weight FB_1, the lowest dose inducing NTD in LM/Bc mice (Gelineau-van Waes *et al.*, 2005), would have provided a dose roughly equivalent to 300 ppm in the diet, assuming gastrointestinal absorption was about 5% (Martinez-Larranaga *et al.* [1999] calculated absorption in orally dosed rats to be 3.5%). A dietary FB_1 concentration of 300 ppm is well above the no-observed-adverse-effect level (NOAEL) of 27 ppm and the lowest-observed-adverse-effect level (LOAEL) of 81 ppm established for female mice in a 90-day feeding study (Voss *et al.*, 1995). However, oral doses of 20 mg/kg body weight FB_1 given to LM/Bc dams on E 7.5–8.5 by gavage induced a 20% incidence of NTDs (Gelineau-van Waes *et al.*, 2005). This dose roughly corresponded to a dietary concentration of 100 ppm FB_1 and is therefore only slightly above the LOAEL.

There are only a few feeding studies on the potential reproductive and developmental toxicity of fumonisins, all of which used *F. verticillioides* culture materials as the fumonisin

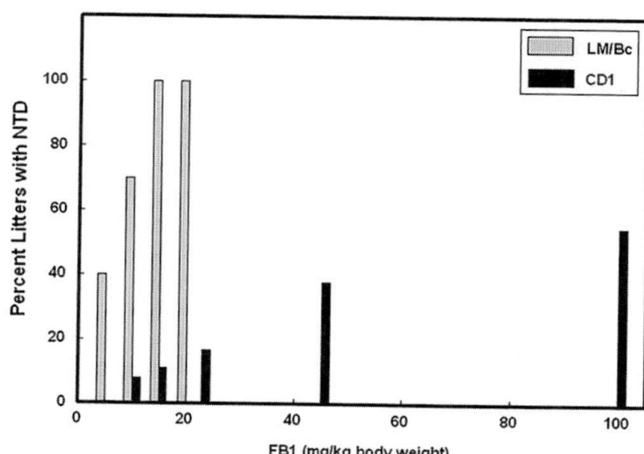

FIGURE 53.5 Dose–response for neural tube defect (NTD) induction by fumonisin B_1 (FB_1) given intraperitoneally to LM/Bc (E 7.5, 8.50) or CD1 (E 7, 8) dams. Bars indicate the percent of litters having at least one NTD (exencephaly)-affected fetus. Adopted from Gelineau-van Waes *et al.* (2005) and Voss *et al.* (2007).

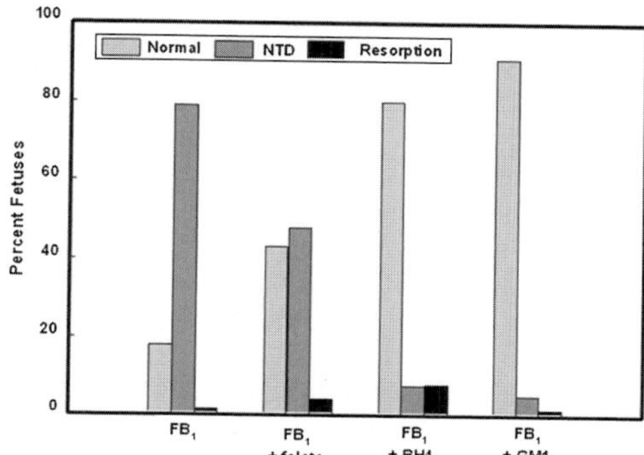

FIGURE 53.6 Protective effect against fumonisin B_1 (FB_1)-induced neural tube defects (NTD) by intraperitoneal injection of folate (50 mg/kg body weight/day, E 0.5–9.5), tetrahydrobiopterin (BH4) (25 mg/kg body weight/day, E 6.5–E9.5) or the complex sphingolipid GM1 (10 mg/kg body weight/day, E 6.5–9.5). Bars denote the percent of fetuses that are phenotypically normal or have NTDs.

source. Male and female rats were continuously fed diets containing up to 55 ppm FB_1 beginning 9 or 2 weeks, respectively, prior to mating. The high dose induced mild maternal toxicity but had no affect on reproductive performance. Sphingoid base and biodistribution studies utilizing radiolabeled FB_1 administered on E 15 indicated that the placenta provided a barrier that prevented *in utero* exposure. However, because placental transfer was evaluated at the end of organogenesis, the possibility that *in utero* exposure occurred earlier should not be ruled out.

LM/Bc and CD1 female mice were fed diets amended with *F. verticillioides* culture material to provide 50 or 150 ppm FB_1 beginning 5 weeks before mating to unexposed males. Dietary exposure continued until the females and their embryos were examined after the conclusion of organogenesis (E 16) (Voss *et al.*, 2006). The high dose diet was mildly hepatotoxic to dams of both strains while no evidence of hepatotoxicity was found at the low dose. The test diets had no effect on overall reproductive performance within each strain. Nonetheless, one of five high dose LM/Bc litters exhibited a 10% incidence of exencephaly. No NTDs were found in CD1 offspring; however, in further contrast to the LM/Bc strain, about 20% of the high dose CD1 litters exhibited elevated fetal death rates of 40 to 70%.

Analysis of fetal livers for sphinganine (Sa) and its Sa 1-phosphate metabolite revealed significantly higher values (more than double those of the controls) only in high dose LM/Bc fetuses. This not only showed that the LM/Bc fetuses were exposed *in utero*, it also confirmed that fumonisins penetrate the placental barrier of LM/Bc mice as was preliminarily shown by the recovery of radiolabel from the embryos of LM/Bc dams injected with $[^{14}C]FB_1$ on E 10.5 (Gelineau-van Waes *et al.*, 2005).

The feeding study was repeated using LM/Bc mice only and experimental diets with 150 or 300 ppm FB_1. While no differences in mean litter weights were found, the diets elicited dose-related trends toward more resorptions and fewer live fetuses per litter. Resorption rates rose from 18% in the controls to 40% at the mid-dose to 52% at the high dose. In contrast to the first feeding study no NTDs were found. Possible explanations for the absence of NTDs in the second study are:

1. The NTD was spontaneous and unrelated to exposure although this seems unlikely as spontaneous NTDs have not been observed in litters of unexposed females.
2. NTDs can be induced by dietary exposure but the slope of the dose–response curve might be low (<1 to <<1). In this case, NTDs would not be consistently found at the lower end of the curve and, accordingly, many additional experimental replicates would be needed to establish the NOAEL. Daily FB_1 intake of dams at 150 ppm FB_1 in the first study was about 25 mg/kg body weight. Assuming gastrointestinal absorption in mice was about 5% or less, internal exposure would have been around 1 mg/kg body weight. Internal exposure in high dose dams from the second study (fed 300 ppm FB_1) would have been higher but still well below the lowest intraperitoneal dose (5 mg/kg body weight) of FB_1 that induced NTDs in LM/Bc mice (Gelineau-van Waes *et al.*, 2005). Daily intakes of 25 mg/kg body weight (first feeding study, high dose group) were only slightly higher than the 20 mg/kg body weight oral dose (gavage) that induced NTDs although gastrointestinal absorption was likely less rapid and peak serum FB_1 concentrations were likely lower when the mycotoxin was given in the diet.
3. The extent to which the culture material added folate, complex sphingolipids or other antagonistic (to FB_1) compounds to the experimental diets is unknown and warrants investigation.
4. Mice might adapt to exposure in one or more ways including up- or downregulation of genes involved in ceramide or complex sphingolipid metabolism, folate uptake and utilization, or signaling pathways to enhance tissue repair. In this regard, six mammalian ceramide synthase genes (CerS1 through CerS6) have been identified (Levy and Futerman, 2010). They differ in their affinities for fatty acids of different chain lengths but at least one gene product, Cers1, showed resistance to inhibition by FB_1 when it was overexpressed in human embryonic kidney cells (Venkataraman *et al.*, 2002). It could be speculated that upregulating the activity of CerS1 or another metabolic pathway could offer some degree of protection against fumonisins.

Additional mechanistic considerations

Nitric oxide (NO) is produced inside cells from L-arginine and O_2. The reaction is catalyzed by one or more nitric oxide synthases (NOS) (Andrew and Mayer, 1999; Mungrue *et al.*, 2003) (Figure 53.7) including endothelial (eNOS), neuronal (nNOS) and inducible (iNOS), three distinct and variably expressed gene products. NO is a signaling molecule that is involved in controlling a spectrum of cellular functions. NOS enzymes have binding sites for L-arginine and

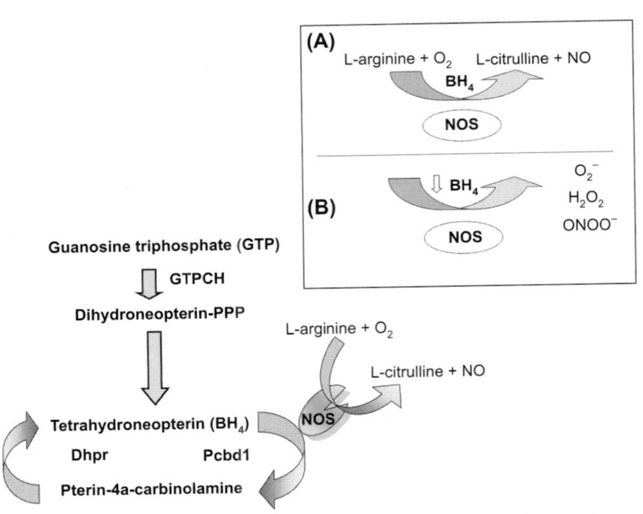

FIGURE 53.7 Simplified depiction of the biosynthetic and salvage pathways for tetrahydrobiopterin. It is synthesized from guanosine triphosphate (first step in the pathway mediated by guanosine triphosphate cyclohydrolase (GTPCH)). Tetrahydrobiopterin is converted to pterin-4a-carbinolamine by pterin-4a-carbinolamine dehydratase (Pcbd1) in a reaction coupled with the synthesis of nitric oxide (NO) and then salvaged in a reaction mediated by dihydropterin reductase (Dhpr). During NO synthesis from L-arginine and O_2 by nitric oxide synthase (NOS) enzymes, tetrahydrobiopterin (BH4) serves as a co-factor for NOS (A). If BH4 levels become limiting (B), NOS becomes "uncoupled" so that NADPH (cofactor for NOS) donates electrons to O_2 rather than L-arginine, leading to production of superoxide, hydrogen peroxide, and/or peroxynitrite and, consequently, oxidative damage in cells.

tetrahydrobiopterin (BH4), as well as for FMN, FAD and NADPH cofactors. BH4 is structurally related to folate and is an essential co-factor for NOS enzymes and NO production (Thony *et al.*, 2000). The *de novo* biosynthesis of BH4 initially involves conversion of guanosine triphosphate (GTP) to 7,8-dihydroneopterin by GTP cyclohydrolase (GTPCH). The 7,8-dihydroneopterin is in turn converted through a series of metabolic steps to BH4 (Figure 53.7). BH4, like folic acid, contains a pteridine moiety and it is predicted on the basis of its structural similarity to 5-methyltetrahydrofolic acid (MTHF) that BH4 can bind the active site of NOS (Hyndman *et al.*, 2002).

BH4 biosynthesis and GTPCH expression have been demonstrated in neural crest cells during early development (Pelletier *et al.*, 2001). BH4 is critical for NOS activity in that it maintains NOS as an NO, rather than superoxide-producing, enzyme (Thony *et al.*, 2000) (Figure 53.7). When BH4 levels are reduced to some critical level, NOS function becomes "uncoupled" so that electrons from NADPH are donated to O_2 rather than to L-arginine. In this uncoupled state, superoxide, hydrogen peroxide and/or peroxynitrite are produced instead of NO, leading to oxidative stress (Vasquez-Vivar *et al.*, 1998; Xia *et al.*, 1998) (Figure 53.7). Coordination of cell cycle progression, mitosis and apoptosis is essential for neural tube closure. In this regard, NOS is constitutively expressed in neuroepithelium during and after neural tube closure and high NO levels trigger entry into S phase and low NO levels facilitate mitosis (Traister *et al.*, 2002). Proper neural tube closure is therefore dependent on NOS activity and its product, NO, affects the critical balance between cell proliferation and apoptosis in the developing neural tube. In this regard, it is important that NOS activity depends upon the availability of endogenous BH4 and extracellular folate (Plachta *et al.*, 2003) and it is possible that fumonisins might indirectly interfere with neural tube closure by disruption of NO homeostasis via a chain of events involving ceramide synthase inhibition, complex sphingolipid depletion, and impaired folate uptake and utilization.

Oxidative stress might also contribute to fumonisin's effects on neural tube closure in mice. *In vitro* and *in vivo* experiments have shown induction of oxidative stress, lipid peroxidation and reduced glutathione by fumonisin exposure (Abel and Gelderblom, 1998; Stockmann-Juvala *et al.*, 2004a,b) and maternal or fetal oxidative stress has been associated with increasing NTD risk in animals (Wells *et al.*, 2005; Yan and Hales, 2006) and humans (Zhao *et al.*, 2006). Oxidative stress related to dietary deficiencies of folate or other antioxidants or diabetes (the effects of diabetes include uncoupling of NOS) are also associated with increased risks of congenital malformation. Tumor necrosis factor α (TNFα) is a multifunctional cytokine that has both pro- and anti-apoptotic properties. Experiments have shown that it modifies the severity of liver injury in fumonisin-exposed mice (Sharma *et al.*, 2002). Expression of iNOS is elicited by TNFα in response to proinflammatory stimuli (Ciesielska *et al.*, 2003; Marion *et al.*, 2003; Serbina *et al.*, 2003) and dose-dependent stimulation of NO production related to enhanced expression of iNOS (Meli *et al.*, 2000) has been observed in response to fumonisin treatment (Rotter and Oh, 1996; Dresden-Osborne and Noblet, 2002).

In addition to inducing iNOS expression, TNFα increases expression of GTPCH (Hukkanen *et al.*, 2003). Upregulation involves generation of intracellular sphingosine-1-phosphate (So 1-P) by sphingosine kinase (Vann *et al.*, 2000, 2002; Spiegel and Milstien, 2003). Basal GTPCH activity and BH4 production are inadequate for optimal iNOS function, meaning that GTPCH induction by cytokines such as TNFα is needed to prevent oxidative stress secondary to uncoupling of the iNOS enzyme (Huang *et al.*, 2005; Peterson and Katusic, 2005).

In summary, induction of NTDs in mice by FB_1 involves multiple interrelated metabolic pathways including ceramide and complex sphingolipid biosynthesis as well as those involving folate, tetrahydrobiopterin and NO (Figure 53.7). These pathways are influenced by cytokines such as TNFα which, in turn, are affected by fumonisin exposure. NTD induction by FB_1 is antagonized by co-exposure to folate, GM1 and tetrahydrobiopterin (Figure 53.7). GM1 has shown the greatest protective effect against NTD induction, presumably by compensating for the loss of complex sphingolipids that result from FB_1 inhibition of ceramide synthase and which in turn lead to reduced folate uptake and utilization.

Hydrolyzed FB1 (HFB1) and NTDs

Hydrolyzed fumonisin is produced during the cooking and steeping of fumonisin-contaminated maize in alkaline water. This process, known as nixtamalization, is used to make masa, tortillas and other foods that are popular in some areas in which NTD incidences are high such as Mexico and Central America, as well as among Hispanic Americans in the USA. Popular snack foods are also made from alkaline cooked maize. During cooking and steeping, fumonisin concentrations are reduced by a combination of extraction into the liquid, conversion to their hydrolyzed forms, or other means such as thermal decomposition or binding to maize matrix components (Humpf and Voss, 2004). Alkaline cooked products contain variable amounts of hydrolyzed fumonisins meaning that it is likely that pregnant women will be exposed to them from time to time.

To study NTD induction potential, cultured rat embryos (E 9.5) were exposed for 45 hours to graded concentrations ranging from 3 to 300 μM HFB_1 (Flynn *et al.*, 1997). Developmental retardation and anomalies occurred at doses ≥100 μM. Twenty-nine percent of the fetuses at 100 μM and 15% at 300 μM had NTDs and other abnormalities were found in 36 and 85% of the fetuses in these two groups, respectively. HFB_1 was therefore about 100-fold less toxic than FB_1 (Flynn *et al.*, 1996) when tested using this experimental model.

Pregnant LM/Bc mice were given doses of HFB_1 ranging from 2.5 to 20 mg/kg body weight on E 7 and E 8 by intraperitoneal injection (Voss *et. al.*, 2009). Vehicle control and positive control (10 mg/kg body weight FB_1) groups were included in the study and as previously shown (Gelineau-van Waes *et al.*, 2005); FB_1 caused a high incidence of fetal mortality and NTDs. It also caused a marked disruption of sphingolipid metabolism in the dams leading to a reduction of complex sphingolipids in maternal liver. In contrast, HFB_1 elicited no adverse effects on fetal development at any dose level. Only minimal changes in the concentrations of sphingoid bases or complex sphingolipids were found in the livers of the dams exposed to the highest dose of 20 mg/kg body weight HFB_1, which is seven-fold greater than the LOAEL for NTD induction by FB_1 in the LM/Bc mouse model (a NOAEL has not been found). Together the *in vivo* (Voss *et al.*, 2009) and *in vitro* findings (Flynn *et al.*, 1997) signify that HFB_1 is not a significant risk factor for NTD.

EFFECT OF COOKING

It is important to understand how thermal processing affects fumonisins during the preparation of maize-based foods that are consumed in large amounts by people likely to be at risk for fumonisin-related health effects. Fumonisins are considered heat stable, although variable amounts of fumonisin "loss" during baking, frying and other cooking processes have been demonstrated (Humpf and Voss, 2004). The amount of "loss" depends upon temperature, cooking time, recipe and other conditions; however, in many cases the reductions are insufficient to meaningfully reduce exposure. For example, fumonisin concentrations were reduced only about 23% in South African stiff porridge prepared from commercially purchased maize meal, and lesser reductions occurred during the preparation of Indian porridge or polenta in Italy (Shephard *et al.*, 2002 and references therein).

Nixtamalization

The effect of alkaline cooking of maize, known as nixtamalization, is of particular interest. This is because alkaline cooked, maize-based foods are consumed in large amounts in Mexico, Central America and among Hispanics in the USA, and because an association between tortilla consumption and NTD risk has been observed (Marasas *et al.*, 2004; Missmer *et al.*, 2006; Gelineau-van Waes *et al.*, 2009). Nixtamalization reduces fumonisin concentrations in the masa or tortilla products from 50 to 80%. Reduction occurs as a combination of extraction into the aqueous cooking/steeping liquid (which is subsequently discarded), conversion to less toxic hydrolyzed forms (Humpf and Voss *et al.*, 2004; Voss *et al.*, 2009), and possibly by binding to the maize matrix.

Reaction with reducing sugars

Fumonisins react with reducing sugars to form products (Humpf and Voss, 2004) that exhibit reduced toxicity when fed to swine (Fernandez-Surumay *et al.*, 2005) or rats (Liu *et al.*, 2001). Binding of the sugar to the primary amine function of FB_1 forms *N*-substituted compounds including *N*-(1-deoxyfructos-1-yl) FB_1 (Poling *et al.*, 2002) and *N*-carboxymethyl FB_1 (Howard *et al.*, 2002), resulting in detoxification. Extrusion cooking combined with glucose supplementation has shown promise as a method for significantly reducing fumonisin concentrations (Bullerman *et al.*, 2008) and toxicity (Voss *et al.*, 2008, 2010). However, the chemical fate of all fumonisins in the uncooked material could not be accounted for after extrusion, suggesting that unknown decomposition or binding products were formed.

Hidden or matrix-bound fumonisins

Emerging evidence indicates that maize and cooked foods can contain so-called "masked", "hidden" or "matrix-bound" fumonisins which are not detected by conventional analyses (Dall'Asta *et al.*, 2009). This was first demonstrated by Kim *et al.* (2003), who reported the recovery of two to three times more bound than free (defined as those fumonisins quantified by conventional means) fumonisins in maize flake cereal. Significant amounts of bound fumonisins have also been found in alkaline cooked products (Humpf and Voss, 2004; Park *et al.*, 2004). The chemical nature of hidden or matrix-bound fumonisins has not been determined but model experiments suggest that when fumonisins are heated, their tricarballylic acid side chains can bind to starch or protein (Humpf and Voss, 2004). Accordingly, four potential outcomes during digestion are possible: (1) release and bioavailability of the parent fumonisin; (2) release and bioavailability of the less toxic hydrolyzed (or partially hydrolyzed) fumonisins; (3) absorption of the intact fumonisins–matrix product; and (4) fecal excretion of the unabsorbed, stable fumonisin–matrix binding product. Indirect evidence infers that fumonisin–maize matrix binding acts to detoxify the mycotoxin. Specifically, fumonisin B_1 concentration and *in vivo* toxicity of *F. verticillioides* culture material to rats were significantly reduced when the culture material was mixed with ground maize prior to alkaline cooking. Nixtamalizing the culture material in the absence of ground maize resulted in a lesser reduction in concentration and only modestly protected against toxicity (Burns *et al.*, 2008).

It remains unknown if the hidden fumonisins found in commercial food products by Kim *et al.* (2003), Park *et al.* (2004) and others (Humpf and Voss, 2004) originated in the raw maize or formed during cooking but it is likely that hidden fumonisins might occur extensively in uncooked maize. This supposition is based on the results of hydrolysis and simulated digestion experiments which revealed that up to about 63% of the total fumonisins in raw maize consisted of hidden forms (Dall'Asta *et al.*, 2009; Motta and Scott, 2009). These "hidden" or matrix-bound fumonisins are problematic because routine analytical procedures detect only free fumonisins and would thereby underestimate the contributions and bioavailability of "hidden" or matrix-bound fumonisins to exposure (Humpf and Voss, 2004; Dall'Aste *et al.*, 2009).

RISK ASSESSMENT AND REGULATORY ACTION

Fumonisin B_1 has been designated as a possible human carcinogen (Group 2B) by the International Agency for Research on Cancer (2001). This signifies that there is sufficient evidence for carcinogenicity in experimental animals but insufficient evidence for carcinogenicity in humans. A provisional maximum tolerated daily intake for fumonisin B_1 of 2 μg/kg body weight has been set by the WHO Joint Expert Committee on Food Additives (JECFA) (Bolger *et al.*, 2001).

The US Food and Drug Administration (Center for Food Safety and Nutrition, 2001) issued an Industry Guidance for fumonisins (sum of fumonisins $B_1+B_2+B_3$) ranging from 2 (degermed dry milled products, fat content <2.25%) to 4 ppm (maize for masa production or whole or partially degermed dry milled products). The maximum allowable fumonisin levels (sum of fumonisins B_1+B_2) in maize and maize products for human consumption set by the Commission of European Communities (2007) range from 0.2 (infant and baby foods) to 1 (maize or maize-based food for direct human consumption) ppm.

CONCLUDING REMARKS AND FUTURE DIRECTIONS

Much has been learned about the general toxicity and carcinogenicity of fumonisins in animals; however, their impact on human health remains unclear. Fumonisin B_1 and other congeners clearly inhibit ceramide synthase and the subsequent disruption of sphingolipid metabolism and function underlies most, if not all, of its toxic, carcinogenic and reproductive effects in animals. The sequence of mechanistic events linking enzyme inhibition to specific toxicities and their relevance for humans remains elusive. The suspicion that fumonisins are a risk factor for NTDs was, like the putative relationship between this mycotoxin and esophageal cancer, initially based on circumstantial and epidemiological observations. NTD etiology is complex and influenced by genetic, environmental and nutritional considerations and, in this regard, there is emerging evidence that fumonisins might be an environmental factor that increases NTD risk in populations heavily dependent on maize as a food staple. This evidence includes *in vivo* induction of NTDs in mice, inhibition of folate uptake and utilization by FB_1 *in vitro* and *in* vivo, and protection against NTD induction in FB_1-exposed mice by folate or the complex sphingolipid GM1. Investigations including epidemiological studies on the relationship between fumonisins exposure and NTD incidence, mechanistic comparisons between sensitive and insensitive animal species and strains, and initiatives to determine the extent to which fumonisins affect sphingolipid metabolism in humans are needed to better understand the extent to which these common mycotoxins found in maize are risk factors for NTD or other birth defects in humans.

REFERENCES

Abel S, Gelderblom WC (1998) Oxidative damage and fumonisin B1-induced toxicity in primary rat hepatocytes and rat liver in vivo. *Toxicology* **131:** 121–31.

Andrew P, Mayer B (1999) Enzymatic function of nitric oxide synthases. *Cardiovasc Res* **43:** 521–31.

Bartók T, Tolgyesi L, Szekeres A, Varga M, Bartha R, Scécsi A, Bartók M, Mesterházy A (2010) Detection and characterization of twenty-eight isomers of fumonisin B_1 (FB_1) mycotoxin in a solid rice culture infected with *Fusarium verticillioides* by reversed-phase high-performance liquid chromatography/electron spray ionization time-of-flight and ion trap mass spectrometry. *Rapid Commun Mass Spectrom* **24:** 35–42.

Bolger M, Coker RD, Dinovi M, Gaylor D, Gelderblom WCA, Paster N, Riley RT, Shephard G, Speijers JA (2001) Fumonisins. In *Safety Evaluation of Certain Mycotoxins in Food (World Health Organization Food Additive Series 47)*. World Health Organization, Geneva. pp. 103–279.

Bullerman LB, Bianchini A, Hanna MA, Jackson LS, Jablonshi J, Ryu D (2008) Reduction of fumonisin B_1 in corn grits by single-screw extrusion. *J Agr Food Chem* **56:** 2400–5.

Burger HM, Abel S, Snijman PW, Swanevelder S, Gelderblom WC (2007) Altered lipid parameters in hepatic subcellular membrane fraction induced by fumonisin B_1. *Lipids* **42:** 249–61.

Burns TD, Snook ME, Riley RT, Voss KA (2008) Fumonisin concentrations and *in vivo* toxicity of nixtamalized *Fusarium verticillioides* culture material: evidence for fumonisin–matrix interactions. *Food Chem Toxicol* **46:** 2841–8.

Burton KE, Steele FM, Jefferies L, Pike OA, Dunn ML (2008) Effect of micronutrient fortification on nutritional and other properties of nixtamal tortillas. *Cereal Chem* **85:** 70–5.

Cárdenas JDF, Godinez MGA, Méndez NLV, Guzmán AL, Acosta LMF, González-Hernández J (2001) Fortificacion y evaluacion de tortillas de nixtamal. *Archivos Latinoamericanos de Nutrición* **51:** 293–302.

Center for Food Safety and Nutrition, US Food and Drug Administration (2001) Background Paper in Support of Fumonisin Levels in Animal Feed: Executive Summary of this Scientific Document (November 9, 2001). http://www.cfsan.fda.gov/~dms/fumonbg4.html

Chang WJ, Rothberg KG, Kamen BA, Anderson RG (1992) Lowering the cholesterol content of MA104 cells inhibits receptor-mediated transport of folate. *J Cell Biol* **118:** 63–9.

Ciesielska A, Joniec I, Przybylkowski A, Gromadzka G, Kurkowska-Jastrzebska I, Czlonkowska A, Czlonkowski A (2003) Dynamics of expression of the mRNA for cytokines and inducible nitric synthase in a murine model of the Parkinson's disease. *Acta Neurobiologiae Experimentalis (Wars)* **63:** 117–26.

Collins TF, Shackelford ME, Sprando RL, Black TN, Laborde JB, Hansen DK, Eppley RM, Trucksess MW, Howard PC, Bryant MA, Ruggles DI, Olejnik N, Rorie JI (1988a) Effects of fumonisin B_1 in pregnant rats. *Food Chem Toxicol* **36:** 397–408.

Collins TF, Sprando RL, Black TN, Shackelford ME, Laborde JB, Hansen DK, Eppley, RM, Trucksess MW, Howard PC, Bryant MA, Ruggles DI, Olejnik N, Rorie JI (1998b) Effects of fumonisin B_1 in pregnant rats: Part 2. *Food Chem Toxicol* **36:** 673–85.

Commission of European Communities (2007) Commission regulation (EC) No 1126/2007 of 28 September 2007 amending Regulation (EC) No. 1881/2006 setting maximum levels for certain contaminants in foodstuffs as regards *Fusarium* in maize and maize products. *Official J Europ Union* 29.9.2007, L255/14.

Constable PD, Smith GW, Rottinghaus GE, Tumbleson ME, Haschek WM (2003) Fumonisin-induced blockade of ceramide synthase in sphingolipid biosynthetic pathway alters aortic input impedence spectrum of pigs. *Am J Physiol – Heart Circ Physiol* **284:** H2034–H2044.

Dall'Asta C, Mangla M, Berthiller F, Molinelli A, Sulyok M, Schuhmacher R, Krska R, Galaverna G, Dossena A, Mitchell R (2009) Difficulties in fumonisin determination: the issue of hidden fumonisins. *Analy Bioanal Chem* **395:** 1335–46.

Dresden-Osborne C, Noblet GP (2002) Fumonisin B_1 affects viability and alters nitric oxide production of a murine macrophage cell line. *Int Immunopharmacol* **2:** 1087–93.

Eaton DL, Beima KM, Bammler TK (in press) Hepatotoxic mycotoxins. In *Comprehensive Toxicology*, 2nd edition (Roth RA, Ganey PE, eds.). Elsevier, New York.

Elortza F, Nuhse TS, Foster LJ, Stensballe A, Peck SC, Jensen ON (2003) Proteomic analysis of glycosylphosphatidylinositol-anchored membrane proteins. *Mol Cell Proteomics* **2:** 1261–70.

Enongene EN, Sharma RP, Bhandari N, Miller JD, Meredith FI, Voss KA, Riley RT (2002) Persistence and reversibility of the elevation in free sphingoid bases induced by fumonisin inhibition of ceramide synthase. *Toxicol Sci* **67:** 173–81.

Fernandez-Surumay G, Osweiler GD, Yaeger MJ, Rottinghaus GE, Hendrich S, Buckley LK, Murphy PA (2005) Fumonisin B-glucose reaction products are less toxic when fed to swine. *J Agr Food Chem* **18:** 4264–71.

Floss A, Casteel SW, Johnson GC, Rottinghaus GE, Krause GF (1994a) Developmental toxicity in hamsters of an aqueous extract of *Fusarium moniliforme* culture material containing known quantities of fumonisin B_1. *Vet Hum Toxicol* **36:** 5–10.

Floss A, Casteel SW, Johnson GC, Rottinghaus GE, Krause GF (1994b) Developmental toxicity of fumonisin in Syrian hamsters. *Mycopathologia* **128:** 33–8.

Flynn TJ, Pritchard D, Bradlaw JA, Eppley R, Page S (1996) *In vitro* embryotoxicity of fumonisin B_1 evaluated with cultured postimplantation staged embryos. *Toxicol in Vitro* **9:** 271–9.

Flynn TJ, Stack ME, Troy AL, Chirtal SJ (1997) Assessment of the embryotoxic potential of the total hydrolysis product of fumonisin B_1 using organogenesis staged rat embryos. *Food Chem Toxicol* **35:** 1135–41.

Foreman JH, Constable PD, Waggoner AL, Levy M, Eppley RM, Smith GW, Tumbleson ME, Haschek WM (2004) Neurologic abnormalities and cerebrospinal fluid changes in horses administered fumonisin B_1 intravenously. *J Vet Intern Med* **18:** 223–30.

Foster LJ, De Hoog CL, Mann M (2003) Unbiased quantitative proteomics of lipid rafts reveals high specificity for signaling factors. *Proc Natl Acad Sci USA* **100:** 5813–8.

Gelderblom WCA, Jaskiewicz K, Marasas WFO, Thiel PG, Horak RM, Vleggaar R, Kriek NP (1988) Fumonisins – novel mycotoxins with cancer promoting activity produced by *Fusarium moniliforme. Appl Environ Microbiol* **54:** 1806–11.

Gelderblom WC, Kriek NP, Marasas WF, Thiel PG (1991) Toxicity and carcinogenicity of the *Fusarium moniiliforme* metabolite, fumonisin B_1, in rats. *Carcinogenesis* **12:** 1247–51.

Gelderblom WC, Sewram V, Shephard GS, Snijman PW, Tenza K, van der Westhuizen L, Vleggaar R (2007) Structure and natural occurrence of sterioisomers of the fumonisin B series mycotoxins. *J Agr Food Chem* **55:** 4388–94.

Gelineau-van Waes JB, Starr L, Maddox JR, Aleman F, Voss KA, Wilberding J, Riley RT (2005) Maternal fumonisin exposure and risk for neural tube defects: mechanisms in an *in vivo* mouse model. *Birth Defects Res (Part A): Clin Mol Teratol* **73:** 487–97.

Gelineau-van Waes JB, Voss KA, Stevens VL, Speer MC, Riley RT (2009) Chapter 5: maternal fumonisin exposure as a risk factor for neural tube defects. *Adv Food Nutr Res* **56:** 145–81.

Gong YY, Torres-Sanchez L, Lopez-Carrillo L, Peng JH, Sulcliffe AE, While KL, Humpf HU, Turner PC, Wild CP (2008) Association between tortilla consumption and human urinary fumonisin B_1 levels in a Mexican population. *Cancer Epidemiol, Biomar Prev* **17:** 688–94.

Harrison LF, Colvin BM, Greene JT, Newman LE, Cole JR Jr (1990) Pulmonary edema and hydrothorax in swine produced by fumonisin B_1, a toxic metabolite of *Fusarium moniliforme*. *J Vet Diagn Invest* **2:** 217–21.

Haschek WM, Voss KA, Beasley VR (2002) Selected mycotoxins affecting animal and human health. In *Handbook of Toxicologic Pathology*, 2nd edition, Volume I (Haschek WM, Rousseaux CG, Wallig MA, eds.) Academic Press, San Diego, pp. 645–99.

Howard PC, Couch LH, Patton RE, Eppley RM, Doerge DM, Churchwell MI, Marques MM, Okerberg CV (2002) Comparison of the toxicity of several fumonisin derivatives in a 28-day feeding study with female $B6C3F_1$ mice. *Toxicol Appl Pharmacol* **185:** 153–65.

Howard PC, Eppley RM, Stack ME, Warbritton A, Voss KA, Lorentzen RJ, Kovach RM, Bucci TJ (2001) Fumonisin B_1 carcinogenicity in a two-year feeding study using F344 rats and B6C3F1 mice. *Environ Health Perspect* **109 (Suppl. 2):** 277–82.

Huang A, Zhang YY, Chen K, Hatakeyama K. Keaney JF Jr (2005) Cytokine-stimulated GTP cyclohydrolase I expression in endothelial cells requires coordinated activation of nuclear factor-kappaB and Stat1/Stat3. *Circ Res* **96:** 164–71.

Hukkanen M, Platts LA, Haralambous S, Ainola M, Konttinen YT, Kollias G, Polak JM (2003) Induction of inducible nitric oxide synthase, argininosuccinate synthase, and GTP cyclohydrolase I in arthritic joints of human tumor necrosis factor-alpha transgenic mice. *J Rheumatol* **30:** 652–9.

Humpf H-U, Voss KA (2004) Effects of food processing on the chemical structure and toxicity of fumonisin mycotoxins. *Mol Nutri Food Res* **48:** 255–69.

Hyndman ME, Verma S, Rosenfeld RJ, Anderson TJ, Parsons HG (2002) Interaction of 5-methyltetrahydrofolate and tetrahydrobiopterin on endothelial function. *Am J Physiol – Heart Circ Physiol* **282:** H2167–H2172.

IARC (International Agency for Research on Cancer) (2002) Fumonisin B_1. In *IARC Monographs on the Evaluation of Carcinogenic Risks to Humans, Vol. 82, Some Traditional Herbal Medicines, Some Mycotoxins, Naphthaline and Styrene.* IARC Press, Lyons, pp. 301–66.

Itikala PR, Watkins ML, Mulinare J, Moore CA, Liu Y (2001) Maternal multivitamin use and orofacial clefts in offspring. *Teratology* **63:** 79–86.

Javed T, Richard JL, Bennett GA, Donbrink-Kurtzman MA, Bunte RN, Koelkebeck KW, Côté LM, Leeper RW, Buck WB (1993) Embryopathic and embryocidal effects of purified fumonisin B_1 or *Fusarium proliferatum* culture material extract on chicken embryos. *Mycopathologia* **123:** 185–93.

Kellerman TS, Marasas WF, Thiel PG, Gelderblom WC, Cawood M, Coetzer JA (1990) Leukoencephalomalacia in two horses induced by oral dosing of fumonisin B_1. *Onderstepoort J Vet Res* **57:** 269–75.

Kim E-K, Scott PM, Lau BP-Y (2003) Hidden fumonisins in cornflakes. *Food Add Contam* **20:** 161–9.

LaBorde JB, Terry KK, Howard PC, Chen JJ, Collins TF, Shackelford ME, Hansen DK (1997) Lack of embryotoxicity of fumonisin B_1 in New Zealand white rabbits. *Fundam Appl Toxicol* **40:** 120–8.

Lebepe-Mazur S, Bal H, Hopmans E, Murphy P, Hendrich S (1995) Fumonisin B_1 is fetotoxic in rats. *Vet Hum Toxicol* **37:** 126–30.

Levy M, Futerman AH (2010) Mammalian ceramide synthases. *Life Sci* **62:** 347–56.

Liu H, Lu Y, Haynes JS, Cunnick JE, Murphy P, Hendrich S (2001) Reaction of fumonisin with glucose prevents promotion of hepatocarcinogenesis in female F344/N rats while maintaining normal hepatic sphinganine/sphingosine ratios. *J Agr Food Chem* **49:** 113–21.

Månsson M, Klejnstrup ML, Phipps RK, Nielsen KF, Frisvad JC, Gotfredsen CH, Larsen TD (2010) Isolation and NMR characterization of fumonisin B_2 and a new fumonisin B_6 from *Aspergillus niger*. *J Agr Food Chem* **27:** 949–53.

Marasas WFO, Kellerman TS, Gelderblom WCA, Coetzer JAW, Thiel PG, van der Lugt JJ (1988) Leukoencephalomalacia in a horse induced by fumonisin B_1 isolated from *Fusarium moniliforme. Onderstepoort J Vet Res* **55:** 197–203.

Marasas WFO (2001) Discovery and occurrence of the fumonisins: a historical perspective. *Environ Health Perspect* **109 (Suppl. 2):** 239–43.

Marasas WFO, Riley RT, Hendricks KA, Stevens VL, Sadler TW, Gelineau-van Waes J, Missmer SA, Cabrera J, Torres O, Gelderblom WCA, Allegood J, Martínez C, Maddox J, Miller JD, Starr L, Sullards MC, Roman AV, Voss KA, Wang E, Merrill AH Jr (2004) Fumonisins disrupt sphingolipid metabolism, folate transport and development of neural crest cells in embryo culture and *in vivo*: a potential risk factor for human neural tube defects among populations consuming fumonisin-contaminated maize. *J Nutr* **134:** 711–16.

Marion R, Coeffier M, Leplingard A, Favennec L, Ducrotte P, Dechelotte P (2003) Cytokine-stimulated nitric oxide production and inducible NO-synthase mRNA level in human intestinal cells: lack of modulation by glutamine. *Clin Nutr* **22:** 523–8.

Martinez-Larranaga MR, Anadon A, Diaz MJ, Fernandez-Cruz ML, Martinez MA, Frejo MT, Martinez M, Fernandez R, Anton RM, Morales ME, Tafur M (1999) Toxicokinetics and oral bioavailability of fumonisin B_1. *Veter Hum Toxicol* **41:** 357–62.

Martinez de Villarreal L, Perez JZ, Vazquez PA, Herrera RH, Campos Mdel R, Lopez RA, Ramirez JL, Sanchez JM, Villarreal JJ, Garza MT, Limon A, Lopez AG, Barcenas M, Garcia JR, Dominguez AS, Nunez RH, Ayala JL, Martinez JG, Gonzalez MT, Alvarez CG, Castro RN (2002) Decline of neural tube defects cases after a folic acid campaign in Nuevo Leon, Mexico. *Teratology* **66:** 249–56.

Meli R, Ferrante MC, Raso GM, Cavaliere M, Di Carlo R, Lucisano A (2000) Effect of fumonisin B1 on inducible nitric oxide synthase and cyclooxygenase-2 in LPS-stimulated J774A.1 cells. *Life Sci* **67(23):** 2845–53.

Miotti S, Bagnoli M, Tomassetti A, Colnaghi MI, Canevari S (2000) Interaction of folate receptor with signaling molecules lyn and G(alpha)(i-3) in detergent-resistant complexes from the ovary carcinoma cell line IGROV1. *J Cell Sci* **113 (Pt 2):** 349–57.

Missmer SA, Suarez L, Felkner M, Wang E, Merrill AH Jr, Rothman KJ, Hendricks KA (2006) Exposure to fumonisins and the occurrence of neural tube defects along the Texas-Mexico border. *Environ Health Perspect* **114:** 237–41.

Motta EL, Scott PM (2009) Bioaccessibility of total bound fumonisin from corn flakes. *Mycotoxin Res* **25:** 229–32.

MRC (1991) Prevention of neural tube defects: results of the Medical Research Council Vitamin Study. MRC Vitamin Study Research Group. *Lancet* **338:** 131–7.

Mungrue IN, Bredt DS, Stewart DJ, Husain M (2003) From molecules to mammals: what's NOS got to do with it? *Acta Physiol Scand* **179:** 123–35.

Palencia E, Torres O, Hagler W, Meredith FI, Williams LD, Riley RT (2003) Total fumonisins are reduced in tortillas using the traditional nixtamalization method of Mayan communities. *J Nutr* **133:** 3200–3.

Park JW, Scott PM, Lau BP-Y, Lewis DA (2004) Analysis of heat-processed corn foods for fumonisins and bound fumonisin. *Food Add Contam* **21:** 1168–78.

Pelletier I, Bally-Cuif L, Ziegler I (2001) Cloning and developmental expression of zebrafish GTP cyclohydrolase I. *Mechan Develop* **109:** 99–103.

Penner JD, Casteel SW, Pittman L Jr, Rottinghaus GE, Wyatt RD (1998) Developmental toxicity of purified fumonisin B_1 in pregnant Syrian hamsters. *J Appl Toxicol* **18:** 197–203.

Peterson TE, Katusic ZS (2005) Transcribing the cross-talk of cytokine-induced tetrahydrobiopterin synthesis in endothelial cells. *Circ Res* **96:** 141–3.

Piedrahita JA, Oetama B, Bennett GD, van Waes J, Kamen BA, Richardson J, Lacey SW, Anderson RG, Finnell RH (1999) Mice lacking the folic acid-binding protein Folbp1 are defective in early embryonic development. *Nature Genet* **23:** 228–32.

Plachta N, Traister A, Weil M (2003) Nitric oxide is involved in establishing the balance between cell cycle progression and cell death in the developing neural tube. *Exp Cell Res* **288:** 354–62.

Poling SM, Plattner RD, Weisleder D (2002) *N*-(1-deoxy-D-fructos-1-yl) fumonisin B_1: the initial reaction product of fumonisin B_1 and D-glucose. *J Agr Food Chem* **27:** 1318–24.

Reddy RV, Johnson G, Rottinghaus GE, Casteel SW, Reddy CS (1996) Developmental effects of fumonisin B_1 in mice. *Mycopathologia* **134:** 161–6.

Rheeder JP, Marasas WFO, Vismer HF (2002) Production of fumonisin analogs by *Fusarium* species. *Appl Environ Microbiol* **68:** 2101–5.

Riley RT, Showker JL, Owens DL, Ross PF (1997) Disruption of sphingolipid metabolism and induction of leukoencephalomalacia by *F. proliferatum* culture material containing fumonisin B_2 or B_3. *Environ Toxicol Pharmacol* **3:** 221–8.

Riley RT, Voss KA (2006) Differential sensitivity of rat kidney and liver to fumonisin toxicity: organ-specific differences in toxin accumulation and sphingoid base metabolism. *Toxicol Sci* **92:** 335–45.

Riley RT, Voss KA, Speer M, Stevens VL, Gelineau-van Waes J (2006) Fumonisin inhibition of ceramide synthase: a possible risk factor for human neural tube defects. In *Sphingolipid Biology* (Hirabayashi Y, Merrill A, Igarashi Y, eds.). Springer Verlag, Tokyo, pp. 345–62.

Rotter BA, Oh YN (1996) Mycotoxin fumonisin B_1 stimulates nitric oxide production in a murine macrophage cell line. *Nat Toxins* **4:** 291–4.

Sadler TW, Merrill AH Jr, Stevens VL, Sullards MC (2002) Prevention of fumonisin B_1-induced neural tube defects by folic acid. *Teratology* **66:** 169–76.

Serbina NV, Salazar-Mather TP, Biron CA, Kuziel WA, Pamer EG (2003) TNF/iNOS-producing dendritic cells mediate innate immune defense against bacterial infection. *Immunity* **19:** 59–70.

Shane B, Stokstad EL (1985) Vitamin B12–folate interrelationships. *Ann Rev Nutr* **5:** 115–41.

Sharma RP, He Q, Meredith FI, Riley RT, Voss KA (2002) Paradoxical role of tumor necrosis factor alpha in fumonisin-induced hepatotoxicity in mice. *Toxicology* **180:** 221–32.

Shephard GS, Leggott NL, Stockenstrom S, Somdyla NIM, Marasas WFO (2002) Preparation of South African maize porridge: effect on fumonisin mycotoxin levels. *South Afr J Sci* **98:** 393–6.

Silani V, Bonifati C, Buscaglia M, Sampietro A, Ghezzi C, Scarlato G (1993) Ganglioside GM1 expression during human spinal cord and neural crest development. *Neuroreport* **4:** 767–70.

Smith GW, Constable PD, Foreman JH, Eppley RM, Waggoner AL, Tumbleson ME, Haschek WM (2002) Cardiovascular changes associated with intravenous administration of fumonisin B_1 in horses. *Am J Vet Res* **63:** 538–45.

Spiegel S, Milstien S (2003) Sphingosine-1-phosphate: an enigmatic signalling lipid. *Nature Rev Mol Cell Biol* **4:** 397–407.

Spiegelstein O, Mitchell LE, Merriweather MY, Wicker NJ, Zhang Q, Lammer EJ, Finnell RH (2004) Embryonic development of folate binding protein-1 (Folbp1) knockout mice: effects of the chemical form, dose, and timing of maternal folate supplementation. *Develop Dyn* **231:** 221–31.

Stevens VL, Tang J (1997) Fumonisin B1-induced sphingolipid depletion inhibits vitamin uptake via the glycosylphosphatidylinositol-anchored folate receptor. *J Biol Chem* **272:** 18020–25.

Stipanuk MH (2004) Sulfur amino acid metabolism: pathways for production and removal of homocysteine and cysteine. *Ann Rev Nutr* **24:** 539–77.

Stockmann-Juvala H, Mikkola J, Naarala J, Loikkanen J, Elovaara E, Savolainen K (2004a) Oxidative stress induced by fumonisin B1 in continuous human and rodent neural cell cultures. *Free Rad Res* **38:** 933–42.

Stockmann-Juvala H, Mikkola J, Naarala J, Loikkanen J, Elovaara E, Savolainen K (2004b) Fumonisin B1-induced toxicity and oxidative damage in U-118MG glioblastoma cells. *Toxicology* **202:** 173–83.

Tang LS, Finnell RH (2003) Neural and orofacial defects in Folp1 knockout mice [corrected]. *Birth Defects Res Part A: Clin Mol Teratol* **67:** 209–18.

Thony B, Auerbach G, Blau N (2000) Tetrahydrobiopterin biosynthesis, regeneration and functions. *Biochem J* **347 (Pt 1):** 1–16.

Traister A, Abashidze S, Gold V, Plachta N, Karchovsky E, Patel K, Weil M (2002) Evidence that nitric oxide regulates cell-cycle progression in the developing chick neuroepithelium. *Develop Dyn* **225:** 271–6.

van der Westhuizen L, Shephard GS, Rheeder JP, Burger HM (2010) Individual fumonisin expsosure and sphingoid base levels in rural populations consuming maize in South Africa. *Food Chem Toxicol* **48:** 1698–703.

Vann LR, Payne SG, Edsall LC, Twitty S, Spiegel S, Milstien S (2002) Involvement of sphingosine kinase in TNF-alpha-stimulated tetrahydrobiopterin biosynthesis in C6 glioma cells. *J Biol Chem* **277:** 12649–56.

Vann LR, Twitty S, Spiegel S, Milstien S (2000) Divergence in regulation of nitric-oxide synthase and its cofactor tetrahydrobiopterin by tumor necrosis factor-alpha. Ceramide potentiates nitric oxide synthesis without affecting GTP cyclohydrolase I activity. *J Biol Chem* **275:** 13275–81.

Vasquez-Vivar J, Kalyanaraman B, Martasek P, Hogg N, Masters BS, Karoui H, Tordo P, Pritchard KA Jr (1998) Superoxide generation by endothelial nitric oxide synthase: the influence of cofactors. *Proc Natl Acad Sci USA* **95:** 9220–5.

Venkataraman K, Riebeling C, Bodennec J, Riezman H, Allegood JC, Sullards MC, Merrill AH Jr, Futerman AH (2002) Upstream of growth and differentiation factor 1 (*uog1*), a mammalian homolog of the yeast longevity assurance gene 1 (LAG1), regulates *N*-stearoyl-sphinganine (C18-(dihydro)ceramide) synthesis in a fumonisin B_1-independent manner in mammalian cells. *J Biol Chem* **277:** 35642–49.

Voss KA, Bacon CW, Norred WP, Chapin RE, Chamberlain WJ, Plattner RD, Meredith FI (1996) Studies on the reproductive effects of *Fusarium moniliforme* culture material in rats and the biodistribution of [^{14}C]fumonisin B_1 in pregnant rats. *Nat Toxins* **4:** 24–33.

Voss KA, Bullerman LB, Bianchini A, Hanna MA, Ryu D (2008) Reduced toxicity of fumonisin B_1 in corn grits by single-screw extrusion. *J Food Protect* **71:** 2036–41.

Voss KA, Gelineau-van Waes JB, Riley RT (2006) Fumonisins: current research trends in developmental toxicology. *Mycotox Res* **22:** 61–8.

Voss KA, Jackson LS, Jablonski JE, Hanna MA, Bullerman LB, Ryu D (2010) Extrusion cooking using a twin-screw apparatus reduces toxicity of fumonisin contaminated corn grits. *Toxicol Sci* **114 (Suppl.):** 247 (abstract).

Voss KA, Plattner RD, Riley RT, Meredith FI, Norred WP (1998) In vivo effects of fumonisin B_1-producing and fumonisin B_1-nonproducing *Fusarium moniliforme* isolates are similar: fumonisins B_2 and B_3 cause hepato- and nephrotoxicity in rats. *Mycopathologia* **141:** 45–58.

Voss KA, Riley RT, Gelineau-van Waes JB (2007) Fetotoxicity and neural tube defects in CD1 mice exposed to the mycotoxin fumonisin B_1. *Mycotoxins* **57 (Suppl.):** 67–72.

Voss KA, Riley RT, Norred WP, Bacon CW, Meredith FI, Howard PC, Plattner RD, Collins TFX, Hansen D, Porter JK (2001) An overview of rodent toxicities: liver and kidney effects of *Fusarium moniliforme* and fumonisins. *Environ Health Perspect* **109:** 259–66.

Voss KA, Riley RT, Snook ME, Gelineau-van Waes J (2009) Reproductive and sphingolipid metabolic effects of fumonisin B_1 and its alkaline hydrolysis product in LM/Bc mice: hydrolyzed fumonisin B_1 did not cause neural tube defects. *Toxicol Sci* **112:** 459–67.

Vudathula DK, Prelusky DB, Ayroud M, Trenholm HL, Miller JD (1994) Pharmacokinetic fate and pathological effects of ^{14}C-fumonisin B_1 in laying hens. *Nat Toxins* **2:** 81–8.

Wang E, Riley RE, Meredith FI, Merrill AH Jr (1999) Fumonisin B_1 consumption by rats causes reversible dose-dependent increases in urinary sphinganine and sphingosine. *J Nutr* **129:** 214–20.

Watanabe R, Funato K, Venkataraman K, Futerman A, Riezman H (2002) Sphingolipids are required for the stable membrane association of glycosylphosphatidylinositol-anchored proteins in yeast. *J Biol Chem* **277:** 49538–44.

Wells PG, Bhuller Y, Chen CS, Jeng W, Kasapinovic S, Kennedy JC, Kim PM, Laposa RR, McCallum GP, Nicol CJ, Parman T, Wiley MJ, Wong AW (2005) Molecular and biochemical mechanisms in teratogenesis involving reactive oxygen species. *Toxicol Appl Pharmacol* **207:** 354–66.

Yan J, Hales BF (2006) Depletion of glutathione induces 4-hydroxynonenal protein adducts and hydroxyurea teratogenicity in the organogenesis stage mouse embryo. *J Pharmacol Exper Ther* **319:** 613–21.

Yates JR, Ferguson-Smith MA, Shenkin A, Guzman-Rodriguez R, White M, Clark BJ (1987) Is disordered folate metabolism the basis for the genetic predisposition to neural tube defects? *Clin Genetics* **31:** 279–87.

Xia Y, Tsai AL, Berka V, Zweier JL (1998) Superoxide generation from endothelial nitric-oxide synthase. A Ca2+/calmodulin-dependent and tetrahydrobiopterin regulatory process. *J Biol Chem* **273:** 25804–8.

Zhao W, Mosley BS, Cleves MA, Melnyk S, James SJ, Hobbs CA (2006) Neural tube defects and maternal biomarkers of folate, homocysteine, and glutathione metabolism. *Birth Defects Res Part A Clin Mol Teratol* **76:** 230–6.

Zitomer NC, Mitchell T, Voss KA, Bondy GS, Pruett ST, Garnier-Amblard EC, Liebeskind LS, Park H, Wang E, Sullards MC, Merrill AH Jr, Riley RT (2009) Ceramide synthase inhibition by fumonisin B1 causes accumulation of 1-deoxysphinganine: a novel category of bioactive 1-deoxysphingoid bases and 1-deoxydihydroceramides biosynthesized by mammalian cell lines and animals. *J Biol Chem* **391:** 2257–63.

CHAPTER

54

Trichothecenes and zearalenone

Michelle Mostrom

INTRODUCTION

Fusarium species of fungi infect a variety of crops, including wheat, corn, barley, oats, rice and forages, that subsequently may enter the food or animal feed chain. *Fusarium* is most commonly found in temperate climates, but contamination of grains is reported worldwide (Placinta *et al.*, 1999; JECFA, 2001; CAST, 2003). While *Fusarium* species may produce a variety of secondary chemical compounds or mycotoxins, this chapter will focus on the trichothecenes, particularly deoxynivalenol (DON) due to extensive contamination of cereals, and zearalenone. More than 150 trichothecene mycotoxins have been recognized in the past 40 years. These fungal metabolites are a group of sesquiterpenoids characterized by a tetracyclic 12,13-epoxytrichothec-9-ene skeleton and a variable number of acetoxy or hydroxyl group substitutions. The epoxy group at C-12 and C-13 is considered essential for toxicity (Figure 54.1). Trichothecenes can be broadly divided into two groups, macrocyclic and non-macrocyclic trichothecenes, based on the presence of a macrocyclic ring linking C-4 and C-15 with diesters (roridin series) and triesters (verrucarin series).

Trichothecenes are potent inhibitors of protein synthesis and toxic to plants and animals. The hallmark clinical sign of trichothecene toxicosis in animals is feed refusal. Additional clinical signs from trichothecene exposure may include emesis, weight loss, immunomodulation, coagulopathy and hemorrhage, and cellular necrosis of mitotically active tissues such as intestinal mucosa, skin, bone marrow, spleen, testis and ovary (CAST, 2003).

Zearalenone is a non-steroidal estrogenic mycotoxin produced by several species of *Fusarium* fungi. The primary producer of zearalenone is *Fusarium graminearum* (teleomorph *Gibberella zeae*). Additional *Fusarium* fungi capable of producing zearalenone include *F. culmorum*, *verticillioides* (*moniliforme*), *sporotrichioides*, *semitectum*, *equiseti* and *oxysporum*. Contamination of cereal grains by zearalenone has been reported worldwide, but primarily occurs in temperate climates. Typically, zearalenone concentrations are low in grain contaminated in the field but increase under storage conditions with moisture greater than 30 to 40%. Zearalenone can bind to tissue estrogen receptors causing morphological and functional changes in reproductive organs (Katzenellenbogen *et al.*, 1979; Shier *et al.*, 2001). Zearalenone may cause major effects on reproduction that can lead to hyperestrogenism, particularly in swine as compared with other species. Prepubertal swine are the most sensitive species. Typical clinical signs of hyperestrogenism are swelling of the vulva, increase in uterine size and secretions, mammary gland hyperplasia and secretion, prolonged estrus, anestrus, increased incidence of pseudopregnancy, infertility, decreased libido and secondary complications of rectal and vaginal prolapses, stillbirths and small litters. Zearalenone contamination of food has been suggested to be a factor in premature thelarche and precocious puberty in young girls (reviewed by Massart and Saggese, 2009).

HISTORICAL BACKGROUND

Mold-infected grains have been associated with ill health in livestock and humans for over a hundred years. In Europe, Russia and Eastern Siberia, "scabby grains" and "moldy hay" have long been recognized as toxic, and a red mold disease or "Akakabi-byo" of Japanese wheat caused gastroenteritis in humans (Saito and Ohtsubo, 1974). Alimentary toxic aleukia (ATA) of human beings and a similar condition (Stachybotryotoxicosis) of horses were associated with overwintered grains and hay during the 1930s and 1940s in the former USSR. Delayed harvest of grain and the cold, wet conditions resulted in the growth of mold on crops and hay. These molds were later identified as *Fusarium sporotrichioides*, *F. poae* and *Stachybotrys alternans* in grain and hay, respectively, and several trichothecene mycotoxins were isolated. The primary toxin associated with ATA was identified as 4β,15-diacetoxy-3α-hydroxy-8α-[3-methylbutyryloxy]-12,13-epoxytrichothec-9-ene or T-2 toxin, which caused epithelial irritation or dermonecrosis, gastrointestinal irritation, immunosuppression and a high mortality rate in affected humans and animals (Joffe, 1974).

The fungus usually involved in scabby grain blights was identified as *Gibberella zeae* (Schwabe) or *Fusarium graminearum*, its asexual or conidial phase (reviewed by Marasas *et al.*, 1984). A trichothecene, chemically described as 3,7,15-trihydroxy-12,13-epoxytrichothec-9-en-8-one, was

Reproductive and Developmental Toxicology, Edited by Ramesh C. Gupta
ISBN: 978-0-12-382032-7

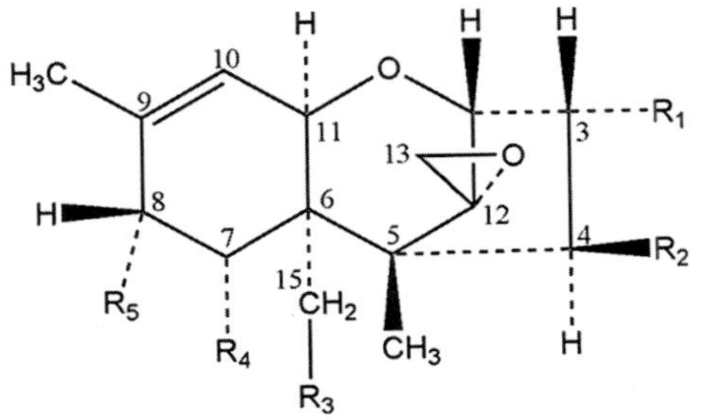

FIGURE 54.1 Chemical structure of Type A trichothecenes. Substitutions R1 through R5 are listed above.

Trichothecene	R1	R2	R3	R4	R5
T-2 toxin	OH	OAc	OAc	H	OCOCH2CH(CH3)2
HT-2 toxin	OH	OH	OAc	H	OCOCH2CH(CH3)2
Diacetoxyscirpenol	OH	OAc	OAc	H	H
Neosolaniol	OH	OAc	OAc	H	OH
Calonectrin	OAC	H	OAc	H	H

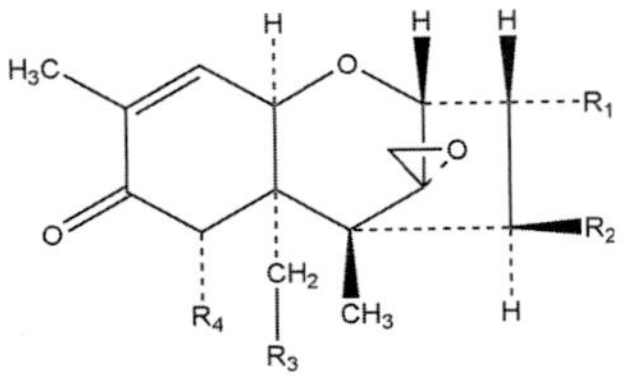

FIGURE 54.2 Chemical structure of Type B trichothecenes. Substitutions R1 through R4 are listed above.

Trichothecene	R1	R2	R3	R4
Nivalenol	OH	OH	OH	OH
Deoxynivalenol	OH	H	OH	OH
Fusarenon-X	OH	OAc	OH	OH
Diacetylnivalenol	OH	OAc	OAc	OH
3-acetyldeoxynivalenol	OAc	H	OH	OH
15-acetyldeoxynivalenol	OH	H	OAc	OH

isolated from barley (Morooka *et al.*, 1972) and field corn infected with *Fusarium graminearum* (Vesonder *et al.*, 1973) and given the trivial name vomitoxin. Vomitoxin, also known as Rd toxin, 4-deoxynivalenol or deoxynivalenol (DON), was demonstrated to be the *Fusarium* toxin responsible for feed refusal and emesis in monogastric animals fed contaminated corn (Vesonder *et al.*, 1976).

Estrogenism in swine was reported in the mid-1920s in the US Mid-West (McNutt *et al.*, 1928). A condition of swelling and eversion of the vagina in young gilts and swelling of the prepuce in males was associated with consuming moldy corn. Prolapse of the vagina and occasionally the rectum were noted as secondary effects. Stob *et al.* (1962) isolated an active metabolite with uterotrophic and anabolic activities from culture of *Gibberella zeae* (*F. graminearum*). The *Fusarium* compound found in corn with uterotrophic activity was eventually named F-2 or zearalenone. Zearalenone has low acute toxicity and displays carcinogenicity, but the majority of clinical signs in animals are related to zearalenone's estrogenic and anabolic properties.

Zearalenone has been speculated as a causative agent in premature thelarche (breast development) and precocious puberty in young girls in Puerto Rico, from 1978 to 1984, and premature thelarche in a school in northern Italy in 1979 (reviewed by Massart and Saggese, 2009). Researchers suggested that food products such as dairy and meat from animals treated with anabolic steroids or growth promoters (zeranol or α-zeralanol used to increase muscle mass in food-producing animals) or grain products contaminated with zearalenone or its analogs were initiating the estrogenic changes. No specific chemicals were identified as the causative agent in these incidents. Following the premature thelarche in northern Italy, the use of anabolic growth promoters in agriculture was banned in 1985 in the European Union.

Sources

Trichothecenes are produced by several genera of fungi, including *Fusarium, Stachybotrys, Myrothecium, Trichothecium* and others (Scott, 1989). Trichothecene mycotoxins (baccharinoids) have also been isolated from Brazilian plants, notably *Baccharis* spp.; however, all medically and economically important sources to date have been fungal, especially *Fusarium. Fusarium* species vary in toxigenic potential by strain, which in turn varies with geographic location. Mycotoxin production by *Fusarium* fungi is heavily dependent on oxygen, environmental pH, osmotic tension and temperature. For example, DON is produced under conditions of low oxygen tension, whereas zearalenone production by the same fungi requires oxygen saturation, usually occurring after field crops senesce (Miller, 2002). *F. graminearum* has an optimum temperature range for growth of 26 to 28°C at a water activity (a_W) greater than 0.88.

Trichothecenes can be chemically classified into four types based upon substitutions at five positions of the trichothecene skeleton, including: Type A which includes T-2 toxin and HT-2 toxin (Figure 54.1); Type B including nivalenol and deoxynivalenol (Figure 54.2); Type C including crotocin (Figure 54.3); and Type D or macrocylics (Figure 54.4). Type A trichothecenes include some of the most toxic trichothecenes, T-2 toxin, its deacetylated metabolite, HT-2 toxin and diacetoxyscirpenol (DAS or anguidine). The Type B trichothecenes are characterized by a keto group at C-8 and hydroxyl group at C-7. These are common natural field contaminants

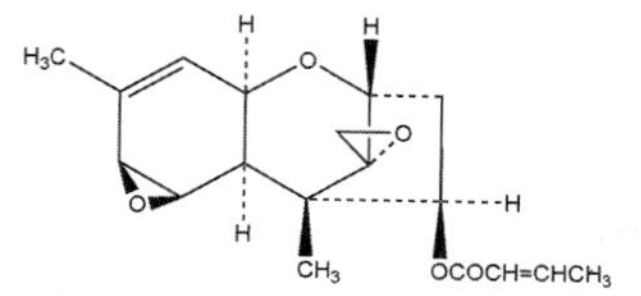

FIGURE 54.3 Chemical structure of Type C trichothecenes.

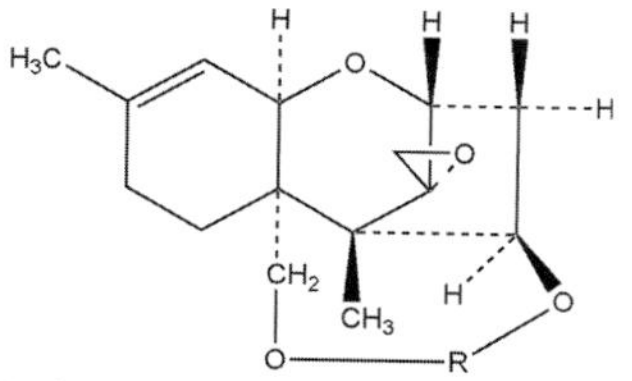

FIGURE 54.4 Chemical structure of Type D trichothecenes and an example of a substitution.

Trichothecene	R
Roridin A	-C(=O)CH(OH)CH(CH3)CH2CH2OC(CHOH) CH=CHCH=CHC(=0)-

of grains and include DON and its acetylated derivatives, nivalenol (3α,4β,7α,15-tetracydroxy-12,13 epoxytrichothec-9-en-8-one), and fusarenon-X (4-acetylnivalenol) produced by *F. culmorum* and *F. graminearum,* and other, closely-related fungi. They are less toxic than the other classes of trichothecenes without the C-8 keto substitution, such as T-2 toxin, diacetoxyscirpenol and the macrocyclic trichothecenes. The Type C trichothecenes typically have a second epoxide ring at C-7,8, and are not produced by *Fusarium,* nor are these trichothecenes associated with adverse effects in livestock. In contrast with Type C trichothecenes, the Type D trichothecenes are potent, cytotoxic compounds with a macrocyclic ring linking C-4 and C-15 on the trichothecene skeleton. The fungus *Stachybotrys alternans* Bonorden (synonyms *S. atra corda* and *S. chartarum* (Ehrenberg ex Link) Hughes) grows worldwide on cellulosic vegetation and wet straw and produces macrocyclic trichothecene mycotoxins (including satratoxins G and H, verrucarin J and roridin E) that are stable, highly toxic and cause characteristic cytotoxic effects (Bata *et al.*, 1985).

Of the trichothecenes, DON is probably the most commonly detected in cereal grains throughout the world (Rotter *et al.*, 1996; CAST, 2003). This mycotoxin is resistant to milling and processing and readily enters the animal feed and human food chains. Foodborne trichothecene contamination, in particular DON, has been linked to acute human toxicoses in China, India and Japan, but little information is available regarding potential health effects from chronic exposure (Bhat *et al.*, 1989; Kuiper-Goodman, 1994; JECFA, 2001).

Zearalenone, commonly found with DON, is chemically described as 6-(10-hydroxy-6-oxo-*trans*-1-undecenyl)-β-resorcyclic acid lactone (Figure 54.5). Zearalenone and active derivatives are produced by *Fusarium* infections of grains and classified as estrogens based on initiation of estrus or cornification of the vagina of adult mice (Mirocha and Christensen, 1974). Alternating moderate and low temperatures and moist weather stimulate zearalenone production by *Fusarium* molds. Zearalenone can be produced fairly quickly in the field during wet weather in the late summer or early fall weather following hail damage to corn. Very high

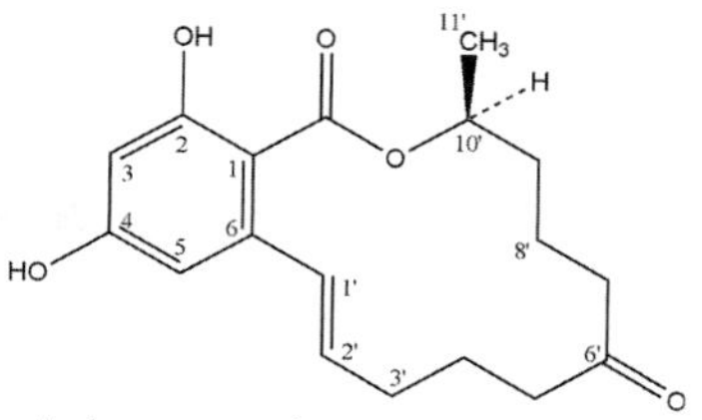

FIGURE 54.5 Chemical structure of zearalenone.

concentrations of zearalenone, which can occur naturally in some field samples, generally resulted from improper storage at high moisture rather than production in the field. Zearalenone is a stable compound that survives food and feed processing; however, extrusion processing can decrease zearalenone concentrations.

TOXICOKINETICS

Understanding the toxicokinetics of trichothecenes is important for understanding potential effects in animals. Trichothecenes undergo all four basic reactions in xenobiotic metabolism. Phase I hydrolysis and oxidation and phase II glucuronide conjugation occur in the body tissues, while reduction of the 12,13-epoxide is thought to occur through microbial action in the gastrointestinal tract. T-2 toxin is the only trichothecene for which all four basic reactions or pathways occur simultaneously in the same animal (Swanson and Corley, 1989). The ability to remove the epoxide oxygen (deepoxidation) is an important step in the detoxification of trichothecenes. Orally administered trichothecenes do not accumulate to a significant extent in the body and are rapidly excreted within a few days in urine and feces (bile) (Swanson and Corley, 1989).

Swine are especially sensitive to deoxynivalenol and kinetic parameters have been studied related to intravenous and acute and chronic oral DON exposures (Coppock *et al.*, 1985; Prelusky *et al.*, 1988, 1990; Prelusky and Trenholm, 1991; Goyarts and Dänicke, 2006). Following an intravenous dose of DON at 1 mg/kg body weight in swine, the mycotoxin distributed rapidly to all tissues and body fluids and declined to negligible levels in all tissues sampled except urine and bile within 24 hours (Prelusky and Trenholm, 1991). DON can be detected very rapidly (less than 2.5 minutes) in the cerebral spinal fluid following intravenous administration in swine; following oral administration of DON in pigs, the plasma DON concentrations correlated closely with cerebral spinal fluid DON levels (Prelusky *et al.*, 1990). Extensive DON tissue accumulation was not detected after dosage, indicating that accumulation of edible tissue residues in swine is unlikely at low-level DON exposure (Prelusky and Trenholm, 1991). Coppock *et al.* (1985) reported no detectable residues of DON in skeletal muscle 24 hours after intravenous DON administration in pigs. The reported half-life of DON in pigs after an intravenous injection of DON at 0.5 mg/kg body weight ranged between 2.08 and 3.65 hours, suggesting that 97% of DON given would be eliminated in 10.1 to 18.3 hours (Coppock *et al.*, 1985). Following a lower intravenous dose of DON in pigs (0.053 mg/kg body weight), serum DON concentrations decreased biphasically with terminal elimination half-lives ($t_{1/2}\beta$) of between 4.2 and 33.6 hours (Goyarts and Dänike, 2006).

After oral exposure, DON is rapidly and nearly completely absorbed in the stomach and proximal small intestine of pigs (Dänicke *et al.*, 2004). Pigs dosed with DON at 5.7 mg DON/kg diet chronically for 4 weeks or with one single oral acute exposure (one feeding) had quick absorption of greater than 50% of the DON administered that was highly distributed, with an apparent volume of distribution (V_d) higher than total body water, and serum elimination half-lives of 6.3 and 5.3 hours in the chronic and acute DON fed pigs, respectively (Goyarts and Dänicke, 2006). A total of 97% of the DON dose (five elimination half-lives) would be eliminated in 31.5 and 26.5 hours after feeding DON chronically or in one single, acute exposure, respectively. The majority of DON ingested from dietary exposure was eliminated in the urine and feces, with urine the main excretory route of DON in an unmetabolized form. The metabolite deepoxy-DON was found in pigs fed the DON contaminated diet chronically or for a period of longer than 4 weeks (Goyarts and Dänicke, 2006). Pregnant swine were fed a *Fusarium*-contaminated ration (4.4 mg DON and 0.048 mg zearalenone/kg diet) on gestation days 35 to 70 and then euthanized on day 70 for tissue harvest and analysis (Dänicke *et al.*, 2006). DON passed the placental barrier in pigs (epitheliochorial placentation in swine as compared with hemochorial placentation of rodents and humans) to a significant extent, but the zearalenone concentrations were too low to demonstrate placental transfer. The *Fusarium*-contaminated diet did not cause adverse effects on performance, organ weights and maintenance of pregnancy of sows nor on fetus weight and length. No teratogenic or embryolethal effects were observed. In a similar study, pregnant swine were fed a *Fusarium*-contaminated wheat ration (9.5 mg DON and 0.358 mg zearalenone/kg diet) from gestation days 75 to 110 and then euthanized on day 110 for tissue harvest and analysis (Dänicke *et al.*, 2007). The spleen weights of fetal piglets were significantly lower in the mycotoxin-fed group. The researchers found that DON and deepoxy-DON passed through the placental barrier and were eliminated via urine and bile of piglets and by the excretory routes (urine, bile, serum) of the dams. As expected, zearalenone and α-zearalenol were detected primarily in the bile of piglets and dams.

In contrast with the poor metabolism of DON by swine, the rumen in livestock is capable of extensive metabolism of DON and other trichothecenes. The major metabolite of oral DON in ruminants is 3α,7α,15-trihydroxytrichothec-9,12-diene-8-one (deepoxydeoxynivalenol or DOM-1). Deepoxidation of DON to DOM-1 is considered a deactivation step resulting in a non-cytotoxic compound; thus, ruminal metabolism serves a protective function. Because biotransformation occurs in the rumen, little parent compound is available for absorption (Prelusky *et al.*, 1986a; He *et al.*, 1992). Côté *et al.* (1986) reported cows fed high concentrations of DON (66 mg/kg diet for 5 days) excreted approximately 20% of the DON fed in urine and feces as unconjugated DOM-1 (96%) and DON (4%). Preliminary data from the study suggested to the authors that a portion of the remaining 80% of the dose was excreted as glucuronide conjugates of DON and DOM-1 in urine.

Poultry have a greater tolerance to trichothecenes than monogastric mammals because of poor absorption following oral exposure, extensive metabolism and rapid elimination from the body (Prelusky *et al.*, 1986b; Gauvreau, 1991). Oral administration of DON in turkeys (*Meleagris gallopava*) revealed that 0.96% of the dose was absorbed from the gastrointestinal tract with rapid excretion of DON and its metabolites in urine and excreta (Gauvreau, 1991). The terminal elimination half-life in turkeys following an intravenous dose of DON was about 44 minutes. Tissue residues of DON and/or metabolites declined rapidly to trace levels.

Lactating cows or laying hens consuming high concentrations of dietary DON (>5 mg/kg) transfer minimal concentrations of DON to the milk or eggs, respectively. Charmley *et al.* (1993) fed 0.59, 42 and 104 mg DON/head/day from contaminated corn and wheat for 10 weeks in a lactation study and found no detectable residues (<1 ng/mL) of DON or DOM-1 in milk. Prelusky *et al.* (1984) evaluated the absorption and distribution of a single large oral dose, 920 mg of DON via rumen intubation, given to each of two lactating cows. Maximum blood levels occurred 4.7 and 3.5 hours after DON administration and were 200 and 90 ng/mL serum (DON and conjugates, respectively). By 24 hours post-dosing only trace levels (<2 ng DON/mL serum) were detected. Free and conjugated DON were detected in cow's milk at low levels (<4 ng/mL) with an estimated 0.0001% of administered dose excreted in milk. Following a 5 day oral exposure trial to high concentrations of DON (~66 mg/kg in the diet), lactating dairy cows excreted unconjugated DOM-1 in the milk at concentrations up to 26 ng/ml (Côté *et al.*, 1986). No DON was detected (detection limit of 10 μg DON/kg tissue) in eggs or tissues of Leghorn chicks and laying hens and broiler chickens fed a ration containing 4 to 5 mg DON/kg for 28 to 160 days (El-Banna *et al.*, 1983). Valenta and Dänicke (2005) did not detect DON, DOM-1 or glucuronide conjugates of these compounds in the yolk or albumen of laying hens fed a maize diet containing 11.9 mg DON/kg dry matter for 16 weeks.

T-2 toxin metabolism has been studied in laboratory and agricultural animals. Metabolism of T-2 toxin generally occurs through deacetylation to HT-2 toxin (at C-4) and additional methabolites. Human and bovine liver homogenates are capable of deacetylating T-2 toxin *in vitro* to HT-2 toxin (Ellison and Kotsonis, 1974). T-2 toxin and metabolites in swine can be eliminated as glucuronide conjugates into bile and undergo deconjugation in the intestinal tract by microbial action and enterohepatic recirculation (Corley *et al.*, 1985).

After receiving three daily oral doses of 180 mg T-2 toxin/day (equivalent to dietary levels of 31 to 35 mg T-2 toxin/kg), a lactating Jersey cow (375 kg) was orally dosed with 156.9 mg of tritium-labeled T-2 toxin (Yoshizawa *et al.*, 1981). The cow showed a good appetite, but milk and urine production decreased by 38 and 50%, respectively, during the experimental period. Plasma concentrations peaked at 8 hours after the tritium-T-2 toxin dose, at 64 ppb (ng/g) T-2 toxin equivalents, and by 72 hours, almost all radioactivity had been eliminated in the urine and feces, in a ratio of 3:7, respectively. About 0.2% of the tritium-T-2 toxin dose was transmitted into the milk with the maximum level of radioactivity in milk at 16 hours post-tritium dose of 37 ppb (T-2 toxin equivalents). The cow was killed and tissues were analyzed to T-2 toxin. T-2 toxin was rapidly metabolized and little T-2 toxin accumulated in organ tissues (muscle, liver, kidney, fat, heart, bile, ovaries and mammary gland), but bile and liver contained higher tritium residues than whole blood. The authors considered that a large amount of the absorbed toxin and its metabolites were eliminated via the bile into the intestinal tract. The delayed elimination of large amounts of radioactivity in the feces indicated that T-2 toxin and its metabolites probably recirculate in the enterohepatic system.

A pregnant Holstein cow was intubated with 182 mg of purified T-2 toxin daily (equivalent to about 0.5 mg T-2 toxin/kg body weight) for 15 consecutive days (Robison *et al.*, 1979). Milk samples collected on days 2, 5, 10 and 12 contained T-2 toxin ranging from 10 to 160 ng/g. The dose given to this cow corresponds to an unusually high feed concentration of 50 mg T-2 toxin/kg; therefore, the authors considered it unlikely that T-2 toxin would be detectable in milk at T-2 toxin concentrations found naturally in feeds. The authors fed a sow (170 kg) T-2 toxin at 12 mg/kg diet (equivalent to 0.5 mg T-2 toxin/kg body weight per day) for 220 days. Six days post-parturition a milk sample was analyzed for T-2 toxin and contained 76 ng/g. Glávits and Ványi (1995) described a "perinatal form of T-2 toxicosis" in swine in Hungary. The authors reported T-2 toxin was excreted in the milk of sows causing lesions, characteristic of T-2, in organs of suckling pigs, including degeneration and necrosis of cells in the bone marrow and death.

Microbial metabolism

In the ruminant, significant metabolism of trichothecenes occurs in the rumen and gastrointestinal tract prior to absorption. King *et al.* (1984) noted almost complete transformation of DON to a deepoxidation product when DON was incubated *in vitro* with rumen fluid for a 24 hour period. Swanson *et al.* (1987) reported DON was partially converted to deepoxidated DON (DOM-1) by rumen microbes. Rumen microbes, in particular protozoa, appear to be active in the deacetylation of the trichothecenes T-2 toxin and DAS to HT-2 and monoacetoxyscirpenol (Kiessling *et al.*, 1984). Microbes in the large intestines of chickens are capable of complete DON transformation *in vitro* to a deepoxy metabolite, whereas no metabolism of DON was reported with the *in vitro* incubation of swine large intestinal contents (He *et al.*, 1992).

Microbial adaptation may require a period of several weeks during which the host animal is exposed to more of the toxic parent trichothecene. The rate and location of deepoxidation of trichothecenes prior to absorption is important in the development of toxic effects. Formation of deepoxides higher in the gastrointestinal tract would reduce the potential toxicity of the trichothecene. Biotransformation of DON is inhibited by low pH *in vitro*, with a pH of 5.2 completely inhibiting DON metabolism either by inactivating the microorganisms or specifically inhibiting the deepoxidation process of DON (He *et al.*, 1992).

Zearalenone

Zearalenone is fairly rapidly absorbed following oral exposure (Dailey *et al.*, 1980). Following a single oral dose of 10 mg zearalenone/kg body weight to 15 to 25 kg pigs, the absorption was approximated to be 80 to 85% (Biehl *et al.*, 1993). Zearalenone and associated metabolites were found in the plasma of a pig in less than 30 minutes after initiating feeding with parent compound. Following zearalenone administration, zearalenone can be localized in reproductive tissues (ovary and uterus), adipose tissue and interstitial cells of the testes (Kuiper-Goodman *et al.*, 1987). The reported biological half-life of total plasma zearalenone radioactivity following the oral dosage in pigs is 86 hours (Biehl *et al.*, 1993). Zearalenone undergoes both phase I and phase II metabolism with involvement of 3α- and 3β-hydroxysteroid dehydrogenase enzymes catalyzing the first biotransformation step. Reduction of the keto group at C-6′ during phase I metabolism results in α- or β-zearalenol. Further reduction of the C11–C12 double bonds results in α- or β-zearalanol. Species differences in zearalenone susceptibility might be related to hepatic biotransformation, with the highest amount of α-zearalenol produced by pig hepatic microsomes, whereas chicken microsomes produced the highest amounts of β-zearalenol (Malekinejad *et al.*, 2005). Humans metabolize zearalenone to α-zearalenol, a more estrogenic compound.

Pigs readily conjugated almost all absorbed zearalenone and α-zearalenol through glucuronidation. While the liver plays a major role in glucuronidation, the intestinal mucosa is active. Zearalenone was reduced to α- and β-zearalenol in sow intestinal mucosa homogenates (duodenum and jejunum) *in vitro* (Olsen *et al.*, 1987). Gastrointestinal flora can aid in the metabolism of zearalenone. Zearalenone can undergo rumen metabolism, with reduction to mostly α-zearalenol and to a lower amount of β-zearalenol (Kiesseling *et al.*, 1984). Whether rumen metabolism will increase or decrease zearalenone toxicity depends on absorption by the gastrointestinal tract, liver metabolism by hydroxysteroid dehydrogenase, and competition at the cytosolic estrogen receptor sites in the animal species.

Zearalenone undergoes extensive enterohepatic circulation and biliary excretion in most species. The major route of excretion for most species is through the feces, although rabbits primarily excrete zearalenone in the urine. Most zearalenone administered in a dose is excreted within a 72-hour period. Approximately 94% of radiolabeled zearalenone, given orally to white Leghorn laying hens at 10 mg/kg body weight, was eliminated through the excreta within 72 hours post-dosing (Dailey *et al.*, 1980). No major retention of radiolabeled activity was found in edible muscle tissue, but lipophilic metabolite(s) were reported in egg yolk (at about 2 mg/kg concentration) 72 hours post-dosing.

Concern has focused on potential residue of zearalenone and its metabolites in milk, eggs and foods, and precocious development of sexual characteristics in young girls (Kuiper-Goodman *et al.*, 1987; JECFA, 2001). Zearalenone and α- and β-zearalenols can be transmitted into the milk of sheep, cows and pigs administered high doses of zearalenone (Hagler *et al.*, 1980; Mirocha *et al.*, 1981). Hyperestrogenism has been reported in lamb and pig nursing dams dosed with zearalenone (Hagler *et al.*, 1980; Palyusik *et al.*, 1980). Dairy cows fed rations with purified zearalenone at 50 mg zearalenone/day and 165 mg zearalenone/day for 21 days had no detectable concentrations of zearalenone or α and β-zearalenol in the milk or plasma (Prelusky *et al.*, 1990). One cow dosed with 544.5 mg zearalenone/day for 21 days had maximum concentrations of 2.5 ng zearalenone/ml and 3.0 ng α-zearalenol/ml in the milk. Cows dosed orally with a one-day dose of 1.8 or 6 g zearalenone had maximum milk levels on day 2 of 4.0 and 6.1 ng zearalenone/ml, respectively. This research indicates that minimal transmission of zearalenone occurs into milk and only for a short period of time after exposure to high concentrations of zearalenone.

Following intubations of tritiated zearalenone into the crops of 7-week-old broiler chickens, the greatest accumulation of radioactivity occurred in the liver 30 minutes post-administration, which became a trace of radioactivity by 48 hours post-administration (Mirocha *et al.*, 1982). Only zearalenone was detected in muscle tissue at approximately 4 ppb at 48 hours post-administration, indicating the zearalenone residues in edible tissue is minimal.

MECHANISMS OF ACTION

Trichothecenes have multiple effects on eukaryotic cells, including inhibition of protein, RNA and DNA synthesis, alteration of membrane structure and mitochondrial function, stimulation of lipid peroxidation, induction of programmed cell death or apoptosis, and activation of cytokines and chemokines. Trichothecenes, types A, B and D, were cytotoxic to a variety of permanent human cell lines and primary cell culture of human endothelial cells, with satratoxins G and H (type D) reported as the most toxic trichothecenes tested and DON (type B) exhibited the lowest cytotoxicity (Nielsen *et al.*, 2009). It is believed that the primary effect of trichothecenes is inhibition of protein synthesis as all of the other reported effects might be secondary to decreased protein synthesis (Rocha *et al.*, 2005).

Protein synthesis inhibition

Trichothecenes bind to ribosomes in eukaryotic cells, in particular to the 60S ribosomal subunits, and interfere with peptidyl transferase activity (McLaughlin *et al.*, 1977). Inhibition of protein synthesis requires an intact 9,10 double bond and the C-12,13 epoxide. Trichothecenes can be divided into two groups based on their site of action on protein synthesis, either preferential inhibition of initiation or inhibition of elongation or termination. Trichothecenes with hydroxyl and acetyl substitutions at both C-3 and C-4, such as T-2 toxin, DAS, scirpentriol and verrucarin A, predominantly inhibit initiation, and compounds such as trichodermin, crotocol, crotocin and verrucarol inhibit elongation or termination (McLaughlin *et al.*, 1977). The cytotoxicity of DON, a trichothecene with a keto group at C-8 and a hydroxyl group at C-7, results from protein synthesis inhibition at the ribosomal level during the elongation and termination step in mammalian cells (Ueno, 1983; Ehrlich and Daigle, 1987). In an *in vivo* low dose DON study in pigs, protein synthesis (using the "flooding dose technique" with radiolabeled phenylalanine as tracer and expressed as fractional synthesis rate) was significantly reduced in kidneys, spleen and ileum of pigs exposed orally to 5.7 mg DON/kg diet for about 4 weeks (Dänicke *et al.*, 2006). Protein synthesis of the liver, skeletal and cardiac muscle, mesenteric lymph nodes, duodenum, jejunum, pancreas and lung were not significantly affected by oral DON exposure.

Trichothecenes inhibit both RNA and DNA synthesis. Using hepatoma cells and phytohemagglutinin-stimulated lymphocytes in an *in vitro* culture, Rosenstein and Lafarge-Frayssinet (1983) reported T-2 toxin inhibited DNA synthesis. DON was demonstrated to inhibit DNA synthesis in splenic lymphocytes and human peripheral blood lymphocytes (Mekhancha-Dahel *et al.*, 1990). Thompson and Wannemacher (1986) reported trichothecenes strongly inhibited RNA synthesis in HeLa cells and had only slight inhibitory effects on Vero cells. The inhibition of nucleic acid synthesis is generally considered secondary to protein synthesis. T-2 toxin inhibited mitochondrial protein synthesis and electron transport action in rat liver cells and *in vivo*, although high doses were used in the studies (Pace, 1983; Pace *et al.*, 1988).

Lipid peroxidation

T-2 toxin is thought to increase production of oxygen radicals, overwhelming the scavenging system for oxygen radicals and resulting in cell injury. Rizzo *et al.* (1994) administered a single oral dose of DON or T-2 toxin at 28 mg/kg body weight or 3.6 mg/kg body weight, respectively, to male Wistar rats on antioxidant deficient diets. Liver peroxides, as measured by thiobarbituric acid-reactive substances, increased 21 and 268% in rats administered DON or T-2 toxin, respectively. Significant decreases in hepatic glutathione concentration and superoxide dismutase activity occurred in the treated rats, as compared with the controls.

Immunotoxicity

Trichothecenes have been shown to both stimulate and impair humoral immunity, cell-mediated immunity and host resistance in experimental and food animals (reviewed by Corrier, 1991; Pestka and Bondy, 1994; Rotter *et al.*, 1996; Bondy and Pestka, 2000; Pestka and Smolinksi, 2005). Immunostimulation after small doses of trichothecenes apparently results from induction of immune- and inflammation-associated genes. Trichothecene doses that partially inhibited translation, upregulated expression of immune-related genes including proinflammatory cytokines and chemokines, cyclooxygenase 2 and inducible nitric oxide synthase (Azcona-Olivera *et al.*, 1995; Ji *et al.*, 1998; Moon and Pestka, 2002; Pestka *et al.*, 2005; Zhou *et al.*, 2005). DON regulated IL-2, a cytokine considered to be a central growth and death factor for antigen-activated T-cells, and IL-8, a pro-inflammatory chemokine that affects host-defense induction of trafficking neutrophils across vascular walls (Pestka *et al.*, 2005). The molecular basis for cytotoxic effects of trichothecenes and immunosuppression is directly or indirectly related to inhibition of protein synthesis. The most potent immunosuppressive trichothecenes are T-2 toxin, DAS, DON and fusarenon-X, which are the most potent protein synthesis inhibitors (Corrier, 1991). Age of exposure is important, as neonatal animals are more sensitive than older animals.

Apoptosis

Apoptosis, a form of programmed cell death, has been proposed to explain the loss of lymphocytes and hematopoietic cells during trichothecene poisoning (Pestka *et al.*, 1994; Shinozuka *et al.*, 1998). Apoptosis normally serves as a self-regulating pathway in the immune system that reduces excessive inflammation and prevents autoimmune disease (Dong *et al.*, 2002); however, inappropriate activation by trichothecenes results in dysfunction. Activation of mitogen-activated protein kinases (MAPKs) by satratoxins and other trichothecenes correlated with and preceded apoptosis (Yang *et al.*, 2000). The authors used two myeloid models, RAW 264.7 murine macrophages and U937 human leukemic cells, in a cleavage assay and determined the potency of cytotoxicity to be satratoxin G, roridin A, verrucarin A>T-2 toxin, satratoxin

F, H>nivalenol and vomitoxin. Using flow cytometry cell cycle analysis and phenotypic staining to study *in vitro* effects, Pestka *et al.* (1994) demonstrated that DON could either inhibit or enhance apoptosis in T, B and IgA+ cells from murine spleen and Peyer's patch. Apoptosis was dependent on lymphocyte subset, source of tissue and glucucorticoid induction.

Cell membrane function

At low concentrations (0.4 pg/ml to 4 ng/ml), T-2 toxin altered several cell membrane functions in L-6 myoblasts, including uptake of calcium, rubidium and glucose, incorporation of thymidine or leucine and tyrosine into DNA or protein, and residual cellular lactate dehydrogenase (Bunner and Morris, 1988). Changes occurred within 10 minutes of exposure, suggesting to the authors that T-2 toxin directly or indirectly affected glucose, nucleotide and amino acid transporters and calcium/potassium channel activities independent of protein synthesis inhibition.

Estrogen receptor binding by zearalenone

Zearalenone and metabolites can interact and bind directly with the cytoplasmic estrogen receptors (ERs), which bind endogenous17β-estradiol, followed by translocation to the nucleus (Katzenellenbogen *et al.*, 1979). The zearalenone estrogen receptor is thought to bind to estrogen responsive elements and activate gene transcription. Stimulation of RNA can lead to protein synthesis and clinical signs of estrogenism. Using *in vitro* cells transfected with human estrogen receptors ERα and ERβ, Kuiper *et al.* (1998) reported that zearalenone binds to both receptors and is a full agonist on ERα and a partial agonist for ERβ; however, at high concentrations zearalenone can act as an ER antagonist on both ERα and ERβ (Mueller *et al.*, 2004). Within the resorcylic acids, α-zearalenol exhibited the greatest binding affinity for cytosolic estrogen receptors, while zearalenone and β-zearalenol displayed much lower binding affinities (Fitzpatrick *et al.*, 1989). The relative estrogenicity of zearalenone and its analogs were evaluated using MCF7 human breast adenocarcinoma cells, with the relative estrogenicity given as (highest to lowest) α-zearalenol > α-zearalanol > β-zearalanol > zearalanone > zearalenone > β-zearalenol (Shier *et al.*, 2001). The 6′ functional group had the largest effect on estrogenicity, with the order of estrogenicity for 6′ substituents given as α-OH >> NH_2 > =O ~ β-OH > β-OAc. The hydroxylation of zearalenone to α-zearalenol apparently is an activation process; whereas the production of β-zearalenol would be a deactivation process. Interspecies variations in sensitivity to zearalenone in the feed could be related to different metabolites produced and the relative binding affinities of zearalenone and metabolites formed. The relative binding affinity of α-zearalenol was greater in the pig than the rat or chicken. The pig and sheep are considered more sensitive to zearalenone than rodents (Zinedine *et al.*, 2007).

Zearalenone can act on the hypothalamic–hypophysial axis. Using 70-day-old Yorkshire gilts (20 to 27 kg) fed 1.5 to 2 mg zearalenone/kg feed for 45 to 90 days, Rainey *et al.* (1990) determined that prepubertal exposure to zearalenone affected the hypothalamic–hypophysial axis and the luteinizing hormone (LH) surges that lasted for at least 44 days post-exposure. However, zearalenone consumption did not delay the onset of pubertal estrus or impair conception rates, ovulation rates or number of fetuses. Slightly older prepubertal gilts (178 days of age and 94 kg) fed 10 mg zearalenone daily for 2 weeks had suppressed mean serum concentrations of luteinizing hormone, but the onset of puberty and subsequent reproduction were not adversely affected (Green *et al.*, 1990). Male rats (70 days old) dosed orally with zearalenone at 20 mg/kg body weight for 35 days had elevated serum prolactin concentrations but showed no changes in serum luteinizing hormone and follicle stimulating hormone concentrations, body and testes weights, or in spermatogonia, spermatocytes and spermatids (Milano *et al.*, 1995). At relatively high concentrations *in vitro*, approximately 400 μM, zearalenone appeared to act directly on interstitial cells from the testes inhibiting steroidogenesis (Fenske and Fink-Gremmels, 1990).

While zearalenone primarily affects reproduction, it may have additional effects. Using *in vitro* cell lines, zearalenone acted as a ligand for human pregnane X receptor (hPXR), which can activate a transcription factor regulating the expression of numerous hepatic drug-metabolizing enzymes, including expression of cytochrome P450 enzymes (Ding *et al.*, 2006). This suggests a potential for zearalenone to induce metabolism of drugs. Clinical trials with pigs of different ages suggest that zearalenone may have diverse biological effects and adverse effects associated with concentrations in feed that do not cause obvious clinical signs (Fink-Gremmels and Malekinejad, 2007).

REPRODUCTIVE TOXICITY

Trichothecenes are toxic to all animal species that have been tested. The Type D trichothecenes, macrocyclics such as the verrucarins and roridin E, are the most acutely toxic trichothecenes, followed by the Type A compounds, DAS, T-2 toxin and HT-2 toxin, Type B, nivalenol, and the lowest acute toxicity is associated with the Type C trichothecene, crotocin (Ueno, 1983). T-2 toxin, the first trichothecene recognized as a naturally occurring mycotoxin, has been studied extensively because of its relative ease of production and its potential as a chemical warfare agent, but T-2 toxicosis is rare in North America. Oral LD_{50} concentrations for T-2 toxin in laboratory animals did not demonstrate marked species differences in sensitivity, but agricultural species do vary in their sensitivity to the different trichothecene toxins. For example, based on toxicity the species susceptibility to DON is ranked as pig (most sensitive), followed by rodent > dog > cat > poulty > ruminants (Prelusky *et al.*, 1994). Neonatal animals are more susceptible. This section will focus on reproductive toxicity.

Friend *et al.* (1986) reported significant weight reductions in young male and female pigs fed DON contaminated feeds at 3.7 and 4.2 mg DON/kg (~0.14 and 0.17 mg/kg body weight/day) feed for 7 weeks; however, no significant histological changes were observed in the testis (seminiferous epithelium) or ovary (follicle). In contrast, several studies indicate that T-2 toxin can affect reproduction. Glávits *et al.* (1983) reported in a field case involving a large swine herd infertility in gilts and sows that coincided with the detection of T-2 and HT-2 toxins at 1 to 2 mg/kg feed. Pathology revealed cystic degeneration of the ovaries and uterine atrophy. Huszenicza *et al.* (2000) evaluated low oral T-2 toxin exposures of 0, 0.3 or 0.9 mg T-2 toxin/day and 9 mg T-2 toxin/day for 3 weeks in ewes and heifers, respectively, on a rich, acidosis-inducing concentrate diet. The results suggested that in ewes and heifers rumen acidosis along with exposure to low oral T-2 toxin intake might delay maturation of the dominant ovarian follicle and ovulation and shorten corpora lutea lifespan (lower plasma progesterone concentrations); although the number of animals in the experiment was small. In an equine study of Trotter mares, the horses were given 7 mg purified T-2 toxin/day in oats (~0.01 mg/kg body weight/day) for 32 to 40 days beginning on estrous cycle day 10 (Juhasz *et al.*, 1997). Skin lesions were noted around the mouth of three horses; however, no adverse effects were noted on the length of the interovulatory interval, luteal and follicular phases of the estrous cycle, plasma progesterone profiles or follicular kinetics. Uterine flushing of five mares in the trial yielded three embryos, suggesting that T-2 toxin had no detrimental effect on ovarian activity, fertilization or oviductal transport.

Sprando *et al.* (2005) reported that male rats gavaged daily for 28 days with DON (0.5, 1.0, 2.5 and 5.0 mg/kg body weight) showed treatment-related effects in the 5 mg/kg body weight group including intense salivation, decreased body weights, sperm counts and serum testosterone concentrations and increased serum follicle stimulating hormone and luteinizing hormone concentrations and sperm tail abnormalities (broken tails). Morphological changes (at the 2.5 and 5 mg DN/kg body weight dosages) were observed in the testis, which included increased testicular germ cell degeneration, failure of sperm release and abnormal germ cell development. The no-observed-effect level (NOEL) for adverse effects of DON on male reproduction in this study was 1.0 mg/kg body weight.

In pregnant rats, T-2 toxin crosses the placenta and is distributed to fetal tissues (Lafarge-Frayssinet *et al.*, 1990). Rousseaux and Schiefer (1987) reported the T-2 toxin caused fetal death at high doses (associated with maternal toxicity), with fetal toxicity primarily in the central nervous system and skeletal system. T-2 toxin administered intravenously at approximately one-third or one-sixth of the LD_{50} (0.41 or 0.21 mg/kg body weight) to sows at the beginning of the third trimester of pregnancy caused vomiting 90 minutes post-injection with the sows becoming listless and aborting their litters 48 to 80 hours later (Weaver *et al.*, 1978a). In another study, three sows were fed purified T-2 toxin in a standard swine ration at 12 mg/kg diet for up to 220 days, causing clinical signs of repeat breeding, small litters (four piglets) and small (0.37 to 0.65 kg) piglets, which had no gross or histological lesions attributable to T-2 toxin (Weaver *et al.*, 1978b). The sows did not develop changes in the complete blood count, total protein or alterations in the bone marrow. These studies used concentrations of T-2 higher than commonly found in feeds screened for visible molds.

Thirty 3-week old single comb white Leghorn hens were fed either purified T-2 toxin or DAS at 2 mg/kg diet for 24 days (Diaz *et al.*, 1994). Egg production dropped about 7% in hens fed either T-2 or DAS on days 13 to 18 of the study, but recovered to near normal by day 24. Shlosberg *et al.* (1984) reported acute, severe reduction in egg production, feed refusal, depression and recumbency, cyanotic appearance of the comb and wattles, and some blue-green discoloration of droppings in a flock of 8-month-old laying hens. Following delivery of new feed, the mean daily egg production dropped from about 2,400 eggs to 150 eggs on day 5 of the new feed (94% drop in production). The feed was changed on day 6 and improvement in clinical signs and normal levels of egg production resumed about 12 days later. Mortality was not changed in the flock; however, necropsies of hens that died after 4 days of the new feed revealed atrophy of the ovaries and abnormally small oviducts. The authors hypothesized that the hens were exposed to a small quantity of highly contaminated trichothecene mycotoxin feed causing direct effects on the female reproductive tract and drop in egg production. The feed sample analyzed for mycotoxins contained T-2 toxin and HT-2 toxin at 3.5 and 0.7 mg/kg, respectively, which the authors thought might be unrepresentatively low. Brake *et al.* (1999) reported that low levels of purified DAS (≤5 mg DAS/kg diet) fed to broiler hens from 67 through 69 weeks of age increased fertility, with little effect on hatchability of fertile eggs. In contrast, DAS fed at 10 or 20 mg/kg diet to broiler males from 25 to 27 weeks of age decreased the hatchability of fertile eggs, which the authors attributed to a direct toxic effect on the testes. Reproductive toxicity associated with trichothecenes generally occurs when exposures reach maternally toxic concentrations, but natural trichothecene-contaminated diets can pose a serious risk to reproductive performance of livestock (Francis, 1989).

When considering the etiology of congenital malformation, the role of maternal toxicity must be evaluated. Maternally toxic doses of trichothecenes can be embryotoxic, with fetal death common in both birds and mammals, generally few frank congenital defects are observed in surviving fetuses, though anomalies in the nervous and skeletal systems have been noted (Francis, 1989). Khera *et al.* (1982) studied the embryotoxicity of DON in pregnant Swiss-Webster mice dosed orally with purified DON at concentrations of 0 to 15 mg DON/kg body weight for 4 days on gestation days 8 through 11. Mice dosed with 5 to 15 mg DON/kg body weight apparently resorbed the embryos, but no adverse effects were noticed in the dams given 2.5 mg DON/kg body weight. A number of skeletal malformations were observed in offspring of mice dosed at 1, 2.5 and 5 mg DON/kg body weight, but no adverse effects were reported in offspring of mice dosed at 0.5 mg DON/kg body weight.

DON fed to rabbits on days 0 through 30 of gestation at increasing levels of 0.3 to 2.0 mg/kg body weight/day caused 100% fetal resorption at 1.8 and 2.0 mg/kg/day and reduced body weight in rabbit does (Khera *et al.*, 1986). Dosages of 0.3 and 0.6 mg DON/kg body weight/day did not produce adverse effects in rabbit fetuses at term and were not maternotoxic. The authors concluded that DON did not produce a teratogenic response in rabbits. Based on an oral gavage study of DON (0, 0.5, 1, 2.5 or 5 mg/kg body weight) in pregnant Sprague-Dawley rats on gestation days 6 to 19, the NOEL for maternal toxicity was 0.5 mg/kg body weight because of dose-related cytoplasmic pallor of hepatocytes and accentuation of the lobular pattern, which was not apparent in control animals, and an increase in liver-body weight ratios at 1 mg/kg body weight (Collins *et al.*, 2006a). The NOEL for fetal toxicity was 1 mg/kg body weight based on a reduction in fetal development at 2.5 and 5 mg/kg body weight. The authors considered DON to be a teratogenic compound at 5 mg/kg body weight due to anomalies, such as fused and misaligned sternebrae and incomplete ossified and bipartite sternebrae. Soft tissue development did not appear to be affected.

A two-generation study of female reproduction and teratology in CD-1 mice fed 0, 1.5 and 3 mg T-2 toxin/kg in a semi-synthetic diet did not reveal any significant differences in major or minor defects among treatment groups (Rousseaux *et al.*, 1986). No long-term reproductive or teratological effects were noted. Minor malformations described as delayed ossification and un-withdrawn yolk sac were reported in chick embryos from hens fed rations containing DON at 2.5 and 3.1 mg DON/kg diet (Bergsjo *et al.*, 1993).

In a documented field case, large numbers of pregnant swine (gilts and sows) were accidentally fed for several months high concentrations of zearalenone and deoxynivalenol at 3 to 5 mg/kg and 6 to 11 mg/kg, respectively, in an ensiled corn cob mixed ration on a dry matter basis (Gutzwiller and Gafner, 2009). Soon after the corn cob mix was introduced into the ration, the animals reduced feed consumption. The reproductive performance data during the 5 months following introduction of the highly contaminated mycotoxin ration (88% non-return rate, no abortions or pseudo pregnancy, 10.2 weaned piglets per litter) were similar to data from the same period of time during the previous year. The authors concluded that the elevated concentrations of deoxynivalenol and zearalenone in the ration chronically fed to pregnant swine had no detectable negative effects on fertility. Exposure of pig oocytes *in vitro* to purified zearalenone or DON (3.12 μmol/L) caused abnormal formation of the meiotic spindle, leading to less fertile oocytes and abnormal ploidy in embryos (Malekinejad *et al.*, 2007). The authors noted that different ratios of zearalenone:DON added to the pig oocytes were additive, rather than synergistic in affecting oocyte maturation and embryo development.

Tiemann and Dänicke (2007) summarized a number of studies of DON and zearalenone on selected reproductive and non-reproductive parameters in swine. The review indicated ingestion of DON caused impairment of porcine oocyte and embryo development, possibly related directly to the toxic effect of DON, and zearalenone affected fertility and reproduction because it exerts estrogenic activity. DON also exerted indirect effects on reproduction through reduced feed intake, resulting in reduced growth and impaired function of liver and spleen. Because swine are physiologically similar to humans (Tumbleson and Schook, 1996), understanding the pathophysiology of DON and zearalenone exposure in pigs may assist understanding potential adverse effects of DON and zearalenone with human exposure.

The NOEL for maternal and fetal toxic effects in pregnant Sprague-Dawley rats gavaged daily on gestation days 6 to 19 with zearalenone in corn oil, at doses of 0, 1 ,2, 4 and 8 mg/kg body weight, was less than 1 mg/kg body weight (Collins *et al.*, 2006b). Decreases in body weight gain and maternal feed consumption were dose related. Fetal body weight was significantly decreased in all treatment groups. At the highest dose of 8 mg/kg body weight, zearalenone delayed skeletal ossification, decreased fetal viability and increased number of litters resorbed. Gonadotropins and sex steroids were analyzed; at the 8 mg zearalenone/kg body weight dosage luteinizing hormone and follicle stimulated hormone were slightly increased, prolactin was significantly increased and progesterone and estradiol were decreased. Zearalenone affected *in utero* development of rats and increased the fetal anogenital index, suggesting a hormonal change and androgenic effect during fetal development, but was not considered a teratogen (Collins *et al.*, 2006b).

Zearalenone has low acute toxicity in most species. In most natural conditions, the concentrations of zearalenone are less than 20 mg/kg (ppm) and generally less than 5 mg zearalenone/kg feed (Sundlof and Strickland, 1986). Prepubertal swine are the most sensitive, cattle may exhibit some adverse affects, and chicken appear to be the least sensitive species. Females are more sensitive than males, and cycling females may be more sensitive than pregnant sows. Pregnant swine may abort. Abortions have been associated in field cases with natural *Fusarium* mold exposure, but have not been reproduced with purified zearalenone (Mirocha and Christensen, 1974). Younger male pigs appear to be more sensitive than older males and can undergo atrophy of the testes and enlargement of mammary glands.

Gilts fed rations with 0, 3, 6 or 9 mg purified zearalenone/kg feed starting the day after they showed the first estrus were bred at subsequent heat periods (Young and King, 1986a). A majority of gilts fed 6 or 9 mg zearalenone/kg feed became pseudopregnant based on examination of their reproductive tract or plasma progesterone levels. Gilts fed rations with 3 mg zearalenone/kg had no reproductive effects. After removal of zearalenone from the diet, approximately half of the gilts fed 6 or 9 mg zearalenone/kg feed returned to estrus spontaneously. No reproductive effects were observed in prepubertal gilts fed a ration with 0.5 mg zearalenone/kg feed (Friend *et al.*, 1990). Young gilts (30 to 35 kg) administered daily 5 mg of purified zearalenone orally developed swelling of the vulva on the fourth day of treatment, an approximate daily dose of 0.167 to 0.143 mg zearalenone/kg body weight (Mirocha and Christensen, 1974). Gilts dosed with 1 mg of purified zearalenone daily for 8 days developed pronounced vulvar swelling. Gilts exposed to higher concentrations of zearalenone may show atrophy of the ovaries along with edema and cellular proliferation of all layers in the uterus. Kuiper-Goodman *et al.* (1987) noted an NOEL for zearalenone in pigs reaching puberty at 0.06 mg/kg body weight/day. Young *et al.* (1990) reported an increased weaning-to-estrus interval and embryonic mortality (measured as a decreased ratio of fetuses to corpora lutea) and a decreased number of fetuses per sow in animals fed 10 mg zearalenone/kg diet.

Male swine fed a high concentration of zearalenone (30 mg/kg feed) appeared to initially have accelerated maturation of spermatogenesis, which occurred 1.5 to 2 months earlier than control animals (Ványi and Széky, 1980). Although germinal epithelium damage was limited to several foci initially, with continued zearalenone exposure the damage became widespread with proliferation of the interstitium around seminiferous tubules. Young and King (1986b) fed lower levels of zearalenone in the diet (0, 3, 6 and 9 mg zearalenone/kg feed) to boars from 32 days of age up to 145 or 312 days of age. Feeding up to 9 mg zearalenone/kg feed to the boars did not affect the libido, but the boars fed the highest dose of zearalenone produced lower total and gel-free volumes of semen with lower total motile sperm. Zearalenone does not appear to affect mature boars. No adverse effects in reproductive parameters, including testicular size, libido, sperm motility and morphology, plasma testosterone and 17β-estradiol concentrations, were reported in mature Yorkshire boars fed increasing concentrations of purified zearalenone at 0, 2, 20 and 200 mg/kg ration for 8 weeks (Ruhr *et al.*, 1983).

Several case reports have associated dairy herd health problems and zearalenone in moldy feed. Young dairy heifers, 6 to 14 months of age, developed slight enlargement of at least one mammary gland quarter while fed moldy corn in a ration (Bloomquist *et al.*, 1982). Following a change in the ration, the heifers returned to normal 7 weeks later.

Zearalenone contamination of the moldy ration was detected by thin-layer chromatography. Roine *et al.* (1971) reported turbid discharge from the vulva, obvious estrous behavior lasting for 1 to 2 weeks, and infertility in dairy cows and heifers. Strains of *Fusarium graminearum* and *culmorum* were isolated from the feed which caused an increase in uterine weight in rats and were capable of producing between 3 and 9.5 mg zearalenone/kg feed. Ványi *et al.* (1974) reported a drop in milk production, feed intake and swelling of the vulva in dairy cows exposed to varying concentrations of zearalenone, ranging from 5 to 75 mg zearalenone/kg feed.

In an experimental study, 18 cycling heifers were dosed with 0 or 250 mg of purified zearalenone daily through one non-breeding estrous cycle and the next two consecutive estrous cycles during which the heifers were bred (Weaver *et al.*, 1986a). The authors calculated that treated heifers were given an average of 250 mg zearalenone/364 kg body weight/day or 0.69 mg zearalenone/kg body weight/day. The control and treated heifers had conception rates of 87 and 62%, respectively, at a statistical probability of $p < 0.065$. Eighteen dairy cows (three cows per group) dosed orally with 0, 31.25, 62.5, 125, 250 and 500 mg of purified zearalenone daily for two consecutive estrous cycles had no changes in serum progesterone concentration, erythrocyte and leucocyte blood counts, packed cell volume, estrous cycle length, clinical health or sexual behavior (Weaver *et al.*, 1986b).

Zearalenone can affect ewe reproduction when ewes are exposed to the mycotoxin prior to mating. Zearalenone, administered orally at concentrations greater than 3 mg/animal/day, given to ewes prior to mating depressed ovulation rates and reduced lambing percentages (Smith *et al.*, 1990). Ewes administered a similar range of oral doses of zearalenone (0, 1.5, 3, 6, 12 and 24 mg/ewe/day) for 10 days, starting 5 days after mating, showed no effect of zearalenone exposure after mating on pregnancy rate or embryonic loss. Breeding rams fed a diet containing 12 mg zearalenone/kg feed for 8 weeks had no significant adverse effects on semen volume, concentration, motility or morphology during the trial and for 6 weeks after zearalenone feeding was ceased (Milano *et al.*, 1991).

In a study of six cycling trotter mares, Juhász *et al.* (2001) determined that daily oral administration of 7 mg purified zearalenone starting 10 days after ovulation until the subsequent ovulation had no adverse effect on reproduction. Zearalenone had no effect on the length of the interovulatory intervals, luteal and follicular phases of the ovary and did not significantly affect uterine edema. However, zearalenone exposure started 10 days after ovulation and the exposure period was short. The dose of purified zearalenone represented a natural contamination of feed of about 1 mg zearalenone/kg feed and ranged between 0.013 and 0.010 mg zearalenone/kg body weight/day for approximately 8 to 10 days. Poultry appear to be fairly resistant to the effects of zearalenone.

RISK ASSESSMENT

A provisional maximum tolerable daily intake for zearalenone in humans was established at 0.5 μg/kg by the Joint Committee FAO/WHO based on the NOEL of 40 μg/kg body weight/day obtained in a 15 day swine study and the LOEL (lowest-observed-effect level) of 200 μg/kg body weight in the study (CCFAC, 2000). The Codex Committee recommended that a total intake of zearalenone and metabolites should not exceed the daily intake level. Zearalenone contamination of cereal grains and forages occurs worldwide and may be a potential danger for animals and humans when the concentrations are elevated in the food or feeds and when the exposure is chronic. Regulations for zearalenone in animal feeds and human foods were reported in 16 countries in 2003 (Zindine *et al.*, 2007). The authors reported limits for zearalenone in various countries for maize, corn, wheat and other commodities to animal and poultry feeds ranged from not detectable to >3,000 μg/kg. Currently, the USA does not have guidelines for zearalenone in foods or feeds. The US Food and Drug Administration (FDA) recently increased advisory levels for DON for dairy and beef cattle rations compared to the European Union guidelines. The FDA reduced the advisory level in raw wheat and wheat by-products to no more than 1 ppm (mg/kg) in finished wheat products, flour, germ and bran. Increased monitoring of mycotoxin contamination of cereal grains going into human food and animal feed chains would generate data for better assessments of exposure risks in different commodities.

TREATMENT

The first action of treatment is to stop exposure to moldy feed or contaminated foods. If using screenings or poor quality grain in animal feeds, cleaning the grain by removing broken, shriveled kernels and washing the grain can lower mycotoxin contamination. Generally, clinical signs of feed refusal will disappear within 7 days after removal of the contaminated feed. Animals may return to production within 14 days. Although in the cases of zearalenone exposures, animals may require 3 to 7 weeks following removal of the contaminated feed to return to normal reproductive status. In naturally contaminated trichothecene feeds and developing mycotoxicosis in livestock, the presence of unidentified mycotoxins or additional fungal metabolites in the ration can complicate clinical signs and diagnosis. The diagnosis may also be frustrated by the difficulty of obtaining a representative feed sample to test and appropriate analytical methodology to identify fungal metabolites.

No specific therapies for trichothecene mycotoxicosis are available. Some trichothecenes undergo enterohepatic recirculation and are excreted in the feces. The use of activated charcoal, which binds toxins within the gastrointestinal tract and prevents toxin reabsorption, plus magnesium sulfate to move the product down the gastrointestinal tract, may be beneficial for acute trichothecene exposures. A number of binders, such as clay and zeolitic products, have been suggested for use with trichothecene-contaminated feed to prevent absorption by animals. Their efficacy has not been proven and marked species variations exist. The US FDA has not approved any ingredient for use as a trichothecene or zearalenone mycotoxin binder.

CONCLUDING REMARKS AND FUTURE DIRECTIONS

Trichothecene mycotoxins occur worldwide; however, both total concentrations and the particular mix of toxins present vary dramatically with environmental conditions. Proper agricultural practices such as avoiding late harvests and reducing overwintered field residue that favors *Fusarium* growth may mitigate trichothecene contamination of grains. Storage of grains at less than 13 to 14% moisture (less than 0.70 α_w) and hay/straw at less than 20% moisture are important in preventing trichothecenes production. Once produced, trichothecenes are stable compounds and can remain present at toxic concentrations in feed for years.

Due to the vague nature of toxic effects attributed to low concentrations of trichothecenes, a solid link between low-level exposure and a specific trichothecene(s) is difficult to establish. Multiple factors, such as nutrition, environmental conditions and chemical exposure to additional xenobiotics or endocrine disruptors, impact health and need to be evaluated with the knowledge of the mycotoxin(s) and concentrations known to cause adverse health effects. Future research particularly focused on mycotoxin metabolism and mechanistic actions would be of immense benefit evaluating the impact(s) of chronic, low-level exposure on human health and livestock performance.

More research data are needed for the metabolism of zearalenone by animals and humans and the potential transfer of zearalenone into consumable animal products, particularly for food typically consumed by infants and young children. In order to evaluate exposure of livestock, more data are needed on the incidence of zearalenone and trichothecenes in animal feeds and guidelines should be established in animal feeds for safe levels of exposure, particularly in young swine.

REFERENCES

Azcona-Olivera JI Ouyang Y, Warner RL, Linz JE, Pestka JJ (1995) Induction of cytokine mRNAs in mice after oral exposure to the trichothecene vomitoxin (deoxynivalenol): relationship to toxin distribution and protein synthesis inhibition. *Toxicol Appl Pharmacol* **133:** 109–20.

Bata A, Harrach B, Ujszaszi K, Kis-Tamas A, Lasztity R (1985) Macrocyclic trichothecene toxins produced by *Stachybotrys atra* strains isolated in middle Europe. *Appl Environ Microbiol* **49:** 678–81.

Bergsjo B, Herstad O, Nafstad I (1993) Effects of feeding deoxynivalenol-contaminated oats on reproductive performance in white leghorn hens. *Br Poultry Sci* **34:** 147–59.

Bhat RV, Beedu SR, Ramakrishna Y, Munshi KL (1989) Outbreak of trichothecene mycotoxicosis associated with consumption of mould-damages wheat production in Kashmir Valley, India. *Lancet* **8628:** 35–7.

Biehl ML, Prelusky DB, Koritz GD, Hartin KE, Buck WB, Trenholm HL (1993) Biliary excretion and enterohepatic cycling of zearalenone in immature pigs. *Toxicol Appl Pharmacol* **121:** 152–9.

Bloomquist C, Davidson JN, Pearson EG (1982) Zearalenone toxicosis in prepubertal dairy heifers. *J Am Vet Med Assoc* **180:** 164–5.

Bondy GS, Pestka JJ (2000) Immunomodulation by fungal toxins. *J Toxicol Environ Health, Part B* **3:** 109–43.

Brake J, Hamilton PB, Kittrell RS (1999) Effects of the trichothecene mycotoxin diacetoxyscirpenol on fertility and hatchability of broiler breeders. *Poultry Sci* **78:** 1690–4.

Bunner DL, Morris ER (1988) Alteration of multiple cell membrane functions in L-6 myoblasts by T-2 toxin: an important mechanism of action. *Toxicol Appl Pharmacol* **92:** 113–21.

CAST (2003) Mycotoxins: Risks in Plant, Animal, and Human Systems. Task Force Report No. 139. Council for Agriculture, Science and Technology, Ames.

CCFAC (2000) Codex Committee on Food Additives and Contaminants. Joint FAO/WHO Expert Committee on Food Additives. Position paper on zearalenone. Publication CCFAC 00/19. Rome, Italy.

Charmley E, Trenholm HL, Thompson BK, Vudathala D, Nicholson JWG, Prelusky DB, Charmley LL (1993) Influence of level of deoxynivalenol in the diet of dairy cows on feed intake, milk production, and its composition. *J Dairy Sci* **76:** 3580–7.

Collins TFX, Sprando RL, Black TN, Olejnik N, Eppley RM, Hines FA, Rorie J, Ruggles DI (2006a) Effects of deoxynivalenol (DON, vomitoxin) on in utero development in rats. *Food Chem Toxicol* **44:** 747–57.

Collins TFX, Sprando RL, Black TN, Olejnik N, Eppley RM, Hamida ZA, Rorie J, Ruggles DI (2006b) Effects of zearalenone on in utero development in rats. *Food Chem Toxicol* **44:** 1455–65.

Coppock RW, Swanson SP, Gelberg HB, Koritz GD, Hoffman WE, Buck WB, Vesonder RF (1985) Preliminary study of the pharmacokinetics and toxicopathy of deoxynivalenol (vomitoxin) in swine. *Am J Vet Res* **46:** 169–74.

Corley RA, Swanson SP, Buck WB (1985) Glucuronide conjugates of T-2 toxin and metabolites in swine bile and urine. *J Agric Food Chem* **33:** 1085–9.

Corrier DE (1991) Mycotoxins: mechanisms of immunosuppression. *Vet Immunol Immunopathol* **30:** 73–87.

Côté L-M, Dahlem AM, Yoshizawa T, Swanson SP, Buck WB (1986) Excretion of deoxynivalenol and its metabolite in milk, urine and feces of lactating dairy cows. *J Dairy Sci* **69:** 2416–23.

Dailey RE, Reese RE, Brouwer EA (1980) Metabolism of [14C]zearalenone in laying hens. *J Agric Food Chem* **28:** 286–91.

Dänicke S, Brüssow K-P, Goyarts T, Valenta H, Ueberschär K-H, Tiemann U (2007) On the transfer of the *Fusarium* toxins deoxynivalenol (DON) and zearalenone (ZON) from the sow to the full-term piglet during the last third of gestation. *Food Chem Toxicol* **45:** 1565–74.

Dänicke S, Goyarts T, Döll S, Grove N, Spolder M, Flachowsky G (2006) Effects of the *Fusarium* toxin deoxynivalenol on tissue protein synthesis in pigs. *Toxicol Lett* **165:** 297–311.

Dänicke S, Valenta H, Döll S (2004) On the toxicokinetics and the metabolism of deoxynivalenol (DON) in the pig. *Arch Anim Nutr* **58:** 169–80.

Diaz GJ, Squires EJ, Julian RJ, Boermans HJ (1994) Individual and combined effects of T-2 toxin and DAS in laying hens. *Br Poultry Sci* **35:** 393–405.

Ding X, Lichti K, Staudiner JL (2006) The mycoestrogen zearalenone induces CYP3A through activation of the pregnane X receptor. *Toxicol Sci* **91:** 448–55.

Dong D, Davis RJ, Flavell RA (2002) MAP kinases in the immune response. *Annu Rev Immunol* **20:** 55–72.

Ehrlich KC, Daigle KW (1987) Protein synthesis inhibition by 8-oxo-12,13-epoxytrichothecenes. *Biochimia et Biophysica Acta* **923:** 206–13.

El-Banna AA, Hamilton RMG, Scott PM, Trenholm HL (1983) Nontransmission of deoxynivalenol (vomitoxin) to eggs and meat in chickens fed deoxynivalenol-contaminated diets. *J Agric Food Chem* **31:** 1381–4.

Ellison RA, Kotsonis FN (1974) *In vitro* metabolism of T-2 toxin. *Appl Microbiol* **27:** 423–4.

Fenske M, Fink-Gremmels J (1990) Effects of fungal metabolites on testosterone secretion *in vitro*. *Arch Toxicol* **64:** 72–5.

Fink-Gremmels J, Malekinejad H (2007) Clinical effects and biochemical mechanisms associated with exposure to the mycoestrogen zearalenone. *Anim Feed Sci Technol* **137:** 326–41.

Fitzpatrick DW, Picken CA, Murphy LC, Buhr MM (1989) Measurement of the relative binding affinity of zearalenone, α-zearalenol and β-zearalenol for uterine and oviduct estrogen receptors in swine, rats and chickens: an indicator of estrogenic potencies. *Comp Biochem Physiol* **94C:** 691–4.

Francis BM (1989) Reproductive toxicology of trichothecenes. In *Trichothecene Mycotoxicosis: Pathophysiologic Effects*, Vol. I (Beasley VR, ed.). CRC Press, Inc., Boca Raton, pp. 143–59.

Friend DW, Thompson BK, Trenholm HL, Hartin KE, Prelusky DB (1986) Effect of feeding diets containing deoxynivalenol (vomitoxin)-contaminated wheat or corn on the feed consumption, weight gain, organ weight and sexual development of male and female pigs. *Can J Anim Sci* **66:** 765–75.

Friend DW, Trenholm HL, Thompson BK, Hartin KE, Fiser PS, Asem EK, Tsang BK (1990) The reproductive efficiency of gilts feds very low levels of zearalenone. *Can J Anim Sci* **70:** 635–45.

Gauvreau HC (1991) Toxicokinetic tissue residue and metabolite studies of deoxynivalenol (vomitoxin) in turkeys, Master Science thesis. Simon Fraser University, Vancouver, BC.

Glávits R, Gabriella S, Sándor S, Ványi A, Gajdás GY (1983) Reproductive disorders caused by trichothecene mycotoxins in a large-scale pig herd. *Acta Vet Hung* **31:** 173–80.

Glávits R, Ványi A (1995) More important mycotoxicoses in pigs. Comprehensive clinico-pathological communication. *Magyar Állatorvosok Lapja* **50:** 407–20.

Goyarts T, Dänicke S (2006) Bioavailability of the *Fusarium* toxin deoxynivalenol (DON) from naturally contaminated wheat for the pig. *Toxicol Lett* **163:** 171–82.

Green ML, Diekman MA, Malayer JR, Scheidt AB, Long GG (1990) Effect of prepubertal consumption of zearalenone on puberty and subsequent reproduction of gilts. *J Anim Sci* 68: 171–8.

Gutzwiller A, Gafner J-L (2009) Fertility of sows exposed to zearalenone and deoxynivalenol – as case report. *Mycotox Res* **25:** 21–4.

Hagler WM, Dankó G, Horvath L, Palyusik M, Mirocha CJ (1980) Transmission of zearalenone and its metabolite into ruminant milk. *Acta Vet Acad Sci Hungarica* **28:** 209–16.

He P, Young LG, Forsberg C (1992) Microbial transformation of deoxynivalenol (vomitoxin). *Appl Environ Microbiol* **58:** 3857–63.

Huszenicza G, Fekete S, Szigeti G, Kulcsar M, Febel H, Kellems RO, Nagy P, Cseh S, Veresegyhazy T, Hullar I (2000) Ovarian consequences of low dose peroral *Fusarium* (T-2) toxin in a ewe and heifer model. *Theriogenology* **53:** 1631–9.

JECFA (2001) Trichothecenes. In *Safety Evaluation of Certain Mycotoxins in Food.* Joint FAO/WHO Expert Committee on Food Additives, FAO Food and Nutrition paper 74/WHO Food Additives Series 47, pp. 419–680. World Health Organization, Geneva.

Ji GE, Park SY, Wong SS, Pestka JJ (1998) Modulation of nitric oxide, hydrogen peroxide and cytokine production in a clonal macrophage model by the trichothecene vomitoxin (deoxynivalenol). *Toxicology* **125:** 203–14.

Joffe AZ (1974) Toxicity of *Fusarium poae* and *F. sporotrichioides* and its relation to alimentary toxic aleukia. In *Mycotoxins* (Purchase IFH, ed.). Elsevier, New York, pp. 229–62.

Juhasz J, Nagy P, Huszenicza G, Szigeti,G, Reiczigel J, Kulcsar M (1997) Long term exposure to T-2 Fusarium mycotoxin fails to alter luteal function, follicular activity and embryo recovery in mares. *Equine Vet J Suppl* **25:** 17–21.

Juhász J, Nagy P, Kulcsár M, Szigeti G, Reiczigel J, Huszenicza G (2001) Effect of low-dose zearalenone exposure on luteal function, follicular activity, and uterine oedema in cycling mares. *Acta Veterinaria Hungarica* **49:** 211–22.

Katzenellenbogen BS, Katzenellenbogen JA, Mordecai D (1979) Zearalenones: characterization of the estrogenic potencies and receptor interactions of a series of fungal resorcylic acid lactones. *Endocrinology* **105:** 33–40.

Khera KS, Whalen C, Angers G (1986) A teratology study on vomitoxin (4-deoxynivalenol) in rabbits. *Food Chem Toxicol* **5:** 421–4.

Khera KS, Whalen C, Angers G. Vesonder RF, Kuiper-Goodman T (1982) Embryotoxicity of 4-deoxynivalenol (vomitoxin) in mice. *Bull Environ Contam Toxicol* **29:** 487–91.

Kiessling K-H, Pettersson H, Sandholm K, Olsen M (1984) Metabolism of aflatoxin, ocratoxin, zearalenone, and three trichothecenes by intact rumen fluid, rumen protozoa, and rumen bacteria. *Appl Environ Microbiol* **47:** 1070–3.

King RR, McQueen RE, Levesque D, Greenhalgh R (1984) Transformation of deoxynivalenol (vomitoxin) by rumen microorganisms. *J Agric Food Chem* **32:** 1181–3.

Kuiper GG, Lemmen JG, Carlsson B, Corton JC, Safe SH, van der Saag PT, van der Burg B, Gustafsson J-A (1998) Interaction of estrogenic chemicals and phytoestrogens with estrogen receptor β. *Endocrinology* **139:** 4252–63.

Kuiper-Goodman T, Scott PM, Watanabe H (1987) Risk assessment of the mycotoxin zearalenone. *Regul Toxicol Pharmacol* **7:** 253–306.

Kuiper-Goodman T (1994) Prevention of human mycotoxicoses through risk assessment and risk management. In *Mycotoxins in Grain. Compounds Other than Aflatoxin* (Miller JD, Trenholm HL, eds.). Eagan Press, St. Paul, pp. 439–69.

Lafarge-Frayssinet D, Chakor K, Lafont P, Frayssinet C (1990) Transplacental transfer of T2-toxin: pathological effect. *J Environ Pathol Toxicol Oncol* **10:** 64–8.

Malekinejad H, Maas-Bakker R, Fink-Gremmels J (2005) Species differences in the hepatic biotransformation of zearalenone. *Vet J* **172:** 96–102.

Malekinejad H, Schoevers EJ, Daemen IJJM, Zijlstra, Colenbrander B, Fink-Gremmels, Roelen BAJ (2007) Exposure of oocytes to the *Fusarium* toxins zearalenone and deoxynivalenol causes aneuploidy and abnormal embryo development in pigs. *Biol Reprod* **77:** 840–7.

Marasas WFO, Nelson PE, Toussoun TA (1984) *Toxigenic Fusarium Species.* The Pennsylvania State University Press, University Park.

Massart F, Saggese G (2009) Oestrogenic mycotoxin exposures and precocious pubertal development. *Int J Androl* **33:** 369–76.

McLaughlin CS, Vaughan MH, Campbell IM, Wei CM, Stafford ME, Hansen BS (1977) Inhibition of protein synthesis by trichothecenes. In *Mycotoxins in Human and Animal Health* (Rodricks JV, Hesseltine CW, Mehlman MA, eds.). Pathotox Publishers Inc., Park Forest South, IL, pp. 263–75.

McNutt SH, Purwin P, Murray C (1928) Vulvovaginitis in swine. *J Am Vet Med Assoc* **26:** 484–92.

Mekhancha-Dahel C, Lafarge-Frayssinet C, Frayssinet C (1990) Immunosuppressive effects of four trichothecene mycotoxins. *Food Addit Contam* **7:** S94–S96.

Milano GD, Becu-Villalobos D, Tapia O (1995) Effects of long-term zearalenone administration on spermatogenesis and serum luteinizing hormone, follicle-stimulating hormone, and prolactin values in male rats. *Am J Vet Res* **56:** 954–8.

Milano GD, Odriozola E, Lopez TA (1991) Lack of effect of a diet containing zearalenone on spermatogenesis in rams. *Vet Rec* **129:** 33–5.

Miller JD (2002) Aspects of the ecology of *Fusarium* toxins in cereals. In *Mycotoxins and Food Safety* (DeVries JW, Trucksess MW, Jackson LS, eds.). *Adv Ex Med Biol* **54:**19–27. Kluwer Academic/Plenum Publishers, New York.

Mirocha CJ, Christensen CM (1974) Oestrogenic mycotoxins synthesized by *Fusarium*. In *Mycotoxins* (Purchase IFH, ed.). Elsevier, New York.

Mirocha CJ, Pathre SV, Robison TS (1981) Comparative metabolism of zearalenone and transmission into bovine milk. *Food Cosmet Toxicol* **19(1):** 25–30.

Mirocha CJ, Robison TS, Pawlosky RJ, Allen NK (1982) Distribution and residue determination of [3H]zearalenone in broilers. *Toxicol Appl Pharmacol* **66:** 77–87.

Moon Y, Pestka JJ (2002) Vomitoxin-induced cyclooxygenase-2 gene expression in macrophages mediated by activation of ERK and p38 but not JNK mitogen-activated protein kinases. *Toxicol Sci* **69:** 373–82.

Morooka N, Uratsuji N, Yoshizawa T, Yamamoto H (1972) [Studies on the toxic substances in barley infected with *Fusarium* spp.] (in Japanese). *J Food Hyg Soc Japan* **13:** 368–75.

Mueller ST, Simon S, Chae K, Metzler M, Korach KS (2004) Phytoestrogens and their human metabolites show distinct agonistic and antagonistic properties on estrogen receptor α (ERα) and ERβ in human cells. *Toxicol Sci* **80:** 14–25.

Nielsen C, Casteel M, Didier A, Dietrich R, Märtlbauer E (2009) Trichothecene-induced cytotoxicity on human cell lines. *Mycotox Res* **25:** 7–84.

Olsen M, Pettersson H, Sandholm K, Visconti A, Kiessling K-H (1987) Metabolism of zearalenone by sow intestinal mucosa in vitro. *Food Chem Toxicol* **25:** 681–3.

Pace JG (1983) Effect of T-2 mycotoxin on the rat liver mitochondria electron transport system. *Toxicon* **21:** 675–80.

Pace JG, Watts MR, Canterbury WJ (1988) T-2 mycotoxin inhibits mitochondrial protein synthesis. *Toxicon* **26:** 77–85.

Palyusik M, Harrach B, Mirocha CJ, Pathre SV (1980) Transmission of zearalenone and zearalenol into porcine milk. *Acta Vet Acad Sci Hungarica* **28:** 217–22.

Pestka JJ, Bondy GS (1994) Immunotoxic effects of mycotoxins. In *Mycotoxins in Grain. Compounds Other than Aflatoxin* (Miller JD, Trenholm HL, eds.). Eagan Press, St. Paul, pp. 339–58.

Pestka JJ, Smolinski AT (2005) Deoxynivalenol: toxicology and potential effects on humans. *J Toxicol Environ Health, Part B* **8:** 39–69.

Pestka JJ, Yan D, King LE (1994) Flow cytometric analysis of the effects of *in vitro* exposure to vomitoxin (deoxynivalenol) on apoptosis in murine T, B and IgA+ cells. *Food Chem Toxicol* **32:** 1125–36.

Pestka JJ, Uzarski RL, Islam Z (2005) Induction of apoptosis and cytokine production in the Jurkat human T cells by deoxynivalenol: role of mitogen-activated protein kinases and comparison to other 8-ketotrichothecenes. *Toxicol* **206:** 207–19.

Placinta CM, D'Mello JPF, Macdonald AMC (1999) A review of worldwide contamination of cereal grains and animal feeds with *Fusarium* mycotoxins. *Anim Feed Sci Technol* **78:** 21–37.

Prelusky DB, Hamilton RMG, Trenholm HL, Miller JD (1986b) Tissue distribution and excretion of radioactivity following administration of 14C-labelled deoxynivalenol to white Leghorn hens. *Fundam Appl Toxicol* **7:** 635–45.

Prelusky DB, Hartin KE, Trenholm HL, Miller JD (1988) Pharmacokinetic fate of 14C-labeled deoxynivalenol in swine. *Fundam Appl Toxicol* **10:** 276–86.

Prelusky DB, Hartin KE, Trenholm HL (1990) Distribution of deoxynivalenol in cerebral spinal fluid following administration to swine and sheep. *J Environ Sci Health B* **25:** 395–413.

Prelusky DB, Rotter BA, Rotter RG (1994) Toxicology of mycotoxins. In *Mycotoxins in Grain. Compounds Other than Aflatoxin* (Miller JD, Trenholm HL, eds.). Eagan Press, St. Paul, pp. 359–403.

Prelusky DB, Trenholm HL (1991) Tissue distribution of deoxynivalenol in swine dosed intravenously. *J Agric Food Chem* **39:** 748–51.

Prelusky DB, Trenholm HL, Lawrence GA, Scott PM (1984) Nontransmission of deoxynivalenol (vomitoxin) to milk following oral administration to dairy cows. *J Environ Sci Health* **B19:** 593–609.

Prelusky DB, Veira DM, Trenholm HL, Hartin KE (1986a) Excretion profiles of the mycotoxin deoxynivalenol, following oral and intravenous administration to sheep. *Fundam Appl Toxicol* **6:** 356–63.

Rainey MR, Tubbs RC, Bennett LW, Cox NM (1990) Prepubertal exposure to dietary zearalenone alters hypothalamo-hypophysial function but does not impair postpubertal reproductive function of gilts. *J Anim Sci* **68:** 2015–22.

Rizzo AF, Atroshi F, Ahotupa M, Sankari S, Elovaara E (1994) Protective effect of antioxidants against free radical-mediated lipid peroxidation induced by DON or T-2 toxin. *Zentralbl Veterinarmed A* **41:** 81–90.

Robison TS, Mirocha CJ, Kurtz HJ, Behrens JC, Chi MS, Weaver GA, Nystrom SD (1979) Transmission of T-2 toxin into bovine and porcine milk. *J Dairy Sci* **62:** 637–41.

Rocha O, Ansari K, Doohan FM (2005) Effects of trichothecene mycotoxins on eukaryotic cells: a review. *Food Addit Contam* **22:** 369–78.

Roine K, Korpinen EL, Kallela K (1971) Mycotoxicosis as a probable cause of infertility in dairy cows. *Nord Vet Med* **23:** 628–33.

Rosenstein Y, Lafarge-Frayssinet C (1983) Inhibitory effect of *Fusarium* T-2 toxin on lymphoid DNA and protein synthesis. *Toxicol Appl Pharmacol* **70:** 283–8.

Rotter BA, Prelusky DB, Pestka JJ (1996) Toxicology of deoxynivalenol (vomitoxin). *J Toxicol Environ Health* **48:** 1–34.

Rousseaux CG, Schiefer HB (1987) Maternal toxicity, embryolethality and abnormal fetal development in CD-1 mice following one oral dose of T-2 toxin. *J Appl Toxicol* **7:** 281–8.

Rousseaux CG, Schiefer HB, Hancock DS (1986) Reproductive and teratological effects of continuous low-level dietary T-2 toxin in female CD-1 mice for two generations. *J Appl Toxicol* **6:** 179–84.

Ruhr LP, Osweiler GD, Foley CW (1983) Effect of the estrogenic mycotoxin zearalenone on reproductive potential in the boar. *Am J Vet Res* **44:** 483–5.

Saito M, Ohtsubo K (1974) Trichothecene toxins of *Fusarium* species. In *Mycotoxins* (Purchase IFH, ed.). Elsevier, New York, pp. 263–81.

Scott PM (1989) The natural occurrence of trichothecenes. In *Trichothecene Mycotoxicosis: Pathophysiologic Effects*, Vol. I (Beasley VR, ed.). CRC Press, Inc., Boca Raton, pp. 1–26.

Shier WT, Shier AC, Xie W, Mirocha CJ (2001) Structure–activity relationships for human estrogenic activity in zearalenone mycotoxins. *Toxicon* **39:** 1435–8.

Shinozuka S, Suzuki M, Noguchi N, Sugimoto T, Uetsuka K, Nakayama H, Doi K (1998) T-2 toxin induced apoptosis in hematopoietic tissues of mice. *Toxicol Pathol* **26:** 674–81.

Shlosberg A, Weisman Y, Handji V (1984) A severe reduction in egg laying in a flock of hens associated with trichothecene mycotoxins in the feed. *Vet Hum Toxicol* **26:** 384–6.

Smith JF, di Menna ME, McGowan LT (1990) Reproductive performance of Coopworth ewes following oral doses of zearalenone before and after mating. *J Reprod Fertil* **89:** 99–106.

Sprando RL, Collins TFX, Black TN, Olejnik N, Rorie JI, Eppley RM, Ruggles DI (2005) Characterization of the effect of deoxynivalenol on selected male reproductive endpoints. *Food Chem Toxicol* **43:** 623–35.

Stob M, Baldwin RS, Tuite J, Andres FN, Gillette KG (1962) Isolation of an anabolic uterotrophic compound from corn infected with *Gibberella zeae*. *Nature* **196:** 1318.

Sundlof SF, Strickland C (1986) Zearalenone and zearanol: potential residue problems in livestock. *Vet Hum Toxicol* **28:** 242–50.

Swanson SP, Corley RA (1989) The distribution, metabolism, and excretion of trichothecene mycotoxins. In *Trichothecene Mycotoxicosis: Pathophysiologic Effects*, Vol. I (Beasley VR, ed.). CRC Press, Inc., Boca Raton, pp. 37–61.

Swanson SP, Nicoletti J, Rood HD, BuckWB, Côte LM, Yoshizawa T (1987) Metabolism of three trichothecene mycotoxins, T-2 toxin, diacetoxyscirpenol, and deoxynivalenol, by bovine rumen microorganisms. *J Chromatogr* **414:** 335–42.

Thompson WL, Wannemacher RW (1986) Structure–function relationship of 12,13-epoxytrichothecene mycotoxins in cell culture: comparison of whole animal lethality. *Toxicon* **24:** 985–94.

Tiemann U, Dänicke S (2007) *In vivo* and *in vitro* effects of the mycotoxins zearalenone and deoxynivalenol on different non-reproductive and reproductive organs in female pigs: a review. *Food Addit Contam* **24:** 306–14.

Tumbleson ME, Schook LB (1996) Advances in swine in biochemical research. In *Advances in Swine in Biochemical Research*. Plenum, New York, pp. 99–112.

Ueno Y (1983) General toxicology. In *Trichothecenes – Chemical, Biological, and Toxicological Aspects* (Ueno Y, ed.). Elsevier, New York, pp. 135–46.

Valenta H, Dänicke S (2005) Study on the transmission of deoxynivalenol and de-epoxy-deoxynivalenol into eggs of laying hens using a high-performance liquid chromatography- ultraviolet method with clean-up by immunoaffinity columns. *Mol Nutr Food Res* **49:** 779–85.

Ványi A, Széky A (1980) Fusariotoxicoses. VI. The effect of F-2 toxin (zearalenone) on the spermatogenesis of male swine. *Magy Állatorv Lapja* **35:** 242–6.

Ványi A, Szemerédi G, Szailer ER (1974) Fusariotoxicoses on a cattle farm. *Magy Állatorv Lapja* **29:** 544–6.

Vesonder RF, Ciegler A, Jensen AH (1973) Isolation of the emetic principle from *Fusarium*-infected corn. *Appl Microbiol* **26:** 1008–10.

Vesonder RF, Ciegler A, Jensen AH, Rohwedder WK, Weisleder D (1976) Co-identity of the refusal and emetic principle from fusarium-infected corn. *Appl Environ Microbiol* **31:** 280–5.

Weaver GA, Kurtz HJ, Bates FY, Ch, MS, Mirocha CJ, Behrens JC (1978b) Acute and chronic toxicity of T-2 mycotoxin in swine. *Vet Rec* **103:** 531–5.

Weaver GA, Kurtz HJ, Behrens JC, Robison TS, Sequin BE, Bates FY, Mirocha CJ (1986a) Effect of zearalenone on the fertility of virgin heifers. *Am J Vet Res* **47:** 1395–7.

Weaver GA, Kurtz HJ, Behrens JC, Robison TS, Sequin BE, Bates FY, Mirocha CJ (1986b) Effect of zearalenone on dairy cows. *Am J Vet Res* **47:** 1826–8.

Weaver GA, Kurtz HJ, Mirocha CJ, Bates FY, Behrens JC, Robinson TS, Gipp WF (1978a) Mycotoxin-induced abortions in swine. *Can Vet J* **19:** 72–4.

Yang G-H, Jarvis BB, Chung Y-J, Pestka JJ (2000) Apoptosis induction by the satratoxins and other trichothecene mycotoxins: relationship to ERK, p38 MAPK, and SAPK/JNK activation. *Toxicol Appl Pharmacol* **164:** 149–60.

Yoshizawa T, Mirocha CJ, Swanson SP (1981) Metabolic fate of T-2 toxin in a lactating cow. *Food Cosmet Toxicol* **19:** 31–9.

Young LG, King GJ (1986a) Low concentrations of zearalenone in diets of mature gilts. *J Anim Sci* **63:** 1191–6.

Young LG, King GJ (1986b) Low concentrations of zearalenone in diets of boars for a prolonged period of time. *J Anim Sci* **63:** 1197–200.

Young LG, Ping H, King GJ (1990) Effects of feeding zearalenone to sows on rebreeding and pregnancy. *Anim Sci* **68:** 15–20.

Zhou H-R, Islam Z, Pestka JJ (2005) Induction of competing apoptotic and survival signaling pathways in the macrophage by the ribotoxic trichothecene deoxynivalenol. *Toxicol Sci* **87:** 113–22

Zinedine A, Soriano JM, Moltó JC, Mañes J (2007) Review on the toxicity, occurrence, metabolism, detoxification, regulations and intake of zearalenone: an oestrogenic mycotoxin. *Food Chem Toxicol* **45:** 1–18.

C H A P T E R

55

Aflatoxins, ochratoxins and citrinin

Ramesh C. Gupta

INTRODUCTION

The occurrence of aflatoxins is ubiquitous, but it is more frequently encountered in tropical countries, such as Africa and Asia. Aflatoxins are produced mainly by *Aspergillus flavus* and *Aspergillus parasiticus*, and very rarely by *Aspergillus nomius* in insignificant amounts. The four major naturally produced aflatoxins are known as aflatoxins B_1, B_2, G_1 and G_2. "B" and "G" refer to the blue and green fluorescent colors produced by these compounds and visualized under UV light on a thin layer chromatography plate. The subscript numbers 1 and 2 indicate major and minor compounds, respectively. AFB_1 and AFB_2 are hydroxylated and excreted in the milk as AFM_1 and AFM_2, which are of a lower toxicity than the parental aflatoxins. Structural formulas of aflatoxins are shown in Figure 55.1. Aflatoxins are both acutely and chronically toxic to humans and animals, causing liver damage, liver cirrhosis, induction of tumors and teratogenic effects. The most common and toxic form of aflatoxins is aflatoxin B_1. Both AFB_1 and AFM_1 are carcinogenic.

Ochratoxins and citrinin are produced by several species of the genera *Aspergillus* and *Penicillium*. Ochratoxin A (OTA) was first described as a metabolite of *Aspergillus ochraceus*, a species with natural habitats in drying and decaying vegetation, fruits, nuts and seeds. Later, it was found in other *Aspergillus* and *Penicillium* species, particularly *Penicillium verrucosum*. *Aspergillus* spp. appears to produce ochratoxins under conditions of high humidity and temperature, whereas *Penicillium* spp. may produce ochratoxins at temperatures as low as 5°C. OTA is a pentaketide-derived dihydroisocoumarin moiety coupled with a 12-carboxy group by a peptide bond to *L*-phenylalanine. There are two commonly recognized OTA analogs, ochratoxin B and C, and of course alkyl esters of ochratoxins. Structural formulas of ochratoxins are shown in Figure 55.2, and the order of their toxicity is OTA > OTB > OTC. OTA and its analogs are the main contaminants of cereals (corn, barley, wheat) and to some extent beans (coffee, soy and cocoa), and the levels are typically less than 200 μg/kg (ppb). Humans are exposed to OTA by consuming contaminated food, particularly pork and grains (Castegnaro *et al.*, 1991; Bretholtz-Emanuelsson *et al.*, 1993). These studies reported OTA levels in human blood and milk up to 35 ppb in wide areas of Europe.

Citrinin was first isolated as a pure compound from a culture of *Penicillium citrinum* in 1931. Later, it was isolated from *A. ochraceus* and *P. verrucosum*, which commonly contaminate grain. Its structural formula is shown in Figure 55.3. In 1951, yellowish colored rice imported from Thailand to Japan was found to be contaminated with *P. citrinum* which contained citrinin. In current molecular biological research, pure synthesized citrinin is used as an inducer of mitochondrial permeability pore opening and inhibits respiration by interfering with complex I of the respiratory chain. Both OTA and citrinin are known to cause nephropathy in animals and Balkan endemic nephropathy (BEN) in humans. Literature reveals that OTA has been studied to a greater extent than citrinin, partly because OTA is at least 10 times more toxic than citrinin.

There are several reports on aflatoxins and ochratoxin, along with a few reports on citrinin, that these mycotoxins produce reproductive and developmental toxicity in humans and animals. This chapter describes in detail the toxicity of these mycotoxins in general, and reproductive and developmental effects in particular.

HISTORICAL BACKGROUND

The fungi producing aflatoxins are commonly found in human food and animal feed around the world. Aflatoxins were isolated about 50 years ago after outbreaks of disease and death in 100,000 turkeys (Blount, 1961), and of cancer in rainbow trout (Halver, 1965) fed rations formulated from peanut and cottonseed meals. The source fungi (*Aspergillus flavus* and *Aspergillus parasiticus*) are ubiquitous, but more frequently encountered in developing countries, affecting dietary staples of rice, corn, cassava, nuts, peanuts and spices. Among the four major aflatoxins (AFB_1, AFB_2, AFG_1 and AFG_2), AFB_1 is the most prevalent and also the most toxic form.

In China, a strong correlation between intakes of aflatoxin-contaminated peanuts, peanut oil and corn and increased mortality rates from liver cancer was reported in five groups of inhabitants from four villages. Exposed individuals had AFM_1 in their urine, which was correlated with a high mortality from

Reproductive and Developmental Toxicology, Edited by Ramesh C. Gupta
ISBN: 978-0-12-382032-7

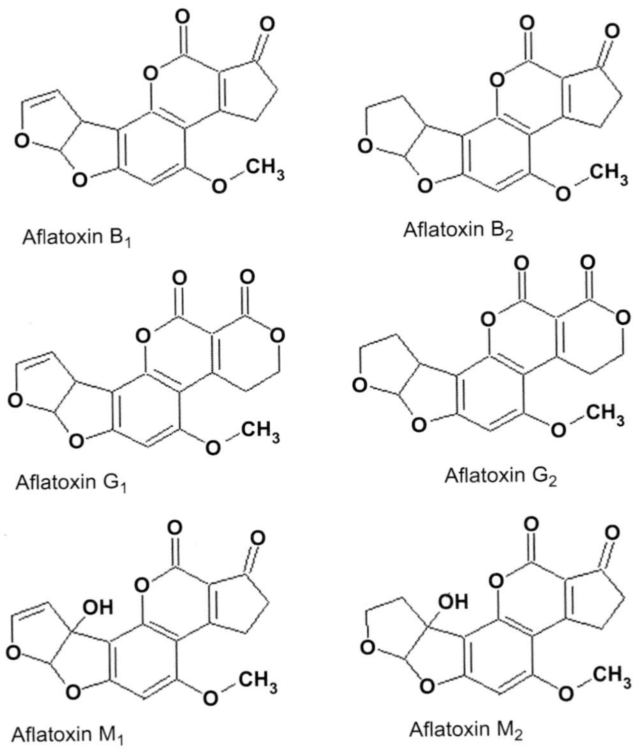

Aflatoxin B_1 Aflatoxin B_2 Aflatoxin G_1 Aflatoxin G_2 Aflatoxin M_1 Aflatoxin M_2

FIGURE 55.1 Structural formulas of aflatoxins.

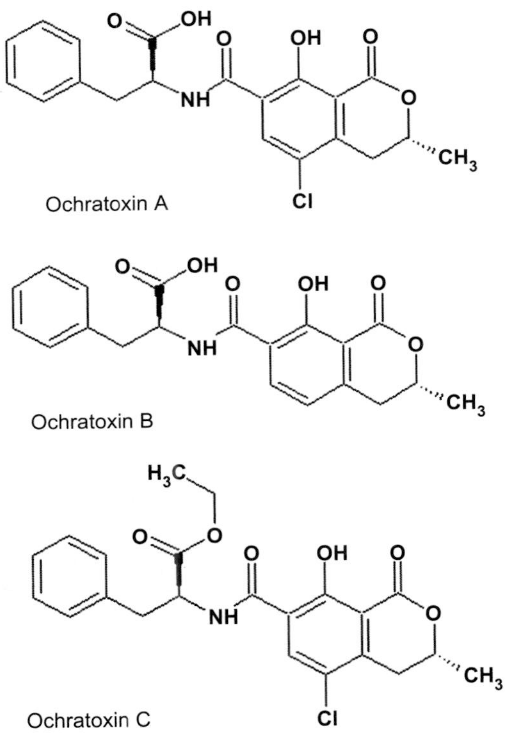

Ochratoxin A Ochratoxin B Ochratoxin C

FIGURE 55.2 Structural formulas of ochratoxins.

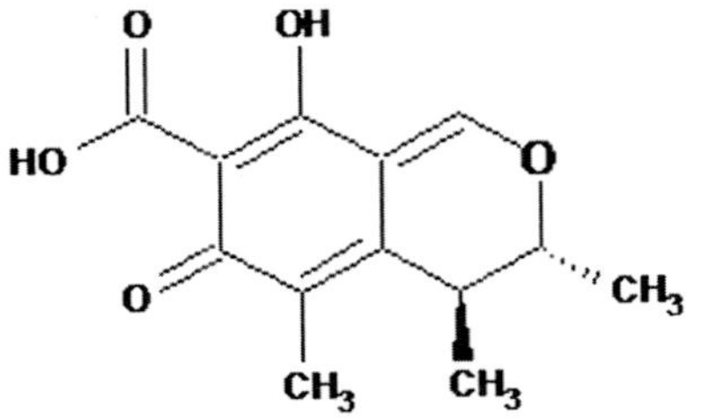

FIGURE 55.3 Structural formula of citrinin.

liver cancer (NLM, 2002a). In 1974, an outbreak of hepatitis, which affected 400 Indian people of whom 100 died by ingesting maize heavily contaminated with *Aspergillus flavus*, had aflatoxin levels up to 15 ppm (Krishnamachari *et al.*, 1975). Consumption of aflatoxin by some of the adults was calculated to be 2–6 mg in a single day, and the acute lethal dose was calculated to be 10–20 mg. According to the report of Lubulwa and Davis (1994), an estimated 20,000 people die from aflatoxin poisoning in Indonesia alone every year. Disease outbreaks due to aflatoxins will continue to be problems of significant public health concern in developing countries as long as people consume contaminated food (Reddy and Raghavender, 2007). In various reports, aflatoxins have also been associated with Reye's syndrome, which is characterized by symptoms of encephalopathy and fatty degeneration of the viscera, in many countries including Europe, Malaysia, Thailand, New Zealand, the USA and Venezuela.

Uriah *et al.* (2001) found that 37% of infertile men in Nigeria had aflatoxin in their blood and semen (700 to 1,392 ng/ml and 60 to 148 ng/ml, respectively), suggesting that aflatoxins may be a contributing factor to the incidence of infertility in Nigerians since the toxin has been shown to produce deleterious effects on the reproductive system. Several studies have revealed that *in utero* exposure to aflatoxins may cause developmental health effects in humans and animals. Gong *et al.* (2002) reported that dietary aflatoxin caused impaired growth in young children in Benin and Togo. In a recent study, Turner *et al.* (2007) reported that a significant number of pregnant women exposed to aflatoxin resulted in growth faltering in the first year of life in Gambian infants. In addition, many experimental studies support the evidence of aflatoxins causing reproductive and developmental toxicity.

The fungi producing ochratoxins and citrinin are commonly encountered in animal feed and human food. They are encountered with great frequency in the Balkan and Scandinavian countries. There are three ochratoxins, but ochratoxin A (OTA) occurs with the greatest frequency naturally in a variety of cereal grains (barley, wheat, oats, corn and beans), peanuts, dried fruits, grapes/resins, cheese and other food products. OTA accumulates in the food chain because of its long half-life. Citrinin usually co-occurs with OTA, and commonly contaminates cereal grains, including wheat, barley, oats, corn and rice. Citrinin also contaminates peanuts and fruits. The levels of OTA and citrinin have been found far lower in human food than in raw animal feed, because during processing and baking human food, citrinin is almost eliminated and OTA is significantly reduced.

Thus far, no cases of acute OTA or citrinin intoxication have been reported in humans. OTA is found more frequently and at higher average concentrations in blood from people living in regions where a fatal human kidney disease (BEN) occurs and is associated with an increased incidence of tumors of the upper urinary tract. However, similar average concentrations have been reported in several other European countries where this disease is not observed. In humans, exposure to OTA and citrinin has been linked with BEN, a chronic kidney disease associated with tumors of the renal system, which can be fatal. Co-occurrence of OTA and citrinin has been implicated in nephropathy of pigs in Denmark, Sweden, Norway and Ireland. These two mycotoxins are also involved in avian nephropathies. Residues of OTA have been detected in the tissues of pigs in slaughterhouses, and it has been shown under experimental conditions that residues can still be detected in tissues 1 month post-exposure. Due to the long half-life of OTA in the feed and body, serious concerns have been raised about animal health, as well as human consumption of meat.

PHARMACOKINETICS/ TOXICOKINETICS

Aflatoxins

Exposure to aflatoxins is typically by ingestion of contaminated foodstuff. Following dermal exposure, absorption is slow but can be significant. In addition, inhalation of aflatoxins has been associated with disease and injury in both humans and animals. Following oral ingestion in the rat, absorption of AFB_1 occurs rapidly in the small intestine and follows first order kinetics (Ramos and Hernandez, 1996). After absorption, 65% of AFB_1 is cleared from the blood in 90 minutes and the plasma half-life is short. The half-life in human liver homogenates is reported to be approximately 13 minutes (Hsieh and Wong, 1982).

Following oral exposure, AFB_1 is metabolized in the intestinal tissue and liver by the microsomal cytochrome P450 (primarily CYP450 $3A_4$ and $1A_2$), resulting in the formation of AFB_1-8,9-epoxide, which binds to DNA and forms AFB_1-guanine adducts (Neal, 1995). *In vitro* metabolism studies have shown the following metabolic reactions for AFB_1: (1) reduction produces aflatoxicol (AFL); (2) hydroxylation produces AFM_1; (3) hydration produces AFB_{2a}; and (4) epoxidation produces AFB_1-2,3-epoxide. The epoxide is the most reactive metabolite and is thought to be responsible for both acute and chronic toxicity of AFB_1 (Hsieh and Wong, 1982).

Furthermore, Kuilman *et al.* (1998) characterized metabolism of aflatoxin B_1 in bovine hepatocytes by measuring total CYP450 content, glutathione S-transferase (GST) activity, ethoxyresorufin *o*-deethylation (EROD), testosterone hydroxylation and α-naphthol glucuronidation. During biotransformation of AFB_1, several metabolites are known to be formed, including AFM_1, AFB_1-dihydrodiol (AFB_1-dhd), AFB_1-glutathione conjugate (AFB_1-GSH) and a polar metabolite. AFB_1-epoxide is detoxified by glutathione conjugation and hydrolysis. The aflatoxin metabolites are excreted mainly in the urine and bile.

Aflatoxin has been shown to cross the placental barrier in humans (Bhat and Moy, 1997). Detection of aflatoxins or their metabolites in cord sera has been used as a biomarker of aflatoxin exposure in women in many countries, including Thailand, Ghana, Nigeria and Gambia. Denning *et al.* (1990) demonstrated transplacental transfer of aflatoxin by quantifying aflatoxins (AFB_1, AFG_1 and AFQ_1) in human cord sera obtained at birth and in serum obtained immediately after birth from mothers in Songkhla, Thailand. Of the 35 samples of cord sera, 17 contained aflatoxin in concentrations ranging from 0.064 to 13.6 nmol/ml, with a mean value of 3.1 nmol/ml. By comparison only two of 35 maternal sera samples contained aflatoxin with a mean value of 0.62 nmol/ml. Recently, Partanen *et al.* (2010) demonstrated placental transfer and metabolism of AFB_1 in human placental perfusions and in *in vitro* studies. Placental perfusion with AFB_1 (0.5 or 5 μM) provided the first direct evidence of the actual transfer of AFB_1 and its metabolism to aflatoxicol (AFL). AFM_1 is also known to cross the placental barrier from the pregnant animal to the fetus. *In vitro* incubations with placental cytosolic fraction confirmed the capacity of human placenta to form AFL. AFL was the only metabolite detected in both perfusions and *in vitro* incubations. It is suggested that AFL is less mutagenic, but putatively as carcinogenic as AFB_1. All these studies suggest that aflatoxin can cross the placental barrier in humans, experimental animals and even the complex placenta of pigs (Peir *et al.*, 1985).

Lamplugh *et al.* (1988) conducted a molecular dosimetry study on women in Gambia and West Africa to establish the relationships between dietary intake of aflatoxins during a 1-week period and a number of aflatoxin biomarkers (aflatoxin metabolite in breast milk). Maxwell *et al.* (1989) detected aflatoxins in 37% of 99 Sudanese, 28% of 191 Kenyan and 34% of 510 Ghanaian breast milk samples. In Ghana, the rate of detection was higher in the wet (41%) than dry (28%) season.

Ochratoxins and citrinin

In most animal species, OTA is absorbed from the stomach because of its lipid soluble, non-ionized and acidic ($pK_a = 7.1$) properties. Based on animal studies, OTA is also absorbed in the duodenum and jejunum, and involved in enterohepatic circulation (Kumagai, 1988; Kumagai and Aibara, 1982). Following oral administration, the overall percentage of OTA absorption is found to be 66% in pigs, 56% in rats, 56% in rabbits and 40% in chickens (Suzuki *et al.*, 1977; Galtier *et al.*, 1981). After a single oral dose, the maximum concentrations of OTA are found within 10–48 h in pigs and rats (Galtier *et al.*, 1979, 1981), 2–4 h in ruminant calves (Sreemannarayana *et al.*, 1988), after 1 h in rabbits and 0.33 h in chickens (Galtier *et al.*, 1981). When absorbed, OTA has shown a high binding affinity for plasma proteins. OTA was found in decreasing order of concentrations in kidney < liver < fat < muscle. The serum half-life of OTA is long and varies widely among various species, i.e., 24–39 h in mice, 35–120 h in rats, 6.7 h in quail, 21–35 days in monkeys (Hagelberg *et al.*, 1989; Kuiper-Goodman and Scott, 1989; Stander *et al.*, 2001), 72–120 h in pigs, 4.1 h in chicken (Galtier *et al.*, 1981) and 840 h in humans (Benford *et al.*, 2001).

Toxicokinetics of OTA in pigs is important from an animal as well as a human health viewpoint. It has been observed that the kidney is the most heavily contaminated with OTA, and that the levels in blood are about five-fold greater than in the kidney. It has been determined that if the level of OTA in swine kidney is 12.1 ng/g (resulting from approximately 1,000 ng/g in the feed), its levels would be 7.8 ng/g in the liver, 4.2 ng/g in the muscle and 2.8 ng/g in the adipose tissue. In ruminants, OTA is usually hydrolyzed in the forestomach by protozoans and bacterial enzymes, and consequently little OTA is found in the tissues (Hult *et al.*, 1976).

It is well established that OTA crosses the placental barrier. Applegreen and Arora (1983a,b) determined distribution of ^{14}C-labeled OTA following its i.v. administration in mice at various stages of pregnancy. Using autoradiography, the highest concentration of radioactivity was found in the bile. Among tissues, the highest concentration was found in the liver, followed by kidney, blood, salivary glands, large vessels, brown fat, myocardium, uterus and lymphatic tissues. OTA was also shown to cross the placental barrier on day 9 of pregnancy, at which time it is most effective in producing fetal malformations.

Literature reveals that residue of OTA can be passed in the milk of rats, rabbits and women, but very little is passed in the milk of ruminants due to its rapid metabolism by ruminal microflora. In many species, including monkeys and humans, the major route of excretion is renal elimination, while in rodents biliary excretion is the major route. Excretion of OTA is influenced by the extent of the enterohepatic circulation and binding to serum albumin and other macromolecules (Galtier *et al.*, 1979). The association constant for the binding of OTA to human albumin is 7.1×10^4 per mole in pigs, 5.1×10^4 per mole in chickens and 4.0×10^4 per mole in rats (Galtier *et al.*, 1981). Elimination half-lives are reported to be 5–6 days in rats and pigs and 19–21 days in vervet monkeys. A human study has revealed a fast distribution phase (half-life about 20 h) and a slow elimination phase (plasma half-life 35 days).

OTA is known to be metabolized in animal tissues to ochratoxin *alpha*, which is the major metabolite. This detoxication process takes place in the cecum of rats and is facilitated by bacterial microflora. The enzymes responsible for hydrolysis to ochratoxin *alpha* are carboxypeptidase A and chymotrypsin. Suzuki *et al.* (1977) demonstrated that rat tissue homogenates of the duodenum, ileum and pancreas also have a high enzyme activity to catalyze this reaction. Activity of these enzymes in liver and kidney is low. Studies in mice suggest that OTA circulates from the liver into the bile and into the intestine, where it is hydrolyzed to ochratoxin *alpha* (Moroi *et al.*, 1985). Following i.p. or p.o. administration of OTA in rats, about 25–27% of the dose is present as ochratoxin *alpha* in the urine. Its presence in the urine can be explained by reabsorption from the intestine. A similar mechanism of intestinal reabsorption of ochratoxin *alpha* has been suggested to occur in ruminant calves (Sreemannarayana *et al.*, 1988). For further details of biotransformation of OTA, readers are referred to an extensive review by Benford *et al.* (2001).

In essence, OTA has a high degree of bioavailability, long-tissue half-life and low plasma clearance rate. OTA excretes mainly in the urine and bile, while its residue can also be detected in the milk. No toxicokinetic data of citrinin are available to describe in this chapter.

MECHANISM OF ACTION

Aflatoxins

Aflatoxins are mutagenic, carcinogenic, teratogenic and immunosuppressive. AFB_1 epoxide is highly electrophilic and reacts with the DNA guanine moiety to form covalent bonds at the *N*-7 guanine residue, leading to "depurination" and carcinogenesis (Smela *et al.*, 2001). "Depurination" is a process in which the purine base of a DNA molecule is lost, potentially leading to a somatic mutation and carcinogenesis. Aflatoxins can damage the mitochondrial membrane by covalent binding to mitochondrial DNA and disruption of energy (ATP) production, and increased cell death by apoptosis. AFB_1 preferentially attacks mitochondrial DNA (mtDNA) vs. nuclear DNA during hepatocarcinogenesis (Niranjan *et al.*, 1982). The concentration of carcinogen adducts in mtDNA remains unchanged even after 24 h, possibly because of lack of excision repair. Similarly, mitochondrial transcription and translation remain inhibited up to 24 h, suggesting long-term effects of AFB_1 on the mitochondrial genetic system. Datta and Kulkarni (2009) reported that AFB_1 is a teratogen in rodents and may be a transplacental carcinogen in humans. Evidence suggests that a mixture of lipoxygenase isoenzymes and AFB_1 adducts are present in human term placenta. Mechanisms involved in reproductive and developmental toxicity may be different than that involved in liver cancer.

Ochratoxins and citrinin

The toxicity of OTA is multifaceted and complex, and as a result multiple mechanisms are involved. In addition to primary toxicity, i.e. nephrotoxicity, OTA is immunotoxic (Stormer and Lea, 1995), teratogenic (Arora *et al.*, 1978) and carcinogenic (Creppy *et al.*, 1985). It is also known to disrupt blood coagulation (Gupta *et al.*, 1979) and glucose metabolism (Pitout, 1968).

OTA is proven genotoxic in both *in vitro* and *in vivo* studies, but the mechanism of genotoxicity is unclear by direct interaction with DNA. Mally *et al.* (2005) suggested that OTA may cause genetic damage in target and non-target tissues, independent of direct covalent binding to DNA. Recent evidence indicates that the site-specific renal toxicity, as well as the DNA damage and genotoxic effects of OTA, is most likely attributable to cellular oxidative damage. OTA, by competing with the phenylalanine aminoacylation reaction catalyzed by Phe-tRNA synthase, caused inhibition of protein, DNA and RNA synthesis (Creppy *et al.*, 1984).

Several lines of experimental observations demonstrate that OTA affects mitochondrial function and causes mitochondrial damage (Wei *et al.*, 1985; Wallace, 1997). OTA impairs mitochondrial respiration and oxidative phosphorylation through interference with the mitochondrial membrane and by inhibition of succinate-supported electron transfer activities of the respiratory chain. OTA also disrupts hepatic microsomal calcium homeostasis by impairing the endoplasmic reticulum membrane via lipid peroxidation (Omar and Rahimtula, 1991).

OTA has been shown to cause pathological changes in the ultrastructure of mitochondria in the liver and in the proximal convoluted tubules and glomeruli of kidneys. These changes include abnormal shapes, enlarged mitochondrial matrix and excessive lipid droplets. OTA has been shown to enhance lipid peroxidation both in *in vitro* and *in vivo* studies (Rahimtula *et al.*, 1988; Omar *et al.*, 1990; Baldi *et al.*, 2004), thereby causing excessive generation of free radicals and oxidative stress. Ultimately, it proceeds to cell death in the hepatocytes and proximal tubules (Hoehler *et al.*, 1997; Gautier *et al.*, 2001). OTA also causes cell death by apoptosis (Seegers *et al.*, 1994), which is mediated through cellular processes involved in the degradation of DNA. The mechanism of action of citrinin is similar to OTA, i.e. mitochondrial damage primarily through oxidative injury in the kidney (Ribeiro *et al.*, 1997).

TOXICITY

Aflatoxins

General toxicity

A variety of toxicological effects are observed in humans and animals following oral, inhalation or dermal exposure to aflatoxin. Following aflatoxin exposure, there can be one of three consequences: (1) large doses lead to an acute illness, followed by death, usually through liver cirrhosis; (2) chronic sublethal doses lead to nutritional and immunologic consequences; and (3) all doses have a cumulative effect and the risk of cancer. The toxicity of aflatoxin can vary between species, within the same species, age and gender, in addition to dose, duration of exposure and nutritional and environmental factors (Howard *et al.*, 1990; Williams *et al.*, 2004).

Rats are found to be the most sensitive mammal with the male Fischer rat being the most sensitive strain. Species differences appear to be due to the differences in the rates and extents of metabolic activation and detoxification. Rabbits and ducks are more susceptible as they have a low median lethal dose (0.3 mg/kg), whereas chickens have a greater tolerance (18 mg/kg). Adult humans usually have a high tolerance of aflatoxin as compared to young children (Williams *et al.*, 2004).

Human studies show a positive correlation between the population exposed to AFB_1 and hepatocellular carcinoma (Wild and Turner, 2002). IARC classified aflatoxins as a human carcinogen (IARC, 1993, 2002) based on experimental evidence for the carcinogenicity of both AFB_1 and AFM_1. Based on studies in rats, FAO/WHO (2001) estimated the potency of AFM_1 to be 10% of that of AFB_1. AFB_1 has also been found as a potent liver carcinogen in a number of animal species and a wide species variability exists. It causes liver tumors in mice, rats, fish, marmosets and monkeys following administration by various routes. The types of cancers described in research animals include hepatocellular carcinoma (rats), colon and kidney (rats), cholangiocellular (hamsters), lung adenomas (mice) and osteogenic sarcoma, adenocarcinomas of the gall bladder and carcinoma of the pancreas (monkeys).

Interestingly, in an *in vitro* study, Cometa *et al.* (2005) examined the effects of AFB_1 on mouse brain acetylcholinesterase (AChE) and specifically on its molecular isoforms (G_1 and G_4). AFB_1 (from 10^{-9} to 10^{-4}M) inhibited mouse brain AChE activity ($IC_{50} = 31.6 \times 10^{-6}$M) and its G_1 and G_4 molecular forms in a dose-dependent manner. Michaelis-Menton parameters indicated that the K_m value increased from 55.2 to 232.2%, whereas V_{max} decreased by 46.2–75.1%. The data suggested that AFB_1-induced AChE inhibition was non-competitive in mouse brain by blocking access of the substrate to the active site or by inducing a defective conformational change in the enzyme through non-covalent binding, interacting with the AChE peripheral binding site, or through both mechanisms. These findings offered an explanation for aflatoxin-induced cholinergic symptoms observed in humans and animals (Hall *et al.*, 1989; Hussein and Brasel, 2001).

Reproductive and developmental toxicity

There are many reports that describe deleterious effects of aflatoxin on the reproductive and developmental systems, such as sexual maturation, growth and maturation of the follicles, levels of hormones, gestation and growth of the fetus (Kourousekos and Lymberopoulos, 2007).

In many *in vivo* and *in vitro* studies, aflatoxin has been investigated for male reproductive toxicity and the principal target organ is the testes and, of course, various aspects of spermatogenesis (Agnes and Akbarsha, 2001, 2003; Ortatatli *et al.*, 2002; Faridha *et al.*, 2006; Tajik *et al.*, 2007; Faisal *et al.*, 2008). In an early study, Egbunike *et al.* (1980) found testicular degeneration, sloughing of germ cells and concomitant reduction in the rate and efficiency of sperm production in rats treated with sublethal doses of AFB_1. Sotomayor *et al.* (1999) investigated the action of AFB_1 on DNA of testes and the consequent germ cell mutagenesis. Agnes and Akbarsha (2001) demonstrated an extensive development of pale vacuolated epithelial cells (PVECs) in all segments of the mouse epididymis as a response to AFB_1 treatment. In a chronic study, Agnes and Akbarsha (2003) treated the Swiss albino mice with AFB_1 (500 µg/kg body weight/day) for 7, 15, 30 and 45 days. AFB_1 caused decreased sperm concentration in the epididymis and sperm motility, increased sperm abnormalities and retention of the cytoplasmic droplet by the sperm, thereby leading to drastically reduced male fertility. With the same AFB_1 treatment, Faridha *et al.* (2006) investigated histopathological and histometric alterations in the testes of Swiss mice. The findings revealed duration-dependent regression of the testis and seminal vesicles, and histopathological changes were observed in both the spermatogenic and androgenic compartments of the testis. Fragmentation of chromatin of pachytene spermatocytes, generation of uni- and multinucleate giant cells, and premature loss of spermatids and spermatocytes occurred, whereas the seminiferous tubules regressed, and the Leydig cells underwent hypertrophy and distortion of shape of the nucleus. Generation of multiple micronucleate giant cells and an extensive loss of germ cells from the seminiferous epithelium were also observed. Treated animals recovered over a period of time since spermatogonia and Sertoli cells are not vulnerable targets to aflatoxin toxicity. In a recent report, Shuaib *et al.* (2010) also reported that AFB_1 caused regression of testis, impairment of spermatogenesis and premature loss of germ cells. Findings revealed the presence of higher concentrations of aflatoxins in the semen of infertile men (40% of cases compared to 8% of controls).

Ibeh and Saxena (1997a,b) reported that AFB_1 impairs the reproductive performance of female animals. Female rats (Druckery Strain) receiving AFB_1 (7.5 and 15 mg/kg, p.o. for 21 days) showed significant reductions in the number of oocytes and large follicles in a dose-related manner. Blood hormone levels and sex organ weights were significantly altered. There were reductions in ovarian and uterine sizes, increases in fetal resorption, implantation loss and intra-uterine death in aflatoxin-exposed female rats. Histopathological examination of the ovaries in aflatoxin exposed mature domestic fowl showed follicular atresia, accompanied by cessation of egg production during the entire feeding period (Hafez *et al.*, 1982). Abd El-Wahhab *et al.* (1996) reported microscopic changes in the ovaries of rabbits treated with 0.15 mg aflatoxin/kg body weight. Pathological alterations in the form of coagulative necrosis appeared mainly in the growing and mature follicles, as well as decreased number and size of Graffian and growing follicles with an increased number of atretic follicles and small areas of degenerative changes. Recently, El-Azab *et al.* (2009) observed that AFB_1-induced infertile females had high levels of LH concentration. This was due to increasing LH basal level from anterior pituitary and/or secretion of gonadotropin releasing hormone (GnRH) from hypothalamus, and lower levels of progesterone synthesis. Furthermore, AFB_1 negatively affects hepatic alpha fetoprotein (AFP) synthesis, which has been shown to cause genital function blockade, leading to reduced levels of hormonal promoters (Castelli *et al.*, 1986).

Deleterious effects of aflatoxin on embryo and the developing fetus have been reported in humans and experimental animals. Abdelhamid (2005) demonstrated that aflatoxin lowered fertility to 13% and significantly increased the mortality of embryos in humans. Following *in utero* exposure to aflatoxin, an increase in fetal resorption, implantation loss and intra-uterine deaths have been observed in experimental animals.

The developmental toxicity of AFB_1 has been studied in various laboratory animal models, and AFB_1 has been found to be embryotoxic and/or teratogenic in rats, mice, hamsters, chick embryos, tadpoles and Japanese medaka eggs. Evidence suggests that aflatoxins are teratogenic to most animal species (WHO, 1990; Wangikar *et al.*, 2005a). Transplacental carcinogenesis by AFB_1 has been reported in rats (Tanaka, 1975; Goettler *et al.*, 1980). Tanimura *et al.* (1982) demonstrated that aflatoxin B_1 induced cleft palate, skeletal malformations and intrauterine growth retardation in mouse fetuses of dams treated with doses of 32 mg/kg, i.p./day for 2 days of gestation day (GD) 6–7, 8–9, 10–11 or 12–13. In a behavioral teratogenicity study, Kihara *et al.* (2000) reported that prenatal exposure of rats to AFB_1 produced a delay of early response development, impaired locomotor coordination and impaired learning ability in the offspring of rats exposed to AFB_1 during mid-pregnancy. This report also noted that early gestational exposure appears to produce more effects than later exposure.

Aflatoxins have been detected in breast milk samples collected in countries of high aflatoxin incidence. Therefore, mother's milk appears to be another route for aflatoxin exposure to a developing organism. Mohiuddin (1972) exposed lactating monkeys with a daily dose of aflatoxin (500 μg) for a period of 18 weeks and found no toxic effects in suckling pups, while mothers showed hepatic lesions. It is important to mention that AFM_1 crosses the placental barrier and thereby reaches the fetus in animals. Human exposure to AFM_1 occurs primarily through the milk and milk products from animals that have consumed AFB_1-contaminated feed (IARC, 1993; Reddy and Raghavender, 2007).

Ochratoxins and citrinin

General toxicity

The acute LD_{50} of OTA, depending on the route of administration, is reported in several animal species and is as follows: female mice (22 mg/kg, i.p.), male rats (30.5 mg/kg, p.o.; 12.6 mg/kg, i.p.), female rats (21.4 mg/kg, p.o.; 14.3 mg/kg, i.p.), chickens (3.3 mg/kg, p.o.), turkeys (5.9 mg/kg, p.o.), quail (16.5 mg/kg, p.o.), 1-day-old chicks (3.6 mg/kg, p.o.), rainbow trout (4.7 mg/kg, i.p.), dog (0.2 mg/kg, p.o.) and female pigs (1 mg/kg, p.o.).

The most sensitive and pivotal effects of OTA are its effects on the kidney in rats and pigs. Pigs appear to be the most sensitive animal species. In a chronic (5-week and 3-month) feeding study conducted on female pigs, a lowest-observed-adverse-effect level (LOAEL) of 8 μg/kg body weight/day was derived based on effects on renal enzymes and renal function tests. No nephropathy was observed at 8 μg/kg body weight/day. In another chronic (2-year) study in female pigs, progressive nephropathy but no renal failure was seen at a dose of 40 μg/kg body weight/day.

OTA has been reported to cause renal toxicity/nephropathy, immunosuppression and neurotoxicity in several species, and is mutagenic, carcinogenic and teratogenic in several experimental animals (Pitt, 2000; Pitt *et al.*, 2000; Gupta, 2007, 2009). Following exposure with a high acute dose, OTA produces necrosis of the renal tubules and periportal liver cells where the main pathological changes are observed.

Target organs for OTA are the kidneys and the developing nervous system (Kuiper-Goodman and Scott, 1989; Krogh, 1992). Other than nephropathy and urinary tumors, the evidence for human toxicity is scant. Balkan endemic nephropathy (BEN) associated with OTA occurs mainly in Europe (Bulgaria, Croatia and Yugoslavia) where OTA is relatively high in the diet and in sera (Radic *et al.*, 1997; Radovanovic, 1989). Similar observations are also made in Egypt and Turkey. Furthermore, the observations suggested that both men and women with urinary tract tumors had elevated levels of OTA in the blood and urine. Approximately one-third of patients dying from BEN have papillomas and/or carcinomas of the renal pelvis, ureter or bladder. Recently, it has been suggested that OTA can cause testicular cancer in humans. The incidence rates of testicular cancer in 20 countries was significantly correlated with the per-capita consumption of coffee and pig meat. Schwartz (2002) demonstrated that OTA is a biologically plausible cause of testicular cancer.

The nephrotoxic effects are related to the fact that OTA interacts with iron, forming a complex and producing hydroxyl radicals that promote lipid peroxidation. Renal damage is morphologically characterized by atrophy of the proximal tubule, fibrosis and sclerosis. It is functionally characterized by incapacity of the tubular function, shown by a reduced ability to concentrate urine (Pitt *et al.*, 2000).

Citrinin toxicity, especially in reference to nephropathy, has been reported in various animal species, including rats (Jordan *et al.*, 1978a; Lockard *et al.*, 1980; Mayura *et al.*, 1984; Singh *et al.*, 2007), hamsters (Jordan *et al.*, 1978b), dogs (Carlton *et al.*, 1974) and poultry (Ahamad and Vairamuthu, 2001). For further details on toxicity of OTA and citrinin, refer to the recent publication of Gupta (2007, 2009).

Reproductive and developmental toxicity

It is well established that OTA crosses the placental barrier and can also be transferred to newborn rats and mice via lactation (Applegreen and Arora, 1983a,b; Fukui *et al.*, 1987; Hallen *et al.*, 1998). In addition, OTA-DNA adducts are formed in the liver, kidney and other tissues of progeny (Pfohl-Leszkowicz *et al.*, 1993; Petkova-Bocharova *et al.*, 1998).

There is strong evidence that OTA causes birth defects in rodents (Hayes *et al.*, 1974; Brown *et al.*, 1976; Wangikar *et al.*, 2004a,b), chickens (Gilani *et al.*, 1978) and pigs (Shreeve *et al.*, 1977). In rodent fetuses, the major target is the developing CNS. In other words, OTA is also considered a neurotoxicant. In mice, damage to the neural plates and folds, midbrain and forebrain was reported in one study, while the second study showed cell death in the telencephalon. Other abnormalities included necrosis of the brain (mice), fetal resorption, visceral and skeletal defects in rats, mice and hamsters (Singh and Hood, 1985; NLM, 2002b), craniofacial (exencephaly, midfacial and lip clefts, hypotelorism and synophthalmia) and body wall malformations in mice (Wei and Sulik, 1993), and a reduction of synapses per neuron in the somatosensory cortex of mice (Fukui *et al.*, 1992). While the mechanism involved in OTA-induced teratogenesis still remains unclear, it seems to directly affect both the progenitor cells and the embryo.

In a dose–response study, Patil *et al.* (2006) observed that a single oral dose of 2.75 mg/kg body weight OTA was found to be the minimum effective teratogenic dose and GDs 6 and 7 were found to be the most critical for the induction of teratogenicity in pregnant Wistar rats.

OTA at 2.75 mg/kg administered on one of the GDs 6–15 caused significant maternal toxicity and various gross, visceral and skeletal anomalies in the fetus. The major gross malformations were external hydrocephaly, incomplete closure of skull and omphalocele. Internal hydrocephaly, microphthalmia, enlarged renal pelvis and renal hypoplasia were the main internal soft tissue anomalies. Major skeletal anomalies were developmental defects in skull bones, sternebrae, vertebrae and ribs. By now, there is compelling evidence that OTA is a teratogen affecting the nervous system, skeletal structures and immune system of research animals. In a teratogenic study in rabbits, Wangikar *et al.* (2005b) found that simultaneous exposure to OTA and AFB_1 produced an antagonistic interaction.

In a recent study, Singh *et al.* (2007) exposed female Wistar rats during GD 6–20 with citrinin at 10 mg/kg food to assess maternal toxicity. The rate of fetal resorptions was 12.5% compared to 3.86% in controls. The histopathological changes were primarily in the kidney. The proximal convoluted tubules (PCT) epithelial cells showed extensive degeneration with vacuolations and desquamation of epithelial cells, and these cells occluded the lumen of the PCT. Large vacuoles were also seen in the epithelial lining cells of the PCT. The cells were swollen with pinkish granular cytoplasm and occasionally karyomegaly of the nuclei. Medullary tubules revealed pinkish, homogeneous proteinaceous materials in their lumina. The intertubular blood vessels were found to be consistently dilated and engorged. Histological changes in the uterus were evident only in cases of abortion or at the resorption sites. The changes included intense congestion of blood vessels both in the endometrium and myometrium. In a follow-up study, using the same treatment regimen, these investigators histopathologically examined the liver and kidneys of rat fetuses (Singh *et al.*, 2008). Evaluation of the fetal liver revealed only sinusoidal dilation and mild vacuolar degeneration, whereas consistent changes in the fetal kidney included tubular degeneration, medullary tubular necrosis, cystic dilatation of tubules, distortion of glomerular capillary tuft and interstitial fibroblastic proliferation. Several investigators have reported similar changes with citrinin in PCT of rats (Jordan *et al.*, 1978a; Lockard *et al.*, 1980), hamsters (Jordan *et al.*, 1978b), dogs (Carlton *et al.*, 1974), mice (Bilgrami and Jeswal, 1993) and poultry (Maryamma *et al.*, 1990; Uma and Vikram Reddy, 1995; Ahamad and Vairamuthu, 2001). Observations of all these studies are consistent with the fact that the kidney is the target organ for citrinin and therefore citrinin is regarded as a nephrotoxic mycotoxin (Ribeiro *et al.*, 1997).

In conclusion, OTA and its analogs can produce a variety of toxic effects, referred to as "ochratoxicosis", including mutagenesis, carcinogenesis, BEN, embryotoxicity, teratogenesis and immune suppression, by damaging mitochondria, DNA, protein and RNA by oxidative injury (lipid peroxidation). OTA causes mitochondrial damage, oxidative burst, lipid peroxidation and interferes with oxidative phosphorylation. In addition, OTA causes cell death by apoptosis.

In contrast to OTA, citrinin is studied to a lesser extent, but citrinin exerts similar toxic effects. Citrinin is embryo/fetotoxic and embryocidal in mice and rats. Yang *et al.* (1993) examined developmental toxicity of citrinin in *Hydra attenuata* (HA) and rat whole embryo culture (WEC). The *Hydra* developmental hazard index (A/D ratio) was equal to 1.5, classifying citrinin as a co-affective developmental toxin. Using whole embryo culture, rat embryos were cultured in homologous (rat) serum containing citrinin at concentrations ranging from 0 to 300 μg/ml for a period of 45 h. The results indicated a concentration-dependent reduction in yolk sac diameter, crown–rump length, somite number, protein and DNA content. Histopathological examination revealed severe diffuse mesodermal and ectodermal necrosis in embryos treated with 250 μg/ml citrinin. Based on both bioassays, citrinin is not found to be a primary developmental mycotoxin.

RISK ASSESSMENT

Aflatoxins

Aflatoxins are potent mutagens and hepatocarcinogens and they have been linked to a wide variety of human health problems (Krishnamachari *et al.*, 1977; Groopman *et al.*, 1996). Interspecies variability in terms of toxicity is large (Wogan, 1992). In both humans and animals, aflatoxin exposure occurs through consumption of contaminated food/feed. In countries with a high dietary aflatoxin intake, a daily exposure of 1.7 μg/kg body weight has been estimated but it could exceed 1 mg/day at certain times of the year (Eaton and Groopman, 1994). Due to the high toxicity of aflatoxins, low limits for aflatoxins in foods have been set by many countries. The US Food and Drug Administration (US FDA) has established maximum allowable levels of total aflatoxin in food at 20 μg/kg (20 ppb) and in milk at 0.5 ppb for human consumption. The total aflatoxin level at 15 ppb is likely to become the maximum level permitted in food commodities in world trade. High levels up to 300 ppb are allowed in feed for cattle, swine and poultry. For immature animals, however, the level is still set at 20 ppb. Realistically, these regulatory guidelines are rarely applied in developing countries.

Currently, there are several biomarkers of aflatoxin exposure that are implemented in humans and animals. Analysis of body fluids for the presence of aflatoxin derivatives is the preferred choice to determine human exposure (Makarananda *et al.*, 1998; Wild and Pisani, 1998). Recent exposure to aflatoxin is reflected in the urine as directly excreted AFM_1 and other detoxication products, but only a small fraction of the dose is excreted this way (NLM, 2002a). The aflatoxin–albumin adduct is measured in peripheral blood, which has a half-life in the body of 30–60 days, and is therefore considered a useful biomarker reflecting long-term exposure to aflatoxins in different populations (Gan *et al.*, 1988). This measure integrates with the exposure over a longer period and hence is a more reliable marker of chronic exposure.

Ochratoxins and citrinin

OTA is the major component of and the most toxic among all ochratoxins. However, it was estimated that an infant could eat up to 10 kg of food contaminated with 20 ppb OTA without significant adverse health effects (Chu, 1974). In later studies, the tolerable dosage in humans was estimated at 0.2 to 0.4 ng/kg body weight based upon the NTP (National Toxicology Program) carcinogenicity study in rats. Given the relatively long half-life of OTA in humans, a tolerable weekly intake (TWI) is determined at 120 ng/kg body weight/week, which equals a total daily intake (TDI) of 17.1 ng/kg body weight/day. However, there are no regulatory levels established for OTA or citrinin.

Negative health effects of mycotoxins are well recognized and are regarded as global issues. Children appear to be an especially vulnerable subgroup, due to their higher food consumption per kg body weight and differences in physiology compared to adults, resulting in relatively higher exposure to toxicants (NRC, 1993). This has been thoroughly described in a recent report published by the Dutch Food and Consumer Product Safety Authority (VMA, 2008). Both national and international authorities on food safety, such as the US FDA, European Food Safety Authority (EFSA) and others, play great roles in preventing adverse health effects by minimizing mycotoxins' exposure.

TREATMENT

There is no specific antidote for toxicity of aflatoxins, ochratoxins and citrinin. Immediate removal of the contaminated food/feed and supplementation with increased levels of protein, vitamins and antioxidants can be rewarding. Recovery is usually slow. Compared to aflatoxins and ochratoxins, citrinin is less of a problem because it is heat unstable, and therefore it is destroyed during the processing and baking of food. Of course, there are some strategic measures to prevent and minimize negative health effects by reducing the levels of these mycotoxins in the food/feed. This is an important global issue rather than a national or regional one. The FDA's goal for aflatoxins has been to minimize contamination by implementing regulations that focus special attention on the management of the problem. Biological exposure of aflatoxins can be minimized by chemoprotection and/or enterosorption. Chemoprevention against aflatoxins has been demonstrated with the use of a number of compounds (such as esterified glucomanoses and other yeast extracts) that either increase detoxification of aflatoxin (Kensler *et al.*, 1993) or prevent the production of the epoxide that leads to chromosomal damage (Hayes *et al.*, 1998). Compounds such as oltipraz and chlorophyll are available to decrease the biologically effective dose (Bolton *et al.*, 1993). Enterosorptive food additives are recommended because they bind aflatoxins and render them biologically unavailable to humans and animals (Williams *et al.*, 2004). These compounds are certain clay minerals that selectively adsorb aflatoxins tightly enough to prevent their absorption from the GI tract (Phillips *et al.*, 1988). In a number of *in vivo* and *in vitro* studies, the use of hydrated sodium calcium aluminosilicates (HSCAS or NovaSil) in contaminated feeds has proven effective in preventing aflatoxicosis in turkeys, chickens, lambs, cattle, pigs, goats, rats and mice. Selected calcium montorilonites have proven to be the most selective and effective of these enterosorbents (Williams *et al.*, 2004). In a detailed study, Mayura *et al.* (1998) investigated preventive effects of HSCAS and zeolitic mineral clinoptilolite in rats exposed to aflatoxin. The study revealed that HSCAS was very effective in reducing bioavailability of AFB_1, while clinoptilolite caused maternal toxicity. It is important to mention that by no means should these binders be considered as mycotoxin eliminators. Also, one disadvantage with these binders is that there can be some interference in the absorption of essential nutrients. This factor should definitely be taken into consideration during pregnancy and developmental period. The strategy involving regular monitoring of mycotoxins residues in feed/food and serum/blood could prevent or minimize the occurrence of mycotoxicosis in humans and animals.

CONCLUDING REMARKS AND FUTURE DIRECTIONS

Aflatoxins, ochratoxins and citrinin are naturally occurring mycotoxins that contaminate food/feed. AFB_1 among aflatoxins and OTA among ochratoxins are the most toxic and occur with greatest frequencies. OTA and citrinin are discussed together because they are both nephrotoxicants. Although these mycotoxins occur ubiquitously, the prevalence of aflatoxins is greater in Africa and Southeast Asia, whereas OTA and citrinin occur mostly in Europe (Balkan and Scandinavian countries). All three mycotoxins have the potential for exerting a variety of toxicological effects in humans and animals. AFB_1 primarily produces hepatic cancer, while OTA and citrinin produce nephropathy. Both AFB_1 and OTA are immunosuppressive, carcinogenic and reproductive and developmental toxicants, and proven teratogens. These mycotoxins have been detected in human blood, semen, placenta and cord blood, and they apparently enter the developing fetus in humans and animals (Applegreen and Arora, 1983a,b; Denning *et al.*, 1990). Aflatoxins have also been detected in human breast milk, cow's milk and dairy products, and infant formula (El-Nezami *et al.*, 1995; Aksit *et al.*, 1997; Srivastava *et al.*, 2001; Elmali *et al.*, 2008). They cause inhibition of protein synthesis and form DNA adducts. Both mycotoxins also cause mitochondrial damage, including mitochondrial DNA, mitochondrial membranes, disruption of energy (ATP) production, and increased cell death by apoptosis. There is wide species variability to these mycotoxins. Male rats (Fischer strain) are most sensitive to aflatoxin, while pigs and dogs are most sensitive to OTA and citrinin. Children and young animals are more sensitive than adults (Cullen and Newberne, 1993; NRC, 1993). In general, aflatoxin is found normally in humans and more frequently in females than in males, although males are more sensitive. The health significance of these mycotoxins is not only for humans and animals, but also for their fetuses and neonates. The health effects of these mycotoxins are potentially profound and therefore deserve further investigations, especially in areas of the developing nervous system, risk assessment, regulatory actions and treatment.

ACKNOWLEDGMENT

I would like to thank Mrs. Kristie M. Rohde and Mrs. Robin B. Doss for their technical assistance in preparation of this chapter.

REFERENCES

Abd El-Wahhab MA (1996) Effect of aflatoxin B treatment on pregnancy, newborn and quality of milk produced from mammals. PhD thesis, Ain Shams University, Faculty of Agriculture, Cairo, Egypt.

Abdelhamid AM (2005) *Carcinogenesis.* 1st edition. Dar Anashr for Universities, Cairo, Egypt.

Agnes VF, Akbarsha MA (2001) Pale vacuolated epithelial cells in epididymis of aflatoxin-treated mice. *Reproduction* **122:** 629–41.

Agnes VF, Akbarsha MA (2003) Spermatotoxic effect of aflatoxin B_1 in the albino mouse. *Food Chem Toxicol* **41:** 119–30.

Ahamad DB, Vairamuthu S (2001) Individual and combined effects of citrinin and aflatoxin B_1 in broiler chicks. *Indian J Vet Pathol* **27:** 32–4.

Aksit S, Caglayan S, Yaprak I, Kansoy S (1997) Aflatoxin: is it neglected threat for formula-fed infants? *Acta Pediatr Jpn* **39:** 34–6.

Applegreen LE, Arora RG (1983a) Distribution studies of ^{14}C-labelled aflatoxin B_1 and ochratoxin A in pregnant mice. *Vet Res Commun* **7:** 141–4.

Applegreen LE, Arora RG (1983b) Distribution of ^{14}C-labelled ochratoxin A in pregnant mice. *Food Chem Toxicol* **21:** 563–8.

Arora RG, Applegreen LE, Bergman A (1978) Distribution of ^{14}C-labelled aflatoxin B_1 in mice. *Acta Pharmacol Toxicol* **43:** 273–9.

Baldi A, Losio MN, Cheli F, Rebucci R, Sangalli L, Fusi E, Bertasi B, Pavoni E, Carli S, Politis I. (2004) Evaluation of the effects of [alpha]-tocopherol and retinol against ochratoxin A cytotoxicity. *Br J Nutr* **91(4):** 507–12.

Benford D, Boyle C, Decant W, Fuchs R, Gaylor DW, Hard G, McGregor DB, Pitt JI, Plestina R, Shepard G, Solfrizzo M, Verger PJP, Walker R (2001) Ochratoxin A. *Joint Expert Food Addit* Rome, 281–418.

Bhat RV, Moy GG (1997) Monitoring and assessment of dietary exposure chemical contaminants. *World Health Statist Quart* **50:** 132–49.

Bilgrani KS, Jeswal P (1993) Control of citrinin caused nephrotoxicosis through aqueous leaf extract of *Vitis vinifera* L. mercurious corrossivus and cortisone. *Indian J Exper Biol* **31:** 482–4.

Blount WP (1961) Turkey "X" disease. *J Br Turk Fed* **9:** 52–4.

Bolton MG, Munoz A, Jacobson LP, *et al.* (1993) Transient intervention with oltipraz protects against aflatoxin-induced hepatic tumorigenesis. *Cancer Res* **53:** 3499–504.

Bretholtz-Emanuelsson A, Olsen M, Oskarsson A, Palminger I, Hult K (1993) Ochratoxin A in cow's milk and human milk with corresponding human blood samples. *JOAC Intl* **76:** 842–6.

Brown MH, Szczeck GM, Purmalis BP (1976) Teratogenic and toxic effects of ochratoxin A in rats. *Toxicol Appl Pharmacol* **37:** 331–8.

Carlton WW, Sansing G, Szczech GM, Tuite J (1974) Citrinin mycotoxicosis in beagle dogs. *Food Cosmet Toxicol* **12:** 479–90.

Castegnaro M, Plestina R, Dirheimer G, Chernozemsky IN, Bartsch H (1991) Mycotoxins, Endemic Nephropathy and Urinary Tract Tumors. IARC Scientific Publications No. 115. World Health Organization/International Agency for Research on Cancer. Lyon, France.

Castelli D, Seralini GE, Lafaurie M, Krebs B, Stora C (1986) Ovarian function during aflatoxin B_1-induced hepatocarcinogenesis in the rat. *Res Commun Chem Pathol Pharmacol* **53(2):** 183–94.

Chu FS (1974) Studies on ochratoxins. *CRC Crit Rev Toxicol* **2(4):** 499–524.

Cometa MF, Lorenzini P, Fortuna S, Volpe MT, Meneguz A, Palmery M (2005) *In vitro* inhibitory effect of aflatoxin B_1 on acetylcholinesterase activity in mouse brain. *Toxicology* **206:** 125–35.

Creppy EE, Kane A, Dirheimer G (1985) Genotoxicity of ochratoxin A in mice: DNA single-stranded break evaluation in spleen, liver, and kidney. *Toxicol Lett* **28:** 29–35.

Creppy EE, Roschenthaler R, Dirheimer G (1984) Inhibition of protein synthesis in mice by ochratoxin A and its prevention by phenylalanine. *Food Chem Toxicol* **22(11):** 883–6.

Cullen JM, Newberne PM (1993) Acute hepatotoxicity of aflatoxins. In *The Toxicology of Aflatoxins: Human Health, Veterinary, and Agriculture Significance* (Eaton DL, Groopman JD, eds.). Academic Press, London, pp. 1–26.

Datta K, Kulkarni AP (2009) Oxidative metabolism of aflatoxin B_1 by lipoxygenase purified from human intrauterine conceptual tissues. *Chem Res Toxicol* **22(5):** 913–7.

Denning DW, Allen R, Wilkinson AP, Morgan MRA (1990) Transplacental transfer of aflatoxin in humans. *Carcinogenesis* **11(6):** 1033–5.

Eaton DL, Groopman JD (1994) *The Toxicology of Aflatoxins: Human Health, Veterinary, and Agricultural Significance.* Academic Press, San Diego, CA.

Egbunike GN, Emerole GO, Aire TA, Ikegwuonu FI (1980) Sperm production rates, sperm physiology and fertility in rats chronically treated with sublethal doses of aflatoxin B_1. *Andrologia* **12:** 467–75.

El-Azab SM, Abdelhamid AM, Shalaby HA, Mehrim AI, Ibrahim AH (2009) Study of aflatoxin B_1 as a risk factor that impairs the reproductive performance in females – Egypt. *The Internet J Toxicol* **6(1):** 1–13.

Elmali M, Yapar K, Kart A, Yaman H (2008) Aflatoxin M_1 levels in milk powder consumed in Turkey. *J Anim Vet Adv* **7(5):** 643–6.

El-Nezami HS, Nicoletti G, Neal GE, Donohue DC, Ahokas JA (1995) Aflatoxin M_1 in human breast milk samples in Victoria, Australia and Thailand. *Food Chem Toxicol* **33:** 173–9.

Faisal K, Faridha A, Akbarsha MA (2008) Induction of micronuclei in spermatocytes *in vivo* by aflatoxin B_1: light and transmission electron microscopic study in Swiss mouse. *Reprod Toxicol* **26:** 303–9.

FAO/WHO (2001) Safety evaluation of certain mycotoxins in food. Prepared for the fifth-sixth meeting of the Joint FAO/WHO Expert Committee on Food Additives (JECFA) WHO Food Additives Series, No. 47/FAO Food and Nutrition paper 74. Rome, Geneva: Food and Agriculture Organization. World Health Organization.

Faridha A, Faisal K, Akbarsha MA (2006) Duration-dependent histopathological and histometric changes in the testes of aflatoxin B_1-treated mice. *J Endocrinol Reprod* **10:** 117–33.

Fukui Y, Hayasaka S, Itoh M, Takeuchi Y (1992) Development of neurons and synapses in ochratoxin A-induced microcephalic mice: a quantitative assessment of somatosensory cortex. *Neurotoxicol Teratol* **14:** 191.

Fukui Y, Hoshino K, Kameyama Y, Yasui T, Toda C, Nagano H (1987) Placental transfer of ochratoxin A and its cytotoxic effect on the mouse embryonic brain. *Food Chem Toxicol* **25(1):** 17–24.

Galtier P, Alvinerie M, Charpenteau JL (1981) The pharmacokinetic profile of ochratoxin A in pigs, rabbits, and chickens. *Food Cosmet Toxicol* **19:** 735–8.

Galtier P, Charpenteau JL, Alvinerie M, Labouche C (1979) The pharmacokinetic profile of ochratoxin A in the rat after oral and intravenous administration. *Drug Metab Disp* **7:** 429–34.

Gan LS, Skipper PL, Peng X, Groopman JD, Chen J-S, Gerald N, Wogan GL, Tannenbaum SR (1988) Serum albumin adducts in the molecular epidemiology of aflatoxin carcinogenesis: correlation with aflatoxin B_1 intake and urinary excretion of aflatoxin M_1. *Oxford J Life Sci Carcinogenesis* **9(7):**1323–5.

Gautier JC, Holzhaeuser D, Marcovic J, Gremaud E, Schilter B, Turesky J (2001) Oxidative damage and stress response from ochratoxin A exposures in rats. *Free Radic Biol Med* **30:** 1089–98.

Gilani SH, Brancroft J, Riley M (1978) Teratogenicity of ochratoxin A in chick embryos. *Toxicol Appl Pharmacol* **46:** 543–6.

Goettler K, Löhrke H, Schweizer H, Hesse B (1980) Effects of aflatoxin B_1 on pregnant inbred Sprague-Dawley rats and their F_1 generation. A contribution to transplacental carcinogenesis. *J Natl Cancer Inst* **64:** 1349–54.

Gong YY, Cardwell K, Hounsa A, Egal S, Turner PC, Hall AJ, Wild CP (2002) Dietary aflatoxin exposure and impaired growth in young children from Benin and Togo: cross sectional study. *Br Med J* **325:** 20–1.

Groopman JD, Wang JS, Scholl P (1996) Molecular biomarkers for aflatoxins: from adducts to gene mutations to liver cancer. *Can J Physiol Pharmacol* **74:** 203–9.

Gupta M, Bandopadhyay S, Paul B, Majumder SK (1979) Hematological changes produced in mice by ochratoxin A. *Toxicology* **14:** 95–8.

Gupta RC (2007) Ochratoxins and citrinin. In *Veterinary Toxicology: Basic and Clinical Principles* (Gupta RC, ed.). Academic Press/Elsevier, Amsterdam, pp. 997–1003.

Gupta RC (2009) Toxicology of the placenta. In *General and Applied Toxicology*, 3rd edition (Ballantyne B, Marrs TC, Syversen T, eds.). John Wiley and Sons, Chichester, pp. 2002–39.

Hafez AH, Megalla SE, Abdel-Fattah HM, Kamel YY (1982) Aflatoxin and aflatoxicosis. II. Effects of aflatoxin on ovaries and testicles in mature domestic fowls. *Mycopathologia* **77(3):** 137–9.

Hagelberg S, Hult K, Fuchs R (1989) Toxicokinetics of ochratoxin A in several species and its plasma-binding properties. *J Appl Toxicol* **9:** 91–6.

Hall RF, Harrison LR, Colvin BM (1989) Aflatoxicosis in cattle pastured in a field of sweet corn. *J Am Vet Med Assoc* **194:** 938.

Hallen IP, Jorhem L, Oskarsson A (1998) Placental and lactational transfer of ochratoxin A in rats: a study on the lactational process and effects on offspring. *Arch Toxicol* **69:** 596–602.

Halver JE (1965) Aflatoxicosis and rainbow trout hepatoma. In *Mycotoxins in Foodstuff* (Wogan GN, ed.). MIT Press, Cambridge, MA, pp. 209–34.

Hayes AW, Hood RD, Lee HL (1974) Teratogenic effects of ochratoxin A in mice. *Teratology* **9:** 93–8.

Hayes JD, Shen X, He X, *et al.* (1998) Regulation of rat glutathione S-transferase A5 by cancer chemopreventive agents: mechanisms of inducible resistance to aflatoxin B_1. *Chem-Biol Interact* **111/112:** 51–67.

Hoehler D, Marqurdt RR, McIntosh AR, Hatch GM (1997) Induction of free radicals in hepatocytes, mitochondria and microsomes of rats by ochratoxin A and its analogs. *Biochim Biophys Acta* **1357:** 225–33.

Howard S, Ramdell D, Eaton DL (1990) Species susceptibility to aflatoxin B_1 carcinogenesis. *Cancer Res* **50:** 615–20.

Hsieh DPH, Wong JJ (1982) Metabolism and toxicity of aflatoxins. *Adv Exp Med Biol* **136(B):** 847–63.

Hult K, Teilling A, Gatenbeck S (1976) Degradation of ochratoxin A by a ruminant. *Appl Environ Microbiol* **32:** 443–4.

Hussein HS, Brasel JM (2001) Toxicity, metabolism, and impact of mycotoxins in humans and animals. *Toxicology* **167:** 101–34.

IARC (1993) Some naturally occurring substances: food items and constituents, heterocyclic aromatic amines and mycotoxins. Monograph 56. International Agency for Research on Cancer. Lyos, France.

IARC (2002) Some traditional herbal medicines, some mycotoxins, naphthalene and styrene. IARC Monograph on the Evaluation of Carcinogenic Risks to Humans. Vol. 82, Lyos, France.

Ibeh IN, Saxena DK (1997a) Aflatoxin B_1 and reproduction. I. Reproductive performance in female rats. *Afr J Reprod Health* **1(2):** 79–84.

Ibeh IN, Saxena DK (1997b) Aflatoxin B_1 and reproduction. II. Gametoxicity in female rats. *Afr J Reprod Health* **1(2):** 85–9.

Jordan WH, Carlton WW, Sansing GA (1978a) Citrinin mycotoxicosis in rats. *Food Cosmet Toxicol* **16:** 431–9.

Jordan WH, Carlton WW, Sansing GA (1978b) Citrinin mycotoxicosis in Syrian hamster. *Food Cosmet Toxicol* **16:** 355–63.

Kensler TW, Davis EF, Bolton MG (1993) Strategies for chemoprevention against aflatoxin-induced liver cancer. In *The Toxicology of Aflatoxins: Human Health, Veterinary, and Agricultural Significance* (Eaton D, Groopman JD, eds.). Academic Press, London, pp. 281–306.

Kihara T, Matsuo T, Sakamoto M, Yasuda Y, Yamamoto Y (2000) Effect of prenatal aflatoxin B_1 exposure on behaviors or rat offspring. *Toxicol Sci* **53:** 392–9.

Kourousekos GD, Lymberopoulos AG (2007) Occurrence of aflatoxins in milk and their effects on reproduction. *J Hellenic Vet Med Soc* **58(4):** 306–12.

Krishnamachari KAVR, Bhat RV, Nagarajan V, Tilak TBG, Tulpule PG (1977) The problem of aflatoxin in human diseases in parts of India: epidemiological and ecological aspects. *Ann Nutr Aliment* **31:** 991–6.

Krishnamachari KAVR, Bhat RV, Nagarajan V, Tilak TBG (1975) Investigation into an outbreak of hepatitis in parts of Western India. *Indian J Vet Res* **63:** 1036–48.

Krogh P (1992) Role of ochratoxin in disease causation. *Food Chem Toxicol* **30:** 213–24.

Kuilman MEM, Maas RFM, Judah DJ, Fink-Gremmels J (1998) Bovine hepatic metabolism of aflatoxin B_1. *J Agr Food Chem* **46(7):** 2707–13.

Kuiper-Goodman T, Scott PM (1989) Risk assessment of the mycotoxin ochratoxin A. *Biomed Environ Sci* **2(3):** 179–248.

Kumagai S, Aibara K (1982) Intestinal absorption and secretion of ochratoxin A in the rat. *Toxicol Appl Pharmacol* **64:** 94–102.

Kumagai S (1988) Effects of plasma ochratoxin A and luminal pH on the jejunal absorption of ochratoxin A in rats. *Food Chem Toxicol* **26(9):** 753–8.

Lamplugh SM, Hendrickse RG, Ageagyei F, Mwanmut DD (1988) Aflatoxins in breast milk, neonatal cord blood and serum of pregnant women (short report). *Br Med J* **296:** 968.

Lockard VG, Phillips RD, Hayes AW, Berndt WO, Neal RM (1980) Citrinin nephrotoxicity in rats: a light and electron microscopic study. *Exp Mol Pathol* **32:** 226–40.

Lubulwa ASG, Davis JS (1994) Estimating the social cost of the impact of fungi and aflatoxins in maize and peanuts. In *Stored Product Protection* (Highly E, Wright EJ, Banks HJ, Champ BR, eds.). CAB International, Wallingford, pp. 1017–42.

Makarananda K, Pengpan U, Srisakulthong M, Yoovathaworn K, Sriwatatanakul K (1998) Monitoring of aflatoxin exposure by biomarkers. *J Toxicol Sci* **23:** 155–9.

Mally A, Pepe G, Ravoori S, Fiore M, Gupta RC, Dekant W, Mosesso P (2005) Ochratoxin A causes DNA damage and cytogenetic effects but no DNA adducts in rats. *Chem Res Toxicol* **18:** 1253–61.

Maryamma KO, Rajan A, Gopalakrishnan MN, Ismail PK, Manmohan CB, Farshid AA (1990) Pathology of citrinin toxicosis in chickens and analysis of residual toxin in tissues. *J Vet Anim Sci* **21:** 67–71.

Maxwell SM, Apeagyei F, De Vries HR, Mwanmut DD (1989) Aflatoxin in breast milk, neonatal cord blood and sera of pregnant women. *Toxin Rev* **8:** 1–2.

Mayura K, Abdel-Wahhab A, McKenzie KS, Sarr AB, Edwards JF, Naguib K, Phillips TD (1998) Prevention of maternal and developmental toxicity in rats via dietary inclusion of common aflatoxin sorbents: potential for hidden risks. *Toxicological Sci* **41:** 175–82.

Mayura K, Parker R, Berndt WO, Phillips TD (1984) Effect of simultaneous prenatal exposure to ochratoxin A and citrinin in the rat. *J Toxicol Environm Health* **13:** 553–61.

Mohiuddin SM (1972) Studies on the effects of aflatoxin on monkeys. PhD thesis, Konkan Krishi Vidyapith, Dapoli, India.

Moroi K, Suzuki S, Kuga T, Yamazaki M, Kanisawa M (1985) Reduction of ochratoxin A toxicity in mice treated with phenylalanine and phenobarbital. *Toxicol Lett* **25:** 1–5.

National Library of Medicine (2002a) Aflatoxins. *Hazardous Substances Data Base.* Toxnet (National Data Network).

National Library of Medicine (2002b) Ochratoxin A, B and C. *Hazardous Substances Data Base.* Toxnet (National Data Network).

National Research Council (1993) *Pesticides in the Diet of Infants and Children.* National Academy Press, Washington DC.

Neal GE (1995) Genetic implications in the metabolism and toxicity of mycotoxin. *Toxicol Lett* **82/83:** 861–7.

Niranjan BG, Bhat NK, Avadhani NG (1982) Preferential attack of mitochondrial DNA by aflatoxin B_1 during hepatocarcinogenesis. *Science* **215:** 73–5.

Omar RF, Hasinoff BB, Mejilla F, Rahimtula AD (1990) Mechanism of ochratoxin A stimulated lipid peroxidation. *Biochem Pharmacol* **40:** 1180–91.

Omar RF, Rahimtula AD (1991) Role of cytochrome P-450 and in ochratoxin A-stimulated lipid peroxidation. *J Biochem Toxicol* **6(3):** 203–9.

Ortatatli M, Ciftci MK, Tuzcu M, Kaya A (2002) The effects of aflatoxin on the reproductive system of rooster. *Res Vet Sci* **72:** 29–36.

Partanen HA, El-Nezami HS, Leppänen JM, Myllynen PK, Woodhouse HJ, Vähäkangas KH (2010) Aflatoxin B_1 transfer and metabolism in human placenta. *Toxicol Sci* **113:** 216–25.

Patil RD, Dwivedi P, Sharma AK (2006) Critical period and minimum single oral dose of ochratoxin A for inducing developmental toxicity in pregnant Wistar rats. *Reprod Toxicol* **22:** 679–87.

Peir AC, McLoughlin ME, Richard JL, Baetz A, Dahfren RR (1985) *In utero* transfer of aflatoxin and selected effects in neonatal pigs. In *Trichothecenes and Other Mycotoxins* (Lacey J, ed.). Wiley, New York, NY, pp. 495–506.

Petkova-Bocharova T, Stoichev II, Chernozemsky IN, Castegnaro M, Pfohl-Leszkowicz A (1998) Formation of DNA adducts in tissues of mouse progeny through transplacental contamination and/or lactation after administration of a single dose of ochratoxin A to the pregnant mother. *Environ Mol Mutagen* **32:** 155–62.

Pfohl-Leszkowicz A, Grosse Y, Kane A, Creppy EE, Dirheimer G (1993) Differential DNA adduct formation and disappearance in three mice tissues after treatment by the mycotoxin, ochratoxin A. *Mutat Res* **289:** 265.

Phillips TD, Kubena LF, Harvey RB, Taylor DR, Heidelbaugh ND (1988) Hydrated sodium calcium aluminosilicates: high affinity sorbent for aflatoxin. *Poult Sci* **67:** 243–7.

Pitout MJ (1968) The effect of ochratoxin A on glycogen storage in the rat liver. *Toxicol Appl Pharmacol* **13:** 299–306.

Pitt JI (2000) Toxigenic fungi: which are important? *Medical Mycol* **38 (Suppl.):** 17–22.

Pitt JI, Basilico JC, Abarca ML, Lopez C (2000) Mycotoxins and toxigenic fungi. *Medical Mycol* **38 (Suppl.):** 41–6.

Radic B, Fuchs R, Peraica M, Lucic A (1997) Ochratoxin A in human sera of endemic nephropathy in Croatia. *Toxicol Lett* **91:** 105–9.

Radovanovic Z (1989) Etiology of Balkan nephropathy: a reappraisal after 30 years. *Eur J Epidemiol* **5:** 372–7.

Rahimtula AD, Bereziat J-C, Bussacchini-Griot V, Bartsch H (1988) Lipid peroxidation as a possible cause of ochratoxin A toxicity. *Biochem Pharmacol* **37:** 4469–77.

Ramos AJ, Hernandez E (1996) *In situ* absorption of aflatoxins in rat small intestine. *Mycopathologia* **134:** 27–30.

Reddy BN, Raghavender CR (2007) Outbreaks of aflatoxicosis in India. *Afr J Food Agr Nutr Develop* **7(5):** 1–15.

Ribeiro SM, Chagas GM, Campello AP, Clupello ML (1997) Mechanism of citrinin induced dysfunction of mitochondria. V. Effect on the homeostasis of the reactive oxygen species. *Cell Biochem Funct* **15:** 203–9.

Schwartz GC (2002) Hypothesis: does ochratoxin A cause testicular cancer? *Cancer Causes Control* **13:** 91–100.

Seegers JC, Bohmer LH, Kruger MC, Lottering ML, de Kock M (1994) A comparative study of ochratoxin A-induced apoptosis in hamster kidney and heLa cells. *Toxicol Appl Pharmacol* **129:** 1–11.

Shreeve BJ, Patterson DP, Pepin GA, Roberts BA, Wzathall AE (1977) Effect of feeding ochratoxin to pig during early pregnancy. *Br J Med* **133:** 412–7.

Shuaib FMB, Ehiri J, Abdullahi A, Williams JH, Jolly PE (2010) Reproductive health effects of aflatoxins: a review of literature. *Reprod Toxicol* **29:** 262–70.

Singh J, Hood RD (1985) Maternal protein deficiency enhances the teratogenicity of ochratoxin A in mice. *Teratology* **32:** 381–8.

Singh ND, Sharma AK, Dwivedi P, Patil RD, Kumar M (2007) Citrinin and endosulfan induced maternal toxicity in pregnant Wistar rats: pathomorphological study. *J Appl Toxicol* **27:** 589–601.

Singh ND, Sharma AK, Dwivedi P, Patil RD, Kumar M (2008) Experimentally induced citrinin and endosulfan toxicity in pregnant Wistar rats: histopathological alterations in liver and kidneys of fetuses. *J Appl Toxicol* **28:** 901–7.

Smela ME, Currier SS, Bailey EA, Essignmann JN (2001) The chemistry and biology of aflatoxin B_1: from mutational spectrometry to carcinogenesis. *Carcinogenesis* **22(4):** 535–45.

Sotomayor RE, Sahu S, Washington M, Hinton DM, Chou M (1999) Temporal patterns of DNA adduct formation and glutathione S-transferase activity in the testes of rats fed with aflatoxin B_1: a comparison with patterns in the liver. *Environ Molec Mutagen* **33:** 293–302.

Sreemannarayana O, Frohlich AA, Vitti TG, Marquardt RR, Abramson D (1988) Studies of the tolerance and disposition of ochratoxin A in young calves. *J Anim Sci* **66:** 1703–11.

Srivastava VP, Bu-Abbas B, Ala-Basuny A, Al-Johar W, Al-Mufti S, Siddiqui MKJ (2001) Aflatoxin M_1 contamination in commercial samples of milk and dairy products in Kuwait. *Food Addit Contam* **18:** 993–7.

Stander MA, Nieuwoudt PS, Steyn GS (2001) Toxicokinetics of ochratoxin A in vervet monkeys (*Cercopithecus aethiops*). *Arch Toxicol* **75:** 262–269.

Stormer FC, Lea T (1995) Effects of ochratoxin A upon early and late events in human T-cell proliferation. *Toxicology* **95:** 45–50.

Suzuki S, Satoh T, Yamazaki M (1977) The pharmacokinetics of ochratoxin A in rats. *Jpn J Pharmacol* **27:** 735–44.

Tajik P, Mirshokraee P, Khosravi A (2007) Effects of different concentrations of aflatoxin B on ram epididymal and ejaculatory sperm viability and motility *in vitro*. *Pak J Biol Sci* **15:** 4500–4.

Tanaka T (1975) Direct and delayed effects of aflatoxin B_1 on rat fetus. *Proc Jpn Assoc Mycotoxicol* **1:** 9–12.

Tanimura T, Kihara T, Yamamoto Y (1982) Teratogenicity of aflatoxin B_1 in the mouse. *Rep Environm Sci Res Instit Kinki Univ* **14:** 247–56.

Turner PC, Collinson AC, Cheung YB, Gong YY, Hall AJ, Prentice AM, Wild CP (2007) Aflatoxin exposure *in utero* causes growth faltering in Gambian infants. *Intl J Epidemiol* **36:** 1119–25.

Uma M, Vikram Reddy M (1995) Citrinin toxicity in broiler chicks: hemato-biochemical and pathological studies. *Indian J Vet Pathol* **19:** 11–14.

Uriah N, Ibeh IN, Oluwafemi F (2001) A study on the impact of aflatoxin on human reproduction. *Afr J Reprod Health* **5(1):** 106–10.

VMA (2008) Exceedances of health based limit values for chemicals present in food for children. Den Haag: Voedsel en Waren Autoriteit, Bureau Risicobeoordeling (www.vwa.nl).

Wallace DC (1997) Mitochondrial DNA in aging and disease. *Scientific Am* **277:** 40–7.

Wangikar PB, Dwivedi P, Sharma AK, Telang AG (2005a) Effects of aflatoxin B_1 on embryo fetal development in rabbits. *Food Chem Toxicol* **43:** 607–15.

Wangikar PB, Dwivedi P, Sinha N, Sharma AK, Telang AG (2005b) Teratogenic effects in rabbits of simultaneous exposure to ochratoxin A and aflatoxin B_1 with special reference to microscopic effects. *Toxicology* **215:** 37–47.

Wangikar PB, Dwivedi P, Sinha N (2004a) Teratogenic effects of ochratoxin A in rabbits. *World Rabbit Sci* **12:** 159–71.

Wangikar PB, Dwivedi P, Sinha N (2004b) Effect in rat of simultaneous prenatal exposure to ochratoxin A and aflatoxin B_1. I. Maternal toxicity and fetal malformations. *Birth Defects Res Part B: Dev Reprod Toxicol* **71:** 343–51.

Wei X, Sulik KK (1993) Pathogenesis of craniofacial and body wall malformations induced by ochratoxin A in mice. *Am J Med Genet* **47:** 862–71.

Wei YH, Lu CY, Lin TN, Wei RD (1985) Effect of ochratoxin A on rat liver mitochondrial respiration and oxidative phosphorylation. *Toxicology* **36:** 119–30.

WHO (1990) World Health Organization Environmental Health Criteria 105. Selected Mycotoxins: Ochratoxins, Trichothecenes, Ergot. World Health Organization, Geneva.

Wild CP, Pisani P (1998) Carcinogen DNA and protein adducts as biomarkers of human exposure in environmental cancer epidemiology. *Cancer Detect Prev* **22:** 273–83.

Wild CP, Turner PC (2002) The toxicity of aflatoxins as a basis for public health decisions. *Mutagenesis* **17:** 471–81.

Williams JH, Phillips TD, Jolly PE, Stiles JK, Jolly CM, Aggarwal D (2004) Human aflatoxicosis in developing countries: a review of toxicology, exposure, potential health consequences, and interventions. *Am J Clin Nutr* **80:** 1106–22.

Wogan GN (1992) Aflatoxin carcinogenesis: interspecies potency differences and relevance for human risk assessment. *Progr Clin Biol Res* **374:** 123–37.

Yang YG, Mayura K, Spainhour CB, Edwards JF, Phillips TD (1993) Evaluation of the developmental toxicity of citrinin using *Hydra attenuata* and postimplantation at whole embryo culture. *Toxicology* **85:** 179–98.

C H A P T E R

56

Zootoxins

Sharon M. Gwaltney-Brant

INTRODUCTION

Poisonous and venomous animals are abundant and include over 400 species of venomous snakes, approximately 1,500 species of toxic marine animals and countless numbers of poisonous or venomous arthropods distributed widely throughout the world (Russell, 2001). Virtually every phylum of the animal kingdom is represented by species that produce toxins, termed *zootoxins*, in the form of either poisons or venoms. *Poisons* are toxins that are produced as secondary metabolic products that accumulate in the host animal tissue or that accumulate in tissues of predators following ingestion of toxin-bearing prey (e.g., ciguatoxin accumulation in predatory fish such as barracuda or jack). *Poisonous* animals exert their toxic effect when their tissues come into contact with another animal, usually via oral contact. *Venoms* are toxins that are produced in specialized tissues and are delivered to the target animal through various *venom apparatuses* (e.g., fangs, stingers, etc.) in a process termed *envenomation*. Therefore, from the standpoint of the toxic animal, poisoning is generally a passive process (e.g., being eaten by a predator) whereas envenomation is an active process whereby the venomous animal intentionally delivers its toxin to the target animal (e.g., bite or sting). Not all exposures to toxic animals result in toxicosis, as variations in toxicity of zootoxins can occur due to host and environmental factors such as age, sex, nutritional status, season, geographic location and toxin composition. Similarly, target animals may vary in their susceptibility to toxins due to factors such as age, size, species and location of bite/sting.

HISTORICAL BACKGROUND

Given the profusion of toxic animals in the environment, it is not surprising that exposure to zootoxins is not uncommon, and the mechanisms by which these toxins exert their effects on the exposed animal have been the subject of study for many years. Many components of animal venoms or their individual components have been studied for their pharmacologic and physiologic effects on animal systems. For instance, venom from the Russell's viper (*Daboia russelii*) possesses such strong thrombotic properties that it has been utilized as a widely used laboratory test of blood clotting. However, the effects of zootoxins on reproduction and development have been less well studied, with the majority of research focusing on snake and scorpion venoms. Although the toxins from many other species have been studied for their physiologic or pharmacologic effects (e.g., extracts of *Heloderma suspectum* (Gila monster) venom have been utilized in the study of pancreatic islet physiology (Ham *et al.*, 2009)), research into the toxic effect of these venoms on reproduction or development is sparse in some areas and completely lacking in others. In many cases the only information available is based on case reports of natural exposures to zootoxins.

As with other toxicants (Haschek, 2010), zootoxins may exert their reproductive or developmental effects at one or more different levels. Toxins may alter fertility by acting on hormones or reproductive organs, interfering with fertilization, or inhibiting blastocyst formation. In those animals that give birth to live young, fetal death, malformation, growth retardation and functional deficit are the potential manifestations of toxic insult during pregnancy. Zootoxins may alter placentation or they may cross the placenta to directly affect the embryo–fetus. Maternal intoxication may result in metabolic abnormalities that interfere with blood or oxygen flow to the fetus, resulting in death or deformity due to hypoxia. In many cases, of maternal intoxication during pregnancy, it may be difficult to determine whether a particular outcome was related to direct action of the venom on the fetus, or whether metabolic aberrations due to maternal toxicosis (e.g., hypotension) produced the adverse effect.

MARINE ZOOTOXINS

Marine zootoxins include toxins from dinoflagellates or algae that accumulate in the tissues of marine animals (e.g., domoic acid, gonyautoxins, ciguatera, etc.), cnidarian (jellyfish, anemones, etc.) toxins, echinoderm (starfish, sea stars, etc.) toxins, mollusk (cone shells, octopus, etc.) toxins and fish toxins (venoms and poisons). Although most of these zootoxins have been studied rather extensively for their acute toxicity and physiological molecular effects, only domoic acid has received much study for its effects on reproduction and development.

Reproductive and Developmental Toxicology, Edited by Ramesh C. Gupta
ISBN: 978-0-12-382032-7

Domoic acid

Domoic acid is a heterocyclic amino acid neurotoxin produced by a variety of marine algae, including *Pseudo-nitzchia australis* and *Chondria armata* (Silvagni *et al.*, 2005), and with a structural similarity to kainic acid (Ramsdell and Zabka, 2008). Domoic acid has been associated with outbreaks of amnesiac shellfish poisoning in humans and with deaths of a variety of sea birds and mammals following algal blooms (FAO/IOC/WHO, 2004; Silvagni *et al.*, 2005; Pulido, 2008; Ramsdell and Zabka, 2008). Since 1998, in addition to acute neurologic dysfunction and degenerative cardiomyopathy, reproductive failure in California sea lions (*Zalophus californianus*) has been associated with *Pseudo-nitzchia australis* algal blooms and domoic acid exposure (FAO/IOC/WHO, 2004; Silvagni *et al.*, 2005; Brodie *et al.*, 2006; Ramsdell and Zabka, 2008).

Toxicokinetics

In adult animals, the oral absorption of domoic acid is 5–10% (FAO/IOC/WHO, 2004). Domoic acid has a low volume of distribution (0.25 L/kg), indicating that it remains primarily in the blood compartment. In animals with mature, intact blood–brain barriers (BBB), domoic acid is largely excluded from the central nervous system; animals with immature or defective BBB are at increased risk of the neurologic effects of domoic acid (FAO/IOC/WHO, 2004; Ramsdell and Zabka, 2008). Domoic acid does cross the placental barrier (Goldstein *et al.*, 2009), and enters the prenatal brain tissue in rats (Tanemura *et al.*, 2009). Domoic acid is not metabolized and is excreted unchanged in the urine. Impaired renal function will result in higher serum concentrations and longer half-lives. The elimination half-life is 20 minutes in rodents and 114 minutes in monkeys (FAO/IOC/WHO, 2004).

Toxicity

Domoic acid toxicosis has been associated with gastrointestinal, cardiovascular and neurologic dysfunction in many species. In humans, a lowest-observed-adverse-effect level (LOAEL) dosage of 1 mg/kg has been identified, with the caveat that pregnant women, infants, children and elderly people may be more susceptible (FAO/IOC/WHO, 2004). Studies of the effects of domoic acid in pregnant humans are lacking, but natural exposures in California sea lions and experimental studies in rodents have shed some light on the mechanisms by which domoic acid may affect reproduction and development.

California sea lions exhibiting reproductive failure from exposure to domoic acid experienced abortion and premature parturition, with placental abruption and brain edema of the fetuses being the primary lesions described (Goldstein *et al.*, 2009). Because many of these pregnant females were themselves showing signs of severe domoic acid toxicosis, the possibility that maternal stress due to manifestations of toxicosis (e.g., seizures) may have contributed must also be considered.

The mechanism by which domoic acid exerts its developmental effects is through the alteration of neurogenesis, particularly within the hippocampus. Exposure of mice on gestation day 13 to 0.6 mg/kg domoic acid *in utero* resulted in no apparent effects in the dams and no apparent abnormalities in the neonates at birth (Ramsdell and Zabka, 2008). Postnatally, EEG irregularities and decreased threshold to domoic acid-induced seizures were noted in the mice. By postnatal day 14, morphologic alterations were noted in the hippocampus and were associated with an increased ratio of glutamate:gamma-aminobutyric acid (GABA) as well as an increased density of domoic acid receptors. Exposure of mice to domoic acid at gestation day 13 (which corresponds to the beginning of neurogenesis in the hippocampus) appears to alter migration and/or differentiation of neuroprogenitor cells, leading to an increase of excitatory (glutaminergic) over inhibitory (GABAergic) circuitry within the hippocampus.

Intrauterine exposure to domoic acid has been shown to cause cognitive and memory dysfunction in adult animals that can appear otherwise normal. Exposure of pregnant rats to 1 mg/kg of domoic acid at gestation days 11.5, 14.5 or 17.5 resulted in transient toxicosis in the dams (which recovered within 24 hours) but no apparent physical or social behavioral abnormalities in the male offspring at birth or up to 11 weeks (Tanemura *et al.*, 2009). Neurobehavioral testing done at 11 weeks, however, revealed severe learning and memory impairment and severe alteration of response to anxiety-inducing stimuli. Morphologically, the brains demonstrated myelin deficiencies and overgrowth of neuronal processes in the limbic cortex neurons.

Risk assessment

Many factors can affect the risk of exposure to and toxicosis from domoic acid, including the season, climactic conditions, water temperature, stage of gestation, duration of exposure and species involved. Conditions favoring the proliferation of dinoflagellates that produce domoic acid include upwelling of nutrient-rich water into euphotic zones in the ocean; wind action can push dinoflagellate blooms into sheltered bays, resulting in the concentration of toxins in the warm, settled water. Concentration of toxin within the gut of planktivorous fish can result in exceptionally high levels of domoic acid, putting predators at risk for toxicosis. For instance, levels of domoic acid in the northern anchovy (*Engraulis mordax*) and Pacific sardine (*Sardinops sagax*), prime prey for California sea lions inhabiting rookeries in and around Monterey Bay, have accumulated levels exceeding one part per thousand (1 mg/g) (Ramsdell and Zabka, 2008).

The manifestations of domoic acid effects on nervous system development also relate to the stage of gestation in which the exposure occurred. Early in fetal life, domoic acid affects the proliferation and migration of hippocampal interneurons and pyramidal cells, resulting in morphologic alterations that become apparent later in life as increased susceptibility to seizures and memory dysfunction (Ramsdell and Zabka, 2008). As development progresses and the formation of synaptic connections occur, domoic acid exposure can result in immature seizure behavior and increased neuronal excitability later in life due to alteration of glutamatergic:GABAergic neuronal ratios. Toward the end of gestation or in early postnatal life, exposure to domoic acid in rodents has resulted in full limbic seizures and increased excitability later in life, again due to alterations in glutamine and GABA ratios within the hippocampus. Table 56.1 summarizes the relative dates for these risks for three species.

TABLE 56.1 Effects of domoic acid on hippocampus in rats, macaque and California sea lions

	Toxic effect		
	Neuronal migration aberration	Hippocampal seizures	Limbic seizures
Rat	G 14–20	G 20–P 7	>P 7
Macaque	G 40–80	G 80–120	G > 120
California sea lion	G 50–120	G 120–200	G > 200

Estimated critical dates of gestation (G) or postnatal (P) for exposure to domoic acid to induce toxic effects within the hippocampus of rats, macaques and California sea lions. The three critical dates correlate with hippocampal neurodevelopmental milestones of neurogenesis, synaptogenesis and peak dendritic spine formation (Ramsdell and Zabka, 2008)

The length of *in utero* exposure will vary with the duration of exposure of the dam to domoic acid as well as the length of pregnancy. Animals with long gestation periods have a higher potential to be exposed repeatedly as environmental domoic acid levels fluctuate over time or to have chronic exposure to persistently low levels of domoic acid in the environment.

Species differences in susceptibility to the reproductive and developmental effects of domoic acid have not been extensively investigated. Many of the differences will likely relate to differences in gestation, including length of gestation, and level of postnatal brain development (i.e., precocity of offspring).

Treatment

No treatment modalities exist to prevent the effects of domoic acid other than to remove the patient from the source of the toxin and provide symptomatic and supportive care. Offspring of pregnant animals exposed to domoic acid may be predisposed to seizure disorders or other neurological effects, depending on the timing and extent of exposure.

OTHER MARINE TOXINS

Ciguatera

Ciguatera fish poisoning results from the ingestion of fish that have accumulated toxins produced by the dinoflagellate *Gambierdiscus toxicus*, and is most commonly associated with the ingestion of predatory reef-fish such as snapper, mackerel and barracuda (Tubaro and Hungerford, 2007). A woman who developed a severe case of ciguatera poisoning during the second trimester of pregnancy experienced increased fetal movements within 1 hour of ingestion of the toxin (Senecal and Osterich, 1991). Although the woman suffered typical ciguatera symptoms (pain, vomiting, paresthesia, abdominal cramping, etc.) for 8 weeks, she delivered a normal infant. In another case, a woman in the third trimester of pregnancy delivered an infant suffering from facial palsy and myotonia of the hands. The difference between these two outcomes may have been due to differences in dose or gestational timing.

Chironex fleckeri

All jellyfish are venomous, utilizing the nematocyst as a venom delivery mechanism to acquire food. The venom of the sea wasp *Chironex fleckeri* produces rapid onset of profound cardiovascular and respiratory effects; the venom also has potent neurotoxic and hemolytic properties (Russell, 1996). A single case report exists of a woman in the third trimester of pregnancy who was stung by a box jellyfish and became unconscious and apneic within minutes (Williamson *et al.*, 1980). The woman was revived by rescuers and transported to a hospital where antivenom was administered; the patient was discharged in 4 days and several weeks later delivered a healthy baby. One of the rescue workers, who was also pregnant, was stung by a tentacle that was adherent on the first victim. This woman also delivered uneventfully 2 weeks after the event.

INSECTS

Hymenoptera

Hymenoptera (bees, wasps, hornets, ants) stings are the leading cause of venomous animal-related death in humans in the USA (Langley, 2004). In spite of the frequency of exposure, case reports and research into the effects of insect stings in pregnant humans are sparse, and information into the effects of insect venoms on reproduction and development of other species is seriously lacking.

Toxicity

Hymenopteran venoms contain a mixture of proteins, peptides and small organic molecules (Gwaltney-Brant *et al.*, 2007). Ant venom tends to have low protein content and is made up primarily of alkaloids, whereas bee venom has much higher protein content. The toxicity of bee venom is heightened by the presence of hyaluronidases and phospholipases, which account for a majority of the allergic responses seen with bee envenomation. Mellitin, a membrane disruptive component of bee venom, can induce hemolysis, increase capillary blood flow, increase cell permeability and enhance the spread of venom within tissue. Apamin is a neurotoxic compound that blocks potassium channels and may be responsible for peripheral nerve dysfunction that occasionally occurs in humans following bee stings. Whole bee venom has been shown to be embryotoxic, but not teratogenic, when injected into pregnant rats between gestation days 6 and 14 (Shkenderov and Todorov, 1979).

Several case reports exist of pregnant women experiencing severe reactions to Hymenopteran stings during pregnancy (Langley, 2004). One case of placental abruption and stillbirth was considered to be directly caused by the ant sting that the mother experienced at 40 weeks of gestation, after which she was treated for anaphylaxis. An infant whose mother suffered severe anaphylaxis following a bee sting in the 30th week of gestation exhibited numerous musculoskeletal abnormalities and died at 64 days of age. Another woman in the 27th week of gestation was treated for anaphylaxis following a wasp (*Paravespula germanica*) sting and had a premature delivery at 35 weeks that was thought to be a post-anaphylactic event.

Multicystic encephalomalacia was identified at autopsy and was considered to be a result of maternal hypotension during the anaphylactic crisis that resulted in fetal hypoxia (Erasmus *et al.*, 1982). The musculoskeletal abnormalities were attributed to lack of fetal movement following the bee sting.

Treatment

Given the frequency of Hymenopteran stings and the scarcity of case reports of adverse events following maternal envenomation, it is likely that most stings result in no fetal harm. However, in cases where anaphylaxis develops secondary to a sting, the risk of adverse effects on the fetus must be considered to be increased, either due to metabolic or cardiovascular derangements during anaphylaxis or the drugs used to manage anaphylaxis. In cases of stings resulting in maternal anaphylaxis, prompt management of signs is essential to minimize risk to the fetus.

Lepidoptera

In 2001, an outbreak of reproductive failure occurred in mares in central Kentucky, with lesser losses in some surrounding states (Sebastian *et al.*, 2003, 2007, 2008). Termed mare reproductive loss syndrome (MRLS), the outbreak was characterized by early fetal losses, late term abortions, fetal pericarditis and fetal unilateral endophthalmitis. Various infectious and toxic etiologies were pursued, but no definitive etiology was found. The outbreaks coincided with an exceptionally high population of Eastern tent caterpillars (ETC, *Malacosoma americanum*) in the environment. Subsequent studies revealed that feeding ETC to pregnant horses resulted in abortions often within 1–7 days of exposure. These experiments showed a dose–response relationship between the ECT and time to abortion (i.e., twice the dose resulted in abortion in half the time), suggesting a toxic etiology, but to date a toxic principle has not been identified.

ARACHNIDA

Spiders

In the USA, two groups of spiders are considered sufficiently venomous to be of importance: the widow spiders (*Latrodectus* spp.) and the recluse spiders (*Loxesceles* spp.) (Gwaltney-Brant *et al.*, 2007). Widow spiders include the black widow spider (*L. mactans*), Western black widow spider (*L. hesperus*), Northern widow spider (*L. variolus*), red widow or red-legged widow spider (*L. bishopi*), and the brown widow spider (*L. geometricus*). The only recluse spider of medical importance in the USA is the brown recluse, *Loxosceles reclusa*.

Toxicity

Widow spiders have an oily venom composed of a mixture of neuroactive proteins, of which α-latrotoxin is the most potent and responsible for most of the signs and symptoms associated with envenomation (Handel *et al.*, 1994; Gwaltney-Brant *et al.*, 2007). Binding of α-latrotoxin to neuronal receptors results in massive release of acetylcholine (ACh) at the neuromuscular junction, resulting in profound muscle contraction. The symptoms of toxicosis relate to this neuromuscular activity and include muscle spasms, muscle pain and abdominal rigidity. Hypertension, tachycardia, hyperesthesia, vomiting and diarrhea may also occur. In pregnancy, the symptoms can resemble those seen in preeclampsia (Sherman *et al.*, 2000). Death is uncommon.

Given the strong muscle contractions that can be induced by *Latrodectus* spp. venom, there could be concerns regarding the potential for strong uterine contractions resulting in spontaneous abortions in pregnant patients. Abortion and fetal expulsion have been reported in mice experimentally envenomated by *Lactrodectus* spiders (Langley, 2004). However, despite intense abdominal cramping in some pregnant women bitten by widow spiders, no abortions have been documented (Russell *et al.*, 1979; Handel *et al.*, 1994; Sherman *et al.*, 2000; Langley, 2004).

Recluse spider venom contains a variety of necrotizing enzymes, of which sphingomyelinase D is the most important (Gwaltney-Brant *et al.*, 2007). The effects of *Loxosceles* spp. toxin are local in nature, causing a spreading necrotic area that may ultimately encompass a large tissue area. Systemic reactions, including hemolysis, dyspnea and coma, can occur but are quite rare.

Because of the local nature of recluse spider venom, adverse effects on fetuses would be considered unlikely. Although experimental data are lacking, case reports of pregnant women bitten by recluse spiders revealed no adverse effect on pregnancy (Anderson, 1991; Langley, 2004).

Treatment

Antivenom is available for management of patients that have been envenomated by widow spiders, and some sources recommend its use in pregnancy to minimize the risk of spontaneous abortion (Sherman *et al.*, 2000). Ancillary treatment of widow spider bites includes calcium gluconate and pain medication (Handel *et al.*, 1994). Treatment of *Loxosceles* envenomation includes local wound management and low dose prednisone therapy (Anderson, 1991).

Scorpions

In many parts of the world scorpion envenomation is a significant public health concern (Barao *et al.*, 2008a; Dorce *et al.*, 2009). In North America members of the genus *Centruroides* inhabit the southwestern states and pose a hazard (Gwaltney-Brant *et al.*, 2007).

Toxicity

Scorpions deliver their venom via a barbed appendage (telson) in their tail that houses two venom glands (Gwaltney-Brant *et al.*, 2007). Scorpion venom contains a variety of compounds that differ among the various scorpion species. Two potent neurotoxins (α-scorpion toxin and β-scorpion toxin) that block voltage-sensitive sodium and potassium channels have been identified in the venom of some of the more toxic scorpion genera. In addition to the neurologic effects, some scorpion venoms produce an inflammatory reaction involving the release of cytokines (Dorce *et al.*, 2009). Envenomated individuals may experience local pain at the sting site along with local edema and pruritus. Systemic effects include paresthesia or numbing of the face, myalgia, cardiac arrhythmias, respiratory depression or seizures. Allergic responses, including vomiting and swelling of eyelids and tongue, may also occur.

A variety of reproductive and developmental effects have been described for the venom of various species of scorpions. Compared to non-pregnant rats, pregnancy appears to increase the rat's susceptibility to scorpion envenomation (Ben Nasr *et al.*, 2008), and epidemiological studies on the effects of scorpion envenomation in pregnant women suggest that the effects of envenomation may be more severe during the second trimester of pregnancy (Ben Nasr *et al.*, 2007a). The venom from several scorpion species, including *Leiurus quinquestriatus*, *Buthus occitanus* and *Tityus serrulatus*, can induce contractions of the uterus in mice and humans (Langley, 2004; Ben Nasr *et al.*, 2007a), and the venom of *Buthus occitanus* induced dynamic dystocia in rats when administered at 0.5 mg/kg on day 22 of gestation (Ben Nasr *et al.*, 2007a,b). These effects on uterine muscle may be mediated by venom components such as 5-hydroxytryptamine found in *L. quinquestriatus* venom and a bradykinin-potentiating peptide found in *Buthus occitanus* venom (Langley, 2004). Contractile effects on the uterus of toxin T1 from *Tityus serrulatus* were found to be due to toxin action on post-ganglionic autonomic nerves causing ACh release and stimulation of muscarinic receptors (Mendonca *et al.*, 1995). Other changes described in late pregnancy scorpion envenomation include fetal death (Barao *et al.*, 2008b; Liebenson *et al.*, 2010), increased blood pressure and increased lipid peroxidation of maternal, placental and fetal tissues (Ben Nasr *et al.*, 2009).

Developmental alterations following *in utero* exposure to *Androctonus amoreuxi* venom on days 9 to 11 of gestation include increased fetal resorption rates in rats exposed to and skeletal defects in viable fetuses (Langley, 2004). Doses of 1 to 2.5 mg/kg of *Tityus serrulatus* venom administered to Wistar rats on days 5, 10 or 16 resulted in minimal to no evidence of fetal or maternal toxicosis (Barao *et al.*, 2008a; Crutterden *et al.*, 2008; Dorce *et al.*, 2009, 2010). However, significant postnatal physical and neurobehavioral alterations were noted, including gender-dependent delays in development of motor skill and reflexes, cognition and learning, and weight gain. Histopathologic examination of several areas within the hippocampus showed gender-dependent decreases in neuronal density.

Risk assessment

The degree of reproductive or developmental injury caused by scorpion venom will depend on the species of scorpion, stage of gestation and degree of envenomation. Exposure to scorpion early in gestation may result in fetal resorption, osseous defects or first trimester abortion (Langley, 2004). Exposure during late term pregnancy may result in spontaneous abortion or dynamic dystocia.

Treatment

Scorpion antivenom is available in most areas where scorpion envenomation is a significant public health problem. Given the potential for scorpion venom to have significant effects on pregnancy, envenomations should be managed through the use of antivenom and symptomatic care. For *L. quinquestriatus* envenomations, the use of drugs such as 5-hydroxytryptamine antagonists, meclofenamic acid or other prostaglandin synthesis inhibitors may be helpful in ameliorating uterine contractions in envenomated pregnant females (Langley, 2004).

REPTILIA

Snakes

Worldwide, venomous snakebites result in tens of thousands of deaths each year, with most fatalities occurring in developing countries with high populations of both humans and venomous snakes and limited access to emergent medical care (Langley, 2010). Epidemiologic surveys of the effects of snake envenomations in pregnant women revealed that overall fetal loss ranged from 20 to 43% and maternal deaths occurred in 4 to 10% of cases (Dunihoo *et al.*, 1992; Langley, 2010).

Venomous snakes are found in the families Colubridae, Crotalidae, Elapidae, Hydrophidae, Laticuldidae and Viperidae, although only members of Crotalidae and Elapidae are native to the USA (Gwaltney-Brant *et al.*, 2007). In the USA, crotalids, also called pit vipers, include rattlesnakes (*Crotalus* and *Sistrus* spp.), copperheads (*Agkistrodon contortrix*) and water moccasins (*A. picivorus*), while elapids are represented by the coral snakes (*Micruroides* spp.).

Toxicokinetics

Crotalids inject their venom through hollow fangs that rotate down and forward in a stabbing motion (Gwaltney-Brant *et al.*, 2007), and subsequent contraction of muscles surrounding the venom glands pump venom through the hollow fangs and into the victim. This muscular action allows the snakes to regulate the amount of venom they inject during a bite; "dry bites", bites that penetrate the skin of the victim but deliver no venom, may occur in up to 25% of snakebites. Once injected, the venom diffuses locally and, if injected in/near a punctured blood vessel, enters the bloodstream.

Elapids deliver their venom through short, non-hinged front fangs that are partially covered by a membrane (Gwaltney-Brant *et al.*, 2007). During a bite, the membrane is pushed away and the venom duct empties at the fang base, bathing the fang with venom which travels through grooves to reach the tissue of the victim. Through chewing actions, the elapid can deliver additional venom to the bite wound.

Toxicity

Crotalid venom contains a complex mixture of enzymes, neurotoxins, cytokines, cardiotoxins, hemolysins, coagulants, anticoagulants, nucleotides/nucleosides, peptides, organic acids and cations (Gwaltney-Brant *et al.*, 2007). The composition of venom varies between species and, within species, may vary considerably with the geographic locality, age of the snake and time of the year (Langley, 2010). Other factors that influence the toxicity of a particular snakebite include amount of venom delivered, location of the bite and age, size and health status of the victim. The toxic effects of crotalid venom can be necrotizing, hemolytic, inflammatory and/or neurotoxic (Gwaltney-Brant *et al.*, 2007). Spreading factors such as hyaluronidase allow the necrotizing effects of crotalid venom to penetrate through tissue. Hemolysins and coagulants/anticoagulants contribute to hematologic abnormalities such as hyper- or hypothrombosis. Cardiotoxins can trigger profound hypotension and neurotoxins can produce muscle fasciculations and/or paralysis.

Elapid venom is primarily neurotoxic, with lesser necrotizing and hemolytic activity (Gwaltney-Brant *et al.*, 2007). The venom causes a non-depolarizing neuromuscular blockade similar to the effects of curare.

Fetal resorptions, deaths and abortions have been reported following maternal exposure to most families of venomous snakes; information regarding reproductive effects of coral snakes is lacking (Langley, 2010). Mechanisms of venom effects on reproduction and development can include fetal hypoxia secondary to maternal hypotension, direct effects of the venom on the fetus, hemorrhages in the placenta and/or uterus resulting in abruptio placentae, venom-induced premature uterine contractions, pyrexia and cytokine release secondary to tissue damage, maternal hemolysis and/or hemorrhage resulting in anemia, and potential maternal anaphylaxis to antivenom (Hanprasertpong and Hanprasertpong, 2008; Otero-Patino, 2009; Pant *et al.*, 2010; Langley, 2010; Spadacci-Morena *et al.*, 2006). Teratogenic effects of experimental exposures of rodents or chicks to various venoms have involved brain, heart, limb, palate and facial abnormalities, depending on the day of gestation upon which the exposure took place and the species of snake (Giacobini *et al.*, 1973; Gabriel-Robez and Clavert, 1980; Al-Humayyd, 1995). In one study, fetal resorptions and teratogenic effects in rat pups were prevented through co-administration of antivenin or indomethacin with crude venom from the Egyptian sand viper (*Cerastes cerastes*) (Al-Humayyd, 1995).

Treatment

Management of venomous snakebite in pregnant patients should follow the same approach as that of the non-pregnant patient (Pantanowitz and Guidozzi, 1996; Langley, 2004). Antivenom should be administered as indicated, as the risks of withholding antivenom far outweigh the risks of proper administration; only one case of serum sickness associated with antivenom use in a pregnant woman has been reported (Langley, 2010). Close monitoring for and treatment of anaphylaxis is essential; the use of ephedrine or phenylephrine rather than epinephrine is recommended to avoid adverse effects on placental blood flow.

CONCLUDING REMARKS AND FUTURE DIRECTIONS

In spite of the relative frequency of human and animal exposures to zootoxins, there is still a large information gap regarding the effects of venoms and poisons on reproduction and development. Information on the effects of zootoxins from venomous marine animals, amphibians, echinoderms, venomous lizards, poisonous birds and venomous or poisonous mammals is lacking. Investigations into the morphologic, physiologic and biochemical mechanisms of the effects of zootoxins could provide the knowledge base needed to determine means of reducing the adverse effects of these toxins.

REFERENCES

Al-Humayyd MS (1995) Toxic effects of the venom from the snake *Cerastes cerastes* (Egyptian sand viper) in pregnant rats. *J Natural Tox* **4:** 35–43.

Anderson PC (1991) Loxosecelism threatening pregnancy: five cases. *Am J Obstet Gynecol* **165:** 454–8.

Barao AA, Bellot RG, Dorce VA (2008a) Developmental effects of *Tityus serrulatus* scorpion venom on the rat offspring. *Brain Res Bull* **76:** 499–504.

Barao AA, Nencioni ALA, Dorce VAC (2008b) Embriotoxic effects of maternal exposure to *Tityus serrulatus* scorpion venom. *J Ven Anim Toxins Trop Dis* **14:** 322–37.

Ben Nasr H, Chaker SH, Riadh B, Zouheir S, Kamel J, Tarek R, Khaled Z (2009) Some biological effects of scorpion envenomation in late pregnant rats. *Expl Toxicol Pathol* **61:** 573–380.

Ben Nasr H, Hammami TS, Sahnoun Z, Rebai T, Bouziziz M, Kassis M, Zeghal KM (2007a) Scorpion envenomation symptoms in pregnant women. *J Venoms Anim Toxins Trop Dis* **12:** 94–102.

Ben Nasr H, Mammami S, Mion G, Sahnoun Z, Chouaiekh F, Rebai T, Kassis M, Goyffon M, Zeghal K (2007b) Effects of *Buthus occitanus tunetanus* envenomation on an experimental murine model of gestation. *Comptes Rendus Biologies* **330:** 890–6.

Ben Nasr H, Serria HT, Selma C, Zouhier S, Tarek R, Mondher K, Kakaria B, Mounir ZK (2008) *In vivo* effects of *Buthus occitanus tunetanus* and *Androctonus australis garzoni* scorpion venoms on pregnant and non-pregnant rats. *J Venoms Anim Toxins Trop Dis* **14:** 366–71.

Brodie EC, Gulland FMD, Greig DJ, Hunter M, Jaakola J, St. Leger J, Leighfield TA, van Dolah FM (2006) Domoic acid causes reproductive failure in California sea lions (*Zalophus californianus*). *Marine Mammal Sci* **22:** 700–7.

Crutterden K, Nencioni AL, Bernardi MM, Dorce VA (2008) Reproductive toxic effects of *Tityus serrulatus* scorpion venom in rats. *Reprod Toxicol* **25:** 497–503.

Dorce ALC, Bellot RG, Dorce VAC, Nencioni ALA (2009) Effects of prenatal exposure to *Tityus bahiensis* scorpion venom on rat offspring development. *Reprod Toxicol* **28:** 365–70.

Dorce AL, Dorce VA, Nencioni AL (2010) Effects of in utero exposure to *Tityus bahiensis* scorpion venom in adult rats. *Neurotoxicol Teratol* **32:** 187–92.

Dunihoo DR, Rush BM, Wise RB, Brooks GG, Otterson WN (1992) Snake bite poisoning in pregnancy. A review of the literature. *J Reprod Med* **37:** 853–8.

Erasmus C, Blackwood W, Wilson J (1982) Infantile multicystic encephalomalacia after maternal bee sting anaphylaxis during pregnancy. *Arch Dis Childh* **57:** 785–7.

FAO/IOC/WHO; Experts Report (2004) Joint ad hoc Expert Consultation on Biotoxins in Bivalve Molluscs. Oslo, Norway; ftp://ftp.fao.org/es/esn/food/biotoxin_report_en.pdf, pp. 11–13.

Gabriel-Robez O, Clavert J (1980) Teratogenic and lethal properties of the various fractions of venom of the viper, *Vipera aspis*. *Acta Anatomica (Basel)* **108:** 225–9.

Giacobini G, Filogamo G, Weber M, Boquet P, Changeux JP (1973) Effects of a snake α-neurotoxin on the development of innervated skeletal muscles in chick embryo. *Proc Natl Acad Sci USA* **70:** 1708–12.

Goldstein T, Zabka TS, Delong RL, Wheeler EA, Yiltalo G, Bargu S, Silver M, Leighfield T, Van Dolah F, Langlois G, Sidor I, Dunn JL, Gulland FM (2009) The role of domoic acid in abortion and premature parturition of California sea lions (*Zalophus californianus*) on San Miguel Island, California. *J Wildlife Dis* **45:** 91–108.

Gwaltney-Brant SM, Dunayer EK, Youssef HY (2007) Terrestrial zootoxins. In *Veterinary Toxicology: Basic and Clinical Principles* (Gupta RC, ed.). Academic Press/Elsevier, Amsterdam, pp. 785–810.

Ham JN, Crutchlow MF, Desal BM, Simmons RA, Stoffers DA (2009) Exendin-4 normalizes islet vascularity in intrauterine growth restricted rats: potential role of VEGF. *Pediatric Res* **66:** 42–6.

Handel CC, Izquierdo LA, Curet LB (1994) Black widow spider (*Lactrodectus mactans*) bite during pregnancy. *Western J Med* **160:** 261–2.

Hanprasertpong J, Hanprasertpong T (2008) Abruptio placentae and fetal death following a Malayan pit viper bite. *J Obstet Gynecol Res* **34:** 258–61.

Haschek WM, Rousseau CG, Wallig MA (2010) Developmental pathology. In *Fundamentals of Toxicologic Pathology*, 2nd edition. Academic Press (Elsevier), New York, pp. 633–72.

Langley RL (2004) A review of venomous animal bites and stings in pregnant patients. *Wilderness Environ Med* **15:** 207–15.

Langley RL (2010) Snakebite during pregnancy: a literature review. *Wilderness Environ Med* **21:** 54–60.

Liebenson L, Liebenson M, Silberstein T (2010) Antepartum fetal death following a yellow scorpion sting. *Arch Gynecol Obstet* **281:** 247–9.

Mendonca M, Da Luz MM, Freire-Maia L, Cunha-Melo JR (1995) Effect of scorpion toxin from *Tityus serrulatus* on the contraction of the isolated rat uterus. *Toxicon* **33:** 355–61.

Otero-Patino R (2009) Epidemiological, clinical and therapeutic aspects of *Bothrops asper* bites. *Toxicon* **54:** 998–1011.

Pant HP, Poudel R, Dsovza V (2010) Intrauterine death following green tree viper bite presenting as antepartum hemorrhage. *Int J Obstet Anesth* **19:** 102–3.

Pantanowitz L, Guidozzi F (1996) Management of snake and spider bite in pregnancy. *Obstet Gynecol Surv* **51:** 615–20.

Pulido OM (2008) Domoic acid pathology: a review. *Marine Drugs* **6:** 180–219.

Ramsdell JS, Zabka TS (2008) *In utero* domoic acid toxicity: a fetal basis to adult disease in the California sea lion (*Zalophus californianus*). *Marine Drugs* **6:** 262–90.

Russell FE (1996) Toxic effects animal toxins. In *Casarett and Doull's Toxicology: The Basic Science of Poisons*, 5th edition (Klaasen CD, ed.). McGraw-Hill, New York, pp. 801–39.

Russell FE (2001) Toxic effects of terrestrial animal venoms and poisons. In *Casarett and Doull's Toxicology: The Basic Science of Poisons*, 6th edition (Klaasen CD, ed.). McGraw-Hill, New York, pp. 945–64.

Russell FE, Marcus P, Streng JA (1979) Black widow spider envenomation during pregnancy: report of a case. *Toxicon* **17:** 188–9.

Sebastian M, Bernard W, Harrison L (2007) Caterpillars and mare reproductive loss syndrome. In *Veterinary Toxicology: Basic and Clinical Principles* (Gupta RC, ed.). Academic Press/Elsevier, Amsterdam, pp. 777–84.

Sebastian MM, Bernard WV, Riddle TW, Latimer CR, Fitzgerald, Harrison LR (2008) Mare reproductive loss syndrome. *Vet Pathol* **45:** 710–22.

Sebastian MM, Gantz MG, Tobin T, Hankins JD, Bosken JM, Hughes C, Harrison LR, Bernard WV, Richter DL, Fitzgerald TD (2003) The mare reproductive loss syndrome and the eastern tent caterpillar: a toxicokinetic/statistical analysis with clinical, epidemiological and mechanistic implications. *Vet Ther* **4:** 324–39.

Senecal PE, Osterich JD (1991) Normal fetal outcome after maternal ciguateric toxin exposure in the second trimester. *J Toxicol Clin Toxicol* **29:** 473–8.

Sherman RP, Groll JM, Gonzalez DI, Aerts MA (2000) Black widow spider (*Lactrodectus mactans*) envenomation in a term pregnancy. *Curr Surg* **57:** 346–8.

Shkenderov S, Todorov S (1979) Effect of bee venom and its low- and high-molecular fractions on embryogenesis in rats. *Eksperimentalna Meditsina Morfologiia* **18:** 160–5.

Silvagni PA, Lowenstine LJ, Spraker T, Lipscomb TP, Gulland FMD (2005) Pathology of domoic acid toxicity in California sea lions (*Zalophus californianus*). *Vet Pathol* **42:** 184–91.

Spadacci-Morena DD, de Tomy SC, Sano-Martins IS, Katz SG (2006) The effect of experimental *Bothrops jararaca* envenomation on pregnant mice. *Toxicon* **47:** 196–207.

Tanemura K, Igarashi K, Matsugami T, Aisaki K, Kitajima S, Kanno J (2009) Intrauterine environment-genome interaction and children's development (2): brain structure impairment and behavioral disturbance induced in male mice offspring by a single intraperitoneal administration of domoic acid (DA) to their dams. *J Toxicol Sci* **34:** SP279–SP286.

Tubaro A, Hungerford J (2007) Toxicology of marine toxins. In *Veterinary Toxicology: Basic and Clinical Principles* (Gupta RC, ed.). Academic Press/Elsevier, Amsterdam, pp. 725–52.

Williamson JA, Callanan VI, Hartwick RF (1980) Serious envenomation by the Northern Australian box-jellyfish (*Chironex fleckeri*). *Med J Aust* **12:** 13–16.

CHAPTER

57

HIV-1 Tat toxin

Shilpa Buch and Honghong Yao

INTRODUCTION

It is estimated that almost 25% of untreated HIV-1-infected individuals and ~7% of HIV-1-infected patients treated with combined antiretroviral therapy develop HIV-associated dementia (HAD) (Budka, 1991; McArthur *et al.*, 1993; Sacktor *et al.*, 2001; Spencer and Price, 1992), a neurodegenerative syndrome that is clinically characterized by progressive cognitive, motor and behavioral abnormalities (Gendelman *et al.*, 1994; Lipton and Gendelman, 1995). Pathological manifestation of HAD, HIV encephalitis (HIVE), is often accompanied by prominent microglial activation, formation of microglial nodules, perivascular accumulations of mononuclear cells, presence of multi-nucleated giant cells, and neuronal damage and loss (Bell, 1998; Gendelman *et al.*, 1994; Nath, 1999). The primary cells infected by HIV-1 in the brain are macrophages/microglia and, to a lesser extent, astrocytes, but not neurons (Kaul *et al.*, 2001). The fact that neuronal death occurs despite the lack of neuronal infectivity leads to the speculation that neurons must be susceptible to toxins released from the infected cells. One broad explanation frequently advocated to explain the loss of neurons in this disease is that cellular (proinflammatory cytokines, chemokine, arachidnoic acid metabolites, etc.) and/or viral proteins (gp120, Tat) released from the infected cells have a direct toxic effect on the neurons (Adamson *et al.*, 1996; Brenneman *et al.*, 1988; Chen *et al.*, 2000; Dreyer *et al.*, 1990; Hof *et al.*, 1998; Kruman *et al.*, 1998b; Patel *et al.*, 2000). Numerous reports have demonstrated the direct toxicity of both HIV envelope gp120 and HIV transactivating (Tat) proteins. Tat is one of the early viral proteins that is expressed during virus replication and is known to play a crucial role in promoting virus replication by transactivating the promoter region of the virus. To date there is no effective treatment that blocks Tat activity.

HIV Tat has diverse but often deleterious effects on various cell types of the CNS. For example, Tat can be toxic for neurons leading to apoptosis. In the glial cells such as astrocytes and microglia, Tat can upregulate expression of various proinflammatory mediators such as cytokines and chemokines, which in turn can result in neuroinflammation and amplification of toxicity to other cell types such as neurons. Additionally, Tat can also have toxic effects on the cells of the blood–brain barrier (BBB), resulting in leakiness of the barrier, which in turn manifests as enhanced influx of inflammatory cells into the central nervous system (CNS). Both cell culture systems and murine animal models have provided valuable tools to explore the role of HIV-1 Tat in the pathogenesis of HIV-associated neurodegenerative disease (HAND). Additionally, in resource-limiting settings, drug abuse, lack of availability of antiretrovirals and perinatal transmission of HIV-1 are major causes of AIDS in children. In such a setting, Tat toxicity could have serious deleterious effects in both the developing fetus and the newborn. This chapter summarizes these findings and the current understanding of the mechanism(s) underlying Tat-induced toxicity.

EFFECT OF HIV TAT IN NEURONS

It is widely accepted that neurodegeneration is one of the hallmark features of HAND. It has been implicated that the viral protein products and but not the virus *per se* can exert neurotoxicity, both *in vitro* and *in vivo* (Bansal *et al.*, 2000; Gurwell *et al.*, 2001; Kaul *et al.*, 2001; Kaul and Lipton, 1999; Lipton *et al.*, 1991; New *et al.*, 1997; Savio and Levi, 1993). HIV Tat, a virus-encoded protein that promotes replication, can be released by HIV-infected cells into the extracellular space and cerebrospinal fluid (CSF). Released Tat is taken up by cells of the CNS resulting in toxic consequences such as neuronal apoptosis (Bonavia *et al.*, 2001; Eugenin *et al.*, 2003; Haughey *et al.*, 2001). Once Tat is taken up by the neurons, it can be transported along the anatomical pathways within the brain, suggesting that sites of neuronal damage may be distant from the site of viral infection (Bruce-Keller *et al.*, 2003). In neurons, Tat internalization occurs primarily through the lipoprotein-related protein receptor (LRP) expressed on the cell surface (Liu *et al.*, 2000). In the brain, LRP is expressed in both neurons and activated astrocytes (Rebeck *et al.*, 1993) and has been shown to bind to at least 16 identified ligands (Herz and Strickland, 2001). Among these, Tat is the only ligand of LRP that has been shown to induce substantial apoptosis. In addition, it has been shown that binding of Tat to LRP and subsequent Tat-induced neuronal apoptosis was mediated by activation of N-methyl-D-aspartic acid (NMDA) receptor, as evidenced by the fact that NMDA receptor antagonist was effective in blocking Tat-induced neurotoxicity. Several groups have

Reproductive and Developmental Toxicology, Edited by Ramesh C. Gupta
ISBN: 978-0-12-382032-7

demonstrated Tat-mediated activation of NMDA receptor by indirect mechanisms (Cheng *et al.*, 1998; Magnuson *et al.*, 1995). It has been reported that Tat mediates activation of the NMDA receptor though the cross-activation of several signaling pathways. For example, following binding of Tat to LRP there is a complex formation between LRP and NMDA receptor, an effect that requires the intracellular scaffolding protein, postsynaptic density protein (PSD-95). In addition to this, both protein kinase C (PKC) and tyrosine kinase were also shown to be involved in Tat-induced NMDA receptor activation (Haughey *et al.*, 2001). Following its uptake through the LRP receptor, Tat escapes the endosomes and localizes to the cytoplasm and the nucleus of the neuronal cells. Intriguingly, Tat-treated neurons have also been shown to display generalized calcium dysregulation (Bonavia *et al.*, 2001). Additionally, activation of nitric oxide synthase (nNOS) and subsequent nitric oxide (NO) production also play a role in Tat-induced neuronal apoptosis.

Furthermore, emerging new *in vitro* data demonstrate Tat-induced neurotoxicity in rat primary neurons. These cells when treated with varying concentrations of Tat 1-72 (50–200 ng/ml) resulted in decreased cell survival (Yao *et al.*, 2009b,c). Specificity of Tat-induced cell death was confirmed by treating the cells with either heat-inactivated or mutant Tat, both of which failed to exert cytotoxicity. Detailed molecular mechanisms underlying neurotoxicity mediated by Tat have implicated the role of extracellular glutamate, levels of which are increased in Tat-treated vs. untreated cells (Zhu *et al.*, 2009). The neurotoxicity elicited by Tat was accompanied by an increase in both caspase-3 activity as well as the release of mitochondrial cytochrome c and endonuclease G (Singh *et al.*, 2004). Activation of nNOS and subsequent NO production also plays a critical role in Tat-induced neurotoxicity (Eugenin *et al.*, 2007). nNOS associates with the NMDA receptor through PSD-95 and is subsequently activated by calcium flux through the NMDA receptor, leading to NO production. Generation of NO involved activation of the p38 MAPK pathway. Interestingly, both p38 and JNK MAPK pathways have been shown to be activated by Tat in primary mouse neurons. However, only p38 MAPK pathway activation has been essential for Tat-induced neurotoxicity (Singh *et al.*, 2004). In addition to the neurotoxicity, Tat exposure also resulted in decreased neural stem cell proliferation implying thereby that fewer progenitor cells were available for differentiation into neurons, thus affecting overall neurogenesis (Kaul *et al.*, 2005).

REVERSAL OF HIV TAT-MEDIATED TOXICITY

In response to cellular damage, the host is also capable of producing trophic growth factors (e.g., platelet derived growth factor-PDGF, brain derived neurotrophic factor-BDNF, fibroblast growth factor-FGF or nerve growth factor-NGF) that can protect neuronal, glial and other resident cells of the brain. Many of these trophic factors provide protection of neurons against various neurotoxins (cytokines, chemokines and viral products). Previous studies have reported that BDNF can prevent HIV Tat-induced neuronal apoptosis via nuclear factor-κB (NF-κB)-dependent mechanism and by regulation of the anti-apoptotic genes including Bcl-2 (Ramirez *et al.*, 2001).

Recent findings also point to the role of PDGF-BB in rescuing dopaminergic neurons against HIV Tat-induced neurotoxicity *in vivo* (Yao *et al.*, 2009c). Confirmation of the neuroprotective role of PDGF against Tat toxicity was also corroborated *in vitro* in primary cultures of rat midbrain neurons. A novel role of the Ca^{2+}-permeable channel-transient receptor potential canonical (TRPC) channels in PDGF-mediated neuroprotection in rat neurons was identified. The mechanism of action involved PDGF-mediated activation of TRPC culminating in amplification of downstream ERK signaling via the Pyk2 pathway, followed by nuclear translocation of CREB, ultimately resulting in neuronal survival (Yao *et al.*, 2009c). These studies implicate the robustness of the neuroprotective action of PDGF against a diverse range of HIV-1 proteins. These findings are given further credence by a recent report indicating the protective role of yet another PDGF isoform. PDGF-CC in various models of neurodegenerative diseases such as Alzheimer's disease, Parkinson's disease and stroke (Tang *et al.*, 2010).

EFFECT OF TAT ON GLIA

Astrocytes

In addition to exerting toxicity on neurons, HIV Tat can also modulate the release of toxic substances from glial cells. For example, it has been shown that intraventricular injection of Tat results in prominent glial cell activation with subsequent infiltration of blood-borne monocytes (Jones *et al.*, 1998). Tat exposure can also impact glial cell function by stimulating the production of proinflammatory cytokines (Chen *et al.*, 1997; Pulliam *et al.*, 2007). In fact, several cell culture studies have suggested that exposure of astrocytes to Tat protein leads to astrocyte activation with the induction of a battery of cytokines and chemokines (D'Aversa *et al.*, 2004; Kutsch *et al.*, 2000; Weiss *et al.*, 1999). Significant among these are tumor necrosis factor-α (TNF-α), monocyte chemoattractant factor-1 (MCP-1)/CCL-2 and CXCL10 (Williams *et al.*, 2009a,b; Eugenin *et al.*, 2005). These findings have tremendous clinical implications since it is becoming increasingly appreciated that the severity of HAD/HIVE correlates more closely with the presence of activated glial cells rather than with the presence and amount of HIV-infected cells in the brain. Thus HIV-1 Tat by its ability to activate astrocytes, the predominant cell types in the CNS, can actually lead to amplification of toxic responses in the CNS. A specific example of this is the induction by astrocytes of the IFN-γ inducible chemokine CXCL10, which is known to recruit both T cells and monocytes into the CNS, resulting in neuroinflammation. It has been demonstrated that the proinflammatory cytokines, IFN-γ and TNF-α, implicated in the pathophysiology of HAD, are markedly increased in the CNS during HIV-1 infection of the brain (Shapshak *et al.*, 2004; Wesselingh *et al.*, 1997). Both of these cytokines via their cooperative actions have also been shown to induce expression of CXCL10 (Majumder *et al.*, 1998). Additional findings have further indicated that HIV-1/HIV-1 proteins can further interact with these cytokines to dramatically induce the expression of CXCL10 in the brain (Asensio *et al.*, 2001; Kutsch *et al.*, 2000; Williams *et al.*, 2009a). This could have deleterious implications for the host resulting in increased brain inflammation. Mechanism of this synergistic interaction of Tat leading to CXCL10 induction involved the JAK, STAT and MAPK (via activation of ERK1/2, p38 and Akt) signaling molecules with the activation of the downstream transcription factor, NF-κB.

Further dissection of mechanisms involved in the synergistic induction of CXCL10 by Tat and cytokines identified oxidative stress as a major player. HIV-1 Tat-induced oxidative stress in astrocytes has been shown to be a critical determinant of the NF-κB targeted genes, specifically CXCL10 (Song *et al.*, 2007). One pivotal mechanism by which oxidative stress is able to impact signaling pathways and their corresponding transcription factors is through a respiratory burst orchestrated by the activation of NADPH oxidase (Adler *et al.*, 1999; Park *et al.*, 2004; Sundaresan *et al.*, 1995; Turchan-Cholewo *et al.*, 2009; Wang *et al.*, 1998). NADPH oxidase, a multi-subunit membrane associated enzyme, is capable of producing superoxide (Babior, 1999; Chanock *et al.*, 1994; El-Benna *et al.*, 2005; Raad *et al.*, 2008). It has recently been demonstrated that treatment of astrocytes with a mixture of Tat and the inflammatory cytokines (IFN-γ and TNF-α) resulted in a respiratory burst, an effect that was abrogated by apocynin, an NADPH oxidase inhibitor. Pretreatment of Tat and cytokine stimulated with apocynin also resulted in a parallel reduction in CXCL10 expression. Synergistic induction of CXCL10 by Tat and cytokines involved activation of the ERK1/2, JNK and Akt pathways with downstream translocation of NF-κB (Figure 57.1) (Williams *et al.*, 2010).

Microglia

Among the diverse cell types in the CNS, microglia, the resident brain microglia, play an important role in various neurodenegerative disorders and most notably HAND (Rock and Peterson, 2006). By elaborating a plethora of cytokines and chemokines, microglia exhibit both protective as well as toxic responses during injury (Rock and Peterson, 2006). More recently numbers of activated microglia are significantly increased following Tat treatment. Microglia are the resident patrol of the CNS that keep the brain environment under constant surveillance. They constitute 10% of the total glial population in the adult CNS (Pessac *et al.*, 2001) and are distributed throughout the brain and the spinal cord. Microglia in the adult mouse brain are derived from the monocyte/macrophage precursor cells that migrate from the yolk sac into the developing CNS where they actively proliferate during development, giving rise to the resident microglial pool (Alliot *et al.*, 1999; Pessac *et al.*, 2001). In the normal mature brain, microglia typically exist in a resting state characterized by ramified morphology, and function to monitor the brain environment (Davalos *et al.*, 2005; Nimmerjahn *et al.*, 2005). In response to certain external insults such as brain injury or infection, however, microglia become rapidly activated (Davalos *et al.*, 2005; Fetler and Amigorena, 2005; Nimmerjahn *et al.*, 2005). These activated microglia undergo a dramatic alteration from their resting ramified state into an ameboid phenotype accompanied by upregulated expression of cell surface markers, including CD11b, CD14, major histocompatibility complex (MHC) molecules and chemokine receptors (Rock *et al.*, 2004). Microglial activation in the context of HIV-1 can be a result of direct infection with the virus or a result of interaction with the viral proteins, such as HIV-1 Tat (D'Aversa *et al.*, 2004) or gp120 (Bonwetsch *et al.*, 1999; Garden *et al.*, 2004; Kong *et al.*, 1996; Kruman *et al.*, 1998a). Several reports have indicated that the treatment of human microglia with Tat induced the release of chemokines such as CCL2, CXCL8, CXCL10, CCL3, CCL4 and CCL5 through activation of MAPK ERK1/2, p38 and PI3K signaling pathways (D'Aversa *et al.*, 2004). Consistent with these findings, recent studies have also reported the effects of drugs of abuse such as morphine and HIV Tat on the activation of both mouse BV-2 microglial cells and primary microglia. The combined effects of HIV Tat and drugs of abuse are covered in greater detail in a separate section below.

In addition to microglial activation, Tat can also induce the migration of human microglial cells, through its impact on autocrine signaling. For example, treatment of microglia with HIV-1 Tat results in increased release of CCL2 leading to activation of the CCL2 receptor CCR2 on these cells (Eugenin *et al.*, 2005). Based on these findings, it is likely that HIV-infected monocytes that transmigrate into the CNS can release both the viral protein products (Tat and gp120) and the chemokine, CCL2, which, in turn, can recruit more infected and uninfected microglia to HIV-infected niches, thereby perpetuating the toxic loops in the CNS.

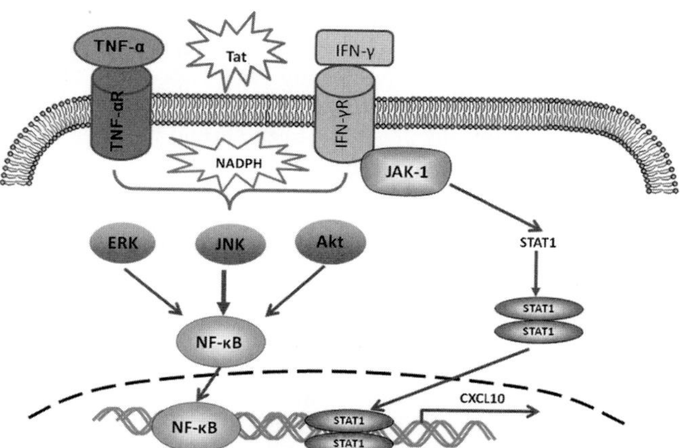

FIGURE 57.1 Schematic of the signaling pathways involved in the increased induction of CXCL10 in astrocytes stimulated with HIV-1 Tat in conjunction with IFN-γ and TNF-α. The major signaling pathways activated include ERK, p38, JNK and Akt, which are able to converge on NF-κB. The activation of NF-κB, along with the activation of STAT-1, results in the transcription of CXCL10 (Williams *et al.*, 2009a,b). Furthermore, it was demonstrated that HIV-1 Tat increases CXCL10 expression in IFN-γ and TNF-α stimulated human astrocytes via NADPH oxidase. NADPH oxides inhibitor was also able to reduce Tat and cytokine-mediated CXCL10 expression and the corresponding signaling molecules ERK, JNK and Akt activation with a concomitant decrease in activation and nuclear translocation of NF-κB, all of which are important regulators of CXCL10 induction (Williams *et al.*, 2010).

EFFECT OF TAT ON MONOCYTES/ MICROPHAGES

Similar to microglia, HIV-1 Tat protein exposure can also lead to dysregulated cytokine/chemokine production in monocytes/macrophages. In fact, enhanced IL-1β production during HIV-1 infection has been attributed partially to HIV protein-Tat in both monocytes/macrophages as well as in T cells (Nath *et al.*, 1999; Pu *et al.*, 2003). IL-1β is one of the key inflammatory cytokines secreted by immune-activated monocytes/macrophages. Detailed mechanisms underlying Tat-mediated increase in IL-1β production by human monocytes has recently been explored. This involves the PLC-PKC pathway dependent phosphorylation of p44/42 ERK and JNK MAP kinases and specific C/EBP and NF-κB transcription factor binding elements within the IL-1β promoter (Yang *et al.*, 2010). It is likely that a similar mechanism could be operating in the neuropathogenesis of HAND. In addition to upregulating the cytokine IL-1β, HIV-1 Tat can also induce the expression of the chemokine CXCL10 in macrophages through its interplay with proinflammatory cytokine, IFN-γ (Dhillon *et al.*, 2008). Synergistic induction of CXCL10 by both Tat and IFN-γ was found to be susceptible to inhibition by the MEK1/2 inhibitor U0126 and the p38 mitogen activated protein kinase (MAPK) inhibitor, thereby underpinning the role of these signaling pathways in the process. In addition, JAK/STAT pathway was also shown to play a major role in Tat/IFN-γ-mediated induction of CXCL10 in macrophages (Dhillon *et al.*, 2008). Thus cooperative interaction of Tat and IFN-γ resulted in enhanced chemokine expression, which in turn can manifest as an amplified inflammatory immune response within the CNS of patients with HAD, by a mechanism involving increased recruitment of lymphocytes/monocytes in the brain.

EFFECT OF TAT ON BLOOD–BRAIN BARRIER

The integrity of the blood–brain barrier (BBB) plays an important role in maintaining a safe neural microenvironment in the brain. BBB normally functions as an interface between the blood and brain parenchyma, acting as a watch guard to inhibit the entry of ions, molecules and infiltrating cells into the CNS. The presence of interendothelial adherens junctions (AJ) and tight junctions (TJ) between endothelial cells (EC) and EC-astrocytes maintains barrier properties (Goldstein, 1988). During the normal immune surveillance, lymphocytes and monocytes cross into the CNS with little or no effect on BBB integrity. However, during progressive HIV-1 infection, there is a breach in this barrier (Avison *et al.*, 2004; Burger *et al.*, 1997; Dallasta *et al.*, 1999; Nottet *et al.*, 1996) leading to influx of inflammatory cells into the brain resulting in clinical and pathological abnormalities, ranging from mild cognitive impairment to frank dementia. Previous studies have demonstrated that HIV infected cells can disrupt an *in vitro* model of the BBB, which was supported by *in vivo* evidence depicting areas of BBB disruption found in regions enriched with activated, infected monocytes/macrophages, thereby leading to the speculation that infected cells themselves could disrupt the BBB.

Although the mechanisms of BBB disruption during HIV-1 infection still remain unclear, alterations in TJ expression have been reported to contribute, at least in part, to this disruption. Hence downmodulation of these tight junction proteins could be considered an indicator of the BBB breach. In brain microvascular endothelial (BMEC) cells it has been shown that Tat treatment resulted in decreased expression and/or distribution of the TJ proteins claudin-1, claudin-5 and zonula occludens (ZO)-2. The decreased claudin-5 expression was further confirmed *in vivo* in mice that were administered Tat into the right hippocampus (Andras *et al.*, 2003). Mechanisms underlying Tat-mediated alteration of TJs involved redox-responsive signal transduction pathways, such as VEGFR-2/Ras/ERK1/2 pathway, PI-3K/Akt/NF-κB pathway and calcium-dependent signaling (Andras *et al.*, 2005). Tat-mediated altered expression of both claudin and ZO-1, -2 could have a significant effect on vascular permeability since claudins are believed to be essential for the structural and functional maintenance of the TJ of BBB and also since ZO-1 proteins mediate interactions of claudins with the actin cytoskeletion and stabilize the claudins in the membrane.

In addition to the direct disruption of the TJ, treatment of BMECs with Tat resulted in increased cellular oxidative stress, decreased levels of intracellular glutathione and activated DNA binding activity and transactivation of transcription factors NF-κB and AP-1. In addition, administration of N-acetylcysteine (NAC), a precursor of glutathione and a potent antioxidant, attenuated both Tat-induced ERK1/2 activation and alterations in ZO-1 expression. These cell culture findings were also corroborated *in vivo* wherein mice injected intracranially with HIV-1 Tat demonstrated increased expression of MCP-1 mRNA and protein in the brain vascular endothelium (Toborek *et al.*, 2003). In addition to the induction of MCP-1, Tat also upregulated expression of cyclooxygenase-2 (COX-2) in HBMECs. Intriguingly, a specific inhibitor of COX-2-rofecoxib attenuated Tat-induced alteration of occludin expression, thus implicating the role of COX-2 in the loss of TJs (Pu *et al.*, 2007).

It is widely recognized that in addition to their role in the maintenance of barrier integrity, BMECs also possess multidrug resistance-associated proteins (MRPs) that are substrates for the efflux transport systems for HIV-1 antiretrovirals. Interestingly, exposure of BMECs to Tat specifically induced MRP1 mRNA and protein expression. These alterations were accompanied by enhanced MRP1-mediated efflux functions. Furthermore, activation of the MAPK signaling cascade was identified as the mechanism critical for Tat-mediated overexpression of MRP1. These results identify yet another mechanism by which Tat exposure can lead to alterations of the BBB functions while decreasing the antiretroviral efficacy in the CNS through overexpression of drug efflux transporters (Hayashi *et al.*, 2006).

Cell adhesion molecules have been shown to play critical roles in leukocyte transmigration across the BBB. Intriguingly, exposure of brain endothelial cells to HIV-1 Tat has been demonstrated to upregulate the expression of endothelial adhesion molecules such as intracellular adhesion molecule-1 (ICAM-1), vascular cell adhesion molecule-1 (VCAM-1) and E-selectin, thereby facilitating transmigration across the endothelial monolayers. HIV Tat mediated increased cell surface expression of VCAM-1 in human pulmonary artery endothelial cells and both the NF-κB and the p38 MAPK inhibitors abolished this effect (Gan *et al.*, 1999; Liu *et al.*, 2005). Additionally, Tat has also been shown to upregulate matrix metalloproteinases (MMPs) in BMVECs, further implicating the involvement of Tat in impairing membrane permeability while facilitating endothelial transmigration of HIV-infected cells (Huang *et al.*, 2009; Nair *et al.*, 2005). More recently, Tat-mediated disruption of TJs has been shown to involve caveolin-1, a lipid raft constituent, which is an early and critical modulator controlling signaling pathways involved in this process (Zhong *et al.*, 2008). Figure 57.2 outlines the molecular pathways affected by HIV Tat in mediating BBB damage.

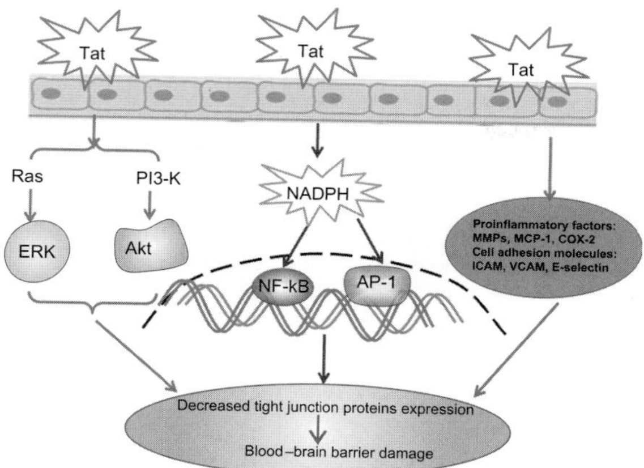

FIGURE 57.2 Schematic of mechanisms underlying Tat-mediated damage to the BBB. Mechanisms underlying Tat-mediated alteration of TJs involve redox-responsive signal transduction pathways, such as Ras/ERK1/2 pathway, PI-3K/Akt/ pathway and calcium-dependent signaling (Andras *et al.*, 2005). Tat exposure resulted in increased cellular oxidative stress, decreased levels of intracellular glutathione and activated DNA binding activity and transactivation of transcription factors NF-κB and AP-1 (Toborek *et al.*, 2003). Tat also induced proinflammatory factors and cell adhesion molecules which contribute to BBB damage (Huang *et al.*, 2009; Liu *et al.*, 2005). Please refer to color plate section.

INTERACTION OF HIV-1 TAT WITH DRUGS OF ABUSE IN MEDIATING NEURONAL INJURY

Drug users represent a significant proportion of the HIV-1-infected and at-risk population. The influence of concurrent drug abuse in HIV neuropathogenesis is also quite significant. The influence of concurrent drug abuse in AIDS is a burning issue, as drug abusers are reported to have higher rates of both HIVE and HAD compared to infected non-drug abusers (Bell *et al.*, 1996; Chiesi *et al.*, 1996; Goodkin *et al.*, 1998; Martinez *et al.*, 1995; Nath *et al.*, 2001). Neuropathologically, drug abusers tend to show greater levels of neuroinflammation as evidenced by microglial activation, astrocytosis and CD8 lymphocytic infiltration (Anthony *et al.*, 2005; Tomlinson *et al.*, 1999). Among the drugs of abuse, alcohol, marijuana, nitrite inhalants, amphetamines, cocaine and hallucinogens are often associated with HIV (Woody *et al.*, 1999). HIV-1 infection and co-morbidities has been the subject of many excellent reviews in recent years (Anthony and Bell, 2008; Nath *et al.*, 2008).

Use of cocaine either by snorting, smoking or by intravenous injection has been known to promote disease progression, including acquisition of secondary opportunistic infections in HIV-1-infected individuals (Fiala *et al.*, 1998; Goodkin *et al.*, 1998). Cocaine synergizes with both HIV-1 Tat and gp120 to aggravate neurotoxic effects of the viral proteins, thus accelerating neuronal apoptosis (Aksenov *et al.*, 2006; Turchan *et al.*, 2001; Yao *et al.*, 2009a). Molecular pathways involved in the combinatorial toxicity of cocaine and Tat on rat dopaminergic neurons include oxidative stress and mitochondrial membrane potential alterations (Aksenov *et al.*, 2006). In addition to cocaine, methamphetamine can also synergize with Tat to elicit increased neurotoxicity (Cai and Cadet, 2008), which has also been confirmed in an *in vivo* study. The mechanism underlying methamphetamine and Tat-mediated synergistic reduction in striatal dopamine involved reduction in dopamine release from the striatum (Cass *et al.*, 2003) and a concomitant decrease in dopamine transporter due to the loss of dopaminergic terminals (Theodore *et al.*, 2006, 2007).

Reactive oxygen species (ROS) are naturally generated in cells as by-products of electron transport in mitochondria and redox enzyme reactions in the cytoplasm. Oxidative stress has been implicated both in the brain and in CSF of HAD patients (Turchan *et al.*, 2003). Oxidative stress is yet another mechanism by which Tat synergizes with methamphetamine or cocaine to mediate toxicity. Boess *et al.* have shown that cocaine exposure in mice resulted in decreased mitochondrial respiration leading to the generation of ROS (Boess *et al.*, 2000). In another study, administration of either Tat or methamphetamine to mice increased markers of oxidative stress in cortical, striatal and hippocampal regions of the brain (Flora *et al.*, 2003). It has also been shown that interactions between Tat and methamphetamine led to deleterious effects on calbindin-positive neurons mainly by dysregulating mitochondrial calcium metabolism, which was also associated with increased levels of oxidative stress (Langford *et al.*, 2004). Tat can thus potentiate the signaling pathways used by drugs of abuse to enhance and amplify toxicity both at the cellular and at the tissue levels.

Similar to methamphetamine and cocaine, Tat can also synergize with morphine, the active metabolite of heroin, to activate glial cells. It has been reported that persistent exposure of astrocyte and glial precursors to both morphine and Tat results in cellular apoptosis, an effect mediated by mu-opioid receptors (MORs) (Khurdayan *et al.*, 2004). Similar findings have also been observed in oligodendrocytes that also express the MOR (Hauser *et al.*, 2009). Intriguingly, recent studies have implicated astroglia as the key mediators for the proinflammatory response that is characteristic of opiate-addicted HIV+ individuals. In fact, combined opiate and Tat exposure synergistically destabilizes levels of intracellular calcium, increases ROS and causes massive release of proinflammatory chemokines in cultured striatal astroglia (El-Hage *et al.*, 2005).

Not only do morphine and Tat upregulate the chemokines, in microglia, combined exposure with both the agents leads to upregulation of the chemokine receptor CCR5, an effect blocked by the opioid receptor antagonist naltrexone. Morphine in combination with Tat also induces morphological changes in the BV-2 microglia from a quiescent to an activated morphology, with a dramatic increase in the expression of the microglial activation marker CD11b. In addition, the mRNA expression of inducible nitric oxide synthase (iNOS), CD40 ligand, interferon-gamma-inducible peptide (IP-10) and the proinflammatory cytokines TNFα, IL-1β and IL-6, which were elevated with Tat alone, were dramatically enhanced with Tat in the presence of morphine (Bokhari *et al.*, 2009). These findings shed light on the cooperative effects of morphine and HIV-1 Tat on both microglial activation and HIV co-receptor upregulation, effects that could result in exacerbated neuropathogenesis.

It should be added that in resource-limiting settings, drug abuse and perinatal transmission of HIV-1 are major causes of AIDS in children. Interestingly, HIV Tat exon I sequences were analyzed from six mother–infant pairs after perinatal transmission and the Tat open reading frame was maintained in 140 of the 154 clones analyzed, with a 90.9% frequency of intact Tat open reading frames. In addition, a low degree of heterogeneity was observed in Tat sequences within mothers, within infants and between epidemiologically linked mother–infant pairs (Husain *et al.*, 2001). These findings can have serious implications on Tat toxicity in both the developing fetus and the newborn.

CONCLUDING REMARKS AND FUTURE DIRECTIONS

CNS disease remains a serious complication in individuals infected with HIV-1. The early viral protein, HIV Tat, has been shown to be a critical determinant for both viral replication and survival. However, in the infected host release of Tat from the infected cells can have serious consequences, as it exerts potent toxicity on various cell types in the brain. In the CNS it can activate monocytes, astrocytes and microglia, which, in turn, leads to a "cytokine/chemokine storm" in the CNS. HIV-1 Tat not only exerts direct toxicity on the neurons, but can also indirectly lead to neuronal apoptosis, via the mediators released from other neighboring cells. These complex cascades of events could be self-propelling, thereby perpetuating a continuum of inflammatory responses in the brain of HIV-1-infected individuals. These are important issues even in the current era of antiretrovirals, since most of the therapeutic drugs do not cross the BBB. HIV Tat can also disrupt the BBB integrity, allowing for increased numbers of inflammatory cells into the CNS. Furthermore, Tat can also cooperate with various drugs of abuse to potentiate toxicity thereby amplifying untoward inflammatory responses in the CNS. HIV Tat thus acts at multiple steps within the CNS to exacerbate disease pathogenesis, and understanding its contributions at various stages of the disease process is crucial for developing strategies that could interfere with disease induction and/or progression.

REFERENCES

Adamson DC, Dawson TM, Zink MC, Clements, JE, Dawson VL (1996) Neurovirulent simian immunodeficiency virus infection induces neuronal, endothelial, and glial apoptosis. *Mol Med* **2:** 417–28.

Adler V, Yin Z, Tew KD, Ronai Z (1999) Role of redox potential and reactive oxygen species in stress signaling. *Oncogene* **18:** 6104–11.

Aksenov MY, Aksenova MV, Nath A, Ray PD, Mactutus CF, Booze RM (2006) Cocaine-mediated enhancement of Tat toxicity in rat hippocampal cell cultures: the role of oxidative stress and D1 dopamine receptor. *Neurotoxicology* **27:** 217–28.

Alliot F, Godin I, Pessac B (1999) Microglia derive from progenitors, originating from the yolk sac, and which proliferate in the brain. *Brain Res Dev Brain Res* **117:** 145–52.

Andras IE, Pu H, Deli MA, Nath A, Hennig B, Toborek M (2003) HIV-1 Tat protein alters tight junction protein expression and distribution in cultured brain endothelial cells. *J Neurosci Res* **74:** 255–65.

Andras IE, Pu H, Tian J, Deli MA, Nath A, Hennig B, Toborek M (2005) Signaling mechanisms of HIV-1 Tat-induced alterations of claudin-5 expression in brain endothelial cells. *J Cereb Blood Flow Metab* **25:** 1159–70.

Anthony IC, Bell JE (2008) The neuropathology of HIV/AIDS. *Int Rev Psychiatry* **20:** 15–24.

Anthony IC, Ramage SN, Carnie FW, Simmonds P, Bell JE (2005) Influence of HAART on HIV-related CNS disease and neuroinflammation. *J Neuropathol Exp Neurol* **64:** 529–36.

Asensio VC, Maier J, Milner R, Boztug K, Kincaid C, Moulard M, Phillipson C, Lindsley K, Krucker T, Fox HS, *et al.* (2001) Interferon-independent, human immunodeficiency virus type 1 gp120-mediated induction of CXCL10/IP-10 gene expression by astrocytes in vivo and in vitro. *J Virol* **75:** 7067–77.

Avison MJ, Nath A, Greene-Avison R, Schmitt FA, Bales RA, Ethisham A, Greenberg RN, Berger JR (2004) Inflammatory changes and breakdown of microvascular integrity in early human immunodeficiency virus dementia. *J Neurovirol* **10:** 223–32.

Babior BM (1999) NADPH oxidase: an update. *Blood* **93:** 1464–76.

Bansal AK, Mactutus CF, Nath A, Maragos W, Hauser KF, Booze RM (2000) Neurotoxicity of HIV-1 proteins gp120 and Tat in the rat striatum. *Brain Res* **879:** 42–9.

Bell DC, Richard AJ, Dayton CA (1996) Effect of drug user treatment on psychosocial change: a comparison of in-treatment and out-of-treatment cocaine users. *Subst Use Misuse* **31:** 1083–100.

Bell JE (1998) The neuropathology of adult HIV infection. *Rev Neurol (Paris)* **154:** 816–29.

Boess F, Ndikum-Moffor FM, Boelsterli UA, Roberts SM (2000) Effects of cocaine and its oxidative metabolites on mitochondrial respiration and generation of reactive oxygen species. *Biochem Pharmacol* **60:** 615–23.

Bokhari SM, Yao H, Bethel-Brown C, Fuwang P, Williams R, Dhillon NK, Hegde R, Kumar A, Buch SJ (2009) Morphine enhances Tat-induced activation in murine microglia. *J Neurovirol* **15:** 219–28.

Bonavia R, Bajetto A, Barbero S, Albini A, Noonan DM, Schettini G (2001) HIV-1 Tat causes apoptotic death and calcium homeostasis alterations in rat neurons. *Biochem Biophys Res Commun* **288:** 301–8.

Bonwetsch R, Croul S, Richardson MW, Lorenzana C, Del Valle L, Sverstiuk AE, Amini S, Morgello S, Khalili K, Rappaport J (1999) Role of HIV-1 Tat and CC chemokine MIP-1alpha in the pathogenesis of HIV associated central nervous system disorders. *J Neurovirol* **5:** 685–94.

Brenneman DE, Westbrook GL, Fitzgerald SP, Ennist DL, Elkins KL, Ruff MR, Pert CB (1988) Neuronal cell killing by the envelope protein of HIV and its prevention by vasoactive intestinal peptide. *Nature* **335:** 639–42.

Bruce-Keller AJ, Chauhan A, Dimayuga FO, Gee J, Keller JN, Nath A (2003) Synaptic transport of human immunodeficiency virus-Tat protein causes neurotoxicity and gliosis in rat brain. *J Neurosci* **23:** 8417–22.

Budka H (1991) Neuropathology of human immunodeficiency virus infection. *Brain Pathol* **1:** 163–75.

Burger DM, Boucher CA, Meenhorst PL, Kraayeveld CL, Portegies P, Mulder JW, Hoetelmans RM, Beijnen JH (1997) HIV-1 RNA levels in the cerebrospinal fluid may increase owing to damage to the blood–brain barrier. *Antivir Ther* **2:** 113–7.

Cai NS, Cadet JL (2008) The combination of methamphetamine and of the HIV protein, Tat, induces death of the human neuroblastoma cell line, SH-SY5Y. *Synapse* **62:** 551–2.

Cass WA, Harned ME, Peters LE, Nath A, Maragos WF (2003) HIV-1 protein Tat potentiation of methamphetamine-induced decreases in evoked overflow of dopamine in the striatum of the rat. *Brain Res* **984:** 133–42.

Chanock SJ, el Benna J, Smith RM, Babior BM (1994) The respiratory burst oxidase. *J Biol Chem* **269:** 24519–22.

Chen P, Mayne M, Power C, Nath A (1997) The Tat protein of HIV-1 induces tumor necrosis factor-alpha production. Implications for HIV-1-associated neurological diseases. *J Biol Chem* **272:** 22385–8.

Chen Z, Huang Y, Zhao X, Skulsky E, Lin D, Ip J, Gettie A, Ho DD (2000) Enhanced infectivity of an R5-tropic simian/human immunodeficiency virus carrying human immunodeficiency virus type 1 subtype C envelope after serial passages in pig-tailed macaques (*Macaca nemestrina*). *J Virol* **74:** 6501–10.

Cheng J, Nath A, Knudsen B, Hochman S, Geiger JD, Ma M, Magnuson DS (1998) Neuronal excitatory properties of human immunodeficiency virus type 1 Tat protein. *Neuroscience* **82:** 97–106.

Chiesi A, Vella S, Dally LG, Pedersen C, Danner S, Johnson AM, Schwander S, Goebel FD, Glauser M, Antunes F, *et al.* (1996) Epidemiology of AIDS dementia complex in Europe. AIDS in Europe Study Group. *J Acquir Immune Defic Syndr Hum Retrovirol* **11:** 39–44.

D'Aversa TG, Yu KO, Berman JW (2004) Expression of chemokines by human fetal microglia after treatment with the human immunodeficiency virus type 1 protein Tat. *J Neurovirol* **10:** 86–97.

Dallasta LM, Pisarov LA, Esplen JE, Werley JV, Moses AV, Nelson JA, Achim CL (1999) Blood–brain barrier tight junction disruption in human immunodeficiency virus-1 encephalitis. *Am J Pathol* **155:** 1915–27.

Davalos D, Grutzendler J, Yang G, Kim JV, Zuo Y, Jung S, Littman DR, Dustin ML, Gan WB (2005) ATP mediates rapid microglial response to local brain injury in vivo. *Nat Neurosci* **8:** 752–8.

Dhillon N, Zhu X, Peng F, Yao H, Williams R, Qiu J, Callen S, Ladner AO, Buch S (2008) Molecular mechanism(s) involved in the synergistic induction of CXCL10 by human immunodeficiency virus type 1 Tat and interferon-gamma in macrophages. *J Neurovirol* **14:** 196–204.

Dreyer EB, Kaiser PK, Offermann JT, Lipton SA (1990) HIV-1 coat protein neurotoxicity prevented by calcium channel antagonists. *Science* **248:** 364–7.

El-Benna J, Dang PM, Gougerot-Pocidalo MA, Elbim C (2005) Phagocyte NADPH oxidase: a multicomponent enzyme essential for host defenses. *Arch Immunol Ther Exp (Warsz)* **53:** 199–206.

El-Hage N, Gurwell JA, Singh IN, Knapp PE, Nath A, Hauser KF (2005) Synergistic increases in intracellular Ca2+, and the release of MCP-1, RANTES, and IL-6 by astrocytes treated with opiates and HIV-1 Tat. *Glia* **50:** 91–106.

Eugenin EA, D'Aversa TG, Lopez L, Calderon TM, Berman JW (2003) MCP-1 (CCL2) protects human neurons and astrocytes from NMDA or HIV-Tat-induced apoptosis. *J Neurochem* **85:** 1299–311.

Eugenin EA, Dyer G, Calderon TM, Berman JW (2005) HIV-1 Tat protein induces a migratory phenotype in human fetal microglia by a CCL2 (MCP-1)-dependent mechanism: possible role in NeuroAIDS. *Glia* **49:** 501–10.

Eugenin EA, King JE, Nath A, Calderon TM, Zukin RS, Bennett MV, Berman JW (2007) HIV-Tat induces formation of an LRP-PSD-95- NMDAR-nNOS complex that promotes apoptosis in neurons and astrocytes. *Proc Natl Acad Sci USA* **104:** 3438–43.

Fetler L, Amigorena S (2005) Neuroscience. Brain under surveillance: the microglia patrol. *Science* **309:** 392–93.

Fiala M, Gan XH, Zhang L, House SD, Newton T, Graves MC, Shapshak P, Stins M, Kim KS, Witte M, *et al.* (1998) Cocaine enhances monocyte migration across the blood–brain barrier. Cocaine's connection to AIDS dementia and vasculitis? *Adv Exp Med Biol* **437:** 199–205.

Flora G, Lee YW, Nath A, Hennig B, Maragos W, Toborek M (2003) Methamphetamine potentiates HIV-1 Tat protein-mediated activation of redox-sensitive pathways in discrete regions of the brain. *Exp Neurol* **179:** 60–70.

Gan X, Zhang L, Berger O, Stins MF, Way D, Taub DD, Chang SL, Kim KS, House SD, Weinand M, *et al.* (1999) Cocaine enhances brain endothelial adhesion molecules and leukocyte migration. *Clin Immunol* **91:** 68–76.

Garden GA, Guo W, Jayadev S, Tun C, Balcaitis S, Choi J, Montine TJ, Moller T, Morrison RS (2004) HIV associated neurodegeneration requires p53 in neurons and microglia. *FASEB J* **18:** 1141–3.

Gendelman HE, Lipton SA, Tardieu M, Bukrinsky MI, Nottet HS (1994) The neuropathogenesis of HIV-1 infection. *J Leukoc Biol* **56:** 389–98.

Goldstein GW (1988) Endothelial cell-astrocyte interactions. A cellular model of the blood–brain barrier. *Ann NY Acad Sci* **529:** 31–9.

Goodkin K, Shapshak P, Metsch LR, McCoy CB, Crandall KA, Kumar M, Fujimura RK, McCoy V, Zhang BT, Reyblat S, *et al.* (1998) Cocaine abuse and HIV-1 infection: epidemiology and neuropathogenesis. *J Neuroimmunol* **83:** 88–101.

Gurwell JA, Nath A, Sun Q, Zhang J, Martin KM, Chen Y, Hauser KF (2001) Synergistic neurotoxicity of opioids and human immunodeficiency virus-1 Tat protein in striatal neurons in vitro. *Neuroscience* **102:** 555–63.

Haughey NJ, Nath A, Mattson MP, Slevin JT, Geiger JD (2001) HIV-1 Tat through phosphorylation of NMDA receptors potentiates glutamate excitotoxicity. *J Neurochem* **78:** 457–67.

Hauser KF, Hahn YK, Adjan VV, Zou S, Buch SK, Nath A, Bruce-Keller AJ, Knapp PE (2009) HIV-1 Tat and morphine have interactive effects on oligodendrocyte survival and morphology. *Glia* **57:** 194–206.

Hayashi K, Pu H, Andras IE, Eum SY, Yamauchi A, Hennig B, Toborek M (2006) HIV-TAT protein upregulates expression of multidrug resistance protein 1 in the blood–brain barrier. *J Cereb Blood Flow Metab* **26:** 1052–65.

Herz J, Strickland DK (2001) LRP: a multifunctional scavenger and signaling receptor. *J Clin Invest* **108:** 779–84.

Hof PR, Lee PY, Yeung G, Wang RF, Podos SM, Morrison JH (1998) Glutamate receptor subunit GluR2 and NMDAR1 immunoreactivity in the retina of macaque monkeys with experimental glaucoma does not identify vulnerable neurons. *Exp Neurol* **153:** 234–41.

Huang W, Eum SY, Andras IE, Hennig B, Toborek M (2009) PPARalpha and PPARgamma attenuate HIV-induced dysregulation of tight junction proteins by modulations of matrix metalloproteinase and proteasome activities. *Faseb J* **23:** 1596–606.

Husain M, Hahn T, Yedavalli VR, Ahmad N (2001) Characterization of HIV type 1 Tat sequences associated with perinatal transmission. *AIDS Res Hum Retroviruses* **17:** 765–73.

Jones M, Olafson K, Del Bigio MR, Peeling J, Nath A (1998) Intraventricular injection of human immunodeficiency virus type 1 (HIV-1) Tat protein causes inflammation, gliosis, apoptosis, and ventricular enlargement. *J Neuropathol Exp Neurol* **57:** 563–70.

Kaul M, Garden GA, Lipton SA (2001) Pathways to neuronal injury and apoptosis in HIV-associated dementia. *Nature* **410:** 988–94.

Kaul M, Lipton SA (1999) Chemokines and activated macrophages in HIV gp120-induced neuronal apoptosis. *Proc Natl Acad Sci USA* **96:** 8212–16.

Kaul M, Zheng J, Okamoto S, Gendelman HE, Lipton SA (2005) HIV-1 infection and AIDS: consequences for the central nervous system. *Cell Death Differ* **12 (Suppl. 1):** 878–92.

Khurdayan VK, Buch S, El-Hage N, Lutz SE, Goebel SM, Singh IN, Knapp PE, Turchan-Cholewo J, Nath A, Hauser KF (2004) Preferential vulnerability of astroglia and glial precursors to combined opioid and HIV-1 Tat exposure in vitro. *Eur J Neurosci* **19:** 3171–82.

Kong LY, Wilson BC, McMillian MK, Bing G, Hudson PM, Hong JS (1996) The effects of the HIV-1 envelope protein gp120 on the production of nitric oxide and proinflammatory cytokines in mixed glial cell cultures. *Cell Immunol* **172:** 77–83.

Kruman II, Nath A, Mattson MP (1998a) HIV-1 protein Tat induces apoptosis of hippocampal neurons by a mechanism involving caspase activation, calcium overload, and oxidative stress. *Exp Neurol* **154:** 276–88.

Kruman I, Guo Q, Mattson MP (1998b) Calcium and reactive oxygen species mediate staurosporine-induced mitochondrial dysfunction and apoptosis in PC12 cells. *J Neurosci Res* **51:** 293–308.

Kutsch O, Oh J, Nath A, Benveniste EN (2000) Induction of the chemokines interleukin-8 and IP-10 by human immunodeficiency virus type 1 Tat in astrocytes. *J Virol* **74:** 9214–21.

Langford D, Grigorian A, Hurford R, Adame A, Crews L, Masliah E (2004) The role of mitochondrial alterations in the combined toxic effects of human immunodeficiency virus Tat protein and methamphetamine on calbindin positive-neurons. *J Neurovirol* **10:** 327–37.

Lipton SA, Gendelman HE (1995) Seminars in medicine of the Beth Israel Hospital, Boston. Dementia associated with the acquired immunodeficiency syndrome. *N Engl J Med* **332:** 934–40.

Lipton SA, Sucher NJ, Kaiser PK, Dreyer EB (1991) Synergistic effects of HIV coat protein and NMDA receptor-mediated neurotoxicity. *Neuron* **7:** 111–18.

Liu K, Chi DS, Li C, Hall HK, Milhorn DM, Krishnaswamy G (2005) HIV-1 Tat protein-induced VCAM-1 expression in human pulmonary artery endothelial cells and its signaling. *Am J Physiol Lung Cell Mol Physiol* **289:** L252–L260.

Liu Y, Jones M, Hingtgen CM, Bu G, Laribee N, Tanzi RE, Moir RD, Nath A, He JJ (2000) Uptake of HIV-1 Tat protein mediated by low-density lipoprotein receptor-related protein disrupts the neuronal metabolic balance of the receptor ligands. *Nat Med* **6:** 1380–7.

Magnuson DS, Knudsen BE, Geiger JD, Brownstone RM, Nath A (1995) Human immunodeficiency virus type 1 Tat activates non-N-methyl-D-aspartate excitatory amino acid receptors and causes neurotoxicity. *Ann Neurol* **37:** 373–80.

Majumder S, Zhou LZ, Chaturvedi P, Babcock G, Aras S, Ransohoff RM (1998) p48/STAT-1alpha-containing complexes play a predominant role in induction of IFN-gamma-inducible protein, 10 kDa (IP-10) by IFN-gamma alone or in synergy with TNF-alpha. *J Immunol* **161:** 4736–44.

Martinez AJ, Sell M, Mitrovics T, Stoltenburg-Didinger G, Iglesias-Rozas JR, Giraldo-Velasquez MA, Gosztonyi G, Schneider V, Cervos-Navarro J (1995) The neuropathology and epidemiology of AIDS. A Berlin experience. A review of 200 cases. *Pathol Res Pract* **191:** 427–43.

McArthur JC, Hoover DR, Bacellar H, Miller EN, Cohen BA, Becker JT, Graham NM, McArthur JH, Selnes OA, Jacobson LP, *et al.* (1993) Dementia in AIDS patients: incidence and risk factors. Multicenter AIDS Cohort Study. *Neurology* **43:** 2245–52.

Nair MP, Mahajan SD, Schwartz SA, Reynolds J, Whitney R, Bernstein Z, Chawda RP, Sykes D, Hewitt R, Hsiao CB (2005) Cocaine modulates dendritic cell-specific C type intercellular adhesion molecule-3-grabbing nonintegrin expression by dendritic cells in HIV-1 patients. *J Immunol* **174:** 6617–26.

Nath A (1999) Pathobiology of human immunodeficiency virus dementia. *Semin Neurol* **19:** 113–27.

Nath A, Conant K, Chen P, Scott C, Major EO (1999) Transient exposure to HIV-1 Tat protein results in cytokine production in macrophages and astrocytes. A hit and run phenomenon. *J Biol Chem* **274:** 17098–102.

Nath A, Maragos WF, Avison MJ, Schmitt FA, Berger JR (2001) Acceleration of HIV dementia with methamphetamine and cocaine. *J Neurovirol* **7:** 66–71.

Nath A, Schiess N, Venkatesan A, Rumbaugh J, Sacktor N, McArthur J (2008) Evolution of HIV dementia with HIV infection. *Int Rev Psychiatry* **20:** 25–31.

New DR, Ma M, Epstein LG, Nath A, Gelbard HA (1997) Human immunodeficiency virus type 1 Tat protein induces death by apoptosis in primary human neuron cultures. *J Neurovirol* **3:** 168–73.

Nimmerjahn A, Kirchhoff F, Helmchen F (2005) Resting microglial cells are highly dynamic surveillants of brain parenchyma in vivo. *Science* **308:** 1314–18.

Nottet HS, Persidsky Y, Sasseville VG, Nukuna AN, Bock P, Zhai QH, Sharer LR, McComb RD, Swindells S, Soderland C, *et al.* (1996) Mechanisms for the transendothelial migration of HIV-1-infected monocytes into brain. *J Immunol* **156:** 1284–95.

Park J, Choi K, Jeong E, Kwon D, Benveniste EN, Choi C (2004) Reactive oxygen species mediate chloroquine-induced expression of chemokines by human astroglial cells. *Glia* **47:** 9–20.

Patel CA, Mukhtar M, Pomerantz RJ (2000) Human immunodeficiency virus type 1 Vpr induces apoptosis in human neuronal cells. *J Virol* **74:** 9717–26.

Pessac B, Godin I, Alliot F (2001) [Microglia: origin and development]. *Bull Acad Natl Med* **185:** 337–346; discussion 346–37.

Pu H, Hayashi K, Andras IE, Eum SY, Hennig B, Toborek M (2007) Limited role of COX-2 in HIV Tat-induced alterations of tight junction protein expression and disruption of the blood–brain barrier. *Brain Res* **1184:** 333–44.

Pu H, Tian J, Flora G, Lee YW, Nath A, Hennig B, Toborek M (2003) HIV-1 Tat protein upregulates inflammatory mediators and induces monocyte invasion into the brain. *Mol Cell Neurosci* **24:** 224–37.

Pulliam L, Sun B, Rempel H, Martinez PM, Hoekman JD, Rao RJ, Frey WH 2nd, Hanson LR (2007) Intranasal Tat alters gene expression in the mouse brain. *J Neuroimmune Pharmacol* **2:** 87–92.

Raad H, Paclet MH, Boussetta T, Kroviarski Y, Morel F, Quinn MT, Gougerot-Pocidalo MA, Dang PM, El-Benna J (2009) Regulation of the phagocyte NADPH oxidase activity: phosphorylation of gp91phox/NOX2 by protein kinase C enhances its diaphorase activity and binding to Rac2, p67phox, and p47phox. *FASEB J* **23:** 1011–22.

Ramirez SH, Sanchez JF, Dimitri CA, Gelbard HA, Dewhurst S, Maggirwar SB (2001) Neurotrophins prevent HIV Tat-induced neuronal apoptosis via a nuclear factor-kappaB (NF-kappaB)-dependent mechanism. *J Neurochem* **78:** 874–89.

Rebeck GW, Reiter JS, Strickland DK, Hyman BT (1993) Apolipoprotein E in sporadic Alzheimer's disease: allelic variation and receptor interactions. *Neuron* **11:** 575–80.

Rock RB, Gekker G, Hu S, Sheng WS, Cheeran M, Lokensgard JR, Peterson PK (2004) Role of microglia in central nervous system infections. *Clin Microbiol Rev* **17:** 942–64, table of contents.

Rock RB, Peterson PK (2006) Microglia as a pharmacological target in infectious and inflammatory diseases of the brain. *J Neuroimmune Pharmacol* **1:** 117–26.

Sacktor N, Lyles RH, Skolasky R, Kleeberger C, Selnes OA, Miller EN, Becker JT, Cohen B, McArthur JC (2001) HIV-associated neurologic disease incidence changes: Multicenter AIDS Cohort Study, 1990–1998. *Neurology* **56:** 257–60.

Savio T, Levi G (1993) Neurotoxicity of HIV coat protein gp120, NMDA receptors, and protein kinase C: a study with rat cerebellar granule cell cultures. *J Neurosci Res* **34:** 265–72.

Shapshak P, Duncan R, Minagar A, Rodriguez de la Vega P, Stewart RV, Goodkin K (2004) Elevated expression of IFN-gamma in the HIV-1 infected brain. *Front Biosci* **9:** 1073–81.

Singh IN, Goody RJ, Dean C, Ahmad NM, Lutz SE, Knapp PE, Nath A, Hauser KF (2004) Apoptotic death of striatal neurons induced by human immunodeficiency virus-1 Tat and gp120: differential involvement of caspase-3 and endonuclease G. *J Neurovirol* **10:** 141–51.

Song HY, Ryu J, Ju SM, Park LJ, Lee JA, Choi SY, Park J (2007) Extracellular HIV-1 Tat enhances monocyte adhesion by up-regulation of ICAM-1 and VCAM-1 gene expression via ROS-dependent NF-kappaB activation in astrocytes. *Exp Mol Med* **39:** 27–37.

Spencer DC, Price RW (1992) Human immunodeficiency virus and the central nervous system. *Annu Rev Microbiol* **46:** 655–93.

Sundaresan M, Yu ZX, Ferrans VJ, Irani K, Finkel T (1995) Requirement for generation of H_2O_2 for platelet-derived growth factor signal transduction. *Science* **270:** 296–9.

Tang Z, Arjunan P, Lee C, Li Y, Kumar A, Hou X, Wang B, Wardega P, Zhang F, Dong L, *et al.* (2010) Survival effect of PDGF-CC rescues neurons from apoptosis in both brain and retina by regulating GSK3beta phosphorylation. *J Exp Med* **207:** 867–80.

Theodore S, Cass WA, Nath A, Maragos WF (2007) Progress in understanding basal ganglia dysfunction as a common target for methamphetamine abuse and HIV-1 neurodegeneration. *Curr HIV Res* **5:** 301–13.

Theodore S, Stolberg S, Cass WA, Maragos WF (2006) Human immunodeficiency virus-1 protein Tat and methamphetamine interactions. *Ann NY Acad Sci* **1074:** 178–90.

Toborek M, Lee YW, Pu H, Malecki A, Flora G, Garrido R, Hennig B, Bauer HC, Nath A (2003) HIV-Tat protein induces oxidative and inflammatory pathways in brain endothelium. *J Neurochem* **84:** 169–79.

Tomlinson GS, Simmonds P, Busuttil A, Chiswick A, Bell JE (1999) Upregulation of microglia in drug users with and without pre-symptomatic HIV infection. *Neuropathol Appl Neurobiol* **25:** 369–79.

Turchan-Cholewo J, Dimayuga VM, Gupta S, Gorospe RM, Keller JN, Bruce-Keller AJ (2009) NADPH oxidase drives cytokine and neurotoxin release from microglia and macrophages in response to HIV-Tat. *Antioxid Redox Signal* **11:** 193–204.

Turchan J, Anderson C, Hauser KF, Sun Q, Zhang J, Liu Y, Wise PM, Kruman I, Maragos W, Mattson MP, *et al.* (2001) Estrogen protects against the synergistic toxicity by HIV proteins, methamphetamine and cocaine. *BMC Neurosci* **2:** 3.

Turchan J, Pocernich CB, Gairola C, Chauhan A, Schifitto G, Butterfield DA, Buch S, Narayan O, Sinai A, Geiger J, *et al.* (2003) Oxidative stress in HIV demented patients and protection ex vivo with novel antioxidants. *Neurology* **60:** 307–14.

Wang X, Martindale JL, Liu Y, Holbrook NJ (1998) The cellular response to oxidative stress: influences of mitogen-activated protein kinase signalling pathways on cell survival. *Biochem J* **333 (Pt 2):** 291–300.

Weiss JM, Nath A, Major EO, Berman JW (1999) HIV-1 Tat induces monocyte chemoattractant protein-1-mediated monocyte transmigration across a model of the human blood–brain barrier and up-regulates CCR5 expression on human monocytes. *J Immunol* **163:** 2953–9.

Wesselingh SL, Takahashi K, Glass JD, McArthur JC, Griffin JW, Griffin DE (1997) Cellular localization of tumor necrosis factor mRNA in neurological tissue from HIV-infected patients by combined reverse transcriptase/polymerase chain reaction in situ hybridization and immunohistochemistry. *J Neuroimmunol* **74:** 1–8.

Williams R, Dhillon NK, Hegde ST, Yao H, Peng F, Callen S, Chebloune Y, Davis RL, Buch SJ (2009a) Proinflammatory cytokines and HIV-1 synergistically enhance CXCL10 expression in human astrocytes. *Glia* **57:** 734–43.

Williams R, Yao H, Dhillon NK, Buch SJ (2009b) HIV-1 Tat co-operates with IFN-gamma and TNF-alpha to increase CXCL10 in human astrocytes. *PLoS One* **4:** e5709.

Williams R, Yao H, Peng F, Yang Y, Bethel-Brown C, Buch S (2010) Cooperative induction of CXCL10 involves NADPH oxidase: implications for HIV dementia. *Glia* **58:** 611–21.

Woody GE, Donnell D, Seage GR, Metzger D, Marmor M, Koblin BA, Buchbinder S, Gross M, Stone B, Judson FN (1999) Non-injection substance use correlates with risky sex among men having sex with men: data from HIVNET. *Drug Alcohol Depend* **53:** 197–205.

Yang Y, Wu J, Lu Y (2010) Mechanism of HIV-1-Tat induction of interleukin-1beta from human monocytes: involvement of the phospholipase C/protein kinase C signaling cascade. *J Med Virol* **82:** 735–46.

Yao H, Allen JE, Zhu X, Callen S, Buch S (2009a) Cocaine and human immunodeficiency virus type 1 gp120 mediate neurotoxicity through overlapping signaling pathways. *J Neurovirol* **15:** 164–75.

Yao H, Peng F, Dhillon N, Callen S, Bokhari S, Stehno-Bittel L, Ahmad SO, Wang JQ, Buch S (2009b) Involvement of TRPC channels in CCL2-mediated neuroprotection against Tat toxicity. *J Neurosci* **29:** 1657–69.

Yao H, Peng F, Fan Y, Zhu X, Hu G, Buch SJ (2009c) TRPC channel-mediated neuroprotection by PDGF involves Pyk2/ERK/CREB pathway. *Cell Death Differ* **16:** 1681–93.

Zhong Y, Smart EJ, Weksler B, Couraud PO, Hennig B, Toborek M (2008) Caveolin-1 regulates human immunodeficiency virus-1 Tat-induced alterations of tight junction protein expression via modulation of the Ras signaling. *J Neurosci* **28:** 7788–96.

Zhu X, Yao H, Peng F, Callen S, Buch S (2009) PDGF-mediated protection of SH-SY5Y cells against Tat toxin involves regulation of extracellular glutamate and intracellular calcium. *Toxicol Appl Pharmacol* **240:** 286–91.

Section 11

Special Topics

C H A P T E R

58

Applications of stem cells in developmental toxicology

Deborah K. Hansen and Amy L. Inselman

Disclaimer. The views expressed are those of the authors and do not reflect the position of the United States Food and Drug Administration.

INTRODUCTION

Three classes of stem cells have been discovered by scientists. While they share the same general properties of self-renewal and the ability to differentiate into specialized cell types, they each represent a unique type of cell. Since the initial discovery and characterization of embryonic stem cells (ESCs) in the early 1980s, they have been heralded for their potential to treat a wide array of debilitating diseases ranging from Alzheimer's to heart disease to diabetes. Embryonic stem cells have been isolated from several species including mice, monkeys and humans and are defined by their ability to continuously self-renew and by their ability to differentiate into specialized cell types representing all three germ layers. In 2006, a groundbreaking discovery by Takahashi (Takahashi and Yamanaka, 2006) led to the development of a new class of stem cells referred to as induced pluripotent stem cells (iPSCs). These specialized adult cells were reprogrammed to assume a stem cell-like state by using a combination of four transcription factors. The developmental and proliferative attributes of ESCs and iPSCs make them a potential *in vitro* model to test drugs and chemicals for reproductive and developmental toxicity as well as for the study of normal growth and developmental mechanisms. Furthermore, the development of human *in vitro* models to determine toxicity could potentially reduce the number of animals used in research while providing a more relevant model system for predicting human susceptibility. Scientists have also identified a third class of stem cells. These cells have been referred to as non-embryonic "adult" stem cells. Unlike their embryonic counterparts, adult stem cells have limited developmental and proliferative potential, but serve a critical role for the repair and replacement of cells that are lost through injury or disease.

EMBRYONIC STEM CELLS

Embryonic stem cells are pluripotent cells capable of giving rise to tissues of the developing embryo, including development of the germ line. Mouse embryonic stem cells (mESCs) were first derived from the inner cell mass of developing blastocysts in 1981 (Evans and Kaufman, 1981; Martin, 1981). However, it would be another 9 years before human embryonic stem cell (hESC) lines would be first reported (Thomas *et al.*, 1998). The first hESC lines were derived from embryos produced through *in vitro* fertilization that were no longer needed by the couples seeking fertility treatment, and for the first time provided unlimited access to human cell lines for potential therapeutic use and for improving product safety through regulatory testing. The successful derivation of hESCs also raised important ethical and legal considerations regarding their use, and to date guidelines and regulations vary from country to country and from state to state. Today, 51 eligible lines have been approved for use in NIH funded research with another 113 lines under review (http://grants.nih.gov/stem_cells/registry/summary_data.htm).

To maintain their pluripotent nature, ES cell lines have traditionally been cultured on a layer of inactivated, mouse primary embryonic fibroblasts in basal medium supplemented with fetal bovine serum. Later it was discovered that the cytokine, leukemia inhibitory factor (LIF), in addition to serum, was sufficient to keep mESCs in a pluripotent, undifferentiated state (Smith and Hooper, 1987; Smith *et al.*, 1988; Williams *et al.*, 1988). While mESCs respond to LIF, hESCs do not (Dahéron *et al.*, 2004; Humphrey *et al.*, 2004), highlighting a critical difference between the culture of mouse and human cell lines. Instead, basic fibroblast growth factor (bFGF) and activin A/nodal/TGF-beta signaling are critical for maintenance of the pluripotent state in hESCs (Beattie *et al.*, 2005; James *et al.*, 2005; Vallier *et al.*, 2005, 2009; Xiao *et al.*, 2006; Greber *et al.*, 2007; Xu *et al.*, 2008). Besides requiring different growth factors, mouse and human ESCs also express different cell surface markers (Draper *et al.*, 2002; Henderson *et al.*, 2002), vary in their ability to differentiate into trophoblast-like

Reproductive and Developmental Toxicology, Edited by Ramesh C. Gupta
ISBN: 978-0-12-382032-7

cells (Niwa *et al.*, 2000; Odorico *et al.*, 2001; Rossant, 2001) and differ in telomerase regulation (Forsyth *et al.*, 2002) as well as expression profiles of cytokines, cell cycle and cell death-regulating genes (Ginis *et al.*, 2004).

The presence of undefined components in the serum or the variability of exogenous factors produced by the feeder layers are a challenge to researchers. Whether ES cells are used in therapy or for toxicological testing, consistent and defined differentiation conditions are needed to help standardize and minimize variation. Standardized protocols for both growth and differentiation will also facilitate comparisons between cell lines and laboratories. Continued improvements and understanding of the pluripotent state has led to the development of mESC and hESC feeder-free, defined culture conditions. Recently, the International Stem Cell Initiative, a consortium of laboratories whose objective is to establish standards for pluripotent stem cell research (Andrews *et al.*, 2005), compared a panel of ten hESC lines and eight previously defined cell culture feeder-free methods (The International Stem Cell Initiative Consortium, 2010). In five separate laboratories the cultures were assessed for up to ten passages for attachment, death and differentiated morphology, for growth by serial counts and for maintenance of stem cell surface marker expression. The consortium found that in addition to the control media and mouse embryonic fibroblast feeder cell layers, only two commercially available-based media (Ludwig *et al.*, 2006a,b; Wang *et al.*, 2007) could support the majority of cell lines for ten passages. This demonstrated that culture of hESCs in defined media is not a trivial undertaking even for those laboratories experienced in hESC culture. Additionally, subtle differences in culturing methods may greatly influence cell pluripotency (The International Stem Cell Initiative Consortium, 2010).

INDUCED PLURIPOTENT STEM CELLS

In 1952 the first nuclear transfer experiments began to ask the fundamental question of whether the nucleus of a differentiated cell was equivalent to that from an early embryo (Briggs and King, 1952). This experiment and many others that followed demonstrated that the nucleus of adult cells maintain plasticity and can be used to reset the cell to an embryonic state. Perhaps the most notable of these experiments was when Dolly the sheep was cloned from an adult cell in 1996 by Wilmut and colleagues (Campbell *et al.*, 1996). Dolly brought cloning and nuclear transfer to the forefront of ethical, moral and legal debates as the ideal of reprogramming cells for therapeutic purposes began to garner attention. The more recent discovery that adult somatic cells could be directly reprogrammed to a stem cell-like state by using a combination of transcription factors without the need for embryos (Takahashi and Yamanaka, 2006; Maherali *et al.*, 2007; Okita *et al.*, 2007; Takahashi *et al.*, 2007; Wernig *et al.*, 2007; Yu *et al.*, 2007; Lowry *et al.*, 2008; Park *et al.*, 2008) has dampened some of these concerns. These iPSCs have once again reenergized the scientific community in hopes that patient-specific cell lines can be created for the study of disease, regenerative medicine, as well as serving as valuable tools for toxicological studies and analysis.

One crucial question that remains is whether iPSCs are identical to hESCs on a genome, transcriptome, epigenome and developmental level (Amabile and Meissner, 2009). Outwardly iPSCs appear indistinguishable from their hESC counterparts. Genomic analysis has shown that while a few karyotypic abnormalities have been observed in iPSC lines, generally they maintain a stable karyotype over prolonged passaging (Takahashi *et al.*, 2007; Wernig *et al.*, 2007; Yu *et al.*, 2007). Recent reports, however, have noted differences in iPSC gene expression patterns and differentiation ability when compared to hESC cultures. A study by Feng *et al.* (2010) compared the ability of iPSCs and hESCs to differentiate into several types of blood and endothelial cells. They found that the hESCs differentiated into the desired cell type more readily than the iPSCs tested. They also noted that the iPSCs began to undergo premature cellular aging and programmed death after only a short time of culture. A similar type of study conducted by Hu and colleagues (2010) compared the differentiation of hESCs and iPSCs into the neuronal lineage. Again the iPSCs were capable of differentiating into the various neuronal types, but differentiation was not as efficient when compared to hESCs, and the iPSC lines displayed greater variability overall.

Extensive genome-wide expression analysis of mouse and human ESCs and iPSCs revealed that although iPSCs are quite similar to their embryonic counterparts, a recurrent gene expression profile appears in iPSCs that is not observed in hESCs. This gene expression signature is independent of origin or method used for iPSC generation and extends to microRNA expression (Chin *et al.*, 2009). Data analysis suggests that the signature pattern of gene expression observed in iPSCs is attributed to differential promoter binding by the factors used for reprogramming, and therefore iPSCs should be considered a unique subtype of embryonic stem cells.

iPSCs, unlike hESCs, enable the creation of patient-specific stem cells to study disease mechanisms, can be customized for patient-specific therapy, and serve as valuable tools for drug discovery and toxicology. However, because variability exists in iPSC reprogramming the biological relevance of the cell lines must be demonstrated through quality standards applicable to hESCs, and need to be agreed upon before cell lines are used to address specific toxicological questions (Vojnits and Bremer, 2010). The guidance for iPSCs should focus on cell morphology, unlimited self-renewal potential, gene and protein expression profiles, as well as lineage-specific marker expression during differentiation. In addition to the quality control standards for hESCs, iPSCs ideally would be evaluated for the factors that define the reprogrammed state. The available methods to generate iPSC lines are inefficient and consist of many uncertainties with largely unknown or poorly understood events. Therefore, variables of the reprogramming technology, including the choice of reprogramming factors, reprogramming factor delivery, selection of target cell type, and culture conditions, should be quality controlled to ensure reproducible results for use in toxicological testing (Maherali and Hochedlinger, 2008).

ADULT STEM CELLS

Adult stem cells have been identified in many tissues of the adult organism where they maintain tissue homeostasis and with limitations are able to replace cells that die due to injury or disease. Unlike ESCs, adult stem cells are multipotent progenitor cells possessing limited differentiation potential or are unipotent, capable of generating only a single specific cell type. Adult stem cells are located in specialized vascular microenvironments, referred to as the stem cell niche. The niche provides intrinsic and extrinsic signals that regulate cell fate and renewal and may explain why adult stem cells, isolated from various tissues, behave differently. The first adult stem cells were identified in the bone marrow in 1961 as cells that were capable of giving rise to multilineage, hematopoietic colonies in the spleen (Till and McCulloch, 1961). However, adult stem cells are rare and difficult to identify with the notable exception being the bone marrow. Experiments have determined that only 1 in 10,000–15,000 cells in the bone marrow are a hematopoietic stem cell. In addition to their small numbers, adult stem cells have limited capacity for division, making generation of large quantities of stem cells difficult for regenerative therapy or *in vitro* toxicological testing.

Typically, adult stem cells are thought to have limited differentiation potential restricted to the cells found in the tissue where the stem cells reside. However, others have reported on a phenomenon referred to as transdifferentiation, whereby an adult stem cell can differentiate into cell types observed in other organs or tissues (i.e., brain stem cell differentiating into a cardiac cell). Whether the phenomenon of transdifferentiation occurs in humans is still the subject of debate. Many questions still surround adult stem cells, including their origin, how they are maintained in the adult organism, how their "niche" controls their behavior, what factors are necessary for proliferation and differentiation, and finally how these factors can be enhanced to promote healing and replacement.

USE OF STEM CELLS IN DEVELOPMENTAL TOXICOLOGY – THE EMBRYONIC STEM CELL TEST (EST)

In the 1980s the concept of the three Rs (reduction, refinement and replacement) gained a foothold in the scientific community in regard to the humane use of animals. ZEBET (National Centre for Documentation and Evaluation of Alternative Methods to Animal Experiments) was established in Berlin in 1989 as the first governmental agency to promote and validate alternative testing methods. In 1993, the European Union established ECVAM (European Centre for the Validation of Alternative Methods); in 1997, the United States government established ICCVAM (Interagency Coordinating Center for the Validation of Alternative Methods), and the Japanese government established JaCVAM (Japanese Centre for the Validation of Alternative Methods). ECVAM held workshops in 1990 (Balls *et al.*, 1990) and 1994 (Balls *et al.*, 1995) to discuss the process for validation of alternative tests. The concepts developed at the second workshop were accepted by ECVAM in 1995 as well as the USA and Organization for Economic Co-operation and Development in 1996 (Spielmann *et al.*, 2008).

Since there is no information on the reproductive and developmental toxicity potential of a large number of chemicals, ECVAM conducted a workshop in 1995 on *in vitro* screening methods for reproductive toxicology (Brown *et al.*, 1995). One of the recommendations of this workshop was to validate and improve existing *in vitro* tests and to develop new tests. Three *in vitro* tests were chosen for validation; these were the rat whole embryo culture test, the rat limb bud micromass test and the embryonic stem cell test (EST).

Freshly isolated embryonic cells were first used to examine teratogenicity by Laschinski *et al.* (1991). The authors examined several of the teratogenic compounds listed by Smith *et al.* (1983) for use in validating *in vitro* test systems as well as a number of antineoplastic compounds. They selected only compounds that did not require metabolic activation. The endpoint of their assay was cytotoxicity as measured with dimethylthiozol-diphenyl tetrazolium (MTT). They compared the cytotoxicity produced in undifferentiated embryonic cells to that produced in differentiated embryonic fibroblasts in order to determine a ratio of cytotoxicity in undifferentiated cells to that in differentiated cells. This was similar to the adult/development ratio proposed for the hydra test (Johnson *et al.*, 1982) and examined whether embryonic cells were more or less sensitive to the cytotoxic effects of chemicals compared to differentiated cells. When comparing the *in vivo* teratogenicity in mice to their *in vitro* results, they found that all six non-teratogenic compounds were negative *in vitro*; however, five of the ten teratogenic compounds were also negative *in vitro*. Although they believed this assay showed promise, they felt that adding the capability of differentiation would enhance the test. Several years later, they described an *in vitro* system in which skeletal muscle and hematopoietic cells were differentiated from D3 mESCs derived from 129/Sv embryos by Doetschman *et al.* (1985). In examining the differentiation of these cells, the authors began to investigate the effect of different culture conditions on the differentiation process (Heuer *et al.*, 1993).

Newall and Beedles (1996) were among the first to test a number of compounds on the differentiation capacity of the D3 mESC line. They used 25 compounds that were the core set used in a multicenter validation study of the rat embryo micromass culture system and evaluated differentiation to an endoderm-like cell type. A range of doses of each compound was used, and the endpoints of the study included cytotoxicity and differentiation assessed after 7 days of culture. The compounds that they tested were assembled into four groups – compounds that were teratogenic at non-maternally toxic doses in all species tested (potent teratogens); compounds that were teratogenic at non-maternally toxic doses in some species, but not all (moderate teratogens); compounds that were teratogenic only at maternally toxic doses (weak teratogens); and compounds that were non-teratogenic in animals (non-teratogens). The test correctly predicted the four potent teratogens and seven of ten non-teratogens. The three false positives were ascorbic acid, diphenyhydramine and furazolidone; the latter two were consistent false positives in the micromass test (Newall and Beedles, 1996). The intermediate groups were the most problematic, with four false negative compounds. Overall, the authors felt that the results of their blinded analysis with mESCs were similar to results with the limb bud micromass test. Since the test used a cell line and no pregnant animals, it had advantages over other *in vitro* test systems.

The EST was modified by Spielmann *et al.* (1997). Differentiation was performed from embryoid bodies (EBs) formed by the aggregation of stem cells for 3 days in small drops of culture medium in the absence of LIF by seeding the mESCs onto the lid of a culture dish in a "hanging drop". EBs resemble cells of the inner cell mass of early embryos in that they are able to differentiate into cells of endodermal, mesodermal and ectodermal origins. Following this initial 3-day culture, EBs were seeded onto bacterial Petri dishes, which prevented adherence and outgrowth of the cells, for an additional 2 days. The cells were then seeded into the wells of a 24-well culture dish for a total of 10 days of culture. At the end of the culture period, the percentage of chemically treated culture wells containing contracting cardiomyocytes was determined and compared to the solvent control wells. A range of concentrations of test articles was tested, and the ID_{50} (concentration of test compound inhibiting cardiomycte differentiation by 50%) was calculated. Additionally, cytotoxicity was determined in the 3T3 fibroblast line as well as in undifferentiated D3 cells. A prediction model was established by ZEBET which allowed the classification of a compound into one of three classes – non-embryotoxic, weakly embryotoxic or strongly embryotoxic.

A prevalidation test was conducted among three laboratories and published in 1999 (Scholz *et al.*, 1999). Results indicated that the testing procedure was able to be transferred to other labs successfully, and the incorporation of an improved prediction model increased the correct classification to an overall 94%. The full validation study was conducted by four laboratories (Genschow *et al.*, 2002). A total of 20 chemicals along with the positive control, 5-fluorouracil, were tested; six of these chemicals were strongly embryotoxic, seven were weakly embryotoxic and seven were non-embryotoxic (Table 58.1). Chemicals were correctly categorized in 78% of experiments using the EST, which was comparable to the 80% observed with whole embryo culture and better than the 70% seen with the rat limb micromass assay. All three assays correctly predicted 100% of strong embryotoxicants. The EST was accepted as a validated *in vitro* assay for developmental toxicity (Spielmann *et al.*, 2008).

USES OF THE EST

The EST is currently being used in some pharmaceutical companies to screen chemicals for developmental toxicity (Marx-Stoelting *et al.*, 2009). A group of scientists at Pfizer Global Research and Development reported that the EST as validated by ECVAM was not adequate for separating non- from weak teratogens, in part due to the cytotoxicity of many of the pharmaceutical agents (Chapin *et al.*, 2007). They were working on two methods to improve this classification. They later reported (Paquette *et al.*, 2008) using a different cell line (derived from DBA/1lacJ mice) and different culture media that they observed about the same relative accuracy as ECVAM had reported with some of the same chemicals (78% for ECVAM and 83% by Paquette *et al.*, 2008). However, the accuracy decreased to 53% when testing 19 in-house compounds, with 50% predictivity for moderate risk and 33% for high risk chemicals. They correctly identified only two of nine candidate compounds as being low risk. They also evaluated 29 commercially available pharmaceutical compounds that were of low or moderate risk. Their overall accuracy was 85% for these compounds. The authors concluded that the results of EST were good and could be used in a pharmaceutical company for making compound-specific decisions; however, they also suggested more work with moderate and high risk compounds as well as other refinements to the assay system were needed.

TABLE 58.1 Chemicals used in the ECVAM full validation study

Chemical (CAS)	*In vivo* teratogenicity class
Acrylamide (79-06-1)	Non-embryotoxic
D-(+)-Camphor (464-49-3)	Non-embryotoxic
Dimethyl phthalate (131-11-3)	Non-embryotoxic
Diphenhydramine hydrochloride (147-24-0)	Non-embryotoxic
Isobutyl-ethyl-valproic acid (–)	Non-embryotoxic
Penicillin G sodium salt (69-57-8)	Non-embryotoxic
Saccharin sodium hydrate (82385-42-0)	Non-embryotoxic
Boric acid (–)	Weakly embryotoxic
Dimehadione (695-53-4)	Weakly embryotoxic
Lithium chloride (7447-41-8)	Weakly embryotoxic
Methoxyacetic acid (625-45-6)	Weakly embryotoxic
Pentyl-4-yn-valproic acid (–)	Weakly embryotoxic
Salicyclic acid sodium salt (54-21-7)	Weakly embryotoxic
Valproic acid (99-66-1)	Weakly embryotoxic
6-Aminonicotinamide (329-89-5)	Strongly embryotoxic
All-trans-Retinoic acid (302-79-4)	Strongly embryotoxic
5-Bromo-2′-deoxyuridine (59-14-3)	Strongly embryotoxic
Hydroxyurea (127-07-1)	Strongly embryotoxic
Methotrexate (59-05-2)	Strongly embryotoxic
Methylmercury chloride (115-09-3)	Strongly embryotoxic

The EST was recently applied to chemicals used in the cosmetic industry; the authors substituted the E14 cell line for the D3 cell line (Chen *et al.*, 2010). Penicillin-G was included as a non-teratogen, and 5-fluorouracil was incorporated as a strong embryotoxicant. The authors examined six chemicals, hydroquinone, eugenol, antimony (III) oxide, melamine, dibutyl phthalate and neodymium (III) nitrate hexahydrate. The first three chemicals were classified as strong embryotoxicants and the other three chemicals as weak embryotoxicants by the test. They claimed that their *in vitro* results were similar to *in vivo* reports of embryotoxicity of these six chemicals. However, catalogs of teratogenic agents (Shepard, 1998; Schardein, 2000), while not categorizing these chemicals as non-, weak or strong embryotoxicants, do not suggest that hydoquinone and antimony are teratogenic.

The EST was also recently utilized to determine potential developmental toxicity of four different sizes of silica nanoparticles (Park *et al.*, 2009). The nanoparticles were specified by the manufacturer to be of average sizes – 10, 30, 80 and 400 nm. Transmission electron microscopy demonstrated that the nanoparticles were taken up by the embryoid bodies. The two smaller nanomaterials both demonstrated developmental toxicity at lower concentrations than those producing cytotoxicity, indicating a specific effect on cardiomyocyte differentiation. There were no cytotoxic or developmental toxic effects of the two large-sized nanoparticles at concentrations up to 100 μg/ml (the highest concentrations tested). These results suggested that the EST could be used to examine the developmental toxicity potential of nanomaterials.

SUGGESTED MODIFICATIONS TO THE EST

A number of modifications for the EST have been suggested by various authors. Peters *et al.* (2008a) recommended a modification to the standard EST protocol using 96 well plates rather than 24 well plates. This simplified moving the EBs to the culture dish, decreased the amount of culture media used (and therefore the expense of the assay) and increased the number of chemicals that could be tested in a single assay.

When they tested their modified protocol to the ECVAM standard protocol using 12 chemicals, they found a difference in ID_{50} with only one chemical.

De Smedt *et al.* (2008) found a great deal of variability when using the standard ECVAM culture procedure. They recommended several modifications to the culture method, including using a non-enzymatic dissociation method rather than the standard trypsin/EDTA to dissociate the cells for subculture, change in the timing of subculture, and modifications in the hanging drop method to standardize EB size. When they tested their modified culture with six chemicals used in the ECVAM validation study, they found no differences in the classifications of the chemicals but much more consistent results.

There are several issues with beating cardiomyocytes as an endpoint. The scoring of this endpoint requires experience and is subject to observer bias, so several groups have suggested molecular endpoints to make this endpoint more objective and more high throughput (reviewed in Buesen *et al.*, 2004). Seiler *et al.* (2004) found that staining EBs with antibodies directed against sarcomeric α-actinin or myosin heavy chain followed by fluorescence-activated cell sorting analysis reduced the time needed for the assay from 10 to 7 days. They stained the cells for intracellular rather than cell surface markers as is usually done for such cell sorting. Comparing this assay to the standard assay using two strong embryotoxicants (5-fluorouracil and all-*trans*-retinoic acid) and penicillin G as a negative embryotoxicant, they found nearly identical ID_{50} values with both methods. In addition to being a shorter assay, this endpoint was also more objective than counting beating cardiomyocytes. They later used this assay to evaluate ten chemicals that were used in the ECVAM validation study representing all three classes of embryotoxicants (Buesen *et al.*, 2009). They observed nearly identical dose–response curves and were able to correctly classify all ten compounds in their study. They suggested these modifications could make the assay shorter, more high throughput and more objective than the standard EST.

Peters *et al.* (2008b) used an automated image analysis and software program approach in an attempt to automate the beating cardiomyocyte endpoint. They compared manual and automated counting using four chemicals and found no significant differences between results. However, there was a large amount of variability using the automated system due to the 3D structure of the EBs. They suggested that further work with this system might help to resolve some of these problems.

It has also been suggested that additional endpoints be added to the test that are able to detect effects on other developing organ systems. Changes in gene expression profiles have been examined by several groups. Rohwedel *et al.* (2001) in reviewing gene expression in embryonic stem cells reported that the early developmental expression of a number of genes was recapitulated during culture of mESCs. Pellizzer *et al.* (2004) used semi-quantitative RT-PCR to follow the expression changes of four genes involved in cardiac differentiation. These genes were POU domain class 5 transcription factor 1 (*Pou5f1*), brachyury (*T*), NK2 transcription factor-related locus 5 (*Nkx2-5*) and α-myosin heavy chain (*Myh6*). They observed that exposure to all-*trans*-retinoic acid or lithium chloride changed the expression of these genes over the 10 days of culture, and that there were differences between the two teratogens. They suggested that analysis of selected key genes could produce more information on the toxicological mechanism of compounds and further suggested that different gene panels could be used for other endpoints of differentiation.

zur Nieden *et al.* (2001) included molecular endpoints for the EST to make the test more quantitative and sensitive. Microscopically they observed immunofluorescence staining for α/β-myosin heavy chain and α-actinin in about 15–25% of cells, which corresponded to the approximate amount of beating cells in these areas. Using semi-quantitative PCR, they examined the expression of the genes for α- and β-myosin heavy chain and found a peak on day 9 of culture. They examined seven chemicals used in the EST validation study and substituted the differentiation portion of the prediction model with the expression of myosin heavy chain and were able to correctly categorize these seven chemicals. They further extended this assay by adding multiple molecular endpoints (zur Nieden *et al.*, 2004). Culture conditions were altered to allow differentiation to osteogenic, chondrogenic and neural cells, and gene expression by PCR was included for each of these cell types. They then compared the beating cardiomyocyte endpoint to expression of myosin heavy chain on day 8 of culture (cardiomyocytes), neurofilament 160 on day 14 of culture (neuronal cells), osteocalcin at day 30 of culture (osteoblasts) and aggrecan on day 32 of culture (chondrocytes). Six chemicals were examined from the three categories of embryotoxicity defined by ECVAM. Penicillin G, the non-teratogen, did not alter expression of any of the genes, and 5-fluorouracil, the strong teratogen, did not demonstrate any target cell specificity. They found that valproic acid which produces neural tube defects specifically affected differentiation of neuronal cells; thalidomide appeared to particularly impair skeletal development. Retinoic acid, another strong teratogen, seemed to affect multiple cell types, and they speculated that a general dysregulation of gene expression might be involved with this agent. Diphenylhydantoin, a weak teratogen, showed differences in gene expression for all cell types at similar concentrations, but the authors suggested that skeletal development might have been more specifically altered. Overall, the authors concluded that the addition of other molecular endpoints and alterations in the culture conditions could make the EST more objective and enhance its predictivity.

Following differentiation, EST cultures consist of a variety of differentiated cell types. Chaudhary *et al.* (2006) developed a method of enriching the population for cardiomyocytes. EBs were cultured in suspension culture for 10 days with cardiomyocyte-specific culture media present for the final 3 days of culture. At day 10, the cells were seeded onto double-membrane culture plates and subjected to laser microdissection and pressure catapulting. On day 12, the areas of beating cardiomyocytes were visualized under the microscope, and these areas were cut by the laser (along with the membrane layer of the culture dish) and catapulted into fresh media. From there, a number of immunohistochemical and RNA assays were performed to examine the presence of cardiac-specific genes and proteins. The authors found that following this procedure, the enriched cultures were viable and retained cardiac functions, and suggested that this method might be useful for cell therapy studies.

Other groups have taken advantage of the multiplicity of cell types in the differentiating embryoid bodies to examine global gene expression profiles. van Dartel *et al.* (2009a), using the EST with modifications, examined the ability of monobutyl phthalate to inhibit cardiomyocyte differentiation.

They observed the dose which produced a 50% inhibition in beating cardiomyocytes; this dose produced only 10% cytotoxicity as measured by resazurin reduction. They then examined global gene expression in embryoid bodies treated with monobutyl phthalate for 6, 12 or 24 hours compared to controls. They found differences in 48 genes after 24 hours of treatment (43 upregulated and 5 downregulated); these genes were enriched for "development", "embryonic development" and "morphogenesis" using an analysis of gene ontology. In order to attempt to detect more subtle gene changes, they used gene set enrichment analysis, which does not initially filter the gene set to examine only those genes which show differential expression. Although treatment with monobutyl phthalate demonstrated no significant gene effects at the individual gene level, the authors could detect changes in cardiomyocyte differentiation as early as 24 hours after the beginning of treatment by changes in the expression of sets of genes. They concluded that this technology could possibly enhance the predictivity of the EST.

The authors extended this observation by exposing EBs to monobutyl phthalate or 6-aminonicotinamide for 24 or 96 hours (van Dartel *et al.*, 2010). RNA was collected from control EBs at 24, 48, 72 and 96 hours and assayed for global gene expression. They observed significant changes by principal component analysis in 1,355 genes over this time period which they referred to as the differentiation track. They also observed significant deviation from this differentiation track at 24 hours after treatment with both compounds. The results with these compounds were somewhat expected, in that both chemicals alter tissues of mesodermal origin. The authors concluded that testing using compounds affecting cells of non-mesodermal origin as well as non-teratogens could help to refine the selection of the gene set.

Attempting to distinguish effects on differentiation from effects on proliferation has been done by examining cytotoxicity in adult as well as embryonic cells. Adler *et al.* (2005) transfected p19 teratocarcinoma cells with green fluorescent protein (GFP) attached to a promoter for murine telomerase which has been shown to be active in embryonic stem cells. They then used this construct to examine the downregulation of expression of GFP when the cells were induced to differentiate with retinoic acid. Later they transfected D3 cells with the same construct (Adler *et al.*, 2006) and demonstrated that the solvent DMSO decreased GFP expression within 2 days of treatment at lower concentrations than those demonstrating cytotoxicity with the MTT assay.

Van Dartel *et al.* (2009b) tried to separate the effects of cytotoxicity from developmental toxicity by changing the exposure window of the EST; they compared the dose–response curves for each of the four chemicals with treatment of EBs on day 0–10 to treatment on day 3–10. Treatment with two cytostatic agents, 5-fluorouracil and bromodeoxyuridine, had greater effects with the longer exposure than did 6-nicotinamide and monobutyl phthalate. The authors determined that this difference was due in part to the anti-proliferative effect of the two cytostatic compounds which produced cytotoxicity at lower concentrations on day 3 than concentrations interfering with differentiation. They suggested that this modification might be considered in future EST designs.

The use of various "-omics" technologies in combination with stem cell growth and differentiation in an effort to understand both requirements for pluripotency as well as differentiation has been suggested (Winkler *et al.*, 2009). Cezar *et al.* (2007) examined metabolomic profiles from hESC lines in the presence and absence of the teratogenic antiepileptic compound, valproic acid. In their proof of concept experiment, they observed differences in molecules in the kynurenine and glutamate metabolic pathways in response to valproate. They suggested that additional advancement of metabolomic technology (over 50% of molecules were not identified in public databases) was needed, but the technology offered the possibility of identifying candidate molecules and pathways associated with developmental abnormalities as well as providing a possible list of candidate biomarkers for preclinical safety evaluation of pharmaceuticals.

USE OF HUMAN STEM CELLS IN THE EST

Current guidelines from the International Conference on Harmonization of Technical Requirements for Registration of Pharmaceuticals for Human Use for fetal/developmental toxicity require testing in two different species, and one species must not be a rodent (http://www.ich.org). One possibility to reduce the number of animals used in developmental toxicity testing would be the inclusion of the EST using human cells in place of the second species required (usually the rabbit). Adler *et al.* (2008) were the first to attempt to use hESCs and human fibroblasts to develop a human EST. They used the H1 stem cell line (from WiCell Research Institute, Inc.) and MRC-5, human embryonic lung fibroblasts to examine cytotoxicity. The hESCs were grown on mouse embryonic fibroblast feeder cells, and EB formation occurred by growth in suspension for 4 days. Although beating cardiomyocytes were observed, there was a great deal of variability in this endpoint, and so molecular markers of differentiation were utilized. After testing differentiation in six different culture media formulations, the medium demonstrating the greatest upregulation of Brachyury (a marker for mesodermal differentiation) and downregulation of Oct-4 (a marker of pluripotency) was selected for further testing of the ability of cardiomyocytes to differentiate. Expression of seven different genes was analyzed after 0, 4, 10, 18 and 25 days of culture. The authors demonstrated a progressive decrease in expression of two markers of pluripotency, Oct-4 and hTERT (human telomerase reverse transcriptase). Brachyury was upregulated at day 4 and decreased at all other times. Two transcription factors expressed during cardiac precursor formation, GATA-4 (GATA binding protein) and Nkx2.5, were upregulated at days 4, 10 and 18, but were decreased by day 25. MHC6 (myosin heavy chain 6) and TNNT2 (troponin T2), both markers of later cardiac differentiation, were upregulated at days 10 and 18 but had decreased by day 25. The authors concluded that although this initial assay showed promise, additional research would be needed to standardize a human EST.

Krtolica *et al.* (2009) speculated that hESC-based *in vitro* systems may have greater potential than do mESC-based systems for modeling early development. They speculated that the differences in DNA methylation and repair enzymes between early mouse and human embryos could play major roles in their responses to drug treatments. The International Stem Cell Initiative (2007) examined the phenotypes of 59 independently derived hESC lines that were derived in different laboratories using various techniques. They concluded that in spite of the different genetic backgrounds and phenotypes in differentiation possessed by these cell lines, there was no evidence of marked differences between the lines from their extensive characterization.

CONSIDERATION OF CULTURE CONDITIONS

Culture conditions for the mouse EST were standardized for the validation study; however, several changes in these conditions or the cell line used have been suggested. Culture conditions can alter the ability of stem cells to differentiate, and in fact different additions need to be made to allow the cells to differentiate along particular pathways. A few culture conditions have been studied for their effect on pluripotency and differentiation capacity.

Although not a culture condition *per se*, the effect of passaging cells has been examined in a few studies, usually by analyzing gene expression changes. Pellizzer *et al.* (2004) examined the effect of passage number of mouse D3 cells on expression of *Oct4*. They observed no differences in expression at passage 3 and 7, but this expression was decreased by about 50% at passage 14. Expression of *Oct4* is generally considered to be a sign of pluripotency, so it is unclear if this cell line was losing this attribute with further passaging.

Baqir and Smith (2003) found that serum starvation of mESCs increased the DNA methylation pattern of two imprinted genes (*Igf2* and *H19*), suggesting decreased expression of these genes in the serum starved cells. Refeeding with serum decreased the methylation pattern suggesting a partial loss of some of the methylation patterns developed during serum starvation. Cell confluency also increased the methylation of these two genes. Passage number also affected gene expression in this study. Examining the same two imprinted genes at different passage numbers (8, 22 or 36) showed a decrease in expression of *Igf2* and *H19* at passage 36 relative to the other two passages. Interestingly, alkaline phosphatase staining, which is used as a marker of pluripotency, was not altered at the later passage time; additionally, *Gadph* and *Oct4* expression were not altered indicating that some of the later passaged cells remained pluripotent.

Baqir and Smith (2006) demonstrated that treatment of two different mESC lines with either 5-azacytidine or trichostatin A altered the transcription of several imprinted genes. These compounds were selected because they are histone deactylase inhibitors, and their activity could alter histones leading to changes in transcription. The pattern of gene changes were different between the two compounds, and many of the gene alterations continued to be expressed following drug removal as well as passaging of the cells, suggesting that the changes were not easily reversible.

Stability of the epigenome can change during culture conditions as well as during line derivation. Allegrucci *et al.* (2007) examined DNA methylation profiles of over 2,000 genomic loci by restriction landmark genome scanning in six independently derived hESC lines. They examined the effects of time in culture and culture conditions on epigenetic stability and observed that culture conditions could produce epigenetic instability and that such instability was more likely to occur in the early phases of culture. They also observed that the unstable loci differed among the cell lines and that the changes were heritable. They concluded that some of these changes may be involved in the varied differentiation potential of various hESC lines (Burridge *et al.*, 2007).

Humpherys *et al.* (2001) demonstrated that subclones derived from V6.5 mESCs cultured with retinoic acid varied a great deal from the parental line in their expression of the gene *H19*. They suggested that the epigenetic status of the cells was altered during culture suggesting that the epigenetic status of ES cells was unstable. Rugg-Gunn *et al.* (2005) observed biallelic expression of imprinted *H19* after prolonged passage. A recent study of expression of imprinted genes in 46 individual hESC lines by Rugg-Gunn *et al.* (2007) suggested that there is greater epigenetic stability among hESC lines than among mouse lines. They examined the expression of ten different imprinted genes which had distinguishing parental single nucleotide polymorphisms from these 46 cell lines. Several of the genes appeared to have very stable epigenetic transmission, but this was not the case for all of the genes. For example, a sample of TE03 from one lab had different allelic expression of *IGF2* than a TE03 sample from another lab; this suggested differences in the culture conditions in the two laboratories. Additionally, cell lines derived and cultured in the same lab demonstrated different epigenetic stability at the *IGF2* locus; this suggested that there could be differences in the blastocysts that were perturbed during hESC derivation. Overall, the authors concluded that epigenetic variation does exist and could play a role in differentiation.

Another culture condition that has been demonstrated to alter proliferation and differentiation of stem cells is the oxygen concentration. In most studies, room air is mixed with CO_2 so that the incubator air is approximately 20% oxygen. However, mean tissue levels of oxygen are around 3% (Csete, 2005). Under low oxygen conditions, spontaneous differentiation of hESCs has been reported to decrease, but the differentiation of particular cell types may be increased making a more homogeneous population (reviewed in Millman *et al.*, 2009). In the presence of LIF, Powers *et al.* (2008) observed a decrease in expression of pluripotency markers (Oct4, Sox2 and Nanog) at 0, 1 and 40% oxygen, but no differences between 5 and 20%. However, they also noted a change in the morphology of the cells at 1% in that more cells appeared to be beginning to differentiate, even though LIF was present. Taken together, these results suggest that culture conditions, particularly the oxygen concentration, may alter the ability of stem cells to proliferate as well as to differentiate.

EB size is also an important factor in the culture and differentiation of mESCs. Valamehr *et al.* (2008) found that intermediate-sized mouse EBs (100–300 μm diameter) had greater proliferative capability, greater differentiation potential and fewer apoptotic cells than either small (<100 μm) or large (>300 μm) EBs. They also observed that a hydrophobic surface, such as polydimethylsiloxane, promoted the formation of this intermediate-sized EB.

CONCLUDING REMARKS AND FUTURE DIRECTIONS

Current experimental paradigms for developmental toxicity testing have remained basically unchanged for nearly 40 years. What will developmental toxicity testing look like in the future? A vision for all toxicity testing, "Toxicity Testing in the 21st Century: A Vision and A Strategy" was put forward by the National Research Council in 2007 (National Research Council, 2007). This vision relies heavily on *in vitro* systems and pathway analysis. The EST could fit well into this plan

(Chapin and Stedman, 2009), but several points need to be considered. Modifications of the assay have been proposed which will make it more objective, more automated, less time consuming and more high throughput. These modifications will need to be agreed upon and validated prior to widespread usage. Also, as currently constructed, the EST examines only a mesodermal derivative; other endpoints may need to be included to cover ectodermal and endodermal derivatives.

Additionally, there appear to be few considerations of characterization of the *in vitro* system. Culture conditions have been shown to alter the epigenome of the cells which changes gene transcription, pluripotency and differentiation capability. Is one cell line sufficient; how many cell lines are needed? There are examples of genetic differences among mouse strains in their response to teratogenic agents; the use of a single cell line from an inbred strain of mouse does not cover all of the genetic variability within the mouse genome. This will be more complicated with the use of human cells which have varied genetic backgrounds.

Human ESCs and iPSCs offer an unprecedented opportunity to use human cell lines to define and classify developmental toxicants. Before the discovery of iPSCs, the proposal to use hESCs for regulatory testing was considered morally or ethically unfavorable. Until now a "normal" unlimited supply of human cell lines was not available. While the potential of hESCs and iPSCs is great, there are many challenges ahead regarding understanding not only the basic biology behind pluripotency and differentiation, but also the regulations and standards that are needed for quality control. Of paramount importance is the reliability and stability of the cell lines. Second to this is the need for reproducible differentiation protocols. Scientists are still working to understand the signals required for differentiating large quantities of cells into pure populations, a large obstacle to overcome for both regenerative medicine and toxicity testing. These cells would then need to recapitulate both *in vivo* and *in vitro* responses that can be independently verified. Additionally, embryonic cells *in vivo* are not in a two-dimensional environment. Therefore, improved culture conditions might include extracellular matrix scaffolds or co-culture with additional cell types as well as the ability to control microenvironmental factors, such as pH and oxygen concentration. Although there is great promise in the utilization of stem cells for a variety of uses, including developmental toxicity testing, there is still much work to be done and much knowledge to be gained before their role in regulatory science can be defined (Hartung and Daston, 2009).

REFERENCES

Adler S, Paparella M, Pellizzer C, Hartung T, Bremer S (2005) The detection of differentiation-inducing chemicals by using green fluorescent protein expression in genetically engineered teratocarcinoma cells. *ATLA* **33:** 91–103.

Adler S, Pellizzer C, Hareng L, Hartung T, Bremer S (2008) First steps in establishing a developmental toxicity test method based on human embryonic stem cells. *Toxicol in Vitro* **22:** 200–11.

Adler S, Pellizzer C, Paparella M, Hartung T, Bremer S (2006) The effects of solvents on embryonic stem cell differentiation. *Toxicol in Vitro* **20:** 265–71.

Allegrucci C, Wu YZ, Thurston A, Denning C, Priddle H, Mummery CL, Ward-van Oostwaard D, Andrews PW, Stojkovic M, Smith N, Parkin T, Jones ME, Warren G, Yu L, Brena RM, Plass C, Young LE (2007) Restriction landmark genome scanning identifies culture-induced DNA methylation instability in the human embryonic stem cell epigenome. *Hum Molec Genet* **16:** 1253–68.

Amabile G, Meissner A (2009) Induced pluripotent stem cells: current progress and potential for regenerative medicine. *Trends Mol Med* **15:** 59–68.

Andrews PW, Benvenisty N, McKay R, Pera MF, Rossant J, Semb H, Stacey GN (2005) The International Stem Cell Initiative: towards benchmarks for human embryonic stem cell research. *Nat Biotechnol* **23:** 795–7.

Balls M, Blaauboer B, Brusik D, Frazier J, Lamp D, Pemberton M, Reinhardt C, Roberfroid M, Rosenkranz H, Schmid B, Speilmann H, Stammati A-L, Walum E (1990) Report and recommendations of the CAT/ERGATT workshop on the validation of toxicity test procedures. *ATLA* **18:** 313–37.

Balls M, Blaauboer BJ, Fentem J, Bruner L, Combes RD, Ekwal B, Fielder RJ, Guillouzo A, Lewis RW, Lovell DP, Reinhardt CA, Repetto G, Sladowski D, Spielmann H, Zucco F (1995) Practical aspects of the validation of toxicity test procedures. The report and recommendations of ECVAM workshop 5. *ATLA* **23:** 129–47.

Baqir S, Smith LC (2003) Growth restricted *in vitro* culture conditions alter the imprinted gene expression patterns of mouse embryonic stem cells. *Cloning Stem Cells* **5:** 199–213.

Baqir S, Smith LC (2006) Inhibitors of histone deacetylases and DNA methyltransferases alter imprinted gene regulation in embryonic stem cells. *Cloning Stem Cells* **8:** 200–13.

Beattie GM, Lopez AD, Bucay N, Hinton A, Firpo MT, King CC, Hayek A (2005) Activin A maintains pluripotency of human embryonic stem cells in the absence of feeder layers. *Stem Cells* **23:** 489–95.

Briggs R, King TJ (1952) Transplantation of living nuclei from blastula cells into enucleated frogs' eggs. *Proc Natl Acad Sci USA* **38:** 455–63.

Brown NA, Spielmann H, Bechter R, Flint OP, Freeman SJ, Jelnick RJ, Koch E, Nau H, Newall DR, Palmer AK, Renault J-Y, Repetto M, Vogel R, Wiger R (1995) Screening chemicals for reproductive toxicity: the current alternatives. The report and recommendations of an ECVAM/ETS workshop (ECVAM workshop 12). *ATLA* **23:** 868–82.

Buesen R, Genschow E, Slawik B, Visan A, Spielmann H, Luch A, Seiler A (2009) Embryonic stem cell test remastered: comparison between the validated EST and the new molecular FACS-EST for assessing developmental toxicity *in vitro*. *Toxicol Sci* **108:** 389–400.

Buesen R, Visan A, Genschow E, Slawik B, Spielmann H, Seiler A (2004) Trends in improving the embryonic stem cell test (EST): an overview. *ALTEX* **21:** 15–22.

Burridge PW, Anderson D, Priddle H, Barbadillo Munoz MD, Chamberlain S, Allegrucci C, Young LE, Denning C (2007) Improved human embryonic stem cell embryoid body homogeneity and cardiomyocyte differentiation from a novel V-96 plate aggregation system highlights interline variability. *Stem Cells* **25:** 929–38.

Campbell KH, McWhir J, Ritchie WA, Wilmut I (1996) Sheep cloned by nuclear transfer from a cultured cell line. *Nature* **380:** 64–6.

Cezar GG, Quam JA, Smith AM, Rosa GJM, Piekarczyk MS, Brown JF, Gage FH, Muotri AR (2007) Identification of small molecules from human embryonic stem cells using metabolomics. *Stem Cells Develop* **16:** 1–14.

Chapin R, Stedman D, Paquette J, Streck R, Kumpf S, Deng S (2007) Struggles for equivalence: *in vitro* developmental toxicity model evolution in pharmaceuticals in 2006. *Toxicol in Vitro* **21:** 1545–51.

Chapin RE, Stedman DB (2009) Endless possibilities: stem cells and the vision for toxicology testing in the 21st century. *Toxicol Sci* **112:** 17–22.

Chaudhary KW, Barrezueta NX, Bauchmann MB, Milici AJ, Beckius G, Stedman DB, Hambor JE, Blake WL, McNeish JD, Bahinski A, Cezar GG (2006) Embryonic stem cells in predictive cardiotoxicity: laser capture microscopy enables assay development. *Toxicol Sci* **90:** 149–58.

Chen R, Chen J, Cheng S, Qin J, Li W, Zhang L, Jiao H, Yu X, Zhang X, Lahn BT, Xiang AP (2010) Assessment of embryotoxicity of compounds in cosmetics by the embryonic stem cell test. *Toxicol Mech Meth* **20:** 112–18.

Chin MH, Mason MJ, Xie W, Volinia S, Singer M, Peterson C, Ambartsumyan G, Aimiuwu O, Richter L, Zhang J, Khvorostov I, Ott V, Grunstein M, Lavon N, Bevenisty N, Croce CM, Clark AT, Baxter T, Pyle AD, Teitell MA, Pelegrini M, Plath K, Lowry WE (2009) Induced pluripotent stem cells and embryonic stem cells are distinguished by gene expression signatures. *Cell Stem Cell* **5:** 111–23.

Csete M (2005) Oxygen in the cultivation of stem cells. *Ann NY Acad Sci* **1049:** 1–8.

Dahéron L, Optiz SL, Zaehres H, Lensch MW, Andrews PW, Itskovitz-Eldor J, Daley GQ (2004) LIF/STAT3 signaling fails to maintain self-renewal of human embryonic stem cells. *Stem Cells* **22:** 770–8.

De Smedt A, Steemans M, De Boeck M, Peters AK, van der Leede P-J, Van Goethem F, Lampo A, Vanparys P (2008) Optimization of the cell cultivation methods in the embryonic stem cell test results in an increased differentiation potential of the cells into strong beating myocard cells. *Toxicol in Vitro* **22:** 1789–96.

Doetschman TC, Eistetter H, Katz M, Schmidt W, Kemler R (1985) The *in vitro* development of blastocyst-derived embryonic stem cell lines: formation of visceral yolk sac, blood islands and myocardium. *J Embryol Exp Morph* **87:** 27–45.

Draper JS, Pigott C, Thomson JA, Andrews PW (2002) Surface antigens of human embryonic stem cells: changes upon differentiation in culture. *J Anat* **200:** 249–58.

Evans MJ, Kaufman MH (1981) Establishment in culture of pluripotential cells from mouse embryos. *Nature* **292:** 154–6.

Feng Q, Lu SJ, Klimanskaya I, Gomes I, Kim D, Chung Y, Honig GR, Kim KS, Lanza R (2010) Hemangioblastic derivatives from human induced pluripotent stem cells exhibit limited expansion and early senescence. *Stem Cells* **28:** 704–12.

Forsyth NR, Wright WE, Shay JW (2002) Telomerase and differentiation in multicellular organisms: turn it off, turn it on, and turn it off again. *Differentiation* **69:** 188–97.

Geneschow E, Spielmann H, Scholz G, Seiler A, Brown N, Piersma A, Brady M, Clemann N, Huuskonen H, Paillard F, Bremer S, Becker K (2002) The ECVAM International Validation Study on *in vitro* embryotoxicity tests: results of the definitive phase and evaluation of prediction models. *ATLA* **30:** 151–76.

Ginis I, Luo Y, Miura T, Thies S, Brandenberger R, Gerecht-Nir S, Amit M, Hoke A, Carpenter MK, Itskovitz-Eldor J, Rao MS (2004) Differences between human and mouse embryonic stem cells. *Develop Biol* **269:** 360–80.

Greber B, Lehrach H, Adjaye J (2007) Fibroblast growth factor 2 modulates transforming growth factor beta signaling in mouse embryonic fibroblasts and human ESCs (hESCs) to support hESC self-renewal. *Stem Cells* **25:** 455–64.

Hartung T, Daston G (2009) Are *in vitro* tests suitable for regulatory use? *Toxicol Sci* **111:** 233–7.

Henderson JK, Draper JS, Baillie HS, Fishel S, Thomson JA, Moore H, Andrews PW (2002) Preimplantation human embryos and embryonic stem cells show comparable expression of stage-specific embryonic antigens. *Stem Cells* **20:** 329–37.

Heuer J, Bremer S, Pohl I, Spielmann H (1993) Development of an *in vitro* embryotoxicity test using murine embryonic stem cell cultures. *Toxicol in Vitro* **7:** 551–6.

Hu BY, Weick JP, Yu J, Ma LX, Zhang XQ, Thomson JA, Zhang SC (2010) Neural differentiation of human induced pluripotent stem cells follows developmental principles with variable potency. *Proc Natl Acad Sci USA* **107:** 4335–40.

Humpherys D, Eggan K, Akutsu H, Hochedlinger K, Rideout III WM, Biniszkiewicz D, Yanagimachi R, Jaenisch R (2001) Epigenetic instability in ES cells and cloned mice. *Science* **293:** 95–7.

Humphrey RK, Beattie GM, Lopez AD, Bucay N, King CC, Firpo MT, Rose-John S, Hayek A (2004) Maintenance of pluripotency in human embryonic stem cells is STAT3 independent. *Stem Cells* **22:** 522–30.

James D, Levine AJ, Besser D, Hemmati-Brivanlou A (2005) TGFbeta/activin/nodal signaling is necessary for the maintenance of pluripotency in human embryonic stem cells. *Development* **132:** 1273–82.

Johnson EM, Gorman RM, Gabel BEG, George ME (1982) The *Hydra attenuata* system for detection of teratogenic hazards. *Teratogen Carcinogen Mutagen* **2:** 263–76.

Krtolica A, Ilic D, Genbacev O, Miller RK (2009) Human embryonic stem cells as a model for embryotoxicity screening. *Regen Med* **4:** 449–59.

Laschinski G, Vogel R, Spielmann H (1991) Cytotoxicity test using blastocyst-derived euploid embryonal stem cells: a new approach to in vitro teratogenesis screening. *Reprod Toxicol* **5:** 57–64.

Lowry WE, Richter L, Yachenchko R, Pyle AD, Tchieu J, Sridharan R, Clark AT, Plath K (2008) Generation of human induced pluripotent stem cells from dermal fibroblasts. *Proc Natl Acad Sci USA* **105:** 2883–8.

Ludwig TE, Bergendahl V, Levenstein ME, Yu J, Probasco MD, Thomson JA (2006a) Feeder-independent culture of human embryonic stem cells. *Nat Methods* **3:** 637–46.

Ludwig TE, Levenstein ME, Jones JM, Berggren WT, Mitchen ER, Frane JL, Crandall LJ, Daigh CA, Conard KR, Piekarczyk MS, Llanas RA, Thomson JA (2006b) Derivation of human embryonic stem cells in defined conditions. *Nat Biotechnol* **24:** 185–7.

Maherali N, Hochedlinger K (2008) Guidelines and techniques for the generation of induced pluripotent stem cells. *Cell Stem Cell* **3:** 595–605.

Maherali N, Sridharan R, Xie W, Utikal J, Eminli S, Arnold K, Stadtfeld M, Yachechko R, Tchieu J, Jaenisch R, Plath K, Hochedlinger K (2007) Directly reprogrammed fibroblasts show global epigenetic remodeling and widespread tissue contribution. *Cell Stem Cell* **1:** 55–70.

Martin GR (1981) Isolation of a pluripotent cell line from early mouse embryos cultured in medium conditioned by teratocarcinoma stem cells. *Proc Nat Acad Sci USA* **78:** 7634–8.

Marx-Stoelting Ph, Adriaens E, Ahr H-J, Bremer S, Garthoff B, Gelbke H-P, Piersma A, Pellizzer C, Reuter U, Rogiers V, Schenk B, Schwengberg S, Seiler A, Spielmann H, Steemans M, Stedman DB, Vanparys P, Vericat JA, Verwei M, van de Water F, Weimer M, Schwarz M (2009) A review of the implementation of the embryonic stem cell test (EST). The report and recommendations of an ECVAM/ReProTect Workshop. *ATLA* **37:** 313–28.

Millman JR, Tan JH, Colton CK (2009) The effects of low oxygen on self-renewal and differentiation of embryonic stem cells. *Curr Opin Organ Transpl* **14:** 694–700.

National Research Council (2007) *Toxicity Testing in the 21st Century: A Vision and A Strategy.* The National Academies Press, Washington DC.

Newall DR, Beedles KE (1996) The stem-cell test: an *in vitro* assay for teratogenic potential. Results of a blind trial with 25 compounds. *Toxicol in Vitro* **10:** 229–40.

Niwa H, Miyazaki L, Smith AG (2000) Quantitative expression of Oct-3/4 defines differentiation, dedifferentiation or self-renewal of ES cells. *Nat Genet* **24:** 372–6.

Odorico JS, Kaufman DS, Thomson JA (2001) Multilineage differentiation from human embryonic stem cell lines. *Stem Cells* **19:** 193–204.

Okita K, Ichisaka T, Yamanaka S (2007) Generation of germline-competent induced pluripotent stem cells. *Nature* **448:** 313–17.

Paquette JA, Kumpf SW, Streck RD, Thomson JJ, Chapin RE, Stedman DB (2008) Assessment of the embryonic stem cell test and application and use in the pharmaceutical industry. *Birth Def Res Pt B* **83:** 104–11.

Park IH, Zhao R, West JA, Yabuuchi A, Huo H, Ince TA, Lerou PH, Lensch MW, Daley GQ (2008) Reprogramming of human somatic cells to pluripotency with defined factors. *Nature* **451:** 141–6.

Park MVDZ, Annema W, Salvati A, Lesniak A, Elsaesser A, Barnes C, McKerr G, Howard CV, Lynch I, Dawson KA, Piersma AH, de Jong WH (2009) *In vitro* developmental toxicity test detects inhibition of stem cell differentiation by silica nanoparticles. *Toxicol Appl Pharmacol* **240:** 108–16.

Pellizzer C, Adler S, Corvi R, Hartung T, Bremer S (2004) Monitoring of teratogenic effects in vitro by analysing a selected gene expression pattern. *Toxicol in Vitro* **18:** 325–35.

Peters AK, Steemans M, Hansen E, Mesens N, Verheyen GR, Vanparys P (2008a) Evaluation of the embryotoxic potency of compounds in a newly revised high throughput embryonic stem cell test. *Toxicol Sci* **105:** 342–50.

Peters AK, Van de Wouwer G, Weyn B, Verheyen GR, Vanparys P, Van Gompel J (2008b) Automated analysis of contractility in the embryonic stem cell test, a novel approach to assess embryotoxicity. *Toxicol in Vitro* **22:** 1948–56.

Powers DE, Millman JR, Huang RB, Colton CK (2008) Effects of oxygen on mouse embryonic stem cell growth, phenotype retention, and cellular energetics. *Biotechnol Bioeng* **101:** 241–54.

Rohwedel J, Guan K, Hegert C, Wobus AM (2001) Embryonic stem cells as an in vitro model for mutagenicity, cytotoxicity and embryotoxicity studies: present state and future prospects. *Toxicol in Vitro* **15:** 741–53.

Rossant J (2001) Stem cells from the mammalian blastocyst. *Stem Cells* **19:** 477–82.

Rugg-Gunn PJ, Ferguson-Smith AC, Pedersen RA (2005) Epigenetic status of human embryonic stem cells. *Nat Genet* **37:** 585–587.

Rugg-Gunn PJ, Ferguson-Smith AC, Pedersen RA (2007) Status of genomic imprinting in human embryonic stem cells as revealed by a large cohort of independently derived and maintained lines. *Hum Molec Genet* **16:** R243–R251.

Schardein JL (2000) *Chemically Induced Birth Defects*, 3rd edition. Marcel Dekker, Inc., New York.

Scholz G, Genschow E, Pohl I, Bremer S, Paparella M, Raabe, H, Southee J, Spielmann H (1999) Prevalidation of the embryonic stem cell test (EST) – a new *in vitro* embryotoxicity test. *Toxicol in Vitro* **13:** 675–81.

Seiler A, Visan A, Buesen R, Genschow E, Spielmann H (2004) Improvement of an in vitro stem cell assay for developmental toxicity: the use of molecular endpoints in the embryonic stem cell test. *Reprod Toxicol* **18:** 231–40.

Shepard TH (1998) *Catalog of Teratogenic Agents*, 9th edition. The Johns Hopkins University Press, Baltimore, MD.

Smith AG, Heath JK, Donaldson DD, Wong GG, Moreau J, Stahl M, Rogers D (1988) Inhibition of pluripotential embryonic stem cell differentiation by purified polypeptides. *Nature* **336:** 688–90.

Smith AG, Hooper ML (1987) Buffalo rat liver cells produce a diffusible activity which inhibits the differentiation of murine embryonal carcinoma and embryonic stem cells. *Develop Biol* **121:** 1–9.

Smith MK, Kimmel GL, Kochhar DM, Shepard TH, Spielberg SP, Wilson JG (1983) A selection of candidate compounds for in vitro teratogenesis test validation. *Teratogen Mutagen Carcinog* **3:** 461–80.

Spielmann H, Grune B, Liebsch M, Seiler A, Vogel R (2008) Successful validation of *in vitro* methods in toxicology by ZEBET, the National Centre for Alternatives in Germany at the BfR (Federal Institute for Risk Assessment). *Exp Toxicol Pathol* **60:** 225–33.

Spielmann H, Pohl I, Doring B, Liebsch M, Moldenhauer F (1997) The embryonic stem cell test (EST), an in vitro embryotoxicity test using two permanent mouse cell lines: 3T3 fibroblasts and embryonic stem cells. *In Vitro Toxicol* **10:** 119–27.

Takahashi K, Tanabe K, Ohnuke M, Narita M, Ichisaka T, Tomoda K, Yamanaka S (2007) Induction of pluripotent stem cells from adult fibroblasts by defined factors. *Cell* **131:** 861–72.

Takahashi K, Yamanaka S (2006) Induction of pluripotent stem cells from mouse embryonic and adult fibroblast cultures by defined factors. *Cell* **126:** 663–76.

The International Stem Cell Initiative (2007) Characterization of human embryonic stem cell lines by the International Stem Cell Initiative. *Nat Biotechnol* **25:** 803–16.

The International Stem Cell Initiative Consortium, Akopian V, Andrews PW, Beil S, Benvenisty N, Brehm J, Christie M, Ford A, Fox V, Gokhale PJ, Healy L, Holm F, Hovatta O, Knowles BB, Ludwig TE, McKay RD, Miyazaki T, Nakatsuji N, Oh SK, Pera MF, Rossant J, Stacey GN, Suemori H (2010) Comparison of defined culture systems for feeder cell free propagation of human embryonic stem cells. *In Vitro Cell Dev Biol Anim* **46:** 247–58.

Thomas JA, Itskovitz-Eldor J, Shapiro SS, Waknitz MA, Swiergiel JJ, Marshall VS, Jones JM (1998) Embryonic stem cell lines derived from human blastocysts. *Science* **282:** 1145–47.

Till JE, McCulloch EA (1961) A direct measurement of the radiation sensitivity of normal mouse bone marrow cells. *Rad Res* **14:** 213–22.

Valamehr B, Jonas SJ, Polleux J, Qiao R, Guo S, Gschweng EH, Stiles B, Kam K, Luo T-JM, Witte ON, Liu X, Dunn B, Wu H (2008) Hydrophobic surfaces for enhanced differentiation of embryonic stem cell-derived embryoid bodies. *Proc Nat Acad Sci USA* **105:** 14459–64.

Vallier L, Alexander M, Pedersen RA (2005) Activin/Nodal and FGF pathways cooperate to maintain pluripotency of human embryonic stem cells. *J Cell Sci* **118:** 4495–509.

Vallier L, Mendjan S, Brown S, Cheng Z, Teo A, Smithers LE, Trotter MW, Cho CH, Martinez A, Rugg-Gunn P, Brons G, Pedersen RA (2009) Activin/Nodal signaling maintains pluripotency by controlling Nanog expression. *Development* **136:** 1339–49.

van Dartel DAM, Pennings JLA, Hendriksen PJM, van Schooten FJ, Piersma AH (2009a) Early gene expression changes during embryonic stem cell differentiation into cardiomyocytes and their modulation by monobutyl phthalate. *Reprod Toxicol* **27:** 93–102.

van Dartel DAM, Pennings JLA, van Schooten FJ, Piersma AH (2010) Transcriptomics-based identification of developmental toxicants through their interference with cardiomyocyte differentiation of embryonic stem cells. *Toxicol Appl Pharmacol* **243:** 420–8.

van Dartel DAM, Zeijen NJL, de la Fonteyne LJJ, van Schooten FJ, Piersma AH (2009b) Disentangling cellular proliferation and differentiation in the embryonic stem cell test, and its impact on the experimental protocol. *Reprod Toxicol* **28:** 254–61.

Vojnits K, Bremer S (2010) Challenges of using pluripotent stem cells for safety assessments of substances. *Toxicology* **270:** 10–17.

Wang L, Schulz TC, Sherrer ES, Dauphin DS, Shin S, Nelson AM, Ware CB, Zhan M, Song CZ, Chen X, Brimble SN, McLean A, Galeano MJ, Uhl EW, D'Amour KA, Chesnut JD, Rao MS, Blau CA, Robins AJ (2007) Self-renewal of human embryonic stem cells require insulin-like growth factor-1 receptor and ERBB2 receptor signaling. *Blood* **110:** 1339–49.

Wernig M, Meissner A, Foreman R, Brambrink T, Ku M, Hochedlinger K, Bernstein BE, Jaenisch R (2007) *In vitro* reprogramming of fibroblasts into a pluripotent ES-cell like state. *Nature* **448:** 318–24.

Williams RL, Hilton DJ, Pease S, Willson TA, Stewart CL, Gearing DP, Wagner EF, Metcalf D, Nicola NA, Gough NM (1988) Myeloid leukaemia inhibitory factor maintains the developmental potential of embryonic stem cells. *Nature* **336:** 684–7.

Winkler J, Sotiriadou I, Chen S, Hescheler J, Sachinidis A (2009) The potential of embryonic stem cells combined with -omics technologies as model systems for toxicology. *Curr Med Chem* **16:** 4814–27.

Xiao L, Yuan X, Sharkis SJ (2006) Activin A maintains self-renewal and regulates fibroblast growth factor, Wnt, and bone morphogenic protein pathways in human embryonic stem cells. *Stem Cells* **24:** 1476–86.

Xu RH, Sampsell-Barron TL, Gu F, Root S, Peck RM, Pan G, Yu J, Antosiewicz-Bourget J, Tian S, Stewart R, Thomson JA (2008) NANOG is a direct target of TGFbeta/activin-mediated SMAD signaling in human ESCs. *Cell Stem Cell* **3:** 196–206.

Yu J, Vodyanik MA, Smuga-Otto K, Antosiewicz-Bourget J, Frane JL, Tian S, Nie J, Jonsdottir GA, Ruotti V, Stewart R, Slukvin II, Thomson JA (2007) Induced pluripotent stem cell lines derived from human somatic cells. *Science* **318:** 1917–20.

zur Nieden NI, Kempka G, Ahr HJ (2004) Molecular multiple endpoint embryonic stem cell test – a possible approach to test for the teratogenic potential of compounds. *Toxicol Appl Pharmacol* **194:** 257–69.

zur Nieden NI, Ruf LJ, Kempka G, Hildebrand H, Ahr HJ (2001) Molecular markers in embryonic stem cells. *Toxicol in Vitro* **15:** 455–61.

CHAPTER

59

Applications of toxicogenomics in reproductive and developmental toxicology

Krishanu Sengupta, Jayaprakash Narayana Kolla, Debasis Bagchi and Manashi Bagchi

INTRODUCTION

Toxicogenomics is a rapidly developing area that promises to aid scientists in understanding the molecular and cellular effects of toxic agents in biological systems. Classically, toxicology is focused on phenotypic changes, i.e. physical or morphological changes observed in an organism resulting from exposure to chemical, physical or biologic agents. Such changes can be either transient or chronic, which leads to death. In a typical whole-animal toxicology study, the toxic effect of a test agent is evaluated by the assessments of clinical signs of toxicity, weight changes in body and vital organs, clinical chemistry and histopathological changes. Over time, increased understanding of the mechanism of action of chemicals or toxicants has increased the efficiency of different tasks such as hazard identification, mechanistic toxicology, risk assessment, etc.

During advancement in medical research, various sophisticated tools and sensitive methods have been implicated in animal toxicology studies. Most importantly, the various state-of-the-art techniques of chemistry, cell biology, molecular biology and genetics are being utilized in a synchronized fashion to assess the adverse effects and identify cellular and molecular targets of toxic agents. These advances have made it feasible to identify adverse effects of the toxic agents at the molecular levels, at the subcellular structures and cellular organelles also. This ability has enhanced etiologic understanding of toxicity and made it possible to assess the relevance of molecular changes in response to toxicity (Christiani, 2007).

DEFINITION OF TOXICOGENOMICS

Toxicogenomics is a field of science that deals with the collection, interpretation and storage of information about gene and protein activity within particular cells or tissues of an organism in response to toxic substances. Toxicogenomics combines toxicology with genomics or other high throughput molecular profiling technologies such as transcriptomics, proteomics and metabolomics. Toxicogenomics endeavors to elucidate molecular mechanisms evolved in the expression of toxicity, and to derive molecular expression patterns (i.e., molecular biomarkers) that predict toxicity or the genetic susceptibility to it (Hamadeh *et al.*, 2002; Christiani, 2007).

According to the National Research Council (NRC) of the USA, "*Toxicogenomics* is defined as the application of genomic technologies (for example, genetics, genome sequence analysis, gene expression profiling, proteomics, metabolomics and related approaches) to study the adverse effects of environmental and pharmaceutical chemicals on human health and the environment. Toxicogenomics combines toxicology with information-dense genomic technologies to integrate toxicant-specific alterations in gene, protein and metabolite expression patterns with phenotypic responses of cells, tissues and organisms. Toxicogenomics can provide insight into gene–environment interactions and the response of biologic pathways and networks to perturbations. Toxicogenomics may lead to information that is more discriminating, predictive and sensitive than that currently used techniques to evaluate exposures to toxicants or to predict effects on human health" (Christiani, 2007).

COMPONENTS OF TOXICOGENOMICS

Toxicogenomics provides an understanding about the molecular and cellular effects of toxic agents in biological systems. This specialized field provides platforms for analysis of genomes, transcripts, proteins and metabolites. The components of toxicogenomics are as follows.

Genomics is the study of the genomes of organisms. The field includes intensive efforts to determine the entire DNA sequence of organisms and fine-scale genetic mapping efforts. The field also includes studies of intragenomic phenomena such as heterosis, epistasis, pleiotropy and other interactions between loci and alleles within the genome. In contrast, the investigation of the roles and functions of single genes is a primary focus of molecular biology or genetics and is a common topic of modern medical and biological

Reproductive and Developmental Toxicology, Edited by Ramesh C. Gupta
ISBN: 978-0-12-382032-7

research. A genome represents the total genes of an individual organism. Thus, genomics is the study of all the genes of a cell, or tissue, at the DNA (genotype), mRNA (transcriptome) or protein (proteome) levels.

Genotyping is the process of elucidating the genotype of an individual with a biological assay. The commonly used genotypic assays or techniques include polymerase chain reaction (PCR), DNA fragment analysis, allele specific oligonucleotide (ASO) probes, DNA sequencing and nucleic acid hybridization to DNA microarrays or beads. Several common genotyping techniques include restriction fragment length polymorphism (RFLP), terminal restriction fragment length polymorphism (t-RFLP), amplified fragment length polymorphism (AFLP) and multiplex ligation-dependent probe amplification (MLPA).

The *transcriptome* is the set of all RNA molecules produced in a single cell or a population of cells. The terminology "transcriptome" can be applied to the total set of transcripts in a given organism, or to the specific subset of transcripts present in a particular cell type. The study of *transcriptomics*, also referred to as expression profiling, examines the expression level of mRNAs in a given cell population, often using high throughput techniques based on DNA microarray technology (Figure 59.1). The use of next-generation sequencing technology to study the transcriptome at the nucleotide level is known as RNA-Seq, also called "Whole Transcriptome Shotgun Sequencing" (WTSS) (Subramanian *et al.*, 2005; Morin *et al.*, 2008; Wang *et al.*, 2009).

Proteomics is the study of proteins, particularly their structures and functions (Anderson and Anderson, 1998; Blackstock and Weir, 1999). The term "proteomics" was first coined in 1997 to make an analogy with genomics, i.e. the study of the genes (James, 1997). The word "proteome" is a blend of "*pro*tein" and "gen*ome*", and was coined by Marc Wilkins in 1994 (Wilkins *et al.*, 1996). The proteome is the entire complement of proteins including the modifications made to a particular set of proteins, produced by an organism or system. It is much more complicated than genomics mostly because while an organism's genome is more or less constant, the proteome differs from cell to cell and from time to time.

It is not always easy to predict or characterize a particular protein based on its mRNA sequence, because many transcripts generate more than one protein through alternative splicing, and a wide variety of proteins are subjected to chemical modifications after translation. These post-translational modifications are critical to the protein's function. Phosphorylation, ubiquitination and other post-translational modifications such as methylation, acetylation, glycosylation, oxidation and nitrosylation modify the functional characteristics of the proteins.

Metabolomics is defined as "the quantitative measurement of the dynamic multiparametric metabolic response of living systems to pathophysiological stimuli or genetic modification" (Nicholson, 2006). The metabolome represents the collection of all metabolites in a biological cell, tissue, organ or organism, which are the end products of cellular processes (Jordan *et al.*, 2009). The most widely used and powerful methods are capillary electrophoresis, high performance liquid chromatography (HPLC), gas chromatography interfaced with mass spectrometry (GC-MS) and nuclear magnetic resonance (NMR) spectroscopy.

Bioinformatics is the application of computer science to the field of molecular biology. The term *bioinformatics* was coined by Paulien Hogeweg in 1979 for the study of informatics processes in biotic systems. Its primary use since at least the late 1980s has been in genomics and genetics, particularly in those areas of genomics involving large-scale DNA sequencing. Bioinformatics now entails the creation and advancement of databases, algorithms, computational and statistical techniques, and theory to solve formal and practical problems arising from the management and analysis of biological data. Over the past few decades rapid developments in genomic and other molecular research technologies and developments in information technologies have combined to produce a tremendous amount of information related to molecular biology (Baldi and Brunak, 2001; Barnes and Gray, 2003; Srinivas, 2006;

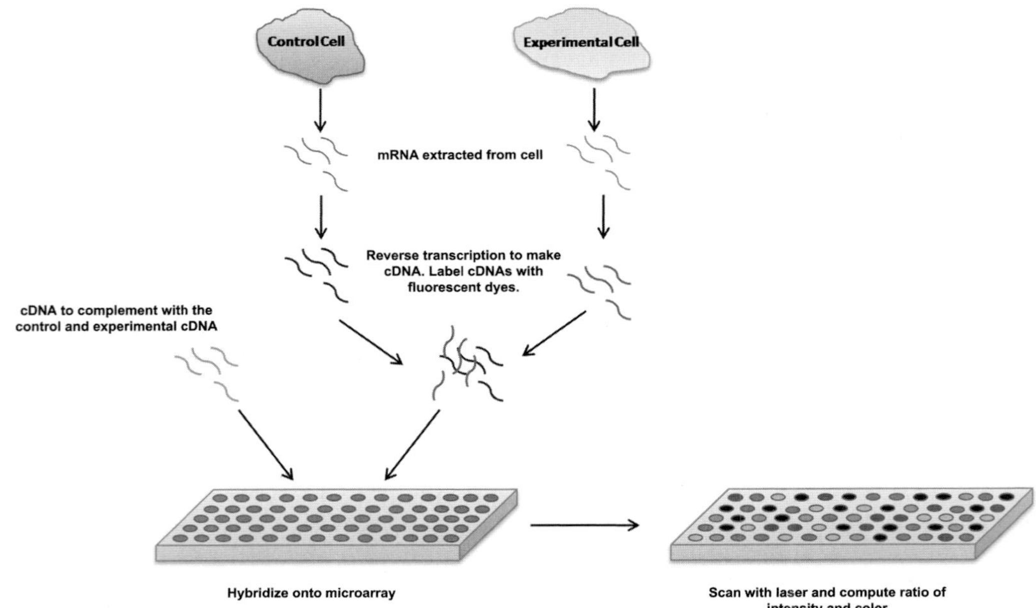

FIGURE 59.1 cDNA microassay for gene expression.

Nair, 2007). It is the name given to these mathematical and computing approaches used to glean understanding of biological processes. Important subdisciplines within bioinformatics and computational biology include:

- the development and implementation of tools that enable efficient access to, and use and management of, various types of information
- the development of new algorithms (mathematical formulas) and statistics with which to assess relationships among members of large data sets, such as methods to locate a gene within a sequence, predict protein structure and/or function, and cluster protein sequences into families of related sequences.

APPLICATIONS OF TOXICOGENOMICS

In general terms, the applications of toxicogenomics can be characterized into two broad and overlapping classes: *mechanistic* or *investigative research* and *predictive toxicology*. The biological relevance of the experimental system for transcript profiling is clearly of major importance where a mechanistic understanding of a toxic process or a mode of action is required. In all likelihood, the toxic endpoint is known in advance (at a physiological, histological and/or biochemical level) and an appropriate test system (*in vitro* or *in vivo*) can be designed to model the endpoint as closely as possible. An example of such an endpoint, non-genotoxic carcinogenesis, is usually evaluated in the context of long-term cancer bioassays in rodents (Chhabra *et al.*, 1990). Toxicogenomic applications may help to identify surrogate markers for the development of phenotype. Using microarray and gel-based expression technologies, the exposure of rodent hepatocytes to the non-genotoxic carcinogen phenobarbital has been studied. In this study, more than 300 genes have been identified which are modulated by phenobarbital (Rodi *et al.*, 1999).

Many other toxic endpoints could be profiled using these methods, with combinatorial approaches such as transgenic or knockout models potentially providing insights into the role of specific genes (Ryffel, 1997). The possibility that a specific group or class of compounds (grouped by toxic endpoint, mechanism, structure, target organ, etc.) may induce signature patterns of gene expression changes is the basis for the application of toxicogenomics to predictive toxicology. The use of these technologies to analyze genome-wide changes in mRNA expression following treatment of *in vitro* systems with known reference toxicants may permit the identification of diagnostic gene expression patterns. Pattern recognition may, in turn, allow the design and construction of *miniarrays*, customized to detect specific toxicity endpoints or pathways. Although *in vitro* systems have practical advantages, there are major drawbacks to consider. Even where appropriate cells *in vitro*, such as primary hepatocytes, are available, compound-induced changes in transcription may not necessarily reflect accurately the response of the corresponding organ *in vivo*. In addition, availability of appropriate cell lines may be limited (although where mechanistic information is not sought, generic cell lines may still be of value), and in some cases metabolism may be required to produce the active chemical reactive species, although often this can be accomplished by pre-incubation with metabolically active cell extracts.

Importantly, where the toxicity is specific to species, strain, sex or route of administration, *in vitro* modeling is unlikely to be fully diagnostic. Nevertheless, even if these systems were able to detect potential adverse health effects of only a small subset of development compounds, their application in predevelopment toxicology screening would be of substantial benefit in providing an early view of compound safety in advance of traditional studies. Development of reference data sets to allow a "pattern recognition" approach to toxicology is likely to require the application of complex computer algorithms and statistical approaches. For example, statistical clustering techniques have been applied to microarray data to analyze the temporal patterns of gene expression that characterize serum responsiveness and wound repair (Iyer *et al.*, 1999), and to distinguish cancerous tissue from normal tissues and cell lines (Alon *et al.*, 1999).

The building of reference data sets, possibly by comparison of microarray output across different laboratories, will require consistency in data analysis and format. A number of resources exist in both the academic and commercial sectors for such purposes (Bassett *et al.*, 1999). One example, the software platform *ArrayDB*, has been developed at the National Human Genome Research Institute. The system facilitates the storage, retrieval and analysis of microarray data along with information linking some 15,000 genes to public domain sequence and pathway databases (Ermolaeva *et al.*, 1998).

TOXICOGENOMICS IN NUTRACEUTICAL RESEARCH

Life and health are heavily influenced by the quality and quantity of the diet. Diet plays an important role on how an individual deals with environmental stressors and toxins to prevent or lessen the impact of diseases. Many components in the diet, either endogenous or exogenous, can modulate the net impact of specific toxicants by acting as inducers, activators, suppressors, inhibitors or substrates of certain toxifying or detoxifying enzymes.

Current developments in genomics and new developments in genetic technologies, such as DNA microarrays, have encouraged the transition of nutrition research from epidemiology and physiology to molecular biology and genetics (IHGSC, 2001; Venter *et al.*, 2001; Waterston *et al.*, 2002). Nutrigenomics includes the study of the genome-wide influences of nutrients at the transcription level. In the past, the effects and mechanisms of dietary components on health and disease have been investigated using functional assays or studies based on single genes or single physiological outcomes of measure. Molecular diagnostics may play a key role in food safety related to genetically modified foods, food-borne pathogens and novel nutraceuticals. Functional outcomes in biology are determined, for the most part, by net balance between sets of genes related to the specific outcome in question.

The DNA microarray technology offers a new dimension of strength in molecular diagnostics by permitting the simultaneous analysis of large sets of genes. Automation of assay and novel bioinformatics tools make DNA microarrays a robust technology for diagnostics. Since its development a few years ago, this technology has been used for the applications of toxicogenomics, pharmacogenomics, cell biology and clinical investigations addressing the prevention and intervention of diseases. Optimization of this technology to specifically address food safety is a vast resource that remains to be mined. Efforts to develop diagnostic custom arrays and simplified bioinformatics tools for field use are warranted. The DNA microarray technology offers substantial versatility to develop powerful diagnostic tools to address issues related to food safety. Since its development a few years ago, this technology has been used for the applications of toxicogenomics, pharmacogenomics, cell biology and clinical investigations addressing the prevention and intervention of diseases.

TOXICOGENOMICS IN DRUG DEVELOPMENT

Toxicogenomics is a new scientific discipline describing the combination of a systematic and comprehensive study of gene expression in response to a drug treatment in a biological system. High expectations are set on this new discipline to fundamentally change the process of drug development, especially in toxicity assessment. The use of expression profiling technologies to mechanistic and predictive toxicology, and biomarker discovery, will enable us to ask detailed questions and generate hypotheses. Ideally, such toxicology research must integrate itself into the discovery phase rather than following it to improve the quality of drug candidates and reduce the overall costs due to attrition during development. However, sound interpretation is required in this new area of data generation to ensure that toxicologically relevant changes are distinguished from those that are not.

The regulatory aspects of toxicogenomics must also be seriously considered. Due to the exploratory and non-validated nature of current gene expression profiling studies, it is not currently an intrinsic part of today's regulatory toxicology. Currently, the value of toxicogenomic data is in mechanistic studies, hypotheses generation, and as a source for providing candidates for validation as biomarkers of toxicity. Toxicogenomics represents a new paradigm in drug development and risk assessment, which promises to generate a wealth of information towards an increased understanding of the molecular mechanisms that lead to drug toxicity and efficacy, and of DNA polymorphisms responsible for individual susceptibility to toxicity.

Gene expression profiling, through the use of DNA microarray and proteomic technologies, will aid in establishing links between expression profiles, mode of action and traditional toxic endpoints. Such patterns of gene expression, or "molecular fingerprints", could be used as diagnostic or predictive markers of exposure, which are characteristic of a specific mechanism of induction of that toxic or efficacious effect. It is anticipated that toxicogenomics will be increasingly integrated into all phases of the drug development process particularly in mechanistic and predictive toxicology, and biomarker discovery.

TOXICOGENOMICS IN REPRODUCTIVE AND DEVELOPMENTAL TOXICOLOGY

Reproductive toxicology is the study of the effects of chemicals on the reproductive and neuroendocrine systems, and also the embryo, fetus, neonate and prepubertal mammal. Recently, there has been serious concern regarding the potential reproductive and health hazards of a range of environmental chemicals known as "endocrine disruptors". An endocrine disruptor is an external agent that interferes with synthesis, secretion, transport, metabolism, binding, action or elimination of natural blood-borne hormones in the body that are responsible for homeostasis, reproduction and developmental processes (Kavlock and Ankley, 1996). As far as endocrine systems are concerned, their activities are basically confined to the hypothalamus–pituitary–gonads and thyroid axis.

These toxicants cause adverse health effects in an intact organism or its progeny. Diverse phenotypic changes that arise from disturbance of the actions of female, male and/or thyroid hormones through agonistic and antagonistic mechanisms or alteration of the homeostatic control balance are clearly concerns for health. In addition to their potential influence on reproductive parameters such as spermatogenesis, the sexual cycle and development of sexual organs, they may affect processes underlying endometriosis, carcinogenesis in hormone-related organs and neurotoxicity leading to intelligence impairment and emotional instability (Table 59.1). These endocrine disruptors may work through by imitating the naturally produced steroid hormones such as estrogen, testosterone, or by blocking the hormone receptor, or by triggering the hormonal pathways and initiating abnormal reactions, such as dioxin and dioxin-like chemicals.

Toxicogenomics, the combined field of toxicology and genomics has become a focus for the research community and regulatory authorities to understand the mode-of-action of a toxicant. With the advent of new genomic technologies, it is now possible to identify, rapidly and holistically, the molecular alterations associated with exposure to toxicants. The simultaneous analysis of expression of thousands of genes as endpoints using cDNA chips or microarrays allows toxicologists a new comprehensive understanding of toxicological issues (Table 59.2). Toxicogenomic tools provide very helpful information relevant to difficult areas such as

TABLE 59.1 Adverse effects of endocrine disruptors

Reproductive dysfunction (spermatogenesis, sexual cycle, endometriosis)
Carcinogenesis (breast, uterus, prostate, testis)
Immune toxicity (loss of resistance to infection)
Developmental disorders of sexual organs (reproductive organ malformation, hypoplasia)
Elevated carcinogenic potential in the second generation (vagina, breast, uterus, prostate, testis)
Neurotoxicity in the second generation (manifested as growth retardation, intelligence impairment, emotional instability)

TABLE 59.2 Advantages of using toxicogenomic tools in toxicology studies

Establish signatures of specific chemically induced altered gene expression
Identify biomarkers of exposure and toxicity
Predict toxicity of unknown agents
Classify and predict phenotypes of toxicity
Delineate models/mechanisms of action
Allow extrapolation from one species to another (from animals to human beings)

dose–response relationships, species-to-species extrapolation and exposure assessment that cannot be resolved with traditional toxicological techniques.

Application of genomic technology to study the reproductive and developmental toxicology overcomes the limitations of conventional or classical toxicological methods. One possibility is that toxicogenomics facilitates differentiation of gene responses specific to endocrine activity from those associated with non-specific general stress. For example, the genomic analysis of transcriptional programs associated with estrogen-induced uterine growth has revealed a wealth of novel information on the molecular events initiated by exposure of the rodent uterus to exogenous estrogen. This approach also allowed a comprehensive analysis of the molecular mechanisms of xenoestrogen (e.g., genistein and diethylstilbesterol) action (Figure 59.2). Furthermore, the identification of co-regulated clusters of estrogen-responsive genes offers the possibility of gaining novel insights into the molecular mechanisms that regulate their expression (Moggs *et al.*, 2003). This could be achieved through extensive bioinformatics analyses of their regulatory regions (Orphanides *et al.*, 2003).

2,3,7,8-Tetrachlorodibenzo-p-dioxin (TCDD, dioxin) causes a diverse spectrum of toxicities in humans and laboratory animals (Couture *et al.*, 1990; Kogevinas, 2001; Ten Tusscher and Koppe, 2004; Mandal, 2005). The fetus is one of the most sensitive targets of dioxins and a broad range of pathophysiological abnormalities, such as disorders of brain development, thyroxin resistance, hepatic damage, hematopoietic disorders and lung dysfunction, are observed in humans after perinatal exposure to dioxins (Ten Tusscher and Koppe, 2004). Dioxins (Figure 59.2) are transferred to fetus and infant through placenta and milk from the mother (Przyrembel *et al.*, 2000). Using DNA microarray and quantitative real-time PCR analyses, Abe *et al.* (2006) identified 38 TCDD-inducible genes in human amniotic epithelial cells.

The Human Genome U133A array (Affymetrix Human Genome U133A) contained 22,277 probe sets including 61 control probe sets, and analyzed the expression level of 18,720 full length transcripts with 13,900 characterized human genes. This study revealed TCDD-inducible genes such as cytochrome P4501A1 and cytochrome P4501B1, interferon-inducible genes and genes related to collagen synthesis or degradation. Interferon-inducible genes were prominently upregulated in TCDD-treated human amniotic epithelial cells, such as IFITM1, G1P2, IFI27 and IFIT1 (Abe *et al.*, 2006). Previously, Mizutani *et al.* (2004) reported that the interferon-related genes were induced in placentas of TCDD-treated Holtzman rats. These investigators speculated that the activation of the interferon signaling pathway impaired the angiogenesis in TCDD-treated rat placentas and brought about a hypoxic state in the placentas.

In addition, it was also an interesting observation through the DNA microarray that the expression of genes related to the synthesis and degradation of collagen, such as MMP9, ITGA2 and ITGA10, were also upregulated by TCDD in human AEC. From this genomic analysis it is speculated that TCDD caused pathological lesions by altering the expression of genes involved in matrix remodeling. Therefore, it is evident that the genomic approach provides a better understanding of genetic basis of the pathology of premature labor by dioxins.

Di-n-butyl phthalate (DBP) is a synthetic phthalic ester often added to hard plastics to make them softer, such as cellulose and some polyvinyl chloride (PVC) plastics. In addition, it is used in the making of adhesives, dyes, personal care products, cosmetics and many more. DBP (Figure 59.2) has potential risk to human health and researchers have evaluated its developmental and reproductive effects, as well as sensitization, systemic effects and genetic toxicity (NTP, 1995; Jiang *et al.*, 2007; Hoppin *et al.*, 2004; Chowdhury and Statham, 2002; Duty *et al.*, 2005; Ema *et al.*, 1995; Jonsson *et al.*, 2005; Reddy *et al.*, 2006).

In a recent study, using high density oligonucleotide DNA microarrays, Gwinn *et al.* (2007) showed altered expression in genes of interest in reproductive toxicity, signal transduction, protein processing, immune response, cell proliferation, organogenesis and oncogenes after 5 or 10 hours of DBP treatment in four strains of normal human mammary epithelial cells. Inhibin A was increased in all cell strains tested. This observation was confirmed with RT-PCR. Mitotic arrest deficient 2 gene (MAD2) is also altered in all cell strains. It is involved in the spindle assembly checkpoint mechanism. MAD2 binds with tumor necrosis factor α convertase (TACE) and MDC9, both of which are implicated in fertilization, sperm migration, myoblast fusion and other developmental processes. The presence of MAD2 has been implicated as a key causal agent in carcinogenesis studies. DNA cystine 5 methyltransferase (DNMT) was also decreased in the DBP-treated human mammary epithelial cells.

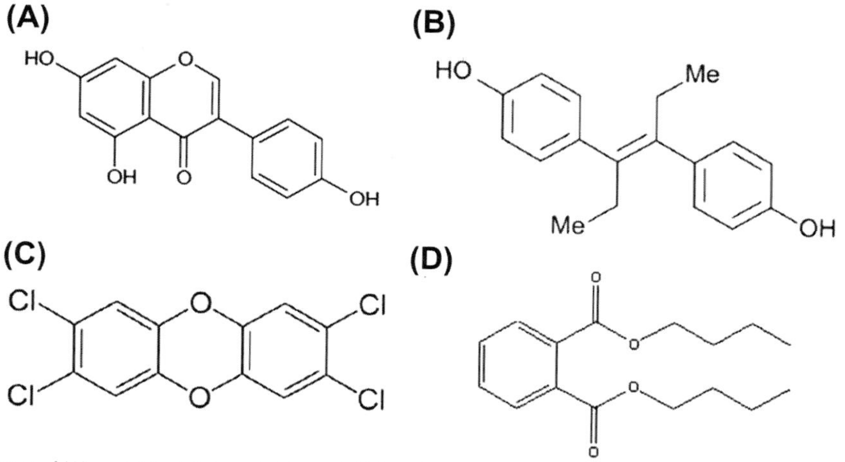

FIGURE 59.2 Chemical structures of (A) genistein, (B) diethylstilbestrol, (C) TCDD (2,3,7,8-tetrachlorodibenzo-*p*-dioxin), and (D) di-*n*-butyl phthalate.

In another study using Gene Fishing PCR on total RNA, Ryu *et al.* (2007) reported that DBP affects the genes involved in xenobiotic metabolism, testis development, sperm maturation, steroidogenesis and immune response, as well as the upregulation of peroxisome proliferation and lipid homeostasis genes in Sprague-Dawley male rats. Using RT-PCR, they found that the LDHA and Spag4 genes were significantly increased, and the PBR gene was significantly decreased in a dose-dependent manner. They also found that at a dose of 750 mg/kg/day DBP significantly increased the steroidogenic-related genes such as SR B1, StAR, P450scc and Cyp17. Ryu *et al.* also evaluated the expression of TR α1, AR and ERβ proteins using Western blot analysis and RT-PCR. They found that the expression of TR α1 was dose dependently increased, while AR and ERβ were significantly decreased. In addition, protein expression of PPARγ was significantly increased, while RXR γ remained unchanged. The authors concluded that DBP can significantly affect the testicular gene expression profiles involved in steroidogenesis and spermatogenesis affecting testicular growth and morphogenesis (Ryu *et al.*, 2007). These genomic studies showed the evidence in favor of toxicity potential of DBP in reproductive and developmental biology by altering the expression of genes that are important in sex hormone synthesis and responsible for reproductive organ development.

CONCLUDING REMARKS AND FUTURE DIRECTIONS

Toxicogenomics is a rapidly developing discipline that provides an understanding of the molecular and cellular effects of various toxicants. Toxicogenomic studies improve our knowledge of the underlying biology and the regulatory networks that integrate the signaling cascades involved in toxicity. Thus, toxicogenomic data advance the introduction of mechanistic insight into risk assessment and fulfill the promise of more accurate and expedited elucidation of class-related biologic effects or predictive toxicity. An urgent need in the field of toxicogenomics is to identify more accurately the orthologous genes or proteins across species. This effort will improve our understanding of conservation of biologic responses to toxic injury and facilitate use of surrogate species that predict the responses in humans.

Although there are important differences in the genomes and proteomes, many responses to chemical and physical stressors are evolutionarily conserved and limitations posed by cross-species extrapolation can be alleviated by focusing analyses on processes conserved across species. However, many genes of experimental animals and humans remain uncharacterized, and divergence can be a major factor in species differences in sensitivity or response. The key goal of toxicogenomic research is to integrate data from multiple sources to produce a comprehensive understanding of the molecular basis of toxicologic responses. Integration of data from different technologies leads to synergistic interpretations beyond what can be resolved when data are analyzed separately or in isolation.

The integration of data from different toxicogenomic technologies has been explored to some extent but these approaches have to be integrated fully. There is also a need to develop mechanisms to better probe the complexity of toxic responses. Toxicologic responses are typically defined by a linear sequence of events. In contrast, a network and system level of organization reflects non-linear cellular states that depict the true complexity of biologic systems. The development of a knowledge base to accurately reflect network-level molecular expression and interpretation requires a new paradigm of data management, integration and computational modeling.

REFERENCES

Abe Y, Sinozaki H, Takagi T, Minegishi T, Kokame K, Kangawa K, Uesaka M, Miyamoto K (2006) Identification of 2,3,7,8-tetrachlorodibenzo-p-dioxin (TCDD)-inducible genes in human amniotic epithelial cells. *Reprod Biol Endocrinol* **4:** 27

Alon U, Barkai N, Notterman DA, Gish K, Ybarra S, Mack D, Levine AJ (1999) Broad patterns of gene expression revealed by clustering analysis of tumor and normal colon tissues probed by oligonucleotide arrays. *Proc Natl Acad Sci USA* **96:** 6745–50.

Anderson NL, Anderson NG (1998) Proteome and proteomics: new technologies, new concepts, and new words. *Electrophoresis* **19:** 1853–61.

Baldi P, Brunak S (2001) *Bioinformatics: The Machine Learning Approach*, 2nd edition. MIT Press, Cambridge, MA, USA.

Bassett DE Jr, Eisen MB, Boguski MS (1999) Gene expression informatics – it's all in your mine. *Nat Genet* **21:** 51–5.

Barnes MR, Gray IC (eds.) (2003) *Bioinformatics for Geneticists*, 1st edition. Wiley Interscience, New York.

Blackstock WP, Weir MP (1999) Proteomics: quantitative and physical mapping of cellular proteins. *Trends Biotechnol* **17:** 121–7.

Chhabra RS, Huff JE, Schwetz BS, Selkirk J (1990) An overview of prechronic and chronic toxicity/carcinogenicity experimental study designs and criteria used by the National Toxicology Program. *Environ Health Perspect* **86:** 313–21.

Christiani DC (*Chair*) (2007) Committee on Applications of Toxicogenomic Technologies to Predictive Toxicology and Risk Assessment, The National Research Council. The National Academic Press, 500 Fifth Street, NW Washington DC, 20001.

Chowdhury MM, Statham BN (2002) Allergic contact dermatitis from dibutyl phthalate and benzalkonium chloride in Timodine cream. *Contact Dermatitis* **46:** 57.

Couture LA, Abbott BD, Birnbaum LS (1990) A critical review of the developmental toxicity and teratogenicity of 2,3,7,8-tetrachlorodibenzo-p-dioxin: recent advances toward understanding the mechanism. *Teratology* **42:** 619–27.

Duty SM, Calafat AM, Silva MJ, Ryan L, Hauser R (2005) Phthalate exposure and reproductive hormones in adult men. *Hum Reprod* **20:** 604–10.

Ema M, Kurosaka R, Amano H, Ogawa Y (1995) Comparative developmental toxicity of n butyl benzyl phthalate and di n butyl phthalate in rats. *Arch Environ Contam Toxicol* **28:** 223–8.

Ermolaeva O, Rastogi M, Pruitt KD, Schuler GD, Bittner ML, ChenY, Simon R, Meltzer P, Trent JM, Boguski MS (1998) Data management and analysis for gene expression arrays. *Nat Genet* **20:** 19–23.

Gwinn MR, Whipkey DL, Tennant LB, Weston A (2007) Gene expression profiling of di n butyl phthalate in normal human mammary epithelial cells. *J Environ Pathol, Toxicol Oncol* **26:** 51–61.

Hamadeh HK, Amin RP, Paules RS, Afshari CA (2002) An overview of toxicogenomics. *Curr Issues Mol Biol* **4:** 45–56.

Hoppin JA, Ulmer R, London SJ (2004) Phthalate exposure and pulmonary function. *Environ Health Perspect* **112:** 571–4.

IHGSC (2001) Initial sequencing and analysis of the human genome. *Nature* **409:** 860–921.

Iyer VR, Eisen MB, Ross DT, Schuler G, Moore T, Lee, JCF, Trent JM, Staudt LM, Hudson J Jr, Boguski MS, Lashkari D, Shalon D, Botstein D, Brown PO (1999) The transcriptional program in the response of human fibroblasts to serum. *Science* **283:** 83–7.

James P (1997) Protein identification in the post-genome era: the rapid rise of proteomics. *Q Rev Biophys* **30:** 279–331.

Jiang J, Ma L, Yuan L, Wang X, Zhang W (2007) Study on developmental abnormalities in hypospadiac male rats induced by maternal exposure to di n butyl phthalate (DBP). *Toxicology* **232:** 286–93.

Jonsson BA, Richthoff J, Rylander L, Giwercman A, Hagmar L (2005) Urinary phthalate metabolites and biomarkers of reproductive function in young men. *Epidemiology* **16:** 487–93.

Jordan KW, Nordenstam J, Lauwers GY, Rothenberger DA, Alavi K, Garwood M, Cheng LL (2009) Metabolomic characterization of human rectal adenocarcinoma with intact tissue magnetic resonance spectroscopy. *Dis Colon Rectum* **52:** 520–5.

Kavlock RJ, Ankley GT (1996) A perspective on the risk assessment process for endocrine-disruptive effects on wildlife and human health. *Risk Analysis* **16:** 731–9.

Kogevinas M (2001) Human health effects of dioxins: cancer, reproductive and endocrine system effects. *Hum Reprod Update* **7:** 331–9.

Mandal PK (2005) Dioxin: a review of its environmental effects and its aryl hydrocarbon receptor biology. *J Comp Physiol [B]* **175:** 221–30.

Mizutani T, Yoshino M, Satake T, Nakagawa M, Ishimura R, Tohyama C, Kokame K, Kangawa K, Miyamoto K (2004) Identification of 2,3,7,8-tetrachlorodibenzo-p-dioxin (TCDD)-inducible and -suppressive genes in the rat placenta: induction of interferon-regulated genes with possible inhibitory roles for angiogenesis in the placenta. *Endocrinology J* **51:** 569–77.

Moggs JG, Deavall DG, Orphanides G (2003) Use of gene expression profiling to understand the transcriptional program associated with estrogen-induced uterine growth. *Pure Appl Chem* **75:** 2429–32.

Morin RD, Bainbridge M, Fejes A, Hirst M, Krzywinski M, Pugh TJ, McDonald H, Varhol R, Jones SJM, Marra MA (2008) Profiling the HeLa S3 transcriptome using randomly primed cDNA and massively parallel short-read sequencing. *BioTechniques* **45:** 81–94.

Nair AS (January 2007) Computational Biology & Bioinformatics – a gentle overview, *Communications of Computer Society of India*.

National Toxicology Program (NTP) (1995) *TOX-30 Toxicity studies of dibutyl phthalate (CAS No. 84-74-2) administered in feed to F344/N rats and B6C3F1 mice* (Report date: April 1995).

Nicholson JK (2006) Global systems biology, personalized medicine and molecular epidemiology. *Mol Syst Biol* **2:** 52.

Orphanides G, Moggs JG, Murphy TC, Edmunds JW, Pennie WD (2003) *Toxicogenomics* (Inoue T, Pennie WD, eds.). Springer, Tokyo, pp. 20–8.

Przyrembel H, Heinrich-Hirsch B, Vieth B (2000) Exposition to and health effects of residues in human milk. *Adv Exp Med Biol* **478:** 307–25.

Reddy B, Rozati R, Reddy B, Raman N (2006) Association of phthalate esters with endometriosis in Indian women. *Int J Obst Gynaecol* **113:** 515–20.

Rodi CP, Bunch RT, Curtiss SW, Kier LD, Cabonce MA, Davila JC, Mitchell MD, Alden CL, Morris DL (1999) Revolution through genomics in investigative and discovery toxicology. *Toxicol Pathol* **27:** 107–10.

Ryffel B (1997) Impact of knockout mice in toxicology. *Crit Rev Toxicol* **27:** 135–54.

Ryu JY, Lee BM, Kacew S, Kim HS (2007) Identification of differentially expressed genes in the testis of Sprague Dawley rats treated with di(n-butyl) phthalate. *Toxicology* **234:** 103–12.

Srinivas A (ed.) (2006) *Handbook of Computational Molecular Biology*. Chapman & Hall/CRC, Boca Raton, FL.

Subramanian A, Tamayo P, Mootha VK, Mukherjee S, Ebert BL, Gillette MA, Paulovich A, Pomeroy SL, Golub TR, Lander ES, Mesirov JP (2005) Gene set enrichment analysis: a knowledge-based approach for interpreting genome-wide expression profiles. *Proc Natl Acad Sci USA* **102:** 15545–50.

Ten Tusscher GW, Koppe JG (2004) Perinatal dioxin exposure and later effects – a review. *Chemosphere* **54:** 1329–36.

Venter JC, Adams MD, Myers EW, Li PW, Mural RJ, Sutton GG, Smith HO, Yandell M, Evans CA, Holt RA (2001) The sequence of the human genome. *Science* **291:** 1304–51.

Wang Z, Gerstein M, Snyder M (2009) RNA-seq: a revolutionary tool for transcriptomics. *Nature Rev Genetics* **10:** 57–63.

Waterston RH, Lindblad-Toh K, Birney E, Rogers J, Abril JF, Agarwal P, Agarwala R, Ainscough R (2002) Initial sequencing and comparative analysis of the mouse genome. *Nature* **420:** 520–62.

Wilkins MR, Pasquali C, Appel RD, Ou K, Golaz O, Sanchez JC, Yan JX, Gooley AA, Hughes G, Humphery-Smith I, Williams KL, Hochstrasser DF (1996) From proteins to proteomes: large scale protein identification by two-dimensional electrophoresis and amino acid analysis. *Biotechnology (NY)* **14:** 61–5.

C H A P T E R

60

Epigenetic regulation of gene and genome expression

Supratim Choudhuri

Disclaimer. The opinions expressed in this article are the author's personal opinions and do not reflect those of the FDA, DHHS or the Federal government

INTRODUCTION

The term epigenetics was coined by Conrad Waddington in early 1940s to indicate developmental events leading from fertilization to mature organism. Waddington defined epigenetics as "the branch of biology which studies the causal interactions between genes and their products, which bring the phenotype into being" (Goldberg *et al.*, 2007). The term was derived by combining two terms, "genetics" and "epigenesis", the latter term means the unfolding of development of an organism from an egg through a sequence of steps. In subsequent expansion of the idea between development and epigenetics, Waddington envisioned that the establishment of cell fates during development is like marbles rolling down a landscape, which he termed epigenetic landscape, to the lowest elevation point from which it cannot revert back to its original state. Hence cell fates, once determined, are irreversible (Goldberg *et al.*, 2007).

Since the coining of the term, epigenetics existed in the shadow of genetics for about 30 years. The true understanding of what we currently define as epigenetics evolved over time as our knowledge on DNA methylation and chromatin modifications and their effects on gene expression increased. The importance of epigenetic factors in gene regulation was first hypothesized decades ago when scientists posited that DNA methylation could heritably alter gene expression (Ginder *et al.*, 2008). Epigenetics can now be defined as the "study of mitotically or meiotically heritable changes in gene function that cannot be explained by changes in the DNA sequence" (Riggs *et al.*, 1996). Epigenetic inheritance involves the transmission of information (epigenetic mark) not encoded in the DNA sequence, from parent cell to daughter cells and from generation to generation. Epigenetic mark is like a bookmark that flags the chromatin state, "on" or "off", "open" or "closed", so it may be identified and maintained in the daughter cells (Choudhuri, 2009a).

Although much needs to be understood in terms of correlative effects vs. causal effects between exposure to various environmental factors and epigenetic changes regulating gene expression, research on epigenetic regulation of gene expression has nonetheless made remarkable progress in recent years. This chapter describes in detail the epigenetic regulation of genes and genome expression.

MOLECULAR MECHANISMS OF EPIGENETIC REGULATION

Epigenetic changes are effected through three major molecular mechanisms: (1) DNA methylation, (2) histone modifications and (3) non-coding RNA (ncRNA) expression. Therefore, it is logical first to describe the chromatin structure, its assembly and remodeling, before discussing the molecular mechanisms of epigenetic regulation.

Chromatin structure, assembly and remodeling

Chromatin is the DNA–histone complex in the nucleus. The structural unit of chromatin is called "nucleosome"; hence chromatin can be envisioned as a repeat of regularly spaced nucleosomes. A nucleosome core particle is composed of a histone octamer and the DNA that wraps around it (Figure 60.1). Histones are globular basic proteins with a flexible N-terminal end (the so-called "tail") that protrudes from the nucleosome. Histones are subject to various covalent modifications that primarily occur on the tail.

The histone octamer is composed of two molecules each of histones H2A, H2B, H3 and H4. DNA wraps around the octamer in a left-handed supercoil of about 1.75 turns that contains approximately 150 bp. Histone H1 is the "linker histone" that, along with "linker DNA", physically connects the adjacent nucleosome core particles. The length of linker DNA varies with species and cell types. A complete nucleosome encompasses approximately 180 and 200 bp of DNA because it includes part of the linker DNA on both sides of the core particle. Figure 60.1 shows different levels of eukaryotic

Reproductive and Developmental Toxicology, Edited by Ramesh C. Gupta
ISBN: 978-0-12-382032-7

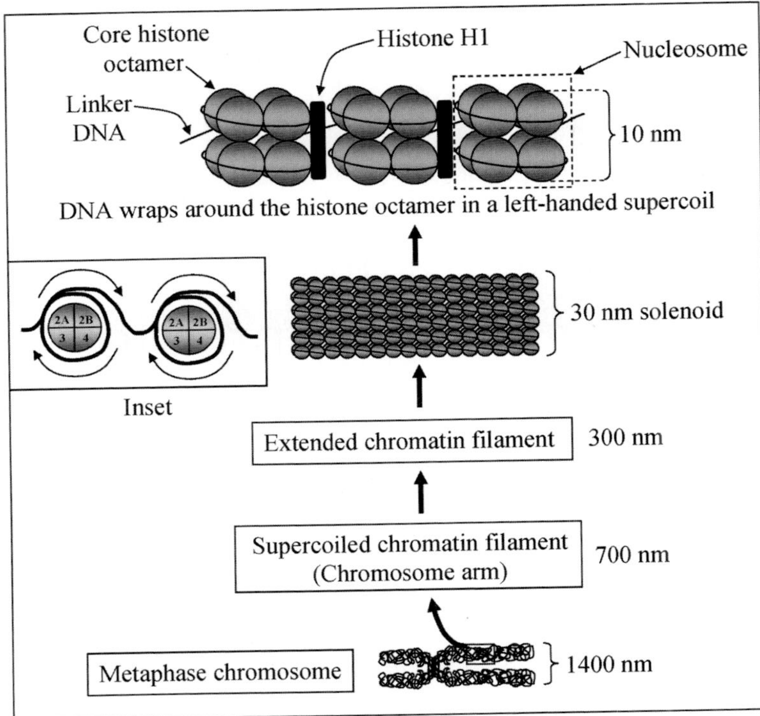

FIGURE 60.1 Nucleosome structure and organization from nucleosome to chromosome. The histone octamer core contains two molecules each of histones H2A, H2B, H3 and H4. The DNA wraps around the octamer in a left-handed supercoil in about 1.75 turns that encloses about 150bp. Histone H1 is the linker histone. Linker histone and linker DNA physically connect adjacent nucleosome core particles. The nucleosomes (10nm each) are condensed into 30nm solenoid fiber structure; 30nm solenoids are condensed into 300nm filament; 300nm filaments are condensed into the 700nm chromosome. During cell division, when the chromosomes duplicate, a 1,400nm metaphase chromosome is produced containing two chromatids, each chromatid being 700nm. The inset shows the position of individual histones with respect to each other as viewed from the top, and the left-handed wrapping of the DNA around each histone octamer core.

genome organization, from chromosome down to the level of nucleosome.

Chromatin can undergo changes in its conformation in response to various cellular metabolic demands. Altered chromatin conformation, in turn, can limit or enhance the accessibility and binding of the transcription machinery, thereby precipitating an epigenetic effect on transcription.

Non-canonical nucleosomes in centromeric chromatin

Nucleosomes may exhibit polymorphism with different histone/DNA stoichiometry and opposite chirality. The existence of half-nucleosomes in the centromeres of *Drosophila* interphase nuclei was previously described. A half-nucleosome is a tetramer that contains one copy each of histones H2A, H2B, H4 and the CenH3 (Cenp-A) variant of histone H3, and is called hemisome. In a more recent study, Furuyama and Henikoff (2009) proposed that these hemisomes wrap DNA in a right-handed manner compared to the canonical nucleosomes that wrap DNA in a left-handed manner. The universality of this finding as well as its genetic significance are yet to be demonstrated.

Chromatin assembly

Chromatin is assembled by proper nucleosome assembly through histone deposition, and is tightly coupled to DNA replication. In the histone deposition process, first the pre-existing core histones are transferred onto the two newly synthesized DNA strands behind the replication fork; the rest of the histones needed to complete chromatin assembly are newly synthesized. The newly synthesized core histones are imported from cytosol to the nucleus by a network of *karyopherins* (*importins*), which bind to the nuclear localization signal in the N-terminal domain of each core histone. These newly synthesized histones are acetylated at lysines 5 and 12 of histone H4 (H4K5ac and H4K12ac, and also H3K14ac in *Drosophila*), but following deposition onto newly replicated DNA, they are rapidly deacetylated by histone deacetylases (Tyler, 2002). The functional significance of such acetylation and subsequent deacetylation is not understood. Acetylation of newly synthesized histone H3 seems to occur at different sites in different species. Acetylation of newly synthesized histones is carried out by cytosolic histone acetyltransferase 1 (HAT1), the only known B-type HAT. In contrast, A-type HATs acetylate chromosomal histones (Parthun, 2007).

During the histone deposition process, $(H3\text{-}H4)_2$ tetramers (formed from H3-H4 heterodimers) first form a stable complex with >120bp of DNA. This is followed by the deposition of H2A-H2B heterodimers. The H2A-H2B heterodimers bind to either side of the $(H3\text{-}H4)_2$ tetramer and extend the wrapping of DNA to >160bp. This creates a structure comprised of the four histone dimers linked end to end in the sequence (H2A-H2B)–(H4-H3)–(H3-H4)–(H2B-H2A) (Wolffe and Hayes, 1999; Verreault, 2000). Figure 60.1 inset shows the position of individual histones with respect to each other as viewed from the top, and the left-handed wrapping of the DNA around each histone octamer core. Reconstitution studies indicate that the wrapping of the $(H3\text{-}H4)_2$ by DNA can be in either direction (right- or left-handed); only the addition of H2A-H2B dimers locks it in the left-handed configuration (Alilat *et al.*, 1999). The positive charge of histones is shielded by various anionic factors to allow chromatin assembly in a regulated and ordered fashion.

A number of histone chaperone proteins aid in the proper deposition of histones, such as chromatin assembly factor-1 (CAF-1), which appears to deposit newly synthesized histones H3 and H4 onto newly replicated DNA via its interactions with proliferating cell nuclear antigen (PCNA). Because PCNA is the processivity factor for the replicating DNA polymerase in eukaryotes, the coupling of CAF-1 with PCNA serves to localize CAF-1 to the sites of DNA synthesis (Ito *et al.*, 1997; Verreault, 2000). Other examples include replication–coupling assembly factor (RCAF), and nucleosome assembly protein-1 (NAP-1) (NAP-2 in humans). Both NAP-1 and human NAP-2 bind to histone H2A-H2B, and with the help of karyopherins, aid in their transport from cytoplasm to nucleus as cells progress from G1 to S phase (Ito *et al.*, 1997; Verreault, 2000).

Although histone chaperones play a crucial role in chromatin assembly, they are not sufficient to generate the typical regular arrays of nucleosomes with 180–200 bp spacing; rather, they lead to the assembly of irregularly spaced nucleosomes. Proper chromatin assembly with regular arrays of nucleosomes requires, in addition to histone chaperones, ATP-dependent chromatin remodeling factors, as discussed below.

Chromatin remodeling

Mature chromatin with regularly spaced nucleosomes is formed in a two-step reaction. In the first step, histone deposition occurs independently of ATP and Mg^{2+} creating irregularly spaced nucleosomes. The second step requires ATP and Mg^{2+} and generates chromatin with properly spaced nucleosomes (Tyler, 2002). Such remodeling involves the use of energy from ATP hydrolysis to induce a net change in the positioning of the histone octamer.

Chromatin remodeling facilitates transcription, too; it involves the breaking and reestablishment of histone–DNA contacts and repositioning of histones from one region of DNA to another through a dissociative pathway or through sliding. At least four major families of chromatin remodeling complexes are known: SWI/SNF (SWI/SNF, RSC, Brahma); Mi-2/CHD (Mi-2 complex, NURD); ISWI (ISW1, ISW2, NURF, ACF, CHRAC, RSF); and INO80, of which the SWI/SNF (switching/sucrose non-fermenting) complex was the first chromatin remodeling complex characterized in budding yeast *Saccharomyces cerevisiae*. The human homolog is referred to as the "hSWI/SNF". The ATPase subunit in yeast SWI/SNF complex is known as "SWI2/SNF2". Mammalian SWI/SNF complex contains either *Brahma-related gene-1* (BRG-1) or *Brahma* (BRM) as its ATPase subunit (Tyler, 2002).

The sliding model of chromatin remodeling involves the breaking of fewer histone–DNA contacts at any given time, and may therefore play a major role in histone repositioning. According to this model, the DNA dissociates from the histone octamer at one edge of the nucleosome, and a neighboring stretch of DNA associates with the octamer to yield a small DNA loop. As this loop spreads along the surface of the octamer, the octamer slides to a new location. Therefore, at any given time, only a small number of histone–DNA contacts are broken during histone sliding (Whitehouse *et al.*, 2000).

Mechanisms of epigenetic regulation

The principal mechanisms that provide the molecular basis of epigenetic regulation of genome expression are (1) DNA methylation, (2) histone modification and (3) regulation of gene expression by ncRNAs.

In addition to these three principal mechanisms, another mechanism that can affect gene expression epigenetically is the physical interaction between two chromosomes, such as the phenomenon of transvection. If a gene has a truncated, non-functional open reading frame (ORF), then it will not be expressed (no product). If its allele in the homologous chromosome has an intact ORF and a functional promoter but a truncated non-functional enhancer, it will also not be expressed or be expressed at a low level. However, when these two alleles are brought in close physical proximity through tight physical pairing (synapsis) of the two homologous chromosomes, the intact enhancer of one allele can interact in *trans* with the intact promoter of the other allele. Such interaction is called intragenic complementation and will cause enhanced gene expression from the allele that has intact promoter but a truncated enhancer (Figure 60.2). Transvection is commonly seen in Dipteran insects and has been well studied in *Drosophila*. The defining feature of transvection is its dependence on homologous chromosomal pairing. Therefore, chromosomal rearrangements that interfere with chromosome pairing also interfere with transvection. There is also a *cis* insulator bypass model of transvection in *Drosophila* (Morris *et al.*, 1998). Transvection can also occur by the action of silencers in *trans*. In mammals, sustained somatic pairing (as seen in *Drosophila*) is generally absent except for some reported examples of tissue- and stage-specific pairing of particular loci, and homologous pairing of oppositely imprinted loci. Nevertheless, recent evidence suggests that regulatory elements might have the capacity to act in *trans* to regulate genes on other chromosomes (Williams *et al.*, 2010).

The three principal mechanisms of epigenetic regulation of genome expression are discussed below.

1. DNA methylation

DNA methylating enzymes

In multicellular eukaryotes, DNA methylation involves covalent modification of cytosine (C) bases at the carbon-5 position of CG dinucleotides, referred to as CpG dinucleotides. The enzyme involved is DNA methyltransferase (DNMT), and the methyl donor is *S*-adenosylmethionine (SAM). The C of CpG is methylated in both strands of DNA. During replication, the parent strand remains methylated, but the newly synthesized daughter strand is not methylated. These hemimethylated segments are recognized by maintenance methyltransferase, which methylates the hemimethylated sites and restores the parental methylation pattern.

There are two types of DNMT enzymes: the *de novo* methyltransferase that establishes the methylation pattern, and the maintenance methyltransferase that maintains the

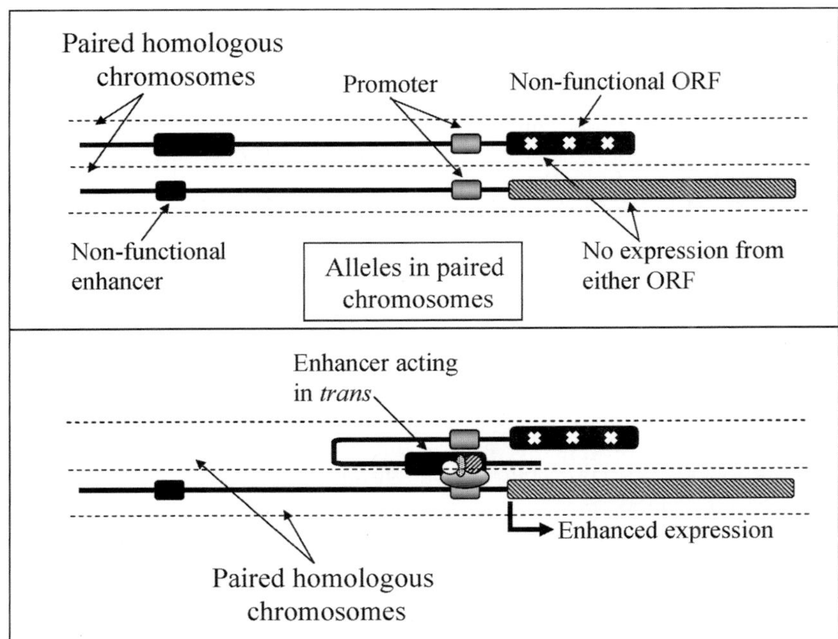

FIGURE 60.2 Transvection and intragenic complementation. Enhancer loops in *trans* and interacts with the intact promoter of the allele that has a functional ORF. As a result, the allele is transcribed, ultimately producing the gene product. Such physical interaction between alleles is only possible because of their physical proximity through homologous chromosome pairing.

methylation pattern once it is established. Mammals have four different DNMTs: DNMT1, 2, 3a and 3b. DNMT3a and 3b are *de novo* DNA methyltransferases, DNMT1 is a maintenance methyltransferase. The true function of DNMT2 is not clear because it has weak methyltransferase activity, and its targeted deletion does not have any impact on the global DNA demethylation in the cell. Based on some recent data, it has been proposed that the original model of discrete *de novo* and maintenance methylation functions by separate enzymes may be an oversimplification. A new model proposed that the *de novo* and maintenance methyltransferases cooperate in creating and maintaining genomic methylation pattern and status (Jones and Liang, 2009).

Transcriptional silencing by DNA methylation

In the genome, CpGs may or may not occur in clusters. CpG clusters, i.e. CpG-rich sequences of the genome, are known as CpG islands. By definition, CpG islands are genomic regions that are at least 200 bp long with 50% or higher G+C content and 60% or higher observed/expected CpG ratio. In mammalian cells, the majority of CpG sites that do not exist as CpG clusters are methylated, such as in satellite DNA, repetitive elements (e.g., transposons), non-repetitive intergenic DNA and exons of genes. However, CpG islands, i.e. CpG clusters, are unmethylated (some could be undermethylated as well). Methylation of the C of CpG is associated with transcriptional silencing, and the absence of methylation is associated with active transcription. Thus, unmethylated CpG islands are associated with the promoters of transcriptionally active genes, such as housekeeping genes and many regulated genes, i.e. genes showing tissue-specific expression. How CpG islands remain unmethylated remains unclear (Li and Bird, 2007).

Transcriptional silencing is the result of a condensed state of chromatin brought about by DNA methylation. It is thought to be achieved by three principal transcription-repressive mechanisms: (1) histone deacetylation, (2) interference with transcriptional activators and (3) repressive histone methylation. Methyl CpG-binding proteins play a crucial role in it. The prototypical methyl CpG-binding protein, which was the first one purified and cloned, was MeCP2 (Nan *et al.*, 1997, 1998; Wakefield *et al.*, 1999). MeCP2 binds 5-methyl cytosine in symmetrically positioned CpG dinucleotides in the mammalian genome; it is also able to bind to a single methylated CpG pair. It contains two functional domains: an 85-amino acid methyl-CpG-binding domain (MBD) essential for binding to 5-methyl cytosine, and a 104-amino acid transcriptional repression domain (TRD). The TRD of MeCP2 interacts with a corepressor complex containing histone deacetylases (HDACs) and transcriptional repressors, such as Sin3a. Recruitment of HDAC causes deacetylation of histones, resulting in a more condensed chromatin conformation and transcriptional silencing (Figure 60.3).

However, HDAC inhibitors (e.g., trichostatin A) do not fully relieve the repressive effects of HDAC recruited by MeCP2, thereby suggesting that mechanisms other than deacetylation also add to the transcription repressive ability of MeCP2. One such mechanism may involve preventing the access of transcriptional activators to the promoter and other regulatory sequences.

Transcriptional suppression by repressive histone methylation was reported by Fuks *et al.* (2003). They studied the role of MeCP2 in murine *H19* gene repression in L929 mouse fibroblast cells. They observed that in addition to recruiting HDAC, MeCP2 also associates with histone methyltransferase activity and methylate Lys9 of histone H3, which is a transcription repressing chromatin modification (Table 60.1). These data demonstrate that MeCP2 reinforces a repressive

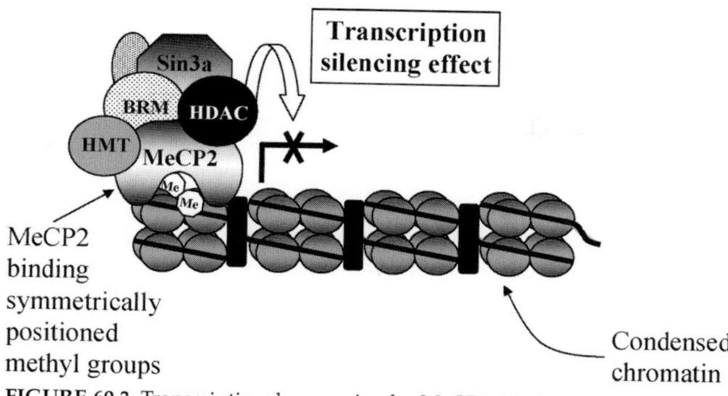

FIGURE 60.3 Transcriptional repression by MeCP2. MeCP2 selectively binds 5-methyl cytosine of the CpG dinucleotides through its methyl-CpG-binding domain (MBD); MeCP2 is able to bind to a single methylated CpG pair. The transcriptional repression domain (TRD) of MeCP2 interacts with a corepressor complex containing histone deacetylases (HDACs), the transcriptional repressor Sin3a and other proteins. HDAC causes deacetylation of histones, resulting in a more condensed chromatin conformation, thereby helping in transcriptional silencing. MeCP2 can also recruit histone methyltransferases (HMTs) that can cause transcription-repressing histone modifications, such as H3K9 methylations.

TABLE 60.1 Some transcriptional activating and repressing histone modifications

Activating modifications	Repressing modifications
Acetylation: Histone H2A: Lysine (K) 5,9,13 Histone H2B: Lysine (K) 5,12,15,20 Histone H3: Lysine (K) 9,14,18,23,56 Histone H4: Lysine (K) 5,8,13,16	
Methylation: Histone H3: Lysine (K) 4,36,79 Histone H3: Arginine (R) 17,23 Histone H4: Arginine (R) 3	Methylation: Histone H3: Lysine (K) 9,27 Histone H4: Lysine (K) 20
Phosphorylation: Histone H3: Threonine (T) 3 Histone H3: Serine (S) 10,28 Histone H3: Tyrosine (Y) 41 Histone H2AX: Serine (S) 139 (for DNA repair)	
Ubiquitination: Histone H2B: Lysine (K) 120, Histone H2B: Lysine (K) 123 (yeast)	Ubiquitination: Histone H2A: Lysine (K) 119
	Sumoylation: Histone H2A: Lysine (K) 126 (yeast) Histone H2B: Lysine (K) 6,7 (yeast) Histone H4: Lysine (K) 5,8,12,16,20

chromatin state by acting as a bridge between two global epigenetic modifications, DNA methylation and repressive histone methylation.

In addition to MeCP2, there are other MBD proteins, such as MeCP1 and MBD1–4. MBD1–MBD4 were all discovered as EST clones with sequence similarity to the MBD motif of MeCP2. Several different experimental approaches strongly suggest a role of these proteins in methylation-dependent transcriptional repression (Choudhuri *et al.*, 2010).

2. *Histone code and various histone modifications*

Histone code hypothesis

Covalent histone modification is reversible; it involves the participation of various proteins and is a precisely regulated phenomenon. In emphasizing the idea that specific histone modifications appear to act sequentially or in combination to form a recognizable "code" that is identified by specific proteins to bring about distinct downstream events like transcriptional activation or repression, Strahl and Allis (2000) coined the term "histone code". The concept of such a code is analogous to the concept of a combination code of numbers in a lock. Only a specific combination of numbers will open a specific lock; changing just one number in that combination will fail to do the job (Choudhuri *et al.*, 2010). For example, trimethylation of histone H3 (H3K4me3) forms a transcription-activating histone code (Vermeulen *et al.*, 2007); likewise, phosphorylation of histone H2AX at serine 139 (H2AXS139ph) forming γ-H2AX forms the histone code for DNA repair (Scully, 2010).

Different types of histone modifications

Histones are subject to many different types of reversible covalent post-translational modifications, such as acetylation, methylation, phosphorylation, ADP-ribosylation, ubiquitination and sumoylation. These modifications impact transcription through chromatin conformation. Table 60.1 shows the histone modifications and their effects on gene expression discussed below and Figure 60.4 shows the (first 20) *N*-terminal amino acid sequence of different histones that are subject to covalent modifications.

Histone acetylation (ac) is a transcription-activating modification that is achieved by the addition of acetyl group (-CH_3CO) from acetyl coenzyme A, to one or more lysine residues at the ε-amino group by histone acetyltransferases (HATs). Acetylation reduces the overall positive charge of histones by neutralizing the positive charge of the target lysine; therefore, it decreases the affinity of histone for the negatively charged DNA. This results in a decondensed, relaxed (i.e., open) chromatin conformation, which allows the transcriptional activators to gain access to their cognate recognition elements and initiate/enhance transcription. Many transcriptional coactivators have HAT activity. Acetylations are removed by histone deacetylases (HDACs).

Histone methylation (mono- (me), di- (me2) or trimethylation (me3)) is catalyzed by histone methyltransferases (HMTs) at lysine and arginine residues, primarily of histone H3 and H4. The methyl group donor is SAM. Methylation increases the bulk but does not interfere with the charge. All known arginine (R) methylations are transcription activating, but lysine (K) methylation can cause either transcriptional activation or repression, depending on which lysine residue is methylated (Table 60.1). Trimethylation of H3K4 (H3K4me3) is transcription activating because it provides a binding site for the general transcription factor TFIID and enhances the recruitment and stability of the transcription preinitiation complex; thus H3K4me3 forms a transcription-activating histone code (Vermeulen *et al.*, 2007). Trimethylation of H3K9 (H3K9me3) is usually transcription repressing, but it can also be associated with transcriptional activation (Vakoc *et al.*, 2005). Histone methylation on lysine is removed

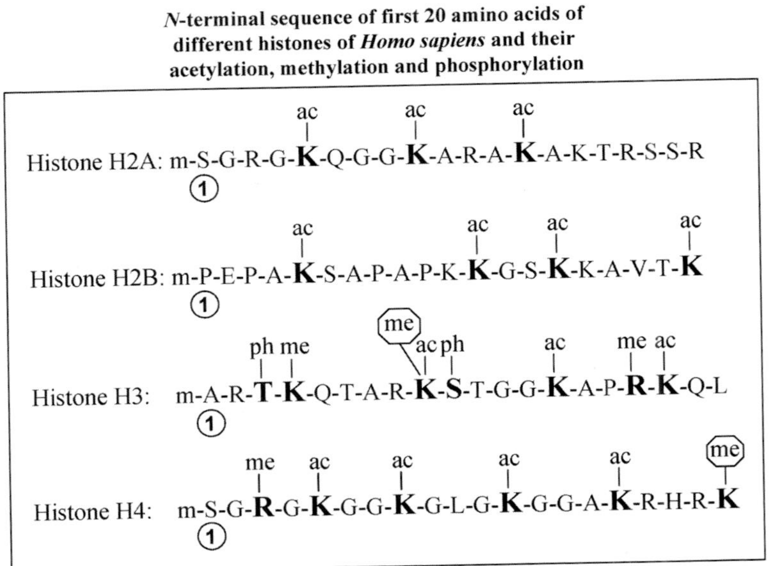

***N*-terminal sequence of first 20 amino acids of different histones of *Homo sapiens* and their acetylation, methylation and phosphorylation**

Histone H2A: m-S-G-R-G-**K**(ac)-Q-G-G-**K**(ac)-A-R-A-**K**(ac)-A-K-T-R-S-S-R

Histone H2B: m-P-E-P-A-**K**(ac)-S-A-P-A-P-K-**K**(ac)-G-S-**K**(ac)-K-A-V-T-**K**(ac)

Histone H3: m-A-R-**T**(ph)-**K**(me)-Q-T-A-R-**K**(me, ac)-**S**(ph)-T-G-G-**K**(ac)-A-P-**R**(me)-**K**(ac)-Q-L

Histone H4: m-S-G-**R**(me)-G-**K**(ac)-G-G-**K**(ac)-G-L-G-**K**(ac)-G-G-A-**K**(ac)-R-H-R-**K**(me)

FIGURE 60.4 The sequence of the first 20 *N*-terminal amino acids of histone H2A, H2B, H3 and H4 are shown. Some of the important amino acid residues in these first 20 amino acids that are subject to frequent activating or repressing modifications are also shown. The methylation within octagon represents repressing methylation (refer to Table 60.1 for a more complete list). The numbering of the amino acids excludes the first methionine encoded by the start codon ATG. In other words, the amino acid next to the first methionine is numbered 1, the next one is 2, and so on.

by demethylases. Methylated arginine is not directly demethylated, but rather converted to citrulline by peptidylarginine deiminase 4 (PAD4/PADI4).

Histone phosphorylation (ph) is a transcription-activating modification. It is achieved by kinase-catalyzed addition of the negatively charged γ-phosphate, usually from ATP or GTP, to one or more serine and/or threonine residues of histone H3. Serine 10 is frequently a target of phosphorylation (H3S10ph). The addition of negatively charged phosphate to the N-terminal histone tails presumably disrupts the electrostatic interactions between histones and DNA, destabilizing local chromatin conformation and triggering transcriptional activation. Phosphorylation of histone H2AX at serine 139 forming γ-H2AX, which accumulates at the site of DNA double-strand breaks and recruits various DNA repair proteins, forms the histone code for DNA repair (Scully, 2010). A recently reported new phosphorylation target is tyrosine 41 on histone H3 (H3Y41ph), by Janus kinase 2 (JAK2) that has translocated to the nucleus (Dawson *et al.*, 2009). Like all other known histone phosphorylations, H3Y41ph is a transcription-activating modification and prevents the binding of heterochromatin protein 1-alpha (HP1-alpha), a transcription repressing protein, to this region of H3. Phosphorylation is removed by specific phosphatases.

Histone H1, H2A, H2B and H3 can all be ubiquitinated at lysine residues, but H2A and H2B ubiquitination are the most common. Table 60.1 shows that ubiquitination can be transcription activating or repressing depending on the lysine residue involved. Ubiquitination of histone H1 results in its release from the DNA, which relieves chromatin condensation and facilitates transcriptional activation. Histone deubiquitination is carried out by ubiquitin proteases.

Histone ADP-ribosylation, like histone ubiquitination, is also less well studied. It involves the transfer of ADP-ribose moiety of NAD^+ to a specific amino acid (arginine, glutamate, lysine), and is catalyzed by ADP-ribosyltransferase. Histones are ADP-ribosylated by poly (ADP-ribose) polymerase-1 (PARP-1) in response to DNA damage. The negative charge of ADP-ribose causes electrostatic repulsion and leads to the pulling of the DNA away from the histones. This relaxes the chromatin structure, making it accessible to repair enzymes.

Histone sumoylation (su) occurs at the lysine residues, and was first reported in 2003 in human cell lines (Shiio and Eisenman, 2003). Small ubiquitin-related modifier (SUMO) is a ubiquitin-like protein; members of this group of proteins are involved in post-translational modifications of many important cellular proteins. Mammalian cells express three major SUMO proteins; SUMO-1, SUMO-2 and SUMO-3. Histone H4 can be conjugated to SUMO-1 and SUMO-3. Of the four major core histones, histone H4 is most efficiently sumoylated both *in vivo* and *in vitro* (Shiio and Eisenman, 2003). Histone sumoylation is a transcription-repressive modification (Table 60.1), and it apparently mediates transcriptional silencing through the recruitment of HDAC and HP1. The extent of histone sumoylation in transcriptional regulation, however, is yet to be determined with certainty (Garcia-Dominiguez and Reyes, 2009). Because SUMO moiety is added through an isopeptide bond (peptide bond involving the ε-amino group of lysine instead of the usual α-amino group), removal of sumoylation requires isopeptidases.

There is cross-talk between chromatin remodeling and histone modification that is vital in transcriptional regulation. A number of histone methyltransferases and demethylases can regulate DNA methylation by either recruiting or regulating the stability of DNMTs, thereby influencing DNMT's ability to recruit HDACs and MBPs to achieve chromatin condensation and gene silencing (Choudhuri *et al.*, 2010).

3. *Non-coding RNA (ncRNA) and epigenetic regulation*

Non-coding RNA (ncRNA)-mediated epigenetic regulation can be mediated by long ncRNAs and small ncRNAs. Some of the long ncRNAs mediating epigenetic effects are

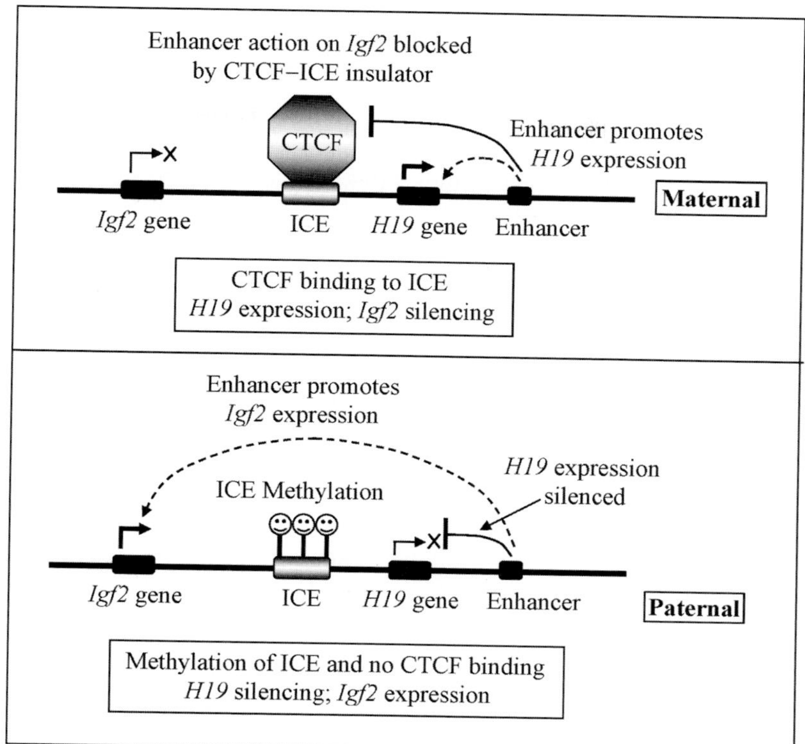

FIGURE 60.5 In mouse, *Igf2* and *H19* genes are on the same chromosome. The *Igf2* gene is located ~80 kb upstream of *H19*. The ICE is located in between *Igf2* and *H19*; it is a ~2.4 kb long region located ~2 kb upstream of *H19*, and it contains an insulator sequence that binds the vertebrate insulator protein CTCF (CCCTC-binding factor). An enhancer region downstream from *H19* can enhance the transcription from both *Igf2* and *H19*. Monoallelic expression of *Igf2* or *H19* is regulated by the methylation status of ICE. Binding of CTCF with the insulator sequence creates a functional insulator. On the maternal chromosome, the ICE-CTCF insulator shields the *Igf2* gene from the enhancer, thus preventing the transcriptional activation of *Igf2*. As a result, *Igf2* expression is silenced. On the paternal chromosome, the ICE is methylated, and thus CTCF cannot bind methylated ICE. As a result, the enhancer can interact with paternal *Igf2* promoter and enhance *Igf2* expression. However, methylation of the ICE causes secondary methylation of the *H19* gene and prevents its expression.

responsible for genomic imprinting and parent-of-origin-specific expression of specific loci. For example, *H19* (2.3 kb) regulating the expression of *Igf2*; *Air* (108 kb) regulating the expression of *Igf2r* cluster; *Kcnq1ot1* (>60 kb) regulating the expression of *Kcnq1* cluster; *Xist* (17 kb) and *Tsix* (40 kb) regulating X-chromosome inactivation in mammals (Choudhuri *et al.*, 2010). One of the best-studied examples of genomic imprinting is that of *Igf2-H19*, in which *H19* is a fetal liver ncRNA, and *Igf2* is the gene encoding insulin-like growth factor 2. In mice, *H19* is paternally imprinted (repressed); hence *Igf2* is paternally expressed. The situation is opposite for the maternal allele. *H19* is maternally expressed; hence *Igf2* is maternally imprinted (repressed). Such imprinted expression is dictated by the methylation status of the imprint control element (ICE). Figure 60.5 shows the mechanism of differential (imprinted) expression of *Igf2-H19* system.

However, in recent years the complexity of ncRNA-mediated epigenetic regulation has expanded with the discovery of various small ncRNAs in animals and plants, such as microRNA (miRNA), small interfering RNA (siRNA), Piwi-interacting RNA (piRNA), repeat-associated siRNA (ra-siRNA), *trans*-acting siRNA (ta-siRNA), natural antisense transcript siRNA (nat-siRNA), heterochromatic siRNA (hc-siRNA), small scan RNA (scnRNA) and qiRNAs (QDE2-interacting small RNAs) (Choudhuri, 2009b). Because the small ncRNAs are ubiquitous and have emerged as powerful epigenetic regulators of gene and genome expression, the following discussion is restricted to miRNA and piRNAs due to their relevance to the current discussion.

Biogenesis and function of miRNA

The first microRNA discovered was *lin-4* in *C. elegans* (Lee *et al.*, 1993). The second microRNA discovered was *let-7*, also in *C. elegans* (Reinhart *et al.*, 2000); but these were not called microRNA, rather they were called small temporal RNA (stRNA) (Pasquinelli *et al.*, 2000) because they control the temporal dimension of development. The term microRNA (miRNA) was coined simultaneously by three groups (Lau *et al.*, 2001; Lagos-Quintana, 2001; Lee and Ambros, 2001) to indicate endogenous small non-coding RNA (ncRNAs) that also include *lin-4* and *let-7*. The shorter designation of individual miRNA and its gene was proposed to be miR-# and *mir-#*, respectively (Lau *et al.*, 2001).

miRNAs are short (~22 nt) ncRNAs that regulate gene expression by binding to their cognate binding sites on the target mRNAs, and inhibiting their translation. The cognate binding sites are mostly at the 3′-end of the mRNA. The inhibition of translation results in the silencing of gene expression, and this phenomenon is called RNA interference (RNAi).

microRNAs are transcribed from miRNA genes into long primary miRNA (pri-miRNA) transcripts that often contain thousands of nucleotides and form stem-loop hairpins.

Pri-miRNAs are transcribed primarily by RNA pol II, but some pri-miRNAs are transcribed by RNA pol III. C19MC (chromosome 19 miRNA cluster), which is the largest known human miRNA gene cluster (100 kb) containing 46 miRNA genes, is transcribed by RNA pol III (Borchert *et al.*, 2006).

The pri-miRNA transcript is processed in the nucleus by Drosha–DGCR8 complex, also called the "microprocessor complex". Drosha processing is called "cropping", which produces 70–80 nt-long precursor miRNA (pre-miRNA). In this process Drosha, which is an RNAse III-type enzyme, actually cleaves the pri-miRNA transcript; and DGCR8 acts as a molecular ruler to determine the Drosha cleavage site, which is at the 11 nt position from the base of the stem structure. The 5′-end of the pre-miRNA has a bias for uridine, and the 3′-end has a 2 nt overhang. Thus, the pre-miRNA has a stem-loop hairpin structure and its 3′-end has a 2 nt overhang (Figure 60.6). Some pri-miRNAs are encoded by introns and are not processed by Drosha; instead they are processed by spliceosome in the nucleus. These intron-derived pri-miRNAs are called mirtrons, and their processing pathway is called mirtron pathway. Because mirtrons are processed by spliceosomes, they contain the signals necessary for spliceosome processing, such as flanking 5′ and 3′ splice sites, as well as branch-point sequence. Following spliceosome processing, the miRNA is released as lariat structure that first undergoes debranching followed by folding to form the pre-miRNA (Figure 60.6; Ruby *et al.*, 2007).

Pre-miRNAs are transported from the nucleus to the cytoplasm by Exportin-5 and Ran-GTP complex. In the cytoplasm, the pre-miRNAs are again processed into ~22 nt-long miRNA/miRNA* duplex by another RNAse III-type enzyme called Dicer. As in Drosha processing, Dicer processing also produces a 2 nt overhang at the 3′-end of each strand of the miRNA/miRNA* duplex. Thus, each strand of the miRNA/miRNA* duplex has a 2 nt overhang at its 3′-end (Figure 60.6).

The duplex undergoes unwinding. One of the two strands, called the guide strand (miRNA), is loaded onto a protein complex called RNA-induced silencing complex (RISC) forming miRISC. The other strand (miRNA*) is not part of the RISC; it is called the passenger strand and is degraded. Guide strand selection is driven by the thermodynamic stability of the miRNA/miRNA* duplex. The unwinding of the duplex by Dicer begins at the 5′-end of the strand that has the lowest thermodynamic stability, and this strand acts as the guide strand (Schwarz *et al.*, 2003).

The guide strand of miRNA binds to its cognate binding site of the target mRNA with a ~2 nt mismatch. The sequence specificity of miRNA guide strand for target recognition is determined by nt 2–8 of its 5′ region, and it is called the "seed sequence". Binding of multiple miRISCs at the 3′-UTR of target mRNA represses its translation, resulting in the silencing of gene expression through RNAi. Of the various proteins present in the miRISC, argonaute2 (Ago2) forms a direct complex with miRNA (as well as with siRNA, discussed below), and Ago2 has endonuclease activity. In the case of miRNAs, the short region of mismatch between the miRNA and the target mRNA prevents Ago2 from cleaving the target mRNA. However, the Ago proteins must remain tightly associated with the target mRNA to keep its translation repressed (Chu and Rana, 2007).

miRNA vs. siRNA

In the context of miRNA, it is worth mentioning the small interfering RNA (siRNA) as well. Like miRNAs, siRNAs are also double-stranded ncRNAs that regulate gene expression by RNAi. There are many common themes in the processing and biogenesis of miRNA and siRNA in the cytoplasm,

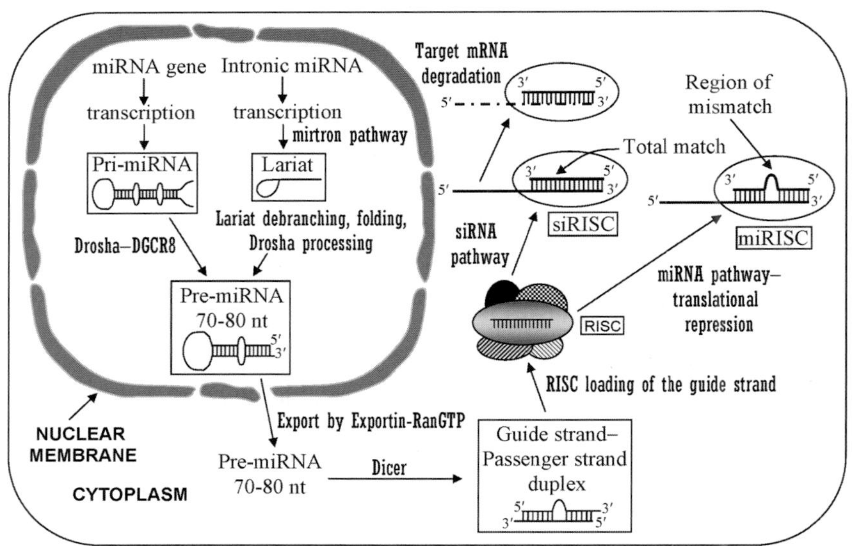

FIGURE 60.6 The pri-miRNA transcript is processed in the nucleus by Drosha–DGCR8 complex to produce a 70–80 nt-long precursor miRNA (pre-miRNA). Pre-miRNA is transported to the cytoplasm by Exportin-5 and Ran-GTP. Some pri-miRNAs that are encoded by introns are processed by spliceosome (the mirtron pathway). Following spliceosome processing, the miRNA is released as lariat structure that first undergoes debranching followed by folding to form the pre-miRNA. In the cytoplasm, the 70–80 nt-long pre-miRNA is further processed into 22 nt-long mature duplex by Dicer. From this duplex, only the guide strand is loaded onto the RISC. If there is a region of mismatch between the target mRNA and the guide strand sequences, the miRNA pathway is activated and the translation of the target mRNA is repressed. If the target mRNA and the guide strand sequences are fully complementary with no mismatch, the siRNA pathway is activated and the target mRNA is degraded.

such as cleavage of a long dsRNA to produce small dsRNA, unwinding of the RNA duplex, RISC (siRISC) loading of only one strand (guide strand), and finally the effector function on the target. However, at the effector step miRNA and siRNA diverge in terms of their mechanism of action. Whereas miRNAs suppress translation of the target mRNA, siRNAs promote the degradation of the target mRNA into pieces. Also, miRNAs bind to their cognate binding site of the target mRNA with a ~2 nt mismatch, but siRNAs bind to their target mRNAs with 100% complementarity. Because of this 100% complementarity, Ago2 which is associated with siRNA in the siRISC, cleaves the target mRNA using its endonuclease activity (Choudhuri, 2010).

siRNAs were originally identified as intermediates in the RNAi pathway after exogenous introduction of long dsRNA. Thus, siRNAs were thought to be primarily exogenous in origin, such as derived directly from virus, transposon or transgene trigger. However, it is now known that dsRNAs are found in cells, which give rise to endogenous siRNAs. dsRNAs form the genetic material of some viruses called dsRNA viruses. Endogenous dsRNAs are produced through conversion of single-stranded RNA into dsRNA by RdRP (RNA-dependent RNA polymerases), or alternatively by transcription of inverted DNA repeats by DNA-dependent RNA polymerases. Endogenous siRNAs have been reported in *C. elegans*, *Drosophila*, as well as in mammals (Ghildiyal and Zamore, 2009).

In mammalian cells, both miRNAs and siRNAs are thought to be loaded into the same RNA-induced silencing complex, where they guide mRNA degradation or translational silencing depending on the complementarity of the target. In contrast, in *Drosophila*, the formation of miRISC and siRISC involves different sets of proteins (Okamura *et al.*, 2004).

Biogenesis and function of piRNA

piRNAs (Piwi-interacting RNAs) are important from the perspective of reproduction and development because they protect the germ-line genome from the onslaught of transposable elements, thereby serving as the guardian of the germ-line genome (Choudhuri, 2009b, 2010). They occur in germ cells as well as in gonadal somatic cells. piRNAs are ~24–30 nt-long; hence slightly longer than a typical miRNA, and are associated with Piwi proteins. They have a 5′ uridine bias and a 2′-O-methylated 3′-end. piRNA genes exist in the genome in clusters that are between 1 and 100 kb long in size and encode between 10 and 4,500 piRNAs. The majority of piRNA clusters are monodirectional, i.e. within a given cluster all piRNAs are derived from one strand of DNA.

The three Piwi proteins that are essential for piRNA function in *Drosophila* are Aub (Aubergine), Piwi and Ago3, and they occur abundantly in germ-line cells. The Piwi homolog found in rat, mouse and zebrafish are called Riwi, Miwi and Ziwi, respectively. Piwi proteins are also expressed in somatic cells that are in close contact with germ-line cells. Piwi mutant animals exhibit defects in germ cell development (Aravin *et al.*, 2007).

About 17% of mammalian piRNAs map to repeat sequences, including LINEs, SINEs and several classes of DNA transposons, and nearly one million piRNA molecules have been reported per spermatocyte or round spermatid. The major sources of piRNAs are discrete heterochromatic piRNA clusters characterized by nested, fragmented and immobilized transposon remnants (Choudhuri, 2009b, 2010).

In *Drosophila*, Piwi and Aub complexes contain piRNAs antisense to a wide variety of transposons. In contrast, Ago3 associates with piRNAs strongly biased toward the sense strand of transposons. piRNAs in Ago3 overlap with piRNAs in Aub by precisely 10 nt at their 5′-ends. Also, the Ago3-bound piRNAs are strongly enriched for "A" at position 10, which is complementary to the 5′ "U" of Aub-bound piRNAs. piRNA biogenesis does not require Dicer because the precursor piRNAs are single-stranded RNAs. However, the processing enzyme that generates piRNA from precursor ssRNA has not been identified yet (Choudhuri 2009b, 2010).

Studies in *Drosophila* revealed that in germ cells and gonadal somatic cells, piRNAs apparently function through slightly different mechanisms.

In germ cells, piRNA transcripts derived from piRNA gene clusters and transcripts from active transposons interact through the action of Piwi proteins to form an adaptive cycle that amplifies piRNAs targeting active mobile genetic elements. The amplification model was termed "ping-pong model" (Brennecke *et al.*, 2007; Gunawardane *et al.*, 2007). According to this model, antisense piRNAs bind to Piwi/Aub and this complex cleaves the sense transposon transcripts (between nucleotides 10 and 11 from the 5′-end) to create sense piRNAs. The sense piRNAs thus generated associate with Ago3 and this complex directs the cleavage of the antisense transcripts, creating antisense piRNAs, which in turn bind to Piwi/Aub. The combination of these steps forms a self-amplifying cycle, and it continues as long as secondary piRNAs are able to recognize and cleave their targets (Figure 60.7).

In gonadal somatic cells, such as follicular cells in the ovary, an Ago3-independent but Piwi-dependent second pathway exists for piRNA biogenesis, as demonstrated in *Drosophila* (Li *et al.*, 2009; Malone *et al.*, 2009). Most of the transposons targeted by this second pathway reside in the *flamenco* piRNA cluster, which was first identified as a repressor of transposon expression in somatic follicular cells. Unlike germ cell-specific piRNAs that contain the ping-pong signatures, somatic cell-specific piRNAs do not contain such ping-pong signatures. In gonadal somatic cells, piRNAs derived from the *flamenco* locus are antisense because they are derived from the plus strand (sense strand) of DNA. These antisense piRNAs can effectively silence target sequences in the absence of an amplification mechanism, such as silencing of transposons like *gypsy*, *ZAM*, *idefix* in somatic follicular cells.

Examples of some epigenetic phenomena

Some epigenetic phenomena that have been well studied are transvection; genomic imprinting; X-chromosome inactivation; paramutation; and heterochromatin spread and position effect variegation. For a brief discussion of these phenomena, see Choudhuri (2009a).

Epigenetic regulation in reproduction and development

The effects of various environmental factors during gestation as well as after birth can bring about epigenetic changes that may have far-reaching consequences in the offspring. These

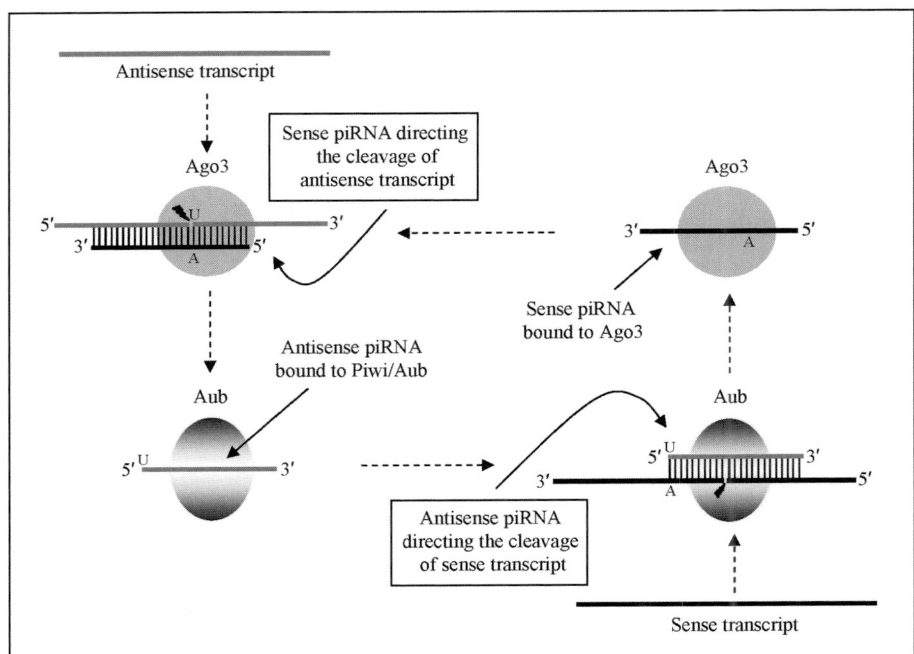

FIGURE 60.7 The ping-pong model of piRNA action for the neutralization of transposons. Precursor sense piRNA transcripts produced from the piRNA gene cluster are cleaved by Piwi/Aub to generate sense piRNAs that associate with Ago3. When encountering a complementary (antisense) target, such as a transposon mRNA, the Ago3-sense piRNA complex directs the cleavage of these antisense transcripts, creating antisense piRNAs. Antisense piRNAs thus generated bind to Piwi/Aub, and the Piwi/Aub-antisense piRNA complex guides the cleavage of more sense target transposon transcripts to further generate sense piRNAs. The combination of these steps forms a self-amplifying loop ("ping-pong"). (Figure reproduced with permission from Choudhuri, 2009b.)

environmental factors range from maternal nutrition during gestation to environmental toxicants.

The influence of epigenetic changes in the prenatal environment may begin as early as in the preimplantation embryo (following fertilization) through the time before birth. Epigenetic changes caused by *in utero* exposure to environmental factors, such as nutritional factors, environmental toxicants, or factors related to lifestyle (such as tobacco smoke, alcohol, chemical carcinogens, infectious agents, UV radiation) can induce alterations in gene expression that may persist throughout life, as well as across multiple generations (Herceg, 2007).

Following fertilization, the parental genomes first undergo demethylation; this is followed by remethylation and reestablishment of the original methylation pattern. *De novo* DNA methylation begins after the formation of the blastocyst. In the blastocyst, the cells that comprise the inner cell mass (ICM) display higher levels of methylation compared to the trophectoderm. For example, pluripotent cells in the ICM show extensive H3K27 methylation, but in the trophectoderm, H3K27 methylation is only detected on the inactive X chromosome. Interestingly, methylation at imprinted loci in oocytes appears to be tied to the methylation status of H3K4. Demethylation of H3K4 plays an important role in establishing imprints during development of the oocyte. Following fertilization, the paternal genome first hyperacetylates histone H4. Subsequently, maternal genome also acetylates both H3 and H4 at several lysine residues (Corry *et al.*, 2009). Obviously, environmental factors that interfere with such normal cycles of epigenetic changes can disrupt the normal developmental process.

The effect of intrauterine environment on the epigenetic state of the genome of the developing embryo continues after fertilization, implantation and through embryogenesis. It was shown that feeding a protein-deficient unbalanced diet to rats during pregnancy caused epigenetic changes in the offspring. This was demonstrated by a ~21–22% lower CpG methylation in the hepatic PPAR-α and glucocorticoid receptor (GR) gene promoters in the offspring, compared to controls (Lillycrop *et al.*, 2005). Gene methylation was determined by methylation-sensitive PCR and mRNA expression was studied by semi-quantitative RT-PCR. Expectedly, lower methylation was associated with the upregulation of both PPAR-α and GR genes. Burdge *et al.* (2007) found that the altered methylation state of PPAR-α and GR promoters can persist through F_2 generation even if F_1 offspring are fed normal diet. The observation on the persistence of undernutrition-induced epigenetic marks in rats for two generations was also corroborated in monkeys (Bertram *et al.*, 2008).

Just as the undernutrition of the mother during pregnancy can cause epigenetic changes in the offspring, overnutrition of the pregnant mother (fed high fat diet) can also cause epigenetic changes in the offsprings. Aagaard-Tillery *et al.* (2008) observed that chronic consumption of high fat diet (35% fat, whereas 13% fat in controls) by mother resulted in significant hyperacetylation of H3K14 in fetal hepatic tissues, and somewhat increased acetylation of H3K9 and H3K18 as well, as revealed by chromatin immunoprecipitation (ChIP) with differential display PCR. The offspring of the obese monkeys were also obese. When the fat content of the diets was altered during pregnancy, maternal obesity was still maintained but the epigenetic changes in offspring were no longer present. Microarray analysis showed that the expression of genes (such as *GPT2*, *Rdh12*, *Npas2*, *Hsp* and *DNAJ2*) involved in metabolism and associated response showed appreciable increase.

Postnatal environmental factors may be as varied as parental care to environmental toxicants. An important role of parental care in shaping up the postnatal epigenome and adulthood behavior was reported in both rats and humans. The degree of licking and grooming (LG), and arched-back nursing (ABN) by the mother (equivalent to different degrees of motherly love and care) during the postnatal period was found to affect behavioral pattern during adulthood through epigenetic modifications of the genome early in life. Differential maternal care was found to result in differences in DNA methylation in the regulatory region of the *glucocorticoid receptor* (*GR*) gene in the hippocampus (GR is involved in stress regulation, and hippocampus is rich in GR); higher methylation was found in pups that received less maternal care and these pups grew into irritable adults, whereas lower methylation was found in pups that received greater maternal care and they grew into calmer adults. A causal relationship was strongly suggested by the fact that these differences emerged over the first week of life, could be reversed with cross-fostering, persisted into adulthood, and were associated with altered histone acetylation and transcription factor (NGFI-A) binding to the GR gene promoter. Significantly higher histone H3K9 acetylation and three-fold higher NGFI-A binding to the hippocampal *GR* gene promoter was found in the adult offsprings that received greater maternal care as pups (Weaver *et al.*, 2004).

A similar observation was made by the same group in human suicide victims. The suicide victims had experienced childhood abuse, which caused an alteration in methylation status in the neuron-specific *GR* gene (*NR3C1*). The authors found increased methylation of the *NR3C1* gene promoter, and concomitant decrease in gene expression resulting in decreased levels of *NR3C1* mRNA. Sequencing of the *NR3C1* gene promoter revealed identical sequence in all subjects, thereby eliminating the possible contribution of nucleotide sequence variations with differential gene expression outcomes (McGowan *et al.*, 2008, 2009).

The similar findings in humans and rats strongly suggest that psychological trauma and recurring negative experiences very early in childhood determine the behavioral pattern in adulthood, and the molecular underpinning of such behavior pattern lies in epigenetic alterations of specific genes (such as the *GR* gene) and their consequent altered expression pattern. These findings also provide clues to how two genetically identical backgrounds can produce different phenotypic outcomes on exposure to different environments.

Developmental toxicity can also be modulated by miRNAs. STS (sodium thiosulfate) is potentially hazardous to human health, especially during embryogenesis. Using zebrafish as a model, Hu *et al.* (2009) studied the expression pattern of brain- and muscle-specific miRNAs detected by whole-mount *in situ* hybridization. The authors found that STS caused developmental abnormalities that resulted in multiple organ malformations. Embryos were more sensitive to STS at 48 hours post-fertilization. STS treatment also resulted in differential expression of miR-124a and miR-133a in the treated embryos. The authors concluded that miR-124a and miR-133a are involved in STS-induced developmental toxicity. This conclusion was based on the observed correlation between the altered miRNA expression profile and the induction of toxicity. Nevertheless, such preliminary findings can be used to design additional studies to investigate potential cause-and-effect relationship (Choudhuri, 2010).

CONCLUDING REMARKS AND FUTURE DIRECTIONS

That the genomic template is not the final be-all-end-all determinant of phenotypic outcome is illustrated by polyphenism. Polyphenism (environmental polymorphism) represents a phenomenon of developmental (and phenotypic) plasticity in which two or more discontinuous phenotypes can be produced in the population in response to environmental cues, such as light, temperature, predator and other factors. For example, *Daphnia* develops sharp head spines in the presence of predators in the environment, but in the absence of predators head spines do not develop. Another example is the honey bee. In honey bees, exclusive exposure to royal jelly during the larval stage induces a queen morph, whereas exposure to other foods induces the worker morph. The phenotypic plasticity observed in polyphenism takes place against the background of a single (same) genomic template in the population. Although an epigenetic basis for polyphenism is yet to be investigated, the phenomenon of polyphenism itself demonstrates that it is the orchestration and regulation of genome expression by environmental cues that contributes to the diversity of phenotypic outcomes. It is tempting to speculate that polyphenism may have a distinct epigenetic component that can orchestrate the environmentally induced temporal regulation of gene expression. Because epigenetic marks can be acquired over a period of time during the life of an individual and then passed on to the offspring, it has brought back Lamarckian flavor to biology. Once established, epigenetic marks can be transmitted to the offspring, and it is this transgenerational persistence of epigenetic changes and its potential impact that make the study of environmental effects on epigenetic regulation an important aspect of environmental and molecular toxicological studies.

Despite recent progress in understanding various molecular aspects of epigenetic regulation of gene expression, a large number of the observed epigenetic changes in various studies have not been functionally linked to observed downstream events. Establishing a cause-and-effect relationship between xenobiotic exposure, epigenetic changes and physiological/pathological consequences becomes further confounded by the fact that epigenetic changes can be acquired over a period of time during the life of an organism. Documented associations between exposure to carcinogens, DNA methylation and the onset of cancers have not always led to any mechanistic insight (Issa, 2004). Also, the differences in global CpG island methylation patterns between normal and cancer cells remain poorly understood (Toyota and Issa, 1999). Thus, even if specific epigenetic changes can be linked to downstream pathological events, it still remains unclear whether there is a temporal switch, or a threshold of epigenetic changes or specific combinations of epigenetic changes (epigenetic code) needed to trigger downstream events leading to specific pathological states. In many instances, an environmental chemical may have paradoxical epigenetic effects. For example, As and Ni deplete cellular SAM levels, reduce DNMT activity and cause global hypomethylation, which can all be mechanistically linked. However, at the same time, they also cause hypermethylation of specific gene promoters. Similarly, acute Cd exposure results in DNA hypomethylation and decreased DNMT activity, whereas chronic Cd exposure results in

DNA hypermethylation and increased DNMT activity. The molecular regulation of such paradoxical effects remains to be explained (Choudhuri *et al.*, 2010b).

From the available evidence, it is also tempting to speculate that chemoepigenomics may help yield more meaningful predictive data. Just as chemogenomics (or chemical genomics) is defined as the study of the effects of chemicals on cell function at the genome level, chemoepigenomics (or chemical epigenomics) can be defined as the study of the effects of chemicals on cell function at the epigenome level. The proof-of-concept for such an approach was successfully demonstrated in the context of genomics, in which gene expression data were used to build a "connectivity map" that connects small molecules, genes, biological pathways and disease (Lamb *et al.*, 2006). Similarly, if chemicals/xenobiotics can be organized by structural, functional or target classes so that their effects on the epigenetic changes can be studied to find out whether structure-specific, function-specific or target-specific epigenetic signatures exist, then that information can be integrated to develop tools that may help predict more accurately the relationships among small molecules, their epigenetic effects and the biological pathways affected by such epigenetic perturbations.

REFERENCES

Aagaard-Tillery KM, Grove K, Bishop J, Ke X, Fu Q, McKnight R, Lane RH (2008) Developmental origins of disease and determinants of chromatin structure: maternal diet modifies the primate fetal epigenome. *J Mol Endocrinol* **41:** 91–102.

Alilat M, Sivolob A, Révet B, Prunell A (1999) Nucleosome dynamics. Protein and DNA contributions in the chiral transition of the tetrasome, the histone (H3-H4)2 tetramer-DNA particle. *J Mol Biol* **291:** 815–41.

Aravin AA, Hannon GJ, Brennecke J (2007) The piwi-piRNA pathway provides an adaptive defense in the transposon arms race. *Science* **318:** 761–4.

Bertram C, Khan O, Ohri S, Phillips DI, Matthews SG, Hanson MA (2008) Transgenerational effects of prenatal nutrient restriction on cardiovascular and hypothalamic–pituitary–adrenal function. *J Physiol* **586:** 2217–29.

Borchert GM, Lanier W, Davidson BL (2006) RNA polymerase III transcribes human microRNAs. *Nat Struct Mol Biol* **13:** 1097–101.

Brennecke J, Aravin AA, Stark A, Dus M, Kellis M, Sachidanandam R, Hannon GJ (2007) Discrete small RNA-generating loci as master regulators of transposon activity in *Drosophila*. *Cell* **128:** 1089–103.

Burdge GC, Slater-Jefferies J, Torrens C, Phillips ES, Hanson MA, Lillycrop KA (2007) Dietary protein restriction of pregnant rats in the F0 generation induces altered methylation of hepatic gene promoters in the adult male offspring in the F1 and F2 generations. *Br J Nutr* **97:** 435–9.

Choudhuri S (2009a) Epigenetic regulation of gene and genome expression. In *Genomics: Fundamentals and Applications* (Choudhuri S, Carlson DB, eds.). Informa Healthcare, NY, pp. 101–28.

Choudhuri S (2009b) Lesser known relatives of miRNA. *Biochim Biophys Res Commun* **388:** 177–80.

Choudhuri S (2010) Small non-coding RNAs: biogenesis, function and emerging significance in toxicology. *J Biochem Mol Toxicol* **24:** 195–216.

Choudhuri S, Cui Y, Klaassen CD (2010) Molecular targets of epigenetic regulation and effectors of environmental influences. *Toxicol Appl Pharmacol* **245:** 378–93.

Chu CY, Rana TM (2007) Small RNAs: regulators and guardians of the genome. *J Cell Physiol* **213:** 412–19.

Corry GN, Tanasijevic B, Barry ER, Krueger W, Rasmussen TP (2009) Epigenetic regulatory mechanisms during preimplantation development. *Birth Defects Res (Part C)* **87:** 297–313.

Dawson MA, Bannister AJ, Göttgens B, Foster SD, Bartke T, Green AR, Kouzarides T (2009) JAK2 phosphorylates histone H3Y41 and excludes HP1alpha from chromatin. *Nature* **461:** 819–22.

Fuks F, Hurd PJ, Wolf D, Nan X, Bird AP, Kouzarides T (2003) The methyl-CpG binding protein MeCP2 links DNA methylation to histone methylation. *J Biol Chem* **278:** 4035–40.

Furuyama T, Henikoff S (2009) Centromeric nucleosomes induce positive DNA supercoils. *Cell* **138:** 104–13.

Garcia-Dominguez M, Reyes JC (2009) SUMO association with repressor complexes, emerging routes for transcriptional control. *Biochim Biophys Acta* **1789:** 451–9.

Ghildiyal M, Zamore PD (2009) Small silencing RNAs: an expanding universe. *Nat Rev Genet* **10:** 94–108.

Ginder GD, Gnanapragasam MN, Mian, OY (2008) The role of the epigenetic signal, DNA methylation, in gene regulation during erythroid development. *Curr Top Dev Biol* **82:** 85–116.

Goldberg AD, Allis CD, Bernstein E (2007) Epigenetics: a landscape takes shape. *Cell* **128:** 635–8.

Gunawardane LS, Saito K, Nishida KM, Miyoshi K, Kawamura Y, Nagami T, Siomi H, Siomi MC (2007) A slicer-mediated mechanism for repeat-associated siRNA 5′-end formation in *Drosophila*. *Science* **315:** 1587–90.

Herceg Z (2007) Epigenetics and cancer: towards an evaluation of the impact of environmental and dietary factors. *Mutagenesis* **22:** 91–103.

Hu W, Cheng L, Xia H, Sun D, Li D, Li P, Song Y, Ma X (2009) Teratogenic effects of sodium thiosulfate on developing zebrafish embryos. *Front Biosci* **14:** 3680–7.

Issa JP (2004) CpG island methylator phenotype in cancer. *Nat Rev Cancer* **4:** 988–93.

Ito T, Tyler JK, Kadonaga JT (1997) Chromatin assembly factors: a dual function in nucleosome formation and mobilization? *Genes Cells* **2:** 593–600.

Jones PA, Liang G (2009) Rethinking how DNA methylation patterns are maintained. *Nat Rev Genet* **10:** 805–11.

Lagos-Quintana M, Rauhut R, Lendeckel W, Tuschl T (2001) Identification of novel genes coding for small expressed RNAs. *Science* **294:** 853–8.

Lamb J, Crawford ED, Peck D, Modell JW, Blat IC, Wrobel MJ, Lerner J, Brunet JP, Subramanian A, Ross KN, Reich M, Hieronymus H, Wei G, Armstrong SA, Haggarty SJ, Clemons PA, Wei R, Carr SA, Lander ES, Golub TR (2006) The Connectivity Map: using gene-expression signatures to connect small molecules, genes, and disease. *Science* **313:** 1929–35.

Lau NC, Lim LP, Weinstein EG, Bartel DP (2001) An abundant class of tiny RNAs with probable regulatory roles in *Caenorhabditis elegans*. *Science* **294:** 858–62.

Lee RC, Ambros V (2001) An extensive class of small RNAs in *Caenorhabditis elegans*. *Science* **294:** 862–4.

Lee RC, Feinbaum RL, Ambros V (1993) The *C. elegans* heterochronic gene *lin-4* encodes small RNAs with antisense complementarity to *lin-14*. *Cell* **75:** 843–54.

Li C, Vagin VV, Lee S, Xu J, Ma S, Xi H, Seitz H, Horwich MD, Syrzycka M, Honda BM, Kittler EL, Zapp ML, Klattenhoff C, Schulz N, Theurkauf WE, Weng Z, Zamore PD (2009) Collapse of germline piRNAs in the absence of Argonaute3 reveals somatic piRNAs in flies. *Cell* **137:** 509–21.

Li E, Bird AP (2007) DNA methylation in mammals. In *Epigenetics* (Allis CD, Jenuwein T, Reinberg D, eds.). CSHL Press, Cold Spring Harbor, NY, pp. 341–56.

Lillycrop KA, Phillips ES, Jackson AA, Hanson MA, Burdge GC (2005) Dietary protein restriction of pregnant rats induces and folic acid supplementation prevents epigenetic modification of hepatic gene expression in the offspring. *J Nutr* **135:** 1382–6.

Malone CD, Brennecke J, Dus M, Stark A, McCombie WR, Sachidanandam R, Hannon GJ (2009) Specialized piRNA pathways act in germline and somatic tissues of the *Drosophila* ovary. *Cell* **137:** 522–35.

McGowan PO, Sasaki A, D'Alessio AC, Dymov S, Labonté B, Szyf M, Turecki G, Meaney MJ (2009) Epigenetic regulation of the glucocorticoid receptor in human brain associates with childhood abuse. *Nat Neurosci* **12:** 342–8.

McGowan PO, Sasaki A, Huang TC, Unterberger A, Suderman M, Ernst C, Meaney MJ, Turecki G, Szyf M (2008) Promoter-wide hypermethylation of the ribosomal RNA gene promoter in the suicide brain. *PLoS One* **3:** e2085.

Morris JR, Chen J-L, Geyer PK (1998) Two modes of transvection: enhancer action in *trans* and bypass of a chromatin insulator in *cis*. *Proc Natl Acad Sci USA* **95:** 10740–5.

Nan X, Campoy FJ, Bird A (1997) MeCP2 is a transcriptional repressor with abundant binding sites in genomic chromatin. *Cell* **88:** 471–81.

Nan X, Ng HH, Johnson CA, Laherty CD, Turner BM, Eisenman RN, Bird A (1998) Transcriptional repression by the methyl-CpG-binding protein MeCP2 involves a histone deacetylase complex. *Nature* **393:** 386–9.

Okamura K, Ishizuka A, Siomi H, Siomi MC (2004) Distinct roles for Argonaute proteins in small RNA-directed RNA cleavage pathways. *Genes Dev* **18:** 1655–66.

Parthun MR (2007) Hat1: the emerging cellular roles of a type B histone acetyltransferase. *Oncogene* **26:** 5319–28.

Pasquinelli AE, Reinhart BJ, Slack F, Martindale MQ, Kuroda MI, Maller B, Hayward DC, Ball EE, Degnan B, Müller P, Spring J, Srinivasan A, Fishman M, Finnerty J, Corbo J, Levine M, Leahy P, Davidson E, Ruvkun G (2000) Conservation of the sequence and temporal expression of let-7 heterochronic regulatory RNA. *Nature* **408:** 86–9.

Reinhart BJ, Slack FJ, Basson M, Squinelli AE, Bettinger JC, Rougvie AE, Horvitz HR, Ruvkun G (2000) The 21-nucleotide *let-7* RNA regulates developmental timing in *Caenorhabditis elegans*. *Nature* **403:** 901–6.

Riggs AD, Martienssen RA, Russo, VEA (1996) Introduction. In *Epigenetic Mechanisms of Gene Regulation* (Russo VEA, *et al.* eds.). CSHL Press, Cold Spring Harbor, NY, pp. 1–4.

Ruby JG, Jan CH, Bartel DP (2007) Intronic microRNA precursors that bypass Drosha processing. *Nature* **448:** 83–6.

Schwarz DS, Hutvágner G, Du T, Xu Z, Aronin N, Zamore PD (2003) Asymmetry in the assembly of the RNAi enzyme complex. *Cell* **115**: 199–208.

Scully R (2010) A histone code for DNA repair. *Nat Rev Mol Cell Biol* **11:** 164.

Shiio Y, Eisenman RN (2003) Histone sumoylation is associated with transcriptional repression. *Proc Natl Acad Sci USA* **100:** 13225–30.

Strahl BD, Allis CD (2000) The language of covalent histone modifications. *Nature* **403**: 41–5.

Toyota M, Issa JP (1999) CpG island methylator phenotypes in aging and cancer. *Semin Cancer Biol* **9:** 349–57.

Tyler JK (2002) Chromatin assembly. Cooperation between histone chaperones and ATP-dependent nucleosome remodeling machines. *Eur J Biochem* **269:** 2268–74.

Vakoc CR, Mandat SA, Olenchock BA, Blobel GA (2005) Histone H3 lysine 9 methylation and HP1gamma are associated with transcription elongation through mammalian chromatin. *Mol Cell* **19:** 381–91.

Vermeulen M, Mulder KW, Denissov S, Pijnappel WW, van Schaik FM, Varier RA, Baltissen MP, Stunnenberg HG, Mann M, Timmers HT (2007) Selective anchoring of TFIID to nucleosomes by trimethylation of histone H3 lysine 4. *Cell* **131:** 58–69.

Verreault A (2000) De novo nucleosome assembly: new pieces in an old puzzle. *Genes Dev* **14:** 1430–8.

Wakefield RI, Smith BO, Nan X, Free A, Soteriou A, Uhrin D, Bird AP, Barlow PN (1999) The solution structure of the domain from MeCP2 that binds to methylated DNA. *J Mol Biol* **291:** 1055–65.

Weaver IC, Cervoni N, Champagne FA, D'Alessio AC, Sharma S, Seckl JR, Dymov S, Szyf M, Meaney MJ (2004) Epigenetic programming by maternal behavior. *Nat Neurosci* **7:** 847–54.

Whitehouse I, Flaus A, Havas K, Owen-Hughes T (2000) Mechanisms for ATP-dependent chromatin remodelling. *Biochem Soc Trans* **28:** 376–9.

Williams A, Spilianakis CG, Flavell RA (2010) Interchromosomal association and gene regulation in *trans*. *Trends Genet* **26:** 188–97.

Wolffe AP, Hayes JJ (1999) Chromatin disruption and modification. *Nucleic Acids Res* **27:** 711–20.

C H A P T E R

61

Mitochondrial dysfunction in reproductive and developmental toxicity

Carlos M. Palmeira and João Ramalho-Santos

INTRODUCTION

In the evolution of eukaryotic cells, mitochondria have for a long time played a prominent role. Nowadays, progress in understanding the structure and function of mitochondria highlighted their integration into a number of cell activities, for example their dynamic behavior as subcellular organelles within a cell and during cell division being a major focus of attention. Besides energy production, mitochondria make an integral contribution to the regulation of several aspects of cell biology such as molecular metabolism, redox status, calcium signaling and programmed cell death (Schatz, 1995). Mitochondria represent one of the main targets of xenobiotic-induced bioenergetic failure (Wallace and Starkov, 2000; Palmeira and Rolo, 2004). It is therefore not surprising that mitochondrial dysfunction can cause cell death through ATP depletion and calcium dysregulation (Di Lisa and Bernardi, 1998). However, the picture is more complex owing to the role played in cell death by proteins released from mitochondria such as cytochrome *c* (Liu *et al.*, 1996) and apoptosis-inducing factor (AIF) (Lorenzo *et al.*, 1999).

MITOCHONDRIAL STRUCTURE

Each mammalian cell contains several hundred to more than a thousand mitochondria, which occupy up to 25% of the volume of the cytoplasm. Mitochondria are among the largest organelles in the cell. Although there is a wide variability in number and morphology (both size and shape) of mitochondria, depending on the cell type, fundamental properties are shared by all tissues. Mitochondria have a double membrane. The outer membrane separates the mitochondrion from the cytosol and defines the smooth outer perimeter of the mitochondrion. The inner membrane is invaginated to form the cristae that protrude and define the matrix of the organelle. Soluble enzymes such as those of the tricarboxylic acid cycle and the β-oxidation pathway are located in the matrix. In recent years, important new insights into the internal organization of the mitochondria have been made (Frey and Manella, 2000; Scheffler, 2001). Cristae are not simple invaginations of the inner membrane, but independent structures that are not always connected with the inner membrane and have an extensively tubular nature. Moreover, the appearance of the cristae is variable with tissues. Tissues requiring periods of higher respiratory activity tend to have a greater surface area of cristae. The outer membrane is permeable to ions and solutes up to 10 kDa, whereas the inner membrane is highly proteinaceous and serves as a permeability barrier. This exceptional low non-specific permeability to protons and other charged solutions, regulated and mediated by proteins, is essential for mitochondrial function. The inner mitochondrial membrane differs from other cellular membranes, since proteins make up to 80% of the inner mitochondrial membrane compared to 50% for most membranes. Some proteins are loosely attached to the surface of the membranes and others are embedded as an integral part of the membrane. The lipid composition of the inner membrane is also unique due to the large content in cardiolipin (diphosphatidylglycerol). The presence of cardiolipin reduces the permeability of the phospholipid bilayer to protons and thus enables a proton-motive force to be established across the inner membrane. Damage to cardiolipin can be particularly detrimental to the mitochondria, because this lipid also plays a critical role in the function of mitochondrial proteins, such as cytochrome *c* oxidase (complex IV) and the adenine nucleotide transporter (ANT) (Paradies *et al.*, 1998). In contrast, the outer membrane is rich in cholesterol and is composed of about half lipid and half protein. The voltage-dependent anion channel (also known as porin, VDAC) is the most abundant protein in the outer mitochondrial membrane and is thought to be a primary pathway for the movement across this membrane (for review see Blachly-Dyson and Forte, 2001). Associated with the outer membrane we also find mitochondrial hexokinase and creatine kinase. Multi-subunit complexes present in both membranes (TIM/TOM complex) mediate the translocation of peptides into mitochondria (for review see Paschen and Neupert, 2001). In the inner mitochondrial membrane, besides the components of the respiratory chain and ATP synthase (Hatefi, 1985), many other proteins are present such as the dicarboxylate and

Reproductive and Developmental Toxicology, Edited by Ramesh C. Gupta
ISBN: 978-0-12-382032-7

tricarboxylate carriers, the phosphate carrier, the ANT and uncoupling proteins.

Among the organelles of animal cells, mitochondria are unique in that they contain their own genome, transcription and translation systems, located in the mitochondrial matrix (Taanman, 1999). However, most of the proteins that reside in the mitochondrion are nuclear gene products. Mitochondrially encoded subunits of components of the respiratory chain (I, III and IV) or ATP synthase (Anderson *et al.*, 1981) are assembled with peptides synthesized in the cytoplasm to produce the functional complexes (Poyton and McEwen, 1996). Gene expression in mitochondria and the nucleus are regulated by environmental and developmental signals, so as to confer on mitochondria the ability to adjust their energy production to meet different energy demands of the cell. Mutations of the mitochondrial DNA have wide-ranging consequences for mitochondrial respiration and bioenergetics, originating cell death and dysfunction as a major aspect to the pathophysiology of mitochondrial DNA diseases (Moraes, 1996; Smeitink *et al.*, 2001; Reinecke *et al.*, 2009).

MITOCHONDRIA AND ENERGY PRODUCTION: OXIDATIVE PHOSPHORYLATION

The inner mitochondrial membrane transduces energy through oxidative phosphorylation, the main process responsible for the production of energy in the form of ATP in eukaryotic cells (Saraste, 1999). The entire general sequence of biochemical events leading to ATP synthesis has been known since Mitchell proposed his chemiosmotic theory (Mitchell, 1966). It elegantly described how mitochondrial respiration creates an electrochemical gradient of protons across the mitochondrial inner membrane, which in turn drives ATP synthesis through the mitochondrial ATP synthase. However, the way in which the oxidative phosphorylation system is regulated in intact tissues still remains a matter of debate. Besides ATP production, other mitochondrial activities that require energy, such as electrophoretic or protonophoric transport of ions, metabolic substrates and proteins for the mitochondrial matrix, are supported by the primary form of energy generated in mitochondria, the electrochemical proton gradient. Interference with the generation of the electrochemical proton gradient or its induced dissipation affects mitochondrial bioenergetics. The initial event of energy conservation is charge separation at the inner mitochondrial membrane. The electrochemical proton gradient is generated by means of electrogenic pumping of protons, from the mitochondrial matrix to the intermembrane space, which is catalyzed by the respiratory chain complexes. Electrons deriving from oxidation of substrates are funneled through the redox carriers of the respiratory chain (for review see Esposti and Ghelli, 1994). This process is coupled to proton ejection at complexes I (NADH:ubiquinone reductase), III (ubiquinol:cytochrome *c* reductase or bc_1-complex) and IV (cytochrome *c* oxidase). The final electron acceptor is molecular oxygen, which through four electron reduction is converted to water. The succession of electron transfer occurs in the following sequence: complex I – ubiquinone – complex III – cytochrome *c* – complex IV – O_2. The amplitude of the electrochemical proton gradient, which is known as respiratory control, regulates the overall rate of electron transport in the respiratory chain.

Ubiquinone is a mobile electron carrier, dissolved in the lipid phase of the membrane, and interacts specifically with complexes I and III (Trumpower, 1990). Succinate dehydrogenase receives electrons from succinate (of the tricarboxylic acid cycle), through the oxidation of $FADH_2$, reducing ubiquinone to ubiquinol. Cytochrome *c*, a mobile protein attached to the cytosolic face of the inner mitochondrial membrane, serves as an electron carrier between complexes III and IV. Energy released from the oxidation of substrates in the matrix is used to reduce NAD^+ and ubiquinone, originating NADH and ubiquinol. NADH is oxidized by complex I, which is composed of more than 40 polypeptides, seven of which are encoded in the mitochondrial genome. Complex I contains a prosthetic flavin mononucleotide and six Fe-S centers. It also contains a binding site for ubiquinone that receives reducing equivalents in steps of one electron forming transient semiquinone radicals. Rotenone is a lipophilic pesticide that binds with high affinity to complex I, specifically inhibiting its catalytic activity, that is, it inhibits the transfer of electrons from complex I to ubiquinone (for review see Esposti, 1998). Since this is the main entry point of the respiratory chain, inhibition of complex I blocks most of the oxidative metabolic reactions conducted by mitochondria. Complex III oxidizes the reduced ubiquinol, being the second entry point of the respiratory chain. Antimycin A inhibits the transfer of electrons from complex II to cytochrome *c*. Cytochrome *b*, one Fe-S protein and a hydrophobic cytochrome c_1 are the main polypeptides that anchor the redox centers. Complex IV (three subunits encoded by mitochondrial DNA) is inhibited by cyanide; $NO^{\bullet}$ inhibits complex IV in a reversible way, through competition with O_2. Complex IV uses more than 90% of the oxygen taken up by the cell (Figure 61.1).

The terminal reduction of O_2 is processed in two steps: (1) transient formations of oxide anions (O^{2-}) in the active site of the enzyme; and (2) the reaction of O^{2-} with matrix protons, promoting the formation of H_2O. This two-step reaction avoids the formation of superoxide radical anion ($O_2{\bullet}^-$), since there is no release of partially reduced oxygen species because of the high binding affinity of cytochrome *c* oxidase. However, during normal metabolism, about 1–5% of the 90% of oxygen is converted into superoxide. The production of toxic reactive oxygen species is significantly increased with inhibition of complex III or IV. The reduction of O_2 to H_2O also induces matrix alkalinization, which helps to establish the transmembrane electrochemical proton gradient. The electrochemical proton gradient, which forms the so-called protonmotive force (Δp), consists of the electrical membrane potential ($\Delta\Psi$) and the pH gradient (ΔpH), across the inner mitochondrial membrane. The magnitude of the electrochemical proton gradient is about −220 mV, and under physiological conditions most of the gradient is in the form of the $\Delta\Psi$ (for review see Azzone *et al.*, 1984). Because the matrix side of the inner mitochondrial membrane is negatively charged and slightly alkaline, mitochondria can accumulate large amounts of positively charged lipophilic compounds and some acids. Complex V or ATP synthase uses the electrochemical proton gradient as the driving force to synthesize ATP from ADP and phosphate (Mitchell, 1966; Abrahams *et al.*, 1994; Capaldi and Aggeler, 2002). Complex V can also operate in reverse, as a proton-translocating ATPase. The ATP synthase complex consists of two assemblies, with a variety of polypeptide subunits (only two encoded by mitochondrial DNA). The extrinsic F_1 contains the catalytic sites. The membrane assembly F_o is a proton channel, specifically inhibited by oligomycin. The

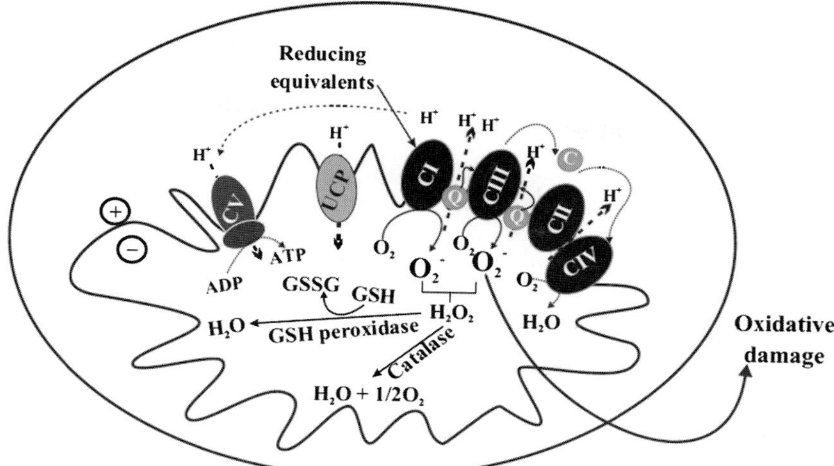

FIGURE 61.1 Electron transport chain ROS generation by mitochondria and dissipation of the proton gradient by UCPs. Scavenging by antioxidant defenses is insufficient to prevent oxidative stress. CI, complex I; CII, complex II; CIII, complex III; CIV, complex IV; CV, ATPsynthase; TCA, tricarboxylic acid cycle; UCP, uncoupling protein.

return of protons through F_o activates the catalytic sites in F_1 to phosphorylate ADP. The rate of mitochondrial ATP synthesis is regulated by alterations in the ATP/ADP ratio (phosphorylation potential) and the $NADH/NAD^+$ ratio (redox potential) (Erecinska and Wilson, 1982).

MITOCHONDRIA, REACTIVE OXYGEN SPECIES (ROS) AND OXIDATIVE STRESS

Generation of reactive, incompletely reduced forms of oxygen (superoxide ($O_2^{\bullet -}$), hydrogen peroxide (H_2O_2), hydroxyl radical ($HO^\bullet$), singlet oxygen ($^1O_2$)) may contribute to the pathophysiology of many diseases (Cadet and Brannock, 1998; Schapira, 1999; Kowaltowski *et al.*, 2009). Mitochondria are an important source of such reactive oxygen species (ROS), being particularly susceptible to damage according to an endogenous and continuous physiological process under aerobic conditions (Boveris and Chance, 1973; Turrens, 1997). Mitochondrial ROS formation occurs in living cells and can contribute to lethal cell injury, since ROS may lead to the oxidative damage of virtually any molecule. This occurs with an excessive accumulation of ROS. Besides being generated in the sequence of a number of metabolic reactions, ROS are also produced in response to various stimuli. ROS are involved in different physiological processes, as mediators in signal transduction pathways activating proteins, or as signaling messengers to activate transcription factors and inducing gene expression (Groeger *et al.*, 2009). Endoplasmic reticulum and nuclear membranes also contain electron transport chains that can lose electrons and generate superoxide radicals. Some fatty acid metabolites, such as those derived from arachidonic acid by the lipoxygenase pathway, are also ROS.

The respiratory chain may produce ROS at complexes I and III (Takeshige and Minakami, 1979; Turrens *et al.*, 1985). Specifically, the ubiquinone site in complex III appears as the major site of mitochondrial ROS production through the conversion of molecular oxygen to the superoxide anion radical ($O_2^{\bullet -}$) by a single electron transfer. Moreover, the inhibition of the respiratory chain, owing to a lack of oxygen or to an inhibitor such as cyanide or antimycin A, increases the ubisemiquinone free radical level in the normal catalytic mechanism of complex III (Turrens *et al.*, 1985). $O_2^{\bullet -}$ is described as a "weak" radical, moderately reactive in aqueous solutions. Enzymatic dismutation by superoxide dismutase (SOD) controls the levels of $O_2^{\bullet -}$ and produces H_2O_2. H_2O_2 is also a weak oxidizing agent and not very reactive (Zhang *et al.*, 1990). However, in the presence of metals (Fe^{2+} or Cu^+), a reductive homolytic cleavage of H_2O_2 produces the highly oxidative and cytotoxic hydroxyl radical ($HO^\bullet$). This highly reactive radical has been shown to play a larger role in producing molecular damage (Halliwell and Gutteridge, 1990). Alternatively, reaction of $O_2^{\bullet -}$ with nitric oxide produces peroxynitrite (Groves, 1999), a potent oxidant, which causes irreversible inhibition of mitochondria respiration and damage to mitochondrial components (complexes I, II, III, IV and V, creatine kinase, aconitase, membranes, DNA, superoxide dismutase, etc.) (Inoue *et al.*, 2000; Riobó *et al.*, 2001). These species deriving from nitrogen are named reactive nitrogen species (RNS).

Because $O_2^{\bullet -}$generation is a continuous and physiological occurrence, mammalian cells developed a complex antioxidant defense system that includes non-enzymatic antioxidants (e.g., glutathione (GSH), thioredoxin), as well as enzymatic antioxidants (e.g., catalase, SOD), to prevent oxidative damage (Sies, 1991). Mitochondria possess an efficient antioxidant system (reviewed in Radi *et al.*, 1991), composed of SOD, glutathione peroxidase, glutathione reductase, GSH, NAD(P) transhydrogenase, NADPH, vitamins E and C, thiol peroxidases and mitochondrial respiration itself (Korshunov *et al.*, 1999). The phenomenon known as mitochondrial mild uncoupling (small decreases in mitochondrial proton gradient) may also counteract excessive production of free radicals by the respiratory chain (Korshunov *et al.*, 1997; Skulachev, 1998). The glutathione redox system allows the reduction of oxidants, such as hydroperoxides. As mitochondria are generally devoid of catalase (catalase has only been detected in rat heart mitochondria), the hydroperoxide detoxification mainly relies on GSH peroxidase. Mitochondrial GSH plays an important role in preserving mitochondria membrane integrity and assuring the reduced state of the intramitochondrial protein thiol groups. Irreversible injury may thus occur following a depletion of the mitochondrial pool of GSH (Reed, 1990).

Under conditions in which mitochondrial generation of ROS is increased, an imbalance between ROS and antioxidants occurs causing oxidative stress, with mitochondrial damage and consequent cell death. Several situations, such as dysfunctional complex I (Robinson, 1998), chemical poisoning and ischemia followed by reperfusion (McDonald *et al.*, 1999) may subject tissues and cells to oxidative stress. Because of the high protein content of the inner mitochondrial membrane, these proteins are one of the primary targets of mitochondrial-generated ROS (Brookes *et al.*, 1999; Poderoso *et al.*, 1999). In membranes, ROS affect cysteine and methionine residues, causing intra-molecular cross-linkings and formation of protein aggregates. Polyunsaturated fatty acids are also main targets for ROS (Paradies *et al.*, 1998). $HO^{\bullet}$ radicals can initiate lipid peroxidation and generate peroxyl and alkoxyl radical intermediates (Uchida *et al.*, 1997; Vieira *et al.*, 2001). The propagation of lipid peroxidation is stopped by the reaction between two radicals or by antioxidants. Mitochondrial membrane lipid peroxidation results in irreversible loss of mitochondrial functions, such as oxidative phosphorylation and ion transport. Oxidants increase the release of calcium from mitochondria, thus stimulating calcium-dependent enzymes, such as proteases, nucleases and phospholipases. Mitochondrial DNA is particularly prone to oxidative damage (Palmeira *et al.*, 1997; Beckman and Ames, 1999; Lu *et al.*, 1999), due to its lack of protective histones, the presence of incomplete repair mechanisms and the proximity of the respiratory chain (Kelly and Scarpulla, 2004).

MITOCHONDRIA AND CALCIUM HOMEOSTASIS

The cytoplasmic pool of calcium is very limited and its free concentration is normally maintained in the region of 0.05–0.5 μM in most cells. The plasma membrane, the endoplasmic reticulum and the mitochondrial inner membrane have calcium transport pathways, which are involved in the regulation of cytoplasmic-free calcium. The evidence of active systems in the inner mitochondrial membrane, which allows the specific transport of calcium both into and out the mitochondrial matrix, suggests that mitochondria play a key role in physiological intracellular calcium homeostasis (Dedkova and Blatter, 2008; Celsi *et al.*, 2009).

The low affinity of the mitochondrial calcium uptake and the normal free calcium concentrations under resting conditions suggested that mitochondrial calcium uptake did not have physiological significance. However, the clear demonstration of calcium uptake into mitochondria, within intact cells, brought a new perspective to this subject. It is possible that mitochondria take up calcium during periodic increases in intracellular calcium concentrations (calcium spikes), or through a close interaction with the endoplasmic reticulum calcium release pathway and plasma membrane channels. Mitochondria are located close to the endoplasmic reticulum, which possess channels sensitive to inositol 1,4,5-trisphosphate ($InsP_3$), a second messenger in the signaling pathway that results in hormone-induced calcium mobilization (Nishizuka, 1992). This indicated a direct link between mitochondria and calcium intracellular stores, suggesting that mitochondria sense microdomains of high calcium, located close to the $InsP_3$-sensitive channels. This allows a more specific and efficient intracellular communication, based on a calcium signal.

Confirming that calcium uptake by mitochondria is important for cell function, mitochondria have developed an elaborate calcium-release system. The physiological role of calcium may be the regulation of respiratory activities. Calcium modulates three intramitochondrial enzymes involved in energy metabolism: the pyruvate dehydrogenase complex, the NAD^+-linked isocitrate dehydrogenase and the 2-oxoglutarate dehydrogenase (McCormack *et al.*, 1990). Since mitochondrial calcium uptake upregulates the activity of these enzymes, it can hardly be doubted that one of the main functions of mitochondrial calcium transport is to increase NADH production following a calcium signal.

THE MITOCHONDRIAL PERMEABILITY TRANSITION

Isolated mitochondria, when exposed to supraphysiological concentrations of calcium, undergo an extensive loss of the characteristic permeability of the inner membrane to ions and molecules (<1,500 Da). This leads to an increase in mitochondrial matrix volume, due to water entry inside mitochondria, resulting in mitochondrial swelling associated with membrane depolarization and uncoupling of the mitochondria, calcium release and unfolding of the inner membrane cristae (Bernardi, 1999; Crompton, 1999). This phenomenon is known as mitochondrial permeability transition. The calcium-induced swelling of mitochondria has been known for a long time (Hunter and Haworth, 1979). Initially, it was explained as the result of non-specific membrane damage by phospholipases (Gunter and Pfeiffer, 1990). The protective effects of phospholipase A_2 inhibitors and the absence of solute selectivity of the permeability pathway reinforced the idea of this being a phenomenon with no role in controlling mitochondrial and cellular function. Since then, many studies have provided evidences for a new dimension in membrane permeability. The MPT is indeed the result of MPTP (mitochondrial permeability transition pores) formation and opening. These pores are described as having 2–3 nm of diameter, with several proteic components and modulated by several agents (for review see Bernardi and Forte, 2007; Halestrap, 2009).

REGULATION AND SIGNIFICANCE OF THE MITOCHONDRIAL PERMEABILITY TRANSITION INDUCTION

Mitochondrial permeability transition is primarily triggered by a rise in matrix calcium. The concentration required is highly variable for different tissues. Additionally, several factors modulate the calcium threshold for MPT induction. Inorganic phosphate is a powerful MPT inducer, whose effect is explained as the result of buffering matrix pH, since the transition is potently inhibited at matrix pH below 7.0. A high membrane potential and a high content in ADP and ATP also prevent MPT induction (Bernardi, 1992; Crompton *et al.*, 1998). Agents that promote an oxidized state of pyridine nucleotides and thiol cross-linkers are inducers of the MPT (Kowaltowski *et al.*, 1995). In contrast, antioxidants have a preventive role (Petronilli *et al.*, 1994). Modulators of mitochondrial calcium matrix, such as Mg^{2+}, are inhibitors. In view of this, conditions and xenobiotics that cause oxidative stress, adenine nucleotide depletion, increased inorganic phosphate concentrations and mitochondrial depolarization will promote the onset of the MPT. Inhibition of MPT can also be observed with bongkrekate, whereas atractylate is an inducer (Crompton *et al.*, 1998). CyA, an immunosuppressive peptide, is a specific MPT inhibitor (Broekemeier *et al.*, 1989). It is now known that increasing calcium concentration can largely relieve inhibition by CyA, while CyA-insensitive permeabilization of the mitochondrial membrane has been described (Sultan and Sokolove, 2001). The proposal of two conformations (low and high conductance) for the MPTP indicated a possible role in normal cell function, besides the involvement in cell death. A state of low conductance, with spontaneous opening and closure, would allow the release of small ions (calcium and protons) from the mitochondrial matrix. In this case, the pore serves as a calcium release channel and a regulator of mitochondrial membrane potential, avoiding membrane hyperpolarization and consequent ROS formation. The stabilization of the pore in the open conformation, the high conductance state, would have drastic consequences for the cell balance (Ichas and Mazat, 1998). A major consequence of MPT induction is inhibition of oxidative phosphorylation, which unrestrained will lead to necrotic cell death. Besides this cell death due to bioenergetic failure, the permeability transition has also been pointed to be involved in the programmed form of cell death (apoptosis), through the release of pro-apoptotic factors.

Taking into consideration the multifaceted role of mitochondria in cell homeostasis and the numerous examples of mitochondria-mediated cell injury, this overview provides an important insight into the role of mitochondrial dysfunction as a primary intracellular target in toxicity.

MITOCHONDRIA IN THE GERM LINE

Male germ cells have 2,000–3,000 mitochondria, although during their differentiation into sperm most are lost in the so-called residual bodies together with much of the cell cytoplasm. Those remaining in sperm (25–75) are rearranged in elongated tubular structures (Ho and Wey, 2007) and are packed helically around the anterior portion of the flagellum. Although sperm mitochondria enter the oocyte during fertilization in mammals (unlike what is often noted in non-specialized literature), they are destroyed in the zygote cytoplasm (Sutovsky *et al.*, 1999), thus ensuring maternal-only mitochondrial inheritance. In fact oocytes in mammals contain 10^5–10^8 mitochondria (Chen *et al.*, 1995; Jansen and de Boer, 1998), and even failure in the destruction of male mitochondria following fertilization would probably result in dilution of paternal mitochondria below detection levels.

During oocyte maturation, and in early embryos, mitochondria are relocated to different regions, probably in response to localized energy demands (Bavister and Squirrell, 2000). However, a recurring theme seems to be that mature oocytes and early embryos maintain an overall low-level (i.e., "quiet") metabolism and low mitochondrial activity, thus minimizing oxidative stress, but generating the necessary ATP to fulfill cellular functions (Leese *et al.*, 2007).

As noted above mitochondrial defects including mtDNA mutations and deletions, and changes to nuclear-encoded mitochondrial proteins are associated with a wide variety of disorders, including infertility (Lee *et al.*, 2001; Balaban *et al.*, 2005; Nakada *et al.*, 2006; Lu *et al.*, 2008). But what is the importance of mitochondrial bioenergetics in reproductive function, and what can we learn from toxicity studies?

TESTIS MITOCHONDRIA AND SPERMATOGENESIS

Although there is a long history of using early embryos, or, more recently, embryonic stem cells, to perform toxicological studies in replacement of adult animals, these studies do not normally focus specifically on mitochondrial function. Moreover, due to biological constraints, the bioenergetics of reproduction are much more widely studied in male gametogenesis, both given the (relative) abundance of material, and the fact that, unlike the ovary, the testis harbors continuous and complete gamete production, from the stem cell spermatogonia to mature sperm (for review see Ramalho-Santos *et al.*, 2009). Energy metabolism and catabolism in the testis involve a unique network of reactions and includes several testis-specific enzymes, hormonal regulation and essential cell-to-cell interactions. The proper functioning of this network is critical for testicular physiology (Bajpal *et al.*, 1998; Erkkila *et al.*, 2006).

Morphology, localization and energy metabolism of testicular mitochondria change markedly during spermatogenesis, and three types of mitochondria are recognizable: orthodox-type mitochondria in Sertoli cells, spermatogonia, preleptotene and leptotene spermatocytes; the intermediate form in zygotene spermatocytes; and the condensed form in pachytene and secondary spermatocytes and early spermatids, a conformation that shifts back to the intermediate form in late spermatids and spermatozoa (De Martino *et al.*, 1979; Figure 61.2). An association between germ cell mitochondrial morphology and metabolic status during spermatogenesis was postulated, in which the "condensed" form presents higher efficiency (De Martino *et al.*, 1979). These morphological changes may be supported/induced by factors released by Sertoli cells. In fact, Activin A was described as an inducer

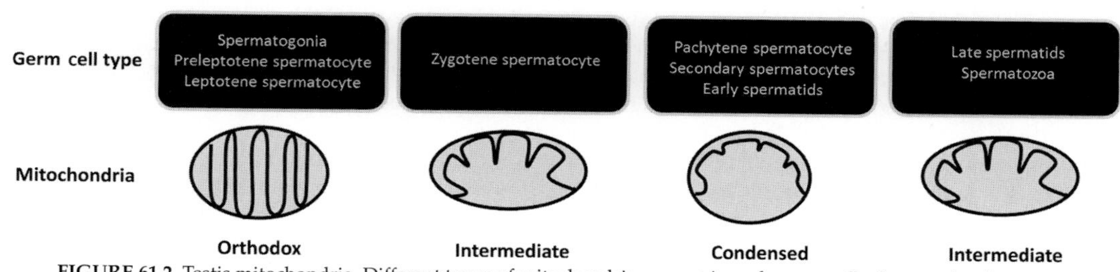

FIGURE 61.2 Testis mitochondria. Different types of mitochondria present in male germ cells. See text for discussion.

of the condensed form, which may be one of the factors contributing to the regulation of the germ cell differentiation by Sertoli cells (Meinhardt *et al.*, 2000). Leydig cell mitochondria present lamellar cristae in close association, with a gap between apposing lamellae of approximately 4 nm, a unique feature of steroid-producing cells. Although the functional significance of these structures is unknown, it was suggested that this component of the cristae is not involved in ATP production since the close apposition of membranes (approximately a 4 nm gap) does not allow for the presence of ATP synthase (Prince, 2002).

Concomitant with the described structural changes, several mitochondrial proteins, such as heat shock protein (hsp) 60 and 70, Lon protease and sulphidryl oxidase (SOx), are known to be expressed and synthesized during distinct phases of spermatogenesis (Meinhardt *et al.*, 1999). Specific isoforms are also found in testicular mitochondria, such as cytochrome *c* and subunit VIb-2 of the cytochrome *c* oxidase (COX) (Hess *et al.*, 1993; Hüttemann *et al.*, 2003). Mutations on the mitochondrial *Drosophila* protein Merlin, common to somatic cells (ortholog in humans is *Neurofibromatosis*), produces viable but sterile males, indicating that the induced deregulation on mitochondrial function, although not affecting somatic cells, has profound implications on germ cell differentiation (Dorogova *et al.*, 2008). However, this is certainly not a general effect, as mice lacking a testis-specific translocase (Tom 34b) are normal and fertile (Terada *et al.*, 2003).

Testis-specific morphogenetic events suggest that male gonads have a higher energy requirement than ovaries, starting early at the time of testis-defining *Sry* activation (Matoba *et al.*, 2008). Because spermatogonial stem cells (SSCs) are slow dividing, it is expected that low mitochondrial membrane potential might be a shared characteristic with other stem cells (for review see Ramalho-Santos *et al.*, 2009). The neonate rat testis cell fraction (0–5 days postpartum – dpp), with the highest concentration of SSCs including gonocytes, exhibited low mitochondrial membrane potential while stem cells in rat pup testes (8–14 dpp) appeared to have more active mitochondria than their gonocyte precursors, which might reflect increased proliferative activity as this population expands to fill the rapidly increasing number of niches (Ryu *et al.*, 2004). Spermatogonia and precursor cells also undergo apoptosis as a natural process to control germ cell number in the testis, and these mechanisms can be exacerbated upon injury (Ramalho-Santos *et al.*, 2009).

THE PARTICULAR CHARACTERISTICS OF TESTICULAR BIOENERGETICS

In the adult testis the survival of germ cells is dependent on carbohydrate metabolism, including both anaerobic (glycolysis) and aerobic (OXPHOS) pathways. However, the different cell types diverge on their favorite substrates (Robinson and Fritz, 1981; Grootegoed *et al.*, 1984; Nakamura *et al.*, 1984; Bajpai *et al.*, 1998; Meinhardt *et al.*, 1999). In fact, the establishment of the blood–testis barrier and the changes in the surrounding medium cause a considerable shift in the energy metabolism of germ cells.

Spermatogonia in the basal compartment are supplied exclusively by blood components; however, after passage to the luminal compartment germ cells rely on the breakdown of lactate and pyruvate provided by Sertoli cells. Therefore, spermatogonia, mature sperm and the somatic Sertoli cells exhibit high glycolytic activity, whereas spermatocytes and spermatids produce ATP mainly by OXPHOS (Robinson and Fritz, 1981; Grootegoed *et al.*, 1984; Nakamura *et al.*, 1984; Bajpai *et al.*, 1998; Meinhardt *et al.*, 1999). This could also be a matter of opportunity: since seminiferous tubule fluid is rich in lactate and poor in glucose, it is hypothesized that, even though spermatocytes have the machinery to produce energy through glycolysis, they rely mostly on lactate (Bajpai *et al.*, 1998). Nonetheless, there are incongruities between availability and usability. Blood vessels, located exclusively between tubules, supply the oxygen needed to perform OXPHOS that only reaches the lumen of the seminiferous tubules by diffusion (Wenger and Katschinski, 2005). The facilitated access of spermatogonia to oxygen would lead us to expect the use of OXPHOS instead of glycolysis. Similarly, having less access to oxygen, spermatocytes were expected to favor mostly glycolysis as an ATP source. However, the substrate availability imposed by seminiferous tubules compartmentalization, together with ATP demand, may prime the cell to different adaptations. It is also possible that stem cells maintain a low metabolism to avoid ROS-related damage (Ramalho-Santos *et al.*, 2009).

One of the main issues to consider when using mitochondrial bioenergetics as a tool for reproductive toxicology is related to the diversity of metabolic solutions for different cell types described above, which result in different types of organelles, likely with distinct properties, being present in a testicular mitochondrial preparation (Figure 61.2). A precise characterization of bioenergetic parameters for mitochondria from each testis-specific cell type is still lacking, and any analysis is carried out on a mixed population, which, although representative of the organ as a whole, prevents more specific characterization of monitored phenomena, for example of the exact mechanisms by which different substances may be affecting mitochondrial bioenergetics, or if they are acting only on a subpopulation of mitochondria.

Regardless, testicular mitochondria have distinct bioenergetic parameters when compared to mitochondria harvested from other tissues. Specifically, testis mitochondria are shown to consume less oxygen to generate approximately the same maximum electric potential as other tissues (Table 61.1) and depict an age-related modification in phosphorylative efficiency with young animals presenting less efficient phosphorylation, which also declines with aging, after a peak during the reproductive period (Amaral *et al.*, 2008; Mota *et al.*, 2009).

There is also the important aspect of proton leak. Although the passage of protons through the inner mitochondrial membrane without synthesis of ATP may seem as a waste of energy, it can have a crucial role in lowering mitochondrial membrane potential in some instances, reducing the tendency of electrons to escape the electron transfer chain, and thus preventing ROS formation. Indeed, testicular mitochondria have the ability to modulate proton leak via uncoupling proteins (Amaral *et al.*, 2008), and use this ability to control ROS production (Rodrigues *et al.*, 2010). Upregulation of uncoupling protein 2 in the testis may constitute a mechanism to protect against the deleterious effects of aging on mitochondrial bioenergetics (Amaral *et al.*, 2008). Following what is a recurring theme, the testis seems to be a unique organelle also in terms of proton leak modulation (Rodrigues *et al.*, 2010), as the uncoupling protein content is intermediate between organs with a high prevalence of uncoupling

TABLE 61.1 Comparative analysis of bioenergetic parameters in different organs

	State3 (natmsO/min/mgprot)	State4 (natmsO/min/mgprot)	RCR	ADP/O	Δψmax (−mV)	Δψrep (−mV)
Brain*	98.82 ± 5.32	47.46 ± 2.63	2.28 ± 0.09	1.27 ± 0.08	177.3 ± 2.2	178.3 ± 1.25
Heart*	145.95 ± 3.56	61.72 ± 6.05	3.38 ± 0.09	1.22 ± 0.03	239.89 ± 0.79	242.13 ± 0.92
Liver+	77.7 ± 7.7	16.9 ± 0.6	4.7 ± 0.5	1.7 ± 0.1	224.0 ± 1.28	221.9 ± 1.63
Kidney*	125.47 ± 13.89	60.51 ± 12.37	2.23 ± 0.28	1.05 ± 0.12	213.09 ± 1.09	213.13 ± 1.95
Testis#	36.78 ± 1.95	24.75 ± 1.06	1.5 ± 0.053	1.74 ± 0.11	206.72 ± 1.74	203.64 ± 2.0

Data show means ± SEM
*According to Moreira *et al.*, 2006
+According to Teodoro *et al.*, 2006
#According to Amaral *et al.*, 2009

proteins (such as the kidney), and organs where they exist in a very low amount (such as the liver). Concomitantly, testicular mitochondria respond less to proton leak agonists and antagonists than kidney mitochondria, but more than liver mitochondria (Rodrigues *et al.*, 2010).

MITOCHONDRIA AND TOXICOLOGY STUDIES IN THE REPRODUCTIVE SYSTEM

The use of mitochondria as tools or markers of injury during toxicity studies has increased recently, with studies involving, among other substances, food additives, pesticides, mycotoxins, cryoprotectants, flame retardants, alcohol, or, more broadly, substances thought to act as endocrine disruptors, especially in male spermatogenesis (reviewed in Tavares *et al.*, 2009)

These studies usually focus on aspects related to both ROS generation and the triggering of mitochondria-based apoptosis mechanisms. Besides the monitoring of biochemical markers for these processes, also evaluated are obvious decreases in gamete production, namely spermatogenesis (i.e., lower sperm counts) or, more indirectly, oogenesis (i.e., decreased presence of functional folicles), changes in testicular or ovarian histological architecture, as well as morphological changes to mitochondria (Talsness *et al.*, 2005; Gupta *et al.*, 2006; Hild *et al.*, 2007; Aly *et al.*, 2009; Faut *et al.*, 2009; Shi *et al.*, 2010; Xu *et al.*, 2010). Membrane damage and swelling are taken as putative gross indicators of induced mitochondrial dysfunction in both the testis (Hild *et al.*, 2007; Zhang *et al.*, 2007; Shi *et al.*, 2010) and the ovary (Talsness *et al.*, 2005; Faut *et al.*, 2009; Xu *et al.*, 2010).

The more common parameters monitored in terms of mitochondria-centered processes relate to ROS formation in the gonads, namely to an increase in oxidative damage following injury, for example monitored via hydrogen peroxide generation and lipid peroxidation products, or with changes in the activity of anti-oxidant defenses. The latter can either be upregulated to respond to increased ROS, or downregulated as a direct effect of the toxicological insult, thus indirectly increasing ROS prevalence in both the testis (Song *et al.*, 2008; Aly *et al.*, 2009; Dhanabalan and Mathur, 2009; Yeh *et al.*, 2009) and ovary (Gupta *et al.*, 2006). In terms of ROS defense mechanisms, enzymatic systems are more routinely monitored. Superoxide dismutase, catalase and, in a fewer number of cases, gluthathione peroxidase and gluthathione reductase are usually targeted for analysis (Gupta *et al.*, 2006; Aly *et al.*, 2009; Dhanabalan and Mathur, 2009). In some cases non-enzymatic anti-oxidants such as vitamin C or gluthathione are also quantified (Aly *et al.*, 2009). In parallel with ROS-related damage, apoptotic markers can be important tools to evaluate mitochondrial function, and recent manuscripts focus on pro-apoptotic modulation of Bcl-2 family proteins, intensification of p53 and Apaf-1, release of mitochondrial cytochrome *c* or activation of caspase-3 (Song *et al.*, 2008; Yeh *et al.*, 2009).

Importantly, the putative protective effects of preventive anti-oxidant and anti-apoptotic treatments against toxic insults can also be evaluated using several of the strategies mentioned, once clear effects are established (Dhanabalan and Mathur, 2009; Yeh *et al.*, 2009).

Although care should be taken in terms of extrapolation to the whole reproductive system, the use of cell cultures can also be extremely useful to pinpoint mitochondrial changes in specific cell types with possible overall negative effects, for example in Sertoli (Song *et al.*, 2008) or Leydig (Zhang *et al.*, 2007) cells.

Concomitantly, testicular mitochondria can also serve as an important and simple tool to monitor the putative toxicological effects of distinct types of substances on reproductive physiology. Again, although in this case mitochondria present in the preparation account for the whole testis, extrapolations to a more complex system must again be done with extreme caution given the diversity of mitochondrial types present, as noted previously. Regardless, testicular mitochondria can serve as a powerful and inexpensive preliminary system either *in vivo* (by isolating mitochondria from treated model animals) or *in vitro* (by adding substances to isolated mitochondria). Several parameters can be precisely monitored using simple biochemical techniques, from mitochondrial membrane potential, to oxygen consumption, to ROS formation, to calcium storage, to apoptotic markers (Amaral *et al.*, 2009).

CONCLUDING REMARKS AND FUTURE DIRECTIONS

In conclusion, available data suggest that testicular mitochondria are functionally unique. Furthermore, recent results (P. Mota, unpublished) clearly show that substances known to interfere with mitochondrial bioenergetics in a defined fashion (such as DDT and its metabolite DDE) act in a very different (sometimes even opposite) way when added to testis mitochondria, in comparison to what is the case for the more classical toxicological model of liver mitochondria. Taken together these observations suggest that, unlike what has been usually the case, testicular mitochondria should be considered as the primary mitochondrial toxicological model to test the effect of distinct substances on male gametogenesis and mammalian reproduction (Tavares *et al.*, 2009).

ACKNOWLEDGMENTS

S. Amaral is thanked for assistance with figures and tables, and P. Mota for sharing unpublished data. M. Sancha Santos, A.S. Rodrigues, P. Oliveira and A. Moreno are thanked for their input in discussions throughout this work.

REFERENCES

Abrahams JP, Leslie AG, Lutter R, Walker JE (1994) Structure at 2.8 A resolution of F1-ATPase from bovine heart mitochondria. *Nature* **370:** 621–8.

Aly HA, Domènech O, Abdel-Naim AB (2009) Aroclor 1254 impairs spermatogenesis and induces oxidative stress in rat testicular mitochondria. *Food Chem Toxicol* **47:** 1733–8.

Amaral S, Mota PC, Lacerda B, Alves M, Pereira MD, Oliveira PJ, Ramalho-Santos J (2009) Testicular mitochondrial alterations in untreated streptozotocin-induced diabetic rats. *Mitochondrion* **9:** 41–50.

Amaral S, Mota P, Rodrigues AS, Martins L, Oliveira PJ, Ramalho-Santos J (2008) Testicular aging involves mitochondrial dysfunction as well as an increase in UCP2 levels and proton leak. *FEBS Lett* **582:** 4191–6.

Anderson S, Bankier AT, Barrell BG, de Bruijn MH, Coulson AR, Drouin J, Eperon IC, Nierlich DP, Roe BA, Sanger F, Schreier PH, Smith AJ, Staden R, Young IG (1981) Sequence and organization of the human mitochondrial genome. *Nature* **290:** 457–65.

Azzone GF, Petronilli V, Zoratti, M (1984) "Cross-talk" between redox- and ATP-driven H+ pumps. *Biochem Soc Trans* **12:** 414–16.

Bajpai M, Gupta G, Setty BS (1998) Changes in carbohydrate metabolism of testicular germ cells during meiosis in the rat. *Eur J Endocrinol* **138:** 322–7.

Balaban RS, Nemoto S, Finkel T (2005) Mitochondria, oxidants, and aging. *Cell* **120:** 483–95.

Bavister BD, Squirrell JM (2000) Mitochondrial distribution and function in oocytes and early embryos. *Hum Reprod* **15 (Suppl. 2):** 189–98.

Beckman KB, Ames BN (1999) Endogenous oxidative damage of mtDNA. *Mutat Res* **424:** 51–8.

Bernardi P (1992) Modulation of the mitochondrial cyclosporin A-sensitive permeability transition pore by the proton electrochemical gradient – evidence that the pore can be opened by membrane depolarization. *J Biol Chem* **267:** 8834–9.

Bernardi P (1999) Mitochondrial transport of cations: channels, exchangers and permeability transition. *Physiol Rev* **79:** 1127–55.

Bernardi P, Forte M (2007) The mitochondrial permeability transition pore. *Novartis Found Symp* **287:** 157–64.

Blachly-Dison E, Forte M (2001) VDAC channels. *IUBMB Life* **52:** 113–18.

Boveris A, Chance B (1973) The mitochondrial generation of hydrogen peroxide. General properties and effect of hyperbaric oxygen. *Biochem J* **134:** 707–16.

Broekemeier KM, Dempsey ME, Pfeiffer DR (1989) Cyclosporin A is a potent inhibitor of the inner membrane permeability transition in liver mitochondria. *J Biol Chem* **264:** 7826–30.

Brookes PS, Bolanos JP, Heales SJ (1999) The assumption that nitric oxide inhibits mitochondrial ATP synthesis is correct. *FEBS Lett* **446:** 261–3.

Cadet JL, Brannock C (1998) Free radicals and the pathobiology of brain dopamine systems. *Neurochem Int* **32:** 117–31.

Capaldi RA, Aggeler R (2002) Mechanism of the $F_{(1)}F_{(0)}$-type ATP synthase, a biological rotary motor. *Trends Biochem Sci* **27:** 154–60.

Celsi F, Pizzo P, Brini M, Leo S, Fotino C, Pinton P, Rizzuto R (2009) Mitochondria, calcium and cell death: a deadly triad in neurodegeneration. *Biochim Biophys Acta* **1787:** 335–44.

Chen X, Prosser R, Simonetti S, Sadlock J, Jagiello G, Schon EA (1995) Rearranged mitochondrial genomes are present in human oocytes. *Am J Hum Genet* **57:** 239–47.

Crompton M (1999) The mitochondrial permeability transition pore and its role in cell death. *Biochem J* **341:** 233–49.

Crompton M, Virji S, Ward JM (1998) Cyclophilin-D binds strongly to complexes of the voltage-dependent anion channel and the adenine nucleotide translocase to form the permeability transition pore. *Eur J Biochem* **258:** 729–35.

De Martino C, Floridi A, Marcante ML, Malorni W, Scorza-Barcellona P, Bellocci M, Silvestrini B (1979) Morphological, histochemical and biochemical studies on germ cell mitochondria of normal rats. *Cell Tissue Res* **196:** 1–22.

Dedkova EN, Blatter LA (2008) Mitochondrial Ca2+ and the heart. *Cell Calcium* **44:** 77–91.

Dhanabalan S, Mathur PP (2009) Low dose of 2,3,7,8 tetrachlorodibenzo-p-dioxin induces testicular oxidative stress in adult rats under the influence of corticosterone. *Exp Toxicol Pathol* **61:** 415–23.

Di Lisa F, Bernardi P (1998) Mitochondrial function as a determinant of recovery or death in cell response to injury. *Mol Cell Biochem* **184:** 379–91.

Dorogova NV, Akhmametyeva EM, Kopyl SA, Gubanova NV, Yudina OS, Omelyanchuk LV, Chang LS (2008) The role of Drosophila Merlin in spermatogenesis. *BMC Cell Biol* **9:** 2–15.

Erecinska M, Wilson DF (1982) Regulation of cellular energy metabolism. *J Membr Biol* **70:** 1–14.

Erkkila K, Kyttanen S, Wikstrom M, Taari K, Hikim AP, Swerdloff RS, Dunkel L (2006) Regulation of human male germ cell death by modulators of ATP production. *Am J Physiol Endocrinol Metab* **290:** 1145–54.

Esposti MD (1998) Inhibitors of NADH-ubiquinone reductase: an overview. *Biochim Biophys Acta* **1364:** 222–35.

Esposti MD, Ghelli A (1994) The mechanism of proton and electron transport in mitochondrial complex I. *Biochim Biophys Acta* **1187:** 116–20.

Faut M, Rodríguez de Castro C, Bietto FM, Castro JA, Castro GD. (2009) Metabolism of ethanol to acetaldehyde and increased susceptibility to oxidative stress could play a role in the ovarian tissue cell injury promoted by alcohol drinking. *Toxicol Ind Health* **25:** 525–38.

Frey TG, Manella CA (2000) The internal structure of mitochondria. *Trends Biochem Sci* **25:** 319–24.

Groeger G, Quiney C, Cotter TG (2009) Hydrogen peroxide as a cell-survival signaling molecule. *Antioxid Redox Signal* **11:** 2655–71.

Grootegoed JA, Jansen R, Van der Molen HJ (1984) The role of glucose, pyruvate and lactate in ATP production by rat spermatocytes and spermatids. *Biochim Biophys Acta* **767:** 248–56.

Groves JT (1999) Peroxynitrite: reactive, invasive and enigmatic. *Curr Opin Chem Biol* **3:** 226–35.

Gunter TE, Pfeiffer DR (1990) Mechanisms by which mitochondria transport calcium. *Am J Physiol* **258:** C755–86.

Gupta RK, Schuh RA, Fiskum G, Flaws JA (2006) Methoxychlor causes mitochondrial dysfunction and oxidative damage in the mouse ovary. *Toxicol Appl Pharmacol* **216:** 436–45.

Halestrap AP (2009) What is the mitochondrial permeability transition pore? *J Mol Cell Cardiol* **46:** 821–31.

Halliwell B, Gutteridge JM (1990) Role of free radicals and catalytic metal ions in human disease: an overview. *Methods Enzymol* **186:** 1–85.

Hatefi Y (1985) The mitochondrial electron transport and oxidative phosphorylation. *Ann Rev Biochem* **54:** 1015–69.

Hess RA, Miller LA, Kirby JD, Margoliash E, Goldberg E (1993) Immunoelectron microscopic localization of testicular and somatic cytochromes c in the seminiferous epithelium of the rat. *Biol Reprod* **48:** 1299–308.

Hild SA, Reel JR, Dykstra MJ, Mann PC, Marshall GR (2007) Acute adverse effects of the indenopyridine CDB-4022 on the ultrastructure of sertoli cells, spermatocytes, and spermatids in rat testes: comparison to the known sertoli cell toxicant Di-n-pentylphthalate (DPP). *J Androl* **28:** 621–9.

Ho HC, Wey S (2007) Three dimensional rendering of the mitochondrial sheath morphogenesis during mouse spermiogenesis. *Microsc Res Tech* **70:** 719–23.

Hunter DR, Haworth RA (1979) The Ca^{2+}-induced membrane transition in mitochondria – I. The protective mechanisms. *Arch Biochem Biophys* **195:** 453–9.

Hüttemann M, Jaradat S, Grossman LI (2003) Cytochrome c oxidase of mammals contains a testes-specific isoform of subunit VIb – the counterpart to testes-specific cytochrome c? *Mol Reprod Dev* **66:** 8–16.

Ichas F, Mazat JP (1998) From calcium signaling to cell death: two conformations for the mitochondrial permeability transition pore. Switching from low- to high-conductance state. *Biochim Biophys Acta* **1366:** 33–50.

Inoue M, Sato EF, Park AM, Nishikawa M, Kasahara E, Miyoshi M, Ochi A, Utsumi K (2000) Cross-talk between NO and oxyradicals, a supersystem that regulates energy metabolism and survival of animals. *Free Radic Res* **33:** 757–70.

Jansen RP, de Boer K (1998) The bottleneck: mitochondrial imperatives in oogenesis and ovarian follicular fate. *Mol Cell Endocrinol* **145:** 81–8.

Kelly DP, Scarpulla RC (2004) Transcriptional regulatory circuits controlling mitochondrial biogenesis and function. *Genes Dev* **18:** 357–68.

Korshunov SS, Krasnikov BF, Pereverzev MO, Skulachev VP (1999) The antioxidant functions of cytochrome c. *FEBS Lett* **462:** 192–8.

Korshunov SS, Skulachev VP, Starkov AA (1997) High protonic potential actuates a mechanism of production of reactive oxygen species in mitochondria. *FEBS Lett* **416:** 15–18.

Kowaltowski AJ, Castilho RF, Vercesi AE (1995) Ca^{2+}-induced mitochondrial membrane permeabilization: role of coenzyme Q redox state. *Am J Physiol* **269:** C141–7.

Kowaltowski AJ, de Souza-Pinto NC, Castilho RF, Vercesi AE (2009) Mitochondria and reactive oxygen species. *Free Radic Biol Med* **47:** 333–43.

Lee CH, Wei YH (2001) Mitochondrial alterations, cellular response to oxidative stress and defective degradation of proteins in aging. *Biogerontology* **2:** 231–44.

Leese HJ, Sturmey RG, Baumann CG, McEvoy TG (2007). Embryo viability and metabolism: obeying the quiet rules. *Hum Reprod* **22:** 3047–50.

Liu X, Kim CN, Yang J, Jemmerson R, Wang X (1996) Induction of apoptotic program in cell-free extracts: requirement for dATP and cytochrome *c*. *Cell* **86:** 147–57.

Lorenzo HK, Susin SA, Penninger J, Kroemer G (1999) Apoptosis inducing factor (AIF): a phylogenetically old, caspase-independent effector of cell death. *Cell Death Diff* **6:** 516–24.

Lu B, Poirier C, Gaspar T, Gratzke C, Harrison W, Busija D, Matzuk MM, Andersson KE, Overbeek PA, Bishop CE (2008) A mutation in the inner mitochondrial membrane peptidase 2-like gene (Immp2l) affects mitochondrial function and impairs fertility in mice. *Biol Reprod* **78:** 601–10.

Lu CY, Lee HC, Fahn HJ, Wei YH (1999) Oxidative damage elicited by imbalance of free radical scavenging enzymes is associated with large-scale mtDNA deletions in aging human skin. *Mutat Res* **423:** 11–21.

Matoba S, Hiramatsu R, Kanai-Azuma M, Tsunekawa N, Harikae K, Kawakami H, Kurohmaru MI, Kanai Y (2008) Establishment of testis-specific SOX9 activation requires high glucose metabolism in mouse sex differentiation. *Dev Biol* **324:** 76–87.

McCormack JG, Halestrap AP, Denton RM (1990) Role of calcium ions in regulation of mammalian intramitochondrial metabolism. *Physiol Rev* **70:** 391–425.

McDonald MC, Filipe HM, Thieme0rmann C (1999) Effects of inhibitors of the activity of poly (ADP-ribose) synthetase on the organ injury and dysfunction caused by haemorrhagic shock. *Br J Pharmacol* **128:** 1339–45.

Meinhardt A, McFarlane JR, Seitz J, de Kretser DM (2000) Activin maintains the condensed type of mitochondria in germ cells. *Mol Cell Endocrinol* **168:** 111–17.

Meinhardt A, Wilhelm B, Seitz J (1999) Expression of mitochondrial marker proteins during spermatogenesis. *Hum Reprod Update* **5:** 108–19.

Mitchell P (1966) Chemiosmotic coupling in oxidative and photosynthetic phosphorylation. *Biol Rev* **41:** 445–502.

Moraes CT (1996) Mitochondrial disorders. *Curr Opin Neurol* **9:** 369–74.

Moreira PI, Rolo AP, Sena C, Seiça R, Oliveira CR, Santos MS (2006) Insulin attenuates diabetes-related mitochondrial alterations: a comparative study. *Med Chem* **2:** 299–308.

Mota PC, Amaral S, Martins L, Pereira ML, Oliveira PJ, Ramalho-Santos J (2009) Mitochondrial bioenergetics of testicular cells from the domestic cat (*Felis catus*) – a model for endangered species. *Reprod Toxicol* **27:** 111–16.

Nakada K, Sato A, Yoshida K, Morita T, Tanaka H, Inoue S, Yonekawa H, Hayashi J (2006) Mitochondria-related male infertility. *Proc Natl Acad Sci USA* **103:** 15148–53.

Nakamura M, Okinaga S, Arai K (1984) Metabolism of pachytene primary spermatocytes from rat testes: pyruvate maintenance of adenosine triphosphate level. *Biol Reprod* **30:** 1187–97.

Nishizuka Y (1992) Intracellular signaling by hydrolysis of phospholipids and activation of proteins kinase-C. *Science* **258:** 607–14.

Palmeira CM, Rolo AP (2004) Mitochondrially-mediated toxicity of bile acids. *Toxicology* **203:** 1–15.

Palmeira CM, Serrano J, Kuehl DW, Wallace KB (1997) Preferential oxidation of cardiac mitochondrial DNA following acute intoxication with doxorubicin. *Biochim Biophys Acta* **1321:** 101–6.

Paradies G, Ruggiero FM, Petrosillo G, Quagliariello E (1998) Peroxidative damage to cardiac mitochondria: cytochrome oxidase and cardiolipin alterations. *FEBS Lett* **424:** 155–8.

Paschen SA, Neupert W (2001) Protein import into mitochondria. *IUBMB Life* **52:** 101–12.

Petronilli V, Constantini P, Scorrano L, Colonna R, Passamonti S, Bernardi P (1994) The voltage sensor of the mitochondrial permeability transition pore is tuned by the oxidation-reduction state of vicinal thiols. *J Biol Chem* **269:** 16638–42.

Poderoso JJ, Carreras MC, Schopfer F, Lisdero CL, Riobo NA, Giulivi C, Boveris AD, Boveris A, Cadenas E (1999) The reaction of nitric oxide with ubiquinol: kinetic properties and biological significance. *Free Radic Biol Med* **26:** 925–35.

Poyton RO, McEwen JE (1996) Crosstalk between nuclear and mitochondrial genomes. *Annu Rev Biochem* **65:** 563–607.

Prince FP (2002) Lamellar and tubular associations of the mitochondrial cristae: unique forms of the cristae present in steroid-producing cells. *Mitochondrion* **1:** 381–9.

Radi R, Turrens JF, Chang LY, Bush KM, Crap JD, Freeman BA (1991) Detection of catalase in rat heart mitochondria. *J Biol Chem* **261:** 14081–24.

Ramalho-Santos J, Varum S, Amaral S, Mota PC, Sousa AP, Amaral A (2009) Mitochondrial functionality and reproduction: from gonads and gametes to embryos and embryonic stem cells. *Hum Reprod Update* **15:** 553–72.

Reed DJ (1990) Glutathione: toxicological implications. *Annu Rev Pharmacol Toxicol* **30:** 603–63.

Reinecke F, Smeitink JA, van der Westhuizen FH (2009) OXPHOS gene expression and control in mitochondrial disorders. *Biochim Biophys Acta* **1792:** 1113–21.

Riobó NA, Clementi E, Melani M, Boveris A, Cadenas E, Moncada S, Poderoso JJ (2001) Nitric oxide inhibits mitochondrial NADH:ubiquinone reductase activity through peroxynitrite formation. *Biochem J* **359:** 139–45.

Robinson BH (1998) Human complex I deficiency: clinical spectrum and involvement of oxygen free radicals in the pathogenicity of the defect. *Biochim Biophys Acta* **1364:** 271–86.

Robinson R, Fritz IB (1981) Metabolism of glucose by Sertoli cells in culture. *Biol Reprod* **24:** 1032–41.

Rodrigues AS, Lacerda B, Moreno A, Ramalho-Santos J (2010) Proton leak modulation in testicular mitochondria affects reactive oxygen species production and lipid peroxidation. *Cell Biochem Funct* **28:** 224–31.

Ryu BY, Orwig KE, Kubota H, Avarbock MR, Brinster RL (2004) Phenotypic and functional characteristics of spermatogonial stem cells in rats. *Dev Biol* **274:** 158–70.

Saraste M (1999) Oxidative phosphorylation at the fin de siècle. *Science* **283:** 1488–93.

Schapira AH (1999) Mitochondrial involvement in Parkinson's disease, Huntington's disease, hereditary spastic paraplegia and Friedreich's ataxia. *Biochim Biophys Acta* **1410:** 159–67.

Schatz G (1995) Mitochondria: beyond oxidative phosphorylation. *Biochim Biophys Acta* **271:** 123–6.

Scheffler IE (2001) Mitochondria make a comeback. *Adv Drug Deliv Rev* **49:** 3–26.

Shi LG, Yang RJ, Yue WB, Xun WJ, Zhang CX, Ren YS, Shi L, Lei FL (2010) Effect of elemental nano-selenium on semen quality, glutathione peroxidase activity, and testis ultrastructure in male Boer goats. *Anim Reprod Sci* **118:** 248–54.

Sies H (1991) Oxidative stress: from basic research to clinical application. *Am J Med* **91:** 31S–38S.

Skulachev VP (1998) Uncoupling: new approaches to an old problem of bioenergetics. *Biochim Biophys Acta* **1363:** 100–24.

Smeitink J, van den Heuvel L, DiMauro S (2001) The genetics and pathology of oxidative phosphorylation. *Nat Rev Genet* **2:** 342–52.

Song Y, Liang X, Hu Y, Wang Y, Yu H, Yang K (2008) p,p′-DDE induces mitochondria-mediated apoptosis of cultured rat Sertoli cells. *Toxicology* **253:** 53–61.

Sultan A, Sokolove PM (2001) Palmitic acid opens a novel cyclosporin A-insensitive pore in the inner mitochondrial membrane. *Arch Biochem Biophys* **386:** 37–51.

Sutovsky P, Moreno RD, Ramalho-Santos J, Dominko T, Simerly C, Schatten G (1999) Ubiquitin tag for sperm mitochondria. *Nature* **402:** 371–2.

Taanman JW (1999) The mitochondrial genome: structure, transcription, translation and replication. *Biochim Biophys Acta* **10:** 103–23.

Takeshige K, Minakami S (1979) NADH- and NADPH-dependent formation of superoxide anions by bovine heart submitochondrial particles and NADH-ubiquinone reductase preparation. *Biochem J* **180:** 129–35.

Talsness CE, Shakibaei M, Kuriyama SN, Grande SW, Sterner-Kock A, Schnitker P, de Souza C, Grote K, Chahoud I (2005) Ultrastructural changes observed in rat ovaries following in utero and lactational exposure to low doses of a polybrominated flame retardant. *Toxicol Lett* **157:** 189–202.

Tavares RS, Martins FC, Oliveira PJ, Ramalho-Santos J, Peixoto FP (2009) Parabens in male infertility – is there a mitochondrial connection? *Reprod Toxicol* **27:** 1–7.

Teodoro J, Rolo AP, Oliveira PJ, Palmeira CM (2006) Decreased ANT content in Zucker fatty rats: relevance for altered hepatic mitochondrial bioenergetics in steatosis. *FEBS Lett* **580:** 2153–7.

Terada K, Ueno S, Yomogida K, Imai T, Kiyonari H, Takeda N, Yano M, Abe S, Aizawa S, Mori M (2003) Expression of Tom34 splicing isoforms in mouse testis and knockout of Tom34 in mice. *J Biochem* **133:** 625–31.

Trumpower BL (1990) The protonmotive Q cycle. Energy transduction by coupling of proton translocation to electron transfer by the cytochrome bc1 complex. *J Biol Chem* **265:** 11409–12.

Turrens JF (1997) Superoxide production by the mitochondrial respiratory chain. *Biosci Rep* **17:** 3–8.

Turrens JF, Alexandre A, Lehninger AL (1985) Ubisemiquinone is the electron donor for superoxide formation by complex III of heart mitochondria. *Arch Biochem Biophys* **237:** 408–14.

Uchida K, Sakai K, Itakura K, Osawa T, Toyokuni S (1997) Protein modification by lipid peroxidation products: formation of malondialdehyde-derived N(epsilon)-(2-propenol)lysine in proteins. *Arch Biochem Biophys* **346:** 45–52.

Vieira HLA, Belzacq AS, Haouzi D, Bernassola F, Cohen I, Jacotot E, Ferri KF, El Hamel C, Bartle LM, Melino G, Brenner C, Goldmacher V, Kroemer G (2001) The adenine nucleotide translocator: a target of nitric oxide, peroxynitrite, and 4-hydroxynonenal. *Oncogene* **20:** 4305–16.

Wallace KB, Starkov AA (2000) Mitochondrial targets of drug toxicity. *Annu Rev Pharmacol Toxicol* **40:** 353–88.

Wenger RH, Katschinski DM (2005) The hypoxic testis and post-meiotic expression of PAS domain proteins. *Semin Cell Dev Biol* **6:** 547–53.

Xu C, Zhang JJ, Chen JA, Cao B, Shu WQ, Cao J (2010) Evaluation of ovotoxicity in female mice caused by organic extracts in tap water from Jialing River in Chongqing, China. *Birth Defects Res B Dev Reprod Toxicol* **89:** 26–33.

Yeh YC, Liu TJ, Wang LC, Lee HW, Ting CT, Lee WL, Hung CJ, Wang KY, Lai HC, Lai HC (2009) A standardized extract of Ginkgo biloba suppresses doxorubicin-induced oxidative stress and p53-mediated mitochondrial apoptosis in rat testes. *Br J Pharmacol* **156:** 48–61.

Zhang SY, Ito Y, Yamanoshita O, Yanagiba Y, Kobayashi M, Taya K, Li C, Okamura A, Miyata M, Ueyama J, Lee CH, Kamijima M, Nakajima T (2007) Permethrin may disrupt testosterone biosynthesis via mitochondrial membrane damage of Leydig cells in adult male mouse. *Endocrinology* **148:** 3941–9.

Zhang Y, Marcillat O, Giulivi C, Ernster L, Davies KJA (1990) The oxidative inactivation of mitochondrial electron transport chain components and ATPase. *J Biol Chem* **265:** 16330–6.

CHAPTER

62

Stress: its impact on reproductive and developmental toxicity

Kavita Gulati and Arunabha Ray

INTRODUCTION

Stress is a phenomenon that is omnipresent in our external and internal environment. Ironically, it is seemingly too well known but too little understood, despite the fact that the knowledge about stress and stress effects have advanced considerably over the last few years. Stress is conceived of as any internal or external stimulus capable of altering/disrupting the physiological milieu and the ability to cope with such aversive situations is a crucial determinant of health and disease. Exposure to such adverse conditions initiates a series of adaptive responses organized to defend the stability of the internal environment and enhance an organism's survival. This orchestrated process, usually referred to as "stress response", involves various mechanisms that allow the body to make the necessary physiological and metabolic adjustments required to cope with the demands of homeostatic challenge (Gold and Chrousos, 2002).

In the 1930s Hans Selye first proposed the concept of stress in biology and medicine and initiated research on stress mechanisms, which helped in understanding the connection between stress and health (Selye, 1936). Selye proposed three universal stages of coping with a stressor – the "General Adaptation Syndrome" (GAS) – comprising (a) an initial "alarm reaction", analogous to "fight or flight" response, (b) a stage of adaptation associated with resistance to the stressor, and eventually (c) a stage of exhaustion and organismic death. It was later demonstrated that these changes are associated with, and to some extent resulted from, activation of the hypothalamic–pituitary–adrenocortical (HPA) axis. It was hypothesized that steroids released into the circulation from adrenal cortex contribute to stress resistance, but may also be responsible for pathological changes. The brain, and some specific areas in it, is the site at which effects of stressors are sensed and appropriate coordinated behavioral and neuroendocrine responses initiated (Ray *et al.* 1987, 1991; Gulati *et al.*, 2009)

STRESSORS AND THEIR IMPACT ON BIOLOGICAL SYSTEMS

In general, stressors can be grouped into three broad categories: (1) psychological stressors – based on a learned response to the threat of an impending adverse condition (fear, anxiety, exposure to a novel or uncontrollable environment); (2) physical stressors – which consist of a physical stimulus and also have a strong psychological component (pain, foot shock, immobilization); (3) stressors that challenge cardiovascular homeostasis (hemorrhage, orthostatic stress/upright tilt, exercise, heat exposure; and (4) environmental stressors. The neuroendocrine responses to stressors are considered important components of survival mechanisms during exposure to life-threatening stimuli (Dayas *et al.*, 2001; Newport and Nemeroff, 2002).

The concept of stress elucidates the behavioral and physiological mechanisms by which genes, early life experiences, living and working environment, interpersonal relationships, diet, exercise, sleep and other lifestyle factors all converge to affect body chemistry, structure and function over a lifetime (McEwen, 2000). Some of the physiological changes associated with the stress response include: (1) mobilization of energy to maintain brain and muscle function, (2) sharpened and focused attention on the perceived threat, (3) increased cerebral perfusion rates and local cerebral glucose utilization, (4) enhanced cardiovascular output and respiration, and redistribution of blood flow, increasing substrate and energy delivery to the brain and muscles, (5) modulation of immune function, (6) inhibition of reproductive physiology and sexual behavior, and (7) decreased feeding and appetite. These orchestrated responses are geared to alter the internal milieu in such a way so as to increase the probability of survival (Goligorsky, 2001). This chapter describes the impact of prenatal stress experienced by the mother on development of the fetus during pregnancy and later in postnatal life.

Reproductive and Developmental Toxicology, Edited by Ramesh C. Gupta
ISBN: 978-0-12-382032-7

STRESS AND DEVELOPMENTAL BIOLOGY

Developmental origins of individual differences

There has been a major paradigm shift in developmental biology regarding fundamental concepts of how the central nervous system and the rest of the organism develops and functions. As thought earlier, development is viewed not just as an expression of information carried in a gene, but rather as a dynamic interdependency of genes and environment. Genes and environment are no longer considered to exert separate influences, characterized by a continuous process of interactions in a place and time – specific manner (Smotherman and Robinson, 1995). This concept also provides evidence and supports the ancient belief, in many cultures, that a mother's emotional state during pregnancy may influence the development of her fetus. Thus the best of physical (including nutrition) and spiritual environment should be provided to the mother. This dynamic gene–environment interaction is affected by evolving various systems during embryonic life to guide development. In the context of this formulation, environment plays a necessary role for development to occur (Gluckman and Hanson, 2004).

Research studies examining the effects of prenatal stress first appeared in the literature in the mid-1950s. In recent years, the topic of stress has gained increasing relevance, both from a basic scientific as well as clinical perspective. There are individual differences in psychoneurobiological processes in health and diseases of the nervous, endocrine, immune, cardiovascular, reproductive, gastrointestinal and musculoskeletal systems (McEwen, 1998; Sapolsky *et al.*, 2000; Lupien and Lepage, 2001). Regarding the origins of individual differences, two kinds of models have been suggested. The first model emphasizes the role of accumulation of adverse social and psychological conditions in producing dysregulation of normally functioning neurobiological processes. The second model emphasizes the developmental origins of individual differences through a series of interactions, or conditional probabilities. This model suggests that the effects of genes, inherited at conception, on fetal developmental and birth outcomes are conditioned by the environment within the fetus and uterus.

The individual differences in psychoneuroendocrine processes during development contribute to the risk of at least three sets of outcomes: prematurity, adverse neurodevelopment and chronic degenerative diseases in adulthood. Each of these distinct classes of adverse health outcomes represents major public health issues, and growing evidence supports a crucial role for early developmental process in their genesis (Gluckman and Hanson, 2004).

Any one influence, such as socioeconomic disadvantage, does not have a single quantifiable risk associated with it. Its risk is conditioned by events and environments at earlier, crucial stages of development (Barker, 2002). This orchestrated response to stress involves various mechanisms that allow the body to make necessary physiological and metabolic adjustments required to cope with the demands of homeostatic challenge (Gold and Chrousos, 2002). Such changes may occur on the physiological (emotional and cognitive), behavioral and biological level (altered autonomic and neuroendocrine function). There is some evidence that preterm parturition is a maternal adaptation to limit the energetic costs of individual pregnancies in case of extreme stress situations at the time of conception (Pike, 2005). A new field of behavioral perinatology has been defined which is an interdisciplinary area of research that involves studies of the dynamic time-, place- and context-dependent interplay between biological and behavioral processes in fetal, neonatal and infant life, i.e. effects of maternal pre- and perinatal stress and maternal–placental–fetal stress physiology. It has been suggested that pre- and perinatal stress play a significant role as an independent risk factor for adverse developmental and health outcomes (Wadhwa, 2005). The most consistently examined psychosocial stress measures include stressful life events and exposure to chronic stressors (Paarlberg *et al.*, 1995). A stressful life event, such as an earthquake, is most likely to result in preterm delivery if it is experienced early in pregnancy (Glynn *et al.*, 2001). Thus, the broader context of women's negative social experiences and emotional state translate into a physiological stress response that influences the risk for poor fetal outcomes.

Neuroanatomy of stress response

Multiple brain structures are involved in the organization of responses to aversive or stressful stimuli. Among them are the hypothalamus, septohippocampal system, amygdala, cingulate and prefrontal cortices, brain regions such as the brainstem catecholamine cell body groups, the parabrachial nucleus, cuneiform nucleus and dorsal raphe nucleus (Van de Kar and Blair, 1999). Most sensory inputs pass through either the reticular activating system or the thalamus, which function as relay stations, to the amygdala and sensory cortex. The amygdala is composed of several nuclei, which perform different functions. The amygdala also innervates and is innervated by the dorsal raphe nucleus and catecholaminergic nuclei located in the brainstem, which, in turn, innervate CRF neurons in the hypothalamic paraventricular nucleus. CRF neurons in the paraventricular nucleus receive input from the central amygdala both directly and through the bed nucleus of the stria terminalis. This amygdala–hypothalamic pathway is believed to play a key role in the adrenocortical response to a number of somatosensory stimuli (Carrasco and Van deKar, 2003; Shekhar *et al.*, 2005). The hypothalamic paraventricular nucleus plays a pivotal role in the adaptive response to stressors. Activation of the parvicellular neurons of the paraventricular nucleus increases the release of CRF and vasopressin and initiates the endocrine response to a stressor, stimulating the release of pro-opiomelanocortin (POMC) products, which include ACTH and β-endorphin. The hypothalamic paraventricular nucleus also contains CRF neurons that project to noradrenergic cell bodies in the locus coeruleus, a norepinephrine system that controls the stress-induced stimulation of the sympatho-adrenal system, and produces an increase in norepinephrine levels in terminal regions such as the frontal cortex (Penalva *et al.*, 2002). ACTH is the key regulator of glucocorticoid secretion from the adrenal cortex. Glucocorticoid hormones, mainly corticosterone in rats and cortisol in humans, are the final effectors of the hypothalamic–pituitary–adrenocortical axis and participate in the control of homeostasis and the response of the organism to stressors (Gesing *et al.*, 2001). The organization of stress response is summarized in Figure 62.1.

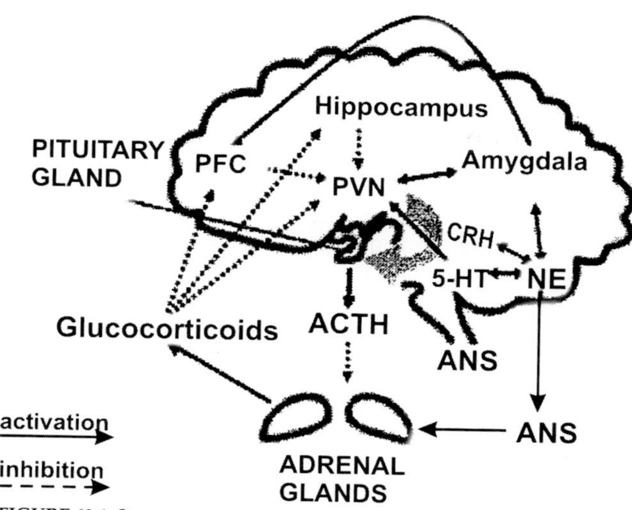

FIGURE 62.1 Stress response system.

Role of the neuroendocrine axis during fetal development

There are many reports suggesting that stress and social factors exert significant influences on physiological processes such as the HPA axis in non-pregnant humans (Chrousos and Gold, 1992; McEwen, 1998). But, *per se*, gestation produces profound alterations in several maternal systems, including the neuroendocrine system (Yen, 1994), that may alter the normal pattern of physiological responses to exogenous stimuli or perturbations such as stress. For instance, pregnancy has been associated with blunted autonomic responses and endocrine responses to a variety of physical and chemical challenges (Schulte *et al.*, 1990). A lot of studies were conducted to determine the effect of maternal stress on the neuroendocrine system and its impact on fetal development. Wadhwa (2005) indicated that despite the pregnancy-associated elevations in baseline concentrations of maternal pituitary–adrenal hormones, maternal stress was associated with enhanced levels of maternal ACTH and cortisol, whereas social support reduced their concentrations. Another study was conducted by the same group to determine whether the application of mild behavioral stress could evoke reliable physiological (i.e., sympathetic–adrenal–medullary/autonomic) responses during different stages of pregnancy, and to determine whether gestational age and baseline pituitary–adrenal stress hormone levels affect the magnitude of autonomic stress reactivity in pregnancy. They found that autonomic reactivity was significantly attenuated in pregnant subjects as compared to non-pregnant controls. Moreover, there was a progressive increase in attenuation of the stress response with advancing gestational age. At rest, there was no association of baseline levels of autonomic and endocrine parameters. However, upon challenge, baseline levels of cortisol accounted for between 30 and 52% of the variance in autonomic responses to stress (higher baseline stress hormone levels were associated with smaller stress responses). It was postulated that maternal pituitary–adrenal hormone concentrations, and not gestational age, *per se*, moderate maternal physiological responses to environmental stress.

As discussed earlier, CRF (or CRH), a 41-amino acid neuropeptide, is hypothesized to be an integrator of multiple components of the stress response. In addition to hypothalamic–pituitary–adrenal regulation, CRF elicits stress-like effects such as the activation of the autonomic nervous system, arousal, anxiety-like behaviors, suppression of the immune system and suppression of eating behavior. It is predominantly of hypothalamic origin. However, during pregnancy, the placenta becomes a major extra-hypothalamic site for CRH production and action. Placental CRH, which has only been found in primates (Smith *et al.*, 1999), is identical to CRH from hypothalamus, but differs markedly in its regulation. Hypothalamic CRH production decreases in a negative feedback loop with increased levels of cortisol, adrenocorticotropin (ACTH), and in an ultrashort loop with circulating CRH (Clifton and Challis, 1997). In contrast, placental CRH production is stimulated by increased glucocorticoids. In contrast to the negative control exerted on the brain and pituitary, cortisol stimulates the production of CRH in the placenta, establishing a positive feedback loop that terminates upon delivery (Clifton and Challis, 1997). The internal environmental cues are delivered via glucocorticoids (stress hormones) in the circulatory system, but fetal responses and the initiation of the final terminal pathway to parturition are regulated by placentally derived CRH. It has been hypothesized that the effects of maternal psychosocial stress and stress-related maternal HPA dysregulation on fetal developmental and health outcomes are mediated, in part, by placental CRH (Vale *et al.*, 1981). It has been implicated as one of the central mediators of the activity of the HPA axis and the physiological responses to stress and inflammation (Vale *et al.*, 1981; Chrousos, 1992). Several studies have demonstrated that placental CRH is involved in the physiology of normal parturition and that elevated CRH concentrations could significantly predict the risk for spontaneous preterm births (Hobel *et al.*, 1999; Erickson *et al.*, 2001; Holzman *et al.*, 2001; Inder *et al.*, 2001; Hoawad *et al.*, 2002). High levels of CRH have been associated with pregnancy-induced hypertension, fetal asphyxia, umbilical vascular insufficiency, preeclampsia, fetal growth restriction, preterm labor and multiple gestation (Perkins *et al.*, 1995; Petraglia *et al.*, 1996; Clifton and Challis, 1997).

Animal studies on developmental biology

Animal models have provided valuable information regarding the role of prenatal stress in negatively influencing critical development of the fetus and health outcomes over their lifespan, including brain structure and function, sexual differentiation, (re)activity of the autonomic nervous, neuroendocrine, immune and reproductive systems, and physical health (Wadhwa *et al.*, 1998; Weinstock, 2001; Kofman, 2002). Prenatal stress in rodents has been found to alter baseline levels and distribution of regulatory neurotransmitters, including norepinephrine, dopamine, serotonin and acetylcholine, as well as stress-induced responsivity of the hypothalamic–pituitary–adrenal (HPA) axis and limbic structures. These prenatal stress-induced alterations have been shown to affect cognition (decreased learning), emotionality (increased anxiety) and social behavior (increased withdrawal) (Kofman, 2002). Similarly, the application of prenatal stress in non-human primates has been shown to alter endocrine, immune and neurobehavioral outcomes in offspring (Coe and Lubach, 2000; Schneider *et al.*, 2001). However, important discrepancies still exist between experimental models and humans, which may be due to the existence of inter-species differences in physiology and the developmental timeline. For example, primates are the only species that produce placental corticotropin-releasing hormone (CRH) during pregnancy. The timing of maturation of the HPA axis relative to birth is also highly species-specific and is closely linked to landmarks of brain development (Dobbing and Sands, 1979). In animals that give birth to precocious offspring (sheep, guinea-pigs, primates), maximal brain growth and a large proportion of neuroendocrine maturation takes place *in utero*. By contrast, in species that give birth to non-precocious offspring (rats, rabbits, mice), much of neuroendocrine development occurs in the postnatal period (Dent *et al.*, 2000).

Wadhwa (2005) proposed that maternal psychosocial stress exerts a significant and independent negative influence on fetal developmental outcomes. It was suggested that these effects are mediated, in part, via maternal–placental–fetal neuroendocrine mechanisms, with a central role for placental CRH. The effects of prenatal stress are also outcome-specific, and are moderated by the nature, timing and duration of stress. The prenatal stress in early gestation exerts a larger impact on outcomes related to the length of gestation and fetal growth as compared to stress exposure in the latter part of gestation. Among spontaneous births prenatal stress directly influences the length of gestation, whereas among elective births, it increases risk of obstetric complications (e.g., preeclampsia) (Wadhwa *et al.*, 1998, 2001, 2002).

Prenatal stress and its impact on fetal growth

A number of studies have been conducted to assess the influence of maternal psychosocial processes on pregnancy outcomes related to the length of gestation and fetal growth and showed that each unit increase of prenatal life event stress was significantly associated with a 55.03 g decrease in infant birth weight and with a 32% increase in the relative risk of low birth weight (<2500 g). Moreover, each unit increase of prenatal pregnancy-specific anxiety was significantly associated with a 3-day decrease in gestational age at birth (Wadhwa *et al.*, 1993). Further, Glynn *et al.* (2001) suggested that psychological responses to a stressor were progressively attenuated as gestation advances, and the timing of stressor in pregnancy could be an important factor in determining its impact on the length of human gestation. Several larger, population-based epidemiological studies of prenatal stress and prematurity-related outcomes have suggested that high levels of maternal psychosocial stress are independently associated with a significant increase in the risk for prematurity. However, the "fetal origins" hypothesis suggests that growth restriction caused by poor maternal dietary intake or inadequate nutrient supply to the fetus during periods of rapid growth may result in preferential allocation of nutrients to energetically expensive functions, such as diverting glucose to the brain as a way of adaptation to the situation (Osmond *et al.*, 1993; Barker *et al.*, 1993; Fowden, 2001). Prolonged nutritional stress during pregnancy results in compromised microvillous structures of the placenta thus further reducing fetal access to nutrients, culminating in delivery of smaller babies (Fowden, 2001; McMillen *et al.*, 2001). The final outcome of each pregnancy is a product of a tug-of-war between maternal limitations placed on fetal growth and coevolved fetal responses to an insufficient environment (Haig, 1993; Wells, 2003). Maternal nutritional status prior to conception, primarily pre-pregnancy body mass index, shows a consistent link to preterm delivery in many nutritional intervention studies (WHO, 1995; Villar *et al.*, 2003).

Prenatal stress and its impact on later life

While the fetal adaptation/adjustments appear to increase the chances of surviving a resource-limited intrauterine environment, they appear to be accompanied by long-term costs to health. There is now considerable evidence that lower birth weight is associated with elevated blood pressure (Huxley *et al.*, 2000), serum cholesterol (Barker *et al.*, 1993) and glucose intolerance (Curhan *et al.*, 1996; Law *et al.*, 2002) later in life. Epidemiological studies have also shown links between lower birth weight and greater risk for adult mortality from cardiovascular disease and non-insulin-dependent diabetes mellitus (NIDDM) (Rasmussen, 2001). Studies regarding mechanism of such effects indicate that the number of nephrons at birth, which is related to fetal nutrition, is linked to increased risk for hypertension later in life (Hinchcliffe *et al.*, 1992; Woods *et al.*, 2001). Major reductions in the size of kidneys resulting from growth restriction are believed to limit sodium excretion, thereby increasing risk for hypertension.

Further, evidence for adjustments of the immune system in response to poor prenatal nutrition or growth has been documented. Several fetal outcomes may be ameliorated by postnatal environmental influences. For example, increase in stress reactivity in early childhood as a result of maternal stress appears to be dampened by a nurturing postnatal psychosocial environment (Brouwers *et al.*, 2001; Monk, 2001). Taken together, fetal responses to a stressful environment appear to permanently alter the function and metabolism of many systems and organs, and persist after birth. Kuzawa (2005) suggested that there may be advantages to buffering against rapid environmental changes by reducing energetic demands across generations when conditions are chronically poor.

In addition to stress as such, other factors like subjective measures of stress perceptions and appraisals, maternal age, body-mass index, occupation, personality and coping styles are more strongly associated with adverse outcomes. In terms of the magnitude of the effect, pregnant women reporting high levels of stress are at approximately double risk for preterm birth or fetal growth restriction compared to women reporting low levels of stress (Hedegaard *et al.*, 1996; Misra *et al.*, 2001; Dole *et al.*, 2003).

The findings of Wadhwa *et al.* (1998) also support the premise that in human pregnancy placental CRH activity is increased by stress-related maternal pituitary–adrenal hormones. Further, Sandman *et al.* (2003) reported that the fetuses of mothers with highly elevated CRH levels did not respond significantly to the presence of the novel stimulus, thereby providing preliminary support for the notion that abnormally elevated levels of placental CRH may play a role in impaired neurodevelopment. Similarly, fetal exposure to relatively high levels of the maternal opiate β-endorphin, relative to ACTH, was associated with a significantly lower rate of habituation – indicative of poor learning and memory. The study further strengthens the role played by the prenatal environment in modulating aspects of human fetal brain development that underlie processes related to recognition, appraisal, response, memory and habituation. Moreover prenatal stress has been shown to affect subsequent infant development. Wadhwa *et al.* (1998) showed that higher levels of prenatal stress and stress hormones significantly increased infant temperamental difficulties. It was found that maternal anxiety and depression during the prenatal, but not the postnatal, period significantly predicted infant behavioral reactivity to novelty.

Maternal neuroendocrine environment and fetal development

As described earlier, there is a surge of stress hormones and altered neuroendocrine environment during prenatal stress of the pregnant mother. The fetal brain and peripheral tissues are very sensitive to a number of agents like growth factors, transcription factors, nutrients, etc. Steroids in particular have powerful organizational effects on the brain and peripheral tissues. Animal studies have demonstrated that during development, fetal exposure to glucocorticoids (GCs) directly affects the development and subsequent function of neurotransmitter systems (and their transporter mechanisms) in the brainstem; the development of GC receptor expression and structural components in the hippocampus; and development and subsequent function of parvocellular neurons (CRH/AVP system). Moreover, because the brainstem neurotransmitter systems project directly to the hippocampus and paraventricular nucleus (PVN), GC-induced changes indirectly impact the function of the hippocampus and PVN (Welberg and Seckl, 2001). Fetal GC exposure also delays axon myelination and affects polyamines, which are the major regulators of neural cell replication and differentiation. The molecular mechanisms of these effects are believed to involve alterations in the set points of HPA axis activity and feedback sensitivity, and alterations of tissue GC receptor expression (Seckl, 2001). Animal studies have shown that antenatal exposure to GCs reduces offspring birth weight and produces permanent hypertension, hyperglycemia, hyperinsulinemia and altered behavior and neuroendocrine responses including increased risk of morbidity and mortality throughout the lifespan (Kramer, 1987; Barker *et al.*, 1993). Preterm delivery of the fetus when it is mature enough to survive in the extrauterine environment may have potential advantages for both the mother and the fetus. For example, avoiding the final few weeks of pregnancy when brain development is most rapid may preserve scarce energy stores for a marginally nourished mother (Peacock, 1991; Haig, 1993). Moreover, the fetus may benefit by avoiding direct competition for limited supplies of glucose and gases. As the demand for glucose and gases to support rapid brain development increases, the fetus may prevent an energy-demanding metabolic crisis by initiating parturition (Ellison *et al.*, 1993).

Endocrine–immune interactions during developmental biology

In addition to maternal–fetal neuroendocrine processes, maternal and fetal proinflammatory immune responses produced by intrauterine or reproductive tract infection play an important role in adverse fetal outcomes (Goldenberg *et al.*, 2000; Romero *et al.*, 2001). As the endocrine and immune systems are known to extensively regulate and counter-regulate one another (McEwen *et al.*, 1997; Elenkov and Chrousos, 1999; Shanks and Lightman, 2001), these interactions are being explored in the context of stress in pregnancy and fetal development. Culhane *et al.* (2001) reported a role for maternal psychosocial stress in the development of reproductive tract infection in human pregnancy in a population of 454 socially disadvantaged, primarily African–American women.

STRESS AND REPRODUCTIVE BIOLOGY

Stress results in a series of complex, interactive, adaptive responses and, when these are inadequate, excessive or prolonged, physiological functions like reproduction are disturbed. The influence of stress on reproduction results from interactions between endocrine, paracrine and neural systems. Stressful stimuli activate the HPA axis and the sympathoadrenal system, the consequences of which have already been discussed in an earlier section. Glucocorticoids are the final effectors of this system. Activation of the sympathoadrenal system evokes the release of noradrenaline from postganglionic nerve terminals, while preganglionic innervation of the adrenal medulla results in increased secretion of catecholamines, principally adrenaline, into the bloodstream. Glucocorticoids and adrenaline act primarily to counteract the effects of stress. The regulation of the reproductive system occurs via by the hypothalamo–pituitatry–gonadal (HPG) axis, and stress can influence reproduction by action at all these three levels, namely the hypothalamus, the pituitary and the gonads. The central nervous system (CNS) is also a key player in reproductive physiology and its dysregulation. A considerable amount of research has been done in the area of stress and reproductive function, and the general consensus is that stress and the neuroendocrine regulation of reproduction are species dependent (Goldstein, 1987; Chatterton, 1990; Tilbrook *et al.*, 1999).

Further, the effects of stress on reproduction depend on the critical timing of stress, the genetic predisposition to stress and the type of stress. The effect of stress on reproduction is also influenced by the duration of the responses induced by various stressors. Acute and chronic stressors induce differential effects on reproductive function. Whereas chronic stress usually consistently inhibits reproductive function, acute (or transient) stress effects could be either stimulatory or inhibitory. Ovulation, expression of sexual behavior and implantation of the embryo are by far the most crucial aspects of reproductive function and neuroendocrine system (Rivier and Rivest, 1991). Thus, plasma gonadotropins assays are a good and sensitive marker/indicator, since the pulsatile secretion of LH is hypothalamus-dependent through GnRH (Clarke and Cummins, 1982; Tilbrook and Clarke, 1995). Like most other neuroendocrine networks, like the HPA axis, the secretion and actions of GnRH are under the feedback regulatory control of gonadal sex steroids and inhibin. Thus, stress may influence the secretion of the gonadotropins through mechanisms that modify the synthesis or the secretion of GnRH, the responsiveness of the gonadotrophs to the actions of GnRH or the feedback actions of gonadal hormones (Figure 62.1). There is an overwhelming body of evidence implicating the hypothalamus and pituitary control of stress but the effects of stress on the feedback actions of gonadal hormones are little understood. The role of the glycoprotein inhibin in such regulation in still unclear, though it is documented that inhibin is a feedback regulator of FSH in both sexes (Clarke *et al.*, 1986; Tilbrook and Clarke, 1995).

Stressor types and reproductive function

A wide variety of stressors are known to influence reproduction. For example, physical stressors (shearing, restraint, foot-shocks, etc.), metabolic stressors (insulin-induced hypoglycemia), immunological stressors (infections and exogenously administered cytokines or endotoxins), cardiovascular stressors (nitroprusside) and psychological stressors (isolation, social interactions, human–animal interactions, etc.) have all been reported to highlight this concept.

A range of other environmental factors, such as nutrition, can also influence reproduction. Interestingly, irrespective of the nature of the stressor, the activation of the HPA axis is the characteristically consistent response and could be associated with reduced LH secretion (Moberg, 1987; Ferin, 1999; Tilbrook *et al.*, 1999). Prolonged stress exposure results in suppressed gonadotropin secretion and reproductive function, whereas the results of studies with acute (short-term) stressors have been equivocal, to say the least. Such variable effects have been found across a variety of species, and there are a number of studies showing fluctuating LH responses to different types of stressors. Some of the short-term stress effects have been replicated by exogenous stress hormone administrations. Thus, while chronic stress consistently inhibits reproduction, the reported effects of acute or repeated acute stress are more variable. Different stressors may stimulate different systems, some being inhibitory and some stimulatory with respect to reproduction. At least some of the variable effects of acute stress may also be explained by differences between the sexes and the influence of sex steroids (Tilbrook *et al.*, 1999).

Stress and reproductive function: role of sex differences

It has been well documented that stress susceptibility is gender-dependent. Recent studies have shown that male and female rats respond in a differential manner to emotional stressors like restraint stress and this is reflected in behavioral, endocrinal and immunological responses, and complex neural pathways and neurohumoral mechanisms may be involved (Chakraborty *et al.*, 2007; Reich *et al.*, 2009). Other studies have shown that these differences may be HPA-axis- and sex-steroid-dependent. The impact of stress on reproduction may also be sex-dependent and is likely to be influenced by the predominance of secretion of a particular sex steroid. For example, the mechanisms of stress-induced LH secretion have been shown to be different in rams and ewes. Studies in gonadectomized male and female sheep showed that the mechanisms of LH suppression in response to experimental stressors were different. It was proposed that a reduction in LH pulse frequency most likely indicated an effect on the secretion of GnRH. Additionally, an alteration in LH pulse amplitude could be a centrally mediated effect to reduce GnRH pulse amplitude or a direct pituitary effect on the gonadotroph. It was concluded that the mechanisms by which isolation and restraint (the stressors used in this study) suppressed LH secretion in males treated with testosterone, and in ewes treated with progesterone, involved a reduction in the secretion of GnRH. These findings also suggest that stress affects reproduction by mechanisms that differ between males and females and with different backgrounds of sex steroids (Tilbrook *et al.*, 1999). Further studies in female rhesus monkeys have shown that ovarian estradiol secretion is a determinant factor on the stress-induced LH profile. Stress-induced LH pulse and hypothalamic electrical activity was detected in ovarioectomized animals – a response that was reversed by estradiol treatment. Similar effects were also seen on exposure to immunological stressors. In ovarioectomized rhesus monkeys, intraventricular injections of interleukin-1α enhanced cortisol levels and lowered LH and FSH, and these responses were normalized after estradiol treatment. It was also shown that the intravenous injection of lipopolysaccharide (LPS, a bacterial endotoxin) resulted in the activation of the HPA axis and increased LH and FSH levels, with either a reduction or no change in estradiol concentrations (Xiao *et al.*, 1998). Gender differences in respect to stress-induced gonadotropin secretion are not reported.

The relationship between stress and human reproduction has also been recognized. Studies have shown that interactions between emotional stress and infertility are possible, and that a bi-directional link could exist between stress and infertility. Most of the investigations indicated that stress may be the effect rather than the cause of infertility. Stress hormones may be acting at the level of the brain to mediate this stress – infertility interaction, especially on the hypothalamus–pituitary and on the female reproductive organs. Catecholamines (adrenalin, nonadrenaline and dopamine) and glucocorticoids may interact with hormones which are responsible for normal ovulatory cycles, i.e. gonadotropin releasing hormone (GnRH), prolactin, LH and FSH. Endogenous opiates (endorphins, enkephalins, dynorphins) and melatonin (a pineal hormone) secretion are altered by stress and could interfere with ovulation. Sympathetic innervation of the female reproductive system provides routes by which stress can influence fertility by acting at the level of the sex organs. Infertility causes stress which compounds with the passage of time. Isolation, emotional unfulfillment, unrealized potential of married life, etc. are among the important causes of this phenomenon (Schenker *et al.*, 1992).

Stress, reproductive function and the neuroendocrine axis: role of glucocorticoids

The CNS and neuroendocrine networking play a crucial role during stress and its depressing influence on reproductive function. GnRH neurons and their connections with other interneurons, as the circulating humoral mediators during stress, play a crucial role in this phenomenon. The responsiveness of the gonadotrophs to GnRH in the pituitary may be under the regulatory influence of various neuromodulators (e.g., neuropeptides) released into the hypophysial portal system during stress. They include CRF, AVP, endogenous opioid peptides, catecholamines, 5-hydroxytryptamine and glucocorticoids. Glucocorticoids, which are synonymous with stress reactions, may act as important regulators of stress-induced suppression of LH. Exogenous administration of natural and synthetic steroids has been shown to lower gonadotropin levels in a variety of species including humans. However, decreased gonadotropin levels have also been reported in response to such drug administration in relation to acute stress. Further, sex and sex steroid status may be determinants for the effects of glucocorticoids on GnRh and gonadotropin secrertion. Further experiments showed that estradiol was able to increase the tissue concentration of GnRH and mRNA encoding the GnRH receptor in ovariectomized ewes and castrated rams and these were differentially attenuated by cortisol injections. These and several other studies led to the hypothesis that cortisol was instrumental in enhancing the effects of estradiol and reducing the stimulation of GnRH receptor expression by estrogen. It was also observed that interactions between cortisol and estradiol and sex differences in such effects were possible (Daley *et al.*, 1999; Tilbrook *et al.*, 1999). Studies in pigs and rhesus monkeys also showed that sustained increased levels of cortisol were needed to suppress reproduction. Exposure to acute stressors and/or infusions of cortisol or ACTH was used as experimental techniques to demonstrate this. In humans, though chronically increased plasma concentrations of cortisol were associated with depressed reproduction (Loriaux and Nieman, 1990), glucocorticoid-induced suppression of gonadotropin secretion has not essentially been a consistent finding. Infusion of cortisol in six men and four women for over 24 h did not affect the mean or pulsatile LH, FSH or α-subunit secretion, and it was proposed that maybe longer exposures to elevated cortisol levels may be required to get the desired effect on reproduction. Alternatively, other mediators released during stress may be involved in such suppression of the gonadal axis. It would be pertinent to mention here that ethical consideration precludes the use of more liberal pharmacological dosing of glucocorticoids in such experimental situations.

Experimental studies to localize the site of such glucocorticoid effects revealed most consistent to less convincing observations in different *in vitro* and *in vivo* set-ups. For example, glucocorticoids were found to decrease the transcriptional activity of the GnRH promoter in GT1 hypothalamic cell lines (Chandran *et al.*, 1994). Studies in rats showed that glucocorticoid receptors could be identified in hypothalamic GnRH neurones (Ahima and Harlan, 1992) and on pituitary gonadotrophs (Kononen *et al.*, 1992). These experimental data support the notion that glucocorticoids act at either of these sites to affect LH secretion in rodents. The results were, however, less confirmatory in nature with pigs and rhesus monkeys, but nevertheless, a hypothalamic site of action for glucocorticoids was contemplated. As mentioned earlier, glucocorticoid feedback action on the brain suppresses overactivity of the hypothalamo–pituitary–adrenal (HPA) axis. In addition, glucocorticoid secretion is also believed to contribute to the stress-induced gonadal suppression by central actions on the pituitary or hypothalamus. Acute or chronic administration of glucocorticoids is known to suppress the activity of the hypothalamo–pituitary–gonadal (HPG) axis. This seems to be a logical effect, because suppression of reproduction would give higher priority to individual survival rather than the maintenance of species (Maeda and Tsukamura, 2006).

Several recent studies contradicted this conventional hypothesis and reported that glucocorticoids could actually be protective during stress-induced inhibition of reproductive function. This effect was prostaglandin mediated and operating at the level of the CNS. Earlier reports had also indicated that glucocorticoids could have similar effects on LH secretion during infectious stress. Interestingly, adrenalectomy resulted in greater suppression of stress-induced LH secretion and that glucocorticoid replacement restored LH secretion (Matsuwaki *et al.*, 2003, 2004, 2006). In non-stressed situations, exogenously administered glucocorticoids do actually suppress LH secretion in a variety of species. However, Matsuwaki *et al.* (2006) proposed that the situation may be different during stress exposures, where this hormone may be protective against stress-induced LH suppression. Thus, endogenously released hormone during stress may act quite differently than the exogenously administered cortisol in non-stressed settings. In fact earlier data had shown that TNF-α (which mimics infectious stress)-induced suppression of LH secretion was attenuated by glucocorticoid administration. Similar findings were shown with the endotoxin (LPS)-induced stress model where glucocorticoids were unable to counteract inhibition of LH secretion in rats and sheep. Such LH suppression was also seen in adrenalectomized and metyrapone (a glucocorticoid synthesis inhibitor)-treated animals. Studies also showed that hypothalamic CRH-mediated GnRH/LH suppression may not be the only answer to this dilemma. Brain prostaglandins (PGs) could be involved in the mediation of this protective effect of glucocorticoids during stress-induced suppression of reproductive function. A variety of stressors like infections, hypoglycemia, restraint-stimulated brain PG synthesis (COX-2 mediated) and indomethacin (a PG synthesis inhibitor) effectively counteracts the stress-induced suppression of LH secretion. It was further speculated that PGs released in the brain could also be responsible for the stress-induced neurobehavioral changes. Thus the role of the HPA axis and its influence on the HPG axis may be different in stressed and non-stressed situations, which could reflect on stress-induced reproductive function.

CONCLUDING REMARKS AND FUTURE DIRECTIONS

The psychoneuroendocrinology of stress and stress-related neuroendocrine dysregulation are important phenomena in fetal outcomes related to prematurity and neurodevelopment. This neuroendocrine response generates life history transitions necessary for survival of the individual. Stressful experiences in early gestation are better predictors of adverse outcomes than the same measures assessed later in gestation. In humans, exposure of the fetus to elevated corticosteroids, either from the mother or the fetal adrenal gland, may predispose individuals to increased health risks throughout life. Inter-individual differences also regulate the risk of developing chronic degenerative diseases in later life. Thus, there are important trade-offs between immediate survival in the developmental habitat vs. long-term phenotypic changes that result in reduced performance as an adult. These neuroendocrine/developmental responses, and their long-term phenotypic consequences, are deeply rooted in the evolutionary history of vertebrate animals.

The clinical application of knowledge about impact of maternal psychosocial stress in pregnancy for risk assessment and intervention has been limited as the commonly used measures of maternal stress have low sensitivity and specificity in predicting adverse outcomes. Thus, there is a need for better methodology to be followed to identify the determinants of inter- and intra-individual variability and form the link between maternal stress and adverse birth outcomes, to identify which subgroup(s) of pregnant women, under what circumstances, and at what stage in pregnancy, are especially susceptible to the deleterious effects of prenatal stress on birth outcomes. The approach to the measurement of maternal stress has relied exclusively on self-report, retrospective recall measures of psychological state or affect over time, which may be prone to numerous biases that undermine validity.

The effects of maternal psychosocial processes are mediated, in part, by the maternal–placental–fetal neuroendocrine axis. The psychoneuroendocrine processes may interact with immune processes to influence the risk of reproductive tract infection and its pathophysiological consequences. Further, stress-related factors in the maternal and intrauterine environment exert a significant influence on the fetal behavior and alter central brain processes related to recognition, memory and habituation. The influence of prenatal stress and maternal–placental hormones on the developing fetus may persist after birth, affecting the temperament and behavioral reactivity in the postnatal life and appear to be accompanied by long-term effects on metabolic and cardiovascular functions.

A variety of stressful conditions are known to suppress reproductive function, such as infection, malnutrition, restraint, exercise, surgical trauma, etc. The HPA axis and its hormones (CRH, ACTH, vasopressin and glucocorticoids) have been shown to inhibit GnRH/gonadotropin secretion by acting at the hypothalamic and/or pituitary levels. CRH, in turn, inhibits GnRH release in hypophyseal portal blood or GnRH pulse generator activity. Arginine vasopressin and ACTH are also reported to inhibit LH secretion by decreasing responsiveness of the pituitary to GnRH as well as decreasing GnRH release. The effects of stress on reproduction depend on the critical timing of stress, the genetic predisposition to stress and the nature of the stressor. The effect of stress on reproduction is also influenced by the duration of the responses induced by various stressors. Chronic stress usually results in inhibition of reproduction, while the effects of acute stress are equivocal – the general trend being inhibitory. The most sensitive of the reproductive processes are ovulation, expression of sexual behavior and implantation of the embryo, since they are directly controlled by the neuroendocrine system. However, for acute stress, which is probably the most commonly experienced form in most species including humans, it is unclear how reproductive function will be affected. Suppression of reproduction is more likely under conditions of chronic stress and may involve action at the hypothalamus or pituitary. Furthermore, there are likely to be species differences in the effect of glucocorticoids on gonadotropin secretion, and the presence of sex steroids and the sex of an individual are likely to be deciding factors. A fresh approach is required to understand the mechanisms by which chronic and acute stress influence reproduction. This approach must consider the stress pathways that are activated by particular stressors and determine how these pathways affect the secretion and actions of various hormones and neuromodulators.

REFERENCES

Ahima RS, Harlan RE (1992) Glucocorticoid receptors in LHRH neurons. *Neuroendocrinology* **56:** 845–50

Barker, DJ (2002) Fetal programming of coronary heart disease. *Trends Endocrinol Metab* **13(9):** 364–8.

Barker D, Gluckman P, Godfrey K, Harding J, Owens J, Robinson J (1993) Fetal nutrition and cardiovascular disease in adult life. *Lancet* **341:** 938–1001.

Brouwers EPM, van Baar AL, Pop VJM (2001) Maternal anxiety during pregnancy and subsequent infant development. *Inf Behav Dev* **24:** 95–106.

Carrasco GA, Van de Kar LD (2003) Neuroendocrine pharmacology of stress. *Eur J Pharmacol* **463:** 235–72.

Chakraborty A, Gulati K, Banerji BD, Ray A (2007) Possible involvement of free radicals in the differential neurobehavioral responses to stress in male and female rats. *Behav Brain Res* **17:** 321–25

Chandran UR, Attardi B, Friedman R, Dong K-W, Roberts JL, DeFranco DB (1994) Glucocorticoid receptor-mediated repression of gonadotropin-releasing hormone promoter activity in GT1 hypothalamic cell lines. *Endocrinology* **134:** 1467–74

Chatterton RT (1990) The role of stress in female reproduction: animal and human considerations. *Int J Fertil* **35:** 8–13

Chrousos GP (1992) Regulation and dysregulation of the hypothalamic–pituitary–adrenal axis. The corticotrophin releasing hormone perspective. *Endocrinol Metab Clin North Am* **21:** 833–58.

Chrousos GP, Gold PW (1992) The concepts and stress and stress systems disorders. *JAMA* **267:** 1244–52.

Clarke IJ, Cummins JT (1982) The temporal relationship between gonadotropin releasing hormone (GnRH) and luteinizing hormone (LH) secretion in ovariectomized ewes. *Endocrinol* **111:** 1737–9.

Clarke IJ, Findlay JK, Cummins JT, Ewens WJ (1986) Effects of ovine follicular fluid on plasma LH and FSH secretion in ovariectomized ewes to indicate the site of action of inhibin. *J Reproduc Fert* **77:** 575–85.

Clifton VL, Challis JG (1997) Placental corticotrophin releasing hormone function during human pregnancy. *Endocrinologist* **7:** 448–58.

Coe CL, Lubach GR (2000) Prenatal influences on neuroimmune set points in infancy. *Ann NY Acad Sci* **917:** 468–77.

Culhane, JF, Rauh V, Farley-McCollum K, Hogan V, Agnew K, Wadhwa PD (2001) Maternal stress is associated with bacterial vaginosis in human pregnancy. *Matern Child Health J* **5:** 127–34.

Curhan G, Chertow G, Willet W (1996) Birth weight and adult hypertension and obesity in women. *Circulation* **94:** 1310–15.

Daley CA, Sakurai H, Adams BM and Adams TE (1999) Effect of stress-like concentrations of cortisol on gonadotroph function in orchidectomized sheep. *Biol Reproduc* **60:** 158–63.

Dayas CV, Buller KM, Crane JW, Day TA (2001) Stressor organization: acute physical and psychological stressors elicit distinctive recruitment patterns in the amygdala and medullary noradrenergic cell groups. *Eur J Neurosci* **14:** 1143–52.

Dent GW, Smith MA, Levine S (2000) Rapid induction of corticotropin-releasing hormone gene transcription in the paraventricular nucleus of the developing rat. *Endocrinol* **141:** 1593–8.

Dobbing J, Sands J (1979) Comparative aspects of the brain growth spurt. *Early Hum Dev* **3:** 79–83.

Dole N, Savitz DA, Hertz-Picciotto I, Siega-Riz AM, McMahon M J, Buekens P (2003) Maternal stress and preterm birth. *Am J Epidemiol* **157:** 14–24.

Elenkov IJ, Chrousos GP (1999) Stress hormones Th1/Th2 patterns, pro/anti-inflammatory cytokines and susceptibility to disease. *Trends Endocrinol Metab* **10(9):** 359–68.

Ellison PT, Panter-Brick C, Lipson SF, O'Rourke MT (1993) The ecological context of human ovarian function. *Hum Reprod* **8:** 2248–58.

Erickson K, Thorsen P, Chrousos G, Grigoriadis DE, Khongsaly O, McGregor J, Schulkin J (2001) Preterm birth: associated neuroendocrine, medical, and behavioral risk factors. *J Clin Endocrinol Metab* **86:** 2544–52.

Ferin M (1999) Stress and the reproductive cycle. *J Clin Endocrinol Metab* **84:** 1768–74.

Fowden A (2001) Growth and metabolism. In *Fetal Growth and Development* (Harding R, Bocking A, eds.). Cambridge University Press, Cambridge, MA, pp. 44–69.

Gesing A, Bilang-Bleuel A, Droste SK, Linthorst ACE, Holsboer F, Reul JMHM (2001) Psychological stress increases hippocampal mineralocorticoid receptor levels: involvement of corticotropin releasing hormone. *J Neurosci* **21:** 4822–9.

Gluckman PD, Hanson MA (2004) Living with the past: evolution, development and patterns of disease. *Science* **305:** 1733–6.

Glynn L, Wadhwa PD, Dunkel-Schetter C, Sandman CA (2001) When stress happens matters: the effects of earthquake timing on stress responsivity in pregnancy. *Am J Obstet Gynecol* **184:** 637–42.

Gold PW, Chrousos GP (2002) Organization of the stress system and its dysregulation in melancholic and atypical depression: high vs low CRH/NE states. *Mol Psychiat* **7:** 254–75.

Goldenberg RL, Hauth JC, Andrews WW (2000) Mechanisms of disease: intrauterine infection and preterm delivery. *N Engl J Med* **342:** 1500–7.

Goldstein DS (1987) Stress-induced activation of the sympathetic nervous system. In *Neuroendocrinology of Stress* (Grossman A, ed.). Bailliere Tindall, London, pp. 253–78.

Goligorsky MS (2001) The concept of cellular "fight-or-flight" reaction to stress. *Am J Physiol Renal Physiol* **280:** F551–61.

Gulati K, Chakraborti A, Ray A (2009) Differential role of nitric oxide (NO) in acute and chronic stress induced neurobehavioral modulation and oxidative injury in rats. *Pharmacol Biochem Behav* **92:** 272–6.

Haig D (1993) Genetic conflicts of pregnancy. *Q Rev Biol* **68:** 495–532.

Hedegaard M, Henriksen TB, Secher NJ, Hatch MC, Sabroe S (1996) Do stressful life events affect duration of gestation and risk of preterm delivery? *Epidemiol* **7(4):** 339–45.

Hinchcliffe S, Lynch M, Sargent P, Howard C, Van Velzen D (1992) The effect of intrauterine growth retardation on the development of renal nephrons. *Br J Obstet Gynaecol* **99:** 296–301.

Hoawad AH, Goldenberg RL, Mercer B, Meis PJ, Iams JD, Das A, Caritis SN, Miodovnik M, Menard MK, Thurnau GR, Dombrowski M, Roberts JM (2002) The preterm prediction study: the value of serum alkaline phosphatase, alpha-fetoprotein, plasma corticotropin-releasing hormone, and other serum markers for the prediction of spontaneous preterm birth. *Am J Obstet Gynecol* **186 (5):** 990–6.

Hobel CJ, Dunkel-Schetter C, Roesch SC, Castro LC, Arora CP (1999) Maternal plasma corticotropin-releasing hormone associated with stress at 20 weeks gestation in pregnancies ending in preterm delivery. *Am J Obstet Gynecol* **180:** S257–63.

Holzman C, Jetton J, Siler-Khodr T, Fisher R, Rip T (2001) Second trimester corticotropin-releasing hormone levels in relation to preterm delivery and ethnicity. *Obstet Gynecol* **97:** 657–63.

Huxley R, Shiell A, Law C (2000) The role of size at birth and postnatal catch-up growth in determining systolic blood pressure: a systematic review of the literature. *J Hypertens* **18:** 815–31.

Inder WJ, Prickett TC, Ellis MJ, Hull L, Reid R, Benny PS, Livesey JH, Donald RA (2001) The utility of plasma CRH as a predictor of preterm delivery. *J Clin Endocrinol Metab* **86(12):** 5706–10.

Kofman O (2002) The role of prenatal stress in the etiology of developmental behavioural disorders. *Neurosci Biobehav Rev* **26(4):** 457–70.

Kononen J, Honkaniemi J, Alho H, Koistinaho J, Iadarola M, Pelto-Huikko M (1992) Fos-like immunoreactivity in the rat hypothalamic–pituitary axis after immobilization stress. *Endocrinology* **130:** 3041–7.

Kramer MS (1987) Determinants of low birth weight: methodological assessment and meta-analysis. *Bull WHO* **65:** 663–737.

Kuzawa C (2005) The origins of the developmental origins hypothesis and the role of postnatal environments: response to Koletzko. *Am J Hum Biol* **17(5):** 662–4.

Law C, Shiell A, Newsome C, Syddall H, Shinebourne E, Fayers P, Martyn C, de Swiet M (2002) Fetal, infant, and childhood growth and adult blood pressure: a longitudinal study from birth to 22 years of age. *Circulation* **105:** 1088–92.

Loriaux L, Nieman L (1990) Stress and reproduction: the role of cortisol. In *Neuroendocrine Regulation of Reproduction* (Yen SSC, Vale WW, eds.). Serono Symposia, Norwell, MA, pp. 307–11.

Lupien SJ, Lepage M (2001) Stress, memory, and the hippocampus: can't live with it, can't live without it. *Behav Brain Res* **127:** 137–58.

Maeda K, Tsukamura H (2006) The impact of stress on reproduction: are glucocorticoids inhibitory or protective to gonadotropin secretion? *Endocrinology* **147(3):** 1085–6.

Matsuwaki T, Kayasuga Y, Yamanouchi K, Nishihara M (2006) Maintenance of gonadotropin secretion by glucocorticoids under stress conditions through the inhibition of prostaglandin synthesis in the brain. *Endocrinology* **147:** 1087–93.

Matsuwaki T, Suzuki M, Yamanouchi K, Nishihara M (2004) Glucocorticoid counteracts the suppressive effect of tumor necrosis factor on the surge of luteinizing hormone secretion in rats. *J Endocrinol* **181:** 509–13.

Matsuwaki T, Watanabe E, Suzuki M, Yamanouchi K, Nishihara M (2003) Glucocorticoid maintains pulsatile secretion of luteinizing hormone under infectious stress condition. *Endocrinology* **144:** 3477–82.

McEwen BS (1998) Protective and damaging effects of stress mediators *N Engl J Med* **338:** 171–9.

McEwen BS (2000) Allostasis and allostatic load: implications for neuropsychopharmacology. *Neuropsychopharmacology* **22:** 108–24.

McEwen BS, Biron CA, Brunson KW, Bulloch K, Chambers WH, Dhabar FS, Goldfarb RH, Kitson RP, Miller A, Spencer RL, Weiss JM (1997) The role of adrenocorticoids as modulators of immune function in health and disease: neural, endocrine and immune interactions. *Brain Res Rev* **23:** 79–133.

McMillen IC, Adams MB, Ross JT, Coulter CL, Simonetta G, Owens JA, Robinson JS, Edwards LJ (2001) Fetal growth restriction: adaptations and consequences. *Reproduction* **122:** 195–204.

Misra DP, O'Campo P, Strobino D (2001) Testing a sociomedical model for preterm delivery. *Paediatr Perinat Epidemiol* **15:** 110–22.

Moberg GP (1987) Influence of the adrenal axis upon the gonads. *Oxford Rev Reprod Biol* **9:** 456–96.

Monk C (2001) Stress and mood disorders during pregnancy: implications for child development. *Psychiat Q* **72:** 347–57.

Newport DJ, Nemeroff CB (2002) Stress. In *Encyclopedia of the Human Brain*, Vol. 4. Elsevier, pp. 449–62.

Osmond C, Barker D, Winter P, Fall C, Simmonds S (1993) Early growth and death from cardiovascular disease in women. *Br Med J* **307:** 1519–24.

Paarlberg K, Vingerhoets AJM, Passchier J, Dekker G, Vangeijn H (1995) Psychosocial factors and pregnancy outcome – a review with emphasis on methodological issues. *J Psychosom Res* **39:** 563–95.

Peacock N (1991) An evolutionary perspective on the patterning maternal investment in pregnancy. *Hum Nat* **2:** 351–85.

Penalva RG, Flachskamm C, Zimmermann S, Wurst W, Holsboer F, Reul JMHM, Linthorst AC (2002) Corticotropin releasing hormone receptor type 1 deficiency enhances hippocampal serotonergic neurotransmission: an in vivo microdialysis study in mutant mice. *Neurosci* **109:** 253–66.

Perkins A, Linton E, Eben F, Simpson J, Wolfe C, Redman C (1995) Corticotrophin-releasing hormone and corticotrophin-releasing hormone binding protein in normal and pre-eclamptic human pregnancies. *Br J Obstet Gynaecol* **102:** 118–22.

Petraglia F, Florio P, Nappi C, Genazzani A (1996) Peptide signaling in human placenta and membranes: autocrine, paracrine, and endocrine mechanisms. *Endocr Rev* **17:** 156–86.

Pike IL (2005) Maternal stress and fetal responses: evolutionary perspectives on preterm delivery. *Am J Human Biol* **17:** 55–65.

Rasmussen KM (2001) The "fetal origins" hypothesis: challenges and opportunities for maternal and child nutrition. *Annu Rev Nutr* **21:** 73–95.

Ray A, Henke PG, Sullivan RM (1987) The central amygdala and immobilization stress induced gastric pathology in rats: neurotensin and dopamine. *Brain Res* **409:** 398–402.

Ray A, Mediratta PK, Puri S, Sen P (1991) Effects of stress on immune responsiveness, gastric ulcerogenesis and plasma corticosterone: modulation by diazepam and naltrexone. *Indian J Exp Biol* **29:** 233–6.

Reich CG, Taylor ME, McCarthy MM (2009) Differential effects of chronic unpredictable stress on hippocampal CB1 receptors in male and female rats. *Behav Brain Res* **203(2):** 264–9.

Rivier C, Rivest S (1991) Effect of stress on the activity of the hypothalamic–pituitary–gonadal axis: peripheral and central mechanisms. *Biol Reprod* **45:** 523–32.

Romero R, Gomez R, Chaiworapongsa T, Conoscenti G, Kim JC, Kim YM (2001) The role of infection in preterm labour and delivery. *Paediatr Perinat Epidemiol* **15(S2):** 41–56.

Sandman CA, Glynn L, Wadhwa PD, Chicz-DeMet A, Porto M, Garite TJ (2003) Maternal HPA dysregulation influences fetal behavior in human pregnancy. *Dev Neurosci* **25(1):** 41–119.

Sapolsky RM, Romero LM, Munck AU (2000) How do glucocorticoids influence stress responses? Integrating permissive, suppressive, stimulatory, and preparative actions. *Endocr Rev* **21(1):** 55–89.

Schenker JG, Meirow D, Schenker E (1992). Stress and human reproduction. *Eur J Obstet Gynecol Reprod Biol* **45(1):** 1–8.

Schneider ML, Moore CF, Roberts AD, Dejesus O (2001) Prenatal stress alters early neurobehavior, stress reactivity and learning in non-human primates: a brief review. *Stress* **4:** 183–93.

Schulte HM, Weisner D, Allolio B (1990) The corticotrophin releasing hormone test in late pregnancy: lack of adrenocorticotrophin and cortisol response. *Clin Endocrinol* **33:** 99–106.

Seckl JR (2001) Glucocorticoid programming of the fetus; adult phenotypes and molecular mechanisms. *Mol Cell Endocrinol* **185(1–2):** 61–71.

Selye H (1936) A syndrome produced by diversal nocuous agents. *Nature* **13:** 32.

Shanks N, Lightman SL (2001) The maternal–neonatal neuroimmune interface: are there long-term implications for inflammatory or stress-related disease? *J Clin Invest* **108(11):** 1567–73.

Shekhar A, Truitt W, Rainnie D, Sajdyk T (2005) Role of stress, corticotrophin releasing factor (CRF) and amygdala plasticity in chronic anxiety. *Stress* **8:** 209–19.

Smith R, Wickings E, Bowman M, Belleoud A, Dubreuil G, Davies J (1999) Corticotropin-releasing hormone in champanzee and gorilla pregnancies. *J Clin Endocrinol Metab* **84:** 2820–5.

Smotherman WP, Robinson SR (1995) Tracing developmental trajectories into the prenatal period. In *Fetal Development: A Psychobiological Perspective* (Lecanuet JP, Fifer WP, Krasnegor NA, Smotherman WP, eds.). Laurence Erlbaum Associates, Hillsdale, NJ.

Tilbrook AJ, Canny BJ, Serapiglia MD, Ambrose TJ, Clarke IJ (1999) Suppression of the secretion of luteinizing hormone due to isolation/restraint stress in gonadectomized rams and ewes is influenced by sex steroids. *J Endocrinol* **160:** 469–81.

Tilbrook AJ, Clarke IJ (1995) Negative feedback regulation of the secretion and actions of GnRH in male ruminants. *J Reprod Fertil Suppl* **49:** 297–306.

Vale W, Spiess J, Rivier C, Rivier J (1981) Characterization of a 41-residue ovine hypothalamic peptide that stimulates secretion of corticotropin and beta-endorphin. *Science* **213:** 1394–7.

Van de Kar LD, Blair ML (1999) Forebrain pathways mediating stress induced hormone secretion. *Front Neuroendocrinol* **20:** 1–48.

Villar J, Merialdi M, Gulmezoglu AM, Abalos E, Carroli G, Kulier R, de Onis M (2003) Nutritional interventions during pregnancy for the prevention or treatment of maternal morbidity and preterm delivery. An overview of randomized controlled trials. *J Nutr* **133:** 1606S–25S.

WHO (1995) Maternal anthropometry and pregnancy outcomes. WHO Collaborative Study. *Bull WHO* **73:** 1–68.

Wadhwa PD (2005) Psychoneuroendocrine processes in human pregnancy influence fetal development and health. *Psychoneuroendocrinology* **30:** 724–43.

Wadhwa PD, Culhane JF, Rauh VA, Barve SS (2001) Stress and preterm birth: neuroendrocrine immune-inflammatory and vascular mechanisms. *Matern Child Health J* **5:** 119–25.

Wadhwa PD, Glynn L, Hobel CJ, Garite TJ, Porto M, Chicz-DeMet A, Wiglesworth A, Sandman CA (2002) Behavioral perinatology: biobehavioral processes in human fetal development. *Regul Pept* **108:** 149–57.

Wadhwa PD, Porto M, Chicz-DeMet A, Sandman CA (1998) Maternal, CRH levels in early third trimester predict length of gestation in human pregnancy. *Am J Obstet Gynecol* **179:** 1079–85.

Wadhwa PD, Sandman CA, Porto M, Dunkel-Schetter C, Garite TJ (1993) The association between prenatal stress and infant birth weight and gestational age at birth: a prospective study. *Am J Obstet Gynecol* **169:** 858–65.

Weinstock M (2001) Alterations induced by gestational stress in brain morphology and behaviour of the offspring. *Prog Neurobiol* **65(5):** 427–51.

Welberg LA, Seckl JR (2001) Prenatal stress, glucocorticoids and the programming of the brain. *J Neuroendocrinol* **13(2):** 113–28.

Wells JCK (2003) The thrifty phenotype hypothesis: thrifty offspring or thrifty mother? *J Theor Biol* **221:** 143–61.

Woods LIJ, Nyengaard J, Rasch R (2001) Maternal protein restriction suppresses the newborn rennin–angiotensin system and programs adult hypertension in rats. *Pediatr Res* **49:** 460–7.

Xiao E, Xia-Zhang L, Barth A, Zhu J, Ferin M (1998) Stress and the menstrual cycle: relevance of cycle quality in the short- and long-term response to a 5-day endotoxin challenge during the follicular phase in the rhesus monkey. *J Clin Endocrinol Metab* **83:** 2454–60.

Yen SC (1994) Endocrinology of pregnancy. In *Maternal–Fetal Medicine: Principles and Practice* (Creasy RK, Resnick R, eds.). WB Saunders, Philadelphia, PA.

CHAPTER

63

Cell signaling mechanisms in developmental neurotoxicity

Chunjuan Song, Arthi Kanthasamy and Anumantha Kanthasamy

INTRODUCTION

Many environmental compounds, including industrial waste, pesticides and heavy metals, are known to cause toxicity in humans. Recent evidence demonstrates that the central nervous system (CNS), particularly during developmental stages, is highly vulnerable to the adverse effects of environmental neurotoxic insult. Specifically, exposure to neurotoxic compounds has been linked to a dramatic increase in a variety of neurodevelopmental disorders such as attention deficit, hyperactivity, learning disability and the autism spectrum (Szpir, 2006). While neurotoxicity evaluations as part of safety assessments are clearly needed (Tilson, 1995, 2000; Eriksson, 1997; Claudio *et al.*, 2000), still fewer than 10% of currently used commercial chemical products have been evaluated, and of those only a small fraction have been assessed for actual developmental neurotoxicity (Landrigan *et al.*, 1994). Among new chemical products released each year, about 70% have never been tested for neurotoxicity, let alone more specifically for developmental neurotoxicity. However, an estimated 25–40% of them will be later proven to be neurotoxic (Claudio *et al.*, 2000; Boyes, 2001; Slotkin *et al.*, 2007b).

Cell signaling cascades that control replication and differentiation of developing neural cells appear to be among the most sensitive targets for developmental neurotoxicity. A growing body of evidence suggests that exposure of developing neural cells to neurotoxic chemicals leads to lasting changes in gene expression, DNA damage, modification of key signaling proteins in pathways, destruction of cell architecture proteins, mitochondrial dysfunction and oxidative stress (O'Callaghan, 1994; Moya-Quiles *et al.*, 1995; Cadenas and Davies, 2000; Garcia *et al.*, 2001; Kobayashi *et al.*, 2010; Lassiter *et al.*, 2009; Slotkin and Seidler, 2010).

This chapter describes key cell signaling mechanisms by which neurotoxic chemicals inflict damage on or induce neurotoxicity to the developing nervous system.

DEVELOPMENTAL NEUROTOXIC CHEMICALS

A large number of neurotoxic compounds selectively target the nervous system. Recently, more than 1,000 neurotoxic chemicals have been identified in laboratory studies, which are far more than the previous estimate of 200 documented human neurotoxins (Grandjean and Landrigan, 2006). Recent studies (Dobbing, 1968; Rodier, 1995; Eriksson, 1997; Rice and Barone, 2000; Tilson, 2000) suggest that most human neurotoxic compounds induce neurotoxicity at very specific and critical developmental stages. Exceptions include chemicals that require metabolic conversion to become neurotoxic; the immature metabolic system does not have these functional pathways (Scheuplein *et al.*, 2002; Ginsberg *et al.*, 2004). In addition, timing of exposure may exempt another subset of neurotoxic compounds that only manifest their deleterious effects on the nervous system during very specific developmental periods (Morell *et al.*, 1994).

Several industrial chemicals, including some metals (e.g., lead, methylmercury), polychlorinated biphenyls, arsenic and toluene, induce subclinical brain dysfunctions and neurodevelopmental disorders. Exposure to these chemicals during early fetal development can cause brain injury at doses much lower than doses that affect adult brain functions. The neurodevelopmental toxicity of manganese (Mn) has recently become a significant public health concern. Epidemiological studies with children have indicated that high levels of Mn exposure, as confirmed by elevated Mn hair levels, are greatly associated with hyperactivity and oppositional behaviors (Pihl and Parkes, 1977; Collipp *et al.*, 1983; Bouchard *et al.*, 2007). Other reports also demonstrate that decreased intellectual functions among children correlate with high concentrations of heavy metals in local drinking water (Wasserman *et al.*, 2006, 2007).

Pesticides make up another large and growing group of chemicals that demonstrate neurotoxic effects. Universally

Reproductive and Developmental Toxicology, Edited by Ramesh C. Gupta
ISBN: 978-0-12-382032-7

valued in agricultural production, pesticides are used extensively in many home landscapes and gardens as herbicides, insecticides and fungicides. Human exposure to pesticides occurs in a variety of other venues. Approximately 300 different pesticides have been reported as contaminants in food products, including baby foods processed in Europe. Contaminated soils and dusts, drinking water and airborne spray drift are also sources of human pesticide exposure (Brussels, 2007). Insecticides that target the neurochemical processes of insects with similar correlates in humans are likely to be neurotoxic in humans. Laboratory studies of model compounds indicate that neurotoxicity might be induced in humans by many pesticides including organophosphates, carbamates, pyrethroids, neonicotinoids, ethylene-bis-dithiocarbamates and chlorophenoxy herbicides (Bjorling-Poulsen *et al.*, 2008).

In addition, evidence shows that the brain is more vulnerable to toxic injury during early stages of development (Rodier, 1995; Kalia, 2008). Thus, some compounds are toxic only to the developing CNS, and cause no toxicity in the mature brain in standard toxicity assays. For example, nicotine is neurotoxic in the developing brain, with vulnerability extending from fetal development through adolescence, whereas nicotine is actually neuroprotective in the adult brain (Berger *et al.*, 1998; Belluardo *et al.*, 2000; Laudenbach *et al.*, 2002; Slotkin, 2002).

VULNERABILITY OF THE DEVELOPING BRAIN

The extreme complexity of brain development, particularly distinct stages, is central to the brain's inherent vulnerability to injury by toxic agents (Rodier, 1995; Kalia, 2008). In the prenatal stage, ectodermal cells of the embryo develop into an exceedingly complex organ composed of billions of accurately located, highly specialized and interconnected cells. Recent studies have demonstrated that both genetic and environmental factors can affect dynamic adaptive changes during this ectodermal cell growth period (Grandjean and Landrigan, 2006; Kalia, 2008). To achieve optimum development, neurons must move to predestined locations from their points of origin along exact pathways, building connections with other cells and establishing communications with other cells via these connections. These processes require precise sequential regulation; however, it may not be possible to subsequently repair or regenerate the developmental process if any stage of the process is delayed or suspended due to toxic insults. Hence, permanent fetal brain damage becomes inevitable following exposure to developmental neurotoxicants (Bjorling-Poulsen *et al.*, 2008). For example, exposure of the developing brains of humans or animals to toxic insults such as X-ray irradiation, methylazoxymethanol, ethanol, lead, methyl mercury or chlorpyrifos has been shown to cause developmental neurotoxicity (Rice and Barone, 2000).

In addition to the need for unusually precise regulation of sequential processes in the developing nervous system, the young brain is also particularly sensitive to early life exposures to neurotoxins as a result of its lower capacity for metabolic detoxification. For instance, several studies have revealed that voltage-gated sodium channels expressed during the embryonic stage are replaced by adult forms as neurodevelopment proceeds; this distinction between the channels might result in different sensitivity to neurotoxicants (Shafer *et al.*, 2005; Bjorling-Poulsen *et al.*, 2008). There is also evidence that early developmental insult may result in latent neurotoxicity that only reveals itself later in life when the environmental neurotoxic exposure is repeated. For example, early life exposure to lead in rodents and primates has been shown to produce Alzheimer's-like pathology (Zawia and Basha, 2005; White *et al.*, 2007; Wu *et al.*, 2008b,a). Also, postnatal exposure of mice to maneb (dithiocarbamate fungicide) and paraquat (a classic bipyridyl herbicide) greatly enhanced the effect of the same pesticides administered later during the adult stage, inducing a loss of dopaminergic neurons in the substantia nigra pars compacta and a decreased dopamine level, consistent with the pathological changes of Parkinson's disease (Cory-Slechta *et al.*, 2005). Recently, developmental exposure to environmental neurotoxic chlorinated biphenyls (PCBs) has been shown to alter ischemic injury at the later stages in a rat model of stroke (Dziennis *et al.*, 2008).

This accumulating body of evidence related to the special susceptibility of the human nervous system to neurotoxic insult during early development demands that a paramount goal of any public health protection program is to eliminate toxic threats to the brain during all stages of development and growth.

CELL SIGNALING MECHANISMS IN DEVELOPMENTAL NEUROTOXICITY

Cell membrane damage

The cell plasma membrane is the first physiological barrier and consequently the primary cell component encountered by biologically active toxins. Changes in membrane properties can bring pronounced downstream cellular effects, such as those leading to altered ion channel properties or interferences with bilayer-embedded receptor proteins following changes in the molecular properties of boundary lipids (Mech *et al.*, 2009). In addition, direct interaction of lead in biological membranes induces lipid peroxidation (Wang *et al.*, 2006). Additionally, several studies have shown that a series of pesticide disturbances interfere with lipid bilayers (Antunes-Madeira and Madeira, 1989; Moya-Quiles *et al.*, 1995; Suwalsky *et al.*, 2003), including the family of phenoxy herbicides, such as 2,4-dichlorophenoxyacetic acid (2,4-D), one of the most efficient and consequently widely used broadleaf herbicides in the world (Bage *et al.*, 1973). This is of special concern because the use of herbicides in agriculture has risen dramatically since the mid-1940s, and recent evidence links herbicide use to toxicological and environment problems. In humans, the central nervous system is one of the targets of chlorophenoxy herbicides (Mori de Moro *et al.*, 1993; Duffard *et al.*, 1996). 2,4-D is reportedly associated with neurobehavioral changes in rats, as well as alterations in the serotonergic and dopaminergic systems (Evangelista de Duffard *et al.*, 1995). Additionally, delayed CNS development along with biochemical and neurobehavioral alterations have been shown in neonatal rats exposed to 2,4-D (Rosso *et al.*, 1997), indicating a developmental toxic effect. While the exact mechanism of phenoxy herbicide neurotoxicity is still not clear, cell membrane damage may be one of the vital components involved (Bradberry *et al.*, 2000). When the concentration of 2,4-D is lower than 0.1 μM, it does not cause significant penetration of lipid monolayers *in vitro* (Rosso *et al.*,

1998), but at higher concentrations (10–100 μM) it induces a deep structural perturbation and increases bilayer width of the hydrophobic section of model membrane systems. This dose-dependent effect on plasma membranes might partly elucidate the dose-dependent CNS toxicity stimulated by chlorophenoxy herbicides (Bjorling-Poulsen *et al.*, 2008).

Instability of cytoskeleton proteins

Microtubules (MTs) are one of the three basic protein filaments found in the cytoskeleton. In neurons, as in other cell types, MTs are responsible for a variety of important cell functions, including maintenance of cell shape and intracellular transport. They are also architecturally unique, being arranged as bundles that parallel the long axis of the cells and extend to both dendrites and axons. Together with microfilaments, MTs are essential to neuronal architecture development, but because of MTs' special vulnerability to toxin-induced destabilization, they are also closely tied to neuronal cell viability. Normal central nervous system development relies on stable MTs to perform cellular functions such as the transportation of substances to the growth cone, neuronal migration and continuance of differentiated neuritic structures, particularly in highly differentiated neurons and in rapidly cycling cells (Wasteneys *et al.*, 1988). Studies have reported that MTs are heterogeneous regarding sensitivity to toxic insult, even in highly differentiated neurons, with the more dynamic MTs being more easily disrupted. Therefore, the dynamic subpopulation of MTs involved in active processes is at greater risk for disturbance when exposed to toxic agents. MTs depolymerize rapidly and are extremely sensitive to the exposure of toxic insults if the cells are in exponential growth phase (Wasteneys *et al.*, 1988). For example, 2,4-D, a potent neurotoxic herbicide, was reported to induce a striking, dose-dependent inhibition of neurite extension, which is associated with reduction of both stable and dynamic MTs in cellular content (Rosso *et al.*, 2000).

Organophosphorus (OP) agents induce depression and cognitive deficits. Chlorpyrifos (O,O-diethyl O-3,5,6-trichloro-2-pyridinyl phosphorothioate; CPF), one of the broad spectrum OP insecticides, remains one of the most widely used pesticides in agriculture. Evidence acquired largely through rodent models indicates that acute or prolonged exposure to CPF and/or its metabolic product(s) produces obvious changes in neuronal function or may injure the central nervous system, especially during the early postnatal period (Zheng *et al.*, 2000; Olivier *et al.*, 2001; Slotkin *et al.*, 2001). A recent report has suggested that microtubule trafficking is affected adversely by exposure to the OP pesticide chlorpyrifos, indicating a novel mode of OP-induced neurotoxicity (Prendergast *et al.*, 2007). Another organophosphate insecticide, dichlorvos, is reported to cause the hyperphosphorylation of tubulin and microtubule-associated protein-2 (MAP-2), which in turn destabilizes the assembly of MTs, impairs axonal transport and ultimately may result in axonal degeneration and delayed neurotoxicity (Choudhary *et al.*, 2001).

Microtubule polymerization disruption in neuronal axons has been suggested as a mechanism causing neurodegenerative diseases (Iqbal *et al.*, 1986; Gendron and Petrucelli, 2009). During the earliest stages of neuronal differentiation or in newly extending neuritis, the MTs are extremely vulnerable to toxicants. Due to the asynchronous development of different brain regions, it is clear that there are various sites and developmental periods where interaction of toxicants with MTs decreases or even prevents the formation of stable MTs, and thus disrupts other processes in which MTs are essential (Falconer *et al.*, 1994).

MITOCHONDRIA DYSFUNCTION, FREE RADICALS GENERATION AND OXIDATIVE STRESS

Overwhelming evidence has accumulated indicating that many chemicals, drugs and physical injuries evoke oxidative stress, which becomes neurotoxic in the developing nervous system. Oxidative stress from the exposure of cells to active extra- or intracellular reactive oxygen species (ROS) is a recognized source of cell injury (Slotkin and Seidler, 2010). The major reservoir of these ROS is the mitochondrion, the principal production site of superoxide radicals (Smith, 2009). Mitochondria have been called "the powerhouses of the cell" because they couple the energy conserving procedure of oxidative phosphorylation with electron transport to release energy and pump protons, to exploit the value of foods in the form of ATP. However, this energetic machinery becomes inefficient due to the somewhat "leaky" electron transport during toxic insults (Cadenas and Davies, 2000). The radicals, as by-products of the electron transport chain, are released from the mitochondria (Smith, 2009). ROS includes nitric oxide (NO), superoxide anions, hydrogen peroxide (H_2O_2), and the highly reactive monoxide and hydroxyl radicals (OH·, NO·) (Apel and Hirt, 2004). ROS are especially active in the neuronal tissue and the brain, where excitatory amino acids and neurotransmitters, which form ROS upon metabolism, are abundant and act as sources of oxidative stress. Glial cells and neurons in the nervous system are post-mitotic cells and are particularly sensitive to the ROS, which cause neuronal damage (Gilgun-Sherki *et al.*, 2001).

A variety of toxins and cellular processes, including toxic xenobiotics, ionizing radiation and inflammation, lead to the generation of ROS (Verity, 1994). ROS generation is believed to result from an imbalance between generation and elimination of ROS, a function performed by antioxidant defenses in the brain. Some neurotoxins induce oxidative stress by producing free radicals as they undergo redox cycling. For example, developmental neurotic insult by the herbicide paraquat or some carbamate pesticides causes cytotoxicity from ROS generation when these compounds undergo redox cycling with the mitochondrial electron transport chain (Cadenas and Davies, 2000; Zhang *et al.*, 2003; Domico *et al.*, 2006; Slotkin and Seidler, 2010). Another subset of neurotoxins increases ROS levels in cells by decreasing activities of free-radical scavenging antioxidant enzymes, instead of generating ROS directly. While any antioxidant enzyme may be a possible target of oxidative neurotoxic insult, the major antioxidant enzymes include: superoxide dismutase (SOD), glutathione-S-transferase (GST), glutathione peroxidase (GSH-Px) and catalase (CAT). For instance, SOD first converts $\bullet O_2^-$ to hydrogen peroxide (H_2O_2), which is subsequently converted into water by glutathione peroxidase (GSH-Px) in the cytosol, or by catalase (CAT) in the peroxisomes (Olsvik *et al.*, 2005; Smith, 2009). Any antioxidant enzyme in the chain is a possible target of oxidative neurotoxic insult. Existing research has shown that carbamates, organic compounds typically used as insecticides, lead to impaired neurobehavioral performance and cognitive deficit in attention, memory, perceptual and motor domains in humans (Roldan-Tapi *et al.*, 2005). They also are known to modify the cellular redox state and accentuate oxidative stress in the rat brain by inducing lipid peroxidation and diminishing the cell's antioxidant defense mechanisms (Delmaestro, 1995; Orrenius *et al.*, 1996; Kamboj *et al.*, 2006). Cytosolic Cu/Zn superoxide dismutase (SOD1), a key enzyme in the antioxidant response, has been reported to be inhibited in mice treated with carbamate diethyldithiocarbamates (DEDC) (Heikkila *et al.*, 1976). Also, glutathione (GSH) levels and catalase activity have been reported to be significantly reduced in rat cerebellar granule cells incubated with chlorophenoxy herbicide *in vitro*, while generation of ROS was augmented (Bongiovanni *et al.*, 2007).

It has been shown that oxidative stress and free radical generation can also be induced by redox metal exposure, such as that associated with lead (Pb) toxicity (Moreira *et al.*, 2001; Emerit *et al.*, 2004; Tamm *et al.*, 2008). A broad range of studies on Pb neurotoxicity have confirmed that this metal is a dangerous toxin, causing a variety of neurobiological disturbances in humans, particularly during pre- and early postnatal stages (Tong *et al.*, 2000; Mendola *et al.*, 2002; Canfield *et al.*, 2003). Research suggests that Pb-induced oxidative stress leads to the accumulation of 5-aminolevulinic acid (ALA), a potential endogenous source of free radicals, induced by inhibiting ALA dehydratase (Nihei and Guilarte, 2001; Wang *et al.*, 2006). Pb exposure also might induce a decrease in activities of antioxidant free radical scavenging enzymes (SOD, GSH-Px and GSH-Re) (Wang *et al.*, 2006; Uttara *et al.*, 2009), which then induces oxidative stress.

Oxidative stress has been suggested to be a shared potential mechanism by which apparently distinct chemicals generate converged and similar developmental neurotoxic effects (Slotkin and Seidler, 2009b), even though the underlying upstream mechanisms of the various neurotoxicants differ (Olanow and Arendash, 1994; Barone *et al.*, 2000; Ohtsuka and Suzuki, 2000; Gitto *et al.*, 2002; Gupta, 2004; Slotkin, 2004; Monnet-Tschudi *et al.*, 2007). When compared with other organs, the brain is particularly vulnerable to oxidant damage due to the many polyunsaturated fatty acids in brain tissue membrane that are easily oxidizable (Gupta, 2004) and also because of the high oxygen consumption in the brain. This vulnerability is exacerbated in the developing brain, which exhibits the typical increased metabolic demand required for growth. The developing brain is additionally threatened because it possesses both fewer antioxidant defenses (Gupta, 2004) and a reduced match of glia, i.e. neuronal cells that protect neurons from oxidative insults (Tanaka *et al.*, 1999).

IMPACTS ON DNA SYNTHESIS

Although replicating cells in development may be less responsive to neurotoxicants than differentiated neurons, the cell replication process is a major target for neurotoxic damage in other ways. For instance, developing cells must maintain a fixed pattern of mitosis until differentiation is triggered by addition of trophic factors. DNA synthesis is then regarded as a marker of cell replication due to its association with cell replication as a macromolecule (Dam *et al.*, 1998; Qiao *et al.*, 2001).

Developing animals recovered more rapidly from neurotoxicant exposure in some studies; however, they were more sensitive to delayed neurotoxicity caused by some neurotoxicants, such as chlorpyrifos. Rats were treated daily on postnatal days 1–4 via low-level chlorpyrifos exposure, which caused no mortality or weight deficits; however, on postnatal day 5 (24h after the last treatment), robust deficits in DNA synthesis were observed in the forebrain and brainstem. The point at which DNA synthesis was inhibited in the brain stem and forebrain indicates the deficit of cell replication (Dam *et al.*, 1998). Various other neurotoxic agents evaluated in *in vitro* models produced consistent results. Organophosphate pesticides (chlorpyrifos, diazinon, parathion), carbamate insecticide (physostigmine), organochlorine pesticide (dieldrin), phenylpyrazole pesticide (fipronil), a metal (divalent nickel; Ni^{2+}) or perfluoroalkyl acids (PFAAS) have inhibited DNA synthesis in undifferentiated neuronotypic PC12 cells (a standard *in vitro* model for neurodevelopmental study) (Slotkin *et al.*, 2007a, 2009; Slotkin and Seidler, 2008; Lassiter *et al.*, 2009). Thus, certain neurotoxicants induce delayed neurotoxicity in developing animals, which is manifested as immediate, direct inhibitory actions on DNA synthesis and then a later effect on neural cell replication or cell proliferation.

GENE EXPRESSION DEREGULATION

Mounting evidence has demonstrated the underlying impact of diverse gene expression on different disease models (Goring *et al.*, 2007; Moffatt *et al.*, 2007; Dermitzakis, 2008; Yang *et al.*, 2009). Environmental chemicals have a potential impact on gene expression at both transcription and translation levels, affecting neuronal development and, in turn, children's health (Royland and Kodavanti, 2008; Kobayashi *et al.*, 2009). In order to elucidate the mechanisms, it is essential to understand the associated alterations in gene expression and find the appropriate molecular markers in the brain.

Propylthiouracil (PTU), a drug frequently prescribed to treat hyperthyroidism, also causes numerous potentially serious side effects (Quax *et al.*, 2009). Studies on PTU have demonstrated its role as a thyroid hormone synthesis inhibitor; PTU affects transcriptomes in the rat cerebral cortex and the hippocampus, as measured by DNA microarrays. After the perinatal administration of PTU, the candidate genes affected are activity-regulated cytoskeleton-associated protein (Arc), Homer 1, early growth response 1 (Egr 1), myelin-associated genes such as myelin-associated oligodendrocytic basic protein (MOBP), myelin basic protein (MBP), proteolipid protein (PLP) and Kcna1. The results indicate that the alterations in gene expression levels may be responsible for the detrimental effects induced by PTU exposure on the nervous system (Kobayashi *et al.*, 2009).

In addition to drugs, environmental toxins such as synthetic pesticides also have a demonstrated ability to affect the expression level of genes, suggesting a causal role in neurodegenerative disease. It has been reported that exposure to low levels of the organochlorine pesticide dieldrin in mice during gestation and lactation changes dopaminergic neurochemistry in their offspring, exacerbating the toxicity from MPTP exposure. One possible mechanism may be that dieldrin perinatal treatment causes an increase in mRNA and protein levels of the dopamine transporter (DAT) and vesicular monoamine transporter 2 (VMAT2), which then induces a greater reduction in striatal dopamine levels and greater DAT: VMAT2 ratios in subsequent MPTP exposures.

In addition, dieldrin exposure during developmental stages also potentiated MPTP-induced increases in GFAP and α-synuclein levels, indicating increased neurotoxicity (Richardson *et al.*, 2006). In contrast, other studies show that dieldrin, as a GABA receptor antagonist, may decrease the expression or change the subunit composition of developing GABA receptor transcripts. If these alterations persist, they might bring long-lasting effects on developing GABAergic neural circuitry, GABA receptor function and GABA-mediated behaviors later in life (Liu *et al.*, 1998). These data suggest that developmental exposure to dieldrin alters the gene expression level as a "silent" state of dopamine dysfunction and might render dopamine neurons more vulnerable in later life (Richardson *et al.*, 2006).

Developmental exposure to heavy metals such as lead also can induce changes in some genes at both mRNA and protein levels. For example, the metabotropic glutamate receptor 5 (mGluR5), which has a functional relationship with learning and memory, has been shown to be the most important target of lead. Investigation of the neurotoxic impact of developmental lead exposure on hippocampal mGluR5 expression revealed that mGluR5 mRNA and protein expression were decreased dose dependently after lead exposure (Xu *et al.*, 2009). Lead has recently been shown to alter amyloid precursor protein (APP) gene expression via activation of sp1 transcription factor (Wu *et al.*, 2008b). Many neurotoxic insults produce up- or downregulation of numerous genes and proteins, affecting gene expression profiles. Most of the genes that are involved can be categorized into three major groups: cell proliferation and differentiation, cell signaling and cell architecture (Lazarov *et al.*, 2005; Ronnback *et al.*, 2005; Costa, 2006; Thiriet *et al.*, 2008).

PROTEIN MODIFICATION

Post-translational modifications of proteins are important regulatory mechanisms in various cellular processes. Protein phosphorylation, a major post-translational mechanism, plays an important role in numerous physiological processes. In the central nervous system, it seems that many extracellular messengers exert their effects by regulating the intracellular concentration of some specific secondary messengers, which in turn further activate kinases to phosphorylate various substrates. Despite the myriad of kinases and phosphatases that regulate the function of neuronal cells, phosphorylation status of specific substrates determines the change in the biological function of the nerve cell. Furthermore, certain phosphoproteins and kinases are actually involved in various aspects and in different cellular procedures, such as gene expression, cellular differentiation and programmed cell death. Moreover, "cross-talk" between distinct signals takes place in diverse brain cells, indicating the intricate relationships between many of the neuronal protein phosphorylation systems (Walaas and Greengard, 1991; He *et al.*, 2006).

In all phosphorylation systems, three basic components are necessary: a protein kinase catalyzing a phosphorylation reaction in the presence of ATP; a specific substrate obtaining phospho- or dephospho- forms; and a protein phosphatase responsible for removing the added phosphate group. A growing body of evidence demonstrates that each of the components could be the putative target for developmental neurotoxicants (O'Callaghan, 1994).

EPIGENETIC MODIFICATIONS

Epigenetics is the study of inherited changes in gene expression that are not coded in the underlying DNA sequences but instead result from non-genetic factors (Wolffe and Guschin, 2000). In the past few years, studies focusing on the relationship between environmental compound exposure and epigenetics have revealed several toxicants capable of making heritable epigenetic marks (Bollati and Baccarelli, 2010). Several types of epigenetic mechanisms have been described, including DNA methylation, histone modifications, nucleosome repositioning, higher-order chromatin remodeling, non-coding RNAs, and RNA and DNA editing (Mehler, 2008). Increasing evidence has shown that environmental influences extend further than the interaction with the DNA sequence, indicating that environmental toxicants can also modify epigenetic states (Bollati and Baccarelli, 2010). Epigenetic modifications have been suggested as a plausible link between environmental exposure and alterations in gene expression that might cause disease phenotypes. Further, environment-induced modifications during early development also might cause permanent changes in patterns of epigenetic modifications. This is suggested by evidence from animal studies indicating that prenatal or early postnatal exposure to environmental insults may cause epigenetic programming alterations, which lead to an increased risk of developing disease (Li *et al.*, 2003; Waterland and Jirtle, 2003; Anway and Skinner, 2006; Koturbash *et al.*, 2006; Waterland, 2006; Fauque *et al.*, 2007). The possibility that environmental effects could be passed on through generations brings additional concern. Additionally, recent studies have shown for the first time that reversible transgenerational alterations in phenotype are actually caused by environmentally induced heritable epigenetic modifications (Jirtle and Skinner, 2007).

There are at least two kinds of important heritable epigenetic modulation mechanisms associated with chromatin: DNA methylation and histone tail modification (Bollati and Baccarelli, 2010). To date, most investigations conducted on environmental exposure-induced developmental epigenetic alterations have focused on DNA methylation. DNA methylation, particularly within promoter regions (CpG islands), always leads to heritable genes silencing without changing the DNA coding sequence (Jirtle and Skinner, 2007; Zhao *et al.*, 2007; Mehler, 2008; Baccarelli and Bollati, 2009). Only a few recent studies have examined the effects of environmental chemicals on histone modifications (Baccarelli and Bollati, 2009). In eukaryotic cells, genomic DNA exists in the form of chromatin, which is composed of DNA molecules, histones and other chromatin-associated proteins. Chromatin is then supercoiled into a highly condensed structure, providing a unique management system for gene expression by controlling access of transcriptional factors (activators and repressors) to DNA molecules (Felsenfeld and Groudine, 2003; Li *et al.*, 2007). Besides functioning as structural proteins, histones have been found to be diversely modified, playing key roles in many cellular processes. In recent years, histone modification, including methylation, phosphorylation, acetylation and ubiquitination, has been linked to many human diseases (Somech *et al.*, 2004; Esteller, 2006). A recent study demonstrated that histone acetylation can regulate neuronal cell death during dieldrin exposure (Song *et al.*, 2010). Chromatin remodeling is regarded as a fundamental cellular

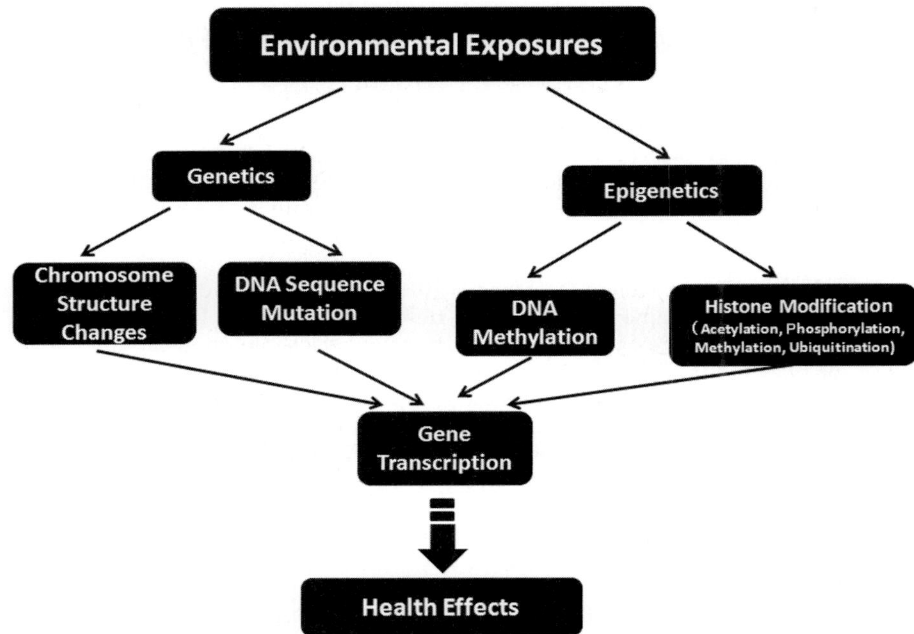

FIGURE 63.1 Environmental exposures induce genetic and epigenetic changes. Different environmental neurotoxins can change gene expression and alter phenotype via both genetic and epigenetic processes. The genetic changes induced by neurotoxins could be the alteration of chromosome structure changes in a large segment of a chromosome or minor changes, such as specific DNA sequence mutation. Whereas epigenetic modification, a more recently recognized mechanism, can also be induced by environmental exposure. There are at least two kinds of important heritable epigenetic modulation mechanisms associated with chromatin: DNA methylation and histone tail modification.

mechanism that integrates various environmental stimuli and chemical exposures with alteration in gene expression (Strahl and Allis, 2000; Tsankova *et al.*, 2007). Epigenetic modulations have been proposed to serve as an intermediate procedure that marks on the "fixed" genome by dynamic environmental experiences, producing stable changes in phenotype (Holliday and Pugh, 1975; Riggs, 1975; Zhao *et al.*, 2007).

Different environmental insults can change gene expression and alter phenotype via both genetic and epigenetic processes (Figure 63.1). However, epigenetic modification, a more recently recognized mechanism, is increasingly the focus of new investigation into environmentally induced change (Jirtle and Skinner, 2007; Bollati and Baccarelli, 2010). Of special concern is the question: If epigenetic adaptations induced by environment occur at early stages of life, could they potentially alter behavior, disease susceptibility and ultimate survival of the individual?

CELL SIGNALING INTEGRATION

Although most laboratory studies tend to focus on outcomes or specific mechanisms of a single agent or class of neurotoxicants, more and more unexpected similarities have been found in effects among apparently unrelated agents, as well as differences between compounds within the same category (Barone *et al.*, 2000; Yanai *et al.*, 2002, 2004; Slotkin, 2004; Szpir, 2006; Monnet-Tschudi *et al.*, 2007; Slotkin and Seidler, 2007, 2009c). This might be, in part, because a wide range of agents may converge on a general set of pathways governing neurodevelopment and neurotoxicity. Several investigations focusing on cell signaling cascades revealed that numerous hormones and neurotransmitters appear to serve as crosstalk points for the integration of diverse signals. For example, key regulators of different cell processes, including cyclic AMP signaling cascade factors, protein kinase A, C and tyrosine kinase families, are important converging points (Nakagawara, 2001; Yanai *et al.*, 2002, 2004, 2006; Reuss and von Bohlen und Halbach, 2003; Slotkin *et al.*, 2003; Kapfhammer, 2004; Meyer *et al.*, 2004, 2005; Aldridge *et al.*, 2005; Slikker *et al.*, 2005; Slotkin and Seidler, 2007, 2008, 2009a).

Hence, cell signaling converging points, which are involved in many cascades controlling neural cell replication and differentiation, appear to be among the most sensitive targets for developmental neurotoxicity induced by environmental toxins such as organophosphate pesticides (OP) (Ward and Mundy, 1996; Song *et al.*, 1997; Schuh *et al.*, 2002; Yanai *et al.*, 2002; Meyer *et al.*, 2003, 2004, 2005; Curtin *et al.*, 2006). Recent research suggests that exposure of developing neurons to OP pesticides leads to long-lasting changes in expression or function level of the key signaling proteins involved in critical pathways that determine essential processes. These include the amount and activity of G protein-coupled receptors, the concentration and function of the G proteins, or the catalytic efficiency or expression level of adenyl cyclase (AC), which generates the second messenger cyclic AMP (cAMP) contributing to both the immediate and long-term effects (Song *et al.*, 1997; Meyer *et al.*, 2003, 2004, 2005; Adigun *et al.*, 2010). During development, levels of cAMP eventually influence cell division, differentiation, neural plasticity, axonal outgrowth and programmed cell death (Shaywitz and Greenberg, 1999; Meyer *et al.*, 2003; Stachowiak *et al.*, 2003). Similarly, PKA and PKC are other converging points for expression of the genes encoding the neurotrophic factors and also mediate neurotoxic effects of

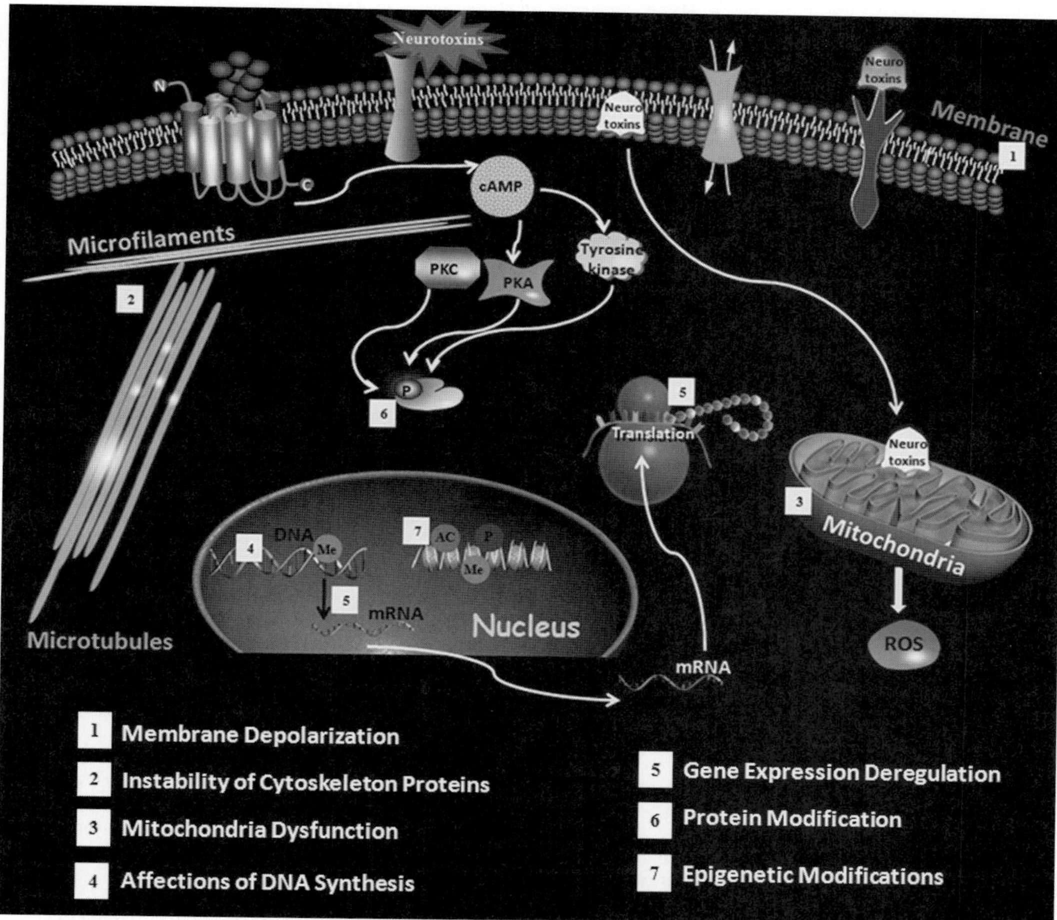

FIGURE 63.2 Cell signaling mechanisms in developmental neurotoxicity. The figure summarizes key cell signaling mechanisms by which neurotoxic chemicals inflict damage or induce neurotoxicity to the developing nervous system. A growing body of evidence suggests that exposure of developing neural cells to neurotoxic chemicals leads to depolarization of cell membranes, destruction of cell architecture proteins, mitochondrial dysfunction and induction of oxidative stress, DNA damage and affection of DNA synthesis, lasting changes in gene expression, modification of key signaling proteins in various pathways, epigenetic changes, and so on. Please refer to color plate section.

metals, environmental tobacco smoke, pesticides and neuroactive drugs in the developing brain (Haykal-Coates *et al.*, 1998; Hilliard *et al.*, 1999; Hasan *et al.*, 2001; Yanai *et al.*, 2002; Reuss and von Bohlen und Halbach, 2003; Li *et al.*, 2005). Reports evaluating effects of exposures to pesticides such as chlorpyrifos, diazinon, dieldrin or the metal Ni^{2+} all affect PKA/PKC, indicating that these divergent neurotoxic agents can nevertheless result in similar developmental outcomes by targeting cell signaling pathways involved in neurodifferentiation during vital developmental periods (Steingart *et al.*, 2000; Beer *et al.*, 2005; Yanai *et al.*, 2006; Slotkin and Seidler, 2007).

Other than the converging signaling cascade points, production of reactive oxygen species is also regarded as another convergent agent, representing a unifying process to account for many of the cellular changes induced by different chemicals (Bagchi *et al.*, 1995; Wright and Baccarelli, 2007; Baccarelli and Bollati, 2009). Furthermore, in a series of recent investigations, direct effects from divergent developmental neurotoxicants on the expression and function of nuclear transcription factors, such as c-fos, p53, AP-1 and CREB, also mediated regulation of numerous pathways, such as the switch from proliferation to differentiation, and are considered important in signal integration (Slotkin, 2004).

CONCLUDING REMARKS AND FUTURE DIRECTIONS

In conclusion, the major mechanisms in cell signaling cascades by which neurotoxicants alter neural cell developmental processes during early life exposure are discussed in this chapter (Figure 63.2). It is important to note that many industrial chemicals, pesticides and heavy metals are capable of inducing neurotoxicity in the human central nervous system, particularly in developing brains. Alterations in cell signaling pathways, perturbations of genomic structure and disruption of the communication process following exposure to neurotoxic compounds are known to cause transient or even permanent cellular functional impairments, and are expected to lead to cell damage or cell death. The cell signaling mechanisms associated with developmental neurotoxicology are not well understood. A detailed understanding of the intricate cell signaling pathways pertaining to developmental neurotoxicity will provide new opportunities for development of rationale-based therapeutic strategies to treat various developmental disorders associated with environmental neurotoxicant exposures.

ACKNOWLEDGMENTS

This study was supported by National Institute of Health (NIH) grants ES10586 and NS65167. The W. Eugene and Linda Lloyd Endowed Chair to AGK is also acknowledged. The authors also acknowledge Ms. Mary Ann deVries for her assistance in the preparation of the manuscript.

REFERENCES

Adigun AA, Seidler FJ, Slotkin TA (2010) Disparate developmental neurotoxicants converge on the cyclic AMP signaling cascade, revealed by transcriptional profiles in vitro and in vivo. *Brain Res* **1316:** 1–16.

Aldridge JE, Meyer A, Seidler FJ, Slotkin TA (2005) Developmental exposure to terbutaline and chlorpyrifos: pharmacotherapy of preterm labor and an environmental neurotoxicant converge on serotonergic systems in neonatal rat brain regions. *Toxicol Appl Pharmacol* **203:** 132–44.

Antunes-Madeira MC, Madeira VM (1989) Membrane fluidity as affected by the insecticide lindane. *Biochim Biophys Acta* **982:** 161–6.

Anway MD, Skinner MK (2006) Epigenetic transgenerational actions of endocrine disruptors. *Endocrinology* **147:** S43–9.

Apel K, Hirt H (2004) Reactive oxygen species: metabolism, oxidative stress, and signal transduction. *Annu Rev Plant Biol* **55:** 373–99.

Baccarelli A, Bollati V (2009) Epigenetics and environmental chemicals. *Curr Opin Pediatr* **21:** 243–51.

Bagchi D, Bagchi M, Hassoun EA, Stohs SJ (1995) In vitro and in vivo generation of reactive oxygen species, DNA damage and lactate dehydrogenase leakage by selected pesticides. *Toxicology* **104:** 129–40.

Bage G, Cekanova E, Larsson KS (1973) Teratogenic and embryotoxic of the herbicides di- and trichlorophenoxyacetic acids (2,4-D and 2,4,5-T). *Acta Pharmacol Toxicol (Copenh)* **32:** 408–16.

Barone S Jr, Das KP, Lassiter TL, White LD (2000) Vulnerable processes of nervous system development: a review of markers and methods. *Neurotoxicology* **21:** 15–36.

Beer A, Slotkin TA, Seidler FJ, Aldridge JE, Yanai J (2005) Nicotine therapy in adulthood reverses the synaptic and behavioral deficits elicited by prenatal exposure to phenobarbital. *Neuropsychopharmacology* **30:** 156–65.

Belluardo N, Mudo G, Blum M, Fuxe K (2000) Central nicotinic receptors, neurotrophic factors and neuroprotection. *Behav Brain Res* **113:** 21–34.

Berger F, Gage FH, Vijayaraghavan S (1998) Nicotinic receptor-induced apoptotic cell death of hippocampal progenitor cells. *J Neurosci* **18:** 6871–81.

Bjorling-Poulsen M, Andersen HR, Grandjean P (2008) Potential developmental neurotoxicity of pesticides used in Europe. *Environ Health* **7:** 50.

Bollati V, Baccarelli A (2010) Environmental epigenetics. *Heredity* **105:** 105–12.

Bongiovanni B, De Lorenzi P, Ferri A, Konjuh C, Rassetto M, Evangelista de Duffard AM, Cardinali DP, Duffard R (2007) Melatonin decreases the oxidative stress produced by 2,4-dichlorophenoxyacetic acid in rat cerebellar granule cells. *Neurotox Res* **11:** 93–9.

Bouchard M, Laforest F, Vandelac L, Bellinger D, Mergler D (2007) Hair manganese and hyperactive behaviors: pilot study of school-age children exposed through tap water. *Environ Health Perspect* **115:** 122–7.

Boyes WK (2001) Neurotoxicology and behavior. In *Patty's Toxicology*, 5th edition (Bingham ECB, Powell CH, ed.). New York, John Wiley & Sons, pp. 55–121.

Bradberry SM, Watt BE, Proudfoot AT, Vale JA (2000) Mechanisms of toxicity, clinical features, and management of acute chlorophenoxy herbicide poisoning: a review. *J Toxicol Clin Toxicol* **38:** 111–22.

Brussels (2007) Monitoring of Pesticide Residues in Products of Plant Origin in the European Union, Norway, Iceland and Liechtenstein 2005. pp. 1–39. Commission of the European Communities. URL: http:/ec.europa.eu/food/fvo/specialreports/pesticide_residues/report_2005_en.pdf.

Cadenas E, Davies KJ (2000) Mitochondrial free radical generation, oxidative stress, and aging. *Free Radic Biol Med* **29:** 222–30.

Canfield RL, Henderson CR Jr, Cory-Slechta DA, Cox C, Jusko TA, Lanphear BP (2003) Intellectual impairment in children with blood lead concentrations below 10 microg per deciliter. *N Engl J Med* **348:** 1517–26.

Choudhary S, Joshi K, Gill KD (2001) Possible role of enhanced microtubule phosphorylation in dichlorvos induced delayed neurotoxicity in rat. *Brain Res* **897:** 60–70.

Claudio L, Kwa WC, Russell AL, Wallinga D (2000) Testing methods for developmental neurotoxicity of environmental chemicals. *Toxicol Appl Pharmacol* **164:** 1–14.

Collipp PJ, Chen SY, Maitinsky S (1983) Manganese in infant formulas and learning disability. *Ann Nutr Metab* **27:** 488–94.

Cory-Slechta DA, Thiruchelvam M, Richfield EK, Barlow BK, Brooks AI (2005) Developmental pesticide exposures and the Parkinson's disease phenotype. *Birth Defects Res A Clin Mol Teratol* **73:** 136–9.

Costa LG (2006) Current issues in organophosphate toxicology. *Clin Chim Acta* **366:** 1–13.

Curtin BF, Pal N, Gordon RK, Nambiar MP (2006) Forskolin, an inducer of cAMP, up-regulates acetylcholinesterase expression and protects against organophosphate exposure in neuro 2A cells. *Mol Cell Biochem* **290:** 23–32.

Delmaestro E (1995) The effects of disulfiram on the hippocampus and cerebellum of the rat brain: a study on oxidative stress. *Toxicol Lett* **75:** 235–43.

Dam K, Seidler FJ, Slotkin TA (1998) Developmental neurotoxicity of chlorpyrifos: delayed targeting of DNA synthesis after repeated administration. *Brain Res Dev Brain Res* **108:** 39–45.

Dermitzakis ET (2008) From gene expression to disease risk. *Nat Genet* **40:** 492–93.

Dobbing J (1968) The development of the blood–brain barrier. *Prog Brain Res* **29:** 417–27.

Domico LM, Zeevalk GD, Bernard LP, Cooper KR (2006) Acute neurotoxic effects of mancozeb and maneb in mesencephalic neuronal cultures are associated with mitochondrial dysfunction. *Neurotoxicology* **27:** 816–25.

Duffard R, Garcia G, Rosso S, Bortolozzi A, Madariaga M, di Paolo O, Evangelista de Duffard AM (1996) Central nervous system myelin deficit in rats exposed to 2,4–dichlorophenoxyacetic acid throughout lactation. *Neurotoxicol Teratol* **18:** 691–96.

Dziennis S, Yang D, Cheng J, Anderson KA, Alkayed NJ, Hum PD, Lein PJ, (2008) Developmental exposure to polychlorinated biphenyls influences stroke outcome in adult rats. *Environ Health Perspect* **116:** 474–80.

Emerit J, Edeas M, Bricaire F (2004) Neurodegenerative diseases and oxidative stress. *Biomed Pharmacother* **58:** 39–46.

Eriksson P (1997) Developmental neurotoxicity of environmental agents in the neonate. *Neurotoxicology* **18:** 719–26.

Esteller M (2006) Cancer epigenomics: DNA methylomes and histone modification maps. *Nature Rev Gen* **8:** 286–98.

Evangelista de Duffard AM, Bortolozzi A, Duffard RO (1995) Altered behavioral responses in 2,4-dichlorophenoxyacetic acid treated and amphetamine challenged rats. *Neurotoxicology* **16:** 479–88.

Falconer MM, Vaillant A, Reuhl KR, Laferriere N, Brown DL (1994) The molecular basis of microtubule stability in neurons. *Neurotoxicology* **15:** 109–22.

Fauque P, Jouannet P, Lesaffre C, Ripoche MA, Dandolo L, Vaiman D, Jammes H (2007) Assisted reproductive technology affects developmental kinetics, H19 imprinting control region methylation and H19 gene expression in individual mouse embryos. *BMC Dev Biol* **7:** 116.

Felsenfeld G, Groudine M (2003) Controlling the double helix. *Nature* **421:** 448–53.

Garcia SJ, Seidler FJ, Crumpton TL, Slotkin TA (2001) Does the developmental neurotoxicity of chlorpyrifos involve glial targets? Macromolecule synthesis, adenylyl cyclase signaling, nuclear transcription factors, and formation of reactive oxygen in C6 glioma cells. *Brain Res* **891:** 54–68.

Gendron TF, Petrucelli L (2009) The role of tau in neurodegeneration. *Mol Neurodegener* **4:** 13.

Gilgun-Sherki Y, Melamed E, Offen D (2001) Oxidative stress-induced neurodegenerative diseases: the need for antioxidants that penetrate the blood brain barrier. *Neuropharmacology* **40:** 959–75.

Ginsberg G, Hattis D, Sonawane B (2004) Incorporating pharmacokinetic differences between children and adults in assessing children's risks to environmental toxicants. *Toxicol Appl Pharmacol* **198:** 164–83.

Gitto E, Reiter RJ, Karbownik M, Tan DX, Gitto P, Barberi S, Barberi I (2002) Causes of oxidative stress in the pre- and perinatal period. *Biol Neonate* **81:** 146–57.

Goring HH, Curran JE, Johnson MP, Dyer TD, Charlesworth J, Cole SA, Jowett JB, Abraham LJ, Rainwater DL, Comuzzie AG, Mahaney MC, Almasy L, MacCluer JW, Kissebah AH, Collier GR, Moses EK, Blangero J (2007) Discovery of expression QTLs using large-scale transcriptional profiling in human lymphocytes. *Nat Genet* **39:** 1208–16.

Grandjean P, Landrigan PJ (2006) Developmental neurotoxicity of industrial chemicals. *Lancet* **368:** 2167–78.

Gupta RC (2004) Brain regional heterogeneity and toxicological mechanisms of organophosphates and carbamates. *Toxicol Mech Methods* **14:** 103–43.

Hasan SU, Simakajornboon N, MacKinnon Y, Gozal D (2001) Prenatal cigarette smoke exposure selectively alters protein kinase C and nitric oxide synthase expression within the neonatal rat brainstem. *Neurosci Lett* **301:** 135–38.

Haykal-Coates N, Shafer TJ, Mundy WR, Barone S Jr (1998) Effects of gestational methylmercury exposure on immunoreactivity of specific isoforms of PKC and enzyme activity during post-natal development of the rat brain. *Brain Res Dev Brain Res* **109:** 33–49.

He K, Huang J, Lagenaur CF, Aizenman E (2006) Methylisothiazolinone, a neurotoxic biocide, disrupts the association of SRC family tyrosine kinases with focal adhesion kinase in developing cortical neurons. *J Pharmacol Exp Ther* **317:** 1320–9.

Heikkila RE, Cabbat FS, Cohen G (1976) In vivo inhibition of superoxide dismutase in mice by diethyldithiocarbamate. *J Biol Chem* **251:** 2182–5.

Hilliard A, Ramesh A, Zawia NH (1999) Correlation between lead-induced changes in cerebral ornithine decarboxylase and protein kinase C activities during development and in cultured PC 12 cells. *Int J Dev Neurosci* **17:** 777–85.

Holliday R, Pugh JE (1975) DNA modification mechanisms and gene activity during development. *Science* **187:** 226–32.

Iqbal K, Grundke-Iqbal I, Zaidi T, Merz PA, Wen GY, Shaikh SS, Wisniewski HM, Alafuzoff I, Winblad B (1986) Defective brain microtubule assembly in Alzheimer's disease. *Lancet* **2:** 421–6.

Jirtle RL, Skinner MK (2007) Environmental epigenomics and disease susceptibility. *Nat Rev Genet* **8:** 253–62.

Kalia M (2008) Brain development: anatomy, connectivity, adaptive plasticity, and toxicity. *Metabolism* **57 (Suppl. 2):** S2–5.

Kamboj A, Kiran R, Sandhir R (2006) Carbofuran-induced neurochemical and neurobehavioral alterations in rats: attenuation by *N*-acetylcysteine. *Exp Brain Res* **170:** 567–75.

Kapfhammer JP (2004) Cellular and molecular control of dendritic growth and development of cerebellar Purkinje cells. *Prog Histochem Cytochem* **39:** 131–82.

Kobayashi K, Akune H, Sumida K, Saito K, Yoshioka T, Tsuji R (2009) Perinatal exposure to PTU decreases expression of Arc, Homer 1, Egr 1 and Kcna 1 in the rat cerebral cortex and hippocampus. *Brain Res* **1264:** 24–32.

Koturbash I, Baker M, Loree J, Kutanzi K, Hudson D, Pogribny I, Sedelnikova O, Bonner W, Kovalchuk O (2006) Epigenetic dysregulation underlies radiation-induced transgenerational genome instability in vivo. *Int J Radiat Oncol Biol Phys* **66:** 327–30.

Landrigan PJ, Graham DG, Thomas RD (1994) Environmental neurotoxic illness: research for prevention. *Environ Health Perspect* **102 (Suppl. 2):** 117–20.

Lassiter TL, MacKillop EA, Ryde IT, Seidler FJ, Slotkin TA (2009) Is fipronil safer than chlorpyrifos? Comparative developmental neurotoxicity modeled in PC12 cells. *Brain Res Bull* **78:** 313–22.

Laudenbach V, Medja F, Zoli M, Rossi FM, Evrard P, Changeux JP, Gressens P (2002) Selective activation of central subtypes of the nicotinic acetylcholine receptor has opposite effects on neonatal excitotoxic brain injuries. *FASEB J* **16:** 423–5.

Lazarov O, Robinson J, Tang YP, Hairston IS, Korade-Mirnics Z, Lee VM, Hersh LB, Sapolsky RM, Mirnics K, Sisodia SS (2005) Environmental enrichment reduces Abeta levels and amyloid deposition in transgenic mice. *Cell* **120:** 701–13.

Li B, Carey M, Workman JL (2007) The role of chromatin during transcription. *Cell* **128:** 707–19.

Li F, Chong ZZ, Maiese K (2005) Vital elements of the Wnt-Frizzled signaling pathway in the nervous system. *Curr Neurovasc Res* **2:** 331–40.

Li S, Hansman R, Newbold R, Davis B, McLachlan JA, Barrett JC (2003) Neonatal diethylstilbestrol exposure induces persistent elevation of c-fos expression and hypomethylation in its exon-4 in mouse uterus. *Mol Carcinog* **38:** 78–84.

Liu J, Brannen KC, Grayson DR, Morrow AL, Devaud LL, Lauder JM (1998) Prenatal exposure to the pesticide dieldrin or the GABA(A) receptor antagonist bicuculline differentially alters expression of GABA(A) receptor subunit mRNAs in fetal rat brainstem. *Dev Neurosci* **20:** 83–92.

Mech A, Orynbayeva Z, Irgebayev K, Kolusheva S, Jelinek R (2009) Screening membrane interactions of pesticides by cells decorated with chromatic polymer nanopatches. *Chem Res Toxicol* **22:** 90–6.

Mehler MF (2008) Epigenetic principles and mechanisms underlying nervous system functions in health and disease. *Prog Neurobiol* **86:** 305–41.

Mendola P, Selevan SG, Gutter S, Rice D (2002) Environmental factors associated with a spectrum of neurodevelopmental deficits. *Ment Retard Dev Disabil Res Rev* **8:** 188–97.

Meyer A, Seidler FJ, Aldridge JE, Slotkin TA (2005) Developmental exposure to terbutaline alters cell signaling in mature rat brain regions and augments the effects of subsequent neonatal exposure to the organophosphorus insecticide chlorpyrifos. *Toxicol Appl Pharmacol* **203:** 154–66.

Meyer A, Seidler FJ, Cousins MM, Slotkin TA (2003) Developmental neurotoxicity elicited by gestational exposure to chlorpyrifos: when is adenylyl cyclase a target? *Environ Health Perspect* **111:** 1871–6.

Meyer A, Seidler FJ, Slotkin TA (2004) Developmental effects of chlorpyrifos extend beyond neurotoxicity: critical periods for immediate and delayed-onset effects on cardiac and hepatic cell signaling. *Environ Health Perspect* **112:** 170–8.

Moffatt MF, Kabesch M, Liang L, Dixon AL, Strachan D, Heath S, Depner M, von Berg A, Bufe A, Rietschel E, Heinzmann A, Simma B, Frischer T, Willis-Owen SA, Wong KC, Illig T, Vogelberg C, Weiland SK, von Mutius E, Abecasis GR, Farrall M, Gut IG, Lathrop GM, Cookson WO (2007) Genetic variants regulating ORMDL3 expression contribute to the risk of childhood asthma. *Nature* **448:** 470–3.

Monnet-Tschudi F, Zurich MG, Honegger P (2007) Neurotoxicant-induced inflammatory response in three-dimensional brain cell cultures. *Hum Exp Toxicol* **26:** 339–46.

Moreira EG, Rosa GJ, Barros SB, Vassilieff VS, Vassillieff I (2001) Antioxidant defense in rat brain regions after developmental lead exposure. *Toxicology* **169:** 145–51.

Morell P, Toews AD, Wagner M, Goodrum JF (1994) Gene expression during tellurium-induced primary demyelination. *Neurotoxicology* **15:** 171–80.

Mori de Moro G, Duffard R, Evangelista de Duffard AM (1993) Neurotoxicity of 2,4-dichlorophenoxyacetic butyl ester in chick embryos. *Neurochem Res* **18:** 353–9.

Moya-Quiles MR, Munoz-Delgado E, Vidal CJ (1995) Effect of the pyrethroid insecticide allethrin on membrane fluidity. *Biochem Mol Biol Int* **36:** 1299–308.

Nakagawara A (2001) Trk receptor tyrosine kinases: a bridge between cancer and neural development. *Cancer Lett* **169:** 107–14.

Nihei MK, Guilarte TR (2001) Molecular changes in glutamatergic synapses induced by Pb2+: association with deficits of LTP and spatial learning. *Neurotoxicology* **22:** 635–43.

O'Callaghan JP (1994) A potential role for altered protein phosphorylation in the mediation of developmental neurotoxicity. *Neurotoxicology* **15:** 29–40.

Ohtsuka K, Suzuki T (2000) Roles of molecular chaperones in the nervous system. *Brain Res Bull* **53:** 141–6.

Olanow CW, Arendash GW (1994) Metals and free radicals in neurodegeneration. *Curr Opin Neurol* **7:** 548–58.

Olivier K Jr, Liu J, Pope C (2001) Inhibition of forskolin-stimulated cAMP formation in vitro by paraoxon and chlorpyrifos oxon in cortical slices from neonatal, juvenile, and adult rats. *J Biochem Mol Toxicol* **15:** 263–9.

Olsvik PA, Kristensen T, Waagbo R, Rosseland BO, Tollefsen KE, Baeverfjord G, Berntssen MH (2005) mRNA expression of antioxidant enzymes (SOD, CAT and GSH-Px) and lipid peroxidative stress in liver of Atlantic salmon (*Salmo salar*) exposed to hyperoxic water during smoltification. *Comp Biochem Physiol C Toxicol Pharmacol* **141:** 314–23.

Orrenius S, Nobel CS, Van Den Dobbelsteen DJ, Burkitt MJ, Slater AF (1996) Dithiocarbamates and the redox regulation of cell death. *Biochem Soc Transact* **24:** 1032–8.

Pihl RO, Parkes M (1977) Hair element content in learning disabled children. *Science* **198:** 204–6.

Prendergast MA, Self RL, Smith KJ, Ghayoumi L, Mullins MM, Butler TR, Buccafusco JJ, Gearhart DA, Terry AV Jr (2007) Microtubule-associated targets in chlorpyrifos oxon hippocampal neurotoxicity. *Neuroscience* **146:** 330–9.

Qiao D, Seidler FJ, Slotkin TA (2001) Developmental neurotoxicity of chlorpyrifos modeled in vitro: comparative effects of metabolites and other cholinesterase inhibitors on DNA synthesis in PC12 and C6 cells. *Environ Health Perspect* **109:** 909–13.

Quax RA, Swaak AJ, Baggen MG (2009) Churg-Strauss syndrome following PTU treatment. *Int J Rheumatol* 2009: 504105.

Reuss B, von Bohlen und Halbach O (2003) Fibroblast growth factors and their receptors in the central nervous system. *Cell Tissue Res* **313:** 139–57.

Rice D, Barone S Jr (2000) Critical periods of vulnerability for the developing nervous system: evidence from humans and animal models. *Environ Health Perspect* **108 (Suppl. 3):** 511–33.

Richardson JR, Caudle WM, Wang M, Dean ED, Pennell KD, Miller GW (2006) Developmental exposure to the pesticide dieldrin alters the dopamine system and increases neurotoxicity in an animal model of Parkinson's disease. *FASEB J* **20:** 1695–7.

Riggs AD (1975) X inactivation, differentiation, and DNA methylation. *Cytogenet Cell Genet* **14:** 9–25.

Rodier PM (1995) Developing brain as a target of toxicity. *Environ Health Perspect* **103 (Suppl. 6):** 73–6.

Roldan-Tapi L, Leyva A, Laynez F, Santed FS (2005) Chronic neuropsychological sequelae of cholinesterase inhibitors in the absence of structural brain damage: two cases of acute poisoning. *Environ Health Perspect* **113:** 762–6.

Ronnback A, Dahlqvist P, Svensson PA, Jernas M, Carlsson B, Carlsson LM, Olsson T (2005) Gene expression profiling of the rat hippocampus one month after focal cerebral ischemia followed by enriched environment. *Neurosci Lett* **385:** 173–8.

Rosso SB, Caceres AO, de Duffard AM, Duffard RO, Quiroga S (2000) 2,4-Dichlorophenoxyacetic acid disrupts the cytoskeleton and disorganizes the Golgi apparatus of cultured neurons. *Toxicol Sci* **56:** 133–40.

Rosso SB, Di Paolo OA, Evangelista de Duffard AM, Duffard R (1997) Effects of 2,4-dichlorophenoxyacetic acid on central nervous system of developmental rats. Associated changes in ganglioside pattern. *Brain Res* **769:** 163–7.

Rosso SB, Gonzalez M, Bagatolli LA, Duffard RO, Fidelio GD (1998) Evidence of a strong interaction of 2,4-dichlorophenoxyacetic acid herbicide with human serum albumin. *Life Sci* **63:** 2343–51.

Royland JE, Kodavanti PR (2008) Gene expression profiles following exposure to a developmental neurotoxicant, Aroclor 1254: pathway analysis for possible mode(s) of action. *Toxicol Appl Pharmacol* **231:** 179–96.

Scheuplein R, Charnley G, Dourson M (2002) Differential sensitivity of children and adults to chemical toxicity. I. Biological basis. *Regul Toxicol Pharmacol* **35:** 429–47.

Schuh RA, Lein PJ, Beckles RA, Jett DA (2002) Noncholinesterase mechanisms of chlorpyrifos neurotoxicity: altered phosphorylation of Ca2+/cAMP response element binding protein in cultured neurons. *Toxicol Appl Pharmacol* **182:** 176–85.

Shafer TJ, Meyer DA, Crofton KM (2005) Developmental neurotoxicity of pyrethroid insecticides: critical review and future research needs. *Environ Health Perspect* **113:** 123–36.

Shaywitz AJ, Greenberg ME (1999) CREB: a stimulus-induced transcription factor activated by a diverse array of extracellular signals. *Annu Rev Biochem* **68:** 821–61.

Slikker W Jr, Xu ZA, Levin ED, Slotkin TA (2005) Mode of action: disruption of brain cell replication, second messenger, and neurotransmitter systems during development leading to cognitive dysfunction – developmental neurotoxicity of nicotine. *Crit Rev Toxicol* **35:** 703–11.

Slotkin TA (2002) Nicotine and the adolescent brain: insights from an animal model. *Neurotoxicol Teratol* **24:** 369–84.

Slotkin TA (2004) Cholinergic systems in brain development and disruption by neurotoxicants: nicotine, environmental tobacco smoke, organophosphates. *Toxicol Appl Pharmacol* **198:** 132–51.

Slotkin TA, Seidler FJ (2007) Developmental exposure to terbutaline and chlorpyrifos, separately or sequentially, elicits presynaptic serotonergic hyperactivity in juvenile and adolescent rats. *Brain Res Bull* **73:** 301–9.

Slotkin TA, Seidler FJ (2008) Developmental neurotoxicants target neurodifferentiation into the serotonin phenotype: chlorpyrifos, diazinon, dieldrin and divalent nickel. *Toxicol Appl Pharmacol* **233:** 211–19.

Slotkin TA, Seidler FJ (2009a) Protein kinase C is a target for diverse developmental neurotoxicants: transcriptional responses to chlorpyrifos, diazinon, dieldrin and divalent nickel in PC12 cells. *Brain Res* **1263:** 23–32.

Slotkin TA, Seidler FJ (2009b) Oxidative and excitatory mechanisms of developmental neurotoxicity: transcriptional profiles for chlorpyrifos, diazinon, dieldrin, and divalent nickel in PC12 cells. *Environ Health Perspect* **117:** 587–96.

Slotkin TA, Seidler FJ (2010) Oxidative stress from diverse developmental neurotoxicants: antioxidants protect against lipid peroxidation without preventing cell loss. *Neurotoxicol Teratol* **32:** 124–31.

Slotkin TA, Auman JT, Seidler FJ (2003) Ontogenesis of beta-adrenoceptor signaling: implications for perinatal physiology and for fetal effects of tocolytic drugs. *J Pharmacol Exp Ther* **306:** 1–7.

Slotkin TA, Cousins MM, Tate CA, Seidler FJ (2001) Persistent cholinergic presynaptic deficits after neonatal chlorpyrifos exposure. *Brain Res* **902:** 229–43.

Slotkin TA, MacKillop EA, Ryde IT, Seidler FJ (2007a) Ameliorating the developmental neurotoxicity of chlorpyrifos: a mechanisms-based approach in PC12 cells. *Environ Health Perspect* **115:** 1306–13.

Slotkin TA, MacKillop EA, Ryde IT, Tate CA, Seidler FJ (2007b) Screening for developmental neurotoxicity using PC12 cells: comparisons of organophosphates with a carbamate, an organochlorine, and divalent nickel. *Environ Health Perspect* **115:** 93–101.

Slotkin TA, Seidler FJ, Wu C, MacKillop EA, Linden KG (2009) Ultraviolet photolysis of chlorpyrifos: developmental neurotoxicity modeled in PC12 cells. *Environ Health Perspect* **117:** 338–43.

Somech R, Izraeli S, Simon AJ (2004) Histone deacetylase inhibitors – a new tool to treat cancer. *Cancer Treat Rev* **30:** 461–72.

Smith DJ (2009) Mitochondrial dysfunction in mouse models of Parkinson's disease revealed by transcriptomics and proteomics. *J Bioenerg Biomembr* **41:** 487–91.

Song C, Kanthasamy A, Anantharam V, Sun F, Kanthasamy AG (2010) Environmental neurotoxic pesticide increases histone acetylation to promote apoptosis in dopaminergic neuronal cells: relevance to epigenetic mechanisms of neurodegeneration. *Mol Pharmacol* **77:** 621–32.

Song X, Seidler FJ, Saleh JL, Zhang J, Padilla S, Slotkin TA (1997) Cellular mechanisms for developmental toxicity of chlorpyrifos: targeting the adenylyl cyclase signaling cascade. *Toxicol Appl Pharmacol* **145:** 158–74.

Stachowiak EK, Fang X, Myers J, Dunham S, Stachowiak MK (2003) cAMP-induced differentiation of human neuronal progenitor cells is mediated by nuclear fibroblast growth factor receptor-1 (FGFR1). *J Neurochem* **84:** 1296–312.

Steingart RA, Silverman WF, Barron S, Slotkin TA, Awad Y, Yanai J (2000) Neural grafting reverses prenatal drug-induced alterations in hippocampal PKC and related behavioral deficits. *Brain Res Dev Brain Res* **125:** 9–19.

Strahl BD, Allis CD (2000) The language of covalent histone modifications. *Nature* **403:** 41–5.

Suwalsky M, Benites M, Norris B, Sotomayor CP (2003) The organophosphorous insecticide chlorpyrifos affects the neuroepithelial junction, the bioelectric parameters of the skin of the frog *Caudiverbera caudiverbera*, and the structure of model cell membranes. *Pest Biochem Physiol* **77:** 44–53.

Szpir M (2006) Tracing the origins of autism: a spectrum of new studies. *Environ Health Perspect* **114:** A412–18.

Tamm C, Sabri F, Ceccatelli S (2008) Mitochondrial-mediated apoptosis in neural stem cells exposed to manganese. *Toxicol Sci* **101:** 310–20.

Tanaka J, Toku K, Zhang B, Ishihara K, Sakanaka M, Maeda N (1999) Astrocytes prevent neuronal death induced by reactive oxygen and nitrogen species. *Glia* **28:** 85–96.

Thiriet N, Amar L, Toussay X, Lardeux V, Ladenheim B, Becker KG, Cadet JL, Solinas M, Jaber M (2008) Environmental enrichment during adolescence regulates gene expression in the striatum of mice. *Brain Res* **1222:** 31–41.

Tilson HA (1995) The concern for developmental neurotoxicology: is it justified and what is being done about it? *Environ Health Perspect* **103 (Suppl 6):** 147–51.

Tilson HA (2000) Neurotoxicology risk assessment guidelines: developmental neurotoxicology. *Neurotoxicology* **21:** 189–94.

Tong S, McMichael AJ, Baghurst PA (2000) Interactions between environmental lead exposure and sociodemographic factors on cognitive development. *Arch Environ Health* **55:** 330–5.

Tsankova N, Renthal W, Kumar A, Nestler EJ (2007) Epigenetic regulation in psychiatric disorders. *Nat Rev Neurosci* **8:** 355–67.

Uttara B, Singh AV, Zamboni P, Mahajan RT (2009) Oxidative stress and neurodegenerative diseases: a review of upstream and downstream antioxidant therapeutic options. *Curr Neuropharmacol* **7:** 65–74.

Verity MA (1994) Oxidative damage and repair in the developing nervous system. *Neurotoxicology* **15:** 81–91.

Walaas SI, Greengard P (1991) Protein phosphorylation and neuronal function. *Pharmacol Rev* **43:** 299–349.

Wang J, Wu J, Zhang Z (2006) Oxidative stress in mouse brain exposed to lead. *Ann Occup Hyg* **50:** 405–9.

Ward TR, Mundy WR (1996) Organophosphorus compounds preferentially affect second messenger systems coupled to M2/M4 receptors in rat frontal cortex. *Brain Res Bull* **39:** 49–55.

Wasserman GA, Liu X, Parvez F, Ahsan H, Factor-Litvak P, Kline J, van Geen A, Slavkovich V, Loiacono NJ, Levy D, Cheng Z, Graziano JH (2007) Water arsenic exposure and intellectual function in 6-year-old children in Araihazar, Bangladesh. *Environ Health Perspect* **115:** 285–9.

Wasserman GA, Liu X, Parvez F, Ahsan H, Levy D, Factor-Litvak P, Kline J, van Geen A, Slavkovich V, LoIacono NJ, Cheng Z, Zheng Y, Graziano JH (2006) Water manganese exposure and children's intellectual function in Araihazar, Bangladesh. *Environ Health Perspect* **114:** 124–9.

Wasteneys GO, Cadrin M, Reuhl KR, Brown DL (1988) The effects of methylmercury on the cytoskeleton of murine embryonal carcinoma cells. *Cell Biol Toxicol* **4:** 41–60.

Waterland RA (2006) Epigenetic mechanisms and gastrointestinal development. *J Pediatr* **149:** S137–42.

Waterland RA, Jirtle RL (2003) Transposable elements: targets for early nutritional effects on epigenetic gene regulation. *Mol Cell Biol* **23:** 5293–300.

White LD, Cory-Slechta DA, Gilbert ME, Tiffany-Castiglioni E, Zawia NH, Virgolini M, Rossi-George A, Lasley SM, Qian YC, Basha MR (2007) New and evolving concepts in the neurotoxicology of lead. *Toxicol Appl Pharmacol* **225:** 1–27.

Wolffe AP, Guschin D (2000) Review: chromatin structural features and targets that regulate transcription. *J Struct Biol* **129:** 102–22.

Wright RO, Baccarelli A (2007) Metals and neurotoxicology. *J Nutr* **137:** 2809–13.

Wu J, Basha MR, Brock B, Cox DP, Cardozo-Pelaez F, McPherson CA, Harry J, Rice DC, Maloney B, Chen D, Lahiri DK, Zawia NH (2008b) Alzheimer's disease (AD)-like pathology in aged monkeys after infantile exposure to environmental metal lead (Pb): evidence for a developmental origin and environmental link for AD. *J Neurosci* **28:**3–9.

Wu J, Basha MR, Zawia NH (2008a) The environment, epigenetics and amyloidogenesis. *J Mol Neurosci* **34:** 1–7.

Xu J, Yan CH, Yang B, Xie HF, Zou XY, Zhong L, Gao Y, Tian Y, Shen XM (2009) The role of metabotropic glutamate receptor 5 in developmental lead neurotoxicity. *Toxicol Lett* **191:** 223–30.

Yanai J, Beer A, Huleihel R, Izrael M, Katz S, Levi Y, Rozenboim I, Yaniv SP, Slotkin TA (2004) Convergent effects on cell signaling mechanisms mediate the actions of different neurobehavioral teratogens: alterations in cholinergic regulation of protein kinase C in chick and avian models. *Ann NY Acad Sci* **1025:** 595–601.

Yanai J, Ben-Shaanan TL, Haimovitch H, Katz S, Kazma M (2006) Mechanism-based approaches for the reversal of drug neurobehavioral teratogenicity. *Ann NY Acad Sci* **1074:** 659–71.

Yanai J, Vatury O, Slotkin TA (2002) Cell signaling as a target and underlying mechanism for neurobehavioral teratogenesis. *Ann NY Acad Sci* **965:** 473–8.

Yang D, Kim KH, Phimister A, Bachstetter AD, Ward TR, Stackman RW, Mervis RF, Wisniewski AB, Klein SL, Kodavani PR, Anderson KA, Wayman G, Pessah IN, Lein PJ (2009) Developmental exposure to polychlorinated biphenyls interferes with experience-dependent dendritic plasticity and ryanodine receptor expression in weanling rats. *Environ Health Perspect* **117:** 426–35.

Zawia NH, Basha MR (2005) Environmental risk factors and the developmental basis for Alzheimer's disease. *Rev Neurosci* **16:** 325–37.

Zhang J, Fitsanakis VA, Gu G, Jing D, Ao M, Amarnath V, Montine TJ (2003) Manganese ethylene-bis-dithiocarbamate and selective dopaminergic neurodegeneration in rat: a link through mitochondrial dysfunction. *J Neurochem* **84:** 336–46.

Zhao X, Pak C, Smart RD, Jin P (2007) Epigenetics and neural developmental disorders: Washington DC, September 18 and 19, 2006. *Epigenetics* **2:** 126–34.

Zheng Q, Olivier K, Won YK, Pope CN (2000) Comparative cholinergic neurotoxicity of oral chlorpyrifos exposures in preweanling and adult rats. *Toxicol Sci* **55:** 124–32.

C H A P T E R

64

Neuroinflammation and oxidative injury in developmental neurotoxicity

Dejan Milatovic, Snjezana Zaja-Milatovic, Rich M. Breyer, Michael Aschner and Thomas J. Montine

INTRODUCTION

Neuroinflammation is a complex response to brain injury involving the activation of glia, release of inflammatory mediators, such as cytokines and chemokines, and generation of reactive oxygen and nitrogen species. The links among risk factors and the development of neuroinflammation are numerous and involve many complex interactions which contribute to vascular compromise, oxidative stress and ultimately brain damage. Once this cascade of events is initiated, the process of neuroinflammation can become overactivated, resulting in further cellular damage and loss of neuronal functions. The immune response is usually activated simultaneously with multiple other stressors and responses to injury, with some aspects proposed to be neurotrophic and others neurotoxic. Inflammatory responses in the brain are also associated with increased levels of prostaglandins (PGs), particularly PGE_2, which plays a central role in brain diseases, including ischemic injury, and several neurodegenerative diseases. PGE_2 signaling is mediated by interactions with four distinct G protein-coupled receptors, EP1–4, which are differentially expressed on neuronal and glial cells throughout the central nervous system (CNS). EP2 activation has been shown to mediate microglial-induced paracrine neurotoxicity, but its role also is dependent on the specific cell type in which EP2 signaling is activated. Neuroinflammation, elevated PGE_2 and inflammatory mediators are also inherent to the aging brain. An increased state of neuroinflammation makes the aged brain more vulnerable to the disruptive effects of both intrinsic and extrinsic factors such as disease, infection, toxicants or stress. This chapter characterizes processes of neuroinflammation and related oxidative injury and discusses alterations associated with developmental neurotoxicity.

NEUROINFLAMMATION AND OXIDATIVE DAMAGE

Neuroinflammation is defined as the activation of the brain's innate immune system in response to an inflammatory challenge and is characterized by a host of cellular and molecular changes within the brain. Aside from neurons, neuroinflammation is also associated with macroglia and microglia, two primary cell types located throughout the nervous system. The macroglia are derived from a nerve cell lineage and are classified into three distinct subtypes: astrocytes, oligodendrocytes and Schwann cells. The astrocytes are the most populous cells of the CNS and support and maintain neuronal plasticity throughout the CNS. Microglia are also interspersed throughout the brain and represent approximately 10% of the CNS population. Microglia differ from the macroglia because they are derived from a monocyte/macrophage cell lineage. Microglia are pivotal in innate immune activation and function to modulate neuroinflammatory signals throughout the brain. In the absence of stimulus, microglia are quiescent and have a ramified morphology (Gonzales-Scarano and Baltuch, 1999). During an innate immune response microglia are activated and become deramified. Active microglia show macrophage-like activities, including scavenging, phagocytosis, antigen presentation, complement activation and release of proinflammatory molecules including cytokines, chemokines and prostanoids. Neuroinflammatory response may also trigger oxidative and nitrosative stress and thus perpetuates the inflammatory cycle. Moreover microglia recruit and activate astrocytes to propagate these inflammatory signals further (Blasko *et al.*, 2004). Astrocytes regulate transendothelial cell migration across the blood–brain barrier (BBB) (Prat *et al.*, 2001) and have an accessory role to neurons, modulating glutamate levels in the extracellular space and preventing glutamate-induced neurotoxicity (Mucke and Eddleston, 1993; Magistretti *et al.*, 1999). Upon activation, astrocytes increase production of glial fibrillary acidic protein (GFAP), and undergo process extension and interdigitation. Activation of these cells may be accompanied by functional deregulation and even degeneration with the consequent disruption of the cross-talk normally occurring between glia and neurons (Peterson and Du, 2009).

The exact pattern of cellular and molecular changes depends largely on the type and duration of the inflammatory challenge experienced by the organism. Neuroinflammation can result from classical injuries such as direct

Reproductive and Developmental Toxicology, Edited by Ramesh C. Gupta
ISBN: 978-0-12-382032-7

insult to the brain that occurs with trauma, encephalitis or ischemia, or from insults such as toxins or infection that follow exposure to bacteria. However, neuroinflammation also occurs following less traditional injuries such as neurodegenerative disorders and even with normal aging and exposure to certain stressors.

Acute neuroinflammatory response resulting in phagocytic phenotype, release of inflammatory mediators such as free radicals, cytokines and chemokines (Tansey *et al.*, 2007; Frank-Cannon *et al.*, 2009) may be generally beneficial to the CNS, since it tends to minimize further injury and contributes to repair of damaged tissue. In contrast, chronic neuroinflammation is a long-standing and often self-perpetuating neuroinflammatory response that persists long after an initial injury or insult. Sustained release of inflammatory mediators and increased oxidative and nitrosative stress activate additional microglia, promoting their proliferation and resulting in further release in inflammatory factors. Owing to this sustained nature of inflammation, the blood–brain barrier (BBB) may be compromised, thus increasing infiltration of peripheral macrophages into the brain parenchyma, further perpetuating the inflammatory process (Rivest, 2009). Rather than serving a protective role as does acute neuroinflammation, chronic neuroinflammation is most often detrimental and damaging to nervous tissue. Thus, whether neuroinflammation has beneficial or harmful outcomes in the brain may depend critically on the duration of the inflammatory response.

Activation of innate immunity occurs simultaneously with several pathogenic processes and responses to stressors and injury, thereby greatly confounding any clear conclusion about cause-and-effect relationships. For these reasons, we have adopted a simple, but a highly specific model of isolated innate immune activation: intracerebroventricular (ICV) injection of low dose lipopolysaccharide (LPS). LPS specifically activates innate immunity through a Toll-like receptor (TLR)-dependent signaling pathway (Imler and Hoffmann, 2001; Akira, 2003). Nine human plasma membrane-spanning TLRs are expressed in many cell types throughout the body and all have been uncovered in the context of innate immune response to micro-organisms. TLR-mediated innate immune response occurs in three phases: an initial signal transduction cascade, secondary signaling cascades and effectors. The initial signaling cascade starts by activation of one of the nine plasma membrane TLRs by a ligand. Response to LPS that also requires another protein, CD14 and adaptor protein MyD88, initiates a bifurcated signal transduction cascade that culminates in altered gene transcription, primarily via NF-κB activation but also through c-Fos/c-Jun-dependent pathways. Some of the activated gene transcripts encode directly for receptor ligands, while others are enzymes that catalyze the formation of receptor ligands that in turn activate secondary autocrine and paracrine signaling cascades. These signaling events culminate in the generation of effector molecules including bacteriocidal molecules, primarily free radicals generated by NADPH oxidase and myeloperoxidase (MPO), as well as cytokines and chemokines that can attract an adaptive immune response (Milatovic *et al.*, 2004).

Within minutes to hours of exposure to LPS, there is increased gene transcription and subsequent translation of cytokines and chemokines, including tumor necrosis factor, interleukin-1 and interferons, as well as several enzymes. Important among these are inducible nitric oxide synthase (iNOS) and cyclooxygenase 2 (COX-2) that catalyze the formation of NO and prostaglandin (PG) H_2, respectively (Palsson-McDermott and O'Neill, 2004). While NO is a potent cell signaling molecule, PGH_2 has relatively low receptor binding affinity, but is rapidly and efficiently converted to multiple PGs or thromboxane A2, each of which is a potent activator of a large family of G protein-coupled receptors (GPCRs) (Hata and Breyer, 2004). The combination of these initial and secondary signaling cascades produces a robust innate immune response.

Recently we have employed the ICV model and identified the molecular and pharmacologic determinants of LPS-initiated cerebral neuronal damage *in vivo* (Montine *et al.*, 2002; Milatovic *et al.*, 2003, 2004). Interestingly, the degree of oxidative damage in this model was equivalent to what we observed in diseased regions of brain from patients with degenerative diseases (Reich *et al.*, 2001). For evaluation of oxidative damage, we used a stable isotope dilution method with gas chromatography and negative ion chemical ionization mass spectrometry (GC-MC/NICI) (Morrow and Roberts, 1997; Milatovic and Aschner, 2009). While numerous methods exist to determine free radical-mediated damage *in vitro*, important limitations arise in living systems where extensive, highly active enzymatic pathways have evolved to metabolize many of the commonly measured products, such as 4-hydroxynonenal (Montine *et al.*, 2002). Therefore, we have applied GC-MS/NICI as a robust quantitative means of measuring free radical damage in vivo and measured F_2-isoprostanes (F_2-IsoPs), products generated from free radical damage to arachidonic acid (AA), which are not extensively metabolized in situ. Since AA is present throughout brain and in different cells in brain at roughly equal concentrations, measurement of cerebral F_2-IsoPs, like all other measures of oxidative damage, reflects damage to brain tissue, but not necessarily to neurons. For these reasons, we developed an assay to measure the analogous products generated from docosahexanoic acid (DHA), F_4-NeuroPs (Roberts *et al.*, 1998). Since DHA is highly concentrated in neuronal membranes, F_4-NeuroPs offer a unique window into free radical damage to neuronal membranes in vivo (Montine *et al.*, 2004). Results from our studies with 2-month-old mice showed that single ICV LPS injections induced delayed, transient elevation in both F_2-IsoPs and F_4-NeuroPs at 24 h after exposure and then returned to baseline by 72 h post-exposure (Table 64.1) (Milatovic *et al.*, 2003). While others have shown that altered gene transcription and increased cytokine secretion occur rapidly and peak within a few hours of LPS exposure, it is likely that delay in neuronal oxidative damage observed in our experiments is related, at least in part, to the time required to deplete antioxidant defenses.

To address if oxidative damage is related to neurodegeneration, we examined directly the dendritic compartment of neurons, which is largely transparent to the standard histological techniques used so far to investigate ICV LPS-induced damage. Using Golgi impregnation and Neurolucida-assisted morphometry of hippocampal CA1 pyramidal neurons (Leuner *et al.*, 2003; Milatovic *et al.*, 2010), we first determined the time course of dendritic structural changes following ICV LPS in mice. Our results show a time course similar to neuronal oxidative damage with maximal reduction in both dendrite length and dendritic spine density at 24 h post-LPS and, remarkably, a return to baseline levels by 72 h (Table 64.1). Thus, these data strongly imply that neuronal oxidative damage is closely associated with dendritic degeneration following ICV LPS. We and others have shown

TABLE 64.1 Cerebral oxidative damage and dendritic degeneration in young mice. Effects of ICV saline (5 µl, control) and ICV LPS (5 µg/5 µl) treatment determined at 24 h and 72 h following exposure

	24 h	24 h	72 h	72 h
	ICV saline	ICV LPS	ICV saline	ICV LPS
F_2-IsoPs (ng/g tissue)	3.26 ± 0.19	4.77 ± 0.26*	3.13 ± 0.11	2.98 ± 0.17
F_4-NeuroPs (ng/g tissue)	13.91 ± 1.17	58.50 ± 5.98*	12.30 ± 1.18	16.80 ± 0.96
Dendritic length (µm)	1018 ± 113	324 ± 37*	848 ± 60	1030 ± 61
Spine density (spine no./ 100 µm dendrite)	16.89 ± 1.67	5.86 ± 0.57*	17.09 ± 1.13	16.77 ± 0.87

Values are means ± SEM
*Significantly different compared to controls ($p < 0.05$)

that primary neurons enriched in cell culture do not respond to LPS (Minghetti and Levi, 1999; Fiebich *et al.*, 2001; Xie *et al.*, 2002), therefore, our results also showed that LPS activated microglial-mediated paracrine oxidative damage to neurons.

Following LPS administration, the animal's immune system recognizes pathogen-associated molecular patterns and stimulates an immediate and robust immune response. In addition to cytokines and chemokines, neuroinflammation is often accompanied by increased productions of PGs. PGs are a class of eicosanoids that are formed by the liberation of AA from phospholipids and a two-step conversion by COX enzymes. COX enzymes are rate-limiting in the formation of PGs. Two main isoforms of the COX enzyme exist, COX-1 and -2, which show 60% homology within a species (O'Banion, 1999; Tanabe and Tohnai, 2002). COX-1 is traditionally thought to have constitutive expression, while COX-2 is highly inducible, although this distinction is not as apparent within the brain. In fact, COX-2 has high basal expression within the brain and particularly the hippocampus, while COX-1 mRNA and protein are increased in the hippocampus by inflammatory stimuli (Bliss *et al.*, 2007). PGs are released by neuronal and glial cells in response to inflammatory challenge. For example, peripheral LPS injection upregulates expression of COX-2 in endothelial cells within the brain vasculature (Quan *et al.*, 1998).

Following cyclization of arachidonic acid to PGG_2 via its bis-oxygenase activity, COX isozymes then catalyze conversion of unstable PGG_2 to PGH_2 by the peroxidase activity (Kaufmann *et al.*, 1997). PGH_2 may be converted to the prostanoids PGD_2, PGE_2, $PGF_2\alpha$, PGI_2 and thromboxane (Tx) A_2 by cell-specific synthases or isomerases. These potent prostanoid signaling molecules exert their effects through autocrine and paracrine stimulation of eight specific GPCRs designated DP, EP1-4, FP, IP and TP, respectively (Hata and Breyer, 2004). Differentially restricted expression of the prostanoid synthases, isomerases and receptors allows these prostanoids to achieve a wide variety of biological actions in different cell types and tissues.

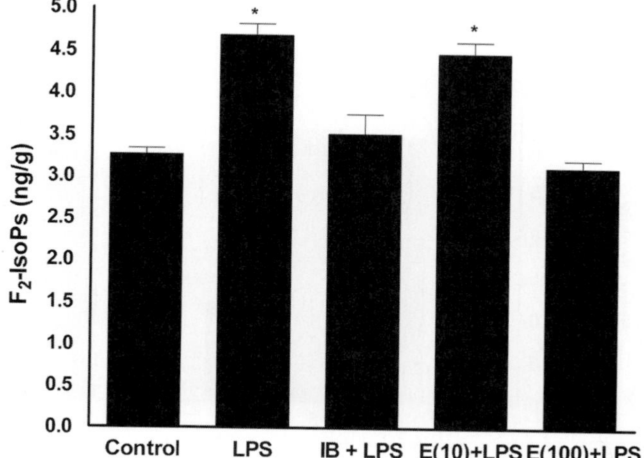

FIGURE 64.1 Ipsilateral cerebral F_2-IsoPs concentrations following ICV saline (control) or LPS (5 µg/5 µl) of young mice with or without systemic pretreatment with ibuprofen (IB, 14 µg/ml) or α-tocopherol injections (E, 10 mg/kg or 100 mg/kg). Brains from mice exposed to LPS were collected 24 hours post-injections. *Significant difference compared to control ($p < 0.01$).

SUPPRESSION OF INNATE IMMUNITY-MEDIATED NEURONAL DAMAGE

We investigated the effectiveness of drugs currently proposed to inhibit COX, and to suppress innate immune response and/or oxidative damage (Stewart *et al.*, 1997; Morris *et al.*, 1998; in'tVeld *et al.*, 2000; Engelhart *et al.*, 2002; Zandi *et al.*, 2002; Lehnardt *et al.*, 2003). Our studies determined if peripheral administration of α-tocopherol (vitamin E), a natural antioxidant product with a number of proposed actions (Brigelius-Flohe and Tabe, 1999) including both antioxidant and anti-inflammatory activities (Li *et al.*, 2001), suppressed oxidative damage following ICV LPS. All measurements for these experiments were done 24 h after ICV LPS. Our results demonstrated that a dose of 10 mg/kg (given for 3 consecutive days before ICV LPS) partially blocked F_2-IsoPs formation (Milatovic *et al.*, 2003), and completely suppressed cerebral oxidative damage at 100 mg/kg (Figure 64.1).

We also determined the effect of α-tocopherol on ICV LPS-induced reduction in hippocampal pyramidal neuron dendritic spine density and dendritic lengths. At 100 mg/kg, α-tocopherol fully suppressed dendritic damage from activated glial innate immune response, corroborating the association between oxidative damage and dendritic degeneration following ICV LPS (Figures 64.2 and 64.3). We have previously shown that α-tocopherol is equally effective in suppressing neuronal oxidative damage from direct excitotoxicity to neurons caused by kainic acid (Milatovic *et al.*, 2005). These data imply that α-tocopherol offers broad protection in the cerebrum from oxidative damage.

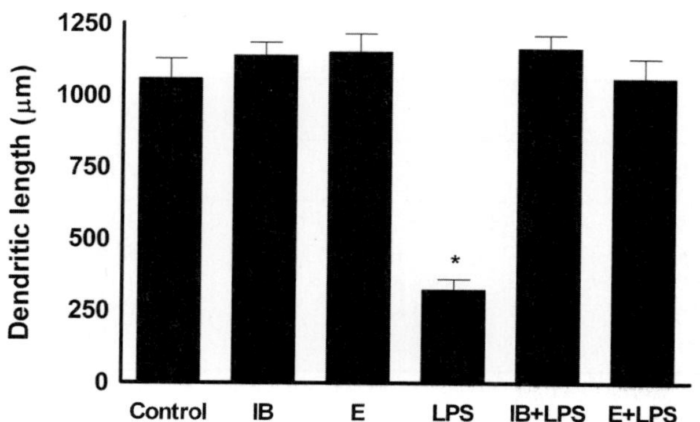

FIGURE 64.2 Dendritic length was determined at 24 hours post-ICV saline (control) or LPS (5 μg/5 μl) injection in CA1 sector hippocampal pyramidal neurons of young mice with or without systemic pretreatment with ibuprofen (IB, 14 μg/ml) or α- tocopherol injections (E, 100 mg/kg). *Significant difference compared to control ($p<0.001$).

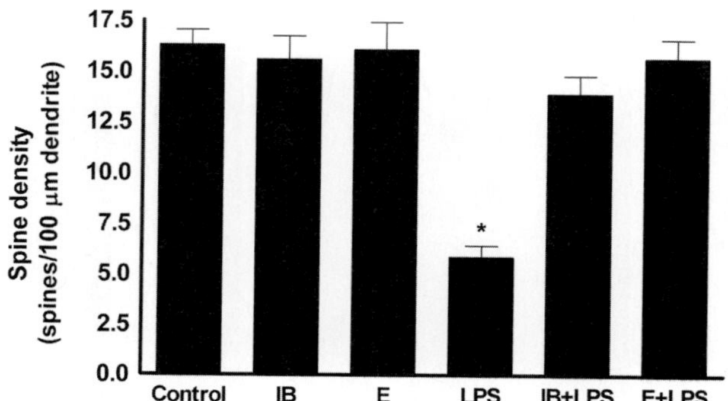

FIGURE 64.3 Spine density was determined at 24 hours post-ICV saline (control) or LPS (5 μg/5 μl) injection in CA1 sector hippocampal pyramidal neurons of young mice with or without systemic pretreatment with ibuprofen (IB, 14 μg/ml) or α-tocopherol injections (E, 100 mg/kg). *Significant difference compared to control ($p<0.001$).

Next, we determined the effectiveness of COX inhibitors and dose–response relationship for the non-steroidal anti-inflammatory drug (NSAID) ibuprofen in our ICV LPS model, utilizing a 2-week pretreatment in drinking water (Milatovic *et al.*, 2003). NSAID alone did not alter basal levels of cerebral F_2-IsoPs or dendritic system of CA1 pyramidal neurons. Ibuprofen at 14 μg/ml drinking water completely suppressed LPS-induced oxidative damage (Figure 64.1) and protected the dendritic system from the degenerative consequences of ICV LPS (Figures 64.2 and 64.3). Others have also shown that NSAIDs can limit oxidative damage in models of neurodegeneration, and that increases in NOS activity and PGE_2 production are associated with oxidative damage (Beal, 1998; Hewett *et al.*, 2000). NSAIDs block COX activity and thereby suppress generation of all COX products including PGE_2, a major signaling molecule, its several eicosanoid derivatives, as well as oxidant by-products. In addition, NSAIDs have several COX-independent actions (Hamburger and McCay, 1990; Asanuam *et al.*, 2001; Weggen *et al.*, 2001).

Recent epidemiological studies demonstrate that chronic COX-2 inhibition can produce adverse cerebrovascular effects, indicating that some PG signaling pathways are beneficial (Egan *et al.*, 2004; Rudic *et al.*, 2005; Funk and FitzGerald, 2007; Andreasson, 2010). Consistent with these concepts, recent studies demonstrate that in the CNS, specific PG receptor signaling pathways mediate toxic effects.

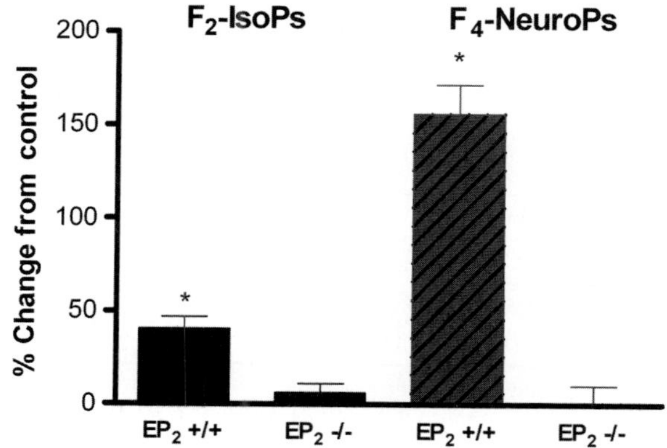

FIGURE 64.4 Ipsilateral cerebral F_2-IsoPs and F_4-NeuroPs concentrations following ICV LPS (5 μg/5 μl) of young wild-type (EP_2 +/+) and EP_2 −/− deficient mice. Brains from mice exposed to LPS were collected 24 hours post-injections. F_2-IsoPs and F_4-NeuroPs data are expressed as % control of mice injected with saline. *Significant difference compared to control ($p<0.05$).

However, complexity is emerging, as exemplified by the PGE_2 EP2 receptor (one of four receptor subtypes for PGE2: EP1, EP2, EP3 and EP4), where cerebroprotective or toxic effects of a particular PG signaling pathway can differ depending on the context of cerebral injury (excitotoxicity vs. inflammation-mediated secondary neurotoxicity) (Montine *et al.*, 2002). We have shown that the EP2 receptor plays a critical role in the generation of ROS in response to ICV LPS (Montine *et al.*, 2002; Milatovic *et al.*, 2005). Following administration of LPS, EP2 deficient (EP2−/−) mice fail to mount the inflammatory oxidative response seen in wild-type mice, as quantified by levels of biomarkers of oxidative damage, F_2-IsoPs and F_4-NeuroPs (Figure 64.4).

In vitro experiments with microglia obtained from EP2−/− mice showed that microglial EP2 was critical to LPS-activated microglia-mediated neurotoxicity (Shie *et al.*, 2005). Pharmacologic suppression of microglia with COX inhibitors (with ibuprofen the most potent, likely due its well-described activities in addition to COX suppression; Insel, 1996) also completely suppressed microglia-mediated neurotoxicity (Shie *et al.*, 2005). Given the concordance between these *in vivo* and *in vitro* findings as well as between our genetic and pharmacologic manipulations with NSAIDs, these data strongly implicate microglial EP2-dependent release of paracrine effectors of neuronal damage following activation by LPS.

Interestingly, the EP2 receptor elicits a very different response in the context of excitotoxicity (Montine *et al.*, 2002). *In vitro* studies of dispersed hippocampal neurons and organotypic hippocampal slices demonstrate that the activation of the EP2 receptor is neuroprotective in paradigms of N-methyl D-aspartate receptor (NMDA) toxicity (McCullough *et al.*, 2004; Liu *et al.*, 2005). In acute glutamate toxicity models, inhibition of protein kinase A (PKA) activation reversed the protective effect of EP2 signaling, indicating that neuronal EP2-mediated protection is dependent on cAMP signaling (McCullough *et al.*, 2004). In contrast to the model of inflammation, genetic deletion of the EP2 receptor in mice did not suppress oxidative damage induced by excitotoxicity (kaininc acid administration) (Montine *et al.*, 2002). Therefore, data suggest a dichotomy of action of the EP2 receptor in the CNS, which is dependent upon type of injury, the specific cell type in which EP2 signaling is activated and the cell-specific and model-specific downstream targets of EP2 signaling in these cells.

AGING

The aging process is defined by a slow deterioration of homeostatic functions throughout the lifespan of an organism. For example, in the adult brain there is a balance between proinflammatory and anti-inflammatory cytokines, but with increased age this balance is shifted towards a proinflammatory state. This increased state of neuroinflammation makes the aged brain more vulnerable to the disruptive effects of both intrinsic and extrinsic factors such as disease, infection, toxicants or stress.

In addition to increased numbers of activated microglia and increased astrocyte expression of GFAP, the aged brain exhibits increased steady-state levels of inflammatory cytokines. For example, circulating levels of interleukin (IL)-6 have been shown to be consistently increased in the elderly population, and in longitudinal studies, increased plasma IL-6 levels were associated with increased chances of cognitive impairment later in life (Weaver *et al.*, 2002; Sparkman and Johnson, 2008). Additionally, increased IL-6 production has been demonstrated in the hippocampus, cerebral cortex and cerebellum of aged mice compared to juvenile mice (Ye and Johnson, 1999). Older mice had elevated tumor necrosis factor-α (TNF-α) production in the brain and plasma after LPS challenge compared with adult controls (Kalehua *et al.*, 2000).

Experiments with 10-month-old senescence-accelerated mice (SAMP8) also showed increased IL-6 levels in the cerebral cortex and hippocampus compared to aged-matched control mice (Tha *et al.*, 2000). *In vitro* experiments with mixed astrocyte and microglial cultures demonstrated that glial cultures from aged mice produced higher steady-state levels of IL-6 mRNA and spontaneously secreted higher levels of IL-6 protein compared to both adult and neonatal cultures (Ye and Johnson, 1999, 2001). Primary mixed glia cultures and coronal brain sections established from the brain of aged rodents were also hyper-responsive to LPS stimulation and produced more inflammatory cytokines (IL-1β and IL-6) than cultures established from adult brains (Ye and Johnson, 2001; Xie *et al.*, 2003). Increase in inflammatory cytokines is also accompanied by reduction of anti-inflammatory molecules such as IL-10 (Ye and Johnson, 2001; Frank *et al.*, 2006) in the brain. Taken together these results suggest that the presence of reactive glia in the aged or diseased brain is permissive to an amplified and prolonged neuroinflammatory response. In addition, altered steady-state levels of proinflammatory and anti-inflammatory mediators may exacerbate the neuroinflammatory status within the CNS and predispose aged individuals to a discordant inflammatory response following immune activation, toxicant exposure or stress.

A previous longitudinal study demonstrated that young individuals exposed to inflammatory events early in life had a higher morbidity and mortality rate as they aged (Finch and Crimmins, 2004). Therefore inflammatory exposure, especially early in life, may predict inflammatory associated complications later in life. Several experimental rodent studies have demonstrated that neonatal exposure to inflammatory stimulus interferes with brain–immune system coordination and may predispose these animals to inflammatory processes later in life (Sternberg *et al.*, 1989; Shanks *et al.*, 2000; Boisse *et al.*, 2004). In a recent study, neonatal rats were challenged with live replicating *E. coli* and then in adulthood were given a secondary challenge with LPS. The secondary challenge with LPS caused a significant increase in astrocyte expression of GFAP in the CA3 region of the hippocampus in rats infected as neonates (Bilbo *et al.*, 2005). Moreover, astrocyte reactivity to secondary challenge of LPS in adulthood was associated with a severe deficit in hippocampal-dependent memory (Bilbo *et al.*, 2005). Although neonatal exposure to a pathogen may interfere with the development of the immune system, this study showed that reactive glia populations are more prevalent with age.

Another possible explanation for the presence of reactive glia in the aged brain is increased oxidative stress. According to the free radical hypothesis of aging, oxidative damage to cell membranes and intracellular proteins increases because of an increase in ROS, a decrease in the capacity of the antioxidant defense mechanisms to scavenge reactive oxygen species, or a combination of these processes (Beckman and Ames, 1998). Several studies showed that oxidative stress contributes to the inflammatory milieu of the aging brain and is associated with the age-related decline in cognitive and motor function (Mattson *et al.*, 2002; Richwine *et al.*, 2005). Increased oxidative stress in aged brain is also supported by evidence from aging rodent studies with the caloric restriction model. It is proposed that increased lifespan is caused by increased DNA repair, increased metabolic efficiency and reduced reactive by-products (Lee *et al.*, 1999). Global evaluations of the inflammatory state of the aged brain using microarray analysis have revealed a gene-expression profile indicative of oxidative stress, complement activation and glial cell reactivity in the neocortex, cerebellum and hippocampus (Lee *et al.*, 2000; Godbout *et al.*, 2005; Blalock *et al.*, 2003). Restricting caloric intake reversed the age-related expression of the oxidative and inflammatory markers (Lee *et al.*, 2004). In fact, calorie restriction both limited the inflammatory profile of the aged brain and enhanced the expression of growth and trophic factors (Lee *et al.*, 2000). In several other models, calorie restriction also reduced other inflammatory markers in the aged rodent brain, including GFAP and CD68 scavenger receptor (Morgan *et al.*, 1999; Wong *et al.*, 2005). Thus, an inflammatory brain profile is detrimental to successful aging, potentially through the reduction of important neurotrophic factors involved in the maintenance of neuronal plasticity.

Given these observations, we investigated if peripheral administration of natural antioxidant α-tocopherol suppresses oxidative damage in aged mice following ICV LPS. All measurements for these experiments were also performed 24 h after ICV LPS. Our results demonstrated that 100 mg/kg α-tocopherol (given for 3 consecutive days before ICV LPS), a dose that fully suppressed cerebral oxidative damage in juvenile mice (Figure 64.1), was ineffective in attenuating LPS-induced F_2-IsoPs formation (Figure 64.5) or restoring hippocampal pyramidal neuron dendritic spine density and dendritic lengths in aged animals (Figures 64.6 and 64.7). Aged mice pretreated with a higher dose of α-tocopherol (500 mg/kg also given for 3 consecutive days before ICV LPS) showed partial protection from LPS-induced oxidative damage and neurodegeneration, corroborating exacerbated neuroinflammatory status that requires a higher dose of antioxidant to suppress oxidative damage and dendritic degeneration in aged mice.

Increased neuroinflammation in aging measured by elevated PGs, particularly PGE_2 (Casolini *et al.*, 2002; Mesches *et al.*, 2004), is often concomitant with hippocampal-dependent memory impairment. Several studies reported

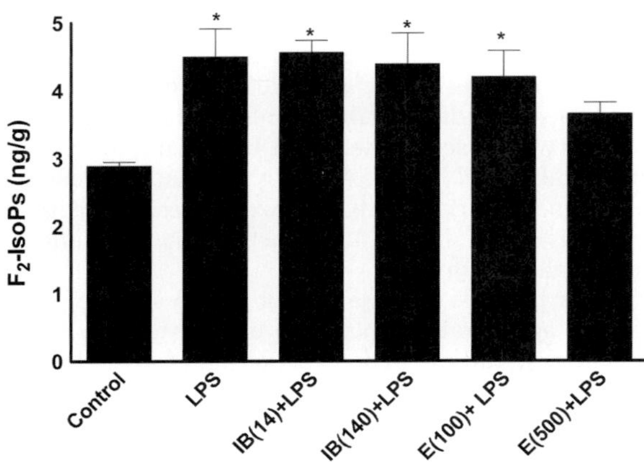

FIGURE 64.5 Ipsilateral cerebral F_2-IsoPs concentrations following ICV LPS (5 μg/5 μl) of aged mice with or without systemic pretreatment with ibuprofen (IB, 14 μg/ml or 140 μg/ml) or α-tocopherol injections (E, 100 mg/kg or 500 mg/kg). Brains from mice exposed to LPS were collected 24 hours post-injections. *Significant difference compared to control ($p < 0.01$).

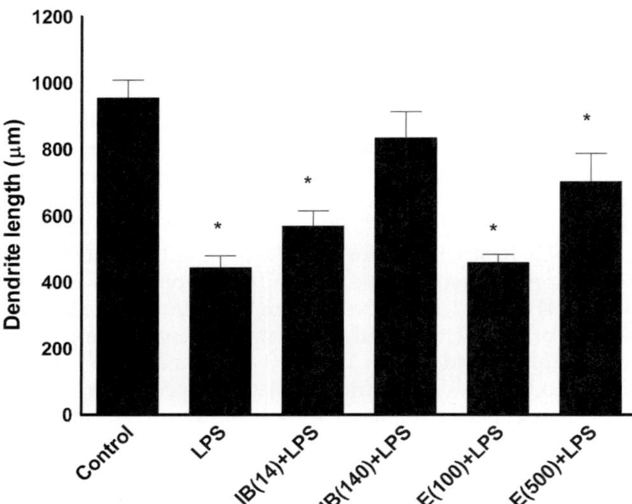

FIGURE 64.6 Dendritic length was determined at 24 hours post-ICV saline (control) or LPS (5 μg/5 μl) injection in CA1 sector hippocampal pyramidal neurons of aged mice with or without systemic pretreatment with ibuprofen (IB, 14 μg/ml or 140 μg/ml) or α-tocopherol injections (E, 100 mg/kg or 500 mg/kg). *Significant difference compared to control ($p < 0.01$).

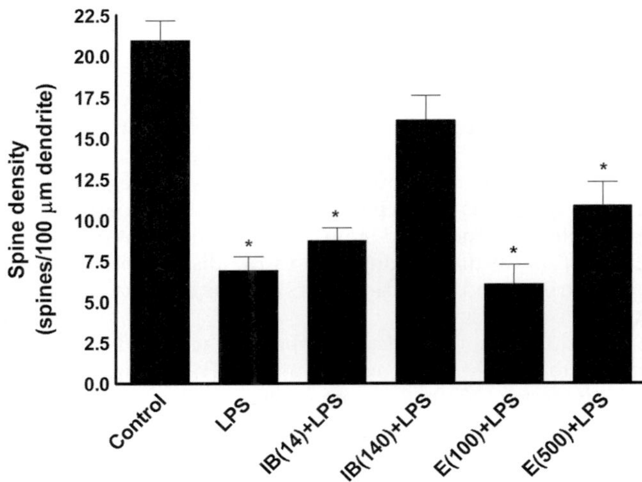

FIGURE 64.7 Spine density was determined at 24 hours post-ICV saline (control) or LPS (5 μg/5 μl) injection in CA1 sector hippocampal pyramidal neurons of aged mice with or without systemic pretreatment with ibuprofen (IB, 14 μg/ml or 140 μg/ml) or α-tocopherol injections (E, 100 mg/kg or 500 mg/kg). *Significant difference compared to control ($p < 0.01$).

memory deficits in aged (16-month-old) compared to young (3-month-old) mice in both passive avoidance task and an elevated plus maze. However, administration of non-selective (naproxen, 6.82 mg/kg), COX-2 preferential (nimesulide, 2.42 mg/kg) and COX-2 selective (rofecoxib, 1.92 mg/kg p.o.) inhibitors for 15 days before training prevented these memory deficits in aged animals (Jain *et al.*, 2002; Bishnoi *et al.*, 2005). Similarly, Casolini *et al.* (2002) found age-related memory deficits in the Morris water maze (MWM). Three-, 16- and 22-month-old rats were trained in the MWM after 4 months of COX-2 selective inhibition (celecoxib, 3 mg/kg twice daily p.o.). Results from the study showed that COX-2 selective inhibition restored performance in the 16-month-old rats to levels seen in the young animals. Within the hippocampus, levels of IL-1β, TNFα and PGE_2 as well as plasma corticosterone levels were elevated in both 16- and 22- compared to 3-month-old animals. COX-2 inhibition also significantly reduced IL-1β, TNFα, PGE_2 and corticosterone levels in 16- but not 22-month-old rats, although levels in aged COX-2-treated animals did not return to those seen in young animals. Together, these data indicate that chronic COX inhibition, particularly during a critical time window (e.g., 18 months), can prevent aging-induced memory deficits, potentially by reducing levels of proinflammatory molecules within the brain.

We have also investigated if NSAID pretreatment suppresses ICV LPS-oxidative damage and neurodegeneration in aged mice. Animals were exposed to ibuprofen at 14 μg/ml or 140 μg/ml in the drinking water for 2 weeks before ICV LPS exposure and levels of F_2-IsoPs, dendritic length and spine density of pyramidal neurons from CA1 hippocampal area were evaluated 24 h after ICV LPS exposure. Analogous to results with antioxidant exposure, ibuprofen at 14 μg/ml in the drinking water that fully suppressed cerebral oxidative damage in juvenile mice (Figure 64.1) was ineffective in attenuating LPS-induced F_2-IsoPs formation (Figure 64.5) or restoring hippocampal pyramidal neuron dendritic spine density and dendritic lengths in aged animals (Figures 64.6 and 64.7). As with α-tocopherol, a higher dose of ibuprofen (140 μg/ml drinking water) afforded protection of the denditic system from the degenerative consequence of ICV LPS (Figures 64.6 and 64.7). Together, our results demonstrate widely differing efficacy of antioxidant and NSAID as *in vivo* neuroprotectants in a model of directly activated glial innate immunity in young and aged mice.

Since a higher dose of antioxidant and NSAID was necessary to suppress oxidative injury in aged mice compared to young mice, we also investigated a potential differential role for EP2 receptor in innate immunity-mediated neuronal damage in these two models. Interestingly, while young EP−/− mice failed to mount the inflammatory oxidative response that is inherent to age-matched wild-type mice following administration of LPS (Figure 64.4), ablation of EP2 in aged animals did not suppress LPS-activated microglia-mediated oxidative injury. Results from our experiment showed no difference in the levels of the biomarker of cerebral oxidative damage (F_2-IsoPs) and neuronal oxidative damage (F_4-NeuroPs) between 21-month-old EP2-deficient and

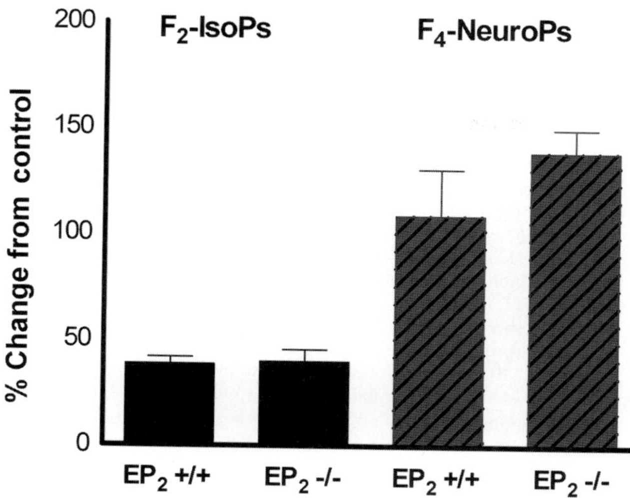

FIGURE 64.8 Ipsilateral cerebral F_2-IsoPs and F_4-NeuroPs concentrations following ICV LPS (5 μg/5 μl) of aged wild-type (EP_2 +/+) and EP_2 −/− deficient mice. Brains from mice exposed to LPS were collected 24 hours post-injections. F_2-IsoPs and F_4-NeuroPs data are expressed as % control of mice injected with saline.

wild-type age-matched controls (Figure 64.8). Together, our data point to a different neuroprotection potential of NSAID and antioxidant as well as the role of microglial EP2 in innate immunity-mediated damage in young and aged animals.

CONCLUDING REMARKS AND FUTURE DIRECTIONS

It is becoming increasingly evident that neuroinflammation and associated oxidative damage play a crucial role in the development and progression of brain diseases. Glia, and in particular microglia, are central to mediating the effects of neuroinflammation. Emerging evidence suggests that the numbers of activated microglia and release of inflammatory mediators from these cells increase with age. This amplified or prolonged exposure to inflammatory molecules, including cytokines, chemokines, ROS and PGs in the aged brain, may impair neuronal plasticity and underlie a heightened neuroinflammatory response. We have shown that a one-time direct activation of glial innate immunity leads to delayed oxidative damage and degeneration of the dendritic system that may be suppressed with antioxidant and NSAID and is dependent of EP2 activation in young but not aged animals. Future studies on differential EP receptor activation and drug efficacy in aged brain are needed not only to provide insight into the pathogenesis of aging, but also to guide the development of selective and efficacious therapies that target neurotoxic mechanisms while maintaining neuroprotective actions.

ACKNOWLEDGMENTS

The authors gratefully acknowledge support by grants from the Department of Defense W81XWH-05-1-0239 (DM, MA) and the National Institute of Health (NIH) NS057223 (DM), R01 10563 and 07331 (MA), and ES16754 and AG05136 (TM).

REFERENCES

Akira S (2003) Toll-like receptor signaling. *J Biol Chem* **278:** 38105–8.

Andreasson K (2010) Emerging roles of PGE2 receptors in models of neurological disease. *Prostaglandins Other Lipid Mediat* **91:** 104–12.

Asanuma M, Nishibayashi-Asanuma S, Miyazaki I, Kohno M (2001) Neuroprotective effects of non-steroidal anti-inflammatory drugs by direct scavenging of nitric oxide radicals. *J Neurochem* **76:** 1895–904.

Beal MF (1998) Excitotoxicity and nitric oxide in Parkinson's disease pathogenesis. *Ann Neurol* **44:** S110–14.

Beckman B, Ames BN (1998) The free radical theory of aging matures. *Physiol Rev* **78:** 547–81.

Bilbo SD, Levkoff LH, Mahoney JH, *et al.* (2005) Neonatal infection induces memory impairments following an immune challenge in adulthood. *Behav Neurosci* **119:** 293–301.

Bishnoi M, Patil CS, Kumar A, Kulkarni SK (2005) Protective effects of nimesulide (COX inhibitor), AKBA (5-LOX inhibitor), and their combination in aging-associated abnormalities in mice. *Methods Find Exp Clin Pharmacol* **27:** 465–70.

Blalock EM, Chen KC, Sharrow K, *et al.* (2003) Gene microarrays in hippocampal aging: statistical profiling identifies novel processes correlated with cognitive impairment. *J Neurosci* **23:** 3807–19.

Blasko I, Stampfer-Kountchev M, Robatscher P, *et al.* (2004) How chronic inflammation can affect the brain and support the development of Alzheimer's disease in old age: the role of microglia and astrocytes. *Aging Cell* **3:** 169–76.

Bliss SP, Shaftel SS, Olschowka JA, Kyrkanides S, O'Banion MK (2007) Chronic hippocampal IL-1β expression elevates PGE2 production in a cyclooxygenase I dependent manner. *Soc Neurosci Abstr* **57:** 17.

Boisse L, Mouihate A, Ellis S, *et al.* (2004) Long-term alterations in neuroimmune responses after neonatal exposure to lipopolysaccharide. *J Neurosci* **24:** 4928–34.

Brigelius-Flohe R, Traber MG (1999) Vitamin E: function and metabolism. *FASEB J* **13:** 1145–55.

Casolini P, Catalani A, Zuena AR, Angelucci L (2002) Inhibition of COX-2 reduces the age-dependent increase of hippocampal inflammatory markers, corticosterone secretion, and behavioral impairments in the rat. *J Neurosci Res* **68:** 337–43.

Egan, KM, Lawson JA, Fries S, *et al.* (2004) COX-2-derived prostacyclin confers atheroprotection on female mice. *Science* 306**(5703):** 1954–7.

Engelhart MJ, Geerlings MI, Ruitenberg A, van Swieten JC, Hofman A, Witteman JC, Breteler MM (2002) Dietary intake of antioxidants and risk of Alzheimer disease. *JAMA* **287:** 3223–9.

Fiebich BL, Schleicher S, Spleiss O, Czygan M, Hull M (2001) Mechanisms of prostaglandin E2-induced interleukin-6 release in astrocytes: possible involvement of EP4-like receptors, p38 mitogen-activated protein kinase and protein kinase C. *J Neurochem* **79:** 950–8.

Finch CE, Crimmins EM (2004) Inflammatory exposure and historical changes in human life-spans. *Science* **305(5691):** 1736–9.

Frank MG, Barrientos RM, Biedenkapp JC, Rudy JW, Watkins LR, Maier SF (2006) mRNA up-regulation of MHC II and pivotal pro-inflammatory genes in normal brain aging. *Neurobiol Aging* **27(5):** 717–22.

Frank-Cannon TC, Alto LT, McAlpine FE, Tansey MG (2009) Does neuroinflammation fan the flame in neurodegenerative diseases? *Mol Neurodegeneration* **4(47):** 1–13.

Funk CD, FitzGerald GA (2007) COX-2 inhibitors and cardiovascular risk. *J Cardiovasc Pharmacol* 50**(5):** 470–9.

Godbout JP, Chen J, Abraham J, *et al.* (2005) Exaggerated neuroinflammation and sickness behavior in aged mice following activation of the peripheral innate immune system. *FASEB J* **19(10):** 1329–31.

Gonzalez-Scarano F, Baltuch G (1999) Microglia as mediators of inflammatory and degenerative diseases. *Annu Rev Neurosci* **22:** 219–40.

Hamburger SA, McCay PB (1990) Spin trapping of ibuprofen radicals: evidence that ibuprofen is a hydroxyl radical scavenger. *Free Rad Res* **9:** 337–42.

Hata AN, Breyer RM (2004) Pharmacology and signaling of prostaglandin receptors: multiple roles in inflammation and immune modulation. *Pharmacol Ther* **103:** 147–66.

Hewett S, Uliasz T, Vidwans A, Hewett J (2000) Cyclo-oxygenase-2 contributes to *N*-methy-d-aspartate-mediated neuronal cell death in primary cortical cell culture. *J Pharm Exp Ther* **293:** 417–25.

Imler JL, Hoffmann JA (2001) Toll receptors in innate immunity. *Trends Cell Biol* **11:** 304–11.

in'tVeld BA, Ruitenberg A, Launer LJ (2000) Duration of non-steroidal anti-inflammatory drug use and risk of Alzheimer's disease. The Rotterdam Study. *Neurobiol Aging* **21:** S204.

Insel PA (1996) Analgesic-antipyretic and anti-inflammatory agents and drugs in the treatment of gout. In *Godman and Gilman's The Pharmacological Basis of Therapeutics* (Hardman JG, Limbird LE, eds.). New York, McGraw-Hill, pp. 617–57.

Jain NK, Patil CS, Kulkarni SK, Singh A (2002) Modulatory role of cyclooxygenase inhibitors in aging- and scopolamine or lipopolysaccharide-induced cognitive dysfunction in mice. *Behav Brain Res* **133(2):** 369–76.

Kalehua AN, Taub DD, Baskar PV, *et al.* (2000) Aged mice exhibit greater mortality concomitant to increased brain and plasma TNF-alpha levels following intracerebro-ventricular injection of lipopolysaccharide. *Gerontology* **46(3):** 115–28.

Kaufmann WE, Andreasson KI, Isakson PC, Worley PF (1997) Cyclooxygenases and the central nervous system. *Prostaglandins* **54:** 601–24.

Lee CK, Klopp RG, Weindruch R, *et al.* (1999) Gene expression profile of aging and its retardation by caloric restriction. *Science* **285(5432):** 1390–3.

Lee CK, Weindruch R, Prolla TA (2000) Gene-expression profile of the ageing brain in mice. *Nat Genet* **25(3):** 294–7.

Lehnardt S, Massillon L, Follett P, Jensen F, Ratan R, Rosenberg P, Volpe J, Vartanian T (2003) Activation of innate immunity in the CNS triggers neurodegeneration through a toll-like receptor 4-dependent pathway. *Proc Natl Acad Sci USA* **100:** 8514–19.

Leuner B, Falduto J, Shors TJ (2003) Associative memory formation increases the observation of dendritic spines in the hippocampus. *J Neurosci* **23:** 6659–65.

Li Y, Liu L, Barger SW, Mrak RE, Griffin WS (2001) Vitamin E suppression of microglial activation is neuroprotective. *J Neurosci Res* **66:** 163–70.

Liu D, Wu L, Breyer R, Mattson MP, Andreasson K (2005) Neuroprotection by the PGE2 EP2 receptor in permanent focal cerebral ischemia. *Ann Neurol* 57**(5):** 758–61.

Magistretti PJ, Pellerin L, Rothman DL, Shulman RG (1999) Energy on demand. *Science* **283(5401):** 496–7.

Mattson M, Chan SL, Duan W (2002) Modification of brain aging and neurodegenerative disorders by genes, diet, and behavior. *Physiol Rev* **82(3):** 637–72.

McCullough L, Wu L, Haughey N, *et al.* (2004) Neuroprotective function of the PGE2 EP2 receptor in cerebral ischemia. *J Neurosci* 24**(1):** 257–68.

Mesches MH, Gemma C, Veng LM, Allgeier C, Young DA, Browning MD, Bickford PC (2004) Sulindac improves memory and increases NMDA receptor subunits in aged Fischer 344 rats. *Neurobiol Aging* **25(3):** 315–24.

Milatovic D, Aschner M (2009) Measurement of isoprostanes as markers of oxidative stress in neuronal tissue. *Curr Prot Toxicol* **12(14):** 1–12.

Milatovic D, Milatovic S, Montine K, Shie FS, Montine TJ (2004) Neuronal oxidative damage and dendritic degeneration following activation of CD14-dependent innate immunity response in vivo. *J Neuroinflammation* **1:** 20.

Milatovic D, Montine KS, Montine TJ (2005b) Suppression of cerebral oxidative damage from excitotoxicity and innate immune response *in vivo* by α- or γ-tocopherol. *J Chromatography B* **827:** 88–93.

Milatovic D, Montine TJ, Zaja-Milatovic S, Madison JD, Bowman A, Aschner M (2010) Morphometric analysis in neurodegenerative disease. *Curr Prot Toxicol* **12(16):** 1–14.

Milatovic D, Zaja-Milatovic S, Montine KS, Horner PJ, Montine TJ (2003) Pharmacologic suppression of neuronal oxidative damage and dendritic degeneration following direct activation of glial innate immunity in mouse cerebrum. *J Neurochem* **87:** 1518–26.

Milatovic D, Zaja-Milatovic S, Montine KS, Nivison M, Montine TJ (2005a) CD14-dependent innate immunity-mediated neuronal damage *in vivo* is suppressed by NSAIDs and ablation of a prostaglandin E_2 receptor, EP2. *Current Medicinal Chemistry-Central Nervous System Agents* **5:** 151–6.

Minghetti L, Levi G (1995) Induction of prostanoid biosynthesis by bacterial lipopolysaccharide and isoproterenol in rat microglial cultures. *J Neurochem* **65:** 2690–8.

Montine KS, Quinn JF, Zhang J, Fessel JP, Roberts L J 2nd, Morrow JD, Montine TJ (2004) Isoprostanes and related products of lipid peroxidation in neurodegenerative diseases. *Chem Phys Lipids* **128:** 117–24.

Montine TJ, Milatovic D, Gupta RC, Valyi-Nagy T, Morrow JD, Breyer RM (2002) Neuronal oxidative damage from activated innate immunity is EP2 receptor-dependent. *J Neurochem* 83**(2):** 463–70.

Morgan TE, Xie Z, Goldsmith S, *et al.* (1999) The mosaic of brain glial hyperactivity during normal ageing and its attenuation by food restriction. *Neuroscience* **89(3):** 687–99.

Morris MC, Beckett LA, Scherr PA, Hebert LE, Bennett DA, Field TS, Evans DA (1998) Vitamin E and vitamin C supplement use and risk of incident Alzheimer disease. *Alzheimer Dis Assoc Disord* **12:** 121–6.

Morrow JD, Roberts LJ (1997) The isoprostanes: unique bioactive products of lipid peroxidation. *Prog Lipid Res* **36:** 1–21.

Mucke L, Eddleston M (1993) Astrocytes in infectious and immune-mediated diseases of the central nervous system. *FASEB J* **7**(13)**:** 1226–32.

O'Banion MK (1999) Cyclooxygenase-2: molecular biology, pharmacology, and neurobiology. *Crit Rev Neurobiol* **13(1):** 45–82.

Palsson-McDermott EM, O'Neill LA (2004) Signal transduction by the lipopolysaccharide receptor, Toll-like receptor-4. *Immunology* **113:** 153–62.

Peterson KE, Du M (2009) Innate immunity in the pathogenesis of polytropic retrovirus infection in the central nervous system. *Immunol Res* **43(1–3):** 149–59.

Prat A, Biernacki K, Wosik K, Antel JP (2001) Glial cell influence on the human blood–brain barrier. *Glia* **36(2):** 145–55.

Quan N, Whiteside M, Herkenham M (1998) Cyclooxygenase 2 mRNA expression in rat brain after peripheral injection of lipopolysaccharide. *Brain Res* **802:** 189–97.

Reich E, Markesbery W, Roberts II L, Swift L, Morrow J, Montine T (2001) Brain regional quantification of F-ring and D/E-ring isoprostanes and neuroprostanes in Alzheimer's disease. *Am J Pathol* **158:** 293–7.

Richwine AF, Godbout JP, Berg BM, *et al.* (2005) Improved psychomotor performance in aged mice fed diet high in antioxidants is associated with reduced ex vivo brain interleukin-6 production. *Brain Behav Immun* **19(6):** 512–20.

Rivest S (2009) Regulation of innate immune response in the brain. *Nat Rev Immunol* **9:** 429–39.

Roberts LJ 2nd, Montine TJ, Markesbery WR, Tapper AR, Hardy P, Chemtob S, Dettbarn WD, Morrow JD (1998) Formation of isoprostane-like compounds (neuroprostanes) in vivo from docosahexaenoic acid. *J Biol Chem* **273:** 13605–12.

Rudic RD, Brinster D, Cheng Y, *et al.* (2005) COX-2-derived prostacyclin modulates vascular remodeling. *Circ Res* 96**(12):** 1240–7.

Shanks N, Windle RJ, Perks PA, *et al.* (2000) Early-life exposure to endotoxin alters hypothalamic–pituitary–adrenal function and predisposition to inflammation. *Proc Natl Acad Sci USA* **97(10):** 5645–50.

Shie FS, Montine KS, Breyer RM, Montine TJ (2005) Microglial EP2 is critical to neurotoxicity from activated cerebral innate immunity. *Glia* **52:** 70–7.

Sparkman NL, Johnson RW (2008) Neuroinflammation associated with aging sensitizes the brain to the effects of infection or stress. *Neuromodulation* **15:** 323–30.

Sternberg EM, Hill JM, Chrousos GP, *et al.* (1989) Inflammatory mediator-induced hypothalamic–pituitary–adrenal axis activation is defective in streptococcal cell wall arthritis-susceptible Lewis rats. *Proc Natl Acad Sci USA* **86(7):** 2374–8.

Stewart WF, Kawas C, Corrada M, Metter EJ (1997) Risk of Alzheimer's disease and duration of NSAID use. *Neurology* **48:** 626–32.

Tanabe T, Tohnai N (2002) Cyclooxygenase isozymes and their gene structures and expression. *Prostaglandins Other Lipid Mediat* **68–69:** 95–114.

Tansey MG, McCoy MK, Frank-Cannon TC (2007) Neuroinflammatory mechanisms in Parkinson's disease: potential environmental triggers, pathways, and targets from early therapeutic intervention. *Exp Neurol* **208:** 1–25.

Tha KK, Okuma Y, Miyazaki H, *et al.* (2000) Changes in expressions of proinflammatory cytokines IL-1beta, TNF-alpha and IL-6 in the brain of senescence accelerated mouse (SAM) P8. *Brain Res* **885:** 25–31.

Weaver JD, Huang MH, Albert M, Harris T, Rowe JW, Seeman TE (2002) Interleukin-6 and risk of cognitive decline: MacArthur studies of successful aging. *Neurology* **59:** 371–8.

Weggen S, Eriksen JL, Das P, Sagi SA, Wang R, Pietzik CU, Findlay KA, Smith TE, Murphy MP, Butler T, Kang DE, Sterling N, Golde TE, Koo EH (2001) A subset of NSAIDs lower amyloidogenic Aβ42 independently of cyclooxygenase activity. *Nature* **414:** 212–16.

Wong AM, Patel NV, Patel NK, *et al.* (2005) Macrosialin increases during normal brain aging are attenuated by caloric restriction. *Neurosci Lett* **390:** 76–80.

Xie Z, Morgan TE, Rozovsky I, *et al.* (2003) Aging and glial responses to lipopolysaccharide in vitro: greater induction of IL-1 and IL-6, but smaller induction of neurotoxicity. *Exp Neurol* **182:** 135–41.

Xie Z, Wei M, Morgan TE, Fabrizio P, Han D, Finch CE, Longo VD (2002) Peroxynitrite mediates neurotoxicity of amyloid beta-peptide1-42- and lipopolysaccharide-activated microglia. *J Neurosci* **22:** 3484–92.

Ye SM, Johnson RW (1999) Increased interleukin-6 expression by microglia from brain of aged mice. *J Neuroimmunol* **93:** 139–48.

Ye SM, Johnson RW (2001) An age-related decline in interleukin-10 may contribute to the increased expression of interleukin-6 in brain of aged mice. *Neuroimmunomodulation* **9:** 183–92.

Zandi PP, Anthony JC, Hayden KM, Mehta K, Mayer L, Breitner JC (2002) Reduced incidence of AD with NSAID but not H(2) receptor antagonists: the Cache County Study. *Neurology* **59**: 880–6.

C H A P T E R

65

Disruption of cholesterol homeostasis in developmental neurotoxicity

Marina Guizzetti, Jing Chen and Lucio G. Costa

INTRODUCTION

Cholesterol is a major component of all membranes. Lipid rafts, organized membrane domains rich in cholesterol, play important roles in the transduction of many signal transduction pathways including signaling pathways involved in morphogenesis. Furthermore, cholesterol is also the precursor of steroid hormones. It is thus not surprising that cholesterol plays an important role during fetal development.

The brain is very rich in cholesterol. Neuronal maturation requires large amounts of cholesterol for neuritogenesis and synaptogenesis; in addition, oligodendrocyte-produced myelin contains massive amounts of cholesterol, and is necessary for the formation of myelinated fibers for the propagation of fast nervous impulses. Important signal transduction pathways involved in the early steps of central nervous system (CNS) development, before neuronal development, such as the sonic hedgehog (SHH) signaling pathway, are also regulated by cholesterol. It is therefore evident that alterations in cholesterol homeostasis (including biosynthesis, trafficking, metabolism and clearance) may result in devastating effects on the developing brain.

This chapter describes the regulation of cholesterol homeostasis in the brain with an emphasis on the regulation of cholesterol homeostasis in neurons and astrocytes. Furthermore, it illustrates the neurodevelopmental effects of the disruption of cholesterol caused by genetic defects in cholesterol biosynthesis and developmental neurotoxicants that affect cholesterol trafficking.

CHOLESTEROL HOMEOSTASIS IN THE BRAIN

The brain is the organ richest in cholesterol in the whole body; indeed, it contains 15–20% of total body cholesterol, but represents only about 5% of total body weight. Most of the brain cholesterol is synthesized *in situ* and for this reason the brain has a high rate of cholesterol synthesis (Dietschy and Turley, 2004). The prevailing hypothesis is that the uptake of cholesterol from the circulation is low, as the blood–brain barrier (BBB) is not permeable to lipoproteins (Bjorkhem and Meaney, 2004), though there is also evidence that cholesterol homeostasis in the brain is affected by plasma cholesterol (Puglielli *et al.*, 2003), and that mechanisms for the uptake of cholesterol by the blood–brain barrier and the blood–cerebrospinal fluid barrier exist (Dehouck *et al.*, 1997; Karasinska *et al.*, 2009).

The better understood mechanism for the control of intracellular cholesterol levels is the regulation of cholesterol synthesis, which occurs in the endoplasmic reticulum from acetylCoA, and involves membrane-bound transcription factors called sterol regulatory element-binding proteins (SREBPs) that activate genes upregulating cholesterol synthesis (Brown and Goldstein, 1999).

Another important mechanism regulating intracellular cholesterol levels is the modulation of cholesterol efflux. This exciting new field of investigation began in 1999 with the identification by three independent groups of the cholesterol transporter ATP-binding cassette A1 (ABCA1), which is involved in cholesterol efflux from cells to lipoproteins (Bodzioch *et al.*, 1999; Lawn *et al.*, 1999; Rust *et al.*, 1999). More recently, two other cholesterol transporters, ABCG1 and ABCG4, have been identified (Wang *et al.*, 2004). These three proteins have been implicated in the regulation of cholesterol levels within a cell, between cells and within a tissue, as they are involved in cholesterol efflux, lipoprotein formation and cholesterol clearance. During high density lipoprotein (HDL) formation, membrane-bound ABCA1 is required for transferring phospholipids and cholesterol from the cell membrane to extracellular lipid-free or lipid-poor apolipoprotein AI or E (apoAI or apoE), causing a decrease in cellular cholesterol and the formation, in the extracellular space, of nascent lipoproteins (cholesterol, apolipoproteins and phospholipids are the main components of lipoproteins) (Oram and Heinecke, 2005). The half-transporters ABCG1 and ABCG4, which may function as homodimers or heterodimers and mediate cholesterol but not phospholipid efflux, are responsible for the further lipidation of these particles, leading to the formation of spherical lipoproteins richer in cholesterol (Vaughan and Oram, 2006).

Reproductive and Developmental Toxicology, Edited by Ramesh C. Gupta
ISBN: 978-0-12-382032-7

In the brain, the major producers of cholesterol are oligodendrocytes, which are responsible for the formation of myelin sheaths; indeed, it has been estimated that myelin contains 70% of the total brain cholesterol (Bjorkhem and Meaney, 2004). Astrocytes are also major producers of cholesterol in the brain; according to *in vitro* studies, they synthesize two or three times more cholesterol than neurons (Bjorkhem and Meaney, 2004). In contrast to oligodendrocytes, which immobilize their cholesterol into myelin, astrocytes produce and release HDL-like particles containing free cholesterol and apoE, and express cholesterol transporters for the release of endogenously synthesized cholesterol (LaDu *et al.*, 1998; Pitas *et al.*, 1987; Wahrle *et al.*, 2004). Astrocyte-produced nascent, lipid-poor and disk-shaped lipoproteins are transformed into spherical particles that are the size and density of plasma HDL by the acquisition of free cholesterol from neurons and from other CNS cells (Kim *et al.*, 2007; LaDu *et al.*, 1998). Lipoproteins can be taken up by axons of neighboring neurons, or can exit the brain through the cerebrospinal fluid (Pitas *et al.*, 1987). The mechanisms of lipoprotein formation in the brain are similar to those described in the periphery. ABCA1, ABCG1 and ABCG4 are highly expressed in the brain (Tachikawa *et al.*, 2005). In astrocytes, ABCA1 has been implicated in cholesterol efflux to lipid-poor apolipoproteins, in lipoprotein formation and in regulating apoE release (Hirsch-Reinshagen *et al.*, 2004; Wahrle *et al.*, 2004). Indeed, in astrocytes derived from ABCA1 null mice, cholesterol accumulates intracellularly as its efflux is inhibited, apoE secretion is reduced and lipoprotein particles contain less cholesterol and ApoE, and are smaller than those present in wild-type astrocytes (Hirsch-Reinshagen *et al.*, 2004; Wahrle *et al.*, 2004). ABCG1 and ABCG4 mediate cholesterol and desmosterol efflux to HDL (Wang *et al.*, 2008), and upregulate cholesterol synthesis through the upregulation of sterol-regulatory element binding protein-2 (Tarr and Edwards, 2008). Neurons also express ABCA1, ABCG1 and ABCG4 cholesterol transporters which, however, do not appear to be involved in cholesterol efflux in these cells (Chen *et al.*, submitted). The transcription of ABCA1 and ABCG1, but not of ABCG4, is under the control of two nuclear receptors, the liver X receptors (LXR) and the retinoic X receptors (RXR); activation of these receptors also inhibits cholesterol synthesis (Tarr and Edwards, 2008).

In contrast to astrocytes, neurons do not secrete lipoproteins, but express numerous low density lipoprotein receptors to acquire lipoproteins (Herz, 2001). Neurons produce enough cholesterol for their survival, but it is believed that cholesterol required for axonal growth and synaptogenesis is provided by surrounding astrocytes (Hayashi *et al.*, 2004; Mauch *et al.*, 2001), although these effects may be specific to some subpopulations of neurons but not others (Ko *et al.*, 2005). In the CNS (as in the periphery) cholesterol exchange between cells is mediated by lipoproteins (LaDu *et al.*, 1998). The main cholesterol carriers in the brain are: apoE, produced by astrocytes (Poirier *et al.*, 1993) and microglia (Nakai *et al.*, 1996), and apoA-I, derived from the systemic circulation or from brain endothelial cells (Panzenboeck *et al.*, 2002). The brain expresses very high levels of apoE, second only to the liver, and apoE mRNA is expressed throughout the whole brain.

The main mechanism of excretion of cholesterol from the brain is through its conversion to 24S-hydroxycholesterol by the enzyme cholesterol 24-hydroxylase, a member of a subfamily of cytochrome P450 enzymes, CYP46, which is expressed in neurons but not in astrocytes (Lund *et al.*, 1999). Brain cholesterol can also exit the brain bound to apoE through the cerebrospinal fluid. 24S-hydroxycholesterol and apoE-bound cholesterol diffuse into the blood and reach the liver for excretion (Raffai and Weisgraber, 2003). 25S-hydroxycholesterol levels in the blood are good indicators of cholesterol metabolism in the brain, as CYP46 is preferentially expressed in the brain, with very low levels detected in the liver (Lutjohann and von Bergmann, 2003).

Figure 65.1 shows a model for cholesterol homeostasis in the brain based on current knowledge.

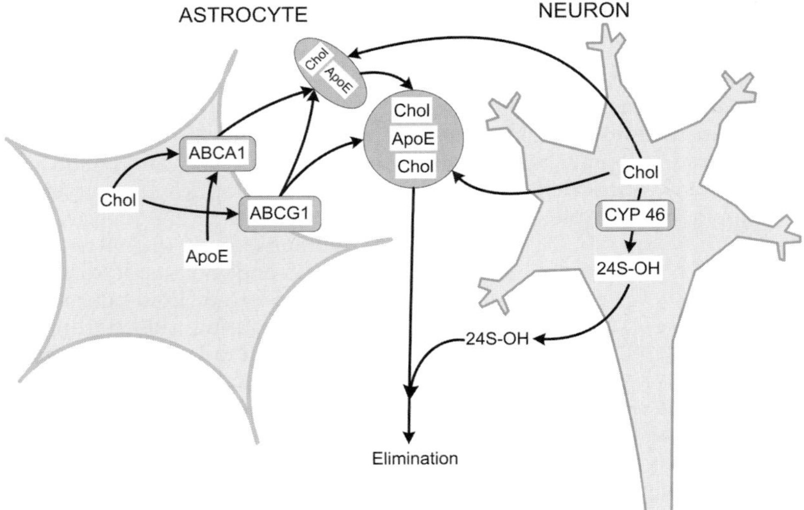

FIGURE 65.1 Model for interactions of astrocytes and neurons in cholesterol homeostasis. Cholesterol is produced by astrocytes and neurons from acetylCoA. Astrocytes produce apoE which, through the interaction with membrane-expressed ABCA1, generates a partially lipidated discoidal complex which, in turn, through an ABCA1- and ABCG1-mediated mechanism, extracts cholesterol from astrocytes and generates spherical lipoprotein particles, enriched in cholesterol. Lipoproteins produced by astrocytes can also extract cholesterol from neurons, through a yet unknown mechanism independent from ABCA1 and ABCG1. Cholesterol can be metabolized to 24S-hydroxycholesterol in neurons (but not in astrocytes) by the neuron-specific CYP46, and exit the brain. Brain cholesterol can also exit the brain when associated to lipoproteins through the cerebrospinal fluid. Chol: cholesterol; 24S-OH: 24S-hydroxycholesterol.

CHOLESTEROL AND BRAIN DEVELOPMENT

The rate of growth of the fetus is faster than of any other stage of life and requires significant amounts of cholesterol. The rates of sterol synthesis are much greater in the fetus than in the adult, and endogenously synthesized cholesterol accounts for the majority of fetal cholesterol, though for fetuses less than 6 months old there is evidence suggesting transport of exogenous cholesterol from the maternal plasma into the fetus (Woollett, 2001). The developing brain also appears to rely almost completely on local synthesis of cholesterol (Jurevics *et al.*, 1997).

Cholesterol is an integral part of every cell membrane, which include neuronal membranes and myelin, to which it confers rigidity and reduces passive permeability. In addition to this "structural" role, cholesterol is essential during development for several other reasons:

1. Cholesterol is a key component of lipid rafts, discrete subcompartments in the exoplasmic leaflet of the plasma membrane in which specific proteins are brought into close proximity to promote their interactions; lipid rafts play an important role in signal transduction (Fielding and Fielding, 2004). Several signaling pathways important for brain development are localized in lipid rafts, including SHH, glia-derived neurotrophic factor (GDNF), and insulin-like growth factor (IGF) signaling (Huo *et al.*, 2003; Simons and Toomre, 2000). Removal of cholesterol from rafts leads to dissociation of the raft proteins from the lipids and inhibition of the signaling pathways localized in the rafts (Simons and Toomre, 2000).
2. Cholesterol is essential for the activation and propagation of the hedgehog signaling that is responsible for patterning and development of the CNS (Marti and Bovolenta, 2002). Inhibition of cholesterol synthesis inhibits the cholesterol-dependent post-translational modification of SHH, disrupts cholesterol-rich plasma rafts involved in SHH signal transduction and interferes with the ability of target tissues to sense or transduce the SHH signaling (Incardona and Roelink, 2000).
3. Cell proliferation requires cholesterol. Cholesterol and by-products of the cholesterol pathway are essential for cell proliferation, particularly early in the G_1 phase of the cell cycle and at the G_1/S interface (Bochelen *et al.*, 1995). Proliferation of astroglial cells is potently inhibited by simvastatin and by phenylacetate, two inhibitors of cholesterol synthesis (Oberdoerster *et al.*, 2000).
4. The ability of CNS neurons to form synapses is limited by the availability of cholesterol, and massive synaptogenesis requires large amounts of cholesterol (Mauch *et al.*, 2001).
5. Inhibition of cholesterol production induces neuronal cell death (Michikawa and Yanagisawa, 1999).
6. Dendrite outgrowth and microtubule stability in cultured neurons depends on cholesterol availability in the medium (Fan *et al.*, 2002), although the optimal amount of cholesterol required to promote the development of one neuronal population can be inhibitory for another type of neuron (Ko *et al.*, 2005), indicating that cholesterol levels in the brain need to be strictly and locally regulated.

In summary, the maintenance of optimal cholesterol levels is essential to brain development. While the regulation of cholesterol synthesis remains the main mechanism by which the brain regulates cholesterol homeostasis, there is evidence that an increase in cholesterol efflux through the upregulation of cholesterol transporters may lead to an increased brain cholesterol clearance, leading to reduced levels of cholesterol in the whole brain.

GENETIC DEFECT IN CHOLESTEROL BIOSYNTHESIS

The importance of cholesterol during development, and particularly during CNS development, is apparent when inborn errors of cholesterol synthesis are considered. To date, six human disorders have been linked to defects in cholesterol biosynthesis (Kelley and Herman, 2001; Nwokoro *et al.*, 2001). The prototype for this group of disorders is the Smith-Lemli-Opitz syndrome (SLOS), which consists in the deficiency of 7-dehydrocholesterol-Δ^7-reductase, the catalyst in the last step of cholesterol synthesis (Nowaczyk *et al.*, 1999). All body tissues of individuals affected by SLOS are deficient in cholesterol. Abnormalities present in SLOS-affected children include microcephaly, mental retardation, growth retardation, holoprosencephaly with agenesis of the corpus callosum, behavioral disorders with autistic characteristics and hyperactivity, and dysmorphic facial features including broad nasal bridge, short nose with anteverted nares, bilateral ptosis, epicanthal folds, micrognathia and cleft palate (Nowaczyk *et al.*, 1999).

Maternal phenylketonuria, a genetic defect in phenylalanine hydrolase, an enzyme that converts phenylalanine to tyrosine, results in abnormal development of the offspring, if not corrected by a diet low in phenylalanine during gestation (Levy and Ghavami, 1996). Phenylacetate, a phenylalanine metabolite which accumulates in people affected by phenylketonuria, is an inhibitor of mevalonate phosphate decarboxylase, an important enzyme in the pathway leading to cholesterol synthesis. Inhibition of mevalonate phosphatase by phenylacetate is considered to be, at least in part, responsible for the effects of phenylketonuria on the developing brain (Wen *et al.*, 1980). The offspring of mothers with phenylketonuria can present microcephaly, mental retardation, seizure, agenesis of the corpus callosum, dysmorphic facial features, growth retardation, behavioral disorders and congenital heart abnormalities, similar to that reported in SLOS (Levy and Ghavami, 1996; Nowaczyk *et al.*, 1999). It is thus conceivable that reduced cholesterol synthesis may be involved in the developmental effects of these two conditions.

In support to this hypothesis, holoprosencephaly, a developmental defect of impaired midline cleavage of the embryonic forebrain, is associated with both SLOS (Cohen and Shiota, 2002) and with maternal phenylketonuria (Keller *et al.*, 2000). The best understood cause of holoprosencephaly is the disruption of SHH signaling network (Cohen and Shiota, 2002), which is regulated by cholesterol.

FETAL ALCOHOL SPECTRUM DISORDERS

In utero alcohol exposure causes a dysmorphogenic neuropathological syndrome (Jones *et al.*, 1973) characterized by craniofacial malformations and a reduced brain mass, which is associated with a variety of neurobehavioral effects including hyperactivity, attention deficit disorder and learning disabilities in childhood (Streissguth and O'Malley, 2000), and depressive and psychotic disorders in adulthood (Famy *et al.*, 1998). While the extreme form of the adverse effects of ethanol on fetal development is known as fetal alcohol syndrome (FAS) (Jones and Smith, 1975), it is now recognized that ethanol can also cause a partial syndrome comprised largely of neurobehavioral disorders, unaccompanied by craniofacial malformations, called alcohol-related neurodevelopmental disorders (ARND), whose incidence may be higher (5/1,000 births) than FAS (0.5–3/1,000 births) (Stratton *et al.*, 1996).

FAS presents similarities with SLOS (see previous section) both in humans and in animal models. In humans similarities include microcephaly, mental retardation, agenesis of the corpus callosum, dysmorphic facial features, growth retardation, behavioral disorders and congenital heart abnormalities (Cohen and Shiota, 2002; Nowaczyk *et al.*, 1999; Streissguth *et al.*, 1980)

Rats in which cholesterol synthesis is inhibited by BM15.766 (an inhibitor of the conversion of 7-dehydrocholesterol to cholesterol) display hypoplasia of the frontal lobes and corpus callosum, anteverted nares, small upturned nose, long upper lip and abnormal cell rounding, similar to that observed in animals treated with ethanol at comparable developmental stages (Dehart *et al.*, 1997; Lanoue *et al.*, 1997).

As observed in SLOS and maternal phenylketonuria, some of the effects of *in utero* alcohol exposure are consistent with holoprosencephaly, which in many cases is a consequence of the disruption of the SHH signaling network (Cohen and Shiota, 2002), which is regulated by cholesterol (Incardona and Roelink, 2000). Ethanol exposure has been shown to inhibit SHH signaling in chicken, zebrafish and mouse embryos (Ahlgren *et al.*, 2002; Chrisman *et al.*, 2004; Li *et al.*, 2007).

CNS development is characterized by vulnerable periods during which exposure to ethanol or other teratogens may result in abnormalities specific to the ontogenic events occurring at the time of exposure. These critical periods of vulnerability have been well characterized in human and rodents (Rice and Barone, 2000).

Ethanol appears to interfere with all the different developmental stages of the CNS. Mental and behavioral abnormalities associated with prenatal alcohol exposure are therefore due to a combination of effects exerted by ethanol at different stages of development (Maier *et al.*, 1999).

A first critical period of development is when organogenesis occurs and the neural tube and crest are formed; this occurs in rats between gestational day (GD) 5 and GD 11, and in humans in the first trimester of pregnancy (Rice and Barone, 2000). During the second week of gestation in rodents (GD 7 in mice and GD 9.5 in rats), and the first month of gestation in humans, specific areas of the CNS begin to form; neurogenesis and migration of cells in the forebrain, midbrain and hindbrain are occurring at this developmental stage (Rice and Barone, 2000). Mice exposed to ethanol at GD 7 or 8 exhibit the craniofacial anomalies associated with FAS, as well as forebrain deficiencies including hypoplasia or aplasia of the corpus callosum, and deficiencies in the hippocampus and the anterior cingulated cortex (Sulik, 2005). These defects are consistent with the holoprosencephaly spectrum of malformations, also observed in animals treated at the same developmental stages with an inhibitor of the cholesterol synthesis (Dehart *et al.*, 1997; Lanoue *et al.*, 1997; Sulik, 2005). In addition, prenatal exposure of primates to ethanol during this period reduces the number of neurons in the somatosensory-motor cortex, and inhibits cortical neural stem cell proliferation (Miller, 2007), an event also inhibited by lack of cholesterol.

The second critical period of development occurs in rats from GD 11–12 to GD 18–21, corresponding to the second trimester of gestation in human (Rice and Barone, 2000). During this period most of the areas of the nervous system are differentiating; this phase is characterized by intense neurogenesis and neuronal migration in the cerebral cortex and hippocampus, two areas greatly affected by *in utero* alcohol exposure (Guerri, 1998). In rats, neurogenesis occurs prenatally in all brain regions, except for the cerebellum and the dentate gyrus of the hippocampus. As soon as neuroblast proliferation stops, differentiation of these cells into neurons and glia begins, followed by the development and elongation of processes that will become axons or dendrites in neurons. At this time of development, neurons from the cerebral cortex leave the germinal zone and migrate using radial glia fibers as scaffolds (Rice and Barone, 2000). Ethanol exposure during this stage alters radial glia and depresses the proliferation, survival and migration of neurons from the neocortex, hippocampus and the principal sensory nucleus (Barnes and Walker, 1981; Miller, 1986, 2007; Miller and Robertson, 1993). Several of the functions characterizing this developmental stage, including cell proliferation and neuronal survival and differentiation, require cholesterol. In addition, neuronal differentiation and migration are promoted by many neurotrophic factors, some of which, such as GDNF or IGF, require cholesterol-rich lipid rafts for the propagation of their signals, and are inhibited in cholesterol-depleted cells (Soscia *et al.*, 2006).

The third critical period in brain development occurs in rats from GD 18 to postnatal day (PND) 9 and is considered the equivalent of the third trimester of pregnancy in humans. Major events during this period include a massive increase in brain size, proliferation of astrocytes and oligodendrocytes, myelination, synaptogenesis and dendritic arborization (Rice and Barone, 2000); all these processes require cholesterol. Ethanol exposure during this developmental stage induces microcephaly and severe neuronal loss, cerebellar and hippocampal abnormalities, and behavioral dysfunctions (Bonthius and West, 1991; Diaz and Samson, 1980; Meyer *et al.*, 1990; West *et al.*, 1986). Administration of ethanol to rats on PND 7 causes severe apoptotic neuronal death in the hippocampus and cerebral cortex (Ikonomidou *et al.*, 2000).

In summary, ethanol interferes with all stages of brain development, and several of the functions affected by ethanol during development require large amounts of cholesterol.

ETHANOL AND CHOLESTEROL

The effects of ethanol on lipids and lipoproteins have been studied in relation to the cardiovascular system, since light to moderate alcohol consumption reduces cardiovascular disease morbidity and mortality, whereas heavy alcohol consumption increases these risks (Hannuksela *et al.*, 2002; van Tol and Hendriks, 2001). An increase in HDL is associated with moderate alcohol intake and appears to account for approximately 50% of alcohol's cardioprotective effect; HDL levels are also elevated in heavy drinkers and alcoholics who, however, are at greater risk for vascular diseases (Frohlich, 1996; Goldberg *et al.*, 1995; Klatsky, 1994).

The effect of alcohol on lipid composition in the brain was the target of intense research until 15 years ago. This research was based on the hypothesis that an important mechanism by which ethanol induced CNS effects in the adult brain may be through the increased fluidity of the cell membranes, resulting in a general "disordering" effect. Lately, the "membrane fluidity" hypothesis has been abandoned, as ethanol has been shown to cause profound changes in protein activation, gene induction, protein–protein interaction, etc., at doses much lower and relevant to human exposure than those affecting the fluidity of the membranes. As a result, investigations of the effects of ethanol on cholesterol homeostasis were abandoned.

Recently, however, cholesterol, as the main constituent of lipid rafts, has been shown to play an important role in the activity of several proteins, including ion channels and signal transduction molecules. An *in vitro* study showed that cholesterol antagonizes the increase in the activity of the neuronal BK_{Ca} channels induced by ethanol (Crowley *et al.*, 2003), suggesting that indeed ethanol may affect cholesterol levels and/or distribution. This effect may be achieved through an increase in cellular cholesterol clearance mediated by the upregulation of cholesterol transporters and brain lipoprotein production (Chen *et al.*, unpublished; Guizzetti *et al.*, 2007).

In the developing brain, exposure to ethanol decreases cholesterol content in the brains of 20-day-old rats whose mothers were fed ethanol during gestation and lactation (Duffy *et al.*, 1991) and in the cerebellum of newborn rats prenatally exposed to ethanol (Soscia *et al.*, 2006). We reported that ethanol upregulates the levels of two cholesterol transporters, ABCA1 and ABCG1, leading to an increase in cholesterol efflux and apoE release from these cells. The increase in cholesterol efflux caused by ethanol is not compensated by an increase in cholesterol synthesis and, consequently, cholesterol content in astrocytes is decreased (Guizzetti *et al.*, 2007). Ethanol also induces the formation of liproproteins in astrocytes, which increase cholesterol efflux from other cell types including neurons (Chen *et al.*, submitted).

In summary, multiple lines of evidence indicate an inverse relationship between ethanol and cholesterol; in the developing brain, disruption of cholesterol homeostasis may play a role in several of the deleterious effects of ethanol. However, the exact mechanisms by which ethanol reduces cholesterol in the developing brain remain to be fully elucidated.

RETINOIC ACID EMBRYOPATHY

Vitamin A (retinol) and its derivatives (retinoids) exert many biological activities and are crucial for the normal development of the embryo. Either an excess or a deficiency of vitamin A and retinoids causes teratogenesis. Retinoids are derived from dietary intake, nutritional supplements and some therapeutic drugs. The vitamin A derivative 13-cis retinoic acid (13-cisRA or isotretinoin), used in the treatment of cystic acne, and the synthetic retinoid eritinate, used in the treatment of psoriasis, are reported human teratogens (Collins and Mao, 1999). 13-cisRA and all-trans retinoic acid (ATRA) have also been shown to cause teratogenesis in animal models (Alles and Sulik, 1989, 1992; Webster *et al.*, 1986).

The developmental effects of excessive retinoic acid present several similarities with alcohol-induced teratogenesis and with the abnormal morphological development observed in individuals with SLOS (Cohen and Shiota, 2002). Similarities include craniofacial abnormalities (holoprosencephaly), microencephaly and cerebellar hypoplasia in humans and limb malformation, craniofacial malformation (holoprosencephaly) and ocular abnormalities in mice (Alles and Sulik, 1989, 1992; Cohen and Shiota, 2002; Lanoue *et al.*, 1997; Porter, 2008; Ruitenberg *et al.*, 2002; Sulik, 2005).

It was recently reported that retinoic acid upregulates ABCA1 levels in macrophages (Costet *et al.*, 2003), and 9-cisRA, in combination with 22R-HC, potently induces ABCA1 and ABCG1 in many cell types including astrocytes. We found that ATRA, 13-cisRA and 9-cisRA, similarly to ethanol, induce ABCA1 and ABCG1 protein levels and reduce cholesterol levels in astrocytes, suggesting that the upregulation of cholesterol transporters may, indeed, be a common mechanism of teratogenesis. Indeed, cholesterol-regulated SHH signaling is altered in retinoic acid embryopathy (Ahlgren *et al.*, 2002; Helms *et al.*, 1997).

Thus, the mechanism of retinoic acid teratogenesis may involve the upregulation of cholesterol transporters, leading to increased lipoprotein size and/or production, and to reduced cholesterol levels in the developing brain, similar to that seen for ethanol.

OPPOSITE EFFECTS OF BRAIN CHOLESTEROL IN DEVELOPMENT AND AGING

Alzheimer's disease (AD), the most common form of dementia, is characterized by extracellular β-amyloid deposits in the brain, intracellular deposition of neurofibrillary tangles in neurons, and loss of neurons and synapses mostly in the neocortex and hippocampus, but also in other brain regions. Several lines of evidence implicate cholesterol metabolism in the pathogenesis of AD (Wolozin, 2004). Apolipoprotein allele ε4, encoding for the isoform 4 of apoE, is a major genetic risk factor for late onset AD; several studies indicate that subjects with elevated mid-life cholesterol are at increased risk for AD, and elevated cholesterol is associated with higher plaque load in AD subjects (Kivipelto *et al.*, 2002). In addition, epidemiological studies indicate that the utilization of 3-hydroxy-3-methylglutaryl coenzyme A reductase inhibitors (statins) to stabilize blood cholesterol levels in mid-life confers some protection against AD later in life (Poirier, 2003). The use of statins during pregnancy is not recommended, because of their potential neurodevelopmental and teratogenic effects; indeed, teratogenic effects from inhibitors of cholesterol synthesis have been reported in animal studies, whether this would occur in humans remains controversial (Edison and Muenke, 2004; Forbes *et al.*, 2008; Kazmin *et al.*, 2007).

The activity of α- and β-secretases, transmembrane proteins that cleave the amyloid precursor protein to generate β-amyloid, is dependent on cholesterol metabolism, as both complexes reside in cholesterol-rich lipid domains in the plasma membrane (Cordy *et al.*, 2003).

The cholesterol transporter ABCA1 has also been implicated in the pathogenesis of AD; two studies have shown that increased ABCA1 reduced the generation of β-amyloid peptides derived from human APP in cell culture models (Koldamova *et al.*, 2003), whereas a third study found that increased ABCA1 increased the generation of rodent β-amyloid (Fukumoto *et al.*, 2002). Recent studies have suggested that members of the ABC transporter family, ABCA1 and ABCG1 in particular, may represent therapeutic targets for the treatment of AD, as they may contribute to the reduction of intracellular cholesterol levels and β-amyloid deposition in brain cells (Hirsch-Reinshagen and Wellington, 2007).

Recent epidemiological studies suggest that moderate ethanol consumption improves cognitive performances in elderly men and women (Bond *et al.*, 2003; Ruitenberg *et al.*, 2002; Stampfer *et al.*, 2005). In addition, several studies have found that light to moderate alcohol consumption is associated with a reduced risk of dementia, including AD (Huang *et al.*, 2002; Mukamal *et al.*, 2003; Ruitenberg *et al.*, 2002). Most studies find an inverse relation between moderate alcohol and vascular dementia (Hebert *et al.*, 2000; Ruitenberg *et al.*, 2002), which is consistent with the known beneficial effects of light-to-moderate alcohol consumption on vascular risk profile (Rimm *et al.*, 1999) and risk of stroke (Reynolds *et al.*, 2003).

Interestingly, ATRA has been investigated recently as a potential treatment for AD; while the mechanism involved in its hypothesized therapeutic effects remains elusive, it is possible that the upregulation of cholesterol transporters and cholesterol efflux may be involved.

Finally, 13-cisRA and ATRA are also in use in the therapy of several tumors, including gliomas (Kaba *et al.*, 1997; Yung *et al.*, 1996). ABCA1 upregulation and cholesterol efflux inhibit cell proliferation and induce cell differentiation; therefore, the effectiveness of retinoic acid in the treatment of brain tumors may be in part due to its effects on cholesterol transporters and cholesterol efflux.

In summary, the reduction of brain cholesterol may be beneficial in the aging brain when high cholesterol is associated with neurodegenerative diseases and brain tumors. A reduction in brain cholesterol, however, may be deleterious for the developing brain when cholesterol is necessary for the proper formation of brain architecture and connections. Ethanol and retinoic acid, therefore, by reducing cholesterol levels through the upregulation of brain cholesterol transporters, may be beneficial to the aging brain but cause damage to the developing brain.

CONCLUDING REMARKS AND FUTURE DIRECTIONS

Cholesterol plays a pivotal role in brain development. Inhibition of cholesterol synthesis, as a consequence of genetic syndromes or exposure to cholesterol inhibitors during gestation, is known to cause neurodevelopmental and teratogenic effects. Recent research demonstrated that cholesterol homeostasis in the brain can be affected by the modulation of ABC cholesterol transporter levels and activity. Altered cholesterol homeostasis through the upregulation of cholesterol transporters appears to be involved in the developmental effects of ethanol and retinoic acid. Any chemical that affects cholesterol homeostasis may therefore be regarded as a potential developmental neurotoxicant.

ACKNOWLEDGMENTS

Work by the authors was supported in part by grant AA17180 from the National Institutes of Health. We thank Mr. Jeff Frkonja for the graphic design of Figure 65.1.

REFERENCES

Ahlgren SC, Thakur V, Bronner-Fraser M (2002) Sonic hedgehog rescues cranial neural crest from cell death induced by ethanol exposure. *Proc Natl Acad Sci USA* **99:** 10476–81.

Alles AJ, Sulik KK (1989) Retinoic-acid-induced limb-reduction defects: perturbation of zones of programmed cell death as a pathogenetic mechanism. *Teratology* **40:** 163–71.

Alles AJ, Sulik KK (1992) Pathogenesis of retinoid-induced hindbrain malformations in an experimental model. *Clin Dysmorphol* **1:** 187–200.

Barnes DE, Walker DW (1981) Prenatal ethanol exposure permanently reduces the number of pyramidal neurons in rat hippocampus. *Brain Res* **227:** 333–40.

Bjorkhem I, Meaney S (2004) Brain cholesterol: long secret life behind a barrier. *Arterioscler Thromb Vasc Biol* **24:** 806–15.

Bochelen D, Mersel M, Behr P, Lutz P, Kupferberg A (1995) Effect of oxysterol treatment on cholesterol biosynthesis and reactive astrocyte proliferation in injured rat brain cortex. *J Neurochem* **65:** 2194–200.

Bodzioch M, Orso E, Klucken J, *et al.* (1999) The gene encoding ATP-binding cassette transporter 1 is mutated in Tangier disease. *Nat Genet* **22:** 347–51.

Bond GE, Burr R, Rice MM, McCurry SM, Graves AB, Teri L, Bowen JD, McCormick WC, Larson EB (2003) Alcohol, aging, and cognitive performance: a cross-cultural comparison. *J Aging Health* **15:** 371–90.

Bonthius DJ, West JR (1991) Permanent neuronal deficits in rats exposed to alcohol during the brain growth spurt. *Teratology* **44:** 147–63.

Brown MS, Goldstein JL (1999) A proteolytic pathway that controls the cholesterol content of membranes, cells, and blood. *Proc Natl Acad Sci USA* **96:** 11041–8.

Chrisman K, Kenney R, Comin J, Thal T, Suchocki L, Yueh YG, Gardner DP (2004) Gestational ethanol exposure disrupts the expression of FGF8 and sonic hedgehog during limb patterning. *Birth Defects Res A Clin Mol Teratol* **70:** 163–71.

Cohen MM Jr, Shiota K (2002) Teratogenesis of holoprosencephaly. *Am J Med Genet* **109:** 1–15.

Collins MD, Mao GE (1999) Teratology of retinoids. *Annu Rev Pharmacol Toxicol* **39:** 399–430.

Cordy JM, Hussain I, Dingwall C, Hooper NM, Turner AJ (2003) Exclusively targeting beta-secretase to lipid rafts by GPI-anchor addition up-regulates beta-site processing of the amyloid precursor protein. *Proc Natl Acad Sci USA* **100:** 11735–40.

Costet P, Lalanne F, Gerbod-Giannone MC, Molina JR, Fu X, Lund EG, Gudas LJ, Tall AR (2003) Retinoic acid receptor-mediated induction of ABCA1 in macrophages. *Mol Cell Biol* **23:** 7756–66.

Crowley JJ, Treistman SN, Dopico AM (2003) Cholesterol antagonizes ethanol potentiation of human brain BKCa channels reconstituted into phospholipid bilayers. *Mol Pharmacol* **64:** 365–72.

Dehart DB, Lanoue L, Tint GS, Sulik KK (1997) Pathogenesis of malformations in a rodent model for Smith-Lemli-Opitz syndrome. *Am J Med Genet* **68:** 328–37.

Dehouck B, Fenart L, Dehouck MP, Pierce A, Torpier G, Cecchelli R (1997) A new function for the LDL receptor: transcytosis of LDL across the blood–brain barrier. *J Cell Biol* **138:** 877–89.

Diaz J, Samson HH (1980) Impaired brain growth in neonatal rats exposed to ethanol. *Science* **208:** 751–3.

Dietschy JM, Turley SD (2004) Thematic review series: brain lipids. Cholesterol metabolism in the central nervous system during early development and in the mature animal. *J Lipid Res* **45:** 1375–97.

Duffy O, Menez JF, Floch HH, Leonard BE (1991) Changes in whole brain membranes of rats following pre- and post-natal exposure to ethanol. *Alcohol Alcohol* **26:** 605–13.

Edison RJ, Muenke M (2004) Mechanistic and epidemiologic considerations in the evaluation of adverse birth outcomes following gestational exposure to statins. *Am J Med Genet A* **131:** 287–98.

Famy C, Streissguth AP, Unis AS (1998) Mental illness in adults with fetal alcohol syndrome or fetal alcohol effects. *Am J Psychiatry* **155:** 552–4.

Fan QW, Yu W, Gong JS, Zou K, Sawamura N, Senda T, Yanagisawa K, Michikawa M (2002) Cholesterol-dependent modulation of dendrite outgrowth and microtubule stability in cultured neurons. *J Neurochem* **80:** 178–90.

Fielding CJ, Fielding PE (2004) Membrane cholesterol and the regulation of signal transduction. *Biochem Soc Trans* **32:** 65–9.

Forbes K, Hurst LM, Aplin JD, Westwood M, Gibson JM (2008) Statins are detrimental to human placental development and function; use of statins during early pregnancy is inadvisable. *J Cell Mol Med* **12:** 2295–6.

Frohlich JJ (1996) Effects of alcohol on plasma lipoprotein metabolism. *Clin Chim Acta* **246:** 39–49.

Fukumoto H, Deng A, Irizarry MC, Fitzgerald ML, Rebeck GW (2002) Induction of the cholesterol transporter ABCA1 in central nervous system cells by liver X receptor agonists increases secreted Abeta levels. *J Biol Chem* **277:** 48508–13.

Goldberg DM, Hahn SE, Parkes JG (1995) Beyond alcohol: beverage consumption and cardiovascular mortality. *Clin Chim Acta* **237:** 155–87.

Guerri C (1998) Neuroanatomical and neurophysiological mechanisms involved in central nervous system dysfunctions induced by prenatal alcohol exposure. *Alcohol Clin Exp Res* **22:** 304–12.

Guizzetti M, Chen J, Oram JF, Tsuji R, Dao K, Moller T, Costa LG (2007) Ethanol induces cholesterol efflux and up-regulates ATP-binding cassette cholesterol transporters in fetal astrocytes. *J Biol Chem* **282:** 18740–9.

Hannuksela ML, Liisanantt MK, Savolainen MJ (2002) Effect of alcohol on lipids and lipoproteins in relation to atherosclerosis. *Crit Rev Clin Lab Sci* **39:** 225–83.

Hayashi H, Campenot RB, Vance DE, Vance JE (2004) Glial lipoproteins stimulate axon growth of central nervous system neurons in compartmented cultures. *J Biol Chem* **279:** 14009–15.

Hebert R, Lindsay J, Verreault R, Rockwood K, Hill G, Dubois MF (2000) Vascular dementia: incidence and risk factors in the Canadian study of health and aging. *Stroke* **31:** 1487–93.

Helms JA, Kim CH, Hu D, Minkoff R, Thaller C, Eichele G (1997) Sonic hedgehog participates in craniofacial morphogenesis and is down-regulated by teratogenic doses of retinoic acid. *Dev Biol* **187:** 25–35.

Herz J (2001) The LDL receptor gene family: (un)expected signal transducers in the brain. *Neuron* **29:** 571–81.

Hirsch-Reinshagen V, Wellington CL (2007) Cholesterol metabolism, apolipoprotein E, adenosine triphosphate-binding cassette transporters, and Alzheimer's disease. *Curr Opin Lipidol* **18:** 325–32.

Hirsch-Reinshagen V, Zhou S, Burgess BL, *et al.* (2004) Deficiency of ABCA1 impairs apolipoprotein E metabolism in brain. *J Biol Chem* **279:** 41197–207.

Huang W, Qiu C, Winblad B, Fratiglioni L (2002) Alcohol consumption and incidence of dementia in a community sample aged 75 years and older. *J Clin Epidemiol* **55:** 959–64.

Huo H, Guo X, Hong S, Jiang M, Liu X, Liao K (2003) Lipid rafts/caveolae are essential for insulin-like growth factor-1 receptor signaling during 3T3-L1 preadipocyte differentiation induction. *J Biol Chem* **278:** 11561–9.

Ikonomidou C, Bittigau P, Ishimaru MJ, *et al.* (2000) Ethanol-induced apoptotic neurodegeneration and fetal alcohol syndrome. *Science* **287:** 1056–60.

Incardona JP, Roelink H (2000) The role of cholesterol in Shh signaling and teratogen-induced holoprosencephaly. *Cell Mol Life Sci* **57:** 1709–19.

Jones KL, Smith DW (1975) The fetal alcohol syndrome. *Teratology* **12:** 1–10.

Jones KL, Smith DW, Ulleland CN, Streissguth P (1973) Pattern of malformation in offspring of chronic alcoholic mothers. *Lancet* **1:** 1267–71.

Jurevics HA, Kidwai FZ, Morell P (1997) Sources of cholesterol during development of the rat fetus and fetal organs. *J Lipid Res* **38:** 723–33.

Kaba SE, Kyritsis AP, Conrad C, Gleason MJ, Newman R, Levin VA, Yung WK (1997) The treatment of recurrent cerebral gliomas with all-trans-retinoic acid (tretinoin). *J Neurooncol* **34:** 145–51.

Karasinska JM, Rinninger F, Lutjohann D, *et al.* (2009) Specific loss of brain ABCA1 increases brain cholesterol uptake and influences neuronal structure and function. *J Neurosci* **29:** 3579–89.

Kazmin A, Garcia-Bournissen F, Koren G (2007) Risks of statin use during pregnancy: a systematic review. *J Obstet Gynaecol Can* **29:** 906–8.

Keller K, McCune H, Williams C, Muenke M (2000) Lobar holoprosencephaly in an infant born to a mother with classic phenylketonuria. *Am J Med Genet* **95:** 187–8.

Kelley RI, Herman GE (2001) Inborn errors of sterol biosynthesis. *Annu Rev Genomics Hum Genet* **2:** 299–341.

Kim WS, Suryo Rahmanto A, Kamili A, Rye KA, Guillemin GJ, Gelissen IC, Jessup W, Hill AF, Garner B (2007) Role of ABCG1 and ABCA1 in regulation of neuronal cholesterol efflux to apolipoprotein-E discs and suppression of amyloid-beta peptide generation. *J Biol Chem* **282:** 2851–61.

Kivipelto M, Helkala EL, Laakso MP, *et al.* (2002) Apolipoprotein E epsilon4 allele, elevated midlife total cholesterol level, and high midlife systolic blood pressure are independent risk factors for late-life Alzheimer disease. *Ann Intern Med* **137:** 149–55.

Klatsky AL (1994) Epidemiology of coronary heart disease – influence of alcohol. *Alcohol Clin Exp Res* **18:** 88–96.

Ko M, Zou K, Minagawa H, Yu W, Gong JS, Yanagisawa K, Michikawa M (2005) Cholesterol-mediated neurite outgrowth is differently regulated between cortical and hippocampal neurons. *J Biol Chem* **280:** 42759–65.

Koldamova RP, Lefterov IM, Ikonomovic MD, Skoko J, Lefterov PI, Isanski BA, DeKosky ST, Lazo JS (2003) 22R-hydroxycholesterol and 9-cis-retinoic acid induce ATP-binding cassette transporter A1 expression and cholesterol efflux in brain cells and decrease amyloid beta secretion. *J Biol Chem* **278:** 13244–56.

LaDu MJ, Gilligan SM, Lukens JR, Cabana VG, Reardon CA, Van Eldik LJ, Holtzman DM (1998) Nascent astrocyte particles differ from lipoproteins in CSF. *J Neurochem* **70:** 2070–81.

Lanoue L, Dehart DB, Hinsdale ME, Maeda N, Tint GS, Sulik KK (1997) Limb, genital, CNS, and facial malformations result from gene/environment-induced cholesterol deficiency: further evidence for a link to sonic hedgehog. *Am J Med Genet* **73:** 24–31.

Lawn RM, Wade DP, Garvin MR, Wang X, Schwartz K, Porter JG, Seilhamer JJ, Vaughan AM, Oram JF (1999) The Tangier disease gene product ABC1 controls the cellular apolipoprotein-mediated lipid removal pathway. *J Clin Invest* **104:** 25–31.

Levy HL, Ghavami M (1996) Maternal phenylketonuria: a metabolic teratogen. *Teratology* **53:** 176–84.

Li YX, Yang HT, Zdanowicz M, Sicklick JK, Qi Y, Camp TJ, Diehl AM (2007) Fetal alcohol exposure impairs hedgehog cholesterol modification and signaling. *Lab Invest* **87:** 231–40.

Lund EG, Guileyardo JM, Russell DW (1999) cDNA cloning of cholesterol 24-hydroxylase, a mediator of cholesterol homeostasis in the brain. *Proc Natl Acad Sci USA* **96:** 7238–43.

Lutjohann D, von Bergmann K (2003) 24S-hydroxycholesterol: a marker of brain cholesterol metabolism. *Pharmacopsychiatry* **36 (Suppl. 2):** S102–6.

Maier SE, Miller JA, Blackwell JM, West JR (1999) Fetal alcohol exposure and temporal vulnerability: regional differences in cell loss as a function of the timing of binge-like alcohol exposure during brain development. *Alcohol Clin Exp Res* **23:** 726–34.

Marti E, Bovolenta P (2002) Sonic hedgehog in CNS development: one signal, multiple outputs. *Trends Neurosci* **25:** 89–96.

Mauch DH, Nagler K, Schumacher S, Goritz C, Muller EC, Otto A, Pfrieger FW (2001) CNS synaptogenesis promoted by glia-derived cholesterol. *Science* **294:** 1354–7.

Meyer LS, Kotch LE, Riley EP (1990) Alterations in gait following ethanol exposure during the brain growth spurt in rats. *Alcohol Clin Exp Res* **14:** 23–7.

Michikawa M, Yanagisawa K (1999) Inhibition of cholesterol production but not of nonsterol isoprenoid products induces neuronal cell death. *J Neurochem* **72:** 2278–85.

Miller MW (1986) Effects of alcohol on the generation and migration of cerebral cortical neurons. *Science* **233:** 1308–11.

Miller MW (2007) Exposure to ethanol during gastrulation alters somatosensory-motor cortices and the underlying white matter in the macaque. *Cereb Cortex* **17:** 2961–71.

Miller MW, Robertson S (1993) Prenatal exposure to ethanol alters the postnatal development and transformation of radial glia to astrocytes in the cortex. *J Comp Neurol* **337:** 253–66.

Mukamal KJ, Kuller LH, Fitzpatrick AL, Longstreth WT Jr, Mittleman MA, Siscovick DS (2003) Prospective study of alcohol consumption and risk of dementia in older adults. *JAMA* **289:** 1405–13.

Nakai M, Kawamata T, Taniguchi T, Maeda K, Tanaka C (1996) Expression of apolipoprotein E mRNA in rat microglia. *Neurosci Lett* **211:** 41–4.

Nowaczyk MJ, Whelan DT, Heshka TW, Hill RE (1999) Smith–Lemli–Opitz syndrome: a treatable inherited error of metabolism causing mental retardation. *Can Med Assoc J* **161:** 165–70.

Nwokoro NA, Wassif CA, Porter FD (2001) Genetic disorders of cholesterol biosynthesis in mice and humans. *Mol Genet Metab* **74:** 105–19.

Oberdoerster J, Guizzetti M, Costa LG (2000) Effect of phenylalanine and its metabolites on the proliferation and viability of neuronal and astroglial cells: possible relevance in maternal phenylketonuria. *J Pharmacol Exp Ther* **295:** 295–301.

Oram JF, Heinecke JW (2005) ATP-binding cassette transporter A1: a cell cholesterol exporter that protects against cardiovascular disease. *Physiol Rev* **85:** 1343–72.

Panzenboeck U, Balazs Z, Sovic A, Hrzenjak A, Levak-Frank S, Wintersperger A, Malle E, Sattler W (2002) ABCA1 and scavenger receptor class B, type I, are modulators of reverse sterol transport at an in vitro blood–brain barrier constituted of porcine brain capillary endothelial cells. *J Biol Chem* **277:** 42781–9.

Pitas RE, Boyles JK, Lee SH, Foss D, Mahley RW (1987) Astrocytes synthesize apolipoprotein E and metabolize apolipoprotein E-containing lipoproteins. *Biochim Biophys Acta* **917:** 148–61.

Poirier J (2003) Apolipoprotein E and cholesterol metabolism in the pathogenesis and treatment of Alzheimer's disease. *Trends Mol Med* **9:** 94–101.

Poirier J, Baccichet A, Dea D, Gauthier S (1993) Cholesterol synthesis and lipoprotein reuptake during synaptic remodelling in hippocampus in adult rats. *Neuroscience* **55:** 81–90.

Porter FD (2008) Smith–Lemli–Opitz syndrome: pathogenesis, diagnosis and management. *Eur J Hum Genet* **16:** 535–41.

Puglielli L, Tanzi RE, Kovacs DM (2003) Alzheimer's disease: the cholesterol connection. *Nat Neurosci* **6:** 345–51.

Raffai RL, Weisgraber KH (2003) Cholesterol: from heart attacks to Alzheimer's disease. *J Lipid Res* **44:** 1423–30.

Reynolds K, Lewis B, Nolen JD, Kinney GL, Sathya B, He J (2003) Alcohol consumption and risk of stroke: a meta-analysis. *JAMA* **289:** 579–88.

Rice D, Barone S Jr (2000) Critical periods of vulnerability for the developing nervous system: evidence from humans and animal models. *Environ Health Perspect* **108 (Suppl. 3):** 511–33.

Rimm EB, Williams P, Fosher K, Criqui M, Stampfer MJ (1999) Moderate alcohol intake and lower risk of coronary heart disease: meta-analysis of effects on lipids and haemostatic factors. *BMJ* **319:** 1523–8.

Ruitenberg A, van Swieten JC, Witteman JC, Mehta KM, van Duijn CM, Hofman A, Breteler MM (2002) Alcohol consumption and risk of dementia: the Rotterdam Study. *Lancet* **359:** 281–6.

Rust S, Rosier M, Funke H, *et al.* (1999) Tangier disease is caused by mutations in the gene encoding ATP-binding cassette transporter 1. *Nat Genet* **22:** 352–5.

Simons K, Toomre D (2000) Lipid rafts and signal transduction. *Nat Rev Mol Cell Biol* **1:** 31–9.

Soscia SJ, Tong M, Xu XJ, Cohen AC, Chu J, Wands JR, de la Monte SM (2006) Chronic gestational exposure to ethanol causes insulin and IGF resistance and impairs acetylcholine homeostasis in the brain. *Cell Mol Life Sci* **63:** 2039–56.

Stampfer MJ, Kang JH, Chen J, Cherry R, Grodstein F (2005) Effects of moderate alcohol consumption on cognitive function in women. *N Engl J Med* **352:** 245–53.

Stratton K, Howe C, Battaglia F (1996) *Fetal Alcohol Syndrome: Diagnosis, Epidemiology, Prevention and Treatment*. National Academy Press, Washington DC.

Streissguth AP, Landesman-Dwyer S, Martin JC, Smith DW (1980) Teratogenic effects of alcohol in humans and laboratory animals. *Science* **209:** 353–61.

Streissguth AP, O'Malley K (2000) Neuropsychiatric implications and long-term consequences of fetal alcohol spectrum disorders. *Semin Clin Neuropsychiatry* **5:** 177–90.

Sulik KK (2005) Genesis of alcohol-induced craniofacial dysmorphism. *Exp Biol Med (Maywood)* **230:** 366–75.

Tachikawa M, Watanabe M, Hori S, Fukaya M, Ohtsuki S, Asashima T, Terasaki T (2005) Distinct spatio-temporal expression of ABCA and ABCG transporters in the developing and adult mouse brain. *J Neurochem* **95:** 294–304.

Tarr PT, Edwards PA (2008) ABCG1 and ABCG4 are coexpressed in neurons and astrocytes of the CNS and regulate cholesterol homeostasis through SREBP-2. *J Lipid Res* **49:** 169–82.

van Tol A, Hendriks HF (2001) Moderate alcohol consumption: effects on lipids and cardiovascular disease risk. *Curr Opin Lipidol* **12:** 19–23.

Vaughan AM, Oram JF (2006) ABCA1 and ABCG1 or ABCG4 act sequentially to remove cellular cholesterol and generate cholesterol-rich HDL. *J Lipid Res* **47:** 2433–43.

Wahrle SE, Jiang H, Parsadanian M, Legleiter J, Han X, Fryer JD, Kowalewski T, Holtzman DM (2004) ABCA1 is required for normal central nervous system ApoE levels and for lipidation of astrocyte-secreted apoE. *J Biol Chem* **279:** 40987–93.

Wang N, Lan D, Chen W, Matsuura F, Tall AR (2004) ATP-binding cassette transporters G1 and G4 mediate cellular cholesterol efflux to high-density lipoproteins. *Proc Natl Acad Sci USA* **101:** 9774–9.

Wang N, Yvan-Charvet L, Lutjohann D, Mulder M, Vanmierlo T, Kim TW, Tall AR (2008) ATP-binding cassette transporters G1 and G4 mediate cholesterol and desmosterol efflux to HDL and regulate sterol accumulation in the brain. *FASEB J* **22:** 1073–82.

Webster WS, Johnston MC, Lammer EJ, Sulik KK (1986) Isotretinoin embryopathy and the cranial neural crest: an in vivo and in vitro study. *J Craniofac Genet Dev Biol* **6:** 211–22.

Wen GY, Wisniewski HM, Shek JW, Loo YH, Fulton TR (1980) Neuropathology of phenylacetate poisoning in rats: an experimental model of phenylketonuria. *Ann Neurol* **7:** 557–66.

West JR, Hamre KM, Cassell MD (1986) Effects of ethanol exposure during the third trimester equivalent on neuron number in rat hippocampus and dentate gyrus. *Alcohol Clin Exp Res* **10:** 190–7.

Wolozin B (2004) Cholesterol and the biology of Alzheimer's disease. *Neuron* **41:** 7–10.

Woollett LA (2001) The origins and roles of cholesterol and fatty acids in the fetus. *Curr Opin Lipidol* **12:** 305–12.

Yung WK, Kyritsis AP, Gleason MJ, Levin VA (1996) Treatment of recurrent malignant gliomas with high-dose 13-cis-retinoic acid. *Clin Cancer Res* **2:** 1931–5.

C H A P T E R

66

Cholinergic Toxicity and the Male Reproductive System

Inbal Mor and Hermona Soreq

INTRODUCTION

Proper function of the male reproductive system requires both continuous proliferation and differentiation of germ cells as well as maintenance of the supporting somatic cells. Toxic agents interfering with either or both of these processes would result in impaired fertility; in addition, certain physiological processes may also exert adverse effects on male reproduction. For example, malnutrition, systemic disease or psychological stress responses may all suppress androgen production and induce direct molecular changes in germ cell production. Key proteins associated with such impairments include signaling factors and, more specifically, proteins involved with acetylcholine signaling (cholinergic signaling). Cholinergic proteins are expressed in various cells of the male reproductive system and are notably involved in both sperm differentiation and sperm function. These include membrane receptors capable of binding the neurotransmitter acetylcholine and the enzyme that hydrolyzes acetylcholine, acetylcholinesterase (AChE). In addition to neurotransmission, cholinergic signaling affects non-neuronal tissues and induces intracellular protein–protein interactions. Disrupted function of any of these cholinergic proteins may induce cholinergic toxicity and exert adverse affects on male fertility. Anticholinesterase agents are commonly used in agriculture as insecticides, resulting in sometimes widespread environmental and occupational exposure. It is noteworthy that psychological stress and anxiety have also been demonstrated to affect cholinergic function in murine testicular tissue, resulting in elevated AChE activity and a shift in AChE subtypes. Other cytotoxic agents such as commonly used chemotherapeutics can affect AChE indirectly, by eliciting a cellular stress response. Moreover, the cytotoxicity of chemotherapeutic drugs can be affected by molecular processes that involve cholinergic proteins. Thus, it is important to understand the role of cholinergic toxicity in the male reproductive system and to address both its direct and indirect effects.

BACKGROUND

Cholinergic molecules in the diverse cell types composing the male reproductive system

Sperm differentiation and the seminiferous tubule histology

The male gonad, the testis, consists mainly of coiled narrow tubules (Figure 66.1A). Male gamete production, spermatogenesis, takes place in the testicular seminiferous tubules (Figure 66.1B).

The hormonal and cellular environment surrounding the germinal cells is created by the Leydig cells found in the interstitium between the tubules (Figure 66.1B) and by the Sertoli cells inside the tubules (Figure 66.1C). In response to gonadotropin, secreted from the pituitary, Leydig cells produce testosterone which affects the Sertoli cells, maintaining the microenvironment of the developing spermatozoa (Leonhardt, 1993; Ross *et al.*, 1995).

Synchronous progression through spermatogenesis is accompanied by advancement of the cells from the tubule periphery toward the central lumen (Figure 66.1C). Spermatogonia, diploid stem cells, are located closest to the basement of the seminiferous epithelium, where these immature cells go through self-renewing proliferative mitotic divisions. A subpopulation of these cells continuously goes through a mitotic division that yields daughter cells named spermatocytes. The two meiotic divisions taking place in primary and then secondary spermatocytes give rise to haploid round spermatids. Spermatids are transformed to spermatozoa through a complex differentiation process, which includes elongation, formation of tail, nuclear condensation, concentration of the mitochondria at the tail mid-piece and loss of cytoplasm. Upon completion of spermatogenesis, the spermatozoa are released from the seminiferous tubules to be carried through the genital duct system.

Reproductive and Developmental Toxicology, Edited by Ramesh C. Gupta
ISBN: 978-0-12-382032-7

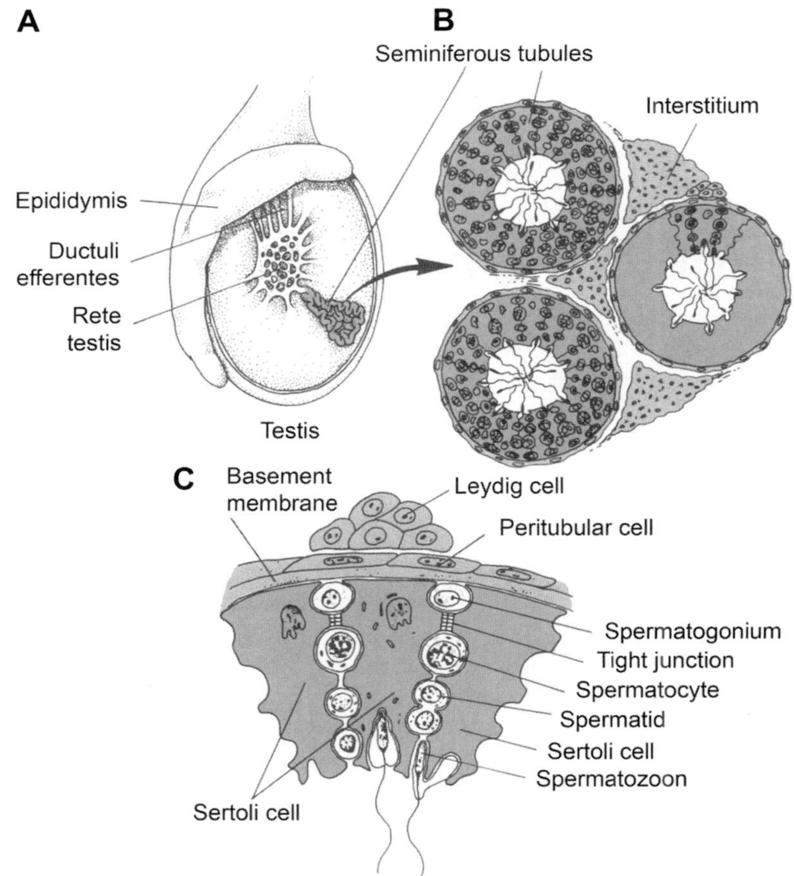

FIGURE 66.1 The testis. (A) Schematic diagram of a longitudinal section through the human testis and the genital duct system. (B) Drawing of a section of human testis; shown are adjacent seminiferous tubules and interstitial tissue between them. (C) Schematic drawing of mouse testicular seminiferous tubule presenting the cell types in spermatogenic differentiation. (From Genuth, 2004.)

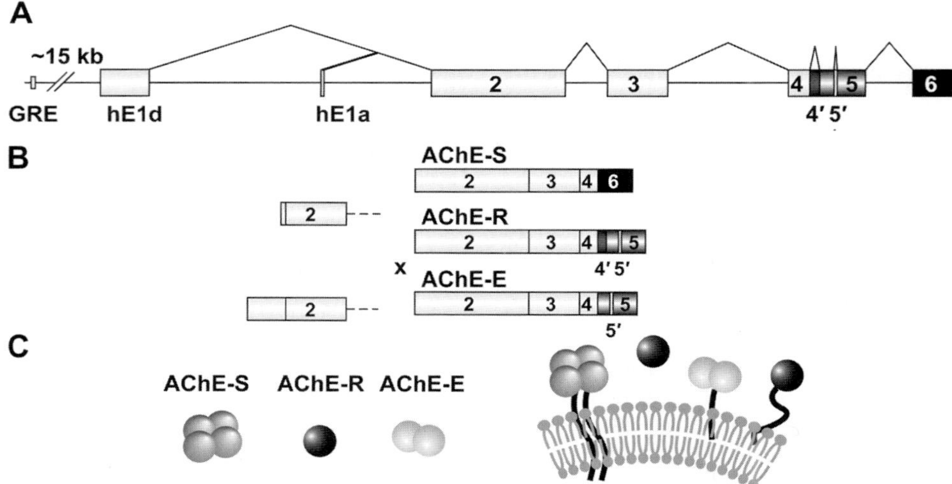

FIGURE 66.2 The AChE gene, alternative transcripts and protein isoforms. (A) Structure of the human AChE gene. Splicing options are shown as lines above the gene. Exon1 (E1) has two versions transcribed from two alternative promoters. 4′ indicates pseudo-intron 4. (B) mRNA transcripts. Each of the alternative human 5′ exons can potentially be combined with the three 3′ alternative transcripts. The C-terminal protein isoform encoded by each 3′ exon is noted. (C) Protein isoforms. Tetrameric globular AChE-S attached to the membrane by the structural anchor proteins ColQ or PRiMA. Monomeric AChE-R is soluble. Dimeric AChE-E is attached to the membrane through a GPi anchor. N-terminally extended N-AChE-R could be attached to the membrane. (From Meshorer *et al.*, 2004.)

Because cells differentiate and progress from the periphery of the tubule to the lumen, particular cell types can be found only in specific combinations in a particular cross-section. Each cellular association is termed a "spermatogenic stage" and a complete set of stages displaying all the different steps of spermatogenesis is termed the "spermatogenic cycle". A specific spermatogonia cell differentiating into a sperm cell would undergo a few cycles, their duration and number depending on the mammalian species.

In an adult testis, the consecutive stages of the spermatogenic cycle are organized along the length of the seminiferous tubule which is termed the "spermatogenic wave". Therefore, a cross-section of the whole testis would provide cross-sections of tubules at all stages of the spematogenic cycle, containing cells at all stages of spermatogenesis. These highly precise changes in cellular association in the seminiferous tubule provide a remarkable display of spatio-temporal organization.

Cholinergic innervation is important for transport of sperm cells along the seminiferous tubules by rhythmic contractions of the surrounding muscles, and thus for male fertility. Additionally, cholinergic molecules are expressed in cells that are unique to the male reproductive system, including Leydig cells (Favaretto *et al.*, 1993) and Sertoli cells (Borges *et al.*, 2001; Lucas *et al.*, 2004). Therefore, sperm production is subject to cholinergic regulation. Cholinergic parasympathetic innervation of smooth muscles is present along the male reproductive tract as in other organs of the body. Cholinergic neurons from the central nervous system release acetylcholine, which activates acetylcholine receptors in the post-synaptic cells (Taylor, 1996). The two types of acetylcholine receptors differ in their mode of action: nicotinic receptors are ion channels whereas muscarinic receptors are G-protein coupled receptors. Nicotinic receptors are mainly localized in parasympathetic ganglia whereas muscarinic receptors are found in the smooth muscles lining the organ (Taylor, 1996). AChE hydrolyzes acetylcholine in the inter-cellular junction, effectively terminating this signaling (Taylor, 1996).

Nicotinic acetylcholine receptors

Nicotinic acetylcholine receptors (nAChR) are found in mammalian sperm (Kumar and Meizel, 2005). This multimeric transmembrane ligand-gated cation channel has been demonstrated to be involved in the sperm acrosome reaction. Upon binding of a glycoprotein in the egg outer membrane, calcium influx through the nAChR and other channels triggers changes in the sperm membrane resulting in release of proteases from the acrosome which allow penetration of the egg membranes and fertilization (Son and Meizel, 2003). nAChRs are also found in differentiating germ cells in the seminiferous tubules (Palmero *et al.*, 1999). Previous evidence further suggests that nAChR molecules along the sperm flagella could be involved in synchronization and regulation of the flagellar beating and therefore in sperm motility (Dwivedi and Long, 1989). Interestingly, additional molecules known to associate with nAChR in muscle and neuronal cells are also found in the sperm (Kumar and Meizel, 2005), suggesting that the modulation of nAChR action which has been described for these tissues could also be relevant for its function in sperm cells. Recently, newly discovered testicular proteins, identified through similarity to venomous toxins, have been identified as nAChR binding proteins that have the potential to modulate the receptor's activity, suggesting an additional level of regulation over the function of this channel (Kaplan *et al.*, 2007; Levitin *et al.*, 2008). nAChRs are also involved in regulation of Leydig cell function. Their expression is elevated following Leydig cell differentiation and maturation (Ge *et al.*, 2005) and both acetylcholine and nicotine have been shown to decrease testosterone secretion from enriched Leydig cell cultures (Favaretto *et al.*, 1993).

Muscarinic acetylcholine receptors

The G-protein coupled muscarinic acetylcholine receptors (mAChR) regulate various intracellular signaling pathways effecting secretion, cell growth, proliferation and death. mAChRs have been located in mature and differentiating sperm (Palmero *et al.*, 1999). Sertoli cells express mAChRs as well; muscarinic agonists have been demonstrated to trigger intracellular signaling cascades and elevate thymidine incorporation (Borges *et al.*, 2001; Lucas *et al.*, 2004). This suggests that activation of mAChRs can modify Sertoli cell function as well as enhance their proliferation. mAChR have further been localized to epithelial cells of the reproductive tract in the efferent duct system and the epididymis (Avellar *et al.*, 2010). There, activation of signal transduction pathways in response to cholinergic innervation results in elevated protein synthesis and secretion, indicating that cholinergic signals are important for the composition of luminal fluid and thus for proper sperm maturation (Avellar *et al.*, 2010).

Acetylcholinesterase splice variants show differential expression patterns in developing germ cells

AChE is classically known to hydrolyze the neurotransmitter acetylcholine in cholinergic synapses (Taylor, 1996). However, extensive research has demonstrated that this enzyme constitutes many isoforms with different C- and N-terminal domains (Meshorer and Soreq, 2006) and that it performs biological functions independent of its catalytic activity (Bigbee *et al.*, 2000; Day and Greenfield, 2002; Johnson and Moore, 2004; Soreq and Seidman, 2001). AChE transcripts undergo alternative splicing at their 3′-end, yielding catalytically active protein isoforms with different C-termini (Figure 66.2A). The transcript containing pseudointron I4 encodes the AChE-R isoform (Figure 66.2A,B). Increases in this variant are characteristic of differentiation processes, such as during neuronal and hematopoietic differentiation (Chan *et al.*, 1998; Dori *et al.*, 2005; Gilboa-Geffen *et al.*, 2007; Grisaru *et al.*, 2006; Shaked *et al.*, 2009, 2008). This soluble monomeric AChE isoform can be either secreted or maintained inside the cell (Meshorer *et al.*, 2004) (Figure 66.2C). Through its unique C-terminus AChE-R can interact with the glycolytic enzyme enolase and elevate its activity (Mor *et al.*, 2008b). Additionally, AChE-R can bind the scaffold protein RACK1 and compete with the pro-apoptotic transcription factor p73, which also binds this protein (Mor *et al.*, 2008a; Ozaki *et al.*, 2003; Sklan *et al.*, 2006). Together, these studies suggest that the R isoform of AChE can participate in different cellular pathways and functions through interaction with various protein partners.

The 5′-end of the AChE pre-mRNA is subject to alternate promoter usage (Figure 66.2A) allowing translation of AChE with an extended N-terminus (N-AChE; Meshorer *et al.*, 2004). The extended N-terminal domain allows localization of AChE to the cell membrane (Mor *et al.*, 2008a; Toiber *et al.*, 2008, 2009). Initiation of transcription from two alternative promoters together with alternative splicing of the 3′ exons therefore yields 5′ and 3′ alternative transcripts encoding AChE proteins containing different combinations of N- and C-terminal domains (Meshorer and Soreq, 2006) (Figure 66.2B).

AChE has long been detected in sperm cells of many animal species (Chakraborty and Nelson, 1976; Egbunike, 1980). As the detection methods used were primarily based on the highly sensitive detection of AChE activity, they could not identify which isoform was expressed. By using specific antibodies, the AChE-R isoform was identified in human and mouse sperm where it localized to the sperm head and tail (Mor *et al.*, 2001). Moreover, detection of AChE-R was positively correlated with sperm motility in humans (Mor *et al.*, 2008b). During spermatogenic differentiation in the human testis, the soluble shorter AChE-R variant is detected in all differentiation stages (Mor *et al.*, 2008a). Interestingly, N-AChE expression was confined to the acrosome of round spermatids (Mor *et al.*, 2008a).

AChE AND MALE FERTILITY

Toxic effects of anti-cholinesterases on sperm differentiation and functioning

Numerous anti-AChE pesticides have been tested for their reproductive toxicity, especially in countries where exposure to such pesticides is widespread. A recent study of early life exposure to the organophosphate (OP) insecticide dimethoate (*O,O*-dimethyl-S-(N-methylcarbamoyl-methyl) phosphorodithioate) exerted pronounced effects on the pituitary–testicular axis of mice (Verma and Mohanty, 2009); in the albino rat, testicular toxicity of another OP pesticide, chlorpyrifos (Joshi *et al.*, 2007), was detected at subacute exposure levels which did not affect body weight. The toxicity biomarkers included reduced epididymal and testicular sperm counts and decreased serum testosterone concentration. Seminiferous tubules showed pathological degeneration, and testicular glycogen and sialic acid content were reduced, whereas cholesterol and protein content were increased in an exposure dose-dependent manner. Malathion was also reported to affect the male reproductive system in rats, with generally similar consequences as those of chlorpyrifos, accompanied by increases in testicular acid phosphatase activities (Choudhary *et al.*, 2008). An intriguing association of cholinergic signaling was indicated by the inhibitory role of cholinergic agonists on testosterone secretion by purified rat Leydig cells (Favaretto *et al.*, 1993).

In-depth studies explored possible connections with the nicotinic and muscarinic signaling systems (Favaretto *et al.*, 1993). Thus, nicotine inhibited whereas the nicotinic antagonist hexamethonium promoted a partial reversal of the nicotine inhibitory effect on basal as well as hCG-stimulated secretion of testosterone. Also, atropine reduced the inhibitory effect of the cholinergic agonist carbachol on the basal levels or stimulated release of testosterone from cultured rat Leydig cells, suggesting that both nicotinic and muscarinic signals were involved. Together, these findings suggest involvement of the parasympathetic system in testicular functioning, which further expands the implications of these findings to other changes in parasympathetic activities (e.g., under physiological stress responses).

Detrimental effects of physiological and psychological stress on testicular tissue and spermatogenesis through modification of cholinergic functioning

Physiological stress responses in the reproductive axis and their effect on spermatogenesis at the cellular level

Systemic stressors have been shown to interfere with normal progression of sperm differentiation. Heat stress reduces sperm production and sperm motility and increases abnormal sperm morphology. Spermatocytes and spermatids are yet more sensitive, so that insults such as exposure to systemic stressors during that stage of spermatogenesis result in the highest proportion of damaged sperm (Lue *et al.*, 1999; Perez-Crespo *et al.*, 2008). Heat stress induces germ cell depletion from the seminiferous tubules and elevation in DNA damage, particularly in spermatocytes (Lue *et al.*, 1999; Paul *et al.*, 2008). Apoptosis, as well as activation of pro-apoptotic proteins such as caspase3 and p38 MAPK, is elevated in germ cells subjected to heat stress (Lizama *et al.*, 2009; Paul *et al.*, 2009). Heat stress also induces elevation of proteins involved in the hypoxic and oxidative stress responses (Paul *et al.*, 2009). Oxidative stress, caused by a wide variety of agents or pathological conditions, is also adversely correlated with sperm quality and male fertility. DNA damage and germ cell apoptosis are common outcomes of oxidative stress during spermatogenesis or sperm maturation (Turner and Lysiak, 2008).

One of the outcomes of the physiological stress response is suppression of the energy-consuming reproductive activity (Sapolsky *et al.*, 2000). Suppression of the HPG (hypothalamic–pituitary–gonadal) axis is directly mediated by action of the stress hormones (McEwen, 1998; Sapolsky *et al.*, 2000). Under normal conditions, the HPG axis is maintained by secretion of gonadotropin releasing hormone (GnRH) from the hypothalamus, which causes a release of LH from the pituitary. This leads to synthesis of testosterone and maintenance of spermatogenesis in the testes. Following stress, suppression by corticotropin releasing hormone (CRH) of GnRH release at the hypothalamus decreases the levels of circulating LH (Jeong *et al.*, 1999; Rivier and Vale, 1985); additionally, induction of a gonadotropin inhibitory hormone would lead to decrease in gonadotropin synthesis (Kirby *et al.*, 2009), though other central stress factors might also be involved. In addition, glucocorticoids disrupt reproductive function by acting directly on the testicular tissue, leading to reduced concentration of LH receptors in the testes (McEwen, 1998; Sapolsky *et al.*, 2000). Leydig cells can also react directly to circulating stress hormones by decreasing testosterone biosynthesis (Dong *et al.*, 2004). Therefore, activation of the HPA (hypothalamic–pituitary–adrenal) axis eventually leads to reduction of testosterone levels, which suppresses spermatogenesis. Decline in testosterone and elevated glucocorticoids have further been shown to induce germ cell apoptosis (Sasagawa *et al.*, 2001). Genes involved in germ cell apoptosis, such as p53 and Bcl family members, are known to be modified by corticosterone and could therefore be involved in stress-induced apoptosis (Sasagawa *et al.*, 2001).

Psychological stress and its effects on spermatogenesis

Reduced male fertility is one of the known consequences of psychological stress (Bigelow *et al.*, 1998; Giblin *et al.*, 1988; Negro-Vilar, 1993). Animal studies have demonstrated impaired sperm properties in stressed animals, e.g. mice subjected to immobilization stress. In addition to elevation of serum corticosterone and decrease of circulating LH and testosterone, such mice displayed a reduction in sperm counts (Almeida *et al.*, 1998; Yazawa *et al.*, 1999). Research on humans further displayed a correlation between various psychological stress parameters and sperm quality. Reduced sperm counts, reduced sperm motility (Clarke *et al.*, 1999; Harlow *et al.*, 1996; Zorn *et al.*, 2008), increases in sperm deformities (Bigelow *et al.*, 1998; Giblin *et al.*, 1988; Negro-Vilar, 1993) and suppression of reproductive hormones have all been found to be correlated with psychological stress (Said, 2008). Additionally, psychological stress has been correlated with oxidative stress markers in seminal plasma (Eskiocak *et al.*, 2005). Thus, different systemic stressors, including psychological stress, could mediate negative effects on sperm quality, similarly to other environmental toxins. Therefore, exploring the molecular aspects of the physiological stress response at the cellular level can help identify molecular processes that participate in the deterioration of germ cells.

The stress-inducible AChE-R variant in spermatogenesis – a case study of the molecular and cellular consequences of psychological stress

AChE gene expression is elevated in various tissues under exposure to different stressors (Zimmerman and Soreq, 2006). In the brain, AChE transcription is elevated following stress (Kaufer *et al.*, 1998). Under stress-induced transcriptional activation, AChE pre-mRNA transcripts further undergo a shift in alternative splicing, leading to pronounced overproduction of the otherwise minor AChE-R isoform in brain (Kaufer *et al.*, 1998), muscle (Brenner *et al.*, 2003), hematopoietic cells (Pick *et al.*, 2006) and the testis (Mor *et al.*, 2001). Mice stressed by confined swimming displayed elevated AChE levels which were localized to maturing spermatozoa in the seminferous tubules. AChE-R overexpressing transgenic mice express AChE-R in meiotic spermatocytes (Figure 66.3A) as well as in maturing spermatozoa, probably modeling the cells that would express this transcript in situations that induce higher levels of AChE expression than forced swimming. Importantly, elevation of AChE-R in transgenic mice was correlated with reduced sperm counts (Figure 66.3B) (Mor *et al.*, 2001). Correspondingly, transgenic pups displayed elevated spermatocyte apoptosis as measured by TUNEL staining (Figure 66.3C) (Mor *et al.*, 2008b).

Examining AChE-R in human sperm cells also suggested that it is correlated with sperm quality and function. The AChE-R subcellular distribution pattern correlated with fertility status (Mor *et al.*, 2001), and cells from patients with unexplained male factor infertility presented reduced AChE-R at the head region. A correlation was also found between sperm motility and the presence of AChE-R (Mor *et al.*, 2008b). Density gradient centrifugation was used to separate sperm samples from sperm-bank donors and infertility patients into three subpopulations according to their motility grade. When cells from all three populations were analyzed by flow

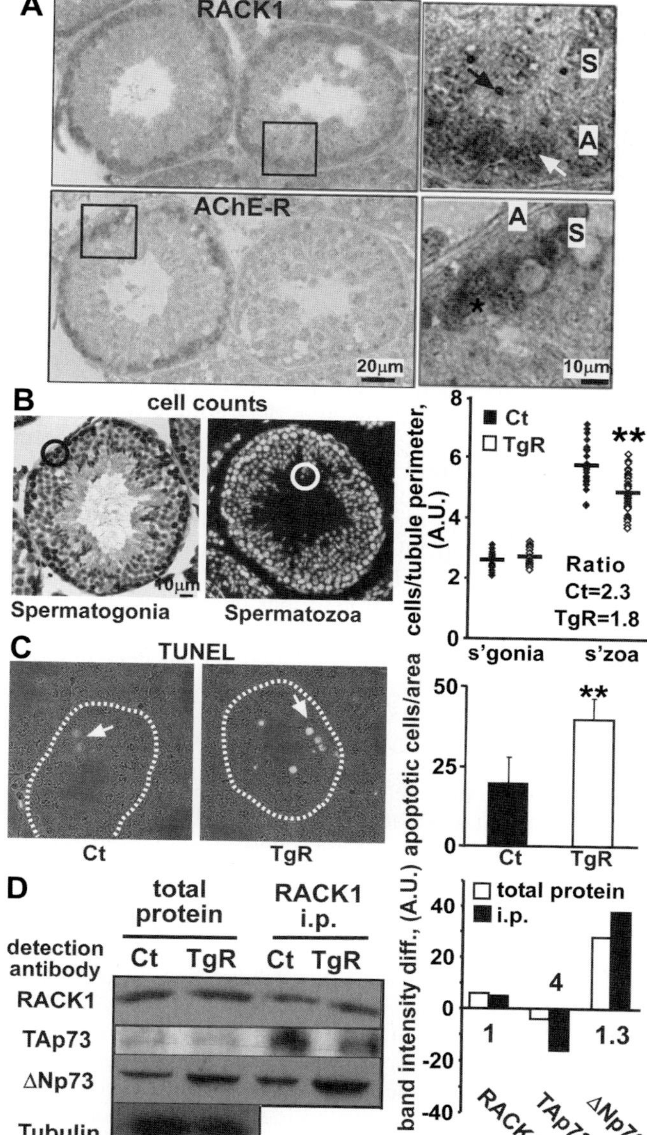

FIGURE 66.3 Apoptosis of meiotic spermatocytes under AChE-R/RACK1 displacement of TAp73. (A) AChE-R and RACK1 co-expression in meiotic spermatocytes of AChE-R transgenic (TgR) mice. Immunostaining in consecutive testicular sections of adult mice. RACK1 is expressed in spermatogonia (A, white arrow), which lack AChE-R, and forms foci in meiotic spermatocytes (S, black arrow), which express AChE-R with both focal (*) and diffuse localization. Squares mark areas of higher magnification. (B) Reduced sperm production in TgR mice engineered to express human AChE-R. Numbers of spermatogonia immunostained by proliferating cell nuclear antigen (PCNA) and DAPI-stained spermatozoa (circles) were normalized per tubule perimeter (arbitrary units, AU; 10 random tubules per animal, 2–4 animals per group). A significant decline in testicular spermatozoa counts occurred in TgR mice as compared to controls (C, $^{**}p<0.001$, Student's *t*-test). Ratio of spermatozoa to spermatogonia counts is presented. (C) Elevated apoptosis in pups of TgR mice. Shown are average numbers of TUNEL-stained cells normalized per tissue area (±SEM) in testicular sections from 20-day old pups, when spermatocytes are the main population in the seminiferous tubule (2–4 sections per mouse, 3 mice per strain, 2 independent experiments). Representative tubules from control and transgenic tissues, arrows mark stained cells (**–$p<0.001$, Student's t-test). (D) Reduced RACK1/TAp73 complexes in 20-day-old TgR pups. Pooled testicular homogenates from 3 TgR or control (Ct) pups were precipitated with anti-RACK1 polyclonal antibody. Homogenates (total protein) and precipitates (RACK1 i.p.) were electroblotted with noted detection antibodies. Bar graph presents the ratio between band intensity of TgR and control samples. Numbers note fold difference. (From Mor *et al.*, 2008b.)

cytometry for the presence of AChE-R, samples from fertile men showed higher percentage of AChE-R-positive cells in the highly motile subpopulation compared with low motility fraction. Patients with unexplained male factor infertility differed from fertile men in that the proportion of AChE-R positive cells was unaltered in all sperm subpopulations and therefore did not correlate with sperm motility. Additionally, highly motile donors' sperm showed higher a proportion of AChE-R positive cells than in patients. Results from human sperm samples and from mouse models suggest that AChE-R expression in early stages of spermatogenesis, as well as its subcellular distribution in mature sperm cells, are related to sperm quality and therefore fertility.

Correspondingly, we wished to find out if indeed changes in AChE-R expression in differentiating germ cells following stress have a causative role in determining sperm quality. Like many other proteins, AChE-R does not operate on its own but rather interacts with other partner proteins (Meshorer and Soreq, 2006). The scaffold protein RACK1 interacts with AChE-R through the C-terminus unique to this AChE isoform (Birikh *et al.*, 2003; Sklan *et al.*, 2006). Both proteins are expressed in spermatocytes (Mor *et al.*, 2008b) (Figure 66.3A). Another protein that interacts with RACK1 is the transcription factor p73 which binds RACK1 through its C-terminus (Ozaki *et al.*, 2003). RACK1 has been demonstrated to negatively regulate p73 function, and translocation of p73 to the nucleus induces apoptosis (Ozaki *et al.*, 2003). In the presence of AChE-R p73 is displaced from RACK1 (Figure 66.3D) (Mor *et al.*, 2008a,b), which would allow to it to translocate to the nucleus. Thus, the detrimental effects of cellular stress on spermatogenesis could be mediated, at least in part by elevation in AChE-R levels which would lead to increased apoptosis (Figure 66.3C).

Sperm cells rely on glycolysis as an energy source to maintain motility (Miki *et al.*, 2004; Storey, 2008). Intriguingly, AChE-R's effects on sperm motility could be mediated through its interaction with the glycolytic enzyme enolase. AChE-R binds enolase and elevates its activity (Mor *et al.*, 2008b). Moreover, sperm cells from AChE-R overexpressing transgenic mice show increased ATP levels (Mor *et al.*, 2008b). Interestingly, transgenic mice show higher proportion of sperm cells with hyperactivated motility, reminiscent of the elevated percentage of AChE-R positive cells in the highly motile subpopulation in human sperm samples.

Changes in AChE-R levels induced by stress could therefore have multifaceted effects on sperm production and function. AChE-R elevation during early stages of spermatogenesis can induce apoptosis, leading to reduced cell counts while modulating motility in surviving sperm by enhancing glycolysis (Figure 66.4).

Because of the dynamic nature of the sperm differentiation process, there could be a wide range of detrimental consequences and levels of severity as a result of exposure to various stressful assaults. Spermatogenic cells at different stages of differentiation display different sensitivities and this can result in different effects on the fertility outcome. This stems from the different molecular processes that occur in the cells as they differentiate, and from their interaction with the supporting somatic cells, which also respond to stressful stimuli. Therefore, the toxicity of physiological and psychological stressors, which results from the molecular processes they elicit, should be considered also in the context of its timing in relation to the cellular stage. Moreover, even when spermatogenesis in itself is complete, exposure to stress can affect the fully mature sperm possibly directly and also indirectly by inducing changes in the luminal fluid. An additional level of complexity exists since molecular events occurring during earlier stages of differentiation could have detectable consequences only in mature sperm cells.

AChE-R modulates the toxicological consequences of chemotherapy

Cis-platinum is a widely used chemotherapeutic agent, employed in the treatment of many cancer types including testicular and ovarian cancer. cis-Platinum induces apoptosis and necrosis by causing DNA damage (Wang and Lippard, 2005). Cholinergic proteins have been demonstrated to participate in the cellular response to cis-platinum and can modify its outcome.

In cell lines derived from non-small cell lung cancer, activation of the nicotinic receptor protects cells from apoptosis induced by cis-platinum (Dasgupta *et al.*, 2006). Nicotine mediates the activation of Akt signal transduction (West *et al.*, 2003) and induces changes in gene transcription which confer resistance to the cytotoxic effect of cis platinum (Dasgupta *et al.*, 2006).

As a general participant in the cellular stress response, AChE is also involved in modulating the toxicity of cis-platinum. Ectopic expression of AChE-R in cultured CHO cells confers greater resistance to cis-platinum as determined by measuring cell viability under increasing cis-platinum concentrations (Mor *et al.*, 2008a). Interestingly, ectopic expression of the synaptic AChE isoform, AChE-S, could not protect the cells (Mor *et al.*, 2008a), testifying to the unique function of the R variant. The effect of AChE-R in transformed cells could be mediated by the displacement of p73 from RACK and the consequence to cell fate would depend on the variant of p73 expressed in the cells. Transcription of the p73 gene

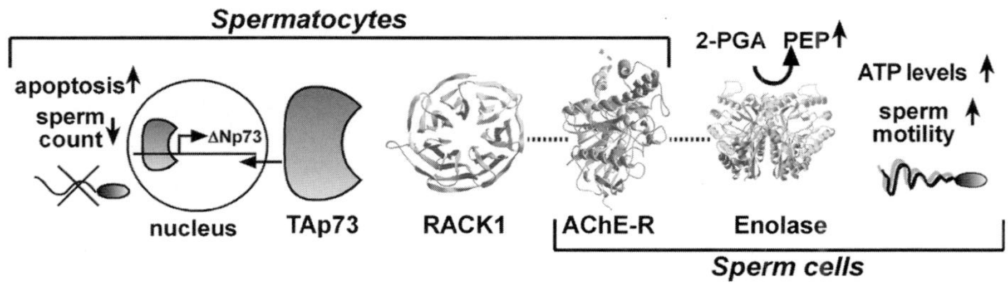

FIGURE 66.4 AChE-R interactions confer dual effect on sperm cells. In meiotic spermatocytes, elevated levels of AChE-R displace p73 from RACK1, resulting in spermatocyte apoptosis and reduced sperm production. In sperm, interaction with AChE-R increases enolase activity and glycolytic activity, which leads to elevated motility. (From Mor *et al.*, 2008b.)

initiates from two alternative promoters, yielding two p73 isoforms: the full length, transcriptionally active protein (TAp73), and the N-terminally truncated dominant negative protein (ΔNp73) which interferes with TAp73 transcriptional activity (Deyoung and Ellisen, 2007). As RACK1 inactivates p73 by binding its C-terminal region, this interaction should be equally available for both p73 variants. Tumor cells are characterized by elevation of the anti-apoptotic ΔNp73 (Coates, 2006; Deyoung and Ellisen, 2007). Also, elevation in ΔNp73 levels has been correlated with increased resistance to cis-platinum treatment in ovarian cancers (Concin *et al.*, 2005). Indeed, AChE-R expressing cells present elevated levels of ΔNp73, explaining their increased resistance to cis-platinum (Mor *et al.*, 2008a). Thus, AChE can modulate the cytotoxicity of cis-platinum by affecting complex molecular pathways.

CONCLUDING REMARKS AND FUTURE DIRECTIONS

Data accumulated over many decades allude to the important role of cholinergic molecules as regulators of different aspects of male fertility. Correspondingly, poisons affecting these molecules cause male infertility. The prominent nature of these effects probably stems from the wide variety of functions played by cholinergic proteins in the male reproductive system, covering spermatogenesis, sperm quality, function of the supporting somatic cells and monitoring the innervation required for sperm transport through the duct system. Thus, factors that dysregulate cholinergic proteins may have potentially complex detrimental consequences to male fertility. Such factors could be environmental, cholinergic toxins, therapeutic (e.g., chemotherapeutic drugs) or even originate from brain-to-body communication such as the physiological stress response. Understanding the complex role of the different cholinergic proteins in regulating male fertility also raises the possibility of using them as biomarkers in male infertility cases, many of which are currently labeled "'unexplained".

Yet, more specifically, overexpression of the AChE-R variant is characteristic of the cellular stress response in the male reproductive system and modulates cell metabolism as well as resistance to chemotherapeutic drugs. This offers a novel reporter for studying the yet incompletely understood connection between stress and cancer. Moreover, being at the crossroads of stress response and cancerous transformation makes targeting of AChE-R (e.g., by synthetic oligonucleotides; Argov *et al.*, 2007; Brenner *et al.*, 2003) a very tempting possibility as it could efficiently affect the detrimental outcomes of both.

REFERENCES

Almeida SA, Petenusci SO, Anselmo-Franci JA, Rosa-e-Silva AA, Lamano-Carvalho TL (1998) Decreased spermatogenic and androgenic testicular functions in adult rats submitted to immobilization-induced stress from prepuberty. *Braz J Med Biol Res* **31:** 1443–8.

Argov Z, McKee D, Agus S, Brawer S, Shlomowitz N, Yoseph OB, Soreq H, Sussman JD (2007) Treatment of human myasthenia gravis with oral antisense suppression of acetylcholinesterase. *Neurology* **69:** 699–700.

Avellar MC, Siu ER, Yasuhara F, Marostica E, Porto CS (2010) Muscarinic acetylcholine receptor subtypes in the male reproductive tract: expression and function in rat efferent ductules and epididymis. *J Mol Neurosci* **40:** 127–34.

Bigbee JW, Sharma KV, Chan EL, Bogler O (2000) Evidence for the direct role of acetylcholinesterase in neurite outgrowth in primary dorsal root ganglion neurons. *Brain Res* **861:** 354–62.

Bigelow PL, Jarrell J, Young MR, Keefe TJ, Love EJ (1998) Association of semen quality and occupational factors: comparison of case–control analysis and analysis of continuous variables. *Fertil Steril* **69:** 11–18.

Birikh KR, Sklan EH, Shoham S, Soreq H (2003) Interaction of "readthrough" acetylcholinesterase with RACK1 and PKCbeta II correlates with intensified fear-induced conflict behavior. *Proc Natl Acad Sci USA* **100:** 283–88.

Borges MO, Abreu ML, Porto CS, Avellar MC (2001) Characterization of muscarinic acetylcholine receptor in rat Sertoli cells. *Endocrinology* **142:** 4701–10.

Brenner T, Hamra-Amitay Y, Evron T, Boneva N, Seidman S, Soreq H (2003) The role of readthrough acetylcholinesterase in the pathophysiology of myasthenia gravis. *FASEB J* **17:** 214–22.

Chakraborty J, Nelson L (1976) Comparative study of cholinesterases distribution in the spermatozoa of some mammalian species. *Biol Reprod* **15:** 579–85.

Chan RY, Adatia FA, Krupa AM, Jasmin BJ (1998) Increased expression of acetylcholinesterase T and R transcripts during hematopoietic differentiation is accompanied by parallel elevations in the levels of their respective molecular forms. *J Biol Chem* **273:** 9727–33.

Choudhary N, Goyal R, Joshi SC (2008) Effect of malathion on reproductive system of male rats. *J Environ Biol* **29:** 259–62.

Clarke RN, Klock SC, Geoghegan A, Travassos DE (1999) Relationship between psychological stress and semen quality among in-vitro fertilization patients. *Hum Reprod* **14:** 753–8.

Coates PJ (2006) Regulating p73 isoforms in human tumours. *J Pathol* **210:** 385–9.

Concin N, Hofstetter G, Berger A, Gehmacher A, Reimer D, Watrowski R, Tong D, Schuster E, Hefler L, Heim K, *et al.* (2005) Clinical relevance of dominant-negative p73 isoforms for responsiveness to chemotherapy and survival in ovarian cancer: evidence for a crucial p53–p73 cross-talk in vivo. *Clin Cancer Res* **11:** 8372–83.

Dasgupta P, Kinkade R, Joshi B, Decook C, Haura E, Chellappan S (2006) Nicotine inhibits apoptosis induced by chemotherapeutic drugs by up-regulating XIAP and survivin. *Proc Natl Acad Sci USA* **103:** 6332–7.

Day T, Greenfield SA (2002) A non-cholinergic, trophic action of acetylcholinesterase on hippocampal neurones in vitro: molecular mechanisms. *Neuroscience* **111:** 649–56.

Deyoung MP, Ellisen LW (2007) p63 and p73 in human cancer: defining the network. *Oncogene* **26:** 5169–83.

Dong Q, Salva A, Sottas CM, Niu E, Holmes M, Hardy MP (2004) Rapid glucocorticoid mediation of suppressed testosterone biosynthesis in male mice subjected to immobilization stress. *J Androl* **25:** 973–81.

Dori A, Cohen J, Silverman WF, Pollack Y, Soreq H (2005) Functional manipulations of acetylcholinesterase splice variants highlight alternative splicing contributions to murine neocortical development. *Cereb Cortex* **15:** 419–30.

Dwivedi C, Long NJ (1989) Effect of cholinergic agents on human spermatozoa motility. *Biochem Med Metab Biol* **42:** 66–70.

Egbunike GN (1980) Changes in acetylcholinesterase activity of mammalian spermatozoa during maturation. *Int J Androl* **3:** 459–68.

Eskiocak S, Gozen AS, Yapar SB, Tavas F, Kilic AS, Eskiocak M (2005) Glutathione and free sulphydryl content of seminal plasma in healthy medical students during and after exam stress. *Hum Reprod* **20:** 2595–600.

Favaretto AL, Valenca MM, Picanco-Diniz DL, Antunes-Rodrigues JA (1993) Inhibitory role of cholinergic agonists on testosterone secretion by purified rat Leydig cells. *Arch Int Physiol Biochim Biophys* **101:** 333–5.

Ge RS, Dong Q, Sottas CM, Chen H, Zirkin BR, Hardy MP (2005) Gene expression in rat Leydig cells during development from the progenitor to adult stage: a cluster analysis. *Biol Reprod* **72:** 1405–15.

Genuth SM (2004) The reproductive glands. In *Physiology* (Levy MN, Berne RM, Koeppen BM, Stanton BA, eds.). St. Louis, Mosby.

Giblin PT, Poland ML, Moghissi KS, Ager JW, Olson JM (1988) Effects of stress and characteristic adaptability on semen quality in healthy men. *Fertil Steril* **49:** 127–32.

Gilboa-Geffen A, Lacoste PP, Soreq L, Cizeron-Clairac G, Le Panse R, Truffault F, Shaked I, Soreq H, Berrih-Aknin S (2007) The thymic theme of acetylcholinesterase splice variants in myasthenia gravis. *Blood* **109:** 4383–91.

Grisaru D, Pick M, Perry C, Sklan EH, Almog R, Goldberg I, Naparstek E, Lessing JB, Soreq H, Deutsch V (2006) Hydrolytic and nonenzymatic functions of acetylcholinesterase comodulate hemopoietic stress responses. *J Immunol* **176:** 27–35.

Harlow CR, Fahy UM, Talbot WM, Wardle PG, Hull MG (1996) Stress and stress-related hormones during in-vitro fertilization treatment. *Hum Reprod* **11:** 274–9.

Jeong KH, Jacobson L, Widmaier EP, Majzoub JA (1999) Normal suppression of the reproductive axis following stress in corticotropin-releasing hormone-deficient mice. *Endocrinology* **140:** 1702–8.

Johnson G, Moore SW (2004) Identification of a structural site on acetylcholinesterase that promotes neurite outgrowth and binds laminin-1 and collagen IV. *Biochem Biophys Res Commun* **319:** 448–55.

Joshi SC, Mathur R, Gulati N (2007) Testicular toxicity of chlorpyrifos (an organophosphate pesticide) in albino rat. *Toxicol Ind Health* **23:** 439–44.

Kaplan N, Morpurgo N, Linial M (2007) Novel families of toxin-like peptides in insects and mammals: a computational approach. *J Mol Biol* **369:** 553–66.

Kaufer D, Friedman A, Seidman S, Soreq H (1998) Acute stress facilitates long-lasting changes in cholinergic gene expression. *Nature* **393:** 373–7.

Kirby ED, Geraghty AC, Ubuka T, Bentley GE, Kaufer D (2009) Stress increases putative gonadotropin inhibitory hormone and decreases luteinizing hormone in male rats. *Proc Natl Acad Sci USA* **106:** 11324–9.

Kumar P, Meizel S (2005) Nicotinic acetylcholine receptor subunits and associated proteins in human sperm. *J Biol Chem* **280:** 25928–35.

Levitin F, Weiss M, Hahn Y, Stern O, Papke RL, Matusik R, Nandana SR, Ziv R, Pichinuk E, Salame S, *et al.* (2008) PATE gene clusters code for multiple, secreted TFP/Ly-6/uPAR proteins that are expressed in reproductive and neuron-rich tissues and possess neuromodulatory activity. *J Biol Chem* **283:** 16928–39.

Lizama C, Lagos CF, Lagos-Cabre R., Cantuarias L, Rivera F, Huenchunir P, Perez-Acle T, Carrion F, Moreno RD (2009) Calpain inhibitors prevent p38 MAPK activation and germ cell apoptosis after heat stress in pubertal rat testes. *J Cell Physiol* **221:** 296–305.

Lucas TF, Avellar MC, Porto CS (2004) Effects of carbachol on rat Sertoli cell proliferation and muscarinic acetylcholine receptors regulation: an in vitro study. *Life Sci* **75:** 1761–73.

Lue YH, Hikim AP, Swerdloff RS, Im P, Taing KS, Bui T, Leung A, Wang C (1999) Single exposure to heat induces stage-specific germ cell apoptosis in rats: role of intratesticular testosterone on stage specificity. *Endocrinology* **140:** 1709–17.

McEwen BS (1998) Protective and damaging effects of stress mediators. *N Engl J Med* **338:** 171–9.

Meshorer E, Soreq H (2006) Virtues and woes of AChE alternative splicing in stress-related neuropathologies. *Trends Neurosci* **29:** 216–24.

Meshorer E, Toiber D, Zurel D, Sahly I, Dori A, Cagnano E, Schreiber L, Grisaru D, Tronche F, Soreq H (2004) Combinatorial complexity of 5′ alternative acetylcholinesterase transcripts and protein products. *J Biol Chem* **279:** 29740–51.

Miki K, Qu W, Goulding EH, Willis WD, Bunch DO, Strader LF, Perreault SD, Eddy EM, O'Brien DA (2004) Glyceraldehyde 3-phosphate dehydrogenase-S, a sperm-specific glycolytic enzyme, is required for sperm motility and male fertility. *Proc Natl Acad Sci USA* **101:** 16501–6.

Mor I, Bruck T, Greenberg D, Berson A, Schreiber L, Grisaru D, Soreq H (2008a) Alternate AChE-R variants facilitate cellular metabolic activity and resistance to genotoxic stress through enolase and RACK1 interactions. *Chem Biol Interact* **175:** 11–21.

Mor I, Grisaru D, Titelbaum L, Evron T, Richler C, Wahrman J, Sternfeld M, Yogev L, Meiri N, Seidman S, Soreq H (2001) Modified testicular expression of stress-associated "readthrough" acetylcholinesterase predicts male infertility. *FASEB J* **15:** 2039–41.

Mor I, Sklan EH, Podoly E, Pick M, Kirschner M, Yogev L, Bar-Sheshet Itach S, Schreiber L, Geyer B, Mor T, *et al.* (2008b) Acetylcholinesterase-R increases germ cell apoptosis but enhances sperm motility. *J Cell Mol Med* **12:** 479–95.

Negro-Vilar A (1993) Stress and other environmental factors affecting fertility in men and women: overview. *Environ Health Perspect* **101 (Suppl. 2):** 59–64.

Ozaki T, Watanabe K, Nakagawa T, Miyazaki K, Takahashi M, Nakagawara A (2003) Function of p73, not of p53, is inhibited by the physical interaction with RACK1 and its inhibitory effect is counteracted by pRB. *Oncogene* **22:** 3231–42.

Palmero S, Bardi G, Coniglio L, Falugi C (1999) Presence and localization of molecules related to the cholinergic system in developing rat testis. *Eur J Histochem* **43:** 277–83.

Paul C, Murray AA, Spears N, Saunders PT (2008) A single, mild, transient scrotal heat stress causes DNA damage, subfertility and impairs formation of blastocysts in mice. *Reproduction* **136:** 73–84.

Paul C, Teng S, Saunders PT (2009) A single, mild, transient scrotal heat stress causes hypoxia and oxidative stress in mouse testes, which induces germ cell death. *Biol Reprod* **80:** 913–19.

Perez-Crespo M, Pintado B, Gutierrez-Adan A (2008) Scrotal heat stress effects on sperm viability, sperm DNA integrity, and the offspring sex ratio in mice. *Mol Reprod Dev* **75:** 40–7.

Pick M, Perry C, Lapidot T, Guimaraes-Sternberg C, Naparstek E, Deutsch V, Soreq H (2006) Stress-induced cholinergic signaling promotes inflammation-associated thrombopoiesis. *Blood* **107:** 3397–406.

Rivier C, Vale W (1985) Effect of the long-term administration of corticotropin-releasing factor on the pituitary–adrenal and pituitary–gonadal axis in the male rat. *J Clin Invest* **75:** 689–94.

Said TM (2008) Emotional stress and male infertility. *Indian J Med Res* **128:** 228–30.

Sapolsky RM, Romero LM, Munck AU (2000) How do glucocorticoids influence stress responses? Integrating permissive, suppressive, stimulatory, and preparative actions. *Endocr Rev* **21:** 55–89.

Sasagawa I, Yazawa H, Suzuki Y, Nakada T (2001) Stress and testicular germ cell apoptosis. *Arch Androl* **47:** 211–16.

Shaked I, Meerson A, Wolf Y, Avni R, Greenberg D, Gilboa-Geffen A, Soreq H (2009) MicroRNA-132 potentiates cholinergic anti-inflammatory signaling by targeting acetylcholinesterase. *Immunity* **31:** 965–73.

Shaked I, Zimmerman G, Soreq H (2008) Stress-induced alternative splicing modulations in brain and periphery: acetylcholinesterase as a case study. *Ann NY Acad Sci* **1148:** 269–81.

Sklan EH, Podoly E, Soreq H (2006) RACK1 has the nerve to act: structure meets function in the nervous system. *Prog Neurobiol* **78:** 117–34.

Son JH, Meizel S (2003) Evidence suggesting that the mouse sperm acrosome reaction initiated by the zona pellucida involves an alpha7 nicotinic acetylcholine receptor. *Biol Reprod* **68:** 1348–53.

Soreq H, Seidman S (2001) Acetylcholinesterase – new roles for an old actor. *Nat Rev Neurosci* **2:** 294–302.

Storey BT (2008) Mammalian sperm metabolism: oxygen and sugar, friend and foe. *Int J Dev Biol* **52:** 427–37.

Taylor P (1996) Agents acting at the neuromuscular junction and autonomic ganglia. In *Goodman and Gilman's The Pharmacological Basis of Therapeutics* (Hardman JG, Limbird LE, Molinoff PB, Ruddon RW, eds.). New York, McGraw-Hill, pp. 177–97.

Toiber D, Berson A, Greenberg D, Melamed-Book N, Diamant S, Soreq H (2008) N-acetylcholinesterase-induced apoptosis in Alzheimer's disease. *PLoS One* **3:** e3108.

Toiber D, Greenberg DS, Soreq H (2009) Pro-apoptotic protein–protein interactions of the extended N-AChE terminus. *J Neural Transm* **116:** 1435–42.

Turner TT, Lysiak JJ (2008) Oxidative stress: a common factor in testicular dysfunction. *J Androl* **29:** 488–98.

Verma R, Mohanty B (2009) Early-life exposure to dimethoate-induced reproductive toxicity: evaluation of effects on pituitary–testicular axis of mice. *Toxicol Sci* **112:** 450–8.

Wang D, Lippard SJ (2005) Cellular processing of platinum anticancer drugs. *Nat Rev Drug Discov* **4:** 307–20.

West KA, Brognard J, Clark AS, Linnoila IR, Yang X, Swain SM, Harris C, Belinsky S, Dennis PA (2003) Rapid Akt activation by nicotine and a tobacco carcinogen modulates the phenotype of normal human airway epithelial cells. *J Clin Invest* **111:** 81–90.

Yazawa H, Sasagawa I, Ishigooka M, Nakada T (1999) Effect of immobilization stress on testicular germ cell apoptosis in rats. *Hum Reprod* 14: 1806–10.

Zimmerman G, Soreq H (2006) Readthrough acetylcholinesterase: a multifaceted inducer of stress reactions. *J Mol Neurosci* **30:** 197–200.

Zorn B, Auger J, Velikonja V, Kolbezen M, Meden-Vrtovec H (2008) Psychological factors in male partners of infertile couples: relationship with semen quality and early miscarriage. *Int J Androl* **31:** 557–64.

Section 12

Endocrine Disruption, Mutagenicity, Carcinogenicity, Infertility and Teratogenicity

CHAPTER

67

Endocrine disruptors

Timothy J. Evans

INTRODUCTION

The relevant and controversial nature of the topic

At the time of the publication of this text, endocrine disruption and its varying connotations are some of the most relevant and contentious topics in environmental science, reproductive and developmental toxicology and endocrinology. Many of the xenobiotics (exogenous chemicals) involved are ubiquitous in the environment and/or have very important roles in agriculture, industry and human health. Wildlife populations, particularly those living in aquatic environments, are usually the first animal species to exhibit adverse xenobiotic-associated effects on reproductive function. Chemical exposures have also been associated with various neoplasias which can affect humans, including those of the breast, uterus, cervix and prostate, as well as birth defects in children, declining sperm numbers in men, endometriosis in women and increasing obesity within the general population. However, interpretations of the experimental data are subject to considerable debate and differences of opinion. Some experimental results have not been reproducible, and others appear to be dependent on the species and strain of animal model being used, as well as the tissue and endpoint being evaluated. Because of the number and volume of chemicals of concern and the importance of environmental and health issues involved, these inconsistencies have resulted in a concerted effort by scientists and health professionals and the expenditure of millions of dollars by government and industry to clarify these issues, especially as they apply to human health.

Some of the information discussed in this chapter will be dealt with in greater detail in other portions of this book. The purpose of this chapter is to define important terms and introduce the reader to key concepts and processes associated with endocrine disruption. The breadth of this subject matter and the risks posed to wildlife populations, domestic animals and humans are in continual flux, especially at the present time. An effort will be made to present this information in a balanced manner and to clearly point out areas where controversies exist and how those might be resolved.

The susceptibility of reproductive processes to "disruption"

The physiological processes, associated behaviors and anatomical structures involved in reproduction in humans and other vertebrates (Figure 67.1) begin with gametogenesis at the time of puberty and sexual maturity and have the immediate, short-term goals of zygote formation and normal embryonic and fetal development (Evans, 2007; Senger, 2003). This integrated system involving at least three separate organisms culminates in the "birth" of a single or multiple offspring, which have the potential to eventually participate in the reproductive process and species survival. In humans, as well as other mammalian species, the initiation and maintenance of lactation for the postpartum nutrition of offspring is also a critical aspect of reproduction (Evans, 2007).

As described in Chapter 2, normal reproduction and development require signaling within and between diverse organs. In sexual reproduction and mammalian pregnancy and parturition, critical communication even takes place between distinctly different organisms (i.e., male and female and mother and offspring, respectively). The dependency of reproductive function on signaling pathways inclusive of gene transcription makes this process especially prone to adverse effects associated with xenobiotic-induced interference with or "disruption" of within-cell, cell-to-cell, organ-to-organ and/or even animal-to-animal communication (Evans, 2007). As scientists continue to investigate the effects of xenobiotics on biological systems, the paradigm of endocrine disruption will continue to "shift", requiring those individuals with any involvement in this area to "step out of the box" and discuss endocrine disruption in a broader context in order to participate in scientific discussions, to design future experiments and/or to make informed, medical or policy decisions based on "good" science (Evans, 2007; Guillette, 2006; McLachlan, 2001).

Reproductive and Developmental Toxicology, Edited by Ramesh C. Gupta
ISBN: 978-0-12-382032-7

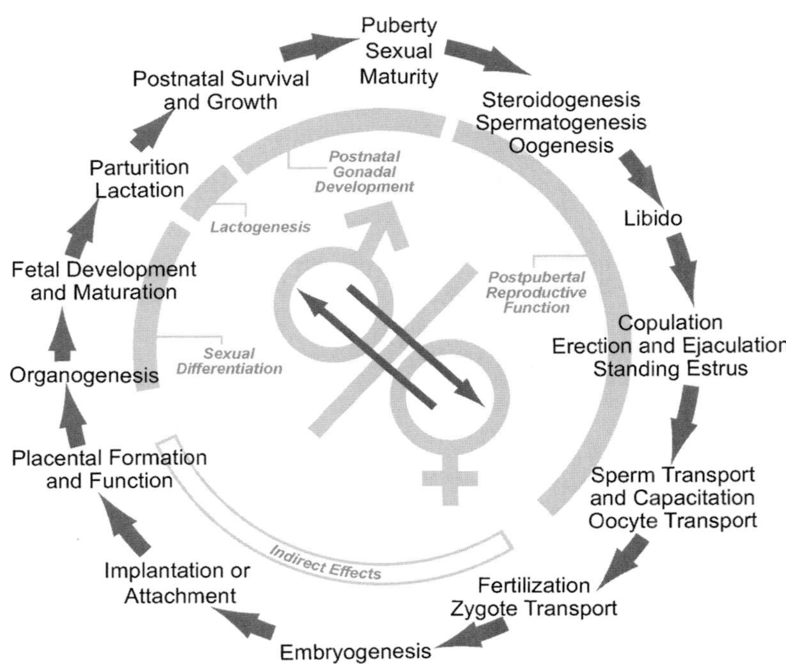

FIGURE 67.1 The continuum of developmental stages and reproductive functions taking place in males and/or females is shown schematically in the outer circle and illustrate the complexity of reproduction in mammalian species, especially in humans, where additional behavioral, psychological, social and environmental factors, as well as eventual senescence (not shown), come into play. The inner gray arcs depict some of specific developmental processes and reproductive functions likely to be directly impacted by mammalian exposures to endocrine-disrupting xenobiotics. Prenatal exposures not only have the potential to affect sexual differentiation, but exposures during this stage of development, particularly if there are associated structural and/or functional abnormalities, can also impact postnatal gonadal development and puberty, as well as postpubertal reproductive function and associated processes. Postnatal/prepubertal exposures can delay puberty, as well as adversely affect reproductive function after the onset of sexual maturity. Postpubertal exposures of non-pregnant animals to endocrine disruptors will most often only directly impact adult reproductive function, although indirect effects (white arc) might be noted on reproduction endpoints, such as fertilization or conception rates, as well as embryogenesis and establishment of pregnancy. Lactogenesis is a reproductive function unique to mammals, and ergot alkaloids suppress the release of prolactin by the anterior pituitary. The arrows in the center demonstrate the potential for masculinization of females and androgynization of males, which might even be progress to sex reversal, especially in wildlife species. This figure was adapted, with permission, from Evans (2007) (modifications and artwork courtesy of Don Connor).

DEFINITIONS AND IMPORTANT CONCEPTS

Hormones and endocrine function

Hormones and hormone receptors play key roles in the aforementioned, reproduction-associated mechanisms for signaling/communication. As described previously in Chapter 2, the term "hormone" traditionally refers to a substance which is secreted into the circulation by a ductless gland and is transported in the circulation to the site or sites where it alters the function of target cells (Evans, 2007; Hodgson *et al.*, 2000). This traditional aspect of hormone action involves organ-to-organ signaling or, even, animal-to-animal signaling, in the case of mammalian pregnancy and parturition, and is specifically described by the term "endocrine". However, it is also recognized that hormones can be involved in "paracrine" and "autocrine" (i.e., cell-to-cell and within-cell, respectively) signaling pathways (Evans, 2007). For the purposes of this chapter, the term "endocrine" will be used very broadly to encompass all aspects of hormone function.

Hormone receptors

The actions of hormones on their targets are frequently mediated through receptors that initiate or inhibit some sort of signal transduction pathway or are required for hormone-induced alterations in gene expression. Hormone–receptor interactions can be modulated by a number of factors, including the amount of hormone present, the affinity of the hormone for the receptor, receptor density and occupancy and interaction with other hormones, receptors and hormone–receptor complexes, as well as a variety of endogenous co-activators and inhibitors (Bigsby *et al.*, 2005; Evans, 2007). It should be clear by the end of this chapter that various xenobiotics are also capable, under certain exposure conditions, of modulating the interactions between endogenous hormones and their receptors. The primary gonadal steroids – i.e., androgens and estrogens (some references also include progesterone) – are referred to as the "sex" steroids, and the imitation and/or inhibition of the actions of these hormones by xenobiotics is what was first referred to as "endocrine disruption" (Krimsky, 2000; McLachlan, 2001). The gonadal steroids interact with receptors which are members of the steroid/thyroid ("nuclear") receptor superfamily, the largest family of transcription factors in eukaryotic systems. While these receptors are often thought of as being exclusively nuclear in their location, they can also be located in the cytoplasm of some cells (Evans, 2007).

Endocrine disruption

"Endocrine disruption" is both a developing, multidisciplinary area of research, involving aspects of both toxicology and endocrinology (McLachlan, 2001), and a potential mechanism of action for many reproductive toxicants. It is critically important for one to carefully define the context in which "endocrine disruption" is being used in order to clearly and accurately discuss one's research findings or opinions with different types of scientists, health professionals, government officials, elected representatives, the popular press and/or the general public (McLachlan, 2001). "Endocrine disruption", as a mechanism of reproductive toxicity, has been defined in a variety of different ways, depending on the circumstances and the intended audience. Endocrine disruption can be defined fairly narrowly with respect to toxicant origin; source or site of toxicant exposure; xenobiotic mechanism of action; and/or the timing of exposure (Evans, 2007; Krimsky, 2000, 2001). While the imitation or inhibition of the actions of androgens or, especially, estrogens by xenobiotics is what was first referred to as "endocrine disruption". However, both the multidisciplinary area of study and the mechanism of xenobiotic action referred to as "endocrine disruption" have now evolved to encompass a wide range of specific mechanisms of action which can ultimately result in adverse effects on invertebrate and/or vertebrate animals (Evans, 2007; McLachlan, 2001; Rogers and Kavlock, 2008).

For the purposes of this chapter "endocrine disruption" will refer to the effects of any synthetic or naturally occurring xenobiotic which can affect the endocrine system of exposed individuals (i.e., the balance of normal hormonal functions) and cause exposure-related physiological alterations (Evans, 2007; Hodgson *et al.*, 2000; Keith, 1997; Rogers and Kavlock, 2008). This definition encompasses any exogenous agents or xenobiotics which interfere with the synthesis, release, transport, distribution, binding, actions, metabolism and/or elimination of endogenous hormones involved in homeostasis or the regulation of developmental processes. Within the broad scope of this definition, reproduction, including prenatal and prepubertal development, is one of the physiological functions most profoundly affected by chemicals capable of endocrine disruption. In fact, it could be argued that the majority of reproductive toxicants, depending on the level of exposure, can interfere with endocrine function in one way or another. However, adverse effects on other, not primarily "reproductive", endocrine systems (e.g., glucocorticoid and thyroid hormone systems) can also be associated with exposures to xenobiotics. These "non-reproductive" effects need to be taken into consideration as well when describing the endocrine disruption associated with exposure to a given chemical. In addition, it should be remembered that reproduction can be significantly impacted as the result of disruption of other endocrine systems (Evans, 2007; Guillette, 2006).

Endocrine-disrupting chemicals, endocrine disruptor and hormonally active agents

Any reproductive toxicant capable of endocrine disruption can be considered an "endocrine-disrupting chemical" ("EDC") or an "endocrine disruptor". Obviously, this includes a large number of xenobiotics which are used in commercially available industrial, agricultural and pharmaceutical products, as well as naturally occurring toxicants produced by plants and fungi. An effort will be made later in this chapter to discuss some of the xenobiotics most often associated with specific endocrine-disrupting mechanisms of action (Evans, 2007).

Another term frequently used with respect to endocrine disruption, especially regarding xenobiotics which interact with endogenous hormone receptors, is "hormonally active agent" or "HAA". "Endocrine-disrupting chemical", "endocrine disruptor" or "hormonally active agent" can often be used interchangeably to discuss the actions of a given xenobiotic (Evans, 2007). However, "endocrine-disrupting chemical" and "endocrine disruptor" generally have negative connotations and imply, by virtue of the inclusion of the term "disrupt", something "dangerous" and the likelihood of adverse or toxic effects. The term "hormonally active agent", on the other hand, is generally more benign and only indicates that a given xenobiotic has the potential to affect a hormonal pathway (Evans, 2007; Krimsky, 2001). As pointed out by Krimsky (2001), a mechanism rather than a specific pathology is inferred by "hormonally active", and "hormonally active agent" is the nomenclature preferred by the National Research Council (Evans, 2007), especially when referring to xenobiotics which interact with endogenous hormone receptors.

It should be remembered that the circumstances and intended audience often dictate the most appropriate terms used to describe xenobiotics suspected of having endocrine activity. "Environmental hormone" and "environmental signal" are examples of other terms which, along with "HAA", "EDC" and endocrine disruptor, have been used to describe xenobiotics capable of interacting with endogenous hormone receptors (McLachlan, 2001). However, the context in which these two terms have been used generally implies environmental contaminants with documented adverse endocrine effects on animal populations or humans (Evans, 2007). In some instances, the term "HAA" might be more "politically correct" (Krimsky, 2001) than "EDC", "endocrine disruptor", "environmental hormone" or "environmental signal" when discussing chemicals with a suspected hormonal activity that has not been proven to be clearly associated with adverse effects on animals in a research and/or clinical setting (Evans, 2007).

Dose and dosage

The terms "dose" and "dosage" are often used interchangeably, and this appears to be particularly true when referring to EDCs. "Dose" generally refers to the total amount of a xenobiotic to which an organism is exposed. "Dosage", on the other hand, in its strictest sense, specifically refers to the amount of a given xenobiotic expressed as some function of the organism and time (Hodgson *et al.*, 2000). An example of a xenobiotic dosage would be mg of xenobiotic per unit of body weight (i.e., kg), usually over a given time period, such as a day. The dosage of xenobiotic A for a 100 kg man, who received a "dose" of 450 mg of xenobiotic A once a day, would be 4.5 mg of xenobiotic A/kg body weight/day.

Route of exposure

The means by which a xenobiotic enters an organism can have a significant impact on which biological functions are affected by a given chemical exposure, as well as the severity of those xenobiotic-induced effects. Oral, respiratory and dermal routes of exposure are very common ways in which animals are "naturally" exposed to xenobiotics. Developing mammals can be exposed prenatally by transplacental diffusion or transport of xenobiotics which have been ingested, inhaled or absorbed through the skin by the mother. Mammalian neonates can also be exposed to chemicals excreted in the milk of their exposed mothers during lactation. Exogenous chemicals can enter the body by intravenous, subcutaneous or intramuscular routes (i.e., parenteral routes of exposure) when administered as part of a therapeutic regimen (Evans, 2006).

The route of exposure determines the bioavailability of a given exogenous chemical (e.g., oral < intramuscular < intravenous route of exposure) and whether a xenobiotic is immediately transported to the liver in the hepatic portal circulation following absorption in the gastrointestinal tract (i.e., oral exposure) or whether the compound initially bypasses the liver and gains entry to the systemic circulation via the other routes of exposure. Depending on the compound, xenobiotics which are transported initially to the liver following oral exposure can be detoxified (i.e., first-past effect), whereby the rest of the body sees very little of the active compound, or these chemicals can be bioactivated into an ultimate toxicant which is distributed throughout the organism (Evans, 2006).

MECHANISMS OF ENDOCRINE DISRUPTION

Critical windows of exposure to endocrine-disrupting chemicals

When discussing the mechanisms of endocrine disruption, it is important to take into consideration the specific reproductive developmental processes and/or reproductive functions which are occurring at the time of exposure. In general, it is these developmental and physiological activities which will most likely be targeted by that specific EDC exposure. However, there are several critical windows of exposure during the gestation and postnatal growth where reproductive development and/or function appear to be particularly susceptible to the adverse effects of endocrine disruption.

The susceptibility of embryonic and fetal development to endocrine disruption

The emphasis with respect to endocrine disruption in humans and one of the bases for the "Theory of Hormone Disrupting Chemicals" (THDC) or the "Environmental Endocrine Hypothesis" (Krimsky, 2000, 2001) has been concern about the enhanced effects of prenatal as compared to postnatal exposures to suspected endocrine disruptors. It is clear from the feminizing effects of prenatal exposures to diethylstilbestrol (DES) (McLachlan, 2001; Newbold *et al.*, 2006) and observations of androgynization in wildlife species (Edwards *et al.*, 2006), that the male fetus is much more sensitive to the adverse effects of endocrine disruptors than male animals during the postnatal period (Hess and Iguchi, 2002). It is also important to remember that both female and even male fetuses have important estrogenic signaling pathways necessary for normal reproductive development and function, which are susceptible to disruption by xenobiotics (Evans, 2007; Hess, 2003). The embryo and fetus, without a developed blood–brain barrier and with only rudimentary DNA repair mechanisms, as well as suboptimal hepatic detoxifying and metabolizing capabilities, are generally considered to be more susceptible to the adverse effects of low-level exposures to xenobiotics than adults (Newbold *et al.*, 2006). It is well understood that there are critical periods of susceptibility of the fetus to the development of specific xenobiotic-induced abnormalities, many of which have an endocrine component (Rogers and Kavlock, 2008). Previous discussions in Chapter 2 describe some the important organizational and formative events taking place during gestation, including those associated with gonadal and phenotypic sexual differentiation. Figure 67.1 illustrates the various components of this cascade of developmental events which might be potentially susceptible to subtle alterations in the normal endocrine milieu (Evans, 2007).

The susceptibility of pre- and peripubertal reproductive development to endocrine disruption

There are important aspects of sexual development and differentiation of sexual behaviors which take place during the postnatal period, even in humans and large domestic mammals (Figure 67.1). The postnatal proliferation of Sertoli cells and Leydig cells, which take place in some mammals, both represent potential targets for endocrine-disrupting xenobiotics. Likewise, early postnatal exposures to estrogenic compounds have been reported to alter the glandular architecture of the uterus, as well as the prostate (Tarleton *et al.*, 2001). While puberty is often described simply in terms of a single, initial reproductive event (e.g., first estrus, ovulation or ejaculation), the attainment of reproductive competency is actually a process which is also very susceptible to the effects of reproductive toxicants. Xenobiotics can interfere with important physiological and morphological transformations necessary for the normal stepwise progression towards reproductive competency. Prepubertal follicular development, as well as the acquisition of the preovulatory LH surge in the female, can both be impaired or delayed by irregularities in the neuroendocrine control or paracrine/autocrine regulation of these processes. Similarly, the transition in testicular estrogen synthesis from the Sertoli cell to the Leydig cell in the males of many species is also susceptible to the adverse effects of xenobiotics (Evans, 2007). Pre- or peripubertal exposure to hormonally active xenobiotics, such as anabolic steroids and antiandrogens, can interfere with postnatal reproductive development and function and can impair an animal's ability to reach its maximum reproductive potential (Evans, 2007).

The susceptibility of postpubertal reproductive function to endocrine disruption

In general, higher doses and longer durations of exposure are required for most EDCs, when comparing the effects of a particular EDC on postpubertal reproductive function to the effects of the same xenobiotic on early postnatal, peripubertal and, especially, prenatal development. As noted previously, the sexually mature animal has a fully developed blood–brain barrier, functional DNA repair mechanisms and adequate detoxifying and metabolizing capabilities within the liver, all of which can make adult animals more resistant to the adverse effects of xenobiotics (Newbold *et al.*, 2006). In males, the blood–testis barrier also becomes more functional as the animal matures and can protect developing germ cell precursors from a variety of xenobiotics.

However, saying that sexually mature animals are most likely more resistant to the effects of endocrine disruption is not the same as saying that adult animals are "immune" to the adverse effects of EDCs. Reproductive function in sexually mature males can potentially be adversely affected by exposures to nuclear estrogen receptor agonists or antagonists, as well as by estrogenic or antiestrogenic EDCs acting independently of receptor-mediated interactions. Follicular development, steroidogenesis, spermatogenesis, libido, erection, ejaculation and epididymal and accessory sex gland function (Figure 67.1), as well as other reproductive processes, are all potentially susceptible to the adverse effects of endocrine-disrupting xenobiotics (Evans, 2007). As shown in Figure 67.1, even sex reversal is possible in adult animals of species of fish and amphibians (Evans, 2007; Hayes *et al.*, 2010; Jobling *et al.*, 2007).

Specific mechanisms for endocrine disruption

Endocrine disruption encompasses a wide range of mechanisms of action which can ultimately result in adverse effects on individual animals or susceptible animal populations. As these mechanisms of action are discussed, it should be noted that some xenobiotics are capable of causing endocrine disruption by functioning as an endogenous hormone receptor ligand, as well as by mechanisms of action which are independent of the formation of a xenobiotic (ligand)–receptor complex. While some exogenous compounds are limited to adverse effects on one endocrine system, other xenobiotics are less discerning and have been associated with impaired function of multiple endocrine organs and/or networks (Evans, 2007; Swedenborg *et al.*, 2009).

"Classic" receptor-mediated endocrine disruption

"Classic" endocrine disruption can involve imitation or mimicry of the interactions between cellular receptors and endogenous hormones (i.e., receptor agonism) and/or a blockade or inhibition of the formation of receptor–hormone complexes (i.e., receptor antagonism) (McLachlan, 2001). With respect to gonadal steroids, both genomic (Warner and Gustaffson, 2006) and physiological responses can be affected by this mimicry or blockade of endogenous hormone receptor-mediated activity (Birkhoj *et al.*, 2004; Thomas and Khan, 2005). Xenobiotics which mimic the actions of endogenous androgens or estrogens (i.e., gonadal steroid receptor agonists) are referred to, respectively, as being either "xenoandrogens" or "xenoestrogens". Conversely, reproductive toxicants which inhibit or block endogenous estrogens or androgens from interacting with their respective receptors (i.e., gonadal receptor antagonists) are generally classified as "antiandrogens" or "antiestrogens". Progestins" ("progestogens" or "progestagens" in some literature) is a generic term for endogenous or synthetic compounds which interact with progesterone receptors, and there is evidence of increasing environmental contamination with these types of EDCs (Evans, 2007; Swedenborg *et al.*, 2009).

Estrogen receptor agonists/antagonists

A wide range of agricultural and industrial chemicals, as well as pharmaceuticals used in birth control preparations, are either estrogen receptor agonists and/or antagonists. Whether there is agonism or antagonism of the estrogen receptor will depend on the prevailing endocrine milieu, the presence or absence of endogenous and exogenous estrogens, the species of exposed animal, the stage of development of the target species at the time of exposure, the type of tissue and physiological response being evaluated, and the distribution of and the relative affinity of the xenobiotic for ERα or ERβ receptors. Some of the synthetic xenoestrogens most commonly discussed with respect to their interactions with estrogen receptors are DES, ethinyl estradiol from birth control pills, *o,p′*-dichlorodiphenyltrichloroethane (DDT) and *o,p′*-dichlorodiphenyldichloroethylene (DDE) and other organochlorine compounds from pesticide use, bisphenol A (BPA) from plastics and epoxy resins and nonylphenol and related compounds from detergents (Bolt *et al.*, 2001; McLachlan, 2001). Naturally occurring estrogen receptor agonists (and occasionally antagonists) include plant xenoestrogens (i.e., phytoestrogens) and a mycotoxin (i.e., zearalenone) (Evans, 2007).

Selective estrogen receptor modulators (SERMs)

As noted previously, xenobiotics can act as receptor agonists or antagonists, depending on the circumstances or tissues involved. The term "selective ER modulators" or "SERMs" was initially used to refer to a class of xenobiotics, which although originally classified as antiestrogens, can function as either estrogen receptor agonists or antagonists, depending on the tissue in which estrogen-dependent responses are being discussed (Dutertre and Smith, 2000; Katzenellenbogen and Katzenellenbogen, 2000). Similar to what was discussed previously for xenoestrogens, these chemicals can have differences in their binding affinities for ERα or ERβ. Several of these specific compounds (i.e., tamoxifen and raloxifen) have been studied for their potential use as therapeutic agents for different types of estrogen-responsive neoplasia (Evans, 2007). It should be noted for the sake of completeness that some authors are now characterizing other xenoestrogens, such as *o,p′*-DDT, *o,p′*-DDE, BPA, nonylphenol-related compounds and phytoestrogens also as SERMs (Safe *et al.*, 2007; Welshons *et al.*, 2006).

Androgen receptor antagonists

Normal phenotypic sexual differentiation of the male fetus, as well as all of the postnatal events which result in the delivery of fertile spermatozoa to the female reproductive tract, is dependent on appropriately timed androgenic stimulation of the male. In recent years, there has been increasing interest in xenobiotics which can interfere with interactions between androgens and their receptors or, in some other way, disrupt androgen-dependent signaling pathways. The dicarboximide fungicides, vinclozolin and procymidone, and/or their metabolites inhibit the binding of androgens to nuclear androgen receptors and can demasculinize and feminize the prenatally exposed male fetus or induce important alterations in pre- or peripubertally exposed offspring (Evans, 2007; Gray *et al.*, 2006). Other EDCs, including the herbicide linuron, *p,p′*-DDE (a metabolite of DDT) and prochloraz (a fungicide), can also function as androgen receptor antagonists (Evans, 2007; Gray *et al.*, 2006). Polybrominated diphenyl ethers (PBDEs) can act as competitive inhibitors of the androgen receptor as well as androgen-induced gene expression (Gray *et al.*, 2006).

Endocrine disruption independent of receptor-mediated interactions

Endocrine disruption which is independent of interactions between xenobiotics and endogenous hormone receptors can occur in a variety of different ways. Xenobiotic exposure can result in alterations in the number of hormone receptor sites (up- or downregulation) or can cause direct or indirect hormone modifications which alter hormonal function (Evans, 2007; Keith, 1997). Xenobiotics can change the rate of synthesis or destruction of endogenous hormones and can alter how hormones are stored, how they are released into and/or transported within the circulation or even how they are eventually cleared from the body (Keith, 1997; Sikka *et al.*, 2005). Any xenobiotic, including various metals or metalloids (e.g., arsenic, cadmium and lead), which is toxic to organs or tissues producing hormones (e.g., testis and ovary) has the potential to decrease hormone synthesis and thereby indirectly cause endocrine disruption (Devine and Hoyer, 2005; Hoyer, 2006). It should also be noted that some of these mechanisms of endocrine disruption are not necessarily exclusive of one another. A given xenobiotic can potentially disrupt the normal balance of hormonal function by more than one mechanism which is independent of direct interactions between the toxicant and an endogenous hormone receptor (Evans, 2007).

Unique receptor-independent antiandrogenic effects of phthalates

Phthalates, which are produced in high volume and are used as plasticizers, are abundant within the environment and share a unique antiandrogenic mechanism. Unlike vinclozolin, phthalates are not androgen receptor antagonists, but it is also clear that they are not uterotropic nor are they capable of inducing a persistent estrus, as would be expected with estrogenic EDCs (Evans, 2007; Gray, *et al.*, 2006). Phthalates actually alter fetal Leydig cell function, resulting in decreased testosterone synthesis and downregulated expression of insulin-like peptide-3, which is required for gubernacular cords formation (Foster and Gray, 2008; Gray *et al.*, 2006). Appropriately timed fetal exposure to di (*n*-butyl) phthalate can result in an abnormal aggregation of Leydig cells in the fetal rat testis, resulting in a failure of Sertoli cell proliferation and functional maturation, similar to what has been proposed as a possible mechanism for the development of gonadal dysgenesis in humans (Mahood *et al.*, 2005, 2006; Sharpe *et al.*, 2003).

"Androgenic" and "estrogenic" effects of xenobiotics

The terms "androgenic" and "estrogenic" and their antonyms "antiandrogenic" and "antiestrogenic" have been used in a number of different contexts. Some authors have used these terms to refer specifically to the agonistic and antagonistic receptor interactions of xenobiotics (Evans, 2007; Hodgson *et al.*, 2000). Because the precise mechanism of endocrine disruption of a given toxicant might not always be known or might involve multiple mechanisms of action, these terms have also been used in a more general sense, especially in livestock and wildlife species, to refer to phenotypic changes which were similar to or the opposite of the effects which would be expected with exposure to endogenous androgens or estrogens (Guillette, 2006). This type of general usage can be helpful in some instances but also has the potential to generate confusion, given that xenoandrogens and progestins frequently have the opposite phenotypic effects as xenoestrogens. For instance, the effects of estrogenic xenobiotics can be described as antiandrogenic or antiprogestagenic in some instances, while the effects of xenoandrogens and progestins can be referred to as being antiestrogenic in nature. Further confusion can be associated with exposures to mixtures of chemicals having different phenotypic effects, as is often the case in instances of environmental contamination, or with exposures to xenobiotics having mixed antiestrogenic and antiandrogenic mixed effects (i.e., methoxychlor). When the terms "androgenic", "estrogenic" or their antonyms are used in this chapter, an attempt is made to denote the intended specific or general meaning of the terms in the context in which they are used. The discretionary use of the terms "feminization" and "masculinization", as well as "defeminization" and "demasculinization", can also, in some instances, help to clarify and/or describe the phenotypic effects of a chemical suspected endocrine disruption (Evans, 2007).

Aryl hydrocarbon receptor-mediated endocrine disruption

The major agonists for the AhR protein belong to a very important class of environmental contaminants referred to collectively as "halogenated or polyhalogenated aromatic hydrocarbons" (HAHs or PAHs, respectively) and includes many highly stable and lipophilic organochlorine industrial chemicals (e.g., polycyclic aromatic hydrocarbons (PAHs), polychlorinated biphenyls (PCBs), polychlorinated dibenzo-*p*-dioxins (PCDDs) and polychlorinated dibenzodifurans (PCDFs)), as well as their metabolites (Safe, 2005). Many of these compounds are very toxic at extremely low dosages, with the LD_{50} expressed in terms of μg/kg. Some aspects of AhR-mediated endocrine disruption are reminiscent of the ligand-induced transcription associated with gonadal steroid receptor function. However, the unique nature of the endogenous AhR and its interactions with primarily xenobiotic agonists warrants additional discussion. Endocrine disruption mediated by the aryl hydrocarbon receptor (AhR) is a relatively complex, species- and tissue-dependent phenomenon, involving several of the previously described mechanisms of EDC action and interactions with many important, environmentally persistent compounds (Evans, 2007). Many of the mechanisms of action mediated by AhR-ligand interactions have been elucidated using 2,3,7,8-tetrachlorodibenzo-*p*-dioxin (TCDD) as a prototypical AhR agonist (Evans, 2007; Safe, 2005). TCDD is considered by many to be the most toxic of all of the HAHs; it is reported to have the highest AhR binding affinity of any of the xenobiotics in that class of chemicals (Safe, 2005); and the AhR has also been referred to as the "dioxin receptor" and is located in the cytoplasm bound to heat shock proteins (Parkinson and Ogilvie, 2008). Following ligand (i.e., TCDD) binding and the subsequent disassociation of the heat shock proteins, the AhR is activated by phosphorylation, and the activated ligand–AhR complex undergoes a rapid sequence of events involving interactions with the AhR nuclear translocator protein (Arnt) and relocation of the ligand–AhR–Arnt complex into the nucleus (Safe, 2005). Within the nucleus, the liganded AhR/Arnt heterodimer can facilitate a variety of endocrine-disrupting mechanisms. This activated heterodimer complex can interact with dioxin/xenobiotic response elements (DREs/XREs), which function in much the same way as the previously discussed HREs, as well as with various co-activators to increase the expression of selected genes (Evans, 2007; Safe, 2005). Depending on the animal species and the tissue, multiple phase I drug-metabolizing enzymes (e.g., cytochrome P450 (CYP) enzymes (CYP1A1, CYP1A2 and CYP1B1)) and enzymes involved in phase II drug-biotransformation reactions (e.g., glutathione-S-transferase and glucuronyl transferase) are induced by TCDD (Safe, 2005).

The antiandrogenic and antiestrogenic properties of TCDD have been associated with the ability of HAHs to induce enzymes involved in androgen and estrogen metabolism. The AhR-mediated effects of TCDD can interfere with the biosynthesis of testosterone and disrupt testosterone signal transduction pathways (Evans, 2007; Sikka, *et al.*, 2005). TCDD can also interact with androgen-, estrogen- and progestin-modulated pathways in a number of different ways, including interference with neuroendocrine development (Petersen *et al.*, 2006). AhR-mediated effects of TCDD can interfere with the biosynthesis of testosterone by a mechanism which alters the regulation of the synthesis and release of LH (Sikka *et al.*, 2005). It has also been shown in cell cultures that TCDD can disrupt testosterone signal transduction pathways (Evans, 2007). The liganded AhR/Arnt heterodimer appears to be able to interact with inhibitory DREs (iDREs) in selected tissues to suppress the expression of some genes induced by estrogens (Safe, 2005). The liganded AhR/Arnt heterodimer is also able to actually block the ability of estrogen-ER complexes to bind to their HREs (Evans, 2007; Thomas and Khan, 2005). A variety of other types of cross-talk between TCDD- and estrogen-mediated signaling pathways probably exist, and in fact TCDD has actually been shown to have the potential for estrogenic activity through interactions between liganded AhR/Arnt heterodimers and unliganded estrogen receptors (both ERα and ERβ) (Bigsby *et al.*, 2005; Evans, 2007; Ohtake *et al.*, 2003; Thomas and Khan, 2005). Ohtake *et al.* (2003) have reported that these novel interactions resulted in the recruitment of unliganded ERs and estrogen-responsive p300 co-activator-to-gene promoters. Based on the experimental results involving TCDD, it is important to remember that the effects of exposures to HAHs and EDCs are frequently dependent on animal species, as well as the type of tissue, organ or physiological response being evaluated.

Epigenetic mechanisms of action of endocrine-disrupting chemicals

In recent years there has been increasing interest in the association between prenatal exposures to some EDCs and the postnatal development of neoplasia (cancer) involving the reproductive tract, as well as the occurrence of transgenerational or vertically transmitted adverse reproductive effects (Birnbaum and Fenton, 2003; Crews and McLachlan *et al.*, 2006; Evans, 2007). These two phenomena are not mutually exclusive of one another, and in fact there is increasing evidence of vertically transmitted reproductive neoplasia (McLachlan *et al.*, 2006). Both tumor formation and transgenerational reproductive abnormalities can occur because of "genetic" mutations or alterations in the genotype (i.e., DNA sequence) or as a result of "epigenetic" changes where there are heritable modifications in the properties of a cell which are not representative of genetic changes (inherited phenotypic alteration without genotypic change) (Crews and McLachlan, 2006; Evans, 2007; McLachlan, 2001).

Epigenetic changes are a normal part of development and probably represent one means for heritable environmental adaptation (Crews and McLachlan, 2006; Evans, 2007). One of the more common mechanisms of epigenetic modification in mammals is DNA methylation of CpG nucleotides in the promoter regions of genes, which results in methylated genes being "turned off" and unmethylated or demethylated genes being "turned on" (Anway and Skinner, 2006; Evans, 2007; McLachlan, 2001). Patterns of DNA methylation are generally established during development at the gastrulation stage (i.e., lineage-specific pattern in somatic cells) and after sex determination (i.e., germ-line-specific lineage pattern in the gonad) (Anway and Skinner, 2006; Evans, 2007). DNA methylation can facilitate "genomic imprinting", a form of epigenetic gene regulation resulting in the expression of the allele from only one parent (i.e., monoallelic expression). The ability of developmental exposures to xenobiotics to provide a basis for adult disease, such as neoplasia, which is also referred to as the "developmental origins hypothesis" (Sharpe and Drake, 2010) could possibly involve epigenetic changes involving methylation or demethylation of the promoters for specific genes (Newbold *et al.*, 2006). While there have been questions about the repeatability of some of the reported xenobiotic-induced epigenetic modifications (Schneider *et al.*, 2008), epigenetic modification by alterations in DNA methylation patterns in the germ-line remains a potential mechanism for observed xenobiotic-induced transgenerational (vertically transmitted) effects associated with male and female infertility and tumor susceptibility in rodents (Anway *et al.*, 2005; Anway and Skinner, 2006; Fenton, 2006; Guerrero-Bosagna and Skinner, 2009; McLaclan *et al.*, 2006; Newbold *et al.*, 2006; Nilsson *et al.*, 2008).

Disruption of "non-reproductive" endocrine systems

Although it can be argued that almost all endocrine systems are "reproductive" at least to some extent, there are multiple systems with primary functions which are not directly related to reproduction, and several of these systems have also been identified as targets of EDCs. In addition, gonadal steroids and xenobiotics which mimic these endogenous hormones are also capable of "non-reproductive" effects. The synthesis of triiodothyronine (T_3) and thyroxine (T_4) by the thyroid gland can be decreased by chemicals which inhibit the uptake of iodine (e.g., perchlorate and thiocyanate) and also by xenobiotics which inhibit thyroperoxidase, such as thiourea, propylthiourea (PTU), some sulfonamides, methimazole, carbimazole, aminotriazole and acetoacetamide (Evans, 2007). The class of compounds known as PBDEs has been shown to interfere with normal thyroid function (Dye *et al.*, 2007; Guillette, 2006), and thyroid hormone secretion can be inhibited by exposure to excessive amounts of iodine or lithium (Evans, 2007). Xenobiotics, such as the *o,p′*-DDD metabolite of DDT, can interfere with glucocorticoid metabolism (Guillette, 2006), and there has been increasing interest in the relationship between gestational and neonatal exposures to xenoestrogens and the development of obesity (Newbold *et al.*, 2006). Some EDCs (e.g., organotin compounds) have even been described as "obesogens" (Grün and Blumberg, 2006). BPA, which is widely used in the plastics industry and other manufacturing processes, can interact with estrogen receptors and has been implicated as a possible cause of obesity and diabetes associated with "Metabolic Syndrome". Recent evidence suggests, however, that, while perinatal administration of BPA can enhance early growth in mice, exposure to this EDC does not result in the eventual development of "Metabolic Syndrome" (Ryan *et al.*, 2010a,b).

EFFECTS OF ENDOCRINE-DISRUPTING CHEMICALS

The scope of the endocrine disruption problem

With a basic understanding of the key terms, concepts and mechanisms of action associated with endocrine disruption, as well as the number of chemicals involved, it should be evident how frequently endocrine-disrupting xenobiotics can interfere with the structural and functional integrity of the multiple organs and tissues, as well as various signaling pathways, involved in normal reproductive function, including embryonic and fetal development (Figure 67.1). As mentioned in the introduction to this chapter, there is currently a great deal of interest in the scope of the endocrine disruption problem, especially as it applies to wildlife populations and human reproduction. Based on traditional toxicological principles and the mechanisms of endocrine disruption which have been discussed, one would expect the observed effects of an EDC exposure to be dependent on amount of specific xenobiotic to which organisms are exposed, the mechanisms of action of the specific chemical involved in the exposure; the reproduction endpoints and target species being evaluated; the habitat in which the animal lives and the route of EDC exposure; and the stage or stages of development of those individual animals or populations exposed to a given EDC. Making the assumption that the specific EDC acts in a traditional dose-dependent, monotonic fashion, the total dose or amount of the endocrine-disrupting xenobiotic to which the individuals or populations are exposed (based on dosage and duration of exposure) will be another important determinant of what reproductive/developmental abnormalities will most likely be observed. This particular approach to evaluating EDC effects is probably applicable for documented instances of endocrine disruption in wildlife populations, particularly fish and amphibians, and in domesticated animals, where, in both instances, exposures often involve relatively high levels of exposure to endocrine-disrupting xenobiotics and the adverse effects are fairly evident. On the other hand, the determination of the scope of endocrine disruption within different human populations, as well as estimation of the actual threat EDCs pose to human reproduction, can be extremely challenging. Large accidental, occupational, or pharmaceutical exposures to EDCs, which are accompanied by obvious clinical signs consistent with hormonal abnormalities, are relatively easy to diagnose as instances of endocrine disruption. Conversely, the direct, adverse effects of often unrecognized, daily, "low dose", environmental exposures to mixtures of chemicals used abundantly in industry, agriculture, and/or medicine can be difficult to assess, and perhaps even harder to replicate in a laboratory setting, especially given the possible different routes and timing of exposure and the use of animal models with varying sensitivities to endocrine disruption, even within tissues and within the same animal. It is with regard to these very low environmental exposures and the experimental results evaluating these effects that toxicologists and endocrinologists often disagree on what represents a significant risk to human health (Diamanti-Kandarkis *et al.*, 2009).

Documented cases of endocrine disruption in wildlife, domestic animals and humans

Examples of EDC-associated effects in wildlife species and domestic animals have been some of the earliest instances of disorders identified as "endocrine disruption" and can serve as a warning for human populations. Several cases of endocrine disruption in humans will also be briefly summarized and will be followed by a discussion of some of the remaining questions regarding endocrine disruption, which are worthy of further investigation. It is hoped that familiarity with the basic facts surrounding these substantiated instances of endocrine disruption, as well as the aspects of endocrine disruption where there remain unanswered questions, will facilitate the reader's accurate interpretation of EDC-related scientific data presented in other chapters of this book, as well as current and future scientific journal articles.

The adverse reproductive effects of endocrine disruption on wildlife species

There have been many, well-documented instances of reproductive abnormalities in species of wildlife living in environments contaminated by industrial and/or agricultural chemicals (Hamlin and Guillette, 2010; Hess and Iguchi, 2002; Jobling *et al.*, 2009; McLaclan, 2001; McLaclan *et al.*, 2006). The deleterious reproductive effects of DDT on birds reported in Rachel Carson's *Silent Spring* resulted from eggshell thinning related to abnormalities in prostaglandins synthesis which were induced by the *p,p′*-DDE metabolite of DDT (Guillette, 2006). Wildlife populations, especially species of fishes and amphibians, are excellent sentinels for endocrine disruption. Their life cycles have been very well understood for over 200 years (Figures 67.2A and 67.2B). Amphibians go through a particularly complicated metamorphosis from a strictly aquatic organism to one which, depending on the species, is amphibious or terrestrial. This process consists of various steps involving various signaling pathways and appears highly susceptible to disruptive effects of xenobiotics and adverse environmental conditions (Hogan *et al.*, 2008) (Figure 67.2B). The dependence of these species on aquatic environments also means that these organisms are likely to encounter water contaminants before other species and increases the number of developmental stages which will be directly in contact with a harmful xenobiotic. Fish and amphibians are exposed to a given aquatic contaminant by multiple routes of exposure, thereby increasing the amount of potential EDCs absorbed by these species (Evans, 2007). In addition, predatory fish and reptiles will have relatively high exposures to organic chemicals which bioaccumulate within the environment (Hess and Iguchi, 2002).

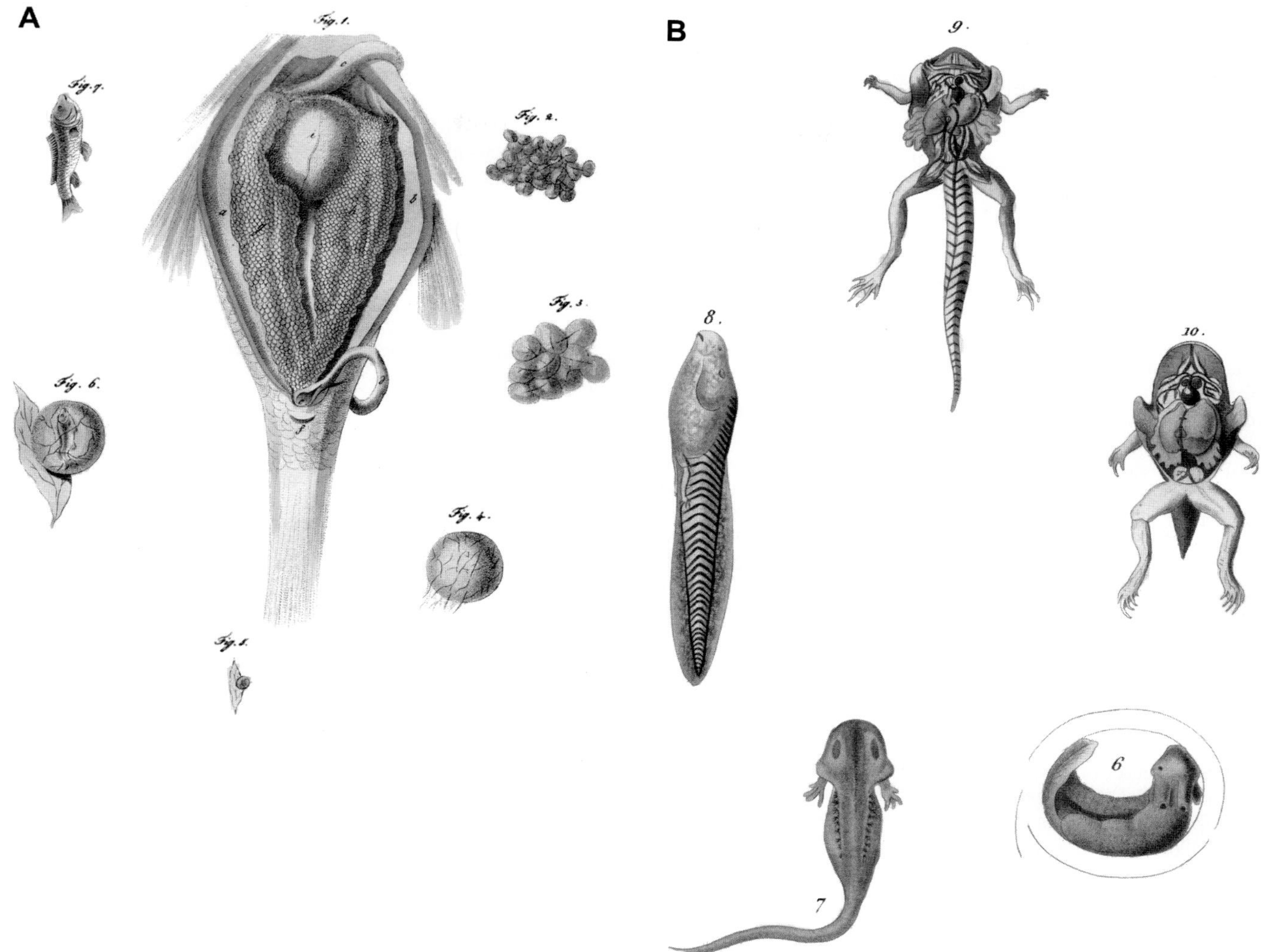

FIGURE 67.2 A and B demonstrate people's understanding of fish and amphibian life cycles 200 years ago. These figures also illustrate the exquisite susceptibility of these life cycles to xenobiotic-induced alterations. It should not be surprising that fish and amphibians are often the first wildlife populations to demonstrate adverse effects from exposure to waterborne contaminants. Fish live their entire lives in an aquatic environment (A; picture adapted by Don Connor from *Porte-Feuille des Enfans* by F.J. Bertuch, 1795), where they are surrounded by exogenous chemicals. It is not hard to imagine diffusion of endocrine-disrupting chemicals into the masses of eggs which are produced, either while they are still within the female, prior to them being deposited (1), or, especially, following direct exposure to xenobiotics, after their release from the female and while they are undergoing developmental changes prior to hatching (2–6). Fish are at additional risk for chemical exposures, compared to air-breathing, terrestrial vertebrates, because they can be exposed to chemicals by a number of different routes of exposure (i.e., ingestion, transport across the gills into the circulation, or, potentially, "dermal" absorption). Like fish, amphibians, such as frogs (B; picture adapted by Don Connor from *Dictionnaire Pittoresque d'Histoire Naturelle et des Phenomenes de la Nature* by Felix Edward Guerin-Meneville, 1839), are also very susceptible to excessive exposures to waterborne xenobiotics during the aquatic stages of their lives, at least in part because of the multiple routes of exposure discussed for fish. However, there are additional xenobiotic-sensitive signaling pathways involved in the development of these species, which take place after the release of the offspring from the egg, because of their metamorphosis from a legless aquatic organism (7) to a four-legged, air-breathing, amphibious or terrestrial animal (10).

Adverse reproductive effects of "androgenic" and "estrogenic" chemicals on wildlife species

Prenatal and postnatal exposures to androgenic and estrogenic environmental contaminants, as well as chemicals classified as having the opposite phenotypic effects, have been associated with various reproductive abnormalities in wildlife. Effluents from pulp and paper mills, as well as runoff from cattle feedlots containing trenbolone used for growth promotion, have been shown to be androgenic and capable of masculinizing female fish (Gray *et al.*, 2006; Orlando *et al.*, 2004). "Androgynization", or a state of indeterminate sexual development encompassing both feminization and demasculinization in males, has been observed in populations of fish, amphibians, reptiles, birds and mammals and is thought to be similar to the testicular dysgenesis syndrome described in humans (Edwards *et al.*, 2006). Ethinyl estradiol is a potent estrogenic compound which is found in many human birth control products and is a common contaminant of raw sewage (Foster and Gray, 2008; McLachlan *et al.*, 2006; Rogers and Kavlock, 2008). An increased incidence in hermaphroditic frogs has been reported in field studies, and adult and immature amphibians exposed to the herbicide atrazine, which has been associated with increased aromatase activity in a number of species, have exhibited various manifestations of feminization in a laboratory setting (Hayes *et al.*, 2006, 2010). Hatchling, juvenile and adult male alligators (*Alligator mississippiensis*), originating from a contaminated Florida lake, have exhibited varying patterns of androgynization, including phallic malformations, resulting from xenobiotic exposures at various stages of development (McLachlan *et al.*, 2006; Milnes *et al.*, 2005). Even mammals such as seals with uterine leiomyomas (fibroids) and hermaphroditic polar bear offspring, found in association with elevated concentrations of xenoestrogens, or cheetahs consuming phytoestrogens in captivity, can exhibit clinical signs of endocrine disruption (McLachlan *et al.*, 2006).

The effects of naturally occurring endocrine-disrupting chemicals on domestic animals

There are many documented cases of endocrine disruption in domestic animals, especially those associated with exposures to naturally occurring xenoestrogens (i.e., phytoestrogens and zearalenone) (Evans, 2007). However, despite the importance of these disorders to human populations consuming the same feedstuffs as their livestock, instances of naturally occurring xenoestrogen exposure in domestic animals often receive relatively cursory treatment in textbooks, as compared to EDC exposures involving wildlife, humans or laboratory species. Just like synthetic xenoestrogens, phytoestrogens and zearalenone can also function as antiestrogens through the inhibition of LH and FSH release from the anterior pituitary and by competing with endogenous estrogens for receptor sites within the tubular genitalia (Cheeke, 1998). The ability of the ergot alkaloids in tall fescue endophyte (*Neotyphodium coenophialum*) or ergot (*Claviceps purpurea*) to inhibit prolactin secretion and, subsequently, lactogenesis and lactation in animal species is clearly another example of endocrine disruption, which has also been observed in women (Evans *et al.*, 2004). More recently, the importance of pets as sentinels for human populations has also been recognized with respect to an apparent relationship between hyperthyroidism in cats and exposure to PBDEs (Dye *et al.*, 2007).

The adverse reproductive effects of phytoestrogens on domestic animals

As covered specifically in Chapter 52, some leguminous plants, including soy beans (*Glycine max*), subterranean clover (*Trifolium subterraneum*), red clover (*Trifolium pratense*), white clover (*Trifolium repens*) and alsike clover (*Trifolium hybridum*), contain phytoestrogens classified as isoflavones (Burrows and Tyrl, 2001; Cheeke, 1998). The isoflavones in soy beans are also consumed in large quantities by human populations. Alfalfa (*Medicago sativa*) is also a legume, but it contains another class of phytoestrogenic compounds referred to as coumestans. Phytoestrogen exposures can result in infertility associated with abnormal estrous cycles and structural and functional changes in the cervix and/or uterus (Burrows and Tyrl, 2001; Cheeke, 1998; Evans, 2007; Ford *et al.*, 2006).

The adverse reproductive effects of zearalenone on domestic animals

The estrogenic mycotoxin zearalenone is produced by *Fusarium graminearum* (formerly *Fusarium roseum*), under certain environmental and storage conditions, in corn, wheat, barley and oats (Cheeke, 1998; Evans, 2007). Swine have been shown to be particularly susceptible to the adverse effects of zearalenone, with prepubertal gilts being affected by concentrations of zearalenone in the feed as low as 1 to 3 ppm (Figures 67.3 and 67.4).

Hyperestrogenism in prepubertal gilts is characterized by swelling of the vulva (Figure 67.3B) and mammary glands, uterine and vaginal enlargement, changes in luminal epithelium of the vagina (Figure 67.4B) and uterus (Figure 67.4D), and ovarian atrophy. Preputial swelling and testicular atrophy have been observed in immature boars, and various ovarian abnormalities, including follicular cysts and prolonged corpora lutea, as well as behavioral abnormalities, have been observed with excessive exposure of cyclic gilts and sows to zearalenone. Human populations on primarily corn diets can also be exposed to zearalenone (Briones-Reyes *et al.*, 2007).

The endocrine-disrupting effects of ergot alkaloids on reproduction in domestic animals

Ergot alkaloids include over 80 indole compounds biosynthesized from L-tryptophan and the isoprene 3R-mevalonic acid derivative of dimethylallyl diphosphate (Roberts *et al.*, 2009). Most naturally occurring ergot alkaloids have been isolated

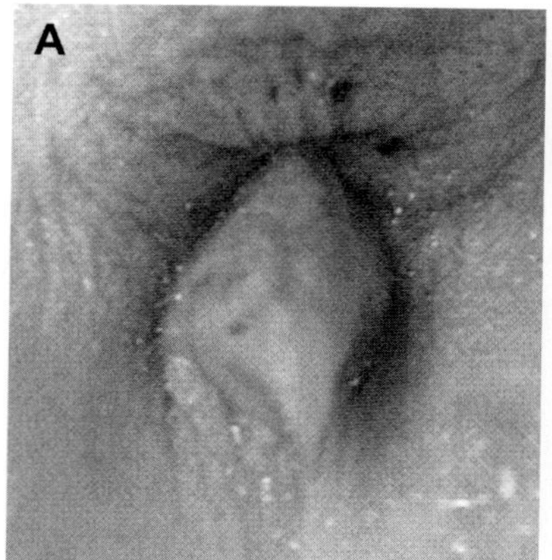

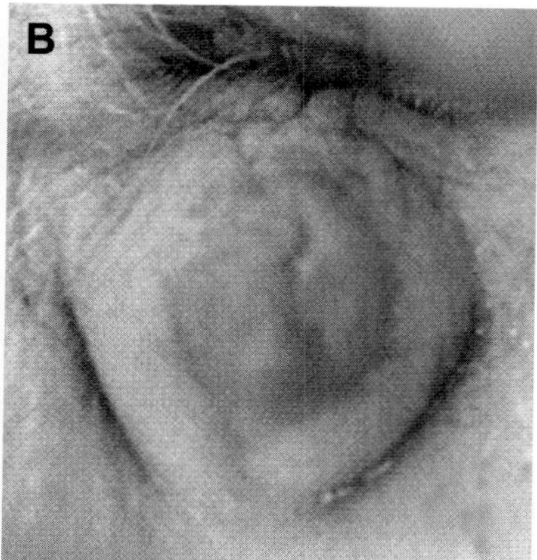

FIGURE 67.3 The vulva of a prepubertal gilt (i.e., young female pig) fed a diet not contaminated by zearalenone is shown in (A). In (B), the vulva of a similarly aged gilt dosed with approximately 100 μg zearalenone/kg body weight/day for 3 weeks is shown. These types of changes in the external genitalia of prepubertal gilts are very typical of what is observed when rations contain 1 to 3 ppm of zearalenone (i.e., 1 to 3 mg of zearalenone/kg of feed).

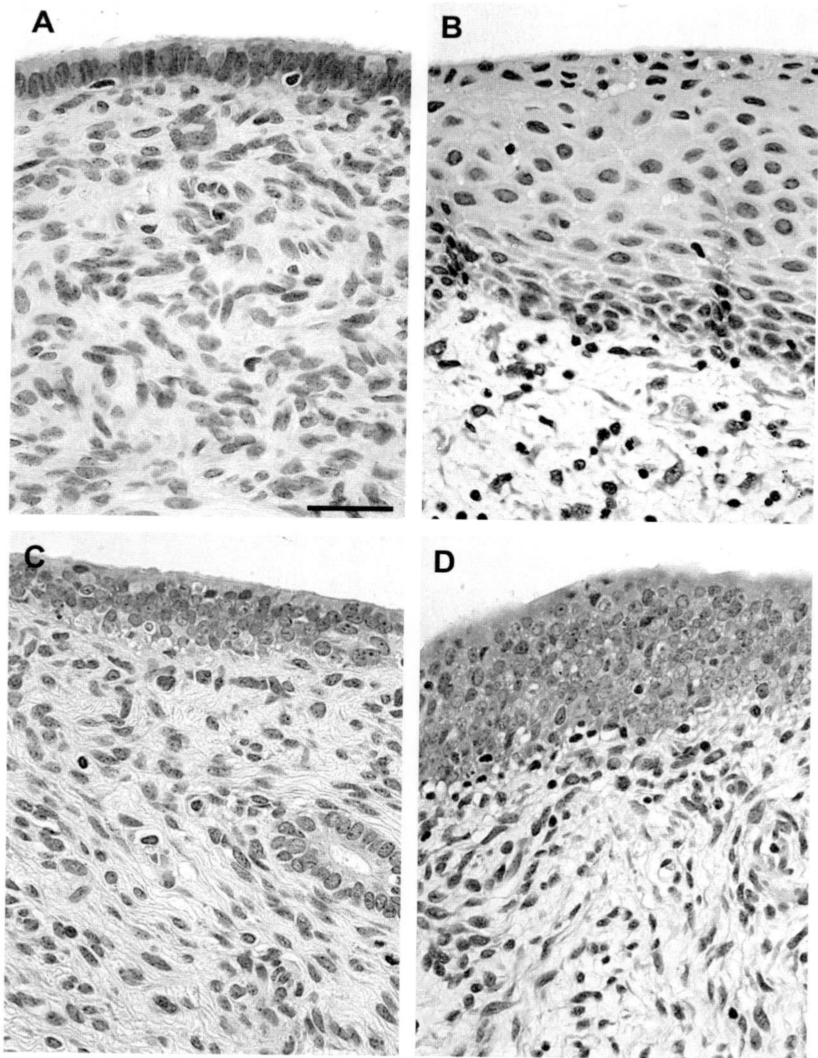

FIGURE 67.4 The transformation of the pseudostratified columnar epithelium normally lining the vaginal lumen of prepubertal gilts (A) into stratified squamous epithelium (i.e., squamous metaplasia), following exposure to approximately 100 μg zearalenone/kg body weight/day for 3 weeks is shown in (B) (400× magnification; bar = 50 μm). The epithelial lining of the uterine lumen of control gilts (C) was noticeably different in histologic appearance from that of the uterine luminal epithelium of the zearalenone-treated prepubertal gilts (D), which demonstrated epithelial (mucosal) hyperplasia as viewed at 400× magnification.

from either fungal sclerotia of *Claviceps purpurea* contaminating small grains or grasses or from the tall fescue endophyte, *Neotyphodium coenophialum* (Burrows and Tyrl, 2001; Cheeke, 1998). Ergot sclerotia, which are also called "ergot" or "ergot bodies" (from the French word "argot", meaning spur), consist of interwoven filamentous fungal hyphae or mycelia, along with the hardened exudate or "honeydew" (Figure 67.5) and contain ergot alkaloids classified primarily as either ergoline alkaloids (e.g., lysergic acid, lysergol, lysergic acid amide and ergonovine) or as ergopeptine alkaloids (e.g., ergotamine, ergocristine, ergosine, ergocryptine, ergocornine and ergovaline) (Evans *et al.*, 2004). Various ergoline alkaloids and ergovaline are the major ergot alkaloids produced by the intercellular endophytic mycelia of *Neotyphodium coenophialum* (Evans *et al.*, 2004). Ergopeptine alkaloids are potent D_2-dopamine receptor agonists which decrease prolactin secretion by the anterior pituitary (Evans *et al.*, 2004), and the most sensitive indicator of ergopeptine alkaloid exposure in animals is hypoprolactinemia. Late-gestational mares exposed to ergopeptine alkaloids from either ergot or fescue endophyte almost always exhibit agalactia, plus varying degrees of prolonged gestation, dystocia, retained fetal membranes and foal dysmaturity (Evans *et al.*, 2004).

Documented adverse reproductive effects of endocrine-disrupting chemicals on humans

With respect to human exposures to EDCs, it can be very difficult to demonstrate a definitive cause-and-effect relationship, based solely on epidemiologic data, when the xenobiotics of concern have weak hormonal activity, the endpoints being evaluated are subtle or only evident long after exposure, and/or a number of different factors can play a causative role in the observed clinical signs. Those reports of xenobiotic-associated effects on human reproduction which are likely to have the most valid conclusions or be the most relevant are those involving retrospective studies of documented exposures to known EDCs contained in medicines or contaminated food or present in an occupational setting

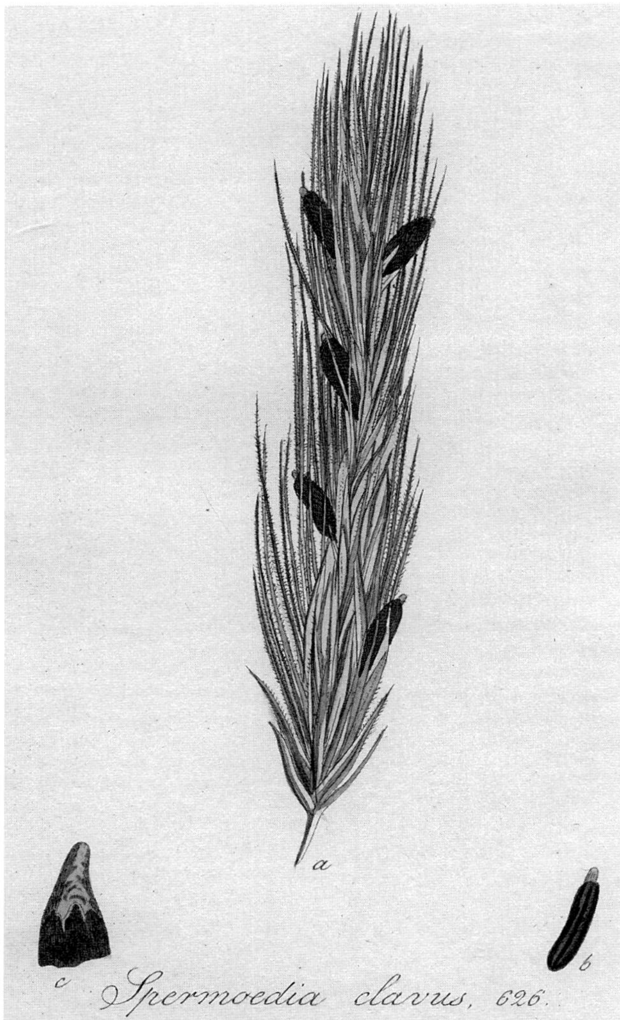

FIGURE 67.5 This is an approximately 170-year-old copper plate showing seed heads of a rye (*Secale cereale*) infected by sclerotia of *Claviceps purpurea* (formerly *Spermoedia clavus*). Pictures of individual ergot bodies are also shown at different magnifications. One of the last recorded, large epidemics of ergotism in humans affected 11,000 people in Russia in 1926. The primary reproductive effects of ergot alkaloids are ecbolic effects and suppression of lactogenesis and lactation (picture adapted by Howard Wilson from *Flora Batava* by J. Kopps, 1844).

(McLachlan *et al.*, 2006; Rogers and Kavlock, 2008). To a somewhat lesser degree, studies presenting epidemiologic evidence of increasing trends of adverse reproductive outcomes, especially in relation to concentrations of confirmed EDCs, can also be of value.

Adverse effects of diethylstilbestrol (DES) on human reproduction

Between 1958 and 1976, DES, a synthetic, non-steroidal xenoestrogen, was prescribed during four to six million pregnancies to prevent miscarriages. Prenatal human exposures to DES have been associated with feminization of male fetuses and an increased incidence of vaginal clear cell adenocarcinoma in the daughters of women treated with DES during pregnancy (McLachlan, 2001; McLachlan *et al.*, 2006; Newbold *et al.*, 2006; Rogers and Kavlock, 2008).

In addition to the postpubertal occurrence of this rare neoplasm, the female offspring of DES-treated women have also been reported to have decreased fertility and an increased likelihood of endometriosis and other adult-onset reproductive abnormalities (McLachlan *et al.*, 2006). The occurrence of these abnormalities in adult women exposed to DES *in utero* has been proposed as an example of xenobiotic-induced epigenetic modifications and transgenerational effects in humans (McLachlan *et al.*, 2006; Newbold *et al.*, 2006).

Adverse reproductive effects of other xenoestrogens on human reproduction

Premature breast development has been observed in prepubertal girls exposed to hair care products or other sources of xenoestrogens. Precocious puberty has also been suspected in young women who consume large amounts of phytoestrogens, especially those in foods consisting primarily of soy (McLachlan *et al.*, 2006), and breast cancer in women is thought to be another potential outcome of early exposures to xenobiotics with estrogenic effects (Fenton, 2006). Menstrual disturbances have historically been reported in female hop pickers, and 8-prenylnaringenin isolated from hops (*Humulus lupulus*) is an extremely potent phytoestrogen (Zanoli and Zavatti, 2008). Recently, concerns have been raised about the additive estrogenic effects of zearalenone in women of lower socioeconomic status eating mycotoxin-contaminated corn, who are also likely to be exposed to other xenoestrogens (Briones-Reyes *et al.*, 2007). Sexual dysfunction in men has also been reported to be associated with occupational BPA exposures in men (Li *et al.*, 2010).

Adverse "antiestrogenic"/"antiandrogenic" effects of heavy metals on human reproduction

A variety of heavy metals and metalloids have been suggested as endocrine disruptors in people. Based on epidemiologic studies evaluating heavy metal burdens in human populations and their correlation with reproductive function, it has been postulated that anterior pituitary release of FSH and LH and ovarian steroidogenesis are inhibited by cadmium in women (Hoyer, 2006). With respect to lead, further evidence suggests that the neuroendocrine function of the hypothalamic–pituitary–gonadal axis appears to be targeted by lead in both men and women (Evans, 2007; Hoyer, 2006; Iavicoli *et al.*, 2009). Occupational exposures to other elements (cadmium, mercury, arsenic, manganese, zinc and iron) have also been associated with reproductive and developmental abnormalities (Iavicoli *et al.*, 2009; Weinberg, 2010).

"Documented" adverse reproductive effects of "antiandrogens" on human reproduction

Although still somewhat controversial, there is a growing body of evidence to support the observation that sperm counts in men within some industrialized regions of the world have been decreasing over the last several decades (Evans, 2007; Skakkebæk *et al.*, 2006; Swan *et al.*, 2000). In conjunction with these alterations in sperm numbers within ejaculates, there appears to have been a concurrent increase in developmental abnormalities within the male reproductive tract consistent with testicular dysgenesis syndrome or TDS (Skakkebæk *et al.*, 2001). Similar to what has been observed in xenobiotic-exposed wildlife, reproductive dysgenesis in human males (i.e., TDS) is associated with reduced semen quality, cryptorchidism, various forms of hypospadias (i.e., incomplete closure of the urethral groove), decreased ano-genital distance (AGD) (normally shorter in females than in males) and testicular cancer (Edwards *et al.*, 2006; Evans, 2007; Skakkebæk *et al.*, 2001). Failure of Sertoli cell proliferation and functional maturation within the seminiferous tubules has been proposed as one mechanism for the pathogenesis of TDS, based on research performed in rodent models using prenatal exposures to phthalates (Mahood *et al.*, 2005, 2006; Sharpe *et al.*, 2003). The findings of an epidemiologic study have suggested a relationship between decreased AGD and prenatal phthalate exposure in male infants (Swan *et al.*, 2005). In other epidemiologic studies, a correlation was shown between reduced semen quality in men within certain regions of the USA and the metabolites of several economically important herbicides (Swan *et al.*, 2003a,b), and a similar relationship has been demonstrated between prostate cancer and certain pesticides (Diamanti-Kandarkis *et al.*, 2009). In addition to these observations, non-occupational exposures to pyrethrin and pyrethroid insecticides, as well as their metabolites, have recently been associated with reduced semen quality and sperm DNA damage in men (Meeker *et al.*, 2008; Xia *et al.*, 2008). One likely mechanism for these pyrethroid-associated sperm abnormalities are recently elucidated "antiandrogenic" effects of this commonly used class of insecticides (Zhang *et al.*, 2008).

"Documented" adverse aryl hydrocarbon receptor-mediated effects on human reproduction

The 1976 release of TCDD near Seveso, Italy, has also been associated with adverse reproductive effects in both men and women. The results of a recently published study showed low endogenous estradiol concentrations in men exposed as either infants or as teenagers. However, while there was decreased semen quality in the men exposed to TCDD during the early postnatal and prepubertal stages of development when Sertoli cell proliferation is testosterone dependent, sperm parameters were improved in men exposed around puberty when Sertoli cell proliferation is dependent on follicle-stimulating hormone, which is likely to be increased in instances where estradiol is decreased (Mocarelli *et al.*, 2008). Boys accidentally exposed to PCBs and PCDFs *in utero* or from the ingestion of contaminated breast milk from exposed mothers have been reported to have various reproductive abnormalities, as well as IQ and behavioral deficits (Foster and Gray, 2008; Rogers and Kavlock, 2008). Several epidemiologic studies have been performed trying to evaluate the incidence of adverse reproductive outcomes associated with dioxin exposure in women. Positive correlations have been reported between serum TCDD concentrations and occurrence of breast cancer (Warner *et al.*, 2002) and the time taken by women desiring to get pregnant to have a confirmed pregnancy (Eskenazi *et al.*, 2010).

The adverse reproductive effects of ergot alkaloids on human reproduction

People, like animals, can also be affected by the ergot alkaloids present in ergot bodies, which replace the seed heads of small cereal grains, such as triticale, wheat, barley, oats and, especially, rye (Figure 67.5) (Burrows and Tyrl, 2001; Cheeke, 1998; Evans *et al.*, 2004). Historically, the most dramatic clinical signs of ergotism in people and animals have been those associated with dry gangrene of the extremities from vasoconstriction and, especially in humans, bizarre behavior related to the lysergic acid diamide (i.e., LSD)-like chemicals present in ergot sclerotia. However, abortion, stillbirths and agalactia have also been very consistent clinical findings in women, particularly in individuals intentionally consuming ergot derivatives to hasten labor or those women forced to eat lower quality grains prior to and after parturition (Lee, 2009). The "oxytocic" effects of ergot can most likely be attributed to the stimulation of α-adrenergic receptors, rather than mimicry of oxytocin, but the pathogenesis of the agalactia, which is so typical of exposures to ergot alkaloids, is via the same D_2 dopamine receptor agonism and endocrine pathways reported in domestic livestock (Evans *et al.*, 2004).

SCREENING FOR ENDOCRINE DISRUPTORS

In 1996, the USEPA was mandated, under the Food Quality Protection and Safe Drinking Water Acts, to develop protocols to screen for endocrine disruption. The Endocrine Disruptor Screening and Advisory Committee was formed in response to this mandate, and a detailed, tiered testing strategy involving multiple *in vitro* and *in vivo* mammalian assays was proposed (Foster and Gray, 2008). Within this testing strategy, rats were selected as the experimental animal of choice and various experiments with a wide range of reproductive endpoints were developed. A variety of other *in vitro* cellular models, as well as *in vivo* animal models using fish, amphibians, avian species and mice, have also been developed and utilized in various academic, industrial and governmental (e.g., FDA) research settings (Rogers and Kavlock, 2008).

REMAINING QUESTIONS/FUTURE DIRECTIONS IN ENDOCRINE DISRUPTION

There should be no doubt in anyone's mind that there are many "real world" examples of endocrine disruption which can impact reproduction of wildlife, domestic animals and/or potentially humans. However, there are still many important questions remaining which need to be answered before we can progress to the next round of environmental policies and research projects related to endocrine disruptors. At the time that this chapter is being written, efforts are being made to answer the questions which follow. Some of these efforts are focusing on one EDC; others are looking at a particular issue from a more general perspective. Much of this type of research has been ongoing for at least 15 years and some of it much longer. There are well-documented differences between laboratory animal species (vom Saal *et al.*, 2010) and between strains within those species, with respect to sensitivity to experimental treatments, and even changes in diet (Ruhlen *et al.*, 2008). As has been alluded to in the introduction to this chapter, efforts to resolve some of the issues which follow will require that regulators, researchers, health professionals and manufacturers "step out of the box" and possibly modify or expand their dosing protocols and routes and timing of xenobiotic exposure, as well as their laboratory animal models and the reproductive endpoints being evaluated. The ultimate goals of our regulatory research and manufacturing efforts should be to establish what chemicals have endocrine-disrupting properties; which of these potential EDCs pose a risk to human and animal populations at environmental, normal domestic and/or occupational levels of exposure; and, finally, how best to remediate these situations, taking into consideration the agricultural, industrial, health and lifestyle issues that will be impacted.

Transgenerational effects of endocrine-disrupting xenobiotics

There is currently great interest in the association between prenatal exposures to some EDCs and the postnatal development of neoplasia (cancer) involving the reproductive tract, as well as the occurrence of transgenerational or vertically transmitted male and female impaired reproductive function (Crews and McLachlan, 2006; Evans, 2007). Both tumor formation and transgenerational reproductive abnormalities could potentially occur because of "epigenetic" changes. DNA methylation of CpG nucleotides in the promoter regions of genes, which results in methylated genes being "turned off" and unmethylated or demethylated genes being "turned on", is one of the more common mechanisms of epigenetic modifications (Anway and Skinner, 2006; Evans, 2007; McLachlan, 2001). These types of epigenetic modification have been proposed as a potential mechanism for vinclozolin-associated transgenerational (vertically transmitted) infertility and tumor susceptibility in rats which have been recently reported (Anway and Skinner, 2006; Guerrero-Bosagna and Skinner, 2009; Nilsson *et al.*, 2008) but, at this point in time, have apparently been difficult to repeat in other laboratories (Schneider *et al.*, 2008).

The effects of mixtures

Other than, possibly, in cases of catastrophic accidents involving single chemicals, medical mishaps, documented mycotoxin-contaminated foods or occupational exposures, it is unrealistic to assume that animals or humans are only exposed to one xenobiotic at a time. Particularly when it comes to daily, low, environmentally relevant exposures to EDCs, target species will almost always be exposed to a mixture of xenobiotics, some of which have the same effects and others which affect an animal in an opposing manner. Given the number of chemicals classified as potential EDCs and the wide array of mechanisms of endocrine disruption, even laboratory animal experiments intended to measure, under controlled conditions, the effects of a specific EDC on reproductive function can inadvertently represent an exposure to more than one endocrine disruptor present in the cages, bedding, food, water or other sources. This is one reason why proper positive controls and large numbers of animals to eliminate litter effects are so critical to the proper design of these types of experiments (Welshons *et al.*, 2003, 2006; Sharpe, 2010). Depending on the activities of the individual chemicals in a mixture, the interactions between those xenobiotics can be additive (i.e., $1+1=2$), subtractive (i.e., $2-1=1$), or, potentially, synergistic (i.e., $1+1=3$). However, some care should be exercised in describing a given chemical interaction as synergistic, when the method of detection for the effect being evaluated is not very sensitive (e.g., $0+0=1$ when it is not possible to detect an effect of $\{1/2\}$). Further translational research needs to be done with mixtures of EDCs to better characterize the types of responses which should be anticipated when the components of a mixture are known.

The "total dose" of endocrine-disrupting chemicals to which populations are exposed

An issue closely related to that of mixtures is how best to determine the total external and, perhaps more importantly, the internal doses of the EDCs to which populations are exposed. Knowing what amounts of endocrine-disrupting xenobiotics are actually bioavailable to an exposed organism can be extremely important when trying to design an experiment to replicate environmental conditions or identify additional, potential sources of a compound. Characterizing the "total" exposure dose can be challenging and comes down to identifying all possible sources of an EDC and improving and standardizing analytical methods for evaluating the concentrations of xenobiotics in different types of matrices, including environmental samples, serum, urine, liver, kidney and fat. This process also needs to take into consideration the route of exposure, and requires an improved understanding of the mechanisms of absorption, distribution, metabolism and elimination of the EDCs of interest within a target species. It is also important to recognize how the toxicokinetics and mechanism of action of a given endocrine-disrupting xenobiotic might vary with dose, route of exposure and even the precise stage of development when an animal is exposed.

Differences in biological activities between metabolites/isomers of a xenobiotic

Even closely related xenobiotics can have very different mechanisms of action and effects on biological systems. A good case in point is DDT and its various metabolites. The endocrine effects of these chemicals appear to be metabolite- and isomer-specific, with *o,p′*-DDT and *p,p′*-DDT both classified as estrogen receptor agonists (sometimes antagonists), *o,p′*-DDD interfering with glucocorticoid metabolism, and *p,p′*-DDE having antiandrogenic activity. Enantioselectivity or stereoselectivity is also clearly evident in chiral, organic compounds, such as *o,p′*-DDT and pyrethroid insecticides, where chemicals which appear essentially identical to one other can vary significantly in their biological activity (Hoekstra *et al.*, 2001; Liu *et al.*, 2008). When interpreting unexpected experimental results involving endocrine-disrupting xenobiotics, one should try to verify whether the effects being measured are those of the parent compound, its metabolites or breakdown products, or isomers or enantiomers of these molecules.

"Low dose effects" of endocrine-disrupting chemicals

The term "low dose effects" can have very different meanings to different groups of scientists. "Low dose effects" can be used to describe adverse outcomes or effects associated with an amount of a particular xenobiotic which approximates environmental concentrations of that chemical. In this sense, the term "low dose effects" is not really controversial, and it would seem relatively plausible that hormonally active xenobiotics can exert effects at very low levels of exposure. In its more controversial usage, "low dose effects" is used to describe adverse outcomes from exposures to dosages of a given EDC which are orders of magnitude less than dosages calculated to be "safe", based on no-observed-adverse-effect levels (NOAELs) or dosages corresponding to concentrations at or, usually, below concentrations of that EDC found in the environment. This aspect of "low dose effects" is closely related to the concept of "non-monotonic" responses to xenobiotics and is discussed in great detail below.

Non-monotonic responses to endocrine-disrupting xenobiotics

"The dose makes the poison"

There continues to be ongoing and frequently acrimonious debate about the various aspects of xenobiotic-induced, abnormal reproductive function. In fact, with respect to endocrine-disrupting xenobiotics, new and conflicting data and exceptions to "classical" mechanisms of toxicity are being reported in the scientific literature and mass media on a regular basis. The origins of some of the current controversy date back approximately 500 years to one of the basic tenets of modern toxicology, which is traditionally credited to a 16th century physician, botanist, alchemist and philosopher named Philippus Aureolus Theophrastus Bombastus von Hohenheim (or, alternatively, Aureolus Philippus Theophrastus Bombastus von Hohenheim or several other permutations and/or spellings of those names), who eventually referred to himself as Paracelsus (i.e., equal to or beyond Celsus, a Roman encyclopedist and physician). Paracelsus stated: "All substances are poisons; there is none which is not a poison. The right dose differentiates a poison from a remedy" (McClellan, 2007). One of the implications of this doctrine is a monotonic dose–response relationship for xenobiotic exposures. In other words, the incidence or severity of the specific effect being evaluated is expected to increase with the amount of the xenobiotic to which a target species is exposed. At some level of exposure, that effect might be therapeutic, but the level of the effect becomes toxic, as it increases with the amount of xenobiotic to which an organism is exposed. This essentially comes down to toxicology being the bigger "evil twin" of pharmacology. Another way to look at these issues is to say that an adverse response being evaluated will decrease as the dose of xenobiotic to which a target species is exposed becomes less. Therefore, if the adverse outcome being evaluated ceases to be observed at a particular dosage of xenobiotic, then the toxicological assumption is made that the adverse effect being evaluated will not be observed at *any* dosage less than that at which the response first disappeared or was no longer observed. This set of ideas has helped establish the premise of there being a "threshold dose" for xenobiotics and their adverse outcomes and is the basis for the majority of modern toxicological testing and risk assessment procedures.

Are we beyond "Paracelsus"?

Species-, strain-, tissue-, stage of development-, time and route of exposure-, xenobiotic- and reproductive endpoint-specific responses have all been reported, with respect to EDC exposures (Evans, 2007). Despite the complex nature of the various interactions involved in exposures to xenobiotics, especially during prenatal development (e.g., stage of fetal development, maternal genetics and nutrition, toxic effects on the mother, placental toxicity), the basic concepts set forth by Paracelsus, including the idea of a threshold response, have, for the most part, stood the test of time (Rogers and Kavlock, 2008). However, exceptions to the typical monotonic dose–response curves predicted by Paracelsus have been observed for several reproductive and other developmental endpoints, such as prostate weight in male offspring, following prenatal exposures, primarily mouse models, to very low doses of xenoestrogens, such as DES and BPA (Judy *et al.*, 1999; Nagel *et al.*, 1997; vom Saal *et al.*, 1997). These "non-monotonic" or U- or inverted U-shaped dose–response curves associated with "low dose" effects of xenoestrogens have been explained, based on endocrinological principles, in part by the estrogenic activity of the specific xenoestrogen involved; the concentration of the unbound, effective xenoestrogen in the serum; partitioning of the xenoestrogen between aqueous and lipid compartments within the body; and the disposition of the xenoestrogen relative to the route of exposure (Judy *et al.*, 1999). More recently, non-genomic estrogenic responses from interactions between BPA and plasma membrane receptors, as well as BPA's reported ability to function as an SERM at concentrations below those reported in humans, have been suggested as other plausible explanations for these observations (Welshons *et al.*, 2006).

Controversy has surrounded these reported "low dose", BPA-induced, non-monotonic dose–response effects, with other scientists not being able to replicate the experimental results, while reportedly using similar experimental protocols (Rogers and Kavlock, 2008; Tyl *et al.*, 2008). Subsequent debate has ensued over a wide range of issues, such as the inclusion of the necessary positive controls in the experiments which did not demonstrate a "low dose", non-monotonic response (Welshons *et al.*, 2003, 2006), as well as the power of the statistical analyses in the experiment demonstrating "low dose", non-monotonic dose–response effects (Owens and Chaney, 2005). Naciff *et al.* (2005) subsequently demonstrated a monotonic dose–response curve for ethinyl estradiol, genistein and BPA, with respect to the expression of 50 different genes in a rat model, and other studies have continued to demonstrate similar types of traditional dose–response relationships for other effects, using various animal models (Sharpe, 2010; Tyl *et al.*, 2008). However, despite these conflicting experimental results, reviews by vom Saal and Hughes (2005) and Welshons *et al.* (2006), as well as a recent scientific statement from the Endocrine Society (Diamanti-Kandarkis *et al.*, 2009), have reiterated concerns about the extremely "low dose", non-monotonic effects of BPA and other EDCs, which have been reported by multiple investigators, and, consequently stress the need to restructure standard risk-assessment procedures, which would have missed these potential effects.

Status of bisphenol A-associated "low dose" and non-monotonic dose–response effects

Regardless of one's thinking on the current controversies surrounding BPA and EDCs, in general, it is important to recognize that exposures to many of these chemicals are widespread, with current estimates of billions of pounds of BPA monomer currently being produced worldwide to manufacture polycarbonate plastics, the epoxy resin linings for most food and beverage cans, dental sealants and additives for other consumer products (vom Saal and Hughes, 2005). The ubiquitous nature and the relative instability of polycarbonate plastics and epoxy resins associated with heat and pH (vom Saal and Hughes, 2005), as well as the conflicting and alarming experimental results surrounding exposures to BPA, are extremely relevant issues to future studies with other EDCs. In addition, it is also critically important to understand and learn from some of the experimental inconsistencies which have been reported during the investigation of BPA. For instance, several questions which can be asked are:

1. Are observed differences between experiments due simply to species variations in reproductive physiology, xenobiotic disposition and/or xenobiotic sensitivity?
2. What roles do diet and xenoestrogens within the diet play in the differences observed between experiments?
3. How many different genomic and non-genomic signaling pathways impact a specific phenotypic change, such as the weight of a particular reproductive organ?
4. Is it reasonable to assume that all of these pathways will respond the same way to different dosing regimens, as well as timing and duration of exposure?
5. Are we comparing "apples to oranges" when making comparisons between "high dose" and "low dose" effects with possibly different mechanisms of action?

These types of questions might be particularly relevant when evaluating endpoints with inputs from both receptor-mediated and non-receptor-mediated pathways (Sharpe, 2010).

The FDA is currently reevaluating the public health risks posed by BPA, and the NIEHS is funding approximately 30 million dollars in research addressing the reported "low dose", non-monotonic effects of BPA, as well as some of the other aforementioned questions and issues surrounding this specific endocrine-disrupting xenobiotic (i.e., transgenerational effects, effects of mixtures and "total" exposure doses). The results of these investigations will be insightful, especially as they are taken into consideration during future risk-assessment decision-making processes for BPA.

It is also of relevance to note that, while these reevaluations and new research initiatives are taking place, other investigators have reported on recently completed experiments, using rat models, which have shed additional light on "low dose" reproductive and developmental neurotoxic effects of BPA and "low dose", non-monotonic, dose–response effects of xenoestrogens (Howdeshell *et al.*, 2008; Ryan *et al.*, 2010a,b; Stump *et al.*, 2010). Thus far, these most recently reported studies have not detected any "low dose" effects of prenatal and lactational exposure to BPA on androgen-dependent reproductive organ weights or sperm numbers in male rats (Howdeshell *et al.*, 2008), sexually dimorphic behavior, puberty, fertility or anatomy in female rats (Ryan *et al.*, 2010a,b), or developmental neurotoxicity endpoints (Stump *et al.*, 2010). Despite objections raised about the estrogenic sensitivity of the rat species used (vom Saal *et al.*, 2010), the Howdeshell and Ryan studies were relatively robust and did include several treatment groups of positive controls, which were treated with a relatively broad range of doses of ethinyl estradiol and which exhibited monotonic, dose-dependent ethinyl estradiol-induced effects on all of the reproductive endpoints evaluated. Efforts were also made in these experiments to include enough experimental animals in each treatment group to account for litter effects.

Based on these most recent reports, including one which did not find a relationship between perinatal exposure to BPA and the development of obesity and diabetes which is characteristic of "Metabolic Syndrome" (Ryan *et al.*, 2010a,b), it is the feeling of some scientists (Sharpe, 2010; Sharpe and Drake, 2010) that sufficient research has been completed to finalize our scientific conclusions, with respect the actual risks to human health posed by BPA. Within the rat models used, this appears be a valid conclusion at the present time. However, given the quantities of BPA present in the environment and the serious health risks which have been suggested by other researchers, it will take additional time to carry out currently funded experiments, evaluate those experimental results, and hopefully reconcile the conclusions of those experiments with those which have already been completed and reported in peer-reviewed journals. It is hoped that by the end of this process there will be answers for some of the more relevant questions regarding BPA and an enhanced understanding of the mechanisms by which endocrine-disrupting xenobiotics interfere with reproductive and developmental signaling pathways.

CONCLUDING REMARKS AND FUTURE DIRECTIONS

We live in a world surrounded by chemicals. Some of these are present only in relatively small quantities, and others are ubiquitous. Many of these compounds and elements can be extremely beneficial or are the by-products of processes of chemicals which improve the quality and convenience of our lives. Unfortunately, some of these same xenobiotics are capable, if present in sufficient quantities, of posing some degree of risk to the reproductive processes of wildlife, domestic animals and/or humans. A common mechanism by which these chemicals can impact reproduction in these species is by, in a multitude of different ways, interfering to some degree with within-cell, cell-to-cell, organ-to-organ or, in mammals, organism-to-organism signaling pathways. It is overly naive to think that any product or activity is going to be completely without risk. We are all different and can vary dramatically in the way we respond to different chemical exposures. The ultimate goal of regulators, with critical input from researchers, as well as manufacturers, should be to make educated decisions regarding environmental stewardship and public health and to invoke precaution as deemed appropriate on a chemical-by-chemical basis.

The knowledge base and scientific and technological resources exist to rationally assess what endocrine disruption risks are real at environmentally relevant concentrations; which xenobiotics are more harmful than beneficial and should be reduced, modified or eliminated; and, finally, how best can industrial, agricultural, health and lifestyle issues be reconciled with the risks posed by some chemicals abundant within our environment. Attempts should be made to constructively explain or resolve discrepancies between experimental results. An accurate assessment of the risk to animal and, ultimately, human reproductive health, from the more potent and/or abundant endocrine-disrupting xenobiotics currently recognized and studied, is critical.

Once appropriately designed and peer-reviewed research projects are completed and the data are evaluated in an objective and balanced fashion, there will eventually have to be some consensus of opinion among regulators, medical professionals, researchers and industry about how human and animal exposures to certain endocrine-disrupting xenobiotics are best going to be addressed. Depending on the specific xenobiotic involved and the overall weight-of-evidence provided, there are going to be at least three different potential outcomes. Some xenobiotics might very well be found not to pose a risk to humans or the animals at the concentrations found in the environment. Other chemicals might require added precautions under certain specific conditions of use or exposure. There will also undoubtedly be circumstances where the use or production of some chemicals will need to be curtailed and new products developed and evaluated.

It is only by reviewing and debating the available evidence and making discerning policy decisions that regulators and researchers, with input from industry, will be able to address future policy and research needs pertaining to endocrine disruption. Environmentally relevant issues and pressing questions will invariably continue to arise pertaining to synthetic and naturally occurring xenobiotics which can potentially interfere with the myriad of homeostatic mechanisms and signaling pathways present in living organisms. Governmental agencies, health professionals, research institutions and chemical manufacturers need to be ready and willing to use the lessons learned, as well as the developed experimental protocols, to prevent, if possible, or quickly investigate future instances of endocrine disruption in animal and human populations.

REFERENCES

Anway MD, Cupp AS, Uzumcu M, Skinner MK (2005) Epigenetic transgenerational actions of endocrine disruptor and male fertility. *Science* **308:** 1466–9.

Anway MD, Skinner MK (2006) Epigenetic transgenerational actions of endocrine disruptors. *Endocrinology* **147 (Suppl.):** S43–S49.

Bigsby RM, Mercado-Feliciano M, Mubiru J (2005) Molecular mechanisms of estrogen dependent processes. In *Endocrine Disruptors: Effects on Male and Female Reproductive Systems*, 2nd edition (Naz RK, ed.). CRC Press and Taylor & Francis Group, LLC, Boca Raton, pp. 217–47.

Birkhoj M, Nellemann C, Jarfelt K, Jacobsen H, Andersen HR, Dalgaard M, Vinggaard AM (2004) The combined antiandrogenic effects of five commonly used pesticides. *Toxicol Appl Pharmacol* **201:** 10–20.

Birnbaum LS, Fenton SE (2003) Cancer and developmental exposure to endocrine disruptors. *Environ Health Perpect* **111:** 389–94.

Bolt HM, Janning P, Michna H, Degen GH (2001) Comparative assessment of endocrine modulators with estrogenic activity: I. Definition of a hygiene-based margin of safety (HBMOS) for xeno-estrogens against the background of European developments. *Arch Toxicol* **74:** 649–62.

Briones-Reyes D, Gómez-Martinez L, Cueva-Rolón R (2007) Zearalenone contamination in corn for human consumption in Tlaxcala, Mexico. *Food Chem* **100:** 693–8.

Burrows, GE, Tyrl RJ (2001) *Toxic Plants of North America*. Iowa State University Press, Ames.

Cheeke PR (1998) *Natural Toxicants in Feeds*, 2nd edition. Interstate Publishers, Inc., Danville, Illinois.

Crews C, McLachlan JA (2006) Epigenetics, evolution, endocrine disruption, health and disease. *Endocrinology* **147 (Suppl.):** S4–S10.

Devine PJ, Hoyer PB (2005) Ovotoxic environmental chemicals: indirect endocrine disruptors. In *Endocrine Disruptors: Effects on Male and Female Reproductive Systems*, 2nd edition (Naz RK, ed.). CRC Press and Taylor & Francis Group, LLC, Boca Raton, pp. 67–100.

Diamanti-Kandarakis E, Bourguignon JP, Giudice LC, Hauser R, Prins GS, Soto AM, Zoeller RT, Gore AC (2009) Endocrine-disrupting chemicals: an Endocrine Society scientific statement. *Endocr Rev* **30:** 293–342.

Dutertre M, Smith CL (2000) Molecular mechanisms of selective estrogen receptor modulator (SERM) action. *J Pharmacol Exper Ther* **295:** 431–7.

Dye JA, Vernier M, Zhu L, Ward CR, Hites RA, Birnbaum LS (2007) Elevated PBDE levels in pet cats: sentinels for humans? *Environ Sci Technol* **41:** 6319–20.

Edwards TM, Moore BC, Guillette LJ Jr (2006) Reproductive dysgenesis in wildlife: a comparative view. Environment, reproductive health and fertility. *Int J Androl* **29:** 109–19.

Eskenazi B, Warner M, Samuels S, Young J, Gerthoux PM, Needham L, Patterson D, Olive D, Gavoni N, Vercellini P, Mocarelli P (2010) Serum dioxin concentrations and time to pregnancy. *Epidemiology* **21:** 224–31.

Evans TJ (2006) Introduction to toxicokinetics and toxicodynamics. In *Small Animal Toxicology*, 2nd edition (Peterson ME, Talcott PA, eds.). Elsevier–Saunders, St. Louis, pp. 18–28.

Evans TJ (2007) Reproductive toxicity and endocrine disruption. In *Veterinary Toxicology: Basic and Clinical Principles* (Gupta RC, ed.). Academic Press/Elsevier, Inc., New York, pp. 206–44.

Evans TJ, Rottinghaus GE, Casteel SW (2004) Fescue. In *Clinical Veterinary Toxicology* (Plumlee KH, ed.). Mosby, Inc., St. Louis, pp. 243–50.

Fenton SE (2009) The mammary gland: a tissue sensitive to environmental exposures. *Rev Environ Health* **24:** 319–25.

Ford JA Jr, Clark SG, Walters EM, Wheeler MB, Hurley WL (2006) Estrogenic effects of genestein on reproductive tissues of ovariectomized gilts. *J Anim Sci* **84:** 834–42.

Foster PMD, Gray LE Jr (2008) Toxic responses of the reproductive system. In *Casarett & Doull's Toxicology: The Basic Science of Poisons*, 7th edition (Klaassen CD, ed.). McGraw–Hill, New York, pp. 761–806.

Gray LE Jr, Wilson VS, Stoker T, Lambright C, Furr J, Noriega N, Howdeshell K, Ankley GT, Luillette L (2006) Adverse effects of environmental antiandrogens and androgens on reproductive development in mammals. Environment, reproductive health and fertility. *Int J Androl* **29:** 96–104.

Grün F, Blumberg B (2006) Environmental obesogens: organotins and endocrine disruption nuclear receptor signaling. *Endocrinology* **147 (Suppl.):** S50–S55.

Guerrero-Bosagna CM, Skinner MK (2009) Epigenetic transgenerational effects of endocrine disruptors on male reproduction. *Semin Reprod Med* **27:** 403–8.

Guillette LJ Jr (2006) Environmental disrupting contaminants – beyond the dogma. *Environ Health Perspect* **114(S-1):** 9–12.

Hamlin HJ, Guillette Jr LJ (2010) Birth defects in wildlife: the role of environmental contaminants as inducers of reproductive and developmental dysfunction. *System Biol Reprod Med* **56:** 113–21.

Hayes TB, Khoury V, Narayan A, Nazir M, Park A, Brown T, Adame L, Chan E, Buchholz D, Stueve T, Gallipeau S (2010) Atrazine induces complete feminization and chemical castration in African clawed frogs (*Xenopus laevus*). *Proc Natl Acad Sci USA* **107:** 4612–17.

Hayes TB, Stuart AA, Mendoza M, Collins A, Noriega N, Vonk A, Johnston G, Liu R, Kpodzo D (2006) Characterization of atrazine-induced gonadal malformations in African clawed frogs (*Xenopus laevis*) and comparisons with effects of an androgen antagonist (cypterone acetate) and exogenous estrogen (17-estradiol): support for the demasculinization/feminization hypothesis. *Environ Health Perspect* **114(S-1):** 134–41.

Hess RA (2003) Estrogen in the adult male reproductive tract: a review. *Reprod Biol Endocrinol* **1:** 52–65.

Hess RA, Iguchi T (2002) Role of herbicides and pesticides on endocrine disruption. In *Proceedings of Annual Conference of the Society for Theriogenology and American College of Theriogenologists*, Colorado Springs, CO, pp. 443–52.

Hodgson E, Mailman RB, Chambers JE, Dow RE (eds) (2000) *Dictionary of Toxicology*, 2nd edition. Grove's Dictionaries Inc., New York.

Hoekstra PF, Burnison BK, Neheli T, Muir DC (2001) Enantiomer-specific activity of o,p′-DDT with the human estrogen receptor. *Toxicol Lett* **125:** 75–81.

Hogan NS, Duarte P, Wade MG, Lean DR, Trudeau VL (2008) Estrogenic exposure affects metamorphosis and alters sex ratios in the northern leopard frog (*Rana pipiens*): identifying critically vulnerable periods of development. *Gen Comp Endocrinol* **156:** 515–23.

Howdeshell KL, Furr J, Lambright CR, Wilson VS, Ryan BC, Gray LE Jr (2008) Gestational and lactational exposure to ethinyl estradiol, but not bisphenol A, decreases androgen-dependent reproductive organ weights and epididymal sperm abundance in the male Long Evans hooded rat. *Toxicol Sci* **102:** 371–82.

Hoyer PB (2006) Impact of metals on ovarian function. In *Metals, Fertility and Reproductive Toxicity* (Golub MS, ed.). CRC Press and Taylor & Francis Group, LLC, Boca Raton, pp. 155–73.

Iavicoli I, Fontana L, Bergamaschi A (2009) The effects of metals as endocrine disruptors. *J Toxicol Environ Health, Part B* **12:** 206–23.

Jobling S, Burn RW, Thorpe K, Williams R, Tyler C (2007) Statistical modeling suggests that antiandrogens in effluents from wastewater treatment works contribute to widespread sexual disruption in fish living in English rivers. *Environ Health Perspect* **117:** 797–802.

Judy BM, Nagel SC, Thayer KA, vom Saal, FS, Welshons WV (indexed in PubMed as Welshons WV, Nagel SC, Thayer KA, Judy BM, vom Saal FS) (1999) Low-dose bioactivity of xenoestrogens in animals: fetal exposure to low doses of methoxychlor and other xenoestrogens increases adult prostate size in mice. *Toxicol Ind Health* **15:** 12–25.

Katzenellenbogen BS, Katzenellenbogen JA (2000) Estrogen receptor transcription and transactivation: estrogen receptor alpha and estrogen receptor beta: regulation by selective estrogen receptor modulators and importance in breast cancer. *Breast Cancer Res* **2:** 335–44.

Keith LH (1997) *Environmental Endocrine Disruptors: A Handbook of Property Data*. John Wiley & Sons, Inc., New York.

Krimsky S (2000) *Hormonal Chaos: The Scientific and Social Origins of the Environmental Endocrine Hypothesis*. Johns Hopkins University Press, Baltimore.

Krimsky S (2001) An epistemological inquiry into the endocrine disruptor thesis. In *Environmental Hormones: The Scientific Basis of Endocrine Disruption* (McLachlan JA, Guillette LJ Jr, Iguchi T, Toscano WA Jr, eds.). *Ann NY Acad Sci* **948:** 130–42.

Lee MR (2009) The history of ergot of rye (*Claviceps purpurea*). I: From antiquity to 1900. *J R Coll Phys Edinb* **39(2):** 179–84.

Li D, Zhou Z, Qing D, He Y, Wu T, Miao M, Wang J, Weng X, Ferber JR, Herrinton LJ, Zhu Q, Gao E, Checkoway H, Yuan W (2010) Occupational exposure to bisphenol-A (BPA) and the risk of self-reported male sexual dysfunction. *Hum Reprod* **25:** 519–27.

Liu H, Zhao M, Zhang C, Ma Y, Liu W (2008) Enantioselective cytotoxicity of the insecticide bifenthrin on a human amnion epithelial (FL) cell line. *Toxicology* **253:** 89–96.

Mahood IK, Hallmark N, McKinnell C, Walker M, Fisher JS, Sharpe RM (2005) Abnormal Leydig cell aggregation in the fetal testis of rats exposed to di (*n*-butyl) phthalate and its possible role in testicular dysgenesis. *Endocrinology* **146:** 613–23.

Mahood IK, McKinnell C, Walker M, Hallmark N, Scott H, Fisher JS, Rivas A, Hartung S, Ivell R, Mason JI, Sharpe R M (2006) Cellular origins of testicular dysgenesis in rats exposed in utero to di(*n*-butyl) phthalate. *Int J Androl* **29:** 148–54.

McClellan RO (2007) Concepts in veterinary toxicology. In *Veterinary Toxicology: Basic and Applied Principles* (Gupta RC, ed.). Academic Press/Elsevier, Inc., New York, pp. 3–24.

McLachlan JA (2001) Environmental signaling: what embryos and evolution teach us about endocrine disrupting chemicals. *Endocrine Res* **22:** 319–41.

McLachlan JA, Simpson E, Martin M (2006) Endocrine disrupters and female reproductive health. *Best Pract Res Clin Endocrinol Metab* **20:** 63–75.

Meeker JD, Barr DB, Hauser R (2008) Human semen quality and sperm DNA damage in relation to urinary metabolites of pyrethroid insecticides. *Hum Reprod* **23:** 1932–40.

Milnes MR, Bermudez DS, Bryan TA, Gunderson MP, Guillette LJ Jr (2005) Altered neonatal development and endocrine function in *Alligator mississippiensis* associated with a contaminated environment. *Biol Reprod* **73:** 1004–10.

Mocarelli P, Gerthoux PM, Patterson DG Jr, Milani S, Limonta G, Bertona M, Signorini S, Tramacere P, Colombo L, Crespi C, Brambilla P, Sarto C, Carreri V, Sampson EJ, Turner WE, Needham LL (2008) Dioxin exposure, from infancy through puberty, produces endocrine disruption and affects human semen quality. *Environ Health Perspect* **116:** 70–7.

Naciff JM, Hess KA, Overmann GJ, Torontali SM, Carr GJ, Tiesman JP, Foertsch LM, Richardson BD, Martinez JE, Daston GP (2005) Gene expression changes induced in the testis by transplacental exposure to high and low doses of 17{alpha}-ethynyl estradiol, genistein, or bisphenol A. *Toxicol Sci* **86:** 396–416.

Nagel SC, vom Saal FS, Thayer KA, Dhar MG, Boechler M, Welshons WV (1997) Relative binding affinity-serum modified access (RBA-SMA) assay predicts the relative in vivo bioactivity of the xenoestrogens bisphenol A and octylphenol. *Environ Health Perspect* **105:** 70–6.

Newbold RR, Padilla-Banks E, Jefferson WN (2006) Adverse effects of the model environmental estrogen diethylstilbestrol are transmitted to subsequent generations. *Endocrinology* **147 (Suppl.):** S11–S17.

Nilsson EE, Anway MD, Stanfield J, Skinner MK (2008) Transgenerational epigenetic effects of the endocrine disruptor vinclozolin on pregnancies and female adult onset disease. *Reproduction* **135:** 713–21.

Owens JW, Chaney JG (2005) Weighing the results of differing "low dose" studies of the mouse prostate by Nagel, Cagen, and Ashby: quantification of experimental power and statistical results. *Regul Toxicol Pharmacol* **43:** 194–202.

Ohtake F, Takeyama K, Matsumoto T, Kitagawa H, Yamamoto Y, Nohara K, Tohyama C, Krust A, Mimura J, Chambon P, Yanaglsawa J, Fuji-Kuriyama Y, Kato S (2003). Modulation of oestrogen receptor signalling by association with the activated dioxin receptor. *Nature* **423:** 545–50.

Orlando EF, Kolok, A, Binzcik GA, Gates JL, Horton MK, Lambright CS, Gray LE Jr, Soto AM, Guillette LJ Jr (2004) Endocrine-disrupting effects of cattle feedlot effluent on an aquatic sentinel species, the fathead minnow. *Environ Health Perspect* **112:** 353–8.

Parkinson A, Ogilvie BW (2008) Biotransformation of xenobiotics. In *Casarett &Doull's Toxicology: The Basic Science of Poisons*, 7th edition (Klaassen CD, ed.). McGraw–Hill, New York, pp. 161–304.

Petersen SL, Krishnan S, Hudgens ED (2006) The aryl hydrocarbon receptor pathway and sexual differentiation of neuroendocrine functions. *Endocrinology* **147 (Suppl.):** S33–S42.

Roberts CA, Kallenbach RL, Hill NS, Rottinghaus GE, Evans TJ (2009) Ergot alkaloid concentrations in tall fescue hay during production and storage. *Crop Science* **49:** 1496–502.

Rogers JM, Kavlock RJ (2008) Developmental toxicology. In *Casarett & Doull's Toxicology: The Basic Science of Poisons*, 7th edition (Klaassen CD, ed.). McGraw–Hill, New York, pp. 415–51.

Ruhlen RL, Howdeshell KL, Mao J, Taylor JA, Bronson FH, Newbold RR, Welshons WV, vom Saal FS (2008) Low phytoestrogen levels in feed increase fetal serum estradiol resulting in the "fetal estrogenization syndrome" and obesity in CD-1 mice. *Environ Health Perspect* **116:** 322–8.

Ryan BC, Hotchkiss AK, Crofton KM, Gray LE Jr (2010a) In utero and lactational exposure to bisphenol A, in contrast to ethinyl estradiol, does not alter sexually dimorphic behavior, puberty, fertility, and anatomy of female LE rats. *Toxicol Sci* **114:** 133–48.

Ryan KK, Haller AM, Sorrell JE, Woods SC, Jandacek RJ, Seeley RJ (2010b) Perinatal exposure to bisphenol-a and the development of metabolic syndrome in CD-1 mice. *Endocrinology* **151:** 2603–12.

Safe SH (2005) 2,3,7,8-tetrachlorodibenzo-*p*-dioxin (TCDD) and related environmental antiandrogens: characterization and mechanism of action. In *Endocrine Disruptors: Effects on Male and Female Reproductive Systems*, 2nd edition (Naz RK, ed.). CRC Press and Taylor & Francis Group, LLC, Boca Raton, pp. 249–87.

Safe SH, Khan S, Wu F, Li X (2007) Chemical-induced estrogenicity. In *Veterinary Toxicology: Basic and Clinical Principles* (Gupta RC, ed.). Academic Press/Elsevier, Inc., New York, pp. 811–22.

Schneider S, Kaufmann W, Buesen R, van Ravenzwaay B (2008) Vinclozolin – the lack of a transgenerational effect after oral maternal exposure during organogenesis. *Reprod Toxicol* **25:** 352–60.

Senger PL (2003) *Pathways to Pregnancy and Parturition*, 2nd edition. Current Conceptions, Inc., Moscow, ID.

Sharpe RM (2010) Is it time to end concerns over the estrogenic effects of bisphenol A? *Toxicol Sci* **114:** 1–4.

Sharpe RM, Drake AJ (2010) Bisphenol A and metabolic syndrome. *Endocrinology* **151:** 2404–7.

Sharpe RM, McKinnell C, Kivlin C, Fisher JS (2003) Proliferation and functional maturation of Sertoli cells, and their relevance to disorders of testis function in adulthood. *Reproduction* **125:** 769–84.

Sikka SC, Kendirci M, Naz R (2005) Endoctine disruptors and male infertility. In *Endocrine Disruptors: Effects on Male and Female Reproductive Systems*, 2nd edition (Naz RK, ed.). CRC Press and Taylor & Francis Group, LLC, Boca Raton, pp. 291–312.

Skakkebæk NE, Rajpert-de Meyts E, Main KM (2001) Testicular dysgenesis syndrome: an increasingly common developmental disorder with environmental aspects. *Hum Reprod* **16:** 972–8.

Skakkebæk NE, Jørgensen N, Main KM, Rajpert-de Meyts E, Leffers H, Andersson A-M, Juul A, Carlsen E, Krog Mortensen G, Kold Jensen T, Toppari J (2006) Is human fecundity declining? *Int J Androl* **29:** 2–11.

Stump DG, Beck MJ, Radovsky A, Garman RH, Freshwater LL, Sheets LP, Marty MS, Waechter JM Jr, Dimond SS, Van Miller JP, Shiotsuka RN, Beyer D, Chappelle AH, Hentges SG (2010) Developmental neurotoxicity study of dietary bisphenol A in Sprague-Dawley rats. *Toxicol Sci* **115:** 167–82.

Swan SH, Brazil C, Drobnis EZ, Liu F, Kruse RL, Hatch M, Redmon JB, Wang C, Overstreet JW (2003a) Geographical differences in semen quality of fertile U.S. males. *Environ Health Perspect* **111:** 414–20.

Swan SH, Elkin EP, Fenster L (2000) The question of declining sperm density revisited: an analysis of 101 studies published 1934–1996. *Environ Health Perspect* **108:** 961–6.

Swan SH, Kruse RL, Liu F, Barr DB, Drobnis EZ, Redmon JB, Wang C, Brazil C, Overstreet JW (2003b) Semen quality in relation to biomarkers of pesticide exposure. *Environ Health Perspect* **111:** 1478–84.

Swan SH, Main KM, Liu F, Stewart SL, Kruse RL, Calafat AM, Mao CS, Redmon JB, Ternand CL, Sullivan S, Teague JL (2005) Decrease in anogenital distance among male infants with prenatal phthalate exposure. *Environ Health Perspect* **113:** 1056–61.

Swedenborg E, Rüegg J, Mäkelä S, Pongratz I (2009) Endocrine disruptive chemicals: mechanisms of action and involvement in metabolic disorders. *J Mol Endocrinol* **43:** 1–10.

Tarleton BJ, Wiley AA, Bartol FF (2001) Neonatal estradiol exposure alters uterine morphology and endometrial transcriptional activity in prepubertal gilts. *Domest Anim Endocrinol* **21:** 111–25.

Thomas P, Khan IA (2005) Disruption of nongenomic steroid actions on gametes and serotonergic pathways controlling reproductive neuroendocrine function by environmental chemicals. In *Endocrine Disruptors: Effects on Male and Female Reproductive Systems*, 2nd edition (Naz RK, ed.). CRC Press and Taylor & Francis Group, LLC, Boca Raton, pp. 3–45.

Tyl RW, Myers CB, Marr MC, Sloan CS, Castillo NP, Veselica MM, Seely JC, Dimond SS, Van Miller JP, Shiotsuka RN, Beyer D, Hentges SG, Waechter JM Jr (2008) Two-generation reproductive toxicity study of dietary bisphenol A in CD-1 (Swiss) mice. *Toxicol Sci* **104:** 362–84.

Warner M, Gustafsson J-A (2006) Nongenomic effects of estrogen: why all the uncertainty? *Steroids* **71:** 91–5.

Warner M, Eskenazi B, Mocarelli P, Gerthoux PM, Samuels S, Needham L, Patterson D, Brambilla P (2002) Serum dioxin concentrations and breast cancer risk in the Seveso Women's Health Study. *Environ Health Perspect* **110:** 625–8.

vom Saal FS, Akingbemi BT, Belcher SM, Crain DA, Crews, D, Guidice LC, *et al.* (2010) Flawed experimental design reveals the need for guidelines requiring appropriate positive controls in endocrine disruption research. *Toxicol Sci* **115:** 612–13

vom Saal FS, Hughes C (2005) An extensive new literature concerning low-dose effects of bisphenol A shows the need for a new risk assessment. *Environ Health Perspect* **113:** 926–33.

vom Saal FS, Timms BG, Montano MM, Palanza P, Thayer KA, Nagel SC, Dhar MD, Ganjam VK, Parmigiani S, Welshons WV (1997) Prostate enlargement in mice due to fetal exposure to low doses of estradiol or diethylstilbestrol and opposite effects at high doses. *Proc Natl Acad Sci USA* **94:** 2056–61.

Weinberg ED (2010) Can iron be teratogenic? *Biometals* **23:** 181–4.

Welshons WV, Nagel SC, vom Saal FS (2006) Large effects from small exposures. III. Endocrine mechanisms mediating effects of bisphenol A at levels of human exposure. *Endocrinology* **147(6) (Suppl.):** S56–S69.

Welshons WV, Thayer KA, Judy BM, Taylor JA, Curran EM, vom Saal FS (2003) Large effects from small exposures. I. Mechanisms for endocrine-disrupting chemicals with estrogenic activity. *Environ Health Perspect* **111:** 994–1006.

Xia Y, Han Y, Wu B, Wang S, Gu A, Lu N, Bo J, Song L, Jin N, Wang X (2008) The relation between urinary metabolite of pyrethroid insecticides and semen quality in humans. *Fertil Steril* **89:** 1743–50.

Zanoli P, Zavatti M (2008) Pharmacognostic and pharmacological profile of *Humulus lupulus L. J Ethnopharmacol* **116:** 383–96.

Zhang J, Zhu W, Zheng Y, Yang J, Zhu X (2008) The antiandrogenic activity of pyrethroid pesticides cyfluthrin and β-cyfluthrin. *Reprod Toxicol* **25:** 491–6.

C H A P T E R

68

Screening systems for endocrine disruptors

Teruo Sugawara

INTRODUCTION

Much interest has recently been shown in endocrine disruptors as environmental pollutants (de Solla *et al.*, 1998; Fry, 1995). "Wingspread Declaration", which was announced in July 1991, encouraged researchers to investigate endocrine disruptors pertaining to hormone problems. Since the presentation of "Our Stolen Future" in 1996, international concern about this problem has been considerably increased. Endocrine disruptors are synthetic chemical substances that can cause adverse effects in organisms or their progeny following the disruption of endocrine systems. Chemical manufacturers produce many products that are used in agriculture, medical healthcare and cosmetic beauty, almost all of which are safe, but some chemical substances seem to cause not only endocrine systems failure, but also homeostasis disturbance. Some researchers have been concerned about the possibilities of endocrine disruptors increasing mental disorders, obesity and type 2 diabetes in children (Newbold *et al.*, 2007, 2009; van den Hazel *et al.*, 2006). Chemical substances that bind to steroid hormone receptors, including estrogen receptors, progesterone receptors or androgen receptors, induce steroid hormone receptor-mediated responses. These compounds include chemicals isolated from plants such as phytoestrogens. Many chemical substances used as pesticides (herbicides, insecticides and fungicides, etc.) have been reported to exert hormonal activities and are thus classified as endocrine disruptors. Although attention has been mainly focused on chemical substances that directly interact with estrogen receptors, chemicals can also affect the endocrine systems by interfering with the synthesis or metabolism of estrogens. Endocrine disruptors have pronounced effects on expression of the steroidogenic acute regulatory protein gene, which is a rate-limiting factor of steroidogenesis (Warita *et al.*, 2006). Disturbance of steroid hormone production in the gonads has become a serious problem because estrogen-like chemicals cause reproductive dysfunction (Safe, 1995a). Hypothalamo-pituitary control of gonadotropin secretion may be affected by smaller concentrations of estrogenic chemicals than reproductive organs. There have been reports of prostatic and testicular cancers, cryptorchism and hypospadias in males who have been exposed to high doses of estrogen (Cocco and Benichou, 1998; Fernandez *et al.*, 2007; Paulozzi, 1999; Sharpe, 1995), and a 50% reduction in human sperm counts in 50 years has also been reported (Carlsen *et al.*, 1992). Another concern is the involvement of xenoestrogens in some common cancers in women. *In utero* exposure to environmental compounds has been thought to be a cause of cancers in children. In early life, exposure to endocrine disruptors affects puberty age and may cause an increase in the risk of breast cancer (Fenton, 2006). It has been reported that diethylstilbestrol (DES), a synthetic estrogen prescribed to pregnant women to prevent spontaneous abortion, caused an increased risk of vaginal cancer in the female progeny of women taking DES (Herbst and Scully, 1970).

The effects of chemical substances on human health are complicated since individuals are exposed to a complex mixture of contaminants. Aromatic hydrocarbons, including dioxin-like compounds (DLCs), disturb endocrine systems of animals and humans and induce reproductive disorders and malignant tumors (Safe, 1995b). DLCs include chemicals with known affinity for the aryl hydrocarbon receptor (AhR), such as polychloro-p-dibenzodioxins (PCDDs), polychloro-p-dibenzofurans (PCDFs), polychlorinated biphenyls (PCBs), polybrominated biphenyls (PBBs), polycyclic aromatic hydrocarbons (PAHs) and other halogenated aromatic hydrocarbons (HAHs). Once discharged, DLCs are concentrated *in vivo* via the food chain, and it is known that DLCs have carcinogenicity and teratogenicity in higher animals and humans (Huff *et al.*, 1994; Kociba and Schwetz, 1982; Kohn, 1995). Although the mechanisms by which DLCs exert toxicity have been extensively studied, much has yet to be learned about the direct effects of dioxin on the female reproductive system. Follicular development in the ovaries, secretion of gonadotropins and steroidogenesis all play important roles in reproductive success and are potentially affected by DLCs (Gao *et al.*, 2000; Son *et al.*, 1999). DLCs are the most potent toxicants of AhR ligands due to their accumulation in the environment, resistance to breakdown and impact on multiple organ systems. Short-term exposure to high doses of DLCs and similar ligands induces endocrine disruption, endometriosis, teratogenesis and abortion; alters sexual behavior; decreases spermatogenesis; and diminishes fertility (Gao *et al.*, 2000).

Reproductive and Developmental Toxicology, Edited by Ramesh C. Gupta
ISBN: 978-0-12-382032-7

It is beyond the scope of this chapter to cover all chemicals that may exert endocrine disruption or screening systems for them. Instead, this chapter describes high throughput screening methods that may enable the researchers to assess a large number of synthetic chemicals for endocrine disruption.

IN VITRO SCREENING ASSAYS

Cell proliferation assays

Currently, the assay methods, which use cells that respond to estrogen, are widely used by researchers. Both proliferation and differentiation of ovary and mammary cells responding to particular hormones are often used in endocrine disruption assays (Popnikolov *et al.*, 2001). Established carcinoma cells from breast cancer or endometrial cancer are used for cell proliferation assays. MCF-7 cells have been established from breast cancer and Ishikawa cells have been established from endometrial cancer (Brooks *et al.*, 1973; Ishiwata *et al.*, 1984). Both MCF-7 and Ishikawa cells are human cells that are highly differentiated carcinoma cell lines and express estrogen receptors. An assay using MCF-7 cells and Ishikawa cells has been widely used for screening endocrine disruptors of chemical class (Fang *et al.*, 2000; Fei *et al.*, 2005; Ohno *et al.*, 2001; Schmitt *et al.*, 2001). This assay, named E-SCREEN, is used to determine whether chemical substances have estrogenic action (Sonnenschein *et al.*, 1995; Soto *et al.*, 1994, 1995). Adding estrogen exogenously causes cells to proliferate and change their shapes (Healicon *et al.*, 1993). The E-SCREEN method detects estrogenic activities using this principle (Fang *et al.*, 2000; Oh *et al.*, 2008; Perez *et al.*, 1998; Rasmussen *et al.*, 2003). This method discovered that certain chemical substances disturb estrogen activities (Fang *et al.*, 2000). For example, alkylphenols, phthalates, PCBs and some insecticides were found to have estrogen-mimicking actions. Briefly, the procedure for E-SCREEN is as follows (Sonnenschein *et al.*, 1995; Soto *et al.*, 1994, 1995). MCF-7 human cells are spread on a 12-well or a 96-well culture plate at a density of 2,000–2,500 cells per well. Phenol-red free DMEM is replaced with charcoal-dextran (CD)-stripped 10% FBS the next day. Then chemical substances to be examined are added to the medium. After 6 days of medium change, the number of cells is counted using cells stained with a dye. Beta-estradiol is used as a control for the assay method. The detection limit of the assay is 10 pg/ml (30 pM) of estradiol, and the concentrations of chemical substances to screen for endocrine disruptors have been reported to be from 10 nM to 10 μM. Toxicity is described in cells, rather than proliferation effect, when chemical substances of high concentration are added to the culture medium (Oh *et al.*, 2006).

Although the cell proliferation assay is very sensitive, assay results are influenced by cell culture conditions. While doing cell culture as a routine work is relevant, it is currently pointed out that some laboratories fail to do so. Cancer cells tend to change their original characters while being subcultured. Expression of the estrogen receptor, which is the basis of the assaying principle, changes and results in alteration of the reactivity of estrogen. The proliferation of MCF-7 cells is affected not only by estrogenic substances but also by growth factors such as EGF and IGF-1 (Stewart *et al.*, 1992; Reddy *et al.*, 1992). The reproducibility of the assay results must be carefully evaluated. Although the assay is effective for screening estrogenic action in humans, we must carefully consider whether the assay is useful for screening estrogenic action in wild animals and aquatic organisms. It is not yet clear whether chemical substances that bind to the human estrogen receptor show estrogenic action in wild animals. Selection of cell lines is important to apply the screening assay to wild animals and aquatic organisms.

A screening procedure (A-SCREEN) for androgenic hormones using the same mechanism as that for E-SCREEN has been reported (Soto *et al.*, 2004). By using the A-SCREEN method, which uses prostate cancer cells, it has been discovered that dichlorodiphenyl dichloroethylene (DDE) has androgenic action in humans. Although A-SCREEN utilizes prostate cancer cell lines, another screening method uses breast cancer MCF-7 cells transfected with androgen receptors (Soto *et al.*, 2004). The existence of androgenic actions among chemical substances is judged by whether it has the effect to repress cell proliferation or not.

Leiomyoma cells have a significantly stronger response to estrogen than do myometrial cells, indicating that leiomyomas may be hypersensitive to estrogen (Andersen *et al.*, 1995). Several estrogen-regulated genes, such as the progesterone receptor and the growth factors IGF-I and EGF and their receptors, have been found to have elevated expression in uterine leiomyomas (Andersen and Barbieri, 1995). The uterus is responsive to estrogen, and the leiomyoma cells are potential targets of endocrine disruptors. Organochlorine pesticides, kepone, TPTE (2,2-bis-(*p*-hydroxyphenyl)-1,1,1-trichloroethane) and endosulfan isomers stimulate proliferation of uterine leiomyoma cells and exhibit agonistic activity (Hodges *et al.*, 2000). Uterine leimyoma cells may be useful for endocrine disruptor screening.

Estrogen-regulated protein assay

Estrogens accelerate activity of cell mitosis and result in proliferation of cancer cells to respond to estrogens. Estrogens have actions not only on cell proliferation but also on specific gene expression. Estrogens bind to their receptors, and then the complex is translocated into the nucleus, where it interacts with the estrogen response element and transcribes the gene. Expression of pS2 is modulated by estrogen in MCF-7 cells (Jakowlew *et al.*, 1984). Estrogenic activity of chemical substances is compared to that of estradiol. Several synthesis estrogens have been investigated by this *in vitro* assay. Briefly, the assay procedure is as follows. MCF-7 cells are cultured for 72 h after addition of chemical substances. The expression level of pS2 is measured by a radioimmunoassay or enzyme-linked immunosorbent assay (ELISA). By using the pS2 assay, some insecticides, dieldrin, endosulfan and toxaphene, were found to have estrogenic activity (Soto *et al.*, 1995). The degree of estrogenic action reflects protein levels in cells. Real-time PCR is useful for measuring expression levels of estrogen-regulated genes. Not only pS2 but also several marker genes have been investigated as candidate genes, and it has been shown that transforming growth factor β3, monoamine oxidase A, and 1-antichymotrypsin are estrogen-regulated genes (Jorgensen *et al.*, 2000). Progesterone receptor (PR) is well known as an estrogen-regulated protein. After exposure to chemical substances for 72 h, the level of PR is measured using ELISA. N-butyl benzyl phthalate has been found to have estrogenic activity (Picard *et al.*, 2001).

Pituitary lactotrophs are well-characterized estrogen-responsive cells. In prolactin (PRL) release assays *in vitro*, primary rat anterior pituitary cells, GH3 cells (somatomammotroph cells) were used to examine the effects of chemical substances (Corcia *et al.*, 1993; Kochukov *et al.*, 2009; Watson *et al.*, 1995). Estrogen binds to estrogen receptors and regulates transcription of PRL through the estrogen response element. The chemical substances, such as xenoestrogens, seem to affect not only proliferation of cells but also PRL production by directly acting on the promoter of the PRL gene. Bisphenol A was found to have an estrogen-mimicking effect on lactotrophs (Steinmetz *et al.*, 1997). Xenoestrogens seem to directly affect endocrine balance and disrupt homeostasis. Exogenous estrogens induce proliferation of anterior pituitary cells and stimulate secretion of PRL in rats (F344 or SD rats) (Chen and Pittman, 1988; Date *et al.*, 2002). To examine whether chemical substances have estrogenic action, PRL production is thought to be a good screening assay both *in vitro* and *in vivo*.

Vitellogenin synthesis in the liver is innate in fish, and the synthesis of vitellogenin is under the control of many hormones, particularly estradiol (Tyler *et al.*, 1991). Vitellogenin synthesis increases with ovary growth in female fish (Hamazaki *et al.*, 1989; Selman and Wallace, 1983). In contrast, there is little vitellogenin synthesis in male fish (Campbell and Idler, 1980). However, if male fish are exposed to exogenous estrogens, including estrogenic chemicals, vitellogenin synthesis will increase. It is thought that vitellogenin synthesis in male fish can be a biomarker for estrogenic chemical contamination in aquatic organisms (Rotchell and Ostrander, 2003). Primary hepatocytes have been cultured to investigate estrogenic chemicals *in vitro* (Hollert *et al.*, 2005; Navas and Segner, 2006). Estrogenic activity of chemical substances was examined using the culture system. The detergents (nonylphenol and octylphenol), pesticides (*o,p′*-DDT and Aroclor) and bisphenol A were found to have estrogenic activity (Celius *et al.*, 1999; Flouriot *et al.*, 1995; Tollefsen *et al.*, 2003). In this screening method, chemicals were exposed for 2 days before evaluation. Evaluated vitellogenin level is not only measurement of protein level but also measurement of vitellogenin gene level using PCR (de Vlaming *et al.*, 2007).

Although all estrogenic chemical substances all have the same effect on proliferation of cells, effects of chemical substances on gene expression are quite different. Different gene expression may depend on the promoter activity of genes, and estrogen response elements of the promoter are thought to be important for genes. If the chemical substances tested have estrogenic activity *in vitro* but not *in vivo*, the test can be used to assay metabolites of chemicals and to examine chemical substances for estrogenic activity (Picard *et al.*, 2001).

Quantitative structure–activity relationships (QSARs)

There are large numbers of chemical substances in our environment to screen for activity of endocrine disruptors. Methods *in silico* are becoming recognized as useful screening systems to prioritize chemical substances (DeLisle *et al.*, 2001; Zauhar and Morgan, 1985; Zauhar *et al.*, 2003). QSAR analyses are applied in chemistry and biological areas. Indeed, in the field of aquatic toxicology, QSAR analyses have been developed as scientifically credible tools for predicting the toxicity of chemicals when little or no empirical data are available (Bradbury, 1995). Analysis of estrogens has been performed for many years and chemical structure and biological function are well known. According to these findings the QSAR of estrogen was applied to analyze the synthetic estrogens (Tong *et al.*, 1997a,b; Waller *et al.*, 1995). QSAR analysis is based on information of chemical structure obtained from a chemical structure database. Structural changes correlate with biological alteration in the estimative method. Several comparative molecular field analysis (CoMFA) models have been developed (Cramer *et al.*, 1989; Loughney and Schwender, 1992; Waller *et al.*, 1996). CoMFA implies structural similarity and diversity from the interaction between estrogen receptors and ligands. Relative binding affinity (RBA) has been predicted by this virtual screening method. Comparison between calculated RBA and experimental RBA using natural estrogens is needed before the QSAR analysis is performed. Using this method prior to *in vivo* assay enables researchers to save time, cost and work. Although QSAR analysis is an efficient method for screening many chemical substances, a large amount of experimental data is required to establish the procedures of QSAR.

Estrogen receptor binding assay

This assay is one of the basic procedures when screening endocrine disruptors, since the method analyzes if the chemical substances are bound to estrogen receptors (Clark and Gorski, 1969; Hahnel, 1971). Cell fractures from cytosol of mammalian uterus, including human uterus, are used as the estrogen receptor source. Radiolabeled estrogens are saturated with estrogen receptors and then mixed with chemical substances to be examined. Chemical substances compete with labeled estrogens to bind sites to estrogen receptors. Using the dextran-charcoal method, the unbound fraction is separated and estrogen bound to the receptor is put into a scintillation counter (Hahnel, 1971; Jungblut *et al.*, 1972). The existence of the estrogen effect among chemical substances can be known by comparing its IC_{50} (the concentration of the test chemical substances that displaces 50% of the reference estrogen from the receptor) with the IC_{50} of 17β-estradiol. Some modified assay methods have been used to evaluate estrogenic activity. Fractions of MCF-7 are used as estrogen receptors, instead of the whole cell (Stoessel and Leclercq, 1986). Estrogen receptor α or β cDNA was cloned into a baculovirus or transfer vectors, and the recombinant baculovirus vectors were transfected into insect Sf9 cells. From these cells, estrogen receptors were purified (Bolger *et al.*, 1998; Kuiper *et al.*, 1998). Estrogen receptors were prepared using *in vitro* translation or glutathione-S-transferase (GST) fusion protein, which consists of human estrogen receptor (Kuiper *et al.*, 1997; Matthews *et al.*, 2000; Matthews and Zacharewski, 2000). For water pollution screening GST fusion protein to fish estrogen receptor is available (Pakdel *et al.*, 1994). A fluorescence polarization (FP) method can be used to measure estrogenic activity to compete with the fluorescent estrogen and recombinant estrogen receptor (Bolger *et al.*, 1998). Several improved assay methods can be eliminated by using either animals or non-radioactive ligands. Non-radioactive ligands are strongly recommended for they are not likely to violate the natural surroundings. These binding assays are used to evaluate the interactions between chemical substances and binding receptors. The assays may give false negative results since this method does not represent the metabolites formed *in vivo*. Although the binding assay is effective for screening estrogenic substances from many chemical substances, the assay does not distinguish agonist and antagonist, since it does not represent transactivity of responder genes to estrogen.

Estrogen receptor transcriptional activation assays in yeast (yeast estrogen screen – YES)

When estrogen binds to the receptor, it becomes active, i.e. conformational changes occur and it enters the nucleus and binds to a specific consensus estrogen receptor response element (ERE). The complex with estrogen and the receptor binds to the ERE and controls the transcription of target genes of estrogen. An estrogen receptor cDNA expression vector and a reporter plasmid in which ERE fused to the *lacZ* gene was inserted were co-transfected into yeast. This yeast estrogen screen (YES) is useful for detecting estrogenic activity of chemical substances (Arnold *et al.*, 1996). Although yeast strains lack endogenous estrogen receptors, yeast has a signal transduction mechanism similar to eukaryotic cells. The yeast screening system implicates not only ligand-binding affinity but also transactivity of estrogenic effects of chemical substances. Several screening systems have been developed and sensitivity of the systems is the pM order (Arnold *et al.*, 1996; Kohno *et al.*, 1994). A recombinant yeast cell bioassay (RCBA) has a detection limit of 0.02 pg/ml of estradiol (Coldham *et al.*, 1997; Klein *et al.*, 1994). Although yeast has a metabolic mechanism that is quite different from that of prokaryotic cells, it does not have the same mechanism of mammalian cells. It is not possible to detect estrogenic activity of chemical substances and metabolite compounds of xenoestrogens in a yeast system without a steroid receptor co-activator. The interaction between estrogens and its receptor, which is the transcriptional steroid receptor co-activator, must be considered when assaying estrogenic activity. Several co-activators of estrogen receptor are known, and steroid receptor co-activator-1 (SRC-1) has been studied by many researchers. The SRC-1 gene is expressed in the same tissues in which the estrogen receptor is expressed. SRC-1 plays important roles in the transduction of estrogen-responsive gene expression in every organ. Reporter yeast strains expressing human estrogen receptors α or β have been developed. These strains contain a reporter plasmid carrying an ERE upstream of the β-galactosidase gene and a plasmid expressing the SRC-1 gene (Chu *et al.*, 2009). A receptor co-activator system of mammalian cells is different from a yeast system. A yeast screening system cannot discriminate an estrogen activator from antiestrogens since yeast lacks a co-activator of the receptor. A yeast two-hybrid system employing the interaction between the human estrogen receptor β ligand-binding domain and the co-activator SRC1 has been reported (Lee *et al.*, 2002; Nishikawa *et al.*, 1999). Anti-estrogenic activity and estrogenic activity of endocrine disruptors were evaluated using this system (Lee *et al.*, 2007, 2006). Although the estrogenic activity of many chemical substances has been examined using a yeast-based screening system, we must understand the character of the system. Generally, the yeast cell wall is thick and several chemical substances cannot penetrate the wall. Some estrogenic substances may not show estrogenic activity because of their inability to penetrate the cell wall. Although a yeast screening system has some disadvantages, yeast strains are easy and inexpensive to maintain, and reporter plasmids in yeast are maintained by a culture medium using a selective medium that is not a mammalian cell culture system. Improved yeast bioassays using a rapid but sensitive screening method for endocrine disruptors have recently been developed with the advent of new chemiluminescent substrates. Due to the high sensitivity (EC_{50} for β-estradiol being approximately 0.7 nM) and very short assay time (2–4 h), environmental water samples can be assayed directly without sterilization, extraction and concentration. These assays are rapid and sensitive methods for determining the presence of chemical substance contamination in environmental samples (Balsiger *et al.*, 2010).

Unlike the yeast two-hybrid system, the yeast one-hybrid system has been used to identify endocrine disruptors (Sugawara *et al.*, 2002; Sugawara and Nomura, 2006). The one-hybrid system is an assay that enables identification of the interaction between DNA and proteins *in vivo* using the yeast host (Fields and Song, 1989; Wei *et al.*, 1999). The principle of the system is that a DNA-binding domain (DNA-BD) and an activation domain (AD) form a complex, resulting in downstream gene transcription. Both *HIS3* and *lacZ* reporter genes are connected to three tandem copies of the estrogen response element. The Gal4-estrogen receptor is a fusion protein made from the AD of the yeast GAL4 transactivator gene and is then incorporated into a plasmid, which is transfected into the YM4271 yeast cell strain. *HIS3* or *lacZ* is activated in the reporter gene when the estrogen receptor is fused with the AD in the presence of an estrogen-like molecule. Then colonies can grow on a minimal culture medium lacking histidine. Interaction of the estrogen receptor with DNA can also be detected using *lacZ* expression with β-galactosidase enzyme. This screening system enabled detection of as little as 10^{-12} mol of β-estradiol. These results show that this newly developed dual assay seems to be useful for the screening of endocrine disruptors that have estrogen-like action. Ten chemicals (dicyclohexyl phathalate, di-*n*-pentyl phthalate, *p*-*n*-pentylphenol, *p*-*t*-octylphenol, *p*-*n*-octylphenol, *p*-*n*-nonylphenol, benzophenone, bisphenol A, *n*-butylbenzene and 1,3-diphenylpropane) have been examined and have been shown to have estrogenic activity.

Mammalian cell reporter gene (MCRG) system

Several advisory committees, including EDSTAC (Endocrine Disruptors Screening and Testing Advisory Committee) and ICCVAM (Interagency Coordinating Committee on the Validation of Alternative Methods), have recommended an assay system that contains stable estrogen-dependent gene expression for detecting estrogenic activity in chemical substances. The assay system using mammalian cells seems to be the best screening system without considering permeability of chemicals through cell walls. An estrogenic signal transducer mechanism seems to be present in mammalians including humans. Basically, several tandem repeats of the estrogen response element are inserted into the reporter gene. Assay of luciferase is convenient and easy for a reporter gene. Mammalian cells and mouse, rat or human cancer cell lines have been used as host cells. In the case of no expression of estrogen receptors in cells, an estrogen receptor expression vector must be transfected into mammalian cells. Since transient cells transfected with a reporter gene need to be prepared every assay time, stable transfected cell lines that have developed seem to provide a much more specific, responsive and quick method for screening chemical substances (Legler *et al.*, 1999). T47D human breast cancer cells transfected with a triplet ERE reporter gene construct have been developed. Assay sensitivity ranged from 1 fM to 100 nM of estradiol. The assay activity was inhibited by ICI 182,780, which is an estrogen antagonist (Wilson *et al.*, 2004). The developed screening system can detect estrogen receptor agonists and antagonists.

Dioxin receptor CALUX assay was also developed for detecting DLCs (Murk *et al.*, 1996). DLCs have an antiestrogenic activity because of the cross-talk between the AhR and estrogen receptor (Safe, 1995b). Indeed, a high expression level of estrogen receptor in host cells brings high sensitivity of the assay. T-47D cells express not only an estrogen receptor but also other nuclear receptors, glucocorticoid, androgen and progesterone receptors. The activation of nuclear receptors, which share common co-activators or co-repressors, is interfered with by competition between these cofactors. Interference between progesterone and estrogen receptors is well known (Kraus *et al.*, 1995). To develop a screening assay system, the cross-talk of a nuclear receptor signal transduction mechanism should be considered. U2-OS human osteosarcoma cells do not express high levels of steroid receptors and lack expression of AhR. A U2-OS-based CALUX assay, which does not reduce the estrogen-induced luciferase activity, has been developed (Sonneveld *et al.*, 2005). These estrogenic activity assay results, which utilize transcriptional activation, are not sometimes consistent with results from other assays, competitive binding assay or uterotropic assay (Shelby *et al.*, 1996). Some chemical substances generally are metabolized in the liver. The established carcinoma cell line may have low expression levels of CYP450 xenobiotic enzymes. The metabolic activation will be needed to consider in the assay system. Reporter gene assay systems can be prepared according to the purpose of screening of hormones. Estrogen and androgen activities were examined in 200 pesticides by *in vitro* reporter gene assays using Chinese hamster ovary cells (Kojima *et al.*, 2004). The assay systems were prepared by temporally transfecting human estrogen α, estrogen β or androgen receptor into CHO cells. Transactivity was assayed using dual luciferase reporter genes. According to their reports, several pesticides had effects of agonists of estrogen receptors α or β, but interestingly, any pesticides did not have effects of agonists of androgen receptor. Androgen-associated transactivity was inhibited by these pesticides. Some of the pesticides were found to have estrogenic activity via the human estrogen receptor and antiandrogenic activity via the human androgen receptor. These chemical substances which have both estrogenic and antiandrogenic activity cause the feminization of animals, including reduced sperm counts.

While hormonal activity of chemical substances is discussed, we need to examine estrogenic or androgenic activity of chemical substances and to determine agonists or antagonists. Estrogens are converted from androgens, i.e. estrogens are synthesized by aromatizing androgen, androstenedione or testosterone. We must consider the aromatizing activity of chemical substances. The induction of imposex in gastropods was allegedly inhibition of aromatization by tributyltin or triphenyltin (Heidrich *et al.*, 2001). Several flavonoid and chemical substances, agriculture chemicals, pesticides and fungicides have been reported as aromatase inhibitors or inducers (Ohno *et al.*, 2004). In an *in vitro* assay, aromatase was measured by the amount of ^{3}H water released from RI-labeled androstenedione (Siiteri and Thompson, 1975). For widespread use of the screening system, a non-RI method is needed. Recently, several assay methods utilizing aromatase activity have been developed. The assay systems were consisted with yeast and an aromatase expression vector (Mak *et al.*, 1999). One of the methods used rat ovarian microsomes (Satoh *et al.*, 2008) and the other used human ovarian granulosa-like tumor cell lines (Ohno *et al.*, 2004).

IN VIVO SCREENING ASSAYS

In vivo assays are needed to validate for *in vitro* assay results. *In vitro* screening systems do not take account of the metabolism of chemical substances because of the presence of xenobiotic metabolic enzymes in the liver. The effects of endocrine activity of some chemical substances are due to metabolites instead of original substances. Chemical substances have weaker hormonal activity than that of natural hormonal substances. Positive data are sometimes obtained at high concentrations of chemical substances. In this situation, the positive results are due to false-positive data. Even if positive results are obtained at higher concentrations of chemicals, the effects of chemical substances are toxic effects to cells rather than endocrine activation. *In vivo* assay is effective in excluding false-positive results in *in vitro* systems.

Uterotropic assays

The uterus is an estrogen-responsive organ and has been used to evaluate estrogenic activity for several decades. Chemical substances suspected of having estrogenic activity or anti-estrogenic activity *in vitro* have been examined using experimental animals. Several assay protocols have been proposed by OECD or US EPA (Combes, 2004; Gelbke *et al.*, 2004; Gray *et al.*, 2004; Kavlock, 1999). Any strain of female rat can be used for this assay. Immature rats or ovariectomized young adult rats are dosed orally or subcutaneously with chemical substances, left for 3 days and then sacrificed. After removing and weighing the uteri, they are soaked in neutral buffered 10% formalin for several days and then embedded in paraffin, and sections stained with hematoxylin and eosin are prepared. The uterine sections are evaluated for uterine gland numbers and for luminal and glandular epithelium cell heights. Using this assay, chemicals have been examined for estrogenic activity. Genistein is a flavonoid from beans with estrogenic activity and has been categorized as a phytoestrogen (Kanno *et al.*, 2002). The pesticide methoxychlor was investigated and found to have estrogenic and antiandrogenic activities (Cupp and Skinner, 2001). Nonyphenol, *o,p′*-DDT, and bisphenol A were also found to be chemical substances with estrogenic activity (Gray *et al.*, 2002, 2004; Shelby *et al.*, 1996).

Pubertal female rat assay

The pubertal female rat assay is an *in vivo* assay using female rats (Clode, 2006; Gray *et al.*, 2002, 2004). The assay sensitivity and reproduction have been reported to be high. The assay endpoints are the age at vaginal opening (VO) and the degree of cornification of vaginal cytology. Several other assays are coupled with the pubertal rat assay. Serum levels of steroid hormones and thyroid hormones can be evaluated for estrogenic activity or anti-steroid action for chemical substances. The assay protocol is briefly as follows: weaning female rats are dosed daily by gavage and the age at VO is monitored. This assay has a major advantage of being able to detect estrogens and antiestrogens. Many data on estrogenic chemicals have been obtained with this assay. Methoxychlor, octylphenol and nonphenol were found to be positive using this assay (Clode, 2006; Gray *et al.*, 2004).

Hershberger assay

In vivo assay of antiandrogenic and androgenic action of chemicals is the Hershberger assay, which examines effects on the androgen-dependent tissues using castrated male rat or intact juvenile male rat (Ashby, 2003; Gelbke *et al.*, 2004; Gray *et al.*, 2004). Castrated rats are treated subcutaneously or orally with chemical substances. At the end of treatment with test compound, which is after 10 days of treatment, autopsy is performed. The endpoints are briefly as follows. The weights of the ventral prostate, seminal vesicles and levator anti muscle are measured. Other endpoints that are measured are the weights of the adrenal gland, liver and kidney and measurement of serum levels of testosterone and luteinizing hormones. This assay has been used for several decades to screen chemical substances and for development of drugs of androgenic hormones (O'Connor *et al.*, 1999; Solo *et al.*, 1975). If assay results of chemical substances are positive, chemicals are suggested to have androgenic activity or antiandrogenic activity. The OECD Hershberger assay has been used to examine several chemicals. Linuron is a herbicide with antiandrogenic activity (Lambright *et al.*, 2000). The *p,p'*-DDE has been found to have antiandrogenic activity in the chemical metabolites (Yamada *et al.*, 2005). Vinclozolin and procymidone were shown to be antiandrogenic fungicides (Ashby *et al.*, 2004; Kang *et al.*, 2004; Lambright *et al.*, 2000).

Fish screening assay

Fish is a popular model in toxicological testing *in vivo* for endocrine disruptors. In the case of fish screening assay not only chemical substances but also their metabolites are examined, as in mammalian models. Fish is cheaper than mammalian animals therefore experimental cost and space are kept to a minimum. Indeed, some chemicals seem to have effects on fish. There have been reports of intersex fish (Burke, 2002; Gercken and Sordyl, 2002; Williams *et al.*, 2009; Woodling *et al.*, 2006). Intersex fish contain male and female tissues in gonads and feminized reproductive ducts. Epidemiological data have demonstrated that intersex is associated with effluent discharge (Kirby *et al.*, 2004). For this reason, fish is a suitable model for screening chemical endocrine disruptors. Since a large number of chemical substances are present in the environment, screening methods are needed that are rapid, easy to use and cost-effective. Biomarkers of fish have been utilized as endocrine-related endpoints of hormonal evaluation, for example secondary sexual characteristics (SSC) and vitellogenin (VTG).

SSC – reproductive endocrinology of the fathead minnow in a 21-day test

A fish screening assay system, which utilizes three kinds of fish, fathead minnow (*Pimephales promelas*), medaka (*Oryzias latipes*) and zebrafish (*Danio rerio*), is popular for the evaluation of endocrine disruptors.

The gross morphological biomarker SCC is utilized in fathead minnow or medaka. The specialized SCC appears on adult fathead minnows in aquarium water containing endocrine disruptors. The number and size of nuptial tubercles are monitored. Nuptial tubercles are located on the head of reproductive-active male fathead minnows. Female and juvenile males and females have no tubercle. The primary observation for SSC is based on the presence and size of tubercles. Androgens cause female fathead minnows to develop nuptial tubercles (Ankley *et al.*, 2001). In contrast, estrogens cause a decrease in the number of tubercles (Miles-Richardson *et al.*, 1999; Weisbrod *et al.*, 2007). This assay protocol has been described as the reproductive endocrinology of the fathead minnow in a 21-day test in the OECD protocol and the US Environmental Protection Agency.

Vitellogenin (VTG)

VTG has been already described in the context of "*in vitro* screening" in this chapter. VTG is a useful biomarker for endocrine disruptors to screen chemical substances in an aquatic ecosystem. The serum levels of VTG or the levels of VTG from homogenate of fish organs are useful for evaluating estrogenic activity. VTG is synthesized in the female liver as the precursor of egg yolk, but neither adult male fish nor juvenile fish produce VTG (Heppell *et al.*, 1995). VTG production increases in male fish when exposed to exogenous estrogen. Antibodies against purified rainbow trout VTG recognized not only fish VTG but also VTG of several other species including amphibians, reptiles and birds. An enzyme-linked immunosorbent assay (ELISA) using the antibody of VTG was developed (Heppell *et al.*, 1995). Measurements of VTG in several species of fish in rivers all over the world have been reported (Zhang *et al.*, 2005). A correlation between endocrine disruptors in sewage effluents receiving waters and plasma VTG concentration in male carp was observed for alkylphenolic compounds in water (Petrovic *et al.*, 2002). The half-life of VTG in plasma of the male flounder is 14 days (Allen *et al.*, 1999; George *et al.*, 2004). VTG protein is stable in fish and is measured in repetitive sampling. High concentrations of VTG protein have some toxic effects in fish, particularly in the kidney. Owing to kidney failure, VTG causes disruption in blood dynamics and function and reduced survival in juvenile fish (Zha *et al.*, 2008). Although endocrine disruptors enhance the production of VTG, endogenous steroid hormones seem to be decreased. Reductions of endogenous steroid levels may have adverse effects on reproduction and fertility (Scott *et al.*, 2006). A relationship between high concentration of VTG and intersex gonads in fish has been reported (Hashimoto *et al.*, 2000). Adult male medaka exposed to octylphenol showed inhibition of spermatogenesis and appearance of intersex, i.e. oocytes were present in their testes (Gronen *et al.*, 1999). Although VTG expression is interpreted as endocrine disruptors, absence of VTG expression cannot be interpreted as absence of warning of reproductive effect in an aquatic ecosystem. Since fertility and hatching success is more sensitive to estrogenic effects than vitellogenin expression, lower doses of the environmental estrogen *o,p'*-DDT had a greater effect in medaka after 8 weeks of exposure (Cheek *et al.*, 2001). Since there is cross-talk between the estrogen receptor and AhR pathways, DLCs strongly inhibited the VTG protein expression in fish (Bemanian *et al.*, 2004). It has recently been reported that chronic exposure of fathead minnow to low concentrations of synthesized estrogens resulted in feminization of males through the production of VTG, which impacts on gonadal development as evidenced by intersex in males and altered oogenesis in females (Kidd *et al.*, 2007). The VTG screening method enables one to estimate risk for aquatic species and identification of the endocrine disruptors.

CONCLUDING REMARKS AND FUTURE DIRECTIONS

There is increasing concern about how many such chemicals are present in our environment. Contamination with endocrine disruptors causes reproductive dysfunction and reproductive failure can have devastating consequences on the population. These chemicals can also easily pass through the placenta during pregnancy and have adverse effects on the normal functioning of neonatal reproductive systems. Potential endocrine disruptors must be fully assessed for reproductive effects, and multigenerational full life cycle exposures are needed to consider hazards assessment.

REFERENCES

Allen Y, Matthiessen P, Scott AP, Haworth S, Feist S, Thain JE (1999) The extent of oestrogenic contamination in the UK estuarine and marine environments – further surveys of flounder. *Sci Total Environ* **233:** 5–20.

Andersen J, Barbieri RL (1995) Abnormal gene expression in uterine leiomyomas. *J Soc Gynecol Investig* **2:** 663–72.

Andersen J, DyReyes VM, Barbieri RL, Coachman DM, Miksicek RJ (1995) Leiomyoma primary cultures have elevated transcriptional response to estrogen compared with autologous myometrial cultures. *J Soc Gynecol Investig* **2:** 542–51.

Ankley GT, Jensen KM, Kahl MD, Korte JJ, Makynen EA (2001) Description and evaluation of a short-term reproduction test with the fathead minnow *(Pimephales promelas).Environ Toxicol Chem* **20:** 1276–90.

Arnold SF, Robinson MK, Notides AC, Guillette LJ Jr, McLachlan JA (1996) A yeast estrogen screen for examining the relative exposure of cells to natural and xenoestrogens. *Environ Health Perspect* **104:** 544–8.

Ashby J (2003) The leading role and responsibility of the international scientific community in test development. *Toxicol Lett* **140–141:** 37–42.

Ashby J, Lefevre PA, Tinwell H, Odum J, Owens W (2004) Testosterone-stimulated weanlings as an alternative to castrated male rats in the Hershberger anti-androgen assay. *Regul Toxicol Pharmacol* **39:** 229–38.

Balsiger HA, de la Torre R, Lee WY, Cox MB (2010) A four-hour yeast bioassay for the direct measure of estrogenic activity in wastewater without sample extraction, concentration, or sterilization. *Sci Total Environ* **408:** 1422–9.

Bemanian V, Male R, Goksoyr A (2004) The aryl hydrocarbon receptor-mediated disruption of vitellogenin synthesis in the fish liver: cross-talk between AHR- and ERalpha-signalling pathways. *Comp Hepatol* **3:** 2.

Bolger R, Wiese TE, Ervin K, Nestich S, Checovich W (1998) Rapid screening of environmental chemicals for estrogen receptor binding capacity. *Environ Health Perspect* **106:** 551–7.

Bradbury SP (1995) Quantitative structure–activity relationships and ecological risk assessment: an overview of predictive aquatic toxicology research. *Toxicol Lett* **79:** 229–37.

Brooks SC, Locke ER, Soule HD (1973) Estrogen receptor in a human cell line (MCF-7) from breast carcinoma. *J Biol Chem* **248:** 6251–3.

Burke M (2002) U.K. fish exhibit intersex traits. *Environ Sci Technol* **36:** 270A.

Campbell CM, Idler DR (1980) Characterization of an estradiol-induced protein from rainbow trout serum as vitellogenin by the composition and radioimmunological cross reactivity to ovarian yolk fractions. *Biol Reprod* **22:** 605–17.

Carlsen E, Giwercman A, Keiding N, Skakkebaek NE (1992) Evidence for decreasing quality of semen during past 50 years. *BMJ* **305:** 609–13.

Celius T, Haugen TB, Grotmol T, Walther BT (1999) A sensitive zonagenetic assay for rapid in vitro assessment of estrogenic potency of xenobiotics and mycotoxins. *Environ Health Perspect* **107:** 63–8.

Cheek AO, Brouwer TH, Carroll S, Manning S, McLachlan JA, Brouwer M (2001) Experimental evaluation of vitellogenin as a predictive biomarker for reproductive disruption. *Environ Health Perspect* **109:** 681–90.

Chen HT, Pittman CS (1988) Effect of estrogen on the expression of a cell-surface antigen associated with rat anterior pituitary somatotrophs. *Mol Cell Endocrinol* **59:** 233–40.

Chu WL, Shiizaki K, Kawanishi M, Kondo M, Yagi T (2009) Validation of a new yeast-based reporter assay consisting of human estrogen receptors alpha/beta and coactivator SRC-1: application for detection of estrogenic activity in environmental samples. *Environ Toxicol* **24:** 513–21.

Clark JH, Gorski J (1969) Estrogen receptors: an evaluation of cytoplasmic-nuclear interactions in a cell-free system and a method for assay. *Biochim Biophys Acta* **192:** 508–15.

Clode SA (2006) Assessment of *in vivo* assays for endocrine disruption. *Best Pract Res Clin Endocrinol Metab* **20:** 35–43.

Cocco P, Benichou J (1998) Mortality from cancer of the male reproductive tract and environmental exposure to the anti-androgen p,p′-dichlorodiphenyldichloroethylene in the United States. *Oncology* **55:** 334–9.

Coldham NG, Dave M, Sivapathasundaram S, McDonnell DP, Connor C, Sauer MJ (1997) Evaluation of a recombinant yeast cell estrogen screening assay. *Environ Health Perspect* **105:** 734–42.

Combes RD (2004) Peer review of validation studies: an assessment of the role of the OECD by reference to the validation of the uterotrophic assay for endocrine disruptors. *Altern Lab Anim* **32:** 111–17.

Corcia A, Steinmetz R, Liu JW, Ben-Jonathan N (1993) Coculturing posterior pituitary and GH3 cells: dramatic stimulation of prolactin gene expression. *Endocrinology* **132:** 80–5.

Cramer RD 3rd, Patterson DE, Bunce JD (1989) Recent advances in comparative molecular field analysis (CoMFA). *Prog Clin Biol Res* **291:** 161–5.

Cupp AS, Skinner MK (2001) Actions of the endocrine disruptor methoxychlor and its estrogenic metabolite on in vitro embryonic rat seminiferous cord formation and perinatal testis growth. *Reprod Toxicol* **15:** 317–26.

Date K, Ohno K, Azuma Y, Hirano S, Kobayashi K, Sakurai T, Nobuhara Y, Yamada T (2002) Endocrine-disrupting effects of styrene oligomers that migrated from polystyrene containers into food. *Food Chem Toxicol* **40:** 65–75.

de Solla SR, Bishop CA, Van der Kraak G, Brooks RJ (1998) Impact of organochlorine contamination on levels of sex hormones and external morphology of common snapping turtles *(Chelydra serpentina serpentina)* in Ontario, Canada. *Environ Health Perspect* **106:** 253–60.

de Vlaming V, Biales A, Riordan D, Markiewicz D, Holmes R, Otis P, Zander R, Lazorchak J (2007) Screening California surface waters for estrogenic endocrine disrupting chemicals (EEDC) with a juvenile rainbow trout liver vitellogenin mRNA procedure. *Sci Total Environ* **385:** 66–79.

DeLisle RK, Yu SJ, Nair AC, Welsh WJ (2001) Homology modeling of the estrogen receptor subtype beta (ER-beta) and calculation of ligand binding affinities. *J Mol Graph Model* **20:** 155–67.

Fang H, Tong W, Perkins R, Soto AM, Prechtl NV, Sheehan DM (2000) Quantitative comparisons of in vitro assays for estrogenic activities. *Environ Health Perspect* **108:** 723–9.

Fei X, Chung H, Taylor HS (2005) Methoxychlor disrupts uterine Hoxa10 gene expression. *Endocrinology* **146:** 3445–51.

Fenton SE (2006) Endocrine-disrupting compounds and mammary gland development: early exposure and later life consequences. *Endocrinology* **147:** S18–24.

Fernandez MF, Olmos B, Granada A, Lopez-Espinosa MJ, Molina-Molina JM, Fernandez JM, Cruz M, Olea-Serrano F, Olea N (2007) Human exposure to endocrine-disrupting chemicals and prenatal risk factors for cryptorchidism and hypospadias: a nested case–control study. *Environ Health Perspect* **115 (Suppl. 1):** 8–14.

Fields S, Song O (1989) A novel genetic system to detect protein–protein interactions. *Nature* **340:** 245–6.

Flouriot G, Pakdel F, Ducouret B, Valotaire Y (1995) Influence of xenobiotics on rainbow trout liver estrogen receptor and vitellogenin gene expression. *J Mol Endocrinol* **15:** 143–51.

Fry DM (1995) Reproductive effects in birds exposed to pesticides and industrial chemicals. *Environ Health Perspect* **103 (Suppl. 7):** 165–71.

Gao X, Petroff BK, Rozman KK, Terranova PF (2000) Gonadotropin-releasing hormone (GnRH) partially reverses the inhibitory effect of 2,3,7,8-tetrachlorodibenzo-p-dioxin on ovulation in the immature gonadotropin-treated rat. *Toxicology* **147:** 15–22.

Gelbke HP, Kayser M, Poole A (2004) OECD test strategies and methods for endocrine disruptors. *Toxicology* **205:** 17–25.

George S, Gubbins M, MacIntosh A, Reynolds W, Sabine V, Scott A, Thain J (2004) A comparison of pollutant biomarker responses with transcriptional responses in European flounders (Platicthys flesus) subjected to estuarine pollution. *Mar Environ Res* **58:** 571–5.

Gercken J, Sordyl H (2002) Intersex in feral marine and freshwater fish from northeastern Germany. *Mar Environ Res* **54**, 651–5.

Gray LE Jr, Ostby J, Wilson V, Lambright C, Bobseine K, Hartig P, Hotchkiss A, Wolf C, Furr J, Price M, *et al.* (2002) Xenoendocrine disrupters-tiered screening and testing: filling key data gaps. *Toxicology* **181–182:** 371–82.

Gray LE Jr, Wilson V, Noriega N, Lambright C, Furr J, Stoker TE, Laws SC, Goldman J, Cooper RL, Foster PM (2004) Use of the laboratory rat as a model in endocrine disruptor screening and testing. *Ilar J* **45:** 425–37.

Gronen S, Denslow N, Manning S, Barnes S, Barnes D, Brouwer M (1999) Serum vitellogenin levels and reproductive impairment of male Japanese Medaka *(Oryzias latipes)* exposed to 4-tert-octylphenol. *Environ Health Perspect* **107:** 385–90.

Hahnel R (1971) Properties of the estrogen receptor in the soluble fraction of human uterus. *Steroids* **17:** 105–32.

Hamazaki TS, Nagahama Y, Iuchi I, Yamagami K (1989) A glycoprotein from the liver constitutes the inner layer of the egg envelope (zona pellucida interna) of the fish, *Oryzias latipes. Dev Biol* **133:** 101–10.

Hashimoto S, Bessho H, Hara A, Nakamura M, Iguchi T, Fujita K (2000) Elevated serum vitellogenin levels and gonadal abnormalities in wild male flounder *(Pleuronectes yokohamae)* from Tokyo Bay, Japan. *Mar Environ Res* **49:** 37–53.

Healicon RM, Westley BR, May FE (1993) Isolation and characterization of an oestrogen-responsive breast-cancer cell line, EFF-3. *Int J Cancer* **53:** 388–94.

Heidrich DD, Steckelbroeck S, Klingmuller D (2001) Inhibition of human cytochrome P450 aromatase activity by butyltins. *Steroids* **66:** 763–9.

Heppell SA, Denslow ND, Folmar LC, Sullivan CV (1995) Universal assay of vitellogenin as a biomarker for environmental estrogens. *Environ Health Perspect* **103 (Suppl. 7):** 9–15.

Herbst AL, Scully RE (1970) Adenocarcinoma of the vagina in adolescence. A report of 7 cases including 6 clear-cell carcinomas (so-called mesonephromas). *Cancer* **25:** 745–57.

Hodges LC, Bergerson JS, Hunter DS, Walker CL (2000) Estrogenic effects of organochlorine pesticides on uterine leiomyoma cells in vitro. *Toxicol Sci* **54:** 355–64.

Hollert H, Durr M, Holtey-Weber R, Islinger M, Brack W, Farber H, Erdinger L, Braunbeck T (2005) Endocrine disruption of water and sediment extracts in a non-radioactive dot blot/RNAse protection-assay using isolated hepatocytes of rainbow trout. *Environ Sci Pollut Res Int* **12:** 347–60.

Huff J, Lucier G, Tritscher A (1994) Carcinogenicity of TCDD: experimental, mechanistic, and epidemiologic evidence. *Annu Rev Pharmacol Toxicol* **34:** 343–72.

Ishiwata I, Ishiwata C, Soma M, Arai J, Ishikawa H (1984) Establishment of human endometrial adenocarcinoma cell line containing estradiol-17 beta and progesterone receptors. *Gynecol Oncol* **17:** 281–90.

Jakowlew SB, Breathnach R, Jeltsch JM, Masiakowski P, Chambon P (1984) Sequence of the pS2 mRNA induced by estrogen in the human breast cancer cell line MCF-7. *Nucleic Acids Res* **12:** 2861–78.

Jorgensen M, Vendelbo B, Skakkebaek NE, Leffers H (2000) Assaying estrogenicity by quantitating the expression levels of endogenous estrogen-regulated genes. *Environ Health Perspect* **108:** 403–12.

Jungblut PW, Hughes S, Hughes A, Wagner RK (1972) Evaluation of various methods for the assay of cytoplasmic oestrogen receptors in extracts of calf uteri and human breast cancers. *Acta Endocrinol (Copenh)* **70:** 185–95.

Kang IH, Kim HS, Shin JH, Kim TS, Moon HJ, Kim IY, Choi KS, Kil KS, Park YI, Dong MS, *et al.* (2004) Comparison of anti-androgenic activity of flutamide, vinclozolin, procymidone, linuron, and p,p′-DDE in rodent 10-day Hershberger assay. *Toxicology* **199:** 145–59.

Kanno J, Kato H, Iwata T, Inoue T (2002) Phytoestrogen-low diet for endocrine disruptor studies. *J Agric Food Chem* **50:** 3883–5.

Kavlock RJ (1999) Overview of endocrine disruptor research activity in the United States. *Chemosphere* **39:** 1227–36.

Kidd KA, Blanchfield PJ, Mills KH, Palace VP, Evans RE, Lazorchak JM, Flick RW (2007) Collapse of a fish population after exposure to a synthetic estrogen. *Proc Natl Acad Sci USA* **104:** 8897–901.

Kirby MF, Allen YT, Dyer RA, Feist SW, Katsiadaki I, Matthiessen P, Scott AP, Smith A, Stentiford GD, Thain JE, *et al.* (2004) Surveys of plasma vitellogenin and intersex in male flounder *(Platichthys flesus)* as measures of endocrine disruption by estrogenic contamination in United Kingdom estuaries: temporal trends, 1996 to 2001. *Environ Toxicol Chem* **23:** 748–58.

Klein KO, Baron J, Colli MJ, McDonnell DP, Cutler GB Jr (1994) Estrogen levels in childhood determined by an ultrasensitive recombinant cell bioassay. *J Clin Invest* **94:** 2475–80.

Kochukov MY, Jeng YJ, Watson CS (2009) Alkylphenol xenoestrogens with varying carbon chain lengths differentially and potently activate signaling and functional responses in GH3/B6/F10 somatomammotropes. *Environ Health Perspect* **117:** 723–30.

Kociba RJ, Schwetz BA (1982) Toxicity of 2,3,7,8-tetrachlorodibenzo-p-dioxin (TCDD). *Drug Metab Rev* **13:** 387–406.

Kohn MC (1995) Biochemical mechanisms and cancer risk assessment models for dioxin. *Toxicology* **102:** 133–8.

Kohno H, Gandini O, Curtis SW, Korach KS (1994) Anti-estrogen activity in the yeast transcription system: estrogen receptor mediated agonist response. *Steroids* **59:** 572–8.

Kojima H, Katsura E, Takeuchi S, Niiyama K, Kobayashi K (2004) Screening for estrogen and androgen receptor activities in 200 pesticides by *in vitro* reporter gene assays using Chinese hamster ovary cells. *Environ Health Perspect* **112:** 524–31.

Kraus WL, Weis KE, Katzenellenbogen BS (1995) Inhibitory cross-talk between steroid hormone receptors: differential targeting of estrogen receptor in the repression of its transcriptional activity by agonist- and antagonist-occupied progestin receptors. *Mol Cell Biol* **15:** 1847–57.

Kuiper GG, Carlsson B, Grandien K, Enmark E, Haggblad J, Nilsson S, Gustafsson JA (1997) Comparison of the ligand binding specificity and transcript tissue distribution of estrogen receptors alpha and beta. *Endocrinology* **138:** 863–70.

Kuiper GG, Lemmen JG, Carlsson B, Corton JC, Safe SH, van der Saag PT, van der Burg B, Gustafsson JA (1998) Interaction of estrogenic chemicals and phytoestrogens with estrogen receptor beta. *Endocrinology* **139:** 4252–63.

Lambright C, Ostby J, Bobseine K, Wilson V, Hotchkiss AK, Mann PC, Gray LE Jr (2000) Cellular and molecular mechanisms of action of linuron: an antiandrogenic herbicide that produces reproductive malformations in male rats. *Toxicol Sci* **56:** 389–99.

Lee HS, Cho EM, Jung JH, Ohta A (2007) Evaluation on antagonist activities of polycyclic aromatic hydrocarbons using the yeast two-hybrid detection system for endocrine disruptors. *Environ Monit Assess* **129:** 87–95.

Lee HS, Miyauchi K, Nagata Y, Fukuda R, Sasagawa S, Endoh H, Kato S, Horiuchi H, Takagi M, Ohta A (2002) Employment of the human estrogen receptor beta ligand-binding domain and co-activator SRC1 nuclear receptor-binding domain for the construction of a yeast two-hybrid detection system for endocrine disrupters. *J Biochem* **131:** 399–405.

Lee HS, Sasagawa S, Kato S, Fukuda R, Horiuchi H, Ohta A (2006) Yeast two-hybrid detection systems that are highly sensitive to a certain kind of endocrine disruptor. *Biosci Biotechnol Biochem* **70:** 521–4.

Legler J, van den Brink CE, Brouwer A, Murk AJ, van der Saag PT, Vethaak AD, van der Burg B (1999) Development of a stably transfected estrogen receptor-mediated luciferase reporter gene assay in the human T47D breast cancer cell line. *Toxicol Sci* **48:** 55–66.

Loughney DA, Schwender CF (1992) A comparison of progestin and androgen receptor binding using the CoMFA technique. *J Comput Aided Mol Des* **6:** 569–81.

Mak P, Cruz FD, Chen S (1999) A yeast screen system for aromatase inhibitors and ligands for androgen receptor: yeast cells transformed with aromatase and androgen receptor. *Environ Health Perspect* **107:** 855–60.

Matthews J, Celius T, Halgren R, Zacharewski T (2000) Differential estrogen receptor binding of estrogenic substances: a species comparison. *J Steroid Biochem Mol Biol* **74:** 223–34.

Matthews J, Zacharewski T (2000) Differential binding affinities of PCBs, HO-PCBs, and aroclors with recombinant human, rainbow trout *(Onchorhynkiss mykiss)*, and green anole *(Anolis carolinensis)* estrogen receptors, using a semi-high throughput competitive binding assay. *Toxicol Sci* **53:** 326–39.

Miles-Richardson SR, Pierens SL, Nichols KM, Kramer VJ, Snyder EM, Snyder SA, Render JA, Fitzgerald SD, Giesy JP (1999) Effects of waterborne exposure to 4-nonylphenol and nonylphenol ethoxylate on secondary sex characteristics and gonads of fathead minnows *(Pimephales promelas)*. *Environ Res* **80:** S122–37.

Murk AJ, Legler J, Denison MS, Giesy JP, van de Guchte C, Brouwer A (1996) Chemical-activated luciferase gene expression (CALUX): a novel in vitro bioassay for Ah receptor active compounds in sediments and pore water. *Fundam Appl Toxicol* **33:** 149–60.

Navas JM, Segner H (2006) Vitellogenin synthesis in primary cultures of fish liver cells as endpoint for in vitro screening of the (anti)estrogenic activity of chemical substances. *Aquat Toxicol* **80:** 1–22.

Newbold RR, Padilla-Banks E, Jefferson WN (2009) Environmental estrogens and obesity. *Mol Cell Endocrinol* **304:** 84–9.

Newbold RR, Padilla-Banks E, Snyder RJ, Jefferson WN (2007) Perinatal exposure to environmental estrogens and the development of obesity. *Mol Nutr Food Res* **51:** 912–7.

Nishikawa J, Saito K, Goto J, Dakeyama F, Matsuo M, Nishihara T (1999) New screening methods for chemicals with hormonal activities using interaction of nuclear hormone receptor with coactivator. *Toxicol Appl Pharmacol* **154:** 76–83.

O'Connor JC, Frame SR, Davis LG, Cook JC (1999) Detection of the environmental antiandrogen p,p-DDE in CD and Long-Evans rats using a tier I screening battery and a Hershberger assay. *Toxicol Sci* **51:** 44–53.

Oh SM, Park K, Chung KH (2006) Combination of in vitro bioassays encompassing different mechanisms to determine the endocrine-disrupting effects of river water. *Sci Total Environ* **354:** 252–64.

Oh SM, Ryu BT, Chung KH (2008) Identification of estrogenic and antiestrogenic activities of respirable diesel exhaust particles by bioassay-directed fractionation. *Arch Pharm Res* **31:** 75–82.

Ohno K, Araki N, Yanase T, Nawata H, Iida M (2004) A novel nonradioactive method for measuring aromatase activity using a human ovarian granulosa-like tumor cell line and an estrone ELISA. *Toxicol Sci* **82:** 443–50.

Ohno K, Azuma Y, Nakano S, Kobayashi T, Hirano S, Nobuhara Y, Yamada T (2001) Assessment of styrene oligomers eluted from polystyrene-made food containers for estrogenic effects in in vitro assays. *Food Chem Toxicol* **39:** 1233–41.

Pakdel F, Petit F, Anglade I, Kah O, Delaunay F, Bailhache T, Valotaire Y (1994) Overexpression of rainbow trout estrogen receptor domains in *Escherichia coli:* characterization and utilization in the production of antibodies for immunoblotting and immunocytochemistry. *Mol Cell Endocrinol* **104:** 81–93.

Paulozzi LJ (1999) International trends in rates of hypospadias and cryptorchidism. *Environ Health Perspect* **107:** 297–302.

Perez P, Pulgar R, Olea-Serrano F, Villalobos M, Rivas A, Metzler M, Pedraza V, Olea N (1998) The estrogenicity of bisphenol A-related diphenylalkanes with various substituents at the central carbon and the hydroxy groups. *Environ Health Perspect* **106:** 167–74.

Petrovic M, Sole M, Lopez de Alda MJ, Barcelo D (2002) Endocrine disruptors in sewage treatment plants, receiving river waters, and sediments: integration of chemical analysis and biological effects on feral carp. *Environ Toxicol Chem* **21:** 2146–56.

Picard K, Lhuguenot JC, Lavier-Canivenc MC, Chagnon MC (2001) Estrogenic activity and metabolism of n-butyl benzyl phthalate in vitro: identification of the active molecule(s). *Toxicol Appl Pharmacol* **172:** 108–18.

Popnikolov N, Yang J, Liu A, Guzman R, Nandi S (2001) Reconstituted normal human breast in nude mice: effect of host pregnancy environment and human chorionic gonadotropin on proliferation. *J Endocrinol* **168:** 487–96.

Rasmussen TH, Nielsen F, Andersen HR, Nielsen JB, Weihe P, Grandjean P (2003) Assessment of xenoestrogenic exposure by a biomarker approach: application of the E-Screen bioassay to determine estrogenic response of serum extracts. *Environ Health* **2:** 12.

Reddy KB, Mangold GL, Tandon AK, Yoneda T, Mundy GR, Zilberstein A, Osborne CK (1992) Inhibition of breast cancer cell growth in vitro by a tyrosine kinase inhibitor. *Cancer Res* **52:** 3636–41.

Rotchell JM, Ostrander GK (2003) Molecular markers of endocrine disruption in aquatic organisms. *J Toxicol Environ Health B Crit Rev* **6:** 453–96.

Safe SH (1995a) Environmental and dietary estrogens and human health: is there a problem? *Environ Health Perspect* **103:** 346–51.

Safe SH (1995b) Modulation of gene expression and endocrine response pathways by 2,3,7,8-tetrachlorodibenzo-p-dioxin and related compounds. *Pharmacol Ther* **67:** 247–81.

Satoh K, Nonaka R, Ishikawa F, Ogata A, Nagai F (2008) In vitro screening assay for detecting aromatase activity using rat ovarian microsomes and estrone ELISA. *Biol Pharm Bull* **31:** 357–62.

Schmitt E, Dekant W, Stopper H (2001) Assaying the estrogenicity of phytoestrogens in cells of different estrogen sensitive tissues. *Toxicol in Vitro* **15:** 433–9.

Scott AP, Katsiadaki I, Kirby MF, Thain J (2006) Relationship between sex steroid and vitellogenin concentrations in flounder *(Platichthys flesus)* sampled from an estuary contaminated with estrogenic endocrine-disrupting compounds. *Environ Health Perspect* **114 (Suppl. 1):** 27–31.

Selman K, Wallace RA (1983) Oogenesis in *Fundulus heteroclitus*. III. Vitellogenesis. *J Exp Zool* **226:** 441–57.

Sharpe RM (1995) Reproductive biology. Another DDT connection. *Nature* **375:** 538–9.

Shelby MD, Newbold RR, Tully DB, Chae K, Davis VL (1996) Assessing environmental chemicals for estrogenicity using a combination of in vitro and in vivo assays. *Environ Health Perspect* **104:** 1296–300.

Siiteri PK, Thompson EA (1975) Studies of human placental aromatase. *J Steroid Biochem* **6:** 317–22.

Solo AJ, Bejba N, Hebborn P, May M (1975) Synthesis and biological activity of some ethers of testosterone. Implications concerning the biological activity of esters of testosterone. *J Med Chem* **18:** 165–8.

Son DS, Ushinohama K, Gao X, Taylor CC, Roby KF, Rozman KK, Terranova PF (1999) 2,3,7,8-Tetrachlorodibenzo-p-dioxin (TCDD) blocks ovulation by a direct action on the ovary without alteration of ovarian steroidogenesis: lack of a direct effect on ovarian granulosa and thecal-interstitial cell steroidogenesis in vitro. *Reprod Toxicol* **13:** 521–30.

Sonnenschein C, Soto AM, Fernandez MF, Olea N, Olea-Serrano MF, Ruiz-Lopez MD (1995) Development of a marker of estrogenic exposure in human serum. *Clin Chem* **41:** 1888–95.

Sonneveld E, Jansen HJ, Riteco JA, Brouwer A, van der Burg B (2005) Development of androgen- and estrogen-responsive bioassays, members of a panel of human cell line-based highly selective steroid-responsive bioassays. *Toxicol Sci* **83:** 136–48.

Soto AM, Calabro JM, Prechtl NV, Yau AY, Orlando EF, Daxenberger A, Kolok AS, Guillette LJ Jr, le Bizec B, Lange IG, *et al.* (2004) Androgenic and estrogenic activity in water bodies receiving cattle feedlot effluent in Eastern Nebraska, USA. *Environ Health Perspect* **112:** 346–52.

Soto AM, Chung KL, Sonnenschein C (1994) The pesticides endosulfan, toxaphene, and dieldrin have estrogenic effects on human estrogen-sensitive cells. *Environ Health Perspect* **102:** 380–3.

Soto AM, Sonnenschein C, Chung KL, Fernandez MF, Olea N, Serrano FO (1995) The E-SCREEN assay as a tool to identify estrogens: an update on estrogenic environmental pollutants. *Environ Health Perspect* **103 (Suppl. 7):** 113–22.

Steinmetz R, Brown NG, Allen DL, Bigsby RM, Ben-Jonathan N (1997) The environmental estrogen bisphenol A stimulates prolactin release in vitro and in vivo. *Endocrinology* **138:** 1780–86.

Stewart AJ, Westley BR, May FE (1992) Modulation of the proliferative response of breast cancer cells to growth factors by oestrogen. *Br J Cancer* **66:** 640–8.

Stoessel S, Leclercq G (1986) Competitive binding assay for estrogen receptor in monolayer culture: measure of receptor activation potency. *J Steroid Biochem* **25:** 677–82.

Sugawara T, Nakajima A, Nomura E (2002) Development of a simple screening system for endocrine disruptors. *Med Sci Monit* **8:** BR431–8.

Sugawara T, Nomura E (2006) Development of a recombinant yeast assay to detect Ah-receptor ligands. *Toxicol Mech Methods* **16:** 287–94.

Tollefsen KE, Mathisen R, Stenersen J (2003) Induction of vitellogenin synthesis in an Atlantic salmon *(Salmo salar)* hepatocyte culture: a sensitive in vitro bioassay for the oestrogenic and anti-oestrogenic activity of chemicals. *Biomarkers* **8:** 394–407.

Tong W, Perkins R, Strelitz R, Collantes ER, Keenan S, Welsh WJ, Branham WS, Sheehan DM (1997a) Quantitative structure–activity relationships (QSARs) for estrogen binding to the estrogen receptor: predictions across species. *Environ Health Perspect* **105:** 1116–24.

Tong W, Perkins R, Xing L, Welsh WJ, Sheehan DM (1997b) QSAR models for binding of estrogenic compounds to estrogen receptor alpha and beta subtypes. *Endocrinology* **138:** 4022–5.

Tyler CR, Sumpter JP, Kawauchi H, Swanson P (1991) Involvement of gonadotropin in the uptake of vitellogenin into vitellogenic oocytes of the rainbow trout, *Oncorhynchus mykiss. Gen Comp Endocrinol* **84:** 291–9.

van den Hazel P, Zuurbier M, Babisch W, Bartonova A, Bistrup ML, Bolte G, Busby C, Butter M, Ceccatelli S, Fucic A, *et al.* (2006) Today's epidemics in children: possible relations to environmental pollution and suggested preventive measures. *Acta Paediatr Suppl* **95:** 18–25.

Waller CL, Juma BW, Gray LE Jr, Kelce WR (1996) Three-dimensional quantitative structure–activity relationships for androgen receptor ligands. *Toxicol Appl Pharmacol* **137:** 219–27.

Waller CL, Minor DL, McKinney JD (1995) Using three-dimensional quantitative structure–activity relationships to examine estrogen receptor binding affinities of polychlorinated hydroxybiphenyls. *Environ Health Perspect* **103:** 702–7.

Warita K, Sugawara T, Yue ZP, Tsukahara S, Mutoh K, Hasegawa Y, Kitagawa H, Mori C, Hoshi N (2006) Progression of the dose-related effects of estrogenic endocrine disruptors, an important factor in declining fertility, differs between the hypothalamo–pituitary axis and reproductive organs of male mice. *J Vet Med Sci* **68:** 1257–67.

Watson CS, Pappas TC, Gametchu B (1995) The other estrogen receptor in the plasma membrane: implications for the actions of environmental estrogens. *Environ Health Perspect* **103 (Suppl. 7):** 41–50.

Wei Z, Angerer RC, Angerer LM (1999) Identification of a new sea urchin Ets protein, SpEts4, by yeast one-hybrid screening with the hatching enzyme promoter. *Mol Cell Biol* **19:** 1271–8.

Weisbrod CJ, Kunz PY, Zenker AK, Fent K (2007) Effects of the UV filter benzophenone-2 on reproduction in fish. *Toxicol Appl Pharmacol* **225:** 255–66.

Williams RJ, Keller VD, Johnson AC, Young AR, Holmes MG, Wells C, Gross-Sorokin M, Benstead R (2009) A national risk assessment for intersex in fish arising from steroid estrogens. *Environ Toxicol Chem* **28:** 220–30.

Wilson VS, Bobseine K, Gray LE Jr (2004) Development and characterization of a cell line that stably expresses an estrogen-responsive luciferase reporter for the detection of estrogen receptor agonist and antagonists. *Toxicol Sci* **81:** 69–77.

Woodling JD, Lopez EM, Maldonado TA, Norris DO, Vajda AM (2006) Intersex and other reproductive disruption of fish in wastewater effluent dominated Colorado streams. *Comp Biochem Physiol C Toxicol Pharmacol* **144:** 10–15.

Yamada T, Sumida K, Saito K, Ueda S, Yabushita S, Sukata T, Kawamura S, Okuno Y, Seki T (2005) Functional genomics may allow accurate categorization of the benzimidazole fungicide benomyl: lack of ability to act via steroid–receptor-mediated mechanisms. *Toxicol Appl Pharmacol* **205:** 11–30.

Zauhar RJ, Morgan RS (1985) A new method for computing the macromolecular electric potential. *J Mol Biol* **186:** 815–20.

Zauhar RJ, Moyna G, Tian L, Li Z, Welsh WJ (2003) Shape signatures: a new approach to computer-aided ligand- and receptor-based drug design. *J Med Chem* **46:** 5674–90.

Zha J, Sun L, Zhou Y, Spear PA, Ma M, Wang Z (2008) Assessment of 17alpha-ethinylestradiol effects and underlying mechanisms in a continuous, multigeneration exposure of the Chinese rare minnow *(Gobiocypris rarus)*. *Toxicol Appl Pharmacol* **226:** 298–308.

Zhang Z, Hu J, An W, Jin F, An L, Tao S, Chen J (2005) Induction of vitellogenin mRNA in juvenile Chinese sturgeon *(Acipenser sinensis Gray)* treated with 17beta-estradiol and 4-nonylphenol. *Environ Toxicol Chem* **24:** 1944–50.

C H A P T E R

69

Developmental and reproductive disorders: role of endocrine disruptors in testicular toxicity

Bashir M. Rezk and Suresh Sikka

INTRODUCTION

The 2010 disaster at the Deepwater Horizon rig and uncontrolled oil leakage into the Gulf of Mexico attracted a great deal of attention and is likely to contribute to major environmental, health and economic impacts. Besides affecting ecosystems, food chains and livelihoods of many individuals, the resultant health issues are a grave concern. Moreover, any such environmental catastrophe will ultimately affect human development, reproductive and general health and lifestyle. During the last five decades, developmental and reproductive toxicity has been recognized as a major concern, mainly due to many such environmental issues and accidents that affect overall health and well-being. Developmental and reproductive toxicologists and epidemiologists identified and classified several environmental chemicals and pharmaceutical products including teratogens and endocrine disruptors that lead to developmental and reproductive disorders. Hence it is highly important to understand the role of such toxicants and environmental endocrine disruptors.

Endocrine disruptors are natural products or synthetic chemicals that interfere with the synthesis, secretion, transport, binding, action or elimination of natural hormones that are responsible for the maintenance of homeostasis, development, reproduction and behavior. Dose, duration and timing of exposure at critical periods of life are important considerations for assessing the adverse effects of endocrine disruptors (Sikka *et al.*, 2004). Effects may be reversible or irreversible, immediate (acute) or latent and not expressed for a period of time. Endocrine disruptors are implicated in the induction of developmental abnormalities and testicular dysgenesis syndrome.

Testicular dysgenesis syndrome is described as demasculinization or feminization. Strikingly, the recent study of Hawass *et al.* (2010) published in *JAMA* speculated that King Tutankhamun and other royalty from this period appear to be somewhat feminized, or at least androgynous. This led to speculation that the royal family tree was riddled with a hormonal disease that caused gynecomastia (excessive breast development in men). On the contrary, CT scans showed no signs of feminization and gynecomastia. Furthermore, the penis of Tutankhamun appeared well developed, thus opening once again a debate on evidence against such feminizing disorders and developmental toxicity.

DEVELOPMENTAL AND REPRODUCTIVE TOXICITY

Developmental toxicity, in general, refers to exposure of either parent to toxicants, teratogens and endocrine disruptors before real conception or during the prenatal or the postnatal development. Embryonic development is a highly specific and programmed process that entails timely and well-measurable proliferation, differentiation and apoptosis to assist normal morphogenesis and organogenesis. Minor alterations in one or more of the embryonic development programs can lead to serious malformation. Reproductive toxicity, on the other hand, is expressed as alterations in gonadal development and function, sexual behavior and performance, ultimately leading to impaired reproduction and infertility. Statistics indicate that 15% of all couples in the USA are infertile, and the male factor is responsible for about 30–40% of these infertility cases (Makker *et al.*, 2009). Reproductive disorders caused by endocrine disruptors may vary from very subtle changes to permanent alterations (Mostafa *et al.*, 2007).

Although disruption of the endocrine balance will adversely affect the adult male reproductive system, the developing male reproductive system pre- and postnatally appears to be particularly susceptible and uniquely sensitive. In mammals, including humans, development of the male phenotype requires activation of the *sry* gene on the Y chromosome. In the absence of expression of that gene,

Reproductive and Developmental Toxicology, Edited by Ramesh C. Gupta
ISBN: 978-0-12-382032-7

the female phenotype develops. The mechanisms of action of the *sry* gene and the cascade of events that follows have not been fully elucidated. However, any interference with Müllerian ducts' ability to regress will result in the presence of rudimentary components of the female reproductive tract in general. Depending on the extent and timing of that interference, the consequences would be complete or partial failure of the development of the male reproductive system, which could limit androgen production, delay or prevent the onset of puberty, and affect sexual behavior in adults (Klyde, 1994).

Testicular differentiation and development

Testicular development requires a cascade of gene activation and differentiation into different cell types. Embryonic stem cells can differentiate to primordial germ cells. Primordial germ cells, subsequently, proliferate and differentiate into pro-spermatogonia (precursor spermatogonia stem cells). Sertoli cells are the first cells to differentiate into the different fetal gonad seminiferous cords surrounded by peritubular myoid cells and enclosing fetal germ cells. Normal Sertoli cell differentiation is important for proper testicular development and function (Sharpe *et al.*, 2003). Recruitment of Sertoli cells is caused by expression of the *sry* gene that works in an autocrine and paracrine signaling way (Brennan and Capel, 2004). Nagamine and co-workers (1999) reported that the number of Sertoli cells is directly proportional to *sry* mRNA levels. In adulthood, the number of Sertoli cells is directly related to production of sperm. Sertoli cells can also differentiate into Leydig cells. The interstitial Leydig cells differentiate and produce testosterone to induce masculinization (Fisher *et al.*, 2003). An interesting recent study by Hu *et al.* (2010) showed that deletion of the insulin-like growth factor 1 (IGF-1) gene resulted in a significant reduction of Leydig cell numbers and reduced levels of testosterone resulting in hypogonadism. This reduction in Leydig cell number and function at least in part is due to alteration in proliferation and differentiation of Sertoli cells but not stem cells that differentiate into these Sertoli cells. Timing of embryonic development is critical, and any delay of maturation of Sertoli cells will reflect on testicular development.

Testicular development and toxicity

Developmental and reproductive epidemiologists reported that exposure of humans to environmental pollutants including teratogens, carcinogens, pesticides, herbicides and toxic metabolites as well as endocrine disrupting chemicals and xenobiotics may interfere with early germ cell development which can induce *testicular dysgenesis syndrome* (TDS) (Skakkebaek *et al.*, 2001) (Figure 69.1). The interesting review of Bonde (2010) emphasized that the reproductive toxicity of many pollutants is by targeting specific cell types of male reproductive tissues (e.g., dibromochloropropane (DBCP) alters spermatogonia cells; ethanol alters Leydig cells; Sertoli cells can be altered by phthalate esters).

A reproductive and developmental study by Cammack *et al.* (2003) showed that Sprague-Dawley rats exposed to phthalates (300 or 600 mg/kg) had depleted germinal tubules and showed reduction in seminiferous tubule diameter. Adverse reproductive effects of phthalates such as atrophy of seminiferous tubules, decrease of testicular weights, sperm count and sperm motility were also observed in the offspring (Lyche *et al.*, 2009).

Importantly, genetic aberrations and chromosomal rearrangements can affect sex-determining genes. Human TDS leads to cryptorchidism, *in situ* germ cell carcinoma of the testis and testicular cancer, reduced sperm quality, hypospadias and microliths in the testis. Additional signs include Sertoli cell-only seminiferous tubules without spermatogenic activity and immature tubules with undifferentiated Sertoli cells (Edward *et al.*, 2006; Skakkebaek *et al.*, 2003). Although these symptoms are developmentally related, their severity can differ. Edwards *et al.* (2006) reported that the sexually undifferentiated embryo can develop into: (1) simultaneous hermaphrodites – expressing functional adult male and female phenotypes at the same time; (2) sequential hermaphrodites – maturing first as one gender and then the other; (3) gonochoristic species – maturing as male or female.

Spermatogenesis

Spermatogenesis is a chronological process spanning about 80 days in man (Figure 69.2) and 40–50 days in the rodent (depending upon species). During this period, the immature germ cells (relatively undifferentiated spermatogonia) develop into highly specialized spermatozoa in a cyclic manner. Spermatogonia undergo several mitotic divisions to generate a large population of primary spermatocytes, which produce haploid spermatids by two meiotic cell divisions. Spermiogenesis is the transformation of spermatids into elongated flagellar germ cells capable of motility. The release of mature germ cells is known as spermiation. Testicular volume consists mainly of these germ cells, which diminish if testicular damage has occurred. During mitotic arrest, the gonocyte becomes acutely sensitive to toxic agents. Low dose irradiation may completely eradicate germ cells while causing little damage to developing Sertoli cells, thus creating a Sertoli-cell-only testis (Mandl, 1964).

Additionally, DNA damage in testis may accelerate the process of germ cell apoptosis, also known as programmed cell death (Sinha-Hikim and Swerdloff, 1999). This can lead to a decline in sperm counts resulting in infertility (Sun *et al.*, 1997). Several studies have indicated a significant increase in the levels of apoptotic spermatozoa in the semen of infertile men (Sakkas *et al.*, 1999, 2002). Patients who were inseminated with samples containing higher degrees of DNA damage (>12%) had poor embryo quality and/or experienced miscarriages (Duran *et al.*, 2002). Sperm, surgically extracted from the epididymis or testicular tissue in patients with obstructive azoospermia undergoing intracytoplasmic sperm injection (ICSI), revealed a significantly high percentage of DNA fragmentation (Sakkas *et al.*, 1999). The oxidative damage to mitochondrial DNA (mtDNA) is also known to occur in all aerobic cells that are rich in mitochondria, including spermatozoa. Multiple mtDNA deletions in spermatozoa could arise through a free radical-driven event occurring at the spermatogonial cell stage and can account for reproductive failure in some men (Kao *et al.*, 1998). Although standard sperm parameters are not predictive of high levels of apoptosis, it may be an independent phenomenon that plays an important role in the pathophysiology of male infertility. It is not clear how ROS-induced DNA-damaged spermatozoa impair the process of fertilization and embryo development.

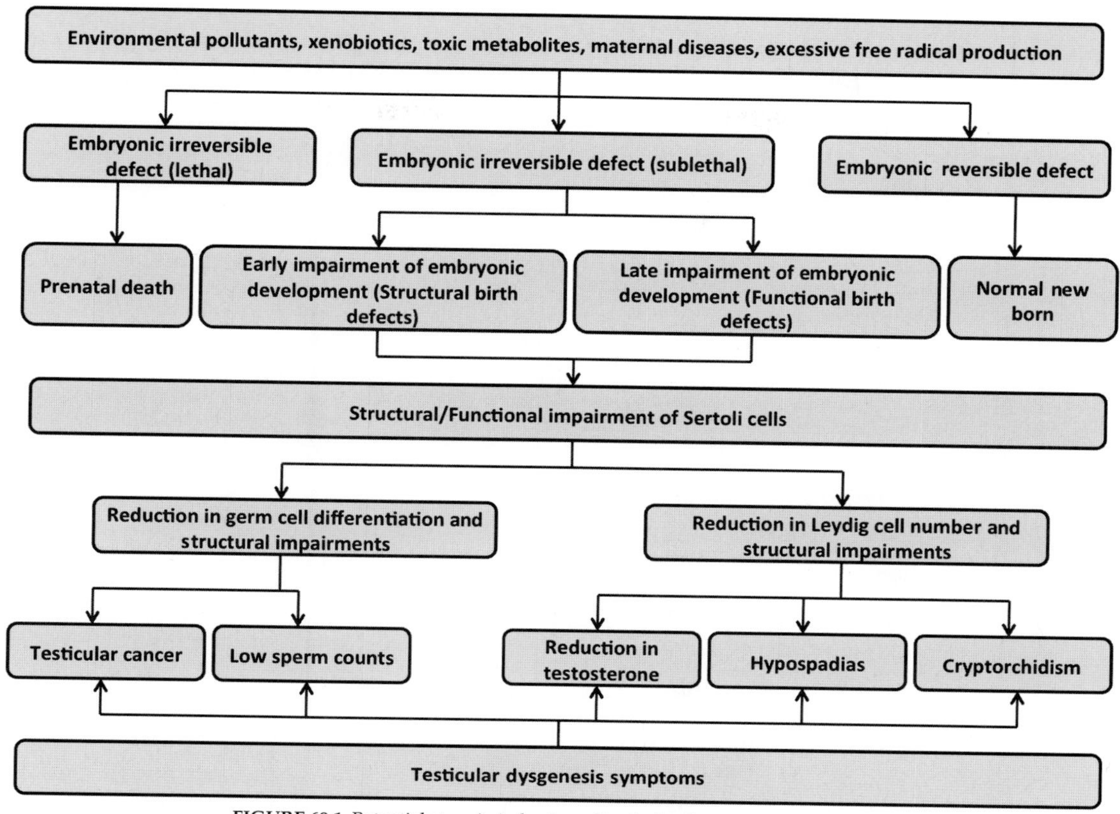

FIGURE 69.1 Potential steps in induction of testicular dysgenesis by toxicants.

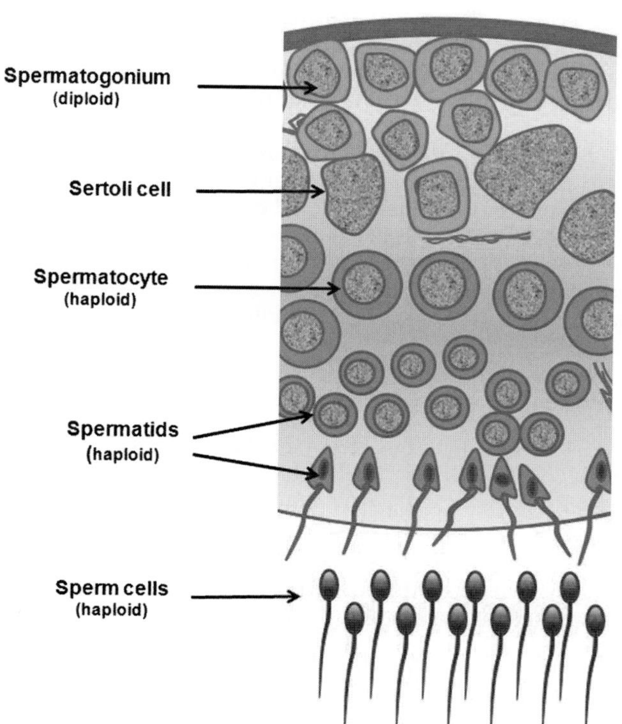

FIGURE 69.2 Graphic representation of spermatogenesis in human testis (80 days).

At present, the key unanswered questions in this direction are the following:

1. Is active apoptosis present in the spermatozoa in semen, and if yes, what is the molecular mechanism of such an apoptotic pathway?
2. Is apoptosis a significant contributor to DNA damage in the seminal spermatozoa?
3. Is this sperm DNA damage via transmembrane receptors and adapter molecules or via mitochondrial membrane damage or both?
4. What is the molecular mechanism(s) of ROS-induced sperm DNA damage? Is it via activation of apoptosis or via some independent action on the DNA integrity?

Considering that oxidative stress plays a significant role in sperm DNA damage and infertility, it becomes even more important to look *in vitro* and *in vivo* into the role of antioxidants that can protect against such oxidative damage to spermatozoa and improve their fertilization potential. Further research is required to elucidate the exact mechanism(s) of association of apoptosis with male factor infertility and the role of antioxidants.

Steroidogenesis

In steroidogenesis the neutral lipid cholesterol is transformed via a series of hydroxylation, oxidation and reduction steps into biologically active compounds including prostagenes, mineralocorticoids, glucocorticoids, androgens and

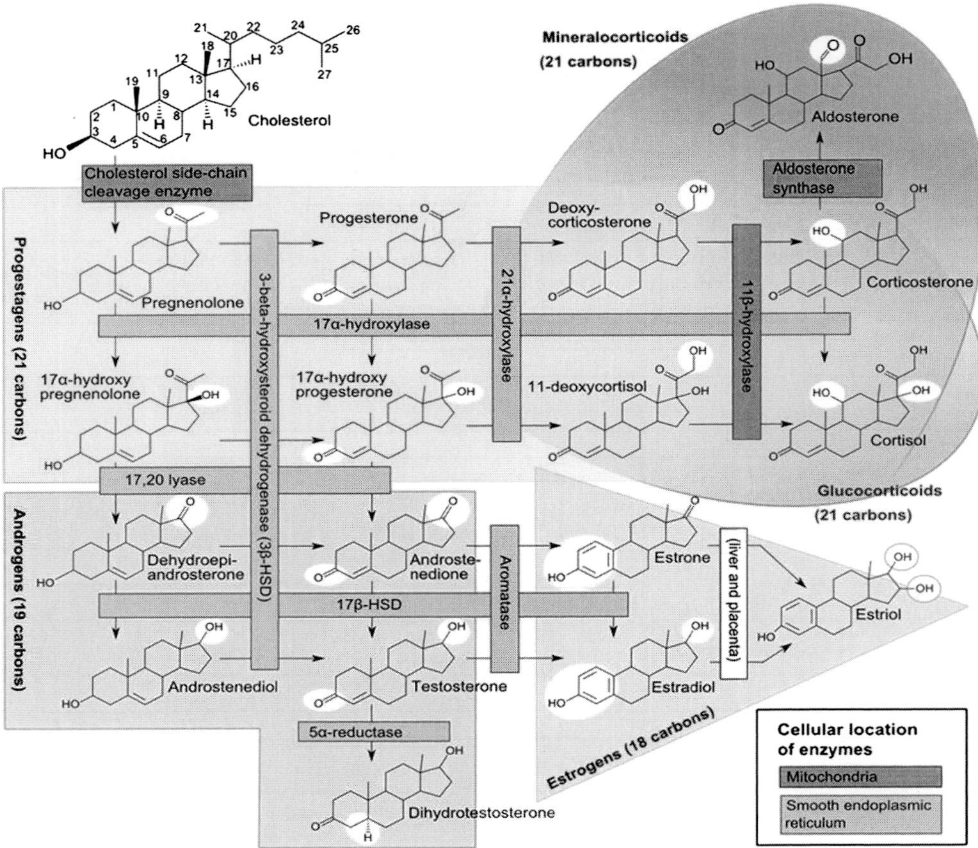

FIGURE 69.3 Graphic representation of testicular steroidogenesis pathway. Cited from http://upload.wikimedia.org/wikipedia/commons/8/84/Steroidogenesis.png.

estrogens (Figure 69.3). Sex hormones such as androgens, estrogens and progestins are fundamental for sex differentiation in the male and support reproduction. A block in the pathway of steroid biosynthesis leads to a lack of hormones downstream and accumulation of the upstream compounds that can activate other members of the steroid receptor family (Biason-Lauber *et al.*, 2010). The response of the steroidogenic targets such as mitochondrial cholesterol transport, CYP11A and CYP17 to endocrine disruptors differs in mammalian species (Scott *et al.*, 2009). However, cholesterol uptake is not susceptible to endocrine disruptors (Scott *et al.*, 2009).

Role of testosterone on male reproduction

As stated above, during embryonic development, testosterone secretion by the fetal testes is responsible for masculinizing the reproductive tract and external genitalia and for promoting descent of the testes into the scrotum. After birth, testosterone secretion ceases, and the testes and the balance of the reproductive system remain small and non-functional until onset of puberty. Environmental chemicals acting as antiandrogen can disrupt this normal sexual development during fetal life (Cheek and McLachlan, 1998).

At the onset of puberty, the Leydig cells once again start secreting testosterone, and spermatogenesis is initiated in the seminiferous tubules for the first time. Testosterone is responsible for the growth and maturation of the entire male reproductive system. Ongoing testosterone secretion is essential for spermatogenesis and for maintaining a mature male reproductive tract throughout adulthood. Potent hormonal disruptors in the environment can impair normal development of these organs of the male reproductive system and can affect sperm production (Thomas and Colborn, 1992).

Other effects of testosterone include development of libido at puberty; maintenance of adult male sex drive; feedback control of the secretion of LH by the anterior pituitary; development and maintenance of male secondary sexual characteristics; and general protein anabolic effects, including bone growth and induction of aggressive behavior. How endocrine disruptors alter these effects in the male is not clearly understood.

ENDOCRINE DISRUPTORS

Several reports suggest that many chemicals released into the environment can affect normal endocrine function (Roa and Schwetz, 1982). Some deleterious effects observed in animals have been attributed to persistent organic chemicals and some pesticides (Cheek and McLachlan, 1998). These chemicals exist in the environment even in minute quantities and if ingested may mimic natural hormones and disrupt bodily functions. Convincing evidence exists that chemical exposures may lead to increased estrogenic activity, reduced androgen levels, or otherwise interfere with the action of androgen during development, thus causing male

TABLE 69.1 Adverse effects of classified and identified endocrine disruptors

Type	Name	Adverse effects
Pesticides	DDT metabolites	Feminization
	Vinclozolin	Feminization
Chemotherapeutics	Cyclophosphamide	Postmeiotic germ cell abnormalities
	Alkylating agents	Complete germinal aplasia
Antimicrobials	Tetracycline derivatives	Impair spermatogenesis and sperm function
Heavy metals	Lead	Suppression of testosterone and spermatogenesis
	Cadmium	Testicular necrosis
	Mercury	Alter spermatogenesis and decrease fertility
Radiation	X-ray	Testicular damage
Smoking	Nicotine, other chemicals	Reduction of sperm quality and bioenergetics

reproductive system abnormalities (Kavlock and Perreault, 1994). Results obtained from the observation of men exposed to DES *in utero* demonstrate that environmental agents may alter neuroendocrine function both during development and in the sexually mature organism (Zaebst, 1980). Tests for the endocrine-disrupting potential of environmental chemicals should include the ability to detect antiandrogenic activity as well as estrogenic activity. Tests also should be able to detect alteration in androgen receptor and other receptor function as reflected in genome expression (Soto *et al.*, 1992). Developmental and reproductive toxicologists classified and identified several endocrine disruptors (Table 69.1).

Pesticides

Vinclozolin, a fungicide used on grapes, and p,p′-DDE, the major persistent metabolite of DDT, have been shown to feminize the reproductive systems of male rat pups born in a multigenerational study (Kelce *et al.*, 1993). These pups had a very small ano-genital distance which is an androgen-dependent measure, and the external genitalia of older animals had female characteristics suggesting that these agents inhibited the action of androgens. For the male reproductive tract to develop, a number of proteins have to be synthesized, and that synthesis depends on androgens secreted by the testes during development. These chemicals interfere with androgens by binding to the androgen receptor and prevent the transcription of DNA. On the other hand, testicular cancer, undescended testis and urethral abnormalities can arise during fetal development. These medical conditions may be due to altered exposure to estrogens during pregnancy and not due to androgen interference. Whereas androgens normally act like keys that open doors to reproductive development, certain androgenic toxicants may act like keys that jam the locks.

Chemotherapeutic agents

As early as 1954, antibacterial agents were reported to be toxic to spermatozoa (Ericsson and Baker, 1967). Antibiotics and cancer chemotherapy usually damage the germinal epithelium (Schlegel *et al.*, 1991; Shalet, 1980). Mechlorethamine, extensively used as nitrogen mustard during the Second World War, causes spermatogenic arrest (Spitz, 1984). Many common cytotoxic agents cause a dose-dependent progressive decrease in sperm count, leading to azoospermia (Meistrich, 1982). Postmeiotic germ cells are specifically sensitive to cyclophosphamide treatment, with abnormalities observed in progeny (Qiu *et al.*, 1992). Chronic low dose cyclophosphamide treatment in men can affect the decondensation potential of spermatozoa due to the alkylation of nuclear proteins or DNA. This is likely to affect pre- and postimplantation loss or contribute to congenital abnormalities in offspring (Trasler, 1987). Combination therapy with alkylating agents has been shown to improve survival in the treatment of Hodgkin's disease, lymphoma and leukemia. However, such combination therapy has induced sterility in most adults, as revealed by complete germinal aplasia in testicular biopsy specimens (Sherins and DeVita, 1973). Many antimicrobials (e.g., tetracycline derivatives, sulfa drugs, nitrofurantoin and macrolide agents, like erythromycin) impair spermatogenesis and sperm function (Ericsson and Baker, 1976; Schlegel, 1991).

In general, the severity of testicular damage is related to the category of chemotherapeutic agent used, the dose and duration of therapy, and the developmental stage of the testis. The recovery of spermatogenesis is variable and depends upon the total therapeutic dose and duration of treatment (Parvinen, 1984). The effects of cytotoxic drugs on the testicular function of children are inconclusive, due to the relative insensitivity in detecting such damage with available technology; however, the prepubertal and adolescent testes show damage to a lesser extent by chemo- and radiation therapy than the postpubertal or older testis (Oats and Lipshultz, 1989). This may be due to rapid turnover and recovery of damaged cells by active spermatogenesis in younger gonads. The use of testicular biopsy, semen analysis and assessment of the hypogonadal–pituitary–gonadal (HPG) axis can commonly achieve the evaluation of testicular toxicity

Heavy metals

Heavy metals (e.g., arsenic, lead, boron, mercury, cadmium, antimony, aluminum, cobalt, chromium, lithium) have been found to exert adverse effects on the reproductive axis of human and experimental animals. More reports are available on lead-induced toxicity than any other heavy metal. Historically, the fall of the Roman Empire has been attributed to lead poisoning (Gilfillan, 1965). Men working in battery plants and exposed to toxic levels of lead demonstrated adverse effects on their reproductive capacity (Lancranjan *et al.*, 1975; Winder, 1989). In animals, lead exposure results in a dose-dependent suppression of serum testosterone and spermatogenesis (Ewing *et al.*, 1981; Foster, 1992). Although testicular biopsies reveal peritubular fibrosis, vacuolation and oligospermia, suggesting that lead is a direct testicular toxicant (Braunstein *et al.*, 1978), some mechanistic studies show that lead exposure can disrupt the hormonal feedback mechanism at the hypothalamic–pituitary level (Sokol, 1987). Animal studies suggest that these effects can be reversed when lead is removed from the system. Such detailed evaluations in humans need further investigations.

Cadmium, another heavy metal, is a testicular toxicant that is used widely in industries like electroplating, battery electrode production, galvanizing, plastics, alloys and paint pigments (Friberg *et al.*, 1974). It is also present in soil, coal, water and cigarette smoke. In animal studies, cadmium has been shown to cause severe testicular necrosis in mice that are also strain-dependent (King *et al.*, 1997). Cadmium–DNA binding and inhibition of sulfhydryl-containing proteins mediate cadmium toxicity directly or through transcription mechanisms. It can also induce the expression of heat shock proteins, oxidative stress response genes and heme oxygenase induction mechanisms (Snow, 1992). Clinical studies have associated cadmium exposure with testicular toxicity, altered libido and infertility. Further studies are needed to delineate the specific gonadotoxic mechanisms involved in cadmium-induced reproductive toxicity. Mercury exposure can happen during the manufacture of thermometers, thermostats, mercury vapor lamps, paint, electrical appliances and in mining. Such exposure can alter spermatogenesis and has been found to decrease fertility in experimental animals.

Radiation

Radiation exposure (X-rays, neutrons and radioactive materials) induce testicular damage that is generally more severe and difficult to recover than that induced by chemotherapy. Radiation effects on the testis depend upon the dose, number and duration of the delivered irradiation, as well as the developmental stage of the germ cell in the testes at the time of exposure (Oats and Lipshultz, 1989). Radiotherapy, which is alternatively used for the treatment of seminomatous germ cell tumors and lymphomas, can be gonadotoxic. In general, germ cells are the most radiosensitive. A direct dose of irradiation to the testes greater than 0.35 Gy causes aspermia. The time taken for recovery increases with larger doses, and doses in excess of 2 Gy will likely lead to permanent azoospermia. At higher radiation doses (>15 Gy), Leydig cells will also be affected (Rowley *et al.*, 1974). Vulnerability of the testis to irradiation depends upon the age and the pubertal status of the male. In addition to direct damage to the testes, whole body irradiation can also damage the hypothalamic–pituitary axis and affect reproductive capability (Ogilvy-Stuart and Shalet, 1993).

Smoking

Cigarette smoke contains over 4,000 chemical constituents and additives including known carcinogens, toxic heavy metals and many chemicals untested for developmental toxicity. Maternal smoking is implicated in the induction of embryonic developmental abnormalities, increased rate of miscarriage, reduced fetal growth and, finally, fetal and neonatal death. A meta-analysis of 12 studies examining the relationship between smoking and risk of infertility found a consistent elevation of risk across studies (Augood *et al.*, 1998). Exposure to tobacco smoke was associated with lower fecundability in both female and male offspring as adults (Rogers, 2009). Smoking is associated with reduced sperm quality and the risk of idiopathic male infertility in men (Colagar *et al.*, 2007). Strikingly, the rate of sperm respiration was significantly lower in smokers (Chohan and Badawy, 2010). This negative impact of cigarette smoking on sperm aerobic metabolism may, in part, explain the lower rate of fertility in smokers. One of the major important mechanisms of deleterious effects of smoking is by generation of free radicals.

MECHANISM OF ACTION OF HORMONAL DISRUPTORS

Natural sex hormones (estrogens or androgens) travel in the bloodstream searching out compatible receptor sites located in the nucleus of specific cells. The hormones enter the cell, lock onto a specific receptor and turn on specific genes. The genes tell the cell to make new proteins or other substances that can change cell functions (grow, divide or make more enzyme). Unlike some hormones that act in seconds or minutes, this process may take hours to complete.

Although natural steroid hormones generally function by binding to specific receptor sites, synthetic environmental estrogens can affect the hormonal system in a number of different ways:

1. They bind to specific receptor sites inside the nucleus of a cell which mimic or evoke a proper hormone response.
2. They block or inhibit a normal hormone response.
3. They mimic and block hormones (PCBs do both).
4. They elicit a weaker or a stronger hormone response, or make a totally new response.
5. They bind to other receptors and create a novel reaction or interfere indirectly with normal hormonal action.
6. They alter production and breakdown of hormone receptors and natural hormones, which change hormonal blood concentrations and endocrine responses.

In addition to previous mechanisms, endocrine disruptors including pesticides, xenobiotics, heavy metals, radiations, smoking and alcohol generate free radicals that can induce developmental and reproductive abnormalities.

FREE RADICALS AND DEVELOPMENTAL TOXICITY

Free radicals can damage DNA and proteins, either through oxidation of DNA bases or through covalent binding resulting in DNA strand breaks and cross-linking. Reactive oxygen species (ROS) can also induce oxidation of critical -SH groups in proteins and DNA, which will alter cellular integrity and function with an increased susceptibility to attack by toxicants.

Free radicals in embryonic development

Free radicals are critical modulators in embryonic development. Very low levels of oxidants enhance embryonic cell proliferation, while mild elevation leads to cell differentiation (Hansen, 2006; Dennery, 2007). Schafer and Buettner (2001) reported that low levels of natural antioxidant reduced glutathione (GSH) induce proliferation, while high levels of oxidized glutathione (GSSG) result in shifting into differentiation and apoptosis. It has been reported that during the early periods of rat embryogenesis the levels of GSH were 17 nmol/mg protein and GSSG concentrations were 1.5 nmol/mg protein (Hiranruengchok and Harris, 1993). However, during the late organogenesis GSH concentrations were 45 nmol/mg protein and the concentrations of GSSG were 7.5 nmol/mg protein (Liu *et al.*, 2006).

Although mitochondria are the main source of free radicals, several xenobiotics, pesticides, herbicides, teratogens and maternal diseases produced excessive oxidant species that are implicated in the induction of embryonic cell apoptosis and teratogenesis (Hansen, 2006; Dennery, 2007). Wells and co-workers (2010) reported that, in humans, 2 weeks after fertilization, toxicity of xenobiotics either results in induction of cell death or has no effect. During early embryonic development, however, toxicity of xenobiotics results in structural birth defects. Moreover, toxic metabolites of xenobiotics induced functional birth defects in the late stage of embryonic development. Studies of Sauer *et al.* (2000) showed that the hypo-sedative drug thalidomide, the most notorious human teratogen, induced elevation of free radicals in murine embryonic stem cells and perturbed vasculogenesis and angiogenesis. Co-administration of hydroxyl radical scavengers restored vasculogenesis and angiogenesis. Additionally, studies of Hansen (2006) showed that thalidomide reduced the GSH/GSSG ratio in limb bud cells isolated from rat and rabbit embryos. Interestingly, in the studies of Parman and co-workers (1999), although thalidomide induced DNA oxidation and subsequently dysmorphogenesis and malformation of rabbit embryos, it had no effect on mice embryos. Pentachlorinated biphenyl 126 (PCB126) is a global environmental contaminant that can induce cellular oxidative stress. Supplementation of vitamin E reduced PCB126-mediated toxicity to zebrafish embryos.

EVALUATION OF MALE REPRODUCTIVE DEVELOPMENT AND TOXICITY

Several methods have evolved for the assessment of toxic effects on the male reproductive system (Table 69.2). Essentially, any risk assessment usually has four components: (1) hazard identification, (2) dose–response assessment, (3) human-exposure assessment, and (4) risk characterization.

TABLE 69.2 Evaluation of effect of hormonal disruptors on the male reproductive axis

Potential sites	Effects	Evaluative tests
Leydig cells	Necrosis	Testes weight, histopathology
	LH/PRL	Receptor analysis and biochemical assays
Sertoli cells	FSH/Steroids	Receptor analysis and biochemical assays
Seminiferous tubules	Spermatogonial mitosis	Germ cell count and percentage of tubules
	Spermatogonial meiosis	Spermatid counts and percentage of tubular with luminal sperm
	Spermatid differentiation	Germ cell culture, morphology
Epididymis	Sperm maturation	Histopathology and biochemical tests
Seminal fluid	Daily sperm production	Spermatid counts and semen analysis
Serum	Hormonal	Biochemical assays

Abbreviations: LH (luteinizing hormone); PRL (prolactin); FSH (follicle stimulating hormone)

The hazard identification and dose–response data are developed from experimental animal studies that may be supplemented with data from *in vitro* studies. This information is then extrapolated and integrated to characterize and assess the risk to the human population. Table 69.2 lists how such effects of endocrine disruptors and other toxicants on specific components of hormones can be evaluated using both *in vivo* and *in vitro* tools.

In vivo systems

In vivo methods are important tools to study the integrated male reproductive system. The complete *in vivo* assessment of testicular toxicity involves multigenerational studies, now required by most regulatory agencies. These multigenerational studies have a complex design, because testicular function and spermatogenesis are very complicated processes. The spermatogenic cycle is highly organized throughout the testis. In the rat, it requires about 50 days. Thus, if a toxicant affects the immature spermatogonia, the effect may not be detectable as a change in mature sperm before 7 to 8 weeks. Effects on more mature germ cells would be detected sooner. To test the sensitivity of all stages of spermatogenesis, the exposure should last the full duration of the cycle. This cannot be achieved *in vitro*, because germ cell differentiation and the physical relationship of stages within the tubules are lost in cell culture systems. The germ cells are entirely dependent upon the Sertoli cells for physical and biochemical support. Complicated endocrine and paracrine systems control Sertoli cells, Leydig cells and germ cells. Besides the loss of paracrine interactions, the altered metabolic activity of target or adjacent cells and difficulty in isolating and testing certain spermatogenic stages are other significant limitations of *in vitro* assessment of testicular toxicity (Lamb and Chapin, 1993). In addition, for accurate identification of stage-specific lesions of the seminiferous epithelium, critical evaluation of morphological structures is very important. Because germ cells are continuously dividing and differentiating, the staging of spermatogenesis has proven to be an extremely sensitive tool to identify and characterize even subtle toxicological changes.

In vitro systems

In vitro systems are uniquely suited to investigate specific cellular and molecular mechanisms in the testis and thus improve risk assessment (Lamb and Chapin, 1993). These *in vitro* models can be used alone or in combination with each other to test hypotheses about testicular toxicity. An original toxicant, its metabolites, the precursors or selective inhibitors can be individually administered to isolated cell types to evaluate specific toxicity mechanisms and to note the interaction of adjacent cell types. Numerous *in vitro* model systems are described in the literature, including Sertoli germ cell co-cultures (Gray, 1988); Sertoli cell-enriched cultures (Chapin, 1990; Steinberger and Clinton, 1993); germ cell-enriched cultures (Foster *et al.*, 1987); Leydig cell cultures (Ewing *et al.*, 1981; Gray, 1988); Leydig–Sertoli cell co-cultures (Chapin *et al.*, 1990); and peritubular and tubular cell cultures (Gray, 1988; Chapin *et al.*, 1990). These *in vitro* systems are the only way to directly compare human and animal responses and to screen a class of compounds for new product development. Though these *in vitro* systems are a valuable adjunct to the *in vivo* test system, they do not replace the *in vivo* data, because they cannot provide all the facts essential for hazard assessment. Moreover, certain dynamic changes associated with spermatogenesis are difficult to model *in vitro*. For example, the release of elongated spermatids by the Sertoli cells (spermiation), which is commonly inhibited by boric acid and methyl chloride, can only be studied at present by specific *in vivo* systems.

Sperm nuclear integrity assessment

Recent attention focuses on assessment of sperm morphology and physiology as important endpoints in reproductive toxicology testing (Darney, 1990). Structural stability of sperm nuclei varies by species, appears to be enhanced by the oxidation of protamine sulfhydryl to inter- and intra-molecular disulfide bonds, and is a function of the types of protamine present. Chemicals may disrupt the structural stability of sperm nuclei, which depend upon their unique packaging either during spermatogenesis or sperm maturation. Decondensation of an isolated sperm nucleus *in vitro* can be induced by exposure to disulfide reducing agents, and the time taken to induce extensive decondensation is considered to be inversely proportional to the stability of the sperm nucleus. Human sperm decondenses most rapidly, followed by that of the mouse and of the hamster, while rat sperm nuclei showed a slower decondensation (Perrault *et al.*, 1988). Such sperm DNA decondensation assay is useful in the evaluation of some cases of unexplained infertility (Zini and Libman, 2006). Evidence suggests that damage to human sperm DNA might adversely affect reproductive outcomes and that the spermatozoa of infertile men possess substantially more sperm DNA damage than do the spermatozoa of fertile men (Zini and Libman, 2006). This is particularly relevant in an era where advanced forms of assisted reproductive technologies are commonly used (technologies that often bypass the barriers to natural selection), because there is some uncertainty regarding the safety of using DNA-damaged spermatozoa. However, sperm head morphology has shown low but significant correlations with the sperm chromatin structure assay (SCSA) variables (Boe-Hansen *et al.*, 2006). Evaluation of damaged sperm DNA seems to complement the investigation of factors affecting male fertility and may prove an efficient diagnostic tool in the prediction of pregnancy outcome (Angelopoulou *et al.*, 2007).

DNA stability assay or SCSA uses direct evaluation of sperm chromatin integrity and may provide information about genetic damage to sperm and predict infertility (Evenson, 1989; Evenson *et al.*, 1991). A shift in DNA pattern (from double-stranded intact DNA to denatured single-stranded DNA) can be induced by a variety of mutagenic and chemical agents and evaluated either by DNA flow cytometry analysis or by sperm chromatin structure assay (Brown, 1995). A modified single cell gel electrophoresis (Comet) assay, which uses a combination of fluorescence intensity measurements by microscopy and image analysis, has been recently validated (Angelopoulou *et al.*, 2007). A shift in the DNA pattern can be evaluated by acridine orange staining, where double-stranded DNA is stained green and single-stranded DNA is stained red. The data are expressed as the DNA Fragmentation Index (DFI). DNA flow cytometry is a very useful tool that permits rapid, objective assessment of a large number of cells, but may not be readily available. Comet assay, when combined with centrifugal elutriation, can provide a useful *in vitro* model to study differences in metabolism and the susceptibility of different testicular cell types to DNA damaging compounds. Thus, new findings through these systems should lead to greater knowledge about effects and mechanism(s) of a chemical or class of chemicals involved in testicular toxicity.

CONCLUDING REMARKS AND FUTURE DIRECTIONS

In summary, a variety of extraneous and internal factors can induce developmental and testicular toxicity leading to teratogenesis, poor sperm quality and male factor infertility. Unfortunately, several of these influences (e.g., glandular infection, environmental toxicants that are mainly estrogenic chemicals, nutritional deficiencies, aging, ischemia and oxidative stress) disrupt the hormonal milieu and have been underestimated. Partial androgen insensitivity mainly due to altered androgen-to-estrogen balance may contribute to significant oligozoospermia. The role of chronic inflammation on the reproductive organs is not completely understood because it is asymptomatic and is difficult to demonstrate objectively. There is an urgent need to characterize all the factors involved and to develop reliable animal models of testicular disease. No major advances have been made for the medical management of poor sperm quality. The application of assisted reproductive techniques such as ICSI to male infertility, regardless of cause, does not necessarily treat the cause and may inadvertently pass on adverse genetic consequences. Clinicians should always attempt to identify the etiology of a possible testicular toxicity, assess the degree of risk to the patient being evaluated for infertility, and initiate a plan to control and prevent exposure to others once an association between occupation/exposure and infertility has been established. Moreover, long-term developmental and reproductive toxic effects to all forms of life due to recent tragic events of oil leaks in Alaska and now in the Gulf of Mexico are yet to be seen.

Humans are experiencing increased incidences of abnormal developmental, reproductive and carcinogenic effects. It appears that these adverse effects may be caused by environmental chemicals acting to disrupt the endocrine system that regulates these processes. This is supported by observations of similar effects in aquatic and wildlife species. In other words, a common theme runs through both human and wildlife reports. In contrast, the hypothesis that the reported increased incidence of human cancers and reproductive abnormalities and infertility can be attributed to an endocrine disruption phenomenon is called into question for several reasons.

First, secretion and elimination of hormones are highly regulated by the body, and mechanisms for controlling modest fluctuations of hormones are in place via negative feedback control of hormone concentrations. Therefore, minor increases of environmental hormones following dietary absorption and liver detoxification of these xenobiotics may be inconsequential in disrupting endocrine homeostasis. Second, low ambient concentrations of chemicals along with low affinity binding of purported xenobiotics to target receptors probably are insufficient to activate an adverse response in adults. Whether the fetus and the young are capable of regulating minor changes to the endocrine milieu is uncertain.

Finally, the data are not available for mixtures of chemicals that may be able to affect endocrine function. At the same time, in the case of environmental estrogens as endocrine disruptors, it is known that competition for binding sites by antiestrogens in the environment may moderate estrogenic effects of some chemicals. Clearly, more research to fill data gaps and to remove the uncertainty in these unknowns is needed.

A causal relationship between exposure to a specific environmental agent and an adverse effect on human health operating via an endocrine disruption mechanism has not been established. Short-term screening studies could be developed and validated in an effort to elucidate a mechanism. Through controlled dose–response studies, it appears that these compounds (e.g., alkyl phenol ethylates and their degradation products, chlorinated dibenzodioxins and difurans, and polychlorinated biphenyls, PCBs) can induce irreversible induction of male sex characteristics on females (imposex), which can lead to sterility and reduced reproductive performance.

REFERENCES

Angelopoulou R, Plastira K, Msaouel P (2007) Spermatozoal sensitive biomarkers to defective protaminosis and fragmented DNA. *Reprod Biol Endocrinol* **5:** 36.

Augood C, Duckitt K, Templeton AA (1998) Smoking and female infertility: a systematic review and meta-analysis. *Hum Reprod* **13:** 1532.

Biason-Lauber A, Boscaro M, Mantero F, Balercia G (2010) Defects of steroidogenesis. *J Endocrinol Invest.* In press.

Boe-Hansen GB, Fedder J, Ersbøll AK, Christensen P (2006) The sperm chromatin structure assay as a diagnostic tool in the human fertility clinic. *Hum Reprod* **6:** 1576.

Bonde JP (2010) Male reproductive organs are at risk from environmental hazards. *Asian J Androl* **12:** 152.

Braunstein GD, Dahlgren J, Loriaux DO (1978) Hypogonadism in chronically lead poisoned men. *Infertility* **1:** 33.

Brennan J, Capel B (2004) One tissue, two fates: molecular genetic events that underlie testis versus ovary development. *Nat Rev Genet* **5:** 509.

Brown DB, Hayes EJ, Uchida T, Nagamani M (1995) Some cases of human male infertility are explained by abnormal in vitro human sperm activation. *Fertil Steril* **64:** 612.

Cammack JN, White RD, Gordon D, Gass J, Hecker L, Conine D, Bruen US, Friedman M, Echols C, Yeh TY, Wilson DM (2003) Evaluation of reproductive development following intravenous and oral exposure to DEHP in male neonatal rats. *Int J Toxicol* **22:** 159.

Chapin RE, Phelps JL, Somkuti SG, Heindel JJ (1990) The interaction of Sertoli and Leydig cells in the testicular toxicity of tri-o-cresyl phosphate. *Toxicol Appl Pharmacol* **104:** 483.

Cheek AO, McLachlan JA (1998) Environmental hormones and the male reproductive system. *J Androl* **19:** 5.

Chohan KR, Badawy SZ (2010) Cigarette smoking impairs sperm bioenergetics. *Int Braz J Urol* **36:** 60.

Colagar AH, Jorsaraee GA, Marzony ET (2007) Cigarette smoking and the risk of male infertility. *Pak J Biol Sci* **10:** 3870.

Darney SP (1991) In vitro assessment of gamete integrity. In *In-vitro Toxicology: Mechanisms and New Toxicology – Alternative Methods in Toxicology,* Vol. 8 (Goldberg AM, ed.). Ann Liebert, Inc. New York, pp. 63–75.

Dennery PA (2007) Effects of oxidative stress on embryonic development. *Birth Defects Res C Embryo Today* **81:** 155.

Duran EH, Morshedi M, Taylor S, Oehninger S (2002) Sperm DNA quality predicts IUI outcome: a prospective cohort study. *Hum Reprod* **12:** 3122.

Edwards TM, Moore BC, Guillette LJ Jr (2006) Reproductive dysgenesis in wildlife: a comparative view. *Int J Androl* **29:** 109.

Ericsson RJ, Baker VF (1967) Binding of tetracycline to mammalian spermatozoa. *Nature* **214:** 403.

Evenson DP (1989) Flow cytometry evaluation of male germ cells. In *Flow Cytometry: Advanced Research and Clinical Applications,* Vol. 1 (Yen A, ed.), CRC Press, Boca Raton FL, pp. 218–46.

Evenson DP, Jost LK, Baer RK, Turner TW, Schrader SM (1991) Individuality of DNA denaturation patterns in human sperm as measured by the sperm chromatin structure assay. *Reprod Toxicol* **5:** 115.

Ewing LL, Zirkin BR, Chubb C (1981) Assessment of testicular testosterone production and Leydig cell structure. *Environ Health Prospect* **38:** 19.

Fisher JS, Macpherson S, Marchetti N, Sharpe RM (2003) Human "testicular dysgenesis syndrome": a possible model using in-utero exposure of the rat to dibutyl phthalate. *Hum Reprod* **18:** 1383.

Foster PMD, Lloyd SC, Prout MS (1987) Toxicity and metabolism of 1,3-dinitrobenzene in rat testicular cell cultures. *Toxicol in Vitro* **1:** 31.

Foster WG, McMahon A, Young-Lai EV, Hughes EG, Rice DC (1992) Reproductive endocrine effects of chronic lead exposure in the male cynomolgus monkey. *Reprod Toxicol* **7:** 203.

Friberg L, Piscator M, Nordberg GF (1974) *Cadmium in the Environment,* 2nd edition. CRC Press, Inc. Cleveland, pp. 37–53.

Gilfillan SC (1965) Lead poisoning and the fall of Rome. *J Occup Med* **7:** 53.

Gray TJB (1988) Application of in vitro systems in male reproductive toxicology. In *Physiology and Toxicology of Male Reproduction* (Lamb JC IV, Foster PMD, eds.). Academic Press, San Diego, pp. 250–53.

Hansen JM (2006) Oxidative stress as a mechanism of teratogenesis. *Birth Defects Res C Embryo Today* **78:** 293.

Hawass Z, Gad YZ, Ismail S, Khairat R, Fathalla D, Hasan N, Ahmed A, Elleithy H, Ball M, Gaballah F, Wasef S, Fateen M, Amer H, Gostner P, Selim A, Zink A, Pusch CM (2010) Ancestry and pathology in King Tutankhamun's family. *JAMA* **303:** 638.

Hiranruengchok R, Harris C (1993) Glutathione oxidation and embryotoxicity elicited by diamide in the developing rat conceptus in vitro. *Toxicol Appl Pharmacol* **120:** 62.

Hu GX, Lin H, Chen GR, Chen BB, Lian QQ, Hardy DO, Zirkin BR, Ge RS (2010) Deletion of the IGF-I gene: suppressive effects on adult Leydig cell development. *J Androl.* In press.

Kao SH, Chao HT, Wei YH (1998) Multiple deletions of mtDNA are associated with decline of motility and fertility of human spermatozoa. *Mol Hum Reprod* **4:** 657.

Kavlock R, Perreault S (1994) Multiple chemical exposure and risks of adverse reproductive function and outcome. In *Toxicological of Chemical Mixtures: From Real Life Examples to Mechanisms of Toxicology Interactions* (Yang RSH, ed.). Academic Press, Orlando, pp. 245–97.

Kelce WR, Monosson E, Gamcsik MP, Laws SC, Gray LE Jr (1994) Environmental hormone disruptors: evidence that vinclozolin developmental toxicity is mediated by antiandrogenic metabolites. *Toxicol Appl Pharmacol* **126:** 276.

King LM, Andrew MG, Sikka SC, George WJ (1997) Murine strain differences in cadmium-induced testicular toxicity. *The Toxicologist* **36:** 186.

Klyde BJ (1994) Hormonal causes of male sexual dysfunction. In *Management of Impotence and Infertility* (Whitehead HM, ed.). J.B. Lippincott Co., Philadelphia, p. 115.

Lamb JC IV, Chapin RE (1993) Testicular and germ cell toxicity: in-vitro approaches. *Reproductive Toxicol* **7:** 17.

Lancranjan I, Popescu HI, Gavanescu O, Klepsch I, Serbanescu M (1975) Reproductive ability of workmen occupationally exposed to lead. *Arch Environ Health* **30:** 396.

Liu JN, Chan HM, Kubow S (2007) Oxidative stress status and development of late organogenesis stage rat whole embryos cultured from gestational days 13.5 to 14.5. *Toxicol in Vitro* **21:** 253.

Lyche JL, Gutleb AC, Bergman A, Eriksen GS, Murk AJ, Ropstad E, Saunders M, Skaare JU (2009) Reproductive and developmental toxicity of phthalates. *J Toxicol Environ Health B Crit Rev* **12:** 225.

Makker K, Agarwal A, Sharma R (2009) Oxidative stress and male infertility. *Indian J Med Res* **129:** 357.

Mandl AM (1964) The radiosensitivity of germ cells. *Biol Reprod* **39:** 288.

Meistrich ML (1982) Quantitative correlation between testicular stem cell survival, sperm production, and fertility in mouse after treatment with different cytotoxic agents. *J Androl* **3:** 58.

Mostafa RM, Mirghani Z, Moustafa KM, El Hefnawi MH (2007) New chapter in old story: endocrine disruptors and male reproductive system. *JMSR* **7:** 33.

Nagamine C, Morohashi K, Carlisle C, Chang D (1999) Sex reversal caused by *Mus musculus domesticus* Y chromosomes linked to variant expression of the testis-determining gene *Sry. Dev Biol* **216:** 182–94.

Oats RD, Lipshultz LI (1989) Fertility and testicular function in patients after chemotherapy and radiotherapy. In *Advances in Urology,* Vol. 2 (Lytton B, ed.). Mosby Year Book, Chicago, pp. 55–83.

Ogilvy-Stuart AL, Shalet SM (1993) Effect of radiation on the human reproductive system. *Environ Health Perspect* **101:** 109.

Parman T, Wiley MJ, Wells PG (1999) Free radical-mediated oxidative DNA damage in the mechanism of thalidomide teratogenicity. *Nat Med* **5:** 582.

Parvinen M, Lahdetie J, Parvinen LM (1984) Toxic and mutagenic influences on spermatogenesis. *Arch Toxicol* **7:** 147.

Perrault SD, Barbee RR, Elstein KH, Zucker RM, Keeler CL (1988) Interspecies differences in the stability of mammalian sperm nuclei assessed in vivo by sperm microinjection and in vitro by flow cytometry. *Biol Reprod* **39:** 157.

Qiu J, Hales BF, Robaire B (1992) Adverse effects of cyclophosphamide on progeny outcome can be mediated through post-testicular mechanisms in the rat. *Biol Reprod* **46:** 926.

Roa KS, Schwetz BA (1982) Reproductive toxicity of environmental agents. *Annu Rev Public Health* **3:** 1.

Rogers JM (2009) Tobacco and pregnancy. *Reprod Toxicol* **28:** 152.

Rowley MJ, Leach DR, Warner GA, Heller CG (1974) Effects of graded doses of ionizing radiation on the human testis. *Radiat Res* **59:** 665.

Sakkas D, Mariethoz E, Manicardi G, Bizzaro D, Bianchi PG, Bianchi U (1999) Origin of DNA damage in ejaculated human spermatozoa. *Rev Reprod* **4:** 431.

Sakkas D, Moffatt O, Manicardi G, Mariethoz E, Tarozzi N, Bizzaro D (2002) Nature of DNA damage in ejaculated human spermatozoa and possible involvement of apoptosis. *Biol Reprod* **66:** 1061.

Sauer H, Günther J, Hescheler J, Wartenberg M (2000) Thalidomide inhibits angiogenesis in embryoid bodies by the generation of hydroxyl radicals. *Am J Pathol* **156:** 151.

Schafer FQ, Buettner GR (2001) Redox environment of the cell as viewed through the redox state of the glutathione disulfide/glutathione couple. *Free Radic Biol Med* **30:** 1191.

Schlegel PN, Chang TSK, Marshall FF (1991) Antibiotics: potential hazards to male fertility. *Fertil Steril* **55:** 235.

Scott HM, Mason JI, Sharpe RM (2009) Steroidogenesis in the fetal testis and its susceptibility to disruption by exogenous compounds. *Endocr Rev* **30:** 883.

Shalet SM (1980) Effects of cancer chemotherapy on testicular function of patients. *Cancer Treatment Rev* **7:** 141.

Sharpe RM, McKinnell C, Kivlin C, Fisher JS (2003) Proliferation and functional maturation of Sertoli cells, and their relevance to disorders of testis function in adulthood. *Reproduction* **125:** 769.

Sherins RJ, DeVita VT Jr (1975) Effect of drug treatment for lymphoma on male reproductive capacity. *Ann Intern Med* **79:** 216.

Sikka SC, Kendirici M, Naz R (2004) Endocrine disruptors and male sexual dysfunction. Endocrine disruptors. In *Effects on Male and Female Reproductive Systems* (Naz RK, ed.). CRC Press, pp. 345–77.

Sinha-Hikim AP, Swerdloff RS (1999) Hormonal and genetic control of germ cell apoptosis in the testis. *Rev Reprod* **4:** 38.

Skakkebaek NE, Rajpert-De Meyts E, Main KM (2001) Testicular dysgenesis syndrome: an increasingly common developmental disorder with environmental aspects. *Hum Reprod* **16:** 972.

Snow ET (1992) Metal carcinogenesis: mechanistic implications. *Pharmacol Ther* **53:** 31.

Sokol RZ (1987) Hormonal effects of lead acetate in the male rat: mechanism of action. *Biol Reprod* **37:** 1135.

Soto A, *et al.* (1992) An "in culture" bioassay to assess the estrogenicity of xenobiotics (E-Screen). In *Chemically-induced Alterations in Sexual and Functional Development: The Wildlife/Human Connection* (Clements TCC, ed.). Princeton Scientific Publishing Co., Princeton, NJ, pp. 295–309.

Spitz S (1984) The histological effects of nitrogen mustards on human tumors and tissues. *Cancer* **1:** 383.

Steinberger A, Clinton JP (1993) Two-compartment cultures of Sertoli cells – applications in testicular toxicology. In *Methods in Toxicology (Part A), Male Reproductive Toxicology* (Chapin RE, Heindel JJ, eds.). Academic Press, New York, pp. 230–45.

Sun J-G, Jurisicova A, Casper RF (1997) Detection of deoxyribonucleic acid fragmentation in human sperm: correlation with fertilization in vitro. *Biol Reprod* **56:** 602.

Thomas KB, Colborn T (1992) Organochlorine endocrine disruptors in human tissue. In *Chemically-induced Alterations in Sexual and Functional Development: The Wildlife/Human Connection* (Clement ETCC, ed.). Princeton Science Publishing Co., Princeton, NJ, pp. 365–94.

Trasler JM, Hales BF, Robaire B (1987) A time course study of chronic paternal cyclophosphamide treatment of rats: effects on pregnancy outcome and the male reproductive and hematologic systems. *Biol Reprod* **37:** 317.

Wells PG, Lee CJ, McCallum GP, Perstin J, Harper PA (2010) Receptor- and reactive intermediate-mediated mechanisms of teratogenesis. *Handb Exp Pharmacol* **196:** 131.

Winder C (1989) Reproductive and chromosomal effects of occupational exposure to lead in males. *Reprod Toxicol* **3:** 221.

Zaebst D, Tanaka S, Haring M (1980) Occupational exposure to estrogens – problems and approaches. In *Estrogens in the Environment* (McLachlan MA, ed.). Elsevier/North-Holland, New York, pp. 377–89.

Zini A, Libman J (2006) Sperm DNA damage: clinical significance in the era of assisted reproduction. [Review] *Can Med Assoc J* **175:** 495.

C H A P T E R

70

Mutagenicity and carcinogenicity: human reproductive cancer and risk factors

Hyung Sik Kim and Byung Mu Lee

INTRODUCTION

There are numerous risk factors for cancer development in reproductive and developmental organs. In general, susceptibility to cancer development may increase in animals and humans exposed to environmental carcinogens during specific embryonic periods. Many carcinogens can cross the placental barrier during pregnancy, resulting in various types of cancer when the exposed fetus reaches adulthood. The scientific literature has demonstrated increases in cancer incidence after prenatal exposure to ionizing radiation, therapeutic drugs and environmental pollutants (McBride, 1998; Wigle *et al.*, 2009). Preconceptional exposure to several types of radiation and a variety of chemical carcinogens during sperm or oocyte maturation can also lead to transgenerational carcinogenesis (Tomatis, 1989; Yamasaki *et al.*, 1992). Tomatis (1989) suggested that prenatal events may contribute to the occurrence of cancer following the direct exposure of embryonic or fetal cells to carcinogenic agents, and prezygotic exposure of the germ cells of one or both parents to a carcinogen/mutagen before mating may lead to deregulation of cellular growth and differentiation.

Furthermore, animal experiments have indicated that prenatal or neonatal exposure to chemicals, including direct- or indirect-acting carcinogens and drugs, increased the incidence of tumor development during adulthood. For example, synthetic or natural estrogens have been classified as human carcinogens: prenatal exposure to these compounds is associated with increases in breast and vaginal cancers in humans, as well as uterine tumors in animals (Herbst and Bern, 1981). In addition, diethylstilbestrol (DES) and radiation were shown to increase cancer risk in humans following their exposure during pregnancy (Weiss *et al.*, 1997). An epidemiological study (3,613 men) suggests that prenatal DES exposure could be associated with testicular cancer (Strohsnitter *et al.*, 2001). The increase in testicular cancer may also be related to early life-stage exposure to environmental estrogens and/or antiandrogens (Skakkebaek *et al.*, 2001). However, there is little epidemiologic evidence for other hormonally mediated cancers after developmental exposure to endocrine-disrupting chemicals (EDCs) or endocrine disruptors. Environmental pollutants were also demonstrated to induce tumors by prenatal exposure in experimental animals. Previous work has shown that exposure to dioxin 2,3,7,8-tetrachlorodibenzo-*p*-dioxin (TCDD) is associated with an increased prevalence and severity of endometriosis in non-human primates (Rier and Foster, 2002). Dioxin alters multiple endocrine systems, and its effects on the developing breast include delayed proliferation and differentiation of the mammary gland, as well as an elongation of the window of sensitivity to potential carcinogens. These new findings suggest that the causes of endocrine-related cancers or susceptibility to cancer may involve developmental exposures rather than exposures at or near the time of tumor detection.

Recently, the transgenerational effect of carcinogens was suggested by an increased incidence of tumors in multiple generations of untreated descendants of females exposed to carcinogen during pregnancy. This inherited change may be an initiating event revealed by exposure to carcinogens during the embryonic stage. In humans, inherited diseases from germ cell mutations due to a spontaneous error in DNA replication and repair or as a consequence of carcinogen exposure can increase the risk of cancer development, including retinoblastoma, familial polyposis of the colon, and others. The transgenerational effects of carcinogenic risk are also demonstrated by cancer-prone families, which are probably more common than originally thought, with a risk that is one order of magnitude higher than in the general population. Familial clustering of cancer may also indicate germ-line mutations in one or more genes. Thus, the inherited predisposition to cancer that is observed today may, at least in part, be explained by exposure to environmental carcinogens in previous generation(s). Since humans are exposed throughout life to many environmental agents, either carcinogenic or able to enhance the progression of cancer, an understanding of the contribution of prenatal exposure to carcinogens could improve the efficacy of prevention.

Reproductive and Developmental Toxicology, Edited by Ramesh C. Gupta
ISBN: 978-0-12-382032-7

MUTAGENESIS AND REPRODUCTIVE ORGAN DISEASES

Prenatal exposure to environmental chemicals has the potential to induce developmental defects through DNA mutation and chromosomal changes. Such changes can occur at the level of both individual genes and chromosomes. Individual gene changes may result in the transmission of altered genetic messages, while changes at the chromosomal level can result in the transmission of abnormalities in chromosomal number or structure. For example, cigarette smoking damages sperm by changing its DNA sequence, resulting in the increased incidence of childhood inheritance of permanent genetic damage, cancer and various diseases (Coelho *et al.*, 2009; Ragheb and Sabanegh, 2009).

Cigarette smoke generates various kinds of mutagens and carcinogens such as reactive oxygen species (ROS) that ultimately lead to DNA damage (Potts *et al.*, 1999). Alcohol and endocrine disruptors also generate ROS and produce oxidative DNA damage, protein carbonylation and lipid peroxidation. DNA damage at the gamete level represents a serious potential risk for transmission of mutations to offspring. This type of alteration may result in sperm DNA mutations, increasing the rates of miscarriage and predisposing offspring to greater hazards of congenital defects, childhood cancer and infertility (Figure 70.1). Several studies indicate that children of men who smoke, but not women who smoke, have an increased risk of childhood cancer. Smoking markedly decreases the levels of antioxidants, vitamins or scavenging enzymes in the body (Lee *et al.*, 1998; Northrop-Clewes and Thurnham, 2007). Interestingly, some of the evidence for chemical exposure involvement in developmental abnormalities comes from paternal exposure. However, some defects of unknown etiology likely involve a genetic component that may be related to parental exposures. Indeed, a few studies have shown a close association between childhood cancers and paternal preconception exposure to physical agents. For example, paternal occupational exposure to ionizing radiation has been associated with an increased risk of neural tube defects and increased risk of childhood leukemia, and several studies have suggested associations between paternal preconception occupational exposure to electromagnetic fields and childhood brain tumors (Gold and Sever, 1994).

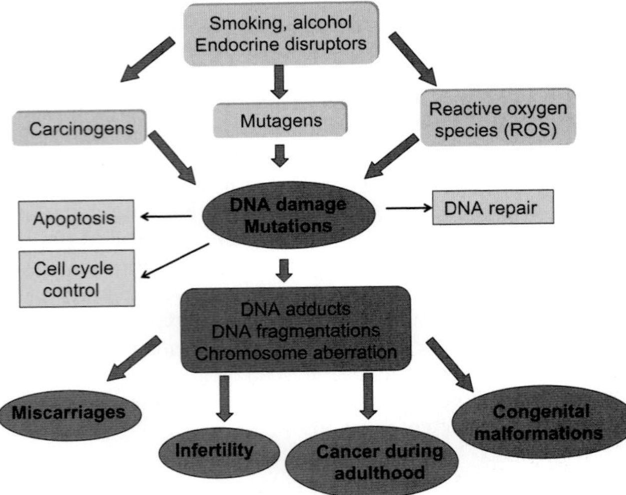

FIGURE 70.1 Schematic representation of reproductive and developmental defects induced by smoking, alcohol and endocrine disruptors in germ cells.

Germ-line mutation by exposure to mutagens is a particular problem in reproductive and developmental toxicology as they can affect both the exposed generation and future generations. This chapter introduces recently identified chemicals in the assessment of adverse reproductive endpoints (Table 70.1).

CARCINOGENICITY AND REPRODUCTIVE DISEASES

Doll and Peto (1981) reported that diet (35%, ranked No. 1) and tobacco smoking (30%, ranked No. 2) were associated with about 65% of all causes of cancer deaths, while reproductive and sexual behavior (7%) and pollution (2%) were less associated with cancer deaths (Figure 70.2). There are other estimates of contributing risk factors for cancer deaths, but the estimate proportions reported by Doll and Peto (1981) have been widely recognized. Carcinogenesis is a multistep process whereby cells may be transformed from a controlled state to an uncontrolled state. There are two key features in this process. First, in the somatic mutation theory of carcinogenesis, the initial step in carcinogenesis induced by a chemical or radiation is a mutation in the DNA of a somatic cell (Stratton *et al.*, 2009; Pleasance *et al.*, 2010). Second, a germ-line mutation in tumor-supressor genes is another aspect of hereditary cancer such as colon cancer in youngsters. Furthermore, a stem cell mutation theory has been considered recently, and other theories may be introduced in the future.

Mechanism of action: biomolecule–adduct, repair, replication and mutation

The integrity of the human genome is continuously affected by endogenous metabolic processes or by exogenous chemical or physical carcinogens that induce covalent binding to DNA, protein and lipids (DeBaun *et al.*, 1970; Weinstein *et al.*, 1976; Lee and Santella, 1988; Kwack and Lee, 2000). The induction of genetic alterations by DNA adduct formation is the major initiating and driving step in the process of multistage chemical carcinogenesis, although epigenetic alterations by protein or lipid adduct formation may also be critically involved (Figure 70.3). The role of protein or lipid adduct formation has not been fully investigated, but such adducts might contribute to alterations of signaling cascades or epigenetic changes during the promotion process. The fundametal mechanism of carcinogenesis involves the basic principles of several cell biological processes including metabolic activation or deactivation of chemical carcinogens, DNA damage, DNA repair, DNA replication and cell cycle regulation, leading to initiation, promotion (stage I (reversible) and stage II (irreversible)) and progression. In terms of the carcinogenesis mechanism, however, attention should also be paid to reactive oxygen species (ROS), reactive nitrogen species (RNS) or free radicals produced by both endogenous and exogenous sources because these free radicals may activate unreactive chemical carcinogens to reactive carcinogens and cause oxidative damage to biomolecules such as DNA, lipid and proteins (Klaunig *et al.*, 1998; Shi *et al.*, 1998; Kim *et al.*, 2000). In the initiation stage of carcinogenesis, ROS mediate carcinogen activation, damage DNA and interfere with repair of damaged DNA (Breimer and Schellens, 1990; Dreher and Junod, 1996; Klaunig *et al.*, 1998; Shi *et al.*, 1998). During the promotion stage of carcinogenesis, ROS contribute to abnormal gene expression, prevent intracellular communication and alter second messenger system functions (Larsson and Cerutti, 1989; Toledano and Leonard, 1991). Furthermore, ROS participate in the progression stage of carcinogenesis by further altering DNA in the initiated cell population (Toyokuni *et al.*, 1995).

Exposure to estrogen or xenoestrogenic substances is a risk factor for development of hormonal carcinogenesis (e.g., breast cancer and endometrial cancer). As is the case in other metabolic activations, estrogen is metabolized to the catechol metabolite 4-hydroxyestrogen, which is further converted to reactive semiquinone or quinone intermediates (Jefcoate *et al.*, 2000; Samuni *et al.*, 2003). Catecholestrogen-quinone intermediates and free radicals produced by redox cycling cause various types of oxidative DNA damage that may subsequently lead to gene mutation and ultimately to tumors from cells that are genetically altered by estrogen-induced genotoxicity. In addition, although tamoxifen has been used as an anticancer agent, tamoxifen is also a carcinogen. Women who take tamoxifen are at significantly increased risk of endometrial cancer. Tamoxifen is also a potent liver carcinogen in male and female rats, and induces endometrial and vaginal tumors when administered to neonatal and adult rats (Carthew *et al.*, 2000; Phillips *et al.*, 2005).

A number of environmental chemicals such as *o,p′*-DDT, some PCB isomers and several polycyclic aromatic hydrocarbons (PAHs) including benzo[a]pyrene induce or promote cancer in animals. Several epidemiologic studies have demonstrated a significant increase in the incidence of prostate, breast, endometrial and testicular cancer in humans during the last 50 years. A large body of evidence demonstrates that human exposure to highly prevalent environmental chemicals with hormonal function may be closely associated with an increase in cancer risk.

TABLE 70.1 Examples of exposures associated with adverse reproductive outcomes

Exposure	Outcomes				
Agents	**Spontaneous abortion**	**Congenital malformation**	**Low birth weight**	**Developmental disabilities**	**Cancer**
Heavy metals	X	X	X	X	X
Organic solvents	X	X	X	X	X
Smoking	X		X	X	X
Alcohol	X	X	X	X	X
Estrogens	X			X	X
Radiation	X	X	X	X	X

X indicates that agent contributes to the specified toxicological outcomes

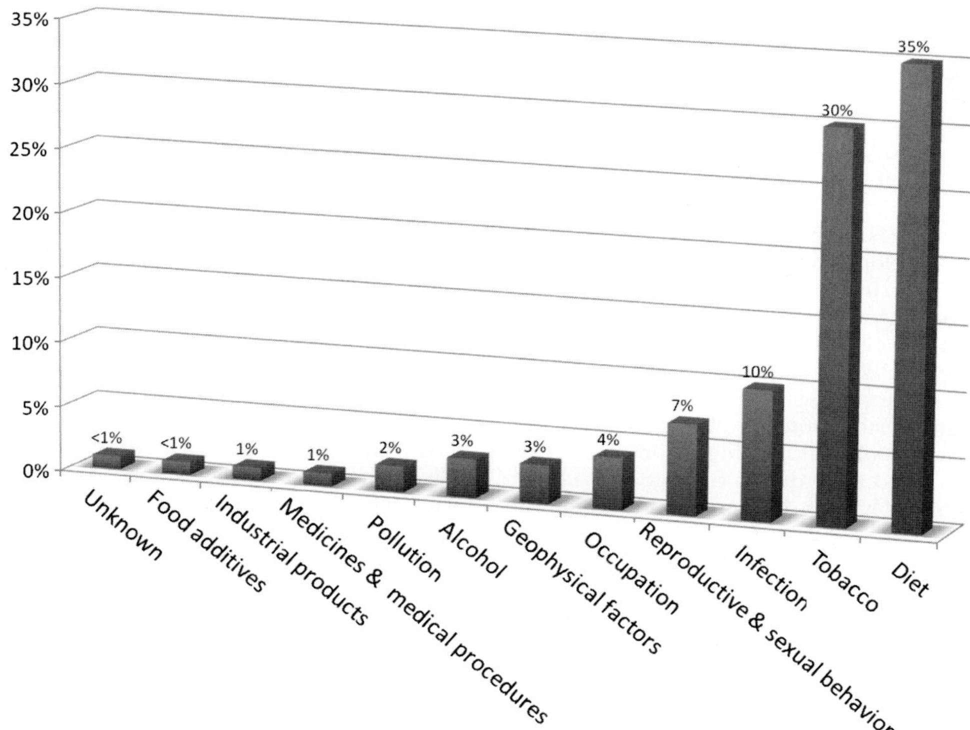

FIGURE 70.2 Best estimate proportions of various risk factors associated with cancer deaths. Sources modified from Doll and Peto (1981) and Lee and Park (2003).

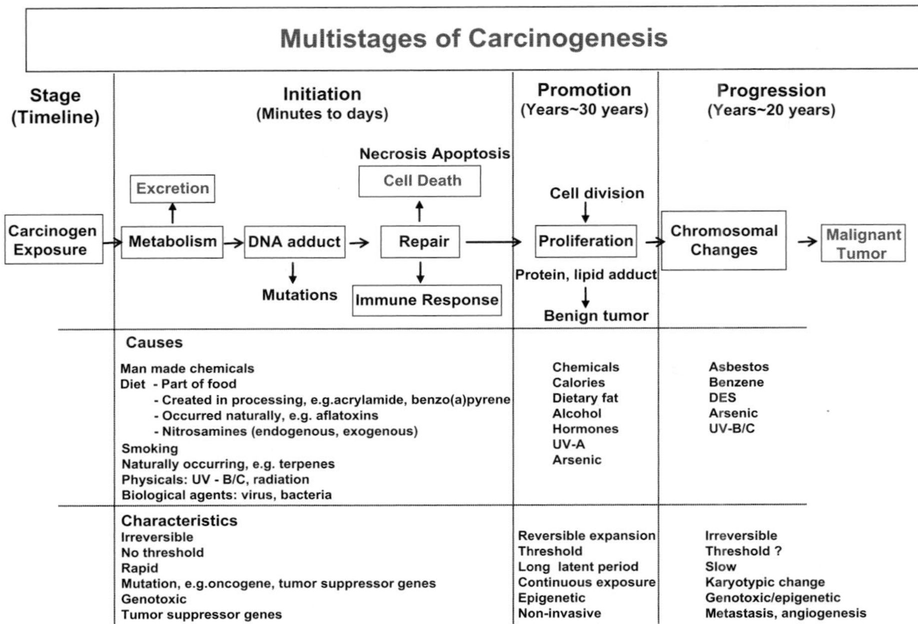

FIGURE 70.3 Multistage chemical carcinogenesis can be conceptually divided into three stages: initiation, promotion and progression. Activation of proto-oncogenes and inactivation of tumor suppressor genes are mutational events that occur as a result of covalent damage to DNA caused by chemical exposures.

Recently, a possible mechanism of cancer development by endocrine disruptors or endocrine disrupting chemicals (EDCs) also has been suggested. EDCs are present in numerous places in our environment such as in food and water (through the use of pesticides) as well as in cosmetics, plastics and other products used daily in the home. Experimental models have been proposed to establish a link between exposure to EDCs and cancer development and to understand other possible mechanisms of EDCs. EDCs disrupt a wide variety of endocrine systems, producing developmental disorders, carcinogenicity and mutagenicity. Moreover, EDCs may adversely impact immunity, fertility and neurobehavior as well as influence susceptibility to cancer.

Ovarian cancer

Ovarian epithelial cancer is the most common cause of death among women who develop gynecologic cancers (Jemal *et al.*, 2007). In particular, ovarian cancer is the second most common gynecologic malignancy, and represents the fifth most common cause of cancer death in women in the USA. Ovarian cancer is rare during childhood and adolescence, accounting for about 1% of cancers in this age group. Of these, 60% are of germ cell origin. Furthermore, the etiology of small cell carcinoma of the ovary is unclear. The high mortality rate of ovarian cancer is believed to be due to the fact that it often goes undetected until it has reached an advanced clinical stage, and the poor prognosis at detection is associated with its metastatic potential (Naora and Montell, 2003). Epithelial ovarian carcinomas are classified into four major categories: serous, mucinous, endometrioid and clear cell. Each subtype of ovarian carcinoma has different clinical characteristics, biological behaviors and responses to chemotherapy.

A possible association between maternal DES exposure and ovarian cancer is speculative. The causative factors of ovarian cancer continue to be elucidated, furthering our understanding of the genesis of ovarian cancer. Genetics, parity, environment, hormonal factors and inflammation all play important and pivotal roles in the development of ovarian cancer. The current understanding of these elements and their respective contribution to the development of this cancer are presented in this chapter.

Although the more established hypotheses that have been proposed to explain increased risk of developing ovarian cancer are related to the number of ovulations or to increased hormone levels, there are additional risk factors that have been identified, including a number of environmental carcinogens. While these factors have been reported to affect the ovarian surface epithelium, they are usually associated with follicular destruction and/or ovotoxicity, so indirect actions due to altered gonadotropin levels cannot be eliminated. Use of perineal talc has been identified as a risk factor, possibly due to its ability to ascend the genital tract and affect the ovarian surface (Hamilton *et al.*, 1984). Indeed, direct exposure of rat ovaries to talc results in focal areas of papillary change in the ovarian surface epithelium, as well as ovarian cysts (Hamilton *et al.*, 1984). Exposure of rhesus and cynomolgus monkeys to the environmental pollutant hexachlorobenzene results in both reproductive failure and notable alterations in the size, shape and degree of stratification of the OSE cell layer (Sims *et al.*, 1991). More recent studies have shown that the insecticide methoxychlor increases both the height of the OSE cell layer and the percentage of atretic follicles in exposed mice (Borgeest *et al.*, 2002). In rodent studies, at least eight chemicals exhibited ovarian carcinogenicity resulting in follicular necrosis, tubular hyperplasia, granulosa cell tumors and benign mixed tumors (Collins *et al.*, 1987; Maronpot *et al.*, 1987). N-ethyl-N-nitrosourea administered to rats intraperitoneally or transplacentally increased the incidence of ovarian tubular adenomas (Stoica *et al.*, 1985). The mechanisms by which these environmental carcinogens enhance the risk of ovarian tumors remain unexplored. The risk factors of ovarian cancer are summarized in Table 70.2.

TABLE 70.2 Summary of ovarian cancer risk factors

Risk factors	Potential adverse outcome	References
Talc (talcum powder)	– Approximately 30% increase in the risk of total epithelial ovarian cancer (EOC) – Glutathione S-transferase M1 (GSTM1) – N-acetyltransferase 2 (NAT2)	Huncharek *et al.* (2003) Cook *et al.* (1997) Gates *et al.* (2008)
Cigarette smoking	– Smoking increased the risk of mucinous tumors	Jordan *et al.* (2006)
Dietary factors	– Red meat increased risk of ovarian cancer – Bread and pasta are associated with an increased risk of breast and ovarian cancer	Bosetti *et al.* (2001)
Alcohol	– Unrelated to ovarian cancer, but positively correlated with breast cancer	Peterson *et al.* (2006)
Overweight	– Associated with an increased risk of ovarian cancer in early adulthood	Olsen *et al.* (2007)

Endometriosis or endometrial cancer

Endometriosis is an estrogen-dependent disease characterized by the presence of endometrial glands and stroma outside the uterine cavity. It is a common gynecological disorder as well as a major cause of infertility (Chedid *et al.*, 1995). There is no single theory to explain all aspects of this multifactored clinical syndrome. While there is a clear association with estrogens, it is accepted that endometriosis is not specifically caused by estrogens but is stimulated by them (Guarnaccia and Olive, 1998). Although epidemiologic data of endometrial cancer induced by EDC exposure are limited, emerging evidence suggests a possible role for ubiquitous environmental contaminants in the pathophysiology of endometriosis. In particular, polyhalogenated aromatic hydrocarbons (PHAH), a class of widespread environmental contaminants including dioxins, have been postulated to be linked to endometriosis (Pauwels *et al.*, 2001; Rier and Foster, 2002). Recently, to evaluate the possible association between PEs and the occurrence of endometriosis, a case–control study was performed (Reddy *et al.*, 2006).

Women with endometriosis had significantly higher concentrations of DBP, BBP, DnOP and DEHP than the control group. Thus, this study suggested that PEs have an etiological association with endometriosis. Additionally, endometriotic women showed significantly higher plasma DEHP concentrations than the control groups, and 92.6% of the detectable DEHP and/or MEHP were in the peritoneal fluid (Luisi *et al.*, 2006). However, no significant differences in either the DEHP/MEHP plasma concentrations or DEHP/MEHP peritoneal fluid concentrations were observed in endometriotic patients as a function of the disease stage at the time of diagnosis. This finding revealed a negative association between DEHP plasma concentrations and endometriosis.

Epidemiologic data on the effects of environmental EDCs on endometrial cancer are limited. Sturgeon *et al.* (1998) found no association between endometrial cancer and 27 PCB congeners, 4 DDT-related compounds and 13 other organochlorine compounds. Several retrospective occupational cohort studies support this (Bertazzi *et al.*, 1987; Brown, 1987). In the Seveso, Italy, industrial accident in 1976, TCDD exposure appeared to reduce the risk of uterine cancer, but the number of cases was too small for a comprehensive evaluation (Bertazzi *et al.*, 1993). It has been implied that higher levels of BPA, which binds estrogen receptor (ER) and plays estrogenic roles, may enhance endometrial hyperplasia. In one study, serum BPA concentrations in healthy subjects with normal endometrium were 2.5 ± 1.5 ng/ml, while BPA levels in patients with simple endometrial hyperplasia of benign nature were 2.9 ± 2.0 ng/ml, which was not significantly different from the controls (Hiroi *et al.*, 2004).

There is some evidence that dietary isoflavones protect women from endometrial proliferation. Specifically, high consumption of soy products and other legumes in US women was associated with a decreased risk of endometrial cancer for the highest quartile of soy intake when compared to the lowest quartile (Goodman *et al.*, 1997; Horn-Ross *et al.*, 2003). Controversially, a recent randomized double-blind, placebo-controlled study on 298 post-menopausal women showed an increased incidence of endometrial hyperplasia following 5 years of treatment with 50 mg of soy isoflavones (Unfer *et al.*, 2004). Thus, phytoestrogenic supplements should be reconsidered, particularly in women at high risk for endometrial cancer.

Vaginal cancer

Vaginal cancer incidence is very low throughout the world. Approximately 6,000 women were diagnosed with vulvar and vaginal cancer and 800 deaths were attributed to each of these cancers in the USA in 2003 (ACS, 2003). Cancer of the vagina is a disease in which malignant cells are found in the tissues of the vagina. According to the American Cancer Society (ACS, 2005), about 2,140 cases of vaginal cancer were diagnosed in the USA in 2005. About 70% of vaginal cancers are squamous cell carcinomas (SCC). These cancers begin in the squamous cells that make up the epithelial lining of the vagina. These cancers are more common in the upper area of the vagina near the cervix. SCC of the vagina often develops slowly. First, some of the normal cells of the vagina develop pre-cancerous changes. Then some of the pre-cancer cells turn into cancer cells.

Risk factors for vaginal cancer include the following: human papilloma virus (HPV) plays a central role in the etiology of a majority of the squamous cell cancers of the vagina. Smoking is another key risk factor for vaginal cancer. A few epidemiological studies on vaginal cancer have been conducted. In the 1950s, the drug DES was given to some pregnant women to prevent miscarriage (premature birth of a fetus that cannot survive), but women who were exposed to DES before birth had an increased risk of developing vaginal cancer. Some of these women developed a rare form of cancer called clear cell adenocarcinoma.

Testicular cancer

Several epidemiological studies indicate that human male reproductive disorders have become more prevalent during the last 50 years (Møller, 2001; McGlynn *et al.*, 2003; Shah *et al.*, 2007). Although testicular cancer is relatively uncommon worldwide, the annual age-adjusted incidence rate of testicular cancer is gradually increasing. The etiology of testicular cancer remains poorly understood, but most of the established risk factors are likely related to disrupting the normal hormonal balance by exposure to endogenous estrogens or environmental xenoestrogens (Bay *et al.*, 2006; Garner *et al.*, 2008).

Scientists have found certain risk factors that make a man more likely to develop testicular cancer. Even if a man has one or more risk factors for this disease, it is impossible to know how much that risk factor contributes to the cancer development. And many men with testicular cancer do not have any of the known risk factors.

Exposure to environmental contaminants has increased over the past century and thus these factors may play an important role in the increasing incidence of testicular cancer. Additionally, epidemiological studies on testicular cancer also indicate that some factors, including exposure to EDCs in postnatal life, are potentially related to testicular cancer (Bay *et al.*, 2006). Furthermore, genetic polymorphisms or aberrations may increase the susceptibility of some individuals to the development of testicular cancer, and this is further compounded by exposure to potential environmental EDCs. There are several male hormonal conditions that are associated with an increased risk of testicular cancer (Swerdlow *et al.*, 1989; Weir *et al.*, 1998; Coupland *et al.*, 2004).

Most testicular cancers occur between the ages of 12 and 50, but this cancer can affect males of any age, including infants and elderly men. About 14% of cases of testicular cancer occur in men with a history of cryptorchidism. In such men, most cancers develop in the testicle that did not descend, but up to 25% of cases occur in the normally descended testicle (ACS, 2003). Based on these observations, some scientists suggest that cryptorchidism may not be the direct cause of testicular cancer, but rather that some other disorder is responsible for increasing the testicular cancer risk and preventing normal positioning of one or both testicles.

A family history of testicular cancer also increases the risk. If a man has the disease, there is an increased risk that one or more of his brothers will also develop it. A recent study found that non-seminoma germ cell tumors occur more frequently among men with certain occupations (e.g., miners, oil and gas workers, leather workers, food and beverage processing workers, janitors and utility workers). Exposure to certain chemicals may contribute to development of the disease, but studies have not clearly identified any specific chemicals as being responsible. No association was found between occupation and risk of seminoma tumors. Only one study found a slightly higher risk of germ cell tumors among men with prolonged occupational exposure to extremely hot or cold temperatures. However, these occupational associations need to be confirmed in other studies before it can be concluded that they represent a significant component of testicular cancer risk.

There is some evidence that men infected with the human immunodeficiency virus (HIV), particularly those with AIDS, are at increased risk. No other infections have been shown to increase testicular cancer risk. Although men whose mothers took the synthetic estrogen diethylstilbestrol (DES) during pregnancy have an increased risk of certain congenital (present at birth) reproductive system malformations, there is no convincing evidence that DES exposure significantly increases a man's risk of developing testicular cancer.

Prostate cancer

Prostate cancer is the most frequently diagnosed cancer and the second leading cause of cancer deaths among males in the USA. It is estimated that over 230,000 men will be newly diagnosed with prostate cancer, and over 30,000 will die of the disease (Hess-Wilson and Knudsen, 2006; Haas *et al.*, 2008). Prostate cancer is dependent on male sex steroid hormone for development, growth and survival. Disruption of the male endocrine system during certain developmental periods may be associated with the development of prostate cancer in animals (Prins *et al.*, 2007). In addition, other hormones, such as insulin-like growth factor and vitamin D, also contribute to the development of prostate cancer. While little is known about the cause of prostate cancer, one possible cause is exposure to EDCs (Ho *et al.*, 2006a,b; Maffini *et al.*, 2006). A recent review addressed the importance of considering the low dose effects of EDCs to clarify their possible role in prostate cancer development (Ho *et al.*, 2006a,b). Developmental exposure to low doses of DES, ethinyl estradiol or BPA has been reported to increase prostate size or weight, suggesting that these agents influence early prostate growth (Prins *et al.*, 2008). These data indicate that the proliferative functions of BPA and DES on the developing prostate can be direct (i.e., do not require androgen stimulation) because a high dose of DES reduced prostate size or weight (Figure 70.4). In conclusion, estrogenic EDCs cause aberrations in the development of the male reproductive tract and could impact prostate cancer initiation.

Although cigarette smoking is a major risk factor of cancer development, most epidemiological studies do not support an association between cigarette smoking and prostate cancer incidence. Smoking is associated with higher plasma testosterone levels in men (Dai *et al.*, 1988; Field *et al.*, 1994), which may enhance tumor progression. Several studies have evaluated the association between alcohol consumption and prostate cancer incidence. Several epidemiologic correlations have also indicated an increased risk of prostate cancer with long-term, high intake of dairy products in male US physicians and males in Sweden. This correlation has been mechanistically associated with high dietary intake of calcium in dairy products. However, the high dietary phosphate in dairy products causes large fluctuations in serum phosphate and is a more likely source of prostate cancer risk from high dietary intake of dairy products.

TRANSGENERATIONAL EFFECTS ON REPRODUCTIVE DISEASES

Environmental toxicants and nutritional status can promote adult-onset diseases (Anway *et al.*, 2005, 2006), ranging from tumors (Yamasaki *et al.*, 1992) to reproductive defects (Ho *et al.*, 2006a,b). Although certain environmental compounds and factors have been shown to influence adult-onset disease, the molecular mechanisms involved are unclear. In particular, exposure to estrogenic chemicals during embryonic or postnatal development may cause transgenerational abnormalities in male reproductive tissues including the testis, seminal vesicles and prostate (Anway and Skinner, 2008a), as well as increased tumor development (Tomatis *et al.*, 1992; Anway *et al.*, 2006; Ho *et al.*, 2006a). The fact that epigenetic mechanisms may play a role in endocrine disruption helps to

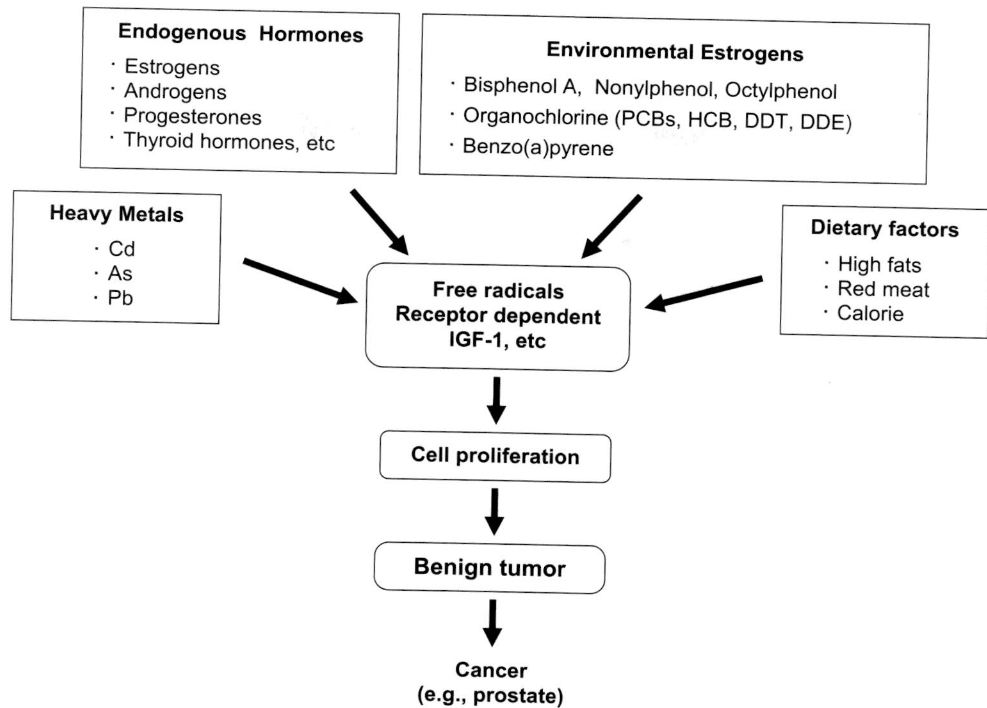

FIGURE 70.4 Illustration of the different sources of environmental chemicals that may affect prostate cancer development and progression. DES, diethylstilbestrol; EE, ethinylestradiol; PCB, polychlorinated bisphenols; HCB, hexachlorobenzene; DDT, dichlorodiphenyltrichloroethane; DDE, dichlorodiphenyltrichloroethylene; IGF, insulin-like growth factor.

explain the transgenerational effects of chemicals. As illustrated, perinatal exposure to carcinogens may contribute to the susceptibility to cancer during adulthood.

Early studies showed that treatment with diethylstilbestrol (DES) during pregnancy resulted in vaginal adenocarcinoma in female offspring in humans (Herbst, 1981) and mice (McLachlan *et al.*, 1977). DES was prescribed to more than 5 million pregnant women from the late 1940s to the early 1970s to prevent abortions and pregnancy complications. After Herbst *et al.* (1972) reported a high incidence of the very rare clear cell adenocarcinoma of the vagina in pubertal girls exposed to DES *in utero*, the use of DES was banned. Structural abnormalities of reproductive organs were also more frequently reported in males exposed to DES than in controls; these abnormalities include hypospadias, epididymal cysts and testicular abnormalities.

These transgenerational phenotypes appear to involve epigenetic reprogramming of male germ-line cells. The altered epigenome provides a potential mechanism for the transgenerational changes in imprinting genes. For example, exposure to the fungicide vinclozolin during embryonic gonadal sex determination alters the epigenetic programming of the male germ line to induce altered DNA methylation in various genes (Birnbaum and Fenton, 2003). Ho *et al.* (2006a,b) demonstrated that exposure to low doses of estradiol or bisphenol A (BPA) during the neonatal developmental period of rats resulted in increased susceptibility to precancerous prostatic lesions in aged animals and sensitized the prostate gland in adult-induced hormonal carcinogenesis. These data thus contribute to the increasing evidence of a correlation between fetal exposure to vinclozoline or benzo(a)pyrene and cancer development (Shibata and Minn, 2000; Birnbaum and Fenton, 2003; Newbold *et al.*, 2006).

The epigenetic mechanism involves the alteration of DNA in the germ line that appears to transmit transgenerational adult-onset disease, including spermatogenic defects, prostate disease, kidney disease and cancer (Anway and Skinner, 2008a,b). These epigenetic changes are brought about by mechanisms such as DNA methylation, histone modifications and non-coding RNAs in the regulation of gene expression patterns. Epigenetic mechanisms are essential to normal development and differentiation, but these can be misdirected, leading to disease, most notably cancer. Indeed, there is now a mounting body of evidence that environmental exposure to EDC, particularly in early development, can induce epigenetic changes that may be transmitted in subsequent generations or serve as the basis of diseases developed later in life. Methylation profiles can be used as molecular markers to distinguish subtypes of cancers and as potential predictors of disease outcome and treatment response. The role of epigenetics in diagnosis and treatment is likely to increase as mechanisms leading to the transcriptional silencing of genes involved in human cancers are revealed (Figure 70.5).

Emerging evidence suggests that epigenetic programming has the potential to affect protein function much later in life and potentially across generations, a factor that adds further complexity to understanding the impact of early life exposure to carcinogens or mutagens on homeostasis across the lifespan and into subsequent generations. The multifactorial nature of chemical-induced carcinogenicity must also be given due consideration in study design and in the selection of appropriate animal models for mechanistic studies.

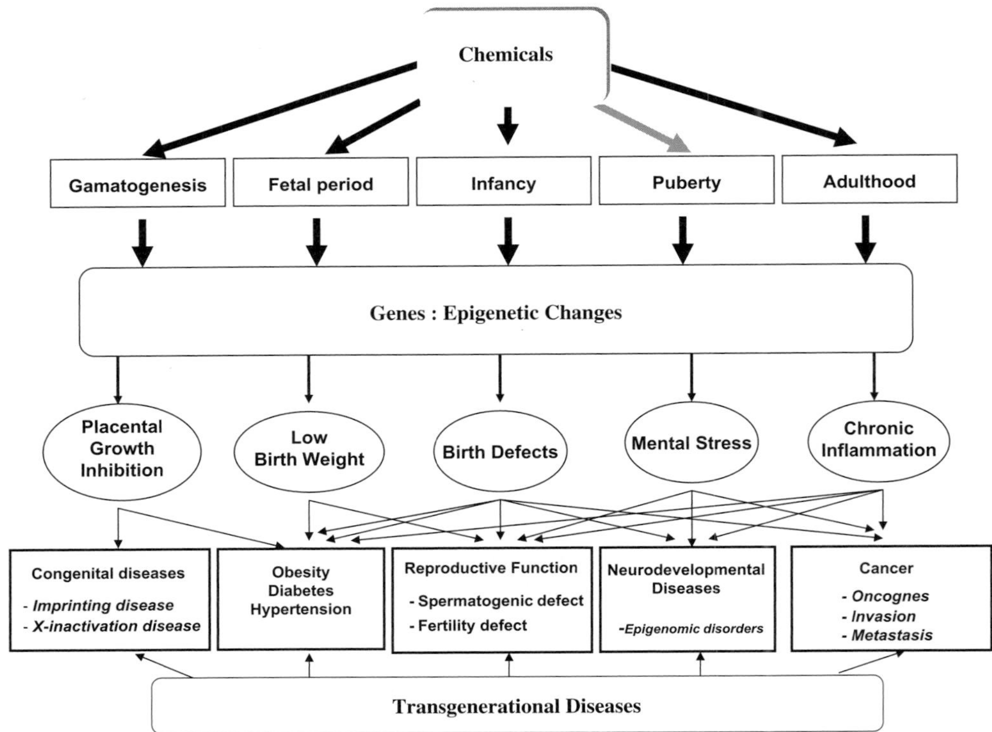

FIGURE 70.5 A model for environmental chemical-induced epigenetic transgenerational diseases. Chemicals reprogrammed the epigenome of developing germ cells during embryonic sex determination, leading to genes and other DNA sequences with altered DNA methylation. These changes are proposed to alter the transcriptomes of the testis and other organs, thereby promoting adult pathologies, some of which are inherited transgenerationally. Epigenetic mechanisms might therefore have a role in the induction of adult-onset disease through environmental exposure early in development.

TABLE 70.3 Multigenerational effects of chemical or physical carcinogens*

Agent	Species (strain)	Treatment schedule	Tumor sites
MCA	Rat (Wistar)	Female F_0 (before and after mating)	Various sites
OATT	Mouse (C3HA)	Pregnant F_0	Liver
DMBA	Mouse (Swiss)	Pregnant F_0	Mammary carcinomas, ovarian tumors, lung adenomas, etc.
DMBA	Mouse (MCA)	Pregnant F_0	Lung adenomas, ovarian tumors, malignant lymphomas, etc.
DES	Mouse (CD-1)	Pregnant F_0	Uterine sarcomas and benign ovarian tumors in F_1 female (treated male F_0 mated with untreated F_0 female)
DES	Mouse (CD-1)	Pregnant F_0	Uterine adenocarcinoma, ovarian tumors
B(a)P	Mouse (A)	Pregnant F_0	Multiple lung adenomas in F_0, F_1, F_2 and F_3
X-ray	Mouse (SHR)	Male F_0 before mating	
			Multiple lung adenomas (urethane treatment in F_1)
			Skin tumor (TPA treatment in F_1)

Abbreviations: MCA, 3-methylcholanthrene; OAAT, o-aminoazotoluene; DMBA, 7,12-dimethylbenz[a]anthracene; DES, diethylstilbestrol; B(a)P, benzo(a)pyrene; TPA, 12-O-tetradecanoylphorbol 13-acetate

*Modified from Yamasaki *et al.* (1992) and Tomatis (1989)

CONCLUDING REMARKS AND FUTURE DIRECTIONS

Many chemicals, including endocrine disruptors, are known to produce various toxicities such as developmental or reproductive toxicity, carcinogenicity, mutagenicity, immunotoxicity and neurotoxicity (Choi *et al.*, 2004). Mechanisms of carcinogenesis due to exposure to endocrine disruptors may be associated with free radical generation and biomolecule (e.g., DNA, protein, lipid) damage after the dysregulation of hormones such as estrogen, testosterone, thyroid and insulin. The hormonal effect on carcinogenesis is receptor dependent or receptor independent, and there is often cross-talk between hormones, and complex signaling cascades may also be involved. During multistage carcinogenesis (i.e., initiation, promotion (stage I (reversible), stage II (irreversible)), progression), genotoxic and epigenetic events are critically associated, which may lead to mutation and cancer. Although genotoxic events are fundamentally the limiting step in carcinogenesis and reproductive disorders, the transgenerational epigenetic role of carcinogens could also be important. Given the unavoidability of human exposure to endocrine disruptors or carcinogens, the application of a chemopreventive strategy that either blocks or retards the process of carcinogenesis might be helpful for public health.

REFERENCES

ACS (American Cancer Society) (2003) Cancer Facts and Figures 2001. Atlanta, Ga: American Cancer Society, 2001.

ACS (American Cancer Society) (2005) Cancer Facts and Figures 2005. American Cancer Society, Inc. Atlanta, GA.

Anway MD, Cupp AS, Uzumcu M, Skinner MK (2005) Epigenetic transgenerational actions of endocrine disruptors and male fertility. *Science* **308:** 1466–9.

Anway MD, Leathers C, Skinner MK (2006) Endocrine disruptor vinclozolin induced epigenetic transgenerational adult-onset disease. *Endocrinology* **147:** 5515–23.

Anway MD, Skinner MK (2008a) Epigenetic programming of the germ line: effects of endocrine disruptors on the development of transgenerational disease. *Reprod Biomed* **16:** 23–5.

Anway MD, Skinner MK (2008b) Transgenerational effects of the endocrine disruptor vinclozolin on the prostate transcriptome and adult onset disease. *Prostate* **68:** 517–29.

Bay K, Asklund C, Skakkebaek NE, Andersson AM (2006) Testicular dysgenesis syndrome: possible role of endocrine disrupters. *Best Pract Res Clin Endocrinol Metab* **20:** 77–90.

Bertazzi PA, Pestori AC, Consonni D (1993) Cancer incidence in a population accidentally exposed to 2,3,7,8-tetrachlorodibenzo-para-dioxin. *Epidemiology* **4:** 398–406.

Bertazzi PA, Riboldi L, Pesatori A, Radice L, Zocchetti C (1987) Cancer mortality of capacitor manufacturing workers. *Am J Ind Med* **11:** 165–76.

Birnbaum LS, Fenton SE (2003) Cancer and developmental exposure to endocrine disruptors. *Environ Health Perspect* **111:** 389–94.

Borgeest C, Symonds D, Mayer LP, Hoyer PB, Flaws JA (2002) Methoxychlor may cause ovarian follicular atresia and proliferation of the ovarian epithelium in the mouse. *Toxicol Sci* **68:** 473–8.

Bosetti C, Negri E, Franceschi S, Pelucchi C, Talamini R, Montella M, Conti E, La Vecchia C (2001) Diet and ovarian cancer risk: a case–control study in Italy. *Int J Cancer* **93:** 911–15.

Breimer DD, Schellens JH (1990) A "cocktail" strategy to assess in vivo oxidative drug metabolism in humans. *Trends Pharmacol Sci* **11:** 223–5.

Brown DP (1987) Mortality of workers exposed to polychlorinated biphenyls – an update. *Arch Environ Health* **42:** 333–9.

Carthew P, Edwards RE, Nolan BM, Martin EA, Heydon RT, White INH, Tucker MJ (2000) Tamoxifen induces endometrial and vaginal cancer in rats in the absence of endometrial hyperplasia. *Carcinogenesis* **21:** 793–7.

Chedid S, Camus M, Smitz J, Van Steirteghem AC, Devroey P (1995) Comparison among different ovarian stimulation regimens for assisted procreation procedures in patients with endometriosis. *Hum Reprod* **10:** 2406–11.

Choi SM, Yoo SD, Lee BM (2004) Toxicological characteristics of endocrine-disrupting chemicals: developmental toxicity, carcinogenicity, and mutagenicity. *J Toxicol Environ Health B* **7(1):** 1–32.

Coelho C, Júlio C, Silva G, Neves A (2009) Tobacco and male infertility: a retrospective study in infertile couples. *Acta Med Port* **22:** 753–8.

Collins JJ, Montali RJ, Manus AG (1987) Toxicological evaluation of 4-vinylcyclohexene. II. Induction of ovarian tumors in female B6C3F1 mice by chronic oral administration of 4-vinylcyclohexene. *J Toxicol Environ Health* **21:** 507–24.

Cook LS, Kamb ML, Weiss NS (1997) Perineal powder exposure and the risk of ovarian cancer. *Am J Epidemiol* **145:** 459–65.

Coupland CA, Forman D, Chilvers CE, Davey G, Pike MC, Oliver RT (2004) Maternal risk factors for testicular cancer: a population-based case–control study (UK). *Cancer Causes Control* **15:** 277–83.

Dai WS, Gutai JP, Kuller LH, Cauley JA (1988) Cigarette smoking and serum sex hormones in men. *Am J Epidemiol* **128:** 796–805.

DeBaun JR, Miller EC, Miller JA (1970) N-hydroxy-2-acetylaminofluorene sulfotransferase: its probable role in carcinogenesis and in protein-(methion-S-yl) binding in rat liver. *Cancer Res* **30:** 577–95.

Doll R, Peto R (1981) The causes of cancer: quantitative estimates of avoidable risks of cancer in the United States today. *J Natl Cancer Inst* **66:** 1193–308.

Dreher D, Junod AF (1996) Role of oxygen free radicals in cancer development. *Eur J Cancer* **32A:** 30–8.

Field AE, Colditz GA, Willett WC, Longcope C, McKinlay JB (1994) The relation of smoking, age, relative weight, and dietary intake to serum adrenal steroids, sex hormones, and sex hormone-binding globulin in middle-aged men. *J Clin Endocrinol Metab* **79:** 1310–16.

Garner M, Turner MC, Ghadirian P, Krewski D, Wade M (2008). Testicular cancer and hormonally active agents. *J Toxicol Environ Health Part B* **11:** 260–75.

Gates MA, Tworoger SS, Terry KL, Titus-Ernstoff L, Rosner B, De Vivo I, Cramer DW, Hankinson SE (2008) Talc use, variants of the GSTM1, GSTT1, and NAT2 genes, and risk of epithelial ovarian cancer. *Cancer Epidemiol Biomarkers Prev* **17:** 2436–44.

Gold EB, Sever LE (1994) Childhood cancers associated with parental occupational exposures. *Occup Med* **9:** 495–539.

Goodman MT, Wilkens LR, Hankin JH, Lyu LC, Wu AH, Kolonel LN (1997) Association of soy and fiber consumption with the risk of endometrial cancer. *Am J Epidemiol* **146:** 294–306.

Guarnaccia MM, Olive DL (1998) Diagnosis and management of endometriosis. In *Textbook of Reproductive Medicine* (Carr BR, Blackwell RE, eds.). Stamford, CT, Appleton & Lange, pp. 112–31.

Haas GP, Delongchamps N, Brawley OW, Wang CY, de la Roza G (2008) The worldwide epidemiology of prostate cancer: perspectives from autopsy studies. *Can J Urol* **15:** 3866–71.

Hamilton TC, Fox H, Buckley CH, Henderson WJ, Griffiths K (1984) Effects of talc on the rat ovary. *Br J Exp Pathol* **65:** 101–6.

Herbst AL (1981) The current status of the DES-exposed population. *Obstet Gynecol Annu* **10:** 267–78.

Herbst AL, Bern H (eds.) (1981) *Developmental Effects of Diethylstilbestrol (DES) in Pregnancy*. New York, Thieme-Stratton.

Herbst AL, Kurman RJ, Scully RE, Poskanzer DC (1972) Clear-cell adenocarcinoma of the genital tract in young females: registry report. N Engl J Med 287: 1259–64.

Hess-Wilson JK, Knudsen KE (2006) Endocrine disrupting compounds and prostate cancer. *Cancer Lett* **241:** 1–12.

Hiroi H, Tsutsumi O, Takeuchi T, Momoeda M, Ikezuki Y, Okamura A, Yokota H, Taketani Y (2004) Differences in serum bisphenol A concentrations in premenopausal normal women and women with endometrial hyperplasia. *Endocrine J* **51:** 595–600.

Ho SM, Leung YK, Chung I (2006a) Estrogens and antiestrogens as etiological factors and therapeutics for prostate cancer. *Ann New York Acad Sci* **1089:** 177–93.

Ho SM, Tang WY, Belmonte de Frausto J, Prins GS (2006b) Developmental exposure to estradiol and bisphenol A increases susceptibility to prostate carcinogenesis and epigenetically regulates phosphodiesterase type 4 variant 4. *Cancer Res* **66:** 5624–32.

Horn-Ross PL, John EM, Canchola AJ, Stewart SL, Lee MM (2003) Phytoestrogen intake and endometrial cancer risk. *J Natl Cancer Inst* **95:** 1158–64.

Huncharek M, Geschwind JF, Kupelnick B (2003) Perineal application of cosmetic talc and risk of invasive epithelial ovarian cancer: a meta-analysis of 11,933 subjects from sixteen observational studies. *Anticancer Res* **23:**1955–60.

Jefcoate CR, Liehr JG, Santen RJ, Sutter TR, Yager JD. Yue W, Santner SJ, Tekmal R, Demers L, Pauley R, Naftolin F, Mor G, Berstein L (2000) Tissue-specific synthesis and oxidative metabolism of estrogens. *J Natl Cancer Inst* **27:** 95–112.

Jemal A, Siegel R, Ward E, Murray T, Xu J, Thun MJ (2007) Cancer Statistics, 2007. *CA Cancer J Clin* **57:** 43–66.

Jordan SJ, Whiteman DC, Purdie DM, Green AC, Webb PM (2006) Does smoking increase risk of ovarian cancer? A systematic review. *Gynecol Oncol* **103:** 1122–9.

Kim HS, Kwack SJ, Lee BM (2000) Lipid peroxidation, antioxidant enzymes, and benzo(a)pyrene quinones in the blood of rats treated with benzo(a) pyrene. *Chem Biol Interact* **127:** 139–50.

Klaunig JE, Xu Y, Isenberg JS, Bachowski S, Kolaja KL, Jiang J, Stevenson DE, Walborg EF Jr (1998) The role of oxidative stress in chemical carcinogenesis. *Environ Health Perspect* **106 (Suppl. 1):** 289–95.

Kwack SJ, Lee BM (2000) Correlation between DNA or protein adducts and benzo[a]pyrene diol epoxide I-triglyceride adduct detected in vitro and in vivo. *Carcinogenesis* **21:** 629–32.

Larsson R, Cerutti P (1989) Translocation and enhancement of phosphotransferase activity of protein kinase C following exposure in mouse epidermal cells to oxidants. *Cancer Res* **49:** 5627–32.

Lee BM, Lee SK, Kim HS (1998) Inhibition of oxidative DNA damage, 8-OHdG, and carbonyl contents in smokers treated with antioxidants (vitamin E, vitamin C, β-carotene and red ginseng). *Cancer Lett* **132:** 219–27.

Lee BM, Park KK (2003) Beneficial and adverse effects of chemopreventive agents. *Mutat Res* **523–524:** 265–78.

Lee BM, Santella RM (1988) Quantitation of protein adducts as a marker of genotoxic exposure: immunologic detection of benzo(a)pyrene-globin adducts in mice. *Carcinogenesis* **9:** 1773–7.

Luisi S, Latini G, de Felice C, Sanseverino F, di Pasquale D, *et al.* (2006) Low serum concentrations of di-(2-ethylhexyl)phthalate in women with uterine fibromatosis. *Gynecol Endocrinol* **22:** 92–5.

Maffini MV, Rubin BS, Sonnenschein C, Soto AM (2006) Endocrine disruptors and reproductive health: the case of bisphenol-A. *Mol Cell Endocrinol* **25:** 254–5.

Maronpot RR (1987) Ovarian toxicity and carcinogenicity in eight recent National Toxicology Program studies. *Environ Health Perspect* **73:** 125–30.

McBride ML (1998) Childhood cancer and environmental contaminants. *Can J Public Health* **89 (Suppl. 1):** S53–S62, S58–S68.

McGlynn KA, Devesa SS, Sigurdson AJ, Brown LM, Tsao L, Tarone RE (2003) Trends in the incidence of testicular germ cell tumors in the United States. *Cancer* **97:** 63–70.

McLachlan JA (1977) Prenatal exposure to diethylstilbestrol in mice: toxicological studies. *J Toxicol Environ Health* **2:** 527–37.

Møller H (2001) Trends in incidence of testicular cancer and prostate cancer in Denmark. *Human Reprod* **16:** 1007–11.

Naora H, Montell DJ (2005) Ovarian cancer metastasis: integrating insights from disparate model organisms. *Nature Rev Cancer* **5:** 355–66.

Newbold RR, Padilla-Banks E, Jefferson WN (2006) Adverse effects of the model environmental estrogen diethylstilbestrol are transmitted to subsequent generations. *Endocrinology* **147:** S11–S17.

Northrop-Clewes CA, Thurnham DI (2007) Monitoring micronutrients in cigarette smokers. *Clin Chim Acta* **377:** 14–38.

Olsen CM, Green AC, Whiteman DC, Sadeghi S, Kolahdooz F, Webb PM (2007) Obesity and the risk of epithelial ovarian cancer: a systematic review and meta-analysis. *Eur J Cancer* **43:** 690–709.

Pauwels A, Schepens PJ, D'Hooghe T, Delbeke L, Dhont M, Brouwer A, Weyler J (2001) The risk of endometriosis and exposure to dioxins and polychlorinated biphenyls: a case–control study of infertile women. *Human Reprod* **16:** 2050–5.

Peterson NB, Trentham-Dietz A, Newcomb PA, Chen Z, Hampton JM, Willett WC, Egan KM (2006) Alcohol consumption and ovarian cancer risk in a population-based case–control study. *Int J Cancer* **119:** 2423–7.

Phillips DH, Hewer A, Osborne MR, Cole KJ, Churchill C, Arlt VM (2005) Organ specificity of DNA adduct formation by tamoxifen and α-hydroxytamoxifen in the rat: implications for understanding the mechanism(s) of tamoxifen carcinogenicity and for human risk assessment. *Mutagenesis* **20:** 297–303.

Pleasance ED, *et al.* (2010) A comprehensive catalogue of somatic mutations from a human cancer genome. *Nature* **463:** 191–6.

Potts RJ, Newbury CJ, Smith G, Notarianni LJ, Jefferies TM (1999) Sperm chromatin damage associated with male smoking. *Mutat Res* **423:** 103–11.

Prins GS, Birch L, Tang WY, Ho SM (2007) Developmental estrogen exposures predispose to prostate carcinogenesis with aging. *Reprod Toxicol* **23:** 374–82.

Prins GS, Tang WY, Belmonte J, Ho SM (2008) Perinatal exposure to oestradiol and bisphenol A alters the prostate epigenome and increases susceptibility to carcinogenesis. *Basic Clin Pharmacol Toxicol* **102:** 134–8.

Ragheb AM, Sabanegh ES Jr (2009) Smoking and male fertility: a contemporary review. *Arch Med Sci* **1A:** S13–S19.

Reddy BS, Rozati R, Reddy S, Kodampur S, Reddy P, Reddy R (2006) High plasma concentrations of polychlorinated biphenyls and phthalate esters in women with endometriosis: a prospective case control study. *Fertil Steril* **85:** 775–9.

Rier S, Foster WG (2002) Environmental dioxins and endometriosis. *Toxicol Sci* **70:** 161–70.

Samuni AM, Chuang EY, Krishna MC, Stein W, DeGraff W, Russo A, Mitchell JB (2003) Semiquinone radical intermediate in catecholic estrogen-mediated cytotoxicity and mutagenesis: chemoprevention strategies with antioxidants. *Proc Natl Acad Sci USA* **100:** 5390–5.

Shah MN, Devesa SS, Zhu K, McGlynn KA (2007) Trends in testicular germ cell tumours by ethnic group in the United States. *Int J Androl* **30:** 206–13.

Shi X, Castranova V, Halliwell B, Vallyathan V (1998) Reactive oxygen species and silica-induced carcinogenesis. *J Toxicol Environ Health B Crit Rev* **1:** 181–97.

Shibata A, Minn AY (2000) Perinatal sex hormones and risk of breast and prostate cancers in adulthood. *Epidemiol Rev* **22:** 239–48.

Sims DE, Singh A, Donald A, Jarrell J, Villeneuve DC (1991) Alteration of primate ovary surface epithelium by exposure to hexachlorobenzene: a quantitative study. *Histol Histopathol* **6:** 525–9.

Skakkebaek NE, Rajpert-DeMeyts E, Main KM (2001) Testicular dysgenesis syndrome: an increasingly common developmental disorder with environmental aspects. *Human Reprod* **16:** 972–8.

Stoica G, Koestner A, Capen CC (1985) Testicular (Sertoli's cell)-like tumors of the ovary induced by N-ethyl-N-nitrosourea (ENU) in rats. *Vet Pathol* **22:** 483–91.

Stratton MR, Campbell PJ, Futreal PA (2009) The cancer genome. *Nature* **458:** 719–24.

Strohsnitter WC, Noller KL, Hoover RN, Robboy SJ, Palmer JR, Titus-Ernstoff L, Anderson D, Hoover RN, Noller KL (2001) Cancer risk in men exposed *in utero* to diethylstilbestrol. *J Natl Cancer Inst* **93:** 545–51.

Sturgeon SR, Sonnenschein C, Chung KL, Fernandez MF, Olea N, Serrano FO (1998) Serum concentrations of organochlorine compounds and endometrial cancer risk (United States). *Cancer Causes Control* **9:** 417–24.

Swerdlow AJ, Huttly SR, Smith PG (1989) Testis cancer: post-natal hormonal factors, sexual behaviour and fertility. *Int J Cancer* **43:** 549–53.

Toledano MB, Leonard WJ (1991) Modulation of transcription factor NF-kappa B binding activity by oxidation-reduction in vitro. *Proc Natl Acad Sci USA* **88:** 4328–32.

Tomatis L (1989) Overview of perinatal and multigeneration carcinogenesis. *IARC Sci Publ* **96:** 1–15.

Tomatis L, Narod S, Yamasaki H (1992) Transgeneration transmission of carcinogenic risk. *Carcinogenesis* **13:** 145–451.

Toyokuni S, Okamoto K, Yodoi J, Hiai H (1995) Persistent oxidative stress in cancer. *FEBS Lett* **358:** 1–3.

Unfer V, Casini ML, Costabile L, Mignosa M, Gerli S, Di Renzo GC (2004) Endometrial effects of long-term treatment with phytoestrogens: a randomized, double-blind, placebo-controlled study. *Fertil Steril* **82:** 145–8.

Weinstein IB, Jeffrey AM, Jennette KW, Blobstein SH, Harvey RG, Harris C, Autrup H, Kasai H, Nakanishi K (1976) Benzo(a)pyrene diol epoxides as intermediates in nucleic acid binding in vitro and in vivo. *Science* **193:** 592–5.

Weir HK, Kreiger N, Marrett LD (1998) Age at puberty and risk of testicular germ cell cancer (Ontario, Canada). *Cancer Causes Control* **9:** 253–8.

Weiss HA, Potischman NA, Brinton LA, Brogn D, Coates RJ, Gammon MD, Malone KE, Schoenberg JB (1997) Prenatal and perinatal risk factors for breast cancer in young women. *Epidemiology* **8:** 181–7.

Wigle DT, Turner MC, Krewski D (2009) A systematic review and meta-analysis of childhood leukemia and parental occupational pesticide exposure. *Environ Health Perspect* **117:** 1505–13.

Yamasaki H, Loktionov A, Tomatis L (1992) Perinatal and multigenerational effect of carcinogens: possible contribution to determination of cancer susceptibility. *Environ Health Perspect* **98:** 39–43.

CHAPTER

71

Genotoxicities and infertility

Tirupapuliyur V. Damodaran

INTRODUCTION

Infertility in humans and animal species has been considered to be an impending health issue of social and economic aspects. The term "infertility" implies that the capacity for producing offspring is diminished or completely lost from a biological point of view and this term includes both subfertility and total sterility. As per the definition of INCIID (International Council on Infertility Information Dissemination), a couple is considered to be infertile if they have not conceived after a year of unprotected intercourse. In a recent estimate, infertility has been found in about 13–18% of couples and growing evidence from clinical and epidemiological studies suggests an increasing incidence of male reproductive problems (Nayernia *et al.*, 2004). According to the American Society for Reproductive Medicine, infertility affects about 6.1 million people in the USA. Female infertility accounts for one-third of infertility cases, male infertility for another third, combined male and female infertility for another 15%, and the remainder of cases is "unexplained".

As a whole, infertility is a very complex problem, which may be the result of malfunctioning of any one or many factors, such as anatomical, physiological, hormonal, psychological, immunological, environmental and genetical factors as well as unknown levels of combinatorial effects of all of these factors.

There have been a number of reports during the last decade emphasizing the need for determining the baseline values for semen parameters, for both fertile and infertile men. The need for demarcating between the baseline values of normal semen parameters, from that of the mild oligozoospermia, can be very well understood because semen parameters, which were concluded as incompatible with the possibility of pregnancy in one geographical region, proved to be good enough, resulting in pregnancy in the other parts of the world (Lewis, 2007). Furthermore, Osser *et al.* (1984) stressed the role of environmental factors in their study on baseline semen data, which showed more severely defective semen parameters in urban areas than in rural areas. These data point to the fact that regional differences in fertility rate could be due to environmental factors, rather than any other differences. Epidemiological factors involved in male infertility may vary from one area to another due to sociomedical and environmental conditions (Osagie *et al.*, 1984).

Recent reports indicate that there has been a steady decline in human male fertility within the past few decades (Carlsen *et al.*, 1992; Parazzini *et al.*, 1998). Even though the direct causes of this remain controversial, the fact that the concurrent increase in the incidence of testicular cancer and cryptorchidism suggests the possibility of environmental factors playing a significant role in complex multifactorial scenarios altering several processes of reproductive fitness in human males (Skakkebaek *et al.*, 1998).

The value of genetic screening in infertile patients with possible genetic factors (both at gene and chromosomal level) has been recognized very well by numerous studies (Matzuk and Lamb, 2008). Research studies about the contribution of environmental factors in several developmental anomalies and/or congenital anomalies affecting reproductive structures of males such as varicocele, undescended testes, Sertoli-only syndrome, hypospadias, testicular dysgenesis and several other syndromes that affect both male and female fertility has been an area of active investigation for several years. Recent advancements in molecular and genetic technology have resulted in identification of several genes that were shown to be involved (when mutated) in the causation of defects in primary and secondary sexual characteristics as well as defective oogenesis and spermatogenesis (Matzuk and Lamb, 2008). Some of these genes were shown to be involved in reproductive toxicologic pathological mechanisms, at least in animal models (Howdeshell *et al.*, 2008; Zhu *et al.*, 2009). Thus, based on these compelling evidences, it may be possible to postulate that parental exposures may result in birth defects (as a worst case scenario) or early onset of adulthood disease (affecting various organ systems including reproductive) as a milder and subtle, yet casting a devastating effect at personal level (such as infertility and impotency) in their children. There were a significant percentage of individuals classified as "unexplained or idiopathic form of infertility" in many epidemiological studies on human infertility. Simple logic can point towards the possibility of unknown genetic mechanisms that may be the result of gene–environment interaction.

Hence, further studies in investigating the role of these newly identified genes are very important not only from

Reproductive and Developmental Toxicology, Edited by Ramesh C. Gupta
ISBN: 978-0-12-382032-7

reproductive fitness point of view, but also from a larger perspective of learning more about birth defects and adult-onset multi-system diseases that cause significant levels of morbidity, mortality and financial burden in families with such individuals. Thus, the genetic basis of infertility and reproductive toxicology becomes an important aspect for clinical assessment and treatment in infertile couples.

A large body of literature, pertaining to the effects of various mutagens on the gametogenic tissues of various species, is available. But the extrapolation to humans from primates (Jagiello and Lin, 1974) and mammals (Anderson, 2001) is not easy. For example, in a recent study, an increase in spermatid micronuclei in mice by treatment with butadiene (BD) and only by its metabolites in rats was noted (Pacchierotti *et al.*, 1998). The cytotoxic response of germ cells in mice was greater than in rats. Dominant lethal mutations have been induced by BD and diepoxybutane, but not by epoxybutene. There was some evidence of congenital malformations in mice after BD exposure and there was a linear concentration-related induction of heritable translocations in mice. There was no induction of dominant lethal mutations or congenital malformations in rats. Using the heritable translocation data in mice, it has been determined that if a worker is continually exposed over 5 or 6 weeks to 20–25 ppm of BD, the risk of producing a child with a balanced reciprocal translocation is twice as high as the background risk. Since genetic damage cannot be measured directly in human germ cells, risk to such cells can also be estimated from germ and somatic cells of the mouse and human somatic cells using the parallelogram approach. In spite of the complexities involved in extrapolating the research data from animal models, the following key conclusions can be made by carefully analyzing the data in the above-mentioned scenario: (1) BD and metabolites are capable of causing mutagenic events (at gene level) as well as clastogenic events (gross chromosomal breakage) and other anomalous events (heritable translocation) in mice. Rats require activation through metabolism to cause clastogenic events leading to aneuploidy. Similarly, humans may have an increased susceptibility for similar genetic damage that may lead to birth defects and other clinical conditions affecting fertility. (2) The existence of other unknown mechanisms such as epigenetic factors that may change the way various organisms respond to toxic stimuli, besides the known physiological differences between species as a function of their proteomic profiles, can be understood. Thus, molecular reproductive toxicology in humans and other important livestocks may very well depend on their inherited normal or abnormal genome (total genetic components) and epigenome (sum of genome-wide epigenetic pattern).

Rapid progress in modern technologies such as toxicogenomics and proteomics has made it possible to study many genes and proteins respectively at global level (Damodaran *et al.*, 2006a,b). This has led to the identification of several biomarkers for a number of toxic chemicals. Besides, candidate gene analysis can be done after careful selection of genes based on their role in the basic structure and function of the cell/tissue/organ/life form under study (Damodaran *et al.*, 2003). Gene expression and regulation as defined by the types and quantities of both mRNAs (transcriptomics) and proteins (proteomics) are regulated at multiple levels. All of these molecular data represent only the response of the static aspect of the genome that follows the central dogma of most of the known life forms, i.e. DNA to RNA to protein. Recent findings clearly establish the fact that there are several other unknown, unexplored and yet to be appreciated mechanisms of gene regulation that constantly monitor and respond appropriately to extrinsic and intrinsic stimuli and record the memories of these responses so that they can be passed on to several generations of cell cycles, life cycles and reproductive cycles in that order.

There are ways, collectively called epigenetic mechanisms, in which life forms (including humans and mammals) regulate their gene expression in response to ever-changing environmental conditions. The epigenetic mechanism encompasses changes (due to environmental exposures including nutritional and dietary products) to mark the genomes that are copied from one cell generation to the next, which may alter gene expression but which do not involve changes in the primary DNA sequence. These marks include DNA methylation (methylation of cytosines within CpG dinucleotides) and post-translational modifications (acetylation, methylation, phosphorylation and ubiquitination) of the histone tails protruding from nucleosome cores. Some of these epigenetic marks are remembered through multiple cell generations and their effects may be revealed in altered gene expression and cell function (Mathers, 2008). Despite their identical genotypes, monozygotic twins show increasing epigenetic diversity with age and with divergent lifestyles. Differences in epigenetic markings may explain some inter-individual variation in disease risk and in response to nutritional and other types of interventions (including antidote therapy to toxicant exposure) (Mathers, 2008).

There are many new opportunities to assess the heritable genetic damaging effects of environmental mutagens on human genomes, especially the sperm genome. The following three are important for immediate use: (1) integration of knowledge on the molecular nature of genetic disorders and the molecular effects of mutagens; (2) the development of more practical assays for germ-line mutagenesis; and (3) the likely use of population-based genetic screening in personalized medicine (Elespura and Sankaranarayanan, 2007).

In this chapter, some of the latest ideas and technology emerging in reproductive toxicology with special reference to infertility are presented. The role of genotoxicity that involves changes in DNA sequence structure as well as the epigenetic changes described above, in affecting all stages of development and function of male and female reproductive system, are discussed.

LATEST METHODOLOGIES APPLIED IN CLINICAL AND MOLECULAR REPRODUCTIVE TOXICOLOGY

Accurate clinical diagnosis can facilitate the process of efficient treatment of the patients with clinical disorders of reproductive failure. Most prominent factors that are routinely seen in an infertility clinic are presented below.

Female infertility: clinical classification

The following are the factors related to female infertility: (1) general factors (diabetes mellitus, thyroid disorders, adrenal disease, significant liver, kidney disease and psychological factors); (2) hypothalamic–pituitary factors (hypothalamic dysfunction, hyperprolactinemia and hypopituitarism); (3) ovarian factors (polycystic ovary syndrome, anovulation, diminished ovarian reserve, luteal dysfunction, premature menopause, gonadal dysgenesis, Turner syndrome, and ovarian tumor); (4) tubal/peritoneal factors (endometriosis, pelvic adhesions, pelvic inflammatory disease (PID, usually due to chlamydia), tubal occlusion; uterine factors (uterine malformations, uterine fibroids (leiomyoma), and Asherman's syndrome); (5) cervical factors (cervical stenosis, antisperm antibodies, and vaginal factors); (6) vaginismus and vaginal obstruction. Both genetic and environmental factors were recorded as etiological factors for the above-mentioned types.

Male infertility: clinical classification

The following are the factors related to male infertility: (1) pretesticular causes including (a) endocrine problems (i.e., diabetes mellitus, thyroid disorders), (b) hypothalamic disorders (i.e., Kallmann syndrome), (c) hyperprolactinemia, (d) hypopituitarism, (e) hypogonadism due to various causes, (f) psychological factors, and (g) drugs, alcohol; (2) testicular factors including (a) genetic causes (e.g., Klinefelter syndrome), (b) neoplasm (e.g., seminoma), (c) idiopathic failure, (d) varicocele, (e) trauma, (f) hydrocele, and (g) mumps; (3) post-testicular causes including (a) vas deferens obstruction, (b) infection, e.g. prostatitis, (c) retrograde ejaculation, (d) hypospadias, and (e) impotence. Both genetic and environmental factors were recorded as etiological factors for the above-mentioned male clinical phenotypes.

Semen evaluation techniques, parameters and definitions

Some causes of male infertility can be determined by analysis of the ejaculate, which contains the sperm. Semen analysis is a good non-invasive technique from which information about the status of the testis, knowledge about accessory reproductive organs such as seminal vesicles, epididymis, sperm chromosome complements, and epigenomic status of the sperms, existing or previous episodes of infection and other pathology can be obtained (Tables 71.1 and 71.2).

TABLE 71.1 Standard parameters of normal semen composition as per WHO (1992) guidelines

Volume (ml)	≥2
pH	7.2–8.0
Sperm concentration (M/ml)	≥20
Total sperm count (M/ejaculate)	≥40
Morphology (% normal)	≥30
Vitality (% live)	≥75
WBC (M/ml)	<1.0
Immunobead test (% sperm with beads)	<20
MAR test (% sperm with RBCs)	<10
Motility within 1 h of ejaculation	
Class a (%)	≥25
Classes a and b (%)	≥50
Neutral alpha-glucosidase (mU/ejaculate)	≥20
Total zinc (μmol/ejaculate)	≥2.4
Total citric acid (μmol/ejaculate)	≥52
Total acid phosphatase (U/ejaculate)	≥200
Total fructose (μmol/ejaculate)	≥13

TABLE 71.2 Nomenclature for semen variables as per WHO guidelines (1992) and from Sun *et al.* (2006)

Medical name	Description
Azoospermia	Complete absence of sperm
Aspermia	Ejaculation does not emit any semen
Oligozoospermia	<10 million sperm/ml of semen
Asthenozoospermia	>40% of sperm have low motility
Teratozoospermia	>40% of sperm with abnormal morphology
Special types of abnormal morphology	
Globozoospermia	Round-headed sperm
Macrocephalic, multinucleated and multiflagellate sperm	Macrocephalic, multinucleated and multiflagellate sperm
Necrospermia	Non-viable/dead sperm
Oligoasthenozoospermia	Motile density <8 million sperm/ml
Hematospermia	Red blood cells present in semen
Pyospermia	White blood cells present in semen
Polyzoospermia	Excessively high sperm concentration

Assessment of viability and motility parameters

In vitro viability is generally assessed both before and after thawing by eosin–nigrosin stain (Damodaran and Marimuthu, 1988; Pintado *et al.*, 2000). Computer-assisted semen analysis (CASA) provides objective and reproducible data on a number of sperm motion parameters and it should enhance the value of motility assessment to fertility prognosis. In recent years there has been an increase in the use of these systems to evaluate semen quality (Holt *et al.*, 1997; Mortimer, 2000; Foote, 2003). Sperm motility parameters are generally assessed using a computer-setting of 25 frames acquired to avoid sperm track overlapping. A minimum contrast of 10, minimum velocity of average path of 30 μm/s, and progressive motility of >80% straightness are required. Sperm motility is essential for normal fertilization, and it is currently the most common parameter of "sperm quality", acting as an indirect measure of metabolic activity and sperm viability (Berlinguer *et al.*, 2009).

Abnormal sperm morphology is classified as defects in the head, midpiece or tail of the sperm (WHO, 1992; Sun *et al.*, 2006). Head defects include large, small, tapered, pyriform, round and amorphous heads, heads with a small acrosomal area (<40% of the head area) and double heads, as well as any combination of these. Globozoospermia, where the sperm head appears small and round due to the failure of the acrosome to develop, is an example of a head defect. Midpiece defects include "bent" neck (where the neck and tail form an angle of greater than 90% to the long axis of the head), asymmetrical insertion of the midpiece into the head, a thick or irregular midpiece, an abnormally thin midpiece (with no mitochondrial sheath), as well as any combination of these types. Tail defects include short, multiple, hairpin, broken or bent (>90°) tails, tails of irregular width, coiled tails, as well as any combination of these (WHO, 1992; Sun *et al.*, 2006).

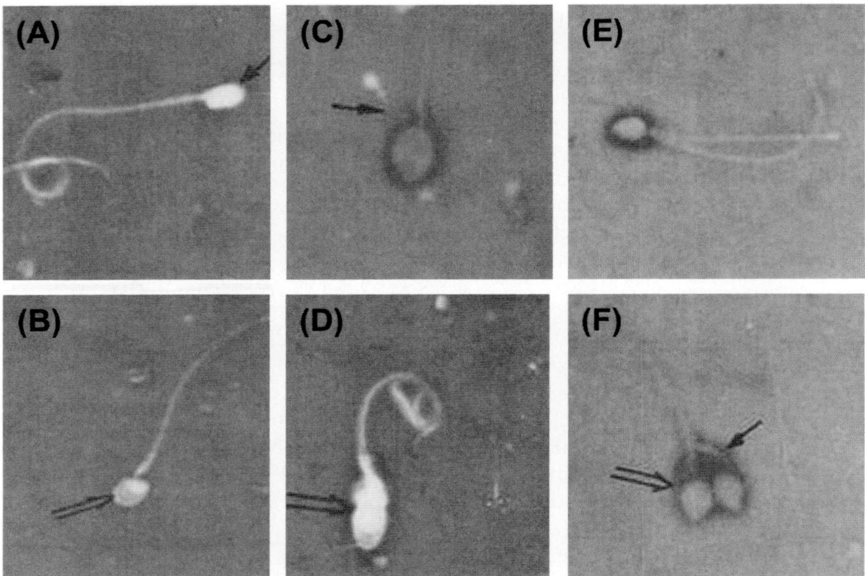

FIGURE 71.1 Eosin–nigrosin staining may show several features of the sperm, including viability, differences in shape of the head and tail and other aspects. (A) Shows a normal oval-shaped sperm that is alive, identified due to the absence of staining, as compared to the dying sperm (B) with dye uptake. Abnormal sperm shapes such as round (C), larger than normal size (D) as well as abnormal tails, such as double tail (E) and combination of both head and tail anomalies (F) may be routinely seen in infertility clinics. (From Damodaran and Marimuthu, 1988.)

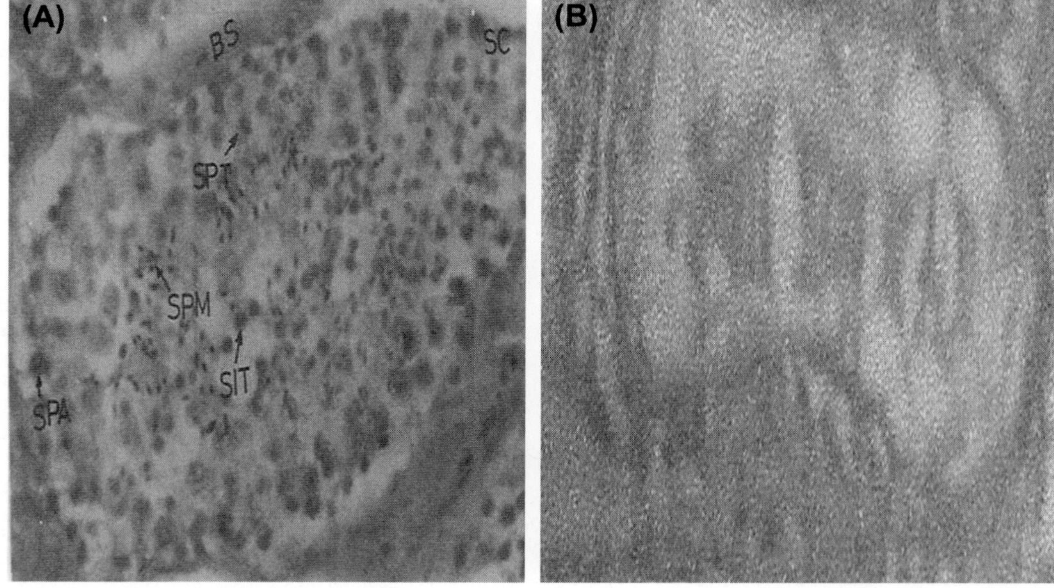

FIGURE 71.2 Histological sections of testicular biopsy specimens reveal a great amount of detail regarding the normal (A) and abnormal (B) spermatogenesis. A shows normal spermatogenesis in a normal human male. BS, SPA, SPT, SIT and SPM denote basement membrane, spermatogonial cells, spermatocyte, spermatids and sperms, respectively. Note the complete absence of any of these cell types in an infertile male with complete hyalinization (B). (From Damodaran and Marimuthu, 1988.)

Figure 71.1 shows representative types of sperm abnormalities (Damodaran and Marimuthu, 1988).

Testicular biopsy and meiotic chromosome analysis

Testicular biopsy is still used for diagnosis, prognosis and treatment options in many countries. Histological evaluation and meiotic chromosome analysis are helpful in identifying the normal or abnormal testicular cell types. Both of these techniques provide valuable qualitative and quantitative data. Figure 71.2 shows the typical histological appearance of normal (A) and abnormal sections of the processed and stained biopsy specimen (Damodaran and Marimuthu, 1988). Figure 71.3 shows the appearance of a normal meiotic metaphase I and II as compared with an abnormal one from various infertile human males. This figure also shows the spermatid micronuclei representing meiotic aneuploidy in infertile human males.

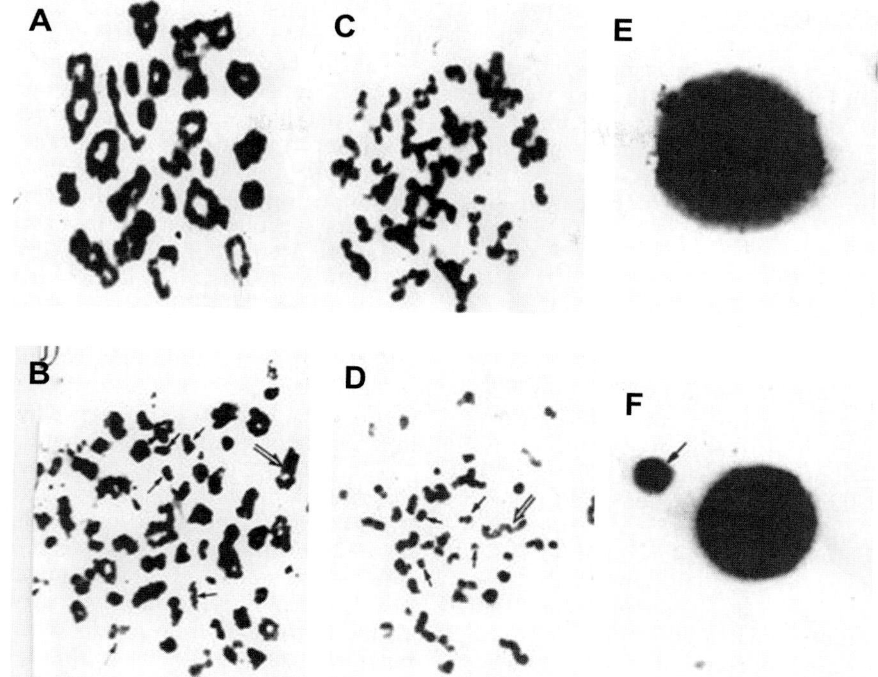

FIGURE 71.3 Meiotic chromosome analyses reveals valuable data from human infertile males. (A) and (B) depict the normal and abnormal meiotic metaphase I, while (C) and (D) show the normal and abnormal meiotic metaphase II. (E) and (F) depict the normal spermatid, while (F) shows the presence of spermatid micronuclei. (From Damodaran and Marimuthu, 1988.)

Extraction and measurement of intracellular ATP

Determination of intracellular ATP concentration can be performed by the enzymatic assay as described by Zinellu *et al.* (2008). Briefly, 50 µl of fresh semen and 150 µl of frozen semen (approximately 1.5*109 cells/ml) can be washed twice with 0.1 ml of cold physiological solution. For the extraction of nucleotides, 0.1 ml of ice-cold 0.6 M perchloric acid can be added to each Eppendorf tube containing spermatozoa and kept for 15 min; after centrifuging in an Eppendorf microfuge (3 minutes at 10,000 rpm) the supernatant can be neutralized with 15 µl of 3.5 M K_2CO_3. ATP levels can be measured spectrophotometrically at 340 nm using NADH-linked enzyme-coupled assays. The enzymatic spectrophotometric ATP assay can be carried out at 37°C with a Beckman DU-7 spectrophotometer, and performed using the coupling enzymes, glucose 6 phosphate dehydrogenase (G6PD) and hexokinase (HK). Addition of excess HK (2 µl from 2 mg/ml) and G6PD (2 µl from 1 mg/ml) in the presence of excess glucose (8 µl from 18 mg/ml) and nicotinamide adenine dinucleotide phosphate (NADP+) (8 µl from 20 mg/ml) to perchloric extract (25 µl) and to 400 µl of TRAP buffer (0.1 M, pH 7.6), the reaction begins and ATP can be determined from the formation of NADPH.

DNA integrity assessment

The comet assay has been adapted to detect germ cell genotoxicity and may be used for demonstrating the ability of a substance or its metabolite(s) to directly interact with the genetic material of gonadal and/or germ cells. Such results are important for the classification of germ cell mutagens, e.g. in the context of the "Globally Harmonized System of Classification and Labelling of Chemicals" (GHS) and male infertility related studies. Tests with cells from the gonads (testis and ovary) seem to be the most appropriate and a promising tool for demonstrating that a test compound reaches the gonads and is able to interact with the genetic material of germ cells. DNA damage was assessed only in frozen/thawed spermatozoa by single-cell gel electrophoresis (comet assay). Analysis of the shape and length of the "comet" tail, just like the DNA content in the tail, gives an assessment of DNA damage. The neutral comet assay allows the detection of double-strand breaks by subjecting lysed cell nuclei to an electrophoretic field at neutral pH (Sakkas *et al.*, 2002; Lewis and Agbaje, 2008). DNA damage can also be assessed by a variety of methods including *in situ* nick translation (Sakkas *et al.*, 1998), TUNEL (Sun *et al.*, 1997; Ahmadi and Ng, 1999) and sperm chromatin structure assay (SCSA) (Saleh *et al.*, 2003; Erenpreiss *et al.*, 2006). Several molecular and cellular markers have been identified as tools to evaluate sperm fertility *in vitro* in raw or processed semen samples (Rodriguez-Martinez and Barth, 2007; Garrido *et al.*, 2008).

Molecular techniques applied DNA and RNA biology

Standard procedures involved in extraction of DNA, RNA, protein are described in detail in several publications (Damodaran *et al.*, 2003, 2006a,b, 2009). Standard gene expression analysis using RT-PCR and toxicogenomics-related techniques are described in several publications (Damodaran *et al.*, 2003, 2006a,b). Extraction from testicular tissue either from testicular biopsy specimens of human beings (in infertility clinics) or from testicular tissues of model organisms like mouse and rats are comparatively easier. RNA and DNA extraction from sperms of the semen samples of human beings and from the epididymal aspirates are relatively challenging, because of the condensed nature of the sperm chromatin. FISH techniques using chromosome and gene-specific probes on sperms and germ cells can be used to detect aneuploidies and synaptonemal complex anomalies (Martin, 2008).

Methylation detection

A number of detection techniques are available to study methylation patterns, which are basically based on enzymatic hydrolysis, digestion with methylation-sensitive restriction enzymes, or bisulfite treatment of genomic DNA prior to downstream analysis (Dahl and Guldberg, 2003; Laird, 2003; Ho and Tang, 2007; Reamon-Buettner and Borlak, 2007). These techniques are used in mapping DNA methylation on individual gene sequences or to detect DNA methylation genome-wide, as a response to the exposure of toxicants. Each method has its strengths and limitations. Recently, another global methylation approach, namely, methyl-DNA immunoprecipitation (mDIP) assay that uses antibodies specific for 5-methyl-cytosine residues, was shown to provide key insights into the mechanisms (Keshet *et al.*, 2006). Most methods involve bisulfite treatment of genomic DNA, which converts cytosine to uracil but ethylated cytosines remain unaltered in this process. After PCR amplification, uracil will be converted to thymidine, which will be determined by direct PCR sequencing (bisulfite sequencing) or methylation-specific PCR (MSP-PCR). In bisulfite sequencing, primers are designed not to contain any CpGs to avoid discrimination against methylated or unmethylated DNA. In MSP-PCR, two pairs of primers are designed; one is specific for (M) methylated DNA and the other for (U) unmethylated DNA. After bisulfite-sequencing or M-specific PCR, amplified fragments are usually cloned to determine the degree of methylation.

BACKGROUND AND BASIC DESCRIPTION OF GENOME

Genome, its regulation, perturbations and responses

Genome is defined as the complete genetic composition (heredity component) of a cell or a species. A gene is defined as a unit of heredity that contributes to the characteristics or traits of an organism. At the molecular level, a gene is composed of organized sequences of DNA. A DNA molecule consists of two strands of nucleotides coiled around each other to form a double helix, held together by hydrogen bonds according to the AT/GC rule. At molecular level, the central dogma of genetics states that most genes (composed of ordered and unique DNA sequence characteristics for each gene) are transcribed into mRNA (transcription), and then the mRNA is translated into polypeptides (translation). Eukaryotes modify their RNA transcripts as well as proteins using processes such as alternate splicing of exons and post-translational modifications respectively to make them functional and more efficient. The promoter of a gene signals the beginning of transcription while the terminator specifies the end of the transcription. Eukaryotic promoters consist of a core promoter and response elements, such as enhancers, that regulate the rate of transcription. Activators and repressors may regulate RNA polymerase II, by interacting with GTFs (general transcription factors) or mediator, a protein complex that wraps around RNA polymerase II. Alternative splicing occurs when a single type of pre-mRNA can be spliced in more than one way, producing polypeptides with different sequences, thereby increasing the size of their proteomes. MicroRNAs (miRNAs) inhibit mRNAs either by inhibiting translation or by promoting the degradation of mRNAs. RNA binding proteins can regulate the transmission of specific mRNAs, for example iron regulatory protein (IRP) regulates the translation of ferritin mRNA. Thus, eukaryotic genes exhibit combinatorial control, meaning that many factors control the expression of a single gene at various levels. This multiple tiers of regulation help life forms to safeguard and faithfully replicate their genome and to perform various biochemical and physiological activities for their survival and propagation. At the same time, these layers of multifactorial and combinatorial control also make the delicate genome and its expression susceptible to perturbations from both intrinsic and extrinsic factors that may be of dietary and environmental origin.

A mutation is a heritable change in the genetic material. Germ-line mutations affect gametes, while somatic mutations affect only a part of the body. Point mutations which affect a single nucleotide can alter the coding sequence of genes in several ways such as silent, missense, nonsense and frameshift mutations. Gene mutations can also alter gene function by changing DNA sequences that are not within the coding region. Spontaneous mutations are the result of errors in natural biological processes, while induced mutations are due to agents in the environment that cause changes in DNA structure. Very often, it is difficult to distinguish whether a mutation is of spontaneous and induced type. DNA repair systems involve proteins that sense DNA damage and repair it before a mutation occurs. Reproductive toxicological outcomes very often depend on the disturbances in the delicate balance between DNA mutation and DNA repair, as many life forms are constantly challenged by chemical, physical and biological agents that can cause significant damage to their genome.

There are four major responses to positional information in developing embryos of eukaryotes such as cell division, cell migration, cell differentiation and apoptosis. These processes define the structure and function of various organ systems of developing embryos and hence a play a major role in the expression of genes (proteins) that define the health and disease symptoms of an adult organism. Any undesirable changes in genes and chromosomes (of the total genetic complement) that carry these genes at basic structural level will result in the disruption of the complex and combinatorial network of activities, resulting in a substantial increase in various forms of birth defects and disease phenotypes of multifactorial origin, causing a considerable amount of escalation in the morbidity and mortality conditions.

Due to the rapid advancements in modern technology related to genetics and molecular biology, several

TABLE 71.3 List of genes identified to be connected to human male sexual differentiation defects (adapted and modified from Matzuk and Lamb, 2008)

Male sexual differentiation-related birth defects are multifactorial in nature and with more studies in this area, it is becoming increasingly apparent that environmental factors play a significant role. The list shown here is the summary of genes (including SNPs and mutations) identified to be involved in human male infertility for most part. For more details of each gene and the associated phenotype, refer to supplement table 2 of the review article by Matzuk and Lamb (2008)
Ambiguous genitalia
(a) Steroid biosynthesis
CYP11A1; CYP11B1; CYP11B2; CYP17; CYP21; CYP21A2; HSD3B2; POR; SRD5A2; StAR
(b) Sex reversal and other related
AMH; AMHR2; AR; ARX; LHCGR; LHR; NRFA1; NR0B1; RSP01; SOX9; SRY; WT1
Gonadal dysgenesis
CYP11A1; NR5A1(Sf1); NR0B1; SRY; SRY promoter; WT1
Hypospadias
AR; ATF3; MAMLD1 (CXorf6); EFNB2; ESR1; ESR2; FGFR2; HOXA13; HOXD11; HOXD13; INSL3; MID1; RXFP2 (LGR8/GREAT)
Micropenis
ALKBH1; AHRR; ALG12; ESR1; GHR; NRSA1; SOX2; TBX3
Cryptorchidism
ARX; CYP19A1; DHH; ESR1; HOXD13; INSL3; KRAS; NRSA1; PTPN11; PWCR; RAF1; RXFP2; SOS1; SOX2; SPAG4L; SPATA12; ZNF214; ZNF215
Testis cancer
AR; BMP; CTNNB1; DIABLO; DND1; EGFR; EEF1A; FOXL2; GNAS; HMGA1; HMGA2; KIT; KND1; KRAS; NANOG; PATZ1; POLG; POU5F1; REG1; SMAD1; SMAD5; SOX2; SOX17; SPATA12. TSPY1; WT1
Defects of vas deferens
CFTR, HNF1B

Note: Micropenis also results in structural and numerical chromosomal alterations in many human chromosomal regions

disease-causing and disease-associated genes, with reference to the biology of reproduction, have been identified in the last several years (Tables 71.3 and 71.5). Identification of ever-increasing numbers of disease phenotype-related genes in mammals and humans has led to development of molecular diagnostic tests, which help monitor the population for early diagnosis, better prognostic and treatment options. The genes listed in the tables were shown to be involved in various general cellular functions as well as reproductive tissue-related functions. Expression of some of these genes was shown to be altered after a toxicant exposure (Table 71.4).

Genetic susceptibility and markers of DNA damage

Most of the metabolic and DNA repair genes carry polymorphisms that are present in the general population at various frequencies. Some of these genetic variations alter the original gene function, thus increasing or decreasing the activity of the corresponding enzyme. Moreover, most of the genetic polymorphisms described in the literature vary in frequency across ethnicity and geographic areas. The function of both metabolic and DNA repair genes may change substantially even in the absence of polymorphisms, and this may happen because of epigenetic changes induced by environmental factors. For example, it has been suggested that the degree of interaction between metabolic genes and tobacco smoke is not linear, but varies with exposure dose, thus making the picture more complex (Taioli *et al.*, 1998). For some genes, a greater degree of gene–environment interaction appears at lower doses of exposure (the interaction follows an inverse dose function), whereas for other genes, a converse high exposure gene effect is observed with the magnitude of interaction that increases as a function of dose. Besides dose levels, types of dosing such as chronic vs. acute exposure, synergistic effects of unlimited types of dosing scenarios with combinatorial effect, and the possibility of more than one factor involved can make the scenario very complex.

Sex determination in the germ cells of mammals

In mammals like mice and probably in humans, the decision to develop as male or female depends on sex-determining signaling molecules in the embryonic gonadal environment rather than the sex chromosome constitution of the germ cells. Germ cells in the female embryos initiate oogenesis and enter meiosis; in males embryos initiate spermatogenesis and inhibit meiosis until after birth. The whole processes of sex determination are still an area of extensive research, because of the fact that knowledge gained from such studies can help prevent several developmental and late-onset human diseases. Both male and female sexual differentiation takes distinctly different courses from the very early stages of embryonic development. Figure 71.4 and 71.5 depict the complex mechanisms involved in such developments.

TABLE 71.4 Selected genes (of sexual differentiation) involved in reproductive toxicological response

The list of genes shown in Table 71.3 was searched for any reports that describe alterations in mRNA or protein expression or any other alterations in gene regulation, using PubMed search. The data collected are presented below

Gene/Chemical studied	Model system	References
1. Genes involved in sexual differentiation		
AMH di(2-ethylhexyl) phthalate (DEHP)	Male rat Fetal testes	Borch *et al.*, 2005
2. Genes involved in ambigous genitalia		
CYP17 fungicides tebuconazole and epoxiconazole	Male and female rats	Taxvig *et al.*, 2007
StAR flutamide and diethylstilbestrol	Male rat	Adamsson *et al.*, 2008
SR-B1, DEHP	Male rat	Borch *et al.*, 2006
StAR, DEHP	Male rat	Borch *et al.*, 2006
PBR DEHP	Male rat	Borch *et al.*, 2006
3. Hypospadias		
ESR1 propyl pyrazole triol	The Japanese quail	Mattsson *et al.*, 2008
ESR2 propyl pyrazole triol	The Japanese quail	Mattsson *et al.*, 2008
FGFR2 DBP	Male rat	Zhu *et al.*, 2009
NSL3 Phthalate esters	Male rat	Howdeshell *et al.*, 2008
NSL3 DEHP	Male rat	Wilson *et al.*, 2007
AR vinclozolin plus procymidone) phthalate esters	Male rat	Rider *et al.*, 2009
4. Cryptorchidism		
CYP19A1 Prochloraz, imazalil, propioconazole, fenarimol, microsomes, triadimenol, triadimefon and dicofol	Human placental	Vinggaard *et al.*, 2000

Consequences of abnormal sexual differentiation

Mutations of genes regulating the germ cell sex determination machinery are first likely to result in agametic gonads and cause infertility in human patients. Second, germ cell sex reversal in humans has been shown to increase the susceptibility of germ cell to develop into tumors. XY female sex-reversed patients exhibit a high incidence of gonadoblastomas, a mixed germ cell-somatic cell tumor that appears to originate from sex-reversed XY oogonia/oocytes (Kocer *et al.*, 2009). Furthermore, carcinoma *in situ*, the non-malignant precursor of seminomatous and non-seminomatous testicular germ cell tumors, has also been proposed to originate from impaired or delayed germ cell differentiation during fetal testis development due to environmental or genetic factors that disrupt the communication between Sertoli cells and germ cells.

Sexual differentiation and aneuploidy in humans

It is well documented that there is a significant difference in frequencies of various types of *de novo* chromosomal abnormalities. For example, aneuploidy leading to miscarriage, infertility and trisomy conditions such as Down syndrome in humans is shown to be present in human oocytes at a 10-fold higher frequency than in human sperm (Kocer *et al.*, 2009). The incidence of aneuploidy in human gametes is also influenced by age in addition to the gender. For example, age-related aneuploidy seen in sperms is increased only by about 2%, while maternal age effect on oocyte aneuploidy rate seems to be about 35%. Aneuploidies arise from errors in chromosome segregation during meiosis, and there are two significant differences. First, male germ cells proceed through meiosis without interruption in adult men, whereas female germ cells initiate meiosis in the embryo and remain arrested in meiotic prophase for decades until hormonal stimulation prior to ovulation. During the oocytes' meiotic arrest, homologous chromosomes are physically held together as bivalents by crossover events and cohesion between the DNA molecules. The gradual loss of these physical connections between homologous chromosomes during the prolonged meiotic arrest, and/or age-dependent defects in the machinery involved in aligning and segregating the homologous chromosomes on the meiotic spindle upon resumption of meiosis could contribute to the high rates of aneuploidy in older females by causing missegregation of meiotic chromosomes. Second, female germ cells appear to respond less stringently than male germ cells to abnormalities that can arise during synapsis and segregation (Kocer *et al.*, 2009).

Spermatogenesis, spermiogenesis and sperm genome

The complex, multistep, highly organized cycles of sperm production involve various factors such as: (1) the hypothalamic–pituitary–gonadal axis, (2) autocrine, paracrine and juxtracrine interactions between the spermatogenic germ cells within the seminiferous tubules, (3) the nurturing somatic cells that reside inside (Sertoli cells), (4) between (Leydig and other interstitial cells) and (5) within the wall of (myoid cells) the tubules. Various factors within the epididymis (a major maturation site for sperm) also play an important role. Spermatogenesis involves the renewal and differentiation of spermatogonial stem cells into rapidly proliferating spermatogonia, meiotic cells (early and late spermatocytes) and haploid cells (round, elongating and elongated spermatids) before release of a sperm into the tubule lumen. Large numbers of genes are specifically expressed in the male germ line, exemplifying the complexity of the spermatogenic process and indicating that mutations in thousands of different genes could cause male infertility. Formation of the acrosome and flagellum of the spermatid contribute to the transformation into sperms by a process called spermiogenesis. Topography of the sperm is unique and complex among all of the known cell types. There are three major distinguishable parts such as: head, midpiece and tail. Normal spermatozoa exhibit an oval-shaped head with a regular outline and an acrosomal cap covering more than one-third of the head surface (Sun *et al.*, 2006). The molecular pathologies resulting in failure of germ cell migration can result in the absence of sperms in the ejaculate which may cause azoospermia. Defects in spermatogonial proliferation, spermatocyte maturation and spermatid maturation can result in maturation arrest at various points mentioned above leading to either azoospermia or oligozoospermia or asthenozoospermia (see Table 71.2 for definitions). Genetically inherited or environmentally

TABLE 71.5 Genes that were shown to be involved in human male infertility defects: spermatogenesis and sperm function (adapted and modified from Matzuk and Lamb, 2008)

For more details of most of the genes and the associated phenotypes, refer to supplement table 2 of the review article by Matzuk and Lamb (2008). Gene entries with bold letters represent new entries in the PubMed database since 2008
Abnormal spermatogenesis
ATM; ATMAC; DAZL; ***EIF4G3****; ERCC2; GTF2A1L; JUN; NLRP14; NRB0B1; POLG; PRM1; PRM2; SDHA; SOX8; XRCC1; YBX2; EIF4G3*
Azoospermia
APOB; ACSBG2; ART3; ATM; BOULE; BPY2; BRCA2; CDY1; CFTR; CREM; DAZ;DDX25; DDX3Y; DRFFY;ERCC1; ERCC2; FASLG; FHL5; FKBP6; ***FKBP52;*** *HNRNPC; HSFY1; KLHL10; LAP3; MBOAT1; MEI1; MLH1; MLH3;MTR; NLRP14; PRDM16; RBMX; RBMY1A1; RBMY1F; SPATA16; SYCP1; SYCP3; TAF7L; TGIF2LX; TSPY;* ***TSSK2****; TSSK4; UBE2B; USP26; UTP14C; USP9Y; UTY; XPC; XPD; XRCC1; YBX2; ZNF230*
Oligospermia
AR*; MT-ATP6; EGF; FASL; H19 and MEST; KLHL10; PIGA; PRM1; PRM2; SHBG; SDHA; TSSK4; UBE2B; VASA*
Asthenozoospermia
AKAP3; AKAP4C; CATSPER2; DNAI1; DNMT3B; DHAH5; DNAH11; DNAL1; PDYN; GNA12; Mitochondrial DNA; ***C14orf104 (KTU), RSPH4A, and RSPH9); Fractalkine;*** *LRRC50; MTHFR; MT-ND4; PIGA; POLG; PPM1G; PRKAR1A;* ***PSA, PAP ;SHBG; SEPT4 and Smcp*** *SPAG16; TEKT1; TEKT2; Tf ; TPN1; TPN2; TXNDC3;* T mt DNA haplotypes
Teratozoospermia
AURKC; PRM1; PVRL2; SPATA16; SP1
Oligoasthenozoospermia
JUND; mt-ND4; NALP14
Oligoasthenoteratozoospermia
MTRR; IL1B; SABP
Acrosome or fertilization
POIA3
DNA damage/infertility
GSTM1 AR; GSTM1 KIT; KITLG; IL1A; OAZ3; PRM1; TSPY; TSSK4; USP26; YBX2
Varicocele effect
MT-ATP6; MT-ATP; CACNA1C; MT-CO1; MT-CO2; MT-ND3

acquired defects in genes required for hormone action, cell proliferation, apoptosis, DNA repair, recombination, chromatin remodeling, cell differentiation, ion channels, motility, cell–cell interactions and function can result in the above-mentioned testicular pathology leading to abnormal semen parameters and consequent infertility. It is obvious that male infertility can result not only from spermatogenesis and sperm function-specific genetic defects but also from defects affecting more basic cellular functions required for mitosis, meiosis and normal differentiated functions of cells that ultimately affect spermatogenesis (Matzuk and Lamb, 2008).

Sperm chromosome anomalies

Aberrations in the genetic information of spermatozoa include numerical and structural chromosome abnormalities (Sun *et al.*, 2006). Numerical abnormalities include aneuploidies and polyploidies, and arise from a missing or extra chromosome(s) due to meiotic non-disjunction. Aneuploidies involve an autosome, a sex chromosome or both; polyploidies have a duplication of all chromosomes. Structural abnormalities include chromosome breaks, gaps, translocations, inversions, insertions, deletions and acentric fragments. The frequency of numerical chromosome abnormalities in sperm of fertile men is 1–2%, and the frequency of structural chromosome abnormalities in sperm varies from 7 to 14% (Martin, 2003). Fluorescence *in situ* hybridization (FISH) analysis of sperm from a large series of infertile men has not generally revealed a specific association between morphologically abnormal sperm and sperm chromosome abnormalities, but has indicated that teratozoospermia, like other forms of abnormal semen profiles (aesthenozoospermia, oligozoospermia), is associated with a modest increase in the frequency of sperm chromosome abnormalities. However, FISH studies on some infertile men and mouse strains have suggested that certain types of morphologically abnormal spermatozoa, such as macrocephalic multitailed spermatozoa, are associated with a very significantly increased frequency of aneuploidy. Thus, there may be an association between sperm morphology and aneuploidy in infertile men with specific abnormalities (Sun *et al.*, 2006).

Sperm chromosome anomalies and DNA damage in individuals exposed to mutagens

Increasing awareness about the harmful effects of pesticides on reproduction and fertility led to sperm chromosome studies. Recio (2001) found that increased levels of

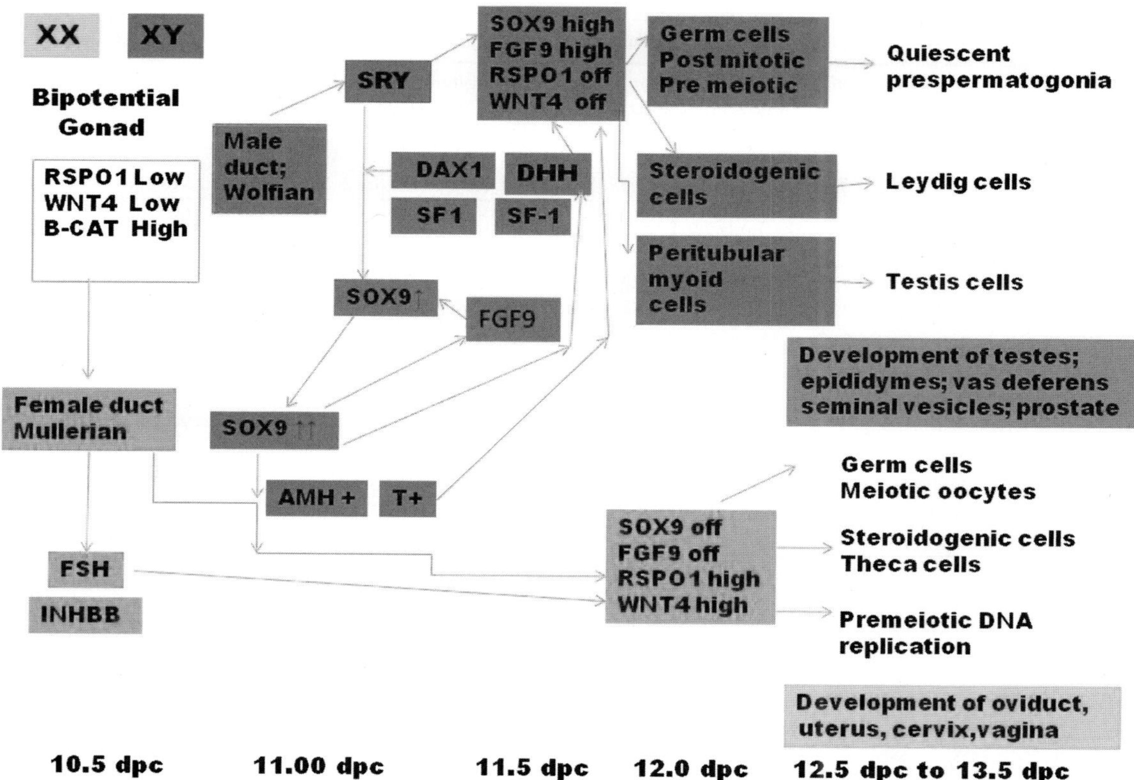

FIGURE 71.4 The complexity of pathways involved in sexual differentiation. The term "dpc" denotes "days post coitum".

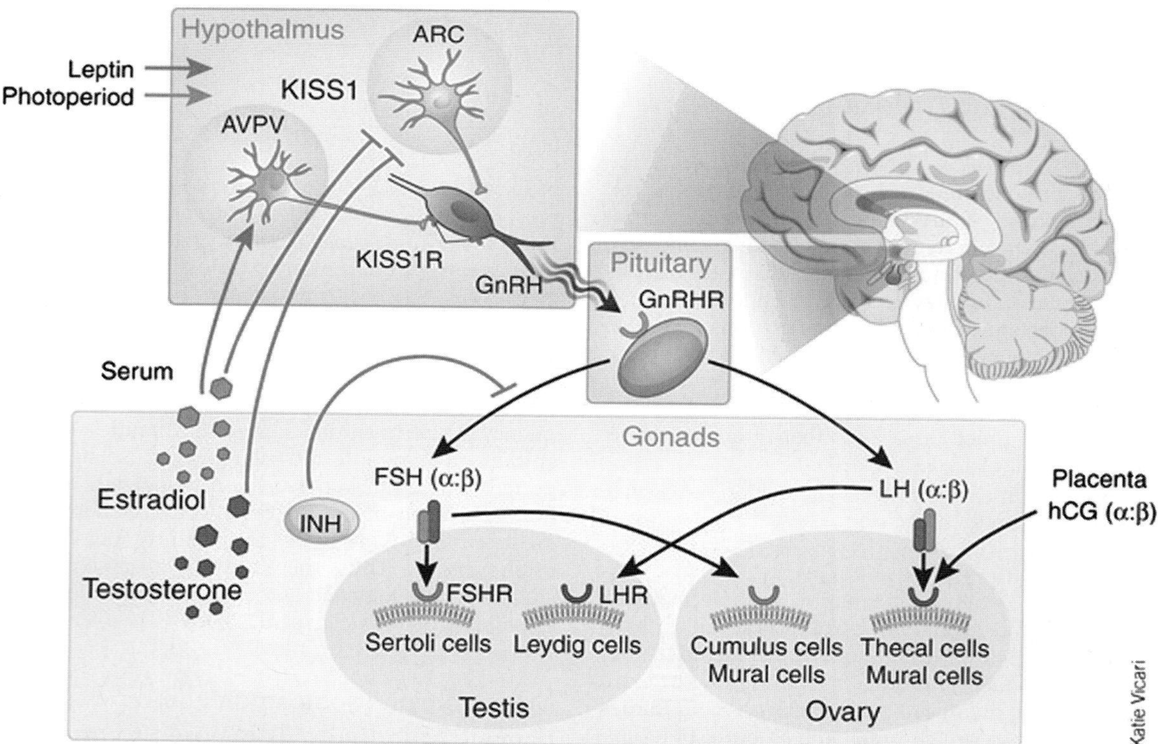

FIGURE 71.5 Neuroendocrine control of pituitary and gonadal function. (From Matzuk and Lamb, 2008, with permission from Macmillan Publishers Ltd.) Please refer to color plate section.

aneuploidies in X, Y and 18 were significantly higher in men exposed to a mixture of parathion, methamidophos, endosulfan and dimethoate. Smith *et al.* (2004) scored aneuploidy and diploidy frequencies for chromosome 13, 21, X and Y using multicolor FISH in more than 800,000 sperm from 20 pesticide appliers whom were exposed to a variety of herbicides, insecticides and fungicides. There was no significant difference between exposed men and control donors. Härkönen *et al.* (1999) studied sperm from 30 Finnish farmers exposed to fungicides and did not find a significant increase in disomy frequencies for chromosome 1 or 7. In contrast, Padungtod *et al.* (1999) studied sperm aneuploidy in 32 pesticide factory workers and found an increase in YY sperm. Similarly, Xia *et al.* (2004) found that fenvalerate significantly increased disomy frequency for chromosome 18, X and Y in 12 men. Xia *et al.* (2005) also found increased sex chromosome disomy in cabaryl-exposed men. The exposed men in both studies were factory workers producing the pesticide; thus, it is likely that they experienced higher levels of pesticide exposure than the farmers working outside in the former two studies. Sanchez-Pena *et al.* (2004) found significantly increased DNA fragmentation in men exposed to organophosphates, carbamates, pyrethroids and organochlorines. Bian *et al.* (2004) noted fenvalerate induced increase in DNA damage in sperm in exposed men. Likewise, Meeker (2004) found a positive correlation of increased sperm DNA damage with exposure to carbaryl and chlorpyrifos.

Sperm chromosome studies in patients treated with radiotherapy and chemotherapy

Martin *et al.* (1986) studied sperm chromosome anomalies using the human sperm/hamster oocyte system on cancer patients treated by radiotherapy (RT) or chemotherapy (CT). The majority of the men had seminoma of the testis and had undergone unilateral orchidectomy. The total body radiation doses were 30–40 Gy, and the testicular radiation doses ranged from 0.4 to 5.0 Gy. The majority of men became azoospermic in the first year after radiotherapy, and some men never regained sperm production throughout the study. Most of the men were producing sperm 2–3 years after RT, but low sperm counts were common. By 36 months post-RT, eight men regained sperm production and had an average sperm chromosome abnormality rate of 20.9%. This was significantly higher than control donors (8.5%). The range in the frequencies of abnormal sperm chromosome complements in individuals at 36 months post-RT was 6–67%, and these frequencies were significantly correlated with the testicular radiation dose. The results demonstrate a significant dose-dependent increase in the frequency of sperm chromosomal abnormalities after RT. Other studies by Jenderny and Röhrborn (1987) did not find a significantly increased frequency of chromosome abnormalities. Genesca *et al.* (1990) found a significant increase in the frequency of structural chromosome abnormalities in the sperm of the two patients. Differences could be due to different treatment regimens, analyzed at different time periods. Recently, Martin *et al.* (1999) using FISH analysis have attempted to examine more homogeneous groups of men with the same type of cancer and treatment. All men had the same treatment with BEP therapy (bleomycin, etoposide, cisplatin). There were no significant differences in the frequencies of numerical abnormalities or structural abnormalities. Patients treated with NOVP therapy (novantrone, oncovin, vinblastine, prednisone), as well as other types of therapy, showed an elevation in aneuploidy frequencies during treatment (Martin *et al.*, 1999; De Mas *et al.*, 2001; Marchetti *et al.*, 2001). Thus, the evidence to date does suggest an increased risk of induced sperm chromosome abnormalities during chemotherapy and up to 18 months following treatment.

Synaptonemal complex analysis

Since infertile men have an increased frequency of aneuploid sperm, decrease in recombination rate has been suggested (Martin, 2003). Sun *et al.* (2005a) studied synaptonemal complexes in pachytene cells from 11 control males with normal spermatogenesis and 23 infertile men: 5 with obstructive azoospermia (OA) and 18 with non-obstructive azoospermia (NOA). Thus, a significant number of men with NOA have abnormalities in chromosome synapsis and an increased frequency of chromosomes with no recombination foci. These meiotic abnormalities could lead to meiotic arrest or an increased frequency of aneuploid sperm. It is possible that various mutagens could affect chromosome recombination by altering the timing of the process or affecting the function of key proteins. Thus analysis of the synaptonemal complex could provide important research clues on the mechanism of potential aneugens (Martin, 2003).

Oogenesis and the role of genome in female reproductive processes

Female reproductive processes are much more complex than male reproductive processes. The following are the main pathways: (1) Several master oocyte-specific transcriptional regulators interact to control primordial follicle formation and follicle maintenance and recruitment into the growing pool, (2) at later steps in folliculogenesis and through ovulation, paracrine factors (such as KIT ligand, GDF9 and BMP15), autocrine factors (such as activins and inhibins) and endocrine hormones (such as FSH, LH, estradiol and progesterone) play key roles. After ovulation, sequential expression of proteins of the zona pellucida and oocyte maternal factors permit proper fertilization and the substantial changes in gene expression necessary for early embryogenesis. Other gene products such as ovarian prostaglandins and steroids are also essential to initiate a cascade of events in the uterus that readies it for implantation of a healthy embryo. Finally, multiple proteins and factors are required for placentation and maternal behavior (Matzuk and Lamb, 2008). Figure 71.6 depicts the complex mechanisms controlled by several pathways (genes) involved in the oogenesis.

Oocyte chromosome anomalies

Asynapsis of homologous chromosomes at the pachytene stage has been associated with gametogenic failure and infertility, but the cellular mechanisms involved are

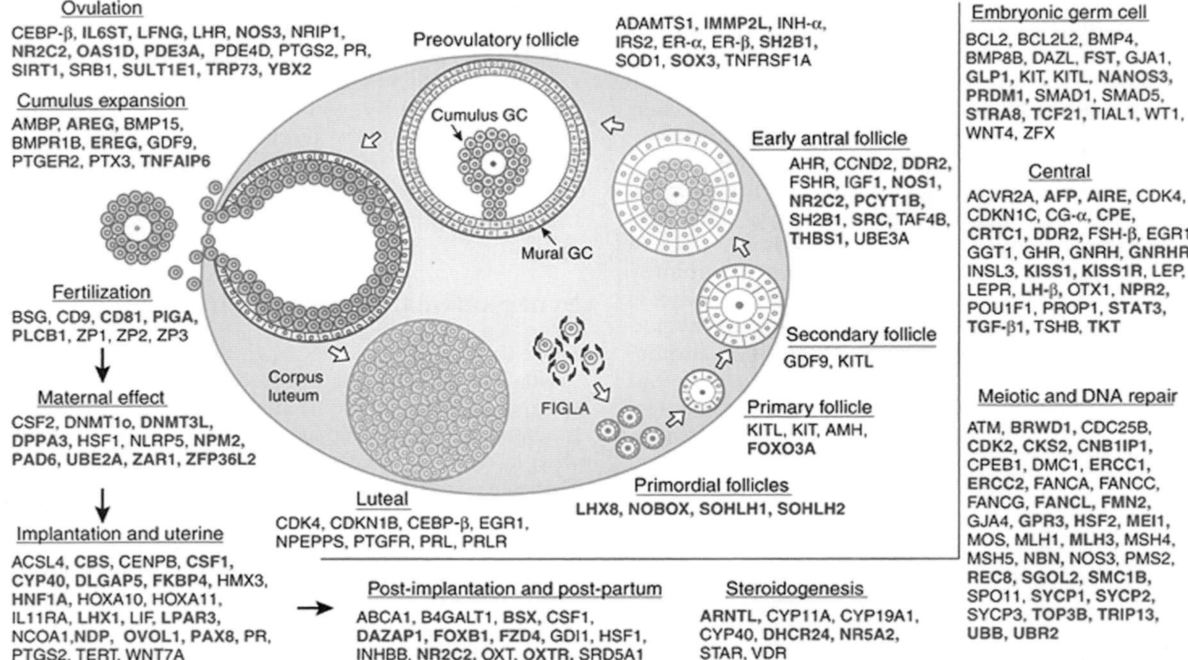

FIGURE 71.6 Genetic dissection of female fertility pathways in mice. (From Matzuk and Lamb, 2008, with permission from Macmillan Publishers Ltd.)

currently unknown in human meiocytes. In mice, the protein encoded by the breast cancer susceptibility gene Brca1 has been described to direct kinase ATR (ataxia telangiectasia and Rad3 related) to any unpaired DNA at the pachytene stage, where ATR triggers H2AX phosphorylation, resulting in the silencing of those chromosomes. In this study, the distribution of ATR, BRCA1 and the phosphorylated histone gammaH2AX is assessed by immunofluorescence in human oocytes and it is found that they localize at unpaired chromosomes at the pachytene stage. Evidence is shown to propose that BRCA1, ATR and gammaH2AX in the human may be part of a system such as the one previously described in mice, which signals unsynapsed chromosomes at pachytene and may lead to their silencing (Garcia-Cruz *et al.*, 2009). Thioglycolic acid has been shown to inhibit mouse oocyte maturation and affect chromosomal arrangement and spindle configuration (Hou *et al.*, 2008). *In vivo* treatment of trichlorfon resulted in polyploid embryos that might have arisen from fertilization of oocytes that were either meiotically delayed and still in metaphase I at fertilization or progressed through anaphase II without cytokinesis. *In vitro* treatment of trichorfon resulted in the induction of aneuploidy and polyploidy at the first meiotic division and of severe morphological alterations of the second meiotic spindle. Butadiene diepoxide treatment resulted in the induction and transmission of chromosome aberrations in mouse oocytes (Tiveron *et al.*, 1997). Acute exposure of female hamsters to carbendazim (MBC) during meiosis resulted in aneuploid oocytes with subsequent arrest of embryonic cleavage and implantation (Jeffay *et al.*, 1996). Carbendazim (MBC) treatment has been shown to disrupt oocyte spindle function and induce aneuploidy in hamsters exposed during fertilization (meiosis II) (Zuelke and Perreault, 1995).

BACKGROUND AND BASIC DESCRIPTION OF EPIGENOME

Epigenome of germ cells and mechanisms of its regulation

Gene regulation without sequence alterations is brought about by epigenetic mechanisms that involve three well-defined mechanisms such as (1) DNA methylation, (2) histone modifications and (3) RNA-associated pathways (Table 71.6). These three epigenetic regulatory pathways are generally associated with the initiation and maintenance of silencing of gene expressions, and cross-talk with each other to effect heritable silencing (Egger *et al.*, 2004). More novel mechanisms of epigenetic pathways affecting gene expression are newly discovered. For example, gene activity can also be induced by direct interactions between chromosomal regions that are positioned at long-distances from one another, resulting in activation or repression (Kiefer, 2007).

DNA methylation

Methylation of DNA, as an epigenetic silencing mechanism of fundamental importance in embryonic development, transcription, chromatin structure, X-chromosome inactivation, genomic imprinting and chromosome instability, has long been known, verified by numerous studies, and has been implicated in several cancer syndromes (involving p14, p15 and p16 locus) as well as human genetic disorders such as Prader–Willi and Angelman syndromes (imprinted regions on human chromosome 15). Modification of DNA by methylation occurs by the covalent addition of

TABLE 71.6 Types of epigenetic modifications and their common mode of action

Epigenetic modification	Role in transcription
DNA methylation	Gene repression
Histone methylation	Gene repression and activation
Histone demethylation	Gene repression and activation
Histone acetylation	Gene activation
Histone deacetylation	Gene repression
Histone phosphorylation	Gene activation and repression
Histone ubiquitylation	Gene repression and activation
Histone sumoylation	Gene repression
Histone biotinylation	Gene repression and activation

a methyl group to position 5 of the cytosine ring, creating 5-methylcytosine (Laird, 2003; Robertson, 2005). Generally, CpG dinucleotides are the sites of almost all methylation in mammalian genomes (Reamon-Buettner and Borlak, 2007). Moreover, these CpG dinucleotides are not equally distributed throughout the genome as they occur in clusters of either large repetitive sequences (such as rDNA, satellite sequences or centromeric repeats) or in short CG-rich DNA stretches, known as CpG islands (CGIs), often found in the promoter region and the first exon of genes. Until recently, these sites were used as landmarks to identify the location of disease causing genes or other genes of importance. Generally, a CpG island is defined as a contiguous window of DNA of at least 500 base-pair-window with a GC content of at least 55% and an observed/expected CpG frequency of at least 0.65% to exclude most Alu repeat sequences (Reamon-Buettner and Borlak, 2007). Generally, CGIs are unmethylated in healthy tissues, while repetitive sequences are highly methylated. Very recently, it has been shown that DNA methylation can affect transcription of genes whose 5-UTRs had low CpG density ("non-CGI promoters") (Eckhardt *et al.*, 2006).

Methylation machinery

The mammalian DNA methylation machinery is mediated by a distinct set of DNA methyltransferases (DNMTs), which establish and maintain DNA methylation patterns; and the methyl-CpG binding proteins (MBDs), which are involved in "reading" methylation marks (Robertson, 2005). DNMT1 is the main enzyme in mammals that preferentially recognizes hemimethylated DNA during replication and thus reestablishes the original methylation patterns after cell divisions, referred to as maintenance methylation. Maintenance of DNA methylation by DNMT1 is crucial for embryonic development, but DNMT1 has also been shown to be required for faithfully maintaining DNA methylation patterns in human cancer cells and is essential for their proliferation and survival (Chen *et al.*, 2007). In contrast, the *de novo* methyltransferases DNMT3a and DNMT3b target new unmethylated DNA sites. Methyl-CpG binding proteins contain the conserved DNA binding motif methyl-cytosine binding domain, which preferentially binds to methylated CpG dinucleotides. These proteins serve as transcriptional repressors, mediating gene silencing via DNA cytosine methylation (Reamon-Buettner and Borlak, 2007).

Methylation in primordial, embryonic germ cells

DNA methylation patterns are reprogrammed in primordial germ cells and in preimplantation embryos by demethylation and subsequent *de novo* methylation. The epigenetic reprogramming may be necessary for the embryonic genome to return to a pluripotent state (Farthing *et al.*, 2008). Genome-wide promoter analysis of DNA methylation in mouse embryonic stem (ES) cells, embryonic germ (EG) cells, sperm, trophoblast stem (TS) cells and primary embryonic fibroblasts (pMEFs). Global clustering analysis shows that methylation patterns of ES cells, EG cells and sperm are surprisingly similar, suggesting that while the sperm is a highly specialized cell type, its promoter epigenome is already largely reprogrammed and resembles a pluripotent state (Farthing *et al.*, 2008) and thus potentially show the same level of vulnerability to environmental insults of all types. There are some key exceptions to this, including high level of methylation of Nanog and Lefty1 in sperm. Thus, environmental exposure can change the methylation of both sperm-specific and other ES and EG cell-specific genes thus altering the gene expression in the offspring.

Some other aspects of DNA methylation

Transcription of gene sequences is influenced by DNA methylation, in which the methyl group that protrudes from the cytosine nucleotide into the major groove of the DNA displaces transcription factors that normally bind to the DNA, or attracts methyl-binding domains, which in turn are associated with gene silencing and chromatin compaction (Fazzari and Greally, 2004). Hence environmental stimuli, either dietary or other types of toxins as well as social environments of life forms, can cause aberrant DNA methylation patterns known as either hypo- or hypermethylation. Both forms can lead to chromosomal instability and transcriptional gene silencing, and both have been implicated in a variety of human malignancies. Aberrant DNA methylation can lead to a number of other human diseases as well (Robertson, 2005). Although both nutrition and chemicals are important environmental factors modulating epigenetic changes, they are commonly studied separately by researchers in different fields. However, these two environmental factors cannot be separated from each other in the real world because a number of chemical agents contaminate food chains. Methyl groups from S-adenosylmethionine (SAM) are needed for DNA methylation. Diets low in sources of methyl groups can lead to global DNA hypomethylation by impairing synthesis of SAM. However, even without nutritional deficiency, an enhanced need to synthesize glutathione (GSH) can impair synthesis of SAM and perturb DNA methylation, because the methylation cycle and the GSH synthesis pathways are biochemically linked. Exposure to environmental chemicals is a common situation in which the need for GSH synthesis is enhanced, because GSH is consumed to conjugate diverse chemicals. Given that GSH conjugation happens at any chemical dose, this hypothesis is relevant even at exposures below the high doses that cause toxicologic responses. At present, general populations are exposed to a large number of chemicals, each at a very low dose. Thus, DNA hypomethylation due to chemical exposure may be common in modern societies and can synergistically interact with nutrition-induced DNA hypomethylation.

Other histone modifications

Epigenetic control of gene expression also involves the proteins (including various types of histones) that package DNA into chromatin. These histones determine whether the chromatin is tightly packed (condensed: heterochromatin), in which case gene expression is silenced, or relaxed (decondensed: euchromatin), in which case gene expression is active. Essentially, eukaryotic chromosomes (chromatin) consist of DNA (deoxyribonucleic acid), histones H1, H2A, H2B, H3, and H4, and non-histone proteins (Grant, 2001; Fischle *et al.*, 2003). DNA and histones form repetitive nucleoprotein units, called the nucleosomal core particles. Each histone consists of a structured domain and an unstructured amino-terminal "tail" of 25–40 residues. The amino-terminal tails of histones protrude from the nucleosomal surface. Covalent modifications of these tails affect the structure of chromatin and form the basis for the epigenetic regulation of chromatin structure and gene function. Amino acid residues in histone tails are modified by covalent acetylation, methylation, phosphorylation, ubiquitination, sumoylation and biotinylation, among others, to regulate gene transcription, mitotic condensation of chromatin and DNA repair (Strahl and Allis, 2000; Grant, 2001; Peterson and Laniel, 2004; Margueron *et al.*, 2005; Kouzarides, 2007). Furthermore, the cross-talk between histone modifications and the specific combinations of histone modifications as a function of histone code specify the structural state of chromatin (Strahl and Allis, 2000). Effector proteins read and carry out the code's instructions to specify the formation of heterochromatin or euchromatin. Heterochromatic DNA is largely inaccessible to transcription factors and chromatin remodelers, making it relatively transcriptionally inert. Specifically, combinations of histone modifications at the N-terminal regions are reversible, and that protein binding to these tails and different histone protein associations bring about a variety of functional outcomes. Although the concept of a heritable epigenetic histone code based on histone modifications is still being tested (thus at level of hypothesis testing), the fact that toxicants either directly or indirectly can affect these modifications may predispose the life forms to possible mutagenic events.

Abnormal methylation patterns affecting reproductive functions

Spermatogenesis is a highly complex process that requires multiple levels of stringent control and synchronization of germ cell development. Because of this complexity, it is also prone to frequent errors, as paternal infertility contributes to 30–50% of all infertility cases (Godmann *et al.*, 2009). There are many mechanisms involving several factors, as the complex interaction of environmental and genetic factors very often results in clinical symptoms that are indistinguishable phenotypically. Aberrant epigenetic profiles, in the form of anomalous DNA and histone modifications, are characteristic of cancerous testis cells (Godmann *et al.*, 2009). Germ cell development is a critical period during which epigenetic patterns are established and maintained. The progression from diploid spermatogonia to haploid spermatozoa involves stage- and testis-specific gene expression and regulation, mitotic and meiotic division, and the histone–protamine transition. All of these processes are postulated to engender unique epigenetic controls (Godmann *et al.*, 2009). It is proposed that exposures to different environmental agents could lead to inter-individual phenotypic diversity as well as differential susceptibility to disease and behavioral pathologies. Inter-individual differences in the epigenetic state could also affect susceptibility to xenobiotics. Although our current understanding of how epigenetic mechanisms impact on the toxic action of xenobiotics is very limited, it is anticipated that in the future, epigenetics will be incorporated in the assessment of the safety of chemicals (Szyf, 2007; Szyf *et al.*, 2008). Human infertile males showed significantly increased methylation alteration at six of seven imprinted loci (LIT1, MEST, SNRPN, PLAGL1, PEG3, H19 and IGF2) tested, with differences in significance observed between oligozoospermic and abnormal protamine patients (Hammoud *et al.*, 2009). The oligozoospermic patients of this study were significantly affected at mesoderm-specific transcript (MEST), whereas abnormal protamine patients were affected at KCNQ1, overlapping transcript 1 (LIT1), and at small nuclear ribonucleoprotein polypeptide N (SNRPN) (Hammoud *et al.*, 2009). In a recent study, an association between abnormal genomic imprinting and hypospermatogenesis, and that spermatozoa from oligozoospermic patients carry a raised risk of transmitting imprinting errors, has been suggested. In a recent study by Boissonnas *et al.* (2010) all normal semen samples showed the expected high global methylation level for all CpGs analyzed. In the teratozoospermia group, 11 of 19 patients presented a loss of methylation at variable CpG positions either in the IGF2 DMR2 or in both the IGF2 DMR2 and the 6th CTCF of the H19 DMR. In the OAT (oligoasthenoteratozoospermia) group, 16 of 22 patients presented a severe loss of methylation of the 6th CTCF, closely correlated with sperm concentration. Recent studies indicate that the active demethylation of male pronuclei occurs in both mouse and human zygotes. It is possible that the abnormal methylation patterns resulting from a dysfunctional cytoplasm may occur in a small number of oocytes and may affect embryonic viability.

Role of endocrine disruptors in transgenerational mutagenesis

Recently, an endocrine disruptor (i.e., vinclozolin) exposure during embryonic gonadal sex determination was shown to induce an adult-onset disease (i.e., male fertility and spermatogenic defect) for multiple generations (i.e., F_1–F_4) and involved epigenetic (i.e., DNA methylation) changes in several genes in the male germ-line (Anway *et al.*, 2005, 2006). This transgenerational phenotype appears to involve altered DNA methylation and epigenetic programming of the male germ-line as the potential causal factor in the phenomenon (Jirtle and Skinner, 2007). Subsequently it has been found that as these trans-generational animals age, multiple adult-onset diseases are observed including tumor development, prostate disease, kidney disease and immune abnormalities (Anway *et al.*, 2006). The ability of an environmental factor (e.g., endocrine disruptor) to promote an epigenetic change in the germ-line is postulated to be a mechanism involved in transgenerational adult onset disease (Anway *et al.*, 2005, 2006; Jirtle and Skinner, 2007). In addition to transgenerational germ-line considerations, the exposure and epigenetic modification of any developing organ system may influence adult-onset disease for the individual and tissue exposed (Skinner, 2008).

These recent studies demonstrating the ability of endocrine disruptors, such as vinclozolin, to induce a transgenerational disease phenotype (Anway *et al.*, 2005, 2006) need to be qualified with respect to conclusions on the toxicology of these compounds. The doses used above were those expected in the environment, such that studies are now needed to compare environmental vs. effective doses. In addition, whether the endocrine disruptor activity or other metabolites may be causal also needs to be assessed. Although caution is needed regarding toxicology conclusions, the phenomenon identified of a transgenerational disease phenotype and relationship with epigenetic modifications does provide a novel etiology to consider for disease. Thus, the role of epigenetic transgenerational phenotypes in adult onset disease needs to be seriously considered (Di Croce, 2004; Egger, 2004; Jiang, 2004; Robertson, 2005; Peaston and Whitelaw, 2006; Skinner, 2008).

Analysis of the transgenerational epigenetic effects on the male germ-line identified 15 candidate genes with altered methylation patterns after embryonic exposure to vinclozolin (Chang *et al.*, 2006). Recently it has been shown that long-term, low dose exposure to arsenic can result in the loss of DNA methylation, as this treatment resulted in the depletion of S-adenosylmethionine, the main cellular methyl donor, and repressed expression of DNA methyltransferase genes, DNMT1 and DNMT3A (Reichard *et al.*, 2007). The list of environmental chemicals and other factors seems to be increasing day by day.

Histone acetylation/deacetylation

Histone acetylation is a reaction where an acetyl group is added usually to lysine residues at the N terminus of histone protein while histone deacetylation is the removal of the acetyl group. There are highly conserved sites of histone H3 lysines at amino-terminal amino-acid positions 9, 14, 18 and 23, and H4 lysines 5, 8, 12 and 16 that are frequently targeted for acetylation-related modifications (Shogren-Knaak, 2006). Histone acetylation is mediated by acetyl-coenzyme A, and in histone deacetylation the acetyl group is transferred to coenzyme A. Histone acetylation is catalyzed by histone acetyltransferases (HATs), while histone deacetylation is catalyzed by histone deacetylases (denoted by HDs or HDACs). There are three major classes of mammalian HDACs: Rpd3 (class 1), Hda1 (class II) and Sir2 (class III). Acetylation removes positive charges thereby reducing the affinity between histones and DNA. Thus, in most cases, histone acetylation enhances transcription while histone deacetylation represses transcription, but the reverse is seen as well (Reamon-Buettner and Borlak, 2007). Histone acetylation is also involved in processes such as replication and nucleosome assembly, higher order chromatin packing and interactions of non-histone proteins with nucleosomes. The neutralization of the basic charge of the histone tails by acetylation is thought to reduce their affinity for DNA and to alter histone–histone interactions between adjacent nucleosomes as well as the interactions of histones with other regulatory proteins (Reamon-Buettner and Borlak, 2007).

Although histone acetylation is broad, studies using HDAC inhibitors have demonstrated that the acetylation process is also necessarily specific. Although treating mice with HDAC inhibitors did not result in hyperacetylation, it did cause severe infertility (Fenic *et al.*, 2004). Trichostatin A (TSA)-treated animals had no evidence of H4 hyperacetylation in the round spermatid, but the number of spermatids was significantly reduced (Fenic *et al.*, 2004, 2008). The inability to detect the hyperacetylation following TSA treatment may be due to an increase in apoptosis in cells with abnormal acetylation levels, or due to a compensatory mechanism involving alternative HDACs that are insensitive to TSA (Pivot-Pajot *et al.*, 2003).

Histone phosphorylation/dephosphorylation

Histone proteins can be modified by the addition or removal of phosphate groups (Aihara *et al.*, 2004; Nowak and Corces, 2004). The addition of negatively charged phosphate groups to histone tails neutralizes their basic charge and is thought to reduce their affinity for DNA. Thus, many enzymes and receptors are switched "on" or "off" by phosphorylation and dephosphorylation (Reamon-Buettner and Borlak, 2007). Phosphorylation is catalyzed by histone kinases whereas dephosphorylation is catalyzed by histone phosphatases (Aihara *et al.*, 2004). Histone phosphorylation influences transcription, chromosome condensation, DNA repair and apoptosis. Among all post-translational modifications that occur on histone tails, phosphorylation is the one that establishes a direct link between chromatin remodeling and intracellular signaling pathways. Phosphorylation of H3 Ser10 is involved in chromosome condensation and subsequent segregation during mitosis/meiosis and in transcriptional activation (Nowak and Corces, 2004). The mechanism by which phosphorylation contributes to transcriptional activation is not fully understood. It has been found that several acetyl transferases have increased HAT activity on serine 10-phosphorylated substrates. Thus, phosphorylation may contribute to transcriptional activation through the stimulation of HAT activity on the same histone tail. Little is also known about gene expression and histone phosphorylation (Kouzarides, 2007).

Energy metabolism is a key factor supporting sperm function. ATP is one of the basic components in a sperm cell and is used not only as an energy source but also for protein phosphorylation in cell signaling and as a cofactor regulating protein function (Miki, 2007). Histone phosphorylation occurs at serine residues of all core histones and is generally associated with gene activation. However, H2Ax phosphorylation (also known as gH2Ax) in germ cells confers the formation of X/Y sex body during spermatogenesis and is a marker for telomere clustering and double-stranded breaks. H2Ax phosphorylation is dependent on the ataxia telangiectasia DNA repair and Rad3-related protein ATR, and on the tumor suppressor BRCA1. Together gH2Ax, ATR and BRCA1 initiate meiotic sex chromosome inactivation (MSCI), but to maintain MSCI throughout the pachytene stage there are many other epigenetic modifications including ubiquinated H2A that are localized to the XY body; however, the exact function each performs is unknown (Hoyer-Fender, 2003).

Recent studies that macrophage migration inhibitory factor (MIF) may play a physiological role in sperm capacitation but may have deleterious effects on sperm function at abnormal pathophysiological levels (due to abnormal phosphorylation events), resulting in endometriosis-associated infertility (Carli *et al.*, 2007)

Polycystic ovary syndrome (PCOS) is a common heterogeneous endocrine disorder associated with amenorrhoea (or oligomenorrhoea), hyperandrogenism, hirsutism, obesity, insulin resistance and an approximately seven-fold increased risk of type 2 diabetes mellitus (NIDDM – non-insulin dependent diabetes mellitus). The multiple biochemical pathways have been implicated in the pathogenesis of PCOS. Abnormal serine phosphorylation in the insulin receptor (IR) and 17,20-lyase activity (CYP17) may impair signal transduction accounting for a post-binding defect in insulin action (Jakubowski, 2005).

Histone ubiquitination/deubiquitination

Histone ubiquitination is a modification mediated by the attachment of ubiquitin (Ub), which is a 76-amino acid protein that is ubiquitously distributed and highly conserved throughout eukaryotic organisms (Zhang, 2003; Kerscher *et al.*, 2006). Ubiquitin has been linked to a variety of cellular processes including protein degradation, stress–response, cell-cycle regulation, protein trafficking, endocytosis signaling and transcriptional regulation. At least four lysine residues (11, 29, 48 and 63) on Ub can serve as attachment sites for further additions of Ub to generate a poly-Ub chain. Attachment of a Ub molecule to the side chain of a lysine residue in the acceptor protein is a complex process involving multi-enzyme-catalyzed steps including E1 activating, E2 conjugating and E3 ligase enzymes. Sequential ubiquitination and deubiquitination are both involved in transcriptional activation, likely mediated through histone methylation (Henry *et al.*, 2003).

The effect of ubiquination generally depends on the core histone modified: ubiquination of H2A associates with transcriptional repression, whereas mono-ubiquination of H2B is linked to transcriptional activation in sperm (Zhu *et al.*, 2005). In male germ cells, recruitment of ubiquinated H2A to the sex body and telomeres occurs long after gH2Ax incorporation, which indicates that H2A-ubiquination may be involved in maintaining silencing in the inactive chromatin, but not establishing MSCI.

Histone sumoylation

Histone proteins are modified by covalent attachment of small ubiquitin-like modifier (SUMO) to lysine residues. SUMO is a member of a growing family of ubiquitin-like proteins involved in post-translational modifications (Johnson, 2004; Iniquez-Lluhi, 2006; Kerscher *et al.*, 2006). Unlike ubiquitination, sumoylation of proteins has not been linked to protein degradation. In mammals, there are three members of the SUMO protein family: SUMO-1, SUMO-2 (SMT3a) and SUMO-3 (SMT3b), which are implicated in regulation of protein–protein interaction and localization, inhibition of ubiquitin-mediated degradation, and enhancement of transcriptional activities, thus participating in diverse cellular processes, including transcriptional regulation, nuclear transport, maintenance of genome integrity and signal transduction (Nathan *et al.*, 2006). Histone sumoylation can mediate gene silencing through recruitment of histone deacetylase and heterochromatin protein 1. Recently, it has been demonstrated that this modification plays important roles in the control of transcription by antagonizing histone acetylation (Nathan *et al.*, 2006). It has been shown that human testicular SUMO-1 has specific functions in heterochromatin organization, meiotic centromere function, and gene expression (Vigodner *et al.*, 2006). SUMO-1 may be involved in maintenance and/or protection of the autosomal SC. SUMO-2/3, though expressed similarly, may function separately and independently during pachytene in men (Brown *et al.*, 2008).

Histone biotinylation

The modification of histones through covalent attachment of the vitamin biotin has been described recently (Kothapalli *et al.*, 2005; Prasanth and Spector, 2007). This modification is mediated by holocarboxylase synthetase and biotinidase. Preliminary studies show that biotinylation of histones plays a role in processes such as cell proliferation, gene silencing and the cellular response to UV-induced DNA damage. Spermatogenesis and oogenesis are complex processes that involve proliferation and differentiation/maturation. These processes also require inactivation (silencing) of one of the two X-chromosomes and XY body during oogenesis and spermatogenesis respectively that may employ biotinylation for these activities. Any perturbations that can dysregulate these functions will eventually lead to development of pathological states.

RNA interference (RNAi) or RNA silencing

A large number of non-coding RNAs (ncRNAs) play an important role in regulating gene expressions, and advances in the identification and function of eukaryotic ncRNAs, e.g. microRNAs and their function in chromatin organization, gene expression, disease etiology, have been recently reviewed (Valencia-Sanchez *et al.*, 2006; Prasanth and Spector, 2007). Indeed, a comprehensive database (RNAdb) of mammalian ncRNAs, including a wide range of mammalian microRNAs, small nucleolar RNAs and larger mRNA-like ncRNAs, has been developed (Pang *et al.*, 2007). The regulatory pathways mediated by small RNAs are usually collectively referred to as RNA interference (RNAi) or RNA-mediated silencing and the subject of recent reviews (Kim and Rossi, 2007). Besides siRNAs and miRNAs, a new RNA silencing pathway involving small RNAs linked to the Argonaute family of proteins has been recently described (Prasanth and Spector, 2007; Carthew-Deutsher, 2009). These small RNAs in the germ-line are called repeat associated (ra) siRNAs in *Drosophila* and their counterpart in mammals is called Piwi-interacting RNAs (piRNAs). In contrast to siRNAs and miRNAs, rasi- and piRNAs do not arise from double-stranded precursors. The key proteins involved in the biosynthesis of the small RNAs localize to ribonucleoprotein particles, including nuage in male germ cells. Consistent with the more ubiquitous nature of Dicer and its microRNA end products, the absence of Dicer results in embryonic lethality, whereas the absence of the germ-line-specific piRNAs family members leads only to male spermatogenic arrest.

The microRNA pathways are crucial for general germ cell growth and differentiation. These pathways have recently been reported as testicular germ cell tumors, the most common cancer in young men. It has been shown that repeat-associated piRNAs suppress retrotransposon mRNAs. Thus, one could speculate that abnormal PIWI activity in the germ-line of a man could increase retrotransposon hopping, resulting in offspring that have an increased susceptibility to diseases, including infertility and testicular cancer, similar to defects observed in other "guardians" of the germ-line (Matzuk and Lamb, 2008).

Dicer1 has been shown to be required for differentiation of the mouse male germ-line (Maatouk *et al.*, 2008). Dicer is also necessary for postnatal differentiation of Müllerian duct mesenchyme-derived tissues of the female reproductive tract. The microRNAs play an important role in the interactions between ovarian germ and somatic cells, and expression of several intraovarian autocrine/paracrine regulators is a major contributing factor in the ovary (Tolubeydukhti *et al.*, 2008). Loss of Dicer within ovarian granulosa cells, luteal tissue, oocyte, oviduct and, potentially, the uterus has been shown to result in female infertility. Transferable quality blastocysts derived from infertile patients were shown to possess aberrant miRNA profiles (McCallie *et al.*, 2010). The development and function of the ovarian CL is a physiological process that appears to be regulated by miRNAs and requires Dicer1 function (Otsuka *et al.*, 2008). MicroRNA-224 was shown to be involved in transforming growth factor-beta-mediated mouse granulosa cell proliferation and granulosa cell function by targeting Smad4 (Yao *et al.*, 2010). MicroRNAs appear to be potent regulators of gene expression in endometriosis and its associated reproductive disorders, raising the prospect of using miRNAs as biomarkers and therapeutic tools in endometriosis (Teague *et al.*, 2010). Very recently, a study has shown bisphenol A (BPA) can alter miRNA expression in placental cells, a potentially novel mode of BPA toxicity (Avissar-Whiting *et al.*, 2010).

Normal and abnormal X chromosome inactivation

X chromosome inactivation is most commonly studied in the context of female mammalian development, where it performs an essential role in dosage compensation. However, another form of X-inactivation takes place in the male, during spermatogenesis, as germ cells enter meiosis. This second form of X-inactivation, called meiotic sex chromosome inactivation (MSCI), has emerged as a novel paradigm for studying the epigenetic regulation of gene expression. New studies have revealed that MSCI is a special example of a more general mechanism called meiotic silencing of unsynapsed chromatin (MSUC), which silences chromosomes that fail to pair with their homologous partners and, in doing so, may protect against aneuploidy in subsequent generations. Furthermore, failure in MSCI is emerging as an important etiological factor in meiotic sterility (James and Turner, 2007). MSCI is believed to result from meiotic silencing of unpaired DNA because the X and Y chromosomes remain largely unpaired throughout first meiotic prophase. However, unlike X-chromosome inactivation in female embryonic cells, where 25–30% of X-linked structural genes have been reported to escape inactivation, X-linked mRNA-encoding genes during spermatogenesis have failed to reveal any X-linked gene that escapes the silencing effects of MSCI in primary spermatocytes; many X-linked miRNAs are transcribed and processed in pachytene spermatocytes. This unprecedented escape from MSCI by these X-linked miRNAs suggests that they may participate in a critical function at this stage of spermatogenesis, including the possibility that they contribute to the process of MSCI itself, and/or that they may be essential for post-transcriptional regulation of autosomal mRNAs during the late meiotic and early postmeiotic stages of spermatogenesis (Song *et al.*, 2009). This also makes them a potential target for alteration by environmental factors.

Fertility therapy and epigenetic modifications

Some of the widely used therapeutic approaches, such as fertility medication (e.g., clomifene citrate) that stimulates the ovaries to "ripen" and release eggs, may result in local changes in the ability of tissues to repair the DNA damage as well as the abnormal methylation events *in situ*. *In vitro fertilization* (IVF), in which eggs are removed from the woman, fertilized and then placed in the woman's uterus, bypassing the fallopian tubes, involve several steps that can increase abnormal methylation and demethylation events. Variations on IVF include the use of donor eggs and/or sperm in IVF. This happens when a couple's eggs and/or sperm are unusable, or to avoid passing on a genetic disease. Intracytoplasmic sperm injection (ICSI) is the method in which a single sperm is injected directly into an egg; the fertilized egg is then placed in the woman's uterus as in IVF. Similarly, zygote intrafallopian transfer (ZIFT) is where eggs are removed from the woman, fertilized and then placed in the woman's fallopian tubes rather than the uterus.

Transgenerational effects of environmental factors on the germ-line in humans

There are several diseases that are caused by aberrant expression of imprinted genes. These include the developmental disorders Prader-Willi syndrome (PWS), Angelman syndrome (AS) and Beckwith–Wiedemann syndrome (BWS). PWS and AS are caused by the disruption of several maternally and paternally imprinted genes located on chromosome 15. The loss of SNRPN expression is most commonly associated with PWS, while the loss of UBE3A is most commonly associated with AS. All causes of BWS to date have been associated with alterations in the methylation state of one or more imprinted genes in the imprinted gene cluster. Assisted reproductive techniques (ART) have been associated with a statistically significant increased risk of AS and BWS in offspring. It is proposed that the frequency of imprinting disorders is increased as a consequence of *in vitro* culturing conditions, or chemical composition of the culture media, which can result in the loss of methylation on imprinted regions in either the oocyte or embryo as opposed to aberrant epigenetic state in male gametes. However, males with oligospermia have an increased frequency of defective methylation compared with normospermic males. This raises the possibility that hypomethylated paternally imprinted genes may contribute to imprinting errors and disease in ART conceived children. Similar to the exposure of rodents to dioxins or caloric restriction, in the human populations there have been many documented cases of changes in sex ratios following chemical exposure or after a natural disaster which may be consistent with altered epigenetic state across a population. For example, in 1976, the population of Seveso in Italy was exposed to the herbicide dioxin. Exposed males produced a higher percentage of female offspring (65%) compared with male offspring. Pesticide workers in several countries are still exposed to high levels of dioxin. An investigation conducted on Russian pesticide workers also found that male exposure to dioxin was associated with an increase in the number of female births (62%). It was proposed that exposure to dioxin affected sperm production in the testis leading to changes in the sex ratio. Similarly, after the Kobe earthquake in Japan, the 10-day war in Slovenia, and in California following the terrorist attacks of September 11, a decline in the sex ratio (male:female) at birth was observed. It has been proposed that stress related to a catastrophic event may have a negative effect on sperm production or function resulting in a decline in sex ratio. Alternatively, it could be interpreted that these studies reveal paternal effects similar to those documented in rodents (Anway *et al.*, 2005). It is of note that within these populations there is no documented evidence of elevated levels of sex reversal or infertility, suggesting that the transmission ratio distortion is a true change in X- vs. Y-bearing sperm (Zamudio *et al.*, 2008).

Other epigenetic mechanisms in female infertility

In endometriosis, altered progesterone receptor expression or diminished activity may lead to attenuated or dysregulated progesterone response and decreased expression of progesterone-responsive genes including HOX genes in the eutopic endometrium. Silencing of progesterone target genes by methylation is an epigenetic mechanism that mediates progesterone resistance. In turn, other mediators of endometrial receptivity that are regulated by HOX (homeodomain transcription factors) genes, such as pinopodes, alphavbeta3 integrin and IGFBP-1, are downregulated in endometriosis. HOXA10 hypermethylation has recently been demonstrated to silence HOXA10 gene expression and account for decreased HOXA10 in the endometrium of women with endometriosis. Since HOX genes are necessary for endometrial growth, differentiation and implantation, their dysregulation by abnormal methylation can affect the above-mentioned functions (Cakmak and Taylor, 2010). Moreover, altered expression of these imprinted genes such as IGF2 and H19 might affect implantation and their timely and appropriate activation (Korucuoglu *et al.*, 2010).

As mentioned earlier, superovulation or ovarian stimulation is currently an indispensable assisted reproductive technology (ART) for human subfertility/infertility treatment. However, recent increased frequencies of imprinting disorders have been attributed to ARTs. Significantly, for Angelman and Beckwith-Wiedemann syndromes, patients have been identified where ovarian stimulation was the only procedure used by the couple undergoing ART. Superovulation in a mouse model has shown to perturb genomic imprinting of both maternally and paternally expressed genes; loss of Snrpn, Peg3 and Kcnq1ot1 and gain of H19 imprinted methylation were observed. This perturbation was dose dependent, with aberrant imprinted methylation more frequent at the high hormone dosage. Superovulation is thought to primarily affect oocyte development; thus, effects were expected to be limited to maternal alleles. However, both maternal and paternal H19 methylation were perturbed by superovulation. Thus, superovulation seems to have dual effects during oogenesis, disrupting acquisition of imprints in growing oocytes, as well as maternal-effect gene products subsequently required for imprint maintenance during preimplantation development (Market-Velker *et al.*, 2010).

ROS (REACTIVE OXYGEN SPECIES)-INDUCED REPRODUCTIVE TOXICITY

ROS include a wide variety of molecules, such as radical (hydroxyl ion, superoxide, nitric oxide, peroxyl, etc.) and non-radical (ozone, singlet oxygen, lipid peroxide, hydrogen peroxide) oxygen derivatives (Agarwal and Prabakaran, 2005). Reactive nitrogen species (nitrous oxide, peroxynitrite, nitroxyl ion, etc.) are also a class of free radicals derived from nitrogen and considered a subclass of ROS (Darley-Usmar *et al.*, 1995). Various cellular components, such as lipids, proteins, nucleic acids and sugars are potential targets of OS. The extent of OS-induced damage depends on the type, duration and amount of ROS involved, and on extracellular factors such as temperature, oxygen tension and the composition of the surrounding environment (Makker *et al.*, 2009).

ROS are toxic to human spermatozoa; however, small amounts of ROS are necessary for spermatozoa to acquire fertilizing capabilities including acrosome reaction, hyperactivation, motility and capacitation (Aitken, 1997, 1999; Gagnon *et al.*, 1991). Immature, morphologically abnormal spermatozoa and seminal leukocytes are the main sources of ROS in human ejaculates (Aitken and West, 1990). Spermatozoa are rich in mitochondria because they need a constant supply of energy for their motility. However, dysfunctional mitochondria can lead to increased production of ROS. Spermatozoa, due to the paucity of cytoplasmic enzymes, are unable to repair oxidative damage (Makker *et al.*, 2009). It has been shown that oxidative stress occurs even in patients with a very low seminal leukocyte count (between 0 and 1×10^6/ml), and a rise in ROS occurs with an increase in leukocyte count. The prostate gland and the seminal vesicles are the main sources of these peroxidase-positive leukocytes in human ejaculate. Leukocytes may be activated in response to various stimuli such as infection and inflammation (Pasqualotto *et al.*, 2005), and these activated leukocytes can produce up to 100-fold higher amounts of ROS compared with non-activated leukocytes (Plante *et al.*, 1994).

ROS in assisted reproductive techniques (ART)

ROS-induced DNA damage may have important clinical implications in the context of ART. Repeated cycles of centrifugation involved in conventional sperm preparation techniques used for ART can increase the production of ROS (Agarwal *et al.*, 1994), thus resulting in high percentage of sperm that may have damaged DNA (Kodama *et al.*, 1997). During procedures like intrauterine insemination (IUI) or *in vitro* fertilization (IVF) any such damage may not be a cause of concern because the collateral peroxidative damage to the sperm plasma membrane ensures that fertilization cannot occur with a DNA-damaged sperm (Makker *et al.*, 2009).

However, in procedures like ICSI (intracytoplasmic sperm injection), this natural selection barrier is bypassed and a spermatozoon with damaged DNA is directly injected into the oocyte. There are number of factors such as oocytes and embryo metabolism, cumulus cells, leukocyte contamination during sperm preparation and culture media in ART procedures that can result in an increase of ROS production (Bedaiwy *et al.*, 2004; Agarwal *et al.*, 2005; Oral *et al.*, 2006).

Smoking, oxidative stress and infertility

Tobacco smoke consists of several (approximately 4,000) compounds such as alkaloids, nitrosamines and inorganic molecules. A significant proportion of these substances are reactive oxygen or nitrogen species. Significant positive association has been reported between active smoking and sperm DNA fragmentation, as well as axonemal damage and decreased sperm count (Makker *et al.*, 2009). Smoking has been shown to affect the quality and quantity of sperm present within a male. Sperm from smokers has been found to be significantly more sensitive to acid-induced DNA denaturation than that from non-smokers because the smokers' sperm has been shown to contain higher levels of DNA strand breaks (Potts *et al.*, 1999). In another study consisting of 655 smokers and 1,131 non-smokers, cigarette smoking was shown to be associated with a significant decrease in sperm density (−15.3%), total sperm count (−17.5%) and total number of motile sperm (−16.6%) (Künzle *et al.*, 2003).

Chemical-induced ROS in infertility

In a transitional epidemiological study on the effect of polycyclic aromatic hydrocarbon conducted on a large population of men, with information on several environmental exposures and measures of both morphological parameters and DNA adducts in sperm, with a follow-up for 1 year, to assess the fertility status, the results indicated that PAH-DNA adducts are a possible marker of fertility, since among the various factors considered (smoking, alcohol, occupational exposure, sperm morphology), DNA adducts was the only parameter significantly associated with the ability to conceive after 1 year (Gaspari *et al.*, 2003). It has been shown that testicular toxicity by nickel compounds may be related to enhanced production of reactive oxygen species, probably mediated through oxidative damage to macromolecules, including damage to DNA (Doreswamy *et al.*, 2004).

ROS-induced sperm DNA damage

Spermatozoa DNA is protected from ROS injury by two factors: (1) characteristic tight packaging of sperm DNA and (2) the antioxidants in seminal plasma (Twigg *et al.*, 1998). Artificially produced ROS in the sperm can cause DNA damage in the form of modification of all bases, production of base-free sites, deletions, frame shifts, DNA cross-links and chromosomal rearrangements (Kemal *et al.*, 2000). Increased ROS production can increase the frequencies of single- and double-strand DNA breaks (Aitken and Krausz, 2001; Spiropoulos *et al.* 2002). Artificially enhanced ROS also can cause various types of gene mutations such as point mutations and polymorphism, resulting in decreased semen quality (Spiropoulos *et al.*, 2002; Sharma *et al.*, 2004). Other mechanisms including denaturation and DNA base-pair oxidation also may be involved (Kodama *et al.*, 1997). If the extent of DNA damage is small, spermatozoa can undergo self-repair; besides the oocyte also is capable of repairing damaged DNA of spermatozoa (Agarwal *et al.*, 2005, 2008a,b). Extensive damage can lead to apoptosis and embryo fragmentation resulting in decreased fertilization rates and poor embryo cleavage (Sakkas *et al.*, 1998). Deletions in the Y chromosome of the offspring can occur if the DNA damage in its component is high and not repairable, leading to infertility (Aitken and Krausz, 2001).

ROS and apoptosis in reproductive tissues

Apoptosis is a genetically controlled, non-inflammatory response to tissue damage characterized by a series of morphological and biochemical changes (Grunewald *et al.*, 2005). It is an important mechanism by which the male reproductive tissue eliminates abnormal spermatozoa, thus maintaining the nursing capacity of the Sertoli cells (Sinha and Swerdloff, 1999). Abnormally high levels of ROS induction can disrupt the inner and outer mitochondrial membranes, inducing the release of the cytochrome-C protein and activating the caspases and apoptosis (Makker *et al.*, 2009). Fas-mediated apoptosis pathway in sperm is another mechanism that is not dependent on ROS induction (Lee *et al.*, 1997). Although the Fas protein often leads to apoptosis, some of the Fas-labeled cells may escape apoptosis through abortive apoptosis. This results in a failure to clear all of the spermatozoa destined for elimination and thus leads to a large population of abnormal spermatozoa in the semen (Makker *et al.*, 2009). This failure to clear Fas-positive spermatozoa may be due to a dysfunction at one or more levels. First, the production of spermatozoa may not be enough to trigger apoptosis in men with hypospermatogenesis. In this case, Fas-positive spermatogonia may escape the signal to undergo apoptosis. Second, Fas-positive spermatozoa also may exist because of problems in activating Fas-mediated apoptosis. In this scenario, apoptosis is aborted and fails to clear spermatozoa that are earmarked for elimination by apoptosis (Makker *et al.*, 2009). In men with abnormal sperm parameters (oligozoospermia, azoospermia), the percentage of Fas-positive spermatozoa can be as high as 50%. Samples with low sperm concentrations are more likely to have a high proportion of Fas-positive spermatozoa (Sakkas *et al.*, 1999). Mitochondrial exposure to ROS results in the release of apoptosis inducing factor (AIF), which directly interacts with the DNA and leads to DNA fragmentation. Activation of caspases 8, 9, 1 and 3 may also be involved (Cande *et al.*, 2002; Makker *et al.*, 2009).

Effect of cell phone use on male reproductive system: ROS connection

A number of recent reports have suggested a possible link between cell phone use and male infertility (Fejes *et al.*, 2005; Wdowiak, 2007; Agarwal *et al.*, 2008a,b; Baste *et al.*, 2008). In addition to the epidemiological studies, the effects of RF-EMW are well studied in animal studies and *in vitro* studies on human semen. Many studies have indicated that EMW decreases the size of the testicular organs. A decrease in the diameter of the seminiferous tubules (Dasdag *et al.*, 1999,

2003) has been reported after exposure to radiofrequency radiations. Ozguner *et al.* (2005) demonstrated a decrease in seminiferous tubular diameter and epithelium thickness after applying RF-EMW of 869 to 894 MHz. These results support the study by Saunders and Kowalczuk (1981) of significant degeneration of the seminiferous epithelium in mice. Wang *et al.* (2008) suggested that RF-EMW might change the permeability of the blood–testis barrier. RF-EMW-mediated ROS formation can lead to heat shock protein (hsp) and phosphorylation, which can alter the secretion of growth factors. This, in turn, can increase the permeability of the blood–brain barrier. The same mechanism might be involved in the RF-EMW-mediated increase in the blood–testis barrier. RF-EMW can lead to ROS. RF-EMW-mediated ROS in semen might be responsible for decline in motility and viability of spermatozoa. De Iuliis *et al.* (2009) reported increase in ROS formation and higher DNA damage due to RF-EMW. Previously, Aitken *et al.* (2005) reported significant damage to the mitochondrial and nuclear genome in epididymal spermatozoa of mice exposed to RF-EMW (900 MHz) for 12 h a day for 7 days.

MOLECULAR TOXICOLOGICAL MECHANISMS OF PATHOGENESIS IN REPRODUCTIVE GENETIC SYNDROMES

Cryptorchidism

Cryptorchidism is one of the most frequent congenital birth defects in male children (2–4% in full-term male births), and it has the potential to impact the health and fertility of the human male, as it can lead to reduced fertility and testicular cancer. There has been a significant increase in the prevalence of cryptorchidism over the last few decades (Foresta *et al.*, 2008). Cryptorchidism is considered a complex disease and is seen as one of the many syndromic features in several syndromes and hence the etiology of cryptorchidism remains for the most part unknown. Testicular descent from intra-abdominal location into the bottom of the scrotum is regulated by the Leydig cell-derived hormones testosterone and insulin-like factor 3. There are abundant amounts of research data from animal studies that support a genetic cause, whereas the genetic contribution to human cryptorchidism is an emerging field of scientific research. Current genetic causes include mutations in the gene for insulin-like factor 3 and its receptor and in the androgen receptor gene. Moreover, some chromosomal alterations, above all the Klinefelter syndrome, are also frequently involved. Environmental factors including endocrine disruptors of testicular descent might also contribute to the etiology of cryptorchidism and its increased incidence in recent years (Foresta *et al.*, 2008). Furthermore, polymorphisms in different genes have recently been investigated as contributing risk factors for cryptorchidism, alone or by influencing susceptibility to endocrine disruptors.

Testicular dysgenesis syndrome (TDS)

There has been a steady decline in semen quality in many Western countries, and part of the explanation may be decreasing male fecundity. A hypothesis has been put forward that decreasing semen quality may be associated with a testicular dysgenesis syndrome (TDS), a spectrum of disorders such as cryptorchidism (undescended testes), penile malformations (e.g., hypospadias, a congenital malformation with abnormal placement of the external urethral orifice) and testicular cancer that may result from an irreversible developmental disorder originating in early fetal life. Thus, TDS comprises various aspects of impaired gonadal development and function (Joensen *et al.*, 2008). A growing body of evidence, including animal models and research in human beings, points to lifestyle factors and endocrine disruptors as risk factors for TDS. The emerging role of Leydig cell dysfunction with subsequent decreased testosterone levels in the pathogenesis of TDS has been advocated (Joensen *et al.*, 2008). Patients with TDS-related symptoms present within a range of severity: at the mild end with slight impairment of spermatogenesis and at the severe end of the range with all of the above-mentioned symptoms. The risk of testicular cancer increases with the severity of symptoms, and an association between decreased male fertility and testicular cancer, as well as its pre-invasive precursor, carcinoma *in situ* (CIS), is now well documented (Berthelsen, 1987; Møller and Skakkebæk, 1999; Baker *et al.*, 2005).

A growing body of evidence, including animal models (Sharpe, 2006) and research in human beings, points to commonly used chemicals ubiquitous in our environment, such as phthalates and persistent pesticides (Sharpe, 2006; Joensen *et al.*, 2008). TDS patients have higher levels of luteinizing hormone (LH) and follicle-stimulating hormone (FSH), as well as a tendency towards lower levels of testosterone indicating Leydig cell dysfunction or defect in Sertoli cells. US and Danish observational studies (Andersson *et al.*, 2007) of population-level serum testosterone and sex hormone-binding globulin (SHBG) concentrations suggested an age-independent decrease in testosterone and SHBG levels over the last 20 years that cannot entirely be explained by health and lifestyle factors.

The clinical symptoms of TDS are thought to originate in early fetal life and share risk factors. Formation of the testis and its early development are both hormone independent, but later testosterone insufficiency may contribute to dysgenetic tubule formation. Various animal models, as well as patients with complete androgen insensitivity syndrome, provide some evidence that androgens are important for early proliferation of Sertoli cells. Most severe forms of TDS observed in patients with disorders of sex differentiation have a genetic cause (e.g., mosaicism for sex chromosome aneuploidy). There are also several epidemiological studies suggesting an association between early phthalate exposure and male reproductive health symptoms, including maternal phthalate exposure during pregnancy and decreased ano-genital length in male infants (Swan *et al.*, 2005) and phthalates in breast milk and changes in the hypothalamic–pituitary–gonadal axis in male offspring (Main *et al.*, 2006). The proposed mechanisms were suppression of gonadotropin secretion via enhanced negative feedback by estrogens, or impairment of Leydig cell development, leading to inadequate testosterone production. More direct antiandrogenic mechanisms have since emerged, namely suppression of androgen production, suppression of androgen receptor expression or suppression of secretion of insulin-like factor-3 by fetal Leydig cells (Sharpe, 2003).

In utero exposure of rats to phthalates such as DBP with a consequential range of dysgenetic features in the male offspring has many similarities with TDS in human beings. This spectrum of disorders in rats has been termed the "phthalate syndrome", first coined in 2003 (Gray and Foster, 2003), and consists of dysgenetic seminiferous tissue, multinucleated gonocytes, as well as reduced androgen production and abnormal Leydig cell aggregation seen in rats when exposed to phthalates in fetal life. These Leydig cell abnormalities are proliferative lesions of developmental origin, as they are seen antenatally in phthalate-exposed male rats. Lesions resembling human Leydig cell adenomas were seen in male rats exposed before birth to DBP, but were dissimilar to traditional Leydig cell adenomas as the Leydig cells were poorly differentiated and the lesions contained aberrant seminiferous tubules (Barlow *et al.*, 2004).

CONCLUDING REMARKS AND FUTURE DIRECTIONS

An accumulation of extensive molecular and genetic data has revolutionized the approaches to diagnostic, prognostic, management and treatment aspects of infertility in humans and livestock. This has also resulted in explosion of scientific research in various research areas pertinent to male and female reproductive biology, reproductive toxicology and clinical practice in andrology, urology and obstetrics and gynecology. At the basic research level, a large body of genetic and molecular data with reference to male and female infertility has resulted in identifying several disease causing genes that affect germ cell migration, germ cell differentiation and viable gamete production. Major genes involved in the initiation, development and proper functioning of both male and female reproductive organ systems were identified. Novel mechanisms of gene regulation called epigenetic control have been identified and their role in altering and transmitting the altered gene expression pattern in successive generations of cell cycles and lifecycles were described. This combined knowledge can used to develop novel approaches for diagnosis and treatment of reproductive toxicology and infertility related clinical scenarios.

With the ever-increasing demand for conceiving healthy biological children in infertility clinics around the globe, more effective screening of the gamete genome of the infertile couples to rule out the possibilities of both static and epigenome abnormalities can be initiated. Drugs targeting epigenetic mechanisms are currently being tested in clinical trials for several disorders (Simonini *et al.*, 2006; McGowan and Szyf, 2010). Better understanding of the mechanisms through which different environmental exposures modify male and female germ cell epigenetic processes may facilitate strategies to prevent and reverse deleterious environmentally driven epigenetic alterations. The dynamic nature of epigenetic regulation, in contrast to the virtually static nature of the gene sequence, provides a mechanism for reprogramming gene function in response to changes in lifestyle activities (McGowan and Szyf, 2010). In this way, epigenetics may provide explanations for well-defined environmental effects on phenotypes.

Assisted reproduction techniques may show significant improvement in reducing the incidence of unpredictable scenarios of unwanted epigenetic changes leading to dysregulated methylation and or imprinting, by *in vitro* supplementation of antioxidants and metal chelators to achieve a better success (Sikka, 2004). Many compounds, like rebamipide, pentoxyfylline, vitamins E and C, SOD, catalase, etc., have been used to protect the sperm genome against ROS damage. Newer sperm preparation techniques such as density gradient centrifugation, glass wool filtration and migration-sedimentation have significantly reduced the level of ROS by removing leucocytes (Makker *et al.*, 2009). Anticipated developments in epigenetics have been described by the National Institutes of Health (Bethesda, MD, USA) as an emerging frontier of science and there is ample evidence of burgeoning interest in the field in many biological sciences and especially research on the biological determinants of health. This aspect is best illustrated by the moves to initiate the Human Epigenome Project, which aims to identify, catalog and interpret genome-wide methylation patterns of all human genes in all major tissues. It is possible that more advanced and different technologies such as positron emission tomography scanning will be sufficiently powerful and sensitive to provide non-invasive whole-body imaging of the methylome in specific tissues. In addition, based on current accumulated evidence, epigenomic marks record a wide variety of environmental exposures which can be used as an epigenetic signature for each individual, so that medical therapy and nutritional benefits can be personalized.

Furthermore, the following future directions can help protect various life forms (including humans and livestock) from accumulating harmful genetic loads both static and epigenomic in origin:

1. Identify more genes that may be involved in normal/abnormal sexual differentiation, germ cell migration, germ cell maturation and function, so that proper diagnostic, prognostic and treatment protocols can be developed. It is well accepted that there are several hundred genes that are involved in reproduction structure and function of which only few are identified and characterized.
2. Identify those genes (from among the gene pool of already discovered and yet to be identified) that may either increase or reduce the pathological outcome after exposures to toxicants.
3. Identify more genes, contributing to altered disease susceptibility, that are epigenetically deregulated by dietary and other environmental exposures.
4. Identify dose levels and time scales for environmental (and nutritional) factors to make the epigenomic and other genomic markings (such as deletions or duplications of seemingly innocuous nature) that may result in disease phenotype after several generations.
5. Identify various periods of the life course (or other circumstances such as infantile, early childhood, reproductively active periods and aging) that make the genome especially vulnerable to altered epigenetic and static markings by environmental and dietary factors.
6. Identify novel modes of interventions to modulate the adverse effects of other environmental exposures, e.g. xenobiotics, or of ageing on reproductive health.

REFERENCES

Adamsson NA, Brokken LJ, Paranko J, Toppari J (2008) In vivo and in vitro effects of flutamide and diethylstilbestrol on fetal testicular steroidogenesis in the rat. *Reprod Toxicol* **25:** 76–83.

Agarwal A, Allamaneni SSR, Nallella KP, George AT, Mascha E (2005) Correlation of reactive oxygen species (ROS) levels with fertilization rate following in vitro fertilization (IVF): a meta-analysis. *Fertil Steril* **84:** 228–31.

Agarwal A, Deepinder F, Sharma RK, Ranga G, Li J (2008a) Effect of cell phone usage on semen analysis in men attending infertility clinic: an observational study. *Fertil Steril* **89:** 124–8.

Agarwal A, Desai NR, Makker K, Varghese A, Mouradi R, Sabanegh E, Sharma R (2008b) Effects of radiofrequency electromagnetic waves (RF-EMW) from cellular phones on human ejaculated semen: an in vitro pilot study. *Fertil Steril* **92:** 1318–25.

Agarwal A, Ikemoto I, Loughlin KR (1994) Relationship of sperm parameters with levels of reactive oxygen species in semen specimens. *J Urol* **152:** 107–10.

Agarwal A, Prabakaran SA (2005) Mechanism, measurement, and prevention of oxidative stress in male reproductive physiology. *Indian J Exp Biol* **43:** 963–74.

Ahmadi A, Ng SC (1999) Developmental capacity of damaged spermatozoa. *Hum Reprod* **14:** 2279–85.

Aihara H, Nakagawa T, Yasui K, Ohta T, Hirose S, Dhomae N, Takio K, KanekoM, TakeshimaY, Muramatsu M, Ito T (2004) Nucleosomal histone kinase-1 phosphorylates H2A Thr 119 during mitosis in the early Drosophila embryo. *Genes Dev* **18:** 877–88.

Aitken RJ (1997) Molecular mechanisms regulating human sperm function. *Mol Hum Reprod* **3:** 169–73.

Aitken RJ (1999) The Amoroso Lecture. The human spermatozoon – a cell in crisis? *J Reprod Fertil* **115:** 1–7.

Aitken RJ, Bennetts LE, Sawyer D, Wiklendt AM, King BV (2005) Impact of radio frequency electromagnetic radiation on DNA integrity in the male germline. *Int J Androl* **28:** 171–9.

Aitken RJ, Krausz C (2001) Oxidative stress, DNA damage and the Y chromosome. *Reproduction* **122:** 497–506.

Aitken RJ, West KM (1990) Analysis of the relationship between reactive oxygen species production and leucocyte infiltration in fractions of human semen separated on Percoll gradients. *Int J Androl* **13:** 433–51.

Anderson D (2001) Genetic and reproductive toxicity of butadiene and isoprene. *Chemico-Biol Interact* **135–136:** 65–80.

Andersson AM, Jensen TK, Juul A, Petersen JH, Jørgensen T, Skakkebæk NE (2007) Secular decline in male testosterone and sex hormone binding globulin serum levels: a study of more than 5000 men participating in Danish population surveys. *J Clin Endocrinol Metab* **92:** 4696–705.

Anway MD, Cupp AS, Uzumcu M, Skinner MK (2005) Epigenetic transgenerational actions of endocrine disruptors and male fertility. *Science* **308:** 1466–9.

Anway MD, Leathers C, Skinner MK (2006) Endocrine disruptor vinclozolin induced epigenetic transgenerational adult-onset disease. *Endocrinology* **147:** 5515–23.

Avissar-Whiting M, Veiga KR, Uhl KM, Maccani MA, Gagne LA, Moen EL, Marsit CJ (2010) Bisphenol A exposure leads to specific microRNA alterations in placental cells. *Reprod Toxicol* Apr 24. [Epub ahead of print]

Baker JA, Buck GM, Vena JE, Moysich KB (2005) Fertility patterns prior to testicular cancer diagnosis. *Cancer Causes Control* **16:** 295–9.

Barlow NJ, McIntyre BS, Foster PM (2004) Male reproductive tract lesions at 6, 12, and 18 months of age following in utero exposure to di(n-butyl) phthalate. *Toxicol Pathol* **32:** 79–90.

Baste V, Riise T, Moen BE (2008) Radiofrequency electromagnetic fields; male infertility and sex ratio of offspring. *Eur J Epidemiol* **23:** 369–77.

Bedaiwy MA, Falcone T, Mohamed MS, Aleem AA, Sharma RK, Worley SE, Thornton J, Agarwal A (2004) Differential growth of human embryos in vitro: role of reactive oxygen species. *Fertil Steril* **82:** 593–600.

Berlinguer F, Madeddu M, Pasciu V, Succu S,Spezzigu A, Satta V, Mereu P, Leoni GG, Naitana S (2009) Semen molecular and cellular features: these parameters can reliably predict subsequent ART outcome in a goat model *Reproduct Biol Endocrinol* **7:** 125.

Berthelsen JG (1987) Testicular cancer and fertility. *Int J Androl* **10:** 371–80.

Bian Q, Xu LC, Wang SL, Xia YK, Tan LF, Chen JF, Song L, Chang HC, Wang XR (2004) Study on the relation between occupational fenvalerate exposure and spermatozoa DNA damage of pesticide factory workers. *Occup Environ Med* **61:** 999–1005.

Boissonnas CC, Abdalaoui HE, Haelewyn V, Fauque P, Dupont JM, Gut I, Vaiman D, Jouannet P, Tost J, Jammes H (2010) Specific epigenetic alterations of IGF2-H19 locus in spermatozoa from infertile men. *Eur J Hum Genet* **18(1):** 73–80.

Borch J, Dalgaard M, Ladefoged O (2005) Early testicular effects in rats perinatally exposed to DEHP in combination with DEHA – apoptosis assessment and immunohistochemical studies. *Reprod Toxicol* **19:** 517–25.

Borch J, Metzdorff SB, Vinggaard AM, Brokken L, Dalgaard M (2006) Mechanisms underlying the anti-androgenic effects of diethylhexyl phthalate in fetal rat testis. *Toxicology* **223:** 144–55.

Brown PW, Hwang K, Schlegel PN, Morris PL (2008) Small ubiquitin-related modifier (SUMO)-1, SUMO-2/3 and SUMOylation are involved with centromeric heterochromatin of chromosomes 9 and 1 and proteins of the synaptonemal complex during meiosis in men. *Hum Reprod* **23(12):** 2850–7.

Cakmak H, Taylor HS (2010) Molecular mechanisms of treatment resistance in endometriosis: the role of progesterone-hox gene interactions. *Semin Reprod Med* **28(1):** 69–74.

Cande C, Cecconi F, Dessen P, Kroemer G (2002) Apoptosis-inducing factor (AIF): key to the conserved caspase-independent pathways of cell death? *J Cell Sci* **115:** 4727–34.

Carli C, Leclerc P, Metz CN, Akoum A (2007) Direct effect of macrophage migration inhibitory factor on sperm function: possible involvement in endometriosis-associated infertility. *Fertil Steril* **88 (4 Suppl.):** 1240–7.

Carlsen E, Giwercman A, Keiding N, Skakkebaek NE (1992) Evidence for decreasing quality of semen during past 50 years. *Bri Med J* **305:** 609–13.

Carthew RW (2006) Molecular biology. A new RNA dimension to genome control. *Science* **313:** 305–6.

Chang HS, Anway MD, Rekow SS, Skinner MK (2006) Transgenerational epigenetic imprinting of the male germline by endocrine disruptor exposure during gonadal sex determination. *Endocrinology* **147:** 5524–41.

Chen T, Hevi S, Gay F, Tsujimoto N, HeT, Zhang B, UedaY, Li E (2007) Complete inactivation of DNMT1 leads to mitotic catastrophe in human cancer cells. *Nat Genet* **39:** 391–6.

Dahl C, Guldberg P (2003) DNA methylation analysis techniques. *Biogerontology* **4:** 233–50.

Damodaran TV, Greenfield ST, Patel AG, Dressman HK, Lin SA, Abou-Donia MB (2006a) Toxicogenomic studies of the rat brain at an early time point following acute sarin exposure. *Neurochem Res* **31:** 361–81.

Damodaran TV, Gupta RP, Attia MK, Abou-Donia MB (2009) DFP initiated early alterations of PKA-p-CREB pathway and differential persistencies of beta tubulin subtypes in the CNS of hens contributes to OPIDN. *Toxicol Appl Pharmacol* **240:** 132–42.

Damodaran TV, Jones HK, Patel AG, Abou-Donia MB (2003) Sarin (nerve agent GB)-induced differential expression of mRNA coding for acetylcholinesterase gene in the rat nervous system. *Biochem Pharmacol* **65:** 2041–7.

Damodaran TV, Marimuthu KM (1988) Human male infertility: study of 190 infertile males by mitotic karyotyping, meiotic analysis, histological evaluation and pedigree analysis. *Genome Research* **(Suppl. 1)**.

Damodaran TV, Patel AG, Greenfield ST, Dressman HK, Lin SA, Abou-Donia MB (2006b) Gene expression profiles of the rat brain immediately and 3 months following acute sarin exposure. *Biochem Pharmacol* **71:** 497–520.

Dasdag S, Akdag MZ, Ulukaya E, Uzunlar AK, Yegin D (2008) Mobile phone exposure does not induce apoptosis on spermatogenesis in rats. *Arch Med Res* **39:** 40–4.

Dasdag S, Ketani MA, Akdag Z, Ersay AR, Sari I, Demirtas OC, Celik MS (1999) Whole-body microwave exposure emitted by cellular phones and testicular function of rats. *Urol Res* **27:** 219–23.

Dasdag S, Zulkuf Akdag M, Aksen F, Yilmaz F, Bashan M, Mutlu Dasdag M, Salih Celik M (2003) Whole body exposure of rats to microwaves emitted from a cell phone does not affect the testes. *Bioelectromagnetics* **24:** 182–8.

De Iuliis GN, Newey RJ, King BV, Aitken RJ (2009) Mobile phone radiation induces reactive oxygen species production and DNA damage in human spermatozoa in vitro. *PLoS One* **4:** e6446.

De Mas P, Daudin M, Vincent M-C, Bourrouillou G, Calvas P, Mieusset R, Bujan L (2001) Increased aneuploidy in spermatozoa from testicular tumour patients after chemotherapy with cisplatin, etoposide and bleomycin. *Hum Reprod* **16:** 1204–8.

Di Croce L, Buschbeck M, Gutierrez A, Joval I, Morey L, Villa R, Minucci S (2004) Altered epigenetic signals in human disease. *Cancer Biol Ther* **3:** 831–7.

Doreswamy K, Shrilatha B, Rajashkumar T, Muralidhara (2004) Nickel-induced oxidative stress in testis of mice: evidence of DNA damage and genotoxic effects. *J Androl* **25:** 996–1003.

Eckhardt F, Lewin J, Cortese R, Rakyan VK, Attwood J, Burger M, Burton J, Cox TV, Davies R, Down TA, Haefliger C, Horton R, Howe K, Jackson DK, Kunde J, Koenig C, Liddle J, Niblett D, Otto T, Pettett R, Seemann S, Thompson C, West T, Rogers J, Olek A, Berlin K, Beck S (2006) DNA methylation profiling of human chromosomes 6, 20 and 22. *Nat Genet* **38(12):** 1378–85.

Egger G, Liang G, Aparicio A, Jones PA (2004) Epigenetics in human disease and prospects for epigenetic therapy. *Nature* **429:** 457–63.

Elespuru RK, Sankaranarayanan K (2007) New approaches to assessing the effects of mutagenic agents on the integrity of the human genome. *Mut Res* **616:** 83–9.

Erenpreiss J, Bungum M, Spano M, Elzanaty S, Orbidans J, Giwercman A (2006) Intra-individual variation in sperm chromatin structure assay parameters in men from infertile couples: clinical implications. *Hum Reprod* **21:** 2061–4.

Farthing CR, Ficz G, Ng RK, Chan CF, Andrews S, Dean W, Hemberger M, Reik W (2008) Global mapping of DNA methylation in mouse promoters reveals epigenetic reprogramming of pluripotency genes. *PLoS Genetics* **4:** e1000116.

Fazzari MJ, Greally JM (2004). Epigenomics: beyond CpG islands. *Nat Rev Genet* 5:446–55.

Fejes I, Zavaczki Z, Szollosi J, Koloszar S, Daru J, Kovacs L, Pal A (2005) Is there a relationship between cell phone use and semen quality? *Arch Androl* **51:** 385–93.

Fenic I, Hossain HM, Sonnack V, Tchatalbachev S, Thierer F, Trapp J, Failing K, Edler KS, Bergmann M, Jung M, Chakraborty T, Steger K (2008) In vivo application of histone deacetylase inhibitor trichostatin-A impairs murine male meiosis. *J Androl* **29:** 172–85.

Fenic I, Sonnack V, Failing K, Bergmann M, Steger K (2004) In vivo effects of histone-deacetylase inhibitor trichostatin-A on murine spermatogenesis. *J Androl* **25:** 811–18.

Fischle W, Wang Y, Allis CD (2003) Histone and chromatin cross-talk. *Curr Opin Cell Biol* **15:** 172–83.

Foote RH (2003) Fertility estimation: a review of past experience and future prospects. *Anim Reprod Sci* **75:** 119–39.

Foresta C, Zuccarello D, Garolla A, Ferlin A (2008) Role of genes and environment in human cryptorchidism. *Endoc Rev* **29:** 560–80.

Gagnon C, Iwasaki A, De Lamirande E, Kovalski N (1991) Reactive oxygen species and human spermatozoa. *Ann NY Acad Sci* **637:** 436–44.

Garcia-Cruz R, Roig I, Robles P, Scherthan H, Garcia Caldés M (2009) ATR, BRCA1 and gammaH2AX localize to unsynapsed chromosomes at the pachytene stage in human oocytes. ATR, BRCA1 and gammaH2AX localize to unsynapsed chromosomes at the pachytene stage in human oocytes. *Reprod Biomed Online* **18:** 37–44.

Garrido N, Remohí J, Martínez-Conejero JA, García-Herrero S, Pellicer A, Meseguer M (2008) Contribution of sperm molecular features to embryo quality and assisted reproduction success. *Reprod Biomed Online* **17:** 855–65.

Gaspari L, Chang SS, Santella RM, Garte S, Pedotti P, Taioli E (2003) Polycyclic aromatic hydrocarbon-DNA adducts in human sperm as a marker of DNA damage and infertility. *Mut Res* **535:** 155–60.

Genesca A, Caballin M, Miro R, Benet J, Bonfill X, Egozcue J (1990) Human sperm chromosomes. Long-term effect of cancer treatment. *Cancer Genet Cytogenet* **46:** 251–60.

Godmann GI, Lambrot RA, Kimmins S (2009) The dynamic epigenetic program in male germ cells: its role in spermatogenesis, testis cancer, and its response to the environment. *Microsc Res Tech* **72:** 603–19.

Grant PA (2001) A tale of histone modifications. *Genome Biol* 2(4). REVIEWS0003.

Gray LE Jr, Foster PMD (2003) Significance of experimental studies for assessing adverse effects of endocrine-disrupting chemicals. *Pure Appl Chem* **75:** 2125–41.

Grunewald S, Paasch U, Said TM, Sharma RK, Glander HJ, Agarwal A (2005) Caspase activation in human spermatozoa in response to physiological and pathological stimuli. *Fertil Steril* **83 (Suppl. 1):** 1106–12.

Hammoud SS, Purwar J, Pflueger C, Cairns BR, Carrell DT (2009) Alterations in sperm DNA methylation patterns at imprinted loci in two classes of infertility. *Fertil Steril* Oct 30. [Epub ahead of print]

Härkönen K, Viitanen T, Larsen S, Bonde J, Lahdetie J (1999) Aneuploidy insperm and exposure to fungicides and lifestyle factors. ASCLEPIOS. A European concerted action on occupational hazards to male reproductive-capability. *Environ Mol Mutagen* **34:** 39–46.

Henry KW, Wyce A, Lo WS, Duggan LJ, Emre NC, Kao CF, Pillus L, Shilatifard A, Osley MA, Berger SL (2003) Transcriptional activation via sequential histone H2B ubiquitylation and deubiquitylation, mediated by SAGA-associated Ubp8. *Genes Dev* **17:** 2648–63.

Ho SM, Tang WY (2007) Techniques used in studies of epigenome dysregulation due to aberrant DNA methylation: an emphasis on fetal-based adult diseases. *Reprod Toxicol* **23:** 267–82.

Holt C, Holt WV, Moore HD, Reed HC, Curnock RM (1997) Objectively measured boar sperm motility parameters correlate with the outcomes of on-farm inseminations: results of two fertility trials. *J Androl* **18:** 312–23.

Hou SY, Zhang L, Wu K, Xia L (2008) Thioglycolic acid inhibits mouse oocyte maturation and affects chromosomal arrangement and spindle configuration. *Toxicol Ind Health* **24:** 227–34.

Howdeshell KL, Rider CV, Wilson VS, Gray LE Jr (2008) Mechanisms of action of phthalate esters, individually and in combination, to induce abnormal reproductive development in male laboratory rats. *Environ Res* **108:** 168–76.

Hoyer-Fender S (2003) Molecular aspects of XY body formation. *Cytogenet Genome Res* **103:** 245–55.

Iniguez-Lluhi JA (2006) For a healthy histone code, a little SUMO in the tail keeps the acetyl away. *ACS Chem Biol* **1:** 204–6.

Jagiello G, Lin JS (1974) Oral contraceptive compounds and mammalian oocyte meiosis. *Am J Obstet Gynecol* **120:** 390–406.

Jakubowski L (2005) Genetic aspects of polycystic ovary syndrome. *Endokrynol Pol* **56:** 285–93.

James M, Turner A (2007) Meiotic sex chromosome inactivation. *Development* **134:** 1823–31.

Jeffay SC, Libbus BL, Barbee RR, Perreault SD (1996) Acute exposure of female hamsters to carbendazim (MBC) during meiosis results in aneuploid oocytes with subsequent arrest of embryonic cleavage and implantation. *Reprod Toxicol* **10:** 183–9.

Jenderny J, Röhrborn G (1987) Chromosome analysis of human sperm. I. First results with a modified method. *Hum Genet* **76:** 385–8.

Jiang YH, Bressler J, Beaudet AL (2004) Epigenetics and human disease. *Annu Rev Genomics Hum Genet* **5:** 479–510.

Jirtle RL, Skinner MK (2007) Environmental epigenomics and disease susceptibility. *Nat Rev Genet* **8:** 253–62.

Joensen UN, Jørgensen N, Rajpert-De Meyts E, Skakkebæk NE (2008) Testicular dysgenesis syndrome and Leydig cell function. *Basic Clin Pharmacol Toxicol* **102:** 155–61.

Johnson ES (2004) Protein modification by SUMO. *Annu Rev Biochem* **73:** 355–82.

Kemal Duru N, Morshedi M, Oehninger S (2000) Effects of hydrogen peroxide on DNA and plasma membrane integrity of human spermatozoa. *Fertil Steril* **74:** 1200–7.

Kerscher O, Felberbaum R, Hochstrasser M (2006) Modification of proteins by ubiquitin and ubiquitin-like proteins. *Annu Rev Cell Dev Biol* **22:** 159–80.

Keshet I, Schlesinger Y, Farkash S, Rand E, Hecht M, Segal E, Pikarski E, Young RA, Niveleau A, Cedar H, Simon I (2006) Evidence for an instructive mechanism of de novo methylation in cancer cells. *Nat Genet* **38:** 149–53.

Kiefer JC (2007) Epigenetics in development. *Dev Dyn* **23:** 1144–56.

Kim DH, Rossi JJ (2007) Strategies for silencing human disease using RNA interference. *Nat Rev Genet* **8(3):** 173–84.

Kocer A, Reichmann J, Best D, Adams IR (2009) Germ cell sex determination in mammals. *Mol Hum Reprod* **15:** 205–13.

Kodama H, Yamaguchi R, Fukuda J, Kasai H, Tanaka T (1997) Increased oxidative deoxyribonucleic acid damage in the spermatozoa of infertile male patients. *Fertil Steril* **68:** 519–24.

Korucuoglu U, Biri AA, Konac E, Alp E, Onen IH, Ilhan MN, Turkyilmaz E, Erdem A, Erdem M, Menevse S (2010) Expression of the imprinted IGF2 and H19 genes in the endometrium of cases with unexplained infertility. *Eur J Obstet Gynecol Reprod Biol* **149:** 77–81.

Kothapalli N, Camporeale G, Kueh A, Chew YC, Oommen AM, Griffin JB, Zempleni J (2005) Biological functions of biotinylated histones. *J Nutr Biochem* **6(7):** 446–8.

Kouzarides T (2007) Chromatin modifications and their function. *Cell* **128:** 693–705.

Künzle R, Mueller MD, Hänggi W, Birkhäuser MH, Drescher H, Bersinger NA (2003) Semen quality of male smokers and nonsmokers in infertile couples. *Fertil Steril* **79:** 287–91.

Laird PW (2003) The power and the promise of DNA methylation markers. *Nat Rev Cancer* **3:** 253–66.

Lee J, Richburg JH, Younkin SC, Boekelheide K (1997) The Fas system is a key regulator of germ cell apoptosis in the testis. *Endocrinol* **138:** 2081–8.

Lewis SEM (2007) Focus on determinants of male fertility. Is sperm evaluation useful in predicting human fertility? *Reproduction* **134:** 31–40.

Lewis SE, Agbaje IM (2008) Using the alkaline comet assay in prognostic tests for male infertility and assisted reproductive technology outcomes. *Mutagenesis* **23:** 163–70.

Maatouk DM, Loveland KL, McManus MT, Moore K, Harfe BD (2008) Dicer1 is required for differentiation of the mouse male germline. *Biol Reprod* **79:** 696–703.

Main KM, Mortensen GK, Kaleva MM, Boisen KA, Damgaard IN, Chellakooty M, Schmidt IM, Suomi AM, Virtanen HE, Petersen DV, Andersson AM, Toppari J, Skakkebaek NE (2006) Human breast milk contamination with phthalates and alterations of endogenous reproductive hormones in three months old infants. *Environ Health Perspect* **114:** 270–6.

Makker K, Agarwal A, Sharma R (2009) Oxidative stress and male infertility. *Ind J Med Res* **129:** 357–67.

Marchetti F, Bishop JB, Lowe X, Generoso WM, Hozier J, Wyrobek AJ (2001) Etoposide induces heritable chromosomal aberrations and aneuploidy during male meiosis in the mouse. *Proc Natl Acad Sci* **98:** 3952–7.

Margueron R, Trojer P, Reinberg D (2005) The key to development: interpreting the histone code? *Curr Opin Genet Dev* **15:** 163–76.

Market-Velker BA, Zhang L, Magri LS, Bonvissuto AC, Mann MR (2010) Dual effects of superovulation: loss of maternal and paternal imprinted methylation in a dose-dependent manner. *Hum Mol Genet* **19:** 36–51.

Martin R, Ernst S, Rademaker A, Barclay L, Ko E, Summers N (1999) Analysis of sperm chromosome complements before, during, and after chemotherapy. *Cancer Genet Cytogenet* **108:** 133–6.

Martin RH (2003) Chromosomal abnormalities in human sperm. In *Advances in Male-Mediated Developmental Toxicity* Vol. 518 (Robaire B, Hales BE, eds.). New York, Plenum Press, pp. 181–8.

Martin RH, Hildebrand K, Yamamoto J, Rademaker A, Barnes M, Douglas G, Arthur K, Ringrose T, Brown IS (1986) An increased frequency of human sperm chromosomal abnormalities after radiotherapy. *Mutat Res* **174(3):** 219–25.

Mathers JC (2008) Personalised nutrition: epigenomics: a basis for understanding individual differences? *Proc Nutr Soc* **67:** 390–4.

Mattsson A, Olsson JA, Brunström B (2008) Selective estrogen receptor alpha activation disrupts sex organ differentiation and induces expression of vitellogenin II and very low-density apolipoprotein II in Japanese quail embryos. *Reproduction* **136:** 175–86.

Matzuk MM and Lamb DJ (2008) The biology of infertility: research advances and clinical challenges. *Nature Med* **14:** 1197–203.

McCallie B, Schoolcraft WB, Katz-Jaffe MG (2010) Aberration of blastocyst microRNA expression is associated with human infertility. *Fertil Steril* **93:** 2374–82.

McGowan PO, Szyf M (2010) The epigenetics of social adversity in early life: implications for mental health outcomes. *Neurobiol Dis.* doi:10.1016/j.nbd.2009.12.026.

Meeker JD, Singh NP, Ryan L, Duty SM, Barr DB, Herrick RF, Bennett DH, Hauser R (2004) Urinary levels of insecticide metabolites and DNA damage in human sperm. *Hum Reprod* **19(11):** 2573–80.

Miki K (2007) Energy metabolism and sperm function. *Soc Reprod Fertil Suppl* **65:** 309–25.

Møller H, Skakkebæk NE (1999) Risk of testicular cancer in subfertile men: case–control study. *Br Med J* **318:** 559–62.

Mortimer ST (2000) CASA – practical aspects. *J Androl* **21:** 515–24.

Nathan D, Ingvarsdottir K, Sterner DE, Bylebyl GR, Dokmanovic M, Dorsey JA, Whelan KA, Krsmanovic M, Lane WS, Meluh PB, Johnson ES, Berger SL (2006) Histone sumoylation is a negative regulator in *Saccharomyces cerevisiae* and shows dynamic interplay with positive-acting histone modifications. *Genes Dev* **20:** 966–76.

Nayernia1 K, Li M, Jaroszynski L, Khusainov R, Wulf G, Schwandt I, Korabiowska M, Michelmann HW, Meinhardt A, Engel W (2004) Stem cell based therapeutical approach of male infertility by teratocarcinoma derived germ cells. *Hum Mol Genet* **13:** 1451–60.

Nowak SJ, Corces VG (2004) Phosphorylation of histone H3: a balancing act between chromosome condensation and transcriptional activation. *Trends Genet* **20(4):** 214–20.

Oral O, Kutlu T, Aksoy E, Ficicioglu C, Uslu H, Turul S (2006) The effects of oxidative stress on outcomes of assisted reproductive techniques. *J Assist Reprod Genet* **23:** 81–5.

Osagie OG, Ogunyemi D, Emuveyan EE, Akinla OA (1984) Etiologic classification and sociomedical characteristics of infertility in 250 couples. *Int J Fertil* **29:** 104–9.

Osser S, Liedholm P, Ranstam J (1984) Depressed semen quality: a study over two decades. *Arch Androl* **12:** 113–16.

Otsuka M, Zheng M, Hayashi M, Lee JD, Yoshino O, Lin S, Han J (2008) Impaired microRNA processing causes corpus luteum insufficiency and infertility in mice. *J Clin Invest* **118:** 1944–54.

Ozguner M, Koyu A, Cesur G, Ural M, Ozguner F, Gokcimen A, Delibas N (2005) Biological and morphological effects on the reproductive organ of rats after exposure to electromagnetic field. *Saudi Med J* **26(3):** 405–10.

Pacchierotti F, Adler ID, Anderson D, Brinkworth M, Demopoulos NA, Lähdetie J, Osterman-Golkar S, Peltonen K, Russo A, Tates A, Waters R (1998) Genetic effects of 1,3-butadiene and associated risk for heritable damage. *Mutat Res* **397:** 93–115.

Padungtod C, Hassold T, Millie E, Ryan L, Savitz D, Christiani D, Ryan LM, Savitz DA, Christiani DC, Xu X (1999) Sperm aneuploidy among Chinese pesticide factory workers: scoring by the FISH method. *Am J Ind Med* **36:** 230–8.

Pang KC, Stephen S, Dinger ME, Engstrom PG, Lenhard B, Mattick JS (2007) RNAdb 2.0–an expanded database of mammalian non-codingRNAs. *Nucl Acids Res* **35:** D178–D182 (database issue).

Parazzini F, Bortolotti A, Colli E (1998) Declining sperm count and fertility in males: an epidemiological controversy. *Arch Androl* **41:** 27–30.

Pasqualotto FF, Sharma RK, Potts JM, Nelson DR, Thomas AJ, Agarwal A (2005) Seminal oxidative stress in patients with chronic prostatitis. *Urology* **55:** 881–5.

Peaston AE, Whitelaw E (2006) Epigenetics and phenotypic variation in mammals. *Mamm Genome* **17:** 365–74.

Peterson CL, Cote J (2004) Cellular machineries for chromosomal DNA repair. *Genes Dev* **18:** 602–16.

Peterson CL, Laniel MA (2004) Histones and histone modifications. *Curr Biol* **14:** R546–R551.

Pintado B, de la Fuente J, Roldan ER (2000) Permeability of boar and bull spermatozoa to the nucleic acid stains propidium iodide or Hoechst 3 or to eosin: accuracy in the assessment of cell viability. *J Reprod Fertil* **118:** 145–52.

Pivot-Pajot C, Caron C, Govin J, Vion A, Rousseaux S, Khochbin S (2003) Acetylation-dependent chromatin reorganization by BRDT, a testis-specific bromodomain-containing protein. *Mol Cell Biol* **23:** 5354–65.

Plante M, de Lamirande E, Gagnon C (1994) Reactive oxygen species released by activated neutrophils, but not by deficient spermatozoa, are sufficient to affect normal sperm motility. *Fertil Steril* **62:** 387–93.

Potts RJ, Newbury CJ, Smith G, Notarianni LJ, Jefferies TM (1999) Sperm chromatin damage associated with male smoking. *Mutat Res* **423:** 103–11.

Prasanth KV, Spector DL (2007) Eukaryotic regulatory RNAs: an answer to the "genome complexity" conundrum. *Genes Dev* **21(1):** 11–42.

Reamon-Buettner ST, Borlak J (2007) A new paradigm in toxicology and teratology: altering gene activity in the absence of DNA sequence variation. *Reprod Toxicol* **24:** 20–30.

Recio R, Robbins WA, Borja-Aburto V, Moran-Martinez J, Froines JR, Hernandez RM, Cebrian ME (2001) Organophosphorous pesticide exposure increases the frequency of sperm sex null aneuploidy. *Environ Health Perspect* **109:** 1237–40.

Reichard JF, Schnekenburger M, Puga A (2007) Long term low-dose arsenic exposure induces loss of DNA methylation. *Biochem Biophys Res Commun* **352(1):** 188–92.

Rider CV, Wilson VS, Howdeshell KL, Hotchkiss AK, Furr JR, Lambright CR, Gray LE Jr (2009) Cumulative effects of in utero administration of mixtures of "antiandrogens" on male rat reproductive development. *Toxicol Pathol* **237:** 100–13.

Robertson KD (2005) DNA methylation and human disease. *Nat Rev Genet* **6:** 597–610.

Rodriguez-Martinez H, Barth AD (2007) In vitro evaluation of sperm quality related to in vivo function and fertility. *Soc Reprod Fertil Suppl* **64:** 39–54.

Sakkas D, Mariethoz E, Manicardi G, Bizzaro D, Bianchi PG, Bianchi U (1999). Origin of DNA damage in ejaculated human spermatozoa. *Rev Reprod* **4:** 31–7.

Sakkas D, Moffatt O, Manicardi GC, Mariethoz E, Tarozzi N, Bizzarro D (2002) Nature of DNA damage in ejaculated human spermatozoa and the possible involvement of apoptosis. *Biol Reprod* **66:** 1061–7.

Sakkas D, Urner F, Bizzaro D, Manicardi G, Bianchi PG, Shoukir Y, Campana A (1998) Sperm nuclear DNA damage and altered chromatin structure: effect on fertilization and embryo development. *Hum Reprod* **13:** 11–19.

Saleh RA, Agarwal A, Nada EA, El-Tonsy MH, Sharma RK, Meyer A, Nelson DR, Thomas AJ (2003) Negative effects of increased sperm DNA damage in relation to seminal oxidative stress in men with idiopathic and male factor infertility. *Fertil Steril* **79:** 1597–605.

Sanchez-Pena LC, Reyes BE, Lopez-Carrillo L, Recio R, Moran-Martinez J, Cebrian ME, Quintanilla-Vega B (2004) Organophosphorous pesticide exposure alters sperm chromatin structure in Mexican agricultural workers. *Toxicol Appl Pharmacol* **196:** 108–13.

Saunders RD, Kowalczuk CI (1981) Effects of 2.45 GHz microwave radiation and heat on mouse spermatogenic epithelium. *Int J Radiat Biol Relat Stud Phys Chem Med* **40:** 623–32.

Sharma RK, Said T, Agarwal A (2004) Sperm DNA damage and its clinical relevance in assessing reproductive outcome. *Asian J Androl* **6:** 139–48.

Sharpe RM. (2003) The "oestrogen hypothesis" – where do we stand now? *Int J Androl* **26:** 2–15.

Sharpe RM (2006) Pathways of endocrine disruption during male sexual differentiation and masculinization. *Best Pract Res Clin Endocrinol Metab* **20:** 91–110.

Shogren-Knaak M, Ishii H, Sun JM, Pazin MJ, Davie JR, Peterson CL (2006) Histone. H4-K16 acetylation controls chromatin structure and protein interactions. *Science* **311(5762):** 844–7.

Sikka SC (2004) Role of oxidative stress and antioxidants in andrology and assisted reproductive technology. *J Androl* **25:** 5–18.

Simonini MV, Camargo LM, Dong E, Maloku E, Veldic M, Costa E, Guidotti A (2006) The benzamide MS-275 is a potent, long-lasting brain region-selective inhibitor of histone deacetylases. *Proc Natl Acad Sci USA* **103:** 1587–92.

Sinha HAP, Swerdloff RS (1999) Hormonal and genetic control of germ cell apoptosis in the testis. *Rev Reprod* **4:** 38–47.

Skakkebaek NE, Rajpert-De Meyts E, Jørgensen N, Carlsen E, Petersen PM, Giwercman A, Andersen AG, Jensen TK, Andersson AM, Müller J (1998) Germ cell cancer and disorders of spermatogenesis: an environmental connection? *APMIS* **106:** 3–11.

Skinner MK (2008) What is an epigenetic transgenerational phenotype? F3 or F2. *Reprod Toxicol* **25:** 2–6.

Smith JL, Garry VF, Rademaker AW, Martin RH (2004) Human sperm aneuploidy after exposure to pesticides. *Mol Rep Dev* **67:** 353–9.

Song R, Ro SS, Michaels JD, Park C, McCarrey JR, Yan W (2009) Many X-linked microRNAs escape meiotic sex chromosome inactivation. *Nat Genet* **41(4):** 488–93.

Spiropoulos J, Turnbull DM, Chinnery PF (2002) Can mitochondrial DNA mutations cause sperm dysfunction? *Mol Hum Reprod* **8:** 719–21.

Strahl BD, Allis CD (2000) The language of covalent histone modifications. *Nature* **403:** 41–5.

Sun F, Greene C, Turek PJ, Ko E, Rademaker A, Martin RH (2005b) Immunofluorescent synaptonemal complex analysis in azoospermic men. *Cytogenet Genome Res* **111:** 366–70.

Sun F, Ko E, Martin RH (2006) Is there a relationship between sperm chromosome abnormalities and sperm morphology? *Reproduct Biol Endocriol* **4:** 1.

Sun F, Trpkov K, Rademaker A, Ko E, Martin RH (2005a) Variation in meiotic recombination frequencies among human males. *Hum Genet* **116:** 172–8.

Sun JG, Jurisicova A, Casper RF (1997) Detection of deoxyribonucleic acid fragmentation in human sperm: correlation with fertilization in vitro. *Biol Reprod* **56:** 602–7.

Swan SH, Main KM, Liu F, Stewart SL, Kruse RL, Calafat AM, Mao CS, Redmon JB, Ternand CL, Sullivan S, Teague JL (2005) Decrease in anogenital distance among male infants with prenatal phthalate exposure. *Environ Health Perspect* **113:** 1056–61.

Szyf M (2007) The dynamic epigenome and its implications in toxicology. *Toxicol Sci* **100:** 7–23.

Szyf M, McGowan P, Meaney MJ (2008) The social environment and the epigenome. *Environ Mol Mutagen* **49:** 46–60.

Taioli E, Zocchetti C, Garte S (1998) Models of interaction between metabolic genes and environmental exposure in cancer susceptibility. *Environ Health Perspect* **106:** 67–70.

Taxvig C, Hass U, Axelstad M, Dalgaard M, Boberg J, Andeasen HR, Vinggaard AM (2007) Endocrine-disrupting activities in vivo of the fungicides tebuconazole and epoxiconazole. *Toxicol Sci* **100:** 464–73.

Teague EM, Print CG, Hull ML (2010) The role of microRNAs in endometriosis and associated reproductive conditions. *Hum Reprod Update* **16:** 142–65.

Tiveron C, Ranaldi R, Bassani B, Pacchierotti F (1997) Induction and transmission of chromosome aberrations in mouse oocytes after treatment with butadiene diepoxide. *Environ Mol Mutagen* **30:** 403–9.

Toloubeydokhti T, Bukulmez O, Chegini N (2008) Potential regulatory functions of microRNAs in the ovary. *Semin Reprod Med* **26:** 469–78.

Twigg J, Irvine DS, Houston P, Fulton N, Michael L, Aitken RJ (1998) Iatrogenic DNA damage induced in human spermatozoa during sperm preparation: protective significance of seminal plasma. *Mol Hum Reprod* **4:** 439–45.

Valencia-Sanchez MA, Liu J, Hannon GJ, Parker R (2006) Control of translation and mRNA degradation by miRNAs and siRNAs. *Genes Dev* **20:** 515–24.

Vigodner M, Ishikawa T, Schlegel PN, Morris PL (2006) SUMO-1, human male germ cell development, and the androgen receptor in the testis of men with normal and abnormal spermatogenesis. *Am J Physiol Endocrinol Metab* **290(5):** E1022–E1033.

Vinggaard AM, Hnida C, Breinholt V, Larsen JC (2000) Screening of selected pesticides for inhibition of CYP19 aromatase activity in vitro. *Toxicol in Vitro* **14:** 227–34.

Wang XW, Ding GR, Shi CH, Zhao T, Zhang J, Zeng LH, Guo GZ (2008) Effect of electromagnetic pulse exposure on permeability of blood–testicle barrier in mice. *Biomed Environ Sci* **21(3):** 218–21.

Wdowiak A, Wdowiak L, Wiktor H (2007) Evaluation of the effect of using mobile phones on male fertility. *Ann Agric Environ Med* **14:** 169–72.

Wilson VS, Howdeshell KL, Lambright CS, Furr J, Earl Gray L (2007) Differential expression of the phthalate syndrome in male Sprague-Dawley and Wistar rats after in utero DEHP exposure. *Toxicol Lett* **170:** 177–84.

World Health Organization (WHO) (1992) *Laboratory Manual for the Examination of Human Semen and Semen-Cervical Mucus Interaction*, 3rd edition. Cambridge, Cambridge University Press.

Xia Y, Bian Q, Xu L, Cheng S, Song L, Liu J, Wu W, Wang S, Wang X (2004) Genotoxic effects on human spermatozoa among pesticide factory workers exposed to fenvalerate. *Toxicology* **203:** 49–60.

Xia Y, Cheng S, Bian Q, Xu L, Collins MD, Chang HC, Song L, Liu J, Wang S, Wang X. (2005) Genotoxic effects on spermatozoa of carbaryl-exposed workers. *Toxicol Sci* **85:** 615–23.

Yao G, Yin M, Lian J, Tian H, Liu L, Li X, Sun F (2010) MicroRNA-224 is involved in transforming growth factor-beta-mediated mouse granulosa cell proliferation and granulosa cell function by targeting Smad4. *Mol Endocrinol* **24:** 540–51.

Zamudio NM, Chong S, O'Bryan MK (2008) Epigenetic regulation in male germ cells. *Reproduct* **136:** 131–46.

Zhang Y (2003) Transcriptional regulation by histone ubiquitination and deubiquitination. *Genes Dev* **17(22):** 2733–40.

Zhu B, Zheng Y, Pham AD, Mandal SS, Erdjument-Bromage H, Tempst P, Reinberg D (2005) Monoubiquitination of human histone H2B: the factors involved and their roles in HOXgene regulation. *Mol Cell* **20:** 601–11.

Zhu YJ, Jiang JT, Ma L, Zhang J, Hong Y, Liao K, Liu Q, Liu GH (2009) Molecular and toxicologic research in newborn hypospadiac male rats following in utero exposure to di-n-butyl phthalate (DBP). *Toxicology* **260:** 120–5.

Zinellu A, Sotgia S, Pasciu V, Madeddu M, Leoni GG, Naitana S, Deiana L, Carru C (2008) Intracellular adenosine 5′-triphosphate, adenosine 5′-diphosphate, and adenosine 5′-monophosphate detection by short-end injection capillary electrophoresis using methylcellulose as the effective electroosmostic flow suppressor. *Electrophoresis* **29:** 3069–73.

Zuelke KA, Perreault SD (1995) Carbendazim (MBC) disrupts oocyte spindle function and induces aneuploidy in hamsters exposed during fertilization (meiosis II). *Mol Reprod Dev* **42:** 200–9.

C H A P T E R

72

Occupational exposure to chemicals and reproductive health

Helena Taskinen, Marja-Liisa Lindbohm and Markku Sallmén

INTRODUCTION

Occupational exposure to some chemical agents may be harmful to the reproductive health, pregnancy and pregnancy outcome of workers. Exposure may affect the reproductive system of men and women and manifest as alterations in sex hormone levels, menstrual disorders, ovarian dysfunction, diminished libido and potency, impairment of semen quality, and infertility or subfertility. Exposure can also induce adverse effects on the developing embryo or fetus. Developmental toxicity may appear as miscarriage, stillbirth, intrauterine growth retardation, toxemia, preterm birth, birth defect, perinatal or postnatal death, disturbances of cognitive development, immunological sensitivity, or childhood cancer.

The recognition of a chemical as a reproductive or developmental toxicant is based on experimental studies or human studies, mainly epidemiological but sometimes case series-type studies. Epidemiological studies provide information on possible effects of occupational exposure to working populations. The advantage of studies in working populations compared to general populations is higher exposure level; this makes it easier to identify potential harmful effects of exposure. This chapter describes the epidemiological studies on the reproductive and developmental effects of occupational exposure to chemical agents.

ORGANIC SOLVENTS

Occupational exposure to various solvents is common. Solvents are used widely in many areas of industry, such as in spray painting, degreasing, furniture manufacture, shoemaking, printing, dry cleaning, in metal industries, reinforced plastics industries and in the production of paints, glues and other chemicals. Usually workers are exposed to a mixture of solvents; exposure to a single solvent is uncommon in the work environment. The main routes of exposure are via inhalation and through the skin. The passage of several solvents through the placenta has been demonstrated in humans and mammals. Some solvents have induced malformations, retarded growth and produced lethal effects to embryos in experiments on animals.

Maternal occupational exposure to high levels of solvents has been associated with reduced fertility, miscarriages, birth defects and low birth weight in several human studies (Lindbohm, 1995; Lindbohm and Taskinen, 2000; Ha *et al.*, 2002; Sallmén *et al.*, 2008; Garlantézec *et al.*, 2009; Table 72.1). In some studies exposure has been related to pregnancy-induced hypertension, preterm birth, poorer neurobehavioral performance and childhood leukemia (Hewitt and Tellier, 1998; Wennborg *et al.*, 2002; Infante-Rivard *et al.*, 2005; McKinney *et al.*, 2008). Some evidence of gene–environment interaction has also been obtained in studies on solvent exposure; combined maternal–infant genotypes were found to modify the effect of exposure on gestational age (Wang *et al.*, 2000; Qin *et al.*, 2008).

Increasing evidence suggests that solvent exposure is associated with delayed conception in women, but the evidence for males is less consistent (Sallmén *et al.*, 1995, 1998, 2008; Correa *et al.*, 1996; Plenge-Bönig and Karmaus, 1999). Data on the effects of solvent exposure on menstrual function, semen characteristics and hormone levels are scarce. The few existing studies on menstruation suggest that exposure may be associated with menstrual disorders (Lindbohm, 1999; Cho *et al.*, 2001). In men, solvent exposure has been associated with reduced semen quality (Figá-Talamanca *et al.*, 2001) and increased follicle-stimulating hormone level (Luderer *et al.*, 2004). In women, preovulatory luteinizing hormone level was significantly lower among those who had higher internal doses of aliphatic hydrocarbons (Reutman *et al.*, 2002).

An increased risk of miscarriage has been observed in industrial populations usually exposed to high levels of solvents. These include employees in manufacturing, dry cleaning, painting, shoe, pharmaceutical, audio speaker, semiconductor and laboratory industries (Lindbohm, 1995). Maternal exposure has also been related to congenital malformations, although the excess of specific malformations among the children of solvent-exposed women has not been systematic. Most often exposure has been linked with oral

Reproductive and Developmental Toxicology, Edited by Ramesh C. Gupta
ISBN: 978-0-12-382032-7

TABLE 72.1 Occupational exposure to metals, pesticides and solvents associated with adverse effects on reproductive health

Hazard	Industry or occupational group	Reported effects, women	Reported effects, men
Inorganic mercury	Lamp industry, chloralkali industry, dental personnel	Reduced fertility,[a] menstrual disorders,[a] fetal loss[a]	Miscarriage[a]
Lead	Battery industry, lead smelting, foundries, pottery industry, ammunition industry and some other metal industries	Reduced fertility,[a] fetal loss,[a] preterm birth,[a] low birth weight,[a] birth defects,[a] impaired cognitive development[a]	Reduced sperm quality, reduced fertility,[a] miscarriage,[a] birth defects[a]
Pesticides[b]	Agriculture, gardening, greenhouse work	Reduced fertility,[a] fetal loss,[a] birth defects,[a] preterm birth,[a] reduced fetal growth,[a] neurodevelopmental effects,[a] childhood leukamia[a]	Reduced sperm quality, reduced fertility,[a] fetal loss,[a] birth defects,[a] childhood cancer[a]
Solvents	Painting, degreasing, shoemaking, printing, dry-cleaning, metal industry and several other fields of industry	Reduced fertility, menstrual disorders, fetal loss, birth defects, preterm birth,[a] pregnancy-induced hypertension,[a] neurodevelopmental effects,[a] childhood leukemia[a]	Delayed conception,[a] reduced semen quality, increased follicle-stimulating hormone level,[a] fetal loss,[a] neural tube defects, childhood leukemia[a]
Benzene	Petrochemical industry, laboratory personnel	Fetal loss,[a] shortened gestation,[a] low birth weight,[a] leukemia[a]	
Carbon disulfide	Viscose rayon industry	Menstrual disorders	Decreased libido and potency
Some ethylene glycol ethers and their acetates	Electronics industry, silk screen printing, photography and dyeing, other industries	Reduced fertility, fetal loss, birth defects, menstrual disorders	Reduced semen quality
Formaldehyde	Mechanical wood industry, pathology laboratories	Reduced fertility,[a] fetal loss[a]	
Tetrachloroethylene	Dry cleaning, degreasing	Reduced fertility,[a] fetal loss	Reduced semen quality[a]
Toluene	Shoe industry, painting, laboratory work	Reduced fertility,[a] fetal loss,[a] leukemia[a]	Fetal loss[a]

[a]Inconclusive evidence
[b]Examples of pesticides with adverse effects in men include dibromochloropropane (DBCP), 2,4-dichlorophenoxyacetic acid (2,4-D), ethylene dibromide, chlordecone and carbaryl

clefts, but also with central nervous system defects and ventricular septal defects (Lindbohm, 1995; Chevrier *et al.*, 2006; Thulstrup and Bonde, 2006). In a recent prospective cohort study maternal exposure was also associated with urinary malformations and male genital malformations (Garlantézec *et al.*, 2009).

The evidence on the developmental effects of paternal solvent exposure is limited and inconsistent. Exposure to solvents in general has been related to early preterm birth in the printing industry, and an increased risk of miscarriage among the wives of exposed workers, in particular among painters and wood workers (Lindbohm, 1995). Children of male painters, printers and occupations exposed to solvents have been repeatedly reported to be associated with birth defects (Chia and Shi, 2002; Hooiveld *et al.*, 2006). A meta-analysis on paternal solvent exposure and pregnancy outcome indicated that exposure in fathers may be associated with an increased risk for neural tube defects but not miscarriage (Logman *et al.*, 2005).

Some studies provide evidence that certain paternal exposures might be related to cancer in their offspring. According to a literature review the evidence is strongest for childhood leukemia and paternal exposure to solvents and paints, and childhood nervous system cancers and paternal exposure to paints (Colt and Blair, 1998). The association between solvent exposure and leukemia was, however, not confirmed in two later studies (Shu *et al.*, 1999; Schüz *et al.*, 2000).

Only a few studies have looked at potential neurodevelopmental toxicity of solvent exposure in children of occupationally exposed mothers. The findings showed that maternal exposure may be associated with neurobehavioral impairments, especially the areas of visual function, motor and verbal skills and attention-deficit-hyperactivity behaviors (Laslo-Baker *et al.*, 2004; Julvez and Grandjean, 2009).

Glycol ethers

Glycol ethers and their acetates are used in a variety of industries and products. Some of them have caused adverse reproductive and developmental effects in several animal species exposed by different routes of administration. Among semiconductor manufacturing workers, exposure to ethylene glycol ethers was related to an increased risk of miscarriage, subfertility and prolonged menstrual cycles (Correa *et al.*, 1996; Chen *et al.*, 2002; Hsieh *et al.*, 2005). In a multicenter case–control study, maternal glycol ether exposure was associated with congenital malformations (Cordier *et al.*, 1997). The association appeared particularly strong in neural tube defects, multiple anomalies and cleft lip.

Exposure to glycol ethers (in particular, 2-methoxyethanol and 2-ethoxyethanol) has been related to reduced semen quality in shipyard painters, metal casters, chemical industry workers and semiconductor industry workers (Figá-Talamanca *et al.*, 2001). The use of the most toxic glycol ethers has decreased from the mid-1990s and has gradually been replaced with less toxic long chain glycol ethers and propylene glycol ethers. The results of a French study are in line with this development (Multigner *et al.*, 2007). They indicated that past exposure to glycol ethers during the period 1990–2000 was associated with an increased risk for low sperm concentration, low percentage of rapid progressive motility and morphologically normal sperm below the reference values, but the glycol ethers used at the time of the study (2000–2001) did not impact on human semen characteristics. In a British study, glycol ether exposure was, however, related to low motile sperm count (Cherry *et al.*, 2008). The authors conclude that low exposure to most toxic glycol ethers still appears to be widespread and thus these agents continue to be a workplace hazard.

Carbon disulfide

Carbon disulfide is used primarily in the production of viscose rayon. Disturbances in sexual function, such as decreased libido and potency, have been reported in several studies on male workers exposed to carbon disulfide. The findings on other reproductive effects are equivocal. Adverse effects have been observed in men chronically poisoned with carbon disulfide, but at lower levels of exposure no significant alterations were noted (Tas *et al.*, 1996). In women, menstrual disorders, including irregular cycles and unusual bleeding, have been related to carbon disulfide exposure (Lindbohm, 1999).

Benzene

Benzene exposure has been suggested as a potential cause of adverse pregnancy outcome in some, although not in all, studies. An increased risk of miscarriage was found among workers of a petrochemical plant exposed to benzene (Xu *et al.*, 1998). Low-level exposure was related to reduced birth weight in children of female petrochemical industry workers, especially in combination with simultaneous exposure to stress (Chen *et al.*, 2000). Benzene exposure was also associated with shortened gestation, but the association was modified by an individual's genotype (Wang *et al.*, 2000). A study among laboratory workers reported an increased risk for neural crest malformations relative to solvents, especially benzene (Wennborg *et al.*, 2002). Environmental exposure to benzene and a mixture of associated traffic-related air pollution was associated with decreases in birth weight and head circumference during pregnancy and at birth (Slama *et al.*, 2009). Another study suggested that living next to a petrol station, with potential for benzene exposure, may be associated with acute childhood leukaemia (Brosselin *et al.*, 2009).

Paternal exposure to benzene has been associated with adverse pregnancy outcome in studies inferring exposure from occupation (Tas *et al.*, 1996). In a study where benzene exposure was defined based on workers' employment history and the results of atmospheric measurements, no association was found between low level of exposure and spontaneous abortion (Stücker *et al.*, 1994).

Toluene

Case reports on toluene abuse during pregnancy indicate that toluene exposure during gestation can cause adverse reproductive outcomes (Wilkins-Haug, 1997). Increased risk of miscarriage has also been observed among shoe workers, audio speaker factory workers and laboratory workers exposed to high levels of toluene (Lindbohm, 1995). Reduced fertility was observed for toluene exposure in women but not in men (Sallmén *et al.*, 1995; Plenge-Bönig and Karmaus, 1999). The findings of one study suggested an increased risk of childhood leukemia for maternal exposure to aromatic hydrocarbons and toluene (Infante-Rivard *et al.*, 2005). Simultaneous exposure to several solvents is, however, common among toluene-exposed workers, making it difficult to attribute adverse effects to any specific solvent. For example, eight different organic compounds were found in air monitoring samples of shoe manufacturing units: n-hexane, hexane isomers and toluene were used in all of them (Sallmén *et al.*, 1998).

Styrene

Exposure to styrene is common in the reinforced plastics industry. Some early studies reported high frequencies of menstrual disturbances, reduced fertility and miscarriage in styrene-exposed women, but the methodological shortcomings of these studies limit the interpretation of their findings. More recent investigations have revealed no difference in menstrual function or pregnancy outcome between exposed and unexposed workers (Lindbohm, 1995, 1999). There has not been any clear association between male or female exposure to styrene and reduced fertility (Sallmén *et al.*, 1995, 1998; Kolstad *et al.*, 2000).

The results on the effects of styrene on sperm quality are conflicting (Tas *et al.*, 1996). An increased proportion of sperm with abnormal morphology was observed in men exposed to styrene and acetone, but no differences in other sperm parameters or gonadal hormones were seen. Overall, there is no clear evidence on the adverse reproductive effects of styrene exposure. Based on human and animal data an expert panel has concluded that there is insufficient evidence to conclude that styrene is a developmental or reproductive toxicant (Luderer *et al.*, 2006).

Tetrachloroethylene

Dry-cleaning work with potential for exposure to tetrachloroethylene has been associated with an increased frequency of miscarriage (Lindbohm, 1995, Figá-Talamanca, 2006). A time-to-pregnancy study suggested decreased fertility in a small group of exposed women (Sallmén *et al.*, 1995). Among men subtle changes in semen quality have been reported from exposure to this agent (Figá-Talamanca *et al.*, 2001). Although the data on the effects of tetrachloroethylene exposure are limited, the findings suggest an association between a high level of exposure to tetrachloroethylene and adverse reproductive outcomes, particularly among women.

Other solvents

Exposure to 2-bromopropane has been associated with adverse reproductive effects in men and women. There are also some reports suggesting that maternal formaldehyde exposure is related to delayed conception and miscarriage, and exposure to trinitrotoluene or trichloroethylene may be harmful for the reproductive health of men (Taskinen *et al.*, 1999b; Figa-Talamanca *et al.*, 2001). Formamide, dimethylformamide and n-methyl-2-pyrrolidone have also been shown to cause fetotoxic and teratogenic effects in laboratory animals, but there are no data on their effects in humans.

In summary, the epidemiologic evidence suggests that high maternal exposure to solvents may represent a hazard for the developing fetus and may impair female fertility. The results for male fertility are less conclusive. The findings on individual solvents must also be interpreted with caution, because coincident exposure to several agents makes it difficult to ascribe adverse effects to a specific compound. Nevertheless, the study results are supportive of adverse effects of some glycol ethers, tetrachloroethylene, toluene, benzene and carbon disulfide on reproduction. It would be prudent to minimize exposure to organic solvents.

METALS

The reproductive toxicity of some metals has been known for a long time, but not all common metals in occupational use have been thoroughly investigated in epidemiological studies. Here we summarize the main findings (see Table 72.1).

Inorganic lead

Occupational exposure to lead and lead compounds may occur when, e.g., lead containing pigments or paints is handled, in production and repair of accumulators, and in production of crystal glass. PVC plastics, brass, soldering metal, bullets and gun powder contain lead compounds. Lead exposure is possible also in the demolition of lead-containing goods or materials, and in inside shooting ranges. Many of the lead compounds are classified as carcinogens or suspected carcinogens.

Exposure to lead at work is followed by biomonitoring, i.e. by measuring the concentration of the lead in the blood (B–Pb). In the literature two units of the concentration of the lead are used: microgram (μg/dl) or micromole (μmol/l):

1 μg/dl = 0.048 μmol/l
1 μmol/l = 20.7 μg/dl

Female-mediated effects

Women's exposure to lead (reviewed in Baranski, 1993) has been reported to have an association with menstrual disorders. Lead may also have an etiologic role in pregnancy-induced hypertension even at low B–Pb levels (Yazbeck *et al.*, 2009).

Lead is transferred across the placenta, and at birth the blood–lead concentration in the umbilical cord is close to that of the mother. The mechanisms of the toxicity of lead to the fetus are mainly unknown. Pilsner *et al.* (2009) found decreased DNA methylation in cord blood with increasing concentration of lead in patella and tibia bones of pregnant women. The finding suggests that the epigenome of the fetus may be influenced by maternal cumulative lead burden, which may influence the disease susceptibility of the offspring. Fetal lead exposure has also an adverse effect on the neurodevelopment of the fetus, and the effect is most pronounced during the first trimester (Hu *et al.*, 2006).

In contradiction to occupational studies, low environmental lead exposure was associated with an increased risk of miscarriage in a small Mexican prospective study (Borja-Aburto *et al.*, 1999). The odds ratio for spontaneous abortion was 1.8 (CI 1.1–3.1) for every 0.24 μmol/l. The mean B–Pb for spontaneous abortion cases was 0.58 μmol/l and that for controls 0.49 μmol/l. Elevated ORs of 2.3, 5.4 and 12.2 were observed in exposure categories 0.24–0.48 μmol/l, 0.49–0.71 and ≥0.72 μmol/l, respectively, as compared with B–Pb <0.24 μmol/l. However, male environmental exposure to lead was not assessed. It is possible that maternal environmental B–Pb is highly correlated with paternal B–Pb. A part of the association could be explained by male exposure to lead or by the combined effects of maternal and paternal exposure. Rather low concentrations of lead in the maternal blood have been associated also with preterm births and small-for-gestational-age babies (B–Pb 0.24–0.5 μmol/l; Torrés-Sanches *et al.*, 1999; Jelliffe-Pawlowski *et al.*, 2006).

Maternal exposure to lead may also affect the child's mental development (reviewed by Bellinger *et al.*, 2005). The maternal plasma lead concentration during the first trimester was a strong predictor of infant mental development at 24 months of age. Lead exposure around 28 weeks' gestation was shown to be the critical period for the child's intellectual development (Schnaas *et al.*, 2006). The exposure levels during pregnancy were moderate, mean B–Pb 8 μg/dl (range 1–33 μg/dl). For the protection of the fetus and especially the child's mental development the occupational limits for reproductively active women should be low enough. A safe level of the B–Pb among pregnant women could be the limit of the unexposed population, which in many countries is B–Pb 0.2–0.3 μmol/l (~4–6 μg/dl). A recommendation of a B–Pb limit of 5 μg/dl for pregnant and lactating women has been suggested (Kosnett *et al.*, 2007).

Male-mediated effects

Occupational exposure to lead has been associated with adverse effects on sperm count and quality. Many different mechanisms and sites of action may play a role in lead toxicity. In men lead may interfere with the reorganization and tight packaging of sperm DNA during spermatogenesis by competition with zinc or protamine-binding sites (Shiau *et al.*, 2004). Apostoli *et al.* (1998) reviewed eight human studies on semen quality, seven on endocrine function, and six studies on trace elements in seminal fluid or blood among the general population. There is evidence that heavy exposure to inorganic lead is detrimental to semen quality. A decrease in various parameters of semen quality and a possible modest effect on the endocrine profile have been observed at B–Pb concentrations >1.9 μmol/l. In one prospective study the adverse effects of lead on sperm were at least partially reversible: average B–Pb decrease from 2 to 1 μmol/l coincided with improvements in the proportion of motile cells, and in penetration.

Male exposure to lead has been connected to decreased fertility rate (occurrence of live birth) showing a tendency toward decreased fertility with increasing duration of exposure. Relatively low exposure to lead (at B–Pb 0.5 μmol/l or above) has been linked with infertility (measured as non-occurrence of a pregnancy during first years of marriage) (Sallmén *et al.*, 2000b). Studies on fertility rates and infertility had no information on family planning, however, and that makes the evidence of these studies inconclusive. Retrospective studies on time to pregnancy have shown conflicting findings: one study reported no adverse effect on male fertility, two studies came up with suggestive findings, and fertility was reduced in a dose–response manner in one study (Shiau *et al.*, 2004). These studies, in turn, have excluded childless couples, and may have underestimated the effect (Sallmén *et al.*, 2000a). Some studies suggest that paternal exposure to lead might also be associated with adverse pregnancy outcome, including miscarriage, birth defects or perinatal deaths, but so far the evidence is weak (Bellinger, 2005).

In summary, lead impairs semen quality at high exposure, say at blood lead levels at or above 1.9 μmol/l. Methodological shortcomings in studies on time to pregnancy and fertility rate make the evidence on these outcomes inconclusive.

Cadmium, mercury and other metals

Workers may be exposed to inorganic mercury in the chlor-alkali industry, in waste management and in recovery of mercury. Smaller exposures may occur in healthcare and in dental care. Inorganic mercury is transferred to the fetus and accumulates in the placenta.

Occupational exposure to mercury, arsenic and manganese has been associated with menstrual disorders (reviewed in Baranski, 1993). Exposure to inorganic mercury from amalgam at a dental assistant's place of work was associated with increased risk of reduced fertility and miscarriage (Rowland *et al.*, 1994).

The effects of methyl mercury are well known as far as fetal effects are concerned; the exposure comes mainly from polluted fish in the diet. Prenatal exposure to methylmercury seems to have stronger adverse effects on the neurobehavioral development of the fetus than postnatal exposure (Grandjean and Landrigan, 2006).

Cadmium and other metallic ions may act as metallo-estrogens and endocrine disruptors. Cadmium is known to accumulate in the placenta, which may decrease the transport of micronutrients, e.g. zinc, to the fetus (Kippler *et al.*, 2010). Cadmium concentration in the placenta of smoking women is double as high as in that of non-smoking women (Stasenko *et al.*, 2010). Cadmium is also reported to have adverse effects on semen quality (reviewed by Wirth and Mijal, 2010).

Men exposed to alkyl mercury had decreased semen counts, and increased teratospermia and astenospermia. Among workers in the explosives industry the concentration of inorganic mercury in semen was 10 times higher than in the serum. Paternal exposure to mercury has also been associated with an increased risk of miscarriage among their wives (reviewed by Lindbohm *et al.*, 1997).

Occupational exposure to manganese may occur in the steel manufacturing, chemical and mining industries, and dry-alkaline battery production. There is evidence suggesting that manganese exposure may have harmful effects on sexual activity of men. The results of studies on male fertility have been contradictory (Tas *et al.*, 1996).

Boron minerals and chemicals are used in the manufacture of glass, ceramics, detergents and bleaches, alloys, metals, fire retardants, fertilizers and wood preservatives. Boron has been shown to adversely affect reproduction in rats, but an overview of male reproductive studies found no indication of impairment of testicular function in boron-exposed workers (Scialli *et al.*, 2010).

Welding

Welding fumes may include many metals with potential reproductive toxicity, e.g. hexavalent chromium, nickel, cadmium, manganese. Carbon monoxide, heat and electromagnetic fields are also possible exposures in welding. Traditionally welders were entirely men, but nowadays women are increasingly to be found in the industry. The research data on the effects on reproduction is mainly of men. A recent study suggests, that maternal exposure during pregnancy to welding fumes or metal dusts or fumes may reduce fetal growth (Quansah and Jaakkola, 2009).

Male welders have been reported to have decreased semen quality (reviewed by Figà-Talamanca *et al.*, 2001). Adverse effects found in cross-sectional studies have not been repeated in follow-up studies (Hjollund *et al.*, 1998a). An association between paternal welding and delayed time to pregnancy has been seen in cross-sectional and case-referent studies, but not in a follow-up study (Hjollund *et al.*, 1998b). However, paternal exposure to stainless steel welding, but not to other metal welding, was associated with an increased risk (adjusted relative risk 3.5, 95% confidence interval 1.3–9.1) for miscarriages among the spouses (Hjollund *et al.*, 2000).

There is suggestive evidence, that paternal exposure to welding fumes may increase the risk of preterm delivery and small-for-gestational-age babies (Quansah and Jaakkola, 2009).

CARBON MONOXIDE

Exposure to carbon monoxide in occupational settings may occur in iron and steel foundries, in welding work, in the alimentary industry in smoking procedures, and in car repair and service stations due to exhaust gases. There is some exposure to carbon monoxide also in the general environment of big cities from traffic.

Carbon monoxide is transported through the placenta and in the fetus the concentration of blood carboxyhemoglobin is 10–15% higher than in the mother's blood. In connection with maternal carbon monoxide intoxications, intrauterine deaths and brain injuries of the child have been reported. Disturbances in the pregnancy and neurological defects and small birth weight of the child have been reported after maternal exposure to 100 ppm concentration of carbon monoxide for 4 hours (Norman and Halton, 1990). Environmental exposure to higher levels of ambient carbon monoxide (>5.5 ppm 3-month average) during the last trimester was associated with a significantly increased risk for low birth weight (OR = 1.22; 95% confidence interval CI, 1.03–1.44) after adjustment for potential confounders, including commuting habits in the monitoring area, sex of the child, level of prenatal care, and age, ethnicity and education of the mother (Ritz and Yu, 1999).

PESTICIDES

Exposure to pesticides may occur in agricultural work, greenhouse work and in the pesticide-producing industry. Typical pesticides are insecticides, herbicides and fungicides. Pesticides enter the body through the skin, via inhaled air or through ingestion. Pesticide formulations may also contain organic solvents. Some pesticides have shown reproductive and/or developmental toxicity (e.g., benomyl, carbaryl, dibromochloropropane, ethylenthiourea, maneb, zineb, thiram) in animals or humans (reviewed by Nurminen, 1995).

Female effects

Several studies have focused on the effects of pesticide exposure on female fertility (Fuortes *et al.*, 1997; Curtis *et al.*, 1999; Abell *et al.*, 2000; Greenlee *et al.*, 2003; Idrovo *et al.*, 2005; Lauria *et al.*, 2006; Bretveld *et al.*, 2006; Hougaard *et al.*, 2009; see Table 72.1). The findings among infertility clinic clients (Fuortes *et al.*, 1997), among Danish greenhouse workers (Abell *et al.*, 2000), workers in flower production (Idrovo *et al.*, 2005) and in women living in an agricultural area (Greenlee *et al.*, 2003) suggest reduced fertility in exposed women. In particular, reduced fecundability has been observed among women, who did not use gloves when handling cultures (Abell *et al.*, 2000). Suggestive evidence was observed in a Dutch study among women working in greenhouses (Bretveld *et al.*, 2006) while some studies have shown no or only weak associations with reduced fertility (Curtis *et al.*, 1999; Lauria *et al.*, 2006; Hougaard *et al.*, 2009). The great variation of the exposure levels and pesticide chemicals in various occupational settings may explain the different results. High exposure is likely to be hazardous.

Increased risk for miscarriage has been observed among women in agricultural occupations, among gardeners who sprayed pesticides during pregnancy (reviewed by Nurminen, 1995) and in greenhouse work (reviewed by Figà-Talamanca, 2006). In one study the increased risk for miscarriage was seen only among those who used pesticides on 3 to 5 days a week during the first trimester of pregnancy. The risk was not increased, however, when a proper respirator or respirator and protective clothing were used (Taskinen *et al.*, 1995, 1999). An increased risk of late miscarriages (OR 1.9, 95% CI 1.6–2.3) among farmers (Kristensen *et al.*, 1997) was also associated with rainy summers, when molds and exposure to mycotoxins (from mold) might be a possible explanation for their finding. Among primigravidous women working in greenhouses an increased crude risk of miscarriages was observed (OR 2.9, 95% CI 0.9–7.6); after correction for confounding the risk was higher (OR 4.0, 95% CI 1.1–14.0) (Bretveld *et al.*, 2008).

Stillbirths without birth defects were increased among women who worked in agriculture or horticulture more than 30 hours/week (McDonald *et al.*, 1987). Women exposed to pesticides had an increased risk for stillbirth (Goulet and Theriault, 1991; Pastore *at al.*, 1997). Environmental exposure to malathion and to insecticides and herbicides has been associated with stillbirths, too (reviewed by Nurminen, 1995).

Several studies have suggested that maternal exposure to several pesticides may increase risk of preterm birth or reduced fetal growth (reviewed by Stillerman *et al.*, 2008). Insecticide (chlorpyrifos) and herbicides (triazine, metolachlor, cyanazine and atrazine) were suggested to have these adverse effects, but in many studies the sample size was limited.

The insecticide DDT (2,2-bis(p-chlorophenyl)-1,1,1-trichloroethane) was banned in industrialized countries in the 1970s, but is still being used in many countries against malaria-transmitting mosquitoes. 1,1-Dichloro-2,2-bis(p-chlorophenyl)ethylene (p,p′-DDE) is a metabolite of DDT. Increased risk of cryptorchidism, hypospadias and polythelia among male offspring was suggested in a study where stored serum samples were used in assessment of the maternal DDE levels during pregnancy. The results were inconclusive (Longnecker *et al.*, 2002). In a retrospective, case–control study the association of the periconceptional exposure to agrichemicals with the development of gastroschisis was investigated. Distance between a woman's residence and site of elevated exposure to agrichemicals was calculated. Maternal exposure to surface water atrazine was associated with fetal gastroschisis (OR 1.6), particularly in spring conceptions (Waller *et al.*, 2010).

An ecologic study, where wheat acreage, low or high, was used as a surrogate measure for exposure to chlorophenoxy herbicides, indicated that infants conceived in spring during the herbicide application season had increased risk for circulatory (other than heart)/respiratory (OR 1.65, 95% CI 1.07–2.55) and musculoskeletal anomalies (1.50, 95% CI 1.06–2.12) (Schreinemachers, 2003). Exposure during pregnancy to p,p′DDE, measured from cord serum, was associated with a delay in mental and psychomotor development at 13 months (Ribas-Fitó *et al.*, 2003).

An association between the use of pesticides and congenital malformations was found in a Mexican study where exposed mothers had a high risk of having a malformed child (OR 3.5, 95% CI 2.0-6.3). Risk was higher if the mother had occupational exposure to pesticides (OR 6.3, 95% CI 3.0–13.7) and in mothers living near areas of pesticides treatment (OR 3.5, 95% CI 1.9–6.3) (Medina-Carrilo *et al.*, 2002). A statistically significant association between birth defects and the exposure of the mothers to certain types of agricultural chemicals was found also in a study in South Africa (Heeren *et al.*, 2003).

The mother's exposure during pregnancy to organophosphate pesticides or pesticide mixtures has been associated with abnormal reflexes of the infant, lower mental development up to 2 years, lower motor skills, communication and problem-solving abilities, creativity and visual acuity up to 5 years (reviewed by Julvez and Grandjean, 2009). Based on a meta-analysis, prenatal occupational pesticide exposure was also related to childhood leukemia (Wigle *et al.*, 2009).

Two earlier reviewers concluded that there is inadequate evidence for either establishing or for rejecting a relationship between pesticides exposure and adverse pregnancy outcome (Nurminen, 1995; García, 1998). More recent studies add evidence of the association with exposure to pesticides and miscarriage, fetal death and congenital malformations, but also negative studies exist. Higher exposure is likely in hot climates, where more pesticides are needed and where the use of the protective clothing and other equipment may be difficult due lack of availability or to heat. The exposure is also highest during spraying in greenhouses or outside. Differences of exposure levels in different countries may explain the different results. However, tasks with high exposure should be avoided during pregnancy. To avoid residues from earlier spraying, workers should have long sleeves and gloves when handling sprayed plants.

Male effects

The nowadays banned pesticide (nematicide) dibromochloropropane (DBCP) is a very hazardous occupational testicular toxin in men causing often irreversible azoospermia or oligospermia due to the atrophy of the seminiferous epithelium only (reviewed by Lähdetie, 1995). Associations between exposure to 2,4-dichlorophenoxyacetic acid (2,4-D) and asthenospermia, necrospermia and teratospermia have been reported. Adverse effects on semen quality have also been observed from exposure to ethylene dibromide (sperm count, viability and motility), chlordecone (Kepone™; estrogenic effect) and carbaryl (sperm morphology) (reviewed by Lähdetie, 1995). A recent review (Jensen *et al.*, 2006) summarizes that ethylene dibromide (EDB), vinclozolin, carbaryl, chlordecone, the herbicides alachlor and atrazine, and the insecticide diazinon have been reported to have adverse effects on semen quality. Also, work at greenhouses has been associated with declined sperm density, motility and morphology. On the other hand, in some Danish studies no significant differences were observed between the semen quality of organic and conventional farmers (reviewed by Jensen *et al.*, 2006).

The findings of the effects of exposure to pesticide on fertility are inconclusive. Prolonged time to pregnancy has been observed among Dutch fruit growers exposed to pesticides (De Cock *et al.*, 1994). However, only suggestive association was found in a time-to-pregnancy study among the families of Finnish greenhouse workers (Sallmén *et al.*, 2003).

Paternal exposure to pesticides as an applicator was associated with increased risk of miscarriage (OR 3.8, 95% CI 1.2–12.0, adjusted for age of the wife and smoking of the parents) in a small size study (Petrelli *et al.*, 2000). In the Ontario Farm Family Health Study, where the data on exposure were collected by questionnaire, 2,110 women provided information on 3,936 pregnancies, including 395 miscarriages. Moderate increases in risk of early abortions were observed for preconception exposures to phenoxy acetic acid herbicides (OR 1.5, 95% CI 1.1–2.1), triazines (OR 1.4, 95% CI 1.0–2.0) and any herbicide (OR 1.4, 95% CI 1.1–1.9). For late abortions, preconception exposure to glyphosate (OR 1.7, 95% CI 1.0–2.9), thiocarbamates (OR 1.8, 95% CI 1.1–3.0) and the miscellaneous class of pesticides (OR 1.5, 95% CI 1.0–2.4) was associated with elevated risks (Arbuckle *et al.*, 2001).

In a review it was concluded that there is inadequate evidence for either establishing a relationship between paternal pesticides exposure and birth defects or for rejecting it (García, 1998). Later studies add evidence of the adverse effects of exposure to pesticides on the male (or parent) to adverse pregnancy outcome. A case–control study showed increased odds ratios for congenital malformations (2.0–2.5, 95% CI included one) for several pesticides; only for pyridyl derivatives was the odds ratio statistically significant (adjusted OR 2.8, 95% CI 1.2–6.4) (García *et al.*, 1998). A combination of herbicide, insecticide and fumigant in the paternal exposure increased the risk of birth defects (OR 2.3, 95% CI 0.9–6.1), but the confidence interval included one (Garry *et al.*, 2002). Paternal occupational exposure to pesticides, as reported by the mother, was associated with increased risk of cleft palate (OR 1.7, 95% CI 0.9–3.4) and for multiple cleft lip with/without cleft palate (OR 1.6, 95% CI 0.7–3.4) (Shaw *et al.*, 1999). Paternal agricultural work in the areas where pesticides are used much, was associated with increased risk of fetal death from congenital anomalies (OR 1.6, 95% CI 1.0–2.6) (Regidor *et al.*, 2004).

Some studies have focused on parental work in agriculture or exposure to pesticides and childhood cancer. The results of a Norwegian study suggest that pesticide exposure is an independent risk factor for paternally mediated childhood brain cancer (Kristensen *et al.*, 1996), although the risk may be partially attributed to other factors in the farming context. Parental exposure to pesticides was in some studies associated with childhood cancer (all sites), leukemia, lymphomas and tumors of the brain and nervous system (reviewed by Gold and Sever, 1994; Efird *et al.*, 2003), but conflicting results have also been presented.

Evidence on the adverse effects of pesticide exposure via males is increasing, and exposure should be minimized by using efficient personal protection.

ANESTHETIC GASES

Occupational exposure to trace concentrations of anesthetic gases may occur in operating rooms, delivery wards, dental offices and veterinary surgeries. Numerous epidemiologic studies have examined the reproductive effects of these gases and yielded conflicting results (Table 72.2). Several studies have shown an increased risk of miscarriage and congenital malformation in the offspring among women occupationally exposed to anesthetic gases, whereas some studies have indicated relative risks close to, or slightly above, unity (Figá-Talamanca, 2000). One possible explanation for the contradictory findings is that the type and level of exposure have varied, due to differences in the substances used in operating rooms, methods of administration and in the scavenging equipment employed. Methodological shortcomings may also have contributed to the reported effects of the positive studies. However, the author of a meta-analysis on miscarriage and exposure to anesthetic gases concludes that a real risk may be present (Boivin, 1997). The conclusion was based on the concordance of findings between animal and human data, and on the most rigorous epidemiologic studies. The results of a recent study among veterinarians also accord with these findings; an increased risk of miscarriage and preterm birth was observed among women exposed to anesthetic gases where these agents were delivered without a gas scavenging system (Shirangi *et al.*, 2008, 2009).

The results of epidemiologic studies on the reproductive effects of exposure to trace concentrations of anesthetic gases in men have been contradictory. Some studies have shown a positive association between paternal exposure to anesthetics and miscarriage or congenital malformations in the offspring, whereas in others there has been no association (Tas *et al.*, 1996). These studies have also been criticized for methodological weaknesses and it remains uncertain whether these agents induce reproductive disorders in men.

With the exception of nitrous oxide, the effects of individual anesthetic gases have not been examined in epidemiologic studies. Exposure to unscavenged nitrous oxide was related to an increased risk of miscarriage in dental personnel (Rowland *et al.*, 1995). A Swedish study showed no increase in risk of miscarriage in midwives (Axelsson *et al.*, 1996), but indicated reduced birth weight and an increased risk of infants being small-for-gestational-age (Bodin *et al.*, 1999). Nitrous oxide exposure has also been associated with reduced fertility. Dental assistants exposed to high levels of unscavenged nitrous oxide, and midwives assisting numerous nitrous oxide deliveries per month, had a longer waiting time to pregnancy as compared with unexposed women (Rowland *et al.*, 1992; Ahlborg *et al.*, 1996).

Occupational exposure of pregnant women and those planning to become pregnant should be reduced by use of protective devices. Efficient scavenging equipment, good ventilation and equipment for the administration of anesthetics are needed to keep the exposure levels low in

TABLE 72.2 Chemical occupational exposures in healthcare work associated with adverse effects on reproductive health of women

Hazard	Industry or occupational group	Reported effects
Anesthetic gases	Hospital, dental and veterinary personnel	Reduced fertility, fetal loss, birth defects,[a] preterm birth[a]
Nitrous oxide	Hospital, dental and veterinary personnel	Reduced fertility, fetal loss,[a] low birth weight, intrauterine growth retardation[a]
Antineoplastic drugs	Hospital and veterinary personnel, pharmaceutical industry, laundries, home care, nursing homes	Reduced fertility,[a] fetal loss, birth defects,[a] preterm birth,[a] low birth weight[a]
Estrogens	Pharmaceutical industry	Fetal loss,[a] hyperestrogenism[a]
Ethylene oxide	Hospital and dental personnel	Fetal loss,[a] preterm birth,[a] postterm birth[a]

[a]Inconclusive evidence

operating rooms, delivery wards, dental offices and veterinary surgeries.

ANTINEOPLASTIC AGENTS AND SOME OTHER DRUGS

Nurses and other hospital workers may be exposed to antineoplastic drugs during preparation, administration, nursing and cleaning activities. Exposure can also occur in laundries, pharmaceutical industries, veterinary clinics, home care and nursing homes (Meijster *et al.*, 2006).

The treatment of patients with antineoplastic drugs has induced gonadal damage and adverse effects on menstrual and ovarian function (Shortridge *et al.*, 1995). In men, cyclophosphamide treatment of patients can induce oligospermia and azoospermia. Some case reports have also described malformations in the offspring of patients when antineoplastic therapy has been given during the first trimester of pregnancy (Hoffman, 1986).

Occupational exposure to antineoplastic drugs has been associated with menstrual dysfunction, infertility and adverse pregnancy outcome (Shortridge *et al.*, 1995; Valanis *et al.*, 1997; Fransman *et al.*, 2007; Table 72.2). An increased risk of miscarriage has been observed in nurses who prepare injectable antineoplastic drug solutions for patients (Figá-Talamanca, 2000). High exposure to these drugs was related to an increased risk of premature delivery and low birth weight (Fransman *et al.*, 2007). An excess of congenital malformations has also been reported in the offspring of exposed women. There are, however, study findings suggesting that safety measures can protect the health personnel against adverse effects of antineoplastic drugs on reproduction (Skov *et al.*, 1992). Exposure to antineoplastic agents should be minimized by the use of protective garments and equipment, and good work practices.

Data on the effects of occupational exposure to other drugs are very scarce, although some drugs have shown adverse effects on the development of the fetus. Excess vitamin A is teratogenic in many species, but the teratogenic dose in humans is unknown. Congenital malformations have been seen in children of women exposed to diethylstilbestrol during pregnancy. Some other sex hormones have induced masculinization of female fetuses and feminization of male fetuses in animal experiments. Occupational exposure to estrogens in the pharmaceutical industry has been related to symptoms of hyperestrogenism in male and female employees and an increased risk of miscarriage (Mills *et al.*, 1984; Taskinen *et al.*, 1986). In a study among pharmacy assistants, handling of unsealed antibiotics was associated with miscarriage and prolonged time to pregnancy (Schaumburg and Olsen, 1990).

Healthcare workers may be exposed to ribavirin, an antiviral drug, which is administered to patients as an aerosol mist in a tent. Ribavirin has been found to be teratogenic and embryolethal in animal experiments, but the absorbed doses among hospital staff are likely to be very small. Some other agents, such as acyclovir, ganciclovir, zidovudine, azathioprine, cyclosporin A and pentamidine, have induced decreased implantation and/or embryolethality in animal experiments. Limited human experience with the use of pentamidine during pregnancy has not suggested adverse effects (Frazier and Hage, 1998).

OTHER CHEMICAL AGENTS

Ethylene oxide is used as a sterilizing agent and in the manufacture of chemicals. In animal experiments, ethylene oxide appears to have reproductive toxic effects at high concentrations. Epidemiologic observations among hospital staff or dental assistants engaged in sterilizing instruments with this agent suggest an association between exposure to ethylene oxide and an increased risk of miscarriage (Hemminki *et al.*, 1982; Rowland *et al.*, 1996; Gresie-Brusin *et al.*, 2007). Exposure to ethylene oxide, also classified as a carcinogen, should be kept to a minimum.

Concentrations of flame retardants and PCBs were analyzed in mid-pregnancy serum samples from 20 women who delivered infants with hypospadias and 28 women who delivered unaffected infants. The concentration means for some pollutants were greater for cases than controls, but none of the differences were statistically significant. The current study adds to a relatively limited knowledge base regarding the potential association of specific contaminants with hypospadias or other birth defects (Carmichael *et al.*, 2010).

Phthalates have been shown to adversely affect reproduction in laboratory animals, but human data on their effects are scarce. A recent study noted an excess of hypospadias associated with maternal occupational exposure to phthalates (Ormond *et al.*, 2009).

CONCLUDING REMARKS AND FUTURE DIRECTIONS

For the prevention of adverse effects, risk management and risk communication are needed at the workplace. Often the adjustment of the work is necessary. International classification of chemicals for reproductive toxicity helps to choose safe chemicals for the production and gives guidelines for their safe use. Occupational health personnel utilize the classification and the warning signs in the risk assessment, but often toxicological consultations are also needed. Legislation on the protection of reproductive and developmental health is based on the scientific evidence of the hazardous exposure, and guidelines on how to implement the legislation should be available for occupational health and safety experts.

The main principle in preventing health hazards from occupational exposure is to avoid harmful exposures. Experimental research is important for identification of the toxic properties of chemicals for the basis of classification of the chemicals according to their safety. In the European Union a system for toxicity assessment was launched in 2007 and it will gradually come into force. The new European Chemicals regulation (REACH) stands for Registration, Evaluation, Authorization and Restriction of Chemicals (REACH, 2006). REACH will require the manufacturers and importers of chemicals to generate data for all chemical substances produced or imported into the EU above one ton per year. Similar activities are current in many other countries, too (Stillerman *et al.*, 2008).

Epidemiological studies are necessary to recognize possible new hazards and to monitor whether the preventive activities are effective enough. Continuous research is needed for the establishment of the evidence base, and regularly conducted critical reviews should collect the evidence for the use of health professionals and administrators.

REFERENCES

Abell A, Juul S, Bonde JPE (2000) Time to pregnancy among female greenhouse workers. *Scand J Work Environ Health* **26:** 131–6.

Ahlborg G Jr, Axelsson G, Bodin L (1996) Shift work, nitrous oxide exposure and subfertility among Swedish midwives. *Int J Epidemiol* **25:** 783–90.

Apostoli P, Kiss P, Porru S, Bonde JP, Vanhoorne M, the ASCLEPIOS study group (1998) Male reproductive toxicity of lead in animals and humans. *Occup Environ Med* **55:** 364–74.

Arbuckle TE, Lin Z, Mery LS (2001) An exploratory analysis of the effect of pesticide exposure on the risk of spontaneous abortion in an Ontario farm population. *Environ Health Perspect* **109:** 851–7.

Axelsson G, Ahlborg G Jr, Bodin L (1996) Shift work, nitrous oxide exposure, and spontaneous abortion among Swedish midwives. *Occup Environ Med* **53:** 374–8.

Baranski B (1993) Effects of the work place on fertility and related reproductive outcomes. *Environ Health Perspect* **101 (Suppl. 2):** 81–90.

Bellinger D (2005) Teratogen update: lead and pregnancy. *Birth Defects Res A Clin Mol Teratol* **73:** 409–20.

Bodin L, Axelsson G, Ahlborg G Jr (1999) The association of shift work and nitrous oxide exposure in pregnancy with birth weight and gestational age. *Epidemiology* **10:** 429–36.

Boivin J-F (1997) Risk of spontaneous abortion in women occupationally exposed to anaesthetic gases: a meta-analysis. *Occup Environ Med* **54:** 541–8.

Borja-Aburto VH, Herz-Picciotto I, Rojas Lopes MR, Farias P, Rios C, Blanco J (1999) Blood lead levels measured prospectively and risk of spontaneous abortion. *Am J Epidemiol* **150:** 590–7.

Bretveld R, Zielhuis GA, Roeleveld N (2006) Time to pregnancy among female greenhouse workers. *Scand J Work Environ Health* **32(5):** 359–67.

Bretveld RW, Hooiveld M, Zielhuis GA, Pellegrino A, van Rooij IA, Roeleveld N (2008) Reproductive disorders among male and female greenhouse workers. *Reprod Toxicol* **25:** 107–14.

Brosselin P, Rudant J, Orsi L, Leverger G, Baruchel A, Bertrand Y, Nelken B, Robert A, Michel G, Margueritte G, Perel Y, Mechinaud F, Bordigoni P, Hémon D, Clavel J (2009) Acute childhood leukaemia and residence next to petrol stations and automotive repair garages: the ESCALE study (SFCE). *Occup Environ Med* **66:** 598–606.

Carmichael SL, Herring AH, Sjödin A, Jones R, Needham L, Ma C, Ding K, Shaw GM (2010) Hypospadias and halogenated organic pollutant levels in maternal mid-pregnancy serum samples. *Chemosphere* **80(6):** 641–6.

Chen D, Cho SI, Chen C, Wang X, Damokosh AI, Ryan L, Smith TJ, Christiani DC, Xu X (2000) Exposure to benzene, occupational stress, and reduced birth weight. *Occup Environ Med* **57:** 661–7.

Chen PC, Hsieh GY, Wang JD, Cheng TJ (2002) Prolonged time to pregnancy in female workers exposed to ethylene glycol ethers in semiconductor manufacturing. *Epidemiology* **13:** 191–6.

Cherry N, Moore H, McNamee R, Pacey A, Burgess G, Clyma JA, Dippnall M, Baillie H, Povey A; participating centres of Chaps-UK (2008) Occupation and male infertility: glycol ethers and other exposures. *Occup Environ Med* **65:** 708–14.

Chevrier C, Dananché B, Bahuau M, Nelva A, Herman C, Francannet C, Robert-Gnansia E, Cordier S (2006) Occupational exposure to organic solvent mixtures during pregnancy and the risk of non-syndromic oral clefts. *Occup Environ Med* **63:** 617–23.

Chia SE, Shi LM (2002) Review of recent epidemiological studies on paternal occupations and birth defects. *Occup Environ Med* **59:** 149–55.

Cho SI, Damokosh AI, Ryan LM, Chen D, Hu YA, Smith TJ, Christiani DC, Xu X (2001) Effects of exposure to organic solvents on menstrual cycle length. *J Occup Environ Med* **43:** 567–75.

Colt JS, Blair A (1998) Parental occupational exposures and risk of childhood cancer. *Environ Health Perspect* **106 (Suppl. 3):** 909–25.

Cordier S, Bergeret A, Goujard J, Ha MC, Aymé S, Bianchi F, Calzolari E, De Walle HE, Knill-Jones R, Candela S, Dale I, Dananché B, de Vigan C, Fevotte J, Kiel G, Mandereau L (1997) Congenital malformation and maternal occupational exposure to glycol ethers. Occupational Exposure and Congenital Malformations Working Group. *Epidemiology* **8:** 355–63.

Correa A, Gray RH, Cohen R, Rothman N, Shah F, Seacat H, Corn M (1996) Ethylene glycol ethers and risks of spontaneous abortion and subfertility. *Am J Epidemiol* **143:** 707–17.

Curtis KM, Savitz DA, Weinberg CR, Arbuckle TE (1999) The effect of pesticide exposure on time to pregnancy. *Epidemiology* **10:** 112–17.

De Cock J, Westweer K, Heederik D, Velde E, Kooij R (1994) Time to pregnancy and occupational exposure to pesticides in fruit growers in the Netherlands. *Occup Environ Med* **51:** 693–9.

Efird JT, Holly EA, Preston-Martin S, Mueller BA, Lubin F, Filippini G, Peris-Bonet R, McCredie M, Cordier S, Arslan A, Bracci PM (2003) Farm-related exposures and childhood brain tumours in seven countries: results from the SEARCH international brain tumour study. *Paediatr Perinat Epidemiol* **17:** 201–11.

Figà-Talamanca I (2000) Reproductive problems among women health care workers: epidemiologic evidence and preventive strategies. *Epidemiol Rev* **22:** 249–60.

Figà-Talamanca I (2006) Occupational risk factors and reproductive health of women. *Occup Med (Lond)* **56:** 521–31.

Figà-Talamanca I, Traina ME, Urbani E (2001) Occupational exposures to metals, solvents and pesticides: recent evidence on male reproductive effects and biological markers. *Occup Med (Lond)* **51:** 174–88.

Fransman W, Roeleveld N, Peelen S, de Kort W, Kromhout H, Heederik D (2007) Nurses with dermal exposure to antineoplastic drugs: reproductive outcomes. *Epidemiology* **18:** 112–19.

Frazier L, Hage M (1998) *Reproductive Hazards of the Workplace*. John Wiley & Sons Inc., New York.

Fuortes L, Clark MK, Kirchner HL, Smith EM (1997) Association between female infertility and agricultural work history. *Am J Ind Med* **31:** 445–51.

García A (1998) Occupational exposure to pesticides and congenital malformations: a review of mechanisms, methods, and results. *Am J Ind Med* **33:** 232–40.

García AM, Benavides FG, Fletcher T, Orts E (1998) Paternal exposure to pesticides and congenital malformations. *Scand J Work Environ Health* **24:** 473–80.

Garlantézec R, Monfort C, Rouget F, Cordier S (2009) Maternal occupational exposure to solvents and congenital malformations: a prospective study in the general population. *Occup Environ Med* **66:** 456–63.

Garry VF, Harkins ME, Erickson LL, Long-Simpson LK, Holland SE, Burroughs BL (2002) Birth defects, season of conception, and sex of children born to pesticide applicators living in the Red River Valley of Minnesota, USA. *Environ Health Perspect* **110 (Suppl. 3):** 441–9.

Gold EB, Sever LE (1994) Childhood cancers associated with parental occupational exposures. *Occup Med* **9:** 495–539.

Goulet L, Thériault G (1991) Stillbirth and chemical exposure of pregnant workers. *Scand J Work Environ Health* **17:** 25–31.

Grandjean P, Landrigan PJ (2006) Developmental neurotoxicity of industrial chemicals. *Lancet* **368:** 2167–78.

Greenlee AR, Arbuckle TE, Chyou PH (2003) Risk factors for female infertility in an agricultural region. *Epidemiology* **14:** 429–36.

Gresie-Brusin DF, Kielkowski D, Baker A, Channa K, Rees D (2007) Occupational exposure to ethylene oxide during pregnancy and association with adverse reproductive outcomes. *Int Arch Occup Environ Health* **80:** 559–65.

Ha E, Cho SI, Chen D, Chen C, Ryan L, Smith TJ, Xu X, Christiani DC (2002) Parental exposure to organic solvents and reduced birth weight. *Arch Environ Health* **57:** 207–14.

Heeren GA, Tyler J, Mandeya A (2003) Agricultural chemical exposures and birth defects in the Eastern Cape Province, South Africa: a case–control study. *Environ Health* **2:** 11.

Hemminki K, Mutanen P, Saloniemi I, Niemi ML, Vainio H (1982) Spontaneous abortions in hospital staff engaged in sterilising instruments with chemical agents. *Br Med J* **285:** 1461–3.

Hewitt JB, Tellier L (1998) Risk of adverse outcomes in pregnant women exposed to solvents. *J Obstet Gynecol Neonatal Nurs* **27:** 521–31.

Hjollund NHI, Bonde JPE, Jensen TK, Ernst E, Henriksen TB, Kolstad HA, Giwercman A, Skakkebaek NE, Olsen J (1998a) Semen quality and sex hormones with reference to metal welding. *Reprod Toxicol* **12:** 91–5.

Hjollund NHI, Bonde JPE, Jensen TK, Henriksen TB, Kolstad HA, Ernst E, Giwercman A, Pritzl G, Skakkebaek NE, Olsen J (1998b) A follow-up study of male exposure to welding and time to pregnancy. *Reprod Toxicol* **12:** 29–37.

Hjollund NHI, Bonde JPE, Jensen TK, Henriksen TB, Andersson A-M, Kolstad HA, Ernst E, Giwercman A, Skakkebaek NE, Olsen J (2000) Male-mediated spontaneous abortion among spouses of stainless steel welders. *Scand J Work Environ Health* **26:** 187–92.

Hoffman DM (1986) Reproductive risks associated with exposure to antineoplastic agents: a review of the literature. *Hosp Pharm* **110:** 930–40.

Hooiveld M, Haveman W, Roskes K, Bretveld R, Burstyn I, Roeleveld N (2006) Adverse reproductive outcomes among male painters with occupational exposure to organic solvents. *Occup Environ Med* **63:** 538–44.

Hougaard KS, Hannerz H, Feveile H, Bonde JP, Burr H (2009) Infertility among women working in horticulture. A follow-up study in the Danish Occupational Hospitalization Register. *Fertil Steril* **91 (4 Suppl.):** 1385–7.

Hsieh GY, Wang JD, Cheng TJ, Chen PC (2005) Prolonged menstrual cycles in female workers exposed to ethylene glycol ethers in the semiconductor manufacturing industry *Occup Environ Med* **62:** 510–16.

Hu H, Téllez-Rojo MM, Bellinger D, Smith D, Ettinger AS, Lamadrid-Figueroa H, Schwartz J, Schnaas L, Mercado-García A, Hernández-Avila M (2006) Fetal lead exposure at each stage of pregnancy as a predictor of infant mental development. *Environ Health Perspect* **114:** 1730–5.

Idrovo AJ, Sanìn LH, Cole D, Chavarro J, Cáceres H, Narváez J, Restrepo M (2005) Time to first pregnancy among women working in agricultural production. *Int Arch Occup Environ Health* **78:** 493–500.

Infante-Rivard C, Siemiatycki J, Lakhani R, Nadon L (2005) Maternal exposure to occupational solvents and childhood leukemia. *Environ Health Perspect* **113:** 787–92.

Jelliffe-Pawlowski LL, Miles SQ, Courtney JG; Materna B, Charlton V (2006) Effect of magnitude and timing of maternal pregnancy blood lead (Pb) levels on birth outcomes. *J Perinatol* **26:** 154–62.

Jensen TK, Bonde JP, Joffe M (2006) The influence of occupational exposure on male reproductive function. *Occup Med (Lond)* **56:** 544–53.

Julvez J, Grandjean P (2009) Neurodevelopmental toxicity risks due to occupational exposure to industrial chemicals during pregnancy *Ind Health* **47:** 459–68.

Kippler M, Hoque AM, Raqib R, Ohrvik H, Ekstroöm EC, Vahter M (2010) Accumulation of cadmium in human placenta interacts with the transport of micronutrients to the fetus. *Toxicol Lett* **192:** 162–8.

Kolstad HA, Bisanti L, Roeleveld N, Baldi R, Bonde JP, Joffe M (2000) Time to pregnancy among male workers of the reinforced plastics industry in Denmark, Italy and The Netherlands. ASCLEPIOS. *Scand J Work Environ Health* **26:** 353–8.

Kosnett MJ, Wedeen RP, Rothenberg SJ, Hipkins KL, Materna BL, Schwartz BS, Hu H, Woolf A (2007) Recommendations for medical management of adult lead exposure. *Environ Health Perspect* **115:** 463–71.

Kristensen P, Andersen A, Irgens LM, Bye AS, Sundheim L (1996) Cancer in offspring of parents engaged in agricultural activities in Norway: incidence and risk factors in the farm environment. *Int J Cancer* **65:** 39–50.

Kristensen P, Irgens LM, Andersen A, Snellingen Bye A, Sundheim L (1997) Gestational age, birth weight, and perinatal death among births to Norwegian farmers, 1967–1991. *Am J Epidemiol* **146:** 329–38.

Lähdetie J (1995) Occupation- and exposure-related studies on human sperm. *J Occup Environ Med* **37(8):** 922–30.

Laslo-Baker D, Barrera M, Knittel-Keren D, Kozer E, Wolpin J, Khattak S, Hackman R, Rovet J, Koren G (2004) Child neurodevelopmental outcome and maternal occupational exposure to solvents. *Arch Pediatr Adolesc Med* **158:** 956–61.

Lauria L, Settimi L, Spinelli A, Figà-Talamanca I (2006) Exposure to pesticides and time to pregnancy among female greenhouse workers. *Reprod Toxicol* **22:** 425–30.

Lindbohm M-L (1995) Effects of parental exposure to solvents on pregnancy outcome. *J Occup Environ Med* **37:** 908–14.

Lindbohm M-L (1999) Effects of occupational solvent exposure on fertility. *Scand J Work Environ Health* **25 (Suppl. 1):** 44–6.

Lindbohm M-L, Sallmén M, Anttila A (1997) Male reproductive effects. In *Occupational Health Practice* (Waldron HA, Edling C, eds.). Butterworth-Heinemann, Oxford, pp. 171–82.

Lindbohm M-L, Taskinen H (2000) Reproductive hazards in the workplace. In *Women and Health* (Goldman MB, Hatch MC, eds.). Academic Press, San Diego, pp. 463–73.

Logman JFS, de Vries LE, Hemels MEH, Khattak S, Einarson TR (2005) Paternal solvent exposure and adverse pregnancy outcomes: a meta-analysis. *Am J Ind Med* **47:** 37–44.

Longnecker MP, Klebanoff MA, Brock JW, Zhou H, Gray KA, Needham LL, Wilcox AJ (2002) Maternal serum level of 1,1-dichloro-2,2-bis(p-chlorophenyl)ethylene and risk of cryptorchidism, hypospadias, and polythelia among male offspring. *Am J Epidemiol* **155(4):** 313–22.

Luderer U, Bushley A, Stover BD, Bremner WJ, Faustman EM, Takaro TK, Checkoway H, Brodkin CA (2004) Effects of occupational solvent exposure on reproductive hormone concentrations and fecundability in men. *Am J Ind Med* **46:** 614–26.

Luderer U, Collins TF, Daston GP, Fischer LJ, Gray RH, Mirer FE, Olshan AF, Setzer RW, Treinen KA, Vermeulen R (2006) NTP-CERHR Expert Panel Report on the reproductive and developmental toxicity of styrene. *Birth Defects Res B Dev Reprod Toxicol* **77(2):** 110–93.

McDonald AD, McDonald JC, Armstrong B, Cherry N, Delorme C, Nolin AD, Robert D (1987) Occupation and pregnancy outcome. *Br J Ind Med* **44:** 521–6.

McKinney PA, Raji OY, van Tongeren M, Feltbower RG (2008) The UK Childhood Cancer Study: maternal occupational exposures and childhood leukaemia and lymphoma. *Radiat Prot Dosimetry* **132:** 232–40.

Medina-Carrilo L, Rivas-Solis F, Fernández-Argüelles R (2002) Risk for congenital malformations in pregnant women exposed to pesticides in the state of Nayarit, Mexico. *Ginecol Obstet Mex* **70:** 538–44. (Article in Spanish)

Meijster T, Fransman W, Veldhof R, Kromhout H (2006) Exposure to antineoplastic drugs outside the hospital environment. *Ann Occup Hyg* **50:** 657–64.

Mills JL, Jefferys JL, Stolley PD (1984) Effects of occupational exposure to estrogen and progestogens and how to detect them. *J Occup Med* **26:** 269–72.

Multigner L, Ben Brik E, Arnaud I, Haguenoer JM, Jouannet P, Auger J, Eustache F (2007) Glycol ethers and semen quality: a cross-sectional study among male workers in the Paris Municipality. *Occup Environ Med* **64:** 467–73.

Norman CA, Halton DM (1990) Is carbon monoxide a workplace teratogen? A review and evaluation of literature. *Ann Occup Hyg* **34:** 335–47.

Nurminen T (1995) Maternal pesticide exposure and pregnancy outcome. *J Occup Environ Med* **37:** 935–40.

Ormond G, Nieuwenhuijsen MJ, Nelson P, Toledano MB, Iszatt N, Geneletti S, Elliott P (2009) Endocrine disruptors in the workplace, hair spray, folate supplementation, and risk of hypospadias: case–control study. *Environ Health Perspect* **117:** 303–7.

Pastore LM, Hertz-Picciotto, Beaumont JJ (1997) Risk of stillbirth from occupational and residential exposures. *Occup Environ Med* **54:** 511–18.

Petrelli G, Figà-Talamanca I, Tropeano R, Tangucci M, Cini C, Aquilani S, Gasperini L, Meli P (2000) Reproductive male-mediated risk: spontaneous abortion among wives of pesticide applicators. *Eur J Epidemiol* **16:** 391–3.

Pilsner JR, Hu H, Ettinger A, Sánchez BN, Wright RO, Cantonwine D, Lazarus A, Lamadrid-Figueroa H, Mercado-García A, Téllez-Rojo MM, Hernández-Avila M (2009) Influence of prenatal lead exposure on genomic methylation of cord blood DNA. *Environ Health Perspect* **117:** 1466–71.

Plenge-Bönig A, Karmaus W (1999) Exposure to toluene in the printing industry is associated with subfecundity in women but not in men. *Occup Environ Med* **56:** 443–8.

Qin X, Wu Y, Wang W, Liu T, Wang L, Hu Y, Chen D (2008) Low organic solvent exposure and combined maternal–infant gene polymorphisms affect gestational age. *Occup Environ Med* **65:** 482–7.

Quansah R, Jaakkola JJ (2009) Paternal and maternal exposure to welding fumes and metal dusts or fumes and adverse pregnancy outcomes. *Int Arch Occup Environ Health* **82:** 529–37.

REACH (2007) Regulation (EC) No 1907/2006 of the European Parliament and of the Council of 18 December 2006 concerning the Registration, Evaluation, Authorization and Restriction of Chemicals. http://eur-lex.europa.eu/LexUriServ/site/en/oj/2007/l_136/l_13620070529en00030280.pdf.

Regidor E, Ronda E, Garcia AM, Domínguez V (2004) Paternal exposure to agricultural pesticides and cause specific fetal death. *Occup Environ Med* **61:** 334–9.

Reutman SR, Lemasters GK, Knecht EA, Shukla R, Lockey JE, Burroughs GE, Kesner JS (2002) Evidence of reproductive endocrine effects in women with occupational fuel and solvent exposures. *Environ Health Perspect* **110:** 805–11.

Ribas-Fitó N, Cardo E, Sala M, Eulàlia de Muga M, Mazón C, Verdú A, Kogevinas M, Grimalt JO, Sunyer J (2003) Breastfeeding, exposure to organochlorine compounds, and neurodevelopment in infants. *Pediatrics* **111(5 Pt 1):** e580–e585.

Ritz B, Yu F (1999) The effect of ambient carbon monoxide on low birth weight among children born in southern California between 1989 and 1993. *Environ Health Perspect* **107:** 17–25.

Rowland AS, Baird DD, Shore DL, Darden B, Wilcox AJ (1996) Ethylene oxide exposure may increase the risk of spontaneous abortion, preterm birth, and postterm birth. *Epidemiology* **7:** 363–8.

Rowland AS, Baird DD, Shore DL, Weinberg CR, Savitz DA, Wilcox AJ (1995) Nitrous oxide and spontaneous abortion in female dental assistants. *Am J Epidemiol* **1416:** 531–8.

Rowland AS, Baird DD, Weinberg CR, Shore DL, Shy CM, Wilcox AJ (1992) Reduced fertility among women employed as dental assistants exposed to high levels of nitrous oxide. *N Engl J Med* **327:** 993–7.

Rowland AS, Baird DD, Weinberg CR, Shore DL, Shy CM, Wilcox AJ (1994) The effects of occupational exposure to mercury vapour on the fertility of female dental assistants. *Occup Environ Med* **51:** 28–34.

Sallmén M, Liesivuori J, Taskinen H, Lindbohm ML, Anttila A, Aalto L, Hemminki K (2003) Time to pregnancy among the wives of Finnish greenhouse workers. *Scand J Work Environ Health* **29:** 85–93.

Sallmén M, Lindbohm ML, Anttila A, Kyyrönen P, Taskinen H, Nykyri E, Hemminki K (1998) Time to pregnancy among the wives of men exposed to organic solvents. *Occup Environ Med* **55:** 24–30.

Sallmén M, Lindbohm M-L, Anttila A, Taskinen H, Hemminki K (2000a) Time to pregnancy among the wives of men occupationally exposed to lead. *Epidemiology* **11:** 141–7.

Sallmén M, Lindbohm M-L, Kyyrönen P, Nykyri E, Anttila A, Taskinen H, Hemminki K (1995) Reduced fertility among women exposed to organic solvents. *Am J Ind Med* **27:** 699–713.

Sallmén M, Lindbohm M-L, Nurminen M (2000b) Paternal exposure to lead and infertility. *Epidemiology* **11:** 148–52.

Sallmén M, Neto M, Mayan ON (2008) Reduced fertility among shoe manufacturing workers. *Occup Environ Med* **65:** 518–24.

Schaumburg I, Olsen J (1990) Risk of spontaneous abortion among Danish pharmacy assistants. *Scand J Work Environ Health* **16:** 169–74.

Schnaas L, Rothenberg SJ, Flores MF, Martinez S, Hernandez C, Osorio E, Velasco SR, Perroni E (2006) Reduced intellectual development in children with prenatal lead exposure. *Environ Health Perspect* **114:** 791–7.

Schreinemachers DM (2003) Birth malformations and other adverse perinatal outcomes in four U.S. wheat-producing states. *Environ Health Perspect* **111:** 1259–64.

Schüz J, Kaletsch U, Meinert R, Kaatsch P, Michaelis J (2000) Risk of childhood leukemia and parental self-reported occupational exposure to chemicals, dusts, and fumes: results from pooled analyses of German population-based case-control studies. *Cancer Epidemiol Biomarkers Prev* **9:** 835–8.

Scialli AR, Bonde JP, Brüske-Hohlfeld I, Culver BD, Li Y, Sullivan FM (2010) An overview of male reproductive studies of boron with an emphasis on studies of highly exposed Chinese workers. *Reprod Toxicol* **29:** 10–24.

Shaw GM, Wasserman CR, O'Malley CD, Nelson V, Jackson RJ (1999) Maternal pesticide exposure from multiple sources and selected congenital anomalies. *Epidemiology* **10:** 60–6.

Shiau CY, Wang JD, Chen PC (2004) Decreased fecundity among male lead workers. *Occup Environ Med* **61:** 915–23.

Shirangi A, Fritschi L, Holman CD (2008) Maternal occupational exposures and risk of spontaneous abortion in veterinary practice. *Occup Environ Med* **65:** 719–25.

Shirangi A, Fritschi L, Holman CD (2009). Associations of unscavenged anesthetic gases and long working hours with preterm delivery in female veterinarians. *Obstet Gynecol* **113:** 1008–17.

Shortridge LA, Lemasters GK, Valanis B, Hertzberg V (1995) Menstrual cycles in nurses handling antineoplastic drugs. *Cancer Nursing* **18:** 439–44.

Shu XO, Stewart P, Wen WQ, Han D, Potter JD, Buckley JD, Heineman E, Robison LL (1999) Parental occupational exposure to hydrocarbons and risk of acute lymphocytic leukemia in offspring. *Cancer Epidemiol Biomarkers Prev* **8:** 783–91.

Skov T, Maarup B, Olsen J, Rorth M, Winthereik H, Lynge E (1992) Leukaemia and reproductive outcome among nurses handling antineoplastic drugs. *Br J Ind Med* **49:** 855–61.

Slama R, Thiebaugeorges O, Goua V, Aussel L, Sacco P, Bohet A, Forhan A, Ducot B, Annesi-Maesano I, Heinrich J, Magnin G, Schweitzer M, Kaminski M, Charles MA; EDEN Mother-Child Cohort Study Group (2009) Maternal personal exposure to airborne benzene and intrauterine growth. *Environ Health Perspect* **117:** 1313–21.

Stasenko S, Bradford EM, Piasek M, Henson MC, Varnai VM, Jurasovi J, Kusec V (2010) Metals in human placenta: focus on the effects of cadmium on steroid hormones and leptin. *Appl Toxicol* **30:** 242–53.

Stillerman KP, Mattison DR, Giudice LC, Woodruff TJ (2008) Environmental exposures and adverse pregnancy outcomes: a review of the science. *Reprod Sci* **15:** 631–50.

Stücker I, Mandereau L, Aubert-Berleur MP, Déplan F, Paris A, Richard A, Hémon D (1994) Occupational paternal exposure to benzene and risk of spontaneous abortion. *Occup Environ Med* **51:** 475–8.

Tas S, Lauwerys R, Lison D (1996) Occupational hazards for the male reproductive system. *Crit Rev Toxicol* **26:** 261–307.

Taskinen H, Chia S-E, Lindbohm M-L, Ching-Ye Hong, Sallmén M, Myint Myint Thein (1999a) Risks to the reproductive health of working women. *People and work. Research Reports* **22**. Finnish Institute of Occupational Health, Helsinki.

Taskinen H, Lindbohm M-L, Hemminki K (1986) Spontaneous abortions among women working in the pharmaceutical industry. *Br J Ind Med* **43:** 199–205.

Taskinen HK, Kyyrönen P, Liesivuori J, Sallmén M (1995) Greenhouse work, pesticides and pregnancy outcome. An abstract. *Epidemiology* **6 (Suppl.):** 109.

Taskinen HK, Kyyrönen P, Sallmén M, Virtanen SV, Liukkonen TA, Huida O, Lindbohm ML, Anttila A (1999b) Reduced fertility among female wood workers exposed to formaldehyde. *Am J Ind Med* **36:** 206–12.

Thulstrup AM, Bonde JP (2006) Maternal occupational exposure and risk of specific birth defects. *Occup Med (Lond)* **56:** 532–43.

Torres-Sánchez LE, Berkowitz G, López-Carrillo L, Torres-Arreola L, Rios C, López-Cervantes M (1999) Intrauterine lead exposure and preterm birth. *Environ Res* **81:** 297–301.

Valanis B, Vollmer W, Labuhn K, Glass A (1997) Occupational exposure to antineoplastic agents and self-reported infertility among nurses and pharmacists. *J Occup Environ Med* **39:** 574–80.

Waller SA, Paul K, Peterson SE, Hitti JE (2010) Agricultural-related chemical exposures, season of conception, and risk of gastroschisis in Washington State. *Am J Obstet Gynecol* **202:** 241.e1–e6.

Wang X, Chen D, Niu T, Wang Z, Wang L, Ryan L, Smith T, Christiani DC, Zuckerman B, Xu X (2000) Genetic susceptibility to benzene and shortened gestation: evidence of gene–environment interaction. *Am J Epidemiol* **152:** 693–700.

Wennborg H, Bonde JP, Stenbeck M, Olsen J (2002) Adverse reproduction outcomes among employees working in biomedical research laboratories. *Scand J Work Environ Health* **28:** 5–11.

Wigle DT, Turner MC, Krewski D (2009) A systematic review and meta-analysis of childhood leukemia and parental occupational pesticide exposure. *Environ Health Perspect* **117:** 1505–13.

Wilkins-Haug L (1997) Teratogen update: toluene. *Teratology* **55:** 145–51.

Wirth JJ, Mijal RS (2010) Adverse effects of low level heavy metal exposure on male reproductive function. *Syst Biol Reprod Med* **56:** 147–67.

Xu X, Cho SI, Sammel M, You L, Cui S, Huang Y, Ma G, Padungtod C, Pothier L, Niu T, Christiani D, Smith T, Ryan L, Wang L (1998) Association of petrochemical exposure with spontaneous abortion. *Occup Environ Med* **55:** 31–6.

Yazbeck C, Thiebaugeorges O, Moreau T, Goua V, Debotte G, Sahuquillo J, Forhan A, Foliguet, Magnin G, Slama R, Charles M-A, Huel G (2009) Maternal blood lead levels and the risk of pregnancy-induced hypertension: the EDEN Cohort Study. *Environ Health Perspect* **117:** 1526–30.

C H A P T E R

73

Teratogenicity

Vincent F. Garry and Peter Truran

INTRODUCTION

Teratology is the study of birth defects, and its goals are (1) to describe and determine etiology, (2) to explore mechanisms involved in the production of birth defects and (3) to devise means of prevention. The concept of "birth defects" has evolved beyond the original emphasis on structural congenital malformations. A current operating definition of birth defects is: "Birth defects are structural or functional abnormalities present at birth that cause physical or mental disability. Some may be fatal" (NICHD, 2010). More broadly, a birth defect may be considered as any structural or functional anomaly manifesting at any age due to causes acting before birth. The validity of this later definition (adapted from the March of Dimes foundation) will be considered in this chapter.

HISTORICAL BACKGROUND

Interest and concern for pregnancy and the fetus is as old as human history. Early on, anatomic abnormalities seen at the birth of a child and thereafter were interpreted as omens, cloaked in mysticism and fear. Perhaps the oldest written records of fetal malformations were scribed some 4,000 years ago on clay tablets (the Tablet of Nineveh) by the Chaldeans, who recorded 62 anatomic malformations. These observations were then used to predict future events. For example, birth of a child with no mouth indicated that the mistress of the house would die soon. On the other hand, if a child had an upper lip that overrode the lower, the people of the world would rejoice (Warkany, 1971). Much of the same pattern of thinking continued well beyond the 16th century. Ambroise Paré (circa 1510–1593), who gained fame as a military surgeon, and whose efforts led to the development of the modern surgical approach to wound care, also dabbled in the study of teratology. In the volume titled "Chyrugery", in his treatise *Monsters and Prodigies* (1573), Paré recorded his thoughts on the causal factors involved in birth defects. These included mechanical, hereditary and intrauterine factors which remain pertinent today. Based on these clinical observations, he came up with 13 "etiologic principles" which provided a rationale for the occurrence of these anatomic abnormalities. The first was the glory of God and the last was the activities of Satan (Warkany, 1977). The impact of these misconceptions persists in parts of world culture even to this day. In parallel with this avenue of the study of developmental abnormalities were works devoted to observations of the patterns of normal development. In this context the contributions of Leonardo da Vinci cannot be overlooked. His anatomic drawings of the normal fetus in the womb (Figure 73.1) led to the beginnings of a revolution in the demystification of pregnancy and development. In the early 19th century, the study of anatomic variables encompassed by anomalies of development took a step forward with the nomenclature and classification scheme developed by Etienne Geoffroy Saint-Hilaire (1772–1844). His initial contributions were based on his observations of mummified fetal specimens during his work as a scientist accompanying Napoleon's Egyptian expedition (Charon, 2004). Later on, his son, Isidore Geoffroy Saint-Hilaire (1805–1861), a noted scientist in his own right, coined the term "teratology" to describe the science of the study of anatomic abnormalities of development (Morin, 1996). Much of the scientific effort in 19th and early 20th century teratology was devoted to the anatomic classification of teratologic findings (Baljet and Heyke, 1992). Overlooked, Gregor Mendel's seminal paper on genetics and heredity, first published 1865, remained in obscurity until his works were rediscovered in 1900 (Allen, 2000). At that point Ballantye (1861–1923) and other prominent teratologists of the day quickly incorporated the genetic paradigm into teratology (Warkany, 1977). More importantly, Ballantyne, a clinician, identified the role of alcohol, mercury and infection in providing links to fetal disease (Reiss, 1999). The formal connection of the science of teratology with experimental embryology and biology has been slow in coming.

August Weismann (1834–1914) made important contributions to the theory of developmental biology. His works laid the framework for the distinction between germ plasm and the soma, and the recognition that germ plasm led to continuity of one generation with the next and to variation between generations. Furthermore, he proposed that changes in external conditions, acting during development, might ultimately cause novel variation in the hereditary material.

Hans Spemann (1869–1941), Nobel laureate in 1935, moved Weismann's concepts into the experimental realm. Together with Hilde Margold, he patiently developed and used microsurgical techniques to transfer early embryonic salamander tissue (gastrula) from the blastopore to the

Reproductive and Developmental Toxicology, Edited by Ramesh C. Gupta
ISBN: 978-0-12-382032-7

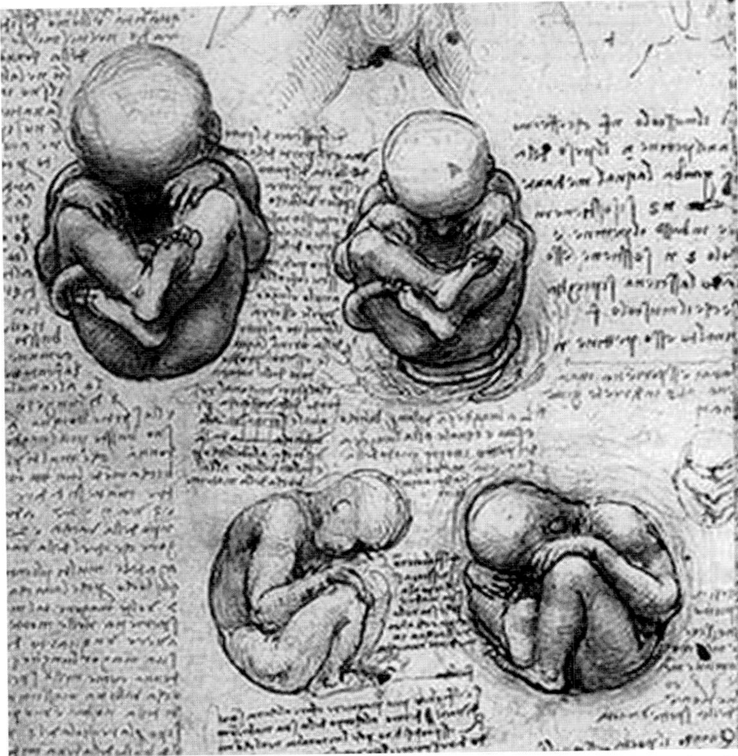

FIGURE 73.1 *Views of fetus and the womb*, Leonardo da Vinci, ca 1510–1512. Please refer to color plate section.

ventral side of another embryo, and grew a new brain and spinal cord. In doing so, he showed that one specific fragment of embryonic tissue was capable of organizing and inducing embryo development and development of specific organs. Sven Otto Horstadius (1898–1996) extended and expanded this concept to explore morphogenesis in echinoderm embryos. In these studies he also explored the effects of pH, temperature and ionic concentrations on development (Jacobson, 2000). At about this time, modern teratology as an experimental and clinical discipline began to take form as a result of the work of Josef Warkany (1902–1992), a pediatrician, described by his peers as the father of modern teratology (Willhite, 2000). His long and productive career began with a series of investigations that marked nutritional and vitamin deficiency as causally related to birth defects. Later works described diabetes as a risk factor for birth defects, and his studies on animals explored the teratologic potential of therapeutic drugs including warfarin, salicylates, thalidomide, methotrexate and aminopterin. He investigated the role of the endocrine system and dysfunctions of the endocrine system in teratogenesis and postnatal development. He took part in the formulation of the central working paradigm of the study of teratology in the 20th century, namely, the principles of teratology (see referenced works in Warkany, 1982).

THE PRINCIPLES OF TERATOLOGY

The six principles of teratology put forward by James G. Wilson (1915–1987) integrated the knowledge gained from developmental biology, genetics, clinical medicine and biochemistry to describe the major factors that can be involved in a teratologic event. These principles (Wilson, 1977), which continue to be relevant today (Kimmel, 2001), are as follows:

1. Susceptibility to teratogenesis depends on the genotype of the conceptus and the manner in which this interacts with environmental factors.
2. Susceptibility to teratogens varies with the developmental stage at the time of exposure.
3. Teratogenic agents act in specific ways on developing cells and tissues to initiate abnormal developmental processes.
4. The final manifestations of abnormal development are death, malformation, growth retardation and functional disorder.
5. The access of adverse environmental influences to developing tissues depends on the nature of the influence.
6. Manifestations of deviant development increase in frequency and in degree as dosage increases from no effect to the 100% lethal (LD_{100}) level.

This chapter will consider each of these principles and illustrate them by specific examples of teratologic agents and their actions. In later parts of the chapter, we will explore the evolution of the study of teratology into the neurobehavioral realm.

BIRTH DEFECT PREVALENCE

More than three in every 100 live births will result in a child with a major structural or genetically based birth defect. Birth defects are a major contributor to infant mortality and result in billions of dollars in healthcare costs (Rynn *et al.*, 2008). In the USA, national estimates of birth defect prevalence are based on birth certificate data (EPA, 2009). Based on these data, the overall birth defect rate per year from 1999 to 2005 was approximately one in 100 live births. However, birth certificate data underestimate the frequency of birth defects, since not all birth defects are apparent and reported at birth or shortly thereafter. To illustrate the point (Garry *et al.*, 2002) examined the relative rate birth defects in a cohort of members of the farming community reported in the first year of life. Comparison of birth defects rates from birth certificate data vs. those confirmed in medical records demonstrated that the relative rates per 1,000 births of CNS (4.6 vs. 1.3), musculoskeletal (9.8 vs. 6.5) and cardiovascular (5.2 vs. 3.7) birth defects were higher in the medical record confirmed dataset. On the other hand, gastrointestinal (2.0 vs. 1.3), urogenital (4.0 vs. 4.4) and genetic/metabolic (0.65 vs. 1.7) birth anomaly rates were nearly equivalent. It is apparent from these data that, although birth anomalies visible at birth or symptomatic shortly thereafter can be captured in birth certificate data, many birth and developmental anomalies, unfortunately, make their appearance well after the newborn period. For example, in the same study, 62% of the birth anomalies reported were identified in the first year of life, another 10% within years 1–3, and 20% in children more than 3 years old. More comprehensive work is ongoing through the Centers for Disease Control (CDC).

For more than 30 years metropolitan Atlanta, Georgia, through the CDC, has engaged and continues to develop an active birth defect reporting system. Medical records of each live birth in the five counties of metropolitan Atlanta are examined and updated through age 5 by trained abstractors. Major structural and/or genetic defects are identified in this group (Rynn *et al.*, 2008). From 1978 to 2005 the overall prevalence of major structural defects was stable, varying from 2.8 to 3.0 per 100 live births. Male children (PR = 1.17) had more defects than females; fewer birth defects were observed among minorities. Issues such as access to care and poverty appear unresolved in these assessments.

Active reporting of birth defect prevalence nationwide is limited to specific major anatomic disorders (US Department of Health and Human Services, 2006). Of more concern, the cause(s) of approximately 70% of birth defects reported are unknown (March of Dimes, 2009). Moreover, frequencies of genetic, environmental, infectious and medication-related causes of birth defects are relatively unknown. To capture the available knowledge base regarding agents linked to human birth defects, Shepard assembled a comprehensive catalog of known human teratogenic agents (Shepard and Lemire, 2004). The spectrum of agents known to cause human birth defects is broad (Table 73.1). Based on our current assessments, it is likely that both the spectrum of agents and frequency of birth defects are wholly underestimated.

TABLE 73.1 Teratogenic agents in human beings

Radiation	*Drugs and environmental chemicals*
Atomic weapons	Aminopterin and methylaminopterin
Radioiodine	Androgenic hormones
Therapeutic	Busulfan
Infections	Captopril (renal failure) Carbamazepine*
Cytomegalovirus (CMV)	Chlorobiphenyls Cigarette smoking Cocaine
Herpes simplex virus 1 and 2	Corticosteroids*
Lymphocytic choriomeningitis	Coumarin anticoagulants Cyclophosphamide
Parvovirus B-19 (Erythema infectiosum)	Diethylstilbestrol
Rubella virus	Diphenylhydantoin Enalapril (renal failure) Etretinate
Syphilis	Fluconazole, high dose Iodides and goiter
Toxoplasmosis	Lithium*
Varicella virus	Mercury, organic
Venezuelan equine encephalitis virus	Methimazole and scalp defects and choanal atresia*
Maternal and metabolic imbalance	Methylene blue via intra-amniotic injection
Alcoholism	Misoprostol*
Amniocentesis, early	Penicillamine
Chorionic villus sampling (before day 60)*	Phenobarbitol*
Cretinism, endemic	1 3..cis-Retinoic acid (Isotretinoin and Accutane) Sartans
Diabetes	Tetracyclines
Folic acid deficiency Hyperthermia	Thalidomide
Myasthenia gravis Phenylketonuria	Toluene abuse
Rheumatic disease and congenital heart block	Trimethadione
Sjogren's syndrome	Valproic acid
Virilizing tumors	

*Denotes agents that produce less than 10 defects in 1,000 exposures
From Shepard and Lemire (2004) with permission

TABLE 73.2 Gestation time frame of humans and experimental animals

	Human	Mouse	Rat	Rabbit
Total gestation time (days)	267d	18–20d	21–22d	31–34d
Implantation	6–7d	3–6d	3–5d	8 d (approx)
Beginning organogenesis	13–14d	6d	8.5d	7.3d
End organogenesis	7–8 wks	15d	15d	18d
Fetuses per litter	1	8–10	12–13	6–9

Adapted from Shepard and Lemire (2004)

THE DEVELOPING EMBRYO

For many years now the primary focus of examination of teratogenic events has been the embryo-sensitive period, the timeframe of organ formation. It is the period in embryonic development where tissue and organ structure are being formed and reformed as development proceeds, a time of rapid cell division, programmed cell death and structural differentiation through cell–cell interaction. Cell movement, timing and cell homing are precisely orchestrated, with each organ system having its critical time of sensitivity to teratogens. Parts of organ building overlap in the timing susceptibility (Table 73.2).

MATERNAL RISK FACTORS

Maternal age

Women who become pregnant beyond age 30 are at increased risk for having a child with a birth defect. Specifically, the risk of chromosomal trisomy and birth defects arising from trisomy, e.g. Down syndrome, rises from about 2–3% to 30% or more for women who become pregnant in their forties. Chromosomal non-disjunctions occurring in the developing ovum either during mitosis or meiosis are major mechanisms leading to the development of fetal trisomy (Hassold and Hunt, 2009). Continued exposures of the ovum to environmental toxicants over time are likely contributors to the increased frequency of ovarian trisomy with age, yet studies to evaluate this concern in humans are non-existent at this writing (Brent, 2004).

Nutrition

The dietary needs of mother and fetus are interrelated. For example, maternal dietary lack of folic acid puts the fetus at special risk for development of a neural tube defect (NTD). The level of risk of NTD is dependent in part on the genotype of the mother, with certain maternal genotypes showing an increased susceptibility to folic acid deficiency (Zhu *et al.*, 2009). Nutritional environments deficient in folic acid, combined with maternal genotypes at special risk, make for an enhanced frequency of NTDs in some racial and ethnic mixes.

Severe maternal starvation during World War 2 led to increased frequency of birth defects and miscarriages (Wynn and Wynn, 1993). However, human adaptation to periods of starvation minimizes the frequency of adverse reproductive outcomes, and results in little or no observable adverse developmental effects (Prentice and Goldberg, 2000).

Morbid obesity and/or gestational diabetes, and diabetes alone, are special risk factors for miscarriage, still births and children with birth defects (Buchanan and Kitzmiller, 1994; Stothard *et al.*, 2009; Biggio *et al.*, 2010). Certain infections, radiation exposure and medications are maternal risk factors with associations to human birth defects (Shepard and Lemire, 2004). However, linkage between exposure and a specific birth defect tends to be more complicated. For example, one or more maternal risk factors (genetics, nutrition, hyperthermia, anticonvulsant medications), alone or together, are linked to the development of neural tube defects (Detrait *et al.*, 2005). The links between environmental chemical exposures including lead, arsenic, cadmium, mercury, PCBs, TCDD, pesticides and solvents and NTDs are less clear.

FETAL ALCOHOL SPECTRUM DISORDER (FASD)

Ethanol readily crosses the placenta. Blood alcohol levels reach equilibrium between mother and fetus within minutes. In early pregnancy (the period of organogenesis) ethanol acts to reduce neural cell proliferation and increase cell death (apoptosis) in a special population of cells (neural crest) that gives rise to facial structures and certain peripheral nerves (Burd *et al.*, 2003). Other mechanisms appear to be more significant later in pregnancy, e.g. the loss of specific brain cells.

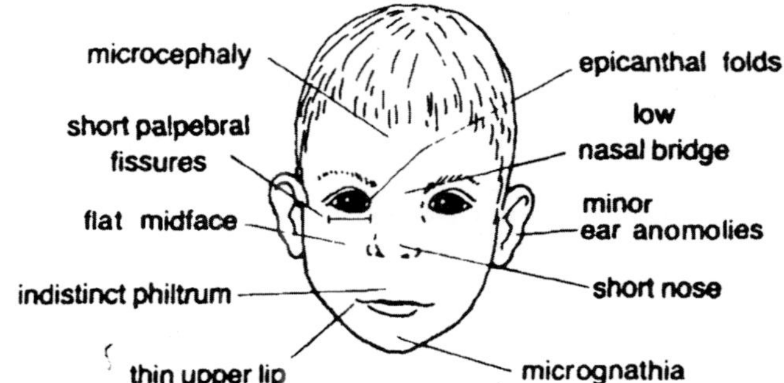

FIGURE 73.2 Facial features in fetal alcohol syndrome. (From Little and Streissguth, 1982. *Alcohol. Pregnancy and the Fetal Alcohol Syndrome.* Slide available from Miller–Fenwick Inc., Timonium, MD 21093.)

By definition, fetal alcohol syndrome (FAS) is a recognized pattern of major and minor malformations, growth deficiency, and neural and neurobehavioral dysfunction. Specific dysmorphic craniofacial anomalies (Figure 73.2), including microcephaly, short palpebral fissures and hypoplastic midface (Jones and Smith, 1973), define the major dysmorphic features in the clinical diagnosis of FAS. For the diagnosis, alcohol-related neurodevelopmental disorders (ARND/FASD) manifest evidence of a characteristic complex behavioral or cognitive abnormalities, inconsistent with normal neurodevelopmental level of the child, e.g. mild to moderate IQ reduction and attention deficit hyperreactivity syndrome (Stromland *et al.*, 2005). In the USA, the prevalence of FAS is estimated at between 2 and 7 per 1,000 in school aged children from mixed socioeconomic groups. Importantly, the prevalence of FASD is estimated to be as high as 2–5% (May *et al.*, 2009). These data make ethanol the most commonly observed, known human teratogen. Risk factors for FAS include maternal age, socioeconomic status, nutrition, ethnicity and genetic factors including those determining variance in maternal metabolism of ethanol. The number of drinks imbibed at one sitting, and their timing during pregnancy (e.g., first trimester), are overriding risks.

METABOLISM OF ETHANOL AND RISK OF FETAL ALCOHOL SYNDROME

Alcohol metabolism involves two key enzymes: alcohol dehydrogenase (ADH) and aldehyde dehydrogenase (ALDH). Both enzymes occur in several forms (isoforms).

Alcohol dehydrogenase (ADH)

ADH is the major enzyme responsible for conversion of ethanol to acetaldehyde. The rate (kinetics) of conversion is dependent on the allelic form of the dimeric enzyme (Edenberg, 2007). The alleles encoding the different ADH and ALDH variants are unevenly distributed among ethnic groups. The mechanism whereby ADH and ALDH variants influence the relative risk of the occurrence of alcoholism, and as a consequence FASD, is thought to involve local elevation of acetaldehyde levels. Higher rates of oxidation of alcohol to acetaldehyde, and/or slower rates of oxidation of acetaldehyde to CO_2 by ALDH, lead to the accumulation of toxic levels of acetaldehyde. The acetaldehyde-induced pathophysiologic (alcohol aversion) reaction is characterized by facial flushing, nausea and rapid heartbeat. One variant of ADH is ADH1B, which is encoded by several alleles. The allele ADH1B3 is unique to people of African descent, and is associated with rapid oxidation of alcohol to acetaldehyde. Approximately 25% of African Americans have this allele. Women and children from families with this allele are at lower risk for alcoholism and FAS (Scott and Taylor, 2007) consistent with their genetic metabolic profile.

Aldehyde dehydrogenase (ALDH)

Two main ALDH enzymes (ALDH1 localized in the cell cytosol; ALDH 2 in the mitochondria) are responsible for conversion of acetaldehyde to acetate. Individuals who carry the ALDH2*2 allele and who are heterozygous show little enzyme activity; those who are homozygous show no oxidant activity for conversion of acetaldehyde to acetate. ALDH 2*2 is relatively common among people of Chinese, Japanese or Korean descent. Twenty to forty percent of mainland and Taiwanese Chinese have at least one allele. The presence of this allele is strongly protective of alcohol dependence (Edenberg, 2007). Registry-based studies (Chavez *et al.*, 1988) suggest that the rate of FAS in Asians residing in the USA is less that 0.03/1,000 live births, consistent with the genetic/metabolic profile of this ethnic group.

CYP2E1

While 90% of ingested alcohol is metabolized to acetaldehyde by ADH enzymes, 10% is metabolized by CYP2E1 enzyme. Interestingly, this polymorphic enzyme is inducible by alcohol itself, and may account for some of the variability of alcohol-related birth defects. Notably, CYP2E1 is inducible in the placenta, and more so in the placenta from alcohol abusers (Gemma *et al.*, 2007).

Finally, twin studies of children of alcoholic mothers show that if one member of a fraternal twin pair has FAS, the second member of the pair is much less likely to have the syndrome. In identical twins, if one member of the twin pregnancy has FAS the second member is highly likely to have FAS, suggesting that both the genotype of the mother and the fetus are linked to the risk of FAS (Streissguth and Dehaene, 1993).

Evidence of variance in susceptibility from animal studies: potential mechanisms of ethanol toxicity

Studies of alcohol teratogenesis in animals are commonly conducted during specific times of heightened susceptibility during pregnancy (period of organogenesis). To demonstrate variance in susceptibility, a study of five strains of mice demonstrated that pregnant females from one strain (B6) showed multiple morphologic malformations in brain, digits, rib and kidney while another showed none (strain 129). The remaining strains showed intermediate frequencies of birth defects. All animals were administered ethanol (5.8 gms/kg) on GD 9. Again, susceptibility to teratogenesis by ethanol depends on the genotype of the mother and timeframe of fetal sensitivity (Downing *et al.*, 2009). In timed studies to focus on forebrain development, alcohol administered during the critical time period GD 7.5 in C57 mice results in prosencephaly. Increased apoptosis-induced inhibition of sonic hedgehog gene expression by ethanol was linked to the occurrence of prosencephaly (Aoto *et al.*, 2008). Minimizing oxidant stress-induced apoptosis (administering antioxidant vitamins C or E) was shown to be a potential preventive therapy. Along these same lines, treatment with different concentrations of alcohol from GD 6 to 15 in C57BL/6 mice resulted in a spectrum of fetal alcohol-related morphologic abnormalities ranging from those of the brain and related neural structures, to abnormalities of heart and limb development. This dose regimen also gave expression to neurobehavioral abnormalities.

In detailed molecular studies, expression of HOXA1 was suppressed in the alcohol-treated animals. HOXA1 is one of several HOX genes involved in development and differentiation, and is involved in hind brain and craniofacial development. The antioxidant folic acid was found to mitigate these effects. In general, the involvement of antioxidants in organogenesis seems to reduce alcohol-induced dysmorphogenesis, and it appears that the developmental effects of alcohol lie in alteration of common signaling pathways for development and differentiation (Green *et al.*, 2007).

ANTIEPILEPTIC DRUGS

Epilepsy affects 1–2% of humans worldwide and has a peak incidence in the first year of life. To prevent or inhibit seizure development, antiepileptic drugs (AEDs) are designed to modify the bursting properties of neurons, inhibit the spread of epileptic activity and alter synchronization of epileptiform neuronal activity. Aside from their therapeutic activities, AEDs, as a drug class, are among the most common causes of fetal malformations. Teratogenic effects have been associated with the use of AEDs, notably, phenytoin, carbamazepine, valproate and phenobarbital (Ikonomidou and Turski, 2009). These effects include major malformations (neural tube defects, congenital heart defects, orofacial clefts and digit anomalies), growth retardation, developmental delay and microcephaly. The cognitive function of children who were exposed to AEDs *in utero* can also be affected. Of the AEDs in human clinical use, valproic acid, is the only AED for which dose-dependent increases in the frequency of malformation have been observed (Perucca, 2005).

Gestation-induced changes in the clearance of AEDs, and subsequent changes in dosing and perhaps poly-therapy with multiple AEDs, are a concern. Increased clearance, together with genetic/metabolic polymorphisms, is a factor affecting the prevalence of AED-associated birth defects (Pennell and Hovinga, 2008; Klotz, 2007). Phenytoin, an effective AED in long-term use, is a prime example of the variance encountered in birth defect frequency due to genetically mediated alteration of drug metabolism. On the other hand, valproate (VPA) rarely shows significant variance in its genetic–metabolic effects.

Comparative findings with AEDs

Valproate (VPA)

Major congenital abnormalities (facial dimorphism, spina bifida, musculoskeletal disorders) have been reported in approximately 11% of VPA-exposed pregnancies in the USA, 6.2–14% in the UK and 17% in Australia through their respective national registries (Smith and Whitehall, 2009). Since VPA is commonly used in epilepsy syndromes with a presumed genetic cause, comparison of patients treated with VPA with and without epilepsy suggests that VPA, and not an underlying epilepsy syndrome, was responsible for the observed increase in birth defects (Bromfield *et al.*, 2008). It is highly probable that intrauterine exposure in the first trimester led to a higher risk of major congenital malformations. Exposure throughout pregnancy was more likely to have adverse behavioral/cognitive outcomes. In this vein, by age 3, children who had been exposed to VPA *in utero* had significantly lower IQ scores than those who had been treated with other AEDs. On average, children of patients receiving VPA had a 7 point lower IQ than those treated with phenytoin (Meador *et al.*, 2009). These findings were adjusted for confounding factors including socioeconomic status and maternal IQ.

While the exact mechanism(s) of VPA's teratogenic effects are uncertain, animal and *in vitro* molecular studies suggest that the inhibition of histone deacetylases (HDAC) is a likely mediator of its fetotoxic effects (Gurvich *et al.*, 2005). This work is further supported by studies of VPA-induced gene activation patterns in the HDAC pathway (Kultima *et al.*, 2004).

Phenytoin (diphenylhydantoin, Dilantin)

Phenytoin (Phn) is an old line anticonvulsant drug in common use from the 1930s to the present day. The drug exerts anti-seizure activity without causing general depression of the CNS. Therapeutically, phenytoin limits sustained firing of the CNS during convulsive episodes. It is also known to have a narrow range of therapeutic efficacy (10 to 20 μg/ml in serum) and is a well-known teratogen. Early studies (Hanson *et al.*, 1976) showed that approximately 5–10% of children exposed to phenytoin *in utero* developed what became known as the fetal hydantoin syndrome (FHS). These children have major craniofacial abnormalities (e.g., cleft lip and palate, microcephaly), underdeveloped nails, and/or mild developmental delays.

Variance in serum concentration and clearance reflected by the polymorphic nature of the enzymes involved in Phn metabolism

These differences are key elements in the fetotoxicity and maternal toxicity of this drug. Phenytoin is almost completely metabolized in the liver by the cytochrome P450 system through CYP2C9 conversion of phenytoin to the arene oxide, followed by hydrolysis to inactive compounds by microsomal epoxide hydrolase (EPHX1). There are over 33 variants of CYP2C9 (Wang *et al.*, 2009). In population studies, mutations of CYP2C9 have been associated with slower Phn metabolism and increased adult toxicity (Klotz, 2007; McCluggage *et al.*, 2009). In regard to fetotoxicity, mothers who had EPHX 1 113H and 139R alleles (relatively rare) more frequently had children with craniofacial abnormalities (Azzato, 2010). The CYP2C9 genotype was not related to these teratogenic effects. Exposure to phenytoin during the 5th or 6th weeks of gestation is the main pharmaceutical cause of cleft lip. Slowing and arrhythmia of the embryonic heart with concurrent hypoxia is thought to be the primary teratogenic mechanism of phenytoin fetotoxicity (Webster *et al.*, 2006; Webster, 2007). Finally, it is often not safe for women who have a seizure disorder to avoid use of AEDs during pregnancy. Seizures and periods of anoxia during seizures are themselves an important risk factor for developmental toxicity.

NEUROBEHAVIORAL TERATOLOGY

This chapter has reported how neurobehavioral teratology plays an important role in the overall developmental toxicity of alcohol and anticonvulsive drugs. In this section, a brief review of the history and conduct of behavioral teratologic studies will be considered, concluding with a few examples of studies conducted in the environmental setting.

The history and purview of neurobehavioral teratology is intertwined with neurodevelopmental toxicology. The broad field of behavioral teratology includes behavioral changes produced by toxicants with documented anatomic neuropathologic findings, for example methylmercury, ethanol and others (e.g., parathion, methyl demeton) where there is significant CNS change but little if any change in the behavior of the offspring of treated animals. In other instances, behavioral changes may be delayed well into the postnatal period and beyond through adulthood, without marked neuroanatomic findings, for example *in utero* lead and PCBs.

As early as 1963 the concept of behavioral teratology was introduced in a review by Werboff and Gottlieb (1963). In that review, the authors described the postnatal behavioral effects of exposure to prenatal X-radiation and to the use of psychoactive drugs in pregnancy. After a period of more than 10 years, Great Britain and Japan incorporated guidelines for neurodevelopmental toxicity testing (DNT) of medicinal products. The 1980s saw the development of the first draft of the US EPA DNT protocol, and over time behavioral testing procedures have evolved as a cooperative effort among agencies and scientists representing the USA, Japan and European Union (Makris *et al.*, 2009). The current US EPA neurodevelopmental toxicity study guidelines for studies in animals are listed in Figure 73.3. The figure outlines parameters of observation and times for specific neurobehavioral examinations for a typical DNT study. The timeframe examined extends from day 6 of gestation to the 60th day after birth. Dosing of animals starts at GD 6 and continues through lactation (PND 21) in the developing/maturing rat (Makris and Raffaele, 2009). Study parameters are comparable to OECD test guideline 426 (adopted October 2007). The dose–response curves produced using the behavioral endpoints specified tend to be complex, and may involve a U-shaped dose–response (e.g., alcohol increases motor activity at low doses with CNS depression, but induces decreased motor activity at high doses). It is of interest that NOEL levels observed in these behavioral studies tend to

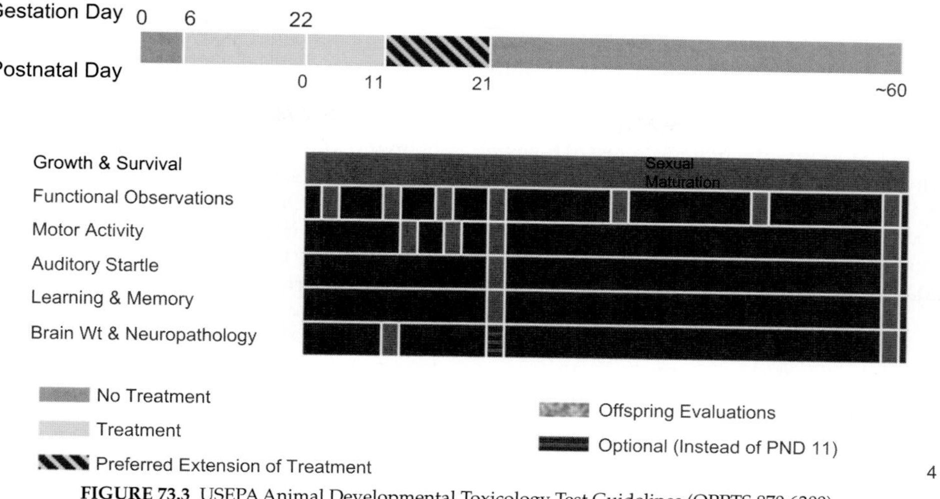

FIGURE 73.3 USEPA Animal Developmental Toxicology Test Guidelines (OPPTS 870.6300).

occur at lower levels than in routine teratologic studies. Conducting these animal studies in a regulatory context is expensive and time consuming (Makris and Raffaele, 2009), but survey of their use and value in safety assessment studies suggests that behavioral parameters can be an improvement over more general toxicologic assessments (Middaugh *et al.*, 2003).

In vivo and *in vitro* screening of potential neurotoxicants, utilizing appropriate biomarkers and toxicant pathway analysis, offers alternatives which allow us to step to the future and address the onslaught of untested chemicals with the potential for harm (Bushnell *et al.*, 2010). While these efforts contribute to our understanding of neurodevelopmental toxicants, the historic insights gained from clinical observation coupled with behavioral biomarker studies should not be overlooked.

ENVIRONMENTAL AGENTS AND BEHAVIORAL TERATOLOGY

Lead

It is well known and accepted that low levels of lead exposure can affect cognition, memory and behavioral control (Needleman, 2009). Higher maternal blood lead levels in the first trimester of pregnancy are a predictor of poorer mental development index (MDI) scores in children at age 24 months. Maternal lead levels in the 2nd and 3rd trimester were not predictive, suggesting that neurodevelopmental events during the first trimester were critical to later cognitive development (Hu *et al.*, 2006). MDI is based on the Bayleys scales of infant development, used routinely to measure mental, motor and relevant child behavior (attention/arousal, engagement, emotional regulation) markers over the first 3 years of life. In another recent study, where the median cord blood lead level was very low (1.21 μg/dl), MDI studies performed at age 3 years detected lower MDI scores among boys even though cord blood lead levels were no different between the sexes. Low lead levels have been associated with lower IQ scores at blood lead levels of less than 10 μg/dl. This finding is much disputed (Ernhart, 2006), but nevertheless, current evidence continues to support the notion that chronic low-level lead exposure *in utero* can have adverse neurodevelopmental effects (Jusko *et al.*, 2008).

PARTICULATE POLLUTION: EXPOSURE TO POLYAROMATIC HYDROCARBONS (PAHs)

PAHs readily cross the placenta (Srivastava *et al.*, 1986; Hatch *et al.*, 1990) and are known to affect neurobehavioral development in experimental animals (Wormley *et al.*, 2004). Recent studies of pregnancy and ambient PAH pollutants conducted in urban environments of New York, Poland and China have documented the effects of airborne PAHs on postnatal neurodevelopment. In the New York studies, the median PAH concentration of the sum of eight selected common PAHs was 2.26 ng/m^3. Prospective studies of minority children residing in the south Bronx, Harlem and Washington Heights, NY, showed that the risk of cognitive development delay by age 3 was almost threefold higher than expected (Perera *et al.*, 2006). By age 5, higher PAH levels (>2.26 ng/m^3) were inversely associated with lower full-scale and verbal IQ scores. Decrements in IQ scores were 4.31 to 4.67 points (Perera *et al.*, 2009). In a parallel study of Caucasian mothers and children residing in Krakow, Poland, the median PAH concentration was 17.96 ng/m^3. In these studies, air monitors were strapped to pregnant women ($N = 550$) for 48 h over different times of the year to establish the ambient PAH norm for the location. Non-verbal measures of reasoning ability were assessed to assure that cultural/linguistic differences between study groups would be minimized (Raven Colored Progressive Matrices test). Studies conducted among the children at age 5 showed a reduction in IQ with higher prenatal (above the median concentration) exposures to PAHs. The average decrease was 3.8 IQ points (Edwards *et al.*, 2010).

The China prospective cohort study took advantage of a planned shutdown of an old coal-fired power plant used to augment power during the local dry season. The municipality is situated in a basin with the power plant located near the center. Two prospective cohorts were identified, one before and one after shutdown. Levels of benzo(a)pyrene-DNA adducts were measured in cord blood regardless of the time of year of delivery. Child development was assessed at age 2 years by the Gesell Developmental Schedule test. This is a preschool test administered individually to children between the ages of 2 and 6. Decreased motor area development was noted in the pre-shutdown cohort when compared to the post-shutdown cohort.

In all, these data show that prenatal exposure to particulate pollutants can have neurodevelopmental consequences. Whether these findings can be considered minor decrements in neurobehavioral development is an unexplored question.

Pesticides

Based on their more obvious toxicant properties, certain classes of pesticides, namely organophosphates and organochlorines, have long been tentatively linked to adverse neurodevelopmental and developmental neurobehavioral effects (Garry *et al.*, 2004). Organophosphates are non-persistent pesticides, and well-known inhibitors of cholinesterase-mediated neurotransmission. Organochlorine insecticides (National Pesticide Information Center (NPIC), 1999) are persistent in tissues with higher lipid content and are stable soil contaminants (half-life: 2–15 years).

Organochlorines

Most insecticides in the organochlorine class have been banned for many years, an exception being DDT use in malarial control. The use and importation of one member of this class, Mirex, has been prohibited in Spain since 1994. However, some 10 or more years later, placental samples obtained at birth still contained Mirex. More importantly, the level of the organochlorine pesticide in the placenta was inversely correlated with cognitive development at age 4 years (Puertas *et al.*, 2010). In contrast with these findings, results from studies of postnatal neurobehavioral development and DDT exposure have been mixed. Few studies performed (children age 4) showed significant decrements of verbal and memory cognitive scale, while other studies of children aged 2 or less showed delayed psychomotor development. Still other neurodevelopmental studies performed in this earlier timeframe (age 2 or less) showed little or no effects on cognition (Jurewicz and Hanke, 2008). Whether these neurobehavioral decrements will be sustained in the long term is not clear.

Organophosphates

As a pesticide class, organophosphates (OPs) are the most widely used insecticides worldwide. OPs are used as part of agricultural practice, in households, public buildings and on stagnant water. They can have moderate to highly acute toxic effects in humans based on the irreversible inhibition of the enzyme cholinesterase, leading to accumulation of the neurotransmitter acetylcholine. Below the level where acute toxicity is observed, gene expression studies show that at least 15 separate toxicity pathways can be affected by the OP chlorpyrifos (CPF) (Bushnell *et al.*, 2010). Repeated low-level treatment with CPF in animals can lead to protracted impairments of sustained attention and an increase in impulsive behaviors (Middlemore-Risher *et al.*, 2010). Studies in neonatal animals further indicate that effects on brain development are separable from systemic OP toxicity (Slotkin *et al.*, 2006). Other neonatal studies show that thyroid function can be impeded with a low level of CPF exposure. Studies on *in utero* exposure to low-level CPFs show (in the postnatal period), abnormal thyroid function and reduced learning ability in female, but not in male mice (Haviland *et al.*, 2010). At sublethal doses of dimethoate given during pregnancy, postnatal studies show adverse effects on the pituitary–testicular axis. Altogether these animal and *in vitro* data show that *in utero* or early postnatal exposure to OPs can have adverse effects on behavior, perhaps on an endocrine basis.

Neurodevelopmental epidemiologic studies of New York City minority newborns who had been exposed *in utero* to low levels of OPs showed an increased level of abnormal reflexes correlated with the level of OP metabolites in the mothers' urine obtained during the prenatal period (Engel *et al.*, 2007). Similar findings were reported in a study of Mexican Americans in California. In these studies, newborns were examined prior to and after the first 3 days of life. Increased abnormal reflexes occurred and were correlated with urinary OPs metabolite levels obtained twice during pregnancy (Young *et al.*, 2005).

Children 3–23 months of age who resided in north Ecuadorian communities engaged in floriculture, and who were consequently exposed to higher levels of OPs, showed decreased fine and gross motor skills (Handal *et al.*, 2006). Similarly, children of mothers employed in floriculture from the same area, studied between 6 and 8 years of age, showed deficits in motor speed, coordination and visual-spatial performance.

The results from animal and human studies seem similar in many respects, giving consistency to the overall data. It is therefore not too surprising that, in a recent US national study (National Health and Nutrition Examination Survey (NHANES), 2000–2004; Bouchard *et al.*, 2010), children with 10-fold increase in urinary OP metabolites were 1.55 times more likely to have ADHD (attention deficit/hyperactivity disorder); children with higher than the median urinary concentration of OP metabolites were twice as likely (OR 1.93; CI 1.23–3.02) to have ADHD (Bouchard *et al.*, 2010). Standardized clinical test procedures (DISC-IV) were employed for the diagnosis of ADHD. It has not been established if these findings arose from *in utero* OP exposure.

In light of all the foregoing animal and human data, the principle "prudence dictates" should be applied with respect to organophosphate use at home and elsewhere.

CONCLUDING REMARKS AND FUTURE DIRECTIONS

In this relatively brief overview of the field of teratology, we explored the scope of this endeavor to include behavioral teratology. Much of the effort utilizes the tools of epidemiology, animal and *in vitro* study. Early on, questions raised by astute clinicians' observations of unusual teratologic events were the key to the initiation of research efforts. Later, regulatory efforts took hold to assure the safety of medications that may be used in pregnancy. More recently, observations in the environmental setting led to a revolution in our understanding of potential teratology events. The work of Theo Colborn, a noted environmental scientist, brought forward the concept of endocrine disruption in deregulation of normal growth and development.

Now the stage is set for the next evolution of this field of study. In this vision, each person will have knowledge of their own genotype, delineating metabolic pathways for processing toxicants and alterations of those pathways through life. Therapeutic intervention will prevent potential teratogenic events, perhaps through pharmacologic treatment or specific gene segment insertion to modify adverse pregnancy outcomes. We will eventually include screening of potential teratogenic agents by gene expression assay with these results being integrated with a personal genotype as a measure of risk. Finally, the delineation of toxicant/metabolic behavioral pathways is in the foreseeable future. However, ethical issues regarding accessing and use of computerized medical records to query genetic profiles, medications and disease burdens as they relate to birth defects are poorly charted waters.

REFERENCES

Allen G (2000) The reception of mendelism in the United States. *CR Acad Sci Paris, Sciences de la vie/Life Sci* **323:** 1081–8.

Aoto K, Shikata Y, Higashiyama D, Shiota K, Motoyama J (2008) Fetal ethanol exposure activates protein kinase A and impairs Shh expression in prechordal mesendoderm cells in the pathogenesis of holoprosencephaly. *Birth Defects Res Part A: Clin Mol Teratol* **82:** 224–31.

Azzato EM (2010) Maternal EPHX1 polymorphisms and risk of phenytoin-induced congenital malformations. *Pharmacogenet Genom* **20(1):** 58–63.

Baljet B, Heyke G (1992) History of classification systems of conjoined twins by specific consideration of the classification systems of Louis Bolk (1866–1930). *Ann Anat* **174(4):** 361–8.

Biggio J, Chapman V, Neely C, Cliver S, Rouse D (2010) Fetal anomalies in obese women: the contribution of diabetes. *Obstet Gynecol* **115(2 Pt 1):** 290–6.

Bouchard M, Bellinger D, Wright R, Weisskopf M (2010) Attention-deficit/hyperactivity disorder and urinary metabolites of organophosphate pesticides. *Pediatrics* **125(6):** e1270–7.

Brent R (2004) Reproductive and genetic risks of preconception exposure to mutagenic agents and reproductive toxins. *Reproduct Toxicol* **19(2):** 242–3.

Bromfield E, Dworetzky B, Wyszynski D, Smith C, Baldwin E, Holmes L (2008) Valproate teratogenecity and epilepsy syndrome. *Epilepsia* **49:** 2122–4.

Buchanan T, Kitzmiller J (1994) Metabolic interactions of diabetes and pregnancy. *Ann Rev Med* **45:** 245–60.

Burd L, Cotsonas-Hassler T, Martsolf JT, Kerbeshian J (2003) Recognition and management of fetal alcohol syndrome. *Neurotoxicol Teratol* **25:** 681–8.

Bushnell P, Kavlock R, Crofton K, Weiss B, Rice D (2010) Behavioral toxicology in the 21st century: challenges and opportunities for behavioral scientists: summary of a symposium presented at the annual meeting of the Neurobehavioral Teratology Society. *Neurotoxicol Teratol* **32(3):** 313–28.

Charon P (2004) Etienne Geoffroy Saint-Hilaire (1772–1844) and anencephaly: contribution of one naturalist to medical knowledge. *Histoire des sciences médicales* **38(3):** 365–83.

Chavez G, Cordero J, Becerra J (1988) Leading major congenital malformations among minority groups in the United States, 1981–1986. *Morb Mort Weekly Report* **37(SS-3):** 17– 24.

Detrait E, George T, Etchevers H, Gilbert JR, Vekemans M, *et al.* (2005) Human neural tube defects: developmental biology, epidemiology, and genetics. *Neurotoxicol Teratol* **27:** 515–24.

Downing C, Balderrama-Durbin C, Broncucia H, Gilliam D, Johnson T (2009) Ethanol teratogenesis in five inbred strains of mice. *Alcoholism: Clin Exp Res* **33:** 1238–45.

Edenberg H (2007) The genetics of alcohol metabolism: role of alcohol dehydrogenase and aldehyde dehydrogenase variants. *Alcohol Res Health* **30(1):** 5–13.

Edwards SC, Jendrychowski W, Butscher M, Camann D, Kieltyka A, Mroz E, *et al.* (2010) Prenatal exposure to airborne polycyclic aromatic hydrocarbons and children's intelligence at age 5 in a prospective cohort study in Poland. *Environ Health Perspect.* In press.

Engel S, Berkowitz G, Barr D, Teitelbaum S, Siskind J, Meisel S, *et al.* (2007) Prenatal organophosphate metabolite and organochlorine levels and performance on the Brazelton Neonatal Behavioral Assessment Scale in a multiethnic pregnancy cohort. *Am J Epidemiol* **165(12):** 1397–404.

EPA (Environmental Protection Agency) (2009) *Birth Defects Prevalence and Mortality*. Retrieved May 26, 2010, from http://cfpub.epa.gov/eroe/index.cfm?fuseaction=detail.viewInd&lv=list.listByAlpha&r=201581&subtop=381.

Ernhart C (2006) Effects of lead on IQ in children. *Environ Health Perspect* **114:** A85–A86.

Garry V (2004) Pesticides and children. *Toxicol Appl Pharmacol* **198:** 152–63.

Garry V, Harkins M, Erickson L, Long-Simpson L, Holland S (2002) Birth defects, season of conception, and sex of children born to pesticide. *Environ Health Perspect* **11 (Suppl. 3):** 441–9.

Gemma S, Vichi S, Testai E (2007) Metabolic and genetic factors contributing to alcohol induced effects and fetal alcohol syndrome. *Neurosci Biobehav Rev* **31:** 221–2.

Green M, Singh A, Zhang Y, Nemeth K, Sulik K, Knudsen T (2007) Reprogramming of genetic networks during initiation of the fetal alcohol syndrome. *Devel Dynam* **236:** 613–31.

Gurvich N, Berman M, Wittner B, Gentleman R, Klein P, Green J (2005) Association of valproate-induced teratogenesis with histone deacetylase inhibition in vivo. *Fed Am Soc Exp Biol J* **19:** 1166–8.

Handal A, Lozoff B, Breilh J, Harlow S (2006) Effect of community of residence on neurobehavioral development in infants and young children in a flower-growing region of Ecuador. *Environ Health Perspect* **115(1):** 128–33.

Hanson J, Myrianthopoulos N, Harvey M, Smith D (1976) Risks to the offspring of women treated with hydantoin convulsants, with emphasis on the fetal hydantoin syndrome. *J Pediatr* **89:** 662–8.

Hassold T, Hunt P (2009) Maternal age and chromosomally abnormal pregnancies: what we know and what we wish we knew. *Curr Opin Pediatr* **21(6):** 703–8.

Hatch M, Warburton D, Santella R (1990) Polycyclic aromatic hydrocarbon-DNA adducts in spontaneously aborted fetal tissues. *Carcinogenesis* **11:** 1673–5.

Haviland J, Butz D, Porter W (2010) Long-term sex selective hormonal and behavior alterations in mice exposed to low doses of chlorpyrifos in utero. *Reprod Toxicol* **29(1):** 74–9.

Hu H, Téllez-Rojo M, Bellinger D, Smith D, Ettinger A, Lamadrid-Figueroa H, *et al.* (2006) Fetal lead exposure at each stage of pregnancy as a predictor of infant mental development. *Environ Health Perspect* **114:** 1730–5.

Ikonomidou C, Turski L (2010) Antiepileptic drugs and brain development. *Epilepsy Res* **88:** 11–22.

Jacobson C-O (2000) Sven Otto Hörstadius. 18 February 1898–16 June 1996. *Biographical Memoirs of Fellows of the Royal Society* **46:** 243–56.

Jones K, Smith D (1973) Recognition of the fetal alcohol syndrome in early infancy. *Lancet* **1:** 999–1001.

Jurewicz J, Hanke W (2008) Prenatal and childhood exposure to pesticides and neurobehavioral development: review of epidemiological studies. *Int J Occup Med Environ Health* **21:** 121–32.

Jusko T, Henderson C, Lanphear B, Cory-Slechta D, Parsons P, Canfield R (2008) Blood lead concentrations <10 µg/dl and child intelligence at 6 years of age. *Environ Health Perspect* **116:** 243–8.

Kimmel C (2001) Overview of teratology. *Current Protol Toxicol* 13.1.1.–13.1.8.

Klotz U (2007) The role of pharmacogenetics in the metabolism of antiepileptic drugs: pharmacokinetic and therapeutic implications. *Clin Pharmacokinetics* **46(4):** 271–9.

Kultima K, Nystrom A-M, Scholz B, Gustafson A-L, Dencker L, Stigson M (2004) Valproic acid teratogenicity: a toxicogenomics approach. *Environ Health Perspect* **112(12):** 1225–35.

Makris S, Raffaele K (2009) Developmental neurotoxicity. In *General and Applied Toxicology* (Ballantyne B, Marrs T, Syversen T, eds.). J. Wiley & Sons Ltd.

Makris S, Raffaele K, Allen S, Bowers W, Hass U, Alleva E, *et al.* (2009) A retrospective performance assessment of the developmental neurotoxicity study in support of OECD test guideline 426. *Environ Health Perspect* **117:** 17–25.

March of Dimes (2009, June) http://search.marchofdimes.com/pnhec/4439_1206.asp. Retrieved May 27, 2010.

May PA, Gossage JP, Kalberg WO, Robinson LK, Buckley D, Manning M, Hoyme HE (2009) Prevalence and epidemiologic characteristics of FASD from various research methods with an emphasis on recent in-school studies. *Develop Disabil Res Rev* **15:** 176–92.

McCluggage L, Voils S, Bullock M (2009) Phenytoin toxicity due to genetic polymorphism. *Neurocritical Care* **10(2):** 222–4.

Meador K, Baker GA, Browning N, Clayton-Smith J, Liporace J, Pennell P, *et al.* (2009) Cognitive function at 3 years of age after fetal exposure to antiepileptic drugs. *New Engl J Med* **360:** 1597–605.

Middaugh L, Dow-Edwards D, Li A, Sandler J, Seed J, Sheets L, *et al.* (2003) Neurobehavioral assessment: a survey of use and value in safety assessment studies. *Toxicol Sci* **76:** 250–61.

Middlemore-Risher M, Buccafusco J, Terry A (2010) Repeated exposures to low-level chlorpyrifos results in impairments in sustained attention and increased impulsivity in rats. *Neurotoxicol Teratol* **32(4):** 415–24.

Morin A (1996) Teratology "from Geoffroy Saint-Hilaire to the present". *Bulletin de l'Association des anatomistes (Nancy)* **80(248):** 17–31.

National Health and Nutrition Examination Survey (NHANES) (2000–2004) *DDT (Technical Fact Sheet).* Retrieved June 9, 2010, from http://npic.orst.edu/factsheets/ddttech.pdf.

Needleman H (2009) Low level lead exposure: history and discovery. *Ann Epidemiol* **19(4):** 235–8.

NICHD (2010, March 24). Retrieved May 26, 2010, from http://www.nichd.nih.gov/health/topics/birth_defects.cfm.

Pennell P, Hovinga C (2008) Antiepileptic drug therapy in pregnancy I: gestation-induced effects on AED pharmacokinetics. *Int Rev Neurobiol* **83:** 227–40.

Perera F, Rauh V, Whyatt R, Tsai W-Y, Tang D, Diaz D, *et al.* (2006) Effect of prenatal exposure to airborne polycyclic aromatic hydrocarbons on neurodevelopment in the first 3 years of life among inner-city children. *Environ Health Perspect* **114:** 1287–92.

Perera F, Zhigang Z, Whyatt R, Hoepner L, Wang S, Camann D, *et al.* (2009) Prenatal airborne polycyclic aromatic hydrocarbon exposure and child IQ at age 5 years. *Pediatrics* **124:** e195–e202.

Perucca E (2005) Birth defects after prenatal exposure to antiepileptic drugs. *The Lancet Neurology* **4(11):** 781–6.

Prentice A, Goldberg G (2000) Energy adaptations in human pregnancy: limits and long-term consequences. *Am J Clin Nutr* **71 (Suppl.):** 1226S–1232S.

Puertas R, Lopez-Espinosa M, Cruz F, Ramos R, Freire C, Pérez-García M, *et al.* (2010) Prenatal exposure to mirex impairs neurodevelopment at age of 4 years. *Neurotoxicology* **31(1):** 154– 60.

Reiss H (1999) Historical insights: John William Ballantyne 1861–1923. *Hum Reprod Update* **5:** 386–9.

Rynn L, Cragan J, Correa A (2008) Update on Overall Prevalence of Major Birth Defects – Atlanta, Georgia, 1978–2005. *Morb Mort Weekly Report* **57(01):** 1–5.

Scott D, Taylor R (2007) Health-related effects of genetic variations of alcohol-metabolizing enzymes in African Americans. *Alcohol Res Health* **30(1):** 18–21.

Shepard T, Lemire R (2004) *Catalog of Teratogenic Agents*, 11th edition. Baltimore: The Johns Hopkins University Press.

Slotkin T, Tate C, Ryde I, Levin E, Seidler F (2006) Organophosphate insecticides target the serotonergic system in developing rat brain regions: disparate effects of diazinon and parathion at doses spanning the threshold for cholinesterase inhibition. *Environ Health Perspect* **114:** 746–51.

Smith J, Whitehall J (2009) Sodium valproate and the fetus: a case study and review of the literature. *Neonatal Network* **28(6):** 363–7.

Srivastavaa V, Chauhana SS, Srivastavaa P, Kumara V, Misra U (1986) Fetal translocation and metabolism of PAH obtained from coal fly ash given intratracheally to pregnant rats. *J Toxicol Environ Health* **18(3):** 459–69.

Stothard K, Tennant P, Bell R, Rankin J (2009) Maternal overweight and obesity and the risk of congenital anomalies. *J Am Med Assoc* **301(6):** 636–50.

Streissguth A, Dehaene P (1993) Fetal alcohol syndrome in twins of alcoholic mothers: concordance of diagnosis and IQ. *Am J Med Genet* **47:** 857–61.

Stromland K, Mattson S, Adnams C, Autti-Ramo I, Warren K (2005) Fetal alcohol spectrum disorders: an international perspective. *Alcoholism: Clin Exper Res* **29(6):** 1121–6.

US Department of Health and Human Services (2006) Improved national prevalence estimates for 18 selected major birth defects – United States, 1999–2001. *Morb Mort Weekly Report* **54/Nos. 51 & 52:** 1301–5.

Wang B, Wang J, Huang S-Q, Su H-H, Zhou S-F (2009) Genetic polymorphism of the human cytochrome P450 2C9 gene and its clinical significance. *Curr Drug Metabol* **10(7):** 781–834.

Warkany J (1971) Syndromes. *Am J Dis Childh* **121(5):** 365–70.

Warkany J (1977) History of teratology. In *Handbook of Teratology*, Vol. 1 (Wilson J, Clark F, (eds.). New York: Springer-Verlag.

Warkany J (1982) Curriculum vitae. *Teratology* **25:** 145–51.

Webster W (2007) The effect of hypoxia in development. *Birth Defects Res Part C: Embryo Today: Reviews* **81(3):** 215–28.

Webster W, Howe A, Abela D, Oakes D (2006) The relationship between cleft lip, maxillary hypoplasia, hypoxia and phenytoin. *Curr Pharmaceut Des* **12(12):** 1431–48.

Werboff J, Gottlieb J (1963) Drugs in pregnancy: behavioral teratology. *Obstet Gynecol Surve* **18:** 420–3.

Willhite C (2000) Josef Warkany. *Toxicol Sci* **58:** 220–1.

Wilson J (1977) In *Handbook of Teratology*, Vol. 1 (Wilson J, Clarke F, eds.). New York: Springer-Verlag, pp. 49–62.

Wormley D, Ramesh A, Hood D (2004) Environmental contaminant – mixture effects on CNS development, plasticity, and behavior. *Toxicol Appl Pharmacol* **197:** 49–65.

Wynn A, Wynn M (1993) The effects of food shortage on human reproduction. *Nutr Health* **9:** 43–52.

Young J, Eskenazi B, Gladstone E, Bradman A, Pedersen L, Johnson C, *et al.* (2005) Association between in utero organophosphate pesticide exposure and abnormal reflexes in neonates. *Neurotoxicology* **26:** 199–209.

Zhu H, Kartiko S, Finnell R (2009). Importance of gene–environment. *Clin Genet* **75:** 409–23.

C H A P T E R

74

Ultrasound and magnetic resonance in prenatal diagnosis of congenital anomalies

Aleksandra Novakov Mikic, Katarina Koprivsek and Dusko Kozic

INTRODUCTION

Ultrasound (US) examination for fetal abnormalities has been a part of the routine antenatal screening programme for many years. Most examinations can be made using a well-designed and structured screening program, with adequate education and follow-up of patients (Novakov *et al.*, 1999). *In utero* brain magnetic resonance imaging (MRI) is now being used increasingly successfully to clarify abnormal ultrasound findings, often resulting in a change of diagnosis or treatment plan. Fetal MR imaging can be a helpful adjunct when sonography analysis is limited, such as in cases of large maternal body habitus, oligohydramnios, low position of the fetal head, or when the fetal spine is positioned posterior. Although future improvements in both US and MR hardware and software will improve the quality of fetal imaging, continued multidisciplinary collaboration among obstetricians, perinatologists, sonographers, child neurologists and pediatric neurosurgeons is critical to ensure maximal growth in the field of fetal imaging.

TERATOGENS AND THEIR EFFECTS

Congenital malformations account for approximately 20% of deaths in the prenatal period. About 65–75% of the causes of congenital malformations are multifactorial or unknown, 20–25% are genetic, while approximately only 10% are environmental (intrauterine infections 3%, maternal metabolic disorders 4%, environmental chemical 4%, drugs and medications <1% and ionizing radiation 1–2%). Teratogens are agents that cause malformations in a developing embryo. Numerous agents exhibit teratogenic effects. The dose and duration of exposure usually are the main determining factors regarding the severity of the damage and the type of defect (Brent *et al.*, 1993; Finnell, 1999).

Among the most researched areas are the effects of epilepsy, diabetes and their therapies, as well as abuse of recreational drugs.

Drugs

Although there are only a few dugs that are associated with a true teratogenic effect in humans, the use of medicinal drugs in pregnancy remains controversial, with many drugs in use having limited safety profiles and even less scientific investigation in pregnancy (Johns *et al.*, 2006). One of the possibilities of contributing to postmarketing surveillance of the teratogenicity of medications is routinely collecting the data in national birth registries and assessing associations between medications and risk for congenital anomalies, which already proved strong associations between valproic acid and spina bifida as well as insulin (as proxy for diabetes) with several types of congenital heart diseases (Lisi *et al.*, 2010)

In the 1960s, thalidomide caused limb deficiencies in thousands of infants worldwide. Either duplication (preaxial polydactyly of hands and feet) or deficiency (absence of thumb) is a common effect of thalidomide; no other human teratogen identified to date has this effect on the developing limb (Holmes, 2002), although limb abnormalities are one of the most common and visible phenotypic effects of several human teratogens (thalidomide, warfarin, phenytoin, valproic acid, misoprostol, chorionic villus sampling and phenytoin).

Sodium valproate is a teratogen responsible for a wide range of abnormalities, including neural tube defects, cleft lip and palate, cardiovascular anomalies, genitourinary defects, developmental delay, limb defects, endocrine abnormalities and autism. It has traditionally been prescribed for epilepsy, but is increasingly used for such psychiatric conditions as bipolar disease. Women of childbearing age taking valproate should be warned of its teratogenicity and advised to plan their pregnancy, take a higher dose of folate, discuss reducing the dose of valproate or changing the drug with their physician, and have detailed antenatal scans (Alsdorf and Wyszinski, 2005; Smith and Whitehall, 2009). The specific inhibition by VPA of histone deacetylase and changes in gene expression may explain the teratogenicity of this drug. Other possible explanations are increased fetal oxidative stress induced by VPA, with the brain being more susceptible to oxidative stress in comparison to other fetal organs, or the folic acid inhibitory action

Reproductive and Developmental Toxicology, Edited by Ramesh C. Gupta
ISBN: 978-0-12-382032-7

of this drug (Ornoy, 2009). In cases of monotherapies, when the effect of valproic acid is compared to carbamazepine, there seems to be a higher risk than exposure to carbamazepine (Wide *et al.*, 2004)

Lithium is a drug used mainly for the treatment of bipolar disorder and there is a possible link with cardiac anomalies, though not as strong as previously thought, and more recent epidemiologic data indicate that teratogenic risk of first trimester lithium is lower than previously suggested so it can be given in pregnancy, with a fetal echocardiography performed in the second trimester (Cohen *et al.*, 1994; Yacobi and Ornoy, 2008). When all drugs used for therapy of bipolar disorder are taken into account, well-characterized risks are associated with valproate, carbamazepine, lamotrigine and lithium (Nguyen *et al.*, 2009).

In the treatment of another psychiatric disorder, depression, potential risk is found in therapy with paroxetine – cardiovascular malformations, and malformations of cranium and abdominal wall (Berard *et al.*, 2007; Diav Citrin *et al.*, 2008).

Benzodiapines readily cross the placenta from early pregnancy and their use has been associated with increased incidence of cleft palate (Johns *et al.*, 2006).

Both maternal asthma status and asthma medication use, particularly bronchodilators, may play a role in cardiac malformations in offspring (Lin *et al.*, 2009).

An increased risk of gastroschisis has been reported due to maternal intake of over-the-counter drugs such as cough and cold medications and analgesics, including aspirin and other NSAIDs during the first trimester of pregnancy (Johns *et al.*, 2006)

Diabetes mellitus

Diabetes is known to carry increased risk of congenital malformations, mainly cardiac malformations and spinal anomalies, and preconception recognition of women at risk is mandatory (Allen *et al.*, 2007).

Recreational drugs

Complications of pregnancy as well as altered fetal behavior are connected with prenatal exposure to cocaine. Other reported problems are reduced head circumference, decreased birth weight and length, a higher incidence of craniofacial abnormalities and cerebral infarction, hydronephrosis, hypospadias and cardiac anomalies, and abnormalities associated with vascular disruption – limb reduction defects and intestinal atresia (Landry and Whitney, 1996; Johns *et al.*, 2006; Salisbury *et al.*, 2007).

Use of alcohol during pregnancy may lead to a broad variety of developmental anomalies – growth deficiency, neurological disorders and craniofacial anomalies. Alcohol-exposed offspring also may have alcohol-related birth defects, when there is limited expression of one or more features associated with FAS – major organ malformation, spontaneous abortion, decreased immune function, hearing impairment and delayed development (Armant and Saunders, 1996). Combination of prenatal use of alcohol and cocaine is more deleterious than use of either of them alone (Randall *et al.*, 1999).

Cigarette smoking

Cigarette smoking is associated with congenital anomalies such as orofacial clefts, limb reduction defects, the Poland sequence of urogenital anomalies (Johns *et al.*, 2006) and anorectal atresia (Miller *et al.*, 2009), and esophageal atresia (Wong Gibbons *et al.*, 2008).
Table 74.1 shows the latest list of additional major potential teratogens.

Prenatal diagnosis

Ultrasound (US) examinations for fetal abnormalities have been a part of the routine antenatal screening program for many years. Most examinations can be made using a well-designed and structured screening program, with adequate education and follow-up of patients (Novakov *et al.*, 1999). *In utero* brain magnetic resonance imaging (MRI) is now being used increasingly successfully to clarify abnormal ultrasound findings, often resulting in a change of diagnosis or treatment plan. Fetal MR imaging can be a helpful adjunct when sonography analysis is limited, such as in cases of large maternal body habitus, oligohydramnios, low position of the fetal head, or when the fetal spine is positioned posterior. Although future improvements in both US and MR hardware and software will improve the quality of fetal imaging, continued multidisciplinary collaboration among obstetricians, perinatologists, sonographers, child neurologists, and pediatric neurosurgeons is critical to ensure maximal growth in the field of fetal imaging.

THE CENTRAL NERVOUS SYSTEM

Cerebral anomalies

Holoprosencephaly

Holoprosencephaly (HPE) is a term used for a group of cerebral anomalies which are the result of a failure or incomplete cleavage of a primitive forebrain – prosencephalon. These cleavage abnormalities can occur both sagittally, resulting in fusion of the cerebral hemispheres, and horizontally, resulting in abnormalities of the optic and olfactory bulbs. There are three types, due to different degrees of failure of cleavage – alobar, semilobar and lobar, alobar being the most severe and lethal (Pilu and Nicolaides, 1999). Known teratogens are alcohol, phenytoin, retinoic acid, maternal diabetes and congenital infections.

Prenatal diagnosis

In the transverse view of the fetal head there is a single midline ventricle replacing the two lateral ventricles or partial segmentation of the ventricles. The alobar and semilobar types are often associated with facial defects (Pilu and Nicolaides, 1999). Facial features include proboscis, midline facial cleft and hypotelorism. Extracranial abnormalities may be found (Nyberg *et al.*, 1987). The alobar type is characterized by a large central cranial fluid collection (a monoventricular cavity lacking ventricular horns and midline structures), a fused thalamus at the floor of this cavity, and characteristic

TABLE 74.1 Updated list of main additional potential teratogens, according to Mountain States Genetics Foundation Newsletter

Medications	
ACE inhibitors (medications for hypertension and congestive heart failure) (Friedman, 2006)	Skull ossification defects, oligohydramnios and renal dysgenesis
Aminopterin	Meroanencephaly, skeletal defects
Busulfan	Cleft palate, corneal opacities, skeletal anomalies
Phenytoin (Dialantin)	Microcephaly, mental retardation, eylide ptosis, phalangeal hypoplasia
Metotrexate	Skeletal anomalies, including vertebral column, face and skull
Tetracycline	Stained teeth, hypoplasia of enamel
Trimethadione	Cleft palate or lip, developmental delay, low-set ears
Large doses of vitamin A (Luo *et al.*, 2004)	Neural tube defects, facial abnormalities
Substances of abuse	
Toluene	Microcephaly, craniofacial abnormalities
Maternal infections	
TORCH (toxoplasmosis, other (varicella, mumps, HIV, coxsackie), rubella, cytomegalovirus, herpes (Lynfield and Eaton, 1995)	Microcephaly, microgyria, cerebral calcifications, cataracts, chorioretinitis, mental retardation, heart defects, deafness
Toxoplasma gondii	Microcephaly, microophthalmia, cerebral calcifications, chorioretinitis
Treponema pallidum	Deafness, abnormal teeth, skeletal anomalies, hydrocephalus
Maternal disorders	
Phenylketonuria	Microcephaly, mental retardation, facial dysmorphism, congenital heart defects
Hypo- and hyperthyroidism	Goiter, growth and developmental retardation
Chemicals	
(Mountain States Genetics Foundation, 1995)	
Lead (exposure common, lead is used in batteries, metals, paint, ceramic glazes, cable covering, some toys) (Woolf *et al.*, 2007)	Central nervous system damage, undescended testicles
Mercury (exposure might happen from broken thermometers, dental fillings, broken fluorescent light bulbs)	Brain atrophy, spasticity, mental retardation
Arsenic (exposure might happen when drinking contaminated well water, living near or working at industrial incinerators or metal smelters)	Low birth weight
Polychlorobiphenyls	Low birth weight
Cobalt (exposure might happen in enamelic industry, during catalytic applications)	Confirmed on animal studies, questionable in humans
Ionizing radiation	Microcephaly, skeletal malformation, mental retardation

facial features (proboscis, single orbit, single nostril or severe hypotelorism) (Filly *et al.*, 1984). The semilobar type is similar, but in a single horseshoe-shaped ventricle there is much mantle. Diagnosis of holoprosencephaly is possible in the first trimester (Souka and Nicolaides, 1997).

Fetal MRI should be considered to confirm and further classify cases of holoprosencephaly (HPE); a false-positive diagnosis of HPE has been reported in cases of hydrocephalus, hydranencephaly, arachnoid or porencephalic cyst, Dandy-Walker malformations with ventriculomegaly, septo-optic dysplasia and other CNS malformations (Simon *et al.*, 2000). Moreover, fetal MRI can provide correct differentiation of the middle intrahemispheric (MIH) variant of HPE from other forms of HPE, and other midline emigrational congenital anomalies. This is particularly important because patients with MIH typically have fewer severe motor and cognitive disabilities than do those with alobar or semilobar HPE. The alobar and semilobar types carry the worst prognoses but are more amenable to reliable prenatal sonographic diagnosis. In general, the long-term outcome in these conditions is significantly better than that of HPE, making the distinction crucial. MRI can provide definitive identification of MIH morphology (widely separated in the most anterior portions of the frontal lobes and deep gray nuclei, absent callosal body, but relatively spared callosal genu and splenium) (Pulitzer *et al.*, 2004) (Figure 74.1).

The incidence of chromosomal abnormality is about 30% and the most frequent ones are trisomy 18, trisomy 13 and triploidy. The anomaly is also associated with toxoplasmosis, intrauterine rubella infection and heavy alcohol exposure and there is a very high increase of the disorder in diabetic mothers.

Porencephaly

Porencephaly is characterized by an intracerebral cyst filled with cerebral fluid, which may or may not be communicating with ventricles and subarachnoid space. There are two types: true porencephaly (agenetic), a developmental anomaly, and pseudoporencephaly (encephaloclastic), which is a destructive condition and a result of vascular, infectious or traumatic incidences.

Porencephaly is prenatally seen as cystic cavities within the brain that usually communicate with the ventricular system, the subarachnoid space or both (Pilu and Nicolaides, 1999). Coronal scans demonstrate loss of cerebral tissue (Romero *et al.*, 1988).

MRI could be used for differentiation of the encephaloclastic porencephaly from agenetic porencephaly and cystic encephalomalacia. Agenetic porencephaly presents as an intraparenchimal cavity, lined by dysplastic gray matter and associated with anomalies of the overlying cortex, usually polymicrogyria. Encephaloclastic porencephaly appears as a smooth wall cavity, i.e. isointense to CSF on all sequences, without internal structure, lined by white matter and the surrounding brain is of normal signal intensity. Cystic encephalomalacia is characterized by irregular cavities with considerable glial septae and astroglial reaction of surrounding brain parenchyma (Prayer *et al.*, 2006; Pistorius *et al.*, 2008) (Figure 74.2).

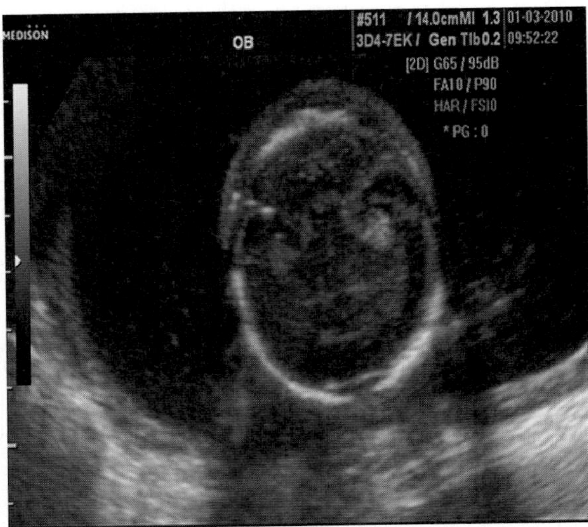

FIGURE 74.1 Holoprosencephaly, US.

Agenesis of corpus callosum

Agenesis of corpus callosum is complete or there is partial failure of the callosal commissural fibers to cross in the midline and from the corpus callosum between the two cerebral hemispheres. This is due to a vascular or inflammatory lesion occurring before the 12th week (between about 8 and 20 weeks gestational age). It may be an isolated finding, but it is also found in association with genetic syndromes and chromosomal abnormality. This condition is associated with a high incidence of other structural anomalies.

Prenatal diagnosis is made on finding the absence of the corpus callosum and septum pellucidum, and the "teardrop" configuration of the lateral ventricles (enlargement of the posterior horns) (see Figures 74.4 and 74.5) (Pilu and Nicolaides, 1999), with the upward displacement of the third ventricle (Romero *et al.*, 1988) and aberrant radial gyri pattern (Figure 74.3).

Direct visualization of the callosum by sonography is difficult and identification of callosal abnormalities relies typically on previously mentioned indirect signs (Callen *et al.*, 2008). Using fetal MRI the corpus callosum can be directly visualized in the sagittal and coronal planes as a curvilinear T2 hypointense structure, located at the superior margin of the lateral ventricles, superior to the fornices. Thin, 3 mm, midline sagittal images are best for assessment of the volume and morphology of all callosal parts (rostrum genu, body and splenium). Fetal MR has been reported to have a greater detection of callosal agenesis as compared with prenatal US (Whitby *et al.*, 2001).

In addition, fetal MR can identify an intact corpus callosum in approximately 20% of cases referred for sonographically suspected callosal agenesis or hypogenesis (Glenn *et al.*, 2005). Although MRI can directly visualize the corpus callosum, it is important to realize that the corpus callosum can be severely stretched in cases of severe ventriculomegaly. In such cases, identifying indirect signs of callosal agenesis might be

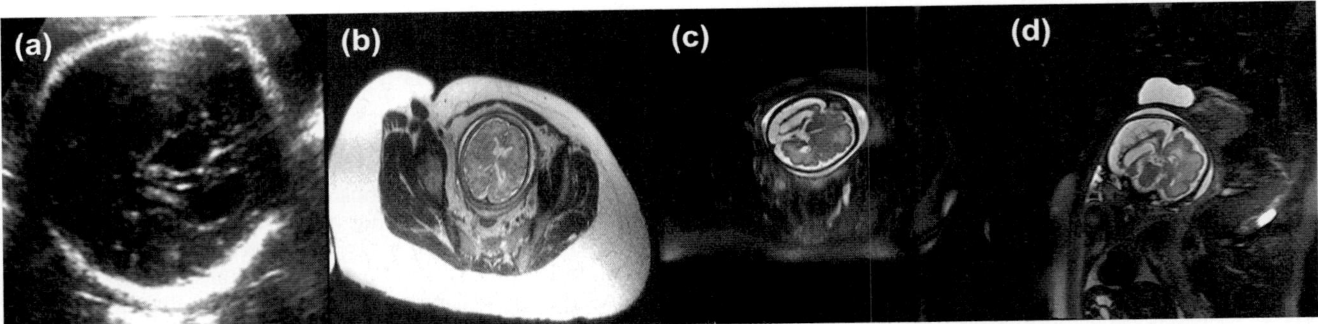

FIGURE 74.2 Porencephaly: (a) US; (b), (c), (d) MRI.

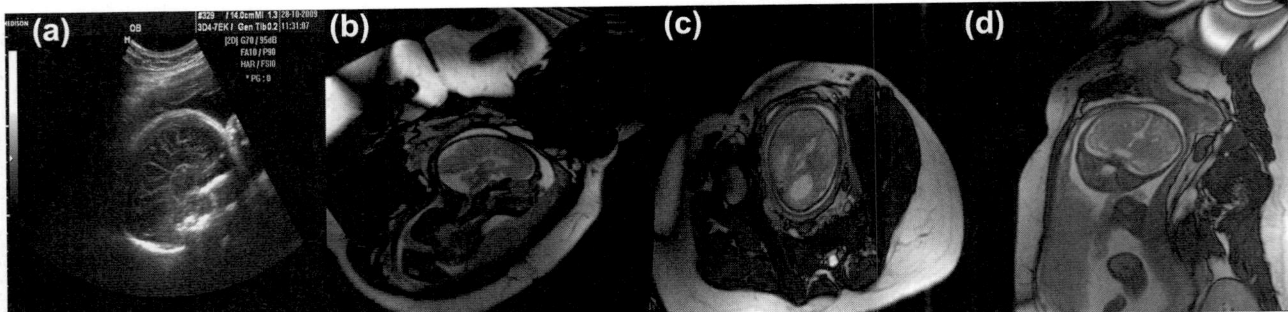

FIGURE 74.3 Agenesis of corpus callosum: (a) US; (b), (c), (d) MRI.

helpful in determining whether the callosum cannot be visualized because it did not form or because it is severely thinned.

Fetal MRI is important in detecting additional abnormalities in cases of callosal agenesis. Indeed, detection of associated brain anomalies by fetal MR is greater than by prenatal sonography in these cases; and additional anomalies are detected by fetal MR in up to 93% of cases (Tang *et al.*, 2009).

In a recent report of callosal agenesis diagnosed by fetal MRI, abnormal sulcation was identified in nearly all fetuses. Posterior fossa abnormalities were identified in one-third to one-half of cases and most commonly included a small and/or dysmorphic cerebellum, followed by small/absent vermis, and dysmorphic or small brainstem (Glenn and Barkovich, 2006).

Dandy-Walker syndrome

The Dandy-Walker malformation is characterised by cystic dilatation in the area of the cisterna magna and partial or complete agenesis of the vermis. It may occur as part of Mendelian disorders (Meckel-Gruber syndrome) and when it is not, there is a certain recurrence risk. There is association with teratogens such as warfarin. Associated intracranial abnormalities occur in about half of the cases and associated extracranial anomalies in 35% – hydrocephalus, agenesis of corpus callosum, encephalocele, neural tube defects, Meckel-Gruber syndrome, trisomy 13 and 18.

Prenatally, a Dandy-Walker malformation is seen as a cystic dilatation of the fourth ventricle with partial or complete agenesis of the vermis (Romero *et al.*, 1988; Pilu and Nicolaides, 1999) (Figure 74.4).

Fetal MRI is helpful in evaluating abnormalities of the posterior fossa. It allows direct visualization of the cerebellar hemispheres, vermis and brainstem in three orthogonal planes. Thus, MRI is useful in clarifying US findings in cystic malformations of the posterior fossa: Dandy-Walker malformation, Dandy-Walker variant, Blake's pouch cyst and retrocerebellar arachnoid cyst (Levine *et al.*, 2003; Adamsbaum *et al.*, 2005; Glenn and Barkovich, 2006; Novakov Mikic *et al.*, 2009).

Ventriculomegaly

Ventriculomegaly is defined as an increased intracranial content of cerebrospinal fluid resulting in the enlargement of the ventricular system. The cause of the abnormality may be congenital infection (toxoplasmosis, rubella, CMV or herpes virus), spina bifida, chromosomal abnormality or genetic defect, but in the majority of cases the etiology is unknown.

Prenatal diagnosis by ultrasound is made on the demonstration of dilated lateral cerebral ventricles, where the lateral ventricle diameter is 10 mm or more. In the cases with chromosomal abnormality ventriculomegaly is usually mild. There is little association between the degree of ventriculomegaly and intellect, because the etiology of the disorder is more important than the severity. In about 10% of cases, there is mild to moderate neurodevelopmental delay (Pilu and Nicolaides, 1999). Fetal mild VM is commonly defined as a ventricular atrial width of 10.0–15.0 mm, and it is considered isolated if there are no associated ultrasound abnormalities. There is no good evidence to suggest that the width of the ventricular atria contributes to the risk of neurodevelopmental outcome in fetuses with mild VM. The most important prognostic factors are the association with other abnormalities that escape early detection and the progression of ventricular dilatation, which are reported to occur in about 13 and 16% of cases, respectively. Most infants with a prenatal diagnosis of isolated mild VM have normal neurological development at least in infancy. The rate of abnormal or delayed neurodevelopment in infancy is about 11%, and it is unclear whether this is higher than in the general population. Furthermore, the number of infants that develop a real handicap is unknown (Melchiorre *et al.*, 2009).

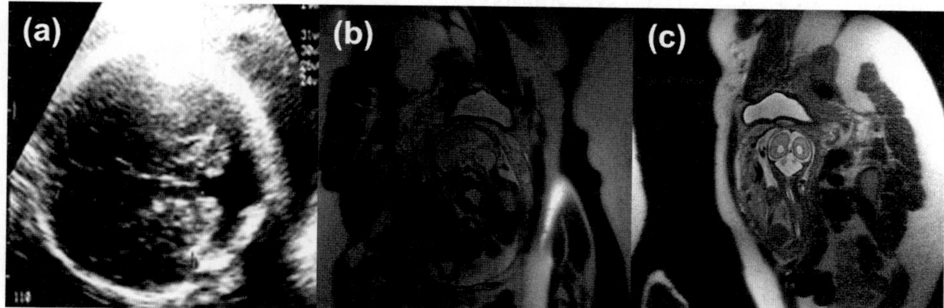

FIGURE 74.4 Dandy-Walker malformation: (a) US; (b), (c) MRI.

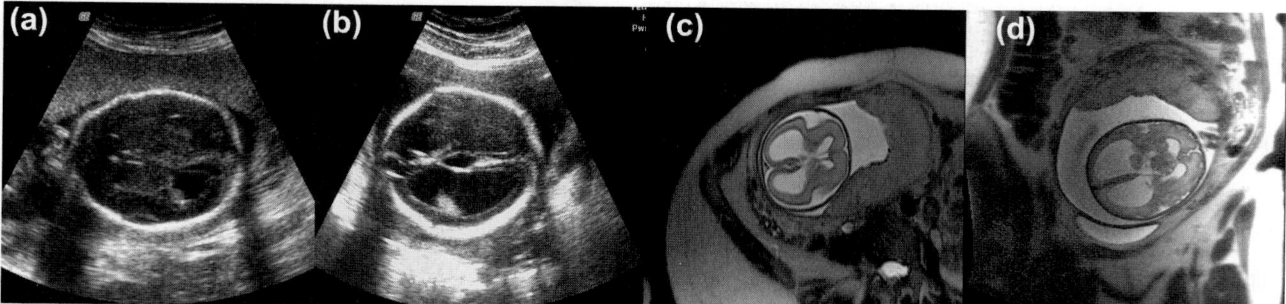

FIGURE 74.5 (a) Ventriculomegaly, US; (b) hydrocephalus, US; (c), (d) ventriculomegaly, MRI.

The presence of additional abnormalities is generally a poor prognostic sign and accompanied by a non-favorable postnatal outcome (Weichert *et al.*, 2010) (Figure 74.5).

Ventriculomegaly detected by US is the most frequent indication for fetal MRI. There are two clinical considerations in a fetus with VM: the degree of ventricular enlargement and the presence or absence of other CNS abnormalities (Levine *et al.*, 2002; Salomon *et al.*, 2006).

Fetal MR does not have a role in assessing the size of the ventricular trigones over and above US. MRI measurement of atrial diameter on axial images is usually within 2 mm of US measurements, even when the MR examination and US are performed on the same day. MRI ventricular measurement should be performed only in cases when the ventricular system could not be assessed on US, due to fetal position or problems caused by calvarial ossification. There is also a specific problem in visualizing the lateral ventricle closest to the sonography probe (near-field effect), which may be of relevance in cases of asymmetric VM (Garel and Alberti, 2006). Fetal MR imaging can be helpful in assessing the additional CNS malformation in fetuses with fetal ventriculomegaly. Studies have shown that MRI can detect additional sonographically occult CNS abnormalities in up to 40–50% of cases. Sonographically occult findings in fetuses with VM include agenesis of the corpus callosum, cortical malformations, periventricular nodular heterotopia, cerebellar dysplasia, partial agenesis of the septum pellucidum, Walker-Warburg syndrome and pontocerebellar dysplasia (Mehta and Levine, 2005).

NEURAL TUBE DEFECTS

Neural tube defects (NTD) and spinal malformations are among the most common congenital malformations. The epidemiology of these anomalies is various – multifactorial inheritance, chromosomal abnormality, teratogens, maternal predisposing factors or they may come as part of a syndrome.

Anencephaly

The anomaly is characterized by the absence of cerebral hemispheres and cranial vault. A vascular membrane covers the crown of the head instead of the skull. The incidence of the anomaly is geographical and population dependent.

The diagnostic ultrasound features are characteristic – the skull never develops, so there is no cranial vault and the brain that is still present up to 14 weeks is gradually eliminated due to the exposure to the amniotic fluid. The face is frog-like with protruding eyes, large tongue and short neck (Romero *et al.*, 1988). Polyhydramnios is present in about two-thirds of cases. Prenatal diagnosis is possible in the first trimester (Souka and Nicolaides, 1997). The anomalies commonly associated with anencephaly are spina bifida, facial clefts, diaphragmatic hernia, hydronephrosis, cardiac anomalies and clubfoot (Figure 74.6).

Iniencephaly

Iniencephaly is a lethal and extremely rare neural tube defect, characterized by fixed retroflexion of the head, cervical dysraphism and occipital bone defect. Iniencephaly is a lethal and extremely rare neural tube defect. Associated anomalies of the nervous and other systems are frequently present. Most cases are diagnosed prenatally by ultrasound.

The characteristic sonographic features are extreme dorsal flexion of the head and very short and deformed spine (Romero *et al.*, 1988). Anencephaly is common as well as an additional lumbosacral meningomyelocele or caudal regression syndrome.

Diagnosis is possible in the first trimester (Souka and Nicolaides, 1997; Gadodia *et al.*, 2010) (Figure 74.7).

Encephalocele

Encephalocele is a protrusion of the intracranial contents through a bony defect on the skull (Romero *et al.*, 1988). In more than two-thirds of cases it is localized in the occipital region, but sometimes it can be found frontal or parietal as well. Meningocele is an anomaly in which only membranes are involved, whereas in encephalocele, the brain tissue can be found in the herniated sac. It may be an isolated condition,

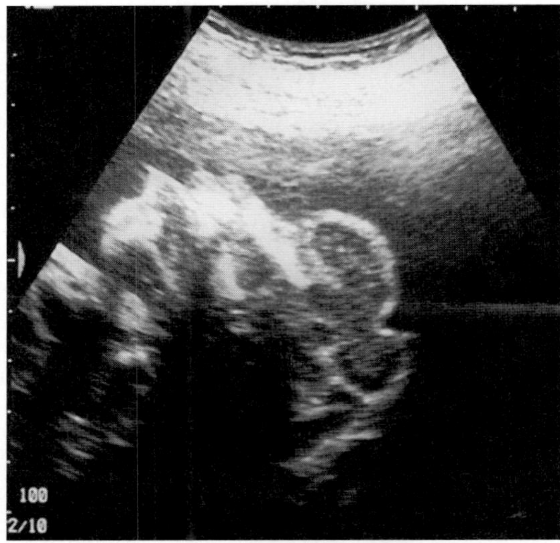

FIGURE 74.6 Anencephaly, US.

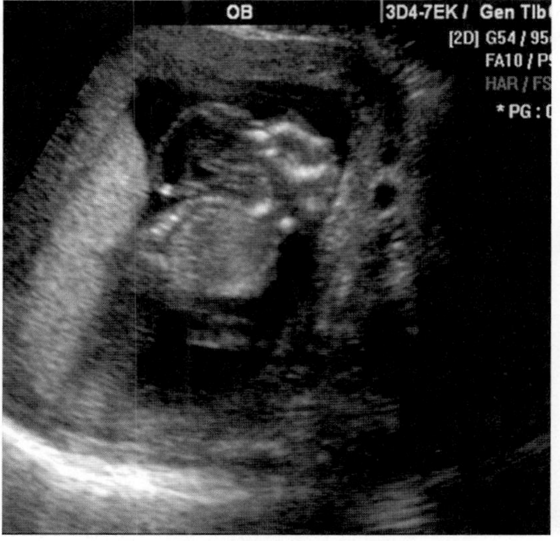

FIGURE 74.7 Iniencephaly, US.

of sporadic occurrence, or it may come as part of a chromosomal and genetic syndrome, including trisomy 13 and Meckel-Gruber syndrome. Known teratogens are cocaine, rubella and maternal hyperthermia.

The prenatal diagnosis is made upon demonstration of a paracranial mass and the defect in the skull should be found in 75% of cases; the mass is occipital, 15% is parietal and 10% is frontal (Romero *et al.*, 1988). Polyhydramnios may be present. The diagnosis is possible in the first trimester (Souka and Nicolaides, 1997).

Fetal MR imaging could be helpful in assessing the content, which protrudes through a calvarial defect, and in distinguishing occipital meningocele from other cystic lesions of the head and neck (e.g., cystic hygroma, teratoma or hemangioma) (Von Koch *et al.*, 2005) (Figure 74.8).

Spina bifida

Spina bifida can be defined as a midline defect of the vertebrae that results in exposure of the contents of the neural canal. Most often, the defect is localized to the posterior arch of the vertebrae. The incidence of this developmental anomaly is geographically dependent, and the highest prevalence is in Great Britain, the lowest in Japan. Known teratogens are valproic acid, folic acid antagonists (methotrexat, aminopterin), vitamin A, thalidomide and maternal diabetes, hyperthermia and folic acid deficiency (Romero *et al.*, 1988).

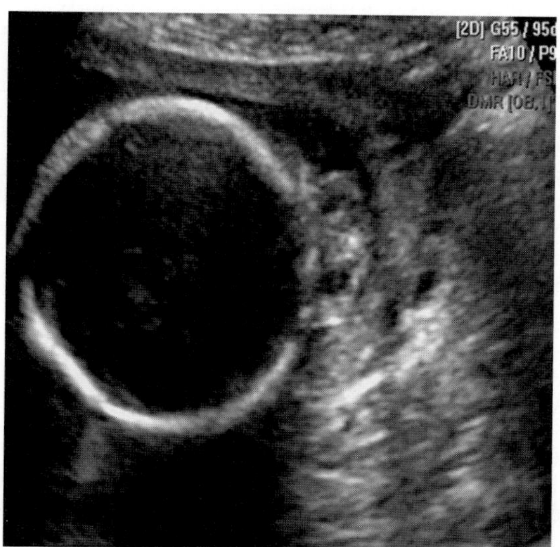

FIGURE 74.8 Meningocoele, US.

The most common are dorsal defects, which can be subdivided into two types – spina bifida occulta (hidden) and aperta (open). The "occulta" type represents about 15% of dorsal defects and is usually a small defect completely covered by skin, or after birth marked as a hypertrichotic place. It is usually asymptomatic. The "aperta" type, on the other hand, represents 85% of the dorsal variation, and the neural canal can either be exposed or covered by a thin meningeal membrane (Romero *et al.*, 1988). Sometimes the lesion appears as a cystic tumor – if there are only meninges within the tumour, it is called "meningocele", and if there is neural tissue, it is "myelomeningocele".

Fetal MRI and US are equally accurate for the detection of closed dorsal defects, but US could be more accurate in assessment of the open neural tube defects in the lumbosacral spine (thin sac of meningocele obscured by amniotic fluid could be easily missed by MRI due to small size and partial volume averaging) (Appasamy *et al.*, 2006).

The prenatal diagnosis is based on characteristic findings that can be divided into (1) soft tissue signs – absence of skin covering the defect/presence of bulging sac (meningocele or myelomeningocele) and (2) bony signs that can be seen in the sagittal, coronal and transverse section. In the sagittal plane, in which the spine appears as two parallel lines converging in the sacrum, there is the disappearance of the posterior line and overlying soft tissue. In the coronal plane, in which the normal spine appears as either two or three parallel lines, there is a widening of the two external lines due to a divergent separation of the lateral processes of the vertebrae. In the transverse, the most important section, in which the neural canal appears as a closed circle, the posterior centers are absent and the lateral ones are set apart. The skin and muscles above the defect are absent.

Cranial findings associated with spina bifida (Nicolaides *et al.*, 1986) are:

1. Ventricular dilatation.
2. The "lemon" sign – a concave deformity of the cranium in the frontal part, at the level of coronal suture. This anomaly is due to the effect of low intraspinal pressure that somehow translates to the soft fetal cranium, which is most susceptible in the frontal part of the skull.
3. The "banana" sign – describes the shape of cerebellum, which resembles a banana curving towards the skull bone. Cerebellum is also smaller in the majority of cases.

See Figure 74.9.

Spina bifida may be associated with other anomalies. The prognosis of spina bifida depends on the location and extent of the spinal defect, whether it is open or closed,

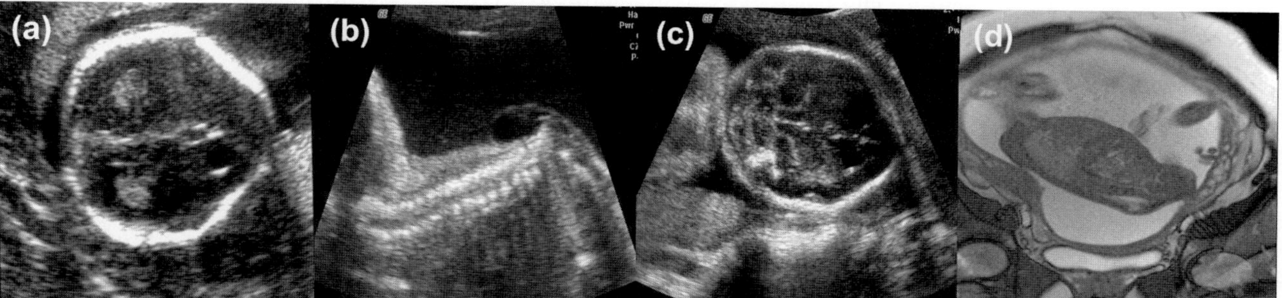

FIGURE 74.9 (a) "Lemon sign", US; (b) spina bifida, US; (c) "banana" sign, US; (d) MRI.

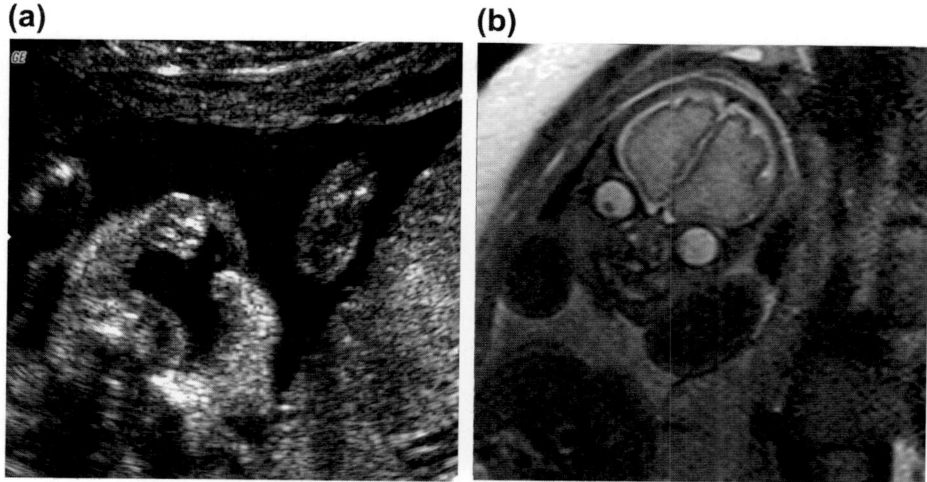

FIGURE 74.10 Cleft lip and palate: (a) US; (b) MRI.

and whether there is hydrocephalus as well as the presence of the associated anomalies. The impairment is worse for proximal and/or open spinal defects and in the presence of hydrocephalus and associated anomalies. Open neuronal tube defects are almost always associated with Arnold Chiary malformation (Chiary II). MRI is more accurate than US in assessment of all the elements of malformation (small posterior fossa, cerebellar herniation through foramen occipitale magnum and open spinal dysraphysm), especially in the cases with oligohydroamnios (Papadias *et al.*, 2008)

There are some indications that diagnosis of spina bifida might be possible in the first trimester (Chaoui and Nicolaides, 2010; Chaoui *et al.*, 2009).

ANOMALIES OF THE FACE

Cleft lip and/or palate

Cleft lip and/or palate are the most common congenital facial deformities at birth and result from failure of fusion of the frontal prominence with the maxillary process during embryogenesis. These deformities account for about 10% of all congenital anomalies. Most medial facial clefts account for less than 1% of all facial clefts. Teratogens known to cause cleft lip/palate are alcohol, maternal phenylketonuria, hyperthermia, hydantoin, trimethadion and methotrexate.

In the vast majority of cases cleft lip and palate have a multifactorial etiology, with both genetic and environmental factors that may influence the development of anomaly. Many syndromes are associated with cleft lip/palate. Associated anomalies are found in 50% of patients with isolated cleft palate and in only 13% of those with cleft lip and palate (Romero *et al.*, 1988).

The sonographic diagnosis of cleft lip/palate depends on the demonstration of a groove extending from one of the nostrils inside the lip and possibly the alveolar ridge (Pilu and Nicolaides, 1999; Romero *et al.*, 1988). The ones that are detected antenatally are usually more severe ones (Figure 74.10).

CARDIAC MALFORMATIONS

Congenital heart disease is a multifactorial disorder and a result of a combined effect of a genetic predisposition and environmental factors in more than 90% of cases.

Maternal diabetes is a well-known cause of fetal cardiac malformations, with an incidence that is five times greater than in healthy populations, and is related to poor glucose control, reflected by hemoglobin A1c levels in the first trimester. Specific cardiac malformations are ventricular septal defects and transposition of the great vessels.

Among teratogens that can cause heart malformations are: alcohol, lithium, vitamin A, antineoplastics, anticonvulsants, steroids, thalidomide, narcotics, amphetamines and oral contraceptives, barbiturates, chlorotheophyline, female sexual hormones, indomethacin, phenothiazines, prochlorperazine, salycylates. Maternal conditions such as diabetes, epilepsy, hyperfenylalaninemia, lupus and phenylketonuria may also cause them.

Ventricular septal defects

Ventricular septal defects (VSD) are by far the most common congenital heart defects. These defects can be in muscular or in membranous parts of the septum (Romero *et al.*, 1988), which influences the chances and the mode of spontaneous closure after the birth, the muscular defects having 65% closure incidence within 5 years, and membranous defects having 25%.

On prenatal ultrasound, the defect is usually visualized as interruption of the interventricular septum and dropout of echoes at the level of IVS (Romero *et al.*, 1988) (Figure 74.11).

Atrioventricular septal defect

Atrioventricular septal defect (AVSD) is one of the most common, serious cardiac defects detected prenatally and occurs in about 0.1/1,000 live births. It is a defect in the atrial and ventricular septa at the cardiac crux and is a result of a persistent primitive atrioventricular canal that is present during embryological development. The anomalies of the AV valves are obligatory (Romero *et al.*, 1988).

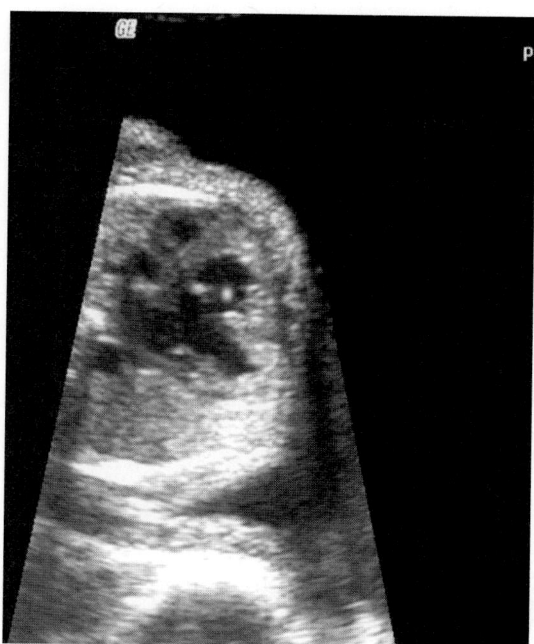

FIGURE 74.11 Ventricular septal defect, US.

In prenatal sonographic appearance of AVSD a large defect is noted at the crux of the heart, with a single AV valve, which has exaggerated excursions. In the incomplete form the only finding may be the defect in the lower portion of the atrial septum. Depending on how much of the cushion is missing, AVSD can be divided into (a) incomplete and (b) complete forms, complete being more common. AVSD is strongly associated with other cardiac anomalies and chromosomal abnormality or in fetuses with cardiosplenic syndromes (Figure 74.12).

With improvement of US equipment as well as routine use of screening for chromosomal abnormalities by nuchal translucency with a detailed anomaly scan at 11–14 weeks, cardiac anomalies have been increasingly diagnosed in the first trimester (Souka and Nicolaides, 1997; Huggon *et al.*, 2002).

ANTERIOR ABDOMINAL WALL DEFECTS

Exomphalos (omphalocele)

Exomphalos is characterized by herniation of the intra-abdominal contents into the base of the umbilical cord, with a covering amnioperitoneal membrane. The most frequently herniated organs are the liver, bowel and stomach.

The characteristic prenatal ultrasound findings are the midline anterior abdominal wall defect, the herniated sac with its visceral contents and the umbilical cord insertion at the apex of the sac (Pilu and Nicolaides, 1999).

Associated chromosomal defects are found in about 30% of the infants with omphalocele, mainly trisomy 18. Chromosomal defects are more common when the sac contains bowel only, rather than liver. Diagnosis is possible in the first trimester (Souka and Nicolaides, 1997) (Figure 74.13).

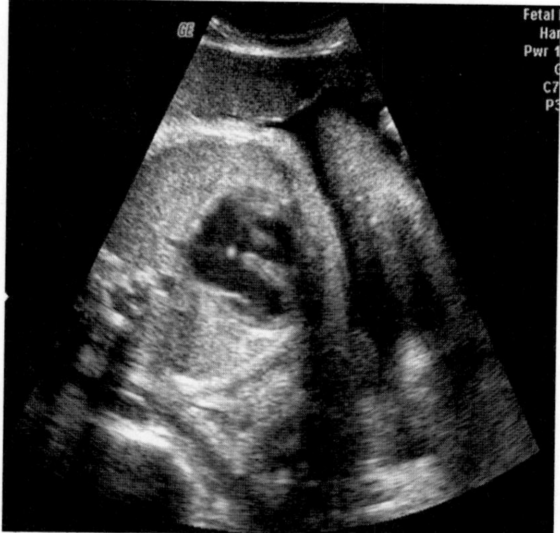

FIGURE 74.12 Atrioventricular septal defect, US.

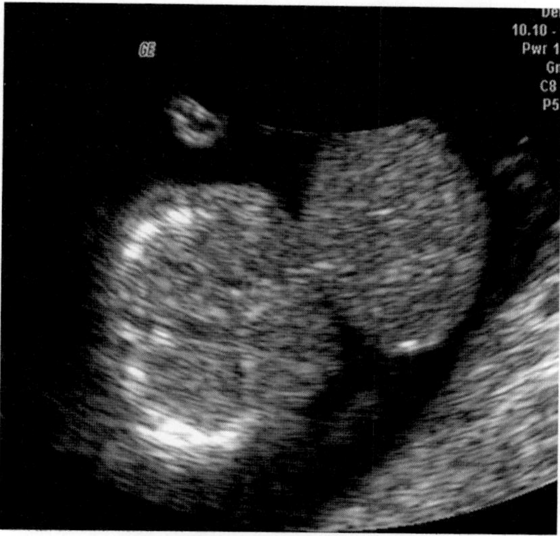

FIGURE 74.13 Omphalocele, US.

Gastroschisis

Gastroschisis is a full thickness defect of the abdominal wall, usually to the right of the umbilicus, allowing intestinal herniation into the amniotic fluid. There is no covering membrane.

Prenatal diagnosis is based on the demonstration of the normally situated umbilicus and the herniated loops of the intestine, which float freely in the amniotic cavity (Pilu and Nicolaides, 1999). Diagnosis is possible in the first trimester (Souka and Nicolaides, 1997). Gastroschisis is usually not associated with chromosomal abnormalities or other structural defects (Figure 74.14).

GASTROINTESTINAL TRACT ANOMALIES

Duodenal atresia

Duodenal atresia or stenosis is the most common of all small bowel obstructions. In most cases the condition is sporadic and the aetiology is unknown, with some cases

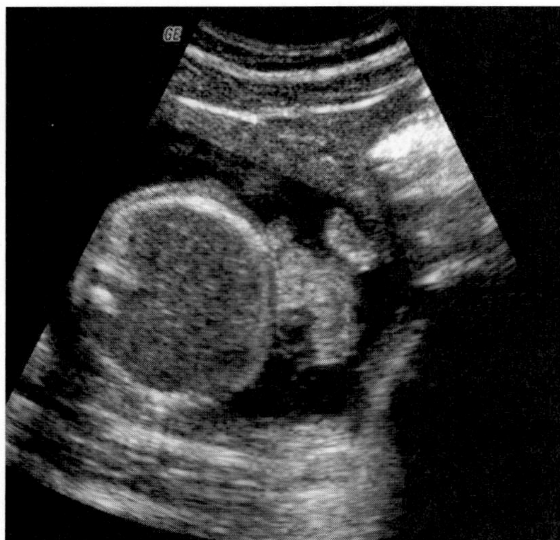

FIGURE 74.14 Gastroschisis, US.

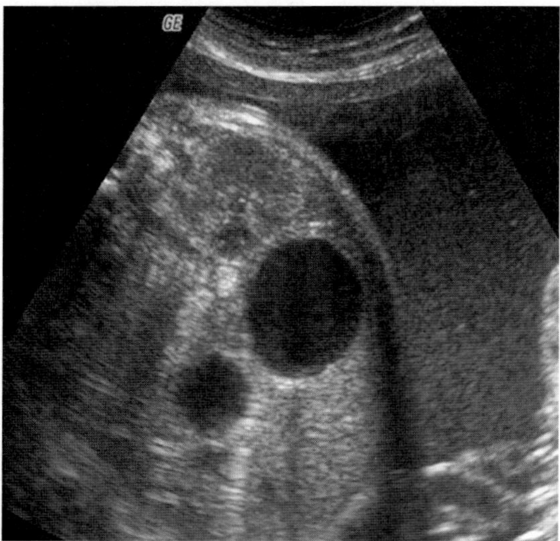

FIGURE 74.15 Duodenal atresia, US.

reported in infants exposed to thalidomide (Romero *et al.*, 1988).

Prenatal diagnosis is based on the demonstration of "double-bubble sign" (the dilated stomach and proximal duodenum) and polyhydramnios. A connection between the two dilated portions can be demonstrated. However, obstruction due to a central web may result in only a single bubble representing the fluid-filled stomach.

Approximately half of the fetuses with duodenal atresia have trisomy 21 and/or cardiac defects. In about 40% of cases there are associated skeletal and vertebral anomalies (Figure 74.15).

FETAL RENAL ABNORMALITIES

Multicystic kidney disease (Potter type II)

Multicystic dysplastic kidney is a congenital dysplasia of the kidneys characterized by large non-homogeneous dilations of the collecting tubules. It may occur segmentally, unilaterally

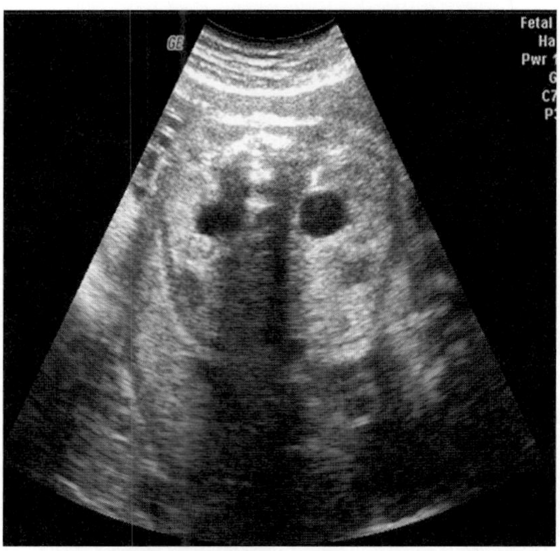

FIGURE 74.16 Hydronephrosis, US.

or bilaterally. Multicystic dysplastic kidneys present usually sporadically, but families with autosomal dominant inheritance have been described. Maternal diabetes is a known teratogen (Romero *et al.*, 1988).

Ultrasound criteria for the diagnosis of MCDK are multiple, peripheral, round renal cysts of variable size, and echogenic renal parenchyma may lie between the cysts (Romero *et al.*, 1988). Kidney size is usually enlarged. There is compensatory hypertrophy; enlargement and hydronephrosis of the contralateral kidney may occur if the condition is unilateral. Amniotic fluid is reduced to absent in bilateral disease and normal in unilateral involvement. The diagnosis is possible in the first trimester (Souka and Nicolaides, 1997).

Obstructive uropathies

The term "obstructive uropathy" encompasses a wide variety of different pathological conditions characterized by dilatation of part or all of the urinary tract. Dilatation of fetal urinary tract frequently, but not absolutely, signifies obstruction. Most common is hydronephrosis, which represents distension of the pelvis and calyces of the kidney, with urine, as a result of ureteral obstruction. It accounts for about 90% of fetal renal anomalies. Obstruction on the level of the ureteropelvic junction is four times more common in males, rather than the level of the ureterovesicular junction in females. Hydronephrosis is thought to be significant if the anterior posterior diameter of the pelvis is >5 mm at any stage of pregnancy. Prenatal diagnosis is based on the findings of dilated renal pelvis with/without dilatation of calyces. Ureters and bladder are normal, as well as the amniotic fluid volume (Figure 74.16).

FETAL SKELETAL ANOMALIES

Skeletal malformations are a heterogeneous group of disorders of bone growth that result in abnormal shape and size of bones. The most common ones are thanatophoric dysplasia, achondroplasia, osteogenesis imperfecta and achondrogenesis (Romero *et al.*, 1988).

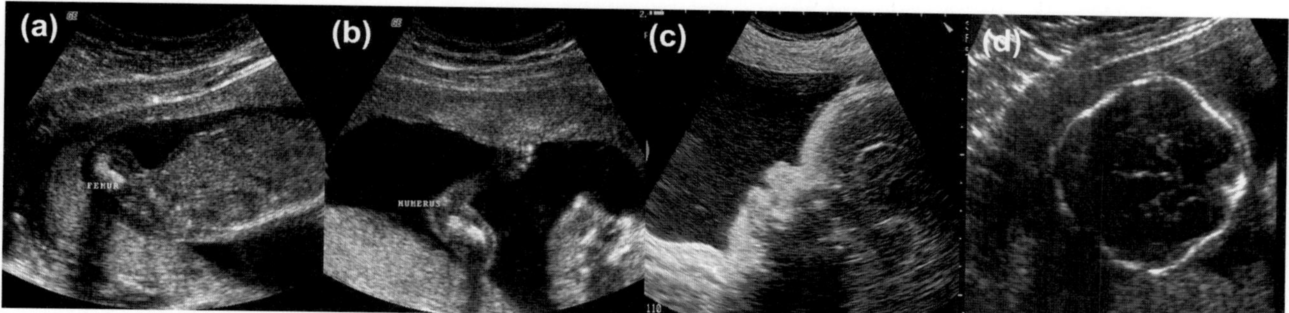

FIGURE 74.17 (a) Short femur, US; (b) short humerus, US; (c) frontal bossing, US; (d) "cloverleaf" skull, US.

Thanatophoric dysplasia

This is a lethal skeletal abnormality with an incidence of about 0.7 in 10,000 births, which makes it the most common skeletal dysplasia. There are two types – type I is of sporadic occurrence and type II is thought to be inherited with an autosomal recessive pattern. The most prenatal ultrasonographic characteristic features are cloverleaf skull, rhizomelia (proximal micromelia) and cranial enlargement. Diagnosis is possible in the first trimester (Souka and Nicolaides, 1997) (Figure 74.17).

CONCLUDING REMARKS AND FUTURE DIRECTIONS

Fetal imaging has become standard in prenatal care. Thorough knowledge of not only pathogenesis but also morphological appearances of different anomalies are mandatory for adequate diagnosis. Detailed anomaly scanning has to give as much information as possible for the parents, regardless of the outcome – if the finding is normal, parents can be reassured, especially if the pregnancy was at increased risk of malformation. If abnormalities are found, the parents need as much accurate information as possible in order to make decisions about the future of the pregnancy. Continuing improvements in prenatal ultrasonography and magnetic resonance imaging, as well as a continued multidisciplinary approach, are mandatory to ensure maximal development in the field of fetal imaging.

REFERENCES

Adamsbaum C, Moutard ML, Andre C, Merzoug V, Ferey S, Quere MP, Lewin F, Fallet Bianco C (2005) MRI of the fetal posterior fossa. *Pediatr Neurol* **35:** 124–40.

Allen VM, Armson BA, Wilson RD, Allen VM, Blight S, Gagnon A, Johnson JA, Langlois S, Summers A, Wyatt P, Farine D, Armson BA, Crane J, Delisle MF, Keenan-Lindsey L, Morin V, Schneider CE, Van Aerde J, Society of Obstetricians and Gynaecologists of Canada (2007) Teratogenicity associated with pre-existing and gestational diabetes. *J Obstet Gynaecol Can* **29(11):** 927–44.

Alsdorf R, Wyszinski DF (2005) Teratogenicity of sodium valproate. *Expert Opin Drug Saf* **4(2):** 345–53.

Appasamy M, Roberts D, Pilling D, Buxton N (2006) Antenatal ultrasound and magnetic resonance imaging in localizing the level of lesion in spina bifida and correlation with postnatal outcome. *Ultrasound Obstet Gynecol* **27(5):** 530–6.

Armant DR, Saunders DE (1996) Exposure of embryonic cells to alcohol: contrasting effects during preimplantation and postimplantation development. *Semin Perinatol* **20(2):** 127–39.

Berard A, Ramos E, Rey E, Blais L, St Andre M, Oraichi D (2007) First trimester exposure to paroxetine and risk of cardiac malformations in infants: the importance of dosage. *Birth Defects Res B Dev Reprod Toxicol* **80(1):** 18–27.

Brent RL, Beckman DA, Landel CP (1993) Clinical teratology. *Curr Opin Pediatr* **5(2):** 201–11.

Callen PW, Callen AL, Glenn OA, Toi A (2008) Columns of the fornix, not to be mistaken for the cavum septi pellucidi on prenatal sonography. *J Ultrasound Med* **279:** 25–31.

Chaoui R, Benoit B, Mitkowska-Wozniak H, Heling KS, Nicolaides KH (2009) Assessment of intracranial translucency (IT) in the detection of spina bifida at the 11–13 weeks scan. *Ultrasound Obstet Gynecol* **34(3):** 249–52.

Chaoui R, Nicolaides KH (2010) From nuchal translucency to intracranial translucency: towards the early detection of spina bifida. *Ultrasound Obstet Gynecol* **35(2):** 133–8.

Cohen LS, Friedman JM, Jefferson JW, Johnson EM, Weiner ML (1994) A reevaluation of risk of in utero exposure to lithium. *JAMA* **27(2):** 146–50.

Diav Citrin O, Shechtman S, Weinbaum D, Wajnberg R, Avgil M, Di Gianantonio E, Clementi M, Weber-Schoendorfer C, Schaefer C, Ornoy A (2008) Paroxetine and fluoxetine in pregnancy: a prospective, multicentre controlled observational study. *Br J Clin Pharmacol* **66(5):** 695–705.

Filly RA, Chinn DH, Callen PW (1984) Alobar holoprosencephaly – ultrasonographic prenatal diagnosis. *Radiology* **151(2):** 455–9.

Finnell RH (1999) Teratology: general considerations and principles. *J Allergy Clin Immunol* **103(2 Pt 2):** S337–S342.

Friedman JM (2006) ACE inhibitors and congenital anomalies. *New Engl J Med* **354:** 2498–500.

Gadodia A, Gupta P, Sharma R, Kumar S, Gupta G (2010) Antenatal sonography and MRI of iniencephaly apertus and clausus. *Fetal Diagn Ther* (Epub ahead of print).

Garel C, Alberti C (2006) Coronal measurement of the fetal lateral ventricles: comparison between ultrasonography and magnetic resonance imaging. *Ultrasound Obstet Gynecol* **27:** 23–7.

Glenn OA, Barkovich J (2006) Magnetic resonance imaging of the fetal brain and spine: an increasingly important tool in prenatal diagnosis: Part 2. *Am J Neuroradiol* **27(9):** 1807–14.

Glenn O, Goldstein RB, Li KC, Young SJ, Norton ME, Busse RF, Goldber JD, Barkovich AJ (2005) Fetal magnetic resonance imaging in the evaluation of fetuses referred for sonographically suspected abnormalities of the corpus callosum. *J Ultrasound Med* **24(6):** 791–4.

Holmes LB (2002) Teratogen induced limb defects. *Am J Med Genet* **112(3):** 297–303.

Huggon IC, Ghi T, Cook AC, Zosmer N, Allan LD, Nicolaides K (2002) Fetal cardiac abnormalities identified prior to 14 weeks of gestation. *Ultrasound Obstet Gynecol* **20(1):** 22–9.

Johns J, Jauniaux E, Burton G (2006) Factors affecting the early embryonic environment. *Rev Gynaecol Perinatal Pract* **6(3–4):** 199–210.

Landry SH, Whitney JA (1996) The impact of prenatal cocaine exposure: studies of the developing infant. *Semin Perinatol* **20(2):** 99–106.

Levine D, Barnes PD, Robertson RR, Wong G, Mehta TS (2003) Fast MR imaging of fetal central nervous system abnormalities. *Radiology* **229:** 51–61.

Levine D, Trop I, Mehta T, Barnes PD (2002) MR imaging appearance of fetal cerebral ventricular morphology. *Radiology* **223:** 652–60.

Lin S, Herdt-Losavio M, Gensburg L, Marshall E, Druschel C (2009) Maternal asthma, asthma medication use, and the risk of congenital heart defects. *Birth Defects Res A Clin Mol Teratol* **85(2):** 161–8.

Lisi A, Botto LD, Robert Gnansia E, Castilla EE, Bakker MK, Bianca S, Cocchi G, de Vigan C, dr Graca Dutra M, Horacek J, Merlob P, Pierini A, Scarano G, Sipek A, Yamanaca M, Mastroiacovo P (2010) Surveillance of adverse fetal effects of medications (SAFE-Med): findings from the International Clearinghouse of Birth Defects Surveillance and Research. *Reprod Toxicol* (Epub ahead of publication).

Luo T, Wagner E, Crandall J, Drager U (2004) A retinoic acid critical period in early postnatal mouse brain. *Biologic Psych* **56:** 971–80.

Lynfield R, Eaton R (1995) Teratogen update: congenital toxoplasmosis. *Teratology* **53:** 176–80.

Mehta TS, Levine D (2005) Imaging of fetal cerebral ventriculomegaly: a guide to management and outcome. *Semin Fetal Neonatal Med* **10:** 421–8.

Melchiorre K, Bhide A, Gika AD, Pilu G, Papagorghiou AT (2009) Counselling in isolated mild fetal ventriculomegaly. *Ultrasound Obstet Gynecol* **34(2):** 212–24.

Miller EA, Manning SE, Rasmussen SA, Reefhuis J, Honein MA: National Birth Defects Study (2009) Maternal exposure to tobacco smoke, alcohol and caffeine, and risk of anorectal atresia: National Birth Defects Prevention Study 1997–2003. *Paediatr Perinat Epidemiol* **23(1):** 9–17.

Mountain States Genetics Foundation (1995) Teratogen update. Newsletter Volume 12.

Nguyen HT, Sharma V, McIntyre RS (2009) Teratogenesis associated with antibipolar agents. *Adv Ther* **26(3):** 281–94.

Nicolaides KH, Campbell S, Gabbe SG, Guidetti R (1986) Ultrasound screening for spina bifida: cranial and cerebellar signs. *Lancet* **2(8498):** 72–4.

Novakov A, Vejnović T, Stojić S, Belopavlović Z (1999) A proposed protocol for obstetrical ultrasound examination. *Med Pregl* **52(9–10):** 351–6.

Novakov Mikic A, Koprivsek K, Lucic M, Belopavlovic Z, Stojic S, Sekulic S (2009) Prenatal diagnosis of posterior fossa anomalies – an overview. *Med Pregl* **62(3–4):** 157–63.

Nyberg DA, Mack LA, Bronstein A, Hirsch J, Pagon R (1987) Holoprosencephaly: prenatal sonographic diagnosis. *AJR Am J Roentgenol* **149(5):** 1051–8.

Ornoy A (2009) Valproic acid in pregnancy: how much are we endangering the embryo and fetus? *Reprod Toxicol* **28(1):** 1–10.

Papadias A, Miller C, Martin WL, Kilby MD, Sgouros S (2008) Comparison of prenatal and postnatal MRI findings in the evaluation of intrauterine CNS anomalies requiring postnatal neurosurgical treatment. *Childs Nerv Syst* **24(2):** 185–92.

Pilu G, Nicolaides KH (1999) *Diagnosis of Fetal Abnormalities – The 18–23 Week Scan*. Diploma in Fetal Medicine Series, Parthenon Publishing, New York.

Pistorius LR, Hellman PM, Visser GH, Malinger G, Prayer D (2008) Fetal neuroimaging: ultrasound, MRI or both? *Obstet Gynecol Surv* **63(11):** 733–45.

Prayer D, Brugger P, Kasprian G, Witzani L, Helmer H, Dietrich W, Eppel W, Langer M (2006) MRI of fetal acquired brain lesion. *Eur J Radiol* **57(2):** 233–49.

Pulitzer SB, Simon EM, Crombleholme TM, Golden JA (2004) Prenatal MR findings of the middle interhemispheric variant of holoprosencephaly. *Am J Neuroradiol* **25:** 1034–6.

Randall CL, Cook JL, Thomas SE, White NW (1999) Alcohol plus cocaine prenatally is more deleterious than either drug alone. *Neurotoxicol Teratol* **21(6):** 673–8.

Romero R, Pilu G, Jeanty P, Ghidini A, Hobbins JC (1988) *Prenatal Diagnosis of Congenital Anomalies*. Appleton and Lange, Norwalk, Connecticut/San Mateo, California.

Salisbury AL, Lester BM, Seifer R, LaGasse L, Bauer CR, Shankaran S, Bada H, Wright L, Liu J, Poole K (2007) Prenatal cocaine use and maternal depression: effects on infant neurobehaviour. *Neurotoxicol Teratol* **29(3):** 331–40.

Salomon LJ, Ouahba J, Delezoide AL, Vuillard L, Oury JF, Sebag G, Garel C (2006) Third trimester fetal MRI in isolated 10- to 12-mm ventriculomegaly: is it worth it? *BJOG* **113:** 942–7.

Simon EM, Hevner R, Pinter JD, Clegg NJ, Miller VS, Kinsman SM, Hahn JS, Barkovich AJ (2000) Assessment of the deep gray nuclei in holoprosencephaly. *Am J Neuroradiol* **21:** 1955–61.

Smith J, Whitehall J (2009) Sodium valproat and the fetus: a case study and review of the literature. *Neonat Netw* **28(6):** 363–7.

Souka AP, Nicolaides KH (1997) Diagnosis of fetal abnormalities at the 11–14 weeks scan. *Ultrasound Obstet Gynecol* **10(6):** 429–42.

Tang PH, Bratha AI, Norton ME, Barkovich AJ, Sherr EH, Glenn OA (2009) Agenesis of the corpus callosum: an MR imaging analysis of associated abnormalities in the fetus. *Am J Neuroradiol* **30(2):** 257–63.

Von Koch CS, Glenn OA, Goldstein RB, Barkovich AJ (2005) Fetal magnetic resonance imaging enhances detection of spinal cord anomalies in patients with sonographically detected bony anomalies of the spine. *J Ultrasound Med* **24:** 781–9.

Weichert J, Hartge D, Krapp M, Germer U, Gembruch U, Axt Fliedner R (2010) Prevalence, characteristics and perinatal outcome of fetal ventriculomegaly in 29,000 pregnancies followed at a single institution. *Fetal Diagn Ther* **27(3):** 142–8.

Whitby E, Paley MN, Davies N, Sprigg A, Griffiths PD (2001) Ultra fast magnetic resonance imaging of central nervous system abnormalities in utero in the second and third trimester of pregnancy: comparison with ultrasound. *BJOG* **108:** 519–26.

Wide K, Windbladh B, Kallen B (2004) Major malformations in infants exposed to antiepileptic drugs in utero, with emphasis on carbamazepine and valproic acid: a nation-wide, population based register study. *Acta Paediatr* **93(2):** 174–6.

Wong Gibbons DL, Romitti PA, Sun L, Moore CA, Reefhuis J, Bell EM, Olshan AF (2008) Maternal periconceptional exposure to cigarette smoking and alcohol and esophageal atresia +/− tracheo-esophageal fistula. *Birth Defects Res A Clin Mol Teratol* **82(11):** 776–84.

Woolf AD, Goldman R, Bellinger DC (2007) Update on the clinical management of childhood lead poisoning. *Pediatr Clin North Am* **54:** 271–94.

Yacobi S, Ornoy A (2008) Is lithium a real teratogen? What can we conclude from the prospective versus retrospective studies? A review. *Isr J Psychiatry Relat Sci* **45(2):** 95–106.

CHAPTER

75

Micro-CT and volumetric imaging in developmental toxicology

Xiaoyou Ying, Norman J. Barlow and Maureen H. Feuston

INTRODUCTION

It has long been desired to visualize fetuses clearly in the womb – imaging and tracking fetal development at the anatomic, molecular, biochemical and genetic levels. Over the last 100 years, especially in the past several decades, many biomedical imaging (bioimaging) technologies have been developed. These bioimaging technologies include various light microscopies, X-ray radiography and fluoroscopy, computed tomography (CT or CAT), magnetic resonance imaging (MRI), positron emission tomography (PET), scintigraphy, single photon emission computed tomography (SPECT), thermography and ultrasound imaging. As these technologies have progressed, many of them have been applied in the study of developmental toxicology.

BIOMEDICAL IMAGING

Although bioimaging technologies have provided many innovative approaches for multidimensional detection, visualization and characterization of biological processes and events, the imaging concept is quite simple and can be described as any technique that can be utilized to obtain biological information within two (x,y) or three (x,y,z) morphological dimensions. For a time-related developmental process or event, time (t) creates a fourth dimension that can be added in a longitudinal study. Although it is often overlooked, there is another important aspect of imaging that in fact may be the most important dimension, the imaging signal wavelength (λ) dimension. Within this critical dimension, namely the electromagnetic spectrum, many special imaging technologies have been developed using different signals along the electromagnetic continuum (Figure 75.1) (Hendee and Ritenour, 2002; Ying and Monticello, 2006). Today, bioimaging approaches are increasingly applied in many types of biological and medical research, including developmental toxicology.

"OF MICE AND MEN" – FROM CLINICAL TO PRECLINICAL IMAGING

With the successful application of modern imaging technologies in the clinical domain, especially tomography imaging approaches such as CT, MRI and ultrasound imaging, scientists immediately began to think about applying these imaging technologies to preclinical toxicology studies. However, the most popular animal species used in preclinical studies are small animals, mostly rodents, and translating the imaging technologies from humans to such a small scale is extremely difficult. For example, the best anatomic resolution a modern clinical CT system can provide is approximately $0.3 \times 0.3 \times 0.3\,mm^3$. To match this resolution, from a human to a rat, or to a mouse, the anatomic resolution of a micro-CT imaging system would need to be approximately $44 \times 44 \times 44\,\mu m^3$ or $20 \times 20 \times 20\,\mu m^3$, respectively. These volumes are approximately 300 (rat) or 3,300 (mouse) times smaller. In addition, as for some imaging modalities such as MRI, this translates to a significant loss in signal due to the reduction of the signal acquiring space. It fact, the signal-to-noise ratio will be very significantly reduced when imaging volume is decreased hundreds or thousands of times. Thanks to modern advancements in preclinical imaging, high resolution versions of all of the major clinical imaging modalities are now available, which enables similar imaging studies on small animals. Furthermore, some new imaging modalities such as *in vivo* whole body bioluminescence imaging and optical tomography, which are currently not available for clinical use, have been developed and help bridge *in vitro* and *in vivo* studies.

The advantages of small animal-based imaging approaches are clear. First, whole body/organ phenotyping with biomedical imaging ensures a better understanding of physiology, pathology, and toxicology, etc. in a complete three-dimensional (3D) anatomic milieu, with more information from the whole body *in vivo* or *ex vivo* organs. Second, it enables greater use of available animal disease models. Third, these technologies allow for *ex vivo* methodologies for correlative imaging studies. A fourth advantage is that

Reproductive and Developmental Toxicology, Edited by Ramesh C. Gupta
ISBN: 978-0-12-382032-7

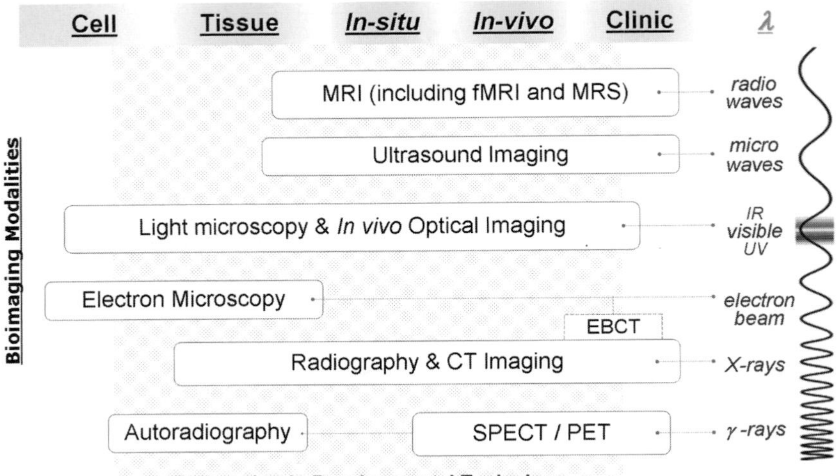

FIGURE 75.1 Commonly used biomedical imaging technologies (MRI = magnetic resonance imaging, fMRI = functional MRI, MRS = MR spectroscopy, CT = computed tomography, EBCT = electron beam CT, PET = positron emission tomography, SPECT = single photon emission computed tomography).

imaging approaches employing small animal imaging technologies greatly aid the potential development of biomarkers for translational studies.

"OF FETUS AND ADULTS" – BIOIMAGING OF SMALL ANIMAL FETUSES

In clinical fetal developmental research, there are severe restrictions on imaging of fetuses *in utero* due to safety concerns. Non-invasive ultrasound imaging is considered safe for the fetus and is routinely applied, although some other imaging modalities such as MRI have also been used. However, in preclinical studies, there is a greater potential to use *in vivo* imaging modalities because restrictions are limited. To take advantage of these evolving technologies in preclinical developmental toxicology, major technical difficulties must be resolved. Difficulties encountered include (1) higher resolution, or ultra-high resolution micro-imaging technologies are required because of such small specimens (see the micro-CT volume measurement in the next sections), and (2) respiration and cardiac contraction, which are much more rapid in small animal species, cause motion artifacts during *in vivo* imaging evaluations. In addition, there are other issues that cannot be ignored, such as the radiation in X-ray imaging, anesthesia, and the imaging recognition and identification of individual fetuses one by one *in utero* in an *in vivo* longitudinal study. That is why, to date, *ex vivo* imaging technologies have been predominantly used in developmental toxicology studies to circumvent these issues. However, all of these difficulties do not override the attractive benefits of imaging during fetal development, especially the investigation of longitudinal embryonic development and organism growth, which opens a new door for obtaining information never available before. In this chapter, with applications in developmental toxicology, the focus will be on micro-volumetric imaging approaches mainly using X-ray-based micro-computed tomography (micro-CT) technologies.

X-RAY MICRO-IMAGING AND MICRO-CT

X-ray properties and imaging

X-rays, an electromagnetic radiation, are emitted by electrons which are outside of the atomic nucleus (unlike other high energy alpha and gamma rays, which are emitted from the atom nucleus). X-rays are similar to visible light but have a much shorter wavelength (from approximately 10 to 0.02 nanometers), and much higher energy (from ~0.12 to ~120 keV). Thus, X-rays can penetrate biological tissues and many other materials that visible light cannot. This high penetrating ability and the different X-ray attenuation coefficients of various body tissues make X-rays a useful signal for biomedical imaging. Generally, X-rays are classified as "soft" or "hard" according to their energy range; "soft" X-ray ranges from ~0.12 to ~12 keV and "hard" X-ray ranges from ~12 to ~120 keV. Understandably, hard X-rays are usually used for solid and/or large objects, and soft X-rays are used for small objects and/or for some special requirements for low energy imaging.

X-ray imaging is not only dependent on the X-ray energy, but also depends on the density of the materials that are to be imaged; the higher the density of the material the more X-ray absorption and less penetration. It is because of these differential absorptions (i.e., X-ray attenuation coefficients) that the different densities of bone, muscle, fat and other soft tissues can be distinguished. This is the physical basis of biomedical X-ray imaging.

Due to the difference between the X-ray attenuation coefficients of various tissues that produce the image contrast, X-ray based technologies are usually good for the imaging of bone and lung. Because bones contain relatively heavy atoms with many electrons that act as absorbers of X-rays, its images are significantly different from surrounding "soft" tissues that mostly consist of water, proteins and other molecules which have lighter atoms. In the lung, air has no absorption of X-rays, so it acts as a "contrast agent" to make lung tissue structure clearly visible due to the contrast differences

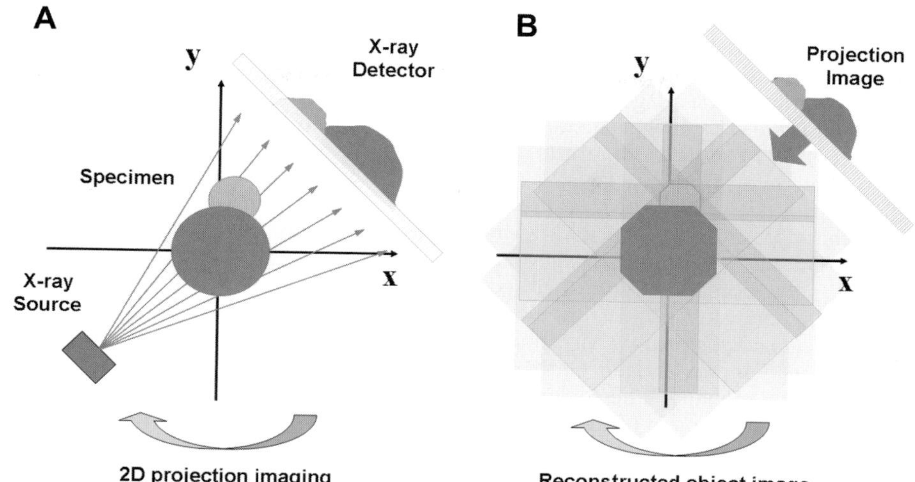

FIGURE 75.2 Illustration of the principle of X-ray projection imaging (A) and computed tomography reconstruction (B). A cone-beam of X-rays travels through the specimen and is projected on an X-ray detector that produces a 2D radiography image. Projection images are generated from many different angles. Using computed tomography processing, the 2D radiography images that are obtained from different angles are used to reconstruct 2D tomography sections and further 3D image datasets. A commonly used reconstruction algorithm in micro-CT is the back-projection method.

TABLE 75.1 Computed tomography scanning models and evolution

CT scan model	Beam	Scan	Detector	Scan time
First generation	Parallel-beam	Translation-rotation	Single paired detector	Long
Second generation	Small fan-beam	Translation-rotation	Multiple detectors (~5–30 detectors)	
Third generation	Large fan-beam (30–60°)	Rotation-rotation (no linear translation)	Multiple detectors (~288–700 detectors)	
Fourth generation	Large fan-beam	Source-rotation only	Multiple detectors (up to ~4,800 detectors)	
Latest	Cone-beam geometry	Continuous spiral/helical scanning	Multiple detectors	Short

between the air and lung tissues. However, for soft tissues and organs, X-ray images produce very poor contrast. Because of this lack of contrast, X-ray-based techniques may not be ideal for soft tissue and organ imaging if no contrast agent is used.

Basic principles of X-ray computed tomography

Planar X-ray imaging, i.e. conventional radiography, produces two-dimensional (2D) projection images of 3D objects; the actual 3D anatomic structure and the related specimen information cannot be accurately presented as the depth information is completely overlapped and mixed. In the early 1970s, Sir Godfrey Newbold Hounsfield and Alan McLeod Cormack developed computed tomography (Hounsfield, 1973; Cormack, 1973). For the first time, thanks to this revolutionary innovation, it became possible to non-invasively obtain *in vivo* quantitative information of tissue X-ray attenuation coefficient differences in uniformly thin cross-sections of tissues, and further 3D whole body volumetric visualization.

There is no fundamental difference between clinical CT and preclinical micro-CT. The CT principles can be defined in three parts: (1) X-ray projection imaging, (2) computer-assisted imaging scan and (3) image reconstruction, and are described below.

Similar to planar X-ray imaging, X-ray projection in a CT scanner also uses a transmission-based technique; X-rays emitted from a source pass through objects and are projected onto a detector(s) (Figure 75.2A). The X-ray source that is used in a micro-CT system can usually produce X-rays ranging from about 20 to 100 keV (hard), and with a single digit micron spot size. Various filters can be inserted into the X-ray pathways to adjust the X-ray "hardness" according to different tissue types. Currently, for achieving high resolution, most modern micro-CT systems employ a large format cooled X-ray digital camera as the detector.

Since the first CT scanner became available in the 1970s, more than four generations of scanning models have been developed (Table 75.1). Newly developed scanning models and techniques significantly reduce CT scanning time, which reduces X-ray exposure, while increasing the scanning resolution and quality.

During a CT scan, hundreds of angular projection images are collected. Once these angular projection images are acquired, a CT image reconstruction algorithm is applied to synthesize the virtual cross-section slices. The mathematical principle of image reconstruction was developed as early as 1917 by Radon (1917). There have been many reconstruction methods developed during the past decades (Herman, 2009; Kak and Slaney, 1988), such as the algebraic reconstruction technique (ART), the Fourier slice theorem, and the filtered-back-projection reconstruction. For example, Figure 75.2B illustrates the principle of the back-projection reconstruction algorithm, as this algorithm is widely used in today's micro-CT image reconstruction. This algorithm simply builds the CT image by essentially reversing the acquisition steps. As data from a large number of X-rays are back-projected onto the image matrix, areas with high X-ray attenuation tend to emphasize one another, as do areas of low attenuation, eventually building the image.

There are some artifacts that are commonly generated in the CT reconstruction process. For example, there are ring artifacts that are caused by defects on the X-ray source window, scintillator or detector window. These defects result in pixel intensity differences that appear as concentric rings in reconstructed slices (Wildenschild *et al.*, 2002). Beam hardening, which is caused by the polychromatic nature of closed X-ray sources that result in higher X-ray attenuation along the sample circumference due to lower energy absorption, is another common artifact (Ketcham and Carlson, 2001). CT image reconstruction is a computationally time-consuming process. For high resolution whole body micro-CT reconstruction, it could take hours to reconstruct 3D volumetric CT datasets. However, high performance computer advances, such as using a computer cluster, can dramatically reduce the reconstruction time from hours to minutes. After CT reconstruction, not only can cross-sectional tissue images be viewed, but interpolating sections along different planes can also be accurately performed thereby enabling a 3D volumetric image dataset to be built. Because the image data are now available in 3D anatomy, not only the internal structure in 3D can be examined, but 3D morphometric parameters can be quantitatively measured and the realistic visual models for virtual travel within the object can also be created with selected simple or complex volumes of interest (Gallagher, 1995; Bonneau, *et al.*, 2006). This is the power of volumetric visualization. With the data obtained in a full 3D anatomic structure, computer assisted volumetric analysis can also be applied.

As stated previously, there is no fundamental difference between clinical CT and micro-CT systems, although a micro-CT system is designed to provide much higher resolution, usually at the single-digit micron level. To obtain these higher resolution CT images, high X-ray dose and long scan time may be required to generate a sufficiently high signal-to-noise ratio. In recent years, there has been a great deal of achievement in developing high resolution micro-CT systems with the advent of better spot size X-ray sources and more sensitive and higher resolution X-ray detectors.

Micro-CT imaging can be conducted in both *in vivo* and *ex vivo* settings. In an *in vivo* system, the X-ray source and camera are usually rotated around the animal(s) to capture projection radiographs. In an *ex vivo* system the sample is usually rotated while the X-ray source and camera are stationary. Either technique can produce similar 3D image data.

Micro-CT systems

Technically, micro-CT systems can be classified depending on the type of X-ray source, camera geometry or scanning methodology (e.g., the fan-beam and cone-beam geometry). In the fan-beam geometry, a point X-ray source and a one-dimensional (1D) X-ray detector array are used to produce 2D radiographs, which are later reconstructed to form the CT images. The fan-beam technique is usually used in clinical CT systems. In the cone-beam geometry, a point X-ray source and a 2D X-ray detector are used to directly generate 2D radiographs. Both *in vivo* and *ex vivo* micro-CT systems can employ either fan-beam or cone-beam geometry for acquisition of 2D radiographs. Today, most micro-CT systems use the cone-beam technology such as the commercial micro-CT systems from GE Healthcare, Scanco Medical, Skyscan, Xradia, etc.

In vivo micro-CT

The architecture of an *in vivo* micro-CT system is usually similar to a clinical CT scanner. An object (patient, animal or other specimen) is placed on a stationary bed and the X-ray source-detector gantry rotates around the object and acquires 2D radiographs from multiple angles starting from 0° to 180 or 360°. A typical example of an *in vivo* scanner is the Skyscan-1076 (Skyscan, Belgium) that uses cone-beam technology for scanning, with a 100 keV X-ray source and a 10 megapixel 2D X-ray detector. When using this technology in preclinical species, respiratory and cardiac gating devices are must-have components to monitor physiological conditions and reduce motion artifacts (Badea *et al.*, 2004).

Ex vivo micro-CT

In most *ex-vivo* micro-CT systems the specimen rotates from 0° to 180 or 360° around the object axis while the X-ray source and X-ray detector are stationary at a fixed distance apart from each other. In modern micro-CT designs, some advanced technologies have been applied to reduce the scan time and improve the image quality such as the use of large format detectors in many commercial micro-CT systems. Some specific techniques have also been developed to further improve imaging speed and flexibility. For instance, the "adaptive geometry" design, in which the distance between the X-ray source and the detector can vary depending on the specimen size, balances scanning resolution and speed (Sasov *et al.*, 2008). To further increase the imaging resolution, nano-CT, namely the CT imaging resolution reaches submicron level, has also been developed.

MICRO-CT IMAGING OF UNSTAINED FETAL SKELETONS

CT imaging can non-invasively and non-destructively produce virtual bone structures in 3D. Since micro-CT can provide single or small double-digit microns spatial resolution that is sufficient for 3D microscopic CT imaging of small size fetuses, utilization of micro-CT in the evaluation of fetal skeletons is a rational choice. Micro-CT imaging studies conducted in our laboratory have confirmed this idea and the results obtained clearly demonstrated the utility of 2D/3D imaging of fetal skeletal structures of mice, rats and rabbits (data not published). In addition, multiple publications have shown that commonly used micro-CT can be successfully applied in the evaluation of fetal skeletal structures. For example, Nuzzo *et al.* (2003) published a micro-CT study on the ossification process in human vertebra during early ossification. They found that the micro-CT volumetric analysis with 3D images at high spatial resolution allows a detailed quantitative description of bone microarchitecture. In 2004, Wolschrijn (2004) reported the use of micro-CT to scan the ulnar medial coronoid process of young dogs to analyze the trabecular structures. Guldberg *et al.* (2004) reviewed micro-CT imaging of skeletal development and growth. Mulder *et al.* (2005) reported a micro-CT study of architecture and mineralization of developing trabecular bone in the pig mandibular condyle. Their results demonstrated that the micro-CT measurement of mineralization was comparable with those obtained with mineral composition analysis. Later, Oest *et al.* (2008) further emphasized that micro-CT evaluation of murine fetal skeletal development yields greater morphometric precision over traditional staining methods. More recently, Wise and Winkelmann (2009a,b) published their investigations of the utility of micro-CT to assess unstained skeletons of rabbit and rat fetuses. Their results indicate that micro-CT imaging with about $100\,\mu m^3$ spatial resolution can effectively assess rabbit and rat fetal skeletal structures. Micro-CT evaluation detected the same skeletal malformations, variations and incomplete ossifications as observed with a traditional staining method, although a few minor specific skeletal abnormalities involving small skeletal elements with minimal ossification did not match exactly. They concluded that micro-CT imaging can effectively be used to assess rat and rabbit fetal skeletal structures, and could significantly reduce the time to skeletal evaluation and data interpretation, as well as reduce the hazardous chemical waste associated with skeletal staining.

Another milestone result was published in 2009 by Winkelmann and Wise concerning the utilization of high-throughput micro-CT imaging of rat and rabbit fetal skeletons to detect abnormalities in developmental toxicity studies (Winkelmann and Wise, 2009). In this study, CT imaging of approximately 400 rat fetuses or approximately 140 rabbit fetuses per hour was achieved using a high speed mini-CT system. However, the high speed mini-CT scanner is not widely available. Utilizing more commonly available micro-CT systems, we have been able to achieve imaging spatial resolutions from ~10 to 50 micron, depending on the study requirements and sample size, while balancing the CT imaging time and the required image resolution. The following are study examples demonstrating this methodology.

Micro-CT imaging of fixed mouse embryonic and fetal skeletons

In this study, four mouse specimens obtained on gestation days 14.5, 15.5, 16.5 and 18.5 were imaged (Figure 75.3A). The specimens were fixed in 95% ethanol. It was possible to image all four specimens in a batch scan because of their small size. A Skyscan 1172 high resolution *ex vivo* micro-CT system (SkyScan, Belgium) was employed.

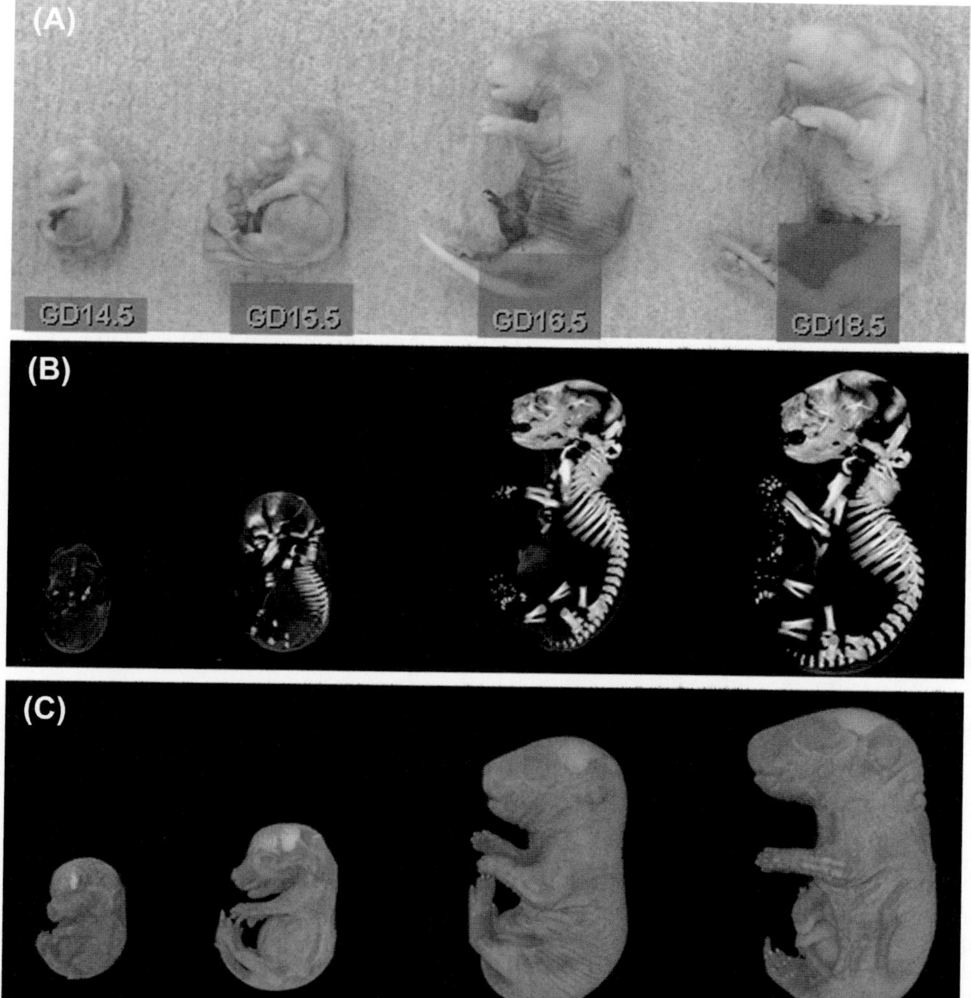

FIGURE 75.3 Unstained mouse specimens on gestation days 14.5, 15.5, 16.5 and 18.5 (A), and 3D volumetric visualization of the CT image data using MIP (maximum intensity projection) (B) and volume rendering (C) techniques. (D, *see next page*) Sample data illustrating the quantitative volumetric analyses of unstained skeletons of the mouse specimens in (A).

(D)

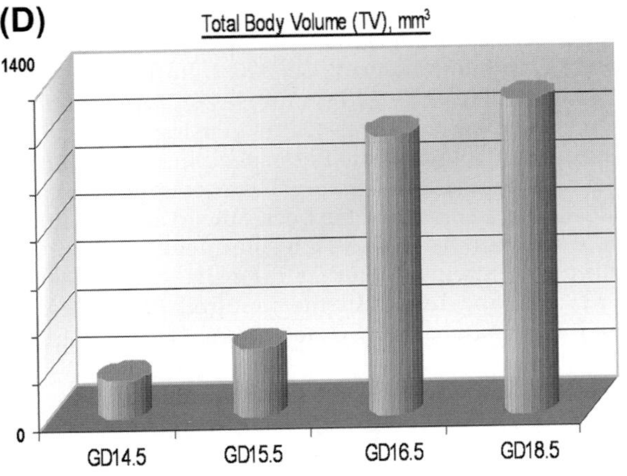

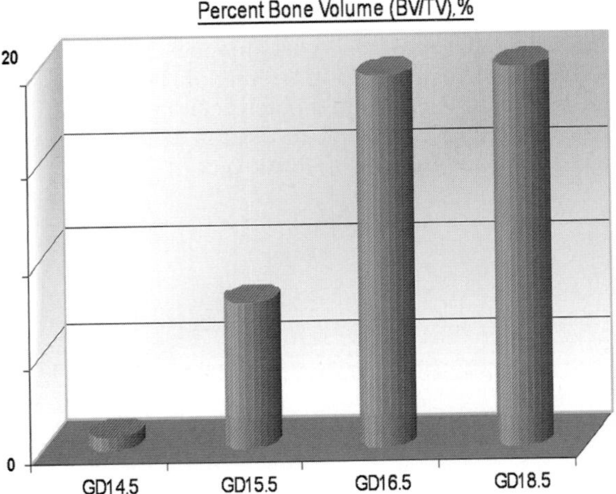

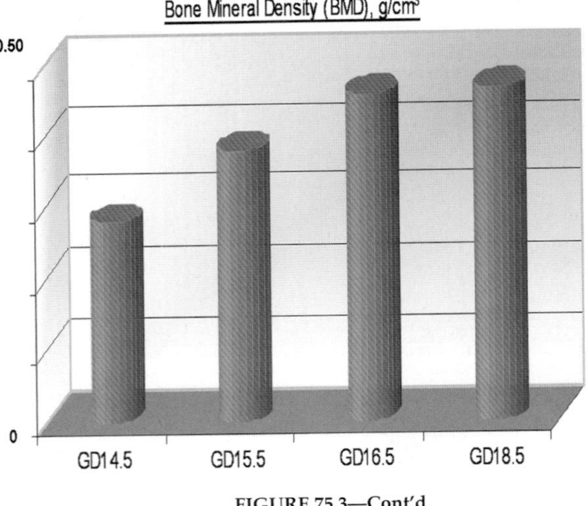

FIGURE 75.3—Cont'd

Scanning and reconstruction protocol

All specimens were scanned at an X-ray source voltage of 50 keV and current of 167 μA for acquiring multiple 2D projection radiographs with a rotation step of 0.5°/180°. Two or four frames raw projection image averaging was used to increase the signal-to-noise ratio. A modified Feldkamp reconstruction algorithm, i.e. multi-slice volumetric cone-beam reconstruction (Feldkamp *et al.*, 1984), was used in the reconstruction to form 2D cross-section CT images from the acquired 2D radiographs. The reconstructed images were generated as 8-bit 256 gray scale BMP images with normalized minimum and maximum values for halftone conversion. During the reconstruction, a correction was also made to reduce the ring artifacts and beam hardening artifacts. The 3D reconstructed CT volumetric image data were reviewed and analyzed using the SkyScan CTAn/CTvol (SkyScan, Belgium) and/or the Amira® (Visage Imaging Inc., CA) software systems (same for other examples shown in this chapter).

2D and 3D mouse images

Figure 75.3B shows visualization with maximum intensity projections, a commonly used volumetric visualization method (Lell *et al.*, 2006; Fishman *et al.*, 2006), for the four specimens. This method would allow for better visualization of differences in mineralized bone formation, compared to CT sectioning display. Figure 75.3C illustrates a volume rendering view, another commonly used volumetric visualization method (Drebin *et al.*, 1988; Fishman *et al.*, 2006), of the four 3D reconstructed specimens. These virtual embryos consist of the digital-CT density data that are related to the tissue X-ray attenuation coefficient data obtained, and represent the exact 3D CT density anatomic structure of the embryos.

Quantitative analysis

Mineralized skeletal structures were virtually isolated by converting gray scale images to binarized images and using global thresholds. Parameters calculated using Skyscan's CTAn software (Skyscan, Belgium), which uses both 2D slice-by-slice and 3D volumetric analyses, include "Total Body Volume", "Bone Mineral Density" and "Average Trabecular Bone Thickness". A sample of data analysis is illustrated in Figure 75.3D. The bone histomorphometry parameters were based on the Report of the ASBMR Histomorphometry Nomenclature Committee (Parfitt *et al.*, 1987).

Micro-CT imaging of skeletons of unstained rat pups

Another example of the utility of bioimaging in development toxicology is in the use of micro-CT analysis of skeletal malformations of rat pups. These rat pups were from a developmental and reproductive toxicity (DART) study in which some structural malformations were observed during the postpartum period. Micro-CT was used to further investigate the findings. The pups were fixed in 4% paraformaldehyde or 95% ethanol. The same SkyScan 1172 micro-CT system was used to image the rat pups.

Scanning and reconstruction protocols

A similar scanning protocol as the one used for the mouse specimens was applied, but the scanning and reconstruction parameters were modified to accommodate the X-ray attenuation from the larger body of the rat pup compared to the

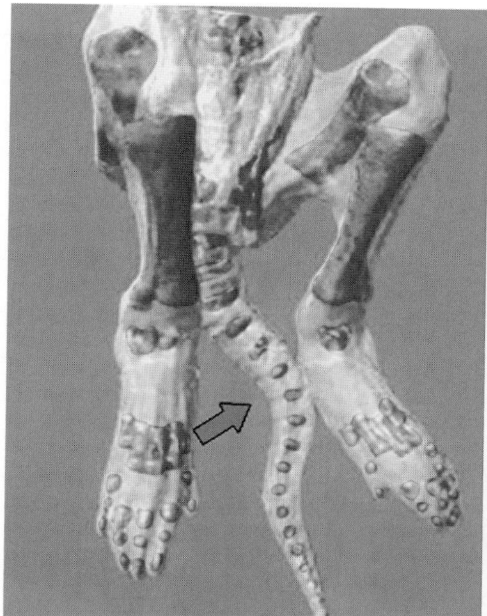

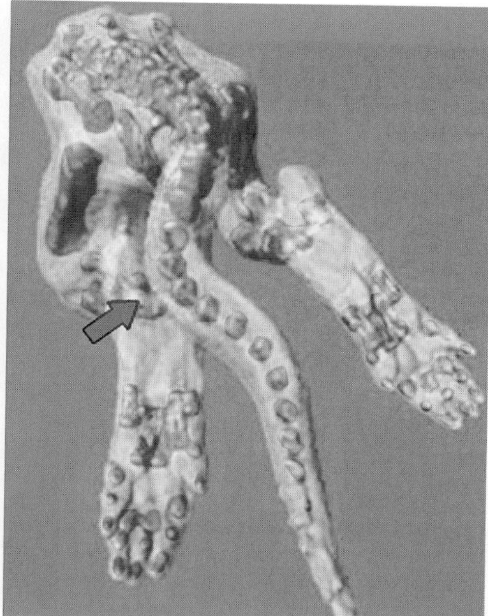

FIGURE 75.4 Example demonstrating the utilization of computer-assisted 3D volumetric visualization and analysis to evaluate a possible skeletal malformation in a rat pup. Arrows indicate the curved tail in the virtual skeletal visualization.

embryo or fetal mouse. Specimens were scanned at an X-ray source voltage of 50 keV and current of 200 μA to acquire multiple 2D radiographs with a rotation step of 0.4°/360° and two frames averaging. Note that a 360° rotation was used as compared to the 180° used in the mouse fetus scanning since more 2D projections result in better signal-to-noise ratio. A 0.5 mm aluminum filter was used to remove the lower energy X-ray spectrum ("soft" X-rays) from the polychromatic X-ray source used in the Skyscan 1172 scanner because the rat specimen had more body mass compared to the mouse specimen. Using a filter also helped reduce the beam hardening artifact produced by the soft X-rays. The same modified Feldkamp reconstruction algorithm (multi-slice volumetric cone-beam reconstruction) was used in the reconstruction of 2D cross-section CT images from the acquired 2D radiographs. During the reconstruction, corrections to reduce the ring-artifact and beam hardening artifact were applied. The reconstructed images were generated as 8-bit 256 gray scale BMP images with normalized minimum and maximum values for halftone conversion.

2D and 3D rat pup images

Figure 75.4 illustrates sample images with the volume rendering display of a rat pup skeletal structure. In the 3D view a bent tail can be clearly seen. In addition, if needed, digital measurement of angles, diameters, length, etc. can be easily applied. The structural malformation appears externally so it can be observed with the naked eye. However, micro-CT imaging provides 3D structure data for skeleton and the surrounding tissues internally. The micro-CT data were collected digitally with 3D volumes. Therefore, structural analyses could be accurately conducted by computer-assisted 3D measurement for parameters such as the length ratio between different land marks, angles, curves, etc., in addition to routine measurement of crown–rump and tail lengths. Visualizing the unprocessed skeletons and surrounding soft tissues together allows for a more accurate evaluation of potential developmental abnormalities.

Micro-CT imaging of unstained fetal skeletons has been practically used in DART studies, even with a high throughput manner (Winkelman and Wise, 2009). In other studies using a common micro-CT system, increased CT imaging throughput can be achieved via specially designed imaging techniques. For example, a 7 to 21 fetus batch scan setup was designed in-house for use in conjunction (Figure 75.5) with a Skyscan 1076 micro-CT system (Skyscan, Belgium). With 36 μm imaging resolution, approximately 80 fetuses per day could be scanned with a 7- or 21-fetus batch scan setup. Furthermore, with a micro-CT scanner with larger object size that will be able to hold more fetuses in one batch scan, higher throughput can be expected.

Summary and discussion

The sample results of unstained rodent embryos, fetuses and pups demonstrates that the micro-CT imaging is able to provide sufficient resolution and image quality for evaluating the skeletal structures of fresh or unstained specimens for studies in developmental toxicology.

The micro-CT method has obvious advantages over the traditional staining process. For example, micro-CT imaging can offer much quicker turnaround time. The traditional staining process takes multiple days to prepare the samples for evaluation. However, micro-CT can produce 3D structural data in minutes to a few hours while maintaining the integrity of the intact specimen. This advantage may allow either some specimens of special interest or selected groups, such as the high dose-treated group, to be scanned for immediate availability of the data.

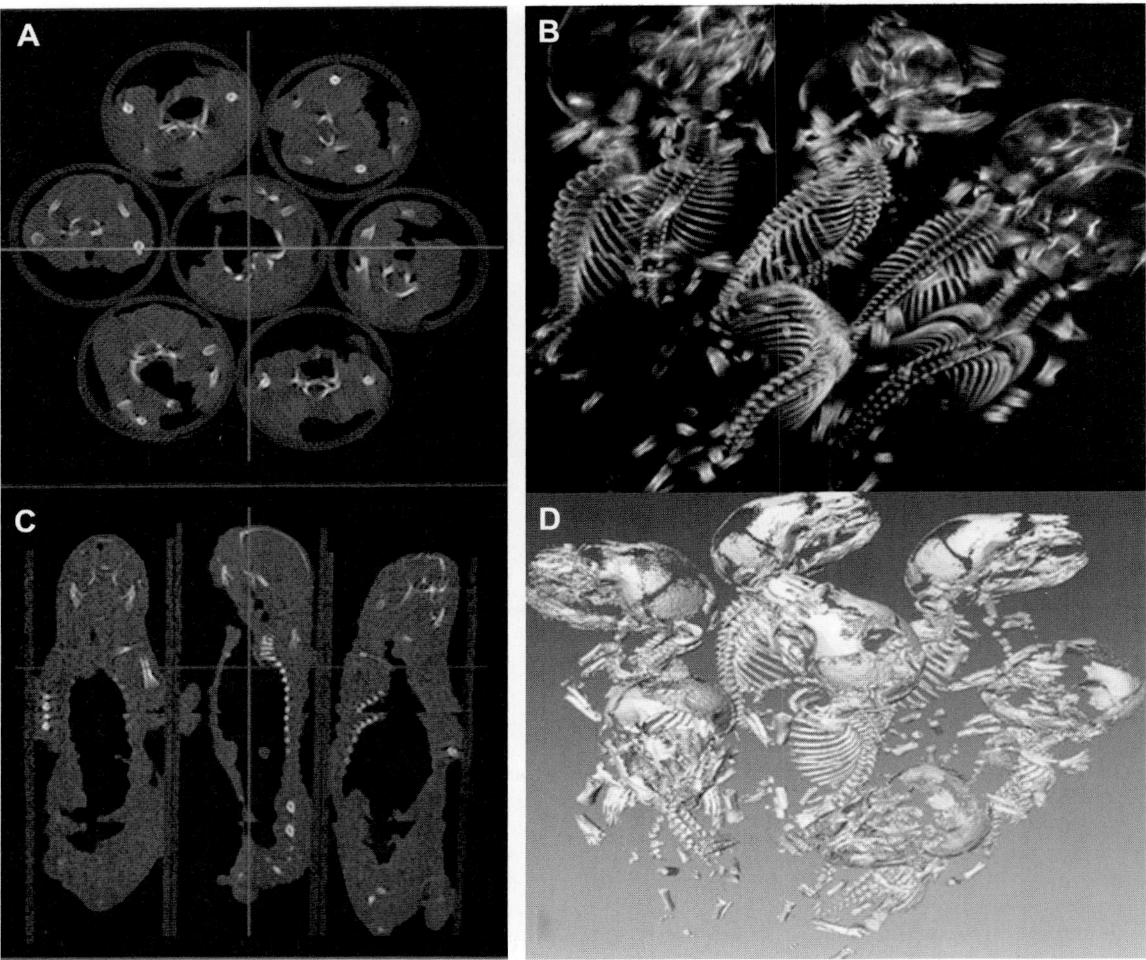

FIGURE 75.5 Increased micro-CT imaging throughput with a simple batch scan of seven rat fetuses. (A) and (C) micro-CT section images of the rat fetuses. (B) MIP display of the fetal skeletons. (D) volume rendering view of the rat fetal skeletons. Please refer to color plate section.

Another unique advantage of micro-CT imaging is its natively digital data format, which enables the direct application of modern digital imaging processing techniques, especially quantitative measurement methods, by employing obtainable computer tools. This approach opens a new door to developmental toxicology since it could result in new analysis methods and novel quantitative data from computer-assisted 3D structure analysis.

Since all data are already in an electronic format, data can be easily shared and managed. With the rapid development of computer technology, this advantage will be increasingly significant. With the advancement of the virtual visualization technologies (Fishman *et al.*, 2006; Peng *et al.*, 2010), novel approaches will become available for DART scientists to assess fetal skeletons in more efficient ways.

MICRO-CT IMAGING OF ALIZARIN RED-S STAINED FETUSES

Traditionally, alizarin red-S-based single-staining is the major method for visualizing the calcified elements of the fetal skeleton, and alizarin red-S with alcian blue-based double-staining is the method for evaluating the cartilage and calcified skeletal structures. These two techniques are still the primary methods for the bone and cartilage examination of fetal skeletons required in preclinical developmental toxicity studies.

However, with these two methods it is difficult to provide accurate information on fetal bone mineralization and density during development. Unquestionably, micro-CT studies on unstained specimens can be conducted to obtain such data. However, scientists may only be interested in bone density measurements after they have already had some initial findings on the stained specimens; or they may not want to change their current workflow to insert a new micro-CT examination. In addition, it may be desirable to re-examine already-stained specimens using the new technology available to obtain more accurate digital 3D skeletal structure and/or ossification analysis. All these needs will require micro-CT imaging of single- and/or double-stained fetuses.

Micro-CT data for previously stained fetal skeletons was not found during a recent literature search. Therefore, a study was conducted to determine if it would be possible to develop a micro-CT assay for skeletal examination on single- and/or double-stained fetuses. The hypothesis was that the CT imaging would be possible because both X-ray micro-CT

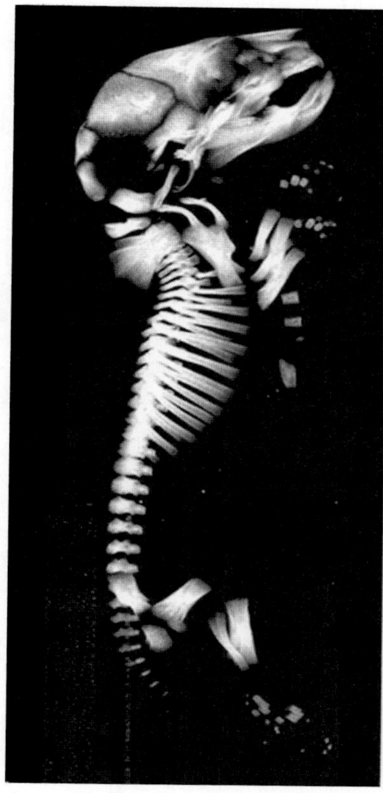
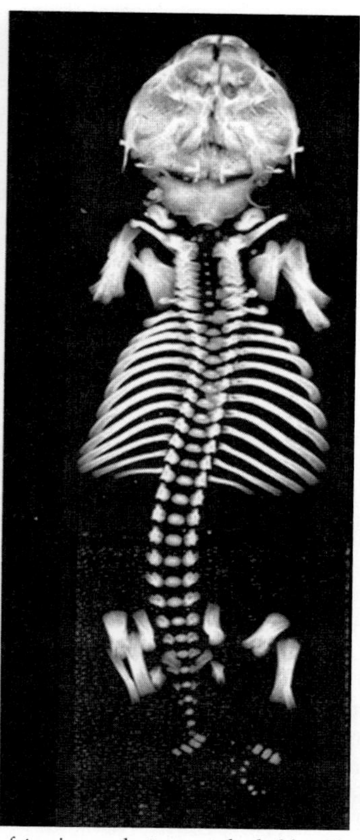

FIGURE 75.6 Digital MIP volumetric visualization of an alizarin red-S-stained rat fetus in a polystyrene tube holder. The images illustrate that the skeletal structure can be clearly visualized, based on the micro-CT images.

and the alizarin red-S staining are positive for calcium mineral deposition and the staining process does not seem to change the calcium in the skeletal structures (Burdan *et al.*, 2002; Gregory *et al.*, 2004).

To develop the micro-CT imaging protocols, single- (alizarin red-S) or double- (plus alcian blue) stained mouse and rat fetuses were used. The fetal specimens were previously eviscerated and skinned, and washed in tap water. In the single-staining process, 95% ethanol was used for dehydration before KOH maceration and alizarin staining (Menegola *et al.*, 2001, 2002). To prevent skull compression, the specimens were processed with graded series (20, 40 and 60% of glycerin) glycerol solution, and finally stored in 80% glycerin with thymol, before the micro-CT imaging.

Micro-CT imaging of stained mouse and rat fetal skeletons

For micro-CT imaging, each specimen was loaded in a custom-made polystyrene tube holder with the micro-CT mounting device. Polystyrene has a very low attenuation for X-rays, thereby making it an ideal sample holder. Since the stained fetuses are pliable, special care was taken to ensure no compression on the specimens and no movement during imaging. A high resolution micro-CT system (SkyScan 1172 or 1173, SkyScan, Belgium) was used for assay development. Settings with 8–25 μm/voxel were used for scanning the fetal specimens, with the size up to about 35 mm diameter, which includes the mouse, rat and some rabbit fetuses (the maximum scanning diameter of 140 mm of the Skyscan 1173 was considered for simultaneous scanning of multiple fetuses to increase the throughput).

Similar scanning and reconstruction protocols as described previously were applied on the stained specimens. Several main parameters were adjusted for differences in the stained tissue characteristics. One major change, for example, was to reduce the electronic voltage for the soft tissues; 40 keV and a current of 200 μA were used to acquire 2D radiographs with a rotation step of 0.4°/180°. Two, four or eight frames averaging were used to increase the signal-to-noise ratio. The reconstructed images were generated as 8-bit 256 gray scale BMP images with normalized minimum and maximum values for halftone conversion.

2D and 3D fetal rat images

The micro-CT imaging results illustrated that the skeletal structures of the stained fetuses were clearly visible on the CT images. The CT densities of the stained skeletons and surrounding soft tissues were significantly different, allowing easy segmentation of the skeletons from the surrounding soft tissues for skeletal analysis. With high resolution CT imaging, the skeletal malformations/variations and incomplete ossifications observed exactly matched the direct observations of the stained specimens. It was also possible to quantitatively measure bone microarchitecture of the stained specimens. For example, a micro-CT image of a single-stained rat fetus is shown in Figure 75.6. Typical outputs of the quantitative analysis of mineralized skeletal structures include bone volume (BV, e.g. 136.68 mm^3 for the sample shown in the figure) and bone surface area (BA, e.g. 1749.68 mm^2 for the sample), etc.

We also scanned double-stained mouse and rat fetuses with the CT imaging method. The skeletal phenotyping was found to be no different than the single-stain, but the alcian blue-stained cartilage could not be clearly distinguished in the CT images in our experiments, although we were able to visualize a part of the cartilaginous skeleton (data not shown).

Micro-CT imaging of stained rabbit fetal skeletons

For large specimens, such as whole rabbit fetuses, the Skyscan 1076 micro-CT system was used, since the scanner can accommodate larger rabbit specimens (< 68 mm diameter). The system employs a microfocus X-ray source of 10 W (20–100 keV) with 5–7 μm resolution and a 10 Mp cooled CCD sensor with optic fiber coupling to an X-ray scintillator. The system has a specimen carriage that is 300 mm long with an effective scannable length of 200 mm, which is suitable for most rabbit fetuses.

As for the CT scan preparation, the rabbit fetus specimens were mounted in polystyrene tube holders, which were subsequently fixed to the specimen bed of the micro-CT. The size of the tubal holders was selected according to the size of the sample. Similar to the scans of mouse- or rat-stained fetuses, special care was taken while mounting the specimens to ensure no pressure was applied on the specimens and that no movement would occur during the CT imaging.

Scanning and reconstruction protocols

The clear-stained rabbit fetus samples were scanned at 35 μm imaging resolution with 60 keV and 167 μA X-ray source settings to acquire 2D radiographs with a rotation step of 0.9°/180°. Four frames averaging was conducted to increase the signal-to-noise ratio. A 0.5 mm aluminum filter was used to reduce the beam hardening effect from the polychromatic nature of the X-ray source and increase the imaging contrast of the bones. Scanning at 35 μm resolution covers a field of view of ~35 mm × 17 mm in a single normal scan. Six continuous scans were automatically conducted to cover the entire length of the rabbit fetus. All segments were automatically stitched after the scans in the reconstruction. No significant difference of the reconstruction protocol was applied to the clear-stained rabbit fetuses. Similar corrections to reduce the ring-artifact and beam hardening artifact were also applied. The reconstructed images were generated as 8-bit 256 gray scale BMP images with normalized minimum and maximum values for halftone conversion.

This newly developed micro-CT assay was used on alizarin red-S-stained rabbit fetuses from a developmental toxicity study to evaluate the CT imaging as compared to observations from traditional examinations. The outcome confirmed that the CT densities of the stained ossified structures were clearly measurable. Based on the CT images, quantitative analysis was also performed. With high resolution CT imaging, the skeletal malformations and/or variations observed were exactly matched with the direct manual observations of the clear-stained specimens (Figure 75.7).

Summary and discussions

The hypothesis that micro-CT imaging should be able to correctly identify the skeletal structures of the single- or double-stained fetuses was confirmed; micro-CT can be used to accurately assess the stained (alizarin red-S with or without alcian blue) bone elements of fetal skeletons of the mouse, rat and rabbit. In addition to skeletal structure analyses, the micro-CT method makes it possible to provide quantitative 3D measurements of skeletal ossification or mineralization and bone microarchitecture on previously stained fetuses. This ability may contribute to the generation of new data by reassessment of existing specimens. This ability also allows

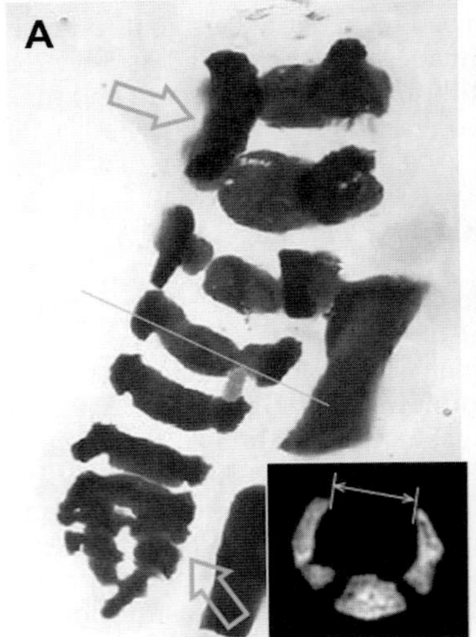

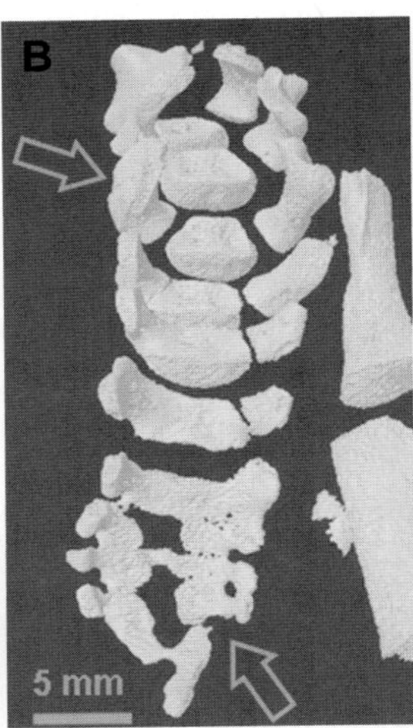

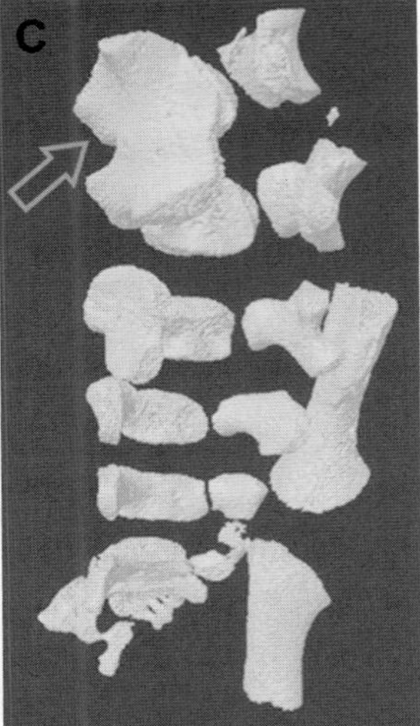

FIGURE 75.7 Micro-CT 3D volumetric imaging and analysis of single-stained vertebral bones of a rabbit fetus. Photo (A) was taken by an independent examiner. The 3D volume rendering visualization (B and C) were based on micro-CT images without prior knowledge malformations. The skeletal malformations and/or variations observed (orange arrows) were exactly matched with the CT data. The small CT image on the photo (A) demonstrates the digital measurement of a vertebral arch.

us to conduct an additional micro-CT study for potentially novel data while not changing the existing workflow, since the study could be carried out after the routine evaluation.

During assay development, it was found that special care was necessary to overcome possible motion during CT scanning since the stained specimens were pliable and imaging was conducted at the level of microns spatial resolution. With different micro-CT systems, the solution may need to be different. For instance, with a high resolution *ex vivo* micro-CT, e.g. the SkyScan 1172, the sample rotates during scanning, so the holder size must be matched with the specimen to restrict possible motion. As for the *in vivo* CT systems, such as the SkyScan 1076, usually the sample is stationary so a slightly larger diameter tube could be selected to hold the specimen, but experience has indicated it is better to wait a few minuets to allow the specimen to settle before starting the CT scan so as to reduce potential motion artifacts. In all cases, the tube should be fully filled with the same storage solution (glycerin in this case) to prevent potential specimen shrinkage during the CT imaging.

HIGH RESOLUTION MICRO-CT IMAGING OF FETAL BONE MICROARCHITECTURE

Bone is a living organ and its microarchitectural development may be more complex than previously realized. The initial ossification, the micro-structure evolution, and the related functions may play critical roles in bone malformation and/or other developmental abnormalities. However, in a recent literature search, there were few high resolution CT imaging studies on the dynamic processes and evolution of microarchitectural structures in fetal bone development. One reason may be the technical limitation. To date, microanatomic analysis at the single micron level is primarily based on histomorphometry techniques. However, histological sectioning is not practical for obtaining the 3D data which are required for accurate analysis of changes in bone microarchitecture. In addition, histology methods cannot directly measure bone ossification and mineralization.

As described in previous sections, regular micro-CT technology has been successfully applied in the evaluation of skeletal structures in developmental toxicology studies, but they have mostly been limited to double-digit micron resolution, which is inadequate for analysis of mouse or rat fetal bone microarchitecture. Therefore, micro-CT assays were developed using high resolution micro-CT technology to obtain 3D bone microarchitecture data from mouse fetuses.

High resolution micro-CT imaging of mouse fetal bones

For this study, a high resolution micro-CT system (SkyScan 1172) with settings of 1.3 or 1.8 μm^3 voxel size for long bones and about 8~10 μm^3 for whole body was used. To determine if the spatial resolution settings were sufficient, a nano-CT system (SkyScan 2011, SkyScan, Belgium) with 800 nm^3 voxel size setting was used in parallel for the long bone scans. The 3D reconstructed CT volumetric image data were reviewed and analyzed using the SkyScan CTAn/CTvol and/or the Amira® software systems.

The long bone specimens were from the gestation day 14.5, 15.5, 16.5 and 18.5 mice, which we used for a previous "non-staining CT study". After the non-destructive whole body micro-CT imaging, the high resolution micro-CT was conducted on the fetal radius and ulna bones.

In the study, both 1.3 and 1.8 μm^3 voxel size resolution CT scans produced clear CT images showing the bone microstructures (Figure 75.8). Especially after 3D reconstruction, the elaborate network of pores and canals within the cortical bone (likely the lacunae–canalicular Haversian system) were obviously visible and even quantitatively measurable. For example, the Haversian canals in the radius and ulna bones of the gestation day 15.5 mouse fetus were mostly open. But, in the radius and ulna bones of the gestation day 18.5 mouse fetus, the Haversian canals were mostly formed (Figures 75.8 and 75.9). Compared with the adult mouse bone, the cortical bone porosity is much higher in fetal bones, which may indicate rapidly developing bone formation in the developmental period (Figure 75.9).

In addition to the microstructure, the 3D microarchitecture of the trabecular bone could also be vividly visualized and measured in 3D. For example, Figure 75.10 shows trabecular bones that are virtually segmented from the fetal mouse ulna. The trabecular microarchitecture CT image data in 3D make it possible to non-destructively quantify the trabecular bone formation or damage, including the bone volume density (BV/TV, i.e. bone volume vs. total volume), trabecular thickness (Tb.Th) and bone surface density (BS/BV, i.e. bone surface vs. bone volume). For example, Table 75.2 shows the data obtained from the bones shown in Figure 75.10.

Ultra-high resolution CT images for the same two bones in this study (data not shown) were also obtained. The comparison with the nano-CT scans and the micro-CT scan indicated that the 1.3 and 1.8 μm^3 resolution settings were sufficient for mouse fetal bone microarchitecture analysis, since there was not much additional structural detail revealed by the nano-CT scans.

Summary and discussion

The results indicate that high resolution micro-CT imaging is a promising method for non-destructive analysis of fetal bone microarchitecture. Since the 3D bone volumetric data obtained after reconstruction reflect 3D anatomy, the bone microarchitecture can be virtually visualized in any plane from any direction, and any portion of the bone can be virtually dissected for quatitative analysis. Obviously this technique could help us to better assess and understand the internal spatial organization. This type of analysis is not available with any conventional histomorphometry techniques.

The information on bone morphological changes and mineralization at a spatial resolution of approximately 1 to 5 microns in 3D provides sufficient detail for investigating bone microarchitecture and any potential changes in developmental toxicology studies. For example, the 3D volumetric images from this study clearly showed the cortical bone porosity. Further quantitative measurement of the porosity might provide additional information on bone formation. In addition, the high resolution CT data could also be utilized to clarify and/or support the relatively lower resolution fetal skeletal abnormality analysis from the higher throughput CT screening.

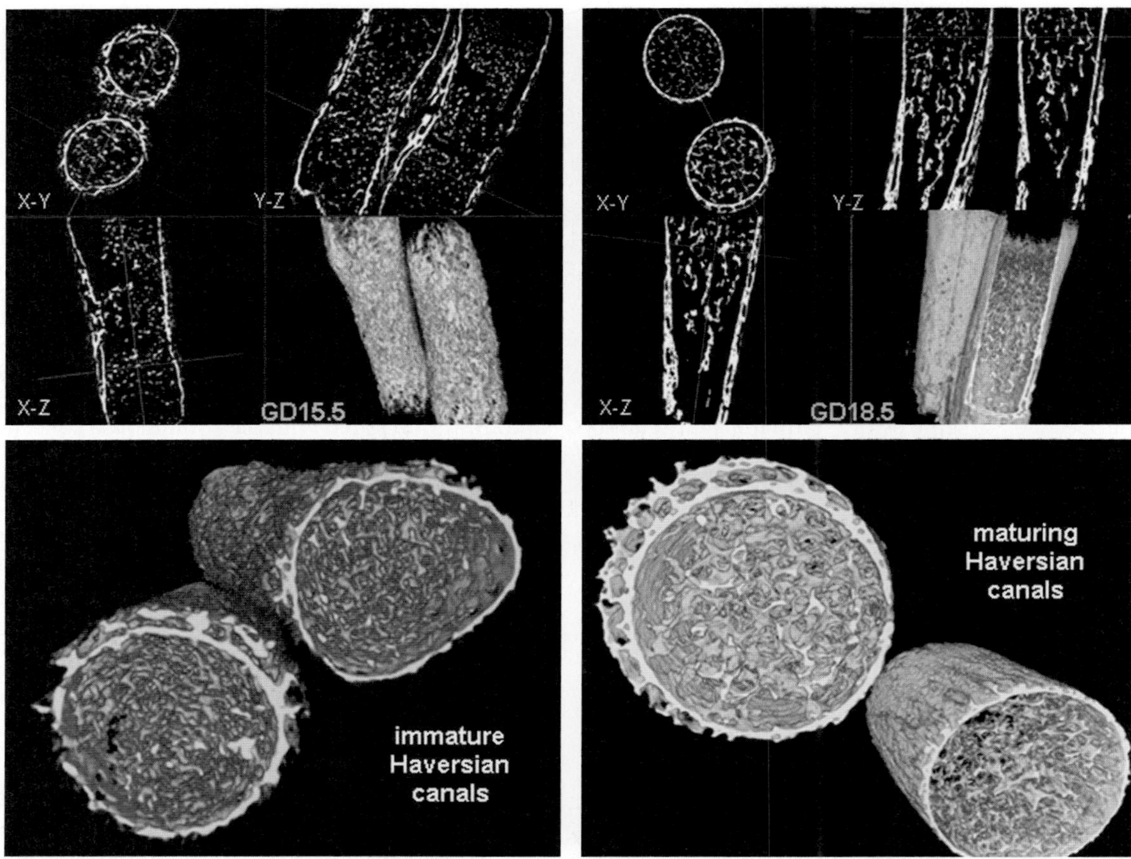

FIGURE 75.8 High resolution micro-CT imaging of unstained embryonic/fetal mouse bones. The images demonstrate 2D micro-CT images (top panels) and 3D volume rendering images (bottom panels) of the radius and ulna of a mouse embryo and fetus.

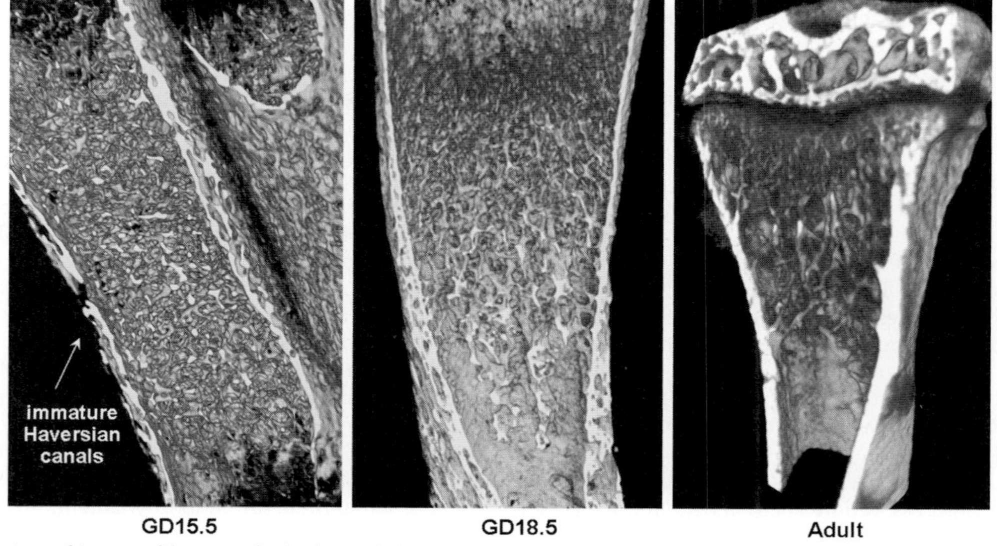

FIGURE 75.9 Bone microarchitecture of the mouse fetal radius and ulna visualized through longitudinal sections by a 3D volume rendering visualization technique (the original CT images were obtained with the CT imaging resolution of 1.3 μm^3 voxel size). An adult mouse long bone is displayed here as reference only (the CT imaging resolution for the adult mouse bone was 10 μm^3 voxel size). The images are not in proportion to the real size.

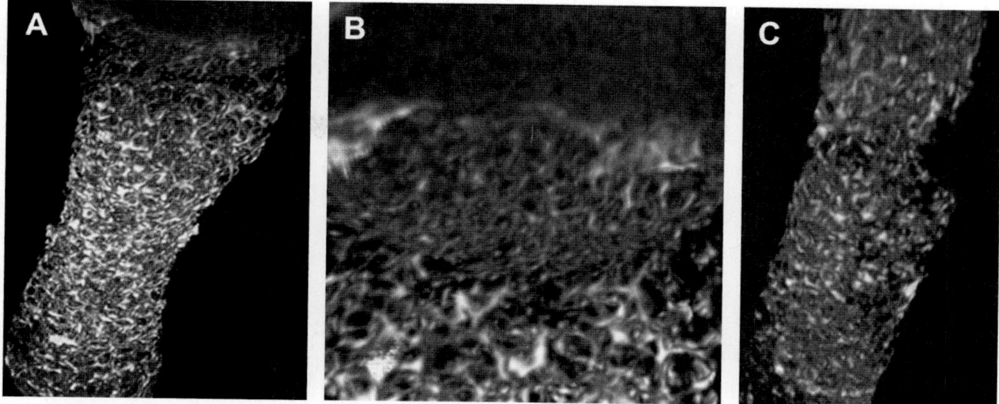

FIGURE 75.10 3D microarchitecture of trabecular bone from a fetal mouse ulna that has been virtually segmented: (A) a complete segment of trabecular bone from an ulna of a mouse embryo (gestation day 15.5); (B) enlarged image of the growth plate of the ulna; (C) 3D view showing a lack of trabecular bone in a local position inside of an ulna.

TABLE 75.2 Sample data from the volumetric analysis of single long bones of mouse specimens by high resolution micro-CT imaging, as shown in Figure 75.8

Parameters	GD 15.5	GD 18.5
Bone volume (BV), mm^3	0.012	0.109
Mean trabecular bone thickness (Tb.Th), mm	0.008	0.014
Bone surface area (BA), mm^2	6.327	27.175
Bone surface-to-volume ratio (BA/BV), 1/mm	529.533	250.189

MICRO-CT IMAGING OF CONTRAST AGENT STAINED SOFT TISSUES AND ORGANS OF FETUSES

As previously described in this chapter, micro-CT technology can be used in developmental toxicology studies to assess bone elements and skeletal structures of rodent embryos, fetuses and pups non-destructively in 3D anatomy. Since most soft tissues are nearly radiotransparent and there are no significant differences in X-ray attenuation coefficients for most major organs and tissues, CT imaging is usually not the primary option for soft tissue and organ evaluations. Exceptions to this general rule are the lung in which air plays a role of contrast agent, the brain in which the CT densities of gray/white matter and some lesions may differ visibly, and tumors or other calcified tissues. However, during the past five years, several encouraging publications have demonstrated some micro-CT imaging results of whole body embryos and/or fetuses with excellent image quality of the internal organs using specific CT contrast-agent staining methods. Johnson *et al.* (2006) published a pioneering article for anatomical phenotyping of mid-gestation embryos using osmium tetroxide staining and micro-CT-based imaging. They claimed that the micro-CT imaging of the osmium tetroxide-stained mid-gestation embryos not only matched or exceeded the tissue contrast achieved by MR microscopy technology, but was faster, less costly, and had a higher resolution. Wirkner and Prendini (2007) reported a micro-CT study on comparative morphology of arthropod vasculature. Mizutani *et al.* (2007, 2008) also reported a micro-CT analysis of the nerve tissues of Drosophila brain with different staining methods. Another study by de Crespigny and coworkers (2008) on 3D micro-CT imaging of mouse and rabbit brains indicated that micro-CT may be a valuable alternative to standard histopathology.

The contrast agent staining process plays a critical role in micro-CT imaging of soft tissue. However, useful staining methods are still lacking although a few staining techniques, such as osmium tetroxide staining, have been successfully used for contrast enhancement (Metscher, 2009a,b). A comprehensive summary table of versatile staining methods is provided in the article (Metscher, 2009b). More recently, Degenhardt and others reported a study on 3D phenotyping of cardiovascular development in mouse embryos by micro-CT with iodine staining (Degenhardt *et al.*, 2010). Those results demonstrated that micro-CT with an iodine staining method produced high quality images and can be used for the characterization of cardiovascular development and analysis of defects in mouse embryos.

Micro-CT imaging of contrast agent-stained mouse embryos

Gestation day 14.5, 15.5, 16.5 and 18.5 mouse specimens were used for assay development. Different fixation methods such as ethanol, paraformaldehyde and 4F1G (4% formaldehyde, 1% gluteraldehyde in 0.1 M phosphate buffer) were tested according to the literature (Metscher, 2009b; Schmidt *et al.*, 2010). Different staining procedures with various stain solutions, such as Lugol's iodine potassium iodide, PTA phosphotungstic acid and osmium tetroxide, were also tried. Considering the toxicity of osmium tetroxide, a relatively low concentration (0.25 to 0.5%, maxium 1%) was used. A high resolution micro-CT system (SkyScan 1172) was used for the imaging, with an approximate setting of 40~50 keV. The spatial resolution was set from about 10 to 25 μm/voxel based on the specimens' size and the details that needed to be visualized. The SkyScan CTvol and the Amira software were used for post-processing for 3D volumetric visualization. One of the preliminary 3D micro-CT images of contrast agent-stained mouse embryos is shown in Figure 75.11.

With whole body 3D data available for embryonic soft tissues/organs, the Wilson procedure (Wilson, 1965; Neubert *et al.*, 1977) can be mimicked by virtually cutting the tissue and displaying the slices on a computer monitor for evaluation of potential teratogenic effects. This volumetric data-based

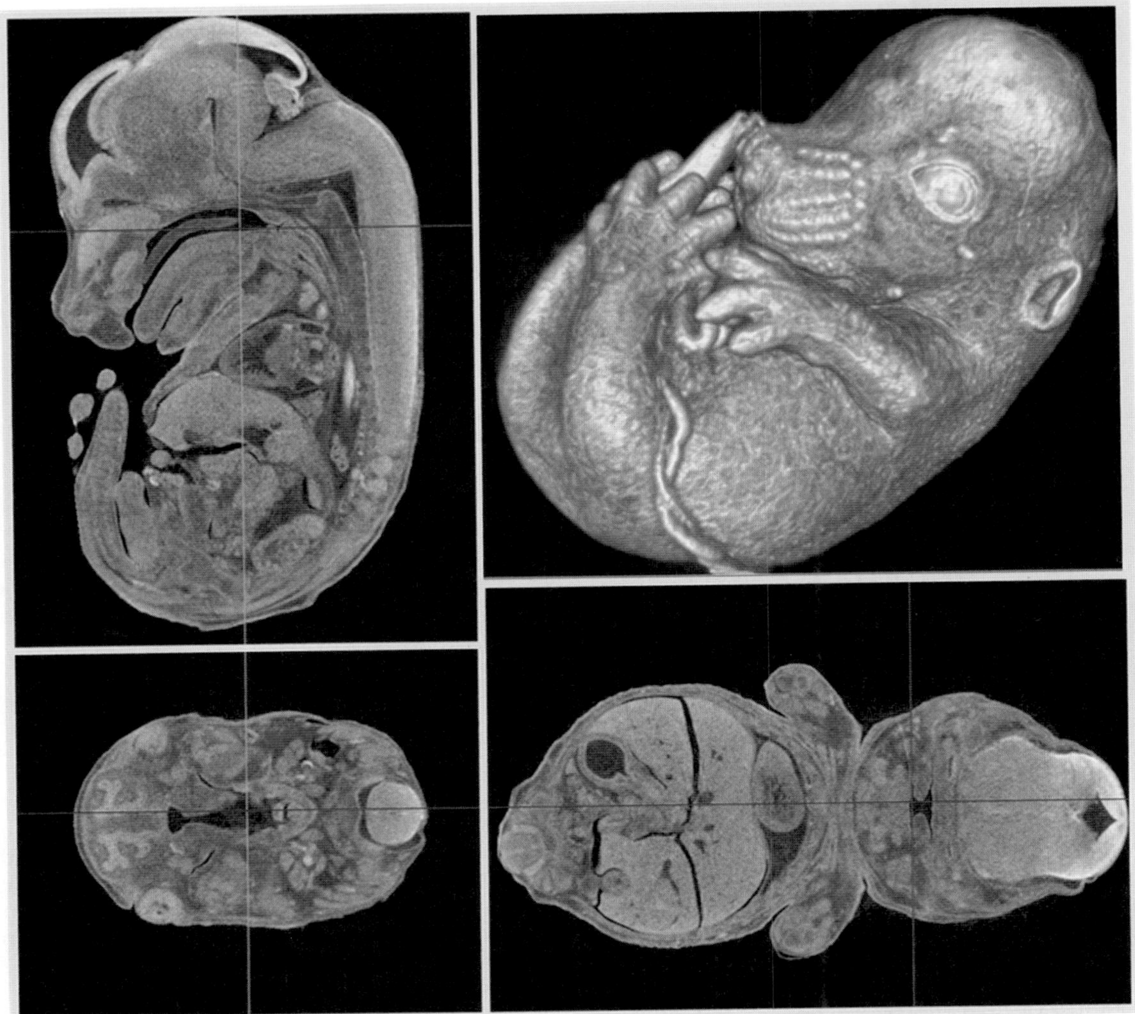

FIGURE 75.11 Micro-CT volumetric imaging of a contrast agent-stained mouse embryo (gestation day 14.5). Please refer to color plate section.

virtual slicing examination has some unique advantages. For example, as demonstrated in the Figure 75.12, not only can the "Wilson slices" be virtually performed, but slices in other planes and from different angles, such as axial, coronal and sagittal views, can be simultaneously viewed. Using this CT-image-based virtual Wilson slicing method one can quickly move the cutting positions for examination of whole embryos.

Summary and discussion

Similar to histological techniques that can provide sufficient details for tissue sections at the micron resolution level, contrast agent-enhanced micro-CT technology has demonstrated the possibility to visualize whole body micro-anatomic changes in 3D. This progress could significantly advance developmental toxicology evaluations, for example the characterization of cardiovascular development in DART studies. Volumetric measurements can more feasibly produce new quantitative data for developmental changes in 3D.

In this technique, contrast agent staining is the key. Although excellent results have been published using inorganic iodine and phosphotungstic acid, osmium tetroxide or iodinated contrast agents, it seems that there is no single optimal set of constants, and local laboratory optimization will be needed to develop the assays further. Namely, each new type of specimen should be tested with different fixatives/stains for the best staining treatment according to the imaging applications.

OTHER VOLUMETRIC IMAGING MODALITIES IN DEVELOPMENTAL TOXICOLOGY

Micro-CT volumetric imaging technology is not all-powerful, it has some significant limitations. The first major disadvantage is the radiation, which may prohibit many translational imaging applications in clinical trials. Second, without contrast agent staining, CT has a poor capacity to differentiate soft tissues/organs. In addition, CT has a low sensitivity for molecular imaging; and limited functional imaging capability. To overcome the limitations, other volumetric imaging technologies such as MRI and ultrasound imaging have been utilized.

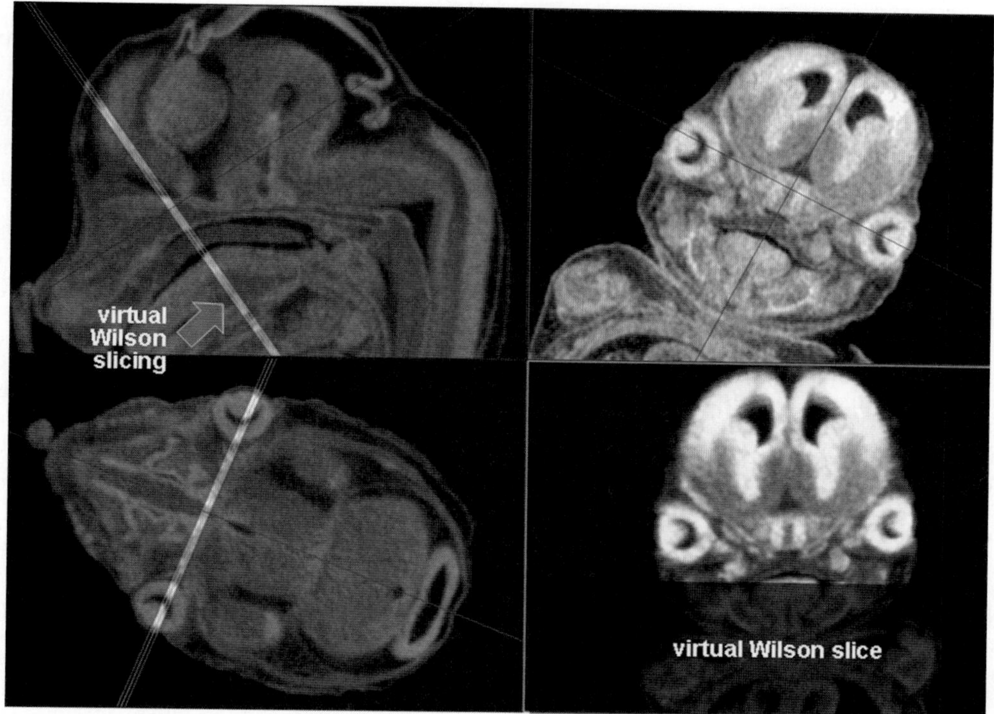

FIGURE 75.12 3D volumetric CT image-based virtual "Wilson slicing". With the 3D CT image dataset, the brain or other anatomic structures could be virtually sliced to assess potential embryotoxic effects. This virtual technique is similar to the original Wilson razor-blade cutting method.

In the clinical setting, MRI is a "safe-to-patient" imaging technology and has been used for human fetal studies (Garel, 2008), mainly for fetal neuroimaging such as using MRI to detect focal ischemic parenchymal and cortical damage in the fetal brain (Garel *et al.*, 2004; Garel, 2006). The imaging principles and methods are exactly the same for clinical and preclinical MRI. However, due to the tremendously smaller body size of animals, fetal MR volumetric imaging requires a high magnetic field animal MRI (MR microscopy) system (Maronpot *et al.*, 2004). Early in the 1980s, Johnson *et al.* (1986) reported the use of MR imaging for reproductive research. Since then, multiple studies using preclinical MR imaging to evaluate the chick, mouse and rat fetuses have been published (Effmann *et al.*, 1988; Hogers *et al.*, 2000, 2001; Maronpot *et al.*, 2004; Danzer *et al.*, 2005; Ahrens *et al.*, 2006; Petiet *et al.*, 2008). More recently, Parnell *et al.* (2009) demonstrated the utility of MR microscopy for quantitative volumetric analysis at the suborgan (brain) level in a developmental toxicity study. To improve the MR imaging resolution, while reducing the scan time, active staining with a MR contrast agent is very useful. Detailed methods and protocols can be found in the literature (Petiet *et al.*, 2007; Petiet and Johnson, 2010). Since current MRI technology requires a long scan time and there is also a high cost to set up such an imaging facility, routine use of MR microscopy in developmental toxicology will likely remain an underutilized approach in the near future. Of course, preclinical fetal MRI could be an ideal translational volumetric imaging tool for detection of fetal soft organ/tissue structure and/or functional abnormalities in some specific developmental toxicity studies.

Ultrasound imaging (UI) is a primary fetal imaging technology in the clinical setting. It is particularly valuable for non-invasively assessing dynamic fetal cardiovascular abnormalities and for real-time visualization of the human fetus (Pugash *et al.*, 2008). High frequency micro-ultrasonography, essentially a small-scaled clinical UI system, is currently available and can achieve approximately 30–40 micron spatial resolution (Spurney *et al.*, 2006). This means it can be applicable to mouse and rat fetal functional and/or structure analyses. Although UI has volumetric imaging capacity that is used for real-time 3D visualization of human fetuses, the use of UI microscopy technology in small animal fetal imaging studies is mainly 2D functional imaging based, which is mostly for analysis of embryonic cardiovascular function and real-time imaging of maternal–fetal interactions in pregnant rodents (Phoon *et al.*, 2006; McQuinn *et al.*, 2007; Hinton *et al.*, 2008; Pallares *et al.*, 2009).

Positron emission tomography (PET) and single photon emission computed tomography (SPECT) are two additional volumetric imaging modalities that have high molecular imaging sensitivity. However, they are limited by their poor spatial resolution (about 1 to 2 mm spatial resolution for preclinical systems) and the requirement for a radioisotope, as well as the complexity of radiopharmaceuticals and maternal–fetal interactions in pregnant rodents. Their application in developmental toxicology is rare at this moment.

Another volumetric imaging technology is optical projection tomography (OPT) imaging. Since it was mainly developed for 3D volumetric visualization and analysis of transparent or near transparent specimens, it can be directly applied to the alizarin red-S- and/or alcian blue-stained embryos and fetuses (Sharpe, 2003, 2004). In fact, the OPT principle is very similar to CT imaging; the major difference being that OPT uses visible light instead of X-rays. OPT possesses some unique advantages such as volumetric visualization and analysis of stained specimens. The utility of this technology is limited because there are only a few suitable applications and not many systems are available. It is worthwhile to note that the OPT equipped with fluorescence capability may play a critical role in accurate 3D volumetric analysis of any fluorescence technique-based molecular imaging (Colas and Sharpe, 2009), such as *in vivo* 3D localization of fluorescence-labeled antibodies.

CONCLUDING REMARKS AND FUTURE DIRECTIONS

Although DART scientists usually deal with small specimens, a large amount of multidisciplinary information may be gathered from the embryos and fetuses to help make decisions in developmental toxicology studies. Non-invasive and non-destructive technologies for 3D volumetric visualization and related tissue/organ characterization of the embryo and fetus are important to promote research in this area. During the past two decades, some bioimaging technologies have advanced to enable the collection of data from inside of embryos and fetuses at the micron resolution level with 3D anatomy, from suborgan to the whole body. Micro-CT is one of the promising technologies. With advanced visualization and analysis technologies, some micro-CT volumetric imaging approaches are practical now for extensive assessment in developmental toxicology studies. Some micro-CT approaches can now even be validated for use in a day-to-day workflow.

In this chapter, starting with a brief introduction of modern bioimaging technologies and their uniqueness when used in DART studies, the focus has been on X-ray micro-CT and volumetric imaging technology, especially for applications in developmental toxicology. For a better understanding of the methodology, special techniques and different systems, X-ray imaging and micro-CT principles, and the advantages and limitations of the X-ray based micro-CT methods were briefly described.

Micro-CT has been applied to developmental toxicology in recent years and has been successfully used in the non-destructive assessment of fetal skeletons. Published studies and our internal experimental results, as exemplified in this chapter, confirm that micro-CT technology is able to obtain 3D volumetric data from unstained fetuses for the assessment of skeletal structure and this non-destructive imaging method offers sufficient 3D volumetric precision. One significant feature is that the micro-CT assessment not only detects skeletal malformations and/or variations in morphology, but can also be used to directly quantitate the level of ossification in developing bones.

Since there is a lack of information in the literature, a study directly imaging single- or double-stained fetuses using micro-CT technology was conducted. The results readily demonstrated that micro-CT imaging can also be used to accurately assess stained fetal skeletons, including quantitative volumetric measurement of the skeletal ossification and mineralization. Though bones and their microarchitecture can be visualized, the detection of cartilage is still problematic and requires special techniques.

To take advantage of the latest high resolution micro-CT technology, another sample study was conducted and has been presented in this chapter to show the micro-CT capability in the assessment of bone microarchitecture in mouse embryonic development. With confirmation using an ultra-high resolution nano-CT, the results showed that bone microstructural details such as the Haversian canals and trabecular bone microstructures can be clearly evaluated in 3D micro-anatomy based on the micro-CT imaging. The results suggest that high resolution micro-CT imaging is a promising method that may provide sufficient detail for investigating bone microarchitecture changes in developmental toxicology studies. This capability could be used to investigate fetal skeletal micro-abnormalities with 3D volumetric analysis.

CT imaging technologies have also demonstrated their potential in 3D non-destructive volumetric analysis of soft tissues and organs of embryos. An experimental sample with a simple staining method was presented in this chapter. The sample vividly showed the 3D resolution that can be achieved from micro-CT volumetric imaging of soft tissues and organs. By staining with special CT contrast agents, it is possible to use the micro-CT methodology for comparative, even functional, studies in developmental toxicology, with the unique advantage of non-destructive high resolution 3D imaging of the whole fetus.

Although micro-CT volumetric imaging technology has been used in developmental toxicology and the value is being increasingly recognized, the application of this methodology in the preclinical setting is still in its infancy. Since the technology and its applications are still rapidly being developed, the full potential of each is yet to be discovered.

From a methodology and application viewpoint, we can definitely envision more studies using validated micro-CT methods for the assessment of skeletal structures in the future, especially with more accurate quantitative measurements for both volumetric anatomic changes and ossification abnormalities. We also expect novel applications using different CT staining techniques on soft tissues and organs for comparative and functional studies, such as volumetric imaging analysis of the entire fetal heart and the intact fetal central nervous system.

Although there are still many issues that need to be resolved, such as radiation dose and live animal handling issues, enhanced *in vivo* micro-CT imaging studies will emerge. For instance, longitudinal monitoring of fetal bone formation in response to maternal treatment with a compound; or using *in vivo* contrast agent staining for an *in vivo* micro-CT functional imaging study. With new 3D micro-anatomic and/or functional measurements of the intact embryo and fetus, we expect novel datasets to improve our visulization and understanding of abnormalities in developmental toxicology.

Besides these new applications and novel datasets, efforts will also be put into developing practical micro-CT assays and/or approaches to match the needs for routine studies. For example, a high throughput micro-CT approach is critical for use on DART studies in the biopharmaceutical industry, since evaluation of a large number of specimens is required. Validation of these new micro-CT imaging assays for GLP studies will also be required in order to get regulatory acceptance.

From micro-CT and volumetric imaging technology perspectives, we can expect new generation micro-CT systems, designed with preclinical applications in mind, to be available in the near future. The directions of technical development are clear. A major one is to significantly increase the CT imaging speed. Although a few systems with high scanning speed already exist, most current micro-CT systems in use are not fast enough with the required resolution for current workflow. For DART studies, we require subminute scans at high image quality with small double-digit micron resolution. For *in vivo* studies, we need continuous image acquisition in near real-time. Thanks to advanced CT scanning technologies, such as the multi-resource and multi-detector design, we could anticipate this kind of high speed micro-CT system to be available in the future.

Besides micro-CT scanning, CT image reconstruction for 3D volumetric visualization will also be improved significantly in the future. Advanced volumetric visualization methods which have already been used in clinical CT systems will become available for preclinical micro-CT systems. We can also expect to have more user-friendly volumetric imaging analysis software and workstations, which are specially designed for preclinical applications. With advancement of preclinical micro-CT imaging, combined with other bioimaging technologies, more applications in developmental toxicology are predicted. In turn, these new applications will promote innovation of the volumetric imaging technologies. This positive loop may result in many innovative approaches and eventually lead to an entire new working environment for development toxicology!

ACKNOWLEDGMENTS

The authors appreciate the invitation of Dr. Ramesh C. Gupta to contribute this chapter. We are grateful for the technical support and contributions from Arun Tatiparthi and Tim Sledz of MicroPhotonics. We thank Jeff Oswald, Michelle Taurino, Corine Trabarel, Isabelle Leconte and Barbara Roe for providing specimens. We also thank Junzhi Ji for assistance with the CT scans. In addition, we are grateful to Bruce Beyer, Anthony DeLise and Peter Glascott for their valuable suggestions and comments. We appreciate the direct support of Marc Bonnefoi and the Disposition, Safety and Animal Research, Scientific Core Platform at sanofi-aventis.

REFERENCES

Ahrens ET, Srinivas M, Capuano S, Simhan HN, Schatten, Gerald P (2006) Magnetic resonance imaging of embryonic and fetal development in model systems. *Methods Mol Med* **124:** 87–101.

Badea C, Hedlund LW, Johnson GA (2004) Micro-CT with respiratory and cardiac gating. *Med Phys* **31:** 3324–9.

Bonneau GP, Ertl T, Nielson GM (eds.) (2006) *Scientific Visualization: the Visual Extraction of Knowledge from Data*. Springer-Verlag, Heidelberg.

Burdan F, Rozylo-Kalinowska I, Rozylo TK, Chahoud I (2002) A new, rapid radiological procedure for routine teratological use in bone ossification assessment: a supplement for staining methods. *Teratology* **66:** 315–25.

Colas JF, Sharpe J (2009) Live optical projection tomography. *Organogenesis* **5(4):** 129–34.

Cormack AM (1973) Reconstruction of densities from their projections, with applications in radiological physics. *Phys Med Biol* **18(2):** 195–207.

Danzer E, Schwarz U, Wehrli S, Radu A, Adzick NS, Flake AW (2005) Retinoic acid induced myelomeningocele in fetal rats: characterization by histopathological analysis and magnetic resonance imaging. *Exp Neurol* **194(2):** 467–75.

de Crespigny A, Bou-Reslan H, Nishimura MC, Phillips H, Carano RA, D'Arceuil HE (2008) 3D micro-CT imaging of the postmortem brain. *J Neurosci Methods* **171:** 207–13.

Degenhardt K, Wright AC, Horng D, Padmanabhan A, Epstein JA (2010) Rapid three-dimensional phenotyping of cardiovascular development in mouse embryos by micro-CT with iodine staining. *Circ Cardiovasc Imaging* **3(3):** 314–22.

Drebin RA, Carpenter L, Hanrahan P (1988) Volume rendering. In Computer Graphics (Proceedings SIGGRAPH '88): 65–74.

Effmann EL, Johnson GA, Smith BR, Talbott GA, Cofer G (1988) Magnetic resonance microscopy of chick embryos in ovo. *Teratology* **38(1):** 59–65.

Feldkamp LA, Davis LC, Kress JW (1984) Practical conebeam algorithm. *J Opt Soc Am A* **1:** 612–19.

Fishman EK, Ney DR, Heath DG, Corl FM, Horton KM, Johnson PT (2006) Volume rendering versus maximum intensity projection in CT angiography: what works best, when, and why. *RadioGraphics* **26:** 905–22.

Gallagher RS (1995) *Computer Visualization*. CRC Press, Boca Raton, FL.

Garel C (2006) New advances in fetal MR neuroimaging. *Pediatr Radiol* **36(7):** 621–5.

Garel C (2008) Fetal MRI: what is the future? *Ultrasound Obstet Gynecol* **31(2):** 123–8.

Garel C, Delezoide AL, Elmaleh-Berges M, Menez F, Fallet-Bianco C, Vuillard E, Luton D, Oury JF, Sebag G (2004) Contribution of fetal MR imaging in the evaluation of cerebral ischemic lesions. *AJNR Am J Neuroradiol* **25:** 1563–8.

Gregory CA, Gunn WG, Peister A, Prockop DJ (2004) An Alizarin red-based assay of mineralization by adherent cells in culture: comparison with cetylpyridinium chloride extraction. *Anal Biochem* **329(1):** 77–84.

Guldberg RE, Lin AS, Coleman R, Robertson G, Duvall C (2004) Microcomputed tomography imaging of skeletal development and growth. *Birth Defects Res C Embryo Today* **72(3):** 250–9. Review.

Hendee, WR, Ritenour ER (2002) *Medical Imaging Physics*, 4th edition. Wiley-Liss, New York.

Herman GT (2009) *Fundamentals of Computerized Tomography: Image Reconstruction from Projections*, 2nd edition. Springer, Berlin.

Hinton RB Jr, Alfieri CM, Witt SA, Glascock BJ, Khoury PR, Benson DW, Yutzey KE (2008) Mouse heart valve structure and function: echocardiographic and morphometric analyses from the fetus through the aged adult. *Am J Physiol Heart Circ Physiol* **294(6):** H2480–8.

Hogers B, Gross D, Lehmann V, Zick K, De Groot HJ, Gittenberger-De Groot AC, Poelmann RE (2000) Magnetic resonance microscopy of mouse embryos in utero. *Anat Rec* **260(4):** 373–7.

Hogers B, Gross D, Lehmann V, de Groot HJ, de Roos A, Gittenberger-de Groot AC, Poelmann RE (2001) Magnetic resonance microscopy at 17.6-Tesla on chicken embryos in vitro. *J Magn Reson Imaging* **14(1):** 83–6.

Hounsfield GN (1973) Computerized transverse axial scanning (tomography). Part 1. Description of system. *Br J Radiol* **46(552):** 1016–22.

Johnson GA, Thompson MB, Gewalt SL, Hayes CE (1986) Nuclear magnetic resonance imaging at microscopic resolution. *J Magn Reson* **68:** 129–37.

Johnson JT, Hansen MS, Wu I, Healy LJ, Johnson CR, Jones GM, Capecchi MR, Keller C (2006) Virtual histology of transgenic mouse embryos for high-throughput phenotyping. *PLoS Genet* **2(4):** e61.

Kak AC, Slaney M (1988) *Principles of Computerized Tomographic Imaging*. IEEE Press.

Ketcham RA, Carlson WD (2001) Acquisition, optimization and interpretation of X-ray computed tomographic imagery: applications to the geosciences. *Comput Geosci* **27:** 381–400.

Lell MM, Anders K, Uder M, Klotz E, Ditt H, Vega-Higuera F, Boskamp T, Bautz WA (2006) Tomandl BF. New techniques in CT angiography. *Radiographics* **26 (Suppl. 1):** S45–S62.

Maronpot RR, Sills RC, Johnson GA (2004) Applications of magnetic resonance microscopy. *Toxicol Pathol* **32 (Suppl. 2):** 42–8. Review.

McQuinn TC, Bratoeva M, Dealmeida A, Remond M, Thompson RP, Sedmera D (2007) High-frequency ultrasonographic imaging of avian cardiovascular development. *Dev Dyn* **236(12):** 3503–13.

Menegola E, Broccia ML, Giavini E (2001) Atlas of the rat fetal skeleton double stained for bone and cartilage. *Teratology* **64:** 125–33.

Menegola E, Broccia ML, Di Renzo F, Giavini E (2002) Comparative study of sodium valproate-induced skeletal malformations using single or double staining methods. *Reprod Toxicol* **16:** 815–23.

Metscher BD (2009a) MicroCT for comparative morphology: simple staining methods allow high-contrast 3D imaging of diverse non-mineralized animal tissues. *BMC Physiol* **9:** 11.

Metscher BD (2009b) MicroCT for developmental biology: a versatile tool for high-contrast 3D imaging at histological resolutions. *Dev Dyn* **238(3):** 632–40.

Mizutani R, Takeuchi A, Hara T, Uesugi K, Suzuki Y (2007) Computed tomography imaging of the neuronal structure of Drosophila brain. *J Synchrotron Radiat* **14(Pt 3):** 282–7.

Mizutani R, Takeuchi A, Akamatsu G, Uesugi K, Suzuki Y (2008) Element-specific microtomographic imaging of Drosophila brain stained with high-Z probes. *J Synchrotron Radiat* **15(Pt 4):** 374–7.

Mulder L, Koolstra JH, Weijs WA, Van Eijden TM (2005) Architecture and mineralization of developing trabecular bone in the pig mandibular condyle. *Anat Rec A Discov Mol Cell Evol Biol* **285(1):** 659–66.

Neubert D, Merker H-J, Kwasigroch TE (eds.) (1977) *Methods in Prenatal Toxicology*. Georg Thieme, Stuttgart.

Nuzzo S, Meneghini C, Braillon P, Bouvier R, Mobilio S, Peyrin F (2003) Microarchitectural and physical changes during fetal growth in human vertebral bone. *J Bone Miner Res* **18(4):** 760–8.

Oest M, Jones JC, Hatfield C, Prater MR (2008) Micro-CT evaluation of murine fetal skeletal development yields greater morphometric precision over traditional clear-staining methods. *Birth Defects Res B* **83:** 582–9.

Pallares P, Fernandez-Valle ME, Gonzalez-Bulnes A (2009) In vivo virtual histology of mouse embryogenesis by ultrasound biomicroscopy and magnetic resonance imaging. *Reprod Fertil Dev* **21(2):** 283–92.

Parfitt AM, Drezner MK, Glorieux FH, Kanis JA, Malluche H, Meunier PJ, Ott SM, Recker RR (1987) Bone histomorphometry: standardization of nomenclature, symbols, and units. *J Bone Miner Res* **2(6):** 595–610.

Parnell SE, O'Leary-Moore SK, Godin EA, Dehart DB, Johnson BW, Johnson GA, Styner MA, Sulik KK (2009) Magnetic resonance microscopy defines ethanol-induced brain abnormalities in prenatal mice: effects of acute insult on gestational day 8. *Alcohol Clin Exp Res* **33(6):** 1001–11.

Peng H, Ruan Z, Long F, Simpson JH, Myers EW (2010) V3D enables real-time 3D visualization and quantitative analysis of large-scale biological image data sets. *Nat Biotechnol* **28(4):** 348–53.

Petiet A, Hedlund L, Johnson GA (2007) Staining methods for magnetic resonance microscopy of the rat fetus. *J Magn Reson Imaging* **25(6):** 1192–8.

Petiet A, Johnson GA (2010) Active staining of mouse embryos for magnetic resonance microscopy. *Methods Mol Biol* **611:** 141–9.

Petiet AE, Kaufman MH, Goddeeris MM, Brandenburg J, Elmore SA, Johnson GA (2008) High-resolution magnetic resonance histology of the embryonic and neonatal mouse: a 4D atlas and morphologic database. *Proc Natl Acad Sci USA* **105(34):** 12331–6.

Phoon CK (2006) Imaging tools for the developmental biologist: ultrasound biomicroscopy of mouse embryonic development. *Pediatr Res* **60(1):** 14–21.

Pugash D, Brugger PC, Bettelheim D, Prayer D (2008) Prenatal ultrasound and fetal MRI: the comparative value of each modality in prenatal diagnosis. *Eur J Radiol* **68(2):** 214–26.

Radon J (1917) Uber die Bestimmung von Funktionen durch ihre Integralwerte langs gewisser Mannigfaltigkeiten. *Ber Verh Sach Akad* **69:** 262–277 (could be viewed via: http://people.csail.mit.edu/bkph/courses/papers/Exact_Conebeam/Radon_Deutsch_1917.pdf).

Sasov A, Nadeem F, Liu X, Verelst K (2008) Adaptive acquisition geometry for micro-CT with large format detectors. *Proc SPIE* Vol. 7078.

Schmidt EJ, Parsons TE, Jamniczky HA, Gitelman J, Trpkov C, Boughner JC, Logan CC, Sensen CW, Hallgrímsson B (2010) Micro-computed tomography-based phenotypic approaches in embryology: procedural artifacts on assessments of embryonic craniofacial growth and development. *BMC Dev Biol* **10:** 18.

Sharpe J (2003) Optical projection tomography as a new tool for studying embryo anatomy. *J Anat* **202(2):** 175–81. Review.

Sharpe J (2004) Optical projection tomography. *Annu Rev Biomed Eng* **6:** 209–28.

Spurney CF, Lo CW, Leatherbury L (2006) Fetal mouse imaging using echocardiography: a review of current technology. *Echocardiography* **23(10):** 891–9.

Wildenschild D, Vaz CMP, Rivers ML, Rikard D, Christensen BSB (2002) Using X-ray computed tomography in hydrology: systems, resolutions, and limitations. *J Hydrology* **267(3–4):** 285–97.

Wilson JG (1965) Methods for administering agents and detecting malformations in experimental animals. In *Teratology: Principles and Techniques* (Wilson JG, Warkany J, eds.). Chicago, University of Chicago Press, pp. 262–77.

Winkelmann CT, Wise LD (2009) High-throughput micro-computed tomography imaging as a method to evaluate rat and rabbit fetal skeletal abnormalities for developmental toxicity studies. *J Pharmacol Toxicol Methods* **59(3):** 156–65.

Wirkner CS, Prendini L (2007) Comparative morphology of the hemolymph vascular system in scorpions – a survey using corrosion casting, MicroCT, and 3D-reconstruction. *J Morphol* **268(5):** 401–13.

Wise LD, Winkelmann CT (2009a) Evaluation of hydroxyurea-induced fetal skeletal changes in Dutch belted rabbits by micro-computed tomography and alizarin red staining. *Birth Defects Res B Dev Reprod Toxicol* **86(3):** 220–6.

Wise LD, Winkelmann CT (2009b) Micro-computed tomography and alizarin red evaluations of boric acid-induced fetal skeletal changes in Sprague-Dawley rats. *Birth Defects Res B Dev Reprod Toxicol* **86(3):** 214–19.

Wolschrijn CF, Weijs WA (2004) Development of the trabecular structure within the ulnar medial coronoid process of young dogs. *Anat Rec A Discov Mol Cell Evol Biol* **278(2):** 514–19.

Ying X, Monticello TM (2006) Modern imaging technologies in toxicologic pathology: an overview. *Toxicol Pathol* **34(7):** 815–26. Review.

Section 13

Toxicologic Pathology

CHAPTER

76

Toxicologic pathology of the reproductive system

Pralhad Wangikar, Tausif Ahmed and Subrahmanyam Vangala

INTRODUCTION

Reproductive organs in humans are subjected to toxic insult (Foster and Gray, 2008) from a variety of environmental agents, including environmental pollutants, drugs (small molecules and biologics), cosmetics, agro-chemicals and pathogens (viruses, bacteria, parasites). Adverse effects of all these agents on male and female reproductive systems are considered to be the major cause of increase in infertility in many countries. In some cases, exposure of pregnant women to chemicals resulted in catastrophic events with children born with congenital malformations, defined as teratogenicity. Tables 76.1 and 76.2 provide a comprehensive list of all male and female anti-fertility agents and teratogens.

Reproductive toxicity refers to the adverse effects of any agent on any aspect of the reproductive cycle, in both genders. These include the impairment of reproductive function (infertility); the induction of adverse effects in the embryo (teratogenicity), such as growth retardation, malformations and death; and the induction of adverse postnatal effects in the off-spring. Toxicity to reproductive organs may occur by a direct action on reproductive organs or by an indirect action via the central nervous system (CNS). Direct effects on the reproductive organs include the gonads (ovaries in the female and testes in the male), the uterus in the female and the prostate gland in the male. Agents that directly act on gonads have to penetrate the blood–testis barrier in males and placental barrier in females. Indirect agents that act on the CNS do so primarily via the disrupting endocrine system (endocrine disruptors). Within the CNS, sensitive sites include the hypothalamus and adjacent areas of the brain, and anterior lobe of the pituitary gland (Foster and Gray, 2008).

The placental barrier in women and the blood–testis barrier in men prevent certain chemicals from entering these organs, although both barriers allow most fat-soluble chemicals to cross (Worth and Balls, 2002). Drugs that are highly water soluble and possess higher molecular weights usually do not to cross these barriers. In addition, drugs highly bound to plasma proteins are less likely to be transported into the testis or across the placental barrier to the fetus. If the fetus is exposed in the uterus to certain chemicals, it may develop abnormalities; this process is known as teratogenesis. Drugs taken by males may be teratogenic if they damage the genetic material (chromosomes) of the spermatozoa, followed by fertilization of the egg by damaged sperm. On the other hand, entry of drugs into semen or secretion of drugs in breast milk appears to have few, if any, barriers.

Reproductive toxicity studies are regulated by several agencies including the FDA (Food and Drug Administration) and the EPA (Environmental Protection Agency) in the USA, the OECD in Europe and equivalent regulatory agencies in other countries. Apart from contraceptive drugs, reproductive toxicity studies are mandated by regulatory agencies before a drug is approved for human use. Environmental pollutants are regulated by EPA guidelines as well. These studies are typically conducted in rodents, e.g. rats or rabbits. The design and conduct of these toxicity studies are conducted under strict compliance with Good Laboratory Practice (GLP) and Animal Welfare Act (AWA) requirements.

During the course of drug development, the effects of novel compounds on the reproductive system are examined in specialized reproductive tests such as segment I, segment II and segment III studies. These studies are aimed to reveal any effect on mammalian reproduction by exposure of mature adult animals to active substances at different stages of reproduction and development. The segment I studies cover effects on male and female fertility and early embryonic development to implantation. Segment II includes studying effects on embryo–fetal development and segment III studies include effects on pre- and postnatal development including maternal function. The details of these segment studies will be covered elsewhere in this chapter. As these studies are infrequently conducted before the first dose of a novel compound to humans, the only assessment of male and female reproductive systems performed prior to the first administration of novel therapeutic agent to humans is histological examination of male and female sex organs in conventional toxicity studies in rodent and non-rodent species. The International Conference on Harmonization (ICH) guidelines agreed that following the studies that showed histopathological examination of the male

Reproductive and Developmental Toxicology, Edited by Ramesh C. Gupta
ISBN: 978-0-12-382032-7

TABLE 76.1 List of environmental and pharmaceutical teratogens

Ionizing radiation	Infectious agents	Drugs	Pollutants and other miscellaneous agents
Radioiodine	Cytomegalovirus	Aminoglycosides	Carbon monoxide
	Herpes Simplex virus I and II	Androgenic hormones	Ethanol
	Parvovirus B-19	ACE inhibitors (enlapril, captopril)	Ethylene oxide
	Rubella virus	AR antagonists (sartans)	Iodides
	Syphilis	Anti-epileptics (carbamazepine, phenytoin, trimethadione, valproic acid)	Lead
	Toxoplasmosis	Busulfan	Lithium
	Varicella virus	Chlorambucil	Mercury, organic
	Venezuelan equine encephalitis virus	Cocaine	Methylene blue
		Coumarins	Polychlorinated biphenyls
		Cyclophosphamide	Tobacco smoke
		Cytarabine	Toluene
		Diethylstilbesterol	Vitamin A (high dose)
		Danazol	
		Ergostamine	
		Fluconazole	
		Folate antagonists (aminopterine, methotrexate)	
		Methimazole	
		Misoprostal	
		Penicillamine	
		Quinine (high dose)	
		Retinoids (accutane, isotretinoin, etretinate, acitretin)	
		Tetracyclines	
		Thalidomide	

TABLE 76.2 List of commonly suspected male and female infertility agents

Agent
Alcohol
Anti-infectives, e.g. metronidazole (male)
Benzene hexachloride (male)
Calcium channel blockers, e.g. nifedipine (male)
Cocaine abuse
Coffee
Cosmetic chemicals (female)
Industrial solvents (acetone, trichloroethylene, xylene)
Glycol ethers (male)
Marijuana abuse
Monosodium glutamate (female)
Nutrasweet (female)
Pesticides
Plastics
Smoking
Vehicle exhaust

reproductive organs in rodents, a 28-day toxicity study was more sensitive in detecting effects than fertility studies (International Conference on Harmonization, 1995; Takayama *et al.*, 1995; Greaves, 2000a).

Effects of xenobiotics on the female reproductive system and the development of the fetus dictate strict regulatory requirements for specific preclinical reproductive safety studies. These studies are usually performed for the novel pharmaceutical agent prior to their widespread use among the women of child-bearing potential or before phase III clinical trials. There are regional differences in the regulations for the inclusion of women of child-bearing potential in the early clinical trials without conducting reproductive toxicity studies. Moreover, clinical trials can be conducted in women not of child-bearing potential without reproductive studies provided the relevant repeated dose toxicity studies are conducted, which include evaluation of reproductive organs (International Conference on Harmonization, 1997).

The main aims of this chapter are to present the pathological changes in the reproductive and developmental systems of the laboratory animals used in toxicological studies and to give a brief overview of potential mechanisms, evaluation of endpoints of toxicity and histopathological lesions of male and female reproductive systems. The principal focus is to highlight the changes in rats and, wherever possible, species differences are presented. Information of some examples of toxicants affecting reproductive and developmental systems and the role of toxicokinetics are also reviewed in this chapter. As an example, the current state of the art in understanding the molecular mechanisms of teratogenesis with thalidomide is also discussed.

HORMONAL REGULATION OF MALE AND FEMALE REPRODUCTION

Hormonal regulation of the estrus cycle

The intrinsic reproductive cycle in female laboratory animals is characterized by regular occurrence of the estrus cycle. During this cycle numerous well-defined and sequential alterations in reproductive tract histology, physiology and cytology occur. These alterations are initiated and regulated by the hypothalamic–pituitary–ovarian (HPO) axis.

It is important to recognize all normal appearances relative to sequential cyclical changes to avoid erroneously labeling them as treatment-related.

There are four stages of the estrous cycle, termed as proestrus, estrus, metestrus and diestrus. Proestrus is first part of the cycle and is characterized by marked changes in the reproductive system, followed by estrus at the end of which ovulation occurs. If conception does not occur, which is the usual situation in toxicity studies, estrus is followed by a short period of metestrus when estrus changes subside. Under some circumstances a longer period, referred to as pseudopregnancy, occurs. Diestrus is the longest period during which the reproductive tract prepares for receipt of the ovum.

The change in the hormones over the cycle results in morphological changes in ovary, uterus and vagina. Folliculogenesis occurs independently of hormonal stimulation until formation of early tertiary follicles. The LHRH (luteinizing hormone releasing hormone), secreted by the hypothalamus, regulates the secretion of LH (luteinizing hormone) and FSH (follicle stimulating hormone) from the anterior pituitary. FSH stimulates development of zona granulosa and triggers expression of LH receptors on the granulosa cells, which synthesize estrogen under the influence of LH.

Just after diestrus, FSH and LH levels begin to increase. The increase in estrogen secretion during proestrus initiates several characteristic morphological changes in the uterus and vagina. This rise in estrogen suppresses release of LHRH from the hypothalamus. However, once the peak estrogen levels are reached its inhibition of LHRH and gonadotropin secretion ceases. At this point estrogen prompts the hypothalamus and anterior pituitary which results in a preovulatory LHRH surge and a corresponding surge in LH results in ovulation. Negative feedback control of pituitary FSH is also achieved by inhibin produced by granulosa cells of maturing follicles. Progesterone levels increase during proestrus and synergize with estrogen for gonadotropin inhibition. After ovulation the corpus luteum secretes progesterone autonomously until it becomes non-functional. Prolongation of corpus luteum function requires continued pituitary secretion of prolactin. Copulation during estrus stimulates twice the daily release of prolactin by anterior pituitary which disrupts normal estrus cyclicity by maintaining the corpus luteum in a functional state. Thus the diestrus phase will be prolonged and the secretion of progesterone will be continued. In the absence of mating the corpus luteum regresses and prolonged diestrus will be terminated and normal reproductive cyclicity will be resumed.

Hormonal regulation of spermatogenesis

The two basic functions of the male reproductive system are production of spermatozoa and production of hormones. Hormone production not only includes production of testosterone and estrogen but a large number of non-steroidal signals are described which have effects on local events, hypothalamic–pituitary axis and even non-reproductive tissues. Understanding the spermatogenesis and its hormonal regulation of the male reproductive system will allow understanding of pathophysiology of reproductive system and detect toxicological effects during preclinical safety studies.

The hypothalamus synthesizes and releases the gonadotropin-releasing hormone (GnRH) that regulates the production and release of the pituitary hormones LH and FSH. LH acts on Leydig cells and stimulates testosterone secretion which exerts its effects on spermatogenesis. FSH predominantly also acts on Sertoli cells and stimulates synthesis of androgen binding protein. Testosterone acts on the male accessory sex glands and helps to maintain their structure and function. It also acts on the hypothalamus and pituitary having negative feedback control on release of FSH and LH. Other hormones such as estradiol, secreted by Leydig cells, also act on the anterior pituitary and control negative feedback for release of FSH and LH. Inhibin secreted by Sertoli cells controls negative feedback for release of FSH (Chapin and Williams, 1989; Ruwanpura *et al.*, 2010).

Morphology of female reproductive tract during the normal estrus cycle

A thorough understanding of the morphology of the female reproductive organs at various phases of the estrus cycle is essential for interpretation of possible induced changes. The following section provides an overview of histological changes observed in the female reproductive tract during the normal estrus cycle. For a detailed description the reader can refer to the guidance documents for histological evaluation of endocrine and reproductive tests and other authoritative texts on this subject in the literature (Greaves, 2000b; Westwood, 2008; OECD, 2008b; Yoshida *et al.*, 2009).

Vagina

During diestrus vaginal mucosa shows three to seven layers of squamous cells (stratum germinativum). The stratum germinativum shows an inner layer of stratum basale consisting of a single layer of columnar cells and outer stratum spinosum multiple layers of polygonal and plump cells reflecting early mucification. Few infiltrated leucocytes are seen in the epithelium. The beginning of proestrus is characterized by formation of stratum granulosum consisting of flattened epithelial cells which contain keratohyalin granules. There are numerous mitotic figures seen throughout the vaginal epithelium. Progressively there is formation of a superficial mucoid layer which consists of many layers of cuboidal cells with mucin-containing cytoplasmic vacuoles. There is the formation of an intensely eosinophilic band of stratum corneum which at the end of the proestrus shows fully cornified epithelial cells along with superfitial mucoid layer.

During estrus no mitotic figures are seen and progressive shedding of the superficial mucoid and cornified layer reduces the height of epithelium and produces cell debris in the lumen. There is progressive infiltration of leucocytes at this stage. During metestrus there is continued desquamation of the remaining cornified epithelium along with loss of stratum granulosum and upper germinativum. A prominent polymorphonuclear cell infiltration is present in superficial epithelial cell layers. Towards the end of metestrus the epithelium reaches its lowest level.

Uterus

The cyclical endometrial changes are characterized histologically by a phase of glandular and stromal proliferation during proestrus and estrus followed by a secretory phase during diestrus. Microscopically, the uterus of the rodent during diestrus is small, poorly vascular, with a slit-like lumen lined with low cuboidal or columnar epithelium. Endometrial glands are inactive initially but towards the end of the phase some activity is seen. Occasional apoptotic epithelial cells and numerous mitotic figures are observed. Slight edema adjacent to the endometrial epithelium is seen towards the end of phase. During proestrus there is slight luminal dilatation and the endometrial lining shows tall cuboidal or columnar epithelium. Frequent mitoses with little infiltration of leucocytes, prominent endometrial vaculature and stromal edema are observed during this stage. The start of estrus is marked with degenerative changes in the endometrial epithelium in glands and lining epithelium. There is loss of mitotic activity and leukocyte infiltration. During metestrus the endometrial degeneration is continued which reduces the height of the endometrial epithelium, but there is a return of mitotic activity and variable infiltration of leukocytes, so both are seen together. Some spontaneous lesions, such as early squamous metaplasia of the endocervix seen during early estrus and marked polymorphonuclear cell infiltration of endometrial glands observed during the late estrus or early metestrus, should be considered while evaluating this tissue microscopically.

Ovary

The ovaries during diestrus show increased numbers of large follicles with a single antral cavity filled with follicular fluid. Increased numbers of atretic follicles are also seen during this phase. Currently formed corpora lutea from previous ovulation which attends the maximum size is the characteristic marker of diestrus. The luteal cells show foamy, eosinophilic cytoplasm and infiltration of fibrous tissue may also be seen at this stage. During proestrus graffian follicles are present at the surface area of the ovary. Most of the follicles are without the cumulus oophorus. The corpora lutea shows degenerative changes characterized by vacuoles in the cytoplasm and increased apoptotic cells. The fibrous tissue formation is evident at the central part. During estrus the degenerating follicles show apoptotic granulosa cells. Both newly formed and degenerating corpora lutea are seen at this stage. Newly formed corpora lutea shows basophilic, small and spindle-shaped luteal cells with capillary formation. The central fluid-filled cavity retained from the follicular stage is seen occasionally. Previously formed corpora lutea shows advanced degenerative process including fibrosis. During metestrus many growing follicles along with atretic follicles are seen. The newly formed corpora lutea contains the fluid-filled cavity of various sizes; the luteal cells are still basophilic with large nuclei. Previously formed corpora lutea shows advanced fibrosis.

POTENTIAL MECHANISMS INVOLVED IN REPRODUCTIVE TOXICITY

After exposure the toxicant is absorbed and distributed to target organs including the hypothalamus, pituitary, liver and male or female reproductive organs where it exerts its adverse effects. The xenobiotics may cause direct toxicity to reproductive organs or may interrupt the reproduction indirectly. The toxicant, either parent or its metabolite(s), interacts with the cellular or subcellular components and disrupts the normal events required for reproductive function. This toxic insult may be very specific, affecting only single cell types, or non-specific, affecting multiple sites in multiple organs. The toxicological mechanisms underlying the male and female reproductive toxicity are complex and involve various factors, such as integration of toxicokinetics, species differences in reproductive toxicology, gender difference and critical period of reproductive development during which sensitivity to toxicity occurs. The potential mechanisms of reproductive toxicity of both male and female are reviewed in the following section.

Directly acting toxicants

Specialized barriers are present in ovaries and testis that restrict the access of water-soluble reproductive toxicants to oocytes and spermatogenic cells. The multiple layers of granulosa cells separate the oocyte in ovaries and tightly joined Sertoli cells supporting spermatogenic cells in the testis. Although the transfer of hydrophilic drugs across these barriers is restricted, they are ineffective against the lipophilic drugs. Directly acting reproductive toxicants may cause damage to the reproductive system by virtue of either structural similarity to endogenous compounds such as hormones and vitamins or because of chemical reactivity. The structural similarity of these drugs to biologically important molecules such as hormones enables easy access to the target sites and misleads the normal biological processes. The xenobiotics in this category are either agonists or antagonists of endogenous hormones. An example of this type of directly acting reproductive toxicant is in oral contraceptives. The chemically reactive compounds such as alkylating agents used in the treatment of neoplastic diseases are cytotoxic, carcinogenic and mutagenic. Reproductive systems are more sensitive to the toxic effects of these compounds than other organ systems. Other examples of direct acting reproductive toxicants in this category include metals such as cadmium, lead and mercury.

Indirectly acting toxicants

Indirectly acting reproductive toxicants may require metabolic activation or they may disrupt the normal physiological control mechanisms such as enzyme modification or the disruption of detoxification or repair mechanisms, thereby causing toxicity to reproductive organs. The ovaries and testis have metabolic activation capabilities that may produce the reactive metabolites responsible for reproductive toxicity. Examples of the xenobiotics in this category are cyclophosphamide and polycyclic aromatic hydrocarbons. As successful reproduction requires hormonal feedback controls, the xenobiotics that alter the rate of steroidogenesis or clearance may alter the reproductive process. Pesticides such as DDT, polychlorinated and polybrominated biphenyls are examples of indirectly acting reproductive toxicants. The availability of the detoxification mechanisms in the biological systems makes the toxicant less toxic or helps in easy excretion. The toxicants may impair the detoxification either by enzyme deficiencies or damaging the organs responsible for detoxification. After toxic damage the repair is possible but some toxicants may impair the repair mechanisms thereby indirectly causing toxicity to reproductive organs.

Potential mechanisms and morphological pattern of female reproductive toxicity

Potential mechanisms

The positive or negative feedback system of hypothalamic, anterior pituitary or gonadal hormones controls the female reproductive tract. There are several sites of action where reproductive toxicants can act and alter the normal function of hypothalamus, anterior pituitary, ovary, uterus, vagina or mammary gland. Table 76.3 shows the site of action of female reproductive organs and the mechanism of action of various toxicants.

The agents acting on the hypothalamus may affect neurotransmitter synthesis or neuropeptide regulation of hypothalamic-releasing factors. The variety of pharmaceuticals modifies the pituitary hormone secretion either by directly acting on the pituitary gland or by acting on pituitary membrane receptors. Thus the compounds targeting central regulation of the neuroendocrine axis and hypothalamic mechanisms can interfere with LH surge, modifying normal feedback, delaying ovulation and exerting adverse effects on fertility (Cooper *et al.*, 1998).

The ovary is a complex tissue which takes care of a set of processes independently and interdependently, therefore any abnormality in these processes may be directly linked to the impairment of female reproductive capacity. Ovarian dysfunction can be induced indirectly by the toxicants that act on the hypothalamic–pituitary axis. The directly acting toxicants may interfere with ovarian function by one of the following mechanisms: irreversible damage to follicles by depleting the follicle population (Mattison, 1983; Plowchalk and Mottison, 1992; Hoyer and Sipes, 1996; Hoyer *et al.*, 2001); altering steroidogenically active follicles (Davis *et al.*, 1994); altering corpus luteum function (Davis *et al.*, 1997). More detailed discussion on the mechanism of action of ovarian toxicants can be found in Mattison and Thomford (1989), Vermeulen (1993) and Davis and Heindel (1998). Table 76.4 depicts examples of some ovarian toxicants, and their mechanism of actions and pathological observations of ovaries due to ovarian toxicants are presented in Table 76.5.

Morphological patterns of female reproductive toxicity

Regardless of the mechanism of toxicity, disruption of hormonal balance will dictate the main morphological features of lesions, and the pattern of changes in various tissues of the female reproductive system will aid in interpretation of the underlying cause of hormonal disruption. The morphological alterations observed in the female rodent reproductive tract following xenobiotic administration are classified by Yuan (1998) and overviewed in detail in the OECD guidance document (2008c). Based on the combined histological appearance of the vagina, uterus and ovary, the morphological responses are classified into three types:

Type I – Atrophic vagina, uterus and ovary.
Type II – Atrophic ovary with hyperplastic/hypertrophic uterus and vagina.
Type III – Hyperplastic/hypertrophic ovary, uterus and vagina.

Type I response is elicited by the compounds that reduce gonadotropin secretion (e.g., stress, reduced food intake), impair follicular development (e.g., cyclophosphamide) or

TABLE 76.3 Site of action of female reproductive organs and mechanism of action of various toxicants

Site of action	Function	Mechanism of action of toxicant – examples
Hypothalamus	• Synthesis and secretion of GnRH • Have receptors for FSH, LH and prolactin	1. Affecting neurotransmitter synthesis 2. Affecting neuropeptide regulation of hypothalamic releasing factors
Anterior pituitary	• Synthesis and secretion of FSH, LH and prolactin • Have receptors for GnRH, FSH, LH and steroids	1. Modification of pituitary hormone secretion – DES 2. Acting on pituitary membrane receptors – bromocriptine inhibition of prolactine release
Ovaries	• Development of follicles (ovum, granulosa cells) • Development of corpus luteum • Synthesis and secretion of estrogen and progesterone • Metabolic processes	1. Hormone analogs – medroxyprogesterone acetate (MPA), mifepristone, tamoxifen 2. Primordial follicle damaging agents – 4-venylcyclohexene diepoxide (VCD-1 & 2), busulfan, cisplatin, cyclophosphamide 3. Metabolite imbalance inducers – anastrozole, di-(2-ethylhexyl) phthalate (DEHP), ethylene glycol monomethyl ether (EGME), endomethacin 4. Endocrine imbalance inducers – atrazine, bromocriptine
Uterus	• Have estrogen and progesterone receptors • Prostaglandin, protein and glycoprotein secretion • Luminal fluid and sperm transport	1. Agents as tamoxifen, toremifene and butyrophenones cause uterine atrophy by loss or suppression of ovarian sex hormone 2. Xenobiotics with estrogenic activity cause endometrial hyperplasia. Ex: oral contraceptives 3. Endometrial metaplasia or endometriosis interfere with sperm transport
Vagina and cervix	• Multiple cell layers and cyclical changes • Responds to hormones • Sperm transport	1. Estrogenic compounds cause hyperkeratosis and hyperplasia 2. Progestational compounds cause increased mucus secretion by endocervical epithelium

TABLE 76.4 Examples of some ovarian toxicants and their mechanism of action

Sr. No	Name of the toxicant	Mechanism of action	Reference
1	Medroxyprogesterone acetate (MPA)	Inhibits the gonadotropin release from pituitary, also possesses antiestrogenic, antiandrogenic and glucocorticoid-like effects	Guthrie and John, 1980; Ohtake *et al.*, 2009
2	Mifepristone	Progesterone receptor antagonist	Gemzell-Danielsson *et al.*, 2004; Tamura *et al.*, 2009
3	Tamoxifen	Selective estrogen receptor modulator	Tsujioka *et al.*, 2009
4	4-Venylcyclohexene diepoxide	Occupational chemical, metabolite of 4-venylcyclohexene. Directly toxicant to small follicles by accelerating the natural process of apoptosis	Smith *et al.*, 1990; Hoyer and Sipes, 1996; Springer *et al.*, 1996; Ito *et al.*, 2009
5	Busulfan	Antineoplastic alkylating agent. Depletion of primordial and primary follicles	Sakurada *et al.*, 2009
6	Cisplatin	Platinum-based antitumor agent. Depletion of primordial and small follicles	Borovskaya *et al.*, 2004; Yeh *et al.*, 2006; Nozaki *et al.*, 2009
7	Cyclophosphamide	Alkylating agent. Depletion of medium–large follicles	Shiromizu *et al.*, 1984; Sato *et al.*, 2009
8	Anastrazole	Potent inhibitor of aromatase, a rate-limiting enzyme in transforming androgen to estrogen. Essential for maturation of follicles	Shirai *et al.*, 2009
9	di(2-ethylhexyl)pthalate (DEHP) and di(2-ethylhexyl) adipate (DEHA)	Plasticizer, inhibits biosynthesis of estradiol through peroxisome proliferator-activated receptor (PPAR) activation and inhibits follicular maturation	Davis *et al.*, 1994; Takai *et al.*, 2009; Wato *et al.*, 2009
10	Indomethacin	Non-steroidal anti-inflammatory drug. Directly and specifically acts on preovulatory follicles	Tsubota *et al.*, 2009
11	PPAR α/γ dual agonist	Inhibits the activation of and expression of aromatase, apoptosis of granulosa cells and decrease in CL	LoveKamp-Swan and Davis, 2003; Sato *et al.*, 2009
12	Atrazine	Herbicide, inhibits the estrogen binding to its receptors and suppresses secretion of LH	Shibayama *et al.*, 2009
13	Bromocriptine	Dopamine agonist, hypoprolactinemia and alters CL formation	Kumazawa *et al.*, 2009
14	Chlorpromazine hydrochloride	Decreased secretion of LH and FSH	Taya *et al.*, 1975; Izumi *et al.*, 2009
15	Sulpiride	D2 antagonist, hyperprolactinemia	Ishii *et al.*, 2009

decrease steroidogenesis in the ovary (e.g., aromatase inhibitors). Type I response is morphologically characterized by atrophy of the vaginal and endometrial epithelium, the endometrial glands are sparse and myometrium is also atrophied. These changes are more easily detected in the vagina than the uterus and ovary. Atrophied ovaries show a reduced number of follicles and corpora lutea and anovulatory follicular cysts may be present. Atrophy of the uterus and vagina is secondary to reduced ovarian steroid hormones (Creasy, 2007; OECD Guidance Document, 2008c).

Type II response is seen when the circulating levels of endogenous or synthetic sex steroids are increased. This results in negative feedback at the hypothalamic–pituitary level which inhibits FSH and LH release inducing ovarian atrophy. Increased levels of circulating sex steroids directly stimulate the uterus and vagina resulting in hyperplasia and hypertrophy. Morphological features depend upon the predominance of type of circulating hormone (estrogen, progesterone or a combination). Under the predominance of estrogen the vagina shows squamous cell hyperplasia and persistent estrus, the uterus shows cystic endometrial hyperplasia, squamous metaplasia in luminal and glandular epithelium and polymorphonuclear infiltration of the endometrium. Under the combined effect of estrogen and progesterone vaginal epithelial mucification is seen and the uterus shows endometrial hyperplasia and pyometra. Ovaries are atrophied with inactive interstitial glands and reduced number of follicles, and corpora lutea with anovulatory follicular cysts may be observed (Long *et al.*, 2001; Tsujioka *et al.*, 2009).

In the case of type III response, the compounds with gonadotropic activity trigger continuous follicle maturation and corpora lutea (CL) formation. Elevated levels of estrogen and progesterone cause hyperplasia/hypertrophy of the uterus and vagina. Effects are dependent on predominance of type of hormone; high levels of FSH and LH cause epithelial hypertrophy and hyperplasia in the vagina; and the vagina and ovaries are enlarged with increased number of CL and follicles. The changes associated with prolactin analogs are mild hypertrophy in the uterus and vagina, hyperplasia of the mammary gland and persistent CL in the ovaries (Creasy, 2007; OECD guidance document, 2008c).

Potential mechanisms and morphological pattern of male reproductive toxicity

Spermatogenesis relies on coordinated support and interactions of the germ cells, Sertoli cells, Leydig cells, peritubular cells, interstitial macrophages and blood vessels. Overall

TABLE 76.5 Pathological observations due to some ovarian toxicants

Category	Name of compound	Pathological observations of ovaries
Hormone analog	MPA	Increased no. of large atretic follicles. Decreased no. of new and old/large or old/small CL
	Mifepristone	Multiple cycts in ovaries. Increased no. of leutinized cysts and enlargement of previously formed CL
	Tamoxifen	Increased no. of large atretic follicles. Increases in interstitial cells and absence of newly formed CL
Primordial follicle damaging agents	4-Vinylcyclohexane diepoxide (VCD-1)	Decrease in no. of small follicles
	4-Vinylcyclohexane diepoxide (VCD-2)	Decrease in no. of small follicles
	Busulfan	Decrease in no. of small follicles
	Cisplatin	Decrease in small and/or large follicle, an increase in atresia of medium and large follicles and/or a decrease in currently formed CL
	Cyclophosphamide	Increased large sized atretic follicles. Atrophy of CL
Metabolite imbalance inducers	Anastrozole	Large abnormal atretic follicles, follicular cysts, decrease in no. of CL
	DEHA	Increase in atresia of large follicles, decrease in no. of currently formed CL and follicular cysts
	DEHP	Vacuolation of stromal cells, increased large atretic follicles. Decreased no. of currently formed CL
	EGME	Hypertrophy of CL with decreased cellular debris indicating apoptosis. Increased no. of large atretic follicles. Decreased no. of currently formed CL
	Indomethacin	Increased no. of leutinized cysts (unruptured follicles)
	PPAR α/γ dual agonist	Increase in atresia of large follicles, granulosa cell exfoliation in the antrum of large follicles. CL with retained oocyte and interstitial gland hyperplasia
Endocrine imbalance inducers	Atrazine	Increase in atresia of large follicles, decreased no. of CL. Swelling of previously formed luteal cells.
	Bromocriptine	Increased no. of CL
	CPZ	Increase in atresia of large follicles
	Sulpride	Increase in atresia of large follicles and increase in follicular cyst

process is regulated by hypothalamic–pituitary–testis endocrine axis and local factors such as paracrine and autocrine control are also involved in regulation of these processes (Creasy, 2001). There are four main cellular target sites for toxicity in testes: Sertoli cells, Leydig cells, germ cells and vascular endothelial cells. It is possible to identify the probable target cell of toxicity by careful examination of early morphological changes and provide critical information for designing additional investigative and mechanistic studies. The examples of toxicants affecting the male reproductive system with their target site and morphological response are presented in Table 76.6.

Pattern of damage associated with Sertoli cell toxicity

Sertoli cells are extremely resistant to cell death; however, depending upon the severity and duration of Sertoli cell damage the morphological changes are seen. The most common morphological response of the Sertoli cells to injury is vacuolization which is described as an early event with many compounds. Subsequent to vacuolization, the changes related to Sertoli cell damage are characterized by multifocal degeneration with formation of multinucleate spermatid aggregates, phagocytosis of spermatocytes, exfoliation of germ cells into the tubular lumen or sloughing of the adluminal portion of Sertoli cells along with its attached germ cells. Another morphological change seen with compounds that reduce the testosterone levels is failure of spermiation and phagocytosis of the sperms by Sertoli cells (Creasy, 1997, 2001).

Although the mechanisms underlying these changes are complex and not known completely, the mechanisms of action reported with Sertoli cell toxicants include change in cytoskeletal function (Boekelheide *et al.*, 1989, 2000) and alteration in the stem cell growth factor secreted by the Sertoli cells (Blanchard *et al.*, 1998). Cytoskeletal functions are central to Sertoli cell activities, including Sertoli-germ cell attachment, germ cell movement from base to tubular lumen and secretory functions (Richburg and Boekelheide, 1996).

Injury to Sertoli cells has potentially serious consequences because of their pivotal role in support of spermatogenesis. Disturbances in structural and metabolic support of germ cells will result in germ cell degeneration and if the injury is sufficiently severe and prolonged Sertoli cell function will be permanently compromised and recovery of spermatogenesis may not be possible.

Pattern of damage associated with germ cell toxicity

Each population of germ cell has its own sensitivity to different chemical toxicants. The stage-specific effects of the chemicals are dependent on the dose and duration of dosing. The early events are characterized by rapid apoptosis and phagocytosis of affected cells by Sertoli cells. The loss of any cell population will result in progressive loss of all later cell types through maturation depletion. This will leave the tubule lined by Sertoli cells and depletion of a single generation of germ cells that are killed by the toxicant. If the injury is stopped, the unaffected cells continue to develop through the next

TABLE 76.6 Examples of toxicants affecting male reproductive tract

Sr. No.	Target site	Chemical affecting	Effect/morphological response	Reference
1	Sertoli cell	2,5-Hexanedione-cyclohexylamine	Vacuolation in cytoplasm, gradual multifocal degeneration of germ cells with formation of multinucleate spermatid aggregates. 2,5-Hexanedione interferes with assembly of microtubules	Chapin *et al.*, 1983; Creasy *et al.*, 1990
		1,3-Dinitrobenzene tri-*o*-cresylphosphate	Rapid degeneration and phagocytosis of spermatocytes	Blackburn *et al.*, 1988; Strandgaard and Miller, 1998
		Phthalate esters	Rapid and extensive exfoliation of germ cells in the tubular lumen	Somkuti *et al.*, 1991
		Colchicine and vinblastine	Sloughing of adluminal portion of Sertoli cells. Colchicines interfere with assembly of microtubules	Russell *et al.*, 1981
		Boric acid, dichloroacetic acid and bromoacetic acid	Failure of spermiation	Chapin and Ku, 1994; Linder *et al.*, 1990, 1994
		Methyldopa, 17 beta estradiol,	Reduces testosterone level and causes failure of spermiation	Dunnick *et al.*, 1986; O'Connor *et al.*, 1998
		Monoethylhexylphthalate	Rapidly alters vimetin and alters cytoskeletal function of Sertoli cells	Richburg and Boekelheide, 1996
2	Germ cells	Glycol ethers	Necrosis of pachytene spermatocytes	Creasy *et al.*, 1985
		Busulfan, bleomycin	Necrosis of spermatogonia	Creasy, 2001
		2-Methoxyethanol, dinitropyrrol	Necrosis of spermatocytes	Ku and Chapin, 1994
		Ethylmethane sulfonate, methyl chloride	Necrosis of round spermatids	Chapin *et al.*, 1984
		Ethane-methane sulfonate	Necrosis of spermatogonia by irreversible DNA damage	Creasy, 2001
3	Effect on interstitial fluid	Estradiol, ethanol	Decreased volume of interstitial fluid	Widmark *et al.*, 1987; Adams *et al.*, 1991
		hCG or LHRH agonist	Increased volume of interstitial fluid	Setchell and Sharpe, 1984; Valenca and Negro-Vilar, 1986
4	Effect on seminiferous tubule fluid	Oxytocin, endothelin 1 and prostaglandins	Effect on contraction of the peritubular myoid cells surrounding thetubules	Maekawa *et al.*, 1996
		Carbendazim	Dilatation of tubular lumen by obstruction of efferent ducts	Nakai *et al.*, 1992
5	Effect on vascular system	Cadmium salts	Endothelial damage and interstitial edema and ischemic necrosis of testis	Aoki and Hoffer, 1978
		5 HT, histamine	Reduced blood flow and focal tubular necrosis	Bocabella *et al.*, 1962; O'Steen 1963
6	Effects on Leydig cell function	Ethanedimethane sulfonate	Leydig cell necrosis	Creasy, 2001
		Lansoprazole	Inhibition of testosterone synthesis	Creasy, 2001
7	Effects on epididymis	α-Chlorohydrin	Inhibition of fluid reabsorbtion, effect on sperm motility and edema of caput	Wong and Yeung, 1977
		Methyl chloride, carbendazim	Epithelial necrosis, sperm granulomas	Nakai *et al.*, 1992
		Deoxychloroglucose	Inhibition of glycolysis and sperm immobility	Creasy, 2001
8	Effects on prostate and seminal vesicle	Flutamide	Atrophy due to androgen receptor blockade	Creasy, 2001
		Finasteride	Atrophy due to inhibition of dihydrotestosterone production from testosterone	Creasy, 2001
9	Effects on vas deferens	Guanethidin	Inhibition of ejaculation due to adrenergic ganglion blockade	Bhatal *et al.*, 1974

stage. The unaffected spermatogonia continue to replenish the germ cell population provided they are associated with functionally competent Sertoli cells. If the cell-specific germ cell toxicant kills the spermatogonia in rats, it will take 8–10 weeks to reflect the effect on fertility. This is the time taken for the unaffected developing spermatids and spermatocytes to complete their development. As the spermatogenesis is species specific, the time delay is obviously dependent upon species; however, these effects can be detected in repeat dose toxicity studies with stage-specific histopathological examination of the testis (Creasy, 1997, 2001).

The molecular mechanisms of germ cell toxicity have also remained elusive. It has been demonstrated that disturbances in the cell–cell communications between Sertoli cells and spermatocytes are important (Ling-Hong *et al.*, 1997). Another mechanism of action well understood is cytotoxic effects of antimitotic agents on rapidly proliferating spermatogonia through irreversible DNA damage (Meistrich, 1986). Most lesions that specifically deplete the germ cell population are reversible; chemicals that damage the stem cell spermatogonia cause irreversible effects.

Pattern of damage associated with Leydig cell toxicity

Since the main function of Leydig cells is steroidogenesis, interference in this function will produce functional disturbances in hormone balance and these changes are difficult to recognize by light microscopy. However, histopathological effects associated with decreased levels of testosterone can be recognized (Russell *et al.*, 1990; Creasy, 2001). Sertoli cell function and germ cell development during stages VII and VIII are dependent on adequate levels of testosterone. Inadequate levels of testosterone will cause degeneration of germ cells passing through these two phases and later this process of maturation depletion results in generalized depletion of all elongating and maturation phase spermatids (Sharpe, 1994). Degenerating pachytene spermatocytes and round spermatids in stages VII and VIII are considered to be the sensitive marker of reduced testosterone production (Russell *et al.*, 1990; Creasy, 2001).

Pattern of damage associated with vascular changes

The seminiferous epithelium is avascular and relies on transport of oxygen and nutrients from the interstitial vasculature. Changes in the blood flow to the testis or damage to the vascular endothelium will reduce oxygen and nutrient movement into the interstitial fluid. Even a mild anoxia or ischemia will cause degeneration and necrosis of testis involving all cell types. Unlike other cases of testicular injury where germ cell death is preceded by apoptosis (Ling-Hong *et al.*, 1997; Strandgaard and Miller, 1998; Lee *et al.*, 1999) and Sertoli cells remain intact, ischemic injury causes oncotic necrosis of germ cells and Sertoli cells. The presence of inflammatory infiltrate that proceeds to fibrosis is a common sequel to this.

Pattern of damage associated with disturbances of fluid balance

Two types of fluid secretion serve an important function in the testis: interstitial fluid transports oxygen and nutrients from blood to tubule and the seminiferous fluid transports sperms and proteins from tubule to rete testis (Setchell, 1990). The volume of interstitial fluid is determined by the permeability of non-fenestrated endothelial cells of the testicular microvasculature, which is regulated by factors secreted by the Leydig cells and seminiferous tubules. The volume of interstitial fluid is decreased after hypophysectomy or by administration of estradiol (Widmark *et al.*, 1987) or ethanol (Adams *et al.*, 1991). The volume of interstitial fluid is increased following administration of hCG or LHRH agonist (Setchell and Shapre, 1984; Valenca and Negro-Vilar, 1986), obstruction of the lymphatic drainage or damage to the endothelium. Increased interstitial fluid is reflected by the increased testicular weight.

Seminiferous tubule fluid is produced by the Sertoli cells and reabsorbed by the rete testis, efferent ducts and caput epididymal epithelium. Movement of fluid from tubule into rete testis is controlled partly by contraction of peritubular myoid cells surrounding the tubules. Production of the fluid by Sertoli cells is androgen dependent and also regulated by germ cell component, particularly the presence of elongating spermatids (Sharpe *et al.*, 1991). Volume of the tubular fluid depends on rate of secretion, rate of transport from the tubule and rate of reabsorbtion in the rete and epididymis. Alteration in function of any of these functions will be reflected by tubular lumen dilatation or contraction. Tubular dilatation can be seen microscopically and it is also reflected as increased testicular weights. Marked tubular dilatation may result in pressure atrophy of the seminiferous epithelium and cause spermatostasis and spermatocele in distended tubules. Tubular contraction represents disturbed Sertoli cell function. As the tubule fluid secretion is an androgen-dependent function, the compounds that reduce the testicular testosterone levels will reduce the fluid secretion and the tubular diameter (Creasy, 2001).

EVALUATION OF REPRODUCTIVE TOXICITY

Regulatory guidelines such as OPPTS (EPA), ICH and OECD define the specific endpoints to detect adverse effects of drugs or chemicals on reproduction and fertility. These guidelines specify only the organs and tissues to be evaluated grossly, weighed and microscopically examined but do not specify sample size and do not indicate parts of appropriate tissues to be examined (Esch *et al.*, 2008). These studies rely primarily on fertility parameters to assess the reproductive performance rather than histopathology. A detailed description of these methods and reproductive indices used during fertility studies is beyond the scope of this chapter and the reader may refer to the specific guidelines. Although general toxicity studies have no such recommendations, it has been shown that reproductive toxicity measures including histopathology from the repeat dose toxicity studies are the most sensitive endpoints in predicting reproductive toxicity (Lanning *et al.*, 2002; Sanbiussho *et al.*, 2009). These endpoints are briefly discussed below.

Reproductive toxicants can affect any part of the reproductive process such as gametogenesis or other signals including multiple steroid or non-steroid hormones, directly or indirectly. These signals impact not only local events but also affect other parts of reproductive tract, hypothalamic–pituitary axis and even non-reproductive tissues. Assessment of various endpoints allows gathering of information on these local and systemic effects. These endpoints include adequate sampling of various reproductive organs, organ weights, their appropriate fixation, processing, slide preparation, staining for microscopic evaluation and microscopic evaluation including testicular or ovarian staging. Along with these pathological parameters, in-life observations such as body weight changes, feed consumption, hormonal analysis and records of estrus cycle are also important.

Endpoints used in the assessment of male and female reproductive toxicity

Clinical pathology

In repeated dose toxicity studies the hematology and clinical chemistry parameters used to assess the organ damage have limited usefulness as far as the assessment of damage to reproductive organs is concerned. However, for damage to the reproductive system, hormonal changes may be detected. Primary hormones that are measured include leutinizing hormone, gonadotropin releasing hormone, follicle stimulating hormone, estradiol, testosterone, progesterone and prolactin. Measurement of circulating 17β-estradiol and progesterone levels can help identify effects of chemicals on the ovary (Hoyer and Devine, 2002) and that of testosterone on the testis (Creasy, 2001). Analysis of creatine kinase, particularly the isoezyme BB, can be of some value to assess the reversible or irreversible damage to the endometrium (Lanning, 2006). For testicular damage, elevated levels of plasma levels of lactate dehydrogenase, isoenzyme LDH-C4 are indicative of acute testicular toxicity (Haqqi and Adhami, 1982; Itoh and Ozasa, 1985; Redear *et al.*, 1991). A urinary marker, a creatinine has been used as a marker of testicular damage, with creatinine appearing more sensitive than plasma LDH-C4, testosterone or testis mass in detection of damage (Moore *et al.*, 1992; Timbrell *et al.*, 1994; Timbrell, 2000).

Dissection

Dissection is an art and knowledge of anatomical arrangements of various components of the reproductive tract is necessary to ensure appropriate sampling. During dissection, weighing and trimming of male reproductive organs care should be taken not to squeeze the testis to prevent artifactual sloughing of germ cells from the seminiferous epithelium. Separation of epididymis from testis should be done carefully to avoid cutting the testicular capsule which will disrupt the tissue architecture (Lanning *et al.*, 2002). In the case of the female reproductive system, the uterus is carefully dissected and fascia and fat trimmed off to avoid loss of luminal contents. The vagina is separated from the uterus at the uterine cervix. Additional guidance for tissue sampling of male reproductive organs is provided by Adkins *et al.* (1982), Lanning *et al.* (2002) and Creasy (2003).

Organ weights

Organ weight changes are very sensitive indicators of chemically induced changes to organs; however, various regulatory guidelines differ regarding the organ weight recommendations. The Society of Toxicologic Pathologists (STP) surveyed regulatory guidelines (Michael *et al.*, 2007) and set the recommendations for evaluation of organ weights in GLP general toxicity studies (Sellers *et al.*, 2007).

It is recommended that in repeat dose GLP toxicity studies in rats, testis, epididymis and prostate gland should be weighed routinely; however, in the case of mice and non-rodents, the epididymis and prostate may be weighed on a case-by-case basis. In the case of female rodents and non-rodents, uterus and ovaries are weighed routinely. The STP recommends that in the case of males weights of reproductive organs should be assessed in mature animals and weighing the ovaries in the case of female rodents is recommended in shorter duration repeat-dose studies (less than 6 months duration), because reproductive senescence starts after 6 months of age (Peluso and Gordon, 1992; Sellers *et al.*, 2007).

Testicular weights are considered valuable in toxicity studies because the changes in the testis weight reflect changes in seminiferous tubules or interstitial edema. Testicular weights revealed sensitivity to toxicity due to perturbations in rapidly dividing cells, physiology and hormones and they aid in the identification of enzyme induction, correlate well with histopathological changes and help in establishing no-observed-effect level (NOEL), even in the absence of morphologic correlate (Michael *et al.*, 2007). Similarly ovarian and epididymal weights are considered useful as they are the common target organs of toxicity; weight variations show correlation with histological observations and are useful in establishing NOEL. The decrement of 10% or greater in the organ weight measures is usually of toxicologic significance; however, because of the remarkable consistency of testicular and epididymal weights, changes of as little as 5% may be an indicator of toxicity, especially when accompanied by correlative macro- or microscopic findings (Holson *et al.*, 2006).

Tissue fixation

For histopathological examination, male and female reproductive tract tissues are best fixed in 10% neutral buffered formalin. However, formalin is not a fixative of choice for testis and most of the regulatory guidelines relating to the reproductive studies recommend that testis should be fixed in Bouin's fluid or in comparative fixative. Due to its picric acid component, Bouin's fluid has a number of disadvantages; therefore modified Davidson's fluid has been reported as an alternative to Bouin's fluid to fix testes for routine histopathological examination. Modified Davidson's fluid is an acetic acid–alcohol–formalin-based fixative and testes fixed in this fixative showed superior overall morphologic details, less shrinkage of germ cells and Sertoli cells and less shrinkage of tubules from interstitial tissue. It also supports staining of spermatid acrosome with Periodic Acid Schiff's (PAS) reagent required for detailed staging of spermatogenic cycle and for immunohistochemical detection of testicular antigens (Lanning *et al.*, 2002; Latendresse *et al.*, 2002).

Tissue sampling/trimming

After fixation of the tissues, sampling of specific structures and tissue orientation of reproductive tissues are important for histological evaluations. A comprehensive set of guidelines for organ sampling and trimming has been devised and published online by the Registry Nomenclature Information System (RENI) and can be readily accessed (http://www.goreni.org/ or http://reni.item.fraunhofer.de/reni/trimming/index.php). For details on dissection and trimming of reproductive organs, the reader can refer to the OECD guidance document for histological evaluation of endocrine and reproductive tests (2008a). Foley *et al.* (2001) advocated observation of two sections of testis, one transverse and one longitudinal, or one section can be used. It is important to include the rete testis while sectioning. Inclusion of rete will allow assessment of obstructive changes in outflow path from the testis and provide evidence of estrogen-induced fluid disturbances in rete and efferent ducts. Transverse sections allow easier stage identification and longitudinal sections assist pathologists in correlating gross testicular observations; also it allows both dorsal and ventral aspects of testis in the section.

For the most effective evaluation of the male reproductive system, the epididymis and testes should be examined concurrently. Epididymal sections are most sensitive in short-term or acute studies in detecting toxicities. For comprehensive evaluation of the epididymis, a longitudinal section of caput and corpus and a transverse section of cauda should be included for examination. A transverse section should be made through the widest part of the seminal vesicle together with the coagulating gland.

Chemically induced or spontaneous proliferative lesions of the rat prostate can be found in all three lobes. The dorsal and lateral lobes exhibit the same spectrum of proliferative lesions; however, they differ from spontaneous and induced lesions in the ventral lobe. Additionally, some strain-specific deviations in the interlobular distribution of benign and malignant neoplasms consequently require the assessment of all compartments. Accordingly, a longitudinal–horizontal section through the dorsolateral and ventral lobes, urethra and, optionally, ureter and ductus deferens represents a less time-consuming method, applicable to routine histological processing and examination of the prostate gland.

For sampling, fixation and sectioning of the uterus and vagina the reader can refer to the OECD report of the initial work towards the validation of the rodent uterotrophic assay – Phase 1 (No. 65: http://www.oecd.org/document). It is recommended to prepare the cross-sections taken midway along the length of each uterine horn. This allows observation of the cell proliferation and histological changes in the uterine components. A section should also be obtained from the uterine cervix. A transverse section should be taken through mid-vagina avoiding vaginal skin. Ovaries should be separated from the oviduct, halved longitudinally and a section obtained from the middle of the organ. While sampling the mammary gland in the case of females it is recommended to use the iliac lymph node and nipple as landmarks.

Embedding and staining

For routine histopathological examination of male and female reproductive organs, paraffin embedded sections stained with hematoxylin and eosin (H&E) provide adequate quality for evaluating screening studies. However, for high resolution light microscopy of testes, which is required during investigative studies, embedding in glycol methacrylate (GMA) resin can be used to prepare semithin sections and embedding in epoxy resin is essential for evaluation of testis by electron microscopy (Lanning *et al.*, 2002). Although regulatory guidelines for general toxicity studies do not include "staging" of testis or ovarian follicular counting, these techniques will help to ensure thorough evaluation that minimizes risk of missing true reproductive toxicants. For studies up to 28 days' duration staining of testis with Periodic Acid Schiff's hematoxylin stain is recommended for spermatogenic staging. To facilitate ovarian follicle counting, immunohistochemical methods using proliferative cell nuclear antigen (PCNA) and cytochrome P450 1B1 (CYP1B1) are recommended (Muskhelishvili *et al.*, 2002, 2005; Picut *et al.*, 2008).

Microscopic evaluation

Testicular staging

While no guidelines require spermatogenic staging, testicular tissues should be examined with knowledge of the testis structure, the process of spermatogenesis and the classification of spermatogenesis. This statement implies that regulatory guidelines do not require quantitative staging but do recommend that pathologists possess stage awareness. The qualitative knowledge of spermatogenic staging aids in recognizing missing germ cells and helps to determine which type of cells (spermatogonia, spermatids, Leydig cells and/or Sertoli cells) are affected due to toxicologic insult. Type of cells affected may provide information regarding the potential reversibility of the effects.

Staging is defined as grouping of germ cell types at a particular phase of development to classify tubular cross-sections into stages of the spermatogenic cycle. In the case of rats the spermatogenic cycle is divided into 14 stages (I to XIV); however, the process and regulation of spermatogenesis applies equally to other species such as mouse, dog and non-human primates.

Four generations of the cells (spermatogonia, spermatocytes, round spermatid and elongating spermatid) develop simultaneously and in precise synchrony with each other. The regulation of spermatogenesis relies not only on the endocrine control of hypothalamic–pituitary–testicular axis but also on the autocrine and paracrine interactions involving Sertoli cells, germ cells, Leydig cells, peritubular cells, interstitial macrophages and endothelial cells (Sharpe, 1988; Heindel and Treinen, 1989; Creasy, 1997).

The cross-section of the seminiferous tubules shows the discrete layers of the germ cells, where spermatogonia lie on the basal lamina and spermatocytes are arranged above them in one or two layers of spermatids. There are two general approaches used to identify the stages of the cycle of seminiferous tubules. One is the "tubular morphology" system based on the changes in the shape of spermatid nucleus, the occurrence of meiotic divisions and arrangement of spermatids within the seminiferous epithelium. This approach is the oldest and used to identify eight stages in rabbits and ram. The other approach is based on changes in the characteristics of the acrosome and morphology of developing spermatids and is called the "acrosomic" system originally developed for rats (Foote and Berndtson, 1992). Based on the changing acrosome structure, in the case of rats the cycle has been divided arbitrarily into 14 stages (Roosen-Runge and Giesel, 1950).

Regulatory guidelines do not require quantitative staging and a detailed description is beyond the scope of this chapter; the reader can refer to Russell *et al.* (1990) and Hess (1990) for an excellent account and practical guide on tubular staging. The following sections describe the use of tubular staging during microscopic examination of the testis to evaluate testicular damage. Table 76.7 shows the morphological characteristics of different types of cells at each spermatogenic stage.

TABLE 76.7 Spermatogenic stages and description of morphological changes seen during each stage

Stage No.	Description
Stage I	Nucleus of elongated spermatids with well-formed hook, acrosome not visible, nucleus of round spermatid is round. Type A1 spermatogonia divide to produce intermediate spermatogonia
Stage II–III	Nucleus of elongated spermatids extend into deeper layers between round spermatids and in round spermatids no clear acrosome but 1 or 2 small granulas seen
Stage IV	Nucleus of elongated spermatids is near to the basal lamina and acrosomes on the round spermatids are covering approximately 30°. At the end of this stage intermediate spermatogenia divides to produce type B spermatogonia
Stage V	Nucleus of the elongated spermatids tending into luminal direction and acrosome on round spermatids is covering approximately 45°
Stage VI	Elongated spermatids are seen on surface of seminiferous tubules and acrosome on the round spermatid covering approximately 80°. At the end of this stage type B spermatogonia divide to produce primary spermatocytes
Stage VII	Spermia along with the residual bodies are seen on the surface of seminiferous tubules. Acrosome or nucleus of round spermatids is round and stains PAS positive and shows abundant cytoplasm
Stage VIII	Characterized by very few spermia in the lumen, prominent residual bodies seen which will be resorbed
Stage IX	No spermatids observed in the lumen of seminiferous tubules, nucleus of the elongated spermatids tends to form ellipsoid and tail starts forming. Type A_1 spermatogonia start dividing at this stage to produce type A_2 spermatogonia
Stage X	Nucleus of the elongated spermatids tends angular and condensation of karyoplasma seen
Stage XI	Nucleus of elongated spermatids becomes rectangular with pronounced condensation
Stage XII	Nucleus of elongated spermatids elongated and more condensed. Acrosome vesicle is large in round and large p-spermatocytes. Each of the type A_2 spermatogonia starts dividing to produce A_3 spermatogonia
Stage XIII	Nucleus of elongated spermatids forming hook-like head and acrosome vesicle is seen in large round di-spermatocytes
Stage XIV	Nucleus of elongated spermatids is completely condensed. The A_3 spermatogonia start dividing to produce type A_4 spermatogonia

Approach for microscopic examination of testis

The aim of the histopathological evaluation of testes in the regulatory studies is to detect the toxic effects and, if damage is seen, to characterize the lesions further. The approach described below will help the pathologist to evaluate the testes histopathologically. Randomly scan the seminiferous tubules at high magnification and check that all layers are present in their approximate normal numbers. Check that the uncommitted, reserve stem cells (type A_0 spermatogonia) are present throughout the cycle; stages I–VIII contain layers of spermatogonia, a layer of pachytene spermatocytes and several layers of round spermatids interspersed with elongated spermatids; stages IX–XIV contain layers of prepachytene spermatocytes, several layers of late pachytene spermatocytes and several layers of elongating spermatocytes; and stage VIII shows spermia in the lumen. This will help to identify when a cell population is missing.

Examine the few tubules between stages IX and XI at high magnification to identify the spermatid retention (delayed spermiation). As all the mature spermatids are released into the tubular lumen during stage VIII, no mature spermatids should be visible during stages IX–XIV. These tubules should contain only a single population of elongating spermatids. Also examine a few tubules at XII stage for sperm head phagocytosis in the basal Sertoli cell cytoplasm. This will help to identify damage to Sertoli cells.

Check the few stage VII tubules for any evidence of degeneration of pachytene spermatocytes and round spermatids, which indicates decreased levels of testosterone. Once identified, the significance of the findings to evaluate the potential effects on overall reproductive function can be interpreted.

Oocyte staging

Guidelines for reproductive toxicity studies recommend qualitative and quantitative evaluation of primordial follicles in the ovary and qualitative assessment for the presence or absence of growing follicles and corpora lutea. Regulatory guidelines for general repeated dose toxicity studies do not include ovarian follicle counting; however, properly conducted follicle counts can supplement qualitative ovarian assessment to characterize ovarian toxicants and understand their site of action (Picut *et al.*, 2008).

Detailed methods of sectioning and counting are given elsewhere (Smith *et al.*, 1991; Bolon *et al.*, 1997; Bucci *et al.*, 1997; Heindel, 1999). The Society for Toxicologic Pathology recommends a two-tier approach for evaluation of rodent ovary. The first-tier evaluation of ovaries should include evaluation of all major components of the ovary, with special attention to qualitative assessment of primordial and primary follicles. The decision to perform second-tier evaluation for quantification of small follicles should be made on a case-by-case basis to characterize the suspected ovarian toxicants (Regan *et al.*, 2005).

As per the Pedersen's follicular classification in rodents, ovarian follicles have been classified into three main categories and further subdivided into eight types according to morphological appearance and follicular size (Table 76.8). The follicles in the first category are non-growing primordial and primary follicles contain the small type 1a to 3a follicles. Category 2 follicles are growing secondary, pre-antral

TABLE 76.8 Oocyte categories and description of morphological characteristics seen

Category	Type	Morphological characteristics
Category 1 Small, non-growing follicles	Type 1	Isolated oocyte
	Type 2	An oocyte surrounded by partial layer of granulosa cells
	Type 3a	An oocyte surrounded by unbroken single layer of granulosa cells (≤20 cells)
	Type 3b	An oocyte surrounded by unbroken single layer of granulosa cells (21–60 cells)
Category 2 Medium growing follicles	Type 4	An oocyte surrounded by two layers of granulosa cells
	Type 5a	An oocyte surrounded by multilayered, solid mantle of granulosa cells. There is no evidence of antrum
	Type 5b	Fully grown preantral oocyte surrounded by many layers of granulosa cells
Category 3 Large antral follicles	Type 6	Small antral with large oocyte surrounded by many layers of granulosa cells and scattered areas of fluid
	Type 7	Antral follicle with single cavity containing follicular fluid. Cumulus oophorus formed without stalk
	Type 8 Graffian follicle	Large antral follicle with single cavity with follicular fluid and a well-formed cumulus stalk

follicles. The follicles in the third category are large antral follicles characterized by a central oocyte and fluid-filled antrum.

The National Institute of Health Sciences (NIHS) and 18 pharmaceutical companies of the Japan Pharmacutical Manufacturers Association (JPMA) have conducted collaborative work to evaluate whether ovarian toxicities are detected by repeated dose general toxicity studies in rats. The results of this study indicated that ovarian toxicity could be detected by careful qualitative histopathological examination conducted in 2- or 4-week repeated dose toxicity studies. The histopathological changes observed demonstrated useful indicators for identification of ovarian toxicity (Sanbuissho *et al.*, 2009). The reduction in the number of small follicles indicates the ovarian atrophy and primordial follicle damaging potential of the agent. A decrease in follicle counts could indicate either direct oocyte toxicity, or an effect on the granulosa or thecal cells that alters the paracrine control of folliculogenesis. The most common finding is increased number of large sized atretic follicles which indicate disturbance of ovulation and large follicle development by ovarian toxicants. The compounds categorized as metabolite imbalance inducers and endocrine imbalance inducers cause follicular cysts. The histopathological changes related to non-ovulated follicles including unruptured follicles, unruptured luteinized follicles, luteal cysts, expansion of cumulus oophorus were caused by compounds categorized as hormonal analogs and metabolite imbalance inducers (Sato *et al.*, 2009; Tamura *et al.*, 2009; Tsubota *et al.*, 2009). A dose–response trend and a statistically significant change in follicle number would indicate a potential effect in humans (OECD Guidance Document, 2008c).

NON-NEOPLASTIC LESIONS OF MALE AND FEMALE REPRODUCTIVE SYSTEMS

Histopathological examination of male and female reproductive organs in repeated dose toxicity studies is a more sensitive indicator to detect the effects of xenobiotics than fertility studies and this is the agreed approach by the International Conference on Harmonization (ICH) guidelines (International Conference on Harmonization, 1995; Takayama *et al.*, 1995; Ubrich and Palmer, 1995; Greaves, 2000a,b). The following section describes the non-neoplastic histopathological lesions induced by various chemicals in the male and female reproductive tract.

Male reproductive system

Lesions of testis

Testicular atrophy

This is the most commonly seen effect in testicular toxicity. The least severe change in the germinal epithelium is the maturation arrest. This is characterized histologically by partial or complete loss of mature spermatids from the lumen of seminiferous tubules. As the degree of atrophy increases, there is progressive loss of deeper layer cells. In marked cases the only discernible cells are a few spermatogonia and Sertoli cells. Other cytological features include vacuolization of germ cell layer and presence of multinucleated giant cells. Germ cell loss progressively causes seminiferous tubules to be shrunken and develop thickened fibrous walls and eventually reach a totally sclerotic end-stage in which only residual interstitial cells remain. Testicular atrophy induced by vitamin E deficiency in rats is irreversible. Various hormonal drugs and their antagonists such as estradiol benzoate (Miyamoto *et al.*, 2000), fadrozole (Kawashita *et al.*, 2000), anticancer agents or nucleic acid modulators such as cyclophosphamide (Watanabe *et al.*, 2000), dopamine antagonist and antidepressant such as reserpine (Yamauchi *et al.*, 2000), dopamine agonist, bromocriptine (Richardson *et al.*, 1984), antihypertensive drugs, methyldopa (Chapin and Williams, 1989), etc. are examples of some of the drugs that cause testicular atrophy.

Necrosis of seminiferous tubules

The necrotic seminiferous tubules show the spermatogenic and spermatocytic cells with pyknotic nuclei. The necrotic cells are sloughed into the lumen forming necrotic debris. Sometimes a patchy dystrophic calcification is also seen. Dietary administration of cobalt induces necrosis of germinal epithelium and Sertoli cells in the seminiferous tubules (Corrier *et al.*, 1985). The agents that cause ischemic injury such as cadmium salts (Aoki and Hoffer, 1978), 5HT and histamine (Creasy, 2001) also cause the oncotic necrosis of germ cells and Sertoli cells which is characterized by the presence of inflammatory infiltrate.

Leydig cell hyperplasia

Histologically, Leydig cell hyperplasia may be diffuse, focal or multifocal in distribution. Although occasionally it is seen as a sporadic finding with normal seminiferous tubules, it is associated with atrophic tubules both in rats and man (Takano and Abe, 1987). Focal hyperplasia in rats is nodular, sometimes displacing the adjacent seminiferous tubules. The nodular foci are composed of Leydig cells with basophilic staining and they represent the earliest stage of Leydig cell tumor in rats. The Society of Toxicologic Pathologists has recommended the criteria for focal hyperplasia as a cell mass of less than the size of three seminiferous tubules and devoid of evidence of compression and significant mitotic activity or endocrine sinusoidal network (McConnell *et al.*, 1992). In rats Leydig cell hyperplasia is the result of age-related changes in the hypothalamic–pituitary axis and local control mechanisms. The drugs that potentiate the Leydig cell hyperplasia include cimetidine, a histamine H_2-receptor blocker (Brimblecombe and Leslie, 1984), buserelin, a synthetic peptide analog of gonadotropin releasing hormone (Donaubauer *et al.*, 1987) and flutamide, a non-steroidal antiandrogen (Physician's Desk Reference, 1999).

Lesions of epididymis

Degeneration

Common degenerative changes in the epididymis epithelium are characterized by vacuolated and basophilic cytoplasm and affected cells may show mineralization of cytoplasm. Stilbesterol treatment causes cyst formation in mice (Gopinath *et al.*, 1987) and butylbenzyle phthalate is associated with necrosis of tubular epithelium of epididymis (Agarwal *et al.*, 1985).

Granulomatous inflammation (sperm granulomas)

Sperm granulomas are composed of a central mass of spermatozoa, some of which are degraded, surrounded by radially arranged epitheloid macrophages and multinucleated giant cells, granulation tissue, lymphocytes and plasma cells (McDonald and Scotome, 1987). It is chronic granulomatous lesion of spermatozoa released into the extra luminal tissue (Sawamoto *et al.*, 2003). Sperm granulomas have been reported in toxicity studies following administration of therapeutic drugs. An adrenergic antagonist, guanethidine derivative was associated with the microdiverticular and fistulae of the vas deferens which resulted in rupture of the vas deferens and leakage of spermatozoa. It was also postulated that guanethidine induced loss of the contractile ability of the epididymis to emit semen (Bhatal *et al.*, 1974). Sperm granulomas were also caused by clostantal salicylanilide antihelminthic (Van Cauteren *et al.*, 1985). L-cysteine, a sulfur containing amino acid, also induces sperm granulomas, which was associated with prolonged maturation of epididymal ducts resulting in obstruction of semen flow, leading to ductal rupture and leakage of spermatozoa into interstitial space (Sawamoto *et al.*, 2003).

Lesions of seminal vesicle and prostate glands

Atrophy

Reduction in size and weight due to glandular atrophy are most common changes seen in the seminal vesicle and prostate during toxicity studies. Since the seminal vesicle and prostate glands are hormone dependent, disturbances in the pituitary–gonadal axis may cause their atrophy. The drugs with antiandrogenic activity, whether acting directly or indirectly, can also produce atrophy. The morphological changes are characterized by reduced secretory activity of glandular epithelium. Acini appear closer together separated by condensed stroma. Some acini contain cell debris or inflammatory cells. These changes are accompanied by loss of weight of seminal vesicle and prostate. The drugs that cause atrophy include goserelin, a synthetic analog of gonadotropin releasing hormone, which produces the effects by suppressing testosterone production (Blask and Leadem, 1987). Flutamide and bicalutamide, potent non-steroidal antiandrogens used in the treatment of prostate cancer, are also reported to produce prostatic atrophy (Chapin and Williams, 1989; Iswaran *et al.*, 1998).

Hypertrophy and hyperplasia of the prostate gland

Glandular prostatic hyperplasia may be seen in dogs involved in chronic toxicity studies. Histologically glandular proliferation with multiple papillary projections into the lumina, the glandular spaces are occupied by complex infolding of the epithelium and lining cells which are often hypertrophic (Gopinath *et al.*, 1987). In the case of rats the focal glandular hyperplasia is characterized by papillomatous cribriform formations which are 3–5 cells thick and are located in one or more acini. The proliferating cells show rounded or oval, hyperchromatic nuclei. Prolonged estrogen or androgen treatment induces hypertrophy and hyperplasia of prostate.

Squamous metaplasia of the prostate

Estrogenic substances influence prostatic growth via their effect on hypothalamic–pituitary–gonadal axis which results in suppression of testosterone production. A metaplastic effect of estrogens involves squamous transformation of the epithelium which is characterized by multilayering of epithelial basal cells which stratify to form multiple layers of squamous cells. Histologically squamous metaplasia is characterized by focal or diffuse replacement of glandular epithelial cells by multilayered cells showing squamous differentiation. A variety of estrogenic substances such as 17β-estradiol and diethylstilbesterol (DES) induces squamous metaplasia in animals. Therefore squamous metaplasia is considered to be a reliable marker or endpoint in assessing estrogenic action of estrogenic compounds (Risbridger *et al.*, 2001).

Female reproductive system

Lesions of ovaries

Oocyte or ovarian follicular degeneration

Oocyte loss has been shown to occur in the ovary following administration of chemotherapeutic agents, antimetabolites, antibiotics, polycyclic aromatic hydrocarbons and ionizing radiations in humans and rodents. Microscopically, the oocyte loss is characterized by pyknosis and cytolysis of oocytes accompanied by focal or diffuse cortical fibrosis, varying degrees of ovarian atrophy or hyperplasia. Damaged oocytes are eliminated primarily through the process of atresia (Nicosia *et al.*, 1985). The stage at which the xenobiotics destroy the ovarian follicle determines the impact on fertility. Agents damaging large growing or antral follicles interrupt the reproduction temporarily; however, xenobiotics damaging oocytes in primordial or primary follicles may lead to infertility which is permanent (Hoyer and Sipes, 1996). There are species differences seen in oocyte sensitivity to ionizing radiation, anticancer drugs or polycyclic hydrocarbons. The mouse oocyte appears to be more sensitive than oocytes of rats or guinea-pigs (Greaves, 2000b). In accurate histological assessment, degree of sampling and plane of section are important and it is proposed that follicular diameter measurement is helpful in assessing follicular maturation (Ataya *et al.*, 1985).

Ovarian atrophy

Typically atrophied ovary is characterized by shrinkage, small size and reduced weight. Microscopically ovaries are devoid of well-developed follicles and corpora lutea. Ovarian stroma is condensed showing hyalinization, or fibrosis residual ova and corpora albicans may be evident. Depending on the species, age, experimental conditions and nature of agents, these basic histological features may be accompanied by increased number of cystic follicles, ceroid and lipid accumulation in interstitial cells or focal interstitial hyperplasia. These features provide important clues to the pathogenesis of ovarian atrophy in toxicity studies. Hormonal compounds such as 17β-estradiol or diethylstilbesterol produce ovarian atrophy (Schardein, 1980), prolonged treatment of rodents, dogs or primates with contraceptive steroids (Fitzgerald *et al.*, 1982), antiestrogen and tamoxifen (Tsujioka *et al.*, 2009). Goserelin, a synthetic analog of leutinizing releasing hormone (Physician's Desk Reference, 1999), also produces ovarian atrophy in rodents.

Cystic changes (follicular cysts, luteal cysts)

Follicular cysts arise in secondary follicles that fail to ovulate and may be single or multiple. Microscopically they have a thin wall lined with cuboidal or flattened granulosa cells, and there is increased amount of follicular fluid and absence of an oocyte. Larger follicular cysts often have a thin fibrous outer layer. Therapeutic agents such as bromocriptine, an ergot compound that stimulates dopamine receptors and inhibits pituitary prolactin secretion, cause follicular cysts in rats (Richardson *et al.*, 1984). Tamoxifen also reduced the number of corpora lutea and induced follicular cyst formation in rats (Tucker *et al.*, 1984).

Lueal cysts (cystic corpora lutea) are microscopically characterized by having a large, fluid-filled central cavity and a wall composed of several layers of luteinized granulosa cells that are polyhedral with foamy, vacuolated, eosinophilic cytoplasm. Progesterone antagonist RU 486 caused an increased number of copora lutea and induced variable-sized luteal cysts which was postulated to be due to inhibition of progesterone giving rise to chronic estrogenic effects (Van der Schoot *et al.*, 1987).

Ovarian hyperplasia

Ovarian hyperplasia observed in preclinical safety studies is a form of interstitial cell or stromal and epithelial hyperplasia. Although these hyperplasias are associated with age-related loss of ovarian function, they are also caused by xenobiotics treatment. The epithelial hyperplasia is characterized by marked and diffuse proliferation of small dark glandular cells in the outer cortex of the ovary. Stromal cell hyperplasias are associated with vacuolization of stromal cells which are enlarged and increased in number. Tamoxifen treatment in dogs caused epithelial hyperplasia (Tucker *et al.*, 1984). Nitrofurantoin, the antibacterial agent, caused stromal hyperplasia showing tubule like differentiation in mice (Maronpot, 1987). Other histological types of hyperplasias include Sertoliform hyperplasia and granulosa cell hyperplasias. Sertoliform hyperplasias have characteristics of tubular or rod-like cells and are similar to those of the Sertoli cells of seminiferous tubules in the testis; they are characterized by focal aggregates of tubular structures. Granulosa cell hyperplasias are occasionally observed and characterized by a thick granulosa cell layer present around large follicles.

Lesions of uterus

Endometrial atrophy

Endometrial atrophy is characterized by reduction in the thickness of the endometrium and loss of endometrial glands, which are inconspicuous and embedded in dense compact stroma. The smooth muscle cells show reduced sarcoplasm and myometrium consists of closely packed cells with elongated nuclei and scanty cytoplasm. The presence of small endometrial cysts is also observed in dogs. Atrophy of uterine endometrium and myometrium is caused by loss or suppression of ovarian sex hormone secretion. The agents such as tamoxifen (Tucker *et al.*, 1984; Tsujioka *et al.*, 2009) and toremifene (Karlsson *et al.*, 1998) typically reduce cell proliferation and produce atrophy of the endometrium and myometrium. Butyrophenones by gonadotropic inhibition caused uterine atrophy in dogs (Gopinath *et al.*, 1987).

Squamous metaplasia of endometrial glands

Although it may develop spontaneously, squamous metaplasia of endometrial columnar epithelium is also induced by administration of estrogenic compounds in rats. Vitamin A deficiency also induces squamous metaplasia of endometrial glands in many species. There is focal or diffuse transformation of glandular epithelial cells into multilayered stratified squamous epithelial cells. Histologically appearances vary based on the epithelium affected, superficial or glandular. Keratinization is not prominent but may develop either by extension of squamous mucosa from cervix into uterine horns or by direct metaplasia of columnar endometrial cells. Diethylestilbesterol treatment in mice during the neonatal period caused squamous metaplasia of the endometrium (Ostrander *et al.*, 1985).

Endometrial hyperplasia

Endometrial hyperplasia is characterized by increase in number of endometrial glands and increase in uterine size. Hyperplasia is associated with age-related decline in the sex hormone levels in which there is relative excess of estrogen levels. Administration of xenobiotics with estrogenic effects or exogenous estrogen also induces endometrial hyperplasia both in humans and in laboratory animals. The responsiveness of the endometrium to estrogen-induced histological changes varies according to compound administered, dose and age among the different species and strains. These factors make extrapolation of findings from laboratory animals to women difficult. Histological changes due to prolonged estrogen or oral contraceptive therapy in humans and non-human primates (Valerio, 1989) are characterized by irregular and cystic dilatation of endometrial glands, which are lined by proliferative, pseudostratified columnar epithelium. Mitotic activity is seen but there is little or no secretory activity and glands are surrounded by dense, highly cellular stroma. In the case of mice the prolonged estrogen administration is characterized by increase in number of dilated or irregular glands, which are lined by hyperchromatic cuboidal or columnar cells. The mitotic activity is increased and the glands are separated by normal appearing stroma. Tamoxifen-induced hyperplasiatic changes in mice appeared more cystic with glandular dilatation than those produced by estrogen (Tucker *et al.*, 1984). In dogs a combination of oral contraceptives caused cystic endometrial hyperplasia (Johnson, 1989).

Endometriosis and adenomyosis

The presence of viable islands of endometrium-like tissue, consisting of glandular and stromal elements, at ectopic sites is known as endometriosis. It is usually confined to pelvic cavity affecting the serous surface of the uterus, ovaries, large intestine, urinary bladder and mesentery. Prolonged treatment of rabbits with stilboesterol induced this condition.

Adenomyosis is the presence of hyperplastic or aberrant endometrial glands and stroma into the hyperplastic myometrial layer. It is associated with hyperprolactinemia in mice (Nagasawa and Mori, 1982) and women (Muse *et al.*, 1982). Long-term treatment of mice and rabbits with estrogen (Mori and Nagasawa, 1983) and progesterone treatment in mice also produced adenomyosis. Rats appear more resistant to the development of this change.

Decidual reaction (deciduoma)

The term deciduoma is defined as proliferation of decidual tissue in the non-pregnant animal. Deciduoma may be single or multiple, unilateral or bilateral and appear as discrete round nodules in the uterine horn. Histologically, deciduoma is characterized by the presence of large, round stromal cells with large round nuclei, prominent nucleoli and abundant eosinophilic cytoplasm containing PAS-positive granules. Instillation of agents such as sesame oil and prostaglandin E2 can induce decidual change in rodents and rabbits (Ohta, 1987). Growth hormone treatment also induced a florid decidual reaction with presence of pleomorphic and bizarre cells in rats. Decidual changes also develop in women and non-human primates following administration of oral contraceptives and at the site of implantation of intrauterine contraceptive devices (Dallenbach-Hellweg and Poulsen, 1996).

Lesions of the vagina and cervix

Vaginal hyperkeratosis and hyperplasia

The hyperkeratosis and hyperplasia of stratified squamous epithelium of the vagina is characterized by thick and leathery appearance of vaginal epithelium with several longitudinal folds in vaginal mucus membrane. Sometimes edema of underlying lamina propria is also seen. It is seen in dogs and primates given estrogenic compounds (Heywood and Wadsworth, 1981) and mice treated with stilboestrol (Greenman *et al.*, 1984). Vaginal keratinization in oophorectomized rats is used as a measure of the estrogenic activity of chemical compounds.

Vaginal mucification

The mucification of the epithelium of the vagina and cervix is characterized by the appearance of columnar cells and the cell cytoplasm contains mucus. The vaginal mucification in rats is caused by the progestational compounds. Long-term treatment of a combination of oral contraceptive steroids to monkeys produces alterations to the endocervix characterized by an increase in viscid mucous secretion by endocervical epithelium (Valerio, 1989).

Squamous metaplasia

The replacement of mature, non-squamous epithelium by stratified squamous epithelium of the endocervical canal is seen in both woman and laboratory animals. Administration of estrogenic compounds in rats and primates are reported to cause squamous metaplasia of the endocervix. Squamous metaplasia appears to develop less readily in the mouse treated with estrogens. Toxicity tests are performed occasionally with a view to evaluate irritancy potential of test substances by scoring the changes in vaginal mucosa. Both macroscopic and microscopic features of irritation are graded such as epithelial exfoliation, hemorrhages, edema, mucosal necrosis and inflammation, ulceration, atrophy and hyperplasia.

Lesions of the mammary gland

Atrophy of the mammary gland

Atrophy of the mammary gland was characterized by reduction in size of mammary ducts that were lined with flattened epithelium and surrounded by a concentric layer of fibrous tissue. Atrophy of the mammary gland was seen following inhibition of its hormonal control. Treatment with the anti-androgen tamoxifen for long periods caused atrophy of the mammary gland in animals (Greaves *et al.*, 1993).

Glandular development and hyperplasia

The epithelial hyperplasia of the mammary gland can be divided into two histological types; duct hyperplasia and lobular hyperplasia. Duct hyperplasia is characterized by epithelial proliferation within the extralobular ducts. There is presence of an increased number of epithelial layers (three or more) above the duct basement membrane. Ductular hyperplasia was reported to be developed by administration of contraceptive steroids containing progestational and estrogenic components in mice, primates and dogs (Gopinath, *et al.*, 1987).

Lobular hyperplasia is characterized by epithelial proliferation in intralobular ductules (acini). In dogs lobular hyperplasia of the mammary gland is well documented where it comprises increased numbers of ductules similar to adenosis in humans (Greaves, 2000b). Repeated administration of dopamine antagonists markedly stimulated the mammary gland, where mammary hyperplasia and excessive secretion are mediated through prolactin production (Gopinath *et al.*, 1987).

ROLE OF TOXICOKINETICS IN MALE AND FEMALE REPRODUCTIVE TOXICITY

Toxicokinetics (TK) is the evaluation of the pharmacokinetics (PK) of a compound at doses used in toxicity studies. An excellent review on toxicokinetic principles and their application to toxicology studies has recently been published (Eichenbaum *et al.*, 2010). Its primary purpose is to correlate the dose administered to the systemic exposure and toxic effects that are observed in all subtypes of non-clinical toxicity studies. According to ICH (International Conference on Harmonization, 1995), TK is defined as the generation of pharmacokinetic data, either as an integral component in the conduct of non-clinical toxicity studies or in specially designed supportive studies, in order to assess systemic exposure. These data may be used in the interpretation of toxicology findings and their relevance to clinical safety issues. ICH guidance states that toxicokinetics should enhance the value of the toxicological data generated, both in terms of interpreting the results of toxicity studies and to allow direct comparison with clinical data as part of the assessment of risk and safety in humans. The assessment of systemic exposure aids the interpretation of dose–response relationships, which can be non-linear due to induction, alteration or saturation of processes involved in the absorption, distribution, metabolism and elimination (ADME) of the compound. Furthermore, TK information may be used to determine that a lack of toxicological response is not due to a lack of drug exposure. For safety assessment, the systemic exposure at the no-observed-adverse-effect level (NOAEL), rather than the administered dose, generally provides more relevant information. These drug exposures can be compared with those determined in humans during clinical studies.

TK data are typically obtained by determining the concentrations of drug/metabolite in plasma, serum, blood or urine samples taken from main toxicology or satellite test animals. The studies are generally designed to determine PK parameters for exposure such as maximum plasma concentration (C_{max}), time of maximum plasma concentration (T_{max}) and area under the plasma (or serum) concentration vs. time curve (AUC). Earlier, the objective of TK studies was simple (i.e., confirmation of the drug administration in toxicity studies); in recent times it has evolved into a powerful tool, which helps to rationalize species, dose selection, dosing vehicles, dosing frequency and ultimately human safety margin assessments (i.e., ratio of AUC or C_{max} in animals at an NOAEL dose to those achieved in humans at therapeutic dose). All this will ensure that the first dose of the new chemical entity (NCE) administered to humans is safe and well tolerated. Hence TK has become an integral part of pharmaceutical safety assessment over the last two decades (Creton *et al.*, 2009).

TK has a major role to play in different types of toxicology studies such as acute, dose range-finding, repeat dose, subchronic, chronic, genetic and reproductive toxicity studies as well as in safety pharmacology, carcinogenicity and bridging studies. It is important to mention that not all ICH guidelines explicitly mention TK as an integral part, and therefore ICH S3A (International Conference on Harmonization, 1995) is generally the most appropriate guideline that should be referred to the role of TK in these different study types. Reproductive toxicity studies are generally conducted after initial phase I safety and tolerability studies and are not typically part of the IND package for seeking approval in human studies. However, many drugs specifically targeting diseases in women require rapid enrollment of women of child-bearing potential in phase I and early phase II studies. Under these conditions, reproductive toxicity studies are conducted pre-FIH, both to ensure safety in the target population and to enable rapid recruitment in the phase II trials. The ICH guidelines mention the following regarding the application of TK evaluations in reproductive toxicity studies (e.g., fertility studies as well as studies in pregnant and lactating animals):

- Maternal toxicity is typically dose limiting for these studies, but plasma concentrations are important for assessing the NOAEL, safety margins and next steps forward.
- Consideration should be given to the possibility that kinetics will often differ in pregnant and non-pregnant animals and therefore must be characterized for both conditions.
- Plasma is the standard matrix. It is also appropriate to study embryo–fetal transfer and secretion in milk not as specific study objectives related to developmental toxicology but as separate programs.

Typically, reproductive toxicity studies are conducted in rats and/or rabbits. Since TK data has already been generated in repeat dose rat studies, it is not essential but "good to have" TK data generated in the fertility and peri- and postnatal studies, to confirm if there is any differences in exposure in pregnant and non-pregnant animals. In practice, many sponsors include TK, either as part of the dose range-finding study or part of the main study, due to observed PK profile differences for some compounds in pregnant animals. Recent regulatory requirements mandate that human metabolites are also present in plasma in at least one reproductive toxicology species to have a valid program for human safety assessment (Schwartz, 2001). The ICH Harmonized Tripartite Guideline, "Detection of toxicity to reproduction for medicinal products", states:

> The limitation of exposure in reproductive toxicity is usually governed by maternal toxicity. Thus, while TK monitoring in reproductive toxicity studies may be valuable in some instances, especially with compounds of low toxicity, such data are not needed for all compounds. Where adequate systemic exposure might be questioned because of absence of pharmacological response or toxic effects, TK principles could usefully be applied to determine the exposures achieved by dosing at different stages of the reproductive process.

The most useful piece of information that can be collected from TK data as a part of reproductive toxicology studies is the relationship between the exposure in the dam and the secondary effects caused in the fetus by the pharmacological action of the drug in the dam. The greatest probability of malformations is during organogenesis, which occurs between days 18 and 60 of gestation in humans and days 6 and 15 in rats. Hence, direct developmental effect on the fetus depends on the relationship between drug exposure in the conceptus and time during the sensitive stages of gestation. In conducting TK during reproductive toxicity studies, one should measure the exposure of drugs in the dam and this can be subsequently related to therapeutic human exposure (AUC or C_{max}). There is a possibility of change in any of the TK parameters between pregnant and non-pregnant dams, due to increase in plasma and total body water, increase in renal plasma flow and glomerular filtration and decrease in concentration of some plasma proteins during pregnancy. The difference in PK of drugs between pregnant and non-pregnant animals provides an indication of the existence of similar differences in humans. However, the best way to find out if such differences in PK really exist is to conduct studies in special human populations such as patients with higher plasma volume, high renal clearance, etc. The TK parameters which should be investigated in reproductive toxicity studies such as embryo–fetal studies depend on which parameter primarily affects the TK. For valproic acid and caffeine, embryo–fetal toxicity is related to C_{max} (Nau, 1985; Sullivan *et al.*, 1987). In the case of retinoids and cyclophosphamide, toxicity is affected by AUC (Reiners *et al.*, 1987; Nau, 1990). Phenytoin is an example where both C_{max} and AUC affect the toxicity. It is important to note that the animals should be sufficiently exposed to the test drug within a dosing interval. In the case where sufficient exposures are not achieved in a dosing interval, one has to dose the animals multiple times in a day or the drug has to be administered as intravenous infusion. It must be noted that any reproductive toxicology studies conducted as per Good Laboratory Practice (GLP), the PK and the bioanalytical phase must also be GLP-compliant.

Fertility and embryo–fetal development study in rats

In a typical embryo–fetal study, male rats are dosed for 4–10 weeks prior to mating. In a 4-week study, it is not necessary to collect blood samples for TK, if the results can be extrapolated from an earlier study of the same duration. For a 10-week study, samples can be collected at the end of week 10 and day 1 data can be extrapolated from previous studies, provided the PK is linear. The treatment period in females is generally 2–4 weeks prior to mating and up to closure of the hard palate. For characterizing the TK, samples can be collected at the end of the study only, as day 1 data can be extrapolated from previous studies.

Pre- and postnatal development studies in rats

In this study, female rats are dosed from implantation to the end of lactation. The exposures in this study can be extrapolated from other studies; hence there is no need for blood collection during this study for studying the TK. However, one should aim to determine the drug exposure in pups via suckling.

Placental transfer studies

Placental transfer studies provide information on placental transfer of drugs by assessing the radioactivity in fetal tissue and maternal blood. There are many morphological differences and similarities in yolk sac and chorioallantoic placenta between rats, rabbits and humans (Garbis-Berkvens and Peters, 1987; Foote and Carney, 2000). For this reason it is unlikely that routine placental transfer studies, in which fetal exposure is determined after closure of the hard palate, would be adequate to correlate embryo–fetal exposure to an NCE with a developmental effect. In spite of the marked differences between placenta of animals, there is not much difference in placental transfer of most chemicals (Mihaly and Morgan, 1984). The relative distribution of a drug between the embryo–fetal and maternal unit is dependent not only on the physico-chemical properties, but also on the physiological parameters and gestational age. Hence placental transfer studies conducted only on one accession during gestation can provide distributional evidence only for this particular period of gestation. Consideration should also be given to the drug protein binding as it is the free drug, which crosses the placenta and is available for distribution.

Milk transfer studies

Drugs that are lipophilic are likely to be excreted in milk of lactating females, and hence the pups will be exposed to the parent or its metabolites during suckling. The drug label should accordingly mention the warning of potential risks from drug consumption via breast milk in human infants. Studies about the excretion of drug in milk in animals cannot provide a quantifiable measure of the extent of milk transfer in humans, and thus the routine conduct of this type of study is questionable. Studies using labeled compounds in rats may provide additional information. Additionally, blood samples can be withdrawn from pups for determining the drug levels due to the potential difference in metabolism between neonates and adults.

TK may be an invaluable tool to aid in assessing the risk of exposure of NCE to the fetus. The main application of TK data in reproductive toxicity studies is through determination of exposure ratios between animals and humans, which ultimately calculates the safety margins. Differences in drug disposition between pregnant and non-pregnant females may help in monitoring more closely the clinical studies conducted in pregnant females or during postmarketing surveillance after drug launch. TK studies should be carefully designed and planned so as to provide maximum information, which would ultimately ensure safety for the humans.

MOLECULAR MECHANISMS OF TERATOGENESIS

Although teratogenesis has been recognized for a long time, the molecular mechanisms of their effects on embryos are only recently being unraveled. A brief description of thalidomide tragedy and induced teratogenesis is provided here. For details, readers are referred to a standalone chapter on thalidomide elsewhere in this book.

Thalidomide was originally marketed as a sedative and anti-hypnotic in 1957 by the German company Chemie-Grunenthal; it was also used as an anti-emetic to relieve morning sickness during early pregnancy (Lenz, 1988; Smithells and Newman, 1992; Stephens *et al.*, 2000; Matthews and McCoy, 2003). It was approved in over 46 countries except the USA but by 1961 it had become clear that thalidomide was the reason for a huge increase in birth defects, principally to the limbs of babies (McBride, 1961; Lenz and Knapp, 1962; Leck and Millar, 1962). Thalidomide has recently been approved to successfully treat leprosy, multiple myeloma, Crohn's disease, AIDS and some cancers, however, with careful controlled guidelines where pregnant woman will be excluded (Calabrese and Fleischer, 2000; Stephens and Fillmore, 2000; Gordon and Goggin, 2003; Bartlett *et al.*, 2004; Franks *et al.*, 2004; Galustian *et al.*, 2004, Teo *et al.*, 2005; Galustian and Dalgleish, 2009). However, thalidomide is poorly controlled in countries like Africa and South America, where leprosy is prevalent and there is poor regulatory handling and lack of understanding of the adverse effects by the patients who ingest these drugs (Vargesson, 2009).

Thalidomide teratogenicity is species specific, occurs in humans and primate species, as well as chickens, but not in rodents (Bauer *et al.*, 1998; Stephens *et al.*, 2000) or hamsters (Fratta *et al.*, 1965; Schumacher *et al.*, 1965, 1968). The reason for this species specificity remains unclear.

Many researchers have focused on unraveling the molecular mechanisms of teratogenesis of thalidomide. Although the story is not completely elucidated the current hypothesis involves blocking angiogenesis of endothelial cells lining the blood vessels leading to growth factor signaling, cell death and mesenchymal loss (Vergesson, 2009).

Thalidomide has both antiangiogenic and anti-inflammatory properties. The antiangiogenic properties have been attributed to its teratogenic actions and anticancer activity. On the other hand, anti-inflammatory properties are considered relevant to treat leprosy, HIV infection-related apthus ulcers, wasting and diarrhea (Knobloch and Rüther, 2008; Vargesson, 2009). To support this theory, the synthetic analogs of thalidomide, antiangiogenic analog CPS49, but not the anti-inflammatory metabolites and analogs of thalidomide, induce limb defects in chicken.

Inhibition of angiogenesis by thalidomide appears to require metabolic activation and is species specific. Bauer *et al.* (1998), using a rat aorta model and human aortic endothelial cells, co-incubated thalidomide in the presence of either human, rabbit or rat liver microsomes. Thalidomide inhibited microvessel formation from rat aortas and slowed human aortic endothelial cell proliferation in the presence of human or rabbit microsomes, but not in the presence of rat microsomes. In the absence of microsomes, thalidomide had no effect on either microvessel formation or cell proliferation, thus demonstrating that a metabolite of thalidomide is responsible for its antiangiogenic effects and that this metabolite can be formed in both humans and rabbits, but not in rodents.

Thalidomide is primarily metabolized by hepatic CYP2C19 and CYP2C6/2C11 to 5-OH-thalidomide in human and rat liver microsomes respectively (Ando *et al.*, 2002a,b). Circular dichroism (CD) spectroscopy used for the stereochemical characterization of the hydroxylated metabolites formed during the *in vitro* biotransformation of (R)- and (S)-thalidomide indicated that the chiral center of thalidomide is unaffected by the stereo-selective biotransformation process (Meyring *et al.*, 2002). (3′R,5′R)-trans-5′-hydroxythalidomide is the main metabolite of (R)-thalidomide, which epimerizes spontaneously to give the more stable (3′S,5′R)-cis isomer. On the contrary, (S)-thalidomide is preferentially metabolized by hydroxylation in the thalidomide moiety, resulting in the formation of (S)-5-hydroxythalidomide. 5-OH thalidomide was subsequently hydroxylated to 5,6-dihydroxythalidomide by CYP2C19, CYP2C9 and CYP1A1 in humans and by CYP2C11, CYP1A1, CYP2C6 and CYP2C12 in rats (Ando *et al.*, 2002).

Gordon *et al.* (1981) suggested that a toxic arene oxide metabolite may be involved in thalidomide teratogenesis. Using cytotoxicity of lymphocytes as a model, it was demonstrated that liver microsomes from rat, rabbit, monkey and human exhibited a good cytotoxic activity in all species except rat. Further, cytotoxic activity in rabbit, monkey and human liver microsomes was enhanced by epoxide hydrolase (an enzyme that detoxifies arene oxides) inhibitors. These studies suggested that metabolic activation of thalidomide to reactive electrophilic arene oxide may be involved in thalidomide teratogenesis.

An alternative mechanism of teratogenesis for thalidomide was proposed by Wells and colleagues (Arlen and Wells, 1996; Parman *et al.*, 1999) where its metabolism may be catalyzed by embryonic prostaglandin H synthase (also known as cyclooxygenase) to reactive free radical intermediates. These free radicals in the presence of cellular glutathione can induce oxidative stress via reactive oxygen species generation. In support of this theory, these authors showed that thalidomide administration to rabbits results in enhanced oxidative DNA damage of embryonic DNA and teratogenesis. Both of these processes were abolished by pretreatment of rabbits with the free radical spin trapping agent alpha-N-tert-butyl phenylnitrone (PBN). In addition, acetyl salicylic acid, a prostaglandin H synthase inhibitor, reduced the thalidomide-induced teratogenicity in rabbits. Interestingly, thalidomide (300% dose given to rabbits) treatment in mice, a species resistant to thalidomide teratogenesis, did not result in enhanced embryonic oxidative DNA damage suggesting that free radicals may play a critical role in thalidomide-induced teratogenesis. It is interesting to note that many human teratogens are metabolized by prostaglandin H synthase to reactive free radical intermediates. These include cyclophosphamide, phenytoin, carbamazepine (Wells *et al.*, 2010). It is perhaps possible that free radical-mediated oxidative damage may play a significant role in teratogenic mechanisms of many xenobiotics.

Thalidomide-induced oxidative stress enhances signaling (Knobloch *et al.*, 2007) through bone morphogenetic proteins (Bmps). This leads to upregulation of the Bmp target gene and Wnt antagonist Dickkopf1 (Dkk1) with subsequent inhibition of canonical Wnt/β-catenin signaling and increased cell death. Thalidomide-induced cell death was dramatically reduced in HEFs and in embryonic limb buds by the use of inhibitors against Bmps, Dkk1 and Gsk3β, a β-catenin antagonist acting downstream of Dkk1 in the Wnt pathway. Moreover, blocking of Dkk1 or Gsk3β dramatically counteracts thalidomide-induced limb truncations and microphthalmia. From these findings, Knobloch *et al.* (2007) concluded that perturbing of Bmp/Dkk1/Wnt signaling is central to the teratogenic effects of thalidomide.

CONCLUDING REMARKS AND FUTURE DIRECTIONS

At the International Conference on Harmonization (ICH) an agreement was reached on the harmonized tripartite guideline, "Timing of non-clinical safety studies for conduct of human clinical trials for pharmaceuticals (M3(R1))". However, several issues remained for further harmonization. The duration of repeated dose toxicity studies in rodents and timing of reproduction toxicity studies to support the inclusion of women of child-bearing potential (WOCBP) are some of them. There are regional variations in conduct of male and female fertility and embyo–fetal development studies in Japan, EU and the USA. Therefore, the only assessment of male and female reproductive organs performed prior to the first administration of a novel pharmaceutical to humans is histopathological examination of sex organs in repeated dose toxicity studies in rodents and non-rodents. Therefore assessment of these organs should be done using meticulous techniques. The collaborative work was organized by NIHS and Japan Pharmaceutical Manufacturer's Association (JPMA) and they concluded that detection of toxic effects on male and female reproductive organs is possible in 2-week repeated dose toxicity studies conducted with careful histopathological examination.

Toxic injury to gonads may be due to either direct or indirect effects of the toxicants. Certain agents exert direct toxicity where some of them are locally metabolized and biotransformed to toxic radicals and other agents mediate toxic injury indirectly through hormonal control. The Society for Toxicologic Pathology has given some recommendations for evaluation of testicular and ovarian toxicity. These recommendations include use of sexually mature animals, organ weights, clinical pathology estimations, consideration of spermatogenic or oocyte staging during microscopic examination and the technical information on tissue sampling, fixation and staining. Addition of reproductive system measures such as testicular homogenization-resistant spermatids and/or epididymal sperm count can also do a good job of predicting reproductive toxicity. Therefore all these methods of toxicologic pathology used for evaluation of male and female reproductive systems along with toxicokinetics and induced histopathology lesions are explained in detail in the present chapter.

In conclusion, meticulous use of different methods of pathology can generate sufficient information for evaluation of reproductive systems during repeated dose toxicity. Further, understanding of various molecular and biochemical mechanisms underlying the pathology of reproductive systems will enable discovery of novel biomarkers of safety including genomics, proteomics and metabonomics (Subrahmanyam and Tonelli, 2007; Williams *et al.*, 2008; Amacher, 2010; Muller and Dieterle, 2010; Scherf *et al.*, 2010; Subrahmanyam, 2010). It is expected that biomarkers in future will help minimize the conduct of long-term studies in animals thus minimizing the use of animals for regulatory reproductive toxicity studies.

REFERENCES

Adams ML, Little PJ, Bell B, Cicero TJ (1991) Alcohol affects rat testicular interstitial fluid volume and testicular secretion of testosterone and beta-endorphin. *J Pharmacol Exp Ther* **258:** 1008–14.

Adkins AG, Alden CL, Kanerva RL (1982) Optimization and standardization of male gonad weight determinations in rats. *Toxicol Pathol* **10:** 33–7.

Agarwal DK, Maronpot RR, Lamb JC, Kluwe WM (1985) Adverse effects of butylbenzyl phthalate on the reproductive and haemopoietic systems of male rats. *Toxicology* **35:** 189–206.

Amacher DE (2010) The discovery and development of proteomic safety biomarkers for the detection of drug-induced liver toxicity. *Toxicol Appl Pharmacol* **245:** 134–42.

Ando Y, Fuse E, Figg WD (2002a) Thalidomide metabolism by CYP2C subfamily. *Clin Cancer Res* **8:** 1964–73.

Ando Y, Price DK, Dahut WL, Cox MC, Reed E, Figg WD (2002b) Pharmacogenetic associations of CYP2C19 genotype with in vivo metabolisms and pharmacological effects of thalidomide. *Cancer Biol Ther* **1:** 669–73.

Aoki A, Hoffer AP (1978). Re-examination of the lesions in the rat testis caused by cadmium. *Biol Reprod* **18:** 579–91.

Arlen RR, Wells PG (1996) Inhibition of thalidomide teratogenicity by acetylsalicylic acid: evidence for prostaglandin H synthase-catalyzed bioactivation of thalidomide to a teratogenic reactive intermediate. *J Pharmacol Exp Ther* **277:** 1649–58.

Ataya KM, McKanna JA, Weintraub AM, Clark MR, Lemaire WJ (1985) A leutinizing hormone-releasing hormone agonist for prevention of chemotherapy-induced ovarian follicular loss in rats. *Cancer Res* **45:** 3651–6.

Bartlett JB, Dredge K, Dalgleish AG (2004) The evolution of thalidomide and its IMiD derivatives as anticancer agents. *Nat Rev Cancer* **4:** 314–22.

Bauer KS, Dixon SC, Figg WD (1998) Inhibition of angiogenesis by thalidomide requires metabolic activation, which is species-dependent. *Biochem Pharmacol* **55:** 1827–34.

Bhatal PS, Gerkens JK, Mashford ML (1974) Spermatic granuloma of epididymis in rats treated with guanethidine. *J Pathol* **112:** 19–26.

Blackburn DM, Gray AJ, Lloyd SC, Sheard CM, Foster PMD (1988) A comparison of the effects of the three isomers of dinitrobenzene on the testis in the rat. *Toxicol Appl Pharmacol* **92:** 54–64.

Blanchard KT, Lee J, Boekelheide K (1998) Leuprolide, a gonadotrophin releasing hormone agonist reestablishes spermatogenesis after 2,5-hexanedione-induced irreversible testicular injury in the rat resulting in normalized stem cell factor expression. *Endocrinology* **139:** 236–44.

Blask DE, Leadem CA (1987) Neuroendocrine aspects of neoplastic growth: a review. *Neuroendocrinol Lett* **9:** 63–73.

Bocabella AV, Salgado ED, Alger EA (1962) Testicular function and histology following serotonin administration. *Endocrinology* **71:** 827–37.

Boekelheide K, Fleming SL, Johnson KJ, Patel SR, Schoenfeld HA (2000) Role of Sertoli cells in injury-associated testicular germ cell apoptosis. *PSEBM* **225:** 105–15.

Boekelheide K, Neely MD, Sioussat TM (1989) The Sertoli cell cytoskeleton: a target for toxicant-induced germ cell loss. *Toxicol Appl Pharmacol* **101:** 373–89.

Bolon B, Bucci TJ, Warbritton AR, Chen JJ, Mattison DR, Heindel JJ (1997) Differential follicle counts as a screen for chemically induced ovarian toxicity in mice: results from continuous breeding bioassays. *Fundam Appl Toxicol* **39:** 1–10.

Borovskaya TG, Goldberg VE, Fomina TI, Pakomova AV, Kseneva SI, Poluektova ME, Goldberg ED (2004) Morphological and functional state of rat ovaries in early and late periods after administration of platinum cytostatics. *Bull Exp Biol Med* **137:** 331–5.

Brimblecombe RW, Leslie GB (1984) Cimetidine. In *Safety Testing of New Drugs: Laboratory Predictions and Clinical Performance* (Laurence DR, McLean AEM, Weatherall M, eds.). Academic Press, London, pp. 65–91.

Bucci TJ, Bolon B, Warbritton AR, Chen JJ, Heindel JJ (1997) Influence of sampling on the reproducibility of ovarian follicle counts in mouse toxicity studies. *Reprod Toxicol* **11:** 689–96.

Calabrese L, Fleischer AB (2000) Thalidomide: current and potential applications. *Am J Med* **108:** 487–95.

Chapin RE, Ku WW (1994) The reproductive toxicity of boric acid. *Environ Health Perspect* **102 (Suppl. 7):** 87–91.

Chapin RE, Morgan KT, Bus JS (1983) The morphogenesis of testicular degeneration induced in rats by orally administered 2,5-hexanedione. *Ex Molec Pathol* **38:** 149–69.

Chapin RE, White RD, Morgan KT, Bus JS (1984) Studies of lesions induced in the testis and epididymis of F344 rats by inhaled methyl chloride. *Toxicol Appl Pharmacol* **76:** 328–43.

Chapin RE, Williams J (1989) Mechanistic approaches in the study of testicular toxicity: toxicants that affect endocrine regulation of testis. *Toxicol Pathol* **17:** 446–51.

Cooper RL, Goldman JM, Tyrey L (1998) The hypothalamus and pituitary as target for reproductive toxicants. In *Reproductive and Developmental Toxicology* (Korach KS, ed.). Marcel Dekker Inc., pp. 195–210.

Corrier DE, Mollenhauser HH, Clark DE, Hare MF, Elissalde MH (1985) Testicular degeneration and necrosis induced by dietary cobalt. *Vet Pathol* **22:** 610–6.

Creasy DM (1997) Evaluation of testicular toxicity in safety evaluation studies: the appropriate use of spermatogenic staging. *Toxicol Pathol* **25:** 119–31.

Creasy DM (2001) Pathogenesis of male reproductive toxicity. *Toxicol Pathol* **29:** 64–76.

Creasy DM (2003) Evaluation of testicular toxicology: a synopsis and discussion of the recommendations proposed by the Society of Toxicologic Pathology. *Birth Def Res (Part B)* **68:** 408–15.

Creasy DM (2007) Female reproductive system II – Toxicological and ageing changes in the female reproductive tract. In *European Course on Toxicologic Pathology Organized by DESV in Veterinary Pathology at Veterinary School of Nantes (France) during April 23–7.*

Creasy DM, Flynn JC, Gray TJB, Butler WH (1985) A quantitative study of stage-specific spermatocyte damage following administration of ethylene glycol monomethyl ether in the rat. *Exp Molec Pathol* **43:** 321–36.

Creasy DM, Ford GR, Gray TJB (1990) The morphogenesis of cyclohexylamine-induced testicular atrophy in the rat: in vivo and in vitro studies. *Exp Molec Pathol* **52:** 155–69.

Creton S, Billington R, Davies W, Dent MP, Hawksworth GM, Parry S, Travis KZ (2009) Application of toxicokinetics to improve chemical risk assessment: implications for the use of animals. *Reg Tox Pharmacol* **55:** 291–9.

Dallenbach-Hellweg G, Poulsen H (1996) *Atlas of Endometrial Pathology*, 2nd edition. Springer-Verlag, Berlin.

Davis B, Almekinder J, Flagler N, Travlos G, Wilson R, Maronpot RR (1997) Ovarian luteal cell toxicity of ethylene glycol monomethyl ether and methoxy acetic acid in vivo and in vitro. *Toxicol Appl Pharmacol* **142:** 328–37.

Davis BJ, Heindel JJ (1998) Ovarian toxicants: multiple mechanisms of action. In *Reproductive and Developmental Toxicology* (Korach KS, ed.). Marcel Dekker Inc., pp. 373–95.

Davis BJ, Maronpot RR, Heindel JJ (1994) Di-(2-ethylhexyl) phthalate suppresses estradiol and ovulation in cycling rats. *Toxicol Appl Pharmacol* **128:** 216–23.

Donaubauer HH, Kramer M, Kreig K, Meyer D, Von Rechenberg W, Sandow J, Schütz E (1987) Investigations of the carcinogenicity of the LH-RH analogue buserelin (HOE 766) in rats using subcutaneous route of administration. *Fundam Appl Toxicol* **9:** 738–52.

Dunnick JK, Harris MW, Chapin RE, Hall LB, Lamb IVJC (1986) Reproductive toxicology of methyldopa in male F344/N rats. *Toxicology* **41:** 305–18.

Eichenbaum G, Subrahmanyam V, Tonelli AP (2010) Chapter 8: Toxicokinetics in support of drug development. In *Early Drug Development: Strategies and Routes to First-in-Human Trials* (Cayen MN, ed.). Wiley, NY, pp. 309–59.

Esch EV, de Rijk EPCT, Buse E, Zöller M, Cline JM (2008) Recommendations for routine sampling, trimming, and paraffin-embedding of female reproductive organs, mammary gland, and placenta in the cynomolgus monkey. *Toxicol Pathol* **36:** 164S–170S.

Fitzgerald J, De La Iglesia F, Goldenthal EI (1982) Ten-year oral toxicity study with norlestrin in rhesus monkeys. *J Toxicol Environ Health* **10:** 879–96.

Foley GL (2001) Overview of male reproductive pathology. *Toxicol Pathol* **29:** 49–63.

Foster PMD, Gray EL (2008). Chapter 20: Toxic responses of the reproductive system. In *Casarette & Doull's Toxicology, The Basic Science of Poisons*, 7th edition (Claassen CD, ed.). McGraw-Hill, New York, pp. 761–806.

Foote RH, Berndtson WE (1992) The germ cells. In *Reversibility in Testicular Toxicity Assessment* (Scialli AR, Clegg ED, eds.). CRC Press, pp. 1–56.

Foote RH, Carney EW (2000) The model as a model for reproductive and developmental toxicity studies. *Reprod Toxicol* **14:** 477–93.

Franks ME, MacPherson GR, Figg WD (2004) Thalidomide. *Lancet* **363:** 1802–11.

Fratta ID, Sigg EB, Maiorana K (1965) Teratogenic effect of thalidomide in rabbits, rats, hamsters and mice. *Toxicol Appl Pharmacol* **7:** 268–86.

Galustian C, Dalgleish A (2009) Lenalidomide: a novel anticancer drug with multiple modalities. *Expert Opin Pharmacother* **10:** 125–33.

Galustian C, Labarthe MC, Bartlett JB, *et al.* (2004) Thalidomide derived immunomodulatory drugs as therapeutic agents. *Expert Opin Biol Ther* **4:** 1963–70.

Garbis-Berkvens JM, Peters PWJ (1987) Comparative morphology and physiology of embryonic and fetal membranes. In *Pharmacokinetics in Teratogenesis*, Vol. 1 (Nau H, Scott WJ, eds.). CRC Press, Inc., Boca Raton, FL, pp. 13–44.

Gemzell-Danielsson K, Marion L (2004) Mechanism of action of mifepristone and levonorgestrel when used for emergency contraception. *Hum Reprod* **10:** 341–8.

Gopinath C, Prentice DE, Lewis DJ (1987) In *Atlas of Experimental Toxicological Pathology* (Gresham GA, ed.). Current Histopathology. MPT Press, pp. 91–103.

Gordon GB, Spielberg SP, Blake DE, Balasubramanian V (1981) Thalidomide teratogenesis: evidence for a toxic arene oxide metabolite. *Proc Natl Acad Sci USA* **78:** 2545–8.

Gordon JN, Goggin PM (2003) Thalidomide and its derivatives: emerging from the wilderness. *Postgrad Med J* **79:** 127–32.

Greaves P (2000a) Male genital tract. In *Histopathology of Preclinical Toxicity Studies – Interpretation and Relevance in Drug Safety Evaluation* (Greaves P, ed.). Elsevier, pp. 627–64.

Greaves P (2000b) Female genital tract. In *Histopathology of Preclinical Toxicity Studies – Interpretation and Relevance in Drug Safety Evaluation* (Greaves P, ed.). Elsevier, pp. 676–726.

Greaves P, Goonetilleke R, Nunn G, Topham J, Orton T (1993) Two-year carcinogenicity study of tamoxifen in Alderley Park Wistar-derived rats. *Cancer Res* **53:** 3919–24.

Greenman DL, Highman T, Kodell RL, Morgan KT, Norvell M (1984) Neoplastic and non-neoplastic responses to chronic feeding of diethyl stilbesterol in C3H mice. *J Toxicol Environ Health* **14:** 551–61.

Guthrie GPJr, John WJ (1980) The in vivo glucucorticoid and antiglucucorticoid actions of medroxyprogesterone acetate. *Endocrinol* **107:** 1393–6.

Haqqi TM, Adhami UM (1982) Testicular damage and change in serum LDH isoenzyme patterns induced by multiple sub-lethal doses of apholate in albino rats. *Toxicol Letters* **12:** 199–205.

Heindel JJ (1999) Oocyte quantitation and ovarian histology. In *An Evaluation and Interpretation of Reproductive Endpoints for Human Health Risk Assessment* (Daston GP, Kimmel CA, eds.). ILSI Press, Washington DC, pp. 57–74.

Heindel JJ, Treinen KA (1989) Physiology of the male reproductive system: endocrine, paracrine and autocrine regulation. *Toxicol Pathol* **17:** 411–45.

Hess RA (1990) Quantitative and qualitative characteristics of the stages and transitions in the cycle of the rat seminiferous epithelium. Light microscopic observation of perdusion-fixed and plastic embedded testes. *Biol Reprod* **43:** 525–42.

Heywood R, Wadsworth PF (1981) The experimental toxicology of estrogens. In *Pharmacology of Estrogens, International Encyclopedia of Pharmacology and Therapeutics*, (Chaudhury RR, ed.). New York, Pergamon Press.

Holson JF, Nemec MD, Stump DG, Kaufman LE, Lindström P, Varsho BJ (2006) Significance, reliability, and interpretation of developmental and reproductive toxicity study findings. In *Developmental and Reproductive Toxicology – A Practical Approach* (Hood RD, ed.). CRC Taylor and Francis, pp. 330–418.

Hoyer PB, Devine PJ (2002) Endocrine toxicology: the female reproductive system. In *Handbook of Toxicology* (Derelanko MJ, Hollinger MA, eds.). Taylor and Francis, pp. 580–603.

Hoyer PB, Devine PJ, Hu X, Thompson KE, Sipes IG (2001) Ovarian toxicity of 4-vinylcyclohexene diepoxide: a mechanistic model. *Toxicol Pathol* **29:** 91–9.

Hoyer PD, Sipes IG (1996) Assessment of follicle destruction in chemical-induced ovarian toxicity. *Ann Rev Pharmacol Toxicol* **36:** 307–31.

International Conference on Harmonization (1995) Reproductive toxicology: toxicity to male fertility. ICH topic S5B, Step 4. Consensus Guideline, November 29, 1995.

International Conference on Harmonization (1997) Non-clinical safety studies for the conduct of human clinical trials for pharmaceuticals. ICH topic M3, Step 4. Consensus Guideline, July 16, 1997.

Ishii S, Ube M, Okada M, Adachi T, Sugimoto J, Inoue Y, Uno Y, Mutai M (2009) Collaborative work on evaluation of ovarian toxicity. 17) Two- or four-week repeated-dose studies and fertility study of sulpiride in female rats. *J Toxicol Sci* **34:** SP175–SP188.

Iswaran TJ, Imai M, Betton GR, Siddall RA (1998) An overview of animal toxicology studies with bicalutamide (ICI 176,334). *J Toxicol Sci* **22:** 75–88.

Ito A, Mafune N, Kimura T (2009) Collaborative work on evaluation of ovarian toxicity. 4) Two- or four-week repeated dose study of 4-vinylcyclohexene diepoxide in female rats. *J Toxicol Sci* **34:** SP52–SP58.

Itoh R, Ozasa HK (1985) Changes in serum lactate dehydrogenase isozyme X activity observed after cadmium administration. *Toxicol Lett* **28:** 151–4.

Izumi Y, Watanabe T, Awasaki N, Hikawa K, Minagi T, Chatani F (2009) Collaborative work on evaluation of ovarian toxicity. 16) Effects of 2 or 4 weeks repeated dose studies and fertility study of chlorpromazine hydrochloride in rats. *J Toxicol Sci* **34:** SP167–SP174.

Johnson AN (1989) Comparative aspects of contraceptive steroids. Effects observed in beagle dogs. *Toxicol Pathol* **17:** 389–95.

Karlsson S, Iatropoulos MJ, Williams GM, Kangas L, Nieminen L (1998) The proliferation in the uterine compartments of intact rats of two different strains exposed to high doses of tamoxifen or toremifene. *Toxicol Pathol* **26:** 759–68.

Kawashita H, Hiratsuka K, Kuroda J, Asada Y, Suzuki T, Muguruma Y, Tomioka S, Tani M, Kondo M, Mineshima H, Nagae Y (2000) Collaborative work to evaluate toxicity on male reproductive organs by repeated dose studies in rats. 4) Fadrozole hydrochloride: an oral 2/4 week male reproductive organ study. *J Toxicol Sci* **25:** 51–62.

Knobloch J, Rüther U (2008) Shedding light on an old mystery: thalidomide suppresses survival pathways to induce limb defects. *Cell Cycle* **7:** 1121–7.

Knobloch J, Shaughnessy JD, Rüther U (2007) Thalidomide induces limb deformities by perturbing the Bmp/Dkk1/Wnt signaling pathway. *FASEB J* **21:** 1410–21.

Ku WW, Chapin RE (1994) Spermatocyte toxicity of 2-methoxyethanol in vivo and in vitro: requirement for an intact seminiferous tubule structure for germ cell degeneration. *Toxicol in Vitro* **8:** 1191–202.

Kumazawa T, Nakajima A, Ishiguro T, Jiuxin Z, Tanaharu T, Nishitani H, Inoue Y, Harada S, Hayasaka I, Tagawa Y (2009) Collaborative work on evaluation of ovarian toxicity. 15) Two- or four-week repeated-dose studies and fertility study of bromocriptine in female rats. *J Toxicol Sci* **34:** SP157–SP165.

Lanning LI, Creasy DM, Chapin RE, Mann PC, Barlow NJ, Regan KS, Goodman DG (2002) Recommended approaches for the evaluation of testicular and epididymal toxicity. *Toxicol Pathol* **30:** 507–20.

Lanning L (2006) Toxicologic pathology assessment. In *Toxicological Testing Handbook – Principles, Applications and Data Interpretation* (Jacobson-Kram D, Keller KA, eds.). Informa Healthcare, pp. 109–30.

Latendresse JR, Warbrittion AR, Jonassen H, Creasy DM (2002) Fixation of testes and eyes using a modified Davidson's fluid: comparison with Bouin's fluid and conventional Davidson's fluid. *Toxicol Pathol* **30:** 524–33.

Leck IM, Millar ELM (1962) Incidence of malformations since the introduction of Thalidomide. *Br Med J* **2:** 16–20.

Lee J, Richburg JH, Shipp EB, Meistrich ML, Boekelheide K (1999) The Fas system a regulator of testicular germ cell apoptosis is differentially up-regulated in Sertoli cell versus germ cell injury of the testis. *Endocrinology* **140:** 852–8.

Lenz WA (1988) A short history of thalidomide embryopathy. *Teratology* **38:** 203–15.

Lenz W, Knapp K (1962) Foetal malformations due to thalidomide. *Ger Med Mon* **7:** 253–8.

Linder RE, Klinefelter GR, Strader LF, Suarez JD, Dyer CJ (1994) Acute spermatogenic effects of bromoacetic acids. *Fundam Appl Toxicol* **22:** 422–30.

Linder RE, Strader LF, Rehnberg GL (1990) Effect of acute exposure to boric acid on the male reproductive system of the rat. *J Toxicol Environ Health* **31:** 133–46.

Ling-Hong L, Wine RN, Miller DS, Reece JM, Smith M, Chapin RE (1997) Protection against methoxyacetic acid induced spermatocytes apoptosis with calcium channel blockers in cultured rat seminiferous tubules: possible mechanisms. *Toxicol Appl Pharmacol* **144:** 105–19.

Long GG, Cohen IR, Gries CL, Young JK, Francis PC, Capen CC (2001) Proliferative lesions of ovarian granulosa cells and reversible hormonal changes induced in rats by a selective estrogen receptor modulator. *Toxicol Pathol* **29:** 403–10.

Lovekamp-Swan T, Davis BJ (2003) Mechanisms of phthalate ester toxicity in the female reproductive system. *Environ Health Perspect* **111:** 139–45.

Maekawa A, Maita K, Harleman JH (1996) Changes in the ovary. In *Pathobiology of the Aging Mouse* (Mohr U, Dungworth DL, Capen CC, Carlton WW, Sundberg JP, Ward JM, eds.). International Life Sciences Institute, Washington DC, pp. 451–67.

Maronpot RR (1987) Ovarian toxicity and carcinogenicity in eight recent National Toxicology Program studies. *Environ Health Perspect* **73:** 125–30.

Mattison DR (1983) Ovarian toxicity: effects on sexual maturation, reproduction and menopause. In *Reproductive and Developmental Toxicity of Fetals* (Clarkson TW, Nordberg GF, Sager PR, eds.). Plenum Press, New York, pp. 41–91.

Mattison DR, Thomford PJ (1989) The mechanism of action of reproductive toxicants. *Toxicol Pathol* **17:** 364–76.

Matthews SJM, McCoy S (2003) Thalidomide: a review of approved and investigational uses. *Clin Ther* **25:** 342–95.

McBride WB (1961) Thalidomide and congenital abnormalities. *Lancet* **2:** 1358.

McConnell RF, Western HH, Ulland BM, Bosland MC, Ward JM (1992) Proliferative lesion of the testis in rats with selected examples from mice. URG-3. In *Guides for Toxicologic Pathology*. STP/ARP/AFIP, Washington DC.

McDonald SW, Scotome RJ (1987) On the mode of sperm autoantigen presentation to the regional lymph node of the testis after vasectomy in rats. *J Anat* **153:** 217–21.

Meistrich MM (1986) Critical components of testicular function and sensitivity to disruption. *Biol Reprod* **34:** 17–28.

Meyring M, Mühlbacher J, Messer K, Kastner-Pustet N, Bringmann G, Mannschreck A, Blaschke G (2002) In vitro biotransformation of (R)- and (S)-thalidomide: application of circular dichroism spectroscopy to the stereochemical characterization of the hydroxylated metabolites. *Anal Chem* **74:** 3726–35.

Michael B, Yano B, Sellers RS, Perry R, Morton D, Roome N, Julie JK, Schafer K (2007) Evaluation of organ weights for rodent and non-rodent toxicity studies: a review of regulatory guidelines and a survey of current practices. *Toxicol Pathol* **35:** 742–50.

Mihaly GW, Morgan DJ (1984) Placental drug transfer: effects of gestational age and species. *Pharmacol* Ther **23:** 253–66.

Miyamoto Y, Ueda K, Oshida K, Ohmori E (2000) Collaborative work to evaluate toxicity on male reproductive organs by repeated dose studies in rats (2). Testicular toxicity in rats treated orally with ethinylestradiol for 2 weeks. *J Toxicol Sci* **25:** 33–42.

Moore NP, Creasy DM, Gray TJB, Timbrell JA (1992) Urinary creatine profiles after administration of cell-specific toxicants to the rat. *Archives of Toxicology* **66:** 435–42.

Mori T, Nagasawa H (1983) Mechanisms of development of prolactin-induced adenomyosis in mice. *Act Anat* **116:** 46–54.

Muller PY, Dieterle F (2009) Tissue-specific, non-invasive toxicity biomarkers: translation from preclinical safety assessment to clinical safety monitoring. *Expert Opin Drug Metab Toxicol* **5:** 1023–38.

Muse K, Wilson EA, Jawad MJ (1982) Prolactin hyperstimulation in response to thyrotropin –releasing hormone in patients with endometriosis. *Fertil Steril* **38:** 419–22.

Muskhelishvili L, Freeman LD, Latendresse JR, Bucci TJ (2002) An immunohistochemical label to facilitate counting of ovarian follicles. *Toxicol Pathol* **30:** 400–2.

Muskhelishvili L, Wingard SK, Latendresse JR (2005) Proliferating cell nuclear antigen – a marker for ovarian follicle counts. *Toxicol Pathol* **33:** 365–8.

Nagasawa H, Mori T (1982) Stimulation of mammary tumerigenesis and suppression of uterine adenomyosis by temporary inhibition of pituitary prolactin secretion during youth in mice. *Proc Soc Exp Biol Med* **171:** 164–7.

Nakai M, Hess RA, Moore BJ, Guttroff RF, Strader LF, Linder RE (1992) Acute and long term effects of a single dose of the fungicide carbendazim on the male reproductive system in the rat. *J Androl* **13:** 507–18.

Nau H (1985) Teratogenic valproic acid concentrations: infusion by implanted minipups vs conventional injection regimen in the mouse. *Toxicol Appl Pharmacol* **80:** 243–50.

Nau H (1990) Correlation of transplacental pharmacokinetics of retinoids during organogenesis with teratogenicity. *Methods Enzymol* **190:** 437–48.

Nicosia SV, Matus-Ridley M, Meadows AT (1985) Gonadal effects of cancer therapy in girls. *Cancer* **55:** 2364–72.

Nozaki Y, Furubo E, Matsuno T, Fukui R, Kizawa K, Kozaki T, Sanzen T (2009) Collaborative work on evaluation of ovarian toxicity. 6) Two- or four-week repeated-dose studies and fertility study of cisplatin in female rats. *J Toxicol Sci* **34:** SP73–SP81.

O'Connor JC, Frame SR, Biegel LB, Cook JC, Davis LG (1998) Sensitivity of a tier I screening battery compared to an in utero exposure for detecting the estrogen receptor agonist 17 beta estradiol. *Toxicol Sci* **44:** 169–84.

O'Steen WK (1963) Serotonin and histamine: effects of a single injection on the mouse testis and prostate gland. *Proc Soc Exp Biol Med* **113:** 161–3.

Ohta Y (1987) Age-related decline in deciduogenic ability of the rat uterus. *Biol Reprod* **37:** 779–85.

Ohtake S, Fukui M, Hisada S (2009) Collaborative work on evaluation of ovarian toxicity. 1) Effects of 2- or 4-week repeated-dose administration and fertility studies with medroxyprogesterone acetate in female rats. *J Toxicol Sci* **34:** SP23–SP29.

Organisation for Economic Co-operation and Development (2008a) Guidance document for histologic evaluation of endocrine and reproductive tests, Endocrine Control of the Oestrous Cycle, Part 2.

Organisation for Economic Co-operation and Development (2008b) Guidance document for histologic evaluation of endocrine and reproductive tests, Endocrine Control of the Oestrous Cycle, Part 3, Section 2.

Organisation for Economic Co-operation and Development (2008c) Guidance document for histologic evaluation of endocrine and reproductive tests, Morphological Patterns of Endocrine Disruption, Part 3, Section 5.

Ostrander PL, Mills KT, Bern HA (1985) Long term responses of the mouse uterus to neonatal diethylstilbesterol treatment and to later sex hormone exposure. *JNCI* **74:** 121–35.

Parman T, Wiley MJ, Wells PG (1999) Free radical-mediated oxidative DNA damage in the mechanism of thalidomide teratogenicity. *Nat Med* **5:** 582–5.

Peluso JJ, Gordon LR (1992) Nonneoplastic and neoplastic changes in the ovary. In *Pathobiology of the Aging Rat* (Mohr U, Dungworth DL, Capen CC, eds.). Iowa State University Press, Ames, IA, pp. 351–2.

Physician's Desk Reference (1999) *Physician's Desk Reference*. 53rd edition. Medical Economics, Montvale, NJ.

Picut CA, Swanson CL, Scully KL, Roseman VC, Parker RF, Remick AK (2008) Ovarian follicle counts using proliferating cell nuclear antigen (PCNA) and semi-automated image analysis in rats. *Toxicol Pathol* **36:** 674–9.

Plowchalk DR, Mottison DR (1992) Reproductive toxicity of cyclophosphamide in the C57BL/6N mouse. I. Effects on ovarian structure and function. *Reproduct Toxicol* **6:** 411–21.

Regan KS, Cline JM, Creasy DM, Davis B, Foley GL, Lanning L, Latendresse JR, Makris S, Morton D, Rehm S, Stebbins K (2005) STP Position Paper: ovarian follicular counting in the assessment of rodent reproductive toxicity. *Toxicol Pathol* **33:** 409–12.

Reiners J, Wittfoht H, Nau H, Vogel R, Tenschert B, Speilmann H (1987) Teratogenesis and pharmacokinetics of cyclophosphamide after drug infusion as compared to injection in the mouse during day 10 of gestation. In *Pharmacokinetics in Teratogenesis*, Vol. 1 (Nau H, Scott WJ, eds.). CRC Press, Inc., Boca Raton, FL, pp. 41–8.

Richardson BP, Turkalj I, Fluckieger E (1984) Bromocriptine. In *Safety Testing of New Drugs: Laboratory Predictions and Clinical Performance* (Laurence DR, McLean AEM, Weatherall M, eds.). Academic Press, London, pp. 19–63.

Richburg JH, Boekelheide K (1996) MEHP rapidly alters both Sertoli cell vimentin laments and germ cell apoptosis in young rat testes. *Toxicol Appl Pharmacol* **137:** 42–50.

Risbridger JP, Wang H, Frydenberg M, Cunha G (2001) The metaplastic effects of estrogen on mouse prostate epithelium: proliferation of cells with basal cell phenotype. *Endocrinol* **142:** 2443–50.

Roosen-Runge EC, Giesel LO Jr (1950) Quantitative studies on spermatogenesis in the albino rat. *Am J Ant* **87:** 1–30.

Russell LD, Ettlin RA, Sinha Hikin AP, Clegg ED (1990) *Histological and Histopathological Evaluation of Testis*. Cache River Press, Clearwater, FL.

Russell LD, Malone JP, Karpas SL (1981) Morphological pattern elicited by agents affecting spermatogenesis by disruption of its hormonal stimulation. *Tissue Cell* **13:** 369–80.

Ruwanpura SM, McLachlan RI, Meachem SJ (2010) Hormonal regulation of male germ cell development. *J Endocrinol* **205:** 117–31.

Sakurada Y, Kudo S, Iwasaki S, Miyata Y, Nishi M, Masumoto Y (2009) Collaborative work on evaluation of ovarian toxicity. 5) Two- or four-week repeated-dose studies and fertility study of busulfan in female rats. *J Toxicol Sci* **34:** SP65–SP72.

Sanbuissho A, Yoshida M, Hisada S, Sagami F, Kudo S, Kumazawa T, Ube M, Komatsu S, Ohno Y (2009) Collaborative work on evaluation of ovarian toxicity by repeated-dose and fertility studies in female rats. *J Toxicol Sci* **34:** SP1–SP22.

Sato M, Shiozawa K, Uesugi T, Hiromatsu R, Fukuda M, Kitaura K, Minami T, Matsumoto S (2009) Collaborative work on evaluation of ovarian toxicity. 7) Effects of 2- or 4- week repeated dose studies and fertility study of cyclophosphamide in female rats. *J Toxicol Sci* **34:** SP83–SP89.

Sawamoto O, Yamate J, Kuwamura M, Kotani T (2003) Age-dependent decrease in incidence of rat sperm granulomas induced by L-cysteine. *J Toxicol Pathol* **16:** 123–7.

Schardein JL (1980) Studies of the components of the oral contraceptive agent in albino rats. II. Progestogenic component and comparison of effects of the components and the combined agent. *J Tox Environ Health* **6:** 895–906.

Scherf U, Becker R, Chan M, Hojvat S (2010) Approval of novel biomarkers: FDA's perspective and major requests. *Scand J Clin Lab Invest Suppl* **242:** 96–102.

Schumacher H, Smith RL, Williams RT (1965) The metabolism of thalidomide: the fate of thalidomide and some of its hydrolysis products in various species. *Br J Pharmacol Chemother* **25:** 338–51.

Schumacher H, Blake DA, Gurian JM, *et al.* (1968) A comparison of the teratogenic activity of thalidomide in rabbits and rats. *J Pharmacol Exp Ther* **160:** 189–200.

Schwartz S (2001) Providing toxicokinetic support for reproductive toxicology studies in pharmaceutical development. *Arch Toxicol* **75:** 381–7.

Sellers RS, Mortan D, Michael B, Roome N, Johnson JK, Yano BL, Perry R, Schafer K (2007) Society of Toxicologic Pathology Position Paper: organ weight recommendations for toxicology studies. *Toxicol Pathol* **35:** 751–5.

Setchell BP (1990) Local control of testicular fluids. *Reprod Fertil Dev* **2:** 291–309.

Setchell BP, Sharpe RM (1984) Effect of injected hCG on capillary permeability, extracellular liquid volume and the flow of lymph in the testes of rats. *J Endocrinol* **91:** 245–54.

Sharpe RM (1988) Endocrinology and paracrinology of the testes. In *Physiology and Toxicology of Male Reproduction* (Lamb JC, Foster PMD, eds.). Academic Press, San Diego, pp. 71–99.

Sharpe RM (1994) Regulation of spermatogenesis. In *The Physiology of Reproduction*, 2nd edition (Knobil E, Neil JD, eds.). Raven Press, New York, pp. 1363–434.

Sharpe RM, Bartlett JMS, Allenby G (1991) Evidence for the control of testicular interstitial fluid volume in the rat by specific germ cell types. *J Endocrinol* **128:** 359–67.

Shibayama H, Kotera T, Shinoda Y, Hanada T, Kajihara T, Ueda M, Tamura H, Ishibashi S, Yamashita Y, Ochi S (2009) Collaborative work on evaluation of ovarian toxicity. 14) Two- or four-week repeated-dose studies and fertility study of atrazine in female rats. *J Toxicol Sci* **34:** SP147–SP155.

Shirai M, Sakurai K, Saitoh W, Matsuyama T, Teranishi M, Furukawa T, Sanbuissho A, Manabe S (2009) Collaborative work on evaluation of ovarian toxicity. 8) Two- or four-week repeated-dose studies and fertility study of Anastrozole in female rats. *J Toxicol Sci* **34:** SP91–SP99.

Shiromizu K, Torgeirsson SS, Mattison D (1984) The effects of cyclophosphamide on oocyte and follicle number in Sprague Dawley Rats, C57BL/CN and DBA /2N mice. *Pediatr Pharmacol* **4:** 213–21.

Smith BJ, Carter DE, Sipes IG (1990) Comparison of the disposition and in vitro metabolism of 4-vinylcyclohexene in the female mouse and rat. *Toxicol Appl Pharmacol* **105:** 364–71.

Smith BJ, Plowchalk DR, Sipes IG, Mattison DR (1991) Comparison of random and serial sections in assessment of ovarian toxicity. *Repro Toxicol* **5:** 379–83.

Smithells RW, Newman CGH (1992) Recognition of thalidomide defects. *J Med Genet* **29:** 716–23.

Somkuti SG, Lapadula DM, Chapin RE, Abou-Donia MB (1991) Light and electron microscopic evidence of tri-*o*-cresyl phosphate (TOCP)-mediated testicular toxicity in F344 rats. *Toxicol Appl Pharmacol* **107:** 35–46.

Springer LN, Flaws JA, Sipes IG, Hoyer PB (1996) Follicular mechanisms associated with 4-vinylcyclohexane diepoxide-induced ovotoxicity in rats. *Reprod Toxicol* **10:** 137–43.

Strandgaard C, Miller MG (1998) Germ cell apoptosis in rat testis after administration of 1,3-dinitrobenzene. *Reprod Toxicol* **12:** 97–103.

Stephens TD, Fillmore BJ (2000) Hypothesis: thalidomide embryopathy – proposed mechanism of action. *Teratology* **61:** 189–95.

Stephens TD, Bunde CJW, Fillmore BJ (2000) Mechanism of action in thalidomide teratogenesis. *Biochem Pharm* **59:** 1489–99.

Subrahmanyam V (2010). Chapter 12: Pathophysiology of endogenous toxins and their relation to inborn errors of metabolism and drug mediated toxicities. In *Endogenous Toxins* (O'Brien PJ, Bruce R, eds.). Wiley-VCH Verlag GmbH & Co. KGaA, pp. 291–316.

Subrahmanyam V, Tonelli AP (2007) Biomarkers, metabonomics, and drug development: can inborn errors of metabolism help in understanding drug toxicity? *AAPS J* **9:** E284–E297.

Sullivan FM, Smith ME, McElhatton PR (1987) Interpretation of animal experiments as illustrated by studies on caffeine. In *Pharmacokinetics in Teratogenesis*, Vol. 1 (Nau H, Scott WJ, eds.). CRC Press, Inc., Boca Raton, FL, pp. 124–7.

Takai R, Hayashi S, Kiyokawa J, Iwata Y, Matsuo S, Suzuki M, Mizoguchi K, Chiba S, Deki T (2009) Collaborative work on evaluation of ovarian toxicity. 10) Two- or four-week repeated dose studies and fertility study of di-(2-ethylhexyl) phthalate (DEHP) in female rats. *J Toxicol Sci* **34:** SP111–SP119.

Takano H, Abe K (1987) Age-related histological changes in the adult mouse testis. *Arch Histol Jpn* **50:** 533–44.

Takayama S, Akaike M, Kawashima K, Takahashi M, Kurokawa Y (1995) Study in Japan on optimal treatment period and parameters for detection of male fertility disorders in rats. *J Toxicol Sci* **20:** 173–82.

Tamura T, Yokoi R, Okuhara Y, Harada C, Terashima Y, Hayashi M, Nagasawa T, Onozato T, Kobayashi K, Kuroda J, Kusama H (2009) Collaborative work on evaluation of ovarian toxicity. 2) Two- or four-week repeated dose studies and fertility study of mifepristone in female rats. *J Toxicol Sci* **34:** SP31–SP42.

Taya K, Sato T, Igarashi M (1975) Effects of prostaglandin F2α upon ovulation and LH, FSH and prolactin secretion in chlorpromazine blocked rats. *Endocrinol Jpn* **22:** 131–6.

Teo SK, Stirling DI, Zeldis JB (2005) Thalidomide as a novel therapeutic agent: new uses for an old product. *Drug Discov Today* **10:** 107–14.

Timbrell JA (2000) *Principles of Biochemical Toxicology*. London, Taylor and Francis.

Timbrell JA, Draper R, Waterfield CJ (1994) Biomarkers in toxicology. New uses for some old molecules. *Toxicol Ecotoxicol News* **1:** 4–14.

Tsubota K, Kushima K, Yamauchi K, Matsuo S, Saegusa T, Ito S, Fujiwara M, Matsumoto M, Nakatsuji S, Seki J, Oishi Y (2009) Collaborative work on evaluation of ovarian toxicity. 12) Effects of 2- or 4-week repeated dose studies and fertility study of indomethacin in female rats. *J Toxicol Sci* **34:** SP129–SP136.

Tsujioka S, Ban Y, Wise LD, Tsuchiya T, Sato T, Matsue K, Ikeda T, Sasaki M, Nishikibe M (2009) Collaborative work on evaluation of evaluation of ovarian toxicity (3) Effects of 2- or 4- week repeated dose toxicity and fertility studies with tamoxifen in female rats. *J Toxicol Sci* **34:** SP43–SP51.

Tucker MJ, Adam HK, Patterson JS (1984) Tamoxifen. In *Safety Testing of New Drugs. Laboratory Predictions and Clinical Performance* (Laurence DR, McLean AEM, Weatherall M, eds.). Academic Press, London, pp. 125–61.

Ubrich B, Palmer AK (1995) Detection of effects on male reproduction. A literature survey. *J Am Coll Toxicol* **14:** 293–327.

Valenca MM, Negro-Vilar A (1986) Propiomelanocortin-derived peptides in testicular interstitial fluid: characterization and changes in secretion after hCG or LHRH analog treatment. *Endocrinology* **118:** 32–7.

Valerio MG (1989) Comparative aspects of contraceptive steroids: effects observed in the monkey. *Toxicol Pathol* **17:** 401–10.

Van Cauteren H, Vandenberghe J, Herin V, Vanparys Ph, Marsboom R (1985) Toxicological properties of closantel. *Drug Chem Toxicol* **8:** 101–23.

Van der Schoot P, Bakker GH, Klijn JGM (1987) Effects of the progesterone antagonist RU 486 on ovarian activity in the rat. *Endocrinology* **121:** 1375–82.

Vargesson N (2009) Thalidomide-induced limb defects: resolving a 50 year old puzzle. *BioEssays* **31:** 1327–36.

Vermeulen A (1993) Environmental, human reproduction, menopause and andropause. *Environ Health Perspect* **101:** 91–100.

Watanabe T, Yamaguchi N, Akiba T, Tanaka M, Takimoto M (2000) Collaborative work to evaluate toxicity on male reproductive organs by repeated dose studies in rats. 12) Effects of cyclophosphamide on spermatogenesis. *J Toxicol Sci* **25:** 129–37.

Wato E, Asahiyama M, Suzuki A, Funyu S, Amano Y (2009) Collaborative work on evaluation of ovarian toxicity. 9) Effects of 2- or 4-week repeated dose studies and fertility study of di(2-ethylhexyl)adipate (DEHA) in female rats. *J Toxicol Sci* **34:** SP101–SP109.

Wells PG, McCallum GP, Lam KC, Henderson JT, Ondovcik SL (2010) Oxidative DNA damage and repair in teratogenesis and neurodevelopmental deficits. *Birth Defects Res C Embryo Today* **90:** 103–9.

Wells PG, Lee CJJ, McCallum GP, Perstin J, Harper PA (2010) Receptor- and reactive-intermediate mediated mechanisms of teratogenesis. In *Adverse Drug Reactions, Handbook of Experimental Pharmacology*, Vol. 196 (Uetrecht J, ed.). Springer-Verlag, Berlin, Heidelberg, pp. 131–62.

Westwood FR (2008) The female rat reproductive cycle: a practical histological guide to staging. *Toxicologic Pathol* **36:** 375–84.

Widmark A, Damber JE, Bergh A (1987) Effects of oestradiol-17-beta on testicular microcirculation in rats. *J Endocrinol* **115:** 489–95.

Williams JA, Andersson T, Andersson TB, Blanchard R, Behm MO, Cohen N, Edeki T, Franc M, Hillgren KM, Johnson KJ, Katz DA, Milton MN, Murray BP, Polli JW, Ricci D, Shipley LA, Subrahmanyam V, Wrighton SA (2008) PhRMA white paper on ADME pharmacogenomics. *J Clin Pharmacol* **48:** 849–89.

Wong PYD, Yeung CH (1977) Inhibition by α-chlorohydrin of fluid reabsorbtion in the rat cauda epididymis. *J Reprod Fertil* **51:** 469–71.

Worth AP, Balls M (eds.) (2002) Chapter 10: Reproductive toxicity. *ATLA* **30 S1:** 95–102.

Yamauchi K, Takaura Y, Noto T, Saegusa T, Nakasuji S, Ohishi Y (2000) Collaborative work to evaluate toxicity on male reproductive organs by repeated dose studies in rats. 7) Effects of reserpine in 2- or 4- weeks studies. *J Toxicol Sci* **25:** 79–85.

Yeh J, Kim B, Liang YJ, Peresie J (2006) Mullerian inhibiting substance as a novel biomarker of cisplatin-induced ovarian damage. *Biochem Biophys Res Commun* **348:** 337–44.

Yoshida M, Sanbuissyo A, Hisada S, Takahashi M, Ohno Y, Nishikawa A (2009) Morphological characterization of the ovary under normal cycling in rats and its viewpoints of ovarian toxicity detection. *J Toxicol Sci* **34:** SP189–SP197.

Yuan Y (1998) Female reproductive system. In *Fundamentals of Toxicologic Pathology* (Haschek WM, Rousseaux CG, eds.). Academic Press, pp. 485–514.

Section 14

Placental Toxicity

C H A P T E R

77

Strategies for investigating hemochorial placentation

Stephen J. Renaud and Michael J. Soares

INTRODUCTION

Viviparity was one of the most significant evolutionary adaptations for vertebrate reproduction because it allowed offspring to develop within the body of the mother removed from predation and environmental pressures. In eutherian mammals including humans, viviparity is dependent on the presence of a placenta. The primary function of the placenta is to support fetal growth and viability. First, the placenta provides a large exchange surface where maternal and fetal circulations closely approach each other, allowing molecules to be transferred between maternal and fetal blood. This exchange is vital to ensure adequate nutritional and gaseous provisions for the fetus. In some species placental cells augment the nutrient supply to the fetus by actively transforming the uterine vasculature. Second, the placenta plays a primary role in the protection of the fetus. The exchange surface of the placenta has specific exclusion principles that ensure potentially teratogenic substances within maternal blood do not enter the fetal circulation. Also, the placenta produces unique immunomodulating agents that actively promote maternal immune acceptance of the conceptus (placenta and fetus) despite its expression of paternal antigens. Third, the placenta provides endocrinological support for the pregnancy by producing various hormones that ensure the maintenance of pregnancy and the modification of maternal metabolism for the advantage of the fetus.

The placenta is a complex structure formed by a heterogeneous population of cells. Cells contributed by the zygote include trophoblast cells, which constitute the epithelial component of the placenta, as well as mesenchyme derived from mesoderm of the allantois. Trophoblast cells are the first cell type to differentiate during embryogenesis and subsequently undergo a multilineage differentiation process, enabling them to form the bulk of the placental architecture and to perform the majority of the aforementioned functions. Allantoic mesoderm, on the other hand, ultimately organizes within the trophoblast-derived placental architecture to develop a circulatory system that connects to the fetal circulation via the umbilical cord. An assorted population of uterine stromal cells adjacent to the developing placenta specializes to form the decidua.

There is diversity in placental structure among eutheria, but there is also remarkable conservation in the basic function of this organ. Anatomically, placentae can broadly be classified into three distinct groups according to the number of intervening layers between maternal blood and trophoblast. Depending on whether the trophoblast lies adjacent to uterine surface epithelium, uterine vascular endothelium or is directly in contact with maternal blood, placentas are categorized as epitheliochorial, endotheliochorial or hemochorial, respectively. Hemochorial placentation occurs in higher primates, including humans, as well as in most rodents. This form of placentation is characterized by a highly erosive trophoblast capable of extensive remodeling of the uterine vasculature thereby permitting the direct flow of maternal blood to the surface of trophoblast cells. The purpose of this chapter is to describe hemochorial placentation and provide strategies and challenges for its investigation. Focus will be placed on hemochorial placentation not only in humans, but also in mice and rats (collectively referred to as rodents hereafter unless otherwise specified) because these rodents are widely used in laboratory settings and because the genetics of these species are becoming increasingly well defined.

EARLY ASPECTS OF PLACENTATION

Even though some aspects of placental architecture differ among species exhibiting hemochorial placentation, the basic foundations underlying formation of the mature placenta are conserved. The following description of the ontogeny of hemochorial placentation is simplified to highlight the parallels among humans and rodents. Only those factors relevant for the formation of the definitive placenta are described. For more detail, the reader is referred to a number of excellent reviews on the comparative anatomy of placentation (Pijnenborg *et al.*, 1981; Georgiades *et al.*, 2002; Carter and Enders, 2004; Enders and Carter, 2004).

Derivation of the trophoblast lineage

Early in embryogenesis, the first cellular specification event results in a polarized epithelial monolayer of trophectoderm surrounding an inner cell mass within a fluid-filled

Reproductive and Developmental Toxicology, Edited by Ramesh C. Gupta
ISBN: 978-0-12-382032-7

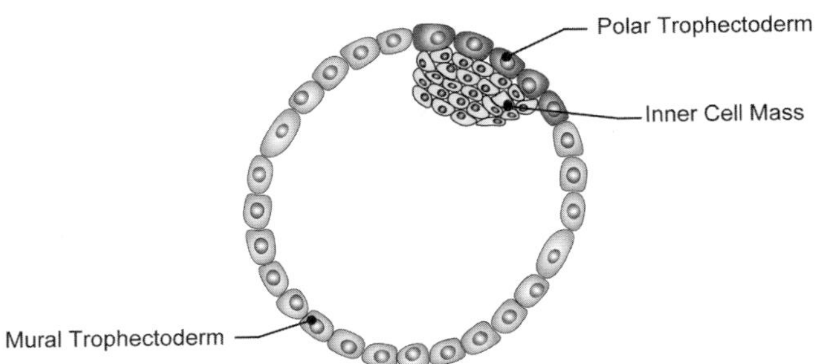

FIGURE 77.1 Illustration depicting the structure of a preimplantation blastocyst. The blastocyst consists of an outer layer of trophectoderm, which is fated to differentiate into trophoblast cells, and an eccentrically placed inner cell mass destined to form the embryo, yolk sac and allantois. The trophectoderm contiguous with the inner cell mass is referred to as the polar trophectoderm, whereas the trophectoderm opposite the inner cell mass is called the mural trophectoderm. Please see color plate section.

blastocoel (Figure 77.1). Although the precise molecular signals that promote this cellular differentiation event are not fully understood, studies in mice have revealed that trophectoderm differentiation is likely spatially regulated, being segregated to peripheral cells of the early embryo, and is associated with repression of the POU-family transcription factor Oct4 and upregulation of the homeodomain-containing transcription factor Cdx2 (Niwa *et al.*, 2005). In humans, reciprocal expression of these transcription factors is thought to similarly regulate trophectoderm specification (Adjaye *et al.*, 2005; Hemberger *et al.*, 2010). The inner cell mass is destined to form the definitive structures of the fetus, as well as the amniotic and yolk sac membranes and allantois, whereas the trophectoderm contains multipotential, self-renewing trophoblast stem (TS) cells fated to progressively differentiate into more specialized populations of trophoblast cells that constitute the epithelial component of the placenta.

Early embryological development occurs within the oviduct and uterine cavity; however, subsequent development requires implantation into a specialized uterine stroma – the decidua – for access to nutritional provisions. In species exhibiting hemochorial placentation, implantation into the decidua begins very soon after blastocyst formation, commencing on embryonic day (E) 5–6 in humans, and E 4–5 in mice and rats. The decidua contiguous with the developing placenta further specializes to form the decidua basalis. For more detailed reviews of embryo implantation, see Cross *et al.* (1994) and Dey *et al.* (2004).

Early trophoblast development

Trophoblast specification along a multilineage differentiation pathway commences around the time of blastocyst implantation. In rodents, the first trophoblast subtype to differentiate is the primary trophoblast giant cell, which is remarkable in that it ceases mitoses but continues to replicate its DNA in a process called endoreduplication, resulting in enormous polyploid cells that arrange into a single layer at the maternal–fetal boundary. These cells first appear within the mural trophectoderm, i.e. opposite the inner cell mass, but inevitably envelop the entire conceptus except for the polar trophectoderm, i.e. trophectoderm contiguous with the inner cell mass (Figure 77.1). The polar trophectoderm expands to form a cylindrical structure containing two separate regions: the proximal extra-embryonic ectoderm and the distal ectoplacental cone. Trophoblast cells within these regions are diploid and progressively differentiate contributing to anatomically and functionally distinct regions of the definitive rodent placenta.

Early trophoblast development in humans exhibits some differences in comparison to rodents. In contrast to rodent placentation, trophectoderm adjacent to the inner cell mass does not organize into a cylindrical structure comprising the ectoplacental cone or extra embryonic ectoderm, but continues to proliferate as mononuclear cytotrophoblast cells that fuse to form an erosive multinucleated syncytiotrophoblast. Overall, the erosive functions of the primordial syncytiotrophoblast in humans are comparable to the functions of the primary trophoblast giant cells in rodents.

THE DEFINITIVE PLACENTA IN HUMANS AND RODENTS

The definitive placenta of humans and rodents contains anatomically and functionally distinct regions. Development of these regions depends on the progressive differentiation of trophoblast cells that specialize depending on proximity to maternal or embryonic tissue. In general, trophoblast cells developing in proximity to the embryo promote the exchange of molecules between maternal and fetal circulations, whereas those cells developing distant from the embryo interact with maternal tissue to promote blood flow to the placenta. A generic illustration depicting the structurally analogous regions of the human and rodent placenta is shown in Figure 77.2A.

Development of the maternal–fetal exchange surface of the placenta

The site of maternal–fetal exchange in rodents, fittingly named the labyrinth zone because of its complex maze-like appearance in cross-section, is architecturally similar and functionally equivalent to that which develops in humans. In both, this region is formed by the fusion of two tissues: trophoblast (referred to as chorion here because it closely opposes the mesothelial membrane surrounding the extra-embryonic cavities), which in rodents is derived from extra-embryonic ectoderm, and the allantois, a vascularized mesoderm emanating from the posterior region of the embryo that will ultimately form the umbilical cord. Hence, placentation in rodents and humans is classified as the chorioallantoic type. In mice, apposition and fusion of the allantois with the chorion occurs around E 8.5. Fetal blood vessels emanate from the allantoic mesoderm and induce chorionic trophoblast cells to undergo extensive branching morphogenesis, producing complex tree-like villous formations that provide an extensive surface area for exchange of materials between maternal and fetal circulations (Figure 77.2B). The most distinctive feature of trophoblast cells lining villi is that they are typically fused, forming a multinucleated syncytiotrophoblast that acts to control the diffusion of materials between circulations. A notable difference in human placental development is that trophoblast syncytialization and primary villous formation precede chorioallantoic fusion, although allantoic mesoderm is still required to complete villous maturation and vascularization.

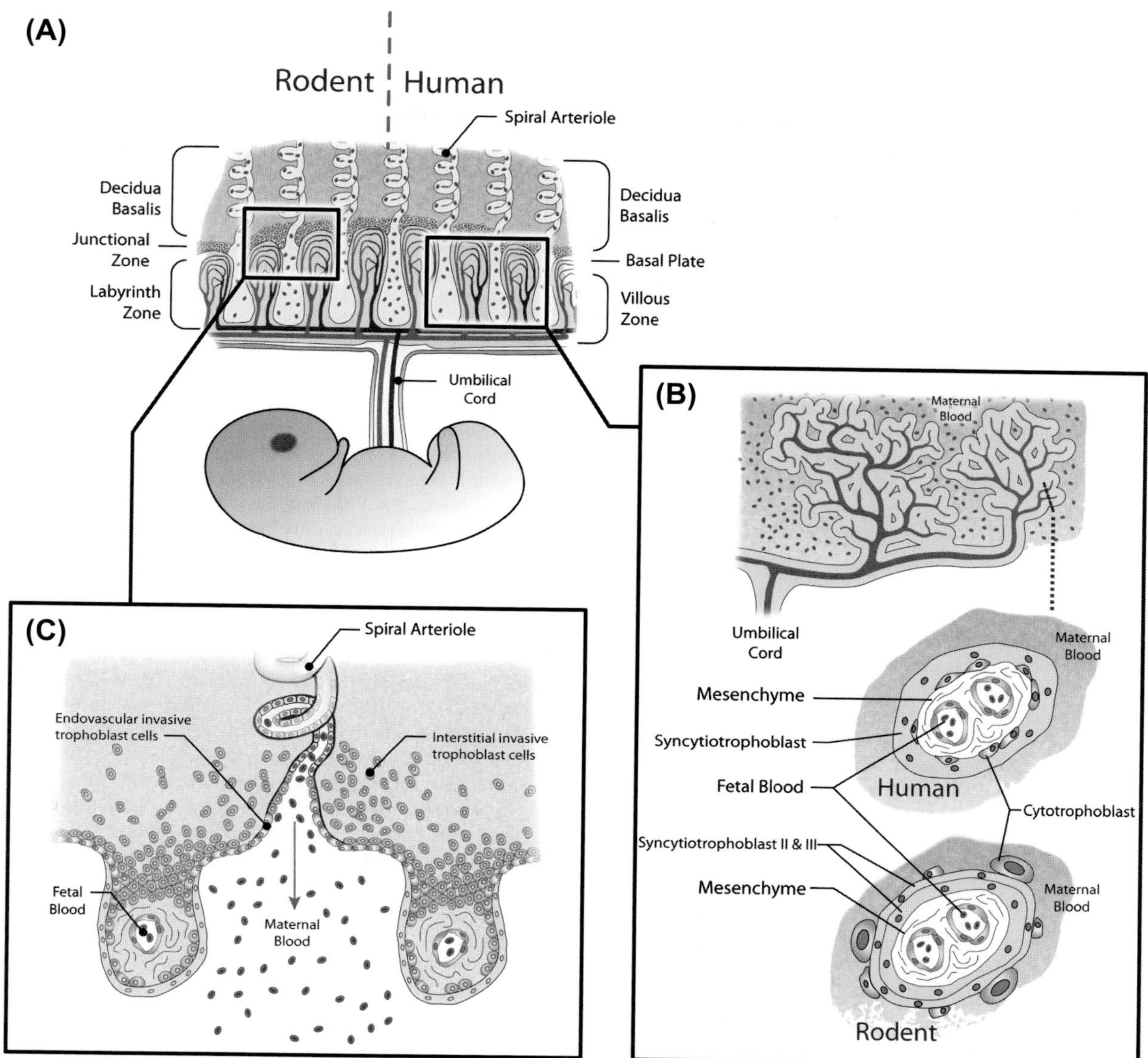

FIGURE 77.2 Schematic representation of analogous structural regions of the definitive human and rodent placenta. (A) Generic structural organization of the rodent and human placenta. Nomenclature associated with rodent placentation is shown on the left, whereas nomenclature related to human placentation is described on the right. (B) Enlarged view of generic maternal–fetal exchange site depicting tree-like villous structures encasing umbilical vessels and bathed in maternal blood. Below, arrangement of villous strata in humans (top) and rodent (bottom) are shown in cross-section. (C) Magnified view of trophoblast–decidual interface, portraying endovascular and interstitial invasive trophoblast cells within the decidua basalis associated with a uterine spiral arteriole. Note the increased internal diameter in the portion of the spiral arteriole lined by trophoblast cells. Please refer to color plate section.

Villous structures are composed of an outer layer of trophoblast bathed in maternal blood surrounding a core of mesenchyme and vessels, which connect to the fetal circulation via the umbilical cord. Therefore, maternal blood is separated from fetal blood by five layers: (1) trophoblast, (2) loosely adherent trophoblast basement membrane, (3) a variable amount of mesenchyme, including fibroblasts and macrophages, (4) endothelial basement membrane, and (5) fetal capillary endothelium. This organization is consistent in species exhibiting hemochorial placentation (Figure 77.2B). Maternal–fetal exchange takes place at the smallest villous branches, sites where fetal capillaries lie in close proximity to the syncytiotrophoblast and, in many cases, the basement membranes of these structures fuse. Larger villi contain the stem branches of fetal vessels and provide structural support for the smaller branches.

Despite similar compositions of villi in rodents and humans, superficial differences exist. For example, the cellular organization of the rodent villous trophoblast differs from its human analog. Rodent villous trophoblast is trilaminar, consisting of a single, outer layer of mononuclear trophoblast cells (layer I) adjacent to maternal blood, and two strata of inner syncytiotrophoblast layers (layers II and III). Thus, rodent placentae are classified as trichorial. Importantly, both layers I and II are in direct contact with maternal blood, whereas layers II and III communicate with each other through gap junctions. Thus, the two layers of syncytiotrophoblast functionally act as a single layer. Human placentae, on the other hand, have a single layer of syncytiotrophoblast outlining the villi and are thus classified as monochorial. However, it should be noted that a second, internal layer of mononuclear cytotrophoblast is present adjacent to the syncytiotrophoblast layer. These underlying villous cytotrophoblast cells are proliferative and act as progenitor cells that fuse with the overlying syncytiotrophoblast for continuous regeneration of the syncytial mass. Villous cytotrophoblast cells form an uninterrupted layer early in pregnancy, but by term these cells exist in discontinuous clusters. A cross-sectional comparison in villous strata between rodents and humans is illustrated in Figure 77.2B.

Despite these anatomical differences, functional analogies can be made between the arrangements of rodent trichorial and human monochorial villi. In both, the syncytiotrophoblast layer(s) act as the barrier to diffusion of materials from maternal blood to the villous core. The functional relevance of the outer mononuclear cytotrophoblast in rodents is not known, but may assist in blood stasis to protect the delicate apical surface of the syncytiotrophoblast and facilitate diffusion of materials. This function is performed by extensive microvilli present on the apical surface of syncytiotrophoblast in humans. Interestingly, during the later stages of pregnancy some of these rodent mononuclear cytotrophoblast cells endoreduplicate and form a type of trophoblast giant cell, albeit with different functional properties than primary trophoblast giant cells (Simmons *et al.*, 2007). Also in both rodents and humans, syncytiotrophoblast is formed through the fusion of mononuclear progenitor cells. These villous cytotrophoblast cells are retained in later pregnancy in humans but not rodents, although small clusters of glycogen-rich mononuclear clusters are present in the murine labyrinth zone that may be vestigial cytotrophoblast cells that failed to undergo fusion. Regardless, the preservation of progenitor cytotrophoblast cells until the later aspects of pregnancy may relate to the much longer duration of pregnancy in humans. The remainder of the villous core consists of a similar composition of allantoic mesenchyme and vasculature in rodents as in humans.

Extravillous trophoblast cells and decidual–trophoblastic interactions

The extravillous portion of the placenta consists of trophoblast cells interacting with uterine decidual cells. These interactions have key roles in the establishment and maintenance of pregnancy, including embryo implantation, anchorage of the placenta to the uterus, hormone secretion, immunological tolerance, and transformation of the uterine vasculature so as to supply the placenta with sufficient maternal blood. The general structure of the extravillous portion of the placenta in relation to the villous zone and decidua basalis is depicted in Figure 77.2C.

Trophoblast cells situated in proximity to the decidua basalis do not undergo branching morphogenesis nor do they associate with fetal vasculature like their counterparts at the site of maternal–fetal exchange. Rather, these cells proliferate and stratify, forming a highly compact cellular region breached only by channels carrying maternal blood to and from the placental exchange surface. In rodents, this region is referred to as the junctional zone because of its location sandwiched between the labyrinth zone and decidua basalis. The junctional zone is comprised of trophoblast cells originating within the ectoplacental cone. In humans, the analogous structure is named the basal plate or cytotrophoblast shell. Unlike the organization of trophoblast lining the villous placenta, trophoblast cells within this region remain mononuclear. In humans, these cells are collectively called extravillous trophoblast cells, aptly named for their external location in relation to the villous structures. Morphologically, two types of extravillous trophoblast cells can be identified, proximal eosinophilic cells and distal glycogen-rich cells. The functional significance of these morphological differences is unclear, although the apical localization of glycogen-containing extravillous trophoblast cells indicates that they may spawn the invasive trophoblast lineage, which will be discussed in the next paragraph. In rodents, three distinct trophoblast cell types can be identified in the junctional zone: secondary trophoblast giant cells, spongiotrophoblast cells and glycogen cells. The phenotypic characteristics of giant cells have previously been introduced, but these secondary giant cells, originating from the periphery of the ectoplacental cone, have some different properties than primary giant cells or labyrinthine giant cells (Simmons *et al.*, 2007). Secondary trophoblast giant cells form a monolayer at the outer regions of the junctional zone, and directly interface with the decidua basalis during early pregnancy. Therefore, it is thought that they play a primary role in the promotion of immunological tolerance via interactions with uterine leukocytes. Secondary trophoblast giant cells are also purported to facilitate implantation, phagocytosis and secretion of cytokines and hormones that promote decidual remodeling during placental expansion. Morphologically it is unclear whether human placentation contains cells comparable to rodent trophoblast giant cells, although given their functions, they have been compared to distal extravillous trophoblast cells interfacing the decidua during early pregnancy (Rossant and Cross, 2001). Spongiotrophoblast cells constitute the majority of the junctional zone, forming a stratified cell layer situated between the labyrinth zone and the secondary trophoblast giant cells. The functional significance of spongiotrophoblast cells is not fully understood, although these cells secrete hormones and cytokines that may be important for decidual remodeling during placental expansion. During the last half of pregnancy, cellular islands containing enormous supplies of glycogen appear within the junctional zone. These cells are appropriately named glycogen cells and appear to give rise to invasive trophoblast cells. Thus, the cellular composition of the rodent junctional zone closely resembles the basal plate in humans.

A separate population of trophoblast cells – the invasive trophoblast lineage – also arises within this region of the placenta, derived from extravillous cytotrophoblast cells and spongiotrophoblast/glycogen cells in humans and rodents, respectively. These invasive trophoblast cells abandon the compact cellular layer where they are derived and migrate into the decidua basalis via two routes: through the uterine parenchyma (interstitial invasion) and within the lumen of the uterine spiral arterioles (endovascular invasion). The different routes of invasion are depicted in Figure 77.2C. The objective of this trophoblast incursion into maternal tissue is to transform the spiral arterioles, the primary feeder vessels of the placenta, into large bore vessels with increased capacity, thus ensuring adequate and consistent blood supply for the exchange surface of the placenta. Altered trophoblast invasion resulting in deficient uteroplacental perfusion is the primary placental defect associated with a number of pregnancy complications, including preeclampsia, fetal growth restriction and the placenta cretas.

The processes regulating rodent and human trophoblast invasion are similar (Pijnenborg *et al.*, 1981). Maturation to an invasive phenotype involves changes in gene expression that promote cessation of proliferation and modification in the expression of cell adhesion molecules and proteases that facilitate cell movement. The rate and depth of invasion is generally most pronounced near the center of the placenta and is significantly less at the periphery. It should be noted, however, that while trophoblast colonization of the decidua occurs during the first half of pregnancy in humans, trophoblast invasion commences at mid-gestation in mice and rats, and continues until near term. In addition, although humans and rodents exhibit both endovascular and interstitial trophoblast invasion, the initial routes of invasion differ between humans and rodents, being primarily interstitial in the former and endovascular in the latter. Interestingly, following the cessation of trophoblast invasion, interstitial trophoblast "giant" cells with high DNA content have been reported within the human decidua basalis. While these giant cells may be comparable to classical trophoblast giant cells in rodents, it is thought that these human "giant" cells arise from fusion of two or more dormant interstitial invasive trophoblast cells rather than through endoreduplication.

Despite these differences, the ultimate goal of spiral arteriole transformation is comparable in humans as in rodents, particularly in larger rodents with more extensive trophoblast invasion such as rats (Ain *et al.*, 2003; Caluwaerts *et al.*, 2005; Vercruysse *et al.*, 2006; Konno *et al.*, 2007). In both, spiral arteriole transformation entails replacement of the endothelium by trophoblast, subsequent development of a pseudoendothelial phenotype, and progressive substitution of the elastic laminae and smooth muscle with a trophoblast-derived fibrous extracellular matrix. This process is likely mediated by deliberate induction of apoptosis and phagocytosis by tumor necrosis factor super family ligands and matrix proteases expressed by trophoblast cells (Ashton *et al.*, 2005), whereas subsequent pseudoendothelialization promotes vascular integrity and discourages maternal immune reactivity and coagulation (Damsky and Fisher, 1998).

Maternal cell populations located at the interface with the placenta are heterogeneous and referred to as the decidua basalis. This structure is situated immediately adjacent to the fetal–maternal boundary and extends as far as the myometrium. In rodents, a specialized extension of the decidua basalis forms between the circular and longitudinal uterine musculature, and is termed the mesometrial triangle or metrial gland. The decidua is formed preemptively in humans as a physiological result of the formation of the corpus luteum and increases in systemic estrogen and progesterone during each menstrual cycle. The human uterus is maximally receptive to blastocyst implantation approximately 6–9 days following ovulation. In rodents, coital stimulation is necessary to activate neuroendocrine signaling required to maintain the corpus luteum and sustain progesterone production. Decidualization is then triggered following blastocyst implantation, which occurs 4–5 days following ovulation. Even though there are species differences regarding the initiation of decidualization, the composition of cells that comprise the decidua is similar between humans and rodents. The main constituents of the decidua are large polygonal endometrial stromal cells with high glycogen and lipid content that facilitate implantation, early embryo nutrition, hormone secretion and regulation of trophoblast invasiveness. Interspersed within the parenchyma are cells associated with endometrial glands and the aforementioned uterine spiral arterioles. A unique assortment of immune cells is also present within the decidua, including macrophages and relatively small numbers of T lymphocytes possessing unusually low alloreactivity, and an immense population of CD56 bright, $CD16^{-}$ natural killer (NK) cells. The latter collection of NK cells is almost exclusively restricted to the uterus. These uterine NK cells localize near spiral arterioles and, in rodents, have been shown to play key roles in pretrophoblastic spiral arteriole modification (Ashkar and Croy, 2001).

Later in gestation, invasive trophoblast cells also colonize the decidua basalis. The depth of trophoblast invasion varies depending on the species, strain and existence of pathological circumstances. Invasive trophoblast cells in mice extend throughout the decidua but not further, whereas in larger rodents such as rats and guinea-pigs, invasive trophoblast cells reach significantly greater depths, expanding well into the mesometrial triangle. In humans, trophoblast cells are highly invasive and can be found throughout the decidua as far as the proximal third of the myometrium, but invasion is significantly shallower in some pregnancy complications, including preeclampsia and fetal growth restriction.

APPROPRIATE MODELS OF HEMOCHORIAL PLACENTATION

The remainder of this chapter is devoted to describing materials and brief methodologies available for the study of hemochorial placentation.

Ex vivo approaches

The placenta is a transient organ that implants within the uterus for a finite period of time, but is expelled at pregnancy termination. Many researchers with access to placental tissues conduct *ex vivo* experiments under controlled culture conditions. Placental tissue from humans is derived from elective termination of pregnancy, Cesarean section, or after labor and delivery, whereas *ex vivo* experimentation in mice and rats is accomplished by removal of preimplantation embryos or dissection of postimplantation placentation sites.

The benefits of *ex vivo* experimentation on discarded placental tissue include the wide availability of tissue, preservation of cell–tissue interactions and the ability to manipulate culture conditions. However, placental tissues collected in this way have been exposed to variable levels of stress associated with expulsion from the uterus, particularly following labored delivery, and thus the condition of the tissue during experimentation may not reflect its appropriate behavior in an *in vivo* setting. Similarly, removal of intact tissue exposed to endogenous hormonal and immunological stimuli and vascular perfusion may affect tissue integrity and cell behavior. Regardless, *ex vivo* experimentation is a valuable resource to gain insight into placental function.

Early embryo culture

Preimplantation embryos can be collected from rodents (mouse: E 3.5; rat: E 4.5) by flushing the uterine horns with an appropriate medium. *In vitro* analysis is also feasible using early human embryos; however, it is regulated under much stricter ethical guidelines and is less commonly used for basic research. Cultured appropriately, preimplantation embryos continue to develop and, if placed on a suitable matrix, recapitulate events associated with blastocyst implantation and early trophoblast invasion (Armant, 2006). Early embryo culture is also used for the isolation of trophoblast stem (TS) and embryonic stem (ES) cells, which will be covered in detail in a later section. Therefore, early embryo culture is a valuable approach to gain insight into molecular events associated with implantation and early trophoblast development.

Placental perfusion

The placenta is a highly vascular organ housing two circulations: maternal and fetal. Separation of the placenta from the mother and fetus during pregnancy termination removes vascular perfusion, which may alter the structural and functional integrity of the placenta. To avoid this, researchers have adopted strategies to perfuse the placenta *ex vivo* by continuous pumping of a perfusate at a specific pressure through catheters inserted within chorionic vessels (for fetal circulation) and within the decidual surface (for maternal circulation) (Schneider, 1991). In humans, this methodology is generally restricted to term placentae due to the fragility of placentae isolated from earlier pregnancy. The uniqueness of this approach is that it enables pharmacological substances to be included with the perfusate, thus allowing researchers to investigate transport properties of the placenta and the effect of these compounds on placental structure and function. This type of methodology is generally not used for murine specimens because of the difficulty in catheterization, and because of the availability of much broader experimental possibilities that allow for pharmacological experimentation *in vivo*. However, vascular corrosion casting of the fetal and maternal aspects of the placenta has been used to study murine placental architecture, indicating that this methodology is feasible in these species (Whiteley *et al.*, 2006).

Placental explants

Placental explants cultured *in vitro* are useful for determining adaptive responses of placental cells to alterations in their milieu. Explants are prepared by dissecting and mincing placental tissue into small masses, followed by plating into appropriate tissue culture wells and incubation for a finite period of time (Miller *et al.*, 2005; Aplin, 2006). Due to the nature of their preparation, explants are essentially a heterogeneous population of placental cells with preservation of some cell–cell and cell–matrix interactions. Therefore, explants are valuable tools for studying placental biology within controlled conditions because they retain some level of tissue integrity. However, because of the heterogeneous nature of placental explants, their variable exposure to maternal factors, and their susceptibility to necrosis, culture durations are generally short and extra caution must be exercised to minimize intra- and inter-experimental variation.

Explants can be prepared from placentas obtained from human or rodent pregnancy. In humans, explants derived from placentae collected from term pregnancy are predominantly used for studying villous function, including transport, viability and expression of hormones, cytokines and growth factors. Controlled environmental pressures can then be used to assess for changes in villous morphology or function. A related methodology involves comparisons in placental function between explants prepared from uncomplicated pregnancies and those prepared from pregnancies with obstetric complications to determine if functional differences exist. Early placental explant cultures can be used to study similar factors associated with villous function, and are also useful to evaluate the biochemistry of cytotrophoblast proliferation, differentiation of extravillous trophoblast cells and extravillous cytotrophoblast invasion through specific matrices. In rodents, placental explants have similarly been used for the study of rodent placental biology *ex vivo*, although these tissue dissections require some skill and considerable practice. Cultures consist of individual regions isolated using a dissecting microscope (ectoplacental cone, junctional zone, metrial gland, labyrinth zone).

In vitro approaches using cell culture models

The ability to study pertinent biological and molecular phenomena *in vitro* has been greatly improved by using isolated cells in culture. Cultured cells are generally homogeneous, abundant and more readily manipulated by simple molecular biological means in comparison to experiments conducted *ex vivo* or *in vivo*. As such, these techniques afford the researcher a wide source of biological material with which to perform mechanistic studies, and greater inter-experimental precision. With respect to placental biology, the use of cultured trophoblast cells has vastly increased our understanding of various aspects of placental development, such as the regulation of cell survival, proliferation and differentiation, and the study of placental physiology including invasive, immunological and signaling functions. Endometrial stromal cells have also been isolated and stimulated to form decidual cells (Ramathal *et al.*, 2010). There are limitations when using *in vitro* models, especially considering that cells in culture are removed from their *in vivo* environment and may thus behave differently. This is especially the case for cells that are cancerous or manipulated to ensure they proliferate and remain viable in culture. Reconstituting the *in vivo* environment through culturing on extracellular matrices or co-culturing with other cell types has merit but also possesses limitations. These limitations should be considered when extrapolating data to the *in vivo* setting.

Primary cell culture

The isolation and enrichment of primary trophoblast cells is a valuable technique that allows for more advanced functional and molecular experiments to be performed. The technique most often used to extract and purify trophoblast cells is based on methodology developed by Kliman and co-workers (Kliman *et al.*, 1986), which uses enzyme-mediated dissociation or phenotypic characteristics to extract individual cells from human placental tissue. Isolated cells are subsequently enriched using density gradient centrifugation and/or positive or negative selection, cultured and used for mechanistic studies while they remain viable. First trimester trophoblast may be advantageous for investigating derivation of both villous and extravillous trophoblast development, whereas term cytotrophoblast may be best suited for examination of villous trophoblast development. Primary trophoblast cells can also be established from cultured human placental explants. As mentioned previously, explants are generally prepared either from first trimester tissue obtained after elective pregnancy termination, or term placenta attained following delivery by Caesarean section. In brief, explants are plated on uncoated wells or wells layered with matrices. After a variable incubation period, non-adherent villous cells and tissue are removed, resulting in a population of adherent cytotrophoblast cells that can be retrieved by trypsinization or matrix digestion. Using this tissue, it is possible to isolate relatively pure populations of extravillous cytotrophoblast cells by exploiting the adhesive and invasive characteristics of these cells. Primary trophoblast cells have also been isolated and cultured from rodent placentae (Thordarson *et al.*, 1987; Lu *et al.*, 1994).

In comparison to *ex vivo* approaches that utilize heterogeneous placental cell populations, the use of primary trophoblast cells allows for enrichment of more homogeneous cell types, thereby facilitating the study of trophoblast physiology in relative isolation. In addition, primary cells are often preferred to transformed or immortalized cell lines because they have undergone few population doublings or manipulations, and are therefore considered more representative of cells *in vivo*. However, there are several difficulties with this technique, including inter-experimental variability, the need for rigorous characterization to avoid contamination with unwanted cell types and changes in cell viability or phenotype throughout the duration of experimentation. In addition, there may be modifications in trophoblast behavior or viability after isolation due to loss of interactions with other placental cells and enzymatic dissociation from extracellular matrices. Finally, it is preferable not to attempt isolation of cells from placentae delivered via vaginal delivery, as cellular phenotypes may change during the labor process and there is an increased risk of contamination with unwanted cell types.

TS cell culture

Pioneering studies in mice showed that TS cells could be isolated from early embryos, and maintained in a diploid, undifferentiated and self-renewing state when cultured in appropriate conditions (Tanaka *et al.*, 1998). Modification of these conditions results in the induction of differentiation into several mature trophoblast subtypes, primarily secondary trophoblast giant cells but also spongiotrophoblast cells and syncytiotrophoblast, with phenotypes comparable to their *in vivo* counterparts. Furthermore, reintroduction of TS cells into early mouse embryos reveals that TS cells are capable of forming all structures of the placenta. Experimentation using mouse TS cells has vastly increased our understanding of TS cell behavior and the molecular regulation of trophoblast differentiation. Recently, rat TS cells cultured using similar conditions as mouse TS cells have also been isolated. When differentiated *in vitro*, rat TS cells are capable of forming all trophoblast subtypes similar to mouse TS cells (Asanoma and Soares, unpublished observations). Additionally, a rat choriocarcinoma (cancerous trophoblast) stem cell line Rcho-1 has also been isolated and well characterized (Faria and Soares, 1991). This cell line can be maintained in proliferative stem conditions and induced to differentiate by removal of growth factor-containing serum. Under these conditions, Rcho-1 stem cells primarily differentiate to trophoblast giant cells, and have been used as a tool to study trophoblast differentiation.

Unlike derivation of mouse and rat TS cells, isolation and characterization of human TS cells has been more difficult due to the limited availability of human embryos and apparently distinct culture requirements for their propagation. Clusters of human TS cells possessing properties similar to their murine counterparts have been identified in first trimester human placentas but have not been successfully cultured (Hemberger *et al.*, 2010).

Human ES cells

Unlike their rodent counterparts, human ES cells spontaneously differentiate into trophoblast-like cells, particularly following induction with bone morphogenetic protein-4 (Xu *et al.*, 2002). Human ES-derived trophoblast cells express many genes characteristic of differentiated human trophoblast. Thus far, appropriate culture conditions have not yet been established to maximize self-renewal of these human ES cell-derived trophoblast cells. Once committed to the trophoblast lineage the cells differentiate. Future studies are required to better understand the biological relevance of human ES cell-derived trophoblast, including a comparison with trophoblast cells derived from early embryos.

Spontaneous, immortalized and transformed trophoblast cell lines

Trophoblast cell lines have become an invaluable tool to study various aspects of trophoblast biology. These cell lines are more resilient when compared to cultures of primary trophoblast cells, including extended lifespans in culture, and are thus advantageous for studies encompassing more detailed investigations of trophoblast function and molecular biology. Trophoblast cell lines can be established from primary cultures by spontaneous *in vitro* selection or by ectopic expression of oncoproteins that confer immortality. Choriocarcinoma cells are transformed populations of trophoblast cells that readily adapt to *in vitro* conditions. However, because of these traits, data obtained from these manipulated or transformed cell lines must be interpreted with caution. These trophoblast cell lines have been removed from their *in vivo* environment for many passages and can be distorted in some of their properties. Regardless, they are commonly used as a convenient and valuable resource to provide insight into trophoblast function. A list of commonly used human trophoblast cell lines is provided in Table 77.1.

In vivo approaches

In vivo models are essential for the study of hemochorial placentation. The following descriptions of *in vivo* models of hemochorial placentation are exclusively based on experimentation in mice and rats (Ain *et al.*, 2006; Natale *et al.*, 2006). In addition to the various parallels between rodent and human placentation presented throughout this chapter, mice and rats are extremely useful for studies in reproduction because they are cost- and space-effective, have relatively short gestations, mature rapidly and exhibit multiparity (more than one conceptus per gestation). In addition, the genetics of these species are becoming increasingly well defined. Mice and rats are also commonly used for modeling

TABLE 77.1 Human trophoblast cell culture models

Name	Source	Method	Reference
Spontaneous			
ED27, ED31	First trimester	Chorionic villous	(Morgan *et al.*, 1998)
ED77	First trimester	Chorionic villous	(Diss *et al.*, 1992)
HT	Term	Chorionic villous	(Ho *et al.*, 1994)
HT-116	First trimester	Extravillous	(Zdravkovic *et al.*, 1999)
HTR-8	First trimester	Extravillous	(Graham *et al.*, 1993)
NHT	First trimester	Chorionic villous	(Nagami *et al.*, 1991)
NPC	First trimester	Chorionic villous	(Rong-Hao *et al.*, 1996)
TL	Term	Chorionic villous	(Ho *et al.*, 1987)
Immortalized			
B6-Tert	NPC	Telomerase	(Wang *et al.*, 2006)
HChEpC1b	Primary first trimester	HPV E6/E7 + Telomerase	(Omi *et al.*, 2009)
HP-A1, A2, W1	Primary term	SV40 T antigen	(Lei *et al.*, 1992)
HTR-8/Svneo	HTR-8	SV40 T antigen	(Graham *et al.*, 1993)
IST-1	Primary first trimester	HPV E6/E7	(Shih *et al.*, 1998)
RSVT-2	HTR-8	RSV	(Khoo *et al.*, 1998)
SGHPL-4, -5	Primary first trimester	SV40 T antigen	(Choy and Manyonda, 1998)
Spa-26	Primary first trimester	SV40 T antigen	(Chou, 1978)
TCL-1	Primary term	SV40 T antigen	(Lewis *et al.*, 1996)
Choriocarcinoma			
AC1-1 to AC1-9	Jeg-3 Mutant		(Funayama, 1997)
ACH-1P to ACH-3P	AC1-1/trophoblast fusion		(Frank *et al.*, 2000)
Bewo	Choriocarcinoma		(Pattillo and Gey, 1968)
Jar	Choriocarcinoma		(Pattillo *et al.*, 1971)
Jeg-3	Choriocarcinoma		(Kohler and Bridson, 1971)

Notes:
HPV E6/E7 = Human papillomavirus-16 early genes E6 and E7
SV40 T antigen = Simian virus-40 large (and small) T antigen
RSV = Rous sarcoma virus

human pregnancy complications such as preeclampsia and fetal growth restriction (Cross, 2003; Podjarny *et al.*, 2004; Banerjee *et al.*, 2009). Most of these models focus on the manifestations of the diseases without addressing the underlying placental pathology. It should also be noted that other *in vivo* models of hemochorial placentation, such as the guinea-pig and non-human primates, have contributed greatly to our understanding of placental development and function. For more information on other animal models of placentation, the reader is referred to Carter (2007).

Transgenesis and gene targeting

Transgenesis is a mode of experimentation involving insertion of a foreign gene into the genome of an organism, followed by germ-line transmission of the gene and analysis of the resulting phenotype in the progeny. Transgenesis can be used to induce the expression of an exogenous gene of interest. Alternatively, gene targeting can be used to interrupt the sequence ("knockout") of a specific endogenous gene. The use of transgenic and gene targeted animals, primarily mice, has significantly increased our understanding of the genetic regulation of placental development; specific knockout mice have been generated that exhibit defective placentation in various stages of placental development, including trophectoderm determination, trophoblast expansion and differentiation, implantation, chorioallantoic fusion, as well as formation and cellular composition of the labyrinth and junctional zones (Simmons and Cross, 2005). Many of these knockouts result in placental phenotypes that interfere with fetal viability. Interestingly, *in situ* and *in vitro* studies using human placental material indicate that many of these mutated genes are involved in human placental development and physiology, providing further evidence of conservation in placental development between mice and humans (Cox *et al.*, 2009). Given the increasing availability of genetically engineered mouse lines and the advent of transgenesis and gene targeting in other mammals including rats, the use of this methodology will be integral to furthering our understanding of placental development.

Lentiviral-mediated gene delivery in trophoblast cells

Lentiviral-mediated gene delivery is a useful approach for manipulating genes specifically within the trophoblast lineage. Unlike transgenesis, which usually modifies genes in all cells of an embryo, lentiviral-mediated gene delivery exploits the peripheral segregation of the trophectoderm and its tight epithelium to specifically infect cells of the trophoblast lineage, sparing the inner cell mass. Lentivirus, in turn, can be manipulated prior to transduction to contain plasmids expressing specific genetic coding regions. These sequences can code for a specific gene of interest, facilitating overexpression in the trophoblast lineage, or alternatively sequences may be designed to code for short hairpin RNA sequences that inhibit the activity of a specific gene (Georgiades *et al.*, 2007; Okada *et al.*, 2007; Lee *et al.*, 2009). Thus, gene expression is modified in all derivatives of the trophectoderm, but not in the embryo or other extra-embryonic membranes.

The methodology of lentiviral-mediated gene delivery involves early embryo culture in the presence of lentiviral particles. Infected blastocysts are then transferred to pseudopregnant females (females mated with vasectomized males), and placental development is assessed throughout gestation. The challenges with this technique are the development of the skill sets required to handle and manipulate early embryos and the requirement of preliminary experimentation to ensure optimal gene delivery and minimal toxicity. Despite these technical requirements, the possibility of trophoblast-specific gene manipulation is powerful; and thus a key research strategy for gaining insight into the regulation of placental development.

In vivo *models of trophoblast invasion*

Studying the regulation of trophoblast invasion has been of immense interest ever since defective trophoblast invasion became linked to preeclampsia and fetal growth restriction decades ago (Robertson *et al.*, 1967). Since *in vivo* analysis of trophoblast invasion in the human is not feasible, the primary methodology to study its regulation is based on *ex vivo* explant outgrowths or *in vitro* invasion assays. While these methods have some merit, trophoblast invasion is a complex process regulated by various *in vivo* factors that cannot possibly be replicated in an *in vitro* setting. In addition, differential factors such as route of invasion (endovascular vs. interstitial) or the process of spiral arteriole remodeling also cannot be assessed. Consequently, the use of animals as models of trophoblast invasion and spiral arteriole remodeling is attractive. Rats, in particular, are promising *in vivo* models for the study of trophoblast invasion, based on the increased depth of invasion and extensive spiral arteriole remodeling compared with mice (Ain *et al.*, 2003; Pijnenborg and Vercruysse, 2004).

Experimentation using rat models is beneficial for understanding both genetic and environmental factors that regulate trophoblast invasion. From a genetics standpoint, considerable information is being garnered from the rat genome, and the availability of rat transgenics is progressively being expanded. Investigation of placentation in transgenics could yield valuable information and provide novel hypotheses on the regulation of trophoblast invasion. In addition, there are strain-specific differences in the depth of invasion, indicating that genetic disparities may be involved in regulating the extent of invasion. For example, trophoblast invasion in the brown Norway rat is much less extensive than in other strains such as Holtzmann, Sprague-Dawley or Wistar, and is associated with poor pregnancy performance (Konno *et al.*, 2007). Analysis of these strain differences may lead to the identification of novel genetic regulatory networks associated with invasion. Finally, altering environmental variables can affect placentation and the capacity of trophoblast cells to invade. An example of this is challenging rats with low oxygen atmospheres, which stimulates robust trophoblast invasion in comparison with rats housed in ambient conditions (Rosario *et al.*, 2008). Future studies using the rat as a model could be beneficial in understanding genetic and environmental factors regulating trophoblast invasion.

CONCLUDING REMARKS AND FUTURE DIRECTIONS

When studying hemochorial placentation, it is vital to establish an appropriate model to address the hypothesis in question. Throughout the first part of this chapter, we described the basic anatomy and physiology of hemochorial placentation in the human and in mice and rats. The goal of this general overview was to provide the reader with a background focusing on similarities and differences with which to determine whether human tissue, an *in vitro* approach or an animal model would be most appropriate for their studies of hemochorial placental development. There are potential limitations to any one experimental approach. Thus, it should be emphasized that the incorporation of multiple model systems in an overall research strategy for investigating hemochorial placentation is meritorious.

ACKNOWLEDGMENTS

We would like to thank Stanton Fenton for illustrative assistance, and all past and current members of our laboratory. SJR is supported by a post-doctoral fellowship awarded by the Lalor Foundation. This work was supported by grants from the National Institutes of Health HD020676, HD048861, HD055523 and HD060115.

REFERENCES

Adjaye J, Huntriss J, Herwig R, BenKahla A, Brink TC, Wierling C, Hultschig C, Groth D, Yaspo ML, Picton HM, Gosden RG, Lehrach H (2005) Primary differentiation in the human blastocyst: comparative molecular portraits of inner cell mass and trophectoderm cells. *Stem Cells* **23:** 1514–25.

Ain R, Canham LN, Soares MJ (2003) Gestation stage-dependent intrauterine trophoblast cell invasion in the rat and mouse: novel endocrine phenotype and regulation. *Dev Biol* **260:** 176–90.

Ain R, Konno T, Canham LN, Soares MJ (2006) Phenotypic analysis of the rat placenta. *Methods Mol Med* **121:** 295–313.

Aplin JD (2006) In vitro analysis of trophoblast invasion. *Methods Mol Med* **122:** 45–57.

Armant DR (2006) Blastocyst culture. *Methods Mol Med* **121:** 35–56.

Ashkar AA, Croy BA (2001) Functions of uterine natural killer cells are mediated by interferon gamma production during murine pregnancy. *Semin Immunol* **13:** 235–41.

Ashton SV, Whitley GS, Dash PR, Wareing M, Crocker IP, Baker PN, Cartwright JE (2005) Uterine spiral artery remodeling involves endothelial apoptosis induced by extravillous trophoblasts through Fas/FasL interactions. *Arterioscler Thromb Vasc Biol* **25:** 102–8.

Banerjee S, Randeva H, Chambers AE (2009) Mouse models for preeclampsia: disruption of redox-regulated signaling. *Reprod Biol Endocrinol* **7:** 4.

Caluwaerts S, Vercruysse L, Luyten C, Pijnenborg R (2005) Endovascular trophoblast invasion and associated structural changes in uterine spiral arteries of the pregnant rat. *Placenta* **26:** 574–84.

Carter AM (2007) Animal models of human placentation – a review. *Placenta* **28 (Suppl. A):** S41–S47.

Carter AM, Enders AC (2004) Comparative aspects of trophoblast development and placentation. *Reprod Biol Endocrinol* **2:** 46.

Chou JY (1978) Establishment of clonal human placental cells synthesizing human choriogonadotropin. *Proc Natl Acad Sci USA* **75:** 1854–8.

Choy MY, Manyonda IT (1998) The phagocytic activity of human first trimester extravillous trophoblast. *Hum Reprod* **13:** 2941–9.

Cox B, Kotlyar M, Evangelou AI, Ignatchenko V, Ignatchenko A, Whiteley K, Jurisica I, Adamson SL, Rossant J, Kislinger T (2009) Comparative systems biology of human and mouse as a tool to guide the modeling of human placental pathology. *Mol Syst Biol* **5:** 279.

Cross JC (2003) The genetics of pre-eclampsia: a feto-placental or maternal problem? *Clin Genet* **64:** 96–103.

Cross JC, Werb Z, Fisher SJ (1994) Implantation and the placenta: key pieces of the development puzzle. *Science* **266:** 1508–18.

Damsky CH, Fisher SJ (1998) Trophoblast pseudo-vasculogenesis: faking it with endothelial adhesion receptors. *Curr Opin Cell Biol* **10:** 660–6.

Dey SK, Lim H, Das SK, Reese J, Paria BC, Daikoku T, Wang H (2004) Molecular cues to implantation. *Endocr Rev* **25:** 341–73.

Diss EM, Gabbe SG, Moore JW, Kniss DA (1992) Study of thromboxane and prostacyclin metabolism in an in vitro model of first-trimester human trophoblast. *Am J Obstet Gynecol* **167:** 1046–52.

Enders AC, Carter AM (2004) What can comparative studies of placental structure tell us?– A review. *Placenta* **25 (Suppl. A):** S3–S9.

Faria TN, Soares MJ (1991) Trophoblast cell differentiation: establishment, characterization, and modulation of a rat trophoblast cell line expressing members of the placental prolactin family. *Endocrinology* **129:** 2895–906.

Frank HG, Gunawan B, Ebeling-Stark I, Schulten HJ, Funayama H, Cremer U, Huppertz B, Gaus G, Kaufmann P, Fuzesi L (2000) Cytogenetic and DNA-fingerprint characterization of choriocarcinoma cell lines and a trophoblast/choriocarcinoma cell hybrid. *Cancer Genet Cytogenet* **116:** 16–22.

Funayama H, Gaus G, Ebeling I, Takayama M, Fuzesi L, Huppertz B, Kaufmann P, Frank HG (1997) Parent cells for trophoblast hybridization II: AC1 and related trophoblast cell lines, a family of HGPRT-negative mutants of the choriocarcinoma cell line JEG-3. *Placenta* **18 (Suppl. 2):** 191–201.

Georgiades P, Cox B, Gertsenstein M, Chawengsaksophak K, Rossant J (2007) Trophoblast-specific gene manipulation using lentivirus-based vectors. *Biotechniques* **42:** 317–318, 320, 322–325.

Georgiades P, Ferguson-Smith AC, Burton GJ (2002) Comparative developmental anatomy of the murine and human definitive placentae. *Placenta* **23:** 3–19.

Graham CH, Hawley TS, Hawley RG, MacDougall JR, Kerbel RS, Khoo N, Lala PK (1993) Establishment and characterization of first trimester human trophoblast cells with extended lifespan. *Exp Cell Res* **206:** 204–11.

Hemberger M, Udayashankar R, Tesar P, Moore H, Burton GJ (2010) ELF5-enforced transcriptional networks define an epigenetically regulated trophoblast stem cell compartment in the human placenta. *Hum Mol Genet* **19:** 2456–67.

Ho CK, Chiang H, Li SY, Yuan CC, Ng HT (1987) Establishment and characterization of a tumorigenic trophoblast-like cell line from a human placenta. *Cancer Res* **47:** 3220–4.

Ho CK, Li SY, Yu KJ, Wang CC, Chiang H, Wang SY (1994) Characterization of a human tumorigenic, poorly differentiated trophoblast cell line. *In Vitro Cell Dev Biol Anim* **30A:** 415–17.

Khoo NK, Bechberger JF, Shepherd T, Bond SL, McCrae KR, Hamilton GS, Lala PK (1998) SV40 Tag transformation of the normal invasive trophoblast results in a premalignant phenotype. I. Mechanisms responsible for hyperinvasiveness and resistance to anti-invasive action of TGFbeta. *Int J Cancer* **77:** 429–39.

Kliman HJ, Nestler JE, Sermasi E, Sanger JM, Strauss JF 3rd (1986) Purification, characterization, and in vitro differentiation of cytotrophoblasts from human term placentae. *Endocrinology* **118:** 1567–82.

Kohler PO, Bridson WE (1971) Isolation of hormone-producing clonal lines of human choriocarcinoma. *J Clin Endocrinol Metab* **32:** 683–7.

Konno T, Rempel LA, Arroyo JA, Soares MJ (2007) Pregnancy in the brown Norway rat: a model for investigating the genetics of placentation. *Biol Reprod* **76:** 709–18.

Lee DS, Rumi MA, Konno T, Soares MJ (2009) In vivo genetic manipulation of the rat trophoblast cell lineage using lentiviral vector delivery. *Genesis* **47:** 433–9.

Lei KJ, Gluzman Y, Pan CJ, Chou JY (1992) Immortalization of virus-free human placental cells that express tissue-specific functions. *Mol Endocrinol* **6:** 703–12.

Lewis MP, Clements M, Takeda S, Kirby PL, Seki H, Lonsdale LB, Sullivan MH, Elder MG, White JO (1996) Partial characterization of an immortalized human trophoblast cell-line, TCL-1, which possesses a CSF-1 autocrine loop. *Placenta* **17:** 137–46.

Lu XJ, Deb S, Soares MJ (1994) Spontaneous differentiation of trophoblast cells along the spongiotrophoblast cell pathway: expression of members of the placental prolactin gene family and modulation by retinoic acid. *Dev Biol* **163:** 86–97.

Miller RK, Genbacev O, Turner MA, Aplin JD, Caniggia I, Huppertz B (2005) Human placental explants in culture: approaches and assessments. *Placenta* **26:** 439–48.

Morgan M, Kniss D, McDonnell S (1998) Expression of metalloproteinases and their inhibitors in human trophoblast continuous cell lines. *Exp Cell Res* **242:** 18–26.

Nagami AI, Kamitani, N, Tominaga T (1991) Establishment of a human trophoblastic cell line (NHT cell line) from normal early pregnancy: formation of pseudovillus structure in vitro. In *Placenta: Basic Research for Clinical Applications* (Soma H, ed.). Karger, Basel.

Natale DR, Starovic M, Cross JC (2006) Phenotypic analysis of the mouse placenta. *Methods Mol Med* **121:** 275–93.

Niwa H, Toyooka Y, Shimosato D, Strumpf D, Takahashi K, Yagi R, Rossant J (2005) Interaction between Oct3/4 and Cdx2 determines trophectoderm differentiation. *Cell* **123:** 917–29.

Okada Y, Ueshin Y, Isotani A, Saito-Fujita T, Nakashima H, Kimura K, Mizoguchi A, Oh-Hora M, Mori Y, Ogata M, Oshima RG, Okabe M, Ikawa M (2007) Complementation of placental defects and embryonic lethality by trophoblast-specific lentiviral gene transfer. *Nat Biotechnol* **25:** 233–7.

Omi H, Okamoto A, Nikaido T, Urashima M, Kawaguchi R, Umehara N, Sugiura K, Saito M, Kiyono T, Tanaka T (2009) Establishment of an immortalized human extravillous trophoblast cell line by retroviral infection of E6/E7/hTERT and its transcriptional profile during hypoxia and reoxygenation. *Int J Mol Med* **23:** 229–36.

Pattillo RA, Gey GO (1968) The establishment of a cell line of human hormone-synthesizing trophoblastic cells in vitro. *Cancer Res* **28:** 1231–6.

Pattillo RA, Gey GO, Delfs E, Huang WY, Hause L, Garancis DJ, Knoth M, Amatruda J, Bertino J, Friesen HG, Mattingly RF (1971) The hormone-synthesizing trophoblastic cell in vitro: a model for cancer research and placental hormone synthesis. *Ann NY Acad Sci* **172:** 288–98.

Pijnenborg R, Robertson WB, Brosens I, Dixon G (1981) Review article: trophoblast invasion and the establishment of haemochorial placentation in man and laboratory animals. *Placenta* **2:** 71–91.

Pijnenborg R, Vercruysse L (2004) Thomas Huxley and the rat placenta in the early debates on evolution. *Placenta* **25:** 233–7.

Podjarny E, Losonczy G, Baylis C (2004) Animal models of preeclampsia. *Semin Nephrol* **24:** 596–606.

Ramathal CY, Bagchi IC, Taylor RN, Bagchi MK (2010) Endometrial decidualization: of mice and men. *Semin Reprod Med* **28:** 17–26.

Robertson WB, Brosens I, Dixon HG (1967) The pathological response of the vessels of the placental bed to hypertensive pregnancy. *J Pathol Bacteriol* **93:** 581–92.

Rong-Hao L, Luo S, Zhuang LZ (1996) Establishment and characterization of a cytotrophoblast cell line from normal placenta of human origin. *Hum Reprod* **11:** 1328–33.

Rosario GX, Konno T, Soares MJ (2008) Maternal hypoxia activates endovascular trophoblast cell invasion. *Dev Biol* **314:** 362–75.

Rossant J, Cross JC (2001) Placental development: lessons from mouse mutants. *Nat Rev Genet* **2:** 538–48.

Schneider H (1991) The role of the placenta in nutrition of the human fetus. *Am J Obstet Gynecol* **164:** 967–73.

Shih I, Wang T, Wu T, Kurman RJ, Gearhart JD (1998) Expression of Mel-CAM in implantation site intermediate trophoblastic cell line, IST-1, limits its migration on uterine smooth muscle cells. *J Cell Sci* **111 (Pt 17):** 2655–64.

Simmons DG, Cross JC (2005) Determinants of trophoblast lineage and cell subtype specification in the mouse placenta. *Dev Biol* **284:** 12–24.

Simmons DG, Fortier AL, Cross JC (2007) Diverse subtypes and developmental origins of trophoblast giant cells in the mouse placenta. *Dev Biol* **304:** 567–78.

Tanaka S, Kunath T, Hadjantonakis AK, Nagy A, Rossant J (1998) Promotion of trophoblast stem cell proliferation by FGF4. *Science* **282:** 2072–5.

Thordarson G, Folger P, Talamantes F (1987) Development of a placental cell culture system for studying the control of mouse placental lactogen II secretion. *Placenta* **8:** 573–85.

Vercruysse L, Caluwaerts S, Luyten C, Pijnenborg R (2006) Interstitial trophoblast invasion in the decidua and mesometrial triangle during the last third of pregnancy in the rat. *Placenta* **27:** 22–33.

Wang YL, Qiu W, Feng HC, Li YX, Zhuang LZ, Wang Z, Liu Y, Zhou JQ, Zhang DH, Tsao GS (2006) Immortalization of normal human cytotrophoblast cells by reconstitution of telomeric reverse transcriptase activity. *Mol Hum Reprod* **12:** 451–60.

Whiteley KJ, Pfarrer CD, Adamson SL (2006) Vascular corrosion casting of the uteroplacental and fetoplacental vasculature in mice. *Methods Mol Med* **121:** 371–92.

Xu RH, Chen X, Li DS, Li R, Addicks GC, Glennon C, Zwaka TP, Thomson JA (2002) BMP4 initiates human embryonic stem cell differentiation to trophoblast. *Nat Biotechnol* **20:** 1261–4.

Zdravkovic M, Aboagye-Mathiesen G, Guimond MJ, Hager H, Ebbesen P, Lala PK (1999) Susceptibility of MHC class I expressing extravillous trophoblast cell lines to killing by natural killer cells. *Placenta* **20:** 431–40.

CHAPTER

78

The placental role in fetal programming

Rohan M. Lewis, Jane K. Cleal and Keith M. Godfrey

INTRODUCTION

The placenta was traditionally envisaged as a "perfect barrier", protecting the fetus from harm, while at the same time allowing transfer of all the nutrients required for fetal growth (Dally, 1998). Sadly this is not the case, and the tragedy of thalidomide demonstrated that the placenta does not always protect the fetus. Furthermore, it is now clear that the placenta does not simply allow the transfer of all the nutrients required by the fetus and that placental nutrient transport capacity is regulated by a complex range of factors. The ability of the placenta to protect the fetus from harmful substances while actively ensuring appropriate nutrient transfer is essential for optimal fetal growth and development. The failure of the placenta to protect or nourish can have significant consequences for the fetus both before birth and throughout its postnatal life.

Over the past 20 years there has been a growing appreciation that how an individual grew in the womb will in part determine their risk of developing disease in adult life. Poor fetal growth, an indication of an impaired intrauterine environment, is associated with increased risk of many common chronic disorders in adult life including coronary heart disease, diabetes and cancer (Gluckman *et al.*, 2008). This phenomenon has been referred to as "fetal programming". The placenta is the interface between the mother and the fetus, influencing both the intrauterine environment and fetal growth. Placental function is therefore likely to be a major determinant of programming effects.

The aim of this chapter is to outline the role of the placenta in fetal programming. In order to understand this, placental function and regulation will be outlined and we will discuss the evidence for placental involvement in programming, together with the maternal and environmental factors which may influence placental function. Finally the implications for the identification of individuals at future risk of disease due to poor placental function and the potential opportunities for interventions will be discussed.

PLACENTAL FUNCTION AND REGULATION

In order to understand the placenta's role in fetal programming it is important to understand its role in sustaining fetal growth. The placenta is the interface between the mother and the fetus. The placental barrier protects the fetus from the substances in maternal blood and controls the flow of maternal nutrients to the fetus. As an endocrine organ the placenta regulates both maternal and fetal physiology. In performing these essential functions the placenta determines the health of the fetus, both *in utero* and in later life.

The placenta is a fetal tissue embedded in the wall of the uterus where it is perfused with maternal blood. It transports maternal nutrients to the fetus and fetal waste products to the mother. Maternal blood enters the placenta from the terminal ends of the uterine spiral arteries and flows around the placental villi before exiting back into the mother's uterine veins. The placental villi contain fetal blood vessels bringing fetal and maternal blood into close proximity but preventing any mixing of the two circulations. This protects the fetus from many unwanted substances but also means that mechanisms must exist to transport the nutrients required by the fetus across the placental barrier (Figure 78.1). This section will outline the roles and functions of the placenta and how it facilitates the transport of substances required by the fetus while preventing the transport of those which are not.

The placental barrier

The placental villi form a physical barrier between the maternal and fetal circulations. Maternal and fetal blood is separated by the syncytiotrophoblast (in direct contact with maternal blood), a discontinuous layer of cytotrophoblast, connective tissue and finally the fetal capillary endothelium (in direct contact with fetal blood). Together these block the transfer of cells and molecules which are not able to diffuse through lipid membranes. However, small lipophilic

Reproductive and Developmental Toxicology, Edited by Ramesh C. Gupta
ISBN: 978-0-12-382032-7

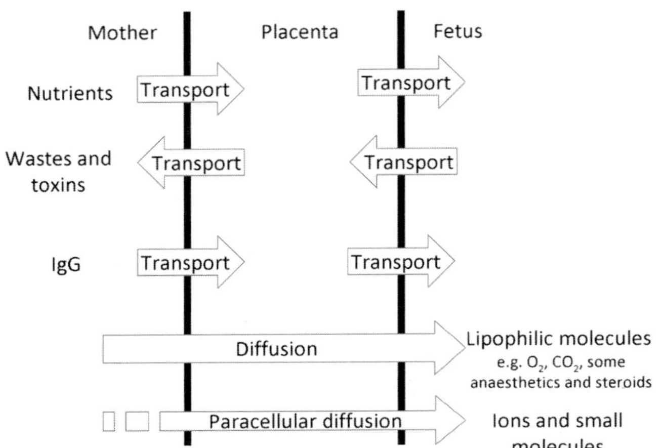

FIGURE 78.1 Nutrients, waste products and IgG must be transported across both the apical and basal membranes of the placental syncytiotrophoblast. Lipophilic molecules may diffuse across the placenta (specific transport mechanisms exist for fatty acids). Ions and molecules may also transfer by paracellular routes. While many molecules may cross the placenta to some degree, the efficiency of transfer will decrease dramatically as molecular size increases.

molecules, such as oxygen and carbon dioxide, can diffuse across the placenta relatively easily.

The primary barrier is the syncytiotrophoblast, a continuous syncytium forming the outer layer of the placental villi. The syncytiotrophoblast is formed by the fusion of cytotrophoblast cells which originate from the embryonic trophectoderm. As well as being the primary barrier between the maternal and fetal circulations the syncytiotrophoblast mediates the transfer of nutrients to the fetus. To this end the maternal facing membrane of the syncytiotrophoblast is covered in microvilli which act to increase the surface area available for nutrient exchange.

Although numerous in early pregnancy, by term cytotrophoblast cells comprise a much smaller proportion of placental volume and form a discontinuous layer underneath the syncytiotrophoblast (Jones *et al.*, 2008). Cytotrophoblast cells are important for the maintenance of the syncytiotrophoblast and continue to fuse with the syncytiotrophoblast throughout gestation.

Lying between the trophoblast and the fetal capillary endothelium is connective tissue. It is thought that relatively free diffusion occurs through the stromal tissue. The fetal capillary endothelium is the final structure that must be crossed before substances reach the fetal blood. The extent to which the capillary endothelium is a barrier to transfer is debated; however, it is clear that there are gaps between endothelial cells through which molecules, including most nutrients, can diffuse (Sibley, 2009). However, this may not always be the case and some substances, for instance lipids and immunoglobin G (IgG), may also need to be transported across this barrier.

Diffusion across the placenta

Passive diffusion across the placenta can occur by transcellular or paracellular routes. Transcellular routes are available to small lipophilic molecules such as O_2 and CO_2. Passive diffusion across the placental syncytiotrophoblast will be proportional to the size of the molecule being transferred. Small lipophilic molecules will diffuse across most easily, whereas larger more hydrophobic molecules will have more difficulty crossing this barrier. That said, it is likely that a little of everything will cross the placenta, although the larger hydrophilic molecules are likely to cross the placenta at very low rates. It is important to note that if a specific transport system exists, as for maternal IgG, or if a molecule is able to use a transporter for a structurally similar molecule then placental transport can be much higher.

The ability of a substance to cross the placenta will depend on its physical characteristics; the smaller and more lipophilic a substance is the more likely that it will reach the fetus. Damage to the integrity of the placental barrier may increase transfer of harmful substances to the fetus and adversely affect fetal development.

Placental transport

Substances which cannot diffuse across the syncytiotrophoblast must be transported across the placenta by specific transport proteins. It is important to note that transport occurs in both the maternal to fetal direction (principally nutrients) and the fetal to maternal direction (principally waste products and toxins).

Transport is mediated by specific transport proteins across both the apical microvillous membrane and the basal membrane of the syncytiotrophoblast. Specific transport proteins exist within the apical and basal syncytiotrophoblast membranes to mediate the transport of both macro and micro nutrients via active transporters (e.g., amino acids, iron) or facilitated diffusion (e.g., glucose, fatty acids). Maternal IgG is transferred across the placenta to the fetus in order to provide an immunological defense mechanism against infection in the first few months of life (Virella *et al.*, 1972).

For optimal fetal growth all nutrients must be available at the required level. Any nutrient can become growth limiting if its levels drop below those required by the fetus. This means that any transport system could potentially become rate limiting for fetal growth.

It should also be considered that the placenta may sometimes transport too much of a particular substance, for instance in maternal diabetes increased glucose transport is associated with fetal overgrowth. Fetal overgrowth is also associated with disease, in particular type 2 diabetes, in later life (Pettitt *et al.*, 1993). Therefore it is not only important that the placenta transports enough nutrients to the fetus, but that it also transports the right balance of nutrients.

Regulation of placental transfer

Placental transport is regulated by signals from both the mother and the fetus. The mechanisms involved are not well understood but may involve hormonal signaling and the placenta sensing plasma nutrient levels. Fetal signals are known to upregulate placental nutrient transport capacity in order to sustain fetal growth. Maternal signals are likely to be more complex as the mother must balance the needs of the fetus against her own ability to support the pregnancy and indeed future pregnancies.

While it is difficult to study fetal signals to the placenta a series of studies in mice has provided clear, though indirect, evidence that the fetus can regulate placental function to sustain its own growth (Dilworth *et al.*, 2010). In this model a placental specific knockout of the gene IGF2 reduced placental size, but in response to fetal signals these placentas transported more nutrients per gram of placental tissue. This increase in placental capacity was, initially at least, able to sustain fetal growth despite reduced placental size. These findings parallel those of observational studies in humans (Godfrey *et al.*, 1998). The mother's ability to limit fetal growth in line with her ability to sustain the pregnancy is referred to as "maternal constraint". It is most elegantly demonstrated by the fact that embryos from large horse breeds are born smaller than their genetic potential when transferred to mothers from smaller breeds (Allen *et al.*, 2002). While the nature of the maternal signals are not yet clear there is evidence from studies of teenage pregnancy that maternal endocrine and metabolic status does affect fetal growth. For example, birth weight has been shown to be greater in teenage pregnancies where the mother continued growing during pregnancy (Jones *et al.*, 2010).

Maternal hormones have been shown to regulate placental nutrient and waste product transport. Hormones including leptin and IGF2 have been demonstrated to increase nutrient uptake by placental tissue (Fowden *et al.*, 2009). The efflux of toxins from the placenta has also been shown to be hormonally regulated. The multidrug resistance gene ABCB1, which transports xenobiotics out of the fetus, is regulated by progesterone and estrogen (Petropoulos *et al.*, 2007).

Placental function may also be regulated in response to plasma nutrient levels, increasing or decreasing in response to maternal availability. Nutrient availability may regulate placental amino acid transporters through the intracellular signaling system mTOR (Roos *et al.*, 2009).

The fact that placental transport capacity can be up- or downregulated means that it does not depend exclusively on placental size. While placental size will provide a guide to transport capacity, regulation of transport capacity means that for a given placental weight actual transport capacity will vary. This has implications for epidemiological studies which use placental weight as an indicator of placental function.

In summary, placental transport has important roles in providing the fetus with nutrients, removing waste products and protecting the fetus from xenobiotics. Poor nutrient supply or inefficient waste product removal could affect fetal development and induce long-term effects on adult physiology.

The placenta as an endocrine organ

The placenta is an important endocrine organ during pregnancy, secreting hormones into both the maternal and fetal circulations. Hormones secreted by the placenta mediate the adaptations in maternal physiology required to support the pregnancy. The first such hormone is human chorionic gonadotropin (HCG), the hormone detected by pregnancy tests. HCG is secreted from the embryonic trophectoderm, the cells which later form the placental trophoblast (Lopata *et al.*, 1997).

Placental hormones such as HCG, placental growth hormone and placental lactogen mediate a wide range of changes in maternal physiology. These include changes to the cardiovascular system, maternal metabolism and the uterus. Levels of placental growth hormone and placental lactogen in maternal blood are positively related to birth weight, indicating their importance to fetal growth (Mannik *et al.*, 2010).

Placental hormone secretion can have negative effects on both the mother and the fetus. In preeclampsia placental factors result in a dangerously high maternal blood pressure, which can only be cured by delivery of the placenta (Young *et al.*, 2010). Placental hormones make the mother more insulin resistant leading some women to develop diabetes during pregnancy which is linked with both fetal growth restriction and macrosomia. This may program the fetus making it more susceptible to disease in later life.

The placenta regulates the transfer of maternal cortisol to the fetus. Cortisol concentrations are higher in the mother than in the fetus, and the hormone can diffuse across cell membranes and so transfer to the fetus. However, the placenta contains an enzyme, 11β-HSD2, which converts cortisol to the inactive metabolite cortisone. In rodents transfer of glucocorticoids across the placenta has been associated with hypertension in humans (Wyrwoll *et al.*, 2009). Babies likely to be delivered prematurely are treated with betamethasone in order to mature the fetal lungs in preparation for birth. Unlike cortisol, betamethasone is not deactivated by 11β-HSD2 and can cross the placenta. It is not yet clear whether this may have long-term effects on the offspring, but in one follow-up study those treated with betamethasone had worse glucose tolerance, possibly a precursor to type 2 diabetes (Dalziel *et al.*, 2005).

In summary, for the fetus to grow the placenta must supply it with nutrients, remove waste products and protect it from harmful substances in maternal blood. In addition the placenta must secrete hormones which adapt the mother's physiology to support the pregnancy. In doing so the placenta is regulated by signals from both the mother and the fetus. If any of these roles are altered this will affect the intrauterine environment and may impair fetal development.

FETAL PROGRAMMING

An individual's risk of developing chronic disease in adult life is in part determined by the way in which they grew *in utero*. The adverse effects of a poor intrauterine environment may be exaggerated when combined with an obesogenic adult lifestyle (Gluckman *et al.*, 2008).

The association between fetal growth and adult disease came to prominence in the 1990s by a series of epidemiological studies which related measurements of size at birth to cardiovascular and metabolic disease 50 or more years later in adulthood (Barker *et al.*, 1990). Extensive work in animal models confirms that a poor intrauterine environment is associated with alterations in adult physiology (McMillen *et al.*, 2005). The long-term effects of developmental exposures within the normal range are referred to as "fetal programming" or the "developmental origins of adult disease".

As the placenta is a central determinant of fetal growth its function would be expected to have an important influence on fetal programming. This section will therefore summarize the evidence for programming in humans and animals, and discuss the evidence for the role of the placenta in fetal programming.

Epidemiological evidence

Numerous epidemiological studies have demonstrated associations between lower birth weight and adult hypertension (Osmond and Barker, 2000), coronary heart disease (CHD) (Barker, 1995) and glucose and insulin metabolism (Newsome *et al.*, 2003).

While the epidemiological evidence focuses on birth weight it is not thought that birth weight itself underlies the relationships. Instead birth weight is regarded as an indicator of the intrauterine environment, with a poor intrauterine environment being associated with lower birth weight. It is also important to note that these relationships are not just seen with low birth weight babies, but occur across the birth weight spectrum (Barker, 1998).

Although there was some inconsistency, most of the initial small studies reported associations between adulthood cardiovascular disease and placental weight or the placental-to-birth weight ratio (Godfrey, 2002). Over the past few years several larger studies have been completed based on records of tens of thousands of births. These larger studies support an association between a higher placental-to-birth weight ratio (a disproportionately large placenta) and higher systolic blood pressure in childhood (Hemachandra *et al.*, 2006) and increased rates of coronary heart disease in adulthood (Risnes *et al.*, 2009). In these pregnancies, despite a relatively large placenta, the fetus has not grown accordingly. It may be the case that in these pregnancies maternal or other environmental factors are decreasing placental efficiency. This adds weight to the notion that it is those babies who grow poorly relative to their growth potential rather than those who are just small who are at risk of later disease. While further large studies would add weight to these findings they do suggest that there is not a simple relationship between placental weight, fetal growth and adult disease.

Given that the placenta is so important for fetal growth it is interesting that the relationships between placental weight and adult outcomes are not stronger. The challenges in making accurate measurements of placental weight may contribute to this weaker than expected relationship. It is more likely that placental weight, and indeed the placental-to-birth weight ratio, are poor indicators of placental function as a result of placental efficiency (transport capacity per gram of placental tissue) being subject to maternal and fetal regulation. It is not easy to measure placental function directly in humans, especially in the context of an epidemiological study. However, it may be possible to identify markers in the placenta which reflect placental function more directly than placental weight. These "placental phenotypes" could prove invaluable, both for future epidemiological studies and for identifying those who may not have received optimal nutrition in the womb.

Animal evidence

Animal models have provided support for the fetal programming hypothesis and are important for understanding the role of the placenta as they provide the opportunity to study placental function.

In contrast to human studies, where a poor intrauterine environment must be inferred indirectly, in experimental studies specific stresses can be imposed during pregnancy and the effects on the offspring and the placenta studied. Many different animal models have been developed to examine these processes. Maternal dietary restriction, either globally or of a specific nutrient, is the most commonly used model but maternal dexamethasone exposure and uterine ligation have also been shown to affect adult physiology in the offspring. Programming effects have been demonstrated in a range of species, including rodents and large animals such as sheep (McMillen *et al.*, 2005).

Placental weight, structure and function have been shown to be altered in these models suggesting a role for the placenta in the pathogenesis of the programming effects. It has been demonstrated that reduced maternal nutrition can either reduce or enhance placental growth, depending on the timing and severity of the challenge (McCrabb *et al.*, 1991). In rats, maternal dietary protein and iron restriction have been shown to affect placental structure (Doherty *et al.*, 2003; Lewis *et al.*, 2001). Changes in placental size and structure demonstrate the placenta's plasticity in response to the maternal environment. However, it is not clear whether these are adaptive changes, which benefit the fetus, or simply part of a pathological process.

Placental function is decreased in maternal nutrient restriction models. Placental transport capacity decreases before fetal growth restriction is seen, providing strong evidence that the placenta has causal effects on fetal development (Jansson *et al.*, 2006). These studies demonstrate how the placenta can alter its function, in response to the maternal environment, in ways which are detrimental to fetal growth. While fetal growth restriction may have adverse long-term consequences, the reduced growth may be a necessary adaptation, as it reduces the demands on the undernourished mother.

Periconceptional influences

Fetal programming may be initiated at the very earliest stages in development, and both maternal nutrition around conception and embryo culture conditions have been shown to have long-term effects on the offspring (Watkins *et al.*, 2008). The placenta develops from the outer cell mass surrounding the early embryo, raising the possibility that placental growth and function may be affected by the early environment.

Mechanisms of programming

The mechanisms by which early development and disease risk in later life are linked have not yet been fully determined. Several explanations have been proposed and more than one underlying mechanism may be responsible for the observations. One hypothesis is that a poor intrauterine environment results in epigenetic changes which persist throughout the lifespan. Alternatively, it has been proposed that altered development of organs and tissues, such as a decreased number of functional units (nephrons) in the fetal kidneys, may play a role.

Epigenetics and programming

Epigenetic regulation affects gene expression without altering the sequence of the genome. Examples include DNA methylation and histone modification. Methylation of cytosines at cytosine–guanine dinucleotides (CpG) within promoter regions of genes is generally associated with transcriptional repression, whereas hypomethylation is associated with transcriptional activity (Razin, 1998). Histone modification affects the packing of DNA within the cell, with more tightly packed genes less accessible to transcription factors and thus less likely to be expressed.

During gametogenesis, and in the preimplantation embryo, there is extensive de-methylation and re-methylation of the genome and these may be critical windows for the laying down of epigenetic modifications (Reik *et al.*, 2001). Epigenetic modification of trophectoderm, which develops into the placenta, is of particular importance as this may affect placental development and function. Altered placental development may, in turn, affect how the fetus develops and program its risk of adult disease.

It is clear from animal studies that the early environment can alter methylation status within the genome (Godfrey *et al.*, 2007). Maternal nutrition and grooming behavior as well as hormone exposure have been shown to alter methylation and phenotype in the offspring. In one mouse strain maternal dietary folate concentration alters the coat color in the offspring through epigenetic modifications (Wolff *et al.*, 1998). Maternal grooming behavior in rats can result in changes in methylation status and expression of glucocorticoid receptor gene in the hippocampus (Weaver *et al.*, 2004).

Placental function will determine the nutrient availability to the fetus, which may then cause epigenetic changes. More specifically the placenta may influence fetal epigenetic programming through its control of the supply of folate to the fetus and its modulation of cortisol transfer. Folate may be a mediator of epigenetic changes as it is an important metabolic source of methyl groups for DNA methylation. A lack of folate in the maternal diet, or impaired placental folate transport, may adversely affect normal epigenetic regulation in the fetus.

The placenta itself is subject to epigenetic regulation in terms of parental imprinting and other epigenetic changes may also occur as a consequence of maternal environment. The early embryonic environment in the fallopian tubes and the uterus may have a particularly important influence on epigenetic processes in the trophophectoderm which mediate placental development and implantation of the embryo.

Developmental alterations

A poor intrauterine environment may impair normal fetal development causing structural changes within organs and tissues which predispose to later disease. If such changes occurred within organs or tissues fully differentiated by birth these changes will therefore persist throughout the individual's postnatal life. It has been suggested that nephron, muscle fiber, adipocyte and pancreatic β-cell number may all be determined by the early environment.

Nephron number is determined *in utero* and in humans is complete by birth. A low nephron number has been linked to adult hypertension (Keller *et al.*, 2003), and impaired kidney development has been suggested as a mediator between the effects of poor *in utero* nutrition and later cardiovascular dysfunction (Moritz *et al.*, 2009). Low birth weight is associated with reduced grip strength in women suggesting the possibility of a persistent *in utero* developmental defect on muscle function (Inskip *et al.*, 2007).

Evolutionary perspectives

There is considerable interest in developmental programming from an evolutionary perspective. While in some cases poor fetal growth may affect adult health simply due to impaired development, other changes may be adaptive, matching the fetus to the environment into which it will be born. If these changes improve offspring survival the mechanisms may have a fitness advantage.

It has previously been proposed that the placenta may be a site of conflict between the maternal and paternal genomes in the form of parental imprinting (Moore *et al.*, 2008). The maternally inherited genome has epigenetic modifications which limit nutrient supply to the fetus (and the demand for maternal resources) while the paternally inherited genome has epigenetic modifications which promote allocation of maternal resources to the fetus (which is at no cost to the father) (Moore *et al.*, 2008). This has been suggested as an example of how the placenta regulates the allocation of nutritional resources between the mother and the fetus and controls fetal growth. However, the importance of maternal–offspring conflict remains intensely debated in evolutionary biology and an alternative interpretation is of a maternal/paternal co-adaptive process, with the matriline being the major player (Keverne *et al.*, 2008).

Predictive adaptive responses (PARs)

Some environmental cues invoke the fetus to make adaptations in prediction of the postnatal environment. These confer no immediate advantage, but may confer a fitness advantage in postnatal life if the prediction is correct (Gluckman and Hanson, 2004). These fetal adaptations have been termed "predictive adaptive responses". There are many examples of predictive adaptive responses in biology. One example is the meadow vole, in which the maternal photoperiod before conception induces pups to be born with the appropriate coat thickness to match the environmental conditions at the time they leave the burrow (Lee *et al.*, 1988).

Predictive adaptive responses may increase overall survival but if the prediction is incorrect then they may be disadvantageous. This may be particularly relevant to human populations where there is significant migration from an undernourished rural setting to urban environments where food is much more available and less physical work is required. Such a mismatch between the pre- and postnatal nutrient environment might, by inappropriate predictive adaptive responses, lead to cardiovascular dysfunction in adulthood (Gluckman and Hanson, 2004).

If predictive adaptations occur in humans the placenta is in the prime position to mediate these effects. The placenta is able to sense the maternal environment and to adjust nutrient transport in order to regulate fetal growth and development.

Programming summary

While the mechanisms underlying fetal programming are not yet fully understood the effects of a poor *in utero* environment on postnatal phenotype can be seen clearly in both human and animal studies. The association between impaired fetal growth and the risk of chronic disease in adult life focuses attention on the determinants of fetal growth.

One of the major determinants of fetal growth is placental function; therefore understanding how the placenta determines fetal growth is central to understanding the causes of programming.

MATERNAL AND ENVIRONMENTAL INFLUENCES ON PLACENTAL FUNCTION AND FETAL DEVELOPMENT

The placenta is subject to a wide range of influences from both the mother and the fetus. Hormonal, nutrient and epigenetic influences on placental function have been discussed above, and in this section broader maternal and environmental influences will be discussed.

Maternal body composition and placental function

Maternal body composition can be seen as a reflection of the mother's ability to support the pregnancy and is an important determinant of fetal growth. Mothers with little adipose or lean mass are less able to provide for the fetus during pregnancy, especially if food becomes scarce during gestation. Epidemiological evidence suggests that maternal body composition is associated with adult health in the offspring and we are now beginning to understand how maternal body composition affects placental function and fetal development.

Aspects of maternal body composition linked with cardiovascular and metabolic disorders in the offspring include the mother's height and adiposity in pregnancy (Fall *et al.*, 1998; Forsen *et al.*, 1997, 2000). Maternal adiposity in pregnancy has also been associated with neonatal bone mass (Godfrey *et al.*, 2001a) and with fat mass in 9-year-old children (Gale *et al.*, 2007). Maternal obesity is associated with upregulation of inflammatory pathways in the placenta which may suggest an underlying mechanism (Zhu *et al.*, 2010). In contrast, maternal thinness and low pregnancy weight gain have been consistently associated with raised blood pressure in the offspring (Adair *et al.*, 2001; Clark *et al.*, 1998; Godfrey *et al.*, 1994; Margetts *et al.*, 1991). Maternal thinness has also been associated with altered blood flow distribution in the fetus, and it has been suggested that changes in fetal blood flow distribution induced by impaired materno-placental nutrient supply could have long-term consequences for cardiovascular and metabolic function (Haugen *et al.*, 2005).

These findings raise the question of how maternal body composition affects the growth of the fetus and its risk of disease in later life. Some affects may act primarily through altered nutrient concentrations in the maternal circulation, with the placenta acting simply as the conduit of the message, while others may involve changes in placental function and the placenta acting as a more active mediator.

Recent data suggest that maternal body composition may affect placental amino acid transport. Maternal upper-arm muscle mass before pregnancy, a proxy indicator of total lean mass, is related to activity of the amino acid transporter System A in the term placenta (Lewis *et al.*, 2010). These studies suggest that placental development and function is affected by pre-pregnant maternal body composition. While it is unlikely that there is a direct relationship between factors such as upper-arm muscle mass and placental function, the relationship may reflect the mother's underlying metabolic capacity. Maternal metabolic capacity may affect protein turnover and inter-organ amino acid exchange. This metabolic environment may therefore alter placental development and function through the action of nutrient sensing pathways, such as the mTOR pathway (Wen *et al.*, 2005).

Maternal diet and dietary balance

Macronutrients

In animal models alterations in the macronutrient content of the maternal diet (carbohydrate, fat and protein) have been shown to have long-term effects on the offspring (McMillen *et al.*, 2005), and there is some evidence from human studies suggesting similar effects (Shiell *et al.*, 2001). Both maternal undernutrition and overnutrition are thought to have short- and long-term consequences.

Effects of maternal diet on placental function could be direct or indirect, and maternal body composition and metabolism will strongly influence the metabolic environment experienced by the placenta in terms of plasma levels of glucose, lipids and amino acids. Body composition will be determined by maternal environment over a much longer time course than current diet and so may be a better indicator of the mother's ability to support the pregnancy.

Micronutrients

The availability of vitamins and minerals may be just as important as macronutrient availability. Placental transfer of micronutrients including zinc, iron, copper, calcium and vitamins A, E and folate have been suggested to play a role in fetal programming (Ashworth *et al.*, 2001). Transfer of folate is a particular focus of interest due to its role in neural tube defects and its role as a methyl donor in DNA methylation and epigenetic programming (Lillycrop *et al.*, 2005).

The placenta is a metabolically active organ and any micronutrient shortage may affect its function directly, impairing its ability to support fetal development. For example, maternal iron restriction has been reported to alter placental structure (Lewis *et al.*, 2001).

Dietary balance

Variation in the nutritional balance of the maternal diet, for instance the ratio of carbohydrate to protein, may affect both placental function and fetal development. In one study pregnant women who reported lower dietary intakes of carbohydrate in early pregnancy had higher placental and birth weights, especially when combined with high intakes of dairy protein in late pregnancy (Godfrey *et al.*, 1996). In the Dutch famine, a period of extreme malnutrition for 5 months in 1944–45, increased placental weight was associated with the combination of famine exposure in early pregnancy and high food intakes in mid–late pregnancy (Lumey, 1998).

In addition to effects on placental size the balance of nutrients in maternal diet has been associated with physiological changes in the offspring. Analysis of the Dutch famine found that there was evidence of an association between raised blood pressure and rations with a low protein density (Roseboom *et al.*, 2001). This is consistent with studies which found that maternal diets with either a low or a high ratio of animal protein to carbohydrate were associated with raised blood pressure in the adult offspring (Campbell *et al.*, 1996). A high protein density in the maternal diet was also associated with insulin deficiency and impaired glucose tolerance in the offspring (Shiell *et al.*, 2000). It is possible that the long-term effects may be a result of the metabolic stress imposed on the mother by an unbalanced diet in which high intakes of essential amino acids are not accompanied by the other micronutrients required to utilize them (Shiell *et al.*, 2000).

Other exposures

Exercise

Moderate exercise is recommended during pregnancy as it is thought to be beneficial for the mother's health and not to be harmful to the fetus (Juhl *et al.*, 2010). During maternal exercise blood flow to the placenta is decreased, which will reduce nutrient availability to the placenta and fetus (Clapp *et al.*, 2000). Moderate exercise does not appear to adversely affect the fetus as it is not associated with any major decrease in fetal or placental weight. Indeed there is some evidence that moderate exercise may be protective against the occurrence of small- and large-for-gestational-age babies (Juhl *et al.*, 2010). Though maternal exercise induces transient reductions in uterine blood flow the improvement in maternal cardiovascular function may increase placental perfusion and be beneficial to the fetus. For continuing, regular, vigorous and sustained exercise throughout pregnancy there is evidence of reduced offspring adiposity both at birth and in later childhood (Clapp, 1996).

Exercise might affect placental function by altering blood flow to the placenta, by altering maternal body composition or by metabolic changes associated with exercise. Some studies have suggested that maternal exercise affects placental structure, with implications for fetal growth. One controlled study found that women who exercised in early pregnancy, but not late pregnancy, had larger placentas and bigger babies (Clapp *et al.*, 2002). However, there is currently little evidence regarding the effects of exercise on placental function.

Sunlight and vitamin D

Placental transport of calcium, vitamin D and protein is essential in enabling optimal fetal bone development. This is important as decreased early bone mass may lead to lower peak bone mass and increase the risk of developing osteoporosis in later life. The regulation of placental calcium transport is not well understood but may be influenced by maternal vitamin D status. Maternal vitamin D insufficiency in late pregnancy has been linked with reduced whole body bone mineral density in the offspring at 9 years of age (Javaid *et al.*, 2006).

Maternal stress and illness

Maternal stress and illness may result in hormonal and/or metabolic imbalances which affect placental function. Stress, either psychological or due to illness, causes cortisol release. As discussed earlier, cortisol may cross the placenta and initiate fetal programming (Cottrell *et al.*, 2009). The extent to which this occurs is determined by expression of 11β-HSD2 in the placenta, which converts cortisol to inactive cortisone. Placental infection is known to decrease the levels of 11β-HSD2 in the placenta potentially allowing more cortisol to cross to the fetus (Johnstone *et al.*, 2005). In addition there is evidence that cortisol may have direct effects on placental amino acid transport (Wyrwoll *et al.*, 2009).

Steroid medications used during pregnancy may influence placental function, and antenatal betamethasone treatment is associated with sex-specific alterations in placental 11β-HSD2 activity (Stark *et al.*, 2009). Furthermore, inhaled steroids used for asthma have been linked with altered placental structure and 11β-HSD2 activity (Clifton *et al.*, 2006; Mayhew *et al.*, 2008).

Environmental toxins

The effects of environmental toxins on the fetus may be due to the placenta's inability to protect the fetus from exposure, or result from indirect effects on the mother or the placenta. For example, nicotine reduces uterine blood flow and nutrient supply to the placenta (Lambers *et al.*, 1996), while also altering placental nutrient transport capacity (Jauniaux *et al.*, 2007). Specific efflux transporters, such as ATP-binding cassette transporters, provide a protective mechanism by transferring harmful substances from the fetal circulation back to the mother. Other transporters, however, may provide a direct means by which the fetus can be exposed to life-threatening substances.

Maternal alcohol consumption during pregnancy can be harmful to the fetus and in some cases result in fetal alcohol syndrome, with growth retardation, facial–cranial and organ anomalies (Kelly *et al.*, 2000) and effects on central nervous system development (Floyd *et al.*, 2005). Alcohol crosses the placenta and may directly affect fetal development. It may also have indirect effects through altered placental function, as some evidence has linked alcohol consumption with decreased placental size, nutrient transport capacity and endocrine function (Burd *et al.*, 2007).

Maternal smoking is a recognized cause of fetal growth restriction and affects placental structure as well as transporter and enzyme activity (Jauniaux *et al.*, 2007). The effects of smoking on placental structure and function may not just make the baby smaller but may have longer-term effects on its health particularly in relation to skeletal development. We have shown that maternal smoking was associated with reduced neonatal bone mass, but not with adipose mass (Javaid *et al.*, 2004). Maternal smoking is reported to decrease bone mass at birth and up until at least 8 years of age (Godfrey *et al.*, 2001b). If this effect persists it could affect the attainment of peak bone mass. Cadmium present in tobacco smoke may affect fetal bone development by competing with calcium for transporters (Lin *et al.*, 1997).

Recreational drug addiction during pregnancy can seriously affect fetal development, with the consequences depending on the drug, dose and gestational age of the fetus. Delta-9-tetrahydrocannabinol in cannabis readily crosses the placenta and so can act on the fetus (Hatch and Bracken, 1986). Cannabinoid receptors are expressed by placental tissue throughout gestation suggesting that the use of this drug may affect placental function directly (Helliwell *et al.*, 2004; Park *et al.*, 2003). The effects of cannabis include fetal growth restriction (Zuckerman *et al.*, 1989), placental abruption, preterm birth, stillbirths and spontaneous miscarriages (Felder *et al.*, 1998; Hatch and Bracken, 1986).

In summary, the maternal environment may influence placental function, with consequences for fetal development. Understanding how the maternal environment affects placental function is particularly important as this could lead to interventions to improve placental function, with long-term benefits for the baby.

THE "PLACENTAL PHENOTYPE", INTERVENTIONS AND TREATMENTS

The association between impaired growth *in utero* and chronic disease in later life means that in assessing an individual's risk of later ill-health it may be important to know how they developed before birth. This would allow the provision of more personalized health advice to those at increased risk. If there were evidence that particular individuals were at greater risk this may encourage them to alter their lifestyles in more healthy ways. Perhaps more importantly it could encourage parents to instill healthier behaviors from an early age.

Birth weight is a poor proxy for fetal undernutrition as some babies will be constitutionally small while others will be small because of an adverse intrauterine environment. One way to determine how the baby grew *in utero* could be to study the placenta. It has been proposed that there may be "placental phenotypes" (identified from a combination of nutrient transporter activity/expression, blood flow and morphology at birth) which would allow us to distinguish those who have been subject to growth restriction *in utero* (Sibley *et al.*, 2005). If these placental biomarkers could be identified and validated they could then be routinely measured to indicate how the fetus grew in the womb. As it is likely to be those who were growth restricted *in utero* who

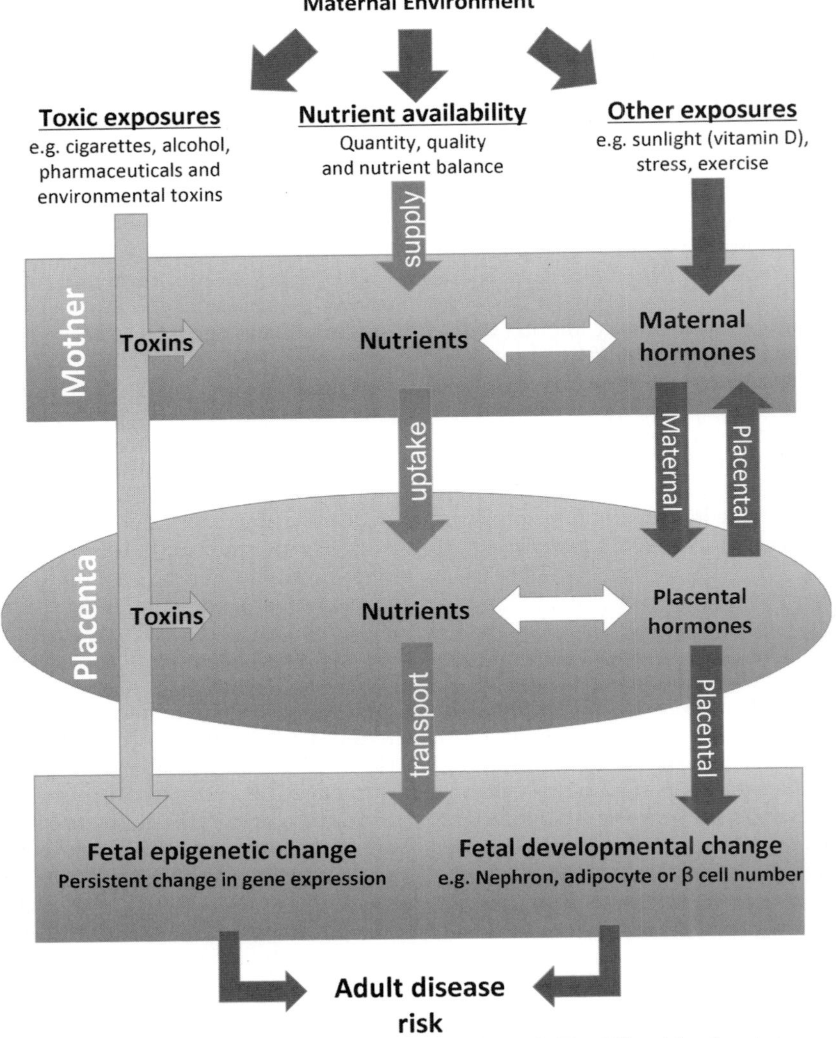

FIGURE 78.2 Fetal programming occurs if the placenta is unable to support normal fetal growth. The ability of the placenta to support fetal growth is determined by its innate properties and interaction with the mother and her environment. Altered placental function may result in fetal epigenetic and developmental changes which predispose to disease in adult life.

will suffer the effects of programming, these biomarkers might provide better information on the risk of ill-health in later life.

Interventions

As our understanding of placental function improves it may become possible to intervene to improve placental function and therefore fetal growth. Identifying placental phenotypes may also allow targeting of exposures which are important for fetal growth. Animal studies demonstrate that interventions are possible to prevent the adverse effects of a poor intrauterine environment. For example, giving rat dams folate during pregnancy prevents some of the adverse long-term effects arising from a low protein maternal diet (Lillycrop *et al.*, 2005). Moreover, a single neonatal treatment with the hormone leptin can prevent effects of maternal undernutrition on adult fat mass and hyperphagia in rats (Vickers *et al.*, 2005). Translating the findings of the animal studies into humans has obvious challenges in terms of demonstration of safety. That said, understanding the causes of placental dysfunction and the consequent fetal programming effects may allow the development of better informed dietary and lifestyle guidelines for women before and during pregnancy.

CONCLUDING REMARKS AND FUTURE DIRECTIONS

The placenta's ability to support fetal growth has long-term health consequences for the offspring. If placental function is inadequate, or if placental efficiency is downregulated to protect maternal reserves, the development of the fetus may be compromised, leading to increased rates of ill-health in later life. The mechanisms by which this occurs are likely to involve epigenetic changes, as well as changes in developmentally determined parameters such as nephron number. These interactions between the environment, mother, placenta and fetus are outlined in Figure 78.2.

The placenta's ability to support fetal growth is not simply a matter of placental sufficiency or insufficiency. Placental function is regulated by both maternal and fetal factors and these can increase or decrease the ability of the placenta to supply nutrients to the fetus. Where the mother has a limited capacity to support the pregnancy limiting fetal growth may be best for both the mother and the fetus.

Poor fetal growth may occur when the mother has a limited ability to support the pregnancy but may also occur when, for some reason, the placenta interprets the maternal environment as insufficient and limits fetal growth accordingly. Maternal dieting or smoking may be examples of situations where the placenta misinterprets the mother's ability to support the pregnancy.

Our current understanding is too limited for us to consider specific interventions or treatments to optimize placental function. However, we now have a greater appreciation of the active role played by the placenta in determining fetal nutrient supply. Future research needs to be targeted on understanding the maternal determinants of placental function.

REFERENCES

Adair LS, Kuzawa CW, Borja J (2001) Maternal energy stores and diet composition during pregnancy program adolescent blood pressure. *Circulation* **104:** 1034–9.

Allen WR, Wilsher S, Turnbull C, Stewart F, Ousey J, Rossdale PD, Fowden AL (2002) Influence of maternal size on placental, fetal and postnatal growth in the horse. I. Development *in utero*. *Reproduction* **123:** 445–53.

Ashworth CJ, Antipatis C (2001) Micronutrient programming of development throughout gestation. *Reproduction* **122:** 527–35.

Barker DJ (1998) In utero programming of chronic disease. *Clin Sci (Lond)* **95:** 115–28.

Barker DJ (1995) Fetal origins of coronary heart disease. *Brit Med J* **311:** 171–4.

Barker DJ, Bull R, Osmond C, Simmonds SJ (1990) Fetal and placental size and risk of hypertension in adult life. *Brit Med J* **301:** 259–62.

Burd L, Roberts D, Olson M, Odendaal H (2007) Ethanol and the placenta: a review. *J Matern Fetal Neonatal Med* **20:** 361–75.

Campbell DM, Hall MH, Barker DJ, Cross J, Shiell AW, Godfrey KM (1996) Diet in pregnancy and the offspring's blood pressure 40 years later. *Br J Obstet Gynecol* **103:** 273–80.

Clapp JF III (1996) Morphometric and neurodevelopmental outcome at age five years of the offspring of women who continued to exercise regularly throughout pregnancy. *J Pediatr* **129:** 856–63.

Clapp JF III, Kim H, Burciu B, Schmidt S, Petry K, Lopez B (2002) Continuing regular exercise during pregnancy: effect of exercise volume on fetoplacental growth. *Am J Obstet Gynecol* **186:** 142–7.

Clapp JF III, Stepanchak W, Tomaselli J, Kortan M, Faneslow S (2000) Portal vein blood flow-effects of pregnancy, gravity, and exercise. *Am J Obstet Gynecol* **183:** 167–72.

Clark PM, Atton C, Law CM, Shiell A, Godfrey K, Barker DJ (1998) Weight gain in pregnancy, triceps skinfold thickness, and blood pressure in offspring. *Obstet Gynecol* **91:** 3–7.

Clifton VL, Rennie N, Murphy VE (2006) Effect of inhaled glucocorticoid treatment on placental 11beta-hydroxysteroid dehydrogenase type 2 activity and neonatal birthweight in pregnancies complicated by asthma. *Aust NZ J Obstet Gynecol* **46:** 136–40.

Cottrell EC Seckl JR (2009) Prenatal stress, glucocorticoids and the programming of adult disease. *Front Behav Neurosci* **3:** 19.

Dally A (1998) Thalidomide: was the tragedy preventable? *Lancet* **351:** 1197–9.

Dalziel SR, Walker NK, Parag V, Mantell C, Rea HH, Rodgers A, Harding JE (2005) Cardiovascular risk factors after antenatal exposure to betamethasone: 30-year follow-up of a randomised controlled trial. *Lancet* **365:** 1856–62.

Dilworth MR, Kusinski LC, Cowley E, Ward BS, Husain SM, Constancia M, Sibley CP, Glazier JD (2010) Placental-specific Igf2 knockout mice exhibit hypocalcemia and adaptive changes in placental calcium transport. *Proc Natl Acad Sci USA* **107:** 3894–9.

Doherty CB, Lewis RM, Sharkey A, Burton GJ (2003) Placental composition and surface area but not vascularization are altered by maternal protein restriction in the rat. *Placenta* **24:** 34–8.

Fall CH, Stein CE, Kumaran K, Cox V, Osmond C, Barker DJ, Hales CN (1998) Size at birth, maternal weight, and type 2 diabetes in South India. *Diabet Med* **15:** 220–7.

Felder CC, Glass M (1998) Cannabinoid receptors and their endogenous agonists. *Ann Rev Pharmacol Toxicol* **38:** 179–200.

Floyd RL, O'Connor MJ, Sokol RJ, Bertrand J, Cordero JF (2005) Recognition and prevention of fetal alcohol syndrome. *Obstet Gynecol* **106:** 1059–64.

Forsen T, Eriksson J, Tuomilehto J, Reunanen A, Osmond C, Barker D (2000) The fetal and childhood growth of persons who develop type 2 diabetes. *Ann Intern Med* **133:** 176–82.

Forsen T, Eriksson JG, Tuomilehto J, Teramo K, Osmond C, Barker DJ (1997) Mother's weight in pregnancy and coronary heart disease in a cohort of Finnish men: follow up study. *Br Med J* **315:** 837–40.

Fowden AL, Sferruzzi-Perri AN, Coan PM, Constancia M, Burton GJ (2009) Placental efficiency and adaptation: endocrine regulation. *J Physiol* **587:** 3459–72.

Gale CR, Javaid MK, Robinson SM, Law CM, Godfrey KM, Cooper C (2007) Maternal size in pregnancy and body composition in children. *J Clin Endocrinol Metab* **92:** 3904–11.

Gluckman PD, Hanson MA (2004) Living with the past: evolution, development, and patterns of disease. *Science* **305:** 1733–6.

Gluckman PD, Hanson MA, Cooper C, Thornburg KL (2008) Effect of *in utero* and early-life conditions on adult health and disease. *N Engl J Med* **359:** 61–73.

Godfrey KM (2002) The role of the placenta in fetal programming – a review. *Placenta* **23 (Suppl. A):** S20–S27.

Godfrey K, Robinson S, Barker DJ, Osmond C, Cox V (1996) Maternal nutrition in early and late pregnancy in relation to placental and fetal growth. *Br Med J* **312:** 410–14.

Godfrey KM, Barker DJ (2001a) Fetal programming and adult health. *Public Health Nutr* **4:** 611–24.

Godfrey KM, Forrester T, Barker DJ, Jackson AA, Landman JP, Hall JS, Cox V, Osmond C (1994) Maternal nutritional status in pregnancy and blood pressure in childhood. *Br J Obstet Gynecol* **101:** 398–403.

Godfrey KM, Lillycrop KA, Burdge GC, Gluckman PD, Hanson MA (2007) Epigenetic mechanisms and the mismatch concept of the developmental origins of health and disease. *Pediatr Res* **61:** 5R–10R.

Godfrey KM, Matthews N, Glazier J, Jackson A, Wilman C, Sibley CP (1998) Neutral amino acid uptake by the microvillous plasma membrane of the human placenta is inversely related to fetal size at birth in normal pregnancy. *J Clin Endocrinol Metab* **83:** 3320–6.

Godfrey KM, Walker-Bone K, Robinson S, Taylor P, Shore S, Wheeler T, Cooper C (2001b) Neonatal bone mass: influence of parental birthweight, maternal smoking, body composition, and activity during pregnancy. *J Bone Miner Res* **16:** 1694–703.

Hatch EE, Bracken MB (1986) Effect of marijuana use in pregnancy on fetal growth. *Am J Epidemiol* **124:** 986–93.

Haugen G, Hanson M, Kiserud T, Crozier S, Inskip H, Godfrey KM (2005) Fetal liver-sparing cardiovascular adaptations linked to mother's slimness and diet. *Circ Res* **96:** 12–4.

Helliwell RJ, Chamley LW, Blake-Palmer K, Mitchell MD, Wu J, Kearn CS, Glass M (2004) Characterization of the endocannabinoid system in early human pregnancy. *J Clin Endocrinol Metab* **89:** 5168–74.

Hemachandra AH, Klebanoff MA, Duggan AK, Hardy JB, Furth SL (2006) The association between intrauterine growth restriction in the full-term infant and high blood pressure at age 7 years: results from the Collaborative Perinatal Project. *Int J Epidemiol* **35:** 871–7.

Inskip HM, Godfrey KM, Martin HJ, Simmonds SJ, Cooper C, Sayer AA (2007) Size at birth and its relation to muscle strength in young adult women. *J Intern Med* **262:** 368–74.

Jansson N, Pettersson J, Haafiz A, Ericsson A, Palmberg I, Tranberg M, Ganapathy V, Powell TL, Jansson T (2006) Down-regulation of placental transport of amino acids precedes the development of intrauterine growth restriction in rats fed a low protein diet. *J Physiol* **576:** 935–46.

Jauniaux E, Burton GJ (2007) Morphological and biological effects of maternal exposure to tobacco smoke on the feto-placental unit. *Early Hum Dev* **83:** 699–706.

Javaid MK, Crozier SR, Harvey NC, Gale CR, Dennison EM, Boucher BJ, Arden NK, Godfrey KM, Cooper C (2006) Maternal vitamin D status during pregnancy and childhood bone mass at age 9 years: a longitudinal study. *Lancet* **367:** 36–43.

Javaid MK, Godfrey KM, Taylor P, Shore SR, Breier B, Arden NK, Cooper C (2004) Umbilical venous IGF-1 concentration, neonatal bone mass, and body composition. *J Bone Miner Res* **19:** 56–63.

Johnstone JF, Bocking AD, Unlugedik E, Challis JR (2005) The effects of chorioamnionitis and betamethasone on 11beta hydroxysteroid dehydrogenase types 1 and 2 and the glucocorticoid receptor in preterm human placenta. *J Soc Gynecol Invest* **12:** 238–45.

Jones CJ, Harris LK, Whittingham J, Aplin JD, Mayhew TM (2008) A re-appraisal of the morphophenotype and basal lamina coverage of cytotrophoblasts in human term placenta. *Placenta* **29:** 215–19.

Jones RL, Cederberg HM, Wheeler SJ, Poston L, Hutchinson CJ, Seed PT, Oliver RL, Baker PN (2010) Relationship between maternal growth, infant birth weight and nutrient partitioning in teenage pregnancies. *Br J Obstet Gynecol* **117:** 200–11.

Juhl M, Olsen J, Andersen PK, Nohr EA, Andersen AM (2010) Physical exercise during pregnancy and fetal growth measures: a study within the Danish National Birth Cohort. *Am J Obstet Gynecol* **202:** 63–8.

Keller G, Zimmer G, Mall G, Ritz E, Amann K (2003) Nephron number in patients with primary hypertension. *N Engl J Med* **348:** 101–8.

Kelly JJ, Davis PG, Henschke PN (2000) The drug epidemic: effects on newborn infants and health resource consumption at a tertiary perinatal centre. *J Paediatr Child Health* **36:** 262–4.

Keverne EB. Curley JP (2008) Epigenetics, brain evolution and behaviour. *Front Neuroendocrinol* **29:** 398–412.

Lambers DS, Clark KE (1996) The maternal and fetal physiologic effects of nicotine. *Semin Perinatol* **20:** 115–26.

Lee TM, Zucker I (1988) Vole infant development is influenced perinatally by maternal photoperiodic history. *Am J Physiol* **255:** R831–R838.

Lewis RM, Doherty CB, James LA, Burton GJ, Hales CN (2001) Effects of maternal iron restriction on placental vascularisation in the rat. *Placenta* **22:** 534–9.

Lewis RM, Greenwood SL, Cleal JK, Crozier SR, Verrall L, Inskip HM, Cameron IT, Cooper C, Sibley CP, Hanson MA, Godfrey KM (2010) Maternal muscle mass may influence system A activity in human placenta. *Placenta* **31:** 418–22.

Lillycrop KA, Phillips ES, Jackson AA, Hanson MA, Burdge GC (2005) Dietary protein restriction of pregnant rats induces and folic acid supplementation prevents epigenetic modification of hepatic gene expression in the offspring. *J Nutr* **135:** 1382–6.

Lin FJ, Fitzpatrick JW, Iannotti CA, Martin DS, Mariani BD, Tuan RS (1997) Effects of cadmium on trophoblast calcium transport. *Placenta* **18:** 341–56.

Lopata A, Oliva K, Stanton PG, Robertson DM (1997) Analysis of chorionic gonadotrophin secreted by cultured human blastocysts. *Mol Hum Reprod* **3:** 517–21.

Lumey LH (1998) Compensatory placental growth after restricted maternal nutrition in early pregnancy. *Placenta* **19:** 105–11.

Mannik J, Vaas P, Rull K, Teesalu P, Rebane T, Laan M (2010) Differential expression profile of growth hormone/chorionic somatomammotropin genes in placenta of small- and large-for-gestational-age newborns. *J Clin Endocrinol Metab* **95:** 2054–7.

Margetts BM, Rowland MG, Foord FA, Cruddas AM, Cole TJ, Barker DJ (1991) The relation of maternal weight to the blood pressures of Gambian children. *Int J Epidemiol* **20:** 938–43.

Mayhew TM, Jenkins H, Todd B, Clifton VL (2008) Maternal asthma and placental morphometry: effects of severity, treatment and fetal sex. *Placenta* **29:** 366–73.

McCrabb GJ, Egan AR, Hosking BJ (1991) Maternal undernutrition during mid-pregnancy in sheep. Placental size and its relationship to calcium transfer during late pregnancy. *Br J Nutr* **65:** 157–68.

McMillen IC, Robinson JS (2005) Developmental origins of the metabolic syndrome: prediction, plasticity, and programming. *Physiol Rev* **85:** 571–633.

Moore T, Mills W (2008) Evolutionary theories of imprinting – enough already! *Adv Exp Med Biol* **626:** 116–22.

Moritz KM, Singh RR, Probyn ME, Denton KM (2009) Developmental programming of a reduced nephron endowment: more than just a baby's birth weight. *Am J Physiol Renal Physiol* **296:** F1–F9.

Newsome CA, Shiell AW, Fall CH, Phillips DI, Shier R, Law CM (2003) Is birth weight related to later glucose and insulin metabolism? – A systematic review. *Diabet Med* **20:** 339–48.

Osmond C, Barker DJ (2000) Fetal, infant, and childhood growth are predictors of coronary heart disease, diabetes, and hypertension in adult men and women. *Environ Health Perspect* **108 (Suppl. 3):** 545–53.

Park B, Gibbons HM, Mitchell MD, Glass M (2003) Identification of the CB1 cannabinoid receptor and fatty acid amide hydrolase (FAAH) in the human placenta. *Placenta* **24:** 990–5.

Petropoulos S, Kalabis GM, Gibb W, Matthews SG (2007) Functional changes of mouse placental multidrug resistance phosphoglycoprotein (ABCB1) with advancing gestation and regulation by progesterone. *Reprod Sci* **14:** 321–8.

Pettitt DJ, Nelson RG, Saad MF, Bennett PH, Knowler WC (1993) Diabetes and obesity in the offspring of Pima Indian women with diabetes during pregnancy. *Diabetes Care* **16:** 310–14.

Razin A (1998) CpG methylation, chromatin structure and gene silencing – a three-way connection. *EMBO J* **17:** 4905–8.

Reik W, Dean W, Walter J (2001) Epigenetic reprogramming in mammalian development. *Science* **293:** 1089–93.

Risnes KR, Romundstad PR, Nilsen TI, Eskild A, Vatten LJ (2009) Placental weight relative to birth weight and long-term cardiovascular mortality: findings from a cohort of 31,307 men and women. *Am J Epidemiol* **170:** 622–31.

Roos S, Powell TL, Jansson T (2009) Placental mTOR links maternal nutrient availability to fetal growth. *Biochem Soc Trans* **37:** 295–8.

Roseboom TJ, van der Meulen JH, van Montfrans GA, Ravelli AC, Osmond C, Barker DJ, Bleker OP (2001) Maternal nutrition during gestation and blood pressure in later life. *J Hypertens* **19:** 29–34.

Shiell AW, Campbell DM, Hall MH, Barker DJ (2000) Diet in late pregnancy and glucose-insulin metabolism of the offspring 40 years later. *Br J Obstet Gynecol* **107:** 890–5.

Shiell AW, Campbell-Brown M, Haselden S, Robinson S, Godfrey KM, Barker DJ (2001) High-meat, low-carbohydrate diet in pregnancy: relation to adult blood pressure in the offspring. *Hypertension* **38:** 1282–8.

Sibley CP (2009) Symposium Report: Understanding Placental Nutrient Transfer – Why Bother? New Biomarkers of Fetal Growth. *J Physiol* **587:** 3431–40.

Sibley CP, Turner MA, Cetin I, Ayuk P, Boyd CA, D'Souza SW, Glazier JD, Greenwood SL, Jansson T, Powell T (2005) Placental phenotypes of intrauterine growth. *Pediatr Res* **58:** 827–32.

Stark MJ, Wright IM, Clifton VL (2009) Sex-specific alterations in placental 11beta-hydroxysteroid dehydrogenase 2 activity and early postnatal clinical course following antenatal betamethasone. *Am J Physiol Regul Integr Comp Physiol* **297:** R510–R514.

Vickers MH, Gluckman PD, Coveny AH, Hofman PL, Cutfield WS, Gertler A, Breier BH, Harris M (2005) Neonatal leptin treatment reverses developmental programming. *Endocrinology* **146:** 4209–10.

Virella G, Silveira Nunes MA, Tamagnini G (1972) Placental transfer of human IgG subclasses. *Clin Exp Immunol* **10:** 475–8.

Watkins AJ, Papenbrock T, Fleming TP (2008) The preimplantation embryo: handle with care. *Semin Reprod Med* **26:** 175–85.

Weaver IC, Cervoni N, Champagne FA, D'Alessio AC, Sharma S, Seckl JR, Dymov S, Szyf M, Meaney MJ (2004) Epigenetic programming by maternal behavior. *Nat Neurosci* **7:** 847–54.

Wen HY, Abbasi S, Kellems RE, Xia Y (2005) mTOR: a placental growth signaling sensor. *Placenta* **26 (Suppl. A):** S63–S69.

Wolff GL, Kodell RL, Moore SR, Cooney CA (1998) Maternal epigenetics and methyl supplements affect agouti gene expression in Avy/a mice. *FASEB J* **12:** 949–57.

Wyrwoll CS, Seckl JR, Holmes MC (2009) Altered placental function of 11beta-hydroxysteroid dehydrogenase 2 knockout mice. *Endocrinology* **150:** 1287–93.

Young BC, Levine RJ, Karumanchi SA (2010) Pathogenesis of preeclampsia. *Annu Rev Pathol* **5:** 173–92.

Zhu MJ, Du M, Nathanielsz PW, Ford SP (2010) Maternal obesity up-regulates inflammatory signaling pathways and enhances cytokine expression in the mid-gestation sheep placenta. *Placenta* **31:** 387–91.

Zuckerman B, Frank DA, Hingson R, Amaro H, Levenson SM, Kayne H, Parker S, Vinci R, Aboagye K, Fried LE (1989) Effects of maternal marijuana and cocaine use on fetal growth. *N Engl J Med* **320:** 762–8.

C H A P T E R

79

The significance of ABC transporters in human placenta for the exposure of the fetus to xenobiotics

Kirsi H. Vähäkangas, Jenni Veid, Vesa Karttunen, Heidi Partanen, Elina Sieppi, Maria Kummu, Päivi Myllynen and Jarkko Loikkanen

INTRODUCTION

Transplacental transport of nutrients and oxygen from the mother to the fetus is the prerequisite of fetal health and growth. On the other hand, the excretion of carbon dioxide and other waste products is necessary. Transplacental transport is, however, not restricted to this physiological exchange of agents, but is believed to extend to the majority of xenobiotics in maternal blood. Although at some stage it was thought that the placenta forms a good barrier against fetal exposure, it is currently understood that most compounds can cross the placenta. Thus both drugs necessary for maternal health during pregnancy (e.g., for epilepsia) and toxic compounds due to occupational or environmental exposure of the mother may reach the fetus. Many xenobiotics go through the placenta very easily by passive diffusion. Passive diffusion is the most common mechanism of transfer and depends on the chemical characteristics of compounds, such as molecular weight, lipid solubility, binding to proteins and the degree of ionization (Sastry, 1999). It is also possible that compounds accumulate in the placenta. For instance, cadmium both accumulates in the human placenta and affects its transport function (Kippler *et al.*, 2010).

The placenta grows and develops throughout the pregnancy. Trophoblastic cells are present already during early development at prelacunar stages making up the outer wall surrounding the blastocystic cavity. The intervillous circulation of maternal blood is likely to be established progressively between the 8th and 12th weeks. Later in pregnancy the exchange between the maternal and fetal circulations takes place in the chorionic villus, which is the functional unit of the human placenta. The structure in the human term placental barrier constitutes syncytiotrophoblast facing maternal blood space, connective tissue and fetal capillary endothelium (Figure 79.1; Benirschke *et al.*, 2006). Under the syncytiotrophoblast some remaining cytotrophoblasts can be found. These cells are the origin of the syncytiotrophoblast. The human placental barrier thins out to about one-tenth of the thickness towards term (50 μm at the end of second month to about 5 μm by the end of week 37).

Two important sets of proteins may affect the transplacental transfer of chemicals, drug metabolism enzymes and transporter proteins (Myllynen *et al.*, 2009). While the selection and activity of the enzymes metabolizing xenobiotics is restricted in the placenta, many transporters are expressed at a high level and their variety in the placenta is large (Vähäkangas and Myllynen, 2009). Transporter proteins play a significant role in transplacental transfer, and some of them have probably developed for the protection of cells and the fetus (Behravan and Piquette-Miller, 2007; Vähäkangas and Myllynen, 2009). The largest superfamily of transporters and one of the most interesting groups with regard to xenobiotics are the ATP-binding cassette (ABC) transporters, because in eukaryotes they are exporters (efflux transporters) with drugs and toxic agents as substrates (Jones *et al.*, 2009; Huls *et al.*, 2009). The efflux ABC transporters were originally found in cancer cells, when an explanation for drug resistance was sought and induction of ABCB1/P-glycoprotein was found in cells and humans treated with cancer medications. The efflux ABC transporters from families ABCB, ABCC and ABCG play a role in transporting xenobiotics and their conjugates, but also endogenous compounds (Borst and Elferink, 2002). Both genetic polymorphisms, endogenous regulation by, e.g., hormones as well as xenobiotics can modify the expression and function of transporters.

In the human placenta, the syncytiotrophoblast, cytotrophoblasts and fetal capillary endothelium express ABC transporters (Figure 79.1). In the syncytiotrophoblast, a different selection of ABC transporters is found in the apical brush-border membrane facing maternal blood and in the basal membrane facing fetal capillaries. The least known is the transporter status of fetal capillary endothelium, but it seems that they also express a unique selection of ABC transporters. This complex organization contributes to polarized transport of compounds to and from the maternal and fetal circulations in the placenta. When estimating the contribution of a specific

Reproductive and Developmental Toxicology, Edited by Ramesh C. Gupta
ISBN: 978-0-12-382032-7

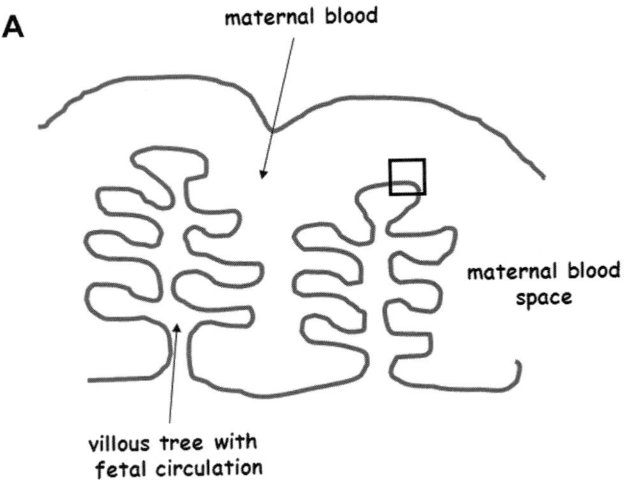

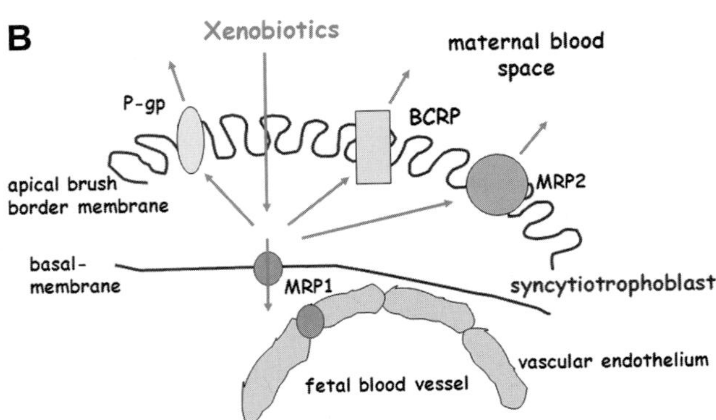

FIGURE 79.1 Human placental structure. (A) Villous trees and circulation in the placenta. The square denotes the site of the structure in (B), which illustrates the placental barrier at term showing the localization of the main ABC transporters in placental membranes.

transporter for fetal exposure both the nature (e.g., uptake vs. efflux) and localization have to be taken into account in addition to the level of expression, functional status and substrate specificity.

STRUCTURE, FUNCTION AND POLYMORPHISMS OF HUMAN EFFLUX ABC TRANSPORTERS

Introduction

The general importance of the ABC transporters is stressed by the fact that they are ubiquitously expressed from bacteria to humans in various organs. This large group of proteins (about 50 members in humans) is divided into subgroups A–G according to their sequence homology. They have a wide selection of substrates including both endogenous compounds and xenobiotics or their conjugates (Table 79.1). ABC transporters are expressed in absorptive, excretory and barrier organs in the human (Schinkel and Jonker, 2003). They require energy for their function provided by binding and hydrolysis of ATP (Rees *et al.*, 2009; Jones *et al.*, 2009). The nucleotide-binding domains of the ABC transporters localized in the cellular part of the proteins are among the most conserved DNA domains. Nucleotide-binding domains consist of 90–110 amino acids and the amino acid sequences are more similar than in the transmembrane domains. The transmembrane domains, on the other hand, are highly variable reflecting the wide variety of substrates. The transmembrane domains consist of membrane-spanning α-helices which give the substrate specificity to the transporter. All transporters may be *N*-glycosylated on the external side of the cell membrane (Schinkel and Jonker, 2003). Depending on the localization, they either prevent or facilitate the transfer of compounds to target organs. In the placenta they are expressed in all membranes of the syncytiotrophoblast and endothelial cells (Figure 79.1).

The expression of ABC transporters is regulated by multiple factors and is induced by many xenobiotics which often are also its substrates. Variation of ABC transporter expression is also caused by genetic factors. Gene polymorphisms have been described in all of the efflux ABC transporters expressed in human placenta (Table 79.1). Some polymorphisms may lead to changes in protein expression and their substrate specificity may also vary (Yanase *et al.*, 2006).

ABCB1/MDR1/P-glycoprotein

The ABCB1/P-glycoprotein (P-gp) is a typical ABC transporter consisting of two transmembrane domains and two nucleotide-binding domains (NBD) (Leslie *et al.*, 2005). Human P-gp contains two subclasses; class I, MDR1/ABCB1, and class II, MDR3/ABCB4 (Syme *et al.*, 2004). The ABCB1/P-gp (170 kDa) is probably the most studied and well-known transporter, because of its numerous interactions with pharmaceutical drugs (Wada, 2006). While the function of ABCB1/P-gp seems to be more concentrated on the transfer of xenobiotics, ABCB4 has also physiological functions in phosphatidylcholine transport and one of its SNPs (single nucleotide polymorphisms) has been reported to associate with intrahepatic cholestasis (Kitsiou-Tzeli *et al.*, 2009). ABCB1/P-gp is downregulated by glucocorticoids in guinea pig placenta (Kalabis *et al.*, 2009). In placenta, expression of ABCB1 decreases when gestation advances (Gil *et al.*, 2005). ABC transporters in basolateral and apical membranes of the placental trophoblast can also be regulated independently (Evseenko *et al.*, 2007)

So far the studies on ABCB1/P-gp polymorphisms in human placenta are at early stages and their final significance remains to be determined. Tanabe and coworkers (2001) found nine SNPs that affect the expression levels of ABCB1/P-gp by decreasing it. Of these, especially the synonymous C1236T and C3435T and the non-synonymous G2677T have been studied in human placenta. Rahi and coworkers (2008) reported the 3435T allele increasing the expression of placental ABCB1/P-gp, while G2677T/A polymorphism did not have any significant effect on transporter expression. According to May *et al.* (2008) polymorphisms of ABCB1/P-gp have no effect on the expression of these transporters in the human placenta. The most recent study (Hemauer *et al.*, 2010) analyzing almost 200 human placentas found all of these polymorphic forms decreasing placental expression of ABCB1/P-gp. Homozygotes for the variant alleles 1236T and 3435T were also associated with increased uptake of paclitaxel into the microvillous membrane vesicles.

TABLE 79.1 ABC-efflux transporters in human placenta. Substrates and inhibitors found in any experimental system are included. Based on reviews by Conseil *et al.* (2005), Vähäkangas and Myllynen (2009) and Mao (2008)

Name	Common alternative names	Polymorphisms in placenta[a]	Cellular localization in placenta[b]	Substrates	Inhibitors
ABCB1	p-gp MDR1	G2677T + C3435T G2677T + C1236T	ST (apic)	Anticancer drugs, protease inhibitors, drugs of abuse, steroids	Verapamil, cyclosporine, PSC833 (valspodar), GG918 GF120918
ABCC1	MRP1		ST (apic), ET	Reduced glutathione, methotrexate and folate analogs, glutathione, glucuronide and sulfate conjugates, heavy metal anionic complexes	Probenecid, cyclosporine, PSC833 MK571
ABCC2	MRP2	G1249A	ST (apic)	Reduced glutathione, methotrexate and folate analogs, glutathione and glucuronide conjugates, heavy metal anionic complexes	Probenecid, cyclosporine, PSC833, MK571
ABCC3	MRP3		ST (apic), ET	Methotrexate and folate analogs, glucuronide glutathione and sulfate conjugates	MK571, benzobromarone
ABCC5	MRP5		ST (basal) ET	cAMP, cGMP, reduced glutathione	
ABCG2	BCRP	C421A	ST (apic)	Anticancer drugs, estrone sulfates, cimetidine, glypuride, nitrofurantoin	GF120918, KO143, Fumitremorgin C, Glucocorticoids, digoxin, novobiocin, nicardipine

[a]With significance on the level of protein in human placenta and/or on the transport function
[b]ST = syncytiotrophoblast; apic = apical; ET = endothelium

ABCG2/BCRP

ABCG2/BCRP (72 kDa) is a so-called half transporter (72 kDa) because it consists of only one transmembrane domain and one nucleotide-binding domain. To become active it probably requires dimerization or oligomeration depending on the function (Robey *et al.*, 2009). ABCG2/BCRP was found relatively recently from MCF-7 breast cancer cells and human placenta (Allikmets *et al.*, 1998; Doyle *et al.*, 1998). It is highly expressed on the apical membrane of the human placental syncytiotrophoblast, but also on the apical membranes of other polarized cells such as kidney excretory epithelia (Vähäkangas and Myllynen, 2009). ABCG2/BCRP has many roles in the transport of essential compounds within the body. For instance, ABCG2/BCRP mediates secretion of urate to urine, and its functional polymorphism may result in gout (Woodward *et al.*, 2009). It is also expressed in the breast tissue, concentrating in mice both harmful xenobiotics, like the heterocyclic amine IQ (Van Herwaarden *et al.*, 2006) and other compounds like vitamin B2, riboflavin (Van Herwaarden *et al.*, 2007), to breast milk. ABCG2/BCRP is commonly believed to protect the fetus from harmful agents because of its localization on the apical, maternal blood facing brush-border membrane of the syncytiotrophoblast and its high expression in the human placenta. Its substrates also include toxic compounds, such as the liver carcinogen aflatoxin B1 (Van Herwaarden *et al.*, 2006) and carcinogenic heterocyclic amines, e.g. PhIP (Pavek *et al.*, 2005).

In human choriocarcinoma BeWo cells ABCG2/BCRP is regulated by estradiol and progesterone (Vore and Leggas, 2008) and ABCG2 promoter has been demonstrated to contain estrogen and hypoxia responsive elements as well as the peroxisome proliferator-activated receptor g (PPARg) response element (Krishnamurthy and Schuetz, 2006; Robey *et al.*, 2009; Vähäkangas and Myllynen, 2009). ABCG2 is also upregulated through the aryl hydrocarbon receptor (AhR) (Ebert *et al.*, 2005). In addition to pregnancy-related steroid hormones and xenobiotics, growth factors also affect ABCG2/BCRP expression. Inflammation seems to decrease the protection of cells by many cytokines and interleukins downregulating ABCG2/BCRP expression (Englund *et al.*, 2007). Contradictory results exist about the expression of human placental ABCG2/BCRP in different stages of pregnancy, one study indicating a decrease by advancing gestation (Meyer zu Schwabedissen *et al.*, 2006) while other studies suggest either no change (Mathias *et al.*, 2005) or rather an increase (Yeboah *et al.*, 2006). Folate seems to affect ABCG2/BCRP expression, but whether it up- or downregulates is still under debate (Ifergan *et al.*, 2004; Lemos *et al.*, 2008).

Over 80 SNPs have been characterized in the ABCG2 gene (Tamura *et al.*, 2007). Among 100 human placentas, Kobayashi *et al.* (2005) found 20 polymorphisms in the ABCG2 gene of which the most common SNPs were G34A or Val112Met (18.0%) and C421A or Gln141Lys (Q141K) (35.5%). Although they did not find any statistically significant genotype-dependent effect on ABCG2 mRNA expression, placentas with the A421 allele had lower ABCG2/BCRP protein levels than those with the C421 allele (Kobayshi *et al.*, 2005). The C421A polymorphism also affects the transport of xenobiotics across the cell membrane, as shown in the accumulation of glypuride in human embryonic kidney cells transfected with the polymorphic allele (Pollex *et al.*, 2010). These SNPs are the most frequent in most ethnic populations (Imai *et al.*, 2002; Kobayashi *et al.*, 2005). The C376T polymorphism is noteworthy, because the T allele does not produce any protein (Imai *et al.*, 2002). However, its significance in the placenta is not known.

ABCC/MRP

The ABCC/MRP transporters are variable in size and structure, but their substrate specificity overlaps. Although they are full transporters with two nucleotide-binding domains ABCC1/MRP1 and ABCC2/MRP2 are structurally different from ABCB1/P-gp. They consist of five domains with an extra aminoterminal transmembrane domain. ABCC1/MRP1 and ABCC2/MRP2 have relevance to detoxification, as they act synergistically with several phase II metabolic enzymes such as GSTs and UGTs (Leslie *et al.*, 2005). Numerous SNPs in human ABCC genes were described by Saito and coworkers (2002) in Japanese individuals, but only some of them probably have clinical significance (Conseil *et al.*, 2005).

ABCC1/MRP1 has a wide range of endogenous substrates, e.g. leukotrienes, and it has been suggested that normally its primary role in the placenta involves these rather than xenobiotics (Atkinson *et al.*, 2003). ABCC2/MRP2 was first detected in a cisplatin-resistant human cancer cell line and transports cytostatics. It is also responsible for transporting many heavy metals such as zinc, copper, manganese, cadmium and arsenic (Leslie *et al.*, 2005). However, according to many publications the substrate specificities of ABCC1/MRP1 and ABCC2/MRP2 are very similar (Table 79.1) but their localization in human placental membranes is different. ABCC1/MRP1 is found on the basal membrane of the syncytiotrophoblast and in endothelial cells. ABCC2/MRP2 is expressed in the apical plasma membrane of the syncytiotrophoblast and its expression in the placenta increases with advancing gestation (Meyer zu Schwabedissen *et al.*, 2005b). ABCC2/MRP2 is also physiologically important for, e.g., liver function and an ABCC2 SNP is responsible for the deficient excretion of bilirubin conjugates causing hyperbilirubinemia in Dubin-Johnson syndrome (Wada, 2006). So far, no effect by ABCC2 polymorphisms on the expression of this transporter in human term placentas have been found while the SNP G1249A lowers the expression in preterm placentas (Meyer zu Schwabedissen *et al.*, 2005b; May *et al.*, 2008).

Like ABCB1/P-gp, the expression of ABCC5/MRP5 also decreases when gestation advances (Meyer zu Schwabedissen *et al.*, 2005a). Important substrates for ABCC5/MRP5 are cyclic nucleotides cAMP and cGMP (Meyer zu Schwabedissen *et al.*, 2005a). Tetramethylpyrazine has been reported to inhibit ABCC5/MRP5 (Wang *et al.*, 2010). It is regulated by human chorionic gonadotropin (hCG) which upregulates ABCC5/MRP5 in human primary trophoblasts (Meyer zu Schwabedissen *et al.*, 2005a).

During the differentiation of cytotrophoblast cells to syncytiotrophoblast the expression of ABCC5/MRP5 (Pascolo *et al.*, 2001; Meyer zu Schwabedissen *et al.*, 2005a) and ABCC2/MRP2 (Meyer zu Schwabedissen *et al.*, 2005b) is increased in the human placenta. While the importance of ABCB1/P-gp and ABCG2/BCRP on transplacental transfer of xenobiotics has been demonstrated (see, e.g., Vähäkangas and Myllynen, 2009), much less is known about ABCC/MRP-transporters and foreign chemicals in the placenta. However, functional inhibition of ABCC2/MRP2 inhibits materno-fetal transfer of talinolol in perfusion of human term placentas (May *et al.*, 2008). In fact it has been suggested by May and coworkers (2008) that the expression of ABCC2/MRP2 increases towards term and that ABCC2/MRP2 may be more important in xenobiotic transfer than ABCB1/P-gp in late pregnancy.

MODELS TO STUDY HUMAN PLACENTAL TRANSPORTERS

Introduction

In vivo numerous endogenous and exogenous compounds may affect the level and functions of transporters making it challenging to determine the role of an individual transporter in xenobiotic transport or drug–drug interactions (Wang *et al.*, 2008). Detailed mechanistic information can be gained from various available *in vitro* models. However, the full complexity of the interactions between substrates, inhibitors and efflux transporters can probably only be seen in situations retaining the whole functional structure of the placenta. The experimental models used to study placental transfer processes *in vitro* include placental perfusion, cultured placental tissue explants or isolated villous trees, primary cell cultures, immortalized or cancer cell lines, placental membrane vesicles and cloned transporters (Table 79.2). *In vivo* data may originate from animal experimentation. Also samples collected from term or preterm deliveries are commonly used when placental transporters are studied.

Placental tissue and tissue preparations

The expression and polymorphisms of placental transporters, and variation in the expression levels of transporters between individuals or during different stages of pregnancy, can be analyzed by utilizing tissue from term placentas after delivery or placentas obtained after elective termination of pregnancy. Several such studies have confirmed the expression of different ABC transporters in human placenta at protein level. These include studies on ABCG2/BCRP (Kobayashi *et al.*, 2005; Myllynen *et al.*, 2008; Vaidya *et al.*, 2009), ABCB1/P-gp (Nagashige *et al.*, 2003; Mölsä *et al.*, 2005; Rahi *et al.*, 2007, 2008; May *et al.*, 2008; Malek *et al.*, 2009; Vaidya *et al.*, 2009), ABCC1/MRP1 (Nagashige *et al.*, 2003; Vaidya *et al.*, 2009) and ABCC2/MRP2 (May *et al.*, 2008; Myllynen *et al.*, 2008; Vaidya *et al.*, 2009). In these studies, immunoblotting, immunohistochemistry and immunofluorescence were utilized to evaluate the expression levels of transporter proteins in placental tissue.

Human placental villous explants can be cultured *in vitro* (Genbacev *et al.*, 1992; Caniggia *et al.*, 1997). Although the structure of tissue in culture is retained, the viability of explant cultures of the placenta is limited (Di Santo *et al.*, 2003). Placental villous explants have been used to study the expression and function of placental transporters (e.g., Atkinson *et al.*, 2006). In addition to term placentas, first-trimester placentas have also been used to establish chorionic villous explant cultures (Cannigia *et al.*, 1997; Ietta *et al.*, 2010). By using this model, Ietta and coworkers (2010) showed that 17β-estradiol reduces the expression of ABCA1 cholesterol transporter both at mRNA and protein levels in first-trimester human cultured villous explants.

Both apical brush-border and basal membrane vesicles have been prepared from human placenta to study the expression and function of transporters. The purity of isolated membrane vesicles can be determined with specific markers. Alkaline phosphatase is a commonly used marker for the apical membrane (Nagashige *et al.*, 2003; Meyer zu Schwabedissen *et al.*, 2005a; Gedeon *et al.*, 2008; Hemauer *et al.*, 2009). Different markers for basal membrane include

TABLE 79.2 Models to study human placental transporters

Type of model	Specific model	Characteristics	Examples of transporter studies
Placental perfusion	Non-recirculating (open/single-pass) perfusion of one cotyledon[1]	Placentas reflect the third trimester of the pregnancy	Role of different transporters and their polymorphisms on transfer kinetics[2,3,4,5,6]
	Recirculating (closed) perfusion of one cotyledon[7]	Placentas reflect the third trimester of the pregnancy	Role of different transporters and their polymorphisms on transfer kinetics[8,9,10]
Placental tissue	Analysis of tissue	Tissue from a born or aborted placenta	Expression, localization and polymorphism of transporters[2,4,6,8,9,11,12,13,14]
Tissue explants	Chorionic villous explant cultures[15,16]	From first to third trimester placentas	Expression and function/activity of transporters[14,17,18]
Primary cell cultures	Human primary cytotrophoblast cells[19,20]	Cytotrophoblast cells from the term placenta; differentiate in culture to form functional syncytiotrophoblast	Expression and activity of transporters, and their effect on trophoblast function[21,22,23,24]
Immortalized cell lines	HChEpC1b[25]	Immortalized primary trophoblast cells from human placenta	No studies on transporters
Cancer cell lines	BeWo (choriocarcinoma)	Cytotrophoblasts; no differentiation to syncytium	Expression and activity of transporters; role of transporters on cellular uptake and efflux[21,23,24,26,27]
	JEG-3 (choriocarcinoma)	Derived from BeWo cells; form large multinucleated syncytia	
	JAr (choriocarcinoma)	Resemble early placental trophoblasts; form syncytia	
Transwell – model	BeWo[*28]	BeWo cells (human choriocarcinoma cells) which form confluent and polarized monolayers	Role of transporters on transcellular transfer[26,29]
Placental membrane vesicles	Placental brush-border and basal membrane vesicles	Useful to study basic transport mechanisms	Expression and localization of transporters; activity of transporters; role of different transporters on transfer kinetics[11,14,22,30,31,32,33]
Cloning	Cloned placental transporters and their promoters	Cloned transporters can be expressed and characterized in various expression systems	Function of cloned transporter; promoter characterization of transporters[34,35,36]

[*]A rat HRP-1 cell line from placenta growing in a monolayer also exists
[1]Schneider *et al.*, 1972; [2]Mölsä *et al.*, 2005; [3]Rahi *et al.*, 2007; [4]Rahi *et al.*, 2008; [5]Rahi *et al.*, 2009; [6]Tertti *et al.*, 2010; [7]Brandes *et al.*, 1983; [8]May *et al.*, 2008; [9]Myllynen et al 2008; [10]Pollex *et al.*, 2008; [11]Nagashige *et al.*, 2003; [12]Kobayashi *et al.*, 2005; [13]Malek *et al.*, 2009; [14]Vaidya *et al.*, 2009; [15]Genbacev *et al.*, 1992; [16]Caniggia *et al.*, 1997; [17]Atkinson *et al.*, 2006; [18]Ietta *et al.*, 2010; [19]Kliman *et al.*, 1986; [20]Petroff *et al.*, 2006; [21]Utoguchi *et al.*, 2000; [22]Meyer zu Schwabedissen 2005a; [23]Evseenko *et al.*, 2006; [24]Evseenko *et al.*, 2007; [25]Omi *et al.*, 2009; [26]Pascolo *et al.*, 2001; [27]Serrano *et al.*, 2007; [28]Bode *et al.*, 2006; [29]Parry and Zhang 2007; [30]Kolwankar *et al.*, 2005; [31]Gedeon *et al.*, 2008; [32]Hemauer *et al.*, 2009; [33]Hemauer *et al.*, 2010; [34]Bailey-Dell *et al.*, 2001; [35]Furesz *et al.*, 2002; [36]Ganapathy *et al.*, 2006

Na^+/K^+-ATPase (Gedeon *et al.*, 2008) and binding activity of ^{3}H-dihyroalprenolol (Nagashige *et al.*, 2003). It is also possible to prepare membrane vesicles overexpressing different transporters to further study their role in transport of potential substrates (Vaidya *et al.*, 2009).

Placental perfusion

Transfer of compounds across the human placenta can be modeled using placental perfusion retaining placental tissue structure and function (Schneider *et al.*, 1972; Ala-Kokko *et al.*, 2000; Vähäkangas and Myllynen, 2006). *In vivo* human studies on new drugs can only be gained in situations where the drug is clinically important for the mother (e.g., Myllynen *et al.*, 2003). Experimental studies on toxic environmental compounds are impossible *in vivo* in humans, but quite a few studies exist where cord blood and maternal concentrations in people exposed in their environment have been compared (Barr *et al.*, 2007). Animal placentas have been perfused also, but it is important to realize that placentas vary more than any other organ between species (Nau, 1986; Leiser and Kaufmann, 1994), making extrapolation from animal studies difficult.

In the most common application of human placental perfusion one cotyledon of the newly born placenta is kept alive with double circulation of fetal and maternal sides (Schneider *et al.*, 1972; Brandes *et al.*, 1983). Perfusion may be either non-recirculating (open/single-pass) or recirculating (closed) perfusion. Samples from maternal and fetal sides, and tissue samples after the perfusion, can be collected. It is also possible to control the conditions of perfusion, e.g. flow rate (Dancis 1985). Human placental perfusion is a versatile model. In addition to the transfer of xenobiotics, DNA adducts (Olivero *et al.*, 1999; Annola *et al.*, 2009) and placental metabolism (Partanen *et al.*, 2010) can be studied in human placental perfusion.

Theoretically, the effect of xenobiotics on placental proteins, e.g. induction of metabolizing enzymes or transporters, can be studied but such studies are restricted by the time of perfusion. The longest human placental perfusion described in the literature lasted 48 hours (Polliotti *et al.*, 1996) but generally placentas are perfused only for a few hours. Still, in a recent placental perfusion study by Malek and coworkers (2009) placental expression level of ABCB1/P-gp was increased in response to methadone alone or in combination with heroin or cocaine. Studies on the role of placental transporters on the transfer of drugs or other xenobiotics across perfused placenta are increasing. However, so far the number of transporters studied is limited and mainly ABCB1/P-gp or ABCG2/BCRP has been studied so far.

Trophoblastic cells

Cell cultures are widely used models to study the function of cells representing different organs including placenta. To study placental transport and transporters with cultured cells, some aspects have to be taken into account before selecting a cell model. Placenta (term or aborted) is a rare example of tissues enabling the establishment of primary cell cultures of human origin. Although methods for isolating and culturing functional primary cytotrophoblasts from human placenta exist (Kliman *et al.*, 1986; Petroff *et al.*, 2006), the establishment of primary placental cell cultures is laborious compared to immortalized or cancer cell lines. On the other hand, cancer cell lines are transformed and thus primary cells clearly have the advantage of representing normal cells.

The most commonly used human placental cell lines derived from choriocarcinoma are BeWo, Jeg-3 and JAr (Table 79.3; Kitano *et al.*, 2004; Vähäkangas and Myllynen, 2006). In addition, Omi *et al.* (2009) have immortalized primary human trophoblast cells to establish a cell line, HChEpC1b, to serve as a model to study the function of trophoblasts. Primary placental cells or continuous cell lines can be utilized to study the expression and cellular localization of transporters. In addition, cultured cells can be used to study cellular uptake or efflux of xenobiotics and physiological compounds, and the role of transporters in these processes. Transcellular transport, however, can only be studied with cells able to form polarized confluent monolayers by using Transwell or side-by-side techniques (Bode *et al.*, 2006).

Kliman *et al.* (1986) showed that isolated cytotrophoblasts from human term placenta differentiate in culture and form a functional syncytiotrophoblast. This is associated with increased expression of ABCC5/MRP5 and production of human chorionic gonadotropin (hCG) in the differentiated multinuclear syncytiotrophoblast (Meyer zu Schwabedissen *et al.*, 2005a). There are also changes in the expression of other ABC transporters during cytotrophoblast differentiation and formation of multinucleated syncytium. Evseenko *et al.* (2006) showed that the expression of ABCB1 and ABCB4 reduced with differentiation while ABCG2 expression strikingly increased both at mRNA and protein levels. Inhibition of ABCG2/BCRP with Ko143 increased cytokine-induced apoptosis in primary trophoblasts and trophoblast-like Bewo cells suggesting a survival role for ABCG2/BCRP in placenta (Evseenko *et al.*, 2007). Utoguchi *et al.* (2000) showed the expression ABCB1/P-gp both in primary human cytotrophoblasts and in BeWo cells. In both cell models, the inhibition of ABCB1/P-gp with cyclosporin A or dipyridamole increased the cellular accumulation of its substrates, calcein-AM and vinblastine (Utoguchi *et al.*, 2000).

All the commonly used choriocarcinoma cell lines (BeWo, Jeg-3, JAr) express ABCB1, several ABCCs and ABCG2 at mRNA level (Table 79.3; Serrano *et al.*, 2007). However, some of these never seem to be translated into proteins to any significant amount. Of these, in BeWo cells ABCB1/P-gp and ABCC2/MRP2 proteins are missing and in JAR cells, ABCC2/MRP2 protein (Evseenko *et al.*, 2006). BeWo cells, despite their limitations, provide a functional model for studies on trophoblastic cell functions, transport and metabolism (Liu *et al.*, 1997). BeWo cells have similar morphological properties and biochemical marker enzymes as normal placental trophoblasts.

TABLE 79.3 The representativeness of human trophoblastic cancer cell lines of human placenta for transporter studies

Placenta, primary trophoblasts	JAr	Jeg-3	BeWo
ABCB1/p-gp[1,3]	mRNA[2], P[2,3]	mRNA[4], P[2]	mRNA[2], P[2], NP[3,5]
ABCG2/ BCRP[1,3]	mRNA[2], P[2,3]	mRNA[2] P[2]	mRNA[2], P[2,3,5]
ABCC1/MRP1[1,3]	mRNA[2], P[3]	mRNA[2]	mRNA[2,7], P[3,7]
ABCC2/MRP2[1,3]	mRNA[2], NP[3]	NDA	mRNA[2,7], NP[3]
ABCC3/MRP3[1]	NDA	NDA	mRNA[7]
ABCC5/MRP5[6]	NDA	NDA	mRNA[7], P[7]

P = protein found, NP = minimal or no protein, mRNA = mRNA found, NDA = no data available
[1]Nishimura and Naito 2005; [2]Serrano *et al.*, 2007; [3]Evseenko *et al.*, 2006; [4]Pavek *et al.*, 2007; [5]Myllynen *et al.*, 2008; [6]Meyer zu Schwabedissen *et al.*, 2005a; [7]Pascolo *et al.*, 2003

Both polarization of the trophoblastic cells (Pascolo *et al.*, 2001) and culture conditions (Immonen *et al.*, 2009) may affect the results of cell culture studies. Pascolo and coworkers (2001, 2003) showed that BeWo cells have strong ABCC1 and weak ABCC5 expression at mRNA and protein level. In these studies, they showed that MK-571, an inhibitor of ABCC/MRP proteins, inhibited the efflux, but not influx, of unconjugated bilirubin from BeWo cells confirming the functionality of ABCCs/MRPs in this cell line (Pascolo *et al.*, 2001). Inhibition was more profound in polarized (Transwell) than in non-polarized BeWo cells (Pascolo *et al.*, 2001). This is in line with the observation that the expression of ABCC1/MRP1 is higher in polarized than non-polarized BeWo cells (Pascolo *et al.*, 2001, 2003). This emphasizes that culture conditions may affect also the expression and thereby the function of other transporters. In addition to human cell lines, immortalized rodent syncytiotrophoblast cell lines, TR-TBTs, have been established. These express several transporters including ABCB1/P-gp and ABCG2/BCRP and can consequently be used in transport studies (for a review, see Kitano *et al.*, 2004).

The prerequisite for reliable studies on transcellular transport in cell cultures is the ability of the cells to form confluent and polarized monolayers with tight junctions. Of the human choriocarcinoma cell lines, only BeWo cells have been reported to fulfill these requirements. A subclone of BeWo cells, BeWo b30, has been published to be usable, albeit with difficulties, in transport studies (Liu *et al.*, 1997; Heaton *et al.*, 2008). Hemmings *et al.* (2001) reported that they have succeeded in culturing primary human cytotrophoblasts on semi-permeable membranes in confluent layers with tight junctions. This model does not seem to be very straightforward either, because it requires several steps for the cells to be seeded and differentiated before confluent layers are formed (Hemmings *et al.*, 2001). However, it may offer an alternative for the studies on transcellular placental transport with the benefit of primary cells of human origin.

It is of interest in this context that a rodent placental trophoblast HRP-1 cell line has been used to study permeability and transport of compounds across polarized monolayers (Shi *et al.*, 1997). Of the ABC transporters, HRP-1 cells express functional Abcg2/Bcrp, but not Abcb1/P-gp (Staud *et al.*, 2006). The presence of other transporters has also been reported in HRP-1 cell line. These include glucose transporter (Das *et al.*, 1998), anionic amino acid uptake proteins (Novak *et al.*, 2001) and transferrin (Morris Buus and Boockfor, 2004). In addition, HRP-1 cells have been used to characterize at least fatty acid transport (Knipp *et al.*, 2000) and organic anion transport (Zhou *et al.*, 2003).

Cloned transporters can be further studied by expressing them either in mammalian cells or in other expression systems. Bailey-Dell *et al.* (2001) characterized genomic organization of the ABCG2 gene by cloning and studied the activity of its promoter by luciferase reporter assay in JAr, Bewo and Jeg-3 choriocarcinoma cell lines. These cells have high endogenous ABCG2/BCRP expression. The function of cloned placental transporters can also be studied in mammalian cells by the vaccinia virus expression system (Ganapathy *et al.*, 2006) or in *Xenopus* oocytes (Furesz *et al.*, 2002; Ganapathy *et al.*, 2006).

STUDIES ON TRANSPLACENTAL TRANSPORT AND PLACENTAL TRANSPORTERS

Introduction

All research models and approaches described have been used to study placental transporters. In addition, there are studies where blood concentrations of environmental and other compounds (e.g., medicinal drugs) have been studied after the birth of babies. These studies give an idea how the compounds reach the fetus and increase understanding of the significance of transplacental transport *in vivo*. Because animal studies, especially transporter knockout mice, have given valuable data about the significance of the role of transporters in fetal exposure and fetotoxicity, some of those data are also included.

In vitro studies

In vitro studies have given valuable information of the expression (both at mRNA and protein level), regulation and substrate specificity of transporters, as well as helped in identification of inhibitors of transporters. Placental tissue preparations, primary trophoblastic cells and trophoblastic cancer cell lines have all been used in these studies.

It has been demonstrated *in vitro* that some estrogenic compounds present in food, like mycotoxin zearalenone (ZEA), bisphenol A (BPA), isoflavone genistein (GEN) and stillbene resveratrol (RES), influence the levels of ABC transporters. Natural estrogens, such as estradiol, as well as xenoestrogens, such as bisphenol A, have been shown to increase the drug efflux activity of ABCB1/P-gp in BeWo cells due to increased protein expression (Jin and Audus, 2005). Also in Bewo cells a 24 h exposure to ZEA induced the expression of ABCC1, ABCC2 and ABCG2 mRNA (Prouillac *et al.*, 2009). Induction of ABCB1/P-gp, ABCC1/MRP1 and ABCC2/MRP2 protein was observed after 48 h of ZEA exposure. Whether the expression is induced or reduced depends on the chemical and concentration used (Hanet *et al.*, 2008).

Atkinson *et al.* (2006) showed that the expression of ABCB1/P-gp is maintained in cultured villous explants from term placentas. In this model, cyclosporin-induced inhibition of ABCB1/P-gp increased intracellular accumulation of ^{3}H-vinblastine. Furthermore, localization of ABCB1/P-gp was found to be similar as it is in an intact placenta, i.e. in the apical microvillous plasma membrane (Atkinson *et al.*, 2006). Vaidya *et al.* (2009) showed the expression of various ABC transporters (ABCC1/MRP1, ABCC2/MRP2, ABCB1/P-gp, ABCG2/BCRP) in term placentas. By exposing cultured human placental villous tissue fragments to 1-chloro-2, 4-dinitrobenzene (CDNB), they showed the formation of 2,4-dinitrophenyl-*S*-glutathione (DNP-SG), a glutathione conjugate of CDNB. The efflux of DNP-SG from cultured villous tissue fragments was partially inhibited by sodium orthovanadate (ATPase inhibitor), MK571 (ABCC/MRP inhibitor), verapamil (ABCB1/P-gp inhibitor) and dipyridamole (inhibitor of ABCG2/BCRP, ABCB1/P-gp and ABCC1/MRP1). Of these inhibitors only orthovanadate marginally reduced the formation of DNP-SG (Vaidya *et al.*, 2009).

In purified membrane vesicles, Nagashige *et al.* (2003) showed that ABCB1/P-gp is observed only in brush-border membrane vesicles. They showed the highest expression of ABCC1/MRP1 in basal membrane vesicles, but this transporter was also found to a lesser extent in brush-border membrane. Immunohistochemistry of placental tissue supported these findings showing ABCB1/P-gp expression in the apical and ABCC1/MRP1 in the basal side of the trophoblast layer (Nagashige *et al.*, 2003). In agreement, Hemauer *et al.* (2009) showed also the expression of ABCB1/P-gp in vesicles of human placental brush-border membrane. According to Hemauer *et al.* (2009), opiates (methadone, buprenorphine, morphine) inhibit the uptake of paclitaxel more potently than a widely used ABCB1/P-gp inhibitor, verapamil, in the vesicles of placental brush-border membrane. In addition, gene polymorphisms of ABCB1 can affect the expression and activity of ABCB1/P-gp (Hemauer *et al.*, 2010). Meyer zu Schwabedissen *et al.* (2005a) showed that the expression and functional activity of ABCC5/MRP5 was mainly localized in basal membrane vesicles although it was also observed, but at lower levels, in vesicles of apical membranes. They showed similar localization of ABCC5/MRP5 in placental tissue by immunofluorescence (Meyer zu Schwabedissen *et al.*, 2005a).

ABCG2/BCRP inhibitor, novobiocin, increased the uptake of ^{3}H-glyburide in human placental brush-border membrane vesicles whereas indomethacin, inhibitor of ABCC/MRP transporters, or verapamil, inhibitor of ABCB1/P-gp, had no effects on uptake of glyburide (Gedeon *et al.*, 2008). This suggests that glyburide is transported by ABCG2/BCRP in human placenta. Vaidya *et al.* (2009) studied the transport of ^{3}H-DNP-SG or ^{3}H-E_217G into Sf9 membrane vesicles individually overexpressing ABCB1/P-gp, ABCG2/BCRP, ABCC1/MRP1, ABCC2/MRP2 or ABCC3/MRP3. According to their results, only ABCC1/MRP1 and ABCC2/MRP2 participate in ATP-dependent transport of DNP-SG. ABCG2/BCRP and ABCC2/MRP2 showed highest activity in the transport of E_217G, although transport in vesicles overexpressing ABCB1/P-gp, ABCC1/MRP1 and ABCC3/MRP3 was significantly higher than in control vesicles (Vaidya *et al.*, 2009).

By using microvillus membrane vesicles isolated from placentas of smokers and non-smokers, Kolwankar *et al.* (2005) showed that smoking has no clear effects on the expression and activity of ABCB1/P-pg or ABCG2/BCRP, although it was clear that CYP1A1 activity was induced in placental microsomes of smokers (Kolwankar *et al.*, 2005) as shown earlier (e.g., Vähäkangas *et al.*, 1989). Of the CYP enzymes, partly regulated by the same factors as the ABC transporters, only CYP1A1 activity has been clearly shown in human placenta (Myllynen *et al.*, 2009). However, xenobiotic metabolism by other enzymes has been shown in human placenta. For instance, cytosolic fraction of human placenta was found to metabolize aflatoxin B1 to aflatoxicol (Partanen *et al.*, 2010).

Animal studies

Human ABCB1/P-gp is encoded by a single ABCB1 gene. However, the mouse has two Abcb1 isoforms of the protein, Abcb1a and Abcb1b, encoded by Abcb1a and Abcb1b genes. The combined distribution and function of Abcb1a and Abcb1b proteins is similar to that of human ABCB1 (Devault and Gros, 1990). In guinea pig placenta the expression of both Abcb1a and Abcb1b mRNA decreases towards the end of gestation similar to human ABCB1 (Kalabis *et al.*, 2009).

The significance of ABCB1/P-gp protein in protecting fetus against xenobiotics has been demonstrated clearly in animal studies. In mouse, inhibition of the placental Abcb1 leads to greatly enhanced transplacental passage of digoxin, saquinavir and paclitaxel into the fetus (Smit *et al.*, 1999). Similar feto-protective functions have also been amply demonstrated in rat placenta (see, e.g., Pavek *et al.*, 2001, 2003). ABCG2/BCRP is a maternally facing efflux transporter similar to ABCB1/P-gp. In mouse Abcg2/Bcrp limits the transfer of nitrofurantoin, topotecan and glyburide from maternal to fetal circulation (for a review see, e.g., Mao, 2008) suggesting that it has also feto-protective functions. In addition, both of these transporters accelerate fetal-to-maternal transport. Cygalova *et al.* (2009) recently showed that they are capable of transporting marker substrates even against concentration gradient from fetal circulation.

The first study to demonstrate the significance of Abcb1/P-gp in the fetal protection against malformations was a mouse study by Lankas and coworkers (1998). In their study the Abcb1 genotype was linked with teratogenicity: 100% of the mouse fetuses with deficient placental Abcb1/P-gp developed cleft palate after exposure to the pesticide ivermectin while wild-type mice with abundant Abcb1 expression in the placenta showed no malformations. Interestingly, the heterozygotes expressing an intermediate level of placental Abcb1 also showed intermediate sensitivity for ivermectin-induced malformations.

Petropoulos *et al.* (2007) demonstrated a significant increase in transplacental transfer of ^{3}H-digoxin in late gestation when compared to earlier embryonic days. Similarly, Coles and coworkers (2009) showed that after repeated dosing more saquinavir reached the fetus at late gestation than in mid-gestation although a similar effect was not seen after a single dose. In a recent study utilizing positron emission tomography (PET) imaging, Chung and coworkers (2010) investigated whether gestational age affects Abcb1 activity in tissue of the pregnant non-human primate *Macaca nemestrina*. Interestingly, their results suggest that Abcb1 activity increases in both the placental barrier and the blood–brain barrier by advancing gestation.

Gestational age is not the only factor affecting the expression of ABC transporters. Petrovic and coworkers (2007) showed in rats that endotoxin-induced inflammation down-regulates mRNA and/or protein expression of several placental transporters (Abcg2, Abcb1a, Abcb1b, Abcc1, Abcc2, Abcc3, Slco1a4, Slco2b1, Slco4a1) which leads to the accumulation of glyburide in the fetus. Environmental and lifestyle factors may also affect placental ABC transporter expression. Interestingly, in a recent study nicotine decreased abcb1a expression during late gestation in the rat while it had no effect on abcb1b mRNA expression. Abcb1/P-gp expression significantly decreased at gestational days 15 and 18 (Wang *et al.*, 2009) which may increase the sensitivity of the fetus for environmental toxins.

Human placental perfusion studies

The main use of human placental perfusion has been to provide information on transfer kinetics of studied compounds. Placental perfusion has been used mainly to characterize transplacental transfer of drugs (e.g., Myllynen *et al.*, 2001, 2003; Myllynen and Vähäkangas, 2002; Mölsä *et al.*, 2005; Rahi *et al.*, 2007, 2008, 2009; May *et al.*, 2008; Pollex *et al.*, 2008, 2010; Earhart *et al.*, 2009; Gavard *et al.*, 2009; Malek *et al.*, 2009; Ueki *et al.*, 2009). So far this model has been utilized less to study the transfer of environmental toxic compounds across the human placenta (e.g., Loibichler *et al.*, 2002; Sörgel *et al.*, 2002; Mose *et al.*, 2007; Myllynen *et al.*, 2008; Annola *et al.*, 2008, 2009; Mathiesen *et al.*, 2009; May *et al.*, 2009; Partanen *et al.*, 2010). Although only term placentas have been studied, implications of the impact by the stage of development have been gained even in perfusion studies. Nanovskaya and coworkers (2008) showed in dual perfused human placenta that the transfer of a known p-glycoprotein substrate, methadone, is 30% higher in term (38–41 weeks) than in pre-term (27–34 weeks) placentas. Important information of the model can be gained by comparing the transfer with available *in vivo* data (Table 79.4). It seems that especially with very lipid soluble compounds there may be a problem with the recovery of the compound in the perfusion system (Myllynen and Vähäkangas, 2002) leading to differences in the transfer in perfusion compared to *in vivo* studies.

Transporter studies in the human placental perfusion model can be conducted in two ways. First, the transfer of a compound from maternal-to-fetal or from fetal-to-maternal circulation can be compared. Such comparison gives an idea whether there may be transporter proteins involved. For example, Mölsä and coworkers noticed that the fetal-to-maternal transfer of saquinavir is 108-fold higher compared with maternal-to-fetal transfer (Mölsä *et al.*, 2005). Second, a specific transporter inhibitor can be used together with the studied substances (Table 79.5). The substance and inhibitor can be added to either the maternal or fetal side. In some cases, the studied substances are added to both fetal and maternal circulations (Kraemer *et al.*, 2006; Pollex *et al.*, 2008). In these cases, inhibitor can be also added to both sides (Kraemer *et al.*, 2006) or only to one side (Pollex *et al.*, 2008). If substances and inhibitors are added to the maternal side, positive results may be seen as an increase in maternal-to-fetal transfer (Myllynen *et al.*, 2008). On the other hand, if substances are added to the fetal side, positive results of an inhibitor may be seen as a decrease of fetal-to-maternal transfer (Rahi *et al.*, 2009).

Indications of the role of several placental transporters in the protection of the human fetus against xenobiotics have been gained in placental perfusion studies. Inhibitors of ABCB1/P-gp, PSC833 (valspodar) and GG918 have been

TABLE 79.4 FM ratios of different xenobiotics *in vivo* and in human placental perfusion

Compound	*In vivo*				Human placental perfusion		
	n	Cord blood	Maternal blood	FM ratio	*n*	Perfusion time	FM ratio
Medicinal drugs							
10-OH-Carbamazepine	12[1]	0.21 ± 0.19 μg/ml	0.19 ± 0.16 μg/ml	1	6[2]	2 h	1
Bupivacaine	11[3]	0.19 μg/ml	0.71 μg/ml	0.27	5[4]	2.5 h	0.25 ± 0.2
					5[5]	2 h	0.56 ± 0.12
Clonidine	5[6]			0.87	4[6]	2 h	0.85
Dexmedetomidine					4[6]	2 h	0.77
Diazepam	30[7](iv)[a]	291 ng/ml	527 ng/ml	0.57	7[7]	2 h	0.48–0.55
	30[7](iv)	449 ng/ml	544 ng/ml	0.84			
	33[7](iv)	940 ng/ml	731 ng/ml	0.82			
	37[7](im)[a]	NA	NA	1.8			
	16[7](im)	57 ng/ml	41 ng/ml	1.3			
Gabapentin	6[8]			1.3–2.1			
Glyburide					5[9]	3 h	0.3 ± 0.5
Indomethacin					4[10]	2 h	0.45 ± 0.16
Lamotrigine	2[11]	7.69/9.45 μM	4.97/9.30 μM	1–1.5	8[11]	2 h	1–1.5
Ropivacaine	11[3]	0.27 μg/ml	0.93 μg/ml	0.29	5[4]	2.5 h	0.25
Sulindac					4[10]	2 h	0.34 ± 0.19
Sulindac sulfide					4[10]	2 h	0.54 ± 0.17
Toxic chemicals							
2-Isopropoxyphenol	180[12]	3.4 ± 3.2 pg/g	3.0 ± 2.5 pg/g	1.1			
Acrylamide	6[13]			[b]0.5	13[14]	4 h	1–1.1
Aflatoxicol					8[15]	4 h	1.1–1.3
Aflatoxin B1	11[16]	3.1 nmol/ml	0.62 nmol/ml	5	8[15]	4 h	0.6
Bendiocarb	180[12]	3.7 ± 2.5 pg/g	4.4 ± 3.0 pg/g	0.8			
Bisphenol A	300[17]	1.1 ± 1.4 μg/l	9.0 ± 14.0 μg/l	0.1	7[18]	3 h	0.8
Chlorpyrifos	180[12]	4.0 ± 6.5 pg/g	4.1 ± 4.5 pg/g	about 1			
Diazinon	180[12]	1.1 ± 1.5 pg/g	1.3 ± 2.2 pg/g	0.9			
Dicloran	180[12]	3.3 ± 3.8 pg/g	3.1 ± 3.5 pg/g	1.1			
Ethanol	6[19]			1	4[20]	2 h	1
Glycidamide					4[14]	4 h	0.9
Methyl mercury				1.8[21]			
Pentachlorphenol	15[22]	1960 pg/g	2830 pg/g	0.7			
Phthalimide	180[12]	25.3 ± 14.3 pg/g	29.0 ± 24.7 pg/g	0.9			
Sum PBDE	15[22]	4.3 ng/g lipid	23.6 ng/g lipid	0.2			
Tetrahydrophthalimide	180[12]	1.9 ± 3.8 pg/g	2.1 ± 3.8 pg/g	0.9			
Total mercury				1[21]			

[a]im = intramuscular, iv = intravenous,
[b]hemoglobin adduct of AA (N-2-carbamoylethylvaline, AAV), NA = not available, FM = feto-maternal
[1]Myllynen *et al.*, 2001; [2]Pienimäki *et al.*, 1995; [3]Ala-Kokko *et al.*, 1997a; [4]Ueki *et al.*, 2009; [5]Ala-Kokko *et al.*, 1995; [6]Ala-Kokko *et al.*, 1997b; [7]Myllynen and Vähäkangas, 2002; [8]Öhman *et al.*, 2005; [9]Kraemer *et al.*, 2006; [10]Lampela *et al.*, 1999; [11]Myllynen *et al.*, 2003; [12]Whyatt *et al.*, 2003; [13]Schettgen *et al.*, 2004; [14]Annola *et al.*, 2008; [15]Partanen *et al.*, 2010; [16]Denning *et al.*, 1990; [17]Lee *et al.*, 2008; [18]Balakrishnan *et al.*, 2010; [19]Idänpään-Heikkilä *et al.*, 1972; [20]Karttunen, Vähäkangas *et al.*, unpublished; [21]Vahter *et al.*, 2000; [22]Guvenius *et al.*, 2003

shown to increase placental transfer of saquinavir (antiretroviral drug) from the maternal to the fetal side (Mölsä *et al.*, 2005) while these same inhibitors did not affect placental transfer of quetiapine, an atypical antipsychotic drug (Rahi *et al.*, 2007). By using an ABCB1/P-gp inhibitor, GF120918, Nanovskaya and coworkers (2005) showed in dual perfused human placenta that the transfer from maternal to fetal circulation of a known ABCB1/P-gp substrate, paclitaxel, was increased by 50% with the use of the inhibitor and the transfer of methadone by 30%.

Inhibitors of ABCC1/MRP1 and OATP transporters expressed on the placental basal membrane, MK-571 and probenecid, decreased the transfer of saquinavir from fetal to maternal circulation to some extent, although the effect was not statistically significant (Rahi *et al.*, 2009). May *et al.* (2008) showed that inhibition of ABCB1/P-gp by valspodar (PSC833) has no effect on transplacental transfer of talinolol whereas its transfer from the maternal to the fetal side increased when ABCC2/MRP2 was inhibited with probenecid during placental perfusion. Inhibition of ABCG2/BCRP transporters by nicardipine seemed to decrease glyburide transfer from fetal to maternal direction in human placenta (Pollex *et al.*, 2008). We have examined the heterocyclic amine, PhIP, which is a food-borne chemical carcinogen together with a specific ABCG2/BCRP inhibitor KO143 (Myllynen *et al.*, 2008). We noticed that inhibition of ABCG2/BCRP transport increases the transfer of PhIP from the maternal to the fetal side. Probenecid, an inhibitor of ABCC1/MRP1 and ABCC2/MRP2 transporters, on the other hand, had no effects on the toxicokinetics of PhIP (Myllynen *et al.*, 2008).

TABLE 79.5 ABC transporter studies with drugs or xenobiotics in human placental perfusion model

Drug/ Xenobiotic	Transporter	Inhibitor	Effect
Digoxin	ABCB1/MDR1/P-gp	Quinidine and verapamil	Neither quinidine nor verapamil affected the maternal-to-fetal transfer of digoxin[1]
Saquinavir	ABCB1/MDR1/P-gp	PSC833 (valspodar) and GG918	Both inhibitors increased the maternal-to-fetal transfer. PSC833 did not affect the fetal-to-maternal transfer[2]
	ABCC1/MRP1	MK-571 and probenecid	Both inhibitors reduced the fetal-to-maternal transfer, although not significantly[3]
Glyburide	ABCB1/MDR1/P-gp	Verapamil	ABCB1 inhibition did not affect glyburide transport[4]
	ABCG2/BCRP	Nicardipine	Inhibition of BCRP decreased the placental transfer from fetal to maternal side[5]
Quetiapine	ABCB1/MDR1/P-gp	PSC833 (valspodar) and GG918	Neither inhibitor increased the transfer from maternal to fetal circulation[6]
PhIP	ABCG2/BCRP	KO143	Inhibition of BCRP increased the placental transport[7]
Talinolol	ABCB1/MDR1/P-gp	PSC833 (valspodar)	Inhibition of ABCB1 had no effect on the transfer from maternal to fetal circulation[8]
	ABCC2/MRP2	Probenecid and verapamil	Inhibition of ABCC2 increased the placental transport from maternal to fetal circulation. Verapamil had stronger effect than probenecid[8]

[1]Holcberg *et al.*, 2003; [2]Mölsä *et al.*, 2005; [3]Rahi *et al.*, 2009; [4]Kraemer *et al.*, 2006; [5]Pollex *et al.*, 2008; [6]Rahi *et al.*, 2007; [7]Myllynen *et al.*, 2008; [8]May *et al.*, 2008

Only some studies on the effect of ABC transporter polymorphisms on xenobiotic or drug transport in human placental perfusion have been published. There is no correlation between the ABCB1 genotype and transplacental transfer of saquinavir (Mölsä *et al.*, 2005; Rahi *et al.*, 2008). Increased transfer of saquinavir due to ABCB1/P-gp inhibition was not affected by ABCB1 polymorphisms C3435T or C2677A/T (Mölsä *et al.*, 2005), although the expression of ABCB1/P-gp was higher in placentas with the 3435T allele (Rahi *et al.*, 2008). This same allele (3435T) in exon 26 was, however, associated with increased placental transfer of quetiapine, although no correlation was observed between its transplacental transfer and placental ABCB1/P-gp expression (Rahi *et al.*, 2007). The 2677G>T/A polymorphism in exon 21 of ABCB1 had no effect on quetiapine transfer (Rahi *et al.*, 2007). Polymorphisms of ABCC2/MRP2 and ABCB1/P-gp had no effect on the transport of talinolol (May *et al.*, 2008). These discrepant results may have an explanation in the result of Sauna and coworkers (2007) who found that combinations of the non-synonymous G2677T with either of the synonymous C1236T or C3435T affect the interaction of the transporter with its substrates. These transfer studies and others showing variation in the expression and function of placental transporter proteins due to gene polymorphisms of ABCB1 (Tanabe *et al.*, 2001, Hitzl *et al.*, 2004) and ABCG2 (Kobayashi *et al.*, 2005) implicate that part of the known individual variation in transplacental transport may well be due to transporter polymorphisms.

Human *in vivo* studies

During pregnancy the mother can be exposed to both drugs and environmental compounds. Indication of fetal exposure to environmental agents *in vivo* has been gained by the measurements of such compounds in meconium, amniotic fluid and cord blood (for an extensive review see Barr *et al.*, 2007). Medicinal drugs, such as antiepileptics (Pienimäki *et al.*, 1997) and anesthetics (Ala-Kokko *et al.*, 1997b) as well as metals and pesticides, have been found in cord blood. While blood concentrations are amenable to change during pregnancy due to elimination through the placenta, meconium accumulates xenobiotics from weeks 12–16 on giving an idea of the exposure during the latter two-thirds of pregnancy (Barr *et al.*, 2007). Pharmaceuticals, illicit drugs and environmental compounds, as well as cotinine as an indication of exposure to smoking, have been detected in meconium. The *in vivo* data confirms what is seen also in human placental perfusion: very few compounds exist that do not cross the placenta to the fetus. It seems that one of the few restrictions is the size of the molecule, so that compounds with very high molecular weight do not get through easily. Such compounds have been used in placental perfusion to probe whether the membrane between maternal and fetal circulation is intact.

In the literature data exist on concurrent analysis of xenobiotics in maternal and cord blood. In some cases there are significant differences between these concentrations. It is possible that at least some of these differences are due to ABC transporters. Comparison of the levels in cord blood and maternal blood at birth gives an indication of the extent of transport (Table 79.4). The ratios give an idea of the distribution but it has to be remembered that the transport may be concentration dependent and that it depends on the biological half-life of the compound, whether measured in cord blood or maternal blood (Barr *et al.*, 2007). So far too few studies exist for final conclusions to be made on the details of placental transport on almost any compound. While it is difficult to study the role of ABC transporters *in vivo* in humans, data are available thanks to other research models (see Table 79.2).

An increasing amount of data shows that many mycotoxins can cross the human placenta. Several studies have reported high levels of aflatoxins and aflatoxin–albumin adducts in maternal and cord blood of mothers living in contaminated areas, proving exposure of the fetus during pregnancy (Denning *et al.*, 1990; Wild *et al.*, 1991; Hsieh and Hsieh, 1993; Abdulrazzaq *et al.*, 2002; Turner *et al.*, 2007). Ochratoxin A has also been detected in cord blood and in maternal and fetal serum, concentrations in fetal blood being higher than in maternal serum which indicates active placental transfer (Zimmerli and Dick, 1995). Increased incidence of neural tube defects in babies after low or moderate consumption by pregnant mothers of corn tortillas contaminated with fumonisin B suggests that it can cross the human placental barrier (Missmer *et al.*, 2006).

Environmental pollutants, such as PBDEs, PCP, PCB and OH-PCB, have been measured in maternal plasma and corresponding cord blood indicating that these environmental toxins can also cross the human placenta (Guvenius *et al.*, 2003; Soechitram *et al.*, 2004; Barr *et al.*, 2007; Park *et al.*, 2009). Because these compounds are endocrine disruptors, exposure during the fetal period may disturb the development of the fetus by disrupting hormonal regulation. Estrogenic bisphenol A, which is also known to act as an endocrine disruptor, has been detected in cord blood, fetal plasma (higher levels than in maternal plasma) and in placental tissue showing that it can cross the human placenta (Schönfelder *et al.*, 2002).

SIGNIFICANCE OF ABC TRANSPORTERS TO FETAL HEALTH AND IMPORTANT TARGETS FOR FUTURE STUDIES

Since ABC transporters take part in important functions in body, it is no wonder that genetic polymorphisms of the transporters are known or suspected to be linked to diseases of many organs. Examples include the suspected link of a low ABCB1/P-gp activity with inflammatory bowel diseases (lower protection against bacterial toxins in the gut) and renal cell carcinoma (lower protection of kidney cells against toxic substances in glomerular filtrate) (Fromm, 2002) and a newly found function of ABCG2/BCRP in urate efflux and a polymorphism with a lower activity linked to gout (Woodward *et al.*, 2009). Fetal health is also affected by transporter status. Recently maternal medication in connection with a maternal 3435TT genotype of ABCB1 was found to increase the risk of cleft lip and cleft palate in children, especially without folate substitution (Bliek *et al.*, 2009), most probably by affecting maternal toxicokinetics of the drugs so that fetal exposure increased. Placental ABC transporters are no less important for fetal health. Theoretically, the ABC efflux transporters may fail their protective function if the activity is decreased by a genetic polymorphism or an inhibitor. Such a situation probably makes the fetus more susceptible to teratogenic agents, as has been demonstrated in transporter knockout mice (Behravan and Piquette-Miller, 2007; Klaassen and Lu, 2008). On the other hand, a decrease would increase the transport of necessary drugs for the fetus.

ABCG2/BCRP is important in cellular folate homeostasis (Ifergan *et al.*, 2004). Folate deprivation has been shown lately to elevate cancer risk. Folate deprivation also impacts ABCG2/BCRP expression, but these results are contradictory (Ifergan *et al.*, 2004; Lemos *et al.*, 2008). In some studies the expression of ABCG2/BCRP is elevated with folate deprivation (Lemos *et al.*, 2008) while other work shows that the expression is decreased (Ifergan *et al.*, 2004). In mice, Abcg2/Bcrp transporter protects fetuses in the womb, e.g. from the heterocyclic amines IQ, PhIP and Trp-P1 exposure (Van Herwaarden *et al.*, 2006), but in mammary gland, the transporter seems to mediate its substrate secretion to breast milk based on studies in Abcg2 knockouts (Jonker *et al.*, 2005; Van Herwaarden *et al.*, 2006). Paulsen and coworkers (1999) have shown a connection between lactational exposure and intestinal neoplasia in mice.

Medical treatment can affect the function of ABC transporters. In many chronic diseases, pharmaceuticals are essential and unavoidable for the welfare of both mother and fetus. A good mini-review by Balayssac and coworkers (2005) lists over 20 drugs, such as verapamil, omeprazole and clarithromycin, that can inhibit ABCB1/P-gp. It is one of the most studied ABC transporters active in the placenta, although its amount decreases during the third trimester of pregnancy (Sun *et al.*, 2006). The usage of ABCB1/P-gp inhibiting drugs during pregnancy will not only affect the concentration of other drugs (such as cyclosporin), but may increase the fetal exposure to xenobiotics as well.

Several ABC transporters are expressed in placental cells. ABCB1/P-gp and ABCG2/BCRP are the most abundant and potentially important in fetal protection due to their localization in the apical brush border of syncytiotrophoblast facing maternal blood. Several ABCC/MRP family members are also expressed in human placenta (Table 79.1) at mRNA and protein levels. They are found in all cell types of the placenta, but the exact localization in many cases is still unclear, especially as to fetal capillaries. The expression of transporter proteins in the human placenta varies depending on the stage of pregnancy. The changes in protein expression, if reflected on the function, have implications both for drug treatment during pregnancy and on the exposure of the fetus to toxic agents. In mouse placenta, the Abcb1/P-gp expression decreases towards term and this is associated with a significant increase in digoxin transfer (Petropoulos *et al.*, 2007). The expression of ABCB1/P-gp decreases with advancing gestation also in human placenta (Mathias *et al.*, 2005; Sun *et al.*, 2006). Discrepant data about the expression of ABCG2/BCRP protein exist with one study indicating a decrease by advancing gestation (Meyer zu Schwabedissen *et al.*, 2006), while other studies suggest either no change (Mathias *et al.*, 2005) or rather an increase (Yeboah *et al.*, 2006). This discrepancy may be partly due to inter-individual variation in the placental expression which also contributes to the difficulties in interspecies extrapolation when, e.g., rodents are used as models. In rodents, Abcg2/Bcrp expression decreases as gestation proceeds (Yasuda *et al.*, 2005; Wang *et al.*, 2006)

Since the placenta is species specific and human placenta thus unique (Benirschke *et al.*, 2006), research models utilizing human placenta and human trophoblastic cells are especially important. More comparison between different models to realize their full potential as putative predictive toxicological test systems is needed as well. All human *in vivo* data of the fetal level of compounds are valuable. Term placenta is, after mothers are convinced to donate it, easy to study, while it is a real challenge to target early placentas, not least due to ethical reasons. Some models, like human placental perfusion, may only be applicable to term placentas, although few attempts to perfuse early placentas have been published.

Transplacental exposure to xenobiotics can be teratogenic and/or carcinogenic as shown by the exposure of pregnant mothers to thalidomide (Ghobrial and Rajkumar, 2003), methylmercury (Castoldi *et al.*, 2008) and diethylstilbestrol (Lynch and Reich, 1985). In addition, there are more recent implications that fetal and early life exposure to xenobiotics may also be responsible for health issues later in adult life (Gluckman *et al.*, 2008). This developmental origin of disease (Wigle *et al.*, 2007; Swanson *et al.*, 2009) stresses the importance of studying more carefully the mechanisms of fetal exposure to xenobiotics, of which the placental transporters play a central role. Studies on gene knockout transgenic mice have clearly shown the importance of placental transporters in the protection against toxic insult to the fetus. Putatively the same is true in humans, but remains to be shown. It is conceivable from the literature that so far little is known about placental transporters, especially their localization. In addition, a better understanding of the expression and function of different transporters and their role in transport of various compounds (nutrients/xenobiotics) is needed to evaluate fetal exposure to all the various potential harmful drugs and environmental compounds.

REFERENCES

Abdulrazzaq YM, Osman, N, Ibrahim A (2002) Fetal exposure to aflatoxins in the United Arab Emirates. *Ann Trop Paediatr* **22:** 3–9.

Allikmets R, Schriml LM, Hutchinson A, Romano-Spica V, Dean M (1988) A human placenta-specific ATP-binding cassette gene (ABCP) on chromosome 4q22 that is involved in multidrug resistance. *Cancer Res* **58:** 5337–9.

Annola K, Heikkinen AT, Partanen H, Woodhouse H, Segerbäck D, Vähäkangas K (2009) Transplacental transfer of nitrosodimethylamine in perfused human placenta. *Placenta* **30:** 277–83.

Annola K, Karttunen V, Keski-Rahkonen P, Myllynen P, Segerbäck D, Heinonen S, Vähäkangas K (2008) Transplacental transfer of acrylamide and glycidamide are comparable to that of antipyrine in perfused human placenta. *Toxicol Lett* **182:** 50–6.

Ala-Kokko TI, Alahuhta S, Jouppila P, Korpi K, Westerling P, Vähäkangas K (1997a) Feto-maternal distribution of ropivacaine and bupivacaine after epidural administration for cesarian section. *Int J Obstet Anesth* **6:** 147–52.

Ala-Kokko TI, Myllynen P, Vähäkangas K (2000) Ex vivo perfusion of the human placental cotyledon: implications for anesthetic pharmacology. *Int J Obstet Anesth* **9:** 26–38.

Ala-Kokko TI, Pienimäki P, Herva R, Hollmén AI, Pelkonen O, Vähäkangas K (1995) Transfer of lidocaine and bupivacaine across the isolated perfused human placenta. *Pharmacol Toxicol* **77:** 142–8.

Ala-Kokko TI, Pienimäki P, Lampela E, Hollmén AI, Pelkonen O, Vähäkangas K (1997b) Transfer of clonidine and dexmedetomidine across the isolated perfused human placenta. *Acta Anaesthesiol Scand* **41:** 313–9.

Atkinson DE, Greenwood SL, Sibley CP, Glazier JD, Fairbairn LJ (2003) Role of MDR1 and MRP1 in trophoblast cells, elucidated using retroviral gene transfer. *Am J Physiol Cell Physiol* **285:** C584–C591.

Atkinson DE, Sibley CP, Fairbairn LJ, Greenwood SL (2006) MDR1 P-gp expression and activity in intact human placental tissue; upregulation by retroviral transduction. *Placenta* **27:** 707–14.

Bailey-Dell KJ, Hassel B, Doyle LA, Ross DD (2001) Promoter characterization and genomic organization of the human breast cancer resistance protein (ATP-binding cassette transporter G2) gene. *Biochim Biophys Acta* **1520:** 234–41.

Balakrishnan B, Henare K, Thorstensen EB, Ponnampalam AP, Mitchell MD (2010) Transfer of bisphenol A across the human placenta. *Am J Obstet Gynecol* **202:** 393.e1–e7.

Balayssac D, Authier N, Cayre A, Coudore F (2005) Does inhibition of P-glycoprotein lead to drug-drug interactions? *Toxicol Lett* **156:** 319–29.

Barr DB, Bishop A, Needham LL (2007) Concentrations of xenobiotic chemicals in the maternal–fetal unit. *Reprod Toxicol* **23:** 260–6.

Behravan J, Piquette-Miller M (2007) Drug transport across the placenta, role of the ABC drug efflux transporters. *Expert Opin Drug Metab Toxicol* **3:** 819–30.

Benirschke K, Kaufmann P, Baergen (2006) *Pathology of the Human Placenta*. New York, Springer.

Bliek BJ, van Schaik RH, van der Heiden IP, Sayed-Tabatabaei FA, van Duijn CM, Steegers EA, Steegers-Theunissen RP (2009) Eurocran Gene-Environment Interaction Group: Maternal medication use, carriership of the ABCB1 3435C>T polymorphism and the risk of a child with cleft lip with or without cleft palate. *Am J Med Genet Part A* **149A:** 2088–92.

Bode CJ, Jin H, Rytting E, Silverstein PS, Young AM, Audus KL (2006) In vitro models for studying trophoplast transcellular transport. *Methods Mol Med* **122:** 225–39.

Borst P, Elferink RO (2002) Mammalian ABC transporters in health and disease. *Ann Rev Biochem* **71:** 537–92

Brandes JM, Tavoloni MN, Potter BJ, Sarkozi L, Shepard MD, Berk PD (1983) A new recycling technique for human placental cotyledon perfusion: application to studies of the fetomaternal transfer of glucose, inulin and antipyrine. *Am J Obstet Gynecol* **146:** 800–6.

Caniggia I, Taylor CV, Ritchie JW, Lye SJ, Letarte M (1997) Endoglin regulates trophoblast differentiation along the invasive pathway in human placental villous explants. *Endocrinology* **138:** 4977–88.

Castoldi AF, Onishchenko N, Johansson C, Coccini T, Roda E, Vahter M, Ceccatelli S, Manzo L (2008) Neurodevelopmental toxicity of methylmercury: laboratory animal data and their contribution to human risk assessment. *Regul Toxicol Pharmacol* **51:** 215–29.

Chung FS, Eyal S, Muzi M, Link JM, Mankoff DA, Kaddoumi A, O'Sullivan F, Hsiao P, Unadkat JD (2010) Positron emission tomography imaging of tissue P-glycoprotein activity during pregnancy in the non-human primate. *Br J Pharmacol* **159:** 394–404.

Coles LD, Lee IJ, Hassan HE, Eddington ND (2009) Distribution of saquinavir, methadone, and buprenorphine in maternal brain, placenta, and fetus during two different gestational stages of pregnancy in mice. *J Pharma Sci* **98:** 2832–46.

Conseil G, Deeley RG, Cole SPC (2005) Polymorphisms of MRP1 (ABCC1) and related ATP-dependent drug transporters. *Pharmacogen Genom* **15:** 523–33.

Cygalova LH, Hofman J, Ceckova M, Staud F (2009) Transplacental pharmacokinetics of glyburide, rhodamine 123, and BODIPY FL prazosin: effect of drug efflux transporters and lipid solubility. *J Pharmacol Exp Ther* **331:** 1118–25.

Dancis J (1985) Why perfuse the human placenta. *Contrib Gynecol Obstet* **13:** 1–4.

Das UG, Sadiq H, Soares MJ, Hay Jr WW, Devaskar SU (1998) Time-dependent physiological regulation of rodent and ovine placental glucose transporter (GLUT-1) protein. *Am J Physiol* **274:** R339–R347.

Denning DW, Allen R, Wilkinson AP, Morgan MR (1990) Transplacental transfer of aflatoxin in humans. *Carcinogenesis* **11:** 1033–5.

Devault A, Gros P (1990) Two members of the mouse mdr gene family confer multidrug resistance with overlapping but distinct drug specificities. *Mol Cell Biol* **10:** 1652–63.

Di Santo S, Malek A, Sager R, Andres AC, Schneider H (2003) Trophoblast viability in perfused term placental tissue and explant cultures limited to 7–24 hours. *Placenta* **24:** 882–94.

Doyle LA, Yang W, Abruzzo LV, Krogmann T, Gao Y, Rishi AK, Ross DD (1998) A multidrug resistance transporter from human MCF-7 breast cancer cells. *Proc Natl Acad Sci USA* **95:** 15665–70.

Earhart AD, Patrikeeva S, Wang X, Abdelrahman DR, Hankins GD, Ahmed MS, Nanovskaya T (2009) Transplacental transfer and metabolism of bupropion. *J Maternal-Fetal Neonatal Med* **31:** 1–10.

Ebert B, Seidel A, Lampen A (2005) Identification of BCRP as transporter of benzo[a]pyrene conjugates metabolically formed in Caco-2 cells and its induction by Ah-receptor agonists. *Carcinogenesis* **26:** 1754–63.

Englund G, Jacobson A, Rorsman F, Artursson P, Kindmark A, Rönnblom A (2007) Efflux transporters in ulcerative colitis: decreased expression of BCRP (ABCG2) and Pgp (ABCB1). *Inflamm Bowel Dis* **13:** 291–7.

Evseenko DA, Murthi P, Paxton JW, Reid G, Emerald BS, Mohankumar KM, Lobie PE, Brennecke SP, Kalionis B, Keelan JA (2007) The ABC transporter BCRP/ABCG2 is a placental survivor factor, and its expression is reduced in idiopathic human fetal growth restriction. *FASEB J* **21:** 3592–605.

Evseenko DA, Paxton JW, Keelan JA (2006) ABC drug transporter expression and functional activity in trophoblast-like cell lines and differentiating primary trophoblast. *Am J Physiol Regul Integr Comp Physiol* **290:** R1357–65.

Fromm MF (2002) Genetically determined differences in P-glycoprotein function: implications for disease risk. *Toxicology* **181–182:** 299–303.

Furesz TC, Heath-Monnig E, Kamath SG, Smith CH (2002) Lysine uptake by cloned hCAT-2B: comparison with hCAT-1 and with trophoblast surface membranes. *J Membr Biol* **189:** 27–33.

Ganapathy V, Fei YJ, Prasad PD (2006) Heterologous expression systems for studying placental transporters. *Methods Mol Med* **122:** 285–300.

Gavard L, Beghin D, Forestier F, Cayre Y, Peytavin G, Mandelbrot L, Farinotti R, Gil S (2009) Contribution and limit of the model of perfused cotyledon to the study of placental transfer of drugs. Example of a protease inhibitor of HIV: nelfinavir. *Eur J Obstet Gynecol Reprod Biol* **147:** 157–60.

Gedeon C, Anger G, Piquette-Miller M, Koren G (2008) Breast cancer resistance protein: mediating the trans-placental transfer of glypuride across the human placenta. *Placenta* **29:** 39–43.

Genbacev O, Schubach SA, Miller RK (1992) Villous culture of first trimester human placenta – model to study extravillous trophoblast (EVT) differentiation. *Placenta* **13:** 439–61.

Ghobrial IM, Rajkumar SV (2003) Management of thalidomide toxicity. *J Support Oncol* **1:** 194–205.

Gil S, Saura R, Forestier F, Farinotti R (2005) P-glycoprotein expression of the human placenta during pregnancy. *Placenta* **26:** 268–70.

Gluckman PD, Hanson MA, Cooper C, Thornburg KL (2008) Effect of in utero and early-life conditions on adult health and disease. *N Engl J Med* **359:** 61–73.

Guvenius DM, Aronsson A, Ekman-Ordeberg G, Bergman A, Nóren K (2003) Human prenatal and postnatal exposure to polybrominated diphenyl ethers, polychlorinated biphenyls, polychlorobiphenyols, and pentachlorophenol. *Environ Health Persp* **111:** 1235–41.

Hanet N, Lancon A, Delmas D, Jannin B, Chagnon MC, Cherkaoui-Malki M, Latruffe N, Artur Y, Heydel JM (2008) Effects of endocrine disruptors on genes associated with 17beta-estradiol metabolism and excretion. *Steroids* **73:** 1242–51.

Heaton SJ, Eady JJ, Parker ML, Gotts KL, Dainty JR, Fairweather-Tait SJ, McArdle HJ, Srai KS, Elliott RM (2008) The use of BeWo cells as an in vitro model for placental iron transport. *Am J Physiol Cell Physiol* **295:** C1445–C1453.

Hemauer SJ, Nonovskaya TN, Abdel-Rahman SZ, Patrikeeva SL, Hankins GD, Ahmed MS (2010) Modulation of human placental P-glycoprotein expression and activity *MDR1* gene polymorphisms. *Biochem Pharmacol* **79:** 921–5.

Hemauer SJ, Patrikeeva SL, Nanovskaya TN, Hankins GD, Ahmed MS (2009) Opiates inhibit paclitaxel uptake by P-glycoprotein in preparations of human placental inside-out vesicles. *Biochem Pharmacol* **78:** 1272–8.

Hemmings DG, Lowen B, Sherburne R, Sawicki G, Guilbert LJ (2001) Villous trophoblasts cultured on semi-permeable membranes form an effective barrier to the passage of high and low molecular weight particles. *Placenta* **22:** 70–9.

Hitzl M, Schaeffeler E, Hocher B, Slowinski T, Halle H, Eichelbaum M, Kaufmann P, Fritz P, Fromm MF, Schwab M (2004) Variable expression of P-glycoprotein in the human placenta and its association with mutations of the multidrug resistance 1 gene (MDR1, ABCB1). *Pharmacogenetics* **14:** 309–18.

Holcberg G, Sapir O, Tsadkin M, Huleihel M, Lazer S, Katz M, Mazor M, Ben-Zvi Z (2003) Lack of interaction of digoxin and P-glycoprotein inhibitors, quinidine and verapamil in human placenta in vitro. *Eur J Obstet Gynecol Reprod Biol* **109:** 133–7.

Hsieh LL, Hsieh TT (1993) Detection of aflatoxin B1-DNA adducts in human placenta and cord blood. *Cancer Res* **53:** 1278–80.

Huls M, Russel FG, Masereeuw R (2009) The role of ATP binding cassette transporters in tissue defense and organ regeneration. *J Pharmacol Exp Ther* **328:** 3–9.

Idänpään-Heikkilä J, Jouppila P, Akerblom HK, Isoaho R, Kauppila E, Koivisto M (1972) Elimination and metabolic effects of ethanol in mother, fetus, and newborn infant. *Am J Obstet Gynecol* **112:** 387–93.

Ietta F, Bechi N, Romagnoli R, Bhattacharjee J, Realacci M, Di Vito M, Ferretti C, Paulesu L (2010) 17β-estradiol modulates the macrophage migration inhibitory factor secretory pathway by regulating ABCA1 expression in human first-trimester placenta. *Am J Physiol Endocrinol Metab* **298:** E411–18.

Ifergan I, Shafran A, Jansen G, Hooijberg JH, Scheffer GL, Assaraf YG (2004) Folate deprivation results in the loss of breast cancer resistance protein (BCRP/ABCG2) expression. A role for BCRP in cellular folate homeostasis. *J Biol Chem* **279:** 25527–34.

Imai Y, Nakane M, Kage K, Tsukahara S, Ishikawa E, Tsuruo T, Miki Y, Sugimoto Y (2002) C421A polymorphism in the human breast cancer resistance protein gene is associated with low expression of Q141K protein and low-level drug resistance. *Mol Cancer Therap* **1:** 611–16.

Immonen E, Serpi R, Vähäkangas K, Myllynen P (2009) Responses of PhIP (2-amino-1-methyl-6-phenylimidazo[4,5-b]pyridine) in MCF-7 cells are culture condition dependent. *Chemico-Biol Interact* **182:** 73–83.

Jin H, Audus KL (2005) Effect of bisphenol A on drug efflux in BeWo, a human trophoblast-like cell line. *Placenta* **26:** S96–S103.

Jones PM, O'Mara ML, George AM (2009) ABC transporters: a riddle wrapped in a mystery inside an enigma. *Trends Biochem Sci* **34:** 520–31.

Jonker JW, Merino G, Musters S, van Herwaarden AE, Bolscher E, Wagenaar E, Mesman E, Dale TC, Schinkel AH (2005) The breast cancer resistance protein BCRP (ABCG2) concentrates drugs and carcinogenic xenotoxins into milk. *Nature Med* **11:** 127–9.

Kalabis GM, Petropoulos S, Gibb W, Matthews SG (2009) Multidrug resistance phosphoglycoprotein (ABCB1) expression in the guinea pig placenta: developmental changes and regulation by betamethasone. *Can J Physiol Pharmacol* **87:** 973–8.

Kippler M, Hoque AM, Raqib R, Ohrvik H, Ekström EC, Vahter M (2010) Accumulation of cadmium in human placenta interacts with the transport of micronutrients to the fetus. *Toxicol Lett* **192:** 162–8.

Kitano T, Iizasa H, Hwang IW, Hirose Y, Morita T, Maeda T, Nakashima E (2004) Conditionally immortalized syncytiotrophoblast cell lines as new tools for study of the blood–placenta barrier. *Biol Pharmaceut Bull* **27:** 753–9.

Kitsiou-Tzeli S, Traeger-Synodinos J, Giannatou E, Kaminopetros P, Roma E, Makrythanasis P, Tsezou A (2009) The c.504T>C (p.Asn168Asn) polymorphism in the ABCB4 gene as a predisposing factor for intrahepatic cholestasis of pregnancy in Greece. *Liver Int*. Epub.

Klaassen CD, Lu H (2008) Xenobiotic transporters: ascribing function from gene knockout and mutation studies. *Toxicol Sci* **101:** 186–96.

Kliman HJ, Nestler JE, Sermasi E, Sanger JM, Strauss JF 3rd (1986) Purification, characterization, and in vitro differentiation of cytotrophoblasts from human term placentae. *Endocrinology* **118:** 1567–82.

Knipp GT, Liu B, Audus KL, Fuji H, Ono T, Soares MJ (2000) Fatty acid transport regulatory proteins in the developing rat placenta and in trophoblast cell culture models. *Placenta* **21:** 367–75.

Kobayashi D, Ieiri I, Hirota T, Takane H, Maegawa S, Kigawa J, Suzuki H, Nanba E, Oshimura M, Terakawa N, Otsubo K, Mine K, Sugiyama Y (2005) Functional assessment of ABCG2 (BCRP) gene polymorphisms to protein expression in human placenta. *Drug Metab Dispos* **33:** 94–101.

Kolwankar D, Glover DD, Ware JA, Tracy TS (2005) Expression and function of ABCB1 and ABCG2 in human placental tissue. *Drug Metab Dispos* **33:** 524–9.

Kraemer J, Klein J, Lubetsky A, Koren G (2006) Perfusion studies of glyburide transfer across the human placenta: Implications for fetal safety. *Am J Obstet Gynecol* **195:** 270–4.

Krishnamurthy P, Schuetz JD (2006) Role of ABCG2/BCRP in biology and medicine. *Ann Rev Pharmacol Toxicol* **46:** 381–410.

Lampela ES, Nuutinen LH, Ala-Kokko TI, Parikka RM, Laitinen RS, Jouppila PI, Vähäkangas KH (1999) Placental transfer of sulindac, sulindac sulfide and indomethacin in human placental perfusion model. *Am J Obstet Gynecol* **180:** 174–180.

Lankas GR, Wise LD, Cartwright ME, Pippert T (1998) Umbenhauer DR: placental P-glycoprotein deficiency enhances susceptibility to chemically induced birth defects in mice. *Reprod Toxicol* **12:** 457–63.

Lee YJ, Ryu HY, Kim HK, Min CS, Lee JH, Kim E, Nam BH, Park JH, Jung JY, Jang DD, Park EY, Lee KH, Ma JY, Won HS, Im MW, Leem JH, Hong YC, Yoon HS (2008) Maternal and fetal exposure to bisphenol A in Korea. *Reprod Toxicol* **25:** 413–19.

Leiser R and Kaufmann P (1994) Placental structure: in a comparative aspect. *Exp Clin Endocrinol* **102:** 122–34.

Lemos C, Kathmann I, Giovannetti E, Dekker H, Scheffer GL, Calhau C, Jansen G, Peters GJ (2008) Folate deprivation induces BCRP (ABCG2) expression and mitoxantrone resistance in Caco-2 cells. *Int J Cancer* **123:** 1712–20.

Leslie EM, Deeley RG, Cole SP (2005) Multidrug resistance proteins: role of P-glycoprotein, MRP1, MRP2, and BCRP (ABCG2) in tissue defense. *Toxicol Appl Pharmacol* **204:** 216–37.

Liu F, Soares MJ, Audus KL (1997) Permeability properties of monolayers of the human trophoblast cell line BeWo. *Am J Physiol* **273:** C1596–C1604.

Loibichler C, Pichler J, Gerstmayr M, Bohle B, Kisst H, Urbanek R, Szepfalusi Z (2002) Materno-fetal passage of nutritive and inhalant allergens across placentas of term and pre-term deliveries perfused in vitro. *Clin Exp Allergy* **32:** 1546–51.

Lynch HT, Reich JW (1985) Diethylstilbestrol, genetics, teratogenesis, and tumor spectrum in humans. *Med Hypotheses* **16:** 315–32.

Malek A, Obrist C, Wenzinger S, von Mandach U (2009) The impact of cocaine and heroin on the placental transfer of methadone. *Reprod Biol Endocrinol* **7:** 61.

Mao Q (2008) BCRP/ABCG2 in the placenta: expression, function and regulation. *Pharmaceut Res* **25:** 1244–55.

Mathias AA, Hitti J, Unadkat JD (2005) P-glycoprotein and breast cancer resistance protein expression in human placentae of various gestational ages. *Am J Physiol Regulat Integr Comp Physiol* **289:** R963–R969.

Mathiesen L, Rytting E, Mose T, Knudsen LE (2009) Transport of benzo[alpha] pyrene in the dually perfused human placenta perfusion model: effect of albumin in the perfusion medium. *Basic Clin Pharmacol Toxicol* **105:** 181–7.

May K, Grube M, Malhotra I, Long CA, Singh S, Mandaliya K, Siegmund W, Fusch C, Schneider H, King CL (2009) Antibody-dependent transplacental transfer of malaria blood-stage antigen using a human ex vivo placental perfusion model. *PLoS One* **4:** e7986.

May K, Minarikova V, Linnemann K, Zygmunt M, Kroemer HK, Fusch C, Siegmund W (2008) Role of the multidrug transporter proteins ABCB1 and ABCC2 in the diaplacental transport of talinolol in the term human placenta. *Drug Metab Dispos* **36:** 740–4.

Meyer zu Schwabedissen HE, Grube M, Dreisbach A, Jedlitschky G, Meissner K, Linnemann K, Fusch C, Ritter CA, Völker U, Kroemer HK (2006) Epidermal growth factor-mediated activation of the map kinase cascade results in altered expression and function of ABCG2 (BCRP). *Drug Metab Dispos: Biol Fate Chem* **34:** 524–33.

Meyer zu Schwabedissen HE, Grube M, Heydrich B, Linnemann K, Fusch C, Kroemer HK, Jedlitschky G (2005a) Expression, localization, and function of MRP5 (ABCC5), a transporter for cyclic nucleotides, in human placenta and cultured human trophoblasts: effects of gestational age and cellular differentiation. *Am J Pathol* **166:** 39–48.

Meyer zu Schwabedissen HE, Jedlitschky G, Gratz M, Haenisch S, Linnemann K, Fusch C, Cascorbi I, Kroemer HK (2005b) Variable expression of MRP2 (ABCC2) in human placenta: influence of gestational age and cellular differentiation. *Drug Metab Dispos: Biol Fate Chem* **33:** 896–904.

Missmer SA, Suarez L, Felkner M, Wang E, Merrill AH Jr, Rothman KJ, Hendricks KA (2006) Exposure to fumonisins and the occurrence of neural tube defects along the Texas–Mexico border. *Environ Health Perspect* **114:** 237–41.

Mölsä M, Heikkinen T, Hakkola J, Hakala K, Wallerman O, Wadelius M, Wadelius C, Laine K (2005) Functional role of P-glycoprotein in the human blood–placental barrier. *Clin Pharmacol Ther* **78:** 123–31.

Morris Buus R, Boockfor FR (2004) Transferrin expression by placental trophoblastic cells. *Placenta* **25:** 45–52.

Mose T, Knudsen LE, Hedegaard M, Mortensen GK (2007) Transplacental transfer of monomethyl phthalate and mono(2-ethylhexyl) phthalate in a human placenta perfusion system. *Int J Toxicol* **26:** 221–9.

Myllynen P, Immonen E, Kummu M, Vähäkangas K (2009) Developmental expression of drug metabolizing enzymes and transporter proteins in human placenta and fetal tissues. *Expert Opin Drug Metab Toxicol* **5:** 1483–99.

Myllynen P, Kummu M, Kangas T, Ilves M, Immonen E, Rysä J, Pirilä R, Lastumäki A, Vähäkangas K (2008) ABCG2/BCRP decreases the transfer of a food-borne chemical carcinogen, 2-amino-1-methyl-6-phenylimidazo(4,5-b)pyridine (PhIP) in perfused term human placenta. *Toxicol Appl Pharmacol* **232:** 210–17.

Myllynen P, Pienimäki P, Jouppila P, Vähäkangas K (2001) Transplacental passage of oxcarbazepine and its metabolites in vivo. *Epilepsia* **42:** 1482–5.

Myllynen PK, Pienimäki PK & Vähäkangas KH (2003) Transplacental passage of lamotrigine in a human placental perfusion system in vitro and in maternal and cord blood in vivo. *Eur J Clin Pharmacol* **58:** 677–82.

Myllynen P, Vähäkangas K (2002) An examination of whether human placental perfusion allows accurate prediction of placental drug transport: studies with diazepam. *J Pharmacol Toxicol Method* **48:** 131–8.

Nagashige M, Ushigome F, Koyabu N, Hirata K, Kawabuchi M, Hirakawa T, Satoh S, Tsukimori K, Nakano H, Uchiumi T, Kuwano M, Ohtani H, Sawada Y (2003) Basal membrane localization of MRP1 in human placental trophoblast. *Placenta* **24:** 951–8.

Nanovskaya TN, Nekhayeva IA, Hankins GD, Ahmed MS (2008) Transfer of methadone across the dually perfused preterm human placental lobule. *Am J Obstet Gynecol* **198:** 126.e1–e4.

Nanovskaya T, Nekhayeva I, Karunaratne N, Audus K, Hankins GD, Ahmed MS (2005) Role of P-glycoprotein in transplacental transfer of methadone. *Biochem Pharmacol* **69:** 1869–78.

Nau H (1986) Species differences in pharmacokinetics and drug teratogenesis. *Environ Health Perspect* **70:** 113–29.

Nishimura M, Naito S (2005) Tissue-specific mRNA expression profiles of human ATP-binding cassette and solute carrier transporter superfamilies. *Drug Metab Pharmacokin* **20:** 452–77.

Novak D, Quiggle F, Artime C, Beveridge M (2001) Regulation of glutamate transport and transport proteins in a placental cell line. *Am J Physiol* **281:** C1014–C1022.

Öhman I, Vitols S, Tomson T (2005) Pharmacokinetics of gabapentin during delivery, in the neonatal period, and lactation: does a fetal accumulation occur during pregnancy? *Epilepsia* **46:** 1621–4.

Omi H, Okamoto A, Nikaido T, Urashima M, Kawaguchi R, Umehara N, Sugiura K, Saito M, Kiyono T, Tanaka T (2009) Establishment of an immortalized human extravillous trophoblast cell line by retroviral infection of E6/E7/hTERT and its transcriptional profile during hypoxia and reoxygenation. *Int J Mol Med* **23:** 229–36.

Olivero OA, Parikka R, Poirier MC, Vähäkangas K (1999) 3′-azido-3′-deoxythymidine (AZT) transplacental perfusion kinetics and DNA incorporation in normal human placentas perfused with AZT. *Mutation Res* **428:** 41–7.

Park HY, Park JS, Sovcikova E, Kocan A, Linderholm L, Bergman A, Trnovec T, Hertz-Picciotto I (2009) Exposure to hydroxylated polychlorinated biphenyls (OH-PCBs) in the prenatal period and subsequent neurodevelopment in eastern Slovakia. *Environ Health Perspect* **117:** 1600–6.

Parry S, Zhang J (2007) Multidrug resistance proteins affect drug transmission across the placenta. *Am J Obstet Gynecol* **196:** 476.e1–476.e6.

Partanen H, El-Nezami H, Leppänen J, Myllynen P, Woodhouse H, Vähäkangas K (2010) Aflatoxin B1 transfer and metabolism in human placenta. *Toxicol Sci* **113:** 216–25.

Pascolo L, Fernetti C, Garcia-Mediavilla MV, Ostrow JD, Tiribelli C (2001) Mechanisms for the transport of unconjugated biliruhin in human trophoplastic BeWo cells. *FEBS Lett* **495:** 94–9.

Pascolo L, Fernetti C, Pirulli D, Crovella S, Amoroso A, Tiribelli C (2003) Effects of maturation on RNA transcription and protein expression of four MRP genes in human placenta and in BeWo cells. *Biochem Biophys Res Commun* **303:** 259–65.

Paulsen JE, Steffensen IL, Andreassen A, Vikse R, Alexander J (1999) Neonatal exposure to the food mutagen 2-amino-1-methyl-6-phenylimidazo[4,5-b] pyridine via breast milk or directly induces intestinal tumors in multiple intestinal neoplasia mice. *Carcinogenesis* **20:** 1277–82.

Pavek P, Cerveny L, Svecova L, Brysch M, Libra A, Vrzal R, Nachtigal P, Staud F, Ulrichova J, Fendrich Z, Dvorak Z (2007) Examination of glucocorticoid receptor alpha-mediated transcriptional regulation of P-glycoprotein, CYP3A4, and CYP2C9 genes in placental trophoblast cell lines. *Placenta* **28:** 1004–11.

Pavek P, Fendrich Z, Staud F, Malakova J, Brozmanova H, Laznicek M, Semecky V, Grundmann M, Palicka V (2001) Influence of P-glycoprotein on the transplacental passage of cyclosporine. *J Pharmacol Sci* **90:** 1583–92.

Pavek P, Merino G, Wagenaar E, Bolscher E, Novotna M, Jonker JW, Schinkel AH (2005) Human breast cancer resistance protein: interactions with steroid drugs, hormones, the dietary carcinogen 2-amino-1-methyl-6-phenylimidazo(4,5-b)pyridine, and transport of cimetidine. *J Pharmacol Exp Ther* **312:** 144–52.

Pavek P, Staud F, Fendrich Z, Sklenarova H, Libra A, Novotna M, Kopecky M, Nobilis M, Semecky V (2003) Examination of the functional activity of P-glycoprotein in the rat placental barrier using rhodamine 123. *J Pharmacol Exp Therap* **305:** 1239–50.

Petroff MG, Phillips TA, Ka H, Pace JL, Hunt JS (2006) Isolation and culture of term human trophoblast cells. *Methods Mol Med* **121:** 203–17.

Petropoulos S, Kalabis GM, Gibb W, Matthews SG (2007) Functional changes of mouse placental multidrug resistance phosphoglycoprotein (ABCB1) with advancing gestation and regulation by progesterone. *Reprod Sci* **14:** 321–8.

Petrovic V, Teng S, Piquette-Miller M (2007) Regulation of drug transporters during infection and inflammation. *Mol Interv* **7:** 99–111.

Pienimäki P, Hartikainen AL, Arvela P, Partanen T, Herva R, Pelkonen O, Vähäkangas K (1995) Carbamazepine and its metabolites in human perfused placenta and in maternal and cord blood. *Epilepsia* **36:** 241–8.

Pienimäki P, Lampela E, Hakkola J, Arvela P, Raunio H, Vähäkangas K (1997) Pharmacokinetics of oxcarbazepine and carbamazepine in human placenta. *Epilepsia* **38:** 309–16.

Pollex E, Lubetsky A, Koren G (2008) The role of placental breast cancer resistance protein in the efflux of glypuride across the human placenta. *Placenta* **29:** 743–7.

Pollex EK, Anger G, Hutson J, Koren G, Piquette-Miller M (2010) Breast cancer resistance protein (BCRP)-mediated glyburide transport: effect of the C421A/Q141K BCRP single-nucleotide polymorphism. *Drug Metab Dispos Biological Fate of Chem* **38:** 740–4.

Polliotti BM, Holmes R, Cornish JD, Hulsey M, Keesling S, Schwartz D, Abramowsky CR, Huddleston J, Panigel M, Nahmias AJ (1996) Long-term dual perfusion of isolated human placental lobules with improved oxygenation for infectious diseases research. *Placenta* **17:** 57–68.

Prouillac C, Videmann B, Mazallon M, Lecoeur S (2009) Induction of cells differentiation and ABC transporters expression by a myco-estrogen, zearalenone, in human choriocarcinoma cell line (BeWo). *Toxicology* **263:** 100–7.

Rahi M, Heikkinen T, Hakkala J, Hakala K, Wallerman O, Wadelius M, Wadelius C, Laine K (2008) Influence of adenosine triphosphate and ABCB1 (MDR1) genotype on the P-glycoprotein-dependent transfer of saquinavir in the dually perfused human placenta. *Hum Exp Toxicol* **27:** 65–71.

Rahi MM, Heikkinen TM, Hakala KE, Laine KP (2009) The effect of probenecid and MK-571 on the feto-maternal transfer of saquinar in dually perfused human term placenta. *Eur J Pharm Sci* **37:** 588–92.

Rahi M, Heikkinen T, Härtter S, Hakkola J, Hakala K, Wallerman O, Wadelius M, Wadelius C, Laine K (2007) Placental transfer of quetiapine in relation to P-glycoprotein activity. *J Psychopharmacol* **21:** 751–6.

Rees DC, Johnson E, Lewinson O (2009) ABC transporters: the power to change. *Nature Rev Mol Cell Biol* **10:** 218–27.

Robey RW, To KK, Polgar O, Dohse M, Fetsch P, Dean M, Bates SE (2009) ABCG2: a perspective. *Adv Drug Deliv Rev* **61:** 3–13.

Saito S, Iida A, Sekine A, Miura Y, Oqawa C, Kawauchi S, Higuchi S, Nakamura Y (2002) Identification of 779 genetic variations in eight genes encoding members of the ATP-binding cassette, subfamily C (*ABCC/MRP/CFTR*). *J Hum Genet* **47:** 147–71.

Sastry BVR (1999) Techniques to study human placental transport. *Adv Drug Del Rev* **38:** 17–39.

Sauna ZE, Kim IW, Ambudkar SV (2007) Genomics and the mechanism of P-glycoprotein (ABCB1). *J Bioenerg Biomembr* **39:** 481–7.

Schettgen T, Kütting B, Hornig M, Beckmann MW, Weiss T, Drexler H, Angerer J (2004) Trans-placental exposure of neonates to acrylamide – a pilot study. *Int Arch Occup Environ Health* **77:** 213–16.

Schinkel AH, Jonker JW (2003) Mammalian drug efflux transporters of the ATP binding cassette (ABC) family: an overview. *Ad Drug Deliv Rev* **55:** 3–29.

Schneider H, Panigel M, Dancis J (1972) Transfer across the perfused human placenta of antipyrine, sodium and leucine. *Am J Obstet Gynecol* **114:** 822–8.

Schönfelder G, Wittfoht W, Hopp H, Talsness CE, Paul M, Chahoud I (2002) Parent bisphenol A accumulation in the human maternal–fetal–placental unit. *Environ Health Perspect* **110:** A703–707.

Serrano MA, Macias RI, Briz O, Monte MJ, Blazquez AG, Williamson C, Kubitz R, Marin JJ (2007) Expression in human trophoblast and choriocarcinoma cell lines, BeWo, Jeg-3 and JAr of genes involved in the hepatobiliary-like excretory function of the placenta. *Placenta* **28:** 107–17.

Shi F, Soares MJ, Avery M, Liu F, Shang X, Audus KL (1997) Permeability and metabolic properties of a trophoblast cell line (HRP-1) derived from normal rat placenta. *Exp Cell Res* **234:** 147–55.

Smit JW, Huisman MT, van Tellingen O, Wiltshire HR, Schinkel AH (1999) Absence or pharmacological blocking of placental P-glycoprotein profoundly increases fetal drug exposure. *J Clin Inv* **104:** 1441–7.

Soechitram SD, Athanasiadou M, Hovander L, Bergman A, Sauer PJ (2004) Fetal exposure to PCBs and their hydroxylated metabolites in a Dutch cohort. *Environ Health Perspect* **112:** 1208–12.

Sörgel F, Weissenbacher R, Kinzig-Schippers M, Hofmann A, Illauer M, Skott A, Landersdorfer C (2002) Acrylamide: increased concentrations in homemade food and first evidence of its variable absorbtion from food, variable metabolism and placental and breast milk transfer in humans. *Chemotherapy* **48:** 267–74.

Staud F, Vackova Z, Pospechova K, Pavek P, Ceckova M, Libra A, Cygalova L, Nachtigal P, Fendrich Z (2006) Expression and transport activity of breast cancer resistance protein (Bcrp/Abcg2) in dually perfused rat placenta and HRP-1 cell line. *J Pharmacol Exp Ther* **319:** 53–62.

Sun M, Kingdom J, Baczyk D, Lye SJ, Matthews SG, Gibb W (2006) Expression of the multidrug resistance P-glycoprotein, (ABCB1 glycoprotein) in the human placenta decreases with advancing gestation. *Placenta* **27:** 602–9.

Swanson JM, Entringer S, Buss C, Wadhwa PD (2009) Developmental origins of health and disease: environmental exposures. *Sem Reprod Med* **27:** 391–402.

Syme MR, Paxton JW, Keelan JA (2004) Drug transfer and metabolism by the human placenta. *Clin Pharmacokin* **43:** 487–514.

Tamura A, Onishi Y, An R, Koshiba S, Wakabayashi K, Hoshijima K, Priebe W, Yoshida T, Kometani S, Matsubara T, Mikuriya K, Ishikawa T (2007) In vitro evaluation of photosensitivity risk related to genetic polymorphisms of human ABC transporter ABCG2 and inhibition by drugs. *Drug Metab Pharmacokin* **22:** 428–240.

Tanabe M, Ieiri I, Nagata N, Inoue K, Ito S, Kanamori Y, Takahashi M, Kurata Y, Kigawa J, Iguchi S, Terakawa N, Otsubo K (2001) Expression of P-glycoprotein in human placenta: relation to genetic polymorphism of the multidrug resistance (MDR)-1 gene. *J Pharmacol Exp Therap* **297:** 1137–43.

Tertti K, Ekblad U, Heikkinen T, Rahi M, Rönnemaa T, Laine K (2010) The role of organic cation transporters (OCTs) in the transfer of metformin in the dually perfused human placenta. *Eur J Pharm Sci* **39:** 76–81.

Turner PC, Collinson AC, Cheung YB, Gong Y, Hall AJ, Prentice AM, Wild CP (2007) Aflatoxin exposure in utero causes growth faltering in Gambian infants. *Int J Epidemiol* **36:** 1119–25.

Ueki R, Tatara T, Kariya N, Shimode N, Tashiro C (2009) Comparison of placental transfer of local anesthetics in perfusates with different pH values in a human cotyledon model. *J Anesth* **23:** 526–9.

Utoguchi N, Chandorkar GA, Avery M, Audus KL (2000) Functional expression of P-glycoprotein in primary cultures of human cytotrophoblasts and BeWo cells. *Reprod Toxicol* **14:** 217–24.

Vähäkangas K, Myllynen P (2009) Drug transporters in the human blood–placental barrier. *Br J Pharmacol* **158:** 665–678.

Vähäkangas K, Myllynen P (2006) Experimental methods to study human transplacental exposure to genotoxic agents. *Mut Res* **608:** 129–35.

Vähäkangas K, Raunio H, Pasanen M, Sivonen P, Park SS, Gelboin HV, Pelkonen O (1989) Comparison of the formation of benzo[a]pyrene diolepoxide–DNA adducts in vitro by rat and human microsomes: evidence for the involvement of P-450IA1 and P-450IA2. *J Biochem Toxicol* **4:** 79–86.

Vahter M, Akesson A, Lind B, Bjors U, Schutz A, Berglund M (2000) Longitudinal study of methylmercury and inorganic mercury in blood and urine of pregnant and lactating women, as well as in umbilical cord. *Environ Res* **84:** 186–94.

van Herwaarden AE, Wagenaar E, Karnekamp B, Merino G, Jonker JW, Schinkel AH (2006) Breast cancer resistance protein (Bcrp1/Abcg2) reduces systemic exposure of the dietary carcinogens aflatoxin B1, IQ and Trp-P-1 but also mediates their secretion into breast milk. *Carcinogenesis* **27:** 123–30.

van Herwaarden AE, Wagenaar E, Merino G, Jonker JW, Rosing H, Beijnen JH, Schinkel AH (2007) Multidrug transporter ABCG2/breast cancer resistance protein secretes riboflavin (vitamin B2) into milk. *Mol Cell Biol* **27:** 1247–53.

Vaidya SS, Walsh SW, Gerk PM (2009) Formation and efflux of ATP-binding cassette transporter substrate 2,4-dinitrophenyl-S-glutathione from cultured human term placental villous tissue fragments. *Mol Pharmaceut* **6:** 1689–702.

Vore M, Leggas M (2008) Progesterone acts via progesterone receptors A and B to regulate breast cancer resistance protein expression. *Mol Pharmacol* **73:** 613–15.

Wada M (2006) Single nucleotide polymorphisms in ABCC2 and ABCB1 genes and their clinical impact in physiology and drug response. *Cancer Lett* **234:** 40–50.

Wang T, Chen M, Yan YE, Xiao FQ, Pan XL, Wang H (2009) Growth retardation of fetal rats exposed to nicotine in utero: possible involvement of CYP1A1, CYP2E1, and P-glycoprotein. *Environ Toxicol* **24:** 33–42.

Wang Q, Strab R, Kardos P, Ferguson C, Li J, Owen A, Hidalgo IJ (2008) Application and limitation of inhibitors in drug-transporter interactions studies. *Int J Pharmaceut* **356:** 12–18.

Wang XB, Wang SS, Zhang QF, Liu M, Li HL, Liu Y, Wang JN, Zheng F, Guo LY, Xiang JZ (2010) Inhibition of tetramethylpyrazine on P-gp, MRP2, MRP3 and MRP5 in multidrug resistant human hepatocellular carcinoma cells. *Oncol Rep* **23:** 211–15.

Wang H, Zhou L, Gupta A, Vethanayagam RR, Zhang Y, Unadkat JD, Mao Q (2006) Regulation of BCRP/ABCG2 expression by progesterone and 17beta-estradiol in human placental BeWo cells. *Am J Physiol Endocrinol Metab* **290:** E798–E807.

Whyatt RM, Barr DB, Camann DE, Kinney PL, Barr JR, Andrews HF, Hoepner LA, Garfinkel R, Hazi Y, Reyes A, Ramirez J, Cosme Y, Perera FP (2003) Contemporary-use pesticides in personal air samples during pregnancy and blood samples at delivery among urban minority mothers and newborns. *Environ Health Perspect* **111:** 749–56.

Wigle DT, Arbuckle TE, Walker M, Wade MG, Liu S, Krewski D (2007) Environmental hazards: evidence for effects on child health. *J Toxicol Environ Health Part B, Crit Rev* **10:** 3–39.

Wild CP, Rasheed FN, Jawla MF, Hall AJ, Jansen LA, Montesano R (1991) In-utero exposure to aflatoxin in west Africa. *Lancet* **337:** 1602.

Woodward OM, Köttgen A, Coresh J, Boerwinkle E, Guggino WB, Köttgen M (2009) Identification of a urate transporter, ABCG2, with a common functional polymorphism causing gout. *Proc Natl Acad Sci USA* **106:** 10338–42.

Yanase K, Tsukahara S, Mitsuhashi J, Sugimoto Y (2006) Functional SNPs of the breast cancer resistance protein-therapeutic effects and inhibitor development. *Cancer Lett* **234:** 73–80.

Yasuda S, Itagaki S, Hirano T, Iseki K (2005) Expression level of ABCG2 in the placenta decreases from the mid stage to the end of gestation. *Biosci Biotechnol Biochem* **69:** 1871–6.

Yeboah D, Sun M, Kingdom J, Baczyk D, Lye SJ, Matthews SG, Gibb W (2006) Expression of breast cancer resistance protein (BCRP/ABCG2) in human placenta throughout gestation and at term before and after labor. *Can J Physiol Pharmacol* **84:** 1251–8.

Zhou F, Tanaka K, Soares MJ, You G (2003) Characterization of an organic anion transport system in a placental cell line. *Am J Physiol* **285:** E1103–E1109.

Zimmerli B, Dick R (1995) Determination of ochratoxin A at the ppt level in human blood, serum, milk and some foodstuffs by high-performance liquid chromatography with enhanced fluorescence detection and immunoaffinity column cleanup: methodology and Swiss data. *J Chromatogr B, Biomed Appl* **666:** 85–99.

CHAPTER

80

Placental toxicity

Ramesh C. Gupta

INTRODUCTION

The placenta is a rapidly developing complex organ which interfaces two separate genomes, mother and fetus. This organ is further complicated by multiple pregnancies, which are rare in human gestation but common in species like cats, dogs, pigs and rodents. The placenta is an evolutionary and unique organ in the sense that it plays multiple roles in the development of the fetus, by serving as the lung, gut, kidney and exocrine/endocrine glands. The most important function of the placenta is to provide oxygen and nutrients to the fetus and a number of factors can influence this process (Mess and Carter, 2007; Carter, 2009). Furthermore, the placenta provides a flow of chemical information between mother and fetus, implantation, cellular growth and maturation, and at the terminal phase of placental life, parturition and delivery.

Placental toxicology is a fascinating subject, as it deals with the toxic effects of chemicals on mother, placenta and fetus. The subject embraces the knowledge of drug- and chemical-induced structural changes in the placenta, placentation, implantation, embryotoxicity, fetotoxicity, growth retardation, teratogenesis and biochemical, neurochemical and functional deficits. The late 19th and early 20th century was a golden age for placental research, and Mathias Duval (1844–1907) was one of the pioneers in elucidating intricate details of the placentas of different mammalian species (Pijnenborg and Vercruysse, 2006). Since the landmark incident of thalidomide in the 1960s, in which >8,000 babies were born with deformities, pharmacologists, toxicologists, teratologists, biologists and regulatory agencies have been actively engaged in evaluating chemicals and drugs for reproductive and developmental toxicity. In several studies, the placenta has been shown to have metabolic and non-metabolic enzymes, ion channels, receptors, transmitters, hormones, growth factors and other molecules of interest (Kanevsky *et al.*, 1997; Rossmanith *et al.*, 1997; Yan *et al.*, 1999; Lips *et al.*, 2005; Hewitt *et al.*, 2006; Pelkonen *et al.*, 2006; Roberts *et al.*, 2008; Setia and Sridhar, 2009; Croy *et al.*, 2009; Gupta, 2009; Riquelme, 2009), thereby receiving enormous attention in the field of reproductive and developmental biology and toxicology. There is mounting evidence that following maternal exposure, the majority of chemicals can cross the placental barrier and reach the fetus, thus producing a variety of adverse effects in the placenta and fetus, as well as the mother. It is noteworthy that certain chemicals can exert toxicity in the placenta or fetus at levels that are not known to produce maternal toxicity, suggesting greater sensitivity of the placenta and fetus.

By now it is well established that the placenta is a target organ for many toxicants. In the assessment of placental toxicity of xenobiotics, there are two major areas of concern: (1) what the placenta does to xenobiotics, and (2) what xenobiotics do to the placenta (Myllynen *et al.*, 2005; Pelkonen *et al.*, 2006; Gupta, 2009). In the former area, the major topics of concern are the entry and possible storage of substances in placental cells and through the placenta, aided perhaps by various transporters and efflux pumps, the distribution and binding of compounds in placental cells and the biotransformation of substances by intracellular enzymes. Metabolic activation and production of reactive intermediates by placental enzymes link these areas with the toxicodynamics of placental toxicants. In the latter area, the effects of compounds on placental blood flow and vasculature and the presence of membrane and intracellular receptors, enzymes and other potential targets for xenobiotics are important areas of placental toxicity. Therefore, by having a wide range of activities, the placenta can modify the outcome of fetal toxicity of chemicals. In the toxicant-exposed mother, the chemical encounters the placenta before it reaches the fetus. The health of the placenta seems as important as the health of the mother or the fetus because the chemical-induced damage in the placenta is likely to appear in the fetus. It is beyond the scope of this chapter to discuss the placental toxicity of every single chemical; instead this chapter is mainly focused on some important drugs and toxicants, while other toxicants are discussed in other chapters of this book.

PLACENTAL STRUCTURE, FUNCTION AND SPECIES DIFFERENCES

Morphologically, the placenta is partly of fetal origin (the trophoblast) and partly of maternal origin (from a transformation of the uterine mucosa). Based on the number of layers between maternal and fetal blood, mammalian

Reproductive and Developmental Toxicology, Edited by Ramesh C. Gupta
ISBN: 978-0-12-382032-7

placentas can be classified as the following types: (1) hemochorial or hemomonochorial in humans and monkeys; (2) hemoendothelial in rats, rabbits, and guinea-pigs; (3) endotheliochorial in cats and dogs; (3) syndesmochorial in sheep, goats and other ruminants; and (4) epitheliochorial in pigs, donkeys and horses. Anatomically, the placenta has also been described as zonary in the dog, bidiscoid in the monkey and multicotyledonary in the sheep. The placental morphology is complex and its thickness depends on the number of fetal and maternal cell layers (Huppertz *et al.*, 2006). For example, the rat and the rabbit have a single layer of cells; primates and humans have three layers of cells; and pigs, donkeys and horses have six layers. The placenta of humans and monkeys is hemochorial, in which the fetal tissue is in direct contact with maternal blood (Figure 80.1). The membrane separating the maternal and fetal compartments is thin and consists of only three layers (syncytiotrophoblast, connective tissue and vascular fetal endothelium).

In humans, there are two stages for the development of the placenta: (1) early embryonic period (2 months), followed by (2) later fetal period (7 months). The placenta is differentiated by the third month of pregnancy. During the embryonic period (the first 2 months) of pregnancy, the embryo acquires a definite form (morphogenesis) and outlines of the main organs (organogenesis). By the end of the second month, the embryo becomes a fetus. During the fetal period (2–9 months), the organs undergo maturation at the histological (histogenesis) and functional levels. During this period, the fetus grows in size (crown–rump length), volume and weight (Figure 80.2). During the embryonic period, there is no placental barrier. Drugs and environmental chemicals have easy access to the developing embryo and interfere with different stages of morphological differentiation. Chemical- or drug-induced dysmorphogenicity has been recognized in experimental animals for many years. The clinical implications of these experimental results have been widely recognized since 1961 due to the discovery of thalidomide-induced phocomelia and other embryopathies. The critical exposure of the embryo occurs *in utero* when the sedative drug thalidomide (100 mg) is ingested by a pregnant woman in the 4th and 6th weeks of pregnancy. About 8,000 victims of this teratogenic substance have been born (Rodin *et al.*, 1962; Taussig, 1962).

During the fetal period, the fully formed placenta plays an important role in the maintenance of nutrition to the fetus and in the secretory and regulatory functions that are essential for the maintenance of pregnancy. All "supplies"

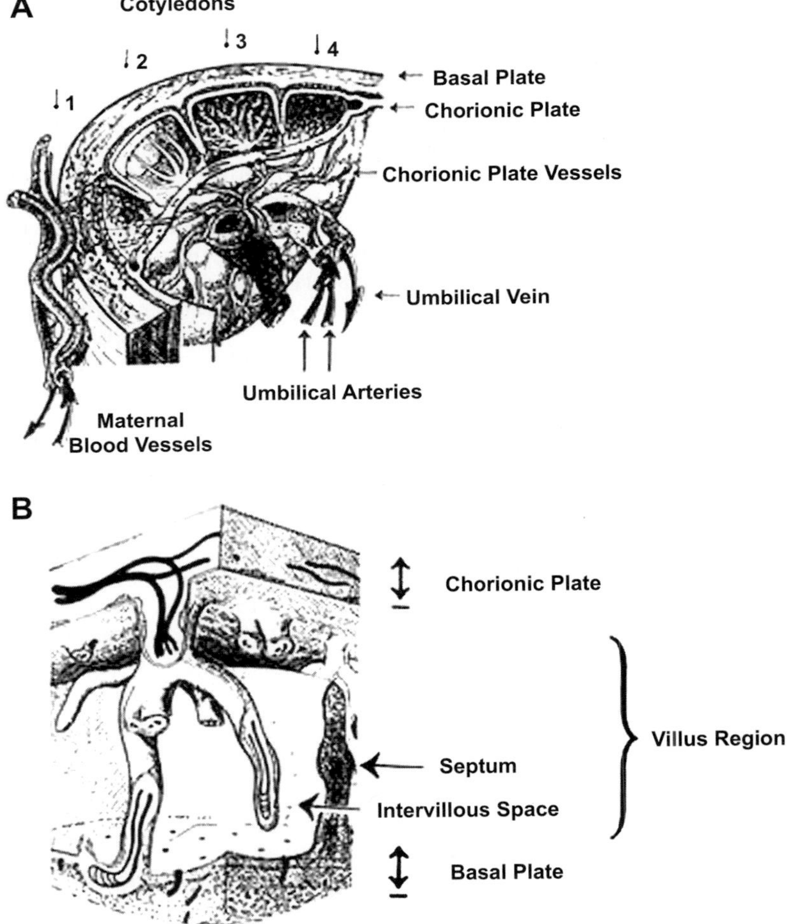

FIGURE 80.1 (A) A cross-section of human term placenta showing four distinct cotyledons. In cotyledon 1, maternal and fetal blood flows are depicted. In cotyledon 2, anchoring villi to basal plate are shown. In cotyledons 3 and 4, all villi and blood flows are shown. (B) Schematic drawing of a single cotyledon, villi and other parts of the placenta. For details of human placental structure, standard books on human embryology should be consulted (Tuchmann-Duplessis *et al.*, 1972; Larsen, 1993).

(oxygen, water, electrolytes, nutrients, hormones, etc.) to the embryo and fetus pass through the placenta. In recent studies, the placenta has been shown to transfer maternal as well as placental antibodies to the fetus (Pentšuk and van der Laan, 2009). Several enzymes involved in drug biotransformation (oxidation, reduction, hydrolysis and conjugation) are present in the placenta. The placenta has a significant role to play in the synthesis of steroid and protein hormones and of several growth and regulatory factors, including acetylcholine, opioids, tachykinins, platelet activating factor, insulin-like growth factors and prostaglandins. If the placenta is not functioning properly, it can be the limiting factor not only for fetal nutrition, but also for the maternal–fetal exchange of physiological constituents as well as waste products that may represent a pathologic risk to the fetus. Some drugs ingested by the mother may enter the placenta and interfere with placental function and, thereby, fetal development. Some of these compounds may enter the placenta, be metabolized into toxic compounds and enter fetal circulation. Therefore, the placenta can be a target organ for drug-/chemical-induced injury by causing alterations in placental structure and functions.

The placenta plays multiple roles, including protection of the fetus, fetal nutrition, respiration, excretion, endocrine and communication between mother and fetus (Rutherford, 2009). The intensity of the passage of substances across the placenta is an important function and is inversely proportional to the thickness of placental membranes. For example, the intensity of Na^+ exchange across different types of placenta can be arranged in the following order: hemochorial > endotheliochorial > syndesmochorial > epitheliochorial. Exchange involves not only physiological constituents, but unfortunately, also substances that represent pathologic risks to the fetus. Therefore, in assessing placental toxicology of chemicals, all physiological and functional variables should be taken into consideration. Due to practical and technical advantages, animal placenta has been used to study placental function and toxicology. Although qualitative similarities among several types of placenta are present, identical function and effects of toxicants should not be assumed (Tsuyoshi, 2007).

PLACENTAL BARRIER

The term "placental barrier" is a widely held false notion, since the placenta is not a true barrier for the transfer of most drugs and toxicants from mother to fetus. The placenta has been characterized as "a lipid membrane that permits bidirectional transfer of substances between maternal and fetal compartments" rather than as a barrier. In humans, the placental barrier consists of the trophoblastic epithelium covering the villi, the chorionic connective tissue and the fetal capillary endothelium. The average thickness of the barrier varies from the 1st trimester (20–30 μm) to 3rd trimester (2–4 μm) (Wloch *et al.*, 2009). At the term, the average exchange area is approximately 11 m^2, and the placental blood flow rate is approximately 450 ml/min (Pacifici and Nottoli, 1995).

The two most important factors involved in transplacental transfer of toxicants are: (1) physico-chemical properties of the chemical, and (2) type of placenta. Any chemical with a molecular weight (MW) <1,000 readily crosses the placenta, and most pesticides, metals, mycotoxins, plant alkaloids and other xenobiotics have a MW <1,000. Hence, these chemicals are not restricted from reaching the fetus. However, the placenta poses a limited permeability barrier to chemicals with a MW >1,000 (Syme *et al.*, 2004; Gupta, 2007, 2009). It is important to mention that metabolic processes in the mother or the placenta can biotransform high MW chemicals into low MW chemicals, thus allowing them to cross the placental barrier. Chemical properties, such as lipophilicity, polarity and degree of ionization, can also affect the placental barrier. Recently, Giaginis *et al.* (2009) described the applicability of a quantitative structure–activity relationship (QSAR) for modeling drugs/chemicals that transport across the human placental barrier. The other factor that predominantly influences the transplacental transfer of chemicals is the type of placenta. From the limited literature available, it appears that the placental barrier is partial and selective to some xenobiotics and is recognized in the simpler choriovitalline type of placenta present in rodents, and also in the chorioallantoic type present in higher mammals (Welsch, 1982; Juchau, 1995). In general, the more complex multilayered placenta of

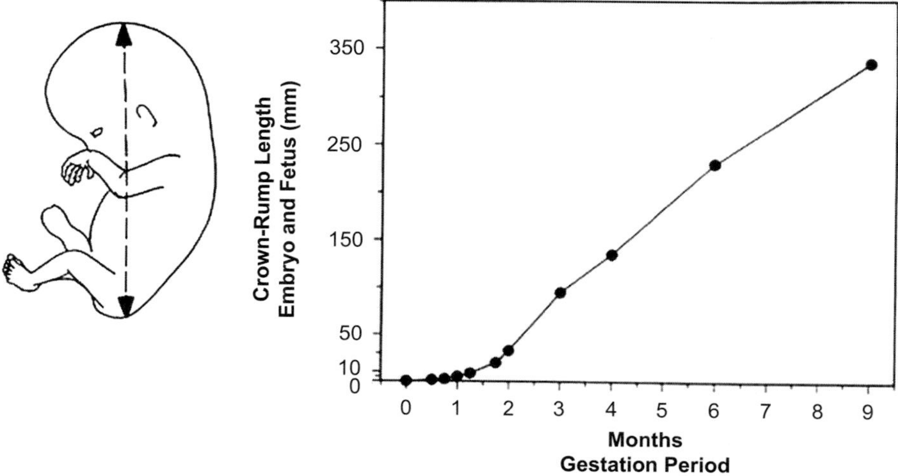

FIGURE 80.2 The relationship between gestation period and crown–rump length of human embryo and fetus. In fetal growth retardation both parameters will decrease.

higher animals can make it more difficult for xenobiotics to gain access to the fetus.

So far, diffusion (simple or facilitated) has been proven to be the only mechanism by which drugs and toxicants cross the human placenta, although several animal studies have suggested a role for active transport or pinocytosis (Mihaly and Morgan, 1984). The rate and extent of transfer differ for various compounds (Welsch, 1982). The rate of diffusion is determined by the maternal–fetal drug gradient, uterine and umbilical blood flow, MW of drug/toxicant, protein binding, lipid solubility and degree of ionization. These factors also determine the time required for maternal–fetal equilibrium.

The evidence for placental transfer of chemicals stems from either direct detection of a chemical residue or its metabolite in the placenta, umbilical cord blood, embryo–fetus or the specific biochemical and morphological changes induced by a chemical toxicant in the placenta–fetus. Placental transfer of various classes of pesticides is described in our previous publications (Gupta, 1995; Pelkonen *et al.*, 2006; Gupta, 2007, 2009). Similar information on placental transfer of metals, mycotoxins and drugs has been reported elsewhere (Eisenmann and Miller, 1996; Rogers, 1996; Gupta, 1998; Pelkonen *et al.*, 2006; Gupta, 2007, 2009).

In essence, the anatomical placental barrier for the majority of toxicants/drugs (including charged molecules such as *d*-tubocurarine, highly ionized salicylates, pesticides, metals, mycotoxins and narcotics) is a widely held false assumption, since they cross the placenta and reach the embryo–fetus and, thereby, produce a variety of toxicological and teratogenic effects (Eisenmann and Miller, 1996; Gupta, 1995, 2007, 2009). Finally, it is noteworthy that since the mid-1990s, another kind of placental barrier (i.e., metabolic barrier) has been recognized by physicians, toxicologists, pharmacologists and others. Human term placenta, by having a significant butyrylcholinesterase (BuChE) activity, metabolizes cocaine and thereby serves as a metabolic barrier to protect the conceptus (Simone *et al.*, 1994; Gupta, 2009).

PLACENTAL SUSCEPTIBILITY TO CHEMICAL TOXICITY

More than one mechanism exists by which toxicants are concentrated in the placenta in greater quantities than in maternal tissues. In general, the large placental surface area comes in contact with a relatively large volume of maternal blood (required for normal placental function), and that makes the placenta vulnerable to toxicants (Eisenmann and Miller, 1996). The placenta has certain biomolecules (proteins, carbohydrates, lipids, nucleic acids/nucleotides and enzymes) which can either be the target of toxicity or can play a role in modification of toxicity. Being rich in proteins, the placenta may bioconcentrate chemical residues by means of protein binding and release them into the placental circulation and ultimately into the fetus. Like the placenta, fetal tissue also accumulates chemical residues because of its inadequate capability for degradation and elimination. An incomplete or partial blood–brain barrier in the fetus is another reason for its greater sensitivity. As a result, birth/congenital defects occur with greater frequency in the central nervous system (CNS) than in any other organ/system when exposed *in utero* to toxicants, such as methyl mercury, lead, thalidomide, retinoids, alcohol and others.

Since the placenta serves as an interface between mother and fetus for nutrients, the health of the fetus seems to be dependent on the health of the mother and the placenta. Unfortunately, certain toxic chemicals are also traversed by similar mechanisms. Eisenmann and Miller (1996) explained the mechanism to support this fact by stating that toxic metals (e.g., cadmium and lead) may enter the placenta and be concentrated there, or may be transferred to the fetus via a mechanism designed to transport nutrients, such as calcium. Further, because fetal demands for nutrients increase with gestation (Haggerty *et al.*, 2002), the potential for placental–fetal intoxication with toxic metals may also increase with gestation (Gupta, 2007, 2009). It is important to mention that pregnancy is a state of oxidative/nitrosative stress arising from increased placental mitochondrial activity and production of reactive oxygen species (ROS) and reactive nitrogen species (RNS). The placental stress level can be further exacerbated by chemicals (e.g., metals, pesticides, mycotoxins, etc.) that are known to produce oxidative/ nitrosative stress.

PLACENTAL TOXICITY MODIFYING FACTORS

During pregnancy, overall toxicity of a chemical can be influenced by the following factors: (1) maternal toxicity, (2) placental transfer and (3) placental–fetal metabolism.

Maternal toxicity

Maternal toxicity can be defined as the transitory or permanent state of alteration in maternal physiology or behavior with a potential to cause adverse effects during embryo–fetal or postnatal development. In contrast, the term "maternotoxic" commonly refers to test dosages, agents, signs/symptoms or data relevant to pregnancy without any connotation to its embryo–fetal implications. Maternal toxicity-related factors, whether intrinsic (homeostasis alterations) or extrinsic (chemical and physical agents) at maternotoxic levels can produce deleterious consequences in fetal development by either altering maternal physiology or causing maternotoxic effects. Some common factors related to maternal toxicity include: (1) route of drug/chemical exposure, (2) maternal drug/chemical distribution, (3) maternal drug/chemical metabolism, (4) uterine blood flow and (5) pH of the blood. Although the exact mechanism by which maternal toxicity factors are responsible for fetal toxicity/teratogenesis remains obscure, alterations in placental function appear to be important. Therefore, it can be suggested that maternal toxicity plays a major role in adverse fetal outcome by modifying placental function.

Placental transfer

Fetal growth directly depends on the nutrients crossing the placenta. Glucose is the principal carbohydrate crossing the placenta and it is transported by facilitated-diffusion glucose transporters, according to concentration-dependent kinetics (Illsley, 2000). Recently, Acevedo *et al.* (2005) demonstrated that insulin and nitric oxide (NO) stimulate glucose uptake in human placenta and suggested that both potential regulators of glucose transport use different signaling pathways. Amino acids are transported through an energy-dependent process via selective amino acid transporters (Battaglia and Regnault, 2001). However, knowledge about placental transport of lipids is still scant. The role and importance of placental transfer in relation to chemical toxicity has already been discussed in the earlier parts of this chapter. Some of the factors that are involved in transplacental transport of chemicals which may alter placental toxicity are discussed here in brief.

The important placental transfer factors include placental blood flow, pH of the blood, placental permeability (passive or active transport system), placental maturity over gestation period (size, surface area and thickness), interspecies variation in placental morphology, lipid–protein content of membranes, placental metabolism, plasma protein binding, lipid solubility and other physico-chemical properties of toxicants (Welsch, 1982; Mihaly and Morgan, 1984; Slikker and Miller, 1994; Andersen *et al.*, 2000; Syme *et al.*, 2004). Factors related to placental morphology, physiology and metabolism seem to be interrelated, and with continuing change, they become more complex as gestation advances.

Plasma protein binding (especially the albumin fraction) appears to be an important factor that can modify placental toxicity. The reason being a chemical in a free form (i.e., unbound) only crosses the placenta. It needs to be mentioned that protein binding is a reversible process and the protein-bound chemical can become a free form and cross the placenta. Once the chemical has reached the fetus, either it remains free to produce deleterious effects or, once again, it can bind to proteins of the blood and fetal tissue, a phenomenon described as the "sink effect". Organophosphate (OP) and carbamate (CM) insecticides as well as cadmium are appropriate examples to substantiate this phenomenon. The protein binding factor has further implications in the potentiation of OP or CM toxicity if the mother is pre-exposed to another OP that binds to esterases or proteins (Pelkonen *et al.*, 2006; Gupta, 1995, 2007).

Placental–fetal metabolism

Placental–fetal metabolism is one of the major factors that can significantly modulate the placental toxicity of certain chemical toxicants (Pasanen and Pelkonen, 1994; Miller *et al.*, 1996; Hakkola *et al.*, 1998; Juchau and Chen, 1998). Metabolism occurs in all maternal, placental and embryo–fetal tissues, but the capacity differs at all stages of gestation. During pregnancy, metabolism of the drug or toxicant is complicated by two major factors: (1) the pregnancy itself, since general metabolic activity is low, which may lower the degradation of drugs or toxicants and thereby increase the toxicity; and (2) pre-exposure or simultaneous exposure to other chemicals or environmental pollutants generally results in either reduced or enhanced metabolism and, consequently, altered placental toxicity. For example, previous exposure to drug-metabolizing enzyme inducers, such as enhanced monooxygenase activity by polychlorinated biphenyls (PCBs), or other similar environmental pollutants, can potentiate the toxicity of the "thioate" type of OP insecticides. Cigarette smoking and chronic consumption of alcohol and drugs of abuse (e.g., steroids, cocaine, cannabis) are additional factors that can modify placental–fetal metabolism and placental toxicity (Sastry and Janson, 1995; Syme *et al.*, 2004; Gupta, 2009).

TOXICITY

Various types of chemicals are known to induce toxicity in the placenta by damaging either structure and/or function. Placental toxicity of some common types of drugs and environmental chemicals is described here in brief.

Abused drugs

The most common drugs used by humans are alcohol, nicotine (tobacco smoking), morphine and cocaine. The common effects of all these drugs are placental function compromise and intrauterine fetal growth retardation (IUGR). There may be direct effects of drugs on the developing fetus, or indirect effects via influence on placental function. In IUGR, there is a decrease in all dimensions of fetal growth, indicating a common cause for the development of all organs of the fetus (Figure 80.2). One of the requirements for the growth and development of fetal organs is essential amino acids for protein synthesis and tissue formation, and therefore effects of abused drugs are evaluated on the placental transport of amino acids. There is enough evidence that abnormalities in the transplacental transport of amino acids may lead to poor fetal growth. Amino acid supply to the fetus and plasma amino acid concentrations are the strongest regulators of amino acid incorporation into protein and the major factors limiting protein breakdown (Pastrakuljek *et al.*, 1999).

Alcohol

Alcohol is a socially acceptable and legal drug often consumed by women prior to and during pregnancy. Alcohol and its major metabolite acetaldehyde readily cross the placenta and blood–brain barrier (BBB). Maternal alcohol consumption, either continuously throughout pregnancy or in a "binge" pattern, can result in an adverse and lasting fatal outcome (Henderson and Schenker, 1995; Isayama *et al.*, 2009). The overall effect of alcohol in the human fetus is described as fetal alcohol syndrome (FAS) characterized by: (1) growth retardation, (2) CNS abnormalities, including abnormal brain morphology, neurological abnormalities and developmental and intellectual impairment, and (3) a characteristic pattern of craniofacial abnormalities (Jones *et al.*, 1973; Larroque, 1992; Stratton *et al.* 1996; Bailey and Sokol, 2008). Preclinical studies indicate that *in utero* exposure to high doses of ethanol results in decreased litter size, decreased size and birth weight of individual offspring, and increased postnatal deaths of neonates. Embryonic and early postnatal alcohol exposures have been investigated experimentally to elucidate the fetal alcohol spectrum disorder (FASD) (Isayama *et al.*, 2009). Experimental studies also indicate that some of the subtle neurochemical, neuroendocrinological and behavioral effects, in addition to improper fetal programming, can persist during adolescence or adulthood (Boksa, 1998; Weinberg *et al.*, 2008; Isayama *et al.*, 2009; Samudio-Ruiz *et al.*, 2009). Epidemiological studies suggest that, even in the absence of growth deficits and developmental delay, subtle but lasting behavioral and intellectual dysfunctions may persist (Committee on Substance and Committee on Children with Disabilities, 1993). FAS and FASD are multifactorial entities with functional and structural abnormalities affecting not only the nervous system but also the whole organism (Isayama *et al.*, 2009). Some of these factors may include neurotransmitters, adhesion molecules, cell death, transcription factors, trophic factors, etc. These "Fetal Alcohol Effects" may include hyperactivity, attention and fine-motor deficits, and a constellation of psychosocial disorders. A question arises about the contribution of the placenta to overall FAS. Alcohol and its metabolite acetaldehyde are known to cause alterations in the primary functions (transport, metabolic and endocrine) of the placenta, in addition to their direct effects on the developing fetus.

Alcoholism is frequently associated with malnutrition, which leads to the lack of normal growth and development of FAS in children. Several studies have focused on the hypothesis that maternal alcohol consumption produces a suboptimal supply of nutrients needed for fetal growth. There is some evidence from animal experiments and *in vitro* experiments using human placental tissues that alcohol affects nutrient transport of amino acids, glucose, some vitamins (vitamin B6, folate and thiamine) and the trace element Zn. Experimental research-based mechanisms involved in FAS and teratogenicity include interference in placental essential amino acids' transport, insufficient oxygen supply due to constriction of umbilical vessels, increased prostaglandins levels, decreased protein synthesis and DNA methylation, free radical damage and decreased ATP levels (Lin, 1981; Nulman *et al.*, 1998; Gupta, 2009). In addition, alcohol influences the effects of biogenic amines on human placental vasculature and therefore placental blood flow. Alcohol also influences fluidity of placental membranes and thereby modulates responsiveness of the placental vasculature to biogenic amines.

Nicotine/tobacco

The use of nicotine and tobacco products constitutes the most significant cause of morbidity and mortality throughout the world. During pregnancy, active smoking or secondhand environmental exposure continue to be a significant health problem. It is well established that the human placenta does not pose a barrier to nicotine and its metabolite (cotinine) transfer from the mother to the developing fetus or in the opposite direction. Maternal smoking during pregnancy can cause: (1) increased spontaneous abortions, (2) reduced fetal breathing movements, (3) fetal growth retardation, (4) abnormal fetal programming for metabolic disorders, (4) reduced postnatal growth and (5) increased risk of sudden infant death syndrome (Seller *et al.*, 1992; Salafia and Shiverick, 1999; England *et al.*, 2001; Zhao and Reece, 2005; Somm *et al.*, 2009). Following prenatal tobacco/nicotine exposure, some of the neurochemical, endocrinal, genetic, reproductive and behavioral effects observed in the fetus may persist until adolescence or adulthood (Holloway *et al.*, 2006; Slotkin, 2008; Gold *et al.*, 2009; Fowler *et al.*, 2009; Somm *et al.*, 2009; Mukhopadhyay *et al.*, 2010; Rückinger *et al.*, 2010).

The findings are consistent that tobacco smoke components influence the process of parturition, and the mechanism involved is described here in brief. Metabolism of nicotine occurs only at very low levels in the human placenta. Nicotine is metabolized to cotinine, which has a long plasma half-life with slow clearance across membrane barriers. In a perfused cotyledon of normal human term placenta, Sastry *et al.* (1998) observed that when nicotine was added on the fetal side, part of it was metabolized to cotinine and its concentration was twice as high on the fetal side as it was on the maternal side. It can be suggested that cotinine accumulation on the fetal side may activate phospholipase A_2-like enzymes and the formation of prostaglandins, which is known to trigger spontaneous abortions in pregnant smokers.

Low birth weight can be attributed to decreased placental functions in smokers. The effects of maternal smoking and nicotine use on placental function have been described by Sastry and Janson (1995) and Shiverick and Salafia (1999). Maternal smoking alters many biochemical parameters in the maternal (increased blood carboxyhemoglobin), placental (lowered oxygen consumption) and fetal (decreased breathing movements) compartments. The final result of all these alterations is fetal growth retardation as indicated by infant birth weight and crown–rump length (Figure 80.2). In general, babies of smokers are 200 g lighter than babies born to comparable non-smokers (Hasselmeyer *et al.*, 1979). The more the mother smokes, the greater the reduction of fetal growth, which is partially due to disturbances in amino acid metabolism as indicated by depressed placental transport of amino acids in smokers.

The placental transfer of amino acids is a two-step process: (1) active uptake of amino acids by placental syncytiotrophoblast cells from the mother's blood; and (2) passive diffusion of amino acids from placental syncytiotrophoblast cells into umbilical blood. The first step is critical, and its efficiency could be compromised, resulting in depressed uptake into the trophoblast under placental hypoxic conditions induced by maternal smoking. Nicotine and tobacco smoke components (carbon monoxide, cyanides and nitrites) reduced active uptake of amino acids by isolated human placental villi (Barnwell and Sastry, 1983). Exposure of human placental villi to nicotine inhibited the uptake of α-aminoisobutyric acid (α-AIB) and decreased maximum velocity (V_{max}, 71%) and Michaelis-Menton constant (K_m, 67%) for its uptake. Part of the inhibition (16%) was not reversible, which may be of significance in chronic smoking. Concentrations of several essential amino acids (Val, Met, Ileu, Leu, Tyr, Phe, His) and non-essential amino acids (Asp, Glu, Gly, Ala, Arg) in the placental villi of non-smoking mothers were about 30–50% higher than those of smokers (Sastry, 1984; Sastry *et al.*, 1989). Concentrations of Thr and Phe were about 14–15% higher in the placental villi of non-smokers than in those of smokers. Four regulatory mechanisms may be involved in the cellular uptake of amino acids in the placenta: (1) gammaglutamyl cycle for the regulation of amino-acid transport; (2) placental ACh release and amino acid transport coupling; (3) phospholipid *N*-methylation in the plasma membrane; and (4) oxidative energy sources (Sastry, 1991). In essence, maternal smoking decreases the uptake of amino acids by the placenta and therefore their transfer from maternal to fetal blood. Further, the placental transfer of all essential amino acids is not affected equally, indicating that the nitrogen balance may be disturbed in the fetus. Thus, fetal undernutrition for amino acids provides partial explanation for tobacco-induced fetal IUGR.

In some animal species, tobacco alkaloids have been studied for pharmacokinetics/toxicokinetics, and are known to cross the placenta and produce teratogenic effects (Suzuki *et al.*, 1974; Sastry and Jansen, 1995; Panter *et al.*, 1999; Czekaj *et al.*, 2002; Avdalovic *et al.*, 2009). In some studies, tobacco components have been shown to produce deleterious effects on embryonic development in the early stages of pregnancy, before the placenta is fully formed. In mice, nicotine increases intracellular Ca^{2+} and reactive oxygen species (ROS) levels, which play a role in nicotine-induced embryonic apoptosis, eventually leading to teratogenesis (Zhao and Reece, 2005). Nulliparous female Wistar rats treated with nicotine bitartrate (1 mg/kg/day, s.c.) for 14 days prior to mating, during pregnancy and throughout lactation until weaning, resulted in: (1) increased time to pregnancy, (2) altered ovarian steroidogenesis and (3) a decreased estrogen:progesterone ratio (Holloway *et al.*, 2006). These observations suggest that fetal and neonatal exposure to nicotine results in delayed ovarian dysfunction in adult female offspring. Swine also appear to be a sensitive species in the context of tobacco-induced teratogenesis. Fetal arthrogryposis occurs without signs of intoxication in the dams and without fetal deaths or abortions, but the deformed piglets usually die shortly after birth. With *Nicotiana glauca*, fetal deformities are preceded by the appearance of signs of acute toxicity in the dam (Keeler *et al.*, 1981). Deformities in the newborn following *in utero* exposure include severe flexure and lateral rotation of the carpal joints, moderate rotation of the fetlocks and, less commonly, spinal malformations, resulting in lordosis or scoliosis and cleft palate (Burrows and Tyrl, 2001). Precisely which component(s), in addition to nicotine, is also involved in inducing teratogenesis is yet to be elucidated.

Morphine

In earlier publications, different aspects of the human placental opioid system have been described (Ahmed and Cemerikic, 1995; Sastry, 1995a). Placental transfer of the three commonly used opioids (fentanyl, alfentanil and sufentanil) was reported by Giroux *et al.* (1997). When ingested by pregnant women, morphine and its analogs are known to retard intrauterine fetal growth, the extent of which is related to the degree of exposure. This raises questions about the role of the placenta in morphine-IUGR and about the occurrence and role of endogenous opioids. Generally, it is believed that enkephalins and endorphins may serve as neuromodulators and may regulate neurotransmitter or hormone release by positive or negative feedback systems. More specifically, enkephalins may regulate neuronal release of acetylcholine (ACh) and norepinephrine by negative feedback systems (Sastry, 1991; Sastry, 1995b). The occurrence of methionine enkephalin and β-endorphin in human placental villi has been demonstrated using sensitive and specific radioimmunoassays and bioassays. Immunoreactive corticotrophin, lipotrophin and β-endorphin occur in whole placental extracts. Dynorphin 1-8 was also identified in placental extracts by mass spectroscopy. The opioid receptor of the placenta was also purified and identified as the kappa subtype (Ahmed *et al.*, 1989). When the floating villi, chorionic plate and basal plate of the same human placenta were extracted and analyzed, the methionine enkephalin concentration was lower in the chorionic and basal plates. This suggests that the distribution of methionine enkephalin is similar to that of ACh in human placenta.

The human placenta is known to have high concentrations of ACh. Inhibition of ACh synthesis in placenta inhibits amino acid uptake. ACh release, activation of a cholinergic receptor, Ca^{2+} influx and amino acid transport are linked to one another in the uptake of amino acids by the human trophoblast (Sastry, 1997). Atropine blocks ACh release and amino acid uptake by placental villi, indicating that ACh stimulates a muscarinic receptor and thereby regulates amino acid uptake by the trophoblast. Amino acid uptake by placental villi is also depressed in a Ca^{2+}-free medium and by morphine (Barnwell and Sastry, 1983). These observations indicate that, in morphine addicts, ACh-facilitated uptake of amino acids by the trophoblast is depressed. Therefore, IUGR in morphine addicts can be partially explained by depressed amino acid transport in the placenta. Some compensatory changes have been reported to occur in the placental opioid systems of mothers who used morphine-like compounds during pregnancy. The number of kappa opiate receptors decreased in the placenta of mothers who used pentazocine or methadone during pregnancy. Morphine did not decrease ACh release from the placenta of these mothers. These observations indicate that the negative feedback mechanism for the release of ACh is depressed or inactivated due to an inadequate number of kappa receptors in the placentas of opiate addicts. This is a compensatory change to improve ACh-facilitated amino acid uptake by the placentas of opiate-addicted mothers. If there are any other compensatory changes (e.g., decrease in the synthesis of opioid peptides) in the opioid systems of opiate addicts, they have yet to be investigated.

Cocaine

Cocaine abuse has become increasingly prevalent among urban as well as rural populations. In inner cities, an estimated 9–18% of pregnant women admitted to large urban hospitals in the USA had used cocaine during their pregnancy. This particular area of research has gained enormous attention since "crack babies" became a sensational media topic during the 1980s. Since then, the effects of cocaine have been extensively studied on mother, placenta, fetus and offspring. The findings and conclusions are ambiguous. According to some reports, cocaine use in pregnancy is associated with a variety of complications (Fantel *et al.*, 1990; Collins *et al.*, 1999; Pastrakuljic *et al.*, 1999; Patel *et al.*, 1999), while according to others reproductive and developmental effects of cocaine appear to be minimal (Coles, 1993; Neuspiel, 1993; Held *et al.*, 1999).

Cocaine and its major metabolites readily cross the placental barrier and enter the fetal circulation with the potential to cause adverse effects on the developing fetus (Dow-Edwards, 1990; Fantel *et al.*, 1990, 1992; Schenker *et al.*, 1993; Collins *et al.*, 1999; Xiao *et al.*, 2000). Studies with the perfused human placental cotyledon showed that rapid cocaine transfer exhibits the characteristic of passive transport, consistent with its high lipid solubility and low molecular weight (Schenker *et al.*, 1993; Simone *et al.*, 1994). As a weak base, cocaine is only 8–10% protein bound in human plasma, suggesting that the majority of the administered dose is available to equilibrate with fetal circulation. Evidence indicates that cocaine decreases uteroplacental blood flow due to its vasoconstrictive effects (Patel *et al.*, 1999; Pastrakuljic *et al.*, 1999). Acute prenatal exposure to cocaine decreases uteroplacental blood flow, and a chronic decrease in uteroplacental blood flow is associated with IUGR (Woods *et al.*, 1987; Plessinger and Woods, 1993). This may be a leading cause for perinatal morbidity and mortality, as well as developmental impairment in later life.

Investigators have focused on various cocaine-induced complications of pregnancy and malformations in infants, but consistent findings are fetal growth retardation and prematurity. Cocaine appears to interfere with normal physiological processes in pregnancy, resulting in a higher incidence of spontaneous abortion, placental abruption and premature labor. Cocaine interferes with placental amino acid transport similar to that described for nicotine and morphine. In *in vitro* studies, Pastrakuljic *et al.* (1999) reported that cocaine decreases the activity of placental amino acid transport systems A, N and possibly systems I and Y^+. In smooth muscle, cocaine acts as a Ca^{2+} antagonist. Cocaine decreases the release of ACh from placental villi due to the blockade of Ca^{2+} influx into the syncytiotrophoblast (Sastry *et al.*, 1977). Ca^{2+} is necessary for the release of ACh and the uptake of amino acids (Sastry *et al.*, 1983). Cocaine depresses the uptake and placental transport of (neutral, acidic and basic) amino acids (Barnwell and Sastry, 1983). This is one of the mechanisms involved in cocaine-induced fetal growth retardation. In addition, cocaine may induce oxidative stress in the fetus secondary to alterations in nutrient and waste exchange at the placenta or perhaps decreases in placental blood flow may release ROS into the fetus (Fantel *et al.*, 1990, 1992). It is interesting to note that prenatal cocaine exposure-induced neurochemical, morphological and behavioral abnormalities may persist during perinatal and postnatal development (Zhen *et al.*, 2001; Richardson *et al.*, 2008, 2009; Frankfurt *et al.*, 2009). In a recent neuroimaging study, evidence suggests that prenatal cocaine exposure results in significant long-term behavioral teratogenic effects (Li *et al.*, 2009).

Metals

Some metals, such as copper, iron, zinc, cobalt, manganese and selenium, are nutritional trace elements, whereas others, such as aluminum, arsenic, cadmium, lead, mercury and nickel, are of toxicological concern. In excessive concentrations, metals from either category can exert a wide range of adverse health effects, including reproductive and developmental toxicity. While these metals have been extensively studied for reproductive toxicity, transplacental transfer and developmental toxicity, very few studies have dealt with placental toxicity *per se*. Placental toxicity of some of these metals is described here in brief.

Aluminum

Aluminum (Al) is used in several forms: chloride, nitrate, hydroxide (in stomach antacids), chlorhydrate (in deodorants), sulfate (in water treatment) and phosphide (in insecticidal grain fumigants). Al is also extensively used in cooking utensils, appliances, automotives, aircraft, construction, etc. In the last two decades, Al has been recognized as an important toxic metal in studies conducted on experimental animals and humans (ATSDR, 2007a).

Al can be absorbed through oral, dermal, inhalation, subcutaneous and other parenteral routes, and with unequal distribution concentrated in the liver, lungs, bone, kidney, spleen, heart, brain and muscles (Yokel and McNamara, 2001). Following prenatal exposure, Al transplacentally traverses and accumulates in the fetal tissues in amounts that can adversely influence fetal development. Studies in mice and rabbits revealed that the placenta contained four- to five-fold higher Al levels than the fetal or maternal tissues (Yokel and McNamara, 1985; Cranmer *et al.*, 1986; Yumoto *et al.*, 2000). However, the placenta of the guinea-pig does not accumulate Al. Furthermore, placental accumulation of Al in mice and rabbits does not preclude accumulation in the fetal tissues. For further details on toxicokinetics of Al, readers are referred to Yokel (1997) and Krewski *et al.* (2007).

Pregnancy in general enhances susceptibility to Al toxicity. There are no reports to describe the effects of Al on the placenta. Reproductive and developmental toxicity of Al is described in detail in a Chapter 32 in this book. In brief, reproductive effects may include decreased testicular and epididymal sperm counts, and necrosis of testes, spermatocytes and spermatids. In developmental studies, Al has been found to cause resorptions, fetal bone abnormalities, including abnormal digits, wavy ribs, missing ribs, absence of xiphoid and poor ossification. This could be due to the binding of Al with phosphate in the tissues, thus reducing the amount of phosphate available for bone formation. Depletion of phosphate has also been linked to Al-induced fetal internal hemorrhage by causing failure of the blood clotting mechanism. The severity of the effects is highly dependent on the form of Al involved. Overall, developing conceptuses or pups are much more sensitive than adults to Al toxicity.

Arsenic

Arsenic (As) occurs in many forms and commonly contaminates the air, food and water. The major sources of human exposure to arsenic include sea food, tobacco and pharmaceutical preparations. Individuals who work in smelters and industries and those involved in the production and use of arsenic-containing pesticides are at especially greater risks. Paint pigments, fly papers and wood preservatives are also potential sources of arsenic.

Both human and animal studies have shown that As crosses the placenta (ATSDR, 2007b; Vahter, 2009). In pregnant mice, Hood *et al.* (1987, 1988) examined the uptake, distribution and metabolism of sodium arsenite (2.5 μg/kg, p.o.) and sodium arsenate (40 μg/kg, p.o.) on GD 18. Maximum concentrations of As in the placenta were noted at 4 and 2 h after administration of arsenite and arsenate, respectively. Corresponding concentrations in the fetal tissues appeared at 24 and 6 h. Regardless of the form of As administered, >80% of the As is methylated (mono- and dimethyl-As) in the fetus. Arsenic is completely eliminated from the placenta and fetus within 24 h of exposure. For some reason organic As does not seem to cross the placenta; instead, it is stored in the placenta.

Epidemiological investigations conducted in a few countries strongly support the evidence of placental toxicity in humans due to As. In a Swedish study, adverse reproductive outcomes (spontaneous abortions, congenital malformations and low birth weights) were observed in populations working in or residing near the Ronnskär copper smelter. Similar findings were observed in a Hungarian study. In a study conducted in Bulgaria, pregnancy complications and rates of mortality at birth (due to malformations) were high in the smelter area. The average concentrations of As in the placenta of exposed populations living near the copper smelter was 26.6 μg/kg, compared with 7.4 μg/kg in the placenta of those living in areas with no industrial sources of metal pollution. In Bangladesh, As ≥0.10 ppm in drinking water was associated with adverse pregnancy outcomes in terms of spontaneous abortion and stillbirth. A study of 202 women from West Bengal, India, revealed that exposure to As concentrations of ≥0.2 ppm in drinking water (approximately 0.02 mg As/kg/day) during pregnancy were associated with a six-fold increased risk of stillbirth.

Although the exact mechanism involved in placental toxicity of As has not been explored, increased lipid peroxidation in the human placenta has been linked to As exposure. Increased lipid peroxidation appears to be due to excess production of superoxide and hydroxyl radicals. Arsenic is known to interact with protein sulfhydryl groups, and thereby inactivate target enzymes. Free sulfhydryls are essential for the function of a wide range of enzymes, including glutamic-oxaloacetic acid transaminase, pyruvate oxidase, monoamine oxidase, choline oxidase, glucose oxidase, urease, oxidoreductases and kinases. Arsenic accumulates in the mitochondria and thereby affects a number of enzymes, including those involved in mitochondrial respiration. As inhibits succinic dehydrogenase activity and uncouples oxidative phosphorylation, which results in ATP declines. Reduced ATP affects virtually all cellular functions (Na^+/K^+ balance, protein synthesis, etc.). In an *in vitro* study, arsenite proved to be teratogenic at concentrations between 3 and 4 μM and embryolethal at higher concentrations, whereas arsenate had similar activity, but at concentrations 10 times higher than arsenite (Chaineau *et al.*, 1990). Induction of stress proteins or heat shock proteins (hsp) synthesis in the embryo has been explained as a common mechanism of teratogenesis by As. In conclusion, inorganic arsenic is much more toxic than organic arsenic. Trivalent As is developmentally more toxic than pentavalent As. For the reproductive and developmental toxicity of As, readers are referred to ATSDR (2007b), as well as Chapter 33 in this book.

Cadmium

The major sources of cadmium (Cd) exposure in humans include contaminated food, cigarette smoke and industrial pollution. Although the biological function of Cd is unknown, its potential for causing placental and developmental toxicity in humans and animals is well established. A correlation between maternal Cd exposure and low fetal birth weight has been established in epidemiological studies conducted in Russia and France.

Cd crosses the placenta in both humans and animals (with similar kinetic characteristics) at minimal levels because much of it accumulates in the placenta, which serves as a remarkable barrier. This is partly due to the ability of Cd to induce synthesis of metallothionein (MT), a small protein rich in sulfur-containing amino acids, and synthesis in maternal tissues, as well as in the placenta. MTs retain Cd in maternal tissues and the placenta and, thereby, reduce Cd transport to the conceptus (Kippler *et al.*, 2010). To date, the best understood mechanism for developmental toxicity is the interaction between Cd and Zn, in which Cd substitutes for Zn in metalloenzymes. Because of the high affinity of MT for Zn, MT sequesters Zn in the placenta, thereby impeding its transfer to the conceptus. Cd inhibits Zn uptake by human placental microvesicles, suggesting that Cd may also compete directly with Zn for membrane transport (Rogers, 1996).

From both human and animal studies, it is clear that the placenta itself is a target organ for Cd toxicity. In low to moderate doses, Cd is sufficiently sequestered in the placenta. But in higher doses, Cd accumulates in the placenta and perturbs the placental transport of essential elements, such as Ca and Zn (Eisenmann and Miller, 1996). Cd also causes placental necrosis and fetal toxicity. Maternal exposure to Cd caused ultrastructural changes in the placenta, initially in the trophoblast cell layer II, and then in the remaining trophoblasts (diSaint' Agnese *et al.*, 1983). Changes included lysosomal vesiculation, nuclear chromatin clumping, nucleolar alterations and apparent mitochondrial calcification. In a recent study, Yang *et al.* (2006) identified a novel molecular mechanism (reduced human placental 11β-HSD2 expression and activity by suppressing HSD11B2 gene transcription) in the placenta by which Cd exerts endocrine disruption, impaired placental function and fetal growth restriction (FGR). In similar experiments, Kawai *et al.* (2002) reported that Cd interferes with placental progesterone production by inhibiting the activity of $P450_{sec}$ enzyme, without affecting cAMP in human trophoblasts.

Subcutaneous administration of Cd chloride acetate or lactate to pregnant rats at a dosage of 0.04 mmol/kg between the 17th and 21st GD resulted in rapid, progressive placental destruction, especially in the pars fetalis (Parizek, 1964). Necrotic changes could often be seen within 6 h. The complete destruction of the pars fetalis resulted in resorptions or delivery of dead conceptuses. Similar effects have been observed with other Cd salts (Rogers, 1996).

In laboratory animals, Cd has been shown to be a developmental toxicant via the oral, inhalation and parenteral routes. Maternal exposure to Cd during pregnancy can cause maternal toxicity, placental damage, impaired implantation, increased resorptions, reduced litter size, fetal growth retardation and congenital malformations in the fetus as well as embryonic/fetal death. The developmental toxicity of Cd during mid to late gestation involves both placental toxicity (reduced blood flow and necrosis) and inhibition of nutrient transport across the placenta. Exposure during late gestation results in fetal death in rats, despite low levels of Cd entering the fetus. The increased toxicity of Cd to the pregnant rat may be due to renal failure subsequent to shock from placental hemorrhage.

In conclusion, reduced uteroplacental blood flow, reduced nutrient transport and placental toxicity by Cd appear to be the major contributing factors for low fetal birth weight, fetal toxicity, malformations and death. Mechanistic studies provide strong evidence that embryotoxicity by Cd (Fein *et al.*, 1997) could be due to inhibition of embryonic DNA and protein synthesis (Holt and Webb, 1987). For details on the reproductive and developmental effects of Cd, readers are referred to Chapter 33 in this book.

Lead

Lead (Pb) occurs naturally in the environment. The common sources of Pb exposure include lead-based paint, batteries, gasoline, ceramics, soil/dust, caulking, roofing, ammunition, and scientific and medical equipment. As a result, the whole environment (including food, water and air) is contaminated with low levels of Pb. Populations at greatest risk to the adverse health effects of Pb have been identified as pregnant women and their unborn children, and preschool-age children.

Lead exposure in the pregnant woman usually occurs through the oral and/or inhalation route. After absorption, Pb is distributed to most of the tissues, but it deposits mainly in the skeleton, kidney and brain (primarily gray matter). Pb is known to cross the placenta in humans and animals, the maternal:cord blood ratio for lead ranges from 0.9 to 0.93 (ATSDR, 2007c). Accumulation of Pb occurs in the fetal brain owing to a partial or complete lack of a blood–brain barrier. The placenta from a Pb-exposed mother can have a greater than three-fold Pb level compared with the placenta from an unexposed mother. In general, cord blood and placenta of exposed women have high Pb levels, which consequently also reflect in the fetus. In fact, prenatal exposure to Pb is generally estimated through maternal and/or cord blood Pb concentrations. Studies suggest that a large maternal–fetal concentration gradient exists and the placenta poses a limited transplacental barrier. Also, a number of adverse maternal health conditions can affect the transfer of Pb to the fetus and/or the retention of Pb by the mother or the fetus. Pb also accumulates in the placenta in times of fetal stress.

At present, the exact mechanism involved in the placental toxicity of Pb remains unknown, although Pb produces intoxication in general by interfering with protein/hemoprotein biosynthesis and by inhibiting membrane and mitochondrial enzymes (Eisenmann and Miller, 1996). Pb is also known to cause deficits in cholinergic, dopaminergic and glutamatergic functions (ATSDR, 2007c).

Following *in utero* exposure, Pb can have a direct effect on the developing conceptus. It has been shown that Pb can interfere with an early stage of development, such as the invasion of the fertilized ovum into the uterine wall. In general, common malformations observed in experimental animals are related to brain defects, neural tube defects and urogenital system and tail defects. Following low levels of Pb exposure in pregnant women, Pb has been associated with increased incidence of preterm births and reduced birth weight (Andrews *et al.*, 1994). Exposure to high levels of Pb can cause infertility, neonatal morbidity, miscarriages, spontaneous abortions and stillbirths. It should be noted that Pb has a greater potential for neurotoxicity than for placental, reproductive or developmental toxicity. Further details on the reproductive and developmental effects of lead can be found in previous publications (Eisenmann and Miller, 1996; Rogers, 1996; Gupta, 1998, 2007; ATSDR, 2007c), and Chapter 33 in this book.

Mercury

Mercury (Hg) is a non-essential metal that occurs naturally in the environment and exists in several forms. The general population is exposed to Hg primarily from food and dental amalgam. In most foodstuffs, Hg is found in the organic form. Fish, marine mammals and some microorganisms convert elemental Hg to organic Hg, which accumulates in the food chain. It is of great interest to note that in humans, organic Hg can be converted to inorganic Hg.

It is now well recognized that Hg (in all forms) is toxic to humans as well as animals. There are numerous incidents in which Hg has been associated with developmental toxicity in humans. The first mass outbreak of methylmercury (MeHg) poisoning occurred in Japan in the 1950s and 1960s following the consumption of heavily contaminated fish. The syndrome was referred to as "Fetal Minamata Disease". An even larger outbreak of MeHg poisoning took place in Iraq in 1971–1972. Poisoning resulted from consumption of bread loaves prepared from wheat seed grain treated with a MeHg-containing fungicide. These incidents, along with others, indicated that prenatal exposure to MeHg caused severe brain damage in the fetus and infants, whereas the mothers were hardly affected. There is mounting evidence which suggests that fetal brain is the target organ for Hg toxicity in humans and animals. In general, pregnant women appear to be more sensitive to MeHg toxicity than non-pregnant women.

MeHg is readily absorbed and distributed throughout the body with various concentrations in different tissues. Hg accumulates in the fetal brain because of the lack of a BBB and the high requirement for protein synthesis. In humans, brain MeHg levels can be as high as six-fold, compared with blood levels. This is in contrast to rats, which have a brain to blood ratio of 0.06, and mice with a ratio of 1.20. There is evidence that human and rodent placenta by having metallothioneins present some barrier to Hg (Yoshida *et al.*, 2002). By using the Gray PBPK model for MeHg, the placenta is modeled as four compartments with separate transfer constants for placental barrier and placental tissue transport. Organic and metallic Hg crosses the placenta more readily than inorganic Hg. Consequently, MeHg and metallic Hg accumulate in the fetus, whereas inorganic Hg concentrates in the placenta. Metallic Hg, after crossing the placenta, can be oxidized to Hg^{2+} in fetal tissues. It has been shown that Hg^{2+} accumulates in the placenta and inhibits the fetal uptake of certain essential metabolites or analogs of these metabolites.

There are no reports describing the effects of Hg on placental structure or function. However, both human and animal studies suggest that MeHg at a moderate to high level of exposure has a strong potential for developmental neurotoxicity. Both the Japan and Iraq incidents provided evidence that Hg-exposed pregnant women delivered infants with severe developmental and behavioral deficits, without any obvious symptoms of Hg poisoning in the mothers during pregnancy. Common developmental defects due to Hg exposure are reduced birth weight, ataxia, retarded walking and limb deformities. At present, human studies with MeHg indicate that maternal hair levels of 10–20 ppm may result in adverse effects on fetal outcome.

Several studies using animal models with a high dose of MeHg exposure have described developmental effects similar to those observed in humans. MeHg has been reported to be embryotoxic, fetotoxic and teratogenic in mice, rats, cats, guinea-pigs and hamsters. In general, resorptions, dead fetuses and cleft palate are the most common findings. Taken together, both human and animal data suggest that prenatal exposure to sufficient amounts of Hg results in endocrine disruption and developmental toxicity (Tan *et al.*, 2009). In addition, Hg has a strong potential for neurotoxicity and neurobehavioral toxicity. For further details, readers are referred to other publications (Eisenmann and Miller, 1996; Gupta, 1998, 2007, 2009; ATSDR, 1999; Castoldi *et al.*, 2008), and Chapter 35 in this book.

Nickel

Nickel (Ni) and its salts are used in alloy steel, stainless steel, cast iron, alkaline batteries, ceramics, electroplating, pigments and catalysts. The general population is exposed to Ni via food, water, air and tobacco smoke, at very low levels. Data suggest that Ni bioconcentrates in fish and aquatic organisms and, therefore, seafood can be a potential source of

Ni exposure. Workers in the industries that produce, process or use Ni are usually exposed to higher levels, and as a result this population group is at greater risk.

Although Ni is an essential element for human and animal health, at higher levels Ni produces deleterious effects, ranging from minor allergic reactions to those as serious as abortions, birth defects and cancer. Epidemiological studies reported inconclusive findings on the developmental toxicity of Ni in humans (Chaschschin *et al.*, 1994). Chen and Lin (1998) reported that Ni crosses the human placenta and produces embryotoxicity and teratogenicity. Ni-induced toxicity was evidenced by significantly increased permeability, lipid peroxidation and Ni concentration, and decreased viability. Exposure of pregnant rats to Ni oxide at a dosage of 1.6 mg/m^{-3} for 23.6 h/day throughout gestation resulted in a decrease in fetal body weight, although the weight of the placenta and the number of fetuses remained unchanged (Weischer *et al.*, 1980). Treatment of pregnant rats during early gestation with Ni chloride (8–16 mg/kg, i.m.) and Ni sulfide (30 mg/kg, i.m.) caused embryolethality at doses that did not cause maternal deaths, suggesting an accumulation of Ni in fetal tissues and a greater sensitivity of the fetal tissue to Ni toxicity (Sunderman *et al.*, 1978). In another study, pregnant rats treated with 4 mg Ni/kg i.p. showed teratogenic malformations (Mas *et al.*, 1985). In a multi-generational and multi-litter study conducted in rats, Ni has been shown to adversely affect the time of gestation, birth weight and the number of pups surviving through lactation (ATSDR, 2005).

Nickel has also been studied for placental toxicity in mice and hamsters. Ni chloride given to pregnant mice on GD 7–11 produces embryotoxic effects such as a higher incidence of resorptions, reduced fetal weight, delayed skeletal ossification and malformations (including acephalia, ankylosis, club foot and skeletal anomalies). Embryonic tissues retained Ni as much as 800 times higher than controls (Lu *et al.*, 1979). With similar findings, Ni has also been proved to be embryotoxic and teratogenic in hamsters. Further details can be found in other publications (Domingo, 1994; ATSDR, 2005).

Insecticides

Four classes of insecticides (organophosphates, carbamates, organochlorines and pyrethroids) are known to adversely affect the mother, placenta and conceptus in laboratory animals (Gupta, 1995, 2007, 2009; Pelkonen *et al.*, 2006). Here, organophosphates and carbamates are discussed together because many of their effects are similar.

Organophosphates and carbamates

Organophosphates (OPs) and carbamates (CMs) are collectively referred to as anticholinesterase compounds. General toxicity as well as reproductive and developmental toxicity of these pesticides have been discussed in Chapter 37 of this book. Recently, Pelkonen *et al.* (2006) described the placental toxicity of anticholinesterase pesticides in detail. By having acetylcholinesterase (AChE) and other cholinergic elements, the placenta remains highly vulnerable to OP and CM toxicity (Koshakji *et al.*, 1974; Cambon *et al.*, 1979; Gupta *et al.*, 1984, 1985; Sastry, 1993; Simone *et al.*, 1994; Pelkonen *et al.*, 2006; Gupta, 2007, 2009). Furthermore, the placenta has drug-metabolizing enzymes (e.g., mixed function oxidase, cytochrome P450 and others), which means that it can transform certain OPs of the "thioate" group (e.g., malathion, parathion, chlorpyrifos, diazinon, guthion and many other) to their "oxon" analogs (e.g., malaoxon, paraoxon, chlorpyrifos oxon, diazoxon, guthoxon, respectively). Similar metabolic pathways, although to a lesser extent, also exist in the fetal tissues (Pelkonen, 1984; Gupta, 1995; Harbison *et al.*, 1995; Juchau, 1995; Buratti *et al.*, 2006; Pelkonen *et al.*, 2006). Therefore, the placenta has the capability of so-called "lethal synthesis", since OPs in the "oxon" form are much more toxic than their parental compounds. The placenta also has an oxidative mechanism, and OPs and CMs are known to exert oxidative stress. In essence, the structure and function of the placenta are so unique that its susceptibility to chemical toxicity seems far greater than that of the mother. Thus, any damage to the placenta caused by anticholinesterase pesticides is likely to reflect in the fetus.

Cholinergic effects

Both OPs and CMs readily cross the placenta and target the cholinergic components of the developing nervous system and other vital organs (Gupta *et al.*, 1984, 1985; Pelkonen *et al.*, 2006; Gupta, 2007, 2009). Inhibition of AChE and butyrylcholinesterase (BuChE) activities can be used as a markers of exposure to OP and/or CM, and AChE can also be used as a marker of effects. Following prenatal exposure to OPs (dicrotophos, diazinon, methyl parathion, quinalphos and several others) significant inhibition of AChE has been demonstrated in maternal, placental, and fetal tissues of rats and mice (Bus and Gibson, 1974; Gupta *et al.*, 1985; Srivastava *et al.*, 1992; Abu-Qare and Abou-Donia, 2001). Similar findings have been reported for CM pesticides, including aldicarb, carbaryl, carbofuran and pirimicarb (Declume and Derache, 1977; Cambon *et al.*, 1979, 1980). Onset and degree of AChE inhibition varied depending on the pesticide used. These studies revealed AChE inhibition as the major biochemical mechanism of toxicity. Furthermore, subchronic prenatal exposure to methyl parathion in rats resulted in altered postnatal development of brain AChE and ChAT activities and selected subtle behavioral deficits (Gupta *et al.*, 1985). It is expected that exposure of a pregnant woman to these pesticides can lead to enhanced levels of ACh, and thereby ACh can influence other components of the cholinergic system in the placenta. In a number of studies, neurotoxic esterase (NTE) enzyme, a putative target for OP-induced delayed neuropathy (OPIDN), has been found in the placenta, although its significance in this tissue is yet to be determined.

Protein synthesis

OPs have been shown to inhibit protein synthesis both *in vivo* (Gupta *et al.*, 1984) and *in vitro* (Welsch and Dettbarn, 1971). The inhibitory effect on *in vivo* protein synthesis of methyl parathion (administered throughout the period of organogenesis) was shown to be dose dependent, greater on day 19 than day 15 of gestation and more pronounced in fetal than in placental or maternal tissues of rats (Gupta *et al.*, 1984).

Endocrinal effects

Human placenta has been recognized as a source of chorionic gonadotropins and steroid hormones. Since the development of the placental cholinergic system follows the development of the syncytiotrophoblast, it is interesting to determine the release of steroid hormones by ACh. Although the cytotrophoblasts, the source of gonadotropins in the placenta, are fully developed in the first 3 months of gestation, some cytotrophobastic cells remain in full-term human placenta (Sastry, 1997). Harbison *et al.* (1975) reported that ACh stimulates placental release of chorionic somatomammotrophin. ACh increases the release of immunoreactive corticotrophin-releasing factor from human placental cell cultures in a dose-related manner, and its effect is reversed by the cholinergic receptor antagonists atropine and hemicholinium.

During pregnancy, the placenta is an important organ for the synthesis of steroid hormones, and it contains two important rate-limiting enzymes: CYP11A1, which catalyzes cholesterol side chain cleavage, and CYP19, an aromatase for the production of estrogens. CYP11A1 seems to be a rather stable and selective enzyme not affected to a great extent by environmental chemicals. On the other hand, CYP19 has a relatively non-discriminatory binding site and a large number of inhibitors have been synthesized, some of which are in use in endocrine cancers. Regarding most anticholinesterase pesticides, it is not known whether they are inhibitors or activators of either one of these two enzymes (Pelkonen *et al.*, 2006). CM pesticides, such as methomyl and pirimicarb weakly stimulated the placental aromatase. The other molecular target of the endocrine effects in the placenta may be intracellular calcium homeostasis since estrogenic pesticides change calcium handling by trophoblasts and this effect may be endocrinally controlled (Derfoul *et al.*, 2003).

Histopathological changes

Levario-Carillo *et al.* (2001) histologically (both light and scanning electron microscope) analyzed the placentas of women living in an agricultural area chronically exposed to parathion. Placentas were characterized with microinfarctions, microcalcifications and increased deposition of fibrinoid material, along with a large proportion of atypical characteristics of villi, such as bullous and balloon-like formations with non-homogeneous surface, and other areas devoid of microvilli. These changes adversely affect fetal biology.

In conclusion, both OPs and CMs have the potential for endocrine disruption, placental toxicity, embryotoxicity, embryolethality, fetotoxicity and teratogenesis. These effects seem to vary depending upon the particular OP or CM involved.

Organochlorines

Organochlorine insecticides are classified into three subgroups: (1) dichlorodiphenylethanes (DDT, dicofol, methoxychlor and perthane); (2) chlorinated cyclodienes (aldrin, dieldrin, endrin, chlordane, endosulfan and heptachlor); and (3) hexachlorocyclohexanes (BHC, chlordane, lindane, mirex and toxaphene). In general, organochlorine insecticides are neurotoxicants. DDT and chlorinated benzene types of insecticides exert paresthesia of the tongue, lips and face, apprehension, tremors and clonic-tonic convulsions. Stimulation of the CNS is the most prominent effect. The acute signs produced by cyclodienes include dizziness, nausea, vomiting, myoclonic jerking, motor hyperexcitability, convulsive seizures and generalized convulsions. It is important to mention that the epoxide metabolites are much more toxic than their parent cyclodiene compounds (Bondy *et al.*, 2003; Silva and Gammon, 2009).

In general, the mechanism of action of organochlorine insecticides is not yet fully understood. The DDT-type insecticides alter the transport of sodium and potassium ions across axonal membranes, resulting in an increased negative after-potential and prolonged action potentials. As a result, repetitive firing and a spontaneous train of action potentials occur. Specifically, DDT inhibits the activation of sodium channels and the activation of potassium conductance. The mechanism of cyclodienes involved in hyperexcitation of the CNS and convulsions has been explained based on their structural resemblance to the bicyclic γ-aminobutyric acid (GABA) receptor antagonist picrotoxin. The mammalian GABA receptor is coupled to an intrinsic chloride ion channel and is the primary mediator of neuronal inhibition in the brain. Like picrotoxin, cyclodienes block the inhibitory action of GABA. Heptachlor (and its toxic metabolite heptachlor epoxide) and related organochlorines are also reported to target dopaminergic neurons in the striatum by releasing dopamine, which appears to play a role in the etiology of idiopathic Parkinson's disease (Kirby *et al.*, 2001).

Some of the organochlorine insecticides have the potential to induce placental toxicity. Many organochlorines and their metabolites are known to be found in the placenta and cord blood and cross the placental barrier (Sala *et al.*, 2001). Shen *et al.* (2005) determined the content of many organochlorine pesticides in human placentas. The average number of pesticides found per placenta was 18.5 from a total of 27. Recently, Wojtowicz *et al.* (2007) reported that DDT and its metabolite DDE (1,1-dichloro-2,2-bis(*p*-chlorophenyl)ethylene) caused inhibition of estradiol secretion (due to direct action on aromatase activity) with concomitant stimulation of progesterone secretion in human term placental explants, which can be attributed to adverse pregnancy outcome.

In animal studies, pregnant Swiss mice exposed to lindane at different stages of pregnancy produced various toxicological effects, including fetotoxicity and reproductive failure (Sircar and Lahiri, 1989). Lindane exposure during early pregnancy (days 1–4) caused total absence of any implantation, during mid-pregnancy (days 6–12) caused total resorption of fetuses, and during late pregnancy (days 14–19) caused the death of all pups within 12 h to 5 days after parturition. In addition, lindane can cause reproductive failure by causing a deficiency of steroid hormones (estrogen and progesterone). Very recently, Di Consiglio *et al.* (2009) reported that following *in utero* exposure of CD1 mice to lindane (25 mg/kg/day, p.o.), during GD 9–16, resulted in an impairment of steroid hormone homeostasis due to CYP-mediated testosterone catabolism modulation without affecting aromatase activity in male offspring. It is interesting to note that the mechanism involved in lindane-induced endocrine disruption differs between males and females.

The organochlorines, in general, are considered to be endocrine-disrupting compounds, and some of them (methoxychlor, *o,p′*-isomers of DDT, DDE, DDD, dieldrin, toxaphene and endosulfan) have been associated with estrogen-like effects in the reproductive system of laboratory animals. In humans, however, the findings are inconsistent (Farhang *et al.*, 2005). In female rodents, methoxychlor mimics estradiol-17β in the reproductive tract. Exposure of rats to methoxychlor before and during pregnancy can cause a blockade of implantation, suppression of uterine decidualization, lack of corpora lutea and atresia of ovarian follicles (ATSDR, 2002). Exposure during the preimplantation period of pregnancy blocks implantation, whereas exposure during the postimplantation period causes fetal resorption. Interference in the requisite hormonal milieu seems to be the major effect. Other effects of methoxychlor include estrogenic influence on uterine preimplantation differentiation, ovum transport rate, luteal regression and postimplantation decidual growth. Hall *et al.* (1997) demonstrated that methoxychlor acts as an estrogen agonist in the uterus and oviduct but as an antiestrogen in the ovary of the mouse. Recently, in an *in vitro* study, Harvey *et al.* (2009) demonstrated that the toxic metabolite 2,2-bis(*p*-hydroxyphenyl)-1,1,1-trichloroethane (HPTE) of methoxychlor significantly inhibited FSH- induced steroid pathway gene expression and steroidogenesis. Furthermore, expression patterns of novel genes regulating signal transduction, transport, cell cycle, adhesion, differentiation, motility and growth, apoptosis, development and metabolism were all altered by HPTE. Literature reveals that dieldrin traverses the placenta by passive diffusion, accumulates in the fetus, and there it produces teratogenic effects, including supernumerary ribs with concomitant decrease in ossification centers (Chernoff *et al.*, 1975, 1979; Jorgenson, 2001).

Exposure of pregnant rats to mirex has been shown to result in perinatal deaths due to persistent cardiovascular problems, such as first- to third-degree fetal heart blockade (Grabowski, 1983). Mirex also causes altered lens growth and cataracts, along with other biochemical, physiological and histological changes (Rogers and Grabowski, 1983).

Pyrethroids

The use of synthetic pyrethroids has increased tremendously in recent years because they possess high insecticidal efficacy and low mammalian toxicity. Still, risks to human and animal health exist from accidental exposure and environmental contamination. These insecticides are of two types. Type I pyrethroids are those which lack α-cyano moiety and give rise to the T-syndrome. This syndrome includes whole body tremors, incoordination, prostration, tonic–clonic seizures and death. Common examples of this type are pyrethrin I, allethrin, tetramethrin, resmethrin and permethrin. Type II pyrethroids are those which contain α-cyano moiety and cause the choreoathetosis/salivation (CS) syndrome. This syndrome is characterized by hyperactive behavior, hunchbacked posture, profuse salivation, tremors and motor incoordination, progressing to sinuous writhing movements. Common examples of this type of pyrethroid include cyphenothrin, cypermethrin, deltamethrin and fenvalerate. Based on symptomatology, Type II syndrome primarily involves action in the CNS, whereas with Type I syndrome, peripheral nerves are also involved. Intoxication by pyrethroids results primarily from hyperexcitation of the nervous system. This hyperexcitation is caused by repetitive firing and depolarization in nerve axons and synapses. Pyrethroids act directly through interaction with the sodium channel gating mechanism, thereby interfering with the generation and conduction of nerve impulses and inducing marked repetitive activity in various parts of the brain. Type I pyrethroids affect sodium channels in nerve membranes, causing repetitive neuronal discharge and a prolonged negative after-potential, the effects being similar to those produced by DDT. Type II pyrethroids produce an even longer delay in sodium channel inactivation, leading to a persistent depolarization of the nerve membrane without repetitive discharge, a reduction in the amplitude of the action potential and eventual failure of axonal conduction and a blockade of impulses. For further details on mechanisms in general toxicity and developmental neurotoxicity of pyrethroids, readers are referred to Shafer and Meyer (2004) and Shafer *et al.* (2005).

Compared to other groups of insecticides, the pyrethroids have not been well studied for placental toxicity because pyrethroids are considered relatively less toxic. For example, permethrin at concentrations of 2,000–4,000 ppm showed only a weak to moderate influence on *in utero* fetal development. Female rats dermally exposed to cyhalothrin throughout pregnancy had offspring with delayed fur development, delayed ear and eye opening and delayed descent of the testes, but with no change in the age of vaginal opening. In adulthood, however, the sexual behavior of both male and female rats exposed to cyhalothrin prenatally is no different from that of control animals (Gomes *et al.*, 1991a,b). Ratnasooriya *et al.* (2003) exposed pregnant rats to lambda cyhalothrin (6.3, 8.3 or 12.5 mg/kg/day, p.o.) during GD 1–7 and noted that the anti-reproductive effects were mainly due to increased preimplantation losses. Enhancement of postimplantation loss played a subsidiary role. The multiple mechanisms involved were maternal toxicity, stress, uterotropic activity and utero-fetotoxicity. Prenatal exposure of rats to a newer pyrethroid, deltamethrin, has been shown to increase early embryonic deaths and fetuses with retarded growth, hyperplasia of the lungs, dilation of the renal pelvis and increase placental weight (Abdel-Khalik *et al.*, 1993). For further details on placental toxicity of pyrethroids, readers are referred to Gupta (2009).

Exposure to pyrethroids during the prenatal or early postnatal stage has been shown to produce significant neurochemical alterations in neonatal rats (Husain *et al.*, 1991, 1992; Malaviya *et al.*, 1993). Delayed maturation of the cerebral cortex occurs due to alterations in key enzymes of the neurotransmission process (monoamine oxidase, AChE and Na^+-K^+ ATPase). Prenatal exposure to these pyrethroids also delays differential responses in the levels of brain regional polyamines and ontogeny of sensory and motor reflexes in offspring. Other biochemical and neurochemical effects of pyrethroids occur due to impairment of the neurotransmitter receptors (dopaminergic, catecholaminergic and cholinergic).

Dioxins and polychlorinated biphenyls (PCBs)

Dioxins

Polychlorinated dibenzo-*p*-dioxins belong to a family of chlorinated aromatic compounds commonly referred to as dioxins. Although there are at least 75 different dioxin congeners, the term dioxin most often refers to 2,3,7,8-tetrachlorodibenzo-*p*-dioxin (TCDD), which is one of the most toxic synthetic chemicals ever known. These compounds are slowly metabolized in the body tissues and, as a result, they persist for a long period of time. It needs to be mentioned that no individual dioxin occurs alone in the environment.

Instead, exposure to dioxins usually occurs with a mixture of dioxin congeners along with dibenzofurans, chlorophenols, polychlorinated biphenyls (PCBs) and other halogenated aromatic compounds. Hence the toxic effects observed in humans and animals are due to a mixture of chemicals, in which TCDD may be only one ingredient (Bursian, 2007). The toxicity of individual congeners varies as much as 1,000-fold.

In animal studies, a variety of toxic effects of TCDD have been reported which include weight loss, hepatotoxicity, porphyria, dermal toxicity, gastric lesions and hemorrhage, thymus atrophy, immunotoxicity, teratogenicity, reproductive failure, enzyme induction and vitamin A depletion (WHO, 1989; Dickson and Buzik, 1993). These effects vary greatly, depending on dose, species, strain, age and gender.

Humans are exposed to dioxins/TCDD by accidental, environmental or occupational means. Contaminated food and water are the major sources of human exposure. So far, there have been only a few studies that have described the placental toxicity of dioxins/TCDD in humans. Human epidemiological studies revealed no clear evidence that TCDD exposure caused birth defects (Mastroiacova *et al.*, 1988; Stockbauer *et al.*, 1988). However, high rates for several malformations (in the genitourinary tract, oral cleft, cardiovascular defects and hip dislocation) have been noted in a few studies (Stockbauer *et al.*, 1988). A study conducted by the CDC (Stellman *et al.*, 1988) revealed that wives of veterans who had been exposed to Agent Orange had significantly higher risks of having children with birth defects, including spina bifida, cleft lip, cleft palate and a variety of neoplasms. Among a variety of adverse effects, chloracne is the only proven consequence to TCDD exposure.

TCDD is considered one of the most potent embryotoxic and teratogenic chemicals in rats and mice. In rats, TCDD is fetotoxic (subcutaneous edema, intestinal hemorrhage, kidney anomalies, reduced fetal weight and increased fetal death rates) rather than teratogenic (WHO, 1989). In mice, however, teratogenic effects (such as cleft palate and hydronephrosis) have been reported with a single or repeated dose as low as 1–10 μg/kg (Skene *et al.*, 1989). In rats and mice, the fetotoxic and teratogenic effects are not observed at 0.1 μg/kg/day. TCDD has also been proven a teratogen in other species, including rabbits, chickens and monkeys (WHO, 1989).

The dioxins and related compounds are proved to be potent reproductive and developmental toxicants by virtue of their ability to disrupt the actions of hormones and growth factors (Gasiewicz, 1997; Petroff *et al.*, 2001; Adamsson *et al.*, 2008). Exposure of pregnant animals to dioxins at extremely low levels (doses that do not adversely affect the mother) leads to alterations in the reproductive system of the pups. Ikeda *et al.* (2002) reported that *in utero* TCDD exposure induces demasculinization in male offspring by inhibiting the aromatase activity in the brain during CNS development. In an *in vitro* study, Augustowska *et al.* (2003) observed disparate findings between the action of pure TCDD and dioxin mixture (polychlorinated dibenzodioxins, PCDDs; and polychlorinated dibenzofurans, PCDFs) on activities of aromatase cytochrome P450 and 3β-hydroxysteroid dehydrogenase in placental cells. More than 50% of the total toxic equivalents in the dioxin mixture was due to the presence of pentachlorodibenzo-*p*-dioxin and pentachlorodibenzofuran. Suzuki *et al.* (2005) correlated the distribution of PCDDs, PCDFs and coplanar-PCBs in human maternal blood, cord blood and placenta, milk and adipose tissue with the average toxic equivalency quantities (TEQs), and found that congeners showing high toxic equivalency factor accumulate in the placenta. Many of the developmental effects are detectable during a very early stage, while other effects are not detectable until the offspring reach puberty. Sperm count is decreased in male offspring and their mating behavior is subtly altered (Gray *et al.*, 1997; Adamsson *et al.*, 2008). Ohsako *et al.* (2002) demonstrated that pregnant Sprague-Dawley rats given a single oral dose of 1 μg TCDD/kg body weight on GD 15 resulted in significant decreases in the urogenital complex and ventral prostate weights and urogenital glans penis length of male rat offspring, when sacrificed on postnatal day 70. Testicular and epididymal weights were also lower than the control group. Anogenital distance was significantly reduced. The same authors also reported that a single oral administration of TCDD (12.5–800 ng/kg) to pregnant Holtzman rats on GD 15 caused a decrease in the androgen receptor (AR) mRNA level in the ventral prostate during the prepubertal period. In severely affected pups, fertility is reduced. These effects have been observed in both rats and hamsters. In another study, adult female rhesus monkeys fed a diet containing 0.5 μg/kg/day TCDD for 6 months suffered hair loss, swelling of the eye lids, loss of lashes, irregularities in menstrual cycle, poor conception and abortion (IARC, 1977).

In addition to the effects described above, the developing immune system appears to be particularly susceptible to TCDD (Skene *et al.*, 1989). The immunosuppressive effects can be mediated through *in utero* exposure or by postnatal exposure via the mother's milk. Evidence suggests that both pre- and postnatal exposure to TCDD can substantially reduce the delayed hypersensitivity and lymphoproliferative response for a prolonged period of time.

There is convincing evidence that all known toxic effects of TCDD are mediated via the aryl hydrocarbon (Ah) receptor. The Ah receptor is present in several tissues, including the liver, lung, kidney and placenta of humans and animals. In rats, the receptor has been detected in the liver, lung, brain, thymus, kidney, skeletal muscle and testes. The Ah receptor has also been detected in human B lymphocytes and tonsils (Dickson and Buzik, 1993). TCDD binds to the Ah receptor–ligand complex. This complex is speculated to transform the receptor to a form that can translocate the nucleus, bind with higher affinity to specific DNA sequences and stimulate transcription (Landers and Brunce, 1991).

Polychlorinated biphenyls (PCBs)

Unlike dioxins, which are unwanted by-products of certain industrial processes and combustion, PCBs are commercially synthesized and used in transformers and capacitors. PCBs represent a complex mixture of 209 unique compounds. Owing to their resistance to thermal degradation and their stability, they persist and bioaccumulate in the environment. Some of these chemicals persist in the environment for tens or hundreds of years, and in the body tissues for many years.

Two major PCB poisoning incidents occurred in the 1970s in which adverse effects were clearly observed in children born to women exposed to high levels of PCBs along with dioxin analogs and polychlorinated dibenzofurans. One incident occurred in Taiwan in 1979, in which many of the babies born had pigmentation abnormalities and problems with their teeth and nails. They were small in size and were developmentally delayed, both physically and mentally. Another incident occurred in Seveso, Italy, in 1976, in which a group of humans were exposed to high levels of dioxin after an explosion at a herbicide plant. The children of these exposed women have not yet been examined for subtle developmental deficits, either structurally or functionally. High concentrations of dioxins and PCBs pose serious health problems in pregnant women and their conceptuses in several other parts of the world, such as the Canadian Great Lakes, South Vietnam, the former Soviet Union and India.

In a recent study, Konishi *et al.* (2009) reported that prenatal exposure to PCBs, dioxin and related compounds at low levels appear to accumulate in the placenta, and thereby retard important placental functions, which result in lower birth weight. In a recent *in vitro* study, Wrobel *et al.* (2009) reported that PCB 77 caused a significant increase of both PGF2α secretion and mRNA expression for COX-2 and PGFS after 6h treatment of myometrial cells. The authors concluded that myometrial synthesis of PGF2α and its further secretion is part of the mechanism by which PCB 77 appears to affect the force of myometrial contractions. In addition, these compounds are known to cause endometriosis (Porpora *et al.*, 2009). A small number of PCBs are dioxin-like in their biological activity and can produce all of the toxic effects mentioned above for dioxin/TCDD. Studies suggest that the unborn may represent a population at special risk because these chemicals disrupt the endocrine system (critical for rapid growth and development), exert neurotoxic and cardiotoxic effects and cause altered behavior in the offspring (Tilson *et al.*, 1990; Cocchi *et al.*, 2009; Colciago *et al.*, 2009; Kopf and Walker, 2009; Mlynarczuk *et al.*, 2009).

CONCLUDING REMARKS AND FUTURE DIRECTIONS

The placenta plays multiple roles by serving as the lung, gut, kidney and endocrine/exocrine gland. It contains metabolic and non-metabolic enzymes, receptors, transmitters, transporters, hormones, prostaglandins, insulin-like growth factors and many other molecules of interest to reproductive biologists and toxicologists. By now, it is well established that the placenta is a target organ for the toxicity of a variety of chemicals. Unlike the toxicology of other organs, placental toxicology is much more complex for three reasons: (1) it deals with three components – mother, placenta and fetus; (2) placental structure and functions vary widely among different species; and (3) continuous changes occur in the structure and function of the placenta throughout gestation. The placental barrier for chemicals appears to be just a widely held false notion. Chemical toxicants and drugs with a molecular weight <1,000 cross the placental barrier with little or no restriction. Some chemicals are found to be detrimental to the placental structure and function because they are concentrated in this tissue. As a result, a variety of abnormalities are seen in the developing conceptus. Furthermore, some of the neurochemical and behavioral deficits observed at birth appear to persist during adolescence and adulthood. This chapter describes in brief the important structural and functional aspects of the placenta, which follows the placental toxicity of commonly abused drugs, heavy metals, insecticides and environmental pesticides. Future studies should explore the novel molecular mechanisms involved in chemical-induced placental toxicity, developmental neurotoxicity and teratogenesis. Additionally, an important area of research in the field of placental toxicology seems to be identification and characterization of the predisposing factors that lead to metabolic and neurological diseases.

ACKNOWLEDGMENT

The author sincerely appreciates Mrs. Robin B. Doss and Mrs. Kristie M. Rohde for their assistance in preparation of this chapter.

REFERENCES

Abdel-Khalik MM, Handfy MS, Abdel-Aziz MI. (1993) Studies on the teratogenic effects of deltamethrin in rats. *Dtsch Tierarztl Wochenschr* **100:** 142–3.

Abu-Qare AW, Abou-Donia MB (2001) Inhibition and recovery of maternal and fetal cholinesterase enzyme activity following a single cutaneous dose of methyl parathion and diazinon, alone and in combination, in pregnant rats. *J Appl Toxicol* **21:** 307–16.

Acevedo CG, Márquez JL, Rojas S, Bravo I (2005) Insulin and nitric oxide stimulates glucose transport in human placenta. *Life Sci* **76:** 2643–53.

Adamsson A, Simanainen U, Viluksela M, Paranko J, Toppari J (2008) The effects of 2,3,7,8-tetrachlorodibenzo-*p*-dioxin on fetal male rat steroidogenesis. *Intl J Androl* **32:** 575–85.

Ahmed MS, Cemerikic B (1995) Opioid receptors in placenta and their functional role. In *Placental Toxicology* (Sastry BVR, ed.). CRC Press, Boca Raton, FL, pp. 107–32.

Ahmed MS, Zhou D, Cavinato AG, Maulik D (1989) Opioid binding properties of the purified kappa receptor from human placenta. *Life Sci* **44:** 867–71.

Andersen HR, Nielsen JB, Grandjean P (2000) Toxicologic evidence of developmental neurotoxicity of environmental chemicals. *Toxicology* **144:** 121–7.

Andrews KW, Savitz DA, Hertz-Picciotto I (1994) Prenatal lead exposure in relation to gestational age and birth weight: a review of epidemiologic studies. *Am J Ind Med* **26:** 13–32.

ATSDR (1999) Agency for Toxic Substances and Disease Registry. *Toxicology Profile for Mercury* 29–357.

ATSDR (2002) Agency for Toxic Substances and Disease Registry. *Toxicology Profile for Methoxychlor*, 19–137.

ATSDR (2005) Agency for Toxic Substances and Disease Registry. *Toxicology Profile for Nickel* 77–155.

ATSDR (2007a) Agency for Toxic Substances and Disease Registry. *Toxicology Profile for Aluminum* 111–240.

ATSDR (2007b) Agency for Toxic Substances and Disease Registry. *Toxicology Profile for Arsenic* 41– 289.

ATSDR (2007c) Agency for Toxic Substances and Disease Registry. *Toxicology Profile for Lead* 149–246.

Augustowska K, Gregoraszczuk EL, Milewicz T, Krzysiek J, Grochowalski A, Chrzaszcz R (2003) Effects of dioxin (2,3,7,8-TCDD) and PCDDs/PCDFs congeners mixture on steroidogenesis in human placenta tissue culture. *Endocr Regul* **37:** 11–19.

Avdalovic M, Putney L, Tyler N, Finkbeiner W, Pinkerton K, Hyde D (2009) *In utero* and postnatal exposure to environmental tobacco smoke (ETS) alters alveolar and respiratory bronchiole (RB) growth and development in infant monkeys. *Toxicol Pathol* **37:** 256–63.

Bailey BA, Sokol RJ (2008) Pregnancy and alcohol use: evidence and recommendations for prenatal care. *Clin Obstet Gynecol* **51:** 436–44.

Barnwell SL, Sastry BVR (1983) Depression of amino acid uptake in human placental villus by cocaine, morphine and nicotine. *Trophoblast Res* **1:** 101–20.

Battaglia FC, Regnault RH (2001) Placental transport and metabolism of amino acids. *Placenta* **22:** 145–61.

Boksa P (1998) Brain insult alters ethanol preference in the adult rat. *Eur J Pharmacol* **348:** 143–53.

Bondy G, Armstrong C, Coady L, Doucet J, Robertson P, Feeley M, Barker M (2003) Toxicity of the chlordane metabolite oxychlordane in female rats: clinical and histopathological changes. *Food Chem Toxicol* **41:** 291–301.

Bursian S (2007) Polychlorinated biphenyls, polybrominated biphenyls, polychlorinated dibenzo-p-dioxins and polychlorinated dibenzofurans. In *Veterinary Toxicology: Basic and Clinical Principles* (Gupta RC, ed.). Academic Press/Elsevier, Amsterdam, pp. 640–59.

Buratti FM, Leoni C, Testai E (2006) Fetal and adult CYP3A isoforms in the bioactivation of organophosphorothionate insecticides. *Toxicol Lett* **167:** 245–55.

Burrows GE, Tyrl RJ (2001) *Toxic Plants of North America.* Iowa State University Press, Ames, IA, pp. 1122–5.

Bus JS, Gibson JE (1974) Bidrin: perinatal toxicity and effects on the development of brain acetylcholinesterase and choline acetyltransferase in mice. *Foo d Cosmet Toxicol* **12:** 313–22.

Cambon C, Declume C, Derache R (1979) Effect of the insecticidal carbamate derivatives (carbofuran, pirimicarb, aldicarb) on the activity of acetylcholinesterase in tissues from pregnant rats and fetuses. *Toxicol Appl Pharmacol* **49:** 203–8.

Cambon C, Declume C, Derache R (1980) Fetal and maternal rat brain acetylcholinesterase. Isoenzymes changes following inseticidal carbamate derivitaves poisoning. *Arch Toxicol* **45:** 257–62.

Carter AM (2009) Evolution of factors affecting oxygen transfer. *Placenta* **30:** S19–S25.

Castoldi AF, Johansson C, Onishchenko N, Coccini T, Roda E, Vahter M, Ceccatelli S, Manzo L (2008) Human developmental neurotoxicity of methylmercury: impact of variables and risk factors. *Reg Toxicol Pharmacol* **51:** 201–14.

Chaineau E, Binet S, Pol D (1990) Embryotoxic effects of sodium arsenite and sodium arsenate on mouse embryo in culture. *Teratology* **41:** 105–12.

Chaschschin VP, Artunina GP, Norseth T (1994) Congenital defects, abortion and other health effects in nickel refinery workers. *Sci Total Environ* **148:** 287–91.

Chen C-Y, Lin T-H (1998) Nickel toxicity to human term placenta: *In vitro* study on lipid peroxidation. *J Toxicol Environ Health Part A* **54:** 37–47.

Chernoff N, Kavlock R J, Katherin JR, Dunn JM, Haseman JK (1975) Prenatal effects of dieldrin and photodieldrin in mice and rats. *Toxicol Appl Pharmacol* **31:** 302–8.

Chernoff N, Kavlock RJ, Hanisch RC, Whitehouse DA, Gray JA Gray LE Jr, Sovocool GW (1979) Perinatal toxicity of endrin in rodents. I. Fetotoxic effects of prenatal exposure in hamsters. *Toxicology* **13:** 155–65.

Cocchi D, Tulipano G, Colciago A, Sibilia V, Pagani F, Vigano D, Rubino T, Parolaro D, Bonfanti P, Colombo A, Celotti F (2009) Chronic treatment with polychlorinated biphenyls (PCB) during pregnancy and lactation in the rat. Part 1. Effects on somatic growth, growth hormone–axis activity and bone mass in the offspring. *Toxicol Appl Pharmacol* **237:** 127–36.

Colciago A, Casati L, Mornati O, Vergoni AV, Santagostino A, Celotti F, Negri-Cesi P (2009) Chronic treatment with polychlorinated biphenyls (PCB) during pregnancy and lactation in the rat. Part 2. Effects on reproductive parameters, on sex behavior, on memory retention and on hypothalamic expression of aromatase and 5alpha-reductases in the offspring. *Toxicol Appl Pharmacol* **239:** 46–54.

Coles CD (1993) Saying "goodbye" to the "crack baby". *Neurotoxicol Teratol* **15:** 290–2.

Collins LM, Pahl JA, Meyer JS (1999) Distribution of cocaine and metabolites in the pregnant rat and fetus in a chronic subcutaneous injection model. *Neurotoxicol Teratol* **21:** 639–46.

Committee on Substance Abuse and Committee on Children with Disabilities (1993) Fetal alcohol syndrome and fetal alcohol effects. *Pediatrics* **91(5):** 1004–6.

Cranmer JM, Wilkins JD, Cannon DJ, Smith L (1986) Fetal–placental–maternal uptake of aluminum in mice following gestational exposure: effect of dose and route of administration. *Neurotoxicology* **7:** 601–8.

Croy BA, Wessels J, Linton N, Tayade C (2009) Comparison of immune cell recruitment and function in endometrium during developmental of epitheliochorial (pig) and hemochorial (mouse and human) placentas. *Placenta* **30** (**Suppl. A**): *Trophoblast Res* **23:** S26–S31.

Czekaj P, Palasz A, Lebda-Wyoborny T, Nowaczyk-Dura G, Karczewska W, Florek E, Kaminski M (2002) Morphological changes in lungs, placenta, liver and kidneys of pregnant rats exposed to cigarette smoke. *Int Arch Occup Environm Health* **75 (Suppl.):** S27–S35.

Declume C, Derache R (1977) Passage placentaire d'un carbamate anticholinestérasique à activité insecticide. Le carbaryl. *Chemosphere* **6:** 141–6.

Derfoul A, Lin FJ, Awumey EM, Kolodzeski T, Hall DJ, Tuan RS (2003) Estrogenic endocrine disruptive components interfere with calcium handling and differentiation of human trophoblast cells. *J Cell Biochem* **89:** 755–70.

Dickson LC, Buzik SC (1993) Health risk of "dioxins": a review of environmental and toxicological considerations. *Vet Hum Toxicol* **35:** 68–77.

Di Consiglio E, De Angelis G, Traina ME, Urbani E, Testai E (2009) Effect of lindane on CYP-mediated steroid hormone metabolism in male mice following *in utero* exposure. *J Appl Toxicol* **29:** 648–55.

diSaint' Agnese PA, Jensen K, Levin AA, Miller RK (1983) Placental toxicity of cadmium in the rat: an ultrastructural study. *Placenta* **4:** 149–63.

Domingo JL (1994) Metal-induced developmental toxicity in mammal: a review. *J Toxicol Environ Health* **42:** 123–41.

Dow-Edwards DL (1990) Maternal and fetal plasma cocaine levels peak rapidly following intragastric administration in the rat. *J Subst Abuse* **2:** 427–37.

England LJ, Kendrick JS, Gargiullo PM, Zahniser SC, Hannon WH (2001) Measures of maternal tobacco exposure and infant birth weight at term. *Am J Epidemiol* **153:** 954–60.

Eisenmann CJ, Miller RK (1996) Placental transport, metabolism, and toxicity of metals. In *Toxicology of Metals* (Chang LW, ed.). CRC Lewis Publishers, Boca Raton, FL, pp. 1003–26.

Fantel AG, Barber CV, Mackler B (1990) Ischemia/reperfusion: a new hypothesis for the developmental toxicity of cocaine. *Teratology* **26:** 285–92.

Fantel AG, Person RE, Burroughs-Gleim CJ, Mackler B (1992) Direct embryotoxicity of cocaine in rats: effects on mitochondrial activity, cardiac function, and growth and development *in vitro. Teratology* **42:** 35–43.

Farhang L, Weintraub JM, Petreas M, Eskenazi B, Bhatia R (2005) Association of DDT and DDE with birth weight and length of gestation in the child health and development studies, 1959–1967. *Am J Epidemiol* **162:** 1–9.

Fein A, Torchinsky A, Pinchasov M, Katz N, Toder V, Herkovits J (1997) Cadmium embryotoxicity: evidence of a direct effect of cadmium on early rat embryos. *Bull Environ Contam Toxicol* **59:** 520–4.

Fowler PA, Bhattacharya S, Gromoll J, Monteiro A, O'Shaughnessy PJ (2009) Maternal smoking and developmental changes in luteinizing hormone (LH) and the LH receptor in the fetal testis. *J Clin Endocrinol Metab* **94:** 4688–95.

Frankfurt M, Wang H-Y, Marmolejo N, Bakshi K (2009) Prenatal cocaine increases dendritic spine density in cortical and subcortical brain regions of the rat. *Dev Neurosci* **31:** 71–5.

Gasiewicz TA (1997) Dioxins and the Ah receptor: probes to uncover processes in neuroendocrine development. *Neurotoxicology* **18:** 393–414.

Giaginis C, Zira A, Theocharis S, Tsantili-Kakoulidou A (2009) Application of quantitative structure–activity relationships for modeling drug and chemical transport across the human placental barrier: a multivariate data analysis approach. *J Appl Toxicol* **29:** 724–33.

Giroux M, Teixera MG, Dumas JC, Desprats R, Grandjean H, Houin G (1997) Influence of maternal blood flow on the placental transfer of three opioids-fantanyl, alfentanil, and sufentanil. *Biol Neonates* **72:** 133–41.

Gold AB, Keller AB, Perry DC (2009) Prenatal exposure of rats to nicotine causes persistent alterations of nicotinic cholinergic receptors. *Brain Res* **1250:** 88–100.

Gomes MDS, Bernardi MM, Spinosa HDS (1991a) Pyrethroid insecticides and pregnancy: effects on physical and behavioral development of rats. *Vet Hum Toxicol* **33:** 315–17.

Gomes MDS, Bernardi MM, Spinosa HDS (1991b) Effect of prenatal pyrethroid insecticide exposure on the sexual development of rats. *Vet Hum Toxicol* **33:** 427–8.

Grabowski CT (1983) Persistent cardiovascular problems in newborn rats prenatally exposed to sub-teratogenic doses of the pesticide, mirex. *Dev Toxicol Environ Sci* **11:** 537–40.

Gray LE Jr, Ostby JS, Kelce WT (1997) A dose response analysis of the reproductive effects of a single gestational dose of 2, 3, 7, 8-tetrachlorodibenzo-*p*-dioxin in male Long Evans hooded rat offspring. *Toxicol Appl Pharmacol* **146:** 11–20.

Gupta RC (1995) Environmental agents and placental toxicity: anticholinesterase and other insecticides. In *Placental Toxicology* (Sastry BVR, ed.). CRC Press, Boca Raton, FL, pp. 257–78.

Gupta RC (1998) Developmental and neurotoxic effects of heavy metals: unusual interactions and biomarkers. In *Heavy Metal: Pollution, Toxication and Chelation* (Sood PP, ed.). Venus Press, New Delhi, pp. 21–66.

Gupta RC (2007) Placental toxicity. In *Veterinary Toxicology: Basic and Clinical Principles* (Gupta RC, ed.). Academic Press/Elsevier, Amsterdam, pp. 245–62.

Gupta RC (2009) Toxicology of the placenta. In *General and Applied Toxicology* (Ballantyne B, Marrs TC, Syversen T, eds.). John Wiley & Sons, Ltd., Chichester, UK, pp. 2003–39.

Gupta RC, Milatovic S, Dettbarn W-D, Aschner M, Milatovic D (2007) Neuronal oxidative injury and dendritic damage induced by carbofuran: protection by memantine. *Toxicol Appl Pharmacol* **219:** 97–105.

Gupta RC, Rech RH, Lovell KD, Welsch F (1985) Brain cholinergic, behavioral, and morphological development in rats exposed *in utero* to methyl parathion. *Toxicol Appl Pharmacol* **77:** 405–13.

Gupta RC, Thornburg JE., Stedman DB, Welsch, F (1984) Effect of subchronic administration of methyl parathion on *in vivo* protein synthesis in pregnant rats and their conceptuses. *Toxicol Appl Pharmacol* **72:** 457–68.

Haggerty P, Allstaff S, Hoad G, Ashton J, Abramovic DR (2002) Placental nutrient transfer capacity and fetal growth. *Placenta* **23:** 86–92.

Hakkola J, Pelkonen O, Pasanen M, Raunio H (1998) Xenobiotic-metabolizing cytochrome P450 enzymes in the human feto-placental unit: role in intrauterine toxicity. *Crit Rev Toxicol* **28(1):** 35–72.

Hall DL, Payne LA, Putnam JM, Huet-Hudson YM (1997) Effect of methoxychlor on implantation and embryo development in the mouse. *Reprod Toxicol* **11:** 703–8.

Harbison RD, Olubadewo J, Dwivedi C, Sastry BVR (1975) Proposed role of a placental cholinergic system in regulation of fetal growth and development. In *Basic and Therapeutic Aspects of Perinatal Pharmacology* (Morselli PL, Garattini S, Serini F, eds.). Raven, New York, pp. 107–17.

Harbison RD, Borgert DJ, Teaf DM (1995) Placental metabolism of xenobiotics. In *Placental Toxicology* (Sastry BVR, ed.). CRC Press, Boca Raton, FL, pp. 213–38.

Harvey CN, Esmail M, Wang Q, Brooks AI, Zachow R, Uzumcu M (2009) Effect of the methoxychlor metabolite HPTE on the rat ovarian granulosa cell transcriptome *in vitro*. *Toxicol Sci* **110:** 95–106.

Hasselmeyer EG, Meyer MB, Catz C, Longo LD (1979) Pregnancy and infant health. In *Smoking and Health: A Report of the Surgeon General* (Pinney JM, ed.). Department of Health, Education and Welfare, Publication No. PHS 79–5006, Washington DC, pp. 81–93.

Held JR, Riggs ML, Dorman C (1999) The effect of prenatal cocaine exposure on neurobehavioral outcome: a meta-analysis. *Neurotoxicol Teratol* **21:** 619–25.

Henderson GI, Schenker S (1995) Alcohol, placental function and fetal growth. In *Placental Toxicology* (Sastry BVR, ed.). CRC Press, Boca Raton, FL, pp. 27–44.

Hewitt DP, Mark PJ, Wadell BJ (2006) Placental expression of peroxisome proliferator-activated receptors in rat pregnancy and the effect of increased glucocorticoid exposure. *Biol Reprod* **74:** 23–8.

Holloway AC, Kellenberger LD, Petrik JJ (2006) Fetal and neonatal exposure to nicotine disrupts ovarian function and fertility in adult female rats. *Endocrine* **30:** 213–16.

Holt D, Webb M (1987) Teratogenicity of ionic cadmium in the Wistar rat. *Arch Toxicol* **59:** 443–7.

Hood RD, Vedel-Macrander GC, Zaworotko MJ, Tatum FM, Meeks RG (1987) Distribution, metabolism and fetal uptake of pentavalent arsenic in pregnant mice following oral or intraperitoneal administration. *Teratology* **35:**19–25.

Hood RD, Vedel-Macrander GC, Zaworotko MJ, Tatum FM, Meeks RG (1988) Uptake, distribution, and metabolism of trivalent arsenic in the pregnant mouse. *J Toxicol Environ Health* **25:** 423–34.

Huppertz B, Burton G, Cross JC, Kingdom JCP (2006) Placental morphology: from molecule to mother – a dedication to Peter Kaufman –a review. *Placenta* **27 (Suppl. A):** S3–S8.

Husain R, Gupta A, Khanna BK (1991) Neurotoxicological effects of a pyrethroid formulation fenvalerate in rat. *Res Commun Chem Pathol Pharmacol* **73:** 111–14.

Husain R, Malaviya M, Seth PK, Husain R (1992) Differential responses of regional brain polyamines following *in utero* exposure to synthetic pyrethroid insecticides: a preliminary report. *Bull Environ Contam Toxicol* **49:** 402–9.

IARC (1977) *Monographs on the Evaluation of the Carcinogenic Risk of Chemicals to Man. Bol. 15. Some Fumigants, the Herbicides 2,4-D and 2,4,5-T, Chlorinated Dibenzodioxins and Miscellaneous Chemicals.* International Agency for Research on Cancer, Lyons, pp. 41–102.

Ikeda M, Inukai N, Mitsui T, Sone H, Yonemoto J, Tohyama C, Tomita T (2002) Changes in fetal brain aromatase activity following *in utero* 2,3,7,8-tetrachlorodibenzo-p-dioxin exposure in rats. *Environm Toxicol Pharmacol* **11:** 1–7.

Illsley NP (2000) Glucose transporters in the human placenta. *Placenta* **21:** 14–22.

Isayama RN, Leite PEC, Lima JPM, Uziel D, Yamasaki EN (2009) Impact of ethanol on the developing GABAergic system. *Anat Record* **292:** 1922–39.

Jones KL, Smith DW, Ulleland CW, Streissguth AP (1973) Pattern of malformation in offspring of chronic alcoholic mothers. *Lancet* **1(815):** 1267–71.

Jorgenson JL (2001) Aldrin and dieldrin: a review of research on their production, environmental deposition and fate, bioaccumulation, toxicology, and epidemiology in the United States. *Environ Health Perspect* **109:** 113–39.

Juchau MR (1995) Placental enzymes: cytochrome P450s and their significance. In *Placental Toxicology* ((Sastry BVR, ed.). CRC Press, Boca Raton, FL, pp. 197–212.

Juchau MR, Chen H (1998) Developmental enzymology. In *Handbook of Developmental Neurotoxicology* (Slikker W, Chang LS, eds.). Academic Press, San Diego, CA, pp. 321–37.

Kanevsky VY, Pozdnyakova LP, Katukov VY, Severin SE (1997) Isolation of the transferrin receptor from human placenta. *Biochem Mol Biol Intl* **42:** 309–14.

Kawai M, Swan KF, Green AE, Edwards DE, Anderson MB, Henson MC (2002) Placental endocrine disruption induced by cadmium: effects of P450 cholesterol side-chain cleavage and 3β-hydroxysteroid dehydrogenase enzymes in cultured human trophoblasts. *Biol Reprod* **67(1):** 178–83.

Keeler RF, Balls LD, Panter KE (1981) Teratogenic effects of *Nicotiana glauca* and concentration of anabasine, the suspect teratogen in plant parts. *Cornell Vet* **71:** 47–53.

Kippler M, Hoque AM, Raqib R, Ohrvik H, Ekström EC, Vahter M (2010) Accumulation of cadmium in human placenta interacts with the transport of micronutrients to the fetus. *Toxicol Lett* **192(2):** 162–8.

Kirby ML, Barlow RL, Bloomquist JR (2001) Neurotoxicity of the organochlorine insecticide heptachlor to murine striatal dopaminergic pathways. *Toxicol Sci* **61:** 100–6.

Konishi K, Sasaki S, Kato S, Ban S, Washino N, Kajiwara J, *et al.* (2009) Prenatal exposure to PCDDs/PCDFs and dioxin-like PCBs in relation to birth weight. *Environ Res* **109:** 906–13.

Kopf PG, Walker MK (2009) Overview of developmental heart defects by dioxins, PCBs, and pesticides. *J Environ Sci Health Part C* **27:** 276–85.

Koshakji RP, Sastry, BVR, Harbison RD (1974) Studies on the levels and nature of cholinesterase in humans and mouse placenta. *Res Commu Chem Pathol Pharmacol* **9:** 181–4.

Krewski D, Yokel RA, Nieboer E, Borchelt D, Cohen J, Harry J, Kacew S, Lindsay J, Mahfouz AM, Rondeau V (2007) Human health risk assessment for aluminium oxide, and aluminum hydroxide. *J Toxicol Environ Health Part B* **10:** 1–269.

Landers JP, Bunce NJ (1991) Review article. The Ah receptor and the mechanism of dioxin toxicity. *Biochem J* **276:** 273–87.

Larroque B (1992) Alcohol and the fetus. *Intl J Epidemiol* **21 (Suppl. 1):** S8–S16.

Larsen WJ (1993) Fetal development and the fetus as patient. In *Human Embryology*. Churchill Livingstone, New York, pp. 435–52.

Levario-Carrillo M, Feria-Velasco A, De Celis R, Ramos-Martinez E, Cordova-Fierro L, Solis FJ (2001) Parathion, a cholinesterase-inhibiting plaguicide induces changes in tertiary villi of placenta of women exposed: a scanning electron miscroscopy study. *Gynecol Obstet Invest* **52(4):** 269–75.

Li Z, Coles CD, Lynch ME, Hamann S, Peltier S, LaConte S, Hu X (2009) Prenatal cocaine exposure alters emotional arousal regulation and its effects on working memory. *Neurotoxicol Teratol* **31:** 342–8.

Lin GWJ (1981) Effect of ethanol feeding during pregnancy on fetal transfer of alpha-amino isobutyric acid in the rat. *Life Sci* **28:** 595–601.

Lips KS, Brüggmann D, Pfeil U, Vollerthun R, Grando SA, Kummer W (2005) Nicotinic acetylcholine receptors in rat and human placenta. *Placenta* **26:** 735–46.

Lu CC, Matsumoto N, Lijima S (1979) Teratogenic effects of nickel chloride on embryonic mice and its transfer to embryonic mice. *Teratology* **19:** 137–42.

Malaviya M, Husain R, Seth PK, Husain R (1993) Perinatal effects of two pyrethroid insecticides on brain neurotransmitter function in the neonate rat. *Vet Hum Toxicol* **35:** 119–22.

Mas A, Holt D, Webb M (1985) The acute toxicity and teratogenicity of nickel in pregnant rats. *Toxicology* **35:** 47–57.

Mastroiacova P, Spagnolo O, Marni E, Meezza L, Bertollini R, Segnei G, Borgna-Pignatti C (1988) Birth defects in the Seveso area after TCDD contamination. *J Am Med Assoc* **259:** 1668–72.

Mess A, Carter AM (2007) Evolution of the placenta during the early radiation of placental mammals. *Comp Biochem Physiol (Part A)* **148:** 769–79.

Mihaly GW, Morgan DJ (1984) Placental drug transfer: effects of gestational age and species. *Pharmacol Ther* **23:** 253–66.

Miller MS, Juchau MR, Guengerich FP, Nebert DW, Raucy JL (1996) Drug metabolizing enzymes in developmental toxicology. *Fund Appl Toxicol* **34:** 165–75.

Mlynarczuk J, Wrobel MH, Kotwica J (2009) The influence of polychlorinated biphenyls (PCBs), dichlorodiphenyltrichloroethane (DDT) and its metabolite-dichlorodiphenyldichloroethylene (DDE) on mRNA expression for NP-I/OT and PGA, involved in oxytocin synthesis in bovine granulosa and luteal cells. *Reprod Toxicol* **28:** 354–8.

Mukhopadhyay P, Horn KH, Greene RM, Pisano MM (2010) Prenatal exposure to environmental tobacco smoke alters gene expression in the developing murine hippocampus. *Reprod Toxicol* **29:** 164–75.

Myllynen P, Passanen M, Pelkonen O (2005) Human placenta: a human organ for developmental toxicology research and biomonitoring. *Placenta* **26:** 361–71.

Neuspiel DR (1993) Cocaine and the fetus: mythology of severe risk. *Neurotoxicol Teratol* **15:** 305–6.

Nulman I, Gladstone J, O'Hayon B, Koren G (1998) The effects of alcohol on the fetal brain. In *Handbook of Developmental Neurotoxicology* (Slikker Jr W, Chang LW, eds.). Academic Press, San Diego, CA, pp. 567–86.

Ohsako S, Miyabara Y, Sakaue M, Ishimura R, Kakeyama M, Izumi H, Yonemoto J, Tohyama C (2002) Developmental stage-specific effects of perinatal 2,3,7,8-tetrachlorodibenzo-p-dioxin exposure on reproductive organs of male rat offspring. *Toxicol Sci* **66:** 283–92.

Pacifici GM, Nottoli R (1995) Placental transfer of drugs administered to the mother. *Clin Pharmacokinet* **28:** 235–69.

Panter KE, James LE, Gardner DR (1999) Lupines, poison-hemlock, and *Nicotiana* spp: toxicity and teratogenicity in livestock. *J Nat Toxins* **8:** 117–33.

Parizek J (1964) Vascular changes at sites of estrogen biosynthesis produced by parenteral injection of cadmium salts: the destruction of placenta by cadmium salts. *J Reprod Fertil* **7:** 263–5.

Pasanen M, Pelkonen O (1994) The expression and environmental regulation of P450 in human placenta. *Crit Rev Toxicol* **24(3):** 211–29.

Pastrakuljic A, Derewlany LO, Koren G (1999) Maternal cocaine use and cigarette smoking in pregnancy in relation to amino acid transport and fetal growth. *Placenta* **20:** 499–512.

Patel TG, Laungani RG, Grose EA, Dow-Edwards DL (1999) Cocaine decreases uteroplacental blood flow in the rat. *Neurotoxicol Teratol* **21:** 559–65.

Pelkonen O (1984) Xenobiotic metabolism in the maternal–placental–fetal unit: implications for fetal toxicity. *Dev Pharmacol Ther* **7 (Suppl. 1):** 11–17.

Pelkonen O, Vahakangas K, Gupta RC (2006) Placental toxicity of organophosphate and carbamate pesticides. In *Toxicology of Organophosphate and Carbamate Compounds* (Gupta RC, ed.). Academic Press/Elsevier, Amsterdam, pp. 463–79.

Pentšuk N, van der Laan JW (2009) An interspecies comparison of placental antibody transfer: new insights into developmental toxicity testing of monoclonal antibodies. *Birth Defects Res (Part B)* **86:** 328–44.

Petroff BK, Roby KF, Gao X, Son D-S, Williams S, Johnson D, Rozman KK, Terranova PF (2001) A review of mechanisms controlling ovulation with implications for the anovulatory effects of polychlorinated dibenzo-*p*-dioxins in rodents. *Toxicology* **158:** 91–107.

Pijnenborg R, Vercruysse L (2006) Mathias Duval on placental development in mice and rats. *Placenta* **27:** 109–18.

Plessinger MA, Woods JR (1993) Maternal, placental and fetal pathophysiology of cocaine exposure during pregnancy. *Clin Obstet Gynecol* **36:** 267–78.

Porpora MG, Medda E, Abballe A, Bolli S, De Angelis I, di Domenico A, Ferro A, Ingelido AM, Maggi A, Panici PE, Felip E (2009) Endometriosis and organochlorinated environmental pollutants: a case–control study on Italian women of reproductive age. *Environ Health Perspect* **117:** 1070–5.

Ratnasooriya WD, Ratnayake SSK, Jayatunga YNA (2003) Effects of Icon®, a pyrethroid insecticide on early pregnancy of rats. *Human Exp Toxicol* **22:** 523–33.

Richardson GA, Goldschmidt L, Willford J (2008) The effects of prenatal cocaine use on infant development. *Neurotoxicol Teratol* **30:** 96–106.

Richardson GA, Goldschmidt L, Willford J (2009) Continued effects of prenatal cocaine use: preschool development. *Neurotoxicol Teratol* **31:** 325–33.

Riquelme G (2009) Placental chloride channels: a review. *Placenta* **30:** 659–69.

Roberts CT, Owens JA, Sferruzzi-Perri AN (2008) Distinct actions of insulin-like growth factors (IGFs) on placental development and fetal growth: lessons from mice and guinea pigs. *Placenta* **22:** S42–S47.

Rodin AE, Koller LA, Taylor JD (1962) Association of thalidomide (Kevadon) with congenital anomalies. *Can Med Assoc J* **86:** 744–6.

Rogers JM (1996) The developmental toxicology of cadmium and arsenic with notes on lead. In *Toxicology of Metals* (Chang LW, ed.). CRC Lewis Publishers, Boca Raton, FL, pp. 1027–45.

Rogers JM, Grabowski CT (1983) Mirex-induced fetal cataracts: lens growth, histology and cation balance, and relationship to edema. *Teratology* **27:** 343–9.

Rossmanith WG, Wolfahrt S, Ecker A, Eberhardt E (1997) The demonstration of progesterone, but not estrogen, receptors in the developing human placenta. *Horm Metab Res* **29:** 604–10.

Rückinger S, Rzehak P, Chen C-M, Sausenthaler S, Koletzko S, Bauer C-P, Hoffmann U, *et al.* (2010) Prenatal and postnatal tobacco exposure and behavioral problems in 10-year-old children: results from the GINI-plus prospective birth cohort study. *Environ Health Perpect* **118:** 150–4.

Rutherford JN (2009) Fetal signaling through placental structure and endocrine function: illustrations and implications from a nonhuman primate model. *Am J Human Biol* **21:** 745–53.

Sala M, Ribas-Fito N, Cardo E, de Muga ME, Marco E, Mazon C, Verdu A, Grimalt JO, Sunyer J (2001) Levels of hexachorobenzene and other organochlorine compounds in cord blood: exposure across placenta. *Chemosphere* **43:** 895–901.

Salafia C, Shiverick K (1999) Cigarette smoking and pregnancy. II. Vascular effects. *Placenta* **20:** 273–79.

Samudio-Ruiz SL, Allan AM, Valenzuela CF, Perrone-Bizzozero NI, Caldwell KK (2009) Prenatal ethanol exposure persistently impairs NMDA receptor-dependent activation of extracellular signal-regulated kinase in the mouse dentate gyrus. *J Neurochem* **109:** 1311–23.

Sastry BVR (1984) Amino acid uptake by human placenta: alterations by nicotine and tobacco smoke components and their implications on fetal growth. In *Physiological and Pharmacological Control of Nervous System Development* (Caciagli F, Giacobini E, Paoletti R, eds.). Elsevier, Amsterdam, pp. 137–40.

Sastry BVR (1991) Placental toxicology: tobacco smoke, abused drugs, multiple chemical interactions and placental function. *Reprod Fertil Dev* **3(4):** 355–72.

Sastry BVR (1993) Placental acetylcholine. In *Molecular Aspects of Placental and Fetal Membrane Autacoids* (Rice GE, Brennecke SP, eds.). CRC Press, Boca Raton, FL, 157pp.

Sastry BVR (1995a) Opioid addiction, placental function and fetal growth. In *Placental Toxicology* (Sastry BVR, ed.). CRC Press, Boca Raton, FL, pp. 83–106.

Sastry BVR (1995b) Neuropharmacology of nicotine: effects on the autoregulation of acetylcholine release by substance P and methionine enkephalin in rodent cerebral slices and toxicological implications. *Clin Exp Pharmacol Physiol* **22(4):** 288–90.

Sastry BVR (1997) Human placental cholinergic system. *Biochem Pharmacol* **53:** 1577–86.

Sastry BVR, Barnwell SL, Moore RD (1983) Factors affecting the uptake of alpha-amino acids by human placental villus: acetylcholine, phospholipid methylation, Ca^{++} and cytoskeletal organization. *Trophoblast Res* **1:** 81–100.

Sastry BVR, Chance MB, Hemontolor ME, Goddijn-Wessel TAW (1998) Formation and retention of cotinine during placental transfer of nicotine in human placental cotyledon. *Pharmacology* **57:** 104–16.

Sastry BVR, Janson, VE (1995) Smoking, placental function and fetal growth. In *Placental Toxicology* (Sastry BVR, ed.). CRC Press, Boca Raton, FL, pp. 45–82.

Sastry BVR, Janson VE, Ahmed M, Knots JA, Schinfeld JS (1989) Maternal cigarette smoking depresses placental amino acid transport which may lower the birth weight of infants. *Ann NY Acad Sci* **562:** 367–9.

Sastry BVR, Olubadewo J, Boehm FH (1977) Effects of nicotine and cocaine on the release of acetylcholine from isolated placental villi. *Arch Int Pharmacodynam Ther* **229:** 23–36.

Seller MJ, Bnait KS, Cairns NJ (1992) Effects of maternal tobacco smoke inhalation on early embryonic growth. In *Effects of Smoking on the Fetus, Neonate and Child* (Poswillo D, Alberman E, eds.). Oxford University Press, Oxford, pp. 45–59.

Setia S, Sridhar MG (2009) Changes in GF/IGF-1 axis in intrauterine growth retardation: consequences of fetal programming? *Horm Metab Res* **41:** 791–8.

Schenker S, Yang Y, Johnson RF, Downing JW, Schenken RS, Henderson GI, Kia TS (1993) The transfer of cocaine and its metabolites across the term human placenta. *Clin Pharmacol Ther* **53(3):** 329–39.

Shafer TJ, Meyer DA (2004) Effects of pyrethroids on voltage-sensitive calcium channels: a critical evaluation of strengths, weaknesses, data needs, and relationship to assessment of cumulative neurotoxicity. *Toxicol Appl Pharmacol* **196:** 303–18.

Shafer TJ, Meyer DA, Crofton KM (2005) Developmental neurotoxicity of pyrethroid insecticides: critical review and future needs. *Environ Health Perspect* **113:** 123–36.

Shen H, Main KM, Kaleva M, Virtanen H, Haavisto A-M, Skakkebaek NE, Toppari J, Schramm, K-W (2005) Prenatal organochlorine pesticides in placentas from Finland: exposure of male infants born during 1997–2001. *Placenta* **26:** 512–14.

Shiverick KT, Salafia C (1999) Cigarette smoking and pregnancy I: Ovarian, uterine and placental effects. *Placenta* **20:** 265–72.

Silva MH, Gammon D (2009) An assessment of the developmental, reproductive and neurotoxicity of endosulfan. *Birth Defects Res (Part B)* **86:** 1–28.

Simone C, Derewlany LO, Oskamp M. Oskamp M, Johnson D, Knie B, Koren G (1994) Acetylcholinesterase and butyrylcholinesterase activity in the human term placenta: implications for fetal cocaine exposure. *J Lab Clin Med* **123:** 400–6.

Sircar S, Lahiri P (1989) Lindane (gamma-HCH) causes reproductive failure and fetotoxicity in mice. *Toxicology* **59:** 171–7.

Skene SA, Dewhurst C, Greenberg M (1989) Polychlorinated dibenzo-*p*-dioxins and polychlorinated dibenzofurans: the risks to human health. A review. *Hum Toxicol* **8:** 173–203.

Slikker W, Miller RK (1994) Placental metabolism and transfer: role in developmental toxicology. In *Developmental Toxicology* (Kimmel CA, Buelke-Sam J, eds.). Raven Press, New York, pp. 245–83.

Slotkin TA (2008) If nicotine is a developmental neurotoxicant in animal studies, dare we recommend nicotine replacement therapy in pregnant women and adolescents? *Neurotoxicol Teratol* **30:** 1–19.

Somm E, Schwitzgebel VM, Vauthay DM, Aubert ML, Hüppi PS (2009) Prenatal nicotine exposure and the programming of metabolic and cardiovascular disorders. *Mol Cell Endocrinol* **304:** 69–77.

Srivastava MK, Raizada RB, Dikshith TS (1992) Fetotoxic response to technical quinalphos in rats. *Vet Hum Toxicol* **34:** 131–3.

Stellman SD, Stellman MJ, Sommer JF (1988) Health and reproductive outcomes among American Legionnaires in relation to combat and herbicide exposure in Vietnam. *Environ Res* **47:** 150–74.

Stockbauer JW, Hoffman RE, Schramm WF Edmonds LE (1988) Reproductive outcomes of mothers with potential exposure to 2,3,7,8-tetrachlorodibenzo-*p*-dioxin. *Am J Epidemiol* **128:** 410–19.

Stratton K, Howe C, Battaglia F (1996) *Fetal Alcohol Syndrome – Diagnosis, Epidemiology, Prevention and Treatment.* National Academy Press, Washington DC.

Sunderman FW, Mitchell JM, Allpas PR, Baselt R (1978) Embryotoxicity and fetal toxicity of nickel in rats. *Toxicol Appl Pharmacol* **43:** 381–90.

Suzuki K, Horiguchi T, Comas-Urrutia AC,Mueller-Heubach E, Morishima HO, Adamsons K (1974) Placental transfer and distribution of nicotine in the pregnant rhesus monkey. *Am J Obstet Gynecol* **119:** 253–62.

Suzuki G, Nakano M, Nakano S (2005) Distribution of PCDDs/PCDFs and co-PCBs in human maternal blood, cord blood, placentas, milk, and adipose tissue: dioxins showing high toxic equivalency factor accumulate in the placenta. *Biosci Biotechnol Biochem* **69(10):** 1836–47.

Syme MR, Paxton JW, Keelan JA (2004) Drug transfer and metabolism by the human placenta. *Clin Pharmacokinet* **43(8):** 487–514.

Tan SW, Meiller JC, Mahaffey KR (2009) The endocrine effects of mercury in humans and wildlife. *Crit Rev Toxicol* **39(3):** 228–69.

Taussig HBA (1962) A study of the German outbreak of phocomelia. *J Am Med Assoc* **180:** 1106–14.

Tilson HA, Jacobson JL, Rogan, WJ (1990) Polychlorinated biphenyls and the developing nervous system: cross-species comparisons. *Neurotoxicol Teratol* **12:** 239–48.

Tsuyoshi N (2007) The problem of species comparison of developmental toxicity: can we extrapolate human developmental toxicity induced by environmental chemicals from the data of rodents. *J Pharmac Soc Japan* **127(3):** 491–500.

Tuchmann-Duplessis H, David G, Haegel P (1972) The placenta: physiology and principal stages of development. In *Illustrated Human Embryology Volume 1, Embryogenesis* (Hurley LS, ed.). Springer Verlag, New York, pp. 73–90.

Vahter M (2009) Effects of arsenic on maternal and fetal health. *Ann Rev Nutri* **29:** 381–99.

Weinberg J, Sliwowska JH, Lan N, Hellemans GC (2008) Prenatal alcohol exposure: fetal programming, the hypothalamic–pituitary–adrenal axis and sex differences in outcome. *J Neuroendocrinol* **20:** 470–88.

Weischer CH, Kordel W, Hockrainer D (1980) Effects of $NiCl_2$ and NiO in Wistar rats after oral uptake and inhalation exposure, respectively. *Zentralbl Bakteriol Mikrobiol Hyg (B)* **171:** 336–51.

Welsch F, Dettbarn W-D (1971) Protein synthesis in lobster walking leg nerves. *Comp Biochem Physiol B* **38:** 393–403.

Welsch F (1982) Placental transfer and fetal uptake of drugs. *J Vet Pharmacol Ther* **5:** 91–104.

WHO (1989) *Polychlorinated dibenzo-para-dioxins and dibenzofurans.* Environmental Health Criteria Document No. 88. World Health Organization, Geneva.

Wloch S, Palasz A, Kaminski M (2009) Active and passive transport of drugs in the human placenta. *Ginekol Pol* **80(10):** 772–7.

Wojtowicz AK, Milewicz T, Gregoraszczuk EL (2007) DDT and its metabolite DDE alter steroid hormone secretion in human term placental explants by regulation of aromatase activity. *Toxicol Lett* **173:** 24–30.

Woods JR, Plessinger MA, Clark KA (1987) Effect of cocaine on uterine blood flow and fetal oxygenation. *J Am Med Ass* **257:** 957–60.

Wrobel MH, Rekawiecki R, Kotwica J (2009) Involvement of prostaglandin F2α in the adverse effect of PCB 77 on the force of contractions of bovine myometrium. *Toxicology* **262:** 224–9.

Xiao Y, He J, Gilbert RD, Zhang L (2000) Cocaine induces apoptosis in fetal myocardial cells through a mitochondria-dependent pathway. *J Pharmacol Exp Ther* **292:** 8–14.

Yan B, Matoney L, Yang D (1999) Human carboxylesterases in term placentae: enzymatic characterization, molecular cloning and evidence for the existence of multiple forms. *Placenta* **20:** 599–607.

Yang K, Julan L, Rubio F, Sharma A, Guan H (2006) Cadmium reduces 11β-hydroxysteroid dehydrogenase type 2 activity and expression in human placental trophoblast cells. *Am J Physiol Endocr Metab* **290:** E135–E142.

Yokel RA (1997) The metabolism and toxicokinetics of aluminum relevant to neurotoxicity. In *Mineral and Metal Neurotoxicology* (Yasui M, Strong MJ, Ota K, Verity MA, eds.). CRC Press, Boca Raton, FL, pp. 81–9.

Yokel RA, McNamara PJ (1985) Aluminum bioavailability and disposition in adult and immature rabbits. *Toxicol Appl Pharmacol* **77:** 344–52.

Yokel RA, McNamara PJ (2001) Aluminum toxicokinetics: an updated minireview. *Pharmacol Toxicol* **88:** 159–67.

Yoshida M, Satoh M, Shimada A, Yamamoto E, Yasutake A, Tohyama C (2002) Maternal-to-fetus transfer of mercury in metallothionein-null pregnant mice after exposure to mercury vapor. *Toxicology* **175:** 215–22.

Yumoto S, Nagai H, Matsuzaki H, *et al.* (2000) Transplacental passage of ^{26}Al transfer through maternal milk to suckling rats. *Nucl Instrum Methods Phys B* **172:** 925–9.

Zhao Z, Reece EA (2005) Nicotine-induced embryonic malformations mediated by apoptosis from increasing intracellular calcium and oxidative stress. *Birth Def Res (Part B)* **74:** 383–91.

Zhen X, Torres C, Wang H-Y, Friedman E (2001) Prenatal exposure to cocaine disrupts D_{1A} dopamine receptor function via selective inhibition of protein phosphatase 1 pathway in rabbit frontal cortex. *J Neurosci* **21:** 9160–7.

CHAPTER

81

Placental pathology

Drucilla J. Roberts

INTRODUCTION

The placenta is a remarkable organ, an adaptation to allow the unique inside development of the mammalian fetus. This organ must facilitate many truly remarkable functions including: seek/find/attach and anchor to a suitable environment in an antigenically foreign "host", control the immune system at the interface with the maternal host, adapt and grow with the growing fetus and its increasing physiologic demands, synthesize and secrete appropriate factors to sustain the pregnancy and control the maternal blood flow to itself, and be able to detach and slough at the appropriate time without causing death of either its fetus or its host. It functions as the fetal lung, kidney, liver, GI tract and endocrine organ. It does all this over 40 short weeks to the incredible disrespect of its host, who often either eats it after delivery, buries it or makes (often rude) remarks about its appearance (most humans). Placentas are, of course, organs unique to mammals and differ between mammalian species in their phenotype; this chapter therefore will focus only on human placentation.

The placenta is a zygotic organ fated very early in gestation, by the morula stage. This early segregation of the extra-embryonic lineage can be beneficial to the embryo in some cases. Chromosomal/genetic mosaicism can result in karyotypically distinct fetal vs. placental tissues (Johnson and Wapner, 1997; Lestou and Kalousek, 1998; Qumsiyeh *et al.*, 1997). The abnormal karyotype can be confined to either the extra-embryonic or embryonic lineage, with quite different phenotypes (Kalousek *et al*, 1989). This same phenomenon may occur for the confinement of other factors (discussed later). The first trimester of human development is focused on both embryonic development and placental function and is arguably more important than that of the embryo; embryonic life will not continue without proper placental development/function. It is clear in humans that the placenta can develop much further without an embryo than the embryo can develop without the placenta! Cross-talk between embryonic and extra-embryonic development, though, is essential for normal development.

One of the important functions of the placenta is to act as a transfer station from mother to fetus *in utero*. It must find and allow passage of needed factors (oxygen, glucose, amino acids, for example) and trap or remove noxious ones (organisms, teratogens). It does so amazingly well, for the most part. The placenta interfaces directly with maternal tissues via its specialized epithelial cells called trophoblast. The maternal flow to the placenta bathes the villous trophoblast (Figure 81.1). These trophoblast cells hold the key to the active, passive (facilitated) and diffusion needed for transfer of materials to, and waste products from, the fetus. Trophoblast shuttles substances between mother and baby between the maternal space (maternal lakes) and the villous vessels (Figure 81.1). The fetal blood flows from arteries in the umbilical cord through the chorionic plate, stem villous, villous vessels and returns through the chorionic plate veins to the umbilical vein to the baby. The two circulations, maternal and fetal, must be uninhibited in the placenta for optimal function.

Placental pathology involves insults in either the maternal or fetal vascular compartments or to the placenta itself. The clinical effects of these pathologies are, for a large part, dependent on placental reserve. Whereas large well-developed placentas can function despite pathologies, a small placenta has little reserve therefore any pathology will likely have clinical effects. This overview of placental pathology will be ordered by compartment – maternal, fetal and placental.

MATERNAL "EFFECT" PATHOLOGIES OF THE PLACENTA

Blood flow to the placenta is ensured via the physiologic conversion of the spiral arterioles which occurs at implantation. The implantation site trophoblast invades the maternal decidualized endometrium and is tropic to its vessels where they invade, colonize and undergo transformation to an endothelial phenotype (Figure 81.2). The vascular walls are altered such that their normally responsive muscular walls are disrupted, ensuring uninterrupted blood flow to the implantation site and therefore to the placenta.

During this process the trophoblast plugs the vessels such that maternal flow to the developing placenta is occluded until the end of the first trimester (Figure 81.2). Early fetal and placental villous development occurs in an anoxic environment. One must assume that the physical force of blood flow and/or the oxygen levels cannot be tolerated by the zygote

Reproductive and Developmental Toxicology, Edited by Ramesh C. Gupta
ISBN: 978-0-12-382032-7

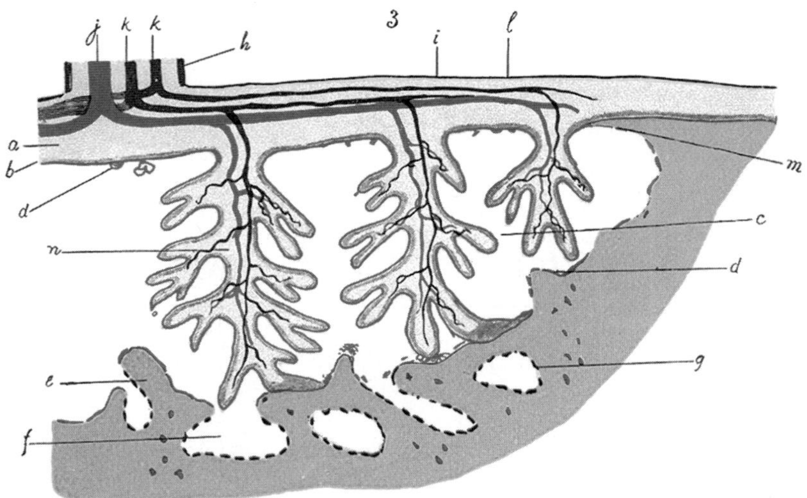

FIGURE 81.1 Placental circulation. Cartoon of placental blood flow (arteries and veins, g,f) showing maternal flow into placental lakes (maternal space, c) and fetal blood flow from umbilical cord (h) arteries (k) into villi (n) and returning in umbilical vein (j). a – Chorionic plate, b – chorion, d – interface, e – decidua, i and l – amniotic epithelium.

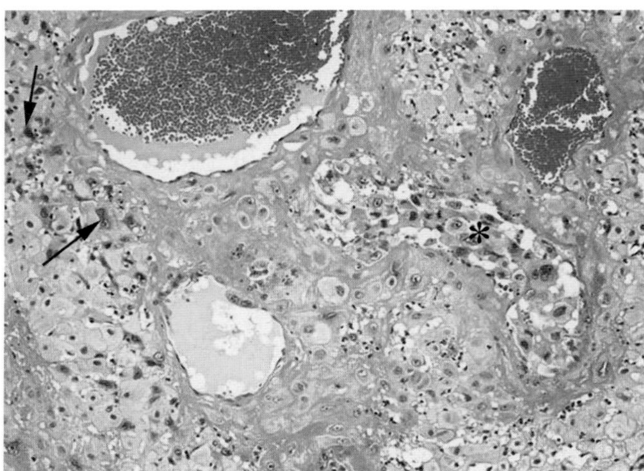

FIGURE 81.2 Implantation site. Ectatic decidual vessels invaded by trophoblast (arrows) plugging lumen (*). H&E 40×.

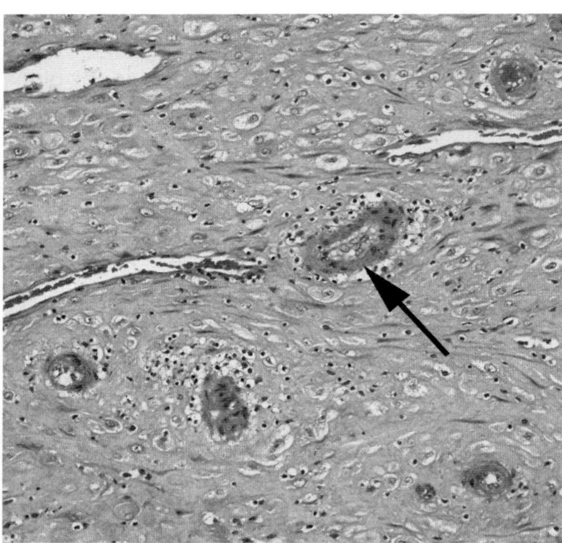

FIGURE 81.3 Unphysiologically altered decidual vessels in decidua basalis demonstrating persistent (inappropriate) muscularization of vessel walls (arrow). H&E 10×.

until after the first trimester (Burton and Jauniaux, 2004; Moffett *et al.*, 2006; Ornoy, 2007). This is an interesting and not well-known phenomenon, especially in teratology circles. As the embryo completes body plan patterning and organogenesis during this time, teratogens which affect early developmental events must gain access to the embryo/placenta via routes other than maternal blood. They likely include secretions from the fallopian tubal epithelium and the endometrial glands (Boomsma *et al.*, 2009; Gray *et al.*, 2001; Scotchie *et al.*, 2009), but they may include factors stored in the ova cytoplasm during oogenesis and meiosis. Evidence for this latter route includes known teratogenic effects of hypovitaminoses and alcohol (Baldwin *et al.*, 1982; Kaminski *et al.*, 1978; Kesmodel *et al.*, 2002; Stoler *et al.*, 1998) that predate conception (Berghella *et al.*, 2010; Bower and Stanley, 1992; Czeizel, 1995; Goldberg *et al.*, 2006; Lewis *et al.*, 2010; Schrander-Stumpel, 1999; Van Dyke *et al.*, 2002; Yerby, 2003).

Most maternal-side pathologies of the placenta involve either alterations in blood flow due to maldevelopment of the placental implantation site or vascular disease, coagulopathies and other (rare) maternal space-occupying lesions.

MALDEVELOPMENT OF THE PLACENTAL IMPLANTATION SITE

Malimplantation must be a defect in the trophoblast biology and results in maladaption of the implantation site vessels. This is evidenced by persistence of the muscularized vascular walls in the decidua and can be diagnosed by placental bed biopsies or decidua which remains on the placenta after deliver (Figure 81.3). The result of these unphysiologically converted vessels is malperfusion of the placenta (Burton

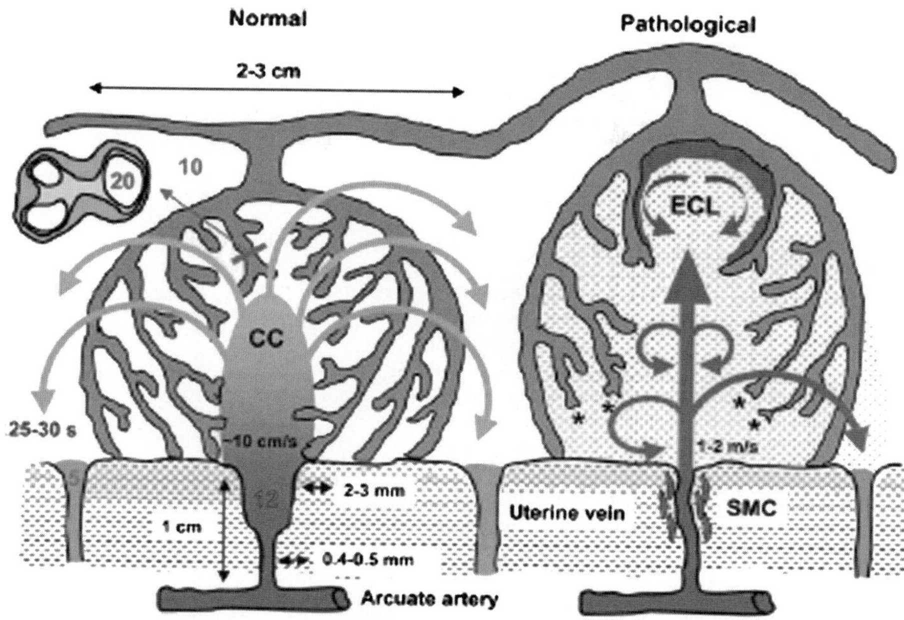

FIGURE 81.4 Cartoon of normal (left panel) and hypertensive (right panel) placenta with increased pressure resulting in increased maternal lakes and villous disruption (echogenic cystic lesions – ECL). CC – central cavity, SMC – smooth muscle cells. (From Burton *et al.*, 2009, with permission.) Please refer to color plate section.

and Jones, 2009; Burton *et al.*, 2009; Goldman-Wohl and Yagel, 2002; Redline *et al.*, 2004). The accepted theory is that this results in placental ischemia, but this has never been proven. Studies have looked at placental oxygen levels and have not detected hypoxia in these cases but may also result in high velocity flow/hypertension and pressure-related damage to the developing placenta (Burton and Jones, 2009; Burton *et al.*, 2009) (Figure 81.4). Whatever the mechanism the result is release of a factor(s) from the placenta which becomes systemic in the mother and likely crosses the placenta to the developing embryo–fetus. Maternal systemic effects include hypertension and all its sequelae, proteinuria, hyper-reflexia – and are diagnosed as pre-eclampsia or toxemia if accompanied by seizures. The fetal phenotype is thought to relate to the placental dysfunction only and includes growth restriction and an increased risk for fetal demise (Altshuler, 1996; Goldenberg *et al.*, 2004; Khong, 2004; Salafia *et al.*, 1995a). Pre-eclampsia/toxemia (PET) occurs at any time during pregnancy from late second trimester to 6 weeks postpartum and is diagnosed by specific clinical findings (Table 81.1). Maternal and fetal sequelae are significant (Table 81.1), which prompts clinical intervention. The placental pathology PET varies with the length of "exposure" *in utero*. Preterm PET (signs and symptoms before 27 weeks gestational age) shows the most dramatic pathologies; term PET placentas are often normal. The constellation of pathologies includes: small placenta by weight (<10th percentile), infarcts (often of unique morphology), chronic abruption, distal villous hypoplasia (accelerated maturation) and maternal vascular pathology (decidual vasculopathy with or without atherosis). Other pathologies may be seen including the fetal response to these pathologies, for example fetal thrombotic vasculopathy and insult-related meconium passage.

Placental size is one of the more reliable indications of well-being *in utero*. If development proceeds without insult then the fetal and placental compartment will grow in parallel and appropriately. Standards for placental weights have been published and are biased for a developed country with good prenatal care and require proper preparation of the placenta for weighing (Pinar *et al.*, 1996, 2002). Placental standards are for placentas weighed trimmed of cord, membranes and loose retroplacental blood (Table 81.2). There are standards for twin and triplet placentas as well. There has been a rather dramatic increase in average placental weight in the past half century

TABLE 81.1 Pre-eclampsia/toxemia

Diagnostic criteria (Bulletins, 2002 #937)
Hypertension: in a woman who was normotensive prior to 20 weeks' gestation with a systolic blood pressure (BP) greater than 140 mm Hg and a diastolic BP greater than 90 mm Hg on two successive measurements 4–6 hours apart. Preeclampsia in a patient with preexisting essential hypertension is diagnosed if systolic BP has increased by 30 mm Hg or if diastolic BP has increased by 15 mm Hg
Proteinuria: defined as 300 mg or more of protein in a 24-hour urine sample. In the emergency department, a urine protein-to-creatinine ratio of 0.19 or greater is somewhat predictive of significant proteinuria (negative predictive value (NPV), 87%) (Rodriguez-Thompson and Lieberman, 2001)
Clinical sequelae (Baumwell and Karumanchi, 2007; Hladunewich *et al.*, 2007)
Maternal: CNS: headache, visual disturbance, seizures, stroke, hemorrhage
Hepatic: bleeding, rupture
Renal: acute tubular necrosis, hemorrhage
Coagulopathies
Death
Fetal: Intrauterine growth restriction
Oligohydramnios
Placental abruption
Encephalopathy
Death

TABLE 81.2 Placental weight standards

GA	Singletons percentiles 10–25–50–75–90%	Twins (combined WT) percentiles 10–25–50–75–90%	Triplets (combined WT) percentiles 10–25–50–75–90%		
12	56				
14	83				
16	110				
18	137.8				
20	145	166–190–218–245–270	226	253	285
22	122–138–157–176–191	191–219–251–282–310	289	319	345
24	145–166–189–212–233	232–267–307–346–382	371	406	445
26	175–200–227–255–280	284–330–380–430–475	444	509	558
28	210–238–270–302–331	345–401–464–527–584	516	621	697
30	249–281–316–352–384	409–478–554–631–700	591	738	849
32	290–325–364–403–438	472–554–644–734–815	674	855	1000
34	331–369–411–453–491	531–624–727–830–923	768	965	1139
36	372–412–457–501–542	582–684–798–912–1014	878	1065	1253
38	409–452–499–547–589	619–728–850–972–1082	1007	1147	1330
40	442–487–537–587–632	638–753–879–1005–1118			

Adapted from Pinar *et al.* (1996) and (2002)

TABLE 81.3 Causes of IUGR (Bane and Gillan, 2003; Cetin *et al.*, 2004; Katzman and Genest, 2002; Khong, 2004; Pham *et al*, 2006; Redline, 2007; Regnault *et al.*, 2002; Tycko, 2006)

Maternal:
- Constitutional
- Tobacco
- Hypertension
- Diabetes complicated with hypertension or renal failure
- Cardiorespiratory diseases
- ETOH abuse
- Anemia
- Infection

Fetal:
- Chromosomal/genetic anomalies
- Structural anomalies
- Infection
- Multiple gestation

Placental:
- Ischemia
- Abnormal placentation
- Massive perivillous fibrin
- Maternal floor infarct
- Massive intervillositis
- Confined placental mosaicism
- Villitis of unclear etiology

which is probably attributed to improved obstetric care and well-being of the population studied (Naeye, 1987; Pinar *et al.*, 1996). Placentas below the 10th percentile suggest a chronic process often due to abnormal maternal perfusion. The biology is similar to the chicken and egg question – which came first, the abnormal implantation resulting in abnormal perfusion (suggesting a developmental defect of the placenta/zygote) or abnormal vasculature resulting in abnormal growth of the placenta (suggesting it is the maternal pathology responsible for the placental size). The answer probably is not as simple as one or the other, and we can avoid the issue in this chapter by just focusing on the pathology! In any case, small placentas are one of the hallmarks of pregnancies complicated with PET, especially preterm PET, although many other pathobiologic scenarios also result in small placentas (Table 81.3).

Maternal vascular disease is a much more specific finding associated with PET. The biology of abnormal implantation results in persistence of the muscularized end arterioles in the decidua, which should all be physiologically altered in the basalis (Figures 81.2 and 81.3). Hypertension leads to vascular damage systemically (or at least locally in the gravid uterus) and is evidenced in the decidual vessels away from implantation, those in the decidua capsularis (Figure 81.5a). These vessels are usually very small unmuscularized structures that become ectatic with fibrinoid necrosis of their walls (Figure 81.5b). In severe cases the walls show "foamy histiocytes" within ("atherosis", Figure 81.5c), likely a degenerative finding (Labarrere, 1988; Redline *et al.*, 2007a; Zhang *et al.*, 2006). The vessels often show a peripheralized clustering of predominantly mononuclear inflammatory cells and may thrombose. This phenotype is similar to the physiologic conversion seen with normal implantation, therefore the diagnosis is made by examination of the decidua away from the disk, the decidua capsularis/parietalis.

Other features include sequelae of the maternal vascular disease including infarcts, abruption and villous damage. Placental infarcts due to maternal vascular events are pyramidal-shaped lesions with the broad end of the pyramid on the maternal floor. The clinical significance of these lesions is a function of the placental reserve. The infarcted parenchyma clearly cannot function for the fetus; so long as there is ample functioning parenchyma the fetus will be unaffected. The fetus with a normal sized or large placenta can withstand the insult of one or even more placental infarcts of this type without sequellae, but the fetus with a small placenta may be significantly affected by a single infarct. The affects may include hypoxic damage to the brain, which has been reported in association with these features as described in PET placentas (Redline *et al.*, 2002), ischemic renal damage leading to oligohydramnios due to renal insufficiency, growth restriction and even fetal death (Chaddha *et al.*, 2004; Gagnon *et al.*, 2002).

In addition to the typical pyramidal-type placental infarcts, placentas damaged by hypertension often show a different type of infarct. These infarcts are central (in the parenchyma by thickness and in the disk by shape), small, round and multiple (Figure 81.6). These "hypertensive-type" infarcts may be due to jet phenomena of the blood flow

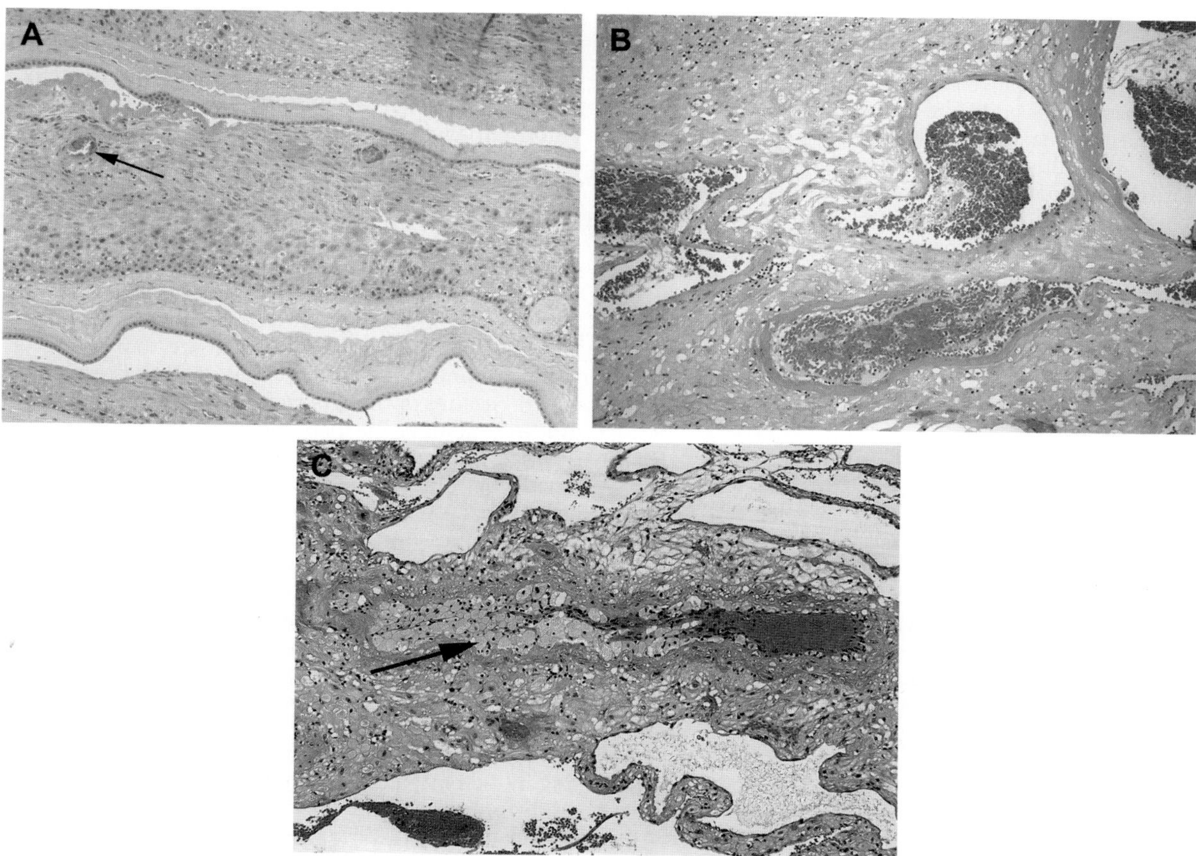

FIGURE 81.5 Decidual vasculopathy. (A) Normal decidua capsularis vasculature. (B) Decidual vasculopathy in decidua capsularis from a placenta complicated with maternal pre-eclampsia at 31 weeks gestational age. Note ectasia and fibrinoid necrosis of vessel walls (compare with those in A). (C) Severe decidual vasculopathy with atherosis (histiocytes, some occluding vessels, arrow). H&E 20×.

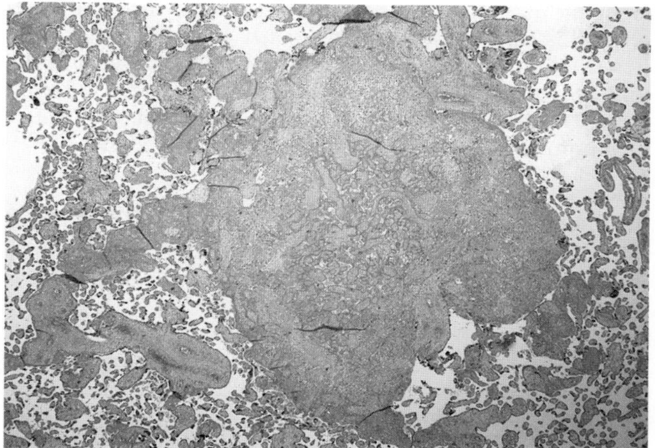

FIGURE 81.6 Hypertensive infarct. Small, round, central infarct, characteristic of prolonged hypertensive/ischemic damage to the placenta. H&E 4×.

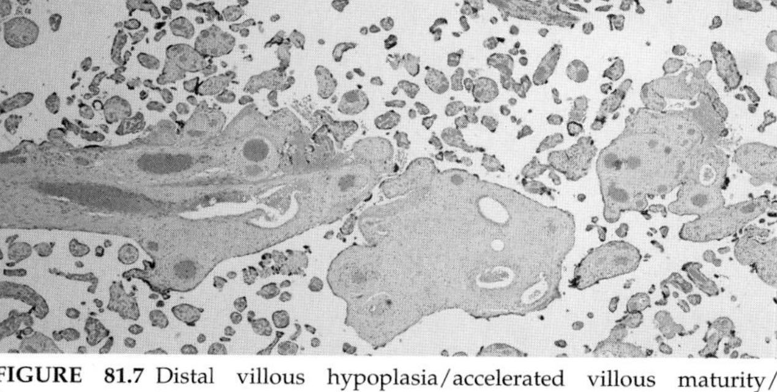

FIGURE 81.7 Distal villous hypoplasia/accelerated villous maturity/hypermature villi – note vast open maternal lakes, small and few distal villi. H&E 4×.

resulting in less flow between the jets, making a watershed zone of relative hypoxia more prone to infarct (Figure 81.4) (Burton *et al.*, 2009).

The pressure may also be the biology behind the characteristic phenotype of the villi in placentas from chronically hypertensive women. The villi show accelerated maturation: are small with large syncytiotrophoblastic knots, widely spaced, have scant stroma and few capillaries (Figure 81.7). This has historically been termed "Tenney–Parker change" after the seminal manuscript in 1940 (Tenney and Parker, 1940) and now replaced by "distal villous hypoplasia" (Redline *et al.*, 2004) and equated with uteroplacental ischemia or malperfusion. It may be that these changes are due to damage from shear stress and pressure not ischemia. Whatever the biology, the histopathologic features are characteristic of severe chronic hypertension in pregnancy.

The features described above are materno-centric (having to do with the maternal to placenta side of the triad). The fetus can respond to insult as well, in its perfusion to the placenta. Neil Sebire has compared the fetal–placental perfusion to pulmonary physiology with the ventilation–perfusion usually matching. In the placenta, with poor perfusion maternally, the fetus (via the vessels in the stem villi as the umbilical cord vessels are poorly innervated; Fox and Khong, 1990) can shunt blood away from the poorly perfused region (when regional, as in the typical type placental infarct) but when the entire placenta is poorly perfused/damaged, the fetus cannot shunt completely away, and therefore suffers globally instead.

INTRAPLACENTAL INTERFERENCE TO MATERNAL FLOW

If the uterine vessels are remodeled appropriately and maternal blood pressure is normotensive, then perfusion to the placenta may still be inhibited by pathologies within the placenta. These include predominantly abnormal fibrin/fibrinoid deposition in the intervillous space. The maternal space is a low resistance, slow flow but large volume space set up for catastrophic hemorrhages by either mother or fetus. Hemorrhage has long been the leading cause of maternal deaths, until modern best obstetric practices available in rich countries changed that. Now the hemostatic tools that trophoblasts have evolved to express cause pathologies.

Fibrin/fibrinoid deposition is common in placentas and is often present at the periphery of the disk (margin) and in the area just beneath the chorionic plate, regions with slow maternal flow. Any damage to the villi, exposing the villous stroma to the maternal blood, results in deposition of perivillous fibrin and is a marker for both slow flow and villous damage (Figure 81.8). The effect of this is related to the pathology of the original insult as well as the space occupying the vascular inhibitory result, and is a function of the placental reserve. Small placentas with lots of fibrin result in fetal compromise, whereas large placentas can accommodate more perivillous fibrin without injury to the fetus. Coagulopathic mothers are at increased risk as well of abnormal fibrin/fibrinoid deposition (Arias *et al.*, 1998; Ariel *et al.*, 2004; Katz *et al.*, 2002; Khong, 2004; Kraus, 2007; Raspollini *et al.*, 2007; Sheppard and Bonnar, 1999; Stella *et al.*, 2006; Waters and Ashikaga, 2006).

There are two entities that involve excess fibrin and have clinical importance: massive intervillositis and maternal floor infarct. These are important clinically because they have a significant recurrence risk and are associated with perinatal morbidity (intrauterine growth restriction, IUGR, and intrauterine fetal demise, IUFD). Both are thought to be somehow immunopathologic (the maternal host rejecting the fetal graft) because of the recurrence risk, but neither have scientific explanations for their etiology.

Massive chronic intervillositis (MCI, also termed chronic histocytic intervillositis) is a lesion that affects the placenta at any gestational age (Boyd and Redline, 2000; Doss *et al.*, 1995; Jacques and Qureshi, 1993; Weber *et al.*, 2006). The intervillous space is filled with fibrin and (usually) admixed maternal cd68 positive histiocytes (Figure 81.9). The result is usually severe IUGR and often IUFD. The fetus is structurally and karyotypically normal. The intervillous space is unusually devoid of maternal red blood cells in this lesion; it is as if they are somehow excluded (shunted) away from the placenta.

Maternal floor infarct (MFI) has a distinctive gross finding in the placental examination (Andres *et al.*, 1990; Bendon and Hommel, 1996; Gersell, 1993; Katzman and Genest, 2002; Mandsager *et al.*, 1994; Naeye, 1985; Vernof *et al.*, 1992). The maternal surface (maternal floor) is significantly effaced by a thick band of fibrin/fibrinoid material (Figure 81.10) said to resemble the rind of an orange. A cut section of this area reveals the band as a thick ribbon that stiffly sits above the spongy normal tissue. Histology shows the fibrin running along the maternal floor encasing the villi (at least three "layers"). It is easy to see how this would affect placental function. Maternal blood cannot get through this layer and the villi are purfused via overflow from adjacent unaffected areas. This is a rare lesion that may be associated with maternal immune phenomena or metabolic disturbances.

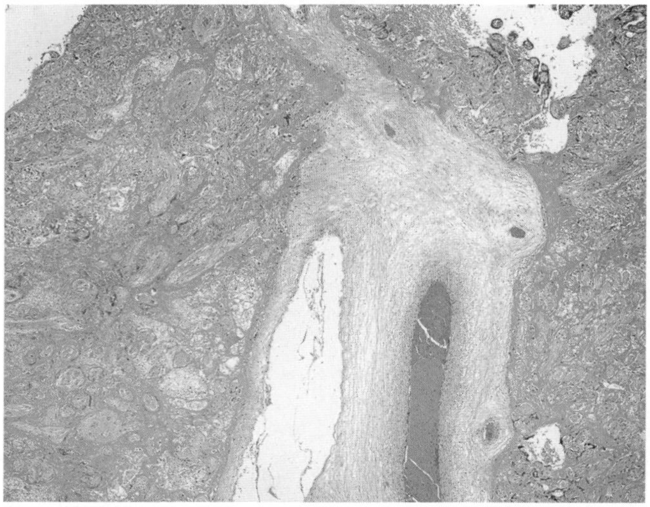

FIGURE 81.8 Massive perivillous fibrin deposition. Notice the maternal lakes are filled with fibrin/fibrinoid material. The fetus is still perfusing the villi (see fetal blood in the stem villous vessel in center). H&E 4×.

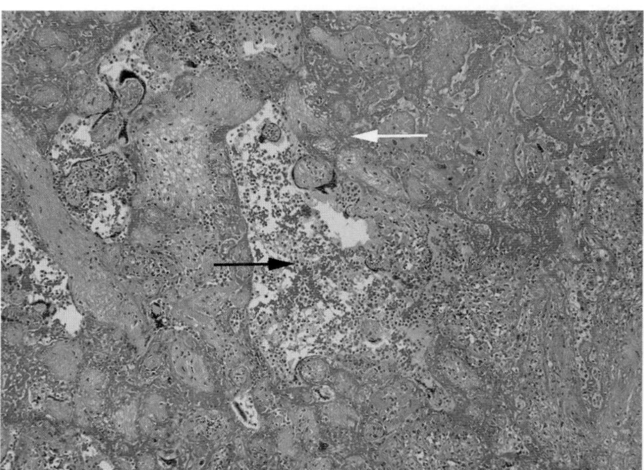

FIGURE 81.9 Massive intervillositis/histiocytic intervillositis. The maternal lakes are filled with histiocytes (black arrow) or fibrin/fibrinoid (white arrow). H&E 4×. Insert shows higher magnification of histiocytic infiltrate. H&E 20×.

Other space occupying lesions can interfere with maternal blood flow within the placenta. These include malignancies, usually hematogenously spread. Any hematogenously metastatic malignancy in the mother can metastasize to the placenta. These present as infarct-like lesions, often small and multiple. Metastatic disease from mother to placenta immediately makes the maternal disease a stage IV (Potter, 1969; Potter and Schoeneman, 1970). The malignancies more common to the reproductive age group published as metastatic lesions in the placenta include malignant melanoma (Altman *et al.*, 2003; Shuhaila *et al.*, 2008), breast (Cross *et al.*, 1951; Eltorky *et al.*, 1995), pulmonary (Folk *et al.*, 2004; Jackisch *et al.*, 2003), pancreatic (Al-Adnani *et al.*, 2007), and other malignancies (I have personally seen an intestinal adenocarcinoma and a large cell lymphoma involving the placenta, in addition to the more common melanoma and breast carcinoma). Hormonally responsive malignancies often "blossom" during pregnancy with widespread metastatic disease. None of these malignancies has been well demonstrated to cross the placenta and metastasize to the fetus. I have seen two cases of leukemia (both of an unusual type, NK cell leukemia) present in both the mother and fetus (Figure 81.11), lethal in both, and it was unclear where the original started.

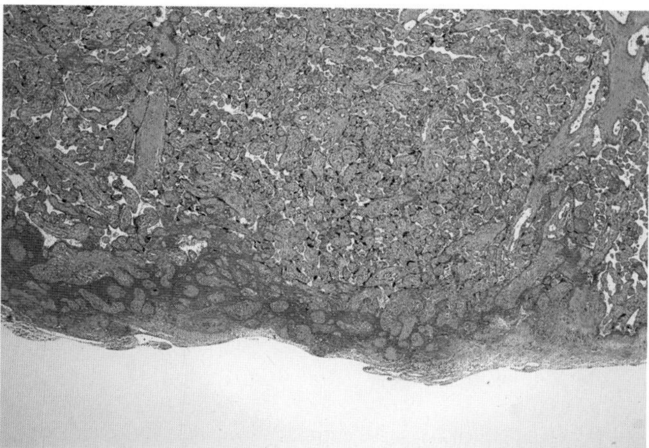

FIGURE 81.10 Maternal floor infarct. The basal plate interface is "infiltrated" by a thick layer of fibrin/fibrinoid material encasing several "layers" of villi. H&E 2×.

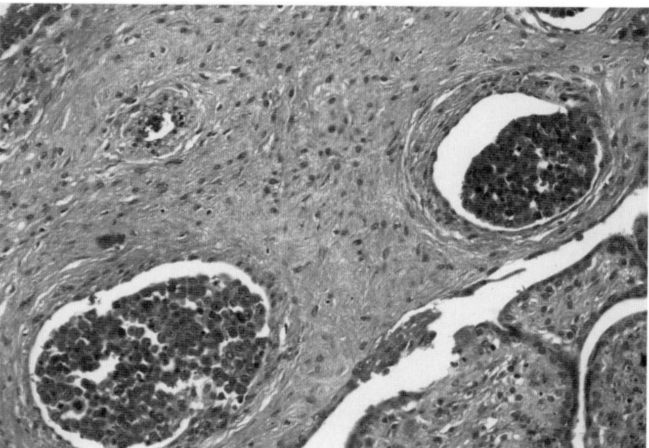

FIGURE 81.11 Congenital leukemia. Fetal blood within villi is nearly all blast forms. H&E 10×.

In all published and in my personal cases of metastatic disease involving the placenta the mothers fared very poorly but the fetus/infants survived.

Other maternal-side pathologies of the placenta

In utero infections occupy a large percentage of placental pathologies and are the focus of much of the anxiety in the clinical setting. In fact, infections of the placenta or infections that gain access to the fetoplacental unit are quite rare. The placenta and all of its tissues act as a very good barrier to most infections yet it is not impervious. Infectious organisms can reach the placenta and have clinical effects whether or not there is true colonization of the placenta or the very rare times infections reach the fetus causing congential infection. There are two routes for placental infection – the "ascending" route via the cervix and the hematogenous route via the maternal circulation within the placenta.

Ascending infections are those caused by organisms that gain access usually through the membranes into the amniotic cavity. These are organisms from the cervico-vaginal environment, whether normal flora or virulent organisms. The result is a local membranous infection which causes either disruption of the membranes and therefore access into the receptive growth environment of the amniotic fluid/cavity or rupture of the membranes and resultant (often preterm) delivery. The organisms reach the fetus through fetal "respiration" of the amniotic fluid, direct colonization of the fetal skin and other contact points with the amniotic fluid, and (theoretically) by swallowing. Common organisms include those typical of the normal vaginal flora (gardineralla, anaerobes, etc.) and virulent "contaminants" (*Mycoplasma, Streptococcal* sp., *E. coli, Candida albicans, Listeria monocytogenes*, etc.). The resultant pathology is chorioamniontitis, inflammation of the membranes of the placenta from maternal margination (Figure 81.12a) with or without a fetal response as well from the fetal vessels in the umbilical cord or chorionic plate (Figure 81.12b,c).

Although fetal infection is rare and is more common in preterm gestations for unclear reasons, fetal sequelae are more common (de Araujo *et al.*, 1994; De Paepe *et al.*, 2004; Holzman *et al.*, 2007; Leviton *et al.*, 2010; Miralles *et al.*, 2005; Onderdonk *et al.*, 2008; Srinivas *et al.*, 2006). The so-termed "fetal inflammatory response syndrome" (FIRS) involves the effects of the fetal inflammatory cells being immature, slowly chemotaxic (therefore locally toxic), more commonly involve eosinophilia and secrete proinflammatory and endothelially damaging cytokines (Il6) resulting in vascular damage and compromise (hypoxia) and endothelial damage (leakiness and visceral damage) (Bashiri *et al.*, 2006; Blackburn, 2008; Gomez *et al.*, 1998; Gotsch *et al.*, 2007; Pacora *et al.*, 2002; Romero *et al.*, 2003; Svigos, 2001; Yoon *et al.*, 2003). FIRS has been associated with neurocompromise primarily in preterm infants (Aaltonen *et al.*, 2005; Andrews *et al.*, 2008; Grether *et al.*, 2003; O'Shea *et al.*, 2009; Schendel, 2001; Svigos, 2001) but also in term infants (Redline, 2008a,b, 2005; Redline and O'Riordan, 2000).

It is now clear that chorioamnionitis (as evidenced by either maternal or fetal inflammation) is not always due to infection in the amniotic cavity but may result from other proinflammatory insults including epidural anesthesia (Lieberman *et al.*, 1997; Philip *et al.*, 1999; Smulian *et al.*, 1999) and likely for some "high responders" labor itself! Documentation of true infection is uncommon but can be diagnosed by placental pathologic examination when bacterial or fungal organisms are visible on the slides (Figure 81.13) or characteristic inflammatory pathology is present, as in listerial placentitis (Figure 81.14; Gersell, 1993; Parkash *et al.*, 1998). True fetal infections are exceptional and clinically serious, but are impossible to predict when acute chorioamnionitis is the only pathologic finding.

Hematogenously spread infections to the placenta have a different placental pathology characterized by a villitis (Figure 81.15a). Chronic villitis is an inflammation of the villi themselves, probably by first infection of the villi (by trophoblast–stroma–endothelial cell infection (Al-Harthi *et al.*, 2002; Csoma *et al.*, 2002; David *et al.*, 1992; Koi *et al.*, 2001; Pereira and Maidji, 2008; Tabata *et al.*, 2007) and then maternal inflammatory migration (Redline and Patterson, 1993), although a fetal response is probably present as well. The villi are damaged by both the infectious agent and the inflammatory response; often this necrosis results in vascular collapse and villous necrosis (which may be a protective mechanism to obviate fetal infection) resulting in placental compromise. Agents responsible for infectious villitis include those common in the population at question. In the eastern USA the most common is CMV (Figure 81.15b) but in other locations might include treponema, HSV, toxoplasmosis, chagas and others.

Maternal sepsis due to bacterial or fungal forms also seeds the placenta hematogenously; however, it does not elicit a chronic villitis but more a septic abortion with purulent intravillositis, placental abcesses and endomyometritis (Heller *et al.*, 2003; Jewett, 1973; Lowenthal *et al.*, 2006; Ooe and Udagawa, 1997).

Most cases of histologically diagnosed chronic villitis are non-infectious (at least in the USA) and are relatively common (Althabe and Labarrere, 1985; Labarrere *et al.*, 1989).

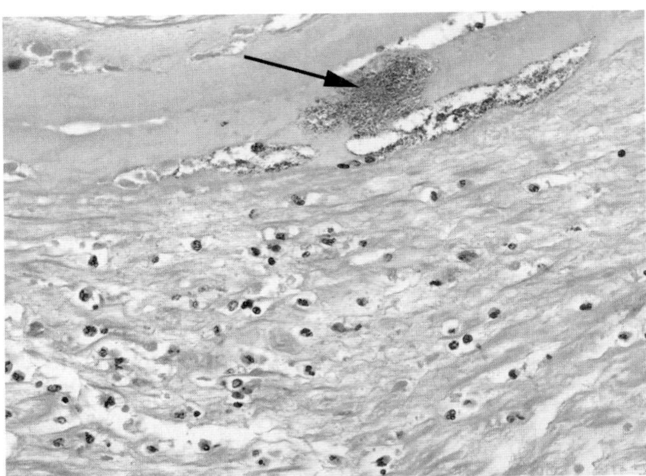

FIGURE 81.13 Chorioamnionitis with abundant bacterial colonies (cocci) present (black arrow). H&E 20×.

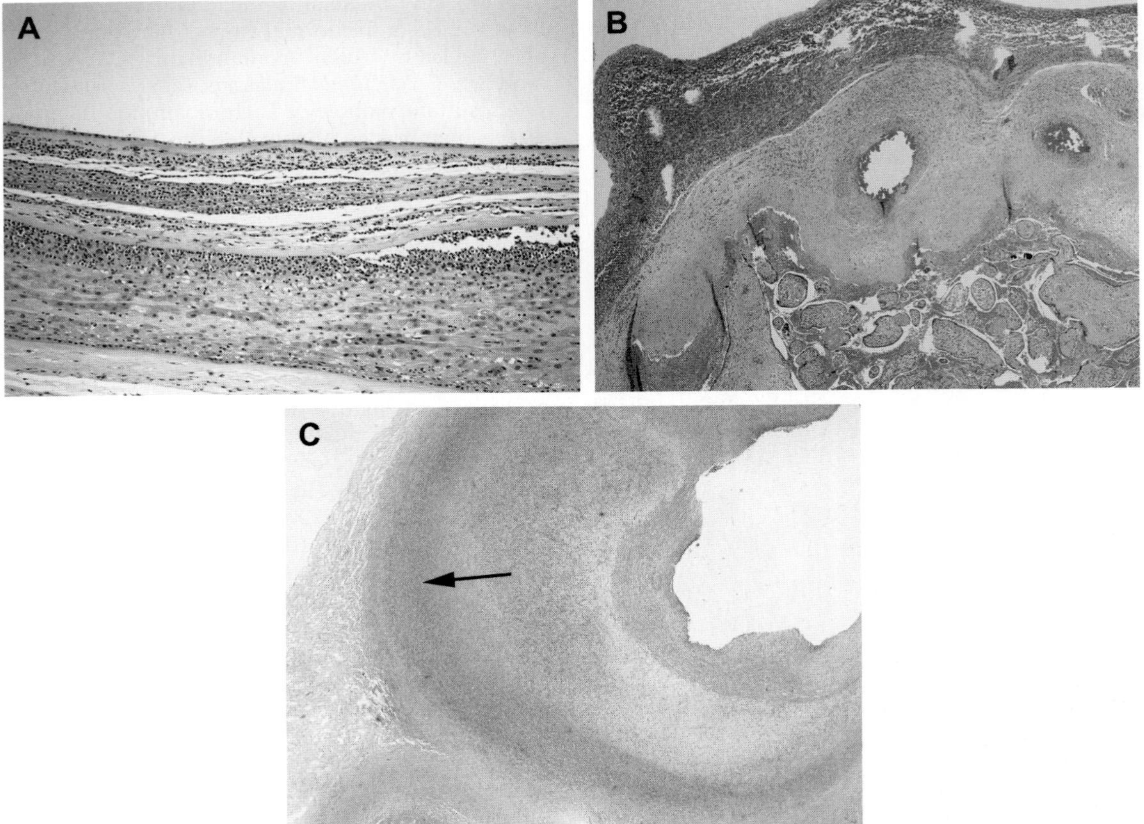

FIGURE 81.12 Acute chorioamnionitis. Membranes (A) and chorionic plate (B) with marked infiltrate of neutrophils. H&E 2×. C. Umbilical vein with necrotizing funisitis (bank of necrotic karyorrhectic debris, black arrow). H&E 2X.

These have been shown to recur (Redline and Abramowsky, 1985), be more common in assisted pregnancies, especially pregnancies conceived by ova-donation (Chan *et al.*, 2007; Gundogan *et al.*, 2009; Styer *et al.*, 2003), and generally be of no clinical significance at term in a placenta with some reserve (normal weight, etc.). For these reasons this typically innocuous chronic villitis is theorized to be a form of immunologically based rejection (maternal vs. fetal allograft). The clinical importance lies in the small recurrence risk (the published recurrence risk of ~30% is much higher than this author's experience of <10%) and related placental insufficiency if diffuse or in an otherwise low placental reserve situation. Usually the relevant villitis is obvious – diffuse, preterm and associated with other signs of fetal compromise like normoblastemia (Redline, 2008c).

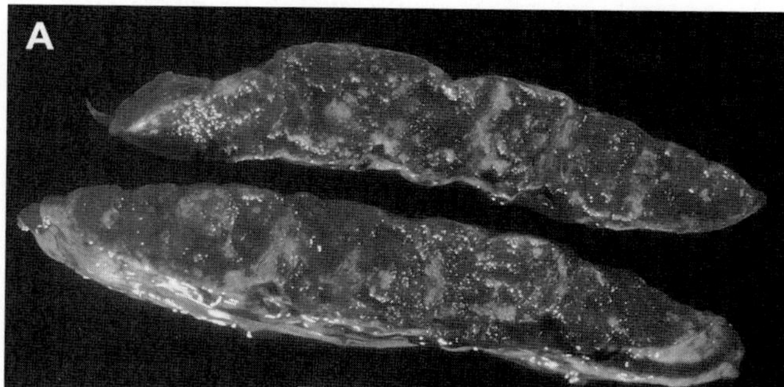

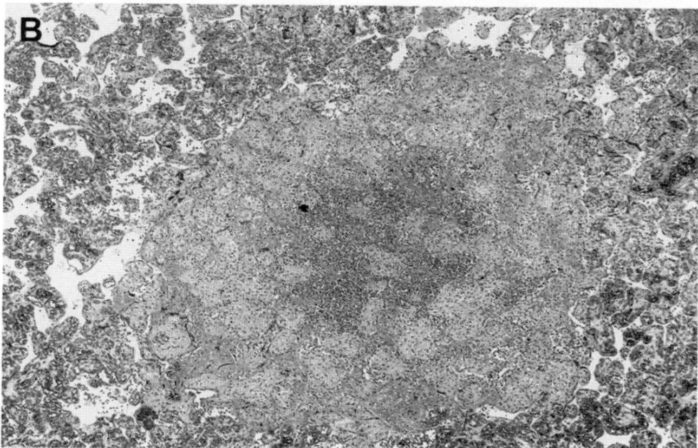

FIGURE 81.14 Placental listeriosis. (A) Gross showing numerous abscesses. (B) Histology with microabscess.

The placental pathology of exposures, whether teratogenic or not, is weak. Most known or suspected teratogens have no effect on placental morphology, therefore the placenta has not helped in suspecting fetal exposures. There are a couple of important exceptions – tobacco inhalation and cocaine.

Maternal tobacco use can affect placental growth and development. The pathologic findings are not characteristic but are highly suggestive and include a small placenta (usually around the 10th percentile for gestational age) with chorangiosis (Figure 81.16). Chorangiosis is an abnormal vascular proliferation in the villi (Altshuler, 1984; Caldarella *et al.*, 2003; Caldwell *et al.*, 1977; De La Ossa *et al.*, 2001; Evers *et al.*, 2003; Gupta *et al.*, 2006; Kaplan, 2007; Ogino and Redline, 2000; Schwartz, 2001; Smith *et al.*, 2003). Most villi at term have 3–5 capillaries and at least one of them is peripheralized and fused to the syncytiotrophoblast. With chorangiosis much more than five vessels are present (I like to use >20 and the villi should be enlarged). Chorangiosis is one of those pathologies that is overdiagnosed. The original manuscript applies a diagnostic rule that the villi in a 10× field have >10 capillaries, there must be at least three fields with the findings and they must be present away from any other relevant pathology (Altshuler, 1984). In my experience, perhaps with the sensationally increased caesarian section rate in the USA, nearly all placentas would meet this criterion. Using a stricter definition – hemangiomatous look to the villi – diffuseness of the finding is needed. Chorangiosis when more strictly applied is most often associated with multigestations, maternal diabetes, high altitude pregnancies, severe and chronic hypoxia, and maternal tobacco use. As most chorangiotic placentas are heavy just due to congestion, a small placenta with chorangiosis is remarkable and suggests maternal tobacco exposure. Maternal smoking has other risks to the fetoplacental unit, including alterations in maternal flow (with a protective effect against the development of pre-eclampsia; Rush *et al.*, 1986; Salafia and Shiverick, 1999; Zhang *et al.*, 1999), increased incidence of abruption (Kaminsky *et al.*, 2007; Lindqvist and Happach, 2006) and other pathologies (Asmussen, 1978; Czekaj *et al.*, 2002; Gupta *et al.*, 1993; Jauniaux and Burton, 2007; Naeye, 1987).

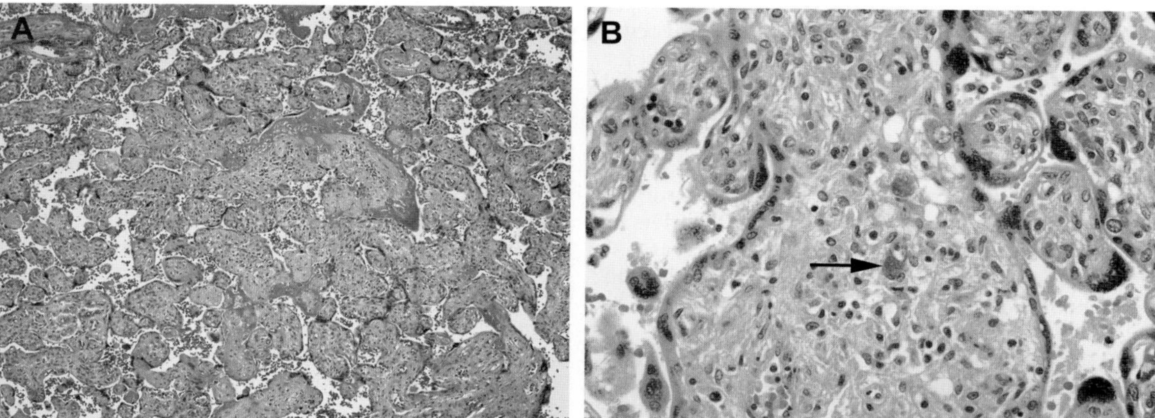

FIGURE 81.15 Chronic villitis. (A) Villitis of unknown etiology: villi with increased mononuclear cells and vascular collapse. H&E 10×. (B) CMV placentitis: chronic villitis, villous expansion, and cytoplasmic inclusions (arrow). H&E 20×.

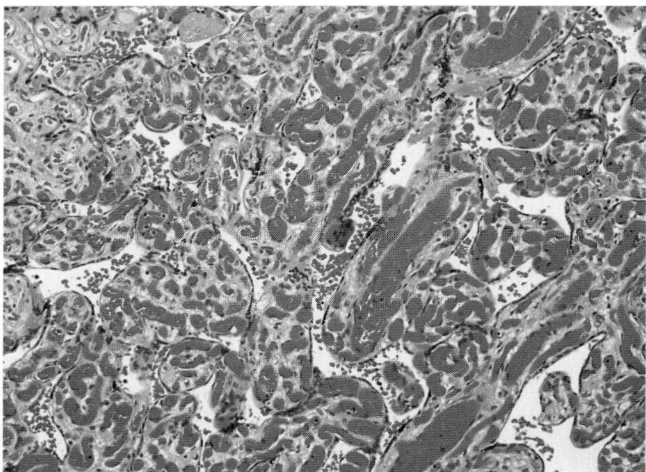

FIGURE 81.16 Chorangiosis. Note the expansion of the villi with numerous small capillaries. H&E 20×.

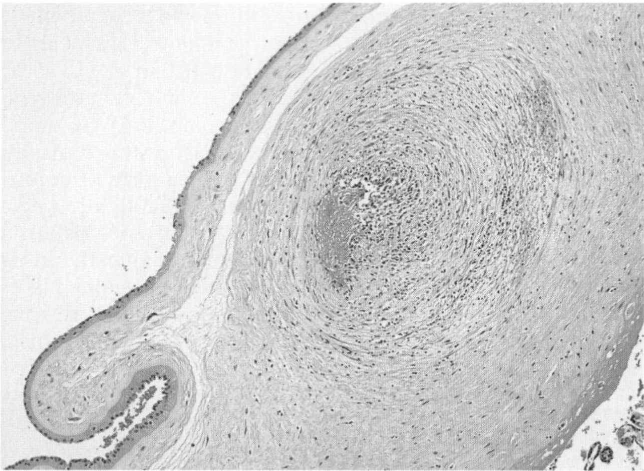

FIGURE 81.17 Eosinophilic T-cell chorionic vasculitis. Chorionic plate vessel with fetal inflammation towards placental disk/away from amniotic cavity. Cells are predominantly mononuclear lymphocytes and eosinophils. H&E 20×.

FETAL PATHOLOGIES OF THE PLACENTA

The fetus can affect the placenta as well, although this has been less well examined. Developmentally – the placenta being a fetal organ – clearly placental maldevelopment can be considered a fetal pathology, but we will discuss this below in the section on primary placental pathologies. Herein we will describe effects from the fetus to the placenta. These are via the umbilical flow to the placenta and involve secondary pathologies of inflammation, fetal heart failure, vascular compromise and hematogenous malignancies.

Evidence of inflammatory pathology of the fetus in the placenta was discussed above and typically is a result of infection of the amniotic fluid or another proinflammatory insult. The pathology is of marginating fetal inflammatory cells directionally from vessels in the umbilical cord and/or chorionic plate (Figure 81.12c). Insults other that infectious organisms include meconium (Api *et al.*, 2001; Burgess and Hutchins, 1996; de Beaufort *et al.*, 2003; Keski-Nisula *et al.*, 2000; Korhonen *et al.*, 2003; Lally *et al.*, 1999; Soukka *et al.*, 2002; Straetemans *et al.*, 2003). Prolonged meconium exposure, or "high-concentration" meconium exposure, may result in fetal inflammation and has been associated with a specific finding in the umbilical cord and chorionic plate vessels of an apoptotic-like necrosis of the vascular myocyte ("meconium associated myonecrosis", MAM). (Altshuler *et al.*, 1992; Altshuler and Hyde, 1989; Rosenfeld *et al.*, 2008; Sienko and Altshuler, 1999; Tessler *et al.*, 2008). MAM is classically associated with post-date deliveries of "normal" infants who then demonstrate early onset neurocompromise. This is a rare finding whose predictive value for neurocompromise is uncertain. Other unusual fetal inflammatory disorders of the placenta include eosinophilic T-cell chorionic vasculitis (Fraser and Wright, 2002) in which fetal eosinophils and T cells are pronounced in a localized few vessels, marginating down towards the placental mass not the amniotic fluid (Figure 81.17). The etiology of this lesion remains obscure as does its clinical relevance, and it may fall into the category of fetal–maternal graft vs. host-like phenomenon.

Fetal heart failure from whatever biology (structural malformations, severe anemia, hypoxia, etc.) may be evidenced by edema of the villi (Figure 81.18). This is an ominous finding and suggests very severe fetal insult and has been associated with sentinel events during labor (for example, abruptio placentae; Elsasser *et al.*, 2010; Salafia *et al.*, 1995b) and the development of significant neurocompromise (Redline, 2008b; Redline *et al.*, 1998, 2007b). The pathology is both evidence of severe heart failure and exacerbation of heart failure by the edematous compression of the placental capillary bed increasing the cardiac afterload (resistance) therefore increasing cardiac failure. Often seen in non-acute situations is a finding termed "hemorrhagic endovasculitis" (HEV) (Altemani and Sarian, 1995; Sander, 1992), in which the placental endothelium sloughs due to hypoxia giving the placental vessels a characteristic look. The result of the sloughed endothelium gives the vessels a false appearance of being recently thrombosed with extravasated red blood cells (Figure 81.19). In stillbirths this finding is diffuse and likely the result of terminal hypoxia and heart failure. In live births it is an ominous finding, which I liken to a near-miss stillbirth.

HEV is a diagnosis in the category of fetal thromboembolic vasculopathy (FEV) (Redline and Pappin, 1995), in which damage to the fetal vessels is the pathology. It is obvious that any compromise to the placental vessels will have an affect on the fetus. The vascular compromise may be evidenced by pathology in either or both the placental venous or arterial tree. One can speculate which side is involved by the pattern of pathology. FEV from arterial thromboembolic pathology is evidenced by sclerotic avascular villi associated sometimes with umbilical arterial pathology (occlusive thrombi, necrosis, etc.) whereas venous pathology is more likely to result in HEV and non-occlusive thrombi in chorionic plate vessels or umbilical vein. In my experience the venous side pathologies are more significant for fetal effects including neural injury and IUFD, whereas arterial pathology affects the placenta, resulting in placental compromise and IUGR.

The biology behind FETV involves a lengthy list, but one that needs to be run through clinically. Inflammatory damage due to meconium or chorioamnionitis and fetal heart failure are both important causes of FETCV and are discussed above. Anatomic compromise of the umbilical cord

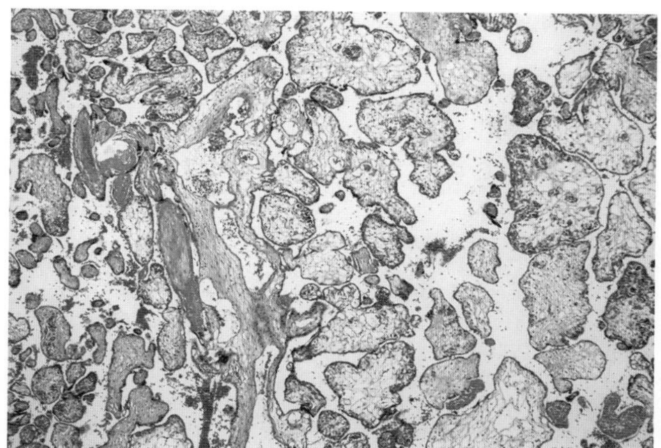

FIGURE 81.18 Marked acute villous edema. H&E 10×.

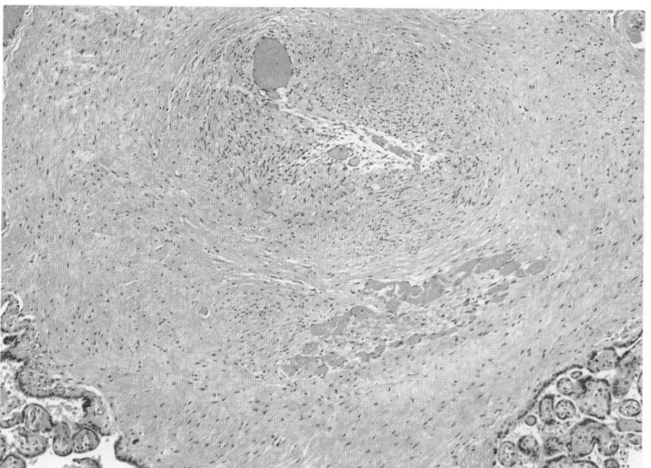

FIGURE 81.19 Hemorrhagic endovasculitis. Stem villous vessels appear re-canalized. H&E 10×.

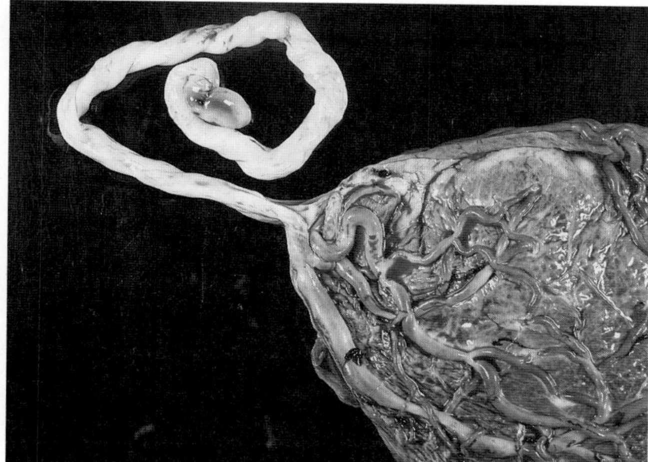

FIGURE 81.20 Gross example of velamentous insertion of the umbilical cord with thrombosed membranous vessels. Please refer to color plate section.

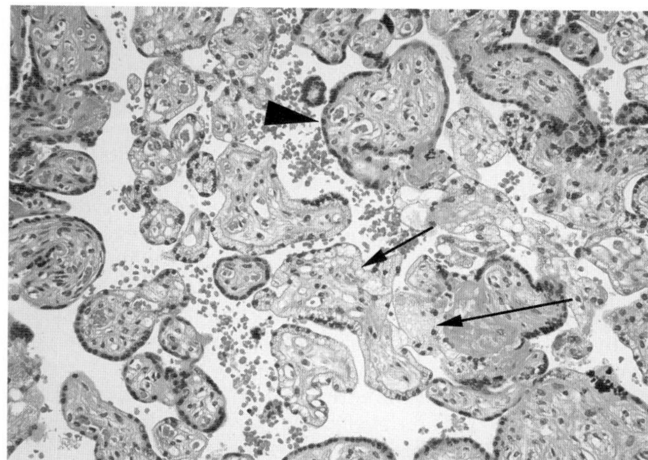

FIGURE 81.21 Inborn error of metabolism. Arrowhead points to normal villous syncytiotrophoblast. Arrows highlight storage material distending the syncytiotrophoblast cytoplasm. H&E 20×. This example was diagnosed after pathologic findings as sialic acid disease.

or velamentous vessels can lead to vascular injury. These include knots of the umbilical cord, cord torsion/kinking and cord prolapse. I would include long umbilical cords in this category as they have more risk for these events as well as increased risk of near failure physically (having to pump and return blood that much further!) (Baergen *et al.*, 2001). Velamenous vessels due to abnormal cord insertion or lobation of the placenta (Figure 81.20) are more easily compressed or damaged by the presenting part and can be the etiology of the FETV. Toxic damage to the vessels via meconium even without the frequently corresponding inflammation can injure the vascular walls, thus their turgidity can lead to vascular compromise and FETV. Fetal hypercoagulable states, for example the high red cell mass occasionally seen in infants of diabetic mothers (Hathaway *et al.*, 1975; Kuhle *et al.*, 2004) or inherited coagulopathies like Factor V Leiden (Vern *et al.*, 2000) may be associated with FETV. Often after exploring this list, the etiology remains obscure. The fetal effects are largely based on the biology behind the FETV, the vascular distribution of the findings (the more diffuse the pathology the more likely the fetal compromise, venous worse than arterial) and the reserve of the placenta itself (small placentas have more significant effects with little pathology or large placentas with multiple pathologies are more likely to affect the fetus).

Fetal constitutional diseases can also manifest in the placenta. Most inborn errors of metabolism present with specific and diagnostic placental findings of foamy storage material in the syncytial trophoblast as well as other cell types in the placenta (Figure 81.21). Placental examination should reveal almost all inborn errors of metabolism and the diagnosis would be made within the first few days of life (Case Records of the Massachusetts General Hospital, 1997; Roberts *et al.*, 1991). The clinical importance cannot be understated. In my experience, these placentally diagnosed cases are index cases without known familial mutations or disease and are the first diagnostic finding.

In some karyotypic anomalies placental findings are characteristic. Certainly in hydatidiform moles, the placenta is diagnostic. Hydatidiform moles are formed by an aberrant fertilization event in which the paternal contribution to the nuclear DNA in the zygote is abnormal. The complete hydatidiform mole results from a meiotic error in the ovum in which meiosis II is abnormal and the maternal pronucleus is lost. The ovum is then fertilized by (usually) two sperm (or theoretically one which endoreduplicates) resulting in a zygote in which all nuclear DNA is paternally derived. This can be demonstrated molecularly (Bifulco *et al.*, 2008; Kihara *et al.*, 2005; Murphy *et al.*, 2009; Sumigama *et al.*, 2007) as well as by immunohistochemistry examining a protein which is normally expressed only off the maternal allele, p57 kip (Castrillon *et al.*, 2001; Chilosi *et al.*, 1998; Fisher *et al.*, 2002; Fukunaga, 2002; Genest *et al.*, 2002; Hoffner *et al.*, 2008; LeGallo *et al.*, 2008; McConnell *et al.*, 2009; Merchant *et al.*, 2005; Sebire *et al.*, 2004). As complete moles do not have maternal DNA, the lack of staining in villous stroma using the antibody is diagnostic. Complete hydatidiform moles are not associated with fetal development and are diagnosed by clinical and pathologic criteria usually in the early first trimester (Table 81.4). The placental tissues are considered malignant due to trophoblastic hyperplasia and atypia and are at significant risk of undergoing transformation to a choriocarcinoma (Sebire *et al.*, 2003). Partial hydatidiform moles are due to polyfertilization or an endoreduplicated sperm which gives a triploid zygote in which the extra-haploid set of nuclear DNA is paternally derived. Although most partial hydatidiform moles are associated with abortive fetal development, live fetuses into the third trimester are known to exist, although dysmorphic with lethal malformations (Figure 81.22a) (Genest, 2001). The placenta in partial hydatidiform moles is maldeveloped with marked irregular dysmorphic villi and syncytiotrophoblastic hyperplasia (Figure 81.22b) (Genest, 2001; Szulman, 1987). The villi have edema and cysternae although not as pronounced as seen in complete hydatidiform moles. Although there is a definite risk for persistence of partial moles (at least chemical – with persistently elevated serum bhcg suggesting persistence of trophoblast) the risk of true malignant behavior is very small (Seckl *et al.*, 2000). Finally, although I believe that the vast majority of partial moles are triploid, not all triploid gestations are partial moles. The development of molar histology and its risk of persistence are limited to those gestations in which the extra-haploid set of nuclear chromosomes is paternal. Maternally derived triploid gestations have a different clinicopathology and are not considered gestational trophoblastic diseases (Chang *et al.*, 2001; Jauniaux, 1999; Murphy *et al.*, 2009; Paradinas, 1998; Rochon and Vekemans, 1990; Sunde *et al.*, 1996).

TABLE 81.4 Molar gestations (Fox, 1997; Fukunaga *et al*, 1995a; Horn and Bilek, 1997)

Complete hydatidiform mole	Partial hydatidiform mole
Diploid or tetraploid	Triploid
Diandric	Extra paternal haploid genome
No fetal development	Fetal development possible – abnormal
Increased risk for choriocarcinoma	Increased risk for persistent bhcg
Excess villous tissue	Excess villous tissue
No umbilical cord/yolk sac	Often yolk sac, rare umbilical cord
Cisterns	Cisterns
Trophoblast hyperplasia all lineages	Trophoblast hyperplasia restricted to syncytiotrophoblast lineage
Round villous contours	Irregular-shaped villous contours
All villi enlarge	Appearance resembling two populations of villi – large and small

Another placental finding that will orient clinical investigation is mesenchymal dysplasia. This is a maldevelopment of the placenta associated with placentomegaly in which the stem villi are enlarged, hydropic (with cisternae), and their vessels are thickened (as are the chorionic plate vessels) (Lage, 1991) (Figure 81.23). The placental findings have been described as a partial hydatidiform mole mimic as there are molar-like enlarged villi and a fetus, yet the fetus/infant does not have the triploid phenotype (Crooij *et al.*, 1985; Feinberg *et al.*, 1988; Teng and Ballon, 1984). This placental phenotype is seen associated with the genetic syndrome Beckwith-Wiedemann (H'Mida *et al.*, 2008; Lage, 1991; Reish *et al.*, 2002; Steele *et al.*, 2002). Beckwith–Weidemann syndrome (BWS) is a non-lethal syndrome comprised of a constellation of features which may include: fetomegaly, macroglossia, omphalocele, hemihypertrophy, congenital and pediatric tumors and adrenal cortical karyomegaly. The genetic disorder is due to overexpression of a maternally imprinted gene/s (therefore paternally expressed) manifested sometime by paternally derived trisomy 11, trisomy 11p or paternal isodisomy 11p (Brown *et al.*, 1992; Junien, 1992; Smith *et al.*, 2007; Waziri *et al.*, 1983). Although not all infants are born with the placental pathology of mesenchymal dysplasia, the association is strong enough that clinical evaluation for the disorder is needed. One of the interesting molecular findings in mesenchymal dysplasia is a paternally enriched placental stromal component (a placental mosaicism in which the villous stromal is diandric) (H'Mida *et al.*, 2008; Kaiser-Rogers *et al.*, 2006).

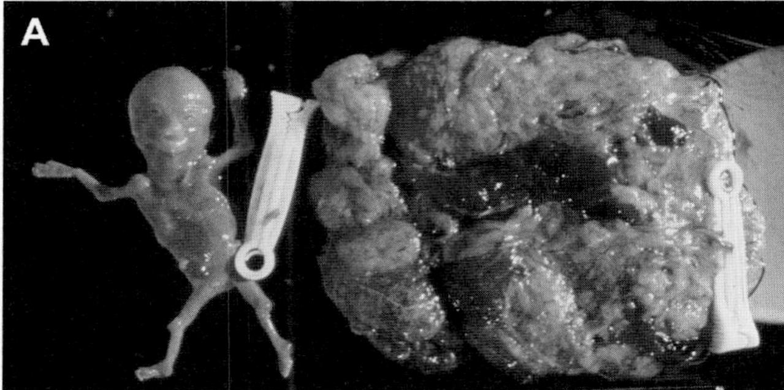

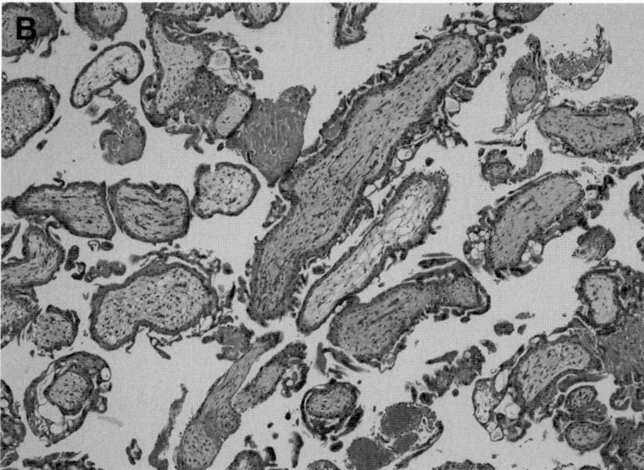

FIGURE 81.22 Triploidy. (A) Gross of a second trimester triploidy/partial hydatidiform mole. Small catechetic fetus with large placenta. Please refer to color plate section. (B) Villi with circumferential syncytiotrophoblastic hyperplasia. H&E 10×.

Trisomy 13 and 18 have also been described as having dysmorphic villi (Cohen *et al.*, 2005; Jauniaux *et al.*, 1998) but these diagnoses are not usually an issue for the placental pathologist. Trisomy 7 and 15 may have some villous dysmorphism (Zaragoza *et al.*, 1998) but since these karyotypes are not associated with fetal development, they present in the first trimester as missed or spontaneous abortions, and are not in the differential diagnosis of placental pathologies at term. Trisomy 21 has been described as having unique placental pathology, with abnormally hypoplastic stem villous vessels leading to an increased risk for hydropic change (Qureshi *et al.*, 1997), although having seen thousands of trisomy 21 placentas I have yet to make this diagnosis. Trisomy 21 fetuses are more likely to have hematopoietic disturbances and these, despite being exceptionally rare, I have seen in the placenta!

Circulating cells at term in the fetal circulation should include only anucleate red blood cells and late stage/immature white blood cells. Anything else is pathology. Hematopoetic malignancies or the pseudo-malignancies seen in association with trisomy 21 can be seen in the placenta. The presence of blast forms in the placenta is often associated with placental and fetal hydrops. The differential diagnosis of any blast forms of circulation includes: severe fetal hypoxic insult, significant fetal anemia (due to a myriad of causes including immune-related, fetal–maternal hemorrhage, parvoviral infection, dyserythropoiesis), and leukemias or leukemoid reactions. The presence of occasional late stage erythroid precursors (normoblasts) is a relatively common finding in any type of significant fetal insult and is therefore non-specific. More than a few normoblasts (10 or more per 10 HPF (Redline, 2008c)) suggests something more ominous. True blast forms of other lineages are distinctly unusual and nearly always associated with a malignancy or trisomy 21. The finding of blasts in the placental circulation is nearly always fatal in my experience. Other congenital malignancies can be hematogenously spread to the placenta, but rarely metastasize (Allen *et al.*, 2007; de Tar and Sanford Biggerstaff, 2006; Doss *et al.*, 1998; Isaacs, 2007; Perkins *et al.*, 1980).

Infants of diabetic mothers in whom insulin resistance is the etiology often have characteristic placental pathologies. The insulin acts as a growth factor to the placenta resulting in heavy placentas (>90th percentile for gestational age) with abnormally prolific vascularization (chorangiosis, Figure 81.16) and moderate villous immaturity with mild dysplasia, so-called distal villous immaturity or delayed villous maturation (Figure 81.24; Burke and Tannenberg, 2007; Kidron *et al.*, 2009; Perez *et al.*, 2009; and see pages 60–61 in Kraus *et al.*, 2004). The increased placental growth and the high glucose load result in fetal overgrowth as well. The diagnosis of diabetic placental pathology can be suggested with these findings even without the clinical diagnosis of maternal diabetes.

PRIMARY PLACENTAL PATHOLOGIES

The placenta itself can be pathologic, although scientists will say that these pathologies can always be partitioned in the maternal or fetal biological camp. I would argue that thinking of them as unique to the placenta is helpful in practice. I would include choriocarcinoma *in situ* and chorangiomas here.

There is one primary malignancy of the placenta – choriocarcinoma. When present only in the placenta it is usually incidental, clinically silent and thus called choriocarcinoma *in situ* (Ariel *et al.*, 2009; Fukunaga *et al.*, 1996, 1995b; Jacques *et al.*, 1998; Jauniaux *et al.*, 1988; Mosher and Genest, 1997; Suh, 1999; Trask *et al.*, 1994). Likely all post-gestational choriocarcinomas are present in the antecedent placenta and if all placentas were examined they would be diagnosed. The presence of malignant trophoblast in infarct-like lesions in the placenta is diagnostic (Figure 81.25) and warrants an investigation into metastatic disease in both the mother and the infant, as it is the only well-documented malignancy that crosses the placenta to the fetus. In my experience, metastatic disease is rare when choriocarcinoma presents in the placenta, but if found is clearly extremely beneficial to the individual. In my experience, these cases are clinically silent and the placenta was examined for independent indications.

Vascular lesions in the placenta are receiving attention as they may have profound implications for the fetus/neonate. The human placental vascular system develops after the villi and vessels form via both vasculogenesis and angiogenesis. Although not experimentally proven, pathologies exist

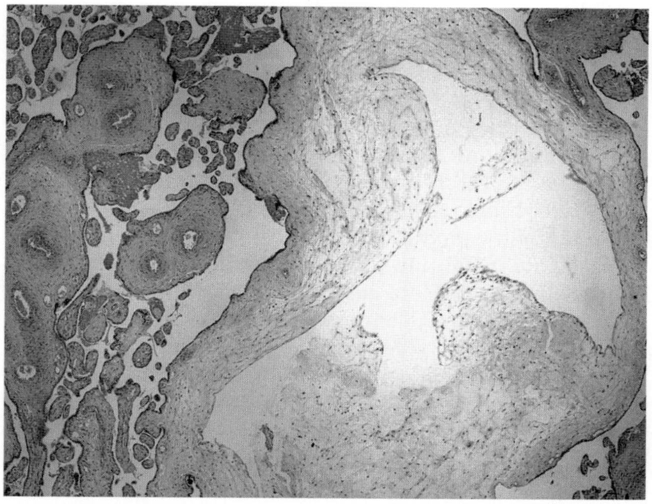

FIGURE 81.23 Mesenchymal dysplasia. Large stem villi with prominent cisternae admixed with normal secondary and tertiary villi. H&E 4×.

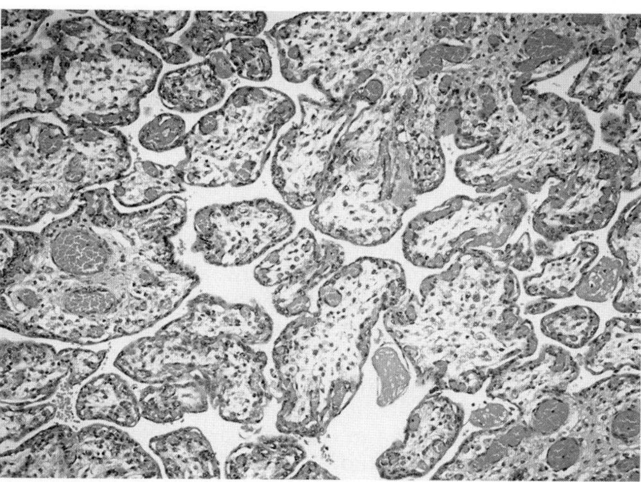

FIGURE 81.24 Diabetic dysplasia. Term placenta with immature appearing large villi. H&E 20×.

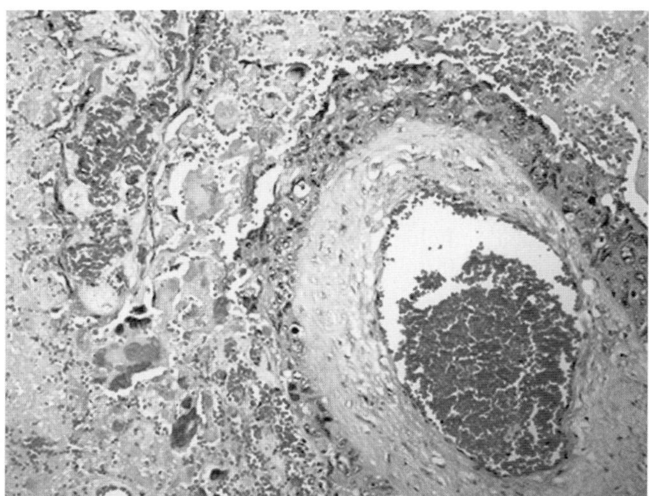

FIGURE 81.25 Choriocarcinoma *in situ*. Malignant circumferential villous trophoblast growing into maternal lakes. Fetal normoblastemia. H&E 20×.

suggestive of placental vascular maldevelopment. Appropriate vascular maturation with the formation of vascular–syncytial membranes between the villous capillary endothelium and the surrounding trophoblastic layer is required for proper placental function. It is likely that primary placental vascular maldevelopment is embryonically lethal.

Probably the best-described vascular lesion of the placenta is the chorangioma, a vascular mass which typically involves a single or a cluster of villi near the chorionic plate (Chopra *et al.*, 2006; Kim *et al.*, 1971; Ogino and Redline, 2000; Sabhikhi *et al.*, 1996). It is unclear if chorangiomas are true neoplasms or maldevelopment (excessive vascular growth without parallel villous growth). These mass-like lesions are associated with vascular lesions in the fetus (Barnes *et al.*, 2007; Hoeger *et al.*, 2009; Lo *et al.*, 2009; Mulliken *et al.*, 2004) as well as morbidity due to flow-related pathologies: anemia, thrombocytopenia and "high output" heart failure. The presence and severity of the fetal consequences are related to the size of the chorangioma, with 5 cm or so being the cut-off (Batukan *et al.*, 2001). There are lesions that suggest a spectrum of associated pathologies with chorangiomatosis and chorangiosis being examples (Ogino and Redline, 2000).

Chorangiomatosis has been defined as stem villous chorangiomas in a large field, not an isolated lesion (Chopra *et al.*, 2006; Ogino and Redline, 2000). The associated morbidity is the same as chorangioma(s) but with the additional, at least potential, compression of the feeding stem villous vessels with the downstream ischemic effect on the associated villi (FETV). A similar lesion, at least in vascular phenotype, is chorangiosis. This is a lesion originally described as affecting distal villi with increased small vessels. Normally the distal/terminal villi have between three and five capillaries. Altschuler's original description of chorangiosis (Altshuler, 1984) describes increased vessel number to more than 10 and provides diagnostic criteria. The etiology of this lesion has been ascribed to a subacute response to placental or fetal hypoxic insult with adaptive angiogenesis. This hypothesis is based on the increase in chorangiosis in placentas from pregnancies in high altitudes (Soma *et al.*, 1995), women with diseases associated with hypoxemia (for example, anemia (Kadyrov *et al.*, 1998), and in my personal experience, the most impressive chorangiosis I diagnosed was in a placenta from a mother with severe peripartum cardiomyopathy presenting with a maternal po2 or 40 and IUFD), and tobacco use during pregnancy (Akbulut *et al.*, 2009; Pfarrer *et al.*, 1999). There is also increased incidence with maternal insulin use (maternal diabetes (Daskalakis *et al.*, 2008)) and in multigestations (Chan *et al.*, 2007; Stroustrup Smith *et al.*, 2003). Perhaps the growth factor effect of insulin is the cause in the former, and the competition for oxygen in multigestations (or a growth factor associated with higher pregnancy factors) for the latter. The finding is relatively common, seen in approximately 10% or so in many series (Redline, 2007) and in my own experience. The original diagnostic criteria may be too generous, and for myself and others, using a more robust increase in vasculature number (more than 20 vessels in most terminal villi) is favored. Diffuse chorangiosis when more strictly defined appears to be a better marker for a significant clinical pathology (usually subacute *in utero* insult, once again from personal experience).

Another primary placental pathology surfacing in the literature includes one which may be important in the still elusively explained etiology for term intrauterine fetal demises (what I like to think of as sudden *fetal* death syndrome – SFDS). Villous maturational arrest/effect (a form of inappropriate villous immaturity) has been associated with SFDS (Burke and Tannenberg, 2007; Kidron *et al.*, 2009; Perez *et al.*, 2009; and see pages 60–61 in Kraus *et al.*, 2004). The hypothesis is that the villous immaturity results in inefficient transfer of gases and nutrients between mother and fetus, such that when the fetal demand exceeds the placental ability to supply, death ensues. As attractive as this theory is, and as desperate as we pathologists are to explain SFDS, the jury is still out both on a reliable and reproducible definition of the placental lesion and on its etiology. The failure of terminal villous maturation may be a maldevelopment of the placenta or may be an adaptation to a teratogen or another insult in the fetal–maternal interaction. We should look forward to more investigation into this lesion in the future.

CONCLUDING REMARKS AND FUTURE DIRECTIONS

The placenta is a still poorly studied organ that may offer significant insights into human reproduction; its immunobiology may answer questions regarding transplant biology (Baricordi *et al.*, 2008; Gorczynski *et al.*, 2002; Mor, 2008; Riley, 2008; Riley and Yokoyama, 2008; Tanaka *et al.*, 2000) and "autoimmune diseases" (Borchers *et al.*, 2010; Klonisch and Drouin, 2009; Lapaire *et al.*, 2007; Lissauer *et al.*, 2007; Reed, 2003; Slavin, 2002), and provide risk assessment into the health of the mother (Eltorky *et al.*, 1995; Folk *et al.*, 2004; Jackisch *et al.*, 2003; Liu and Guo, 2006; Roberts and Oliva, 2006), neonatal (Nelson, 2007; Redline, 2006; Roberts, 2008; Roberts and Oliva, 2006), and the adult outcome from the neonate (Gluckman, 2004; Godfrey, 2000; Henriksen, 2002; Stocker, 2005; Wu, 2004) is broadly defined. One of the hardest issues in placental pathology is determining its pathobiology, with experimentation being frowned on in human reproduction, and human placentation differing so significantly from other mammals that analogies from other mammalian model systems are not that helpful. For example, there does not appear to be any other mammalian animal that develops trophoblastic malignancies and pre-eclampsia/toxemia still has no animal model that recapitulates all the important symptoms seen in humans. We are left with translational studies, and even these are limited. Examination of the placenta is still rare, even in developed countries, therefore we do not have an ongoing set of "normal" placentas for correlative controls, and probably most limiting is that medical/behavioral/educational follow-up on the infant is very difficult to obtain. Given these complications, studies are biased by ascertainment and by lack of appropriate controls. Let us hope that the future brings a revitalized interest in the placenta and novel approaches to its investigation.

REFERENCES

Aaltonen R, Heikkinen T, Hakala K, Laine K, Alanen A (2005) Transfer of proinflammatory cytokines across term placenta. *Obstet Gynecol* **106:** 802–7.

Akbulut M, Sorkun HC, Bir F, Eralp A, Duzcan E (2009) Chorangiosis: the potential role of smoking and air pollution. *Pathol Res Pract* **205:** 75–81.

Al-Adnani M, Kiho L, Scheimberg I (2007) Maternal pancreatic carcinoma metastatic to the placenta: a case report and literature review. *Pediatr Dev Pathol* **10:** 61–5.

Al-Harthi L, Guilbert LJ, Hoxie JA, Landay A (2002) Trophoblasts are productively infected by CD4-independent isolate of HIV type 1. *AIDS Res Hum Retroviruses* **18:** 13–17.

Allen AT, Dress AF, Moore WF (2007) Mirror syndrome resulting from metastatic congenital neuroblastoma. *Int J Gynecol Pathol* **26:** 310–12.

Altemani AM, Sarian MZ (1995) Hemorrhagic endovasculitis of the placenta. A clinical–pathological study in Brazil. *J Perinat Med* **23:** 359–63.

Althabe O, Labarrere C (1985) Chronic villitis of unknown aetiology and intrauterine growth-retarded infants of normal and low ponderal index. *Placenta* **6:** 369–73.

Altman JF, Lowe L, Redman B, Esper P, Schwartz JL, Johnson TM, Haefner HK (2003) Placental metastasis of maternal melanoma. *J Am Acad Dermatol* **49:** 1150–4.

Altshuler G (1984) Chorangiosis. An important placental sign of neonatal morbidity and mortality. *Arch Pathol Lab Med* **108:** 71–4.

Altshuler G (1996) Role of the placenta in perinatal pathology (revisited). *Pediatr Pathol Lab Med* **16:** 207–33.

Altshuler G, Arizawa M, Molnar-Nadasdy G (1992) Meconium-induced umbilical cord vascular necrosis and ulceration: a potential link between the placenta and poor pregnancy outcome. *Obstet Gynecol* **79:** 760–6.

Altshuler G, Hyde S (1989) Meconium-induced vasocontraction: a potential cause of cerebral and other fetal hypoperfusion and of poor pregnancy outcome. *J Child Neurol* **4:** 137–42.

Andres RL, Kuyper W, Resnik R, Piacquadio KM, Benirschke K (1990) The association of maternal floor infarction of the placenta with adverse perinatal outcome. *Am J Obstet Gynecol* **163:** 935–8.

Andrews WW, Cliver SP, Biasini F, Peralta-Carcelen AM, Rector R, Alriksson-Schmidt AI, Faye-Petersen O, Carlo W, Goldenberg R, Hauth JC (2008) Early preterm birth: association between in utero exposure to acute inflammation and severe neurodevelopmental disability at 6 years of age. *Am J Obstet Gynecol* **198:** 466 e1–466 e11.

Api A, Olguner M, Hakguder G, Ates O, Ozer E, Akgur FM (2001) Intestinal damage in gastroschisis correlates with the concentration of intraamniotic meconium. *J Pediatr Surg* **36:** 1811–15.

Arias F, Romero R, Joist H, Kraus FT (1998) Thrombophilia: a mechanism of disease in women with adverse pregnancy outcome and thrombotic lesions in the placenta. *J Matern Fetal Med* **7:** 277–86.

Ariel I, Anteby E, Hamani Y, Redline RW (2004) Placental pathology in fetal thrombophilia. *Hum Pathol* **35:** 729–33.

Ariel I Boldes R, Weintraub A, Reinus C, Beller U, Arbel R (2009) Chorangiocarcinoma: a case report and review of the literature. *Int J Gynecol Pathol* **28:** 267–71.

Asmussen I (1978) Arterial changes in infants of smoking mothers. *Postgrad Med J* **54:** 200–5.

Baergen RN, Malicki D, Behling C, Benirschke K (2001) Morbidity, mortality, and placental pathology in excessively long umbilical cords: retrospective study. *Pediatr Dev Pathol* **4:** 144–53.

Baldwin VJ, MacLeod PM, Benirschke K (1982) Placental findings in alcohol abuse in pregnancy. *Birth Defects Orig Artic Ser* **18:** 89–94.

Bane AL, Gillan JE (2003) Massive perivillous fibrinoid causing recurrent placental failure. *Bjog* **110:** 292–5.

Baricordi OR, Stignani M, Melchiorri L, Rizzo R (2008) HLA-G and inflammatory diseases. *Inflamm Allergy Drug Targets* **7:** 67–74.

Barnes CM, Christison-Lagay EA, Folkman J (2007) The placenta theory and the origin of infantile hemangioma. *Lymphat Res Biol* **5:** 245–55.

Bashiri A, Burstein E, Mazor M (2006) Cerebral palsy and fetal inflammatory response syndrome: a review. *J Perinat Med* **34:** 5–12.

Batukan C, Holzgreve W, Danzer E, Bruder E, Hosli I, Tercanli S (2001) Large placental chorioangioma as a cause of sudden intrauterine fetal death. A case report. *Fetal Diagn Ther* **16:** 394–7.

Baumwell S, Karumanchi SA (2007) Pre-eclampsia: clinical manifestations and molecular mechanisms. *Nephron Clin Pract* **106:** c72–c81.

Bendon RW, Hommel AB (1996) Maternal floor infarction in autoimmune disease: two cases. *Pediatr Pathol Lab Med* **16:** 293–7.

Berghella V, Buchanan E, Pereira L, Baxter JK (2010) Preconception care. *Obstet Gynecol Surv* **65:** 119–31.

Bifulco C, Johnson C, Hao L, Kermalli H, Bell S, Hui P (2008) Genotypic analysis of hydatidiform mole: an accurate and practical method of diagnosis. *Am J Surg Pathol* **32:** 445–51.

Blackburn S (2008) Cytokines in the perinatal and neonatal periods: selected aspects. *J Perinat Neonatal Nurs* **22:** 187–90.

Boomsma CM, Kavelaars A, Eijkemans MJ, Lentjes EG, Fauser BC, Heijnen CJ, Macklon NS (2009) Endometrial secretion analysis identifies a cytokine profile predictive of pregnancy in IVF. *Hum Reprod* **24:** 1427–35.

Borchers AT, Naguwa SM, Keen CL, Gershwin ME (2010) The implications of autoimmunity and pregnancy. *J Autoimmun* **34:** J287–J299.

Bower C, Stanley FJ (1992) Periconceptional vitamin supplementation and neural tube defects; evidence from a case–control study in Western Australia and a review of recent publications. *J Epidemiol Community Health* **46:** 157–61.

Boyd TK, Redline RW (2000) Chronic histiocytic intervillositis: a placental lesion associated with recurrent reproductive loss. *Hum Pathol* **31:** 1389–96.

Brown KW, Gardner A, Williams JC, Mott MG, McDermott A, Maitland NJ (1992) Paternal origin of 11p15 duplications in the Beckwith-Wiedemann syndrome. A new case and review of the literature. *Cancer Genet Cytogenet* **58:** 66–70.

Burgess AM, Hutchins GM (1996) Inflammation of the lungs, umbilical cord and placenta associated with meconium passage in utero. Review of 123 autopsied cases. *Pathol Res Pract* **192:** 1121–8.

Burke CJ, Tannenberg AE (2007) Intrapartum stillbirths in hospital unrelated to uteroplacental vascular insufficiency. *Pediatr Dev Pathol* **10:** 35–40.

Burton GJ, Jauniaux E (2004) Placental oxidative stress: from miscarriage to preeclampsia. *J Soc Gynecol Investig* **11:** 342–52.

Burton GJ, Jones CJ (2009) Syncytial knots, sprouts, apoptosis, and trophoblast deportation from the human placenta. *Taiwan J Obstet Gynecol* **48:** 28–37.

Burton GJ, Woods AW, Jauniaux E, Kingdom JC (2009) Rheological and physiological consequences of conversion of the maternal spiral arteries for uteroplacental blood flow during human pregnancy. *Placenta* **30:** 473–82.

Caldarella A, Buccoliero AM, Taddei GL (2003) Chorangiosis: report of three cases and review of the literature. *Pathol Res Pract* **199:** 847–50.

Caldwell C, Purohit DM, Levkoff AH, Garvin AJ, Williamson HO, Horger EO (1977) Chorangiosis of the placenta with persistent transitional circulation. *Am J Obstet Gynecol* **127:** 435–36.

Case Records of the Massachusetts General Hospital (1997) Weekly clinicopathological exercises. Case 23-1997. A premature newborn infant with congenital ascites. *N Engl J Med* **337:** 260–7.

Castrillon DH, Sun D, Weremowicz S, Fisher RA, Crum CP, Genest DR (2001) Discrimination of complete hydatidiform mole from its mimics by immunohistochemistry of the paternally imprinted gene product p57KIP2. *Am J Surg Pathol* **25:** 1225–30.

Cetin I, Foidart JM, Miozzo M, Raun T, Jansson T, Tsatsaris V, Reik W, Cross J, Hauguel-de-Mouzon S, Illsley N, *et al.* (2004) Fetal growth restriction: a workshop report. *Placenta* **25:** 753–7.

Chaddha V, Viero S, Huppertz B, Kingdom J (2004) Developmental biology of the placenta and the origins of placental insufficiency. *Semin Fetal Neonatal Med* **9:** 357–69.

Chan OT, Mannino FL, Benirschke K (2007) A retrospective analysis of placentas from twin pregnancies derived from assisted reproductive technology. *Twin Res Hum Genet* **10:** 385–93.

Chang SD, Chu DC, Chen DP, Lin PY, Soong YK (2001) Phenotype II triploid pregnancy and study of the parental origin of the extra set of chromosomes with fluorescence microsatellite analysis: case report. *Chang Gung Med J* **24:** 258–62.

Chilosi M, Piazzola E, Lestani M, Benedetti A, Guasparri I, Granchelli G, Aldovini D, Leonardi E, Pizzolo G, Doglioni C, *et al.* (1998) Differential expression of p57kip2, a maternally imprinted cdk inhibitor, in normal human placenta and gestational trophoblastic disease *Lab Invest* **78:** 269–76.

Chopra A, Iyer VK, Thapar R, Singh N (2006) Diffuse multifocal chorangiomatosis of the placenta with multiple intestinal stenosis of the fetus: combination of rare causes for nonimmune hydrops fetalis. *Indian J Pathol Microbiol* **49:** 600–2.

Cohen MC, Roper EC, Sebire NJ, Stanek J, Anumba DO (2005) Placental mesenchymal dysplasia associated with fetal aneuploidy. *Prenat Diagn* 25: 187–92.

Crooij MJ, Van der Harten JJ, Puyenbroek JI, Van Geijn HP, Arts NF (1985) A partial hydatidiform mole, dispersed throughout the placenta, coexisting with a normal living fetus. Case report. *Br J Obstet Gynaecol* **92:** 104–6.

Cross RG, O'Connor MH, Holland PD (1951) Placental metastasis of a breast carcinoma. *J Obstet Gynaecol Br Emp* **58:** 810–1.

Csoma E, Bacsi A, Liu X, Szabo J, Ebbesen P, Beck Z, Konya J, Andirko I, Nagy E, Toth FD (2002) Human herpesvirus 6 variant a infects human term syncytiotrophoblasts in vitro and induces replication of human immunodeficiency virus type 1 in dually infected cells. *J Med Virol* 67: 67–87.

Czeizel AE (1995) Primary prevention of birth defects by periconceptional care, including multivitamin supplementation. *Baillieres Clin Obstet Gynaecol* **9:** 417–30.

Czekaj P, Palasz A, Lebda-Wyborny T, Nowaczyk-Dura G, Karczewska W, Florek E, Kaminski M (2002) Morphological changes in lungs, placenta, liver and kidneys of pregnant rats exposed to cigarette smoke. *Int Arch Occup Environ Health* **75 (Suppl.):** S27–S35.

Daskalakis G, Marinopoulos S, Krielesi V, Papapanagiotou A, Papantoniou N, Mesogitis S, Antsaklis A (2008) Placental pathology in women with gestational diabetes. *Acta Obstet Gynecol Scand* **87:** 403–7.

David FJ, Autran B, Tran HC, Menu E, Raphael M, Debre P, Hsi BL, Wegman TG, Barre-Sinoussi F, Chaouat G (1992) Human trophoblast cells express CD4 and are permissive for productive infection with HIV-1. *Clin Exp Immunol* **88:** 10–6.

de Araujo MC, Schultz R, Vaz FA, Massad E, Feferbaum R, Ramos JL (1994) A case–control study of histological chorioamnionitis and neonatal infection. *Early Hum Dev* **40:** 51–8.

de Beaufort AJ, Bakker AC, van Tol MJ, Poorthuis BJ, Schrama AJ, Berger HM (2003) Meconium is a source of pro-inflammatory substances and can induce cytokine production in cultured A549 epithelial cells. *Pediatr Res* **54:** 491–5.

De La Ossa MM, Cabello-Inchausti B, Robinson MJ (2001) Placental chorangiosis. *Arch Pathol Lab Med* **125:** 1258.

De Paepe ME, Friedman RM, Gundogan F, Pinar H, Oyer CE (2004) The histologic fetoplacental inflammatory response in fatal perinatal group B-streptococcus infection. *J Perinatol* **24:** 441–5.

de Tar M, Sanford Biggerstaff J (2006) Congenital renal rhabdoid tumor with placental metastases: immunohistochemistry, cytogenetic, and ultrastructural findings. *Pediatr Dev Pathol* **9:** 161–7.

Doss BJ, Greene MF, Hill J, Heffner LJ, Bieber FR, Genest DR (1995) Massive chronic intervillositis associated with recurrent abortions. *Hum Pathol* **26:** 1245–51.

Doss BJ, Vicari J, Jacques SM, Qureshi F (1998) Placental involvement in congenital hepatoblastoma. *Pediatr Dev Pathol* **1:** 538–42.

Elsasser DA, Ananth CV, Prasad V, Vintzileos AM (2010) Diagnosis of placental abruption: relationship between clinical and histopathological findings. *Eur J Obstet Gynecol Reprod Biol* **148:** 125–30.

Eltorky M, Khare VK, Osborne P, Shanklin DR (1995) Placental metastasis from maternal carcinoma. A report of three cases. *J Reprod Med* **40:** 399–403.

Evers IM, Nikkels PG, Sikkema JM, Visser GH (2003) Placental pathology in women with type 1 diabetes and in a control group with normal and large-for-gestational-age infants. *Placenta* **24:** 819–25.

Feinberg RF, Lockwood CJ, Salafia C, Hobbins JC (1988) Sonographic diagnosis of a pregnancy with a diffuse hydatidiform mole and coexistent 46,XX fetus: a case report. *Obstet Gynecol* **72:** 485–8.

Fisher RA, Hodges MD, Rees HC, Sebire NJ, Seckl MJ, Newlands ES, Genest DR, Castrillon DH (2002) The maternally transcribed gene p57(KIP2) (CDNK1C) is abnormally expressed in both androgenetic and biparental complete hydatidiform moles. *Hum Mol Genet* **11:** 3267–72.

Folk JJ, Curioca J, Nosovitch JT, Jr, Silverman RK (2004) Poorly differentiated large cell adenocarcinoma of the lung metastatic to the placenta: a case report. *J Reprod Med* **49:** 395–7.

Fox H (1997) Differential diagnosis of hydatidiform moles. *Gen Diagn Pathol* **143:** 117–25.

Fox SB, Khong TY (1990) Lack of innervation of human umbilical cord. An immunohistological and histochemical study. *Placenta* **11:** 59–62.

Fraser RB, Wright JR Jr (2002) Eosinophilic/T-cell chorionic vasculitis. *Pediatr Dev Pathol* **5:** 350–5.

Fukunaga M (2002) Immunohistochemical characterization of p57(KIP2) expression in early hydatidiform moles. *Hum Pathol* **33:** 1188–92.

Fukunaga M, Endo Y, Ushigome S (1995a) Flow cytometric and clinicopathologic study of 197 hydatidiform moles with special reference to the significance of cytometric aneuploidy and literature review. *Cytometry* **22:** 135–8.

Fukunaga M, Nomura K, Ushigome S (1996) Choriocarcinoma in situ at a first trimester. Report of two cases indicating an origin of trophoblast of a stem villus. *Virchows Arch* **429:** 185–8.

Fukunaga M, Ushigome S, Ishikawa E (1995b) Choriocarcinoma in situ: a case at an early gestational stage. *Histopathology* **27:** 473–6.

Gagnon R, Harding R, Brace RA (2002) Amniotic fluid and fetal urinary responses to severe placental insufficiency in sheep. *Am J Obstet Gynecol* **186:** 1076–84.

Genest DR (2001) Partial hydatidiform mole: clinicopathological features, differential diagnosis, ploidy and molecular studies, and gold standards for diagnosis. *Int J Gynecol Pathol* **20:** 315–22.

Genest DR, Dorfman DM, Castrillon DH (2002) Ploidy and imprinting in hydatidiform moles. Complementary use of flow cytometry and immunohistochemistry of the imprinted gene product p57KIP2 to assist molar classification. *J Reprod Med* **47:** 342–6.

Gersell DJ (1993) Chronic villitis, chronic chorioamnionitis, and maternal floor infarction. *Semin Diagn Pathol* **10:** 251–66.

Gluckman PD, Hanson MA (2004) Maternal constraint of fetal growth and its consequences. *Semin Fetal Neonat Med* **9(5):** 419–25.

Goldberg BB, Alvarado S, Chavez C, Chen BH, Dick LM, Felix RJ, Kao KK, Chambers CD (2006) Prevalence of periconceptional folic acid use and perceived barriers to the postgestation continuance of supplemental folic acid: survey results from a Teratogen Information Service. *Birth Defects Res A Clin Mol Teratol* **76:** 193–9.

Goldenberg RL, Kirby R, Culhane JF (2004) Stillbirth: a review. *J Matern Fetal Neonatal Med* **16:** 79–94.

Goldman-Wohl D, Yagel S (2002) Regulation of trophoblast invasion: from normal implantation to pre-eclampsia. *Mol Cell Endocrinol* **187:** 233–8.

Gomez R, Romero R, Ghezzi F, Yoon BH, Mazor M, Berry SM (1998) The fetal inflammatory response syndrome. *Am J Obstet Gynecol* **179:** 194–202.

Gorczynski RM, Hadidi S, Yu G, Clark DA (2002) The same immunoregulatory molecules contribute to successful pregnancy and transplantation. *Am J Reprod Immunol* **48:** 18–26.

Gotsch F, Romero R, Kusanovic JP, Mazaki-Tovi S, Pineles BL, Erez O, Espinoza J, Hassan SS (2007) The fetal inflammatory response syndrome. *Clin Obstet Gynecol* **50:** 652–83.

Gray CA, Bartol FF, Tarleton BJ, Wiley AA, Johnson GA, Bazer FW, Spencer TE (2001) Developmental biology of uterine glands. *Biol Reprod* **65:** 1311–23.

Grether J.K, Nelson KB, Walsh E, Willoughby RE, Redline RW (2003) Intrauterine exposure to infection and risk of cerebral palsy in very preterm infants. *Arch Pediatr Adolesc Med* **157:** 26–32.

Gundogan F, Bianchi DW, Scherjon SA, Roberts DJ (2009) Placental pathology in egg donor pregnancies. *Fertil Steril* **93(2):** 397–404.

Gupta I, Hillier VF, Edwards JM (1993) Multiple vascular profiles in the umbilical cord; an indication of maternal smoking habits and intrauterine distress. *Placenta* **14:** 117–23.

Gupta R, Nigam S, Arora P, Khurana N, Batra S, Mandal AK (2006) Clinicopathological profile of 12 cases of chorangiosis. *Arch Gynecol Obstet* **274:** 50–3.

H'Mida D, Gribaa M, Yacoubi T, Chaieb A, Adala L, Elghezal H, Saad A (2008) Placental mesenchymal dysplasia with Beckwith-Wiedemann syndrome fetus in the context of biparental and androgenic cell lines. *Placenta* **29:** 454–60.

Hathaway WE, Mahasandana C, Makowski EL (1975) Cord blood coagulation studies in infants of high-risk pregnant women. *Am J Obstet Gynecol* **121:** 51–7.

Heller DS, Moorehouse-Moore C, Skurnick J, Baergen RN (2003) Second-trimester pregnancy loss at an urban hospital. *Infect Dis Obstet Gynecol* **11:** 117–22.

Hladunewich M, Karumanchi SA, Lafayette R (2007) Pathophysiology of the clinical manifestations of preeclampsia. *Clin J Am Soc Nephrol* **2:** 543–9.

Hoeger PH, Maerker JM, Kienast AK, Syed SB, Harper JI (2009) Neonatal haemangiomatosis associated with placental chorioangiomas: report of three cases and review of the literature. *Clin Exp Dermatol* **34:** e78–e80.

Hoffner L, Dunn J, Esposito N, Macpherson T, Surti U (2008) P57KIP2 immunostaining and molecular cytogenetics: combined approach aids in diagnosis of morphologically challenging cases with molar phenotype and in detecting androgenetic cell lines in mosaic/chimeric conceptions. *Hum Pathol* **39:** 63–72.

Holzman C, Lin X, Senagore P, Chung H (2007) Histologic chorioamnionitis and preterm delivery. *Am J Epidemiol* **166:** 786–94.

Horn LC, Bilek K (1997) Histologic classification and staging of gestational trophoblastic disease. *Gen Diagn Pathol* **143:** 87–101.

Isaacs H Jr (2007) Fetal and neonatal hepatic tumors. *J Pediatr Surg* **42:** 1797–803.

Jackisch C, Louwen F, Schwenkhagen A, Karbowski B, Schmid KW, Schneider HP, Holzgreve W (2003) Lung cancer during pregnancy involving the products of conception and a review of the literature. *Arch Gynecol Obstet* **268:** 69–77.

Jacques SM, Qureshi F (1993) Chronic intervillositis of the placenta. *Arch Pathol Lab Med* **117:** 1032–5.

Jacques SM, Qureshi F, Doss BJ, Munkarah A (1998) Intraplacental choriocarcinoma associated with viable pregnancy: pathologic features and implications for the mother and infant. *Pediatr Dev Pathol* **1:** 380–7.

Jauniaux E (1999) Partial moles: from postnatal to prenatal diagnosis. *Placenta* **20:** 379–88.

Jauniaux E, Burton GJ (2007) Morphological and biological effects of maternal exposure to tobacco smoke on the feto–placental unit. *Early Hum Dev* **83:** 699–706.

Jauniaux E, Halder A, Partington C (1998) A case of partial mole associated with trisomy 13. *Ultrasound Obstet Gynecol* **11:** 62–4.

Jauniaux E, Zucker M, Meuris S, Verhest A, Wilkin P, Hustin J (1988) Chorangiocarcinoma: an unusual tumour of the placenta. The missing link? *Placenta* **9:** 607–13.

Jewett JF (1973) Septic induced abortion. *N Engl J Med* **289:** 748–9.

Johnson A, Wapner RJ (1997) Mosaicism: implications for postnatal outcome. *Curr Opin Obstet Gynecol* **9:** 126–35.

Junien C (1992) Beckwith-Wiedemann syndrome, tumourigenesis and imprinting. *Curr Opin Genet Dev* **2:** 431–8.

Kadyrov M, Kosanke G, Kingdom J, Kaufmann P (1998) Increased fetoplacental angiogenesis during first trimester in anaemic women. *Lancet* **352:** 1747–9.

Kaiser-Rogers KA, McFadden DE, Livasy CA, Dansereau J, Jiang R, Knops JF, Lefebvre L, Rao KW, Robinson WP (2006) Androgenetic/biparental mosaicism causes placental mesenchymal dysplasia. *J Med Genet* **43:** 187–92.

Kalousek DK, Barrett IJ, McGillivray BC (1989) Placental mosaicism and intrauterine survival of trisomies 13 and 18. *Am J Hum Genet* **44:** 338–43.

Kaminski M, Rumeau C, Schwartz D (1978) Alcohol consumption in pregnant women and the outcome of pregnancy. *Alcohol Clin Exp Res* **2:** 155–63.

Kaminsky LM, Ananth CV, Prasad V, Nath C, Vintzileos AM (2007) The influence of maternal cigarette smoking on placental pathology in pregnancies complicated by abruption. *Am J Obstet Gynecol* **197:** 275 e1–e5.

Kaplan CG (2007) Fetal and maternal vascular lesions. *Semin Diagn Pathol* **24:** 14–22.

Katz VL, DiTomasso J, Farmer R, Carpenter M (2002) Activated protein C resistance associated with maternal floor infarction treated with low-molecular-weight heparin. *Am J Perinatol* **19:** 273–7.

Katzman PJ, Genest DR (2002) Maternal floor infarction and massive perivillous fibrin deposition: histological definitions, association with intrauterine fetal growth restriction, and risk of recurrence. *Pediatr Dev Pathol* **5:** 159–64.

Keski-Nisula L, Aalto ML, Katila ML, Kirkinen P (2000) Intrauterine inflammation at term: a histopathologic study. *Hum Pathol* **31:** 841–6.

Kesmodel U, Wisborg K, Olsen SF, Henriksen TB, Secher NJ (2002) Moderate alcohol intake in pregnancy and the risk of spontaneous abortion. *Alcohol Alcohol* **37:** 87–92.

Khong TY (2004) Placental vascular development and neonatal outcome. *Semin Neonatol* **9:** 255–63.

Kidron D, Bernheim J, Aviram R (2009) Placental findings contributing to fetal death, a study of 120 stillbirths between 23 and 40 weeks gestation. *Placenta* **30:** 700–4.

Kihara M, Matsui H, Seki K, Nagai Y, Wake N, Sekiya S (2005) Genetic origin and imprinting in hydatidiform moles. Comparison between DNA polymorphism analysis and immunoreactivity of p57KIP2. *J Reprod Med* **50:** 307–12.

Kim CK, Benirschke K, Connolly KS (1971) Chorangioma of the placenta. Chromosomal and electron microscopic studies. *Obstet Gynecol* **37:** 372–6.

Klonisch T, Drouin R (2009) Fetal-maternal exchange of multipotent stem/progenitor cells: microchimerism in diagnosis and disease. *Trends Mol Med* **15:** 510–8.

Koi H, Zhang J, Parry S (2001) The mechanisms of placental viral infection. *Ann NY Acad Sci* **943:** 148–56.

Korhonen K, Soukka H, Halkola L, Peuravuori H, Aho H, Pulkki K, Kero P, Kaapa PO (2003) Meconium induces only localized inflammatory lung injury in piglets. *Pediatr Res* **54:** 192–7.

Kraus FT (2007) Clinical syndromes with variable pathologic features. *Semin Diagn Pathol* **24:** 43–7.

Kraus FT, Redline RW, Gersell DJ, Nelson M, Dicke JM (2004) Placental Pathology: Armed Forces Institute of Pathology.

Kuhle S, Massicotte P, Chan A, Mitchell L (2004) A case series of 72 neonates with renal vein thrombosis. Data from the 1-800-NO-CLOTS Registry. *Thromb Haemost* **92:** 729–33.

Labarrere CA (1988) Acute atherosis. A histopathological hallmark of immune aggression? *Placenta* **9:** 95–108.

Labarrere CA, Faulk WP, McIntyre JA (1989) Villitis in normal term human placentae: frequency of the lesion determined by monoclonal antibody to HLA-DR antigen. *J Reprod Immunol* **16:** 127–35.

Lage JM (1991) Placentomegaly with massive hydrops of placental stem villi, diploid DNA content, and fetal omphaloceles: possible association with Beckwith-Wiedemann syndrome. *Hum Pathol* **22:** 591–7.

Lally KP, Mehall JR, Xue H, Thompson J (1999) Meconium stimulates a proinflammatory response in peritoneal macrophages: implications for meconium peritonitis. *J Pediatr Surg* **34:** 214–17.

Lapaire O, Hosli I, Zanetti-Daellenbach R, Huang D, Jaeggi C, Gatfield-Mergenthaler S, Hahn S, Holzgreve W (2007) Impact of fetal-maternal microchimerism on women's health – a review. *J Matern Fetal Neonatal Med* **20:** 1–5.

LeGallo RD, Stelow EB, Ramirez NC, Atkins KA (2008) Diagnosis of hydatidiform moles using p57 immunohistochemistry and HER2 fluorescent in situ hybridization. *Am J Clin Pathol* **129:** 749–55.

Lestou VS, Kalousek DK (1998) Confined placental mosaicism and intrauterine fetal growth. *Arch Dis Child Fetal Neonatal Ed* **79:** F223–F226.

Leviton A, Allred EN, Kuban KC, Hecht JL, Onderdonk AB, O'Shea TM, Paneth N (2010) Microbiologic and histologic characteristics of the extremely preterm infant's placenta predict white matter damage and later cerebral palsy. The ELGAN study. *Pediatr Res* **67:** 95–101.

Lewis S, Lucas RM, Halliday J, Ponsonby AL (2010) Vitamin D deficiency and pregnancy: From preconception to birth. *Mol Nutr Food Res* **54:** 1092–102.

Lieberman E, Lang JM, Frigoletto F Jr, Richardson DK, Ringer SA, Cohen A (1997) Epidural analgesia, intrapartum fever, and neonatal sepsis evaluation. *Pediatrics* **99:** 415–19.

Lindqvist PG, Happach C (2006) Risk and risk estimation of placental abruption. *Eur J Obstet Gynecol Reprod Biol* **126:** 160–4.

Lissauer D, Piper KP, Moss PA, Kilby MD (2007) Persistence of fetal cells in the mother: friend or foe? *BJOG* **114:** 1321–5.

Liu J, Guo L (2006) Intraplacental choriocarcinoma in a term placenta with both maternal and infantile metastases: a case report and review of the literature. *Gynecol Oncol* **103:** 1147–51.

Lo K, Mihm M, Fay A (2009) Current theories on the pathogenesis of infantile hemangioma. *Semin Ophthalmol* **24:** 172–7.

Lowenthal A, Katz M, Almog Y (2006) Severe reversible myocardial depression in septic abortion. *Acta Obstet Gynecol Scand* **85:** 502–3.

Mandsager NT, Bendon R, Mostello D, Rosenn B, Miodovnik M, Siddiqi TA (1994) Maternal floor infarction of the placenta: prenatal diagnosis and clinical significance. *Obstet Gynecol* **83:** 750–4.

McConnell TG, Murphy KM, Hafez M, Vang R, Ronnett BM (2009) Diagnosis and subclassification of hydatidiform moles using p57 immunohistochemistry and molecular genotyping: validation and prospective analysis in routine and consultation practice settings with development of an algorithmic approach. *Am J Surg Pathol* **33:** 805–17.

Merchant SH, Amin MB, Viswanatha DS, Malhotra RK, Moehlenkamp C, Joste NE (2005) p57KIP2 immunohistochemistry in early molar pregnancies: emphasis on its complementary role in the differential diagnosis of hydropic abortuses. *Hum Pathol* **36:** 180–6.

Miralles R, Hodge R, McParland PC, Field DJ, Bell SC, Taylor DJ, Grant WD, Kotecha S (2005) Relationship between antenatal inflammation and antenatal infection identified by detection of microbial genes by polymerase chain reaction. *Pediatr Res* **57:** 570–7.

Moffett AE, Loke CE, McLaren AE (2006) *The Biology and Pathology of the Trophoblast*. Cambridge, Cambridge University Press.

Mor G (2008) Inflammation and pregnancy: the role of toll-like receptors in trophoblast-immune interaction. *Ann NY Acad Sci* **1127:** 121–8.

Mosher R, Genest DR (1997) Primary intraplacental choriocarcinoma: clinical and pathologic features of seven cases (1967–1996) and discussion of the differential. *J Surg Pathol* **2:** 83–98.

Mulliken JB, Anupindi S, Ezekowitz RA, Mihm MC Jr (2004) Case records of the Massachusetts General Hospital. Weekly clinicopathological exercises. Case 13–2004. A newborn girl with a large cutaneous lesion, thrombocytopenia, and anemia. *N Engl J Med* **350:** 1764–75.

Murphy KM, McConnell TG, Hafez MJ, Vang R, Ronnett BM (2009) Molecular genotyping of hydatidiform moles: analytic validation of a multiplex short tandem repeat assay. *J Mol Diagn* **11:** 598–605.

Naeye RL (1985) Maternal floor infarction. *Hum Pathol* **16:** 823–8.

Naeye RL (1987) Do placental weights have clinical significance? *Hum Pathol* **18:** 387–91.

Nelson KB (2007) Perinatal ischemic stroke. *Stroke* **38:** 742–5.

O'Shea TM, Allred EN, Dammann O, Hirtz D, Kuban KC, Paneth N, Leviton A (2009) The ELGAN study of the brain and related disorders in extremely low gestational age newborns. *Early Hum Dev* **85:** 719–25.

Ogino S, Redline RW (2000) Villous capillary lesions of the placenta: distinctions between chorangioma, chorangiomatosis, and chorangiosis. *Hum Pathol* **31:** 945–54.

Onderdonk AB, Hecht JL, McElrath TF, Delaney ML, Allred EN, Leviton A (2008) Colonization of second-trimester placenta parenchyma. *Am J Obstet Gynecol* 199: 52 e1–52 e10.

Ooe K, Udagawa H (1997) A new type of fulminant group A streptococcal infection in obstetric patients: report of two cases. *Hum Pathol* **28:** 509–12.

Ornoy A (2007) Embryonic oxidative stress as a mechanism of teratogenesis with special emphasis on diabetic embryopathy. *Reprod Toxicol* **24:** 31–41.

Pacora P, Chaiworapongsa T, Maymon E, Kim YM, Gomez R, Yoon BH, Ghezzi F, Berry SM, Qureshi F, Jacques SM, *et al.* (2002) Funisitis and chorionic vasculitis: the histological counterpart of the fetal inflammatory response syndrome. *J Matern Fetal Neonatal Med* **11:** 18–25.

Paradinas FJ (1998) The diagnosis and prognosis of molar pregnancy: the experience of the National Referral Centre in London. *Int J Gynaecol Obstet* **60 (Suppl. 1):** S57–S64.

Parkash V, Morotti RA, Joshi V, Cartun R, Rauch CA, West AB (1998) Immunohistochemical detection of Listeria antigens in the placenta in perinatal listeriosis. *Int J Gynecol Pathol* **17:** 343–50.

Pereira L, Maidji E (2008) Cytomegalovirus infection in the human placenta: maternal immunity and developmentally regulated receptors on trophoblasts converge. *Curr Top Microbiol Immunol* **325:** 383–95.

Perez MH, Boulos T, Stucki P, Cotting J, Osterheld MC, Di Bernardo S (2009) Placental immaturity, endocardial fibroelastosis and fetal hypoxia. *Fetal Diagn Ther* **26:** 107–10.

Perkins DG, Kopp CM, Haust MD (1980) Placental infiltration in congenital neuroblastoma: a case study with ultrastructure. *Histopathology* **4:** 383–9.

Pfarrer C, Macara L, Leiser R, Kingdom J (1999) Adaptive angiogenesis in placentas of heavy smokers. *Lancet* **354:** 303.

Pham T, Steele J, Stayboldt C, Chan L, Benirschke K (2006) Placental mesenchymal dysplasia is associated with high rates of intrauterine growth restriction and fetal demise: a report of 11 new cases and a review of the literature. *Am J Clin Pathol* **126:** 67–78.

Philip J, Alexander JM, Sharma SK, Leveno KJ, McIntire DD, Wiley J (1999) Epidural analgesia during labor and maternal fever. *Anesthesiology* **90:** 1271–5.

Pinar H, Stephens M, Singer DB, Boyd TK, Pflueger SM, Gang DL, Roberts DJ, Sung CJ (2002) Triplet placentas: reference values for weights. *Pediatr Dev Pathol* **5:** 495–8.

Pinar H, Sung CJ, Oyer CE, Singer DB (1996) Reference values for singleton and twin placental weights. *Pediatr Pathol Lab Med* **16:** 901–7.

Potter JF (1969) Metastasis of maternal cancer to placenta and fetus. *Am J Obstet Gynecol* **105:** 645.

Potter JF, Schoeneman M (1970) Metastasis of maternal cancer to the placenta and fetus. *Cancer* **25:** 380–8.

Qumsiyeh MB, Adhvaryu SG, Peters-Brown T, Fry-Mehltretter L, Kath SM, Kay HH (1997) Discrepancies in cytogenetic findings in chorionic villi. *J Matern Fetal Med* **6:** 351–5.

Qureshi F, Jacques SM, Johnson MP, Hume RF Jr, Kramer RL, Yaron Y, Evans MI (1997) Trisomy 21 placentas: histopathological and immunohistochemical findings using proliferating cell nuclear antigen. *Fetal Diagn Ther* **12:** 210–15.

Raspollini MR, Oliva E, Roberts DJ (2007) Placental histopathologic features in patients with thrombophilic mutations. *J Matern Fetal Neonatal Med* **20:** 113–23.

Redline R (2008a) Cerebral palsy in term infants: a clinicopathologic analysis of 158 medicolegal case reviews. *Pediatr Dev Pathol* **11:** 456–64.

Redline R, Minich N, Taylor H, Hack M (2007a) Placental lesions as predictors of cerebral palsy and abnormal neurocognitive function at school age in extremely low birth weight infants (<1 kg). *Pediatr Dev Pathol* **10(4):** 282–92.

Redline RW (2005) Severe fetal placental vascular lesions in term infants with neurologic impairment. *Am J Obstet Gynecol* 192: 452–7.

Redline RW (2006) Placental pathology and cerebral palsy. *Clin Perinatol* **33:** 503–16.

Redline RW (2007) Villitis of unknown etiology: noninfectious chronic villitis in the placenta. *Hum Pathol* **38:** 1439–46.

Redline RW (2008b) Cerebral palsy in term infants: a clinicopathologic analysis of 158 medicolegal case reviews. *Pediatr Dev Pathol* 11: 456–64.

Redline RW (2008c) Elevated circulating fetal nucleated red blood cells and placental pathology in term infants who develop cerebral palsy. *Hum Pathol* **39:** 1378–84.

Redline RW, Abramowsky CR (1985) Clinical and pathologic aspects of recurrent placental villitis. *Hum Pathol* **16:** 727–31.

Redline RW, Boyd T, Campbell V, Hyde S, Kaplan C, Khong TY, Prashner HR, Waters BL (2004) Maternal vascular underperfusion: nosology and reproducibility of placental reaction patterns. *Pediatr Dev Pathol* **7:** 237–49.

Redline RW, Minich N, Taylor HG, Hack M (2007b) Placental lesions as predictors of cerebral palsy and abnormal neurocognitive function at school age in extremely low birth weight infants (<1 kg). *Pediatr Dev Pathol* **10:** 282–92.

Redline RW, O'Riordan MA (2000) Placental lesions associated with cerebral palsy and neurologic impairment following term birth. *Arch Pathol Lab Med* **124:** 1785–91.

Redline RW, Pappin A (1995) Fetal thrombotic vasculopathy: the clinical significance of extensive avascular villi. *Hum Pathol* **26:** 80–5.

Redline RW, Patterson P (1993) Villitis of unknown etiology is associated with major infiltration of fetal tissue by maternal inflammatory cells. *Am J Pathol* **143:** 473–9.

Redline RW, Wilson-Costello D, Borawski E, Fanaroff AA, Hack M (1998) Placental lesions associated with neurologic impairment and cerebral palsy in very low-birth-weight infants. *Arch Pathol Lab Med* **122:** 1091–8.

Redline RW, Wilson-Costello D, Hack M (2002) Placental and other perinatal risk factors for chronic lung disease in very low birth weight infants. *Pediatr Res* **52:** 713–19.

Reed AM (2003) Microchimerism in children with rheumatic disorders: what does it mean? *Curr Rheumatol Rep* **5:** 458–62.

Regnault TR, Galan HL, Parker TA, Anthony RV (2002) Placental development in normal and compromised pregnancies – a review. *Placenta* **23 (Suppl. A):** S119–S129.

Reish O, Lerer I, Amiel A, Heyman E, Herman A, Dolfin T, Abeliovich D (2002) Wiedemann-Beckwith syndrome: further prenatal characterization of the condition. *Am J Med Genet* **107:** 209–13.

Riley JK (2008) Trophoblast immune receptors in maternal–fetal tolerance. *Immunol Invest* **37:** 395–426.

Riley JK, Yokoyama WM (2008) NK cell tolerance and the maternal–fetal interface. *Am J Reprod Immunol* **59:** 371–87.

Roberts DJ (2008) Placental pathology, a survival guide. *Arch Pathol Lab Med* **132:** 641–51.

Roberts DJ, Ampola MG, Lage JM (1991) Diagnosis of unsuspected fetal metabolic storage disease by routine placental examination. *Pediatr Pathol* **11:** 647–56.

Roberts DJ, Oliva E (2006) Clinical significance of placental examination in perinatal medicine. *J Matern Fetal Neonatal Med* **19:** 255–64.

Rochon L, Vekemans MJ (1990) Triploidy arising from a first meiotic nondisjunction in a mother carrying a reciprocal translocation. *J Med Genet* **27:** 724–6.

Rodriguez-Thompson D, Lieberman ES (2001) Use of a random urinary protein-to-creatinine ratio for the diagnosis of significant proteinuria during pregnancy. *Am J Obstet Gynecol* **185:** 808–11.

Romero R, Chaiworapongsa T, Espinoza J (2003) Micronutrients and intrauterine infection, preterm birth and the fetal inflammatory response syndrome. *J Nutr* **133:** 1668S–1673S.

Rosenfeld CR, Zagariya AM, Liu XT, Willis BC, Fluharty S, Vidyasagar D (2008) Meconium increases type 1 angiotensin II receptor expression and alveolar cell death. *Pediatr Res* **63:** 251–6.

Rush D, Kristal A, Blanc W, Navarro C, Chauhan P, Campbell Brown M, Rosso P, Winick M, Brasel J, Naeye R, *et al.* (1986) The effects of maternal cigarette smoking on placental morphology, histomorphometry, and biochemistry. *Am J Perinatol* **3:** 263–72.

Sabhikhi AK, Chaudhury MC, Singh D, Raja LN (1996) Chorangioma of the placenta with hydrops fetalis. *Indian Pediatr* **33:** 520–1.

Salafia C, Shiverick K (1999) Cigarette smoking and pregnancy II: vascular effects. *Placenta* **20:** 273–9.

Salafia CM, Ernst LM, Pezzullo JC, Wolf EJ, Rosenkrantz TS, Vintzileos AM (1995a) The very low birthweight infant: maternal complications leading to preterm birth, placental lesions, and intrauterine growth. *Am J Perinatol* **12:** 106–10.

Salafia CM, Minior VK, Lopez-Zeno JA, Whittington SS, Pezzullo JC, Vintzileos AM (1995b) Relationship between placental histologic features and umbilical cord blood gases in preterm gestations. *Am J Obstet Gynecol* **173:** 1058–64.

Sander CM (1992) Hemorrhagic endovasculitis of the placenta. *Am J Obstet Gynecol* **167:** 1483.

Schendel DE (2001) Infection in pregnancy and cerebral palsy. *J Am Med Womens Assoc* **56:** 105–8.

Schrander-Stumpel C (1999) Preconception care: challenge of the new millennium? *Am J Med Genet* **89:** 58–61.

Schwartz DA (2001) Chorangiosis and its precursors: underdiagnosed placental indicators of chronic fetal hypoxia. *Obstet Gynecol Surv* **56:** 523–5.

Scotchie JG, Fritz MA, Mocanu M, Lessey BA, Young SL (2009) Proteomic analysis of the luteal endometrial secretome. *Reprod Sci* **16:** 883–93.

Sebire NJ, Makrydimas G, Agnantis NJ, Zagorianakou N, Rees H, Fisher RA (2003) Updated diagnostic criteria for partial and complete hydatidiform moles in early pregnancy. *Anticancer Res* **23:** 1723–8.

Sebire NJ, Rees HC, Peston D, Seckl MJ, Newlands ES, Fisher RA (2004) p57(KIP2) immunohistochemical staining of gestational trophoblastic tumours does not identify the type of the causative pregnancy. *Histopathology* **45:** 135–41.

Seckl MJ, Fisher RA, Salerno G, Rees H, Paradinas FJ, Foskett M, Newlands ES (2000) Choriocarcinoma and partial hydatidiform moles. *Lancet* **356:** 36–9.

Sheppard BL, Bonnar J (1999) Uteroplacental hemostasis in intrauterine fetal growth retardation. *Semin Thromb Hemost* **25:** 443–6.

Shuhaila A, Rohaizak M, Phang KS, Mahdy ZA (2008) Maternal melanoma with placental metastasis. *Singapore Med J* **49:** e71–e72.

Sienko A, Altshuler G (1999) Meconium-induced umbilical vascular necrosis in abortuses and fetuses: a histopathologic study for cytokines. *Obstet Gynecol* **94:** 415–20.

Slavin S (2002) Maternal–fetal relationship, natural chimerism and bilateral transplantation tolerance as the basis for non-myeloablative stem cell transplantation. *Int J Hematol* **76 (Suppl. 1):** 172–5.

Smith AC, Choufani S, Ferreira JC, Weksberg R (2007) Growth regulation, imprinted genes, and chromosome 11p15.5. *Pediatr Res* **61:** 43R–47R.

Smith AS, Huang WY, Wong G, Levine D (2003) Placental chorangiosis associated with markedly elevated maternal chorionic gonadotropin. A case report. *J Reprod Med* **48:** 827–30.

Smulian JC, Shen-Schwarz S, Vintzileos AM, Lake MF, Ananth CV (1999) Clinical chorioamnionitis and histologic placental inflammation. *Obstet Gynecol* **94:** 1000–5.

Soma H, Watanabe Y, Hata T (1995) Chorangiosis and chorangioma in three cohorts of placentas from Nepal, Tibet, and Japan. *Reprod Fertil Dev* **7:** 1533–8.

Soukka HR, Ahotupa M, Ruutu M, Kaapa PO (2002) Meconium stimulates neutrophil oxidative burst. *Am J Perinatol* **19:** 279–84.

Srinivas SK, Ma Y, Sammel MD, Chou D, McGrath C, Parry S, Elovitz MA (2006) Placental inflammation and viral infection are implicated in second trimester pregnancy loss. *Am J Obstet Gynecol* **195:** 797–802.

Steele EK, Johnston KM, Parker MJ (2002) A rare but distinctive placental lesion associated with Beckwith-Wiedemann syndrome. *J Obstet Gynaecol* **22:** 90–1.

Stella CL, How HY, Sibai BM (2006) Thrombophilia and adverse maternal–perinatal outcome: controversies in screening and management. *Am J Perinatol* **23:** 499–506.

Stoler JM, Huntington KS, Peterson CM, Peterson KP, Daniel P, Aboagye KK, Lieberman E, Ryan L, Holmes LB (1998) The prenatal detection of significant alcohol exposure with maternal blood markers. *J Pediatr* **133:** 346–52.

Straetemans M, Schonbeck Y, Engel JA, Zielhuis GA (2003) Meconium-stained amniotic fluid is not a risk factor for otitis media. *Eur Arch Otorhinolaryngol* **260:** 432–5.

Stroustrup Smith A, Huang WY, Wong G, Levine D (2003) Placental chorangiosis associated with markedly elevated maternal chorionic gonadotropin. A case report. *J Reprod Med* **48:** 827–30.

Styer AK, Parker HJ, Roberts DJ, Palmer-Toy D, Toth TL, Ecker JL (2003) Placental villitis of unclear etiology during ovum donor in vitro fertilization pregnancy. *Am J Obstet Gynecol* **189:** 1184–6.

Suh YK (1999) Placental pathology casebook. Choriocarcinoma in situ of placenta associated with transplacental hemorrhage. *J Perinatol* **19:** 153–4.

Sumigama S, Itakura A, Yamamoto T, Nagasaka T, Yamamoto E, Ino K, Kikkawa F (2007) Genetically identified complete hydatidiform mole coexisting with a live twin fetus: comparison with conventional diagnosis. *Gynecol Obstet Invest* **64:** 228–31.

Sunde L, Mogensen B, Olsen S, Nielsen V, Christensen IJ, Bolund L (1996) Flow cytometric DNA analyses of 105 fresh hydatidiform moles, with correlations to prognosis. *Anal Cell Pathol* **12:** 99–114.

Svigos JM (2001) The fetal inflammatory response syndrome and cerebral palsy: yet another challenge and dilemma for the obstetrician. *Aust NZ J Obstet Gynaecol* **41:** 170–6.

Szulman AE (1987) Clinicopathologic features of partial hydatidiform mole. *J Reprod Med* **32:** 640–3.

Tabata T, McDonagh S, Kawakatsu H, Pereira L (2007) Cytotrophoblasts infected with a pathogenic human cytomegalovirus strain dysregulate cell-matrix and cell–cell adhesion molecules: a quantitative analysis. *Placenta* **28:** 527–37.

Tanaka A, Lindor K, Ansari A, Gershwin ME (2000) Fetal microchimerisms in the mother: immunologic implications. *Liver Transpl* **6:** 138–43.

Teng NN, Ballon SC (1984) Partial hydatidiform mole with diploid karyotype: report of three cases. *Am J Obstet Gynecol* **150:** 961–4.

Tenney B, Parker F (1940) The placenta in toxemia of pregnancy. *Am J Obstet Gynecol* **39:** 1000–5.

Tessler R, Pan J, Fiori HH, Belik J (2008) Human meconium has a pulmonary vascular and airway smooth muscle relaxant effect. *Pediatr Res* **64:** 24–8.

Trask C, Lage JM, Roberts DJ (1994) A second case of “chorangiocarcinoma” presenting in a term asymptomatic twin pregnancy: choriocarcinoma in situ with associated villous vascular proliferation. *Int J Gynecol Pathol* **13:** 87–91.

Tycko B (2006) Imprinted genes in placental growth and obstetric disorders. *Cytogenet Genome Res* **113:** 271–8.

Van Dyke DC, Stumbo PJ, Mary JB, Niebyl JR (2002) Folic acid and prevention of birth defects. *Dev Med Child Neurol* **44:** 426–9.

Vern TZ, Alles AJ, Kowal-Vern A, Longtine J, Roberts DJ (2000) Frequency of factor V(Leiden) and prothrombin G20210A in placentas and their relationship with placental lesions. *Hum Pathol* **31:** 1036–43.

Vernof KK, Benirschke K, Kephart GM, Wasmoen TL, Gleich GJ (1992) Maternal floor infarction: relationship to X cells, major basic protein, and adverse perinatal outcome. *Am J Obstet Gynecol* **167:** 1355–63.

Waters BL, Ashikaga T (2006) Significance of perivillous fibrin/oid deposition in uterine evacuation specimens. *Am J Surg Pathol* **30:** 760–5.

Waziri M, Patil SR, Hanson JW, Bartley JA (1983) Abnormality of chromosome 11 in patients with features of Beckwith-Wiedemann syndrome. *J Pediatr* **102:** 873–6.

Weber MA, Nikkels PG, Hamoen K, Duvekot JJ, de Krijger RR (2006) Co-occurrence of massive perivillous fibrin deposition and chronic intervillositis: case report. *Pediatr Dev Pathol* **9:** 234–8.

Yerby MS (2003) Clinical care of pregnant women with epilepsy: neural tube defects and folic acid supplementation. *Epilepsia* **44 (Suppl. 3):** 33–40.

Yoon BH, Park CW, Chaiworapongsa T (2003) Intrauterine infection and the development of cerebral palsy. *BJOG* **110 (Suppl. 20):** 124–7.

Zaragoza MV, Millie E, Redline RW, Hassold TJ (1998) Studies of non-disjunction in trisomies 2, 7, 15, and 22: does the parental origin of trisomy influence placental morphology? *J Med Genet* **35:** 924–31.

Zhang J, Klebanoff MA, Levine, RJ, Puri M, Moyer P (1999) The puzzling association between smoking and hypertension during pregnancy. *Am J Obstet Gynecol* **181:** 1407–13.

Zhang P, Schmidt M, Cook L (2006) Maternal vasculopathy and histologic diagnosis of preeclampsia: poor correlation of histologic changes and clinical manifestation. *Am J Obstet Gynecol* **194:** 1050–6.

Section 15

Domestic, Wildlife and Aquatic Species

CHAPTER

82

Reproductive and developmental toxicity in avian species

Robert W. Coppock and Margitta M. Dziwenka

INTRODUCTION

Wild birds are exposed to environmental chemicals that alter reproductive performance and cause terata (Bosveld and van den Berg, 2002; Ottinger *et al.*, 2009). Birds, especially migratory birds, can feed over a wide geographic area. Wild birds are sentinels of environmental safety because they share our environment and many are high trophic feeders. Birds have developed different strategies to allow them to use a variety of habitats. They use unique physiological mechanisms for sexual differentiation, reproduction and ontogenic differences, for example the differences in maturity at hatching for precocial and altricial birds. Persistent organic pollutants (POPs) have been shown to be endocrine disrupting substances (EDCs) and teratogenic in wild birds. Reproduction in birds is both metabolically and physically demanding. During the nesting season many birds must also deal with the dynamics of climate, and temporal changes in the kinds and supply of feedstuffs available. The timing of migration, establishing nesting areas, courtship, nest building, mating and egg laying is important for successful reproductive outcomes. The endocrine system of birds, like other vertebrate species, is highly integrated and disruption of one component has significant consequences on homeostasis. Disruption of thyroid function during incubation can cause terata. Reproductive disruptions in birds can affect all stages of reproduction starting with behavioral changes, production of abnormal eggs, eggshell thinning, and epigenetic and teratogenic effects that persist into adult life (Giesy *et al.*, 1994; Fry, 1995; Jenssen *et al.*, 2010).

SKELETAL DEFECTS

Skeletal defects in birds can affect mobility, feeding and possibly durability in combat and defense. Abnormalities were observed in the chicks of fish-eating birds and linked to certain POPs especially the polyhalogenated aromatic hydrocarbons (Giesy *et al.*, 1994). Thyroid function in birds and other vertebrate species is important in reproduction and development (McNabb, 2007). Brain and skeletal development can be impaired with POPs that target thyroid function. The wildlife annual performance reports noted a decline in the Foster's turn (*Sterna forsteri*) population in Green Bay, Lake Michigan, and scientific studies were subsequently reported (Hoffman *et al.*, 1987; Kubiak *et al.*, 1989). The terns at the Green Bay sites had decreased populations without eggshell thinning, a decrease in hatchability and an increase in congenital defects. Increases in congenital deformities in chicks of fish-eating birds were reported in the 1960s and 1970s (Gilbertson, 1983; Gilbertson *et al.*, 1991). Fish-eating birds in the lower Great Lakes showed abnormally large occurrences of congenital deformities in chicks of black-crowned night-herons (*Nycticorax nycticorax*), herring gulls (*Larus argentatus*), ring-billed gulls (*L. delawarensis*), common terns (*Sterna hirundo*) and Caspian terns (*Hydroprogne caspia*) (Gilbertson *et al.*, 1976, 1991). There was a shift from low reproductive success due to DDE-linked eggshell thinning to a syndrome resembling chick edema. In areas contaminated with PCBs, reproductive success decreased and congenital defects in chicks and unhatched embryos increased. Studies of herring gull chicks from areas with high POPs found that congenital defects were increased 100 to 200 times (Peakall and Fox, 1987). Congenital defects in chicks included beak and mandibular defects, eye defects, skull defects, leg abnormalities, inability to walk and other musculoskeletal deformities, and altered feather growth. Edema and other pathology, growth retardation, cytochrome p450 enzyme induction, were observed. These observations were similar to chick edema disease observed in domestic poultry, which had been linked to TCDD, PCDF and PCBs in poultry feed (Firestone, 1973; McKinney *et al.*, 1976). The disease syndrome in fish-eating birds was named Great Lakes embryo mortality, edema and deformities syndrome (Gilbertson *et al.*, 1991). A rickets-like syndrome was observed in gray heron nestlings (Thompson *et al.*, 2006). The heron nestlings showed fractures of the tarsus and tibia due to low mineralization. Tissue levels of TCDD, PCBs and PCDFs were high.

High selenium in agricultural water used for wetland management was identified as the most likely cause of embryonic mortality and terata in nesting aquatic birds (Ohlendorf *et al.*, 1986, 1988). Malformations observed were anophthalmia and microphthalmia, micromelia and amelia,

Reproductive and Developmental Toxicology, Edited by Ramesh C. Gupta
ISBN: 978-0-12-382032-7

ectrodactyly and clubfoot, beaks that were missing, reduced or crossed, other skeletal defects, and hydrocephaly and exencephaly. The hearts in some embryos were considered to be abnormal. Species studied were American coot (*Fulica americana*), mallard (*Anas platyrhynchos*), northern pintail (*A. acuta*), cinnamon teal (*A. cyanoptera*), gadwall (*A. strepera*), black-necked stilt (*Himantopus mexicanus*), American avocet (*Recurvirostra americana*) and eared grebe (*Podiceps nigricollis*). The species with the most reduction in viable hatchlings were eared grebe and American coot.

Species differences exist in sensitivity of birds to TCDD. The wood duck is reasonably tolerant to TCDD (Augspurger *et al.*, 2008). Debates also exist as to the causation of skeletal defects in birds. Screech owls have been observed to have congenital leg defects (Albers *et al.*, 2001). The owls had increased radioactivity from the uptake of radioactive cesium. The female had a leg deformity and this trait was also passed on to some of the owlets when the female was mated with a different male. The trait was considered to be heterozygous dominant and not related to radiation. The owls were not tested for thyroid function and POPs. Inheritable radiation-induced mutation may also have occurred. There is evidence to support that the majority of skeletal deformities are not compatible with survival in wild birds.

SOFT TISSUE DEFECTS

Nervous system

The PCBs, PCDDs and PCDFs are known to cause neurologic terata in wild birds. These POPs have been associated with brain asymmetry in herons and cormorants (Henshel *et al.*, 1995, 1997; Custer *et al.*, 2001). Brain symmetry was studied in wild blue heron in British Columbia. A high occurrence of intercerebral asymmetry was observed. Intercerebral asymmetry was significantly correlated with TCDD and TCDD-TEQs (toxic equivalence factors) levels in eggs taken from the same nest. The occurrences of intercerebral asymmetry decreased with decreasing levels of TCDD and TCDD-TEQs. The TEQ correlated best with depth measurements that included the anterior hypothalamus. Preliminary histological evaluation of heron hatchling brains showed that cell density in the pyriform cortex increased with increasing TCDD levels (Henshel, 1998). Brain asymmetry was studied in double-crested cormorant hatchlings in nesting areas known to have low, moderate and high levels of PCBs, TCDD, TCDF and PHAHs. Increasing natural exposure *in ovo* to PCBs, PCDD and PCDF increased the likelihood for chicks to hatch with asymmetric brains. The effect of TCDD on brain symmetry was studied in chicken embryos (Henshel *et al.*, 1997). The authors found that TCDD caused the brain asymmetry terata that were similar to the terata observed in eagles, herons and cormorants. In chick embryos, TCDD and PCB congener CB-126 were shown to alter lipid synthesis, which was related to changes in brain symmetry (Stanton *et al.*, 2003). A dose response to TCDD was found for occurrences and severity of brain terata. Demyelination of the spinal cord was determined by immunohistochemical analysis (Henshel, 1998). It is likely that thyroid dysfunction could be one of the mechanisms (McNabb, 2007), but measurements of thyroid hormones were not included in the studies. Female zebra finches with known fertility were administered four doses of 10 μg Aroclor 1248 *per os* every 5 days (Hoogesteijn *et al.*, 2008). Controls were females administered corn oil. After treatment, the females were placed with the paired male and allowed to nest. One egg was removed from each nest and tested for PCBs. No signs of toxicity were observed in the hens. Both male and female progeny of PCB-treated hens had significantly smaller robustus arcopallialis nuclei than control birds. The higher vocal center did not differ in either sex between exposed and control groups. These data provide evidence that mating songs may be altered by PCBs and likely by endocrine disruption. High environmental selenium has been reported to cause hydrocephaly and exencephaly in aquatic birds (Ohlendorf *et al.*, 1986, 1988).

Soft tissue other than brain

Changes in heart measurements and observations in nestling passerines were associated with PCB contamination (DeWitt *et al.*, 2006). For house wrens (*Troglodytes aedon*) and tree swallows the heart somatic index was decreased at the more contaminated sites. For Carolina chickadee (*Parus carolinesis*) and tree swallow, the heart somatic index significantly decreased with log PCB levels, and in tree swallow the heart somatic index decreased with increasing log TCDD TEQ toxic equivalents. Abnormal air sacs were reported in a swallow in the Chernobyl study (Moller *et al.*, 2007).

EGGSHELL THINNING AND PRODUCTIVITY

A bird egg is a self-contained protective system for the developing embryo that ensures aerobic metabolism, regulates water and storage of waste, and manages nutrients. The parents ensure incubation temperature and other factors are maintained within a critical window to guarantee successful embryonating processes. Studies on declining populations of birds have shown that eggshell thinning and desiccation can be a cause of reduced reproductive performance. The cause of decreased reproductive performance in white-tailed sea eagle (*Haliaeetus albicilla*) was studied in Sweden (Helander *et al.*, 1982, 2002). The occurrences of undeveloped eggs, the strongest correlation with the desiccation index (water loss during development), was correlated to DDE. The levels of 2,2-bis(4-chlorophenyl)-1,1-dichloroethene (DDE) decreased five-fold from 1964 to 1999 and the PCB levels decreased three-fold from the mid-1980s. There was a trend for the PCB congeners to shift towards higher levels of chlorination. The TEQ of PCBs expressed as 2,3,7,8-tetrachlorodibenzo-*p*-dioxin remained constant due to the primary contribution from CB-126. Eggs containing dead embryos had higher levels of PCB, but not DDE, implying lethal concentrations of PCBs.

The factors affecting the reproductive successes of bald eagles have been reviewed (Bowerman *et al.*, 1995). The reproductive success of bald eagles is inverse with levels of *p,p′*-DDE, PCBs and TEQ for TCDDs. The concentrations of *p,p′*-DDE and PCBs in abandoned eggs and plasma of nesting eagles correlated with decreased reproductive performance. The occurrences of egg shell thinning have decreased with decreasing *p,p′*-DDE. Decreased hatching has increased with increasing levels of PCBs. Mercury is not correlated with bald eagle productivity. The effects of dieldrin may be co-correlated to the effects of PCBs and DDT complex. A study on DDE and dieldrin in captive barn owls showed that DDE was associated with eggshell thinning, subsequent egg breakage and embryo mortality (Mendenhall *et al.*, 1983). Dieldrin alone caused a smaller significant eggshell thinning, but did not reduce breeding success. These observations suggest that toxicologic interactions between DDE and dieldrin may exist.

Electromagnetic fields have been shown to alter eggshell thickness (Fernie *et al.*, 2000b). American kestrels exposed to EMFs laid larger eggs with decreased eggshell thickness. Measurements were taken at the time the egg was laid.

TERATOGENIC ENDOCRINE DISRUPTION

Endocrine disruptions can alter the ability to respond to stress and changes in metabolic demands and reproductive successes (Tyler *et al.*, 1998; Lorenzen *et al.*, 1999; Mayne *et al.*, 2005). A study in herring gull embryos found that basal corticosterone levels were negatively correlated with yoke sac PCDDs, PCDFs, PCBs and non-*ortho* PCBs (Lorenzen *et al.*, 1999). This study shows that *in ovo* exposure to EDCs has the potential of compromising the ability of birds to adapt to physiologic distress. Mayne *et al.* (2005) in 2000 and 2001 studied the effects of orchard spraying on thyroid function in tree swallow and eastern bluebird nestlings. Based on the type and consumption of pesticides, the orchards were assumed to use endocrine disrupting pesticides. Parameters reported were thyroid hormones and histopathology. Individual nests were exposed to as many as seven individual non-target pesticide applications and up to five non-target pesticide mixtures. Thyroid specimens collected in 2000 from chicks in the reference area had predominantly large, round, colloid-filled follicles covered by a single layer of flattened or low-cuboidal epithelial cells. The thyroid glands from chicks in orchard sites had smaller, irregularly shaped or collapsed follicles with little colloidal material and hypertrophy of thyroid follicular epithelia. A positive correlation existed between follicular epithelial cell height and pesticide exposures. In 2001, tree swallow chicks from reference sites had thyroid follicles containing predominantly non-uniformly stained colloid and tall columnar epithelial cells. In contrast, orchard chicks had follicles with lumens containing uniform dark colloid and low cuboidal epithelium, and focal hypertrophy of epithelial cells was observed. Chicks from sprayed orchards had a significantly higher proportion of focal or diffuse hypertrophic thyroid epithelia when compared to chicks from non-sprayed orchard sites. A positive correlation was found between thyroxin (T_4) and *p,p′*-DDE in the eggs. The Ontario study on the effects of orchard spraying in tree swallows found a significant increase in triiodothyronine (T_3) and increasing number of mixtures of orchard sprays to which the chicks were exposed (Bishop *et al.*, 1998). Historically, goiterogenic chemicals were found in Great Lake Pacific salmon that caused thyroid lesions in rats, and it was later found that herring gulls had a high occurrence of thyroid lesions (Moccia *et al.*, 1986). The lesion was considered to be due to goiterogenic material in the food web.

The *in ovo* effects of PBDE congeners on thyroid function were studied in American kestrels (Fernie *et al.*, 2005). Eggs were injected at 19 days of incubation with a 1,500 ng mixture of PBDEs. The PBDE mixture consisted of 56.4% of DE-47; 27.2% of DE-99; 24.8% of DE-100; and 0.6% of DE-153. For 29 days the nestlings were exposed to 100 ng/g PBDE mixture. Treatment with PBDE congeners lowered plasma T_4, and did not change T_3 concentrations and thyroid glandular structure. Congeners DE-47, DE-100 and DE-99 were negatively associated with T_4. Hepatic oxidative stress was increased in the females as shown by increased GSSG:GSH and a marginal increase in lipid peroxidation and increased oxidized glutathione.

PCB residues in eggs of wild birds have been linked with reduced reproductive success and embryonic deformities (Fernie *et al.*, 2000a and references cited). A controlled study of captive American kestrels exposed to 7 mg PCBs/kg body weight/day via the food for 1 month prior to pairing and exposure was continued until the end of the incubation period (Fernie *et al.*, 2000a). The mean total PCB level in the eggs was 34.1 μg/g of egg wet weight (ww). The egg size was more variable in the PCB exposed group, but absolute egg mass and volume did not differ. For the PCB-treated birds, the yolks were heavier and there was less wet and dry albumen. Water content and eggshell thickness were not affected by PCB treatment. The results from this study show that PCB exposure results in eggs with more lipid and less protein available for embryonic development. The effect of *in ovo* exposure has also been studied where the parental generation was fed PCB-spiked feed for 100 days during the first breeding season and were not exposed to PCBs during the second breeding season. In the first year, the adults laid eggs with 34.1 μg PCBs/g whole egg (ww). Altered growth was observed in the first year nestlings (Fernie *et al.*, 2003a). The higher toxic equivalent exposures of PCBs were linked with nestlings that were lighter and had longer bones and feathers, females who grew at a faster rate (mass and bone) and males who grew at a slower rate (mass). The authors concluded that physiological, biochemical and behavioral changes are likely mechanisms. In a follow-up study, the effects on the second year nestlings were also examined and the offspring from the first study were paired with unexposed birds (Fernie *et al.*, 2003b). Maternal-to-egg-exposed F_2 females were larger, showed altered growth rates and delayed maximal growth and fledging as compared to controls. The maternal-to-egg-exposed males were heavier, had shorter bones, grew faster and fledged approximately 2 days later when compared to the control males. The maternally exposed F_2 females had elevated plasma T_3 levels, but the F_2 males had suppressed T_3 levels. The paternally exposed F_2 generation was comparable in size to the controls, but had longer tarsi bones and showed slower, delayed growth in both sexes and delayed fledging in the females. There were also lower T_4 levels in the F_2 males. The developmental changes in the nestlings were linked to several possible mechanisms by the authors which included maternal PCB deposition, parental behavior, neurobehavioral and endocrine–thyroid function in the nestlings. Another study found that the second generation females had suppressed egg laying and delays in clutch initiation and smaller clutch sizes for the PCB-exposed pairs (Fernie *et al.*, 2001b). There was no evidence found regarding effects on fertility or hatching success but reduced reproductive outcomes were noted, particularly reduced fledging success and an increased complete brood mortality. The effects on mortality, deformities and post-hatch immune function following *in ovo* exposure to PCB were studied in white leghorn chicken eggs (Lavoie and Grasman, 2007). This study showed that *in ovo* exposure suppressed antibody responses in the juvenile chickens.

There is increasing evidence that eggshell thinning is a teratogenic effect due to female birds being exposed to EDCs that mimic estrogens. During the 1950s and 1960s an increase in egg loss was observed especially in birds feeding at the higher trophic levels. The increase in egg loss was shown to be due to eggshell thinning resulting in increased egg breakage (Ratcliffe, 1970). The cause of eggshell thinning was attributed to chlorinated pesticides, especially DDT. Bitman *et al.* (1968) and Bitman and Cecil (1970) demonstrated the estrogenic effects of *p,p′*-DDT and analogs in chickens and quail. The model proposed that the endocrine disruption was occurring as primary toxicity in adult females due to endocrine disruption of carbonic anhydrase-mediated deposition of eggshell. Studies in chickens, reported in the 1930s, showed that *in ova* exposure to estrogens produced hens that laid soft-shelled eggs (Fry and Toone, 1981 and references therein). Studies in Japanese quail showed that *in ovo* exposure to ethynylestradiol caused teratogenic changes in the reproductive organs (Berg *et al.*, 2001). The effects observed were retention of the right oviduct, reduction in size of the left oviduct and increased length of the uterovaginal junction. Altered cytology was observed in the uterus (shell gland), magnum and the uterovaginal junction. Treatment of Japanese quail *in ovo* with ethynylestradiol (20 ng/g of egg) caused disruption of carbonic anhydrase (CA) expression in the shell gland (Holm *et al.*, 2001). Control birds had carbonic anhydrase located in the membranes of the tubular gland cells of the uterus and surface epithelium was always devoid of CA. The ethynylestradiol resulted in disruption of the CA distribution in the tubular glands. Chicken hens were exposed *in ovo* to 20 ng ethynylestradiol/g of egg (Berg *et al.*, 2004). The exposed hens produced eggs with thinner eggshells and reduced deformation strength than controls. The *in ovo* treatment with ethynylestradiol decreased the number of uterine capillaries and decreased the occurrences of shell gland capillaries with carbonic anhydrase activity. Domestic hens were exposed *in ovo* to 37 or 75 mg of *o,p′*-DDT/g of egg (Holm *et al.*, 2006). Hens from eggs treated *in ovo* with *o,p′*-DDT laid thin-shelled eggs. They also had reduced occurrences of shell gland capillaries with CA activity. Egg laying was not affected by the *o,p′*-DDT dosage levels. These studies provide insight into the mechanism of action for eggshell thinning and show that eggshell thinning can be terata due to *in ovo* exposure of females to estrogenic EDCs.

Genetic sex determination in birds shows that the female is the heterogametic sex (ZW) and the male is homogametic (ZZ) (Fry, 1995). The homogametic sex is generally considered to be the "default" sex because in the absence of hormonal and other influences the sexual phenotype is the homogenetic sex. In birds, the default phenotype sex in the absence of estradiol is male. Endocrine changes during embryological development are important in the development of sex-specific neurocircuits (Panzica *et al.*, 2007). In many male birds, the testosterone-dependent neurocircuits can be "turned off" by caponization. Treating females with testosterone does not "turn on" the sex-specific neurocircuits observed in the male. These effects can render the birds as non-breeders or compromised breeders may compete for mates. A reduction in the number of male gulls was observed in the Channel Islands off the coast of California (Fry and Toone, 1981). The sex ratio of males to females on Santa Barbara Island was observed to skew to ~3.8 females for each male. Some of the females were pairing with females. Contamination of the eggs with DDT was proposed as a possible cause. To test the effects of xenoestrogens, gull eggs were injected with xenoestrogens. Injecting gull eggs with DDT, using doses comparable to those found in contaminated seabird eggs, induced anatomical feminization of male birds and abnormal development of the oviduct in females. Gulls were found to be more resistant to EDC-induced eggshell thinning. The Ontario orchard spray study in tree swallows found a trend for the increased occurrence of testicular Sertoli cell disruptions with increasing number of mixtures to which the male chicks were exposed (Bishop *et al.*, 1998). Key enzymes in the metabolic pathways of steroid hormones can be the target of xenobiotics and by this mechanism cause or contribute to hormonal disruption with reproductive and developmental toxicities as outcomes (Sanderson, 2006).

The effects of penta-BDE congeners were studied in incubating and nesting captive American kestrels (Fernie *et al.*, 2006). In each clutch, the eggs were divided between groups by laying sequence. At the nineteenth day of incubation, the eggs were injected with oil (control) or 18.7 μg penta-BDE congeners. The congeners' profile was 56.4% DE-47; 27.2% DE-99; 24.8% DE-100; and 0.6% DE-153. After hatching, the nestlings were administered *per gavage* 15.6 ng of penta-BDE congeners/g body of weight/day for 29 days. Treatment of the embryonating eggs and nestlings with penta-PBDE congeners did not affect hatching or fledging success. However, the exposed nestlings had increased food consumption, increased rate of weight gain and were larger (mass, bones, feathers). The increased food consumption was associated with increased body burdens of penta-BDE congeners. Interesting associations with penta-BDE congeners were found. DE-100 was associated with growth and was positively associated with body size, increase in body mass, and increased mass of food consumed. The increased DE-183 and DE-153 were associated with increased bone length, and DE-99 was associated with increased feather length. The increase in body size could alter hunting agility, energy requirements and overall survival.

There were increased diversity and frequency of congenital abnormalities in barn swallows from the Chernobyl study area as compared to control areas (Moller *et al.*, 2007). The number of nestlings with abnormalities was more frequent than abnormalities observed in the parents, suggesting abnormalities reduced the survival of the nestlings.

BEHAVIORAL CHANGES AND NESTING SUCCESS

Birds have many different mating strategies dependent on male and female behaviors. These behaviors are endocrine driven and the timing of onset of the events is important. In some species, the female is dependant on supplemental feeding by the male to achieve energy stores for egg production. The timing of reproductive behavior is important and interactive timing of male and female reproductive behavior is essential for successfully sequencing reproductive events. Nest building in some species is important for containment of the eggs and nestlings, and the nest also provides protection from adverse environmental conditions. The quality of the nest build by swallows (*Tachycinetbai color*) influences reproductive outcomes (McCarty and Secord, 1999). The female builds the grass matt and the quality of the grass matt effects egg hatch. The male builds the feather matt and the number of feathers influences growth rate of nestlings and level of ectoparasite infestation. Swallows breeding in PCB-contaminated areas built smaller nests of lower quality compared with those in uncontaminated areas. Captive European starlings were implanted with a device to slowly release 150 µg penta-PBDE (Van den Steen *et al.*, 2009). The data suggested a trend for a penta-PBDE reduction in the number of egg-laying females. Females implanted with penta-PBDE implants produced eggs with increased mass and volume. These effects could be due to endocrine disruption. The effects of PCBs were studied in wild European starlings at a Superfund site (IL, USA) (Arenal *et al.*, 2004). Nest boxes were placed at two study and two reference sites. Starling productivity and adult provisioning behavior were monitored. Differences did not exist among study and reference sites for the number of eggs laid and the percent of eggs hatched. At the PCB-contaminated sites, there was reduced nest provisioning behavior and decreased chick survival.

An increase in environmental POPs is associated with a decrease in reproductive outcomes in predatory birds. Reduction in successful reproductive outcomes was reduced in white-tailed sea eagles by increasing egg levels of DDE and PCB (Helander *et al.*, 1982). A study found that herring gulls in Lake Ontario had decreased nest defense and were less attentive to their eggs (Fox *et al.*, 1978). Incubating Lake Ontario gulls appeared to apply less heat to their eggs as required by ambient conditions. Other studies found that nesting herring gulls with high POPs were more aggressive towards human intruders and towards each other (Peakall and Fox, 1987). Decreased nest defense and decreased successful reproductive outcomes were observed. These abnormalities have been linked to POP-induced endocrine dysfunction. Breeding behavior in American kestrels is essential for successful reproductive outcomes (Fernie *et al.*, 2008 and references cited therein). The breeding behavior of kestrels, under experimental conditions, can be altered by DE-71 (Fernie *et al.*, 2008). Adult American kestrels in a captive research colony were orally exposed to safflower oil (controls), or technical DE-71 at 0.3 or 1.6 ppm, for 75 days. Exposure to DE-71 started 21 days before breeding. The kestrels at both DE-71 exposure levels had different timing of mating behaviors. The DE-71-treated groups also copulated less, spent less time in their nest boxes and participated in fewer pair-bonding behaviors. The effects of hexabromocyclododecane (HBCD) and PBDEs on reproduction were studied in captive American kestrels (Fernie *et al.*, 2009). Dose regimens resulted in kestrels producing eggs that contained similar PBDE and HBCD concentrations reported for the eggs from wild herring gulls and peregrine falcons. Egg laying was delayed in treated birds and the treated birds also produced smaller eggs. The overall reproductive outcome was reduced fertility and reproductive success. Increased levels of PBDEs in osprey eggs in Washington and Oregon have a negative effect on reproductive (Henny *et al.*, 2009). This study found that when ΣPBDEs levels in osprey eggs were >1,000 ng/g of egg (ww) reproductive outcomes were decreased. The PBDEs did not affect eggshell thickness.

The effect of exposure to PCBs on courtship behavioral and hormonal alterations was studied in captive male and female American kestrels (Fisher *et al.*, 2001). Birds were exposed via the diet to 7 mg/kg body weight/bird/day of a 1:1:1 mixture of Aroclors 1248, 1254 and 1260. This resulted in a mean residue of 34.1 µg/g of egg (ww), considered by the authors to be environmentally relevant. One week after pairing, no differences were found between treated and control birds in circulating total androgens or 17β-estradiol levels. The authors concluded that the treated and control birds were all in the same endocrine phase of the breeding season. The PCB-exposed males showed significantly more sexual and flight behaviors when compared to control males. Sexual behaviors were defined as nest box inspections, solicitation of copulation, and food offering and giving to the female. Fight behaviors included flying from one perch to another and aerial displays. The frequency of the male sexual behaviors was correlated to the total PCB residues in the eggs of the mates and the data showed there was a delay in clutch initiation and a greater number of completely infertile clutches. The reproductive success of wild birds generally considered to be affected by a number of environmental contaminants. Breeding pairs of captive American kestrels were fed PCB spiked food prior to and during the breeding season (Fernie *et al.*, 2001a). The reproductive changes that were noted during the PCB exposure included smaller clutches laid later in the season and increased number of infertile clutches. Hatching success was also reduced and in the PCB-exposed group, 50% of the nestlings died within 3 days of hatching. Approximately 60% of the PCB-exposed pairs, which had hatchlings, did not produce fledglings. Many birds during the egg incubation season develop bare areas of skin called brood patches. The brood patches allow heat to be transferred to the eggs during incubation. It is theorized that the size of the brood patch could influence hatching success or that it may be a factor in the relationship between poor incubation behavior and hatching failure. In a controlled study of American kestrels, birds were exposed to a mixture of PCBs (Aroclor 1248, 1254, 1260) via the diet. Treated birds were exposed to approximately 7 mg/kg body weight/day while a similar sized group remained unexposed and served as controls (Fisher *et al.*, 2006). Brood patch sizes were not related to total PCB residue levels in the eggs of the exposed birds; however, PCB exposure was linked to the variation in the patch size found in both the male and female birds. The brood patches were not related to the various incubation behaviors or hatching success in any of the study birds. The authors concluded that PCBs are EDC substances and the observed changes in brood patches were an EDC response to PCB exposure. PCB exposure has been shown to result in longer incubation periods and altered incubation behaviors (Fisher *et al.*, 2006).

Debate exists on the effects of EMFs on bird physiology, behavior and reproduction. There are issues and debates regarding the effects of electromagnetic fields (EMFs) on the nervous system in birds. Fernie and Bird (1999) and Fernie *et al.* (1999) found that EMFs mimicked increased photoperiod in male kestrels by altering melatonin and advancing the onset of molt. Male kestrels also increased in body mass. The exposure to EMF was equivalent to a 735 kV 60 hertz transmission line. Fledglings from parents exposed to EMFs for two breeding seasons had reduced serum melatonin levels.

The effects of electromagnetic fields on the behavior of birds have been studied (Fernie *et al.*, 2000b,c; Doherty and Grubb, 1998). Fernie *et al.* (2000b) observed wild kestrels in nest boxes which were located approximately 1 m below a transmission line and were exposed to a 1.2 µT magnetic field and 0.05 ± 0.01 kV/m electric field. The kestrels were observed during courtship, incubation, brooding and the fledgling phase. They also conducted a controlled study where 20 pairs of kestrels were exposed to either a 30 ± 0.03 μT magnetic field and a 10 ± 0.04 kV/m electric field or control conditions. On a 24h basis, the wild kestrels were exposed to the electromagnetic fields from 71% (during courtship) to 90% (during incubation) of the time. The controlled study allowed for 88% exposure in a 24h period. In the controlled study, the EMF-exposed females were significantly more active, alert and perched on the roof more frequently during courtship as compared to the control females. The EMF exposed males were also significantly more active than the control males but there were no significant differences in perching distance between mates, aggression or courtship feeding. The behavior of the EMF-exposed females was unaffected during incubation but the EMF-exposed males were significantly more alert than the control males during this period. During the brood rearing period, the EMF-exposed females preened and rested significantly less as compared to the controls. Feeding rates of the nestlings and other observed behaviors were unaffected by exposure to EMFs. The study concludes that the behavioral changes noted occurred predominantly in the courtship and brood rearing phases and had no effect on egg laying, clutch size and incubation of eggs.

Tree swallows had lower reproductive success (fledglings/clutch size) when nesting under power lines (Doherty and Grubb, 1998). House wrens were not affected. Fernie *et al.* (2000c), in a 2-year study, found that fertility of American kestrels was increased by EMFs equivalent to a 735kV 60 hertz power line. Egg size was larger for the EMF-exposed birds which had thinner eggshells. For the EMF-exposed kestrels, hatching success was decreased and the number of fledglings was decreased in the second year. In the first year the number of fledglings was increased. Eggshells were thinner in the EMF-exposed birds laying larger eggs.

CONCLUDING REMARKS AND FUTURE DIRECTIONS

Birds are generally regarded as sensitive sentinels of environmental safety. In many ways birds of flight live a delicate balance of reserve body mass and flight endurance. Birds must respond to many environmental stressors including ambient weather conditions, availability of feed and water, and the metabolic stress of reproduction. Exposure to POPs has been shown to cause abnormal skeletal development as well as affecting the development of the nervous system. The integrity of the eggshell and composition of the egg are crucial to the successful development of the embryo. Exposure to POPs has also been linked to eggshell thinning and desiccation which has led to a reduction in reproductive performance in some species. Embryonic deformities have also been linked to environmental pollutant exposure. Studies have shown that birds consuming feedstuffs contaminated with POPs and nesting in areas with high POPs can cause endocrine disruption and decreased reproductive successes. The timing of reproductive behavior in male and female birds needs to be coordinated with each other and with the season. Endocrine disruption that occurs during embryonation often results in terata of the endocrine system. Birds are exposed to mixtures of POPs in the environment, and these mixtures can be more toxic than the parent material or mixtures released into the environment. Reproductive success of birds relies on many integrated processes ranging from courtship to fledging success. It has also been demonstrated that the effects of exposure can have a detrimental impact on subsequent generations without further exposure. Disruption at any one these multiple processes can have a significant negative impact on the survival of the species.

REFERENCES

Albers PH, Hoffman DJ, Brisbin IL Jr (2001) Unusual leg malformations in screech owls from a South Carolina Superfund site. *J Toxicol Environ Health A* **63(2):** 89–99.

Arenal CA, Halbrook RS, Woodruff M (2004) European starling (*Sturnus vulgaris*): avian model and monitor of polychlorinated biphenyl contamination at a Superfund site in southern Illinois, USA. *Environ Toxicol Chem* **23(1):** 93–104.

Augspurger TP, Tillitt DE, Bursian SJ, Fitzgerald SD, Hinton DE, Di Giulio RT (2008) Embryo toxicity of 2,3,7,8-tetrachlorodibenzo-*p*-dioxin to the wood duck (*Aix sponsa*). *Arch Environ Contam Toxicol* 659–69.

Berg C, Blomqvist A, Holm L, Brandt I, Brunstrom B, Ridderstrale Y (2004) Embryonic exposure to oestrogen causes eggshell thinning and altered shell gland carbonic anhydrase expression in the domestic hen. *Reproduction* **128(4):** 455–61.

Berg C, Holm L, Brandt I, Brunstrom B (2001) Anatomical and histological changes in the oviducts of Japanese quail, *Coturnix japonica*, after embryonic exposure to ethynyloestradiol. *Reproduction* **121(1):** 155–65.

Bishop CA, Van Der Kraak GJ, Ng P, Smits JE, Hontela A (1998) Health of tree swallows (*Tachycineta bicolor*) nesting in pesticide-sprayed apple orchards in Ontario, Canada. II. Sex and thyroid hormone concentrations and testes development. *J Toxicol Environ Health A* **55(8):** 561–81.

Bitman J, Cecil HC, Harris SJ, Fries GF (1968) Estrogenic activity of *o,p'*-DDT in the mammalian uterus and avian oviduct. *Science* **162(851):** 371–2.

Bitman J, Cecil HC (1970) Estrogenic activity of DDT analogs and polychlorinated biphenyls. *J Agric Food Chem* **18(6):** 1108–12.

Bosveld AT, van den Berg M (2002) Reproductive failure and endocrine disruption by organohalogens in fish-eating birds. *Toxicology* **181–182:** 155–9.

Bowerman WW, Giesy JP, Best DA, Kramer VJ (1995) A review of factors affecting productivity of bald eagles in the Great Lakes region: implications for recovery. *Environ Health Perspect* **103 (Suppl. 4):** 51–9.

Custer TW, Custer CM, Hines RK, Stromborg KL, Allen PD, Melancon MJ, Henshel DS (2001) Organochlorine contaminants and biomarker response in double-crested cormorants nesting in Green Bay and Lake Michigan, Wisconsin, USA. *Arch Environ Contam Toxicol* **40(1):** 89–100.

DeWitt JC, Millsap DS, Yeager RL, Heise SS, Sparks DW, Henshel DS (2006) External heart deformities in passerine birds exposed to environmental mixtures of polychlorinated biphenyls during development. *Environ Toxicol Chem* **25(2):** 541–51.

Doherty Jr PF, Grubb Jr TC (1998) Reproductive success of cavity-nesting birds breeding under high-voltage powerlines. *Am Midl Natural* **140(1):** 122–8.

Fernie KJ, Bird DM (1999) Effects of electromagnetic fields on body mass and food-intake of American kestrels. *Condor* **101(3):** 616–21.

Fernie KJ, Bird DM, Dawson RD, Lague PC (2000c) Effects of electromagnetic fields on the reproductive success of American kestrels. *Physiol Biochem Zool* **73(1):** 60–5.

Fernie KJ, Bird DM, Petitclerc D (1999) Effects of electromagnetic fields on photophasic circulating melatonin levels in American kestrels. *Environ Health Perspect* **107(11):** 901–4.

Fernie K, Bortolotti G, Drouillard K, Smits J, Marchant T (2003b) Developmental toxicity of in ovo exposure to polychlorinated biphenyls: II. Effects of maternal or paternal exposure on second-generation nestling American kestrels. *Environ Toxicol Chem* **22(11):** 2688–94.

Fernie KJ, Bortolotti GR, Smits JE, Wilson J, Drouillard KG, Bird DM (2000a) Changes in egg composition of American kestrels exposed to dietary polychlorinated biphenyls. *J Toxicol Environ Health A* **60(4):** 291–303.

Fernie KJ, Leonard NJ, Bird DM (2000b) Behavior of free-ranging and captive American kestrels under electromagnetic fields. *J Toxicol Environ Health A* **59(8):** 597–603.

Fernie KJ, Smits JE, Bortolotti GR, Bird DM (2001a) Reproduction success of American kestrels exposed to dietary polychlorinated biphenyls. *Environ Toxicol Chem* **20(4):** 776–81.

Fernie KJ, Smits JE, Bortolotti GR, Bird DM (2001b) *In ovo* exposure to polychlorinated biphenyls: reproductive effects on second-generation American kestrels. *Arch Environ Contam Toxicol* **40(4):** 544–50.

Fernie K, Smits J, Bortolotti G (2003a) Developmental toxicity of in ovo exposure to polychlorinated biphenyls: I. Immediate and subsequent effects on first-generation nestling American kestrels (*Falco sparverius*). *Environ Toxicol Chem* **22(3):** 554–60.

Fernie KJ, Shutt JL, Mayne G, Hoffman D, Letcher RJ, Drouillard KG, Ritchie IJ (2005) Exposure to polybrominated diphenyl ethers (PBDEs): changes in thyroid, vitamin A, glutathione homeostasis, and oxidative stress in American kestrels (*Falco sparverius*). *Toxicol Sci* **88(2):** 375–83.

Fernie KJ, Laird Shutt J, Ritchie IJ, Letcher RJ, Drouillard K, Bird DM (2006) Changes in the growth, but not the survival, of American kestrels (*Falco sparverius*) exposed to environmentally relevant polybrominated diphenyl ethers. *J Toxicol Environ Health A* **69(16):** 1541–54.

Fernie KJ, Shutt JL, Letcher RJ, Ritchie IJ, Sullivan K, Bird DM (2008) Changes in reproductive courtship behaviors of adult American kestrels (*Falco sparverius*) exposed to environmentally relevant levels of the polybrominated diphenyl ether mixture, DE-71. *Toxicol Sci* **102(1):** 171–8.

Fernie KJ, Shutt JL, Letcher RJ, Ritchie IJ, Bird DM (2009) Environmentally relevant concentrations of DE-71 and HBCD alter eggshell thickness and reproductive success of American kestrels. *Environ Sci Technol* **43(6):** 2124–30.

Firestone D (1973) Etiology of chick edema disease. *Environ Health Perspect* **5:** 59–66.

Fisher SA, Bortolotti GR, Fernie KJ, Bird DM, Smits JE (2006) Brood patches of American kestrels altered by experimental exposure to PCBs. *J Toxicol Environ Health A* **69(17):** 1603–12.

Fisher SA, Bortolotti GR, Fernie KJ, Smits JE, Marchant TA, Drouillard KG, Bird DM (2001) Courtship behavior of captive American kestrels (*Falco sparverius*) exposed to polychlorinated biphenyls. *Arch Environ Contam Toxicol* **41(2):** 215–20.

Fox GA, Gilman AP, Peakall DB, Anderka FW (1978) Behavioural abnormalities of nesting Lake Ontario herring gulls. *J Wildl Manage* **42(3):** 477–83.

Fry DM, Toone CK (1981) DDT-induced feminization of gull embryos. *Science* **213(4510):** 922–4.

Fry DM (1995) Reproductive effects in birds exposed to pesticides and industrial chemicals. *Environ Health Perspect* **103 (Suppl. 7):** 165–71.

Giesy JP, Ludwig JP, Tillitt DE (1994) Deformities in birds of the Great Lakes region: assigning causality. *Environ Sci Technol* **28(3):** 128a–135a.

Gilbertson M (1983) Etiology of chick-edema disease in herring gulls in the lower Great Lakes. *Chemosphere* **12(3):** 357–70.

Gilbertson M, Kubiak T, Ludwig J, Fox G (1991) Great Lakes embryo mortality, edema, and deformities syndrome (GLEMEDS) in colonial fish-eating birds: similarity to chick-edema disease. *J Toxicol Environ Health* **33(4):** 455–520.

Gilbertson M, Morris RD, Hunter RA (1976) Abnormal chicks and PCB residue levels in eggs of colonial birds on the Lower Great Lakes. *AUK* **93(3):** 434–42.

Helander B, Olsson A, Bignert A, Asplund L, Litzen K (2002) The role of DDE, PCB, coplanar PCB and eggshell parameters for reproduction in the white-tailed sea eagle (*Haliaeetus albicilla*) in Sweden. *Ambio* **31(5):** 386–403.

Helander B, Olsson M, Reutergardh L (1982) Residue levels of organochlorine and mercury compounds in unhatched eggs and the relationships to breeding success in white-tailed sea eagles *Haliaeetus albicilla* in Sweden. *Holarctic Ecol* **5(4):** 349–66.

Henny CJ, Kaiser JL, Grove RA, Johnson BL, Letcher RJ (2009) Polybrominated diphenyl ether flame retardants in eggs may reduce reproductive success of ospreys in Oregon and Washington, USA. *Ecotoxicology* **18(7):** 802–13.

Henshel D (1998) Developmental neurotoxic effects of dioxin and dioxin-like compounds on domestic and wild avian species. *Environ Toxicol Chem* **17(1):** 88–98.

Henshel DS, Martin JW, Norstrom R, Whitehead P, Steeves JD, Cheng KM (1995) Morphometric abnormalities in brains of great blue heron hatchlings exposed in the wild to PCDDs. *Environ Health Perspect* **103 (Suppl. 4):** 61–6.

Henshel DS, Martin JW, Norstrom RJ, Elliott J, Cheng KM, DeWitt JC (1997) Morphometric brain abnormalities in double-crested cormorant chicks exposed to polychlorinated dibenzo-*p*-dioxins, dibenzofurans, and biphenyls. *Great Lakes Res* **24(1):** 11–26.

Hoffman DJ, Rattner BA, Sileo L, Docherty D, Kubiak TJ (1987) Embryotoxicity, teratogenicity, and aryl hydrocarbon hydroxylase activity in Forster's terns on Green Bay, Lake Michigan. *Environ Res* **42(1):** 176–84.

Holm L, Berg C, Brunstrom B, Ridderstrale Y, Brandt I (2001) Disrupted carbonic anhydrase distribution in the avian shell gland following in ovo exposure to estrogen. *Arch Toxicol* **75(6):** 362–8.

Holm L, Blomqvist A, Brandt I, Brunstrom B, Ridderstrale Y, Berg C (2006) Embryonic exposure to *o,p'*-DDT causes eggshell thinning and altered shell gland carbonic anhydrase expression in the domestic hen. *Environ Toxicol Chem* **25(10):** 2787–93.

Hoogesteijn AL, Kollias GV, Quimby FW, De Caprio AP, Winkler DW, DeVoogd TJ (2008) Development of a brain nucleus involved in song production in zebra finches (*Taeniopygia guttata*) is disrupted by Aroclor 1248. *Environ Toxicol Chem* **27(10):** 2071–5.

Jenssen BM, Aarnes JB, Murvoll KM, Herzke D, Nygard T (2010) Fluctuating wing asymmetry and hepatic concentrations of persistent organic pollutants are associated in European shag (*Phalacrocorax aristotelis*) chicks. *Sci Total Environ* **408(3):** 578–85.

Kubiak TJ, Harris HJ, Smith LM, Schwartz TR, Stalling DL, Trick JA, Sileo L, Docherty DE, Erdman TC (1989) Microcontaminants and reproductive impairment of the Forster's tern on Green Bay, Lake Michigan – 1983. *Arch Environ Contam Toxicol* **18(5):** 706–27.

Lavoie ET, Grasman KA (2007) Effects of in ovo exposure to PCBs 126 and 77 on mortality, deformities and post-hatch immune function in chickens. *J Toxicol Environ Health A* **70(6):** 547–58.

Lorenzen A, Moon TW, Kennedy SW, Glen GA (1999) Relationships between environmental organochlorine contaminant residues, plasma corticosterone concentrations, and intermediary metabolic enzyme activities in Great Lakes herring gull embryos. *Environ Health Perspect* **107(3):** 179–86.

Mayne GJ, Bishop CA, Martin PA, Boermans HJ, Hunter B (2005) Thyroid function in nestling tree swallows and eastern bluebirds exposed to non-persistent pesticides and *p,p'*-DDE in apple orchards of southern Ontario, Canada. *Ecotoxicology* **14(3):** 381–96.

McCarty JP, Secord AL (1999) Nest-building behavior in PCB contaminated tree swallows. *Auk* **116(1):** 55–63.

McKinney JD, Chae K, Gupta BN, Moore JA, Goldstein HA (1976) Toxicological assessment of hexachlorobiphenyl isomers and 2,3,7,8 tetrachlorodibenzofuran in chicks. I. Relationship of chemical parameters. *Toxicol Appl Pharmacol* **36(1):** 65–80.

McNabb FM (2007) The hypothalamic–pituitary–thyroid (HPT) axis in birds and its role in bird development and reproduction. *Crit Rev Toxicol* **37(1–2):** 163–93.

Mendenhall VM, Klaas EE, McLane MAR (1983) Breeding success of barn owls (*Tyto alba*) fed low levels of DDE and dieldrin. *Environ Contam Toicol* **12(7):** 235–40.

Moccia RD, Fox GA, Britton A (1986) A quantitative assessment of thyroid histopathology of herring gulls (*Larus argentatus*) from the Great Lakes and a hypothesis on the causal role of environmental contaminants. *J Wildl Dis* **22(1):** 60–70.

Moller AP, Mousseau TA, de Lope F, Saino N (2007) Elevated frequency of abnormalities in barn swallows from Chernobyl. *Biol Lett* **3(4):** 414–17.

Ohlendorf HM, Hoffman DJ, Saiki MK, Aldrich TW (1986) Embryonic mortality and abnormalities of aquatic birds – apparent impacts of selenium from irrigation drainwater. *Sci Total Environ* **52:** 49–63.

Ohlendorf HM, Kilness AW, Simmons JL, Stroud RK, Hoffman DJ, Moore JF (1988) Selenium toxicosis in wild aquatic birds. *J Toxicol Environ Health* **24(1):** 67–92.

Ottinger MA, Lavoie ET, Abdelnabi M, Quinn Jr MJ, Marcell A, Dean K (2009) An overview of dioxin-like compounds, PCB, and pesticide exposures associated with sexual differentiation of neuroendocrine systems, fluctuating asymmetry, and behavioral effects in birds. *J Environ Sci Health C Environ Carcinog Ecotoxicol Rev* **27(4):** 286–300.

Panzica GC, Viglietti-Panzica C, Mura E, Quinn MJ Jr, Lavoie E, Palanza P, Ottinger MA (2007) Effects of xenoestrogens on the differentiation of behaviorally-relevant neural circuits. *Front Neuroendocrinol* **28(4):** 179–200.

Peakall DB, Fox GA (1987) Toxicological investigations of pollutant-related effects in Great Lakes gulls. *Environ Health Perspect* **71:** 187–93.

Ratcliffe DA (1970) Changes attributable to pesticides in egg breakage frequency and eggshell thickness in some British birds. *J Appl Ecol* **7(1):** 67–115.

Sanderson JT (2006) The steroid hormone biosynthesis pathway as a target for endocrine-disrupting chemicals. *Toxicol Sci* **94(1):** 3–21.

Stanton B, DeWitt J, Henshel D, Watkins S, Lasley B (2003) Fatty acid metabolism in neonatal chickens (*Gallus domesticus*) treated with 2,3,7,8-tetrachlorodibenzo-*p*-dioxin (TCDD) or 3,3',4,4',5-pentachlorobiphenyl (PCB-126) in ovo. *Comp Biochem Physiol C Toxicol Pharmacol* **136(1):** 73–84.

Thompson HM, Fernandes A, Rose M, White S, Blackburn A (2006) Possible chemical causes of skeletal deformities in grey heron nestlings (*Ardea cinerea*) in North Nottinghamshire, UK. *Chemosphere* **65(3):** 400–9.

Tyler CR, Jobling S, Sumpter JP (1998) Endocrine disruption in wildlife: a critical review of the evidence. *Crit Rev Toxicol* **28(4):** 319–61.

Van den Steen E, Eens M, Covaci A, Dirtu AC, Jaspers VL, Neels H, Pinxten R (2009) An exposure study with polybrominated diphenyl ethers (PBDEs) in female European starlings (*Sturnus vulgaris*): toxicokinetics and reproductive effects. *Environ Pollut* **157(2):** 430–6.

CHAPTER

83

Endocrine disruption in wildlife species

Robert W. Coppock

INTRODUCTION

There are >4,500 species of mammals and a diversity of reproductive strategies to optimize successful outcomes (Damstra *et al.*, 2002). Additionally, wild mammals have developed strategies to live in hostile environments with adverse conditions varying from extreme heat to intense cold. The endocrine adaptations for these environments have not been well studied. Wild mammals are exposed to environmental chemicals, including endocrine disrupting chemicals (EDCs) that have been shown to cause endocrine disruption in laboratory studies. There is a growing concern and increasing scientific evidence that environmental exposure to xenobiotics alters physiologic processes by disrupting endocrine homeostats (Gee, 2006). Many endocrine disruptors are persistent organic pollutants (POPs), including polyhalogenated aromatic hydrocarbons (PHAHs) and chlorinated organics (COs), and the majority of these chemicals are also bioconcentrated in body fat. These compounds pass from the placenta into the fetus, and are also excreted in milk fat. Disruptions of the endocrine system cause multifactorial disease because of the interrelationship of the endocrine system (Capen, 2001). The endocrine system is difficult to study in total because of the inherent interrelated complexity. The majority of studies, especially in wild animals, have been limited to specific components. Findings from these studies have raised concerns regarding the effects of pollutants in the environment.

Studies have shown that the long-term effects of POPs in wild mammals can or have affected population dynamics. Stakeholders have taken actions that include raising concerns, enacting guidelines and legalization, funding research and creating educational opportunities for development of expertise (Damstra *et al.*, 2002; Horrigan *et al.*, 2002; Lyons, 2006; Jenssen, 2006; Jobling and Tyler, 2006). The Scientific Committee on Toxicity, Ecotoxicity and the Environment (CSTEE) defined endocrine disruptor as follows: "An endocrine disrupter is an exogenous substance or mixture that alters function(s) of the endocrine system and consequently causes adverse health effects in an intact organism, or its progeny, or (sub)populations" (Vos *et al.*, 2000). Endocrine-disrupting chemicals express effects by various mechanisms. These mechanisms include receptor agonists, receptor antagonists, up- and downregulation of hormone synthesis and metabolism, and alteration of hormone regulator feedback mechanisms and paraendocrine functions (Hansen, 1998; Damstra *et al.*, 2002; Guillette, 2006). Compounds such as triclocarban and triclosan have limited endocrine effects, but have the potential to enhance the actions of endogenous steroid hormones (Ahn *et al.*, 2008). For example, triclocarban has been shown to amplify the receptor-mediated response to testosterone (Chen *et al.*, 2008). In the real world, mammals including humans are exposed to a mixture of EDCs. Mixtures of EDCs are found in effluents and, once released into the environment, the effects can be difficult to predict (Thorpe *et al.*, 2006). Most studies in marine mammals relate, by statistical methods, the endocrine disrupting effects to observed tissue levels of selected POPs. Age of exposure to EDCs can be important. The reversibility of EDC-induced endocrine disruption is generally much less when it occurs in the embryo–fetus and can have life-long effects (Magnusson, 2005). Endocrine disruption in the fetus can cause congenital misprogramming of the endocrine system and may not be expressed until puberty and adult life (Damstra *et al.*, 2002). Congenital changes to the endocrine system also can cause unexpected sensitivity to environmental stimuli and endocrine disrupting chemicals. Stakeholders, which include scientists, physicians and veterinarians and governmental agencies, are raising concerns because of the known and potential short- and long-term effects of EDCs to quality of life and population dynamics. Specific disease syndrome (Baltic Seal Disease Complex) is considered to be caused by POPs and endocrine disruption is a prominent component of the disease (Bergman, 2007).

NEUROENDOCRINE DISRUPTION

The hypothalamus is the interface between the nervous system and the pituitary gland (Diamanti-Kandarakis *et al.*, 2009; Gore, 2010). Hypothalamic nerve cells release hormones into a portal system that flows to the anterior pituitary gland (Table 83.1). The hypothalamus regulates through the hypothalamic–pituitary–gonadal, hypothalamic–pituitary–thyroid and hypothalamic–pituitary–adrenal gland axes. There is feedback from the peripheral organs to the hypothalamus (long-loupe feedback) and from the peripheral organ to the pituitary gland (short-loupe feedback). All of these axes

Reproductive and Developmental Toxicology, Edited by Ramesh C. Gupta
ISBN: 978-0-12-382032-7

TABLE 83.1 Hormonal regulation by the hypothalamus–pituitary axis

Hypothalamic releasing hormone	Effect on pituitary	Target endocrine gland	Effect
Corticotropin-releasing hormone (CRH)	Releases adrenocorticotropic hormone (ACTH)	Adrenal gland	Production of glucocorticoids
Thyrotropin-releasing hormone (TRH)	Release of thyroid stimulating hormone (TSH)	Thyroid gland	Release of T_3 and T_4; effect on basal metabolism
Gonadotropin-releasing hormone (GnRH)	Release of follicle stimulating hormone (FSH) and luteinizing hormone (LH)	Ovary or testicle	Ovulation, production of estrogens and progesterone; production of spermatozoa and androgens
Dopamine	Prolactin	Mammary gland	Milk production

are susceptible to EDCs through a number of mechanisms. The timing of exposure to EDCs in terms of age-live-stages generally produces different outcomes. Endocrine disruptors can alter sexual differentiation of the brain during fetal development. Normal sexual differentiation in mammals is the net effect of fetal and maternal hormones acting on the fetal brain. The most studied effect is the impact on sexual functions and behaviors. Changes that occur during fetal development may not be expressed until after puberty. Long-term effects can be changes in mating and parental behavior, and cross-gender behavior has been observed. The cause of endocrine disruption during fetal development is generally considered to be xenobiotic interactions with steroid hormones in the fetal brain. The brain also has p450 aromatase and EDCs can alter fetal metabolism of endogenous steroid hormones. EDC-induced apoptosis of endocrine-active hypothalamic neurons in the fetus is considered to be a possible mechanism of action. Disruption of pituitary–adrenal gland and hypothalamic–pituitary–thyroid axes can have an effect on metabolism and stress tolerance.

ADRENAL GLAND

The adrenal cortex produces steroid hormones that are vital for health, and the adrenal gland is a common sensitive target to toxic insult (Capen, 2001; Rosol *et al.*, 2001; Harvey and Everett, 2003; Hinson and Raven, 2006; Ulleras *et al.*, 2008). Disruption of the self-regulating hypothalamic–pituitary–adrenal axis (HPA axis) is understudied and underappreciated (Capen, 2001). Anatomically, mammals have adrenal glands and the avian and teleost species have interrenal glands. The adrenal and interrenal glands secrete sterane core hormones, for example glucocorticoids such as cortisol. Production of the steroid hormones is primarily under the control of adrenocorticotrophin hormone (ACTH) from the anterior pituitary. The synthesis and release of ACTH is regulated by hypothalamic corticotrophin-releasing hormone and arginine vasopressin. This dynamic system is self-regulated by negative feedback from cortisol on both the hypothalamus and pituitary. The HPA axis responds to physiologic stress, and ACTH-induced hyperplasia of the adrenal gland can be caused by intoxication. The adrenal cortex is sensitive to direct toxic insult because it has a disproportionately large blood supply in ml of blood/g of tissue, it has lipophilicity and a high concentration of cytochrome p450 (CYP) and other enzymes normally utilized in steroidogenesis, and the adrenal gland can bioactivate toxicants (Harvey and Everett, 2003; Hinson and Raven, 2006). The HPA axis has high compensatory capacity to deal with toxic insults. Studies to monitor the HPA axis need to include blood levels of adrenal steroids and ACTH, and pathology of the adrenal or interrenal glands. The adrenal gland stores cholesterol and essentially synthesizes steroid hormones from cholesterol *pro re nata*. The rate-limiting step is cholesterol transported to the inner mitochondrial membrane; a process dependent on steroidogenic acute regulatory protein (StAR). Endocrine disrupting chemicals can by altering the activities of adrenal CYP enzyme activities disrupt synthesis of hormones in the adrenal cortex. The adrenal gland can synthesize all classes of steroids. Corticosterone is the principal glucocorticoid of rats, mice, birds, reptiles and amphibians (Rosol *et al.*, 2001). In hamsters, dogs, cats, non-human primates, humans and fish, cortisol is the primary glucocorticoid. Aldosterone is the principal mineralocorticoid produced in the adrenal gland (Rosol *et al.*, 2001). The production of aldosterone is stimulated by angiotensin II and potassium ions. The juxtaglomerular apparatus of the kidney produces renin that cleaves angiotensinogen to produce angiotensin II. The liver produces angiotensinogen. Aldosterone acts in the kidney to conserve sodium ions, excrete potassium ions and increase blood volume. Decreased adrenal function compromised the ability to survive distress and maintain homeostasis. Death caused by adrenal gland insufficiency is less overt than endocrine disruptions that produce more explicit features. Lesions in the adrenal gland are likely under-reported in wildlife and other species (Rosol *et al.*, 2001).

A number of xenobiotics have been shown to disrupt the adrenal gland. The use of *in vitro* studies provides insight into the mechanisms of xenobiotics targeting the adrenal gland. Mercury causes disruption of adrenal and interrenal gland function in a number of species (Tan *et al.*, 2009). These effects are considered to compromise response to stress. Dichlorodiphenyltrichloroethane (DDT) metabolized to *o,p′*-DDD [1,1-dichloro-2,2-bis(4-chlorophenyl)ethane] is known to disrupt adrenal steroidogenesis in some mammalian species, including humans. The mechanism of action is by damage of the mitochondria (Rosol *et al.*, 2001). Harding *et al.* (1999) studied wild mink in British Columbia, and reported that there was no correlation between adrenal gland mass and liver levels of selected POPs, namely organochlorine pesticides, PCBs, TCDDs and TCDFs. Histopathology and other examinations were not reported. The levels of POPs in British Columbia min were lower than in other studies. Mohr *et al.* (2008), reporting a study on the toxicity of bunker C fuel oil in mink, was of the opinion that the adrenal gland was a target organ for petroleum. Hypertrophy of the zona fasciculata and reticularis was observed along with an increase in cytoplasmic vacuoles. In a study on TCDD in domestic mink, the mass of the adrenal gland was increased (Hochstein *et al.*, 1998). Lindane, carbofuran and pentachlorophenol were observed to cause changes in adrenal gland mass in mink (Benimetskii Iu and Klochkov, 1979). In a two-generation study, mink were fed feed treated with lindane at 1 mg/kg/day, carbofuran at 0.05 mg/kg/day, pentachlorophenol (PCP) at 1 mg/kg/day or a control diet. In the F_1 generation, lindane and PCP increased the adrenal gland mass in females. In the F_2 generation, the adrenal gland mass was decreased by carbofuran. There was no difference across treatments for adrenal gland mass for the F_1 and F_2 male mink. Amyloidosis of the adrenal gland has been observed in two Stejneger's beaked whales (Tajima *et al.*, 2007). Amyloidosis was also observed in the heart, spleen, pancreas, liver and kidney. The diffuse amyloidosis may have been triggered by an inflammatory reaction. The adrenal glands of beluga whales including whales killed by hunters and whales found stranded were examined by histopathology (Lair *et al.*, 1997). Cysts of various sizes were observed in mature animals and the occurrence increased with age. The occurrences of macroscopic cysts also increased with age. Hyperplastic nodules were observed in whales from the St. Laurence estuary. It is not known if these lesions are an aging process or caused by EDCs.

A study was done in free-ranging polar bears in the Svalbard region of Norway (Oskam *et al.*, 2004). The auxiliary girth and body mass together accounted for >50% of the variation in plasma cortisol concentration. The summation (Σ) of pesticides combined with ΣPCBs accounted for 25% of the variation in plasma cortisol levels. The Σpesticides had a negative contribution to cortisol levels and the ΣPCBs contributed positively to plasma cortisol. The overall contribution of OCs to the plasma cortisol variation was negative. Bergman (2007) considered adrenal hyperplasia to be a significant aspect of Baltic seal disease complex. All gray and female ringed seals ≥10 years of age had some degree of cortical hyperplasia. Gray seals >15 years of age also had cortical hyperplasia ≥ grade 2. Adrenal adenomas were also observed.

Maternal exposure to environmental levels of PCBs can have sex-specific effects on adrenal function in the offspring and the effects are delayed until puberty. Goats, from day 60 of gestation until parturition, were administered PCBs (PCB congener marked as CB) in the form of 49 µg CB-126/kg body weight/day, 98 µg CB-153/kg body weight/day, or corn oil for 3 days a week (Zimmer *et al.*, 2009). This study suggests that low-level exposure to CB-153 and CB-126 during pregnancy does not affect maternal basal cortisol concentrations, and also does not affect the overall basal cortisol concentrations in the kids. However, at puberty, the males exposed *in utero* to CB-153 had reduced basal cortisol levels during the main part of the reproductive season. During the reproductive season, the effects linked to CB-126 were not as consistent as the group exposed to CB-153. When the males matured, both CB-126 and CB-153 caused stress-induced prolonged peak cortisol levels.

Studies have shown that the HPA axis is an underappreciated target for POPs. Exposure *in utero* to EDCs that target the HPA axis later in life and sex differences can occur. The HPA axis can be compromised and the compromised effect can be influenced by activity in the HPA axis. Compromises in the HPA axis can result in decreased ability to adapt to dynamic environmental stressors and have the potential for serious consequences in many wildlife populations (Jenssen, 2006; Noyes *et al.*, 2009).

THYROID

The hypothalamic–pituitary–thyroid axis (HPT axis) is sensitive to disruption by EDCs and the EDCs can act through different mechanisms (Tyler *et al.*, 1998; Diamanti-Kandarakis *et al.*, 2009; Boas *et al.*, 2009; Zoeller, 2010). The homeostasis of thyroid hormones (THs) is highly regulated by the interactions of regulatory processes (Diamanti-Kandarakis *et al.*, 2009). Thyroid hormones in the blood are regulated within a relatively narrow range primarily by negative feedback relationship with the release of TSH (Zoeller, 2010). The thyroid gland takes up iodine using the sodium/iodine transporter. Iodination of thyroglobulin reaction is catalyzed by thyroid peroxidase as the first step in the production of THs (tetraiodothyronine or T_4 and 3,5,3′-triiodothyronine or T_3). Upon release into the blood from the thyroid gland, THs are free in blood or bound to transport proteins. Important differences for blood transporter mechanisms exist between mammalian species. The thyroid receptor TRβ2, expressed in the pituitary gland and hypothalamic paraventricular nucleus, appears to be the predominant mediator of the negative feedback action of THs on TSH release. The THs are metabolized in peripheral tissues that include the conversion of T_4 to T_3 by deiodinases. Cell transporters move T_3 and T_4 in and out of the somatic cells. The liver also regulates THs through up- and downregulation of catabolic reactions that remove THs from the blood. The THs are conjugated and excreted in bile. The THs, especially T_3, are important in thermoregulation and regulation of metabolism. The developing brain is susceptible to hypothyroidism (Gilbert and Zoeller, 2010). Normal thyroid function is essential for fetal development. Endocrine fetal hypothyroidism, regardless of the cause, is a teratogen. (see Chapter 84). Radioactive iodine is an EDC because it causes pathology in the thyroid gland (Barsano, 1981).

A number of mechanisms have been identified for EDCs that target thyroid homeostasis (Builee and Hatherill, 2004; Crofton, 2008; Diamanti-Kandarakis *et al.*, 2009; Zoeller, 2010). Studies in immature rats provide evidence that CB-95 reduces the response of the pituitary gland to thyroid releasing hormone (Khan and Hansen, 2003). Perchlorate (ClO_4^{-1}), thiocyanates (SCN^{-1}) and nitrates (NO_3^{-1}) impede the uptake of iodine by the thyroid gland by interference with the sodium/iodide transporter. Thyroid peroxidase can be inhibited and thus block the iodination of thyroglobulin. Thionamides, aniline derivatives, substituted phenols, the herbicide amitrole and the fungicide metabolite ethylenethiourea inhibit thyroperoxidase (Crofton, 2008). Chemicals that up- and downregulate hepatic Phase II reactions, especially conjugation reactions, can alter the half-life of T_4. Transport of THs in the blood can be altered by xenobiotics competing for the transporter proteins. Studies (*in vitro*) have shown that specific congeners in brominated fire retardant metabolites have affinity for the transthyretin TH transporter (Hamers *et al.*, 2008). Thyroid disruption may occur when the xenobiotic interferes with the movement of TH into and out of cells. Another target is deiodinases and xenobiotics that target this enzyme to block the conversion of T_4 to T_3. The binding of

T_3 to the receptor is essential for physiologic activity, and xenobiotics that are T_3 receptor antagonists block the physiologic action of T_3 and xenobiotics that are thyroid receptor agonist upregulate the T_3 activity in the cell. Xenobiotics that act on the AhR, the pregnane X-receptor and other receptors upregulate uridine diphosphate glucuronyl transferase can alter the catabolism of THs. Pathologic changes can occur in the thyroid gland. Histopathology can be an indicator of thyroid gland dysfunction. Hypertrophy can be an indicator of disruption of long- and short-loupe inhibition with hypertrophy being caused by TSH stimulation. Another cause of hypertrophy is decreased production of THs by the thyroid gland increasing the release of TSH. Atrophy of the thyroid gland can occur and decreased release of TSH by the pituitary can be one of the causes.

Thyroid histopathology and dysfunction have been observed in wild mammalian species and these changes have been linked to dietary organochlorine contaminants (OCs). A chronic study was done in arctic fox (male) to determine the effects of OCs in blubber on thyroid function and histopathology (Sonne *et al.*, 2009). The foxes were fed a diet containing minke whale blubber or a diet containing pork fat (control). The foxes were 8 weeks old at the start of the experiment and ~2 years old at study termination. Dietary OCs (as fed) were 171 ng PCBs/g, 62 ng DDT/g, 42 ng CHL/g, 2 ng HCH/g, 3 ng CBZ/g and 23 ng dieldrin/g. Thyroid histopathology attributed to the OCs was observed, namely hyperplasia of the thyroid-C cells. Similar changes have been observed in polar bears (Sonne, 2010). The histopathology of thyroid glands from beluga whales taken from the St. Laurence estuary (SLE) and Hudson Bay was studied (Mikaelian *et al.*, 2003). Nine of 16 whales from the SLE and 6/14 whales from Hudson Bay were observed to have adenomatous hyperplasia of the thyroid. Thyroid follicular cysts were found in 9/16 whales from SLE and 4/17 of the whales from Hudson Bay. Cysts were found in belugas as young as 2.5 years old (age determined by tooth dentine growth layers). Pituitary tumors were not observed in the SLE whales.

The effect of pesticides and a wood preservative on thyroid function have been studied in mink. Lindane, carbofuran and pentachlorophenol were studied in a two-generation study in mink (Benimetskii Iu and Klochkov, 1979). The mink were fed feed treated with lindane at 1 mg/kg/d, carbofuran at 0.05 mg/kg/d, pentachlorophenol (PCP) at 1 mg/kg/d or a control diet. In the PCP group, male mink in F_1 and F_2 generations and female mink in the F_2 generation had a decrease in serum T_4. In the lindane and carbofuran groups, the F_1 males also had significantly decreased T_4. No changes in maternal T_4 and T_3 were observed. All of the mink in the lindane, PCP and carbofuran groups had a decrease in thyroid mass and this effect was statistically significant in the F_2 females. Genotype can influence seasonal thyroid response in mink (Benimetskii Iu and Klochkov, 1979). A study in humans suggests that females exposed to chlorinated dioxins can, 25 years post-exposure, give birth to babies with neonatal thyroid dysfunction (Baccarelli *et al.*, 2008). Using a multigenerational design, ocean fish or Saginaw Bay carp were fed to ranch mink to give dietary levels of 0.0 ppm, 0.25, 0.5 or 1.0 ppm PCBs (Restum *et al.*, 1998). Serum T_4 levels increased in the parental males and females in the 1.0 ppm group. At the 1.0 ppm level, the T_3 levels were unchanged or increased in females and males, respectively. In F_1 female mink, T_4 levels were not changed and there was a decrease in T_3 levels. A remarkable decrease in the survival of the F_2 kits did not allow additional multigenerational evaluations of thyroid function. Mink in the 1.0 ppm group had increased thyroid mass.

Studies in Alaskan northern fur seals suggest that high levels of specific PCB congeners could be targeting the thyroid gland (Wang *et al.*, 2010). Studies in harbor seals showed that seasonal trends occurred in circulating total T_4 (tT_4) levels with the peak tT_4 being in the summer months (Hall and Thomas, 2007). In the same study, log PCB levels in blubber was a predictor of increased total T_3 (tT_3) and males had the highest PCB and tT_3 levels. The best indicator of tT_3 was the ΣPCBs in blubber. The relationship between blubber PCBs and THs and the thyroid receptor (TR) gene expression was studied in harbor seals (Tabuchi *et al.*, 2006). Negative correlations were found between tT_4 and free T_4 and ΣPCBs in blubber. Increased levels of PCBs in blubber increased the expression of *TR-α*. In another study fish from areas of the ocean that have high PCBs (Wadden Sea) and fish from areas of the ocean (Atlantic Ocean) with low PCB contamination were fed to common seals (Brouwer *et al.*, 1989). Total T_4, free T_4 (fT_4) and tT_3 in blood were lower in seals fed fish from the Wadden Sea. Colloid depletion and fibrosis of the thyroid gland has been observed in an epidemic die-off of harbor seals (Schumacher *et al.*, 1993). The effects of EDCs on thyroid function during infectious disease are not well understood.

Studies have been done correlating the levels of OCs in polar bears (Skaare *et al.*, 2001). Blood was collected from 101 polar bears in eastern Svalbard and the age determined by a tooth examination (counts of cementum growth layer groups). Blood was assayed for selected OCs and T_4 and T_3. Females had significantly higher levels of THs, and the levels of THs in females did not change with age. The concentrations of THs were negatively correlated with age in male bears. The tT_4/fT_4 and tT_3/fT_3 ratios were significantly higher in males than in females. The tT_4/fT_4 ratio decreased linearly with increasing concentrations of PCBs and hexachlorobenzene (HCB). The T_4/fT_4 ratio was positively associated with DDE. The ΣOCs were found to explain 30 and 7% of the variation of the tT_4/fT_4 and tT_3/fT_3 ratios, respectively, after correcting for age and sex.

Thyroid dynamics from birth to weaning has been reported for gray seal pups (Woldstad and Jenssen, 1999). Two days following birth tT_4 was high and then dropped to a lower stable level. Gray seal pups for body size have a high metabolic rate at birth and then the metabolic rate decreases. The tT_3 concentrations were lowest in neonatal pups then increased as a function of age. This likely was due to upregulation of deiodination increasing as a function of age. Free thyroxine (fT_4) did not vary as a function of age. In a study of gray seal pups in the Baltic Ocean and Norwegian Atlantic, gender, age, body mass and population were not predictors of plasma tT_4 and fT_4 (Sormo *et al.*, 2005). Gray seal pups from the Baltic Ocean had lower plasma tT_3 and fT_3. The blubber concentrations of OCs were higher in the pups residing in the Baltic Ocean. The PCB congeners CB-99, CB-118, CB-138, CB-153, CB-170, CB-183 and *p,p′*-DDE were correlated negatively with plasma tT_3 concentrations. These results suggest that specific PCBs used in the model may have more significance on thyroid function than the total concentration of the congeners in a particular group. A Japanese study in large seals collected in costal waters of Hokkaido found that tT_3 and fT_3 were negatively correlated with OCs (Chiba *et al.*, 2001). For ribbon seals, tT_3 levels significantly decreased with an increase of CB-170 and CB-18 congeners.

Ring and gray seals from the Baltic Sea and reference areas of Svalbard (Norway) and Sable Island (Canada) were studied for the effects of OCs on thyroid and vitamin D (Routti *et al.*, 2008). For the seals from the Baltic Sea, the ΣPCB was >80 times higher, and the total DDT was >100-fold higher than for the Svalbard seals. The geographical differences in gray seals from the Baltic Sea were 2.5 higher for ΣPCBs and four-fold higher for total DDT than Sable Island seals. The Baltic ring seals had a negative correlation between plasma tT_4 and fT_4 and age. Body condition in the Baltic ringed seals showed a positive relationship with tT_3 level and the tT_3/tT_4 ratio. In the gray seal the fT_3/tT_3 ratio showed a strong positive correlation with ΣOC load. The plasma tT_4, tT_3, fT_4 and fT_3 levels were strongly correlated with plasma retinol levels in the gray seals. For the Baltic ringed seals, a significant negative correlation was shown for tT_4, tT3 and ΣPCBs and between tT4 and total DDT, whereas the fT_4/tT_4 ratio and total DDT were positively correlated. In ringed seals the plasma levels of 1,25-dihydroxyvitamin D3 were negatively correlated with PHAHs. This observation is interesting because Sonne *et al.* (2009) reported hyperplasia of the thyroid-C cells in Arctic fox fed a diet containing blubber contaminated with PHAHs.

A study on the relationship between plasma PCBs and THs and retinol was conducted in free-ranging female polar bears (Braathen *et al.*, 2004). There were females with cubs of the year (FWCOY) and females without cubs of the year (FWOCOY), and a group of males. The PCB congeners CB-99, CB-153, CB-156, CB-180 and CB-194 were correlated with each other and the concentrations of CB-118 did not correlate with the other congeners. The FWCOY group had negative correlations between ΣPCBs and fT_4, fT_3 and the tT_4:t/tT_3 ratio. For the FWOCOY group, the ΣPCBs were negatively correlated to tT_4 and positively correlated to the tT_3/Ff_3 ratio, and CB-118 was positively correlated to fT_3 and negatively correlated to the tT_3/fT_3 ratio. For males, ΣPCBs were negatively correlated to fT_3 and positively correlated to fT_4/fT_3 whereas CB-118 was negatively correlated to the fT_4/fT_3 ratio. This study suggests that PCBs could target thyroid function in female polar bears.

The polybrominated diphenylethers (PBDEs) target the thyroid gland (Zoeller, 2010). The PBDEs have been shown to disrupt thyroid function in mink (Zhang *et al.*, 2009). In a reproductive study female mink were fed a diet containing 0, 0.1, 0.5 and 2.5 ppm (wt/wt) in feed of a technical pentabrominated diphenyl ether mixture (DE-71). The offspring were exposed until they were 33 weeks old. There was an increase in vacuolization in the thyroid gland of the dams and T_4 was significantly reduced in the 2.5 ppm DE-71 group. Female juveniles had a significant increase in tT_4. The overall trend was an increase in T_4 and a decrease in T_3 with significance differences occurring in the 2.5 ppm group in dams and juveniles in the 0.5 ppm group. In the 0.5 ppm group, follicular cell height was increased in juveniles. The T_4 outer ring deiodinase activity (primarily type II deiodinases) was not affected at any dose or life stage. There was a significant increase in hepatic ethoxyresorufin *o*-deethylase activity in all offspring at 33 weeks. Wild mink, based on tissue levels of PBDEs, could exceed the NOAE defined in this study. Studies in sheep have shown that *in utero* exposure to PBDE (DE-47) can alter thyroid function in lambs (Abdelouahab *et al.*, 2009). Pregnant ewes were given weekly intravenous injections of DE-47 at 0.2, 2 and 20 µg/kg body weight from the 5th to 15th week of gestation. The lambs exposed to DE-47 *in utero* had a significant decrease in T_4 and T_3 at the 135th day of gestation. A study in young (≤1 year of age) gray seals showed that PBDEs in blubber and age were a good predictor of serum levels of tT_4 and tT_3 (Hall *et al.*, 2003). The tT_4 and tT_3 increased with increasing levels of PBDEs in blubber.

Hexabromocyclododecane (HBCD) has been shown to target the thyroid gland in rats (van der Ven *et al.*, 2006). Rats were administered a dose range from 0 to 200 mg HBCD/kg body weight/day for 28 days. In the female rats there was a decrease in serum tT_4, an increase in pituitary mass, increased pituitary immunostaining for TSH, increased thyroid mass and thyroid follicle cell activation. Induction of T_4-glucuronyl transferase was observed suggesting upregulation of T_4 catabolism. Data modeling showed that thyroid mass was the most sensitive parameter with thyroid mass being increased at 1.6 mg/kg body weight/day. Since HBCD has the potential of being a persistent bioaccumulation compound, it is reasonable that HBCD could target the thyroid gland in wildlife species.

SEX HORMONES AND REPRODUCTION

A brief overview of the dynamic and intricate regulation of the hypothalamus–pituitary–gonadal axis (HPG axis) has recently been reviewed (Damstra *et al.*, 2002; Diamanti-Kandarakis *et al.*, 2009; Gore, 2010). The HPG axis has four components. These are the GnRH-secreting neurons located in the medial preoptic nucleus of the hypothalamus, the hypothalamic–pituitary portal system, the gonadotropic cells in the anterior pituitary gland (adenohypophysis) that secrete luteinizing hormone (LH) and follicle stimulating hormone (FSH), and hormone-secreting cells in the gonads (ovary – theca and granulosa cells, testicle – Leydig and Sertoli cells). Neurons in the hypothalamus release pulses of GnRH into the hypothalamic portal system which in turn stimulates the release of FSH and LH from the pituitary gland. The gonadotropic cells are sensitive to the pulses of GnRh with irregular low amplitude pattern stimulating FSH release and high frequency inducing LH release (Knobil, 1988). In the gonads, LH acts on ovarian theca and testicular Leydig cells and FSH on ovarian granulosa and testicular Sertoli cells. Gonadotropin synthesis and release is highly modulated by complex feedback mechanisms. Gonadal sex steroids, stimulated by LH, and inhibin A (female) and inhibin B (male), stimulated by FSH, via the blood, provide feedback to the hypothalamus and pituitary gonadotropes to reduce the secretion of GnRH, LH and FSH. The inhibins selectively inhibit FSH and the sex steroids inhibit LH secretion. Sex steroids, primarily testosterone in the male and estradiol in female, negatively regulate LH secretion via effects on both GnRH secretion and gonadotrope function. Testosterone and estradiol also exert some negative feedback on FSH secretion; in contrast, inhibin selectively inhibits FSH secretion. In a similar manner, the sex steroids, primarily testosterone in the male and estradiol in the female, negatively modulate LH secretion by effects on both GnRH secretion and gonadotrope function. Paracrine interactions occur. In females, androgen produced in the thecal cells is converted to estradiol by the granulosa cells. Testosterone produced by the Leydig cells is converted to estradiol, which also has negative feedback on the pituitary and hypothalamus. Important in the paracrine and feedback mechanisms is the ability of cells to up- and downregulate the expression of enzymes that transform sex steroids and by this mechanism can alter HPG and paracrine homeostasis. Enzyme induction by EDCs can alter homeostasis of enzymes that transform sex steroids.

There are concerns that endocrine disruption can alter reproduction in wildlife species. These concerns are increased in species that have declining numbers, and wildlife species that have critical numbers (Derocher *et al.*, 2003). The Arctic is a sink for POPs and these pollutants are biomagnified in predators that are at the top of the food chain (Ropstad *et al.*, 2006). These species have evolved reproductive mechanisms and temporal strategies that ensure succus. A study in the Svalbard region of Norway found that testosterone was the highest in adult male polar bears from April to May and in August (Oskum *et al.*, 2003). Axial girth had a positive relationship with extractable fat in plasma and a negative relationship with plasma testosterone. The plasma Σchlorinated pesticides and ΣPCB congener levels were negatively correlated with plasma testosterone. A study in harvested immature and mature male polar bears from east Greenland provided more evidence on the relationship between chlorinated organic compounds and testosterone (Letcher *et al.*, 2009). These findings suggest that in immature males, contaminants such as transchlordane, CB-118, dieldrin and CB-153 influence the variation in testosterone levels. In adult males, compounds such as transchlordane, *p,p′*-DDE, DE-47 and CB-128 appear to be important determinants in the variation of testosterone. A study in live captured female polar bears in the Svalbard region of Norway correlated progesterone and 17β-estradiol (E_2) with CB-congeners (Haave *et al.*, 2003). Progesterone was the lowest in females with offspring. In females with offspring there was a positive correlation of progesterone with ΣPCB congener levels with the ΣPCB congener levels explaining 27% of the variation. The ΣPCB congeners were not correlated with E_2 and cortisol. Reproductive organs from 55 male and 44 female polar bears from Scoresby Sound in east Greenland were studied (Sonne *et al.*, 2006). Multiple regression analyses showed a significant inverse relationship between organochlorine pollutants (OCPs) and baculum length and baculum weight. Baculum densities decreased with increasing chlordanes, DDTs and HCB. In females, a significant inverse relationship was found between ovary length and ΣPCB and ΣCHL. There also was an inverse relationship between ovary mass and ΣPBDE, and inverse relationship between uterine horn length and HCB levels.

The Baltic seal disease syndrome in gray and ringed seals is linked to high body burdens of OCPs (Vos *et al.*, 2000). Bergman (2007) had reported on reproductive pathology and pregnancy for the 1977 to 1996 interval. Stenosis of the uterus was observed in 42% of the gray seals in the 1987 to 1996 study period and a trend likely exists for decreased occurrences. Baltic gray seals have been observed to have uterine leiomyomas in senility with an age shift trend over the last 9 study years for uterine leiomyomas to occur more frequently in younger females. The observed pregnancies in gray seals increased from 9 to 60%. A controlled reproductive performance study was done in common seals (Reijnders, 1986). Seals in group 1 were fed fish taken from the Wadden Sea and group 2 was fed fish from the northeast Atlantic. Fish from the Wadden Sea were remarkably higher in PCBs and *p,p′*-DDE. Males on the Atlantic diet were allowed to inseminate females. Females in group 1 had significantly lower successful pregnancies. In group 1, there was a decreased follicular-associated estradiol in the non-pregnant females and for this group there was an overall decrease in estradiol. Methylmercury accumulates in the gonads of harp seals and alters steroid biosynthesis (Tan *et al.*, 2009).

Mink, with some disagreement, are generally considered an indicator species for environmental safety (Brunstrom *et al.*, 2001; Basu *et al.*, 2007; Bowman and Schulte-Hostedde, 2009). Ranch-raised mink fed Great Lakes fish contaminated with PCBs, or treated with PCBs directly, have demonstrated reproductive impairment including anovulation, fetal resorption, delayed ovulation, increased gestation and decreased litter size. Studies in mink have shown that POPs in feedstuffs can impair reproduction and cause changes in reproductive organs (Hornshaw *et al.*, 1983). The research group at Michigan State University (Aulerich *et al.*, 1971) showed that coho salmon from the Great Lakes impaired reproductive function in mink. The reproductive effects were linked to POPs in the fish. Feeding studies showed that cattle and fish tissue containing PCBs were more toxic to mink than equivalent mass of Aroclor 1254, and cattle and fish tissues also impaired reproductive success (Platonow and Karstad, 1973; Hornshaw *et al.*, 1983). Wren *et al.* (1987a,b) showed that PCBs (Aroclor 1254) in combination with methylmercury (Methyl-Hg) decreased the survival of mink kits, and a reduction in kit survival was not observed with PCBs or Methyl-Hg treatments. Examination of data from areas known to have high environmental levels of POPs suggested there was a decrease in mink populations (Wren, 1991). The reproductive toxicology of PCBs in carp from Saginaw Bay on Lake Huron, USA, was studied in ranch mink (Heaton *et al.*, 1995). Marine fish was substituted for Lake Huron fish to give 0, 10, 20 or 40% dietary levels of Lake Huron carp. Dietary levels were 0.015, 0.72, 1.53 and 2.56 mg PCBs/kg diet, or 1.03, 19.41, 40.02 and 80.76 ng TEQs/kg diet, respectively. Mink were exposed 85 days inclusive before and throughout the reproductive period. Total PCBs consumed by feeding mink 0, 10, 20 or 40% carp were 0.34, 13.2, 25.3 and 32.3 mg PCBs/mink, respectively. And the TEQs ingested were 23, 356, 661 and 1,019 ng TEQs/mink, respectively. Reduction in feed consumption was inversely proportional to the ΣPCB and ΣTEQ in the diet. Time-of-birth body masses of kits were reduced in the 20 and 40% carp groups. The kit body weights and survival in the 10 and 20% carp groups were significantly reduced at 3 and 6 weeks of age. Females in the 40% carp group whelped the fewest number of kits and these kits were stillborn or died ≤24 h post-whelping. Mink in a multigenerational study were fed ocean fish or Saginaw Bay carp to give dietary levels of 0.0, 0.25, 0.5 or 1.0 ppm PCBs (Restum *et al.*, 1998; Shipp *et al.*, 1998). The concentration of hepatic estrogen binding generally decreased with increasing dietary PCB concentrations and uterine estrogen binding site concentration was unchanged. Testicular volume was not changed in the parental and F_1 generation, and there was no difference in male libido. In the females in the 0.25 ppm group, the onset of estrus was delayed and whelping rate was decreased. Kits born to females in the 0.5 ppm and higher exposure groups had decreased body mass and increased kit mortality was observed. A British Columbia study in wild mink found that baculum length was negatively correlated with PCB levels in body fat (Harding *et al.*, 1999). This observation is in contrast to the report of Aulerich *et al.* (2000) that feeding Aroclor 1254 (2 mg/kg of feed) to 12-week-old male mink kits for 20 weeks caused a weak correlation with baculum length and mass. These observations suggest that multiple chemical interactions could be causing the effect or the effect is due to specific CB congeners.

Under laboratory conditions, fish from the Housatonic River were shown to decrease kit survival in mink (Bursian *et al.*, 2006). The toxic equivalence (TEQ) (Van den Berg *et al.*, 1998) contributions from PCDDs, PCDFs, non-*ortho*-PCBs and mono-*ortho*-PCBs in the treatment diets averaged 2.8 ± ±0.8%, 6.8 ± ±1.9%, 59.1 ± 1.4% and 32.1 ± 0.3%, respectively. The total PCBs in the diet were 3.7 µg/g of feed or 68.5 pg TEQ. Mature female mink were fed 0.0006 (control), 0.016, 0.053, 0.180 or 1.40 ppb 2,3,7,8-tetrachlorodibenzo-p-dioxin (TCDD) for 131 to 132 days (Hochstein *et al.*, 2001). A dose-dependent reduction in birth weight and kit survival was observed. A reproduction study was done on Clophen A50 (CA50) in female mink (Brunstrom *et al.*, 2001). The dose levels for technical CA50 were 0.0 (fish oil), 0.1 or 0.3 mg/animal/day. Other treatment groups received 0 to 1-*ortho*-CBs extracted from 0.3 mg of CA50 (could contain dicyclic aromatic contaminants), 2 to 4-*ortho*-CBs extracted from 0.3 mg of CA50 and an acetonitrile extract from Baltic gray seal blubber that contained 0.064 mg ΣPCB and 0.021 mg ΣDDT. The aryl methyl sulfones had been removed from the blubber extract. All the groups were given the CA50 or extracts for 3 days/week for 18 months over two breeding seasons. Females in the 0.3 mg CB50 group had reduced whelping frequency and in the second reproductive season and all birthed kits died ≤24 h. Females in the 0.1 mg CB50 group had impaired reproductive performance. The group receiving the 0 to 1-*ortho*-CBs extract had severely reduced kit survival. The groups administered the 2 to 4-*ortho*-CBs seal blubber extract did not have a significant decrease in reproductive performance. Previous studies have reported that estrogen and progesterone levels are unaltered in mink treated with PCBs (Shipp *et al.*, 1998).

Sheep and other domestic ruminants can likely be used to predict the effects of POPs in wild ruminants. The EDCs in sewage sludge spread on pasturelands were shown to cause endocrine disruption in sheep (Paul *et al.*, 2005; Fowler *et al.*, 2008; Bellingham *et al.*, 2009). These studies, described in Chapter 84, show that exposure *in utero* to mixtures of environmental chemicals may have long-term effects on the reproductive capacity of sheep. A histopathological study provides evidence that POPs may decrease the reproductive capacity of free roaming male elands (Borman *et al.*, 2010). The animals were taken from the Rietvlei Nature Reserve, the Suikerbosrand Nature Reserve and the Molopo Nature Reserve close to the Kalahari Desert. In 24 elands from the Rietvlei and Suikerbosrand Nature Reserves all the testicles were abnormal. Lesions observed were multiple intratubular dystrophic calcifications, focal areas of spermatozoa stasis and fibrosis accompanied by interstitial cell infiltrates. Also observed were vacuolization of Sertoli cells and sloughing of the seminiferous epithelium. In the rete testis, adenomatous changes were observed and overall spermatogenesis was generally impaired. In the three elands taken from the Molopo Natural Reserve one animal had a few focal testicular lesions. Eleven of 17 elands taken from the Rietvlei Nature Reserve had p-nonylphenol in fat at 84.8 ± 24.6 µg/kg, 6/17 had detectable levels of p-nonylphenol below the quantification level and OCs were not detected. Analyses of fat from the elands taken from the Suikerbosrand Nature Reserves showed: 5/7 had detectable octylphenol residues averaging 50 ± 30.1 µg/kg fat, 3/7 had detectable p-nonylphenol averaging 140 ± 78 µg/kg fat, 3/7 had *o,p′*-DDT averaging 115 ± 30 µg/kg fat, 3/7 had *p,p′*-DDT averaging 130 ± 50 µg /kg fat, 5/7 had *o,p′*-DDE averaging 28 ± 10 µg/kg fat, 7/7 had *o,p′*-DDD averaging 80 ± 30 µg/kg fat, and *p,p′*-DDE was not detected. Fat samples from the Molopo Nature Reserve showed 1/3 had *p,p′*-DDE at 60 µg/kg fat, and 1/3 had *p,p′*-DDT at 71 µg/kg fat. A study in domestic goats showed that exposure *in utero* to environmental levels of PCBs can affect pituitary and gonadal hormones in female offspring (Lyche *et al.*, 2004). Pregnant goats were administered PCBs in the form of 49 µg CB-126/kg body weight/day, 98 µg CB-153/kg body weight/day, or corn oil for 3 days/week from day 60 of gestation until parturition. In the female kids exposed *in utero* to CB-153, prepubertal plasma levels of LH were lower. Also, the females exposed *in utero* to CB-153 had delayed onset of puberty, and higher progesterone levels during luteal phase of the estrous cycles. Plasma levels of prolactin and FSH were not affected. Exposure *in utero* to CB-126 did not alter age of puberty, prolactin, FSH, LH or prolactin parameters.

Sonne *et al.* (2008) proposed that diet high in seal blubber containing polyhalogenated aromatic hydrocarbons consumed by a pregnant bitch could be linked to perineal and penile hypospadias in a pup. Pregnant bitches fed minke blubber gave birth to pups with reduced testicular size (Letcher *et al.*, 2009). Chlormequat (2-chloroethyltrimethyl ammonium chloride), a plant growth regulator, has been reported (contaminated grain feeding study) to suppress behavioral and physical signs of estrus in domestic pigs (Sorensen and Danielsen, 2006). In a laboratory study on chlormequat in male laboratory mice, there was a reduction of *in vitro* fertility, but *in vivo* fertility was not impaired (Torner *et al.*, 1999). The reason for this discrepancy is not understood. The effects of chlormequat in wildlife have not been reported.

Mycotoxins have been shown to cause endocrine disruption in mink (Yamini *et al.*, 1997; Sharma *et al.*, 2002). Zearalenone (ZEA) was fed at 20 mg ZEA/kg from ~2 months before mating until kits were 3 weeks old. All female mink fed ZEA mated and 25% whelped. Histopathology was mild to severe endometrial hyperplasia, endometritis to metritis, and ovarial follicles were atrophied and degenerated. Oat-derived ergot alkaloids were studied in mink (Sharma *et al.*, 2002). Female mink (four groups of 12 mink) were fed diets containing 0, 3, 6 or 12 ppm ergot alkaloids from 2 weeks prior mating until the kits were ~1 month old. Dietary ergot alkaloids at the 6 ppm dietary level caused a longer gestation period. The number of kits whelped decreased with increasing dietary ergot. Ergot caused a decrease in serum prolactin levels.

ECOLOGICAL EFFECTS

The endocrine system in wildlife species is well adapted for their environment. Their endocrine system responds to environmental changes to maintain physiologic homeostasis and ensure reproductive success. Chemical hormonal disruption can alter homeostasis and have long-term impact on the population, and a unique disease syndrome linked to POPs can emerge (Vos *et al.*, 2000). Female fecundity is generally considered to be more sensitive in terms of environmental levels of EDCs required to lower the total lifetime progeny as compared to the environmental level of EDCs that would decrease the fecundity of males (Gurney, 2006). If a large number of males in a critical population are affected, the fertility of the males can have an impact on the population. Cryptorchidism has increased in the critical population of Florida panther, and questions are being raised if this condition is linked to environmental EDCs (Facemire *et al.*, 1995). If this link is established, the Florida panther male could be more sensitive to EDCs than females. The toxicokinetics of bioaccumulation of persistent organic pollutants (POPs) is different in males and reproducing females. Females transfer POPs to the fetus and excrete POPs in milk. Studies in bottlenose dolphins have shown that the POPs in the body fat of males is accumulated linearly with age (Wells *et al.*, 2005; Yordy *et al.*, 2010). Lactation is important in decreasing maternal burdens of POPs in body fat. The levels of POPs are higher in females before parturition and depurate with subsequent parturitions. The survivability of first-born can be decreased and the first-born has higher levels of POPs. The *in utero* endocrine disruptive effects could also be higher in offspring born to younger females. Mercury can alter sex ratios in rats and reduce male survival (Tan *et al.*, 2009). A debate exists on the effects of EDCs on sex ratio.

Chemicals are being released into the environment before the long-term impact is fully appreciated. For example, the results of *in vitro* screening indicated that brominated fire retardants (BFRs) have endocrine-disrupting potencies (Hamers *et al.*, 2006). The test material consisted of 27 individual BFRs consisting of 19 polybrominated diphenyl ether congeners, tetrabromobisphenol-A, hexabromocyclododecane, 2,4,6-tribromophenol, *ortho*-hydroxylated brominated diphenyl ether 47 and tetrabromobisphenol-A-bis(2,3) dibromopropyl ether. The endocrine-disrupting activities observed were androgen receptor antagonism, progesterone receptor antagonism, inhibition of estradiol sulfotransferase, inhibition and potentiation of T_3-mediated cell proliferation. The potency of some BFRs was higher than the potency for natural ligands or clinical drugs used as positive controls.

CONCLUDING REMARKS AND FUTURE DIRECTIONS

EDCs have been shown to work through a variety of mechanisms. The endocrine system is in a dynamic state of homeostasis interrelated with hepatic, renal, neural and immune functions. Small changes in endocrine function can have long-reaching consequences on the status of health and longevity. The food web contains a complex mixture of POPs and the observed endocrine effects are likely the effect of complex biologic interactions of EDCs in the mixture. It is likely that genetic selection of wildlife for tolerance to EDCs has occurred. In small or decreasing populations, the genetic diversity available for selection within the population could also be decreasing. The interactions of EDCs with infectious diseases are essentially unknown. The EDCs can also be impinging on the ability of wildlife to adapt to environmental dynamics and habitat encroachments (Jenssen, 2006).

REFERENCES

Abdelouahab N, Suvorov A, Pasquier JC, Langlois MR, Praud JP, Takser L (2009) Thyroid disruption by low-dose BDE-47 in prenatally exposed lambs. *Neonatology* **96(2):** 120–4.

Ahn KC, Zhao B, Chen J, Cherednichenko G, Sanmarti E, Denison MS, Lasley B, Pessah IN, Kultz D, Chang DP, Gee SJ, Hammock BD (2008) In vitro biologic activities of the antimicrobials triclocarban, its analogs, and triclosan in bioassay screens: receptor-based bioassay screens. *Environ Health Perspect* **116(9):** 1203–10.

Aulerich RJ, Ringer RK, Seagran HL, Youatt WG (1971) Effects of feeding coho salmon and other Great Lakes fish on mink reproduction. *Can J Zool* **49(5):** 611–16.

Aulerich RJ, Bursian SJ, Napolitano AC, Oleas T (2000) Feeding growing mink (*Mustela vison*) PCB Aroclor 1254 does not affect baculum (os-penis) development. *Bull Environ Contam Toxicol* **64(3):** 443–7.

Baccarelli A, Giacomini SM, Corbetta C, Landi MT, Bonzini M, Consonni D, Grillo P, Patterson DG, Pesatori AC, Bertazzi PA (2008) Neonatal thyroid function in Seveso 25 years after maternal exposure to dioxin. *PLoS Med* **5(7):** e161.

Barsano CP (1981) Environmental factors altering thyroid function and their assessment. *Environ Health Perspect* **38:** 71–82.

Basu N, Scheuhammer AM, Bursian SJ, Elliott J, Rouvinen-Watt K, Chan HM (2007) Mink as a sentinel species in environmental health. *Environ Res* **103(1):** 130–44.

Beard AP, Rawlings NC (1998) Reproductive effects in mink (*Mustela vison*) exposed to the pesticides Lindane, Carbofuran and Pentachlorophenol in a multigeneration study. *J Reprod Fertil* **113(1):** 95–104.

Bellingham M, Fowler PA, Amezaga MR, Rhind SM, Cotinot C, Mandon-Pepin B, Sharpe RM, Evans NP (2009) Exposure to a complex cocktail of environmental endocrine-disrupting compounds disturbs the kisspeptin/GPR54 system in ovine hypothalamus and pituitary gland. *Environ Health Perspect* **117(10):** 1556–62.

Benimetskii IS, Klochkov DV (1979) [Functional state of the thyroid gland in the postnatal period in mink of different genotypes]. *Ontogenez* **10(4):** 410–13.

Bergman A (2007) *Pathological Changes in Seals in Swedish Waters: The Relation to Environmental Pollution.* Department of Biomedical Sciences and Veterinary Public Health, Swedish University of Agricultural Sciences, Uppsala: Doctoral Thesis.

Boas M, Main KM, Feldt-Rasmussen U (2009) Environmental chemicals and thyroid function: an update. *Curr Opin Endocrinol Diabetes Obes* **16(5):** 385–91.

Bornman MS, Barnhoorn IE, de Jager C, Veeramachaneni DN (2010) Testicular microlithiasis and neoplastic lesions in wild eland (*Tragelaphus oryx*): possible effects of exposure to environmental pollutants? *Environ Res* **110(4):** 327–33.

Bowman J, Schulte-Hostedde AI (2009) The mink is not a reliable sentinel species. *Environ Res* **109(7):** 937–9; discussion 940–1.

Braathen M, Derocher AE, Wiig O, Sormo EG, Lie E, Skaare JU, Jenssen BM (2004) Relationships between PCBs and thyroid hormones and retinol in female and male polar bears. *Environ Health Perspect* **112(8):** 826–33.

Brouwer A, Reijnders PJH, Koeman JK (1989) Polychlorinated biphenyl (PCB)-contaminated fish induces vitamin A and thyroid hormone deficiency in the common seal (*Phoca vitulina*). *Aquatic Toxicol* **15:** 99–106.

Brunstrom B, Lund BO, Bergman A, Asplund L, Athanassiadis I, Athanasiadou M, Jensen S, Orberg J (2001) Reproductive toxicity in mink (*Mustela vison*) chronically exposed to environmentally relevant polychlorinated biphenyl concentrations. *Environ Toxicol Chem* **20(10):** 2318–27.

Builee TL, Hatherill JR 2004 The role of polyhalogenated aromatic hydrocarbons on thyroid hormone disruption and cognitive function: a review. *Drug Chem Toxicol* **27(4):** 405–24.

Bursian SJ, Sharma C, Aulerich RJ, Yamini BR, Mitchell RR, Orazio CE, Moore DR, Svirsky S, Tillitt DE (2006) Dietary exposure of mink (*Mustela vison*) to fish from the Housatonic River, Berkshire County, Massachusetts, USA: effects on reproduction, kit growth, and survival. *Environ Toxicol Chem* **25(6):** 1533–40.

Capen CC (2001) Overview of structural and functional lesions in endocrine organs of animals. *Toxicol Pathol* **29(1):** 8–33.

Chen J, Ahn KC, Gee NA, Ahmed MI, Duleba AJ, Zhao L, Gee SJ, Hammock BD, Lasley BL (2008) Triclocarban enhances testosterone action: a new type of endocrine disruptor? *Endocrinology* **149(3):** 1173–9.

Chiba I, Sakakibara A, Goto Y, Isono T, Yamamoto Y, Iwata H, Tanabe S, Shimazaki K, Akahori F, Kazusaka A, Fujita S (2001) Negative correlation between plasma thyroid hormone levels and chlorinated hydrocarbon levels accumulated in seals from the coast of Hokkaido, Japan. *Environ Toxicol Chem* **20(5):** 1092–7.

Crofton KM (2008) Thyroid disrupting chemicals: mechanisms and mixtures. *Int J Androl* **31(2):** 209–23.

Damstra T, Barlow S, Bergman A, Kavlock R, Van Der Kraak G (2002) *Global Assessment of the State-of-the-Science of Endocrine Disruptors.* Geneva, Switzerland, WHO.

Derocher AE, Wolkers H, Colborn T, Schlabach M, Larsen TS, Wiig O (2003) Contaminants in Svalbard polar bear samples archived since 1967 and possible population level effects. *Sci Total Environ* **301(1–3):** 163–74.

Diamanti-Kandarakis E, Bourguignon JP, Giudice LC, Hauser R, Prins GS, Soto AM, Zoeller RT, Gore AC (2009) Endocrine-disrupting chemicals: an Endocrine Society scientific statement. *Endocr Rev* **30(4):** 293–342.

Facemire CF, Gross TS, Guillette Jr LG (1995) Reproductive impairment in the Florida panther: nature or nurture? *Environ Health Perspect* **103 (Suppl. 4):** 79–86.

Fowler PA, Dora NJ, McFerran H, Amezaga MR, Miller DW, Lea RG, Cash P, McNeilly AS, Evans NP, Cotinot C, Sharpe RM, Rhind SM (2008) In utero exposure to low doses of environmental pollutants disrupts fetal ovarian development in sheep. *Mol Hum Reprod* **14(5):** 269–80.

Gee D (2006) Late lessons from early warnings: toward realism and precaution with endocrine-disrupting substances. *Environ Health Perspect* **114 (Suppl. 1):** 152–60.

Gilbert ME, Zoeller RT (2010) Thyroid hormones – impact on the developing brain: possible mechanisms of neurotoxicity. In *Neurotoxicology* (Harry GJ, Tilson HA, eds.). New York, Informa Healthcare.

Gore AC (2010) Neuroendocrine targets of endocrine disruptors. *Hormones (Athens)* **9(1):** 16–27.

Guillette LJ Jr (2006) Endocrine disrupting contaminants – beyond the dogma. *Environ Health Perspect* **114 (Suppl. 1):** 9–12.

Gurney WS (2006) Modeling the demographic effects of endocrine disruptors. *Environ Health Perspect* **114 (Suppl. 1):** 122–6.

Haave M, Ropstad E, Derocher AE, Lie E, Dahl E, Wiig O, Skaare JU, Jenssen BM (2003) Polychlorinated biphenyls and reproductive hormones in female polar bears at Svalbard. *Environ Health Perspect* **111(4):** 431–6.

Hall AJ, Kalantzi OI, Thomas GO (2003) Polybrominated diphenyl ethers (PBDEs) in grey seals during their first year of life – are they thyroid hormone endocrine disrupters? *Environ Pollut* **126(1):** 29–37.

Hall AJ, Thomas GO (2007) Polychlorinated biphenyls, DDT, polybrominated diphenyl ethers, and organic pesticides in United Kingdom harbor seals (*Phoca vitulina*) – mixed exposures and thyroid homeostasis. *Environ Toxicol Chem* **26(5):** 851–61.

Hamers T, Kamstra JH, Sonneveld E, Murk AJ, Kester MH, Andersson PL, Legler J, Brouwer A (2006) *In vitro* profiling of the endocrine-disrupting potency of brominated flame retardants. *Toxicol Sci* **92(1):** 157–73.

Hamers T, Kamstra JH, Sonneveld E, Murk AJ, Visser TJ, Van Velzen MJ, Brouwer A, Bergman A (2008) Biotransformation of brominated flame retardants into potentially endocrine-disrupting metabolites, with special attention to 2,2′,4,4′-tetrabromodiphenyl ether (BDE-47). *Mol Nutr Food Res* **52(2):** 284–98.

Hansen LG (1998) Stepping backward to improve assessment of PCB congener toxicities. *Environ Health Perspect* **106 (Suppl. 1):** 171–89.

Harding LE, Harris ML, Stephen CR, Elliott JE (1999) Reproductive and morphological condition of wild mink (*Mustela vison*) and river otters (*Lutra canadensis*) in relation to chlorinated hydrocarbon contamination. *Environ Health Perspect* **107(2):** 141–7.

Harvey PW, Everett DJ (2003) The adrenal cortex and steroidogenesis as cellular and molecular targets for toxicity: critical omissions from regulatory endocrine disrupter screening strategies for human health? *J Appl Toxicol* **23(2):** 81–7.

Heaton SN, Bursian SJ, Giesy JP, Tillitt DE, Render JA, Jones PD, Verbrugge DA, Kubiak TJ, Aulerich RJ (1995) Dietary exposure of mink to carp from Saginaw Bay, Michigan. 1. Effects on reproduction and survival, and the potential risks to wild mink populations. *Arch Environ Contam Toxicol* **28(3):** 334–43.

Hinson JP, Raven PW (2006) Effects of endocrine-disrupting chemicals on adrenal function. *Best Pract Res Clin Endocrinol Metab* **20(1):** 111–20.

Hochstein JR, Bursian SJ, Aulerich RJ (1998) Effects of dietary exposure to 2,3,7,8-tetrachlorodibenzo-p-dioxin in adult female mink (*Mustela vison*). *Arch Environ Contam Toxicol* **35(2):** 348–53.

Hochstein Jr MS, Render JA, Bursian SJ, Aulerich RJ (2001) Chronic toxicity of dietary 2,3,7,8-tetrachlorodibenzo-p-dioxin to mink. *Vet Hum Toxicol* **43(3):** 134–9.

Hornshaw TC, Aulerich RJ, Johnson HE (1983) Feeding Great Lakes fish to mink: effects on mink and accumulation and elimination of PCBS by mink. *J Toxicol Environ Health* **11(4–6):** 933–46.

Horrigan L, Lawrence RS, Walker P (2002) How sustainable agriculture can address the environmental and human health harms of industrial agriculture. *Environ Health Perspect* **110(5):** 445–56.

Jenssen BM (2006) Endocrine-disrupting chemicals and climate change: a worst-case combination for arctic marine mammals and seabirds? *Environ Health Perspect* **114 (Suppl. 1):** 76–80.

Jobling S, Tyler CR (2006) Introduction: the ecological relevance of chemically induced endocrine disruption in wildlife. *Environ Health Perspect* **114 (Suppl. 1):** 7–8.

Khan MA, Hansen LG (2003) Ortho-substituted polychlorinated biphenyl (PCB) congeners (95 or 101) decrease pituitary response to thyrotropin releasing hormone. *Toxicol Lett* **144(2):** 173–82.

Knobil E (1988) The neuroendocrine control of ovulation. *Hum Reprod* **3(4):** 469–72.

Lair S, Beland P, De Guise S, Martineau D (1997) Adrenal hyperplastic and degenerative changes in beluga whales. *J Wildl Dis* **33(3):** 430–7.

Letcher RJ, Bustnes JO, Dietz R, Jenssen BM, Jorgensen EH, Sonne C, Verreault J, Vijayan MM, Gabrielsen GW (2009) Exposure and effects assessment of persistent organohalogen contaminants in Arctic wildlife and fish. *Sci Total Environ*. In press.

Lyche JL, Oskam IC, Skaare JU, Reksen O, Sweeney T, Dahl E, Farstad W, Ropstad E (2004) Effects of gestational and lactational exposure to low doses of PCBs 126 and 153 on anterior pituitary and gonadal hormones and on puberty in female goats. *Reprod Toxicol* **19(1):** 87–95.

Lyons G (2006) Viewpoint: policy requirements for protecting wildlife from endocrine disruptors. *Environ Health Perspect* **114 (Suppl. 1):** 142–6.

Magnusson U (2005) Can farm animals help to study endocrine disruption? *Domest Anim Endocrinol* **29(2):** 430–5.

Mikaelian I, Labelle P, Kopal M, De Guise S, Martineau D (2003) Adenomatous hyperplasia of the thyroid gland in beluga whales (*Delphinapterus leucas*) from the St. Lawrence Estuary and Hudson Bay, Quebec, Canada. *Vet Pathol* **40(6):** 698–703.

Mohr FC, Lasley B, Bursian S (2008) Chronic oral exposure to bunker C fuel oil causes adrenal insufficiency in ranch mink (*Mustela vison*). *Arch Environ Contam Toxicol* **54(2):** 337–47.

Noyes PD, McElwee MK, Miller HD, Clark BW, Van Tiem LA, Walcott KC, Erwin KN, Levin ED (2009) The toxicology of climate change: environmental contaminants in a warming world. *Environ Int* **35(6):** 971–86.

Oskam IC, Ropstad CE, Dahl E, Lie E, Derocher AE, Wiig O, Larsen S, Wiger R, Skaare JU (2003) Organochlorines affect the major androgenic hormone, testosterone, in male polar bears (*Ursus maritimus*) at Svalbard. *J Toxicol Environ Health A* **66(22):** 2119–39.

Oskam I, Ropstad E, Lie E, Derocher A, Wiig O, Dahl E, Larsen Skaare JU (2004) Organochlorines affect the steroid hormone cortisol in free-ranging polar bears (*Ursus maritimus*) at Svalbard, Norway. *J Toxicol Environ Health A* **67(12):** 959–77.

Paul C, Rhind SM, Kyle CE, Scott H, McKinnell C, Sharpe RM (2005) Cellular and hormonal disruption of fetal testis development in sheep reared on pasture treated with sewage sludge. *Environ Health Perspect* **113(11):** 1580–7.

Platonow NS, Karstad LH (1973) Dietary effects of polychlorinated biphenyls on mink. *Can J Comp Med* **37(4):** 391–400.

Reijnders PJ (1986) Reproductive failure in common seals feeding on fish from polluted coastal waters. *Nature* **324(6096):** 456–7.

Restum JC, Bursian SJ, Giesy JP, Render JA, Helferich WG, Shipp EB, Verbrugge DA, Aulerich RJ (1998) Multigenerational study of the effects of consumption of PCB-contaminated carp from Saginaw Bay, Lake Huron, on mink. 1. Effects on mink reproduction, kit growth and survival, and selected biological parameters. *J Toxicol Environ Health A* **54(5):** 343–75.

Ropstad EI, Oskam C, Lyche JH, Larsen HJ, Lie E, Haave M, Dahl E, Wiger R, Skaare JU (2006) Endocrine disruption induced by organochlorines (OCs): field studies and experimental models. *J Toxicol Environ Health A* **69(1–2):** 53–76.

Rosol TJ, Yarrington JT, Latendresse J, Capen CC (2001) Adrenal gland: structure, function, and mechanisms of toxicity. *Toxicol Pathol* **29(1):** 41–8.

Routti H, Nyman M, Jenssen BM, Backman C, Koistinen J, Gabrielsen GW (2008) Bone-related effects of contaminants in seals may be associated with vitamin D and thyroid hormones. *Environ Toxicol Chem* **27(4):** 873–80.

Schumacher U, Zahler S, Horny HP, Heidemann G, Skirnisson K, Welsch U (1993) Histological investigations on the thyroid glands of marine mammals (*Phoca vitulina*, *Phocoena phocoena*) and the possible implications of marine pollution. *J Wildl Dis* **29(1):** 103–8.

Sharma C, Aulerich RJ, Render JA, Reimers T, Rottinghaus GE, Kizilkaya K, Bursian SJ (2002) Reproductive toxicity of ergot alkaloids in mink. *Vet Hum Toxicol* **44(6):** 324–7.

Shipp EB, Restum JC, Bursian SJ, Aulerich RJ, Helferich WG (1998) Multigenerational study of the effects of consumption of PCB-contaminated carp from Saginaw Bay, Lake Huron, on mink. 3. Estrogen receptor and progesterone receptor concentrations, and potential correlation with dietary PCB consumption. *J Toxicol Environ Health A* **54(5):** 403–20.

Skaare JU, Bernhoft A, Wiig O, Norum KR, Haug E, Eide DM, Derocher AE (2001) Relationships between plasma levels of organochlorines, retinol and thyroid hormones from polar bears (*Ursus maritimus*) at Svalbard. *J Toxicol Environ Health A* **62(4):** 227–41.

Sonne C (2010) Health effects from long-range transported contaminants in Arctic top predators: An integrated review based on studies of polar bears and relevant model species. *Environ Int*. In press.

Sonne C, Dietz R, Born EW, Leifsson PS, Andersen S (2008) Is there a link between hypospadias and organochlorine exposure in East Greenland sledge dogs (*Canis familiaris*)? *Ecotoxicol Environ Saf* **69(3):** 391–5.

Sonne C, Leifsson PS, Dietz R, Born EW, Letcher RJ, Hyldstrup L, Riget FF, Kirkegaard M, Muir DC (2006) Xenoendocrine pollutants may reduce size of sexual organs in East Greenland polar bears (*Ursus maritimus*). *Environ Sci Technol* **40(18):** 5668–74.

Sonne C, Wolkers H, Leifsson PS, Iburg T, Jenssen BM, Fuglei E, Ahlstrom O, Dietz R, Kirkegaard M, Muir DC, Jorgensen EH (2009) Chronic dietary exposure to environmental organochlorine contaminants induces thyroid gland lesions in Arctic foxes (*Vulpes lagopus*). *Environ Res* **109(6):** 702–11.

Sorensen MT, Danielsen V (2006) Effects of the plant growth regulator, chlormequat, on mammalian fertility. *Int J Androl* **29(1):** 129–33.

Sormo EG, Jussi I, Jussi M, Braathen M, Skaare JU, Jenssen, BM (2005) Thyroid hormone status in gray seal (*Halichoerus grypus*) pups from the Baltic Sea and the Atlantic Ocean in relation to organochlorine pollutants. *Environ Toxicol Chem* **24(3):** 610–16.

Tabuchi M, Veldhoen N, Dangerfield N, Jeffries S, Helbing CC, Ross PS (2006) PCB-related alteration of thyroid hormones and thyroid hormone receptor gene expression in free-ranging harbor seals (*Phoca vitulina*). *Environ Health Perspect* **114(7):** 1024–31.

Tajima Y, Shimada A, Yamada TK, Cowan DF (2007) Amyloidosis in two Stejneger's beaked whales (*Mesoplodon stejnegeri*) stranded at the Sea of Japan. *J Zoo Wildl Med* **38(1):** 108–13.

Tan SW, Meiller JC, Mahaffey KR (2009) The endocrine effects of mercury in humans and wildlife. *Crit Rev Toxicol* **39(3):** 228–69.

Thorpe KL, Gross-Sorokin M, Johnson I, Brighty G, Tyler CR (2006) An assessment of the model of concentration addition for predicting the estrogenic activity of chemical mixtures in wastewater treatment works effluents. *Environ Health Perspect* **114 (Suppl. 1):** 90–7.

Torner H, Blottner S, Kuhla S, Langhammer M, Alm H, Tuchscherer A (1999) Influence of chlorocholinechloride-treated wheat on selected *in vitro* fertility parameters in male mice. *Reprod Toxicol* **13(5):** 399–404.

Tyler CR, Jobling S, Sumpter JP (1998) Endocrine disruption in wildlife: a critical review of the evidence. *Crit Rev Toxicol* **28(4):** 319–61.

Ulleras E, Ohlsson A, Oskarsson A (2008) Secretion of cortisol and aldosterone as a vulnerable target for adrenal endocrine disruption – screening of 30 selected chemicals in the human H295R cell model. *J Appl Toxicol* **28(8):** 1045–53.

Van den Berg M, Birnbaum L, Bosveld ATC, Brunstrom B, Cook P, Feeley M, *et al.* (1998) Toxic equivalency factors (TEFs) for PCBs, PCDDs, PCDFs for humans and wildlife. *Environ Health Perspect* **106(12):** 775–92.

van der Ven LTM, Verhoef A, van de Kuil T, Slob W, Leonards PEG, Visser TJ, *et al.* (2006) A 28-day oral dose toxicity study enhanced to detect endocrine effects of hexabromocyclododecane in Wistar rats. *Toxicol Sci* **94(2):** 281–92.

Vos JG, Dybing E, Greim HA, Ladefoged O, Lambre C, Tarazona JV, Brandt I, Vethaak AD (2000) Health effects of endocrine-disrupting chemicals on wildlife, with special reference to the European situation. *Crit Rev Toxicol* **30(1):** 71–133.

Wang D, Shelver WL, Atkinson S, Mellish JA, Li XQ (2010) Tissue distribution of polychlorinated biphenyls and organochlorine pesticides and potential toxicity to Alaskan northern fur seals assessed using PCBs congener specific mode of action schemes. *Arch Environ Contam Toxicol* **58(2):** 478–88.

Wells RS, Tornero V, Borrell A, Aguilar AA, Rowles TK, Rhinehart HL, Hofmann S, Jarman WM, Hohn AA, Sweeney JC (2005) Integrating life-history and reproductive success data to examine potential relationships with organochlorine compounds for bottlenose dolphins (*Tursiops truncatus*) in Sarasota Bay, Florida. *Sci Total Environ* **349(1–3):** 106–19.

Woldstad S, Jenssen BM (1999) Thyroid hormones in grey seal pups (*Halichoerus grypus*). *Comp Biochem Physiol A Mol Integr Physiol* **122(2):** 157–62.

Wren CD (1991) Cause–effect linkages between chemicals and populations of mink (*Mustela vison*) and otter (*Lutra canadensis*) in the Great Lakes basin. *J Toxicol Environ Health* **33(4):** 549–85.

Wren CD, Hunter DB, Leatherland JF, Stokes PM (1987a) The effects of polychlorinated biphenyls and methylmercury, singly and in combination, on mink. I: Uptake and toxic responses. *Arch Environ Contam Toxicol* **16(4):** 441–7.

Wren CD, Hunter DB, Leatherland JF, Stokes PM (1987b) The effects of polychlorinated biphenyls and methylmercury, singly and in combination on mink. II: Reproduction and kit development. *Arch Environ Contam Toxicol* **16(4):** 449–54.

Yamini B, Bursian SJ, Aulerich RJ (1997) Pathological effects of dietary zearalenone and/or tamoxifen on female mink reproductive organs. *Vet Hum Toxicol* **39(2):** 74–8.

Yordy JE, Wells RS, Balmer BC, Schwacke LH, Rowles TK, Kucklick JR (2010) Life history as a source of variation for persistent organic pollutant (POP) patterns in a community of common bottlenose dolphins (*Tursiops truncatus*) resident to Sarasota Bay, FL. *Sci Total Environ* **408(9):** 2163–72.

Zhang S, Bursian SJ, Martin PA, Chan HM, Tomy G, Palace VP, Mayne GJ, Martin JW (2009) Reproductive and developmental toxicity of a pentabrominated diphenyl ether mixture, DE-71, to ranch mink (*Mustela vison*) and hazard assessment for wild mink in the Great Lakes region. *Toxicol Sci* **110(1):** 107–16.

Zimmer KE, Gutleb AC, Lyche JL, Dahl E, Oskam IC, Krogenaes A, Skaare JU, Ropstad E (2009) Altered stress-induced cortisol levels in goats exposed to polychlorinated biphenyls (PCB 126 and PCB 153) during fetal and postnatal development. *J Toxicol Environ Health A* **72(3–4):** 164–72.

Zoeller TR (2010) Environmental chemicals targeting thyroid. *Hormones (Athens)* **9(1):** 28–40.

CHAPTER

84

Teratogeneses in livestock

Robert W. Coppock and Margitta M. Dziwenka

INTRODUCTION

There are multiple agents that cause teratogenic effects in livestock. These range from viruses, chemicals, poisonous plants and nutrient deficiencies to manipulation of embryos. It is estimated that the majority of teratogenic effects in livestock go undiagnosed. The teratogens which have been identified have generally been endemic in an area or have been reproduced under laboratory conditions. For example, many of the congenital defects of the central nervous system of calves are not diagnosed (Leipold, 1993). Many congenital defects, regardless of the cause, are not compatible with life. Dennis (1993) reported that congenital defects in sheep occur in 0.2 to 2% of the lambs born and of these, 50% are stillbirths. In horses, it is estimated that 2 to 3% of aborted fetuses and stillborn foals have anomalous development of embryonic structures (Whitwell, 1980). Many animal breeders assume that the birth defects are genetic in origin resulting in under-reporting. Reporting congenital defects is essential if the etiology is to be established. Teratogenic substances are expressed differently in different species. For a particular teratogen, some species are resistant and others are sensitive. This likely reflects differences in xenobiotic metabolism and embryologic factors. The stage of gestation in which the insult occurs is important in determining the organ systems damaged. Chemicals and viruses that decrease fetal mobility generally cause deformations of the skeleton. It is estimated that many teratogenic effects are not compatible with fetal life and end in abortion. The majority of pharmaceutics and biologics used in livestock have disclaimers for safety in pregnant females and have not been tested for teratogenic effects.

EMBRYOLOGY OF DOMESTIC ANIMALS

It is important to have an understanding of the embryological development of a fetus in order to understand the malformations which may occur due to teratogen exposure. The gestational stage at which the exposure occurs can determine the terata observed in the fetus. Early in development, vertebrate embryos pass through a stage where they are all anatomically similar and only later in development do the species-specific differences become apparent (Table 84.1). Prenatal development is divided into four main periods: fertilization, blastogenesis, embryogenesis and fetogenesis (Szabo, 1989). Fertilization is the union of the male and female germ cells to form a zygote. The zygote undergoes a series of rapid cell divisions known as cleavage and then develops into a hollow blastocyst that implants in the uterine endometrium. The timing and process of implantation varies between species. In the majority of domestic species, such as the cat, dog, cattle, horse, sheep and swine, the blastocyst develops to a point where it fills the majority of the uterine cavity. This is known as central or superficial implantation. Embryogenesis is the period when organ formation and differentiation occurs. All vertebrate embryos develop into three sheets of cells or germ layers and it is from these that all tissues and organs later develop. The outermost layer is the ectoderm from which will develop the neural tissues, epidermis and some of the bony and connective tissue structures of the head. The middle layer or mesoderm consists of a more loose population of cells that will eventually form the majority of the muscles, skeletal structures and urogenital and cardiovascular systems. The endoderm is the deepest layer and forms the lining of the digestive tract and respiratory system, and the organs related to digestion. It is important to note that almost all of the organs or tissues in the body develop from more than one germ layer or from different parts of the same germ layer (de Lahunta and Noden, 1985).

Embryonic development proceeds in a rostral to caudal fashion therefore many of the organs/tissues present in early organogenesis are associated with the head and neck (de Lahunta and Noden, 1985). Many vertebrate embryos are very similar at the stage of development when the primordial structures of the majority of the organ systems are present. Differences in developmental rates between the various species may be responsible for the species' different responses to the same environmental insult (Szabo, 1989). The body of the embryo is covered by the ectodermal epithelium and beneath this layer is the hollow neural tube which runs down the dorsal midline (de Lahunta and Noden, 1985). The neural tube has a number of enlarged vesicles located rostrally which are the early manifestations of the brain. Another hollow tube is located near the ventral midline and will develop into the gastrointestinal system, and layers of endoderm and ectoderm close the rostral and

Reproductive and Developmental Toxicology, Edited by Ramesh C. Gupta
ISBN: 978-0-12-382032-7

TABLE 84.1 Comparison of major prenatal events in domestic animals (day post-conception)

Event	Cat	Dog	Cattle	Horse	Sheep	Swine
Morula	–	–	5 to 7	3 to 8	3 to 4	3 to 4
Blastula	6 to 8	8 to 10	8 to 10	13 to 14	5 to 8	5 to 10
Implantation	12 to 14	13 to 14	11 to 13	–	10 to 14	10 to 12
Primitive streak	12 to 14	14 to 15	14 to 18	14 to 15	13 to 14	11 to 12
First somites	13 to 14	14 to 16	18 to 20	15 to 17	14 to 15	13 to 15
First brachial arches	14 to 15	–	22 to 24	220 to 21	17 to 18	15 to 17
Neuropore (anterior) closed	–	17 to 18	23 to 25	20 to 22	18 to 19	5 to 16
Optic vesicle	14 to 15	14 to 15	23 to 24	–	19 to 20	16 to 18
Heart beat	21 to 22	23 to 25	21 to 24	22 to 25	18 to 20	19 to 24
Lens and optic cup	21 to 22	–	–	26 to 30	23 to 25	19 to 20
Neuropore (posterior) closed	–	18 to 19	24 to 25	22 to 24	19 to 20	15 to 16
Forelimb buds	17 to 18	21 to 22	24 to 25	26 to 28	21 to 22	16 to 18
Olfactory pits	20 to 21	22 to 23	30 to 31	–	23 to 25	20 to 21
Tail buds	–	19 to 20	26 to 30	–	22 to 23	15 to 18
Hind limb buds	18 to 19	21 to 22	26 to 28	28 to 30	22 to 23	18 to 20
Intestinal loops herniate into umbilical cord	20 to 21	30 to 32	–	–	–	20 to 21
Pigment in eye	21 to 22	25 to 26	30 to 31	31 to 36	24 to 25	20 to 21
Tongue	26 to 27	25 to 27	44 to 45	–	–	25 to 28
Auditory meatus	21 to 22	24 to 25	34 to 35	36 to 37	25 to 27	23 to 26
Vibrissary papillae	23 to 24	28 to 30	44 to 45	–	38 to 42	28 to 30
Eyelids forming	24 to 25	30 to 32	38 to 39	38 to 40	27 to 28	36 to 38
Nasomaxillary process	22 to 24	–	34 to 35	30 to 36	30 to 34	24 to 28
Pinna	23 to 24	25 to 28	38 to 40	35 to 40	27 to 28	28 to 30
Forelimbs digits separate	24 to 26	30 to 35	33 to 34	35 to 36	35 to 38	30 to 32
Hind limbs digits separate	26 to 27	32 to 36	36 to 38	38 to 40	–	32 to 34
Hair follicles on trunk	27 to 28	42 to 43	70 to 76	–	–	55 to 56
Eyelid closure	30 to 31	39 to 40	58 to 60	60 to 63	43 to 45	40 to 50
Palate closure	31 to 32	30 to 35	54 to 56	46 to 48	35 to 38	34 to 36
Intestinal withdrawal into abdomen	–	35 to 40	–	–	–	45 to 50
Hair around eyes and muzzle	35 to 37	37 to 38	70 to 76	96 to 110	80 to 90	32 to 36
External genitalia differentiate	–	33 to 35	56 to 60	43 to 45	41 to 43	36 to 55
Birth	60 to 65	60 to 65	280 to 340	330 to 340	145 to 155	112 to 116

Adapted with permission from Szabo (1989)

caudal ends of this tube (de Lahunta and Noden, 1985). The more rostral end is the pharynx and is already specialized in the embryo with lateral outpouchings that extend to the ectoderm and are known as pharyngeal pouches. The remaining tissues present at this stage in the embryo are mesodermal. Future body segments, known as somites, develop in a craniocaudal direction until approximately 40 pairs are formed. The head and tail folds are evident at the 7 somite stage and by the 10 somite stage, the first mandibular process arch and developing pericardium are evident. The second hyoid arches as well as maxillary and mandibular features are seen in the 14 somite embryo and the anterior neuropore is closed in the 20 somite embryo. The posterior neuropore closes by the 25 to 28 somite stage and the third pharyngeal arch, optic vesicles and umbilical cord all develop in the later stages. The parts and regions of the body are clearly recognizable as embryogenesis continues and the limb buds subdivide and future digits become evident. The facial processes gradually increase in size and the snout begins to form with closed external nares. The future lens and pigment become evident in the optic vesicle as well as recognizable eyelids and external ears. By the end of embryogenesis, all of the species recognizable features are present (Szabo, 1989).

The next period is termed fetogenesis and is defined by rapid growth; however, not all regions of the body grow at the same rate. For example, at the beginning of the fetal period, the head is approximately one-half of the total body length while by the end of the period it is only one-fourth of the length (Szabo, 1989). During this period, the features and structures of the fetus develop and move into their final shape and positions. A comparison of the major prenatal events in domestic animals is presented in Table 84.1.

TERATOGENIC VIRUSES

Introduction

Teratogenic viruses can be an important cause of terata in livestock. The majority of the teratogenic viruses have been studied in livestock species (Table 84.2). Teratogenic viruses as a cause of congenital defects generally can be determined by virological and serological methods. The interactions of teratogenic viruses with chemical teratogens have not been studied in livestock.

TABLE 84.2 Summary of teratogenic viruses

Virus	Species	Terata	Gestation day	Reference
Aino	Cattle	Arthrogryposis, hydranencephaly and cerebellar hypoplasia	132 to 156	Tsuda *et al.*, 2004
Akabane	Cattle Sheep Goats	Arthrogryposis, hydranencephaly Hydranencephaly Porencephaly	76 to 173	Charles, 1994; Oberst, 1993; Kono *et al.*, 2008
Blue tongue	Cattle Sheep	Hydranencephaly, retinal dysplasia	30 to 105 50 to 55	Maxie and Youssef, 2007; Oberst, 1993; Vercauteren *et al.*, 2008; Dal Pozzo *et al.*, 2009; Dennis, 1993.
Border disease	Sheep Goats	Scoliosis, brachygnathism, prognathism, arthrogryposis, hydranencephaly, cerebellar hypoplasia and hairy fleece	First and second trimester	Oberst, 1993; Nettleton *et al.*, 1998
BVD	Cattle	Hydrocephalus, hydranencephaly, porencephaly cerebellar hypoplasia, microencephaly, demyelination and brachygnathism, retinal dysplasia and atrophy, optic atrophy, cataract, microphthalmia and persistent pupillary membrane, brachygnathism, retarded growth and growth arrest lines, thymic aplasia, pulmonary hypoplasia, hypotrichia to alopecia	75 to 170	Blanchard *et al.*, 2010; Schlafer and Miller, 2007; Dubovi, 1994; Maxie and Youssef, 2007

Bunyaviruses

Aino virus

Experimental studies have shown that the Aino virus is teratogenic in cattle. Fetuses injected with Aino virus on days 132 to 156 of pregnancy had arthrogryposis, hydranencephaly and cerebellar hypoplasia at birth (Tsuda *et al.*, 2004).

Akabane virus

Akabane virus is in the genus *Orthobunyavirus* and is a member of the *Bunyaviridae* family. It is widely distributed in temperate to tropical regions of the world. Akabane virus is a recognized teratogen in cattle, sheep and goats (Charles, 1994; Oberst, 1993). These reports are primarily from Japan, Korea, Taiwan, Australia, Israel and Turkey. The virus replicates first in the placentome and then in the fetus. The teratogenic effects of *in utero* Akabane virus infection are secondary to the effects of the virus on the developing nervous system (Swinyard and Bleck, 1985). The affected conceptus show severe muscle atrophy and fixation of the joints by tendon contracture. The teratogenic mechanism for arthrogryposis is considered to be decreased limb movement (Van Vleet and Valentine, 2007). Akabane virus can cause arthrogryposis–hydranencephaly syndrome in calves (Charles, 1994; Kono *et al.*, 2008). Timing of infection is important in expression of teratogenic effects. Hydranencephalic and porencephaly effects generally occur when the cow is infected on days 76 to 104 of gestation. The arthrogryposis deformity (multiple congenital contracture) occurs when the cow is infected on days 103 to 173 of pregnancy. Vertebral deformities can occur, which include torticollis and scoliosis; these can occur with and without deformed limbs. The association between infection with Akabane virus and teratogenic effects is generally based on serologic evidence. In pregnant cows infected with Akabane virus, fetal infections occur in 20 to 40% of the cow infections.

The Akabane virus is teratogenic in lambs and kids. In sheep and goats, a high prevalence of abortions can occur and lambs are born with arthrogryposis accompanied with hydranencephaly and hydrencephalus. The most sensitive time for teratogenic effects is during the first and second trimester of pregnancy. Prolonged gestation can also be observed and be an effect of fetal endocrine dysfunction.

Cache Valley virus

The Cache Valley virus (CVV) has been shown to cause hydranencephaly, hydrocephalus, porencephaly, microencephaly, arthrogryposis, torticollis and scoliosis in sheep (Chung *et al.*, 1990; Oberst, 1993; Edwards, 1994). The most sensitive interval is gestation days 36 to 46. The CVV has been identified in malformed lambs in Texas. The LaCross, San Angelo and Main Drain viruses produce identical congenital defects as the CVV (Edwards *et al.*, 1997).

Rift Valley fever virus

Rift Valley fever virus is considered to be teratogenic in sheep (Oberst, 1993). Vaccination at 30 to 105 days of pregnancy with MLV has been reported to cause hydrops amnii, arthrogryposis and hydranencephaly in sheep (Bird *et al.*, 2009).

Flaviviridae

Bovine virus diarrhea virus

Bovine virus diarrhea virus (BVDV) is in the family Flaviviridae, genus Pestivirus and is known to be teratogenic (Oberst, 1993; Baker, 1995; Maxie and Youssef, 2007). Both the cytopathic and non-cytopathic strains of the virus are considered to be teratogenic. Exposure of susceptible dams to the virus during days 75 to 170 of gestation can result in skeletal and neurologic defects (Maxie and Youssef, 2007; Blanchard *et al.*, 2010). Neurological and skeletal defects include hydrocephalus, brachygnathism, hydranencephaly, porencephaly, cerebellar hypoplasia, microencephaly, demyelination and brachygnathism, retarded growth and growth arrest lines, thymic aplasia and pulmonary hypoplasia. Ocular defects observed with BVD are retinal dysplasia and atrophy, optic atrophy, cataract, microphthalmia and persistent pupillary membrane in the eye, and hypotrichia to alopecia.

Border disease virus

Border disease virus is teratogenic in sheep (Oberst, 1993; Nettleton *et al.*, 1998). Teratogenic lesions reported are scoliosis, brachygnathism, prognathism, arthrogryposis, hydranencephaly, cerebellar hypoplasia and hairy fleece.

Hog cholera virus

The hog cholera virus is considered to cause teratogenic effects when the fetus is infected on gestation days 13 to 14. Teratogenic effects are cerebellar and spinal hypoplasia, hydrocephalus, arthrogryposis and piglets born with congenital tremors (Oberst, 1993).

Japanese B encephalitis virus

The Japanese B encephalitis virus has been reported to cause birth defects in piglets (Radostits *et al.*, 2007).

Orbivirus

Blue tongue virus is considered to be a teratogenic virus in cattle and sheep (Dennis, 1993; Maxie and Youssef, 2007; Vercauteren *et al.*, 2008; Dal Pozzo *et al.*, 2009). The congenital defects observed are hydranencephaly (hydrocephalus internus). This lesion is considered to be a type 1 proencephaly. In addition to hydranencephaly, retinal dysplasia has been observed in sheep (Oberst, 1993). The sensitive period for fetal infection is 30 to 105 days of gestation in cattle and 50 to 55 days of pregnancy in sheep.

Parvovirus

Feline panleukopenia virus infection can cause renal dysplasia in cats (Maxie and Newman, 2007).

TERATOGENIC PLANTS

Introduction

Chemicals found in plants can be teratogenic in livestock (Burrows and Tyrl, 2001). The majority of teratogenic effects of poisonous plants have been demonstrated in laboratory animals. A few plants have been shown to be teratogenic in livestock species and other plants are suspected of being teratogenic in livestock species. Plants of different species that contain the same toxins can produce similar teratogenic effects (Panter *et al.*, 1999; Molyneux *et al.*, 2007). The stage of gestation when exposure occurs is important as teratogenic effects may only be expressed at a specific stage of embryologic development (Binns *et al.*, 1964). Plants contain mixtures of phytotoxins and the multiple chemical interactions involved in the expression of teratogenic effects are not well understood. Some phytotoxins may be inherently teratogenic and others undergo biotransformation to the ultimate teratogen. The phytotoxins in plants can vary with season, geographical area and stages of growth. Additionally, the concentration of phytotoxins can be distributed unevenly between roots, fleshy parts and seeds.

Apiaceae

Poison hemlock (*Conium maculatum*), in North America, is a non-native teratogenic plant (Burrows and Tyrl, 2001). *C. maculatum* is teratogenic in cattle, pigs and sheep (Edmonds *et al.*, 1972; Keeler, 1974; Keeler and Balls, 1978; Panter *et al.*, 1985a,b). Coniine and gamma coniceine are considered the teratogenic agents (Burrows and Tyrl, 2001). Coniine predominates in the mature plant and seeds and gamma coniceine predominates in early growth (Panter *et al.*, 1988b). Ewes administered *C. maculatum* at doses sufficient to cause material toxicity gave birth to lambs that had contracture and lateral deviation of the carpal joint (Panter *et al.*, 1988a). The deviation and flexure of the carpal joint generally resolved with growth of the lamb. Sows administered *C. maculatum* seeds or plants, dose ≥1.07 mg of gamma-coniceine/kg body weight, from gestation day 30 to 45 give birth to piglets with lesions of cleft palate and brachygnathia (Panter *et al.*, 1985a). Sows administered *C. maculatum* seed or plant materials on gestation days 43 to 61 gave birth to piglets showing arthrogryposis and twisted and malaligned bones in the limbs, and thoracic cage deformity can occur (Panter *et al.*, 1985b). Teratogenic effects consisting of arthrogryposis and spinal curvature were observed in calves when cows were administered *C. maculatum* on gestation days 50 to 75 of gestation (Keeler and Balls, 1978). Administering *per gavage* fresh poison hemlock or gamma coniine to cattle on gestation days 40 to 75 caused teratogenic lesions of arthrogryposis and scoliosis in live calves. Teratogenic effects were not observed in foals born to mares administered coniine on gestation days 45 to 75 (Keeler *et al.*, 1980). The plant tissue and seeds from *C. maculatum* administered on gestation days 30 to 60 were observed to be teratogenic in goats with the seeds remarkably producing more teratogenic effects (Panter *et al.*, 1990a). The congenital effects observed were multiple congenital contractures that included torticollis, scoliosis, lordosis, arthrogryposis, over extension, and flexure and rigidity of the joints. Ribcage abnormalities were also observed.

Dennstaedtiaceae

The ingestion of bracken fern (*Pteridium* spp.) by pregnant dams has been associated with retarded fetal development in rats and mice (Burrows and Tyrl, 2001). This effect does not appear to have been reported for livestock species.

Fabaceae

Genera that contain teratogenic species include *Astragalus*, *Oxytropis* and *Lupinus*. *Astragalus lentiginosus*, *A. pubentissimus* and *Oxytropis sericea* are teratogenic in sheep and cattle, and *A. mollissimus* has been incriminated as a teratogen in horses (James *et al.*, 1969; McIlwraith and James, 1982; Panter *et al.*, 1989; Panter and Keeler, 1990; James *et al.*, 1994a; Radostits *et al.*, 2007). Skeletal defects and limb contractures were observed in lambs born to ewes fed *Astragalus* and *Oxytropis* spp. at various times from gestation days 1 to 120 (James *et al.*, 1967, 1969; Keeler *et al.*, 1967). Other teratogenic effects in lambs are weak lambs with decreased nursing vigor, and decreased cardiac function (James, 1972; Panter *et al.*, 1987, 1999; James *et al.*, 1994a). Neuroaxonal dystrophy, neurovisceral cytoplasmic vacuolization, vacuolization of the thyroid acinar epithelium, kidney proximal tubular cells, hepatocytes and adrenal cortical cells have been observed in fetuses from ewes fed *A. lentiginosus* (James, 1972; Hartley and James, 1973, 1975). *Astragalus lentiginosus* and *A. pubentissimus* have been observed to be teratogenic in cattle. The teratogenic substance in species of *Astragalus* and *Oxytropis* is reported by some authors to be swainsonine. However, plants in Australia that contain swainsonine have not been reported to be teratogenic in sheep and cattle suggesting that a mixture of compounds may be required for the teratogenic effect (Keeler, 1988). Studies were done that showed the teratogenic effects of aminoacetonitrile and α,γ-diaminobutyric acid in sheep and aminoacetonitrile in cattle are similar to teratogenic effects of *Astragalus* and *Oxytropis* spp. (Keeler *et al.*, 1967; Keeler and James, 1971).

Species of *Lupinus* are teratogenic and cause "crooked calf disease" characterized by arthrogryposis, kyphosis, scoliosis torticollis and cleft palate (Shupe *et al.*, 1967, 1968; Panter *et al.*, 2002). Species shown to be teratogenic are *L. arbustus*, *L. caudatus*, *L. formosus*, *L. sericeus* and *L. laxiflorus* (Panter and Keeler, 1990; Panter *et al.*, 1998). The most sensitive period for teratogenic effects in cattle is gestation days 40 to 70, and limb contractures can occur at later times in gestation (Shupe *et al.*, 1967; Panter *et al.*, 1998). A number of compounds have been proposed as being the teratogenic agents, but rather than a specific chemical, the overall effect of a mixture of plant chemicals decreasing fetal movement could be the mechanism of action (Keeler *et al.*, 1969; Keeler and Panter, 1989; Burrows and Tyrl, 2001). The putative teratogens are anagyrine and ammodendrine and a recent study has shown that body condition of the cow can alter their toxicokinetics (Keeler and Panter, 1989; Lee *et al.*, 2008). The alkaloid profile of *L. sulphureus* was reported as varying between geographic regions (Cook *et al.*, 2009). Thus a number of variables can affect the teratogenic effects of lupines. Milk from goats feeding on lupine has been incriminated as a teratogen causing bilateral radial hemimelia, red cell aplasia and persistent azygous vein in a human baby (Ortega and Lazerson, 1987). The mother, during pregnancy, was sick on several occasions after drinking goat's milk. One goat gave birth to a kid with deformities similar to crooked calf disease, and a pregnant bitch that drank goat's milk subsequently gave birth to pups with abnormal limbs.

The leaves of *Leucaena leucocephala*, a tropical shrub legume, are high in protein and are used as forage. In a feeding trial in pigs, *L. leucocephala* at 10% of the diet was considered to cause abortions and polypodia of pectoral limbs (Wayman *et al.*, 1970).

Liliaceae

Plants in the Liliaceae family (lily) are known or suspected to be teratogenic (Burrows and Tyrl, 2001). Western false hellebore (*Veratrum californicum*) fed to ewes on gestation days 10 to 15 caused cyclopian-type teratological effects (Binns *et al.*, 1962, 1964; Shupe and James, 1983). Cyclopian terata has been observed in foals born to mares that graze *V. eschscholtzii* (Shupe and James, 1983). Prolonged gestation may occur and is considered due to absence of a fetal pituitary gland (Burrows and Tyrl, 2001). Deformities of the limbs can occur in lambs if the ewes are exposed on gestation days 28 to 32. Lambs may also be born with tracheal stenosis. Feeding *V. californicum* after gestation day 15 can cause abnormal brain development in sheep (James, 1974). Species of *Veratrum* contain the alkaloids jervine, cyclopamine (11-deoxojervine) and cycloposine (3-glucosyl-11-deoxojervine), and these compounds are known to be teratogenic (Keeler, 1984). The primary teratogen is cyclopamine (Figure 84.1), and the critical exposure time is gestation days 13 to 15 (Molyneux *et al.*, 2007; Welch *et al.*, 2009). Jervine has been identified in species of *Zigadenus* giving this species teratogenic potential (Burrows and Tyrl, 2001).

Under field conditions, *V. californicum* consumed by pregnant ewes causes early embryonic death and the only clinical sign is the rancher observing open ewes (Keeler, 1990).

Pinaceae

Pregnant cows consuming ponderosa pine (*Pinus ponderosa*), in addition to abortion, can give birth to small and sickly calves (James *et al.*, 1994b; Burrows and Tyrl, 2001). The mechanism of action is considered to be alterations in steroid metabolism and necrosis of luteal cells. Long-term endocrine disruptions in the offspring, if they occur, are not known.

Poaceae

Six of eight heifers grazing a regrowth of drought-stressed Sudex (*Sorghum* spp.) gave birth to calves with rigid flexion of the rear limbs. Wallerian degeneration of the spinal cord and ventral and lateral tracts in the medulla and pons were also affected (Seaman *et al.*, 1981). *Sorghum* spp. have also been associated with musculoskeletal defects in foals. Burrows and Tyrl (2001) were not able to repeat this condition in horses by administering cyanide to pregnant mares. Additional observations are required to define the teratogenic effects of *Sorghum* spp.

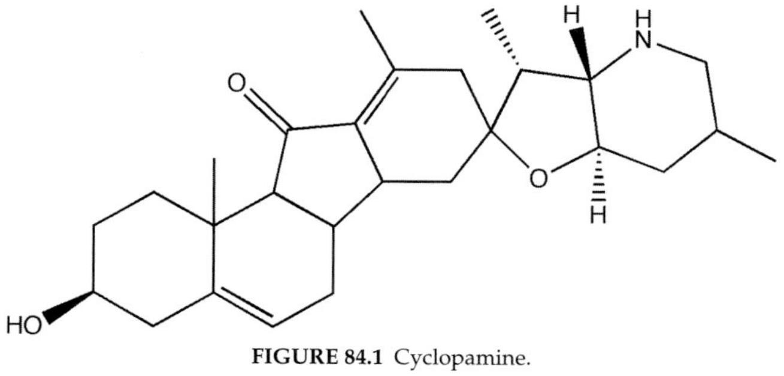

HO O H H N O H

FIGURE 84.1 Cyclopamine.

Rosaceae

Pregnant sows consuming black cherry (*Prunus serotina*) were observed to give birth to piglets with deformed limbs and agenesis of the tail and anus (Selby *et al.*, 1971; Molyneux *et al.*, 2007). The pregnant dams were eating leaves and bark from black cherry trees.

Solanaceae

Plants in the genera *Nicotiana* have been shown to be teratogenic. *Nicotiana tabacum* was associated with an epidemic outbreak of congenital defects in piglets fed tobacco stalks and was later shown to be teratogenic in pigs (Menges *et al.*, 1970; Crowe and Pike, 1973; Crowe and Swerczek, 1974). Wild tree tobacco (*Nicotiana glauca*) is teratogenic in calves when cows were administered *N. glauca* on gestation days 45 to 75 (Keeler, 1979; Keeler *et al.*, 1981a,b). The teratogenic effects were moderate to severe arthrogryposis of the pectoral limbs, abnormal spinal curvature and rib cage deformity. *Nicotiana glauca* and anabasine-rich extracts have been shown to be teratogenic in goats when administered on gestation days 32 to 41 (Panter *et al.*, 1990b; Weinzweig *et al.*, 1999). The teratogenic lesion was cleft palate and decreased fetal movement; hyperflexion of the neck and wedging of the tongue obstructing migration of the palatal shelves were observed (Panter *et al.*, 1990b; Weinzweig *et al.*, 2008). Ewes administered *N. glauca* on gestation days 34 to 55 gave birth to lambs that had moderate to severe flexure of the carpal and metacarpal joints, abnormal rotation of the limbs and some lambs had lordosis (Keeler and Crowe, 1984). The less severe flexure resolved within 4 to 6 weeks. Arthrogryposis has been observed in piglets born to sows administered *N. glauca* on gestation days 16 to 68 (Keeler *et al.*, 1981a,b).

NUTRITION AND TERATOLOGY

Minerals and vitamins

Manganese deficiency

Manganese (Mn) deficiency has been reported to cause congenital defects in calves (Rojas *et al.*, 1965; Hansen *et al.*, 2006). Pregnant cows and heifers deficient in Mn generally do not show clinical signs of deficiency. A study in beef heifers on the long-term effects of Mn deficiency showed that 17-month-old heifers (bred at 13 months of age) on a diet containing 15.8 mg of Mn/kg of dry matter (DM) gave birth to calves with limb and facial deformities (Hansen *et al.*, 2006). Blood levels of Mn in pregnant heifers on the 15.8 mg of Mn/kg DM ration were not different from pregnant heifers receiving a diet containing 50 mg Mn/kg DM. Congenital defects in the calves were smaller stature and some calves had superior brachygnathism. Calves born to heifers on the 15.8 mg of Mn/kg DM diet had lower blood Mn levels. In another study, pregnant Hereford cows (4 years old) were fed a diet containing 16.6 ppm Mn for the proceeding 12 months (Rojas *et al.*, 1965). The cows required four services/conception. The calves born to cows on the low Mn diet showed enlarged joints, stiffness, twisted legs and a general physical weakness. The calves also had shortened humeri that had a remarkable reduction in breaking strength. Neonatal knuckling of the pelvic limbs was also observed. Neonatal hepatic Mn levels were 11.84 and 6.94 ppm, respectively, for calves born to control and deficient cows. Neonatal renal levels of Mn were 2.52 and 1.17 ppm, respectively, for calves born to the control and deficient cows. Authors in South Africa, New Zealand, Australia and Canada reporting field observations have described putative Mn deficiency of pregnant cows causing skeletal deformations in calves (Ribble *et al.*, 1989; Hidiroglou *et al.*, 1990; Staley *et al.*, 1994; McLaren *et al.*, 2007; Cave *et al.*, 2008). Calves showed disproportionate limb to body trunk length (McLaren *et al.*, 2007). The pathology has been described as brachygnathism, bilateral valgus deformity of the forelimbs, fetlock overextension, disproportionate shortening of length-to-epiphyseal diameter of predominantly the proximal limb bones, reduced range of joint movement, and the vertebral column showed variable kyphosis and lordosis. Carpal bones can be malformed and disorganization of the growth plates was observed. The mandible showed decreased trabecular bone. Similar observations were described in calves deficient in liver Mn and grazing forage from soil repetitively contaminated with sea water and high in strontium (Staley *et al.*, 1994). Availability of Mn in the diet should be assessed if Mn deficiency is suspected.

Vitamin A

Vitamin A deficiency (hypovitaminosis A) during pregnancy causes congenital defects in pigs and cattle (Done, 1968; Szabo, 1989; Wilcock, 2007; Maxie and Newman, 2007; Thompson, 2007). In cattle, abnormal development of the cranial bones occurs as well as hydrocephalus with herniation of the cerebellum vermis. Congenital blindness can occur and failure of the optic nerve foramen to remodel causes contracture of the optic nerve. In pigs, hypovitaminosis A during pregnancy causes congenital defects including hydrocephalus, compression and herniation of the spinal cord, hypoplasia of eye structures and microphthalmia, supernumerary ears, cleft palate, arthrogryposis and dysmorphogenesis of skeletal muscle. Additionally renal dysplasia, pulmonary hypoplasia, diaphragmatic hernia, hepatic cysts, and cardiac and genital malformations can be observed. Pups born to a bitch with hypovitaminosis A can have abnormal skeletal development of the head and spinal column, and nervous system deficiencies including deafness and blindness.

Iodine – thyroid

Congenital goiter can be observed and generally is caused by dietary deficiency in iodine and dietary substances that interfere with iodine metabolism. In herds where congenital dietary iodine deficiency is observed, the addition of iodine to the diet stops calves being born with congenital goiter (Andrews *et al.*, 1948; Wither, 1997). Brassica plants can be teratogenic in terms of causing congenital goiter in calves. Iodine deficiency during pregnancy causes alopecia or abnormal hair growth, skin edema and other skeletal terata. There is putative evidence that high nitrate levels in forage fed to mares can be teratogenic and mimics congenital iodine deficiency (Allen *et al.*, 1996). Full term and prolonged gestation with immature foals was observed. Pathology observed in foals included hyperplastic thyroid, prognathic mandibulae, osteochondrosis consisting of incorrectly ossified carpal and tarsal bones, flexural deformities of the forelimbs, rupture of common digital extensor tendons and incomplete closure of the abdominal wall. Signs of immaturity included short hair and pliable ears. Thyroid lesions have been observed in the fetuses of ewes that have ingested locoweeds (Hartley and James, 1973). A number of polyhalogenated aromatic hydrocarbons can cause endocrine disruption of the thyroid gland.

Copper

Extreme copper (Cu) deficiency has been linked to a congenital defect in lambs known as swayback (Radostits *et al.*, 2007). The Cu deficiency stops the formation of myelin as well as causing demyelination and may start as early as mid-gestation. Lambs may be affected at birth or there may be a delay in the clinical signs. These may be linked to peaks in myelin development at day 90 of gestation and then again around day 20 of the postnatal period. Lambs born severely deficient in Cu can develop swayback in the critical postnatal period (progressive spinal swayback). Lesions are found in the white matter of the cerebrum in lambs affected at birth and in the spinal cord in the delayed occurrences. Lambs may be stillborn or born small and weak with fine tremors of the head. Some lambs may be bright and alert but will be uncoordinated with hind end weakness.

MYCOTOXINS

There are few reports of mycotoxin-linked congenital defects in livestock. Griseofulvin, used as a drug, was found to be teratogenic in cats. Dacasto *et al.* (1995) reported that pregnant sows exposed to zearalenone in the feed give birth to female piglets with abnormal external genitalia. Mares grazing endophyte-infected fescue can have prolonged gestation and give birth to large weak foals (Porter and Thompson, 1992; Coppock and Jacobsen, 2009).

PESTICIDES

Teratogenic effects of pesticides in farm animals have been reviewed (Szabo, 1989). Carbaryl is teratogenic to dogs (Smalley *et al.*, 1968). Beagle bitches in a feeding study received doses of 50, 25, 12.5, 6.25 and ~3.13 mg of carbaryl/kg body weight. The terata observed in all but the 3.13 mg/kg dose were abdominal and thoracic fissures and varying degrees of intestinal agenesis and displacement. Also observed were skeletal defects including brachygnathia, ecaudate pups and superfluous phalanges. Several of the pups had multiple defects that were difficult to categorize. Dystocia was observed due to uterine atony. Carbaryl has been shown to be teratogenic in pigs. When administered to pregnant pigs at dietary levels of 4 to 16 mg/kg, carbaryl caused stillbirths and malformations in piglets. Diazinon administered to pregnant bitches causes increased stillbirths and neonatal deaths in dogs, but was not teratogenic. Diazinon is teratogenic in swine.

DRUGS

Some drugs have been reported to be teratogenic in domestic animals. Aspirin had been shown to be teratogenic in cats and dogs (Khera, 1976; Robertson *et al.*, 1979). Aspirin administered *per os* at 25 and 50 mg/kg body weight to pregnant queens on gestation days 10 to 20 increased the non-specific terata in kittens. In dogs, the terata, primarily consisting of cleft palate, micrognathia, anasarca, cardiovascular malformations and tail anomalies, were observed in pups after the bitch was administered *per os* 400 mg of aspirin bid/kg body weight on gestation days 15 to 22. No terata in pups were observed born to bitches given 100 mg of aspirin/kg body weight. Pregnant mares treated with sulfonamides, pyrimethamine, folic acid and vitamin E gave birth to foals with bone marrow aplasia and hypoplasia, lymphoid hypoplasia, renal hypoplasia and nephrosis (Toribio *et al.*, 1998). The breeds were Quarter Horse, Thoroughbred and Tennessee Walking Horse. Methallibure causes embryo death and is teratogenic in pigs (King, 1969; Akpokodje, 1971; Akpokodje and Barker, 1971). Methallibure fed to pregnant gilts during gestation days 29 to 50 caused skeletal defects consisting of fixed flexion due to contracted tendons and the long bones of the limbs were shorter and thicker than normal (King, 1969; Akpokodje, 1971). The heads were disproportionately short, with distorted mandible and dorsolateral side of the cranium; the scalp was devoid of hair. Details of cranial terata in porcine embryos showed the frontal and parietal bones to be affected (Akpokodje, 1971). Arthrogryposis has also been reported for methallibure.

Griseofulvin is both a drug and a mycotoxin and is teratogenic in cats (Scott *et al.*, 1975; Coppock and Jacobsen, 2009). Pregnant queens in a cat colony and in homes were administered 500 to 1,000 mg griseofulvin *per os* weekly for a dermatophyte (Scott *et al.*, 1975). The terata observed included exencephaly, malformed prosencephalon and hydrocephalus. Skeletal malformations included cranium bifidum, spina bifida, abnormal atlantooccipital articulation, cleft palate, absence of maxillae, absence of tail vertebrae and cyclopia. Anophthalmia accompanied with absence of optic nerves and rudimentary optic tracts were also observed. Visceral terata were atresia ani, atresia coli and absence of atrioventricular valves in the heart.

Parasiticides

Some members of the benzimidazole group of parasiticides are teratogenic (Radostits *et al.*, 2007). Parbendazole was studied in several countries and generally concluded to be teratogenic in sheep at 60 mg/kg body weight and was not teratogenic at 30 mg/kg body weight (Szabo, 1989). The teratogenic effects include limb contractures, excessive flexion and extension of the joints, absence of the femur, humerus, ulna, hypoplasia of the digits, and hip displacement (Saunders *et al.*, 1974). Parbendazole was not teratogenic in cattle at 60 mg/kg body weight (Szabo, 1989). Cambendazole is teratogenic in sheep at 50 mg/kg body weight. At four times the therapeutic dose, albendazole is teratogenic in sheep (Radostits *et al.*, 2007). Apholate is an insect chemosterilant and alkylating agent was suspected of being teratogenic in sheep (Younger, 1965). There is putative and experimental evidence that trichlorfon is teratogenic in pigs (Bolske *et al.*, 1978; Knox *et al.*, 1978; Fatzer *et al.*, 1981). Pregnant sows were treated *per os* with trichlorfon during pregnancy. Piglets were born with cerebellar hypoplasia. The teschen/talfan virus was isolated from liver and spleen in one of the piglets. A diagnostic laboratory observed that treatment of sows with trichlorfon during gestation days 45 to 63 caused an increase in a syndrome in piglets characterized as ataxia and tremor, a pronounced cerebellar hypoplasia and a reduction in the size of the spinal cord. This condition was also produced experimentally.

ENVIRONMENTAL CHEMICALS AND FACTORS

Polyhalogenated aromatic hydrocarbons

Contaminants in the environment and feedstuffs are of concern. Hyperplasia of the thyroid gland has been observed in piglets born to sows fed polybrominated biphenyls (Werner and Sleight, 1981). Polychlorinated biphenyl (PCB) congeners have been shown to be teratogenic in goats (Lyche, 2006; Gutleb *et al.*, 2010). Exposure of does to PCB-153 and PCB-126 during gestation was shown to affect the maternal immunity in the kids. Does were exposed orally from gestation day 60 until delivery at dosages of 98 μg of PCB 153/kg body weight or 49 ng PCB 126/kg body weight. The effects of the exposure on the postnatal humoral immune responses were assessed by determining the levels of total immunoglobulin G and immunoglobulins to predetermined microbes at weeks 0, 1, 2, 4, 6 and 8 of age. The kids were also immunized at 2 weeks of age and the immune responses analyzed. The toxic effects of PCB-153 were studied in pregnant ewes (Gutleb *et al.*, 2010). The ewes were dosed *per os* with a corn oil control or PCB-118 49 μg/kg body weight/day and PB-153 98 μg/kg body weight/day every 3 days starting on the first day of gestation and continuing to gestation day 134. The trabecular bone mineral content at the metaphysis in male fetuses was ~30% lower in the PCB-118 group compared to male fetuses in the control group. In the PCB-153 group, the female fetuses showed a 19% reduction in the metaphyseal trabecular cross-sectional area. For the PCB-153 group, the diaphysis marrow cavity was smaller in female and male fetuses. This study shows that PCB-153 has an effect of developing bone in sheep. No report was given on thyroid gland histopathology. In Greece, semen from ovine, caprine, bovine and porcine species was assayed for persistent organic pollutants (POPs) (Kamarianos *et al.*, 2003a). The most common POPs were *p,p'*-DDE (80–100% of samples), HCB (73.9–100%) and gamma-HCH (69.6–100%). The follicular fluid of ovine, caprine, bovine and porcine species was also assayed in Greece for POPs (Kamarianos *et al.*, 2003b). The most commonly detected POPs were gamma-HCH (90–100% of samples) followed by HCB (80–100%), and *p,p'*-DDE (75–90.91%). These studies show that gametes are exposed to POPs before fertilization occurs.

Mercury

Methyl mercury had been reported to be teratogenic in cats (Khera, 1973). The teratogenic lesions are abnormalities of the spinal column, abnormal limbs, umbilical hernias and decreased cell density in the external granular layer of the cerebellum. Elevated levels of mercury were observed in fetal blood and brain.

Fetal endocrine disruption

Long-term studies have been done in sheep on the endocrine and teratogenic effects of exposure to multiple POPs after the spreading of sewage sludge on pasture lands. During mating and gestation sheep were pastured on lands that had received municipal sewage sludge and control sheep were pastured on lands that had received equivalent fertilization without sewage sludge (Paul *et al.*, 2005, Fowler *et al.*, 2008; Bellingham *et al.*, 2009). Decreased fetal body weight was observed at 110 days' gestation in both male and female fetuses (Paul *et al.*, 2005). There was a reduction in testicular mass, a reduction in Sertoli and Leydig cell numbers, and a reduction in fetal blood testosterone and inhibin A. Blood levels of follicle stimulating and luteinizing hormones were not decreased. Using the same experimental design, a study was done on the effect of sewage sludge on fetal ovarian parameters (Fowler *et al.*, 2008). Treatment reduced numbers of growth differentiation factor (GDF9) and induced myeloid leukemia cell differentiation protein (MCL1) positive oocytes by 25 to 26%. There was an increase in pro-apoptotic Bax by 65%, and 42% of protein spots in the treated ovarian proteome were differently expressed. A decrease in fetal body mass of female and male fetuses was observed, but there was no difference between treatment and control sheep for ovarian mass. Serum prolactin levels were decreased. In a subsequent study using the same experimental design, fetal body weights between treatment and control groups were not changed, but there was a reduction in GnRH mRNA expression in the hypothalamus. The hypothalamus and pituitary gland had reduced GnRH receptor (GnRHR) and galanin receptor (GALR) mRNA expression (Bellingham *et al.*, 2009). These studies show that mixtures of environmental chemicals may have long-term effects on reproductive capacity. The studies also show there is a likelihood that real world exposure to chemical mixtures can produce effects that would be different to knowledge gained from laboratory exposure to single chemicals. Sonne *et al.* (2008) proposed that a diet high in seal blubber containing polyhalogenated aromatic hydrocarbons (PAHs) consumed by a pregnant bitch could be linked to perineal and penile hypospadias in a pup. Concerns are being expressed regarding the potential teratogenic effects of environmental perchlorate, polybrominated diphenyl ethers and other PAHs (Crofton and Zoeller, 2005; Kirk, 2006; Mastorakos *et al.*, 2007). The interactions of different environmental chemicals on the developing thyroid gland are not well understood and need to be considered in risk models used to assess the impact of POPs in cattle (Crofton *et al.*, 2005; Crofton, 2008; Gilbert and Zoeller, 2010).

In vitro fertilization systems

The *in vitro* systems for fertilization can result in bovine congenital defects (Farin *et al.*, 2006). During early embryologic development, abnormalities that are not compatible with fetal life result in abortion. Congenital defects associated with *in vitro* production and somatic cell nuclear transfer methods are altered fetal body weight, abnormally increased duration of gestation, increased perinatal mortality, increased occurrences of male fetuses, increased fetal edema, altered growth of heart, brain, spinal cord and skeletal muscle, abnormal biochemical parameters, defects in fetal membranes including abnormal development of the chorioallantoic membranes and blood vessels, alterations in placentome morphology and feto-maternal contact, and increased occurrences of hydrallantois and hydramnios. The "abnormal offspring syndrome" (AOS) has been proposed to more accurately assess the congenital defects from *in vitro* production and somatic cell nuclear transfer methods to produce bovine embryos. The four types of AOS proposed are:

Type I: abnormal development and death of the embryo or early conceptus (early embryonic death/abortion) prior to completion of organogenesis (approximately day 42 of gestation in cattle).

Type II: abnormal development of the placental membranes and fetus; fetus dies (fetal death/abortion) between completion of organ differentiation and full term (day 42 to day 280 of gestation in cattle).

Type III: a full-term fetus and/or placenta with severe developmental abnormalities and no evidence of compensatory response by the fetus/placenta. Parturition is normal (eutocia) or difficult (dystocia). The calves are severely compromised with altered clinical, hematological or biochemical parameters; death occurs around the time of parturition or during the neonatal period.

Type IV: a full-term fetus and/or placenta with moderate abnormalities; however, the feto-placental unit compensates and adapts to the compromising genetic or physiological insults and survives. Parturition is normal (eutocia) or difficult (dystocia). The calves may be normal or abnormal in size for their breed, and they may have clinical, hematological or biochemical abnormalities.

DIAGNOSIS

The diagnosis of teratogen exposure as the cause of a congenital defect can be challenging for a variety of reasons. Causal links between the observed congenital defect and a causative agent are often not considered. An accurate history may be difficult to establish as the pregnant females may have moved locations or changed ownership during the time between exposure and the recognition of the abnormalities. Representative feed from the suspect source may have been given and is no longer available for chemical and biological testing, etc. Exposure parameters may be difficult to establish, especially for environmental substances. The teratogenic effect may be livestock species specific and has not been reported in laboratory animals. The specimens that would provide accurate descriptions of the defects were not presented for professional examination. A differential diagnosis is important to establish and specimens for virology may not be available. Serology can be used and monitoring titer changes is important.

CONCLUDING REMARKS AND FUTURE DIRECTIONS

Congenital defects in livestock are generally under-reported. It is likely that under-reporting of congenital defects associated with chemical agents occurs. A number of agents have been reported as being teratogenic in livestock species and these links have been established when veterinarians and livestock specialists have established causal links. Species differences in terata are not well understood. It is likely there is genetic predisposition between and within species. New studies on endocrine disruption in sheep suggest that teratogenic endocrine dysfunctions and some causes of reproductive soundness could be teratogenic in origin. Few pharmaceutical biologics used in livestock species have been tested for teratogenic effects. Compared to rodent studies, teratogenic studies in livestock species are expensive and labor intensive. It is important that research groups continue to study the teratogenic effects of plants and other substances in livestock species. The interactions between natural toxins, environmental chemicals, especially POPs, and viruses need further study.

REFERENCES

Akpokodje JU (1971) Further observations on the teratogenic effect of methallibure in swine. *Can Vet J* **12(6):** 125–8.

Akpokodje JU, Barker CA (1971) Embryonic deaths in gilts fed methallibure during gestation. *Can Vet J* **12(6):** 121–4.

Allen AL, Townsend HG, Doige CE, Fretz PB (1996) A case–control study of the congenital hypothyroidism and dysmaturity syndrome of foals. *Can Vet J* **37(6):** 349–51; 354–8.

Andrews FN, Shrewbury CL, Harper C, Vestal CM, Doyle LP (1948) Iodine deficiency in newborn sheep and swine. *J Anim Sci* **7(3):** 298–310.

Baker JC (1995) The clinical manifestations of bovine viral diarrhea infection. *Vet Clin North Am Food Anim Pract* **11(3):** 425–45.

Barker CA (1971) Embryonic deaths in gilts fed methallibure during gestation. *Can Vet J* **12(6):** 121–4.

Bellingham M, Fowler PA, Amezaga MR, Rhind SM, Cotinot C, Mandon-Pepin B, Sharpe RM, Evans NP (2009) Exposure to a complex cocktail of environmental endocrine-disrupting compounds disturbs the kisspeptin/GPR54 system in ovine hypothalamus and pituitary gland. *Environ Health Perspect* **117(10):** 1556–62.

Binns W, James LF, Shupe JL (1964) Toxicosis of *Veratrum californicum* in ewes and its relationship to a congenital deformity in lambs. *Ann NY Acad Sci* **111:** 571–6.

Binns W, James LF, Shupe JL, Thacker EJ (1962) Cyclopian-type malformation in lambs. *Arch Environ Health* **5:** 106–8.

Bird BH, Ksiazek TG, Nichol ST, Maclachlan NJ (2009) Rift Valley fever virus. *J Am Vet Med Assoc* **234(7):** 883–93.

Blanchard PC, Ridpath JF, Walker JB, Hietala SK (2010) An outbreak of late-term abortions, premature births, and congenital deformities associated with a bovine viral diarrhea virus 1 subtype b that induces thrombocytopenia. *J Vet Diagn Invest* **22(1):** 128–31.

Bolske G, Kronevi T, Lindgren NO (1978) Congenital tremor in pigs in Sweden. A case report. *Nord Vet Med* **30(12):** 534–7.

Burrows GE, Tyrl JR (2001) *Toxic Plants of North America*. Ames, IA: Iowa State University Press.

Cave JG, McLaren PJ, Whittaker SJ, Rast L, Stephens A, Parker EM (2008) An extended outbreak of congenital chondrodysplasia in calves in South East Australia. *Aust Vet J* **86(4):** 130–5.

Charles JA (1994) Akabane virus. *Vet Clin North Am Food Anim Pract* **10(3):** 525–46.

Chung SI, Livingston Jr CW, Edwards JF, Crandell RW, Shope RW, Shelton MJ, Collisson EW (1990) Evidence that Cache Valley virus induces congenital malformations in sheep. *Vet Microbiol* **21(4):** 297–307.

Cook D, Lee ST, Gardner DR, Pfister JA, Welch KD, Green BT, Davis TZ, Panter KE (2009) The alkaloid profiles of *Lupinus sulphureus*. *J Agric Food Chem* **57(4):** 1646–53.

Coppock RW, Jacobsen BJ (2009) Mycotoxins in animal and human patients. *Toxicol Ind Health* **25(9–10):** 637–55.

Crofton KM (2008) Thyroid disrupting chemicals: mechanisms and mixtures. *Int J Androl* **31(2):** 209–23.

Crofton KM, Craft ES, Hedge JM, Gennings C, Simmons JE, Carchman RA, Carter Jr WH, DeVito MJ (2005) Thyroid-hormone-disrupting chemicals: evidence for dose-dependent additivity or synergism. *Environ Health Perspect* **113(11):** 1549–54.

Crofton KM, Zoeller RT (2005) Mode of action: neurotoxicity induced by thyroid hormone disruption during development – hearing loss resulting from exposure to PHAHs. *Crit Rev Toxicol* **35(8–9):** 757–69.

Crowe MW, Pike HT (1973) Congenital arthrogryposis associated with ingestion of tobacco stalks by pregnant sows. *J Am Vet Med Assoc* **162(6):** 453–5.

Crowe MW, Swerczek TW (1974) Congenital arthrogryposis in offspring of sows fed tobacco (*Nicotiana tabacum*). *Am J Vet Res* **35(8):** 1071–3.

Dacasto M, Rolando P, Nachtmann C, Ceppa L, Nebbia C (1995) Zearalenone mycotoxicosis in piglets suckling sows fed contaminated grain. *Vet Hum Toxicol* **37(4):** 359–61.

Dal Pozzo F, Saegerman C, Thiry E (2009) Bovine infection with bluetongue virus with special emphasis on European serotype 8. *Vet J* **182(2):** 142–51.

De Lahunta A, Noden DM (1985) *The Embryology of Domestic Animals – Developmental Mechanisms and Malformations*. Williams & Wilkins, Baltimore.

Dennis SM (1993) Congenital defects of sheep. *Vet Clin North Am Food Anim Pract* **9(1):** 203–17.

Done JT (1968) Congenital nervous diseases of pigs: a review. *Lam Anim* **2:** 207–17.

Dubovi EJ (1994) Impact of bovine viral diarrhea virus on reproductive performance in cattle. *Vet Clin North Am Food Anim Pract* **10(3):** 503–14.

Edmonds LD, Selby LA, Case AA (1972) Poisoning and congenital malformations associated with consumption of poison hemlock by sows. *J Am Vet Med Assoc* **160(9):** 1319–24.

Edwards JF (1994) Cache Valley virus. *Vet Clin North Am Food Anim Pract* **10(3):** 515–24.

Edwards JF, Karabatsos N, Collisson EW, de la Concha Bermejillo A (1997) Ovine fetal malformations induced by *in utero* inoculation with Main Drain, San Angelo, and LaCrosse viruses. *Am J Trop Med Hyg* **56(2):** 171–6.

Farin PW, Piedrahita JA, Farin CE (2006) Errors in development of fetuses and placentas from *in vitro*-produced bovine embryos. *Theriogenology* **65(1):** 178–91.

Fatzer R, Hani H, Scholl E (1981) [Congenital tremor and cerebellar hypoplasia in piglets following treatment of sows with Neguvon during pregnancy.] *Schweiz Arch Tierheilkd* **123(1):** 29–36.

Fowler PA, Dora NJ, McFerran H, Amezaga MR, Miller DW, Lea RG, Cash P, McNeilly AS, Evans NP, Cotinot C, Sharpe RM, Rhind SM (2008) In utero exposure to low doses of environmental pollutants disrupts fetal ovarian development in sheep. *Mol Hum Reprod* **14(5):** 269–80.

Gilbert ME, Zoeller RT (2010) Thyroid hormones – impact on the developing brain: possible mechanisms of neurotoxicity. In *Neurotoxicology* (Harry GH, Tilson HA, eds.). New York, Informa Healthcare.

Gutleb AC, Arvidsson D, Orberg J, Larsson S, Skaare JU, Aleksandersen M, Ropstad E, Lind PM (2010) Effects on bone tissue in ewes (*Ovies aries*) and their foetuses exposed to PCB 118 and PCB 153. *Toxicol Lett* **192(2):** 126–33.

Hansen SL, Spears JW, Lloyd KE, Whisnant CS (2006) Feeding a low manganese diet to heifers during gestation impairs fetal growth and development. *J Dairy Sci* **89(11):** 4305–11.

Hartley WJ, James LF (1973) Microscopic lesions in fetuses of ewes ingesting locoweed (*Astragalus lentiginosus*). *Am J Vet Res* **34(2):** 209–11.

Hartley WJ, James LF (1975) Fetal and maternal lesions in pregnant ewes ingesting locoweed (*Astragalus lentiginosus*). *Am J Vet Res* **36(6):** 825–6.

Hidiroglou M, Ivan M, Bryan MK, Ribble CS, Janzen ED, Proulx JG, Elliot JI (1990) Assessment of the role of manganese in congenital joint laxity and dwarfism in calves. *Ann Rech Vet* **21(4):** 281–4.

James JF (1974) Diet-related birth defects. *Nut Today* July/Aug: 4–11.

James LF (1972) Effect of locoweed on fetal development: preliminary study in sheep. *Am J Vet Res* **33(4):** 835–40.

James LF, Keeler RF, Binns W (1969) Sequence in the abortive and teratogenic effects of locoweed fed to sheep. *Am J Vet Res* **30(3):** 377–80.

James LF, Molyneux RJ, Panter KE, Gardner DR, Stegelmeier BL (1994b) Effect of feeding ponderosa pine needle extracts and their residues to pregnant cattle. *Cornell Vet* **84(1):** 33–9.

James LF, Panter KE, Stegelmeier BL, Molyneux RJ (1994a) Effect of natural toxins on reproduction. *Vet Clin North Am Food Anim Pract* **10(3):** 587–603.

James LF, Shupe JL, Binns W, Keeler RF (1967) Abortive and teratogenic effects of locoweed on sheep and cattle. *Am J Vet Res* **28(126):** 1379–88.

Kamarianos A, Karamanlis X, Theodosiadou E, Goulas P, Smokovitis A (2003a) The presence of environmental pollutants in the semen of farm animals (bull, ram, goat, and boar). *Reprod Toxicol* **17(4):** 439–45.

Kamarianos A, Karamanlis X, Theodosiadou E, Goulas P, Smokovitis A (2003b) The presence of environmental pollutants in the follicular fluid of farm animals (cattle, sheep, goats, and pigs). *Reprod Toxicol* **17(2):** 185–90.

Keeler RF (1974) Coniine, a teratogenic principle from *Conium maculatum* producing congenital malformations in calves. *Clin Toxicol* **7(2):** 195–206.

Keeler RF (1979) Congenital defects in calves from maternal ingestion of *Nicotiana glauca* of high anabasine content. *Clin Toxicol* **15(4):** 417–26.

Keeler RF (1984) Teratogens in plants. *J Anim Sci* **58(4):** 1029–39.

Keeler RF 1988 Livestock models of human birth defects, reviewed in relation to poisonous plants. *J Anim Sci* **66(9):** 2414–27.

Keeler RF (1990) Early embryonic death in lambs induced by *Veratrum californicum*. *Cornell Vet* **80(2):** 203–7.

Keeler RF, Balls LD (1978) Teratogenic effects in cattle of *Conium maculatum* and conium alkaloids and analogs. *Clin Toxicol* **12(1):** 49–64.

Keeler RF, Balls LD, Shupe JL, Crowe MW (1980) Teratogenicity and toxicity of coniine in cows, ewes, and mares. *Cornell Vet* **70(1):** 19–26.

Keeler RF, Balls LD, Panter K (1981b) Teratogenic effects of *Nicotiana glauca* and concentration of anabasine, the suspect teratogen in plant parts. *Cornell Vet* **71(1):** 47–53.

Keeler RF, Binns W, James LF, Shupe JL (1969) Preliminary investigation of the relationship between bovine congenital lathyrism induced by aminoacetonitrile and the lupine induced crooked calf disease. *Can J Comp Med* **33(2):** 89–92.

Keeler RF, Crowe MW (1984) Teratogenicity and toxicity of wild tree tobacco, *Nicotiana glauca* in sheep. *Cornell Vet* **74(1):** 50–9.

Keeler RF, James LF (1971) Experimental teratogenic lathyrism in sheep and further comparative aspects with teratogenic locoism. *Can J Comp Med* **35(4):** 332–7.

Keeler RF, James LF, Binns W, Shupe JL (1967) An apparent relationship between locoism and lathyrism. *Can J Comp Med Vet Sci* **31(12):** 334–41.

Keeler RF, Panter KE (1989) Piperidine alkaloid composition and relation to crooked calf disease-inducing potential of *Lupinus formosus*. *Teratology* **40(5):** 423–32.

Keeler RF, Shupe JL, Crowe MW, Olson A, Balls LD (1981a) *Nicotiana glauca*-induced congenital deformities in calves: clinical and pathologic aspects. *Am J Vet Res* **42(7):** 1231–4.

Khera KS (1973) Teratogenic effects of methylmercury in the cat: note on the use of this species as a model for teratogenicity studies. *Teratology* **8(3):** 293–303.

Khera KS (1976) Teratogenicity studies with methotrexate, aminopterin, and acetylsalicylic acid in domestic cats. *Teratology* **14(1):** 21–7.

King GJ (1969) Deformities in piglets following administration of methallibure during specific stages of gestation. *J Reprod Fertil* **20(3):** 551–3.

Kirk AB (2006) Environmental perchlorate: why it matters. *Anal Chim Acta* **567(1):** 4–12.

Kitano Y, Yamashita S, Makinoda K (1994) A congenital abnormality of calves, suggestive of a new type of arthropod-borne virus infection. *J Comp Pathol* **111(4):** 427–37.

Knox B, Askaa J, Basse A, Bitsch V, Eskildsen M, Mandrup M, Ottosen HE, Overby E, Pedersen KB, Rasmussen F (1978) Congenital ataxia and tremor with cerebellar hypoplasia in piglets borne by sows treated with Neguvon vet (metrifonate, trichlorfon) during pregnancy. *Nord Vet Med* **30(12):** 538–45.

Kono R, Hirata M, Kaji M, Goto Y, Ikeda S, Yanase T, Kato T, Tanaka S, Tsutsui T, Imada T, Yamakawa M (2008) Bovine epizootic encephalomyelitis caused by Akabane virus in southern Japan. *BMC Vet Res* **4:** 20.

Lee ST, Panter KE, Pfister JA, Gardner DR, Welch KD (2008) The effect of body condition on serum concentrations of two teratogenic alkaloids (anagyrine and ammodendrine) from lupines (*Lupinus* species) that cause crooked calf disease. *J Anim Sci* **86(10):** 2771–8.

Leipold HW, Hiraga T, Dennis SM (1993) Congenital defects of the bovine central nervous system. *Vet Clin North Am Food Anim Pract* **9(1):** 77–91.

Lyche JL, Larsen HJ, Skaare JU, Tverdal A, Johansen GM, Ropstad E (2006) Perinatal exposure to low doses of PCB 153 and PCB 126 affects maternal and neonatal immunity in goat kids. *J Toxicol Environ Health A* **69(1–2):** 139–58.

Mastorakos G, Karoutsou EI, Mizamtsidi M, Creatsas G (2007) The menace of endocrine disruptors on thyroid hormone physiology and their impact on intrauterine development. *Endocrine* **31(3):** 219–37.

Maxie MG, Newman SJ (2007) Urinary system. In *Jubb, Kennedy and Palmer's Pathology of Domestic Animals* (Maxie MG, ed.). Toronto, ON, Elsevier.

Maxie MG, Youssef S (2007) Nervous system. In *Jubb, Kennedy and Palmer's Pathology of Domestic Animals*, (Maxie MG, ed.). Toronto, ON, Elsevier.

McIlwraith CW, James LF (1982) Limb deformities in foals associated with ingestion of locoweed by mares. *J Am Vet Med Assoc* **181(3):** 255–8.

McLaren PJ, Cave JG, Parker EM, Slocombe RF (2007) Chondrodysplastic calves in Northeast Victoria. *Vet Pathol* **44(3):** 342–54.

Menges RW, Selby LA, Marienfeld CJ, Aue WA, Greer DL (1970) A tobacco related epidemic of congenital limb deformities in swine. *Environ Res* **3(4):** 285–302.

Molyneux RJ, Lee ST, Gardner DR, Panter KE, James LF (2007) Phytochemicals: the good, the bad and the ugly? *Phytochemistry* **68(22–24):** 2973–85.

Nettleton PF, Gilray JA, Russo P, Dlissi E (1998) Border disease of sheep and goats. *Vet Res* **29(3–4):** 327–40.

Oberst RD (1993) Viruses as teratogens. *Vet Clin North Am Food Anim Pract* **9(1):** 23–31.

Ortega JA, Lazerson J (1987) Anagyrine-induced red cell aplasia, vascular anomaly, and skeletal dysplasia. *J Pediatr* **111(1):** 87–9.

Panter KE, Bunch TD, James LF, Sisson DV 1987 Ultrasonographic imaging to monitor fetal and placental developments in ewes fed locoweed (*Astragalus lentiginosus*). *Am J Vet Res* **48(4):** 686–90.

Panter KE, Bunch TD, Keeler RF (1988a) Maternal and fetal toxicity of poison hemlock (*Conium maculatum*) in sheep. *Am J Vet Res* **49(2):** 281–3.

Panter KE, Bunch TD, Keeler RF, Sisson DV, Callan RJ (1990a) Multiple congenital contractures (MCC) and cleft palate induced in goats by ingestion of piperidine alkaloid-containing plants: reduction in fetal movement as the probable cause. *J Toxicol Clin Toxicol* **28(1):** 69–83.

Panter KE, Gardner DR, Molyneux RJ (1998) Teratogenic and fetotoxic effects of two piperidine alkaloid-containing lupines (*L. formosus* and *L. arbustus*) in cows. *J Nat Toxins* **7(2):** 131–40.

Panter KE, James LF, Gardner DR (1999) Lupines, poison-hemlock and *Nicotiana* spp: toxicity and teratogenicity in livestock. *J Nat Toxins* **8(1):** 117–34.

Panter KE, James LF, Gardner DR, Ralphs MH, Pfister JA, Stegelmeier BL, Lee ST (2002) Reproductive losses to poisonous plants: influence of management strategies. *J Range Manage* **55(3):** 301–8.

Panter KE, James LF, Hartley WJ (1989) Transient testicular degeneration in rams fed locoweed (*Astragalus lentiginosus*). *Vet Hum Toxicol* **31(1):** 42–6.

Panter KE, James LF, Stegelmeier BL, Ralphs MH, Pfister JA (1999) Locoweeds: effects on reproduction in livestock. *J Nat Toxins* **8(1):** 53–62.

Panter KE, Keeler RF (1990) *Conium*, *Lupinus*, and *Nicotiana* alkaloids: fetal effects and the potential for residues in milk. *Vet Hum Toxicol* **32 (Suppl.):** 89–93; discussion 93–4.

Panter KE, Keeler RF, Baker DC (1988b) Toxicoses in livestock from the hemlocks (*Conium* and *Cicuta* spp.). *J Anim Sci* **66(9):** 2407–13.

Panter KE, Keeler RF, Buck WB (1985a) Induction of cleft palate in newborn pigs by maternal ingestion of poison hemlock (*Conium maculatum*). *Am J Vet Res* **46(6):** 1368–71.

Panter KE, Keeler RF, Buck WB (1985b) Congenital skeletal malformations induced by maternal ingestion of *Conium maculatum* (poison hemlock) in newborn pigs. *Am J Vet Res* **46(10):**2064–6.

Panter KE, Keeler RF, Bunch TD, Callan RJ (1990b) Congenital skeletal malformations and cleft palate induced in goats by ingestion of *Lupinus*, *Conium* and *Nicotiana* species. *Toxicon* **28(12):** 1377–85.

Paul C, Rhind SM, Kyle CE, Scott H, McKinnell C, Sharpe RM (2005) Cellular and hormonal disruption of fetal testis development in sheep reared on pasture treated with sewage sludge. *Environ Health Perspect* **113(11):** 1580–7.

Porter JK, Thompson Jr FN (1992) Effects of fescue toxicosis on reproduction in livestock. *J Anim Sci* **70(5):** 1594–603.

Radostits OM, Gay CC, Hinchcliff KW, Constable PD (2007) *Veterinary Medicine. A Textbook of the Diseases of Cattel, Horses, Sheep, Pigs and Goats*, 10th edition. Toronto, Saunders.

Ribble CS, Janzen ED, Proulx JG (1989) Congenital joint laxity and dwarfism: a feed-associated congenital anomaly of beef calves in Canada. *Can Vet J* **30(4):** 331–8.

Robertson RT, Allen HL, Bokelman DL (1979) Aspirin: teratogenic evaluation in the dog. *Teratology* **20(2):** 313–20.

Rojas MA, Dyer IA, Cassatt WA (1965) Manganese deficiency in the bovine. *J Anim Sci* **24:** 664–7.

Saunders LZ, Shone DK, Philip JR, Birkhead HA (1974) The effects of methyl-5(6)-butyl-2-benzimidazole carbamate (parbendazole) on reproduction in sheep and other animals. I. Malformations in newborn lambs. *Cornell Vet* **64 (Suppl. 4):** 7–40.

Schlafer DH, Miller RB (2007) Female genital system. In *Jubb, Kennedy and Palmer's Pathology of Domestic Animals* (Maxie MG, ed.). Toronto, ON, Elsevier.

Scott FW, LaHunta A, Schultz RD, Bistner SI, C Riis RC (1975) Teratogenesis in cats associated with griseofulvin therapy. *Teratology* **11(1):** 79–86.

Seaman JT, Smeal MG, Wright JC (1981) The possible association of a sorghum (*Sorghum sudanese*) hybrid as a cause of developmental defects in calves. *Aust Vet J* **57(7):** 351–2.

Selby LA, Menges RW, Houser EC, Flatt RE, Case AA (1971) Outbreak of swine malformations associated with the wild black cherry, *Prunus serotina*. *Arch Environ Health* **22(4):** 496–501.

Shupe JL, Binns W, James LR, Keeler RF (1967) Lupine, a cause of crooked calf disease. *J Am Vet Med Assoc* **151(2):** 198–203.

Shupe JL, Binns W, James LR, Keeler RF (1968) A congenital deformity in calves induced by the maternal consumption of lupin. *Aus J Agric Res* **19(2):** 335–40.

Shupe JL, James LF (1983) Teratogenic plants. *Vet Hum Toxicol* **25(6):** 415–21.

Smalley HE, Curtis JM, Earl FL (1968) Teratogenic action of carbaryl in beagle dogs. *Toxicol Appl Pharmacol* **13(3):** 392–403.

Sonne C, Dietz R, Born EW, Leifsson PS, Andersen S (2008) Is there a link between hypospadias and organochlorine exposure in East Greenland sledge dogs (*Canis familiaris*)? *Ecotoxicol Environ Saf* **69(3):** 391–5.

Staley GP, van der Lugt JJ, Axsel G, Loock AH (1994) Congenital skeletal malformations in Holstein calves associated with putative manganese deficiency. *J S Afr Vet Assoc* **65(2):** 73–8.

Swinyard CA, Bleck EE (1985) The etiology of arthrogryposis (multiple congenital contracture). *Clin Orthop Relat Res* **194:** 15–29.

Szabo KT (1989) *Congenital Malformations in Laboratory and Farm Animals*. San Diego: Academic Press.

Thompson K (2007) Bones and joints. In *Jubb, Kennedy and Palmer's Pathology of Domestic Animals* (Maxie MG, ed.). Toronto, ON, Elsevier.

Toribio RE, Bain FT, Mrad DR, Messer IV NT, Sellers RS, Hinchcliff KW (1998) Congenital defects in newborn foals of mares treated for equine protozoal myeloencephalitis during pregnancy. *J Am Vet Med Assoc* **212(5):** 697–701.

Tsuda T, Yoshida K, Ohashi S, Yanase T, Sueyoshi M, Kamimura S, Misumi K, Hamana K, Sakamoto H, Yamakawa M (2004) Arthrogryposis, hydranencephaly and cerebellar hypoplasia syndrome in neonatal calves resulting from intrauterine infection with Aino virus. *Vet Res* **35(5):** 531–8.

Van Vleet JF, Valentine BA (2007) Muscle and tendon. In *Jubb, Kennedy and Palmer's Pathology of Domestic Animals* (Maxie MG, ed.). Toronto, ON, Elsevier.

Vercauteren G, Vandenbussche CF, Ducatelle R, Van der Heyden S, Vandemeulebroucke E, De Leeuw I, Deprez P, Chiers K, De Clercq K (2008.) Bluetongue virus serotype 8-associated congenital hydranencephaly in calves. *Transbound Emerg Dis* **55(7):** 293–8.

Wayman O, Iwanaga II, Hugh WI (1970) Fetal resorption in swine caused by *Leucaena leucocephala* (Lam.) de Wit. in the diet. *J Anim Sci* **30(4):** 583–8.

Weinzweig J, Panter KE, Pantaloni M, Spangenberger A, Harper JS, Lui F, Gardner D, Wierenga TL, Edstrom LE (1999) The fetal cleft palate: I. Characterization of a congenital model. *Plast Reconstr Surg* **103(2):** 419–28.

Weinzweig J, Panter KE, Patel J, Smith DM, Spangenberger A, Freeman MB (2008) The fetal cleft palate: v. elucidation of the mechanism of palatal clefting in the congenital caprine model. *Plast Reconstr Surg* **121(4):** 1328–34.

Welch KD, Panter KE, Lee ST, Gardner DR, Stegelmeier BL, Cook D (2009) Cyclopamine-induced synophthalmia in sheep: defining a critical window and toxicokinetic evaluation. *J Appl Toxicol* **29(5):** 414–21.

Werner PR, Sleight SD (1981) Toxicosis in sows and their pigs caused by feeding rations containing polybrominated biphenyls to sows during pregnancy and lactation. *Am J Vet Res* **42(2):** 183–8.

Whitwell KE (1980) Investigations into fetal and neonatal losses in the horse. *Vet Clin North Am Large Anim Pract* **2(2):** 313–31.

Wilcock BP (2007) Eye and ear. In *Jubb, Kennedy and Palmer's Pathology of Domestic Animals* (Maxie MG, ed.). Toronto, ON, Elsevier.

Wither SE (1997) Congenital goiter in cattle. *Can Vet J* **38(3):** 178.

Younger RL (1965) Probable induction of congenital anomalies in a lamb by apholate. *Am J Vet Res* **26(113):** 991–5.

C H A P T E R

85

Mare reproductive loss syndrome

Manu Sebastian

INTRODUCTION

Mare reproductive loss syndrome (MRLS) can be described as an epidemic of early fetal loss and late fetal loss (EFL/LFL) which can occur with smaller numbers of fibrinous pericarditis (FP), unilateral uveitis (UU) and *Actinobacillus* encephalitis (AE). MRLS occurred during the spring of 2001 at horse farms in and around central Kentucky. EFL and LFL were identified during the last week of April, peaked on May 5th and declined rapidly thereafter. Fibrinous pericarditis and unilateral uveitis were identified during the same time period. The same pattern of abortion and pericarditis, but in lesser numbers, was observed in 2002 (Harrison, 2001; Kane and Kilby, 2001; Powell, 2001; Sebastian, 2008b).

The risk factors identified by the four epidemiological investigations of this syndrome included: exposure to moderate to high concentrations of eastern tent caterpillars (*Malacosoma americanum*, ETCs) (Figure 85.1) in the pastures, the presence of cherry trees, ≥50 broodmares/farm, feeding hay in pasture, greater than usual amounts of white clover in pastures, abortion during a previous pregnancy, being fed on pastures exclusively during the 4-week period prior to abortion, access to pasture after midnight during the 4-week period prior to abortion, drinking from a water trough, or not, access to water buckets or automatic water taps, etc. Risk factors associated with fibrinous pericarditis included: being from a farm with mares and foals affected by MRLS, exposure to ETCs in or around the pastures, younger age, shorter duration of residence in Kentucky, being fed hay grown outside Kentucky, lack of access to pond water and a lack of direct contact with cattle (Cohen *et al.*, 2003a,b; Dwyer *et al.*, 2003; Seahorn *et al.*, 2003).

Approximately 14,980 foals of all breeds were lost due to MRLS in 2001. Similar fetal losses, abortions and stillbirths were reported from southern Ohio, West Virginia and Tennessee during the same time period, indicating that MRLS was not limited to Kentucky. A lesser incidence of MRLS was recorded in central Kentucky in 2002, and few cases were reported in 2003. At least 17 breeds of horses were affected. The abortions were heavily concentrated in central Kentucky but aborted equine fetuses from 32 counties in Kentucky were submitted to the University of Kentucky diagnostic laboratory for necropsy. The specific number of LFL and EFL abortions in the field was not recorded. MRLS was also reported from Florida in 2006. The economic loss due to MRLS in 2001 was estimated at $336 million. The combined losses from MRLS in 2001 and 2002 were estimated at approximately $500 million. MRLS was therefore one of the most economically devastating acute diseases to strike the livestock industry (Paulick, 2001).

A similar equine abortion storm was observed in Australia during the winter of 2004. These abortions had an unusual and consistent clinical and pathological appearance. Abortions were observed at mid term to later stages of pregnancy. Pathological findings included inflammation of the amnion and amniotic portion of the umbilical cord extending to the allantois and in chronic cases inflammation extending through the allantois to the chorion around the site of the attachment of the umbilical cord. The aborted fetuses showed variable non-specific inflammatory changes. The bacteria isolated from the stomach content or lung or amnion/umbilical cord included *Cellulomonas* spp., *Microbacterium aggregans*, *Arthrobacter* spp., *Curtobacterium* spp., non-beta hemolytic slow-growing *Streptococci*, other coryneform bacteria, and some Gram-negative non-fermenting rods. ETCs are not present in Australia but other caterpillar species with setae or hairs are reported to occur in EFL-affected regions. Processionary caterpillars (*Ochragaster lunifer*) were reported to be the most abundant species reported in regions where these abortion cases had occurred. Experimental administration of 5 g of macerated exoskeleton of processionary caterpillars, daily for 5 days by nasogastric tubing, resulted in abortion of two out six treated animals (Perkins *et al.*, 2007; Cawdell-Smith *et al.*, 2009).

CLINICAL FINDINGS

Fetal loss

Early fetal loss was observed in the first trimester and LFL was observed in the last trimester of gestation. Very few clinical signs were observed in mares which had EFL. The clinical signs observed included sero-sanguineous or purulent vulvar discharge, and fetal membranes protruding from their vulva with fetuses located either in the vagina or vulva. Few mares (approximately <15%) showed mild colic signs, abdominal straining or low-grade fever (101.0–101.5°F) 1 to 3 days before EFL. In dead fetuses the typical ultrasound

Reproductive and Developmental Toxicology, Edited by Ramesh C. Gupta
ISBN: 978-0-12-382032-7

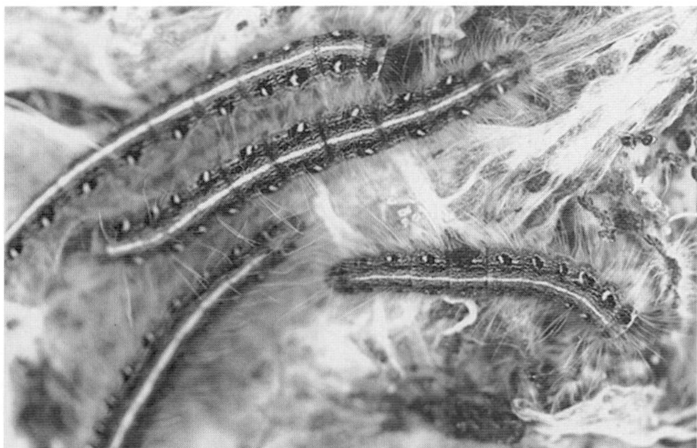

Figure 85.1 Eastern tent caterpillars, *Malacosoma americanum*, in their nest. (From Gupta, 2007, p. 777. Reproduced with permisssion from Elsevier.)

presentation was a dead fetus (i.e., no heartbeat), surrounded by echogenic allantoic fluid and a more echogenic amniotic fluid. In live fetuses ultrasound examination showed a fetus with slow heart rate and slow movements, suspended in an amniotic fluid which was echogenic, either "cloudy" or "flocculent". The majority of EFL cases occurred between days 40 and 80 of gestation, with few cases up to 140 days.

Allantoic fluid was aspirated from three EFL mares and culture of this aspirate allantoic fluid grew alpha *Streptococcus* bacteria in two cases and *E. coli* in one case. Complete blood counts and blood chemistry panel evaluation from these mares did not show any significant abnormalities. Microscopic examination of uterine biopsies from EFL mares within 7 days of abortion showed moderate to severe inflammation (Riddle and LeBlanc, 2003). Clinical observation associated with LFL included explosive parturition, dystocia, foaling while standing, premature placental separation ("red bag delivery") stillbirth, foals born weak and agalactic mares. The foals born to these mares were weak and many required resuscitation. These weak foals, which were admitted to local equine veterinary hospitals, survived for up to 4 days. These foals were dehydrated, hypothermic and tachycardic with irregular respiration. Leucopenia, hypoglycemia and acidosis were also observed. Bilateral hyphema was observed in many of these foals at birth. Blood cultures from these foals were rarely positive for bacteria. The most frequently isolated bacteria were alpha *Streptococcus* and *Actinobacillus* spp. (Byars and Seahorn, 2002).

Fibrinous pericarditis (FP)

Clinical presentation of the pericarditis cases included ultrasonographic evidence of effusive fibrinous pericarditis, tachycardia, muffled heart sounds, hyperfibrinogenemia, lethargy, tachypnea, jugular pulse distention and pleural effusion and/or ascitis. Analysis of fluid from the pericardial sac of most cases demonstrated a low white cell count and high protein content. This fluid was mostly sterile exudate, but in cases where bacteria grew, they were similar to those observed in EFL/LFL abortions. In 2001, 38 cases of FP were admitted to two large central Kentucky referral veterinary clinics. These cases occurred in horses of all ages, breeds and sexes including non-pregnant mares. Less than 15 confirmed cases of pericarditis were recorded in 2002 and two cases were reported associated with MRLS in 2003 (Bolin *et al.*, 2004).

Unilateral uveitis (UU)

Unilateral uveitis was an exclusive clinical finding associated with MRLS. In 2001, 40 UU cases were observed in foals, yearlings and adult horses of all breeds, ages and sexes. The clinical signs were per acute, with profound exudative ophthalmitis occurring within the first 12-hour period. The other consistent changes with these cases included corneal edema and exudates in the anterior and posterior chambers. The anterior chamber exudates were tan yellow, presumably a proteinaceous and often accompanied by hemorrhage from the surface of the iris. A markedly turbid yellow vitreous was visible through a mid-range pupil, and this was confirmed by ultrasound. These cases were refractive to treatment resulting in blindness followed by various degrees of global atrophy. Fewer cases were reported in 2002. Histopathological examination was not conducted on the affected eye as none of the affected eyes was enucleated (Latimer, 2002).

During the period of MRLS in 2001, three cases of meningoencephalitis (age >4 years), caused by the same organism, *Actinobacillus* sp. associated with the EFL/LFL/FP cases, were diagnosed on necropsy. Similar *Actinobacillus* sp. associated meningoencephalitis were not observed during MRLS in 2002 (Sebastian *et al.*, 2002a, 2003a).

PATHOLOGICAL FINDINGS

Most of the EFL placentas and fetuses submitted for examination were in a state of severe autolysis. Varying degrees of neutrophils infiltration were observed in the placental membranes, and the amniotic and allantoic fluids indicating a bacterial placentitis. Bacterial organisms isolated from EFL were similar to those isolated from LFL and funisitis was not observed in EFL. LFL was separated from the EFL aborted fetuses and no funisitis was observed in these.

In LFL fetuses gross pathological lesions included pale brown placenta, in sharp contrast to its normal dark reddish brown color, with a thick, dull, edematous yellowish umbilical cord, hemorrhage in the eyes, marked placental thickening, placental edema and intact cervical star ("red bag"). Lung lobes of few fetuses had edema. Histopathological findings associated with LFL included placentitis, funisitis and perinatal pneumonia. In lungs, alveoli contained free bacterial colonies with and without inflammatory response and numerous free squamous epithelial cells. One of the most important lesions of LFL was funisitis (inflammation of umbilical cord) and was mostly confined to the amniotic segment of the umbilical cord. The inflammatory cells were mostly confined to the surface of the neutrophils admixed with bacterial colonies. In allantochorion, the inflammatory cells, predominantly neutrophils, were confined to the coelomic space in the subchorionic stroma, mostly around vessels in the stroma. The distribution of inflammatory cells in the placenta was therefore distinguishable from the ascending placentitis by the pattern of distribution of inflammatory cells. No single lesion was pathognomonic for LFL-MRLS. The diagnosis depended on the history, clinical signs, pathological and microbiological findings (Williams *et al.*, 2002; Cohen *et al.*, 2003c).

Ten different bacterial species were isolated from lung, stomach fluid, allantochorion and placental fluid of LFL 2001 cases. The majority of them were non-beta hemolytic

Streptococci (51%) and/or *Actinobacillus* spp. (13%) (Donahue *et al.*, 2002).

Fibrinous pericarditis cases were characterized by large quantities of sero-fibrinous fluid (up to 3 liters) in the pericardial cavity. The characteristic histopathological finding was fibrinopurulent inflammation of the visceral pericardium with extension of this inflammation into the myocardium. In 31% of these cases *Actinobacillus* spp. was isolated and the remaining cases had no bacterial isolates. *Actinobacillus* spp. was isolated from a total of 10 non-treated horses out of 32 cases submitted for necropsy during MRLS 2001 (Bolin *et al.*, 2004). No eyes from the unilateral uveitis cases were submitted for pathological examination. Virological and serological examinations conducted on the fetal and placental samples by different referral laboratories in the USA did not identify any viral agents.

INVESTIGATION OF ETIOLOGIC AGENTS

A variety of tests were conducted to rule out toxic etiological agents like nitrate/nitrite, ergot alkaloid/fescue toxicosis, phytoestrogens and other mycotoxins, and none of these agents were identified in the tissue or fluid samples evaluated.

Epidemiological investigations identified multiple risk factors including the presence of ETCs associated with the syndrome. The presence of ETCs had both spatial and temporal association with MRLS abortions. This epidemiological finding led to a search for a toxin associated with the ETC habitat. The principal food of ETCs is black cherry tree leaves, which contain organic cyanide prunasin, which is digested and metabolized to mandelonitrile. Mandelonitrile, which spontaneously hydrolyzes to yield cyanide, is also present in the regurgitated materials of ETCs and is used by the ETC as a defensive chemical against predators (Fitzgerald, 2002). Considering the role of cyanide as a probable etiological agent related to the relationship with ETCs, several experimental studies were conducted in pregnant mares by exposing them to variable cyanide doses which were not lethal to mares and none of the studies could induce abortion. Detailed experimental studies conducted by administration of mandelonitrile at a dose of 2mg/kg/horse twice a day in feed, for 14 days to six late term pregnant mares, did not yield any abortions (Harkins *et al.*, 2002). No abortions were observed in a pilot study conducted by exposing mandelonitrile vapor to pregnant mares for 6 hours for 3 consecutive days. Thus the role of mandelonitrile and cyanide as a primary cause of MRLS was ruled out.

CATERPILLAR STUDIES

The first experiments designed to replicate the natural exposure of mares to ETCs were carried out in spring of 2002. Pregnant mares were exposed to live ETCs or their frass (feces) for 6 hours each day for a maximum of 10 days or until they aborted. In this experiment pregnant mares exposed to ETCs and frass aborted; however, no abortions occurred in the frass-only group. Bacteria similar to natural cases of MRLS were cultured from most of the fetal/placental tissues. This experiment established that ETC exposure can cause EFL/MRLS abortions (Webb *et al.*, 2003).

In another experiment, pregnant mares in the first trimester of pregnancy were administered ETCs and frass by gastric gavage for 10 days. The experiment comprised five control mares (administered saline), five mares administered 2.5g/day of frass (by gastric tube) that had been stored at –80°C and five mares administered 50g/day homogenized ETCs, by nasogastric tube. The mares were confined to the stalls during the entire period of the experiment and were fed with hay from Nevada. This experimental study thus confirmed the cause–effect relationship of ETC exposure to EFL and also ruled out involvement of Kentucky hay or pastures (Bernard *et al.*, 2004).

Experimental studies for replicating LFL were conducted by gastric gavage of homogenized ETCs to late-term pregnant mares. The experiment consisted of six pregnant mares administered 50g/day of ETCs for 9 days and control mares gavaged with saline. The ETCs for this experiment were collected from Michigan and were maintained live by feeding fresh Kentucky black cherry leaves. All mares exposed to ETCs aborted and none of the control mares aborted. No abnormal clinical signs, blood chemistry panel changes or blood cultures were recorded throughout the entire experiment. The placentas of aborted fetuses had intact cervical star. The role of ETCs in LFL was confirmed by this experiment and experiment also demonstrated that ETCs from a region other than central Kentucky are capable of causing MRLS (Sebastian *et al.*, 2002b).

An experiment was conducted to determine the abortifacient potential in different body components of ETCs in which pregnant mares were exposed to different anatomical components/fractions and filtrates of ETCs. This experiment consisted of seven groups of five early pregnant mares, and the ETCs used in the experiments were preserved at –80°C. Group 1, the positive controls, were fed 50g ETC homogenate mixed in sweet feed. Group 2, the negative controls, were fed saline mixed sweet feed. Groups 3, 4, 5 and 6 were fed specific parts, extracts, filtrates and retentates of ETCs. For this experiment, ETCs were dissected into three distinct body parts: exoskeleton, gut and internal contents. All three components were fed to pregnant mares in early stages of gestation. Other early-term mares were fed filtrates of a phosphate buffered saline homogenate of ETCs that had been filtered (<45 microns) and the retentate from this preparation was fed to two groups of mares in early stages of gestation. Positive and negative control groups were also maintained in the experiment. All five mares in the positive control group aborted. Three out of five mares in the group fed with exoskeleton aborted and one mare in the group fed with retentate aborted. No other groups were affected. This experiment suggested that ETC exoskeleton has abortifacient potential compared with other components of the body (Webb *et al.*, 2003).

The abortifacient potential of frozen ETCs, autoclaved ETCs and gypsy moth caterpillars (GMCs), a hairy caterpillar, were investigated in detail. Three out of five mares fed frozen ETCs (maintained at –80°C) aborted; none of the five mares administered ETCs that were autoclaved before administration aborted. One of the four GMC-treated mares aborted; however, the abortion was considered atypical for MRLS and as such was excluded from the analysis. This experiment suggested that freezing will not reduce the abortifacient potential of ETCs but autoclaving will lead to loss of abortifacient potential (Webb *et al.*, 2003). GMCs which have many hairs similar to ETCs did not induce abortion in pregnant mares, suggesting that hair of caterpillars may not play a role in the pathogenesis of MRLS. Similarly another experiment was conducted using forest tent caterpillars (*Malacosoma distria,* FTCs) which are closely related to ETCs as they both are of the same genus. Early term mares were administered 100 g of FTC homogenate/mare for 5 days (the FTCs were raised/hatched out in laboratory), by stomach tube. A second group of early term mares served as controls. No abortions were observed in the FTC challenge group or the controls. This experiment suggests that the abortifacient potential is not uniformly present in all *Malacosoma*/tent caterpillar species and also hair/setae of caterpillars may not play a role in the pathogenesis of MRLS. Multiple experiments were conducted to rule out the role of bacteria and viral agents in MRLS. To rule out the role of bacteria ETCs were sterilized with alcohol by blending with 95% ethanol in a mechanical blender for 5 minutes and allowed to sit at room temperature for 2 hours. The absence of bacteria was confirmed by culturing the homogenate. The test group of pregnant mares was administered 50 g of alcohol-treated homogenate for 10 consecutive days via a nasogastric tube. The negative control mares received 200 ml of 10% ethanol. Two of the five mares that received the ethanol-treated ETC homogenate aborted. These abortions were considered typical of MRLS.

No abortions were observed in the ethanol-only administered control group. This experiment suggested that the causative agent is not an ETC associated bacterium. Ethanol has bactericidal property but may not have the potency to destroy viruses and hence the role of viruses in MRLS was not ruled out by this experiment. Irradiation has been proven to destroy virus and bacteria and hence an experiment was conducted using irradiated ETCs to evaluate the role of virus in MRLS. Homogenate of ETCs was prepared in normal saline and was exposed to 30 kGy cobalt irradiation, a level demonstrated to destroy/inactivate marker bacteria and viruses while not significantly altering the activity of enzymatic or chemical markers. The experiment consisted of three groups with group A mares administered 100 g non-irradiated fresh frozen ETCs by gastric gavage, group B mares 100 g of irradiated fresh frozen ETCs and group C mares served as negative controls which were administered saline; all mares administered for 10 days or until abortion. Three of the group B mares administered 100 g irradiated ETCs aborted. All group B mares administered 100 g fresh frozen ETCs aborted within 32 to 120 hours after the onset of treatment. All group C mares maintained their pregnancy. The aborted fetuses from group A mares had gross and histopathological changes similar to those observed in the natural MRLS cases. *Actinobacillus* spp. and *Streptococcus* spp. were isolated from these fetoplacental units. This was the first experiment in which the typical MRLS funisitis has been demonstrated in experiment, funisitis being a typical and to some extent defining lesion in many field MRLS cases. The results of this experiment demonstrated that frozen ETCs from 2003 preserved at −80°C will induce abortion in late gestation mares. This experiment ruled out the role of naturally occurring virus or bacteria in ETCs. It was interpreted that irradiation markedly reduced the abortifacient capabilities of the 2003 ETCs but did not eliminate altogether their capability to induce abortion (Sebastian *et al.*, 2003a).

LABORATORY ANIMAL MODELS

Administration of ETCs in different doses, different routes and different stages of pregnancy in pregnant mice did not result in any statistically significant number of abortions. Experimental studies in rats using ETC-mixed feed, fed from day 4 of gestation through to the end of gestation, did not yield a statistically significant number of abortions. A pilot study was conducted to evaluate the abortifacient potential of ETCs by feeding them to pregnant pigs. Two out of five gilts fed ETC aborted their litters, while none of the controls aborted. The pilot study in pigs suggests that ETCs have an abortifacient potential in species other than equine. Experiments conducted in pregnant goats administered 50 g of homogenized ETCs (same dose administered to the late-term pregnant mares) did not result in abortions (Sebastian *et al.*, 2002c, 2008a).

PATHOGENESIS AND OTHER OBSERVATIONS

There was no substantial evidence to suggest that MRLS had a long-term effect on fertility. Mares which aborted in 2001 conceived in 2002 and maintained their pregnancies at rates consistent with prior years. Blood collected from pregnant mares after administration of irradiated and non-irradiated ETCs were tested for immune status and no definitive evidence of an immunosuppression was observed (Flaminio *et al.*, 2005). In a study conducted in EFL mares in central Kentucky equine farms, it was observed that one farm had fewer fetal losses, suggesting that management or environmental factors may have an effect. The study also ruled out the association of any specific sire used for mating in the stud farm (Morehead *et al.*, 2002).

In a study conducted to compare the effect of different doses of ETCs administered to late-term mares, the statistical analysis suggested that ETC-induced abortions are characterized by a dose-dependent lag time, followed by initiation of the abortions, which occur at a rate that is also dose dependent. Using this analysis, the estimated rates of ETC exposure occurring during the MRLS 2001 in central Kentucky could be calculated. Based on this study, it was estimated that during MRLS 2001 mares had an initial exposure to about 5 g ETCs/day, increasing to about 30 g/day at the peak of the outbreak (Sebastian *et al.*, 2003b).

Similar abortion storms had been recorded from Kentucky during the spring of 1981 and 1982, and there was anecdotal evidence of an ETC population explosion during the same period in central Kentucky. No experimental or detailed epidemiological studies were conducted to confirm the role of ETC in that episode

There were several unique features of MRLS, which included the absence of significant clinical signs and abnormalities in clinical chemistry panels, or complete blood counts, specific location of lesion in fetoplacental units, pathological lesions confined to pericardium, eye and bacteriological findings. Hence the specific pathogenesis of this syndrome cannot be defined. The histopathological studies conducted on LFL fetuses and placentas are indicative of the absence of the classic routes of entry of pathogenic organisms into the fetal membranes, via the cervix, or hematogenously. In LFL placentas the inflammatory infiltrates observed in the allantochorion were generally confined to the coelomic space in the subchorionic stroma and very closely associated with blood vessels suggesting a primary vascular involvement. The distribution of inflammatory cells was similar in experimental cases, suggesting a similarity in the pathogenesis. In the LFL fetuses submitted to the Livestock Disease Diagnostic Center no single pathological finding was identified as being specific for MRLS, although a characteristic finding was funisitis. Funisitis, inflammation of the umbilical cord, has not previously been reported in the veterinary literature as a primary lesion, although inflammatory cell infiltrates of the umbilical cord have been reported. The intact cervical star area and minimal inflammation on the chorionic surface of the allantochorion suggests that pathogenic organisms especially bacteria may not be the primary etiological agent. *Actinobacillus* spp. and *Streptococcus* spp. were the two bacterial species isolated from the fetoplacental units in the majority of LFL cases. Recently it was reported that MRLS-like *Streptococcus* spp. were found in the alimentary tract of mares with a greater concentration in the upper part of the tract, the tongue, tonsillar area and esophagus. Comparison of isolates from different mares demonstrates dissimilarities suggesting that the source of fetal and placental infection in each mare is derived from its own bacterial population and that this bacterium may not be the primary etiological agent. The pathogenesis of FP and UU is unknown.

TREATMENT AND PREVENTION

Several therapeutic strategies were attempted but none of them was found to have any significant effect. Mares which aborted by MRLS were lavaged (uterine) and treated with antibiotics based on culture and sensitivity and in the subsequent heat most of the mares had normal uterine cytological findings. Sulfonamide–trimethoprim combinations and other broad spectrum antibiotics were administered to combat the bacterial infections. Foals born with MRLS were treated by supportive care with fluids, resuscitation and antibiotics, but the majority of these foals did not survive. The FP was treated with antibiotics (Ceftiofur sodium, Ampicillin) after drainage of pericardial fluid. Unilateral uveitis cases were treated with systemic and topical antibiotics, non-steroidal anti-inflammatory drugs (NSAID and corticosteroid), atropine, tissue plasminogen activator, mycotoxin binders and cyclosporine. Other medications administered include Domperidone to treat possible ergotoxin involvement, mycotoxin binders to eliminate possible mycotoxins in feed, non-steroidal anti-inflammatory drugs such as Flunixin meglumine to reduce inflammatory responses and Pentoxifylline to improve the blood supply to the fetus, all with no obvious therapeutic effect. Prevention of ETCs included cutting down cherry trees, spraying of ETC nests with insecticides and muzzling of mares when out in pasture. These preventive measures reduced the incidence of MRLS in subsequent years, in farms which adopted the ETC control measures (Riddle and LeBlanc, 2003).

CONCLUDING REMARKS AND FUTURE DIRECTIONS

MRLS was a unique disease syndrome characterized by early-term and late-term abortions in equines during a specific period of time with few cases of FP and UU during the same period. Extensive microbiological and toxicological evaluation of affected mares, aborted fetuses and their placenta did not yield any specific causative agent(s). Multiple risk factors were identified by epidemiological studies and the presence of ETCs in pasture was one of the risk factors. Experimental studies using ETCs by exposure in the field or gastric gavage induced abortion in early-term and late-term pregnant mares. The experimental studies conducted with gypsy moth and laboratory raised forest tent caterpillars, both species having hairs (setae), did not induce abortions in pregnant mares. Experimental studies also suggest that irradiation partially reduced the abortifacient potential of ETCs and abortion is not caused by the direct effect of virus or bacteria in ETCs. In the studies using irradiated ETCs, the bacteria isolated from the aborted fetuses and their fetal membranes did not originate from the ETCs. Results of that experiment strongly suggest that an ETC resident virus is not the cause of MRLS and the abortifacient appears to be a factor other than bacteria and virus in the ETCs. The placentitis observed in field and experimental MRLS cases appears to be different from typical ascending placentitis associated with bacteria and hence bacteria observed in the fetoplacental units of aborted fetuses may be secondary invaders. The observations of experiments with irradiated ETCs suggest that MRLS may be caused by an unidentified toxin present in ETCs which leads to the separation of placenta from the uterus leading to hypoxia with secondary invasion of bacteria found in the oral and gastrointestinal tract of the mare. The statistical analysis of the results of experiments defining the correlation between abortion time and dose supports the hypothesis that MRLS is caused by an unknown toxin (Sebastian *et al.*, 2003b). The specific pathogenesis of MRLS is still unknown. Elimination of ETCs in horse pastures and avoiding direct exposure to ETCc appear to prevent MRLS. A similar abortion storm in equine species was recently reported from Australia and processionary caterpillars were identified in numerous pastures used by the aborted mares. A pilot study conducted with the gastric administration of exoskeleton of these caterpillars resulted in abortion of two mares out of six.

REFERENCES

Bernard WV, LeBlanc MM, Webb BA, *et al.* (2004) Evaluation of early fetal loss induced by gavage with eastern tent caterpillars in pregnant mares *J Am Vet Med Assoc* **225:** 717–21.

Bolin DC, Donahue M, Vickers ML, *et al.* (2004) Microbiologic and pathologic findings in an epidemic of equine pericarditis. *J Vet Diagn Invest* **17:** 38–44.

Byars TD, Seahorn TL (2002) Clinical observations of mare reproductive loss syndrome in critical care mares and foals. *Proceedings First Workshop on Mare Reproductive Loss Syndrome*, University of Kentucky, Lexington, KY, USA, pp. 15–6.

Cawdell-Smith AJ, Todhunter KH, Perkins NR, Bryden WL (2009) Stage of pregnancy and foetal loss following exposure of mares to processionary caterpillars. *J Equine Vet Sci* **29(5):** 339–40.

Cohen ND, Carey VJ, Donahue JG *et al.*, (2003a). Case–control study of late-term abortions associated with mare reproductive loss syndrome in central Kentucky. *J. Am. Vet. Med. Assoc.* **222**, 199–209.

Cohen ND, Carey VJ, Donahue JG, *et al.* (2003c) Descriptive epidemiology of late-term abortions associated with the mare reproductive syndrome loss in central Kentucky. *J Vet Diagn Invest* **15:** 295–7.

Cohen ND, Donahue JG, Carey VJ, *et al.* (2003b) Case–control study of early-term abortions (early fetal losses) associated with mare reproductive loss syndrome in central Kentucky. *J Am Vet Med Assoc* **222:** 210–17.

Donahue JM, Sells S, Giles RC, *et al.* (2002) Bacteria associated with mare reproductive loss syndrome. *Proceedings First Workshop on Mare Reproductive Loss Syndrome*, University of Kentucky, Lexington, KY, USA, pp. 27–9.

Dwyer RM, Lindsey PG, Traub-Dargatz JL, *et al.* (2003) Case–control study of factors associated with excessive proportions of early fetal losses associated with mare reproductive loss syndrome in central Kentucky during 2001. *J Am Vet Med Assoc* **222:** 613–19.

Fitzgerald TD (2002) The biology of tent caterpillars as it relates to mare reproductive loss syndrome. *Proceedings First Workshop on Mare Reproductive Loss Syndrome*, University of Kentucky, Lexington, KY, USA, pp. 84–7.

Flaminio JF, Nydam DV, Sebastian MM, *et al.* (2005) The Mare Reproductive Loss Syndrome (MRLS) and the Eastern Tent Caterpillar: immunological testing of aborting mares. *Intl J Appl Res Vet Med* **3:** 207–16.

Gupta RC (2007) *Veterinary Toxicology: Basic and Clinical Principles*. Elsevier, New York.

Harkins JD, Dirikolu L, Sebastian M, *et al.* (2002) Cherry trees, plant cyanogens, caterpillars, and the Mare Reproductive Loss Syndrome (MRLS): toxicological evaluation of a working hypothesis. *Proceedings First Workshop on Mare Reproductive Loss Syndrome*, University of Kentucky, Lexington, KY, USA, pp. 68–74.

Harrison LR (2001) Kentucky abortion storm and related conditions (2001). *Proceedings US Animal Health Association* **105:** 227–9.

Kane E, Kilby E (2001) Death in the bluegrass: an epidemic of lost pregnancies, dead foals and sick horses strikes central Kentucky and beyond, challenging researchers and veterinarians to identify the cause and staunch the unprecedented loss of equine lives. *Equus* **287:** 60–8.

Latimer C (2002) Endophthalmitis syndrome: spring 2001, 2002. *Proceedings First Workshop on Mare Reproductive Loss Syndrome*, University of Kentucky, Lexington, KY, USA, pp. 26–8.

Morehead JP, Blanchard TL, Thompson JA, Brinsko SP (2002) Evaluation of early fetal losses on four equine farms in central Kentucky: 73 cases (2001). *J Am Vet Med Assoc* **220:** 1828–30.

Paulick R (2001) MRLS Kentucky economic impact: $336 million. *The Horse* **18(12):** 15.

Perkins NR, Sebastian M, Todhunter KH, Wylie RM, Begg AP, Gilkerson JR, Racklyeft DJ, Chicken C, Wilson MC, Cawdell-Smith AJ, Bryden WL (2007) Chapter 26: Pregnancy loss in mares associated with exposure to caterpillars in Kentucky and Australia. In *Poisonous Plants: Global Research and Solutions* (Panter KE, Wierenga TL, Pfister JA, eds.). CABI Publishing, Wallingford, Oxford, UK, pp. 165–9.

Powell DG (2001) Mare reproductive loss syndrome (MRLS). *Equine Dis Q* **9(4):** 5–7.

Riddle WT, LeBlanc MM (2003) Update on mare reproductive loss syndrome. *Proceedings Society for Theriogenology and Symposium*, Columbus, OH, USA, pp. 85–99.

Seahorn JL, Slovis N, Reimer J (2003) Case–control study of factors associated with fibrinous pericarditis among horses in central Kentucky during spring 2001. *J Am Vet Med Assoc* **223:** 832–8.

Sebastian M, Bernard W, Harrison L, *et al.* (2003a) Experimental induction of mare reproductive loss syndrome with irradiated eastern tent caterpillar to assess whether the primary pathogen in mare reproductive loss syndrome is a toxic molecule or a microorganism. *Proceedings Workshop on the Equine Placenta*, University of Kentucky, Lexington, KY, USA, pp. 27–8.

Sebastian M, Bernard W, Riddle T, Latimer C, Fitzgerald TD, Harrison LR (2008b) Mare Reproductive Loss Syndrome – a review. *Vet Pathol* **45:** 710–22.

Sebastian M, Gantz MG, Tobin T, *et al.* (2003b) The mare reproductive syndrome and the eastern tent caterpillars: a toxicokinetic/statistical analysis with clinical, epidemiologic, and mechanistic implications. *Vet Therap* **4:** 324–39.

Sebastian M, Giles R, Donahue J, *et al.* (2002a) Encephalitis due to *Actinobacillus* species in three adult horses. *Vet Pathol* **39:** 630.

Sebastian M, Harkins JD, Jackson C, *et al.* (2002c) Preliminary evaluation of a mouse model of MRLS. *Proceedings First Workshop on Mare Reproductive Loss Syndrome*, University of Kentucky, Lexington, KY, USA, pp. 51–3.

Sebastian M, Pence ME, Hines II ME, Watson C (2008a) Mare Reproductive Loss Syndrome: eastern tent caterpillars do not induce abortion in goats. American College of Veterinary Pathologist, 58th meeting, Savannah, November 5–9. *Vet Pathol* **44(5):** 750.

Sebastian M, Williams D, Harrison L, *et al.* (2002b) Clinical and pathological features of experimentally induced MRLS late-term abortion with eastern tent caterpillar. *Proceedings First Workshop on Mare Reproductive Loss Syndrome*, University of Kentucky, Lexington, KY, USA, pp. 80–1.

Webb BA, Barney WE, Dahlman DL, *et al.* (2003) Eastern tent caterpillars (*Malacosoma americanum*) cause mare reproductive loss syndrome. *J Inst Physiol* **50:** 185–93.

Williams NM, Bolin DC, Donahue JM, *et al.* (2002) Gross and histopathological correlates of MRLS. *Proceedings First Workshop on Mare Reproductive Loss Syndrome*, University of Kentucky, Lexington, KY, USA, p. 29.

CHAPTER

86

Reproductive and developmental toxicity in fishes

Helmut Segner

INTRODUCTION

Ecotoxicology deals with the fate and effects of contaminants in the biosphere (Newman, 1998). Contrary to human toxicology, which is concerned with effects of chemicals on the individual organism, ecotoxicology is concerned with toxic effects on ecological entities, i.e. populations, communities or ecosystems. In practice, however, ecotoxicology builds on conventional toxicological endpoints which are determined in selected sentinel species or in species representing trophic levels in a food chain, and infers from these individual-level effects to processes at higher levels of biological organization. This approach inherently suffers from uncertainty and ignorance (Calow and Forbes, 2003; Segner, 2007).

Changes of developmental and reproductive parameters can be major drivers of alterations in population growth (Gleason and Nacci, 2001; Newman, 2001; Grist *et al.*, 2003; Gurney, 2006). Therefore, toxicant effects on development and reproduction are of particular relevance when assessing the risk of environmental pollution to ecological structures and functions. This chapter will discuss recent progress and current knowledge on the developmental and reproductive toxicity of fishes as they are a key group in aquatic ecosystems. The field has taken an impressive development over the last years, which has been stimulated at least in part by the emergence of the endocrine disruption issue. There is compelling evidence that hormonally active substances have adverse impacts on wild fish populations (Sumpter and Johnson, 2006), and since endocrine-disrupting chemicals (EDCs) affect particularly developmental and reproductive properties, this has necessitated, on the one hand, a better understanding of the involved mechanisms and, on the other hand, the development of appropriate testing methodologies and assessment strategies. A further momentum to the recent progress of developmental and reproductive toxicity of fishes comes from the increasing use of small laboratory fish species as models in biomedical, toxicological and pharmacological research – a development ecotoxicology is clearly taking advantage of this approach.

REPRODUCTIVE AND DEVELOPMENTAL PHYSIOLOGY OF TELEOST FISH

The hypothalamus–pituitary–gonad (HPG) axis

The physiological regulation of reproduction of adult fish is mediated through the hypothalamus–pituitary (hypophysis)–gonad (HPG) axis (Figure 86.1). This axis integrates information from external (e.g., social stimuli from potential mating partners) and environmental (e.g., water temperature) cues with internal signals (e.g., nutritional status of the animal) to promote or suppress gonad maturation, spermatogenesis/oogenesis, reproductive behavior and spawning. Basic features of the reproductive endocrine system are similar among teleost fish – despite their wide spectrum of reproductive strategies and tactics of breeding – and they are similar between teleost fish and tetrapods. However, there also exist significant differences (McNabb *et al.*, 1999; Rocha and Rocha, 2006; Zohar *et al.*, 2010). The hypothalamus integrates the incoming external and internal signals into the synthesis of neurotransmitters and neurohormones which then orchestrate the pituitary activity. The pituitary consists of a glandular part, the adenohypophysis, and a neurosecretory part, the neurohypophysis. In contrast to tetrapods, teleosts lack a portal system connecting the hypothalamus and hypophysis, instead the neurons containing the neurohormones have long axons that extend into the pituitary and release their contents in close proximity to their hypophyseal target cells.

The hypothalamus synthesizes gonadotropin-releasing hormone (GnRH), the primary neurohormone that controls reproduction. Vertebrates typically have two forms of GnRH, whereas in most teleost orders there occur species which express three forms of GnRH (Zohar *et al.*, 2010). Each of the three forms display specific neuroanatomical distribution patterns in the brain and their expression is regulated by complex interactions of multiple neurotransmitters and environmental cues (Zohar *et al.*, 2010). For instance, Okuzawa *et al.* (2003) demonstrated seasonal variation of the

Reproductive and Developmental Toxicology, Edited by Ramesh C. Gupta
ISBN: 978-0-12-382032-7

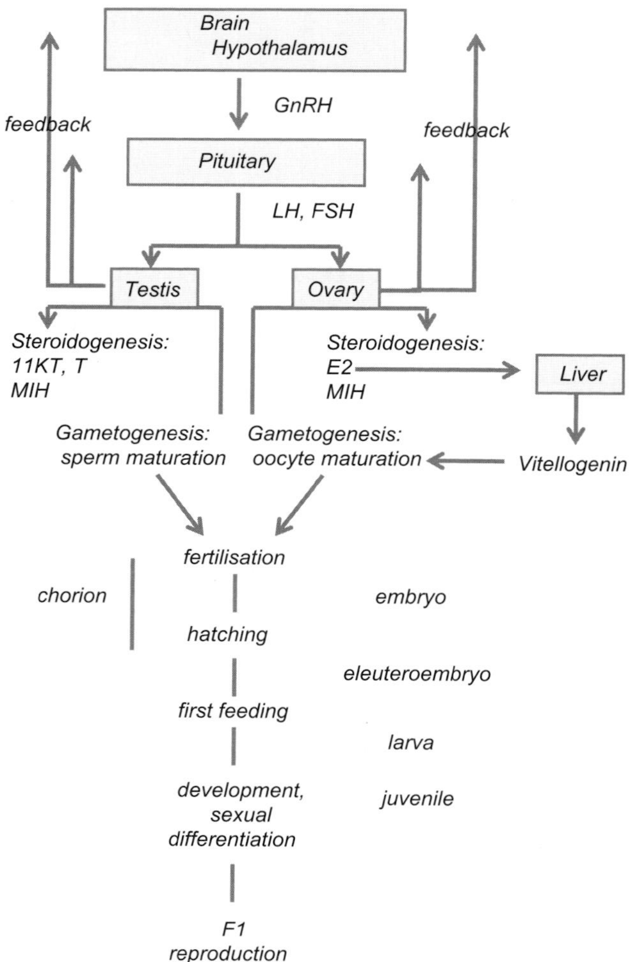

FIGURE 86.1 Schematic graphical presentation of the reproductive axis and development in teleost fish. Abbreviations: E2 = 17β-estradiol, FSH = follicle stimulating hormone, LH = luteinizing hormone, MIH = matruation inducing hormone, T = testosterone, 11KT = 11-ketotestosterone.

expression of the three GnRH forms in the hypothalamus of red seabream, *Pagrus major*. The physiological actions of the GnRHs are pleiotropic and involve several classes of receptors (Kah *et al.*, 2007; Okubo and Nagahama, 2008).

The hypothalamic GnRHs are centrally involved in the control of gonadotropin (GTH) secretion in the anterior part of the pituitary. This has been functionally established in all orders of teleosts (Yaron *et al.*, 2003; Zohar *et al.*, 2010). Gonadotropin production is stimulated via Ca^{2+}/PKC signaling pathways which are activated upon binding of GnRHs to the GnRH receptors in the pituitary (Khan and Thomas, 1999). Fish produces two forms of GTH, GTH-I and GTH-II, which correspond to the mammalian follicle-stimulating hormone (FSH) and luteinizing hormone (LH), respectively. The hypophyseal gonadotropins act on the steroid synthesis of gonads, but at the same time the gonadotropins as well as the GnRHs and GnRH receptors are under feedback control by the gonad-secreted sex steroids. GnRH receptor expression varies with sex and reproductive stage, and attains a maximum at the time the gonads are fully grown (Clelland and Peng, 2009). Sexual steroids inform the brain/pituitary complex on the sexual status of the organism, and modulate expression of reproduction-related neuropeptides and neurotransmitters in the brain and pituitary (Zohar *et al.*, 2010). In principal, the feedback effects of sex steroids on GnRH and gonadotropin secretion result from hormone binding to the respective receptors in brain and pituitary, but the detailed mechanisms of how sex steroids influence the brain neurohormone status of fish are not understood yet. Interestingly, the GnRH-producing neurons do not possess estrogen receptors (ERs) (Navas *et al.*, 1995) so that a direct negative feedback of estrogen on brain GnRH production appears to be not likely, but the feedback appears to be mediated though other, indirect processes. For androgens, aromatization to estrogens may be needed to exert their effects on gonadotropin secretion. The teleostean brain is characterized by a remarkably high capacity to convert androgens into estrogens (Callard *et al.*, 1990). This conversion is mediated by a specific brain aromatase gene, *cyp19a1b*, which is different to the aromatase gene expressed in the gonads, *cyp19a1a* (Cheshenko *et al.*, 2008). Interestingly, the teleostean brain aromatase possesses an estrogen-responsive element (ERE) in the promoter region – in contrast to *cyp19a1a* – and indeed can be upregulated by experimental estrogen treatment (cf. Cheshenko *et al.*, 2008). Brain aromatase is found exclusively in radial glial cells – which are progenitors of neurons – but is not found in neurons as is the case in mammals (Menuet *et al.*, 2003; Pellegrini *et al.*, 2007).

Gonadotropin release from the pituitary is regulated, in addition to GnRH and sex steroids, by a variety of signal molecules including neuropeptide Y (NPY), dopamine, gamma-aminobutyric acid (GABA), gonadotropin-inhibitory hormone as well as peptides of the KiSS system (van der Kraak *et al.*, 1997; Zohar *et al.*, 2010). Furthermore, there exists evidence for interactions with other endocrine systems such as the glucocorticoid/stress system, the growth hormone (GH)/insulin-like growth factor (IGF) system, the leptin system or the melatonin system. An example is the expression of glucocorticoid receptors in GnRH neurons (Teitsma *et al.*, 1999). Interactions may be also more indirect, as discussed, e.g., for melatonin, which has been shown to modulate GTH release despite the lack or low expression of melatonin receptors in the pituitary (Khan and Thomas, 1996). While the feedback of gonad steroids to the brain–pituitary complex ensures a coordinated regulation within the reproductive axis, the interference with the other endocrine systems ensures an integration of the reproductive activity into the overall physiological status of the organisms, e.g. nutritional and energetic status, or with environmental cues such as photoperiod.

Gonad maturation and gametogenesis

The gonadotropins released from the pituitary function in regulating gonad development and maturation. They primarily influence sex steroid hormone synthesis and gametogenesis. In the testis, spermatogenesis starts with a self-renewing stem cell population, the primordial or primary spermatogonia, which are held within cysts formed by Sertoli cells (Schulz *et al.*, 2000; Fishelson, 2003; Rocha and Rocha, 2006). The spermatogonia develop through a species-specific number of mitotic cell cycles (for instance, 14 in the guppy, 10 in the Japanese eel) into pimary spermatocytes, which undergo a first meiotic division to generate the secondary spermatocytes. These cells complete the secondary meiotic division and form the spermatids. In a cellular restructuring process known as spermiogenesis, the haploid spermatids differentiate into flagellated spermatozoa. The mature sperm cells enter the lumen of the seminiferous tubules, then the efferent ducts where they are mixed with secretion fluid and finally they are released via the urogenital papilla. Sperm cell development is tightly regulated by endocrine and paracrine factors. The pituitary gonadotropins regulate mainly the testicular Leydig and Sertoli cells, thereby paving the way for germ cell differentiation. While GTH-II/LH targets mainly the steroidogenic Leydig cells, GTH-I/FSH targets the Sertoli cells. Androgens originating from the Leydig cells (being themselves under LH regulation) stimulate spermatogenesis, with their effect apparently being mediated through the Sertoli cells. Growth factors such as IGF-I have been shown to stimulate sperm cell proliferation and maturation, a process that is under the control of growth hormone (GH) (LeGac *et al.*, 1996). Also, LH-triggered increase of maturation inducing hormone (MIH; see below) is an important factor for sperm maturation, as well as the production of seminal plasma for the milt (Rocha and Rocha, 2006).

In females, oogenesis starts with oogonia that multiply by mitosis to form oogonial nests (Selman *et al.*, 1993; Lubzens *et al.*, 2010). The transition from oogonia into primary oocytes is characterized by the initiation of meiosis. The meiotic division is then arrested at the end of the prophase in the diplotene stage. The next steps in oocyte development – often designated as (internal and external) vitellogenesis (Mommsen and Korsgard, 2008) – are characterized by a pronounced growth in size. Initially, this growth is due to formation of cortical alveolar vesicles. In parallel, a differentiated follicular layer consisting of theca and granulosa cells starts to surround the oocyte. The cortical alveoli contain oocyte-produced glycoproteins which are released to the egg surface as part of the "cortical reaction" at fertilization, thereby triggering the restructuring of egg envelope proteins in order to form the chorion. The oocyte growth phase following the cortical alveolar stage is dominated by the incorporation of exogenous nutritional materials, mainly liver-derived vitellogenin to produce the yolk reserves needed for the development of the embryo. Finally, oocyte maturation takes place, a phase that is characterized by reduced yolk accumulation, resumption of meiosis, migration of the nucleus to the oocyte periphery, germinal vesicle breakdown and hydration. At the end of the maturation process, ovulation takes place and follicular cells degenerate. The hormonal mechanisms controlling oogonia proliferation and oocyte recruitment in teleosts are incompletely understood; however, pituitary gonadotropins are primary regulators, either directly or indirectly (e.g., via paracrine growth factors) of oocyte vitellogenesis and maturation (Clelland and Peng; 2009; Lubzens *et al.*, 2010). Comparable to male fish, sex steroids and growth factors appear to be involved in gametogenesis also in female fish (Ge, 2005; Berishvili *et al.*, 2006; Lubzens *et al.*, 2010). GTH-I/FSH binds to receptors in the membrane of theca cells and thereby stimulates steroidogenesis. The female sex steroids are produced in the follicular epithelial cells, with the theca cells supplying androgens to the granulosa cells. These cells express the ovarian isoform of aromatase, *cyp19a1a*, which catalyzes the conversion of the androgens into estrogens (two-cell hypothesis; Clelland and Peng, 2009). Importantly, gonadotropin receptor expression and activity of steroidogenic enzymes vary with developmental stage of the oocyte, for instance in zebrafish the FSH expression and activity are low in primary oocytes, increase in cortical alveolar oocytes, reach their maximum in vitellogenic oocytes and decline again during maturation (Kwok *et al.*, 2005). High estrogenic activity during the vitellogenic stage is important as the circulating E2 induces synthesis of vitellogenin protein in the liver, which travels via the bloodstream to the ovary and is incorporated by receptor-mediated pinocytosis into the developing oocyte (Tyler and Sumpter, 1996). Another important group of proteins synthesized in the liver under the influence of estrogens are the egg envelope or zona radiata proteins (Lubzens *et al.*, 2010). Towards the end of the reproductive cycle, a surge of circulating GTH-II/LH takes place and this plays a prominent role in final oocyte maturation. LH stimulates a shift in follicular production from E2 to maturation-inducing hormone (MIH), and this increase of MIH then activates via membrane progestin receptors the synthesis of maturation promotion factor (MPF), which finally releases the follicles from the prophase I arrest (Clelland and Peng, 2009). The MIH of teleosts is either 17,20β-dihydroxy-4-pregnen-3-one (17,20β) (salmonids, cyprinids, etc.) or 17,20β-21-trihydroxy-4-pregnen-3-one (many perciforms and flatfishes) (Clelland and Peng, 2009). The ability of follicle cells to synthesize MIH must be paralleled by the ability of the oocytes to respond to MIH ("maturational competence"), and indeed they express an increasing number of MIH receptors on their surface (Lubzens *et al.*, 2010). The LH/MIH/MPF-triggered oocyte maturation can be modulated by a variety of additional factors, for instance a prominent role of activin has been demonstrated in zebrafish (Ge, 2005). Finally, the mature egg is ovulated from the ovarian follicle into the ovarian cavity or into the abdominal cavity (e.g., salmonids). The ovulation process is stimulated by prostaglandins, and in some species also by MIH, with both of them acting as pheromones to influence reproductive behavior and synchronization of spawning.

A common event in fish ovaries is follicular atresia (Lubzens *et al.*, 2010): atretic follicles undergo prominent morphological changes such as disintegration of oocyte nucleus and hypertrophy of follicle cells. Phagocytic immune cells invade the sites with atretic follicles to remove the degenerating cells. Atresia may represent an apoptotic process, but this remains to be verified. The factors initiating oocyte atresia in teleosts are poorly known; however, it needs to be emphasized that follicular atresia is not only occurring under conditions of adverse stress, but also under physiological conditions, for instance to regulate oocyte recruitment in species spawning in several batches over the year (McNabb *et al.*, 1999).

The description of egg and sperm formation and the involved hormonal processes as given above are generalizations, with numerous variations existing among species. Overall, the picture that is emerging from the studies on hormonal regulation of testicular and ovarian development and maturation is that pituitary gonadotropins and sex steroids are indeed key regulatory factors; however, there exists a complex cross-talk between various hormonal factors and systems ensuring integration of reproduction with other physiological process in the animal, e.g. growth and energy status, and with environmental cues, e.g. photoperiod.

Despite using the same molecular, cellular and physiological elements for regulating reproduction, reproductive strategies of teleost fish are highly diverse, representing the diverse evolutionary adaptations to their ecological conditions. For instance, while the majority of teleosts are oviparous, some species such as the guppy show viviparity, with embryos developing within the female reproductive system (Jalabert, 2005). Variation occurs also in the frequency of spawning – it may be once in the life span (semelpar), as it is the case for Atlantic salmon (semelpar), or several times during the life span (iteropar), e.g. like zebrafish. Pronounced species differences exist also with respect to ovarian development, which can show synchronous development (all oocytes develop synchronously), group synchronous (at least two groups of oocytes – vitellogenic and maturing – coexist in the ovary) or asynchronous (oocytes of all stages are present, without a dominant stage; e.g. zebrafish) (Rocha and Rocha, 2006). Accordingly, spawning patterns can vary, with synchronous spawners releasing all eggs in one batch at one time, or fractional spawners releasing batches of eggs over extended time periods.

Fertilization and egg/sperm quality

The egg is bounded by a series of membranes, with an outer, relatively tough one (chorion), and the vitelline membrane around the yolk. It must contain all the nutrients required by the developing embryo from fertilization until start of exogenous feeding. The egg yolk has to support both fueling of embryonic development as well as building up of the tissues. The yolk material has been deposited in the growing oocyte by the mother, with liver-derived vitellogenin being the major precursor (Hiramatsu *et al.*, 2005). The ovulated eggs contain water (between 60 and 90%, depending on whether the eggs are buoyant or demersal), proteins and amino acids, lipids and lipoproteins, micronutrients such as vitamins, as well as hormones such as estradiol or thyroid hormones. Deficiencies in egg composition can have adverse effects on development, as it is exemplified by the M74 syndrome. This syndrome, which leads to high mortalities among early life stages of Baltic salmon, is associated with low thiamine levels in salmon eggs and yolk sac fry (Börjeson and Norrgren, 1997).

Mature sperm cells, in order to be able to fertilize the eggs, have to acquire motility. In salmonids, the spermataozoa in the lumen of the seminiferous tubulus are not yet mobile. They acquire the potential for motility only during migration down the sperm ducts, and this is caused by an increase of semen pH (Morisawa, 1994). Sperm motility is then actually realized upon release into the aquatic environment, and the trigger for this are extracellular ionic and osmotic changes (Morisawa, 1994). To sustain flagellar movement, the spermatozoa face a huge energy demand. In species with external fertilization, this is usually provided from endogenous substrates, while species with internal fertilization appear to utilize also exogenous substrates (Ingermann, 2008). Survival time of the sperm cells in the water is generally very short and rarely exceeds 2 minutes (Kime, 1998). In contrast to mammals, fish sperm fertilizes the egg not by penetrating the oocyte wall but fertilization takes place through a funnel-like micropyle located at the animal pole of the egg. After the egg is activated by the sperm, the micropyle closes thereby preventing polyspermy. Furthermore, the egg envelope or chorion undergoes hardening and separates from the vitelline membrane leading to the formation of the perivitelline space. This includes also protection against pathogens, as the egg shell contains anti-microbial factors (Modig *et al.*, 2007).

The vast majority of teleost species have external fertilization; however, a few species such as guppy, *Poecilia reticulata*, have internal fertilization. In most species with internal fertilization, the fertilized eggs are retained and undergo development in the maternal body. Hatching either precedes or coincides with parturition, i.e. the females give birth to free-living young fish.

Egg and sperm quality may be defined as the ability to fertilize or to be fertilized, respectively. The quality is determined by the intrinsic properties of the gametes themselves as they have been provided by the parents. Numerous factors such as broodstock nutrition or stress can influence egg and sperm quality (Bobe and Labbé, 2010). The question what makes a good egg or sperm quality and how this can be assessed has been debated for a long time but has yet to be answered. Egg size, weight and morphology can provide estimates on the developmental potential of eggs, but the parameters show huge variation and the relation with egg quality is not simple and straightforward (Kjorsvik *et al.*, 1990). In fractional spawners, the quality of eggs produced in different batches over a spawning season may vary considerably, even if the husbandry conditions are apparently equivalent over the whole period (Kjesbu *et al.*, 1996). Much attention has been given on the role of maternal nutrition on egg quality; however, the evidence that diet can directly affect egg quality is limited. On the sperm side, motility, together with morphology, appear to be useful parameters, but it still can be difficult to correlate sperm quality parameters to the fertilization rate obtained with the same sperm (Bobe and Labbé, 2010). One of the more meaningful quality parameters which reflect both egg and sperm is fertilization success. There have been also numerous attempts to use molecular and biochemical parameters to estimate egg and sperm quality. For instance, high expression of apoptosis-related markers, or high cathepsin enzymatic activities, may be indicative of eggs with low viability (e.g., Carnevali, 2007). Also maternal mRNA transcripts have been evaluated for their utility as egg/sperm quality indicators (Aegerter *et al.*, 2005). Transcriptomic and proteomic profiling of eggs and sperm may be able to identify sets of quality-indicating genes or protein sets; however, the analysis gets complicated due to the rapid temporal changes of gene and protein expression in developing embryos (Ziv *et al.*, 2008).

Post-fertilizational development

Key steps in the early life development of fish are cleavage and embryogenesis, hatching, first feeding and metamorphosis. Cleavage and embryonic pattern formation have been intensively studied in fish (see a recent review by Hall, 2008) as in many species these processes can be observed directly under the microscope. Cleavage follows a discoideal meroblastic pattern, where the large yolk volume restricts cell division to a small area at the animal pole. Immediately after fertilization, egg cytoplasm and yolk begin to separate, forming a single blastomer at the animal pole, and from there the first vertical and then horizontal divisions start. Organogenesis occurs during the embryonic stage and continues in the larval stage. Hormones and growth factors, initially of maternal origin and later of embryonic origin, play key roles in control of tissue differentiation and growth. Critical processes in the ontogenetic differentiation of structures and function may occur during specific periods or "windows" of development, and disturbances of these critical processes can lead to persisting structural and functionl changes (McLachlan, 2001).

The freshly fertilized egg is composed predominantly of maternal components. They play a pivotal role in early embryo development until activation of zygotic transcription (Bobe and Labbé, 2010). For instance, the spatial distribution of specific maternal mRNA within the oocyte is important to specify the dorso-ventral axis of the embryo (Howley and Ho, 2000). It is only after activation of zygotic gene expression that the embryo no longer solely relies on maternally provided transcripts. Activation of zygotic transcription occurs during the "mid blastula transition" stage, which, for instance, in zebrafish occurs at cycle 10 (Kane and Kimmel, 1993).

Hatching is the developmental period during which the fish is very sensitive to environmental stressors, probably because of leaving the relatively protected environment of the egg (Rosenthal and Alderdice, 1976). It requires the breakdown of the chorion layers, and this is achieved by specific hatching enzymes secreted by the embryo (Jobling, 1995). The degree of differentiation of the larvae at hatch varies with species: for instance, in many marine species the larvae hatch after only a few days of embryonic development at very small size, with a number of organs such as stomach, jaws, etc. not fully developed yet, whereas salmonids hatch at a rather advanced stage of differentiation (Jobling, 1995). Hatching does not imply that the young fish immediately starts with external feeding, but for a certain period they still rely on the endogenous yolk reserves. This period is designated as the "eleutheroembryo" or "free embryo" period (Belanger *et al.* 2010) and its length depends on how long the yolk reserves can still nourish the developing organism. The transition to exogenous feeding is again a critical period, often accompanied by high mortalities, as many larvae may fail to take external food, or, in the natural environment, they may be unable to find sufficient food and therefore die by starvation (Jobling, 1995). The final transition from larval stages to the adult form takes place during metamorphosis. In a number of teleost species such as flatfishes, this period involves pronounced structural and functional changes in a number of organs, while in other species it is more gradual and not clearly evident (Segner *et al.* 1993, 1994).

The nomenclature of fish early life stages is confusing, which may be related to the fact that fish show rather diverse developmental trajectories or life history strategies through which adulthood can be achieved. Depending on timing and pattern of differentiation, often "altricial" and "precocial" modes of development are distinguished (Belanger *et al.*, 2010): precocial species develop directly from the embryo stage by gradual transition into the juvenile stage – an example are the salmonids – while altricial species possess a distinct larval stage before they develop into the juvenile stage – an example are flatfishes. The separation line between embryo and larval/juvenile periods is the mode of feeding: embryos rely on endogenous feeding, while larvae and juveniles rely on exogenous feeding. Therefore, the terms "eleutheroembryo" or "free embryo" should be preferred over terms such as "yolk-sac larvae". The juvenile period lasts until sexual maturation of the fish, i.e. the onset of the adult stage. While the terminology as described above is rather straightforward, there are numerous other terms in use, and this may be related, e.g., to specific life history traits – for instance, the life stage of salmon undergoing seaward migration is called "smolt" – or to ecological age classes, e.g. the term "young-of-the-year".

Developmental rates are determined by intrinsic factors, but also by environmental factors. For instance, for fish as poikilotherms, temperature has a key influence on developmental rates. Generally, the rates increase with increasing water temperature, at least up to an optimum temperature. In order to make results from studies with different temperature regimes comparable, the concept of "day-degrees" has been developed (Jobling, 1995). This concept assumes that the product of incubation temperature (°C) and the time (days) required to reach any particular stage of development is constant. For instance, hatching would occur at the same time if a fish embryo is incubated either for 10 days at 10°C or for 20 days at 5°C.

Sexual development

The gonads develop from primordial germ cells (PGCs) and somatic cells. The mechanisms controlling PGC specification in fish are not fully understood to date, but recent evidence indicates that it is dependent on the asymmetrical distribution of maternally inherited material in the developing embryo (Raz, 2003). The PGCs emerge in extragonadal areas and migrate to the germinal ridges where they coalesce with somatic elements to form the early, still undifferentiated gonads (Patiño and Takashima, 1995; Devlin and Nagahama, 2002). Subsequently, the gonads undergo a period of growth, with proliferation of both somatic and germ cells. This period can last for days, months or even years, depending on the species (Piferrer, 2001; Devlin and Nagahama, 2002) as well as on growth rates (van Aerle *et al.*, 2004; Lawrence *et al.*, 2008).

The sexually undifferentiated gonads may develop directly into either ovaries or testes. This mode of sexual development is called differentiated gonochorism and is widespread among teleosts. Alternatively, the developing gonads may initially go through a phase when the gonads of all individuals, irrespective of their genetic sex, display immature oocytes, and only after this non-functional female stage may they differentiate into functional male or female gonads. This mode of sexual development is called undifferentiated gonochorism or non-functional hermaphroditism; an example is provided by zebrafish (*Danio rerio*) (Takahashi, 1977; Maack and Segner, 2004). A number of teleost species develop as functional hermaphrodites, either synchronously, i.e. one individual contains simultaneously functional male and female gonads, or sequentially (Devlin and Nagahama, 2002). Protandric fish species such as seabream, *Sparus aurata*, develop first as males, while protogynic species such as many coral reef-inhabiting Serranidae develop first as females.

Morphological signs of the onset of ovarian differentiation are entry of germ cells into meiosis and alterations of somatic cell arrangement that eventually lead to formation of the ovarian cavity (Strüssmann and Nakamura, 2002). In males, an early morphological sign of testicular differentiation is appearance of the efferent duct as a slit-like space in the stromal tissue; further indications are intensive germ cell mitosis and formation of germ cell cysts (Strüssmann and Nakamura, 2002). Following phenotypic sexual differentiation of the gonads, the next stages in sexual development are puberty (Okuzawa, 2002), and, finally, the mature, reproductively active stage.

Ontogenetic changes of sex steroid synthesis and the activity of steroidogenic enzymes, in particular of aromatase, are considered to direct the phenotypic differentiation of the early, non-differentiated gonads into either tesis or ovary, and probably they are also involved in the maintenance of the differentiated phenotype (Devlin and Nagahama, 2002; Guiguen *et al.*, 2010). The hypothesis of sex steroids as organizers of gonadal sex differentiation in fish has been put forward by

Yamamoto (1969), who found that sex differentiation of medaka can be shifted by estrogen treatment into the female phenotype, and by androgens into the male phenotype, irrespective of genetic sex determination, differentiation to the female phenotype, and by androgen treatment to the male phenotype. Since then, numerous studies including recent molecular work have corroborated and extended the original hypothesis of Yamamoto (1969). The role of sex steroids as morphogenic factors of gonadal differentiation implicates that sex-specific synthesis of steroid hormones has to start before morphological differentiation of the gonads. In fact, this has been demonstrated for a number of species (van den Hurk *et al.*, 1982; Kobayashi *et al.*, 1998; Govoroun *et al.*, 2001).

The factors triggering onset of gonad sexual differentiation and of sex-specific gonadal steroidogenesis in developing fish are little understood to date. A number of genes that are known to be involved in sex differentiation in mammals have been discussed; however, the available evidence on their functional role is equivocal (Rodriguez-Mari *et al.*, 2005; von Hofsten and Olson; 2005; Orban *et al.*, 2009). Studies with zebrafish and medaka point to a role of the germline in directing sexual differentiation (Slanchev *et al.*, 2005; Kurokwa *et al.*, 2007; Siegfried and Nüsslein-Volhard, 2008). Also the neuroendocrine/hypothamalus–pituitary system is likely to play a role in controlling onset and direction of gonadal steroidogenesis of developing fish, but again available information is fragmentary (Parhar, 1997; Devlin and Nagahama, 2002: Strüssmann and Nakamura, 2002). These deficiencies in knowledge of the regulating processes of sexual development in fish handicap the understanding of disrupting effects of toxicants.

The ontogenetic period when endogenous synthesis of sex steroids increases and gonad development is directed into the female or male direction represents a critical window of sexual differentiation, as during that period the sexually still undifferentiated gonads are susceptible to the organizational effect of steroids, regardless of whether they are of endogenous or of environmental origin (Baroiller and D'Cotta, 2001; Piferrer, 2001). Thus, exposure of developing fish during the critical period to compounds with sex steroid activity, or to compounds that change endogenous sex steroid synthesis, can induce an irreversible change of phenotypic sex, overriding genetic sex determination (Segner *et al.*, 2006).

TOXIC IMPACT ON THE REPRODUCTIVE LIFE STAGES OF FISH

Adverse effects of chemical compounds on reproductive parameters of adult fish

Field and laboratory studies have shown that a wide variety of chemical substances, both inorganic and organic ones, interfere with reproductive performance of adult fish (for reviews see Kime, 1998; Tyler *et al.*, 1998; Fairbrother *et al.*, 1999; Arcand-Hoy and Benson, 2001; Lawrence and Hemingway, 2003; Bernanke and Köhler, 2008, Johnson *et al.*, 2008; Tillitt *et al.*, 2008). The complexity of reproductive physiology in fish, involving the precise physiological coordination of a wide variety of reproductive and endocrine processes by diverse tissues, makes it particularly vulnerable to interference by contaminants and other environmental factors. Reproductive peculiarities that make fish particularly vulnerable to toxic impact are ovipary and external fertilization (Fairbrother *et al.*, 1999). Also vitellogenesis, a process associated with ovipary, has been found to be highly responsive to toxicants. A number of further distinguishing features of fish reproduction exist, for instance the use of 11-ketosterone rather than testosterone as major androgen by many teleostean species, or the presence of multiple isoforms of sex steroid receptors; however, the relevance of these physiological specificities for toxicological processes is not well understood.

Endpoints typically measured to assess reproductive toxicity of chemicals to mature fish include fecundity (number of eggs ovulated per female, possibly corrected for female size), clutch size, spawning frequency, age to maturation, fertilization success, reproductive behavior, or gonadosomatic index (the ratio of gonad to body weight). In addition to these apical endpoints, also molecular and physiological parameters are frequently measured, e.g. circulating levels of reproductive hormones, vitellogenin levels, or gonad histopathology. Each of these parameters may vary with the species-specific reproductive strategy. For instance, fecundity can vary from a few eggs per female in one species up to thousands of eggs per female in another species. Fish may reproduce as fractional or as periodic spawners, they may produce yolk-rich or yolk-poor eggs, they may rely on brood care or not, etc. In addition, many natural factors such as genetic variation, body size or nutrition modulate fecundity among individuals of a given species (Sumpter and Johnson, 2006). Thus, reproductive parameters often show high natural variability, which requires considerable knowledge of intra- and inter-specific background variability of reproductive parameters to enable the detection of toxic impacts on fish reproduction. This applies not only for field studies, where it is often difficult to obtain information on baseline variability of reproductive parameters of the species of interest (Sumpter and Johnson, 2006; Bittner *et al.*, 2009), but also for widely used laboratory model species such as zebrafish (*Danio rerio*), Japanese medaka (*Oryzias latipes*) or fathead minnow (*Pimephales promelas*) (Grim *et al.*, 2007; Watanabe *et al.*, 2007; Paull *et al.*, 2008). As pointed out by Paull *et al.* (2008), this variability necessitates high levels of replication when testing for chemical effects on fish reproductive parameters.

Chemical substances often affect not only a single but multiple reproductive parameters at the same time. For instance, a chemical may cause reduced egg production, and at the same time it may alter reproductive behavior (Nakayama *et al.*, 2004; Weis, 2009). *Vice versa*, a toxicant-induced change in a particular reproductive endpoint could arise from multiple processes, for instance reduced fecundity could be the consequence of impaired gonadal maturation, reduced spawning ability, decreased egg production, and, in species with size-dependent fecundity as is the case with many teleosts, it could also be indirectly affected due a chemical-induced reduction of growth rate.

As fish are a vertebrate group with external fertilization, waterborne toxicants can directly influence this process. Particularly the released sperm cells appear to be sensitive to the presence of toxicants in the water, be it through cytotoxic effects or through both genomic and non-genomic endocrine-dusrupting actions (Kime, 1998; Thomas and Doughty, 2004). As summarized by Kime (1998), fish sperm differ in three aspects from sperm of mammals: (1) they are immotile within the testis or sperm ducts, and attain motility only on ejaculation when the milt is mixed with water, (2) the motility is often of only short duration and rarely exceeds 2 minutes, and (3) they do not penetrate the oocyte wall, but enter the oocyte via a special channel, the micropyle. A sperm property that is particularly sensitive to toxic exposure is sperm motility. Due to the rapid decrease of sperm motility within a short time period, measurement of fish sperm motility is difficult (Kime, 1998). Nowadays, computer-assisted sperm analysis (CASA) is often the method of choice to achieve an objective and quantitative assessment of sperm motility. Using this methodology, it could be clearly shown that numerous chemical compounds including metals, pesticides or endocrine active compounds are able to alter fish sperm motility. The question is whether altered sperm motility indeed affects the fertilizing ability. One of the few studies that have addressed this question is that of Hashimoto *et al.* (2009), which showed that the negative impact of ethinylestradiol on sperm motility is indeed associated with reduced fertilization success. A *caveat*, however, is that the spermiotoxicity of a pollutant can depend on the egg:sperm ratio (Rurangwa *et al.*, 1998).

Apart from gamete production and fertilization success, toxicants can also affect reproductive behavior, in particular courtship behavior and parental care (Jones and Reynolds, 1997; Patisaul and Adewale, 2009). Toxicants can cause behavioral modifications through affecting neuronal signaling, for instance, organophosphates inhibit acetylcholinesterase activity, as well as through influencing endocrine signaling and hormone levels. An example comes from the study of Salierno and Kane (2009) who showed that ethinylestradiol altered the reproductive behavior in fathead minnow, together with changes in circulating levels of sex steroids and with reduced development of breeding tubercles on male fish. Likewise, Coe *et al.* (2008) observed that exposure of breeding colonies of zebrafish to ethinylestradiol disrupted reproductive hierarchies, and this effect was expressed at concentrations that did not affect egg production. The behavioral change was associated with suppression of the male sex hormone, 11-ketotestosterone. Also, Larsen *et al.* (2008) studied behavioral effects of ethinylestradiol on zebrafish, but in contrast to Coe *et al.* (2009), they measured courtship behavior and exposed the fish not only during the breeding phase but from the egg stage until sexual maturity. Under these conditions, courtship behavior was altered at a high concentration (5 ng/l) which induced a drastic change of sex ratio in the population, while at low ethinylestradiol concentrations (0.05 and 0.5 ng/l), courtship behavior did not change – although secondary sexual characteristics (urogenital papillae, body color) were affected. Another relevant question of reproductive behavior is whether toxicants are able to modulate chemical communication between sexual partners. For instance, several fish species use degradation products of MIH as pheromones to synchronize the spawning of male and female fish. Given this prominent role of MIH metabolites in coordinating spawning, what would happen if a toxicant changes MIH synthesis? Contaminant effects on chemical communication may also be manifest on the receptor side, for instance through adverse effects on development or functioning of chemosensory cells (Froehlicher *et al.*, 2009). Unfortunately, the impact of toxicants on chemical communication during reproduction of fish has been rarely studied to date.

Reproductive toxicity of chemicals in fish can be species specific (highlighting how cautiously the word "fish" in this chapter has to be interpreted). An interesting example is provided by the studies on the impact of pulp mill effluents, which are known to have the potential to alter reproductive capabilities of fish (Rolland, 2000). Canadian investigations on two fish species, longnose sucker (*Catostomus catostomus*) and lake whitefish (*Coregonus clupeaformes*), living in the vicinity of a pulp mill effluent in Jackfish Bay at the Great Lakes, revealed that both species display similar responses of the endogenous steroid hormone titers to effluent exposure but the consequences of the effluent-induced physiological changes to reproductive fitness strongly varied between the two species: while in the longnose sucker there was no impairment of gonad development and reproductive potential, lake whitefish suffered from reduced ovarian and testicular development, with more than 90% of the population not developing gonads for the upcoming spawning season (van der Kraak *et al.*, 1992).

The mechanisms that underly chemical-induced reproductive impairment of fish are manifold. Reproductive toxicity can arise from both indirect and direct effects of chemicals on reproductive performance. Indirect effects of chemicals on reproduction could arise from a reallocation of the available energy resources (Heath, 1995; Kooijman 1998). Acclimation to toxic stressors is associated with increased metabolic rates, and this extra expenditure of energy reduces – in the sense of a trade-off – the available energy resources for reproduction. Direct effects of chemicals may take place through the modulation of endocrine processes in a series of target organs such as brain/pituitary, gonads, liver, etc. The integrative nature of the reproductive system involving numerous feedback loops complicates investigations of the primary targets and mechanisms of chemical interference because changes at one site will ultimately affect the activities of other sites or levels (van der Kraak *et al.*, 1992). It also complicates the understanding of how molecular, cellular and physiological changes translate into a change of reproductive output. Therefore, it is difficult to sort out the role of individual processes and targets. Still, two modes of action appear to play key roles in the direct effects of environmental chemicals on fish reproduction: (1) effects mediated through agonistic or antagonistic modulation of receptor signaling and the receptor-regulated pathways, and (2) effects mediated through modulation of hormone metabolism, i.e. hormone synthesis, transport and catabolism/excretion. These mechanisms are discussed in more detail in the following paragraphs on two well-documented examples of reproductive toxicants in fish, namely polyaromatic hydrocarbons (PAHs) and endocrine-disrupting compounds (EDCs).

Reproductive toxicity of PAHs

The PAH example may illustrate the complexity of toxicant effects on fish reproduction. Both laboratory and field studies have consistently shown that exposure of maturing or spawning fish to PAHs negatively affects fish reproduction, leading to decreased spawning success, decreased gonadosomatic index, or to lower circulating levels of sex steroid hormones and vitellogenin (Fairbrother *et al.*, 1999; Hoffmann and Oris, 2006; Johnson *et al.*, 2008). For instance, in the Puget Sound, USA, female English sole (*Parophrys vetulus*) from sites with high PAH concentrations in the sediment suffer from increased ovarian atresia, reduced vitellogenin synthesis, lower levels of plasma E2 and reduced fertilization success compared to sole from reference sites (Johnson *et al.*, 2008, and references therein). When gravid English sole were brought from the Puget Sound into the laboratory and artificially induced to spawn, spawning success was significantly lower in fish from PAH-contaminated sites than from reference sites (Casillas *et al.*, 1991). Although effects of PAH on reproduction have not been studied as extensively in male as in female English sole, available evidence suggests that also males show PAH-related reproductive dysfunctions, e.g. lower circulating levels of androgens (Johnson *et al.*, 2008). Reproductive abnormalities similar to those described for English sole have also been reported for other fish species living in the Puget Sound. For instance, winter flounder (*Pleuronectus americanus*) from PAH-contaminated sites in Boston Harbor displayed depressed plasma vitellogenin levels, increased ovarian atresia, reduced egg size and 10–30% declines in fertilization success and percent in comparison to reference fish (Fairbrother *et al.*, 1999, and references therein). Congruent findings have been described for PAH-exposed starry flounder (*Platichthys stellatus*) from San Francisco Bay (Spies and Rice, 1988) and white croaker (*Genyonemus lineatus*) from the Los Angeles area (Cross and Hose, 1988). Furthermore, a number of laboratory studies documented suppressive effects of PAHs on fish reproduction (cf. Fairbrother *et al.*, 1999).

The mechanisms through which PAHs affect reproductive performance of sexually mature fish appear to involve multiple processes and pathways. One mode of action that has been described repeatedly is that cytochrome P4501A (CYP1A)-inducing PAHs such as benzo(a)pyrene can modulate the expression and/or activity of steroidogenic enzymes eventually leading to altered steroid synthesis (Afonso *et al.*, 1997; Hoffman and Oris, 2006; Dong *et al.*, 2008). Steroidogenic genes such as cytochrome P45019 (*cyp19*), possess putative AhR-responsive elements in their promoter region (Cheshenko *et al.*, 2007, 2008) and therefore could be directly affected via PAH-induced AhR activation. However, an effect of AhR-activating PAHs on gonadal steroidogenesis may also be mediated through a modulation of pituitary gonadotropin release and/or an attenuation of gonadotropin responsiveness of the gonads (Pocar *et al.*, 2005; Heiden *et al.*, 2008). An alternative mechanism would be that PAHs reduce the levels of circulating steroid hormones by enhancing their catabolism (Navas and Segner, 1998). Many PAHs are able to induce the expression of cytochrome p450 enzymes which are involved in endogenous steroid degradation and, indeed, increased estrogen catabolism in PAH-treated fish has been demonstrated experimentally (Förlin and Haux, 1985). Reduced levels of E2 may then lead to changes in the hypothalamus–pituitary axis, and this again may have consequences on oocyte maturation/atresia as well as on egg number and spawning. In this context, two published reports are of interest: Casillas *et al.* (1991) observed that English sole from PAH-contaminated sites was significantly less responsive to LH treatment than fish from reference sites. Likewise, Navas *et al.* (2004) found that exposure of seabass (*Dicentrarchus labrax*) to CYP1A-inducing β-naphthoflavone suppressed the LH surge preparing the fish for spawning. These effects may arise from the PAH impact on gonadal steroid synthesis and circulating sex hormone levels, but they may also arise from direct PAH effects in the neuroendocrine system, as both hypothalamus and pituitary of fish express inducible CYP1A (Andersson *et al.*, 1993; Ortiz-Delgado *et al.*, 2002). These observations indicate that PAHs can interfere at several points with the reproductive feedback systems of fish. Finally, the ability of PAHs to activate the arylhydrocarbon receptor (AhR) is associated with an anti-estrogenic capacity, probably through a cross-talk between the AhR and ER pathways (Anulacion *et al.*, 1997; Navas and Segner, 2000; Kirby *et al.*, 2007; Bugel *et al.*, 2010). The impaired vitellogenin production can have consequences for oocyte maturation, fecundity and egg quality.

PAH impact on fish reproduction depends on timing of exposure. This is suggested by the observation of Anderson *et al.* (1996) that anti-estrogenic actvity of CYP1A-inducing PAHs in rainbow trout was low during those periods of the reproductive cycle when E2 levels were high. Similarly, Navas *et al.* (2004) found that CYP1A-inducing β-naphthoflavone suppressed circulating LH levels of seabass only during the spawning period, but not during periods of gonadal recrudescence.

Reproductive toxicity of EDCs

EDCs are environmental substances that interfere with the endogenous hormone system of exposed organisms, be it by altering hormone signaling or by altering endogenous hormone synthesis, transport and catabolism. Most intensively studied are EDCs that behave as estrogen mimics, i.e. they activate as ligands the ERs and thereby modulate ER-regulated gene expression. Much of the original evidence for endocrine disruption came from studies on aquatic wildlife (Tyler *et al.*, 1998; Vos *et al.*, 2000; Sumpter, 2005), which may be related to the fact that the aquatic environment is the ultimate sink for hormonally active substances, including natural and synthetic estrogens, industrial chemicals, pesticides, organochlorine compounds, pharmaceuticals or phytoestrogens. Effects that have been frequently observed in wild fish populations as a consequence of exposure to estrogen-active compounds include elevated levels of vitellogenin in male fish, development of intersex gonads, i.e. gonads containing both male and female germ cells, or alterations of sex steroid levels (Purdom *et al.*, 1994; Jobling *et al.*, 1998; Larsson *et al.*, 1999; Vermeirssen *et al.*, 2005; Tyler *et al.*, 2008). While the causative link between these pathophysiological changes of the reproductive system of fish and exposure to estrogenic EDCs is well established, the evidence that they translate into reduced reproductive capabilities of wild fish populations is less convincing (Mills and Chichester, 2005; Segner, 2005; Tyler and Jobling, 2008). In a study on roach (*Rutilus rutilus*), from UK rivers, the majority of intersex fish with elevated vitellogenin levels was able to produce viable male gametes; however, they were of poorer quality than those from males of reference sites (Jobling *et al.*, 2002). Also fertilization capability of intersex roach was compromised, and this effect was inversely related to the severity of gonadal intersex. In an experimental lake study in Canada, ethinylestradiol was added over a prolonged period at a low concentration (5–6 ng/l, nominal) to the water. Indigenous fathead minnow responded to this exposure by elevation of vitellogenin levels, gonad histopathological changes and ultimately by near extinction of the species from the lake (Kidd *et al.*, 2007).

In contrast to the scarce evidence of adverse effects of EDCs on fish reproductive output and recruitment in the field, laboratory studies have unequivocally demonstrated that estrogenic EDCs at environmentally realistic concentrations can significantly impair reproductive performance of adult fish (Caldwell *et al.*, 2008). Many of these studies have been performed with small laboratory fish species, in particular zebrafish (*Danio rerio*), fathead minnow (*Pimephales promelas*) and Japanese medaka (*Oryzias latipes*). The advantages of these species for assessing reproductive toxicity include that they are fractional spawners and provide eggs throughout the year for easy experimentation, that there exist protocols for their maintenance in continuous culture in a laboratory setting, that they develop from the fertilized egg into the mature adult stage within a few months, that their reproductive biology is fairly well known and that a number of EDC biomarkers are established for these species (Ankley and Johnson, 2004; Scholz and Mayer, 2008; Segner, 2009). Consequently, the three species are also candidate species for the EDC test guidelines currently under development by the OECD (OECD, 2004, 2009).

A selection of studies on the effects of estrogen-active compounds on reproductive output (fecundity, fertility) of adult, sexually mature fish and associated changes in physiological parameters is given in Table 86.1 (for more literature see Mills and Chichester, 2005; OECD, 2004, 2009). What is clearly evident is that the potencies of natural and synthetic estrogens differ by orders of magnitude from those of xenoestrogens. Responses at the suborganism level, for instance VTG induction, can have lower threshold concentrations than responses at the organism level, i.e. fecundity and fertility; however, this is not always the case, but sensitivities may be identical at both biological levels. Whether there exist consistent species differences in the sensitivity to estrogenic compounds is difficult to deduce from the available data owing to the inter-study variations of experimental conditions and protocols (compare, for instance, the test protocol used for fathead minnow by Harries *et al.*, 2000 vs. that of Ankley *et al.*, 2001). The comparison is further complicated by the generally high variability of reproductive parameters in fish (see above) together with the statistically probably not optimally design of many protocols for adult reproductive tests (cf. Melvin *et al.*, 2009). However, even when comparing different species under identical experimental conditions, the conclusions concerning species differences in sensitivity remain equivocal. Oern *et al.* (2006) observed that when developing zebrafish and Japanese medaka were exposed to 10 ng/l ethinylestradiol, only zebrafish showed a significant elevation of whole body VTG levels. When exposure concentration was increased to 100 ng/l ethinylestradiol, there occurred 100% mortality in zebrafish, while medaka were surviving now displaying a significant induction of VTG. In contrast, Seki *et al.* (2006) who exposed adult zebrafish, medaka and fathead minnow for 21 days to (measured) E2 concentrations between 8.77 and 86 ng/l found medaka to be most sensitive: significant induction of hepatic VTG occurred in medaka at ≥8.94 ng/l E2, while in fathead minnow and zebrafish, VTG was significantly elevated only at 86 ng/l E2. However, it must be kept in mind that the two studies used different life stages, different exposure durations, and different substances and analyzed compartments (whole body VTG in the study of Örn *et al.*, 2006; blood levels of VTG in the study of Seki *et al.*, 2006). A parameter that appears to respond in a species-specific way is gonadal intersex. This appears to be a typical – and highly sensitive – response of medaka to estrogenic exposure, while it appears to be absent in zebrafish and fathead minnow (Table 86.1).

The adverse effects of environmental estrogen-active compounds on reproductive output of fish can be mediated through several target sites and processes (Figure 86.2). The initial event of the mechanism(s) through which environmental estrogen-active compounds eventually disrupt the endocrine homeostasis of fish is agonistic binding to ERs. In the classical ER pathway, the hormone or xenobiotic ligand binds to the ER that induces conformation changes in the receptor leading to the formation of a homodimer and to the phosphorylation of the receptor at specific tyrosine and serine residues. The activated receptor can now bind to DNA sequences responsive to estrogens, the so-called estrogen-responsive elements (ERE), giving rise to transcriptional activation of cis-linked target genes (Tsai and O'Malley, 1994; Couse and Korach, 1999). Ligand-dependent ER activation also triggers recruitment of a number of co-activators which alter chromatin structure and facilitate recruitment of the RNA polymerase II transcriptional machinery (Heldring *et al.*, 2007). There are several physiological factors of relevance for the activation of the ER pathway (Rooney and Guillette, 2000): (1) number of ERs in a given tissue; importantly, the expression of ERs can be upregulated by their own ligands, which has been demonstrated in fish both for the natural ligand, E2, and for xenoestrogens (Nimrod and Benson, 1997; Sabo-Attwood *et al.*, 2007); (2) tissue-specific expression of ERs; and (3) expression of receptor subtypes. Within a single species, several ER subtypes can exist, for instance in rainbow trout, four ER subtypes have been identified (Nagler *et al.*, 2007). They show differential tissue distribution, but the functional implications of this are not yet understood. In addition to the nuclear/cytoplasmic ERs which mediate genomic actions of estrogens, estrogen signaling may occur also through membrane-bound ERs. In fish, the presence of such rapid, non-genomic pathways of estrogen action has been demonstrated, for instance in the gonads (Loomis and Thomas, 2000; Garcia-Reyero *et al.*, 2009). In addition to activation by their endogenous, natural ligands, a broad variety of environmental substances can act as ligands of ERs (Rooney and Guillette, 2000).

Uptake of (xeno)estrogens from the environment into the organism changes internal hormone equilibria and, consequently, hormone signaling. Activation of estrogen signaling by (xeno)estrogen binding to ERs leads to distinct gene expression changes, which may vary with species and tissues as well as with duration and dose of exposure. A prototypic response of fish to activation of ER signaling is the induction of hepatic VTG synthesis (Hiramatsu *et al.*, 2005). This is a rapid response, which, particularly in male fish with low or zero baseline VTG levels, shows a high induction amplitude. As fish species possess multiple VTG isoforms, the individual isoforms may vary in their response to estrogens. While female fish use VTG to produce egg yolk, male fish have no physiological usage for VTG. At high exposure concentrations, VTG can accumulate in tissues and the circulatory system of male fish, eventually giving rise to pathological alterations (Folmar *et al.*, 2001; Zaroogian *et al.*, 2001).

In the gonads, (xeno)estrogens, i.e. environmental compounds that behave as ER ligands, have been shown to target the steroid biosynthesis pathway. Estrogen treatment down-regulated expression of StAR (steroidogenic acute regulatory protein), cytochrome P450 side-chain cleavage enzyme (P450ssc), cytochrome P450 17 (CYP17) and 11β-hydroxysteroid dehydrogenase 2 (11β-HSD) in the ovaries of cod (*Gadus morhua*) and fathead minnow (Filby *et al.*, 2007; Kortner and Arukwe, 2007; Garcia-Reyero *et al.*, 2009). These enzymes play key roles in steroidogenesis, for instance StAR regulates the delivery of cholesterol for steroid synthesis, and their down-regulation implicates a reduced capacity for

Table 86.1 Examples of laboratory studies on the effect of estrogen-active compounds on reproductive output and physiological parameters of fish

Compound	Fish species	Exposure duration and route	Exposure concentration(s)	Effect(s)	Reference
17beta-estradiol (E2)	*Oryzias latipes*	21 d, water, flow-through	29.3–463 ng/l (measured)	Reduced fecundity at >= 463 ng/l Reduced fertility at Y=463 ng/l Increased testis-ova at >=29.3 ng/l Increased VTG at >=55 ng/l	Kang *et al.*, 2002
17beta-estradiol(E2)	*Oryzias latipes*	14 d, static renewal	272–27, 200 ng/l (nominal)	Reduced fecundity at >=816 ng/l	Shioda *et al.*, 2002
17beta-estradiol(E2)	*Pimephales promelas*	21 d, static renewal	316 ng/l (measured; nominal: 500 ng/l)	Reduced fecundity Reduced GSI Reduced oocyte/sperm maturation Reduced SSC Increased VTG	Bringolf *et al.*, 2004
17beta-estradiol(E2)	*Danio rerio*	21 d, static renewal	27–272 ng/l (nominal)	No effect on fecundity Increased VTG at >=86 ng/l No intersex	van der Ven *et al.*, 2004
Ethinyl-estradiol	*Oryzias latipes*	21 d, flow through, pair-breeding,	32.6–488 ng/l (measured)	Reduced fecundity at 488 ng/l Increased VTG at >=63.9 ng/l Increased intersex at >=63.9 ng/l	Seki *et al.*, 2002
Ethinyl-estradiol	*Pimephales promelas*	21 d, flow through	0.1–100 ng/l (nominal)	Increased fecundity at >=0.1 ng/l Reduced fecundity at >=10 ng/l Reduced fertilization at >=10 ng/l Reduced GSI at >=1 ng/l Reduced sperm no. at >=10 ng/l Reduced SSC at >=1 ng/l Increased VTG at >=1 ng/l	Pawlowski *et al.*, 2004
Ethinyl-estradiol	*Danio rerio*	21 d, static renewal	5-50 ng/l (nominal)	Reduced spawning at >=10 ng/l Increased VTG at >=5 ng/l	van den Belt *et al.*, 2001
Ethinyl-estradiol	*Fundulus heteroclitus*	21-28 d, static renewal	0.1–100 ng/l (nominal)	Reduced fecundity at 100 ng/l Reduced fertility at 100 ng/l Increased GSI at 100 ng/l Reduced sex steroid level at 100 ng/l Increased VTG at 100 ng/l No intersex	Peters *et al.*, 2007
4-nonylphenol	*Oryzias latipes*	21 d, flow-through	2,500–184,000 ng/l	Reduced fecundity at >=101,000 ng/l Reduced fertility at 184,000 ng/l Increased intersex at >=2500 ng/l Abnormal spermatogenesis at 184,000 ng/l	Kang *et al.*, 2003
4-nonylphenol	*Pimephales promelas*	6 weeks (3 weeks pre-exposure to determine baseline values, 3 weeks exposure), flow-through	650–82,000 ng/l (measured)	Reduced fecundity at 8,100–57,700 ng/l Increased VTG at 650–8,100 ng/l No intersex	Harries *et al.*, 2000
4t-octylphenol	*Danio rerio*	21 d, static renewal	1,300–10,0000 ng/l (nominal)	No effect on fecundity No effect on fertility No effect on VTG	van den Belt *et al.*, 2001
4t-pentylphenol	*Pimephales promelas*	6 weeks (3 weeks pre-exposure to determine baseline values, 3 weeks exposure), flow-through	5,600–56,000 ng/l (nominal)	Reduced fecundity at >=5,600 ng/l Increased VTG at 560,000 ng/l No intersex	Panter *et al.*, 2010
Bisphenol A	*Oryzias patipes*	21 d, flow-through	837,000–3,120,000 ng/l (measured)	No effect on fecundity No effect on fertility Increase testis-ova at >=837,000 ng/l Increased VTG at 312,000 ng/l	Kang *et al.*, 2002

The described effects represent statistically significant changes
VTG = vitellogenin
"Fertility" refers to fertilization success, i.e. the percentage of eggs successfully fertilized
"Fecundity" refers to egg production per female (partly measured as cumulative egg number, partly as eggs per day)
SSC = secondary sex characteristics

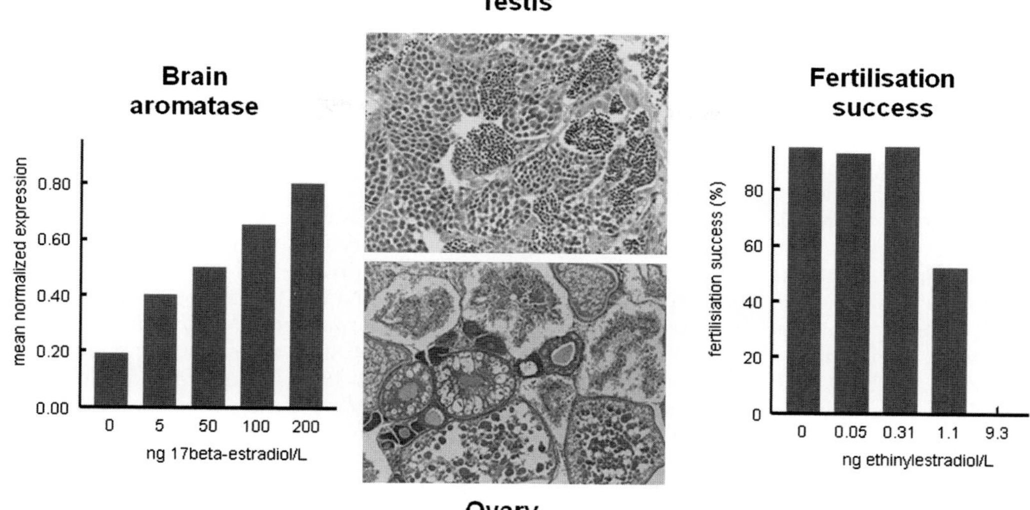

FIGURE 86.2 Associated effects of environmental estrogen-active compounds (here: 17β-estradiol and ethinylestradiol) at several levels of fish reproduction (brain aromatase, gamete maturation, fertilization success), exemplified for zebrafish. Left figure: exposure of zebrafish to increasing concentrations of 17β-estradiol results in a concentration-dependent induction of brain aromatase, cyp19a1b, expression (data from Kallivretaki *et al.*, 2006). Middle figure: exposure of zebrafish to 10ng/l ethinylestradiol reduces sperm maturation in testsis (top micrograph: few mature sperm cells, and dominance of early maturation stages, i.e. spermatocytes and spermatogonia), and enhances oocyte atresia (bottom micrograph) (Rossteuscher and Segner, unpublished). Right figure: exposure of zebrafish to increasing concentrations of ethinylestradiol results in a concentration-dependent decrease of fertilization success (data from Schäfers *et al.*, 2007).

ovarian androgen and estrogen synthesis. The estrogenic effects on gene expression may be mediated through ERE in the promoter regions of these genes. An argument supporting this interpretation would be the finding of Garcia-Reyero *et al.* (2009) that ovarian aromatase, *cyp19a1a*, which has no ER in the promoter (Cheshenko *et al.*, 2008), undergoes no downregulation in estrogen-exposed fathead minnow. However, mechanisms other than ER signaling may be involved as well, in particular as Filby *et al.* (2007) observed a down-regulation of ERα expression in the gonads of ethinylestradiol-treated fathead minnow. In females, such an alternative mechanism could be a shift in the relative share of the individual oocyte maturation stages within the ovary, as these stages have different expression levels of steroidogenic genes (Ge, 2005). In line with this, a long-term exogenous estrogen supply may disrupt the endogenous E2 cycle during reproduction which is characterized by a peak of ovarian estrogen synthesis during oocyte vitellogenesis and a decline with final oocyte maturation (Kobayashi *et al.*, 1988). Finally, gonadotropin responsiveness of estrogen-exposed gonads may be altered, and as the gonadotropins orchestrate gonadal maturation and spawning (see above), this could have implications on gametogenesis. This mechanism may then be involved in the enhanced frequency of atretic follicles in the ovaries of estrogen-exposed fish (van der Ven *et al.*, 2003; Wolf *et al.*, 2004; Leino *et al.*, 2005) as well as in the decreased presence of mature sperm stages in the testis of male fish (Figure 86.2) – both changes eventually leading to reduced fecundity and fertilization success. An interesting aspect to the discussion on the impact of (xeno)estrogens on fish gonad functioning is provided by a global gene expression analysis of the gonads of zebrafish exposed to ethinylestradiol (Santos *et al.*, 2007). In this analysis, 379 genes were differently expressed between control and exposed females, while control and exposed males differed by 114 genes. Among the genes differently regulated by ethinylestradiol in females, the biological processes over-represented included mitochondrion organization and biogenesis, as well as energy pathways. The mitochondria are involved in energy pathways and in steroidogenesis, indicating that the steroid exposure disturbs orderly biosynthetic processes required for oogenesis. This interpretation is further supported by the over-representation of genes involved in protein transport in the estrogen-treated females, as protein transport is central to oocyte growth. These findings highlight that estrogenic effects on reproductive functions are not only a matter of interference with specific targets in hormonal pathways but involve also overall biosynthesis and energy processes required for the successful building up of gametes.

Another potential target of (xeno)estrogen actions in the organism is the brain, in particular the hypothalamus and pituitary (see above). Particular attention has been given to the influence of (xeno)estrogens on the brain aromatase, *cyp19a1b*, which is known to oscillate with reproductive cycles of fish (Gonzalez and Piferrer, 2003; Villeneuve *et al.*, 2006). Indeed, a relation between brain aromatase and pituitary LH or FSH production has been observed in some teleosts (Antonopoulou *et al.*, 1999) and it has been demonstrated that xenoestrogens are able to modulate pituitary LH synthesis (Yadetie and Male, 2002). Brain aromatase of fish is inducible by (xeno)estrogens (Figure 86.2) (Kishida *et al.*, 2001; Melo and Ramsdell, 2001; Hinfray *et al.*, 2006) which agrees with the presence of putative ERE in its promoter (Cheshenko *et al.*, 2008). The functional implications of this induction are not clear to date, but it may be speculated that the effects of estrogenic exposure on reproductive performance of adult fish are at least in part mediated through modulating brain aromatase activity and expression. Overall, although estrogen receptor activation is well established as the primary biological effect in disruption of adult fish reproduction by environmental estrogens, surprisingly little is known of the mechanisms by which this initial event translates into impaired fecundity or fertility.

Endocrine disruption of adult reproduction is not only a matter of chemicals acting as ER ligands, but occurs also through chemicals acting as ER antagonists, as ligands of other hormone receptors, in particular androgen receptors, or as modulators of steroid synthesis (Ankely *et al.*, 2003; Jensen *et al.*, 2004; OECD, 2004, 2009; Sharpe *et al.*, 2004; Andersen *et al.*, 2006). An excellent body of information has been generated concerning the mechanisms by which aromatase-inhibiting substances such as fadrozole impair reproduction of fathead minnow (see Ankley *et al.*, 2009). This work includes studies from the measurement of phenotypic responses in adult reproductive tests (Ankely *et al.*, 2002) up to graphical models utilizing transcriptomic data to model chemical-induced gene expression changes in the HPG axis (Villeneuve *et al.*, 2007; Zhang *et al.*, 2008). It is this kind of systematic approach that should increasingly be used in future studies to reveal the mechanisms underlying reproductive toxicity of environmental chemicals in fish.

As discussed above, the issue of endocrine disruption is usually connected with exposure to chemical substances. However, it has been shown that also other environmental factors can act as endocrine disruptors. For instance, hypoxia disrupts sexual development and reproduction of fish (Wu *et al.*, 2003; Shang *et al.*, 2006, Thomas *et al.*, 2007). Hypoxia interferes with the reproductive axis at the brain level, changing neuorendocrine parameters such as hypothalamic serotonin (5-HT) content and the activity of the 5-HT biosynthetic enzyme, tryptophan hydroxylase (Rahman and Thomas, 2009), and hypoxia interferes with the reproductive axis at the gonad level by decreasing the levels of the gamete maturation-inducing hormone progestin, and, as a consequence, impairing gamete maturation (Thomas and Rahman, 2009). Interestingly, at least part of the hypoxia effects on fish reproduction appears to be mediated through non-genomic signaling pathways (Thomas and Rahman, 2009).

TOXIC IMPACT ON THE DEVELOPING LIFE STAGES OF FISH

Developmental toxicity due to maternal transfer of toxicants

Toxic exposure of adult fish can have indirect consequences for the offspring in that the exposure modifies the reproductive physiology of the parents and this can result in impaired quality of eggs and sperm (see above). Due to the oviparous mode of reproduction of fish, adult exposure can also have direct consequences for the offspring through the transfer of chemicals from the contaminated parent fish into the eggs (e.g., Ostrach *et al.*, 2008). An early example of adverse effects in early life stages of fish evoked by toxicants that passed from the parent through the yolk is the heavy mortality of trout fry observed in lakes in the New York area following excessive use of DDT for insect control between 1951 and 1957 (Burdick *et al.*, 1964). A close relationship was found between early life stage mortality and the DDT content of the eggs. This relationship could be confirmed by laboratory studies demonstrating that eggs obtained from parents fed with a DDT-containing diet suffered significantly higher mortalities than eggs from unexposed parents (Burdick *et al.*, 1972). Maternally transmitted DDT was able to induce early life stage mortality at concentrations that do not impair maternal fecundity (Allison *et al.*, 1963). Adverse consequences of maternally transferred toxicants on development and survival of early life stages are not restricted to DDT, but have been shown for other chemical classes as well (Westerlund *et al.*, 2000). Importantly, the toxic consequences of maternal toxicant deposition may become evident during the early life stages; however, delayed effects may also occur. This has been nicely illustrated by the work of Papoulias *et al.* (2003), who in order to simulate maternal transfer, injected medaka embryos with a DTT metabolite, *o,p*-DDE, and this early life exposure had consequences for gonadosomatic index and gonad histopathology of adult, 107-day-old fish.

Maternal transfer of toxicants into the eggs has been intensively studied for salmonid populations at the Great Lakes (Niimi, 1983; Miller, 1993). For organic contaminants such as DDT, chlordane, Mirex, endrin and dieldrin, no large concentration differences were found between the whole body of the parents and the eggs, with the lipid content in the fish and the egg markedly influencing this distribution. For inorganic mercury, burdens were much higher in the fish than in eggs, indicating that transmittance of this metal is low. One group of chemicals that has attracted particular attention with respect to parent–egg transfer are dioxins and polychlorinated biphenyls (Peterson *et al.*, 1993; Walker *et al.*, 1994) as these compounds are causally involved in the decline of certain salmonid species in the Great Lakes. As shown by Giesy *et al.* (2002) for rainbow trout, dietary 2,3,7,8-tetrachlorodibenzo-p-dioxin (TCDD) is accumulated in a dose-dependent manner into tissues of the parent fish, and it is also transferred into the eggs. A 300-day exposure of the adults to diets containing 1.8, 18 or 90 ng TCDD/kg food resulted in TCCD concentrations in the eggs of 0.3 ng/kg, 2.3 ng/kg and 19.5 ng/kg, respectively. TCDD treatment reduced survival of the adults, but surprisingly had no effect on total number of eggs or parameters of egg quality such as egg weight, diameter, lipid content or caloric content. However, survival of eggs and fry were significantly reduced in a dose-dependent manner. Accumulation, maternal transfer and effects of dietary TCDD were also studied by Heiden *et al.* (2005). Chronic dietary exposure of zebrafish resulted in the dose-dependent accumulation of 1.1–36 ng TCDD/g fish. TCDD accumulation had no effects on survival or spawning activity, but it significantly decreased the ovarian-somatic index and induced ovarian necrosis and altered follicular development. The ovarian changes appear to be related to an attenuated gonadotropin responsiveness of the gonads and/or decreased ovarian E2 biosynthesis under TCDD exposure (Heiden *et al.*, 2008). Maternal transfer resulted in the accumulation of 0.094–1.2 ng TCDD/g egg, which was sufficient to induce the typical signs of larval TCDD toxicity, commonly referred to as blue sac syndrome (see below). Thus, TCCD concentrations that remained without overt effects on survival and reproduction of adults had a marked influence on offspring health at all TCDD concentrations tested.

Developmental toxicity due to chemical exposure of fish embryos, larvae and juveniles

Fish early life stages have been used as vertebrate models in developmental biology for a long time (Mullins and Nüsslein-Volhard, 1993), but they are now gaining increasing importance as toxicological models. There are mainly three motivations behind the enhanced use of fish early life stages for toxicological purposes:

1. The developmental formation of the organism body plan and functions requires orderly and integrated expression of genes involving complex regulatory and signaling networks. It is self-evident that these processes are vulnerable to the interference of exogenous chemicals with gene expression and/or chemical signaling (McNabb *et al.*, 1999; McLachlan, 2001). While this is true for developing stages of all vertebrate classes, early life stages of fish have several features that make them particularly vulnerable to toxicants, including the development outside the mother in direct exposure to environmental toxicants, and the lipid-rich yolk material which favors the accumulation of lipophilic xenobiotics into the egg. For developing stages of invertebrates like seastar nauplii, it has been shown that the activity of xenobiotic transporters of the ABC family reduce bioaccumulation of certain chemical groups (Epel, 1998); however, whether such transporters are expressed and active on the chorion of fish eggs remains to be investigated.
2. Developmental stages of fish offer a number of technical advantages for toxicological screening and testing (Hill *et al.*, 2005). They develop outside the mother (in contrast to the *in utero* development of mammals) which facilitates exposure and experimental manipulation, including the possibility of microinjection of chemicals as well as of experimental tools such as morpholinos into the egg (Hill *et al.*, 2005; Nassef *et al.*, 2010). The eggs of many fish species are transparent enabling direct observation of toxicant-induced phenotypic malformations, visual tracing of individual cell fates during organogenesis, or whole mount staining of the expression of target genes and proteins. When using small laboratory fish species such as zebrafish, whole-year round production of eggs is possible. In addition, embryonic development of these species is rapid so that toxic effects on organogenesis can be studied within a short observational period. Finally, as fish eggs and early life stages are usually small, the use of microplate formats is possible, which supports high throughput phenotypic screening. Taken together, these advantages have promoted the increasing usage of fish early life stages in pharmacological drug discovery (e.g., Goldsmith, 2004; Hill *et al.*, 2005; Zon and Peterson, 2005), and as both a fish and general vertebrate toxicological model (Spitsbergen and Kent, 2003; Hill *et al.*, 2005, Carvan *et al.*, 2005; Ankley and Villeneuve, 2006).
3. Another line of reasoning that has promoted the use of toxicity tests with fish early life is the 3R discussion on reducing, replacing and refining *in vivo* testing (see below, and Braunbeck *et al.*, 2005; Embry *et al.*, 2010).

There is a growing body of literature on the toxicity of industrial chemicals, pesticides and pharmaceuticals to developing life stages of fish, addressing a wide variety of questions such as the relation between toxicity, tissue pathology and gene expression (Volz *et al.*, 2006), investigation of toxic mechanisms (Tilton *et al.*, 2008; Li *et al.*, 2009), identification of vulnerable windows for developmental chemical toxicity (e.g., Oxendine *et al.*, 2006), or assessing the protective role of toxicant-induced molecular and cellular responses (Volz *et al.*, 2008). Two aspects, however, have attracted surprisingly little attention: one aspect is the importance of

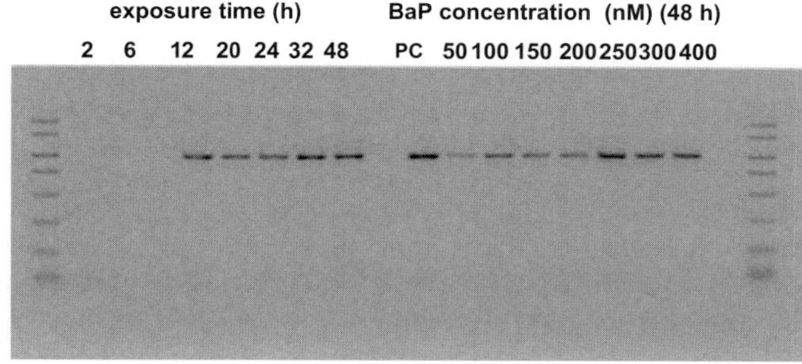

FIGURE 86.3 Induction of cytochrome P4501A (CYP1) mRNA in zebrafish embryos by benzo(a)pyrene. On the left side, the gel shows the induction response in relation to hours post-fertilization (2–48 hours), on the right side the induction in relation to exposure concentration (50–400 nM). PC = positive control. The levels of mRNA were measured by means of RT-PCR (Segner, unpublished).

biokinetics and biotransformation in toxicity to fish early life stages – what metabolic capabilities are present at what stages of development and what are the uptake and excretion pathways and processes in a fish embryo, etc.? There exists evidence that fish embryos and eleutheroembryos express inducible activities of phase I and phase II biotransformation enzymes, e.g. CYP1A (Figure 86.3) and glutathione-S-transferase (Binder and Stegeman, 1984; Guiney *et al.*, 1997; Wang *et al.*, 1998, 2006; Kopponen *et al.*, 2000), and that fish embryo stages are able to metabolize and excrete endogenous and exogenous substrates (Wiegand *et al.*, 2000; Petkam *et al.*, 2003). A more systematic investigation of the metabolic capabilities and capacities of fish embryos should be of relevance considering the current discussion on using fish embryos as alternative test systems in regulatory risk assessment (see below). A second, to date largely neglected aspect of fish developmental toxicity is that of delayed or persisting effects of early life exposure. In this case, toxic effects of chemical exposure are not evident in the exposed developmental stages, but are manifest only later in life. Ottinger and Kaatari (2000) have shown that exposure of rainbow trout embryos to aflatoxin leads to long-term immune dysfunction. Similarly, Milston *et al.* (2003) observed that short-term early life exposure of Chinook salmon (*Oncorhynchus tshawytscha*) to *o,p′*-DDE or DMSO caused long-term humoral immunosuppression. Tiedeken and Ramsdell (2007) demonstrated that *in ovo* exposure of zebrafish embryos to domoic acid resulted in increased susceptibility of larval fish to another toxicant. Such findings are not only relevant with respect to fish toxicity, but may also contribute to the ongoing discussion in mammalian toxicology on fetal origin of adult disease.

Developmental toxicity of dioxin-like chemicals

The case of developmental toxicity of dioxins and PCBs to fish was highlighted by the decline of lake trout (*Salvelinus namaycush*) stocks in Lake Ontario during the 20th century. There is compelling evidence, both from ecoepidemiological criteria and from mechanistic research, that this is related to the accumulation of persistent chemicals, including dioxins, furans and PCBs (Rolland, 2000; Cook *et al.*, 2003; Carney *et al.*, 2006). Lake trout have been shown to bioaccumulate higher levels of these substances than most other fish species in the Great Lakes because of their long life span, relatively high fat content and their position in the food chain. In addition to direct uptake from water, eggs accumulate significant levels of lipophilic chemicals from the mother (Miller, 1993). Lake trout embryos were found to be extremely sensitive to toxicity induced by TCDD and related dioxins, furanes and PCB. These chemicals induce in lake trout sac fry the blue sac disease, which consists of yolk sac and pericardial edema, hemorrhages, impaired heart and vasculature development, and jaw malformations secondary to inhibited chondrogenesis; the disease signs are followed by mortality of the sac fry prior to swim-up (Spitsbergen *et al.*, 1991; Walker *et al.*, 1991; Peterson *et al.*, 1993). Maternal transfer of TCDD to lake trout eggs results in sac fry mortality when concentrations in the eggs exceed 30 pg/g wet weight. The TCDD-induced phenotype is not restricted to early life stages of lake trout but can be induced in all freshwater fish species (Hill *et al.*, 2005; Carney *et al.*, 2006).

The TCDD toxicity to fish embryos is mediated through the AhR pathway. While the understanding of the physiological role of this receptor in early development is only emerging (e.g., Vuori *et al.*, 2008), its involvement in xenobiotic toxicity has been known for a long time. Evidence for a role of AhR signaling in dioxin toxicity to fish early life stages came from the finding that TCDD and other AhR-binding chemicals interact in an additive fashion to cause blue sac disease (Zabel *et al.*, 1995). Further evidence came from experiments with zebrafish embryos using morpholinos to knock down the expression of AhR and the associated aryl hydrocarbon receptor nuclear translocator (ARNT) (Carney *et al.*, 2006). As fish express different isoforms of both proteins, subsequent research examined which specific isoform is responsible for the TCDD effect, and could demonstrate that zebrafish AHR2 and ARNT1 are required for mediating the hallmark endpoints of TCDD toxicity in developing zebrafish (Carney *et al.*, 2006, and references therein). Although considerable evidence has now accumulated that the AhR pathway is mediating early life stage toxicity of dioxin-like chemicals to fish, the way in which activation of this pathway leads to toxicity is still under discussion. It has been hypothesized that induction of AhR-regulated biotransformation enzymes such as CYP1A plays a role in causing toxic effects, for instance by causing oxidative stress which could damage the vascular endothelia (Guiney *et al.*, 1997). However, morpholino knockdown of the *cyp1a* gene in zebrafish embryos did not protect against TCDD-induced embryotoxicity (Carney *et al.*, 2004) which makes a causative role of CYP1A unlikely. Ongoing research is using microarray approaches to identify new candidate genes with relevance for TCDD embryotoxicity, and is exploring a possible role of receptor cross-talks. The example of the research on blue sac disease may illustrate the power of fish early life stages as models for studying developmental toxicity of chemicals.

Disruption of sexual development of fish by EDCs

EDCs can modulate sexual differentiation of developing fish. This effect is different from the influence of EDCs on reproductive physiology of adult fish (see above). In the latter case, EDCs interfere with the normal functioning of the already differentiated sexual status that can lead to, e.g., regression of gametogenesis, or expression of female-specific vitellogenin in male fish. EDC exposure of developing fish, with a yet undifferentiated sexual status, however, can lead to a permanent change of phenotypic sex (Devlin and Nagahama, 2002; Segner *et al.*, 2006).

As laid out above, sex steroids act as organizers of phenotypic sexual differentiation of fish gonads. Thus, any exogenously induced disturbance in the endogenously programmed ratios of the steroid hormones has the potential to change the direction and progression of sexual differentiation in the developing fish. Timing of exposure is a crucial factor: endogenous regulation of sexual differentiation occurs during a specific developmental period, and it is particularly this "critical period" when the developing fish is sensitive to the disrupting effect of exogenous signals (Piferrer, 2001). EDC exposure before or after the critical window will have no or little effect on sexual differentiation (Blazquez *et al.*, 1998, Gray *et al.*, 1999; Maack and Segner, 2004; van Aerle *et al.*, 2002, 2004). The developmental timing of the critical period varies with species (Piferrer, 2001).

The impact of estrogen-active EDCs on gonad sexual differentiation during ontogeny has been studied for a number of fish species developing as differentiated gonochorists. An illustrative example of how the impact of EDCs on sexual differentiation of fish can vary with the endocrine potency of the chemical compounds is provided by the study of Gimeno *et al.* (1998). These authors exposed genetically male carp during the critical period to either the weak estrogen, 4-tert-pentylphenol (36, 90 or 256 μg TPP/l) or to the strong estrogen, E2 (9 or 23 μg E2/l). After 20 days of exposure, the gonads of control and TPP-exposed fish were yet at an undifferentiated stage, whereas fish exposed to 9 or 23 μg E2/l already displayed oviducts, indicating the onset of phenotypic feminization of the genetically male carp. In TPP-treated fish, oviduct formation started after 30 days of exposure, while gonads of control fish were still undifferentiated at that time. After 90 days of treatment, 100% of the E2-exposed carp possessed oviducts, i.e. were phenotypic females, while in the TPP groups, the percentage of feminized fish varied with exposure concentration: in the groups exposed to 90 or 256 μg TPP/l, all individuals had developed oviduct and oocytes, while only 50% of the individuals of the 36 μg TPP/l group were feminized.

Laboratory studies have shown that environmentally realistic concentrations of EDCs are able to induce phenotypic sex change of developing fish, when applied during the appropriate developmental period. For instance, in medaka – a differentiated gonochorist – the critical period of gonad sexual differentiation takes place around and shortly after hatching. Papoulias *et al.* (1999) administered EE2 by microinjection into the egg. The injected EE2 was present for 8 days before and 4 days after hatch, i.e. during the critical period. Microinjection of 0.5–2.5 ng EE2/egg caused phenotypic sex reversal of genetic males into females, with 2.5 ng/egg being the most effective dose. Hartley *et al.* (1998) exposed medaka shortly after hatch for only 48 h to 4 or 29.4 μg E2/l which led to increased percentages of females after a 2-week grow-out period. Koger *et al.* (2000) treated medaka embryos of stage 10 or 1-, 7- and 21-day-old larvae for 6 days with 15 μg E2/l and measured the sex ratios after a 5-month rearing in control water. Sex ratios were significantly biased towards females when estrogen exposure had taken place during the embryo stage 10 or the 1- or 7-day post-hatch period, while exposure of 21-day-old medaka induced no alteration of sexual differentiation. Testis–ova were observed in all treatments, including the 21-day post-hatch group. Nimrod and Benson (1998) exposed medaka to 0.01–1.66 μg E2/l from hatch until the first month of age and found that all concentrations led to exclusively female populations – while expsoure to the weak ER agonist, nonylphenol, at concentrations up to 1.9 μg/l had no effect on the sex ratio. Gray *et al.* (1999) exposed male medaka to 100 μg octylphenol/l, with the treatments starting at 1, 3, 7, 21 or 35 dph, respectively. They observed no change in sex ratio, but increased incidence of testis–ova, which was highest in the groups exposed at 1 to 3 dph, but declined when exposures were initiated with older fry.

The impact of EDCs on development of phenotypic sex of fish may vary with the pattern of sexual differentiation. This has been exemplified for zebrafish (Brion *et al.*, 2004; Nash *et al.*, 2004; Fenske *et al.*, 2005; Segner *et al.*, 2006; Segner, 2009; Schäfers *et al.*, 2007). This species develops as undifferentiated gonochorist or non-functional hermaphrodite. When juvenile zebrafish are exposed to estrogens during the period of gonad differentiation, all fish develop gonads with ovarian morphology. If estrogen exposure continues until adulthood, ovarian morphology is maintained and they at least partly develop into mature ovaries. If, however, estrogen exposure stops after the critical period, then a bisexual male/female population develops, i.e. about half of the individuals with ovarian-type gonads at the end of the exposure period convert into individuals with testes (Hill and Janz, 2003; Fenske *et al.*, 2005; Schäfers *et al.*, 2007). A likely mechanism explaining this effect is that administration of exogenous estrogens during zebrafish development could inhibit transition of the early, non-functional ovary into testicular tissue, i.e. testicular differentiation is arrested at the non-functional ovarian-like stage. When estrogen exposure is stopped, the arrested male gonads undergo transition from ovarian-like into a testicular morphology, i.e. the EDC effect proves to be reversible (Fenske *et al.*, 2005; Segner, 2009). The reversibility of EDC-induced gonadal feminization appears to depend on the concentration and duration of estrogen exposure, and it may also differ for morphologcial and fucntional parameters (Maack and Segner, 2004; Schäfers *et al.*, 2007; Larsen *et al.*, 2009).

The mechanisms of action of exogenous EDCs on gonad differentiation in fish are not well understood, but in principal they could be mediated through the same mechanisms as EDC effects on adult reproductive physiology, i.e. through binding to endogenous hormone receptors or through modulation of steroid synthesis. Both mechanisms will result in altered levels and ratios of sex steroids in the developing organism, and this then can have consequences on the process of sexual differentiation. Exposure to environmental estrogens or androgens could alter the endogenous hormone levels during the critical developmental period, and this altered estrogen/androgen ratio would then modulate the relevant signaling events in the differentiation process. An alternative process by which environmental substances can lead to altered endogenous hormone levels and ratios is inhibition of steroidogenesis, as it has been shown for compounds like fadrozole, prochloraz or tributyltin which inhibit CYP19 aromatase (McAllister and Kime, 2003; Shimasaki *et al.*, 2003; Fenske and Segner, 2004; Kinnberg *et al.*, 2004). An interesting question concerning the mechanisms underlying altered gonad sexual differentiation is to what extent the EDC effects arise from a direct impact on the gonads (Schulz *et al.*, 2007) or if they become effective through modulating the HPG axis. As reviewed by Guiguen *et al.* (2010), ovarian aromatase, *cyp19a1a*, plays a pivotal role in the development of an ovarian or testicular phenotype; questions, however, exist with respect to the upstream regulation of the ovarian aromatase. One speculation is that the brain isoform of aromatase (which is estrogen-sensitive – which may provide the link to the feminizing activity of environmental estrogens) could play a role in triggering and/or directing gonadal aromatase activity and sexual differentiation (Trant *et al.*, 2001; Matsuoka *et al.*, 2006), i.e. the brain would sex the gonads, a model that deviates from the mammalian model. However, findings from recent studies do not support this hypothesis (Kuhl and Brouwer, 2006; Kallivretaki *et al.*, 2007).

Reproductive and developmental toxicity arising from life-cycle and/or multigenerational exposure of fish

Life-cycle tests refer to exposure of fish from fertilization until adulthood and possibly partial or full next generation (multigeneration tests). They are able to indicate toxicant-induced changes in adult reproductive output and in recruitment, including changes in egg and embryo survival and differentation, in hatching success, in larval and juvenile growth and survival, or in sexual differentiation. Life-cycle tests cover all modes of toxic action, regardless if the chemical toxicity occurs as, e.g., altered fecundity of adult females or a shift in sex ratio during development. If performed as multigeneration tests, they can reveal potential changes in biological parameters and toxicant sensitivity of the F_1 and F_2 generations that have not yet been expressed in the parent generation (Foran *et al.*, 2002; Nash *et al.*, 2004; Zha *et al.*, 2008; Cripe *et al.*, 2009). As such, these tests provide the most comprehensive assessment of long-term chemical toxicity to fish development, growth, recruitment and reproduction. Particularly if life-cycle tests are not restricted to the measurement of apical endpoints, such as survival or fecundity, but are complemented with molecular, histopathological and/or physiological endpoints, they are powerful tools to inform on the ecotoxicological hazards of chemicals (Braunbeck *et al.*, 1990; Bresch *et al.*, 1990; Hinton, 1993). This advantage of life-cycle tests also explains their preferred application for the asssessment of EDCs (Yokota *et al.*, 2001; Seki *et al.*, 2003, 2004, 2005; Nash *et al.*, 2004; Fenske *et al.*, 2005; Schäfers *et al.*, 2007; OECD, 2008; Zha *et al.*; 2008; Cripe *et al.*; 2009; Deng *et al.*, 2010).

Life-cycle tests, to keep them feasible, are primarily performed with short-lived species such as fathead minnow, medaka and zebrafish. Still, these tests are laborious and costly, which motivates the ongoing discussion on whether partial life-cycle tests are able to substitute for full life-cycle tests, i.e. if the partial life-cycle tests would provide comparable sensitivity and information as the full or multigeneration life-cycle test. A partial life-cycle test restricts exposure, for instance, to the reproducing adult fish prior and during spawning, plus a short-term exposure of F_1 embryos and juvenile fish (van der Ven *et al.*, 2007). Duration of the F_1 exposure depends on the intended information – is the aim to measure toxic effects on F_1 embryo viability and hatching success or on F_1 sexual development? This depends on the biology and physiology of the test species, for instance the timing of the critical window of sexual differentiation. The strengths and weaknesses of partial vs. full life-cycle tests with resepct to regulatory hazard assessment of chemicals has been recently discussed by the OECD (2008).

Regulatory tests on reproductive and developmental toxicity of fish

Both at the national and international level, there exist guidelines and test protocols for early life stage tests with fish, for instance the OECD Test Guideline 210 on Fish Early Life Stage Toxicity. This test intends to determine lethal and sublethal effects of chemicals on early life stages of fish, with the exposure covering the period from fertilization through embryonic development until the fish are free-feeding. Effects are assessed at the levels of abnormal appearance and behavior, hatching success and survival. Effects on fish development beyond the embryo exposure period are not measured. Recently, fish early life stage tests have attracted increasing attention, not primarily to assess developmental toxicity *per se*, but as substitutes for acute fish lethality tests (Embry *et al.*, 2010).

Standardized guidelines exist also for fish reproductive tests. The OECD, for instance, has developed the Test Guideline 229 (Fish Short Term Reproduction Test) which is intended as a screening assay to explore the consequences of a 21-day exposure on vitellogenin, secondary sexual characteristics and possibly gonad histopathology. Adult reproductive tests measuring chemical toxicity to fecundity and/or fertilization success are currently not validated for regulatory purposes. Also for life-cycle tests, an OECD guideline currently does not exist, but the US EPA has published a guideline (US EPA, 1996). If and to what extent an extended fish early life stage test assessing chemical effects on sexual differentiation may substitute for a full life-cycle test is an ongoing debate (Holbech *et al.*, 2006; Panter *et al.*, 2006).

CONCLUDING REMARKS AND FUTURE DIRECTIONS

While research and knowledge on developmental and reproductive toxicity of chemicals in fish has made substantial progress over recent years, there remain several areas where there is a paucity of information. One of these areas is the still poorly developed understanding of the ecological meaning of toxic effects on fish development and reproduction. The textbook approach to this question is to assume a linear translation of changes in developmental and reproductive rates into changes of population growth. However, this view appears to be too simplistic (Hutchinson *et al.*, 2006; Segner, 2007). Translation across biological levels depends on a variety of factors, for instance one and the same decrease of embryo survival may have different population-level consequences in two species with contrasting life history strategies. Further, what must not be neglected are the compensatory processes as well as the fact that each level of biologcial organization possesses emerging properties not predictable from the levels below. Here, future research must invest substantial efforts to better understand the factors and processes that decide on whether and how a toxic effect translates into an ecological effect.

A second area that has attracted surprisingly little attention is the question of persisting effects of early life exposure to toxic chemicals. For instance, standard fish early life stage toxicity tests assess adverse effects occurring until the end of the exposure period – however, what if effects become manifest only later in life? This "early basis of late disease" issue is intensively discussed in mammalian toxicology, but has not yet found much echo in the ecotoxicology world – although, given the reproductive and developmental peculiarities of fish, such delayed toxicity effects should be common. One example is endocrine disruption which brought an awareness of the possibility of transgeneration effects as well as the fact that exposure during a restricted period of life can have long-term consequences, e.g., on sexual differentiation. Further, as discussed above, there exist a few studies reporting that short-term early life exposure of fish impaired parameters such as immune functions later in life. In this context, the possibility of epigenetic effects, i.e. heritable changes in gene expression and gene function without accompanying alterations in DNA sequence, has to be addressed – again an aspect that to date has attracted by far too little attention in ecotoxicology (Legler, 2010). Better understanding of delayed and transgenerational toxicity is not a matter of academic curiosity, but it has direct and practical implications for ecological risk assessment.

REFERENCES

Aegerter S, Jalabert B, Bobe J (2005) Large scale real time PCR analysis of mRNA abundance in rainbow trout eggs in relationship with egg quality and postovulatory ageing. *Mol Reprod Dev* **72:** 377–85.

Afonso LOB, Campbell PM, Iwama GK, Devlin RH, Donaldson EM (1997) The effect of the aromatase inhibitor fadrozole and two polynuclear aromatic hydrocarbons on sex steroid secretion by ovarian follicles of coho salmon. *Gen Comp Endocrinol* **106:** 169–74.

Andersen L, Goto-Kazeto R, Trant JM, Nash JP, Korsgaard B, Bjerregard P (2006) Short-term exposure to low concentrations of the synthetic androgen methyltestosterone affects vitellogenin and steroid levels in adult male zebrafish (*Danio rerio*). *Aquat Toxicol* **76:** 342–52.

Anderson MJ, Miller MR, Hinton DE (1996) In vivo modulation of 17β-estradiol-induced vitellogenin synthesis and estrogen receptor in rainbow trout (*Oncorhynchus mykiss*) liver cels by β-naphthoflavone. *Toxicol Appl Pharmacol* **137:** 210–17.

Andersson T, Förlin L, Olsen S, Fostier A, Breton B (1993) Pituitary as a target organ for the toxic effect of P4501A1-inducing chemicals. *Mol Cell Endocrinol* **91:** 99–105.

Ankley GT, Bencic DC, Breen MS, Collette TW, Conolly RB, Denslow ND, Edwards SW, Ekman DR, Garcia-Reyero N, Jensen KM, Lazorchak JM, Martinovic D, Miller DH, Perkins EJ, Orlando EF, Villeneuve dL, Wang RL, Watanabe KH (2009) Endocrine disrupting chemicals in fish: developing exposure indicators and predictive models of effects based on mechanisms of action. *Aquat Toxicol* **92:** 168–78.

Ankley GT, Jensen KM, Makynen EA, Kahl MD, Korte JJ, Hornung MW, Henry TR, Denny JS, Leino RL, Wilson VS, Cardon MC, Hartig PC, Gray EL (2003) Effects of the androgenic growth promoter 17beta-trenbolone on fecundity and reproductive endocrinology of the fathead minnow. *Environ Toxicol Chem* **22:** 1350–60.

Ankley GT, Johnson RD (2004) Small fish models for identifying and assessing the effects of endocrine disrupting chemicals. *ILAR J* **45:** 469–83.

Ankley GT, Kahl MD, Jensen KM, Hornung MW, Korte JJ, Makynen EA, Leino RL (2002) Evaluation of the aromatase inhibitor fadrozole in a short-term reproduction assay with the fathead minnow (*Pimephales promelas*). *Toxicol Sci* **67:** 121–30.

Ankley GT, Villeneuve DL (2006) The fathead minnow in aquatic toxicology: past, present and future. *Aquat Toxicol* **78:** 91–102.

Anulacion BF, Lomax DP, Bill DD, Johnson LL, Collier TK (1997) Assessment of anti-estrogenic activity in CYP1A induction in English sole exposed to environmental contaminants. Society of Environmental Toxicology and Chemistry (SETAC). 18th Annual Meeting; 16–20 November 1997, San Francisco. SETAC Press, Pensacola, FL, p. 137.

Antonopoulou E, Swanson P, Mayer I, Borg B (1999) Feedback control of gonadotropins in Atlantic salmon, *Salmo salar*, male parr. II Aromatase inhibitor and androgen effects. *Gen Comp Endocrinol* **114:** 142–50.

Baroiller JF, D'Cotta H (2001) Environment and sex determination in farmed fish. *Comp Biochem Physiol* **130C:** 399–409.

Belanger SE, Balon EK, Rawlings JM (2010) Saltatory ontogeny of fishes and sensitive early life stages for ecotoxicological tests. *Aquat Toxicol* **97:** 88–95.

Berishvili G, D'Cotta H, Baroiller JF, Segner H, Reinecke M (2006) Differential expression of IGF-I mRNA and peptide in the male and female gonad during early development of a bony fish, the tilapia *Oreochromis niloticus*. *Gen Comp Endocrinol* **146:** 204–10.

Bernanke J, Köhler HR (2008) The impact of environmental chemicals on wildlife vertebrates. *Rev Environ Contam Toxicol* **198:** 1–47.

Binder RL, Stegeman JJ (1984) Microsomal electron transport and xenobiotic monooxygenase activities during the embryonic period of development in the killifish, *Fundulus heteroclitus*. *Toxicol Appl Pharmacol* **73:** 432–43.

Bittner D, Bernet D, Wahli T, Segner H, Küng C, Largiader CR (2009) How normal is abnormal? Discrimination between deformations and natural variation in gonad morphology of European whitefish *Coregonus lavaretus*. *J Fish Biol* **74:** 1594–614.

Börjeson H, Norrgren L (1997) M/4 syndrome: a review of potential etiological factors. In *Chemically Induced Alterations in Functional Development and Reproduction of Fishes* (Rolland RM, Gilbertson M, Peterson RE, eds.). SETAC, Pensacola, USA, pp. 153–60.

Blazquez M, Zanuy S, Carillo M, Piferrer F (1998) Structural and functional effects of early exposure to estradiol 17β and 17α-ethynylestradiol on the gonads of the gonochoristic teleost *Dicentrachus labrax*. *Fish Physiol Biochem* **18:** 37–47.

Bobe J, Labbé C (2010) Egg and sperm quality in fish. *Gen Comp Endocrinol* **165:** 535–48.

Braunbeck T, Böttcher M, Hollert H, Kosmehl T, Lammer E, Leist E, Rudolf M, Seitz N (2005) Towards an alternative for the acute fish LC50 test in chemical assessment: the fish embryo toxicity test goes multi-species – an update. *ALTEX* **22:** 87–102.

Braunbeck T, Storch V, Bresch H (1990) Species-specific reaction of liver ultrastructure in zebrafish and trout after prolonged exposure to 4-chloroaniline. *Arch Environ Contam Toxicol* **19:** 405–18.

Bresch H, Beck H, Ehlermann D, Schlaszus H, Urbanek M (1990) A long-term toxicity tests comprising reproduction and growth of zebrafish with 4-chloroaniline. *Arch Environ Contam Toxicol* **19:** 419–37.

Bringolf RB, Belden JB, Summerfelt RC (2004) Effects of atrazine on fathead minnow in a short-term reproduction assay. *Environ Toxicol Chem* **23:** 1029–35.

Brion F, Tyler CR, Palazzi X, Laillet B, Porcher JM, Garric J, Flammarion P (2004) Impacts of 17β-estradiol, including environmentally relevant concentrations, on reproduction after exposure during embryo-larval, juvenile and adult life stages in zebrafish (*Danio rerio*). *Aquat Toxicol* **68:** 193–217.

Bugel SM, White SA, Cooper KR (2010) Impaired reproductive health of killifish (*Fundulus heteroclitus*) inhabiting Newark Bay, NJ, a chronically contaminated estuary. *Aquat Toxicol* **96:** 182–93.

Burdick GE, Dean HJ, Harris EJ, Skea J, Karcher R, Frisa C (1972) Effect of rate and duration of feeding on the reproduction of salmonid fishes reared and held under controlled conditions. *NY Fish Game J* **19:** 97–115.

Burdick GE, Harris EJ, Dean HJ, Walker TM, Skea J, Colby D (1964) The accumulation of DDT in lake trout and the effect on reproduction. *Trans Am Fish Soc* **93:** 127–36.

Caldwell DJ, Mastrocco F, Hutchinson, TH, Länge R, Heijerick D, Janssen C, Anderson PD, Sumpter JP (2008) Derivation of an aquatic predicted no-effect concentration for the synthetic hormone, 17α-ethinylestradiol. *Environ Sci Technol* **42:** 7046–54.

Callard G, Schlinger B, Pasmanik M (1990) Non-mammalian vertebrate models in studies of brain-steroid interactions. *J Exp Zool* **(Suppl. 4):** 6–16.

Calow P, Forbes VE (2003) Does ecotoxicology inform ecological risk assessment? *Environ Sci Technol* **37:** 146A–151A.

Carney SA, Peterson RE, Heideman W (2004) 2,3,7,8-tetrachlorodibenzo-p-dioxin activation of the aryl hydrocarbon receptor/aryl hydrocarbon receptor nuclear translocator pathway causes developmental toxicity through a CYP1A-independent mechanism in zebrafish. *Molec Pharmacol* **66:** 512–21.

Carney SA, Prasch AL, Heideman W, Peterson RE (2006) Understanding dioxin developmental toxicity using the zebrafih model. *Birth Defects Res A* **76:** 7–18.

Carnevali E (2007) Reproductive endocrinology and gamete quality. *Gen Comp Endocrinol* **153:** 273–4.

Carvan MJ, Heiden TK, Tomasiewicz H (2005) The utility of zebrafish as a model for toxicological research. In *Biochemistry and Molecular Biology of Fishes*, Vol. 6 (Mommsen TP, Moon TW, eds.). Elsevier, Amsterdam, pp. 3–41.

Casillas E, Misitano DA, Johnson LL, Rhodes SD, Collier TK, Stein JE, McCain BB, Varanasi U (1991) Inducibility of spawning and reproductive success of female English sole (*Parophrys vetulus*) from urban and non-urban areas of Puget Sound, Washington. *Mar Environ Res* **31:** 99–122.

Cheshenko K, Brion F, Le Page Y, Hinfray N, Pakdel F, Kah O, Segner H, Eggen RIL (2007) Expression of zebrafish aromatase *cyp19a* and *cyp19b* genes in response to the ligands of estrogen receptor and aryl hydrocarbon receptor. *Toxicol Sci* **96:** 255–67.

Cheshenko K, Pakdel F, Segner H, Kah O, Eggen RE (2008) Interference of endocrine disrupting chemicals with aromatase CYP19 expression or activity, and consequences for reproduction of teleost fish. *Gen Comp Endocrinol* **155:** 31–62.

Clelland E, Peng C (2009) Endocrine/paracrine control of zebrafish ovarian development. *Mol Cell Endocrinol* **312:** 45–52.

Coe TS, Hamilton PB, Hodgson D, Paull GC, Stevens JR, Sumner K, Tyler CR (2008) An environmental estrogen alters reproductive hierarchies disrupting sexual selection in group spawning fish. *Environ Sci Technol* **42:** 5020–5.

Cook PM, Robbins JA, Endicott DD, Lodge KB, Guiney PD, Walker MK, Zabel EW, Peterson RE (2003) Effects of aryl hydrocarbon receptor-mediated early life stage toxicity to lake trout populations in Lake Ontario during the 20th century. *Environ Sci Technol* **37:** 3864–77.

Couse JF, Korach KS (1999) Estrogen receptor null mice: what have we learned and where will they lead us? *Endocr Rev* **20:** 358–417.

Cross JN, Hose JE (1988) Evidence for impaired reproduction in white croaker (*Genyonemus lineatus*) from contaminated areas of Southern California. *Mar Environ Res* **24:** 185–8.

Deng J, Liu C, Yu L, Zhou B (2010) Chronic exposure to environmental levels of tribromophenol impairs zebrafish reproduction. *Toxicol Appl Pharmacol* **243:** 87–95.

Devlin RH, Nagahama Y (2002) Sex determination and sex differentiation in fish: an overview of genetic, physiological and environmental influences. *Aquaculture* **208:** 191–364.

Dong W, Wang L, Thornton C, Scheffler BE, Willett KL (2008) Benzo(a)pyrene decreases brain and ovarian aromatase mRNA expression in *Fundulus heteroclitus*. *Aquat Toxicol* **88:** 289–300.

Embry MR, Belanger SE, Braunbeck T, Galay-Burgos M, Halder M, Hinton DE, Leonard MA, Lillicrap A, Norberg-King T, Whale G (2010) The fish embryo toxicity test as an animal alternative method in hazard and risk assessment and scientific research. *Aquat Toxicol* **97:** 79–87.

Epel D (1998) Use of multidrug transporters as first line of defense against toxins in aquatic organisms. *Comp Biochem Physiol* **120A:** 23–8.

Fairbrother A, Ankley GT, Birnbaum LS, Bradbury SP, Francis B, Gray ET, Hinton DE, Johnson LL, Peterson RE, van der Kraak G (1999) Reproductive and developmental toxicology of contaminants in oviparous animals. In *Reproductive and Developmental Effects of Contaminants in Oviparous Vertebrates* (DiGiullio RT, Tillitt DE, eds.). SETAC Press, Pensacola, FL, USA, pp. 283–361.

Fenske M, Maack G, Schäfers C, Segner H (2005) An environmentally relevant concentration of ethinylestradiol induces arrest of male gonad development in zebrafish, *Danio rerio*. *Environ Toxicol Chem* **24:** 1088–98.

Fenske M, Segner H (2004) Aromatase modulation alters gonadal differentiation in developing zebrafish (*Danio rerio*). *Aquat Toxicol* **67:** 105–26.

Fishelson L (2003) Comparison of testes structure, spermatogenesis, and spermacytogenesis in young, aging and hybrid cichlid fish. *J Morphol* **256:** 285–300.

Folmr LC, Gardner GR, Schreibman MP, Magliulo-Cepnao L, Mills MJ, Zaroogian G, Gutjahr-Gobell R, Haebler R, Horowitz DB, Denslow ND (2001) Vitellogenin-induced pathology in male summer flounder (*Paralichthys dentatus*). *Aquat Toxicol* **51:** 431–41.

Förlin L, Haux C (1985) Increased excretion in the bile of 17β-3H-estradiol-derived radioactivity in rainbow trout treated with β-naphthoflavone. *Aquat Toxicol* **6:** 197–208.

Froehlicher M, Liedtke A, Groh KJ, Neuhauss SCF, Segner H, Eggen RI (2009) Zebrafish (*Danio rerio*) neuromast: promising biological endpoint linking developmental and toxicological studies. *Aquat Toxicol* **95:** 307–19.

Garcia-Reyero N, Kroll KJ, liu L, Orlando EF, Watanabe KH, Sepulveda MS, Villeneuve DL, Perkins EJ, Ankely GT, Denslow ND (2009) Gene expression responses in male fathead minnows exposed to binary mixtures of an estrogen and antiestrogen. *BMC Genomics* **10:** 308.

Ge W (2005) Intrafollicular paracrine communication in the zebrafish ovary: the state of the art of an emerging model for the study of vertebrate folliculogenesis. *Mol Cell Endocrinol* **237:** 1–10.

Giesy JP, Jones PD, Kannan K, Newsted JL, Tillitt DE, Williams LL (2002) Effects of chronic dietary exposure to environmentally relevant concentrations of 2,3,7,8-tetrachlorodibenzo-p-dioxin on survival, growth, reproduction and biochemical responses of female rainbow trout (*Oncorhynchus mykiss*). *Aquat Toxicol* **59:** 35–53.

Gimeno S, Komen H, Gerritsen AGM, Bowmer T (1998) Feminisation of young males of the common carp, *Cyprinus carpio*, exposed to 4-tert-pentylphenol during sexual differentiation. *Aquat Toxicol* **43:** 77–92.

Gleason TR, Nacci DE (2001) Risks of endocrine-disrupting compounds to wildlife: extrapolating from effects on individuals to population response. *Hum Ecol Risk Assess* **7:** 1027–42.

Goldsmith P (2004) Zebrafish as a pharmacological tool: the how, why, and when. *Curr Opin Pharmacol* **4:** 1–9

Gonzaelz A, Piferrer F (2003) Aromatase activity in the European sea bass (*Dicentrachus labrax*) brain. Distribution and changes in relation to age, sex and the annual reproductive cycle. *Gen Comp Endocrinol* **132:** 223–30.

Govoroun M, McMeel OM, D'Cotta H, Ricordel MJ, Smith T, Fostier A, Guiguen Y (2001) Steroid enzyme gene expressions during natural and androgen-induced gonadal differentiation in the rainbow trout, *Oncorhynchus mykiss*. *J Exp Zool* **290:** 558–66.

Gray MA, Niimi AJ, Metcalfe CD (1999) Factors affecting the development of testis–ova in medaka exposed to octylphenol. *Environ Toxicol Chem* **18:** 1835–42.

Grim KC, Wolfe M, Hawkins W, Johnson R, Wolf J (2007) Intersex in Japanese medaka (*Oryzias latipes*) used as negative controls in toxicological bioassays: a review of 54 cases from 41 studies. *Environ Toxicol Chem* **26:** 1636–43.

Grist EPM, Wells MC, Whitehouse P, Brighty G, Crane M (2003) Estimating the effects of 17alpha-ethynylestradiol on popuations of fathead minnow: are conventional toxicological endpoints adequate? *Environ Sci Technol* **27:** 1609–16.

Guiguen Y, Fostier A, Piferrer F, Chang CF (2010) Ovarian aromatase and estrogens: a pivotal role for gonadal sex differentiation and sex change in fish. *Gen Comp Endocrinol* **165:** 352–66.

Guiney PD, Smolowitz RM, Peterson RE, Stegeman JJ (1997) Correlation of 2,3,7,8-tetrachlorodibenzo-p-dioxin induction of cytochrome P4501A in vascular endothelium with toxicity in early life stages of lake trout. *Toxicol Appl Pharmacol* **143:** 256–73.

Gurney WSC (2006) Modeling the demographic impact of endocrine disruptors. *Environ Health Persp* **114 (Suppl. 1):** 122–6.

Hashimoto S, Watanabe E, Ikeda M, Tearo Y, Strüssmann CA, Inoue M, Hara A (2009) Effects of ethinylestradiol on medaka (*Oryzias latipes*) as measured by sperm motility and fertilization success. *Arch Environ Contam Toxicol* **56:** 253–9.

Hall CE (2008) Pattern formation. In *Fish Larval Physiology* (Finn RN, Kapoor BG, eds.). Science Publishers, Enfield (NH), pp. 3–26.

Hartley WR, Thiyagarajah A, Anderson MB, Broxson MW, Major SE, Zell SI (1998) Gonadal development in Japanese medaka (*Oryzias latipes*) exposed to 17β-estradiol. *Mar Environ Res* **46:** 145–8.

Heath AG (1995) *Water Pollution and Fish* Physiology, 2nd edition. Lewis Publishers, Boca Raton, FL.

Heiden TK, Hutz RJ, Carvan MJ (2005) Accumulation, tissue distribution and maternal transfer of dietary 2,3,7,8-tetrachlorodibenzo-p-dioxin; impacts on reproductive success of zebrafish. *Toxicol Sci* **87:** 497–502.

Heiden TK, Struble CA, Rise ML, Hessner MJ, Hutz RJ, Carvan MJ (2008) Molecular targets of 2,3,7,8-tetrachlorodibenzo-p-dioxin (TCDD) within the zebrafish ovary: insights into TCDD-induced endocrine disruption and reproductive toxicity. *Reprod Toxicol* **25:** 47–57.

Heldring N, Pike A, Andersson S (2007) Estrogen receptors: how do they signal and what are their targets? *Physiol Rev* **87:** 905–31.

Hill RL, Janz DM (2003) Developmental estrogenic exposure in zebrafish (*Danio rerio*). I. Effects on sex ratio and breeding success. *Aquat Toxicol* **63:** 417–29.

Hill AJ, Teraoka H, Heideman W, Peterson RE (2005) Zebrafish as a model vertebrate for investigating chemical toxicity. *Toxicol Sci* **86:** 6–19.

Hinfray N, Palluel O, Turies C, Cousin C, Porcher JM, Brion F (2006) Brain and gonadal aromatase as potential targets of endocrine disrupting chemicals in a model species, the zebrafish (*Danio rerio*). *Environ Toxicol* **21:** 332–7.

Hinton DE (1993) Cells, cellular responses and their markers in chronic toxicity of fishes. In *Aquatic Toxicology: Molecular, Biochemical and Cellular Perspectives* (Malins DC, Ostrander GK, eds.). Lewis Publishers, London, pp. 207–39.

Hiramatsu N, Cheek AO, Sullivan CV, Matsubara T, Hara A (2005) In *Environmental Toxicology. Biochemistry and Molecular Biology of Fishes*, Vol. 6 (Mommsen TP, Moon TW, eds.). Elsevier, Amsterdam, pp. 432–72.

Holbech H, Kinnberg K, Petersen GI, Jackson P, Hylland K, Norrgren L, Bjerregrad P (2006) Detection of endocrine disrupters: evaluation of a fish sexual development test (FSDT). *Comp Biochem Physiol* **144C:** 57–66.

Hontela A (1998) Interrenal dysfunction in fish from contaminated sites: in vivo and in vitro assessment. *Environ Toxicol Chem* **17:** 44–8.

Howley C, Ho RK (2000) mRNA localization patterns in zebrafish oocytes. *Mech Dev* **92:** 305–9.

Hutchinson T, Ankley GT, Segner H, Tyler CR (2006) Screening and testing for endocrine disruption in fish – biomarkers as "signposts" not "traffic lights" in risk assessment. *Environ Health Perspect* **114 (Suppl. 1):** 106–14.

Ingermann RL (2008) Energy metabolisms and respiration in fish spermatozo. In *Fish Spermatology* (Alavi SMH, Cosson JJ, Coward K, Raffiee G, eds.). Alpha Science International, Oxford, UK, pp. 241–66.

Jalabert B (2005) Particularities of reproduction and oogenesis in teleost fish compared to mammals. *Reprod Nutr Dev* **45:** 261–79.

Jalabert B, Baroiller JF, Breton B, Fostier A, Le Gac F, Guiguen Y, Monod G (2000) Main neuro-endocrine, endocrine and paracrine regulations of fish reproduction, and vulnerability to xenobiotics. *Ecotoxicology* **9:** 25–40.

Jensen KM, Kahl MD, Makynen EA, Korte JJ, Leino RL, Butterworth BC, Ankley GT (2004) Characterization of responses to the anti-androgen flutamide in a short-term reproduction assay with fathead minnow. *Aquat Toxicol* **70:** 99–110.

Jobling M (1995) *Environmental Biology of Fishes*. Chapman & Hall, London.

Jones JC, Reynolds JD (1997) Effect of pollution on reproductive behaviour of fishes. *Rev Fish Biol Fisheries* **7:** 463–91.

Kah O, Lethimonier C, Somoza G, Guilgur LG, Vaillant C, Lareye JJ (2007) GnRH and GnRH receptors in metazoan: a historical, comparative and evolutive perspective. *Gen Comp Endocrinol* **153:** 346–64.

Kallivretaki E, Eggen R, Neuhauss S, Alberti M, Kausch U, Segner H (2006) Aromatase in zebrafish: a potential target for endocrine disrupting chemicals. *Mar Environ Res* **62:** S187–S190.

Kallivretaki E, Eggen RIL, Neuhauss SCF, Kah O, Segner H (2007) The zebrafish brain-specific aromatase, *cyp19a2*, is neither expressed nor distributed in a sexually dimorphic manner during sexual differentiation. *Develop Dyn* **236:** 3155–66.

Kane DA, Kimmel CB (1993) The zebrafish midblastula transition. *Development* **119:** 447–56.

Kang IK, Yokota H, Oshima Y, Tsuruda Y, Oe T, Imada N, Tadokoro H, Honjo T (2002) Effects of bisphenol A on the reproduction of Japanese medaka (*Oryzias latipes*). *Environ Toxicol Chem* **21:** 2394–400.

Kang IK, Yokota H, Oshima Y, Tsuruda Y, Hano T, Maeda M, Imada N, Tadokoro H, Honjo T (2003) Effects of 4-nonylphenol on the reproduction of Japanese medaka (*Oryzias latipes*). *Environ Toxicol Chem* **22:** 2438–45.

Khan IA, Thomas P (1996) Melatonin influences gonadotropin II secretion in the Atlantic croaker, *Micropogonias undulatus*. *Gen Comp Endocrinol* **104:** 231–42.

Khan IA, Thomas P (1999) Ovarian cycle in teleost fish. In *Fish Physiology* (Knobil E, Neil JD, eds.). Academic Press, New York, pp. 552–64.

Kime DE (1998) *Endocrine Disruption in Fish*. Kluwer Academic Publishers, Boston.

Kinnberg K, Holbech H, Petersen GI, Bjerregard P (2007) Effects of the fungicide prochloraz on the sexual development of zebrafish (*Danio rerio*). *Comp Biochem Physiol* **145C:** 165–70.

Kirby MF, Smith AJ, Rooke J, Neall P, Scott AP, Katsiadaki I (2007) Ethoxyresorufin-O-deethylase (EROD) and vitellogenin (VTG) in flounder (*Platichtyhs flesus*): system interaction, crosstalk and implications for monitoring. *Aquat Toxicol* **81:** 233–44.

Kishida M, Mclellan M, Miranda JA, Callard GV (2001) Estrogen and xenoestrogens upregulate the brain aromatase isoform (P450aromB) and perturb markers of early development in zebrafish (*Danio rerio*). *Comp Biochem Physiol* **129B:** 261–8.

Kjesbu OS, Solemdal P, Bratland P, Fonn M (1996) Variation in annual egg production in individual captive Atlantic cod, *Gadus morhua*. *Can J Fish Aquat Sci* **53:** 610–20.

Kjorsvik E, Mangorjensen A, Holmefjord I (1990) Egg quality in fishes. *Adv Mar Biol* **26:** 71–113.

Kobayashi M, Aida K, Hanyu I (1988) Hormone changes during the ovulatory cycle in goldfish. *Gen Comp Endocrinol* **69:** 301–7.

Kobayashi T, Nakamura M, Kajiura-Kobayashi H, Young G, Nagahama Y (1998) Immunolocalization of steroidogenic enzymes (P450scc, P450c17, P450arom, and 3beta-HSD) in immature and mature testes of rainbow trout (*Oncorhynchus mykiss*). *Cell Tiss Res* **292:** 573–7.

Koger CS, Teh SJ, Hinton DE (2000) Determining the sensitive developmental stages of intersex induction in medaka (*Oryzias latipes*) exposed to 17β-estradiol or testosterone. *Mar Environ Res* **50:** 201–6.

Kooijman SALM (1998) Process-oriented descriptions of toxic effects. In *Ecotoxicology – Ecological Fundamentals, Chemical Exposure and Biological Effects* (Schüürmann G, Markert B, eds.). John Wiley & Sons/Spektrum Akademischer Verlag, New York/Heidelberg, pp. 483–520.

Koponen K, Lindström-Seppä P, Kukkonen JVK (2000) Accumulation pattern and biotransfromation enzyme induction in rainbow trout embryos exposed to sublethal aqueous concentrations of 3,3′,4,4′-tetrachlorbiphenyl. *Chemosphere* **40:** 245–53.

Kortner TM, Arukwe A (2007) The xenoestrogen, 4-nonylphenol, impaired steroidogenesis in previtellogenic oocyte culture of Atlantic cod (*Gadus morhua*) by targeting the StAR protein and P450scc expression. *Gen Comp Endocrinol* **150:** 419–29.

Kuhl AJ, Brouwer M (2006) Antiestrogens inhibit xenoestrogen-induced brain aromatase activity but do not prevent xenoestrogen-induced feminization in Japanese medaka (*Oryzias latipes*). *Environ Health Persp* **114:** 500–6.

Kurokawa H, Saito D, Nakamura S, Katoh-Fukui Y, Ohta K, Baba T, Morohashi KI, Tanaka M (2007) Germ cells are essential for sexual dimorphism in the medaka gonad. *Proc Natl Acad Sci USA* **104:** 16958–63.

Kwok HF, So WK, Wang Y, Ge W (2005) Zebrafish gonadotropins and their receptors. I. Cloning and characterization of zebrafish follicle-stimulating hormone and luteinizing hormone receptors – evidence for their distinct functions in follicle development. *Biol Reprod* **72:** 1370–81.

Larsen MG, Bilberg K, Baatrup E (2009) Reversibility of estrogenic sex changes in zebrafish (*Danio rerio*). *Environ Toxicol Chem* **28:** 1783–5.

Larsen MG, Hansen KB, Henriksen PG, Baatrup E (2008) Male zebrafish (*Danio rerio*) courtship behaviour resists the feminising effects of 17α-ethinylestradiol – morphological sexual characteristics do not. *Aquat Toxicol* **87:** 234–44.

Lawrence C, Ebersole JP, Kesseli RV (2008) Rapid growth and out-crossing promote female development in zebrafish. *Environ Biol Fish* **81:** 239–46.

Leatherland JF (2000) Contaminant-altered thyroid function in wildlife. In *Environmental Endocrine Disrupters. An Evolutionary Perspective* (Giulette L, Cairns DA, eds.). Taylor & Francis, New York, pp. 155–81.

LeGac F, Loir M, LeBail PY, Ollitrault M (1996) Insulin-like growth factor (IGF-I) mRNA and IGF-I receptor in trout testis and in isolated spermatogenic and Sertoli cells. *Molec Reprod Develop* **44:** 23–35.

Legler J (2010) Epigenetics: an emerging field in environmental toxicology. *Integr Environ Assessm Manag* **6:** 314–15.

Leino RL, Jensen KM, Ankley GTR (2005) Gonadal histiology and characteristic histopathology associated with endocrine disruption in the adult fathead minnow (*Pimephales promelas*). *Environ Toxicol Pharmacol* **19:** 85–98.

Li D, Lu C, Wang J, Cao Z, Sun D, Xia H, Ma X (2009) Developmental mechanisms of arsenite toxicity in zebrafish (*Danio rerio*) embryos. *Aquat Toxicol* **91:** 229–337.

Loomis AK, Thomas P (2000) Effects of estrogens and xenoetsrogens on androgen production by Atlantic croajer testes in vitro: evidence for a nongenomic action mediated by an estrogen membrane receptor. *Biol Reprod* **62:** 995–1004.

Lubzens E, Young G, Bobe J, Cerda J (2010) Oogenesis in teleosts: how fish eggs are formed. *Gen Comp Endocrinol* **165:** 367–89.

Maack G, Segner H (2003) Morphological development of the gonads of zebrafish. *J Fish Biol* **62:** 895–906.

Maack G, Segner H (2004) Life stage-dependent sensitivity of zebrafish (*Danio rerio*) to estrogen exposure. *Comp Biochem Physiol* **139C:** 47–55.

Matsuoka MP, van Nes S, Andersen O, Benfey TJ, Reith M (2006) Real time PCR analysis of ovary- and brain-type aromatase gene expression during Atlantic halibut (*Hippoglossus hippoglosus*) development. *Comp Biochem Physiol* **144B:** 128–35.

McAllister BG, Kime DE (2003) Life exposure to environmental levels of the aromatase inhibitor tributyltin causes masculinisation and irreversible sperm damage in zebrafish (*Danio rerio*). *Aquat Toxicol* **65:** 309–16.

McLachlan JA (2001) Environmental signaling: what embryos and evolution teach us about endocrine disrupting chemicals. *Endocr Rev* **22:** 319–41.

McNabb A, Schreck C, Tyler CR, Thomas P, Kramer V, Specker J, Mayes M, Selcer K (1999) Basic physiology. In *Reproductive and Developmental Effects of Contaminants in Oviparous Vertebrates* (DiGiulio RT, Tillitt DE, eds.). SETAC Press, Pensacola (FL), pp. 113–222.

Melo AC, Ramsdell JS (2001) Sexual dimorphism of brain aromatase activity in medaka: induction of a female phenotype by estradiol. *Environ Health Persp* **109:** 257–64.

Melvin SD, Munkittrick KR, Bosker T, MacLatchy DL (2009) Detectable effect size and bioassay power of mummichog (*Fundulus heteroclitus*) and fathead minnow (*Pimephales promelas*) adult reproductive tests. *Environ Toxicol Chem* **28:** 2416–25.

Menuet A, Anglade I, Le Guevel R, Pellegrini E, Pakdel F, Kah O (2003) Distribution of aromatase mRNA and protein in the brain and pituitary of female rainbow trout: comparison with estrogen receptor alpha. *J Comp Neurol* **462:** 180–93.

Miller M (1993) Maternal transfer of organochlorine compounds in salmonines to their eggs. *Can J Fish Aquat Sci* **50:** 1405–15.

Milston RH, Fitzpatrick MS, Vella AT, Clements S, Gundersen D, Feist G, Crippen TL, Leong J, Schreck CB (2003) Short-term exposure of chinook salmon (*Oncorhynchus tshawytscha*) to o,p′-DDE or DMSO during early life history stages causes long-term humoral immunosuppression. *Environ Health Persp* **111:** 1601–7.

Modig C, Westerlund L, Olson PE (2007) Oocyte zona pellucida proteins. In *The Fish Oocyte: From Basic Studies to Biotechnological Applications* (Babin CJ, Cerda J, Lubzens E, eds.). Springer, Dordrecht, NL, pp. 113–39.

Mommsen T, Korsgaard B (2008) Vitellogenesis. In *Fish Reproduction* (Rocha MJ, Arukew A, Kapoor BG, eds.). Science Publishers, Enfield, pp. 1–36.

Morisawa M (1994) Cell signalling mechanisms for sperm motility. *Zool Sci* **11:** 647–62.

Mullins M, Nüsslein-Volhard C (1993) Mutational approaches to studying embryonic pattern formation in the zebrafish. *Curr Opin Genet Develop* **3:** 648–54.

Nagler JJ, Cavileer T, Sullivan J, Cyr DG, Rexroad C (2007) The complete nuclear estrogen receptor family in the rainbow trout: discovery of the novel ERα2 and both ERβ isoforms. *Gene* **392:** 164–73.

Nakayama K, Oshima Y, Yamaguchi T, Tsuruda Y, Kang IJ, Kobayashi M, Imada N, Honjo T (2004) Fertilization success and sexual behaviour in male medaka, *Oryzias latipes*, exposed to tributyltin. *Chemosphere* **55:** 1331–7.

Nash JP, Kime DE, van der Ven LT, Wester PW, Brion F, Maack G, Stahlschmid-Allner P, Tyler CR (2004) Long-term exposure to environmental concentrations of the pharmaceutical ethynylestradiol causes reproductive failure in zebrafish. *Environ Health Perspect* **112:** 1725–33.

Navas JM, Anglade I, Bailhache T, Pakdel F, Breton B, Jego P, Kah O (1995) Do gonadotropin-releasing hormone neurons express estrogen receptors in the rainbow trout? A double immunohistochemical study. *J Comp Neurol* **363:** 461–74.

Navas J, Segner (1998) Antiestrogenic activity of anthropogenic and natural chemicals. *Environ Sci Poll Res* **5:** 72–81.

Navas JM, Segner H (2000) Antiestrogenicity of β-naphthoflavone and PAHs in cultured rainbow trout hepatocytes: evidence for a role of the arylhydrocarbon receptor. *Aquat Toxicol* **51:** 79–92.

Navas JM, Zanuy S, Segner H, Carillo M (2004) β-naphthoflavone alters normal plasma levels of vitellogenin, 17β-estradiol and luteinizing hormone in sea bass broodstock. *Aquat Toxicol* **67:** 337–45.

Newman MC (1998) *Fundamentals of Ecotoxicology*. Sleeping Bear/Ann Arbor Press, Chelsea, USA.

Newman MC (2001) *Population Ecotoxicology*. John Wiley & Sons, New York.

Niimi AK (1983) Biological and toxicological effects of environmnetal contaminants in fish and their eggs. *Can J Fish Aquat Sci* **40:** 303–10.

Nimrod AC, Benson WH (1997) Xenobiotic interaction with and alteration of channel catfish estrogen receptor. *Toxicol Appl Pharmacol* **147:** 381–90.

Nimrod AC, Benson WH (1998) Reproduction and development of Japanese medaka following an early life stage exposure to xenoestrogens. *Aquat Toxicol* **44:** 141–56.

OECD (2008) *Detailed review paper on fish life-cycle tests*. Series on Testing and Assessment, No. 95, Paris.

Oern S, Yamani S, Norrgren L (2006) Comparison of vitellogenin induction, sex ratio, and gonad morphology between zebrafish and Japanese medaka after exposure to 17alpha-ethinylestradiol and 17beta-trenbolone. *Arch Environ Contam Toxicol* **51:** 237–43.

Okubo K, Nagahama Y (2008) Structural and functional evolution of gonadotropin-releasing hormone in vertebrates. *Acta Physiol (Oxf)* **193:** 3–15.

Okuzawa K (2002) Puberty in teleosts. *Fish Physiol Biochem* **26:** 31–41.

Okuzawa K, Gen K, Bruysters M, Bogerd J, Gothilf Y, Zohar Y, Kagawa H (2003) Seasonal variation of the three native gonadotropin-releasing hormone messenger ribonucleic acid levels in the brain of red seabream. *Gen Comp Endocrinol* **130:** 324–32.

Orban L, Sreenivasan R, Olsson PE (2009) Long and winding roads: testis differentiation in zebrafish. *Mol Cell Endocrinol* **312:** 35–41.

Ortiz-Delgado JB, Sarasquete C, Behrens A, Gonzalez de Canales ML, Segner H (2002) Expression, cellular distribution and inducibility of cytochrome P4501A (CYP1A) in gilthead seabream, *Sparus aurata*, brain. *Aquat Toxicol* **60:** 269–83.

Ostrach DJ, Low-Marchelli JM, Eder KJ, Whiteman SJ, Zinkl JG (2008) Maternal transfer of xenobiotics and effects on larval striped bas in the San Francisco estuary. *Proc Natl Acad Sci USA* **105:** 19354–9.

Ottinger CA, Kaatari SL (2000) Long-term immune dysfunction in rainbow trout (*Oncorhynchus mykiss*) exposed as embryos to aflatoxin B_1. *Fish Shellfish Immunol* **10:** 101–6.

Oxendine SL, Cowden J, Hinton DE, Padilla S (2006) Vulnerable windows for developmental toxicity in the Japanese medaka fish (*Oryzias latipes*). *Aquat Toxicol* **80:** 396–404.

Panter GH, Hutchinson TH, Hurd KS, Bamforth J, Stanley RD, Dufell S, Hargreaves A, Gimeno S, Tyler CR (2006) Development of chronic tests for endocrine active chemicals. Part I. An extended fish early life stage test for oestrogenic active chemicals in the fathead minnow. *Aquat Toxicol* **77:** 279–90.

Panter GH, Hutchinson TH, Hurd KS, Bamforth J, Stanley RD, Wheeler JR, Tyler CR (2010) Effects of a weak oestrogenic active chemical (4-*tert*-pentylphenol) on pair-breeding and F1 development in the fathead minnow (*Pimephales promelas*). *Aquat Toxicol* **97:** 314–23.

Papoulias DM, Noltie DB, Tillitt DE (1999) An in vivo model fish system to test chemical effects on sexual differentiation and development: exposure to ethynyl estradiol. *Aquat Toxicol* **48:** 37–50.

Papoulias DM, Villalobos SA, Meadows J, Noltie DB, Giesy JP, Tillitt DE (2003) In ovo exposure to o,p-DDE affects sexual development but not sexual differentiation in Japanese medaka (*Oryzias latipes*). *Environ Health Persp* **111:** 29–32.

Parhar IS (1997) GnRH in tilapia: three genes, three origins and their roles. In *GnRH Neurons: Gene to behaviour* (Parhar IS, Sakuma Y, eds.). Brain Shuppan, Tokyo, pp. 99–122.

Patiño R, Takashima F (1995) Gonads. In *An Atlas of Fish Histology. Normal and Pathologic Features*, 2nd edition (Takashima F, Hibiya T, eds). Kodansha Ltd, Tokyo, Gustav Fischer Verlag Stuttgart, New York, pp. 128–53.

Patisaul AB, Adewale HB (2009) Long-term effects of environmental endocrine disruptors on reproductive physiology and behavior. *Front Behav Neurosci* **3:** 10.

Paull GC, van Look KJ, Santos EM, Filby AL, Gray DM, Nash JP, Tyler CR (2008) Variability in measures of reproductive success in laboratory-kept colonies of zebrafish and implications for studies addressing population-level effects of environmental chemicals. *Aquat Toxicol* **87:** 115–26.

Pawloski S, van Aerle R, Tyler CR, Braunbeck T (2004) Effects of 17alpha-ethinylestradiol in a fathead minnow (*Pimephales promelas*) gonadal recrudescence assay. *Ecotox Environ Safety* **57:** 330–45.

Pellegrini E, Mouriet K, Anglade I, Menuet A, Le Page Y, Guguen MM, Marmignon MH, Brion F, Pakdel F, Kah O (2007) Identification of aromatase-positive radial glial cells as progenitor cells in the ventricular layer of the forebrain in zebrafish. *J Comp Neurol* **501:** 150–67.

Peters REM, Courtenay SC, Capamgan S, Hewitt ML, MacLatchy DL (2007) Effects on reproductive potential and endocrine status in the mummichog (*Fundulus heteroclitus*) after exposure to 17alpha-ethinylestradiol in a short-term reproductive assay. *Aquat Toxicol* **85:** 154–66.

Peterson RE, Theobald HM, Kimmel GL (1993) Developmental and reproductive toxicity of dioxins and related compounds. *Crit Rev Toxicol* **23:** 283–335.

Petkam R, Renaud RL, Leatherland JF (2003) The role of CYP1A1 in the in vitro metabolisms of pregnenolone by the liver of rainbow trout embryos. *Comp Biochem Physiol* **135C:** 277–84.

Piferrer F (2001) Endocrine sex control strategies for the feminization of fish. *Aquaculture* **197:** 229–81.

Pocar P, Fischer B, Klonisch T, Hombach-Klonisch S (2005) Molecular interactions of the aryl hydrocarbon receptor and its biological and toxicological relevance for reproduction. *Reproduction* **129:** 379–89.

Rahman RS, Thomas P (2009) Molecular cloning, characterization and expression of two tryptophan hydroxylase (TPH-1 and TPH-2) genes in the hypothalamus of Atlantic croaker: down-regulation after chronic exposure to hypoxia. *Neuroscience* **158:** 751–65.

Raz E (2003) Primordial germ cell development: the zebrafish perspective. *Nature Rev Genetics* **4:** 690–700.

Rocha MJ, Rocha E (2006) Morphofunctional aspects of reproduction from synchronous to asynchronous fishes – an overview. In *Fish Endocrinology*, Vol. 2 (Reinecke M, Zaccone G, Kapoor BG, eds.). Science Publishers, Enfield (NH), pp. 571–663.

Rodriguez-Mari A, Yan YL, Miller RA, Wilson C, Canestro C, Postlethwait JH (2005) Characterization and expression pattern of zebrafish anti-Müllerian hormone (amh) relative to sox9a, sox9b, and cyp19a1a, during gonad development. *Gene Expr Pattern* **5:** 655–67.

Rolland RM (2000) Ecoepidemiology of the effects of pollution on reproduction and survival of early life stages in teleosts. *Fish Fisheries* **1:** 41–72.

Rosenthal H, Alderdice DF (1976) Sublethal effects of environmental stressors, natural and pollutional, on marine fish eggs and larvae. *J Fish Res Board Can* **33:** 2047–65.

Rurangwa E, Roelants I, Huskens G, Ebrahimi M, Kime DE, Ollevier F (1998) The minimum effective spermatozoa to egg ratio for artificial insemination and the effects of mercury on sperm motility and fertilization ability in the African catfish (*Clarius gariepinus*). *J Fish Biol* **53:** 402–13.

Sabo-Attwood T, Blum JL, Kroll KJ, Patel V, Birkholz D, Szabo NJ, Fisher SZ, McKenna R, Campbell-Thompson M, Denslow ND (2007) Distinct expression and activity profiles of largemouth bass (*Micropterus salmoides*) estrogen receptors in response to estradiol and nonylphenol. *J Molec Endocrinol* **39:** 223–37.

Salierno JD, Kane AS (2009) 17α-ethinylestradiol alters reproductive behaviours, circulating horones, and sexual morphology in male fathead minnows (*Pimephales promelas*). *Environ Toxicol Chem* **28:** 953–61.

Schäfers C, Teigeler M, Wenzel A, Maack G, Fenske M, Segner H (2007) Concentration- and time-dependent effects of the synthetic estrogen, 17α-ethynylestradiol, on reproductive capabilities of the zebrafish, *Danio rerio*. *J Toxicol Environ Health A* **70:** 768–79.

Scholz S, Mayer I (2008) Molecular biomarkers of endocrine disruption in small model fish. *Mol Cell Endocrinol* **293:** 57–70.

Schulz RW, Boger J, Goos HJTh (2000) Spermatogenesis and its endocrine regulation. In *Reproductive Physiology of Fish* (Norberg B, Kjesbu OS, Taranger GL, Andersson E, Stefansson SO, eds.). University of Bergen, Bergen, Norway, pp. 225– 32.

Schulz RW, Boger J, Male R, Ball J, Fenske M, Olsen LC, Tyler CR (2007) Estrogen-induced alterations in *amh* and *dmrt1* expression signal for disruption in male sexual development in the zebrafish. *Environ Sci Technol* **41:** 6305–10.

Segner H (2005) Developmental, reproductive, and demographic alterations in aquatic wildlife: establishing causality between exposure to endocrine-active compounds (EACs) and effects. *Acta Hydrochim Hydrobiol* **33:** 17–26.

Segner H (2007) Ecotoxicology – how to assess the impact of toxicants in a multifactorial environment. In *Multiple Stressors: A Challenge for the Future* (Mothersill C, Mosse I, Seymour C, eds). NATO Advanced Workshop, Environmental Security. Springer, Heidelberg–New York, pp. 39–56.

Segner H, Eppler E, Reinecke M (2006) The impact of environmental hormonally active substances on the endocrine and immune systems of fish. In *Fish Endocrinology* (Reinecke M, Zaccone G, Kapoor BG, eds.). Science Publishers, Enfield (NH), pp. 809–65.

Segner H, Rösch R, Verreth J, Witt U (1993) Larval nutritional physiology: studies with *Coregonus lavaretus*, *Clarias gariepinus* and *Scophthalmus maximus*. *J World Aquacult Soc* **24:** 121–34.

Segner H, Storch V, Reinecke M, Kloas W, Hanke W (1994) The development of functional digestive and metabolic organs in turbot, *Scophthalmus maximus*. *Mar Biol* **119:** 471–86.

Seki M, Fujishima S, Nozaka T, Maeda M, Kobayashi K (2006) Comparison of responses to 17beta-estradiol and 17beta-trenbolone among three small fish species. *Environ Toxicol Chem* **25:** 2742–52.

Seki M, Yokota H, Matsubara H, Tsuruda Y, Maeda M, Tadokoro H, Kobayashi K (2002) Effect of ethinylestradiol on the reproduction and induction of vitellogenin and testis–ova in medaka (*Oryzias latipes*). *Environ Toxicol Chem* **21:** 1692–8.

Seki M, Yokota H, Matsubara H, Maeda M, Tadokoro H, Kobayashi K (2003) Fish full life-cycle testing for the weak estrogen 4-*tert*-pentylphenol on medaka (*Oryzias latipes*). *Environ Toxicol Chem* **22:** 1487–96.

Seki M, Yokota H, Matsubara H, Maeda M, Tadokoro H, Kobayashi K (2004) Fish full life-cycle testing for androgen methyltestosterone on medaka (*Oryzias latipes*). *Environ Toxicol Chem* **23:** 774–81.

Seki M, Yokota H, Maeda M, Kobayashi K (2005) Fish full life-cycle testing for 17beta-estradiol on medaka (*Oryzias latipes*). *Environ Toxicol Chem* **24:** 1259–66.

Selman S, Wallace RA, Sarka A, Qi X (1993) Stages of oocyte development in the zebrafish, *Brachydanio rerio*. *J Morphol* **218:** 203–24.

Shang EHH, Yu RMK, Wu RSS (2006) Hypoxia affects sex differentiation and development, leading to a male-dominated population in zebrafish (Danio rerio). *Environ Sci Technol* **40:** 3118–22.

Sharpe RL, MacLatchy DL, Courtenay SC, van der Kraak GL (2004) Effetcs of a model androgen (methyl testosterone) and a model anti-androgen (cyproterone actetate) on reproductive endocrine endpoints in a short-term adult mummichog (*Fundulus heteroclitus*) bioassay. *Aquat Toxicol* **67:** 203–15.

Shimasaki Y, Kitano T, Oshima Y, Inoue S, Imada N, Honjo T (2003) Tributyltin causes masculinization in fish. *Environ Toxicol Chem* **22:** 141–4.

Shioda T, Wakabayashi M (2000) Effect of certain chemicals on the reproduction of medaka (*Oryzias latipes*). *Chemosphere* **40:** 239–43.

Siegfried KR, Nüsslein-Volhard C (2008) Germ line control of female sex differentiation in zebrafish. *Dev Biol* **324:** 277–87.

Slanchev K, Stebler J, de la Cueva-Mendez G, Raz E (2005) Development without germ cells: the role of the germ line in zebrafish sex differentiation. *Proc Natl Acad Sci USA* **102:** 4074–9.

Spies RW, Rice JWD (1988) Effects of contaminants on reproduction of starry flounder, *Platichthys stellatus*, in San Francisco Bay, California. II. Reproductive success of fish captured in San Francisco Bay and spawned in the laboratory. *Mar Biol* **98:** 191–200.

Spitsbergen JM, Kent ML (2003) The state of the art of the zebrafish model for toxicology and toxicopathology research – advantages and current limitations. *Toxicol Pathol* **31 (Suppl.):** 62–87.

Spitsbergen JM, Walker MK, Olson JR, Peterson RE (1991) Pathologic lesions in early life stages of lake trout, *Salvelinus namaycush*, exposed to 2,3,7,8-tetrachlorodibenzo-p-dioxin as fertilized eggs. *Aquat Toxicol* **19:** 41–72.

Strüssmann CA, Nakamura M (2002) Morphology, endocrinology, and environmental modulation of gonadal sex differentiation in teleost fishes. *Fish Physiol Biochem* **26:** 13–29.

Sumpter JP, Johnson AP (2006) Lessons from endocrine disruption and their applications to other issues concerning trace organics in the aquatic environment. *Environ Sci Technol* **39:** 4321–32.

Takahashi H (1977) Juvenile hermaphroditism in the zebrafish, *Brachydanio rerio*. *Bull Fac Fish Hokkaido Univ* **28:** 57–65.

Teitsma CA, Anglade I, Lethimonier C, Le Drean G, Saligaut D, Ducouret B, Kah O (1999) Glucocorticoid receptor immunoreactivity in neurons and pituitary cells implicated in reproductive functions in rainbow trout: a double immunohistochemical study. *Biol Reprod* **60:** 642–50.

Thomas P, Doughty K (2004) Disruption of rapid, nongenomic steroid actions by environmental chemicals: interference with progestim stimulation of sperm motility in Atlantic croaker. *Environ Sci Technol* **38:** 6328–32.

Thomas P, Rahman MS, Khan IA, Kummer JA (2007) Widespread endocrine disruption and reproductive impairment in an estuarine fish population exposed to seasonal hypoxia. *Proc R Soc B* **274:** 2693–701.

Tiedeken JA, Ramsdell JS (2007) Embryonic exposure to domoic acid increases the susceptibility of zebrafish larvae to the chemical convulsant pentylenetetrazole. *Environ Health Persp* **115:** 1547–52.

Tilton F, Du JKL, Tanguay RL (2008) Sulfhydryl systems are a critical factor in the zebrafish developmental toxicity of the dithiocarbamate sodium metam. *Aquat Toxicol* **90:** 121–7.

Trant JM, Gavasso S, Ackers J, Chung BC, Place AR (2001) Developmental expression of cytochrome P450 aromatase genes (CYP19a and CYP19b) in zebrafish fry (*Danio rerio*). *J Exp Zool* **290:** 475–83.

Tsai MJ, O'Malley BW (1994) Molecular mechanisms of action of steroid/thyroid receptor superfamily members. *Annu Rev Biochem* **63:** 451–86.

Tyler CR, Jobling S, Sumpter JP (1998) Endocrine disruption in wildlife: a critical review of evidence. *Crit Rev Toxicol* **28:** 319–61.

Tyler CR, Sumpter JP (1996) Oocyte growth and development in teleosts. *Rev Fish Biol* **6:** 287–318.

US EPA (1996) *Ecological Effects Test Guidelines*. Office of Prevention, Pesticides and Toxic Substances 850.1500. Fish life-cycle toxicity. EPA 712–C-96-122. Washington DC.

Van Aerle R, Pounds N, Hutchinson TR, Maddix S, Tyler CR (2002) Window of sensitivity for the estrogenic effects of ethynylestradiol in early life stages of fathead minnow, *Pimephales promelas*. *Ecotoxicology* **11:** 423–34.

Van Aerle R, Runnals TJ, Tyler CR (2004) Ontogeny of gonadal sex development relative to growth in fathead minnow. *J Fish Biol* **64:** 355–69.

Van den Belt K, Verheyen R, Witters H (2001) Reprodctive effects of ethinylestradiol and 4-t-octylphenol on the zebrafish. *Arch Environ Contam Toxicol* **41:** 458–67.

Van den Hurk R, Lambert JGD, Peute J (1982) Steroidogenesis in the gonads of rainbow trout (*Salmo gairdneri*) fry before and after the onset of gonadal sex differentiation. *Reprod Nutr Dev* **22:** 413–25.

Van der Kraak G, Chang JP, Janz DM (1997) Reproduction. In *The Physiology of Fishes*, 2nd edition (Evans DH, ed.). CRC Press, Boca Raton, pp. 465–88.

van der Kraak GL, Munkittrick KR, McMaster ME, Portt CB, Chang JP (1992) Exposure to bleached kraft pulp mill effluent disrupts the pituitary–gonadal axis of white sucker at multiple sites. *Toxicol Appl Pharmacol* **115:** 224–33.

Van der Ven LTM, van den Brandhof EJ, Vos JH, Wester PW (2007) Effects of the estrogen agonist 17beta-estradiol and antagonist tamoxifen in a partial life-cycle assay with zebrafish (*Danio rerio*). *Environ Toxicol Chem* **26:** 92–9.

Van der Ven LTM, Wester PW, Vos JG (2003) Histopathology as a tool for the evaluation of endocrine disruption in zebrafish (*Danio rerio*). *Environ Toxicol Chem* **22:** 908–13.

Vermeirssen ELM, Burki R, Joris C, Peter A, Segner H, Suter M, Burkhardt-Holm P (2005) Characterization of the estrogenicity of Swiss midland rivers using recombinant yeast bioassay and plasma vitellogenin concentration of feral male brown trout. *Environ Toxicol Chem* **24:** 2226–33.

Villeneuve DL, Knoebl I, Kahl MD, Jensen KM, Hammermeister DE, Greene KJ, Blake LS, Ankley GT (2006) Relationship between brain and ovary aromatase activity and isoform-specific aromatase mRNA expression in the fathead minnow (*Pimephales promelas*). *Aquat Toxicol* **76:** 353–68.

Villeneuve DL, Larkin P, Knoebl I, Miracle AL, Kahl MD, Jensen KM, Makynen EA, Durhan EI, Carter BI, Denslow ND, Ankley GT (2007) A graphical systems model to facilitate hypothesis-driven ecotoxicogenomics research on the teleost brain–pituitary–gonadal axis. *Environ Sci Technol* **41:** 321–30.

Volz DC, Hinton DE, Law JM, Kullman SW (2006) Dynamic gene expression changes precede dioxin-induced liver pathogenesis in medaka fish. *Toxicol Sci* **85:** 572–84.

Volz DC, Kullman SW, Howarth DL, Hardman RC, Hinton DE (2008) Protective response of the Ah receptor to ANIT-induced biliary epithelial cell toxicity in see-through medaka. *Toxicol Sci* **102:** 262–77.

Von Hofsten J, Olsson PE (2005) Zebrafish sex determination and differentiation: involvment of FTZ-FI genes. *Reprod Biol Endocrinol* **3:** 63.

Vos JG, Dybing E, Greim HA, Ladefoged O, Lambre C, Tarazona JV, Brandt I, Vethaak AD (2000) Health effects of endocrine-disrupting chemicals on wildlife, with special reference to the European situation. *Crit Rev Toxicol* **30:** 71–133.

Vuori KA, Nordlund E, Kallio J, Salakoski T, Nikinmaa M (2008) Tissue specific expression of aryl hydrocarbon receptor and putative developmental regulatory modules in Baltic salmon yolk-sac fry. *Aquat Toxicol* **87:** 19–27.

Walker MK, Cook PM, Batterman AR, Butterworth BC, Berini C, Libal JJ, Hufnagle LC, Peterson RE (1994) Translocation of 2,3,7,8-tetrachlorodibenzo-p-dioxin (TCDD) from adult female lake trout (*Salvelinus namaycush*) to oocytes: effects on early life stage development and sac fry survival. *Can J Fish Aquat Sci* **51:** 1410–19.

Walker MK, Spitsbergen JM, Olson JR, Peterson RE (1991) 2,3,7,8-tetrachlorodibenzo-p-dioxintoxicity during early life stage development of lake trout (*Salvelinus namaycush*). *Can J Fish Aquat Sci* **48:** 875–83.

Wang WD, Chen YM, Hu CH (1998) Detection of Ah receptor and Ah receptor nuclear translocator mRNAs in the oocytes and developing embryos of zebrafish (*Danio rerio*). *Fish Physiol Biochem* **18:** 49–57.

Wang L, Scheffler BE, Willett KL (2006) CYPC1 messenger RNA expression is inducible by benzo(a)pyrene in *Fundulus heteroclitus* adults and embryos. *Toxicol Sci* **93:** 331–40.

Watanabe KH, Jensen KM, Orlando EF, Ankley GT (2007) What is normal? A characterization of the values and variability in reproductive endpoints of the fathead minnow, *Pimephales promelas*. *Comp Biochem Physiol* **146C:** 348–56.

Weis JS (2009) Reproductive, developmental, and neurobehavioural effects of methylmercury in fishes. *J Environ Sci Health C* **27:** 212–25.

Westerlund L, Billsso K, Andersson PL, Tysklind M, Olsson PE (2000) Early life stage mortality in zebrafish (*Danio rerio*) following maternal exposure to polychlorinated biphenyls and estrogen. *Environ Toxicol Chem* **19:** 1582–8.

Wiegand C, Pflugmacher S, Giese M, Frank H, Steinberg C (2000) Uptake, toxicity, and effects on detoxication enzymes of atrazine and trifluoroacetate in embryos of zebrafish. *Ecotox Environ Safety* **45:** 122–31.

Wolf JC, Dietrich DR, Friederich U, Caunter J, Brown AR (2004) Qualitaive and quantitative histomorphological assessment of fathead minnow *Pimephales promelas* gonads as an endpoint for evaluating endocrine-active compounds: a pilot methodology study. *Toxicol Pathol* **32:** 600–12.

Wu RSS, Zou BS, Woo NYS, Lam PKS (2003) Aquatic hypoxia is an endocrine disruptor and impairs fish reproduction. *Environ Sci Technol* **37:** 1137–41.

Yadetie F, Male R (2002) Effects of 4-nonylphenol on gene expression of pituitary hormones in juvenile Atlantic salmon (*Salmo salar*). *Aquat Toxicol* **58:** 113–29.

Yaron Z, Gur G, Melamed P, Rosenfeld H, Elizur A, Levavic-Sivan B (2003) Regulation of fish gonadotropins. *Int Rev Cytol* **225:** 131–85.

Yokota H, Seki M, Maeda M, Oshima Y, Tadokoro H, Honjo T, Kobayashi K (2001) Life-cycle toxicity of 4-nonylphenol to medaka (*Oryzias latipes*). *Environ Toxicol Chem* **20:** 2552–60.

Zabel EW, Cook PM, Peterson RE (1995) Toxic equivalency factors of polychlorinated dibenzo-p-dioxin, dibenzofuran, and biphenyl congeners based on early life stage mortality in rainbow trout (*Oncorhynchus mykiss*). *Aquat Toxicol* **31:** 315–28.

Zaroogian G, Gardner G, Horowitz DB, Gutjahr-Gobell R, Haebler R, Mills L (2001) Effect of 17beta-estradiol, o,p′-DDT, octylphenol and p,p′-DDE on gonadal development and liver and kidney pathology in juvenile male summer flounder (*Paralichthys dentatus*). *Aquat Toxicol* **54:** 101–12.

Zhang X, Hecker M, Park JW, Tompsett AR, Jones PD, Newsted J, Au DW, Kong R, Wu RS, Giesy JP (2008) Time-dependent transcriptional profiles of genes of the hypothalamic–pituitary–gonadal axis in medaka (*Oryzias latipes*) exposed to fadrozole and 17beta-trenbolone. *Environ Toxicol Chem* **27:** 2504–11.

Ziv T, Gattegno T, Chapotevsky V, Wolf H, Barnea E, Lubzens E, Admon A (2008) Comparative proteomics of the developing fish (zebrafish and gilthead seabream) oocytes. *Comp Biochem Physiol* **3D:** 12–35.

Zohar Y, Munoz-Cueto JA, Elizur A, Kah O (2010) Neuroendocrinology of reproduction in teleost fish. *Gen Comp Endocrinol* **165:** 438–55.

Zon LI, Peterson RT (2005) In vivo drug discovery in the zebrafish. *Nature Rev Drug Discovery* **4:** 35–44.

Index

C

D

E

G

H

M

N

O

P

Q

R

S

Y

Z

Color Plates

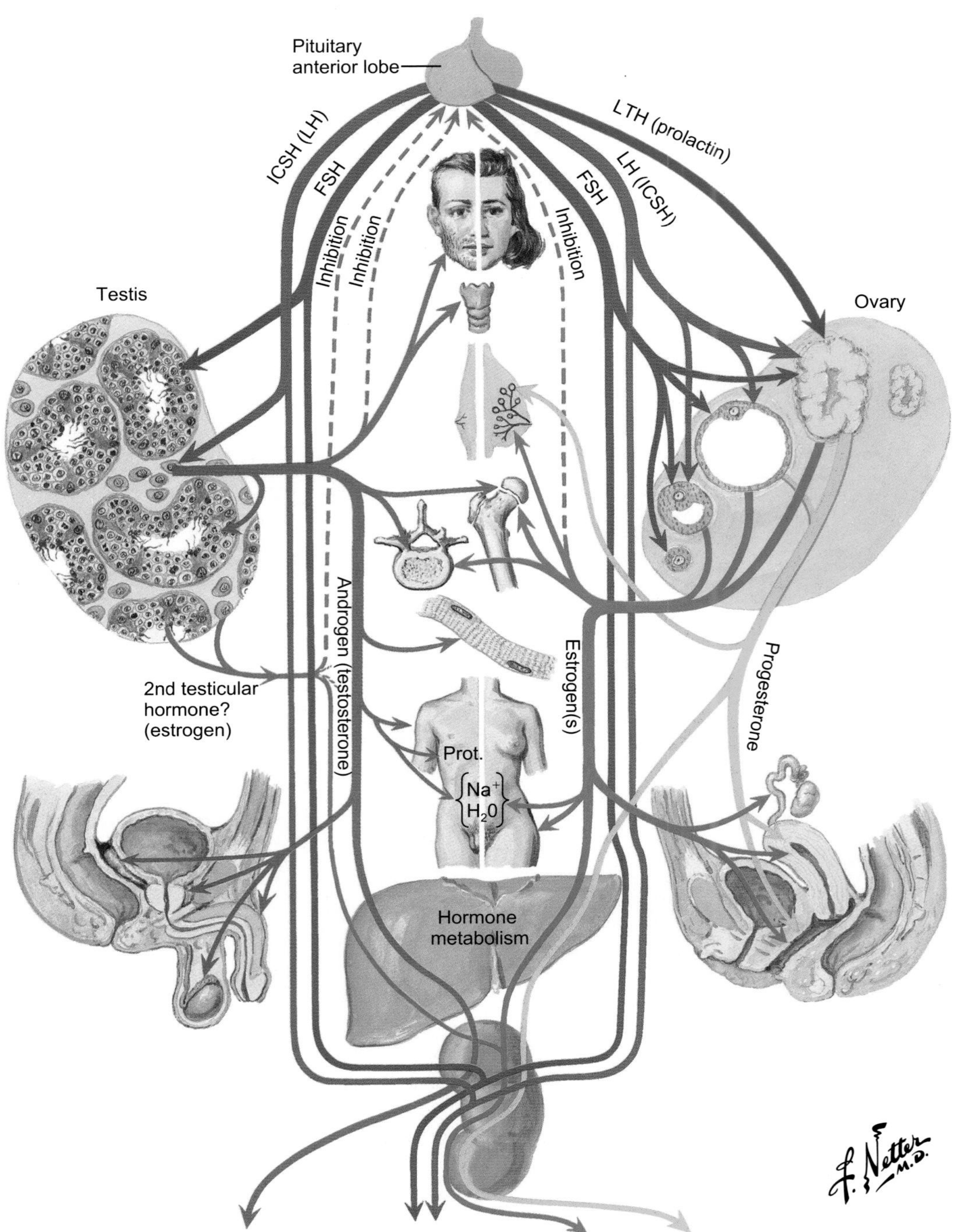

FIGURE 2.3 The basic gonadal steroidogenic pathways, target sites, feedback loops and routes of excretion for the adult male and female human are summarized in this figure. Positive and negative feedback mechanisms involving gonadal steroids help maintain an endocrine environment which is conducive to normal male and female reproductive function. Figure was obtained, with permission, from Netter (1997).

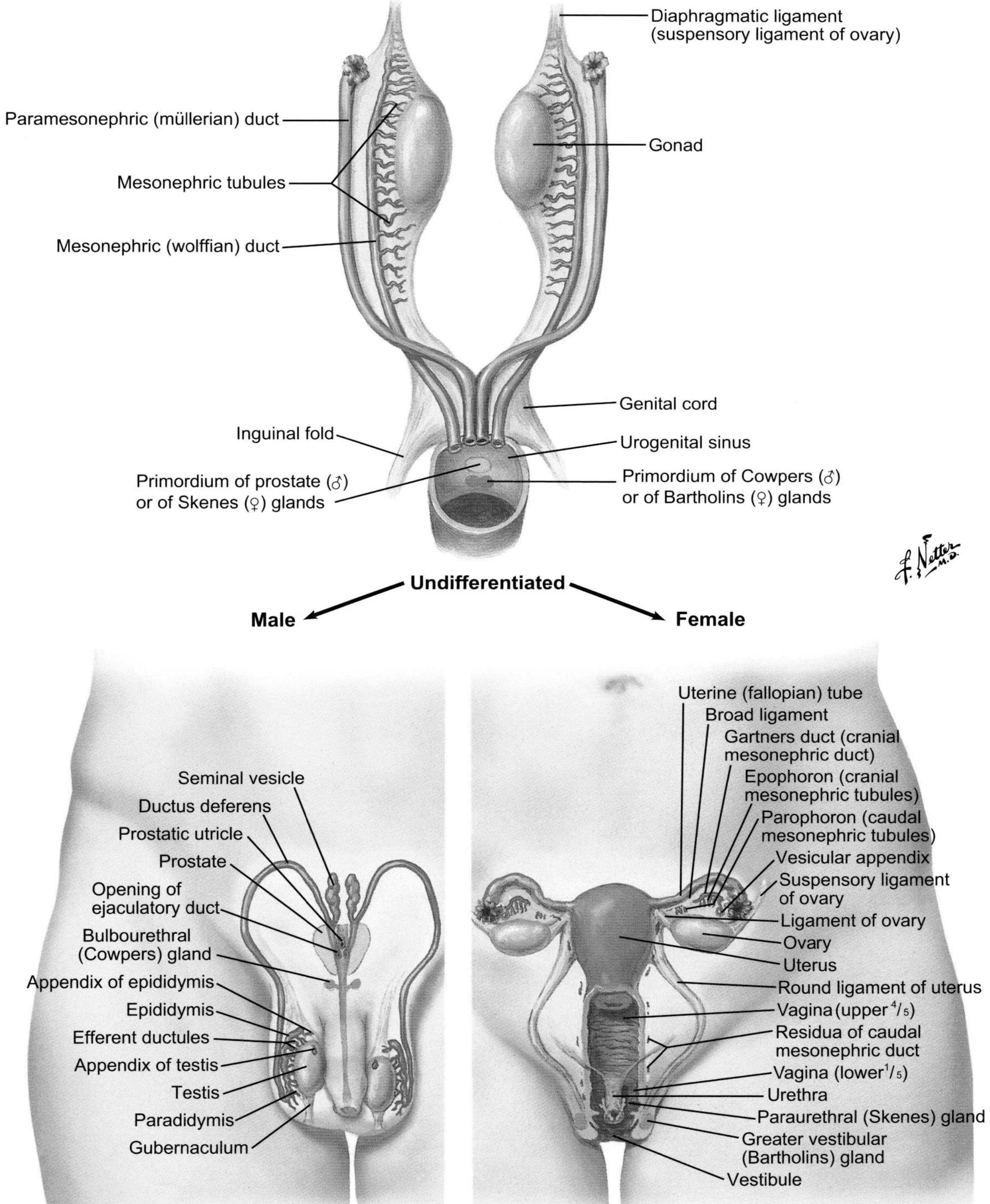

FIGURE 2.4 The "undifferentiated" stage observed in the fetus, regardless of genotypic sex, early in gestation prior to gonadal sexual differentiation, as well as the gonads, internal genitalia and other associated anatomical structures of the sexually mature male and female are shown in **A**. **B** illustrates the standard sequence of events in the development of the external genitalia of men and women, as well as other mammalian species. The failure of the urethral groove to close at any point during this sequence results in various degrees of hypospadias, which is a relatively common congenital birth defect in male offspring and one which has been induced in laboratory species by prenatal exposure to a number of xenobiotics. Figures were obtained, with permission, from Netter (1997).

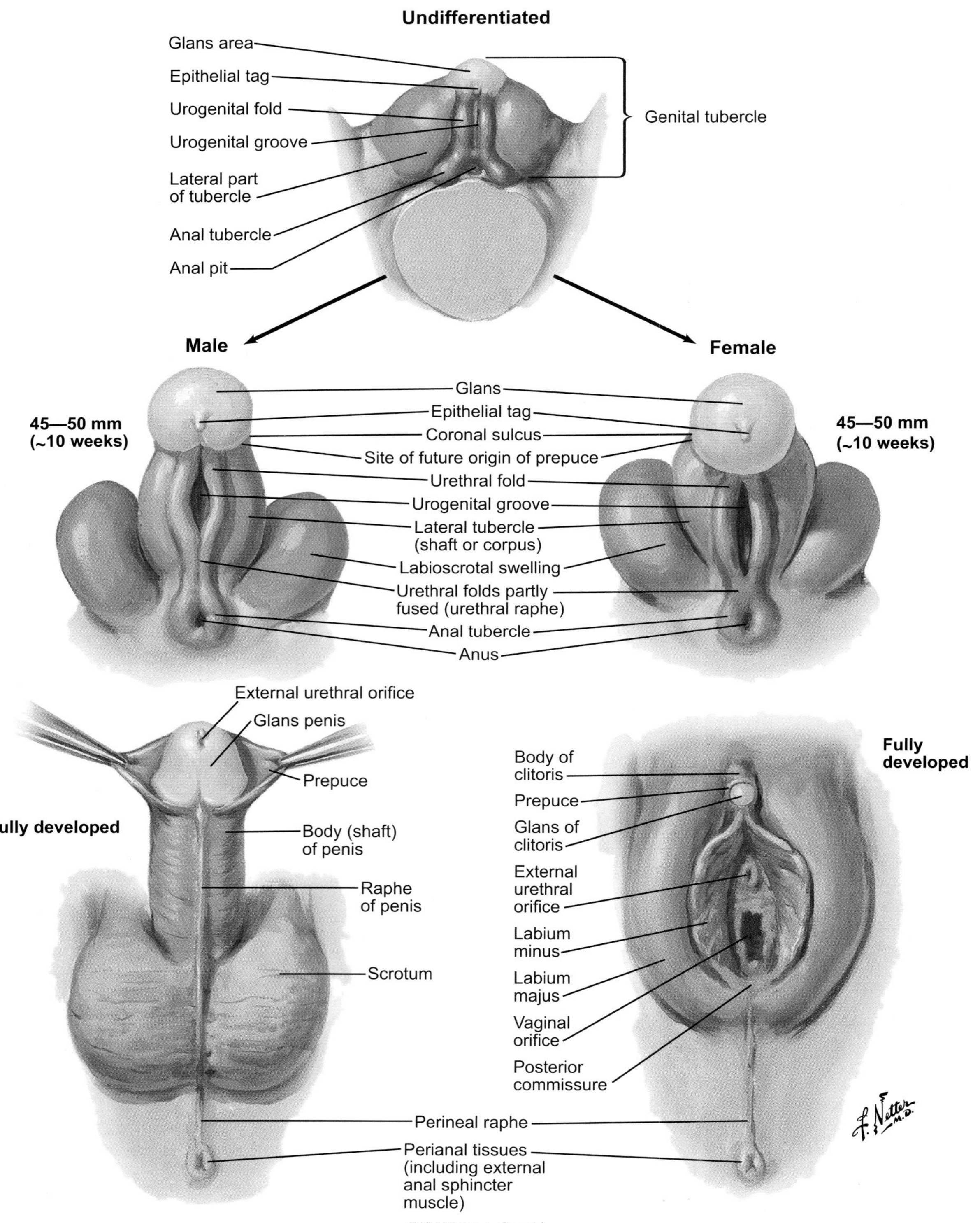

FIGURE 2.4 Cont'd

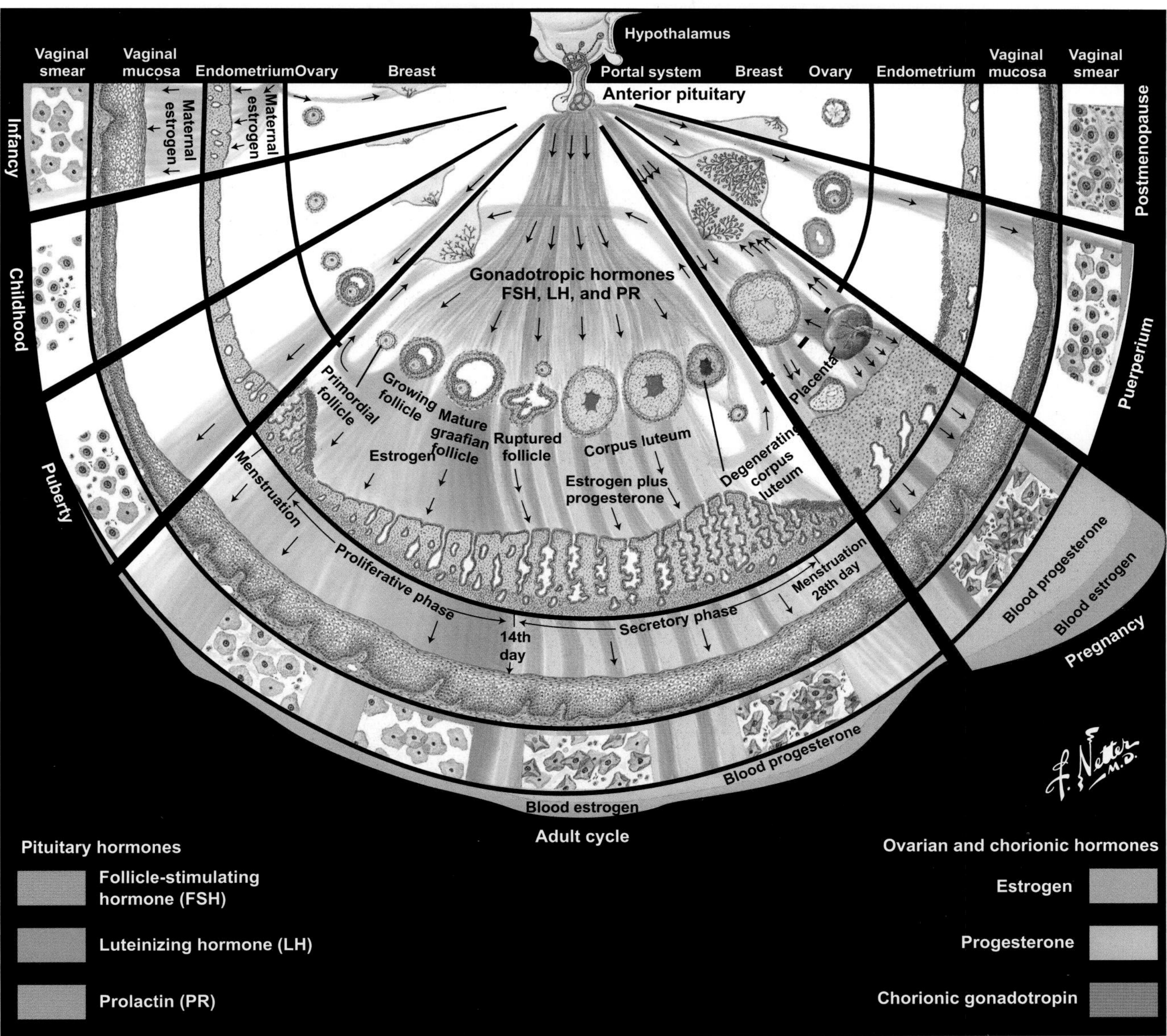

FIGURE 2.8 In humans, chemical exposures can take place over an entire lifetime, and early xenobiotic exposures have the potential to affect reproductive events occurring later in life. This figure clearly and comprehensively summarizes all of the anatomical and physiological reproductive changes which can take place in women's lives between infancy and menopause, including those associated with puberty and the various stages of the menstrual cycle, as well as periods of pregnancy and lactation. The transition between the various aspects of a woman's reproductive activity involves alterations in anterior pituitary hormone secretion and structural and functional modifications in the ovaries, endometrium, vaginal epithelium and the mammary glands. Figure was obtained, with permission, from Netter (1997).

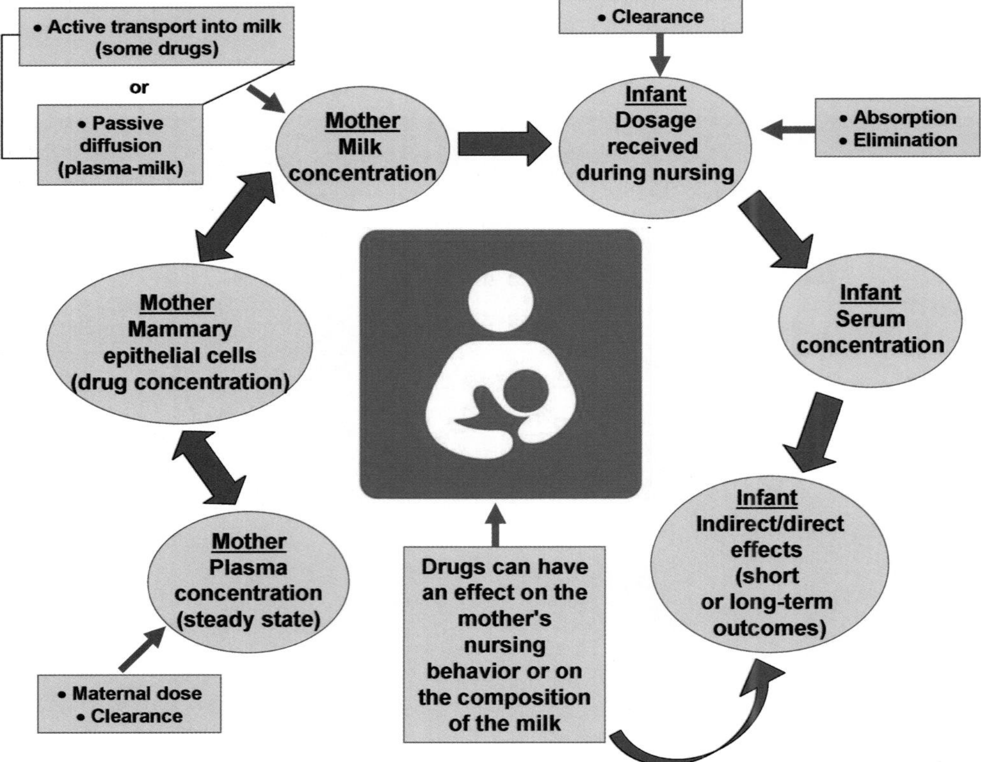

FIGURE 6.1 Infant drug exposure through breastfeeding.

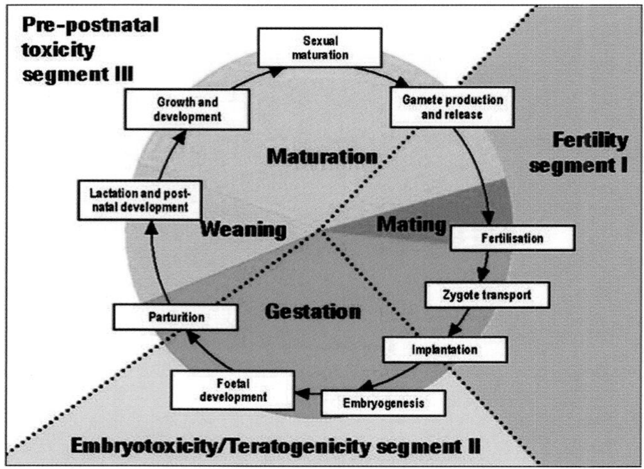

FIGURE 8.2 Segment 1, 2 and 3 studies of drug testing according to ICH. (Adapted with author's permission from Spielmann, 2009.)

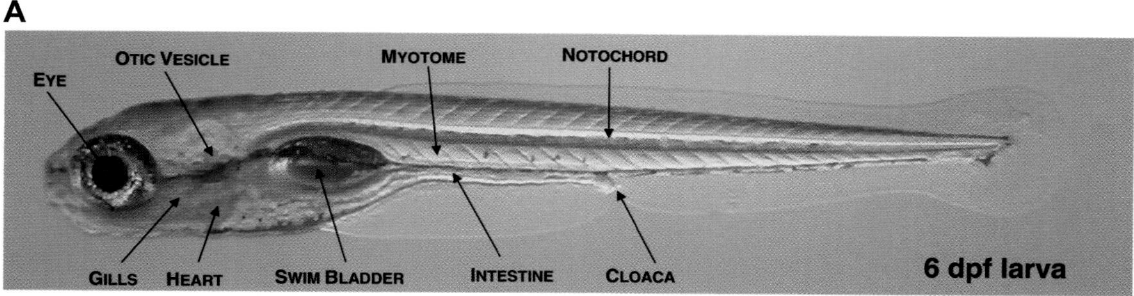

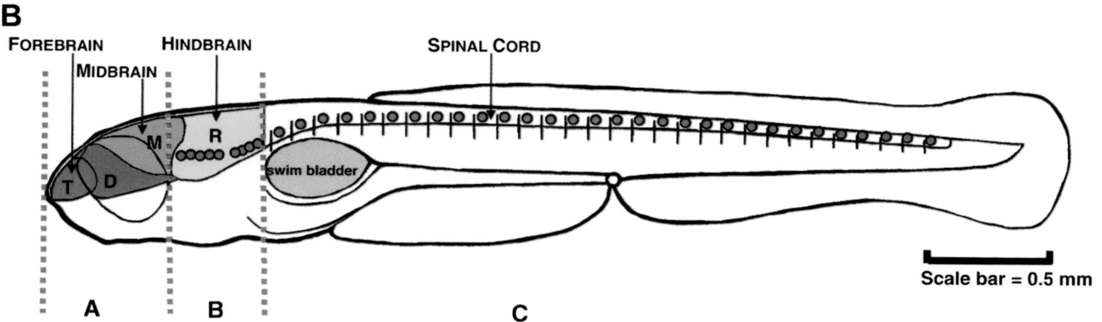

FIGURE 15.1 Photograph and schematic depicting the major anatomical features of the 6-day-old zebrafish larva. T: telencephalon; D: diencephalon; M: mesencephalon; and R: rhombencephalon. Vertical red dotted lines represent convenient dissection locations for obtaining fore- and mid-brain vs hindbrain samples using the eye and swim bladder as landmarks. Filled red circles represent the superior and inferior serotonergic raphe neurons in the hindbrain and the ventromedial serotonergic neurons in the spinal cord. Reprinted from Airhart *et al.* (2007), with permission from Elsevier.

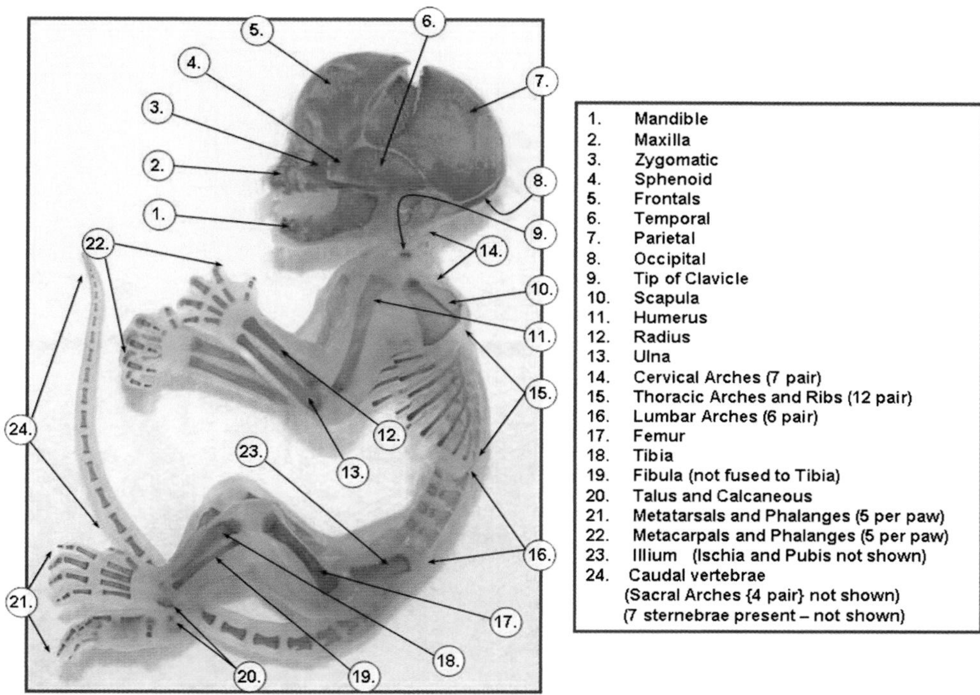

FIGURE 17.7 Alizarin stained fetal skeletal of cynomolgus monkey (GD 100).

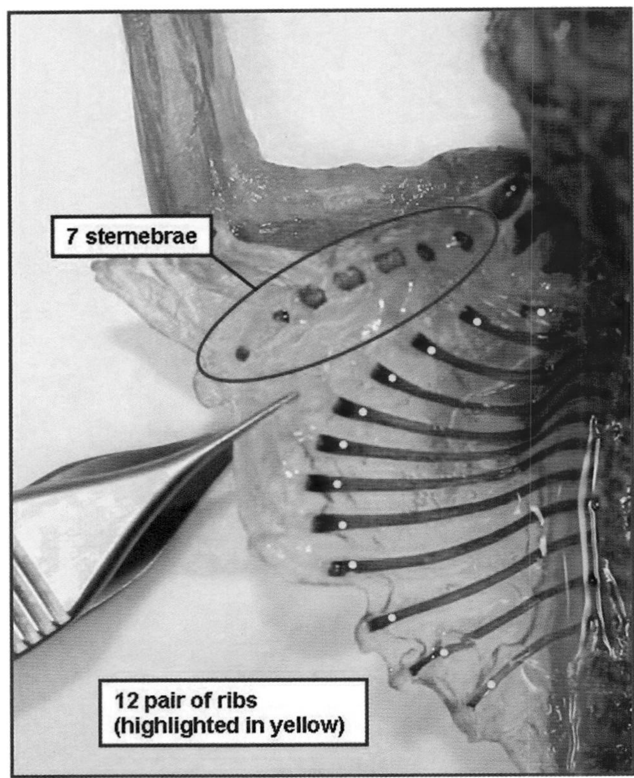

FIGURE 17.8 Fetus with normal sternebrae and ribs.

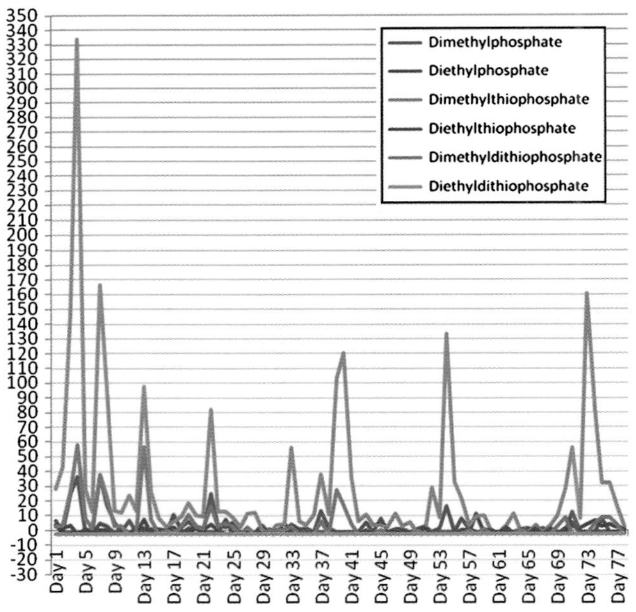

FIGURE 20.1 The intraperson temporal (over 71 days) variability of excretion of six dialkylphosphate metabolites of OP pesticides is shown.

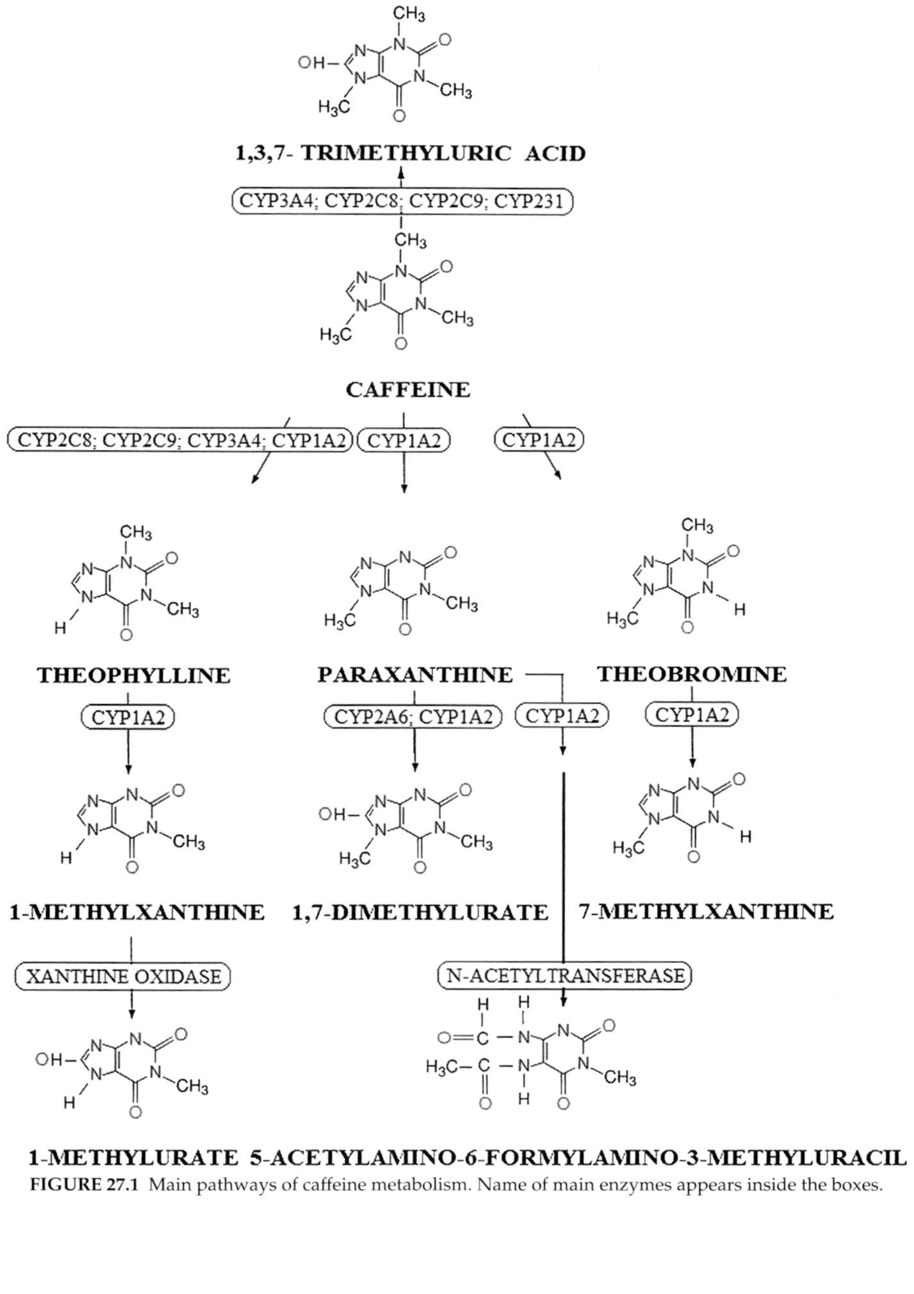

1,3,7- TRIMETHYLURIC ACID

CYP3A4; CYP2C8; CYP2C9; CYP231

CAFFEINE

CYP2C8; CYP2C9; CYP3A4; CYP1A2

CYP1A2

CYP1A2

THEOPHYLLINE

PARAXANTHINE

THEOBROMINE

CYP1A2

CYP2A6; CYP1A2

CYP1A2

CYP1A2

1-METHYLXANTHINE

1,7-DIMETHYLURATE

7-METHYLXANTHINE

XANTHINE OXIDASE

N-ACETYLTRANSFERASE

1-METHYLURATE

5-ACETYLAMINO-6-FORMYLAMINO-3-METHYLURACIL

FIGURE 27.1 Main pathways of caffeine metabolism. Name of main enzymes appears inside the boxes.

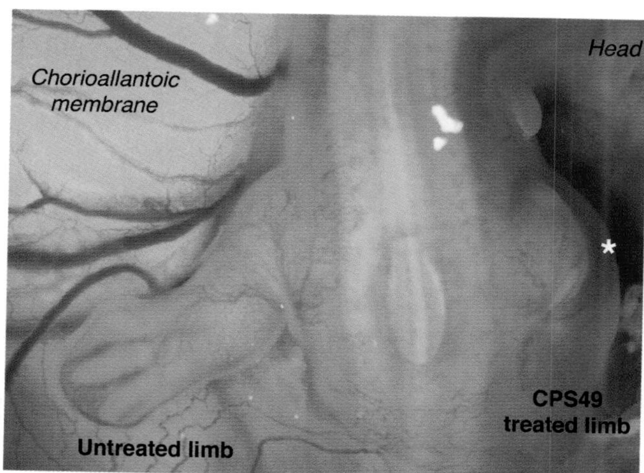

FIGURE 31.4 CPS49 induces limb defects. Chick embryo, 3 days after CPS49 exposure at day 2.5, as the limb is starting to develop. Note the right limb is truncated and just a stump remains (asterisk denotes missing limb). The rest of the embryo appears normal – this is due to vessel immaturity in the limb at the time of drug exposure.

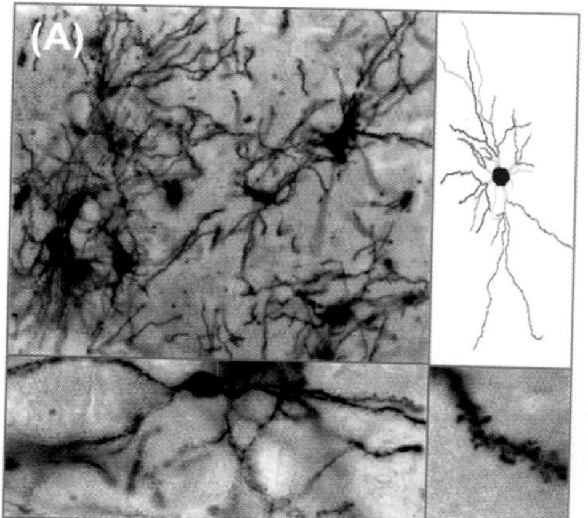

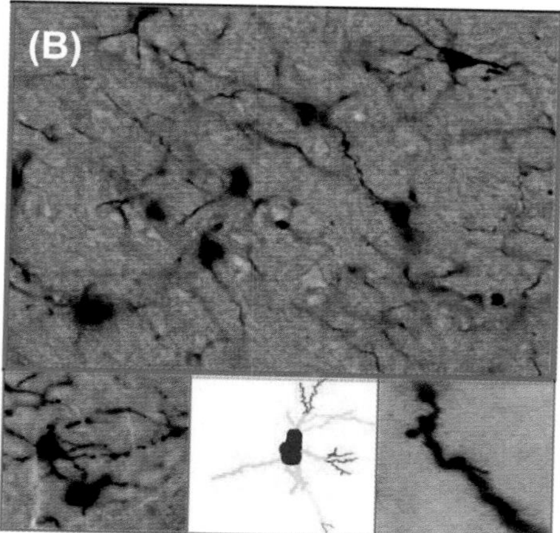

FIGURE 34.3 Photomicrographs of mouse striatal sections with representative tracings of medium spiny neurons (MSNs) from mice treated with saline (control) (A) or $MnCl_2$ (100 mg/kg, s.c.) (B). Brain from mouse exposed three times (day 1, 4 and 7) to $MnCl_2$ was collected 24 h post last injection. Treatment with Mn-induced degeneration of striatal dendritic system, decrease in total number of spines and length of dendrites of MSNs. Tracing and counting are done using a Neurolucida system at 100× under oil immersion (MicroBrightField, VT). Colors indicate the degree of dendritic branching (yellow = 1°, red = 2°, purple = 3°, green = 4°, turquoise = 5°).

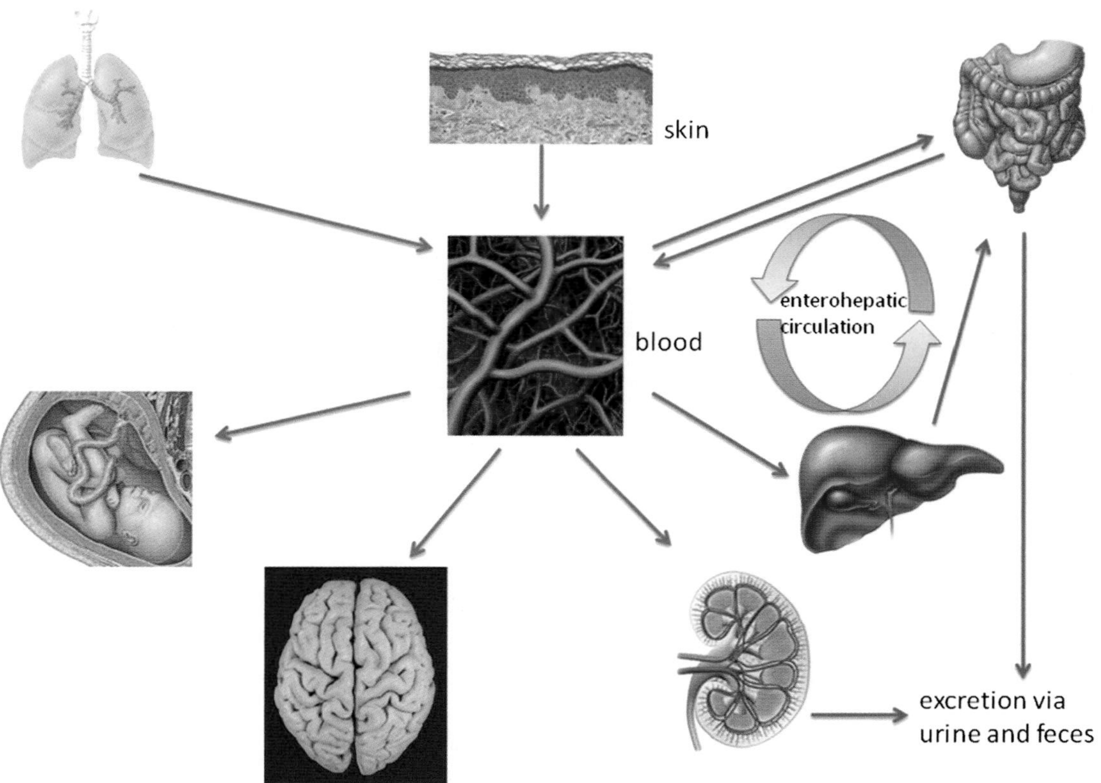

FIGURE 35.1 The distribution of MeHg in the human body. MeHg is readily absorbed by the lung, skin and gastrointestinal tract. Once in the circulation, MeHg predominantly accumulates in red blood cells and is slowly redistributed to other organ systems, including the CNS (major), kidneys and liver. MeHg can cross the placental–blood barrier and it accumulates in the fetus at higher concentrations compared to the mother.

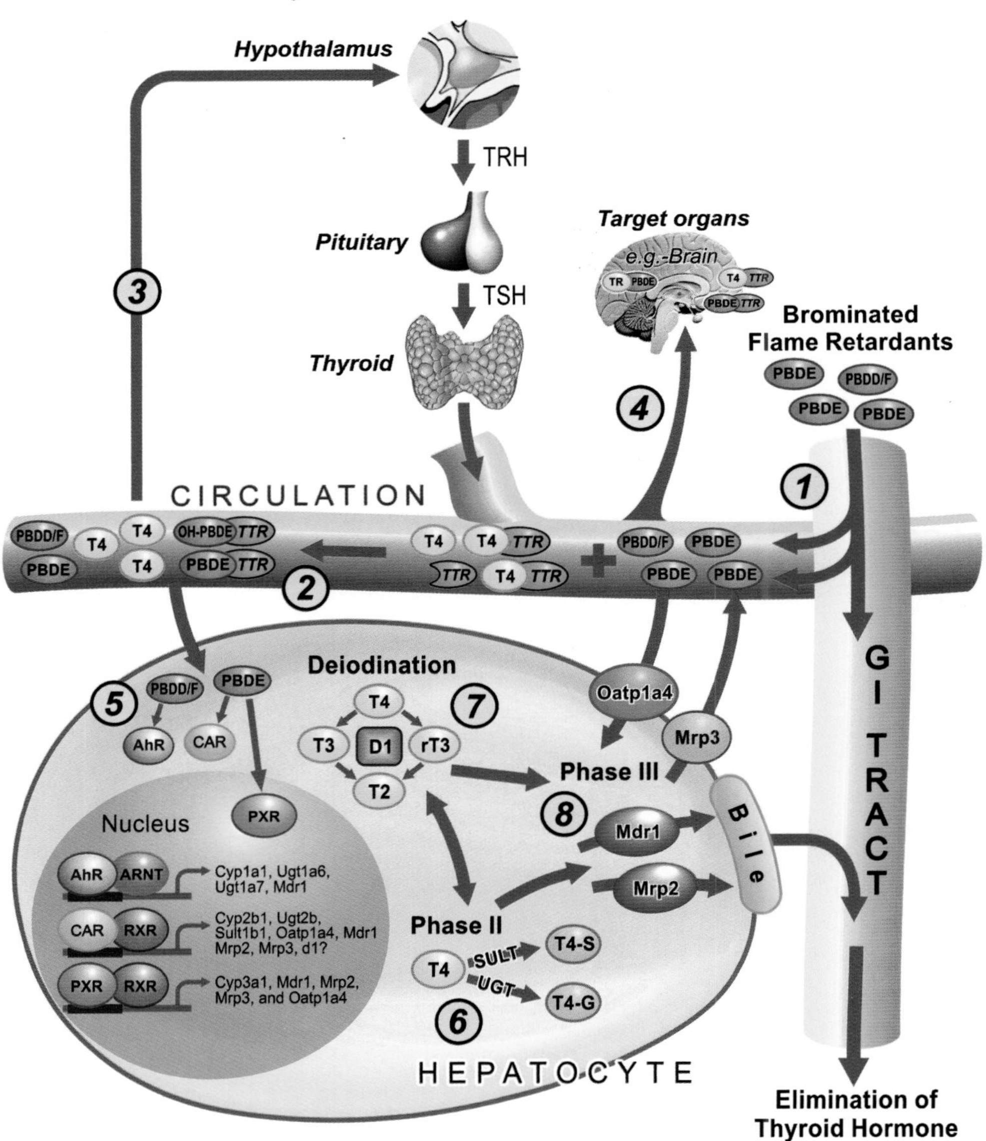

FIGURE 40.2 Possible mechanism(s) of disruption of thyroid hormone homeostasis following developmental exposure to commercial PBDE mixtures. (1) PBDEs as well as PBDD/Fs enter the circulation from gastrointestinal (GI) tract. (2) PBDEs in the parent or hydroxylated form can displace thyroxine (T_4) from serum binding proteins such as transthyretin (TTR). The resulting free T_4 will be subjected to hepatic metabolism and elimination. (3) Reduced circulating T_4 levels trigger the hypothalamic–pituitary axis to synthesize and secrete more T_4 by thyroid. (4) PBDEs bound to TTR along with T_4 will reach target organs including brain, where it can bind to thyroid hormone receptor to elicit a biological/toxicological effect. (5) PBDEs and PBDD/Fs activate nuclear receptors in hepatocytes initiating transcription of xenobiotic metabolizing enzymes (XMEs) for T_4 elimination. (6) XMEs consequently conjugate T_4 by phase II enzymes, uridine diphosphate glucuronyl transferase (UGT) and sulfotransferase (SULT). (7) Deiodinase 1 (D1) deiodinates T_4 to its metabolites. (8) Influx transporters (Oatp1a4) further increase the T_4 uptake for metabolism. Efflux transporters eliminate T_4 or its conjugates from hepatocytes into either the serum (Mrp3) or the bile (Mrp2). (Adapted from Szabo *et al.*, 2009; Kodavanti and Curras-Collazo, 2010.)

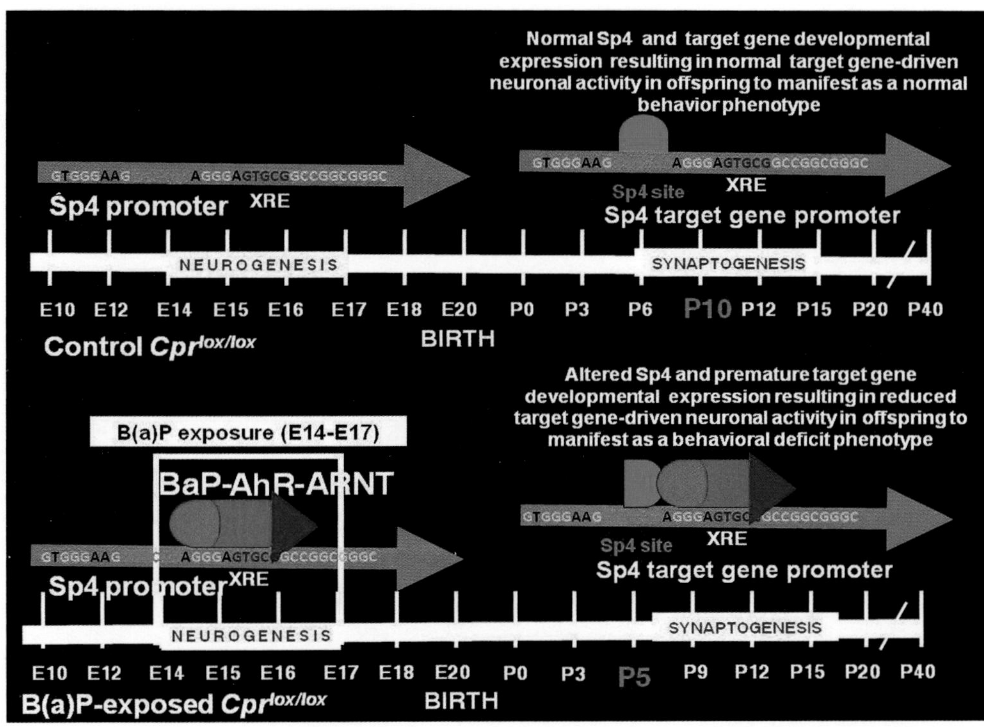

Figure 44.6 Proposed signaling subsequent to *in utero* B(a)P exposure. *Top panel*: normal homeostasis; normal temporal activation of Sp4 expression and of its target genes during embryonic development in timed-pregnant control *Cpr*$^{lox/lox}$ mice is depicted from E 10 to 20 (birth). During the early postnatal period, target gene expression is necessary for the establishment of glutamatergic (NMDA) circuits and synapses. Sp4 target genes facilitate in establishing glutamatergic currents that are key to enhancing the strength of synaptic connections. Temporal Sp4 and target gene expression is key to glutamatergic-driven neuronal activity during the period from P 7 to 15 in *Cpr*$^{lox/lox}$ offspring to give a normal behavioral phenotype. *Bottom panel*: dysregulated homeostasis; *Cpr*$^{lox/lox}$ mice exposed to B(a)P aerosol from E14 to 17 give birth to offspring on E 20. B(a)P-exposed *Cpr*$^{lox/lox}$ offspring demonstrate a premature peak of Sp4 expression and altered target gene expression. The resulting target gene subunit is predicted to exhibit altered glutamatergic-driven neuronal activity that manifests as a behavioral deficit phenotype.

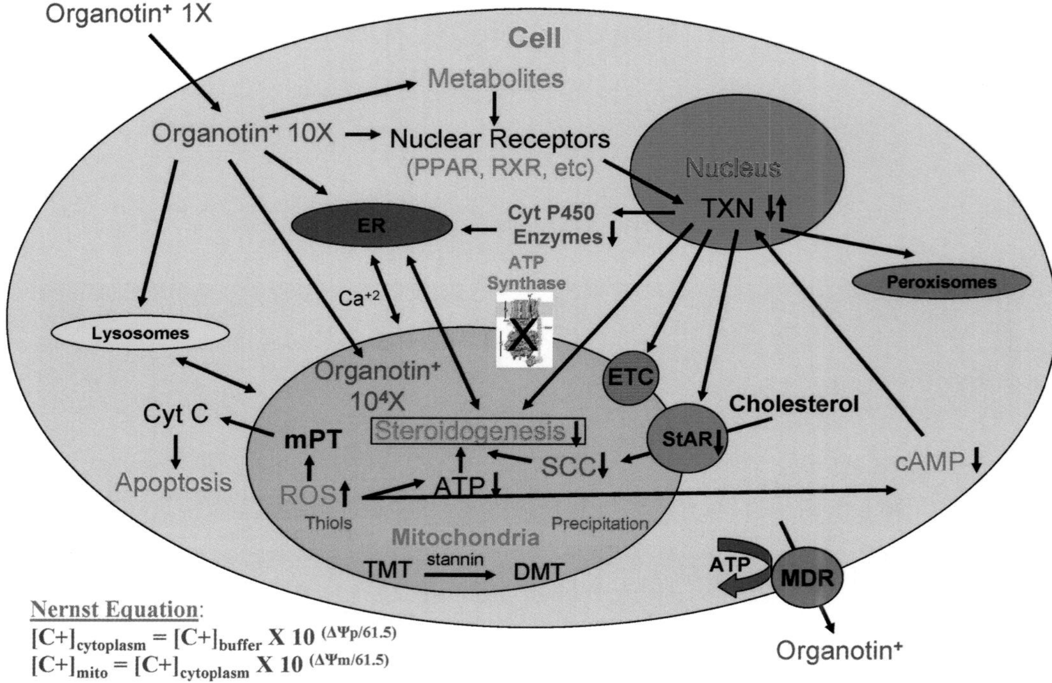

FIGURE 49.1 Organotin integrative model of toxicity. Organotins and their metabolites have effects on cells at multiple levels, including nuclear receptors, gene transcription, enzyme inhibition, free radical production, ATP generation, steroid production and apoptosis. Organotin cations can be bio-accumulated into the cells according to the Nernst equation, by a factor of 10 into the cytosol and by a factor of 10,000 into the mitochondria. Abbreviations: Cyt C – cytochrome C; SCC – side chain cleavage enzyme or desmolase; ROS – reactive oxygen species; ATP – adenosine triphosphate; TXN – transcription; mPT – mitochondrial permeability transition (swelling); ETC – electron transport chain; StAR – steroid hormone acute regulatory protein; Cyt P450 – cytochrome P450 enzymes; cAMP – cyclic adenosine monophosphate; TMT – trimethyltin; DMT– dimethyltin; $\Delta\Psi_p$ – plasma membrane potential in mV; $\Delta\Psi_m$ – mitochondrial potential; ER – endoplasmic reticulum; MDR – multi-drug resistance xenobiotic pumps.

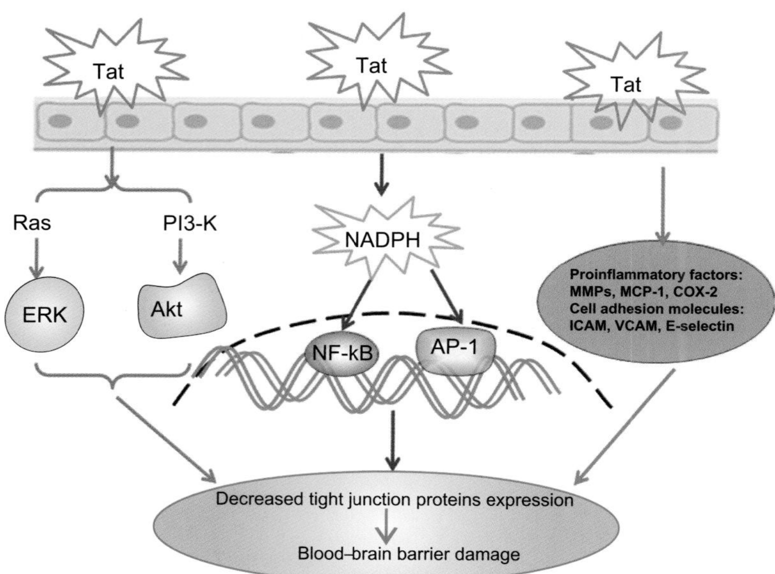

FIGURE 57.2 Schematic of mechanisms underlying Tat-mediated damage to the BBB. Mechanisms underlying Tat-mediated alteration of TJs involve redox-responsive signal transduction pathways, such as Ras/ERK1/2 pathway, PI-3K/Akt/ pathway and calcium-dependent signaling (Andras *et al.*, 2005). Tat exposure resulted in increased cellular oxidative stress, decreased levels of intracellular glutathione and activated DNA binding activity and transactivation of transcription factors NF-κB and AP-1 (Toborek *et al.*, 2003). Tat also induced proinflammatory factors and cell adhesion molecules which contribute to BBB damage (Huang *et al.*, 2009; Liu *et al.*, 2005).

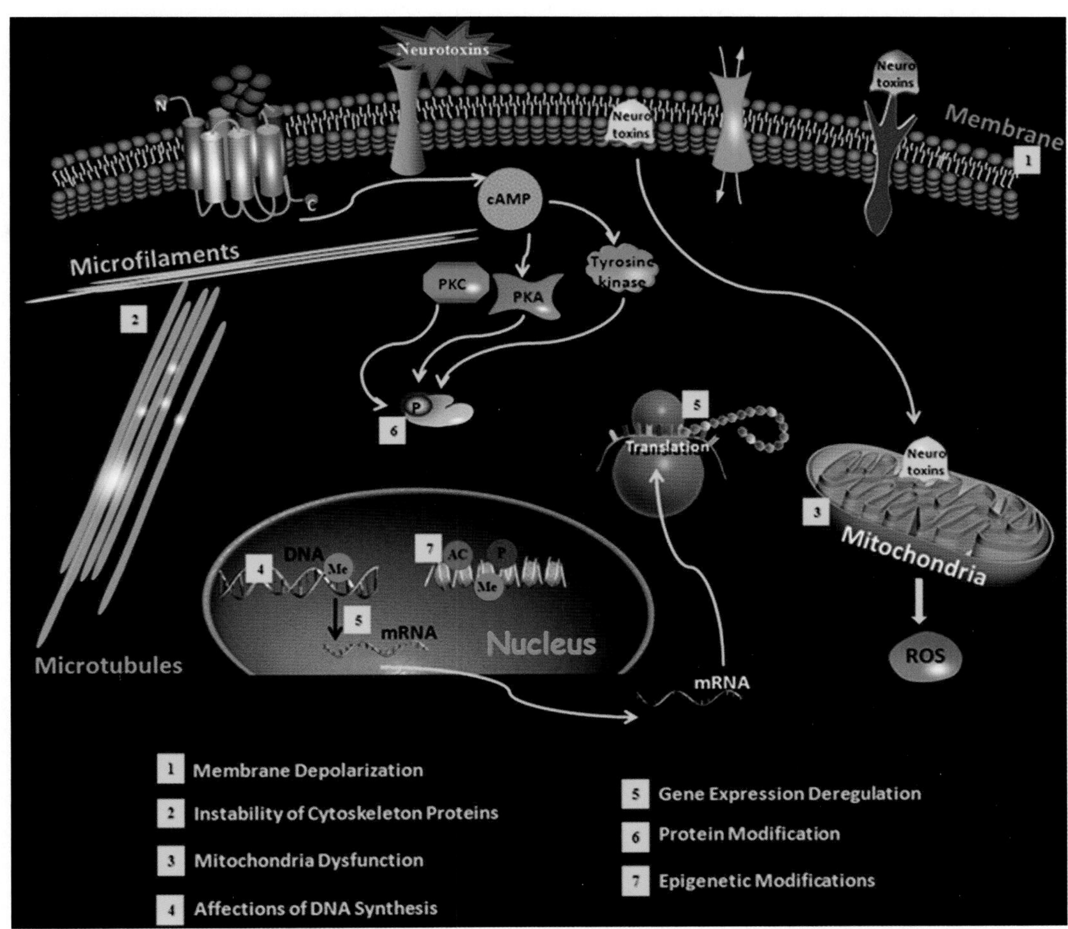

FIGURE 63.2 Cell signaling mechanisms in developmental neurotoxicity. The figure summarizes key cell signaling mechanisms by which neurotoxic chemicals inflict damage or induce neurotoxicity to the developing nervous system. A growing body of evidence suggests that exposure of developing neural cells to neurotoxic chemicals leads to depolarization of cell membranes, destruction of cell architecture proteins, mitochondrial dysfunction and induction of oxidative stress, DNA damage and affection of DNA synthesis, lasting changes in gene expression, modification of key signaling proteins in various pathways, epigenetic changes, and so on.

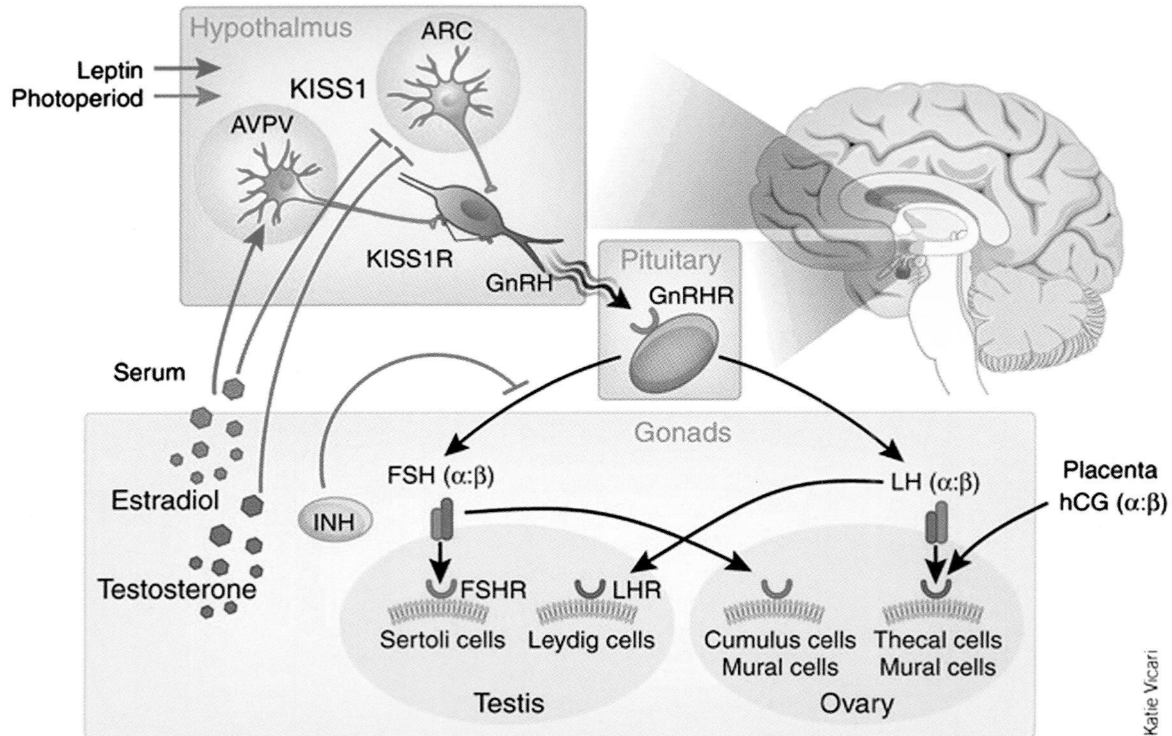

FIGURE 71.5 Neuroendocrine control of pituitary and gonadal function. (From Matzuk and Lamb, 2008, with permission from Macmillan Publishers Ltd.)

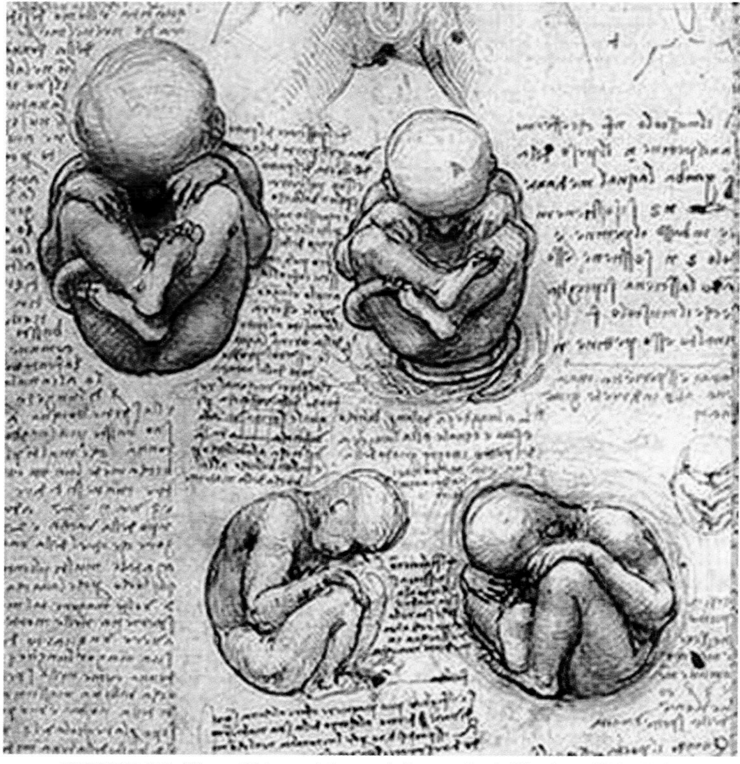

FIGURE 73.1 *Views of fetus and the womb*, Leonardo da Vinci, ca 1510–1512.

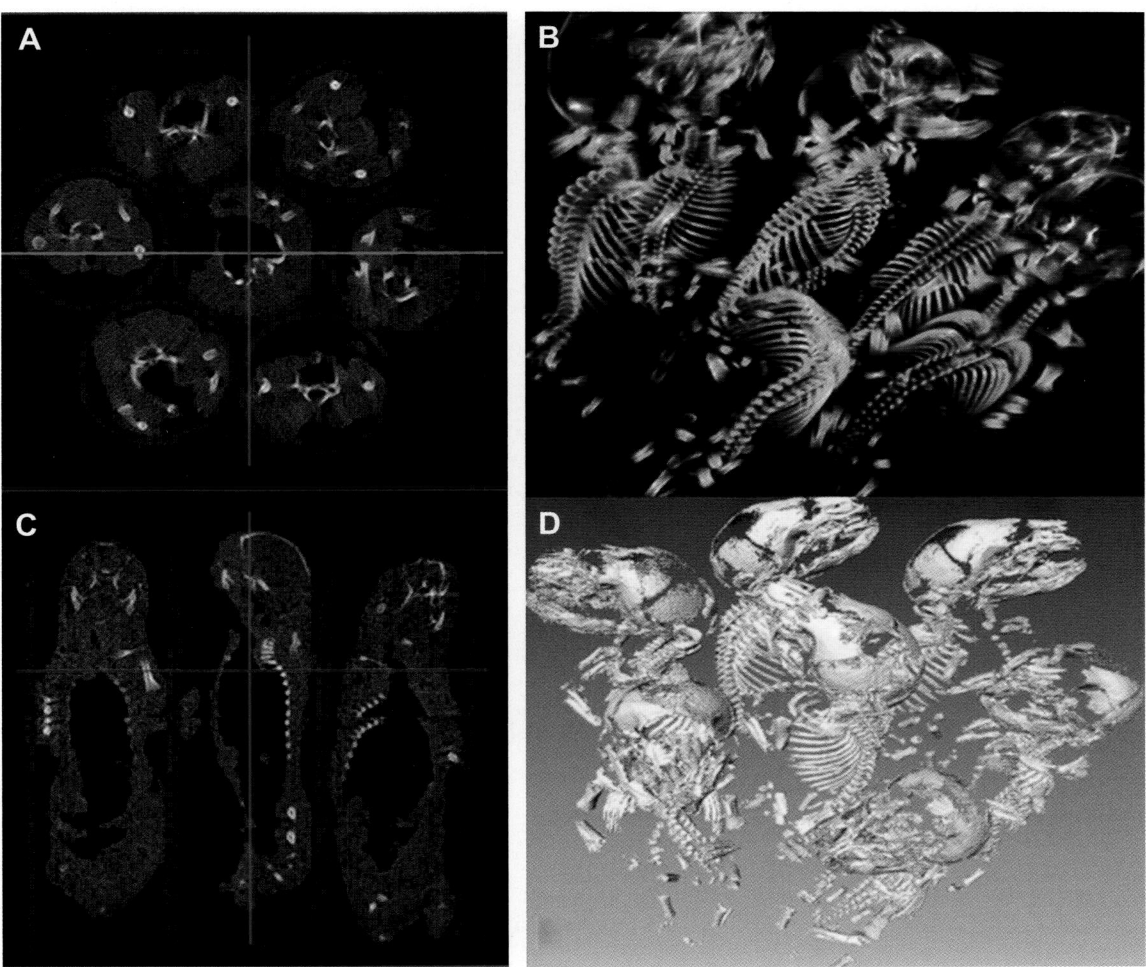

FIGURE 75.5 Increased micro-CT imaging throughput with a simple batch scan of seven rat fetuses. (A) and (C) micro-CT section images of the rat fetuses. (B) MIP display of the fetal skeletons. (D) volume rendering view of the rat fetal skeletons.

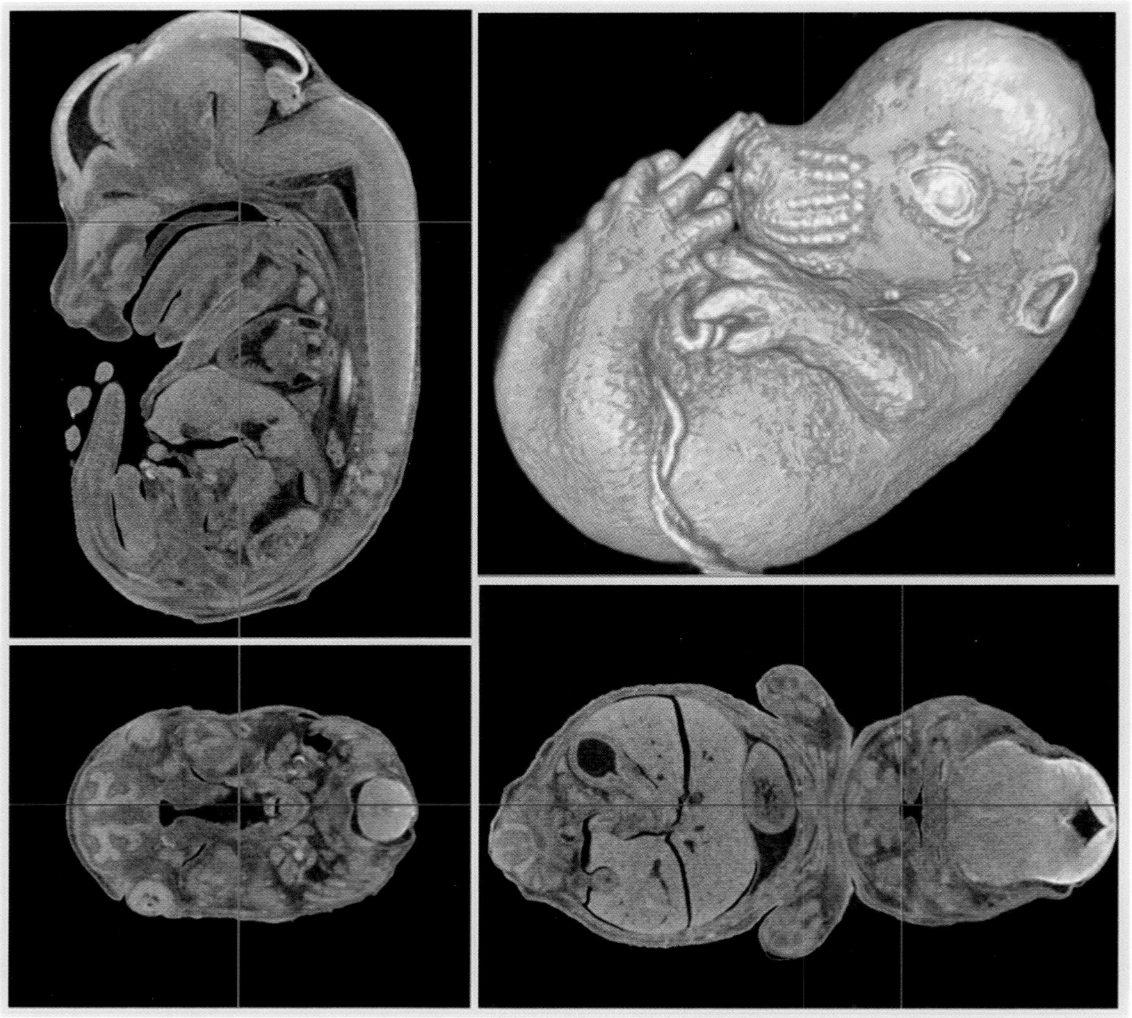

FIGURE 75.11 Micro-CT volumetric imaging of a contrast agent-stained mouse embryo (gestation day 14.5).

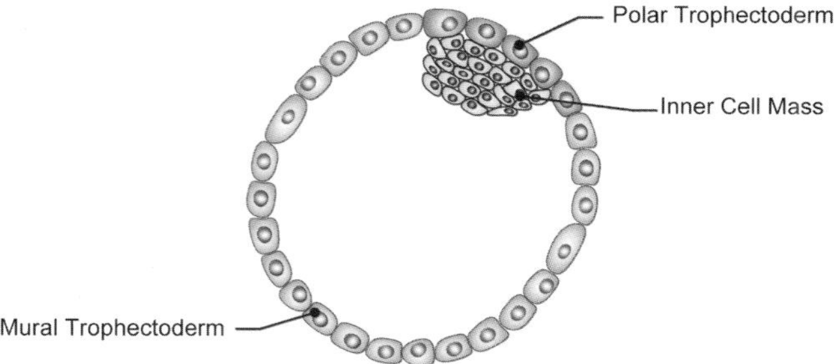

FIGURE 77.1 Illustration depicting the structure of a preimplantation blastocyst. The blastocyst consists of an outer layer of trophectoderm, which is fated to differentiate into trophoblast cells, and an eccentrically placed inner cell mass destined to form the embryo, yolk sac and allantois. The trophectoderm contiguous with the inner cell mass is referred to as the polar trophectoderm, whereas the trophectoderm opposite the inner cell mass is called the mural trophectoderm.

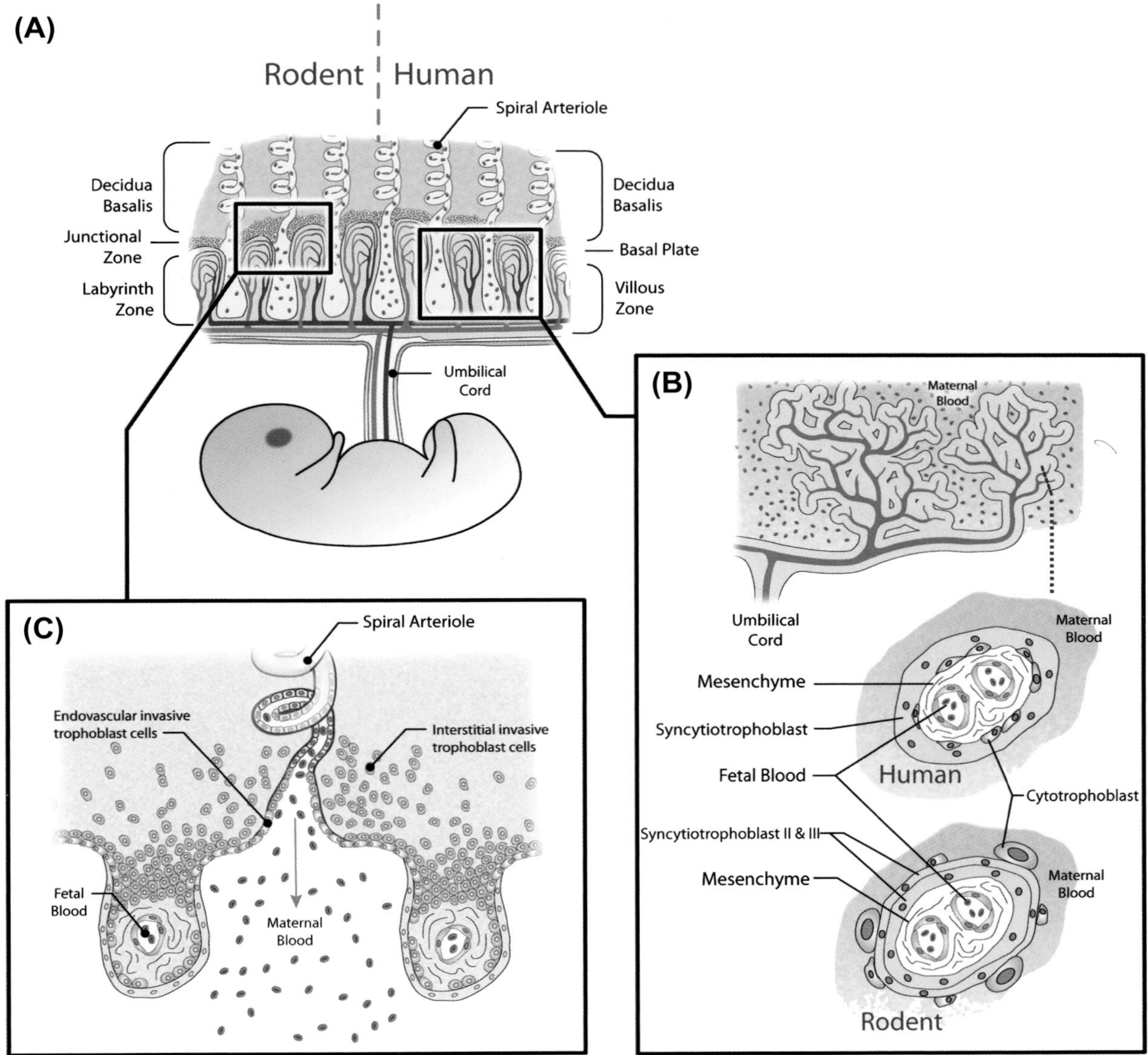

FIGURE 77.2 Schematic representation of analogous structural regions of the definitive human and rodent placenta. (A) Generic structural organization of the rodent and human placenta. Nomenclature associated with rodent placentation is shown on the left, whereas nomenclature related to human placentation is described on the right. (B) Enlarged view of generic maternal–fetal exchange site depicting tree-like villous structures encasing umbilical vessels and bathed in maternal blood. Below, arrangement of villous strata in humans (top) and rodent (bottom) are shown in cross-section. (C) Magnified view of trophoblast–decidual interface, portraying endovascular and interstitial invasive trophoblast cells within the decidua basalis associated with a uterine spiral arteriole. Note the increased internal diameter in the portion of the spiral arteriole lined by trophoblast cells.

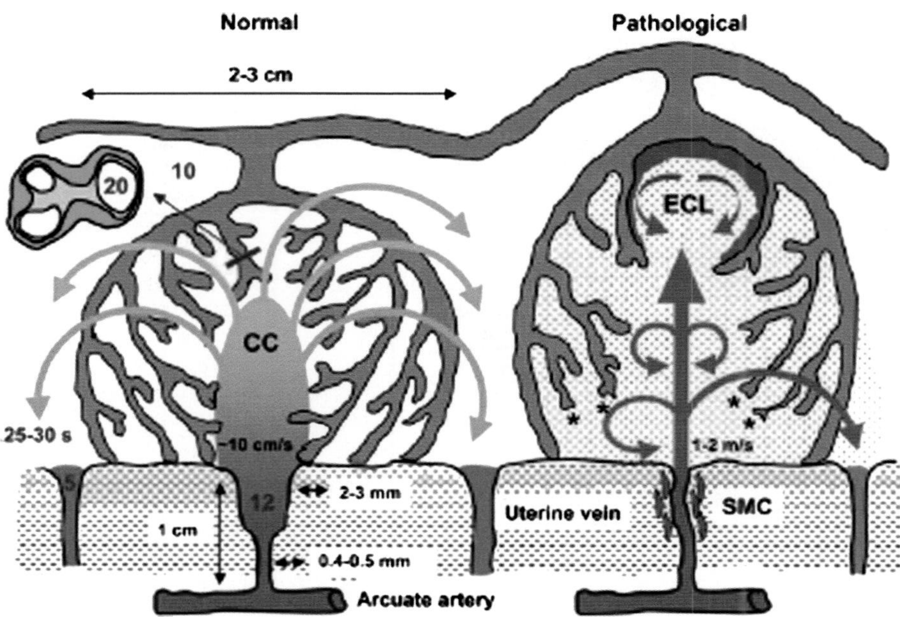

FIGURE 81.4 Cartoon of normal (left panel) and hypertensive (right panel) placenta with increased pressure resulting in increased maternal lakes and villous disruption (echogenic cystic lesions – ECL). CC – central cavity, SMC – smooth muscle cells. (From Burton *et al.*, 2009, with permission.)

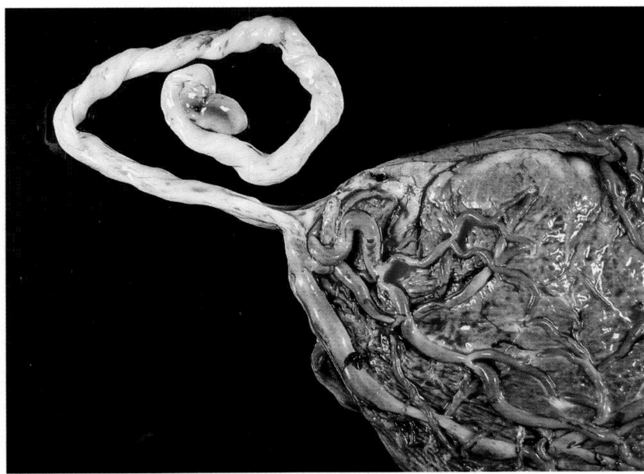

FIGURE 81.20 Gross example of velamentous insertion of the umbilical cord with thrombosed membranous vessels.

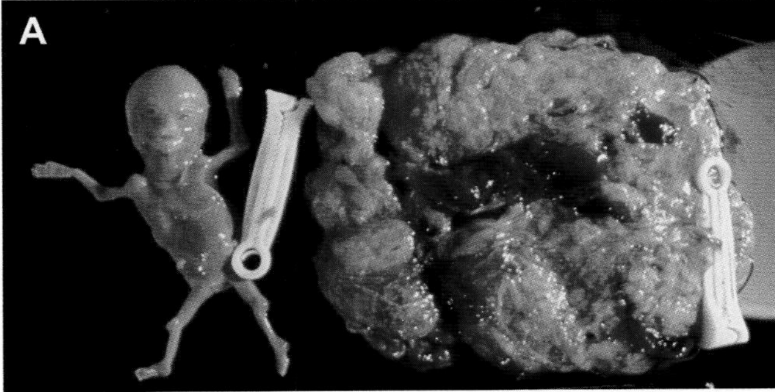

FIGURE 81.22A Triploidy. Gross of a second trimester triploidy/partial hydatidiform mole. Small catechetic fetus with large placenta.